SCHMIDEK & SWEET

Operative Neurosurgical Techniques

INDICATIONS, METHODS, AND RESULTS

Sixth Edition

Volume 1

Alfredo Quiñones-Hinojosa, MD

Associate Professor of Neurological Surgery and Oncology
Department of Neurosurgery
The Johns Hopkins University
Neuroscience and Cellular and Molecular Medicine
Director, Brain Tumor Surgery Program, Johns Hopkins Bayview
Director, Pituitary Surgery Program, Johns Hopkins Hospital
Baltimore, Maryland

ELSEVIER
SAUNDERS

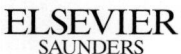
ELSEVIER
SAUNDERS

1600 John F. Kennedy Blvd.
Ste 1800
Philadelphia, PA 19103-2899

SCHMIDEK & SWEET OPERATIVE NEUROSURGICAL TECHNIQUES:
INDICATIONS, METHODS, AND RESULTS,   ISBN: 978-1-4160-6839-6
SIXTH EDITION
Copyright © 2012, 2006, 2000, 1995, 1988, 1982 by Saunders, an imprint of Elsevier Inc.

Notices

Knowledge and best practice in this field are constantly changing. As new research and experience broaden our understanding, changes in research methods, professional practices, or medical treatment may become necessary.

Practitioners and researchers must always rely on their own experience and knowledge in evaluating and using any information, methods, compounds, or experiments described herein. In using such information or methods they should be mindful of their own safety and the safety of others, including parties for whom they have a professional responsibility.

With respect to any drug or pharmaceutical products identified, readers are advised to check the most current information provided (i) on procedures featured or (ii) by the manufacturer of each product to be administered, to verify the recommended dose or formula, the method and duration of administration, and contraindications. It is the responsibility of practitioners, relying on their own experience and knowledge of their patients, to make diagnoses, to determine dosages and the best treatment for each individual patient, and to take all appropriate safety precautions.

To the fullest extent of the law, neither the Publisher nor the authors, contributors, or editors, assume any liability for any injury and/or damage to persons or property as a matter of products liability, negligence or otherwise, or from any use or operation of any methods, products, instructions, or ideas contained in the material herein.

Library of Congress Cataloging-in-Publication Data
Schmidek & Sweet operative neurosurgical techniques : indications, methods, and results. -- 6th ed. / [edited by] Alfredo Quiñones-Hinojosa.
    p. ; cm.
  Schmidek and Sweet operative neurosurgical techniques
  Operative neurosurgical techniques
  Rev. ed. of: Schmidek & Sweet operative neurosurgical techniques / [edited by] Henry H. Schmidek, David W. Roberts. 5th ed. c2006.
  Includes bibliographical references and index.
  ISBN 978-1-4160-6839-6 (set : hardcover : alk. paper) -- ISBN 978-9996086854 (v. 1) -- ISBN 9996086852 (v. 1) -- ISBN 978-9996086915 (v. 2) -- ISBN 9996086917 (v. 2)
  I. Quiñones-Hinojosa, Alfredo. II. Schmidek, Henry H., [date]. III.
Title: Schmidek and Sweet operative neurosurgical techniques. IV. Title:
Operative neurosurgical techniques.
  [DNLM: 1. Neurosurgical Procedures--methods. 2. Brain
Neoplasms--surgery. 3. Craniocerebral Trauma--surgery. 4. Nervous System
Diseases--surgery. WL 368]
  617.4'8--dc23   2012005310

Content Strategist: Julie Goolsby
Content Development Specialists: Agnes Byrne and Lisa Barnes
Publishing Services Manager: Pat Joiner-Myers
Senior Project Manager: Joy Moore
Designer: Lou Forgione

Printed in China

Last digit is the print number: 9 8 7 6 5 4 3 2 1

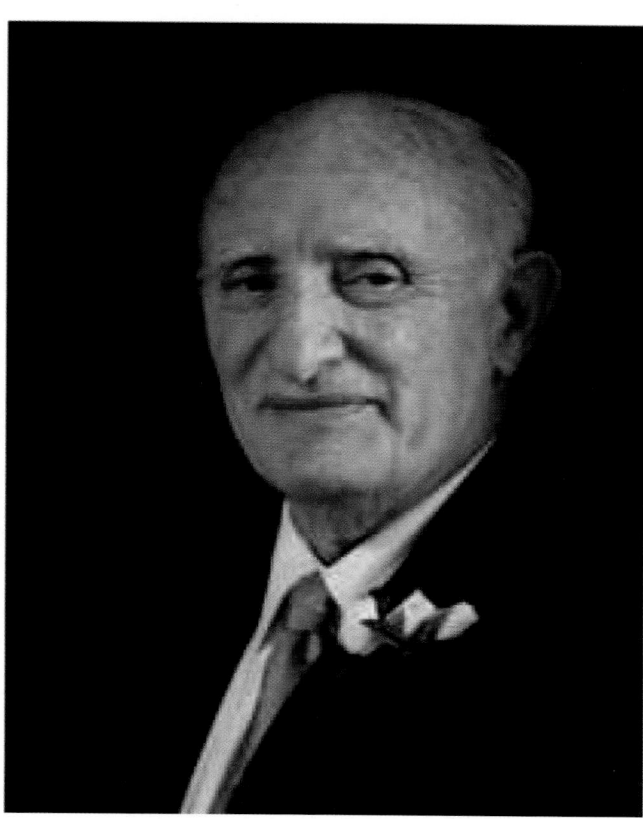

Henry Schmidek was undoubtedly an extraordinary man. He was intellectually gifted with a voracious curiosity and neverending gusto for knowledge and life. His immense love of his family was apparent to everyone who had the pleasure of his company. By trade he was a neurosurgeon, author, mentor, cattle farmer, and naval officer, but he took the time to enjoy the simple pleasures of sailboat racing and fly-fishing and was a loving husband, father, and grandfather. He did all of these things with impeccable perfection. I heard the shocking news that Dr. Schmidek had suddenly died in the fall of 2008. Our field lost a hero, but he has left behind a legacy of many contributions to the field of neuroscience, neurosurgery, and medicine.

Born in China on September 10, 1937, Dr. Schmidek studied medicine at the University of Western Ontario, where he was awarded all of their gold medals for his year. He then continued at McGill University and the University of London. He completed his residency in neurosurgery at the Massachusetts General Hospital under his mentor, Dr. William H. Sweet. At Hahnemann Medical College in Philadelphia, he became the youngest chairman of a neurosurgical department in its history. This was followed by the Chairmanship at the University of Vermont College of Medicine and then the esteemed positions of Chief of the Neurosurgical Service at The New England Deaconess Hospital and an Associate Professor of Surgery at the Harvard Medical School. Dr. Schmidek authored or edited 10 neurosurgical texts, most notably five editions *of Schmidek & Sweet Operative Neurosurgical Techniques.* This book is currently the most universal text in neurosurgery. He retired in 2001 in Vermont, where he became the CEO of Brigadoon Farm and raised prized Kobe cattle.

In 1984, Dr. Schmidek initiated a course, *Review and Update on Neurobiology for Neurosurgeons,* at the Marine Biological Laboratories in Woods Hole, Massachusetts. Designed to inspire all neurosurgeons in cutting-edge research in the field, this course has been proven to be extremely successful and has motivated many residents to pursue careers in academic surgery and beyond.

This new edition of *Schmidek & Sweet Operative Neurosurgical Techniques* is part of Dr. Schmidek's legacy. I tried to keep the same spirit that characterized the prior editions of this book and made it a favorite among students, residents, and faculty alike since its first printing. As I edited this text with the help of a superb team of section editors and contributors, I reflected on the life of Dr. Schmidek and came to realize that it is not about how long we live but the contributions we make to this world, the people we touch, and the legacy we leave behind.

Alfredo Quiñones-Hinojosa

SECTION ONE: SURGICAL MANAGEMENT OF BRAIN AND SKULL BASE TUMORS; SECTION SEVEN: TRAUMA

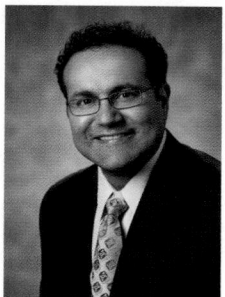

Alfredo Quiñones-Hinojosa, MD
EDITOR-IN-CHIEF
Associate Professor of Neurological Surgery and Oncology
Department of Neurosurgery
The Johns Hopkins University
Neuroscience and Cellular and Molecular Medicine
Director, Brain Tumor Surgery Program, Johns Hopkins Bayview
Director, Pituitary Surgery Program, Johns Hopkins Hospital
Baltimore, Maryland

SECTION TWO: OPERATIVE TECHNIQUES IN PEDIATRIC NEUROSURGERY

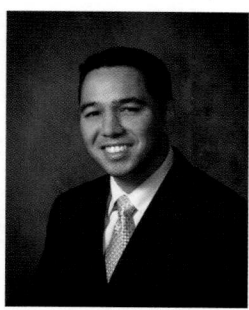

Kurtis Auguste, MD
Assistant Professor
Director, Pediatric Epilepsy Surgery
Department of Neurological Surgery
UCSF Children's Hospital
Children's Hospital Oakland
Oakland, California

SECTION THREE: VASCULAR DISEASES

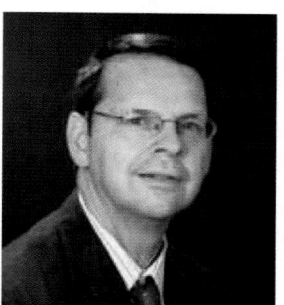

Christopher S. Ogilvy, MD
Director, Endovascular and Operative Neurovascular Surgery
Massachusetts General Hospital
Robert G. and A. Jean Ojemann Professor of Neurosurgery
Harvard Medical School
Boston, Massachusetts

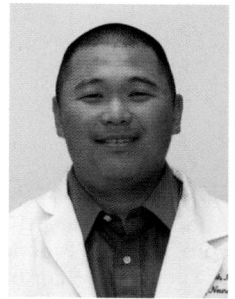

Brian L. Hoh, MD, FACS, FAHA, FAANS
William Merz Associate Professor
Department of Neurosurgery
University of Florida
Gainesville, Florida

SECTION FOUR: HYDROCEPHALUS;
SECTION FIVE: STEREOTACTIC RADIOSURGERY

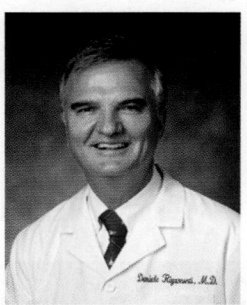

Daniele Rigamonti, MD, FACS
Professor of Neurosurgery, Oncology, and Radiation
Departments of Oncology and Molecular Radiation Sciences
Director, Stereotactic Radiosurgery
Director, Hydrocephalus and Pseudotumor Cerebri Program
Departments of Neurosurgery and Radiation Oncology
Johns Hopkins School of Medicine
Baltimore, Maryland

SECTION SIX: FUNCTIONAL NEUROSURGERY

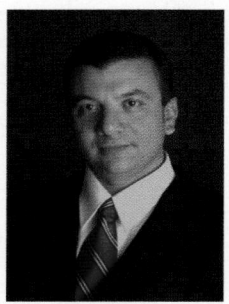

Emad Eskandar, MD
Director, Neurosurgical Residency Program
Director, Functional Neurosurgery
Massachusetts General Hospital
Associate Professor
Harvard Medical School
Boston, Massachusetts

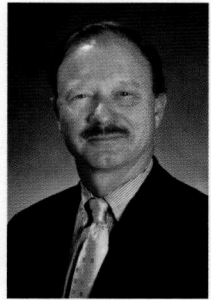

G. Rees Cosgrove, MD, FRCSC
Stoll Professor and Chairman
Department of Neurosurgery
The Warren Alpert Medical School of Brown University
Chief of Neurosurgery
Rhode Island Hospital and Miriam Hospital
Providence, Rhode Island

SECTION SEVEN: TRAUMA;
SECTION EIGHT: SURGICAL MANAGEMENT OF NERVOUS SYSTEM INFECTIONS

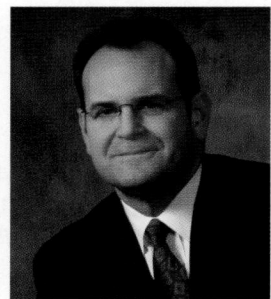

Geoffrey T. Manley, MD, PhD
Professor and Vice Chairman
Department of Neurological Surgery
University of California, San Francisco
Chief of Neurosurgery
Co-Director
Brain and Spinal Injury Center (BASIC)
San Francisco General Hospital
San Francisco, California

SECTION NINE: NEUROSURGICAL MANAGEMENT OF SPINAL DISORDERS

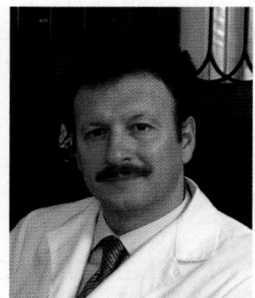

Ziya L. Gokaslan, MD, FACS
Danlin M. Long Professor of Neurosurgery, Oncology,
and Orthopedic Surgery
Vice Chairman
Department of Neurosurgery
Director
Johns Hopkins Hospital Neurosurgical Spine Program
Baltimore, Maryland

SECTION TEN: SURGICAL MANAGEMENT OF THE PERIPHERAL NERVOUS SYSTEM

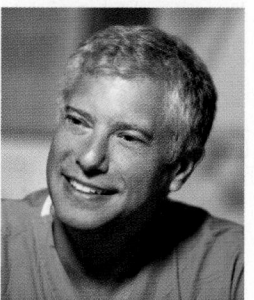

Allan J. Belzberg, MD, FRCSC
Associate Professor of Neurosurgery
The Johns Hopkins University School of Medicine
Director, Peripheral Nerve Surgery
Johns Hopkins Hospital
Baltimore, Maryland

Frank L. Acosta, MD
Assistant Professor
Department of Neurological Surgery
Director of Spinal Deformity
Cedars–Sinai Medical Center
Los Angeles, California
Spinal Infections: Vertebral Osteomyelitis and Spinal Epidural Abscess
Anterior Lumbar Interbody Fusion: Indications and Techniques
Surgical Management of Cerebrospinal Fluid Leakage after Spinal Surgery

P. David Adelson, MD
Director of Neurosciences and Neurosurgery
Department of Neurosurgery
Phoenix Children's Hospital
Phoenix, Arizona
Management of Pediatric Severe Traumatic Brain Injury

John R. Adler, Jr., MD
Dorothy and TK Chan Professor
Department of Neurosurgery
Stanford University Medical Center
Stanford, California
CyberKnife Radiosurgery for Spinal Neoplasms
Radiation Therapy and Radiosurgery in the Management of Craniopharyngiomas

Kamran V. Aghayev, MD
Spine Fellow
Department of Neurosurgery
University of South Florida
Neuro-Oncology
H. Lee Moffitt Cancer Center and Research Institute
Tampa, Florida
Transtemporal Approaches to Posterior Cranial Fossa

Manish K. Aghi, MD, PhD
Assistant Professor in Neurological Surgery
University of California, San Francisco
San Francisco, California
Cerebellar Tumors in Adults
Surgical Management of Intracerebral Hemorrhage

Basheal M. Agrawal, BS, MD
Department of Neurological Surgery
University of Wisconsin Hospital and Clinics
Madison, Wisconsin
Transforaminal Lumbar Interbody Fusion: Indications and Techniques

Manmeet S. Ahluwalia, MD
Section Head
Neuro-Oncology Outcomes
Brain Tumor and Neuro-Oncology Center
Neurological Institute
Associate Staff
Taussig Cancer Institute
Cleveland Clinic
Assistant Professor
Department of Medicine
Cleveland Clinic
Lerner College of Medicine of Case Western University
Cleveland, Ohio
Chemotherapy for Brain Tumors

Faiz Ahmad, MD
Fellow
University of Miami
Miami Children's Hospital
Jackson Memorial Hospital
Management of Nerve Sheath Tumors Involving the Spine

Ellen Air, MD, PhD
Assistant Professor
Director of Epilepsy Surgery
Department of Neurosurgery
University of Cincinnati College of Medicine and Mayfield Clinic
Cincinnati, Ohio
Radiation Therapy of Epilepsy

Pablo Ajler, MD
Department of Neurosurgery
Hospital Italiano de Buenos Aires
Assistant Professor
Department of Surgery
Instituto Universitario del Hospital Italiano de Buenos Aires
Buenos Aires, Argentina
Management of Shunt Infections

Felipe C. Albuquerque, MD
Assistant Director of Endovascular Neurosurgery
Barrow Neurological Institute
Phoenix, Arizona
Embolization of Tumors: Brain, Head, Neck, and Spine

Arun P. Amar, MD
Associate Professor
Department of Neurosurgery
University of Southern California
Los Angeles, California
Prolactinomas

Luca Amendola, MD
Department of Orthopedics and Traumatology
Spine Surgery
Ospedale
Bologna, Italy
*Management of Primary Malignant Tumors of the Osseous
    Spine*

Christopher Ames, MD
Director
University of California Spine Center
University of California, San Francisco
San Francisco, California
*Anterior Lumbar Interbody Fusion: Indications
    and Techniques*

Beejal Y. Amin, MD
Fellow
Department of Neurosurgical Surgery
University of California, San Francisco
San Francisco, California
Surgical Management of Posterior Fossa Meningiomas

Sepideh Amin-Hanjani, MD, FAANS, FACS, FAHA
Professor and Program Director
Co-Director of Neurovascular Surgery
Department of Neurosurgery
University of Illinois at Chicago
Chicago, Illinois
*Surgical Management of Cavernous Malformations
    of the Nervous System*

Joshua M. Ammerman, BS, MD
Assistant Clinical Professor
Department of Neurosurgery
George Washington University School of Medicine
Washington, District of Columbia
*Video-Assisted Thoracoscopic Discectomy: Indications
    and Techniques*

William S. Anderson, PhD, MD
Assistant Professor of Neurosurgery
The Johns Hopkins University School of Medicine
Department of Neurosurgery
Johns Hopkins Hospital
Baltimore, Maryland
Dorsal Root Entry Zone Lesions

Ronald I. Apfelbaum, MD
Professor
Department of Neurosurgery
University of Utah
Salt Lake City, Utah
*Neurovascular Decompression in Cranial Nerves V, VII, IX,
    and X*

Michael L. J. Apuzzo, MD, PhD
Edwin Todd/Trent H. Wells, Jr. Professor of Neurological
    Surgery and Radiation Departments of Oncology,
    Biology, and Physics
University of Southern California, Los Angeles
Keck School of Medicine
Director of Neurosurgery
Director of the Cyber Knife Unit
University of Southern California Kenneth Norris, Jr. Cancer
    Hospital
Director, Center for Stereotactic Neurosurgery
    and Associated Research
Clinical Director of Surgical Neuro-Oncology
Director of the Gamma Unit Facility
University of Southern California Hospital
Editor in Chief
World Neurosurgery
Los Angeles, California
*Transcallosal Surgery of Lesions Affecting the Third
    Ventricle: Basic Principles*

Rocco Armonda, MD
Director
Cerebrovascular Surgery, Interventional Neuroradiology,
    and Neurotrauma
Department of Neurosurgery
Walter Reed Military Medical Center
Director
Department of Neurosurgery
Uniformed Services University of the Health Sciences
Bethesda, Maryland
Management of Penetrating Brain Injury

Paul M. Arnold, MD
Professor of Neurosurgery
University of Kansas Medical Center
Kansas City, Kansas
Thoracolumbar Anterolateral and Posterior Stabilization

Harel Arzi, MD
Spine Fellow
Department of Neurosurgery
University of Kansas Medical Center
Kansas City, Kansas
Thoracolumbar Anterolateral and Posterior Stabilization

Ashok R. Asthagiri, MD
Staff Neurosurgeon
National Institutes of Health
Bethesda, Maryland
*Surgical Management of Parasagittal and Convexity
    Meningiomas*

Kurtis Auguste, MD
Assistant Professor
Director, Pediatric Epilepsy Surgery
Department of Neurological Surgery
UCSF Children's Hospital
Children's Hospital Oakland
Oakland, California
*Contemporary Dorsal Rhizotomy Surgery for the Treatment
    of Spasticity in Childhood*

Tariq E. Awad, MD, MSc, PhD
Assistant Professor
Department of Neurosurgery
Suez Canal University
Assistant Professor
Department of Neurosurgery
Suez Canal University Hospital
Ismailia, Egypt
Dynamic Stabilization of the Lumbar Spine: Indications and Techniques

Khaled M. Aziz, MD, PhD
Assistant Professor of Neurosurgery
Director of the Division of Complex Intracranial Surgery
Department of Neurosurgery
Allegheny General Hospital
Drexel Medical School
Pittsburgh, Pennsylvania
Surgical Management of Petroclival Meningiomas
Management of Cranial Nerve Injuries

Tipu Aziz, FRCS(SN), D.Med.Sci
Head of Oxford Functional Neurosurgery
Nuffield Department of Neurosurgery
University of Oxford
Department of Neurological Surgery
John Radcliffe Hospital
Oxford, United Kingdom
Cervical Dystonia and Spasmodic Torticollis: Indications and Techniques

Joachim M. Baehring, MD, DSc
Associate Professor
Departments of Neurology, Medicine, and Neurosurgery
Yale University School of Medicine
New Haven, Connecticut
Surgical Approaches to Lateral and Third Ventricular Tumors

Mirza N. Baig, MD, PhD
Neurosurgeon
Department of Neurological Surgery
Mercy Brain and Spine Center
Des Moines, Iowa
Cerebellar Tumors in Adults

Roy Bakay, MD
The A. Watson Armor III and Sarah Armour Presidential Chair and Residency Research Director
Rush University Medical Center
Chicago, Illinois
Brain–Computer Interfacing Prospects and Technical Aspects

Perry A. Ball, MD, FACS
Neurosurgeon
Departments of Medicine and of Orthopedics
Section of Neurosurgery
Dartmouth-Hitchcock Medical Center
The Dartmouth Institute for Health Policy and Clinical Practice
Lebanon, New Hampshire
Spinal Cord Stimulation and Intraspinal Infusions for Pain

Stefano Bandiera, MD
Attending Surgeon
Department of Oncologic and Degenerative Spine Surgery
Rizzoli Institute
Bologna, Italy
Management of Primary Malignant Tumors of the Osseous Spine

Nicholas M. Barbaro, MD
Professor and Chair
Department of Neurological Surgery
University of Indiana School of Medicine
Medical Director
Indiana University Health Neuroscience Center
Indianapolis, Indiana
Radiation Therapy of Epilepsy
Corpus Callosotomy: Indications and Techniques

Frederick G. Barker II, MD
Associate Professor of Surgery
Department of Neurosurgery
Harvard Medical School
Associate Visiting Neurosurgeon
Neurosurgical Service
Massachusetts General Hospital
Boston, Massachusetts
Surgical Approach to Falcine Meningiomas

Daniel L. Barrow, MD
MBNA/Bowman Professor and Chairman
Department of Neurosurgery
Emory University School of Medicine
Atlanta, Georgia
Surgical Management of Terminal Basilar and Posterior Cerebral Artery Aneurysms

Sachin Batra, MD, MPH
Research Fellow
Department of Neurological Surgery
Johns Hopkins Hospital
Baltimore, Maryland
Adult Pseudotumor Cerebri Syndrome
Stereotactic Radiosurgery for Pituitary Adenomas

Joshua Bederson, MD
Professor and Chair
Department of Neurosurgery
FPA Neurosurgery Department
The Mount Sinai Hospital
New York, New York
Management of Spinal Cord Tumors and Arteriovenous Malformations

Kimon Bekelis, MD
Resident
Department of Neurosurgery
Dartmouth-Hitchcock Medical Center
Lebanon, New Hampshire
Ensuring Patient Safety in Surgery—First Do No Harm
Surgical Management of Infratentorial Arteriovenous Malformations

Carlo Bellabarba, MD
Director
Orthopaedic Spine Service
Department of Orthopaedics and Sports Medicine
University of Washington/Harborview Medical Center
Professor
Department of Orthopaedics and Sports Medicine
University of Washington School of Medicine
Seattle, Washington
Management of Sacral Fractures

Lorenzo Bello, MD
Associate Professor of Neurosurgery
Neurological Sciences and Istituto Clinico Humanitas
Università degli Studi di Milano
Milano, Italy
Surgical Management of Low-Grade Gliomas

Allan J. Belzberg, MD, FRCSC
Associate Professor of Neurosurgery
The Johns Hopkins University School of Medicine
Director
Peripheral Nerve Surgery
Johns Hopkins Hospital
Baltimore, Maryland
Dorsal Root Entry Zone Lesions
Peripheral Nerve Tumors of the Extremities

Bernard R. Bendok, MD
Associate Professor of Neurological Surgery and Radiology
Department of Neurosurgery
Northwestern University
Chicago, Illinois
Endovascular Management of Spinal Vascular
  Malformations

Ludwig Benes, MD
Vice Chairman
Department of Neurosurgery
Philipps University Hospital
Marburg, Germany
Surgical Management of Aneurysms of the Vertebral
  and Posterior Inferior Cerebellar Artery Complex

Edward C. Benzel, MD
Chairman
Department of Neurosurgery
Staff, Center for Spine Health
Neurological Institute
Cleveland Clinic
Cleveland, Ohio
Management of Cervical Spondylotic Myelopathy

Helmut Bertalanffy, MD
Professor and Chairman
Department of Neurosurgery
University Hospital
Zurich, Switzerland
Surgical Management of Aneurysms of the Vertebral
  and Posterior Inferior Cerebellar Artery Complex

Chetan Bettegowda, MD, PhD
Resident
Department of Neurosurgery
The Johns Hopkins University School of Medicine
Baltimore, Maryland
Supratentorial Tumors in the Pediatric Population:
  Multidisciplinary Management

Ravi Bhatia, MS, MCh
Professor and Head of the Department of Neurosurgery
  (Retired)
All India Institute of Medical Sciences, New Delhi
New Delhi, India
Management of Tuberculous Infections of the Nervous System

Sanjay Bhatia, MBBS, MS, MCh
Assistant Professor
Department of Neurosurgery
West Virginia University
Assistant Professor
Department of Neurosurgery
Ruby Memorial Hospital
Morgantown, West Virginia
Surgical Management of Petroclival Meningiomas

Allen T. Bishop, MD
Professor
Department of Orthopedics
Mayo Clinic College of Medicine
Mayo Clinic
Rochester, Minnesota
Nerve Transfers: Indications and Techniques

Keith L. Black, MD
Chairman and Professor
Department of Neurosurgery
Director
Maxine Dunitz Neurosurgical Institute
Cedars-Sinai Medical Center
Los Angeles, California
Current Surgical Management of High-Grade Gliomas

Lewis S. Blevins, MD
Medical Director
California Center for Pituitary Disorders at University
  of California, San Francisco
Department of Neurological Surgery
University of California, San Francisco
San Francisco, California
Multimodal Assessment of Pituitary and Parasellar Lesions

George T. Blike, MD
Medical Director, Patient Safety and Training Center
Dartmouth-Hitchcock Medical Center
Lebanon, New Hampshire
Ensuring Patient Safety in Surgery—First Do No Harm

Ari Blitz, MD
Assistant Professor
Department of Radiology and Radiological Science
Division of Neuroradiology
The Johns Hopkins University and Medical Center
Baltimore, Maryland
Adult Pseudotumor Cerebri Syndrome

Göran C. Blomstedt, MD, PhD
Assistant Professor
Department of Neurosurgery
Helsinki University Hospital
Helsinki, Finland
Management of Infections After Craniotomy

Benjamin Blondel, MD
Spine Division
Department of Orthopedic Surgery
Hospital for Joint Diseases
New York, New York
Université de la Méditerranée
Orthopedic Surgery Department
Marseille, France
*Management of Degenerative Lumbar Stenosis
and Spondylolisthesis*

Kofi Boahene, MD, FACS
Assistant Professor
Department of Otolaryngology, Head, and Neck Surgery
The Johns Hopkins School of Medicine
Baltimore, Maryland
Management of Cerebrospinal Fluid Leaks

Bernardo Boleaga, MD
Department of Magnetic Resonance Imaging
Clinica Londres
Mexico City, Mexico
*Presurgical Evaluation for Epilepsy Including Intracranial
Electrodes*

Markus Bookland, MD
Resident
Department of Neuroscience
Center for Neurovirology
Temple University School of Medicine
Philadelphia, Pennsylvania
Surgical Management of Extracranial Carotid Artery Disease

Stefano Boriani, MD
Head
Department of Oncologic and Degenerative Spine Surgery
Rizzoli Institute
Bologna, Italy
*Management of Primary Malignant Tumors of the Osseous
Spine*

Christopher M. Boxell, MD
Neurosurgeon
Department of Neurological Surgery
University of Oklahoma
Oklahoma City, Oklahoma
Tulsa Spine and Specialty Hospital
Tulsa, Oklahoma
Cervical Laminoplasty: Indications and Techniques

Henry Brem, MD
Harvey Cushing Professor of Neurosurgery
Departments of Ophthalmology and Oncology
The Johns Hopkins Medical Institutions
Director
Hunterian Neurosurgical Laboratory
Department of Neurosurgery
Chairman
Department of Neurosurgery
The Johns Hopkins University School of Medicine
Baltimore, Maryland
Transcranial Surgery for Pituitary Macroadenomas

Albino Bricolo, MD
Professor and Chairman
Department of Neurosurgery
University of Verona Medical School
University Hospital of Verona
Verona, Italy
Surgical Management of Petroclival Meningiomas

Jason A. Brodkey, MD, FACS, FIPP
Neurosurgeon
Ann Arbor Spine Center
Ann Arbor, Michigan
Transtemporal Approaches to Posterior Cranial Fossa

Jacques Brotchi, MD, PhD
Emeritus Professor and Honorary Chairman
Department of Neurosurgery
Erasme Hospital
Brussels, Belgium
*Surgical Management of Intramedullary Spinal Cord Tumors
in Adults*

Jeffrey N. Bruce, MD
Professor of Neurological Surgery
Edgar M. Housepian Professor of Neurological Surgery
Columbia University College of Physicians and Surgeons
Attending Neurosurgeon
New York Presbyterian Medical Center
New York, New York
Management of Pineal Region Tumors

Michael Bruneau, MD
Neurosurgeon
Department of Neurosurgery
Erasme Hospital
Brussels, Belgium
*Surgical Management of Intramedullary Spinal Cord Tumors
in Adults*

Bradley R. Buchbinder, MD
Director
Clinical Functional Magnetic Resonance Imaging
Staff Neuroradiologist
Division of Neuroradiology
Massachusetts General Hospital
Boston, Massachusetts
Motor Cortex Stimulation for Intractable Facial Pain

Kim J. Burchiel, MD
John Raaf Professor and Chairman
Oregon Health and Science University
Portland, Oregon
Deep Brain Stimulation in Movement Disorders: Parkinson's Disease, Essential Tremor, and Dystonia

Timothy G. Burke, MD
Neurosurgeon
Department of Neurosurgery
Anne Arundel Medical Center
Annapolis, Maryland
Circumferential Cervical Spinal Fusion

Ali Bydon, MD
Assistant Professor
Department of Neurosurgery
The Johns Hopkins University
Clinical Director of Spinal Surgery
Department of Neurosurgery
The Johns Hopkins Bayview Medical Center
Baltimore, Maryland
Posterior Lumbar Fusion by Open Technique: Indications and Techniques

Francesco Cacciola, MD
Walton Centre for Neurology and Neurosurgery
Liverpool, United Kingdom
Anterior Approaches for Multilevel Cervical Spondylosis

Kevin Cahill, MD, PhD, MPH
Spine Fellow
Department of Neurosurgery
University of Miami Miller School of Medicine
Miami, Florida
Dorsal Root Entry Zone Lesions

Paolo Cappabianca, MD
Professor and Chairman
Department of Neurological Sciences
Division of Neurosurgery
Università degli Studi di Napoli Federico II
Naples, Italy
Endocrinologically Silent Pituitary Tumors

Anthony J. Caputy, MD
Professor and Chairman
Department of Neurosurgery
The George Washington University
Washington, District of Columbia
Video-Assisted Thoracoscopic Discectomy: Indications and Techniques

Francesco Cardinale, MD
Neurosurgeon
Centre Claudio Munari for Epilepsy and Parkinson Surgery
Niguarda Hospital
Milan, Italy
Multilobar Resection and Hemispherectomy in Epilepsy Surgery

Ricardo L. Carrau, MD
Professor of Otolaryngology-Head and Neck Surgery and Neurosurgery
Director of the Maxillofacial Trauma Service
Director of the Consult Service
Director of the Tracheotomy and Swallowing Unit
University of Pittsburgh Medical Center
Pittsburgh, Pennsylvania
Endoscopic Endonasal Approach for Craniopharyngiomas

Benjamin S. Carson, MD
Professor and Director
Department of Pediatric Neurosurgery
Professor of Neurosurgery, Oncology, Plastic Surgery, and Pediatrics
The Johns Hopkins Medical Institutions
Department of Neurosurgery
The Johns Hopkins Medical Institutions
Baltimore, Maryland
Neurosurgical Problems of the Spine in Achondroplasia

Bob S. Carter, MD
Professor and Chief
Department of Neurosurgery
University of California, San Diego
San Diego, California
Surgical Management of Intracerebral Hemorrhage

Giuseppe Casaceli, MD
Resident in Neurosurgery
Neurological Sciences and Istituto Clinico Humanitas
Università degli Studi di Milano
Milano, Italy
Surgical Management of Low-Grade Gliomas

Laura Castana, MD
Epilepsy and Parkinson Surgery Centre
C. Munari Ospedale Niguarda Ca'Granda
Milan, Italy
Multilobar Resection and Hemispherectomy in Epilepsy Surgery

Gabriel Castillo, MD
Associate Neurosurgeon
Puerta de Hierro Medical Center
Guadalajara, Mexico
Surgical Treatment of Paraclinoid Aneurysms

Luigi M. Cavallo, MD, PhD
Neurosurgeon
Department of Neurological Sciences
Division of Neurosurgery
Università degli Studi di Napoli Federico II
Naples, Italy
Endocrinologically Silent Pituitary Tumors

C. Michael Cawley, MD
Associate Professor
Departments of Neurosurgery and Radiology
Emory University School of Medicine
Atlanta, Georgia
Surgical Management of Terminal Basilar and Posterior Cerebral Artery Aneurysms

Aabir Chakraborty, MD
Honorary Senior Lecturer
Neurosciences
Institute of Child Health
University College, London
Consultant
Pediatric Neurosurgery
Great Osmond Street Hospital for Children
London, United Kingdom
*Methods for Cerebrospinal Fluid Diversion in Pediatric
Hydrocephalus: From Shunt to Scope*

Edward F. Chang, MD
Chief Resident
Department of Neurological Surgery
University of California, San Francisco
San Francisco, California
Corpus Callosotomy: Indications and Techniques

Eric C. Chang, BS, MD
Resident
Department of Neurosurgery
Massachusetts General Hospital
Harvard University
Boston, Massachusetts
Surgical Approach to Falcine Meningiomas

Steven D. Chang, MD
Robert C. and Jeannette Powell Professor
Department of Neurosurgery
Stanford University
Stanford, California
CyberKnife Radiosurgery for Spinal Neoplasms
*Radiation Therapy and Radiosurgery in the Management
of Craniopharyngiomas*

Jens R. Chapman, MD
Professor
Department of Orthopaedics and Sports Medicine
University of Washington
Seattle, Washington
Management of Sacral Fractures

E. Thomas Chappell, MD
Neurosurgeon
Department of Neurosurgery
University of California, Irvine
Irvine, California
*Neurosurgical Management of HIV-Related Focal Brain
Lesions*

Neeraj Chaudhary, MD, MRCS(UK), FRCR(UK)
Assistant Professor
Fellowship Program Co-Director
Division of Neurointerventional Surgery
Departments of Radiology and Neurosurgery
University of Michigan Health System
Ann Arbor, Michigan
Endovascular Management of Intracranial Aneurysms

Douglas Chen, MD, FACS
Co-Director, Hearing and Balance Center
Adjunct Associate Professor of Surgery
(Otolaryngology and Neurosurgery)
Allegheny University of the Health Sciences
Pittsburgh, Pennsylvania
Management of Cranial Nerve Injuries

James Chen, BS
Division of Interventional Neuroradiology
Department of Radiology
Johns Hopkins Hospital
Baltimore, Maryland
*Imaging Evaluation and Endovascular Treatment
of Vasospasm*

Linda C. Chen, BS
Medical Student
Department of Neurosurgery
The Johns Hopkins University
Baltimore, Maryland
*Supratentorial Tumors in the Pediatric Population:
Multidisciplinary Management*

Boyle C. Cheng, PhD
Associate Professor
Department of Neurosurgery
Drexel University College of Medicine
Director
Department of Neurosurgery
Division of Research
Allegheny General Hospital
Pittsburgh, Pennsylvania
*Dynamic Stabilization of the Lumbar Spine: Indications
and Techniques*

Joshua J. Chern, MD, PhD
Neurosurgeon
Children's Healthcare of Atlanta
Atlanta, Georgia
*Instrumentation and Stabilization of the Pediatric Spine:
Technical Nuances and Age-Specific Considerations*

John H. Chi, MD, MPH
Assistant Professor
Department of Neurosurgery
Brigham and Women's Hospital
Harvard Medical School
Boston, Massachusetts
*Lateral Lumbar Interbody Fusion: Indications
and Techniques*

Wade W. Chien, MD
Clinical Fellow
Division of Otology/Neurotology
Department of Otolaryngology
The Johns Hopkins School of Medicine
Baltimore, Maryland
Hearing Prosthetics: Surgical Techniques

E. Antonio Chiocca, MD, PhD
Chairman
Department of Neurological Surgery
Dardinger Family Professor of Oncologic Neurosurgery
Physician Director
OSUMC Neuroscience Signature Program
Co-Director
Dardinger Center for Neuro-Oncology and Neurosciences
Co-Director
Viral Oncology Program of the Comprehensive Cancer
    Center
James Cancer Hospital and Solove Research Institute
The Ohio State University Medical Center
Columbus, Ohio
Cerebellar Tumors in Adults

Rohan Chitale, MD
Neurosurgeon
Department of Neurosurgery
Thomas Jefferson University Hospital
Philadelphia, Pennsylvania
*Endovascular Treatment of Cerebral Arteriovenous
    Malformations*

Bhupal Chitnavis, BSc(Hons) MBBS, FRCS(Eng), FRCS(SN)
Consultant Neurosurgeon
Department of Neurosurgery
London Bridge Hospital
London, United Kingdom
*Disc Replacement Technologies in the Cervical and Lumbar
    Spine*

Lana D. Christiano, MD
Department of Neurological Surgery
University of Medicine and Dentistry of New Jersey
Newark, New Jersey
Surgical Management of Tumors of the Jugular Foramen

Ray M. Chu, MD
Neurosurgeon
Department of Neurosurgery
Cedars–Sinai Medical Center
Los Angeles, California
Current Surgical Management of High-Grade Gliomas

Elisa F. Ciceri, MD
Director
Department of Interventional Neuroradiology
Fondazione
Milan, Italy
Endovascular Management of Dural Arteriovenous Fistulas

Michelle J. Clarke, MD
Assistant Professor of Neurosurgery
Mayo Clinic
Rochester, Minnesota
Management of Penetrating Injuries to the Spine

Alan Cohen, MD, FACS, FAAP
Robert and William Reinberger Chair in Pediatric
    Neurological Surgery
Professor
Departments of Neurological Surgery and Pediatrics
Director
Neurological Surgery Residency Program
Case Western Reserve University School of Medicine
Cleveland, Ohio
Management of Tumors of the Fourth Ventricle

Annamaria Colao, MD, PhD
Professor of Endocrinology
Chief of the Neuroendocrine Unit
University Federico II
Naples, Italy
Endocrinologically Silent Pituitary Tumors

Geoffrey P. Colby, MD, PhD
Neurosurgeon
The Johns Hopkins Medical Center
Baltimore, Maryland
Endovascular Management of Dural Arteriovenous Fistulas

Massimo Collice, MD[†]
Former Professor and Chairman
Department of Neurological Sciences
A.O. Niguarda
Chief
Department of Neurosurgery
Niguarda Ca'Granda Hospital
Milan, Italy
Management of Traumatic Intracranial Aneurysms

Daniel Condit, BS
ThedaCare Behavioral Health–Midway
Menasha, Wisconsin
Deep Brain Stimulation for Pain

Alexander L. Coon, MD
Assistant Professor of Neurosurgery, Neurology,
    and Radiology
Director, Endovascular Neurosurgery
Johns Hopkins Hospital
Department of Neurosurgery
Baltimore, Maryland
Endovascular Management of Dural Arteriovenous Fistulas

Cassius Vinícius Corrêa Dos Reis, MD
Assistant Professor of Neurosurgery
Medical School
Universidade Federal de Minas Gerais
Belo Horizonte, Brazil
Surgical Management of Tumors of the Foramen Magnum

[†]Deceased.

G. Rees Cosgrove, MD, FRCSC
Stoll Professor and Chairman
Department of Neurosurgery
The Warren Alpert Medical School of Brown University
Chief of Neurosurgery
Rhode Island Hospital and Miriam Hospital
Providence, Rhode Island
Temporal Lobe Operations in Intractable Epilepsy
Cingulotomy for Intractable Psychiatric Illness

Massimo Cossu, MD
Claudio Munari Epilepsy Surgery Center
Niguarda Hospital
Milan, Italy
Multilobar Resection and Hemispherectomy in Epilepsy
* Surgery*

William T. Couldwell, MD, PhD
Professor and Chairman of Neurosurgery
Department of Neurosurgery
University of Utah Health Science Center
Salt Lake City, Utah
Prolactinomas

William T. Curry, MD
Attending Neurosurgeon
Department of Neurosurgery
Massachusetts General Hospital
Assistant Professor
Department of Surgery
Harvard Medical School
Boston, Massachusetts
Surgical Approach to Falcine Meningiomas

Guilherme Dabus, MD
Associate Professor
Departments of Radiology and Neurological Surgery
Wertheim College of Medicine–Florida International
  University
Director, Fellowship Program
Department of Neurointerventional Surgery
Baptist Cardiac and Vascular Institute
Miami, Florida
Endovascular Management of Spinal Vascular
* Malformations*

Teodoro Forcht Dagi, MD, DMedSC
Chief Medical Officer
AventuraHQ Inc.
Denver, Colorado
Management of Cerebrospinal Fluid Leaks

Giuseppe D'Aliberti, MD
Department of Neurosurgery
Niguarda Ca'Granda Hospital
Milan, Italy
Management of Traumatic Intracranial Aneurysms

Moise Danielpour, MD
Director
Pediatric Neurosurgery Program
Department of Neurosurgery
Cedars-Sinai Medical Center
Los Angeles, California
Contemporary Dorsal Rhizotomy Surgery for the Treatment
* of Spasticity in Childhood*

Mark J. Dannenbaum, MD
Clinical Instructor/Cerebrovascular Fellow
Departments of Neurosurgery and Radiology
Emory University
Atlanta, Georgia
Surgical Management of Terminal Basilar and Posterior
* Cerebral Artery Aneurysms*

Ronan M. Dardis, MD, MPhil, FRCSI(Neuro Surg)
Consultant Neurosurgeon
Department of Neurosurgery
University Hospitals Coventry and Warwickshire
Honorary Associate Clinical Professor
University of Warwick
Warwickshire, United Kingdom
Disc Replacement Technologies in the Cervical and Lumbar
* Spine*

Hormuzdiyar H. Dasenbrock, MD
Department of Neurosurgery
Brigham and Women's Hospital
Children's Hospital of Boston
Harvard Medical School
Boston, Massachusetts
Posterior Lumbar Fusion by Open Technique: Indications
* or Techniques*

Reza Dashti, MD, PhD
Associate Professor
Department of Neurosurgery
Istanbul University
Cerrahpasa Medical Faculty
Istanbul, Turkey
Endovascular Neurosurgery Fellow
Department of Neurosurgery
University of Illinois at Chicago
Chicago, Illinois
Surgical Management of Aneurysms of the Middle Cerebral
* Artery*

Arthur L. Day, MD
Professor and Chairman
Harvard Medical School
Brigham and Women's Hospital
Boston, Massachusetts
Management of Unruptured Intracranial Aneurysms
Surgical Management of Cerebellar Stroke—Hemorrhage
* and Infarction*

John Diaz Day, MD
Associate Professor
Director
Cranial Base Surgery Program
Department of Neurosurgery
University of Texas Health Science Center at San Antonio
San Antonio, Texas
Tumors Involving the Cavernous Sinus

Vedran Deletis, MD, PhD
Associate Professor
Institute for Neurology and Neurosurgery
Roosevelt Hospital
New York, New York
Intraoperative Neurophysiology: A Tool to Prevent and/or
* Document Intraoperative Injury to the Nervous System*

Ramiro Del-Valle, MD
Chairman
Gamma Knife Neurosurgery Center
Mèdica Sur Clinical Foundation
Mexico City, Mexico
*Role of Gamma Knife Radiosurgery in the Management
    of Arteriovenous Malformations*

Franco DeMonte, MD
Professor
Mary Beth Pawelek Chair
Department of Neurosurgery
The University of Texas MD Anderson Cancer Center
Houston, Texas
Spheno-Orbital Meningioma

Francesco Dimeco, MD
Department of Neurological Surgery
Fondazione Istituto Neurologico
Milan, Italy
Surgical Management of Low-Grade Gliomas

Robert Dodd, MD, PhD
Assistant Professor
Department of Neurosurgery
Stanford University School of Medicine
Stanford, California
CyberKnife Radiosurgery for Spinal Neoplasms

Francesco Doglietto, MD, PhD
Department of Neurosurgery
Catholic University School of Medicine
Rome, Italy
Surgical Management of Lesions of the Clivus

Lutz Dörner, MD
Department of Neurosurgery
Universitätsklinikum
Kiel, Germany
*Surgical Navigation with Intraoperative Imaging: Special
    Operating Room Concepts*

Michael J. Dorsi, MD
Chief Resident
Department of Neurosurgery
The Johns Hopkins School of Medicine
Baltimore, Maryland
Peripheral Nerve Tumors of the Extremities

Gaby D. Doumit, MD, MSc
Staff
Department of Plastic Surgery
Cleveland Clinic
Cleveland, Ohio
*Principles of Scalp Surgery and Surgical Management
    of Major Defects of Scalp*

James M. Drake, MSc, FRCS(C), MBBCh
Professor
Department of Surgery
Division of Neurosurgery
University of Toronto
Pediatric Neurosurgeon
Hospital for Sick Children
Toronto, Canada
*Methods for Cerebrospinal Fluid Diversion in Pediatric
    Hydrocephalus: From Shunt to Scope*

Doniel Drazin, MD, MA
Department of Neurosurgery
Cedars-Sinai Medical Center
Los Angeles, California
*Contemporary Dorsal Rhizotomy Surgery for the Treatment
    of Spasticity in Childhood*
*Spinal Infections: Vertebral Osteomyelitis and Spinal
    Epidural Abscess*
*Anterior Lumbar Interbody Fusion: Indications
    and Techniques*
*Surgical Management of Cerebrospinal Fluid Leakage after
    Spinal Surgery*

Rose Du, MD, PhD
Instructor
Department of Neurosurgery
Brigham and Women's Hospital
Harvard Medical School
Boston, Massachusetts
Management of Intracranial Aneurysms Caused by Infection

Thomas B. Ducker, MD
Professor
Department of Neurological Surgery
The Johns Hopkins School of Medicine
Baltimore, Maryland
Circumferential Cervical Spinal Fusion

Hugues Duffau, MD, PhD
Professor and Chairman
Department of Neurosurgery
Hôpital Gui de Chauliac
CHU de Montpellier
Montpellier, France
Cortical and Subcortical Brain Mapping

Bradley S. Duhon, MD
Neurosurgeon
Gordon Spine & Brain Associates
Tyler, Texas
Lumbar Microdiscectomy: Indications and Techniques

Paula Eboli, MD
Resident
Department of Neurological Surgery
Cedars–Sinai Medical Center
Los Angeles, California
*Spinal Infections: Vertebral Osteomyelitis and Spinal
    Epidural Abscess*

Mohamed Samy Elhammady, MD
Instructor of Clinical Neurological Surgery
Department of Neurological Surgery
University of Miami Miller School of Medicine
Miami, Florida
*Far Lateral Approach and Transcondylar and Supracondylar
    Extensions for Aneurysms of the Vertebrobasilar Junction*

Pamela Ely, MD, PhD
Associate Professor of Medicine, Emeritus
Section of Hematology/Oncology
Dartmouth Medical School
Hanover, New Hampshire
*Management of Primary Central Nervous System
    Lymphomas*

Nancy E. Epstein, MD
Clinical Professor of Neurological Surgery
The Albert Einstein College of Medicine
Bronx, New York
Chief of Neurosurgical Spine and Education
Winthrop University Hospital
Mineola, New York
Management of Far Lateral Lumbar Disc Herniations

Kadir Erkmen, MD
Associate Professor
Department of Neurosurgery
Dartmouth-Hitchcock Medical Center
Lebanon, New Hampshire
Ensuring Patient Safety in Surgery—First Do No Harm

Thomas Errico, MD
Professor and Chief
Division of Spine Surgery
Departments of Orthopedic Surgery (Ortho Spine Surgery
    Division Director) and Neurosurgery
New York University Langone Medical Center
New York, New York
*Management of Degenerative Lumbar Stenosis
    and Spondylolisthesis*

Emad N. Eskandar, MD
Director, Neurosurgical Residency Program
Director, Functional Neurosurgery
Massachusetts General Hospital
Associate Professor
Harvard Medical School
Boston, Massachusetts
*Temporal Lobe Operations in Intractable Epilepsy
Motor Cortex Stimulation for Intractable Facial Pain*

Clifford J. Eskey, MD, PhD
Associate Professor of Radiology and Surgery
Department of Radiology
Dartmouth-Hitchcock Medical Center
Lebanon, New Hampshire
Vertebroplasty and Kyphoplasty: Indications and Techniques

Felice Esposito, MD, PhD
Division of Neurosurgery
Division of Maxillo-Facial Surgery
Università degli Studi di Napoli Federico II
Napoli, Italy
Endocrinologically Silent Pituitary Tumors

Camilo E. Fadul, MD
Professor
Departments of Medicine and Neurology
Dartmouth Medical School
Hanover, New Hampshire
Director of Neuro-Oncology Program
Norris-Cotton Cancer Center
Dartmouth-Hitchcock Medical Center
Lebanon, New Hampshire
*Management of Primary Central Nervous System
    Lymphomas*

Gilbert J. Fanciullo, MD, MS
Director
Section of Pain Medicine
Dartmouth-Hitchcock Medical Center
Lebanon, New Hampshire
Professor of Anesthesiology
Dartmouth Medical School
Hanover, New Hampshire
Spinal Cord Stimulation and Intraspinal Infusions for Pain

Kyle M. Fargen, MD, MPH
Resident
Department of Neurosurgery
University of Florida
Gainesville, Florida
Endovascular Treatment of Stroke

Gidon Felsen, PhD
Departments of Physiology and Biophysics
University of Colorado School of Medicine
Aurora, Colorado
*Novel Targets in Deep Brain Stimulation for Movement
    Disorders*

Dong Xia Feng, MD, PhD
Department of Neurosurgery
University of Arkansas College of Medicine
Department of Neurosurgery
Little Rock, Arkansas
Tumors Involving the Cavernous Sinus

Richard G. Fessler, MD, PhD
Professor of Neurological Surgery
Northwestern University Feinberg School of Medicine
Chicago, Illinois
Surgical Approaches to the Cervicothoracic Junction

Aaron G. Filler, MD, PhD, FRCS
Medical Director
Institute for Nerve Medicine
Santa Monica, California
Imaging for Peripheral Nerve Disorders

John C. Flickinger, MD, FACR
Professor of Radiation Oncology and Neurological Surgery
University of Pittsburgh School of Medicine
Pittsburgh, Pennsylvania
Vestibular Schwannomas: The Role of Stereotactic Surgery

John R. Floyd, MD
Assistant Professor of Neurological Surgery
Department of Neurological Surgery
University of Texas Health Science Center, San Antonio
San Antonio, Texas
Spheno-Orbital Meningioma

Kevin T. Foley, MD
Professor
Department of Neurological Surgery
Semmes-Murphey Neurologic and Spine Institute
Memphis, Tennessee
*Percutaneous Placement of Lumbar Pedicle Screws:
    Indications and Techniques*

Kostas N. Fountas, MD, PhD
Associate Professor of Neurosurgery
Department of Neurosurgery
University Hospital of Larissa School of Medicine
University of Thessaly
Larissa, Greece
*Mesencephalic Tractotomy and Anterolateral Cordotomy
    for Intractable Pain*

Howard Francis, MD
Associate Professor
The Johns Hopkins University
Baltimore, Maryland
Hearing Prosthetics: Surgical Techniques

James L. Frazier, MD
Chief Resident
Department of Neurosurgery
Johns Hopkins Hospital
Baltimore, Maryland
Surgical Management of Brain Stem Tumors in Adults

Kai Frerichs, MD
Director of Endovascular Neurosurgery
Neuro-Oncology
Harvard Medical School
Dana-Farber Cancer Center Institute
Boston, Massachusetts
Management of Unruptured Intracranial Aneurysms

David M. Frim, MD, PhD
Ralph Cannon Professor and Chief
Section of Neurosurgery
The University of Chicago
Chicago, Illinois
*Surgical Management of Neurofibromatosis Types 1 and 2
Surgical Management of Hydrocephalus in the Adult*

Sebastien Froelich, MD
Department of Neurosurgery
Strasbourg University Hospital
Strasbourg, France
Surgical Management of Petroclival Meningiomas

Takanori Fukushima, MD
Consulting Professor of Surgery
Department of Surgery
Division of Neurosurgery
Duke University Medical Center
Durham, North Carolina
*Tumors Involving the Cavernous Sinus
Surgical Management of Tumors of the Jugular Foramen*

Philippe Gailloud, MD
Director of the Division of Interventional Neuroradiology
Director of the Endovascular Surgical Neuroradiology
    Program
Co-Director of The Johns Hopkins Center for Pediatric
    Neurovascular Diseases
Johns Hopkins Hospital
Baltimore, Maryland
*Surgical Management of Infratentorial Arteriovenous
    Malformations
Adult Pseudotumor Cerebri Syndrome*

Sergio Maria Gaini, MD
Professor in Neurosurgery
Department of Neurological Sciences
Università degli Studi di Milano
Milano, Italy
Surgical Management of Low-Grade Gliomas

Chirag D. Gandhi, MD
Assistant Professor of Neurological Surgery and Radiology
Director of Endovascular Neurosurgery Fellowship Program
Director of Undergraduate Neurosurgical Education
Director of Traumatic Brain Injury Basic Science Laboratory
Neurological Institute of New Jersey
Newark, New Jersey
Endovascular Treatment of Head and Neck Bleeding

Dheeraj Gandhi, MD, MBBS
Director, Interventional Neuroradiology
The Johns Hopkins Bayview
Associate Professor
Departments of Radiology, Neurosurgery, and Neurology
The Johns Hopkins School of Medicine
Baltimore, Maryland
*Imaging Evaluation and Endovascular Treatment of
    Vasospasm*

Gale Gardner, MD
Professor
Department of Otology/Neurotology
Louisiana State University Shreveport
Shreveport, Louisiana
Transtemporal Approaches to Posterior Cranial Fossa

Paul Gardner, MD
Assistant Professor
Department of Neurosurgery
University of Pittsburgh
Pittsburgh, Pennsylvania
Endoscopic Endonasal Approach for Craniopharyngiomas

Mark Garrett, MD
Neurosurgical Resident
Division of Neurological Surgery
Barrow Neurological Institute
St. Joseph's Hospital and Medical Center
Phoenix, Arizona
Posterior Lumbar Interbody Fusion

Tomás Garzón-Muvdi, MD, MS
Postdoctoral Fellow
Department of Neurosurgery
The Johns Hopkins Medical Institutions
Baltimore, Maryland
*Surgical Management of Infratentorial Arteriovenous
    Malformations
Management of Neurocysticercosis*

Alessandro Gasbarrini, MD
Medical Director
Istituto Ortopedico Rizzoli
Bologna, Italy
*Management of Primary Malignant Tumors of the Osseous
    Spine*

Fred H. Geisler, MD, PhD
Founder
Illinois Neuro Spine Center
Aurora, Illinois
Lumbar Spinal Arthroplasty: Clinical Experiences of Motion Preservation

Joseph J. Gemmete, MD
Associate Professor of Radiology
Departments of Radiology, Neurosurgery,
    and Otolaryngology
University of Michigan Hospitals
Ann Arbor, Michigan
Endovascular Management of Intracranial Aneurysms

Massimo Gerosa, MD
Professor of Neurosurgery
University of Verona
Chairman
Department of Neurosurgery
University Hospital
Verona, Italy
Stereotactic Radiosurgery Meningiomas

Atul Goel, MCh
Residency Program Director
Neurosurgery Department Chairman
Consulting Surgeon
Seth Medical College
Mumbai, India
Anterior Approaches for Multilevel Cervical Spondylosis

Ziya L. Gokaslan, MD, FACS
Danlin M. Long Professor of Neurosurgery, Oncology,
    and Orthopedic Surgery
Vice Chairman
Department of Neurosurgery
Director
Johns Hopkins Hospital Neurosurgical Spine Program
Baltimore, Maryland
Surgery for Metastatic Spine Disease
Surgical Resection of Sacral Tumors

L. Fernando Gonzalez, MD
Thomas Jefferson University
Jefferson Medical College
Assistant Professor
Department of Neurological Surgery
Division of Neurovascular Surgery and Endovascular
    Neurosurgery
Philadelphia, Pennsylvania
*Endovascular Treatment of Cerebral Arteriovenous
    Malformations*

C. Rory Goodwin, BS
Resident
Johns Hopkins Hospital
UNCF/Merck Postdoctoral Fellow
Baltimore, Maryland
Transcranial Surgery for Pituitary Macroadenomas

Takeo Goto, MD
c/o Kenji Ohata, MD
*Orbitozygomatic Infratemporal Approach to Parasellar
    Meningiomas*

Grahame C. Gould, MD
Resident
Department of Neurological Surgery
Yale University
Yale New Haven Hospital
New Haven, Connecticut
Surgical Approaches to Lateral and Third Ventricular Tumors

M. Sean Grady, MD
Chairman and Professor
Department of Neurosurgery
University of Pennsylvania School of Medicine
Philadelphia, Pennsylvania
*Surgical Management of Major Skull Defects and Potential
    Complications*

Andrew W. Grande, MD
Assistant Professor
Department of Neurosurgery
University of Minnesota
Minneapolis, Minnesota
*Percutaneous Stereotactic Rhizotomy in the Treatment
    of Intractable Facial Pain*

Ramesh Grandhi, MD
Resident
University of Pittsburgh Medical Center
Pittsburgh, Pennsylvania
*Perioperative Management of Severe Traumatic Brain Injury
    in Adults*

Alexander L. Green, FRCS(SN), MD, BSc, MBBS
Spalding Senior Lecturer
Consultant Neurosurgeon
John Radcliffe Hospital
Oxford, United Kingdom
*Functional Tractography, Diffusion Tensor Imaging,
    Intraoperative Integration of Modalities,
    and Neuronavigation*
Surgical Management of Extratemporal Lobe Epilepsy

Jeffrey P. Greenfield, MD, PhD
Assistant Professor of Neurological Surgery
Department of Neurological Surgery
Weill Cornell Medical College
Assistant Member
Department of Neurosurgery
Memorial Sloan-Kettering Cancer Center
New York, New York
Endoscopic Approach to Intraventricular Brain Tumors

Bradley A. Gross, MD
Resident
Harvard Medical School
Resident
Department of Neurosurgery
Brigham and Women's Hospital
Boston, Massachusetts
Management of Intracranial Aneurysms Caused by Infection

Rachel Grossman, MD
Neurosurgical Oncology Fellow
Department of Neurosurgery
The Johns Hopkins University
Baltimore, Maryland
Management of Suppurative Intracranial Infections

Mari Groves, MD
Neurosurgical Resident
Johns Hopkins Hospital
Baltimore, Maryland
Neurosurgical Problems of the Spine in Achondroplasia

Gerardo Guinto, MD
Professor and Chairman
Department of Neurosurgery
Hospital de Especialidades Centro Medico Siglo XXI
Mexico City, Mexico
Surgical Management of Sphenoid Wing Meningiomas

Richard Gullan, BSc, MBBS, MRCP, FRCS
Consultant Neurosurgeon
BMI Healthcare
London, United Kingdom
Disc Replacement Technologies in the Cervical and Lumbar Spine

Gaurav Gupta, MD
Senior Fellow
Department of Neurosurgery
University of Medicine and Dentistry of New Jersey
New Jersey Medical School
Newark, New Jersey
Surgical Management of Tumors of the Jugular Foramen
Management of Ulnar Nerve Compression

Nalin Gupta, MD, PhD
Associate Professor
Neurological Surgery and Pediatrics
Chief, Division of Pediatric Neurosurgery
University of California, San Francisco
San Francisco, California
Fetal Surgery for Open Neural Tube Defects

Todd C. Hankinson, MD, MBA
Assistant Professor
Department of Neurosurgery
Children's Hospital Colorado
University of Colorado, Denver
Aurora, Colorado
Surgical Decision-Making and Treatment Options for Chiari Malformations in Children

Ake Hansasuta, MD
Neurosurgeon
Ramathibodi Hospital
Bangkok, Thailand
CyberKnife Radiosurgery for Spinal Neoplasms

James S. Harrop, MD
Associate Professor of Neurologic and Orthopedic Surgery
Jefferson Medical College
Philadelphia, Pennsylvania
Management of Injuries of the Cervical Spine and Spinal Cord

Griffith R. Harsh IV, MD, MA, MBA
Professor
Stanford Medical School
Stanford, California
Management of Recurrent Gliomas

Alia Hdeib, MD
Department of Neurological Surgery
University Hospitals Case Medical Center
Cleveland, Ohio
Management of Tumors of the Fourth Ventricle

Stefan Heinze, MD
Neurosurgeon
Department of Neurosurgery
Philips University Marburg
Marburg, Germany
Surgical Management of Aneurysms of the Vertebral and Posterior Inferior Cerebellar Artery Complex

John Heiss, MD
Head, Clinical Unit
Surgical Neurology Branch
National Institute of Neurological Disorders and Stroke
National Institutes of Health
Bethesda, Maryland
Management of Chiari Malformations and Syringomyelia

Dieter Hellwig, MD, PhD
Head, Stereotactic and Functional Neurosurgery
International Neuroscience Institute
Hanover, Germany
Arachnoid, Suprasellar, and Rathke's Cleft Cysts

Juha Hernesniemi, MD, PhD
Professor and Chairman
Department of Neurosurgery
University Hospital of Helsinki
Helsinki, Finland
Surgical Management of Aneurysms of the Middle Cerebral Artery

Roberto C. Heros, MD
Professor
Co-Chairman and Program Director of Neurological Surgery
University of Miami
Miami, Florida
Far Lateral Approach and Transcondylar and Supracondylar Extensions for Aneurysms of the Vertebrobasilar Junction

Todd Hillman, MD
Otolaryngologist
Pittsburgh Ear Associates
Co-Director of the Hearing and Balance Center
Pittsburgh, Pennsylvania
Surgical Management of Petroclival Meningiomas

Jose Hinojosa, MD, PhD
Servicio de Neurocirugìa Peditrica
Hospital Universitario Infantil
Madrid, Spain
Methods of Cranial Vault Reconstruction for Craniosynostosis

Girish K. Hiremath, MD
Chief Resident
Department of Neurosurgery
Cleveland Clinic
Cleveland, Ohio
Fellow
Minimally Invasive Spine Surgery
William Beaumont Hospital
Royal Oak, Michigan
*Minimally Invasive Posterior Cervical Foraminotomy
and Microdiscectomy*

Brian L. Hoh, MD, FACS, FAHA, FAANS
William Merz Associate Professor
Department of Neurosurgery
University of Florida
Gainesville, Florida
*Management of Dissections of the Carotid and Vertebral
Arteries*
Endovascular Treatment of Stroke

L. Nelson Hopkins, MD
Professor of Neurosurgery and Radiology
Director
Toshiba Stroke Research Center
State University of New York at Buffalo
Buffalo, New York
Endovascular Treatment of Intracranial Occlusive Disease

Wesley Hsu, MD
Assistant Professor
Departments of Neurosurgery and Orthopedic Surgery
Wake Forest Baptist Health
Winston-Salem, North Carolina
Transoral Approaches to the Cervical Spine
Surgical Resection of Sacral Tumors

Yin C. Hu, MD
Fellow
Barrow Neurosurgical Associates
Phoenix, Arizona
Embolization of Tumors: Brain, Head, Neck, and Spine

Jason H. Huang, MD
Associate Professor
Department of Neurosurgery
University of Rochester
Rochester, New York
Peripheral Nerve Injury

Judy Huang, MD
Associate Professor
Department of Neurosurgery
Johns Hopkins Hospital
Baltimore, Maryland
*Surgical Management of Posterior Communicating, Anterior
Choroidal, Carotid Bifurcation Aneurysms*

**Peter J. Hutchinson, BSc(Hons), MBBS, PhD, FRCS(Surg
Neurol)**
Senior Academy Fellow
Reader and Honorary Consultant Neurosurgeon
Academic Division of Neurosurgery
Addenbrooke's Hospital and University of Cambridge
Cambridge, United Kingdom
*Surgical Management of Chronic Subdural Hematoma in
Adults*

Jonathan A. Hyam, MBBS, BSc, MRCS
Neurosurgery Specialist Registrar
Oxford Functional Neurosurgery
John Radcliffe Hospital
Clinical Researcher
Department of Physiology, Anatomy, and Genetics
Tutor in Basic Medical Sciences
Lincoln College
University of Oxford
Oxford, United Kingdom
*Functional Tractography, Diffusion Tensor Imaging,
Intraoperative Integration of Modalities,
and Neuronavigation*

Adriana G. Ioachimescu, MD, PhD
Assistant Professor
Medicine and Neurological Surgery
Emory School of Medicine
Co-Director
Department of Neurological Surgery
Emory Neuroendocrine Pituitary Center
Emory University Hospital
Atlanta, Georgia
Growth Hormone–Secreting Tumors

Pascal M. Jabbour, MD
Assistant Professor
Department of Neurosurgery
Thomas Jefferson University Hospital
Philadelphia, Pennsylvania
*Endovascular Treatment of Cerebral Arteriovenous
Malformations*

Juan Jackson, MD
Clinical Dosimetrist
The Johns Hopkins University
Baltimore, Maryland
Stereotactic Radiosurgery for Pituitary Adenomas

George I. Jallo, MD
Professor of Neurosurgery, Pediatrics, and Oncology
The Johns Hopkins University School of Medicine
Baltimore, Maryland
Surgical Management of Brain Stem Tumors in Adults
*Supratentorial Tumors in the Pediatric Population:
Multidisciplinary Management*
Endoscopic Third Ventriculostomy

Ivo P. Janecka, MD, MBA, PhD
Director
Foundation for Surgical Research and Education
New York, New York
Anterior Midline Approaches to the Skull Base

Mohsen Javadpour, MB, BCh, FRCS(SN)
Consultant Neurosurgeon
Walton Centre for Neurology and Neurosurgery
Liverpool, United Kingdom
*Surgical Management of Cranial Dural Arteriovenous
Fistulas*

Andrew Jea, MD
Assistant Professor
Department of Neurosurgery
Baylor College of Medicine
Staff Neurosurgeon
Department of Pediatric Neurosurgery
Texas Children's Hospital
Houston, Texas
Instrumentation and Stabilization of the Pediatric Spine: Technical Nuances and Age-Specific Considerations

Sunil Jeswani, MD
Resident
Department of Neurosurgery
Cedars–Sinai Medical Center
Los Angeles, California
Spinal Infections: Vertebral Osteomyelitis and Spinal Epidural Abscess
Anterior Lumbar Interbody Fusion: Indications and Techniques
Surgical Management of Cerebrospinal Fluid Leakage after Spinal Surgery

David H. Jho, MD, PhD
Neurosurgery Resident
Department of Neurosurgery
Massachusetts General Hospital
Harvard Medical School
Boston, Massachusetts
Endoscopic Endonasal Pituitary and Skull Base Surgery
Anterior Cervical Foraminotomy (Jho Procedure): Microscopic or Endoscopic

Diana H. Jho, MD, MPH
Neurosurgery Resident
Department of Neurosurgery
Allegheny General Hospital
Pittsburgh, Pennsylvania
Endoscopic Endonasal Pituitary and Skull Base Surgery
Anterior Cervical Foraminotomy (Jho Procedure): Microscopic or Endoscopic

Hae-Dong Jho, MD, PhD
Professor and Chairman
Department of Neuroendoscopy
Jho Institute, Allegheny General Hospital
Pittsburgh, Pennsylvania
Endoscopic Endonasal Pituitary and Skull Base Surgery
Anterior Cervical Foraminotomy (Jho Procedure): Microscopic or Endoscopic

Bowen Jiang, MD
Stanford University
School of Medicine
Stanford, California
Radiation Therapy and Radiosurgery in the Management of Craniopharyngiomas

Tae-Young Jung, MD, PhD
Associate Professor
Department of Neurosurgery
Chonnam National University Hwasun Hospital
Chonnam National University Medical School
Hwasun-Gun Jeonnam, Korea
Posterior Fossa Tumors in the Pediatric Population: Multidisciplinary Management

M. Yashar S. Kalani, MD, PhD
Neurosurgical Resident
Division of Neurological Surgery
Barrow Neurological Institute
St. Joseph's Hospital and Medical Center
Phoenix, Arizona
Posterior Lumbar Interbody Fusion

Hideyuki Kano, MD, PhD
Research Assistant Professor of Neurological Surgery
University of Pittsburgh
Pittsburgh, Pennsylvania
Vestibular Schwannomas: The Role of Stereotactic Radiosurgery

Silloo B. Kapadia, MD
Professor
Department of Pathology
Penn State College of Medicine
Director, Surgical Pathology
Department of Anatomic Pathology
Penn State
Milton S. Hershey Medical Center
Hershey, Pennsylvania
Anterior Midline Approaches to the Skull Base

Michael G. Kaplitt, MD, PhD
Vice Chairman for Research
Department of Neurological Surgery
Weill Cornell Medical College
New York, New York
Molecular Therapies for Movement Disorders

Christoph Kappus, MD
Department of Neurosurgery
University of Marburg UKGM
Marburg, Germany
Arachnoid, Suprasellar, and Rathke's Cleft Cysts

Eftychia Z. Kapsalaki, MD
Professor of Diagnostic Radiology
Department of Radiology
University Hospital of Larissa
University of Thessaly School of Medicine
Larissa, Greece
Mesencephalic Tractotomy and Anterolateral Cordotomy for Intractable Pain

Yuval Karmon, MD
Department of Neurosurgery
State University of New York at Buffalo
Buffalo, New York
Endovascular Treatment of Intracranial Occlusive Disease

Amin B. Kassam, MD
Professor and Chairman
Department of Neurological Surgery
University of Pittsburgh School of Medicine
Director
Minimally Invasive Endoneurosurgery Center
University of Pittsburgh Medical Center
Pittsburgh, Pennsylvania
Endoscopic Endonasal Approach for Craniopharyngiomas

Sudhir Kathuria, MD, MBBS
Assistant Professor
Department of Radiology
Assistant Professor
Department of Neurosurgery
Johns Hopkins Hospital
Baltimore, Maryland
*Imaging Evaluation and Endovascular Treatment
of Vasospasm*

Takeshi Kawase, MD, PhD
Honorary Professor
Department of Neurosurgery
Keio University School of Medicine
Tokyo, Japan
Surgery for Trigeminal Neurinomas

Alexander A. Khalessi, MD
Co-Director of Neurovascular Surgery and Neurosurgical
   Director of NeuroCritical Care
Division of Neurological Surgery
University of California, San Diego
San Diego, California
Endovascular Treatment of Intracranial Occlusive Disease

Kathleen Khu, MD
Clinical Associate Professor
Section of Neurosurgery
Department of Neurosciences
University of the Philippines–Philippine General Hospital
Manila, Philippines
Management of Adult Brachial Plexus Injuries

Daniel H. Kim, MD
Professor
Director, Spinal Neurosurgery and Reconstructive
   Peripheral Nerve Surgery
Department of Neurosurgery
Baylor College of Medicine
Houston, Texas
Surgical Approaches to the Cervicothoracic Junction

Matthias Kirsch, PD Dr. med.
Department of Neurosurgery
Carl Gustav Carus University Hospital
Dresden, Germany
*Surgical Management of Midline Anterior Skull Base
   Meningiomas*

Riku Kivisaari, MD, PhD
Neurosurgeon and Radiologist
Department of Neurosurgery
Helsinki University Central Hospital
Helsinki, Finland
*Surgical Management of Aneurysms of the Middle Cerebral
   Artery*

Angelos G. Kolias, BM, MSc, MRCS
Academic Clinical Registrar in Neurosurgery
Academic Division of Neurosurgery
Addenbrooke's Hospital and University of Cambridge
Cambridge, United Kingdom
*Surgical Management of Chronic Subdural Hematoma
   in Adults*

Douglas Kondziolka, MD, MSc, FRCSC
Peter J. Jannetta Professor of Neurological Surgery
Department of Neurological Surgery
University of Pittsburgh
Pittsburgh, Pennsylvania
*Vestibular Schwannomas: The Role of Stereotactic
   Radiosurgery*

Marcus C. Korinth, MD, PhD Professor Dr. med.
Department of Neurosurgery
Medizinisches Zentrum Stadteregion Aachen
Aachen, Germany
*Treatment Evolution in Management of Cervical Disc
   Disease*

Dietmar Krex, MD
Department of Neurosurgery
Carl Gustav Carus University Hospital
University of Technology
Dresden, Germany
*Surgical Management of Midline Anterior Skull Base
   Meningiomas*

Mark D. Krieger, MD
Associate Professor
Department of Neurological Surgery
University of Southern California
Los Angeles, California
Prolactinomas

Kartik G. Krishnan, MD, PhD
Department of Neurosurgery
Center for Clinical Neurosciences
Johann Wolfgang Goethe University
Frankfurt, Germany
Management of Median Nerve Compression

Ajit A. Krishnaney, MD
Staff
Center for Spine Health
Department of Neurosurgery
Cleveland Clinic
Cleveland, Ohio
Management of Cervical Spondylotic Myelopathy

Maureen Lacy, PhD
Associate Professor of Psychiatry, Behavioral Neurosciences,
   and Surgery
Department of Psychiatry
University of Chicago Medical Center
Chicago, Illinois
Surgical Management of Hydrocephalus in the Adult

Santosh D. Lad, MS, MRSH
Senior Consultant Neurosurgeon
Department of Anesthesiology and Intensive Care
   and Neurosurgery
Khoula Hospital
Muscat, Oman
Fungal Infections of the Central Nervous System

Jose Alberto Landeiro, MD, PhD
Neurosurgery Clinic
Hospital da Força Aérea do Galeão
Rio de Janeiro, Brazil
Surgical Management of Tumors of the Foramen Magnum

Frederick F. Lang, MD
Professor
The University of Texas MD Anderson Cancer Center
Houston, Texas
Surgical Management of Cerebral Metastases

Shih-Shan Lang, MD
Resident
Department of Neurosurgery
University of Pennsylvania
Philadelphia, Pennsylvania
*Surgical Management of Major Skull Defects and Potential
    Complications*

Françoise LaPierre, MD
Professor Emeritus
Department of Neurosurgery
Poitiers University Medical School
Poitiers, France
Management of Cauda Equina Tumors

Paul S. Larson, MD
Associate Professor
Department of Neurological Surgery
University of California, San Francisco
Chief, Neurosurgery
Surgical Section
San Francisco VA Medical Center
San Francisco, California
Deep Brain Stimulation for Intractable Psychiatric Illness

Michael T. Lawton, MD
Professor
University of California, San Francisco
San Francisco, California
*Surgical Management of Anterior Communicating
    and Anterior Cerebral Artery Aneurysms*

Marco Lee, MD
Clinical Assistant Professor
Department of Neurosurgery
Stanford University School of Medicine
Stanford, California
*Radiation Therapy and Radiosurgery in the Management
    of Craniopharyngiomas*

Martin Lehecka, MD, PhD
Consultant Neurosurgeon
Department of Neurosurgery
Helsinki University Central Hospital
Helsinki, Finland
*Surgical Management of Aneurysms of the Middle Cerebral
    Artery*

Allan Levi, MD, PhD
Professor
Departments of Neurological Surgery, Orthopedics,
    and Rehabilitation
Chief of Neurospine Service
Jackson Memorial Hospital
University of Miami
Miami, Florida
Management of Nerve Sheath Tumors Involving the Spine

Elad I. Levy, MD
Associate Professor
Department of Neurosurgery
Associate Professor
Department of Radiology
State University of New York at Buffalo
Buffalo, New York
Endovascular Treatment of Intracranial Occlusive Disease

Robert E. Lieberson, MD
Assistant Professor of Neurosurgery
Department of Neurosurgery
Stanford University
Stanford, California
CyberKnife Radiosurgery for Spinal Neoplasms

Michael Lim, MD
Assistant Professor
Department of Neurosurgery
Assistant Professor
Department of Oncology
The Johns Hopkins University
Baltimore, Maryland
Stereotactic Radiosurgery for Trigeminal Neuralgia

Ning Lin, MD
Clinical Fellow in Surgery
Department of Neurosurgery
Brigham and Women's Hospital
Boston, Massachusetts
Management of Intracranial Aneurysms Caused by Infection

Göran Lind, MD
Consultant Neurosurgeon
Department of Neurosurgery
Karolinska University Hospital
Stockholm, Sweden
Retrogasserian Glycerol Rhizolysis in Trigeminal Neuralgia

Bengt Linderoth, MD, PhD
Professor of Neurosurgery
Karolinska Institutet
Stockholm, Sweden
Professor of Physiology
Oklahoma University Health Sciences Center
Oklahoma City, Oklahoma
Retrogasserian Glycerol Rhizolysis in Trigeminal Neuralgia
Spinal Cord Stimulation for Chronic Pain

Timothy Lindley, MD, PhD
Department of Neurosurgery
University of Iowa
Iowa City, Iowa
*Craniovertebral Abnormalities and Their Neurosurgical
    Management*

Antoine Listrat, MD
Neurosurgeon
Department of Pediatric Neurosurgery
University Hospital
Poitiers, France
Management of Cauda Equina Tumors

Charles Y. Liu, MD, PhD
Associate Professor
Department of Neurological Surgery
University of Southern California
Keck School of Medicine
Los Angeles, California
*Transcallosal Surgery of Lesions Affecting the Third
Ventricle: Basic Principles*

James K. Liu, MD
Assistant Professor
Director of Skull Base and Pituitary Surgery
Department of Neurological Surgery
University of Medicine and Dentistry of New Jersey
New Jersey Medical School
Newark, New Jersey
Prolactinomas
Surgical Management of Tumors of the Jugular Foramen

John C. Liu, MD
Vice Chair Spine Surgery
Department of Neurosurgery
Cedars–Sinai Medical Center
Los Angeles, California
*Anterior Lumbar Interbody Fusion: Indications
and Techniques*

Giorgio Lo Russo, MD
Chief Epilepsy Neurosurgeon
Epilepsy Surgery Centre
Niguarda Hospital
Milan, Italy
*Multilobar Resection and Hemispherectomy in Epilepsy
Surgery*

Christopher M. Loftus, MD, DHC(Hon), FACS
Chairman
Department of Neurosurgery
Temple University Hospital
Philadelphia, Pennsylvania
Surgical Management of Extracranial Carotid Artery Disease

Russell R. Lonser, MD
Chief
Surgical Neurology Branch
National Institute of Neurological Disorders and Stroke
National Institutes of Health
Bethesda, Maryland
*Surgical Management of Parasagittal and Convexity
Meningiomas*
*Neurovascular Decompression in Cranial Nerves V, VII, IX,
and X*

Daniel C. Lu, MD, PhD
Assistant Professor
Department of Neurosurgery
University of California, Los Angeles
Los Angeles, California
*Percutaneous Placement of Lumbar Pedicle Screws:
Indications and Techniques*

Yi Lu, MD, PhD
Department of Neurosurgery
Brigham and Women's Hospital
Harvard Medical School
Boston, Massachusetts
Lateral Lumbar Interbody Fusion: Indications and Techniques

L. Dade Lunsford, MD
Lars Leksell and Distinguished Professor of Neurological
Surgery
University of Pittsburgh Medical Center
Pittsburgh, Pennsylvania
*Vestibular Schwannomas: The Role of Stereotactic
Radiosurgery*

M. Mason Macenski, PhD
Masonovations Medical Consulting
Minneapolis, Minnesota
*Dynamic Stabilization of the Lumbar Spine: Indications
and Techniques*

Jaroslaw Maciaczyk, MD
Laboratory of Molecular Neurosurgery
Department of Stereotactic and Functional Neurosurgery
Neurocenter
University of Freiburg
Freiburg, Germany
Interstitial and LINAC-Radiosurgery for Brain Metastases

Joseph R. Madsen, MD
Director
Epilepsy Surgery Program
Director
Neurodynamics Laboratory
Department of Neurosurgery
Children's Hospital Boston
Associate Professor of Surgery
Department of Surgery
Harvard Medical School
Boston, Massachusetts
*Treatment of Intractable Epilepsy by Electrical Stimulation
of the Vagus Nerve*

Subu N. Magge, MD
Department of Neurosurgery
Spine Center
Lahey Clinic Medical Center
Burlington, Massachusetts
Thoracoscopic Sympathectomy for Hyperhidrosis

Giulio Maira, MD
Director
Università Cattolica del Sacro Cuore
Institute of Neurosurgery
Catholic University School of Medicine
Rome, Italy
Surgical Management of Lesions of the Clivus

Martijn J. A. Malessy, MD, PhD
Department of Neurosurgery
Leiden University Medical Center
Leiden, The Netherlands
*Nerve-Grafting Procedures for Birth-Related Peripheral
Nerve Injuries*

David G. Malone, MD
Oklahoma Spine and Brain Institute
Tulsa, Oklahoma
Cervical Laminoplasty: Indications and Techniques

Allen Maniker, MD
Chief
Department of Neurosurgery
Beth Israel Medical Center
New York, New York
Management of Ulnar Nerve Compression

Geoffrey T. Manley, MD, PhD
Professor and Vice Chairman
Department of Neurological Surgery
University of California, San Francisco
Chief of Neurosurgery
Co-Director
Brain and Spinal Injury Center (BASIC)
San Francisco General Hospital
San Francisco, California
Decompressive Craniectomy for Traumatic Brain Injury
Management of Penetrating Brain Injury

Jotham Manwaring, BS, MD
Physician
Department of Neurosurgery
University of South Florida
Tampa, Florida
Management of Pediatric Severe Traumatic Brain Injury

Mitchell Martineau, MS
Oklahoma Spine and Brain Institute
Tulsa, Oklahoma
Cervical Laminoplasty: Indications and Techniques

Robert L. Martuza, MD
Chief of Neurosurgery Service
Department of Neurosurgery
Massachusetts General Hospital
William and Elizabeth Sweet Professor of Neuroscience
Department of Surgery
Harvard Medical School
Boston, Massachusetts
Suboccipital Retrosigmoid Surgical Approach for Vestibular Schwannoma (Acoustic Neuroma)

Marlon S. Mathews, MD
Resident
Department of Neurological Surgery
State University of New York at Buffalo
Buffalo, New York
Neurosurgical Management of HIV-Related Focal Brain Lesions

Nestoras Mathioudakis, BA, MD
Clinical Fellow
Department of Endocrinology and Metabolism
The Johns Hopkins University School of Medicine
Baltimore, Maryland
Medical Management of Hormone-Secreting Pituitary Tumors

Paul McCormick, MD, MPH
Herbert and Linda Gallen Professor of Neurological Surgery
Department of Neurosurgery
Columbia University College of Physicians and Surgeons
New York, New York
Intradural Extramedullary Tumors

Michael W. McDermott, MD
Professor in Residence of Neurological Surgery, Halperin Endowed Chair
Neurosurgical Director
UCSF Gamma Knife® Radiosurgery Program
Vice Chairman
Department of Neurological Surgery
University of California, San Francisco
San Francisco, California
Craniopharyngiomas

Cameron G. McDougall, MD, FRCSC
Director of Endovascular Neurosurgery
Barrow Neurological Institute
Phoenix, Arizona
Embolization of Tumors: Brain, Head, Neck, and Spine

H. Maximilian Mehdorn, MD, PhD
Professor and Chairman
Department of Neurosurgery
University Hospital Schleswig-Holstein
Kiel, Germany
Surgical Navigation with Intraoperative Imaging: Special Operating Room Concepts

Vivek A. Mehta, MD
Neurosurgery Resident
Department of Neurosurgery
University of Southern California
Neurosurgery Resident
Department of Neurosurgery
University of Southern California
Los Angeles, California
Supratentorial Tumors in the Pediatric Population: Multidisciplinary Management

Arnold Menezes, MD
Professor and Vice Chairman
University of Iowa Carver College of Medicine
Professor of Neurosurgery
University of Iowa Hospitals and Clinics
Iowa City, Iowa
Craniovertebral Abnormalities and Their Neurosurgical Management

Patrick Mertens, MD
Department of Neurosurgery
Hôpital Neurologique
Lyon, France
Surgery for Intractable Spasticity

Frederic B. Meyer, MD
Chair, Neurosurgery
Department of Neurosurgery
Mayo Clinic
Rochester, Minnesota
Tumors in Eloquent Areas of Brain

444

4444

Matthew K. Mian, BSE
Medical Student
Division of Health Sciences and Technology
Harvard Medical School
Department of Neurosurgery
Massachusetts General Hospital
Boston, Massachusetts
Temporal Lobe Operations in Intractable Epilepsy
Motor Cortex Stimulation for Intractable Facial Pain

Rajiv Midha, MD, MSc, FRCSC
Professor
Department of Neurosurgery
University of Calgary
Calgary, Canada
Management of Adult Brachial Plexus Injuries

Diego San Millán Ruíz, MD
Neuroradiology Unit
Department of Diagnostic and Interventional Radiology
Hospital of Sion
Sion, Switzerland
Adult Pseudotumor Cerebri Syndrome

Jonathan Miller, MD
Director, Functional and Restorative Neurosurgery
Assistant Professor of Neurological Surgery
Case School of Medicine
University Hospitals Case Medical Center
Cleveland, Ohio
Management of Tumors of the Fourth Ventricle

Neil R. Miller, MD
Professor of Ophthalmology, Neurology, and Neurosurgery
Frank B. Walsh Professor of Neuro-Ophthalmology
The Johns Hopkins University
Baltimore, Maryland
Adult Pseudotumor Cerebri Syndrome

Zaman Mirzadeh, MD, PhD
Department of Neurological Surgery
University of California, San Francisco
San Francisco, California
Surgical Management of Anterior Communicating and Anterior Cerebral Artery Aneurysms

Ganpati Prasad Mishra, MS, MCh
c/o Shrikant Rege, MD
Fungal Infections of the Central Nervous System

Symeon Missios, MD
Resident
Department of Neurosurgery
Dartmouth-Hitchcock Medical Center
Lebanon, New Hampshire
Ensuring Patient Safety in Surgery—First Do No Harm

James B. Mitchell, BS, MSN
Service Manager
Department of Pediatric Neurosurgery
Kaiser Permanente
Oakland, California
Surgical Management of Spinal Dysraphism

Alim Mitha, MD, SM
Assistant Professor
Clinical Neurosciences and Radiology
University of Calgary
Cerebrovascular/Endovascular/Skull Base Neurosurgeon
Department of Neurosurgery
Foothills Medical Centre
Calgary, Canada
Surgical Management of Midbasilar and Lower Basilar Aneurysms

J. Mocco, MD, MS
Associate Professor
Department of Neurological Surgery
Vanderbilt University Medical Center
Nashville, Tennessee
Endovascular Treatment of Stroke

Abhay Moghekar, MD
Assistant Professor of Neurology
The Johns Hopkins Hospital
Baltimore, Maryland
Adult Pseudotumor Cerebri Syndrome

Jacques J. Morcos, MD, FRCS(Eng), FRCS(Ed)
Professor of Clinical Neurosurgery and Otolaryngology
Department of Neurological Surgery
University of Miami
Miami, Florida
Far Lateral Approach and Transcondylar and Supracondylar Extensions for Aneurysms of the Vertebrobasilar Junction

Chad J. Morgan, MD
Cox Monett Hospital
Monett, Missouri
Percutaneous Stereotactic Rhizotomy in the Treatment of Intractable Facial Pain

John F. Morrison, MD, MS
Department of Surgery
Boston University School of Medicine
Boston, Massachusetts
Thoracoscopic Sympathectomy for Hyperhidrosis

Henry Moyle, MD
Neurosurgery Associates
New York, New York
Endovascular Treatment of Extracranial Occlusive Disease

Carrie R. Muh, MD, MSc
Pediatric Neurosurgical Associates
Children's Healthcare of Atlanta
Atlanta, Georgia
Growth Hormone–Secreting Tumors

Debraj Mukherjee, MD, MPH
Resident
Department of Neurosurgery
Cedars–Sinai Medical Center
Los Angeles, California
Spinal Infections: Vertebral Osteomyelitis and Spinal Epidural Abscess

Arya Nabavi, MD, MaHM, PhD
Professor
Vice Chairman
Department of Neurosurgery
University-Hospital Schleswig-Holstein, Campus Kiel
Kiel, Germany
Surgical Navigation with Intraoperative Imaging: Special Operating Room Concepts

Michael J. Nanaszko, BA
Department of Neurosurgery
Weill Cornell Medical College
New York, New York
Molecular Therapies for Movement Disorders

Dipankar Nandi, MBBS, MChir, DPhil, FRCS
Honorary Senior Lecturer
Imperial College
Consultant Neurosurgeon
Charing Cross Hospital
London, United Kingdom
Cervical Dystonia and Spasmodic Torticollis: Indications and Techniques

Raj Narayan, MD, FACS
Senior Vice President of Neurosurgery
North Shore–LIJ Health System
Chairman of Neurosurgery
North Shore University Hospital and LIJ Medical Center
Manhassett, New York
Management of Penetrating Injuries to the Spine

Sabareesh K. Natarajan, MD, MBBS, MS
Department of Neurosurgery
State University of New York at Buffalo
Buffalo, New York
Endovascular Treatment of Intracranial Occlusive Disease

Edgar Nathal, MD, DMSc
Head
Department of Neurosurgery
Instituto Nacional de Ciencias Médicas y de la Nutrición
Professor of Vascular Neurosurgery
Division of Neurosurgery
Instituto Nacional de Neurología y Neurocirugía
Coordinator of Neurosurgery
Medical Sciences
Medica Sur, Hospital and Foundation
Titular Professor
Vascular Neurosurgery
Universidad Nacional Autónoma de México (UNAM)
Mexico, Distrito Federal, Mexico
Surgical Treatment of Paraclinoid Aneurysms

Vikram V. Nayar, MD
Department of Neurosurgery
Georgetown University Hospital
Washington, DC
Management of Unruptured Intracranial Aneurysms
Surgical Management of Cerebellar Stroke—Hemorrhage and Infarction

Audumbar Shantaram Netalkar, MD
Consultant Neurosurgeon
Apollo Victor Hospitals
Goa Medical College
Goa, India
Fungal Infections of the Central Nervous System

C. Benjamin Newman, MD
Resident Physician and Surgeon
Department of Neurosurgery
University of California, San Diego
San Diego, California
Embolization of Tumors: Brain, Head, Neck, and Spine

Trang Nguyen, MD
Department of Neurosurgery
Johns Hopkins Hospital
Baltimore, Maryland
Stereotactic Radiosurgery for Trigeminal Neuralgia

Laura B. Ngwenya, MD, PhD
Department of Neurological Surgery
The Ohio State University Medical Center
Columbus, Ohio
Cerebellar Tumors in Adults

Antonio Nicolato, MD
Department of Neurosurgery
University of Verona and University Hospital
Verona, Italy
Stereotactic Radiosurgery Meningiomas

Mika Niemelä, MD, PhD
Associate Professor
Head of Section (Neurosurgical OR)
Head of Neurosurgery Research Group at Biomedicum Helsinki
Department of Neurosurgery
Helsinki University Central Hospital
Helsinki, Finland
Surgical Management of Aneurysms of the Middle Cerebral Artery

Guido Nikkhah, MD, PhD
Department of Stereotactic and Functional Neurosurgery
Hospital of the Albert-Ludwigs-University
Freiburg, Germany
Interstitial and LINAC-Radiosurgery for Brain Metastases

Anitha Nimmagadda, MD
Department of Neurological Surgery
Rockford Health Physicians
Rockford, Illinois
Endovascular Management of Spinal Vascular Malformations

John K. Niparko, MD
Professor of Otolaryngology-Head and Neck Surgery
Director
Otology, Neurotology, Skull Base Surgery
Director
The Hearing Center
Director
The Listening Center
The Johns Hopkins Hospital
Baltimore, Maryland
Hearing Prosthetics: Surgical Techniques

Ajay Niranjan, MBBS, MCh
Associate Professor of Neurosurgery
University of Pittsburgh
Pittsburgh, Pennsylvania
Vestibular Schwannomas: The Role of Stereotactic Radiosurgery

Richard B. North, MD
Professor (retired)
Departments of Neurosurgery, Anesthesiology, and Critical Care Medicine
The Johns Hopkins University School of Medicine
Director
Neuromodulation, Surgical Pain Management, and Surgical Spine Pain Program
Berman Brain and Spine Institute
Sinai Hospital
Baltimore, Maryland
Spinal Cord Stimulation for Chronic Pain

José María Núñez, MD, MSc
Neurosurgeon
Epilepsy Clinic
Mexico General Hospital
Mexico City, Mexico
Presurgical Evaluation for Epilepsy Including Intracranial Electrodes

W. Jerry Oakes, MD
Professor
Departments of Surgery and Pediatrics
Division of Neurosurgery
University of Alabama Health System
Birmingham, Alabama
Surgical Decision-Making and Treatment Options for Chiari Malformations in Children
Management of Occult Spinal Dysraphism in Adults

Christopher S. Ogilvy, MD
Director, Endovascular and Operative Neurovascular Surgery
Massachusetts General Hospital
Robert G. and A. Jean Ojemann Professor of Neurosurgery
Harvard Medical School
Boston, Massachusetts
Management of Dissections of the Carotid and Vertebral Arteries
Surgical Management of Intracerebral Hemorrhage
Surgical Management of Cavernous Malformations of the Nervous System

Kenji Ohata, MD, PhD
Professor and Chairman
Department of Neurosurgery
Osaka City University
Osaka, Japan
Orbitozygomatic Infratemporal Approach to Parasellar Meningiomas

Jeffrey G. Ojemann, MD
Professor
Department of Neurological Surgery
University of Washington
Center for Integrative Brain Research
Seattle Children's Research Institute
Seattle, Washington
Mapping, Disconnection, and Resective Surgery in Pediatric Epilepsy

Steven Ojemann, MD
Department of Neurological Surgery
University of California, San Francisco
San Francisco, California
Novel Targets in Deep Brain Stimulation for Movement Disorders

David O. Okonkwo, MD, PhD
Chief of Neurotrauma
University of Pittsburgh Medical Center
Pittsburgh, Pennsylvania
Perioperative Management of Severe Traumatic Brain Injury in Adults

Edward H. Oldfield, MD
Professor of Neurosurgery and Internal Medicine
University of Virginia
Charlottesville, Virginia
Cushing's Disease
Management of Chiari Malformations and Syringomyelia

Brent O'Neill, MD
Department of Neurosurgery
University of Colorado
Aurora, Colorado
Mapping, Disconnection, and Resective Surgery in Pediatric Epilepsy

Nelson M. Oyesiku, MD, PhD, FACS
Professor of Neurological Surgery
Director of the Laboratory of Molecular Neurosurgery and Biotechnology
Emory University
Atlanta, Georgia
Growth Hormone–Secreting Tumors

Roberto Pallini, MD, PhD
Assistant Professor
Department of Neuroscience
Institute of Neurosurgery
Catholic University School of Medicine
Rome, Italy
Surgical Management of Lesions of the Clivus

Aditya S. Pandey, MD
Assistant Professor of Neurosurgery
Department of Neurosurgery
University of Michigan
Ann Arbor, Michigan
Endovascular Management of Intracranial Aneurysms

Dachling Pang, MD, FRCSC, FACS
Professor of Pediatric Neurosurgery
Department of Neurological Surgery
University of California, Davis
Sacramento, California
Chief of Pediatric Neurosurgery
Department of Pediatric Neurosurgery
Kaiser Permanente Hospitals
Oakland, California
Surgical Management of Spinal Dysraphism

Kyriakos Papadimitriou, MD
Postdoctoral Fellow
Department of Neurosurgery
Johns Hopkins Hospital
Baltimore, Maryland
*Surgical Management of Posterior Communicating, Anterior
    Choroidal, Carotid Bifurcation Aneurysms*

José María Pascual, MD
c/o Ruth Prieto
*Surgical Management of Severe Closed Head Injury
    in Adults*

Aman Patel, MD
Professor of Neurosurgery and Radiology
Department of Neurosurgery
Mount Sinai School of Medicine
New York, New York
Endovascular Treatment of Extracranial Occlusive Disease

Anoop P. Patel, MD
Resident
Department of Neurosurgery
Massachusetts General Hospital
Boston, Massachusetts
*Surgical Management of Cavernous Malformations
    of the Nervous System*

Toral R. Patel, MD
Neurosurgery Resident
Department of Neurosurgery
Yale University School of Medicine
New Haven, Connecticut
Surgical Approaches to Lateral and Third Ventricular Tumors

Vincenzo Paterno, MD
Department of Neurosurgery
International Neurosurgery Institute
Hanover, Germany
Arachnoid, Suprasellar, and Rathke's Cleft Cysts

Rana Patir, MS, MCh
Director
Department of Neurosurgery
Max Super Speciality Hospital
New Delhi, India
Management of Tuberculous Infections of the Nervous System

Alexandra R. Paul, MD
Department of Neurosurgery
Johns Hopkins Hospital
Baltimore, Maryland
Endovascular Management of Dural Arteriovenous Fistulas

Sanjay J. Pawar, MBBS, MS, MCh
Neurosurgeon
Department of Neurosurgery
Khoula Hospital
Muscat, Oman
Fungal Infections of the Central Nervous System

Richard Penn, MD
Professor
Department of Surgery
University of Chicago
Chicago, Illinois
Surgical Management of Hydrocephalus in the Adult

Erlick A. C. Pereira, MA, DM, BCh, MRCS(Eng)
Neurosurgery Specialty Registrar
Nuffield Department of Surgery
University of Oxford
Oxford, United Kingdom
*Functional Tractography, Diffusion Tensor Imaging,
    Intraoperative Integration of Modalities,
    and Neuronavigation*
Surgical Management of Extratemporal Lobe Epilepsy

Mick J. Perez-Cruet, MD, MSc
Vice Chairman, Neurosurgery
Director, Spine Program
Department of Neurosurgery
William Beaumont Hospital
Royal Oak, Michigan
*Minimally Invasive Posterior Cervical Foraminotomy
    and Microdiscectomy*

Eric C. Peterson, MD
Resident in Neurological Surgery
University of Washington
Seattle, Washington
*Far Lateral Approach and Transcondylar and Supracondylar
    Extensions for Aneurysms of the Vertebrobasilar Junction*

Mark A. Pichelmann, MD
Assistant Professor of Neurosurgery
Department of Neurosurgery
Mayo Clinic
Rochester, Minnesota
Tumors in Eloquent Areas of Brain

Joseph M. Piepmeier, MD
Nixdorff-German Professor of Neurosurgery
Vice Chair of Clinical Affairs, Neurosurgery
Section Chief
Department of Neuro-Oncology
Director
Department of Surgical Neuro-Oncology
Yale School of Medicine
New Haven, Connecticut
*Surgical Approaches to Lateral and Third Ventricular
    Tumors*

Marcus O. Pinsker, MD
Department of Stereotactic and Functional Neurosurgery
University Medical Center Freiburg
Freiburg, Germany
Interstitial and LINAC-Radiosurgery for Brain Metastases

Lawrence H. Pitts, MD
Professor of Neurosurgery
University of California, San Francisco
San Francisco, California
Decompressive Craniectomy for Traumatic Brain Injury

Rick J. Placide, MD
Chief of Orthopedic Surgery
Spine Surgeon and Orthopaedic Surgeon
Chippenham Medical Center
Richmond, Virginia
Management of Cervical Spondylotic Myelopathy

Willem Pondaag, MD
Department of Neurosurgery
Leiden University Medical Center
Leiden, The Netherlands
Nerve-Grafting Procedures for Birth-Related Peripheral Nerve Injuries

Kalmon Post, MD
Professor and Chairman
Department of Neurosurgery
Mount Sinai School of Medicine
New York, New York
Management of Spinal Cord Tumors and Arteriovenous Malformations

Matthew B. Potts, MD
Resident
Department of Neurological Surgery
University of California, San Francisco
San Francisco, California
Decompressive Craniectomy for Traumatic Brain Injury

Lars Poulsgaard, MD
Consultant Neurosurgeon
University Clinic of Neurosurgery
The Neuroscience Center
University Hospital of Copenhagen, Rigshospitalet
Copenhagen, Denmark
Translabyrinthine Approach to Vestibular Schwannomas

Gustavo Pradilla, MD
Resident
Department of Neurosurgery
The Johns Hopkins University School of Medicine
Baltimore, Maryland
Surgical Management of Infratentorial Arteriovenous Malformations

Charles J. Prestigiacomo, MD, FACS
Associate Professor
Department of Neurological Surgery
Associate Professor
Department of Radiology
New Jersey Medical School
University of Medicine and Dentistry of New Jersey
Research Professor
Department of Biomedical Engineering
New Jersey Institute of Technology
Newark, New Jersey
Endovascular Treatment of Head and Neck Bleeding

Daniel M. Prevedello, MD
Assistant Professor
Department of Neurological Surgery
University of Pittsburgh
Pittsburgh, Pennsylvania
Endoscopic Endonasal Approach for Craniopharyngiomas

Ruth Prieto, MD
Department of Neurosurgery
Clinico San Carlos University Hospital
Madrid, Spain
Surgical Management of Severe Closed Head Injury in Adults

Alfredo Quiñones-Hinojosa, MD
Associate Professor of Neurological Surgery and Oncology
Department of Neurosurgery
The Johns Hopkins University
Neuroscience and Cellular and Molecular Medicine
Director, Brain Tumor Surgery Program, Johns Hopkins Bayview
Director, Pituitary Surgery Program, Johns Hopkins Hospital
Baltimore, Maryland
Transcranial Surgery for Pituitary Macroadenomas
Supraorbital Approach Variants for Intracranial Tumors
Multimodal Treatment of Orbital Tumors
Management of Cerebrospinal Fluid Leaks
Management of Suppurative Intracranial Infections

Leonidas M. Quintana, MD
Professor
Neurosurgical Department
Valparaíso University School of Medicine
Valparaíso, Chile
Surgical Treatment of Moyamoya Disease in Adults

Scott Y. Rahimi, MD
Assistant Professor
Department of Neurosurgery
Georgia Health Sciences University
Augusta, Georgia
Surgical Management of Terminal Basilar and Posterior Cerebral Artery Aneurysms

Rudy J. Rahme, MD
Postdoctoral Research Fellow
Department of Neurological Surgery
Northwestern University Feinberg School of Medicine
Chicago, Illinois
Endovascular Management of Spinal Vascular Malformations

Rodrigo Ramos-Zúñiga, MD, PhD
Chairman
Department of Neurosciences
Universidad de Guadalajara
Guadalajara, Mexico
Supraorbital Approach Variants for Intracranial Tumors
Management of Neurocysticercosis

Nathan J. Ranalli, MD
Senior Resident
Department of Neurosurgery
University of Pennsylvania
Philadelphia, Pennsylvania
Management of Median Nerve Compression

Shaan M. Raza, MD
Neurosurgery Resident
Department of Neurosurgery
Johns Hopkins Hospital
Baltimore, Maryland
Supraorbital Approach Variants for Intracranial Tumors
Multimodal Treatment of Orbital Tumors

Pablo F. Recinos, MD
Resident
Department of Neurosurgery
The Johns Hopkins University School of Medicine
Baltimore, Maryland
Transcranial Surgery for Pituitary Adenomas
Endoscopic Third Ventriculostomy
Stereotactic Radiosurgery for Trigeminal Neuralgia

Violette Renard Recinos, MD
Neurosurgery Resident
Department of Neurosurgery
Johns Hopkins Hospital
Baltimore, Maryland
Endoscopic Third Ventriculostomy

Shrikant Rege, MD
Neurologist
Tukoganj, South Indore
Fungal Infections of the Central Nervous System

Thomas Reithmeier, MD
Department of Neurosurgery
University of Cologne
Cologne, Germany
Interstitial and LINAC-Radiosurgery of Brain Metastases

Katherine Relyea, MS
Medical Illustrator
Department of Pediatric Neurosurgery
Baylor College of Medicine
Houston, Texas
Instrumentation and Stabilization of the Pediatric Spine: Technical Nuances and Age-Specific Considerations

Daniel Resnick, MD, MS
Associate Professor and Vice Chairman
Department of Neurosurgery
University of Wisconsin
Madison, Wisconsin
Transforaminal Lumbar Interbody Fusion: Indications and Techniques

Daniele Rigamonti, MD, FACS
Professor of Neurosurgery, Oncology, and Radiation
Departments of Oncology and Molecular Radiation Sciences
Director, Stereotactic Radiosurgery
Director, Hydrocephalus and Pseudotumor Cerebri Program
Departments of Neurosurgery and Radiation Oncology
The Johns Hopkins School of Medicine
Baltimore, Maryland
Adult Pseudotumor Cerebri Syndrome
Stereotactic Radiosurgery for Pituitary Adenomas

Philippe Rigoard, MD, PhD
Neurosurgeon
Department of Spine Neurosurgery
University Hospital
Poitiers, France
Management of Cauda Equina Tumors

Jaakko Rinne, MD, PhD
Associate Professor
Department of Neurosurgery
University of Eastern Finland
Director
KUH Neurocenter
Kuopio University Hospital
Kuopio, Finland
Surgical Management of Aneurysms of the Middle Cerebral Artery

Jon H. Robertson, MD
Professor and Chairman
Department of Neurosurgery
University of Tennessee Health Science Center
Memphis, Tennessee
Transtemporal Approaches to Posterior Cranial Fossa

Shimon Rochkind, MD
Director
Division of Peripheral Nerve Reconstruction
Tel Aviv Sourasky Medical Center
Tel Aviv, Israel
Management of Adult Brachial Plexus Injuries
Management of Thoracic Outlet Syndrome

Jack P. Rock, MD
Residency Program Director
Department of Neurosurgery
Henry Ford Hospital
Detroit, Michigan
Surgical Management of Posterior Fossa Meningiomas

Rossana Romani, MD
Department of Neurosurgery
Helsinki University Central Hospital
Helsinki, Finland
Surgical Management of Aneurysms of the Middle Cerebral Artery

Guy Rosenthal, MD
Department of Neurosurgery
Hadassah-Hebrew University Medical Center
Jerusalem, Israel
Department of Neurosurgery
San Francisco General Hospital
University of California, San Francisco
San Francisco, California
Management of Penetrating Traumatic Brain Injury

Robert H. Rosenwasser, MD, FACS, FAHA
Professor and Chairman
Department of Neurological Surgery
Professor
Department of Radiology
Thomas Jefferson University
Philadelphia, Pennsylvania
Endovascular Treatment of Cerebral Arteriovenous Malformations

Nathan C. Rowland, MD, PhD
Resident
Department of Neurological Surgery
University of California, San Francisco
San Francisco, California
Corpus Callosotomy: Indications and Techniques

James T. Rutka, MD, PhD, FRCSC
Professor
Department of Surgery
Division Neurosurgery
University of Toronto
Toronto, Canada
Posterior Fossa Tumors in the Pediatric Population:
  Multidisciplinary Management
Supratentorial Tumors in the Pediatric Population:
  Multidisciplinary Management

Samuel Ryu, MD
Radiation Oncologist
Henry Ford Health System
Detroit, Michigan
Surgical Management of Posterior Fossa Meningiomas

Francesco Sala, MD
Assistant Professor of Neurosurgery
Department of Neurological Sciences and Vision
University Hospital
Verona, Italy
Intraoperative Neurophysiology: A Tool to Prevent and/or
  Document Intraoperative Injury to the Nervous System

Roberto Salvatori, MD
Associate Professor
Department of Medicine
The Johns Hopkins University
Baltimore, Maryland
Medical Management of Hormone-Secreting Pituitary Tumors
Stereotactic Radiosurgery for Pituitary Adenomas

Kari Sammalkorpi, MD
c/o Göran Blomstedt, MD
Management of Infections After Craniotomy

Nader Sanai, MD
Director, Division of Neurosurgical Oncology
Director, Barrow Brain Tumor Research Center
Barrow Neurological Institute
St. Joseph's Hospital and Medical Center
Phoenix, Arizona
Surgical Management of Midbasilar and Lower Basilar
  Aneurysms

Thomas Santarius, MD, PhD, FRCS(Surg Neurol)
Specialist Registrar in Neurosurgery
Academic Division of Neurosurgery
Addenbrooke's Hospital and University of Cambridge
Cambridge, United Kingdom
Surgical Management of Chronic Subdural Hematoma
  in Adults

Amar Saxena, MBBS, MS, MCh(Neurosurgery), FRCS(Eng), FRCS(Surg Neurol)
Chairman
Higher Surgical Committee in Neurosurgery
  for West Midlands
University Hospitals Coventry and Warwickshire
Coventry, United Kingdom
Disc Replacement Technologies in the Cervical and Lumbar
  Spine

Gabriele Schackert, Professor Dr. med.
Department of Neurosurgery
University Hospital
Dresden, Germany
Surgical Management of Midline Anterior Skull Base
  Meningiomas

Uta Schick, MD, PhD, Priv.-Doz. Dr. med.
Department of Neurosurgery
University of Heidelberg
Heidelberg, Germany
Surgical Approaches to the Orbit

Thomas A. Schildhauer, MD, PhD
BG-Kliniken Bergmannsheil
Ruhr-Universitat
Bochum, Germany
Management of Sacral Fractures

Alexandra Schmidek, MD
Division of Plastic Surgery
Beth Israel Deaconess Medical Center
Harvard Medical School
Boston, Massachusetts
Principles of Scalp Surgery and Surgical Management
  of Major Defects of Scalp

Henry H. Schmidek, MD, FACS†
Formerly Visiting Professor in Neurosurgery
Nuffield Department of Surgery
Lecturer in Neuroscience
Balliol College
Oxford University
Oxford, England
Management of Suppurative Intracranial Infections

Meic H. Schmidt, MD
Chief
Division of Spine Surgery
Associate Professor of Neurosurgery
Director, Spinal Oncology Service, Huntsman Cancer
  Institute
Director, Neurosurgery Spine Fellowship
Department of Neurosurgery
University of Utah
Salt Lake City, Utah
Lumbar Microdiscectomy: Indications and Techniques

Paul Schmitt, MD
New Jersey Medical School
University of Medicine and Dentistry of New Jersey
Newark, New Jersey
Endovascular Treatment of Head and Neck Bleeding

†Deceased.

Johannes Schramm, MD
Professor and Chairman
Department of Neurosurgery
University of Bonn
Bonn, Germany
*Mapping, Disconnection, and Resective Surgery in Pediatric
  Epilepsy*

Joseph Schwab, MD
Massachusetts General Hospital
Boston, Massachusetts
*Management of Primary Malignant Tumors of the Osseous
  Spine*

Theodore H. Schwartz, MD, FACS
Professor of Neurosurgery, Otorhinolaryngology, Neurology,
  and Neuroscience
Weill Cornell Medical College
New York Presbyterian Hospital
New York, New York
Endoscopic Approach to Intraventricular Brain Tumors

Patrick Schweder, MD
Department of Neurosurgery
The Royal Melbourne Hospital
Parkville, Australia
Cingulotomy for Intractable Psychiatric Illness

Daniel M. Sciubba, BS, MD
Assistant Professor of Neurosurgery, Oncology,
  and Orthopaedic Surgery
Director of Spine Research
Department of Neurosurgery
The Johns Hopkins Institutions
Baltimore, Maryland
*Management of Injuries of the Cervical Spine and Spinal
  Cord*
Management of Degenerative Scoliosis
Surgery for Metastatic Spine Disease

R. Michael Scott, MD
Professor of Surgery (Neurosurgery)
Harvard Medical School
Neurosurgeon-in-Chief
The Children's Hospital Boston
Boston, Massachusetts
*Revascularization Techniques in Pediatric Cerebrovascular
  Disorders*

Raymond F. Sekula, Jr., MD
Surgical Director
Microvascular and Skull Base Neurosurgery Program
  and the Cranial Nerve Disorders Program
Department of Neurosurgery
UPMC Hamot
Associate Professor
Co-Director, Center for Cranial Nerve Disorders
Director, Chiari Clinic
Allegheny Neuroscience Institute
Drexel University College of Medicine
Pittsburgh, Pennsylvania
Surgical Management of Petroclival Meningiomas
Management of Cranial Nerve Injuries

Patrick Senatus, MD, PhD
Assistant Professor
Department of Neurosurgery
University of Connecticut
Farmington, Connecticut
Deep Brain Stimulation for Pain

Amjad Shad, MBBS, FRCS(Ed), FRCS(SN)MR
Department of Neurosurgery
Radcliffe Infirmary
Oxford, United Kingdom
*Disc Replacement Technologies in the Cervical and Lumbar
  Spine*

Ali Shaibani, MD
Associate Professor in Radiology and Neurological Surgery
Northwestern University Feinberg School of Medicine
Chicago, Illinois
*Endovascular Management of Spinal Vascular
  Malformations*

Manish S. Sharma, MBBS, MS, MCh
Fellow
Department of Neurological Surgery
Mayo Clinic
Rochester, Minnesota
Assistant Professor
Department of Neurosurgery
All India Institute of Medical Sciences
New Delhi, India
Nerve Transfers: Indications and Techniques

**Rewati Raman Sharma, MBBS, MS(Neurosurgery),
DNB(Neurosurgery)**
Senior Consultant Neurosurgeon
National Neurosurgical Centre
Department of Neurosurgery
Chairman
Hospital Staff Development: CME, RESEARCH,
  CPD activities
Khoula Hospital
Senior Consultant Neurosurgeon
Department of Neurosurgery
Al Raffah Hospital
Senior Consultant Neurosurgeon
Department of Neurosurgery
Muscat Private Hospital
Muscat, Oman
Fungal Infections of the Central Nervous System

Sameer A. Sheth, MD, PhD
Resident
Department of Neurosurgery
Massachusetts General Hospital
Boston, Massachusetts
Temporal Lobe Operations in Intractable Epilepsy
Motor Cortex Stimulation for Intractable Facial Pain

Alexander Y. Shin, MD
Professor of Orthopedic Surgery
Department of Orthopedic Surgery
Mayo Clinic College of Medicine
Rochester, Minnesota
Nerve Transfers: Indications and Techniques

Ali Shirzadi, MD
Senior Resident, Neurological Surgery Residency Program
Department of Neurosurgery
Cedars–Sinai Medical Center
Los Angeles, California
Spinal Infections: Vertebral Osteomyelitis and Spinal Epidural Abscess
Surgical Management of Cerebrospinal Fluid Leakage after Spinal Surgery

Adnan H. Siddiqui, MD, PhD
Assistant Professor of Neurosurgery
Assistant Professor of Radiology
Director of Neuroendovascular Critical Care
Director of Neurosurgical Research
Department of Neurosurgery
State University of New York at Buffalo
Buffalo, New York
Endovascular Treatment of Intracranial Occlusive Disease

Roberto Leal Silveira, MD, PhD
Neurosurgeon in Chief
Department of Neurosurgery
Hospital Madre Teresa
Belo Horizonte, United Kingdom
Surgical Management of Tumors of the Foramen Magnum

Nathan E. Simmons, MD
Assistant Professor of Neurosurgery
Dartmouth-Hitchcock Medical Center
Lebanon, New Hampshire
Surgical Techniques in the Management of Thoracic Disc Herniations

Marc Sindou, MD, DSc
Professor of Neurosurgery
University Claude Bernard de Lyon
Chairman
Department of Neurosurgery
Hôpital Neurologique P. Wertheimer PH.D
Neurophysiology
Lyon, France
Surgery for Intractable Spasticity

Marco Sinisi, MD
Consultant Neurosurgeon
Peripheral Nerve Injury Unit
Royal National Orthopaedic Hospital
Honorary Senior Lecturer
Department of Nerve Surgery
Imperial College of London
London, United Kingdom
Management of Entrapment Neuropathies

Timothy Siu, MBBS, FRACS, PhD
Clinical Senior Lecturer
Australian School of Advanced Medicine
Macquarie University
Sydney, Australia
Surgical Management of Cerebral Metastases

Edward Smith, MD
Staff Neurosurgeon
Department of Neurosurgery
Children's Hospital Boston
Boston, Massachusetts
Revascularization Techniques in Pediatric Cerebrovascular Disorders

Joseph R. Smith, MD, FACS
Professor Emeritus
Department of Neurosurgery
Medical College of Georgia
Augusta, Georgia
Mesencephalic Tractotomy and Anterolateral Cordotomy for Intractable Pain

Patricia Smith, MD
Postdoctoral Research Fellow
Department of Neurosurgery
Strong Hospital
University of Rochester Medical Center
Rochester, New York
Peripheral Nerve Injury

Matthew Smyth, MD
Associate Professor of Neurosurgery and Pediatrics
Department of Neurological Surgery
Washington University
Director, Pediatric Epilepsy Surgery Program
Neurosurgeon, Craniofacial Surgery Program
St. Louis Children's Hospital
St. Louis, Missouri
Mapping, Disconnection, and Resective Surgery in Pediatric Epilepsy

Domenico Solari, MD
Department of Neurological Sciences
Università degli Studi di Napoli Federico II
Naples, Italy
Endoscopic Endonasal Approach for Craniopharyngiomas

David Solomon, MD, PhD
Assistant Professor of Neurology and Otolaryngology—Head and Neck Surgery
Department of Neurology
Johns Hopkins Hospital
Baltimore, Maryland
Adult Pseudotumor Cerebri Syndrome

Adam M. Sonabend, MD
Department of Neurological Surgery
Columbia University Medical Center
New York, New York
Peripheral Nerve Injury

Mark M. Souweidane, MD
Vice Chairman and Professor
Director
Pediatric Neurosurgery
Department of Neurological Surgery
Weill Cornell Medical College
Associate Attending Neurosurgeon
Department of Pediatric Neurosurgery
New York Presbyterian Hospital
Associate Attending Surgeon
Department of Pediatric Neurosurgery
Memorial Hospital for Cancer and Allied Diseases
Assistant Attending Orthopedic Surgeon
Department of Neurosurgery
Hospital for Special Surgery
New York, New York
Endoscopic Approach to Intraventricular Brain Tumors

Edgardo Spagnuolo, MD
Assistant Professor
Chief of Neurosurgical Department
Surgical Department Teaching Unit
School of Medicine
Universidad de la República
Maciel Hospital
Montevideo, Uruguay
Chief of Neurosurgical Department
Neurosurgical Departments of Private Institutions
Montevideo, Uruguay
Chief of Vascular Committee, Southern Chapter
Vascular Committee
Federación Latinoamericana de Neurocirugía
Montevideo, Uruguay
*Surgical Management of Cerebral Arteriovenous
    Malformations*

Robert F. Spetzler, MD
Director and J. N. Harber Chair of Neurological Surgery
Division of Neurological Surgery
Barrow Neurological Institute
Phoenix, Arizona
Professor
Department of Surgery
Section of Neurosurgery
University of Arizona College of Medicine
Tucson, Arizona
*Surgical Management of Midbasilar and Lower Basilar
    Aneurysms*

Robert J. Spinner, MD
Professor
Departments of Neurologic Surgery, Orthopedics,
    and Anatomy
Mayo Clinic
Rochester, Minnesota
Nerve Transfers: Indications and Techniques

Andreas M. Stark, MD
Department of Neurosurgery
Universitätsklinikum Schleswig-Holstein, Campus Kiel
Kiel, Germany
*Surgical Navigation with Intraoperative Imaging: Special
    Operating Room Concepts*

Philip A. Starr, MD, PhD
Associate Professor of Neurosurgery
University of California, San Francisco
San Francisco, California
Deep Brain Stimulation for Intractable Psychiatric Illness

Ladislau Steiner, MD, PhD
Professor
Lars Leksell Center for Gamma Surgery
Professor of Neurosurgery and Radiology
University of Virginia
Charlottesville, Virginia
*Gamma Knife Surgery for Cerebral Vascular Malformations
    and Tumors*
Gamma Surgery for Functional Disorders

Michael P. Steinmetz, MD
Chairman, Department of Neuroscience
MetroHealth Medical Center
Associate Professor
Case Western Reserve University School of Medicine
Cleveland, Ohio
Management of Cervical Spondylotic Myelopathy

Shirley I. Stiver, MD, PhD
Assistant Professor of Neurological Surgery
Principal Investigator, Brain and Spinal Injury Center
University of California, San Francisco
San Francisco, California
Decompressive Craniectomy for Traumatic Brain Injury
Management of Skull Base Trauma

Prem Subramanian, MD, PhD
Associate Professor of Ophthalmology, Neurology,
    and Neurosurgery
Wilmer Eye Institute
The Johns Hopkins University School of Medicine
Baltimore, Maryland
Associate Professor of Surgery
Division of Ophthalmology
Uniformed Services University of the Health Sciences
Bethesda, Maryland
Multimodal Treatment of Orbital Tumors
Adult Pseudotumor Cerebri Syndrome

Michael E. Sughrue, MD
Department of Neurological Surgery
University of California, San Francisco
San Francisco, California
Craniopharyngiomas
Decompressive Craniectomy for Traumatic Brain Injury

Ian Suk, BScBMC, CMI
Associate Professor of Neurosurgery and Art as Applied
    to Medicine
Department of Neurosurgery
Johns Hopkins Hospital
Baltimore, Maryland
*Posterior Lumbar Fusion by Open Technique: Indications
    and Techniques*

Daniel Q. Sun, MD
Department of Neurosurgery
The Johns Hopkins University School of Medicine
Baltimore, Maryland
Stereotactic Radiosurgery for Pituitary Adenomas

Ulrich Sure, MD
Neurosurgeon
Department of Neurosurgery
Philipps University
Marburg, Germany
*Surgical Management of Aneurysms of the Vertebral
and Posterior Inferior Cerebellar Artery Complex*

Oszkar Szentirmai, MD
Chief Resident
Department of Neurosurgery
University of Colorado
Aurora, Colorado
*Novel Targets in Deep Brain Stimulation for Movement
Disorders*

Alexander Taghva, MD
Department of Neurological Surgery
University of Southern California
Keck School of Medicine
Los Angeles, California
*Transcallosal Surgery of Lesions Affecting the Third
Ventricle: Basic Principles*

Giuseppe Talamonti, MD
Department of Neurosurgery
Niguarda Ca'Granda Hospital
Milan, Italy
Management of Traumatic Intracranial Aneurysms

Rafael J. Tamargo, MD, FACS
Walter E. Dandy Professor of Neurosurgery
Director, Division of Cerebrovascular Neurosurgery
Professor of Neurosurgery and Otolaryngology
Vice Chairman
Department of Neurosurgery
Neurosurgery Co-Director
Neurosciences Critical Care Unit
Department of Neurosurgery
Johns Hopkins Hospital
Baltimore, Maryland
*Surgical Management of Infratentorial Arteriovenous
Malformations*

Richard J. Teff, MD
Neurological Surgeon
Department of Surgery
San Antonio Military Medical Center
San Antonio, Texas
*Management of Penetrating and Blast Injuries
of the Nervous System*

John M. Tew, Jr., MD
The Neuroscience Institute
University of Cincinnati College of Medicine
and the Mayfield Clinic
Cincinnati, Ohio
*Percutaneous Stereotactic Rhizotomy in the Treatment
of Intractable Facial Pain*

Nicholas Theodore, MD, FAANS, FACS
Chief, Spine Section
Division of Neurological Surgery
Barrow Neurological Institute
Phoenix, Arizona
Clinical Professor
Department of Surgery
Creighton University School of Medicine
Omaha, Nebraska
Posterior Lumbar Interbody Fusion

Philip V. Theodosopoulos, MD
Associate Professor
Residency Program Director
Department of Neurosurgery
University of Cincinnati
Cincinnati, Ohio
Craniopharyngiomas

B. Gregory Thompson, Jr., MD
Professor and Vice-Chair
Department of Neurosurgery
University of Michigan
Ann Arbor, Michigan
Endovascular Management of Intracranial Aneurysms

Wuttipong Tirakotai, MD, MSc
Doctor
Department of Neurosurgery
Prasat Neurological Institute
Bangkok, Thailand
Arachnoid, Suprasellar, and Rathke's Cleft Cysts
*Surgical Management of Aneurysms of the Vertebral
and Posterior Inferior Artery Complex*

Stavropoula I. Tjoumakaris, BS, MD
Instructor
Department of Neurosurgery
Thomas Jefferson University Hospital
Philadelphia, Pennsylvania
*Endovascular Treatment of Cerebral Arteriovenous
Malformations*

James H. Tonsgard, MD
Associate Professor
Department of Pediatrics and Neurology
Director
Neurofibromatosis Program
The University of Chicago
Chicago, Illinois
Surgical Management of Neurofibromatosis Types 1 and 2

David Trejo, MD
Unit of Stereotactic, Functional Neurosurgery
and Radiosurgery
Hospital General de México
Mexico City, Mexico
*Presurgical Evaluation for Epilepsy Including Intracranial
Electrodes*

Michael Trippel, MD, Dipl.-Ing.
Stereotactic Neurosurgery
University Hospital
Freiburg, Germany
Interstitial and LINAC-Radiosurgery for Brain Metastases

R. Shane Tubbs, MS, PA-C, PhD
Associate Professor
Departments of Cell Biology and Surgery
Division of Neurosurgery
University of Alabama at Birmingham
Director, Anatomical Donor Program/Gross Anatomy
    Laboratory
University of Alabama at Birmingham School of Medicine
Director of Research in Pediatric Neurosurgery
Children's Hospital of Alabama
Birmingham, Alabama
*Surgical Decision-Making and Treatment Options for Chiari
    Malformations in Children*
Management of Occult Spinal Dysraphism in Adults

Luis M. Tumialan, MD, LCDR MC(DMO) USN
Department of Neurosurgery
Naval Medical Center San Diego
San Diego, California
*Minimally Invasive Lumbar Microdiscectomy: Indications
    and Techniques*

Andreas Unterberg, MD, PhD
Professor of Neurosurgery
Universitätsklinikum Heidelberg
Neurochirurgische Universitätsklinik
Heidelberg, Germany
Surgical Approaches to the Orbit

Michael S. Vaphiades, DO
Professor
Department of Ophthalmology
University of Alabama at Birmingham
Birmingham, Alabama
Multimodal Assessment of Pituitary and Parasellar Lesions

T. Brooks Vaughan, MD
Assistant Professor
Department of Medicine and Pediatrics
The University of Alabama at Birmingham
Birmingham, Alabama
Multimodal Assessment of Pituitary and Parasellar Lesions

Anand Veeravagu, MD
Stanford University
School of Medicine
Stanford, California
*Radiation Therapy and Radiosurgery in the Management
    of Craniopharyngiomas*

Ana Luisa Velasco, MD, PhD
Head of Epilepsy Clinic
Functional Neurosurgery Unit
General Hospital of Mexico
Mexico City, Mexico
*Presurgical Evaluation for Epilepsy including Intracranial
    Electrodes*

Francisco Velasco, MD
Senior Investigator
Department of Neurology and Neurosurgery
General Hospital of Mexico
Mexico City, Mexico
*Presurgical Evaluation for Epilepsy including Intracranial
    Electrodes*

Gregory J. Velat, MD
Clinical Lecturer
Department of Neurological Surgery
University of Florida
Gainesville, Florida
*Management of Dissections of the Carotid and Vertebral
    Arteries*
Endovascular Treatment of Stroke

Angela Verlicchi, MD
Neurologist
Free University of Neuroscience Anemos
Reggio Emilia, Italy
Stereotactic Radiosurgery for Meningiomas

Frank D. Vrionis, MD, MPH, PhD
Senior Member and Director, Spinal and Skull Base
    Oncology
Department of Neuro-Oncology
H. Lee Moffitt Cancer Center
Professor of Neurosurgery, Orthopaedics, and Oncology
Department of Neurosurgery
University of South Florida
Tampa, Florida
Transtemporal Approaches to Posterior Cranial Fossa

Michel Wager, MD, PhD
Professor of Neurosurgery
Department of Neurological Surgery
University Hospital
Poitiers, France
Management of Cauda Equina Tumors

M. Christopher Wallace, MD, FACS, FRCSC
Professor
Department of Neurosurgery
University of Toronto
Toronto, Canada
*Surgical Management of Cranial Dural Arteriovenous
    Fistulas*

Gary S. Wand, MD
Professor of Medicine and Psychiatry
The Johns Hopkins University School of Medicine
Baltimore, Maryland
Multimodal Assessment of Pituitary and Parasellar Lesions

Benjamin C. Warf, MD
Department of Neurosurgery
Children's Hospital Boston/Harvard Medical School
Boston, Massachusetts
*Methods for Cerebrospinal Fluid Diversion in Pediatric
    Hydrocephalus: From Shunt to Scope*

Michael F. Waters, MD, PhD
Assistant Professor
Departments of Neurology and Neuroscience
Stroke Program Director
University of Florida
Gainesville, Florida
Endovascular Treatment of Stroke

Joseph Watson, MD
Associate Professor
Department of Neurosurgery
Virginia Commonwealth University
Director Inova Regional Neurosurgery Service
Department of Neuroscience
Inova Health System
Falls Church, Virginia
Cushing's Disease

Martin H. Weiss, MD
Professor of Neurological Surgery
University of Southern California
Los Angeles, California
Prolactinomas

Nirit Weiss, MD
Department of Neurosurgery
Mount Sinai Hospital
New York, New York
Management of Spinal Cord Tumors and Arteriovenous Malformations

William Welch, MD, FACS, FICS
Department of Neurosurgery
University of Pennsylvania
Chief of Neurosurgery
Pennsylvania Hospital
Philadelphia, Pennsylvania
Dynamic Stabilization of the Lumbar Spine: Indications and Techniques

J. Kent Werner, Jr., BS
MD, PhD Candidate
Department of Neuroscience
The Johns Hopkins University School of Medicine
Baltimore, Maryland
Ensign
Medical Corps, United States Navy
Bethesda, Maryland
Management of Penetrating Brain Injury

Louis A. Whitworth, MD
Assistant Professor in Neurosurgery
Director of Functional and Stereotactic Neurosurgery
University of Texas Southwestern Medical Center at Dallas
Dallas, Texas
Deep Brain Stimulation in Movement Disorders: Parkinson's Disease, Essential Tremor, and Dystonia

Christopher Winfree, MD, FACS
Assistant Professor of Neurological Surgery
Department of Neurological Surgery
Neurological Institute
Columbia University Medical Center
New York, New York
Peripheral Nerve Injury

Timothy F. Witham, BS, MD
Assistant Professor of Neurosurgery
Department of Neurosurgery
The Johns Hopkins University School of Medicine
Baltimore, Maryland
Management of Penetrating Injuries to the Spine

Jean-Paul Wolinsky, MD
Associate Professor of Neurosurgery and Oncology
Department of Neurosurgery
The Johns Hopkins University
Baltimore, Maryland
Transoral Approach to the Cervical Spine
Atlantoaxial Instability and Stabilization

Judith M. Wong, MD
Department of Neurosurgery
Brigham and Women's Hospital
Harvard Medical School
Boston, Massachusetts
Lateral Lumbar Interbody Fusion: Indications and Techniques

Shaun Xavier, MD
New York Hospital for Joint Diseases
New York, New York
Management of Degenerative Lumbar Stenosis and Spondylolisthesis

Bakhtiar Yamini, MD
Assistant Professor of Surgery
University of Chicago Medical Center
Chicago, Illinois
Surgical Management of Neurofibromatosis Types 1 and 2

Claudio Yampolsky, MD
Department of Neurosurgery
Muñiz Infectious Diseases Hospital
Buenos Aires, Argentina
Management of Shunt Infections

Michael J. Yaremchuk, MD, FACS
Craniofacial Surgery Fellow
Professor of Surgery
Harvard School of Medicine
Assistant in Surgery
Plastic and Reconstructive Surgery
Director, Craniofacial Surgery
Plastic and Reconstructive Surgery
Massachusetts General Hospital
Boston, Massachusetts
Principles of Scalp Surgery and Surgical Management of Major Defects of Scalp

Reza Yassari, MD, MS
Section of Neurosurgery
Department of Surgery
University of Chicago Hospital
Chicago, Illinois
Atlantoaxial Instability and Stabilization
Neurologic Problems of the Spine in Achondroplasia

Chun-Po Yen, MD
Department of Neurological Surgery
University of Virginia
Charlottesville, Virginia
Gamma Knife Surgery for Cerebral Vascular Malformations and Tumors
Gamma Surgery for Functional Disorders

John Yianni, MD, MBBS, BSc, FRCS
Department of Neurosurgery
John Radcliffe Hospital
Oxford, United Kingdom
Cervical Dystonia and Spasmodic Torticollis: Indications and Techniques

Alexander K. Yu, MD, MSBE, MS
Chief Resident
Department of Neurosurgery
Allegheny General Hospital
Pittsburgh, Pennsylvania
Surgical Management of Petroclival Meningiomas
Management of Cranial Nerve Injuries

Eric L. Zager, MD
Professor of Neurosurgery
University of Pennsylvania
Philadelphia, Pennsylvania
Management of Median Nerve Compression
Management of Thoracic Outlet Syndrome

Bruno Zanotti, MD
Neurosurgeon and Neurologist
Unit of Neurosurgery
Azienda Ospedaliero-Universitaria S.M. della Misericordia
Udine, Italy
Stereotactic Radiosurgery for Meningiomas

Marco Zenteno, MD
Department of Neurological Endovascular Therapy
Instituto Nacional de Neurología y Neurocirugía
Universidad Nacional Autonoma de Mexico
Comprehensive Stroke Center, Hospital
Mexico City, Mexico
Role of Gamma Knife Radiosurgery in the Management of Arteriovenous Malformations

Mehmet Zileli, MD
Professor of Neurosurgery
Department of Neurosurgery
Ege University Faculty of Medicine
Izmir, Turkey
Stabilization of the Subaxial Cervical Spine (C3–C7)

Alexandros D. Zouzias, MD
Resident
Neurological Institute of New Jersey
Newark, New Jersey
Endovascular Treatment of Head and Neck Bleeding

Drs. Schmidek and Sweet co-edited the first single volume entitled *Current Techniques in Operative Neurosurgery* in 1977. At the time, this first edition reflected their own interests in contemporary neurosurgical procedures. This book has continued the same tradition in the subsequent editions: to provide the working neurosurgeon with information that would be useful when taking a patient to the operating room. The chapters provided an overview of the topic, a discussion of available options, and results. In many cases, alternative surgical and nonsurgical options were included for dealing with a particular clinical situation. The goal from the first edition has been to provide a single source that would allow a neurosurgeon to develop a surgical plan for the patient. The chapter references would be up to date and allow further immersion in the topic as needed. The success of these volumes places *Operative Neurosurgical Techniques: Indications, Methods, and Results* among the most widely used neurosurgical texts worldwide. Now in its sixth edition, this title is dedicated to Dr. Schmidek's unending effort to advance the knowledge and expertise of medical students throughout the world. The field of neurological surgery has experienced a tremendous evolution during the last decade, and I have added multiple section editors to keep the current edition as modern as possible.

The sixth edition continues to reflect the same underlying vision for the book and attempts to keep up to date with the rapidly evolving changes in neurosurgery. This new and improved edition consists of 10 sections and 206 chapters authored by 510 contributors representing neurosurgical services from several different countries. It was the intention of Dr. Schmidek in the previous editions to reflect the ongoing worldwide changes, to include contributions of internationally renowned doctors, and to perpetuate the idea of a worldwide text in neurosurgery. This edition has lived up to that goal. Approximately 43% of the chapters deal with material not previously addressed in this text, including the topics of pediatric neurosurgery, endovascular surgery, new spine and skull base minimally invasive techniques, and the study of peripheral nerves. Where appropriate, chapters published in earlier editions have been extensively rewritten. All the chapters have been reviewed by myself and my co-editors to ensure that they reflect the current state of the art.

This edition could not have been accomplished without the enthusiastic participation of the section editors and contributors who put in extraordinary efforts to complete their chapters in time. Every effort has been made to produce a product worthy of the contributions. This could only have been accomplished with the professionalism of Julie Goolsby, Agnes Hunt Byrne, and Lisa Barnes at Elsevier; my staff Colleen Hickson and Caitlin Rogers; and Cassie Carey at Graphic World Publishing Services. I extend to all of the section editors, contributors, and staff members from Elsevier, Graphic World, and Hopkins my most sincere thanks for a tremendous job, which was incredibly well done.

Alfredo Quiñones-Hinojosa, MD

CONTENTS

Section Two

OPERATIVE TECHNIQUES IN PEDIATRIC NEUROSURGERY

Section Three

VASCULAR DISEASES

OPEN TREATMENT

ENDOVASCULAR TREATMENT

Section Four

HYDROCEPHALUS

Section Five

STEREOTACTIC RADIOSURGERY

Volume Two

Section Six

FUNCTIONAL NEUROSURGERY

SURGICAL MANAGEMENT OF MEDICALLY INTRACTABLE EPILEPSY

SURGICAL MANAGEMENT OF PSYCHIATRIC AND MOVEMENT DISORDERS

Section Seven

TRAUMA

Section Eight

SURGICAL MANAGEMENT OF NERVOUS SYSTEM INFECTIONS

VASCULAR DISEASES/ENDOVASCULAR TREATMENT

HYDROCEPHALUS

STEREOTACTIC RADIOSURGERY

TRAUMA

SURGICAL MANAGEMENT OF NERVOUS SYSTEM INFECTIONS

NEUROSURGICAL MANAGEMENT OF SPINAL DISORDERS/DEGENERATIVE SPINE DISORDER/CERVICAL SPINE

NEUROSURGICAL MANAGEMEMENT OF SPINAL DISORDERS/DEGENERATIVE SPINE DISORDER/LUMBAR SPINE

NEUROSURGICAL MANAGEMENT OF SPINAL DISORDERS/CONGENITAL AND DEVELOPMENTAL SPINAL ABNORMALITIES

CHAPTER 1

Ensuring Patient Safety in Surgery— First Do No Harm

SYMEON MISSIOS • KIMON BEKELIS • GEORGE T. BLIKE • KADIR ERKMEN

Primum non nocere—first do no harm. This often-quoted phrase epitomizes the importance the medical community places on avoiding iatrogenic complications.[1] In the process of providing care, patients, physicians, and the entire clinical team join to use all available medical weapons to combat disease to avert the natural history of pathologic processes. Iatrogenic injury or, simply, "treatment-related harm" occurs when this implicit rule to "first do no harm" is violated. Both society and the medical community have historically been intolerant of medical mistakes, associating them with negligence. The fact is that complex medical care is prone to failure. Medical mistakes are much like "friendly-fire" incidents in which soldiers in the high-tempo, complex fog of war mistakenly kill comrades rather than the enemy. Invariably, medical error and iatrogenic injury are associated with multiple latent conditions (constraints, hazards, system vulnerabilities, etc.) that predispose front-line clinicians to err. This chapter will review the science of human error in medicine and surgery. The specific case of wrong-sided brain surgery will be used as an illustration for implementation of emerging new strategies for enhancing patient safety.

The Nature of Iatrogenic Injury in Medicine and Surgery

The earliest practitioners of medicine recognized and described iatrogenic injury. Iatrogenic (Greek, iatros = doctor, genic = arising from or developing from) literally translates to "disease or illness caused by doctors." Famous examples exist of likely iatrogenic deaths, such as that of George Washington, who died while being treated for pneumonia with blood-letting. The Royal Medical and Surgical Society, in 1864, documented 123 deaths that "could be positively assigned to the inhalation of chloroform."[2] Throughout history, physicians have reviewed unexpected outcomes related to the medical care they provided to learn and improve that care. The "father" of modern neurosurgery, Harvey Cushing, and his contemporary Sir William Osler modeled the practice of learning from error by publishing their errors openly so as to warn others on how to avert future occurrences.[3-5] However, the magnitude of iatrogenic morbidity and mortality was not quantified across the spectrum of health care until the Harvard Practice Study, published in 1991.[6] This seminal study estimated that iatrogenic failure occurs in approximately 4% of all hospitalizations and is the eighth leading cause of death in America—responsible for up to 100,000 deaths per year in the United States alone.[7]

A subsequent review of over 14,700 hospitalizations in Colorado and Utah identified 402 surgical adverse events, producing an annual incidence rate of 1.9%.[8] The nature of surgical adverse events were categorized by type of injury and by preventability (Table 1-1).

These two studies were designed to characterize iatrogenic complications in health care. While not statistically powered to allow surgical subspecialty analysis, it is likely that the types of failures and subsequent injuries that this study identified can be generalized to the neurosurgical patient population. More recent literature supports the findings of these landmark studies.[9-11]

The Institute of Medicine used the Harvard Practice Study as the basis for its report, which endorsed the need to discuss and study errors openly with the goal of improving patient safety.[7] The Institute of Medicine report on medical errors, "To Err Is Human: Building a Safer Health System," must be considered a landmark publication.[12] It was published in 1999 and focused on medical errors and their prevention. This was followed by the development of other quality improvement initiatives such as the Joint Commission on the Accreditation of Healthcare Organizations (JCAHO) Sentinel Events Program.[12]

One might argue that morbidity and mortality reviews already achieve this aim. The "M&M" conference has a long history of reviewing negative outcomes in medicine. The goal of this traditional conference is to learn how to prevent future patients from suffering similar harm, and thus incrementally improve care. However, frank discussion of error is limited in M&M conferences. Also, the actual review practices fail to support deep learning regarding systemic vulnerabilities[13]; indeed, since M&M conferences do not explicitly require medical errors to be reviewed, errors are rarely addressed. One prospective investigation of four U.S. academic hospitals found that a resident vigilantly attending weekly internal medicine M&M conferences for an entire year would discuss errors only once. The surgical version of the M&M conference was better with error discussion. However, while surgeons discussed adverse events associated with error 77% of the time, individual provider error was the focus of the discussion and cited

Table 1-1   Surgical Adverse Events Categorized by Type of Injury and Preventability

Type of Event	Percentage of Adverse Events	Percentage Preventable
Technique-related complication	24	68
Wound infection	11	23
Postoperative bleeding	11	85
Postpartum/neonatal related	8	67
Other infection	7	38
Drug-related injury	7	46
Wound problem (noninfectious)	4	53
Deep venous thrombosis	4	18
Nonsurgical procedure injury	3	59
Diagnostic error/delay	3	100
Pulmonary embolus	2	14
Acute myocardial infarction	2	0
Inappropriate therapy	2	100
Anesthesia injury	2	45
Congestive heart failure	1	33
Stroke	1	0
Pneumonia	1	65
Fall	0.5	50
Other	5.5	32

as causative of the negative outcome in 8 of 10 conference discussions.[13] Surgical conference discussion rarely identified structural defects, resource constraints, team communication, or other system problems. Further limiting its utility, the M&M conference is reactive by nature and highly subject to hindsight bias. This is the basis for most clinical outcome reviews, focusing solely on medical providers and their decision making.[14] In their report, titled "Nine Steps to Move Forward from Error" in medicine, human factors experts Cook and Woods challenged the medical community to resist the temptation to simplify the complexities that practitioners face when reviewing accidents post hoc. Premature closure by blaming the closest clinician hides the deeper patterns and multiple contributors associated with failure, and ultimately leads to naive "solutions" that are weak or even counterproductive.[15] The Institute of Medicine has also cautioned against blaming an individual and recommending training as the sole outcome of case review.[7] While the culture within medicine is to learn from failure, the M&M conference does not typically achieve this aim.

A Human Factors Approach to Improving Patient Safety

Murphy's law—that whatever can go wrong will—is the common-sense explanation for medical mishaps. The science of safety (and how to create it), however, is not common sense. The field of human factors engineering grew out of a focus on human interaction with physical devices, especially in military or industrial settings. This initial focus on how to improve human performance addressed the problem of workers that are at high risk for injury while using a tool or machine in high-hazard industries. In the past several decades, the scope of this science has broadened. Human factors engineering is now credited with advancing safety

and reliability in aviation, nuclear power, and other high hazard work settings. Membership in the Human Factors and Ergonomics Society in North America alone has grown to over 15,000 members. Human factors engineering and related disciplines are deeply interested in modeling and understanding mechanisms of complex system failure. Furthermore, these applied sciences have developed strategies for designing error prevention and building error tolerance into systems to increase reliability and safety, and these strategies are now being applied to the healthcare industry.[16-21] The specialty of anesthesiology has employed this science to reduce the anesthesia-related mortality rate from approximately 1 in 10,000 in the 1970s to over 1 in 250,000 three decades later.[22] Critical incident analysis was used by a bioengineer (Jeffrey Cooper) to identify preventable anesthesia mishaps in 1978.[23] Cooper's seminal work was supplemented by the "closed-claim" liability studies, which delineated the most common and severe modes of failure and factors that contributed to those failures. The specialty of anesthesiology and its leaders endorsed the precepts that safety stems more from improved system design than from increasing vigilance of individual practitioners. As a direct result, anesthesiology was the first specialty to adopt minimal standards for care and monitoring, preanesthesia equipment checklists similar to those used in commercial aviation, standardized medication labels, interlocking hardware to prevent gas mix-ups, international anesthesia machine standards, and the development of high-fidelity human simulation to support crisis team training in the management of rare events. Lucien Leape, a former surgeon, one of the lead authors of the Harvard Practice Study, and a national advocate for patient safety, has stated, "Anesthesia is the only system in healthcare that begins to approach the vaunted 'six sigma' (a defect rate of 1 in a million) level of clinical safety perfection that other industries strive for. This outstanding achievement is attributable not to any single practice or development of new anesthetic agents or even any type of improvement (such as technological advances) but to application of a broad array of changes in process, equipment, organization, supervision, training, and teamwork. However, no single one of these changes has ever been proven to have a clear-cut impact on mortality. Rather, anesthesia safety was achieved by applying a whole host of changes that made sense, were based on an understanding of human factors principles, and had been demonstrated to be effective in other settings."[24] The Anesthesia Patient Safety Foundation, which has become the clearinghouse for patient safety successes in anesthesiology, was used as a model by the American Medical Association to form the National Patient Safety Foundation in 1996.[25] Over the subsequent decade, the science of safety has begun to permeate health care.

The human factors psychologist James Reason has characterized accidents as evolving over time and as virtually never being the consequence of a single cause.[26,27] Rather, he describes accidents as the net result of local triggers that initiate and then propagate an incident through a hole in one layer of defense after another until irreversible injury occurs (Fig. 1-1). This model has been referred to as the "Swiss cheese" model of accident causation. Surgical care consists of thousands of tasks and subtasks. Errors in the execution of these tasks need to be prevented, detected, and managed, or tolerated. The layers of Swiss cheese

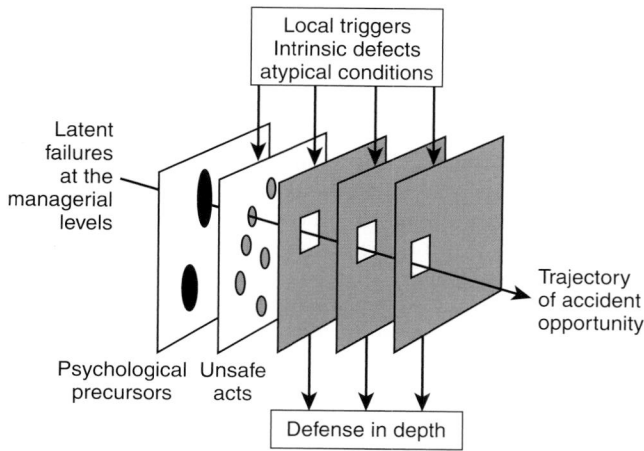

FIGURE 1-1 Reason's model of accident causation. Accidents (adverse outcomes) require a combination of latent failures, psychological precursors, event triggers, and failures in several layers of the system's "defense in depth." *(Copyright Dr. Reason.)*

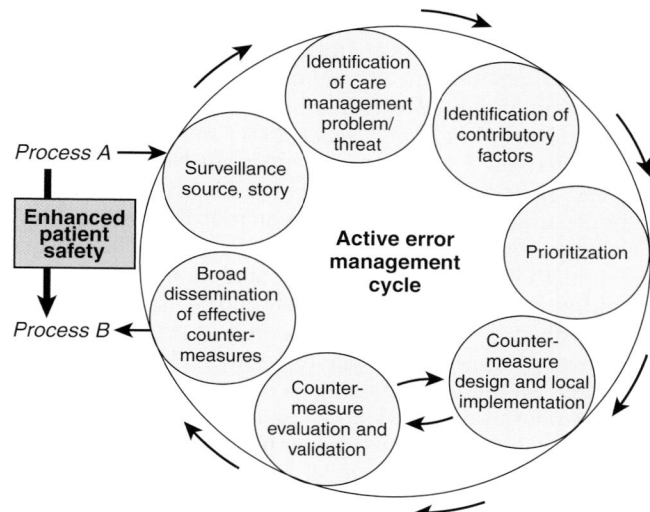

FIGURE 1-2 Sequence of steps for identifying vulnerabilities and then implementing corrective measures. *(Copyright Blike 2002.)*

represent the system of defenses against such error. *Latent conditions* is the term used to describe "accidents waiting to happen" that are the holes in each layer that will allow an error to propagate until it ultimately causes injury or death. The goal in human factors system engineering is to know all the layers of Swiss cheese and create the best defenses possible (i.e., make the holes as small as possible). This very approach has been the centerpiece of incremental improvements in anesthesia safety.

One structured approach designed to identify all holes in the major layers of cheese in medical systems has been described by Vincent.[28,29] He classifies the major categories of factors that contribute to error as follows:

1. Patient factors: condition, communication, availability, and accuracy of test results and other contextual factors that make a patient challenging
2. Task factors: using an organized approach in reliable task execution, availability, and use of protocols, and other aspects of task performance
3. Practitioner factors: deficits and failures by any individual member of the care team that undermines management of the problem space in terms of knowledge, attention, strategy, motivation, physical or mental health, and other factors that undermine individual performance
4. Team factors: verbal/written communication, supervision/seeking help, team structure, and leadership, and other failures in communication and coordination among members of the care team such that management of the problem space is degraded
5. Working conditions: staffing levels, skills mix and workload, availability and maintenance of equipment, administrative and managerial support, and other aspects of the work domain that undermine individual or team performance
6. Organization and management factors: financial resources, goals, policy standards, safety culture and priorities, and other factors that constrain local microsystem performance
7. Societal and political factors: economic and regulatory issues, health policy and politics, and other societal factors that set thresholds for patient safety

If this schema is used to structure a review of a morbidity or mortality, that review will be extended beyond myopic attention to the singular practitioner. Furthermore, the array of identified factors that undermine safety can then be countered systematically by tightening each layer of defense, one hole at a time. I have adapted active error management as described by Reason and others into a set of steps for making incremental systemic improvements to increase safety and reliability. In this adaptation, a cycle of active error management consists of (1) surveillance to identify potential threats, (2) investigation of all contributory factors, (3) prioritization of failure modes, (4) development of countermeasures to eliminate or mitigate individual threats, and (5) broad implementation of validated countermeasures (Fig. 1-2).

The goal is to move from a reactive approach based on review of actual injuries toward a proactive approach that anticipates threats based on a deep understanding of human capabilities and system design that aids human performance rather than undermines it.

A comprehensive review of the science of human factors and patient safety is beyond the scope of this chapter; neurosurgical patient safety has been reviewed, including ethical issues and the impact of legal liability.[30] Safety in aviation and nuclear power has taken over four decades to achieve the cultural shift that supports a robust system of countermeasures and defenses against human error. However, it is practical to use an example to illustrate some of the human factors principles introduced. Consider this case example as a window into the future of managing the most common preventable adverse events associated with surgery (see Table 1-1).

EXAMPLE OF MEDICAL ERROR: "WRONG-SIDED BRAIN SURGERY"

Wrong-site surgery is an example of an adverse event that seems as though it should "never happen." However, given over 40 million surgical procedures annually, we should not be surprised when it occurs. The news media has diligently reported wrong-site surgical errors, especially when they involve neurosurgery. Headlines such as "Brain Surgery Was Done on the Wrong Side, Reports Say" (*New York Daily News*, 2001) and "Doctor Who Operated on the Wrong Side of Brain Under Scrutiny" (*New York Times*, 2000), are inevitable when wrong-site brain surgery occurs.[31-33] As predicted, these are not isolated stories. A recent report from the state of Minnesota found 13 instances of wrong-site surgery in a single year during which time approximately 340,000 surgeries were performed.[34] No hospital appeared to be immune to what appears on the surface to be such a blatant mistake. Indeed, an incomplete registry collecting data on wrong-site surgery since 2001 now includes over 150 cases. Of 126 instances that have been reviewed, 41% relate to orthopedic surgery, 20% relate to general surgery, 14% to neurosurgery, 11% to urologic surgery, and the remaining to the other surgical specialties.[35] In a recent national survey,[36] the incidence of wrong-sided surgery for cervical discectomies, craniotomies, and lumbar surgery was 6.8, 2.2, and 4.5 per 10,000 operations, respectively.

The sensational "front-page news" media fails to identify the deeper second story behind these failures and how to prevent future failures through creation of safer systems.[37] In this example, we provide an analysis of contributory factors associated with wrong-site surgery to reveal the myriad of holes in the defensive layers of "cheese." These holes will need to be eliminated to truly impact the frequency of this already rare event and create more reliable care for our patients.

Contributory Factor Analysis

PATIENT FACTORS ASSOCIATED WITH WRONG-SITE SURGERY

Patient Condition (Medical Factors That If Not Known Increase the Risk for Complications)

Neurosurgical patients are at higher risk for wrong patient surgery than average. Patients and their surgical conditions contribute to error. When patients are asked what surgery they are having done on the morning of surgery, only 70% can correctly state and point to the location of the planned surgical intervention.[38] Patients are a further source of misinformation of surgical intent when the pathology and symptoms are contralateral to the site of surgery, a common condition in neurosurgical cases. Patients scheduled for brain surgery and carotid surgery often confuse the side of the surgery with the side of the symptoms. Patients with educational or language barriers or cognitive deficits are more vulnerable since they are unable to accurately communicate their surgical condition or the planned surgery.

Certain operations in the neurosurgical population pose higher risk for wrong-site surgery. While left–right symmetry and sidedness represents one high-risk class of surgeries, spinal procedures in which there are multiple levels is another.[39]

Patients with anatomy and pathology that disorient the surgical team to side or level are especially at risk. Anterior cervical discectomies can be approached by surgeons from either side. This lack of a consistent cue for the rest of

the surgical team as to the approach for the same surgery makes it unlikely anyone would trap an error in positioning or draping. It is known that patient position and opaque draping can remove external cues as to left and right orientation of the patient and thus predispose surgeons to wrong-sided surgery. When a patient is lateral, fully draped, and the table rotated 180 degrees prior to the attending surgeon entering the operating theater, it is difficult to verify right from left. Furthermore, the language for positioning creates ambiguity since the terminology of left lateral decubitus, right side up, and left side down are used interchangeably by the surgical team to specify the position. A patient with bilateral disease, predominant right-sided symptoms, and left-sided pathology having a left-sided craniotomy in the right lateral decubitus position with the table turned 180 degrees and fully draped obviously creates more confusion than a gallbladder surgery in the supine position.

Communication (Factors That Undermine the Patient's Ability to Be a Source of Information Regarding Conditions That Increase the Risk for Complications and Need to Be Managed)

Obviously, patients with language barriers or cognitive deficits represent a group that may be unable to communicate their understanding of the surgical plan. This can increase the chance of patient identification errors that lead to wrong-site surgery. In a busy practice, patients requiring the same surgery might be scheduled in the same operating room (OR). It is not uncommon to perform five carotid endarterectomies in a single day.[40] When one patient is delayed and the order switched to keep the OR moving, this vulnerability is expressed. Patients with common names are especially at risk. A 500-bed hospital will have approximately 1,000,000 patients in the medical record system. About 10% of patients will have the same first and last names. Five percent will have a first, middle, and last name in common with one other individual. Only by cross-checking the name with one other patient identifier (either birth date or a medical record number) can wrong-patient errors be trapped.[41]

Another patient communication problem that increases risk for wrong-site surgery consists of patients marking themselves. Marking the skin on the side of the proposed surgery with a pen is now common practice by the surgical team and part of the Universal Protocol. However, some patients have placed an X on the site not to be operated on. The surgical team has then confused this patient mark with their own in which an X specifies the side to be operated on. Patients are often not given information of what to expect and will seek outside information. For example, a neurosurgeon on a popular daytime talk show discussing medical mistakes stated incorrectly that patients should mark themselves with an X on the side that should not be operated on.[42] This error in information reached millions of viewers, and was in direct violation of recommendations for marking provided by the Joint Commission on Accreditation of Healthcare Organizations (and endorsed by the American College of Surgeons, American Society of Anesthesiology, and Association of Operating Room Nurses). Patients who watched this show and took the advice of the physician are now at higher risk than average for a wrong-sided surgical error.

Availability and Accuracy of Test Results (Factors That Undermine Awareness of Conditions That Increase the Risk for Complications and Need to Be Managed)

Radiologic imaging studies can be independent markers of surgical pathology and anatomy. However, films and/or reports are not always available. Films may be lost or misplaced. Also, they may be unavailable because they were performed at another facility. New digital technology has created electronic imaging systems that virtually eliminate lost studies. However, space constraints have led many hospitals to remove old view boxes to make room for digital radiologic monitors. When patients bring films from an outside hospital, this decision to eliminate view boxes prevents effective use of the studies. Even when available, x-rays and diagnostic studies are not labeled with 100% reliability. Imaging studies have been mislabeled and/or oriented backward, leading to wrong-sided surgery.[43]

TASK FACTORS ASSOCIATED WITH WRONG-SITE SURGERY

Tasks are the steps that need to be executed to accomplish a work goal. It is especially important to structure tasks and task execution procedures when work domains are complex, the task must be executed under time pressure, and the consequences of errors in task execution are severe. Typical tools for structuring task execution are protocols, checklists, and algorithms.

Task Design and Clarity of Structure (Consider This to Be an Issue When Work Is Being Performed in a Manner That Is Inefficient and Not Well Thought Out)

In large hospitals, ORs do not execute a consistent set of checks and balances to verify that the right patient, the surgical intent, and critical equipment and implants are present. If surgical team members think that they can announce the patient name and procedure aloud and that this will reliably prevent wrong-site surgery, they are mistaken. Structuring tasks for reliability such that current failure rates will be moved from approximately 1 in 30,000 to 1 in 1 million will take the kind of task structure and consistency seen on the flight decks of commercial planes. For decades, pilots have used well-organized preflight checklists to perform the tasks to start up an engine and verify that all mission-critical equipment is present and functional.

An example of a mature use of checklists exists in anesthesiology. An anesthesia machine (and other critical equipment) must be present and functional prior to the induction of anesthesia and initiation of paralysis so that a patient can have an airway as well as breathing and circulatory support provided within seconds to avoid hypoxia and subsequent cardiovascular complications. Until 1990, equipment failures were a significant problem leading to patient injury in anesthesia, even though anesthesia machines and equipment had been standardized and were being used on thousands of patients in a given facility.[44] At this time, a preanesthesia checklist was established to structure the verification of mission critical components required to provide the anesthetic state and to verify that

these components functioned nominally.[45] This checklist includes over 40 items and has included redundancy for checking critical components. It has been introduced as a standard operating procedure for the discipline of anesthesia and is now mandated by the U.S. Food and Drug Administration[46] (Fig. 1-3).

Availability and Use of Protocols (If Standard Protocols Exist, Are They Well Accepted and Are They Being Used Consistently?)

The first attempts to establish standardized protocols for patient safety began with JCAHO.[35] The JCAHO Sentinel Event system began monitoring major quality issues in the late 1980s about the same time the original AAOS Sign Your Site program launched. A sentinel event was defined as "an unexpected occurrence involving death or serious physical or psychological injury, or the risk thereof."[35] In addition to the reporting aspect of the program, a quality review is triggered that requires a root cause analysis to try to determine factors contributing to the sentinel event.

The Universal Protocol was a logical extension of the Sentinel Events quality improvement program. Wrong-site surgery is considered a sentinel event. Because of the mandatory reporting of Sentinel Events, some of the best data on the incidence and anatomic location of wrong-site surgeries come from the JCAHO. Before implementation of the Universal protocol, the JCAHO analyzed 278 reports of wrong-site surgery in the Sentinel Events database up to 2003.[47] This review showed that in 10% of the cases the wrong procedure had been performed, in 12% surgery had been performed on the wrong patient, and a further 19% of the reports characterized miscellaneous wrongs. Thus it was felt that a protocol to address this issue must include provisions to avoid wrong patient, wrong procedure, as well as wrong-site surgery.

In May 2003, the JCAHO convened a "Wrong Site Surgery Summit" to look into possible quality initiatives in this area. The three most effective measures identified were patient identification, surgical site marking, and calling a "time out" before skin incision to verify factors such as the initial patient identification, patient allergies, completion of preoperative interventions such as intravenous antibiotics, the procedure to be performed, available medical records, imaging studies, equipment etc. When correlated to Sentinel Event Data, it was found that only 12% of wrong-site surgeries occurred in institutions with two of three protocols applied.[48] More importantly, no incidences of wrong-sided surgery were detected in institutions with all three measures in place. Therefore, these three key processes became the Core Elements of the Universal Protocol, which is a mandatory quality screen in all JCAHO-certified hospitals since July 1, 2004.[48]

The universal protocol for preventing wrong-patient, wrong-site errors is based on checklist principles; but it is not yet a validated comprehensive checklist that will trap errors in the way aviation checklists do. This is largely due to the lack of consistent execution of the checklists in a challenge-response format that is identical in procedure and practice throughout a single hospital's ORs.[49,50] This protocol is a first step, but the barriers to effective implementation are extensive at present and hinder improved safety.[51,52]

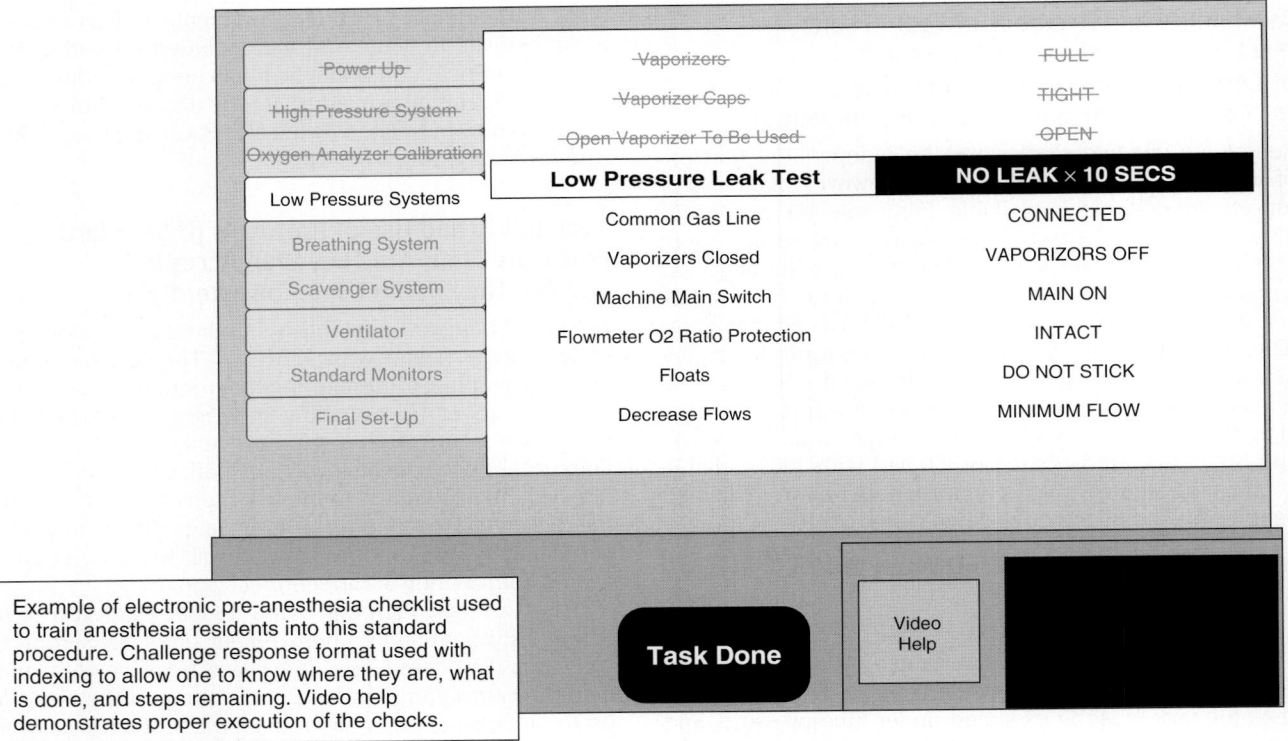

Example of electronic pre-anesthesia checklist used to train anesthesia residents into this standard procedure. Challenge response format used with indexing to allow one to know where they are, what is done, and steps remaining. Video help demonstrates proper execution of the checks.

FIGURE 1-3 Example of computer implementation.

Another hazard is the lack of clarity for marking surgical sites. Marking the surgical site has been endorsed to improve safety and is a major component of the Universal Protocol. However, as described previously, the mark can be a source of error when placed inappropriately by the patient or any other member of the surgical team. Some specifics regarding the details of what, when, and how to mark are lacking. Do you mark the incision site or the target of the surgery? What constitutes a unique and definitive mark? What shape and color should be used? What type of pen should be used? Does the ink pose any risk for infection or is it washed off during the course of preparation? Who should place the mark? What are the procedures that get marked and which should not? Are there any patients for whom the mark is dangerous? How do you mark for a left liver lobe resection or other procedures like brain surgery in which there is a single organ but still sidedness that is critical? I worked with over 10 surgical specialties to develop specific answers to these questions. Multiple marks and pens were tested. Not all symbols and pens were equally effective. Many inks did not withstand preparation and remain visible in the operative field. We now use specific permanent pens (Carter fine and Sharpie very fine) and a green circle to mark only "sided" procedures. We specified that the target is marked rather than the incision, the mark must be done by the surgeon, and the mark must be placed in a manner in which it is visible during the preincision check after the position, preparation, and drape have been completed. For example, a procedure requiring cystoscopy to inject the right ureteral orifice to treat reflux is now marked on the right thigh so that the green circle mark is a cue to all members of the surgical team and can be

seen even when the patient is prepared and draped. Again, we used the mark to specify the target, not the incision or body entry point. In addition, we have had every procedure in our booking system labeled as "mark required" or "mark not required," because this was not always clear. Even with this level of specificity, we have found marking to be erroneous and inconsistent during our initial implementation. Marking the skin for spine surgery to indicate the level may increase the risk of wrong-site errors.[53] A superior method for "marking" to verify the correct spinal level to be operated upon is to perform an intraoperative radiologic study with a radiopaque marker. We expect that many revisions to this type of safety measure will be needed before the marking procedure is robust and truly adds safety value. Cross-checking procedures in aviation were developed and matured over decades to achieve the reliability and consistency now observed.[54]

Statistics for the first two quarters after implementation of the Universal Protocol were encouraging.[55] It appeared that reports of wrong-site surgeries had declined below the rate of approximately 70 cases per year for the previous 2 years. However, after a full year's statistics had been accumulated, it was found that the incidents of wrong-site surgery had actually increased to about 88 for 2005.[12] Overall, wrong-site surgery had climbed to the number 2 ranking in frequency of sentinel events. Whether these data represent a true increase in the frequency of wrong-site surgery or are simply explained by better awareness and reporting is unclear at this time.

Currently the direction in patient safety is more toward a holistic surgical checklist, including all aspects of a patient visit to the hospital and not only the limited time out before surgery.[56] A number of studies have been conducted that evaluated the use of checklists in medicine and their effect in behavior modification.[56] To that effect, the WHO surgical checklist has been developed.[57] The features of the Universal Protocol have been integrated in this checklist with the addition of preprocedural and postprocedural checkpoints. Results from the implementation of the WHO checklist are encouraging. These initial attempts have been extended to the development of checklists, like the SURPASS checklist,[58] that cover the whole surgical pathway from admission to discharge. Overall, although it has been shown that aviation based team training elicits initially sustainable responses, effects may take years to be part of the surgical culture.[59]

PRACTITIONER FACTORS ASSOCIATED WITH WRONG-SITE SURGERY

Knowledge, Skills, and Rules (Individual Deviation from Standard of Care Due to Lack of Knowledge, Poor Skills, or a Failure to Use Rules Associated with Best Practice)

Knowledge deficits are often due to over-reliance on memory for information used rarely. Measures that increase availability of referent knowledge when needed would be helpful. Unfortunately, references at the point of care on the day of surgery are not standard or reliable. Three descriptions of the surgery often exist. The operative consent lists the planned surgery in lay language patients should be able to understand. The surgical preoperative note may provide a technical description of the planned surgery but often is incomplete, failing to include such information as the specific reason for surgery, sidedness, target, approach, position, need for implants, and/or special equipment. The booking system will often use a third nomenclature to describe the planned surgery that is administrative and linked to billing codes. The use of three different references for the same surgical procedure creates ambiguity. A "right L3–L4 facetectomy in the prone position" may be listed on the consent form as a "right third lumbar vertebrae joint surgery" on the consent and a CPT code "LUMBAR FACETECTOMY 025-36047."[60]

Subtle knowledge deficits are more likely to reach a patient and cause harm when individuals are charged to do work that is at the limits of their competency. The culture of medicine does not encourage *knowledge calibration*, the term used to describe how well individuals know what they know and know what they do not know.[61] At our institution, when preoperative nurses were assigned the role of marking patients to identify sidedness, they routinely marked the wrong site or marked in a manner such that the mark was not visible after the position, prep, and drape. These nurses accepted this assigned role because our medical culture encourages guessing and assertiveness. On further review, we have found that only the surgeon has the knowledge required to specify the surgical plan in detail and to mark patients correctly. Other members of the surgical team often have subtle knowledge deficits regarding surgical anatomy, terminology, and technical requirements such that they are prone to err in marking or positioning patients. Similarly, nurses and anesthesiologists in the presurgical areas are not able to verify or reconcile multiple differing sources of information as to the surgical plan. Instead, they often propagate errors and/or enter new misinformation into scheduling systems and patient records.

Attention (Factors That Undermine Attention)

Task execution is degraded when attention is pulled away from the work being performed. Distraction and noise are significant problems in the operating theater that can dramatically affect performance and vigilance. Because the wall and floor surfaces are designed to be cleaned easily, noise levels in the OR are similar to those on a busy highway.[62,63] The preincision interval is a very active time, when the patient is being given anesthesia, being positioned, and being prepared. These parallel activities represent competing priorities that conflict with a coordinated effort by the entire surgical team to verify surgical intent.

Strategy (Given Many Alternatives, Was the Strategy Optimized to Minimize Risks through Preventive Measures and through Recovery Measures That Use Contingency Planning and Anticipatory Behaviors?)

Strategic planning is not a major contributory factor for wrong-site surgery in my opinion. However, we have found that our initial attempts to use the exact same preincision checklist for all types of surgical populations was a strategic error and overly simplistic.

Motivation/Attitude (Motivational Failures and Poor Attitudes Can Undermine Individual Performance—the Psychology of Motivation Is Complex)

Because wrong-site surgery is a rare event, motivating the operative team to invest significant energy into preventive measures can be challenging. Even though the career risk for performing a wrong-site surgery is significant, the rarity of this complication predisposes surgeons to deny this complication as a significant problem. Part of the problem is that surgeons do not have an adequate understanding of human vulnerabilities and the potential for error. Many surgeons see wrong-site surgery as purely a failure in vigilance by an individual surgeon. The motivation to lead a team effort and accept cross-checking is therefore low. Human error training in surgery is just now beginning to address the decreased performance associated with fatigue, personal stress, production pressure, and so forth. Motivational barriers are not limited to the surgeon. Many nurses and anesthesiologists see wrong-site surgery as an isolated surgeon failure and believe that they should have no responsibility for verifying patient and/or procedure. Individual training about human error is needed across all members of the operative team to increase motivation to change behavior and use new methods (such as a team-executed checklist) to prevent wrong-site surgery.

Physical/Mental Health (Provider Performance Deviations from Standard "Competencies" Can Be Due to Physical or Mental Illness)

Industries that have come to accept the human component as having requirements for optimal human–machine system performance have thus promoted regular "fit-for-duty" examinations.[64] In the aviation industry, job screening includes a "color-blindness" test for air traffic controllers since many of the monitors encode critical information in color.[65] Some specific provider health conditions can predispose to wrong-site surgery. Surgeons and other members of the perioperative team with dyslexia and related neuropsychiatric deficits have particular difficulty with sidedness and left–right orientation.

TEAM FACTORS ASSOCIATED WITH WRONG-SITE SURGERY

A complex work domain will overwhelm the cognitive abilities of any one individual and not permit expertise of the entire field of practice. A common strategy for managing the excess demands that complex systems (like that of human physiology and pathophysiology) place on any individual is to subspecialize. Breaking a big problem into smaller parts that are then more manageable by a group of individuals is rational. However, by "fixing" the problem of individual cognitive work overload, a new class of problems manifests— those due to team communication and coordination failure. Many human factors experts consider team failures to be the most common contributory factor associated with error in complex sociotechnical work systems.[66] Crisis resource management training and team training in aviation is considered to have played a major role in improving aviation safety.[67] These methods are just now being applied in medicine.[68]

Verbal/Written Communication (Any Communication Mode That When It Fails Leads to a Degradation in Team Performance)

Verbal communications fail due to noise (just do not hear) or content comprehension (mismatch between what was intended and what was understood). Noise should be minimized to support verbal communication in the OR. Comprehension problems have many mechanisms. Human-to-human communication requires "grounding," which is the process whereby both parties frame the communication episode based on how the one conveying a message discovers the frame of reference of the one receiving the message. This activity represents a significant part of effective communication. Agreeing on a common language and structuring communication goes a long way toward increasing accuracy and speed of communication of mission-critical information.[17,18,69] While isolated examples of structured communication across members of the operative team exist, it is usually confined to individuals knowledgeable in safety science and the use of structured communication in the military and in aviation.

Supervision/Seeking Help (Any Member of the Team Who Fails to Mobilize Help When Getting into a Work Overload Situation, or a Team Member in a Supervisory Role Failing to Provide Adequate Oversight, Especially in Settings in Which There Are Learners and/or Transient Rotating Team Members)

True team performance is only realized when a group of individuals share a common goal, divide work tasks between individuals to create role delineation and role clarity within the team, and know each other's roles well enough to provide cross-checks of mission-critical activities.[70] On medical teams, data gathering and treatment implementation tend to be nursing roles, and diagnostic decision making and treatment selection tend to be physician roles.[71] A myriad of supporting clinicians and nonclinicians are vital in medical teams. The nurse, nurse practitioner, medical student, physicians, and others must be able to detect problem states or deviations from the "expected course" and activate control measures. When a practitioner fails to work within his or her competencies or is on the learning curve for his or her role on the team, failure to get or provide supervision comes into play. For wrong-site surgery errors, this issue manifests when one surgeon does the preoperative consultation and operative planning and the other starts the surgery with incomplete knowledge. For example, a resident or fellow may fail to call an attending physician to seek clarification of the operative plan.

Team Structure and Leadership (Teams That Do Not Have Structure, Role Delineation, and Clarity, and Methods for Flattening Hierarchy While Resolving Conflict Will Have Suboptimal Team Performance)

Teams will inevitably have to face ambiguous situations that need immediate action. Authority gradients prevent junior members of the team from questioning the decision making and action planning of the leader (a nurse might be hesitant to tell a senior surgeon that he or she is violating a safety procedure, and/or the surgeon might disregard the nurse).[70] Methods for flattening hierarchy will lead to more robust team situational awareness and support cross-checking behavior. In contrast, it is essential to have efficient ways of resolving conflict, especially under emergency conditions. Some surgeons view the Universal Protocol as a ridiculous requirement forced upon them by regulatory bodies responding to liability pressure. This can create a void in leadership regarding team behaviors that would otherwise help to trap errors that predispose to wrong-site surgery.

Working Conditions Associated with Wrong-Site Surgery

Individuals and teams cannot perform optimally when they have inadequate resources to manage the work at hand. Typically, workers have little control over the conditions in which they are required to work. Managers make decisions that ultimately aid or constrain practitioners in terms of ratios of patients per provider, the physical space available, and the tools and/or technology available to front-line workers.

Staffing Levels, Skills Mix, and Workload (Managers Facing Financial Pressures, a Nursing Shortage, and Increasing Patient Acuity Can Choose to Institute Hiring Freezes and Reduce Staffing Ratios to Decrease the Costs Associated with Care)

While institutions and providers that have high surgical case volumes have been noted to have the best surgical outcomes, medical mishaps occur even in these institutions. Providing exceptional care to a few patients is easier than providing reliable care to everyone.[72] Indeed, excessive production pressure and patient volumes are associated with safety violations due to cutting corners when productivity goals are unrealistic. Over two thirds of wrong-site surgeries occurred in ambulatory surgery settings in which patient acuity is the lowest but productivity pressures are high.[73] Financial constraints have forced more ORs to be staffed by temporary traveling position nurses, have resulted in nursing orientations that have been reduced, and have increased production pressure on surgeons to increase their utilization of OR time. Unfortunately, such aggressive measures to utilize all the capacity of the OR resources conflicts with the need for some reserve capacity to manage the inherent uncertainty and variability associated with medical disease and surgical care. As a result, emergency situations can easily overwhelm care systems that lack reserve resources. Providers calling in sick during flu season and/or a flurry of surgical emergencies can create dangerous conditions for elective surgery due to the need to redirect those resources that might otherwise be available.

Availability and Maintenance of Equipment (Technology and Tools Vary in their Safety Features and Usability: Equipment Must Be Maintained or It Can Become a Liability)

For preventing wrong-site surgery, we have found that the specific marking pen we are utilizing needs to be stocked and available throughout the hospital to allow surgeons to perform the safety practices we have required. Surgeons unable to find a green marker will use alternative pens, resulting in a variation in practice that degrades the value of the safety measure. Other aspects of our wrong-site surgery safeguards have proved difficult to maintain. A computerized scheduling system had triggers to cue the operative team as to the marking protocol and special equipment needs. When a new procedure was added to the scheduling system, the programmers overlooked the "needs to be marked" trigger, and for a period of time these patients were not marked. The operative team had been using technology designed to support their work, but that technology was not maintained. The best team of practitioners can perform even better when provided state-of-the-art working conditions. For example, patient identification technology that utilizes bar coding and radiofrequency identification tags will virtually eliminate wrong patient errors.[74] Although this technology is currently available, few organizations have been able to afford this technology to prevent wrong-site errors due to patient misidentification.

Administrative and Managerial Support (In Complex Work Settings, Domain Experts That Perform the Work Need to Be Supported by Personnel Who Are Charged with Managing Resources, Scheduling, Transcription, Billing, etc.)

Clinical information systems (e.g., an OR scheduling system) are not reliable or robust at confirming operative intent early in the process or planning for surgery.[51] Busy surgical clinics often do not have efficient and reliable mechanisms for providing a scheduling secretary with the information they need or for verifying that booking information is accurate. Secretaries may be using a form that is illegible or may simply be working from a verbal description of the planned surgery. Because these support personnel may not understand the terminology, errors are common. In addition, busy surgeons may forget that other information,

such as the operative position required, the need for surgical implants, or the requirement for special equipment, is not obvious, and thus fail to be explicit. In addition, this work and the expertise required are often undervalued. The result can be to hire inexperienced secretaries and accept high support staff turnover.

ORGANIZATIONAL FACTORS ASSOCIATED WITH WRONG-SITE SURGERY

Organizations must make safety a priority. If production pressure and economic goals are in conflict with safety, organizations must have structure and methods for ensuring safety as the priority.[75] Independent offices of patient safety and patient safety officers with the authority to stop operations when necessary are examples of organizational structures designed to maintain safety in the face of economic pressure.

Financial Resources (Safety Is Not Free: The Costs Associated with Establishing Safe Practices and Acquiring Safety Technology May Be Prohibitive)

Many organizations have implemented the Universal Protocol, but have done so in an incomplete manner, performing the minimum to pass a regulatory review. Given the rarity of wrong-site surgery, the cost of preventing each instance would appear significant (although good safety habits or practice can or should be generalizable). The financial impact of correcting computer system flaws, improving secretarial support, and slowing down throughput to perform safety checks is unknown. Costs are a significant barrier to implementing safeguards robustly.

Goals and Policy Standards (Practice of Front-Line Workers Is Shaped by Clear Goals and Consistent Policies That Are Clinically Relevant)

Policies and procedures regarding prevention of wrong-site surgery are difficult to develop. Legal liability tends to constrain medical policymakers to be purposely vague. Explicit procedures that are standardized would be helpful. Unfortunately, newly developed procedures may be recommended as policy prior to proper testing and validation for effectiveness. For example, the Universal Protocol has not been fully validated and yet this protocol has been mandated.

Safety Culture and Priorities (A Safety Culture of an Organization May Be Pathologic, Reactive, Proactive, or Generative)

Most hospitals today are reactive in their culture of safety.[27] The result is that those institutions that have had the most public wrong-site surgeries have done the most to establish safety countermeasures to prevent future wrong-site surgery. Proactive action to invest in creating safeguards was beyond the capability or commitment of most healthcare organizations as of 2005.

SOCIOPOLITICAL FACTORS ASSOCIATED WITH WRONG-SITE SURGERY
Economic, Regulatory Issues, Health Policy, and Politics

We practice medicine within large national healthcare systems. Currently, third-party payers wish for safety to be a priority. However, organizations that invest in safety

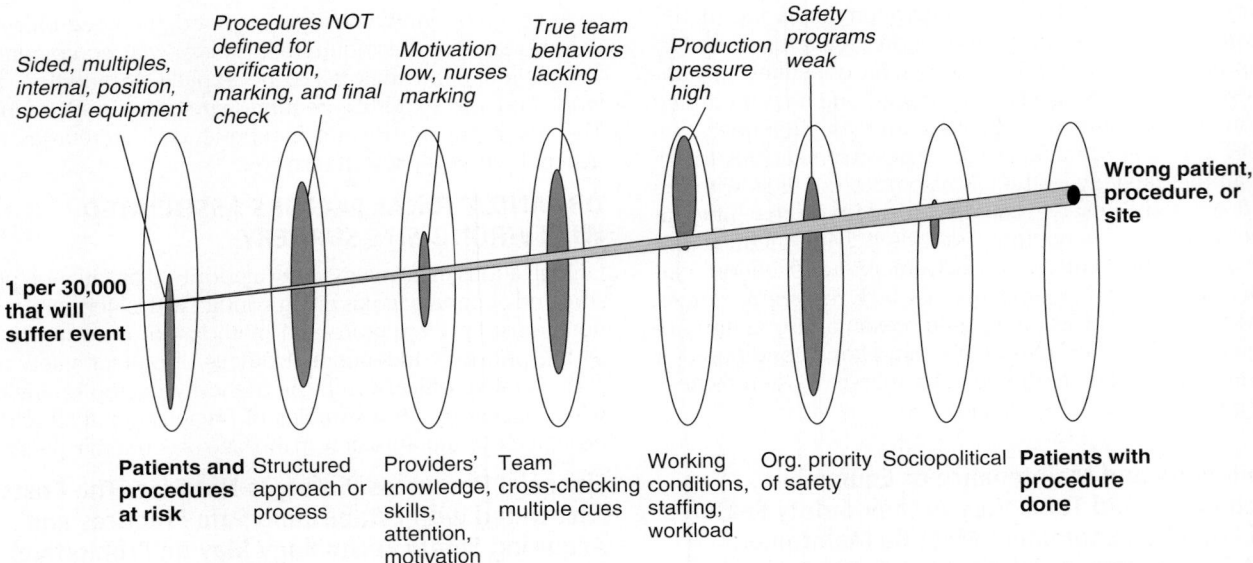

FIGURE 1-4 This graphic summarizes the major vulnerabilities identified as contributory toward wrong-site surgical error.

technologies to avert error do not typically get a return on that investment. In fact, hospital investment to prevent iatrogenic injury directly benefits third-party payers, not the hospital. Similarly, our legal system does not serve as a strong incentive for safety because jury verdicts do not accurately identify and punish negligent care. Rather, patients with negative outcomes that were not preventable still win jury verdicts, while patients that truly suffered a preventable adverse event commonly fail to seek legally allowed compensation.[76]

SUMMARY OF CONTRIBUTORY FACTOR ANALYSIS

This example of wrong-site surgery was used to illustrate the multiple contributory factors that allow error to propagate and evolve into an injury-causing accident. Even with an error as blatant as wrong brain surgery, one can identify multiple vulnerabilities in the multiple layers of our complex medical care systems (Fig. 1-4). While hindsight bias tempts one to blame the individuals involved as the sole causative factor, it is clear that the individuals are part of a complex system with multiple latent conditions (hazards and "accidents waiting to happen"). High-reliability organizations are notable for their dedication to systematically identify all hazards and then counter each one. These organizations understand that failure is multidimensional and so is maximizing safety.

Perspective

The plethora of factors associated with breaches in patient safety underline the complexity of this phenomenon and the protean solutions required to address it. This need is now more imperative than ever, especially in the face of the adoption by the Centers for Medicare and Medicaid Services (CMS) of a nonreimbursement policy for certain "never events."[77] This initiative has been powered by the trend to motivate hospitals to improve patient safety by implementing standardized protocols. These newly defined "never events" limit the ability of the hospitals to bill Medicare for

adverse events and complications. The nonreimbursable conditions apply only to those events deemed "reasonably preventable" through the use of evidence-based guidelines. The need to address this problem effectively and to verify the solution through double-blind, placebo-controlled randomized trials is therefore imperative.

Summary

Reducing iatrogenic injury has become a priority in health care. The scientific disciplines that have advanced safety in other high-hazard industries such as aviation and nuclear power are just beginning to be used to help advance safety in health care. The causes of iatrogenic injury are complex, as are robust solutions. Success in other industries has been achieved through the use of a global strategy based on small incremental changes to identify threats and then systematically counter each one. Aviation started using this approach over 40 years ago. This strategy appears viable in health care but requires a long-term commitment. In addition, the battle to improve reliability and safety will be ongoing. Eliminating one set of vulnerabilities always reveals new ones that did not previously exist. Thus, the goal is to trade in the old problems for new ones that are more bearable. The future is hopeful as new safety sciences support medicine's quest to "first do no harm."

KEY REFERENCES

Bernstein M, Hebert PC, Etchells E. Patient safety in neurosurgery: detection of errors, prevention of errors, and disclosure of errors. *Neurosurg Q.* 2003;13(2):125-137.

Blike G, Biddle C. Preanesthesia detection of equipment faults by anesthesia providers at an academic hospital: comparison of standard practice and a new electronic checklist. *AANA J.* 2000;68:497-505.

Brennan TA, Leape LL, Laird NM, et al. Incidence of adverse events and negligence in hospitalized patients—results of the Harvard Medical Practice Study I. *N Engl J Med.* 1991;324(6):370-376.

Cook RI, Woods DD, Miller C. A tale of two stories: contrasting views of patient safety. Chicago: National Patient Safety Foundation; 1998. Available at http://www.npsf.org/exec/front.html.

de Vries EN, Hollmann MW, Smorenburg SM, et al. Development and validation of the SURgical PAtient Safety System (SURPASS) checklist. *Qual Saf Health Care.* 2009;18(2):121-126.

Gawande AA, Thomas EJ, Zinner MJ. The incidence and nature of surgical adverse events in Colorado and Utah in 1992. *Surgery.* 1999;126(1):66-75.

Helmreich RL, Foushee HC. Why crew resource management? The history and status of human factors training programs in aviation. In: Wiener E, Kanki Helmreich R, eds. *Cockpit Resource Management.* New York: Academic Press; 1993.

Jhawar BS, Mitsis D, Duggal N. Wrong-sided and wrong-level neurosurgery: a national survey. *J Neurosurg Spine.* 2007;7(5):467-472.

Joint Commission on Accreditation of Healthcare Organizations. Lessons learned: wrong site surgery, sentinel event, No. 6. 2001. Available at http://www.jcaho.org/edu_ pub/sealert/sea6.html.

Joint Commission on Accreditation of Healthcare Organizations. *Joint Commission on the Accreditation of Healthcare Organizations.* Oakbrook, IL: Sentinel Event Alert; 2003.

Joint Commission on Accreditation of Healthcare Organizations. Sentinel Event Alert: Follow-up Review of Wrong Site Surgery. No. 24, 2001.

Joint Commission on Accreditation of Healthcare Organizations. Sentinel Event Statistics. 2003. Available at: http://www.jcaho.org/accredited+organizations/hospitals/sentinel+events/sentinel+events+ statistics.htm.

Joint Commission on Accreditation of Healthcare Organizations. *Joint Commission on the Accreditation of Healthcare Organizations.* Oakbrook, IL: Universal Protocol Toolkit; 2004.

Kohn LT, Corrigan JM, Donaldson MS, eds. *To Err Is Human: Building a Safer Health System.* Washington, DC: National Academy Press; 2000.

Leape LL, Berwick DM, Bates DW. What practices will most improve safety? *JAMA.* 2002;288:501-507.

Leape LL, Rennan Ta, Laird N, et al. The nature of adverse events in hospitalized patients. Results of the Harvard Medical Practice Study II. *N Engl J Med.* 1991;324:377-384.

Lembitz A, Clarke TJ. Clarifying "never events" and introducing "always events." *Patient Saf Surg.* 2009;3(1):26.

Makary MA, Mukherjee A, Sexton JB, et al. Operating room briefings and wrong-site surgery. *J Am Coll Surg.* 2007;204(2):236-243.

National Patient Safety Foundation. The NPSF is an independent, nonprofit research and education organization. Available at http://www.npsf. org/html/research/rfp.html.

Sax HC, Browne P, Mayewski RJ, et al. Can aviation-based team training elicit sustainable behavioral change? *Arch Surg.* 2009;144(12):1133-1137.

Smith CM. Origin and uses of primum non nocere—above all, do no harm! *J Clin Pharmacol.* 2005;45:371-377.

Vincent N, et al. Patient safety: Understanding and responding to adverse events. *N Engl J Med.* 2003;348(11):1051-1056.

Wilson I, Walker I. The WHO Surgical Safety Checklist: the evidence. *J Perioper Pract.* 2009;19(10):362-364.

Wong DA. The Universal Protocol: A one-year update. AAOS Bulletin. *American Academy of Orthopedic Surgeons.* 2005;53:20.

Wong DA, Watters 3rd WC. To err is human: quality and safety issues in spine care. *Spine (Phila Pa 1976).* 2007;32(suppl 11):S2-S8.

Numbered references appear on Expert Consult.

CHAPTER 2

Surgical Navigation with Intraoperative Imaging: Special Operating Room Concepts

ARYA NABAVI • ANDREAS M. STARK • LUTZ DÖRNER • H. MAXIMILIAN MEHDORN

One of the most challenging technological innovations in neurosurgery encompasses the interdisciplinary effort to integrate microneurosurgery and imaging. Neurosurgical techniques have reached a high level of sophistication. Increasing understanding of neurophysiology as well as neuropathology, precise preoperative imaging, small tailored approaches, and specialized instruments, as well as detailed monitoring techniques have led to improved results, and generated higher standards for safety and outcome.

However, the means to confirm the surgeon's intraoperative evaluation, whether or not the desired surgical objective was achieved, were limited. Postoperative imaging for neurooncologic, neurovascular, and instrumented spine surgery supported the ambition to obtain intraoperative quality insurance.

For high-grade gliomas, in 1994 Albert reported that post-operative imaging showed tumor remnants in 77% of patients who were presumed to have undergone gross total resection.[1] In 2006,[2] Stummer et al. published a multicenter randomized study, which, as a byproduct, showed residual tumors in 64% of the patients undergoing conventional microsurgical tumor resection (only patients with high-grade gliomas were included, which was deemed—by imaging criteria—to be fully resectable). With the importance of the extent of resection for high-[1,2] as well as low-grade gliomas,[3,4] these findings emphasize the need for improvement.

In neurovascular surgery the routine use of intraoperative angiography has been advocated to avoid undetected residual disease.[5,6] In spinal surgery, the significant percentage of misplaced screws could be reduced from 10%, but still occurs with approximately 5%, even with modern navigation techniques.[7] These findings underscored the desire to complement advanced preoperative evaluation with intraoperative quality control. Thus various surgical groups proceeded to integrate imaging into their procedures.

The earliest attempts were made with ultrasound (US) and computed tomography (CT). The immediate impact on surgical procedures was small, due to limited resolution (US and CT) and cumbersome integration into the operating room (CT). Another avenue opened with the introduction of image-guided neuronavigation (IGN) systems.[8,9] These systems allowed the transfer of increasingly refined presurgical image information into the operating theater to guide surgical procedures. However, intraoperative changes ("brain shift") critically limited their application

accuracy.[10,11] The concept of intraoperative imaging resurfaced. With magnetic resonance imaging (MRI) becoming the method of choice for the imaging of the central nervous system, pioneering efforts to introduce this modality into surgery provided proof of the concept.[12-14] These initial experiences with intraoperative MRI (iMRI)[15-17] ignited diversification into a variety of approaches.

The integration of surgery and imaging technology, especially MRI, demands consideration of safety, as well as procedural and architectural issues. In this chapter, we focus on those imaging technologies that have resulted in modified operating room (OR) designs and changes in the surgical workflow.

Computer-Assisted, Image-Guided Neuronavigation

The major link between imaging and integration of this information into surgery is provided by navigation systems. Diagnostic computer-based image-analysis and three-dimensional (3D) modeling facilitated the spatial definition of complex pathologic processes. The desire to use this information directly in the surgical field led to the introduction of IGN systems in the mid-1980s[8,9] and their commercial availability in the early 1990s. These systems provided the surgeon with a tool that allowed the transfer of presurgical image information in an intuitive and interactive fashion into the surgical field (see Chapter 3 for more detail on neuronavigation).

By combining a computer with a detection system (at present, generally light-emitting diodes [LEDs]), the location of a pointer tip (or likewise registered tool) within the surgical field can be viewed on a computer display. This is achieved by registering "physical" (the surgical field) with "image" (the preoperative images within the computer) space. The surgeon uses the pointer like a 3D mouse to scroll through the images. Pointing at specific areas within the surgical field, the correlating location in the preoperative images is displayed on the computer screen in its anatomic context. Generally this method is an asset in planning approaches and verifying various internal landmarks.

Meanwhile, the technology has proceeded from being a novelty to an established asset for neurosurgical procedures. Questions of prior consideration, that is, application accuracy and integration of instruments, were overcome. However, the major shortcoming was the dependence on preoperative image data. Since intraoperative changes (e.g., CSF drainage, tumor resection, sagging of the cortex, swelling of underlying tissue, summarized as "brain shift"), accumulate throughout surgery, preoperative data become invalidated.[10,11,18] This has particular influence on glioma surgery. While enabling precise approach planning and localization, resection control is generally beyond the capacity of these systems, since they cannot account for intraoperative changes. Intraoperative imaging resolved this issue directly. It enables continued use of these systems with newly acquired accurate data.

A different avenue investigates mathematical models to compensate for brain shift. Various algorithms can characterize and calculate deformation matrixes.[10,11,19] Various brain shift patterns were identified. A multimodal approach appears potentially useful, which uses intraoperative "sparse" US data[20-22] to calculate a deformation matrix, which is then used to elastically deform preoperative MRI images. Albeit all these efforts advances were meager and the only option to provide precise updated navigation remains the integration of intraoperative images.

Intraoperative Imaging

We provide an overview and comprehensive organizational framework for imaging modalities that influence surgical work flow and OR-suite design. While this relates to CT and primarily MRI, recent multimodal imaging implemented in OR suites includes US and fluoroscopy, and these will be addressed as well.

INTRAOPERATIVE FLUOROSCOPY

Operating theaters for stereotactic neurosurgery had built-in biplane x-ray to eliminate parallax artifacts in imaging of electrode placement. With the limited scope of this application, these ORs remained rare and have largely been replaced by standard fluoroscopy, or more recently intraoperative MRI.[23,24]

In instrumented spinal surgery, fluoroscopy is used as an online imaging modality for planning and verifying screw positioning. Combinations with navigation systems have been propagated. Intraoperative angiography has been employed by major vascular centers for quality insurance in aneurysm and AVM surgery.[5,6]

For both angiography and spinal instrumentation, a major shortcoming was the planar imaging, providing indirect spatial information. While the integration of IGN added this dimension, reservations about accuracy led to reevaluation of CT for spinal instrumentation. A more recent development allowing 3D rotation fluoroscopy may result in an easier way to obtain spatial information. Initial questions as to the spatial accuracy of these systems have been addressed in more recent generations. Recently hybrid angiography ORs combining neurointervention and neurosurgery for neurovascular cases have been introduced.

INTRAOPERATIVE ULTRASOUND

Intraoperative US (IoUS) was one of the first to be employed as an intraoperative imaging modality in neurosurgery.[25] With subsequent new generations, image quality improved

and miniaturization of the hand-pieces enhanced applicability. Advantages are the dynamic, surgeon-driven, on-line character of the information.[26] Particularly in vascular surgery, the flow-related analysis of duplex sonography provides additional flexibility. Further major developments were the introduction of spatially accurate 3D ultrasound,[27] of contrast agents[28] and the integration of US into navigation systems.[26,29-31] In particular, the last aspect provided the means for easier interpretation of the images, which generally demands experience.

For the last 20 years, IoUS has been regarded as the most promising system for online information acquisition in neurosurgery. Still, these systems remain limited in their distribution. Potential reasons may be the unfamiliarity with the technique of ultrasound and its limitations in tissue differentiation,[32] differing from the most widely distributed primary diagnostic modality of MRI.[33]

Major indications are circumscribed lesions, such as metastasis, cavernomas, vascular pathologies, and for spinal intradural lesions. With its integration into conventional navigation systems and in combination with iMRI[34] the unfamiliarity with this modality might potentially be overcome.

INTRAOPERATIVE COMPUTED TOMOGRAPHY

Shalit and Lunsford first reported the integration of a stationary CT into OR.[35,36] The next generation of CTs was mobile, permitting shared application in the OR and the ICU. However, image quality and radiation exposure limited the application and further implementation of this modality. Further advances in CT- and OR-table technology and integration with navigation systems have led to a reappraisal.

Modern CT-OR (Fig. 2-1) solutions use a rail system to move the CT between a parking position and the patient for scanning,[37] which provides full access to the patient. In spine surgery, intraoperatively acquired images can be used to update navigation systems to provide additional image guidance for screw placement, as well as verification of correct positioning. For neurovascular surgery, intraoperative

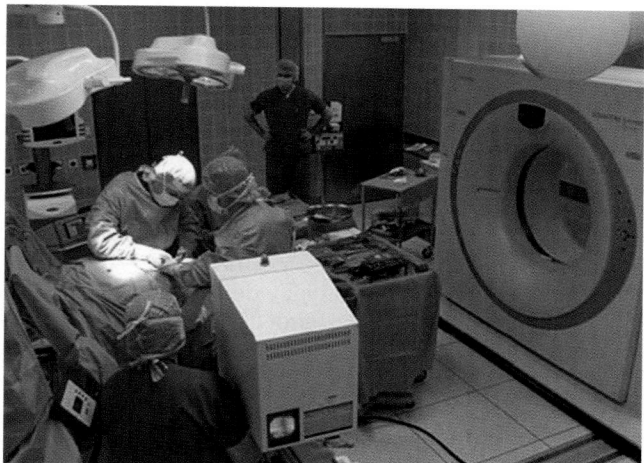

FIGURE 2-1 Overview of iCT unit. The CT is moved along the patient axis on a rail system. Navigation system in the left corner of the image is mobile. *(From Uhl E, Zausinger S, Morhard D, Heigl T, Scheder B, Rachinger W, Schichor C, Tonn JC. Intraoperative computed tomography with integrated navigation system in a multidisciplinary operating suite. Neurosurgery. 2009;64:231-239, Fig. 1D.)*

CT-angiography has the potential to provide information on obtained occlusion of vascular pathologies, but also with perfusion CT on potential vascular compromise.

For the definition of brain tumors—particularly low-grade lesions, but also high-grade gliomas—the intraoperative imaging quality remains less informative. Gross total surgical resection may be documented, but the sensitivity to detect residual tumor, even with the present CT generation, remains inferior to MRI. Furthermore, cumulative radiation exposure limits the number of potential intraoperative scans.

INTRAOPERATIVE MAGNETIC RESONANCE IMAGING

MRI is the diagnostic standard for lesions of the central nervous system. Its imaging capability extends beyond pure anatomic resolution into function (fMRI) and connectivity (DTI), as well as pathophysiologic conditions (spectroscopy, perfusion).

Postoperative MRI remains the gold-standard for defining the extent of resection in neurooncology[1,2] and pituitary lesions.[38]

The desire to employ the potential of MRI to monitor open neurosurgical procedures, as means to quality insurance, resection control, and complication detection led to the combination of MRI and surgery.[13] Presently intraoperative MRI is used primarily for gliomas and pituitary lesions,[38-40] but also for vascular[41] and epilepsy surgery.[42]

In the mid-1990s, two major approaches spearheaded the implementation of intraoperative MRI for neurosurgical procedures and forecast the future direction of this emerging specialty.

The "twin operating theater"[14,16] combined surgery and imaging (low-field, open 0.2 T MR system with a horizontal opening) by using two adjacent rooms. The patient was transferred between surgical and imaging site. Thus conventional OR equipment could be used without MR-safety or compatibility issues. To minimize the time for the transfer, this approach was modified by operating in the vicinity of the MRI, the "fringe field."[43,44]

The open magnet design ("double doughnut")[12,13,17] aimed at a full integration of surgery and MRI. The vertical opening provided the surgeon with access to the patient. Surgical and imaging site were merged, a transfer was unnecessary. For practical reasons, surgery was discontinued during scanning. However, this design held the potential to provide real-time imaging, such as in biopsies, or through "continuous imaging" protocols.[45] Furthermore, a navigation system was an integral part of the MRI. With a localizer, the surgeon controlled the scanning plane of the MRI interactively.[46,47] Specially developed software for intraoperative navigation extended the functionality.[48,49] This solution is closest to the symbiosis of surgery and imaging. However, by operating in a magnetic field, constraints in regards to technical equipment, in particular the microscope, the 56-cm gap for the surgeon, and the need for nonferromagnetic instruments, microneurosurgical standards were difficult to uphold.

These pioneering clinical experiences proved that the vision[50] to bring MRI into the surgical surrounding could be realized. Biopsies as well as interstitial therapies could be blended with MRI into a novel procedure. However, it became evident, that the synthesis of open surgery and MRI into a comprehensive new method proved too complex. Either imaging potential, in comparison to preoperative high-field diagnostic scans, patient access or both, were restricted.

While various systems of low- and mid-field range persist, the limitations of the prototypes, in regards to field strength and thus image quality as well as patient access, have led development in different directions. Installations with various MR designs and a wide, increasing range of field strength (0.15–3.0 Tesla) are currently in use.

With emphasis on accessibility, a minimized, compact open MRI (0.12 T, 0.15 T) was introduced, which fit beneath the surgical table.[51,52] To integrate high-field (1.5 T and higher) imaging, while providing ample patient access and only minimal influence on microneurosurgical instruments and techniques, surgical and imaging sites were separated. This can be achieved within an integrated OR-MR design ("dedicated"),[15,40,53] or by arranging MR and OR into separate adjacent modules/rooms[41,54-56] ("shared resources").

A comprehensive classification, which encompasses present arrangements and accommodates potential future developments and expansions, cannot be based on variable characteristics such as field-strength and MR-design. Since the original concept was to merge surgery and imaging, it is reasonable to use work flow to distinguish among different installations. Specific issues for the integration of MRI into the surgical surrounding such as MR safety and compatibility of equipment, field strength, shielding, MR design,[47,57,58] and imaging characteristics will be outlined before discussing various MR-OR integrations.

MR Safety, Compatibility, and Shielding

The introduction of a magnet into a surgical surrounding raises safety issues pertaining to interaction of the magnetic field and OR equipment.[47,58-61] The magnet can exert a pull on ferromagnetic instruments. Generally the strength of the pull is related to field strength (and MR shielding) and distance to the MRI. The so-called 5-gauss line demarcates the inner area, in which the pull increases and the outer zone, in which ferromagnetic instruments can be safely used without being drawn into the MRI. In most MR-ORs, this demarcation is indicated on the floor. The immediate area around the 5-gauss line, which is within the magnetic field but still has no significant pull, is called the "fringe" field.

Instruments and equipment that are nonferromagnetic, and can be used in either area without being drawn into the MR, are called MR-safe. However, contrary to MR-compatible equipment, they cause image artifacts when left in the imaging field during scanning, or as with electrical equipment, cause interference with the imaging. Thus, equipment that is neither magnetic nor interferes with the imaging is called MR-compatible.

Shielding is necessary to prevent the interaction of the magnet with radio-frequency (RF) technology. Normally the entire room is shielded to prevent the magnet's influence on electrical devices and vice versa. Alternatively, a specific shielding can be laced around the patient for scanning. While all nonessential electrical equipment can be turned off during scanning, or is primarily based outside the shielded room (e.g., the computer for image guided navigation), special anesthesia equipment is used to prevent RF noise (artifacts) in the images.

MR Design ("Open-Bore" and "Closed-Bore" Systems) and Field Strength

The static magnetic field of the MRI is generated within its bore. In open-bore (i.e., open-magnet) systems, the magnet is divided into two poles. The gap can be horizontal or vertical ("double doughnut"),[59] resulting in different access to the patient.

In diagnostic high-field scanners, the bore is a closed tunnel. With improved MR design, so-called "short-bore" systems, with shorter tunnel length, became available, providing some access to the patient. Thus smaller operations like biopsies or deep brain stimulation (DBS) electrode placement can be performed within the bore ("in-bore" procedures).

Generally the open-magnet design has lower field strength than the "short-bore" closed systems. Higher field strength generally promotes acquisition speed (temporal resolution) as well as quality of the subsequently acquired images (spatial resolution). A wider range of image sequences is available (e.g., spectroscopy, DTI, fMRI, dynamic scanning).[15,62,63] Furthermore, the homogeneity of the magnetic field increases, reducing geometric distortions. This issue is of major importance in low- and mid-field scanners. Phantom studies performed on the compact 0.12 T system provided acceptable application accuracy.[52] However, studies in a stronger magnetic field (mid-field 0.5 T, open MR system) have shown that significant geometric distortions are present,[64] which are machine- and patient-induced. These findings have to be considered when using non–high-field MR units (below 1 T) for resection control and updated neuronavigation.

Imaging

Which imaging to choose depends on the lesion's imaging characteristics in diagnostic studies. Enhanced and non-enhanced T1WI, T2, and occasionally FLAIR answer most questions.[39,40,53,54,62,65] For low-grade lesions, T2 and FLAIR images are the most appropriate.[40,53,54] For enhancement, pre- and post-contrast T1 images are acquired.

Further sequences may potentially yield additional information,[53] such as location of functional centers or fiber tracts. Both features can be extracted from intraoperative MRI, especially the latter.[66]

The intraoperative MRI is essentially a surgical tool. It is implemented to support surgical decision making. Thus the surgeon has to define his or her intention and the subsequent question, which primarily relates to the achieved extent of resection (residual tumor and its localization) and complication avoidance (distance to critical structures). It is essential that the surgeon acquires a good working knowledge of MRI to compile the individual imaging protocol and analyze the images according to surgical objectives.[40,41,53,62]

Practical challenges in interpreting intraoperative images largely pertain to nonspecific contrast enhancement ("spread enhancement"). The surgical result is described by "removed percent of contrast-enhancing lesion." Since contrast enhancement merely reflects the local breakdown of the blood–brain barrier, it is unsurprising that contrast spreads into surrounding regions over time. While almost inconsequential in diagnostic imaging, acknowledging this phenomenon is of major importance for intraoperative MRI (iMRI) to avoid over-resection. Thus scans for the initial neuronavigation-assisted resection should be acquired prior to surgery. When imaging is for resection control, pre- and post-contrast T1 images and subtraction are compared to identify residual contrast enhancement. New sequences capturing the dynamic nature of neovascularized areas, in particular dynamic susceptibility contrast-weighted perfusion MRI (DSC-MRI), provide more accurate intraoperative information than conventional contrast-enhanced T1WI.[67] Future development of specific contrast media may lead to a resolution of this problem.[68,69]

Integration of Intraoperative Navigation and MRI

The shortcomings of image-guided navigation in detecting intraoperative changes were a major motivation to implement intraoperative imaging. Since surgery and imaging take place in different coordinate systems, the transfer of the images between these venues represents the crucial integrating step. IGN provides this essential link.[40,70,71]

In most MRI-installations, navigation systems are ceiling mounted. Initial navigation is performed with preoperative images until the surgeon deems an update necessary to regain accurate navigation. The intraoperative images are sent directly from the scanner console to the navigation system. The images are fused (automated image fusion algorithm) to the already registered preoperative images and shown on the display (Fig. 2-2). With the DRF reattached in its original position, the images can be used for updated navigation without additional re-referencing. Thus intraoperative updates for neuronavigation can be acquired at the surgeon's discretion, and used for updated navigation.

OR-MR INTEGRATIONS

The horizontal systems were mostly adjacent to a conventional OR.[14,16] The patient was moved from the surgical site to the imaging site. An improved workflow left the patient within the fringe field to shorten the transfer.[43,44]

The vertical units (i.e., "double doughnut") had the advantage, that patient transport was not necessary because imaging and surgical sites were the same. The vertical orientation of the gap between the poles gave, however confined, acceptable access to the positioned patient. This facilitated the workflow but posed high demands on the equipment and surgical workflow.[17,47,50]

The basic concept of these original designs persists in current solutions. In the shared-resource and more elaborate multimodal imaging OR concepts, surgical site and imager are separated into adjacent rooms. In "dedicated, integrated MR-OR" environments, surgical and imaging sites are separated but in the same specially planned room.

The pivotal links are the physical arrangement between surgical and imaging sites (patient or MR transport) and the information transfer (updated imaging for neuronavigation).

Shared Resources and Multimodal Imaging OR Concepts

The separated room concept for surgical and imaging sites was developed to allow the unimpeded usage of surgical tools as well as perfect imaging. An additional economic aspect was that while surgery was progressing, the idle MRI could be used for routine imaging—hence, the notion

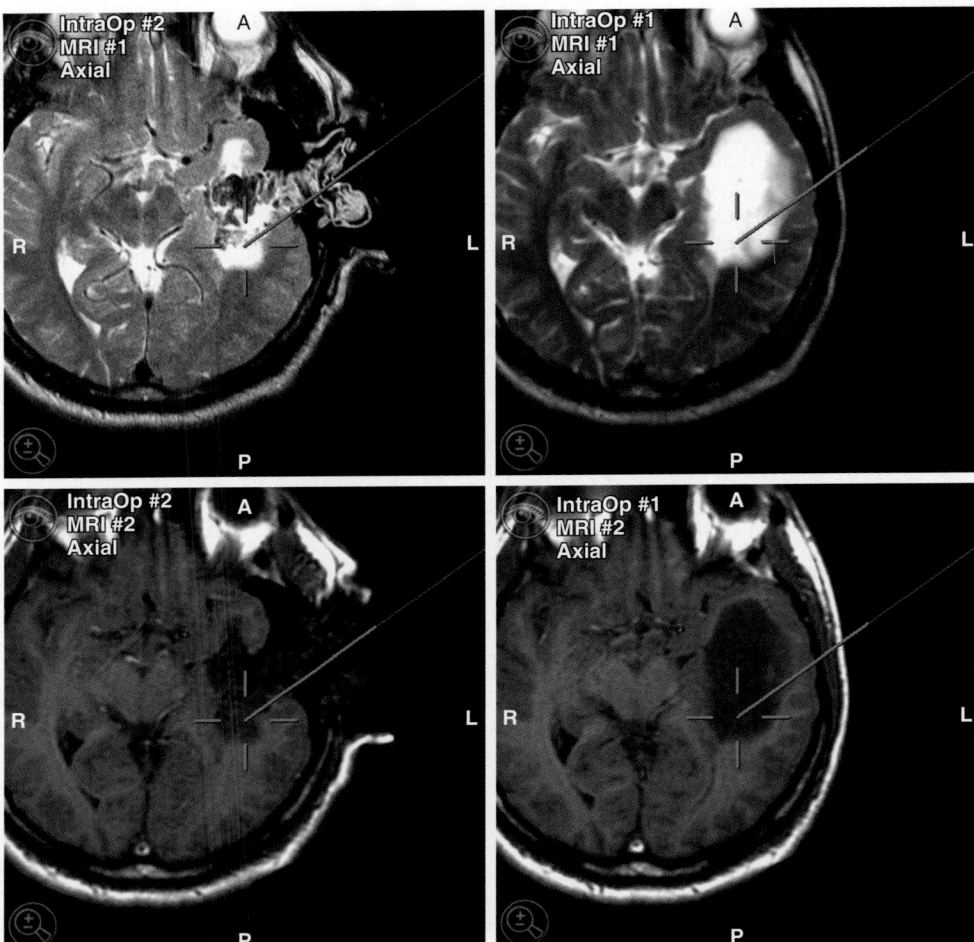

FIGURE 2-2 Updated navigation with intraoperative images (screen shot of navigation system display). Images were acquired after tumor (anaplastic astrocytoma) bulk resection for localization of residual tumor. T2 and T1WI intra- and preoperative for comparison.

of shared resources. However, this demanded special arrangements for connecting surgical and imaging sites. Potentially, the patient can be brought to the MRI or the MRI to the patient.

The first mobile MRI (Fig. 2-3) was developed and installed in Calgary.[41] The 1.5-T unit is mounted on a ceiling rail system, which permits transporting the MRI into the surgical area (overhead crane technology). The specially designed operating table is MR-compatible, as patient positioning can be adjusted hydraulically. Furthermore, the RF coils are integrated into the surgical table. The upper detachable portion can be repositioned for imaging. The MRI usually resides in a separate room. On its way in and during scanning, ferromagnetic instruments have to be removed from its path and beyond the 5-gauss line. If not needed during the procedure, the magnet can be potentially used as a shared resource for conventional scanning, or serve adjacent ORs connected by a common rail system.

Stationary MRIs in separated rooms are presently 3-T MRI units, where the higher field necessitates more elaborate shielding (Fig. 2-4). The 5-gauss line extends farther away from the MRI, raising demands on MR-safe and compatible equipment and instruments. This and the fact that 3-T systems are not yet widely used led to implementation as separated rooms, permitting shared imaging resources between surgery and radiology.[54,56]

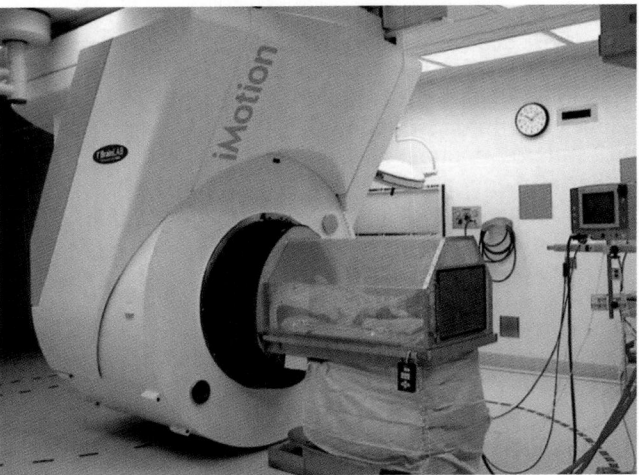

FIGURE 2-3 Ceiling-mounted, mobile MRI (1.5 T) in Calgary. Overhead crane technology permits the transfer of the MRI to the surgical site. *(From Kaibara T, Saunders JK, Sutherland GR. Advances in mobile intraoperative magnetic resonance imaging. Neurosurgery. 2000;47:131-138, Fig. 4.)*

The surgical site is a conventional operating theater. The patient is positioned on a surgical OR table with a floating top, which can be connected to the MR system. Either a rail system[56] or a wheeled transfer table[54] is used. The headholder can be either separated from flexible surface coils,[56]

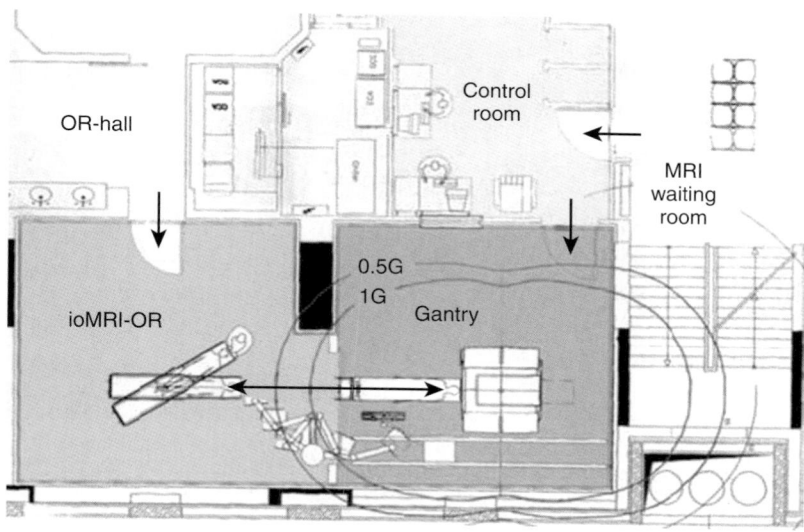

FIGURE 2-4 Example of shared-resources layout. *(From Pamir MN, Ozduman K, Dincer A, Yildiz E, Peker S, Ozek MM. First intraoperative, shared-resource, ultra-high-field 3-Tesla magnetic resonance imaging system and its application in low-grade glioma resection. J Neurosurg. 2010;112:57-69, Fig. 1.)*

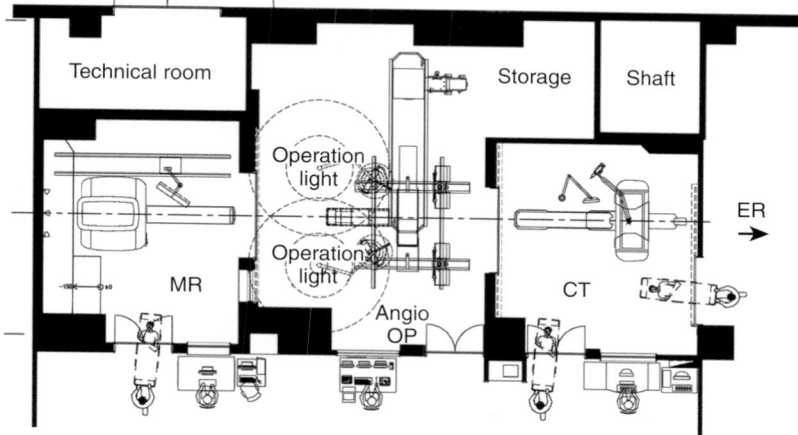

FIGURE 2-5 Multimodality imaging OR layout for the modular expansion of shared-resources twin-OR. Due to the modular design, various modalities can be used. *(From Matsumae M, Koizumi J, Fukuyama H, et al. World's first magnetic resonance imaging/x-ray/operating room suite: A significant milestone in the improvement of neurosurgical diagnosis and treatment. J Neurosurg. 2007;107:266-273, Fig. 1.)*

or integrated into the rigid imaging coils.[54] In the latter case, a removable sterile top portion is disconnected for surgery and replaced for scanning.

The rooms have additional entrances to provide access to the MR while surgery progresses in the adjacent room. Thus during the surgical time, routine diagnostics can be performed. Costs and function can be shared between neurosurgery and radiology. While the economic aspect is appealing, the concept of obtaining image-information on demand for surgical decision making is impeded. If the MR is occupied, the surgical patient has to wait. Presently the transfer distance, as well as the preparations to provide safety, represents an additional delay.[56] It becomes cumbersome, and thus less likely, that repeated intraoperative scans are obtained.

The separation of imaging and surgery into adjacent rooms establishes a modular design. Accordingly separate modules can be added to extend the single-modality imaging OR. Such a multimodal-imaging OR concept is based on a conventional OR with fluoroscopy at its core. US can be added. Ceiling-mounted navigation systems are the connecting link to the imaging units. The moveable OR table has a floating top, which can be connected to either imaging gantry.

In the MRXO[55] concept (Fig. 2-5), the central OR-angiography room is connected to a 1.5-T MRI and a CT suite. Both suites have separate entrances to admit patients from radiology (MRI) and the emergency room (CT), adherent to the shared-resources concept. This setup is primarily designed for neurosurgical applications.

In the planned AMIGO (advanced multimodality image guided operative)[72] design, the fully equipped surgical room (fluoroscopy, US, navigation system) will be flanked by a 3-T MRI unit and a PET-CT. With this design, the applicability of the suite is not only as a shared resource in regards to simultaneous imaging of other patients during surgery, but also expandable to an interdisciplinary suite serving different specialties.

Dedicated OR-MR Environment

Dedicated systems realize the close integration of MRI and surgery within one OR-MR environment.

Dedicated Low-Field System

The 0.15-T MRI (previous generation 0.12 T) is an open-bore system with two poles.[51,52,73] The MRI is positioned beneath the patient's head (Fig. 2-6). On demand the magnet is raised to place the surgical field in the imager. Images are acquired and transmitted to the connected navigation unit for updated navigation. The OR has to be shielded to avoid RF interference, and all other nonessential equipment has to be turned off. Alternatively, the patient and the scanner can be shielded separately.[74] This compact MRI provides the closest approximation to the original concept of merging imaging and surgery in space. The application can be integrated into a conventional OR, provided shielding is implemented and used on demand by raising the poles to imaging level. Despite the application comfort, the low field holds challenges in regards to homogeneity (spatial resolution and geometric distortions) and field of view (120–160 mm vs. 220 mm in high-field systems). These systems are used for intraoperative imaging in glioma[51,52] and pituitary surgery.[75,76]

Dedicated High-Field System

These installations combine a fully equipped neurosurgical OR with a high-field scanner, primarily 1.5-T MR units, into a comprehensive unit.[15,40,53] Two main setups provide this dedicated environment.[15,40,53] The 5-gauss border represents a demarcation that permits the spatial division of the OR-MR suite.[40,53,60] Surgical and imaging site are connected by a surgical table, which attaches directly to the scanner. The surgical area is reached by disconnecting the table and rotating it either by 30 degrees[15,40] (Fig. 2-7) or 160 degrees[53] (Fig. 2-8) away from the MR axis, to place the operating field outside the 5-gauss line.

The primary fully equipped surgical site for microneurosurgery is outside the 5 gauss line, where ferromagnetic tools and equipment (e.g., microscope, ultrasonic aspirator, bipolar coagulation, and cortical stimulation) can be used unimpeded. The rigid head fixation has to be fully MR compatible. The material of the pins has no influence on the overall imaging (local artifacts with metal pins). The head fixation can be integrated into the rigid RF coil with restricted degrees of freedom.[53] More flexibility for positioning is achieved by a modified carbon-fiber, MR-compatible Mayfield clamp attached to the table top used with surface coils.[40] One coil is positioned below the patient's head, within the Mayfield clamp, while the top coil is removed during surgery and replaced for scanning.

For surgical navigation, the dynamic reference frame (DRF) is attached to the head-holder. The navigation system is registered, the craniotomy planning finalized. In integrated MR-OR solutions the navigation system is ceiling

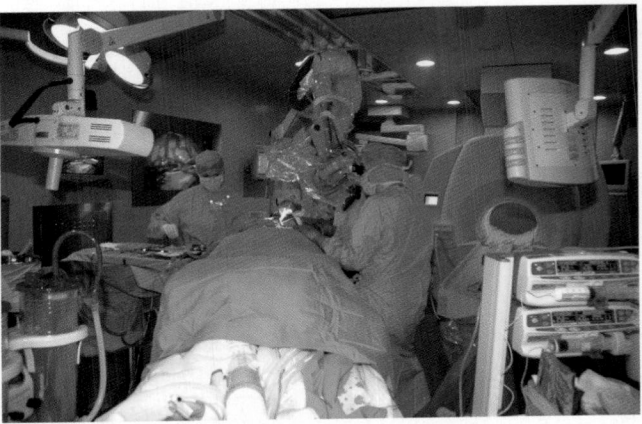

FIGURE 2-7 Fully integrated OR-MR (1.5 T) environment at the authors' institution. Patient is turned away from MR axis by 30 degrees to position the head into the primary surgical area outside the 5-gauss line. Ceiling-mounted navigation system. Open procedure for left frontal glioma. *(OR-MR setup in Kiel/Germany.)*

mounted, with the computer placed outside the shielded room. After craniotomy, the operation is performed, using state-of-the art microneurosurgical techniques. For lesions in eloquent areas the authors' group utilizes the technique of awake craniotomy with cortical stimulation.[77]

Imaging can be initiated at every point the surgeon deems feasible. Ferromagnetic material is removed and the surgical field covered with additional sterile drapes. The table is returned into the MR axis, connected, and the patient transferred to the imaging site.

In both arrangements,[40,53] the interval from stopping the surgery to initial scanning commonly takes about 3 to 5 min.

The surgeon determines the imaging protocols based on presurgical imaging characteristics. The images are transferred to the navigation system as soon as they are acquired for updated accurate navigation.[40,71]

The surgical field is redraped on top of the previous draping. If residual tumor is identified, updated neuronavigation allows the precise localization for resection. If no

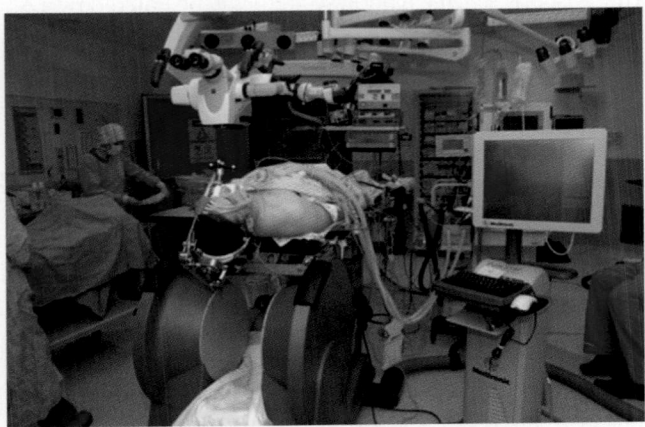

FIGURE 2-6 Compact low-field MRI (0.12-15 T). Position before draping. Ceiling-mounted navigation system. Special headrest with integrated coil and flexible coil positioned for pituitary surgery. *(Courtesy of M. Hadani, Sheba Medical Center; Tel Hashomer, Israel.)*

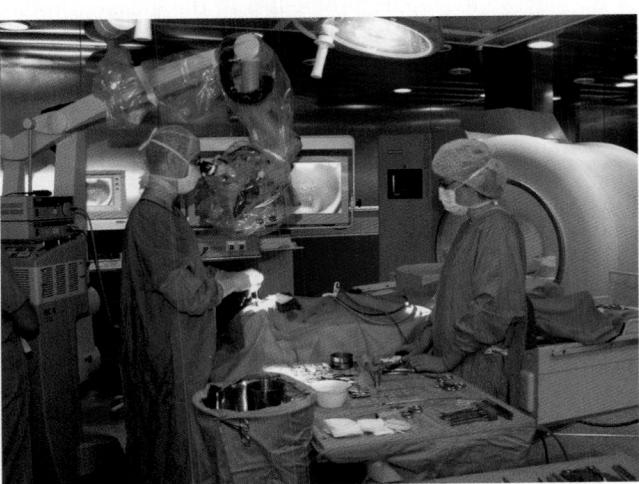

FIGURE 2-8 Depiction of the system with table turned away 160 degrees from MR axis, to position head outside 5-gauss line (1.5 T MR). Pituitary surgery. *(Courtesy Prof. C. Nimsky, OR-MR setup in Erlangen, Germany.)*

further resection is necessary or deemed feasible, surgery is concluded.

Biopsies and burr-hole procedures in a dedicated, high-field MRI can be performed in the primary surgical site outside the 5-gauss line with standard equipment (conventional stereotactic frames; computer-guided, navigated free-hand biopsies; navigated endoscopy).[40] More sophisticated in-bore procedures use the capacity of real-time imaging. Burr-hole and dural opening are performed outside the 5-gauss line with standard equipment. After a MR-compatible burr hole mounted device is attached, the patient is transferred into the MR for scanning. The mounted guide is fixed to preserve the planed trajectory. During the probe's advance in-plane imaging (1–3 images/second) provides real-time control and final image confirmation of the target point.[78] With short-bore MRs, the needle can be advanced by the surgeon reaching into the bore. However, remote control or robotic devices provide more comfortable reach and can be potentially employed within MRIs with less access.[78,79] Current studies discuss in-bore procedures for deep brain stimulation.[24]

Within the integrated system originally described by Hall et al.[15] a secondary surgical site can be used for specific tasks.[40,65] When the MRI table is extended beyond the back of the MRI, the patient's head can be accessed freely for surgery. This area is within the 5-gauss line, thus necessitating the use of MR-safe equipment. While ultrasonic aspirator and bipolar coagulation can be used in this site, microscopes which provide familiar illumination and magnification qualities are not available. The transfer to the MRI is much shorter, repeated imaging becomes easier. This secondary surgical site returns to the idea of a close interlacing of imaging and surgery. However, as long as microneurosurgical techniques are hampered, the utility of this area is limited to smaller interventions.

Interestingly despite this restrain, this secondary surgical site allowed a major development: the inception of an integrated, dedicated 3-T system within an operating theater.[80,81] Contrary to shared-resources solutions, this setup is the only one to attempt the combination of intraoperative 3-T system and surgery. While there are still significant drawbacks, this installation provides the proof of concept, that dedicated high-field OR-MR rooms for biopsies and open craniotomies can be realized.[80-82]

Summary

Intraoperative imaging addresses the crucial need to support surgical decision making with online information to improve quality control and complication avoidance. The main modalities are US, fluoroscopy, CT, and MRI.

Ultrasound can be easily integrated into the surgical workflow. Combination with navigation systems facilitates interpretation. The capacity to simultaneously capture flow and structure is particularly useful in vascular malformations. Resection control for gliomas is of limited use, even with the most recent contrast-enhanced US.

Mobile fluoroscopy has been integrated into conventional ORs for spinal surgery and DBS. The biplane representation has been extended to a 3D perspective by rotating units. This enhances their potential application for vascular neurosurgery and spinal instrumentation, where 3D rotational fluoroscopy may become a competitor for intraoperative CT.

The evolution of IoUS and fluoroscopy has facilitated integration into the surgical surrounding. Current-generation equipment has been reduced in size, while significant improvements have been achieved in functionality.

CT and MRI are less prone to undergo simultaneous miniaturization and improvement. These cut-plane imaging modalities are primarily integrated through workflow and suite design.

The latest iCT generation shows significant improvement in image quality and integration into the surgical workflow. Spinal instrumentation and vascular neurosurgery are the main indications. In brain tumor surgery, the use of iCT is less conclusive, albeit there have been significant improvements, in particular for low-grade gliomas.

In iMRI suites, intraoperative imaging has taken its most elaborate form. Despite its cost, special demands, and labor intensiveness, this field keeps expanding, due to the unparalleled imaging capabilities for the analysis of structural pathology as well as physiologic investigations of the central nervous system (e.g., neurooncology, epilepsy surgery). Various groups reported more complete resections for high-grade gliomas and pituitary lesions employing intraoperative low-,[52,83] mid-,[84,85] and high-field systems.[39,86] Increased resection percentages were also shown for low-grade lesions.[53,87]

The attempt to decrease MRI size to facilitate integration, resulted in a compact low-field system, albeit with limited imaging potential.[51] Higher-field MRIs providing diagnostic imaging capability are integrated primarily through their suite design, which separates surgical and imaging site within the same (dedicated systems) or adjacent rooms (twin operating theater, shared resource). In dedicated systems, the transfer between surgical and imaging site can be achieved swiftly.[40,53] In shared resource concepts, transfer is longer. Furthermore potential conflicts in using the imaging for surgery and routine diagnostics may lead to prolonged waiting periods before intraoperative imaging can be commenced.[54,56]

Long envisioned intraoperative MRI has been successfully combined with standard microneurosurgical and navigation techniques into comprehensive units for neurosurgical procedures.[50,88] High-field MRI and its intraoperative application represent a major interdisciplinary challenge and opportunity. Further refinements may lead back to the original concept of merging therapy and MRI, with robotic devices for surgery, focused US for noninvasive ablative procedures[88] or open high-field magnet designs.

Multimodal imaging OR concepts (MRXO and AMIGO) extend the modular arrangement as realized by the shared-resources concept. Additional modalities have been integrated into adjacent rooms (CT, PET-CT, and high-field MRI) of a hybrid neurointerventional-neurosurgical OR (angiography and US). The modular shared-resources design provides the structural framework for integrating otherwise incompatible units. Such installations represent a major research effort to evaluate the impact and value of different imaging modalities.

The essential link between imaging and surgery is the computer-assisted IGN system. It represents the platform on which the pre- and intra-operative multimodal imaging information coalesces to enable surgical decision making.[71,88-90]

In current systems, imaging interrupts surgery for various periods of time. While microneurosurgical techniques remain unrestricted, the surgical workflow is disrupted and the procedure prolonged. Thus intraoperative imaging represents a compromise balancing the additional value of the imaging information versus timely conclusion of the surgery.

Especially for MRI, the overabundance of high-quality image information becomes a challenge in its own right. Fiber tracking has been employed in sophisticated ways, delineating the major fiber connections.[91,92] Spectroscopy has been used to guide stereotactic biopsies,[93] and with further refinement may yield information on resection borders in open surgery.[54]

Intraoperative imaging has to be carefully balanced to minimize delay while obtaining the best information possible. Any device used for intraoperative imaging becomes a surgical tool, and has to be employed with the same scrutiny and deliberation. It remains the surgeon's obligation to decide, ideally in close communication with neuroradiologists, when to obtain which information as a basis for surgical decision making.

Conclusion

Intraoperative imaging and navigation have developed from a vision[50] to a neurosurgical reality. The development of various OR designs to accommodate intraoperative imaging and surgery has accelerated. Solutions apparently prohibitive in scope and cost 10 years ago have been implemented and surpassed. The higher the expectation of image information, the more complex the resulting design. The most intricate, but at present also the most flexible and informative modality for cranial neurosurgery, is intraoperative MRI. The multitude of designs, implementations, and field strengths make this a most multifaceted area of expertise. Incorporation of magnets with increasing field strengths and multimodal imaging concepts (MRXO) including metabolic information (AMIGO) represent the next challenges.

Technological advances almost appear to gain autonomous momentum. It is essential to ensure that surgical needs remain at the core of this multidisciplinary effort.

KEY REFERENCES

Black PM, Moriarty T, Alexander 3rd E, et al. Development and implementation of intraoperative magnetic resonance imaging and its neurosurgical applications. *Neurosurgery*. 1997;41:831-842.

Claus EB, Horlacher A, Hsu L, et al. Survival rates in patients with low-grade glioma after intraoperative magnetic resonance image guidance. *Cancer*. 2005;103:1227-1233.

Hadani M, Spiegelman R, Feldman Z, et al. Novel, compact, intraoperative magnetic resonance imaging-guided system for conventional neurosurgical operating rooms. *Neurosurgery*. 2001;48:799-807.

Hall WA, Galicich W, Bergman T, Truwit CL. 3-Tesla intraoperative MR imaging for neurosurgery. *J Neurooncol*. 2006;77:297-303.

Hall WA, Martin AJ, Liu H, et al. High-field strength interventional magnetic resonance imaging for pediatric neurosurgery. *Pediatr Neurosurg*. 1998;29:253-259.

Jankovski A, Francotte F, Vaz G, et al. Intraoperative magnetic resonance imaging at 3-T using a dual independent operating room-magnetic resonance imaging suite: development, feasibility, safety, and preliminary experience. *Neurosurgery*. 2008;63:412-424.

Jolesz FA, Nabavi A, Kikinis R. Integration of interventional MRI with computer-assisted surgery. *J Magn Reson Imaging*. 2001;13:69-77.

Matsumae M, Koizumi J, Fukuyama H, et al. World's first magnetic resonance imaging/x-ray/operating room suite: a significant milestone in the improvement of neurosurgical diagnosis and treatment. *J Neurosurg*. 2007;107:266-273.

Nabavi A, Black PM, Gering DT, et al. Serial intraoperative magnetic resonance imaging of brain shift. *Neurosurgery*. 2001;48:787-797.

Nabavi A, Dorner L, Stark AM, Mehdorn HM. Intraoperative MRI with 1.5 Tesla in neurosurgery. *Neurosurg Clin North Am*. 2009;20:163-171.

Nabavi A, Goebel S, Doerner L, et al. Awake craniotomy and intraoperative magnetic resonance imaging: patient selection, preparation, and technique. *Top Magn Reson Imaging*. 2009;19:191-196.

Nimsky C, Fujita A, Ganslandt O, et al. Volumetric assessment of glioma removal by intraoperative high-field magnetic resonance imaging. *Neurosurgery*. 2004;55:358-370.

Nimsky C, Ganslandt O, Cerny S, et al. Quantification of, visualization of, and compensation for brain shift using intraoperative magnetic resonance imaging. *Neurosurgery*. 2000;47:1070-1079.

Nimsky C, Ganslandt O, Kober H, et al. Intraoperative magnetic resonance imaging combined with neuronavigation: a new concept. *Neurosurgery*. 2001;48:1082-1089.

Nimsky C, Ganslandt O, Von Keller B, et al. Intraoperative high-field-strength MR imaging: implementation and experience in 200 patients. *Radiology*. 2004;233:67-78.

Pamir MN, Ozduman K, Dincer A, et al. First intraoperative, shared-resource, ultrahigh-field 3-Tesla magnetic resonance imaging system and its application in low-grade glioma resection. *J Neurosurg*. 2010; 112:47-69.

Schulder M. Intracranial surgery with a compact, low-field-strength magnetic resonance imager. *Top Magn Reson Imaging*. 2009;19:179-189.

Steinmeier R, Fahlbusch R, Ganslandt O, et al. Intraoperative magnetic resonance imaging with the magnetom open scanner: concepts, neurosurgical indications, and procedures: A preliminary report. *Neurosurgery*. 1998;43:739-747.

Sutherland GR, Kaibara T, Louw D, et al. A mobile high-field magnetic resonance system for neurosurgery. *J Neurosurg*. 1999;91:804-813.

Sutherland GR, Latour I, Greer AD. Integrating an image-guided robot with intraoperative MRI: a review of the design and construction of neuroarm. *IEEE Eng Med Biol Mag*. 2008;27:59-65.

Tronnier VM, Wirtz CR, Knauth M, et al. Intraoperative diagnostic and interventional magnetic resonance imaging in neurosurgery. *Neurosurgery*. 1997;40:891-900.

Uhl E, Zausinger S, Morhard D, et al. Intraoperative computed tomography with integrated navigation system in a multidisciplinary operating suite. *Neurosurgery*. 2009;64:231-239.

Numbered references appear on Expert Consult.

SURGICAL MANAGEMENT OF BRAIN AND SKULL BASE TUMORS

ALFREDO QUIÑONES-HINOJOSA

Functional Tractography, Diffusion Tensor Imaging, Intraoperative Integration of Modalities, and Neuronavigation

JONATHAN A. HYAM • ALEXANDER L. GREEN • ERLICK A.C. PEREIRA

Diffusion tensor imaging (DTI) with functional tractography is a noninvasive MRI modality which depicts the probable location and orientation of subcortical white matter tracts *in vivo*. DTI offers a variety of possible applications for neurosurgeons and neuroscientists to help further the understanding of neurologic organization and function and to advance patient care which explains the enthusiasm and optimism with which it has been received. Potential clinical applications for individual patients include prediction of neurologic outcome from tumor[1] and stroke,[2-4] targeting for functional and stereotactic neurosurgery[5-7] and pre- and intra-operative planning for the surgical resection of space-occupying lesions. This chapter shall focus on the application of DTI in the surgical resection of intra-axial brain tumors.

Surgery occupies a vital place in the management of intra-axial brain tumors by virtue of providing symptom relief, recovery of pathologic tissue for diagnosis and beneficial influence on long-term outcome. The ultimate aim of resection of intra-axial brain tumors is to achieve as complete excision of neoplastic tissue as possible. A substantial body of evidence exists to suggest that a greater extent of resection results in extended mean survival time in low-grade and high-grade glioma.[8-17] However, the neurosurgeon is limited in the scope of surgical resection possible by the imperative to avoid injury to eloquent brain tissue and therefore the development of post-operative neurologic deficits. Knowledge of which tissue is functionally important in the individual patient is therefore crucial in pre-operative and intra-operative decision making. Although imaging in the form of computerized tomography (CT) and MRI can define structural anatomy, they do not provide reliable information on functional anatomy in the individual. Other modalities need to be employed by the neurosurgeon to delineate areas of functional importance. This functional mapping can be performed by invasive and non-invasive methods. Invasive examinations include pre-operative cortical electrode grid recordings and intra-operative cortical and subcortical stimulation. Non-invasive examinations include functional MRI and magnetoencephalography (MEG). Of those studies performed pre-operatively, none provide information on subcortical functional anatomy.

Despite great care taken by the neurosurgeon to avoid injury to eloquent cortex through careful pre-operative and intra-operative functional mapping and meticulous surgical technique, straying into critical subcortical white matter tracts can still result in devastating deficits. There is concern that localization using subcortical white matter stimulation is less reliable and safe than cortical stimulation.[18,19] By visually representing white matter tracts to the surgeon, DTI promises to improve the safety of tumor resections, especially when involving subcortical areas.

Scientific Principles of DTI

Diffusion MRI scans image the molecular diffusion of water at the same scale as cellular dimensions and therefore allow the microarchitecture of the brain to be investigated. The constant random motion of molecules is described by Brownian motion and is exploited by diffusion imaging to specifically detect the displacement of water molecules through the brain tissue medium. Diffusion-weighted scanning consists of a T2-weighted spin-echo sequence with the addition of two diffusion-sensitizing gradients applied before and after the 180° refocusing pulse, through an identical axis. Therefore, there is a loss of signal intensity as a result of incomplete rephasing of water proton spins after they have moved during the time elapsed between the two diffusion-sensitizing gradients.[20] Diffusion times in the region of 10 to 50 ms are used which provides microscopic detail, capturing average molecular displacements of 10 μm.[20] Scan acquisition using standard MRI systems takes 3 to 10 min,[21] and therefore is minimally burdensome on patient, radiographer, or scanner time.

The direction of the passage of water is different depending on the nature of tissue in which it is found. Where no structural boundaries exist nearby, the molecular motion of water is unimpeded and equal in all directions. This is known as isotropic diffusion. This is exhibited within the cerebrospinal fluid spaces of the brain, with the exception of sites of bulk flow such as the aqueduct of Sylvius or foramen of Munro.[20] Isotropic diffusion is also believed to occur in grey matter.[22,23] In contrast, myelinated white matter fiber tracts are arranged into parallel, densely packed bundles that impede the diffusion of water molecules perpendicular to the fibers' direction. Therefore, diffusion of water molecules in this situation is not equal in all directions and is defined as anisotropic diffusion. Detection of water molecule anisotropy is the basis of diffusion tensor imaging and tractography.

The diffusion tensor is a 3 × 3 matrix of vectors which mathematically describes the three-dimensional (3D) directionality and magnitude, or diffusion anisotropy, of water molecules.[20,21,24] The three principal axes of the diffusion tensor are termed eigenvectors. When plotted as an ellipsoid, isotropic diffusion is a sphere whereas anisotropic diffusion forms an elongated ellipsoid, becoming a prolate (cigar) shape when the eigenvector of greatest magnitude is much larger than the other two. Prolate diffusion within a brain voxel is assumed to represent a white matter fiber bundle where the primary eigenvector is aligned with the axonal axis. Tracing of white matter tracts to produce functional tractograms uses each voxel's diffusion tensor to link it to adjacent voxels and in this way trace out the likely path of a fiber bundle in 3D space (Fig. 3-1).

DTI fiber tract data can be presented in two forms. Functional anisotropy maps provide information on fiber anatomy in cross-sectional two-dimensional (2D) images with color-coded axes where the brightness is proportional to the degree of anisotropy (see Fig. 3-1). By convention, the anteroposterior axis is represented by green, left-right by red, and up-down by blue. Therefore, the corpus callosum will appear red, for example. Alternatively, deterministic or probabilistic[25] functional tractography performs a 3Ddimensional reconstruction and portrayal of the fiber pathways based on following a white matter tract from voxel to voxel as described above (Fig. 3-2). Specified anatomic points, known as "seeds" (see Fig. 3-1), can be selected by the user from where the tractogram can be plotted by the processing software to delineate proposed neural connectivity with the selected site. Alternatively, larger volumes of brain can be selected as regions of interest or "masks." To reduce dependence on the user and therefore the inherent subjectivity of seed selection while also increasing the likelihood of depicting functionally relevant tracts, Schonberg et al. used functional MRI to define where seed points

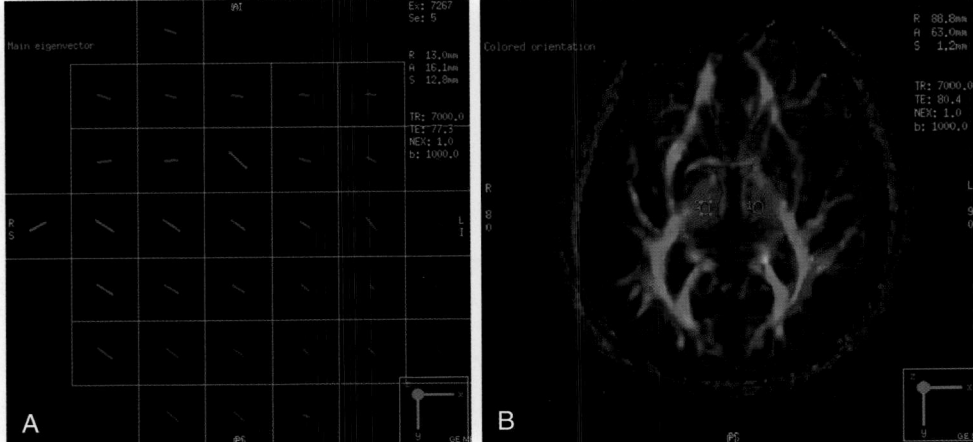

FIGURE 3-1 Main eigenvectors in adjacent voxels providing the basis for tractogram construction (A). Fractional anisotropy map derived from diffusion tensor image (B). Examples of seed points are seen overlying both thalami.

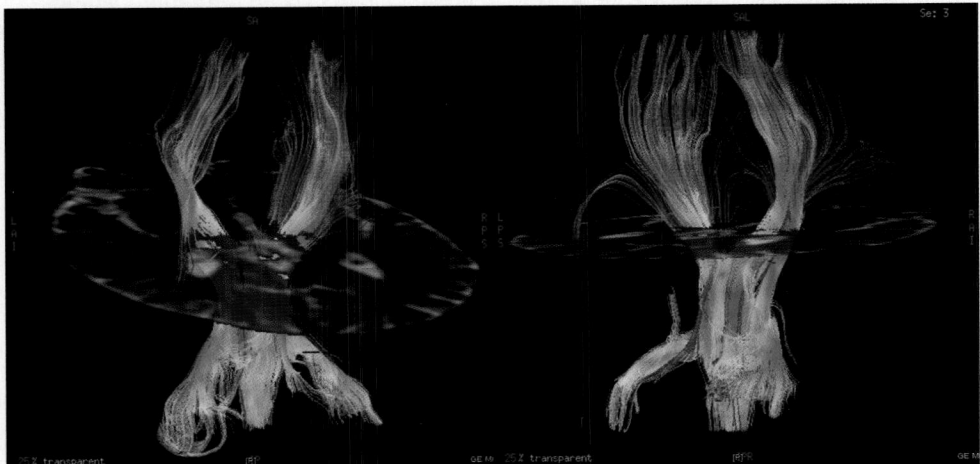

FIGURE 3-2 Tractogram representing the ascending and descending pathways among cortex, brainstem, and cerebellum after seed selected in pons. *(Courtesy of Prof. Peter Silburn and Dr. Terry Coyne, University of Queensland, Brisbane, Australia.)*

should be sited.[26] Although this represents an extra stage of patient assessment, they found that it enabled a more comprehensive mapping of fiber systems such as the pyramidal tract and the superior longitudinal fasciculus. See glossary of terms in Table 3-1.

Preoperative Planning Applications

DTI shows the surgeon the relationship of the intra-axial tumor to local white matter tracts in multiple planes. A variety of aspects of the tumor–tract relationship can therefore be demonstrated. The identity of the tract can be surmised from its position and course, such as the corticospinal tract and optic radiations. The proximity of the tumor to the tract can be appreciated. Also the position of the tumor can be seen in relation to the tract, for example superior, lateral, medial etc., allowing optimal approach to be determined to highly eloquent and complex areas such as the pons.[27] Displacement of the tract by the tumor or edema can also be demonstrated.[28,29] This is crucial information when planning a surgical trajectory in order to avoid eloquent tissue. DTI has been found to provide important preoperative warning of this surgical hazard in situations where a precisely planned trajectory is imperative such as during resection of thalamic juvenile pilocytic astrocytoma with displacement of the posterior limb of the internal capsule.[30] Incorporation of white matter fibers within the tumor mass, seen especially in low-grade tumors,[31] and destruction of white matter fibers by the tumor can also be depicted. These features will have profound implications for the extent of resection amenable for the individual tumor.

DTI can also help elucidate the anatomy of poorly described pathways in vivo in the human to inform and advance established surgical strategies. Resection strategies that aim to excise normal as well as neoplastic tissue with a view to minimizing the likelihood of recurrence such as frontal and temporal lobectomy can be enhanced by DTI to maintain safety. The anatomico-functional connectivity of the dominant temporal lobe, for example, was reviewed by Duffau et al. using a combination of DTI and subcortical intraoperative stimulation studies to elucidate the white matter pathways, which should represent the resection boundaries of temporal lobectomy such as the pyramidal tract and the anterior wall of the temporal part of the superior longitudinal fasciculus.[32] Indeed, DTI has

been proposed as the preoperative investigation to assess individual patients' risk of visual field defect prior to anterior temporal lobe resection as it images the Meyer loop of the optic radiation as it courses anteriorly from the lateral geniculate nucleus and around the tip of the temporal horn before projecting to the visual cortex. The individual variation of this white matter pathway[33] increases the risk of a deficit which can permanently disqualify the patient from holding a driving license. Therefore, preoperative warning of a more ventral position of the Meyer loop along its course anterior to the temporal horn should identify those with a higher likelihood of postoperative deficit.[34,35]

Although DTI visualizes white matter tracts, it is possible to extrapolate these projections and therefore visualize their grey matter cortical projections/origins. Kamada et al. applied this technique to map the primary motor area (PMA) preoperatively in thirty patients with supratentorial lesion affecting the motor system.[36] By selecting seed points within the corticospinal tract at the cerebral peduncle, plus the medial lemniscus to differentiate from somatosensory projections, a PMA map was produced that was successfully validated against subsequent intraoperative cortical somatosensory evoked potentials. Indeed, fMRI failed to identify the PMA in eight patients. The reasons for this were inherent in the patients' pathology through its effect on the motor system in that they were incapable of successfully completing the self-paced finger tapping task required to elicit the blood oxygenation level dependent signal that fMRI detects. In contrast, DTI requires no patient tasks to acquire its data and therefore offers an important alternative for preoperative noninvasive cortical mapping in patients who, for whatever reason, cannot complete them.

DTI has been applied in neuro-oncology beyond not only functional mapping but for noninvasive assessment of tumor architecture in terms of cell density, white matter invasion and even histologic discrimination such as the distinction between primary and secondary intra-axial tumors.[37-41] It has been proposed that DTI can distinguish between vasogenic edema and tumor-infiltrated edema. Edematous tissue surrounding glioma is generally accepted to be infiltrated by tumor cells. In contrast, edema surrounding cerebral metastases or meningioma is considered to be vasogenic.[40,42] Therefore, hyperintensity surrounding tumor on T2-weighted MRI may reflect any of glioma, metastasis or meningioma. However, as the FA at the voxels corresponding to the site of edema has been shown in some studies to be of a lower value in infiltrative pathologies such as glioma, a tumor infiltration index was derived by Lu et al. to help distinguish against pathologies producing only vasogenic edema.[39] There have been contradictory reports including a PET-labeling study questioning whether this DTI analysis is specific enough to differentiate between tumor-infiltrated edema and vasogenic edema.[41,43] Further investigation will determine whether DTI can fulfill this potential and provide reliable presurgical histologic tumor characterization.

Therefore, DTI provides advanced warning of potential intraoperative misadventures to help surgeons adapt their approach subsequently in theater to minimize these. Even prior to this stage, DTI can inform the surgeon of how amenable the tumor is to surgery by virtue of its relationship to eloquent brain and even potentially its histologic nature,

Table 3-1	Glossary of Diffusion Tensor Imaging Terms
Isotropic diffusion	Motion of Molecules Being Equal in all Directions
Anisotropic diffusion	Motion of molecules not being equal in all directions
Fractional anisotropy	Directionally averaged diffusion of water molecules within a voxel measured as its deviation from isotropic diffusion
Diffusion tensor	Matrix of vectors which mathematically describe anisotropic diffusion within a 3D space
Tractography	Representation of white matter fiber tracts produced by following eigenvectors of adjacent voxels in 3D space

and therefore what surgery can offer in terms of likely benefits and associated risk of adverse effects.

Intraoperative Neuronavigation

The prospect of intraoperative tract navigation is possibly the most exciting application of DTI for the surgeon. It is logical to expect that an intraoperative map of functionally important subcortical tracts should reduce the likelihood of inadvertent straying into white matter pathways, reassure the surgeon to be more aggressive allowing optimization of resection limits or, conversely, restraint when critical tracts are close leading to an associated reduction in the incidence of postoperative neurologic deficits and increase in tumor volume reduction. A number of studies have sought to establish whether current DTI techniques fulfill this promise.

Various neuronavigation systems capable of integrating DTI with frameless stereotaxy exist. The DTI FA sequence can be subjected to predefined thresholds to delineate in three dimensions the white matter tracts of interest and the surgeon can then also manipulate the final renditions using the drawing tools available in the software. A standard 3D stereotactic neuronavigational MRI sequence is selected to provide the reference images for navigating and the DTI sequence is selected to provide the working images to be merged with it. The intensity of the tractograms can be altered to optimize the prominence of the tracts with respect to the structures of interest, usually the tumor, and the surgeon's preference. Standard patient registration and navigating strategies are then employed as in conventional navigation. Depending on the surgeon's preferences and the particular software and hardware facilities available, the navigational display can be presented on the workstation beside the patient or projected through the microscope's heads-up display.

The feasibility of intraoperative guidance by incorporation of DTI fiber tracking into neuronavigation systems has been demonstrated by a number of investigators within the last decade.[44-49] White matter pathways such as the pyramidal tract and the optic radiation were successfully portrayed in relation to intra-axial tumors such as cavernoma and glioma. Coenen et al. were the first to report the use of intraoperative neuronavigation with 3D tract reconstruction to assist the resection of glioblastoma associated with the pyramidal tract. They found fiber tract navigation to be a helpful adjunct to resection in the four patients in whom it was applied. Subsequent studies have also underlined its potential for efficiency and patient safety.[47,48] The ability of DTI to reliably predict the true location of critical white matter pathways intraoperatively is crucial for the technique to be applied with confidence during surgery. Investigators have evaluated intraoperative DTI's accuracy in depicting motor pathways by comparing it to intraoperative electrophysiologic methods, in particular cortical stimulation.[50,51] One particular study of 13 patients employed electrical motor cortex stimulation to verify the location of the precentral gyrus and indirectly the pyramidal tract, DTI neuronavigation correctly predicted the principal motor pathways' position in 92%.[51] DTI has not only been applied to surgery for supratentorial tumors but also to the resection of brainstem lesions such as cavernoma with promise of improving operative safety.[52]

The perceived benefits of fiber tract neuronavigation need to be translated into objective improvements in aspects of patient care; however, few studies have addressed this rigorously with objective endpoints. Notably, Wu et al. performed a prospective, randomized controlled trial to attend to this deficiency in the literature.[53] They studied 238 patients undergoing resection for high- and low-grade supratentorial glioma involving the pyramidal tracts over 4 years. A total of 118 patients underwent preoperative DTI scanning to aid preoperative planning and integration by rigid registration into the neuronavigation system for intraoperative image guidance. This cohort was compared to 120 similar controls undergoing resection aided by standard neuronavigation. Multiple outcome measures were improved by the implementation of fiber tracking. Gross total resection of high-grade glioma in the DTI group was achieved in more than twice the number of cases than in the control group (74.4% vs. 33.3%). Median survival was 21.2 months in the DTI group compared to 14 months and DTI neuronavigation estimated hazard ratio was 0.570, conferring a 43% reduction in mortality risk. With respect to neurologic function, 6-month Karnofsky Performance Scale score was significantly better in the DTI group (32.8% vs. 15.3%). A criticism of this investigation was the lack of physician blinding in the nonradiologic assessments. However, it provides Class I evidence that fiber tract neuronavigation can improve patient mortality and morbidity in glioma surgery, and that this technology can be successfully integrated into a routine neurosurgical practice.

The promising results of these investigations need to be repeated, particularly as scanner technology, analysis techniques, and intraoperative imaging advances. The impact on preservation of other tracts such as the optic radiations and language pathways also warrants examination.

Limitations of DTI

Although DTI promises to be an effective tool in the surgeon's armamentarium, its limitations must be borne in mind so that it is appropriately interpreted in individual patients. DTI does not directly trace fibers unlike tracer injection studies, which remain the gold standard for defining neural connectivity. Rather it produces representations of white matter tracts based on the fundamental assumption that the dominant direction of water movement is aligned with the predominant direction of white matter fiber bundles within each voxel.[21,54] This is closer to the biological reality in some circumstances more than others. Neuronal axons are micrometers wide but the voxels used are in the order of a few millimeters in each plane; therefore, one voxel may contain some tens of thousands of axons. If a voxel contains groups of nearby axons with differing longitudinal axes such as are found at sites where different tracts cross or axons whose path is tortuous and change course within a very short distance, their anatomy will be misrepresented by current DTI methods. Advances in resolution and modeling of water diffusion are improving this limitation such that complex fiber architectural relationships can be depicted more reliably and accurately in the future.[55-61] In larger, densely packed parallel fiber bundles such as the corpus callosum, this is much less of a problem.

Other limitations include the inability to decipher whether a tract is projecting retrograde or anterograde,[55] which hampers neuroscientific investigation. However, in the context of surgical planning and intraoperative neuronavigation, the presence and location of major white matter tracts is the critical information rather than the direction in which they project.

A further limitation is that tractography is a user-dependent technique. The ultimate results of fiber tracking reflect the chosen thresholding of the functional anisotropy, the site and size of selected seed areas, and which algorithm is used.[62] A threshold value of 0.15 to 0.2 has been suggested by a rigorous, albeit retrospective, comparison of DTI tract representation and stereotactic biopsy histologic findings, although the functionality of the tracts was not evaluated.[40] Therefore, interuser variation can produce important differences in the tractogram generated.

Acquisition and processing of DTI images is affected by multiple sources of spatial inaccuracy therefore allowances need to be made when interpreting tractograms during surgical resection to maintain patient safety. During the scanning process, static and encoding direction-dependent distortions occur due to factors such as magnetic field inhomogeneity, imperfections in gradient waveforms, and eddy currents.[52] Although progress has been made in minimizing the impact of these by correcting for the resulting misrepresentations,[63,64] some inaccuracy remains in the current DTI technique. The integration of DTI images with neuronavigation systems produces further discrepancy with an image registration error in the region of 2 to 3 mm, although this is comparable to the error encountered when integrating functional MRI data.[48]

Neuronavigation using functional tractography also suffers from the same limitations as conventional neuronavigation. Patient registration error must be factored in to the overall inaccuracy.[48] Further, any change in patient position with respect to the registration landmarks will severely diminish accuracy. As neuronavigation images are acquired preoperatively, they do not respond in real-time to the changing anatomy and brain shifts of cranial surgery. Therefore, head positioning, continuing resection, cerebrospinal fluid loss, breach of the ventricles and brain retraction, for example, will diminish the accuracy. However, with the advent of intraoperative MRI, this limitation could in future be overcome. Nimsky et al.[47] successfully applied preoperative and intraoperative DTI and stereotactic MRI acquisition with a 1.5-Tesla scanner in 37 patients undergoing glioma surgery. They first demonstrated that it was feasible to perform intraoperative DTI in all patients and that the encountered brain shift was reflected in DTI white matter tract shifts of up to 15 mm.

The multiple sources of spatial inaccuracy described above must be taken into consideration when employing DTI during tumor resection in patients. Animal, phantom, and patient studies have attempted to quantify this discrepancy.[65-67] Berman et al. compared the location of DTI-imaged fiber tracts to intraoperative subcortical stimulation and found a mean distance between stimulation sites and imaged tracts of 8.7 mm.[65] Investigators therefore advise a safety margin of up to 1 cm to be maintained around the depicted white matter pathways, such as the corticospinal tract, during surgery.[31,48,65]

Intraoperative Integration of Modalities

In view of the limitations of DTI described above and the complementary information that can be provided by other techniques, integration of DTI with other modalities has been implemented in the hope of harnessing all of their advantages to enhance neuronavigation. Some modalities, such as CT and MEG, can be integrated directly with the neuronavigation images while others, such as subcortical stimulation, are used alongside the neuronavigation system.

The term "functional neuronavigation" has been coined to describe the incorporation of MEG and fMRI data into frameless stereotactic neuronavigation systems.[48] This has been an important adjunct to modern tumor surgery and has been demonstrated to reduce morbidity during resection of lesions adjacent to eloquent brain.[68] These modalities provide truly functional information generated preoperatively during series of patient tasks, whereas DTI provides only structural information. All three imaging modalities can be incorporated into the neuronavigation system to provide simultaneous representations of the cortical and subcortical functionally important tissue which is then displayed on the workstation or heads-up display. Successful incorporation and navigation using fMRI and DTI together has been reported to be user-friendly and suitable for routine use within a neurosurgical service[69] and to help facilitate maximal tumor resection,[70] although there has been no control group to compare outcomes with. Other imaging modalities such as CT or MR angiography can also be incorporated within the neuronavigation system providing the surgeon with the optimal anatomic and functional representation of the intracranial cavity.

If preoperative imaging, such as MEG, fMRI, and angiography, are integrated with DTI and stereotactic images and intraoperative MRI is performed then registration will be lost due to the brain shift associated with surgery.[71] There are potential solutions to this problem whereby the preoperative data are registered with the intraoperative data; however, as brain shift is complex and difficult to predict reliably,[47] suitable algorithms to make this correction are some way off. Therefore, as intraoperative DTI has been shown to be a more reliable possibility in responding to brain shift,[47] this may be the most accurate intraoperative functional imaging modality once the resection has advanced.

An alternative solution to the brain shift problem during surgery is the use of intraoperative 3D ultrasound scanning (3D USS). It has the advantage over intraoperative MRI of not requiring modifications to the operating theater and it is much less expensive. 3D USS acquired intraoperatively can be used to update preoperative stereotactic MRI images, allowing continued navigation with fMRI and DTI data throughout the resection.[72] Two studies of patients undergoing resection of cavernoma or glioma have found that intraoperative updates of fMRI and DTI neuronavigation by 3D USS has been feasible,[69,70] and that the combination facilitates maximal tumor resection.[70]

Subcortical stimulation has been used in trials to verify the reliability of depicted DTI fiber tracts; however, it can be used in tandem with DTI to confirm functional tissue location. Bello et al. reported the accurate identification of eloquent fiber tracts using a combination of DTI

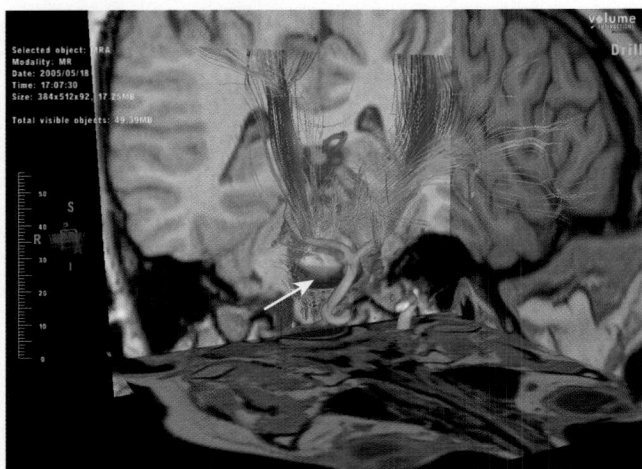

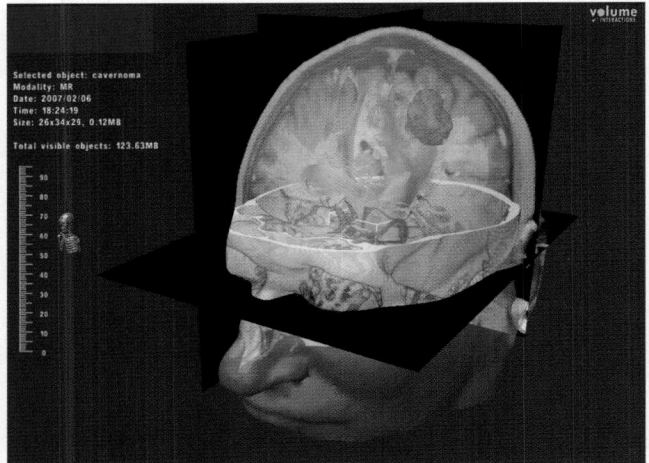

FIGURE 3-3 Example of a brainstem cavernoma (*white arrow*) depicted on a virtual reality workstation by incorporation of T1-weighted MRI, DTI tractography, and MR angiography. The cavernoma is intimate to the posterior circulation which lies against its anterior and superior surfaces, but the tumor is predominantly anterior to white matter tracts. (*Courtesy of Dr. Ralf A. Kockro, University Hospital of Zurich, Switzerland, and Volume Interactions PTE Ltd.*)

FIGURE 3-4 Example of a subcortical cavernoma (*red*) represented on a virtual reality workstation. Integration of T1-weighted MRI and DTI tractography demonstrates distortion of the left pyramidal tract by the cavernoma. (*Courtesy of Dr. Ralf A. Kockro, University Hospital of Zurich, Switzerland, and Volume Interactions PTE Ltd.*)

neuronavigation and subcortical electrical stimulation during resection of low- and high-grade glioma in 64 patients.[31] They concluded that surgery safety was improved with a shorter operative time and fewer intraoperative seizures. The use of combined intraoperative recorded motor-evoked potentials with neuronavigation has been supported by other investigators with reported benefits such as real-time demonstration of spatial relationships, less injury to eloquent tracts and optimal tumor resections.[73,74] Again, no controlled trials currently exist; however, the addition of direct functional monitoring would be expected to increase the likelihood of identifying eloquent pathways. Intraoperative DTI has been successfully coregistered with the electrical stimulation probe to facilitate both navigation and stimulation of cortical and subcortical tracts during resection of recurrent glioblastoma beside eloquent brain.[75] Therefore, it is possible for both of these modalities to be truly integrated in the operating theater.

Virtual reality technology in neurosurgery has emerged during the last decade as a viable complement to surgical planning and intraoperative performance.[76-79] It is possible to integrate the variety of imaging modalities including fiber tracking into the virtual display (Figs. 3-3 and 3-4). Intraoperative neuronavigation using this technology has also been achieved.[80] This therefore allows a preoperative "dry run" of surgery in the virtual world using multiple anatomic and functional image data followed by the retracing of the same operative steps stereotactically in the operating theater. Virtual neurosurgery may be an important platform in which DTI fiber tracking is employed in the future.

Postoperative Evaluation

There is scope for DTI to answer important surgical questions postoperatively. Duffau et al. suggest postoperative check DTI to compare with preoperative DTI to help establish whether eloquent tracts have been interrupted.[32] In the case of new deficits occurring postoperatively, interruption of pre-existing functional tracts would imply that direct surgical injury had been the cause. Alternatively, an intact pathway in the presence of a novel deficit may suggest that there had been indirect injury to eloquent tissue from interruption of the white matter bundles' blood supply such as the perforators to the pyramidal tract.[81]

Just as DTI has been shown to predict functional outcome after stroke,[2-4] it may provide prognostic information with regard to postoperative deficits. If relevant tracts are spared this may suggest a more favorable prognosis with function potentially returning in some degree with time. It is important to bear in mind, however, that intact tract anatomy alone does not guarantee functional recovery as DTI describes the tissue architecture but does not provide information on the level of physiologic performance.

Summary

Diffusion tensor imaging is an exciting and developing non-invasive modality, which has the potential to help surgical decision making and improve safety for patients. It can be applied in diagnosis, preoperative planning, intraoperative navigation with or without other complementary modalities, and in postoperative assessment. DTI does have a number of limitations which the neurosurgeon must keep in mind when treating patients, although several of these may be addressed by advances in the state of the art.

KEY REFERENCES

Behrens TE, Johansen-Berg H, Woolrich MW, et al. Non-invasive mapping of connections between human thalamus and cortex using diffusion imaging. *Nat Neurosci.* 2003;6:750-757.

Berman JI, Berger MS, Chung SW, et al. Accuracy of diffusion tensor magnetic resonance imaging tractography assessed using intraoperative subcortical stimulation mapping and magnetic source imaging. *J Neurosurg.* 2007;107:488-494.

Berman JI, Berger MS, Mukherjee P, et al. Diffusion-tensor imaging-guided tracking of fibers of the pyramidal tract combined with intraoperative cortical stimulation mapping in patients with gliomas. *J Neurosurg.* 2004;101:66-72.

Ciccarelli O, Catani M, Johansen-Berg H, et al. Diffusion-based tractography in neurological disorders: concepts, applications, and future developments. *Lancet Neurol.* 2008;7:715-727.

Coenen VA, Huber KK, Krings T, et al. Diffusion-weighted imaging-guided resection of intracerebral lesions involving the optic radiation. *Neurosurg Rev.* 2005;28:188-195.

Coenen VA, Krings T, Mayfrank L, et al. Three-dimensional visualization of the pyramidal tract in a neuronavigation system during brain tumor surgery: first experiences and technical note. *Neurosurg.* 2001;49(1):84-92:(discussion 92).

Duffau H, Thiebaut de Schotten M, Mandonnet E. White matter functional connectivity as an additional landmark for dominant temporal lobectomy. *J Neurol Neurosurg Psychiatry.* 2008;79(5):492-495.

Ganslandt O, Fahlbusch R, Nimsky C, et al. Functional neuronavigation with magnetoencephalography outcome in 50 patients with lesions around the motor cortex. *J Neurosurg.* 1999;91(1):73-79.

Gasco J, Tummala S, Mahajan NM, et al. Simultaneous use of functional tractography, neuronavigation-integrated subcortical white matter stimulation and intraoperative magnetic resonance imaging in glioma surgery: technical note. *Stereotact Funct Neurosurg.* 2009;87: 395-398.

Gulati S, Berntsen EM, Solheim O, et al. Surgical resection of high-grade gliomas in eloquent regions guided by blood oxygenation level dependent functional magnetic resonance imaging, diffusion tensor tractography, and intraoperative navigated 3D ultrasound. *Minim Invasive Neurosurg.* 2009;52:17-24.

Johansen-Berg H, Behrens TEJ. Just pretty pictures? What diffusion tractography can add in clinical neuroscience. *Curr Opin Neurol.* 2006;19:379-385.

Kamada K, Todo T, Masutani Y, et al. Combined use of tractography-integrated functional neuronavigation and direct fiber stimulation. *J Neurosurg.* 2005;102:664-672.

Kinoshita M, Hashimoto N, Goto T, et al. Fractional anisotropy and tumor cell density of the tumor core show positive correlation in diffusion tensor magnetic resonance imaging of malignant brain tumors. *Neuroimage.* 2008;43:29-35.

Kinoshita M, Yamada K, Hashimoto N, et al. Fiber-tracking does not accurately estimate size of fiber bundle in pathological condition: initial neurosurgical experience using neuronavigation and subcortical white matter stimulation. *Neuroimage.* 2005;25:424-429.

Mukherjee P, Berman JI, Chung SW, et al. Diffusion tensor MR imaging and fiber tractography: theoretic underpinnings. *Am J Neuroradiol.* 2008;29:632-641.

Nimsky C, Ganslandt O, Fahlbusch R. Implementation of fiber tract navigation. *Neurosurgery.* 2006:58(ONS Suppl 2):ONS-292–304.

Nimsky C, Ganslandt O, Hastreiter P, et al. Preoperative and intraoperative diffusion tensor imaging-based fiber tracking in glioma surgery. *Neurosurgery.* 2005;56(1):130-138.

Nimsky C, Ganslandt O, Merhof D, et al. Intraoperative visualization of the pyramidal tract by diffusion-tensor-imaging-based fiber tracking. *Neuroimage.* 2006;30(4):1219-1229.

Okada T, Mikuni N, Miki Y, et al. Corticospinal tract localization: integration of diffusion-tensor tractography at 3-T MR imaging with intraoperative white matter stimulation mapping — preliminary results. *Radiology.* 2006;240(3):849-857.

Rasmussen Jr I-A, Lindseth F, Rygh OM, et al. Functional neuronavigation combined with intra-operative 3D ultrasound: initial experiences during surgical resections close to eloquent brain areas and future directions in automatic brain shift compensation of preoperative data. *Acta Neurochir (Wien).* 2007;149:365-378.

Schonberg T, Pianka P, Hendler T, et al. Characterization of displaced white matter by brain tumors using combined DTI and fMRI. *Neuroimage.* 2006;30:1100-1111.

Stadlbauer A, Nimsky C, Buslei R, et al. Diffusion tensor imaging and optimized fiber tracking in glioma patients: histopathologic evaluation of tumor-invaded white matter structures. *Neuroimage.* 2007;34: 949-956.

Wu J-S, Mao Y, Zhou W-J, et al. Clinical evaluation and follow-up outcome of diffusion tensor imaging-based functional neuronavigation: a prospective, controlled study in patients with gliomas involving pyramidal tracts. *Neurosurgery.* 2007;61(5):935-948:(discussion 948-949).

Yogarajah M, Focke NK, Bonelli S, et al. Defining Meyer's loop-temporal lobe resections, visual field deficits and diffusion tensor tractography. *Brain.* 2009;132:1656-1668.

Numbered references appear on Expert Consult.

CHAPTER 4

Intraoperative Neurophysiology: A Tool to Prevent and/or Document Intraoperative Injury to the Nervous System

VEDRAN DELETIS • FRANCESCO SALA

Over the past 25 years, intraoperative neurophysiology (ION) has established itself as a clinical discipline that uses neurophysiologic methods—especially developed or modified from existing methods of clinical neurophysiology—to detect and prevent intraoperatively induced neurologic injuries. Recent developments have solidified its role in neurosurgery and other surgical disciplines. Ideally, ION not only predicts but serves to prevent intraoperatively induced injury to the nervous system. Furthermore, ION can be used to document the exact moment when the injury occurred. As a result, it can be used for both educational and medicolegal purposes.

Generally, ION techniques can be divided in two groups: mapping and monitoring. Neurophysiologic mapping is a technique that, when applied intraoperatively, enables us to identify anatomically indistinct neural structures by their neurophysiologic function. This allows the surgeon to avoid lesioning critical structures in the course of the surgical procedure. In essence, the information gained from neurophysiologic mapping allows the surgeon to operate more safely.

The following procedures use a neurophysiologic mapping technique: identification of the primary motor cortex with direct cortical stimulation, identification of the cranial nerve motor nuclei on the surgically exposed floor of the fourth ventricle, mapping of the corticospinal tract (CT) subcortically (i.e., at the level of the cerebral peduncle or at the spinal cord), mapping of the pudendal afferents in the sacral roots, before selective dorsal rhizotomy, and so on.

Neurophysiologic monitoring is a technique that continuously evaluates the functional integrity of nervous tissue and gives feedback to the (neuro)surgeon. This feedback can be instantaneous, as in a recently developed technique of monitoring motor-evoked potentials (MEPs) from the epidural space of the spinal cord or limb muscles. If the surgical procedure allows us to combine monitoring with mapping techniques, then optimal protection of nervous tissue can be achieved during neurosurgery.

Furthermore, ION uses provocative tests to examine their influence on neurophysiologic signals before the surgical procedure. A temporary clamping of the carotid artery during endarterectomy with monitoring of somatosensory-evoked potentials (SEPs) or electroencephalography is a typical example of a provocative test that measures the ability of the collateral cerebral circulation to supply a potentially ischemic hemisphere. Endovascular injection of a short-acting barbiturate or lidocaine into a vascular malformation of the spinal cord, before embolization, and observation of its influence on the neurophysiologic signals is another example of a provocative test.

Supratentorial Surgery

Surgery for brain gliomas has become more and more aggressive. This is based on clinical data that support better patient survival and quality of life after gross total removal of both low- and high-grade lesions.[1,2]

However, the resection of tumors located in eloquent brain areas, such as the rolandic region and frontotemporal speech areas, requires the identification of functional cortical and subcortical areas that must be respected during surgery. Moreover, the dogmatic assumption that tumoral tissue could not retain function has been repeatedly questioned by neurophysiologic and functional magnetic resonance imaging studies.[3-5] In response to the need for a safe surgery in eloquent brain areas, the past decade has seen the development of a number of techniques to map brain functions, including, but not limited to, functional magnetic resonance imaging, magnetoencephalography, and positron emission tomography.[6-11]

The neurophysiologic contribution to brain mapping has been evident since the late 19th century with the pioneering work of Fritsch and Hitzig[12] and Bartholow.[13] In the 20th century, Penfield and colleagues[14,15] made invaluable contributions through intraoperative mapping of the sensorimotor cortex, whose findings have been substantiated by a number of recent studies.[16-18]

SOMATOSENSORY-EVOKED POTENTIAL PHASE-REVERSAL TECHNIQUE

To indirectly identify the central sulcus, SEPs can be recorded from the exposed cerebral cortex by using the phase-reversal technique. SEPs are elicited by stimulation of the median nerve at the wrist and the posterior tibial nerve at the ankle (40-mA intensity, 0.2-msec duration, 4.3-Hz repetition rate). Recordings are performed from the scalp at CZ'-FZ (for legs) and C3'/C4'-CZ' (for arms) according to the 10–20 International Electroencephalography System. After craniotomy, a strip electrode is placed across the exposed motor cortex and primary somatosensory cortex, transversing the central sulcus. This technique is based on the principle that an SEP, elicited by median nerve stimulation at the wrist, can be recorded from the primary sensory cortex.[19] Its mirror-image waveform can be identified if some of the contacts of the strip electrode are placed on the opposite side of the central sulcus, over the motor cortex[20-22] (Fig. 4-1). For phase reversal, a strip electrode with four to eight stainless steel contacts with an intercontact distance of 1 cm is used. In the literature, the success rate of the phase reversal technique to indirectly localize the primary motor cortex ranges between 91%[20,21] and 97%.[18] Interestingly, identification of the central sulcus by magnetic resonance imaging provided contradictory results when compared with intraoperative phase reversal.[20] Although it is expected that ongoing progress in the field of functional magnetic resonance imaging will eventually replace the need for neurophysiologic tests, ION still retains the highest reliability in mapping of the motor cortex and language areas when compared with functional neuroimaging.[23-26]

DIRECT CORTICAL STIMULATION (60-HZ PENFIELD TECHNIQUE)

Once the motor strip has indirectly been identified by the phase reversal technique, direct cortical stimulation is needed to confirm the localization of the motor cortex. Most current methods are based on the original Penfield technique. This calls for continuous direct cortical stimulation over a period of a few seconds with a frequency of

stimulation of 50 to 60 Hz and observation of muscle movements.[14,16,27] An initial current intensity of 4 mA is used and, if no movements are elicited in contralateral muscles of the limbs and face, stimulation is increased in steps of 2 mA to the point at which movements are elicited.[16] Muscle responses can either be observed visually or documented by multichannel electromyography, which appears to be more sensitive.[28] If no response is elicited with an intensity as high as approximately 16 mA, that area of cortex is considered not functional and can therefore be removed.[29] It should be emphasized that a negative mapping does not always ensure safety. To increase the chances of obtaining a positive mapping result, technical and anesthesiologic drawbacks have to be carefully ruled out and cortical exposure should be generous.

More in general, a limitation to the reliability of cortical mapping is the large variability of threshold for a positive mapping response across and within individuals.[30] A motor response from the same muscular group can be elicited from more than one cortical site, using different stimulation intensities.

Therefore, function localization may vary in different studies as a result of stimulation parameters and mapping strategies. Mapping strategies appear as one of the main variables that may affect the results of stimulation. Two different theories underline the choice of one or the other strategy:

1. Some authors apply the concept that thresholds (the minimum stimulation current required to induce functional changes) vary across the exposed cortex depending on the task being assessed and the location being maped. This is in keeping with the observation that even afterdischarge (AD) thresholds can vary significantly, not only across the population but in the same subject at different cortical sites.[30,31] Accordingly, they attempt to

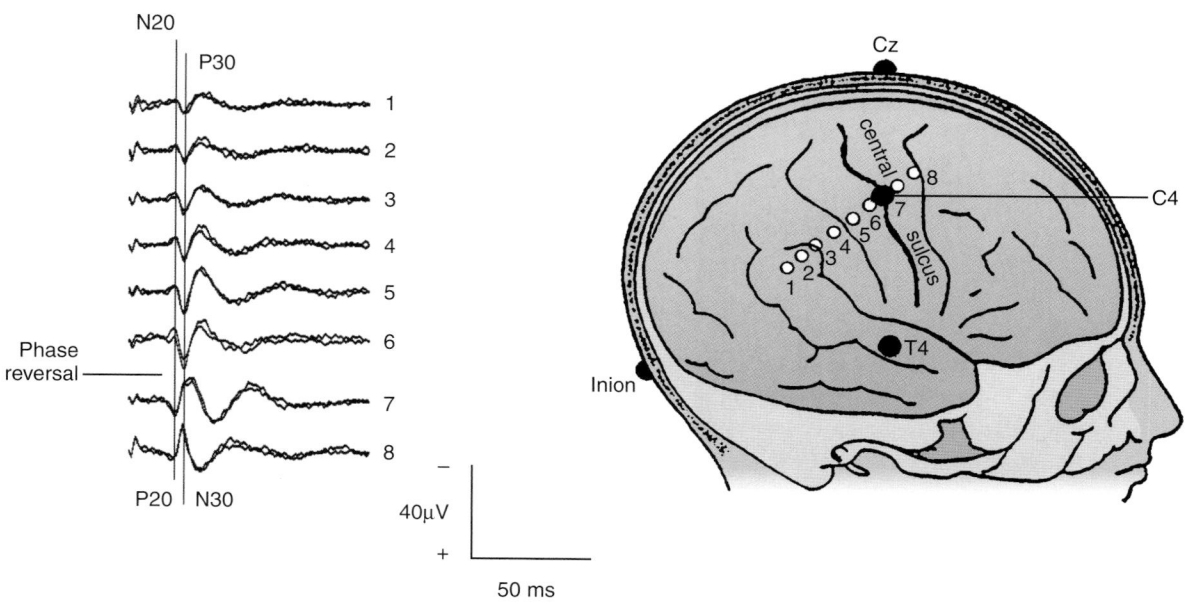

FIGURE 4-1 Identification of the central sulcus by phase reversal of median nerve cortical somatosensory-evoked potentials. To the right is a schematic drawing of the exposed brain surface with a grid electrode position orthogonally to the central sulcus. On the left are the recorded evoked potentials phase reversed between electrode 6 and 7, showing a mirror image of the evoked potential between the motor and sensory cortices, depicting the central sulcus lying between electrodes 6 and 7. *(From Deletis V. Intraoperative neurophysiological monitoring. In: McLone D, ed. Pediatric Neurosurgery: Surgery of the Developing Nervous System, 4th ed. Philadelphia: WB Saunders; 1999:1204-1213.)*

maximize stimulation currents at each cortical site to ensure the absence of eloquent function. Doing so, it is more common to exceed AD thresholds in adjacent cortices, and there is a higher risk of distal activation due to current spreading to adjacent sites.

2. Other authors[29,32,33] keep stimulation intensity constant while mapping the entire cortex and set threshold just below the lowest current observed to induce AD. This strategy is aimed to minimize the risk of inducing ADs (which may invalidate the results) and clinical seizures, but may miss the identification of eloquent cortical sites.

Spreading of the current using the 60-Hz stimulation technique is limited to 2 to 3 mm as detected by optical imaging in monkeys.[34] Accordingly, one can assume that using this technique is safe for removal of tumors very close to the motor and sensory pathways as long as stimulation is repeated whenever a 2- to 3-mm section of tumoral tissue is removed.[29] Similarly, this technique allows us to map motor pathways subcortically while removing tumors that arise or extend to the insular, subinsular, or thalamic areas.[27,35] At the subcortical level, the stimulation intensity required to elicit a motor response is usually lower than that required for cortical mapping. When performing subcortical mapping, however, we have

to keep in mind that a distal muscle response after stimulation of subcortical motor pathways can be misleading. Although this stimulation activates axons distal to the stimulation point, the possibility of damage to the pathways proximal to that point cannot be ruled out. This is a concern, especially when dealing with an insular tumor where there is a risk of cortical or subcortical ischemia induction secondary to manipulation of perforating vessels (Fig. 4-2).

Despite its popularity in the past, this 60-Hz Penfield technique has some disadvantages. With the exception of speech mapping, it is our opinion that these disadvantages should prevent its use as a motor cortex/pathways mapping technique. First, this technique can induce seizures in as many as 20% of patients, despite therapeutic levels of anticonvulsants and regardless of whether there is a preoperative history of intractable epilepsy.[36,37] Second, in children younger than 5 years old, direct stimulation of the motor cortex for mapping purposes may not yield localizing information because of the relative unexcitability of the motor cortex.[19,38] Third, because this is a mapping and not a monitoring technique, no matter how often cortical or subcortical stimulation is repeated, the functional integrity of the motor pathways cannot be assessed continuously during surgery.

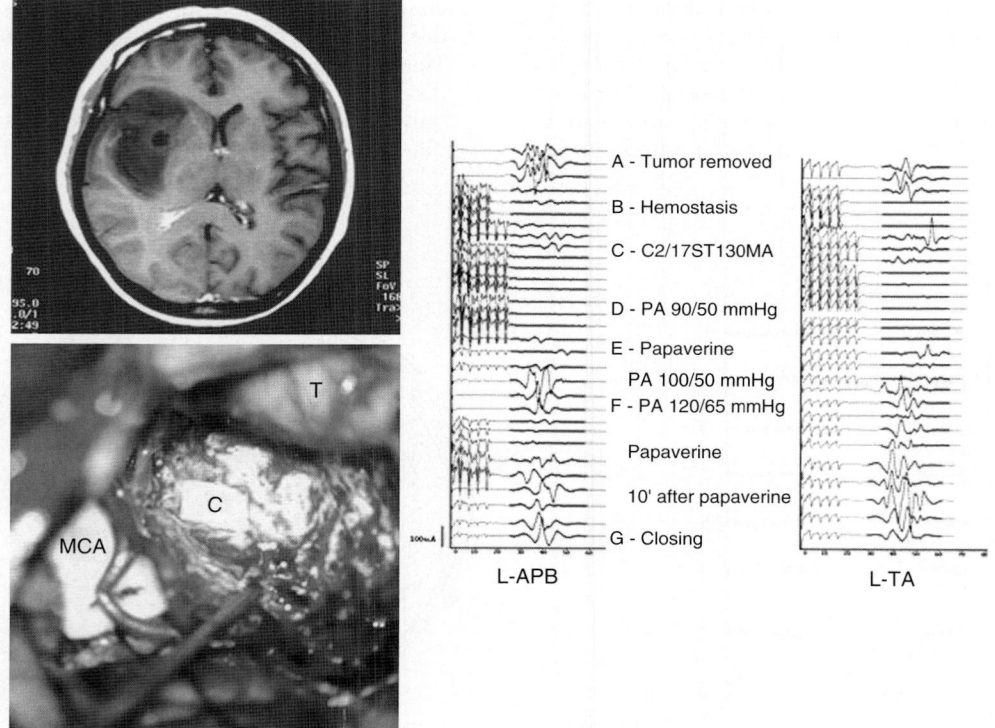

FIGURE 4-2 *Upper left*: Preoperative axial contrast-enhanced, magnetic-resonance, T1-weighted image of a right frontotemporoinsular anaplastic astrocytoma that was removed with the assistance of intraoperative neurophysiologic monitoring. *Lower left*: Intraoperative view at the end of tumor resection. The internal capsule (*C*) has been identified using mapping of the subcortical motor pathways with the short train of stimuli technique. The temporal lobe (*T*) and branches of the middle cerebral artery (*MCA*) are on view. *Right*: Motor-evoked potentials (MEPs) recorded intraoperatively from the left abductor brevis pollicis (*L-APB*) and tibialis anterior (*L-TA*) muscles. MEP recordings at the end of tumor removal (*A*); MEP loss during hemostasis (*B*); transitory MEP reappearance by increasing stimulation to seven stimuli and 130-mA intensity (*C*); new disappearance of MEPs despite increased stimulation (*D*); progressive MEP reappearance after papaverine infusion and increased systemic blood pressure (*E* and *F*); MEPs at the end of the procedure (*G*). *(Modified from Sala F, Lanteri P. Brain surgery in motor areas: The invaluable assistance of intraoperative neurophysiological monitoring. J Neurosurg Sci. 2003;47:79-88.)*

DIRECT CORTICAL STIMULATION AND MOTOR-EVOKED POTENTIAL MONITORING (SHORT TRAIN OF STIMULI TECHNIQUE)

Recently, mapping techniques have integrated monitoring techniques to continuously assess the functional integrity of the motor pathways and therefore increase the safety of these procedures.[20,39-41] The following is a description of the technique that we use at our institutions and have found suitable for both mapping and monitoring.

Muscle MEPs are initially elicited by multipulse transcranial electrical stimulation (TES). Short trains of five to seven square-wave stimuli of 500-μsec duration with an interstimulus interval of 4 msec are applied at a repetition rate of as high as 2 Hz through electrodes placed at C1 and C2 scalp sites, according to the 10–20 International Electroencephalography System. The maximum stimulation intensity should be as high as 200 mA, which is strong enough for most cases. Muscle responses are recorded via needle electrodes inserted into the contralateral upper and lower extremity muscles. We usually monitored the abductor pollicis brevis and the extensor digitorum communis for the upper extremities and the tibialis anterior and the abductor hallucis for the lower extremities. For the face area, the orbicularis oculi and orbicularis oris muscles are typically used.

After exposure of the cortex and once phase reversal has been performed, direct cortical stimulation of the motor cortex can be achieved by using a monopolar-stimulating probe to identify the cortical representation of contralateral facial and limb muscles. The same parameters of stimulation used for TES, except for a much lower intensity (≤20 mA), can be used.[39] Sometimes the short train of stimuli technique requires slightly higher current intensities than those required by the Penfield technique. However, by using a very short train, the charge applied to the brain is significantly reduced[42] and, consequently, the risk of inducing seizures. The number of pulses in the short-train technique is five to seven pulses per second, whereas in the Penfield technique, there are 60 pulses per second. The effect of stimulation on the cerebral cortex, from a neurophysiologic point of view, differs between the Penfield technique and the short train of stimuli technique. The Penfield technique delivers one stimulus every 15 to 20 msec continuously for a couple of seconds. The short train of stimuli technique delivers five to seven stimuli in a period of approximately 30 msec with a long pause between trains (470 to 970 msec, which depends on train repetition rate—1 or 2 Hz). Therefore, the Penfield technique is more prone to produce seizures, activating the cortical circuitry more easily than short-train stimuli do. Furthermore, compared with the Penfield technique, the short-train technique does not induce strong muscle twitches that may interfere with the surgical procedure. Responses are usually recorded from needle electrodes used to record muscle MEPs elicited by TES. However, any combination of recording muscles can be used, according to the tumor location. The larger the number of monitored muscles, the lower the chance of a false-negative mapping result. We suggest that stimulation of the tumoral area should always be performed to rule out the presence of some functional cortex. As already described, this is especially true in the case of low-grade gliomas.[3-5]

In the illustrative case presented in Fig. 4-2,[39] an impairment of muscle MEPs occurred at the end of tumor removal when opening and closing mapping procedures had already been done and confirmed the integrity of motor pathways distal to the stimulation point at the level of the internal capsule. However, ischemia of the pyramidal tracts secondary to severe vasospasm of the main perforating branches of the middle cerebral artery occurred during hemostasis and was detected by muscle MEP monitoring. If not detected in time, this event would have likely resulted in an irreversible loss of muscle MEPs and, consequently, a permanent motor deficit. Mapping techniques are unlikely to detect these events because they do not allow a continuous "online" assessment of the functional integrity of neural pathways.

In our experience with using the short-train technique, a threshold lower than 5 mA for eliciting muscle MEPs usually indicated proximity to the motor cortex. When muscle responses are elicited through higher stimulation intensities, activation of the CT is of less localizing value because of the possibility of spreading of the current to adjacent areas.[39]

Once mapping of the cortex has clarified the relationship between eloquent motor areas and the lesion, continuous MEP monitoring of the contralateral muscles can be sustained throughout the procedure to assist during the surgical manipulation. To do so, one of the same contacts of the strip electrode can be used as an anode for stimulation while the cathode is at Fz. The stimulation point on the motor cortex with the lowest threshold used to elicit muscle MEPs from contralateral limbs or face usually corresponds with the contact from which the largest amplitude of the mirror-image SEPs was obtained. The same stimulation parameters as those used for the short-train mapping technique can be used.

When removing a tumor that extends subcortically, preservation of muscle MEPs during monitoring from the strip electrode will guarantee the functional integrity of motor pathways and avoid the need for periodic remapping of the cortex at known functional sites.[39]

For insular tumors where the motor cortex is not exposed by the craniotomy, a strip electrode can still be gently inserted into the subdural space to overlap the motor cortex. Phase reversal and/or direct cortical stimulation can be used to identify the electrode with the lowest threshold to elicit muscle MEPs. The use of MEPs during surgery for insular tumors has proved very useful to identify impending vascular derangements to subcortical motor pathways in time for corrective measures to be taken. In spite of the observation that intraoperative MEP changes occurred in nearly half of the procedures, these were reversible in two thirds of the cases.[43]

WARNING CRITERIA AND CORRELATION WITH POSTOPERATIVE OUTCOME

Still debated are the warning criteria for changes in muscle MEPs that are used to inform the surgeon about an impending injury to the motor system. It should be stressed that although for spinal cord surgery, a "presence/absence" of muscle MEPs criterion has proved to be reliable and strictly correlates with postoperative results,[44,45] there are not definite MEP parameters indicative of significant impairment during supratentorial surgery.[46] We believe that the predictive value of muscle MEPs is different for supratentorial and spinal cord surgeries. As such, different warning criteria must be employed. This judgment is based on the difference in types of CT fibers in supratentorial portion of the CT as compared with the spinal cord. Different groups with established experience in this field have proposed similar criteria,[40,46] suggesting that a shift in latency between 10% and 15% and a decrease in amplitude of more than 50% to 80% correlate with some degree of postoperative motor deficit. However, a permanent new motor deficit has consistently correlated only with irreversible complete loss of muscle MEPs.[46]

A persistent increase in the threshold to elicit muscle MEPs or a persistent drop in muscle MEP amplitude, despite stable systemic blood pressure, anesthesia, and body temperature, represents a warning sign. However, it should be noted that muscle MEPs are easily affected by muscle relaxants, bolus of intravenous anesthetics and high concentrations of volatile (and other) anesthetics such that wide variation in muscle MEP amplitude and latency can be observed.[47] Due to this variability, the multisynaptic nature of the pathways involved in the generation of muscle MEPs, and the nonlinear relationship between stimulus intensity and the amplitude of muscle MEPs, the correlation between intraoperative changes in muscle MEPs (amplitude and/or latency) and the motor outcome are not linear. Further clinical investigation is needed to clarify sensitive and specific neurophysiologic warning criteria for brain surgery.

Brain Stem Surgery

The human brain stem is a small and highly complex structure containing a variety of critical neural structures. These include sensory and motor pathways; sensory and motor cranial nerve nuclei; cardiovascular and respiratory centers; neural networks supporting swallowing, coughing, articulation, and oculomotor reflexes; and the reticular activating system. In such a complex neural structure, even small lesions can produce severe and life-threatening neurologic deficits.

The neurosurgeon faces two major problems when attempting to remove brain stem tumors. First, if the tumor is intrinsic and does not protrude on the brain stem surface, approaching the tumor implies a violation of the anatomic integrity of the brain stem. Knowledge of the location of critical neural pathways and nuclei is mandatory when considering a safe entry into the brain stem,[48,49] but may not suffice when anatomy is distorted. Morota and colleagues[50] reported that visual identification of the facial colliculus based on anatomic landmarks was possible in only three of seven medullary tumors and was not possible in five pontine tumors. The striae medullares were visible in four of five patients with pontine tumors and in five of nine patients with medullary tumors.

Therefore, functional rather than anatomic localization of brain stem nuclei and pathways should be used to identify safe entry zones.

MAPPING TECHNIQUES

Neurophysiologic mapping techniques have been increasingly used to localize CT and cranial nerve motor nuclei on the lateral aspect of the midbrain and on the floor of the fourth ventricle.[50-54]

MAPPING OF THE CORTICOSPINAL TRACT AT THE LEVEL OF THE CEREBRAL PEDUNCLE

This is a recently described technique used to map the CT tract within the brain stem at the level of the cerebral peduncle.[54,55] To identify the CT, we use a hand-held monopolar-stimulating probe (0.75-mm tip diameter) as a cathode, with a needle electrode inserted in a nearby muscle as an anode. If the response (D wave) is recorded from an epidural electrode, a single stimulus is used. Conversely, if the response is recorded as a compound muscle action potential from one or more muscles of contralateral limbs, a short train of stimuli should be used.

We usually increase stimulation intensity to 2 mA. When a motor response is recorded, the probe is then moved in small increments of 1 mm to find the lowest threshold to elicit that response.

This technique is particularly useful for midbrain tumors that have displaced the CT tract from its original position. Usually, the so-called midbrain lateral vein described by Rhoton[56] represents a useful anatomic landmark because it allows an indirect identification of the CT tract, located anterior to the vein. However, when an expansive lesion distorts anatomy, only neurophysiologic mapping allows the identification of the CT and, consequently, a safe entry zone to the lateral midbrain.

In the case of a cystic midbrain lesion, sometimes mapping of the CT is negative at the beginning of the procedure, but a positive response can be recorded when mapping from within the cystic cavity toward the anterolateral cystic wall.[57]

MAPPING OF MOTOR NUCLEI OF CRANIAL NERVES ON THE FLOOR OF THE FOURTH VENTRICLE

This technique is based on intraoperative electrical stimulation of the motor nuclei of the cranial nerves on the floor of the fourth ventricle, using a hand-held monopolar stimulating probe. Compound muscle action potentials are then elicited in the muscles innervated by the cranial motor nerves. A single stimulus of 0.2-msec duration is delivered at a repetitive rate of 2.0 Hz. Stimulation intensity starts at approximately 1 mA and is then reduced to determine the point with the lowest threshold that elicits muscle responses corresponding with the mapped nucleus (Fig. 4-3). No stimulation intensity higher than 2 mA should be used.[50,51] To record the responses from cranial motor nerves VII, IX/X, and XII, wire electrodes are inserted into the orbicularis oculi and orbicularis oris muscles, the posterior wall of the pharynx, and the lateral aspect of the tongue muscles, respectively. Based on mapping studies, characteristic patterns of motor cranial nerve displacement, secondary to tumor growth, have been described (Fig. 4-4).[58] The case described in Fig. 4-5 is consistent with this observation.

A similar methodology can be applied to identify the motor nuclei of cranial nerves innervating ocular muscles (nerves III, IV, and VI) during a dorsal approach to midbrain lesions as well as quadrigeminal plate, tectal, and pineal region tumors.[59,60]

Despite the relative straightforwardness of the fourth ventricle mapping technique and its indisputable usefulness in planning the most appropriate surgical strategy to enter the

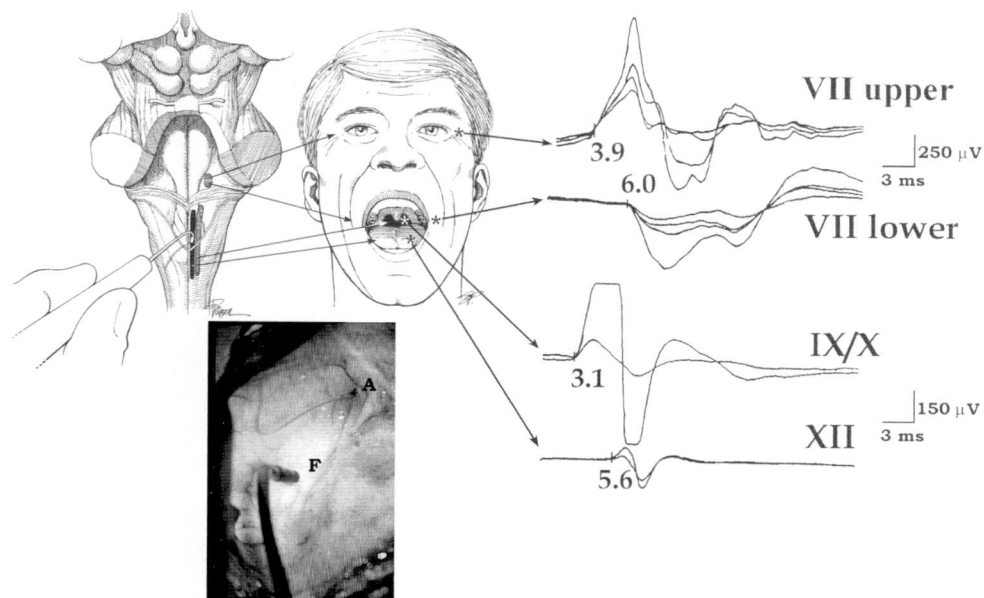

FIGURE 4-3 Mapping of the brain stem cranial nerve motor nuclei. *Upper left*: Drawing of the exposed floor of the fourth ventricle with the surgeon's handheld stimulating probe in view. *Upper middle*: The sites of insertion of wire hook electrodes for recording the muscle responses are depicted. *Far upper right*: Compound muscle action potentials recorded from the orbicularis oculi and oris muscles after stimulation of the upper and lower facial nuclei (upper two traces) and from the pharyngeal wall and tongue muscles after stimulation of the motor nuclei of cranial nerves IX/X and XII (*lower two traces*). *Lower left*: Photograph obtained from the operating microscope shows the hand-held stimulating probe placed on the floor of the fourth ventricle (*F*). *A*, aqueduct. *(Reproduced from Deletis V, Sala F, Morota N. Intraoperative neurophysiological monitoring and mapping during brain stem surgery: A modern approach. Oper Tech Neurosurg. 2000;3:109-113.)*

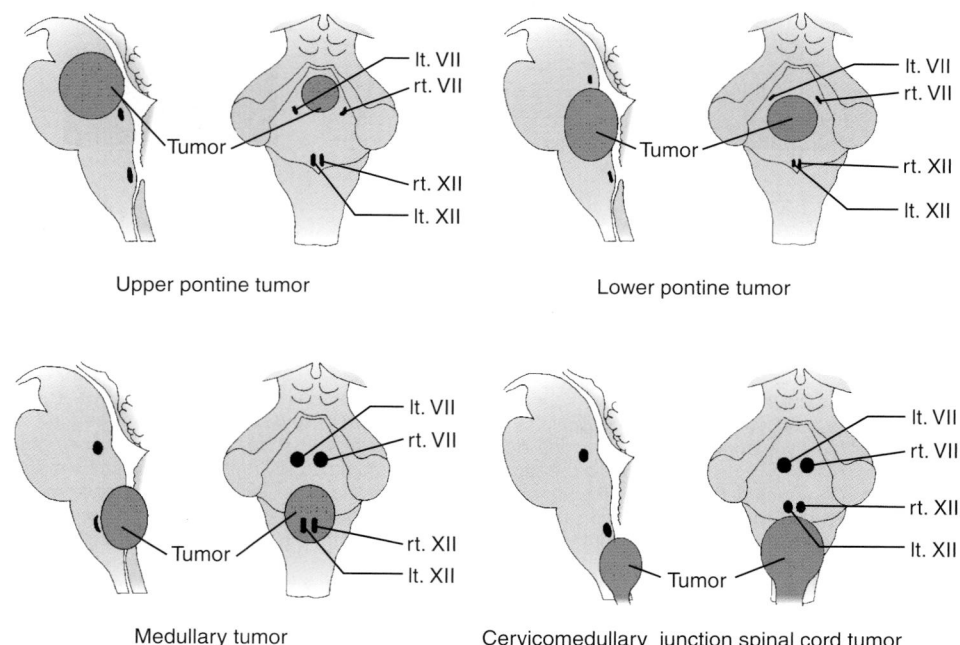

FIGURE 4-4 Typical patterns of cranial nerve motor nuclei displacement by brain stem tumors in different locations. *Upper and lower pontine tumors*: Pontine tumors typically grow to push the facial nuclei around the edge of the tumor, suggesting that precise localization of the facial nuclei before tumor resection is necessary to avoid their damage during surgery. *Medullary tumors*: Medullary tumors typically grow more exophytically and compress the lower cranial nerve motor nuclei ventrally; these nuclei may be located on the ventral edge of the tumor cavity. Because of the interposed tumor, in these cases mapping before tumor resection usually does not allow identification of cranial nerve IX/X and XII motor nuclei. Responses, however, could be obtained close to the end of the tumor resection when most of the tumoral tissue between the stimulating probe and the motor nuclei has been removed. At this point, repeat mapping is recommended because the risk of damaging motor nuclei is significantly higher than at the beginning of tumor debulking. *Cervicomedullary junction spinal cord tumors*: These tumors simply push the lower cranial nerve motor nuclei rostrally when extending into the fourth ventricle. *(Reproduced from Morota N, Deletis V, Lee M, et al. Functional anatomic relationship between brain stem tumors and cranial motor nuclei. Neurosurgery. 1996;39:787-794.)*

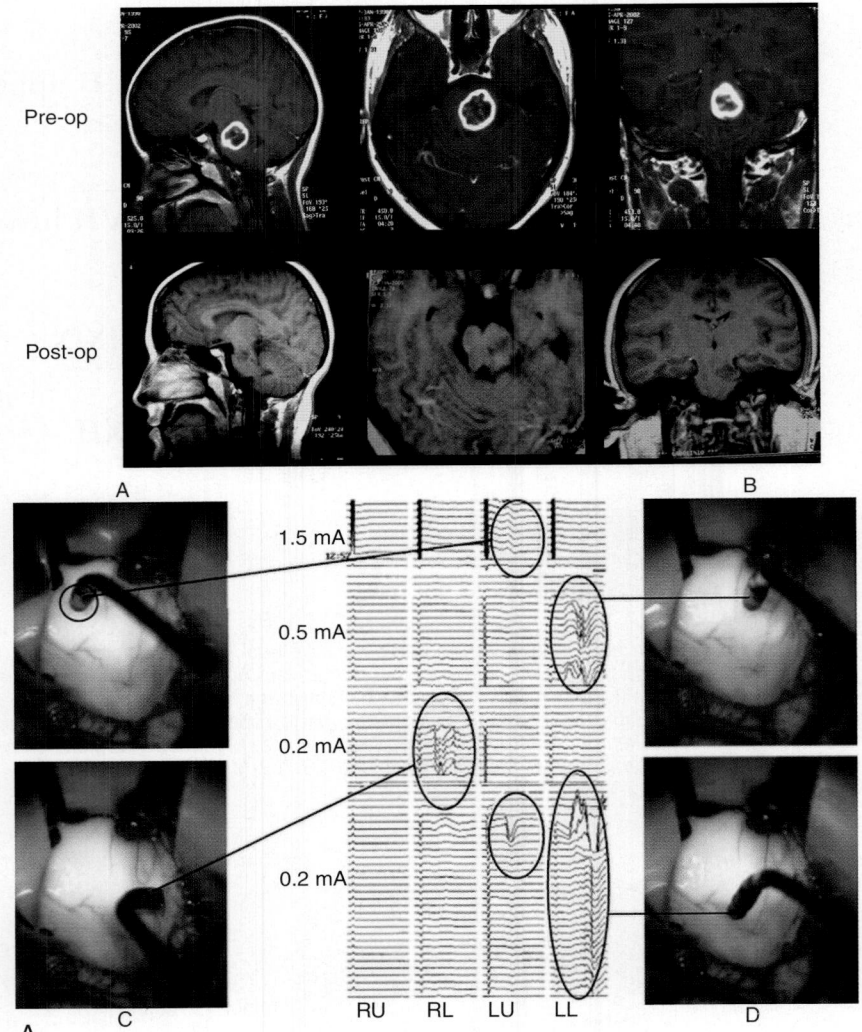

FIGURE 4-5 *Upper panel: (Top):* Preoperative contrast-enhanced, T1-weighted magnetic resonance imaging (MRI) of an upper left pontine low-grade astrocytoma in a 16 year old female. *Bottom:* Postoperative MRI study showing complete tumor removal. Surgery was performed under neurophysiologic guidance. *Middle panel:* Direct mapping of the facial nerve motor nuclei on the floor of the fourth ventricle. The tumor was approached through a median suboccipital craniectomy. When the floor of the fourth ventricle was exposed, the median sulcus appeared dislocated to the right and the left median eminence was expanded. Electromyographic wire electrodes were inserted bilaterally in the left (*LU*) and right (*RU*) orbicularis oculi and left (*LL*) and right (*RL*) orbicularis oris muscles for mapping and monitoring of the seventh nerve, and in the abductor pollicis brevis (*LA* and *RA*) for continuous monitoring of the corticospinal tract integrity. We initially stimulated on the left side, approximately 1.5 cm rostral to the striae medullares, where the motor nuclei were expected to be according to normal brain stem functional anatomy. A response was obtained from the left orbicularis oculi (*LU*) at a stimulation intensity of 1.5 mA (*A*). By moving the stimulating probe caudally and to the right, a consistent response from the left orbicularis oris (*LL*) was recorded at a stimulation intensity of 0.5 mA (*B*). At this point, we moved the stimulation probe more laterally to the right side, approximately 1 cm above the striae medullares, and a clear response was recorded from the right orbicularis oris (*RL*) at the lowest threshold intensity of 0.2 mA (*C*). Finally, by moving the stimulating probe paramedially to the left side, a few millimeters above the striae medullares, a consistent response was recorded from both the left orbicularis oris (*LL*) and orbicularis oculi (*LU*), using the same low threshold (0.2 mA) (*D*). The conclusion was drawn that the tumor displaced caudally the facial nerve motor nuclei, especially on the left side. Based on mapping results, the surgeon decided to enter the brain stem on the left side in correspondence with the higher threshold stimulating point (*A*).

Continued

brain stem, postoperative functional outcome is not always predicted by postresection responses.[50] In the case of mapping of the motor nuclei of the seventh cranial nerve, brain stem mapping cannot detect injury to the supranuclear tracts originating in the motor cortex and ending on the cranial nerve motor nuclei. Consequently, a supranuclear paralysis would not be detected, although lower motoneuron integrity has been preserved. Similarly, the possibility of stimulating the intramedullary root more than the nuclei itself exists.

This could result in a false-negative peripheral response still being recorded despite an injury to the motor nuclei.[50]

Mapping of the glossopharyngeal nuclei is also of limited benefit. Recording activity from the muscles of the posterior pharyngeal wall after stimulation of the ninth cranial nerve motor nuclei on the floor of the fourth ventricle assesses the functional integrity of the efferent arc of the swallowing reflex. This technique, however, does not provide information on the integrity of afferent pathways and

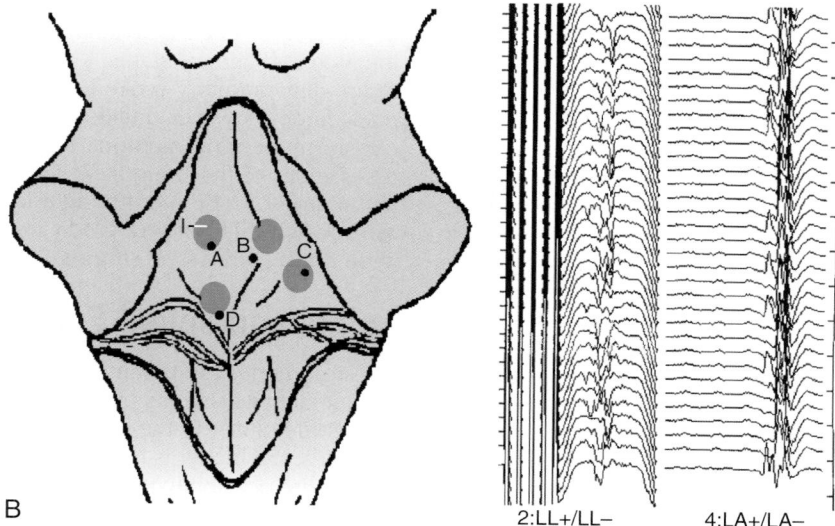

B

2:LL+/LL−   4:LA+/LA−

FIGURE 4-5, cont'd *Lower left*: Schematic summary of mapping results. *A* and *B* represent the original position of the left and right facial colliculi, as expected according to brain stem anatomy. *A, B, C,* and *D* correspond to the stimulating point illustrated in the upper panel. *C* and *D* also correspond to the lower threshold to elicit a consistent response from, respectively, the right and left muscles innervated by the facial nerve. The conclusion was made that real location of facial nerve motor nuclei (*C* and *D*) was more caudal than expected, especially on the left side, due to the tumor mass effect. Accordingly, initial incision (*I*) was carried on transversely in correspondence with stimulating point *A*. *Lower right*: Continuous neurophysiologic monitoring of muscle motor-evoked potentials during tumor removal. Electromyographic wire electrodes were inserted in the left orbicularis oris (*LL*) and abductor pollicis brevis (*LA*) muscles for continuous monitoring of, respectively, the corticobulbar and corticospinal tract integrity, after transcranial electrical stimulation (electrode montage C4/Cz; short train of four stimuli; intensity 50 mA). *(Modified from Sala F, Lanteri P, Bricolo A. Intraoperative neurophysiological monitoring of motor evoked potentials during brain stem and spinal cord surgery. Adv Tech Stand Neurosurg. 2004;29:133-169.)*

afferent/efferent connections within brain stem, which are indeed necessary to provide functions involving reflexive swallowing, coughing, and the complex act of articulation. Recently, however, Sakuma and colleagues[61] succeeded in monitoring glossopharyngeal nerve compound action potentials after stimulation of the tongue in dogs, opening the possibility of a new field of investigation in humans. Functional magnetic resonance imaging of the brain stem has also provided a new, yet experimental, tool to localize cranial nerve nuclei in humans.[62]

An intrinsic limitation of all mapping techniques, however, is that these do not allow the continuous evaluation of the functional integrity of a neural pathway. The identification of the safe entry zone for approaching a pontine astrocytoma, as in Fig. 4-5, does not provide any information on the well-being of the adjacent corticospinal, corticobulbar, sensory, and auditory pathways during the surgical manipulation aimed to remove the tumor. Therefore, it is essential to combine mapping with monitoring techniques.

MONITORING TECHNIQUES

SEPs and brain stem auditory-evoked potentials have been extensively used to assess the functional integrity of the brain stem, and we refer the reader to the related literature for a review of these classic techniques. Unfortunately, SEPs and brain stem auditory-evoked potentials can evaluate only approximately 20% of brain stem pathways.[63] As a result, their use is of limited valued when the major concern is related to corticospinal and cranial nerve motor function. Still, brain stem auditory-evoked potentials can provide useful information on the general well-being of the brain stem, especially during those procedures in which a significant surgical

manipulation of the brain stem and/or of the cerebellum is expected. When interpreting brain stem auditory-evoked potential recordings, a thoughtful analysis of the waveform and of their correlation with neural generators provides useful information about the localization of the changes.

When an initial myelotomy is performed at the region of dorsal column nuclei of the medulla, further monitoring with SEPs is compromised due to limitations similar to those related to intramedullary spinal cord tumor surgery after myelotomy.[54] For pontine and midbrain tumors, SEPs have little localizing value but can still be used to provide nonspecific information about the general functional integrity of the brain stem (because it is expected that a major impending brain stem failure will be detected by changes in SEP parameters).

Similar to what has occurred for brain and spinal cord surgery, the major breakthrough in modern ION of the brain stem has been the advent of MEP-related techniques.

With regard to motor function within the brain stem, standard techniques for continuously assessing the functional integrity of motor cranial nerves relies on the recording of spontaneous electromyographic activity in the muscles innervated by motor cranial nerves.[60,64,65] Several criteria have been proposed to identify electromyographic activity patterns that may anticipate transitory or permanent nerve injury, but these patterns are not always easily recognizable and criteria remain vague or at least subjective. Overall, convincing data regarding a clinical correlation between electromyographic activity and clinical outcomes is still lacking.[60,64]

Seeking more reliable techniques in the neurophysiologic monitoring of motor cranial nerve integrity, the possibility of extending the principles of CT monitoring to the corticobulbar tracts is currently under investigation.[57,66]

Monitoring of Corticobulbar (Corticonuclear) Pathways

For this purpose, TES with a train of four stimuli, with an interstimulus interval of 4 msec, and a train-stimulating rate of 1 to 2 Hz, intensity between 60 and 100 mA can be used. The stimulating electrode montage is usually C3/Cz for right-side muscles and C4/Cz for left-side muscles. For recording muscle MEPs, electromyographic wire electrodes are inserted in the orbicularis oris and orbicularis oculi muscles for nerve VII, in the posterior pharyngeal wall for the cranial motor nerves IX and X, and in the tongue muscles for the hypoglossal nerve (i.e., in the same manner as described for mapping of motor nuclei of the cranial nerves). Reproducible muscle MEPs can be continuously recorded from the facial, pharyngeal, and tongue muscles while the brain stem is surgically manipulated (see Fig. 4-5). This technique allows one to monitor the entire pathway, from the motor cortex down to the neuromuscular junction so that a supranuclear injury can be detected. However, the corticobulbar tract monitoring technique is still far from becoming standardized due to some theoretical and practical drawbacks. First, from a neurophysiologic perspective, use of the lateral montage as an anodal stimulating electrode (C3 or C4) increases the risk that strong TES may not activate the corticobulbar pathways but the cranial nerve directly. Accordingly, an injury to the corticobulbar pathway rostral to the point of activation may be masked by a misleading preservation of the muscle MEP. To minimize this risk, stimulation intensity should be kept as low as possible. One of the ways to recognize structure generating this response is as follows; 90 msec after delivering train of stimuli a single stimulus was delivered through the same stimulating montage. The rationale for this kind of stimulation is the fact that in most patients under general anesthesia, only a short train of stimuli can elicit "central" responses generated by the motor cortex or subcortical part of corticobulbar tract (CBT). If a single stimulus elicits a response, this should be considered a "peripheral" response which activates the cranial nerve directly by spreading current more distally.[67]

Furthermore, given the continuous fluctuations in the threshold required to elicit muscle MEPs intraoperatively (i.e., due to variability in room temperature, anesthesiologic regimen, and physiologic variability in muscle MEP threshold, and so on), the appropriate threshold for monitoring corticobulbar pathways should be rechecked throughout the surgical procedure. Another limitation of this technique is that spontaneous electromyographic activity can sometimes hinder the recording of reliable muscle MEPs from the same muscles. In our experience, this spontaneous activity appears to be more common in the pharyngeal muscles as compared with the facial and tongue muscles. Further experience with this technique will indicate the extent to which monitoring of the corticobulbar tract predicts postoperative function and allows an impending injury to the motor cranial nerves to be recognized in time to be corrected (see Fig. 4-5).

Due to the complexity of the brain stem's functional anatomy, the more neurophysiologic techniques that can be rationally integrated, the better the chances for successful monitoring.[68] The battery of techniques to be used should be tailored to each individual patient according to tumor location and clinical status. Keeping this in mind, SEPs and brain stem auditory-evoked potentials should always be considered. However, unlike in the past decade when these classic monitoring methods allowed only a very limited assessment of the brain stem functional integrity, current techniques of MEP monitoring and motor nuclei mapping are receiving increasing credit in assisting the neurosurgeon during brain stem surgery.

Spinal and Spinal Cord Surgery

These surgeries are potentially burdened with serious neurologic deficits such as para- or quadri-plegia (paresis). As a rule, the closer to the spinal cord that the neurosurgeon operates, the higher is the risk of injury. Of course, there is always the possibility that surgeries on the bony structures of the spinal cord can result in paraplegia.[69,70] Furthermore, long-lasting intraoperative hypotension can be disastrous for the spinal cord if neurophysiologic monitoring has not been used because no other routine methods are available to evaluate the functional integrity of the spinal cord during hypotension.

It has been shown that the use of SEPs to monitor the functional integrity of the spinal cord is inadequate and can result in false-negative results (i.e., no changes in SEP parameters intraoperatively, but the patient wakes up paraplegic after surgery[69,70]). Therefore, it is mandatory that during spinal and spinal cord surgeries, monitoring of both sensory and motor modalities of evoked potentials is conducted. Each of these methods evaluates different long tracts; SEPs evaluate the dorsal columns, whereas MEPs evaluate CT If a lesion to the spinal cord is diffuse in nature, affecting both long tracts, monitoring one of them may suffice. Unfortunately, this is not always the case. A typical example is anterior spinal cord artery syndrome with preservation of SEPs and disappearance of MEPs.[70]

Surgery for intramedullary spinal cord tumors requires a special approach concerning monitoring with MEPs. During this type of surgery, very precise surgical instruments are used, such as the Contact Laser System (SLT, Montgomeryville, PA),[71] and a very selective lesion within the spinal cord can occur. Therefore, monitoring this type of surgery using only MEPs recorded from limb muscles can be insufficient. Monitoring the D wave (i.e., recording descending activity of the CT using catheter electrodes placed over the exposed spinal cord) should be combined with MEP recording from limb muscles. Combining both of these techniques proved highly effective in preventing paraplegia/quadriplegia. This gives the neurosurgeon the opportunity to be more radical in tumor resection. This combined type of monitoring can precisely predict transient postoperative motor deficits[45,72] and clearly distinguish them from permanent ones.

NEUROPHYSIOLOGIC MONITORING OF THE SPINAL CORD AND SPINAL SURGERIES WITH MOTOR-EVOKED POTENTIALS

A schematic drawing of techniques for eliciting MEPs by TES or direct electrical stimulation of the exposed motor cortex while recording them from the spinal cord (D wave) or limb muscles (muscle MEPs) is presented in Fig. 4-6.

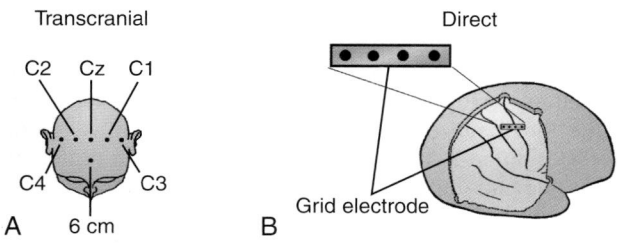

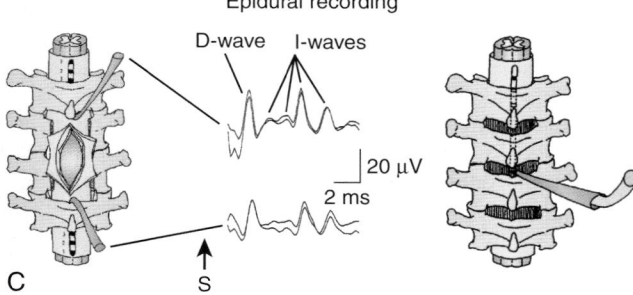

Epidural recording

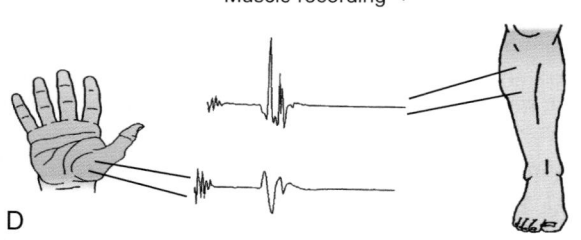

Muscle recording

FIGURE 4-6 A, Schematic illustration of electrode positions for transcranial electrical stimulation of the motor cortex according to the 10-20 International Electroencephalography System. The site labeled *6 cm* is 6 cm anterior to Cz. B, Illustration of grid electrode overlying the motor and sensory cortexes. C, Schematic diagram of the positions of the catheter electrodes (each with three recording cylinders) placed cranial to the tumor (control electrode) and caudal to the tumor to monitor the descending signal after passing through the site of surgery (*left*). In the middle are *D* and *I waves* recorded rostral and caudal to the tumor site. On the right is depicted the placement of an epidural electrode through a flavectomy/flavotomy when the spinal cord is not exposed. D, Recording of muscle motor-evoked potentials from the thenar and tibial anterior muscles after eliciting them with short train of stimuli applied either transcranially or over the exposed motor cortex. (*Modified from Deletis V, Rodi Z, Amassian VE. Neurophysiological mechanisms underlying motor evoked potentials in anesthetized humans. Part 2: Relationship between epidurally and muscle recorded MEPs in man. Clin Neurophysiol 2001;112:445-452.*)

Table 4-1 summarizes the results from the combined use of D-wave and muscle MEP recordings during surgery for intramedullary spinal cord tumors. The neurosurgeon can proceed with the surgery aggressively, without jeopardizing the patient's motor status despite the complete disappearance of the muscle MEPs during surgery. This is only allowed when the D-wave amplitude does not decrease more than 50% from the baseline amplitude. After disappearance of muscle MEPs, patients will have only transient postoperative motor deficits, with a full recovery of muscle strength later on. Therefore, to achieve a good postoperative motor outcome, it is imperative that the critical decrement in D-wave amplitude not be permitted. The neurophysiologic

Table 4-1   Principles of Motor-Evoked Potential Interpretation

D Wave	Muscle MEP*	Motor Status
Unchanged or 30%–50% decrease	Preserved	Unchanged
Unchanged or 30%–50% decrease	Lost uni- or bilaterally	Transient motor deficit
>50% decrease	Lost bilaterally	Long-term motor deficit

*In the tibial anterior muscle(s).
Source: Deletis V. Intraoperative neurophysiological monitoring. In: McLone D. Pediatric Neurosurgery: Surgery of the Developing Nervous System, 4th ed. Philadelphia: WB Saunders; 1999:1204-1213.

explanation for transient paraplegia is that the D wave is generated exclusively by the descending activity of the transcranially activated fast neurons of the CT, whereas muscle MEPs are generated by the combined action of the fast neurons of the CT and propriospinal and other descending tracts within the spinal cord (of course, with consecutive activation of alpha motoneurons, peripheral nerves, and muscles). The selective lesion to the propriospinal and other descending tracts can occur with the use of precise neurosurgical instruments (e.g., contact laser with a tip of 200 μm, producing minimal collateral damage).[71] Lesioning of the propriospinal system and other descending tracts can be functionally compensated postoperatively, whereas a lesion to the fast neurons of the CT cannot. Empirically, we have discovered that decrements in the amplitude of the D wave occur in a stepwise fashion (except in the case of anterior spinal artery lesion). Therefore, the neurosurgeon has enough time to make a decision and can immediately stop the surgery when a critical decrement in D-wave amplitude occurs. The previous statement has been tested in 100 surgeries for intramedullary spinal cord tumors performed by one neurosurgeon and using a combined monitoring method. This approach showed a sensitivity of 100% and a specificity of 91%.[45] Based on these results, Table 4-1 was produced to explain the meaning and predictive features of combined monitoring of the spinal cord surgery using muscle MEPs and D wave.

Combined monitoring of MEPs in one typical patient with an intramedullary spinal cord tumor showed a disappearance of muscle MEPs and a sustained D wave. This resulted in a transient postoperative paraplegia, with a complete recovery from paraplegia, as presented in Fig. 4-7.

MAPPING OF THE CORTICOSPINAL TRACT WITHIN THE SURGICALLY EXPOSED SPINAL CORD

Further improvement in the prevention of lesioning of the CT during spinal cord surgery has been achieved by introducing a neurophysiologic method of mapping the CT by using a D-wave collision technique. This technique has recently been developed by our group and has allowed us to precisely map the anatomic location of the CT when the anatomy of the spinal cord has been distorted.[73,74] The anatomic position of the CT is difficult to determine by visual inspection alone. D-wave collision is accomplished by simultaneously stimulating the exposed spinal cord (with a small handheld probe delivering a 2-mA intensity stimulus), with TES to elicit a D wave. Because the resulting signals are

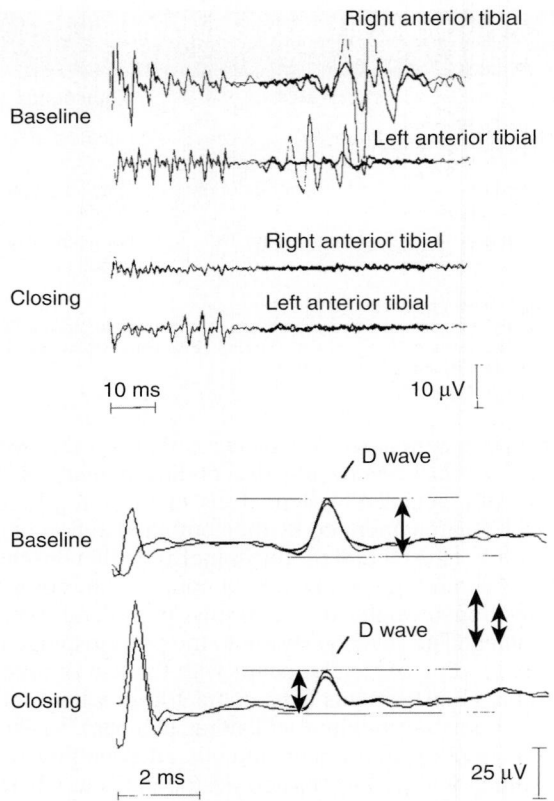

FIGURE 4-7 A 9-year-old boy underwent gross total resection of a pilocytic astrocytoma of the thoracic spinal cord that spanned four spinal segments. Preoperatively, there were no motor deficits. During surgery, the muscle motor-evoked potentials from the left and right tibial anterior muscles were lost (*upper*) and the *D wave* decreased, although not less than 50% of baseline value (*lower*). Postoperatively, the patient was paraplegic. Within 1 week, he regained antigravity force in both legs, and by 2 weeks he walked again. *(Reproduced from Kothbauer K, Deletis V, Epstein FJ. Intraoperative spinal cord monitoring for intramedullary surgery: An essential adjunct. Pediatr Neurosurg. 1997;26:247-254.)*

transmitted along the same axons, the descending D wave collides with the ascending signal carried antidromically along the CT (Fig. 4-8). This results in a decrease in the D-wave amplitude recorded cranially to the collision site. This phenomenon indicates that the spinal cord-stimulating probe is in close proximity to the CT. This could potentially guide surgeons to stay away from the "hot spot." Mapping of the CT is now in the process of a technical refinement. Its initial use indicates an impressive ability to selectively map the spinal cord for the CT's anatomic location. Using this method, the CT can be localized within 1 mm. This is in concordance with the other CT mapping techniques used within the brain stem that show the same degree of selectivity.[50]

MAPPING OF THE DORSAL COLUMNS OF THE SPINAL CORD

To protect the dorsal columns from lesioning during myelotomy, a novel neurophysiologic technique has been developed. To approach an intramedullary tumor, accepted neurosurgical techniques require a midline dorsal myelotomy. Distorted anatomy, however, often does not allow a precise determination of the anatomic midline by visual inspection and anatomic landmarks. Therefore, to facilitate the precise determination of the medial border between the left and right dorsal columns of the spinal cord, a technique for dorsal column mapping has been developed.[75] Dorsal column mapping is based on two basic principles. First, after stimulation of the peripheral nerves, evoked potentials traveling through the dorsal columns can be recorded. Second, the area over the dorsal columns of the spinal cord where the maximal amplitude of the SEPs is recorded represents the point on the recording electrode in closest proximity to the dorsal columns. For recording these traveling waves, a miniature multielectrode is placed over the surgically exposed dorsal columns of the spinal cord. This electrode consists of eight parallel wires, 76 μm in diameter and 2 mm in length, placed 1 mm apart and embedded in a 1-cm² (approximately) silicone plate (Fig. 4-9). An extremely precise amplitude gradient of the SEPs is recorded as the conducted potentials pass beneath the electrodes after alternating stimulation of the tibial nerves.

The amplitude gradient of the conducted potentials indicates the precise location of the functional midline corresponding to the dorsal fissure of the spinal cord (i.e., the optimal site for myelotomy). These data can be used by the neurosurgeon to prevent injury to the dorsal columns that could occur through an imprecise midline myelotomy. This is especially useful during surgery for intramedullary spinal cord tumors or during the placement of a shunt to drain syringomyelic cysts (see Fig. 4-9).[74]

NEUROPHYSIOLOGIC MONITORING DURING SPINAL ENDOVASCULAR PROCEDURES

Endovascular procedures for the embolization of spinal and spinal cord vascular lesions carry the risk of spinal cord ischemia.[76] Whenever these procedures are performed under general anesthesia, only neurophysiologic monitoring can provide an "online" assessment of the functional integrity of sensory and motor pathways. Monitoring of SEPs and muscle MEPs is performed in the same fashion as described for monitoring of intramedullary spinal cord tumor surgery.[77,78] The D wave, in contrast, is usually not monitored during these procedures because these patients receive a considerable amount of heparin in the perioperative period and the percutaneous placement of the recording epidural electrode would expose the patient to the risk of an epidural bleed. Besides safety issues, there is also no evidence that monitoring the D wave is an essential adjunct to muscle MEPs during these endovascular procedures. Both peripheral and myogenic MEPs have, in fact, been proven to be more sensitive than the D wave in detecting spinal cord ischemia. Similar results have been consistently reported both in experimental and clinical studies, supporting the hypothesis that whenever the mechanism of spinal cord injury is purely ischemic, muscle MEPs may suffice.[79-82] Given the complexity of spinal cord hemodynamics, which is even more unpredictable in the presence of a spinal cord hypervascularized lesion, it is mandatory to perform both SEP and MEP monitoring to enhance the safety of these risky procedures.[78]

A critical step regarding neurophysiologic monitoring during these procedures consists of the provocative tests.[78,83,84] These tests rely on the properties of two drugs,

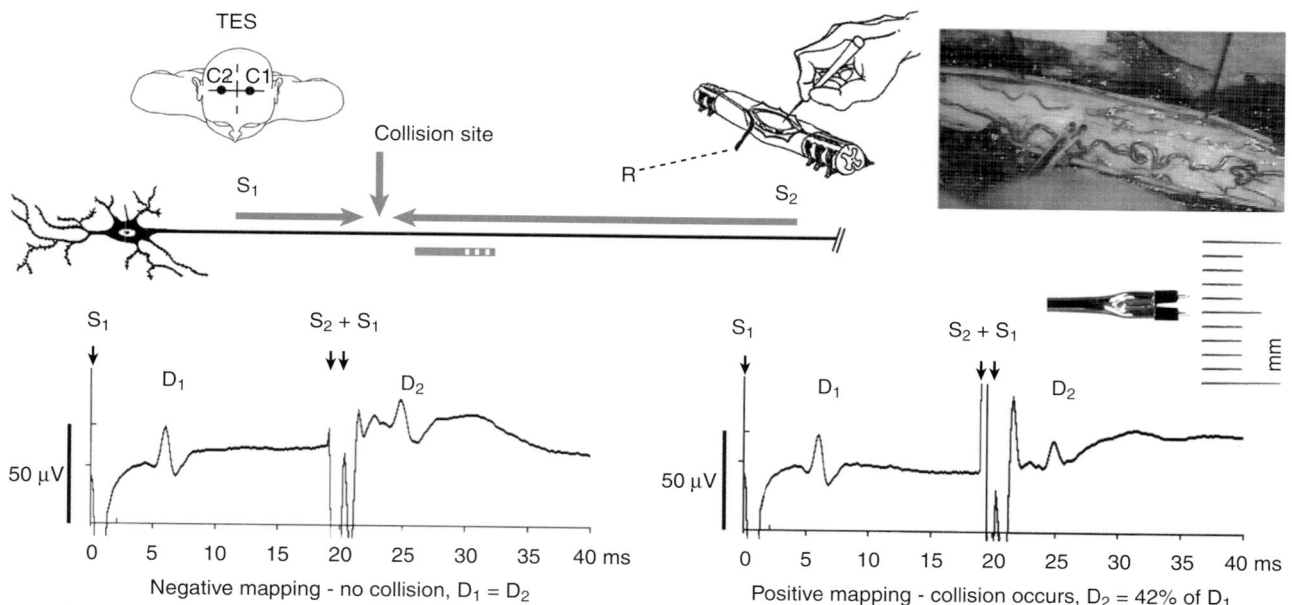

FIGURE 4-8 The neurophysiologic basis for intraoperative mapping of the corticospinal tract (CT). Mapping of the CT by the D-wave collision technique (see text for details). S_1, transcranial electrical stimulation (TES); S_2, spinal cord electrical stimulation; D_1, control D wave (TES only); D_2, D wave after combined stimulation of the brain and spinal cord; R, the cranial electrode for recording D wave in the spinal epidural space. *Lower left*: Negative mapping results ($D_1 = D_2$). *Lower right*: Positive mapping results (D_2-wave amplitude significantly diminished after collision). *Inset*: Handheld stimulating probe over the exposed spinal cord. *(Modified from Deletis V, Camargo AB. Interventional neurophysiological mapping during spinal cord procedures. Stereotact Funct Neurosurg. 2001;77:25-28.)*

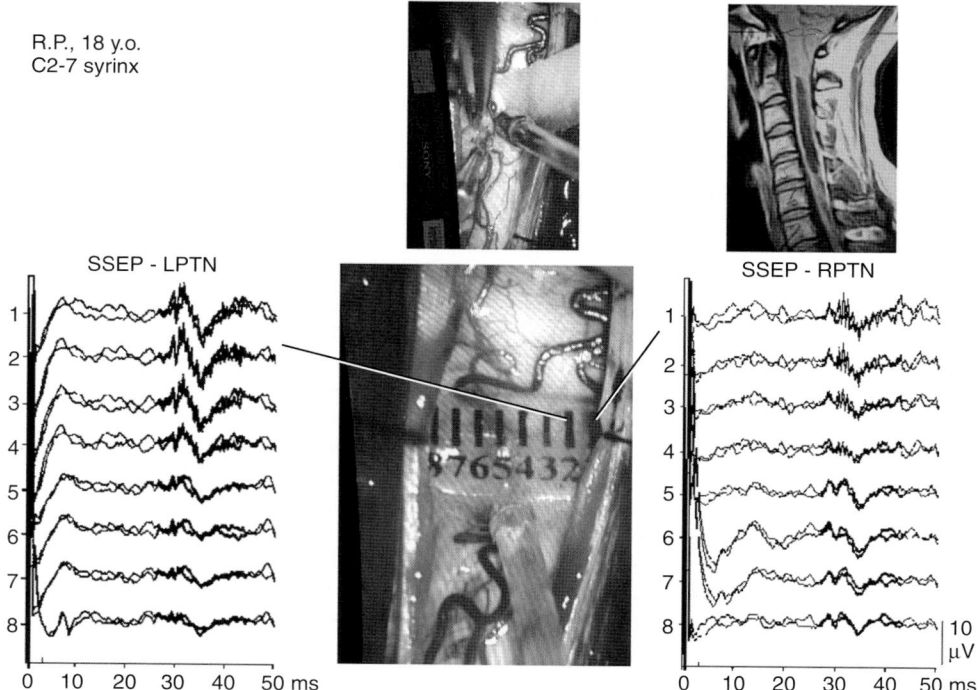

FIGURE 4-9 Dorsal column mapping in an 18-year-old patient with a syringomyelic cyst between the C2 and C7 segments of the spinal cord. *Upper right*: Magnetic resonance imaging shows the syrinx. *Lower middle*: Placement of miniature electrode over surgically exposed dorsal column; vertical bars on the electrode represent the location of the underlying exposed electrode surfaces. Sensory-evoked potentials after stimulation of the left and right tibial nerves showing maximal amplitude between electrodes 1 and 2 (*lower left and right*). These data strongly indicate that both dorsal columns from the left and right lower extremities have been pushed to the extreme right side of the spinal cord. Using these data as a guideline, the surgeon performed the myelotomy using a YAG laser through the left side of the spinal cord and inserted the shunt to drain the cyst (*upper middle*). The patient did not experience a postoperative sensory deficit. *(Reproduced from Krzan MJ. Intraoperative neurophysiological mapping of the spinal cord's dorsal column. In: Deletis V, Shils JL, eds. Neurophysiology in Neurosurgery. A Modern Intraoperative Approach. San Diego: Academic Press; 2002:153-164.)*

lidocaine and amobarbital, to selectively block axonal and neuronal conduction (respectively) when injected intra-arterially in the spinal cord.[85] Provocative tests are usually performed once the endovascular catheter has reached the embolizing position, before any embolizing material is injected. If that specific vessel not only feeds the target of the embolization (e.g., spinal cord arteriovenous malformation, hemangioblastoma, arteriovenous fistula) but also perfuses normal spinal cord, it is expected that the provocative drug will block the white and/or gray matter conduction, and this will be reflected in neurophysiologic tests. Criteria for positive provocative tests are the disappearance of the MEPs and/or a 50% decrease in SEP amplitude. If the test is positive, embolization from that specific catheter position is not performed and embolization from a different feeder or from a more selectively advanced catheter position is attempted. Provocative tests mimic the effect of the embolization and select those patients amenable to a safe embolization. Although the specificity of provocative tests has not been tested (because the procedure is abandoned whenever provocative tests are consistently positive), their sensitivity has proven to be very high and no false-negative results (i.e., new postoperative neurologic deficit despite embolization performed after a negative provocative test) have so far been reported.[78]

Surgery of the Lumbosacral Nervous System

Intraoperative monitoring during surgery of the lumbosacral nervous system is a very demanding task and is still not developed in comparison with monitoring of the surgeries for other parts of the central and peripheral nervous systems. The neurophysiologic techniques used to monitor the lumbosacral nervous system are dependent on the pathology and structures involved. Generally, monitoring of the lumbosacral system involves the epiconus, conus, and cauda equina. These structures are essential in both voluntary and reflexive control of micturition, defecation, and sexual function as well as somatosensory and motor innervation of the pelvis and lower extremities. So far, only methodologies for monitoring and mapping of the somatomotor and somatosensory components of the lumbosacral nervous system have been developed. Intraoperative monitoring of the vegetative component of the lumbosacral nervous system is still in the embryonic stage.[86]

One of the most widely used applications of intraoperative monitoring of the lumbosacral nervous system, at least in the pediatric population, is for patients undergoing surgery for a tethered spinal cord. During these procedures, the surgeon cuts the filum terminale or removes the tethering tissue that envelopes the conus and/or the cauda equina roots. In a large series of patients operated on for tethered spinal cords, permanent neurologic complications have been described in as many as 4.5%.[87,88] The rate increased to 10.9% when transient complications were considered. Due to the tethering, the lumbosacral nerve roots leave the spinal cord in different directions than in a healthy spinal cord. Furthermore, the cord may be skewed and sometimes a nerve root may pass through a lipoma. Nerve roots may also be involved in the thickened filum terminale that is cut during untethering. Direct electric stimulation of these structures in the surgical field or direct recording from them after peripheral nerve stimulation has proven helpful. Using mapping techniques, functional neural structures of the lumbosacral region can be correctly identified and thus possibly preserved. In Fig. 4-10, schematic drawings of the most important neurophysiologic techniques for monitoring afferent and efferent events (i.e., recording and monitoring neurophysiologic signals from sensory or motor parts of the lumbosacral system) are presented. During intraoperative testing with these techniques, it has been found that some of them are more important than others, from pragmatic point of view. Only these are described.

PUDENDAL DORSAL ROOT ACTION POTENTIALS

In the treatment of spasticity (e.g., in cerebral palsy), sacral roots are increasingly being included during rhizotomy procedures.[89] Children who underwent L2–S2 rhizotomies had an 81% greater reduction in plantar/flexor spasticity compared with children who underwent only L2–S1 rhizotomies. However, as more sacral dorsal roots have been included in rhizotomies, neurosurgeons have experienced an increased rate of postoperative complications, especially with regards to bowel and bladder functions.

To spare sacral function, we have attempted to identify those sacral dorsal roots carrying afferents from pudendal nerves using recordings of dorsal root action potentials after stimulation of dorsal penile or clitoral nerves. Patients were anesthetized with isoflurane, nitrous oxide, fentanyl, and a short-acting muscle relaxant introduced only at the time of intubation. The cauda equina was exposed through a T12–S2 laminotomy/laminectomy, and the sacral roots were identified using bony anatomy. The dorsal roots were separated from the ventral ones, and dorsal root action potentials were recorded by a hand-held sterile bipolar hooked electrode (the root being lifted outside the spinal canal) (Fig. 4-11). The dorsal root action potentials were evoked by electrical stimulation of the penile or clitoral nerves. One hundred responses were averaged together and filtered between 1.5 and 2100 Hz. Each average response was repeated to assess its reliability. Afferent activity from the right and left dorsal roots of S1, S2, and S3 were always recorded, along with occasional recordings from the S4–S5 dorsal roots. Of special relevance was the finding that in 7.6% of these children, all afferent activity was carried by only one S2 root (see Fig. 4-11C and F). These findings were confirmed by a later analysis of results of mapping in 114 children (72 male, 42 female; mean age, 3.8 years).[90] Mapping was successful in 105 of 114 patients. S1 roots contributed 4%, S2 roots 60.5%, and S3 roots 35.5% of the overall pudendal afferent activity. The distribution of responses was asymmetrical in 56% of the patients (see Fig. 4-11B, C, and F). Pudendal afferent distribution was confined to a single level in 18% (see Fig. 4-11A) and even to a single root in 7.6% of patients (see Fig. 4-11C and F). Fifty-six percent of the pathologically responding S2 roots during rhizotomy testing (using electrical stimulation of dorsal roots with spreading activity in adjacent myotomes) were preserved because of the significant afferent activity (as demonstrated during pudendal mapping). None of the 105 patients developed long-term bowel or bladder complications.

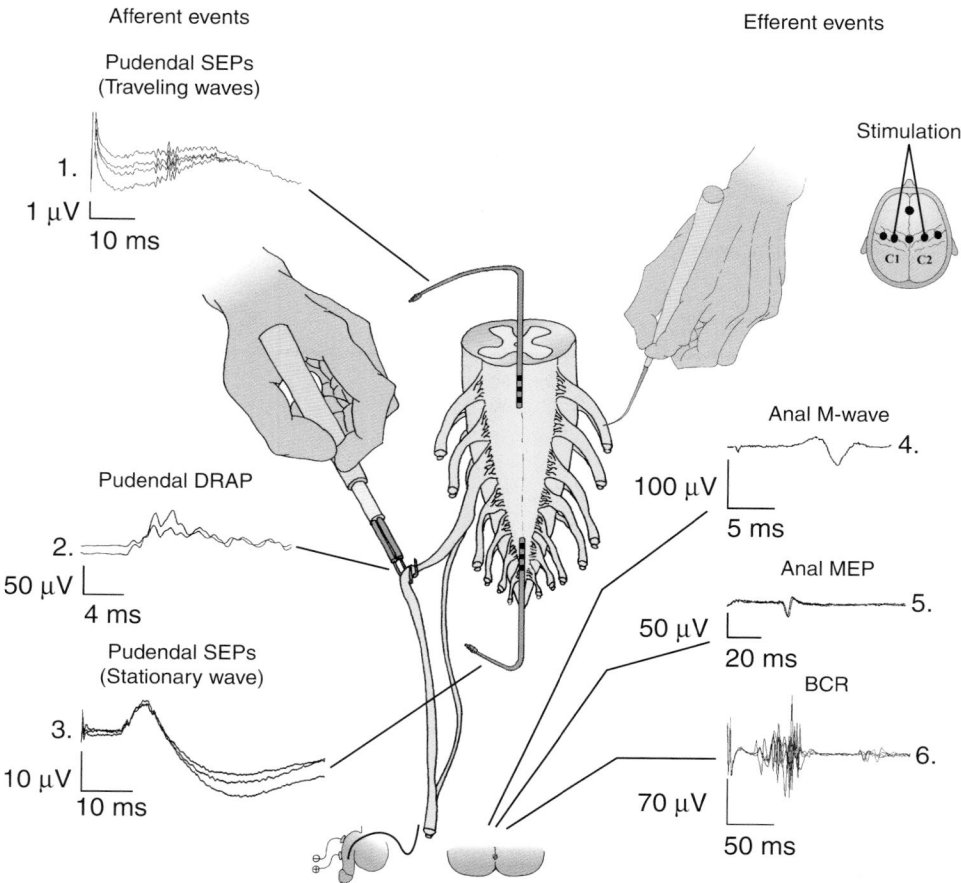

FIGURE 4-10 Neurophysiologic events used to intraoperatively monitor the sacral nervous system. *Left*: Afferent events after stimulation of the dorsal penile/ clitoral nerves and recording over the spinal cord: 1, pudendal somatosensory-evoked potentials (SEPs), traveling waves; 2, pudendal dorsal root action potential; and 3, pudendal SEPs, stationary waves recorded over the conus. *Right*: Efferent events: 4, anal M wave recorded from the anal sphincter after stimulation of the S1–S3 ventral roots; 5, anal motor-evoked potentials recorded from the anal sphincter after transcranial electrical stimulation of the motor cortex; 6, bulbocavernosus reflex obtained from the anal sphincter muscle after electrical stimulation of the dorsal penile/ clitoral nerves. *BCR*, bulbocavernosus reflex; *DRAP*, dorsal root action potentials; *MEP*, motor-evoked potential. *(From Deletis V. Intraoperative neurophysiological monitoring. In: McLone D, ed. Pediatric Neurosurgery: Surgery of the Developing Nervous System, 4th ed. Philadelphia: WB Saunders; 1999:1204-1213.)*

All our results in the early series of dorsal root mapping with 19 patients have been confirmed by analysis of the larger series of 105 patients.[90] With this series, we showed that selective S2 rhizotomy can be performed safely without an associated increase in residual spasticity while preserving bowel and bladder function by performing pudendal afferent mapping.[89] Therefore, we suggest that the mapping of pudendal afferents in the dorsal roots should be employed whenever these roots are considered for rhizotomy in children with cerebral palsy without urinary retention. In children with cerebral palsy with hyper-reflexive detrusor dysfunction, in whom sacral rhizotomy may be considered to alleviate the problem, preoperative neurologic investigation of the child should help in making appropriate decisions. In any case, intraoperative mapping of sacral afferents should make selective surgical approaches possible and provide the maximal benefit for children with cerebral palsy. Mapping of pudendal afferents has been further expanded by introducing methodology that maps afferents from the anal mucosa by stimulating them using anal plug electrodes and recording them in the same way as penile/clitoral afferents.[91]

MAPPING AND MONITORING OF MOTOR RESPONSES FROM THE ANAL SPHINCTER

These responses can be elicited by direct stimulation of the S2 to S5 motor roots and recording from the anal sphincters, after surgical exposure of the cauda equina, or by TES of the motor cortex. The first method of cauda equina stimulation, using a small hand-held monopolar probe, is easy to perform with recording of responses from each anal hemisphincter with intramuscular wire electrodes identical to the ones used to record the bulbocavernosus reflex.[92] This mapping method is very useful when it becomes necessary to identify roots within the cauda equina during tethered cord or tumor surgeries in which the normal anatomy is distorted. To perform mapping, the surgeon must stop surgery and map the roots with a monopolar probe. To continuously monitor the functional integrity of parapyramidal motor fibers (for volitional control of the anal sphincters)

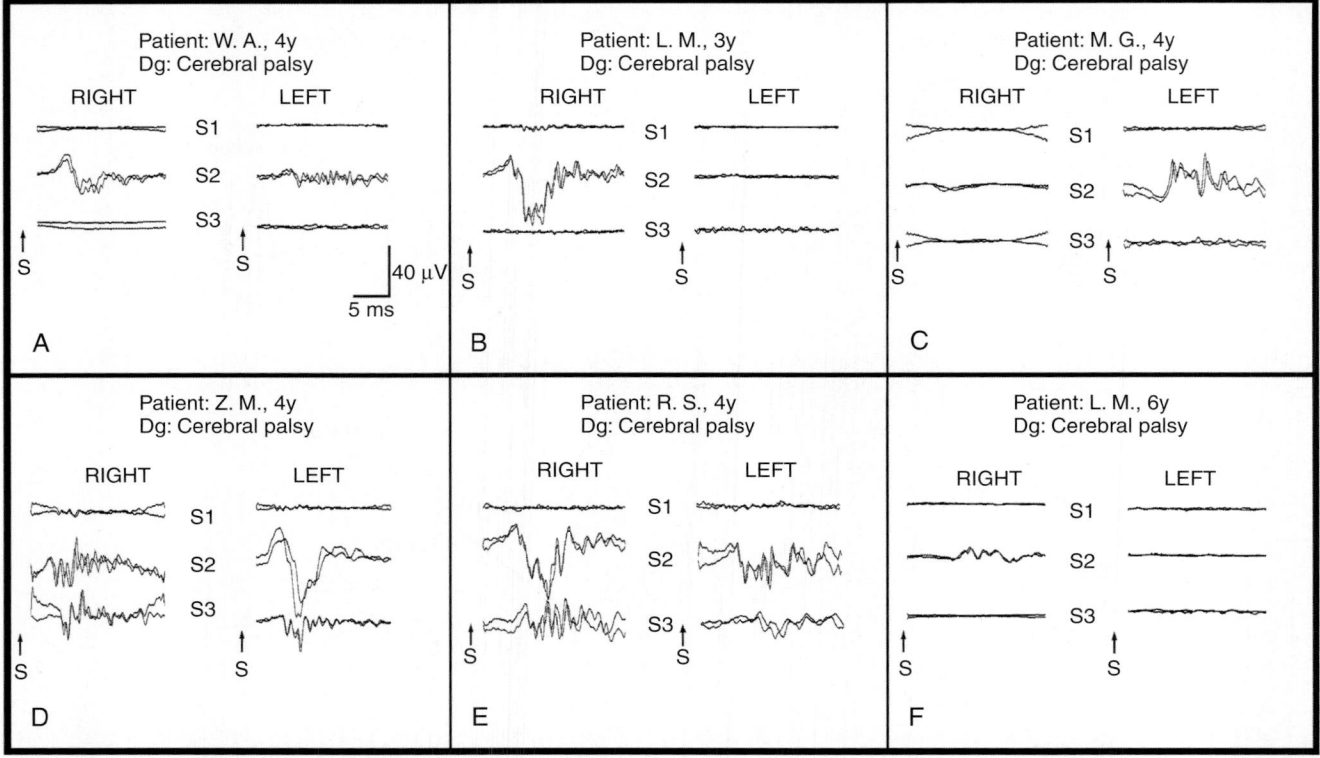

FIGURE 4-11 Six characteristic examples of dorsal root action potentials showing the entry of a variety of pudendal nerve fibers to the spinal cord via S1–S3 sacral roots. A, Symmetrical distribution of dorsal root action potentials confined to one level (S2) or three levels (D). Asymmetrical distribution of dorsal root action potentials confined to the one side (B), only one root (C or F), or all roots except right S1 (E). Recordings were obtained after electrical stimulation of bilateral penile/clitoral nerves. *(From Vodušek VB, Deletis V. Intraoperative neurophysiological monitoring of the sacral nervous system. In: Deletis V, Shils J, eds. Neurophysiology in Neurosurgery: A Modern Intraoperative Approach. San Diego: Academic Press; 2002:197-217.)*

and the motor aspects of the pudendal nerves from the anterior horns to the anal sphincters, the method of TES and recording of anal responses was introduced. Because the response recorded from the anal sphincter after TES has to pass multiple synapses at the level of the spinal cord, this method is moderately sensitive to anesthetics and rather light anesthesia should be maintained. So far no clinical correlation using this method has been published.

MONITORING OF THE BULBOCAVERNOSUS REFLEX

The bulbocavernosus reflex is an oligosynaptic reflex mediated through the S2–S4 spinal cord segments that is elicited by electrical stimulation of the dorsal penis/clitoris nerves with the reflex response recorded from any pelvic floor muscles. The afferent paths of the bulbocavernosus reflex are the sensory fibers of the pudendal nerves and the reflex center in the S2–S4 spinal segment. The efferent paths are the motor fibers of the pudendal nerves and anal sphincter muscles. In neurophysiologic laboratories, the bulbocavernosus reflex is usually recorded from the bulbocavernosus muscles, and this is where it gets its name. We have described an intraoperative method for recording the bulbocavernosus reflex from the anal sphincter muscle, with improvement in methodology reported by others.[92–94] The advantage of bulbocavernosus reflex monitoring is that it tests the functional integrity of the three different anatomic structures: the sensory and motor fibers of the pudendal

nerves and the gray matter of the S2–S4 sacral segments (see Fig. 4-10). Because of a lack of published statistical data collected for large groups of patients, the reliability of monitoring for conus and cauda equina surgeries remains unclear.

Special Consideration for ION in Children

ION techniques are extensively used in adult neurosurgery and, in their principles, can be applied to the pediatric population. However, especially in younger children, the motor system is still under development, making both mapping and monitoring techniques more challenging.

With regard to D-wave monitoring, Szelenyi et al. reviewed D-wave data from 19 children aged 8 to 36 months operated on for intramedullary spinal cord tumors.[95] The D-wave was present in 50% of children aged 21 months or older but was never recorded in children younger than 21 months. Although the preoperative neurologic status of these children was not specified, a 50% D-wave monitor ability rate compares unfavorably to the data reported in adults, where mean monitor ability rate is around 66% and reaches 80% in patients in McCormick grade I.[45] This is likely due to the immaturity of the CT in younger children where incompletely myelinated fibers have variable conduction velocities resulting in desynchronization.[96] A few studies have recently looked at the feasibility of muscle MEP monitoring in children after TES, and consistently reported higher threshold in younger children.[95,97,98] Our data are in agreement with those reported by Journee et al., who suggested preconditioning TES to overcome some of the limitations in eliciting MEPs in this subgroup of patients. [96,99]

According to Nezu, electrophysiologic maturation of the CT innervating hand muscles is complete by the age of 13 and the CT appears to be the only spinal cord pathway with incomplete myelination at birth.[100,101] There is likely a discrepancy between the anatomic and neurophysiologic development of the CT. Cortico-motoneuronal connections reach sacral levels between 18 and 28 weeks PCA, and are completed at birth.[102] Myelination of the lumbar spinal cord occurs between 1 and 2 years of age, with a slower development for lower extremities than for upper extremities.[103] However, the neurophysiologic maturation of the CT progresses throughout childhood and adolescence with myelogenesis and synaptogenesis that continues in to the second decade of life. Overall, a transition from development to motor control function exists for the CT.[104] In conclusion, in Pediatric Neurosurgery essentially the same techniques used in adults can be applied to map and monitor the motor system. Yet, younger children have less excitable motor cortex and pathways due to their neurophysiologic—rather than anatomic—immaturity. Different stimulating parameters may be required to overcome these limitations.

KEY REFERENCES

Bricolo A, Turazzi S. Surgery for gliomas and other mass lesions of the brainstem. In: Symon L, ed. *Advances and Technical Standards in Neurosurgery.* vol 22. Vienna: Springer-Verlag; 1995:261-341.

Cedzich C, Taniguchi M, Schafer S, et al. Somatosensory evoked potential phase reversal and direct motor cortex stimulation during surgery in and around the central region. *Neurosurgery.* 1996;38:962-970.

Deletis V. Intraoperative neurophysiology and methodology used to monitor the functional integrity of the motor system. In: Deletis V, Shils JL, eds. *Neurophysiology in Neurosurgery: A Modern Intraoperative Approach.* San Diego: Academic Press; 2002:25-51.

Deletis V, Vodusek DB. Intraoperative recording of the bulbocavernosus reflex. *Neurosurgery.* 1997;40:88-92.

Dong CC, Macdonald DB, Akagami R, et al. Intraoperative facial motor evoked potential monitoring with transcranial electrical stimulation during skull base surgery. *Clin Neurophysiol.* 2005;116(3):588-596.

Duffau H, Capelle L, Sichez JP, et al. Intra-operative direct electrical stimulations of the central nervous system: the Salpetrière experience with 60 patients. *Acta Neurochir (Wien).* 1999;141:1157-1167.

Eyre JA. Development and plasticity of the corticospinal system in man. *Neural Plast.* 2003;10:93-106.

Huang JC, Deletis V, Vodusek DB, et al. Preservation of pudendal afferents in sacral rhizotomies. *Neurosurgery.* 1997;41:411-415.

Jones SJ, Buonamassa S, Crockard HA. Two cases of quadriparesis following anterior cervical discectomy, with normal perioperative somatosensory evoked potentials. *J Neurol Neurosurg Psychiatry.* 2003;44:273-276.

Kothbauer K, Deletis V, Epstein FJ. Motor evoked potential monitoring for intramedullary spinal cord tumor surgery: correlation of clinical and neurophysiological data in a series of 100 consecutive procedures. *Neurosurg Focus.* 1998;4:1-9.

Minahan RE, Sepkuty JP, Lesser RP, et al. Anterior spinal cord injury with preserved neurogenic "motor" evoked potentials. *Clin Neurophysiol.* 2001;112:1442-1450.

Morota N, Deletis V, Epstein FJ, et al. Brain stem mapping: neurophysiological localization of motor nuclei on the floor of the fourth ventricle. *Neurosurgery.* 1995;37:922-930.

Morota N, Deletis V, Lee M, et al. Functional anatomic relationship between brain stem tumors and cranial motor nuclei. *Neurosurgery.* 1996;39:787-794.

Neuloh G, Pechstein U, Schramm J. Motor tract monitoring during insular glioma surgery. *J Neurosurg.* 2007;106:582-592.

Neuloh G, Schramm J. Mapping and monitoring of supratentorial procedures. In: Deletis V, Shils JL, eds. *Neurophysiology in Neurosurgery: A Modern Intraoperative Approach.* San Diego: Academic Press; 2002:339-401.

Ojemann GA. Functional mapping of cortical language areas in adults. Intraoperative approaches. *Adv Neurol.* 1993;63:155-163.

Penfield W, Boldrey E. Somatic motor and sensory representation in the cerebral cortex of man as studied by electrical stimulation. *Brain.* 1937;60:389-443.

Pouratian N, Cannestra AF, Bookheimer SY, et al. Variability of intraoperative electrocortical stimulation mapping parameters across and within individuals. *J Neurosurg.* 2004;101:458-466.

Rodi Z, Vodusek DB. Intraoperative monitoring of bulbocavernous reflex—the method and its problems. *Clin Neurophysiol.* 2001;112:879-883.

Sala F, Krzan MJ, Deletis V. Intraoperative neurophysiological monitoring in pediatric neurosurgery: why, when, how? *Childs Nerv Syst.* 2002;18:264-287.

Sala F, Manganotti P, Grossauer S, et al. Intraoperative neurophysiology of the motor system in children: a tailored approach. *Child's Nerv Syst.* 2010;26:473-490.

Strauss C, Romstock J, Fahlbusch R. Pericollicular approaches to the rhomboid fossa. Part II: Neurophysiological basis. *J Neurosurg.* 1999;91:768-775.

Vodušek DB, Deletis V. Sacral roots and nerves, and monitoring for neuro-urologic procedure. In: Nuwer M, ed. *Monitoring neural function during surgery.* Elsevier; 2007:423-433.

Yingling CD, Ojemann S, Dodson B, et al. Identification of motor pathways during tumor surgery facilitated by multichannel electromyographic recording. *J Neurosurg.* 1999;91:922-927.

Numbered references appear on Expert Consult.

CHAPTER 5

Gamma Knife Surgery for Cerebral Vascular Malformations and Tumors

CHUN-PO YEN • LADISLAU STEINER

The gamma knife is a neurosurgical tool used either as a primary or adjuvant procedure for intracranial pathologies. It was developed in the late 1960s as an alternative to open stereotactic lesioning for functional disorders. Variations in anatomy and needs for physiologic confirmation of the target limited its usefulness for these indications at that time. However, the technology was found to be efficacious in the management of structural disorders later on. The limited scope of the pathologies treated with the gamma knife (intracranial) and unique technology make the gamma knife an extension of the neurosurgeons' therapeutic armamentarium and not a separate specialty. It should not be mistaken for a form of radiation therapy, for it differs in concept from the radiation oncologists' idea of tumor treatment that is based on variable tissue response to fractionated radiation. It is a single session, stereotactically guided procedure for various neurosurgical pathologic processes limiting exposure to radiation as much as possible to the lesion only.

Recently it has been shown that the gamma knife can palliate some ocular tumors. In a more limited application of the concept, the treatment of extracranial tumors in abdominal and thoracic locations has evolved with the use of the various stereotactic body radiation therapy machines.[1-4] Obviously, lesions that lie outside the central nervous system will not be treated by a neurosurgeon. However, when it is used for neurosurgical pathology, no one is more qualified to apply it. It is the operator and the pathology that define the use of a technology. When Walter Dandy placed a cystoscope in a ventricle for the first time, he was not performing a urologic procedure.[5] The microscope when used by the neurosurgeon, ophthalmologist, or otolaryngologist is a neurosurgical, ophthalmologic, or otolaryngologic instrument, respectively.

It is remarkable how difficult it was, and still is for some neurosurgeons, to accept the use of gamma knife as a neurosurgical tool. Some of the causes of this reticence can be identified:

1. Lack of historic perspective makes it difficult for some neurosurgeons to realize that Leksell's concept was rooted in the philosophy of the founders of neurosurgery, that is, recognition of technological advances and their application to neurosurgical practice. The early adoption by Cushing of the x-ray machine, his use of the "radium bomb" in glioma treatment,[6] and the introduction, also by Cushing, of radiofrequency treatment of lesions are just a few examples of "technology transfer."

2. The difficulty of accepting a neurosurgical procedure without opening the skull, despite the fact that every neurosurgeon knows that trephination is itself a minor part of the neurosurgical act. The laser beam, the bipolar coagulator, and the ultrasound probe are accepted without resistance because they are used after trephining the skull. The recently introduced "photon radiosurgery" with its limited scope compared to gamma surgery is accepted widely as "neurosurgery" because it reaches the target through a small burr hole.

3. The loss of the thrill and glamor provided by open surgery.

4. The deeply rooted acceptance of the dogma that where ionizing beams are involved a radiotherapist is needed. The last 40 years have demonstrated that a neurosurgeon can acquire the necessary knowledge of radiophysics and radiobiology to handle ionizing beams. This is much easier than for a radiation oncologist to master neuroanatomy and management of neurosurgical lesions, and thus to exclude bias when deciding whether to use the microscope or the gamma knife in each particular case.

The trend in cranial as well as spinal neurosurgery has been minimally invasive approaches. These may be achieved with the increasing skill of the operators and by new technology. If the result of these changes in the procedure, aspects are modified or even eliminated, the procedure is still neurosurgical. To relegate less-invasive procedures to non-surgeons is to argue that the only aspect of a patient's care that is unique to a surgeon is purely technical. This is patently untrue; it is the surgeon's responsibility to maintain surgical care standards by adapting to new technologies.

There is no substitute at this time for the physical extirpation of a mass lesion in terms of cure or control of either vascular or oncologic pathologies. The attractiveness of radiosurgery is not that it supplants open neurosurgical procedures, but that it allows treatment of pathologies only treated earlier with unacceptable morbidity or mortality. There is, and likely always will be a gray area where the benefits of various modalities are debated. It will only be through evaluation of long-term results of these various therapies as well as their availability, cost, experience of the operators and individual patient preferences that the "best" therapy in any given case is decided.

In this chapter we describe the results of our experience with the gamma knife as well as published results of other centers where required.

Table 5-1 lists all the cases treated with the gamma knife worldwide through 2006. It should be kept in mind that many of the indications listed are not universally accepted as appropriate for gamma surgery. In this chapter we will give our version of the facts for each indication.

History

Clarke and Horsley developed the first stereotactic system,[7] and the method was first applied clinically by Spiegel et al.[8] This system allowed for the localization of intracranial structures by their spatial relationship to Cartesian coordinates relative to a ring rigidly affixed to the skull. This was a prerequisite to the development of radiosurgery by Lars Leksell. His ambition was to develop a method of destroying localized structures deep within the brain without the degree of coincident brain trauma associated with open procedures. The convergence of multiple ionizing beams at one stereotactically defined point was the result. A nominal dose is delivered to the paths of each incident beam. However, at the point of intersection of the beams, a dose proportional to the number of individual beams is delivered. The physical specifications of the device would be designed to ensure steep drop-off of delivered radiation at the edge of the intersection point. This would allow precise selection of the targeted lesion and minimization of trauma to surrounding tissue. He named this concept *radiosurgery* in 1951.[9]

Various sources of ionizing radiation were tried. Leksell first used an orthovoltage x-ray tube coupled to a stereotactic frame in the treatment of trigeminal neuralgia and for cingulotomy in obsessive compulsive disorders.[9] A cyclotron was then used as an accelerated proton source and used to treat various pathologies.[10,11] The cyclotron was too cumbersome and expensive for widespread application. A linear accelerator was evaluated but found at that time to lack the inherent precision necessary for this work. Fixed gamma sources of cobalt-60 and a fixed stereotactic target fulfilled the requirements of precision and compactness. The first gamma knife was built between 1965 and 1968.

The use of a single high dose of ionizing beams to treat neurosurgical problems was a novel and creative concept 40 years ago, which changed the direction of development in many fields of neurosurgery. However, a creative innovation is not perfect in its inception. The gamma knife was not an exception. Contributions of excellence by numerous neurosurgeons and physicists, and utilizing advances in computer technology to improve the software used in planning have over the years defined the present use of the tool. For instance improvements in the planning system now allow for systematic shielding of the optic apparatus from exposure during treatment of parasellar masses. In lesions only 2 to 5 mm away, the dose to sensitive structures can be limited to less than 2% to 7% of the maximum dose. However, in spite of all the changes in application of gamma surgery the underlying concepts behind it have not changed since its inception. This speaks for the sagacity of Lars Leksell and his invention.

Doses delivered and indications for the various pathologies treated were all empiric initially. In the subsequent discussions this should be considered when doses, both minimal and maximal are discussed, as well as results.

Pathophysiology

The effects of single high-dose gamma radiation on pathologic and normal tissue have been studied on clinical human and experimental animal tissue. These studies are incomplete because the human material tends to come from treatment failures and the experimental material is from normal animals. However some conclusions as to the method of effectiveness and of tissue tolerances can be drawn.

NORMAL TISSUE

The relative radioresistance of normal brain relates to its low mitotic activity. Also, the rate at which a total dose of radiation is applied affects the damage caused by the dose. This is due to the ability of the cell to effect repairs during

Table 5-1 Cases Treated with Gamma Knife Worldwide through December 2008		
Diagnosis	*n*	**Percentage**
Vascular	**65,084**	**12.95**
Arteriovenous malformation	57,136	11.37
Cavernous angioma	3,258	0.65
Other vascular	4690	0.93
Tumor	**397,215**	**79.01**
Benign	176,319	35.07
Vestibular schwannoma	46,835	9.32
Trigeminal schwannoma	2,822	0.56
Other schwannoma	1,590	0.32
Meningioma	64,115	12.75
Pituitary tumor	38,553	7.67
Pineal tumor	3,540	0.70
Craniopharyngioma	4,053	0.81
Hemangioblastoma	2,056	0.41
Chordoma	1,911	0.38
Hemaniopericytoma	1,151	0.23
Benign glial tumors	3,594	0.71
Other benign tumors	6,099	1.21
Malignant	**220,896**	**43.94**
Metastasis	185,070	36.81
Malignant glial tumors	26,437	5.26
Chondrosarcoma	775	0.15
Nasopharyngeal carcinoma	1,454	0.29
Other malignant tumors	7,160	1.42
Ocular Disorder	**1,966**	**0.39**
Functional	**38,461**	**7.65**
Intractable pain targets	622	0.12
Trigeminal neuralgia	32,798	6.52
Parkinson's disease	1,473	0.29
Obsessive compulsive disorder	154	0.03
Epilepsy	2,399	0.48
Other functional targets	1,015	0.20
Total indications	502,726	100.0

Note: These figures include cases treated at gamma knife sites throughout the world from 1968 through December 2008.
Source: Elekta Radiosurgery Inc.

the actual time of irradiation. A higher dose rate (same total dose applied over a shorter period of time) consequently increases the lethality of the dose. The normal tissue surrounding the stereotactically targeted pathologic tissue receives a markedly lower dose but over the same time. Therefore, not only is the total dose lower, but the dose rate is lower as well. The radiation effect is seen most clearly at doses above and below 1 Gy/min.[12] This radiobiological phenomenon explains part of the relative safety of single dose radiation with steep gradients at the edge of targeted tissue on the surrounding structures. There are likely additional mechanisms of such sparing.

The steep gradient of dose and consequently dose rate described above does not exist in conventional radiotherapy. When treating tumors the radiation oncologist uses "fractionation" or dividing the total dose into smaller portions, which allows repair of normal tissue as well as transition of dormant cells within the target to cells in division (at which time they are more sensitive to radiation). Creating a dose gradient at the lesion's margin not only eliminates the need for fractionation but also improves the effectiveness of the delivered dose within the target (high-dose rate zone) 2.5 to 3 times that of the same dose delivered in a fractionated manner. The gamma knife stereotactically excludes normal tissue from the high-dose rate zone as much as possible. It may also take advantage of the natural difference in susceptibility of pathologic versus normal tissue.

In order to understand the radiobiology of a single high-dose of radiation on normal brain the parietal lobe of rats treated by a gamma knife was studied at our center. It was found that a dose of 50 Gy caused astrocytic swelling without changes in neuronal morphology or breakdown of the blood–brain barrier at 12 months. There was fibrin deposition in the walls of capillaries. At 75 Gy, necrosis was seen at 4 months as was breakdown of the blood–brain barrier. More vigorous morphological changes were seen in astrocytes and hemispheric swelling coincident with the necrosis occurred at 4 months. With the dose increased to 120 Gy, necrosis was seen at 4 weeks but not associated with hemispheric swelling. Astrocytic swelling occurred at only 1 week postirradiation.[13] These findings are consistent with earlier reports on the effective dose to produce well-defined lesions in the thalamus in patients treated with the gamma knife.[14,15]

TUMOR RESPONSE

Little is known about the pathophysiologic changes induced by gamma surgery at the cellular level in tumors. Division of tumor cells is presumably inhibited by radiation induced damage to DNA. Also it has been shown that the microvascular supply to tumors is inhibited by changes resulting from gamma surgery. In meningiomas studied after this treatment there was reduction of blood flow over time.[16] Tumors responding early showed the greatest reduction in blood flow. Other authors have proposed that the induction of apoptosis by gamma radiation to proliferating cells may be responsible for at least a portion of the effect of gamma surgery on tumors.[17,18] Although such contentions may be premature they may point the direction to future research.

Thus the pathophysiologic effect of gamma surgery seems not to be tumor necrosis. For this, higher doses than typically used would be required. Necrotic doses are rarely used for gamma surgery (e.g., in functional cases). Ideally following gamma surgery, tumors begin to shrink without changes in the normal tissue. The rate of shrinkage in general is slower in more benign tumors.

The effectiveness of the therapy is most dependent on the ability to define and treat the entire lesion. However, the result can also be obtained at times by treating the nutrient or feeding vessels of tumors (e.g., meningiomas). Malignant gliomas do poorly with any surgical technique, including gamma surgery because of the inability to include all of the microscopic disease within the treated area. Individual metastatic deposits and small benign tumors are adequately handled with both open resection and with the gamma knife because the tumor margin can be well-defined intraoperatively or on neuroimaging studies.

In order to conformally cover the target more than one isocenter is nearly always utilized. When multiple radiation fields are made to overlap the radiation dose distribution becomes inhomogeneous. The resulting areas of local maxima are called "hot spots." Controversy exists as to whether the presence of "hot spots" in gamma surgery is beneficial or detrimental. An even dose distribution is an essential and basic concept in radiotherapy. There is some evidence that these areas may be of benefit in gamma surgery. The factors to keep in mind to understand this line of reasoning are as follows: due to radiation geometry hot spots are usually located in the deep portions of the target. In tumors this is usually the area that receives the poorest blood supply and is therefore relatively hypoxic and radioresistant. Furthermore the ability of a cell to respond to otherwise sublethal dosages of radiation can be affected by its own condition as well as the state of the cells near it. Cells that are sublethally injured and are in the vicinity of similar cells recover more often than cells that are in the vicinity of lethally injured cells. The hot spots therefore create islands of lethally injured cells that will enhance the cell kill in the sublethal injury zone.[19] Oxygen is a radiosensitizer, and the relatively high-dose rate of the hot spots will act to offset any loss of efficacy in the hypoxic core of the target. This position is supported by the work of other authors.[20]

CRANIAL NERVES

The susceptibility of cranial nerves to injury from gamma surgery is of great interest. Tolerance is dependent on the particular nerve and the individual nerves involvement by the pathologic process requiring treatment. Because of these it is difficult to extrapolate exact numbers in many instances. Some statements can be made with some certainty.

The optic and acoustic nerves are the most sensitive to radiation of the cranial nerves. Being central nervous system tracts, containing oligodendrocytes, and carrying complex information is thought to be the source of their vulnerability. These tracts are unable to regenerate following injury. Optic neuropathy has been reported as a complication following single doses greater than 8 Gy.[21] The tolerable level of radiation to the optic apparatus is still a subject of debate. Some advocate that the optic apparatus can tolerate doses as high as 12 to 14 Gy.[22-24] Others recommend an upper limit of 8 Gy.[21,25] Small volumes of the optic apparatus exposed to doses of 10 Gy or less may be acceptable in some cases.[26,27] Both the tolerable absolute dose and volume undoubtedly vary from patient to patient. This degree of variability likely depends upon the extent of damage to the optic apparatus by pituitary adenoma compression, ischemic changes, type and timing of previous interventions (e.g., fractionated radiation therapy and surgery), the patient's age, and the presence or absence of other co-morbidities (e.g., diabetes).

On the other hand the trigeminal and facial nerves are significantly more resilient. Few developed profound hypoesthesia in trigeminal neuralgia patients treated with gamma knife using doses of 80 to 90 Gy. Vey few facial pareses were reported in several large groups of vestibular schwannomas treated with radiosurgery.

The cranial nerves in the cavernous sinus are relatively robust. Low incidence of neuropathies has been reported with doses up to 40 Gy.[21] We have not observed any neuropathies of CN IX through XII in the treatment of glomus jugulare tumors.

NORMAL CEREBRAL VASCULATURE

There is both clinical and experimental data regarding the effect of single high-dose gamma irradiation of normal cerebral vasculature. In treating 1,917 arteriovenous malformations we have seen only two incidences of clinical syndromes possibly associated with the stenosis of normal vessels. This low incidence has occurred even though occasionally normal vessels are included in the treatment field. One case was reported after treating a glioma with 90 Gy gamma surgery followed by 40 Gy of fractionated whole brain irradiation of a middle cerebral artery occlusion. Steiner et al. described two cases in which disproportionate white matter changes might have been ascribed to venous stenosis and occlusion.[28] Another case, of a diencephalic AVM, demonstrated marked edema associated with venous outflow occlusion. This patient suffered visual and cognitive deficits but over the course of months his neurologic status returned to baseline (Fig. 5-1).

In our treatment of pituitary adenomas with cavernous sinus extension or parasellar meningiomas, we have not observed occlusion of normal vasculature. This absence of stenosis is noted even though the internal carotid artery or portions of the circle of Willis, or its proximal branches, are often included in the treatment field. The only incidence of treating an intracranial aneurysm by us with a gamma knife did lead to narrowing and eventual occlusion of the adjacent small posterior communicating artery segment.[29] Whether this was associated with the obliteration of the aneurysm neck or primary changes in the artery is unknown. It is possible that the incidence of occlusion of smaller vessels is more common than recognized as the occlusion would occur slowly and compensatory changes could take place preventing clinical syndromes from occurring. Regardless, the clinical impact is minimal. Others have noted injury to the cavernous segment of the carotid artery following radiosurgery for pituitary adenomas. A total of four cases have been reported and in only two of these cases were the patients symptomatic from carotid artery stenosis.[30-32] Pollock et al. have recommended that the prescription dose should be limited to less than 50% of the intracavernous carotid artery vessel diameter.[32] Shin et al. recommended restricting the dose to the internal carotid artery to less than 30 Gy.[33]

Experimental studies done on normal vasculature in the brains of rats and cats showed similar findings.[34,35] The primary injury was endothelial necrosis and desquamation, muscular coat hypertrophy and fibrosis at lower doses (25 to 100 Gy). At doses up to 300 Gy necrosis of the muscular layer was seen in cats. In only one instance, a rat anterior cerebral artery treated with 100 Gy was occlusion of a vessel seen. Similar studies on hypercholesterolemic rabbits treated with 10 to 100 Gy showed no histologic changes in the basilar arteries and no instances of occlusion after 2 to 24 months.[36]

ARTERIOVENOUS MALFORMATIONS

The minimal clinical and only moderate histologic change in the normal cerebral vasculature after high doses of gamma radiation is in sharp contrast to the response of the vessels of an arteriovenous malformation (AVM). Complete radiographic obliteration can be achieved after appropriate gamma surgery. The effects of ionizing radiation and a role in the management of AVMs was first reported in 1928 by Cushing and Bailey.[37] During craniotomy for an AVM he had to interrupt surgery due to major hemorrhage from the lesion. He then treated the patient with fractionated radiation. At reoperation 5 years later only an obliterated avascular mass was discovered. This early success was overshadowed by numerous series of failures.[38-40] In this early period, Johnson was the only one to report reasonable results with a 45% angiographic obliteration.[41] The introduction of the gamma knife rekindled interest in the treatment of AVMs with radiation.[42]

The pathologic changes in AVMs treated with the gamma knife have been described by several authors.[43-45] The earliest change is damage to the endothelium with swelling of the endothelial cells and subsequent denudation or separation of the endothelium from the underlying vessel wall. The most important changes are seen later in the intima with the appearance of loosely organized spindle cells (myofibroblasts) and an extracellular matrix containing collagen type IV, not seen in the intima of untreated vessels. Expansion of the extracellular matrix and cellular degeneration define the final stage prior to luminal obliteration. The occlusion of the vessels is not a thrombotic process but rather the culmination of concentric narrowing of the vessel by an expanding vessel wall.

Gamma Surgery Procedure

PERIOPERATIVE MANAGEMENT

Patients are routinely evaluated the day prior to gamma surgery. Preoperative consults are obtained as necessary including evaluation by the neuroradiology service. The patients are loaded with anti-seizure medications and levels drawn prior to therapy. Patients already on medication for seizures also have their levels evaluated. Although we have never had a patient have a seizure during therapy, the small but serious risk of a generalized seizure while the patient is secured within the gamma unit makes every precaution reasonable. Patients are also started on systemic dexamethasone the evening prior to therapy and this is continued until the following evening. The use of high-dose peri-operative dexamethasone is empiric. Although

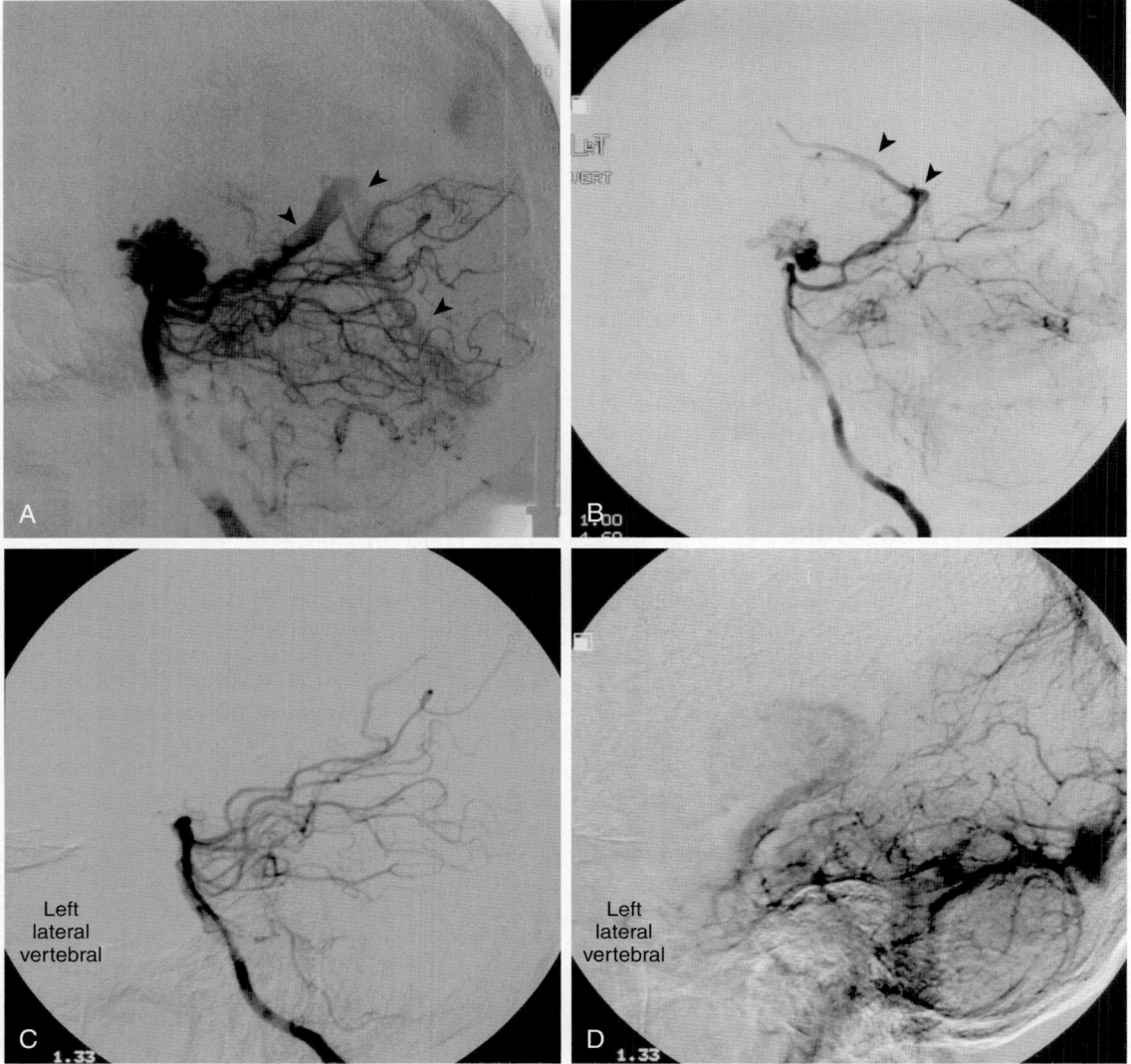

FIGURE 5-1 A, Thalamic AVM shown with lateral vertebral arteriography. B, Similar view obtained 17 months after gamma surgery shows partial obliteration of the nidus. The basal vein of Rosenthal, the vein of Galen, and the straight sinus were not visualized. Venous drainage of the residual AVM appears to be through ascending choroidal veins and the internal cerebral veins. Early (C) and late (D) filling vertebral arteriogram obtained 37 months after gamma surgery shows obliteration of the AVM and complete absence of the deep venous system.

we have used steroids throughout our experience with the gamma knife, their original purpose, to minimize vasogenic edema at the time of therapy, has never been documented as a problem. Hence its prophylactic use is debatable.

FRAME PLACEMENT

The placement of the head frame is done in the operating room at our institution. The patient is given intravenous sedation, usually short acting narcotics (e.g., fentanyl) and propofol, until they are no longer responsive to verbal or moderate physical stimuli. The anesthesia service monitors the patient throughout the procedure. We have found this far superior to the previous practice of applying the frame using only local anesthesia. Patients that were treated both before and since we have applied the frame in this way have provided clear feedback preferring frame placement under anesthesia.

We have fashioned a simple strap with Velcro ends that is placed across the patients head and then fastened above the frame after it has been lowered into the desired position. This holds the frame in position while the pins are secured. This eliminates the need for the earplugs in the auditory canal, which can be painful.

The space available within the gamma knife is limited as is the three dimensional coordinate system within the frame itself. For these reasons care must be taken to skew the placement of the frame in the direction of the pathology if it is far off the center of the brain. The shifting of the frame is of less importance with the latest gamma knife model, Perfexion, which has a much larger radiation cavity.

IMAGING AND DOSE PLANNING

The accuracy of a gamma surgery is ultimately dependent on the neurosurgeon's ability to visualize the intended target. Thus, the technique would be impossible without imaging studies that allow three-dimensional views of anatomic structures in the brain. Magnetic resonance image (MRI) is the most used imaging modality because of its superior visualization of soft tissue structures and solid tumors. Typical MRI protocols include T1-weighted pre- and postcontrast (Gadolinium-enhanced) images through the entire volume of the head. Sequences may be a collection of 2D image slices, or a true 3D acquisition such as the MP-RAGE or its successors. Specialized sequences such as constructive interference in steady state (CISS) protocols may be used for circumstances such as visualization of the internal auditory canals, the cerebellopontine angle, and parasellar regions.

In planning the treatment of an AVM, digital subtraction angiography remains the imaging modality of choice. As with the MRI and computed tomography (CT), images are acquired using a fiducial system. However the digital subtraction angiography is based on projections rather than tomographic information. Images need to be geometrically corrected to account for the curvature of the image intensifier screen before importing the images into the treatment planning system. Gadolinium-enhanced MRI is currently often used to correlate the extent of the AVM nidus with angiography. It helps to define the shape of the AVM and confirms angiographically obtained information. However, it is sometimes difficult to differentiate the nidus from the feeding arteries and draining veins so the MRI tends to overestimate the size of the AVM. The capability to incorporate CTA and MRA data into the planning process is under investigation.

THE GAMMA KNIFE

The gamma knife assembly is comprised of unit that contains the radiation source and treatment couch that delivers the patient into the unit. Within the unit are 201 cobalt-60 source capsules aligned with two internal collimators that direct the gamma radiation toward the center of the unit. A third external collimator helmet is attached to the treatment couch. Four external collimator helmets are provided, and they have fixed diameter apertures that create a 4-, 8-, 14-, or 18-mm diameter isocenter. By changing external collimator helmets, the diameter of the roughly spherical isocenter can be varied. The 201 individual collimators within the helmet are machined to exact standards to direct the 201 beams of gamma radiation to a common point where they intersect, creating the isocenter. The frame attached to the patient's head is adjusted within the collimator helmet so that the area to be treated is at that point of intersection.

In the new gamma knife model, Perfexion, the central body contains 192 cobalt-60 sources that are grouped into eight independent source sectors and collimators are entirely internal to the radiation body. Each source sector is housed in an aluminum frame that is attached to sector drive motors at the rear of the radiation body via linear graphite bushings. There are 576 collimators machined into 12 cm-thick tungsten in five concentric rings to align with the source assembly configurations. Each source has three available collimators (4, 8, and 16 mm) as well as shielded positions ("blocked") to shield a critical structure. To achieve a particular collimation, the sector drive motors move the sources along their bushings to the correct position over the appropriate collimator opening.

These changes allow a single isocenter composed of different beam diameters to optimize dose distribution shape for each individual shot.

TREATMENT EXECUTION

After the treatment plan has been made the patient is moved on to the gamma knife couch and the y and z coordinates for the first exposure are set on the frame attached to the patient's head. The patient's head is then placed within the collimator helmet and secured on either side by trunions and the x coordinate is set. The head at this point is suspended by the frame within the helmet. The exposure time of the corresponding isocenter is entered at the control panel twice for confirmation and the session then commences with the entire couch being mechanically pulled into the body of the unit. The external collimator helmet locks into place with the internal collimators. After each exposure the patient is withdrawn from the collimator helmet and the process is repeated. Necessary changes of the collimator helmet are made as needed according to the plan. The introduction of the Automatic Positioning System (APS), a system that sets the coordinates by six independent motors just outside the irradiation field, has led to shorter treatment times, enhanced selectivity, and better physician work-flow. In the gamma knife Perfexion, the treatment table itself acts as a positioning device (the Patient Position System, or PPS). The stereotactic frame is attached to the treatment table via a removable frame adapter that attaches to the frame and acts as an interface with the treatment table. Treatment execution with Perfexion is a fully automated process including set up of the stereotactic coordinates, alignment of different sector positions and set up of exposure times. Obviously these changes will not affect the efficacy of the treatment but will make the process simpler for the operator.

At the end of the treatment the frame is removed from the head within the suite. There is usually a sensation of tightening and discomfort reported by the patient during removal. At least two pairs of hands should be available to steady the frame and prevent injury by a pin as they are removed. Venous bleeding when it occurs can be controlled with hand held pressure for a few minutes. The occasional arterial bleeder might require a suture. After frame removal the pin sites are dressed in a sterile fashion, steri-strips are used to oppose the skin edges for optimal cosmesis, and a modest head wrap applied.

Indications

VASCULAR MALFORMATION

Arteriovenous Malformations

The indications for gamma surgery of arteriovenous malformations (AVMs) versus other treatment options are in many cases unclear at best. Small asymptomatic inoperable AVMs are clearly best treated with the gamma knife while AVMs with a large symptomatic hemorrhage in noneloquent superficial brain are best treated with open surgery. The reason for this is that the risk-benefit value is clear in both of these situations. In other situations it is more ambiguous. Knowledge of the capabilities of various treatments to effect cure, the associated morbidity and mortality associated with the treatment and the natural history of the disease following various treatments must be known to accurately prescribe the most efficacious treatment plan. Unfortunately these are in most instances not known. The natural history of AVMs is not fully understood. Some authors believe that size matters, with smaller AVMs bleeding at a higher rate than larger ones or at a lower rate.[46-49] There is also evidence that size is independent of the hemorrhage rate.[50-52] Similarly the rate of hemorrhage of an AVM following a previous hemorrhage is thought to be higher than the rate in unruptured AVMs by some authors[46,52,53] but not by others.[47,54,55] The effects of age, gender, pregnancy and AVM location also confound the question of risk of rupture.[50-52,56-58]

The results of microsurgery published in the literature tend to come from centers of excellence and the patients they treat with open surgery are, by definition more amenable to this treatment. The effectiveness of the treatment by this manner and its co-morbid results are known shortly after surgery. The short-term morbidity of treatment with the gamma knife approaches zero but because the benefit and potential complications require time to become apparent follow-up of these patients is problematic. The quality of the AVMs treated with the gamma knife also varies in large series with those treated by microsurgery. All of these make comparison of the modalities difficult. Add to that the additional risks and benefits of preoperative embolization and the matter is that much less clear. It is paramount to the physician treating a patient harboring an AVM to be aware, as much as possible, of the options that are available and the magnitude of the risks and benefits associated with each.

Early Experience

Since the first AVM case treated by Steiner et al. in 1972,[42] we have treated over 2500 AVMs with the gamma knife. As experience with this tool grows the capabilities and limitations of the gamma knife are being defined.

Serendipitously the first AVM was treated by prescribing a 25 Gy peripheral dose. Subsequent changes in protocol showed a significant decrease in success with doses less than 23 Gy and small improvements in obliteration rates but with significantly more radiation associated complications with higher doses. Optimally, therefore, we treat most AVMs with 23 to 25 Gy at the margin. While more patients with relatively large AVMs were treated, dose lower than 23 Gy was quite often used in hopes of achieving a total obliteration with reasonable risk of complications.

As in microsurgery, also when performing gamma surgery, feeding arteries or draining veins should be left alone and only the nidus should be treated. In very large AVMs, only partially treated due to the excessive dose necessary to treat optimally, occasional cures have been achieved. This is thought to be due to fortuitous inclusion of all the pathologic shunts within the higher dose treatment field. Targeting only the feeding vessels to the AVM have had very limited success because of recruitment of small angiographically occult feeding arteries. Interestingly, the first patient ever treated had only the feeding vessels targeted and a cure was obtained.[42] The early success with this strategy has not been reproduced.

The results of gamma surgery on AVMs is affected by the minimum dose applied to the AVM and the size of the AVM. These two factors are interdependent. It has been shown that the limitation of the allowed margin dose by the size of the malformation decreases the rate of obliteration. There are reports contending that low-dose gamma surgery with large malformations results in obliteration rates that are comparable to smaller lesions treated with a larger margin dose. It is doubtful that these results will hold up with larger series. Thus far at our center, larger AVMs have had a lower obliteration rate.

Between 1970 and 1990, 880 AVM patients were optimally treated. Optimally is defined as at least 25 Gy at the margin of the entire nidus of the AVM. Of these patients the age range was 3 to 76 years. Approximately 15% were pediatric patients (<18 years old). The presenting symptoms were hemorrhage (70%), seizures (16%), headache (5%), neurologic deficits not associated with acute hemorrhage (4%), and other symptoms (5%). The majority of referrals were for AVMs deemed operable only with unacceptable morbidity explaining the fact that 73% of the AVMs were located in deep areas of the brain or within eloquent cortex. Patients treated earlier were subjected to a vigorous protocol of repeated angiograms. Later with the introduction of CT and then MRI, angiography was not performed until nidus was no longer evident on these screening examinations. The angiogram should be complete, of high quality, and should be reviewed by an experienced and interested neuroradiologist or neurosurgeon.

Imaging Outcomes. Following gamma surgery, angiography reveals hemodynamic changes occur before changes in the size and shape of an AVM.[59] First, the flow rate decreases progressively. This may be related to the changes in the sizes of the feeding arteries and outflow veins. The outcome of an AVM following radiosurgery may be a total, subtotal, or partial obliteration of the nidus.

Total obliteration of the AVM after radiosurgery was defined as "complete absence of former nidus, normalization of afferent and efferent vessels, and a normal circulation time on high-quality rapid serial subtracted angiography"[59] (Fig. 5-2). Any remaining nidus, regardless of its size, is considered partial obliteration (Fig. 5-3). Subtotal obliteration of an AVM means the angiographic persistence of an early filling draining veins without demonstrable nidus (Fig. 5-4).[60]

Of the 880 patients treated 461 had adequate angiographic follow-up. Of these 461 patients, 80% were found to be cured within 2 years. At the time of the last evaluation of the results only 5% of patients had no change in the status of their AVMs. Ten percent had subtotal obliteration and 5% were partially obliterated. In this group of patients obliteration rates were affected by the size of the nidus. The rate for AVMs less than 1 cm^3 in volume was 88%. For 1 to 3 cm^3 it was 78% and for greater than 3 cm^3 it was 50%.

No patient that was harboring an angiographically proven obliterated AVM has ever hemorrhaged in our experience. Nor has a patient with a subtotally obliterated AVM sustained a postradiosurgery hemorrhage. Regardless of this we do not consider a patient cured until he has total obliteration of the AVM. The early draining vein represents persistence of the shunt.

Clinical Outcomes. A review of the long-term clinical outcomes following gamma surgery was carried out on 247 patients we treated between 1970 and 1983.[61] The presenting

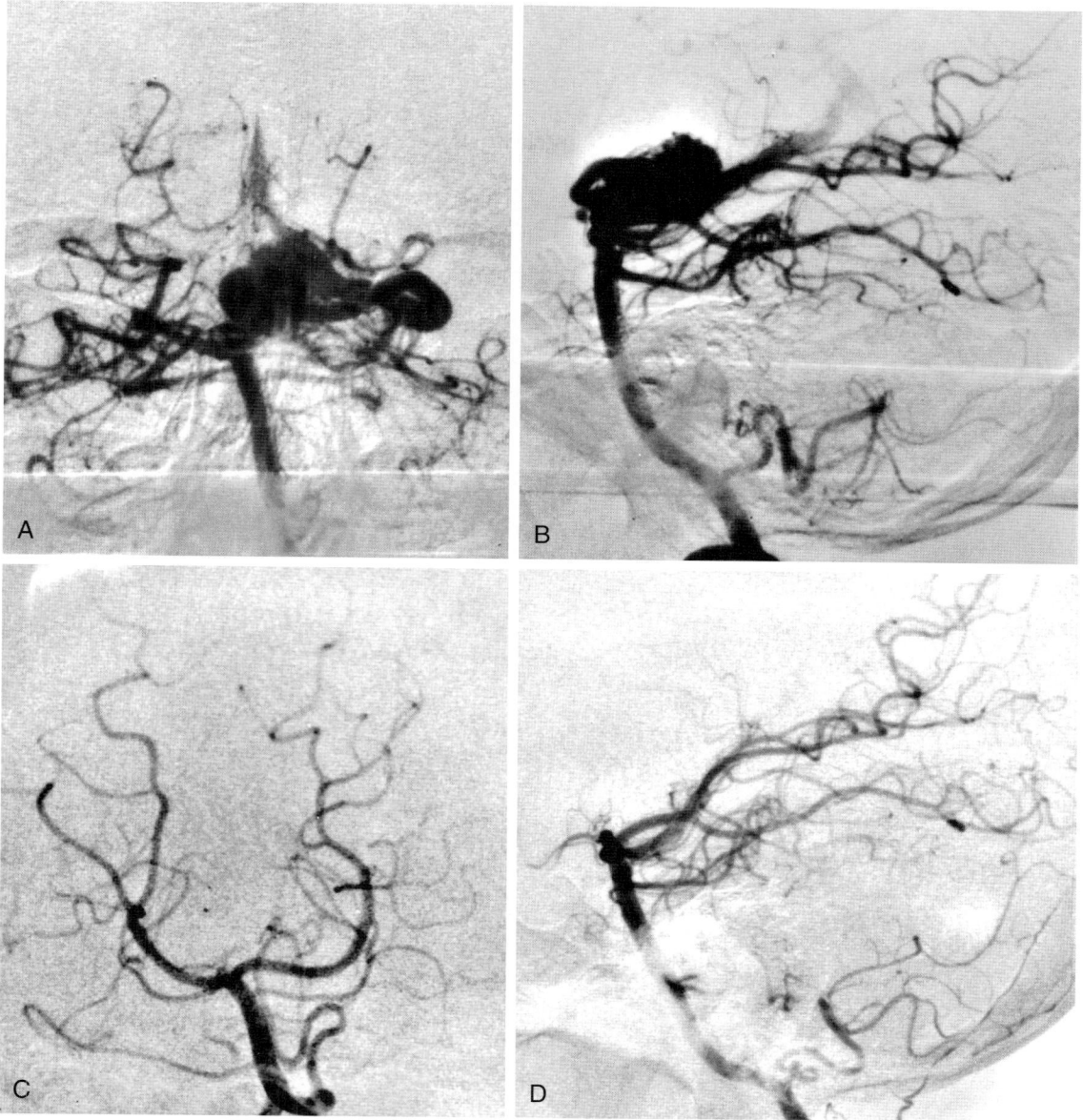

FIGURE 5-2 Obliteration of a midbrain AVM. Vertebral arteriogram showing (A) frontal and (B) lateral views before and (C and D) two years after gamma surgery. There was no neurologic deficit.

symptoms widely varied and 94% of the patients had hemorrhaged prior to therapy. Ninety-eight of these patients had chronic headaches and 66% had complete relief following gamma surgery. An additional 9% improved. Twenty-six percent had seizures prior to therapy and 19% of these became seizure free and 51% improved. Eleven patients (5%) without prior seizures had at least one seizure following therapy. Resolution or significant improvements were also seen in 53 of 74 patients with motor deficits (72%), 19 out of 46 with a sensory deficit (41%), 23 out of 44 with memory disturbance (52%), and 26 out of 35 with language dysfunction (74%).

The cause for clinical improvement following gamma surgery in such a large number of patients is unknown. The natural history of neurologic deficits to improve over time must be presumed to play a major role. The improvement in regional blood flow following AVM obliteration may also be

responsible for a portion of the gains made by the patients. Whatever the reason is, significant improvement is seen in many patients.

Outcomes of Gamma Surgery for Arteriovenous Malformations after 1989. Since 1989, a total of 1350 AVM patients were treated with gamma surgery at the Lars Leksell center for Gamma Surgery, University of Virginia, Charlottesville. Excluding 82 patients completely lost to follow-up, 139 patients with follow-up of less than 2 years and additional 106 patients with large AVMs undergoing only partial treatment, we analyze the outcome of 1023 AVMs. There were 523 males and 500 females with a mean age of 34 years (range 4–82 years). The presenting symptoms leading to the diagnosis of AVMs was hemorrhage in 529 (52%), seizure in 237 (23%), headache in 133 (13%), and

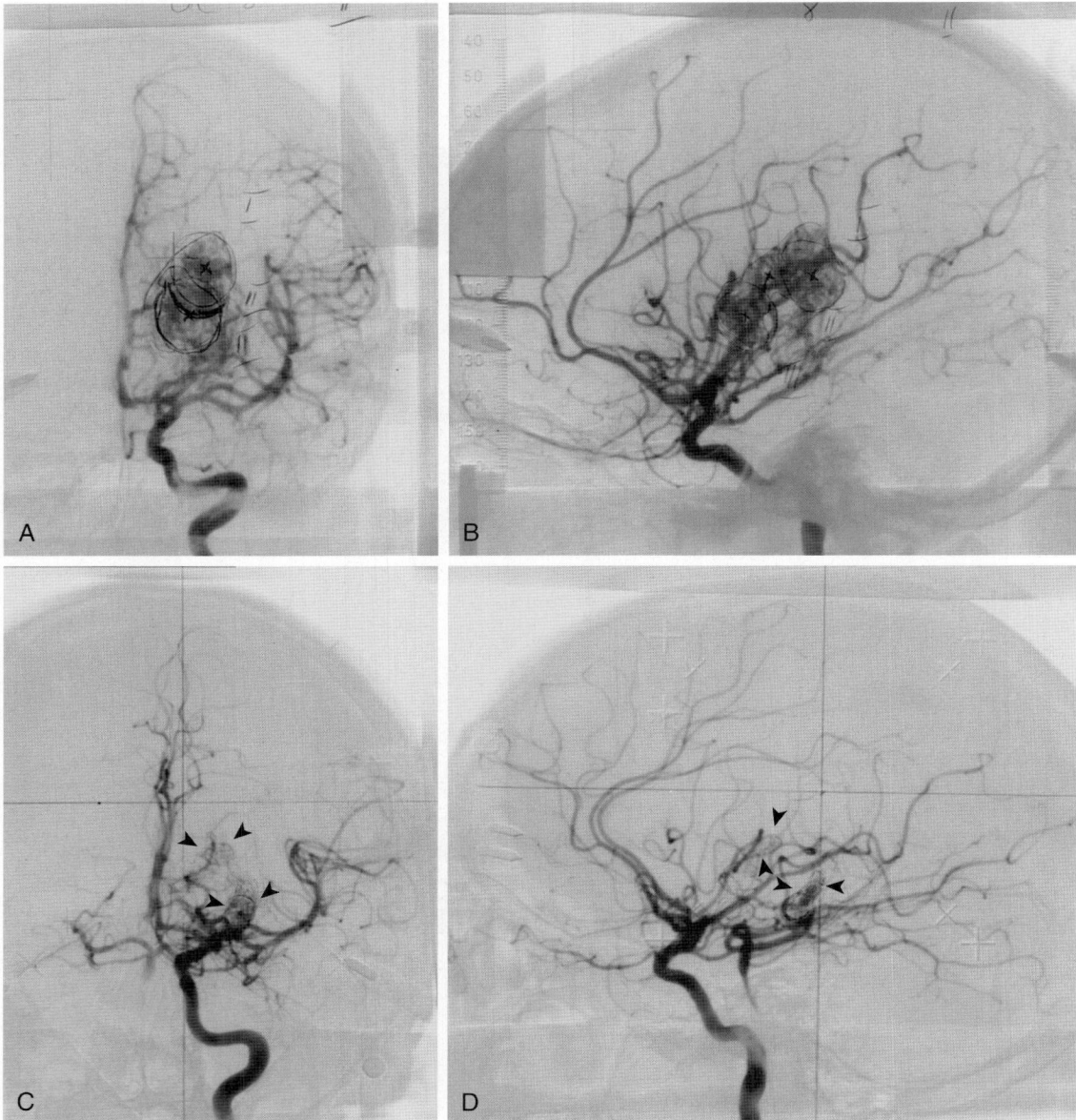

FIGURE 5-3 Partial obliteration of an AVM. Left sylvian AVM shown in anteroposterior (A) and lateral (B) views of a left carotid angiogram. Same views 4 years later (C and D) show a decrease in the size of the nidus but persistent shunting of blood through the partially obliterated malformation *(arrowheads)*. The residual AVM was recently retreated.

neurologic deficits in 94 (9%). In 30 patients (3%), the AVMs were incidental findings. The locations of the AVMs were in the cerebral hemispheres in 630 (62%), basal ganglion in 96 (9%), thalamus in 82 (8%), corpus callosum in 38 (4%), brain stem in 84 (8%), cerebellum in 68 (7%), and insula in 25 patients (2%). The Spetzler-Martin grading of the AVMs were Grade I in 174 (17%) patients, grade II in 328 (32.1%), Grade III in 440 (43%), Grade IV in 78 (7.6%) and grade V in three (0.3%). One hundred and twenty-two patients (12%) had previous partial resection of the nidi, and 244 patients (24%) underwent preradiosurgical embolization. The nidus volume ranged from 0.1 to 33 cm^3 (mean 3.5 cm^3). The mean prescription dose was 21.1 Gy (range 5–36 Gy), and the mean maximum dose was 39.0 Gy (range 10–60 Gy). The mean number of isocenters was 2.7 (range 1–22).

The mean follow-up was 80 months. Gamma surgery yielded a total angiographic obliteration in 552 (54%) and subtotal obliteration in 42 (4%) patients. In 290 (28%) patients, the AVMs remained patent and in 139 patients (14%) no flow voids were observed on the MRI. The angiographic total obliteration was achieved in 66% of patients with nidus less than 3 cm^3; 44% between 3 and 8 cm^3, and 28% with nidus volume larger than 8 cm^3. Small nidus volume, high prescription dose, and low number of isocenters are predictive of obliteration. Preradiosurgical embolization has a negative effect on obliteration.

The reported obliteration rate following radiosurgery varied greatly.[62-65] One should be cautious when interpreting the results owning to the biases injected from different cut-off time and imaging modality used to conclude total

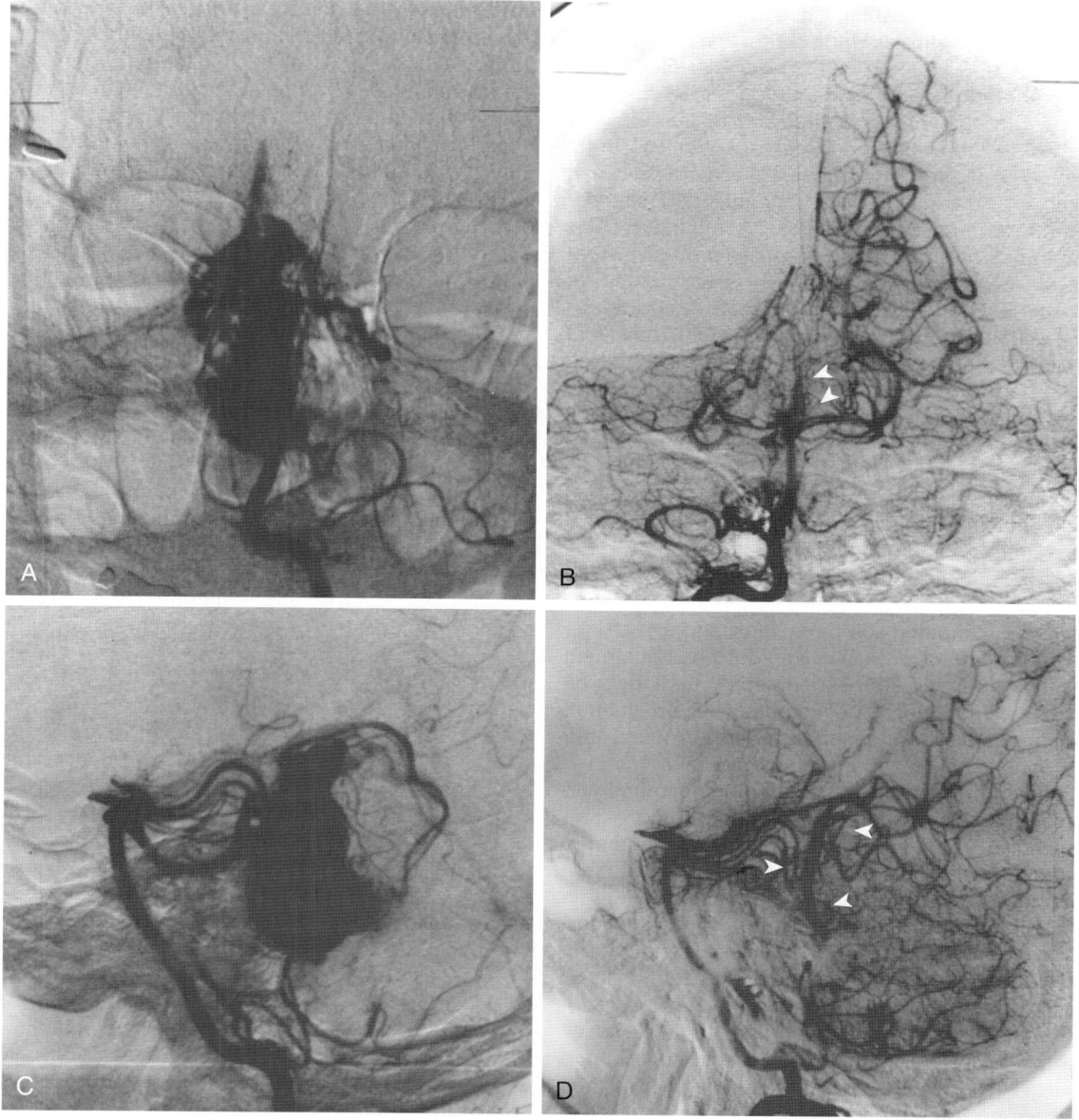

FIGURE 5-4 Subtotal obliteration of an AVM after gamma surgery. Anteroposterior (A) and lateral (C) vertebral angiograms demonstrating AVM located within the vermis of the cerebellum. Control angiography with the same views (B and D) obtained 3 years after gamma surgery shows no demonstrable nidus but the presence of an early filling vein *(arrowheads)*.

obliteration. Studies only including patients with long follow-up, reporting only patients undergoing angiography or including MRI as imaging study to conclude obliteration tend to overestimate the success rate of radiosurgery.[63,66,67]

Gamma Surgery for AVMs in Pediatric Patients.
Between 1989 and 2007, we treated 200 AVM patients less than 18 years of age. Fourteen cases with follow-up less than 2 years were excluded, leaving 186 patients for analysis. There were 98 males and 88 females with a mean age of 12.7 years (range 4–18 years). The presenting symptoms leading to the diagnosis of AVMs were hemorrhage in 133 (72%) patients, seizure in 29 (16%), headache in 11 (6%), and neurologic deficits in 8 (4%). Five (3%) patients were asymptomatic. Thirty-eight patients underwent embolization prior

to gamma surgery. Incomplete surgical resection was carried out in 24 patients. Five patients had partial resection and embolization before undergoing gamma surgery.

The locations of the AVMs were hemispheric in 101 (54%) patients, thalamus in 24 (13%), basal ganglia in 23 (12%), corpus callosum in 9 (5%), brain stem in 18 (10%), insula/sylvian fissure in 5 (3%), and cerebellum in 6 (3%). The nidus volumes ranged from 0.1 to 24 cm^3 (mean 3.2 cm^3). The treatment parameters were: mean prescription dose 21.9 Gy (range 7.5–35 Gy); mean maximum dose 40.1 Gy (range 20–50 Gy).

Following gamma surgery, a total obliteration was confirmed in 109 (59%) and subtotal obliteration in 9 (5%). Forty-nine (26%) patients still had patent residual nidus. In 19 (10%) patients, obliteration was confirmed on MRI only. The actuarial angiographic obliteration rate was 34% at 2 years, 46% at 3 years, and 51% at 5 years. In general, the imaging outcome of pediatric patients is similar to that observed in adult population. A negative history of preradiosurgical embolization and a high prescription dose were significantly associated with increased rate of obliteration.

Only a small series of children went through a systemic psychological test analyzing the cognitive deficits after gamma surgery. However, yearly follow-ups including questioning the parents, the patients, and the referring doctors about the intellectual development and possible cognitive or endocrinologic deficits were conducted. According to this information, 95% of the children had normal intellectual development after radiosurgery with satisfactory or good school performance. As adults, they performed from average to excellent and were socially well-adjusted.

Some studies had proposed that in pediatric patients the response to radiosurgery seems to be less favorable.[66] Hypotheses such as the immature vessels in pediatric cases more likely to recover from radiation induced damage and neovascularization in response to radiation have been proposed. Our experience show comparable result in children compared to adults. Additionally, we observe that adverse radiation induced damage seems to be more tolerable for kids, which proves that radiosurgery has a favorable benefit risk profile in the management of pediatric AVMs. However, the risk of hemorrhage remained in pediatric patients and the development of secondary tumor cannot be overlooked.

Gamma Surgery following Embolization of Arteriovenous Malformations.

The effectiveness of partial embolization followed by gamma surgery in the management of relatively large AVMs still remains controversial. When comparing the outcome in patients treated with gamma knife alone to those with combined embolization and gamma knife treatment, recent studies reported less favorable outcome in patients with preradiosurgical embolization.[65,68]

Between 1989 and 2007, a total number of 217 AVMs with prior partial embolization were treated with gamma surgery at the Lars Leksell center. There were 107 males (49%) and 110 females (51%) with a mean age of 32.8 years. Most of the AVMs were embolized with liquid embolics such as NBCA or ethanol. In 167 patients the nidus was compact after the embolization, whereas the angiogram of 50 cases revealed that the nidus was broken apart after the endovascular procedures. The mean volume of the nidus at the time of GKS was 5.1 cm^3 (range 0.02–24.9 cm^3). The mean prescription dose was 19.6 Gy (range 10–28.0 Gy) and the mean maximum dose was 37.2 Gy (range 20–50 Gy).

After gamma surgery an angiographically confirmed total obliteration of the AVMs was achieved in 71 patients (27%) (Fig. 5-5). A total obliteration on MRI was observed in 26 patients (10%). In 157 patients (60%) only a partial obliteration could be obtained after a follow-up period of at least 2 years. Eight patients (3%) presented with a subtotal obliteration. The outcome after gamma surgery in embolized AVMs (obliteration rate 27%) is much less favorable than AVMs treated with gamma knife only (obliteration rate 72%).

Recanalization of previously embolized parts of the nidus,[69] difficulty in nidus delineation following previous embolization,[65] and attenuation of radiation dose by embolization materials[70] have been proposed to explain the less

favorable outcome in patients with preradiosurgical embolization. Theoretically, volume reduction following embolization affords a lower chance of radiosurgery-related adverse effect; however, our data do not show this. Additionally, the complications from embolization are not negligible. Therefore, the use of embolization before gamma knife treatment remains problematic and awaits further investigation.

Gamma Surgery for Large Arteriovenous Malformations.

Recently, there has been much discussion of gamma surgery for large AVMs. The main problem with large AVMs is due to the dependence of the obliteration response on dose and volume; this dependency requires a delicate balance in deciding an efficient dose but low enough to avoid adverse neurologic deficits.

The following strategies are currently available to treat large AVMs with radiosurgery.
1. Embolization of a portion of the AVMs then performing radiosurgery if the nidus shrinks to a size manageable with radiosurgery. However, embolization should effectively shrink the nidus for radiosurgery to achieve good results; otherwise fragmentation of the nidus into a number of segments will make the radiosurgical planning difficult and increasing the probability of radiosurgery failure.
2. Staged radiosurgery to selected volumes of the AVMs. Sirin et al.[71] used staged volumetric radiosurgery in 28 large AVMs. Out of the 21 patients, seven underwent repeat radiosurgery and were eliminated from outcome analysis. Of the remaining 14 patients, three had total obliteration on angiograms, and 4 had no flow voids on MRI but had no follow-up angiography. Four patients had hemorrhages after radiosurgery resulting in two deaths. Worsened neurologic deficits occurred in one patient.
3. Treating the whole nidus in one session with low-dose radiosurgery. Pan et al.[72] reported an obliteration rate of 25% for AVMs with volume larger than 15 cm^3. The obliteration rate increased to 50% at 50 months follow-up. The morbidity was 3.3%. Post-treatment hemorrhage occurred in 9.2% of cases.
4. At Lars Leksell center, we evaluated a protocol using combined radiosurgery and microsurgery for the management of large AVMs. Gamma surgery was performed for the deep medullary portion of the AVMs as a first step. The second step was planned as microsurgical extirpation of the superficial segment if the goal of the first step, obliteration of the deep segment of the AVM, was achieved. However, in less than 5% of the patients, this goal was achieved.

The management of large AVMs demonstrates that every treatment has its limitations. In an effort to solve the problems of the management of large AVMs, a cautious approach is warranted pending the development of new techniques and agents for embolization.

Hemorrhage Risk in the Treatment–Response Interval

Whether gamma surgery without obliteration of the nidus provides partial protection from hemorrhage is still controversial. It has been demonstrated by some authors that there may be some degree of protective effect.[73-75] Because the

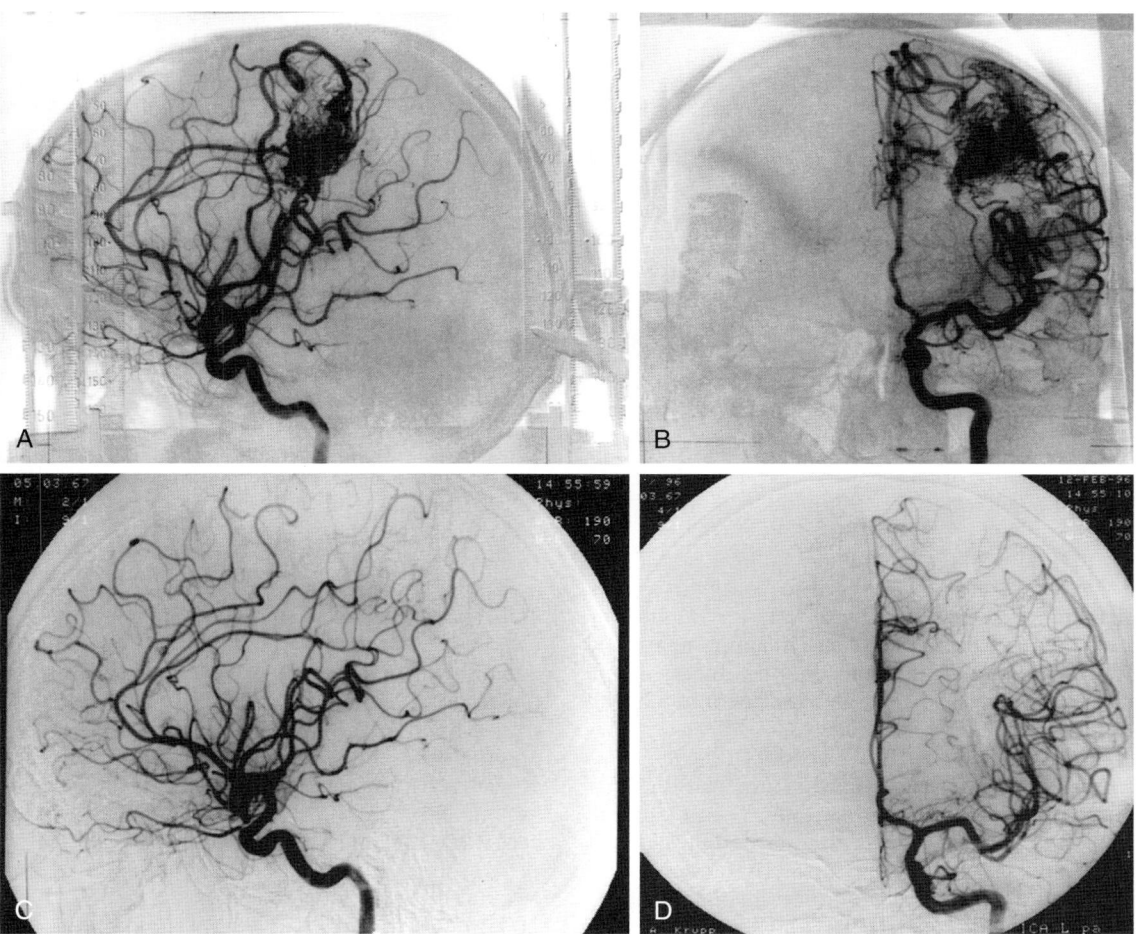

FIGURE 5-5 Gamma surgery following a partial embolization of the AVM. A 24-year-old male diagnosed with a left-sided AVM at the left sensorimotor cortex following a hemorrhage (A and B lateral and frontal projections of angiograms). The patient underwent a partial embolization. The nidus obliterated completely 3 years following gamma surgery (C and D).

incidence of hemorrhage in a matched group of untreated patients will likely never be known and the timing of obliteration is not known except as being between diagnostic scans, it is a difficult position to support.

The incidence of hemorrhage following gamma surgery during the first 2 years was studied in 1604 of our patients and reported by Karlsson et al.[76] There were 49 hemorrhages for an annual incidence of 1.4%. This is slightly lower than the generally accepted rate of 2% to 4% per year but includes all 1604 patients, consisting of those known and not known to have obliterated AVMs. Of these hemorrhages, 14 were fatal (annual rate of 0.4%) and 9 had permanent neurologic deficits (annual rate of 0.3%).

Repeat Gamma Surgery for Incompletely Obliterated Arteriovenous Malformations. In general, the risk of hemorrhage persists as long as the AVM nidus is still patent. This provided the rationale for retreatment of still patent AVMs following the initial gamma surgery.

In our experience, 74 males and 66 females with a mean age of 33 years underwent repeat gamma surgery for still-patent AVMs following initial gamma surgery from 1989 to 2007. Causes of initial treatment failure included inaccurate nidus definition in 14, failure to fill part of the nidus due to hemodynamic factors in 16, recanalization of embolized AVM compartments in 6, and suboptimal dose (<20 Gy) in 23 patients. Nineteen patients had repeat gamma surgery for subtotal obliteration of AVMs. In 62 patients, the AVMs failed to obliterate in spite of correct target definition and adequate dose. At the time of retreatment, the nidus volume ranged from 0.1 to 6.9 cm^3 (mean 1.4 cm^3) and the mean prescription dose was 20.3 Gy. Clinical follow-up ranged from 15 to 220 months with a mean of 84.2 months after repeat gamma surgery.

Repeat treatment yielded a total angiographic obliteration in 77 (55%) (Fig. 5-6) and subtotal obliteration in 9 (6.4%) patients. In 38 (27.1%) patients, the AVMs remained patent. In 16 patients (11.4%) no flow voids were observed on the MRI. High prescription dose, small nidus volume, nidi with only superficial venous drainage, and a negative history of prior embolization were significantly associated with increased rate of AVM obliteration. Clinically, 126 patients improved or remained stable and 14 experienced deterioration (8 due to a rebleed, 2 caused by persistent arteriovenous shunting, and 4 related to radiation induced changes).

We advise repeat gamma surgery in cases with still patent nidi 3 to 4 years after initial gamma surgery when open

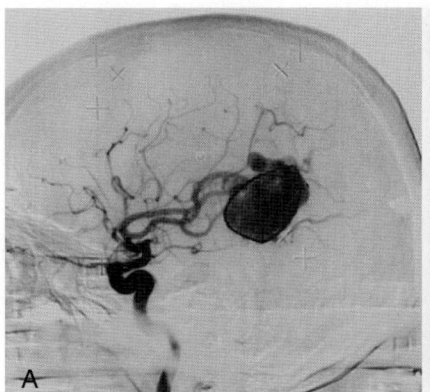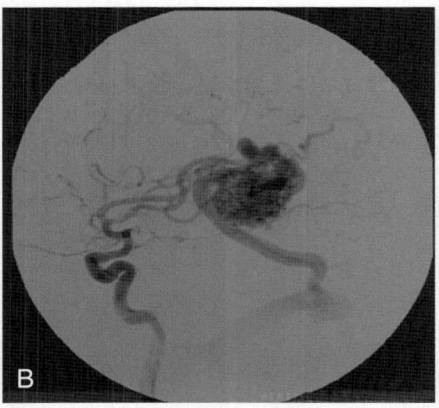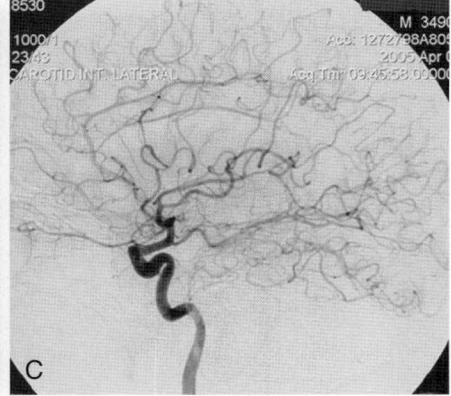

FIGURE 5-6 Repeat gamma surgery for AVM. A 33-year-old male with a left parietal AVM presenting with seizure. The patient underwent first gamma surgery with a prescription of 20 Gy in 1991 (A). The flow of the nidus seemed to be reduced but the overall size of the nidus had not changed (B). He had a repeat gamma surgery in 2002 with 18 Gy as a prescription dose and the nidus completely obliterated in 2005 (C). His seizure frequency decreased significantly.

surgery or endovascular procedures were expected to yield higher risk of complications than gamma surgery. Our experience showed that when repeating gamma knife treatment a dose of at least 20 Gy led to a higher chance of subsequent nidus obliteration (77% vs. 47% with prescription dose less than 20 Gy).

Hemorrhage from Angiographically Confirmed Obliterated Arteriovenous Malformations. Some studies have noted AVM reappearance after apparent gamma knife surgery obliteration.[77] In our histopathologic analysis, gamma surgery of AVMs caused endothelial damage, proliferation of smooth muscle cells, and the elaboration of extracellular collagen by these cells, which led to progressive stenosis and obliteration of the AVM nidus.[43] In this same report, there was evidence of small trapped vessels that would have very little blood flow. It is unclear what histopathologic process would permit the formation of new vessels following radiosurgical-induced obliteration of the AVM nidus. However, it is clear that the infrequent and small trapped vessels observed by Schneider et al.[43] could not explain the angiographic findings reported by Linqvist et al.[78] Such inconsistent findings following radiosurgical treatment of AVMs suggest the need for further clinical and histopathologic investigation and the continued follow-up of patients, particularly pediatric ones, following gamma surgery.

In our series of AVMs treated with gamma surgery, we observed no recurrent hemorrhage after angiographically confirmed obliteration of the AVMs. In one case reported by Guo et al., a rebleed occurred after angiographic documentation of nidus obliteration.[79] The MRI findings suggested that hemorrhage possibly resulted from radiation-induced tissue damage. Furthermore, the histologic examination of the suspected recanalized AVM revealed channels that were one-fiftieth the size of the smallest vascular channels in AVMs, making it unlikely that these were vessels with significant blood flow. This view has been further confirmed by the fact that a repeat angiogram revealed no evidence of residual malformation or recanalization. Rebleeding, in spite of post-treatment angiograms interpreted as normal, may be explained by unsatisfactory quality of the neuroimaging studies or inadequate interpretation leading to the misdiagnosis of angiographic cure.

Subtotal Obliteration of Arteriovenous Malformations. Subtotal obliteration of an AVM following gamma surgery has been reported sporadically. This angiographic phenomenon implies a complete disappearance of AVM nidus but persistence of early filling drainage veins (see Fig. 5-4). Theoretically, the early filling venous drainage suggests that some shunting still persists.

We reported a series of 159 patients with subtotal obliteration of AVMs (SOAVMs).[60] The incidence of SOAVMs was 7.6% from a total of 2093 AVM patients who were treated with gamma surgery and had angiographic follow-up available. The diagnosis was made after a mean of 29.4 months (range 4–178 months) following gamma surgery.

During the cumulative period of 767 patient-years (a mean of 4.9 years per patient) after the diagnosis of SOAVMs, no SOAVMs had ruptured. Follow-up angiography was performed in 90 of 136 patients in whom SOAVMs had no further treatment. These studies showed a total obliteration of the original AVMs as well as disappearance of the early filling vein in 66 patients (73%). Twenty-four patients (27%) had persistent SOAVMs. Twenty-three patients with SOAVMs were treated with gamma knife targeting the proximal end of the early filling veins. In this group, follow-up angiography was performed in 19 patients, confirming disappearance of the early filling vein in 15 patients (79%) and persistent SOAVMs in four patients (21%). None of the patients suffered a rupture of the lesion. This suggests that the protection from rebleeding at the stage of subtotal obliteration is significant.

Our series shows that subtotal obliteration of the AVMs did not necessarily prove to be a premature stage of an ongoing obliteration, and instead might be the end point of the obliteration process. Earlier in our series, we repeated gamma surgery for SOAVMs, targeting the proximal segment of the early filling vein. After repeat treatment, 79% SOAVMs were obliterated. However, the necessity of retreatment remains to be determined given the fact that in the whole group no hemorrhage occurred and that 73% of SOAVMs obliterated spontaneously.

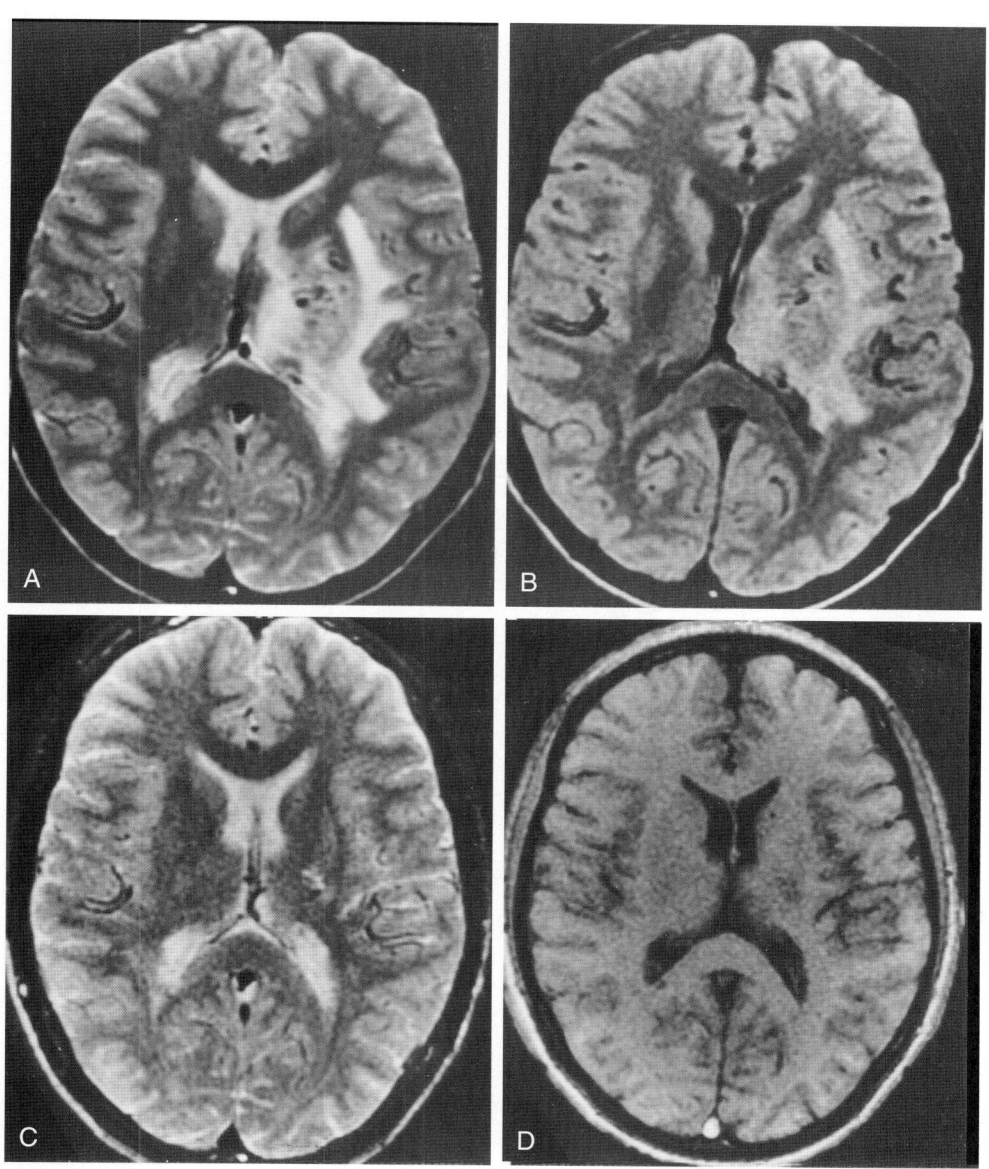

FIGURE 5-7 Onset and resolution of radiation-induced changes of normal brain tissue. Radiation-induced changes 6 months following radiosurgical treatment of a left basal ganglia arteriovenous malformation with a margin dose of 20 Gy. Appearance on (A) T2- and (B) T1-weighted MRI. These changes showed progressive regression and complete disappearance at 2 years following onset (C and D). Angiography documented total obliteration of the arteriovenous malformation.

Complications

Radiation-Induced Changes

Radiation-induced change is an increased T2 signal around the AVMs on MRI following radiosurgery (Fig. 5-7). Radiation damage of glial cells, endothelial cells damage followed by breakdown of blood–brain barrier, excessive generation of free radicals or release of vascular endothelial growth factors have been proposed to explain this imaging finding. The severity of radiation-induced changes on images and associated neurologic deficits varied ranging from asymptomatic, a few millimeters increased T2 signal surrounding the treated nidus to massive brain edema with symptoms and signs of increased intracranial pressure. From our 1500 gamma knife procedures performed for AVM patients with follow-up MRI available for analysis, 34% of patients developed radiation-induced changes. Among them, 60% had mild (a few millimeters of increased T2 signal surrounding the nidus), 33% had moderate (compression of ventricle and effacement of

sulci) and 7% had severe (midline shift) radiation-induced changes. The mean time to the development of radiation-induced changes was 13 months after gamma surgery. Resolution of these changes was the usual course and the mean duration of the changes was 22 months. Large nidus volumes, high prescription doses, history with preradiosurgical embolization, and nidus without previous hemorrhage were associated with higher risk of radiation-induced changes.

Of the patients who developed radiation-induced changes, 122 (8.7%) patients had headache, worsening or new seizures, or neurologic deficits. Patients with severe radiation induced changes and nidus at eloquent areas were more likely to develop symptoms. Twenty six patients (1.8%) had permanent neurologic deficits.

Cyst Formation

A rare occurrence following gamma surgery for AVMs is the development of an expansive cyst at or adjacent to an obliterated AVM (Fig. 5-8). Cyst developed after resolution of

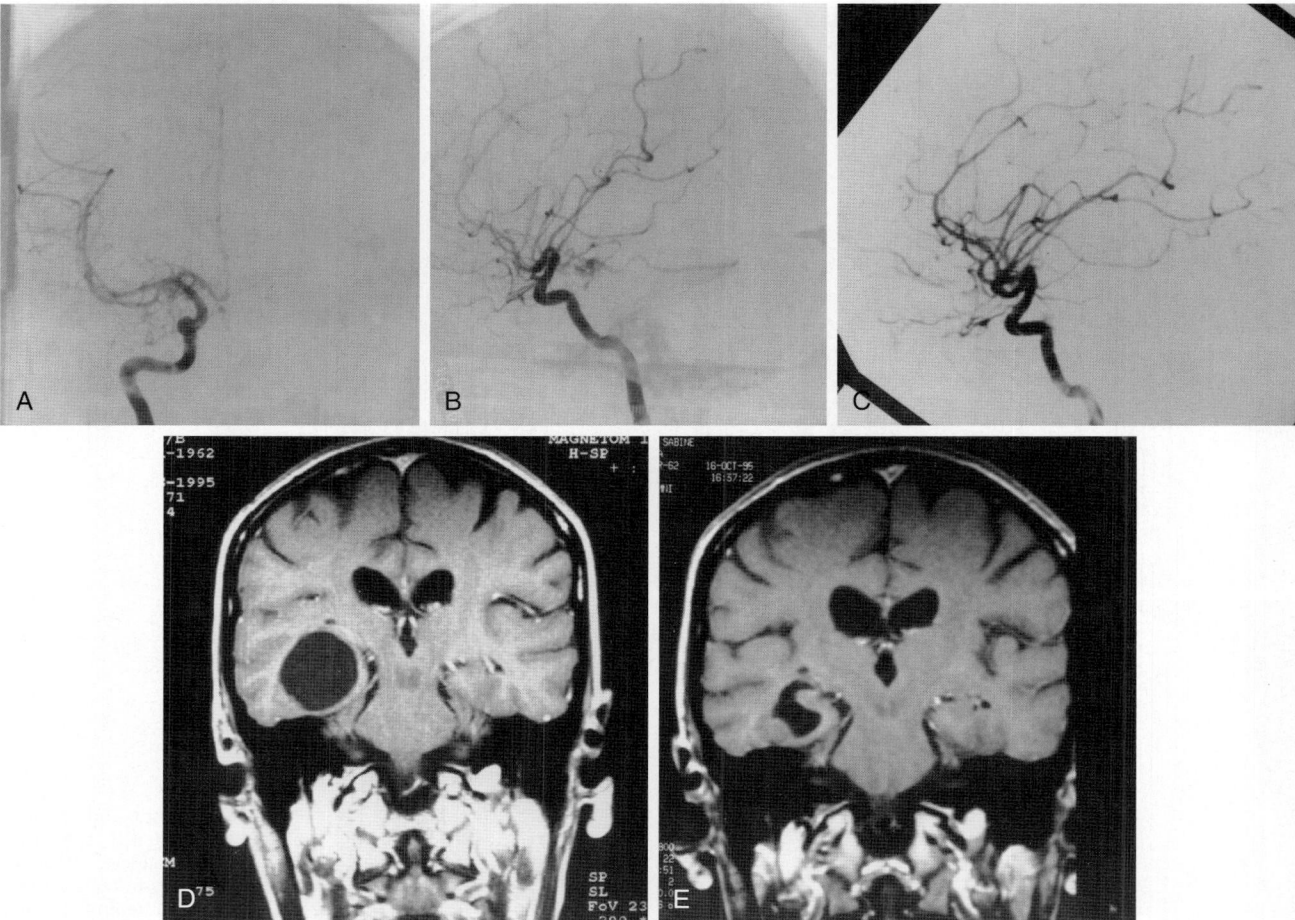

FIGURE 5-8 Delayed occurrence of cyst formation following gamma surgery for an AVM. This small, right-sided AVM visualized on anteroposterior (A) and lateral carotid arteriography (B) was cured as shown on this control angiogram obtained 2 years after gamma surgery (C). The development of headaches and personality changes prompted an MRI examination 7 years after gamma surgery (D and E). This cyst was surgically decompressed. Biopsy of the cyst wall did not reveal any evidence of tumor. (Follow-up MRI courtesy of Professor J. Camaert, Chairman, Department of Neurosurgery, Gent, Belgium.)

previous hemorrhages or fluid cavities from encephalomalacia after surgeries should not be considered as complications related to gamma surgery. First reported in 1992[45] in two patients out of a series of forty, we found a total of 20 patients (1.6%) developing a cyst after a mean of 8.1 years postradiosurgery from our 1272 patients with follow-up MRI available.[80] Six patients had large cysts and three of them were symptomatic requiring surgery. Two cases underwent craniotomy and drainage of the cyst. The cyst wall showed no evidence of neoplasia. Direct radiation injury to the perilesional brain tissue, increased permeability of the blood–brain barrier with accumulation of the exudative fluid, hemodynamic perturbations during gradual obliteration of the nidus with subsequent ischemic tissue damage, and tissue destruction due to subclinical perilesional hemorrhages have been proposed as the possible mechanisms of cyst formation.

Radiosurgery-Induced Neoplasia

We found two meningiomas from 1333 AVM patients treated with gamma surgery (Fig. 5-9); however, follow-up imaging was performed over a period of at least 10 years in only 288 of these patients.[81] If we conservatively estimate that radiosurgery-induced lesions would be evident within a 10-year time interval, then our incidence of radiosurgery-induced neoplasia is 2 in 2880 person-years or 69 in 100,000 person-years. Thus, there is a 0.7% chance that a radiation-induced tumor may develop within 10 years following gamma surgery. The long latency and relative rarity of these lesions following radiosurgery may defy a conclusive determination of the true incidence.

Dural Arteriovenous Fistulas

Although dural arteriovenous fistulas (dAVFs) comprise approximately 15% of all intracranial vascular malformations, the precise mechanism of formation remains unknown. The leading theories include adjacent venous sinus stasis as well as alterations in local expression of vasogenic factors, such as vascular endothelial growth factor and fibroblastic growth factor.[82,83]

From a treatment standpoint, experience with dAVFs is distinct from AVMs. Studies have established that the flow dynamics of dAVFs are the most important indicator of the need to treat and modality to choose, be it embolization, open microsurgery, or radiosurgery. As the aggressive natural history of lesions with cortical venous reflux differs significantly from lesions without angiographic evidence of

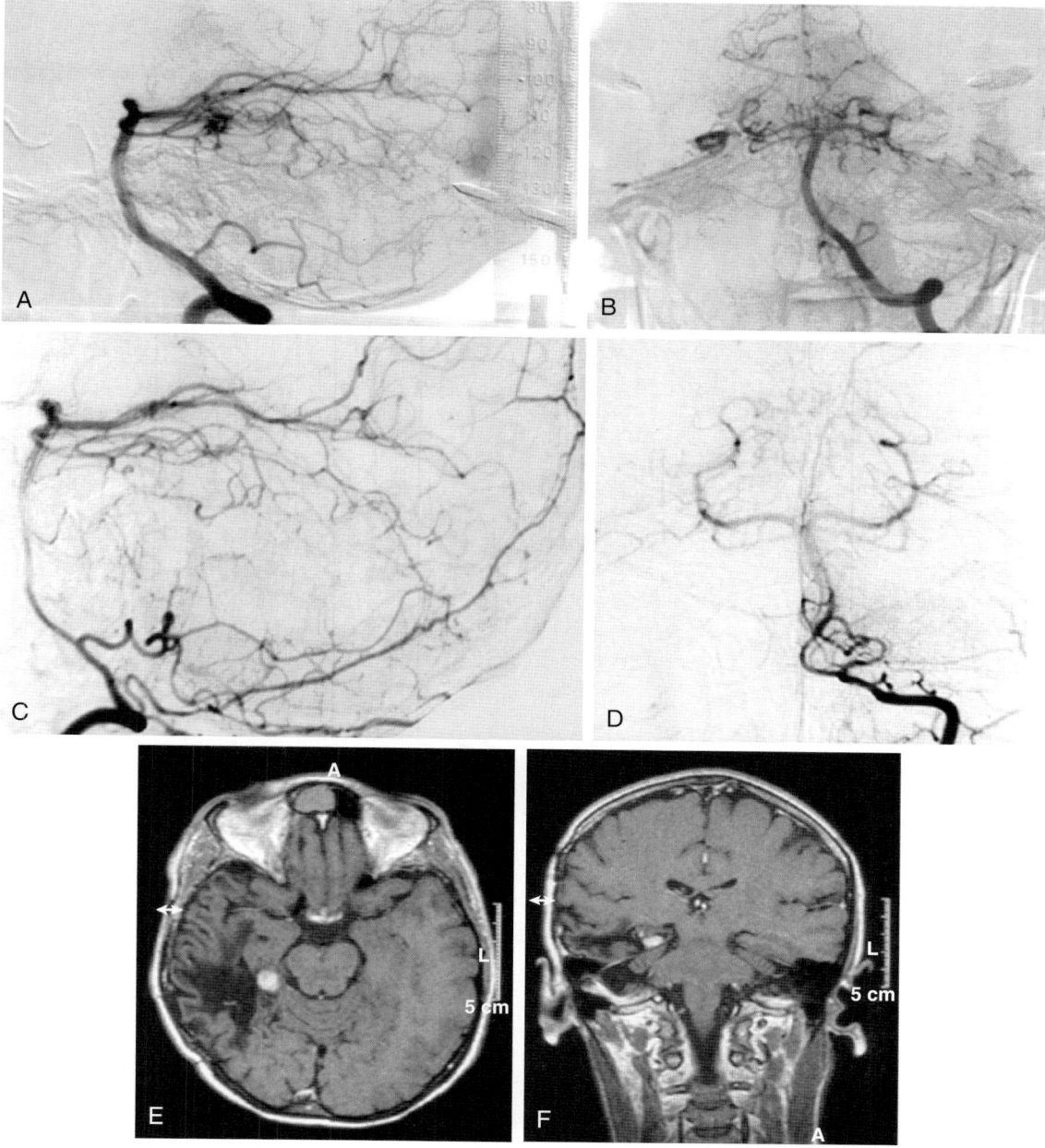

FIGURE 5-9 Radiation-induced neoplasia. Anteroposterior (A) and lateral (B) views of vertebral angiograms demonstrate a right temporal AVM before gamma surgery. Two years after treatment the nidus obliterated completely (C and D). Axial and coronal contrast-enhanced, T1-weighted MRI (E and F) obtained 10 years postradiosurgery show a meningioma adjacent to the superior surface of tentorium. It is located in the area where the previous AVM was situated.

cortical venous reflux, early definitive therapy via endovascular procedures or open surgical resection appears to be preferable to radiosurgery as a first-line treatment. Although radiosurgery is thought to be an effective agent for decreasing neovascularization in dAVFs, the time interval needed for the desired effect is too great to justify radiosurgery as a first-line therapy.[84]

The long-term analysis of radiosurgery for dAVFs over 25 years at the Karolinska University Hospital in Stockholm, Sweden included 52 patients treated between 1978 and 2003. The obliteration rate reported in this study was 68% with 16 dAVFs presenting as less aggressive Borden I or Cognard I/IIa lesions.[85] In a similar institutional experience at the Lars Leksell center between 1989 and 2005, 55 patients with dAVFs were treated with gamma surgery, primarily as an adjunct to surgery or embolization. Obliteration rates measured by angiography at 3 years ranged from 54% to 65%, with the 16 patients classified as Borden I lesions (Fig. 5-10). Unlike the Karolinska study, the majority of patients treated at the Lars Leksell center received gamma surgery as a secondary therapy, with 41 of the 54 patients receiving surgical or endovascular intervention prior to radiosurgery. Regardless of the difference in utilization of radiosurgery as a primary or secondary treatment modality, the results of these long-term studies indicate that gamma knife is an effective and safe treatment for intracranial dAVFs.

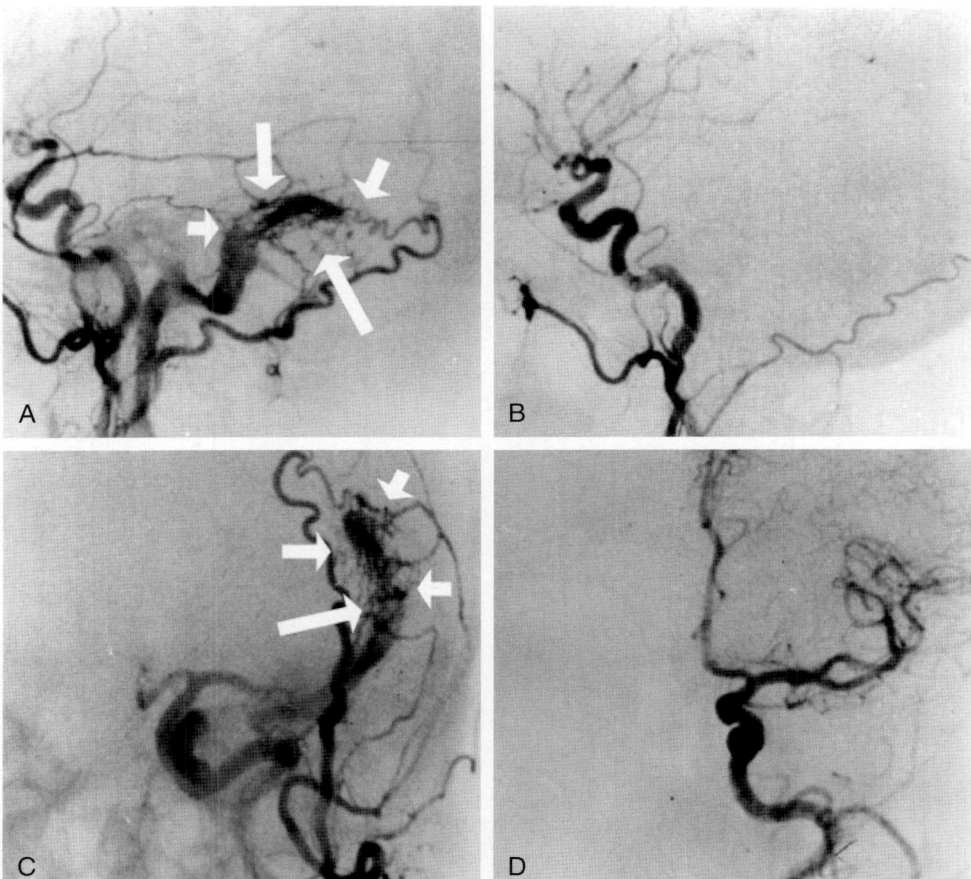

FIGURE 5-10 Total obliteration of dural arteriovenous fistula following gamma surgery. Left common carotid angiogram lateral (A) and (C) frontal projections of a dural arteriovenous fistula in the region of the left transverse sinus. Complete obliteration is demonstrated at 2 years following gamma surgery in the (B) lateral and (D) frontal projections.

Vein of Galen Malformations

We have treated nine patients with vein of Galen malformations. The patients ranged in age from 4 to 72 years of age. Among these patients, there were three with Yasargil Type I, one with Type II, two with type III, and three with type IV malformations. Prior embolization had failed in four of the cases. Three of the vein of Galen malformations were treated twice with radiosurgery. Follow-up angiograms were obtained in eight of the patients treated.[86] Four malformations were completely obliterated (Fig. 5-11). Another one seems to be obliterated but definitive confirmation could not be obtained as the patient refused a final angiogram. Another patient has some residual fistula not in the initial radiosurgical treatment field and has been retreated. Two other patients had marked reduction of flow through their malformations.

Cavernous Malformations

The success of treating AVMs prompted the treatment of cavernous malformations (CMs) with the gamma knife. Their tendency to be small in size, with the lack of intervening normal brain tissue and relatively low rate of clinically significant hemorrhage made CMs a natural target for the gamma knife. The rate of hemorrhage for cavernomas is widely disparate in the neurosurgical literature reported as between 0.1% and 32%.[87-90] This is largely due to semantic differences in defining a hemorrhage with some authors counting the presence of a hemosiderin ring on MRI as

evidence of a hemorrhage as well as in determining the date from which patients were at risk for hemorrhages.

Gamma surgery of CMs appears to have a histologic effect on them, which is not evident on imaging studies. In a case reported earlier,[29] a gamma surgery treated CM followed for 5 years showed no change on MRI studies. Histologic examination following surgical removal of the lesion showed it to be partially obliterated (Fig. 5-12).

A total of 23 patients have been treated by us for CMs between 1985 and 1996, 22 of which are available for follow-up evaluation.[91] Maximum treatment dose varied from 11 to 60 Gy (mean 33 Gy). Peripheral dose varied from 9 to 35 Gy (mean 18 Gy). Nine symptomatic hemorrhages occurred in this group after therapy for an annual incidence of 8%. Four of these patients were subsequently operated upon. Six patients suffered neurologic decline secondary to radiation-induced changes, five of which were permanent. Two patients subsequently underwent surgery. Thus the permanent radiation-induced complication rate is 22%, nearly 12 times higher than expected for a similarly treated group of AVM patients. The high incidence of post-treatment hemorrhage and radiation-induced complications is greater than the expected morbidity from an untreated group. For this reason the routine use of the gamma knife in the treatment of CMs cannot be supported at this time.

There have been observations in literature that demonstrate a protective effect of gamma surgery on the rate of hemorrhage in these lesions. Based on 38 cases,

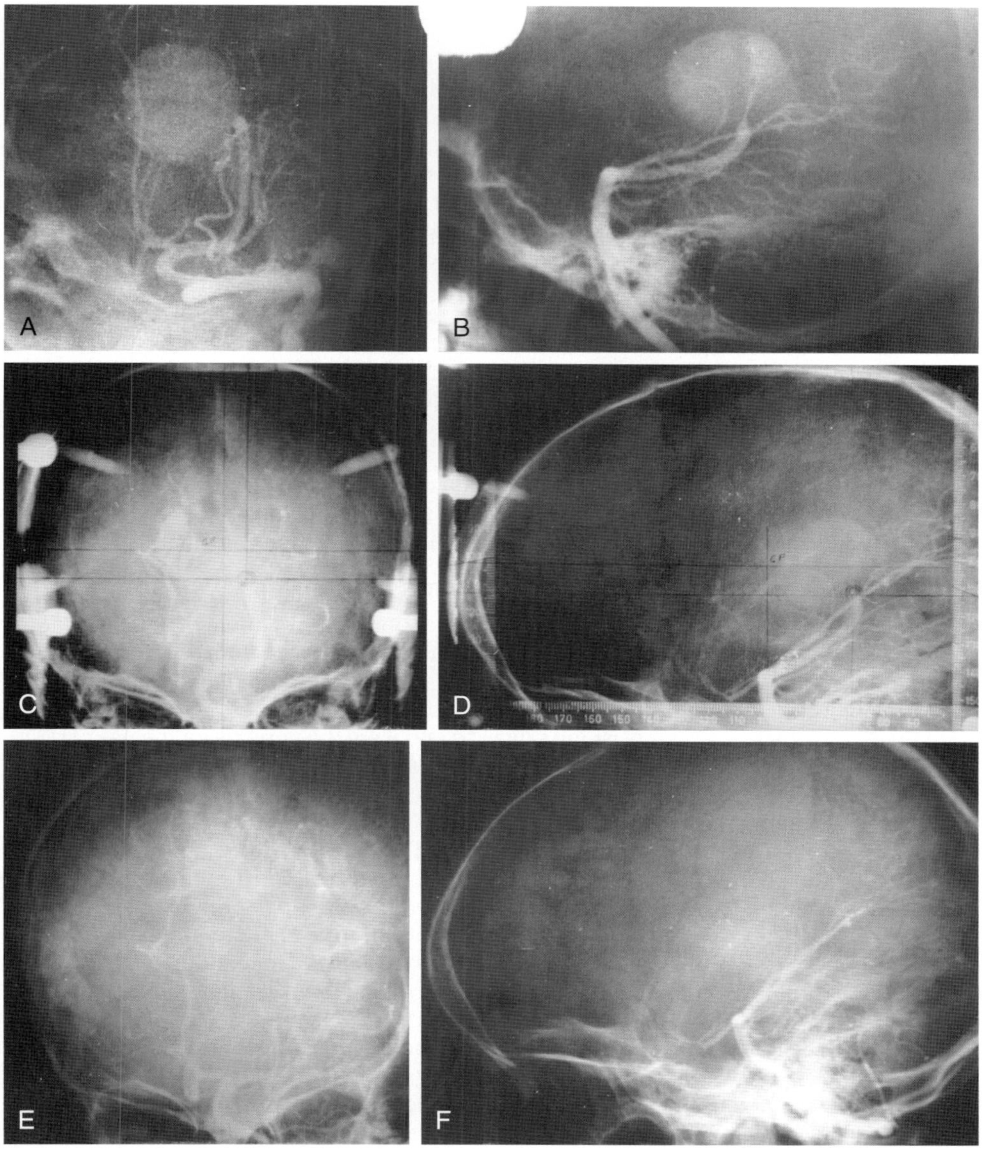

FIGURE 5-11 Gamma surgery for a vein of Galen malformation. A-P (A) and lateral (B) vertebral angiograms show direct shunting of blood into the primitive precursor (promesencephalic vein) of the vein of Galen. C and D, Stereotactic angiogram obtained at the time of treatment. E and F, Control angiography obtained 1 year later demonstrate cure of the malformation. (Courtesy of Hernan Bunge, MD, Clinica del Sol, Buenos Aires, Argentina.)

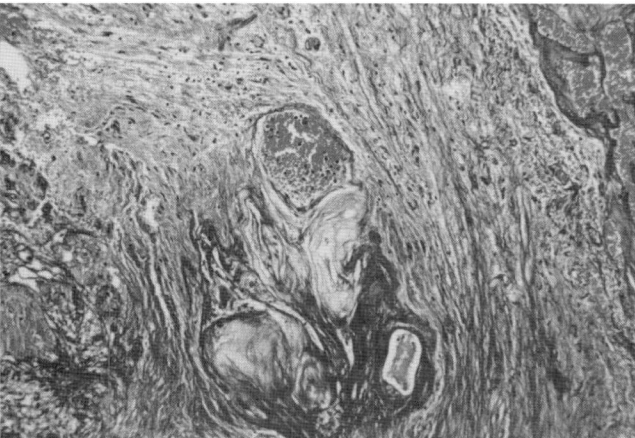

FIGURE 5-12 Hematoxylin and eosin stained histologic section of a cavernous malformation that was treated with gamma surgery. Because no change was observed on serial MRI examinations over 5 years, the lesion was excised. Except for a single persistent capillary channel, the malformation was obliterated.

Kondziolka et al.[92] maintain that radiosurgery offers benefit to these patients. They reported that 6 patients (15%) had significant reduction in size with a 13% hemorrhage rate; 10 of the patients (26%) developed neurologic deficits, 2 of these underwent surgery and succumbed to the illness. The rate of complications reported by them in the face of the fact that only 15% of the patients in this series had any reduction in the size of the lesion does not, in our opinion, constitute grounds for justifying radiosurgery for CMs. Furthermore, their contention that the complications reported by us may in part be due to the high doses used in treatment does not get support from their statistics with a lower dose. These 38 patients were a part of a later report on 47 patients from the same authors detailing the outcome. They found a postradiosurgery annual hemorrhage rate of 8.8%, which is high when compared to the risk reported by the same authors at 0.6% to 4.5%, even if the difference is not statistically significant. They chose, however, to compare their postradiosurgery hemorrhage rates with the preradiosurgery rate in the same subjects, making the assumption that the rate could be based on an epoch starting from first observation or first hemorrhage. This is fallacious since the malformation was present before the presenting hemorrhage and most likely from birth. Recomputed on this basis the preradiosurgery annual bleed rate comes to 5.9%, which is more congruent with expected natural history. Once again the incidence of hemorrhages postradiosurgery seems spuriously higher.

During the past decade, gamma knife has been widely used in some centers to treat CMs. Since the lesions cannot be precisely visualized by any imaging studies, the outcome of radiosurgery was universally evaluated based on the hemorrhage rate before and after radiosurgery using the same group of patients as control. There are methodological flaws in such study design. As been demonstrated in publications,[93] patients with previous hemorrhages tend to bleed more often. By calculating the clustering number of hemorrhages in the short period of follow-up time, which was prematurely terminated by radiosurgery prompted by the hemorrhage, the preradiosurgical hemorrhage rate was erroneously high ranging from 17% to 36%.[64,88,94-96] The hemorrhage rate after gamma surgery is these series ranged from 2% to 4%, which seems to be significantly low compared to the preradiosurgical bleeding rate but actually is not much different while comparing to the number reported in series studying natural course of CMs. Of note, the complications in these series remained to be high.

Developmental Venous Anomalies

The natural history of developmental venous anomalies (previously named venous angiomas) is benign[97] and clearly not a surgical lesion. Prior to clear elucidation of this prognosis, 19 patients were treated for this entity by us.[98] One patient was cured and three were partially obliterated. Three patients suffered radionecrosis, and one had symptomatic edema. One patient with radionecrosis underwent subsequent debridement. A 5% cure incidence with a 30% complication incidence for a benign entity is unacceptable.

TUMORS

Treatment of tumors with gamma surgery introduces a new approach to the evaluation of the endpoint of the treatment. Unlike microsurgery no actual debulking of tissue occurs, and, in the short term, there are no visible changes. However, in the long term, the tumors often shrink, and some even disappear entirely on follow-up neuroimaging studies. Success is therefore established by a pattern of reducing tumor size over serial follow-up studies or the lack of growth. With benign tumors, the natural history may be one of no growth for many years. As such, longer follow-up is necessary to ascertain whether gamma surgery affords true tumor volume control in slow growing tumors.

In an attempt to eliminate some of the subjectivity of naked eye observations and the obvious fallacy resulting from the estimation of a three dimensional object on the basis of three linear measurements in orthogonal planes, we have developed software that allows estimation of lesion volume based on MRI or CT.[99] The procedure involves scanning the study into a computer program and outlining the pathology in each slice. The computer then measures the area within the contour and calculates a volume based on slice thickness, the process is repeated for each slice and the total volume calculated by integrating the individual slice volumes. The error of this method was determined by comparing various hand-partitioned volumes with volumes estimated using polyhedrons to approximate the regions of interest on each slice. The average relative error is strongly dependent on the number of axial slices obtained through the object of interest and is fairly independent of the size of the object itself. For objects varying in volume from 0.1 to 10 cc, the average relative errors per number of slices through the object have been computed as follows: 3% for 7 slices, 4% for 6 slices, 6% for 5 slices, 11% for 4 slices, and 21% for 3 slices. Volumetric estimation based on 1 or 2 slices through the region of interest produces unacceptable average relative errors of more than 40%. We now require all follow-up studies to be performed with a slice thickness of 3 mm with zero overlap or gap between adjacent slices. Such a protocol generally helps ensure the acquisition of 3 or more slices through the region of interest. Even though the technique of volume estimation has an acceptable level of accuracy, we prefer to ignore changes of less than 15%.

Pituitary Adenomas

The efficacy of radiation in the treatment of pituitary adenomas was well-documented before gamma surgery was used for this disease.[100,101] Reduced fractionation techniques had been shown to have effectiveness in the treatment of Cushing's disease and were the impetus for the use of radiosurgery. MRI has replaced less exact invasive localization procedures such as cisternography and CT in the planning of gamma surgery in patients with pituitary adenomas. There still remain difficulties with the use of gamma surgery. The peripheral dose that can be delivered for macroadenomas is limited if the optic apparatus is in proximity with the tumor. Localization of microadenomas can be difficult with even the best MRI examinations (e.g., a fat suppression MRI protocol) and amelioration of hypersecretory syndromes is delayed.

One of the best indications for gamma surgery of secretory or nonsecretory pituitary adenomas is residual tumor that is not removable with microsurgical techniques (i.e., tumors within the cavernous sinus). If it is known before microsurgery that the cavernous sinus is involved and a debulking procedure is considered, then every effort to clear the tumor away from the optic nerves and chiasm should be made in order to make gamma surgery postoperatively more effective. A suprasellar approach should be considered if there is doubt that this can be accomplished through a trans-sphenoidal approach. There is some difficulty in differentiating residual tumor from postoperative changes on MRI. A thorough operative note concerning any foreign material or grafts left behind is important, as well as a high-quality preoperative scan for comparison.

Another indication for gamma surgery is persistence or recurrence of elevated hormone levels after microsurgery. In the presence of residual or recurrent tumor that is not readily amenable to further extirpation, either because of its location or the inability to localize the tumor within the sella, gamma surgery can be applied. Tumor within the cavernous sinus can be treated. Difficulty in localizing the tumor usually requires radiosurgical targeting of all the contents within the sella, and such an approach carries a fair risk of postradiosurgical hormonal insufficiency.[102] If the patient has a secretory microadenoma but the symptomatology is not urgent and microsurgery is for some reason not considered, then gamma surgery can be used as the primary therapy.

In preparation for treatment with high-dose, narrow beam radiation, many centers have recommended a temporary cessation of antisecretory medications in the peritreatment time period. In 2000, Landolt et al. first reported a significantly lower hormone normalization rate in acromegalic patients who were receiving antisecretory medications at the time of radiosurgery.[103] Since then, this same group as well as others has documented a counterproductive effect of antisecretory medications on the rate of hormonal normalization following gamma surgery.[32,104] The degree to which and the mechanism by which antisecretory medications lower hormonal normalization rates is unknown, but Landolt et al. have hypothesized that these drugs lower the tumor's metabolic rate and decrease their radiosensitivity.[105,106] Moreover, the optimal time period to hold antisecretory medications in conjunction with gamma surgery is not clear. Landolt and Lomax recommend that dopamine agonists be withheld 2 months prior to the procedure.[104] For acromegalics, they recommend altering antisecretory medication administration as early as 4 months prior to radiosurgery and completely halting all antisecretory medications 2 weeks prior to radiosurgery.[103] Although many centers have incorporated such methodology into their treatment regimen, the potential risk and benefits of halting antisecretory medication administration should be weighed. The functional adenoma may be more likely to respond to gamma surgery. However, in the absence of antisecretory medication control, it may also enlarge thereby risking adjacent structures (e.g., the optic apparatus), necessitating a lower prescription dose, and making effective treatment more difficult.

Most centers have observed effective growth control of pituitary adenomas following gamma surgery. However, there have been a wide range of outcomes with regard to hormonal normalization of secretory adenomas. The varied outcome results for hormonal normalization may arise from the following reasons:[105] early studies utilized CT rather than more precise MRI for dose planning;[106] different criteria for defining an endocrinologic cure have been applied in various studies and there is little consensus even within the neuro-endocrinologic community for precise defining criteria[107]; and many studies had short or intermediate follow-up periods and may not have been long enough to observe patients with an endocrinologic recurrence following an initial remission.

Nonsecretory Tumors

We have treated 100 patients with nonsecretory pituitary tumors, 90 of which have imaging and endocrinologic follow-up of a minimum of 6 months and an average of 45 months[108] (Tables 5-2 and 5-3). Of these, 59 (65.6%) had a decrease in the volume of their tumors (Fig. 5-13) and 24 (26.7%) had no change in the size. In seven (7.8%) patients, the tumors increased in size. Of note, among 61 tumors involving the cavernous sinus, 39 shrank, 17 remained unchanged, and five increased in size. The minimal effective peripheral dose was 12 Gy; peripheral doses greater than 20 Gy did not seem to provide additional benefit. In 61 patients with residual pituitary function at the time of gamma surgery, new hormone deficiency occurred in 12 patients (20%).

Growth Hormone–Secreting Tumors (Table 5-4)

We have performed gamma knife procedures on 137 patients with growth hormone secreting adenomas (Table 5-4). Follow-up of at least 18 months was available for 95 of these patients. There was normalization of IGF-1 in 53% of cases at an average time of 30 months after radiosurgery. Three patients developed recurrence of their acromegaly after initial remission, with a mean time to recurrence of

Table 5-2 Gamma Surgery for Pituitary Adenomas Outcomes at University of Virginia

Tumor Type	Patient No.	TUMOR SIZE Decreased (%)	Unchanged (%)	Increased (%)	Endocrine Remission (%)
Nonsecretory	90[a]	66	27	7	n/a
Acromegaly	90[a]/95[b]	92	6	2	53
Prolactinomas	23[a]/28[b]	46	43	11	26
Cushing's	67[a]/90[b]	80	14	6	53
Nelson's	22[a]/15[b]	55	46	9	20

[a]Numbers of patients available for imaging evaluation.
[b]Numbers of patients available for endocrinologic evaluation.

Table 5-3 Imaging Outcomes of Radiosurgery for Nonsecretory Pituitary Adenomas

Author	Year	Patient No.	F/U (Months)	Peripheral Dose (Gy)	TUMOR SIZE (%) Decreased	Unchanged	Increased	New Hormone Deficit (%)	Visual Complication (%)
Pollock et al.[170]	2008	62	44.9	16	60	37	3	25	0
Mingione et al.[108]	2006	90	44.9	18.5	65.6	26.7	7.8	25	0
Iwai et al.[171]	2005	34	59.8	14	58.1	29	12.9	6.5	0
Losa et al.[172]	2004	54	41.1	16.6	96.1	NR	3.9	9.6	0
Sheehan et al.[173]	2002	42	31.2	16	42.9	54.8	2.4	0	4.8

F/U, follow-up; NR, not reported.

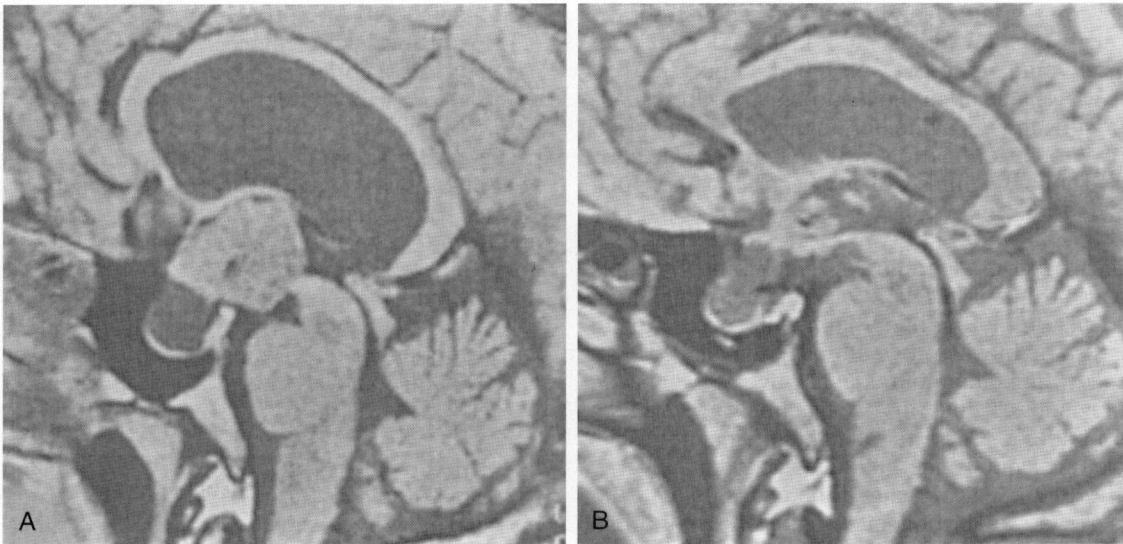

FIGURE 5-13 Nonsecretory pituitary adenoma treated with gamma surgery following three microsurgical resections. Sagittal T1-weighted MRI of a nonsecretory pituitary adenoma in a 34-year-old man (A), demonstrating marked reduction at 30 months after radiosurgery (B). Patient recovered his visual acuity and had resolution of his visual field defect, and returned to his job as a policeman.

Table 5-4 Hormone and Imaging Outcome of Radiosurgery for Growth Hormone–Secreting Pituitary Adenomas

Author	Year	Patient No.	F/U (Months)	Peripheral Dose (Gy)	IGF-1 Normalization (%)[a]	TUMOR VOLUME CHANGE (%)			New Hormone Deficit (%)	Visual Complication (%)
						Decreased	Unchanged	Increased		
Jagannathan	2008	95	57	22	53	92	6	2	34	4
Losa et al.[174]	2008	83	69	21.5	60.2	45.8	51.8	2.4	8.5	0
Vik-Mo et al.[175]	2007	53	66	26.5	58	41.5[b]	47.2[b]	0	23	3.8
Pollock et al.[176]	2007	46	63	20	50	70	30	0	33	0
Jezkova et al.[177]	2006	96	53.7	32	50	62.3	37.7	0	27.1	0
Voges et al.[c178]	2006	64	54.3	15.3	49.8	23.4	73.5	3.1	12.3	1.4
Castinetti et al.[179]	2005	82	49.5	12-40	40	NR	NR	NR	17.1	0
Attanasio	2003	30	46	20	23	58	42	0	6.7	0

F/U, follow-up; IGF-1, insulin-like growth factor-1; NR, not reported.
[a]Includes patients on and off medications.
[b]Tumor volume unavailable for six patients.
[c]Linac radiosurgery.

42 months. New endocrinologic deficiencies developed in 34% of patients, with hypothyroidism and low testosterone levels being the most common new endocrinopathies.

In five patients the tumors could not be identified on MRI and the whole sella was targeted. Of the remaining 90 tumors treated with gamma surgery, a decrease in tumor size was seen after 83 (92%) gamma procedures. Tumor growth was seen after 2 (2%) procedures. No change in tumor volume was seen after 5 (6%) procedures. Four patients developed the new-onset of visual acuity deficits; three of these patients had received prior conventional fractionated radiation therapy and their vision recovered following a short course of steroids. One patient developed deterioration in visual fields secondary to tumor growth. His vision continued to deteriorate in spite of repeat trans-sphenoidal surgery. One patient developed temporal lobe epilepsy 15 months following radiosurgery with MRI showing temporal enhancement. She is free of seizure with normal MRI scans and off antiepileptics 45 months after gamma surgery. No instance of ophthamoplegia occurred in any patients.

Prolactin-Secreting Tumors

Prolactinomas are usually well-controlled by dopamine agonists (Table 5-5). Nonetheless, this medication occasionally fails to achieve remission and is not tolerated by all patients. Alternative for these patients not responding to medical therapy is surgery. Patients who are refractory to medical and/or surgical therapy may be treated with gamma surgery. Of the 37 prolactin secreting tumors treated by us at the Lars Leksell gamma knife center,[109] 28 have imaging follow-up of 1 year or more. Thirteen (46%) had a decrease in the size, 12 (43%) were unchanged and three (11%) were increased. Excluding patients with normal prolactin level before gamma surgery and those with normal level at the last follow-up while still receiving dopamine agonists, endocrine follow-up was available for 23 patients. There was remission (serum prolactin level <20 ng/ml) in 26% of cases. New onset endocrine deficiency developed in 29% of patients. Two patients had new onset extraocular movement problems; one developed an oculomotor and the other an abducens nerve palsy. In both cases, the

Table 5-5	Hormone and Imaging Outcome of Radiosurgery for Prolactin-Secreting Pituitary Adenomas										
						TUMOR VOLUME CHANGE (%)			**New**	**Visual**
Author	**Year**	**Patient No.**	**F/U (Months)**	**Peripheral Dose (Gy)**	**Hormone Remission**	**Decreased**	**Unchanged**	**Increased**	**Hormone Deficit (%)**	**Complication (%)**
Pouratian et al.[109]	2006	23	58	18.6	24	46	43	11	28	7
Choi et al.[180]	2003	21	42.5	28.5	24	50	50	0	0	0
Pan et al.[181]	2000	128	33	31.5	52	57.8	40.6	1.6	NR	0
Landolt and Lomax[104]	2000	20	29	25	25	NR	NR	NR	NR	5
Mokry et al.[182]	1999	21	31	14	21	NR	NR	NR	NR	NR
Levy et al.[183]	1991	20	12	NR	60	NR	NR	NR	NR	NR

F/U, follow-up; NR, not reported.

Table 5-6	Hormone and Imaging Outcome of Radiosurgery for ACTH-Secreting Pituitary Adenomas										
					24-Hour UFC Normaliza-tion (%)	**TUMOR VOLUME CHANGE (%)**			**New**	**Visual**
Author	**Year**	**Patient No.**	**F/U (Months)**	**Peripheral Dose (Gy)**		**Decreased**	**Unchanged**	**Increased**	**Hormone Deficit (%)**	**Complication (%)[a]**
Jagannathan et al.[110]	2007	90	41.3	23	54	92	3	5	22	5.6
Castinetti et al.[184]	2007	40	54.7	29.5	42.5	NR	NR	NR	15	0
Kobayashi et al.[185]	2002	20	63.6	28.7	35[b]	85	15	0	NR	NR
Hoybye et al.[186]	2001	18	204	60–100[c]	83	NR	NR	NR	69	0
Levy et al.[183]	1991	64	NR	NR	86	NR	NR	NR	NR	NR

ACTH, adrenocorticotropic hormone; F/U, follow-up; NR, not reported; UFC, urine-free cortisol.
[a]Visual field defect or CN 3,4,6 palsy.
[b]ACTH <50 pg/ml; cortisol <10 mg/dl.
[c]Range of maximal doses.

cavernous sinus was involved and both cases received a prescription dose of 25 Gy.

ACTH-Secreting Tumors

A total of 107 patients with Cushing's disease underwent gamma surgery at our institution (Table 5-6). Seventeen patients who had less than 12 months follow-up were excluded, leaving 90 patients evaluable.[110] All but one patient had undergone previous trans-sphenoidal operations. Of note, in 23 patients in which no tumor can be identified on planning MRI, the entire sellar content and adjacent cavernous sinuses were targeted. The mean prescription dose of gamma surgery was 23 Gy (range 8–30 Gy). Of 67 patients with visible tumors, imaging follow-up demonstrated a decrease in the size of the tumor in 62 cases (92%), no change in 2 (3%), and an increase in size in 3 (5%). However since the hypercortisolism defines the dangerous character of the ACTH-secreting tumor, the control of endocrine abnormalities is the true measure of tumor control. Normal 24-hour, urine-free cortisol levels were achieved in 49 patients (44%), at an average time of 13 months post-treatment (range 2–67 months). Ten patients who achieved remission after gamma surgery suffered a recurrence. Seven of these patients had repeat gamma knife procedures, with three patients achieving another remission. New endocrine deficiencies developed in 20 patients (22%), with hypothyroidism being the most commonly found new endocrinopathy. Five patients developed new-onset ophthalmoplegia (four of them with visual acuity deficits). One of them had received prior conventional fractionated radiation therapy, three had two gamma knife surgeries, and one had fractionated radiotherapy and subsequently two gamma procedures. Evidence of radiation-induced changes presenting as increased enhancement of parasellar area was seen in three patients but only one had symptoms attributable to these changes.

The results of 35 patients treated at the Karolinska Institute have been reported.[111] Of the 29 patients that had follow-up of up to 9 years, 22 (76%) had normalization of their endocrine abnormalities, 10 within 1 year and the remainder within 3.

Nelson's Syndrome

Patients with an ACTH-secreting pituitary tumor may require a bilateral adrenalectomy to treat their Cushing's disease when surgical extirpation and radiosurgery for the pituitary tumor failed to normalize hormonal production (Table 5-7). Approximately one third of these patients will experience Nelson's syndrome, namely, enlargement of residual pituitary adenoma, developing hyperpigmentation and/or having an elevated level of serum ACTH. At the Lars Leksell center, we have performed gamma surgery on 23 Nelson's patients. Five patients had previously received conventional fractionated radiation therapy, and two patients had received prior gamma surgery for Cushing's disease. Median prescription dose to the tumor margin was 25 Gy (range 4–30 Gy). Twenty two patients had imaging follow-up and the mean imaging follow-up was 20 months (range 125–124 months). Fifteen patients had elevated ACTH level before gamma surgery and follow-up ACTH level was available. The mean endocrine follow-up was 50 months (range 13–166 months). Tumors decreased in 12 (55%) patients, remained unchanged in 8 (36%), and increased in 2 (9%). ACTH levels decreased in 10 patients (67%) with a median decrease of 75% (range 29%–93%). Three patients (31%) achieved normal ACTH levels with a mean time to remission of 9.4 months postradiosurgery. New endocrinopathies were seen in 4 out of 10 patients with residual pituitary function before gamma knife procedures, growth hormone deficiency being the most common new hormonal deficit. One patient suffered from a permanent oculomotor nerve palsy.

It is worth noting that there is a wide variation in both the rates of endocrinologic cure and hypopituitarism following gamma surgery. The difference in cure rates between modern radiosurgical series is likely due to the definition of cure employed and the length of follow-up. However, the discrepancy in the reported rates of hypopituitarism is more likely a function of the degree to which there is rigorous endocrinologic follow-up testing.

Craniopharyngiomas

Craniopharyngiomas are very difficult tumors to treat. Their benign histology is misleading. The near impossibility to resect completely and usual location in and about the hypothalamus make them difficult to cure. Microsurgery, intracystic instillation of radioisotopes, radiation therapy, and now radiosurgery have all been used. Long-term evaluation of patients with craniopharyngiomas is available after various treatment protocols.[112,113] The general consensus is that as complete a surgical resection as possible, without creating significant morbidity, should be performed; this is followed by radiation therapy and gives reasonable long-term survival. The ill effects on children after receiving fractionated brain irradiation are well-known.[114,115] Good results with resection alone have been achieved but only in the hands of a few neurosurgeons. Even so, long-term results of children with subtotal resection followed by radiation therapy has been shown to be superior to complete resection alone[116] and the deficits incurred with aggressive surgery can be considerable.

Gamma surgery as an adjunct to microsurgical resection has been used in lieu of radiation therapy, or in addition to it, at several centers. The instillation of radioisotopes (e.g., P32) into large, nonloculated cystic components of the tumor and gamma surgery for the solid portion is the treatment policy for craniopharyngiomas at our center.

We treated 37 craniopharyngiomas in 35 patients. The prescription doses ranged from 6 to 25 Gy (mean 13.3 Gy). The follow-up ranged between 8 and 212 months with a mean of 62.5 months. Four tumors increased in size. A decrease in the solid component of the tumor was seen in 29 (Fig. 5-14) and no change was seen in 4. However, of the patients whose solid tumors decreased or remained unchanged, 10 developed new or enlarged cystic component with 4 of them requiring further surgical resection and 4 receiving intracavitary P32 instillation. In total, 23 patients improved or remained stable clinically. Twelve deteriorated and 10 of them died from complications of disease or surgeries. The mean 5-year survival rate was 71%.

Several other series have been reported in the use of gamma surgery in the treatment of craniopharyngiomas[117,118] with results similar to ours. As larger series with longer follow-up become available it is likely that gamma surgery will either take the place of less discriminate radiation therapy, or be a useful adjunct to it.

Meningiomas

Meningiomas are usually benign, circumscribed tumors that arise from the coverings of the central nervous system and therefore tend to be superficial. Because of these attributes microsurgical extirpation of the entire tumor as well as any involved meninges is the treatment of choice.

Table 5-7	Hormone and Imaging Outcome of Radiosurgery for Nelson's Syndrome									
					Hormone	TUMOR VOLUME CHANGE (%)			New	Visual
Author	Year	Patient *n*	F/U (Months)	Peripheral Dose (Gy)	Remission (%)	Decreased	Unchanged	Increased	Hormone Deficit (%)	Complication (%)
Mauerman et al.[187]	2007	23	20/50[a]	25	20	54.5	36.4	9.2	40	4
Voges[b178]	2006	9	63/47[a]	15.3	16.7	44.4	44.4	11.2	NR	NR
Pollock and Young[188]	2002	11	37	20	24	82[c]		18	9	27

[a]Mean imaging follow-up/mean endocrine follow-up.
[b]Linac radiosurgery.
[c]Tumor under control.
F/U, follow-up; NR, not reported.

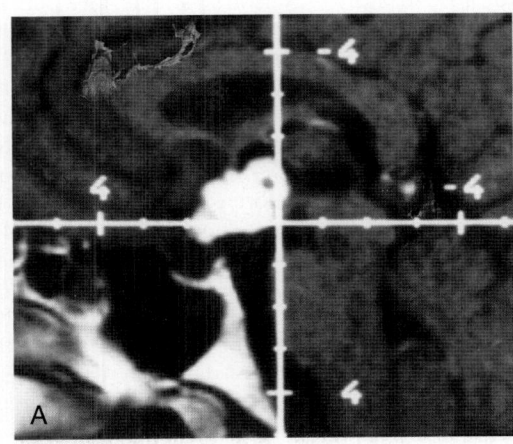
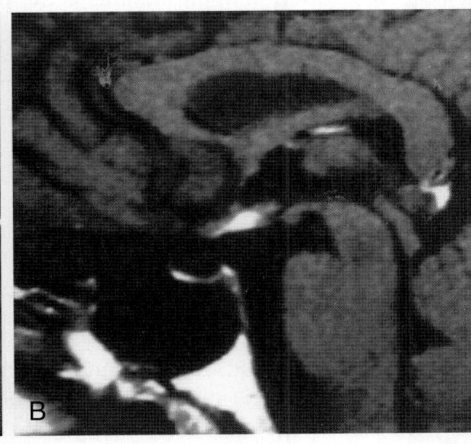

FIGURE 5-14 Reduction in size of craniopharyngioma treated with gamma surgery. Residual craniopharyngioma following microsurgery treated with the gamma knife. Contrast-enhanced T1-weighted images before (A) and 4 months after treatment (B). Marked reduction in tumor size. Patient has a normal neurologic examination and endocrine profile.

Unfortunately many meningiomas do not have one or more of the mentioned attributes. Aggressive, locally invasive tumors, especially those invading or involving critical or difficult to control neural or vascular structures and those at the skull base can be problematic in their complete removal. The use of radiation to lower the recurrence rate following microsurgical removal of meningiomas was shown to be beneficial.[118-120] Recurrence rates were found to be dramatically decreased, and for patients with residual tumor following surgery the progression of tumor growth was significantly decreased.

We have treated 750 meningiomas at the Lars Leksell center since 1989. The most recent evaluation of our material was for 206 patients with a follow-up of 1 to 6 years. Tumor volume ranged from 1 to 32 cm³. These patients received an average of 38 Gy maximum dose (range 20–60 Gy) and an average peripheral dose of 14 Gy (range 10–20 Gy). There were 142 patients treated for residual tumor and 64 treated with gamma surgery primarily. Imaging follow-up was available for 151 patients. Of the evaluated patients 94 (63%) showed a decrease in the volume of their tumor greater than 15%. No change in size was seen in 40 (26%) and an increase in size in 17 (11%).

Tumors within the parasellar compartment, which is a part of the extradural neural axis compartment, can be difficult to remove with microsurgery without significant morbidity.[121,122] Residual tumor attached to still patent vascular or critical neural structures can be targeted with gamma surgery and allows less radical microsurgical resection and a lower incidence of morbidity.

We have recently reviewed the central skull base meningiomas involving the sellar-parasellar space in 138 patients. There were 107 females (78%) and 31 (22%) males. The mean age was 54 years (range 19–85). Mean tumor volume at the time of radiosurgery was 7.5 cm³ (range 0.2–55 cm³). Eighty-four patients had prior microsurgery with partial resection of the tumor. Fifty-four had an upfront gamma procedure. In our assessment, the gamma treatment was optimal in 109 (79%) and nonoptimal in 29 cases (21%). We defined nonoptimal treatment as follows: the part of the tumor close to the optic apparatus did not receive the desired prescription dose, typically because there was no distance between the tumor and the visual pathways. The mean prescription dose used in this series was 13.7 Gy (range 4.8–30 Gy). The mean maximum dose was 34.2 Gy (range 16–60 Gy). The mean MRI follow-up was 82.4 months (range 24–216 months). Sixty-six tumors (48%) shrank (Fig. 5-15), 52 (38%) remained unchanged and 20 (14%) increased in size. Fourteen patients developed new or deteriorated cranial nerve deficits; 11 due to tumor progress and 3 in spite of good tumor control. There was no mortality. Young age, optimal treatment, and smaller tumor size were correlated with better outcome. The tumor progression–free survival at 5 years was 95.4% and at 10 years was 71%.

We have long-term follow-up of 10 to 21 years for 31 meningiomas treated with the gamma knife. Two thirds of these tumors have either shrunk significantly or remained stable, and among these were cases where only the vascular supply for the tumor was targeted (Fig. 5-16). This has resulted in significant tumor shrinkage and lasting effect even in the long term. Our practice has been to obtain a stereotactic angiogram prior to gamma surgery for large tumors. This allows treatment to include the vascular supply when ideal treatment is not possible because of radiation dose constraints imposed by the treatment volume or proximity of the tumor to the optic apparatus. Recently we have used MRA source images instead of angiograms to conduct treatment planning. Using MRI, the group from Heidelberg proved that radiation occluded small nutrient vessels of meningiomas providing the rationale for the treatment we have used since 1976.

The primary therapy for meningiomas is microsurgery. The advantage of histologic diagnosis, debulking and reasonable chance of cure secures surgical extirpation as the procedure of choice for this tumor. The tumors most amenable to gamma surgery treatment are less than 10 to 15 cm³ in volume. The ability of gamma surgery to effectively treat small tumors with low morbidity argues strongly, however, for minimizing morbidity during open procedures. The option to treat residual tumor in critical or hard to reach locations should temper the ambition of total surgical removal. This is especially true in locations where complete meningeal resection is impossible and thus the chance of recurrence is high.

Vestibular Schwannomas

Historically and incorrectly referred to as an acoustic neuroma, we prefer the designation of vestibular schwannoma, which recognizes the anatomic and histologic origins of these tumors.[123] There may be no other intracranial neuropathology about which the proper treatment arouses as much controversy as the vestibular schwannoma. Neurosurgeons cite the series of surgeons with enormous experience removing these tumors to justify suboccipital removal, while otolaryngologists sacrifice the inner ear during the translabyrinthine approach in an attempt to better expose and preserve the facial nerve. Radiosurgery's proponents cite excellent tumor control and low morbidity but must acknowledge that although the tumor often shrinks, it is still there. Therefore it is in the best interest of our patients that long-term outcome in patients treated with these three modalities be thoroughly evaluated.

The first vestibular schwannomas treated with the gamma knife were by Leksell and Steiner in 1969.[124] Since then more than 36,843 have been treated around the world through 2006. The indications for gamma surgery for this tumor vary. Some physicians advocate gamma surgery in medically high risk patients, patients who refuse microsurgery, and in patients with postoperative residual tumors. However, others advocate gamma surgery as the treatment of choice in nearly all cases of vestibular schwannomas. The usefulness of irradiation in the postoperative period was shown by Wallner in 1987 where external beam irradiation lowered the recurrence rate from 46 to 6% in Boldrey's surgical series at the University of California at San Francisco.[125] By then, gamma surgery was already being widely applied to this disease under many circumstances. The fact is that for a number of reasons few neurosurgeons acquire the necessary competency to satisfactorily extirpate these tumors. This situation may change if a method to improve the acquisition of skills required for extirpation of these lesions is found.

The advent of MRI has made planning for gamma procedures much more exact. With a high-quality MRI scan

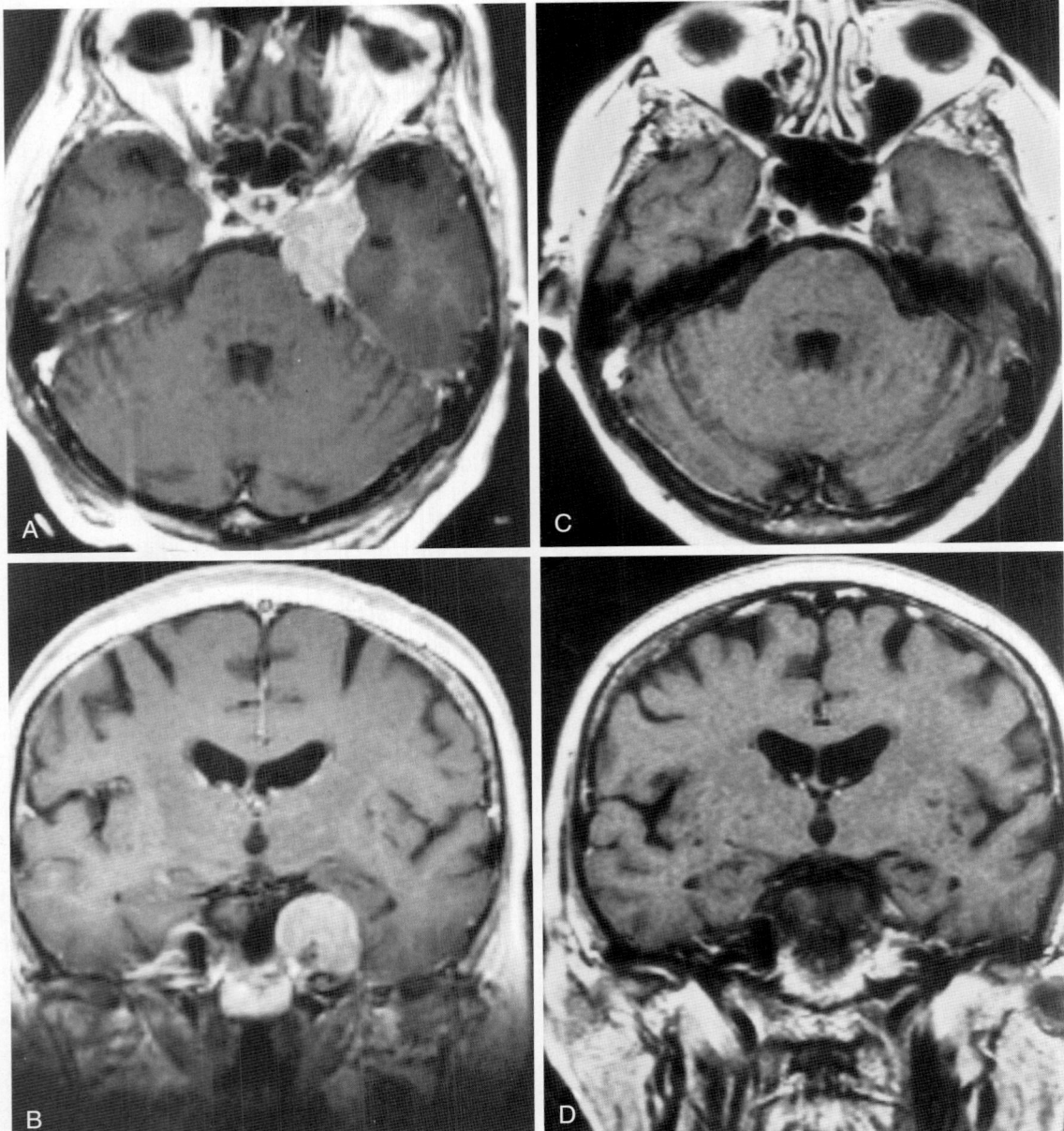

FIGURE 5-15 Large left parasellar meningioma residual following microsurgery visualized on postcontrast, T1-weighted axial (A) and coronal (B) MRI. MRI obtained 6 months following gamma surgery shows that the tumor has disappeared (C and D). Repeated control MRI examinations at 5 years show no recurrence of the tumor.

and a relatively small tumor, the seventh cranial nerve can occasionally be visualized and carefully excluded from the treatment field. The trigeminal nerve can nearly always be identified except with the largest tumors, which in most cases should not be treated primarily with gamma surgery.

Small collimators are used to better match the isodose configuration to the size and shape of the tumor. We have had no brain stem–related complications. Previously we used minimum peripheral doses up to 20 Gy and maximum doses up to 70 Gy. Presently, we use a margin dose of 11 to 13 Gy at the 30% to 50% isodose curve. The incidence of cranial nerve palsies rose considerably at the higher doses without significant improvement in the degree of tumor control.

At the Lars Leksell center, we have treated 470 patients with vestibular schwannomas. A total of 153 of these patients with more than 12 months of follow-up have been reported.[126] Radiosurgery was the primary treatment for 96 of such patients and was the adjutant (following microsurgery) in 57. The volume of the treated tumors ranged from 0.02 to 18.3 cm^3.

Of the patients treated primarily with gamma surgery a decrease in tumor size was seen in 81% (78 patients), no change in 12%, and an increase in size in 6%. Among those 78 patients with a decrease in the size of their tumors, the decrease was greater than 50% in 20 patients. It is our policy to not consider decreases in volume of less than 15% as significant. This is true of all tumors that we

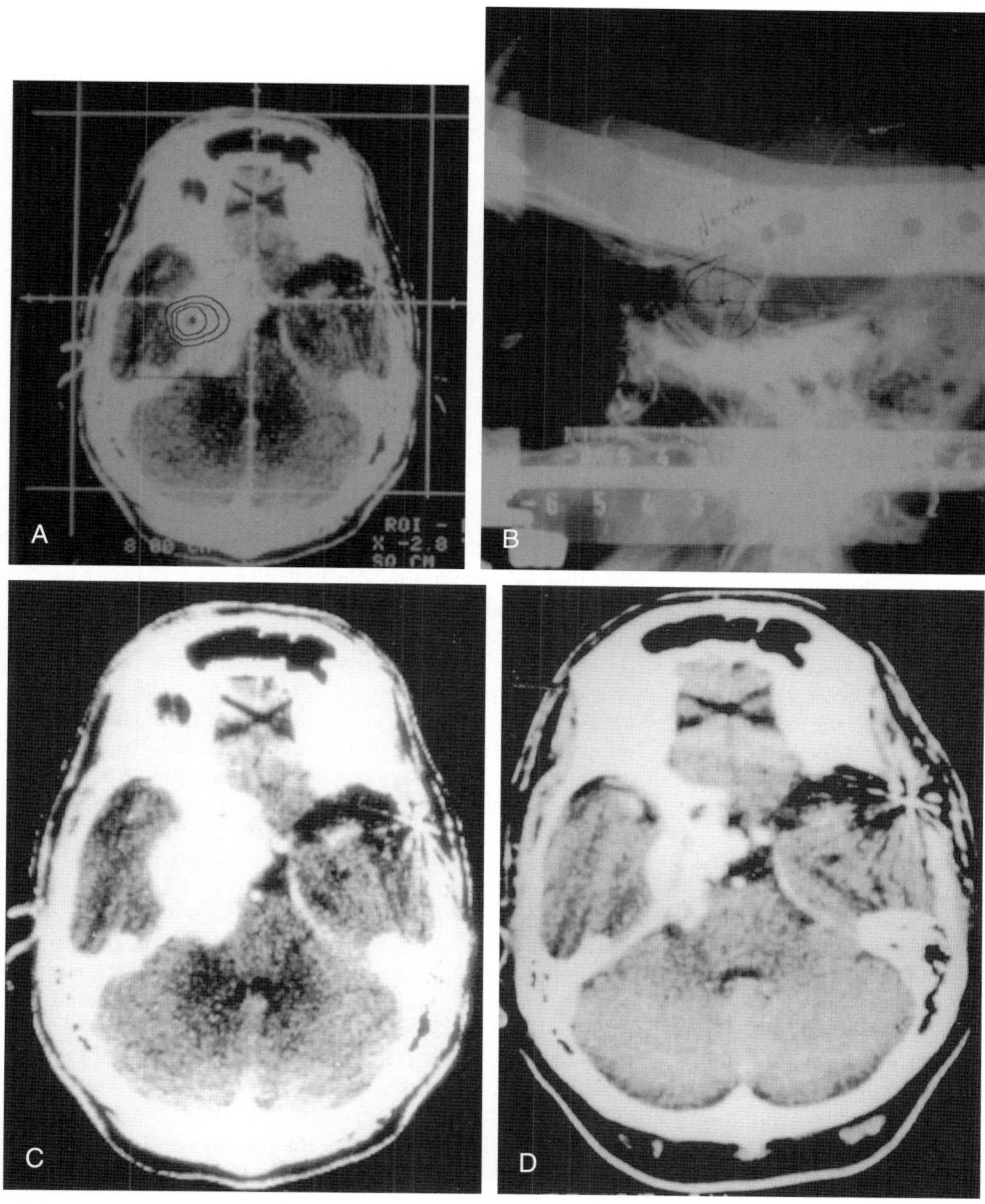

FIGURE 5-16 Long-term result of gamma surgery for meningioma. CT scans of a right parasellar meningioma treated with radiation to the nutrient vessels as defined by a CT and angiogram (A and B, respectively). The original size of the tumor is depicted in the pre–gamma surgery axial CT (C), and the last follow-up at 18 years after gamma surgery is shown (D). The tumor has substantially decreased in size.

treat. Imaging follow-up for these patients ranged from 1 to 10 years.

Of the 57 patients treated with gamma surgery after microsurgery, a decrease in tumor size was seen in 65%, no change in 25%, and an increase in size in 10%. Among the 37 patients with a decrease in tumor size, the decrease was greater than 50% in 12 patients. The outcome in terms of postradiosurgical volume reduction in patients who had prior microsurgery is worse than those who were primarily treated with gamma surgery. This difference is likely a result of the increased difficulty with accurate targeting in those who have undergone prior microsurgery. Of note, although our experience with treating large vestibular schwannomas is small (*n* = 19), we have observed a 95% tumor control rate in these following gamma surgery.

In our patients, there were five with transient changes in trigeminal sensation and three with facial paresis. In

the first patient, the facial paresis occurred 6 months after the gamma surgery. Unnecessary surgery was performed without asking for our advice and the facial nerve was cut during surgery. Another patient recovered completely in six weeks, and the third has nearly completely recovered at 10 months. Of the patients with useful hearing prior to gamma surgery, 58% retained their hearing following radiosurgery. The majority of hearing changes were observed at the 2-year checkup, and additional auditory changes were observed as late as eight years postradiosurgery.

Other centers report similar rates of tumor control (i.e., with no change or decrease in the size of the tumor) seen in 89% to 100% of patients.[127-129]

Evaluation of the material from the Karolinska group included evaluation of radiographic changes besides size.[130] The most common change was loss of central enhancement within the tumor on either contrasted MRI or

CT studies. This occurred in 70% of patients and typically was observed within 6 to 12 months of treatment. However, these changes were reversible. Another change that was observed and that we have often seen is a transient increase in the size of the tumor during the first 6 months after gamma surgery. This is commonly seen in tumors that then regress to their original size or smaller (Fig. 5-17).

We have not seen an instance of cerebellar edema or hydrocephalus requiring spinal fluid diversion following gamma surgery for vestibular schwannomas, but both of these have been reported elsewhere.[130,131]

Astrocytomas

The treatment of astrocytomas, whether low or high grade, is largely defined by the ability to effectively reduce the tumor burden as much as possible and to lessen the rate of recurrence. Except in the case of pilocytic astrocytoma cure is rare. Classically the goal of reducing tumor burden is obtained by gross total resection with a margin of "normal" brain when possible and postoperative radiation in the case of more malignant tumors. The indication for radiation therapy for intermediate grade tumors, chemotherapy, repeat surgical debulking, and other therapies is dependent on several factors, many of which are not clearly defined. Into this cornucopia of choices, gamma surgery has been introduced. Intellectually, we have difficulty accepting the application of a focused technique for an infiltrative process. Nevertheless, recent results showing improved survival indicate that this negative attitude may be inappropriate.

In the case of low-grade tumors, gamma surgery can be used in place of surgical resection when the tumor is in an inaccessible location (e.g., brain stem) or when the patient opts for this alternative. Their small size and relative circumscription make planning straightforward, and fairly good results have been obtained.

For high-grade tumors, gamma surgery may be employed in several ways. If the tumor is small and in an inaccessible location (e.g., thalamus), gamma surgery is used to treat the tumor primarily. Focal or whole brain irradiation is also used as an adjunct therapy. The incidence of radionecrosis is relatively high when aggressive protocols are used and differentiating recurrence from this phenomenon

can be problematic. Gamma surgery can also be used as an adjunct to surgical resection. The incidence of residual postoperative tumor is unfortunately not uncommon after "total" surgical resections and care is often taken when the tumor abuts eloquent brain so as not to leave neurologic deficit even at the expense of incomplete gross tumor resection. In these cases, gamma surgery can be used to treat the residual tumor. Whole or focal radiation therapy has been used to lower the recurrence rate after these surgical therapies have been undertaken.

Low-Grade Astrocytomas

We treated 21 pilocytic tumors, 2 subependymal giant cell astrocytomas (Grade II), and 26 Grade II astrocytomas with gamma surgery between 1989 and 2003 at the Lars Leksell center. The median treatment volume was 2.4 cm^3 with a range of 0.5 to 36.0 cm^3. The median prescription dose was 15 Gy. The mean clinical follow-up was 63 months. Median clinical progression-free survival was 44 months (range 0–118 months). The 5-year clinical progression-free survival was 41%. Eight patients died of disease progression. No information on the cause of the death was available for one patient. The duration of imaging follow-up was 59 months (range 2–118 months). Median imaging progression-free survival was 37 months (range 0–80 months). Five-year, imaging progression-free survival was 37%. At the last imaging follow-up, 37 tumors decreased or remained unchanged and 12 tumors increased in size. Three patients experienced transitory neurologic deficits associated with increased T2 signal on MRI.

Yen et al. reported on a series of 20 patients with brainstem gliomas presenting with clinical or imaging progression treated with gamma surgery.[132] Sixteen tumors were located in the midbrain, four in the pons and one in the medulla oblongata. The mean tumor volume at the time of gamma surgery was 2.5 cm^3. Tissue diagnosis was available in only 10 cases (50%). The cases without histology were treated based upon appearance on imaging as well-defined small tumors. Mean prescription dose was 15 Gy (range 10–18 Gy). The tumor disappeared in 4 patients (20%) (Fig. 5-18) and shrank in 12 patients (60%) after a minimal of 12 months of follow-up (mean follow-up 78 months). Transitory extrapyramidal symptoms and fluctuating times

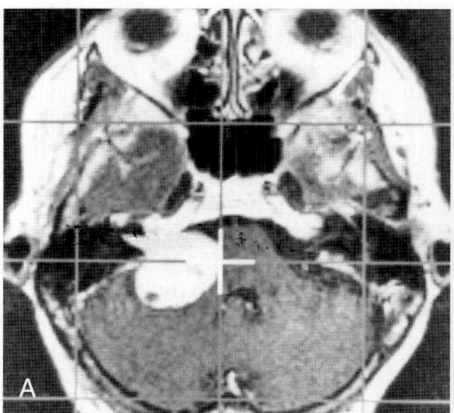
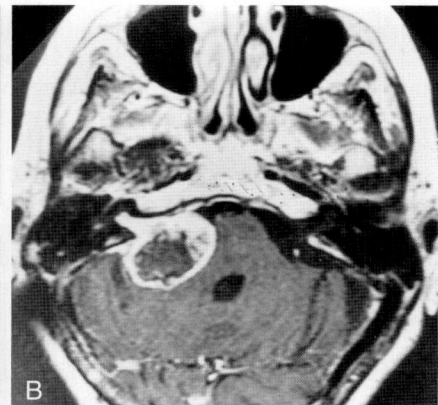
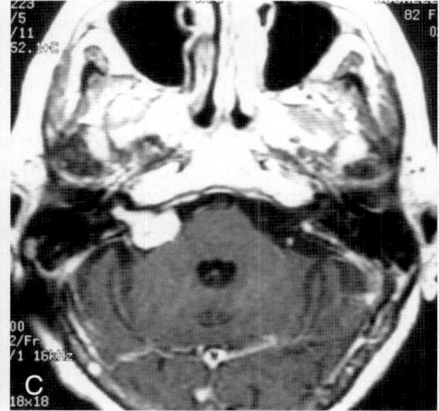

FIGURE 5-17 A right vestibular schwannoma with a volume of 9.3 cm^3 shown on a postcontrast, T1-weighted axial MRI prior to gamma surgery (A). Same lesion 6 months after treatment shows central nonenhancement and no change in size (B). At 36 months after treatment, the lesion is again homogeneously enhancing and is significantly smaller (69%) (C). Control MRI examinations for 6 years show that lesion has remained stable.

of consciousness occurred in one patient. Tumor progression occurred in four patients. One of these four patients required a ventriculoperitoneal shunt for hydrocephalus, two experienced neurologic deterioration, and one died of tumor progression.

High-Grade Astrocytomas

From an intellectual standpoint, it is difficult to understand how a patient with a highly invasive and diffuse tumor like a high-grade glioma can benefit from such a focused treatment as gamma surgery. However, when coupled with chemotherapy and fractionated radiation therapy, the gamma knife can be used to treat the largest concentration of the

residual tumor based upon the neuroimaging studies. It seems clear that no single treatment modality in the neuro-oncology armamentarium is a magic bullet for such tumors, and, as such, this multimodality approach to high-grade gliomas is prudent.

We have treated 56 malignant astrocytomas. Our experience has been similar to other reported series[133-135] with the majority of patients showing initial decrease in size or remaining stable for a period of time (Fig. 5-19); however, recurrence and progression is the rule with these tumors and no therapy is curative. Because of the differences in histology and the wide variety of therapies and protocols available for these tumors it is difficult to judge the benefit of

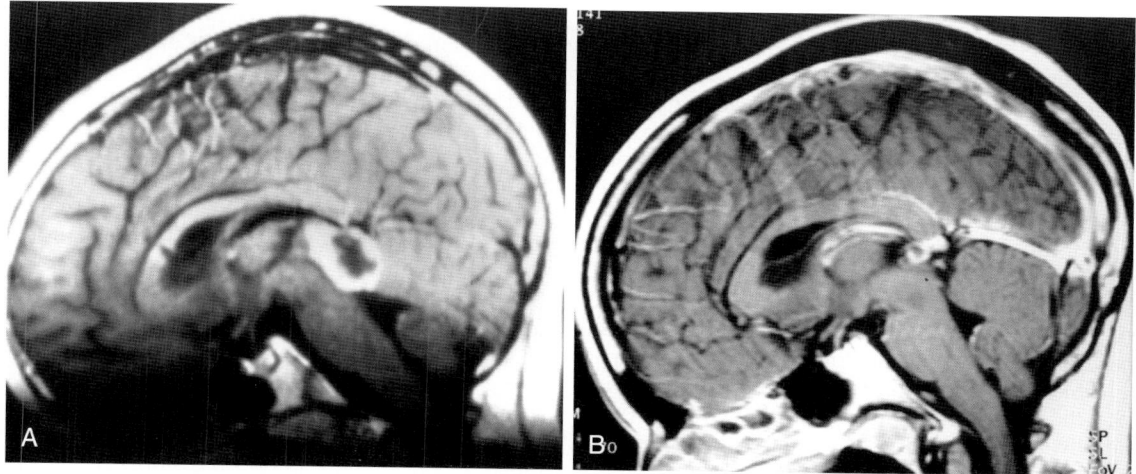

FIGURE 5-18 A pilocytic astrocytoma shown on a postcontrast, T1-weighted sagittal MRI image (A). Annual control MRI examinations were obtained and the latest made 9 years following gamma surgery is shown (B).

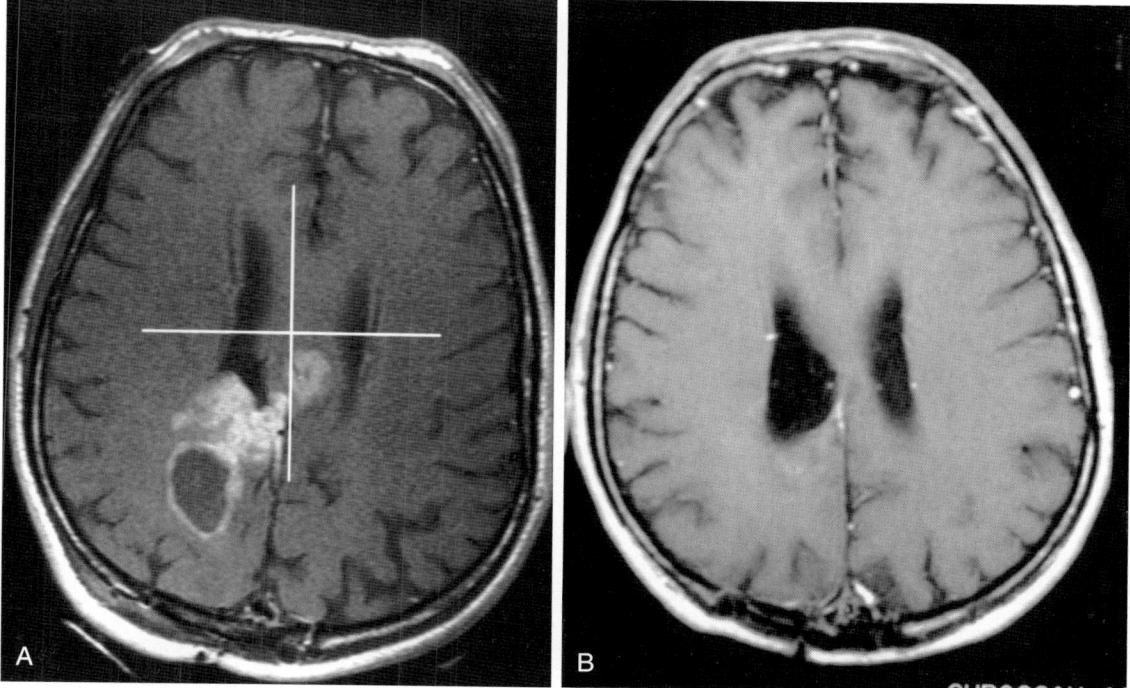

FIGURE 5-19 Postcontrast, T1-weighted axial MRI demonstrating a right parietal glioblastoma multiforme and associated cyst on postcontrast, T1-weighted axial MRI (A). Same patient 11 months after gamma surgery shows complete radiographic disappearance of lesion (B).

gamma surgery. Although our group and Nwokedi et al.[136] have observed a statistically significant prolongation of life expectancy in the group of patients undergoing aggressive multi-modality treatment (e.g., including some or all of the following: radical tumor debulking, radiation therapy, chemotherapy, and gamma surgery), it remains to be seen if these findings will be borne out in larger, better controlled studies. The limit of the benefit that radiation can contribute to the treatment of these lesions seems to have been reached, hence it may be stated that the dose escalation with the gamma knife in the treatment protocol of this disease will change only marginally the clinical outcome. It is also conceivable that targeting tumor angiogenesis and finding ways to induce apoptosis will have some impact on the management of these cases.

Neurocytomas

Central neurocytomas were described by Hassoun et al. in 1982.[137] According to Brandes et al., 210 cases were reported in the literature.[138] The histology, biological behavior and clinical course of central neurocytomas may vary from benign to more aggressive patterns.[139] Surgical resection is the first choice of treatment. Rades and Fehlhauer compared 108 and 74 patients who underwent complete or incomplete resection.[140] At 5 years tumor control rates were 85% and 46%, respectively. If the surgical resection is not total, the residual tumor should be irradiated. The 5-year tumor control rate with postoperative radiotherapy increased from 46% to 83% after incomplete resection but radiotherapy did not seem to improve survival rate.[140]

With the advent of radiosurgery, it was used as upfront or adjunct therapy following surgery. We used the gamma knife in 7 patients with a total of 9 neurocytomas.[141] The mean tumor volume at the time of the gamma procedures ranged from 1.4 to 19.8 cm³ (mean 6.0 cm³). A mean prescription dose of 16 Gy (range 13–20 Gy) was used. After a mean follow-up period of 60 months, 4 tumors disappeared and 5 shrank significantly (Fig. 5-20). One patient had a

hemorrhage in the tumor 1 year after gamma surgery and the tumor had decreased significantly at the last follow-up. This patient had a new tumor at some distance of the successfully treated one. Four patients were asymptomatic during the follow-up period and a patient with hemiparesis caused by a previous transcortical resection was stable. A patient died of sepsis due to a shunt infection.

Chordoma

Skull base chordomas are a rare neoplasm arising from the remnants of notochord. Although histologically benign, these tumors are locally invasive and present significant management challenges. There is consensus that surgical debulking should be performed. Proton radiotherapy has been the mainstay of treatment for recurrent or residual tumors.[142,143]

Fifteen patients (8 males and 7 females) had undergone gamma surgery between 1990 and 2007 at Lars Leksell center. The median age was 46 years (range 13–80). Twelve patients had undergone tumor resection. Mean tumor volume was 5.8 cm³ (range 1.03–15.6 cm³). The tumors were treated with a mean prescription dose of 12.7 Gy (range 12–20 Gy) and a mean maximal dose of 36.7 Gy (range 28–50 Gy).

Imaging follow-up was available for all patients with a median time of 88 months (range 8–167), and clinical follow-up was available for 11 patients with a median of 70 months (range 8–132). At the last follow-up, tumor control was achieved in five out of 15 patients (33.3%) after initial GKS (Fig. 5-21). Actuarial 5- and 10-year tumor control rates after one gamma surgery was 42.6% and 34%, respectively. Three patients who underwent a second gamma surgery achieved good tumor control. Actuarial 5- and 10-year tumor control rates after one or more gamma procedures improved to 50.3%. Symptomatic progression was seen in 75% of the patients.

For the management of intracranial chordoma, surgery as radical as possible is the main treatment alternative—a goal frequently not achieved and some forms of radiation have to be used as an adjunct. Chordoma is relatively radioresistant and respond best to high doses of fractionated proton

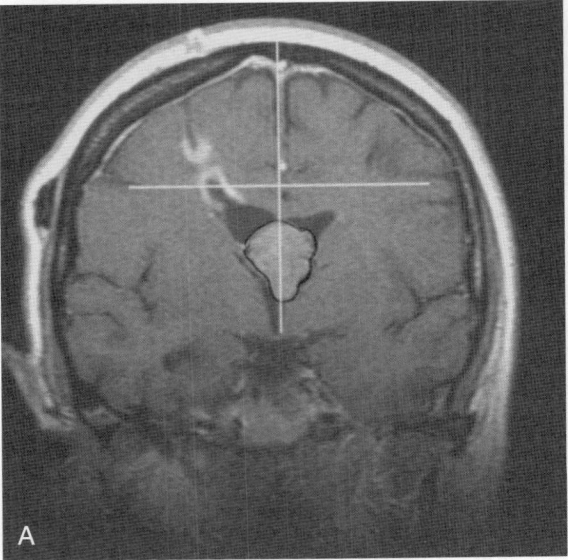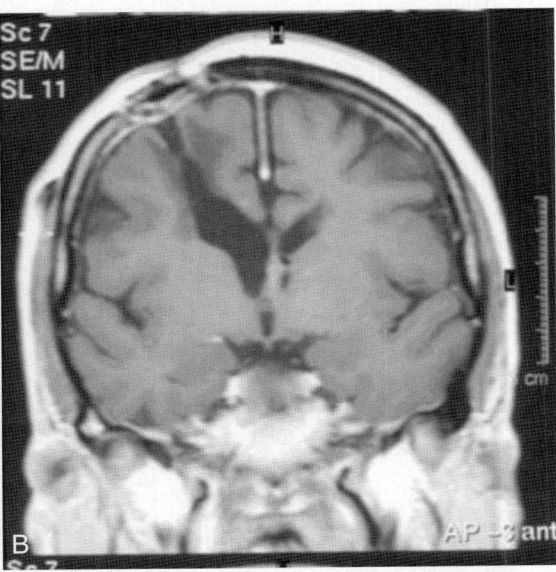

FIGURE 5-20 Gamma surgery for central neurocytoma. T1-weighted, contrast-enhanced MRI reveals a moderately enhancing neurocytoma spanning both lateral ventricles (A). The last follow-up image obtained 14 years following gamma surgery shows that the tumor decreased in size significantly with only some residual tissue in the septum pellucidum (B).

radiotherapy. The physical and biological properties of the proton—it carries higher kinetic energy and as they slow down a higher release of energy (Bragg peak)—make it an excellent source of radiation for chordomas. Amichetti et al. in a review article presented the current data on the treatment of skull base chordomas with proton beam and compared the outcomes to those obtained with fractionated photon radiation, ion therapy, fractionated stereotactic photon therapy, and radiosurgery.[142] With proton therapy, doses above 70 cobalt Gray equivalent can be applied safely, achieving local control rates at 3 years of 67.4% to 87.5%, at 5 years of 46% to 73%, and at 10 years of 54%. The estimated overall survival rates are 66.7% to 80.5% at 5 years and 54% at 10 years.

Chondromas and Chondrosarcomas

These are rare tumors in the skull base. We have treated four chondromas and eight chondrosarcomas with gamma surgery. More than 50% shrinkage was observed in two cases of chondrosarcomas and three tumors shrank 25% to 50%. None progressed at follow-up, ranging from 1 to 5 years (median 3.5 years).

Muthukumar et al. treated 15 patients (nine with chordomas and six with chondrosarcomas) with gamma surgery and reported their results with an average follow-up of 4 years. Four of their patients had died; only two deaths were related to progression of disease and both of these had progression outside of the treated area. Only one of the surviving 11 had tumor progression, and five had shrunk.[144] Gamma surgery seems to be a reasonable treatment alternative for these tumors, but longer follow-up and larger series are required before definitive statements can be made.

Hemangioblastomas

The gold standard treatment for hemangioblastomas is the surgical resection of the solid component of the tumor. It is not necessary to resect, if present, the cystic portion of the tumor. Similarly with gamma surgery only the solid portion of these tumors were targeted. We treated 16 hemangioblastomas with the gamma procedure. Five of them had von Hippel-Lindau disease. The mean prescription dose was 15 Gy. The patients were followed for an average of 21 months. In 12 patients (75%), the solid component of the tumor targeted did decrease in size. In 4 patients, it remained unchanged. It was not uncommon, however, for the cystic portion of the tumor to grow larger regardless of the behavior of the solid portion. During the follow-up, 6 of 16 patients (42%) required surgical drainage for expanding cysts. Although several patients responded well, the high incidence of second, open procedures indicates that the microsurgical removal of hemangioblastomas is in most cases the initial procedure of choice.

Hemangiopericytomas

Hemangiopericytomas are tumors of mesenchymal origin. They are recognized for their aggressive clinical behavior, high recurrence rates, and tendency for distant metastases even after a gross total resection. Initial treatment is usually resection. Upon recurrence, adjuvant treatment is frequently used. Chemotherapy has provided only marginal benefit.[145] Radiosurgery or fractionated radiotherapy has been used as alternatives.

Between 1989 and 2008, we treated 28 recurrent or residual hemangiopericytomas in 21 patients with gamma surgery. The median age was 47 years (range 31–61 years). Eight patients had prior fractionated radiotherapy. The mean prescription and maximum radiosurgical doses to the tumors were 17 and 40 Gy, respectively. Thirteen tumors had undergone repeat gamma surgery. The median follow-up period was 68 months (range 2–138 months). At the last follow-up, local tumor control was demonstrated in 10 of 21 patients (47.6%). Of the 28 tumors treated, 8 decreased in size on follow-up imaging (28.6%), 5 remained unchanged (17.9%), and 15 ultimately progressed (53.6%). The progression free

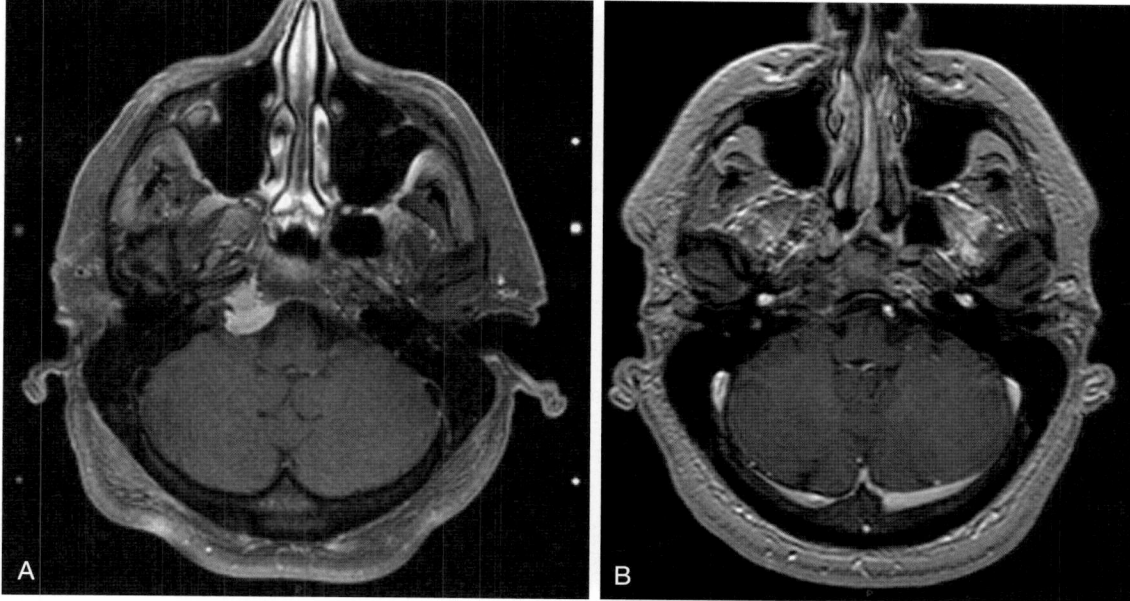

FIGURE 5-21 Gamma surgery for chordoma. A 45-year-old male with chordoma was treated with gamma surgery. The size of the tumor progressively decreased. However, after 5 years, recurrence occurred. At the time of retreatment with gamma surgery, the tumor measured 3 cm³ on enhanced, T1-weighted MRI (A). It shrank progressively and, after close to 9 years, measured 0.1 cm³ (B).

survival rates were 90%, 60%, and 29% at 1, 3, and 5 years after initial gamma surgery. The progression free survival rate improved to 95%, 72%, and 72% at 1, 3, and 5 years after one or multiple gamma surgery. The 5-year survival rate after radiosurgery was 81%. In 4 (19%) of 21 patients, extracranial metastases developed.

Metastatic Tumors

Surgical extirpation of a solitary brain metastasis has been shown to significantly prolong survival if the primary disease is controlled. Likewise whole brain irradiation has been show to be of benefit for some tumor types. These conclusions and the well-defined limits on neuroimaging studies of most metastatic lesions make them very amenable to gamma surgery. Because of this as well as the high incidence of these lesions, the treatment of metastatic tumors is presently the most frequent indication for gamma surgery worldwide.

Except for solitary lesions causing mass effect, the treatment of metastatic brain tumors is primarily palliative. In the instance of solitary metastasis the occurrence of long-term survival is not unheard of; however, in general the guiding philosophy is palliation, reversal of neurologic deficits and maintenance of quality of life. There has been some disagreement regarding the total number and volume of tumors that can be treated with gamma surgery in the instance of multiple metastases. Our general guideline is not to treat more than five if that is known to be the case. We have treated more but usually when additional lesions were discovered on the treatment MRI. With the gamma knife model C, if metastatic deposits are located very far from one another in space the ability to treat them all with the same frame placement may be difficult due to the limitation of the space within the treatment helmet. Such consideration makes frame placement for widely separated metastases a challenge at times. The large radiation space within the gamma knife model Perfexion basically eliminates this concern.

Most reports regarding gamma surgery for metastatic tumors report a 7- to 15-month survival following treatment. Local tumor control rates range from 71% to 98.5%. The histology, dosages, and previous treatments vary considerably through the literature. Most centers are using a peripheral dose of 18 to 22 Gy. These doses are adjusted down if whole brain irradiation has been given previously. The reduction of dose in the instance of tumors that appear after whole brain irradiation is possibly not necessary or desirable. In a study comparing the efficacy of surgery plus whole brain radiotherapy with radiosurgery alone in the treatment of solitary brain metastases less than or equal to 3.5 cm in diameter, local tumor control and 1-year death rates did not statistically differ between the two groups.[146] In a large, multi-institutional study, the omission of upfront fractionated radiation therapy did not compromise the overall length of survival in brain metastasis patients who had undergone radiosurgery.[147] Radiosurgery even appears to be efficacious for treating traditionally relatively "radioresistant" brain metastases such as melanoma and renal cell carcinoma.

We have treated more than 1,000 patients for metastatic tumors to the brain. Evaluation of our series demonstrated an 81% to 97% control rate of treated lesions (disappeared, shrank, or did not change) and a median survival of 8 to 14 months. The usual cause of death was systemic disease.

LUNG CARCINOMA

Lung carcinoma is the leading cause of death from cancer and the most common source of brain metastases (Table 5-8). Depending on the actual histologic subtypes, lung carcinoma metastasizes intracranially between 13% and 54% of the time. The overall frequency of brain metastasis in patients with lung carcinoma is approximately 32% and between 54% and 64% of patients with lung carcinoma metastatic to the brain harbor or eventually develop multiple lesions.[148,149] Treatment options include symptomatic medical management with corticosteroids and whole-brain radiation therapy, which lead to a median survival of 3 to 6 months. Patient with small cell lung cancer developed metastases quite early and adjuvant chemotherapy has also become well-accepted for the treatment of extracranial disease in small cell lung cancer. We have treated 903 metastases in 262 patients with lung carcinoma. The median survival was 15.4 months. Age of less than 65 years, a Karnofsky performance score of greater than 70, and controlled extracranial disease were associated with increased survival.

Table 5-8	Outcome of Radiosurgery for Metastatic Lung Carcinoma					
	Patients/ tumors *n*	Prescription Dose Mean (Range)	Imaging Follow-up (Mean/Range)	Tumor Control	Survival (Mean)	Factors Associated with Prolonged Survival
Sheehan et al.[a] (2002)[189]	273/627	16(11–22.5) Gy	NS	84%	7 months	Female Higher KPS Adenocarcinoma Absence of active systemic disease ↓ Interval from primary to brain metastases
Jawahar et al.[b] (2004)[190]	44/91	15.4 (11–22) Gy	18.3 months	73%	4.5 months	Controlled primary disease Good response to radiosurgery
Sheehan et al.[c] (2005)[191]	27/47	16 (13–20) Gy	NS	81%	18 months	Higher KPS Smaller tumor volume ↓ Interval from primary to brain metastases
UVA[b] (2008)[192]	267/903	19 (3–25) Gy	12[1-150] months	90%	14 months	Higher KPS Control of lung primary

[a]Non–small cell lung carcinoma only.
[b]Small and non–small cell lung carcinoma.
[c]Small cell lung carcinoma only.
KPS, Karnofsky performance score; NS, not stated.

BREAST CARCINOMA

While improved neuroimaging enable early diagnosis of brain metastases, better treatment of systemic disease increased the frequency of the diagnosis of intracranial metastases as well. Breast cancer is a paradigm in this regard (Table 5-9). The advent of an effective targeted therapy, such monoclonal antibody against HER-2, allows patients to survive much longer than before, thus increased likelihood of central nervous system relapse.

Breast cancer is the second most common cause of cerebral metastases. Incidences of metastasis to the central nervous system ranging from 10% to 20% have been reported in clinical series and 30% in autopsy series.[150,151] Breast cancer is considered to be a relatively radiosensitive tumor and radiosurgery in the treatment of breast carcinoma that has metastasized to the brain has shown its effectiveness in prolonging overall survival.

We have treated 43 patients with a total of 84 metastatic lesions from breast carcinoma. Overall median survival was 13 months after gamma surgery.[152] Analysis revealed that a high Karnofsky performance score and a single lesion correlated with increased survival. Overall median time to local tumor control failure was 10 months. The tumor control rate from the literature ranged from 81% to 94% and the median survival ranged from 13 to 19 months.[105,152,153]

MELANOMA

The incidence of melanoma has progressively risen over the decades (Table 5-10). Melanoma is now the third most common primary tumor associated with central nervous system metastasis. Brain metastases were found in up to 75% of melanoma cases at autopsy and involvement of the central nervous system is the cause of the death in approximately one third of all patients.[106] Radiosurgery seems to overcome the problem of radioresistance observed in melanoma. With a single high radiosurgical dose, the tumor control rate following radiosurgery for cerebral metastatic melanoma seems favorable ranging from 61 to 90%. However, the prolongation of survival is not promising with most series reporting median survival in the range of 5.7 to 7.1 months.[154–157]

Table 5-9 Outcome of Radiosurgery for Metastatic Breast Carcinoma

	Patients/ Tumors n	Prescription Dose (Mean/Range)	Imaging Follow-up (Mean/Range)	Tumor Control	Survival (Mean)	Factors Associated with Prolonged Survival
Firlik et al. (2000)[153]	30/58	12–20 Gy	9 (1–31) months	93%[a]	13 months	Solitary metastasis Small lesion (<4 cm)
Amendola et al. (2000)[106]	68/518	15–24 Gy	NS	94%[a]	7.8 months	NS
Lederman et al.[b] (2001)[193]	60/246	12–25 Gy (1 fraction) 6 Gy (4 fractions)	NS	82%[a]	7.5 months	Solitary metastasis Absence of visceral diseases
Akyurek et al. (2007)[105]	49/84	18 (14–20) Gy	NS	78% at 1 year 48% at 2 years	19 months	High KPS High SIR Postmenopausal status Positive estrogen receptor
UVA (2008)[152]	86/166	18 (16–24) Gy	10 (3–54) months	81%[a]	13 months	High KPS High SIR Patient age >60 years

[a]Based on the last image follow-up.
[b]71% had fractionated radiosurgery (4 × 600c Gy).
KPS, Karnofsky performance score; SIR, score index for radiosurgery.

Table 5-10 Outcome of Radiosurgery for Metastatic Melanoma

	Patients/ Tumors n	Prescription Dose (Mean)	Imaging Follow-up (Mean/Range)	Tumor Control	Survival (Mean)	Factors Associated with Prolonged Survival
Mathieu et al. (2008)[154]	244/754	18 (10–22) Gy	8.1 (0.3–114.3) months	86.2[a]	5.3 months	Solitary metastasis Small lesion (<8 cm³) Absence of active systemic disease Non-cerebellar lesions
Christopoulou et al. (2006)[194]	29/105	25.3 (15–30) Gy	NS	61[a]	5.7 months	Decreased numbers ↓ Interval from primary to brain metastases
Radbill et al. (2004)[155]	51/188	17.3 (10–21) Gy	NS	81[a]	6.1 months	RPA class 1 Solitary metastasis Noncerebellar lesions
Selek et al. (2004)[156]	103/153	18 (10–24) Gy	NS	49% at 1 year	6.7 months	High SIR
Yu et al. (2002)[157]	122/332	20 (14–24) Gy	6.8 months	90[a]	7.0 months	Total tumor volume <3 cm³ Inactive systemic disease
UVA (2008)[195]	90/130	21 (18–24) Gy	9 (3–78) months	81[a]	10.4 months	Solitary metastasis Absence of visceral metastases

[a]Based on the last image follow-up.
RPA, recursive partitioning analysis; SIR, score index for radiosurgery.

Table 5-11   Outcome of Radiosurgery for Metastatic Renal Cell Carcinoma

	Patients/ Tumors *n*	Prescription Dose (Mean/Range)	Imaging Follow-up Mean (Range)	Tumor Control	Survival (Mean)	Factors Associated with Prolonged Survival
Shuto et al. (2006)[161]	69/314	8–30[21.8] Gy	7.1 (3–39) months	82.8%	9.5 months	Low number of metastases High KPS High RPA class
Muacevic et al. (2004)[196]	85/376	21 Gy	NS	94%	11.1 months	KPS > 70 RPA class I
Sheehan et al. (2003)[160]	69/146	16 (12.5–20) Gy	NS	96%	15 months	Younger patient age High KPS 2 months from primary to brain metastases Higher marginal dose Higher maximal dose Higher treatment isodose
Hoshi et al. (2002)[197]	42/113	25 (20–30) Gy	12.5 (0.2–88) months	93%	12.5 months	KPS ≥ 80 Treated by GK more than once Obtained complete/partial response GK
Goyal et al. (2000)[198]	29/66	18 (7–24) Gy	NS	91%	10 months	None
UVA (2008)[159]	65/40	21 (18–24) Gy	10 (3–54) months	97	8 months	None

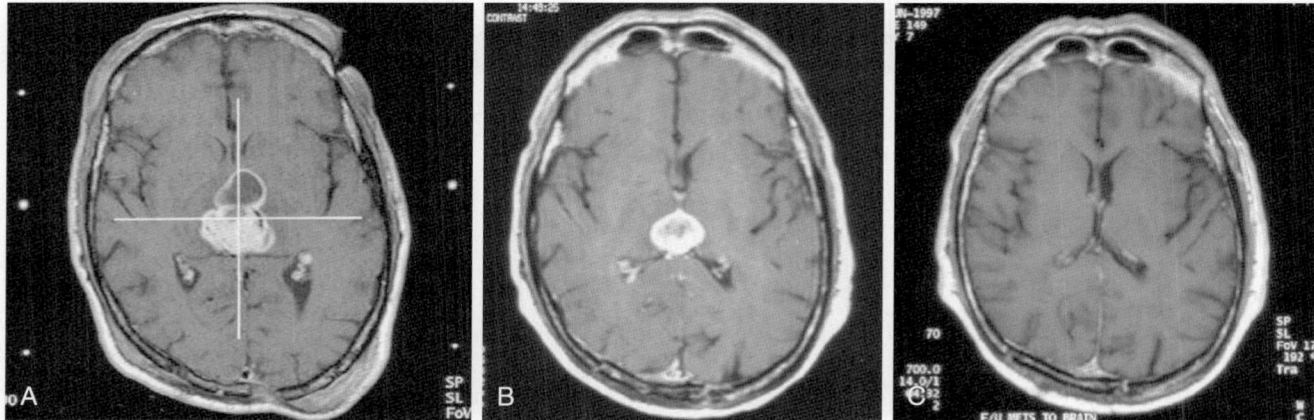

FIGURE 5-22 Gamma surgery for renal cell carcinoma. Postcontrast, axial T1-weighted MRI at time of treatment (A), and at 3 months (B) and 1 year (C) following gamma surgery. This patient developed two additional metastases that were subsequently successfully treated with gamma surgery. The patient survived 17 months before succumbing to metastatic deposits outside the brain.

We have treated 90 melanoma patients with a total of 133 tumors. Forty tumors (30%) disappeared, 45 tumors (34%) shrank, 23 tumors (17%) remained unchanged in size, and 25 tumors (19%) grew. Mean prescription dose to the tumor margin was 19 Gy (range 12–23 Gy). The median survival was 10.4 months. A single metastasis and absence of extracranial disease correlated with improved prognosis.

RENAL CELL CARCINOMA

Renal cell carcinomas are responsible for approximately 2% of cancer deaths in the United States annually, and they have a 10% incidence of developing into brain metastases[158] (Table 5-11). The resistance to fractionated radiation therapy and a tendency for limited numbers of metastases make radiosurgery a rational alternative in the management of renal cell carcinoma metastases to the brain. The reported tumor control rate following radiosurgery for metastatic renal cell carcinoma ranged from 83% to 96%.[151,159-161]

A series of 40 patients with 65 renal cell carcinoma brain metastases was treated by us. The average survival was 9.2 months after radiosurgery. A total of 41 tumors decreased in volume, 6 tumors disappeared, and 16 tumors remained unchanged in size (Fig. 5-22). Only 2 tumors increased in size following treatment. An unmatched control group of 119 patients that received external brain radiation therapy had an average survival of 4.4 months.[162] Factors associated with longer survival in the group treated with gamma surgery included a higher Karnofsky performance status, absence of extracranial metastases, adjuvant whole brain radiation therapy and prior surgical resection. The size and number of metastases did not have a significant effect on survival, although in cases of single metastasis with controlled local disease long-term survival could be achieved.

UVEAL MELANOMAS

The most common surgical treatment for uveal melanomas is enucleation, but several centers have relatively large series in the treatment of these tumors with gamma surgery.[163-166] Other therapeutic options include radium plaque therapy, and proton beam therapy. The first uveal melanoma treated with gamma surgery was in Buenos Aires[167] and gamma surgery has become a more frequently used procedure for this unusual pathology (Fig. 5-23). The use of gamma surgery and its stereotactic technique requires that the eyeball be fixated relative to the stereotactic frame. This is accomplished with retrobulbar blocks and external fixative sutures that are attached to the frame.

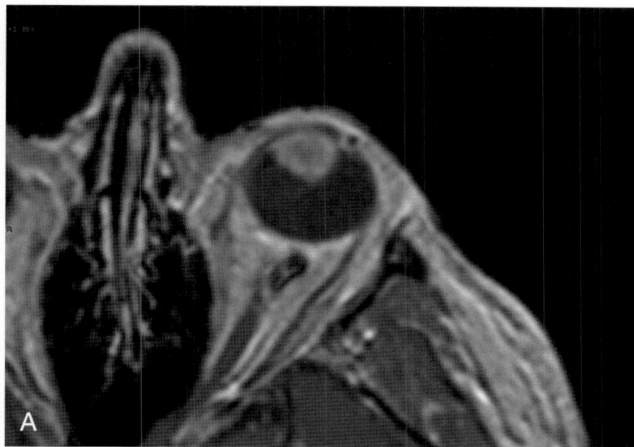
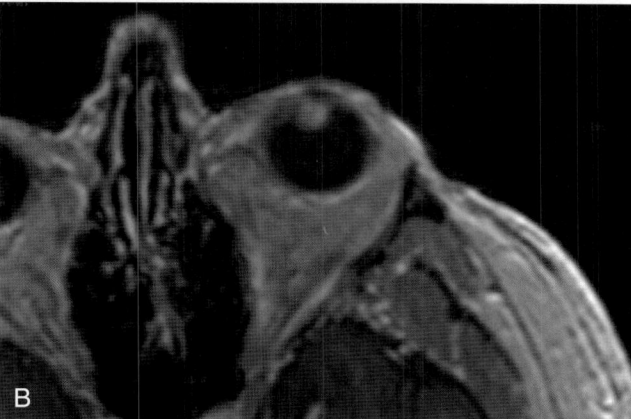

FIGURE 5-23 Gamma surgery for ocular melanoma. Postcontrast, axial T1-weighted MRI at time of treatment (A) and at 16 months (B) following gamma surgery. The tumor shrank significantly.

The Sheffield group reported a series of 29 patients treated and followed for an average of 14 months. The average peripheral dose was 73 Gy, corresponding to the 50% isodose line.[163] The dose was delivered in two sessions not more than 8 days apart. All but two patients had good local control. The two failures required later enucleation. Three patients died of metastatic disease. More recent work suggests that a lower margin dose of 41.5 Gy may be just as effective in terms of tumor control but be associated with a lower risk of neovascular glaucoma.[168] In a series of 75 patients with uveal melanoma followed for a minimum of 10 months, Simonova et al. reported 84% local tumor control and secondary glaucoma in 25%.[169]

Conclusions

Technical advances and improvements of the Gamma unit will increase the ease of use of the machine and better defined protocols should improve the clinical results obtained with its use. Other advances in fields such as pharmacology may allow the selective sensitization of tumors or provide protective effect to normal tissue increasing the efficacy and safety in vascular malformation and tumor treatment. In the first stage of development of gamma surgery, it is mandatory to define its usefulness in various pathologies. The elimination of its use when not clinically indicated and to expand its use into new areas when it has been shown to have efficacy are important goals. The rapidly accumulating material from patients that have been treated will define the place of the gamma knife in the armory of neurosurgery.

KEY REFERENCES

Amichetti M, Cianchetti M, Amelio D, et al. Proton therapy in chordoma of the base of the skull: a systematic review. *Neurosurg Rev.* 2009;32:403-416.

Andrade-Souza YM, Ramani M, Scora D, et al. Embolization before radiosurgery reduces the obliteration rate of arteriovenous malformations. *Neurosurgery.* 2007;60:443-451:discussion 451-442.

Jagannathan J, Sheehan JP, Pouratian N, et al. gamma knife surgery for Cushing's disease. *J Neurosurg.* 2007;106:980-987.

Johnson R. *Radiotherapy of cerebral angiomas with a note on some problems in diagnosis Berlin.* Springer-Verlag; 1975.

Karlsson B, Kihlstrom L, Lindquist C, et al. Radiosurgery for cavernous malformations. *J Neurosurg.* 1998;88:293-297.

Kobayashi T, Kida Y, Mori Y, Hasegawa T. Long-term results of gamma knife surgery for the treatment of craniopharyngioma in 98 consecutive cases. *J Neurosurg.* 2005;103:482-488.

Kondziolka D, Lunsford LD, Kestle JR. The natural history of cerebral cavernous malformations. *J Neurosurg.* 1995;83:820-824.

Leksell L. The stereotaxic method and radiosurgery of the brain. *Acta Chir Scand.* 1951;102:316-319.

Lindquist C, Guo WY, Karlsson B, Steiner L. Radiosurgery for venous angiomas. *J Neurosurg.* 1993;78:531-536.

Mingione V, Yen CP, Vance ML, et al. Gamma surgery in the treatment of nonsecretory pituitary macroadenoma. *J Neurosurg.* 2006;104:876-883.

Pan DH, Guo WY, Chung WY, et al. Gamma knife radiosurgery as a single treatment modality for large cerebral arteriovenous malformations. *J Neurosurg.* 2000;93(Suppl 3):113-119.

Pan L, Zhang N, Wang EM, et al. Gamma knife radiosurgery as a primary treatment for prolactinomas. *J Neurosurg.* 2000;93(Suppl 3):10-13.

Prasad D, Steiner M, Steiner L. Gamma surgery for vestibular schwannoma. *J Neurosurg.* 2000;92:745-759.

Schneider BF, Eberhard DA, Steiner LE. Histopathology of arteriovenous malformations after gamma knife radiosurgery. *J Neurosurg.* 1997;87:352-357.

Sheehan J, Yen CP, Steiner L. Gamma knife surgery-induced meningioma. Report of two cases and review of the literature. *J Neurosurg.* 2006;105:325-329.

Sirin S, Kondziolka D, Niranjan A, et al. Prospective staged volume radiosurgery for large arteriovenous malformations: indications and outcomes in otherwise untreatable patients. *Neurosurgery.* 2006;58:17-27:discussion 17-27.

Snell JW, Sheehan J, Stroila M, Steiner L. Assessment of imaging studies used with radiosurgery: a volumetric algorithm and an estimation of its error. Technical note. *J Neurosurg.* 2006;104:157-162.

Stafford SL, Pollock BE, Leavitt JA, et al. A study on the radiation tolerance of the optic nerves and chiasm after stereotactic radiosurgery. *Int J Radiat Oncol Biol Phys.* 2003;55:1177-1181.

Steiner L, Forster D, Leksell L, et al. Gammathalamotomy in intractable pain. *Acta Neurochir (Wien).* 1980;52:173-184.

Steiner L, Leksell L, Greitz T, et al. Stereotaxic radiosurgery for cerebral arteriovenous malformations. Report of a case. *Acta Chir Scand.* 1972;138:459-464.

Steiner L, Yen CP, Jagannathan J, et al. Gamma Knife: clinical aspect. In: Lozano AM, Gildenberg PL, Tasker RR, eds. *Textbook of Stereotactic and Functional Neurosurgery.* New York. Springer; 2009:1037-1085.

Tishler RB, Loeffler JS, Lunsford LD, et al. Tolerance of cranial nerves of the cavernous sinus to radiosurgery. *Int J Radiat Oncol Biol Phys.* 1993;27:215-221.

Tsuzuki T, Tsunoda S, Sakaki T, et al. Tumor cell proliferation and apoptosis associated with the gamma knife effect. *Stereotact Funct Neurosurg.* 1996;66(Suppl 1):39-48.

Yen CP, Sheehan J, Steiner M, et al. Gamma knife surgery for focal brainstem gliomas. *J Neurosurg.* 2007;106:8-17.

Yen CP, Varady P, Sheehan J, et al. Subtotal obliteration of cerebral arteriovenous malformations after gamma knife surgery. *J Neurosurg.* 2007;106:361-369.

Numbered references appear on Expert Consult.

CHAPTER 6

Cortical and Subcortical Brain Mapping

HUGUES DUFFAU

The first goal of brain surgery, especially in neuro-oncology, is to optimize the extent of resection (EOR) of the lesion. Indeed, maximal resection of glioma, when possible, is currently the first treatment to consider, both in low-grade gliomas (LGGs)[1] and in high-grade gliomas.[2] In the recent series measuring *objectively* the EOR on repeated postoperative MRI, all of them supported EOR as a statistically significant predictor of overall survival. In WHO grade II gliomas, when no signal abnormality was visible on control MRI, especially on FLAIR-weighted imaging (i.e., the so-called "complete resection"), patients had a significantly longer overall survival compared with patients having any residual abnormality. Interestingly, even in cases of incomplete tumor removal, patients with a greater percentage of resection had a significantly longer overall survival. In addition to the percentage of resection, the postoperative tumor volume is also a predictor of survival, with a significantly longer overall survival when the residue is less than 10 ml ("subtotal resection") compared with more than 10 ml ("partial resection").[3] In glioblastomas, it was also shown that the complete removal of the enhanced part of the tumor controlled on postsurgical MRI increased the median survival around 17 months, instead of only 12 months if a residual enhancement was left.[2]

Therefore, the dilemma of cerebral surgery is to maximize the EOR while preserving brain functions. Nonetheless, due to the frequent location of supratentorial gliomas near or within the so-called "eloquent" areas, and due to their infiltrative feature (poorly demarcated), for a long time chances of performing an extensive glioma removal were considered low, whereas the risk of generating postoperative sequelae was high. Indeed, many surgical series have reported a rate of permanent and severe deficit between 13% and 27.5% following removal of intra-axial tumors (for a review, see ref. 4).

Consequently, to optimize the benefit-to-risk ratio of surgery, an increasing number of authors used functional mapping methods over the last decade. Indeed, considerable interindividual anatomofunctional variability was demonstrated in healthy volunteers.[5] Furthermore, this variability is increased in cases of gliomas, due to cerebral plasticity, explaining why many patients have no or only a mild deficit before surgery, especially in slow-growing tumor such as LGG.[6] It is thus mandatory, for every patient, to study the cortical functional organization, effective connectivity, and brain plastic potential, in order to tailor the resection according not only to oncologic but also to cortico–subcortical functional boundaries.

The goal of this article is to review how, in addition to functional neuroimaging, the method of intraoperative electrostimulation mapping (IESM), at both the cortical and subcortical levels, has enabled significant improvement in the results of glioma surgery, with regard to the impact on the natural history of the tumor as well as on preservation of quality of life. The fundamental implications of IESM will also be considered, especially in the cognitive neurosciences.

Presurgical Functional Brain Mapping: Advances and Pitfalls

PREOPERATIVE NEUROCOGNITIVE ASSESSMENT

Gliomas, especially LGG, are usually revealed by inaugural seizures in young patients who have had a normal life, with no or only a mild neurologic deficit. However, recent extensive neuropsychological examinations have demonstrated that most of patients had cognitive disturbances, especially concerning working memory and executive functions.[7] This is the reason why a systematic preoperative neurocognitive assessment is now recommended to search the possible neuropsychological deficit not identified by a standard neurologic examination, to adapt the surgical methodology (e.g., functional mapping under local anesthesia) to the results of this assessment, to benefit from a presurgical baseline allowing a comparison with the postsurgical evaluation, and to plan specific functional rehabilitation.

It is nonetheless puzzling to note that these deficits are not more pronounced, despite the frequent location of LGG in the so-called "eloquent areas." This can be explained by mechanisms of brain reshaping allowing functional compensation in cases of slow-growing lesions. Indeed, it was shown that cerebral remapping was possible, with a recruitment of perilesional or remote areas within the ipsilesional hemisphere and/or recruitment of contra-hemispheric homologous areas. The recent integration of these concepts into the therapeutic strategy has resulted in dramatic changes in the surgical management of LGG patients, with an increase of surgical indications in eloquent regions classically considered "inoperable".[6]

PREOPERATIVE FUNCTIONAL NEUROIMAGING: A NECESSARY BASELINE

In this context, advances in functional neuroimaging (FNI), namely functional MRI (fMRI), positron emission tomography and magnetoencephalography, have enabled to perform a non-invasive cortical mapping of the whole brain, and is currently a standard before resection of gliomas. FNI gives an estimation of the location of the eloquent areas (e.g., regions involved in sensorimotor, language, visual, and even higher cognitive function) in relation to the tumor, and provides information with regard to the hemispheric language lateralization. Thus, these methods may be useful for surgical indications, partly depending on the location of the tumor and its relationships with eloquent areas detected by FNI (allowing an estimation of the tumor resectability); surgical planning, namely the selection of the surgical approach and the delineation of the limits of resection; and selection of surgical technique, especially the decision to wake up the patient intraoperatively if the glioma is close to language or cognitive areas—on the basis of the laterality index on FNI in addition to the handedness of the patient provided by the neuropsychological examination.

However, it is worth noting that FNI methods are not yet reliable enough *at the individual scale*, despite constant improvement efforts, mainly because the results depend on biomathematical models used for reconstruction. Regarding fMRI, correlations with intraoperative electrophysiology demonstrated that the sensitivity of fMRI was currently only around 71% for movement, and from 59% to 100% for language (specificity from 0% to 97%).[8] Such discrepancies can be explained by a neurovascular decoupling in cases of glioma (blood-oxygen–level dependence response in the vicinity of gliomas does not reflect the neuronal signal as accurately as it does in healthy tissue), by inadequate tasks (not adapted to the location of the glioma and/or to the neurologic status of the patient), or to methodological problems (e.g., selection of the threshold). As a consequence, there is a risk of false negative and then to operate a patient without intraoperative mapping, although the glioma is actually located in crucial areas for the function, but not detected by preoperative FNI. Moreover, an erroneous interpretation of brain reshaping ("pseudoreorganization") can be made. Finally, these methods are not able to differentiate the structures essential for the function, which should be surgically preserved, from those which can be functionally compensated and so potentially resected without permanent deficit. Thus, there is a double risk: first, failure to select a patient for surgery while the tumor was operable, and second, to stop the resection prematurely with a lower impact on the natural history of the glioma (or both).

The recent development of the diffusion tensor imaging (DTI) has also allowed the identification of the main bundles and their location in relation to the tumor. However, this new method needs to be validated before it can be used routinely for surgical planning, especially due to the fact that results of DTI, as FNI, strongly depend on the biomathematical models used for the fiber tracking. Indeed, comparison of distinct fiber-tracking software tools found different results, showing that neurosurgeons have to be cautious about applying tractography results intraoperatively, especially when dealing with an abnormal or distorted fiber tract anatomy. Furthermore, correlations between DTI and intrasurgical subcortical stimulation demonstrated that, despite good correspondence, DTI is not yet optimal for mapping language tracts in patients. Negative tractography does not rule out persistence of a fiber tract, especially when invaded by a glioma.[9] Moreover, DTI enables study of the sole anatomy of the subcortical pathways, but not their function.

With the aim of overcoming these pitfalls, one can currently consider performing longitudinal studies based on pre-, intra-, and post-operative mapping rather than relying exclusively on static information based on a unique presurgical functional neuroimaging analysis. Consequently, the additional use of invasive electrophysiological investigations is highly recommended for surgery in eloquent structures.

INTRASURGICAL FUNCTIONAL BRAIN MAPPING: TOWARD A HODOTOPIC VIEW OF BRAIN PROCESSING

Intraoperatively, the integration of multimodal imaging into frameless stereotactic surgery was extensively used in the past decade and referred to as "functional neuronavigation." However, a randomized trial failed to demonstrate significant impact of navigation on postoperative results.[10] It can be explained by the limitations of the presurgical neuroimaging detailed above, as well as to the high risk of intraoperative brain shift, due to surgical retraction, mass effect, gravity, extent of resection (especially for voluminous tumors), and cerebrospinal fluid leakage. Several technical improvements have been proposed to reduce the effects of this shift, but their reliability has still to be optimized: combination with intraoperative ultrasound, producing real-time imaging; use of mathematical models based on data from ultrasonography or digital images that track cortical displacement; and intraoperative MRI. Nevertheless, their actual value on the improvement of EOR and preservation of quality of life remains to demonstrate. As a consequence, invasive electrophysiologic investigations currently remain the "gold standard" when operating in eloquent brain structures.

First, the technique of somatosensory- and motor-evoked potentials was extensively used in the past decades for intraoperative identification of the central region. However, its reliability regarding the localization of the rolandic sulcus is not optimal, with accurate localization of the central sulcus reported only 91% to 94%. Estimation of the overall sensitivity and negative predictive value of this method is around 79% and 96%, respectively. Moreover, phase reversal recording identifies only the central sulcus itself, but offers no direct information on the particular distribution of motor function on the adjacent exposed cerebral structures. Also, whereas the method of motor evoked potentials was improved, when recording compound muscle action potentials, only the monitored muscles can be controlled, that is, there is an inability to detect and possibly avoid motor deficits in nonmonitored muscles. Next, monitoring of muscle action potentials does not mean monitoring of complex movements and action adapted to the environment, which is nonetheless the ultimate goal for the patient. Above all, intraoperative-evoked potentials cannot currently be used to map language, memory or other higher functions crucial for patients' quality of life (for a review, see ref.11).

Numerous authors have also promoted the use of extra-operative electrophysiologic recordings and stimulations via the implantation of subdural grids. Using this method, the patient is in optimal conditions, in his or her room, to perform the tasks; this point is particularly important for children. Moreover, recent advances in the interpretation of the electrophysiologic signal, such as electrocorticographic spectral analysis evaluating the event-related synchronization in specific bands of frequency, have allowed a better understanding of the organization of the functional cortex, and a study of the connectivity, in particular via the recording of "cortico-cortical evoked potential." However, extraoperative electrophysiologic mapping, typically in grids with 1-cm-spaced electrodes, has limited accuracy. Also, it is necessary to perform two surgical procedures, one to implant grids and a second to remove the lesion. In addition, there is a risk of infectious complications due to the presence of subdural grids over several days. Although this method was extensively advocated in epilepsy surgery, because it also allows detection of the seizure foci, only the cortex can be mapped. It provides no information about the axonal connectivity, that is, mapping of subcortical structures is not possible.

INTRASURGICAL CORTICAL AND SUBCORTICAL ELECTROSTIMULATION MAPPING METHODS

Taking into account the advantages and the limits of these different mapping techniques, more and more neurosurgeons advocate the additional use of intrasurgical electrostimulation mapping (IESM), under general or local anesthesia during surgery in eloquent areas.[12,13] Indeed, except for tumors located within the motor structures, the mapping is performed in awake patients. However, as previously mentioned, since movements and action are more complex than single muscle contractions, it is also currently proposed to map the motor function under local anesthesia with active participation of the patient.[14] The principle is to use IESM as a focal and transitory virtual lesion to obtain an individual functional map both at cortical and subcortical levels, and to test if a structure involved by a lesion is still crucial for the function—which is, for instance, observed in 15% to 20% of LGG cases. Stimulation of an essential area generates a transient disruption of the task performed by the patient, and this area should be preserved. An individual cortical mapping is thus obtained before the resection, which can be tailored according to functional boundaries (Fig. 6-1). Practically, a bipolar electrode tip spaced 5 mm apart and delivering a biphasic current (pulse frequency 60 Hz, single-pulse phase duration 1 millisecond) is applied to the brain. The current intensity adapted to each patient is determined by progressively increasing the amplitude in 1-mA increments from a baseline of 2 mA until a functional response is elicited, with 6 mA as the upper limit under local anesthesia, and with 16 mA as the upper limit under general anesthesia—with the goal of avoiding the generation of seizures. The patient is never informed when the brain is stimulated. At least one picture presentation without stimulation must separate each stimulation, and no site is stimulated twice in succession to avoid seizures. Each cortical site (size 5 × 5 mm, due to the spatial resolution of the probe) of the entire cortex exposed by the bone flap is tested three times. Indeed, it is admitted nowadays

that three trials are sufficient to ensure whether an area is crucial for language, by generating disturbances during its three stimulations, and with normalization of the function as soon as the stimulation is stopped. This limitation of trials and tasks is required by the timing of the surgical procedure, because the patient is awake and can be tired at the end of the resection.

Interestingly, recent series show that the surgical procedure can be simplified by avoiding the use of intraoperative electrocorticography despite an equivalent reliability of electrical mapping and without increasing the rate of seizures.[12] However, in cases of stimulation-induced seizures, the use of cold Ringer's lactate is recommended to abrogate the seizure activity. In addition, some authors emphasized the value of "negative mapping" (no identification of eloquent sites) in the setting of a tailored cortical exposure.[13] Although such recommendation is acceptable for high-grade gliomas, since the surgical goal is mainly to remove the enhanced part of the tumor, a negative mapping can be dangerous in surgery of diffuse LGG, especially in nonexpert hands. Indeed, due to the fact that LGG is poorly delineated, the limit of the resection will be essentially guided according to functional criteria. Because negative mapping can be due to false negative for methodologic reasons, it does not guarantee the absence of eloquent sites. In the experience reported by Sanai et al., all four patients with permanent postoperative deficits had no positive sites detected prior to their resections.[12] Therefore, other authors continue to promote a wider bone flap, in order to obtain a systematic positive mapping before performing the resection.[11,12] *Moreover, a positive mapping might also allow an optimization of the EOR, since the resection can be pursued until eloquent areas are encountered, that is, with no margin around the functional structures.* A recent study demonstrated that in a consecutive and homogeneous series of 115 LGG in the left dominant hemisphere, the rate of permanent deficit remained lower than 2% despite the absence of margin around the language sites.[12]

IESM allows the mapping of motor function (possibly under general anesthesia, by inducing involuntary motor response, but also in awake patient by eliciting a disturbance of the movement), somatosensory function (by eliciting dysesthesias described by the patient himself intraoperatively), visual function (by eliciting phosphenes and/or visual field deficit described by the patient), auditivo-vestibular function (by inducing vertigo), language (spontaneous speech, counting, object naming, comprehension, writing, reading, bilingualism, switching from one language to another), and also the mapping of higher-order functions such as calculation, memory, spatial cognition, cross-modal judgment or even emotional processing, by generating transient disturbances if the electrical stimulation is applied at the level of a functional "epicenter."[14] It is crucial that a speech therapist/neuropsychologist/neurologist be present in the operative room, in order to interpret accurately the kind of disorders induced by IESM, for instance speech arrest, anarthria, speech apraxia, phonological disturbances, semantic paraphasia, perseveration, anomia, dysculia, and so on. *Thus, IESM is able to identify in real-time the cortical sites essential for the function before the beginning of the resection, in order to both select the best surgical approach and to define the cortical limits of the lesion removal.*

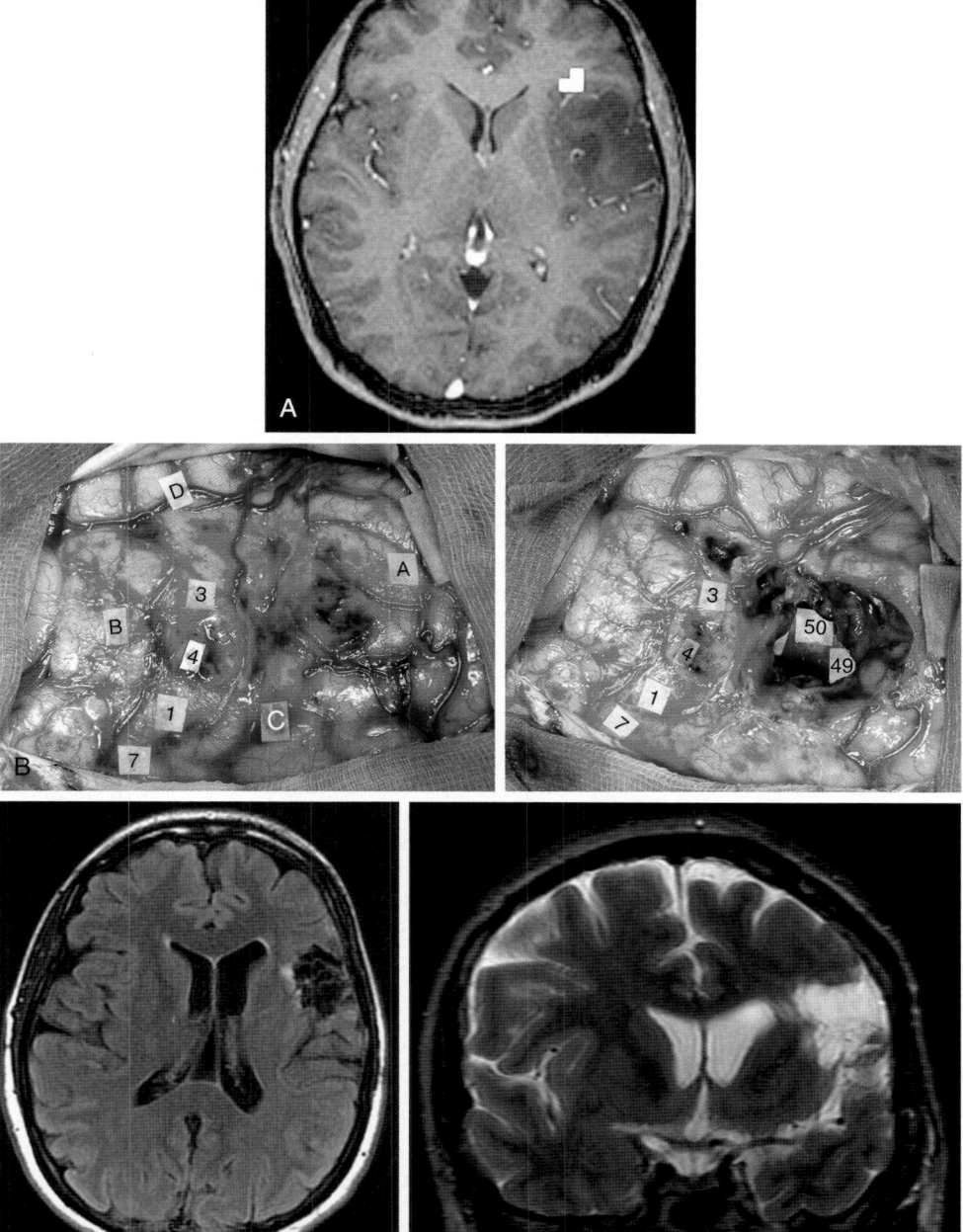

FIGURE 6-1 A, Preoperative language fMRI in a patient with no deficit, showing an LGG that involves the left inferior frontal gyrus (Broca's area), with an activation immediately in front of the tumor (within the anterior insula). B, Intraoperative views before (*left*) and after (*right*) glioma resection, delineated by letter tags. IESM shows a reshaping of the eloquent maps, with a recruitment of perilesional language sites located behind the glioma. There was no crucial site within the left inferior frontal gyrus. Thus, an extensive resection of Broca's area was possible, by preserving the subcortical connectivity in the depth of the cavity (50, corresponding to the anterior part of the arcuate fasciculus). Stimulation of the anterior insula-generated anomia.[49]C, Postoperative axial FLAIR- (left) and coronal T2-weighted MRI, demonstrating a complete resection of the glioma, in a patient with no deficit.

Another major issue is the use of subcortical mapping throughout the resection, in addition to the cortical mapping before the lesion removal.[11,12] Brain lesion studies have taught that damage of the white matter pathways generated more severe deficit than cortical injury. Therefore, the subcortical tracts subserving motor, somatosensory, visual, auditivovestibular, language, and cognitive functions must be detected during the lesion removal, in order to preserve anatomofunctional connectivity while optimizing the EOR, that is, to pursue the resection until eloquent pathways are detected. Interestingly, according to the same principle as that described at the cortical level, IESM can also identify eloquent subcortical structures. It allows the study of anatomofunctional connectivity by directly and regularly stimulating the white matter tracts and deep gray nuclei throughout the resection, and by eliciting functional response when in contact with deep crucial areas (Fig. 6-1). Furthermore, IESM enables a better understanding of the brain connectivity, showing that dynamic cerebral processing is underlain by parallel distributed and interactive networks, the so-called "hodology."[15] This connectionist view also opens the door to the concept of cerebral plasticity, crucial in LGG surgery.

One of the major advantages of IESM for brain mapping in adult patients is that it *intrinsically* does not cause any false negatives—if the methodology is rigorously applied as detailed previously. Indeed, IESM is highly sensitive for detecting the cortical and axonal eloquent structures, and it also provides a unique opportunity to study brain connectivity, since each area responsive to stimulation is in fact an input gate into a large-scale network, rather than an isolated discrete functional site. IESM, however, also has a limitation, as its specificity is suboptimal. Indeed, IESM may lead to interpretation that a structure is crucial, due to the induction of a transient functional response when stimulated, whereas this effect is caused by backward spreading of the electrostimulation along the network to an essential area, and/or the stimulated region can be functionally compensated thanks to long-term brain plasticity mechanisms. In brief, although IESM is still the gold standard for brain mapping, due to the risk of "false positives," its combination with new methods such as perioperative FNI and biomathematical modeling is now mandatory, to clearly differentiate those networks that are actually indispensable to function from those that can be compensated.[16]

IESM: NEW INSIGHTS INTO DYNAMIC FUNCTIONAL ORGANIZATION OF THE BRAIN

Complementary methods of functional mapping are used to better understand the pathophysiology of functional areas, and thus to improve surgical planning in various eloquent regions.

Anatomofunctional Organization of Supplementary Motor Area

The supplementary motor area (SMA), namely the front-omesial area located in front of the primary motor area of the inferior limb, is involved in the planning of the movement. Its resection induces the classical "SMA syndrome." This syndrome is characterized by a complete akinesia and even mutism in cases of lesions of the left dominant SMA, which occurs approximately 30 min following the end of the resection, as observed in awake patients. Then, this syndrome suddenly and spontaneously resolves around the 10th day following surgery, even if some rehabilitation is often needed during 1 to 3 months in order to allow a truly complete functional recovery. Using preoperative fMRI, it has been shown that the occurrence of this syndrome was not related to the volume of the frontal resection, but directly to the removal of a specific structure called the "SMA-proper," detectable on the preoperative FNI. Thus, on the basis of the presurgical fMRI, it is now possible to predict, before surgery, if an SMA syndrome will occur or not postoperatively, and to inform the patient and his family.[17] Moreover, by coupling preoperative fMRI, the pattern of clinical deficit after surgery, and the extent of resection on the postoperative MRI, the existence of a somatotopy within the SMA-proper has been demonstrated—namely, from anterior to posterior: the representation of language (at least in the dominant hemisphere), of the face, then the superior limb, and then the inferior limb (immediately in front of the paracentral lobule). As a consequence, it is also possible to predict before SMA resection the severity and the pattern of the postoperative transient deficit (e.g., only mutism, or mutism and akinesia of the superior limb, or akinesia of the entire hemibody). This has an important impact in planning rehabilitation.

Role of Insula in Language and Swallowing

Although the insular lobe is also frequently involved in tumors, particularly LGGs, this structure was poorly studied over a long period of time for technical reasons. In fact, the insula is an anatomical, cytoarchitectonic, and functional interface between the allocortex and neocortex. Recent FNI studies have enhanced understanding of this multimodal lobe in many functions, in particular in language. Indeed, preoperative fMRI has regularly showed an activation of the anterior insular cortex in the dominant hemisphere during language tasks, as reported in healthy volunteers. Moreover, these results were confirmed by IESM, which induced language disorders, and more specifically articulatory disturbances when applied on the insular cortex, supporting the role of this structure in the complex planning of speech, as previously suggested in stroke studies.[18] These data have important implications for the neurosurgeon, since in left dominant (frontotemporo) insular lesions, resection carries a high risk of being incomplete. Moreover, following resection of LGG involving the right nondominant insulo-opercular structures, the induction of a transient Foix-Chavany-Marie syndrome can be observed, that is, a bilateral facio-linguo-pharyngo-laryngal palsy, with a reversible inability for the patient to speak and swallow.

Functional Organization of Broca's Area

Using IESM, it was shown that the classical "Broca's area" was not basically involved in speech production, but was in fact implied in several language processings: its posterior part (pars opercularis) is more involved in phonological processing, its superior part (pars triangularis) is implied in syntactic processing, and its anterior part (pars orbitaris) is more involved in a large semantic network that overlays the inferior fronto-occipital fasciculus.[19] Interestingly, these results provided by IESM are in accordance with those obtained using fMRI, as shown in a recent meta-analysis of the literature.[5]

Role of Premotor Cortex in Language

Although many studies have allowed a better clarification of the implication of this structure in motor function, its participation in language remains poorly understood. Interestingly, it has demonstrated using IESM that stimulation of the dominant dorsal premotor area (namely the structure lateral to the SMA, in front of the primary motor area of the hand), induced anomia when stimulated. On the other hand, stimulation of the dominant ventral premotor cortex regularly elicited anarthria.[12] These results give strong arguments in favor of the involvement of the dorsal premotor cortex in the naming network, in accordance with fMRI studies which have suggested that this region could participate to lexical retrieval and that its engagement might be related to conceptual category; and the involvement of the ventral premotor cortex in the planning of articulation, explaining why lesion studies have reported that damage of the "lower motor cortex" induced speech apraxia (i.e., aphemia).

Functional Organization of Wernicke's Area

Concerning lesions located within dominant temporal posterior areas, tasks adapted to test comprehension during IESM have been developed. For instance, a triad of pictures is shown, and the patient is asked to pair them by naming two pictures with conceptual links, such as a pyramid and a palm tree. Interestingly, several sites within the posterior part of the superior temporal gyrus specifically elicited an anomia without comprehension disorders when stimulated, although other sites within the same gyrus elicited only comprehension disorders with preservation of the ability to name, and other areas generated only phonological disturbances. These results give some arguments in favor of the complexity of the functional organization of Wernicke's area (in accordance with fMRI results) with its participation not only in comprehension, but also in naming phonological processing.[5]

Role of Angular Gyrus in Calculation

The supramarginal and angular gyri in the dominant hemisphere are known to participate to complex cognitive functions, such as calculation. In patients harboring left posterior parietal LGG, both multiplication and subtraction have been tested using IESM. Interestingly, it was found that functional epicenters more involved in arithmetic facts such as rote multiplication, with tables learned by heart, were located immediately above the posterior end of the sylvian fissure, and thus very close to the language sites. On the other hand, actual calculation such as subtraction recruited functional sites located in the superior part of the angular gyrus, immediately below the intraparietal sulcus, namely close to the areas involved in working memory. These results suggest the existence of a "calculotopy" within the angular gyrus. Despite a transient dyscalculia following surgery, the patients recovered.

Role of Frontal Eye Field and Cingulate Eye Field in Oculomotor Behavior

The functional anatomy of the frontal eye field has also been studied using both preoperative fMRI and IESM. This is a region located laterally and in front of the primary motor area of the face, implied in the regulation of the voluntary and involuntary ocular saccades. Indeed, IESM of this area evoked contraversive smooth eye movements recorded electro-oculographically. Moreover, stimulation of an anterior subregion of this electrically determined frontal eye field disclosed both smooth eye movement and interfered with oculomotor behavior, suppressing self-paced saccades in the awake patient. It is worth noting that the posterior part of the anterior cingulum, namely the "cingulate eye field," could also play a role in suppression of unwanted saccades (i.e., antisaccades).

Role of the Right Supramarginal Gyrus and Posterior Temporal Areas in Spatial Awareness

The use of a line bisection task during awake surgery in patients with a lesion involving the right parietotemporal junction enables the mapping the areas involved in the spatial awareness. A significant rightward deviation is usually observed during the stimulation of the anteroinferior part of the supramarginal gyrus and the caudal part of the superior temporal gyrus. In other words, a transient and reproducible left neglect is induced by electrical inactivation of cortical sites essential for the visuospatial integration, at the level of the right parietotemporal junction. If these eloquent areas are preserved, the patients show no signs of neglect when examined a few days after surgery. These findings demonstrate that the supramarginal gyrus and the caudal part of the superior temporal gyrus in the right hemisphere, are critical to the symmetrical processing of the visual scene in humans.[20]

Role of the Left Dorsolateral Cortex in Judgment

For lesions located within the left dominant prefrontal cortex, tasks of cross-modal (visual-verbal) congruent and incongruent judgment have been performed in awake patients. Visual and auditory stimuli were presently simultaneously, both referring to the same item (congruence condition), or not (semantic or phonemic incongruent condition). It was shown that brain areas not involved in naming processing elicited a reproducible deficit of incongruent judgment when stimulated, especially at the level of the left dorsolateral prefrontal region, even if an interindividual variability was observed, as for other functions.[21] Preservation of such executive functions is essential for the daily life, in particular regarding decision making and planning of complex strategy.

Interestingly, other anatomofunctional correlations can also be made using functional mapping in patients operated on for brain lesions, in particular with regard to writing, reading, bilingualism and language switching, memory, emotional processing, or even control of micturition.

In summary, the neurosurgeon must adapt his treatment strategy, and in particular the surgical technique (especially concerning the selection of the functional tasks in order to optimize the reliability of the intraoperative mapping, and then the precise boundaries of the resection) to the better knowledge of the functional organization of the brain applied to each patient.

IESM: STUDY OF THE SUBCORTICAL CONNECTIVITY

As previously mentioned, the study of individual anatomofunctional connectivity underlying the eloquent networks is mandatory in brain surgery, to avoid postoperative permanent neurologic deficit.

Subcortical Motor Pathways

In precentral lesion, after detection and preservation of the primary motor cortical areas using IESM, it is also important to detect the corresponding descending motor pathways using subcortical stimulation, and their somatotopy, that is, the different fibers of the corona radiata, with the pyramidal bundles of the lower limb medially, of the upper limb and of the face more laterally. As at the cortical level, these subcortical motor fibers constitute the posterior and deep functional limits of the resection, until the opening of the ventricle. The pyramidal pathways may also be identified at the level of the posterior limb of the internal capsule, in particular in cases of (fronto-temporo-)insular lesion, in which the deep boundaries of the resection are given when subcortical stimulation induce motor responses in the inferior part of the corona radiata up to the superior part of the mesencephalic peduncles.[11]

Subcortical Somatosensory Pathways

In the same way, the thalamo-cortical somatosensory pathways and their somatotopy can be identified by IESM, which induces dysesthesias in awake patients in cases of retrocentral tumors.[11]

Subcortical Visual Pathways

Subcortical visual pathways can be mapped in patients who undergo surgery in awake conditions for temporo-occipito-parietal lesion, with induction of a transient "shadow" and/or phosphenes in the contralateral visual field during stimulation of the posterosuperior and deep part of the surgical cavity, sometimes with also metamorphopsia (i.e., visual illusion). Thus, if resection is stopped at this level, patients are left with only a residual quadrantanopsia without any consequence on the quality of life.

Subcortical Language Pathways

In left dominant precentral lesion, after identification of the motor and language cortical sites within the prerolandic and inferior frontal gyri (Broca's area), IESM also enables detection of different language pathways.[12] Medially, IESM can identify the fasciculus subcallosal medialis (running from the SMA and cingulate gyrus to the head of the caudate nucleus), which elicits transient transcortical motor aphasia during its stimulation; this tract is involved in the initiation of language. Posteriorly, the fibers coming from the premotor ventral cortex must be detected, inducing anarthria when stimulated: this pathway is crucial for speech production. More laterally, the operculo-insular connections should also be detected, by generating a complete speech arrest during stimulation; these connections are particularly involved in speech planning.

In addition to these locoregional language pathways, IESM also allows the detection of long-distance–association pathways, with first of all, the deep part of the superior longitudinal fasciculus, namely the arcuate fasciculus (AF). Indeed, in patients with a lesion involving the left insula and/or left inferior frontal gyrus, it is possible to identify the anterior part of AF, located within the anterior floor of the external capsule (under the superior part of the insula) and also under the posterior part of the so-called Broca's area (namely the pars opercularis and pars triangularis of the inferior frontal gyrus). Stimulation induces transient symptoms classically observed in conduction aphasia, associating phonemic paraphasia and repetition disorders. In the same way, AF must also be detected at the level of its posterosuperior loop, located under the supramarginal gyrus, in patients operated on for a left posterior parietal lesion. The same symptoms associating phonemic paraphasias and repetition disorders are induced during stimulation. Again, AF is detected in posterior temporal lesions, the posterior part of its posterior funiculus corresponding to the anterior functional limit of the resection. Finally, the anterior part of the anterior funiculus of AF must also have been used as the posterior functional boundary of left dominant anterior and mid-temporal lobectomy.[12] Interestingly, AF seems also to subserve a wide network involved in language switching (from a native language to another language or vice versa): IESM can disrupt such function, crucial to detection and preservation in bilingual patients.

In addition to the AF, there is a lateral part of the superolongitudinal fasciculus. In particular, in patients harboring a left retrocentral supra-sylvian lesion, IESM detects not only the language cortical sites at the level both of the ventral premotor cortex in front of the tumor and of the supramarginal gyrus and/or angular gyrus behind it, but also a fronto-parietal subcortical network inducing speech apraxia when stimulated. This operculo-opercular loop might underlie the anatomofunctional connectivity of the working memory circuit. Indeed, as recently demonstrated by DTI, this loop corresponds to the anterior segment of an indirect pathway of the classical superior longitudinal fasciculus, which runs parallel and lateral to the AF, by connecting Broca's territory with the inferior parietal lobe. It seems that this tract might be involved in the vocalization of semantic content. Therefore, this example illustrates well that IESM and DTI can be combined in order to better understand the anatomofunctional connectivity of the brain.[15]

In addition to this "dorsal phonological root," IESM has provided arguments supporting the likely role of the inferior fronto-occipital fasciculus (IFOF) in the semantic system, that is, the "ventral semantic root." Indeed, in patients with a lesion involving the frontal structures immediately in front and above the Broca's area—namely, the pars orbitaris of the left inferior frontal gyrus and the dorsolateral prefrontal area—the anterior part of the IFOF has been identified under these regions, by eliciting semantic paraphasias during subcortical stimulation. In the same way, IFOF has also been detected, by inducing the same symptoms (i.e., semantic paraphasias) when stimulated, in its intermediate part located within the anterior floor of the internal capsule (in front and inferiorly to the AF, and behind and superiorly to the uncinate fasciculus), in surgery for left insular lesion. Again, IFOF has been detected in left temporal LGG, by eliciting semantic disorders when stimulated, and it constituted the deep limit of the resection (above the roof of the temporal horn of the ventricle).[19]

Interestingly, it was demonstrated that stimulation of the anterior part of the inferior longitudinal fasciculus, in front of the visual word form area (i.e., the basal part of the temporo-occipital junction, involved in high-level visual processing such as reading), as well as stimulation of the uncinate fasciculus, never generated transient language disturbances, and thus could be removed with no aphasia. It seems that this indirect pathway from the temporo-occipital areas to the prefrontal region, with a relay at the level of the temporal pole (temporo-occipital area, inferior longitudinal fasciculus, temporal pole, uncinate fasciculus, orbito-frontal and prefrontal areas) can be compensated by the direct pathways constituted by the IFOF.[12]

In addition, IESM also allows the mapping of the deep gray nuclei, sometimes invaded by tumors such as LGG. Indeed, stimulation of the head of the dominant caudate in patients harboring a frontomesial LGG coming in contact of the striatum in the depth, generally generates perseverations namely the repetition of the previous item while the next item is presented to the patient. These results give further arguments in favor of an inhibitor role of the caudate in the control of cognition. Equally, it is important to map the lateral part of the dominant lentiform nucleus, at the end of the resection of insular tumors. Lentiform stimulation induces anarthria, supporting the likely role of this structure in the planning of articulation, in association with the insula and ventral premotor cortex.[12]

Finally, it is also important to use IESM for language, both at cortical and subcortical levels, for lesion involving the right hemisphere in right-handed or even ambidextrous patients, due to the bilateral distribution of language.

In all cases, these language bundles should systematically constitute the subcortical functional limits of the resection.

Subcortical Pathway Involved in Spatial Awareness

Using a task of line bisection during awake surgery in patients harboring a lesion within the right parieto-temporal junction (as previously described at the cortical level), IESM must also detect the white matter tracts implied in spatial processing, in order to avoid postoperative left neglect. During the stimulation of part II of the superior longitudinal fasciculus, a significant rightward deviation is regularly observed.[20] As a consequence, it seems that this parieto-frontal pathway subserves spatial awareness, and that a lesion at its level may generate a permanent left neglect. Stimulation of the right superior longitudinal facsiculus may also induce vertigo by disrupting a large network between the parieto-insular vestibular cortex and the visual and the sensory-motor areas.

These results suggest that damage to restricted regions of white matter can cause the dysfunction of large-scale cognitive networks. Also, these illustrations show that it is possible to adapt the intraoperative testing to each patient with the goal of mapping the subcortical pathway underlying other cognitive functions than language. Interestingly, although IESM of the interhemispheric white matter pathways has been performed, no functional responses were elicited by stimulating the corpus callosum. Such results have allowed resection of LGGs involving this structure without any consequence on the quality of life, whatever the location of the "callosectomy."

In summary, the vision of the neural basis of cognition begins to shift from a localizationist and then an associationist view toward a "hodologic" organization (i.e., dynamic parallel large-scale networks able to compensate themselves). Indeed, from Lichtheim to Geschwind, cognitive functions such as language were conceived in associationist terms of centers and pathways, the general assumption being that visual and auditory linguistic information were processed in localized cortical regions with the serial passage of information between regions through white matter tracts. *Currently, an alternative hodologic account is proposed, in which language is conceived as resulting from parallel distributed processing performed by distributed groups of connected neurons rather that individual centers.*[15] In contrast to the serial model of language in which one processing must be finished before the information enters another level of processing, these new models of "independent networks" state that different processing can be performed simultaneously with interactive feedback. Interestingly, the recent methodologic advances in DTI as well as intraoperative cortico-subcortical electrical mapping have enabled direct observation in humans of the anatomofunctional connectivity that underlies linguistic functions, supporting and completing Mesulam's large-scale neural network model of language. In particular, it seems that there are at least two parallel pathways, namely the dorsal phonologic stream and the ventral semantic stream, which converge to a common final tract allowing speech production. Furthermore, this entire network is modulated by cortico-striato-pallido-thalamo-cortical loops. Of course, it is worth noting that the goal of this new concept is not to substitute the "cortical centers"

(topology) with "subcortical pathways" (hodology), but rather to envision the common interactive processing of both gray and white matters ("hodotopy").[15] The next step to progress in the understanding of brain connectivity might be a more accurate analysis of the interactions between the language circuit and networks underlying other cognitive functions, in particular the visuospatial component in which the role of the superior longitudinal fasciculus has been emphasized, as well as emotional and behavioral aspects. Such a multimodality approach seems to represent a unique opportunity to move toward an integrative model of the various functions. In this way, recent advances in biomathematical modeling of the electrophysiologic and hemodynamic signals, which allow a reliable study of the activity time course within the neuronal networks via the analysis of the synchrony (the so-called "chrono-architecture"), may open a new door to the effective connectivity, that is, the influence that one neural system exerts over another.

Consequently, it is crucial for neurosurgeons to improve their knowledge of anatomofunctional connectivity, and thus to integrate more easily and more systematically the concept of subcortical mapping in surgical strategy. This is desirable because the gliomas, in essence, involve both cortical and subcortical structures, and thus they may alter connectivity. Next, lesions of the white matter may elicit more severe permanent deficits than cortical damage. In addition, such a hodologic view may explain why some epicenters considered essential for language in a localizationist model—for instance, Broca's area—can be in certain conditions involved by a tumor (or even surgically removed) with no aphasia due to a functional compensation within a large distributed network (i.e., so-called brain plasticity).[22]

IESM: NEW INSIGHTS INTO BRAIN PLASTICITY

As early as the beginning of the 19th century, two opposing perspectives on central nervous system function were suggested. First, the theory of equipotentiality hypothesized that the entire brain, or at least one complete hemisphere, was implied in the practice of a functional task. Conversely, the theory of "localizationism," in which each part of the brain was supposed to correspond to a specific function, was built following the seminal description of "phrenology." Progressively, frequent reports of lesional studies led into an intermediate view, namely a brain organized in highly specialized functional areas, called "eloquent" regions (such as the central, Broca's, and Wernicke's areas), for which any lesion gives rise to major irrevocable neurologic deficits, and in "nonfunctional" structures, with no clinical consequences when injured. Based on these first anatomofunctional correlations, and despite descriptions by certain pioneers of postlesional recovery, the dogma of a static functional organization of the brain was dominant for a long time, that is, inability to compensate any injury involving the so-called eloquent areas. However, through regular reports of improvement in functional status following damage to cortical and/or subcortical structures considered as "critical," this view of a "fixed" central nervous system was called into question. Consequently, many investigations were performed, initially in vitro and in animals, and then more recently in humans since the development of FNI, in order to study the mechanisms underlying these compensatory phenomena, known as cerebral plasticity.

Cerebral plasticity can be defined as the continuous processings that allow short-, middle-, and long-term remodeling of neuronosynaptic organization, in order to optimize the functioning of the networks of the brain during phylogenesis, ontogeny, physiological learning and following lesions involving the peripheral as well as the central nervous system. Several hypotheses about the pathophysiologic mechanisms underlying plasticity have been considered. At a microscopic scale, these mechanisms seem to be essentially represented by synaptic efficacy modulations, unmasking of latent connections, phenotypic modifications, synchrony changes, and neurogenesis. At a macroscopic scale, diaschisis, functional redundancies, crossmodal plasticity with sensory substitution and morphologic changes may be involved. Moreover, the behavioral consequences of such cerebral phenomena have been analyzed in humans in the last decade, both in physiology (ontogeny and learning) and in pathology. In particular, the ability to recover after a lesion of the nervous system, and the patterns of functional reorganization within an eloquent area and/or within distributed networks, allowing such compensation have been extensively studied.[23]

Interestingly, the field of slow-growing cerebral tumors such as LGGs, has demonstrated that large amounts of cerebral tissue could be removed, inside or outside the so-called eloquent areas, with impressive recovery, with no permanent detectable functional consequences.[6,22] Such knowledge combined to the use of IESM allows better study of the dynamic reorganization of the eloquent maps induced by LGGs at the individual scale, and thus opens new surgical indications in classically "inoperable" areas.

Preoperative Plasticity

As already mentioned, it could seem surprising that numerous patients harboring a brain tumor, especially an LGG, typically have only mild functional deficits, in spite of the frequent invasion of eloquent structures. This means that these slow-growing lesions have likely induced progressive functional brain reshaping, as suggested by preoperative FNI. Interestingly, reorganization patterns may differ among patients, a very important concept for the neurosurgeon with the goal to optimize both indications of surgery and surgical planning.[6,23] Indeed, despite the limitations of the preoperative FNI previously detailed, these methods have shown that three kinds of preoperative functional redistribution are possible in patients without any deficit. In the first, due to the infiltrative feature of gliomas, function still persists within the tumor, thus with a very limited chance to perform a fair resection without inducing postoperative sequelae. In the second, eloquent areas are redistributed around the tumor, thus with a reasonable chance to perform at least a near-total resection despite a likely immediate transient deficit, but with secondary recovery within a few weeks to months. In the third, a preoperative compensation by remote areas already exists within the lesional hemisphere and/or by the contralateral homologous; consequently, the chance of performing a real total resection of this kind of glioma is very high, with only a slight and very transient deficit. Therefore, in cases of brain lesions involving eloquent areas, plasticity mechanisms seem to be based on an hierarchically organized model: first, with intrinsic reorganization within injured areas (indice of favorable outcome); and second, when this reshaping is not sufficient, other regions implicated in the functional network are recruited, in the ipsilateral hemisphere (close and even remote to the damaged area) and then in the contralateral hemisphere if necessary.[23]

Intraoperative Plasticity

Intraoperative stimulation before any resection has allowed the confirmation of the existence of a functional reshaping induced by brain lesions, notably with a possible remapping of the motor homunculus and also a reorganization of the language sites. Moreover, acute reorganization of functional maps was equally observed during the resection, likely due to the surgical act itself which can generate a locoregional hyperexcitability, as has been demonstrated in head injury.[6] Indeed, in several patients harboring a frontal lesion, although stimulation of the precentral gyrus induced motor responses only at the level of a limited number of cortical sites before resection, an acute unmasking of redundant motor sites located within the same precentral gyrus and eliciting the same movements than the previous adjacent sites when stimulated, was observed immediately following lesion removal. Acute unmasking of redundant somatosensory sites was also regularly observed within the retrocentral gyrus in patients operated on for a parietal glioma. Furthermore, it was equally possible to detect a redistribution within a more larger network involving the whole rolandic region, that is, with unmasking of a functional homologous area located in the precentral gyrus for the first cortical representation and in the retrocentral gyrus for its redundancy (or vice versa). Finally, intraoperative mapping also has a prognostic value concerning the postoperative recovery: a positive response means that the patient will recover.

Postoperative Plasticity

The mechanisms of such a plasticity induced by surgical resection within eloquent areas were also studied by performing postoperative FNI once patients had recovered preoperative functional status. In particular, several patients were examined following resection of gliomas involving the SMA, which elicited a transient postsurgical SMA syndrome (see above). Functional MRI showed, in comparison to the preoperative FNI, the occurrence of activations of the SMA and premotor cortex contralateral to the lesion: the contrahemispheric homologous area thus participated to the postsurgical functional compensation.[17]

IESM: THERAPEUTIC IMPLICATIONS IN ONCOLOGIC NEUROSURGERY

Incorporating individual plastic potential in surgical strategy for gliomas, especially LGGs, has the following goals: extend the indications of resection in eloquent structures previously considered inoperable; maximize the extent of glioma removal, by performing the resection according to (dynamic) functional boundaries, and minimizing the risk of postoperative permanent neurologic deficits or even improving quality of life.[23]

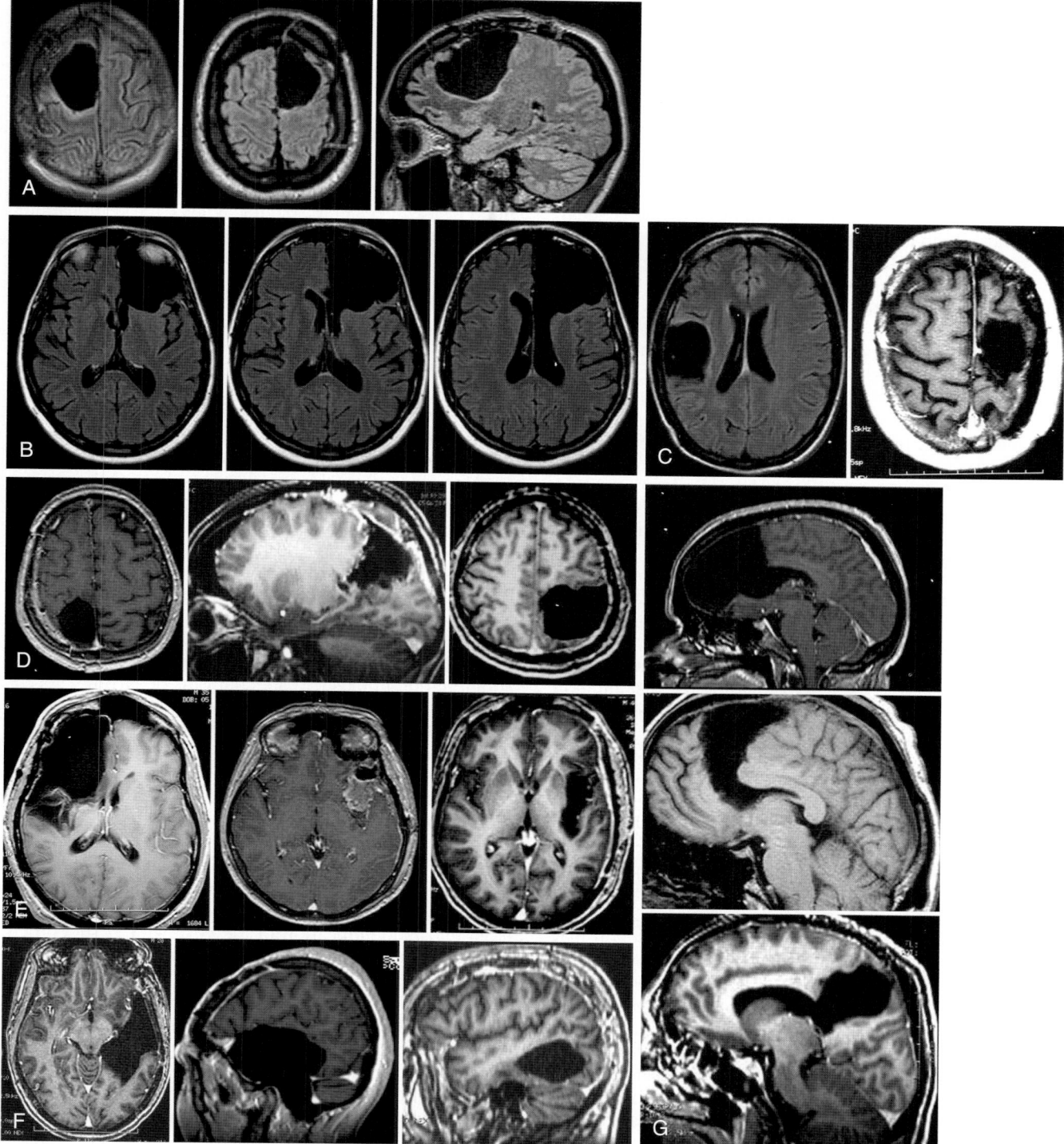

FIGURE 6-2 Examples of extensive glioma resection performed within eloquent areas using IESM, with preservation the quality of life thanks to brain plasticity. A, Right and left SMA. B, Entire left frontal lobe including Broca's area. C, Primary sensorimotor area of the face and primary motor area of the hand. D, Primary somatosensory area and parietal lobe. E, Right paralimbic system and left insula. F, Anterior/mid and posterior left dominant temporal lobe. G, Corpus callosum.

Consequently, several surgical series showed that it was possible to remove LGGs invading the following eloquent brain structures (Fig. 6-2):

- SMA resection: As previously mentioned, all patients recover, and postoperative fMRI has supported functional compensation by the contralateral SMA and premotor cortex as well as by the ipsilesional primary motor cortex.[17]

- Insular resection: Despite hemiparesis after right insula removal, likely because this region is a nonprimary motor area, and transient speech disturbances following left dominant insula resection, all patients recover—except in rare cases of deep stroke.[18] Moreover, it was possible in right nondominant fronto-temporo-insular LGGs involving the deep gray nuclei, to remove the clautrum without any cognitive disorders (despite its suggested role in consciousness), and also to remove the invaded striatum without inducing motor deficit or movement disorders. This compensation can be explained by a recruitment of parallel subcortical circuits such as pallido-luyso-pallidal, strio-nigro-striate, cortico-strio-nigro-thalamo-cortical, and cortico-luysal networks.

- S1 resection: The first results using pre- and postoperative FNI have suggested the possible recruitment of "redundant" eloquent sites around the cavity within the postcentral gyrus. In accordance with IESM data, results show unmasking of redundant somatosensory sites during resection, likely explained by the decrease of the cortico-cortical inhibition. The recruitment of the second somatosensory area or posterior parietal cortex, primary motor area (M1) (due to strong anatomofunctional connections between the pre- and retro-central gyri), and contralateral primary somatosensory area are also possible factors in recovery.
- Resection of the (dominant) parietal posterior lobe can be performed without inducing any sequelae, and even with a possible improvement in comparison to preoperative status, especially using the pointing task.[22]
- Resection of nondominant M1 of the face: Recovery of the usual transient central facial palsy, with a potential Foix-Chavany-Marie syndrome when the insula is also involved, is likely explained by the disinhibition of the contralateral homologous sites, via the transcallosal pathways.[6]
- Resection of M1 of the upper limb: On the basis of the existence of multiple cortical motor representations in humans using fMRI and IESM, the compensation of the motor function could be explained by the recruitment of parallel networks within M1, allowing the superior limb area removal, eventually using two consecutive surgeries in order to induce durable remapping following the first one.
- Broca's area resection: Language compensation may be rooted in the recruitment of adjacent regions, and in particular the pars orbitaris of the inferior frontal gyrus, the dorsolateral prefrontal cortex, and the insula.[23]
- Temporal language area resection: Language compensation following left dominant temporal resection could be explained by the fact that this function seems to be organized with multiple parallel networks.[5] Consequently, beyond the recruitment of areas adjacent to the surgical cavity, the long term reshaping could be related to progressive involvement of (1) remote regions within the left dominant hemisphere, such as the posterior part of the superior temporal gyrus, the pars triangularis of inferior frontal gyrus, or other left frontolateral regions; and (2) the contralateral right nondominant hemisphere due to a transcallosal disinhibition phenomenon.[2]

It has also been shown that other "eloquent" areas involved by LGG could be resected without inducing postoperative permanent deficit, such as the frontal eye field or the corpus callosum.

Postoperative Functional Mapping: Toward Multiple-Stages Surgical Approach

POSTOPERATIVE FUNCTIONAL AND ONCOLOGIC RESULTS

A dramatic improvement of the surgical results was provided by advances in IESM. First, it has been demonstrated that the use of IESM has allowed to significantly increase the surgical indications in eloquent areas which were classically considered as "inoperable."[4]

In addition, despite a frequent transitory neurologic worsening in the immediate postoperative period (due to the attempt to perform a maximal tumor removal according to cortico-subcortical functional limits using IESM), leading to a specific functional rehabilitation, *more than 98% of patients recovered the same status than before surgery after glioma resection within eloquent brain areas guided by functional mapping, and returned to a normal social and professional life*.[12,13] Even more, at least in LGG, 15% to 20% of patients can improve in comparison to their preoperative neurologic and neuropsychological assessment, and 80% of patients with presurgical intractable epilepsy can benefit from relief of seizures.[18] In other words, LGG surgery is currently not only able to preserve brain functions but may also improve patients' quality of life as demonstrated by extensive neurocognitive assessment performed after the surgical resection. These data support the existence of additional brain plasticity mechanisms occurring after the operation, likely facilitated by a systematic and adapted rehabilitation.[23] Interestingly, this rate of less than 2% of sequelae is very reproducible among the teams using IEMS worldwide. In comparison, in series that did not use IEMS, the rate of sequelae ranged from 13% to 27.5%, with a mean around 19% (for a review, see ref. 4).

Finally, *a comparative of LGG resection performed without or with IESM showed that the EOR was significantly increased thanks to IESM, along with better functional results following resection within eloquent areas*.[3,4] Indeed, since IESM allows identification of the cortical and subcortical eloquent structures individually, it seems logical to perform a resection according to *functional boundaries*. The resection is continued until the functional structures are detected by IESM, *and not before*, in order to optimize the EOR without increasing the risk of permanent deficit.

Moreover, while extensive resection is still controversial in neuro-oncology, especially concerning LGG, current surgical results support the positive impact of such a "maximal" treatment strategy, with a benefit in the natural history of the tumors that seems to be directly related to the EOR.[1-4]

MULTIPLE-STAGES SURGICAL APPROACH AND THE ROLE OF SERIAL MAPPING

However, the price to pay to obtain such favorable functional results is sometimes to perform incomplete resection of the glioma when the tumor has invaded areas still crucial for the function. A new concept recently proposed is to use postoperative FNI—since it can be easily repeated due to its noninvasive feature—when the patient has totally recovered, in order to compare the new maps to those obtained before surgery. Indeed, even if this method has the limitations detailed previously, subtraction between a pre- and post-operative acquisition may nonetheless show a possible additional functional reshaping due to the (1) resection itself, (2) rehabilitation, and (3) regrowth of the residual tumor (as before surgery).

Interestingly, recent series have demonstrated that such remapping was not a theoretical concept, but a concrete reality. Postoperative FNI performed some months or years following the surgery clearly showed a new recruitment of perilesional areas and/or remote regions within the ipsilesional hemisphere and/or a recruitment of contralateral structures.[17] On the basis of these data, a second surgery was proposed in patients who continued to lead a normal life, before the occurrence of new symptoms (except possible seizures), only because of an increase in glioma size. The second surgery was also conducted using intraoperative cortical and subcortical mapping, in order to validate the mechanisms of brain reshaping hypothesized but not proven by preoperative FNI, before performing the additional resection[24] (Fig. 6-3). *Preliminary results supported the efficacy and the safety of such reoperation for LGGs not totally removed during a first surgery, due to their location within eloquent areas.* Indeed, in this recent experience, 74% of resections were complete or subtotal (less than 10 ml of residue) following the second operation, despite no additional serious neurologic deficit; on the contrary, there was improvement of neurologic status in 16% of cases. Again, the seizures were reduced or disappeared in 82% of patients with epilepsy before the second operation. The median time between the two operations was 4.1 years, and all patients were still alive with a median follow-up of 6.6 years despite an initial incomplete resection. Therefore, these original data demonstrated that thanks to mechanisms of cerebral plasticity, it is possible to reoperate patients with an LGG involving eloquent areas with minimal morbidity and increased EOR. However, 58% of tumors had already progressed to high-grade glioma at the time of the second surgery, raising the problem of the timing of reoperation. It was thus suggested to "over-indicate" an early reintervention in order to anticipate the second surgery before anaplastic transformation.[25]

Interestingly, one can currently consider to perform postoperative FNI after rehabilitation and recovery following a second surgery in order to open the door to a possible third or even fourth resection several years after the previous operations. The goal is both to allow the patient to enjoy a normal life as well as to increase overall survival. It is also possible to integrate surgeries within a dynamic therapeutic strategy, including chemotherapy and radiotherapy, especially when a wide removal is not possible for functional reasons.[3] To this end, neoadjuvant chemotherapy was recently advocated for LGGs, with the goal of inducing tumor shrinkage before an operation or a reoperation.[3]

Conclusions and Perspectives

Brain surgery may now benefit from important technical developments in the field of functional mapping, using complementary noninvasive methods of FNI and invasive IESM. Such recent advances have enabled better understanding of

the eloquent brain organization for each patient, in order to integrate the concept of inter-individual anatomofunctional variability in surgical strategy. Furthermore, intraoperative real-time subcortical stimulation, in association with cortical mapping, gives a unique opportunity to study the so-called "effective connectivity," since it allows on-line correlations between discrete and transient "virtual" lesions, which can be performed at each place of a distributed network (each cortical and subcortical sites being perfectly identified anatomically using 3D MRI) and their functional consequences (accurately analyzed by a speech therapist along the surgical procedure). Combination of these intraoperative anatomofunctional data with those provided by DTI (subcortical anatomic data), magnetoencephalography (temporal data), and fMRI (perioperative functional data) could enable one to elaborate individual and predictive models of the functioning of neurono-synaptic circuits, that is, to open a new door to hodotopy.[15] Such correlations with IESM, which remains the gold standard regarding functional brain mapping, can also enable to validate the noninvasive method of neuroimaging, especially the new technique of DTI.[9]

Moreover, such connectionist models may lead to a better knowledge of the dynamic potential of spatiotemporal reorganization of the parallel and interactive networks, namely the mechanisms of brain plasticity, thought to play a major role of functional compensation in slow-growing tumors and in their surgical resection. In this way, individual plastic potential could be better understood using repeated intraoperative mappings combined to postsurgical NFI, and then possibly guiding specific postoperative rehabilitation program in order to optimize the quality of functional recovery.[6,22-24]

In addition to its fundamental implications, IESM also allows to perform tumor resection according to functional boundaries, therefore, leading to the optimization of the benefit-to-risk ratio of surgical removal in cerebral glioma. Indeed, these new techniques (serial brain mappings) and concepts (hodology and plasticity) have allowed significant extension of resection indications in eloquent areas classically considered as "inoperable," such as Broca's area, the insula, and even in the left dominant hemisphere, the central area or the left posterior temporal regions; a significant decrease in the rate of permanent deficit at less than 2%, instead of 13% to 27% (mean 19%) without mapping; improvement in the quality of life, thanks to seizures control (in around 80% of cases, especially in insular and/or temporal LGG) and to cognitive rehabilitation; and a significant increase in the EOR compared with the series without brain mapping, thus with an increased impact on median survival.

In practice, in order to evolve toward a multistage surgical approach (i.e., second or third surgery more extensive than the first one in cases of initial incomplete resection within crucial areas), a dynamic strategy has to be envisaged for functional neuroimaging.[24,25] The goal is to switch from a "static" use of a unique preoperative FNI assessment (limited technique with lack of reliability), to longitudinal studies based on repetition of the FNI before and after surgical resection(s), with the goal to analyze a possible brain reshaping at the individual scale, and to select the candidates to reoperation(s). The next step is now to

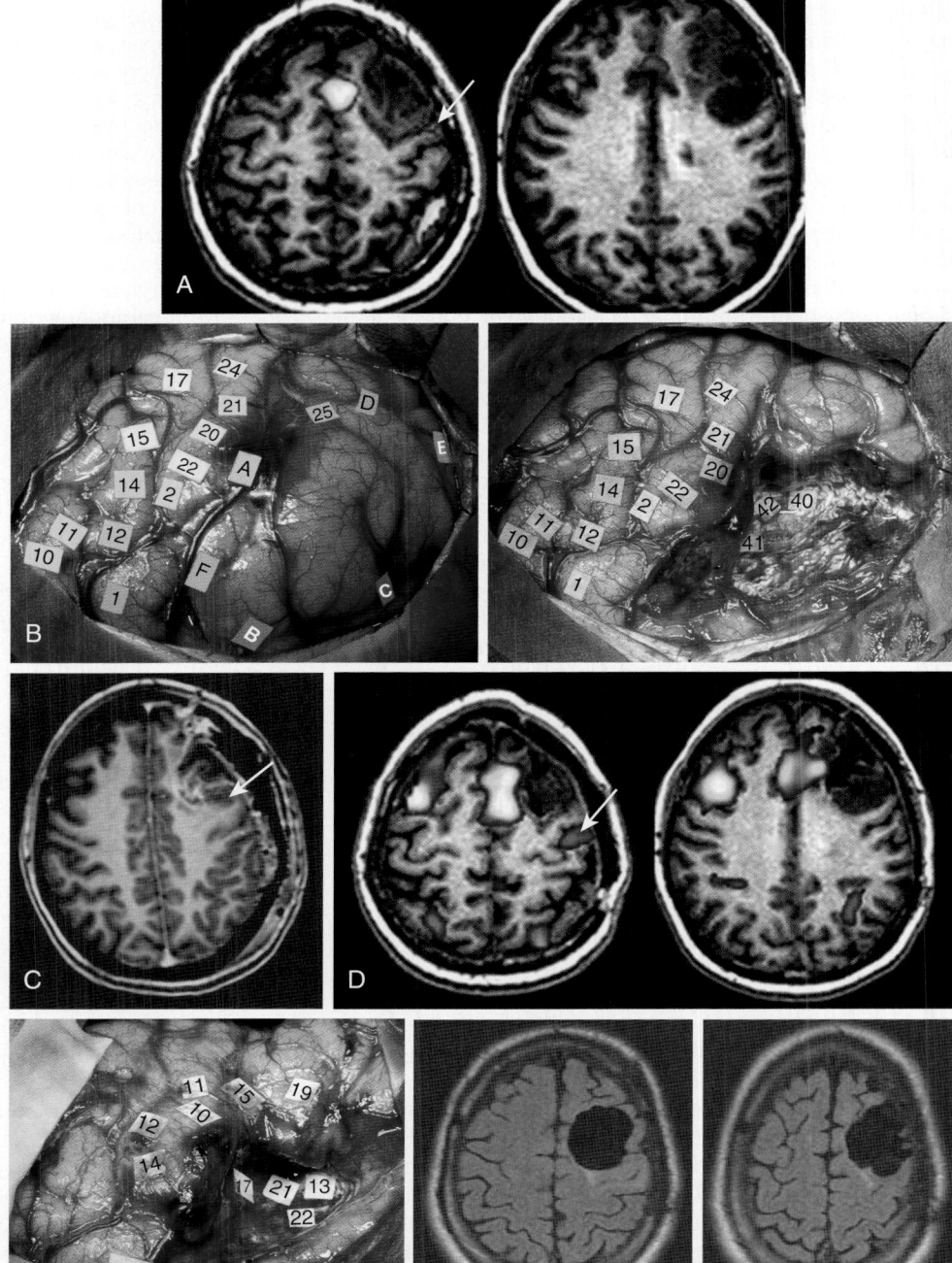

FIGURE 6-3 Illustration of the multiple-stages surgical approach. A, Preoperative language fMRI in a patient without deficit, bearing an LGG involving the left premotor area: language activation was very close to the posterior part of the tumor (*arrow*). B, Intraoperative views before (*left*) and after (*right*) resection of the glioma, delineated by letter tags. IESM shows a reshaping of the eloquent maps, with a recruitment of perilesional language sites, allowing a subtotal resection with nevertheless a posterior residue due to invasion of crucial areas (number tags). C, Immediate postoperative enhanced T1-weighted MRI showing the residue. D, Postoperative language fMRI 4 years after the first fMRI, showing recruitment of the contralateral hemisphere, and the posterior displacement of activation previously located at the posterior border of the tumor. E, Intraoperative view during the second surgery, confirming the remapping, and allowing a more extensive tumor resection with no permanent deficit. F, Postoperative, axial FLAIR-weighted MRI showing the improvement of the extent of resection thanks to functional reshaping.

use biomathematical models able to examine brain functional interaction through effective connectivity, in order to attempt to predict *before surgery* the patterns of postsurgical remapping at the individual scale on the basis of the data provided by the preoperative FNI.

KEY REFERENCES

Desmurget M, Bonnetblanc F, Duffau H. Contrasting acute and slow growing lesions: a new door to brain plasticity. *Brain*. 2007;130:898-914.

Duffau H. Lessons from brain mapping in surgery for low-grade glioma: insights into associations between tumour and brain plasticity. *Lancet Neurol*. 2005;4:476-486.

Duffau H. Brain plasticity and tumors. *Adv Tech Stand Neurosurg*. 2008; 33:3-33.

Duffau H. The anatomo-functional connectivity of language revisited: new insights provided by electrostimulation and tractography. *Neuropsychologia*. 2008;4:927-934.

Duffau H. A personal consecutive series of surgically treated 51 cases of insular WHO Grade II glioma: advances and limitations. *J Neurosurg*. 2009;110:696-708.

Duffau H. Surgery of low-grade gliomas: towards a "functional neurooncology." *Curr Opin Oncol*. 2009;21:543-549.

Duffau H. Awake surgery for nonlanguage mapping. *Neurosurgery*. 2010;66:523-528.

Duffau H, Capelle L, Denvil D, et al. Usefulness of intraoperative electrical subcortical mapping during surgery for low-grade gliomas located within eloquent brain regions: functional results in a consecutive series of 103 patients. *J Neurosurg.* 2003;98:764-778.

Duffau H, Gatignol P, Mandonnet E, et al. New insights into the anatomo-functional connectivity of the semantic system: a study using cortico-subcortical electrostimulations. *Brain.* 2005;128:797-810.

Duffau H, Gatignol P, Mandonnet E, et al. Contribution of intraoperative subcortical stimulation mapping of language pathways: a consecutive series of 115 patients operated on for a WHO grade II glioma in the left dominant hemisphere. *J Neurosurg.* 2008;109:461-471.

Duffau H, Lopes M, Arthuis F, et al. Contribution of intraoperative electrical stimulations in surgery of low grade gliomas: a comparative study between two series without 1985-96 and with 1996-2003 functional mapping in the same institution. *J Neurol Neurosurg Psychiatry.* 2005;76:845-851.

Gil Robles S, Gatignol P, Lehéricy S, et al. Long-term brain plasticity allowing multiple-stages surgical approach for WHO grade II gliomas in eloquent areas: a combined study using longitudinal functional MRI and intraoperative electrical stimulation. *J Neurosurg.* 2008;109:615-624.

Giussani C, Roux FE, Ojemman J, et al. Is preoperative functional magnetic resonance imaging reliable for language areas mapping in brain tumor surgery? Review of language functional magnetic resonance imaging and direct cortical stimulation correlation studies. *Neurosurgery.* 2010;66:113-120.

Krainik A, Duffau H, Capelle L, et al. Role of the healthy hemisphere in recovery after resection of the supplementary motor area. *Neurology.* 2004;62(8):1323-1332.

Leclercq D, Duffau H, Delmaire C, et al. Comparison of diffusion tensor imaging tractography of language tracts and intraoperative subcortical stimulations. *J Neurosurg.* 2010;112:503-511.

Mandonnet E, Winkler PA, Duffau H. Direct electrical stimulation as an input gate into brain functional networks: principles, advantages and limitations. *Acta Neurochir (Wien).* 2010;152:185-193.

Martino J, Taillandier L, Moritz-Gasser S, et al. Re-operation is a safe and effective therapeutic strategy in recurrent WHO grade II gliomas within eloquent areas. *Acta Neurochir (Wien).* 2009;151:427-436.

Plaza M, Gatignol P, Cohen H, et al. A discrete area within the left dorsolateral prefrontal cortex involved in visual-verbal incongruence judgment. *Cereb Cortex.* 2008;18:1253-1259.

Sanai N, Mirzadeh Z, Berger MS. Functional outcome after language mapping for glioma resection. *N Engl J Med.* 2008;358:18-27.

Smith JS, Chang EF, Lambom KR, et al. Role of extent of resection in the long-term outcome of low-grade hemispheric gliomas. *J Clin Oncol.* 2008;26:1338-1345.

Stummer W, Pichlmeier U, Meinel T, et al. Fluorescence-guided surgery with 5-aminolevulinic acid for resection of malignant glioma: a randomised controlled multicentre phase III trial. *Lancet Oncol.* 2006;7:392-401.

Teixidor P, Gatignol P, Leroy M, et al. Assessment of verbal working memory before and after surgery for low-grade glioma. *J Neurooncol.* 2007;81:305-313.

Thiebaut de Schotten M, Urbanski M, Duffau H, et al. Direct evidence for a parietal-frontal pathway subserving spatial awareness in humans. *Science.* 2005;309:2226-2228.

Vigneau M, Beaucousin V, Herve PY, et al. Meta-analyzing left hemisphere language areas: phonology, semantics, and sentence processing. *Neuroimage.* 2006;30:1414-1432.

Willems PW, Taphoorn MJ, Burger H, et al. Effectiveness of neuronavigation in resecting solitary intracerebral contrast-enhancing tumors: a randomized controlled trial. *J Neurosurg.* 2006;104:360-368.

Numbered references appear on Expert Consult.

CHAPTER 7

Chemotherapy for Brain Tumors

MANMEET S. AHLUWALIA

Factors Influencing Delivery of Chemotherapy to the Brain

BLOOD–BRAIN BARRIER

Treatment of brain tumors with systemic chemotherapy poses challenges unique to brain tumors. Concentrations of chemotherapeutic agents within central nervous system (CNS) depends on multiple factors, including ability of the agents to cross the blood–brain barrier (BBB), the volume of distribution of the drug in the brain parenchyma and the extent to which the drug is actively transported out of the brain.[1] Therefore many promising compounds fail in CNS drug development due to limited access to the target sites in the brain. Foremost is the BBB, which impedes delivery of adequate concentrations of most chemotherapeutic agents to the tumor; others include the brain tumor barrier (BTB), blood–cerebrospinal fluid (CSF) barrier, and brain–CSF barrier.[2] Paul Ehrlich first described the BBB in 1985 when he noted that all body tissues except the brain were stained when certain vital dyes were injected intravenously into animals.[3]

The BBB critically controls the passage of drugs or other compounds from the blood to the CNS and protects the brain from the foreign and undesirable molecules. The major component of the BBB is a monolayer of brain capillary endothelial cells. The restriction of brain penetration arises from the presence of tight junctions between adjacent endothelial cells and interaction between astrocytes and endothelial cells.[4] In contrast to other blood vessels in the body, the endothelial cells of brain capillaries lack intercellular fenestrations, and have high electrical resistance and low ionic permeability rendering them relatively impermeable to many water-soluble compounds.[2,4] The principal route to cross the BBB is via the lipid-mediated transport of small nonpolar molecules through the BBB by passive diffusion or less frequently by catalyzed transport.[5] For a drug to successfully reach the brain parenchyma requires uptake across the luminal (blood-facing) membrane into the endothelial cells, transport across the transcellular membrane, and finally efflux across the abluminal side (brain parenchyma–facing membrane) into the interstitial fluid. The key to successful chemotherapy of brain tumors is adequate drug delivery to the tumor-infiltrated brain around the tumor and the individual tumor cells. To cross the BBB, chemotherapeutic drugs administered systemically must be less than approximately 200 daltons in size, lipid soluble, not bound to plasma proteins, and minimally ionized.[2,4] As a result, there is a positive correlation between lipophilicity of the drug and its ability to cross the BBB.

ROLE OF STEROIDS

Steroids are important in the management of patients with brain tumors particularly in patients with bulky disease and those who have hydrocephalus. Dexamethasone has the best CNS penetration of all the steroids and is most commonly used in practice.[6] Steroids decrease CSF production and cerebral blood flow and help to reduce vasogenic edema associated with the tumor. However, the steroid can impair delivery of the chemotherapeutic agents to the tumor.[7] The assessment of response to treatment can also be affected by steroid use. Steroids can potentially decrease the degree of gadolinium enhancement that is a surrogate for the leakiness of the blood vessels and decrease the measurable volume of the tumor.[8] Guidelines for determining response criteria to chemotherapy now require that the patient be on the same or a lower steroid dose as compared to baseline before determining an objective response.[9,10]

Mechanisms of Drug Resistance and Strategies to Overcome Resistance

EFFLUX TRANSPORTERS

However, uptake can be lower than predicted for drugs as they are subject to extrusion from the brain by active BBB efflux transporters. Drug transporters belong to two major superfamilies, ABC (adenosine triphosphate binding cassette) and SLC (solute carrier) transporters.[11,12] ABC transporters are integral membrane proteins, many of which are located in the plasma membrane are primary active transporters, and they couple ATP hydrolysis to active efflux of their substrates against concentration gradients.[13] The most extensively studied BBB transporter of the ABC family is P-glycoprotein (P-gp) initially discovered in 1976,[14] but members of the multidrug resistance-associated proteins (MRP),[15] family and breast cancer resistance protein (BCRP)[16] have also been identified in brain endothelial cells and choroid plexus epithelial cells. Anticancer agents were among the first drugs identified to be substrates of BBB efflux transporters, that is, of Pgp as well as MRPs and BCRP.

DNA REPAIR ENZYMES

Methyl guanine methyl transferase (MGMT) is an enzyme that removes chloroethylation or methylation damage from the O(6) position of guanine following alkylating chemotherapy, and hence is involved in DNA-repair.[17] Clinical response to alkylating agents such as temozolomide (TMZ) in GBM patients has been correlated to the activity of the MGMT repair enzyme.[18] The MGMT gene may be silenced by methylation of its promoter that prevents repair of DNA damage and increases the lethal effect of chemotherapy. O(6)-benzylguanine (O(6)-BG) is an AGT substrate that inhibits AGT by suicide inactivation, and based on these findings, clinical trials with agents such as O6-benzylguanine (O6BG) added to alkylating agents have been pursued that deplete MGMT.[19,20] Unfortunately, this approach has been limited by systemic toxicities to date, as the combined toxicity of O6BG and TMZ has required significant dose reductions in TMZ, the presumed active agent for cancer cell death.[20]

Poly (ADP-ribose) polymerase-1 (PARP-1) is an enzyme that catalyzes the transfer of β-nicotinamide adenine dinucleotide (NAD+) to poly(ADP-ribose).[21] PARP-1 enzyme catalyzes the synthesis of polymers for DNA repair after injury, and PARP-1 influences both direct repair and base excision repair of DNA after injury from alkylating agents or ionizing radiation and is a key enzyme in the DNA repair pathways complementary to and downstream of MGMT.[21] Hence, the PARP-1 enzyme inhibition is an attractive target for glioma therapy. PARP-1 inhibitors have also been shown to overcome resistance to TMZ in both mismatch repair-proficient and -deficient glioma cells in culture, and numerous PARP-1 inhibitors are in clinical trials in patients with high-grade gliomas.[22,23]

Strategies to Improve Drug Delivery to Treat Brain Tumors

Most cytotoxic agents do not cross BBB, and conventional methods of drug delivery often results in low levels of drug to the brain; therefore, innovative treatments and alternative delivery techniques are needed. These have included intra-arterial drug administration, high-dose chemotherapy, the use of drug embedded in a controlled-release, biodegradable matrix delivery system, disruption of the BBB by hyperosmolar solutions or biomolecules and convection enhanced delivery.

INTRA-ARTERIAL CHEMOTHERAPY

The goal of this approach is to deliver chemotherapy intra-arterially so that the tissue perfused by that artery is exposed to higher plasma concentrations of the drug during the first passage through the circulation. The principal advantage to this approach is to maximize the amount of drug crossing through the BBB and minimize systemic side effects. Theoretical modeling suggests that intra-arterial infusion can produce a 10-fold increase in peak drug concentrations as compared to intravenous infusion.[24] However, two phase-III trials failed to show a survival benefit for intra-arterial chemotherapy (IAC).[25,26] A large trial of over 300 patients with newly diagnosed malignant glioma was conducted by the Brain Tumor Study Group (BTSG) trial to assess the efficacy of IAC chemotherapy in which nutrients were randomly assigned to IAC or intravenous (IV) BCNU with or without IV 5-fluorouracil (5-FU) and radiation therapy (RT). This study was closed early when an interim analysis showed shorter survival times in patients receiving IAC.[26] The side effects of the IAC in these two studies included catheter-related complications such as bleeding, infection, thrombosis, treatment-related neurotoxicity, leukoencephalopathy, cortical necrosis, and ipsilateral blindness.[25,26]

INTRA–CEREBROSPINAL FLUID CHEMOTHERAPY

Intra-CSF chemotherapy involves administration of drugs either into the lateral ventricle, usually through a surgically implanted subcutaneous device, such as an Ommaya reservoir[27] or instilling the drug into the lumbar subarachnoid space (i.e., intrathecal therapy). The benefit of this approach is that small doses of chemotherapeutic agents given intrathecally can produce high concentrations within the CSF with minimal systemic toxicity. However, abnormal CSF flow and obstruction due to tumor or scarring from prior surgical interventions impair its utility in the treatment for primary brain tumors. Intrathecal administration of drugs has limited penetration into the brain parenchyma, and is generally employed in treatment or prophylaxis of leptomeningeal disease.[28] Side effects include increased risks of neurotoxicity (especially with radiation) and chemical meningitis.

MANIPULATING BBB PERMEABILITY OR METHODS TO CAUSE BBB DISRUPTION

Various agents have been used to modify BBB and/or BTB in an attempt to increase the drug concentration in the tumor.[29] Drug delivery to brain tumors can potentially be improved by increasing the permeability of the BBB with hyperosmolar solutions such as mannitol and vasoactive compounds such as bradykinin analogues that induce an osmotic opening of the BBB and BTB.[29,30] Hyperosmolar solutions increase capillary permeability by temporarily opening the intercellular tight junctions of the brain endothelium that results in increased movement of water soluble substances. Complications with this approach include increased risk of stroke and seizures,[31] and no clinical benefit has been demonstrated with this approach so far.[32]

HIGH-DOSE CHEMOTHERAPY

High-dose chemotherapy (HDCT) is theoretically promising as increases the peak concentration of unbound drug in the circulation and can result in greater transfer of drug across the BBB. The associated myelosuppression seen with this approach requires use of autologous hematopoietic cell rescue and treatment-related morbidity is substantial. The survival using this approach is similar to that achieved by conventional chemotherapy or targeted therapy and its use remains investigational.[33,34]

WAFERS/IMPLANTABLE POLYMERS

Surgical implantation of solid-phase reagents permits constant drug delivery into the tumor without significant systemic or local side effects. The most commonly used "wafer" is a copolymer matrix with carmustine that is implanted directly into the tumor resection cavity at the time of surgical intervention and has been approved for use in patients with malignant gliomas. This therapy has been approved for patients with newly diagnosed and recurrent high-grade gliomas.[35,36]

CONVECTION-ENHANCED DELIVERY

Convection-enhanced delivery (CED) involves direct intra-tumoral infusion with various chemotherapeutic drugs and has been designed to use pharmacological agents that would not normally cross the BBB, and this approach is particularly useful for the delivery of large molecules.[37] Drugs are delivered through one to several catheters placed stereotactically directly within the tumor mass or around the tumor or the resection cavity and it allows distribution of substances throughout the interstitium via positive-pressure infusion.[38] Several classes of drugs are amenable to this technology including chemotherapeutics or targeted drugs.[39] Two multicenter randomized controlled trials in patients with recurrent GBM (PRECISE and TransMID) demonstrated that CED of agents was safe and well tolerated.[40] However, no survival benefit was seen in PRECISE, a phase III trial to assess the efficacy of this approach in patients with GBM upon first relapse compared to treatment with carmustine wafers.[40] Results of the TransMID trial have not been presented or published yet.

Various CNS Tumors

LOW-GRADE GLIOMAS

Low-grade gliomas (LGGs) comprise approximately 20% of CNS glial tumors with approximately 1800 new cases diagnosed each year in the United States.[41] Oligodendrogliomas represent 3.7% of all primary brain and CNS tumors.[41] Patients with LGGs typically present between the second and fourth decades of life. The optimal role of surgical resection in the long-term outcome of patients with LGG remains controversial, and the debate about the effect on outcome of its timing and extent persists. Nevertheless, surgery continues to be indispensable to provide tissue for histopathologic diagnosis and importantly molecular characterization that is prognostic and helps determine therapy approach. Retrospective studies have shown that more extensive resection rather than simple debulking is more beneficial and that greater than 99% resection yields improved overall survival (OS) and progression-free survival (PFS).[42]

Radiation Therapy

The value of RT in managing LGGs is controversial. This is due to prolonged natural history of LGGs and these patients are more likely to live long enough to suffer from the late effects of RT. In addition, dose of RT to treat LGGs is not clear. The most commonly used RT for the treatment of LGGs is 54 Gy with a range of 45 to 60 Gy, based on results of the European Organization for Research and Treatment of Cancer (EORTC) trial 22844[43] and the North Central Cancer Treatment Group/Radiation Therapy Oncology Group(RTOG)/Eastern Cooperative Oncology Group study.[44]

In the EORTC trial, there was no significant difference in OS and PFS in patients of LGG treated with 59.4 Gy in 33 treatments or 45 Gy in 25 treatments.[43] In the multigroup trial there was no survival benefit of using 64.8 Gy compared to 50.4 Gy.[44] A higher dose of RT (64.8 Gy) resulted in higher rates of radiation necrosis, and consequently doses above 60 Gy are avoided in this patient group.[44]

Moreover, the benefit of RT is limited to improvement in PFS without translating into any improvement in OS as was demonstrated by the EORTC trial 22845.[45] This study evaluated the role of up-front RT versus observation in LGG. A total of 311 patients were treated with immediate RT (54 Gy in 6 weeks) or no therapy until progression.[45] Up-front RT significantly prolonged the median PFS (5.4 years vs. 3.7 years), but did not result in improvement in OS (7.4 years vs. 7.2 years).[45] This suggests that radiation may have a comparable effect whether it is administered early or at subsequent tumor progression.

Chemotherapy

There is no level 1 evidence that postoperative chemotherapy significantly prolongs survival in patients with LGGs. The RTOG 98-02 was a three-arm trial in which 111 patients with a favorable prognosis (age <40 years and gross tumor resection) were followed with observation following surgery. A total of 251 patients with an unfavorable prognosis (age ≥40 years or those who had subtotal resection or biopsy only) were randomized to receive RT (54 Gy in 30 fractions) followed by six cycles of procarbazine, lomustine, and vincristine (PCV), or the same dose of RT only. At the last update of the trial presented at the American Society of Clinical Oncology meeting in 2008, PFS was increased with adjuvant PCV chemotherapy; however, the OS was similar in the two groups.[46] However, after 2 years, the addition of chemotherapy to RT did result in a significant OS and PFS advantage suggesting a delayed advantage to chemotherapy.[46]

Recently, TMZ has been increasingly been used to treat this patient population. In a retrospective review of 149 patients with LGGs treated with TMZ, a partial response (PR) rate of 15% and a minor response (MR) rate of 38% were reported.[47] In addition stable disease (SD) was seen in 37% and PD in 10% with a median PFS of 28 months. Tissue from 86 patients showed that codeletion of 1p/19q was associated with a significantly higher response rate (RR), a longer response to TMZ, especially with 1p/19q codeletion improved PFS and OS.[47] These results provide strong evidence that LGGs respond to TMZ. Besides LOH 1p/19q, methylation status of the MGMT promoter (MGMTP) predicts response to TMZ in LGG.[48] The LGG patients with methylation of MGMTP had an improved PFS compared to those with unmethylated MGMTP when treated with TMZ ($p < 0.0001$).[48]

MALIGNANT GLIOMA

Malignant gliomas (MG) or high-grade gliomas (HGG) include WHO grade IV gliomas, also known as GBM, and WHO grade III gliomas referred to as anaplastic gliomas (AG) (anaplastic astrocytoma [AA], anaplastic oligodendroglioma [AO], and anaplastic oligoastrocytoma [AOA]).[49] The goals of surgery are to establish a histological diagnosis and relieve mass effect. Biopsy alone is used in situations where the lesion is not amenable to resection, or the patient's overall clinical condition will not permit surgery. However, maximal surgical resection while preserving neurological function is preferred.

GLIOBLASTOMA

Radiation

Even patients who undergo a gross total resection of their glioblastoma (GBM) have a high recurrence rate, and for over three decades adjuvant radiation therapy has been the standard approach for GBMs. The efficacy of radiation was initially established in the 1970s in a trial of over 300 patients with an AG addition of adjuvant whole-brain radiation therapy (WBRT) to surgical resection resulted in increased median survival from 14 to 36 weeks.[50] A seminal analysis of patients treated in the previous Brain Tumor Cooperative Group Trials had established the standard radiation dose to be 60 Gy in the late 1970s,[51] and dose escalation above 60 Gy with WBRT has not been shown to provide further additional benefit.[52,53] Predominant mode of recurrence in patients with high-grade gliomas treated with radiation has been local failure within 2 cm of the enhancing tumor.[54-56] Serious side effects of WBRT such as progressive and irreversible radiation necrosis, with accompanying small blood vessel injury, and demyelination led to the utilization of involved field radiation therapy (IFRT) as the standard approach for adjuvant RT to minimize toxicity. The pattern of treatment failure seen with IFRT are similar to those seen with WBRT and are mostly local failures within 2 cm of the initial tumor.[55] In the United States, the RTOG treatment volumes generally used that deliver a 46-Gy dose to the peritumoral edema with a 2-cm margin and a 14-Gy boost to the enhancing tumor with a 2.5-cm margin. In Europe, a full 60 Gy are delivered to a 2- to 3-cm margin around the enhancing tumor without any field reduction. At present, T2 or fluid-attenuated, inversion-recovery magnetic resonance imaging (MRI) sequences are used to identify peritumoral edema, and the T1 sequence with contrast images is used to identify the enhancing portion of the tumor. If the tumor margin is defined upon contrast enhancement, typically a margin of 2.0 to 3.0 cm is used, and a margin of 1.0 to 2.0 cm is used if the RT field is defined by the T2-weighted MRI abnormality. Use of metabolic imaging such as positron emission tomography (PET), MR diffusion and MR perfusion, and MR spectroscopy are promising as they represent areas of activity that may need different treatment planning as compared to that defined by the traditional MRI sequences.[57,58] However, they are still largely investigational at present, and are employed to define boost volumes rather than primary target volumes. Further advances in imaging will likely change the method of tumor delineation.

Intensity-modulated RT (IMRT) is a technique that utilizes software and modification of standard linear accelerator output to deliver varied intensity of radiation across each treatment field. IMRT is beneficial especially when the tumor is juxtaposed to radiation-sensitive structures. IMRT is increasingly used these days as it may reduce radiation-related adverse effects[59] and can escalate the radiation dose delivered to the tumor. However, as of this writing, no proven benefit has been demonstrated by delivering doses in excess of 60 Gy.[59,60]

Chemotherapy

The benefit of adjuvant temozolomide (Stupp regimen) was established in a seminal phase III trial, when 573 patients with newly diagnosed GBM were randomly assigned to postoperative involved-field RT (60 Gy in daily 30 fractions) versus the RT plus concurrent temozolomide (TMZ) (75 mg/m^2 daily up to 49 days) followed by up to six cycles of adjuvant TMZ (150 to 200 mg/m^2 daily for 5 days, every 28 days).[61] This study demonstrated a benefit with adjuvant TMZ with a 2.5-month median improvement of OS (12.1 months for RT alone vs. 14.6 months for RT plus TMZ). At 2 years, 26.5% of patients treated with TMZ plus RT were alive, compared with 10.4% of patients treated with RT alone. This benefit was even more impressive at 5 years when 9.8% of patients treated with TMZ plus RT were alive compared to 1.9% patients treated with RT alone.[62] However, this study did not include patients older than 70 years of age, which constitutes 20% of all patients with newly diagnosed GBMs (discussed below). It also excluded patients with low performance status who were not independent in activities of daily living, a group constituting at least 10% of all newly diagnosed patients with GBMs in which the treatment plan needs to be tailor made according to the patient's ability to tolerate RT and or chemotherapy.

As previously mentioned, MGMT is an enzyme responsible for DNA repair following alkylating chemotherapy. During the course of tumor development, the MGMT gene may be silenced by methylation of its promoter, which prevents repair of DNA damage and increases the effectiveness of alkylating agents such as TMZ. MGMT was determined retrospectively from the tumor tissue of 206 patients and appeared to be a prognostic factor for improved survival and was predictive of benefit from chemotherapy.[18] For those with MGMT methylation, the 2-year survival rates were 49% and 24% with combination therapy and with RT alone, respectively, while for those without MGMT methylation, the 2-year survival rates were 15% and 2%, respectively. Biodegradable wafers impregnated with carmustine (Gliadel® wafer) that function as a slow-release carrier system for local drug delivery implanted at the time of resection are approved therapy for patients with newly diagnosed MG.[35,36] In a phase III trial, 240 newly diagnosed malignant glioma patients were randomized to placement of up to eight carmustine wafers or a placebo, followed by standard RT.[35,36] Patients receiving carmustine polymer had a statistically significant increase in median survival (13.9 vs. 11.6 months). This difference in survival, however, was not statistically significant when the analysis was restricted to GBM.[35,36] Additional toxicities with Gliadel included increase in the incidence of CSF leak and intracranial hypertension compared to placebo.[35,36]

Bevacizumab is a monoclonal antibody that binds vascular endothelial growth factor (VEGF), which plays a critical role in the development of the abnormal vasculature observed in tumors including malignant gliomas.[63] Two phase II trials that have been reported evaluating the addition of Bevacizumab to standard RT and TMZ (Stupp regimen).[64,65] In a study conducted at Duke, a total of 125 patients with newly diagnosed GBM received standard radiation therapy, TMZ, and bevacizumab. At a 21-month follow-up, the median PFS of 13.8 months and median OS of 21.3 months was reported.[65] These results are similar to the median PFS and OS of 13.6 and 19.6 months, respectively, in a phase II trial of bevacizumab plus TMZ and RT in patients with newly diagnosed GBM reported by Albert Lai and colleagues.[64] These compare with PFS and OS of

7.6 and 21.1 months in the University of California, Los Angeles/KPLA control cohort.[64] These two studies demonstrate that patients treated with BEV and TMZ during and after RT may show improved PFS without improved OS compared to the historical control group. The two phase III ongoing studies, RTOG 0825 (NCT00884741) and Hoffmann-La Roche Study (NCT00943826) will help answer the question of whether adding bevacizumab to TMZ and radiotherapy will improve survival of patients with GBM.

Recurrent Glioblastoma

Progression versus Pseudoprogression

Despite recent advances in therapeutics, most patients with GBM develop tumor recurrence after the above therapy. Recurrence is suspected when a previously stable patient develops new neurologic signs and symptoms or when surveillance MRI with gadolinium imaging shows increased tumor size or new enhancement usually accompanied with increased edema. However, clinical and imaging changes may be due to complications such as infection, a decrease in steroid use or radiation necrosis (also referred to as "pseudoprogression"). Radiation necrosis is a well-known late effect of RT of the brain that can mimic tumor recurrence. Pseudoprogression is a similar effect of transient increase in tumor enhancement that has been described after combined chemoradiotherapy and that occurs more rapidly and dramatically than after radiation alone. Pseudoprogression has been noted to occur between 20% and 30% of the cases in recent series.[66-68] It has been suggested that "pseudoprogression may occur more frequently in patients with methylation of the MGMT promoter as it increases the effect of chemoradiotherapy on residual tumor and that this translates to the transient worsening of imaging characteristics.[69] In the same series, survival in patients with pseudoprogression was significantly better than survival in those whose scans were initially stable (38 months vs. 20.2 months).[69] Various novel imaging modalities such as magnetic resonance perfusion with or without spectroscopy, and PET are used to help distinguish between pseudoprogression and true early progression of disease, but are not always reliable, and none has yet been widely accepted as standard practice. In most cases, repeat imaging is helpful to distinguish between the two, while in select cases surgery may be necessary to relieve mass effect and obtain a tissue diagnosis.

Therapeutic Options

When a tumor reaches a certain size, the requirements for oxygen and nutrients lead to the growth of new blood vessels and tumors can promote the formation of new vessels through the process of angiogenesis.[70] GBMs are among the most vascular tumors known and hence therapy directed against tumor-associated vasculature is a promising strategy.[70] Bevacizumab is a monoclonal antibody directed toward VEGF, and is the prototype of antiangiogenic agents in clinical use for treatment of GBM. Bevacizumab was approved by the Food and Drug Administration (FDA) for recurrent GB in the United States based on two trials of bevacizumab as a single agent or combined with irinotecan in recurrent GBM patients after initial treatment with chemoradiation and adjuvant TMZ. In a randomized, phase II clinical trial, 167 patients with recurrent GBM were treated with bevacizumab alone or bevacizumab in combination with irinotecan; there was no statistically significant difference in the median OS in the group treated with bevacizumab alone (9.2 months) compared to the those treated with combination of bevacizumab and irinotecan (8.7 months).[71] The objective response rate was 25.9% in patients who received bevacizumab monotherapy, and there were no complete responses per the outside review. Median duration of response was 4.2 months among the responders and the 6-month PFS (PFS-6) was 36%. The second study by the National Cancer Institute involved 48 recurrent high-grade glioma heavily pretreated patients treated with bevacizumab alone.[10] The objective response as determined by independent review was 19.6% and median duration of response was 3.9 months in responders.[72] The FDA approved bevacizumab as a single agent based on improvement in objective response rate in these studies, although no increased survival was seen.

Potent anti-VEGF activity of bevacizumab results in normalization of permeable tumor vessels producing rapid and marked reduction in edema and contrast enhancement on neuroimaging.[73] This effect of rapid and dramatic improvements in MRI can occur within days of initiation of treatment with antiangiogenic agents such bevacizumab, cediranib, sunitinib, sorafenib, and aflibercept, and is partly a result of reduced vascular permeability to contrast agents rather than a true antitumor effect. These imaging changes can make evaluation of tumor response and progression difficult if one relies on commonly used MacDonald criteria of two-dimensional measurement of enhancing disease. In addition, a subset of patients treated with bevacizumab develop tumor recurrence observed as an increase in the nonenhancing component on T2-weighted/fluid-attenuated inversion recovery (FLAIR) sequences. This likely reflects a phenotypically invasive tumor recurrence pattern due to co-option of normal cerebral vessels and diffuse perivascular spread of tumor cells. Hence, the Response Assessment in Neuro-Oncology Working Group proposed a new standardized response criterion that takes into consideration the challenges of nonenhancing signal abnormality changes, pseudoprogression, and pseudoresponse.[10]

Carmustine polymer wafers (Gliadel) may prolong survival and has been approved for use after surgery in locally recurrent high-grade glioma.[74] A prospective, randomized phase-III trial demonstrated a modest increase in OS from 23 weeks in those patients who received placebo wafers compared to 31 weeks receiving Gliadel.[74] However, the study included recurrent low- and higher-grade gliomas, and the benefit in the GBM subgroup was smaller than in the whole cohort. This study predated the use of chemoradiation and adjuvant TMZ, and the benefit of this approach in recurrent GBM patients treated with prior TMZ is unclear.

Other options for patients who have contraindication to bevacizumab or prior to therapy with bevacizumab include rechallenge with alternative dosing schedules of TMZ.[75] One of the mechanisms of resistance to TMZ occurs through direct repair of DNA damage by MGMT enzyme, and an effective strategy to overcome such form of resistance is to deplete tumor cell MGMT. TMZ rechallenge with alternative doses and dosing schedules that deliver higher cumulative doses over prolonged periods of time can result in depletion of MGMT,[76] and has been shown to be directly toxic to endothelial cells.[77] Commonly used TMZ dosing schedules are 75 to 100 mg/m^2 (21 days on/7 days off), 150 mg/m^2 (7 days on/7 days off), and 50 mg/m^2 daily dosing. Similar responses seen in patients with high and low levels of tumor MGMT support the rationale that these regimens may overcome MGMT-mediated resistance.[78]

Other chemotherapy options for recurrent GBM include nitrosoureas (e.g., carmustine, fotemustine) either as single agent or in combination (most commonly used regimen, PCV) that have shown activity in previously treated patients.[79-81] Other chemotherapeutic agents used in this patient population includes carboplatin, etoposide, and irinotecan, which have demonstrated modest efficacy as single agents or in combination regimens.[82-85] Recently in a randomized phase III trial of 325 recurrent GBM patients, lomustine was found to be superior to the pan-VEFG receptor inhibitor, cediranib.[86]

Molecularly Targeted Therapy

In the past decade there has been substantial growth in the number of novel therapies due to increased understanding of the molecular pathways involved in glioma formation and progression. Malignant transformation in gliomas is often the result of the sequential accumulation of genetic aberrations and proliferation of growth factor signaling pathways that include the vascular endothelial growth factor (VEGF), epidermal growth factor (EGF), and platelet-derived growth factor (PDGF).[87]

A number of agents that target VEGF have been developed including **bevacizumab.** Tyrosine kinase inhibitors that target VEGF pathway include cediranib,[88,89] and adnectin.[90-92] Small-molecule EGFR inhibitors such as gefitinib and erlotinib are well tolerated in patients with recurrent HGG, but responses have been disappointing.[93,94] There are a number of agents that target different signal transduction pathways including PI3K/AKT/mTOR,[95,96] RAF-MEK-ERK,[97,98] PDGF,[99,100] SRC,[101] and PKC[102] pathways are undergoing trials in patients with high-grade gliomas (Table 7-1). Results from clinical trials with most of these molecular-targeted therapies with the exception of bevacizumab have been disappointing so far. This is likely due to the complexity of the molecular abnormalities in recurrent high-grade gliomas, the redundancy of the signaling pathways, and the inability of many of these agents to cross the BBB.

ELDERLY PATIENTS

The incidence of elderly patients with high-grade gliomas is increasing. The optimal treatment for this group of patients is unknown as they tend to respond less well to standard chemotherapy and have poorer prognosis than younger patients. A recent population-based analysis of GBM patients aged 65 years and older showed a median survival of only 4 months.[103]

The optimal dose and schedule of RT in the elderly has not been determined. RT benefit in the elderly was demonstrated in a prospective randomized clinical trial in which 85 patients aged 70 and older with grade-III or -IV gliomas had good performance status. Patients treated with IFRT (50 Gy in 1.8-Gy fractions) had a modest survival benefit over those who received supportive care alone (median survival of 29.1 weeks vs. 16.9 weeks).[104] No further deterioration in performance status, quality of life, or cognitive function was seen in the patients treated with radiation.[104]

Table 7-1   Selected Molecularly Targeted Agents in Clinical Trials in High-Grade Gliomas

Drug Name	Type of Drug	Targets
ABT-888	Tyrosine kinase inhibitor	PARP-1, PARP-2
Aflibercept	Soluble decoy receptor	VEGF-A,B, PlGF
AMG 102	Thrombospondin-1 mimetic peptide	FGFR, VEGFR2
Bevacizumab	Monoclonal antibody	VEGF-A
Brivanib	Monoclonal antibody	FGF pathway
Cediranib	Tyrosine kinase inhibitor	VEGFR1–3, PDGFRβ, c-Kit
Cetuximab (Erbitux)	Monoclonal antibody	EGFR
CT-322	Fibronectin (adnectin)-based inhibitor	VEGFR1–3
Dasatinib	Immunomodulatory and anti-inflammatory	PDGFRβ, BCR-ABL, c-Kit
Erlotinib (OSI-774)	Tyrosine kinase inhibitor	EGFR
Everolimus (RAD-001)	Tyrosine kinase inhibitor	mTOR
Gefitinib (ZD1839)	Tyrosine kinase inhibitor	EGFR
Imatinib	Tyrosine kinase inhibitor	PDGFRβ, Flt3, c-Kit
IMC-1121B	Monoclonal antibody	VEGR
Lapatinib (GW-572016)	Tyrosine kinase inhibitor	EGFR
Lenalidomide	Tyrosine kinase inhibitor	PDGFRβ, Src, BCR-ABL, c-Kit, EphA2
Lonafarnib (SCH-66336)	Farnesyl tranferase inhibitor	Ras
Pazopanib (GW786034)	Tyrosine kinase inhibitor	VEGFR1–3, PDGFRβ, c-Kit
Sorafenib	Tyrosine kinase inhibitor	VEGFR2,3, BRAF, PDGFRβ, c-Kit, Ras, p38α
Sunitinib	Tyrosine kinase inhibitor	VEGFR2, PDGFRβ, Flt3, c-Kit
Tandutinib (MLN518)	Tyrosine kinase inhibitor	COX-2
Temsirolimus (CCI-779)	Tyrosine kinase inhibitor	mTOR
Tipifarnib (R115777)	Farnesyl tranferase inhibitor	Ras
Vandetanib (ZD6474)	Tyrosine kinase inhibitor	VEGFR2, EGFR, RET
Vatalanib (PTK787)	Tyrosine kinase inhibitor	VEGFR1–3, PDGFRβ, c-Kit
XL-184	Tyrosine kinase inhibitor	VEGFR2, Met, RET, c-Kit, Flt3, Tie-2
XL-765	Tyrosine kinase inhibitor	mTOR, PI3K

Source: Modified from Ahluwalia MS, Gladson CL. Progress on antiangiogenic therapy for patients with malignant glioma. J Oncol. 2010;2010:689018.

An abbreviated course of RT may be appropriate treatment in select groups of elderly patients, especially for those with poor performance status. This was demonstrated in a prospective randomized study of 100 patients with GBM aged 60 years and older who were either randomized to treatment with 40 Gy in 15 fractions over 3 weeks or 60 Gy in 30 fractions over 6 weeks. There was no difference in median survival between the two groups, 5.6 months in the short-course RT group versus 5.1 months in the 6-week RT group, fewer patients discontinued the abbreviated RT schedule (10% vs. 26%), and the short-course RT was better tolerated—only 23% of patients required corticosteroid increases, compared with 49% in the 6-week RT.[105]

As previously mentioned, the EORTC/NCIC study that established the current standard of care for GBM, RT with concomitant TMZ followed by adjuvant TMZ, excluded patients aged more than 70 years. Due to concerns regarding increased toxicity with combined chemoradiation therapy in older patients, chemotherapy with TMZ has been studied as an alternative to RT.[106] At the American Society for Clinical Oncology (ASCO) meeting in 2010, the Nordic Elderly Trial reported that 342 GBM patients aged 60 years and older were randomly assigned to either receive 60 Gy in 30 fractions or 34 Gy in 10 fractions RT or chemotherapy with TMZ (200 mg/m^2 for 5 days with cycles repeated every 28 days).[107] There was no significant difference in OS between the three treatment arms, with median survival being 8 months for TMZ, 7.5 months for hypofractionated RT, and 6 months for 6-week RT ($p = 0.14$). The study suggested that hypofractionated RT is preferable to standard 6-week RT in elderly patients, which is consistent with a previous Canadian study.[105]

The Neurooncology Working Group (NOA) of the German Cancer Society randomized 373 anaplastic astrocytoma or GBM patients aged 65 years and older and Karnofsky performance status (KPS) of 60 or higher to treatment with (1) IFRT of 54 to 60 Gy or (2) TMZ 100 mg/m^2 in a 1 week on/1 week off[108] regime. The primary aim of the trial was to demonstrate that TMZ treatment is comparable to RT. Longer OS was seen in patients initially managed with RT (median survival 293 vs. 245 days in those treated with dose-dense TMZ).[108] The patients in the TMZ arm had an increased risk of death compared with patients in the RT arm, as well as an increased incidence of adverse events, suggesting that RT is preferable in this population.

Another reasonable alternative for treating elderly patients with GBM and poor performance status is therapy with TMZ as demonstrated by the ANOCEF "TAG" trial, a phase II trial of TMZ in elderly patients with GBM and poor performance status (KPS < 70).[109] In this multicenter, prospective phase-II trial, 70 patients (10 centers) with a median age of 77 years were treated with TMZ. A PFS-6 of 29% and median OS of 25 weeks observed in this study compared favorably with an expected 12 to 16 weeks from a purely supportive approach.

ANAPLASTIC ASTROCYTOMA
Chemotherapy
The role of adjuvant chemotherapy following surgery in patients with AA is less clear, as there is no level 1 evidence that such treatment improves survival. The EORTC/NCIC phase III trial that established the survival benefit with TMZ excluded patients with AA and no randomized trial has evaluated the benefit of adjuvant chemotherapy in addition to RT in patients with AA. TMZ has been shown to be active in patients with AA in a retrospective analysis of 109 patients from two consecutive trials; adjuvant TMZ was as effective and less toxic than PCV.[110] In the analysis, outcomes of 49 patients treated with PCV and 60 with TMZ were compared, and there was no significant difference in the 2-year PFS and the median PFS and

OS between the two groups. Adjuvant chemotherapy was discontinued prematurely less often with TMZ than PCV because of toxicity (0% vs. 37%). Due to its better toxicity profile, TMZ has replaced PCV as the treatment regimen for these patients.

Adjuvant Chemotherapy versus Adjuvant RT
A German phase III trial (NOA-4) compared adjuvant chemotherapy to adjuvant RT in a phase III trial of 318 patients with grade III gliomas.[111] Following surgical resection, the patients were randomized to adjuvant RT with chemotherapy on progression or to adjuvant chemotherapy (either PCV or TMZ) with RT on progression of the disease. There was no difference in time to treatment failure in the different groups. Similar outcomes were seen in the patients treated with TMZ or PCV.[111]

Recurrent Anaplastic Astrocytoma
TMZ has demonstrated good single-agent activity with an acceptable safety profile, and improved QOL in patients with recurrent AA.[112] In a multicenter phase II trial of recurrent AA treated with TMZ demonstrated a PFS-6 of 46% and objective response rate of 35%.[112] Other options for these patients include treatment with bevacizumab and irinotecan.[113,114] In phase II trials, this regimen has a demonstrated RR of 55% to 66% with a median PFS-6 of 56% to 61% with an acceptable safety profile.[113,114]

OLIGODENDROGLIAL TUMORS
Oligodendroglial tumors constitute 5% to 20% of all glial tumors.[115] Oligodendroglial tumors exhibit more sensitivity to chemotherapy as compared to nonoligodendroglial tumors. This chemosensitivity was initially reported in 1988 when Cairncross and Macdonald reported dramatic responses to chemotherapy in eight consecutive patients with recurrent AO.[116] TMZ is preferred over the PCV regimen these days due to better patient tolerance, ease of administration, and improved patient compliance. There are no randomized trials comparing PCV and TMZ for efficacy in oligodendroglial tumors. Molecular genetic studies have revealed an association between radiographic responses and allelic loss of chromosome 1p, often in association with loss of chromosome 19q.[117] The 1p/19q codeletion that is associated with sensitivity to chemotherapy is mediated by an unbalanced translocation of 19p to 1q. Randomized studies have shown that 1p/19q codeletion is associated with a better outcome with RT. Multiple studies have established the activity of PCV in patients with both low-grade and anaplastic oligodendroglial tumors.[118-120]

Two prospective, randomized, controlled trials of AO and AOA patients have shown that PCV chemotherapy prior to RT does not result in a survival benefit, although it does lead to a longer PFS time. In the RTOG 94-02 trial, patients were randomized to either four cycles of up-front intensified PCV chemotherapy followed by RT or RT only.[121] In the second trial, EORTC 26951, patients were randomized to RT followed by adjuvant PCV or RT alone.[122] In both the trials, there was improvement in the PFS that did not translate to a survival benefit. In both trials, most of the patients randomized to the RT arm received PCV at progression, which helps explain the longer PFS without improvement in survival time.

MEDULLOBLASTOMA

Primitive neuroectodermal tumors (PNET) are highly malignant, small, round, densely cellular, blue cell tumors of the CNS, which have a propensity to disseminate throughout the neuraxis. PNETs can originate anywhere within the CNS, although the posterior fossa is the most common site of origin. Posterior fossa PNETs are called medulloblastomas.

Medulloblastomas are the most common malignant brain tumors in children and account for approximately 20% of all pediatric CNS tumors and 40% of all posterior fossa tumors.[123] The peak incidence of medulloblastoma is between 5 and 9 years of age,[123] with 10% of cases diagnosed within the first year of life, and the incidence decreases with age. Medulloblastomas account for 1% to 3% of all brain tumors in adults.

Dissemination throughout the cerebrospinal fluid, at least at the microscopic level, is assumed for all PNETs, and craniospinal RT is an integral component of the initial management of patients with medulloblastoma, both to control residual posterior fossa disease and to treat any disease that has spread along the craniospinal axis. However, toxicity to the brain and spinal cord limits the doses used.[124] Medulloblastoma are quite chemosensitive and respond to a variety of cytotoxic drugs.[125] The most active agents include cisplatin, cyclophosphamide, carboplatin, and methotrexate (MTX). However, since chemotherapy is generally administered after craniospinal RT, the use of MTX has largely been abandoned outside of the infant population because of neurologic complications of leukoencepalopathy.[126,127]

The medical treatment of children with medulloblastoma can be divided into 3 main categories: standard risk medulloblastoma in patients older than 3 years of age, high-risk medulloblastoma in patients older than 3 years of age, and medulloblastoma in infants and young children. The average-risk medulloblastoma are children aged 3 years and older who have undergone a complete or near complete resection, have negative cerebrospinal fluid cytology, and have no evidence of distant metastases. In absence of a clinical trial which is preferred, children are treated with a radiation (23.4 Gy to the craniospinal axis with a posterior fossa boost for a total dose of 55.8 Gy). RT is typically followed by eight cycles of adjuvant chemotherapy with cisplatin, vincristine, and either cyclophosphamide or lomustine.[128] This is based on the 5-year, event-free and OS rates of 81% and 86%, respectively, of 379 evaluable children with average-risk medulloblastomas who were treated with this regimen in a phase II trial.[128]

Craniospinal RT is best avoided in children aged 3 years or younger with medulloblastoma due to high risk of severe neurologic impairment. These patients are treated with combination chemotherapy to either delay or obviate the need for craniospinal RT. The optimal treatment for children with metastatic, unresectable, or recurrent medulloblastoma is unknown; these patients should be included on a clinical protocol whenever possible. In the absence of a suitable clinical study, they are treated with craniospinal RT followed by combination chemotherapy.

In adults, the clinical experience with medulloblastoma is limited, and treatment is done based on experience in children. The optimal treatment for adults with metastatic, unresectable, or recurrent medulloblastoma is unknown, and these patients should be treated in a clinical trial whenever possible. If a clinical trial is not available, a combined modality treatment including craniospinal RT and adjuvant chemotherapy is used. A phase II study involving 95 adults with medulloblastoma patients over a 20-year period was reported recently at ASCO 2010 meeting.[129] In this study, low-risk patients defined as no residual disease following surgery were treated only with craniospinal RT while high-risk patients (residual disease following surgery or distant metastases) treated with two cycles of "up-front chemotherapy" (cisplatin, etoposide, and cyclophosphamide) before craniospinal radiation followed by maintenance chemotherapy. For low-risk patients, 10-year PFS and OS rates of 46% and 65%, respectively, were observed, whereas in those with high-risk disease, the 10-year PFS and OS rates were 36% and 45%, respectively.[129] The value of adjuvant chemotherapy in low-risk patients and benefits of preirradiation chemotherapy compared with postirradiation chemotherapy is unknown.

Recurrent Disease

Most patients with medulloblastoma that relapse do so within 2 years of completing therapy, and a significant proportion of them relapse with disseminated disease. It is imperative to perform CSF cytology and MRI of the brain and entire spine with and without gadolinium at the time of relapse to determine the full extent of disease. Bone scan and bone marrow examination should be considered in appropriate cases. For infants and young children treated with chemotherapy only at the time of up-front therapy, radiation therapy is an option for patients with local recurrence, albeit at a high cost. High-dose chemotherapy followed by autologous stem cell rescue has also been used effectively as a salvage option.[130,131]

MENINGIOMAS

Meningiomas are the most common type of primary brain tumors in adults, accounting for one third of total brain tumors.[132] Current management for meningiomas consists of surgery, RT, and stereotactic radiosurgery. These approaches are effective in achieving tumor control for most of patients with WHO grade I tumors and a subset of patients with WHO grade II tumors. However, there are limited treatment options for patients with inoperable or higher grade meningiomas who develop recurrent disease following surgery and RT. Chemotherapy use in meningioma is mostly limited to patients who have exhausted all surgical and radiotherapy options.[132] The most commonly used agents in treatment of meningiomas include hydroxyurea,[133,134] somatostatin analogues,[135] and hormonal agents, such as progesterone receptor inhibitors.

Hydroxyurea is an oral ribonucleotide reductase inhibitor that arrests meningioma cell growth in the S phase of the cell cycle.[136] Despite initial promising preliminary data, response rates have generally been less than 5%.[133,134,137] Chamberlain and colleagues treated 16 patients with recurrent meningiomas with monthly injections of a sustained-release somatostatin preparation (sandostatin LAR).[135] Approximately 60% of the patients either had a partial response or achieved stable disease.[135] This study has generated considerable interest in the therapeutic potential of somatostatin analogues and a clinical trial involving pasireotide (SOM230), a novel somatostatin analog with a wider somatostatin receptor spectrum (including subtypes 1, 2, 3, and 5) and higher affinity (particularly for subtypes 1, 3, and 5) than sandostatin, is being evaluated in patients with recurrent meningiomas. Although initial studies of the anti-progesterone mifepristone (RU486) were encouraging,[138] a prospective randomized SWOG multicenter study failed to demonstrate any benefit.[139] In this study of 180 patients, treatment with mifepristone did not result in any improvement in PFS or OS compared to placebo.[139]

The importance of dysregulated cell signaling as a cause of neoplastic transformation is increasingly apparent and recent studies have identified aberrant expression of critical signaling molecules in meningioma cells. Hence a number of targeted agents have been evaluated in meningiomas. A phase II trial of PTK787 (vatalanib) in 25 patients with recurrent or progressive meningiomas demonstrated partial response in 1 patient (4.0%) and stable disease in 15 patients (60.0%).[140] Overall PFS-6 was 57.2% and median time to progression was 7.5 months (intent to treat). Median OS was 26.9 months. A phase II trial of sunitinib (SU011248) of 50 patients with recurrent meningiomas showed a median PFS of 5.1 months and PFS-6 of 36%.[141] These studies with targeted therapy suggest that targeted therapy may have a better role than cytotoxic therapies. More studies are warranted as it is likely that these novel therapies will complement traditional approaches such as surgery and radiotherapy and lead to more effective treatments for patients with meningiomas.

BRAIN METASTASIS

The main goals of systemic therapy in patients of brain metastasis (BM) includes control of the existing BM (local brain control), prevention of future BM (distant brain control), and control of the systemic disease (systemic control). Systemic therapies are used either alone or in combination with radiation and generally selected based on their efficacy in specific tumor histology and their ability to successfully penetrate the BBB. Most commonly utilized drugs include cytotoxics like TMZ,[142] methotrexate,[143] capecitabine,[144] topotecan,[145] and targeted agents such as lapatinib[146] given their ability to cross the BBB and the sensitivity of tumors that commonly metastasize to the brain to these agents. Complications of systemic chemotherapy include myelosuppression, fatigue, immune suppression, gastrointestinal dysfunction, or drug-specific toxicities. Currently, the role of chemotherapy in the management of brain metastases is limited. Many commonly seen brain metastases (from melanoma and non–small-cell lung cancer (NSCLC), are relatively chemoresistant, and the patients often develop BM after use of the most effective chemotherapeutic agents (Table 7.2).

NON–SMALL-CELL LUNG CANCER

Response rates of patients with non–small-cell lung cancer (NSCLC) with BM chemotherapy are highest in patients without any prior history of systemic treatment or RT. Chemotherapeutic agents commonly used in this patient population include platinum agents (cisplatin[147]), premetexed,[148] TMZ,[149] topotecan,[150] and targeted agents such as gefitinib[151] and erlotinib.[152] The response rates to these chemotherapies range between 5% and 38%.[148] Increasingly, targeted therapies such as gefitinib and erlotinib are being used in the treatment of NSCLC patients with BM. In a prospective study of 41 consecutive NSCLC patients with measurable BM, four patients treated with gefitinib (250 mg daily) demonstrated partial response (PR; 10%) and SD in seven patients (17%).[151] Median duration of PR was 13.5 months and a median PFS of 3 months was observed.[151] Patients who are more likely to have an activating mutation of the EGFR have reported substantially higher response rates to these therapies.[152] In a study of the 23 Korean patients, never-smokers with adenocarcinoma of the lung, 16 (69.6%) achieved a PR, and 3 experienced SD.

Table 7-2   Selected Trials with Chemotherapeutic Agents in Patients with Brain Metastasis

Cancer (Histology)	Chemotherapy Regimen	No. of Pts	Objective Response Rate (%)	Median Overall Survival (Months)
Non–small-cell lung cancer	Temozolomide + cisplatin + WBRT[175]	50	16	5
	Gefitinib[176]	76	33.3	9.9
	Gefitinib[151]	41	9.7	5
	Vinorelbine, gemcitabine, carboplatin[177]	22	45	8.2
	Cisplatin + vinorelbine[178]	76	27	6
	Cisplatin + etoposide[159]	43	30	8
Small-cell lung cancer	Teniposide[179]	80	33	2.9
	Topotecan[180]	30	33	3.6
Breast cancer	Topotecan[181]	24	33.3	6.3
	Patupilone[182]	45	19	–
	CMF (or CAF)[183]	22	59	5.8
	Cisplatin + etoposide[159]	56	38	8
	Various chemotherapy regimens (CFP, CFPMV, MVP, CA)[160]	100	50	NR
	Capecitabine and temozolomide[157]	24	18	3
Melanoma	Temozolomide + thalidomide + WBRT[184]	39	76	4
	Temozolomide + docetaxel[148]	10	24	4.7
	Temozolomide + cisplatin[148]	9	24	4.7

CA, cyclophosphamide-adriamycin; CAF, cyclophosphamide-adriamycin-5-fluorouracil; CFP, cyclophosphamide-5-fluorouracil-prednisone; CMF, cyclophosphamide-methotrexate-5-fluorouracil; MV, methotrexate-vincristine; MVP, methotrexate-vincristine-prednisone; NR, not reported; WBRT, whole-brain radiotherapy.
Source: Modified from Ranjan T, Abrey LE. Current management of metastatic brain disease. Neurotherapeutics. 2009;6(3):598-603.

SMALL-CELL LUNG CANCER

Varied response rates between 27% to 82% have been reported when previously untreated patients of small-cell lung cancer (SCLC) that present with BM are treated with chemotherapy.[153-155] Response rates in previously treated patients with brain metastases are considerably lower and comparable to the response rates seen with extracranial disease in patients with SCLC with second-line chemotherapy.[153] To further improve the response rates, combination approach of chemotherapy and RT was compared to chemotherapy alone.[156] In a phase III EORTC trial, 120 patients with BM from SCLC were randomized to treatment with teniposide alone or teniposide and RT. Although the response rate in the combined modality group was significantly higher (57%) than in the teniposide-alone group (22%), this did not result in a prolongation of survival, likely due to progression of disease outside the brain.

BREAST CANCER

Chemotherapeutic agents used in the treatment of brain metastases in patients with breast cancer include capecitabine,[157] TMZ,[158] etoposide,[159] and platinum agents.[159] One hundred consecutive breast cancer patients treated with different combinations of chemotherapy showed an objective response rate of 50% and a median duration of response of 7 months.[160] However, in this study less than 10% of patients had received adjuvant chemotherapy and approximately half had not received chemotherapy for metastatic disease, and hence it is difficult to extrapolate these response rates today, as most of the patients with breast cancer have been heavily pretreated by the time they develop brain metastasis. Recently targeted agents such as lapatinib are increasingly being used in the treatment of HER2 positive breast cancer patients. Two single-arm clinical trials have shown promising outcomes in these traditionally poor-prognosis patients when treated with lapatinib, an orally active, small-molecule inhibitor of epidermal growth factor receptor (EGFR) and HER2, in patients with refractory CNS metastases.[161,162] An objective RR of 20% was seen in patients who entered the lapatinib-plus-capecitabine extension.[161]

MELANOMA

Brain metastasis from melanoma is generally resistant to cytotoxic chemotherapy, and systemic treatment has been ineffective in the management of melanoma BM until recent approval of ipilimumab in patients with metastatic melanoma. In a phase II trial of metastatic melanoma patients with brain metastasis, impressive activity was seen with ipilimumab. In this phase II trial, 51 patients were treated in Arm 1, of which five patients had a global PR and four SD, for an overall global disease control rate of 17.6% in this cohort of patients. Similar response rates were seen in patients with CNS disease compared to systemic disease. This offers an exciting option for these patients with dismal outcomes. TMZ has systemic activity in patients with advanced melanoma, and although objective responses to TMZ have been reported, the overall response rate is less than 10%.[163,164] A combination approach of chemotherapy and RT was compared to chemotherapy alone in a prospective randomized phase III trial of fotemustine plus WBRT versus fotemustine alone in patients with BM from malignant melanoma.[165]

Although the addition of fotemustine to WBRT significantly increased the median time to progression of BM, it did not improve the RR or OS.[165]

Defining chemotherapy's role in BM management is made challenging by the limited number of studies conducted. Many trials have included patients with various tumor types, and there is no restriction to the number of prior therapies, a majority of these patients have uncontrolled systemic disease which are responsible for the death in these patients. A chemotherapeutic agent of choice should be chosen based on a patient's functional status, extent of disease, ability of the drug to cross the BBB, volume and number of metastases, previous therapies, type of primary cancer, and the molecular characteristics of the tumor. More clinical trials using chemotherapy in patients with BM are desperately needed, and it is crucial to enroll these patients in clinical trials if available.

LEPTOMENINGEAL METASTASIS

Leptomeningeal metastasis (LM) or neoplastic meningitis (NM) refers to the dissemination of cancer to the arachnoid mater, CSF, and pia mater, which occurs in approximately 2% to 8% of all patients with cancer.[166] LM is diagnosed in 1% to 5% of patients with solid tumors, 5% to 15% of patients with leukemia (often referred to as leukemic meningitis), and lymphoma (called lymphomatous meningitis), and 1% to 2% of patients with primary brain tumors.[167] Breast, lung, and melanoma are the most common cancers that metastasize and involve the leptomeninges. LM usually occurs in patients with progressive systemic cancer (>70%), but can be the first manifestation of cancer in ~5% of the patients.[168]

Radiotherapy

External beam radiotherapy (RT) is often used in patients with LM.[169] RT is used for palliation of symptoms (cauda equina syndrome), correction of CSF flow abnormalities and if bulky disease is present when IFRT is the modality used. RT is used to treat bulky disease as intrathecal chemotherapy is limited by diffusion to 3-mm penetration into tumor nodules and is not effective in bulky disease.[170]

Intrathecal Chemotherapy

Intrathecal (IT) chemotherapy is the mainstay of treatment of LM. The most commonly used IT chemotherapeutic agents for LM methotrexate (MTX),[171] cytarabine (Ara-C),[172] depocyt ®,[173] and less commonly, thiotepa.[174] Usual schedule includes induction phase (4–6 weeks), followed by consolidation phase and maintenance phase. Complications of IT include those related to the ventricular reservoir and due to chemotherapy itself.[170] Chemical aseptic meningitis is the most frequent complication observed, and leukoencephalopathy can occur, especially when the combination of RT and IT is used.[173]

KEY REFERENCES

Brandes AA, Franceschi E, Tosoni A, et al. Efficacy of tailored treatment for high- and low-risk medulloblastoma in adults: a large prospective phase II trial. *ASCO Meeting Abstracts*. 2010;28:2003.

Brem H, Piantadosi S, Burger PC, et al. Placebo-controlled trial of safety and efficacy of intraoperative controlled delivery by biodegradable polymers of chemotherapy for recurrent gliomas. The Polymer-Brain Tumor Treatment Group. *Lancet*. 1995;345:1008-1012.

Cairncross G, Berkey B, Shaw E, et al. Phase III trial of chemotherapy plus radiotherapy compared with radiotherapy alone for pure and mixed anaplastic oligodendroglioma: Intergroup Radiation Therapy Oncology Group Trial 9402. *J Clin Oncol.* 2006;24:2707-2714.

Chamberlain MC, Glantz MJ, Fadul CE. Recurrent meningioma: salvage therapy with long-acting somatostatin analogue. *Neurology.* 2007; 69:969-973.

Friedman HS, Prados MD, Wen PY, et al. Bevacizumab alone and in combination with irinotecan in recurrent glioblastoma. *J Clin Oncol.* 2009;27:4733-4740.

Glantz MJ, Jaeckle KA, Chamberlain MC, et al. A randomized controlled trial comparing intrathecal sustained-release cytarabine (DepoCyt) to intrathecal methotrexate in patients with neoplastic meningitis from solid tumors. *Clin Cancer Res.* 1999;5:3394-3402.

Hegi ME, Diserens AC, Gorlia T, et al. MGMT gene silencing and benefit from temozolomide in glioblastoma. *N Engl J Med.* 2005;352:997-1003.

Karim AB, Maat B, Hatlevoll R, et al. A randomized trial on dose-response in radiation therapy of low-grade cerebral glioma: European Organization for Research and Treatment of Cancer (EORTC) Study 22844. *Int J Radiat Oncol Biol Phys.* 1996;36:549-556.

Kreisl TN, Kim L, Moore K, et al. Phase II trial of single-agent bevacizumab followed by bevacizumab plus irinotecan at tumor progression in recurrent glioblastoma. *J Clin Oncol.* 2009;27:740-745.

Lin NU, Carey LA, Liu MC, et al. Phase II trial of lapatinib for brain metastases in patients with human epidermal growth factor receptor 2-positive breast cancer. *J Clin Oncol.* 2008;26:1993-1999.

Lin NU, Dieras V, Paul D, et al. Multicenter phase II study of lapatinib in patients with brain metastases from HER2-positive breast cancer. *Clin Cancer Res.* 2009;15:1452-1459.

Macdonald DR, Cascino TL, Schold Jr SC, Cairncross JG. Response criteria for phase II studies of supratentorial malignant glioma. *J Clin Oncol.* 1990;8:1277-1280.

Muldoon LL, Soussain C, Jahnke K, et al. Chemotherapy delivery issues in central nervous system malignancy: a reality check. *J Clin Oncol.* 2007;25:2295-2305.

Packer RJ, Gajjar A, Vezina G, et al. Phase III study of craniospinal radiation therapy followed by adjuvant chemotherapy for newly diagnosed average-risk medulloblastoma. *J Clin Oncol.* 2006;24:4202-4208.

Shaw E, Arusell R, Scheithauer B, et al. Prospective randomized trial of low- versus high-dose radiation therapy in adults with supratentorial low-grade glioma: Initial report of a North Central Cancer Treatment Group/Radiation Therapy Oncology Group/Eastern Cooperative Oncology Group study. *J Clin Oncol.* 2002;20:2267-2276.

Shaw EG, Wang M, Coons S, et al. Final report of Radiation Therapy Oncology Group (RTOG) protocol 9802: radiation therapy (RT) versus RT + procarbazine, CCNU, and vincristine (PCV) chemotherapy for adult low-grade glioma (LGG). *ASCO Meeting Abstracts.* 2008;26:2006.

Stupp R, Hegi ME, Mason WP, et al. Effects of radiotherapy with concomitant and adjuvant temozolomide versus radiotherapy alone on survival in glioblastoma in a randomised phase III study: 5-year analysis of the EORTC-NCIC trial. *Lancet Oncol.* 2009;10:459-466.

Stupp R, van den Bent MJ, Hegi ME. Optimal role of temozolomide in the treatment of malignant gliomas. *Curr Neurol Neurosci Rep.* 2005;5: 198-206.

van den Bent MJ, Afra D, de Witte O, et al. Long-term efficacy of early versus delayed radiotherapy for low-grade astrocytoma and oligodendroglioma in adults: the EORTC 22845 randomised trial. *Lancet.* 2005;366:985-990.

van den Bent MJ, Carpentier AF, Brandes AA, et al. Adjuvant procarbazine, lomustine, and vincristine improves progression-free survival but not overall survival in newly diagnosed anaplastic oligodendrogliomas and oligoastrocytomas: a randomized European Organisation for Research and Treatment of Cancer phase III trial. *J Clin Oncol.* 2006;24:2715-2722.

Vredenburgh JJ, Desjardins A, Herndon II JE, et al. Phase II trial of bevacizumab and irinotecan in recurrent malignant glioma. *Clin Cancer Res.* 2007;13:1253-1259.

Wen PY, Kesari S. Malignant gliomas in adults. *N Engl J Med.* 2008;359: 492-507.

Wen PY, Macdonald DR, Reardon DA, et al. Updated response assessment criteria for high-grade gliomas: response assessment in neuro-oncology working group. *J Clin Oncol.* 2010;28:1963-1972.

Westphal M, Hilt DC, Bortey E, et al. A phase 3 trial of local chemotherapy with biodegradable carmustine (BCNU) wafers (Gliadel wafers) in patients with primary malignant glioma. *Neuro Oncol.* 2003;5:79-88.

Wick W, Hartmann C, Engel C, et al. NOA-04 randomized phase III trial of sequential radiochemotherapy of anaplastic glioma with procarbazine, lomustine, and vincristine or temozolomide. *J Clin Oncol.* 2009; 27:5874-5880.

Numbered references appear on Expert Consult.

CHAPTER 8

Current Surgical Management of High-Grade Gliomas

RAY M. CHU • KEITH L. BLACK

The malignant glioma has been the neurosurgeon's eternal hydra, continually growing despite treatment. The category "high-grade glioma" (HGG) is heterogeneous, including mainly anaplastic astrocytoma (AA), glioblastoma multiforme (GBM), gliosarcoma, and anaplastic oligodendroglioma (AO). The incidence of new primary brain tumors in the United States is estimated to be 18 per 100,000, resulting in approximately 40,000 new primary brain tumors per year, 22,000 of which are high grade.[1] A total of 12,920 deaths in 2008 were attributed to primary malignant brain tumors.[2] Despite continually renewed efforts at treating HGGs, the odds of significant long-term survival have remained poor and stable for the past three decades with 2% to 4% of patients with GBM surviving to the 5-year point.[3]

Preoperative Workup

Magnetic resonance imaging (MRI) with and without gadolinium is essential for preliminary differential diagnosis, decision for surgery, and operative planning. Thallium SPECT scan, PET scan, or MR spectroscopy may help in determination of high grade versus low grade tumor, although none of these studies is definitive, and differentiation between HGGs and metastases is difficult.[4] These studies are more helpful in cases with previous surgery and radiation in determining recurrent tumor vs. radiation effect, especially MR spectroscopy and MR perfusion. For selected patients who cannot undergo MRI (e.g., patients with a cardiac pacemaker), CT with and without contrast provides similar, albeit less detailed information. CT perfusion may be an aid in better defining the tumor from cerebral edema as well as help with the potential for post-treatment radiation effects.

A Wada (intracarotid amobarbital) test is the definitive, albeit invasive, method to establish cerebral hemispheric dominance for language and memory. It is required for procedures in patients with a seizure disorder with tumor in whom a formal temporal lobectomy is planned. A Wada may be useful in selected other patients, such as patients with a dominant hemisphere temporal lobe tumor in whom tumor resection without temporal lobectomy is planned. Although both functional MRI and a Wada test offer similar information about cerebral dominance,[5,6] a Wada test does not offer anatomic localization of critical areas for language as MRI does nor truly investigates the potential bilaterality of language.[7,8] Functional MRI is more useful than a Wada test for lesions of the dominant hemisphere near the motor cortex, frontal lobe pars triangularis and opercularis (Broca's area), or Wernicke's area. With changes in metabolic activity and blood flow demand, an active area of the brain during a silent speech or motor task becomes infused with more oxygenated blood; this change can be detected since oxygenated blood carries a different paramagnetic signal than deoxygenated (blood oxygen level–dependent or BOLD signal) (Fig. 8-1).[9,10] One limitation of functional MRI is that it becomes less useful in patients with a recurrent tumor because of altered vascular patterns and MR artifacts from the previous surgery. Some patients require both a Wada and a functional MRI as part of preoperative planning.

Cytoreduction

Although decompression of mass effect is a surgical goal and influences symptomatic survival, controversy exists over whether the extent of resection influences survival or time to progression for HGGs. Dandy originally proposed hemispherectomy for selected patients with malignant tumors, but there was no significant effect on mortality.[11] Next, there were data suggesting that for GBMs, biopsy and resection were equivalent in terms of survival, and that it was really postoperative radiation that had a meaningful effect on survival. More recently, the Glioma Outcomes Project reported a statistically significant extension of survival for patients with HGGs who undergo resection over biopsy (median survival 51.6 weeks vs. 27.1 weeks, respectively).[12] This study was limited by lack of central pathologic review, lack of quantification of amount of resection, sampling error from a biopsy, and selection bias in biopsy vs. resection. Other surgeons have also reported extension of survival for patients with 90% or better resection; resection better than 98% was associated with a median survival of 13 months versus 8.8 months with less than 98% in one study.[13] In a recent series focused on the GBM population for patients given aggressive (but not always gross total) resection, Gliadel chemotherapy wafers, radiation, and Temodar, median survival was 20.7 months, and the 2-year survival rate was 36%.[14] Additionally, subtotal resection, the volume of residual tumor at the time of first recurrence, may negatively influence response to chemotherapy in terms of time to progression and overall survival.[15] Thus, it is not

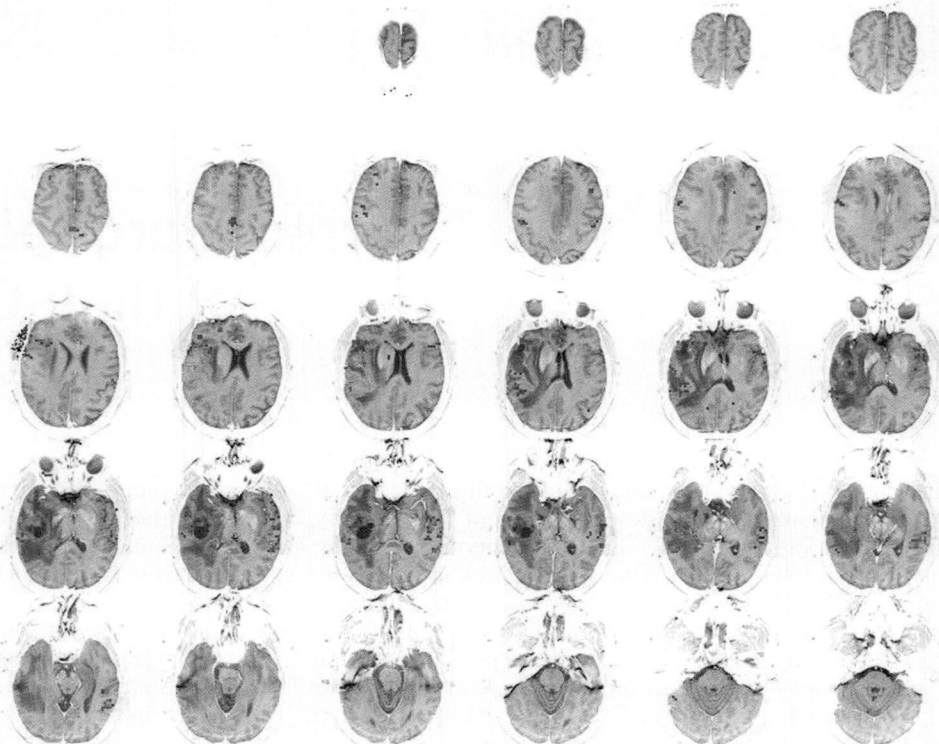

FIGURE 8-1 Functional MRI during a silent speech task in a patient with a glioblastoma of the left temporal glioblastoma (left and right are reversed).

clear that only a biopsy should be performed if a surgeon is facing a tumor that cannot totally be resected. However, even gross total resection does not truly address the diffuse nature of malignant gliomas.

Intraoperative Imaging

Even with continual improvements with operating microscopes, some form of intraoperative imaging or navigation is useful. A high-quality intraoperative ultrasound assists in many types of surgeries, but cannot aid in incision and craniotomy planning. Also, many tumors, especially lower-grade tumors, may not be dense enough compared to the normal brain to be visualized adequately by this method. Ultrasound is more helpful when the density difference is greater, such as if there is a hematoma to evacuate in addition to the tumor, if there is a cystic component, or if there is a need for ventricular access.

Frameless stereotactic navigation is very helpful in a craniotomy for tumor resection—some would say essential. This technology incorporates a preoperatively obtained MRI with fiducial markers that are left in place on the scalp. In the operating room, these markers or contours of the face can be registered in reference to a frame that is visualized by a computer via an optical apparatus, electromagnetic waves, or mechanical arms. This technology allows the surgeon to visualize points on the scalp and skull and compare them to the MRI, aiding in planning of a small, localized incision and craniotomy as well as ensuring that the exposure of the lesion is adequate. Surgical navigation can be performed intracranially with a localizing probe or with image fusion into the operating microscope based on focus depth. Because frameless navigation is based on a

preoperative set of images without updating in the operating room, the surgeon needs to account for brain shift during the procedure. Brain shift up to 2 cm can occur, and is more common with increased patient age, cortical rather than subcortical structures, larger tumor volume, and lesions far from some point of tethering such as the skull base or falx.[16] Once brain shift is taken into account, resection to the imaging abnormality borders (when safe) assists in the goal of cytoreduction.

Intraoperative MRI systems are available as well. Low-field (<0.5-T) systems allow most normal operating room equipment to be used throughout the case except right at the point of imaging.[17,18] Because the imaging can be updated, the surgeon does not need to account for brain shift. For craniotomies, once resection is deemed complete by the surgeon, an MRI can be performed to assess whether there is occult residual tumor, aiding in the aim of cytoreduction. These systems offer a smaller field of view, less detailed images, longer acquisition time, and fewer types of imaging options than conventional diagnostic MRIs.

High-field (1.5-T) systems exist, which offer all the imaging capabilities of a standard, diagnostic MRI.[19] A biopsy needle can be watched in near–real time as it is passed to target and verified at the target before samples are taken. With craniotomies, intraoperative imaging can confirm completeness of tumor resection, which is especially helpful in cases of low-grade gliomas when the distinction between tumor and normal brain is less apparent. At closure, an MRI can be performed to exclude hemorrhage; for patients with a biopsy or simple craniotomy, excluding the hemorrhage may allow a patient to be transferred to a step-down unit instead of the ICU. These systems, however, require construction of an operating room suite specifically designed for an intraoperative MRI to provide adequate shielding and safety measures. The high-field strength requires a larger magnet than the low-field systems, limiting access to the patient. Normal operating room equipment can be used outside the 5-gauss line (several feet from the center of the bore of the magnet); inside that line, only MRI-compatible (titanium or surgical-grade stainless steel) instruments can be used.

Motor Strip Mapping

Surgery in the parietal lobe or the posterior frontal lobe may require motor strip mapping. Short-acting muscle relaxants are used during induction, and anesthetics are lightened for the mapping, but the patient does not need to emerge from anesthesia fully. Rather than identification of the motor cortex itself, this technique relies on identification of the sensory cortex by looking for somatosensory-evoked potentials (SSEPs). A 1 × 8 or other sized subdural electrode is used. By noting the electrodes with a positive (precentral) as opposed to a negative (postcentral) amplitude and noting the two electrodes between which there is phase reversal, the primary motor cortex can be identified and protected. This technique has good correlation to magnetoencephalography when integrated into the surgical navigation system.[20]

Awake Craniotomy

Awake craniotomy with cortical mapping affords the ultimate protection for surgery in or near language areas. In one option, patients are never intubated—they are merely sedated with an agent like Propofol, which takes effect quickly and wears off quickly; proponents of this pattern espouse that patients' airways are less irritated and that language testing is better quality. The other way to accomplish the anesthesia is for patients to be nasotracheally intubated so that the endotracheal tube can later be withdrawn out of the vocal cords and language tasks can be performed. In addition to a local anesthetic to the incision, a field block to the scalp in the area of the incision as well as the Mayfield pins is performed with a long-acting anesthetic such as bupivicaine. Muscle relaxants may be used at induction, but they must be short-acting. Draping is per routine except that the face needs to have an unobstructed view so visual naming and interaction with the neuropsychologist are possible, so one must be careful that the head frame and subsequent retractor bars do not obscure vision. Once the craniotomy is created, anesthetics are lightened, the endotracheal tube is withdrawn from the vocal cords, and a handheld bipolar stimulator is used to stimulate areas likely to have language function or areas of planned resection to determine the effect. Continuous language testing can be performed during resection to reconfirm safety. Once resection is complete, the endotracheal tube is replaced and general anesthesia is reinstated for closure.

Frontal Lobe

High-grade gliomas are most common in the frontal lobe, as it occupies one third of the surface of the brain and is the largest lobe.[21] The frontal lobe tolerates unilateral surgical resection very well as long as the motor cortex and Broca's area are respected. Frontal lobe tumors are often amenable to image-complete resection. For tumors with significant growth into the corpus callosum and across the midline, surgical resection is unlikely to provide significant cytoreduction, and therefore a biopsy may be the more prudent choice.

MOTOR CORTEX

For lesions in the posterior frontal lobe, operative anatomy and imaging are not always sufficient to make adequate surgical plans. Functional MRI can reliably identify the motor strip, but even with modern neuronavigation systems, surgical resection is safer with some type of functional evaluation. Two current ways to identify motor cortex include intraoperative cortical stimulation mapping (discussed above) and placement of a subdural grid for mapping out of the operating room.

Proponents of subdural grid placement argue that electrocorticography out of the operating room and without sedation is superior. Time is not limited, and residual effects of anesthetics and narcotics can be minimized. Operating-room time at resection is minimized, but the patient requires two surgeries. The additional risks of the second surgery for grid removal and surgical resection are minimal. However, some surgeons prefer intraoperative testing to subdural grid placement. Intraoperative mapping may gain an extra margin of safety from continuous testing during surgical resection.

BROCA'S AREA

Approximately 95% of right-handed, 85% of ambidextrous, and 75% of left-handed persons will have left-sided cerebral dominance for language.[22] Broca's area encompasses the middle and posterior parts of the inferior frontal gyrus, that is, the pars opercularis and the pars triangularis. Protection of language area via awake craniotomy and intraoperative corticography or subdural electrode placement for cortical mapping is essential for tumors adjacent to Broca's area (Fig. 8-2).

PREMOTOR AREA

Deficits from surgical resection in the premotor area generally recover over a period of weeks to months through reorganization. Premotor weakness generally shows a better response to stimulation than to voluntary initiation.

SUPPLEMENTARY MOTOR AREA

The supplementary motor area (SMA) occupies the posterior one third of the superior frontal gyrus and is responsible for planning of complex movements of contralateral extremities but ipsilateral planning to a small effect.[23] The full "SMA syndrome" involves speech arrest, contralateral weakness, and near-total recovery in weeks to months. For tumors involving the SMA, functional MRI shows ipsilateral decreased SMA activity compensated by increased contralateral activity.[24] After resection in the SMA, the motor deficit is further compensated by recruitment of activity in the contralateral SMA and premotor cortex. Typically, leg weakness improves followed by the arm and then speech. There are patients who have reported even 6 months of significant speech trouble before returning to almost normal speech.

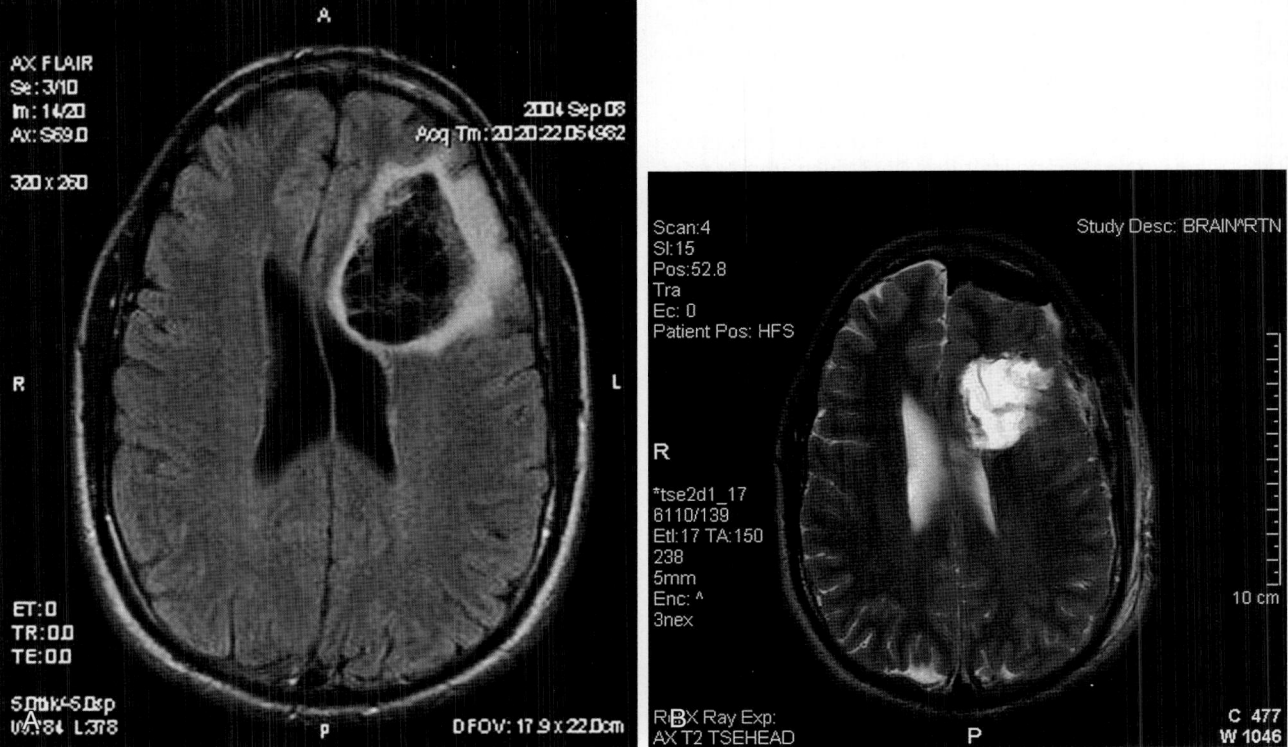

FIGURE 8-2 Preoperative (A) and postoperative (B) brain MRI in a patient with seizures, revealing a heterogeneous lesion of mixed signal on FLAIR that was nonenhancing (not shown). Surgery with awake craniotomy was performed; an image-complete resection was achieved. Pathology revealed an anaplastic oligodendroglioma, and the patient was referred for chemotherapy.

Temporal Lobe

Anterior temporal lobe lesions are amenable to surgical resection. Decompression of mass effect in this area is especially important due to proximity to the brainstem. Resection is generally safe back to 4 cm back from the temporal tip on the dominant hemisphere and 6 cm back on the nondominant side. Removal of temporal lobe back to 6 cm is often associated with at least a rim of visual defect in the contralateral superior quadrant, but this deficit is generally well tolerated. On the dominant side, resection at or behind 4 cm back from the tip of the middle cranial fossa requires either intraoperative electrocorticography or subdural grid placement for identification of Wernicke's area (Fig. 8-3). When a lesion involves the hippocampus, it is most likely that the contralateral hippocampus is compensating for function, but for the dominant hemisphere, this is best proven with a Wada test before surgery.

Parietal Lobe

Complete lesions of the dominant parietal lobe can be characterized by Gerstmann's syndrome, which consists of left/right confusion, digit agnosia, acalculia, and agraphia.[25] Even with a large parietal lobe neoplasm, the deficit is usually incomplete. Lesions of the dominant superior parietal lobule alone rarely cause the full syndrome; the angular gyrus has to be involved.[26] Low-grade gliomas are more likely than HGGs to have infiltrated into still functioning cortical areas; HGGs tend more to displace and destroy

function. Restoration of a preoperative dominant parietal deficit is unlikely unless there is a cystic component, a hematoma to evacuate, or significant mass effect from edema that resolves with surgery and radiation (Fig. 8-4). Surgery within the nondominant parietal lobe is generally tolerated well as long as there is not a large parietal stroke that can lead to significant neglect of the contralateral side. Motor strip mapping adds an extra layer of safety as described above.

Occipital Lobe

Occipital lobe surgery almost invariably results in some form of visual field cut, although most high-grade tumors that present in this location have already caused a visual defect. It is very difficult to improve visual symptoms with resection in this area. Some tumors that present more laterally may leave less visual field disturbance but may cause occipital association symptoms such as visual auras, color agnosia, or episodic blindness. Some researchers have described the use of visual-evoked potentials during occipital tumor resections, but the potentials are generally thought to be unreliable.

Prognosis

Outcome from diagnosis for an HGG depends on several factors. Precise pathologic diagnosis contributes a significant impact, as approximately 30% of patients with GBM survive to the 1-year point versus 60% of patients with anaplastic astrocytoma.[27] However, glioblastoma and the rare gliosarcoma do not differ significantly in behavior, response to

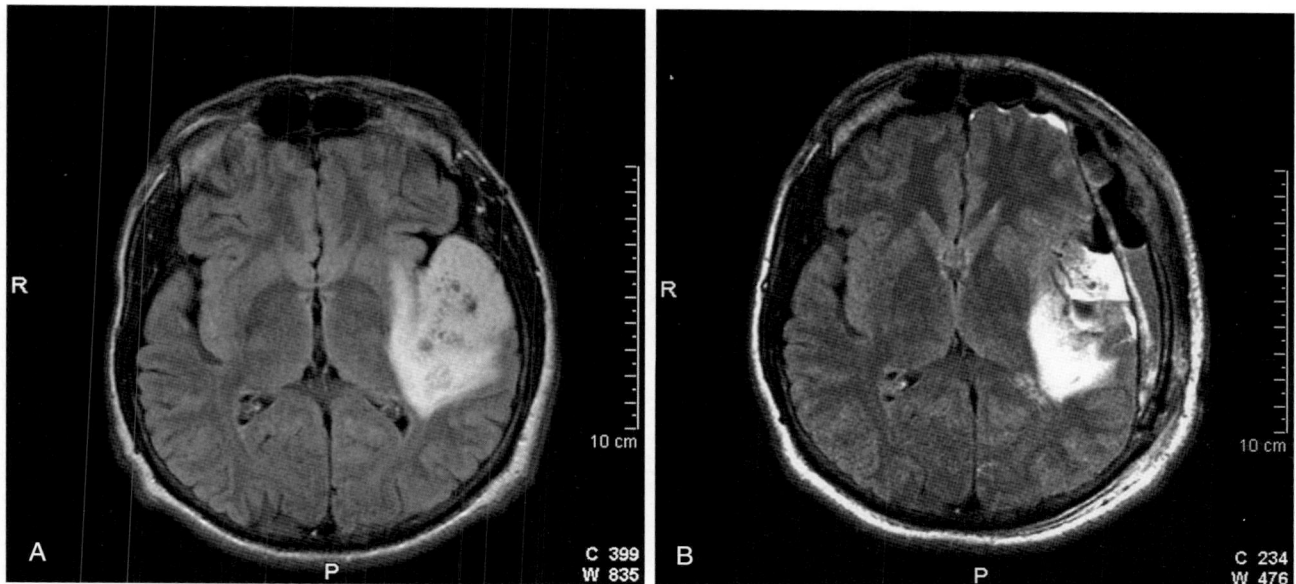

FIGURE 8-3 A 40-year-old, right-handed man presented with seizures. Preoperative brain MRI (A) was remarkable for a nonenhancing left temporal lesion. Functional imaging revealed language posterior to the lesion (not shown). Craniotomy for gross total resection was performed. Postoperative imaging (B) showed resection of the lesion with residual FLAIR abnormality posteriorly. Pathology showed mixed oligoastrocytoma.

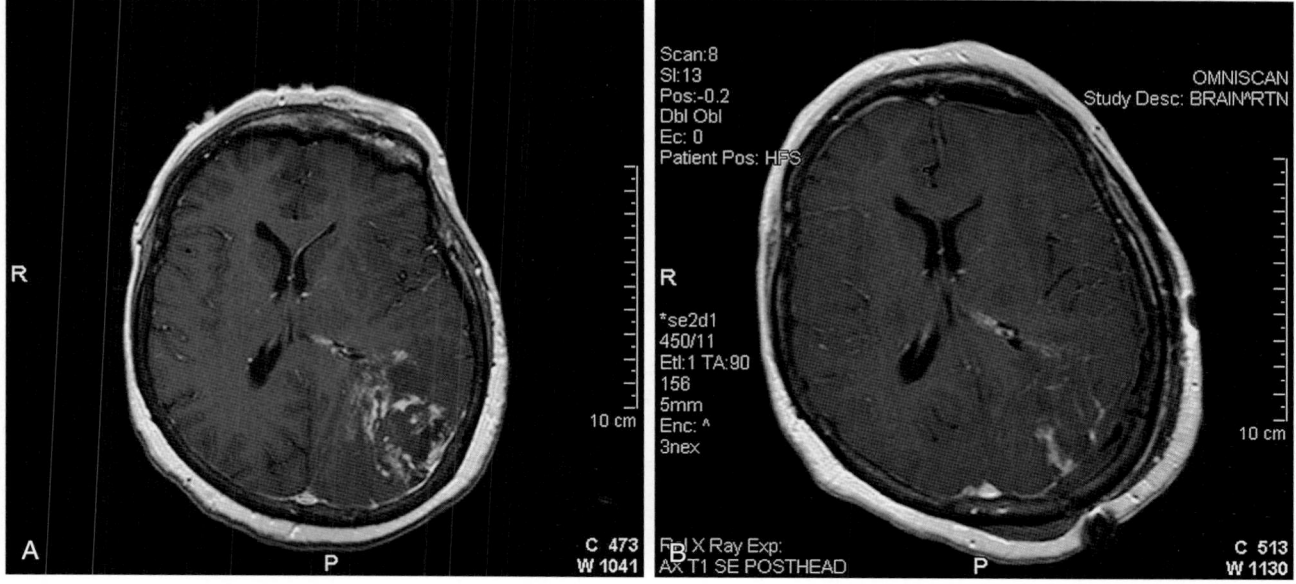

FIGURE 8-4 A 60-year-old, right-handed woman presented with increasing word-finding difficulty and right-sided hemiparesis. A brain MRI (A) revealed an enhancing left parietal mass with edema. At awake craniotomy, there was no involvement of the language area by tumor, and an image-complete resection was achieved (B). Pathology demonstrated glioblastoma, and the patient underwent radiation therapy and chemotherapy. Her speech improved after surgery, possibly because of resolution of mass effect and little direct involvement of the speech area by tumor.

therapy, or cytogenetics.[28] According to recently published data from the Glioma Outcomes Project, resection instead of biopsy, age less than or equal to 60, and Karnofsky Performance Scale of 70 or greater were all significantly correlated with outcome.[12]

New Directions

Certainly, surgery alone for HGGs will not provide a cure or have the largest long-term effect for patients with an HGG. Surgeons also have impact on radiation and chemotherapy

delivery to the brain. Besides local chemotherapy with BCNU-impregnated wafers,[29] other avenues proposed to effect change in the local tumor environment include convection-enhanced delivery (CED) of chemotherapy or targeted toxins.[30] An option for increasing the local dose of radiation is an implantable balloon system for radioactive iodine,[31] but it is unclear if this method of radiation delivery is clearly better than focused conventional radiation to the area. To date, there have been no convincing data that have driven an intracavity therapy to be widely accepted. Overall, these local delivery approaches to HGGs raise interesting questions but also battle with the notion over whether malignant glioma is a focal or diffuse disease.

An approach that attacks the diffuse nature of gliomas is immunotherapy. One option involves creation of a subcutaneous vaccine specific to the patient's resected tumor using tumor lysate–pulsed dendritic cells.[32,33] Vaccinated patients demonstrate an antigen-specific T-cell response and survival benefit as well as increased responsiveness to chemotherapy.[34] Other potential strategies include interleukin gene introduction via viral vectors,[35] vaccination with dendritic–glioma cell fusions using interleukin-12,[36] or scores of other targets to immunotherapy. What additional therapies will be useful over the next 10 years are unpredictable.

Summary

Craniotomy for tumor resection is a mainstay of current treatment for high-grade gliomas when it can be done safely. Neuroanatomy is the foundation that allows safe surgical resection. Newer technologies allow ever-improving levels of surgical safety. Overall, surgical resection alone will not cure malignant brain tumors unless coupled with other strategies that address the diffuse nature of the disease such as novel chemotherapy delivery options or immunotherapy.

KEY REFERENCES

Barnholtz-Sloan JS, Sloan AE, Schwartz AG. Relative survival rates and patterns of diagnosis analyzed by time period for individuals with primary malignant brain tumor, 1972-1997. *J Neurosurg.* 2003;99: 458-466.

Benbadis SR, Binder JR, Swanson SJ, et al. Is speech arrest during wada testing a valid method for determining hemispheric representation of language? *Brain Lang.* 1998;65(3):441-446.

Binder JR, Swanson SJ, Hammeke TA, et al. Determination of language dominance using functional MRI: a comparison with the Wada test. *Neurology.* 1996;46:978-984.

Chu RM, Tummala RP. Hall WA: intraoperative magnetic resonance imaging-guided neurosurgery. *Neurosurg Q.* 2003;13:234-250.

Galanis E, Buckner JC, Dinapoli RP, et al. Clinical outcome of gliosarcoma compared with glioblastoma multiforme: north Central Cancer Treatment Group results. *J Neurosurg.* 1998;89:425-430.

Keles GE, Lamborn KL, Chang SM, et al. Volume of residual disease as a predictor of outcome in adult patients with recurrent supratentorial glioblastomas multiforme who are undergoing chemotherapy. *J Neurosurg.* 2004;100:41-46.

Knecht S, Drager B, Deppe M. Handedness and hemispheric language dominance in healthy humans. *Brain.* 2000;123:2512-2518.

Krainik A, Duffau H, Capelle L, et al. Role of the healthy hemisphere in recovery after resection of the supplementary motor area. *Neurology.* 2004;62:1323-1332.

Kunwar S. Convection-enhanced delivery of IL13-PE38QQR for treatment of malignant glioma: presentation of interim findings from ongoing phase 1 studies. *Acta Neurochir Suppl.* 2003;88:105-111.

Lacroix M, Abi-Said D, Fourney DR, et al. A multivariate analysis of 416 patients with glioblastoma multiforme: prognosis, extent of resection, and survival. *J Neurosurg.* 2001;95:190-198.

Laws ER, Parney IF, Huang W, et al. Survival following surgery and prognostic factors for recently diagnosed malignant glioma: data from the Glioma Outcomes Project. *J Neurosurg.* 2003;99(3):467-473.

McGirt MJ, Than KD, Weingart JD, et al. Gliadel (BCNU) wafer plus concomitant temozolomide therapy after primary resection of glioblastoma multiforme. *J Neurosurg.* 2009;110:583-588.

McLendon RE, Halperin EC. Is the long-term survival of patients with intracranial glioblastoma multiforme overstated? *Cancer.* 2003;98: 1745-1748.

Reinges MH, Nguyen HH, Krings T, et al. Course of brain shift during microsurgical resection of supratentorial cerebral lesions: limits of conventional neuronavigation. *Acta Neurochir (Wien).* 2004;146(4): 369-377.

Romstock J, Fahlbusch R, Ganslandt O, et al. Localisation of the sensorimotor cortex during surgery for brain tumors: feasibility and waveform patterns of somatosensory evoked potentials. *J Neurol Neurosurg Psychiatry.* 2002;72:221-229.

Roux F, Boetto S, Sacko O, et al. Writing, calculating, and finger recognition in the region of the angular gyrus: a cortical stimulation study of Gerstmann syndrome. *J Neurosurg.* 2003;99:716-727.

Russell SM, Kelly PJ. Incidence and clinical evolution of postoperative deficits after volumetric stereotactic resection of glial neoplasms involving the supplementary motor area. *Neurosurgery.* 2003;52: 506-516.

Sabsevitz DS, Swanson SJ, Hammeke TA, et al. Use of preoperative functional neuroimaging to predict language deficits from epilepsy surgery. *Neurology.* 2003;60:1788-1792.

Steinmeier R, Fahlbusch R, Ganslandt O, et al. Intraoperative magnetic resonance imaging with the Magnetom open scanner: concepts, neurosurgical indications, and procedures: a preliminary report. *Neurosurgery.* 1998;43:739-748.

Tatter SB, Shaw EG, Rosenblum ML, et al. An inflatable balloon catheter and liquid ^{125}I radiation source (GliaSite Radiation Therapy System) for treatment of recurrent malignant glioma: multicenter safety and feasibility trial. *J Neurosurg.* 2003;99:297-303.

Westphal M, Hilt DC, Bortey E, et al. A phase 3 trial of local chemotherapy with biodegradable carmustine (BCNU) wafers (Gliadel wafers) in patients with primary malignant glioma. *Neuro-Oncology.* 2003; 5(2):79-88.

Wheeler CJ, Das A, Liu G, et al. Clinical responsiveness of glioblastoma multiforme to chemotherapy after vaccination. *Clin Cancer Res.* 2004; 10:5316-5326.

Yu JS, Liu G, Yong WH, et al. Vaccination with tumor lysate-pulsed dendritic cells elicits antigen-specific, cytotoxic T-cells in patients with malignant glioma. *Cancer Res.* 2004;64:4973-4979.

Numbered references appear on Expert Consult.

CHAPTER 9

Surgical Management of Low-Grade Gliomas

LORENZO BELLO • FRANCESCO DIMECO • GIUSEPPE CASACELI • SERGIO MARIA GAINI

The term "low-grade glioma" refers to a series of primary brain tumors characterized by benign histology (low proliferation, low neoangiogenesis phenomena) and aggressive behavior related to the slowly progressive tendency to invade the normal brain parenchyma.[1-4] These neoplasms are classified as grade II (out of IV) by the World Health Organization classification of brain tumors and include the following entities: grade II astrocytoma (further divided in fibrillary and protoplasmic), grade II oligoastrocytoma, and grade II oligodendroglioma.[5] Pilocytic astrocytomas, or grade I astrocytomas, are occasionally referred to as low-grade gliomas but due to their peculiar behavior, require separate considerations. In this chapter, low-grade gliomas refer only to WHO grade II tumors.

Low-grade gliomas are slow growing tumors, typically affecting younger individuals (median age 35), and mainly males (male/female ratio 1.5) who clinically present with seizures (often partial seizures).[6] Headache, personality changes, and focal neurologic deficits represent the other most common symptoms. The neurologic symptoms include motor/sensory deficits, dysphasia/aphasia, disinhibition, apathy, and visuospatial disturbances according to tumor location and size.[1,7,8] Interestingly, some authors report the tendency of low-grade gliomas to occur in eloquent areas or in their proximity.[9]

Overall, the median survival of low-grade gliomas is about 10 years and well-defined negative prognosticators include older age (>40 years), larger size (>5-cm diameter), eloquent location, and reduced Karnofsky performance status.

The optimal treatment for low-grade gliomas has yet to be determined. Watchful observation, needle biopsy, and open biopsy, as well as surgical resection have all been advocated by different authors.[2,10-16] No evidence of class I or II exists regarding the optimal management of these patients, even if the more modern tendency is to obtain at least some type of tissue diagnosis.[17,18] The rationale behind the observational or "wait-and-see" policy was the occasionally indolent or very slowly progressive behavior of these tumors.[14,16] On the other hand, following the modern oncologic concepts, some authors proposed performing a biopsy to obtain a histopathologic confirmation of the nature of the neoplasm before deciding on further management. Surgical resection of low-grade gliomas is still matter of debate, although recent studies are increasingly supporting its role.[10,13,17,18-22] Surgery can in fact achieve multiple aims: more reliable histologic diagnosis with eventual

molecular profile (e.g., 1p/19q loss and MGMT status), symptom relief; beneficial effect on seizure control, and lower rate of recurrence and malignant transformation.[13,18,20] Nevertheless, surgery carries unavoidable (albeit low) risks that can potentially and permanently affect the patient's quality of life.

Given this general information on low-grade glioma behavior and the possibility of treatment, it is clear that a modern surgical approach to these tumors has the goal of maximal resection of the mass and minimizing postoperative morbidity to preserve the patient's functional integrity.[13,18-20,23] Since the natural history of the tumor can be relatively long (with or without surgery), the conservation of simple and complex neurologic functions of patients is mandatory. To achieve the goal of a satisfactory tumor resection associated with full preservation of the patient's abilities, a series of neuropsychological, neurophysiologic, neuroradiologic, and intraoperative investigations must be performed. In this chapter, we will describe the rationale, indications, and modality for performing a safe and rewarding surgical removal of low-grade gliomas.

Rationale and Indications

The major aims of surgical treatment are[1] obtaining adequate specimens and representative tissue to reach a correct histologic and molecular diagnosis;[2] achieving cytoreduction to decrease rate of recurrence and malignant transformation, possibly prolonging survival;[3] improving patient neurologic symptoms; and[4] obtaining better seizure control. These goals can be reached by tailoring the surgical approach on location, modality of growth, and biological behavior of the tumor, as well and patient characteristics.

HISTOLOGIC AND MOLECULAR DIAGNOSIS

It is well known that astrocytomas represent a challenge for the neuropathologist, mainly in terms of grading the tumor. The size or number of needle biopsy specimens does not always permit all tests eventually required for immunohistochemical or molecular analysis. In addition, the biopsy site can significantly change the final results because gliomas are typically very heterogeneous with areas of different malignity. Recently, proton MR spectroscopy or MR perfusion has been used to partially overcome the latter problem, providing information on the presence of choline peaks (index of membrane production and malignancy) or areas of increased angiogenesis that can guide the surgeon in identifying the best location for performing the biopsy.[24-26] In any case, the risk of underestimating, or more rarely overestimating, the grade is a distinct possibility for needle and even open biopsies eventually resulting in significant changes in the choice of the most appropriate treatment.

Molecular markers have become a standard in determining the type of low-grade glioma. In fact, chromosome 1p/19q loss of heterozygosity plays a very important role in the distinction between oligodendrogliomas or astrocytomas. This molecular marker is relevant not only in the histotype definition but also in therapeutic implications.[18,27,28] In fact, 1p/19q loss as well as MGMT methylation (another important marker) facilitate predicting the response to certain chemotherapeutic agents. More recently, unexpected mutations affecting the isocitrate dehydrogenase (IDH1) gene at codon 132 have been found in 77% of grade II gliomas, and it was found associated with 1p19q deletions and MGMT methylated status, and with a better outcome.[29] Obviously, inadequate or incorrect sampling of the tumor can dramatically impair the possibility of a molecular analysis.

SIZE, LOCATION, AND GROWTH

Most of low-grade gliomas are localized close or within the so-called eloquent areas, such as the areas of the brain that control motor, language, or visuospatial functions. In a recent series, as well as in the experience of our group, 82.6% of tumors were located within eloquent motor or language areas (27.3% of cases within the SMA, 25.0% in the insula, 18.9% in language centers, 6.0% in the primary somatosensory area, 4.5% in the primary motor area).[9,30,31] As for the modality of growth, these tumors are characterized by a prevalent diffusive pattern of growth.[9,32] Groups of tumor cells or single tumor cells diffuse away from the main tumor mass along vessels or short and long white matter tracts. These features are responsible for the typical aspect of low-grade gliomas seen in MR images, which is characterized by a morphology strictly resembling that of white matter tracts along which the tumor grows and diffuses. In addition, despite their occasional apparently indolent behavior, low-grade gliomas are characterized by a continuous growth, with periods of faster and lower rates of growth during the entire time of the natural history of the tumor.[32] Most of the lesions judged as stable actually did show various degrees of growth; minor changes in the diameter (e.g., 1 to 2 mm) reflect a significant cellular growth in terms of volume.[32] For the sake of simplicity, the rate of growth of a tumor can be quantified by measuring the maximal diameter onto FLAIR MR images. Repetitive measurement on representative sections demonstrated that the tumor continuously grows and that the mean increase of the tumor diameter is around 4 mm/year. Furthermore, an increase in tumor diameter larger than 8 mm/year, even in the absence of contrast enhancement or modification of T2 or FLAIR images, is associated with a high tendency toward malignant transformation and aggressive biological behavior. These data stress the point that serial measurements of tumor volumes are an important tool to determine the biological behavior of the tumor. At the same time, it is clear that tumor volume is an important prognostic factor, able to determine per se the biological behavior of the tumor overtime. In fact, larger tumor volumes are more frequently

associated with a higher risk of malignant transformation and shorter patient survival.[18] Tumor volume is associated with the risk of developing neurologic symptoms, increase in the risk of seizures, and probability of impacting in the social and professional life of patients.

NEUROLOGIC SYMPTOMS

The majority of patients who are diagnosed with low-grade gliomas usually come to medical attention because of sudden occurrence of seizures.[7,18] These patients are generally intact at the gross neurologic examination, but they frequently present more subtle symptoms affecting complex neurologic functions (memory, language, character, visuospatial orientation, etc.) that require a specific testing by a neuropsychologist.[31,33,34] As will be detailed below, this type of testing is mandatory when considering surgery for this type of lesion because it allows tailoring the intraoperative testing to the patient and permits finely assessing the impact of surgery on the patients' superior neurologic functions.[35]

Those patients who present with frank neurologic deficits (e.g., hemiparesis, ataxia, aphasia) are usually candidates for surgery because their symptoms are related to direct mass effect of the tumor on the cortex or on the subcortical white matter tracts. In this case, tumor removal can significantly relieve symptoms depending on the degree of the preoperative impairment as well as on the degree of parenchymal disruption. This category of patients carries higher surgical risks in terms of morbidity and mortality than that of neurologically intact patients. Nevertheless, in terms of surgery, the presence of a mass effect is a straightforward indication for tumor resection since a waiting policy will quickly result in further neurologic deterioration.

SEIZURES

Large tumors and insular locations are usually associated with a higher risk of developing seizures, which are difficult to be controlled by antiepileptic drugs, requiring the administration of multiple medications. Despite polytherapy, seizure control can still be very poor. In these latter cases, surgery becomes an appealing option to improve seizure control. It has been clearly shown that surgical resection is associated with a marked improvement in terms of seizure occurrence. In other cases, patients might be severely disabled by the side effects of multiple antiepileptic medications and again surgery can allow reduction of drug administration. It is a matter of debate whether surgical resection of low-grade gliomas for seizure control should be performed in an epilepsy surgery setting (with surface and eventually deep-electrode recordings, with resection of all the foci) or in a purely oncologic setting (with neurophysiologic monitoring, including electrocorticography, but no deep electrodes and no resection of normal brain foci).

As mentioned above, surgery for gliomas aims to maximally remove the tumor mass and at the same time to preserve the patient's functional integrity. This policy applies to the resection of any glioma but more specifically to those located close or within eloquent areas. The concept of eloquence refers not only to areas involved in motor, language, or visuospatial functions, but also, more widely, to any area affecting the well being of the individual (e.g., memory, socioaffective behavior, specific tasks performance, etc.).

In all these cases, extensive resection and maximal functional integrity can still be achieved through the intraoperative use of brain mapping techniques.[11,18,19,30,36-38]

Intraoperative Mapping

The term "intraoperative mapping" refers to a group of techniques that allow safe and effective removal of lesions that are located in so-called eloquent or functional areas. This can be achieved by the identification and preservation at time of surgery of cortical and subcortical sites that are involved in specific functions. The concept of detecting and preserving the essential functional cortical and subcortical sites has been recently defined as surgery according to functional boundaries, and it is performed by using the so-called brain mapping technique.

Performing brain mapping requires a series of preoperative evaluations and intraoperative facilities that involve different specialists. A complete neuropsychological evaluation is generally the first step of the process permitting to select the suitable patients and to individualize the intraoperative testing. Then, sophisticated imaging techniques including fMRI and DTI-FT (diffuse tensor imaging–fiber tracking techniques) give the opportunity to attentively plan surgical strategies. In addition, these images can be loaded into the neuronavigation system becoming thus available peri- and intra-operatively for orientation. Intraoperative MR or ultrasound can be used as well, if available. Finally and most importantly, a series of neurophysiologic techniques are employed at the time of surgery to precisely guide the surgeon in the tumor removal. These include cortical and subcortical direct electrical stimulation (DES), motor-evoked potentials (MEP), multichannel EMG, EEG and ECoG recordings.

NEUROPSYCHOLOGICAL EVALUATION

Neuropsychological evaluation comprises a large number of tests to assess various neurologic functions such as cognitive, emotional, intelligence, and basic language functions. Such a broad-spectrum evaluation provides information on how the tumor has impacted on the social, emotional, and cognitive life of the patient. It is important that the testing be the most extensive possible because the tumor that grows along fiber tracts may alter connectivity between separate areas of the brain, resulting in impairment of functions that may not be documented in the case of a neuropsychological examination limited to testing of functions strictly related to the area of the brain in which the tumor has grown.[13,30,31,38] When this extensive testing is administered, changes can be documented in more than 90% of patients.[13,30,31] These data represent the baseline with which the effect of surgical and future treatment should be compared. Additionally, when the tumor involves language or visuospatial areas or pathways, a more extensive specific evaluation should be added.

The neuropsychological assessment also allows one to build up a series of tests composed of various items that will be used intraoperatively for the evaluation and mapping of various functions, among which memory, language in its various components, and visuospatial orientation are some of the most important. For language evaluation, a battery of preoperative tests evaluates verbal language production

and comprehension, together with repetition.[30,39-41] Hemispheric language dominance is evaluated through the Edinburgh Inventory Questionnaire and fMRI. Most tests generally used have been standardized on the normal population. In addition, various tests can be adjusted according to the nationality of the patient. It is important to include in the battery both qualitative and quantitative tests, and normative data must be available for the quantitative procedure. It is also important that a speech therapist and a (neuro) psychologist manage patient assessments.

Preoperative language evaluation is also used to prepare a series of tests that will be used intraoperatively for assessing language during surgery. Among these tests, object naming is probably the most important. In the case of a tumor located in the dominant or parietal areas, number recognition and reading, as well as calculations or writing should be added to preoperative testing and considered for intraoperative evaluation.[9,42,43] When the patient is bilingual or speaks more than two languages, it is important to include evaluation of these languages in the preoperative testing.[32,44-48] In any case, bi- or multi-lingual assessment is generally recommended also intraoperatively.[44] Visuospatial functions are usually evaluated for tumor located in the parietal lobe, generally on the right side.[13] Unilateral spatial neglect is a complex and disabling syndrome that typically results from right hemisphere damage, and it is characterized by impaired awareness of the contralesional left half of space, objects, and mental images. In this case, the patient is presented with various tests such as the line bisection test or star cancellation test to evaluate spatial awareness.

NEURORADIOLOGIC EVALUATION

The neuroradiologic examination consists of basic exams, such as morphologic T1, T2, and FLAIR images, as well as postcontrast T1 images. These images together with volumetric sequences provide information on the site and location of the tumor, and allows to determine its relationship with various structures, such as major vessels, and to measure tumor volume, and when performed at different time points to establish the speed of growth. Further MR studies include MR spectroscopy, which allows designing a map of areas within the tumor in which tumor metabolism is more or less pronounced (multipixel MR spectroscopy map).[25,26] This is of great assistance in tissue sampling at the time of surgery for histologic and molecular purposes. Perfusion MR studies are useful for designing perfusion maps,[49,50] which provide additional and complementary information of the biological behavior of the tumor and help in the tissue collection for histologic and molecular purposes at the time of surgery.[24] Metabolic information may be also obtained by performing SPECT or PET, and these data may be incorporated into the navigation system for surgical guidance as well.[51,52]

The neuroradiologic investigations include functional studies, such as fMRI, and anatomic studies such as DTI-FT. The former provides functional information on the location of cortical sites, which activates in response to motor or various language tasks. Motor fMRI is generally used to design a map of the cortical motor sites and to establish their relationship with the tumor.[53] fMRI for language provides a map of the cortical sites that activate during language tasks, such as denomination (object naming), famous face naming, verb generation, and verbal fluency.[48,54] All these data form a complex map of how the various components of language are organized at the cortical level and allow establishment of spatial relationship between these cortical areas and the tumor mass. It is usually recommended that language fMRI be performed with the same tests that are used for language evaluation to increase its reliability.

DTI-FT techniques allow depicting the connectivity around and inside a tumor, by reconstructing and visualizing the fiber tracts, which run around or inside the tumor mass[55] (Fig. 9-1). DTI-FT provides anatomic information on the location of motor tracts, mainly the corticospinal tract (CST), and various language tracts, involved either in the phonologic or semantic components of language.[56-59] For a better visualization of tracts in low-grade gliomas, an FA (fraction of anisotropy) of 0.1 should be used, and additional regions of interest (ROIs) for a particular tract such as the anterior part of the superior longitudinalis or the SMA portion of the CST can be added.[56,60,61] The basic DTI-FT map includes the CST for the motor part, and the superior longitudinalis (SLF), which includes the fasciculus arcuatus, and the inferior fronto-occipital (IFO) tract for the language part.[38,39,56] The SLF is the basic tract involved in the phonologic component of language; the IFO is the basic tract involved in the semantic component of language. Additional tracts that can be reconstructed are the uncinatus (UNC) and the inferior longitudinalis (ILF) tracts, which provide information on the semantic

and phonologic component of language in the frontal and temporal lobe, or the subcallosum fasciculus, involved in the phonologic component of language, sited in the lateral border of the lateral ventricle.[56,60,62] Preoperative neuroimaging produces an impressive amount of information concerning the anatomic and functional boundaries of the lesion to be resected. Together with the volumetric morphologic images, the DTI-FT images are usually loaded into the neuronavigation system and help in the perioperative period in performing the resection. However, the imaging gives information based on probabilistic measurements, and although they may have a relatively high sensitivity or specificity, they still carry a certain amount of mistake, which cannot, at least nowadays, be considered as sufficient for performing a safe and effective resection.

ANESTHESIOLOGIC EVALUATION

Besides the standard anesthesiologic work-up, the patient should be examined for his or her ability to experience intraoperative awake monitoring when needed. Preparation and selection of patients by anesthesiologists with expertise in awake surgery is recommended.[63,64] In our institution, the only absolute contraindications to awake surgery are the lack of cooperation, age older than 70 years, obesity, and difficult airway or airway affected by severe cardiovascular or respiratory diseases. In addition, common contraindications to any general anesthesia regimen,

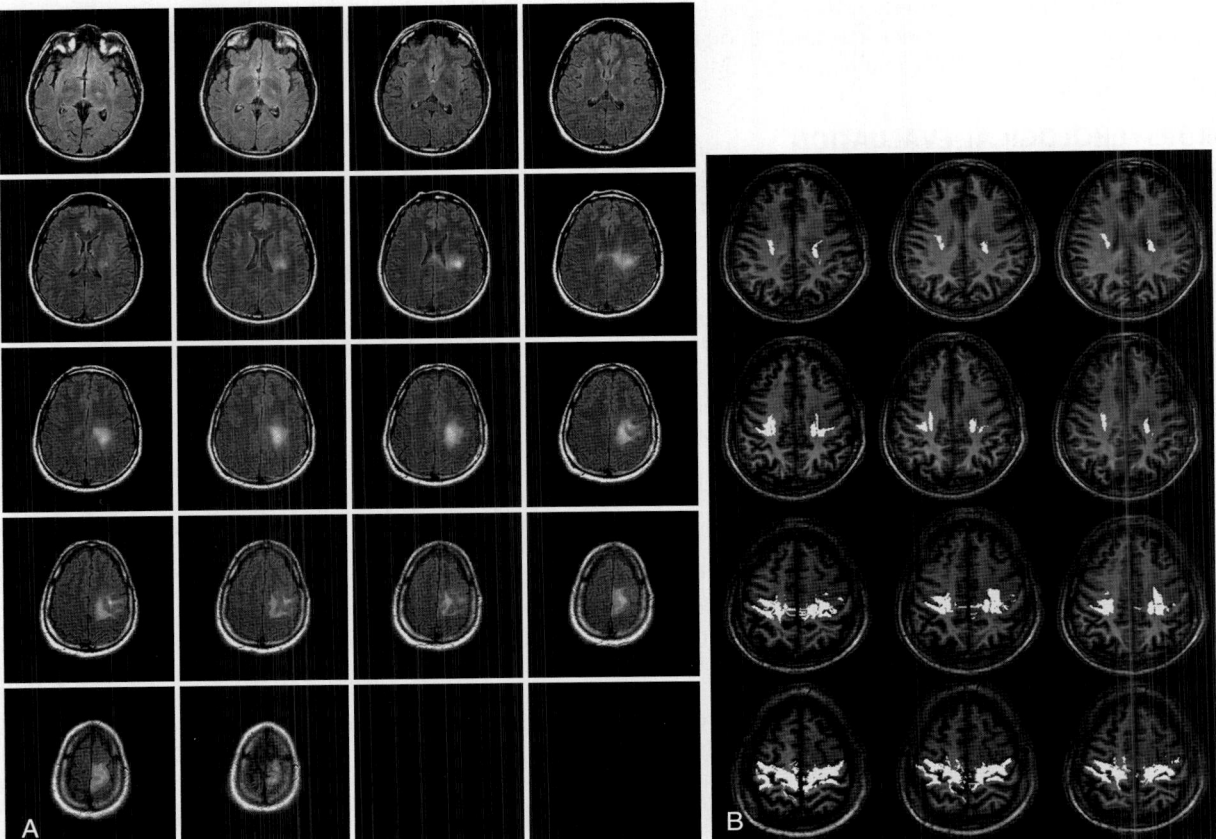

FIGURE 9-1 (A) FLAIR MR images showing a rolandic diffuse low-grade glioma (low-grade astrocytoma). (B) DTI-FT reconstruction for CST (*white*) superimposed to MR T1-weighted images showing that the CST is strictly intermingled with the tumor.

communication difficulties (moderate to severe aphasia), psychological imbalance (extreme anxiety), prone position, and inability to lie still for many hours are also included.

Once the preoperatory work-up is completed according to the site and the characteristics of the tumor, and the results of neuropsychological evaluation and functional and anatomic imaging obtained, each patient is offered an individualized surgical and monitoring strategy, which can be summarized as follows:

- Lesions in the nondominant hemisphere, away from eloquent areas and without relationship with areas of activation according to fMRI: motor monitoring (optional)
- Lesions in the nondominant hemisphere, in central or precentral area or in relationship with the CST (e.g., insular, temporomesial tumors) and small central lesions in the dominant hemisphere: motor mapping and monitoring
- Lesions in the nondominant hemisphere, in postcentral region: motor mapping and monitoring, visuospatial mapping
- Lesions in the dominant hemisphere: motor mapping and monitoring, language mapping more or less visuospatial mapping for parietal lesions

Intraoperative Protocol

The intraoperative protocol includes anesthesia modalities, neurophysiology, neuropsychology, and intraoperative imaging.

ANESTHESIA

Total intravenous anesthesia with propofol and remifentanil is used in our institution for performing these procedures. Newer drugs, such as dexmedetomidine, are emerging as effective and safe in producing sedation without inducing respiratory depression and without affecting electrophysiologic monitoring. In patients requiring only motor mapping, the patient is intubated through the nose and a light surgical anesthesia is maintained throughout the procedure. No muscle relaxants are employed during surgery to allow neurophysiologic assessment. When language or the visuospatial functions have to be tested during surgery, the patient can be maintained either awake during the entire surgery, or awakened for the phase of the surgery during which the mapping is performed.[18,30,36,39,44,56,63-65] In our institution, patients receive a laryngeal mask that is maintained until after the craniotomy and dural opening. At this point, the patient is awakened, while adequate analgesia is maintained to allow function monitoring. Time for awakening varies between 20 to 50 minutes, depending on the ability of the patient to metabolize the anesthetics. The anesthesiologist should be able to keep the patient awake for the entire time of subcortical mapping, which may be required particularly during long-lasting operations to alternate rest periods with those awake and responsive periods. Fatigue is observed in most of the patients, and its appearance correlates with duration of mapping, and the test difficulties (extensive language and visuospatial mapping).[25,44] Five percent of patients require suspension of mapping for a period longer than 20 minutes. The occurrence of seizures is the most important complication during the awake time of surgery, and can be controlled either by cold saline irrigation or by the infusion of a small bolus (1 ml) of propofol. Partial seizures occurred in our series in 4% of patients during surgery, and were related to mapping. Generalized seizures occurred in two patients at the end of the craniotomy. These two patients required reintubation. Vomiting is a rare complication, and can be controlled by the administration of antiemetics at the beginning of the mapping phase.

NEUROPHYSIOLOGY

The major components of the neurophysiologic protocol are monitoring (EEG, ECoG, EMG, MEP) and mapping (DES) procedures[11,31,60,66-68] (Table 9-1).

EEG activity is recorded bilaterally by four subdermal needle electrodes, providing four bipolar leads. EEG is registered to monitor brain activity when EcoG is not available, that is, at the beginning and the end of surgery, when titrating the level of anesthesia is particularly useful. It also allows assessing brain activity at a distance from the operating field, such as in the contralateral hemisphere.

The EcoG activity is recorded from a cortical region adjacent to the area being stimulated, by means of subdural strip electrodes with four to eight contacts in a monopolar array, referred to a *midfrontal electrode*. Cerebral activity is recorded with a bandpass of 1.6 to 320 Hz, and displayed with a sensitivity of 50 to 100 microns per centimeter for EEG and 200 to 400 microns per centimeter for EcoG. Continuous electrocorticographic recordings (Comet, Grass) are used during the entire duration of the procedure to monitor the brain basal electrical activity and the level of anesthesia, to define the working current, and to monitor for the occurrence of afterdischarges, electrical seizures or even clinical seizures during the resection. Because of this, EEG and ECoG recordings should be kept during the entire duration of the operation.

Continuous multichannel EMG recording (Comet, Grass, or Inomed ISIS) is used throughout the entire procedure. Several separate muscles (agonist and antagonist muscles) can be monitored, either in the contralateral or ipsilateral body. Motor responses are collected by pairs of subdermal hooked needle electrodes inserted into the contralateral muscles from face to foot. The most used setting is comprehensive of face (upper and lower face), neck, arm, forearm, hand, upper leg, and lower leg. In addition to EMG recordings, motor activity is also evaluated clinically.

MEP recording allows continuous monitoring of motor function. The "train of five technique," which was introduced for surgery in anesthetized patients, has been described as sensitive in detecting imminent lesions of the motor cortex and the pyramidal pathways.[69] For this purpose, a strip containing four to eight electrodes is placed over the precentral gyrus. A single stimulus or a double pulse stimulus (individual pulse width 0.3–0.5 millisecond, anodal constant current stimulation, interstimulus interval 4 milliseconds, stimulation intensity close to motor threshold) is usually delivered. MEP recording is usually alternated with direct cortical and subcortical motor mapping. MEP monitoring is very useful because it provides real-time information on the integrity of the motor pathways during the resection of large parts of the tumor not closely related to the functional structures. In addition, MEP provides warnings of impending brain ischemia, due

Table 9-1	Summary of Clinical Experience for 503 Patients with Low-Grade Gliomas Treated at University of Milan		
Location	**Type of Monitoring**	**Immediate Deficits**	**Permanent Deficits**
Rolandic (nondominant) 73 patients	MEP, EEG, ECoG, DES (Motor mapping)	Motor (48 patients, 65.7%)	Motor (2 patients, 2.7%)
Rolandic (dominant) 15 patients			
Small lesions* 7 patients (all asleep)	MEP, EEG, ECoG, DES (Motor mapping)	Motor (7 patients, 100%)	Motor (no patients, 0%)
Medium to large lesions 8 patients (all awake)	MEP, EEG, ECoG, DES (Motor and language mapping)	Motor (8 patients, 100%) Language (6 patients, 75%)	Motor (no patients, 0%) Language (no patients, 0%)
SMA (nondominant) 33 patients	MEP, EEG, ECoG, DES (Motor mapping)	Motor (25 patients, 75.7%)	Motor (no patients, 0%)
SMA (dominant) 41 patients (all awake)	MEP, EEG, ECoG (Motor and language mapping)	Motor (36 patients, 87.8%) Language (36 patients, 87.8%)	Motor (1 patient, 2.4%) Language (2 patients, 4.8%)
Frontal (nondominant) 32 patients	MEP, EEG, ECoG (Monitoring)	Motor (no patients, 0%)	Motor (no patients, 0%)
Frontal (dominant) 100 patients (all awake)	MEP, EEG, ECoG, DES (Motor and language mapping)	Motor (30 patients, 30.0%) Language (72 patients, 72.0%)	Motor (no patients, 0%) Language (2 patients, 2.0%)
Temporal (dominant)	MEP, EEG, ECoG, DES (Motor and language mapping)	Motor (2 patients, 1.7%) Language (94 patients, 81.7%)	Motor (no patients, 0%) Language (2 patients, 1.7%)
Parietal (nondominant) 14 patients (10 awake for involvement of second branch of SLF)	MEP, EEG, ECoG, DES (Motor mapping; visuospatial mapping in awakened)	Motor (3 patients, 21.4%) Visuospatial (2 patients, 14.2%)	Motor (no patients, 0%) Visuospatial (no patients, 0%)
Parietal (dominant) 18 patients (all awake)	MEP, EEG, ECoG, DES (Motor, language and visuospatial mapping)	Motor (4 patients, 22.2%) Language (9 patients, 50%) Visuospatial (2 patients, 11.1%)	Motor (no patients, 0%) Language (1 patient, 5.5%) Visuospatial (no patients, 0%)
Paralimbic (nondominant) 29 patients	MEP, EEG, ECoG, DES (Motor mapping)	Motor (6 patients, 20.7%)	Motor (1 patient, 3.4%)
Paralimbic (dominant) 33 patients (all awake)	MEP, EEG, ECoG, DES (Motor and language mapping)	Motor (2 patients, 9%) Language (21 patients, 63.6%)	Motor (1 patient, 3 %) Language (no patients, 0%)

Notes: Patients are divided according to tumor location. The type of monitoring used and the occurrence of immediate (within 1 week) and permanent (after 3 months) deficits are reported. For each location the number of patients treated and the number of awake patients are reported. For immediate and permanent deficits, the number and the relative percentage of patients are also indicated. Overall mortality was 0.4% (2 patients) (1 case of pulmonary embolia and 1 case of infection).
SLF, superior longitudinalis fasciculus; SMA, supplementary motor area.
*Small lesions are defined those that involved only the corticospinal tract, as defined by DTI FT images. In these cases, only a motor mapping in sleeping patients was performed. The patient is awakened in all cases in which the dominant SLF is involved.

to critical vessel interruption, mostly in deep temporal or insular regions.[52]

Direct electrical stimulation (DES) for cortical and subcortical mapping is usually performed by the use of a bipolar handheld stimulator with a 1-mm electrode-delivered stimulation, tips 5 mm apart, connected to an Ojemann Cortical Stimulator (Integra Neuroscience) or an Osiris or ISIS stimulator (Inomed, Germany), which delivers biphasic square-wave pulses, each phase lasting 1 millisecond, at 60 Hz in trains lasting 1 to 2 seconds for cortical mapping and 1 to 4 seconds for subcortical mapping. Subcortical mapping is alternated with the resection in a back-and-forth fashion. Subcortical mapping is performed by using the same current threshold applied for cortical mapping. Alternatively, monopolar stimulation can be used, either cortically or subcortically, by delivering a single- or double-pulse stimulus, according to the train-of-five technique.

To start the mapping procedure, the working current is established. As movement is easy to observe, it is advisable to start the procedure with motor function mapping. Once the intensity of the current for stimulation is determined, the same is used in most cases throughout the procedure. Initially, a low current intensity (2 mA) is used, which is then progressively increased until a movement is induced. A stimulus duration of 1 or 2 seconds is usually enough to generate a motor response. At this point, it is good practice to stimulate the areas close to that in which the current induced the movement, map them, and check whether the current is able to evoke motor responses in these zones as well. If not, the current intensity may be increased and adjusted to evoke appreciable motor responses. It is also recommended to check with the ECoG if the applied current may induce afterdischarges in nearby brain areas. Only the current immediately below those inducing afterdischarges have to be used for mapping. If afterdischarges are seen, the current should be set up at least 0.5 mA under the previous one. In any case, ECoG recording is used to detect the appearance of afterdischarges during mapping in order to keep the test reliable. In fact, only the responses evoked in the absence of afterdischarges are considered trustworthy.

For language mapping, the initial test used is counting. The current is usually applied to the premotor cortex related to the face, and the test is aimed at determining whether the current stops the patient from counting. This has to be repeated several times and counting stopped at least three times in order to be reliable.[41] If not, the current intensity is increased until these results are produced. When the current is established, DES is applied to the entire exposed surface of the brain, and the occurrence of afterdischarges checked in the ECoG. The stimulus duration is between 1 to 4 seconds. Only the current that is not inducing afterdischarges in the entire stimulated cortex is used for mapping.

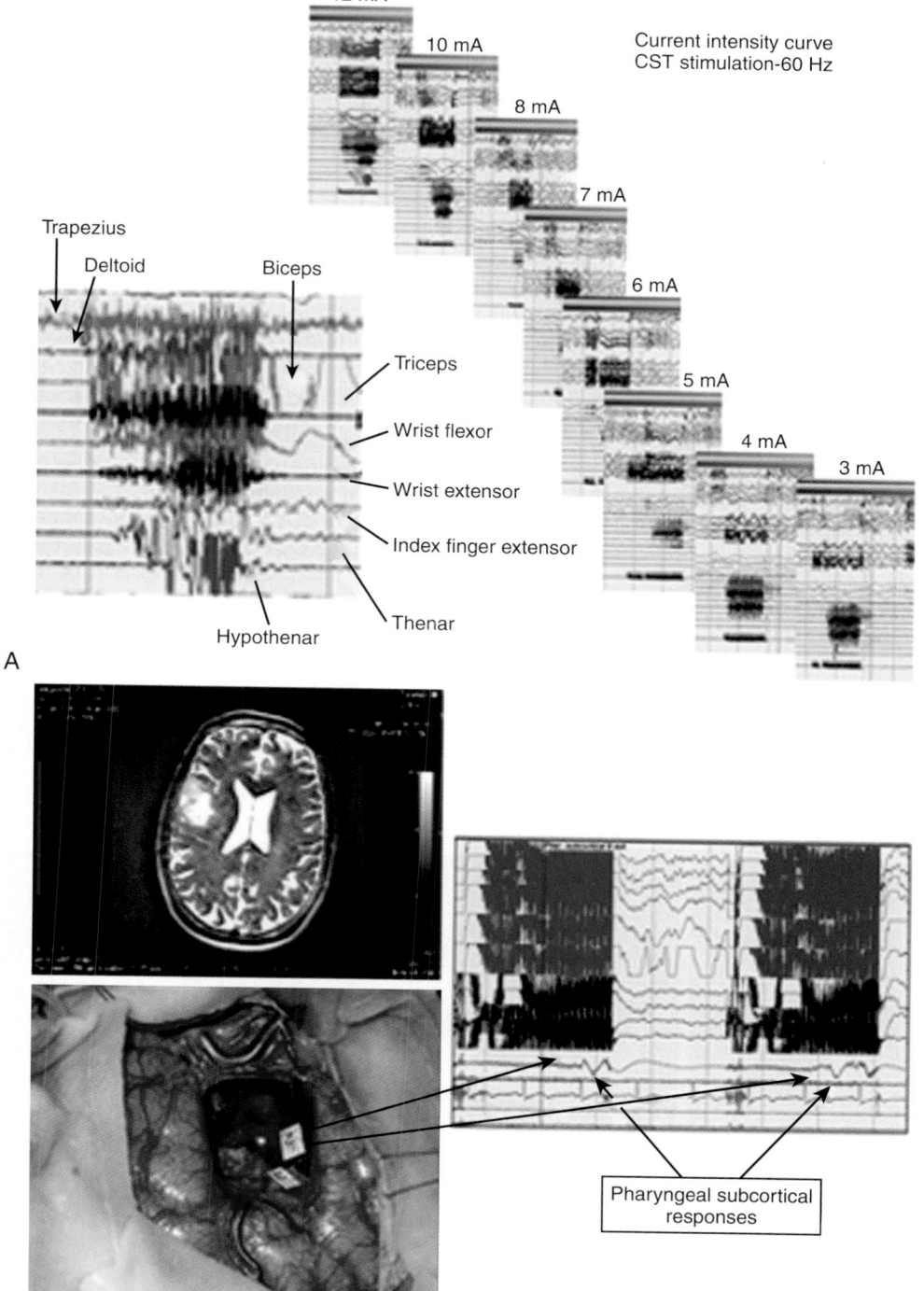

FIGURE 9-2 (A) Current intensity curve. When during subcortical stimulation a motor response is evoked, a curve intensity curve is performed by progressively decreasing the intensity of the current. The motor response is maintained till the current of 3 mA indicates that stimulation is very close to the CST. (B) The placement of electrodes in the soft palate and in the tongue allows detecting motor response from fibers to pharyngeal muscles during subcortical stimulation, in a case of right precentral low-grade glioma. The *upper left panel* shows a T2-weighted MR image of the tumor mass. The *lower left panel* shows the intraoperative picture of the surgical fields, with the resection cavity. The location in the resection cavity where subcortical stimulation evoked pharyngeal muscle responses is marked with sterile tags.

In case of afterdischarges, the current intensity is decreased by at least 0.5 mA.

For subcortical mapping, either the same current used for cortical mapping or a current raised to 2 mA is applied, and the stimulus is continuously alternated with the resection. When a response was induced at a subcortical level, performing an intensity–response curve is recommended to assess maintenance of the response either at very low current-intensity levels. This can help in estimating the distance between the point of stimulation and the functional tract (Fig. 9-2). Also, during subcortical mapping, ECoG is continuously monitored to look for the occurrence of afterdischarges and seizures, in order to verify reliability of responses.

MEP monitoring is typically used at the beginning of the procedure, and helps in identifying the location of the motor strip. During resection, MEP recording is alternated with subcortical motor mapping and provides additional information on the integrity of motor pathways.[70]

The resection margin is usually kept at least 5 mm away from functional areas, and may come very close to subcortical pathways

RESULTS OF MAPPING OR MONITORING PROCEDURES

Motor Mapping

We usually map motor responses in patients with tumors located in rolandic or premotor or parietal regions. Motor mapping is also applied at cortical and subcortical levels for lesions located in the insula or deep temporal region, in which motor pathways can be encountered during resection. For lesions located in the nondominant hemisphere, the patient is kept under general anesthesia. The placement of a series of electrodes in the inner palate and pharyngeal muscles, as well as in the tongue, is useful to detect responses from these muscles. For lesions close or within visuospatial or language areas of pathways, the patient is always awakened during the procedure. In both awake and asleep settings, a stimulation duration of 1 or 2 seconds is usually enough to generate a motor response. At cortical stimulation, we observed various morphologies of EMG responses: cortically evoked responses showed great variations in amplitude, but they appeared always as continuous tonic bursts of activity, often incrementing during stimulation. The smallest amplitudes were observed in the neck and the shoulder or in the mouth.

Occasionally, in patients under general anesthesia and receiving a large amount of antiepileptic medications, it might be difficult to evoke cortical motor responses, even after the current intensity has been increased until that which might induce the appearance of afterdischarges. In these patients, the use of monopolar stimulation can be useful for identifying the location of the motor cortex and to plan the site of incision, allowing continuing resection. During subcortical stimulation, motor responses appeared as focal (few muscles) when the tract is stimulated in close vicinity to the surface, while they appeared on multiple muscle groups with deep stimulation (Figs. 9-3 and 9-4). For resection of tumors located in the premotor cortex, the placement of electrodes in the ipsilateral muscles allows detection of responses coming from these segments during resection. In addition, when resection is approaching the deep portion of the tumor, subcortical stimulation permits detection of small motor responses without overt muscle activity, which indicate that the resection is getting close to motor pathways. When these warning responses are identified, resection should proceed carefully in this region until more pronounced motor responses are identified, usually when the tip probe is touching and stimulating the motor pathways. This can be confirmed by performing a current intensity curve.

The simultaneous use of CUSA and DES at the subcortical level in proximity to the corticospinal tract may result in the abolition of previously evident motor responses. This abolition is generally fully reversible after turning the CUSA off. An analogous pattern of inhibition of motor responses can also be evident when the DES is applied cortically and CUSA is used subcortically when close to motor pathways. This interference with motor mapping may be interpreted as a transitory inhibition of axonal conduction. This should be kept in mind by the surgeon when using both tools during resection.[67]

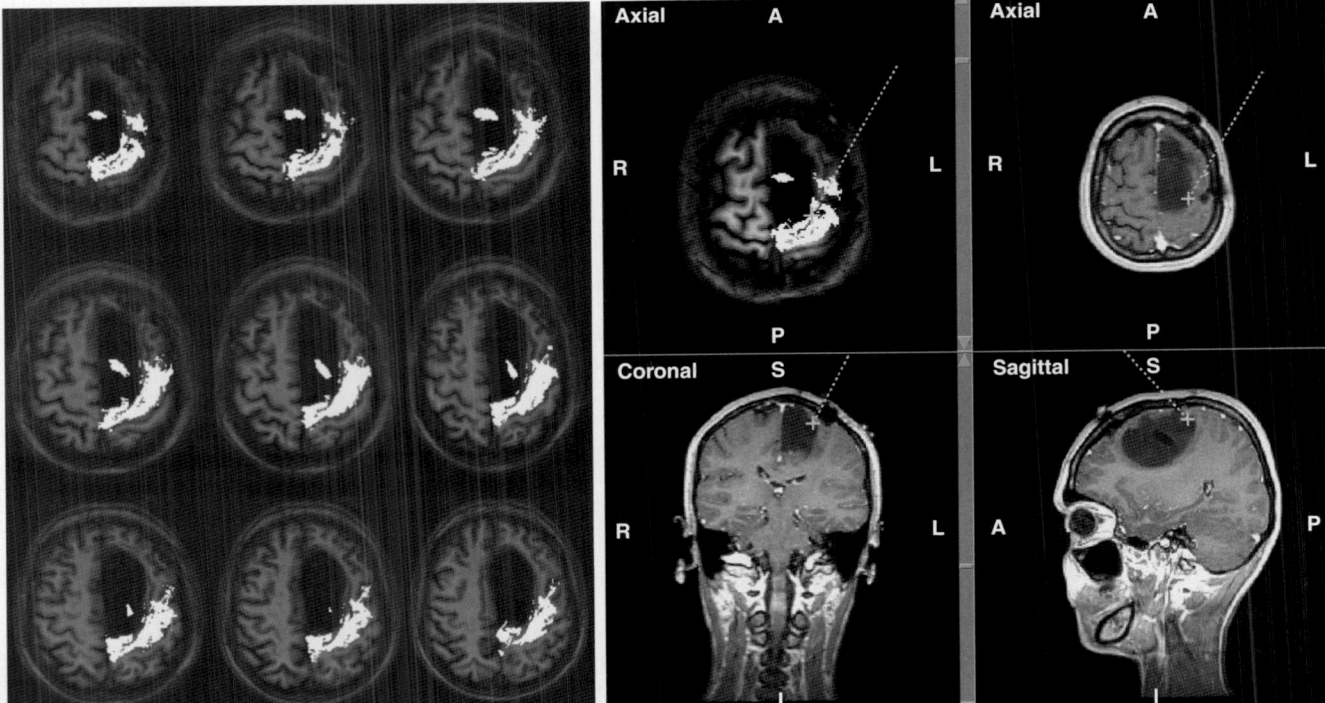

FIGURE 9-3 *Right panel*: DTI-FT reconstruction of CST (*white*) in a case of rolandic and SMA low-grade oligodendroglioma. And DES data for CST in case of rolandic tumors. DTI reconstructed the CST (*bright white tract*) at the posterior border and partially infiltrating the tumor mass. The fibers were reconstructed with an FA of 0.1. The *left panels* show intraoperative snapshots, taken where DES, performed in site indicated by the center of the green cursors, located motor responses at the beginning of resection, by subcortical stimulation.

Motor Monitoring

For continuous motor monitoring with MEP, a strip electrode is placed over M1, delivering monopolar pulses to elicit motor-evoked potentials (MEPs) in a few target muscles. MEPs are monitored throughout the surgery, except when the surgeon needs direct subcortical mapping. MEP monitoring is very useful because it provides on-line information of the motor pathway integrity during resection of a large part of the tumor not closely located to functional structures. MEP provides warnings of impending brain ischemia due to critical vessel interruption, mostly in deep temporal or insular regions.[70]

Language and Visuospatial Monitoring

Each stimulation should start before presentation of the material, and should be followed by at least a task without stimulation (two tasks are standard). The stimulus is applied immediately before the item is presented to the patient, and a neuropsychologist in the operating room (OR) is evaluating patient performance during various tests administered at both cortical and subcortical levels.

Various types of errors are possible during test administration. During the administration of each test, the ECoG and EEG must be checked for afterdischarges or electrical seizures. Only errors in the absence of ECoG disturbances are reliable. A site can be defined as essential for language when it produces language disturbances at least three times during various nonconsecutive stimulations. Cortical language sites coding for object naming, verb generation, face naming, word or sentence comprehension, numbers, or colors can be identified in several regions in the frontal, temporal, or parietal lobes, which differ according to patient gender and other characteristics.[18,30] For subcortical language mapping, the patient is asked to perform an object-naming and a verb-generation task during which the surgeon can continue to perform resection, which is alternated with stimulation. When a language disturbance is produced, the site is then carefully tested for the occurrence of semantic or phonemic paraphasia. Each tract can be recognized at a subcortical level by the appearance of semantic (inferior fronto-occipital tract, uncinatus), or phonemic (superior longitudinalis, inferior longitudinalis) paraphasia associated with typical language disturbances,

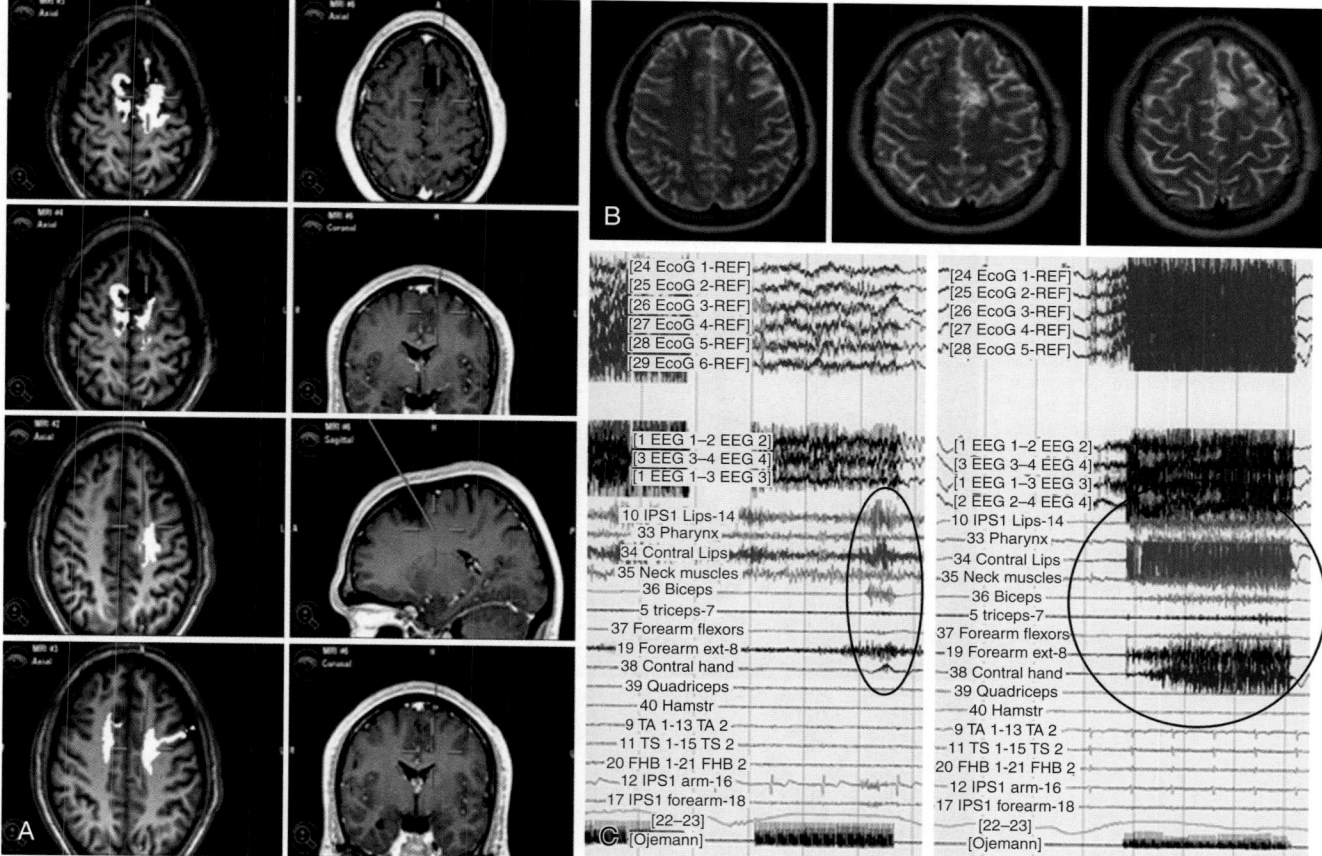

FIGURE 9-4 DTI-FT and DES data in a case of oligodendroglioma grade II involving the left preSMA, in which DTI-FT data for SLF, SMA, CST fibers, highlighted as bright white ROI, were fused with T1-weighted images, fused with volumetric postcontrast T1-weighted images, and were loaded into the neuronavigation system and available intraoperatively. Resection was performed with the aid of motor and language cortical and subcortical mapping in awake patient, which was continuously alternated with the tumor resection. Resection was stopped when language responses (phonemic paraphasias) or motor responses were encountered. (A) Panels show intraoperative snapshots were subcortical stimulation evoked phonemic paraphasia (SLF, *upper panel*), complex leg motor responses (SMA), and upper limb responses (CST, *lower two panels*). The intraoperative snapshots were taken where DES, performed in site indicated by the center of the green cursors, identified such a response. (B) Postoperative T2-weighted images showing the resection of the tumor. (C) *Right lower panels* report EMG findings obtained during subcortical stimulation of the CST. Activation of the upper limb is indicated with a *black circle*.

such as speech arrest in proximity to the subcallosum (Figs. 9-4 and 9-5).

Visuospatial mapping is typically performed in patients with lesions located in the parietal lobe, and in cases of dominant location, it is combined with language mapping. The patient is usually requested to look at a line in a touchscreen and to bisect it by touching its center with a pen. A deviation over 2 cm to the right or left is usually considered as pathologic, and is associated with interference in the visuospatial function. Subcortical visuospatial mapping identifies a small and discrete tract, usually running at the lateral midborder of the tumor that is involved in this function. Preservation of this tract as well as cortical sites prevents the occurrence of neglect during the postoperative course.

EEG and ECoG Monitoring

EEG and ECoG recordings should be kept during the entire duration of the procedure because they permit monitoring for the occurrence of afterdischarges, electrical seizures, and even clinical seizures. The occurrence of afterdischarges is quite common during these procedures, and the main objective of monitoring is to recognize those that occur in response to stimulation, in order to maintain testing reliability. Groups of ECoG spikes or electrical seizures occur in up to 30% to 40% of cases, and may be related to stimulation. In any case, when they appear irrigating the cortex and surgical cavity with cold saline is recommended, as in most instances this results in control and reversal of the situation. Clinical seizures occur in 4% of cases, and most of them are focal. In these cases, the EEG is useful to look for diffusion of the seizure, either in the same or the contralateral hemisphere. In selected cases, ECoG can be used to detect the generation of spikes in specific areas of the cortex, either near or distant from the tumor mass, that are responsible for sustained electrical activity. ECoG is also used to titrate and monitor the level of anesthesia, particularly in sleeping patients. A continuous trace recording is usually recommended in this setting

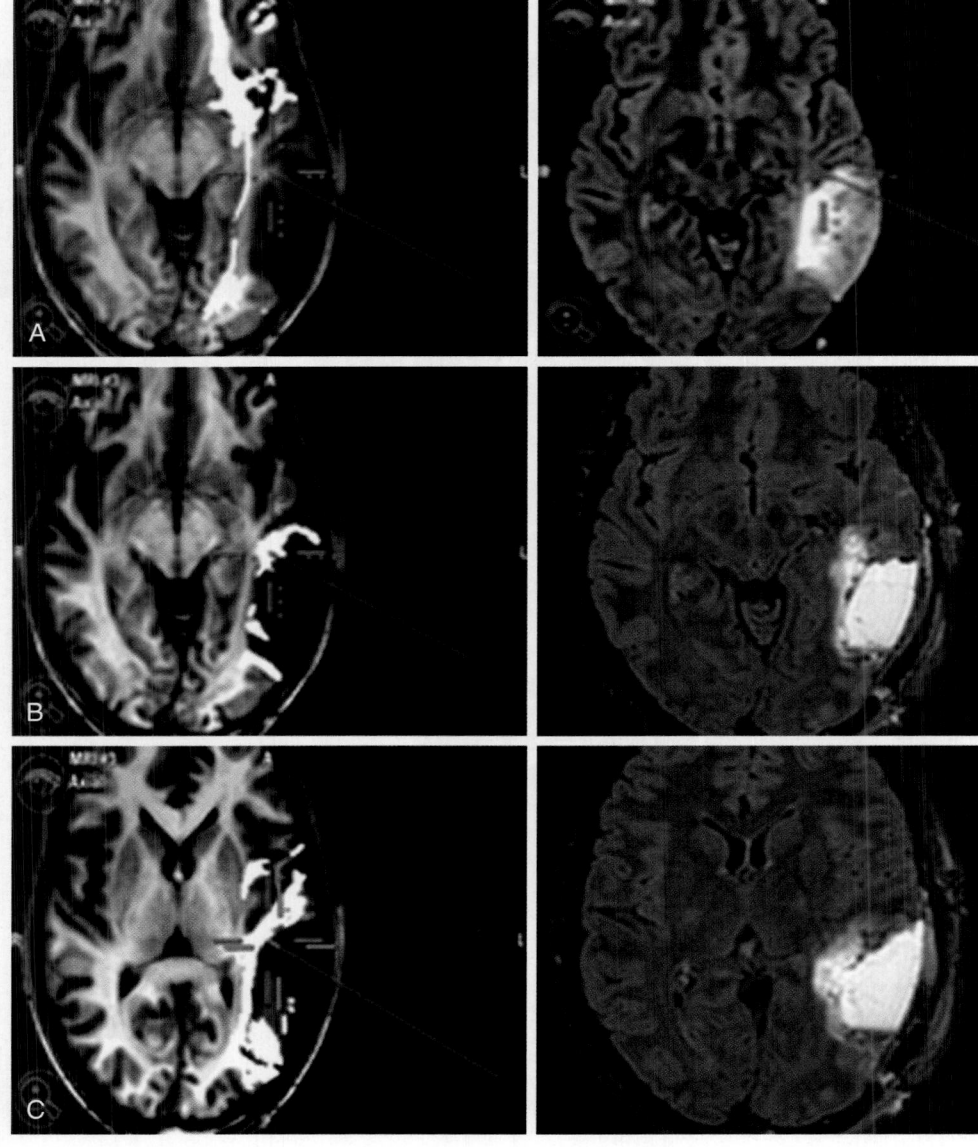

FIGURE 9-5 A case of left temporal oligodendroglioma. DTI-FT data for IFO, ILF, and SLF, highlighted as bright white ROI, were fused with T1-weighted images, fused with volumetric postcontrast T1-weighted images, and were loaded into the neuronavigation system and available intraoperatively. Resection was performed with the aid of motor and language cortical and subcortical mapping in awake patient, which was continuously alternated with the tumor resection. Resection was stopped when language responses (phonemic or semantic paraphasias) or motor responses were encountered. The *left panels* show intraoperative snapshots where subcortical stimulation evoked semantic paraphasia (SLF, A), phonemic paraphasia followed by speech arrest (ILF, B), and phonemic paraphasia (SLF, C). The intraoperative snapshots were taken where DES, performed in site indicated by the center of the red cursor, identified such a response. The *middle* and *lower* panels show postoperative FLAIR images showing that the margins of resection were coincident with location of the tracts.

to ensure optimal response to cortical and subcortical stimulation.

Results of Intraoperative Imaging

Both morphologic volumetric T1, T2, or FLAIR images, along with motor and language fMRI and DTI-FT images, are usually loaded into the neuronavigation system. Neuronavigation helps during surgery to localize the tumor, and to define the relationship between the tumor and the surrounding functional and anatomic structures, both at cortical and subcortical levels. To estimate clinical navigation accuracy, the target registration error localizing a separate fiducial (not used for registration) is usually performed at the beginning of surgery. The target registration error should be less than 2 mm. The main limitation in using a neuronavigation system, particularly for large tumors, is the occurrence of brain shift, which occurs already at the beginning of surgery when the dura is opened, and increases with the progress of tumor removal.[53,56,71-73] To reduce the problem of brain shift during resection, repeated landmark checks are performed during surgery to ensure overall ongoing clinical navigation accuracy. Using a craniotomy limited to the minimum necessary to expose the tumor area and a small portion of the surrounding brain, minimizes brain shift. For frontal tumors located in proximity of the CST, resection is started from the posterior border where the CST is located and, after its identification, the tract is followed inside the tumor mass. Afterward, the remaining anterior part of the tumor is removed. Similarly, in the case of parietal tumors, resection is started from the anterior border following the same principle.

When preoperative fMRI is correlated with intraoperative findings, motor fMRI usually matches with data obtained via DES, although the extent of the functional activations is larger than the area defined with intraoperative mapping, and results are strictly dependent on the type of task used for testing.[19,74,75] In any case, motor fMRI can be safely used for planning surgery. For language correlation, the results are variable and different according to series. Naming and verb generation tasks are most widely used for language fMRI studies. Language fMRI data obtained with naming or verb generation tasks are imperfectly correlated with intraoperative brain mapping results (sensitivity 59% and specificity 97% when the two fMRI are combined).[48,54,76] fMRI shows greater activation than observed with direct cortical mapping, which on the contrary, demonstrates only essential language sites. In our experience, sensitivity can be increased up to 72% by using the same figures in fMRI naming tasks as employed during surgery. Nevertheless, false negatives have been documented in up to 8% of patients, even when using the same naming tasks. Therefore, language fMRI cannot be used to make critical decisions in the absence of direct brain mapping. Language fMRI is useful to establish language laterality and can effectively replace the Wada test.

In low-grade gliomas, preoperative DTI-FT shows that the tracts were mostly infiltrated and interrupted or dislocated by the tumor mass. In addition, a large portion of the tracts were documented inside the tumor mass.[61] As for the correspondence with DES and their clinical use, we have to remember that DTI-FT is providing anatomic information, whereas subcortical mapping provides functional data.[56,57,61,62] This is of relatively less importance for CST, but of particular relevance for language tracts, in which the anatomic distribution of the tract as depicted by DTI is greater than the functional distribution obtained with mapping. Therefore, large portions of tracts as depicted by DTI-FT can be removed because they are not pertinent to the function tested at that time.

Additional problems may derive from the FA used for tract reconstruction, which can vary inside the same tumor according to its grade of heterogeneity. In cases of rolandic tumors, DTI reconstructs the CST mainly inside the tumor mass (98% of cases). In the majority of bulky tumors, the tract is displaced anteriorly (22%), or more frequently posteriorly (78%), and highly infiltrated by the tumor mass. Less frequently, and in case of highly infiltrating and diffuse low-grade gliomas, the tract is depicted inside the tumor mass and as highly infiltrated. In the first tumor group, subcortical DES locates the tract in the same position where it is depicted by DTI-FT (Figs. 9-3 and 9-4). Some discrepancies are observed only in the superior portion of the tract, close to the cortical surface, where DTI-FT fails to reconstruct fibers, and instead DES locates motor responses. Even the placement of additional ROIs does not improve the fiber reconstruction. More problematic are cases of highly diffuse low-grade gliomas, where DTI-FT usually reconstructs the tract as highly infiltrated and inside the tumor mass.

Particularly in cases with a long history of seizures, and at the beginning of the resection when 60-Hz stimulation is applied over the regions of the tumor where DTI-FT depicted the location of the upper portion of tract, DES usually fails to locate overt motor responses. When the current intensity is progressively increased to induce responses, this usually results in seizures without overt movements. In these cases, electrical identification of the CST requires the use of monopolar stimulation, which is associated with a lower incidence of seizures. However, as in previous cases, DTI-FT fails to show fibers close to the more lateral portion of the *homunculus*, probably due to the presence of crossing fibers that cannot be depicted by the simple tensor model used here for tractography, where DES (generally with monopolar stimulation) induces laryngeal or upper or lower face responses.

When a portion of the tumor is removed, and the CST partially decompressed, the 60-Hz stimulation starts again to identify motor responses, usually in the same location where DTI-FT reconstructs the deeper portion of the CST. As for the SLF, the anatomic distribution of this tract is usually larger than the functional distribution when language subcortical mapping is performed. This is particularly the case for frontal and temporal tumors. As for the IFO tract, its anatomic distribution is small and usually corresponds to the functional one depicted by subcortical mapping (Figs. 9-4 and 9-5). Some problems may occur for F3 low-grade gliomas in which DTI-FT fails in reconstructing the more superior part of the tract at the inferior border of the tumor, when the tumor infiltration in this area is quite extensive.

The anatomic distribution of the UNC tract is small and usually corresponds to the functional one depicted by subcortical mapping. The reconstruction of this tract in F3 tumors requires placement of an additional ROI at this level. In F3 low-grade gliomas, the tract is usually inside the tumor mass, and the depicted fibers are typically identified as functional by subcortical mapping.

In temporal LGG tumors, the tract is still described as inside the tumor mass, but the fibers are extensively infiltrated and interrupted, and not functional. Our experience on a large number of patients showed that the combined use of DTI-FT and DES is a feasible approach that can be effectively and safely applied in routine clinical activity.[56,61] When available and loaded into the neuronavigation system, DTI-FT can help in reducing time spent in surgery by helping the surgeon locate where in the tract to start subcortical stimulation and thus proceed with a careful resection. This may result in a smaller number of stimulations needed to safely locate a tract, fewer seizures, and less patient fatigue.

Apart from cases in which DTI-FT data can be obtained intraoperatively by the intraoperative MR system, in most settings DTI-FT data are usually loaded into the neuronavigation system and combined with preoperative MR images. For correct use of DTI-FT data in this setting, two points appear to be critical: transfer of the data to the neuronavigation system, and the use of technical adjustments during surgery to maintain global accuracy of the information. In our center, DTI-FT data are saved as a compatible format (DICOM) by using Medx Software (Medical Numerics, Inc.), which permits the images to be transferred and loaded onto the neuronavigation system. The neuronavigational system performs an automatic coregistration between DTI-FT data sets and preoperative MR images acquired with references applied on the skull of the patient by a voxel-by-voxel, intensity-matching nonlinear algorithm. For the second point, resection should be performed to maintain the maximal accuracy of the neuronavigation system to reduce the problem of brain shift, as already discussed.

Intraoperative MR has been more widely used for surgical treatment of low-grade gliomas[20,71,77] by using both low (0.2 or 0.5) or high[1.5] magnetic fields. The advantage of using intraoperative MR images is to have a precise judgment of surgical removal while the patient is still in the operating room. In addition, by performing repeated images during surgery, it is possible to update morphologic images and transfer them into the neuronavigation system to overcome the problem of brain shift. Progression of surgery can be followed and the occurrence of intraoperative complications monitored. In at least 20% of cases of low-grade gliomas, remnants of the tumor can be visualized in the field and further removed.

The major limitation of the intraoperative MR system is cost of the machine and instruments. Lower magnetic fields may permit the use of nonmagnetic surgical instruments, and thus lower cost of machine and installation. Various lower-field machines are available, such as the 0.2 Polestar or the 0.5 GE. The 0.5 GE prototype allows on-time intraoperative images during surgery,[20] but is limited by the restricted surgical room and by the need to use nonmagnetic surgical tools. In addition, low magnetic fields do not permit fMRI or DTI-FT studies. The intraoperative high-field magnetic resonance (MR) system provides high-quality images and offers various modalities beyond standard anatomic imaging, such as MR spectroscopy, diffusion tensor imaging, and functional MR imaging, providing not only data on the extent of resection and localization of tumor remnants but also on metabolic changes, tumor invasion, and localization of functional eloquent cortical and deep-seated brain areas. Various systems have been developed and used. In most of them, the patient is located in a bed and moved into the magnet for MR images. Recently 3T MR systems have been put in place, or are under construction, including in our institution (University of Milan).

Ultrasound is another imaging option used for intraoperative visualization of low-grade gliomas. Advances in ultrasound technology have made the image quality of the ultrasound comparable to intraoperative MR.[78] Recent studies and the experience of our center showed that the integration of intraoperative ultrasound with neuronavigation represents an efficient and inexpensive tool for intraoperative imaging and surgical guidance. Brain shift detected with intraoperative ultrasound could be used to update preoperative image data such as fMRI and DTI-FT in order to increase the value of this information through the operation. However, intraoperative MR systems are superior to ultrasound methods in revealing tumor remnants.

The Concept of Subpial Resection

Surgical removal is usually performed via tailored craniotomy exposing the tumor area and limited surrounding cortex. In the case of temporal or frontal tumors in the dominant hemisphere, the craniotomy should expose the face premotor cortex to allow testing at the beginning of resection to establish in the awakened patient the current intensity to be used. In other cases, the placement of a subdural strip permits reaching the motor cortex and performing MEP monitoring. When the relationship between the tumor and the functional areas is established and the point of entry identified, resection begins using a transcortical subpial approach. This allows removal of nonfunctional tumor tissue until functional borders are identified and preservation of arteries and veins. Resection cavities are eventually connected to one another, maintaining the vasculature skeleton. The safety of this microsurgical strategy is indicated by the patient morbidity profile.[13,18,31,37,56,61]

Functional Results of Surgery

Resection margins are usually kept 5 mm apart from essential cortical sites, and are usually coincident with subcortical sites (Tables 9-2 and 9-3). When this is achieved, motor or language deficits develop in the immediate postoperative period in 72.8% and 65.4% of cases, respectively. When no subcortical sites are identified, this risk is very low (3%–5%).[12,30,38,39,56,77,79,80] In our experience, most of the deficits were transient and disappeared within 1 month from surgery. Overall, in the group of patients in which a subcortical functional site was identified during the resection, the likelihood of developing a permanent deficit was less of 4%, independent of histology and location. This percentage reached 7% in patients with a pre-existing motor or language deficit.

In contrast, when no subcortical sites were found at the time of surgery, the likelihood of inducing a permanent deficit was even lower (2%). These results further reinforce the concept that when a subcortical site is found, the surgeon is very close to the subcortical pathway. Therefore, when a subcortical response is reliably detected, the resection

Table 9-2   Neurophysiologic Protocol

Technique	Aim	Modality	Rationale	Indication
EEG	Monitoring of basal brain activity	Bilateral recording, four bipolar leads	Monitoring of brain areas not covered by ECoG and of contralateral hemisphere, seizure surveillance at beginning and end of surgery, monitoring of level of anesthesia	Each case undergoing cortical stimulation (MEP, DES)
ECoG	Direct monitoring of cortical activity	Subdural strip/grid electrodes adjacent to craniotomy site	Detection of: afterdischarges, electrical/clinical seizures related to stimulation, epileptogenic foci	Each case undergoing cortical stimulation (MEP, DES), epilepsy surgery
EMG	Monitoring/mapping of motor activity	Subdermal hooked-needle electrodes, extensive insertion in several contra- and ipsi-lateral muscles from face to foot	High sensitivity and specificity in detecting subclinical responses to MEP/DES, allows use of lower stimulation intensity	Each case undergoing cortical and subcortical electrical stimulation, MEP
MEP	Real-time continuous monitoring of motor activity	Train-of-five technique, cortical strip electrodes (never transcranial)	Complementary to direct bipolar stimulation, allows continuous monitoring of motor pathways when DES is not performed, can detect impending brain ischemia	Identification of central sulcus and monitoring of motor pathways
DES	Mapping of cortical and subcortical functions	Direct electrical bipolar stimulation	Allows direct identification of cortical and subcortical functional areas	Accurate and reliable testing of motor, language, and cognitive functions

Table 9-3   Functional Borders Encountered during Resection According to Tumor Location

Location	Functional Borders
Rolandic or SMA nondominant	Posteriorly: CST and leg component of SMA fibers
Rolandic or SMA dominant	Posteriorly: CST and leg component of SMA fibers
	Laterally: SLF
	Inferiorly: IFO, subcallosum
Precentral nondominant	Posteriorly: CST (if reachable)
Precentral dominant	Posteriorly: SLF
	Laterally and inferiorly: SLF, IFO, UNC
Parietal nondominant	Anteriorly: CST
	Laterally: second branch SLF
Parietal dominant	Anteriorly: CST
	Laterally: SLF
	Inferiorly: IFO, visual pathways
Temporal dominant	Medial: UNC, IFO, ILF
	Posteriorly: SLF
Insular dominant	Anteriorly: IFO, SLF, UNC
	Medially: IFO, CST
	Posteriorly: CST, SLF

CST, corticospinal tract; IFO, inferior longitudinalis fasciculus; SLF, superior longitudinalis fasciculus; SMA, supplementary motor area; subcallosum, subcallosum fasciculus; UNC, uncinatus fasciculus.

must be stopped and then continued in adjacent structures because there is a great potential for damage to functional structures.[21,30,77,80] If no subcortical structures are found, the resection can be continued because the probability of injury to essential structures is low. These data indicate subcortical stimulation as a reliable tool for guiding surgical resection, as well as for predicting the likelihood of developing a deficit postoperatively.

The low incidence of postoperative deficits in patients in whom no subcortical tracts were identified is usually due to vascular damage and the development of ischemic areas. MEP monitoring can help in preventing motor deficits due to vascular injury.[52] Long-term postoperative neuropsychological evaluation found that 79.5% of patients had long-term postoperative normal language, 18.6% showed mild disturbances but still compatible with normal daily life, and only 2.3% showed long-term impairment. Similar figures were observed for the resection of low-grade gliomas close to motor areas or pathways. These functional results were totally different from those obtained when subcortical stimulation was not applied. Analysis of patients with high- or low-grade gliomas operated on in our institution before the use of direct electrical stimulation showed 23% with permanent language or motor deficits, in accordance with results reported in other series.[12,30,81]

Oncologic Results of Surgery

Surgery performed with the aid of brain mapping techniques permits attainment of several oncologic objectives. It permits collection of a large amount of material, which helps the pathologist the histologic and molecular diagnosis. It increases the number of cases submitted to surgical treatment: in accordance with previous reports in the literature, this percentage in our series moved from 11% of cases when mapping was not available, to 81% when mapping was applied, with a significant decrease in the number of cases that were submitted to biopsy only.[12,18,30,81] Moreover, it reduces the percentage of postoperative permanent deficits, which fell from 33% to 2.3% for language or motor functions. Another important effect is the decline in the incidence of seizures, particularly in low-grade glioma patients with a long epileptic history and affected by insular tumors.

Seizure control is more likely to be achieved after gross total resection than after subtotal resection/biopsy alone. In fact when total or subtotal resection is achieved, in more than 80% of cases a positive impact on seizures is documented, with reduction in the number of antiepileptic drugs (AEDs) administered. In addition, suppression of AEDs is possible in 30% of cases.[40] Lastly, and most important, is the impact that these techniques have on the extent of resection.

The use of brain mapping techniques increased the percentage of patients in which a total and subtotal resection was achieved. In our series of low-grade gliomas, the percentage of total and subtotal resections was 11% in the period in which no mapping was available, and 69.8% in the time in which brain mapping techniques were applied. These figures are in accordance with the results of other groups.

A large number of class III and II studies suggests that more extensive resection at the time of initial diagnosis may be a favorable prognostic factor for this type of tumors.[12,17-22,31,38,77,82] The evaluation of resection extent is usually performed on postoperative FLAIR volumetric images with the aid of semiautomatic segmentation software.[21,71] The ability to achieve a complete resection (no abnormalities seen on postoperative FLAIR images) or subtotal resection (a postoperative volume on volumetric postoperative FLAIR images of less than 10 ml) is influenced by both preoperative tumor volume and tumor involvement of eloquent tissue, particularly at the subcortical level.[18] Preoperative tumor volume is a significant predictor of patient survival and progression-free survival per se, as well as the involvement of subcortical tracts. Extent of resection as well as pre- and post-operative tumor volume strongly influence progression-free survival and time to malignant transformation. In addition, extent of resection has also an influence of patient survival. Total resection (no abnormalities in postoperative FLAIR volumetric images) is seen in 37.5% of patients in our series, and can usually be reached in small or well-demarcated tumors. In addition, no tumor recurrence is found in these patients at 5 years follow-up. Because tumor size is inversely related to patient outcome, delaying surgical intervention may increase the risk of malignant transformation. Moreover, all efforts made to increase the extent of resection are warranted.[18]

Strategy for Large Diffuse or Recurrent Tumors: The Concept of Brain Plasticity

Low-grade gliomas present as a variable type of tumors ranging from discrete and apparently well defined lesion, to either diffuse or less discrete lesion. The therapeutic strategies for the more defined type of tumors are those we previously described. Large diffuse tumors still represent a challenge. Most of them are histologically diffuse astrocytoma, and contain functional subcortical tracts. In these cases, a total or subtotal resection as initial strategy is quite difficult to be achieved. Although partial removal may still be beneficial,[18] particularly in cases where a mass effect is present, the majority of these patients underwent stereotactic biopsy only, usually guided by spectroscopy MR images, followed by adjuvant treatments. A recent strategy to increase the rate of resection in these tumors is represented by the use of up-front preoperative chemotherapy. TMZ administered up front for a period of up to 6 months in a limited group of patients resulted in a decrease in tumor cell invasion, and reduced tumor cell infiltration along large fiber tracts, which help in reaching a larger proportion of tumor removal (ref. 80, Soffietti et al., 2010 in press). Alternatively, chemotherapy may be used as adjuvant treatment after partial removal, and in these cases it may further decrease postoperative tumor volume.[27,28,83] In addition, in the case of large tumors, a two-time surgical strategy may be chosen, particularly in cases involving language areas or pathways. In these instances, the initial surgery is continued as long as patient collaboration and responsiveness are maintained, and then is resumed from 1 week to several months later. In our institution, the patient is subjected to a second surgery 4 to 6 months later, which permits patient recovery from the initial surgery, and brain plasticity to occur.[40]

Cerebral plasticity could be defined as the continuous processing allowing short-, middle-, and long-term remodeling of the neurono-synaptic organization.[13] Plasticity may occur in the preoperative period in low-grade gliomas and in this case, is the results of the progressive functional brain reshaping induced by these slow growing lesions.[13,84,85] Brain plasticity also occurs in the postoperative period. This has been shown by submitting patients that have recovered from postoperative deficit status, to functional neuroimaging studies some months after surgery and when a recovery has occurred, demonstrating the activation of different areas of the brain, close or remote to those were involved in the preoperative period. Plasticity may occur at a cortical level or (less frequently) at a subcortical level, where it can be explained by the recruitment or unmasking of parallel and redundant subcortical circuits.[38] The occurrence of such phenomenon of compensation is of particular relevance because it allows extending surgical indications. It allows extending the initial surgery until functional boundaries are encountered, which allows the patient to recover in the postoperative period due to activation of redundant functional areas when the essential are preserved at the cortical or subcortical levels. Second, the functional reshaping induced by the initial surgery can be used to perform a second surgery with the aim of removing areas of the brain initially essential for function, and that due to the functional reshaping induced by the initial surgery or to the continuous slow growth of the tumor, have lost their essential nature in terms of function. This functional reshaping phenomenon can be observed up to a period of 6 months after the initial surgery, and allows performing a more radical second surgery with an increase in oncologic benefit for the patient.

Despite aggressive and early treatment, low-grade gliomas recur. As already discussed, the rate of recurrence is influenced by the preoperative tumor volume and to a lesser extent by the extent of surgical removal.[10,18,23,38] The duration of the longest-lasting symptom, tumor size, and presence of preoperative contrast enhancement are associated with tumor recurrence at last follow-up. A diagnosis of FA does not have a statistical association with tumor recurrence.[86] A tumor recurrence may still retain the morphologic feature of low-grade gliomas, or may show signs of tumor progression, such as contrast enhancement. The appearance of contrast enhancement is usually associated with a large preoperative volume, and with the presence of limited or focal enhancement in the preoperative MR images. Generally, when total or subtotal removals were achieved at the time of initial surgery, the recurrent tumor has a greater chance of recurring as a low-grade one. When only a partial removal was obtained, the potential for recurrence toward a higher grade is much greater. When a tumor recurs, various therapeutic options are available: surgery, chemotherapy, radiotherapy, or a wait-and-see policy.[13,83]

Surgery usually is intermingled with the other therapeutic modalities, and is the treatment of choice when a subtotal or even a total removal can be predicted, such as for discrete lesions. When this is feasible, the prognosis of the patient is still favorable. Brain mapping techniques can still be applicable in cases of recurrent tumors, even after radiotherapy. Alternatively, surgery may be used to decrease tumor volume to enhance the effect of chemo- or radiotherapy. Generally, a patient with low-grade gliomas may undergo several surgeries during the entire time of the disease, and surgery is used for various objectives and strictly associated with the other therapeutic modalities. Up to 30% of patients in our series underwent four surgeries, and 12% had up to five operations. We observed a decrease in the extent of resection with the increase in the number of surgeries, but this was not associated with an increase in the occurrence of transient and permanent postoperative deficits.

Conclusive Remarks

The purpose of brain mapping techniques is to identify and preserve at the time of surgery the cortical and subcortical sites essential to retain function. In our experience, in most low-grade gliomas, motor or language disturbances were induced either inside the tumor mass or at the tumor margins, because most of the essential sites, particularly at the subcortical level, were located within the tumor or adjacent to it. Resection was stopped when language, motor or visuospatial, cortical, and subcortical areas were encountered. Consequently, we have experienced an extremely low percentage of postoperative permanent neurologic deficits. The systematic use of brain mapping techniques reduced the incidence of postoperative deficits to less than 3%, much lower than the 23% obtained in our institution when these techniques were not applied. In addition, brain mapping did not negatively affect our ability to perform extensive resections in a large percentage of cases—on the contrary, the percentage of total and subtotal resections significantly improved in comparison to the time in which DES was not applied. This further influences seizure outcome and various oncologic endpoints, such as progression-free survival, overall survival, and malignant transformation.

Brain mapping and monitoring are demanding techniques. Especially in the case of awake surgery, these require close collaboration among neurosurgeon, neuropsychologist, and neurophysiologist. The latter two should be present in the operating room and work as a team to assist the surgeon to combine neurophysiologic information with the interpretation of language disturbances and compare these data with surgical anatomy. In addition, a well-trained anesthesiologist is essential, because sedation and analgesics must be titrated to keep the patient calm and without pain, but fully awake and able to reliably perform tasks. Excessive sedation or anxiety and pain, in fact, may reduce patient compliance and compromise test results. It is also worth mentioning that in the case of awake anesthesia, the patient needs to be prepared in advance to the awakening phase and to the performance of tasks in the operating room. As a matter of fact, brain mapping can be a significantly time-consuming procedure, in particular when the results of mapping are unsatisfactory and additional or repeated testing is required. This may obviously result in greater burden for the patient and need for rest, with further prolongation of surgical time. If patient compliance is compromised due to excessive duration of the procedure, stopping surgery with plans for a second intervention in 2 to 3 months is recommended. This can also be scheduled in advance according to tumor preoperative size and characteristics.

Along with the above described issues, brain mapping is intrinsically limited by the fact that only the functions that are specifically tested are preserved. If this is of relative importance for simple functions, such as motor functions, it is particularly relevant for complex cognitive functions. Time strongly affects mapping quality and that means only a limited number of well-selected tests can be administered to the patient: This should be kept in mind when dealing with large tumors located in the dominant hemisphere in areas densely filled with functional sites, such as the temporoparietal junction or the precentral area. In such regions, a careful selection of the tasks and a systematic execution of the mapping are crucial to save the basic cognitive functions, but may not be able to investigate other superior functions, such as calculation, writing, reading, and second languages. The surgeon has therefore to plan preoperatively, according to tumor size and location, which information should be obtained through the mapping procedure, and to inform the patient about the possible limitations of each approach.

Another critical technical issue is the relationship between stimulating current intensity and distance from the functional site, in particular when subcortical mapping is performed. In the literature, there are no available works studying the penetration distance of subcortical bipolar stimulation in the white matter, while the range of bipolar stimulation on the cortex has been observed to be approximately 2 to 10 mm.[11,33,66] When a response was induced at a subcortical level, we always performed an intensity–response curve, in order to assess the maintenance of the response at very low current intensity levels. This can help in estimating the distance between the point of stimulation and the functional tract. In addition, we commonly observed that as we approximated the end of the resection, a lower current intensity was needed to induce a response. Functional structures probably regain their normal excitability threshold once the mass effect exerted by the tumor is relieved. Anesthesiologic factors may also play a role (e.g., progressive clearance of anesthetic drugs). In order to maintain mapping reliability and to avoid false-positive findings that could lead to premature interruption of the resection, verifying and eventually decreasing the working current once a large part of the tumor has been removed are recommended. Nevertheless, further studies are needed to clarify this point.

Globally considered, surgery accomplished according to functional and anatomic boundaries allows maximal resection of the tumor and maximal preservation of patient functional integrity. This can be reached at the time of the initial surgery, depending on the functional organization of the brain, or may require additional surgeries, eventually intermingled with adjuvant treatments. The use of brain mapping techniques extends surgical indications with greater oncologic impact.

KEY REFERENCES

Bello L, Castellano A, Fava E, et al. Intraoperative use of DTI FT and subcortical mapping for surgical resection of gliomas: technical considerations. *Neurosurg Focus.* 2010;28:E6.

Bello L, Fava E, Carrabba G, et al. Present day's standards in microsurgery of low-grade gliomas. *Adv Tech Stand Neurosurg.* 2010;35:113-157.

Bello L, Gallucci M, Fava M, et al. Intraoperative subcortical language tract mapping guides surgical removal of gliomas involving speech areas. *Neurosurgery.* 2007;60:67-80:discussion 80-82.

Bello L, Gambini A, Castellano A, et al. Motor and language DTI fiber tracking combined with intraoperative subcortical mapping for surgical removal of gliomas. *Neuroimage. Jan.* 2008;1(39):369-382:Epub August 29, 2007.

Berger MS, Deliganis AV, Dobbins J, et al. The effect of extent of resection on recurrence in patients with low grade cerebral hemisphere gliomas. *Cancer.* 1994;74:1784-1791.

Bertani G, Fava E, Casaceli G, et al. Intraoperative mapping and monitoring of brain functions for the resection of low-grade gliomas: technical considerations. *Neurosurg Focus.* 2009;27:E4.

Capelle L, Duffau H, Lopes M, et al. Recurrence and malignant degeneration after resection of adult hemispheric low grade gliomas. *J Neurosurg.* 2010;112:10-17.

Claus EB, Horlacher A, Hsu L, et al. Survival rates in patients with low-grade glioma after intraoperative magnetic resonance image guidance. *Cancer.* 2005;103:1227-1233.

Desmurget M, Bonnetblanc F, Duffau H. Contrasting acute and slow-growing lesions: a new door to brain plasticity. *Brain.* 2007;130(Pt 4): 898-914.

Duffau H. Lessons from brain mapping in surgery for low-grade glioma: insights into associations between tumour and brain plasticity. *Lancet Neurol.* 2005;4:476-486.

Duffau H, Capelle L, Sichez N, et al. Intraoperative mapping of the subcortical language pathways using direct stimulations. An anatomo-functional study. *Brain.* 2002;125:199-214.

Duffau L, Capelle L. Preferential brain locations of low-grade gliomas. *Cancer.* 2004;100:2622-2626.

Hoang-Xuan K, Capelle L, Kujas M, et al. Temozolomide as initial treatment for adults with low-grade oligodendrogliomas or oligoastrocytomas and correlation with chromosome 1p deletions. *J Clin Oncol.* 2004;22:3133-3138.

Kaloshi G, Benouaich-Amiel A, Diakite F, et al. Temozolomide for low-grade gliomas: predictive impact of 1p/19q loss on response and outcome. *Neurology.* 2007;22(68):1831-1836.

Keles GE, Chang EF, Lamborn KR, et al. Volumetric extent of resection and residual contrast enhancement on initial surgery as predictors of outcome in adult patients with hemispheric anaplastic astrocytoma. *J Neurosurg.* 2006;105:34-40.

Keles GE, Lamborn KR, Berger MS. Lowgrade hemispheric gliomas in adults: a critical review of extent of resection as a factor influencing outcome. *J Neurosurg.* 2001;95:735-745.

Keles GE, Lundin DA, Lamborn KR, et al. Intraoperative subcortical stimulation mapping for hemispherical perirolandic gliomas located within or adjacent to the descending motor pathways: evaluation of morbidity and assessment of functional outcome in 294 patients. *J Neurosurg.* 2004;100:369-375.

Klein M, Heimans JJ. The measurement of cognitive functioning in low-grade glioma patients after radiotherapy. *J Clin Oncol.* 2004;22:966-967.

Lote K, Egeland T, Hager B, et al. Survival, prognostic factors, and therapeutic efficacy in low-grade glioma: a retrospective study in 379 patients. *J Clin Oncol.* 1997;15:3129-3140.

Mandonnet E, Jbabdi S, Taillandier L, et al. Preoperative estimation of residual volume for WHO grade II glioma resected with intraoperative functional mapping. *Neuro-oncology.* 2007;9:63-69.

Mokhtari K, Poirier J, Sahel M, et al. WHO grade 2 gliomas in adults: a study of prognostic factors with special emphasis on the role of surgery. *J Neurooncol.* 2002;4:S17-S69.

Pignatti F, van den Bent M, Curran D, et al. European Organization for Research and Treatment of Cancer Brain Tumor Cooperative Group; European Organization for Research and Treatment of Cancer Radiotherapy Cooperative Group: Prognostic factors for survival in adult patients with cerebral low-grade glioma. *J Clin Oncol.* 2002;20: 2076-2084.

Ricard D, Kaloshi G, Amiel-Benouaich A, et al. Dynamic history of low-grade gliomas before and after temozolomide treatment. *Ann Neurol.* 2007;61:484-490.

Sanai N, Berger MS. Glioma extent of resection and its impact on patient outcome. *Neurosurgery.* 2008;62:753-764:discussion 264-266. Review.

Smith JS, Chang EF, Lamborn KR, et al. Role of extent of resection in the long-term outcome of low-grade hemispheric gliomas. *J Clin Oncol.* 2008;26:1338-1345.

Numbered references appear on Expert Consult.

CHAPTER 10

Management of Recurrent Gliomas

GRIFFITH R. HARSH IV

Introduction

Renewed growth of a mass at the site of a previously treated glial tumor raises the issues of indications for and choices of treatment. Important considerations include the following:

1. Is the mass a recurrence of the original tumor?
2. Why did the tumor regrow?
3. What threat to the patient's neurologic function and survival does this regrowth pose?
4. What additional therapy is appropriate?

Confirmation of Recurrence

When recurrent growth of a glioma is suspected clinically or radiographically, the full set of imaging studies should be reviewed with careful attention directed toward detecting any change of imaging signals and documenting the size of the lesion. The original pathology specimen should be reviewed.

DIFFERENTIAL DIAGNOSIS

An enlarging lesion at the site of a previously treated tumor likely represents renewed growth of an incompletely eradicated initial tumor rather than the development of a new pathologic entity. Exceptions are infrequent but those in the following list need to be considered:

- A distinctly new tumor may arise at the site of an eradicated tumor. This is more likely to occur if there is a genetic predisposition to tumor development shared by cells in the area; for example, multiple gliomas may occur in a patient with tuberous sclerosis.
- A tumor of related histology may supplant the original tumor; for example, the astrocytic component may replace the oligodendrocytic component as the predominant subtype of a mixed glioma, or a gliosarcoma may arise from a previously treated glioblastoma.
- The initial therapy may induce a secondary tumor of a different type; for example, a glioblastoma in the radiation field of a low-grade glioma.
- Non-neoplastic lesions may mimic tumor growth; for example, an abscess or granuloma at the site of resection of a tumor induced by treatment of the original tumor, or radiation necrosis following focal high-dose irradiation.[1,2]

These alternative diagnoses must be excluded before prognosis is addressed and therapy is chosen. Neurodiagnostic imaging usually permits accurate prediction of the diagnosis. Generally, recurrent tumors have imaging features similar to those of the original lesion. A recurrent malignant glioma will likely have central low intensity, rim enhancement, and hypointense surround on enhanced T1-weighted magnetic resonance imaging (MRI). In some cases, however, attention to subtle differences may be required: a more spherical, sharply demarcated shape may suggest abscess rather than recurrent malignant glioma; and a diffuse, irregularly marginated pattern of surrounding edema may indicate radiation necrosis rather than recurrent tumor.

Two scenarios, malignant progression and radiation effects, often pose particular diagnostic difficulty. In each case, alternative diagnoses are often impossible to distinguish using current imaging modalities alone. Thus, biopsy for histologic evaluation and confirmation may be necessary.

MALIGNANT PROGRESSION

The first scenario is the renewed growth of a low grade tumor. When low grade gliomas regrow after therapy, approximately half remain nonanaplastic, but the other 50% have progressed to a more malignant form.[3] Molecular analyses have delineated genetic correlates of this progression.[4] Enlarging low grade tumors will usually resemble the original tumor on imaging studies. When progression in grade has occurred, the new tumor may also resemble the old one, especially if the original tumor enhanced with contrast. Enhancement is highly predictive of likelihood of recurrence; low grade enhancing tumors are 6–8 times more likely to recur than nonenhancing ones.[3] Most commonly, new malignant growth in a previously nonenhancing glioma enhances and thus is readily identified. In one study, only 30% (16/42) of low-grade tumors enhanced initially, but 92% (22/24) enhanced at recurrence.[3] Occasionally, an enlarging malignant focus may not enhance. It might, however, be apparent as a region of hypermetabolism on a 2-deoxyglucose or 11-C methionine PET study, or have an increased rate of enhancement on a dynamic MRI scan, increased activity on a dual-isotope, single-photon emission computerized tomogram (SPECT), or increased choline signal on magnetic resonance spectroscopy (MRS).[5-7] The differential specificity of each of these new modalities is approximately 80% to 90%. Usually, however, histologic analysis after biopsy or resection is warranted to verify malignant transformation.[8]

RADIATION EFFECTS

The second scenario that causes diagnostic difficulty is renewed enlargement of a tumor mass following radiation. Often, CT and MR imaging inadequately distinguish recurrent tumor from radiation-induced enlargement. Usually only large, very malignant tumors grow sufficiently fast to show significant enlargement during, or within 3 months of completing, a course of radiation. When this does occur, the prognosis is particularly poor.[9]

Radiation can cause tumor enlargement in three ways:[1] through an early reaction, occurring during or shortly after irradiation, which is likely to be edema;[2] through an early delayed reaction arising a few weeks to a few months after radiation which involves edema and demyelination; and[3] through a late delayed reaction that occurs 6 to 24 months after radiation and reflects radiation-induced necrosis.[10] Regional teletherapy to a dose of 60 Gy is the current standard radiation treatment for most gliomas.[11] Although these doses have a low risk of inducing radiation necrosis, regional early and early delayed effects are relatively common. In most cases, tissue swelling represents edema and is transient. Acute symptoms from early and early delayed effects of radiation usually respond quickly to a short course of corticosteroids. The low density, T1 hypointense, T2 hyperintense regions of edema correspond to the area irradiated. Chronically, these volumes of brain will demonstrate parenchymal atrophy, enlargement of subarachnoid spaces, and ex vacuo ventricular dilatation. Dementia with apathy, inanition, and memory loss and decline in fine motor control are the clinical correlates. In the absence of new tumor growth, enhancement on CT and MRI beyond the initial resection margin is infrequent; when it does occur, it is patchy, irregularly marginated, and it can be distinguished from the more focal appearance of recurrent tumor.

In contrast, the late delayed effect of radiation-induced necrosis appears at about the time malignant tumors might be expected to recur.[12] It is thus more likely to be mistaken for recurrent tumor growth. The risk of radiation necrosis increases with the volume of tissue treated, the dose delivered, and the fraction size.[13] Radiation necrosis following fractionated treatment to doses less than 70 Gy is rare, but it is much more common following brachytherapy or radiosurgery, which deliver high doses of radiation to relatively small volumes over a short time period.[12,14,15] A common protocol for brachytherapy is a 50- to 60-Gy boost (to 60 Gy of regional external beam radiotherapy) to a 0- to 5-cm tumor delivered over approximately 1 week. The radiosurgery equivalent is a 10- to 20-Gy boost to a 0- to 3-cm diameter tumor delivered in less than 1 hour.[16] Necrosis is radiographically and pathologically evident in almost all cases and symptomatic in about half.

Whether it arises from higher doses of fractionated radiotherapy, brachytherapy, or radiosurgery, radiation necrosis is often difficult to distinguish from recurrent tumor. It forms a ring contrast-enhancing mass that resembles a malignant tumor. It has a CT hypodense, T1 hypointense, T2 hyperintense center; an enhancing annular region; and a hypodense, T1 hypointense, T2 hyperintense surround. The surround corresponds to edema that strikingly radiates along white matter tracts. The similarity of this appearance to that of recurrent tumors and the time course of its occurrence frequently necessitates additional measures to differentiate radiation-induced necrosis from recurrent tumor. A variety of functional neurodiagnostic imaging techniques attempt to distinguish between these two possibilities. These include PET scans, SPECT studies, cerebral blood volume mapping, and MRS. Regions of high activity are thought to distinguish recurrent tumor from relatively metabolically inactive and hypovascular radiation necrosis.[6] Although specificity in differentiating tumor from radiation necrosis of up to 100% has been claimed, in many cases these studies are inconclusive and the diagnosis is revealed either by the clinical course or by analysis of a pathology specimen.

When an enlarging mass, which is either recurrent tumor, radiation necrosis, or both, becomes symptomatic, corticosteroid therapy is required.[17] Up to half the patients receiving brachytherapy and radiosurgery for a malignant glioma develop symptoms that either prove refractory to corticosteroids or require debilitating long-term steroid use.[12,18,19] Surgery for resection of an enlarging, symptomatic mass is needed in 20% to 40% of cases following brachytherapy or radiosurgery of a malignant glioma. At reoperation for presumed radiation necrosis following focal radiation treatment of a malignant glioma, necrosis without tumor was found in 5% of cases, tumor alone in 29%, and a mixture of radiation necrosis and tumor in 66%.[12] In almost all cases, the tumor that is seen is of reduced viability.[20,21]

Causes of Recurrence

Renewed growth of a brain tumor following surgery and possibly radiation and chemotherapy indicates failure of these therapies to reduce the tumor mass to a size and cell number that would permit its eradication by the patient's immune system (Fig. 10-1).[22] Failure arises from a number of factors that limit the efficacy of each modality.

RECURRENCE AFTER SURGERY

Surgery may fail because of anatomic considerations, pathologic features, or errors in judgment or technique. The involvement of critical structures may limit the initial resection: involvement of the optic pathways, diencephalon, internal capsule, brain stem, or eloquent cortex by a glioma often precludes complete removal. Tumor recurrence, despite removal of all macroscopically evident tumor, can occur if there is microscopic infiltration of adjacent

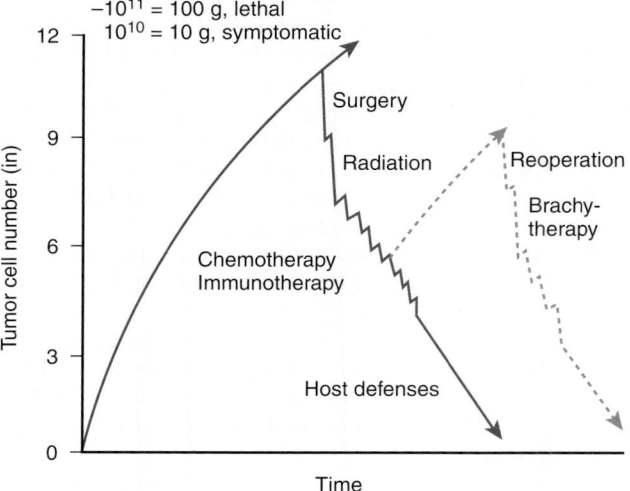

FIGURE 10-1 Multimodality therapy of malignant gliomas. Various therapeutic methods, including reoperation, are used in the attempt to reduce the number of tumor cells.

structures. Even low grade cerebral gliomas are usually infiltrative. Anaplastic astrocytomas characteristically are widely invasive. Finally, errors in judgment, such as preoperatively underestimating the amount of tumor that can be safely removed or intraoperatively failing to remove tumor that was targeted, result in potentially resectable tumor being left as a nidus of regrowth.

RECURRENCE AFTER RADIATION

Radiation therapy may fail because of inadequate targeting, underutilization of tolerable dose, or radiation resistance of the tumor cells. Proximity to critical anatomical structures can also limit maximal allowable radiation dosage. Furthermore, the correlations between imaging abnormality and tumor extent are incomplete. Pathologic studies have shown that individual tumor cells can be found throughout and even beyond CT hypodense and MRI T2 hyperintense areas of malignant glioma.[23,24] For each individual case, the extent of brain invasion from the contrast-enhancing margin of a malignant glioma is incompletely known. The choice of field size for irradiation of such lesions is difficult and relies as much on the trade-off between target volume and tolerable dose as on the accurate delineation of tumor boundaries. Failure to include an adequate annulus of tissue about the tumor to accommodate imaging uncertainty and technical error may leave tumor cells incompletely irradiated.

Even if the maximal dose tolerated by infiltrative surrounding brain is delivered, tumor cells may remain viable. Hypoxic, nonproliferating cells and tumor stem cells are particularly radioresistant; with time or change in the physiologic conditions following therapy, re-entry of cells into the cell cycle permits the proliferation that results in clinically apparent tumor recurrence.[25,26] Analysis of patterns of failure demonstrates that, even with maximal tolerable doses of photon radiation of 70 to 80 Gy, almost all malignant astrocytomas fail centrally.[27] A study of high dose fractionated proton irradiation following radical resection of glioblastomas showed the following:[1] a dose between 80 and 90 Gy is sufficient to prevent tumor regrowth;[2] outside of this high dose volume, tumor regrows, usually in areas receiving between 60 and 70 Gy;[3] enlargement of the high dose volume to include more peripheral areas is likely to induce unacceptably high levels of symptomatic radiation-related necrosis.[28]

RECURRENCE AFTER CHEMOTHERAPY

Chemotherapy fails as a result of inadequate drug delivery, toxicity, or cell resistance. The blood–brain barrier is deficient in the contrast-enhancing region of the tumor, but surrounding brain usually has an intact blood–brain barrier; lipid-insoluble drugs thus have limited access to tumor cells infiltrating peripheral regions. The margin between drug efficacy and neurotoxicity, bone marrow suppression, pulmonary injury, and gastrointestinal side-effects is often narrow. Non-cycling cells and tumor stem cells are resistant to cell-cycle specific drugs, and potentially vulnerable cells often rapidly develop biochemical means of resistance to chemotherapeutic agents.[25,26,29]

Even if these therapies significantly reduce the tumor burden, the patient's immune response may be rendered ineffective by chemotherapy and by the tumor's secretion of factors antagonistic to immune function, such as IL-10, prostaglandin E2, and transforming growth factor (TGF)-beta 2, and its expression of apoptosis-inducing molecules, such as Fas ligand (FasL) and galectin-1.[30] Each of these limitations of each component of multimodality therapy may contributes to failure to prevent tumor regrowth. At the time of tumor recurrence, consideration of these reasons for failure is essential to assessment of prognosis and to the choice of subsequent therapy.

Prognostic Implications of Residual and Recurrent Tumor

In the management of a recurrent glioma, consideration of the prognostic implications of regrowth is essential. The presence of residual tumor and the occurrence of tumor regrowth likely have different prognostic implications.

RESIDUAL TUMOR

Radiologic demonstration of residual tumor after initial treatment may be consistent with preoperative goals and expectations; the prognosis would be that originally formulated. If, however, residual tumor is identified unexpectedly, the prognosis may need to be altered. The prognostic import of residual tumor is best seen in the relationship between extent of resection and likelihood of tumor recurrence.

Cytoreductive surgery is a fundamental part of the treatment of most systemic malignancies.[31] In most cases, there is a strong relationship between the extent of resection and outcome. For gliomas, correlation between extent of resection or, more significantly, size of residual tumor, and outcome measures, such as interval to tumor progression and survival, has been strongly suggested by retrospective and prospective series, but not by randomized clinical trials.[32] More recently, one study, reported a significant survival advantage when 98% or greater resection is achieved.[33]

Correlation of survival with extent of resection for low grade gliomas has been suggested by retrospective uncontrolled reviews and comparisons with historical controls.[3,34-36] One study of 461 adult patients with low grade cerebral gliomas found that gross total surgical removal correlated with length of survival.[37] Another reported median survival duration of 7.4 years following maximal surgical resection. The median survival of a subgroup patients with hemispheric tumors compared favorably (10 years vs. 8 years) with that of a comparable series treated with biopsy and radiation alone.[3,35] Additional studies have demonstrated that extensive resection of low grade gliomas delays tumor recurrence.[36,38]

For high grade gliomas, the correlations between the extent of resection at the initial operation and[1] the time to tumor recurrence and[2] the duration of patient survival have been disputed.[39] Historical reports and reviews of large series have noted the association of survival and extent of resection for both astrocytomas and oligodendrogliomas.[11,40-43] Extensive reviews of the literature, however, have failed to locate randomized, controlled clinical trials comparing survival after biopsy with that after radical resection of malignant gliomas.[44,45] Nevertheless, the benefit of surgical cytoreduction has been strongly suggested by the following findings:

1. Reviews of multicentered trials have shown that the more complete the resection, the longer the patient lived.[46-48]

2. In a study of 243 patients, multivariate regression analysis identified extent of resection as an important prognostic factor ($p < 0.0001$) for survival.[49]

3. In a retrospective review of 1215 patients with WHO grade III or IV, increasing extent of surgical resection was associated with improved survival independent of age, degree of disability WHO grade, or subsequent treatment modalities used.[50]

4. Single center studies have confirmed this relationship: in one study containing 21 glioblastomas and 10 anaplastic astrocytomas, median duration of survival after gross total resection was 90 weeks versus only 43 weeks following subtotal resection, and the 2-year survival rates were 19% and 0%, respectively, even though the two groups were well matched for other prognostically significant variables;[34,51] in another study, patients with gross total resection of malignant glioma lived longer (76 vs. 19 weeks) than those who underwent only a biopsy, even after correction for tumor accessibility and all other prognostically significant variables[52] and one large recent series showed that GTR (>98%) significantly increases the duration of survival.[33]

5. In two larger series, patients with resected cortical and subcortical grade IV gliomas lived longer (50.6 vs. 33.0 weeks[53] and 39.5 vs. 32.0 weeks[54] after surgery and radiation than those who underwent biopsy and radiation.

6. Small postoperative tumor volume has been shown to correlate with longer time to tumor progression after surgery[55] and longer patient survival.[56,57]

Although less than ideal, the data that exist for gliomas and experience with tumors outside the central nervous system suggest the benefit of cytoreduction when a near-total removal (2 log reduction of tumor cell number) of a glial tumor can be achieved. Thus, failure to identify and remove readily accessible tumor mass at an initial operation might warrant reoperation before regrowth occurs.

RECURRENT TUMOR

Regrowth of tumors after an initial response (diminution or stability) to surgery and radiation therapy is ominous. This is particularly true if the growth is more rapid or more infiltrative than that of the original tumor. Such growth often exhibits changes in the basic biology of the tumor that make it less responsive to subsequent therapy. A short interval between initial treatment and recurrence of symptoms often indicates rapid regrowth and a poor prognosis. Factors to be considered in estimating prognosis include the biology of the tumor (its pathology, growth rate, and invasiveness), its resectability, its prior response to radiation and chemotherapy, and the age and performance status of the patient.[58] Estimates of the recurrent tumor's size, growth rate, invasiveness, and location must be made in assessing its potential for causing both neurologic deficit and death. Reappearance of a slowly growing, well-demarcated frontal convexity oligodendroglioma with deletions of chromosomes 1p and 19q in a middle-aged patient of good

neurologic condition after a 10-year interval of postsurgical quiescence clearly carries a prognosis very different from that of diffuse diencephalic spread of a glioblastoma multiforme in an elderly patient with a poor performance status 3 months after treatment with surgery, radiation, and chemotherapy.[59]

Therapy of Recurrent Glial Tumors

The choice of therapy of a recurrent tumor is based upon a comparison of the natural history of the regrowing tumor with the risk–benefit calculus of potential therapies.

THERAPY OF RECURRENT GLIOMAS

The choice of therapy of a recurrent glioma is based on a comparison of the natural history of the regrowing tumor with the risk–benefit ratio of potential therapies. Recurrent gliomas warrant aggressive multimodality therapy if the patient is in good neurologic and general medical condition and therapeutic options offer a realistic chance for significant improvement in neurologic status or extension of survival.[60]

PATTERNS OF RECURRENCE OF GLIOMAS

When gliomas recur, most do so locally. Historically, more than 80% of recurrent glioblastoma multiforme arose within 2 cm of the original margin of contrast-enhancing tumor.[61,62] In one series, over 90% of glioma cases showed recurrence at the original tumor location, while 5% developed multiple lesions after treatment.[63] In another study of 36 patients with malignant gliomas receiving 70 to 80 Gy of fractionated radiation, 32 (89%) had central (at least 95% of the recurrent tumor within the volume receiving at least 95% of the maximum dose) or in-field (at least 80% of tumor within this highest dose volume) recurrence, and 3 (8%) had marginal recurrence. Only one (3%) fell predominantly outside the high dose range. Seven patients had multiple sites of recurrence, but only one had a large recurrence outside the high dose volume.[27] This tendency to recur locally is a function of tumor cell distribution. There is a gradient of tumor cell density in which tumor cell number decreases rapidly at increasing distances from the contrast-enhancing rim of solid tumor. Thus, although individual tumor cells spread through the brain at great distances from the primary site, there are so many more cells locally that the odds favor local reaccumulation of tumor mass.[23,24]

Factors contributing to the likelihood of local recurrence include the following:

1. Relative predominance of tumor cell mass in the region
2. Statistical likelihood that a local cell will be the cell that first develops a competitive proliferative advantage
3. Possibility that the physiologic milieu (hypervascularity and increased permeability, disrupted tissue architecture, and paracrine growth factor stimuli) at the site is particularly conducive to regrowth.

As tumor cell proliferation resumes at the initial tumor site, cells again spread rapidly and diffusely. Tumor cell proliferation resumes at distant sites as a result of the influx of these new, mitotically active cells or the renewed growth of cells that spread before the initial treatment.[63] Biologic therapeutic agents may also affect the pattern of recurrence; recent experience with bevacizumab (Avastin) suggests that tumors treated with this inhibitor of VEGF are more likely to recur as diffusely infiltrative lesions distant from the original site of tumor.[64] Consequently, treatments targeting local recurrence alone will, at best, be briefly palliative. Treatment of tumor recurrence thus usually involves a combination of modalities aimed at both local and distant disease.

EPIDEMIOLOGY OF RECURRENT GLIOBLASTOMA

The heterogeneity in defining recurrence and the variability of treatment algorithms employed at different institutions result in a vague profile of recurrent glioblastoma multiforme.[65] In a multi-center trial of reoperation for resection and placement of cavitary biodegradable BCNU-wafer in 222 patients with recurrent glioblastoma and a Karnofsky Performance Score of at least 60, the median interval from initial diagnosis to tumor recurrence was 12 months.[66] Among a cohort of 301 patients with GBM, 223 patients had tumor recurrence at a median interval from initial diagnosis of 4.9 months;[67] 64% of these had a Karnovsky Performance Score greater than 70 at the time of recurrence.

Glioblastoma recurrence is demonstrated on imaging obtained in routine surveillance or in response to new or recurring symptoms. In a questionnaire-based study of patients with recurrent glioblastoma or anaplastic astrocytoma and a KPS >70, self-reported symptoms included fatigue, uncertainty about the future, motor difficulties, drowsiness, communication difficulties, and headache.[68] While most symptoms likely reflected tumor recurrence, confounding factors such as radiation necrosis and steroid treatment may have contributed to generalized fatigue, and pain and uncertainty about the future may have resulted from the diagnosis alone, independent of current tumor status. Incoordination, weakness, visual loss, and pain were reported more frequently by patients with recurrent glioblastoma than by those with anaplastic astrocytoma, providing evidence that more aggressive disease will cause greater neurological deficit.

THERAPY OF RECURRENT MALIGNANT GLIOMA

Choice of therapy for a recurrent glioma must consider the tumor's current and previous histology, previous treatment, and location and the patient's age, medical and neurologic conditions, and preferences. An enlarging lesion that was originally a low grade glioma should undergo biopsy (stereotactically or, if resection is anatomically feasible, by open craniotomy) to confirm histology (Fig. 10-2). If the tumor remains low grade and a large part of the lesion can be resected without inflicting significant neurologic deficit, it should be removed; if previously irradiated to significantly less than maximal tolerable dose, the tumor bed and surrounding area should receive fractionated radiotherapy. The longer the interval since the initial radiotherapy, the higher the dose that can be given safely at recurrence. If the tumor is inaccessible to surgery, radiation alone should be prescribed. If a low grade tumor previously irradiated to a maximal tolerable dose recurs as a low grade glioma, it should be resected, if possible. If it is inaccessible, stereotactically delivered focal radiation is an attractive option.[69,70]

Surgery

If the low grade tumor recurs as a high grade tumor or if a high grade tumor recurs, reoperation should be attempted if the patient has a Karnofsky score of at least 70 and removal of all or almost all of the contrast-enhancing tumor is potentially attainable, or if the tumor mass is causing neurologic symptoms that might be palliated by its reduction. Removal of tumor may improve the patient's quality of life by alleviating neurologic deficit or permitting reduction of steroid dose. It may also prolong survival by reducing tumor burden and improving response to radiation, chemotherapy, immunotherapy, or biologic therapy.[71,72]

Radiation Therapy

If the tumor was not irradiated previously, the tumor bed and its annular margin should receive regional radiotherapy. Even when radiotherapy has been used initially, it is an option at recurrence, but doses permitted under standard guidelines for conventional fractionation and volumes are unlikely to be high enough to be effective. Other possibilities include highly conformal conventionally fractionated radiotherapy (e.g., IMRT, intensity modulated radiation therapy), hypofractionated stereotactic radiotherapy, interstitial brachytherapy, and stereotactic radiosurgery.[72-76] In one study, the use of highly conformal teletherapy for re-irradiation of recurrent gliomas (mean re-irradiation dose of 38 Gy, range 30.6–59.4 Gy) at a median time of 38 months (range 9–234 months) produced radiographic stability or regression and neurologic improvement in two thirds of the patients.[75] In another study, 10 patients with recurrent malignant gliomas treated with intensity-modulated radiation therapy (daily fractions of 5 Gy to a total median dose of 30 Gy) demonstrated median overall survival duration of 10.1 months from the time of treatment, with 1- and 2-year survival rates of 50% and 33%, respectively.[76]

Hypofractionated stereotactic radiotherapy (SRT) combines high dose per fraction with stereotactic targeting. Hypofractionated SRT (e.g., 20–30 Gy in 2–5-Gy fractions) of recurrent malignant gliomas resulted in a median duration of subsequent survival of 9.3 months (15.4 months for grade III tumors and 7.9 months for grade IV tumors) in one study.[77] Another protocol that delivered 20 to 50 Gy in 5-Gy fractions to 29 patients with recurrent high grade astrocytomas resulted in a median duration of survival after retreatment of 11 months.[78] Steroid dependent toxicity occurred in 36% of patients, reoperation was required in 6%, and a total dose in excess of 40 Gy predicted radiation damage ($p < 0.005$). Another study used 24 Gy in 3 Gy fractions, 30 Gy in 3 Gy fractions, and 35 Gy in 3.5 Gy fractions to boost previously irradiated residual or recurrent malignant gliomas at a mean of 3.1 months (range 1–46 months) after standard treatment to 60 Gy. Sixty percent of patients required less steroid and 45% improved neurologically. Eighty percent of those receiving 30 or 35 Gy responded. The median duration of survival was 10.5 months. No grade 3 toxicity occurred. Reoperation was not performed.[79] A fourth protocol combined fractionated stereotactic radiosurgery and taxol as a radiosensitizer for recurrent malignant gliomas. It resulted in median survival duration of 14.2 months in 14 selected patients.[80] These four studies suggest that hypofractionated SRT has moderate efficacy and acceptable safety in selected patients.

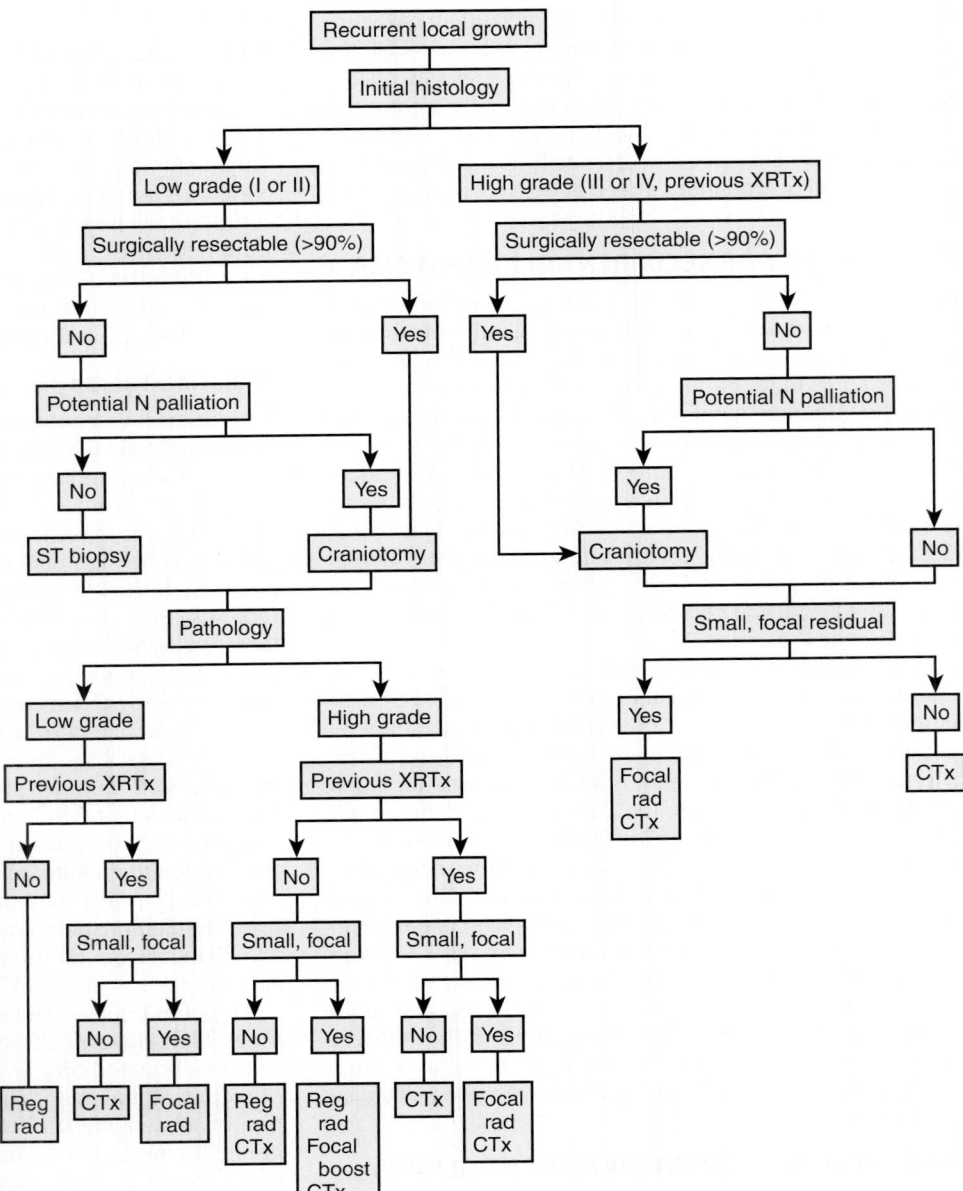

FIGURE 10-2 Recurrent glioma. Decisions in the management of a recurrent tumor should consider grade, resectability, and prior therapy. N, neurologic; reg rad, regional fractionated radiation therapy; focal rad/boost, stereotactic radiosurgery, brachytherapy, or radiotherapy; small, focal, less than 10 cm³, radiographically demarcated; CTx, chemotherapy; ST, stereostatic; XRTx, radiotherapy.

Although several studies suggested promise for brachytherapy in treating glioblastomas, both initially and at the time of recurrence, tumors in these studies were highly selected for small size and focality, two features that would make them appropriate for stereotactic radiosurgery or radiotherapy, less invasive techniques with equivalent results.[12,81,82] In a retrospective comparison of interstitial brachytherapy and radiosurgery for recurrent glioblastomas, the median durations of survival in the two groups were similar (11.5 months and 10.2 months, respectively). Patterns of failure were similar. The actuarial risks of reoperation for necrosis at 12 and 24 months were 33% and 48% respectively, after radiosurgery, and 54% and 65%, respectively, after brachytherapy, with the caveat that the brachytherapy group had larger tumors and longer follow-up.[83,84]

Other forms of focal radiation therapy of recurrent gliomas such as photodynamic therapy (PDT), boron neutron capture therapy (BNCT), intraoperative radiation (IORT),

and radiolabeled monoclonal antibodies to tumor cells' surface receptors have been studied.[85-90] A dozen clinical trials have measured the safety and efficacy of irradiation of a tumor's resection cavity by 131I-labeled mAb 81C6 (anti-tenascin C). Promising results for this technique during initial resection suggest its potential utility during reoperation as well.[90]

Although some of these studies report modest benefit, the diffuse infiltration of malignant tumors at the time of recurrence and the dose-limiting toxicity that occurs after 60-70 Gy of radiation frustrate focal therapies and warrant more systemic approaches such as chemotherapy and biologic and immune therapies.

Chemotherapy

Chemotherapy of infiltrative gliomas at diagnosis and at recurrence is often valuable. Temozolamide (Temodar, TMZ), an oral DNA-methylating agent with a benefit-toxicity profile superior to that of antecedent alternative intravenous alkylating agents such as BCNU and CCNU, has become the drug of choice. TMZ is appropriate for those low grade tumors not treated by chemotherapy at the time of initial presentation; one study reported a response rate of 47%.[91] If the tumor recurs despite TMZ, a protracted schedule of TMZ administration or strategies using CCNU alone, PCV, bevacizumab (Avastin) alone or bevacizumab combined with other drugs (e.g., Irinotecan) can be given.[64,92-95]

For Grade III tumors, TMZ is also recommended.[96] Perhaps reflective of the favorable biology of the tumor, TMZ of anaplastic oligodendrogliomas with deletions of chromosomes 1p and 19q is particularly effective.[59,97] In the initial treatment of patients with GBM, the addition of TMZ to radiotherapy increases the percentage of patients surviving at 2 years to 26.5% from 10.4% for radiotherapy alone and the median duration of survival to 14.6 months from 12.1 months.[98] At the time of renewed growth of a high grade tumor, if the tumor has not previously been exposed to TMZ, TMZ should be given. If TMZ had been used but it was discontinued prior to either tumor progression or treatment-limiting toxicity occurring, rechallenge with TMZ or a single nitrosurea agent would be appropriate.[99] Patients treated for recurrent or progressive GBM with TMZ showed an overall response rate of 19% and mean time to progression of 11.7 weeks.[99] Similarly, treatment of recurrent GBM with a standard TMZ regimen (150 to 200 $mg/m^2 \times 5$ days in 28-day cycles) produced a progression-free survival rate of 6 months (PFS-6) of 21% vs. 8% following procarbazine.[100] A more intensive regimen (150 mg/m^2 daily on a week on/week off cycle) yielded a PFS-6 of 48% with an overall PFS-12 of 81%[101] and combinations of TMZ with the matrix metalloproteinase inhibitor, marimastat, or 13-cis-retinoic acid, produced rates of PFS-6 of 39% and 32%, respectively.[102] If TMZ was used to treat the primary tumor and toxicity occurred, then an agent with a different toxicity risk profile should be used.[95]

Limitations of the efficacy of TMZ and related alkylating agents (BCNU, CCNU) reflect cellular drug resistance mechanisms, including the suppression of DNA repair mechanisms. The MGMT cytoprotective repair protein removes TMZ-induced methyl adducts at the O6-guanine in DNA.[103,104] Administration of O6-benzlguanine to suppress this DNA repair has increased the cytotoxicity of TMZ in preclinical models.[105]

Intracavitary implantation of wafers of drug polymers attempts to enhance local drug delivery while avoiding systemic side effects. The initial randomized, double blinded clinical trial with intracavitary BCNU wafers showed longer median survival (31 vs. 23 weeks) and improved survival rates 6 months after treatment of recurrent GBM in the BCNU arm relative to the placebo arm, but the survival curves converged at longer follow-up, and higher rates of symptomatic edema, infection (3.6% vs. 0.9%) and seizures (37.3% vs. 28.6%) were noted.[66]

Chemotherapy offers little benefit to patients whose tumors recur a second time.[106] Nor is multiagent chemotherapy more beneficial than single-agent chemotherapy.[107] And hematologic toxicity is worse with more complex combinatorial agents.[108-110]

For cancer patients, quality of life is an important consideration. Patients suffering from recurrent GBM reported greater satisfaction and a higher health-related quality of life (HRQOL) when treated with TMZ than with PCV.[68] Choice of chemotherapy should consider such findings as well as efficacy, toxicity, and cost.

Biologic and Immune Therapies

Delineation of the molecular pathways of glial tumorigenesis has fostered development and testing of small molecule inhibitors and monoclonal antibodies targeting their components. Erlotinib and gefitinib, inhibitors of the epidermal growth factor receptor (EGFR)—a tyrosine kinase amplified or mutated in a high percentage of glioblastomas—are two examples of such molecular-based therapeutic agents. However, recent phase II trials have failed to demonstrate convincing effect. Gefitinib provided rates of progression-free survival at 8 months (PFS-6) of 14% in a prospective study of 28 patients with recurrent or progressive high-grade glioma and of 13% in 53 patients with recurrent glioblastoma.[111,112] A randomized, phase II trial conducted by the European Organization for Research and Treatment of Cancer found a PFS-6 of 12%, for patients with recurrent glioblastomas treated with gefitinib compared to a PFS-6 of 24% for the control group treated with either BCNU or TMZ.[113] Disappointment over the failure of EGFR inhibitors as single agents has not dimmed optimism that they may be more valuable when used in conjunction with other therapeutic agents.

EGFRvIII, a constitutively active form of the receptor resulting from its most common deletion (found in each 30% of GBM), has been targeted by small inhibitory molecules and monoclonal antibodies specific for the mutated receptor. Tyrphostin, an inhibitor of EGFR more active against the mutated than against the wild-type receptor, has significantly delayed tumor recurrence in animal models and is entering the clinical phase of trials.[114] And mAbs raised against the variant receptor have shown antitumor effects in cell culture.[115]

Since EGFR is an initial component of the PI3Kinase pathway, which is crucial to cell survival, proliferation and motility, tumor cells, when chronically activated by the EGFRvIII mutation, become dependent on PI3k, and thus potentially sensitized to its disruption.[116,117] Interestingly, the PTEN tumor–suppressor protein, an inhibitor of the P13K pathway, is often lost in glioblastoma.[118] Based on these observations, it has been hypothesized that while possession of the EGFRvIII mutation would sensitize tumors to EGFR kinase inhibitors, loss of PTEN would mitigate this effect by disassociating EGFR inhibition from inhibition of the downstream P13K pathway. Coexpression of EGFRvIII and PTEN at both mRNA and protein levels was significantly associated with a clinical response in glioblastomas treated with EGFR kinase inhibitors.[117] Thus, although inhibition of EGFR activity and the PI3K pathway may not be effective against all GBM, it may hold promise against tumors, at diagnosis or at recurrence, selected for having predisposing molecular lesions.

Targeting the tumor's vasculature is another promising strategy.[119] Bevacizumab (Avastin), an inhibitor of vascular endothelial growth factor (VEGF) with antiangiogenic and antiedema effects, rapidly reduces contrast enhancement at the site of tumor. This response is associated with increased time to tumor progression: bevacizumab and

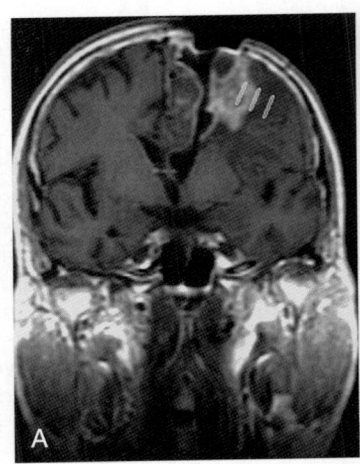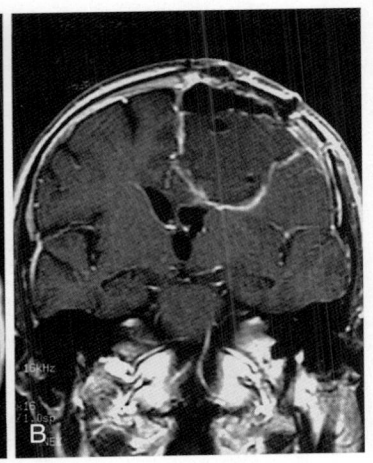

FIGURE 10-3 Adjuvant therapy. Reoperation provides the opportunity to implant drug polymers, immune stimulants, toxins, viruses, radioisotpoes, therapeutic cells, and infusion catheters for subsequent delivery of therapeutic agents. A 39-year-old man developed marginal recurrence about the cystic resection cavity left after removal and irradiation of an anaplastic astrocytoma 3 years previously. As part of a gene-therapy trial, three columns of vector-producing cells were infused within the tumor, at the tumor margin, and in the surrounding tumor-infiltrated brain. A, Coronal MRI. Five days later, the tumor and the infused tissue to be analyzed were removed. Care was taken to extend the resection to the margin of eloquent areas and to achieve watertight closure. B, Coronal, immediately postoperative MRI.

irinotecan produced a PFS-6 rate of 46% in patients with recurrent glioblastoma.[120] Despite other similarly impressive bevacizumab-induced increases in time to local recurrence of contrast-enhancing tumor, lengthened overall survival has not been observed. This suggests that the rapid, often substantial, reduction of contrast enhancement induced by bevacizumab may reflect decreases in vascular permeability rather than true regression of tumor. Furthermore, there is increasing concern both that the suppression of angiogenesis during treatment is transient and that treatment may favor more diffuse, initially hypoangiogenic growth.[64] Despite these concerns, an advisory committee to the Food and Drug Administration recently unanimously recommended approval of bevacizumab for treatment of glioblastoma.

Immunotherapy also holds great promise for patients with malignant gliomas.[121] Efforts to enhance the immune response to tumors include both passive and active strategies.[122] Passive approaches include implantation of modified immune cells into a resection cavity. One early study employing lymphokine-activated killer (LAK) cells and IL-2 reported a median duration of survival of 53 weeks after reoperation and implantation compared with 26 weeks following reoperation and chemotherapy.[123] Another implanting the LAK cells without the IL-2 in 40 patients with recurrent glioblastomas reported a median duration of survival of 9 months and a 1-year survival rate of 34%.[124] Adoptive immunotherapy, a variety of passive immunotherapy, is receiving great interest. Tissue harvested at surgery is disaggregated and various constituents (simple lysate, DNA, proteins, etc.) are used to prime dendritic cells harvested from the patient's blood or tumor.[125,126] Active immune strategies employ vaccination. Clinical testing of a vaccine to EGFR vIII has progressed to a phase III trial based on safety and efficacy against newly diagnosed GBM in phase I and II trials.[127] Confirmation of the actual clinical benefit of these and other efforts to enhance the immune response awaits completion of phase III trials.

Monoclonal antibodies to other tumor cell surface receptors have also been used to block other components of growth factor signaling pathways (e.g., PDGF), to deliver toxins specifically to tumor cells (e.g., toxin linked to EGF or IL-13), and, as mentioned above, to selectively irradiate tumor sites (e.g., I131-mAb).[90,128] For example, *Pseudomonas* exotoxin has been targeted to the IL-13 receptors highly expressed on malignant glioma cells by injecting the toxin conjugated to IL-13 into the resection cavity of recurrent, malignant glioma. *Pseudomonas* exotoxin conjugated to TGFalpha also has been investigated in a phase I trial, with relative safety but mixed results in terms of efficacy. Overall, toxin delivery by cytokines has demonstrated relative safety and variable efficacy.

Cells carrying therapeutic genes have also been used. Preliminary gene therapy studies using ganciclovir activated by a thymidine kinase gene delivered by a retrovirus produced by a modified mouse fibroblast packaging cell line have proved feasibility and safety but have not yet achieved proof of mechanism or demonstrated efficacy.[129,130] In a small study that examined the effects of an intratumoral injection of retroviral vector-producing cells combined with intravenous ganciclovir, the authors obtained a 1-year survival rate of 25% with tumor response in 50% of the cases.[131]

Numerous such strategies utilize reoperation to harvest tissue for molecular analysis or to guide tumor specific therapies and as a source of agents for vaccination. Reoperation also presents an opportunity to implant drug polymers, immune stimulants, toxins, viruses, radioisotopes, therapeutic cells, and infusion catheters for subsequent delivery of therapeutic agents (Fig. 10-3).[66,123,128,129,131]

Reoperation for Malignant Glioma

RATIONALE FOR REOPERATION

Early reoperation, within months of the initial procedure, might be indicated for complications such as intracerebral, subdural, or epidural hematoma, wound dehiscence and infection, or hydrocephalus and CSF leakage. Occasionally, failure to identify and remove readily accessible tumor mass might warrant reoperation. In the Royal Melbourne Hospital experience, 5 of 200 patients underwent early reoperation.[132] More frequently, true tumor recurrence after an interval of response to the initial therapy is the reason for considering reoperation. Reoperation is justified if it produces sustained improvement of neurologic condition and quality of life or significant increase of response rates to adjuvant therapy. Palliation of neurologic symptoms by surgery results from reduction of the local mass effect produced by the tumor and tumor-induced edema. Steroid dose may be able to be reduced and steroid side effects diminished.

Multiple studies have shown that initial surgical cytoreduction of a malignant glioma can both improve neurologic deficits and promote maintenance of high-performance status. One review of 82 patients examined five categories of neurologic function in each patient. Preoperatively, 191 neurologic deficits were noted. Postoperatively, 151 deficits were improved or stable and 40 were worse.[133] Another study showed that patients undergoing gross total resection of their malignant gliomas were likely to have improved neurologic function (97% of 36 patients had either improved or stable neurologic examinations), higher functional status (mean KPS score improvement of 6.8%), and extended maintenance of good functional status (185 weeks).[34,51] A third study confirmed that more extensive resection was correlated with better immediate postoperative performance, lower 1-month mortality rate, and longer survival: 43% of patients with malignant gliomas improved, 50% remained unchanged, and 7% suffered deterioration in their neurologic condition following resection of at least 75% of their tumor. A more limited resection proved inferior (28% improved, 51% were unchanged, and 21% were worse).[49]

Similar results can be achieved by reoperation. In one series, 45% of patients had an improved Karnofsky score following reoperation.[108] In another series focusing on reoperation, when gross tumor resection was achieved, 82%[32,39] of patients had improvement or stability in their Karnofsky score.[134] In a third, patients with Karnofsky scores of 50 or less also underwent reoperation. Two-thirds improved from a dependent to an independent state and the median duration of survival was similar to that for all patients undergoing reoperation.[135]

The doubling rate of malignant gliomas is so high, however, that the benefit from reoperation will be very brief unless adjuvant therapies are able to induce remission of tumor growth. Surgical resection is especially beneficial when reduction of tumor burden improves the response rate to such adjuvant therapies. One early study of multidrug chemotherapy following reoperation for recurrent malignant gliomas used multivariate analysis to identify prognostic factors. During chemotherapy, disease stabilization or partial response occurred in 29 of 51 (57%) patients. Median time to tumor progression was 19 weeks for all pathologies; it was 32 weeks for patients with anaplastic astrocytomas and 13 weeks for those with glioblastoma multiforme. Median survival time was 40 weeks for all pathologies; it was 79 weeks for patients with anaplastic astrocytoma and 33 weeks for those with glioblastoma multiforme. Thirty-five percent of patients had serious chemotoxicity, but none had permanent morbidity or mortality. Factors associated with a longer median time to tumor progression included a higher Karnofsky score, lower grade of initial histology, lack of prior chemotherapy, less myelotoxicity, smaller postoperative tumor volume, greater extent of resection, and a local rather than diffuse pattern of recurrence. Those associated with a longer median survival time were a higher Karnofsky score, anaplastic astrocytoma rather than glioblastoma at recurrence, greater and myelotoxicity, and lobar rather than central location of the tumor.[72]

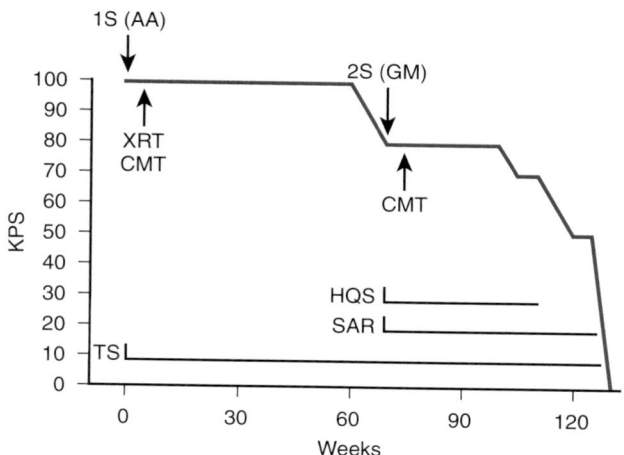

FIGURE 10-4 Quality-of-life considerations in the management of patients with malignant gliomas. Maintenance of high-performance status is a critical feature of outcome. The Karnofsky score (KPS) as a function of time indicates the quality of survival time that follows each intervention. 1S, initial surgery; XRT, radiation therapy; CMT, chemotherapy; 2S, reoperation; TS, total survival; HQS, high-quality survival (K = ≥70); SAR, survival after reoperation; AA, anaplastic astrocytoma; GBM, glioblastoma multiforme.

More recent studies from the University of California-San Francisco (UCSF), Memorial Sloan-Kettering, the University of Washington, and Johns Hopkins University have shown that reoperation followed by chemotherapy leads to stabilization of performance score for significant intervals.[66,108,136,137] At UCSF, 44% of patients with glioblastomas maintained a performance level of at least 70 (a level consistent with self care and judged to be survival of high quality (58%)) for at least 6 months after reoperation; 18% maintained this level for at least a year; and 3 patients did so for longer than 3 years. Most (52% of 31) patients with anaplastic astrocytomas maintained this performance level for at least 12 months after reoperation; 13% had more than 4 years of high quality survival. Approximately 90% of the survival after reoperation for anaplastic astrocytoma was of high quality[136] (Fig. 10-4). In the Memorial Sloan-Kettering group, the median duration of maintenance of independent status (Karnofsky score of at least 80) was 34 weeks. In the Seattle series, patients with a Karnofsky score of at least 70 maintained this high level of function for an average of 37 weeks after reoperation for glioblastoma and for 70 weeks after reoperation for anaplastic astrocytoma.[137]

A more complete resection of recurrent tumor increases the duration as well as the quality of patient survival.[60,134] Support for reoperation is found in comparisons of the outcomes in cases in which different degrees of tumor removal were accomplished and in comparisons of the survival of patients following reoperation with that of historical controls not receiving reoperation. Patients in whom gross total resection of a glioblastoma is achieved survive longer (45.6 vs. 25.6 weeks) than do those receiving near-total or subtotal resections; for anaplastic astrocytomas, the effect of extent of resection is similar (87.5 vs. 55.7 weeks).[137] Comparable results were obtained by another group in which the median duration of survival for GBM patients after gross total resection was 76 weeks and for anaplastic astrocytoma was 33 months.[138] In the Sloan-Kettering

Table 10-1	Karnofsky Performance Status	
Definition	**Percent**	**Criteria**
Able to carry on normal activity and to work. No special care is needed	100	Normal; no complaints; no evidence of disease.
	90	Able to carry on normal activity; minor signs or symptoms of disease.
	80	Normal activity with effort; some signs or symptoms of disease.
Unable to work. Able to live at home, care for most personal needs. A varying amount of assistance is needed.	70	Cares for self. Unable to carry on normal activity or to do active work.
	60	Requires occasional assistance, but is able to care for most of his or her needs.
	50	Requires considerable assistance and frequent medical care.
Unable to care for self. Requires equivalent of institutional or hospital care. Disease may be progressing rapidly.	40	Disabled; requires special care and assistance.
	30	Severely disabled; hospitalization is indicated although death is not imminent.
	20	Very sick; hospitalization necessary; active supportive treatment necessary.
	10	Moribund; fatal processes progressing rapidly.
	0	Dead.

From Karnofsky D, Burchenal JH, Armistead GC Jr, et al. Triethylene melamine in the treatment of neoplastic disease. Arch Intern Med. 1951;87:477-516.

series that grouped glioblastomas and anaplastic astrocytomas together, a similar difference was found (51.2 vs. 23.3 weeks).[108] In the UCSF series, survival of patients undergoing reoperation and chemotherapy for either anaplastic astrocytoma or glioblastoma was longer than that of patients receiving chemotherapy alone at the time of tumor recurrence.[136]

A later study from UCSF[67] evaluated 46 patients (15.3%) who underwent reoperation among a group of 301 patients with glioblastoma multiforme. The actuarial rate of reoperation was 15% at 1 year and 31% at 2 years after the initial diagnosis. Patients who were younger ($p = 0.01$) and who had received an extensive resection initially were more likely to undergo reoperation. KPS scores after reoperation were improved in 28% of patients, unchanged in 49%, and worse in 23%. There was no perioperative mortality. Eight (17.4%) underwent a third operation. A high preoperative KPS score was the only factor predictive of longer survival after reoperation. Similar to the earlier study, the median duration of survival after reoperation was 36 weeks: 61% were alive at 6 months and 24% at 21 months after reoperation. The median period of high-quality survival was 18 weeks (Table 10-1). A subset of 32 patients who underwent reoperation within 45 days of first tumor recurrence was compared with a control group of 141 patients who did not. The median duration of survival after recurrence was 18.7 weeks longer (42.4 vs. 23.7 weeks) in the group undergoing reoperation ($p < 0.05$, hazard ratio = 0.67, 95% confidence interval = 0.44–1.00) even when controlled for age and KPS score at the time of recurrence. The 13-week difference in survival was potentially due to selection bias. Adjusting for resectability by eliminating from the control group those who underwent biopsy only as the first operation and those whose recurrent tumor was separate from the original tumor reduced the statistical significance of this difference ($p = 0.12$; hazard ratio = 0.71, 95% confidence interval = 0.46–1.09). The Cox multivariate proportional hazards model adjusted for resectability predicted that a typical 55-year-old man with a KPS score of 80 likely would survive 8 weeks longer (35 vs. 27 weeks) with reoperation than without it. Selection bias was also reduced by stratifying

reoperation and control groups by propensity to undergo reoperation. This analysis identified reoperation ($p = 0.03$, hazard ratio = 0.64, 95% confidence interval = 0.42–0.96) as well as KPS score as statistically significant predictors of longer survival.[67]

The benefit of reoperative surgery is also suggested by experience with brachytherapy. Patients undergoing reoperation for tumor recurrence and/or radiation necrosis following brachytherapy for glioblastomas, either initially or at first recurrence, survived longer than those not receiving reoperation (median total survival of 120 vs. 62 weeks for patients with primarily treated tumors and 90 vs. 37 weeks for patients treated with brachytherapy at the time of first recurrence).[12]

Reoperation as a part of the multimodality treatment of recurrent gliomas is further supported by study of long-term survivors of glioblastoma multiforme. A review of the UCSF experience identified 22 of 449 (5%) patients with glioblastomas who survived at least 5 years after diagnosis. Sixteen of 22 had tumor recurrence that was treated; and 9 underwent between one and three reoperations. For 8 of the 16 patients with treated recurrence, survival after treatment of recurrence (median of 4.5 years) was longer than the remission produced by the initial treatment.[138]

The benefit to survival from reoperation is not above dispute. As noted above, multivariate analyses of chemotherapy studies have found that extent of resection and smaller postoperative volume are associated with prolongation of time to tumor progression but not of survival.[32] A similar study of survival after progression of malignant gliomas identified high KPS score and age less than 50 years as independent prognostic factors.[139] Those who underwent reoperation (58/143 patients) lived longer (median of 35 weeks vs. 16 weeks, $p < 0.005$ in univariate analysis) after tumor recurrence than those treated without reoperation, but multivariate analysis identified only a trend toward reduction of risk of death (hazard ratio = 0.74; 95% confidence interval = 0.50–1.11; $p = 0.014$) following reoperation. Randomized controlled trials using prognostic indices for analysis of outcomes are needed to evaluate definitively the benefits of reoperation.[140]

Table 10-2 Reoperation for Recurrent Gliomas

Author	Pt #	Path	SAR	HQS	Morb	Mort	↑K	Px Relations	Weeks
Young et al.[141]	24	GBM	14		52%	17%	25%	K≥60 → SAR II > 12 m → SAR	22 vs. 9 16.5 vs. 8.5
Salcman[60]	40	MG	37			0%		Age <40 → SAR	57 vs. 36
Ammirati et al.[34]	55	64%Gm$$	36	34	16%	64%	45%	K>70 → SAR Grade → SAR Ext. resect. → SAR	48.5 vs. 19 61 vs. 29 51.2 vs. 23.3
Harsh et al.[136]	49	GBM	36	10	8%	5%	5%	Age → SAR K≥70 → HQS	
Harsh et al.[136]	21	AA	88$$	83$$	3%	3%	10%	Age → HQS Grade → SAR	
Berger et al.[137]	56	GBM						K≥70 → SAR K≥70 → SQE Age ≤60 → SQE II > 12 m → SAR	70.7 vs. 36.5 36.6 vs. 8.4 35.1 vs. 9.4 150 vs. 48 99.5 vs. 22.4
Berger et al.[137]	14	AA						II > 12 m → SQE	
Kaye[132]	50	GBM				16%	0%	Age → SAR Grade → SAR II → SAR Age → HQS Grade → HQS II → HQS	
Barker et al.[67]	46	GBM	36	18	23%	0%	28%	K → SAR	

Path, pathology; pt, patient; GBM, glioblastoma multiforme; AA, anaplastic astrocytoma; SAR, survival after reoperation; HQS, high-quality survival (K≥70); morb, morbidity; mort, mortality; ↑K, increased performance (Karnofsky) score; Px relations, statistically significant relationship; II, interoperative interval; ext resect, extent of resection; SQE, same quality existence.

SELECTION OF PATIENTS FOR REOPERATION

Case selection is critical to outcome. The patient's profile of prognostic factors, the predicted tolerance of the procedure, and the feasibility of extensive tumor resection without undue risk of new neurologic morbidity must all be considered. Multiple characteristics have been identified as predictive of a good response to reoperation (Table 10-2). Foremost among these are tumor histology, patient age, performance status, interoperative interval, and extent of resection.

The prognostic significance of tumor grade is evident in most series. Median duration of survival after reoperation was 88 weeks for patients with anaplastic astrocytomas but only 36 weeks for those with glioblastomas at UCSF, and 61 weeks and 29 weeks, respectively, at Sloan-Kettering.[108,136]

The effect of age may overwhelm that of tumor grade. In one series, survival after reoperation was 57 weeks for those younger than 40 years but only 36 weeks for older patients.[60] Other authors found an association between youth and total survival duration after diagnosis and between youth and quality of survival after reoperation, but not between youth and duration of survival after reoperation.[108,136]

Preoperative performance score significantly affects outcome. At Kentucky, median duration of survival after reoperation was 22 weeks for patients with performance scores of at least 70 but only 9 weeks for more disabled patients.[141] In the Seattle series, for glioblastomas, survival after reoperation was almost twice as long (71 vs. 36 weeks) for patients with Karnofsky scores of at least 70 than for those with lower scores.[137]

The prognostic importance of the interval between initial treatment and recurrence is disputed.[142] The Kentucky series found survival to be twice as long if the interval between operations exceeded 6 months. In Seattle, a threefold difference (150 vs. 48 weeks for glioblastoma, and 164 vs. 52 weeks for anaplastic astrocytomas) was noted when the time to progression exceeded 3 years.[137] Others, however, have found either no relation, or an inverse relation, between the interoperative interval and duration of survival after reoperation.[60,108,136]

The likelihood of substantial resection must also be anticipated. The ability to remove sufficient tumor mass to reduce intracranial pressure and palliate neurologic symptoms depends on the location of the tumor and its physical characteristics. Removal is facilitated by a more superficial location in noneloquent areas, a discrete pseudoencapsulated mass is more easily removed than a less well-marginated diffuse one, drainage of a cystic component will often provide immediate reduction of mass, as well as an avenue for further tumor resection.

During the interval between initial surgery and tumor recurrence, the patient will usually undergo therapy that might affect tolerance of surgery. The decision to reoperate must consider overall physical condition, tissue viability, blood coagulability, hematologic reserve, and immune function following surgery, radiation, corticosteroids, and chemotherapy. A high risk of multisystem failure, failure to thrive, intracranial hemorrhage, anemia, wound infection, pneumonia, and neurologic damage may exist. This risk should be assessed for each patient by obtaining preoperative chemical, hematologic, and radiographic studies.

In choosing patients for reoperation and subsequent therapy, consideration of the individual patient's profile of these prognostically significant factors permits a reasonable estimate of the likelihood of benefit from the procedure. Quality of life is a very important determinant of benefit as perceived by the patient, family, and society. Reoperation and subsequent multimodal therapy should be chosen only if maintenance of a reasonable level of function is anticipated (Figure 10-4).

PREPARATION FOR REOPERATION

Before surgery, the patient is likely to be receiving corticosteroids; these should be continued. At the time of induction of anesthesia, the patient is fitted with thigh-high intermittent-compression air boots. Additional steroids, prophylactic antibiotics, and osmotic and loop diuretics are given and the patient is hyperventilated. In positioning the patient, the likelihood of elevated intracranial pressure makes attention to elevation of the head above the level of the heart particularly important.

REOPERATIVE EXPOSURE

In planning the needed exposure, the tumor can be located by its relationship to the margins of the craniotomy and to the cortical pattern of gyri and sulci on the preoperative MRI scan, by intraoperative frameless stereotaxy, or by intraoperative MRI.[143,144] The procedure should be planned in advance to ensure adequate skin opening, craniotomy, and durotomy to expose the recurrent mass. All may need enlarging because of the increased extent of the tumor or a desire to perform corticography for mapping of motor or speech function.

The skin incision from the previous operation is usually used. The skin opening can be increased by additional incisions. They should be external to the previous flap, avoid its base and other vascular pedicles, and intersect the previous incision at right angles. The margins of the prior craniotomy flap should be defined. Generally, this is best accomplished with a curette, beginning at the prior trephination. Depending on the interoperative interval, the prior flap may need to be recut. Dissection in the epidural plane can be begun with a curette followed by a No. 3 and then a No. 2 Penfield dissector. The craniotomy plate is further elevated as the dura is stripped from its inner surface with a dissector. Epidural adhesions fixing dura to the craniotomy margin should be preserved as prophylaxis against postoperative extension of an epidural fluid collection unless the craniotomy needs to be enlarged. In this case, these adhesions are dissected with a curette and trimmed. After the dura is stripped from the undersurface of the cranial plate, an additional segment of bone can be removed with a craniotome.

The durotomy may need to be enlarged, but often it can be limited to part of the dural exposure. It should be planned to minimize traverse of cortical adhesions. For instance, in re-exposing a temporal lesion, the durotomy can be placed over the cyst remaining from the prior resection. Flapping the dura superiorly then allows adhesions to be put on traction such that they may be dissected from cortex, coagulated, and sharply divided. Extending a durotomy along an old incision line should be avoided. The old incision line should be traversed perpendicularly and as infrequently as possible in that it is often the site of the densest adhesions. Microdissection of larger vessels from dural attachments may be necessary. Once the dura is opened and retracted, the exposed cortex is inspected for the surface presentation of the tumor, apparent as abnormal color, consistency, and vascularity.

Localization of the subcortical extent of the tumor is then undertaken. Again, the preoperative imaging studies and stereotactic techniques are of value.[145] Brain shift occurring during dural opening and tumor resection must be considered when using these techniques. Intraoperative MRI or ultrasonography may help correct for this.[144,146,147] Tumor may also be found by locating a cystic resection cavity or encephalomalacic brain left after the previous operation. In that almost all tumors recur within 2 cm of the original tumor's margin, exposure of the initial tumor's surgical bed will usually reveal at least part of the recurrent mass.

Electrocorticographic mapping of motor, sensory, and speech areas may reduce the chance of inflicting neurologic deficit and may encourage a more extensive resection by revealing the relationship of the site of cortical traverse and of the subsequent subcortical dissection to eloquent brain (Fig. 10-5). This technique is often more difficult at the time of reoperation because of cortical disruption by the tumor and prior surgery.[148] However, long term reshapings of language, sensory, and motor maps in some patients have allowed gross total resection of recurrent gliomas without neurologic sequelae.[149,150]

Generally, the appearance of the tumor itself is the best guide to its extent. Tumor-infiltrated cortex is likely to have increased vascular markings, a pink to gray color, and a firm consistency. Its central core may vary from yellow cystic fluid of low viscosity to high viscosity, soupy, white necrosis which resembles pus, to a yellow-gray, granular, honeycomb-like material. Typically, the center is relatively avascular although it may be traversed by thrombosed blood vessels.

Some advocate incision into the tumor mass and internal debulking with an ultrasonic aspirator or laser as an initial step; however, this often induces significant hemorrhage. Enucleation by circumferential dissection in the pseudoplane about the rim of solid tumor is usually more satisfactory. Arteries supplying the tumor and veins draining it can be coagulated and divided as they enter the tumor mass, much as the vascular supply of an arteriovenous malformation is handled. In areas of noneloquent brain in particular, the softened, necrotic, highly edematous white matter around the tumor provides an excellent plane of dissection. The use of bipolar cautery forceps and suction together accomplishes this dissection while reducing local mass. Beyond the encephalomalacic brain lies more normal brain which, although edematous and possibly injured by prior retraction and radiation therapy, is often functional and should be preserved.

Often the tumor can be removed as a single specimen without the need for significant retraction of surrounding brain. In general, gentle, transient gentle pressure on a cottonoid paddy lying on the margin of resection provides sufficient exposure of the dissection plane that fixed self-retaining retractors are unnecessary. Retraction of the tumor mass is preferable to retraction of surrounding brain. Often, identification of the appropriate plane for the circumferential dissection is facilitated by this retraction on the tumor; coherence of the tumor mass helps delineate the plane between solid tumor and tumor-infiltrated brain.

Once the tumor mass has been removed, the margins of resection should be inspected to verify completeness of the excision. The margins should be free of tumor that is more firm, glassy, opaque, and hypervascular. Biopsies of

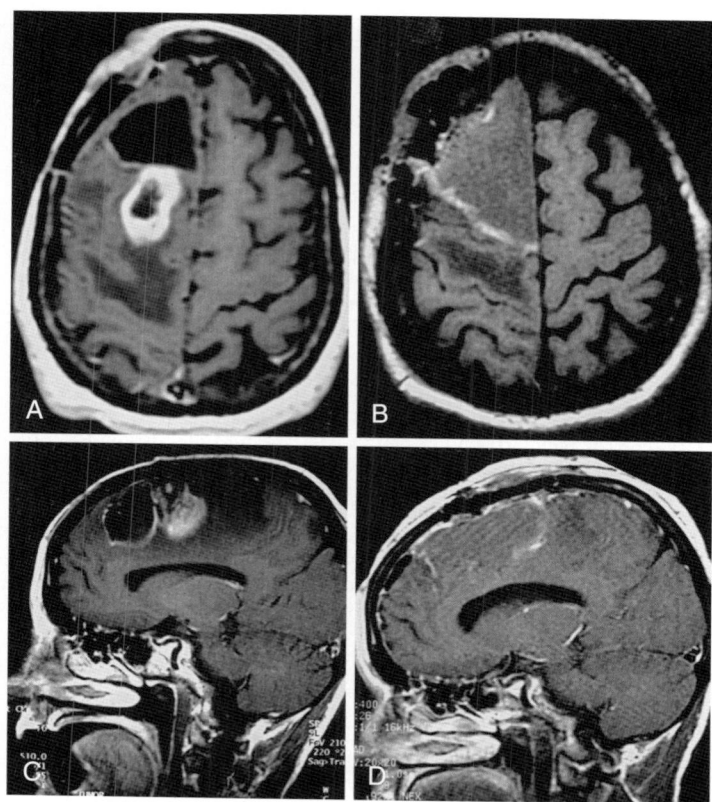

FIGURE 10-5 Recurrent malignant glioma. A 43-year-old woman developed right arm and leg weakness 11 months following complete resection and irradiation (60 Gy) of a right frontal glioblastoma. Pre-reoperative axial (A) and sagittal (C) MR scans showing contrast enhancement just posterior to the resection cavity. Reoperation, guided by intraoperative electrocorticographic mapping of the primary motor area, accomplished gross total removal of the recurrent tumor and surrounding frontal lobe back to the precentral sulcus, as seen on postoperative axial (B) and sagittal (D) images. After resolution of perioperative edema, full extremity strength returned.

the surrounding edematous brain should be sent for frozen-section analysis to verify absence of tumor. If solid tumor or tumor infiltrating into noneloquent areas remains, it should be removed. In some cases, extension of tumor into eloquent areas or diencephalic structures will preclude resection of the entire mass. In such cases, the tumor should be divided. This often entails coagulation of numerous strands of small, thin-walled blood vessels. This is particularly true if the extension is in the direction of the vascular supply, such as medial extension of a temporal lobe tumor toward the posterior aspect of the sylvian fissure. Particular care should be taken to coagulate and sharply divide these vessels. Tearing them without prior coagulation will leave a loose end that will retract and continue to bleed. Such loose ends should be directly coagulated rather than tamponaded with hemostatic packing, which may encourage deeper dissection of a hematoma.

After the resection has been completed, hemostasis should be confirmed by filling the tumor cavity with saline and, during a Valsalva maneuver, observing for wisps of continuing hemorrhage. This should be performed with the patient's blood pressure at least as high as the normal pressure. The cavity is then aspirated, lined with a single layer of oxidized cellulose, and filled again with irrigation fluid. Hyperventilation is then reversed to permit expansion of the brain during closure.

Watertight dural closure is essential. Often, this can be attained by primary suturing, given the decompression from the operation. If the dura is incompetent, it may be supplemented by a pericranial graft or a synthetic dural replacement. Peripheral and central dural tacking sutures are placed. The bone fragments are wired together, and the

craniotomy plate is then fixed with titanium miniplates. The wound is irrigated repeatedly with antibiotic solution and then closed in layers with 2-0 absorbable suture in muscle, fascia, and galea. The galeal sutures should be inverted and the knots should be cut short to avoid erosion superficially. They should be placed in sufficient proximity that tension-free closure of the skin is possible. Staples or simple running 4-0 nylon skin sutures usually provide adequate closure except at sites of attenuation, where horizontal mattress sutures may be preferred.

Postoperatively, the patient should be closely monitored for signs of increased intracranial pressure from hematoma or edema. Fluid restriction, dehydration, and corticosteroids should usually be continued. The patient should be mobilized as soon as possible and a gadolinium enhanced MRI scan should be obtained as soon as it is tolerable to assess extent of tumor resection.

KEY REFERENCES

Ammirati M, Galicich JH, Arbit E, Liao Y. Reoperation in the treatment of recurrent intracranial malignant gliomas. *Neurosurgery.* 1987;21: 607-614.

Ammirati M, Vick N, Liao YL, et al. Effect of the extent of surgical resection on survival and quality of life in patients with supratentorial glioblastomas and anaplastic astrocytomas. *Neurosurgery.* 1987;21: 201-206.

Barker II FG, Chang SM, Gutin PH, et al. Survival and functional status after resection of recurrent glioblastoma multiforme. *Neurosurgery.* 1998;42:709-720:discussion 709-723.

Barker II FG, Prados MD, Chang SM, et al. Radiation response and survival time in patients with glioblastoma multiforme. *J Neurosurg.* 1996;84:442-448.

Berger MS, Tucker A, Spence A, Winn HR. Reoperation for glioma. *Clin Neurosurg.* 1992;39:172-186.

Brandes AA, Tosoni A, Franceschi E, et al. Recurrence pattern after temozolomide concomitant with and adjuvant to radiotherapy in newly diagnosed patients with glioblastoma: correlation with MGMT promoter methylation status. *J Clin Oncol.* 2009;27:1275-1279.

Brem H, Piantadosi S, Burger PC, et al. Placebo-controlled trial of safety and efficacy of intraoperative controlled delivery by biodegradable polymers of chemotherapy for recurrent gliomas. The Polymer-Brain Tumor Treatment Group. *Lancet.* 1995;345:1008-1012.

Cairncross JG, Ueki K, Zlatescu MC, et al. Specific genetic predictors of chemotherapeutic response and survival in patients with anaplastic oligodendrogliomas. *J Natl Cancer Inst.* 1998;90:1473-1479.

Chandler KL, Prados MD, Malec M, Wilson CB. Long-term survival in patients with glioblastoma multiforme. *Neurosurgery.* 1993;32:716-720:discussion 720.

Coffey RJ, Lunsford LD, Taylor FH. Survival after stereotactic biopsy of malignant gliomas. *Neurosurgery.* 1988;22:465-473.

Fitzek MM, Thornton AF, Rabinov JD, et al. Accelerated fractionated proton/photon irradiation to 90 cobalt gray equivalent for glioblastoma multiforme: results of a phase II prospective trial. *J Neurosurg.* 1999;91:251-260.

Harsh IV GR, Levin VA, Gutin PH, et al. Reoperation for recurrent glioblastoma and anaplastic astrocytoma. *Neurosurgery.* 1987;21:615-621.

Hochberg FH, Pruitt A. Assumptions in the radiotherapy of glioblastoma. *Neurology.* 1980;30:907-911.

Kelly PJ, Daumas-Duport C, Scheithauer BW, et al. Stereotactic histologic correlations of computed tomography- and magnetic resonance imaging-defined abnormalities in patients with glial neoplasms. *Mayo Clin Proc.* 1987;62:450-459.

Kim HK, Thornton AF, Greenberg HS, et al. Results of re-irradiation of primary intracranial neoplasms with three-dimensional conformal therapy. *Am J Clin Oncol.* 1997;20:358-363.

Liau LM, Prins RM, Kiertscher SM, et al. Dendritic cell vaccination in glioblastoma patients induces systemic and intracranial T-cell responses modulated by the local central nervous system tumor microenvironment. *Clin Cancer Res.* 2005;11:5515-5525.

McGirt MJ, Chaichana KL, Gathinji M, et al. Independent association of extent of resection with survival in patients with malignant brain astrocytoma. *J Neurosurg.* 2009;110:156-162.

Nazzaro JM, Neuwelt EA. The role of surgery in the management of supratentorial intermediate and high-grade astrocytomas in adults. *J Neurosurg.* 1990;73:331-344.

Norden AD, Young GS, Setayesh K, et al. Bevacizumab for recurrent malignant gliomas: efficacy, toxicity, and patterns of recurrence. *Neurology.* 2008;70:779-787.

Rostomily RC, Spence AM, Duong D, et al. Multimodality management of recurrent adult malignant gliomas: results of a phase II multiagent chemotherapy study and analysis of cytoreductive surgery. *Neurosurgery.* 1994;35:378-388:discussion 388.

Salcman M, Kaplan RS, Ducker TB, et al. Effect of age and reoperation on survival in the combined modality treatment of malignant astrocytoma. *Neurosurgery.* 1982;10:454-463.

Shrieve DC, Alexander III E, Wen PY, et al. Comparison of stereotactic radiosurgery and brachytherapy in the treatment of recurrent glioblastoma multiforme. *Neurosurgery.* 1995;36:275-282:discussion 282-284.

Smith JS, Tachibana I, Passe SM, et al. PTEN mutation, EGFR amplification, and outcome in patients with anaplastic astrocytoma and glioblastoma multiforme. *J Natl Cancer Inst.* 2001;93:1246-1256.

Stupp R, Mason WP, van den Bent MJ, et al. Radiotherapy plus concomitant and adjuvant temozolomide for glioblastoma. *N Engl J Med.* 2005;352:987-996.

Yu JS, Liu G, Ying H, et al. Vaccination with tumor lysate-pulsed dendritic cells elicits antigen-specific, cytotoxic T-cells in patients with malignant glioma. *Cancer Res.* 2004;64:4973-4979.

Numbered references appear on Expert Consult.

CHAPTER 11

Tumors in Eloquent Areas of Brain

MARK A. PICHELMANN • FREDERIC B. MEYER

Lesions presenting themselves in close proximity to eloquent cortex and underlying white matter tracts provide a challenging subset of disorders for the neurosurgeon. Advances over the last 40 years in the ability to localize functional parenchyma by a variety of means have facilitated a more aggressive approach to the management of these lesions from a surgical standpoint. Neuronavigational systems in combination with anatomic and functional imaging advances as well as electrophysiologic study have greatly advanced the neurosurgeon's ability to effectively and safely treat these lesions. The goals of surgery for tumors located in eloquent areas of the brain are to maximize the extent of resection, minimize neurologic morbidity, and potentially treat intractable tumor-related epilepsy.

This chapter will focus on lesions juxtaposed or involving eloquent areas of the brain. Any number of pathologic entities can potentially manifest in functionally eloquent regions; however, gliomas will be a particular focus because of their more invasive nature compared with more focal lesions as well as the potential for eloquent cortical and subcortical white matter to be located within the tumor mass.

Rationale for Aggressive Resection

Resection of focal tumors in theory involves resection of the tumor mass without disruption of adjacent functional brain, since these tend to displace rather than invade. In the absence of the tumor presenting to the cortical surface, however, identifying eloquent cortex in an effort to safely approach deep seated lesions is of prime importance. Circumscribed lesions such as gangliogliomas, metastases, cavernomas, and arteriovenous malformations (AVMs) are examples of more focal masses that are usually more amenable to complete resection with less risk to adjacent cortex and white matter when compared with infiltrating gliomas. The exception to this may be epileptogenic zones that can be separate from the tumor mass or gliotic tissue that is not easily distinguishable from tumor-involved brain.

Surgery for diffuse tumor masses such as oligodendrogliomas and astrocytomas involves consideration of another dimension, that being resection of tumor infiltrating functional brain. It is well recognized that these diffuse tumors extend into otherwise grossly normal-appearing or slightly gliotic and potentially eloquent areas.[1-3] The identification of this functional brain within the tumor margin is important for ensuring continued neurologic function. The topic concerning the benefits of extent of resection with respect to high- and low-grade gliomas is controversial. Unfortunately, there are no prospective, randomized controlled trials to specifically address the benefits of radical resection. We are thus restricted to considering nonrandomized, retrospective data in an effort to guide clinical therapy. It cannot be overemphasized that decision making must be individualized and is best undertaken with a multidisciplinary approach to each patient considering the risks and benefits of each specific treatment option. Any benefit of surgery will come only by way of minimizing operative and neurologic morbidity related to the treatment.

The literature, overall, supports a positive effect of surgery on the natural history of low-grade gliomas. In a number of studies, gross or near-gross total resection of low-grade astrocytomas was correlated with lower recurrence rates and longer times to progression as compared with subtotal resection.[4-10] Fewer studies have correlated extent of resection with a survival advantage.[11] The rationale for aggressive resection is based on the assumption that small tumors will with time progress to larger tumors and become potentially either more difficult to resect or nonresectable. There is also good evidence to suggest that the potential for malignant degeneration is related to the tumor size and length of time the mass has been present.[4,12] Malignant degeneration has been variously reported, and probably occurs in about 50% of patients harboring these lesions.[13,14] An exhaustive review of this literature is beyond the scope of this chapter, and the reader is referred to a recent review by Keles and colleagues.[15] Surgery for high-grade gliomas is less controversial. Several studies not only indicate a benefit for time to progression and improved neurologic performance, but also improved survival.[16-26] Newer evidence, however, emphasizes that acquired motor or speech deficits may negatively impact overall survival.[27]

Therefore, the advantages to utilizing a maximal tumor resection strategy include less likelihood of tissue sampling error, an immediate reduction in signs and symptoms of mass effect, improved control of intractable seizures with dedicated seizure monitoring, and the potential positive effects in decreasing the risk of malignant dedifferentiation through cytoreduction and influencing outcome as it pertains to delaying progression.

Definitions of Eloquent Cortex

The concept of cortical localization with respect to language dates back to Broca's seminal report of two patients with nonfluent aphasia after having suffered autopsy-proven left inferior frontal strokes.[28] Wernicke subsequently added the description of another form of aphasia, variously termed *fluent aphasia*, in 1874 under similar circumstances.[29] These experiments of nature have opened the door to extensive research efforts at anatomically localizing various aspects of language and motor function to specific regions of the cerebral cortex. Numerous types of language deficit can result from injury both to cortical and subcortical regions. The focus here will be directed toward those regions essential for language and motor function as it applies to neurosurgical procedures and practice.

Sir Victor Horsley[30] performed the first stimulation mappings of the cerebral cortex in a series of patients when he stimulated the motor and somatosensory cortex producing contralateral limb movement and paresthesias. About 50 years later, Penfield and Boldrey detailed their results in stimulation of the precentral and postcentral gyri and noted that primary motor and sensory function is reliably located in these regions, although they may be displaced from their usual anatomic location as a result of mass effect from adjacent tissue.[31] They found these areas to be indispensable for movement and emphasized that during surgery every effort to preserve their structural integrity should be made. An exception to this general rule may be the face region, which is represented bilaterally, and resection of lesions in the nondominant motor cortex have been described.[32] This is not advocated in the dominant hemisphere because of the close proximity of language areas and the greater role the face motor region may play as association cortex with the language areas.

The most extensive work done on mapping primary essential language areas up to recent years was done by Penfield and colleagues as well.[33,34] Penfield tested naming, counting, spelling, and reading in patients during awake craniotomy and documented these areas on maps of the lateral and superior cortical surface. Three main areas were identified as being essential for language function. These were the inferior frontal opercular area (corresponding to Broca's area), the posterior temporal area (corresponding to Wernicke's area), and a third area located on the medial and superior surfaces of the superior frontal gyrus (the supplementary motor area). They also noted that these sites had relative importance in subserving language function, with the posterior temporal and inferior frontal regions being unresectable if language function was to be preserved. They also noted that the mesial frontal region was associated with severe expressive deficits postoperatively but that these deficits gradually disappeared in the weeks following surgery. Numerous others have confirmed this observation, indicating that resection of the supplementary motor area does not generally lead to permanent deficits as long as the more posterior primary motor cortex is spared.[35,36]

The standard technique for intraoperative stimulation mapping was also developed by Penfield to a large extent and later refined by Ojemann et al.[37] Of note in Penfield's stimulation maps is that errors in naming and object recognition were indeed clustered in the classical Broca's and Wernicke's areas, but a significant number of sites occurred outside of these traditional boundaries. In classic mapping studies done by Ojemann and colleagues on 117 patients, 67% had more than one distinct essential language area and 24% had three or more distinct areas subserving

language function in the dominant hemisphere peri-sylvian region. There was also greater variability in the temporal language area as compared with the frontal region. Additionally, essential language sites were found to be confined to an area of 2.5 cm^2 or less in about 50% of people, with only 16% of patients having an area equal to or larger than 6 cm^2.[37] Seldom are the entire extents of classical language areas essential for language function thus allowing potentially aggressive resection of lesions in eloquent areas.

To summarize, motor and sensory cortex are reliably localized to the precentral and postcentral gyri, respectively, in both hemispheres and are often readily identified on magnetic resonance imaging (MRI). The majority of essential motor neurons are located in the posterior portion of the precentral gyrus adjacent to the central sulcus. Compartmentalization of language functions is less precise based on cortical anatomy alone. In contrast to classic views of motor and sensory localization, language does not provide the surgeon with the same degree of certainty based on anatomic landmarks. There is wide variability in both the number and location of essential language sites within individual patients as evidenced by Ojemann's work. Language sites cannot be accurately defined with anatomic imaging only, and other means, such as functional imaging and/or direct negative stimulation mapping, must be used to minimize patient morbidity when considering resection of lesions in the peri-sylvian region of the dominant hemisphere. It must be kept in mind that language functions as a network of interconnected areas involved in parallel and serial processing to accomplish a task, although it is convenient to think of these areas as having discrete anatomic boundaries for the purposes of surgical planning and resection.

Testing of Cerebral Dominance

The evaluation of cerebral dominance has interested scientists since the time of Broca. It is well established that the vast majority of right-handed individuals are left brain dominant for speech and language function, while fewer left-handed individuals are left brain dominant, but still a majority. Efforts at finding out which patients may have atypical language localization (i.e., bilateral or right sided) is of great importance to the neurosurgeon particularly when operating in the peri-sylvian region of the right hemisphere. Strauss and Wada evaluated patients for various lateralized preferences, including hand, foot, eye, and ear, and found that taken together, these had a higher correlation with cerebral dominance than any one did alone. Perhaps more revealing in this study was that only 3% of patients with all left-sided preferences were left hemisphere dominant, indicating a high-risk group for undergoing right-sided surgical procedures.[38] Noninvasive means of testing for dominance offer clues about the lateralization of cerebral dominance, but application to a broad population base is problematic. These evaluations alone cannot be used to predict cerebral dominance reliably in individual patients, especially those with any left-sided preference. The intracarotid amobarbital procedure is the method of choice for the determination of dominance in this setting.

The intracarotid amobarbital procedure was initially developed by Wada in 1949[39] and later applied to a larger number of patients in reports by Wada and Rasmussen[40] and Branch and colleagues[41] for determining cerebral dominance with respect to language function. Milner and colleagues applied the technique to study the dominance of memory in patients undergoing resection of mesial temporal lobe structures for epilepsy.[42] There have been numerous other applications of this technique, but the focus of this chapter will be on testing for language and memory dominance as it applies to lesions in eloquent cortex.

Tumors involving peri-sylvian and mesial temporal structures are often in close proximity to potentially essential language cortex and the hippocampus, which has been shown to be of prime importance in memory processing. It is also well established that memory in addition to language tends to lateralize in individuals. It is important for the surgeon to know to which hemisphere language is dominant and in certain circumstances, as with medial temporal lobe lesions, to know potential memory lateralization before embarking on aggressive resection. Wada testing can add light to the decision about whether or not more detailed preoperative or intraoperative study is necessary in individual patients. At a minimum, patients with planned peri-sylvian or medial temporal resections without strict left-sided preferences should be considered for Wada testing or undergo functional imaging because these individuals will often have atypical language representation.

Anatomic Localization of Eloquent Areas

Several methods have been described for localizing the central sulcus based on external (skull) landmarks. This gives the surgeon a general idea of where the precentral and postcentral gyri are located preoperatively and can help in planning the craniotomy in the absence of neuro-navigational aids. These techniques are based on Taylor-Haughton lines.[43] The motor strip is typically located 4 to 5 cm posterior to the coronal suture in the midsagittal plane.[44]

The central sulcus is often readily identified on preoperative imaging. Berger and colleagues correlated intraoperative stimulation mapping of motor cortex with preoperative MRI scans and found that the central sulcus is reliably identified on high-vertex axial T2-weighted imaging as transverse sulci with the motor cortex located immediately anterior (Fig. 11-1). Additionally, it was found less reliably on slightly parasagittal images using the termination of the cingulate sulcus in the marginal sulcus with the sensorimotor cortex anterior to this.[45] Efforts at localizing language areas have been less certain, although for Broca's area, which is more constant in location, Quiñones-Hinojosa and colleagues have demonstrated 87% to 89% accuracy when the frontal opercular area is categorized in specific anatomic subtypes when compared to intraoperative stimulation mapping.[46] This may be readily identified on sagittal imaging as an "M-shaped" gyrus representing the pars orbitalis, triangularis, and opercularis (Fig. 11-2).

Though attractive, this method may be most useful for identifying lesions that are in proximity to the rolandic sulcus and thus require more invasive testing either preoperatively with functional imaging and/or with intraoperative mapping.

Intraoperative Stimulation Mapping

Localization of eloquent areas of the brain during surgery is of paramount importance both in preserving function and in ensuring the most radical resection possible when lesions are in close proximity to them. Furthermore, tumors may abut eloquent cortex, displacing it and making landmarks more difficult to identify, or they may invade critical

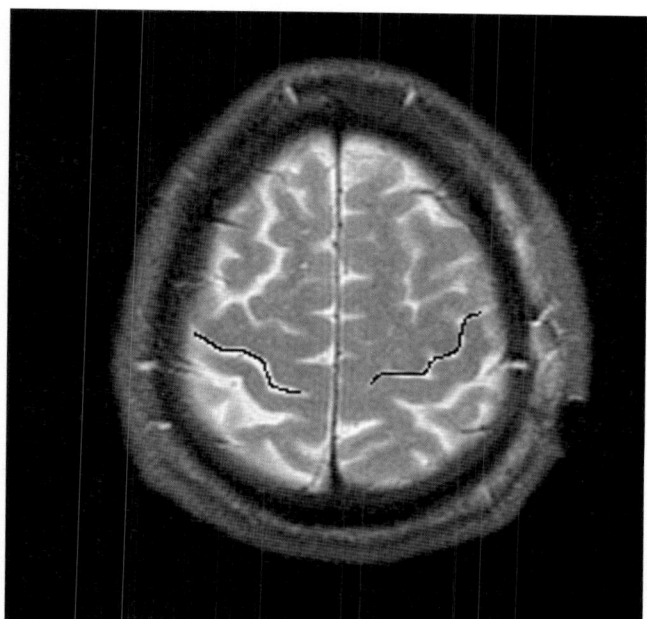

FIGURE 11-1 High vertex axial imaging can be used to locate the central sulcus (black line) on most patients as a transversely oriented sulcus posterior to the end of the superior frontal sulcus.

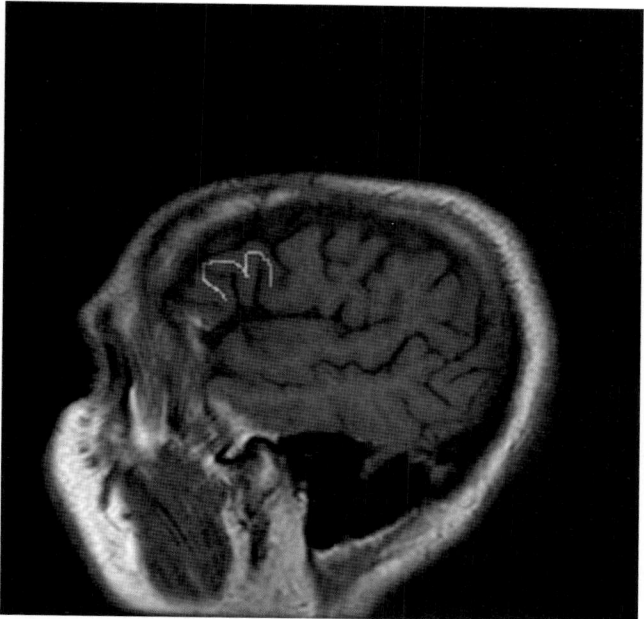

FIGURE 11-2 The frontal operculum can often be identified as an M-shaped gyrus (*gray line*) on lateral sagittal imaging just superior to the sylvian fissure.

structures. Intraoperative cortical stimulation is widely used and has been validated in numerous studies. It is currently the "gold standard" in the identification and preservation of eloquent areas to which all other modalities such as functional imaging should be compared.

LOCALIZATION OF PRIMARY MOTOR AND SENSORY CORTEX

The method of using somatosensory evoked potentials to identify the sensorimotor cortex was introduced by Goldring in treating pediatric epilepsy patients.[47] It has since broadened to include use in patients having tumors in the rolandic region.[48,49] Somatosensory evoked potential mapping is quick and reliable in identifying the somatosensory region. Typically, an eight-contact strip electrode array is placed over the region of interest in a transverse orientation, and stimulation of the median or tibial nerve, depending on the lesion location, is done with recording of the contralateral cortical surface, either epidurally or subdurally. The somatosensory cortex is located at the point of phase reversal between two adjacent contacts. The array of electrodes may then be repositioned to confirm the location of the central sulcus superiorly or inferiorly.

The advantages of this procedure over stimulation mapping are that the risk for inducing seizures is significantly less, and it may be performed epidurally, thus potentially limiting exposure of eloquent cortex through a tailored dural opening suitable for the needs at hand. Additionally, electrodes may be placed beneath the adjacent bone not involved in the craniotomy flap to localize sensorimotor cortex.

Motor-evoked potentials have more recently been used to identify motor cortex specifically and allow direct stimulation monitoring of motor cortex and subcortical pathways with a high-frequency stimulator in patients under general anesthetic by observing limb movements or with electromyography.[48,50,51]

Cortical stimulation mapping can be used to map the rolandic cortex with great precision (Figs. 11-3 to 11-5). Mapping of the motor cortex can be done with the patient either awake or under general anesthesia. Somatosensory stimulation can only be done with the patient awake. Stimulation may involve the cortex or subcortical white matter, which may be especially advantageous for tumors that extend deeply into the hemisphere or in the region of the internal capsule in the case of insular masses. Notably, children may have relatively inexcitable cortex as compared to adults, making stimulation mapping more difficult.[52]

LOCALIZATION OF LANGUAGE CORTEX

Permanent language dysfunction, even relatively minor, can be of considerable distress to the patient and family. Identification of essential language sites is of great importance during lesion resection in the peri-sylvian region of the dominant hemisphere. Language mapping, in contrast to mapping motor cortex, must be done with the patient awake and cooperative. If speech function, reading, or comprehension is impaired because of the location of the mass, intraoperative stimulation mapping for language function will not usually be helpful. Additionally, adults with neurologic, psychiatric, or significant medical comorbidities such as obesity or pulmonary problems may not be able to tolerate an awake procedure. Prior to surgery, the patient is counseled by the surgeon, anesthesiologist, and speech pathologist or neurologist about the nature of the procedure, the environment, and their expected duties. It is crucial to assess a patient's language function prior to surgery to obtain a baseline against which to compare intraoperative testing. It is often more labor intensive and time consuming for the surgical team and requires perseverance in identifying essential language regions.

STIMULATION MAPPING TECHNIQUE

Patient positioning is of great importance to balance the requirements of a multidisciplinary team during the surgical procedure. The patient must be comfortable enough with respect to head position and padding of pressure

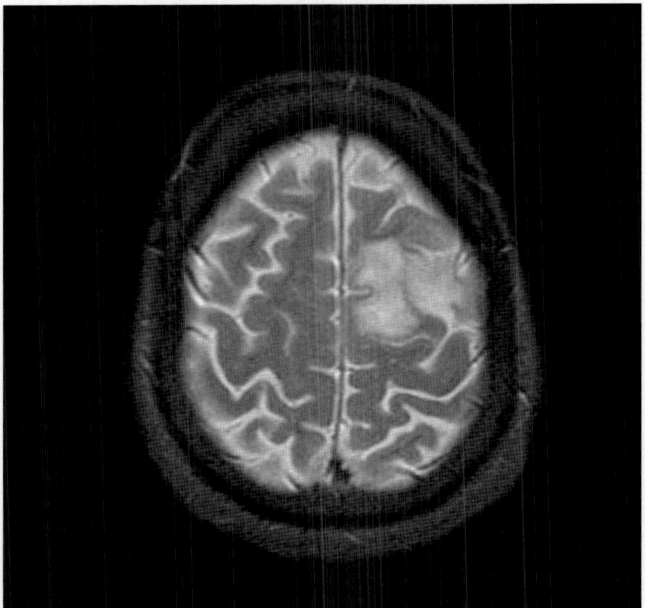

FIGURE 11-3 Preoperative T2-weighted magnetic resonance imaging revealing a low-grade glial tumor adjacent to the motor cortex in the supplementary motor area.

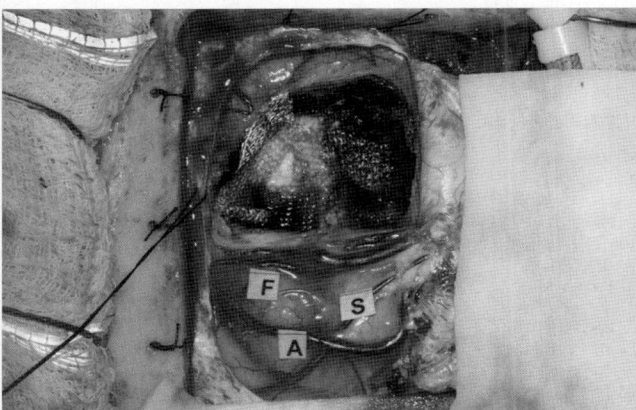

FIGURE 11-4 Intraoperative photograph of the patient in Figure 11-3 showing stimulation mapping of the right upper arm and leg region done before tumor removal. The resection was done with stereotactic guidance and ongoing neurologic examinations, both motor and speech, to protect the radiating white matter tracts during the resection of the deeper components of the tumor. A, arm; F, face; S, shoulder.

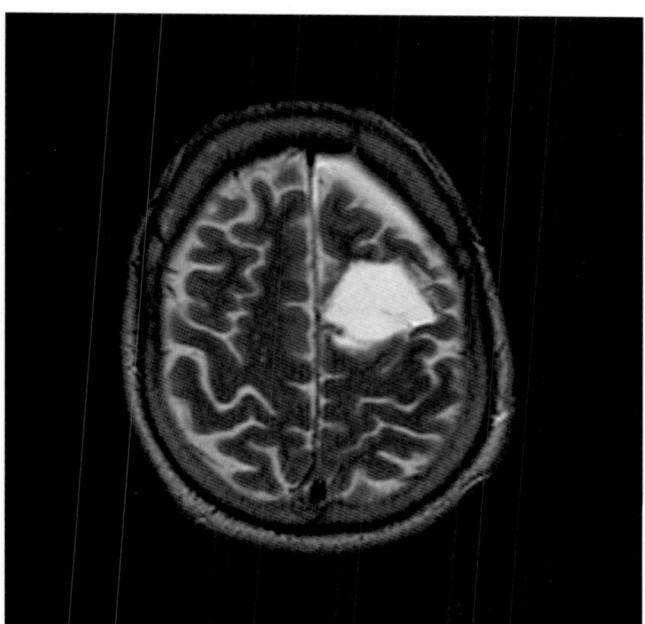

FIGURE 11-5 Postoperative T2-weighted magnetic resonance imaging of the patient in Figure 11-3 revealing complete removal of all T2 signal abnormality.

points to allow cooperation for often extended periods of time. He or she must have an unobstructed view of the examiner so as to participate fully in testing during the procedure. The anesthesiologist must also have ready access to the airway for emergency intubation as well as monitoring during pin placement and craniotomy, when the patient is under more sedation. In our practice, frameless stereotaxis is often used and, therefore, patient positioning must also consider line-of-sight issues of the infrared camera and stereotactic equipment.[53] With these issues in mind, the surgeon must often determine if there will be adequate access to the lesion. Often, optimal positioning from the surgical standpoint is somewhat compromised, and judgment must be exercised about the feasibility of doing an awake procedure as opposed to using alternative methods such as extraoperative mapping. Usually, however, a satisfactory solution can be found, facilitating safe tumor resection.

The patient is given fentanyl and propofol for conscious sedation for placement of the pinion, scalp incision, and craniotomy, and then awakened for the cortical and/or subcortical mapping. A mixture of bupivacaine (0.25%) and lidocaine (0.5%) that is pH-adjusted is used to infiltrate the pin sites and subsequently the scalp incision when the head has been positioned. Intraoperative stereotactic neuronavigation is useful to plan the craniotomy and scalp incision as well as to allow necessary exposure of the tumor and for mapping of adjacent language or sensorimotor cortices. This will also allow for feedback intraoperatively with respect to tumor volume excision, as discussed further later. Preoperatively, the maximum volume of local anesthetic that can be safely used throughout the procedure is calculated based on the patient's weight (2-3 mg/kg of bupivacaine or 4-6 mg/kg of lidocaine). A reserve of 10 to 15 ml is kept on hand for application to the dura after the craniotomy as well as for additional discomfort the patient may

have during the stimulation mapping portion of the procedure. After the mapping has been completed, the patient may again be sedated to finish the necessary resection and closure.

The stereotactic navigation system can be used to outline the tumor and identify possible motor and sensory cortex to minimize the amount of time spent mapping as well as serving as a useful guide about the extent of tumor resection. Intraoperatively, the main concern with stereotaxis and the use of preoperative imaging is brain shift. As the operation progresses, this distortion increases as cerebrospinal fluid is lost and the tumor is resected. This distortion is accentuated when the tumor is large or when the ventricle is entered. Intraoperative ultrasound is an alternative method to ensure maximal resection after mapping has been done to localize the tumor boundaries as well as potentially allowing correction due to brain shift.[54] Small tickets or catheters may be used to outline the depth of the tumor around the periphery in a "picket fence" arrangement, with resection proceeding up the edge of each catheter. This minimizes the chance that brain shift will have an adverse effect on tumor resection. Ultrasound has shown good correlation to T2 signal abnormality on MRI.[55]

Standard cortical mapping is then done with the Ojemann stimulator, as has been described previously.[52] An established anesthesia protocol should be in place in anticipation of the rare instance that stimulation induces a seizure, especially if the patient's head is fixed in a pinion. To minimize induction of intraoperative seizure activity, a surface electrocorticography strip is placed outside the resection field on the cortical surface to monitor for afterdischarges. Stimulation current is selected to be less than that which results in 1 or 2 afterdischarges. If there is evidence of cortical irritability following stimulation, the brain's surface is irrigated with ice-cooled saline. A low setting (2–5 mA) constant current, 60-Hz biphasic square wave stimulus with a 1-msec duration is used to stimulate various regions of interest. Motor stimulation may have to be higher than sensory stimulation. If no response is elicited at 16 mA, then no functional cortex is located in the stimulated area. A quick test of the temporalis muscle reflected from the craniotomy site can confirm that the equipment is functional in sleeping patients. Electromyography can be used when performing mapping of the motor cortex to provide greater sensitivity and lessen the chances of stimulation induced seizure activity.[56] Contact of the bipolar stimulator, parallel to the adjacent sulci, should last 1 to 2 seconds, and no two stimulation trials should be attempted in succession in one area. Current may need to be increased to identify certain areas such as the face motor region and depends on the anesthesia used if the patient is asleep. Pediatric patients also may require higher stimulation current to elicit a response, as noted earlier. The patient is assessed for motor or sensory findings with each stimulus when mapping the perirolandic areas. The cortex is stimulated in stepwise fashion at 1.5-cm intervals, with two to three positive stimulations defining functional cortex.[53] A numbered tag is then placed on the brain surface at these sites. Subcortical tracts may also be stimulated similarly during tumor resection with the same or slightly higher current parameters.[57-60] This may be particularly useful for insular gliomas adjacent to the internal capsule or medial temporal tumors growing over the tentorial edge to identify the cerebral peduncle at the medial extent of the resection.

Language mapping is done similarly, with a speech pathologist examining the patient with confrontational naming, spelling, counting, reading, or other site-specific test. The patient is shown objects or assessed every 4 seconds with any errors, anomia, dysnomia, hesitation, or speech arrest being noted. After each stimulation trial, the patient is allowed to name an object without stimulation to ensure recovery of function. Afterdischarges are allowed to dissipate prior to the next stimulation. It is important to note when stimulating the posterior inferior frontal lobe that speech arrest is not caused by oropharyngeal motor arrest, as occurs when stimulating the precentral gyrus, by observing the patient as well as listening. Stimulation of the postcentral gyrus may aid in this distinction, because the patient is able to note oropharyngeal sensory stimuli. Cortical sites essential for language function have been found to be located on the crests of gyri and not generally in sulci unless continuous with an adjacent gyrus, according to Ojemann and co-workers.[37]

Most stimulation-induced seizures last only 10 to 30 seconds, and cold saline can be applied to the cortical surface to abort the majority of these. Seizures lasting longer than this should be treated more aggressively with benzodiazepines, because generalization of a focal seizure can lead to an unsafe situation with a patient in pinions and limited access to the airway. Again, every effort should be made to use low stimulation current as well as meticulous monitoring of afterdischarges to prevent this complication.

A limitation of intraoperative cortical mapping is that high-intensity stimulation may inhibit or activate functional areas whereas low-intensity stimulation may not identify intended target areas.[61] Other pitfalls to be aware of are that more than two language areas can exist, and thus the inability to identify any eloquent cortex should raise caution that the stimulation is not working rather than lead to the conclusion that none exists in a given area. Also, preservation of cortex with disruption of subcortical tracts by undercutting gyri may lead to permanent morbidity.

It is often straightforward to identify by MRI the central sulcus or to map eloquent motor and language cortex as just described. However, it is more difficult to map the subcortical white matter tracts. One technique to minimize the risk of injury to radiating white matter tracts is to conduct repetitive neurologic and speech examinations during the ongoing tumor resection. This obviously requires a coordinated team approach, which includes having both a neurologist and speech pathologist, possibly with interpreters for mapping multiple language regions available in the operating room. With ongoing examinations, the surgeon is able to be more aggressive and proceeds with resection until the onset of neurologic deficits. In this circumstance, a maximum neurologically permissible resection of infiltrative tumors can be performed with a risk of significant neurologic injury that approximates 15%.[53]

There is evidence that epilepsy associated with slow-growing low-grade neoplasms resides in adjacent tumor-free cortex.[62] Epilepsy associated with AVMs may be similar.[63] With respect to lesions in eloquent cortex, this epileptogenic zone may also reside in functional cortex, hence the need to perform either extraoperative mapping as described later, or intraoperative electrocorticography to define this area. Multiple studies have shown that resection of adjacent electrocorticography-active foci results in improved seizure control as compared with resection of the tumor mass alone.[62] Children may fare better in this regard than adults.[64] Combining an epilepsy operation with an oncologic operation may provide the best chance at tumor and seizure control. It is also important to monitor for epileptic discharges after resection to ensure that additional seizure foci are not left behind.

Intraoperative cortical mapping combined with appropriate functional imaging and stereotactic neuronavigation should theoretically protect the patient from iatrogenic neurologic morbidity. This, however, is not always the case, and there are several possible reasons. First, patients with lesions in eloquent areas already have some degree of neurologic impairment, and manipulation or close resection to critical areas may worsen the neurologic condition. Additionally, maximizing resection by removing tumor until a deficit becomes apparent is a strategy sometimes used.[8,52] Second, regional ischemia and peritumoral edema may become manifest after an apparently uneventful resection.[65] Third, a lack of specificity of the testing paradigm to the area of resection may miss potentially eloquent areas. This is minimized by using naming as a part of language evaluation, as the majority of aphasias have anomia as a component of the syndrome. More specific tests, however, can be done when there is concern about important association cortex or functions such as calculation.[66] Complex language functions may in time be better identified with more specific testing paradigms used after assessment with functional MRI (fMRI), evaluating the specific functional modalities at risk during lesion resection.[67]

Resection of gliomas to within 2 cm of eloquent tissue used in naming carries a risk of persistent postoperative deficit, as noted by Ojemann and Dodrill.[68] Haglund and colleagues later reported on a series of patients undergoing temporal glioma resection that a margin of greater than 8 mm was associated with no postoperative deficits lasting more than 30 days.[69] In general, it is best to keep a margin of about 1 cm between resection and eloquent cortex. Subcortical pathways from sensorimotor and language areas are thought to descend perpendicular to gyri; therefore, undercutting identified eloquent cortex should be avoided.

The majority of the deficits induced during awake craniotomy are temporary in nature and lasting major neurologic morbidity relatively rare. Patients must be counseled preoperatively of this risk and the expected temporary nature of the postoperative deficits.

Functional Imaging

There has been an explosion in recent years in the research and application of functional imaging to neurosurgery. These techniques are based on identifying regions of the brain that are "active" relative to other regions of the brain during a specific testing algorithm. This technology is extremely helpful in that it offers the possibility of localizing eloquent areas of cortex with respect to a mass lesion preoperatively, determining the best surgical approach, and potentially guiding the decision to use intraoperative mapping in a given patient.

Functional MRI (fMRI) and positron emission tomography (PET) scanning are being used more frequently in the preoperative assessment of eloquent areas of the brain. Functional MR signal changes are believed to be a result of local blood oxygenation differences between activated and, therefore, more metabolically active, brain and relatively silent areas. This has been termed the blood oxygen level-dependent (BOLD) contrast method and requires no contrast agent[70] (Fig. 11-6). Various paradigms exist for testing certain areas of the brain. All are dependent on a comparison with the performance of a task and a resting state or alternate task. fMRI studies and their interpretation, therefore, are extremely dependent on the tasks and comparisons used. While fMRI measures the changes in deoxyhemoglobin levels reflecting oxygen consumption, PET measures regional differences in cerebral blood flow through use of an injected radioisotope, most commonly $[^{15}O]H_2O$ or $2-[^{18}F]-2$-desoxy-D-glucose (FDG). Despite the inherent differences in the physiologic basis for the imaging modalities, concordance between them when compared to intraoperative stimulation mapping has been good.[71,72] In the future, fMRI may have more efficacy in comparison with PET because of its noninvasive nature and more widespread availability.

Maps of eloquent areas identified on fMRI or PET can be coregistered or "fused" to standard MRI scans, slice by slice manually or with fusion software, to give better anatomic detail in most neuronavigational systems.[73,74] This coregistration can in turn be applied in planning the surgical procedure, as well as during the formal operation. The potential benefit to using fMRI data is that it preoperatively determines the general location of eloquent cortex with respect to the lesion in question, allowing for preprocedural

planning of the craniotomy and the approach to the tumor, as well as aiding in the decision whether to apply intraoperative stimulation. It may further reduce the size of the craniotomy, thus minimizing both surgical morbidity and the amount of time spent performing intraoperative mapping.[75]

More recently there has been interest in combining fMRI with diffusion-weighted MR images (diffusion tensor imaging [DTI]) to identify the motor cortex and pyramidal tracts with respect to space-occupying lesions.[76,77] This may also provide additional insight into the preoperative planning and again reduce the time needed for intraoperative stimulation of subcortical tracts, which can be tedious and time consuming. It may also shed light on specific areas where the tumor mass may invade deep white matter tracts that must be spared during resective surgery. This information may be coregistered with MRI or fMRI imaging sets using neuronavigation at the time of surgery to maximize safety.

Several potential pitfalls should be taken into account when relying on fMRI, DTI, or PET data. There can be significant technical issues in integrating functional scans with a neuronavigational system with respect to echo-planar image distortion and complementary slice integration. This may lead to functional mislocalization of eloquent tissue.[78] The areas identified by fMRI or PET utilized for a specific task are often much larger than those identified at surgery with electrical mapping. This poses a problem in deciphering on fMRI the areas that are essential for a given task and the areas that simply participate in a task but are nonessential. This has been more problematic in mapping language areas than in mapping sensorimotor regions.[79,80] Additionally, local vasoreactivity in peritumoral brain may distort results that rely on vasoreactivity and oxygen consumption for producing data maps.[81] A recent review by Giussani and colleagues nicely illustrates these complex issues.[82]

Intraoperative stimulation mapping remains the gold standard for identifying and preserving functional cortex and subcortical white matter; however, noninvasive methods such as fMRI are desirable, and further research and paradigm validation may improve the usefulness of this technique in the future.

Conclusions

Surgery of lesions or epileptic foci located in eloquent areas of the brain provides a unique challenge to the neurosurgeon. The goals are to maximize resection and minimize neurologic morbidity. Several techniques for achieving these goals have been presented. A multidisciplinary approach to treating these patients is the standard, and it should be kept in mind that these techniques should be viewed as complementary to each other, with no single approach serving as a stand-alone method of ensuring safe removal of lesions in eloquent brain.

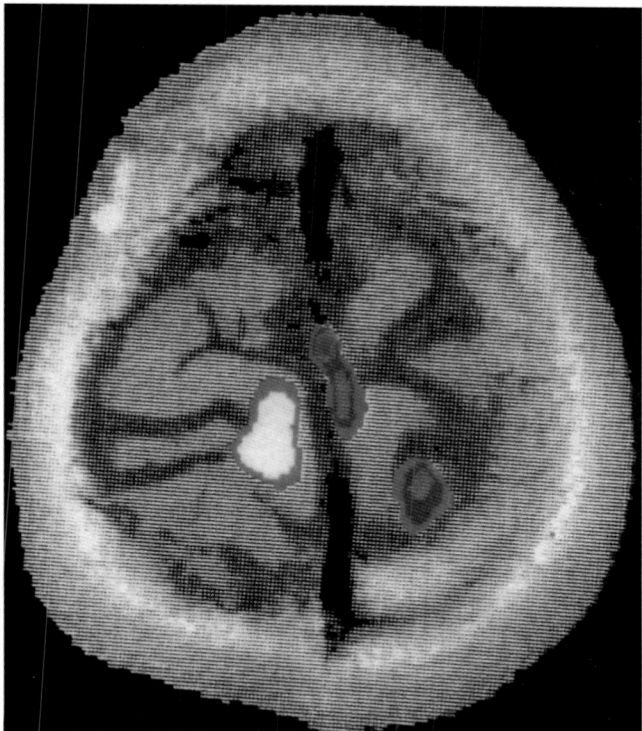

FIGURE 11-6 Functional magnetic resonance image using the BOLD technique for identifying motor cortex preoperatively.

KEY REFERENCES

Bello L, Gallucci M, Fava M, et al. Intraoperative subcortical language tract mapping guides surgical removal of gliomas involving speech areas. *Neurosurgery.* 2007;60:67-80.
Berger MS, Cohen WA, Ojemann GA. Correlation of motor cortex brain mapping data with magnetic resonance imaging. *J Neurosurg.* 1990;72:383-387.

Berger MS, Kincaid J, Ojemann GA, et al. Brain mapping techniques to maximize resection, safety, and seizure control in children with brain tumors. *Neurosurgery.* 1989;25:786-792.

Bittar RG, Olivier A, Sadikot AF, et al. Presurgical motor and somatosensory cortex mapping with functional magnetic resonance imaging and positron emission tomography. *J Neurosurg.* 1999;91:915-921.

Boling W, Olivier A, Fabinyi G. Historical contributions to the modern understanding of function in the central area. *Neurosurgery.* 2002;50:1296-1310.

Coenen VA, Krings T, Weidemann J, et al. Sequential visualization of brain and fiber tract deformation during intracranial surgery with three-dimensional ultrasound: an approach to evaluate the effect of brain shift. *Neurosurgery.* 2005;56(Suppl 1):133-141.

Duffau H, Capelle L, Denvil D, et al. Usefulness of intraoperative electrical subcortical mapping during surgery for low-grade gliomas located within eloquent brain regions: functional results in a consecutive series of 103 patients. *J Neurosurg.* 2003;98:764-778.

Duffau H, Lopes M, Denvil D, et al. Delayed onset of the SMA syndrome after surgical resection of the mesial frontal lobe: a time course study using intraoperative mapping in an awake patient. *Stereotact Funct Neurosurg.* 2001;76:74-82.

Giussani C, Roux FE, Ojemann J, et al. Is preoperative functional magnetic resonance imaging reliable for language areas mapping in brain tumor surgery? Review of language functional magnetic resonance imaging and direct cortical stimulation correlation studies. *Neurosurgery.* 2010;66:113-120.

Keles GE, Lamborn KR, Berger MS. Low-grade hemispheric gliomas in adults: a critical review of extent of resection as a factor influencing outcome. *J Neurosurg.* 2001;95:735-745.

Lacroix M, Abi-Said D, Fourney DR, et al. A multivariate analysis of 416 patients with glioblastoma multiforme: prognosis, extent of resection, and survival. *J Neurosurg.* 2001;95:190-198.

Laws ER, Parney IF, Huang W, et al. Survival following surgery and prognostic factors for recently diagnosed malignant glioma: data from the glioma outcomes project. *J Neurosurg.* 2003;99:467-473.

LeRoux P, Berger MS, Wang K, et al. Low grade gliomas: comparison of intraoperative ultrasound characteristics with preoperative imaging studies. *J Neurosurg.* 1992;13:189-198.

McGirt MJ, Chaichana KL, Attenello FJ, et al. Extent of surgical resection is independently associated with survivial in patients with hemispheric infiltrating low-grade gliomas. *Neurosurgery.* 2008;63:700-708.

McGirt MJ, Mukherjee D, Chaichana KL, et al. Association of surgically acquired motor and language deficits on overall survival after resection of glioblastoma multiforme. *Neurosurgery.* 2009;65:463-469.

Meyer FB, Bates LM, Goerss SJ, et al. Awake craniotomy for aggressive resection of primary gliomas located in eloquent brain. *Mayo Clin Proc.* 2001;76:677-687.

Nimsky C, Ganslandt O, Hastreiter P, et al. Preoperative and intraoperative diffusion tensor imaging-based fiber tracking in glioma surgery. *Neurosurgery.* 2005;56:130-137.

Ojemann G, Ojemann J, Lettich E, et al. Cortical language localization in left, dominant hemisphere. *J Neurosurg.* 1989;71:316-326.

Proescholdt MA, Macher C, Woertgen C, et al. A level of evidence in the literature concerning brain tumor resection. *Clin Neurol Neurosurg.* 2005;107:95-98.

Quiñones-Hinojosa A, Ojemann SG, Sanai N, et al. Preoperative correlation of intraoperative cortical mapping with magnetic resonance imaging landmarks to predict localization of the Broca area. *J Neurosurg.* 2003;99:311-318.

Romstock J, Fahlbusch R, Ganslandt, et al. Localization of the sensorimotor cortex during surgery for brain tumours: feasibility and waveform patterns of somatosensory evoked potentials. *J Neurol Neurosurg Psychiatry.* 2002;72:221-229.

Roux FE, Boulanouar K, Lotterie JA, et al. Language functional magnetic resonance imaging in preoperative assessment of language areas: correlation with direct cortical stimulation. *Neurosurgery.* 2003;52:1335-1347.

Sawaya R. Extent of resection in malignant gliomas: a critical summary. *J Neurooncol.* 1999;42:303-305.

Schmidt MH, Berger MS, Lamborn KR, et al. Repeated operations for infiltrative low-grade gliomas without intervening therapy. *J Neurosurg.* 2003;98:1165-1169.

Skirboll SS, Ojemann GA, Berger MS, et al. Functional cortex and subcortical white matter located within gliomas. *Neurosurgery.* 1996;38:678-685.

Numbered references appear on Expert Consult.

CHAPTER 12

Management of Primary Central Nervous System Lymphomas

CAMILO E. FADUL • PAMELA ELY

The phrase "primary central nervous system lymphoma" (PCNSL) is used to designate an extranodal lymphoma restricted to the nervous system, which account for about 3% of all brain tumors. Most are large B-cell lymphomas but a few cases of T-cell lymphomas have been reported. A common location is the brain parenchyma surrounding the ventricular system, but any craniospinal structure, in addition to the eye, can be involved. Although not as common, isolated spinal cord, meningeal, or ocular PCNSL can also occur. On the other hand, brain lesions are not infrequently accompanied by leptomeningeal and ocular dissemination. This chapter does not cover nervous system involvement as the first manifestation of systemic lymphoma, which can masquerade as PCNSL.

Among brain tumors, PCNSL has gained notoriety because, although still rare, it has recently increased in incidence and, unlike other brain tumors, has a high response rate to chemotherapy and radiation therapy. Before 1980, PCNSL would occur in a few individuals who were immune suppressed, usually after kidney transplant. The advent of the acquired immunodeficiency syndrome (AIDS) epidemic brought a steep increase in the frequency of this tumor. Nevertheless, the increased incidence was also seen in individuals without AIDS or other known immunosuppressive states, except for older age. Pathogenesis, diagnostic approach, treatment, and prognosis differ according to the patient's immune state; thus when there is a suspicion of PCNSL, establishing an individual's immunocompetency is of fundamental importance in deciding the most appropriate management.

At some point in his or her career, the neurosurgeon will be required to decide about surgery for a lesion suspected of being PCNSL by imaging studies. Unfortunately, the appearance is not specific, making it necessary to have this entity in mind as part of the differential diagnosis of any mass lesion. Because this tumor is highly responsive to nonsurgical forms of therapy, the role of surgery has to be tempered accordingly. In some cases, it will entail the deferral of surgical resection of a mass until the pathologic result of a diagnostic biopsy is available for review. In others, it involves refraining from the use of steroids until after the biopsy is performed to ensure the best diagnostic yield from the specimen. Moreover, placement of a reservoir with intraventricular catheter for chemotherapy administration may be required as part of the treatment. Therefore, it is important for the neurosurgeon to be aware of the clinical and diagnostic characteristics suggestive of PCNSL while actively participating in the subsequent therapeutic antineoplastic phase.

This chapter describes concepts pertaining to PCNSL of relevance for the neurosurgical practice taking into account, where appropriate, differences according to the patient's immune state. Initial consideration will be given to the pathogenesis, etiology, and epidemiology of this type of lymphoma. Clinical presentation and diagnostic approach when the suspicion of PCNSL arises will be reviewed. Finally, therapeutic interventions, complications, and prognostic factors will be described in detail, insofar as they are important to understanding the surgical role in the overall interdisciplinary treatment approach of PCNSL.

Pathogenesis and Molecular Pathology

PCNSLs are almost exclusively of B-cell origin with only 2% of T-cell origin. The most common histologic subtype is the CD20-positive, diffuse, large-cell, B-cell, non-Hodgkin's lymphoma (NHL), with a smattering of other more indolent B-cell lymphomas reported. The disease is more common in the immunocompromised than in the immunocompetent, but the pathogenesis of these disorders is uncertain regardless of the immunocompetency of the patient.[1,2]

Normal B cells arise from the hematopoietic stem cell and initially undergo antigen-independent differentiation, with immunoglobulin rearrangement in the bone marrow prior to emerging from the marrow as mature but naive B cells. These B cells move to secondary lymphoid organs where, upon encountering antigen, they undergo somatic hypermutation of the immunoglobulin variable region in the germinal center microenvironment. The presence of T cells, antigen presenting cells and the appropriate cytokine milieu are generally considered a requirement for somatic hypermutation with subsequent affinity maturation.[3] B cells displaying the highest affinity for antigen are rescued from apoptosis and become either a memory cell or the terminally differentiated plasma cell.

Malignant B cells can be viewed as B cells arrested at a certain stage of differentiation. The developmental state of the cell will be reflected in its morphologic attributes, the degree of immunoglobulin rearrangement, the expression

HISTOGENESIS OF PCNSL

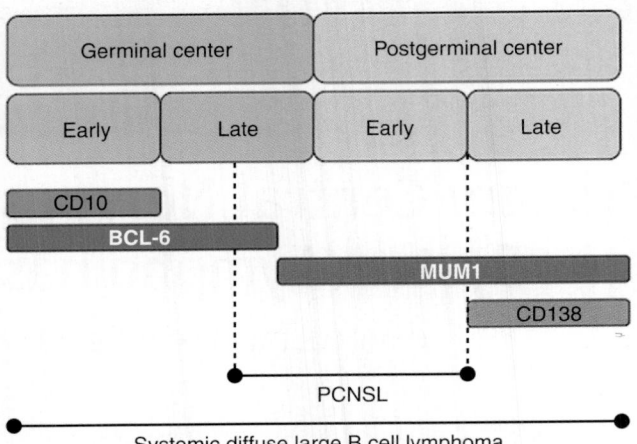

FIGURE 12-1 A model for the histogenesis of PCNSL based on the developmental stage of B-cell arrest as indicated by antigen expression. (Adapted from Camilleri-Broet S, Criniere E, Broet P, et al. A uniform activated B-cell-like immunophenotype might explain the poor prognosis of primary central nervous system lymphomas: analysis of 83 cases. Blood 2006;107:190-196.)

of surface molecules including CD10, BCL-6, MUM-1, and CD138 (which serve as markers of the B cell's transition through the germinal center), and the presence of intraclonal heterogeneity. In the majority of PCNSLs, the malignant cells are BCL-6 positive (60%–100%), MUM-1 positive (90%–100%), and have undergone immunoglobulin rearrangement with somatic hypermutation. These findings suggest that the malignant cell has seen antigen, passed through the germinal center but has not yet become a plasma B cell, that is, the cell of origin in most PCNSLs is a B cell on the verge of exiting the germinal center (Fig. 12-1).[4-6] Because there are no germinal centers in the brain, the B cell has, in all likelihood, migrated from a node to the CNS, probably in response to an antigen.[7] It is unclear, however, whether the malignant transformation of B cell occurs prior to or following migration into the CNS.

A rat model of the disease, developed by Knopf and colleagues,[8] suggests that PCNSL arises in response to an antigenic stimulus, an infection perhaps, where the antigen has moved into a draining lymph node and serves to recruit naive B cells. Presumably, antigen retained in the CNS as well as the expression of specific chemokines prompts trafficking of B cells back into the CNS. Although this hypothetical scenario is compatible with the pathologic stage of development and differentiation of the malignant cell, several questions remain unanswered, including identification of the site of malignant transformation as mentioned above, the complete lack of involved lymph nodes, and the identification of the intracerebral antigen driving the process.

Certainly, there is abundant data that Epstein-Barr virus (EBV) is involved in the pathogenesis of PCNSL in the HIV-positive patient. There are, however, equally compelling data that EBV positivity is a rarity in PCNSL occurring in the immunocompetent individual.[3,9,10] Thus, it is quite possible that the underlying pathogenesis differs, depending on the immunocompetency of the patient.

Epidemiology

PCNSL was considered a rare tumor occurring in a few immunosuppressed organ transplant recipients until the early 1980s when, coinciding with the AIDS epidemic, there was a marked increase in its frequency. The increase in incidence was seen in all age groups but was more evident in men than in women.[11] At its peak, prior to the highly active antiretroviral therapy (HAART) era, the relative-risk in HIV-infected individuals was 1000- to 3600-fold higher than in immunocompetent individuals; this has declined dramatically, essentially by an order of magnitude, since the introduction of HAART.[12,13] However, a definite and persistent rise in incidence in the immunocompetent population has been observed.[14,15] Patients without immune suppression are usually older, and the male-to-female ratio is 1.2 to 1.7:1.[11] Most studies corroborate that this change in the incidence of PCNSL is independent of trends in the incidence of brain tumors and in NHL.[16]

Clinical Manifestations

The clinical effects of PCNSL are indistinguishable from those associated with other brain tumors. In addition to the routine medical history, special care should be taken to elicit information about the possibility of immune suppression, especially HIV infection. PCNSL usually occurs several years after the diagnosis of HIV infection has been made.[17] Because PCNSL only occurs in about 3% of all AIDS patients,[18] infections like toxoplasmosis are a more likely diagnosis in this setting. It should be noted, however, that as a cause of intracranial mass lesions in an individual with AIDS, PCNSL is second only to toxoplasmosis.[12]

Approximately 8% of immunocompetent patients will have a history of successful treatment of a non–nervous system malignancy prior to the diagnosis of PCNSL.[19] In these cases, the diagnosis is even more challenging and might be delayed because of the concern of secondary nervous system involvement from the previous malignancy. When the previous malignancy is an extraneural NHL, absence of systemic disease on diagnostic workup and comparison of gene rearrangement studies on the biopsy specimens of both lymphomas can demonstrate that they are separate entities. Whether these patients have an increased predisposition to multiple neoplastic processes, or the PCNSL is the result of the antineoplastic treatment for the first tumor, is unknown.[19]

The relative frequency of clinical manifestations of PCNSL does not differ greatly between immunosuppressed and immunocompetent individuals. Nevertheless, there are some differences that might be of clinical relevance when considering the diagnosis. In immunocompetent patients, the median age at presentation is in the sixth decade of life, whereas the median age for AIDS patients is in the fourth decade of life. Patients with AIDS more often have multiple lesions than do immunocompetent individuals, making the clinical topographic diagnosis difficult, and the latency between the onset of symptoms and diagnosis seems to be shorter.[18]

The clinical course is usually subacute, with a few months elapsing between the onset of symptoms and the diagnosis of a mass lesion by imaging studies. There are several reports of spontaneous transient remission of symptoms associated with PCNSL.[20] The most common symptoms associated with PCNSL are focal neurologic deficit, increased intracranial pressure, alteration of mental function, or a combination of these manifestations. At the time of initial presentation, approximately one third will have symptoms of increased intracranial pressure, about 50% will have behavioral changes, and approximately 10% will have seizures.[18] Between 30% and 42% of patients will experience a combination of focal and nonfocal symptoms at the time of diagnosis. The neurologic examination will yield a variety of signs that can be localizing or nonlocalizing (e.g., increased intracranial pressure or alteration in the mental function). Hemiparesis and ataxia are the most common focal neurologic signs, but aphasia, acalculia, visual field defects, and cranial nerve palsies are also common.[18] Cranial-spinal nerve palsies and hydrocephalus might be secondary to lymphomatous meningeal infiltration, which is present in up to 42% of all patients with PCNSL.[18] Visual symptoms might precede or follow the diagnosis of PCNSL and will depend on the ocular structure affected by the tumor. However, 50% of the patients with PCNSL and ocular involvement detected by slit-lamp examination are asymptomatic.[21] Clinically apparent ocular involvement at presentation is found in about 8% to 10% of PCNSL patients,[18] but vitreous involvement of the eye occurring prior to or during the course of CNS lymphoma has been noted in up to 25% of patients.[22] In about half of the cases with ocular involvement, visual symptoms can be the first manifestation of PCNSL, preceding neurologic symptoms by several months. Decreased visual acuity or floaters may prompt the patient to seek medical attention, and any nonspecific uveitis refractory to topical or systemic steroids should bring ocular PCNSL to mind.[21]

Rare clinical syndromes that sometimes are associated with PCNSL include those where the tumor location is restricted to the spinal cord, the leptomeninges, and the hypothalamus. These are especially challenging cases because, in addition to other neoplastic diseases, benign inflammatory entities can have a similar clinical and radiologic presentation. Isolated spinal cord involvement occurs in 1% to 2% of all PCNSL[18] and can be associated with syringomyelia.[23] The level and extent of myelopathic involvement will guide the clinical presentation. Secondary involvement of the spinal cord in patients with cerebral lesions is not a rare occurrence.[24] PCNSL may also present as hypothalamic dysfunction causing diabetes insipidus,[18] as pituitary apoplexy with bitemporal hemianopsia or as isolated third nerve palsy.[25]

A variant of PCNSL, clinically presenting with progressive cognitive decline and gait disorder and associated with diffuse white matter abnormality without enhancement on MRI was initially described in 1999.[26] The term "lymphomatosis cerebri" has been used to describe this uncommon condition, which can be difficult to diagnose because of the nonspecific clinical and imaging findings;[26-30] it can be erroneously diagnosed as vascular leukoencephalopathy, multiple sclerosis (MS), or gliomatosis cerebri.

Diagnosis

A definitive diagnosis of PCNSL cannot be made on clinical or imaging grounds, and histologic confirmation is essential. CT scan or MRI will initially establish the presence of

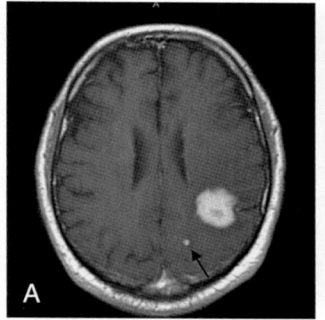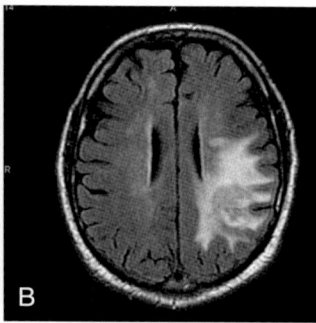

FIGURE 12-2 T1-enhanced (A) and FLAIR (B) MRI showing the infiltrative character of PCNSL. *Arrow* shows small satellite area of enhancement that on the FLAIR seems to be connected to the larger lesion.

a mass lesion with characteristics that, although suggestive of PCNSL, are not specific for this entity (Fig. 12-2). CSF analysis helps in the differential diagnosis and in some cases makes the diagnosis by the demonstration of malignant B lymphocytes.[18] HIV testing is required in all patients suspected of having PCNSL. In spite of the information obtained from these studies, tissue diagnosis is required in most circumstances.

IMAGING STUDIES

There are some characteristics on imaging studies that, although not pathognomonic, would strongly suggest that the mass lesion identified might be of lymphomatous origin. In the immunocompetent host a higher level of suspicion is required. Head CT scan shows a hyperdense or isodense mass, solitary in 86% of the cases,[31] that usually exhibits homogenous enhancement after the administration of iodinated contrast.[32] Lesions are usually supratentorial and localized in the deep periventricular areas.[31] Because of their infiltrative nature, the lesions might have indistinct borders and result in minimal surrounding edema or compressive effect (see Fig. 12-2). Occasionally it can appear as a ring-enhancing lesion with a hypodense, necrotic core, indistinguishable from a high-grade glioma. Lesions can be multiple, suggestive of metastatic disease or infection, but the scarce perilesional edema should raise the suspicion of PCNSL. In about 10% of the cases the lesions are localized in the posterior fossa.

On MRI, most of the lesions are hypointense or isointense on T1-weighted images, and only about 40% are hyperintense on T2-weighted images.[32] Although most lesions enhance after the administration of gadolinium exceptions include cases when the study follows the administration of steroids or when there is a diffuse infiltrating lymphoma (lymphomatosis cerebri) (Fig. 12-3). The appearance of PCNSL is of such heterogeneity that it should be considered in the differential diagnosis of any mass lesions detected on imaging studies (Fig. 12-4).

PCNSL in the immunocompromised patient may have a more variable appearance on imaging studies.[33] Infection is more likely to be responsible for a mass or enhancing lesion on imaging studies than PCNSL in this population, but no specific pattern has been established that can be used to distinguish between CNS lymphoma, toxoplasmosis, or other CNS diseases that occur in patients with AIDS.[18] Unlike immunocompetent patients, AIDS-associated PCNSL

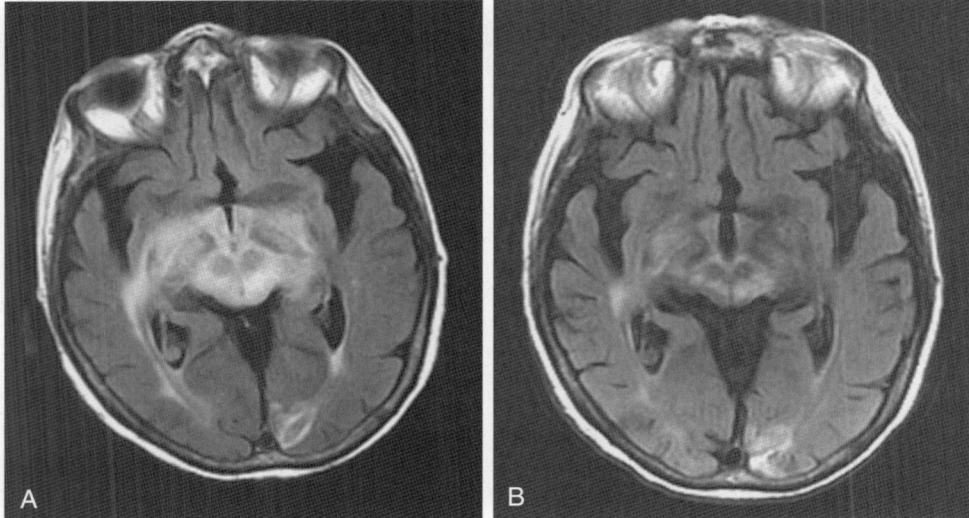

FIGURE 12-3 FLAIR MRI prior to (A) and after (B) treatment of lymphomatosis cerebri.

has been reported to present with multiple lesions in 71% to 80% of cases, to show ring-like enhancement in 50% of cases, and to lack enhancement in about 10% to 27% of the lesions.[33] Spontaneous hemorrhage, a nonenhancing lesion, or diffuse white matter changes do not exclude lymphoma in an immunocompromised patient.

Advanced MRI techniques may be helpful to pre-operatively suggest PCNSL. Magnetic resonance spectroscopy (MRS) shows massively elevated lipid resonances in PCNSL; although this may also be present in glioblastoma, the

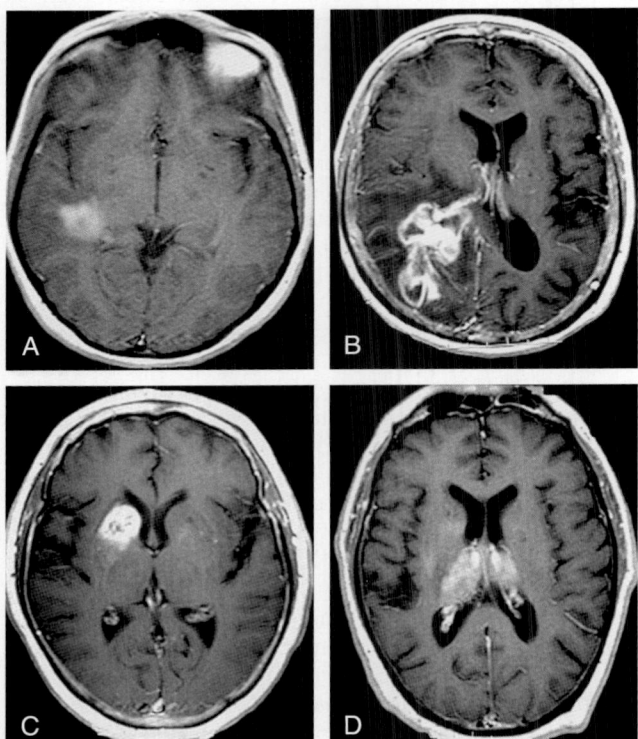

FIGURE 12-4 T1-enhanced MRI of entities mimicking PCNSL on imaging studies: (A) multiple sclerosis, (B) toxoplasmosis in a patient with a history of renal transplant, (C) stroke, and (D) arteriovenous malformation.

finding of elevated lipid resonances in combination with a markedly elevated choline/creatine ratio, may improve the preoperative differentiation of PCNSL and glioma.[34] Dynamic susceptibility contrast-enhanced perfusion MRI reveals that the relative cerebral blood volume ratio is lower for PCNSL, correlating with the lower microvessel density by immunohistochemistry, than high grade gliomas.[35] Using diffusion tensor imaging, with the enhancing lesion as the region of interest and comparing to the contralateral normal-appearing white matter, the fractional anisotropy and the apparent diffusion coefficient (ADC) ratios can be measured. Both parameters are significantly lower in lymphomas than glioblastoma and may assist in differentiating between these two entities.[36] The ADC ratios, however, do not allow a reliable distinction between toxoplasmosis and lymphoma.[37]

Nuclear medicine has also been suggested as a possible method to discriminate between PCNSL and other types of malignant as well as nonmalignant pathologies without resorting to histologic diagnosis. In a study comparing N-isopropyl-p-(^{123}I)-iodoamphetamine (^{123}I-IMP) single photon emission computerized tomography (SPECT) in patients with malignant glioma, PCNSL and meningioma, the ^{123}I-IMP retention uptake in the 6-hour to 24-hour SPECT images were significantly higher in PCNSL than in those of both malignant gliomas and meningiomas.[38] In patients with AIDS, the thallium[201]-SPECT delayed retention index may be useful to discriminate PCNSL from infectious lesions with high sensitivity and specificity.[39] The diagnostic utility of these techniques has yet to be determined in larger series, and histologic confirmation is still considered the gold standard for diagnosis of PCNSL.

Tumor infiltration of the nervous system can be more diffuse than is appreciated on imaging studies. Correlation of autopsy and MRI findings in 10 patients who died with PCNSL showed that all had tumor infiltration in CNS regions that were normal radiographically, including T2 sequences.[40] Therefore, the infiltrative microscopic tumor burden of PCNSL renders futile any attempt to resect these lesions. The surgical role is restricted to a tissue biopsy for histologic diagnosis.

TABLE 12-1	Differential Diagnosis of PCNSL
Disease	**Diagnostic Studies**
Multiple sclerosis	Past medical history, CSF
High-grade glioma	SPECT-MRS
Infection	HIV infection, CSF
Sarcoidosis	ACE level, calcium
Meningioma	MRS
Vascular	Cerebral angiogram, MRI DWIs

ACE, angiotensin-converting enzyme; CSF, cerebrospinal fluid; DWI, diffusion-weighted images; HIV, human immunodeficiency virus; MRS, magnetic resonance spectroscopy; SPECT, single photon emission computerized tomography.

TISSUE DIAGNOSIS AND STAGING

While the diagnosis of PCNSL is usually suggested by the appearance of a focal lesion on CT or MRI, confirmation of the diagnosis of PCNSL in the immunocompetent requires tissue to definitively differentiate PCNSL from metastatic disease, glioma, sarcoidosis, and inflammatory lesions (Table 12-1). Because the CSF is involved at diagnosis 20% of the time, a brain biopsy can be avoided if malignant cells can be obtained from the CSF.[41] Similarly, malignant (though often asymptomatic) uveitis is apparent in 10% to 20% of patients with PCNSL at presentation and may serve as the source of cells on which the diagnosis may be based.[42,43] Cytologic examination of cells, as the sole parameter by which the diagnosis is made, is not optimal because it cannot determine monoclonality, a condition that is necessary though not sufficient for the diagnosis of lymphoma. In the case of B-cell lymphoma, monoclonality can be determined by flow cytometric detection of light-chain restriction if there are sufficient cells available. In T-cell disease, and when there are inadequate numbers of malignant B cells for flow cytometry, the diagnosis can be established by polymerase chain reaction (PCR) studies on the basis of T-cell receptor or immunoglobulin rearrangement, respectively. This technique is susceptible to false positives if too few cells are present and to false negatives if the DNA is highly degraded.[44] It is important to underscore the fact that most lymphomas, including PCNSL, are quite sensitive to steroids. Cell death and tumor regression may occur as early as 24 hours after initiation of therapy. If tissue or a specimen for cytology is obtained following initiation of steroids, the result may be nondiagnostic because of cell death and tissue necrosis. Unless the patient is showing evidence of rapid neurologic deterioration or impending herniation, tissue should be obtained prior to starting any steroid therapy.[45,46] Although a retrospective study exists challenging this concept,[47] it seems prudent to avoid the unnecessary use of corticosteroids prior to diagnostic biopsy for PCNSL.

Once the diagnosis is made, patients generally undergo staging to determine the extent of involvement. Baseline evaluations include a physical and a neurologic exam, as well as cognitive function assessment. Because systemic involvement tends to occur more commonly at relapse, and because evidence of systemic disease is found in less than 5% at diagnosis, the necessity for a full lymphoma staging has been called into question.[48] There is general agreement that, besides a complete history and physical, a CBC, standard chemistries with an LDH, HIV status, chest x-ray,

CSF examination, and slit-lamp examination are absolutely required. A full staging would also include CT of the chest, abdomen, and pelvis, as well as bilateral bone marrow biopsies. Finally, testicular ultrasound should be considered in all elderly men. Full staging is inevitably required for any patient enrolled in a clinical trial and is recommended for all patients with PCNSL in the published guidelines for standardization of baseline evaluations.[49]

The role of ^{18}F-fluorodeoxyglucose (FDG) PET to rule out systemic disease in the initial evaluation of patients presenting with PCNSL is uncertain. Two retrospective studies using PET in the initial staging of immunocompetent patients have revealed abnormalities (e.g., other malignancies, systemic sites of lymphoma as well as concurrent sites within the nervous system) undetected by other diagnostic studies in 19% and 28% of patients respectively.[50,51] It remains to be determined if FDG PET is needed in all patients with the presumptive diagnosis of PCNSL (Fig. 12-5).

The approach to a focal brain lesion in the HIV population is slightly different. The detection of EBV DNA by PCR in the CSF was initially found to be a sensitive (80% to 84%) and highly specific (100%) diagnostic marker of AIDS-related PCNSL, thus potentially obviating the need for a biopsy; these results, however, could not be confirmed in a later study.[52-54] A brain biopsy in the AIDS patient carries a significant morbidity (8.4%) and mortality (2.9%),[55] but is recommended when the CSF is negative for lymphoma, the focal lesion is atypical for toxoplasmosis, there is progression on a brief trial of antitoxoplasmosis therapy, toxoplasma serologies are negative, there is a rapid neurologic decline, or there are discordant CSF EBV and thallium^{201}-SPECT results.[12,17] It is noteworthy that a pre-HAART retrospective study of presumed or confirmed PCNSL in HIV-positive patients revealed there was no difference in the overall survival (1.2 months) between the two groups, presumptive and biopsy-confirmed, leading the authors to conclude there may be little benefit in subjecting the patient to the diagnostic procedure given the dismal outcome.[56] The use of HAART and its impact on the CD4 count has allowed the use of more aggressive chemotherapeutic regimens without undue toxicity, and resulted in improved life expectancy for these patients. These changes will undoubtedly influence the algorithm, and they suggest that earlier diagnostic procedures may be in order for this patient population.

DIFFERENTIAL DIAGNOSIS

PCNSL may present with a variety of signs and symptoms and has a capacity to mimic many other nonmalignant neurologic conditions.[57] It can be confused with multiple sclerosis (MS) in patients who present with neurologic dysfunction, a nonenhancing periventricular lesion, and CSF pleocytosis. Administration of corticosteroid causes clinical improvement and regression of PCNSL in some patients; this may be interpreted as a steroid-induced remission from an exacerbation of MS. Sustained clinical dependence on corticosteroid is unusual in MS, and should lead to consideration of PCNSL. Repeat CSF examination and gadolinium-enhanced MRI scan obtained off corticosteroid should differentiate between the two diagnostic possibilities.[58] PCNSL cortical lesions may be difficult to distinguish from extra-axial masses such as meningioma on imaging studies (Fig. 12-6). In the case of immunocompromised

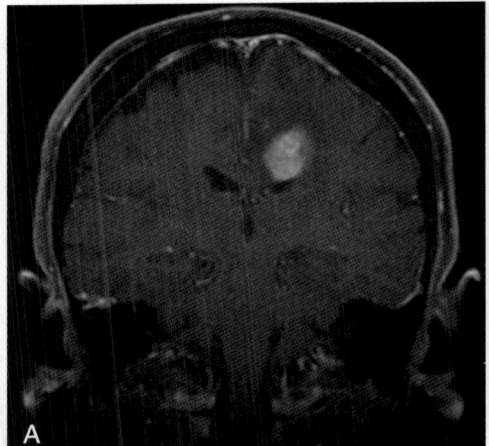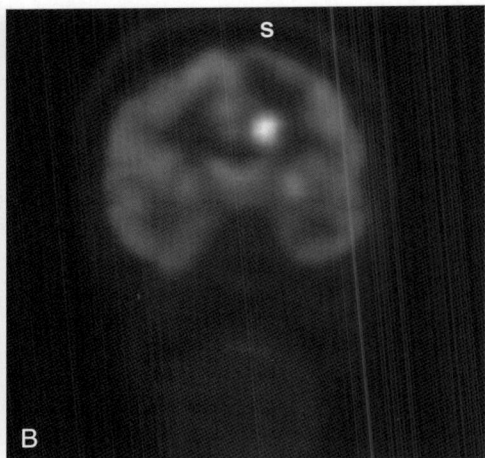

FIGURE 12-5 Coronal T1-enhanced MRI (A) and 18-fluoro-2-deoxyglucose (FDG) PET image (B) of patient with PCNSL at the time of diagnosis.

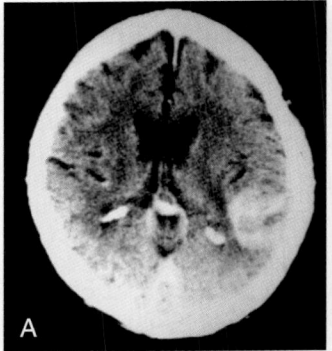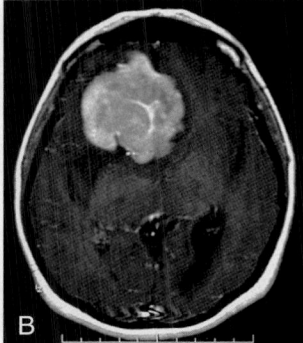

FIGURE 12-6 A, Head CT scan with contrast demonstrating left temporal-parietal enhancing mass. Biopsy revealed PCNSL. B, T1-enhanced MRI showing a right frontal PCNSL. The lesion was dural-based, infiltrating brain parenchyma, and malignant meningioma was considered in the differential diagnosis before surgery.

individuals, infections such as *Toxoplasma gondii* should always be included in the differential diagnosis.

Treatment

In spite of its infiltrative nature, PCNSL is one of the few brain tumors in which a durable remission can be achieved with appropriate treatment. Unfortunately, this sometimes is at the expense of significant treatment-related toxicity. Because PCNSL is rare, and because the disease behaves in an aggressive manner (with a life expectancy of less than 5 months if left untreated), the design of and accrual to large clinical trials has been limited. These hindrances to progress notwithstanding, there are now several interventions with varying toxicities available that can result in an increased disease-free, as well as overall, survival. An interdisciplinary, multimodality therapeutic strategy can, therefore, be designed to accommodate specific patient characteristics such as age, comorbid conditions, and immune status.

STEROIDS

Steroids induce apoptosis of lymphoid cells and can result in complete disappearance of the clinical and imaging manifestations associated with PCNSL.[59] Although reduced edema plays a role, most of the rapid and dramatic

responsiveness to corticosteroids is mediated by their cytotoxic activity. Because of the exquisite sensitivity of lymphoma cells to steroids, their administration to the patient with PCNSL carries important diagnostic and therapeutic implications. In 40% of patients, a rapid and dramatic regression of PCNSL follows their administration.[60] Further, there can be a complete response after steroids in about 15% of the cases, resulting in the complete disappearance of the target for the biopsy.[59] In another series, however, the majority of immunocompetent PCNSL patients received steroids before biopsy and had neither significant MRI change nor required of second biopsy for diagnosis.[47] A dramatic clinical and MRI improvement would make the diagnosis of PCNSL very likely, although as previously mentioned there are other entities that exhibit similar steroid-responsiveness.

Even when a complete response is obtained on steroids alone, the disease will recur either at the same or in a remote site within the nervous system. Due to the potential development of steroid resistance, their use as monotherapy for PCNSL is not recommended, though they are usually used in combination with chemotherapy as part of the therapeutic regimen. It has been shown that the addition of corticosteroids to the first course of methotrexate chemotherapy was associated with a higher rate of complete responses.[61]

Steroids are known immune suppressants that, in combination with chemotherapy or in patients already immunocompromised, may lead to opportunistic infections such as *Pneumocystis (jiroveci) carinii* pneumonia (PCP), listeriosis, and fungal infections. PCP prophylaxis is routinely used while patients are on steroids and chemotherapy.

SURGERY

PCNSL is an infiltrative tumor, usually localized in the deep periventricular regions, and is highly responsive to radiation and chemotherapy. Therefore, surgical resection is of limited benefit and can carry significant morbidity. In a retrospective study including 248 immunocompetent patients with PCNSL, 132 underwent stereotactic biopsy for diagnosis of PCNSL, resulting in a procedure-related morbidity of 3.7% and no mortality. The remaining 116 underwent surgical resection (because imaging studies were not suggestive of lymphoma) with a mortality rate of 3.4%. Multivariate analysis revealed that surgical resection was an unfavorable prognostic factor[31] and may increase functional deficit.[18]

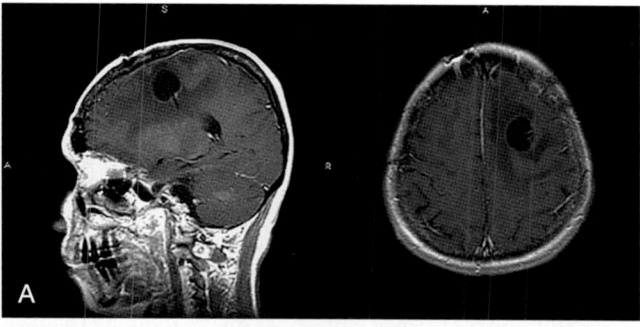
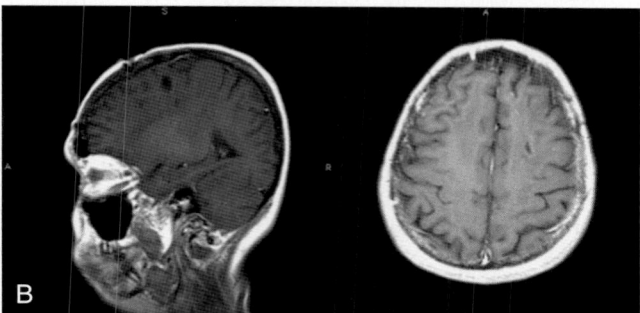

FIGURE 12-7 T1-enhanced sagittal and axial MRI of a patient with PCNSL who developed a porencephalic cyst surrounding a reservoir catheter (A) and that decreased in size after removal of the device (B).

When there is the suspicion of PCNSL, the role of surgery is restricted to a stereotactic biopsy to provide tissue for diagnostic purposes.

In AIDS patients, the diagnosis of PCNSL is extremely likely in patients with hyperactive lesions on thallium[201]-SPECT and a CSF positive for EBV-DNA. If the lesion is hypoactive on SPECT, with negative CSF EBV-DNA, the recommendation is empiric antitoxoplasma therapy. If there is disagreement between the SPECT and CSF PCR results, a brain biopsy is advisable.[53]

Despite common contiguity with the ventricular system, only 7% of the patients have hydrocephalus requiring shunting.[31] When leptomeningeal lymphomatous spread is documented, intraventricular chemotherapy is often recommended. An intraventricular catheter with a subgaleal reservoir for ease of administration is usually placed. Before therapeutic use of the reservoir, a nuclear medicine flow study is performed to ensure correct catheter placement as well as good distribution of the chemotherapy agent. Reservoirs have been associated with complications necessitating removal of the device (Fig. 12-7). Infection is the most common complication, occurring in about 15% of patients with PCNSL.

RADIATION THERAPY

Radiotherapy was the first intervention to have a significant impact on PCNSL survival, with an increased median survival of 12 to 18 months.[31,46,62] Like systemic lymphomas, PCNSLs are considered to be extremely radiosensitive as was exemplified in a study in which a 40-Gy dose to the whole brain (WB) followed by a 20-Gy boost to the lesion(s) yielded an 83% complete remission rate. Unfortunately, the remissions were not durable; the median survival from the start of radiation therapy (RT) was only 11.6 months.[62]

Unlike other tumors, there is no classic dose–response curve for radiation in PCNSL, but there does appear to be a threshold dose of 50 Gy. A review of the literature, including patients receiving only RT, found a 42.3% 5-year survival for patients receiving greater than 50 Gy, as compared with a 12.8% 5-year survival for those receiving less than 50 Gy.[62]

A devastating and irreversible complication, treatment-related delayed neurotoxicity occurs most commonly following radiation or combination chemoradiation therapy (particularly when radiation precedes the chemotherapy) and only rarely following chemotherapy alone. The elderly are particularly vulnerable with an incidence of 80% in those surviving more than 5 years. It manifests as cognitive dysfunction early on followed by motor and autonomic dysfunction.[63] While consolidation with WBRT after chemotherapy does improve the failure-free survival, it does not improve overall survival.[64] For patients who are 60 years or older, current clinical trials rarely include radiation as initial treatment because of the high risk of severe cognitive impairment and neurotoxicity-related mortality. Recent trial designs have deferred RT or recommended the use of low-dose RT consolidation after chemotherapy. RT deferred until relapse yields a response rate (79%) and overall survival rate (32 months from diagnosis) comparable to those obtained when RT was included in the initial treatment plan.[65] Reduced-dose RT (40 to 45 Gy) in patients younger than 60 years who achieve a complete response with aggressive chemotherapy may decrease the occurrence of severe cognitive impairment, but the cost is an extremely high incidence of chemotherapy-related toxicity and lower response rates.[66] Recently, response-adapted therapy adjusting the radiation dose to less than 24 Gy for patients who achieved a complete remission with immunochemotherapy has resulted in excellent disease control (the increased incidence of neutropenia notwithstanding) and no decline in cognitive testing though median follow-up is only 37 months.[67]

RADIOSURGERY

Although PCNSL is a diffuse disease frequently with multiple enhancing lesions, CSF dissemination and ocular involvement, treatment with radiosurgery has been utilized. Two small studies have reported excellent initial local control of disease with gamma knife radiosurgery but, as expected, the majority of patients develop new lesions in other locations.[68,69] Therefore, the potential benefit and long-term neurotoxicity of this therapeutic modality in the management of PCNSL is uncertain and possibly limited for symptom control of localized recurrent disease.

METHOTREXATE-BASED CHEMOTHERAPY

The use of combined modality chemoradiation therapy is generally considered to yield improved outcomes over radiation therapy alone, although this consensus is based on retrospective studies only (Fig. 12-8).[60] Further, regimens containing either high-dose methotrexate (defined as more than 1.5 gm/m^2 per cycle) or high-dose cytarabine are associated with improved survival though only the use of high-dose methotrexate appears to be an independent favorable prognostic factor.[70] These two chemotherapeutic agents are commonly used in lymphoma therapy and have excellent penetration into the CNS, even in the presence of an intact blood-brain barrier (BBB). Importantly, early studies

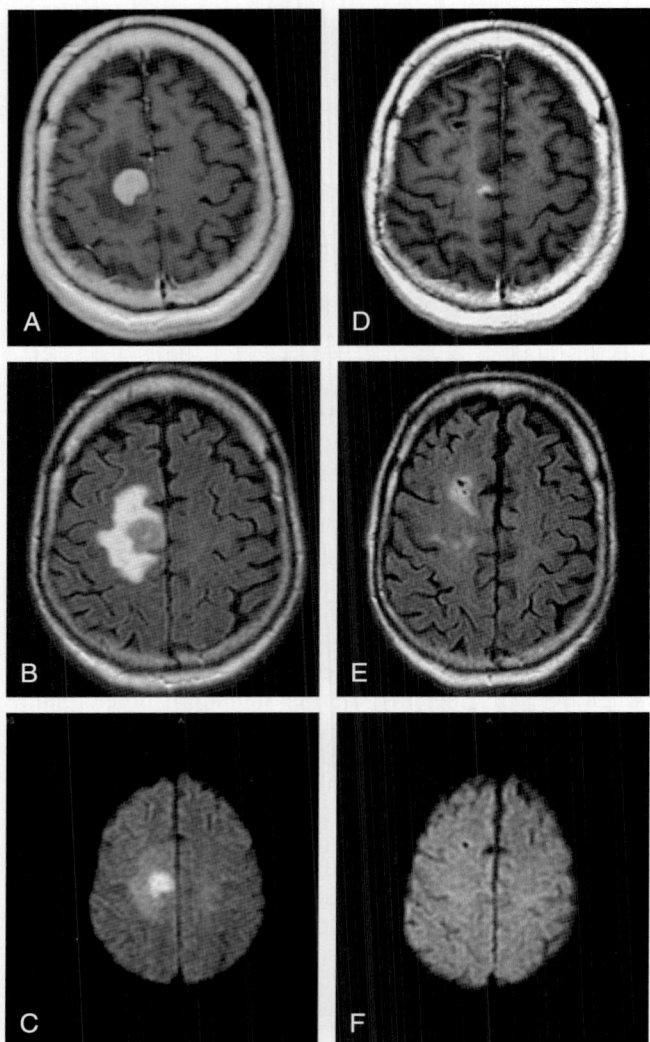

FIGURE 12-8 T1-enhanced (A), FLAIR (B), and DWI (C) MRI of patient with PCNSL at the time of diagnosis (A, B, C) and after five cycles of chemotherapy (D, E, F).

established that neither route of administration (intrathecal versus intravenous) nor chemotherapeutic agent, regardless of age, is correlated with increased neurotoxicity.[70] Multiple studies have confirmed these findings over the past decade, with median survivals ranging from 33 months to 60 months when a high-dose methotrexate regimen was used with or without subsequent WBRT (Table 12-2).[70-82]

In the elderly, studies using high-dose methotrexate-based regimens without RT have resulted in lower response rates and shorter durability of remission than in younger patients with PCNSL. The event-free survival of 5.9 to 15 months and the overall survival of 14 to 34 months are disappointing but the low incidence of both treatment-related mortality and neurotoxicity as well as a plateau in the survival curves suggests that, even in this population usually exhibiting both poor prognostic features (age and poor performance status), durable remissions with acceptable toxicity are possible.[73,74,79,82]

The use of high-dose methotrexate, therefore, has emerged as the standard of care for PCNSL. Although

questions of optimal chemotherapeutic combination and the role of post-chemotherapy radiation remain unanswered, they have given rise to the development of risk- and response-adapted interventions. Determining optimal drug combination turns on the balance of increased toxicity versus increased remission durability. Acutely, high-dose methotrexate and high-dose cytarabine carry extensive toxicity profiles that include significant bone marrow suppression, mucositis, dermatitis, and neurotoxicity. The extent and severity of toxicity for both drugs depends on rapid and reliable renal excretion and, in the case of methotrexate, restoration of the intracellular stores of reduced folate in normal cells by the administration of leucovorin (5-formyl-tetrahydrofolic acid). Thus aggressive hydration, alkalinization of the urine, initiation of leucovorin rescue within 24 to 48 hours following the methotrexate infusion, and close monitoring of renal function and methotrexate level are imperative when giving methotrexate. Infection secondary to neutropenia will remain a significant problem, particularly as more aggressive chemotherapeutic regimens are used. The addition of steroids to high-dose methotrexate renders these patients increasingly susceptible to opportunistic infections.

INTRATHECAL THERAPY

High-dose intravenous (IV) methotrexate, which penetrates an intact BBB and results in therapeutic levels of drug in the CSF, has brought into question the routine use of intrathecal (IT) therapy for patients with PCNSL. Based on retrospective data, there is a growing consensus that outside of a clinical trial, IT therapy should be used only in the setting of a positive CSF cytology, if at all, in up-front treatment.[83] Of note, however, a phase II trial of patients treated without IT therapy was stopped following interim analysis due to a high rate of early relapse when compared to the results of a previous trial of comparable PCNSL patients who received the same chemotherapy regimen but with the addition of IT therapy[84] further supporting the need for randomized trials to answer this pressing question. IT therapy is routinely used at relapse or if leptomeningeal disease persists after initiation of systemic high-dose methotrexate therapy.[83,85] Methotrexate, cytarabine, and hydrocortisone have all been used singly or in combination for IT therapy. Rituximab, an anti-CD20 monoclonal antibody beneficial in systemic large-cell B-cell lymphoma but which does not penetrate the BBB when given IV, has been shown to be well tolerated and effective when given intrathecally.[86-88]

OTHER THERAPEUTIC OPTIONS

Durable remissions and cure rates are distinctly lower in diffuse large-cell lymphoma of the CNS than in systemic diffuse large-cell, B-cell NHL. This is, in part, because of the difficulty in obtaining adequate drug levels when given systemically across an intact BBB. The chemotherapeutic regimens for systemic diffuse large-cell lymphoma routinely utilize only a few drugs, specifically those of the alkylator class, that are known to penetrate the CNS. Within this class, penetration varies from drug to drug (Table 12-3). Other strategies to increase the uptake of drugs include the use of a lipid-soluble drug (i.e., temozolomide), increased plasma concentrations, intra-arterial drug injection, and osmotic disruption of the BBB.[89] The results of a multi-institutional

TABLE 12-2 Response Rates, Overall and Progression-Free Survival, and Toxicity to PCNSL Treatment Regimens with and without Radiation, for Patients of All Ages Including Elderly

Study	n	Therapy	WBRT	IT	ORR(%)	OS (mo)	PFS	Delayed Neurotoxicity and Treatment-Related Mortality
High-dose MTX-based chemotherapy with radiation								
Abrey 2000	52	MTX 3.5 g/m² multiagent	yes	yes	94	60	NA	Neurotoxicity: 25% overall, 83% in patients aged >60 years receiving WBRT
O'Brien 2000	46	MTX 1 g/m² single agent	yes	yes	45	33	17	Neurotoxicity: 14%
Ferreri 2001	13	MTX 3 g/m² multiagent	yes	no	92	25+	NA	Neurotoxicity: 15%
DeAngelis 2002	102	MTX 2.5 g/m² multiagent	yes	yes	94	36+	24	Neurotoxicity: 15%
Poortmans 2003	52	MTX 3 g/m² multiagent	yes	yes	81	46	NA	Non-neurologic TRM: 10%
Omura 2005	17	MTX 1 g/m² multiagent	yes	yes	88	32	18	Neurotoxicity: 29%
High-dose MTX-based chemotherapy without radiation								
Schlegel 2001	20	MTX 5 g/m² multiagent	no	yes	70	54	20.5	Neurotoxicity: 5%
Pels 2003	65	MTX 5 g/m² multiagent	no	yes	71	50	21	Neurotoxicity: 3%
Batchelor 2003	25	MTX 8 g/m² single agent	no	no	74	22+	12.8	Neurotoxicity: 0%
High-dosed MTX-based chemotherapy without radiation in the elderly								
Abrey 2000	22	MTX 3.5 g/m² multiagent	no	yes	NA	33	10	Non-neurologic TRM: 0% Neurotoxicity: 5%
Pels 2003	32	MTX 5 g/m² multiagent	no	yes	56	34	15	Non-neurologic TRM: 13%
Hoang-Xuan 2003	50	MTX 1 g/m² multiagent	no	yes	48	14	10	Non-neurologic TRM: 2% Neurotoxicity: 2%
Omura 2007	23	MTX 3 g/m² multiagent	no	no	55	35	8	Non-neurologic TRM: 4%
Illerhaus 2009	30	MTX 3 g/m² multiagent	no	no	70	15.4	5.9	Non-neurologic TRM: 7% Neurotoxicity: 0% in MTX only, 100% in 2 patients unable to tolerate MTX receiving WBRT

IT, intrathecal; mo, months; MTX, methotrexate; ORR, overall response rate; OS, overall survival; PFS, progression-free survival; TRM, treatment-related mortality; WBRT, whole-brain radiation therapy.

trial using intra-arterial delivery following osmotic BBB disruption has resulted in an excellent overall response rate (81%) but significant toxicity was incurred with a combined procedural and chemotherapeutic complication rate of 33%.[90] High-dose IV therapy, which results in better penetration, is limited by systemic toxicity. However, if the dose-limiting toxicity of the agents is bone marrow suppression or ablation, stem cell rescue can be used to overcome that particular toxicity. On the assumption that there is no significant difference in the biologic behavior between systemic and CNS-isolated large-cell B-cell lymphoma, stem cell transplant, which is routinely used in systemic lymphoma,[91,92] has been proposed as a potentially curative intervention in PCNSL. Initially trialed in young PCNSL patients with poor prognostic indicators or relapsed/refractory disease,[93-95] the results were so encouraging that high-dose therapy with autologous stem cell rescue has

been moved up to first-line therapy by several groups.[96-100] Results in newly diagnosed patients using high-dose methotrexate, ablative chemotherapy with stem cell rescue, and, finally, WBRT post-transplant yielded OS of 87% at 5 years, but unacceptable neurotoxicity rates of 24%.[96] A revised protocol using radiation in the post-transplant period only when a complete response was not obtained following chemotherapy, has given very encouraging results: the disease free and overall survival at 3 years is 77% without evidence of significant neurotoxicity to date.[96]

THERAPY FOR INTRAOCULAR LYMPHOMA

The therapy for intraocular lymphoma, whether it occurs in isolation or in the presence of other CNS lesions, deserves separate mention. Neither involved field irradiation nor systemic chemotherapy alone results in durable remissions in the eye, but the addition of orbital radiation to a high-dose, methotrexate-based regimen has been associated with both a higher response rate and decreased intraocular relapse rate.[21] No difference in outcome has been found between patients treated with local (RT or intravitreal chemotherapy) as opposed to systemic chemo- or chemoradiation therapy.[101] When used, radiation to both orbits is recommended due to the fact that bilateral eye involvement occurs in almost 80% of cases.[21] Ocular RT carries a substantial morbidity including radiation retinitis, dry eye syndrome, corneal erosions, glaucoma, and cataracts. Intravitreal methotrexate (400 μg on a once or twice weekly basis with or without monthly maintenance) has been used with success.[102-104] A retrospective interinstitutional study of intravitreal methotrexate in patients with intraocular lymphoma revealed resolution of intraocular disease in all

TABLE 12-3 Systemic Antineoplastic Agents Used in Lymphoma Therapy That Penetrate the Blood–Brain Barrier

Methotrexate
Cytosine arabinoside
Procarbazine
BCNU
CCNU
Thiotepa
Temozolomide
Mercaptopurine (low concentrations)
Melphalan (low concentrations)
Cyclophosphamide (low concentrations)

patients for whom there is complete information. No patient in this study relapsed in the eye; complications included keratopathy, cataract formation or acceleration and rarely, neovascularization.[102] The optimal therapy for PCNSL with intraocular involvement remains to be defined. At present, combined chemotherapy followed by ocular irradiation appears to give the best results.

TREATMENT FOR AIDS-RELATED PCNSL

Treatment of AIDS-related lymphomas in general has been discouraging. Full-dose chemotherapy in the immunocompromised host results in an unacceptable morbidity and mortality, whereas dose reduction results in inadequate therapy, with tumor progression and drug resistance. Standard therapy has been palliative, using corticosteroids and WBRT, with only 10% of patients surviving more than 1 year. Less aggressive chemotherapy (procarbazine, CCNU, vincristine [PCV]) does appear to increase the median survival from 4 months with radiation alone to 13 months in one small study.[105] The benefit of combined modality therapy over radiotherapy has been confirmed in other studies.[56] The decision to treat with combined modality, as opposed to radiation alone, should be based on the patient's performance status, extent of disease, comorbid conditions, projected prognosis, and the patient's desire for aggressive therapy.[105] However, a linked SEER-Medicare database search of AIDS patients with PCNSL revealed that 46% of patients received RT alone and 40% received no treatment at all with the result that the prognosis for AIDS-related PCNSL remains dismal.[106] Given that AIDS-associated PCNSL is uniformly EBV+, hydroxyurea, which at a low dose can deplete deoxyribonucleotide reserves exerting an antiviral effect, has been trialed in this population.[107] To date there are only case reports of regression of PCNSL following initiation of HAART and improvement in the CD4+ cell count.[108] Further study will be needed to establish a causal link between lymphoma remission and restoration of immunocompetency.

TREATMENT OF RECURRENT PCNSL

In spite of the improved outcomes, the recurrence rates for PCNSL after first-line treatment remain high. Once the tumor recurs, diverse strategies have been proposed though most remain unstudied in a rigorous manner. The treatment in these cases is palliative and therefore the potential benefit in prolonging survival has to be tempered by the potential for toxicity.

In patients who only received chemotherapy initially, WBRT has been used as salvage therapy for refractory/relapsing PCNSL with a 58% complete response rate reported in one study, though neurotoxicity occurred in 29% within a median of 7 months following RT.[65] As noted above, high-dose chemotherapy with hematopoietic stem cell rescue was initially studied in relapsed or refractory patients younger than 65 years and has yielded encouraging results.[109]

Other chemotherapy options that have been used include topotecan, PCV, high-dose cytarabine and rechallenge with high-dose methotrexate-based regimen with variable results.[110-113] Temozolomide, an oral alkylating agent with good nervous system penetration and a favorable side effect profile, has been examined in a trial of recurrent PCNSL resulting in a 31% overall response rate and minimal toxicity.[114] A retrospective analysis of patients receiving IV rituximab in conjunction with temozolomide, followed by single agent temozolomide, revealed an objective response rate of 53% with an acceptable toxicity profile.[115] Nonetheless, the majority of responders relapsed with a median survival of only 14 months.

Prognosis

At present, regardless of immunocompetency, the primary cause of death for patients with PCNSL is their disease. For the patient with AIDS-related PCNSL, until immunocompetency can be restored, the prognosis will remain grim; the best survival results obtained with current therapeutic strategies are no more than 1 year. In the immunocompetent population, if PCNSL is untreated, the median survival is less than 5 months. Treated with radiation alone, median survival is approximately 1 year. However, median survival has improved dramatically as combination modality therapies have been introduced; median survivals of 2 to 5 years are now routinely being reported using high-dose methotrexate regimens. Given that systemic, diffuse, large-cell B-cell lymphoma is a curable disease in a significant percentage of patients, there is no theoretical reason why some patients with PCNSL of the diffuse, large-cell, B-cell subtype cannot be cured.

The ability to determine which patients will likely do well would be of great benefit and would aid in tailoring therapy to the patient. There is general agreement that age and performance status are the most important predictors of outcome.[77,79,116] In a multicenter retrospective study of 378 immunocompetent patients, Ferreri and colleagues have attempted to identify other factors that may predict response. Besides age and performance status, serum LDH, CSF protein concentration, and involvement of the deep structures of the brain were independent predictors of survival.[117] Survival, of course, is not the only endpoint worthy of measure, and chronic toxicity to the CNS, resulting in an unacceptable quality of life, must be factored into the equation. The opportunity to study, for the first time, PCNSL patients surviving for more than 5 years, has revealed that in patients under 60 years of age, combination chemoradiation therapy yields a superior overall survival to chemotherapy alone but the price is a 26% incidence of debilitating and irreversible neurotoxicity. In patients over 60 years of age, overall survival was identical in the two groups (with and without WBRT) but the cause of death in those receiving WBRT was neurotoxicity while in those who did not, the cause of death was relapse.[63] Although the optimal therapy for PCNSL has not yet been determined, it does appear that PCNSL may, like its systemic counterpart, be a potentially curable malignancy. Current therapies hold the hope that the price of cure will not include unacceptable cognitive dysfunction.

KEY REFERENCES

Abrey LE, Batchelor TT, Ferreri AJ, et al. Report of an international workshop to standardize baseline evaluation and response criteria for primary CNS lymphoma. *J Clin Oncol.* 2005;23:5034-5043.

Abrey LE, Yahalom J, DeAngelis LM. Treatment for primary CNS lymphoma: the next step. *J Clin Oncol.* 2000;18:3144-3150.

Angelov L, Doolittle ND, Kraemer DF, et al. Blood-brain barrier disruption and intra-arterial methotrexate-based therapy for newly diagnosed primary CNS lymphoma: a multi-institutional experience. *J Clin Oncol.* 2009;27:3503-3509.

Antinori A, De Rossi G, Ammassari A, et al. Value of combined approach with thallium-201 single-photon emission computed tomography and Epstein-Barr virus DNA polymerase chain reaction in CSF for the diagnosis of AIDS-related primary CNS lymphoma. *J Clin Oncol.* 1999;17:554-560.

Bataille B, Delwail V, Menet E, et al. Primary intracerebral malignant lymphoma: report of 248 cases. *J Neurosurg.* 2000;92:261-266.

DeAngelis LM, Seiferheld W, Schold SC, et al. Combination chemotherapy and radiotherapy for primary central nervous system lymphoma: radiation Therapy Oncology Group Study 93-10. *J Clin Oncol.* 2002;20:4643-4648.

Ekenel M, Iwamoto FM, Ben-Porat LS, et al. Primary central nervous system lymphoma: the role of consolidation treatment after a complete response to high-dose methotrexate-based chemotherapy. *Cancer.* 2008;113:1025-1031.

Ferreri AJ, Blay JY, Reni M, et al. Prognostic scoring system for primary CNS lymphomas: the International Extranodal Lymphoma Study Group experience. *J Clin Oncol.* 2003;21:266-272.

Ferreri AJ, Abrey LE, Blay JY, et al. Summary statement on primary central nervous system lymphomas from the Eighth International Conference on Malignant Lymphoma, Lugano, Switzerland, June 12 to 15, 2002. *J Clin Oncol.* 2003;21:2407-2414.

Gavrilovic IT, Hormigo A, Yahalom J, et al. Long-term follow-up of high-dose methotrexate-based therapy with and without whole brain irradiation for newly diagnosed primary CNS lymphoma. *J Clin Oncol.* 2006;24:4570-4574.

Grimm SA, Pulido JS, Jahnke K, et al. Primary intraocular lymphoma: an International Primary Central Nervous System Lymphoma Collaborative Group Report. *Ann Oncol.* 2007;18:1851-1855.

Herrlinger U, Schabet M, Bitzer M, et al. Primary central nervous system lymphoma: from clinical presentation to diagnosis. *J Neurooncol.* 1999;43:219-226.

Hoang-Xuan K, Taillandier L, Chinot O, et al. Chemotherapy alone as initial treatment for primary CNS lymphoma in patients older than 60 years: a multicenter phase II study (26952) of the European Organization for Research and Treatment of Cancer Brain Tumor Group. *J Clin Oncol.* 2003;21:2726-2731.

Hottinger AF, DeAngelis LM, Yahalom J, Abrey LE. Salvage whole brain radiotherapy for recurrent or refractory primary CNS lymphoma. *Neurology.* 2007;69:1178-1182.

Jahnke K, Thiel E, Martus P, et al. Relapse of primary central nervous system lymphoma: clinical features, outcome and prognostic factors. *J Neurooncol.* 2006;80:159-165.

Kasamon YL, Ambinder RF. AIDS-related primary central nervous system lymphoma. *Hematol Oncol Clin North Am.* 2005;19:665-687;vi-vii.

Knopf PM, Harling-Berg CJ, Cserr HF, et al. Antigen-dependent intrathecal antibody synthesis in the normal rat brain: tissue entry and local retention of antigen-specific B cells. *J Immunol.* 1998;161:692-701.

Kreisl TN, Panageas KS, Elkin EB, et al. Treatment patterns and prognosis in patients with human immunodeficiency virus and primary central system lymphoma. *Leuk Lymphoma.* 2008;49:1710-1716.

Nelson DF. Radiotherapy in the treatment of primary central nervous system lymphoma (PCNSL). *J Neurooncol.* 1999;43:241-247.

Omuro AM, DeAngelis LM, Yahalom J, Abrey LE. Chemoradiotherapy for primary CNS lymphoma: an intent-to-treat analysis with complete follow-up. *Neurology.* 2005;64:69-74.

Schlegel U, Schmidt-Wolf IG, Deckert M. Primary CNS lymphoma: clinical presentation, pathological classification, molecular pathogenesis and treatment. *J Neurol Sci.* 2000;181:1-12.

Shah GD, Yahalom J, Correa DD, et al. Combined immunochemotherapy with reduced whole-brain radiotherapy for newly diagnosed primary CNS lymphoma. *J Clin Oncol.* 2007;25:4730-4735.

Siegal T, Zylber-Katz E. Strategies for increasing drug delivery to the brain: focus on brain lymphoma. *Clin Pharmacokinet.* 2002;41:171-186.

Soussain C, Hoang-Xuan K, Taillandier L, et al. Intensive chemotherapy followed by hematopoietic stem-cell rescue for refractory and recurrent primary CNS and intraocular lymphoma: societe Francaise de Greffe de Moelle Osseuse-Therapie Cellulaire. *J Clin Oncol.* 2008;26:2512-2518.

Sparano JA. Clinical aspects and management of AIDS-related lymphoma. *Eur J Cancer.* 2001;37:1296-1305.

Numbered references appear on Expert Consult.

CHAPTER 13

Surgical Management of Brain Stem Tumors in Adults

JAMES L. FRAZIER • GEORGE I. JALLO

Brain stem tumors account for 1.5% to 2.5% of all intracranial tumors in adults while comprising 10% to 20% of all pediatric tumors.[1-4] These tumors are less common in adults and, therefore, more clinical studies have been conducted in children with brain stem tumors, specifically brain stem gliomas, since they are more common in this patient population.[3-10] Adults with brain stem gliomas have a median survival of 5 to 7 years which is longer than that of children.[2-5] Historically, brain stem tumors were treated as a homogenous group of lesions with radiotherapy, which usually proceeded without histopathologic confirmation. Surgery for these tumors was rare and typically limited to biopsy, extirpation of cystic lesions, and the placement of shunts for obstructive hydrocephalus. However, Pool documented one of the first surgical resections of a brain stem tumor located in the area of the cerebral aqueduct in 1968.[11] This reported case led to the advent of further investigation and development of surgical techniques to treat lesions located in the brain stem.

Although brain stem tumors were thought to be homogeneous, the advent of computed tomography (CT) and magnetic resonance imaging (MRI) changed this belief, and imaging of the brain provided evidence that these lesions comprised a heterogeneous group. Detailed imaging allowed distinction among different tumor types according to location and growth pattern. This tumor heterogeneity would be confirmed by histopathologic examination as surgery was increasingly used as neurosurgical operative techniques, including stereotactic biopsies, and perioperative care significantly evolved.

Imaging and Classification

Prior to the advent of MRI, CT was utilized to assess the pathology of brain stem lesions and biopsy was often needed to guide management. MRI has become the primary diagnostic modality for patients with brain stem tumors because it has advanced the diagnosis and categorization of these lesions by providing superior anatomic detail of the brain stem and posterior fossa.[12-16] T1- and T2-weighted MR imaging have provided the ability to differentiate the tissue characteristics of tumors in many cases. In adults, the differential diagnosis for brain stem lesions may be broad and may include such pathologic entities like metastatic tumors, demyelinating processes, infectious processes, granulomas, cavernous malformations, hemangioblastomas, or hematomas that should be differentiated from gliomas.

Based upon MRI and CT data, classification schemes have been developed for grouping brain stem tumors according to growth patterns and the feasibility of surgical resection (Table 13-1).[13,14,17-21] The earliest classification schemes were based on CT images and surgical observation.[17,19,21] Later schemes relied on MR imaging, in which better neuroanatomic details were made available.[13,14,18] The most recently developed classification system relied on both CT and MRI.[20] All of these schemes classify the tumor into either a focal or diffuse growth pattern, while the more complex classifications further subdivide the tumors into location within the brain stem, presence or absence of an exophytic component, and the presence of hydrocephalus or hemorrhage. The more complex schemes were developed in an attempt to predict tumor behavior and guide operative versus nonoperative management. In general, tumors with a focal growth pattern have been considered amenable to surgical extirpation in contrast to those with a diffuse growth pattern.

FOCAL TUMORS

Focal tumors are intrinsic to the brain stem and may be cystic or solid (Fig. 13-1). They are typically not associated with edema and contrast enhancement may be variable. A majority of these tumors are low-grade gliomas, but some malignant tumors, such as a World Health Organization (WHO) grade-IV astrocytoma, may imitate a focal one, known as a pseudofocal tumor. In pseudofocal tumors, MRI and CT imaging demonstrate focal enhancement after the administration of contrast with normal signal characteristics from the peritumoral area that imitates the focal lesion.

Furthermore, the majority of cervicomedullary gliomas are low-grade, noninfiltrative tumors, and their growth is usually confined rostrally by the white matter of the corticospinal tract and medial lemniscus.[22]

EXOPHYTIC TUMORS

Focal brain stem tumors with an exophytically growing component are usually low-grade and well circumscribed (Fig. 13-2). They are typically dorsally exophytic tumors growing into the fourth ventricle or cervicomedullary tumors with exophytic growth into the cisterna magna and fourth ventricle (Fig. 13-3). It should be mentioned that, in

Table 13-1	**Classification Schemes for Brain Stem Tumors**	
Author	**Method Used to Create System**	**Classification System**
Epstein[21]	CT	Intrinsic
		Diffuse
		Focal
		Cervicomedullary
		Exophytic
		Anterolateral into cerebello-pontine angle
		Posterolateral and into brachium pontis
		Disseminated
		Positive cytology
		Positive myelography
Epstein and McCleary[19]	CT, MRI, and surgical observation	Diffuse
		Focal
		Cervicomedullary
Stroink et al.[17]	CT	Group I—dorsal exophytic glioma
		Group IIa—intrinsic brain-stem tumors
		Hypodense, no enhancement
		Group IIb—intrinsic brain-stem tumors
		Hyperdense, contrast enhancing exophytic
		Group III—focal cystic tumor with contrast enhancement
		Group IV—focal intrinsic isodense contrast enhancement
Barkovich et al.[14]	MRI	Location (midbrain, pons, medulla)
		Focality (diffuse or focal)
		Direction and extent of tumor growth
		Degree of brainstem enlargement
		Exophytic growth
		Hemorrhage or necrosis
		Evidence of hydrocephalus
Albright[18]	MRI	Focal (midbrain, pons, medulla)
		Diffuse
Fischbein et al.[13]	MRI	Midbrain
		Diffuse
		Focal
		Tectal
		Pons
		Diffuse
		Focal
		Medulla
		Diffuse
		Focal
		Dorsal exophytic
Choux et al.[20]	CT and MRI	Type I—diffuse
		Type II—intrinsic, focal
		Type III—exophytic, focal
		Type IV—cervicomedullary

addition to focal tumors, some diffuse tumors may cause bulging into the fourth ventricle, cerebellopontine angle, and prepontine and other cisterns.

DIFFUSE TUMORS

Diffuse brain stem tumors appear hypo- to iso-intense and hyper-intense on T1-weighted and T2-weighted MR images, respectively (Fig. 13-4). There is variable enhancement with contrast administration, and contrast enhancement in these tumors may be indicative of malignant degeneration. Moreover, the tumor boundaries are not able to be delineated on MRI, and the brain stem is typically enlarged and deformed.

Additional Imaging Modalities

Imaging of the central nervous system has evolved with the continual development of more sophisticated techniques. Positron emission tomography (PET) has been used in an attempt to differentiate low-grade from high-grade brain stem gliomas, particularly in the pediatric population.[23-26] Although the MR imaging characteristics of gliomas may be highly diagnostic in the pediatric population allowing for the potential use of PET imaging to attempt to determine the degree of malignancy, the heterogeneity of lesions in the adult population may not allow for the procurement of useful data until studies are conducted correlating preoperative PET imaging with histologic diagnosis. One study utilized PET imaging in two adults with dorsal midbrain lesions and obstructive hydrocephalus.[27] The lesions were hyperintense on T2-weighted images and partial contrast enhancement was observed in one patient. The patients underwent preoperative PET studies followed by an endoscopic third ventriculostomy combined with endoscopic biopsy sampling of the lesions. Glial proliferation, which contained the partial enhancement with contrast, and a possible low-grade glioma were diagnosed in the two patients, respectively. Results of the PET imaging in both patients suggested that the lesions had nontumorous characteristics and portended a good prognosis. With larger-scale studies, PET imaging may someday prove to be more informative and predictive of the biological behavior of dorsal midbrain lesions than a biopsy.

Magnetic resonance spectroscopy (MRS) is a noninvasive imaging modality used for tissue characterization and complements data obtained from MRI. The concentrations of creatine, phosphocreatine, choline, N-acetylaspartate, lactate, and lipids are analyzed in an effort to differentiate various pathologic processes. It has been used to distinguish between normal and abnormal tissues and grading of brain tumors. Inflammation, infectious processes, and tumors may potentially be distinguished with MRS.[28] Studies have been conducted with MRS to investigate brain stem lesions with histologic correlation in some cases.[28-31] MRS can provide additional information on brain stem lesions, but further studies are needed with histologic confirmation given the broad differential diagnosis of brain stem lesions in adults.

Diffusion tensor imaging (DTI) is an imaging modality that demonstrates white matter tracts. The relationship of sensory and motor tracts to brain stem tumors has been investigated in pediatric patients.[32,33] With further studies and evolution of this technique for use in the brain stem, DTI may play a role in assisting the treatment planning for brain stem lesions in adults.

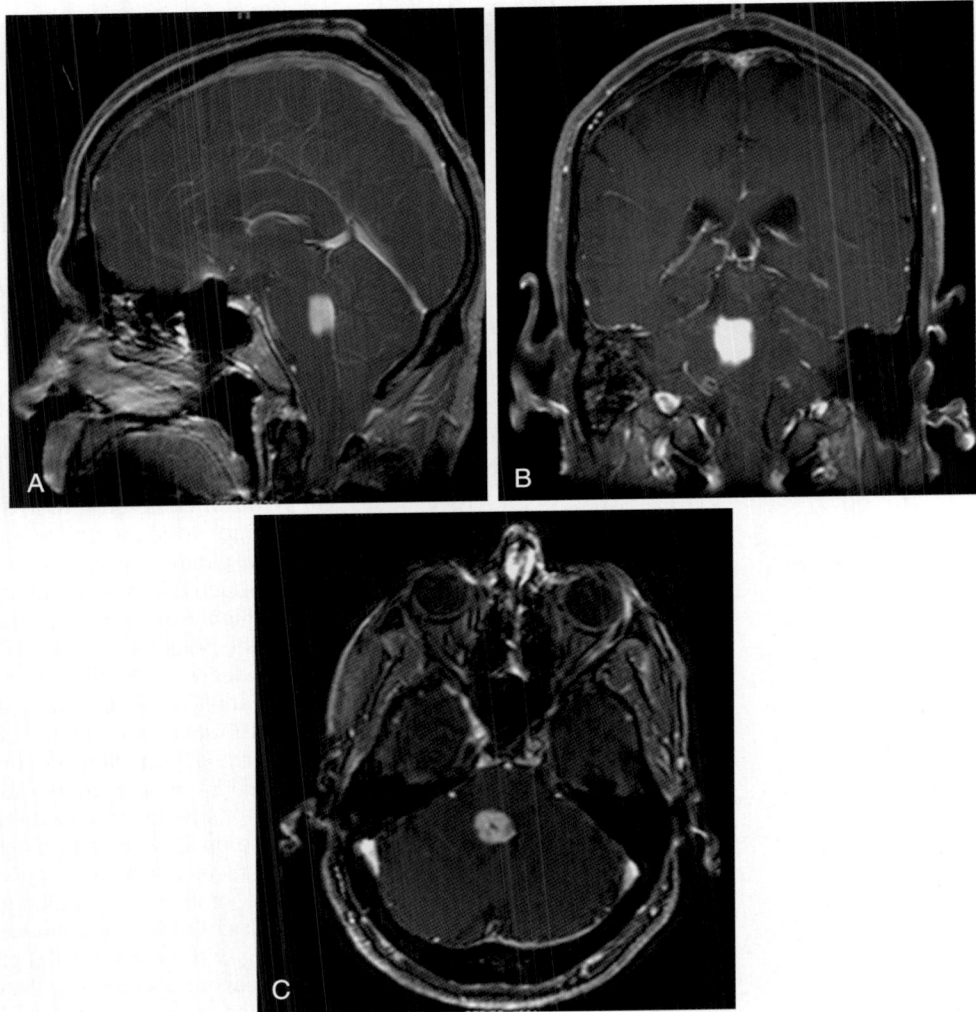

FIGURE 13-1 Focal pontine glioma. A, Post-contrast sagittal MRI demonstrates an enhancing mass in the pons. B, Post-contrast coronal MRI. C, Post-contrast axial MRI.

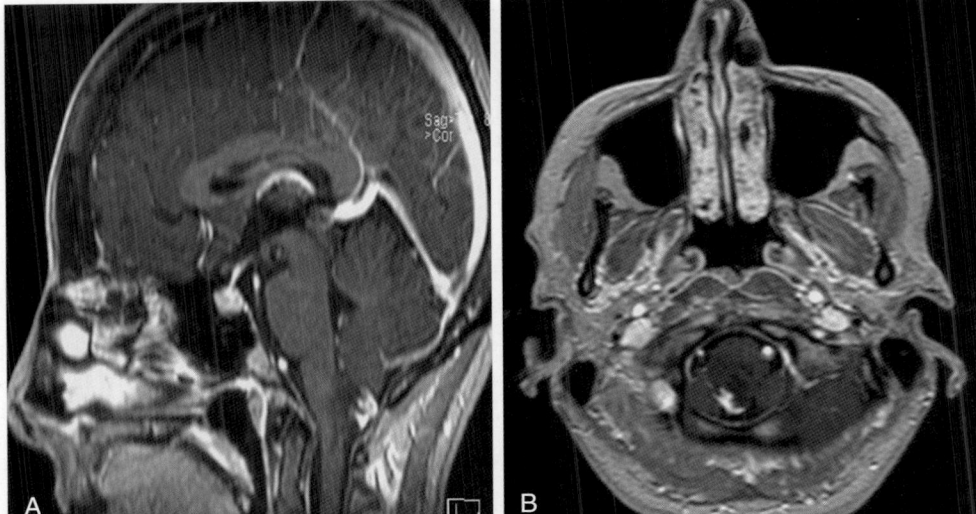

FIGURE 13-2 Dorsal exophytic cervicomedullary glioma. A, Post-contrast sagittal MRI demonstrates a hypointense lesion with enhancement in the posteriocaudal part. B, Post-contrast axial MRI.

Clinical Manifestations

The clinical presentation of brain stem tumors varies and has been correlated with the growth pattern, location, and degree of malignancy. Focal tumors tend to have a slow progression to neurologic signs in contrast to diffuse malignant tumors, which have a fast progression to neurologic signs. The manifestations include headaches, nausea, vomiting, diplopia, weakness, ataxia, numbness, cranial neuropathies, and/or vertigo. Pontine and cervicomedullary

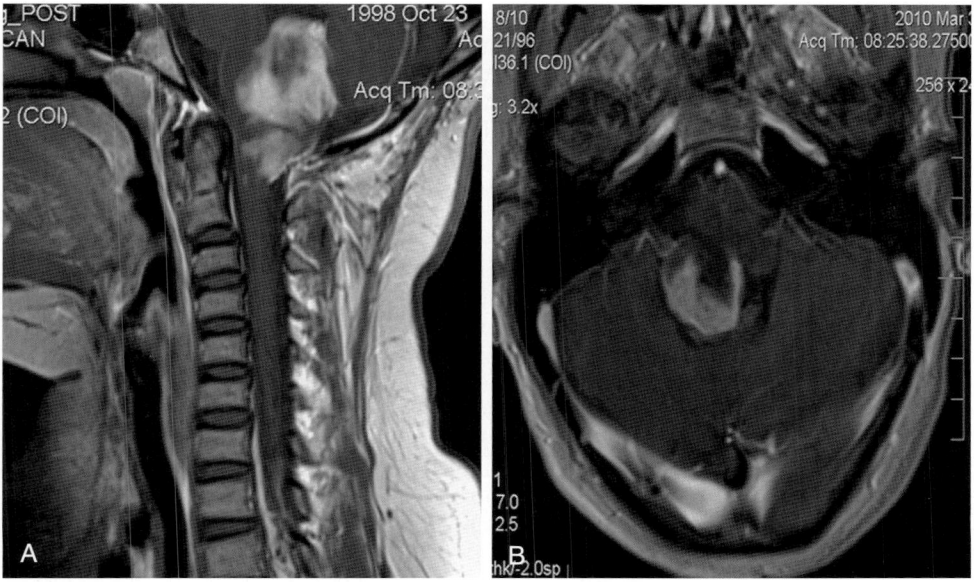

FIGURE 13-3 Cervicomedullary glioma with dorsal exophytic component. A, Post-contrast sagittal MRI demonstrates enhancing mass. B, Post-contrast axial MRI.

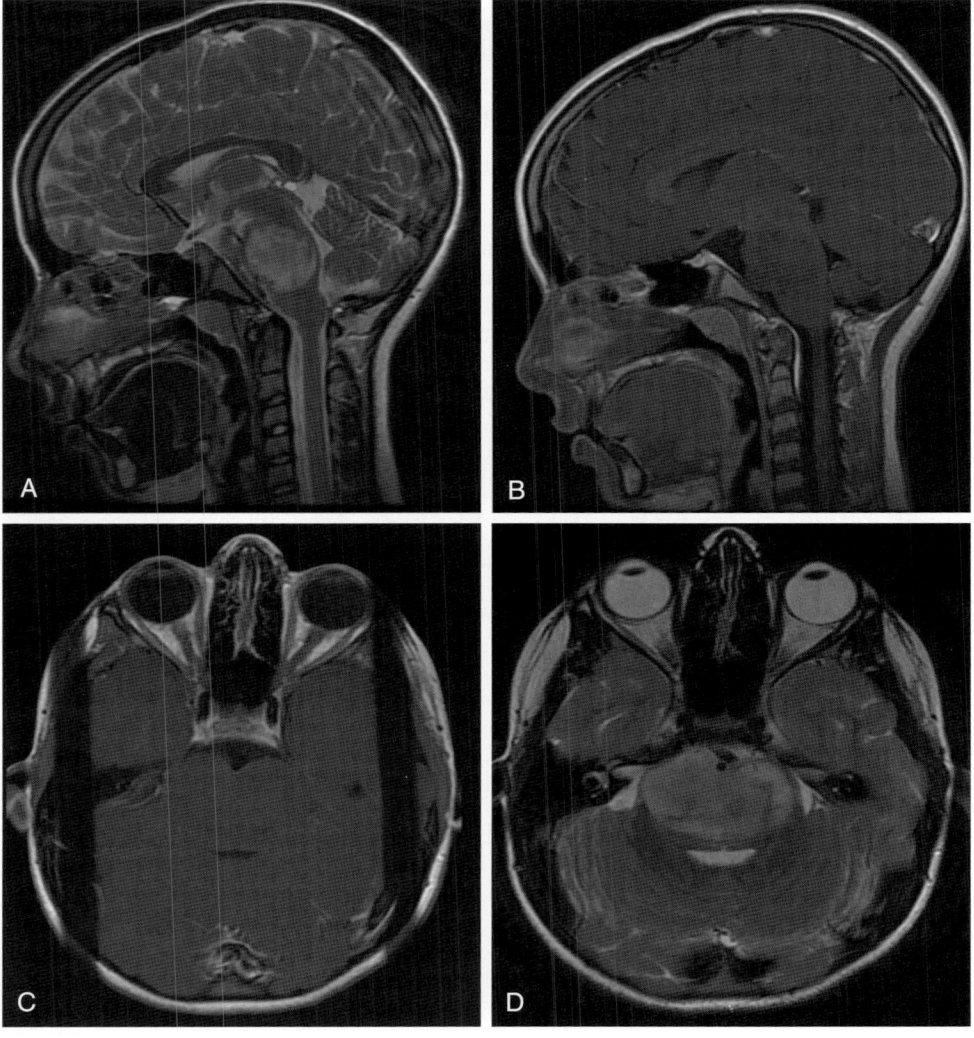

FIGURE 13-4 Diffuse pontine glioma. A, T2-weighted sagittal MRI demonstrating hyperintense mass in the pons. B, Hypointense, nonenhancing pontine mass on post-contrast sagittal T1-weighted MRI. C, Hypointense, nonenhancing pontine mass on post-contrast axial T1-weighted MRI. D, T2-weighted axial MRI demonstrating hyperintense pontine mass.

tumors typically present with cranial neuropathies and long tract signs. Midbrain tumors can present with obstructive hydrocephalus, oculomotor deficit, hemiparesis, and ataxia, while dorsally exophytic tumors typically present with signs of obstructive hydrocephalus.

Stereotactic Biopsy

Since the late 1970s, stereotactic biopsies of brain stem lesions have been performed and account for 5% to 12% of all brain biopsies.[34-56] This procedure was not used widely in the pediatric population because it was reported that characteristic MRI features were sufficient to diagnose diffuse brain stem gliomas without the need for a biopsy.[14,57-59] Biopsies of brain stem lesions are not as common as other brain biopsies because of the risk involved in obtaining tissue. However, studies have shown that stereotactic brain stem biopsies can be routinely performed in a safe and effective manner.[34,40,42-46,51-56] In some published series, the reported rate of complications has ranged between 2.5% and 7.7%.[54,56,60]

In adults with contrast-enhancing brain stem lesions, other pathologic processes must be considered in the differential diagnosis because studies have demonstrated preoperative radiographic diagnoses to be incorrect in 10% to 25% of cases in patients over 20 years of age presenting with a contrast-enhancing lesion in the brain stem.[60,61] In addition to malignant glioma, the differential diagnosis may include infectious processes, such as abscess, tuberculomas, and toxoplasmosis, demyelinating disease, sarcoidosis, progressive multifocal leukoencephalopathy, metastasis, lymphoma, and vascular processes, such as vasculitis and infarction (Figs. 13-5, 13-6, and 13-7).[2] This heterogeneity of brain stem lesions in adults makes it difficult to make a diagnosis on the basis of imaging alone. Therefore, image-guided stereotactic biopsies are indicated in many adult brain stem lesions that enhance with contrast and generally in cases in which the diagnosis of the lesion is in doubt to determine the histology of the abnormal process.

Stereotactic biopsies of the brain stem are performed with image guidance utilizing either CT or MRI. Approaches used include the transfrontal, transtentorial, and transcerebellar routes depending on the location of the lesion within the brain stem. The transtentorial approach, which is really not used, places vital vasculature and cranial nerves at risk and may cause pain with tentorial puncture.[62,63] In addition, this route crosses the pia two additional times above and below the tentorium. The ipsilateral transfrontal route frequently requires traversing the lateral ventricle and is limited to midline regions of the pons and medulla by the tentorial incisura.[41,51,64,65] Moreover, the suboccipital transcerebellar approach has been used for lesions in the lower midbrain, pons, middle cerebellar peduncle, and rostral medulla.[34,46,47,54,66,67] Due to patient positioning, intubation and general anesthesia is generally required although the use of local anesthesia has been reported.[54,67] With this approach, a potential drawback is the discomfort associated with muscle dissection prior to placement of the twist-drill hole.

An alternative contralateral, transfrontal, extraventricular approach using a Leksell stereotactic frame system has been described for reaching lesions in the lateral pons and middle cerebellar peduncle (Fig. 13-8).[53] The needle's trajectory crosses only one pial surface and avoids the ventricle and tentorium. In a reported series of six patients, diagnostic samples were obtained in all patients and there was no surgical morbidity.[53]

Indications for Surgery

In general, patients with a clinical presentation and imaging consistent with a diffuse glioma will not benefit from surgical intervention, although experimental studies are being conducted for the local intracranial delivery of therapeutic agents to these lesions.[1,68-72] Focal brain stem tumors are considered amenable to surgical resection, which is often the primary treatment of choice. Dorsal midbrain tumors, such as tectal gliomas known to be indolent and stable clinically and radiographically for many years, may

FIGURE 13-5 Pontine glioblastoma that extends into the right midbrain and thalamus. A, Post-contrast coronal MRI demonstrating the ring-enhancing cystic lesion. B, Post-contrast sagittal MRI.

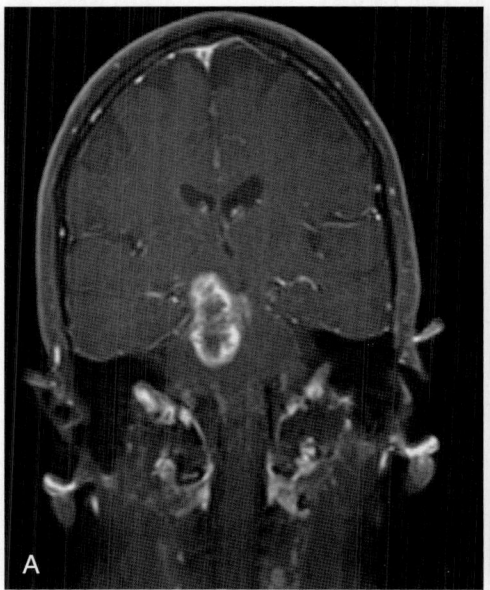
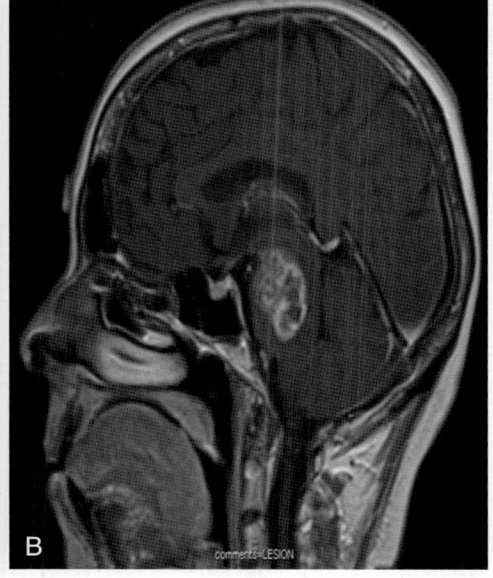

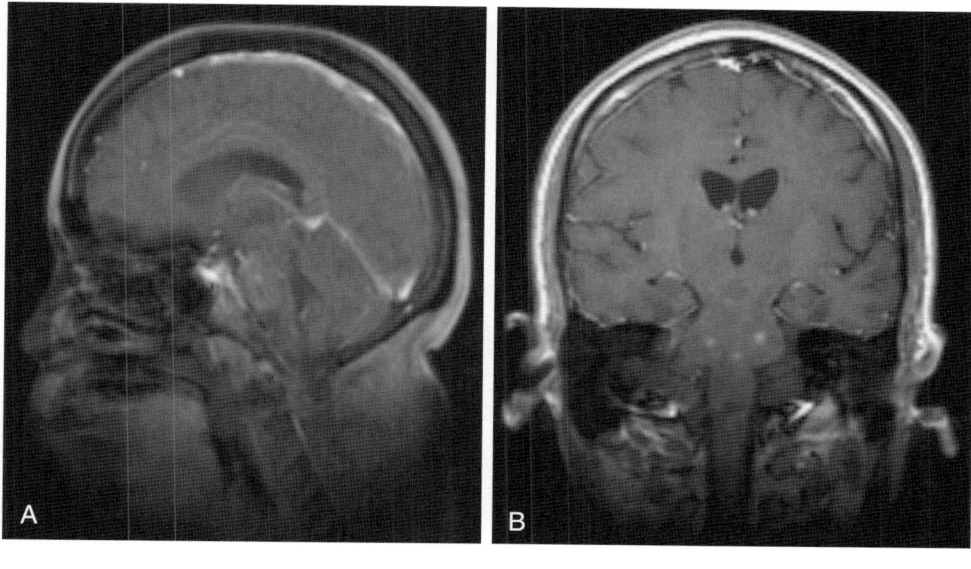

FIGURE 13-6 Contrast-enhancing pontine lesions. A biopsy revealed an inflammatory process. A, Post-contrast sagittal MRI. B, Post-contrast coronal MRI.

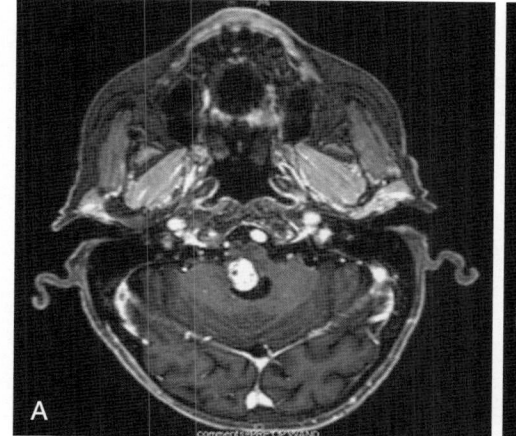
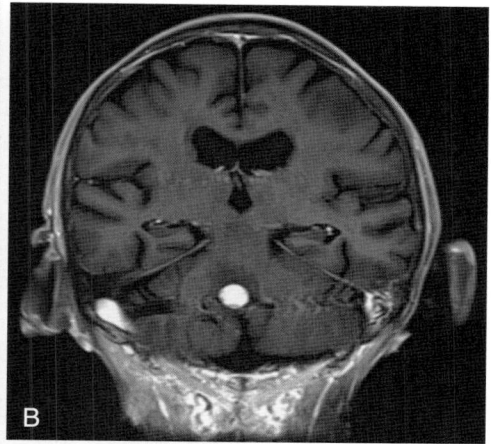
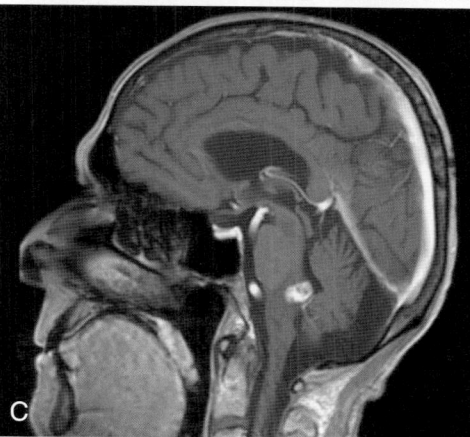

FIGURE 13-7 Non–small cell carcinoma metastases in the medulla. A, Post-contrast axial MRI demonstrates the enhancing lesion in the medulla. B, Post-contrast coronal MRI. C, Post-contrast sagittal MRI.

be initially managed in a nonoperative manner with serial imaging, and surgery is performed in cases of tumor progression on MRI.[73] Obstructive hydrocephalus, if present, may be treated with an endoscopic third ventriculostomy and the tumor can be followed with serial MR imaging.

For those undergoing brain stem surgery, patients should be informed that there may be a transient or permanent worsening of their neurologic condition.

Intraoperative Neurophysiologic Monitoring and Mapping

The complex neuroanatomic organization of the brain stem presents a formidable challenge to neurosurgeons when operating on lesions in this complex, small structure. Within the brain stem, cranial nerve nuclei and ascending

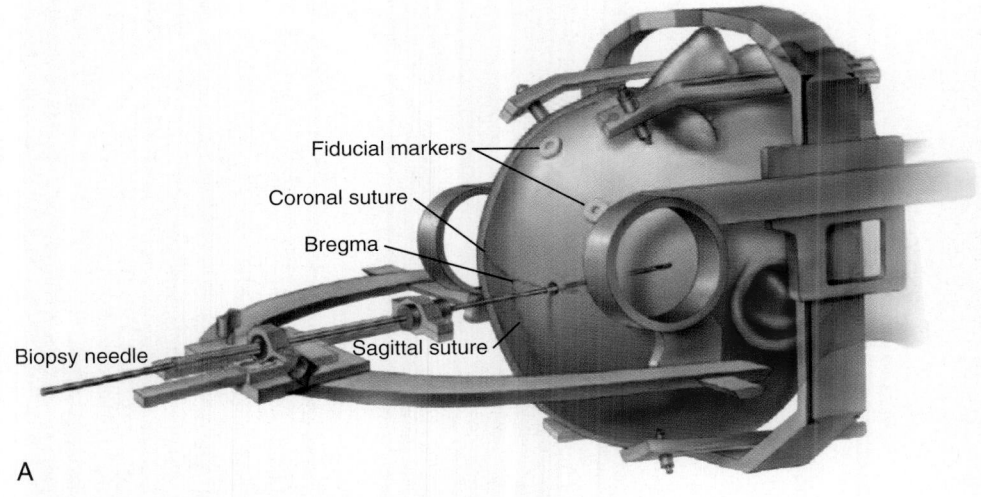

A

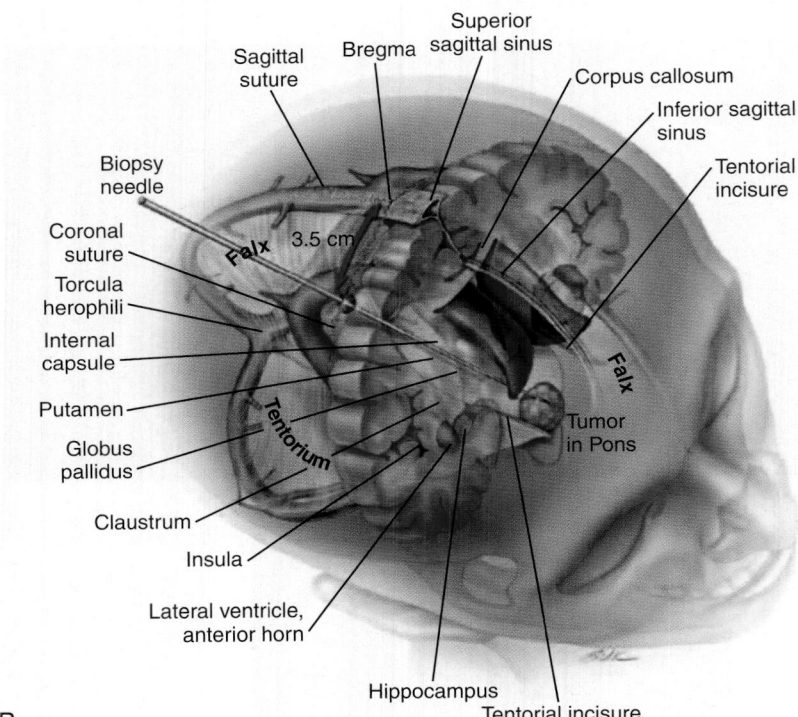

B

FIGURE 13-8 A and B, Illustration depicting the contralateral, transfrontal, extraventricular approach to an infratentorial lesion .with the aid of a Leksell stereotactic frame system. (Reproduced with permission from Amundson EW, McGirt MJ, Olivi A. A contralateral, transfrontal, extraventricular approach to stereotactic brainstem biopsy procedures. J Neurosurg 2005;102:565-570, by the American Association of Neurosurgeons. Copyright by Ian Suk.)

and descending pathways are contained here. Tumors can distort the normal anatomy of the brain stem, such as anatomic landmarks on the floor of the fourth ventricle like the facial colliculus and striae medullares, and make surgery even more challenging. The introduction of intraoperative neurophysiologic monitoring and mapping has allowed for safer surgery and assisted in formulating the operative plan while minimizing risk to critical brain stem structures.

Brain stem auditory, somatosensory, and motor-evoked potentials are utilized to monitor their corresponding pathways during surgery. This form of monitoring does not help to prevent the injury of vital brain stem structures because functional mapping is not taking place to identify danger zones during surgery.

Functional mapping of the fourth ventricular floor has allowed the identification of brain stem cranial nerve motor nuclei and their relationship to the tumor.[74-76] The responses from muscles innervated by cranial nerves VII, IX, X, and XII can be recorded during surgery as the neurosurgeon stimulates the floor of the fourth ventricle with a hand-held monopolar probe. To prevent the occurrence of damage to the floor of the fourth ventricle during stimulation, the tip of the probe is round and approximately 0.75 mm in size. Muscle action potentials, through the utilization of EMG, can be recorded from the orbicularis oculi and oris muscles (CN VII), posterior pharyngeal wall (CN IX, X), and tongue muscles (CN XII). Confirmation should be obtained that the muscle relaxant does not interfere with EMG recordings. Moreover, the extent of brain stem compression, pathology, and distance to the cranial nerve motor nuclei play important roles in determining the threshold intensity, which can be as low as 0.2 mA for a hematoma, while brain stem tumors usually require higher threshold intensities up to 2.0 mA. After a muscle response is recorded, utilization of the threshold intensity allows for localization of the nuclei by moving the stimulation probe every 1 mm. This information allows for a safe site for an incision and attempts to minimize injury during tumor removal.[74-76] If muscle responses are not detected, technical problems with the stimulator and/or recording system may be present, or the cranial nerve motor nuclei may be located ventral to the pathology. If the nuclei are located ventral to the brain stem pathology, then repeated stimulation would be required through the lesion for detection of the nuclei.

Moreover, the corticospinal tracts can be mapped at the level of the cerebral peduncles.[77] A Kartush handheld stimulator (Medtronic Xomed, Inc.) is used to focally stimulate the midbrain with EMG monitoring of specific muscles. This intraoperative modality allows the surgeon to determine the location of the aforementioned pathways in relation to the tumor and safely make an incision in the midbrain. Localization of the corticospinal tracts assists the surgeon in an endeavor to protect them during the dissection around and mobilization of the lesion.

Surgical Approaches

The location and size of the tumor within the brain stem dictates the surgeon's operative approach for resection. The complex neuroanatomic structure of the brain stem and surrounding vasculature must be taken into consideration when formulating the surgical strategy. MRI is utilized to localize the tumor and plan the most optimal route to the tumor that will minimize the risk of injury to neurovascular structures.

For tumors in the dorsal pons, fourth ventricular floor, dorsal medulla, and posterior cervicomedullary junction, we prefer the suboccipital approach with the patient placed in the prone position. Tumors in the midline tectal region can be reached by the supracerebellar-infratentorial approach, and we also perform this procedure with the patient in the prone position. Lesions in the posterolateral pons, lateral middle cerebellar peduncle, superior lateral medulla, and cerebellopontine angle can be accessed through a retrosigmoid approach, and the far-lateral approach, which provides an anterolateral trajectory to the brain stem, is utilized for lesions in the inferolateral pons and anterolateral medulla. We use the park-bench position for both the retrosigmoid and far-lateral approaches.

The subtemporal approach provides access to lesions of the lateral midbrain. An orbitozygomatic approach provides additional access to the rostral pons, interpeduncular region, and pontomesencephalic junction in addition to the lateral midbrain.[78-80] These approaches may be combined with an anterior petrosectomy for lesions located more inferior in the ventral pons.

Surgical Techniques

The complex neuroanatomic structure of the brain stem requires very careful microsurgical technique when resecting tumors. The small dimensions of the brain stem demand precise movements and good intraoperative judgment at all times. An optimally functioning surgical microscope is vital to operations in and around the brain stem.

Intrinsic tumors necessitate an incision in the surface of the brain stem and require a thorough understanding of the anatomy. Although many tumors can be accessed where it is closest to the surface, it must bear in mind that this may not be the optimal route in some cases. The incision is usually small and less than 1 cm, which typically provides enough space for the resection of large tumors. Tumors in the vicinity of the corticospinal tracts in the cerebral peduncles can be mapped for a safe entry point. For tumors approached through the fourth ventricular floor, mapping of the floor is extremely important for placement of the incision to avoid cranial nerve nuclei, such as VII, IX, X, and XII. In addition, there are areas of the brain stem that can be entered relatively safely. Dorsal pontine tumors approached through the fourth ventricular floor can be entered through the median sulcus above the facial colliculus, suprafacial, infrafacial, and area acoustica. Tectal mesencephalic tumors can be accessed through the supracollicular, infracollicular, and lateral mesencephalic sulcus, while longitudinal myelotomies can be performed in the posterior median fissure below the obex, posterior intermediate sulcus, and posterior lateral sulcus for medullary and cervicomedullary tumors.[81]

Once the tumor has been reached, its consistency is evaluated and will determine the method of extirpation according to the surgeon's preference. A tumor specimen should be submitted as soon as possible for determination of the histology. The histology will determine if a gross-total resection is feasible, which is more likely in the case of benign tumors. Depending on the surgeon's preference, microretractors may be used. Tumors should be removed in a piecemeal fashion and not en bloc. If a cyst is associated with the tumor, removal of the cystic fluid aids in tumor debulking by providing additional space for manipulation. Ultrasonic aspiration set at a low intensity and suction rate and/or microscissors are more effective for solid tumors. Microbipolar coagulation and simultaneous aspiration of coagulated tissue may be used for soft tumors. The surgical resection must be confined to the inside of the tumor to avoid injury to normal surrounding structures. After a majority of the tumor is debulked, a normal boundary between the tumor and normal brain is sought. When delineation between tumor and normal brain is identified, gross-total resection is feasible in most cases. Tumor resection should be stopped when an interface between the two cannot be visualized because the decision to continue with debulking the lesion may increase the chances of postoperative neurologic morbidity. In addition, some tumors may be highly vascular and the vessels must be coagulated during tumor debulking, which may cause ischemic damage to surrounding normal brain.

For focal tumors with an exophytic component, this protruding aspect of the tumor provides an avenue for surgical access to the tumor. Moreover, tumors that penetrate the subarachnoid space may contact or encase vital arteries, and those that penetrate the ventral brain stem may contact the vertebral or basilar arteries and their branches; therefore, these tumors must be approached with extreme caution. Tumors arising from the subependymal aspect of the pons or medulla with no or minimal brain stem invasion and protruding into the fourth ventricle comprise a subgroup of dorsally exophytic tumors that are benign and can be resected with success.[22,82,83]

Postoperative Care

After undergoing brain stem surgery, patients require very close observation in the immediate postoperative period. Patients should at least remain intubated overnight in the intensive care unit, and a CT scan may be performed to identify hemorrhage and/or hydrocephalus. The surgeon should be prepared to place an intraventricular catheter for the possible development of obstructive hydrocephalus, especially for tumors in the fourth ventricle. Extubation may be performed when the CT does not reveal anything concerning, the patient regains consciousness, and the ventilatory parameters demonstrate the patient can successfully breathe on his/her own. Some patients operated on for midbrain lesions may experience an extended comatose or stuporous state before regaining full consciousness. Surgery for lower brain stem tumors may cause dysphagia, vocal cord paresis, and/or loss of the cough and gag reflex and should be anticipated. Some patients may have dysphagia preoperatively, which may worsen after surgery. These patients must be observed with great vigilance as they may be at risk for aspiration.

Conclusion

Brain stem surgery can present a formidable challenge to the neurosurgeon but advances in imaging, surgical approaches, and intraoperative neurophysiologic monitoring have decreased the risk and morbidity associated with these operations. Focal intrinsic brain stem tumors with or without an exophytic component and primarily exophytic lesions are indicated and amenable to surgical resection. Although there have been advances in microsurgical techniques for brain stem surgery, continual evolution of these techniques are needed to provide the best care possible for patients.

Furthermore, brain stem gliomas in adults are poorly understood since they account for less than 3% of gliomas, and there is a paucity of studies when compared to the pediatric population. However, the few reported studies have shown that survival in adults is longer than that of children. More studies are needed to assess the natural history of these tumors and operative outcomes.

KEY REFERENCES

Abernathey CD, Camacho A, Kelly PJ. Stereotaxic suboccipital transcerebellar biopsy of pontine mass lesions. *J Neurosurg.* 1989;70:195-200.

Amundson EW, McGirt MJ, Olivi A. A contralateral, transfrontal, extraventricular approach to stereotactic brainstem biopsy procedures. Technical note. *J Neurosurg.* 2005;102:565-570.

Barkovich AJ, Krischer J, Kun LE, et al. Brain stem gliomas: A classification system based on magnetic resonance imaging. *Pediatr Neurosurg.* 1990;16:73-83.

Numbered references appear on Expert Consult.

CHAPTER 14

Cerebellar Tumors in Adults

LAURA B. NGWENYA • MIRZA N. BAIG • MANISH K. AGHI • E. ANTONIO CHIOCCA

Many lesions affect the posterior fossa, and the cerebellum in particular. Some tumors, such as brain stem gliomas, cerebellar pontine angle tumors, fourth ventricle tumors, and pineal area tumors extend into the cerebellum from surrounding areas. Metastatic lesions to the cerebellum are also common. However, tumors intrinsic to the cerebellum are less frequent. Primary cerebellar tumors represent only 3.5% of all primary brain and central nervous system (CNS) tumors.[1] In children, infratentorial lesions are more prevalent, comprising 16.6% of CNS tumors, while only 6% of primary CNS tumors are found in the cerebellum of adults.[1] In this chapter, we will focus only on intrinsic cerebellar tumors.

Clinical Presentation, Diagnosis, and Preoperative Management

Patients with a cerebellar lesion often present with a headache and signs of cerebellar dysfunction. Clinical signs of these deficits are detected by the presence of dysmetria in finger-to-nose or heel-to-shin testing, and dysdiadochokinesis demonstrated by testing of rapid alternating movements. Patients may also present with ataxic tremor, dysarthria, postural instability, or gait disturbances. The cerebellum demonstrates functional localization; cerebellar signs often correlate with the location of the cerebellar lesion.[2] The deep cerebellar nuclei have specific deficits when damaged. The midline fastigial nuclei play a role in postural ataxia, whereas globus, embolliform, and dentate nuclei are important for limb ataxia. Injury to the dentate nuclei can lead to dysarthria and mutism in some patients. Midline lesions, affecting the cerebellar vermis and midline cerebellar nuclei, are more likely to demonstrate truncal instability. Lesions involving the cerebellar hemispheres are more likely to show limb ataxias and associated dysmetria.

Patients with a cerebellar mass may also present with symptoms related to compression. Depending on tumor location, large cerebellar tumors can cause compression of the brain stem, which can cause obstruction of the fourth ventricle and various cranial nerve signs, depending on tumor location. Patients may present with hydrocephalus and increased intracranial pressure. Accordingly, headache, nausea, and vomiting are common presenting symptoms for patients with cerebellar tumors.[3,4] When a patient presents with signs and symptoms of obstructive hydrocephalus, such as lethargy or coma, an emergent externalized ventricular catheter should be placed prior to surgical planning. In patients with long-standing ventriculomegaly and minimal clinical symptoms, intravenous steroids may alleviate symptoms and obviate the need for an externalized ventricular catheter.

In adult patients that present with a suspected cerebellar mass, an appropriate work-up should be done to obtain as much information as possible prior to surgery. Neuroimaging typically involves computed tomography (CT) and magnetic resonance imaging (MRI). CT scans have the advantage that they can be done rapidly, and thus help determine immediate treatment upon initial presentation of the patient. MRI gives better visualization of the posterior fossa, and is thus the imaging modality of choice for patients with a suspected cerebellar lesion. The appearance of the lesion in the MRI sequences can help narrow the differential diagnosis of the lesion. Cerebellar tumors can be identified as solid or cystic. Solid components of tumors can be evaluated with T1 and T2 MRI sequences. Most solid components are isointense to gray matter on T1 and T2; however, tumors such as pilocytic astrocytomas can appear isointense to cerebrospinal fluid (CSF) on T2.[5,6] For tumors that are highly vascular, such as hemangioblastomas, diffusion-weighted imaging (DWI) will show low signal, and apparent diffusion coefficient (ADC) will show increased signal within the solid vascular portion of the tumor. This imaging pattern contrasts with tumors that are highly cellular, such as medulloblastoma, that will have high DWI and low ADC signal.[6] Tumors that have abnormal vessels, such as in Lhermitte-Duclos, or tumors with evidence of prior hemorrhage, will benefit from susceptibility-weighted imaging (SWI) sequences, which are sensitive to venous blood and hemorrhage.[7] Cystic portions of tumors are generally hypointense on T1 and hyperintense on T2 due to the liquid component; fluid attenuation inversion recovery (FLAIR) sequences can be helpful in tumors such as hemangioblastomas where the cystic component is different from CSF.[6] Tumors with a large percentage of fat-containing substance, such as in cerebellar liponeurocytomas, can be identified by hyperintense streaks on T1, and fat suppression sequences can aid in their diagnosis.[8] The pattern of contrast enhancement after the administration of gadolinium is also useful, as some cerebellar tumors enhance strongly and homogeneously, whereas others show heterogeneous enhancement patterns.

Patients, especially adults, with a cerebellar mass should also receive screening scans to evaluate for possible metastatic disease to the cerebellum. Such a workup should include imaging of the chest (via chest x-ray and/or CT scan of the chest) and also CT of the abdomen and pelvis. The treatment of metastatic lesions to the cerebellum is often dictated by a number of factors, including the identity of the tumor of origin, the size, location, and number of metastases. Please refer to the subsequent chapter on metastatic lesions for further details.

Intrinsic Cerebellar Tumors in Adults

CEREBELLAR ASTROCYTOMAS

Gliomas represent 36% of all primary brain and CNS tumors; of these, 3% are located in the cerebellum.[1] Gliomas of the cerebellum are frequently astrocytomas. The most common is the pilocytic astrocytoma, which represents between 70% to 90% of cerebellar astrocytomas.[3,9] Pilocytic astrocytomas are low-grade, World Health Organization (WHO) classification grade I tumors that represent 5% to 6% of all gliomas.[10] In children they are the most common glioma, of which 67% occur in the cerebellum. In adults, the location of pilocytic astrocytomas is evenly distributed between supra- and infra-tentorial lesions.[9,11]

Cerebellar pilocytic astrocytomas demonstrate consistent imaging features. These tumors are found equally in the cerebellar vermis or hemispheres. They appear as well-circumscribed, unencapsulated lesions that often have cyst formation and a solid mural nodule. The solid component of the tumor is often isointense to CSF on T2 MRI and shows strong contrast enhancement.[5] Tumor necrosis is not evident in histopathologic evaluation. Classically, pilocytic astrocytomas show regions with compact bipolar cells that alternate with microcystic, loosely organized regions. Eosinophilic granular bodies and Rosenthal fibers are commonly present.

These tumors generally have a good prognosis after surgical resection with an 85% to 100% 5-year survival rate.[1,9,10] The favorable prognosis in these patients has been attributed to the low-grade nature of cerebellar pilocytic astrocytomas and the ability to achieve a gross total resection. It has been documented that surgeons tend to overestimate the degree of tumor resection.[12] As most tumor recurrence is related to residual tumor,[12,13] it is recommended that within 48 to 72 hours after surgery an MRI, with and without gadolinium, be obtained to determine if gross total resection has occurred. Rarely, malignant transformation of pilocytic astrocytomas can occur.[14] Adjuvant therapy, either radiation or chemotherapy, is not indicated for patients with cerebellar pilocytic astrocytomas, as gross total resection alone yields excellent prognosis.[9,11] The characteristics of cerebellar astrocytomas are summarized and compared to other intrinsic cerebellar tumors in Table 14-1.

Not all astrocytomas found in the cerebellum are low-grade pilocytic astrocytomas. The pilomyxoid astrocytoma (PMA) is an astrocytoma that shows similarities to the pilocytic astrocytoma, but histopathology confirms it lacks Rosenthal fibers, has a mucoid matrix, and shows an angiocentric arrangement of tumor cells, making it a distinct entity. Additionally, PMA is more aggressive, defined as WHO grade II, and often shows CSF dissemination at presentation.[10,15] The PMA is found most frequently in children; however, cases have been reported in adults, and PMAs have been detected in the cerebellum.[16,17] It has been demonstrated that up to 6% of astrocytomas presenting in the cerebellum are WHO grade III, and 17% exhibit the more malignant features of glioblastoma multiforme.[3] Radiographic features of these tumors include heterogeneous contrast enhancement and significant edema; leptomeningeal spread is common.[18] Because of the infiltrating nature, or the involvement of deep-seated tissues, these tumors are not cured by surgery and recur with higher frequency. For this subset of high-grade cerebellar astrocytomas, additional treatment modalities such as radiation, chemotherapy,[19,20] and/or radiosurgery have been performed.[21,22]

MEDULLOBLASTOMAS

Embryonal tumors, including medulloblastoma, represent 1.5% of primary CNS tumors.[1] Medulloblastomas are malignant WHO grade IV tumors of the cerebellum, of which 70% occur in children under the age of 16 years. They are fairly common in children, representing 20% to 30% of all

Table 14-1	**Tumors in Adult Cerebellum**					
Tumor Type	**WHO Grade**	**Percentage of All CNS Tumors**	**Location of Tumor**	**Imaging Characteristics**	**5-Year Overall Survival**	**Recommended Treatment**
Pilocytic astrocytoma	I	2.1%	Vermis = hemispheres	Well circumscribed, contrast enhancing; often with cystic formation and mural nodule	85%–100%	GTR
Medulloblastoma	IV	1.5%	Hemispheres > vermis	Variable definition, variable enhancement; may have cystic or necrotic foci	64%–84%	GTR plus craniospinal XRT with posterior fossa boost
Cerebellar lipo-neurocytoma	II	N/A	Hemispheres > vermis	Minimal heterogeneous enhancement; mottled areas of hyperintensity	N/A	GTR
Hemangio-blastoma	I	0.8%	Hemispheres > vermis	Intense enhancement, flow voids; solid or cystic with mural nodule	>50%[a]	GTR with close follow-up and screening for VHL
Lhermitte-Duclos	I	N/A	Hemispheres	CT—low density with occasional calcifications; MR—"tiger stripe" nonenhancing	N/A	GTR with screening for Cowden syndrome

[a]The exact 5-year survival rate is unknown. Patients with sporadic hemangioblastoma have excellent prognosis postresection; however, those with VHL have significant morbidity and early mortality associated with their systemic disease.
GTR, gross total resection; XRT, radiation therapy; N/A, data not available; VHL, Von-Hippel Lindau.

intracranial neoplasms in the pediatric sector, whereas in adults there is an incidence of approximately 0.5 per million.[23,24] In adults, medulloblastomas are rarely seen beyond the fifth decade of life. Eighty percent occur in patients aged 21 to 40 years.[10] Most childhood medulloblastomas are found in the vermis. With increasing age, there is a progressive involvement of the cerebellar hemispheres, thus the majority of adult medulloblastomas are hemispheric. Additionally, there are radiographic differences in the appearance of childhood and adult medulloblastomas. In children, the classic radiographic appearance is that of a well-defined homogenous tumor that shows marked contrast enhancement and is without cystic or necrotic degeneration. In comparison, adult medulloblastomas are more variable in appearance (see case report 1). They are not as well defined, the degree of contrast enhancement varies, and there are often small cystic or necrotic foci.[25,26] Adult patients are also more likely to exhibit the desmoplastic nodular subtype of histopathology. Nodular, reticular free regions of neuronal maturation surrounded by densely packed proliferative cells that produce an intercellular reticulin fiber network characterizes this subtype. It is thought that this desmoplastic subtype may contribute to some of the variety seen on radiographic imaging, but it is unclear whether this subtype affects prognosis.[26-28]

Despite the differences in childhood and adult medulloblastoma, the recommended treatment regimen is similar. Standard treatment involves gross total resection followed by craniospinal irradiation. Given this treatment, the 5-year overall survival for adult medulloblastomas is 64% to 84%.[23,29-31] Many factors influence the outcome of adult patients with medulloblastoma. Approximately 18% to 33% of patients have metastatic disease at presentation including spinal cord, CSF, and extraneural metastases. Metastasis has been shown to be a poor prognostic indicator, as has involvement of the brain stem, involvement of the floor of the fourth ventricle, radiation dose less than 50 Gy, and large-cell variant histopathologic subtype.[23,29,32,33] In contrast, patient age less than 20, gross total resection of tumor, and completion of radiation treatment within 48 days are known to be positive prognostic indicators.[23,30]

Recent studies have explored the role of adjuvant chemotherapy for patients with adult medulloblastoma. The benefit of chemotherapy is still unclear in the adult medulloblastoma population so there are no universal guidelines for administration of chemotherapy. Gross total resection and radiation are the most important factors in preventing recurrence, and primary adjuvant chemotherapy has not been shown to have a significant association with survival.[33,34] However, for high-risk patients, it appears that chemotherapy may delay the risk of recurrence by approximately 3 years, and thus, there may be a role for chemotherapy in a subpopulation of adult patients with medulloblastoma.[32,35] For patients with widely metastatic medulloblastoma who have failed multiple treatment options, new chemotherapy techniques that target tumor-specific mutations show promise as future treatment modalities.[36]

Case Report 1: Medulloblastoma

A 22-year-old female, without a significant past medical history, presented to the emergency department with 2 weeks of occipital headache and blurry vision. Ophthalmology evaluation revealed papilledema and dysconjugate gaze. On examination she was sleepy, but arousable, and able to follow simple commands. Head CT revealed a cerebellar lesion with mass effect causing some effacement of the fourth ventricle and hydrocephalus (Fig. 14-1A).

The patient was admitted to the intensive care unit and an externalized ventricular catheter was placed. The patient underwent MRI of the brain that revealed a 2×1 cm cystic lesion that was hyperintense on T2 (B), hypointense on T1, and showed heterogeneous enhancement with gadolinium (C, arrow). Subsequent MRI of cervical, thoracic, and lumbar spine revealed increased disease burden involving areas of diffuse leptomeningeal enhancement and nodular lesions throughout the spine (D, arrowheads).

The patient was brought to the operating room and underwent a prone position suboccipital craniectomy for resection of tumor. Postoperative imaging revealed a gross total resection of the tumor, demonstrated in T2 (E) and T1 with gadolinium (F). Postoperatively, the patient failed challenging of her extraventricular catheter. Therefore, she eventually underwent a subsequent operation for placement of a ventriculoperitoneal shunt.

Final pathology revealed medulloblastoma, WHO grade IV. Within 1 month of surgery, she received craniospinal irradiation with a posterior fossa boost. After radiation, she was noncompliant with follow-up for some time. At 1 year postop she is stable, with resolution of her diplopia and dysconjugate gaze, and no progression of disease on subsequent imaging. She is scheduled to receive post radiation lomustine (CCNU) and cisplatin chemotherapy.

CEREBELLAR LIPONEUROCYTOMA

Cerebellar liponeurocytoma is a rare cerebellar neoplasm found primarily in adults.[10] It has previously been named in the literature as lipomatous medulloblastoma, neurolipocytoma, medullocytoma, and lipomatous glioneurocytoma. The now widely accepted name is cerebellar liponeurocytoma. Initially, this entity was thought to hold similarities to medulloblastomas, but the cerebellar liponeurocytoma is distinct. It is found primarily in adults and typically presents in the fifth or sixth decade, which is substantially older than the age of presentation for medulloblastomas. Additionally, cerebellar liponeurocytomas have a low proliferative index, and therefore a favorable prognosis. Although they do not exhibit malignant transformation, they have a recurrence rate of approximately 50%, with a mean time to recurrence of approximately 10 years.[37,38] Because of the propensity for recurrence, cerebellar liponeurocytomas are designated as WHO grade II.[10]

On neuroimaging, cerebellar liponeurocytomas can be difficult to distinguish from other more common cerebellar tumors. They are prevalent in the cerebellar hemispheres as compared to the vermis. MRI T1 imaging usually demonstrates a hypointense lesion with mottled or streaked areas of hyperintensities that correspond to adipose containing areas. These lesions are usually associated with a minimal amount of heterogeneous enhancement, and minimal associated edema.[8,10] The main criterion distinguishing this tumor type from others in the cerebellum is the presence of intratumoral areas of fat. Histologically, this is represented by cells showing advanced neuronal differentiation and areas of focal accumulation of mature lipidized tumor.

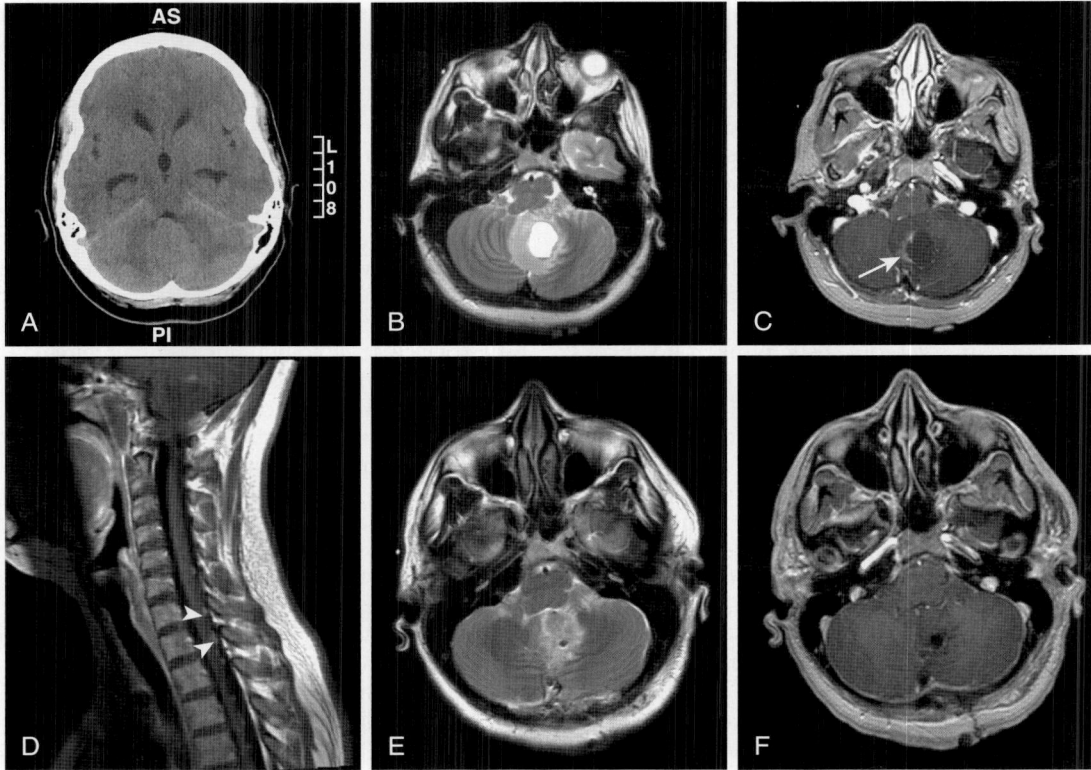

FIGURE 14-1 Medulloblastoma. A, Head CT demonstrates some fourth ventricular effacement and ventricular enlargement. B, T2 MRI shows a cystic cerebellar lesion with T2 hyperintensity. C, T1 MRI with gadolinium shows some enhancement (*arrow*). D, T1 MRI with gadolinium of cervico-thoracic spine demonstrates nodules of enhancement consistent with disseminated disease. E, Post-operative T2 MRI shows expected postsurgical changes. F, Postoperative T1 MRI with gadolinium is consistent with gross total resection of lesion.

Similarly to other cerebellar neoplasms, treatment is gross total resection. Cerebellar liponeurocytomas have a tendency for exophytic growth into CSF spaces and gross total resection is not always obtainable. Yet, the role of adjuvant radiotherapy or chemotherapy has not been established. Some authors believe that due to the nature of these tumors to recur, it is feasible to consider adjuvant radiotherapy to the posterior cranial fossa immediately after the initial surgery.[39] Yet others suggest that radiation therapy is best reserved for evidence of recurrence.[38] Regardless, most are in agreement that due to the nonmalignant nature of these tumors, aggressive radiotherapy, as is standard for medulloblastomas, is not necessary for cerebellar liponeurocytomas.

HEMANGIOBLASTOMAS

Hemangioblastomas represent about 1% of all intracranial tumors,[1] but about 8% of posterior fossa tumors in adults. They are slow-growing, highly vascular tumors that are classified as WHO grade I.[10] Hemangioblastomas occur most frequently in the cerebellum; however, they can also be found in the brain stem or spinal cord.

Cerebellar hemangioblastomas are distinct on neuroimaging. Classically, they can be solid, solid with cystic component, or cystic with nodule (see case report 2). They are found more commonly in cerebellar hemispheres as compared to the vermis.[40,41] Due to the highly vascular nature of these tumors, flow voids are usually present. In addition, these tumors are heterogeneous in T2, and show intense

contrast enhancement.[42] Angiography is useful to evaluate the tumor feeding vessels prior to surgical intervention.

Approximately 30% of patients with cerebellar hemangioblastomas have the multisystem cancer syndrome Von-Hippel Lindau (VHL). Patients with VHL develop numerous visceral lesions including renal cell carcinoma, pancreatic islet cell tumors, pheochromocytoma, and papillary cystoadenomas of the epididymis and broad ligament. CNS manifestations include endolymphatic sac tumors and multiple hemangioblastomas. The hemangioblastomas typically occur in the retina, brain stem, cerebellum, spinal cord, and nerve roots. Patients with VHL tend to be younger, and have multiple hemangioblastomas at presentation.[41,43-45]

Sporadic, compared to VHL-associated cerebellar hemangioblastomas, are not significantly different in location within the cerebellum, solid versus cystic type, or surgical outcomes. Treatment of cerebellar hemangioblastoma involves gross total resection and typically has a favorable prognosis. However, VHL patients have significant morbidity related to their systemic disease, and are more likely to develop additional hemangioblastomas, with an average of one every 2.1 years.[43] Thus, the subgroup of patients with VHL must be recognized. Any patient with a cerebellar hemangioblastoma should undergo appropriate screening for VHL. At a minimum, this should include neuroimaging of the neuraxis to look for additional hemangioblastomas. Because patients with VHL often have multiple hemangioblastomas, it is important to have thresholds for treatment of these lesions. Tumors that need resection are generally

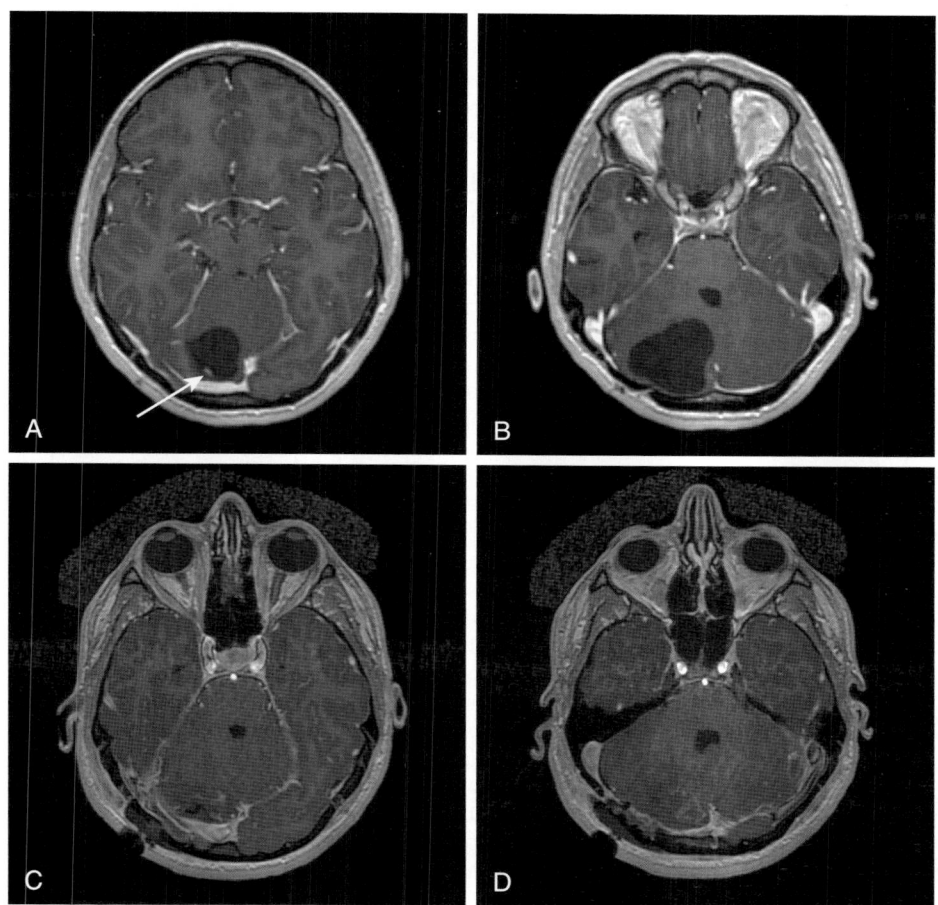

FIGURE 14-2 Hemangioblastoma. A, T1 MRI with gadolinium shows a hypointense cerebellar lesion with a small enhancing mural nodule (*arrow*). B, The lesion is primarily cystic, with minimal fourth ventricular effacement. C, D, Postoperative T1 MRI with gadolinium demonstrates gross total resection, including resection of the mural nodule.

those that are, or will become, symptomatic. The strongest predictors of symptomatic progression are tumor/cyst growth greater than 112 mm^3 per month and tumor/cyst size greater than 69 mm.[3,41] Hemangioblastomas in VHL can be asymptomatic, and these patients require long-term follow-up with imaging every 6 to 12 months.

Adjuvant radiotherapy has been considered in some cases of hemangioblastomas. Given that gross total resection gives a favorable prognosis, cases of stereotactic radiosurgery or fractionated external beam radiotherapy are generally preserved for those patients with subtotal resection or tumor recurrence.[46] For patients receiving adjuvant stereotactic radiosurgery, better progression-free survival has been associated with smaller tumor volumes, solid tumor type, and margin dose of 15 Gy or more.[47]

Case Report 2: Hemangioblastoma

A 25-year-old female presented to an outside facility with positional headaches. The headaches were associated with nausea, vomiting, and dizziness. She was found to have a cerebellar lesion and underwent a suboccipital craniotomy for resection of a hemangioblastoma. She initially had resolution of her symptoms; however, 2 years later she had return of her positional headaches and was referred to our neurosurgical service. On exam, she had slight dysmetria with finger-to-nose, but was otherwise neurologically intact.

Imaging revealed an enhancing mural nodule near the torcula (Fig. 14-2A, arrow) within a large cystic lesion

(B). Imaging of the neuraxis did not reveal any additional lesions.

The patient was brought to the operating room for an elective suboccipital craniotomy for resection of the cystic lesion. Upon exposure of the suboccipital surface of the cerebellum, the large cystic lesion was encountered and the cyst was perforated to allow for cerebellar relaxation. The mural nodule was resected.

Postoperative imaging demonstrated a total resection of the lesion (C, D). The pathology was consistent with hemangioblastoma. The patient received additional imaging of the chest, abdomen, and pelvis that revealed multiple pancreatic cysts and kidney lesions, suspicious for Von-Hippel Lindau.

The patient had resolution of her symptoms, and was discharged with close follow-up and referral for her likely new diagnosis of Von-Hippel Lindau disease.

LHERMITTE-DUCLOS DISEASE

Lhermitte-Duclos disease (LDD) is a rare dysplastic gangliocytoma of the cerebellum that is associated with Cowden syndrome (CS). It is unclear whether LDD is hamartomatous or neoplastic, but if considered neoplastic it is WHO Grade I due to its low proliferative index.[10] In support of the neoplastic nature of LDD, a recent case report, in which a patient was initially thought to have cerebellar abnormality on imaging from a head injury, was diagnosed with LDD 5 years later. In this case, the tumor showed a doubling time of approximately 42 months, which is consistent with that of a low-grade tumor.[48]

CS is an autosomal dominant disorder characterized by multiple hamartomas and high risk for breast, nonmedullary thyroid, and endometrial cancers. Along with mucocutaneous lesions such as trichilemmomas, LDD is a pathognomonic lesion for the diagnosis of CS.[49] Virtually all cases of adult LDD are associated with CS. Cowden syndrome is caused by a mutation in the phosphatase and tensin homologue (PTEN) gene found on chromosome ten. Decreased amounts of PTEN have been found in LDD tissue, further supporting the association between CS and LDD.[50]

Neuroimaging of LDD is distinct, because it shows a hemispheric cerebellar mass on CT that is hypointense and may have areas of calcification. On MRI, the mass appears as alternating linear bands of hyperintense and isointense areas on T2. This pattern, often referred to as "tiger-stripe," can also be seen in T1 imaging. The striated appearance correlates with the gross pathology of expanded cerebellar folia. LDD is characterized by having thinned white matter, a widened granule cell layer, and dysplastic molecular layer.[7,51] Also apparent on imaging of LDD is a high PET uptake, which does not correlate with tumor proliferative activity. Additionally, MR spectroscopy shows a high lactate peak with decreased choline, N-acetyl aspartate, and creatinine levels. Despite these distinct features, there have been reported cases of adult medulloblastoma mimicking LDD on imaging, thus making intraoperative pathology extremely important, since the management of these two entities is strikingly different.[52]

Treatment of LDD, as with all cerebellar tumors, is gross total resection. The gross appearance of LDD is usually a pale area with thickened folia, yet the border with surrounding cerebellum is often indistinct (see case report 3). Since LDD is associated with Cowden syndrome, it is important that all patients presenting with LDD be appropriately screened for other systemic cancers, as these are the hallmark of CS and contribute to the morbidity of this disease.[53,54]

Case Report 3: Lhermitte-Duclos Disease

A 61-year-old obese female, with past medical history significant for mild mental retardation, presented with a 4-week history of headache, truncal ataxia, instability, and multiple falls. There was associated nausea, and worsening of headaches with coughing and straining. CT scan of the head showed hypodensity and mass effect in the right cerebellar hemisphere, with mild ventriculomegaly. Subsequent MRI of the brain indicated a hypertrophy of the right cerebellar hemisphere with mass effect on the fourth ventricle. An MRI of the brain with contrast did not show any enhancement. T2 sequence of the cerebellar region indicated exaggerated folia in the right hemisphere.

The patient underwent external ventriculostomy placement, suboccipital craniectomy, C-1 laminectomy, debulking of right cerebellar lesion, and duraplasty (video 1). The ventriculostomy was discontinued on postoperative day 1, and the patient advanced in activity and diet with an uneventful postoperative course. Her headache resolved and she underwent outpatient physical therapy for her gait and balance.

Surgical Approaches to the Cerebellum

The majority of tumors found in the cerebellum are amenable to gross total resection. Therefore, the surgical management of such tumors varies more according to the tumor location than to the presumed tumor diagnosis. Vermian and hemispheric tumors that are close to the surface are easier to access surgically. Deep-seated anterior tumors are often more difficult to reach, and may require complicated operative approaches.

SUBOCCIPITAL CRANIOTOMY

Most cerebellar tumors can be approached via a suboccipital craniotomy or craniectomy. This midline or paramedian approach allows access to lesions in the cerebellar vermis and cerebellar hemispheres. In cases where the tumor extends into venous sinuses, brain stem, or deep cerebellar nuclei, complete resection may not be possible without disabling deficits, and surgical debulking for decompression and relief of symptoms may be more appropriate. Stereotactic navigation may be useful in assisting with localization of the lesion and avoidance of venous sinuses, but unless a small deep-seated lesion is being approached, it is not necessary since the anatomy is clear.

Patients may be positioned in a prone, lateral decubitus, or sitting position. The choice of position is dictated by the neurosurgeon's preference and experience. The head is placed in three-point fixation, with careful attention to ensure padding of all pressure points. The prone position has the advantage that there is a lower risk of venous air embolism. However, blood may pool in the surgical field and obscure view. Additionally, there is increased pressure on facial structures in this position. In the lateral decubitus position, there is also a decreased risk of air embolism, and the advantage of good airway access. The disadvantage of the lateral position is that the weight of the upper cerebellar hemisphere may interfere with the surgical approach. The sitting position has the advantages of drainage of CSF and blood out of the surgical field by gravity, and excellent visibility of the superior vermis. However, the sitting position confers some surgeon discomfort because of the requirement of operating with arms outstretched; in addition, the sitting position is associated with a higher risk of venous air embolism. Thus, for the sitting position many additional precautions must be taken such as preoperative transesophageal echocardiogram with bubble study to assess for a patent foramen ovale, precordial Doppler during the procedure for detection of venous air embolism, and placement of a central venous catheter to allow for aspiration of air embolism should one occur.

Consideration is given to possible placement of a ventricular catheter for CSF diversion prior to surgery. This depends on the size of the tumor, its mass effect, the status of the fourth ventricle, and the need for CSF diversion for brain relaxation intraoperatively or during the postoperative period. If indicated, an external ventricular catheter may be placed on the operating table after induction of anesthesia via an occipital burr hole. The burr hole is placed 3 to 4 cm from the midline and 6 to 7 cm above the inion. The catheter is then inserted with a trajectory parallel to the skull base, aiming for the middle of the forehead. In adults, an insertion length of approximately 10 to 12 cm will reach the foramen of Monro. Sometimes, as a precaution, a burr hole can be drilled without placement of a catheter, allowing the ability to place a ventricular catheter in an acute situation.

Prior to incision, the patient is usually given decadron, mannitol, and lasix. This is particularly important in cases where there is significant edema. This will help decrease the swelling of brain tissue and prevent herniation once the dura is opened. Also, perioperative antibiotics are given to protect against infiltration of skin flora.

If stereotactic navigation is employed, registration and verification of accuracy can be done prior to draping and prepping the patient. One advantage of frameless stereotactic navigation is that it may guide the surgeon's ability to minimize the size of skin incision and bony removal, particularly for small lesions. Frameless stereotaxy can also be incorporated into intraoperative MRI, if available. Intraoperative MRI can be useful to detect residual tumor, and has been shown to increase the extent of tumor resection from 83% to 98%.[55,56] However, it is necessary that appropriate precautions are taken by the anesthesia team and operating room staff to ensure that the patient can be monitored safely during the surgical procedure.[57]

For a suboccipital approach, the inion is located and the incision is made inferiorly until the spinous process of C2 is reached. Raney clips can be placed on the skin edges to provide hemostasis. Midline incisions should be continued along the avascular median raphe, and tissue is reflected from the cranium with a periosteal elevator. Self-retaining retractors are used to maximize surgical exposure. The size and extent of tumor resection will determine whether the arch of C1 needs to be exposed completely. For tumors away from the midline, this same approach is done, but with a paramedian incision. Paramedian incisions necessitate cautery of muscle. Venous bleeding from emissary veins and diploic veins need to be addressed and controlled meticulously with bone wax during periosteal exposure and bony removal.

The size of the craniotomy or craniectomy is often dictated by the size and location of the tumor. When making burr holes there are many important considerations. Anatomically, the suboccipital space is just below the transverse sinus, in the midline lies the confluence of sinuses, and far laterally the transverse-sigmoid sinus junction is encountered. It is advantageous to avoid making a burr hole directly over the sinuses. Traditionally, the superior nuchal line has been used to estimate the intracranial course of the transverse sinus, and the inion has been used as a marker for the torcular herophili. Yet, neither superficial landmark is always reliable in marking the location of the sinuses. The insertion point of the semispinalis capitus muscles has been shown to be a better landmark for identification of the medial transverse sinus.[58] Stereotactic navigation can aid in mapping out the location of the sinuses, and some studies suggest that a faster craniotomy is possible, and that complications such as venous air embolism are decreased with navigation-assisted surgery.[59]

Once the craniotomy is open, the dura is incised in a Y-shaped fashion. The midline incision of the dura will usually cut into the occipital sinus with fairly extensive hemorrhage. This can be controlled by cutting the dura and then employing surgical clips on either side of the midline sinus prior to the final dural cut. The suboccipital surface of the cerebellum will then be facing the surgeon. If indicated, the arachnoid covering the cisterna magna can be incised allowing for CSF drainage and brain relaxation.

Sometimes, a shortened ventriculostomy catheter can be sutured to the dura and left in the cisterna magna, in order to allow for CSF drainage during the operation, particularly with paramedian or lateral approaches where the inferior lobe or tonsil of the cerebellum can block continuous drainage of the cisterna magna. This catheter is then removed at the conclusion of the intracranial part of the surgery, before dural closure. Careful dissection in this area is necessary, as branches of the posterior inferior cerebellar artery course along this surface. Stereotactic navigation as well as intraoperative ultrasound can be used to aid in location of tumors that are not seen readily at the surface. A small corticectomy parallel to the cerebellar folia is often necessary to reach tumors that do not reach the pial surface. Once the tumor is reached, it is carefully dissected from the surrounding normal tissue and removed with a combination of aspiration, cautery, and microdissection experiments. Ultrasonic aspiration is helpful for debulking large tumors necessitating piecemeal removal. When deciding on a method of resection, it is important to bear in mind that some studies suggest that piecemeal removal of tumors is associated with increased risk of recurrence, and thus en bloc resection may be preferable, particularly for metastatic lesions.[60,61]

Certain tumor types require specific resection techniques to ensure the best resection. Cerebellar pilocytic astrocytomas have a fleshy appearance, are well demarcated from surrounding cerebellar tissue, and often have a cystic component with a mural nodule. The cyst should be aspirated, and the mural nodule should be removed. The cyst wall need not be removed, as it is usually not a separate capsule, but instead displaced portions of normal brain tissue. Medulloblastomas tend to be friable, thus careful dissection and prudent hemostasis are necessary. Cerebellar liponeurocytomas are yellowish on gross appearance due to the high content of fat cells. This distinct coloration aids in the total resection of this tumor type. Hemangioblastomas are often red in appearance due to their vascularity, and often benefit from preop angiography, which allows the surgeon to identify the main feeding arteries. Careful attention must be made to cauterize feeding vessels as the tumor is removed.[44] In cases of cystic hemangioblastoma, the cyst wall should be evaluated for signs of tumor, as failure to remove intramural tumor has been associated with recurrence.[62] In cases of Lhermitte-Duclos, the indistinct border between abnormal and normal cerebellum is challenging. Care must be taken to avoid resection of normal cerebellar tissue since too wide of a surgical excision has been shown to be associated with lingering cerebellar signs.[54]

Meticulous hemostasis is needed in the postoperative tumor cavity prior to closure, especially in the posterior fossa. Bipolar electrocautery, with different sizes of cottonoids, cotton balls, and other hemostatic products are essential. The tumor cavity can be also lined with a single layer of oxidized cellulose or other hemostatic product; however, care must be taken that such product is not able to float away in the postoperative period, potentially causing problems with normal flow of CSF pathways. In cases of doubt, it is preferable not to leave such products. Closure of the surgical site involves a watertight dural closure. If the native dura is not amenable to this, nuchal ligament harvested during exposure, pericranium from the occipital area or a dural substitute can be used. The patient should be given a Valsalva maneuver to test for CSF leakage. The surgical wound is closed in multiple layers to help prevent formation of a pseudomeningocoele.

OTHER SURGICAL APPROACHES TO THE POSTERIOR FOSSA

Lesions located anteriorly on the tentorial surface of the cerebellum are often difficult to reach by the standard suboccipital approach. Normal cerebellar tissue can be at risk of injury during attempts to gain access to this region.

A modification to the suboccipital craniotomy, the supracerebellar infratentorial approach can be used to resect anterior cerebellar tumors, especially those at the posterior incisura space and within the culmen of the vermis. For this approach, the skin incision is made approximately 2 cm superior to the inion and extends to the posterior cervical region. A midline or U-shaped incision can be used. The craniotomy should extend from just above the torcular herophili superiorly, to the foramen magnum inferiorly. Ideally, the craniotomy allows the inferior border of the superior sagittal sinus, and the medial edges of the transverse sinuses to be clearly viewed. The dura is opened in a Y- or U-shaped fashion. Bridging veins from the cerebellum to the tentorium are cauterized. Gentle retraction on the tentorium allows the tentorial surface of the cerebellum to come into view facilitating resection of lesions on this surface. This approach accesses lesions at the cerebellar-brain stem junction, and is a traditional approach used to resect pineal lesions.[63,64] Adjustment of this approach to a paramedian or lateral craniotomy allows progressively further anterior lesions to be reached.[65]

The occipital transtentorial approach is another alternative when resecting anterosuperior cerebellar lesions. In this approach, the patient is prone and a curved or a U-shaped skin incision is made over the confluence of sinuses. Craniotomy location is dictated by exact tumor location, but in general, burr holes are placed adjacent to the venous sinuses. Upon removal of the bone flap, a curved dural incision is made and the occipital pole is retracted rostrally with caution not to injure any nearby bridging veins. The tentorium is then visualized with the tentorial surface of the cerebellum lying beneath. Care is taken with manipulation of this surface, as it can lead to significant transient bradycardia in some patients. An incision in the tentorium is made parallel to the straight sinus, and then peaked to allow access to the anterosuperior cerebellar tumor. For this approach, intraoperative drainage of CSF by incision of cisternal arachnoid membranes is often useful to promote brain relaxation. With the use of image guidance and sometimes endoscopy, this approach has been shown to be a safe and effective approach for anterosuperior cerebellar lesions.[66] The disadvantages of this approach are that the tumor is at a far working distance, and significant retraction of the occipital pole may be necessary to reach the tumor edge.

An additional tactic to tumors in this region is the posterior subtemporal transtentorial approach. For this method the patient is positioned supine with the head turned to the side. An extraventricular catheter or lumbar drain is usually placed prior to incision to allow adequate drainage of CSF during the case. A U-shaped incision is made in the parietotemporal region beginning approximately 5 mm anterior to the tragus and ending 10 mm posterior to the mastoid notch. A temporal craniotomy is made, and the dura is opened in a U-shaped fashion. At this point, the vein of Labbe is encountered and precautions are made to avoid injury to this vessel. The temporal lobe is gently retracted. Patient positioning that allows gravity to gently elevate the temporal lobe, CSF diversion, and patient diuresis can facilitate the necessary retraction of temporal lobe. Once the temporal lobe is sufficiently elevated from the floor of the temporal fossa, the tentorium is encountered and incised, with careful adherence to the course of the trochlear nerve. The tentorium is tacked up, and the tumor can be reached and resected. The advantages of this approach are the short working distance and avoidance of unnecessary damage to the cerebellum.[67,68] However, disadvantages include the significant risks encountered such as potential injury to the vein of Labbe and the risk of temporal lobe edema or injury from retraction.

In cases where a cerebellar lesion extends to the anterior inferomedial region, a far lateral approach can be used. In this approach, an inverted L- or J-shaped incision is made. This incision begins approximately 5 cm below the inion, extends superiorly to the superior nuchal line and laterally to the mastoid, staying just in front of the posterior border of the sternocleidomastoid muscle. The muscular anatomy is important for this approach, as is the vascular anatomy, because after craniectomy the vertebral artery and its branches are exposed.[69] Careful dissection of the vertebral artery is done, as this allows better mobilization of the artery. If desired, the occipital condyle can be drilled with attention to the anatomy of the underlying hypoglossal canal. The amount of condyle that is drilled depends on surgeon's preference and degree of exposure needed; however, with greater than 50% of unilateral occipital condyle resection, hypermobility is noted, thus atlanto-occipital fusion should be considered.[70,71] With the far lateral approach, lesions that extend to the skull base and craniocervical junction can be resected.

There are numerous surgical approaches to the posterior fossa and the cerebellum, and none have been shown to be superior.[72-74] Ultimately, choice of approach to tumors in this region is dictated by surgeon's experience and preference.

Postsurgical Complications and Management

Surgery in the posterior fossa has been reported to have a complication rate as high as 32% in a series of 500 patients,[75] although with modern techniques this rate may have become much lower. Of surgeries exclusive to resection of cerebellar tumors, complications included cerebellar edema (5%), hydrocephalus (5%), cerebellar hematomas (3%), and cerebellar mutism (1%).[75]

CSF leaks are the most common surgical complication in the posterior fossa. They can be minimized with watertight dural closure. Dural closure is best when using native dura or harvested autologous material. A dural substitute can be used as on onlay or suturable material when a watertight closure cannot otherwise be obtained. However, recent studies suggest that these dural substitutes may increase complication rates. A suturable bovine matrix dural substitute was associated with a 50% risk of complications, such as CSF leak, aseptic meningitis, hydrocephalus, and symptomatic pseudomeningocoele, compared to 18% of cases where no dural substitute was used.[76] Ideally, surgeons should strive to achieve primary dural closure whenever possible.

The need for permanent CSF diversion is associated with CSF leak and hydrocephalus. Approximately 35% of children that have undergone posterior fossa surgery require either ventriculoperitoneal shunting or endoscopic third ventriculostomy.[77,78] This requirement has been associated with younger age and midline tumors in children, but factors predicting need for CSF diversion in adults have not been established.

Cerebellar mutism is a rare postoperative complication seen with resection of cerebellar tumors. This complication occurs in about 1% of cases, and is observed more commonly in children, although cases have been reported in adults. Cerebellar mutism is considered a severe form of dysarthria; it manifests as hesitant slow speech, or frank mutism. In all documented cases it is transient and associated with vermal tumors.[79,80] Cerebellar mutism is believed to be related to post surgical edema or ischemia involving the dentate nucleus or pathways of the dentatorubrothalamic tract.

KEY REFERENCES

Abel TW, Baker SJ, Fraser MM, et al. Lhermitte-Duclos disease: a report of 31 cases with immunohistochemical analysis of the PTEN/AKT/mTOR pathway. *J Neuropathol Exp Neurol.* 2005;64:341-349.

Ammerman JM, Lonser RR, Dambrosia J, et al. Long-term natural history of hemangioblastomas in patients with von Hippel-Lindau disease: implications for treatment. *J Neurosurg.* 2006;105:248-255.

Ammerman JM, Lonser RR, Oldfield EH. Posterior subtemporal transtentorial approach to intraparenchymal lesions of the anteromedial region of the superior cerebellum. *J Neurosurg.* 2005;103:783-788.

Ammirati M, Bernardo A, Musumeci A, et al. Comparison of different infratentorial-supracerebellar approaches to the posterior and middle incisural space: a cadaveric study. *J Neurosurg.* 2002;97:922-928.

Bonneville F, Savatovsky J, Chiras J. Imaging of cerebellopontine angle lesions: an update. Part 2: intra-axial lesions, skull base lesions that may invade the CPA region, and non-enhancing extra-axial lesions. *Eur Radiol.* 2007;17:2908-2920.

Central Brain Tumor Registry of the United States. *Primary Brain Tumors in the United States, Statistical Report 2000-2004.* CBTRUS; 2008.

Conway JE, Chou D, Clatterbuck RE, et al. Hemangioblastomas of the central nervous system in von Hippel-Lindau syndrome and sporadic disease. *Neurosurgery.* 2001;48:55-62:discussion 62-63.

Dubey A, Sung W, Shaya M, et al. Complications of posterior cranial fossa surgery—an institutional experience of 500 patients. *Surg Neurol.* 2009;72:369-375.

Hirschl RA, Wilson J, Miller B, et al. The predictive value of low-field strength magnetic resonance imaging for intraoperative residual tumor detection. Clinical article. *J Neurosurg.* 2009;111:252-257.

Jackson TR, Regine WF, Wilson D, et al. Cerebellar liponeurocytoma. Case report and review of the literature. *J Neurosurg.* 2001;95:700-703.

Jagannathan J, Lonser RR, Smith R, et al. Surgical management of cerebellar hemangioblastomas in patients with von Hippel-Lindau disease. *J Neurosurg.* 2008;108:210-222.

Kunschner LJ, Kuttesch J, Hess K, et al. Survival and recurrence factors in adult medulloblastoma: the M.D. Anderson Cancer Center experience from 1978 to 1998. *Neuro-oncology.* 2001;3:167-173.

Lai R. Survival of patients with adult medulloblastoma: a population-based study. *Cancer.* 2008;112:1568-1574.

Lanzino G, Paolini S, Spetzler RF. Far-lateral approach to the craniocervical junction. *Neurosurgery.* 2005;57:367-371:discussion 367-371.

Linscott LL, Osborn AG, Blaser S, et al. Pilomyxoid astrocytoma: expanding the imaging spectrum. *AJNR Am J Neuroradiol.* 2008;29:1861-1866.

Louis DN, Ohgaki H, Wiestler OD, et al. *WHO classification of tumours of the central nervous system.* France: international Agency for Research on Cancer Lyon; 2007.

Meltzer CC, Smirniotopoulos JG, Jones RV. The striated cerebellum: an MR imaging sign in Lhermitte-Duclos disease (dysplastic gangliocytoma). *Radiology.* 1995;194:699-703.

Morreale VM, Ebersold MJ, Quast LM, et al. Cerebellar astrocytoma: experience with 54 cases surgically treated at the Mayo Clinic, Rochester, Minnesota, from 1978 to 1990. *J Neurosurg.* 1997;87:257-261.

Moskowitz SI, Liu J, Krishnaney AA. Postoperative complications associated with dural substitutes in suboccipital craniotomies. *Neurosurgery.* 2009;64:28-33.

Patel AJ, Suki D, Hatiboglu MA, et al. Factors influencing the risk of local recurrence after resection of a single brain metastasis. *J Neurosurg.* 2009:doi:10.3171/2009.11.JNS09659.

Riffaud L, Saikali S, Leray E, et al. Survival and prognostic factors in a series of adults with medulloblastomas. *J Neurosurg.* 2009;111:478-487.

Robinson S, Cohen AR. Cowden disease and Lhermitte-Duclos disease: an update. Case report and review of the literature. *Neurosurg Focus.* 2006;20:E6.

Sherman JH, Sheehan JP, Elias WJ, et al. Cerebellar mutism in adults after posterior fossa surgery: a report of 2 cases. *Surg Neurol.* 2005;63:476-479.

Shirane R, Kumabe T, Yoshida Y, et al. Surgical treatment of posterior fossa tumors via the occipital transtentorial approach: evaluation of operative safety and results in 14 patients with anterosuperior cerebellar tumors. *J Neurosurg.* 2001;94:927-935.

Numbered references appear on Expert Consult.

CHAPTER 15

Surgical Management of Cerebral Metastases

TIMOTHY SIU • FREDERICK F. LANG

Cerebral metastases are a leading cause of morbidity and mortality for patients with systemic cancer and are among the most common tumors encountered by neurosurgeons. The contemporary neurosurgical management of brain metastases has become progressively more complex as the number of available treatment options increases. For half a century, corticosteroids and whole-brain radiation therapy (WBRT) were regarded as the standard of care for patients with brain metastases. However, due to technological advances in operative neurosurgery and radiation therapy over the last two decades, surgical resection and stereotactic radiosurgery (SRS) have become integral parts of the management armamentarium. Additionally, with modern advances in neuro-imaging, the detection of small, asymptomatic metastases has become increasingly frequent, allowing for the performance of highly controlled surgical resections with minimal morbidity, yet at the same time deepening the controversy surrounding the optimal roles of surgery versus SRS in the management of brain metastases. The increasing trend toward aggressive and novel systemic therapy for both early and late stage cancer has also led to the expectation that the treatment of brain metastases should not excessively delay or interfere with treatment of the systemic disease. Modern neurosurgeons, therefore, are faced with complex treatment decisions when encountering patients with brain metastases and must be familiar with the risks and benefits of all available management options in order to integrate the appropriate surgical interventions into the overall treatment plan of the cancer patient.

This chapter provides an overview of the currently available neurosurgical treatments for cerebral metastases, with a particular focus on defining the role of surgical resection in the cancer patient. Specific attention is given to patient selection, operative techniques, surgical outcomes, as well as treatment alternatives.

Magnitude of the Problem

Cerebral metastases are the most common brain tumors in adults.[1] Approximately 20% to 40% of patients with cancer develop brain metastases during the course of their illness.[2-5] It has been estimated that of more than 560,000 patients in the United States dying each year of cancer, approximately 19%, or more than 100,000 patients, will have brain metastases.[6-8] Most brain metastases arise from lung, breast, and renal cell tumors; however, melanoma, followed by lung, breast, and renal cell carcinoma, has the greatest propensity to develop brain metastases (Table 15-1). Characteristically, breast and renal cell carcinomas tend to present as a single metastasis within the brain, while melanoma and lung cancers have an increased incidence of multiplicity.[3,9,10] In addition, the interval between the diagnosis of the primary cancer and the brain metastasis depends on the histology of the primary cancer, with breast cancer generally exhibiting the longest interval (mean, 3 years) and lung cancer the shortest (mean, 4 to 10 months).[11] The highest incidence of brain metastases is seen in the fifth to seventh decades of life and is equally common among males and females. However, lung carcinoma is the source of most brain metastases in males, and breast carcinomas the most common source of metastases in females. Males with melanoma are more likely to develop brain metastases than are females.[10]

Treatment Goals: Advantages of Surgical Resection

The goals of treating brain metastases are (1) to establish a histologic diagnosis, (2) to relieve neurologic symptoms, and (3) to provide long-term local disease control. Compared with other treatment options (i.e., corticosteroids, WBRT, and SRS), surgical resection has distinct advantages for achieving these goals.

First, surgery is the only treatment modality that can provide a histologic diagnosis. Although progress in imaging techniques such as magnetic resonance (MR) spectroscopy may allow for precise determination of tumor pathology in the future, surgery remains the only established method for achieving this goal at present. The importance of tissue diagnosis is paramount when the diagnosis of brain metastasis is in question. This occurs most commonly in patients without a diagnosis of primary cancer, or rarely in patients with two known primary tumors. Nevertheless, even for patients with a single known systemic cancer, failure to obtain histologic confirmation may still lead to erroneous diagnosis in 5% to 11% of the cases.[12,13] Therefore, it is important not to omit tissue sampling when clinical features raise suspicion of other disease processes such as cerebral abscess or primary lymphoma, whose imaging findings may be indistinguishable from metastatic tumors.

Second, compared with other modalities, surgery is most effective in immediately relieving symptoms caused by the mass effect of the lesion. Although corticosteroids reduce the effects of vasogenic edema, they do not alter the

Table 15-1 Proportion of Brain Metastases and Propensity to Metastasize to Brain According to Primary Tumor			
OVERALL INCIDENCE (%)		**PROPENSITY TO METASTASIZE (%)***	
Lung carcinoma	45	Melanoma	50
Breast carcinoma	20	Lung carcinoma	25
Melanoma	15	Breast carcinoma	25
Renal cell carcinoma	10	Renal cell carcinoma	15
Colon carcinoma	5	Colon carcinoma	5
Other	5		

*Proportion of patients with primary cancer developing brain metastases.

pressure exerted from the lesion itself, and their side effects preclude long-term use. Radiation treatment, including SRS, may reduce the tumor mass, but the effect is delayed.

Third, surgical resection is well documented to result in long-term local control of metastatic lesions with minimal morbidity. Although WBRT and SRS may provide local control, eradication of the lesion, as objectively demonstrated on imaging studies, is less predictable for these modalities when compared with surgery. In contrast, with modern techniques, complete resection can be achieved in nearly all cases. The certainty in predicting such an immediate outcome is a major advantage over radiation-based modalities.

Patient Selection

Patient selection is the cornerstone of surgical management. Not all patients with brain metastases are candidates for resection, and decisions to operate should be based on a firm understanding of the variables influencing surgical outcomes. Determining whether surgical resection is the best option for a particular patient requires a careful consideration of a number of parameters, including the multiplicity, the location, and the size of the lesion(s), in the context of the clinical status of the patient as well as the histology of the primary tumor. The decision for surgical resection must be weighed against and integrated with other treatment options, namely WBRT and SRS.

RADIOGRAPHIC ASSESSMENT

Preoperative studies, particularly MR imaging, are used to determine the number, location, size, and resectability of intracranial metastases. These tumor features are critical in selecting patients for surgery.

NUMBER OF LESIONS

A primary consideration in deciding to operate is the number of lesions. MR imaging is more sensitive than computed tomography (CT) for the detection of small metastases or those within the posterior fossa[14-16] and is thus recommended for definitively establishing the number of intracranial metastases. The term "single" cerebral metastasis is used to describe one metastasis to the brain in the face of other systemic metastases, whereas "solitary" cerebral metastasis indicates that the brain is the only site of metastatic disease within the body.[17] Although single cerebral metastases constitute approximately 30% of all cases of patients with brain metastases, solitary metastases are rare.[18] To determine management options, patients should

be divided into two broad categories: patients with single/solitary metastases or with multiple brain metastases.

SINGLE AND SOLITARY BRAIN METASTASIS

Patients with single/solitary brain metastases are the best candidates for surgery. It has been demonstrated by class I evidence that surgical resection of single or solitary brain metastases is superior to treatment with WBRT alone. The evidence is derived from three randomized controlled trials reported in the 1990s comparing surgical resection plus WBRT with WBRT alone, of which two showed a significant reduction of recurrence and extension of survival with surgical treatment.[12,19,20]

Patchell and colleagues reported the first study comparing surgical resection plus WBRT with WBRT alone.[12] The authors included patients ($n = 47$) with single brain metastases, good performance status (Karnofsky Performance Scale [KPS] score ≥ 70), and limited extent of disease. They found that the rate of local recurrence was significantly ($p < 0.02$) lower in the surgical group (20%) compared with the WBRT group (52%). Likewise, the overall length of survival was significantly longer ($p < 0.01$) following surgical resection plus WBRT (median, 40 weeks) compared with WBRT alone (median, 15 weeks). Importantly, the improved survival was accompanied by maintenance of functional independence (38 weeks in the surgical group vs. 8 weeks in the WBRT group, $p < 0.005$). A multivariate analysis further indicated that surgical resection ($p < 0.0001$) and the absence of disseminated disease ($p < 0.0004$) were predictors of better outcome. These results provided, for the first time, class I evidence in support of surgical resection plus WBRT in lieu of WBRT alone as the gold standard for treatment of single/solitary brain metastases.

In a second prospective randomized study, Vecht and colleagues also compared surgery plus WBRT with WBRT alone in patients with single brain metastases. Like Patchell et al., they included only patients with good performance status and reported a significantly longer median survival time after surgery plus WBRT (43 weeks) compared with WBRT alone (26 weeks, $p = 0.04$).[20] A major difference from the trial of Patchell and colleagues, however, was that the investigators stratified the patients by site (lung cancer vs. non-lung cancer) and by status of extracranial disease (progressive vs. stable). Importantly, they found that the benefits of surgery were most evident in patients with limited systemic disease. Specifically, patients with stable extracranial disease had a more prolonged survival when treated with surgical resection and WBRT (median, 12 months) than when treated with WBRT alone (median, 7 months, $p = 0.04$). In contrast, patients with progressive extracranial disease generally fared worse and the survival was independent of whether or not surgical resection was performed (median survival time of 5 months in both combined treatment and WBRT alone groups). The tumor type, lung versus non-lung histology, was not a strong predictor of survival.

In a third study, Mintz et al. reported a multicenter prospective trial that randomized 84 patients to either surgery plus WBRT or WBRT alone.[19] In contrast to the previous two trials, there was no difference in the median survival time of the surgery plus WBRT group (24 weeks) compared with the WBRT alone group (27 weeks, $p = 0.24$). Likewise, the duration of time that patients maintained a KPS score ≥ 70 was not different between the two groups. However, the data did support previous findings that extra-cranial metastases were an important predictor of mortality. One key difference between the study of Mintz et al. and the other two randomized trials was that Mintz et al. included patients with lower performance status (inclusion criterion was KPS score ≥ 50, compared with > 70 in the other studies). Consequently, 21% of their study population had a KPS score < 70, and 45% of patients suffered from extracranial metastases. In contrast, patients with active extracranial disease comprised only 37% of patients in the study of Patchell et al. and 32% of patients in the study of Vecht et al. Because low KPS scores and active extracranial disease are associated with poor survival, the differences between these trials suggest that the benefits of surgery may diminish in patients with more advanced disease as the systemic tumor burden predominates in the clinical course. Such differences also highlight the influence of study populations in altering the overall outcome of clinical trials.

On the basis of these three randomized controlled trials, a Cochrane meta-analysis concluded that for patients with good performance status (KPS score ≥ 70) and controlled systemic disease, surgical resection plus WBRT provides the best outcome for patients with single brain metastases.[21] This same conclusion was also reached in recently published guidelines.[22] The collective data suggest that the benefits of surgery extend not only to prolongation of overall survival but also to maintenance of functional independence and local disease control, by reducing deaths and disabilities from neurologic causes. For patients with lower performance status (KPS score < 70), the evidence is less clear, as the burden of the extracranial disease is likely to outweigh the influence of the cerebral pathology. However, when considering the implications of these data in clinical practice, it is important to note that the benefits of surgical resection are not limited to the outcome measures examined in these clinical trials, and the role of surgery in reversing neurologic symptoms and deficits by immediate decompression of local mass effects and prevention of death from brain herniation cannot be overemphasized. For example, a drowsy patient harboring a large posterior fossa single metastasis may be unjustly denied a life-saving operation should the decision to operate be based solely on performance status. Therefore, recommendation for surgery requires not only justification from sound literature-based evidence but also the exercise of good clinical judgment, with an ultimate goal of maximizing the clinical outcome of each individual patient.

MULTIPLE BRAIN METASTASES

The traditional treatment of multiple brain metastases is with WBRT, and the presence of multiple metastases has been considered in the past a contraindication to surgery, even when the tumors are surgically accessible.[23-26] However, an increasing volume of literature in recent years has suggested that surgery may have a role in the treatment of multiple metastases for a defined patient population. In a retrospective analysis, Bindal et al. reported the outcome of 56 patients who underwent resection for multiple brain metastases. Patients were divided into those who had one or more lesions left unresected (group A, $n = 30$), and those who had undergone resection of all lesions (group B, $n = 26$).[27] These patients were compared with a group of matched controls who had single metastases that were surgically resected (group C, $n = 26$). There was no difference in surgical mortality (3%, 4%, and 0% for groups A, B, and C, respectively) or morbidity (8%, 9%, and 8% for groups A, B, and C, respectively) regardless of treatment group. Most importantly, patients with multiple metastases who had all the lesions resected (group B) had a significantly longer survival (median, 14 months) than patients who had some lesions left unresected (group A; median, 6 months; $p = 0.003$). The survival time of patients who had all lesions removed (group B) was similar to that of patients with resected single metastases (group C; median, 14 months). It was concluded that removal of multiple metastatic lesions is as effective as resection of single metastases, with the important caveat that all lesions had to be removed.[27]

In support of the above findings, Iwadate and colleagues reported a median survival time of 9.2 months following resection of multiple brain metastases in 61 patients; this was similar to the survival time of 8.7 months following resection of a single brain metastasis in 77 contemporary patients.[28] Predictors of shorter survival were age greater than 60 years, KPS score < 70, incomplete surgical resection, and the presence of extensive systemic cancer. Similarly, in a recent single surgeon retrospective series of 208 patients, resection of one or more symptomatic tumors in 76 patients harboring multiple brain metastases achieved a median survival time of 11 months.[29] This outcome compared favorably with the median survival time of 8 months in the 132 patients with surgically resected single metastases.[29]

Based on these studies, patients with multiple metastases should not be excluded a priori from surgery. However, it should be noted that the definition of "multiple" in most reported studies was three to four tumors, and in practice, patients with more than four lesions are generally not considered good surgical candidates and are conventionally treated with WBRT alone. Nevertheless, with the advent of SRS, a multimodal treatment model that includes surgical resection for larger (>3 cm in maximal diameter) lesions and SRS for smaller lesions has made it more feasible to offer local treatment for even more than four lesions. For example, resection of one or two larger symptomatic lesions and providing SRS for two or three smaller (1–2 mm in maximal diameter) metastases is becoming an increasingly accepted approach.

LOCATION

Resectability (i.e., whether a tumor can be removed with minimal morbidity) is dictated primarily by tumor location. With modern microneurosurgical techniques there are very few, if any, regions within the brain that are inaccessible to the neurosurgeon. However, accessibility and resectability are not the same. The most important features that determine resectability are whether the tumor is deep or superficial and whether the tumor is within or near "eloquent" brain. Stereotactic image-guided surgical techniques and skull base exposures have made previously unreachable tumors resectable. A variety of techniques help to preserve functionally important brain regions during resection. Nevertheless, lesions that are deeply located and within "eloquent areas" are inevitably associated with slightly higher surgical morbidity than those within noneloquent and superficial areas. In this context, Sawaya and colleagues studied 400 consecutive patients undergoing craniotomies for brain tumor resection.[30] They found that major neurologic complications occurred in 13% of patients undergoing resection of tumors from "eloquent" brain regions, whereas the incidence was 5% and 3%, respectively, for patients undergoing resection of tumors located within "near-eloquent" and "noneloquent" brain regions. The potential morbidity (hence, recovery time) associated with surgical removal must therefore be weighed against the limited survival expectancy of this patient population. Patients with metastases to the brain stem, thalamus, and basal ganglia are generally not considered surgical candidates, except in rare circumstances. Treatment of lesions in these locations with noninvasive modality such as SRS may be warranted. However, it must be noted that significant morbidity could also develop with SRS when treating lesions near the eloquent brain or cranial nerves, and no study to date has convincingly showed that the morbidity of surgery is more than that of SRS in these circumstances.

LESION SIZE

The size of the lesion is another factor that must be considered when choosing therapy. For lesions that are greater than 3 cm in maximum diameter, surgical resection is the primary option because surgery rapidly relieves the mass effect that commonly occurs with these larger, often symptomatic lesions. In contrast, SRS is generally not applicable for tumors >3 cm in diameter because SRS typically results in an unacceptably high radiation dose to the surrounding normal brain due to the limited degree of conformity that can be achieved for large volume tumors.[31,32] However, for lesions <1 cm in maximum diameter, radiosurgery is often the ideal treatment because most of these tumors are asymptomatic, and localizing small lesions at surgery, even with MR imaging guidance, may be difficult, especially when deep in the brain.

The most difficult lesions for which to decide an optimal treatment are those between 1 and 3 cm in maximum diameter. For these lesions, either surgery or radiosurgery can be applied. Currently, there is limited evidence available demonstrating the superiority of one treatment over the other (see the following). For these patients, other factors such as the resectability, extent of the systemic disease, and the presence of comorbidities may influence the final decision.

CLINICAL ASSESSMENT

The status of the patient's systemic disease (i.e., the extent of the primary tumor and of noncerebral metastases) is a critical consideration in the decision to resect a brain metastasis because advanced systemic disease is a major predictor of short-term survival, whereas limited systemic disease is associated with long survival in patients undergoing surgery for cerebral metastases (see previous).[12,20,27,33-35] Indeed, after resection of a single brain metastasis, up to 70% of patients will succumb to their systemic disease and not to their brain disease.[12] In this context, most patients with absent systemic disease are surgical candidates, whereas most patients with widely disseminated cancer are not. Decision making in patients with significant systemic cancer burden that is responding to therapy poses a challenge. One practical approach is to determine the expected survival time for the patient, excluding the presence of

Table 15-2 Considerations in Patient Selection for Surgical Removal of Brain Metastases

Factor	Requirement for Surgery
Status of Systemic Disease	
Control of primary cancer	Expected survival >3 months
General medical condition	Able to withstand surgery/anesthesia
Neurologic status	KPS score ≥ 70
Resectability	
Accessibility	Not brain stem, basal gangila, thalamus
Size	>1 cm in maximal diameter

KPS, Karnofsky Performance Scale.

cerebral metastases. At many centers, patients who are expected to survive for more than 3-4 months are usually candidates for surgical resection.

In addition, the preoperative neurologic status should be considered, because patients with marked neurologic deficits have been shown to have a shorter median survival time than patients who are neurologically intact.[35,36] However, as alluded to previously, it is important not to exclude patients from surgery on this basis alone, because there are many patients whose neurologic deficits improve following resection of the offending tumor. One way to determine the potential for recovery is to assess the response of the deficit to corticosteroid administration. Patients whose neurologic deficits are likely to improve after resection usually demonstrate an improvement after treatment with corticosteroids, whereas patients who will not improve postoperatively do not have such a response to corticosteroids. In general, a surgical patient should have an expected survival of at least 3 months, be able to withstand anesthesia, and have a KPS score ≥ 70 (Table 15-2). Patients who have major cardiac, pulmonary, renal, or hematologic diseases may be better suited for nonsurgical treatment.

To assist in treatment decision, several investigators have advocated dividing patients into prognostic categories based on clinical features as determined from prospective clinical trials. One of the most widely recognized predictive models was developed by Gaspar and colleagues, who identified three prognostic groups of patients with brain metastases based on a recursive partitioning analysis (RPA) of 1200 patients enrolled in three consecutive Radiation Therapy Oncology Group (RTOG) trials conducted between 1979 and 1993 that were originally designed to evaluate radiation fractionation paradigms and radiation sensitizers.[37] The analysis identified three prognostic categories: class I included patients with a KPS score > 70, age <65 years, controlled primary cancer, and no extracranial metastases; class III was defined by patients with a KPS score < 70; and class II included all other patients. These RPA groups correlated with survival as the median survival time of class I, II, and III patients were 7.1 months, 4.2 months, and 2.3 months, respectively. Based on this analysis, it has been suggested that class I patients are good candidate for aggressive treatment including surgery whereas class III patients are not. Although in practice, these RPA classes have not been adopted into clinical use, they are commonly used as a research tool in designing, stratifying, and assessing treatment results of clinical trials. An understanding of

Table 15-3 Radiosensitivity of Brain Metastases to Conventional Fractionated Radiotherapy

Highly Sensitive	Intermediately Sensitive	Poorly Sensitive
Lymphoma	Breast cancer	Melanoma
Germinoma	Lung (non–small cell) cancer	Renal cancer
Lung (small cell) cancer	Colon cancer	Sarcoma

Data from JG Cairncross, JH Kim, JB Posner. Radiation therapy for brain metastases. Ann Neurol. 1980;7:529-541; and FF Lang, R Sawaya. Surgical management of cerebral metastases. Neurosurg Clin North Am. 1996;7:459-484.

this classification is, therefore, important in critically evaluating the current neuro-oncology literature.

HISTOLOGIC ASSESSMENT

The type of primary cancer, particularly its relative radiosensitivity, is an important consideration in treatment decision making (Table 15-3). In this context, primary treatment with WBRT is strongly considered for patients with highly radiosensitive tumors, such as lymphoma, germ cell tumors, and small cell lung cancer. The most common types of tumors to metastasize to the brain, namely breast and non–small cell lung cancer, are intermediately sensitive to conventional fractionated radiotherapy, and surgery will have a role in many cases. For radioresistant tumors (e.g., melanoma, renal cell carcinoma, and sarcomas), surgical resection is often the treatment of choice. Although this categorization is useful for conventional fractionated radiotherapy, the same does not necessarily hold true for SRS, as melanoma, renal cell carcinoma, and sarcomas may respond well to radiosurgery. The reason behind this difference in response to WBRT and SRS is not entirely clear, but it has been postulated that SRS is tumoricidal because it affects tumor vasculature differently from WBRT.[38]

Surgical Technique

Successful extirpation of cerebral metastases is based on good basic neurosurgical techniques in conjunction with technologies for tumor localization and functional brain mapping. A clear understanding of the surgical anatomy of these lesions results in safe and effective tumor removal.

SURGICAL ANATOMY

Cerebral metastases consist of solid tumor without intervening brain tissue. Although there may be some infiltration of tumor cells into the surrounding brain, this is usually less than 5 mm deep.[8] Typically, the mass of tumor cells is surrounded by a gliotic rim that separates the tumor from the surrounding edematous brain. The lesions commonly arise at the gray-white matter junction, where a reduction in blood vessel diameter causes the embolic tumor to become trapped.[39]

In the supratentorial space, metastases may be classified based on their relationship to adjacent sulci and gyri.[39,40] Metastases may occur just under the cortex and fill a gyrus (subcortical), deep within a gyrus adjacent to a sulcus (subgyral), below a sulcus (subsulcal), deep within the hemispheric white matter (lobar), or within the ventricle (intraventricular).[41] In the posterior fossa, cerebellar metastases can be categorized as occurring in either deep or hemispheric locations; hemispheric lesions can be considered as lateral or medial. A subset arises directly within the vermis. Knowledge of the relationship to the sulcus is particularly important because this may determine the appropriate surgical path to the tumor (see the following).

Another important aspect of the surgical anatomy is the location of blood vessels. "Arterialized" veins that drain the lesion are often evident on the brain surface, and surgeons must carefully consider the venous drainage when resecting the lesion. More importantly, the arterial supply to most metastases comes from vessels parasitized from branches of larger vessels that arise within the sulci.

RESECTION METHODS

Careful planning and meticulous attention to detail are necessary to minimize surgical complications. The surgeon must devote appropriate attention to each stage of the operative procedure, including positioning, opening, tumor resection, and closure. The technique must result in complete removal of the lesion, with preservation of neurologic function and minimal disruption of the surrounding brain.

POSITIONING

After careful review of the preoperative imaging and correlation with known anatomic landmarks, it should be possible to identify and mark the location of the tumor as it projects onto the scalp and to tentatively define the incision prior to immobilization of the head and final positioning of the patient. This is a useful exercise not only as a check of the neuronavigation system (see the following) and to decrease total reliance on such devices but also to aid in proper placement of the head immobilizer and to determine the most appropriate position for the patient. Typically, patients are positioned with the guiding principle that the lesion should be at the top of the operative field. After selection of the most appropriate position for the patient, the head is rigidly fixed in a neurosurgical head-holder (e.g., the Mayfield 3-pin clamp) and then secured to the operating table. The tumor can then be marked out on the scalp using the neuronavigation system, if available. After the location of the tumor has been determined, a final appropriate skin incision is planned. The authors generally prefer linear skin incisions, where possible, because the risk of compromising the vascular supply to the scalp is decreased as compared with utilization of flaps.

EXPOSURE AND OPERATIVE APPROACH

Standard neurosurgical principles of preservation of blood supply and minimal injury to tissues guide the operation. Frameless stereotaxy is preferred because it allows for smaller cranial and dural openings with minimal exposure of normal brain and because it assists in determining the optimal trajectory to the tumor. However, unless intraoperative imaging with CT or MR (and, in some cases, ultrasound) is available, the system cannot be updated during the operative procedure.

Surgical approaches to a brain metastasis are based on its anatomic location.[39] Supratentorial subcortical lesions are best resected by an incision in the apex of the sulcus and circumferential dissection of the tumor (transcortical approach) (Fig. 15-1). Removal of a cortical plug above the lesion improves exposure; this may be problematic when

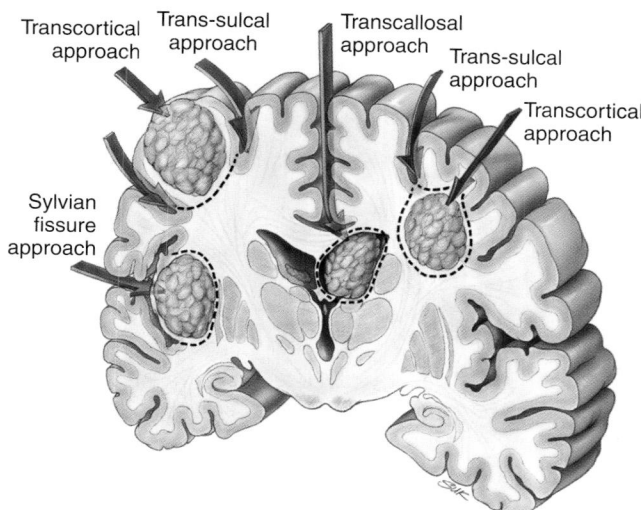

Transcortical approach
Trans-sulcal approach
Transcallosal approach
Trans-sulcal approach
Transcortical approach
Sylvian fissure approach

FIGURE 15-1 Surgical approaches to supratentorial metastases: transsylvian approach to a metastasis of the external capsule; transcortical and trans-sulcal approaches to a subcortical metastasis, which is shown filling the gyrus; transcallosal approach to an intraventricular tumor. *(Modified from Lang FF, Chang EL, Suki D, et al. Metastatic brain tumors. In: Winn HR, ed. Youmans Neurological Surgery, 5th ed. Philadelphia: WB Saunders;2004.)*

the lesion arises within eloquent cortex. In such a situation, a longitudinal incision dictated by local functional mapping performed with direct brain stimulation (see the following) may minimize injury to the surrounding brain.

Lesions in subgyral or subsulcal locations are best approached by splitting the sulcus leading to the lesion. Subgyral tumors are removed by making an incision in the side of the split sulcus, whereas subsulcal lesions are entered at the sulcal base (transsulcal approach) (see Fig. 15-1). Metastases located deep within the white matter, independent of a single sulcus or gyrus (lobar), may be approached either transcortically or trans-sulcally (see Fig. 15-1). Tumors in the subinsular cortex may be approached by splitting the sylvian fissure. Midline metastases are best approached by splitting the interhemispheric fissure; tumors may then be resected by further splitting or entering a deep gyrus (see Fig. 15-1). Intraventricular lesions may be approached transcallosally or transcortically (Fig. 15-2; see Fig. 15-1).

Cerebellar tumors are best approached along the shortest transparenchymal route to the lesion. Superior hemispheric lesions are approached via the supracerebellar cistern and then incising the cerebellum at the closest point to the tumor. This requires a high suboccipital craniotomy with exposure of the transverse sinus. Lateral hemispheric lesions are approached directly from a posterior trajectory. Inferior cerebellar tumors require opening of the foramen magnum. Midline tumors can be resected after splitting the vermis.

LESION EXTIRPATION

Once the lesion is reached, resection is usually performed in a circumferential, en bloc fashion by dissection in the gliotic pseudocapsule surrounding the lesion (Fig. 15-3). Circumferential dissection is carried out in this gliotic plane

without violating the wall of the tumor. Such an approach ensures gross-total resection (because tumor cells rarely infiltrate beyond the gliotic plane) and also reduces spillage of cells into the surrounding area. For lesions located directly in the eloquent brain (e.g., motor strip or speech centers), a longitudinal incision parallel to the orientation of the gyrus can be made and the tumor resected in an "inside-out," piecemeal fashion, rather than en bloc. Piecemeal removal may also be preferred for very large lesions in difficult areas (e.g., within the ventricle).

The importance of performing an en bloc resection has been highlighted in a retrospective study conducted by Suki et al., in which 260 patients with 1-2 posterior fossa metastases were analyzed based on the type of resection for the development of leptomeningeal disease (LMD, i.e., carcinomatous meningitis).[42] Whereas only 6% of 123 patients who underwent en bloc resection developed LMD, 14% of 137 patients who had a piecemeal resection developed LMD. In a related study of 542 patients with supratentorial metastatic tumors from the same investigators, similar results were noted.[43] Specifically, of 191 patients who underwent piecemeal resection, 9% developed LMD, whereas LMD developed in only 3% of 351 patients who had en bloc resections. These results remain significant even after controlling for other covariates including tumor volume, tumor type, extent of resection, and patient characteristics such as age, KPS score, and extracranial disease burden. Although these findings have yet to be confirmed in a prospective manner, it is prudent to conclude that en bloc resection should be performed whenever feasible.

When resecting cerebral metastases, particularly during en bloc resections, care must be taken also to preserve the main arteries that lie within sulci. Most metastases receive their blood supply from several small branches arising from the main vessel. It is critical to identify these branches and to individually coagulate and cut them. This step reduces bleeding during resection and ensures that the main artery is not damaged. Likewise, particular care should be taken to preserve all surface veins so that the drainage of the normal brain is not disrupted.

TECHNICAL ISSUES IN RESECTING MULTIPLE METASTASES

When resecting multiple brain metastases, special attention must be given to planning the operation. Resection of multiple metastases can be performed via one craniotomy that encompasses all the lesions or via multiple, separate craniotomies. The decision to perform multiple craniotomies is determined by the proximity of the lesions to each other: lesions that are some distance apart generally require separate craniotomies. When multiple craniotomies are required, it is usually possible to perform all the craniotomies simultaneously without having to redrape the patient. The patient may be placed in a neutral position and turned from side to side on the operating table so that the lesion that is being operated on is positioned at the top of the operative field. Linear skin incisions are particularly effective when performing multiple craniotomies, and they also reduce the risk of compromising the vascular supply to the scalp. To maximize efficiency, each step of the operation (i.e., skin incision, bone flap elevation, dural opening, tumor removal, hemostasis, and closure) is performed

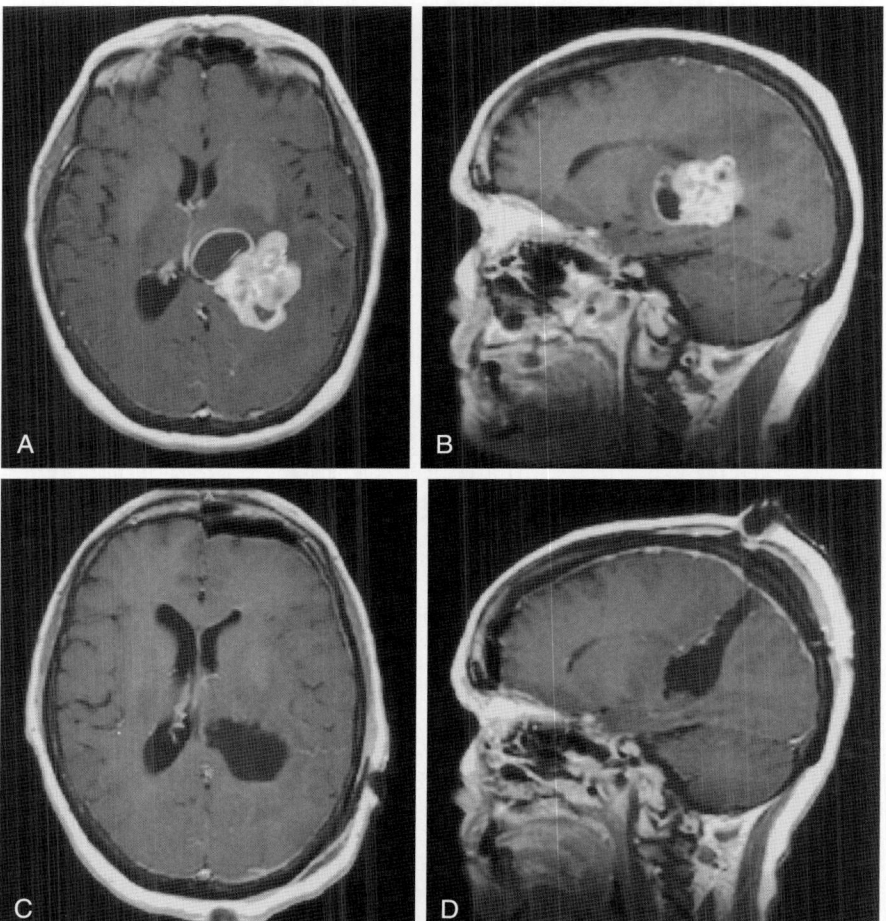

FIGURE 15-2 Intraventricular metastatic renal cell carcinoma. Preoperative axial (A) and sagittal contrast-enhanced (B) MR images showing a metastasis in the atrium of the left lateral ventricle. The lesion was completely resected utilizing a transcortical approach through the superior parietal lobule (C and D). *(From Vecil GG, Lang FF. Surgical resection of metastatic intraventricular tumors. Neurosurg Clin North Am. 2003;14:593-606.)*

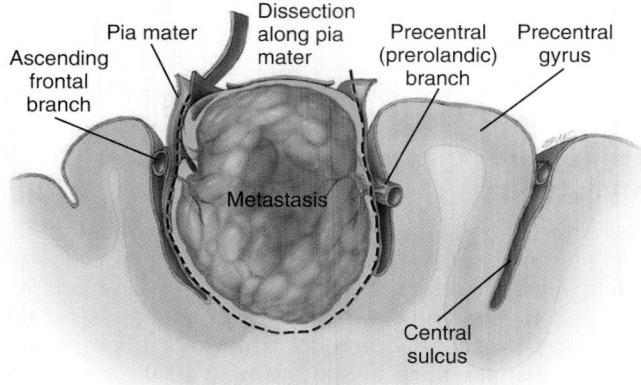

FIGURE 15-3 En bloc technique of metastasis resection. A metastasis filling a gyrus is pictured. The tumor is removed en bloc after dissection in the adjacent sulci and deep to the lesion through the base of the sulci. All but those vessels directly supplying the tumor are preserved. *(Modified from Hentschel SH, Lang FF. Current surgical management of glioblastoma. Cancer J. 2003;9:113-126.)*

at each location before the next step is performed. This approach is preferred to removing one lesion at one site and closing that wound and then removing one lesion at another site, not only because it is more efficient, but also because it minimizes the time between hemostasis and

patient awakening. Thus any untoward events (e.g., hematoma formation) do not go undetected while the patient is under anesthesia.

SURGICAL ADJUNCTS

Safe and effective resection of cerebral metastases requires accurate identification of the location of each lesion and the surgical corridor through which it can be resected. The ability to identify the lesion is enhanced by the use of computer-assisted image-guided stereotaxis, intraoperative ultrasonography, and (in some centers) intraoperative MR imaging. Other useful adjuncts include somatosensory evoked potentials (SSEPs) and intraoperative direct brain stimulation, both of which allow for identification of functional (eloquent) brain regions.

ULTRASOUND

Intraoperative ultrasound is a valuable adjunct available to the surgeon that provides a relatively low-cost method for visualizing tumors below the surface of the brain. Most brain metastases appear homogeneously hyperechogenic, although those with necrotic centers or cysts may be hypoechoic centrally (Fig. 15-4). Compared with other methods of localization, ultrasound has the advantage of real-time imaging; therefore, changes in the tumor, as well as brain shift, are readily identifiable as the resection proceeds. Ultrasound also allows for visualization of

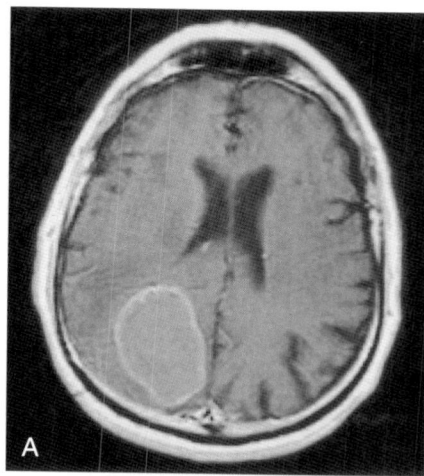
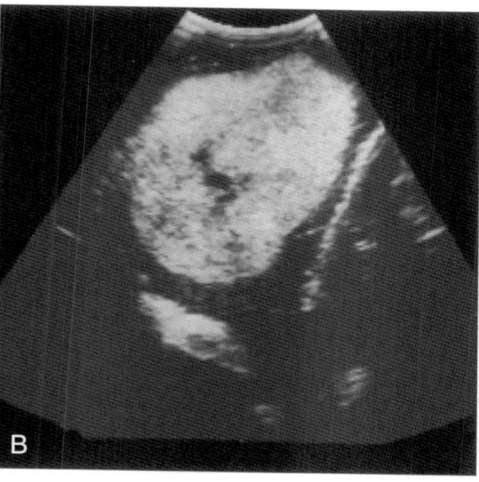

FIGURE 15-4 Occipital lobe metastasis. The contrast-enhanced MR image (A) and the intraoperative ultrasound image (B) are shown. The central hypodensity on the ultrasound image represents necrosis within the tumor.

the adjacent sulci and other intracranial landmarks (e.g., the ventricle), thus assisting in selection of a corridor of approach to the tumor. Ultrasound can assist in the determination of the extent of tumor resection because gross-total resection corresponds to complete removal of the echogenic mass, in most cases. However, in cases of recurrent tumors after radiotherapy, radiation necrosis may obscure the boundaries of the lesion, making determination of the extent of resection more difficult.[44]

STEREOTAXIS

Advances in localization technology have allowed for the evolution of rigid frame-based stereotaxy into frameless systems. These "neuronavigation" devices allow neurosurgeons to navigate the brain based on the preoperative images. These systems are particularly useful for planning the skin incision and craniotomy and the initial trajectory to the lesion. However, they suffer from the inability to compensate for intraoperative changes such as brain shift unless they can be updated with intraoperative imaging (usually MR images or even ultrasonography).[45] Thus the authors generally rely on ultrasound as the resection proceeds.

INTRAOPERATIVE MR IMAGING

The inability of neuronavigation systems to track intraoperative changes in real time has led to the development of intraoperative MR imaging systems. Surgery may be performed within the magnet itself or outside of it, necessitating that the patient be brought into the unit or that the unit be brought to the patient. The main uses of these systems are to update the neuronavigation system during the operation, to confirm the extent of tumor resection, and to rule out intracranial complications prior to leaving the operating room. The cost of current systems has precluded widespread application, particularly for well-demarcated lesions such as brain metastases.

FUNCTIONAL MAPPING

When resecting metastases within eloquent areas of the brain, mapping the location of the critical functions is vital to safe tumor resection. Preoperative identification of sensory, motor, and language cortices is possible with functional MR imaging,[46] and diffusion-tensor imaging allows for

identification of important white matter tracts (e.g., internal capsule).[47] These preoperative studies, however, are only a general guide, and precise localization of function usually requires verification during the surgical resection. Consequently, functional mapping methods have been used to precisely define eloquent brain regions intraoperatively.

Neurophysiologic techniques, such as SSEPs, can be utilized to identify the reversal of phase that occurs between the motor and sensory cortices. A strip electrode is placed on the cortical surface, and stimulation of median, ulnar, or posterior tibial nerves results in cortical potentials that are detected by the electrodes. A "reversal of phase" is seen when the electrode covers both the motor and the sensory cortex, because the motor potentials are typically positive, and sensory potentials are typically negative. This permits an intraoperative indirect identification of motor and sensory cortices. The technique has also been used to continuously monitor the potentials throughout the operative procedure so as to guide resections adjacent to the primary somatosensory cortex.[48]

Direct cortical electrical stimulation can be used to identify eloquent cortex and is particularly useful in the localization of language areas. The technique involves stimulation of the cerebral cortex at a frequency of 60 Hz for 1 millisecond with biphasic square wave pulses and a current of 1 to 15 mA (Fig. 15-5).[49-51] Stimulation of the motor cortex elicits a motor response in the patient, thus resulting in an objective response, which is an advantage over the SSEP technique. Stimulation of subcortical motor pathways can also be performed in a similar manner; however, the results are somewhat less reliable than with cortical stimulation.[52]

Although motor mapping can be performed with patients under general anesthesia, language mapping requires an awake patient. The authors' current method of awake craniotomy employs intubation with a laryngeal mask and short-duration anesthetics, along with a local anesthetic scalp block prior to placement of the three-point head fixator.[53] The muscle (if exposed) and dura are carefully infiltrated with local anesthetic. Once the craniotomy is completed, the patient is awakened, and the laryngeal mask is removed. Cortical stimulation with mapping of speech may then commence. Speech areas are usually defined as sites where electrical stimulation elicits speech arrest. In addition, patients

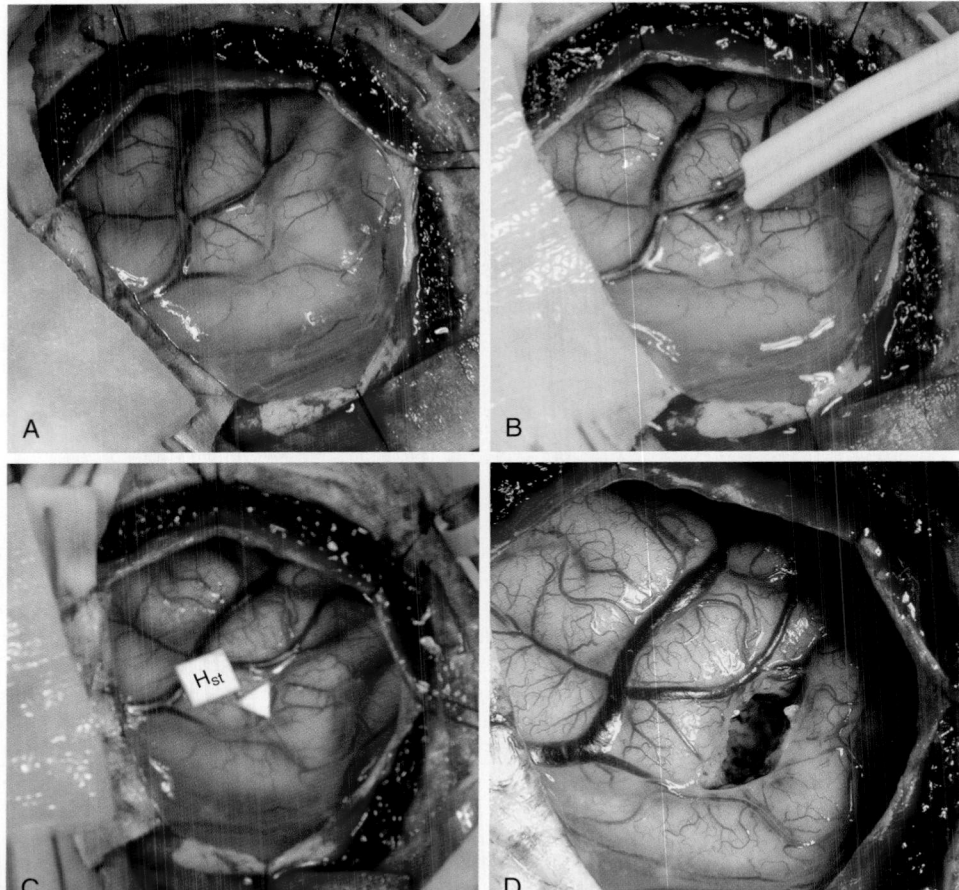

FIGURE 15-5 Intraoperative photographs depicting removal of a metastasis from the motor area of the brain. A, The brain prior to resection demonstrating slightly clouded leptomeninges along with an enlarged gyrus. B, A bipolar cortical stimulator was used to electrically stimulate the cerebral cortex, and a motor response was elicited. C, The cortical stimulation resulted in hand movement in the area marked by the white label (Hst). The white arrowhead marks a sulcus overlying the tumor. D, The tumor has been completely resected and all vascular structures preserved utilizing a trans-sulcal approach through the sulcus identified in C. The patient experienced no permanent alteration of neurologic function.

can freely converse during the resection of the tumor in order to avoid loss of function as the resection proceeds. Once the resection is completed, the laryngeal mask may be replaced and the patient anesthetized, if required; or a short-acting sedative, along with a narcotic, may be given during the closure. This awake method allows for the safe removal of the tumor from eloquent brain and provides the patient with maximal comfort.

Outcomes after Surgical Resection

SURGICAL MORTALITY

Most studies define surgical mortality as death that occurs within 30 days of operation, although some of the earlier surgeons used shorter intervals.[54-56] Other series include deaths after 30 days if the patient did not leave the hospital.[34,57] Surgical mortality has decreased dramatically since the earliest reports. For example, Cushing found that the mortality after resection of brain metastases was quite high (38%).[57] In contrast, over the last two decades, using modern techniques, surgical mortalities of 3% or less have often been reported (Table 15-4). In fact, some of the more recent series report no mortality after surgery for brain metastases.[33,44,58,59] In the randomized trial of Patchell and colleagues,[12] the 30-day operative mortality and the 30-day postradiotherapy mortality were both 4%. In a comprehensive analysis of 400 craniotomies for all types of

brain tumors, the overall 30-day mortality for patients with cerebral metastases was 2% (4/194), with the cause of death being sepsis in two patients and progressive leptomeningeal carcinomatosis in two others.[30]

SURGICAL MORBIDITY

Postoperative morbidity after surgery for brain metastases includes those related to neurologic changes and those related to non-neurologic problems (e.g., postoperative hematoma, wound infection, deep venous thrombosis, pneumonia, and pulmonary embolism). Some studies separate these two aspects of morbidity;[27,29,33,35] others consider them together,[12,20,24] a few report only neurologic morbidity;[36,54,60-62] and many do not report morbidity at all (see Table 15-4).[26,34,55,56,63,64]

One of the most comprehensive analyses of postoperative complications for brain metastases was conducted by Sawaya and colleagues.[30] This series from a large tertiary cancer center reviewed the complications that occurred after 194 craniotomies for brain metastases performed using all the modern technologies described above. Importantly, complications were categorized as either neurologic (directly producing neurologic compromise), regional (at the surgical site), or systemic (more generalized medical problems). Complications were considered to be minor (not life threatening and not prolonging the length of the hospital stay) when they resolved within a few days to 30 days without surgical intervention. They were considered to be

Table 15-4	Results of Surgical Resection of Single Brain Metastases, Including Mortality and Morbidity						
						SURVIVAL	
Study	No.	Histology	WBRT	Mortality	Morbidity	Median (Months)	1 Year
Ferrara et al. (1990)[60]	100	Mixed	71%	6%	N/A	13	N/A
Patchell et al. (1990)[12]	25	Mixed	100%	4%	8%	10	45%
Bindal et al. (1993)[27]	26	Mixed	54%	0%	8% (0% neuro)	14	50%
Vecht et al. (1993)[20]	32	Mixed	100%	9%	41% total 13% (major)	10	41%
Wronski et al. (1995)[86]	231	Lung	84%	3%	17% (neuro)	11	46%
Bindal et al. (1996)[58]	62	Mixed	66%	0%	5%	16.4	58%
Pieper et al. (1997)[87]	63	Breast	86%	5%	N/A	16	62%
Muacevic et al. (1999)[88]	52	Mixed	100%	1.6%	7.7%	17	53%
Wronski et al. (1999)[89]	73	Colon	43.8%	4%	N/A	8.3	31.5%
Schoggl et al. (2000)[90]	66	Mixed	100%	0%	4.5%	9	83%
O'Neill et al. (2003)[91]	74	Mixed	82%	N/A	13.5% (neuro) 9.5% (systemic)	N/A	62%
Paek et al. (2005)[29]	132	Mixed	19%	N/A	5.3% (neuro) 9.1% (non-neuro)	8	N/A
Overall	936		71%	3%	15%	11.5	53%

N/A, not available; WBRT, whole-brain radiation therapy.

major when they persisted for more than 30 days (reducing the quality of life) or required aggressive treatment because of their life-threatening nature. The rates of major neurologic, regional, and systemic complications were 6%, 3%, and 6%, respectively. In a critical analysis of factors contributing to complications, the authors reported that the most important variable affecting the frequency of neurologic complications was the relationship of the tumor to functional (eloquent) brain. Specifically, tumors located within or near eloquent brain had more neurologic complications than did those in noneloquent areas. Nevertheless, the risk of major neurologic complications, even when the lesion was within eloquent areas, was low (13%). Based on their extensive data, the authors used a statistical model to predict the risk of major complications from any source. They found that patients who were relatively young (age 40 years), with a KPS score of 100 and a metastasis in noneloquent brain, had a 5% risk of a major complication, whereas, at the opposite extreme, for a relatively old patient (age 65 years) with a low KPS score (of 50) and a tumor in eloquent brain, this risk rose to 23%.

RECURRENCE

Recurrence is fairly easily measured after resection because surgery typically removes the entire gadolinium contrast-enhancing tumor mass (as visualized by MR imaging) and causes regression of the secondary brain edema. Thus, reappearance of a contrast-enhancing mass and edema on an MR image can be determined, although minimal postoperative contrast enhancement may be present for up to 3 months after surgery. In addition, one must distinguish between recurrence at the surgical site (i.e., local recurrence) and the development of new lesions in the brain at sites outside the initial resection site (i.e., distant recurrence). These events represent two distinct biologic processes. Local recurrence represents regrowth of microscopic residual disease after surgery, whereas distant recurrence is believed to arise from hematogenous dissemination of tumor cells to the brain from the primary

site. When evaluating rates of local and distant tumor recurrence, it is important to know whether the patients received adjunctive WBRT. In the prospective study by Patchell and colleagues of patients with single brain metastases who were then randomized either to receive or not to receive WBRT after surgery,[65] the local recurrence rate after surgery alone was 46% (21 of 46 patients), whereas the distant recurrence rate was 37% (17 of 46 patients). This high rate of local recurrence is not consistent with the results of other studies, which suggest recurrence rates of 10% to 15%.[66] Table 15-5 lists the local and distant recurrence rates in recent surgical series of brain metastases.

SURVIVAL

Most series from the modern neurosurgical era that include metastases with different tumor histologies indicate a median patient survival time of 11 months and a 1-year survival rate of 53% (see Table 15-4). Kelly and colleagues[39] reported a 1-year survival rate of 63% using computer-assisted stereotactic craniotomy. Studies from a large tertiary cancer center reported a median survival time of 14 months, with a 1-year survival rate of 50% for patients with single brain metastases.[27,33] Similar median (14 months) and 1-year (55%) survival values were observed in patients with multiple metastases in whom all the lesions were removed.[27] In most studies, variables associated with poor survival are the presence of multiple metastases, extensive and progressive systemic cancer, and a poor KPS score.

Role of Stereotactic Radiosurgery

Stereotactic radiosurgery in the form of gamma knife or linear accelerator methods delivers a single large dose of focused radiation, with rapid falloff in the surrounding tissue through cross-firing from many directions, to destroy lesions localized by stereotaxy. A major advantage of this technique over conventional surgery is that it can treat surgically inaccessible tumors, especially where eloquent brain would be transgressed during surgery to reach the lesion. Many brain

Table 15-5   Local and Distant Recurrence following Resection of Single Brain Metastasis

Study	No.	Local Recurrence	Distant Recurrence	Both	Latency (Median)
Patchell et al. (1990)[12]	25	20%	20%	12%	15 months (l)
Bindal et al. (1993)[27]	26	16%	27%	8%	25% at 6 months
Wronski et al. (1995)[86]	231	23.8%	36.6%	3%	N/A
Bindal et al. (1996)[58]	62	13%	26%	5%	N/A
Pieper et al. (1997)[87]	63	17%	16%	N/A	15 months
Muacevic et al. (1999)[88]	52	25% at 1 year	10% at 1 year	N/A	N/A
Wronski et al. (1999)[89]	73	49.3%	Overall		3.6 months
Schoggl et al. (2000)[90]	66	16.7%	15.2%	N/A	3.9 months (l) 3.7 months (d)
O'Neill et al. (2003)[91]	74	18%	18%	5.4%	N/A
McPherson et al. (2010)[82]	358	19%	44%	N/A	11.1 months (l) 8.7 months (d)
Overall	1030	22%	26%	5%	9.7 months

l, local; d, distant recurrence; N/A, not available.

metastases that in the past could only be treated with WBRT can now be directly targeted by SRS. Other advantages compared with surgery are that SRS is less costly, less invasive (requiring only placement of a stereotactic head frame under local anesthesia), requires shorter hospital stays because only a single fraction of radiation is given, and can be offered to patients who cannot tolerate surgery. Based on early retrospective reports, SRS has been shown to be effective in treating cerebral metastases, with local control rates ranging from 85% to 95% and a patient median survival time of 7 to 13 months.[63-65] These results compare favorably with a local recurrence rate of 10% to 15% reported after surgical resection.[66] Nevertheless, SRS has several important limitations compared with surgery. First, due to aforementioned dosing limitations, treatment is restricted to small lesions, usually to those not exceeding 3 cm in maximum diameter (volume <10–12 cm[3]).[28,29] Second, no histologic verification of the metastatic nature of the lesion can be obtained with SRS, which is important considering that 5% to 11% of patients with systemic cancer are found to have nonmetastatic brain lesions (e.g., primary brain tumors or abscesses).[8,12,13] Third, because SRS does not have the immediate effect of tumor extirpation, patients may have to remain on high steroid doses for longer intervals, and the mass effects of tumors (e.g., neurologic deficits and raised intracranial pressure) are not immediately relieved.

To define the role of SRS in the management of cerebral metastases, several randomized controlled trials have been conducted in recent years. In order to determine the benefits of adding SRS to standard WBRT, Kondziolka et al. randomized 27 patients with two to four cerebral metastases (≤2.5 cm) to receiving either WBRT alone or WBRT plus SRS.[67] They found that the addition of SRS (16 Gy) to the standard 30 Gy WBRT dose significantly prolonged the median time to local control failure from 6 months to 36 months ($p = 0.0005$). However, the median survival time of patients receiving WBRT plus SRS (11 months) was not found to be significantly longer than in those having WBRT alone (7.5 months, $p = 0.22$). Notably, the power of this study was grossly limited by its small sample size.

In another prospective study, Andrews et al. addressed the same question, comparing the treatment outcome of WBRT with or without an SRS boost.[68] In this multicenter study

carried out under the auspices of the RTOG, 333 patients with one to three brain metastases (≤4 cm in maximal diameter) were randomized to receive either WBRT alone or WBRT plus SRS. In the primary analysis of all 333 patients, there was no difference in survival between the patients who received WBRT plus SRS and those who received WBRT alone (6.5 months for WBRT plus SRS vs. 5.7 months for WBRT alone, $p = 0.14$). However, when analyzing the data in terms of secondary outcomes, patients treated with the combined approach were more likely to have stable or improved performance status (43% for WBRT plus SRS vs. 27% for WBRT alone, $p = 0.03$) and decreased steroid use at the 6-month follow-up evaluation. Most importantly, in a subset analysis that included only patients with single metastases ($n = 186$), there was a small but significant improvement in median survival time in the WBRT plus SRS group (6.5 months) when compared with the WBRT alone group (4.9 months, $p = 0.04$). This study represents the first large-scale randomized trial of SRS as an adjuvant to WBRT and has provided vital data in support of the positive impact of SRS in the treatment of single, small brain metastases.

The minimally invasive nature of SRS has led to the important question of whether SRS should replace surgery as the primary treatment of brain metastases, particularly single metastases. To date there is only one published randomized trial[69] that has attempted to compare SRS with conventional surgery in treatment efficacy. Specifically, Muacevic et al. conducted a multicenter randomized clinical trial in which patients with small (<3 cm maximal diameter) single metastases, good performance status (KPS score ≥ 70), and stable systemic disease were randomized to receive either SRS or conventional surgery plus WBRT. This study was initially designed to recruit 240 patients in order to achieve enough statistical power to detect a 15% difference in 1-year survival. However due to poor patient accrual, the study was aborted, and only 64 patients were randomized in this trial. The results showed that the median survival time was 9.5 months in the surgery plus WBRT group and 10.3 months in the SRS group, the difference between which did not reach statistical significance ($p = 0.8$). Although the investigators concluded that the results supported SRS and surgery as being essentially equivalent treatments, because the study was aborted before the accrual goal was reached, it did not have the power to demonstrate equivalence. Because of this weakness, the validity of the statistical evaluation is questionable, and the claim for equivalence based on the negative comparisons was unsound.[70]

In a separate effort to address the same question, the group at The University of Texas MD Anderson Cancer Center (MD Anderson) has also undertaken a prospective randomized trial comparing SRS with conventional surgery, but preliminary results have only been reported in abstract form.[71] In this clinical trial, patients >16 years old, with newly diagnosed, single brain metastases, and receive a KPS score > 70were randomly assigned to receive conventional surgery or SRS. Similar to the trial of Muacevic et al., this MD Anderson trial also suffered from poor accrual. However, in the MD Anderson trial eligible patients who refused randomization were allowed to choose their treatment and were then followed identically to patients who accepted randomization. Thus this trial included both randomized and nonrandomized arms. Outcome measures were local recurrence, distant recurrence, and overall survival. Fifty-nine patients were entered in the randomized arm (30 received surgery and 29 received SRS), and 155 patients were entered in the nonrandomized arm (89 chose surgery and 66 chose SRS). In the preliminary analysis, treatment with SRS had a statistically significant increased risk of local recurrence compared with surgery in both the randomized and nonrandomized arms of the trial. Based on multivariate analyses which took into account the randomized and nonrandomized populations, and adjusted for confounding covariates (age, gender, WBRT, primary tumor type, extent of disease, tumor volume and location, KPS score, and RPA class) and randomization effects, SRS was associated with a nearly threefold increased risk of local recurrence compared with surgery. For overall survival, the smaller randomized trial showed no difference between surgery and SRS, but there was a significant advantage of surgery over SRS in the larger nonrandomized arm. As a measure of baseline heterogeneity, there was no difference in distant recurrence rates between the groups in both the randomized and nonrandomized arms of the trial, suggesting that the patients in the SRS group and the surgery group were similar in both arms of the trial. Therefore, in this prospective trial characterized by the inclusion of randomized and nonrandomized arms, conventional surgery appeared to provide a significant advantage over SRS in terms of local recurrence and suggests that surgery may also provide an advantage in terms of overall survival. On the basis of these data, the investigators recommended that surgery should be the treatment of choice for brain metastases that are amenable to either treatment. SRS, on the other hand, can be adopted as the primary modality for treatment of small (<1 cm) lesions, especially if they are multiple, surgically inaccessible, and located deep within the brain. Patients with multiple medical comorbidities who cannot tolerate conventional surgery are also candidates for SRS.

Another consideration in deciphering the role of SRS compared with surgery in the management of brain metastases is that local tumor control rates after SRS fall sharply when the maximum diameter of the tumor exceeds 1 to 1.5 cm, as demonstrated in two retrospective series.[72,73] Consequently, it has been argued that the upper size limit of a 3-cm maximal diameter may be too high for adequate

SRS treatment,[74] and it has been suggested that a lower threshold (e.g., 2–2.5 cm maximal diameter) may be more appropriate as the upper limit for applying SRS. More careful studies of the issue of tumor size and the efficacy of radiosurgery are needed.

Role of Whole-Brain Radiation Therapy

Whole-brain radiation therapy has traditionally been considered the standard treatment for patients with cerebral metastases, particularly multiple brain metastases. Based on the results of multiple RTOG trials conducted in the 1970s and 1980s, it is established that patient survival is prolonged from 1 to 2 months with supportive care alone to 3-6 months with a standard regime of 30 Gy delivered in 10 fractions.[62,75,76]

After surgery or SRS, adjuvant WBRT is often recommended on a routine basis in an effort to eradicate residual cancer cells at the resection site and to eliminate microscopic foci at distant sites within the brain.[22] However, the benefit of this practice has been questioned in recent years as improvement in systemic cancer treatment has resulted in more patients surviving long enough to be exposed to the debilitating neurocognitive side effects of WBRT. This has particularly become an issue for patients with good KPS scores as these patients are most affected by radiation-induced neurocognitive sequelae emerging 6 to 12 months post treatment, which may critically outweigh the intended therapeutic benefits of WBRT.[77] Several authors have, therefore, suggested that WBRT should be withheld, especially for radioresistant tumors such as melanoma and renal cell carcinoma, and only be considered when local treatment fails.[78,79]

In order to clarify whether routine adjuvant WBRT is of benefit after surgical resection of single brain metastases, Patchell and colleagues randomized 95 patients with single metastasis to WBRT or observation after conventional surgery.[65] The patients who received WBRT showed a significant reduction in tumor recurrence, both at the site of the surgery and at distant sites in the brain, compared with the observation group. Specifically, whereas the overall recurrence rate was 70% in the observation group, it was only 18% in the adjuvant WBRT group ($p < 0.001$). However, this decrease in recurrence in the WBRT group did not translate into a statistically significant improvement in survival, as the median survival time of the adjuvant WBRT group was 12 months and that of the observation group was 10.8 months ($p = 0.39$). However, it must be noted that the trial was not sufficiently powered to detect a difference in survival between the groups. In addition, 61% of the patients in the observation group eventually crossed over to the WBRT group and received salvage WBRT for recurrence. Therefore, the lack of a significant difference in overall survival between the groups must be interpreted with caution. Also, because neurocognitive function was not assessed, the functional effects of routine adjuvant WBRT were not addressed in this study.

In a related study, Aoyama and coworkers from the Japanese Radiation Oncology Study Group investigated the impact of withholding adjuvant WBRT following SRS.[80] In this randomized trial, patients with one to four cerebral metastases were randomized to either WBRT or observation after SRS. Similar to the study by Patchell et al.,[65] in this study of 132 patients, the rate of local tumor control at 1 year was superior in the WBRT group (88.7%) compared with the observation group (72.5%). However, the median survival times were similar in both groups (7.5 months in the WBRT group vs. 8 months in the observation group, p = 0.42), with only 16% of patients in the observation group crossing over to receive salvage WBRT. Of patients who survived for more than 12 months, functional assessment was performed using KPS scores. The rate of functional status preservation (KPS score $\geq$ 70) was not significantly different at 1 year between the two groups (33.9% in the adjuvant WBRT group vs. 26.9% in the observation group). Nevertheless, it should be noted that the KPS score is a measure primarily of physical functions, not of cognitive functions and the preservation in KPS score cannot be interpreted as preservation of neurocognitive abilities, such as learning and verbal skills.

In a recently reported prospective randomized trial, Chang et al. investigated the neurocognitive effects of WBRT based on serial examinations of cognitive functions across several domains using validated assessment tools.[81] In this trial, patients with one to three newly diagnosed brain metastases were randomized to receive either SRS plus WBRT (n = 28) or SRS alone (n = 30). Patients were evaluated before treatment and then monthly afterwards. By 4 months, patients receiving WBRT suffered a significantly greater decline in memory and learning ability compared with patients receiving SRS alone. These results, obtained from an interim analysis, were so significant that the study was terminated before the targeted enrollment of 90 patients was reached. Interestingly, although the 1-year local tumor control rate was lower in patients in the observation group (67%) when compared with the WBRT group (100%, p = 0.012), the overall median survival time in the observation group (15.2 months) was superior to that of the WBRT group (5.7 months, p = 0.003). As a secondary finding, such a marked difference in survival between the two groups is difficult to account for post hoc, but as suggested by the authors, significant differences in the use of salvage and systemic therapies between the two groups, which were not stratified and controlled a priori, may play a role.

Taken together, these randomized trials have provided corroborative evidence that although adjuvant WBRT reduces the risk of tumor recurrence, this benefit may not translate into improvements in survival or functional status. Conversely, the strategy of omitting adjuvant WBRT and applying salvage therapy when recurrence occurs appears not only effective in maintaining overall survival but also significantly avoids the deleterious neurocognitive side effects of WBRT.

Given that adjuvant WBRT reduces recurrence but is not innocuous, it has become increasingly desirable to define subsets of patients who are at higher risk of experiencing early local or distant recurrence after surgical resection or SRS and who would, therefore, potentially benefit from adjuvant WBRT, despite the potential risk for developing neurocognitive dysfunction in the long term. To this end, McPherson et al.[82] analyzed the outcomes of 358 patients with single brain metastases originating from a wide range of primary sites, all of whom were treated with microsurgical resection without or with the standard dose adjuvant WBRT. In a multivariate analysis, it was found that tumors >3 cm in maximal diameter that did not receive adjuvant WBRT had a significantly increased risk of recurring locally (HR = 3.14, CI 1.02–9.69, p = 0.05). Additionally, patients whose primary disease was progressing and who did not receive WBRT had a significantly increased risk of distant recurrence (HR = 2.16, CI 1.01–4.66, p = 0.05). There was no effect of WBRT based on tumor type. Based on this retrospective report, it has been suggested that after surgical resection of a single metastasis, adjuvant WBRT may be most beneficial in patients in whom the resected metastasis was large (>3 cm) or in whom the systemic disease is active. Conversely, adjuvant WBRT may be withheld in patients whose resected metastasis was small and in whom the systemic disease is controlled.

As a substitute for adjuvant WBRT after resection of a single metastasis, it has been suggested that SRS can be applied to the tumor resection cavity in order to decrease the chance for local tumor recurrence following surgery, while avoiding the adverse effects of WBRT.[83,84] Supported by the observation in melanoma brain metastases that the presence of intratumoral hemorrhage was associated with increased recurrence,[85] the role of treating the resection cavity with SRS has been particularly advocated in tumors that have hemorrhaged, as it is hypothesized that during hemorrhage the normally defined tumor–brain interface characteristic of cerebral metastases are inevitably violated, resulting in widely dispersed micrometastases that are not amenable to surgical resection alone. Despite the theoretical appeal of this approach, the current data supporting postresection SRS are limited to few small retrospective series.[83,84] Although favorable local disease control rates (>94%) have been reported, further validation from clinical trials is required. In light of this, a randomized controlled trial was opened at MD Anderson in August 2009 to evaluate the efficacy of postoperative SRS treatment the resection bed in reducing the risk of local tumor recurrence. This trial, expected to be completed in 2014, will provide important data to clarify the proper use of this adjunctive treatment.

KEY REFERENCES

Andrews DW, Scott CB, Sperduto PW, et al. Whole brain radiation therapy with or without stereotactic radiosurgery boost for patients with one to three brain metastases: phase III results of the RTOG 9508 randomised trial. *Lancet.* 2004;363:1665-1672.

Aoyama H, Shirato H, Tago M, et al. Stereotactic radiosurgery plus whole-brain radiation therapy vs. stereotactic radiosurgery alone for treatment of brain metastases: a randomized controlled trial. *JAMA.* 2006;295:2483-2491.

Chang EL, Hassenbusch 3rd SJ, Shiu AS, et al. The role of tumor size in the radiosurgical management of patients with ambiguous brain metastases. *Neurosurgery.* 2003;53:272-280:discussion 280-281.

Chang EL, Wefel JS, Hess KR, et al. Neurocognition in patients with brain metastases treated with radiosurgery or radiosurgery plus whole-brain irradiation: a randomised controlled trial. *Lancet Oncol.* 2009;10:1037-1044.

DeAngelis LM, Delattre JY, Posner JB. Radiation-induced dementia in patients cured of brain metastases. *Neurology.* 1989;39:789-796.

Gaspar L, Scott C, Rotman M, et al. Recursive partitioning analysis (RPA) of prognostic factors in three Radiation Therapy Oncology Group (RTOG) brain metastases trials. *Int J Radiat Oncol Biol Phys.* 1997;37:745-751.

Hart MG, Grant R, Walker M, et al. Surgical resection and whole brain radiation therapy versus whole brain radiation therapy alone for single brain metastases. *Cochrane Database Syst Rev.* 2005:CD003292.

Kondziolka D, Patel A, Lunsford LD, et al. Stereotactic radiosurgery plus whole brain radiotherapy versus radiotherapy alone for patients with multiple brain metastases. *Int J Radiat Oncol Biol Phys.* 1999;45: 427-434.

Lang FF: Conventional surgery versus stereotactic radiosurgery in the treatment of single brain metastases: a prospective study with both randomized and nonrandomized arms. (clinicaltrails.gov: NCT00460395), Seventy-sixth Annual Meeting of the American Association of Neurological Surgeons (AANS), 2008.

Lang FF, Sawaya R. Surgical management of cerebral metastases. *Neurosurg Clin N Am.* 1996;7:459-484.

Lang EF, Slater J. Metastatic brain tumors. Results of surgical and nonsurgical treatment. *Surg Clin N Am.* 1964;44:865-872.

McPherson C, Suki D, Feiz-Erfan I, et al. Adjuvant whole brain radiation therapy after surgical resection of single brain metastases. *Neuro-oncology E-pub ahead of print.* 2010.

Mintz AH, Kestle J, Rathbone MP, et al. A randomized trial to assess the efficacy of surgery in addition to radiotherapy in patients with a single cerebral metastasis. *Cancer.* 1996;78:1470-1476.

Muacevic A, Wowra B, Siefert A, et al. Microsurgery plus whole brain irradiation versus gamma knife surgery alone for treatment of single metastases to the brain: a randomized controlled multicentre phase III trial. *J Neurooncol.* 2008;87:299-307.

Paek SH, Audu PB, Sperling MR, et al. Reevaluation of surgery for the treatment of brain metastases: review of 208 patients with single or multiple brain metastases treated at one institution with modern neurosurgical techniques. *Neurosurgery.* 2005;56:1021-1034:discussion 1021-1034.

Patchell RA, Tibbs PA, Walsh JW, et al. A randomized trial of surgery in the treatment of single metastases to the brain. *N Engl J Med.* 1990;322:494-500.

Patchell RA, Tibbs PA, Regine WF, et al. Postoperative radiotherapy in the treatment of single metastases to the brain: a randomized trial. *JAMA.* 1998;280:1485-1489.

Sawaya R. Surgical treatment of brain metastases. *Clin Neurosurg.* 1999;45:41-47.

Sawaya R, Bindal R, Lang F. Metastatic brain tumors. In: Kaye AH, Laws ER, eds. *Brain tumors: an encyclopedic approach.* ed 2nd. New York: Churchill Livingstone; 2001:999-1026.

Sawaya R, Hammoud M, Schoppa D, et al. Neurosurgical outcomes in a modern series of 400 craniotomies for treatment of parenchymal tumors. *Neurosurgery.* 1998;42:1044-1055:discussion 1055-1056.

Sawaya R, Wildrick DM. Metastatic brain tumors: surgery perspective. In: Chin LS, Regine WF, eds. *Principles and practice of stereotactic radiosurgery.* New York: Springer; 2008:193-199.

Selek U, Chang EL, Hassenbusch 3rd SJ, et al. Stereotactic radiosurgical treatment in 103 patients for 153 cerebral melanoma metastases. *Int J Radiat Oncol Biol Phys.* 2004;59:1097-1106.

Suki D, Abouassi H, Patel AJ, et al. Comparative risk of leptomeningeal disease after resection or stereotactic radiosurgery for solid tumor metastasis to the posterior fossa. *J Neurosurg.* 2008;108:248-257.

Suki D, Hatiboglu MA, Patel AJ, et al. Comparative risk of leptomeningeal dissemination of cancer after surgery or stereotactic radiosurgery for a single supratentorial solid tumor metastasis. *Neurosurgery.* 2009;64:664-674:discussion 674-676.

Vecht CJ, Haaxma-Reiche H, Noordijk EM, et al. Treatment of single brain metastasis: radiotherapy alone or combined with neurosurgery? *Ann Neurol.* 1993;33:583-590.

Numbered references appear on Expert Consult.

CHAPTER 16

Multimodal Assessment of Pituitary and Parasellar Lesions

T. BROOKS VAUGHAN • LEWIS S. BLEVINS • MICHAEL S. VAPHIADES • GARY S. WAND

Pituitary and parasellar lesions represent a unique variety of neoplasms and other disease processes that are best addressed employing a multidisciplinary approach to assessment and treatment. Their close proximity to critical structures, potential association with endocrine dysfunction, and their propensity for recurrence or persistence after initial therapy often demands the skills of an experienced neurosurgeon, endocrinologist, radiologist, ophthalmologist, and radiation oncologist. Further, multiple tools, including laboratory tests, radiologic studies, and other specialized investigations are indispensable aids to patient care. This chapter will emphasize the need for a multimodal initial evaluation and a team approach to assessment.

Background and Epidemiology

The most common lesion encountered in the sella will be a pituitary adenoma. Estimates of the prevalence of pituitary adenomas vary widely between studies, which are performed using either MRI or autopsy findings. A recent meta-analysis found a prevalence of 22.5% in imaging studies (range 1%–40%) and 14.4% in postmortem studies (range 1%–35%), for an overall prevalence of 16.7%.[1] The vast majority of pituitary adenomas are microadenomas (diameter <1 cm). Macroadenomas are far less common, and their prevalence in the population is estimated to be approximately 0.2%.[1] Macroadenomas make up a much larger proportion of adenomas that come to clinical attention, however. A cross-sectional study of 81,149 patients in Banbury, UK found the overall prevalence of known pituitary tumors to be 77.6 cases per 100,000 inhabitants (or 63 total cases). Of these, only 7 were found incidentally. The others presented with some sort of clinical symptomatology, and of those, 41% were macroadenomas.[2]

The prevalence of "functional tumors"—adenomas that hypersecrete hormones resulting in a clinical syndrome—is in the range of 50% to 60% of all clinically apparent pituitary tumors. The most common functional or secretory tumors are prolactinomas (approximately 40%), followed by ACTH-secreting tumors (14%), growth hormone (GH)–secreting tumors (5%), and TSH-secreting tumors and mixed tumors (both under 1%).[3] Many "nonfunctional" tumors are clinically silent gonadotroph adenomas, while a small proportion of these produce but do not secrete ACTH, GH, or TSH.

The majority of pituitary tumors remain stable after their initial detection. In one meta-analysis of eight studies including 144 patients who were followed from 2 to 8 years, 84% of microadenomas of the pituitary gland remained stable in size. A few (6%) regressed and approximately 10% increased in size. In contrast, 20% of macroadenomas grew (11% of those were due to apoplexy), 11% diminished in size, and 69% remained stable.[4]

Pathogenesis

A great deal has been learned about the pathogenesis of some pituitary lesions but the pathogenesis of the majority of pituitary and parasellar lesions is still unknown. It is clear there are a variety of molecular mechanisms responsible for neoplastic transformation. Pituitary adenomas arise from adenohypophysial cells of the anterior pituitary. The vast majority of pituitary tumors are thought to be benign. Adenomas can, however invade local structures including the dura of the sella, local bony structures, and the sphenoid sinus cavity. Pituitary carcinoma, defined by the presence of local discontinuous or systemic spread, is extremely rare and probably represents approximately 0.2% to 0.5% of all pituitary lesions.[5] Pituitary neoplasms are monoclonal, and outside of defined genetic syndromes, their cause is not well understood.

At least five genes have been identified as causes of pituitary adenomas with four of them comprising familial pituitary tumor syndromes: MEN1, PRKAR1A, CDKN1B, and AIP. Genetic disorders such as MEN1 (a mutation in the MENIN protein that reverses function of tumor suppressor gene), and Carney's complex (PRKAR1A, insufficient activity of protein kinase-A regulatory subunit 1) are examples of models for pituitary tumor development. The CDKN1B gene causes a MEN-like syndrome (MEN4) associated with hyperparathyroidism and other rare tumors.[6] Another recently discovered mutation is located in the AIP (aryl hydrocarbon receptor–interacting protein) gene (11q13).[7,8] This appears to act as a tumor suppressor gene and mutations predispose to GH-secreting pituitary tumors.[7,9,10] Approximately 40% of sporadic GH-secreting adenomas are associated with a somatic mutation in the Gs alpha gene.[11,12] The mutation results in constitutive activation of the cAMP/PKA signal transduction pathway and leads to neoplastic transformation of somatotroph cells of the pituitary.[13,14]

Clinical Presentation

Pituitary and parasellar lesions may come to attention in a variety of ways. They may be detected incidentally on radiographic scans obtained for unrelated reasons, or as a result of clinical symptoms and signs attributable to either endocrine dysfunction or to mass effect. Clinical syndromes of hormone excess result from hypersecretion of prolactin, growth hormone, ACTH or TSH causing the amenorrhea/galactorrhea syndrome, acromegaly, Cushing's disease, or secondary hyperthyroidism, respectively. Rarely, patients have clinical features of gonadotropin excess. Mass effect symptoms and signs may include headache, visual field loss, diplopia, facial pain, and epistaxis, as well as CSF leaks. Further, varying degrees of hypopituitarism due to compressive injury may result in partial or complete loss of pituitary function. Thus, careful hormonal, neuroradiologic, and ophthalmologic assessments are essential in the evaluation of patients affected by these tumors.

The Initial Evaluation

The initial evaluation of patients with pituitary tumors begins with a general history and physical examination in order to determine if there are co-morbidities or other medical issues that will affect the evaluation and management of the pituitary patient. Surgical risk is determined and appropriate consultations are obtained when necessary. For example, patients with acromegaly and sleep apnea may require evaluation by a pulmonologist prior to surgery. Diabetes and hypertension in acromegalic and Cushingoid patients may require treatment to decrease surgical morbidity. A thorough assessment of the clinical manifestations of the disease process may guide the selection of subsequent laboratory and radiological studies. Laboratory assessment of the hormonal status of affected patients allows for determination of a specific diagnosis, subsequent treatment planning, and permits decisions as to whether or not hormone replacements are necessary.

Laboratory Investigations

The most appropriate screening tests for an incidentally discovered pituitary lesion are the topic of much debate.[15,16] A survey of endocrinologists in the United States and United Kingdom suggested that, when confronted with a microadenoma, a range of 0 to 16 tests would be ordered (median 7).[16,17] Most experts would advocate screening for both pituitary insufficiency and hormone excess as both states are relevant in the initial decision-making and also the long term follow-up of patients. This information is particularly important in the context of a preoperative evaluation. Clinical findings should guide medical decision-making. For example, patients who are obviously Cushingoid will require specific testing of adrenal function that may not be conducted in those who appear to have acromegaly.

HYPOPITUITARISM

One or more pituitary deficiencies will be present in 70% to 90% of patients with macroadenomas.[18] Microadenomas rarely cause pituitary insufficiency. Other tumors in the area of the sella, including tuberculum sellae and cavernous sinus meningiomas, craniopharyngiomas, and Rathke's cleft cysts may also cause pituitary insufficiency. A uniform approach to screening for pituitary dysfunction is useful since symptoms and signs can be vague as many patients have adapted over time to a state of chronic pituitary dysfunction and may not perceive their symptoms as abnormal. Pituitary deficiency tends to manifest in the following order of frequency: loss of GH, followed by gonadotrophins, followed by loss of adrenal and then thyroid function.[4] Diabetes insipidus is the least common deficiency in a typical pituitary adenoma. A typical screening panel therefore will include the following, with interpretation discussed below: serum IGF-1, estradiol, or testosterone levels (depending on sex) in conjunction with an FSH and LH level, TSH and free T4, and a cortisol stimulation test. A prolactin level should always be drawn as well and is discussed in the section on pituitary hypersecretion. Table 16-1 summarizes typical signs and symptoms of pituitary insufficiency.

Growth Hormone Deficiency

A serum IGF-1 is the best initial screening test for GH deficiency. We suggest this test in the preoperative setting so that the adequacy of pituitary function can be documented. An IGF-1 below the age-adjusted normal range indicates GH deficiency. Otherwise, if the IGF-1 is low or even in the lower quartile of the normal range, current guidelines suggest the use of a diagnostic stimulation test to determine if GH deficiency is present. While the insulin tolerance test is the gold standard test, the arginine and glucagon stimulation tests are acceptable surrogate tests provided they are interpreted in the proper clinical context. Growth hormone replacement is usually only addressed in the postsurgical patient.

Central Hypogonadism

Hypogonadism is the second most common hormone-deficient state in patients with partial hypopituitarism. In most cases, this disorder does not need to be addressed preoperatively. In fact, the addition of estrogen replacement therapy in women may raise the risk of venous thrombosis. To assess gonadal function in men, a serum leuteinizing hormone (LH) and testosterone level are usually indicated. In women, the presence of normal menses usually obviates the need for laboratory testing of the gonadal axis. In amenorrheic women of reproductive age, a follicle stimulating hormone (FSH) level and a serum estradiol may be useful. In postmenopausal women, FSH levels are usually elevated so a low or normal level may be taken to indicate significant pituitary dysfunction.

Central Hypothyroidism

Central hypothyroidism is common in patients with pituitary lesions. Mistakes can be made if TSH values are incorrectly interpreted, as they may be low, normal, or even slightly elevated. The defining characteristic of central hypothyroidism in patients with pituitary disease is a low free T4. Clearly, levels below the normal range are abnormal, but some experts will consider thyroid hormone replacement if levels are in the lower quartile of the normal range.

It is critical to ensure adequate adrenal function (see below) prior to the initiation of thyroid hormone replacement. Thyroid hormone administration will increase

Table 16-1   Signs and Symptoms of Pituitary Deficiency

Hormonal Deficiency	Signs and Symptoms	Diagnosis	Treatment
Growth hormone (GH)	Fatigue, weight gain, diminished exercise tolerance, osteoporosis, hyperlipidemia	Screen with IGF-1, consider confirmatory tests if IGF-1 subnormal or in lowest quartile for age Confirmatory tests include arginine-GHRH stimulation tests, insulin tolerance tests, glucagon stimulation test Reassess after any pituitary surgery	Daily SC injections of growth hormone Treatment not required in preoperative phase
Gonadotrophins (LH/FSH)	Impotence, diminished libido, osteoporosis, hot flashes, mood lability, vaginal dryness, testicular atrophy, loss of axillary/pubic hair in men, change in shaving habits	LH/FSH levels in conjunction with testosterone levels in men, estradiol levels in women	Testosterone via patch, gel, injection in men (can be addressed postoperatively) Cyclic estrogen and progesterone in women (may raise risk for thrombosis in perioperative phase)
Adrenal insufficiency (ACTH) *Should be addressed and treated prior to surgery	Weight loss, nausea, anorexia, hyponatremia, hypoglycemia, hypotension (which, if critically ill, may not respond to fluid or pressors)	Morning cortisol less than 5 µg/dl Low dose ACTH stimulated cortisol <18 µg/dl at 30 minutes (standard-dose test may be an acceptable alternative)	Hydrocortisone 15–30 mg per day divided into two doses, two thirds given in morning, one third given at approximately 4 p.m. (nonstressed) Prednisone approximately 5 mg daily (nonstressed) Dexamethasone 0.125–0.375 mg nightly (nonstressed)
Hypothyroidism (TSH) *Should be addressed and treated (after adrenal replacement) prior to surgery	Weight gain, constipation, fatigue, cold intolerance, bradycardia, dry skin, delayed relaxation of deep tendon reflexes	Free T4 subnormal, or consider if in the lowest quartile. TSH most often normal, but can be low or even slightly elevated	Levothyroxine orally, 1.6 µ/kg is typically full-replacement dose Start more slowly in elderly or in presence of cardiovascular disease (25–50 µg/day) Ensure that the adrenal axis is assessed and insufficiency treated prior to initiating treatment
Diabetes insipidus *Should prompt close attention to fluid in electrolyte status if known prior to surgery	Polyuria, polydipsia, hypernatremia Questioning regarding noctural symptoms useful Not often seen in typical pituitary adenoma	Water deprivation test if necessary 24-hr urine collection to document volume	DDAVP in nasal, oral, or subcutaneous forms Starting dose 1–2 µg subcutaneous, 10 µg nasal, or 0.1 mg oral In ambulatory outpatient, typically dose first at night to address nocturia, then reassess daytime symptoms

metabolic demand for cortisol while at the same time increasing its clearance, and might precipitate overt adrenal insufficiency in a patient deficient in cortisol. Chronic replacement can be accomplished in most adults with approximately 1.6 µg of levothyroxine per kilogram lean body weight per day. In the elderly, or those with significant cardiac morbidities, most experts recommend initiating levothyroxine replacement with 25 to 50 µg daily. To address severe hypothyroidism in the preoperative setting, in the absence of contraindications, 200 to 400 µg of levothyroxine may be administered IV, followed by oral administration of a usual replacement dose. When patients are unable to take their medication orally the intravenous administration of 85% of a typical oral dose daily until the patient can take oral medications will meet their needs. There is no clear evidence that T3 replacement is beneficial.

Central Adrenal Insufficiency

Undiagnosed central adrenal insufficiency represents the most significant danger to the patient with hypopituitarism. The best test to assess the integrity of pituitary-adrenal function has been the subject of significant controversy. While insulin-induced hypoglycemia is the gold standard, the procedure is time consuming and sometimes risky. However, stimulation with ACTH 1-24 best combines high accuracy with practicality and is felt to best correlate with the results

of an insulin tolerance test.[19,20] There is debate on whether one should conduct this test with 1 or 250 µg of ACTH 1-24. One caveat of the ACTH 1-24 stimulation test is its accuracy is limited until about 6 weeks following a pituitary insult; despite the limitations of the cosyntropin-stimulation tests, there is little evidence that clinically significant adrenal insufficiency will be missed by either test.[21]

Oral regimens for adrenal hormone replacement in a non-stressed patient include hydrocortisone 15 to 30 mg daily, usually in divided doses, dexamethasone 0.25 mg at bedtime, or prednisone 5 mg daily.[22] Adjustments in dosing are based on clinical symptoms and signs of either glucocorticoid excess or deficiency, as there is, at this point, no reliable, reproducible laboratory test to assess the adequacy of treatment. The HPA axis is usually reassessed 6 to 8 weeks after surgery to determine if ongoing chronic treatment is necessary. Many patients will experience improvement in pituitary function after surgery and their glucocorticoid replacement may be abruptly discontinued. Patients with Cushing's disease may experience a period of temporary adrenal insufficiency of 6 to 18 months due to suppression of normal corticotroph cells by pre-existing hypercortisolism. They must be reassessed at regular intervals to determine the need for ongoing steroid replacement.

Treatment with replacement doses of glucocorticoids is indicated in all patients with documented central adrenal

Table 16-2 Signs and Symptoms of Pituitary Excess

Hormonal Excess	Signs and Symptoms	Diagnosis	Treatment Options
ACTH (Cushing's disease)	Moon facies, buffalo hump, supraclavicular fullness, purple striae, central obesity, proximal muscle weakness, ecchymosis, osteopenia, hyertension, insulin resistance, mood disorders	Screening tests include 24-hr urine cortisol above upper limit of normal, 1 mg dexamethasone suppression test (1.8 µg/dl most sensitive and 5 µg/dl most specific), and salivary cortisol (over 4 nmol/l) tests Confirmatory tests include CRH/dex test (see text)	Surgical cure if achievable Medical therapy with ketoconazole, mitotane, mifepristone Radiotherapy *See dedicated chapter on Cushing's disease
GH (acromegaly)	Skeletal and soft tissue overgrowth, carpal tunnel syndrome, hyperhidrosis, hypertension, congestive heart failure, obstructive sleep apnea, insulin resistance, colon polyps	IGF-1 above age-adjusted normal range Failure to suppress below 1 µg/l on a growth hormone suppression test	Surgical cure if achievable Somatostatin analogues and GH receptor antagonists Radiotherapy *See dedicated chapter on acromegaly
Prolactinoma	Menstrual irregularities in women, infertility, decreased libido, impotence, galactorrhea, weight gain	Elevated prolactin levels, typically above 200 in prolactin-secreting macroadenomas	Dopamine agonists bromocriptine and cabergoline *See dedicated chapter on prolactinomas
Thyrotropin (TSH-secreting adenoma)	Goiter, moist skin, palmar erythema, weight loss, tachycardia, palpitations, irregular menses, insomnia, fine tremor, brisk deep tendon reflexes	Inappropriately normal or elevated TSH in setting of elevated FT_4	Surgical cure if achievable Somatostatin analogues Radiotherapy Acute control of hyperthyroidism with thionamides and use of beta blockers may be required before surgery

insufficiency. Empiric treatment prior to surgery is acceptable in the setting of pituitary apoplexy, especially in the setting of large space occupying lesions, and when an urgent or emergent procedure is indicated even in the absence of documented adrenal dysfunction. A reasonable therapeutic regimen when the patient is under significant physiological stress is 25 mg of intravenous hydrocortisone every 8 hours. In a crisis, one may want to initiate intravenous glucocorticoid replacement with 100 mg initially and 50 mg every 8 hours thereafter. Mineralocorticoid replacement is not necessary in secondary adrenal insufficiency.[23]

Diabetes Insipidus

Diabetes insipidus (DI), due to arginine-vasopressin (AVP) deficiency, is uncommon in pituitary adenomas. If present on the initial evaluation, consideration should be given to alternative diagnoses such as infiltrative lesions (hypophysitis, sacrcoidosis), metastatic lesions, craniopharyngiomas and other tumors. Cardinal features of DI include polyuria (more than 30 ml of urine per kilogram of body weight in 24 hr) in the presence of hyperosmolality, inappropriately dilute urine, dehydration, and subsequent thirst. When obtaining a history, it is helpful to inquire specifically about nocturnal symptoms, since many normal patients may perceive what they feel is excessive thirst or urination during the day. If their symptoms resolve overnight DI is unlikely. If DI is noted preoperatively, patients will require very close monitoring of fluid intake and urine output along with serum sodium levels.

PITUITARY HYPERSECRETION

Pituitary adenomas can secrete hormones in excess resulting in particular clinical syndromes. Other sellar and parasellar tumors will not present in this fashion, although mild prolactin elevations can be seen with many large tumors due to compression of the infundibulum. The major hypersecretory states are discussed individually in other

chapters, but all should be considered in the initial evaluation of a pituitary mass. Table 16-2 summarizes some of the possible signs and symptoms associated with various hypersecretory states.

Prolactinoma

Prolactinomas represent approximately 40% of pituitary tumors.[1] They are more common in women with a gender ratio of 10:1.[24] Women usually present when their tumors are microadenomas. Men are more likely to present with macroadenomas. Whether this is function of delayed presentation (women may present quickly with menstrual irregularities) or of unique biological properties of tumors in men is unclear.[25]

A serum prolactin should be obtained in all patients with pituitary tumors, as this information will affect treatment decisions. Prolactin levels of greater than 200 µg/l are almost always associated with a prolactin-secreting macroadenoma. Prolactin levels less than 200 µg/l can be caused by microprolactinomas and also a variety of parasellar lesions (pseudoprolactinoma), infiltrative processes, as well as physiologic and pharmacologic causes.[24] Any tumor or infiltrative process that interferes with the delivery of dopamine, which inhibits prolactin production, to the normal lactotrophs can cause hyperprolactinemia that is often referred to as "stalk-effect hyperprolactinemia." Pregnancy should be excluded in any woman with hyperprolactinemia and amenorrhea. A variety of drugs can cause hyperprolactinemia. If medications are suspected as a cause of hyperprolactinemia, they should be discontinued if possible, and the prolactin level reevaluated 1 month thereafter. Severe primary hypothyroidism can cause hyperprolactinemia. Thus, a serum TSH level is valuable during an initial evaluation of hyperprolactinemic patients.

The clinician must be aware that the differential diagnosis for hyperprolactinemia is large encompassing pathological and physiological causes. Defining the cause of

Table 16-3   Differential Diagnosis of Hyperprolactinemia

Physiologic

Stress
Pregnancy
Coitus
Nursing
Exercise
Sleep

Pathologic

Prolactinomas: micro- and macro-adenomas
Subset of growth hormone–secreting adenomas
Miscellaneous causes
Hypothyroidism
Idiopathic
Chronic renal failure
Chronic liver failure
Polycystic ovarian syndrome

Elevation without Clinical Symptomatology

Macroprolactinemia

Medications

Antihypertensives (methyldopa, reserpine, verapamil)
Antipsychotics (phenothiazines, butyrophenonones)
Antidepressants (tricyclics, occasional reports with SSRIs)
GI medications (metoclopramide, domperidone)
Narcotics
Estrogens
Protease inhibitors

Effects on the Pituitary Stalk

Mass effect from any sellar mass
Infiltrative disease (Histiocytosis, sacrcoidosis, metatasis, tuberculosis)
Sectioning of stalk from basal skull fracture, iatrogenenic surgical injury, facial trauma

Neurogenic

Chest wall injury
Chest wall lesion

Source: Adapted from Mancini T, Casanueva FF, Giustina A. Hyperprolactinemia and prolactinomas. Endocrinol Metab Clin North Am. 2008;37:67-99, viii.

hyperprolactinemia is crucial since true prolactinomas are treated medically with dopamine agonists, pseudo-prolactinomas are surgically removed and other causes have their own unique treatments. Table 16-3 presents a summary of the differential diagnosis of hyperprolactinemia.

A small subset of extremely large prolactinomas can produce enormous amounts of prolactin that overwhelm antibodies used in the assay resulting in a false lowering of prolactin levels.[26] This is known as the "hook effect." In the setting of a macroadenoma, when a prolactinoma is suspected, prolactin levels should be performed on diluted serum samples to avoid this error in laboratory diagnosis. Most modern radioimmunoassays are able to detect prolactin levels as great as 4000 µg/l without being subject to the "hook effect." We recommend that treating physicians being aware of the prolactin test performance in the laboratories they employ to evaluate their patients.[27]

On occasion a patient will be found to have an elevated prolactin but without symptoms of hyperprolactinemia. This is often due to a condition known as macroprolactinemia. In this disorder, prolactin aggregates with circulating IgG antibodies resulting in decreased clearance of the complex and thus elevated prolactin levels.[28-30] However, the prolactin-IgG complex is devoid of biological activity and thus the absence of symptoms. This condition does not require treatment and needs to be distinguished from true hyperprolactinemia. Incubating the serum with polyethylene glycol, which removes the prolactin-IgG complex prior to performing the assay, can identify the phenomenon.

Cushing's Disease

Cushing's disease is a term applied to a specific form of Cushing's syndrome (pathological hypercortisolism) caused by an ACTH-secreting pituitary tumor. Cushing's syndrome may be due to a variety of other disorders including the syndrome of ectopic ACTH secretion, adrenal tumors, and exogenous glucocorticoid therapy for non-endocrine disease processes. Due to the risks that hypercortisolism can pose in the perioperative period, including deep venous thrombosis, pneumocystis pneumonia and other infections, poor wound healing as well as steroid hormone withdrawal in the postoperative period, most would have a low threshold to screen for Cushing's prior to pituitary surgery.

Recent guidelines review proposed diagnostic approaches to the evaluation of patients with suspected Cushing's syndrome.[31] The inclusion of an endocrinologist experienced with this disorder to establish and confirm the diagnosis is strongly advised. Generally speaking, and depending on the clinical situation, one should start with screening tests, then proceed to diagnostic or confirmatory tests, and finally, to differential diagnostic tests.

There are at least three reliable screening tests to evaluate patients with suspected hypercortisolism. Keep in mind that screening tests are designed to be sensitive but not specific. Thus, there will be false positive tests and not everyone with a positive screening test will be ultimately diagnosed with pathologic hypercortisolism. Appropriate screening tests include the overnight 1 mg dexamethasone suppression test, the 24-hour urine collection for free cortisol and creatinine, and the midnight salivary cortisol collection.[32-36] For most patients who require screening only, performance of one of these tests is indicated. The salivary cortisol and 24-hour urine free cortisol collection should be done at least twice to confirm abnormal initial findings. A positive dexamethasone suppression test is identified when an 8 a.m. cortisol is greater than 1.8 µg/dl following administration of 1 mg of dexamethasone at 11 p.m. the prior night. Using this cutoff gives the test a sensitivity of approximately 95% with specificity of 80%. To enhance specificity to over 95%, a cutoff of 5 µg/dl may be used, which will sacrifice sensitivity (falling to 85%).[31] A 24-hour urine cortisol above the upper limits of normal may be considered a positive screening test, along with a late-night salivary cortisol level of 4 nmol/l or greater.[31]

Diagnostic tests are designed to balance sensitivity and specificity. They are used to confirm the diagnosis of pathologic hypercortisolism. Diagnostic tests for hypercortisolism include the 24-hour urine cortisol, the dexamethasone suppressed CRH stimulation test, (CRH/Dex test) and the formal low-dose dexamethasone suppression test.[37,38] A 24-hour urine cortisol excretion rates greater than two to three times the upper limit of normal is generally considered to be a positive test. The CRH/Dex test is performed by administering dexamethasone, 0.5 mg every 6 hours for 2 days followed by CRH stimulation on the morning of the third day. A cortisol value greater than 1.4 µg/dl 15 minutes after CRH administration indicates an abnormal result.[39] Treating physicians are encouraged to review the performance of tests employed by their laboratory and draw upon their own experiences to determine what constitutes an abnormal response to a formal dexamethasone suppression test.

Once Cushing's syndrome is established, the cause must be identified: ACTH-secreting pituitary adenoma (Cushing's disease), ectopic ACTH production or an adrenal tumor. Differential diagnostic tests for hypercortisolism include the plasma ACTH level, the overnight high-dose dexamethasone suppression test, and inferior petrosal sinus sampling. The first step in identifying the cause of Cushing's syndrome is to obtain a random ACTH level and perform a high-dose dexamethasone test. If the plasma ACTH levels are low (levels depend upon the assay employed), then an ACTH-secreting tumor is ruled out. If ACTH levels are normal or elevated the result indicates that Cushing's syndrome could be secondary to a pituitary tumor or ectopic production of ACTH by tumors located below the neck.

The high-dose dexamethasone suppression test is often, but not always useful in distinguishing these two entities. Generally cortisol levels do not suppress substantially when the cause of the Cushing's is an ectopic tumor; however there are many exceptions. On the other hand, cortisol levels in the setting of an ACTH-secreting adenoma generally suppress by greater than 50% from baseline values. When the suppression does not approach or exceed 90%, or when the results are difficult to interpret, inferior petrosal sinus sampling is indicated. Patients thought to have Cushing's disease should undergo an MRI scan of the pituitary gland.

Inferior Petrosal Sinus Sampling

Inferior petrosal sinus sampling is a procedure that may be required to confirm the source of ACTH-dependent Cushing's syndrome. Lab studies can often differentiate ectopic from pituitary ACTH-driven Cushing's syndrome, but it is clear that the levels, even on dynamic testing, may have some overlap. IPSS may be particularly useful when the lab evaluation suggests a pituitary source for ACTH but none can be identified by MRI scanning. Studies have varied in their estimation of the sensitivity and specificity of the test. Earlier studies have shown it to be very sensitive (96%) and specific (100%), but there have been recent studies questioning these estimates.[40,41] It is clear that the experience of the practitioner has an effect on the utility of the test, and even some large medical centers may not be able to perform the procedure reliably.

The technique is performed by cannulation of the bilateral femoral veins, and advancing catheters into the inferior petrosal sinuses via the internal jugular veins. Baseline ACTH values are obtained from the periphery and the inferior petrosal sinuses both before and after CRH stimulation (1 µg/kg of body weight). A ratio of 2.0 from the petrosal sinus to the periphery before CRH stimulation, or 3.0 afterward is felt to be consistent with pituitary Cushing's disease. In ectopic disease, the ratio is typically less than 2.0 both before and after CRH stimulation.[42]

False negative tests have been described in several situations. Ectopic pituitary tumors can render it inaccurate, as can hypoplastic or anomalous inferior petrosal sinuses. While IPSS results can lateralize, those findings may be misleading and are not highly specific. One study suggested that a gradient of 1.4 across sides was able to predict tumor location 78% of the time.[42]

Acromegaly

Growth hormone–secreting pituitary tumors account for 95% of acromegaly. Rarely, ectopic GH- or GH-releasing-hormone (GHRH)–secreting tumors are a cause. Most pituitary tumors are macroadenomas at the time of diagnosis. Approximately one third of tumors secrete additional pituitary hormones such as prolactin or TSH.[43]

In most patients, screening with an IGF-1 level is sufficient to establish the diagnosis. IGF-1 levels are reported as age-adjusted and attention should be paid to where the level falls within the normal range. When the IGF-1 levels are slightly elevated, an oral glucose suppression test is indicated. This test is performed by the oral administration of 75 grams of glucose and the measurement of serum GH levels every 30 minutes for 2 hours. Using the modern ultrasensitive assay, a normal individual will suppress GH levels to below 1 µg/l.[44]

Hyperthyroidism

TSH-secreting adenomas are uncommon and account for less than 1% of all pituitary adenomas. These aggressive tumors usually present as macroadenomas with a goiter and clinical features of hyperthyroidism. Generally, the free T4 and T3 levels are elevated in the setting of an inappropriately normal or elevated serum TSH concentration. TSH-secreting tumors often co-secrete other hormones; therefore measurement of PRL, GH and alpha subunit should be performed.[45,46] The alpha subunit can be useful in distinguishing TSH-secreting pituitary adenomas from thyroid hormone resistance (either pituitary, peripheral or generalized types). A suggested method to confirm the presence of a TSH-secreting tumor is to calculate the molar ratio of alpha subunit to TSH: (alpha subunit in nmol/l)/(serum TSH in µIU/l) × 10. A ratio exceeding 1.0 is found in 80% of patients with TSH-secreting adenomas.[45] Preoperative control of the hyperthyroidism is necessary and can be achieved with somatostatin analogs or the brief use of antithyroid medication, possibly in combination with beta-blockade.

Radiologic Studies

The differential diagnosis of sellar and parasellar neoplasms is quite large (Table 16-4). In many cases, an accurate diagnosis may be arrived at based on clinical symptoms and signs, and specific radiographic features. Occasionally, however, sellar lesions mimic one another and the actual diagnosis may only be resolved by histologic examination of resected tissue. Magnetic resonance imaging (MRI) is the primary modality employed in imaging of sellar and parasellar neoplasms. A typical MRI protocol calls for sagittal and coronal imaging, with thin-sectioned (2-3 mm) T1-weighted images with and without contrast. Some disease processes have very well defined characteristics on MRI that permit their identification prior to surgery. Computed tomography has a role in the evaluation for calcifications within the lesion and in defining the integrity of the parasellar bony anatomy. It may also be acutely useful in suspected apoplexy to identify hemorrhage.

Table 16-4	Lesions of Sella and Parasellar Region	
Type of Lesion	**MRI/CT Findings**	**Clinical Clues**
Physiologic enlargement of the pituitary	Larger than average gland without discrete tumor seen	Pregnancy, primary hypothyroidism, hypogonadism and adrenal insufficiency, normal variant May return to normal size after underlying endocrine cause is treated/resolves
Pituitary microadenoma	Hypointense lesion when compared to normal gland on postcontrast T1 images	Pituitary insufficiency rare. May be nonsecretory or secrete prolactin, ACTH, GH, or very rarely TSH
Pituitary macroadenoma	May see sellar expansion, deviation of the stalk away from the tumor, elevation of optic chiasm, occasional invasion into cavernous sinuses, sphenoid sinuses, suprasellar cistern or pterygopalatine fossa	Pituitary insufficiency common in non-secretory lesion. May secret prolactin, ACTH, GH or rarely TSH. Multiple hormones can be secreted, and insufficiency of some hormones may accompany excess of others
Pituitary apoplexy	CT scan may be initially useful revealing hemorrhage. Hemorrhage initially hyperintense on T1 images, hypointense on T2. Eventually hyperintense on both types of images	Sudden headache, signs and symptoms of acute central adrenal insufficiency, cranial nerve palsy, visual compromise
Cystic pituitary lesions: Rathke's cleft cysts Pars intermedia cysts Arachnoid cysts	Cyst fluid often dark on T1 imaging and bright on T2 imaging, but if fluid is proteinaceous, can be dark on both. Arachnoid cysts usually suprasellar, but can be intrasellar and displace gland posteriorly	Headaches, pituitary insufficiency possible
Empty sella	Small gland may be present on floor of sella. "Sword sign" seen as stalk transverses empty sella	Pituitary insufficiency possible, but function usually normal
Craniopharyngioma	Cystic lesion. Calcification on CT high specific, not sensitive. Can be cystic, solid, or both. Solid component may be bright on T1, cystic component bright on T2	Diabetes insipidus, pituitary insufficiency common. More common than pituitary adenoma in children
Meningioma	Uniform appearance on CT and MRI with similar appearance to gray matter. May lateralize within sella. Tuberculum sellae meningioma may have tail ("bird's beak"). May encase vessels and narrow lumen	Lateralizing visual symptoms
Chordomas/chondrosarcomas	May be calcified on CT. May be quite invasive. May destroy rather than expand sella	Visual symptoms most likely complaint. Pituitary insufficiency rare
Gliomas	May arise from optic tract or nerves. May be hypointense on T1 images and hyperintense on T2.	Visual symptoms most likely complaint Pituitary insufficiency rare
Germ-cell tumors (teratomas, germinomas, choriocarcinomas)	Enhance with CT contrast, isointense to brain on T1 images, hyperintense on T2	Most common in children and adolescents. DI and pituitary insufficiency common
CNS lymphomas	Contrast enhancing, contact subarachnoid space, can be necrotic	Possibly in context of disseminated lymphoma and immunocompromise. Can be seen as sole lesion and in immunocompetent
Inflammatory/infectious lesions	Thickening of stalk, loss of posterior pituitary bright spot	Diabetes insipidus common along with other pituitary deficiencies Evaluate for signs and symptoms of TB, sarcoidosis, Wegener's granulomatosis, histiocytosis
Vascular lesions	Black on MRI, homogeneous blush on contrast CT. MRA diagnostic	

Source: Adapted from Kaltsas GA, Nomikos P, Kontogeorgos G, Buchfelder M, Grossman AB. Clinical review: diagnosis and management of pituitary carcinomas. J Clin Endocrinol Metab. 2005;90:3089-3099.

PITUITARY HYPERPLASIA

The normal pituitary gland is 9 to 10 mm in greatest dimension. It is rectangular on coronal section and somewhat semilunar on sagittal section. Physiologic enlargement of the pituitary gland, as can be seen in young menstruant women, and hyperplasia that can be seen during pregnancy, in the setting of primary hypothyroidism, primary adrenal insufficiency, or hypogonadism, can lead to a trapezoidal shape of the gland on coronal sections and a globular shape on sagittal sections. These entities should be considered prior to assuming that pituitary enlargement represents a pituitary tumor.[4,47]

PITUITARY ADENOMAS

Microadenomas of the pituitary gland typically show diminished enhancement on postcontrast T1 images through the sella. The normal pituitary will appear hyperintense in relationship to the tumor. The pituitary stalk will often deviate laterally towards the contralateral side from the tumor on coronal imaging. Occasionally, however, postcontrasted images fail to delineate the tumor. In this setting, and when there is obvious evidence for a syndrome of hormone hypersecretion, serial dynamic contrast-enhanced images often delineate a microadenoma. Macroadenomas of the gland are obvious. On occasion, these lesions are hypodense. The normal pituitary is often displaced laterally or superiorly and will enhance. Occasionally, tumors invade the cavernous sinuses or extend inferiorly into the sphenoid sinuses, inferiorly and laterally into the pterygopalatine fossa and related spaces, or extend superiorly into the suprasellar cistern and elevate the optic chiasm. Magnetic resonance imaging provides for excellent definition of the limits of growth of a pituitary macroadenoma in most cases.

The syndrome of pituitary apoplexy can result from either hemorrhage or infarction of a pre-existing pituitary tumor. It has some unique presenting characteristics that are quite different from other pathology in the region. Early during the initial event, CT may be helpful, but if not directed at the sella details may be missed. MRI of the hemorrhage in the first few days will be hyperintense on T1 weighted imaging and hypointense on T2. As time progresses, hemorrhage will be hyperintense on T1 and T2 weighted imaging as hemoglobin degrades to methemoglobin, and fluid levels may begin to be seen as sedimentation begins. In the case of visual loss, more rapid surgical intervention may lead to better outcomes.[48]

PITUITARY CYSTIC LESIONS

Some pituitary adenomas undergo degenerative change and may present as predominately cystic or solid and cystic lesions within the sella. The cyst fluid is usually hypointense on T1 images with or without contrast. Cystic adenomas may be hyperintense on T2 imaging. Occasionally, hemorrhage is seen within pituitary tumors. Blood products are usually hyperintense on T1 images. Primary pituitary cysts, such as pars intermedia cysts and Rathke's cleft cysts are usually hypointense on T1 imaging. The latter lesions, however, may mimic a pituitary tumor. These lesions may not be hyperintense on T2 imaging if the fluid is very proteinaceous. Arachnoid cysts are most commonly suprasellar, but can be intrasellar and are often hypointense and distort the sellar contents and displace the pituitary stalk posteriorly.[47,49] Patients who have primary or secondary empty sella often have a small gland, usually situated in the floor of the sella, and the pituitary stalk traverses the empty sella as it passes to the residual or remnant gland. In many patients, the stalk is straight and tapered and has the appearance of a sword leading to the well known "sword sign" taken to confirm the presence of an empty sella and exclude the diagnosis of an intrasellar cyst.

CRANIOPHARYNGIOMAS

Craniopharyngiomas are epithelial tumors that arise along the path of the craniopharyngeal duct. They are the most common lesions of the parasellar area in children. There is a bimodal age distribution, with peak prevalence seen in children 5 to 14 years old and adults 50 to 74 years old.[50] They can have imaging characteristics in common with cystic pituitary lesions. CT scanning may be useful when a craniopharyngioma is suspected, and the presence of calcium within the lesion on CT is highly suggestive, but is only seen in 50% of such tumors. The tumors may be solid, cystic, or both. The solid component will often enhance with contrast on T1 weighted MRI imaging and the cystic component will usually be hyperintense on T2 weighted imaging.[51] Craniopharyngiomas may also be located in the region of the pituitary stalk or situated with an epicenter in the hypothalamus. The majority will be between 2 and 4 cm in diameter, but they can be bigger.[50] Suprasellar craniopharyngiomas may result in mass effect on the ventricular system and are often accompanied by a high rate of hypopituitarism and diabetes insipidus.

MENINGIOMAS

Meningiomas are usually benign neoplasms of the dura mater. The majority are WHO grade I, but atypical (WHO II) and anaplastic (WHO III) lesions are described.[52] Peak incidence is in the 4th to 7th decade.[53] In adults, they are the second most common lesion encountered in the parasellar area after pituitary adenomas.[54] Parasellar meningiomas include those that arise from the diaphragma sella, tuberculum sella, or the dura overlying the medial walls of the cavernous sinuses. They are often diagnosed based on imaging characteristics. They tend to have very uniform enhancement with gadolinium contrast and their appearance is similar to gray matter both on CT and MRI.[47] A gnarled appearance is often seen in cavernous sinus meningiomas. Tuberculum sellae meningiomas often have a dural tail that extends over the planum sphenoidale, which distinguishes them from pituitary adenomas.[49] On coronal sections, this tail often gives the appearance of a bird's beak. Adjacent bone may be thickened or sclerotic. Meningiomas often encase arterial vessels and narrow their lumen, which is again atypical of pituitary adenomas.[51]

CHORDOMAS AND CHONDROSARCOMAS

Chordomas and chondrosarcomas are cartilaginous tumors arising from the notochord remnant in the skull base. Chordomas are low-grade tumors, but can be quite destructive and have a significant mortality risk (5-year survival 65%).[55] Intracranial chondrosarcomas are far less common than chordomas and fewer than 200 are described in the literature.[56] These lesions grow in all directions and can efface normal anatomic structures, compress the brainstem, and obliterate the sella. They tend to invade and destroy the sella rather causing the expansion one may see with a typical pituitary adenoma. They often cause bony destruction and may contain calcifications best seen on CT. They tend to be hyperintense on T2 weighted imaging and enhance with contrast. Like craniopharyngiomas, these lesions may be calcified on CT scanning.

Initial presenting complaints are likely to be related to visual symptoms or headaches. Diplopia is more likely than visual field defects, reflecting their propensity to affect the cranial nerves within the cavernous sinuses.[51] They are not likely to be associated with pituitary insufficiency, but it has been described, particularly in association with chondrosarcoma.[56]

OTHER MALIGNANT LESIONS OF THE SELLA

Parasellar gliomas, malignant lesions that can range from low to high grade, arise from glial tissue located in the hypothalamus, optic chiasm, optic nerves, or the optic tracts. Examples include pilocytic astrocytomas, a low-grade (WHO I) lesion, that is often associated with neurofibromatosis type 1 (NF-1). Higher-grade gliomas in the parasellar region include astrocytomas (WHO II) and anaplastic astrocytomas. Occasionally astrocytomas will progress to gliobastomas (WHO grades III-VI).[51] These lesions tend to be large, potentially infiltrative, suprasellar masses. They tend to be hypointense to brain on T1- weighted images and hyperintense on T2 weighted images. They may demonstrate heterogeneous enhancement with contrast.[5]

Germ-cell tumors (germinomas, choriocarcinomas, teratomas) are most commonly seen in childhood and adolescence. There are often synchronous lesions located in the suprasellar region, the vicinity of the third ventricle, and in the area of the pineal gland. These lesions often are suspected based on the radiographic characteristics in conjunction with the clinical presentation characterized by profound hypopituitarism and diabetes insipidus. These lesions tend to enhance with CT contrast and be isointense to brain on T1-weighted images and hyperintense on T2-weighted images.

Primary CNS lymphomas in the parasellar region have been described in both immunocompromised and immunocompetent patients. Presenting features include including diabetes insipidus, pituitary stalk thickening, and fever.[57] Synchronous lesions are not uncommon and there may be evidence of disseminated lymphoma. Contrast-enhancing lesions in contact with the subarachnoid space and without necrosis are characteristic of parasellar lymphomas.

Metastases to the parasellar region may mimic a lesion of the pituitary stalk or of the sella. In most cases, there is additional evidence for intracranial metastases or distant metastases to other sites including the skeletal system and the liver. Melanoma and carcinomas of the breast and lung account for most cases of metastases to the pituitary stalk. Imaging characteristics may mimic a primary stalk tumor such as a glioma or choristoma or an infiltrative process causing thickening of the pituitary stalk.[5] These tumors tend to have irregular borders.

INFLAMMATORY LESIONS

A variety of infiltrative and inflammatory lesions may affect the parasellar region. Many of these disorders will manifest in the context of systemic symptoms of the underlying disease process. While radiographic and clinical features may be pathognomonic, in many cases, a diagnosis of infiltrative disease is secured by a response to steroid or antibiotic therapy and in some cases, only after surgery has been performed and the biopsy evaluated.

Sarcoidosis may present as a sellar mass, as thickening of the pituitary stalk, or even as a hypothalamic mass. Some patients may have communicating hydrocephalus and leptomeningeal enhancement. The disorder may be limited to the central nervous system or may be seen in association with the typical pulmonary or skin findings of sarcoidosis. Hyperprolactinemia due to stalk effect, DI, and hypopituitarism are not uncommon. An elevated serum or CSF ACE level may be helpful in securing the diagnosis but biopsy is often required. The pituitary "bright spot" on T1 weighted imaging may not be seen in patients who have resultant diabetes insipidus. Sarcoid granulomata tend to be isointense on T1 weighted imaging and will often enhance with gadolinium.[58]

Lymphocytic hypophysitis is characterized by either focal or diffuse infiltration of the pituitary by lymphocytes with accompanying inflammation and is felt to be an autoimmune disorder. Hypophysitis often mimics a pituitary tumor. The inflammatory mass is often diffuse and hyperintense on postcontrast T1 images. Patients usually have profound degrees of hypopituitarism that are not usually seen when similar degrees of enlargement of the sellar contents are seen in other disorders such as meningiomas, pituitary adenomas, and so on.[49] Lymphocytic neuroinfundibulohypophysitis is associated with diabetes insipidus and loss of the pituitary bright spot on MRI. Xanthomatous hypophysitis is described as a reaction to ruptured cyst components.[58] The appearance on MRI may be indistinguishable from sarcoidosis, and clinical manifestations are similar.

Wegener's granulomatosis may affect the pituitary and mimic an inflammatory condition. Most patients have evidence of coexisting renal and pulmonary disease. MRI often reveals a thickened infundibulum, but will not reliably distinguish this lesion from other inflammatory processes.[58]

Langerhan's cell histiocytosis is characterized by proliferation of specific dendritic cells of the reticuloendothelial tissue. This disorder is more common in children (70%) than it is in adults (30%) and is quite rare. Diabetes insipidus is one of the more common early manifestations of the disorder. A thickened pituitary stalk and lack of a posterior pituitary bright spot on MRI may be seen.[58] Occasionally patients also have lesions involving the skin, liver, lungs, spleen, and bone marrow.

INFECTIOUS DISORDERS

Pituitary abscesses may be seen in the setting of a pituitary tumor and are more common in the setting of a pre-existing Rathke's cleft cyst. These infections may also be seen in patients with sphenoid sinusitis. On MRI, a pituitary abscess is typically cystic, hypo- or iso-intense on T1 weighted imaging and hyper or iso-intense on T2 imaging. Ring enhancement is often seen. Fever is not reliably present. Pituitary abscesses are often first diagnosed at the time of pituitary surgery when the surgeon encounters pus. Cultures should be obtained to permit appropriate identification of the infectious agent and directed antibiotic therapy.[59,60]

Intracranial tuberculosis is uncommon. The prevalence depends upon the underlying prevalence of tuberculosis in particular patient populations. Affected patients usually have systemic manifestation of the disease process but pituitary and suprasellar lesions have been described as the sole or presenting feature of the infection. A recent report illustrates a case where a tuberculoma was misdiagnosed as idiopathic granulomatous hypophysitis for which steroid treatment was initiated. The patient developed tuberculous meningitis, illustrating the need to maintain a degree of suspicion and to ensure antibiotic therapy is provided when indicated.[61]

VASCULAR DISORDERS

Intrasellar aneurysms arise from the carotid arteries but can arise from the anterior communicating arteries. These lesions often mimic pituitary adenomas but can usually be readily distinguished by appropriate imaging techniques. They may appear black on conventional MRI and show homogenous blush on contrasted CT images.[58] MRA or conventional angiogram may confirm the diagnosis, and should be considered if an aneurysm is suspected.

Ophthalmologic Studies

The ophthalmologic exam and associated testing is a critical component of the evaluation of the patient with a sellar or parasellar lesion. In many cases these patients may present with visual complaints that ultimately lead to the discovery of their lesion. An experienced neuro-opthalmologist can often discern a great deal about a tumor's location and some clues about its etiology from a detailed exam. Alternatively, the lesion may be discovered by other means, and the ophthalmologic exam may reveal previously unknown visual symptomatology that may influence the treatment plan, particularly in regards to surgery.

The optic chiasm is typically few millimeters above the diaphragma sellae separated by the suprasellar cistern. However, the chiasm can occupy both a "prefixed" or "post-fixed" relationship to the diaphragma sellae (each in about 5% of the population). In the prefixed position, the chiasm is placed more anteriorly, with a shorter length of the optic nerves traveling over the pituitary gland and any potential associated pathology. In the postfixed position, the chiasm is more posterior, and a longer section of optic nerve is above the gland. The position of the chiasm will produce differing clinical manifestations when compression occurs from below. Lateral to the pituitary gland cranial nerves III, IV, V_1, V_2, and VI traverse the cavernous sinus.[62]

To review, the chiasm represents the junction the optic nerves. The temporal fibers come from each optic tract, do not cross the chiasm, and travel anteriorly to innervate the ipsilateral eye. The nasal fibers cross the chiasm and travel to the contralateral eye. Therefore visual information from the left visual space is transmitted to the right cerebral cortex, and information from the right visual space is transmitted to the left visual cortex. The nasal fibers are arranged such that the upper quadrant fibers remain superior and cross posteriorly in the chiasm. The lower quadrant fibers remain inferior, and cross anteriorly in the chiasm. Thus, visual findings may differ depending on whether compression comes from above or below the chiasm.

The first step for the examining neuro-ophthalmologist is a thorough history and physical exam. This will include the formal ophthalmologic testing discussed below, but also vital signs, investigation of the integrity of the cranial nerves, and attention to the overall physical appearance of the patient, who may exhibit signs or symptoms of an underlying endocrine disorder. The manner in which the symptoms presented (sudden vs. gradual) and the exact nature of the symptoms are critical. Patients may present with visual field loss and complaints related to bumping into objects or difficulties while driving. The loss may manifest itself simply as a subtraction of the visual field, not blackness, which is more suggestive of optic nerve or retinal pathology. Changes in color vision may be noted, along with headache, diplopia, or ptosis.

A thorough ophthalmologic examination is extremely important. This is performed preferably with the patient's own corrective lenses, or if unavailable, with manifest refraction or correction by pinhole. Usually, in early chiasmal compression from a pituitary tumor, visual acuity and visual fields will be normal or near normal. Loss of visual acuity may suggest a very large pituitary tumor or pathology other than a typical pituitary lesion. Visual testing should also include color vision testing with pseudoisochromatic plates and formal visual field testing. Desaturation of color vision may be one of the earliest signs of a chiasmal lesion, preceding actual field deficits.[63]

All patients suspected of having a visual problem should have confrontational field testing. However, in the ophthalmologist's office, automated visual fields, usually by Humphrey automated perimetry, should be performed. This testing is critical, as it may be used as a baseline against which to compare future examinations and is often the first clue to the examining physician that the patient may have a pituitary tumor large enough to cause a visual field deficit. The most typical initial visual field defect associated with a pituitary adenoma is a bitemporal superior quadrantic defect, produced due to pressure from below on the chiasm. A bitemporal inferior quadrantic defect is suggestive of pressure from above, as might be seen from a craniopharyngioma growing downward onto the chiasm. More severe pressure from either direction can produce a dense bitemporal hemianopsia.[62,63]

The pattern of visual field deficit may vary depending upon whether the chiasm is prefixed, postfixed, or normal. Pressure upon a prefixed chiasm, especially if not exactly midline, may result in a homonymous hemianopia on the side contralateral to the tumor. A postfixed chiasm may allow for minimal visual loss despite a very large tumor, or may manifest with symptoms mimicking optic neuritis with pain on eye movement, monocular visual acuity loss, and a central scotoma on visual field testing. A Marcus-Gunn pupil or relative afferent pupillary defect (RAPD) is predicated upon inter-eye luminance disparity. Its presence indicates that the amount of illumination reaching the midbrain from each retina and optic nerves is unequal. It will appear to be a paradoxical dilation of the abnormal eye when viewing each eye as it is illuminated. An RAPD is an indication of more marked chiasmal compression and visual field loss.

Formal testing of ocular motility, including ductions, saccades, pursuit, and alternate cover tests may reveal pathology related to the compression of cavernous sinuses and CN III, IV, and VI. Pathology in this area should certainly lead to consideration of cavernous sinus extension of a pituitary tumor, but also to alternative pathology. Involvement of CN III may result in a unilateral dilated pupil, ptosis, and a globe that is deviated inferiorly and laterally. Involvement of CN IV will result in vertical diplopia and upward deviation. Involvement of CN VI will result in horizontal diplopia due to the inability to abduct the involved eye. It is likely that deficits will be seen in combination. Horner's syndrome may develop due to compression of the sympathetic neurons in the cavernous sinus.[62,63]

The fundoscopic exam may provide clues as to the duration of the deficit. Papilledema is almost never seen in the setting of a pituitary lesion, but could result if the tumor blocks the foramina of Monro. More typically, optic atrophy may be seen, which is felt to take at least 4 to 6 weeks to develop. Retinal processes, which may at times mimic chiasmal disease, should be excluded, as well as optic disc anomalies.

It is important to form a differential diagnosis during the exam, which will typically be supplemented by MRI scanning, preferably of the brain and orbits with and without fat suppression and gadolinium. Chiasmal findings, which respect the midline, are suggestive of pituitary adenomas, suprasellar meningiomas or aneurysms, and craniopharyngiomas. Para-chiasmal findings suggest alternate pathology and potentially lateralization and may be seen with other tumors such as optic gliomas, or sphenoid wind meningiomas. Multiple cranial nerve involvement can exist in the presence of malignancy or apoplexy.

Coordination of Care

The diseases discussed in this chapter are uncommon and complex. Several studies illustrate that experienced pituitary neurosurgeons obtain greater likelihoods of surgical success and have lower rates of surgical morbidity and mortality.[64] Neuroradiologists play a key role in providing expert interpretation of radiographic images and in establishing a differential diagnosis. When indicated, neuro-ophthalmologists conduct in-depth evaluations to document whether pituitary and parasellar lesions have affected the visual pathways. Radiation oncologists are essential in the management of patients with residual tumors, and in particular those with residual hormone-secreting neoplasms.

Logistically, it is best if this evaluation can happen in a coordinated fashion in a single day. This is easiest in a dedicated pituitary clinic, but could be done in separate clinics with close communication between physicians. Due to the low prevalence of the diseases described in this chapter, patients are often forced to travel long distances to reach an experienced center. It is very helpful if there is a designated coordinator to ensure appropriate labs and images are conducted and available at the time of the visit. Treatment requires constant communication between physicians, often accomplished electronically. A periodic case conference where involved specialists can discuss challenging cases, jointly review imaging and pathology, and clarify treatment plans is extremely helpful. Much of the endocrine testing described above is highly technical, carries some risk, and is best accomplished in a dedicated infusion center.

Endocrinologists play an essential role in the evaluation and management of patients with pituitary tumors and related disorders. They are often called upon to coordinate the care amongst the subspecialists involved in the case. Endocrinologists conduct postoperative assessments of the adequacy of pituitary function and of the biochemical status of residual disease in patients with hormone-secreting neoplasms. Endocrinologists are essential in the medical management of persistent hormone hypersecretion and in the coordination of adjuvant therapy including reoperation and radiotherapy, adrenalectomy, and so on. In the event that an endocrinologist is unavailable, it behooves the treating neurosurgeon to play the role of assessor of the medical and endocrine status of the patient or to work with a designated primary care physician.

KEY REFERENCES

Bertherat J, Chanson P, Montminy M. The cyclic adenosine 3',5'-monophosphate-responsive factor CREB is constitutively activated in human somatotroph adenomas. *Mol Endocrinol.* 1995;9: 777-783.

Buchfelder M, Schlaffer S. Surgical treatment of pituitary tumours. *Best Pract Res Clin Endocrinol Metab.* Oct 2009;23(5):677-692.

Buurman H, Saeger W. Subclinical adenomas in postmortem pituitaries: classification and correlations to clinical data. *Eur J Endocrinol.* May 2006;154(5):753-758.

Castro M, Elias PC, Quidute AR, et al. Out-patient screening for Cushing's syndrome: the sensitivity of the combination of circadian rhythm and overnight dexamethasone suppression salivary cortisol tests. *J Clin Endocrinol Metab.* Mar 1999;84(3):878-882.

DiGiovanni R, Serra S, Ezzat S, Asa SL. AIP Mutations are not identified in patients with sporadic pituitary adenomas. *Endocr Pathol.* Summer 2007;18(2):76-78.

Elston M, McDonald K, Clifton-Bligh R, Robinson B. Familial pituitary tumor syndromes. *Nat Rev Endocrinol.* Aug 2009;5(8):453-461.

Ezzat S, Asa SL, Couldwell WT, et al. The prevalence of pituitary adenomas: a systematic review. *Cancer.* Aug 1 2004;101(3):613-619.

Fernandez A, Karavitaki N, Wass JA. Prevalence of pituitary adenomas: a community-based, cross-sectional study in Banbury (Oxfordshire, UK). *Clin Endocrinol (Oxf).* 2010;72:377-382.

FitzPatrick M, Tartaglino LM, Hollander MD, et al. Imaging of sellar and parasellar pathology. *Radiol Clin North Am.* Jan 1999;37(1):101-121:x.

Georgitsi M, Heliovaara E, Paschke R, et al. Large genomic deletions in AIP in pituitary adenoma predisposition. *J Clin Endocrinol Metab.* Oct 2008;93(10):4146-4151.

Glezer A, Paraiba DB, Bronstein MD. Rare sellar lesions. *Endocrinol Metab Clin North Am.* Mar 2008;37(1):195-211:x.

Hamacher C, Brocker M, Adams EF, et al. Overexpression of stimulatory G protein alpha-subunit is a hallmark of most human somatotrophic pituitary tumours and is associated with resistance to GH-releasing hormone. *Pituitary.* Apr 1998;1(1):13-23.

Heliovaara E, Raitila A, Launonen V, et al. The expression of AIP-related molecules in elucidation of cellular pathways in pituitary adenomas. *Am J Pathol.* 2009;175:2501-2507.

Kaltsas GA, Evanson J, Chrisoulidou A, Grossman AB. The diagnosis and management of parasellar tumours of the pituitary. *Endocr Relat Cancer.* Dec 2008;15(4):885-903.

Kaltsas GA, Nomikos P, Kontogeorgos G, et al. Clinical review: diagnosis and management of pituitary carcinomas. *J Clin Endocrinol Metab.* May 2005;90(5):3089-3099.

King Jr JT, Justice AC, Aron DC. Management of incidental pituitary microadenomas: a cost-effectiveness analysis. *J Clin Endocrinol Metab.* Nov 1997;82(11):3625-3632.

Krikorian A, Aron D. Evaluation and management of pituitary incidentalomas—revisiting an acquaintance. *Nat Clin Pract Endocrinol Metab.* Mar 2006;2(3):138-145.

Lanzino G, Dumont A, Lopes M, Laws EJ. Skull base chordomas: overview of disease, management options, and outcome. *Neurosurg Focus.* 2001;10(3):E12.

Melmed S, Colao A, Barkan A, et al. Guidelines for acromegaly management: an update. *J Clin Endocrinol Metab.* May 2009;94(5):1509-1517.

Molitch ME. Nonfunctioning pituitary tumors and pituitary incidentalomas. *Endocrinol Metab Clin North Am.* Mar 2008;37(1):151-171:xi.

Powell M, Lightman SL, Laws ER. *Management of Pituitary Tumours: the Clinician's Practical Guide.* 2nd ed. Totowa, NJ: Humana Press; 2003.

Vance ML. Perioperative management of patients undergoing pituitary surgery. *Endocrinol Metab Clin North Am.* Jun 2003;32(2):355-365.

Vierimaa O, Georgitsi M, Lehtonen R, et al. Pituitary adenoma predisposition caused by germline mutations in the AIP gene. *Science.* 2006;312(5777):1228-1230:May 26.

Yanoff M, Duker JS, Augsburger JJ. *Ophthalmology.* 3rd ed. Edinburgh: Mosby Elsevier; 2009.

Zee CS, Go JL, Kim PE, Mitchell D, Ahmadi J. Imaging of the pituitary and parasellar region. *Neurosurg Clin North Am.* Jan 2003;14(1):55-80:vi.

Numbered references appear on Expert Consult.

CHAPTER 17

Medical Management of Hormone-Secreting Pituitary Tumors

NESTORAS MATHIOUDAKIS • ROBERTO SALVATORI

The majority of pituitary tumors are hormone-secreting.[1] With the exception of prolactinomas, surgery has historically been the mainstay of treatment for hormone-secreting as well as non-functioning pituitary tumors. In recent years, however, medical therapy has assumed an increasingly important role in the management of hormone-secreting pituitary adenomas. In addition to being the primary treatment for prolactinomas, medical therapy can serve an adjunctive role in the treatment of growth-hormone (GH) secreting tumors, refractory Cushing's disease, and the rare thyroid-stimulating-hormone (TSH)-secreting adenomas. In a subset of patients with acromegaly, medical therapy can be the primary treatment approach. This chapter will review the pharmacological profile, therapeutic efficacy, safety, and side effects of the most common medications used in the treatment of pituitary tumors. In addition, the role of medical therapy in relation to neurosurgical management will be emphasized.

Prolactinomas

GENERAL CONSIDERATIONS

The decision of whether to initiate medical therapy in a patient with a prolactinoma should take into account the size of the tumor, fertility status of the patient, and the presence of symptoms related to hyperprolactinemia. In general, therapy is indicated for macroadenomas. A premenopausal woman with a microprolactinoma who does not have bothersome galactorrhea and does not wish to become pregnant may be reassured and treated with estrogen replacement. Likewise, a post-menopausal woman with a microprolactinoma may not require any treatment. This conservative approach is justified by the observation that approximately 90% of microprolactinomas will not grow in size over a 4- to 6-year period.[2] In these patients, monitoring with periodic prolactin measurements and MRI's is appropriate. While it is unlikely for a prolactinoma to grow without a concurrent rise in serum prolactin levels, this occurrence has been reported, and therefore some clinicians will monitor with periodic MRI's even if prolactin levels are stable. Significant increases in serum prolactin levels or evidence of growth of a microprolactinoma are indications for treatment, given the possibility that such a tumor represents one of the small minority that will grow to become a macroadenoma. Alternatively, given the high

surgical cure rate of microprolactinomas (up to 75%), surgery may be considered upfront in lieu of medical treatment in those patients who are interested in permanent and immediate cure.[3]

In the evaluation of hyperprolactinemia, it is important to recognize the phenomenon of macroprolactinemia, a laboratory finding that does not require any treatment. Patients with elevated prolactin levels who have either mild or no symptoms of hyperprolactinemia may, in fact, have large circulating complexes of the prolactin protein (more than 150 kDa), called macroprolactin. This larger prolactin protein, which can spuriously elevate serum prolactin levels, can be recognized by a simple laboratory method using PEG precipitation.[4] As many as 10% to 26% of patients with idiopathic hyperprolactinemia have macroprolactinemia, and this entity should be suspected particularly in patients with discordant laboratory findings and clinical symptoms.[4]

DOPAMINE AGONISTS

In the majority of cases, dopamine receptor agonists are the mainstay of treatment for prolactinomas. These drugs inhibit prolactin secretion by binding to the D2 receptor of tumoral lactotrophs, which leads to decreased formation of prolactin secretory granules and thus reduced tumor volume. There may also be a cytocidal effect of dopamine agonist treatment on tumor cells resulting in tumor shrinkage and fibrosis.[5] Among these drugs, cabergoline and bromocriptine are the most commonly used in practice today, as their use is substantiated by the greatest amount of clinical experience and evidence. The other dopamine agonists include quinagolide, a non-ergot derivative not available in the United States, and pergolide, an ergot derivative previously used to treat Parkinson's disease that was removed from the U.S. market due to an increased risk of cardiac valvular disease.

Pharmacologic Aspects

There are currently three dopamine agonists available in the treatment of prolactinomas: cabergoline, bromocriptine, and quinagolide (Table 17-1).

The semisynthetic ergot derivative, bromocriptine, a D2 agonist and weak D1 antagonist, was the first available medical treatment for prolactinomas. Administered orally, bromocriptine has a relatively short half-life (7 hours), often necessitating two to three daily doses, although once daily

Table 17-1 Dopamine Agonist Treatment of Prolactinomas

Dopamine Agonist	Dosage Forms	Typical Starting Dose	Dosing Frequency	Titration Schedule	Mean Effective Dose
Bromocriptine	Capsule: 5 mg Tablet: 2.5 mg	1.25 mg/day	One to three times daily	Increase by 1.25 mg weekly	7.5 mg
Cabergoline	Tablet: 0.5 mg	0.25 mg/1–2 times weekly	Once or twice weekly	Increase by 0.25 mg increments at 2- to 3-month intervals	0.5 to 3.5 mg
Quinagolide*	Tablet: 0.025 mg Tablet: 0.05 mg Tablet: 0.075 mg	0.025 mg/day × 3 days, then 0.05 mg/day × 3 days	Daily	Increase by 0.025 mg increments weekly	0.075 to 0.5 mg

*Not available in United States.
Source: UpToDate, Inc. Bromocriptine: Drug Information, Cabergoline: Drug Information, Quinagolide: Drug Information. Available at www.uptodate.com. Waltham, MA: UpToDate;2009.

dosing may occasionally be effective. The standard dosage is 2.5 to 15 mg per day, and most patients are successfully treated with 7.5 mg or less.[6] Since gastrointestinal side effects are common, it is usually recommended to start with very low doses (1.25 mg/day) and gradually titrate upward by 1.25 mg increments weekly until a dose of 7.5 mg is reached.[6] In resistant patients, doses as high as 20 to 30 mg per day may be necessary.

Cabergoline, a preferential D2-receptor agonist, has largely supplanted bromocriptine as the first-line treatment of prolactinomas due to its superior efficacy, longer half-life, and greater tolerability. Its half-life of 2.5 to 4.5 days allows for once or twice weekly administration.[7] The typical starting dose of cabergoline is 0.25 mg orally once or twice weekly, with escalation of dosing by 0.25-mg increments at 2- to 3-month intervals if plateau effect is reached, until prolactin levels normalize. In most patients, the therapeutic dose range is 0.5 to 3.5 mg weekly. A recent study found that more than 95% of patients are able to achieve normal prolactin levels with high-dose treatment (from 6 to 11 mg/wk).[8]

Quinagolide is a non-ergot derivative D_2-receptor agonist commonly used to treat prolactinomas in Europe and Canada. The half-life of quinagolide is 22 hours, which allows for a once-daily dosing regimen. As with cabergoline, the simpler dosing regimen and reduced side effect profile of quinagolide allows for better patient compliance compared with bromocriptine. Typical doses are 0.075 mg to 0.4 mg daily, and most patients are effectively treated with 0.1 mg/day. This drug can be rapidly titrated to therapeutic doses in just 7 days: a starting dose of 0.025 mg is given for 3 days and is titrated by 0.025 mg every 3 days until a dose of 0.075 mg is achieved.

Therapeutic Efficacy

For microprolactinomas, bromocriptine is 80% to 90% effective at normalizing prolactin levels and shrinking tumor mass, whereas the success rate is around 70% for macroprolactinomas.[2] The improvement in headache and visual field defects is rapid and dramatic in most patients, occurring within a few days after the first dose. These changes often precede radiographic evidence of tumor shrinkage. Likewise, gonadal and sexual function may improve even before complete normalization of serum prolactin levels, although sometimes normalization of testosterone may require several months of normal prolactin levels[2]. The degree of tumor shrinkage seen with bromocriptine does not necessarily correlate with the nadir prolactin level or the extent of decline in prolactin levels.[2]

Table 17-2 Efficacy of Cabergoline in Treatment of Microprolactinomas

Study Author (Year)	Reference	No. of Patients	Proportion of Patients with Prolactin Normalization (%)
Ciccarelli et al. (1997)	86	25	96
Colao et al. (1997)	32	8	100
Muratori et al. (1997)	87	26	96
Cannavo et al. (1999)	88	26	88
Verhelst et al. (1999)	89	174	93
De Luis et al. (2000)	90	8	100
Di Sarno et al. (2000)	91	23	95
Pinzone et al. (2000)	92	12	83
DiSarno et al. (2001)	93	60	90
Colao et al. (2003)	94	97	86
Colao et al. (2004)	15	10	80
Vilar et al. (2008)	11	121	83–91 in naïve patients 81–88 in BCR-intolerant patients 50–61 BCR-resistant 100 BCR-responsive
Ono et al. (2008)	8	93	99
All studies combined		683	91*

*Calculation derived from sum of responders/sum of all patients studied.

Although most prolactinomas remain responsive to bromocriptine over time, the drug is generally not curative, as hyperprolactinemia and tumor growth will often recur after withdrawal of therapy. Prolonged use of bromocriptine has been associated with perivascular fibrosis and increased tumor consistency in prolactinomas that ultimately are surgically removed; the extent of fibrosis seems to correlate with the duration of pre-surgical treatment with bromocriptine and may impact the technical ease of surgical resection.[9]

Early studies found cabergoline to be 80% to 95% effective at normalizing prolactin levels, with varying degrees of tumor reduction seen in 70% to 90% of patients.[10] The efficacy of cabergoline in normalizing prolactin levels in micro- and macro-prolactinomas is shown in Tables 17-2 and 17-3, respectively. Although there is considerable variability among studies with respect to tumor shrinkage, a recent large study showed a significant (>50%) tumor shrinkage in 80% of patients, and complete disappearance of the tumor mass in 57% of patients.[11] Cabergoline is able to

Table 17-3   **Efficacy of Cabergoline in Treatment of Macroprolactinomas**

Study Author (Year)	Reference	No. of Patients	Proportion of Patients with Prolactin Normalization (%)
Biller et al. (1996)	95	15	73
Ciccarelli et al. (1997)	86	9	78
Colao et al. (1997)	32	19	79
Colao et al. (1997)	96	23	78
Cannavo et al. (1999)	88	11	100
Verhelst et al. (1999)	89	181	77
Colao et al. (2000)	33	110	81 of naive patients 82 in BRC-responsive 95 in BRC-intolerant 51 in BRC-resistant
Pontikides et al. (2000)	97	12	100
Di Sarno et al. (2001)	93	56	82
Pinzone et al. (2001)	92	34	79
Sibal et al. (2002)	98	35	83
Bolko et al. (2003)	99	6	83
Colao et al. (2003)	94	107	64
Colao et al. (2004)	15	10	76
De Rosa et al. (2004)	100	41	73
Ono et al. (2008)	8	57	98
Vilar et al. (2008)	11	117	78
All studies combined		843	79*

*Calculation derived from sum of responders/sum of all patients studied.

induce tumor shrinkage more effectively in dopamine agonist naïve patients compared with those who have received prior dopamine agonist treatment (Fig. 17-1). Furthermore, cabergoline offers the potential for cure after several years of treatment, allowing for withdrawal of therapy.[12, 13]

The beneficial effects of cabergoline on gonadal function are well documented in both sexes. Compared with bromocriptine, cabergoline is more effective at normalizing prolactin levels and restoring ovulation and is associated with fewer, milder, and shorter-lived side effects.[14] Serum testosterone levels have been shown to normalize in the majority of patients, with concurrent improvement in sperm count and parameters.[15]

Quinagolide normalized prolactin levels in 73% of patients with microadenomas and 67% of patients with macroadenomas.[16] Tumor reduction was seen in 55% of patients with microadenomas and 75% of patients with macroadenomas.[16] Although cabergoline has been found to be more effective at normalizing prolactin levels and reducing tumor size compared with quinagolide, both drugs show similar efficacy on reproductive function.

Pergolide, a semisynthetic ergoline derivative, was initially approved in the United States only for the treatment of Parkinson's disease. Typical doses used in the treatment of hyperprolactinemia range from 0.05 mg to 0.5 mg/day, whereas higher doses (>3 mg/day) have been used in Parkinson's patients.[17] Although pergolide has been found to be effective at normalizing prolactin levels and reducing the size of macroprolactinomas, this drug was withdrawn from the U.S. market in 2007 due to the increased risk of valvular heart disease in Parkinson's patients receiving high daily doses.

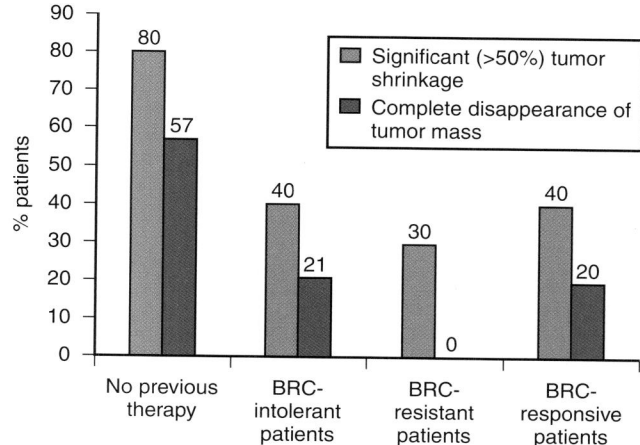

FIGURE 17-1 Efficacy of cabergoline on tumor shrinkage in patients with macroprolactinomas. BRC, bromocriptine. (From Vilar L, Freitas MC, Naves LA, et al. Diagnosis and management of hyperprolactinemia: results of a Brazilian multicenter study with 1234 patients. J Endocrinol Invest. 2008;31:436-444. Editrice Kurtis.)

Tolerability and Side Effects

The most common side effects of dopamine agonists include gastrointestinal, cardiovascular, and neurologic symptoms (Table 17-4). In general, if a patient cannot tolerate the first dopamine agonist administered, a trial of a second drug should be given.

Among the dopamine agonists, bromocriptine is the least well tolerated, with up to 12% of patients being unable to tolerate therapeutic doses.[2] Up to one third of patients will experience nausea and vomiting, an effect that can be minimized by initiating a low dose and titrating very slowly.[2] Taking the medication with a small snack may also reduce these symptoms.[2] A gradual dose titration and taking the medication at bedtime may also help reduce postural hypotension and dizziness experienced by as many as 25% of patients.[2] Syncope is rare but has been reported even with small initial doses.[18] Tolerance to postural hypotension usually develops rapidly.[18] Drowsiness, headache, and nasal congestion are common complaints. The safety of bromocriptine in psychiatric patients has not yet been established; there are case reports of onset or exacerbation of preexisting psychosis. Other psychiatric

Table 17-4   **Side Effects of Dopamine Agonists**

Common Side Effects of Dopamine Agonists

Gastrointestinal
  Nausea
  Vomiting
Cardiovascular
  Postural hypotension
  Dizziness
  Syncope (rare)
Neurologic
  Headache
  Drowsiness
  Exacerbation of pre-existing psychosis (rare)
  Dyskinesias (high-dose treatment)

symptoms associated with high doses of bromocriptine include anxiety, depression, insomnia, paranoia, and hyperactivity.[18] At higher doses used in the treatment of Parkinson's disease, reversible pleuro-pulmonary changes and retroperitoneal fibrosis have been reported, but these changes are unlikely to occur at the doses used to treat prolactinomas.[2]

While cabergoline and bromocriptine have similar side effect profiles, cabergoline has been shown to be better tolerated in several large comparative studies.[11, 19] Compared with bromocriptine, the side effects of cabergoline are generally less frequent, milder, and of shorter duration.[2] Nausea and vomiting are most commonly observed, followed by headache and dizziness.[2] In a multi-center randomized trial of hyperprolactinemic women, 3% could not tolerate cabergoline compared with 12% who had to stop taking bromocriptine.[14] It has been proposed that fluctuations in concentrations of dopamine agonists are the main cause of side effects; cabergoline would be better tolerated due to its long half-life and relatively steady plasma concentration.[18]

Quinagolide has also shown better tolerability compared with bromocriptine. In a double-blind comparative study of 47 hyperprolactinemic patients, quinagolide was tolerated by 90% of patients versus 75% of patients treated with bromocriptine.[20] As with the other dopamine agonists, the most frequent side effects include nausea, vomiting, headache, and dizziness. These effects are transient and occur within the first few days of starting therapy or during dose adjustments.[18]

Dopamine Agonists and Valvular Heart Disease

Recently, the safety of dopamine agonists has been brought into question after two large population-based studies showed an increased risk of cardiac valvular disease in Parkinson's disease patients being treated with high doses of these drugs, and particularly cabergoline and pergolide.[21, 22] It is now recognized that one of the "off target" effects of dopamine agonists is activation of the serotonin (5-HT) receptor, of which there are 7 distinct subtypes.[23] High concentrations of the subtype 5-HT2B receptor are found on cardiac valves and the pulmonary arteries.[23] Both pergolide and cabergoline have been implicated in the development of cardiac valvular fibrosis because of their agonist effects at the 5-HT2B receptor.[23] Bromocriptine, which is only a partial agonist at the 5-HT2BR, had until recently not been thought to pose an increased risk of cardiac valvular disease, as there had only been a single case report suggesting an association.[23] However, a recent prospective study suggests that bromocriptine may, in fact, be equally associated with the development of cardiac valvulopathy at high cumulative doses.[24]

Several studies have recently examined the effect of cabergoline on cardiac valvular disease in patients with prolactinomas.[25] These patients typically receive much lower doses (10–20 times less) than in Parkinson's disease. Only one of seven studies available to date showed an association between cabergoline use and valvular regurgitation. In this study, there was an increased risk of moderate tricuspid regurgitation in patients who had received cumulative cabergoline doses greater than 280 mg.[26] However, in another study, patients receiving cabergoline (0.25–4 mg/wk) for 3 to 4 years (mean cumulative dose of 311 mg), had no increased

prevalence of clinically significant valvular heart disease.[16] Even in patients treated with cabergoline for 8 years who received cumulative doses as high as 1728 mg, there was no increased risk of clinically relevant heart disease.[28]

Therefore, conventional doses of cabergoline used to treat prolactinoma patients do not currently appear to pose an increased risk of cardiac valvular disease. However, until larger prospective studies clarify the issue, it may be prudent to monitor patients requiring higher doses of cabergoline (>2 or 3 mg/wk) with serial echocardiograms. If valvulopathy develops, it may be reasonable to switch to bromocriptine. Alternatively, surgical resection may be appropriate. This issue underscores the importance of using the smallest effective dose and attempting withdrawal from cabergoline treatment in patients who achieve normalization of prolactin levels and significant tumor shrinkage to minimize their cumulative lifetime exposure to the drug.[25]

Dopamine Agonists and Pregnancy

Two principal considerations arise in the management of women with prolactinomas who either desire fertility or who become pregnant: (1) the risk of tumor growth due to physiologic stimulation of tumoral lactotrophs induced by pregnancy, and (2) the effects of dopamine agonists on fetal development. These two considerations should be weighed against each other on an individualized basis, taking into account the size of the patient's initial tumor, response to treatment, and the patient's ability to tolerate side effects of treatment. It has been estimated that the risk for significant tumor enlargement during pregnancy is 1.6% to 5.5% in microprolactinomas and 15.6% to 35.7% in macroprolactinomas.[18]

Generally, discontinuation of dopaminergic therapy is recommended at the time of diagnosis of pregnancy in patients with microadenomas because the risk of tumor growth overall is quite low. Visual field exams should be performed each trimester and the patient should be told to report any new headache pattern or visual disturbances; dopamine agonists should be resumed and titrated up rapidly if there is MRI evidence of significant tumor growth.

For patients with macroadenomas, especially those in close proximity to the optic chiasm or cavernous sinuses, contraception should be encouraged while attempting to reduce the size of the tumor prior to pregnancy. If a patient with a macroprolactinoma becomes pregnant, there are several different therapeutic approaches that can be offered: (1) dopamine agonists may be stopped after conception with neuro-ophthalmological exams performed throughout pregnancy, (2) dopamine agonists may be continued throughout pregnancy, (3) trans-sphenoidal surgery may be performed in later stages of pregnancy if the enlarged tumor does not respond to resumption of dopamine agonists, or (4) delivery if tumor growth cannot be controlled and the pregnancy is advanced enough.[2]

Bromocriptine has conventionally been the drug of choice in women with prolactinomas who desire fertility or who become pregnant. There is substantial evidence showing that exposure to bromocriptine at the time of conception does not cause birth defects or increase the risk of spontaneous abortions, ectopic pregnancies, trophoblastic disease, or multiple pregnancies.[29] However, evidence is also accumulating to show that cabergoline may have an equally good safety record in terms of pregnancy outcomes.[30] A recent 12-year prospective study of cabergoline use in 329 pregnancies showed no increased risk of miscarriage or fetal malformation.[30]

Dopamine Agonist Resistance

A subset of patients with prolactin-secreting pituitary tumors demonstrate "biochemical" resistance (failure to normalize prolactin levels) or "mass" resistance (absence of tumor shrinkage) to dopamine agonists.[2] Resistance to dopamine agonists occurs in both micro and macro-adenomas and is believed to be mediated by the downregulation of pituitary D2 receptors.[31] Biochemical resistance has been estimated to occur in approximately 10% to 20% of patients on dopamine agonists. Mass resistance has been estimated to occur in approximately 30% to 40% and 15% of patients to bromocriptine and cabergoline, respectively.[2, 31] The prevalence of resistance to quinagolide is unclear given the lack of data regarding its use in dopamine-agonist naïve patients.[6]

Most tumors resistant to bromocriptine will respond to cabergoline. When switched to cabergoline, 85% of patients resistant to bromocriptine and quinagolide achieved normal prolactin levels, and 70% had some change in tumor size.[32] A recent large study showed that cabergoline normalized prolactin levels in 61% and 50% of bromocriptine-resistant microprolactinomas and macroprolactinomas, respectively.[11]

Therapeutic options in the management of dopamine-resistant prolactinomas include (1) increasing the dose of the dopamine agonist, (2) switching to an alternative dopamine agonist, (3) trans-sphenoidal surgery, and (4) radiation therapy. In most cases, the resistance to dopamine agonist is partial, and a response can be achieved by progressively increasing the dose of the drug. A recent study showed that in more than 95% of patients resistant to bromocriptine prolactin normalized with individualized high-dose cabergoline treatment (mean dose 5.2 mg/wk).[8] Bromocriptine-resistant patients generally require higher doses of cabergoline and have less tumor shrinkage compared to treatment-naïve patients.[33] In general, switching from cabergoline to bromocriptine is unlikely to be efficacious.

While trans-sphenoidal surgery is never a first-line treatment for macroprolactinomas, it remains an important option for patients who cannot tolerate dopamine agonists or when medical therapy is ineffective at controlling symptoms or restoring reproductive function. There is little long-term outcome data regarding patients with macroprolactinomas treated with dopamine agonists who subsequently proceed to surgery. In a recent study of 72 patients, 35% of patients required trans-sphenoidal surgery due to resistance and/or intolerance of dopamine agonists.[34] This study, which an outlier given the disproportionately high number of dopamine agonist resistant patients, showed that additional tumor shrinkage was achieved in 57% of operated patients, while only 22% were able to attain normoprolactinemia without dopamine agonists following surgery.[34] Surgery was associated with a high incidence of hypopituitarism regardless of whether patients received subsequent radiotherapy.[35] The remission rate for surgery when used as second-line treatment for prolactinomas is quite low (around 22%). As opposed to its curative role in the other

secretory macroadenomas, surgery plays only a "debulking" role in macroprolactinomas, and therefore should be reserved for patients who, despite maximal medical therapy, have progressive tumor enlargement and are at risk of visual compromise or neurological deficits.[35]

Conventional fractionated radiation therapy should be considered a last-line option in the management of dopamine-resistant prolactinomas given the delayed treatment effects and the high rate of panhypopituitarism. On the other hand, radiosurgery may be an effective treatment in secretory pituitary adenomas, with a lower risk of long-term hypopituitarism.[36]

Dopamine Agonist Withdrawal

The optimal duration of therapy for patients with prolactinomas is uncertain. Until recently, dopamine agonist treatment had been considered a "lifelong" requirement. However, after a landmark study by Colao et al. demonstrated disease remission in a considerable proportion of patients following withdrawal from cabergoline, attention shifted towards defining selection criteria for withdrawal and identifying predictors of long-term remission.[12, 37] Defining the optimal timing and appropriate candidates for withdrawal is difficult because of the heterogeneity of studies that have examined this issue, which differ with respect to the causes of hyperprolactinemia (idiopathic vs. micro/macroprolactinoma), the type and duration of dopamine agonist treatment, and the treatment prior to the start of dopamine agonist therapy.[38] Despite the inherent difficulty in extrapolating from these disparate studies, the Pituitary Society has proposed certain criteria for withdrawal, including (1) normoprolactinemia and (2) tumor absence or markedly reduced tumor volume after a minimum of 1 to 3 years of dopamine agonist treatment.[39] A recent study tested the applicability of these criteria and found a recurrence rate of 54% after withdrawal of long-term cabergoline treatment.[13] In this study, most patients had recurrence of disease within 1 year of discontinuation, and a similar recurrence rate (52% vs. 55%) was seen in patients with microprolactinomas and macroprolactinomas.[13] The size of the tumor remnant prior to withdrawal appears to be predictive of recurrence risk.[13]

A recent meta-analysis showed that long-term remission occurs in only 21% of patients following dopamine agonist withdrawal.[38] The best chance for a long-term remission is seen in patients treated with cabergoline for more than 2 years, with a mean remission rate around 54%, whereas remission is seen in only 20% of patients withdrawn from bromocriptine.[38] Considering the financial burden, occasional problems with tolerability, and potential risk of valvulopathy with long-term dopamine agonist treatment, it is reasonable to attempt withdrawal in patients who have been on a dopamine agonist (particularly if cabergoline) for 2 years or more.

Acromegaly

GENERAL CONSIDERATIONS

Trans-sphenoidal surgery is currently the first treatment approach in acromegaly when a definitive cure can be expected, as is the case with microadenomas, where cure rates are as high as 80% in the hands of an experienced neurosurgeon.[38] Surgery is also indicated for decompressive

Table 17-5   Drugs Used in Treatment of Acromegaly

Drug	Brand Name	Dosage Forms	Typical Starting Dose	Dosing frequency	Usual effective dose
Octreotide	Sandostatin®	SubQ, IV inj: 0.05 mg/ml; 0.1 mg/ml; 0.2 mg/ml; 0.5 mg/ml; 1 mg/ml	50 µg 3 times/day	Daily	100–200 µg 3 times/day
	Sandostatin LAR®	IM depot inj: 10 mg, 20 mg, 30 mg	20 mg I.M. every 4 wks	Monthly	10–40 mg daily
Lanreotide	Somatuline Depot®	IM inj: 60 mg/0.4 ml, 90 mg/0.4 ml, 120 mg/0.5 ml	90 mg every 4 weeks for 3 months	Monthly	60–120 mg every 4 weeks
Pegvisomant	Somavert®	SubQ inj: 10, 15, 20 mg	40 mg loading dose, followed by 10 mg daily	Daily	Increase by 5-mg increments every 4–6 weeks

subQ, subcutaneous; inj, injection; IM, intramuscular.
Source: Pegvisomant: Drug Information, Octreotide: Drug Information, Lanreotide: Drug Information, Pegvisomant: Drug Information. Available at www.uptodate.com. Waltham, MA: UpToDate; 2009.

purposes in the cases of large tumors that cause chiasmatic compression. Since the biochemical cure rate of macroadenomas following surgery is less than 50% (particularly if extrasellar extension of the tumor is present), many patients will require some form of adjuvant treatment following surgical resection.[40] In addition, medical therapy should be considered as primary approach for patients without vision compromise who either have higher than normal surgical risk or whose tumor is deemed not to be surgically curable.[41] Finally, two recent studies have suggested an increase in surgical cure rate in macroadenomas when they are pretreated for 4 to 6 months with a long-acting somatostatin analog. If confirmed, this may expand the role of these drugs to all macroadenomas before surgical attempt.[42, 43] The estimated benefit of postsurgical radiotherapy is often outweighed by the delayed onset of effects and the risk of panhypopituitarism.

There are three classes of medications used in the treatment of acromegaly, each with different receptor target actions:

1. Somatostatin analogues, octreotide and lanreotide, inhibit somatotroph cell proliferation and GH secretion by binding to the somatostatin receptors on tumoral cells.
2. Dopamine agonists bind to dopamine D2 receptors expressed on both somatotroph and mammotroph cells, exerting negative control.
3. The GH receptor antagonist Pegvisomant blocks the effect of GH. Somatostatin analogues are often considered first-line treatment.

SOMATOSTATIN ANALOGUES: PHARMACOLOGIC ASPECTS

The presently commercially available somatostatin analogues act on two of the five somatostatin receptors existing in nature. The dosing frequencies of the somatostatin analogues are summarized in Table 17-5.

Octreotide was the first available somatostatin analogue. It has a relatively short half-life of 2 hours after subcutaneous injection, which requires a three times daily dosing to maintain therapeutic concentrations. The starting dose is usually 100 to 250 µg three times daily up to a maximum of 1500 µg daily.[40] Nowadays, this formulation has been substituted by octreotide LAR (long-acting release), a long-acting depot formulation administered

as an intramuscular injection every 4 weeks. The starting dose is 20 mg increasing or decreasing by 10 mg increments (maximal dose 40 mg) based on clinical and biochemical response.[40]

Lanreotide SR (sustained release) is a biodegradable polymer microparticle that allows a slow release following subcutaneous injection every 7 to 14 days.[40] Lanreotide autogel is a longer-acting depot formulation that allows for injections every 28 days.[40] In the United States, only the latter formulation is available.

SOMATOSTATIN ANALOGUES: THERAPEUTIC EFFICACY

Somatostatin analogues are 40% to 60% effective at achieving biochemical control. Improvements in acromegaly symptoms generally correlate with the degree of IGF-1 reduction. In terms of tumor shrinkage, these drugs are 50% to 75% effective at reducing tumor size when used as primary treatment, whereas the effectiveness decreases to around 20% when used as secondary treatment.[40, 44] The degree of tumor shrinkage is by no means as dramatic as the one seen with dopaminergic agents in prolactinomas. The primary treatment efficacy results are comparable to those observed in patients with macroadenomas previously treated by trans-sphenoidal surgery or pituitary irradiation,[45, 46] validating the use of somatostatin analogues as a first-line modality in certain patients.

Biochemical Control

Within the class of somatostatin analogues, prospective studies have shown octreotide LAR to be modestly superior to lanreotide SR both with respect to biochemical normalization and tumor shrinkage, although the reliable interpretation of some of these studies may be compromised by a selection bias as patients were pre-selected according to sensitivity to somatostatin analogues (Fig. 17-2).[47] In patients who had not been selected for somatostatin analogue responsiveness before study entry, octreotide LAR has been found to be 54% and 63% effective at normalizing GH and IGF-1 levels, respectively, whereas the efficacy rate for lanreotide SR is 48% and 42%, respectively.[48] Higher-dose lanreotide SR, at 60 mg every 21 to 28 days, appears to be as effective as octreotide LAR at achieving biochemical normalization when pre-selection bias is not

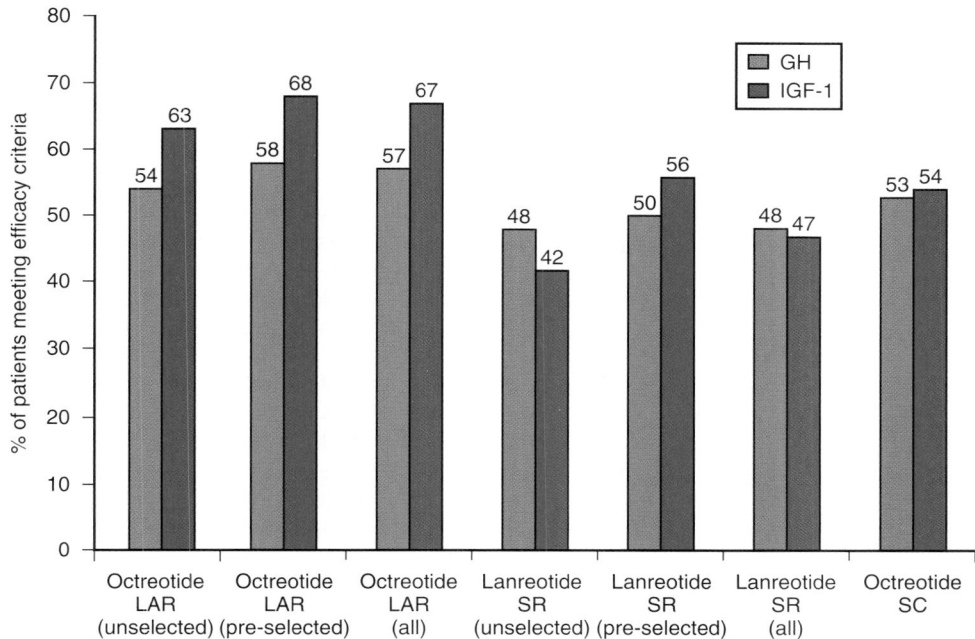

FIGURE 17-2 Biochemical efficacy of somatostatin analogue therapy for acromegaly. Unselected, patients who had not been selected for somatostatin analogue responsiveness before study entry. Preselected, patients who were selected for somatostatin analogue responsiveness before study entry. All, all patients. GH, growth hormone. IGF-1, insulin-like growth factor. LAR, long-acting release. SR, sustained release. SC, subcutaneous. (Data from Freda PU, Katznelson L, van der Lely AJ, et al. Long-acting somatostatin analog therapy of acromegaly: AA meta-analysis. J Clin Endocrinol Metab. 2005;90:4465-4473.)

Table 17-6	Efficacy of Long-Acting Somatostatin Analogues in Treatment of Acromegaly			
Somatostatin Analogue	**References**	**GH ≤ 2.5 µg/l (%)**	**IGF-1 Normalization (%)**	**Tumor Shrinkage >20% (%)**
Octreotide LAR 10–40 mg q28d	43, 46, 102–123	57 (648/1139)	58 (644/1115)	62 (273/439)
Lanreotide SR 30 mg q7/10/14d	108, 112, 119, 123–127	33* (134/411)	49 (202/411)	29 (45/153)
Lanreotide SR 60 mg q21/28d	128–130	61 (73/120)	60 (72/120)	43 (33/77)
Lanreotide autogel 60, 90, 120 mg q28d	50-52, 131–138	59 (331/559)	47 (262/559)	75 (36/48)
All treatments combined		53 (1186/2229)	54 (1180/2205)	54 (387/717)

Note: Percentages derived from calculation of weighted mean percent (sum of responders/sum of participants studied for given outcome). Data include the use of somatostatin analogues as both primary and secondary treatment, and both unselected and preselected (known sensitivity to somatostatin analogues) patients.
*One trial of 112 patients had GH cut-off of ≤3.0 mg/l.

taken into account (Table 17-6). The depot formulation lanreotide autogel also appears to be as effective as octreotide LAR at lowering GH and IGF-1 levels, even though there is only a single randomized trial comparing the two drugs.[49-55] Recent studies suggest that lanreotide autogel may be effective at tumor shrinkage in as many as 75% of patients (Table 17-6). The lanreotide autogel preparation has the advantage of being self- or partner-administered at home avoiding the need of monthly traveling to the doctor's office.[56] The relative efficacies of the somatostatin analogues are shown in Fig. 17-3.

Tumor Shrinkage

The effects on tumor size have been shown to be slightly higher in naïve patients.[47] A recent meta-analysis including treatment naïve and previously operated patients showed that 33% of patients treated with lanreotide SR or autogel experienced a variable tumor shrinkage (ranging from 10% to 77%).[44] In three studies that included groups of treatment naïve patients, Lanreotide Autogel induced tumor shrinkage

in 71% to 77% of patients.[44] Thus far, the only predictor of response to tumor shrinkage appears to be the timing of somatostatin analogue therapy (primary vs. secondary), and data are conflicting with respect to other variables such as tumor size (micro. vs. macroadenoma), biochemical responsiveness, or dose of somatostatin analogues.

SOMATOSTATIN ANALOGUES: PRIMARY VERSUS SECONDARY THERAPY

Weighing the relative merits of surgical and medical treatment in acromegaly has proven to be difficult. The first randomized trial of medical treatment versus surgery showed a comparable success rate between octreotide LAR and trans-sphenoidal surgery, with both groups showing significant (>20%) shrinkage and similar biochemical response.[57] Although this study was not powered to show superiority of medical vs. surgical treatment, it suggests that medical therapy may be used safely in patients who are not surgical candidates. Another argument for primary somatostatin treatment is the potential beneficial effect of pre-surgical treatment on surgical cure. Two recent prospective studies suggest that pre-operative treatment with somatostatin analogues may improve the chance of surgical cure in patients with macroadenomas.[42, 43] Finally, the potential for reduced perioperative cardiovascular complications due to GH excess may be another reason to consider pre-operative somatostatin treatment.[58] A general approach to the treatment of acromegaly is shown in Fig. 17-4.

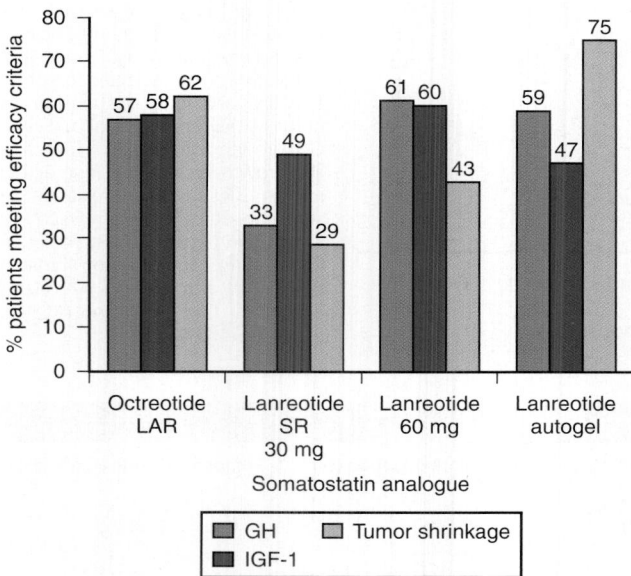

FIGURE 17-3 Efficacy of long-acting somatostatin analogues in acromegaly (data derived from Table 17-6). Studies include both preselected (sensitive to somatostatin therapy) and unselected (somatostatin analogue naive) patients, and combined primary (without surgical intervention) and secondary (following surgery or radiation) treatment outcome data. Efficacy criteria include GH ≤ 2.5 mg/l, IGF-1 normalization, and tumor volume reduction greater than 20%. LAR, long-acting release; SR, sustained release.

SOMATOSTATIN ANALOGUES: TOLERABILITY AND SIDE EFFECTS

Somatostatin analogues are generally well tolerated. The most common side effects are gastrointestinal symptoms, such as abdominal cramps, flatulence, diarrhea or constipation, and nausea (Table 17-7).[59] Biliary tract abnormalities, such as gallstones, sediment and sludge, and dilatation, are fairly common, occurring in as many as 50% of patients during the first 2 years of treatment, although they tend not to progress thereafter.[59] Local skin irritation and pain at the injection site is mild and usually dose-dependent. Rarely, patients who require frequent injections or who are treated for long duration (i.e., metastatic carcinoid) may develop subcutaneous nodules in the gluteal area, believed to be a granulomatous reaction to the drug.[60] Sinus bradycardia and conduction abnormalities have been described in 10% to 25% of patients, and medications that prolong the QT interval should not be used with somatostatin analogues.[59] Impairment of pancreatic insulin secretion by somatostatin analogues may result in mild hyperglycemia, particularly in patients who have pre-existing glucose intolerance, although a clear diabetogenic effect of these medications has not been found.[61] Data on the safety of somatostatin analogues during pregnancy are scarce, but there are case reports of octreotide LAR use in pregnant acromegalic women resulting in uneventful pregnancies and healthy babies.[62]

DOPAMINE AGONISTS IN ACROMEGALY: THERAPEUTIC EFFICACY

As monotherapy, dopamine agonists have a limited role in acromegaly given their inferior efficacy compared with somatostatin analogues. Bromocriptine is only 15% effective at normalizing GH levels when used in high doses in acromegalic patients.[40] Initial studies with cabergoline as primary treatment in acromegaly showed biochemical efficacy of 27% to 39% and suggested a higher likelihood of success in pituitary tumors that co-secrete GH and prolactin.[63, 64]

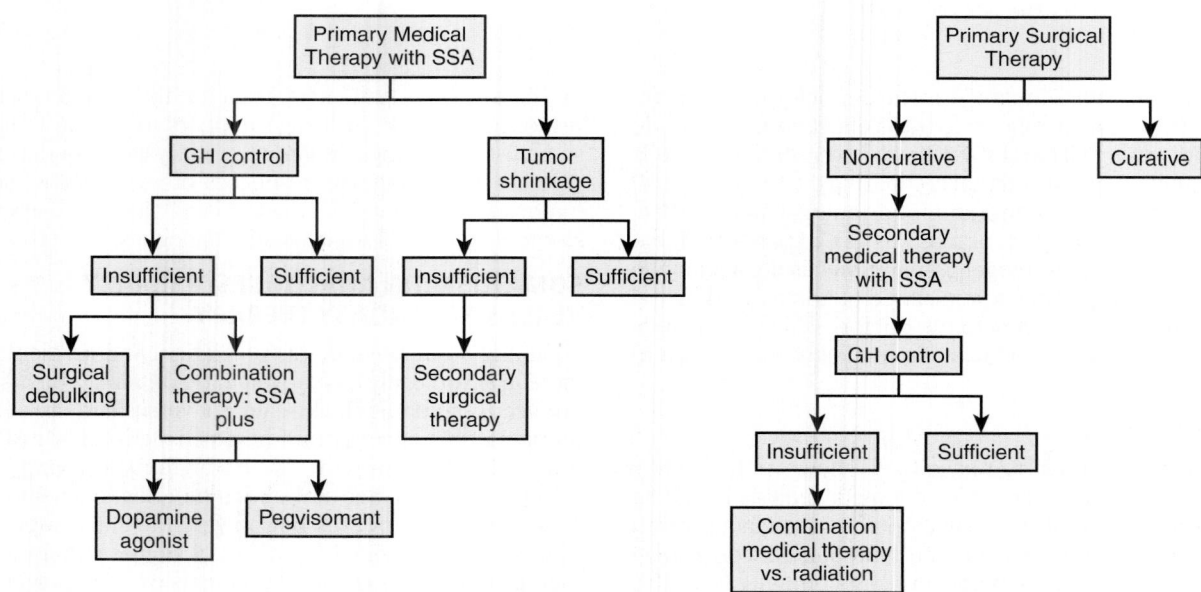

FIGURE 17-4 Approach to the treatment of acromegaly. SSA, somatostatin analogue; GH, growth hormone. (Adapted from Feelders RA, Hofland LJ, van Aken MO, et al. Medical therapy of acromegaly: efficacy and safety of somatostatin analogues. Drugs. 2009;69:2207-2226.)

Table 17-7 Common Side Effects of Somatostatin Analogues

Gastrointestinal (common)
Nausea
Flatulence
Abdominal cramps
Diarrhea
Constipation
Nausea
Gallbladder abnormalities (sediment, sludge, microlithiasis, gallstones)
Dermatologic
Local injection site irritation and pain
Cardiovascular
Asymptomatic sinus bradycardia
Conduction abnormalities
Endocrinologic
Impaired glucose tolerance
Hyperglycemia
Hypoglycemia (rarely)

Table 17-8 Common Side Effects of Pegvisomant

Gastrointestinal
Hepatic impairment
Diarrhea
Nausea
Dermatologic
Injection site pain or skin irritation
Infection
Cardiovascular
Hypertension
Chest pain
Peripheral edema
Neurologic
Dizziness
Risk of progressive pituitary tumor growth

Interestingly, however, recent studies show that neither basal prolactin concentrations nor co-immunostaining of GH and prolactin predicts a more favorable response.[65, 66] Instead, prior radiotherapy appears to be associated with an enhanced efficacy of GH response to dopamine agonists compared with somatostatin analogues.[65] In general, dopamine agonists are reserved as adjuvant treatment to optimize medical therapy in partially somatostatin-resistant acromegalic patients; in these patients, the addition of cabergoline to a somatostatin analogue normalized IGF-1 levels in 42% of cases.[66]

PEGVISOMANT: PHARMACOLOGIC ASPECTS

Pegvisomant, a genetically engineered GH analogue, is a competitive inhibitor acting at the receptor level that prevents that action of native GH. The drug is administered as a subcutaneous injection, with an initial loading dose of 40 mg, followed by an initial dose of 10 mg daily (Table 17-5). Since pegvisomant typically causes elevations in serum GH levels, only serum IGF-1 levels can be used as markers of effective dose response. Doses are adjusted by 5 mg increments at 4- to 6-week intervals according to IGF-1 levels.

PEGVISOMANT: THERAPEUTIC EFFICACY

Pegvisomant was found in initial trails to be highly effective at normalizing IGF-1 levels (90%–97% patients) and controlling acromegalic symptoms; however, because of its mechanism of action at the peripheral level, this drug does not reduce tumor size or GH levels.[67] A large post-marketing study has placed it efficacy in IGF-1 normalization at 70%, possibly in part due to failure of dose titration.[68]

PEGVISOMANT: TOLERABILITY AND SIDE EFFECTS

Pegvisomant is usually well tolerated, with the most common side effects listed in Table 17-8. The main concern is the risk of liver damage, with up to 9% of patients reported to have elevated transaminases, sometimes as high as 8-10 times the upper limit of normal.[40] Liver function tests should be assessed before treatment and monthly for the first 6 months of treatment, quarterly for the next 6 months, and biannually the following year.[69]

Whether pegvisomant poses an increased risk of tumor growth via blockage of negative feedback by IGF-1 on the pituitary gland is uncertain. A 5-year observational study found a risk of tumor growth in 5% of patients treated with pegvisomant, which is higher than the expected 2.2% risk of continuous tumor progression during somatostatin analogue treatment.[70] Another 5-year observational study found a 2.8% incidence of increased tumor growth, which appears reassuring; however this study had a lower biochemical normalization rate raising the possibility that the lower rate of tumor growth may be influenced by failure to titrate to therapeutic dose ranges.[68] Given the uncertainty about tumor growth related to pegvisomant, it is recommended that patients on this drug be followed with serial MRI studies every 6 months.[40]

In acromegalic patients who are partially resistant to treatment with somatostatin analogues alone, the addition of once weekly subcutaneous pegvisomant injections normalized IGF-1 concentrations in 90% to 95% of cases.[71] This reduced frequency dosing offers a financial advantage in patients who might otherwise require high-dose pegvisomant monotherapy. Combination therapy with pegvisomant is currently reserved for those patients who achieve insufficient control after somatostatin therapy and surgical treatment.

EMERGING THERAPIES IN ACROMEGALY

Pasireotide (SOM230), a novel somatostatin analogue with affinity for multiple somatostatin receptor subtypes is a promising emerging therapy for acromegaly. Initial studies have shown this drug to be as effective as the currently available somatostatin analogues.[72] The effect on IGF-1 levels by pasireotide appears to be more sustained compared with octreotide, suggesting a longer half-life.[72] Further long-term studies examining the effect on tumor shrinkage and sustained biochemical response are presently under way to determine whether pasireotide is a reasonable chronic treatment option in acromegaly. In addition, a newer chimeric molecule, BIM-23A387, directed towards both somatostatin and dopamine receptors, may offer improved efficacy in acromegaly due to its proposed synergistic receptor activation.[73]

Cushing's Disease

GENERAL CONSIDERATIONS

Trans-sphenoidal surgery is the definitive treatment in Cushing's disease; in the hands of an experienced neurosurgeon, the cure rate of ACTH-secreting pituitary microadenomas is high.[74] However, approximately 10% to 30% of patients will not be cured and will require some form of adjuvant treatment, including conventional radiotherapy, stereotactic radiosurgery, medical therapy, and bilateral adrenalectomy.[75] This subset of patients with refractory or residual Cushing's disease poses a significant management challenge, as each of these secondary therapeutic options carries adverse risks. These patients are best managed in a multidisciplinary setting, such as in dedicated pituitary centers, where there is close collaboration between experienced neurosurgeons, endocrinologists, and radiation therapists.

Criteria for Cure and Remission

A step-wise approach should be taken in the postoperative evaluation of Cushing's disease patients to assess their response to surgery.[75] An expert consensus statement published in 2008 recommends assessment of remission by measurement of morning serum cortisol during the first postoperative week, either by withholding exogenous glucocorticoids or by using low dose dexamethasone testing.[76] Given the likelihood of central adrenal insufficiency in patients who are surgically cured, close monitoring for signs of hypoadrenalism is necessary if glucocorticoid treatment is not empirically initiated following surgery. Persistent postoperative morning serum cortisol levels of less than 2 µg/dl are associated with remission, and a 10-year recurrence rate of approximately 10%.[76] A persistent serum cortisol level above 5 µg/dl at 6 weeks following surgery requires evaluation for persistent hypercortisolemia. Biochemical evidence of pathologic ACTH hypersecretion following surgery may be indicated by repeatedly elevated urine free cortisol levels, abnormal diurnal variation patterns in serum or salivary cortisol levels, or an abnormal cortisol response to dexamethasone suppression.

Persistent Disease after Surgery

Once the diagnosis of residual (or recurrent) Cushing's disease is confirmed, treatment options should be considered in the context of the individual patient. Repeating trans-sphenoidal surgery should be considered in most patients, especially those with accessible tumor visible on MRI. Cure rates for repeated surgery range from approximately 40% to 70%.[75] The main risk associated with repeated surgery is the development of hypopituitarism. Conventional radiotherapy may not be effective until months to years following treatment, which is often not acceptable in a patient with persistent, severe hypercortisolemia. Single-treatment stereotactic radiosurgery offers the advantage of minimized radiation to normal pituitary or adjacent structures, and has been reported to have a remission rate of 50%.[36] A recent study using stereotactic radiosurgery as either primary or adjuvant therapy in the treatment of secretory pituitary adenomas (acromegaly, Cushing's disease, prolactinomas)

found a 23% incidence of hypopituitarism at 4- to 8-year follow-up.[36]

Medical therapy is generally a temporizing measure in patients with residual Cushing's disease. The goal of medical therapy is to attain control of hypercortisolemia and thereby minimize the associated negative health consequences (hypertension, hyperglycemia, gastrointestinal ulcerations, infection, osteoporosis, etc.) of patients awaiting the therapeutic effects of radiation treatment or planning to undergo repeat surgery. Medications used to treat hypercortisolemia include inhibitors of adrenal steroid production, such as ketoconazole and metyrapone, and mitotane, an adrenolytic agent. Although these medications may be highly effective in the control of hypercortisolemia, they have no effect on tumor size and do not restore the normal function of the hypothalamic-pituitary-adrenal axis.

ADRENAL INHIBITORS: PHARMACOLOGIC ASPECTS, THERAPEUTIC EFFICACY, AND SIDE EFFECTS

Ketoconazole is the first-line drug used to lower cortisol levels in Cushing's disease patients. This oral antifungal agent, at higher doses, blocks cortisol production by inhibiting two enzymes in the glucocorticoid synthesis pathway, 17 alpha-hydroxylase and 17,20 lyase.[67] Typical starting doses are 200 mg twice daily, titrated up to a maximal dose of 400 mg four times daily based on serum cortisol levels and 24-hour urine free cortisol levels.[67] Although remission rates on ketoconazole have been reported in 25% to 76% of patients, the medication is generally poorly tolerated, and carries a high risk of hepatitis at the chronically high doses often required to treat hypercortisolemia.[67] Hepatitis occurs in as many as 12% of patients and therefore close monitoring of liver function tests is required. The increased risk of hypogonadism in men may be a reason to consider metyrapone as an alternative in this patient population. In order to be absorbed, ketoconazole requires low gastric pH. Absorption is therefore reduced in patients with achlorhydria or on proton pump inhibitors or H2 blockers. The use of acidic drinks such as coca cola improves absorption of the drug.[77]

Although no longer commercially available in the United States, metyrapone can be provided on a compassionate basis by contacting the manufacturer (Novartis) directly.[76] This drug, which works by blocking the final step in cortisol synthesis, is 80% effective at controlling hypercortisolemia.[78] Cortisol suppression can be maintained chronically with doses of 500 to 2000 mg/day.[79] Nausea, vomiting, and dizziness may occur with metyrapone, possibly due to sudden cortisol withdrawal and relative adrenal insufficiency.[79] Another adverse side effect is acne and hirsutism (in women), which results from shunting of steroidogenic precursors towards the androgen pathway. This side effect may be a reason to favor ketoconazole in female patients.

Mitotane, a cytotoxic drug primarily used in the treatment of patients with adrenocortical carcinoma, can be used at lower doses to control hypercortisolemia. The mechanism of the adrenolytic effect is postulated to involve covalent

Table 17-9	Drugs Used in Treatment of Refractory Cushing's Disease			
Drug	**Dosage Form**	**Typical Starting Dose**	**Maximum Dosage**	**Side Effects (Frequencies Reported When Available)**
Ketoconazole	Tablet: 200 mg	200 mg twice daily	400 mg 3 times daily	1%–10% Pruritis (2%) Nausea (3%–10%) Vomiting (3%–10%) Abdominal pain (1%) <1% Diarrhea Fever Headache Gynecomastia Hemolytic anemia Hepatotoxicity Hypogonadism/impotence Leukopenia Thrombocytopenia Somnolence
Metyrapone	Capsule: 250 mg	250 mg four times daily	1500 mg four times daily	CNS: Headache, dizziness, sedation Allergic rash Nausea, vomiting, abdominal discomfort pain Bone marrow suppression (rare)
Mitotane	Tablet: 500 mg	500 mg three times daily	3000 mg three times daily	CNS depression (32%) Lethargy/somnolence (25%) Dizziness/vertigo (15%) Skin rash (15%) Anorexia (25%) Nausea (39%) Vomiting (37%) Diarrhea (13%) Weakness (12%) Headache (5%) Confusion (3%) Muscle tremor (3%)
Etomidate	Injection 2 mg/ml	Bolus of 0.03 mg/kg IV	Infusion of 0.1 mg/kg/hr	>10% Nausea Pain at injection site Myoclonus 1%–10% Hiccups <1% Apnea Arrhythmia Bradycardia/tachycardia Hypertension Hyper/hypoventilation Laryngospasm

Sources: Biller BM, Grossman AB, Stewart PM, et al. Treatment of adrenocorticotropin-dependent Cushing's syndrome: A consensus statement. J Clin Endocrinol Metab. 2008;93:2454-2462; Ketoconazole: Drug Information, Metyrapone: Drug Information, Mitotane: Drug Information, Etomidate: Drug Information. Available at www.uptodate.com. Waltham, MA: UpToDate;2009.

binding to target proteins within adrenal cells resulting in oxidative damage and adrenal cortical atrophy.[79] Typical therapeutic doses range from 2 to 4 g, with the maximum daily dose of 9 g.[76] The main drawbacks to this medication are its slow onset of action (weeks to months) and poor tolerability due to gastrointestinal and central nervous system side effects. Careful monitoring of drug and cortisol levels is required.[76]

Intravenous etomidate therapy is reserved for situations where rapid control of cortisol levels is required and there are barriers to oral therapy.[76] The drug lowers cortisol and aldosterone levels by blocking 11-β-hydroxylase. Short-term continuous infusions of etomidate reduce serum cortisol in 11 to 24 hours.[79]

The pharmacologic aspects and side effects of the adrenal inhibitors[76,139] are summarized in Table 17-9.

EXPERIMENTAL TREATMENTS IN CUSHING'S DISEASE

There are currently no medical therapies that are effective at shrinking ACTH-secreting pituitary tumors, and many tumor-targeted drugs are being investigated. The dopamine receptors, D2 and D4, are expressed in about 75% of ACTH-pituitary adenomas, making dopamine agonists appealing experimental agents. Cabergoline may be partially effective in controlling the hypercortisolemia in patients with Cushing's disease, but the long-term efficacy and the effects on tumor shrinkage remain to be seen.[80] The newer somatostatin analogue, pasireotide (SOM230), has been shown to reduce ACTH secretion in vitro; early clinical studies show promising results in patients with de novo, persistent, or recurrent Cushing's disease.[81] Studies of patients with ectopic ACTH syndrome suggest that the combination of somatostatin analogues and dopamine agonists may offer additional therapeutic benefit in patients with pituitary-dependent Cushing's disease.[10]

TSH-Secreting Pituitary Adenomas

TSH-secreting pituitary adenomas are exceedingly rare. The goals of therapy include tumor removal and restoration of the euthyroid state. While trans-sphenoidal surgery is the first approach, because most patients are diagnosed when adenomas are macros, the reported cure rate is only around 38%.[82] For those patients who do not achieve surgical remission, adjuvant medical therapy offers promising results. Medical treatment relies mainly on the use of somatostatin analogues, which inhibit thyrotroph cell growth by binding to the somatostatin receptor found on both normal pituitary and tumoral cells. Octreotide is 90% effective at normalizing thyroid hormone levels and 50% effective at reducing tumor size.[10] As with growth-hormone secreting tumors, there is evidence that pre-surgical treatment with somatostatin analogues may impact the ease of surgical removal.[83] Typically, the doses of somatostatin analogues required to normalize TSH levels are lower than the doses used in the treatment of GH-secreting tumors: octreotide SC (300 mg/day), lanreotide SR (30 mg every 14 days), and octreotide LAR (10 mg/day).[10] However, due to the rarity of this disease, it is difficult to make generalizations about dose requirements, so each patient's response and tolerance to somatostatin therapy should be considered individually.

Clinically Nonfunctioning Pituitary Tumors

Nonfunctioning pituitary tumors are usually not amenable to medical treatment. However, because the absence of hormonal hypersecretion frequently leads to a delayed diagnosis, complete surgical cure may not always be possible due to the large size of these tumors at presentation. Radiotherapy may be offered to prevent tumor regrowth. Recently, medical treatment with dopamine agonists, somatostatin analogues, or a combination of the two has been explored as adjuvant treatment in nonfunctioning tumors. Treatment with these drugs relies on the fact that many nonfunctioning adenomas express dopamine and somatostatin receptors. Improvements in visual field were seen in 20% and 32% of tumors treated with dopamine agonists and somatostatin analogues, respectively; tumor shrinkage was seen in 28% and 5%, respectively.[84] Larger controlled trials are still needed to determine the effectiveness of medical therapy in this tumor type.

KEY REFERENCES

Beck-Peccoz P, Persani L. Thyrotropinomas. *Endocrinol Metab Clin North Am*. 2008;37:123-134:viii-ix.
Ben-Shlomo A, Melmed S. Acromegaly. *Endocrinol Metab Clin North Am*. 2008;37:101-122:viii.

Blevins Jr LS, Sanai N, Kunwar S, Devin JK. An approach to the management of patients with residual Cushing's disease. *J Neurooncol*. 2009 Sep;94(3):313-319.
Brue T. ACROSTUDY: Status update on 469 patients. *Horm Res*. 2009 Jan;71(Suppl 1):34-38.
Carlsen SM, Lund-Johansen M, Schreiner T, et al. Preoperative octreotide treatment in newly diagnosed acromegalic patients with macroadenomas increases cure short-term postoperative rates: a prospective, randomized trial. *J Clin Endocrinol Metab*. 2008 Aug;93(8):2984-2990.
Casanueva FF, Molitch ME, Schlechte JA, et al. Guidelines of the Pituitary Society for the diagnosis and management of prolactinomas. *Clin Endocrinol (Oxf)*. 2006 Aug;65(2):265-273.
Chanson P, Boerlin V, Ajzenberg C, et al. Comparison of octreotide acetate LAR and lanreotide SR in patients with acromegaly. *Clin Endocrinol (Oxf)*. 2000 Nov;53(5):577-586.
Colao A, Pivonello R, Di Somma C, et al. Medical therapy of pituitary adenomas: effects on tumor shrinkage. *Rev Endocr Metab Disord*. 2009 Jun;10(2):111-123.
Dekkers OM, Lagro J, Burman P, et al. Recurrence of hyperprolactinemia after withdrawal of dopamine agonists: systematic review and meta-analysis. *J Clin Endocrinol Metab*. 2010;95:43-51.
Freda PU, Katznelson L, van der Lely AJ, et al. Long-acting somatostatin analog therapy of acromegaly: a meta-analysis. *J Clin Endocrinol Metab*. 2005 Aug;90(8):4465-4473.
Kharlip J, Salvatori R, Yenokyan G, Wand GS. Recurrence of hyperprolactinemia after withdrawal of long-term cabergoline therapy. *J Clin Endocrinol Metab*. 2009 Jul;94(7):2428-2436.
Maiza JC, Vezzosi D, Matta M, et al. Long-term (up to 18 years) effects on GH/IGF-1 hypersecretion and tumour size of primary somatostatin analogue (SSTa) therapy in patients with GH-secreting pituitary adenoma responsive to SSTa. *Clin Endocrinol (Oxf)*. 2007 Aug;67(2):282-289.
Mancini T, Casanueva FF, Giustina A. Hyperprolactinemia and prolactinomas. *Endocrinol Metab Clin North Am*. 2008 Mar;37(1):67-99:viii.
Mao ZG, Zhu YH, Tang HL, et al. Preoperative lanreotide treatment in acromegalic patients with macroadenomas increases short-term postoperative cure rates: a prospective, randomised trial. *Eur J Endocrinol*. 2010 Apr;162(4):661-666.
Mazziotti G, Giustina A. Effects of lanreotide SR and Autogel on tumor mass in patients with acromegaly: a systematic review. *Pituitary*. 2010;13(1):60-67.
Molitch ME. Pituitary disorders during pregnancy. *Endocrinol Metab Clin North Am*. 2006 Mar;35(1):99-116:vi.
Ono M, Miki N, Kawamata T, et al. Prospective study of high-dose cabergoline treatment of prolactinomas in 150 patients. *J Clin Endocrinol Metab*. 2008 Dec;93(12):4721-4727.
Pascal-Vigneron V, Weryha G, Bosc M, Leclere J. [Hyperprolactinemic amenorrhea: treatment with cabergoline versus bromocriptine. Results of a national multicenter randomized double-blind study]. *Presse Med*. 1995 Apr 29;24(16):753-757.
Schteingart DE. Drugs in the medical treatment of Cushing's syndrome. *Expert Opin Emerg Drugs*. 2009 Dec;14(4):661-671.
Valassi E, Klibanski A, Biller BM. Clinical review: potential cardiac valve effects of dopamine agonists in hyperprolactinemia. *J Clin Endocrinol Metab*. 2010 Mar;95(3):1025-1033.
Vilar L, Freitas MC, Naves LA, et al. Diagnosis and management of hyperprolactinemia: results of a Brazilian multicenter study with 1234 patients. *J Endocrinol Invest*. 2008 May;31(5):436-444.
Webster J, Piscitelli G, Polli A, et al. A comparison of cabergoline and bromocriptine in the treatment of hyperprolactinemic amenorrhea. Cabergoline Comparative Study Group. *N Engl J Med*. 1994 Oct 6;331(14):904-909.

Numbered references appear on Expert Consult.

CHAPTER 18

Growth Hormone–Secreting Tumors

CARRIE R. MUH • ADRIANA G. IOACHIMESCU • NELSON M. OYESIKU

Hypersecretion of growth hormone (GH) from a functioning pituitary tumor before the closure of the epiphyseal plates of long bones results in gigantism, while hypersecretion after closure leads to acromegaly.

Phenotypic features of acromegaly include acral enlargement; coarse facial features with frontal bossing, prognathism, diastema and macroglossia; skin thickening, hypertrichosis, malodorous hyperhidrosis, and acanthosis nigricans; and deepening of the voice due to laryngeal hypertrophy. Other manifestations include headaches, lethargy, obstructive sleep apnea, peripheral neuropathies such as carpal tunnel syndrome, and bony deformation including bone thickening and vertebral osteophyte formation. Other consequences include abnormal carbohydrate metabolism and diabetes mellitus; cardiovascular diseases including hypertension, atherosclerosis, and cardiomyopathy; and an increased risk of other neoplasms including colon cancer.[1-6] Patients with acromegaly have a two- to three-fold increase in mortality due to cardiovascular and cerebrovascular diseases. Normalization of GH levels may decrease this risk substantially to levels comparable to the general population.[7,8] Other clinical manifestations are related to mass effect of the pituitary tumor, including headaches, visual loss (classically bitemporal hemianopia), and hormonal deficiencies (hypogonadism, hypothyroidism, and hypoadrenalism).

The disease is insidious, which leads to a delayed diagnosis, often seven to ten years after onset of symptoms.[9] Recently, this lag has shortened significantly, likely due to the increase in magnetic resonance imaging.[10] Patients with acromegaly generally present in the third to fifth decade, and both sexes are affected equally.[11]

The average annual incidence of acromegaly is three to four per million, and the prevalence is 40 to 70 cases per million people.[7,10] The vast majority of cases, 95% to 98%, are due to a GH-secreting pituitary adenoma.[9,10,12] Pituitary adenomas from somatotroph cells may lead to excessive secretion of GH, while adenomas from acidophil stem cells or mammosomatotrophs often secrete both GH and prolactin (PRL).[9,12] Most GH-secreting tumors (75%–80%) are macroadenomas (>1 cm in diameter),[7] and 20% to 50% co-secrete PRL or other pituitary hormones.[13] Rare causes of acromegaly include ectopic GH-secreting tumors such as bronchial carcinoid or pancreatic islet cell tumors; hypothalamic GH-releasing hormone (GHRH)-secreting tumors; exogenous administration of GH; or familial syndromes such as McCune-Albright syndrome, multiple endocrine neoplasia I (MEN-I) or Carney complex.[9]

Growth Hormone

Growth hormone is required for normal growth, and its role is increasingly important after the first year of life, with a GH peak achieved during puberty. GH release is stimulated by GHRH from the hypothalamus, and is inhibited by somatostatin. Pituitary somatotroph cells secrete GH in periodic bursts. GH stimulates the liver's production of somatomedin-C, also known as insulin-like growth factor 1 (IGF-1), which stimulates somatostatin release at the hypothalamus and inhibits GH release at the pituitary.

There is some heterogeneity in GH due to differential splicing and post-translational modification.[14-16] Two main forms of GH are found in the circulation: the 22K form comprises 90% of serum GH, and the 20K form makes up 5%.[16] This heterogeneity may explain differences between levels measured by radioimmunoassays and actual biological activity in some patients.

GH and IGF-1 levels are highest in children and young adults, then decrease with age. In normal subjects, serum GH levels are very low or undetectable during most of the day. GH has a half life of 20 to 30 minutes and is secreted in short pulses, peaking two to seven times each day. GH secretion is increased by sleep, exercise, stress, and hypoglycemia, and decreased by obesity, hyperglycemia, and excess glucocorticoids. IGF-1 has a much longer half-life, between two and 18 hours, and serum levels are significantly more stable throughout the day.

Diagnosis

The evaluation of patients for acromegaly involves multidisciplinary collaboration between neurosurgeons, neuroendocrinologists, neuro-ophthalmologists, and neuro radiologists.

The suspicion of acromegaly is usually based on physical examination, while incidental radiologic detection in patients without typical manifestations is rare. Laboratory testing is needed to prove GH excess, while radiology techniques are used to visualize the tumor (Fig. 18-1). Screening laboratory tests include measurement of basal GH and IGF-1, and laboratory confirmation occurs when GH fails to suppress with oral glucose tolerance testing.

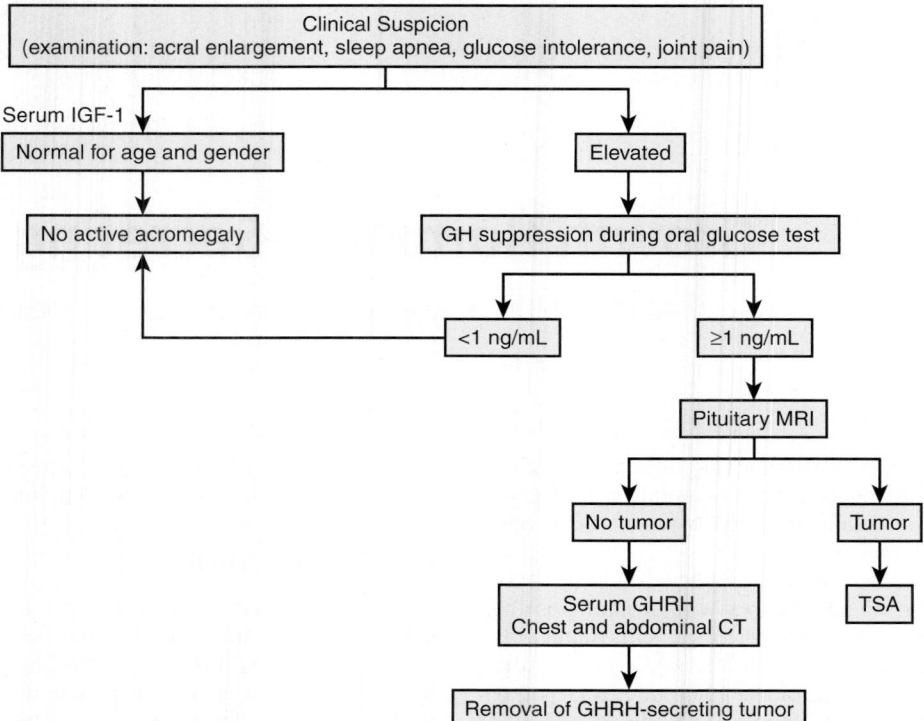

FIGURE 18-1 Algorithm for diagnosis and treatment of acromegaly.

LABORATORY DIAGNOSIS

Random Serum GH Measurement

In healthy subjects, random GH levels are less than 5 ng/ml while most acromegalic patients have levels greater than 10 ng/ml. In active acromegaly, the normal episodic GH pattern is replaced by a constantly elevated GH level throughout the day.[1] However, GH levels fluctuate widely and GH has a short half-life, so some acromegalic patients have normal GH levels on initial testing. Serum GH levels may be elevated in other conditions including uncontrolled diabetes mellitus, renal failure, malnutrition and during physical or emotional stress, even in the absence of acromegaly.[13] Therefore, random GH measurement is not the preferred screening test for acromegaly.

IGF-1 Measurement

Serum IGF-1 measurement is the best single test for screening. The measurement of IGF-1 is used to provide an indicator of the body's overall exposure to GH. Normal ranges for IGF-1 vary between different assays and are age- and gender-dependent.[13] IGF-1 is increased in nearly all acromegalic patients, even those in whom random single GH levels are within the normal range. IGF-1 is also a reliable indicator for post-treatment hormonal remission, as it reflects GH secretion over the prior 24 hours.[4] One of the IGF-1 binding proteins (IGFBPs) can be measured to assist in the diagnosis of acromegaly. The level of IGFBP-3 correlates directly with GH, but the overlap with normal persons limits its use.

GH Suppression to Hyperglycemia

The oral glucose suppression test (75 g) is used to confirm a diagnosis of acromegaly. In a normal control, GH decreases to below 1 ng/ml after a glucose load, whereas in an acromegalic patient, this suppression fails to occur.[17] This test is useful to document biochemical remission after surgical removal of the pituitary tumor,[18] but does not appear to be useful to assess control in patients receiving therapy with somatostatin analogues.[17]

Other Dynamic Tests

Other dynamic tests are rarely needed to diagnose acromegaly. Thyrotropin-releasing hormone (TRH) stimulation leads to a significant increase in GH in untreated acromegalics, although it does not cause a significant change in GH levels in normal subjects. This response may also occur in the setting of liver disease, renal failure, or depression. TRH-stimulation may identify patients who, despite a normal postsurgical GH level, have residual GH-secreting tumor.[19] Administration of oral L-Dopa or bromocriptine, a dopamine agonist, to a fasting normal subject increases GH secretion, though it paradoxically decreases GH levels in a fasting acromegalic patient.[20]

GHRH

GHRH levels should not be routinely used in diagnosis of acromegaly. However, they are useful in patients with confirmed acromegaly who do not harbor a pituitary tumor. Ectopic acromegaly, due to non-central nervous system tumors such as a pancreatic islet cell tumor or a bronchial carcinoid, results in a significantly elevated serum GHRH, whereas GHRH is usually low with a GH-secreting adenoma.[21]

Other Hormones

Hormonal assessments are needed to measure prolactin co-secretion, although moderately elevated prolactin can be due to stalk effect. Pituitary hormone deficiencies may be measured by ACTH, cortisol, TSH, free T4, FSH, LH levels in both genders, estradiol in women, and testosterone in men.

RADIOLOGIC EVALUATION

Plain x-rays of the skull are not required, though they may demonstrate an enlarged, rounded sella, and the sellar floor may appear doubled due to a thinned, asymmetrically worn laminar dura. A high resolution, contrast-enhanced MRI through the sellar region is the preferred modality to delineate the tumor and its anatomical relationships. This is essential for surgical planning as it will show the precise size and location of the lesion. A CT scan may be helpful for sphenoid sinus anatomy.

Those rare patients with acromegaly but without a pituitary lesion on MRI, should undergo a workup to find a GHRH-secreting tumor with abdominal and chest imaging.

OTHER INVESTIGATIONS NECESSARY IN PATIENTS WITH ACROMEGALY

Neuro-ophthalmologic examination, including visual field testing and visual acuity, should be obtained before and after treatment to determine specific deficits and monitor changes. Sleep studies are necessary to assess for sleep apnea in patients with excessive daytime sleepiness. Because of an increased prevalence of colon polyps in patients with acromegaly, a colonoscopy is recommended for all patients at diagnosis and every 3 to 5 years thereafter, if polyps are found.

Treatment

Treatment for acromegaly is intended to normalize GH and IGF-1 levels, and to remove the tumor while preserving normal pituitary function.

SURGERY

Surgical adenomectomy by an experienced neurosurgeon remains the first-line treatment for most patients with acromegaly.[22,23] The goals of surgical resection are to eliminate mass effect, preserve or restore pituitary and visual function, and obtain tissue for histopathologic analysis.[24]

Most of these tumors are sellar or suprasellar lesions that may be removed trans-sphenoidally using a direct endonasal, sublabial, or trans-septal approach with an endoscope or microscope. The first trans-sphenoidal resection of a pituitary lesion was performed by Hermann Schloffer in 1907; the procedure was popularized by Harvey Cushing in the two decades that followed.[25,26] Neurosurgeons have been improving the trans-sphenoidal adenomectomy (TSA) since. A craniotomy may rarely be necessary when a tumor has extensive suprasellar or parasellar extension.

Endonasal Trans-Sphenoidal Approach

Typically, the approach is begun with the patient supine and his head in a Mayfield pin head-holder. The neck is slightly extended and the head is gently turned to the right to face the surgeon, to permit a good view through the nares.

In an endonasal approach, the surgeon enters directly into the sphenoid sinus though the sphenoid ostium. In a microscopic unilateral trans-septal approach, a small incision is made in the mucosa of the right nostril. A submucosal plane is developed along the septum until the anterior wall of the sphenoid sinus is reached. A speculum is then inserted and the septum is subluxed and deviated. The operating microscope is brought into the field. An osteotome and Kerrison rongeur are used to open the sphenoid sinus and enlarge it until the surgeon can visualize the lateral portion of the sella. Fluoroscopy or neuro-navigation may then be obtained to confirm the sella's position; however, direct visualization is usually sufficient.

The sellar floor is opened with an osteotome and enlarged with an up-biting Kerrison rongeur, revealing the dura. A midline or lateral vertical incision is made in the dura with a number 11 blade, and is enlarged using up-angled scissors. A sellar adenoma will generally be exposed at this point. An extracapsular plane may be developed along the pseudocapsule, or the tumor may be debulked intracapsularly, and curettes, pituitary rongeurs, gentle suction, and irrigation may be used to extract the tumor piecemeal. Good suction is necessary, as adenomas can be quite bloody, and at times, only tumor removal will stop the bleeding.

Once the tumor is resected, the sellar floor may be repaired with a variety of options such as Duraform, fascia, fat, bone, cartilage, or prosthesis. The sphenoid sinus may be left open or closed with Duraform, DuraSeal, or a piece of fat harvested from the patient's abdomen. The speculum is removed and the patient's septum is repositioned in the midline. Absorbable suture is used to seal the mucosa at the inside edge of the nare. Mucosal secretions may necessitate a nasal trumpet overnight to improve nasal respirations.

Endoscopy

In recent years, endoscopes have replaced microscopes at many centers. The patient is positioned in the same manner as that described previously for the microscopic approach. The endoscope is used to visualize the sphenoethmoid recess. The bilateral sphenoid ostia are widened using a mushroom punch, and then the posterior nasal septum is incised and resected using straight through-cutting instruments and a microdebrider. The anterior wall of the sphenoid sinus and the intersinus septum are resected using Kerrison punches and straight through-cutting instruments.

The lesion is removed in the same manner as described with the microscopic approach. Duraform is then placed over the sella, and the sphenoid sinus is packed using Gelfoam. NasoPore is laid over the posterior septectomy site and the sphenoethmoid recesses bilaterally. A mucosal septal flap may be used if a CSF leak is present. A speculum is not needed with this approach.[27,28]

The straight surgical endoscope provides a wide field of view, while angled scopes permit enhanced visualization of the sellar wall, suprasellar, retrosellar, or parasellar regions. Three-dimensional endoscopes have been recently introduced and provide a stereoscopic, nondistorted view of the regional anatomy in contrast to older two-dimensional endoscopes (Figure 18-2).

Sublabial Trans-Sphenoidal Approach

Sublabial may be the appropriate approach for patients with large tumors or pediatric patients with small nares. The upper lip is retracted, an incision is made horizontally in the gingival mucosa, and the maxilla and nasal cavity floor are accessed. A vertical incision is made to separate

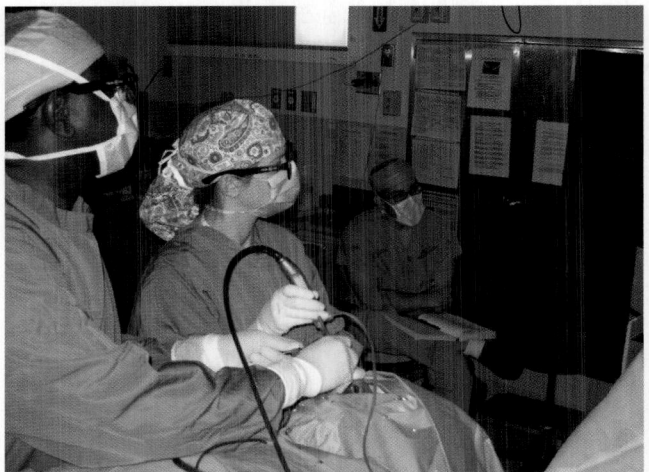

FIGURE 18-2 The endoscope allows a surgeon to use a "three-handed" technique, with an assistant driving the endoscope in one nare while the primary surgeon has an instrument in each side. The three-dimensional (3D) endoscope provides a more anatomically realistic view of the operative field than does the traditional two-dimensional endoscope. The required 3D glasses are seen in this photograph.

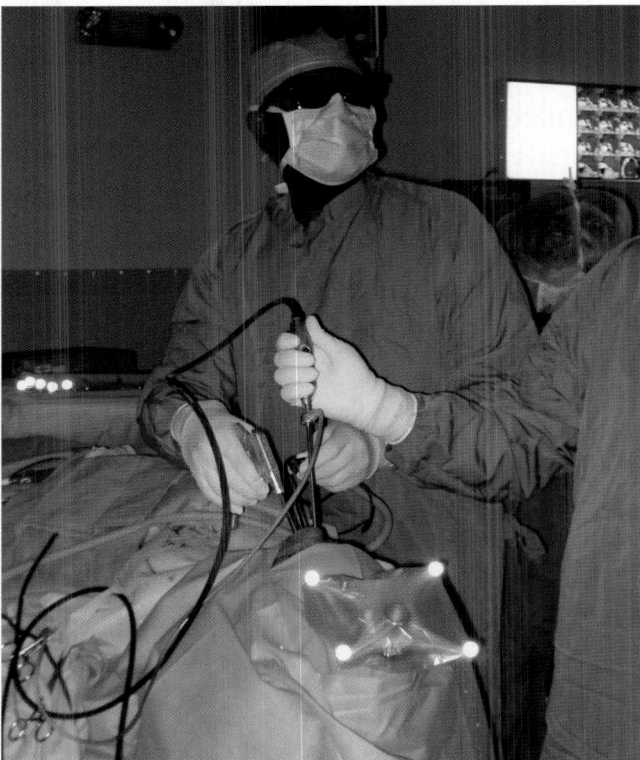

the nasal mucosa from the septum, and the anterior septum is subluxed and deviated. The speculum is inserted and the microscope or endoscope is brought into the field. The operation continues in the same manner as described above.[29]

Neuronavigation

Frameless stereotactic neuronavigation permits the surgeon to confirm his position at any point during the TSA to assess the proximity of surrounding structures or determine when he is approaching the limits of the tumor (Figure 18-3). Navigation may be used to assist with large lesions that involve the carotid arteries or recurrent lesions where the normal anatomy has been altered by a prior operation.[30,31]

Outcomes of Trans-Sphenoidal Surgery

Clinical Outcomes

Following operative decompression, visual field defects improve in 70% to 89% of patients,[32,33] remain unchanged in 7% percent, and rarely worsen (<4%).[34] Headaches usually improve in a few days, while soft-tissue swelling and glucose and blood pressure control improve progressively in the next few weeks postoperatively. Bony abnormalities persist, while joint symptoms often improve, although complete resolution is unlikely.

Postoperative Biochemical Outcome

Plasma GH levels rapidly decrease within hours after surgery,[35] while IGF-1 levels improve over the next several weeks to months.[22]

The success rate in achieving biochemical control of GH levels varies widely due to the diverse criteria used by different authors and changes in hormonal assays.[36] Recent studies have established more stringent criteria for "biochemical cure" or remission, requiring a random GH less than 2.5 µg/l, GH nadir less than 0.4 µg/l after an oral glucose tolerance test, as well as a normal IGF-1.[36,37] Until 2010,

FIGURE 18-3 The localizer for the Stealth neuronavigation system can be seen at the superior aspect of the patient's head, where it is connected via the Mayfield headframe. Neuronavigation may be used in conjunction with the microscopic or endoscopic trans-sphenoidal approaches.

GH nadir used as the threshold during oral glucose tolerance testing was 1.0 µg/l. Using these criteria, a 2003 study of 59 patients followed for an average of more than 13 years after TSA showed that 52% achieved long-term biochemical remission after surgery alone.[38] Overall, the postoperative remission rate is 80% for patients with GH-secreting microadenomas and less than 50% in macroadenomas, while long-term recurrence rate is 3% to 10%.

The factors predictive of surgical outcome include: tumor size, extrasellar growth, dural invasion, and preoperative GH level.[18,22,23,35,39,40] More than 40% of acromegalic patients treated with surgery initially will require additional treatment.[41-43] Reoperation for acromegaly has a lower success rate and higher complication rate than does the initial surgery. Reoperation is generally reserved for patients unresponsive to other forms of therapy or who have progressive visual impairment despite medical therapy.[43]

Complications

Potential complications from trans-sphenoidal surgery include hemorrhage, carotid artery injury, ischemic stroke, visual impairment, cerebrospinal fluid leak, nasal septal perforation, and epistaxis. The risk of stroke or death is less than 1%, while the risk of CSF rhinorrhea is 5%. Postoperative hypopituitarism may occur in 3% to 15% patients. In the first few days postoperatively, morning serum cortisol levels should be measured. Patients with symptoms of hypocortisolemia and a morning serum cortisol less than 10 µg/dl usually receive glucocorticoid replacement upon discharge. A full evaluation of pituitary hormones should be repeated at six to 12 weeks postoperatively to determine need for replacement.

Diabetes insipidus (DI) and the syndrome of inappropriate antidiuretic hormone secretion (SIADH) are potential transient postoperative complications after trans-sphenoidal surgery, occurring in 30% of patients, while permanent DI occurs in fewer than 10%. It is very important to monitor fluid balance, serum sodium and urine specific gravity postoperatively.

Mortality for patients undergoing trans-sphenoidal surgery is very low, approximately 0.5%. Among patients with giant macroadenomas, the mortality is approximately 1%. Following resection of a giant macroadenoma, when some residual tumor may remain, a rare but potentially fatal postoperative complication is apoplexy. In one study of 134 surgically resected giant adenomas, four patients suffered fatal postoperative pituitary apoplexy.[44] These patients must be closely watched.

Trans-sphenoidal pituitary exploration for patients with acromegaly with no pituitary tumor seen on MRI and a negative workup for an ectopic GHRH-secreting lesion is controversial. Surgical exploration may rarely reveal a small lesion hidden by the wall of the cavernous sinus or along the sellar floor.[45]

PHARMACOLOGIC THERAPY

There are three main categories of pharmacologic treatment of acromegaly: Somatostatin analogues, growth hormone-receptor antagonists, and dopamine agonists.[46]

Somatostatin Analogues

Somatostatin analogues (octreotide and lanreotide) should be considered in patients with abnormal GH or IGF-1 levels postoperatively, either alone or while awaiting the effects of radiation. They are also recommended for patients who are medically unstable for surgery (e.g., those with uncontrolled hypertension, diabetes mellitus, or sleep apnea), or patients in whom tumors are clearly invasive and complete surgical removal is unlikely.[6,47] Poor-risk patients may be reconsidered for surgery if their medical condition improves after treatment with somatostatin analogues.[48]

Most acromegalic patients treated with somatostatin analogues achieve a significant decrease in serum GH and IGF-1 levels.[49,50] A double-blind, randomized, multi-center study of 115 acromegalic patients showed that octreotide, at a dose of 100 µg three times per day for six months, reduced mean GH levels by 70% and IGF-1 levels by 60%.[51] Tumor size shrinks by 25% to 50% in 20% to 47% of patients with acromegaly on chronic octreotide therapy.[47,48,51-53] Eight to 12 weeks of preoperative somatostatin analogue therapy shrinks GH-secreting macroadenomas by about 40%,[54] and short-term preoperative octreotide administration decreases surgical risk in patients who have cardiac and metabolic complications of acromegaly.[48,55] It is debatable, however, whether this affects surgical outcome. Two prospective, randomized studies demonstrated no benefit of preoperative octreotide on rate of hormone normalization postoperatively or on duration of hospital stay.[56,57]

With somatostatin analogues, relief of clinical symptoms is often seen immediately after starting the injections and before serum GH levels have declined. Many clinicians

discontinue somatostatin analogues in patients who are undergoing radiation therapy, as there is a theoretical concern that it may be radioprotective, based on the experience with dopamine agonists in prolactinomas.[58] Side effects associated with the long-term administration of somatostatin analogues are relatively minor and include pain at the injection site, nausea, abdominal cramps, mild steatorrhea, hyperglycemia, and cholesterol gallstones.[51,52,59] Discontinuation of medical therapy may result in rebound of pretreatment hormone levels and tumor size.[54,60]

Growth Hormone–Receptor Antagonist

Pegvisomant is an alternative for patients in whom surgery and medical therapy with somatostatin analogues are ineffective or poorly tolerated.[61] Pegvisomant, a mutated derivative of GH, is a highly effective antagonist of GH action in patients with acromegaly, and normalizes IGF-1 in more than 90% of patients.[6,46] The inhibition of GH action, rather than pituitary GH secretion, represents a paradigm shift in the medical management of acromegaly.[46,62-64] Pegvisomant does not act directly on the adenoma, and there is a potential risk of increase in GH secretion and tumor enlargement due to a loss of negative feedback from serum IGF-1. Early results, however, suggest that while there is some increase in GH level with pegvisomant therapy, it is not progressive and does not lead to a significant increase in tumor growth in up to two years of follow-up.[46,62-65] Nevertheless, serial MRI scans to monitor tumor size are recommended. IGF-1 and not GH levels should be followed to monitor treatment with pegvisomant. Combined therapy with somatostatin analogues and pegvisomant normalized IGF-1 in most patients.[66]

Side effects from pegvisomant are generally minor. Some patients have asymptomatic hepatic enzyme elevation after initiation of pegvisomant, which normalizes after the stopping the drug,[46,67] but few serious cases of hepatitis were reported.[6]

Dopamine Agonists

Therapy with dopamine agonists may be attempted for tumors that co-secrete prolactin. Bromocriptine is effective in lowering GH and IGF-1 levels in only 20% of patients, with only 10% achieving normalization.[6,68,69] Side effects include nausea, vertigo, hypotension, and nasal stuffiness. The newer generation of long-acting D2-receptor agonists, including cabergoline and quinagolide, appear to be more effective and better tolerated than bromocriptine.[48,70,71] Long-term administration of cabergoline to 64 patients normalized plasma IGF-1 levels in 39% of patients and decreased IGF-1 modestly in another 28%.[71] It is most effective for patients with less active disease (IGF-1 < 750 ng/ml) and those with mixed GH and prolactin-secreting tumors.[68]

RADIATION THERAPY

Radiotherapy is indicated for patients who are unsuitable for or have failed surgery, and in whom medical therapy with somatostatin analogues and dopamine agonists has failed to achieve biochemical remission. In the first two years after radiation, a significant decrease in GH levels is usually achieved, followed by a slow decline for years thereafter.[72-77] GH concentrations of approximately 5 µg/l are achieved in 80% of patients, though this may take 10 to

15 years to achieve. Few patients are actually "cured" if one applies strict criteria.[61,78]

Risks of conventional radiotherapy include visual changes from radiation damage to the optic nerve or chiasm, cognitive and neurologic deficits from radiation necrosis in adjacent brain, and a small risk for the development of secondary brain tumors such as gliomas.[72-74,77,79] Hypopituitarism occurs in 30% to 70% of patients within 10 years.[72,80,81] Stereotactic radiosurgery, such as the gamma knife or linear accelerator, is replacing conventional radiotherapy at most medical centers.[77,80,82,83] In one study, gamma knife radiosurgery (GKS) was used as the primary procedure in 68 of 79 patients with GH-secreting tumors. All patients saw a decline in GH levels within six months.[83] In a small series using CyberKnife, 44% of patients achieved biochemical remission after an average 25 months of follow-up.[84]

The major risk from SRS is radiation damage to the visual pathways, but this can be decreased by limiting the radiation dose to the optic chiasm to less than 10 Gy. Structures in the cavernous sinus are less radiosensitive, so an ablative dose may be administered to tumors with lateral invasion or impingement on the cranial nerves. This allows SRS to function as an adjuvant to surgical resection in patients with tumors that have invaded the cavernous sinus. Stereotactic radiosurgery has lower long-term risks of developing cognitive changes or a second neoplasm than does conventional radiation, and SRS appears to induce remission more rapidly than does fractionated radiotherapy.[80,83] As with conventional radiotherapy, approximately 30% of patients develop new hormone deficiencies after SRS.[80,84] In patients who cannot safely undergo SRS due to the proximity of the visual pathways to the tumor margin, fractionated stereotactic radiotherapy may be a safer and more effective alternative to conventional radiotherapy.[80,83]

Pediatric

GH-secreting tumors in children and adolescents with gigantism are more often aggressive and invasive than in adults.[85] Trans-sphenoidal resection of GH-secreting tumors is safe in pediatric patients. For patients with small nares, a sublabial approach may be used. The risk of recurrence after surgical resection is higher in pediatric than in adult patients, however. The rate of postoperative complications including DI is higher in a series of pediatric patients than in adult series, and the likelihood of achieving biochemical remission is lower, 60% versus 78%.[85]

Although there are less data than for adults, medical therapy with somatostatin analogues decreases serum IGF-1 levels in children. A small study of children treated with pegvisomant decreased IGF-1 levels, decreased somatic growth, and improved acromegalic features in all three patients.[86] Radiotherapy has special risks in the pediatric population because of the danger of panhypopituitarism and its effects on growth and puberty. The years-long delay in effectiveness with radiation may preclude any effect on the rapid growth seen in children with gigantism. Generally, the risks of pituitary radiotherapy outweigh the potential benefits in children.[85]

KEY REFERENCES

Abe T, Tara LA, Lüdecke DK. Growth hormone-secreting pituitary adenomas in childhood and adolescence: features and results of transnasal surgery. *Neurosurgery.* 1999;45(1):1-10.

Abosch A, Tyrrell JB, Lamborn KR, et al. Transsphenoidal microsurgery for growth hormone-secreting pituitary adenomas: initial outcome and long-term results. *J Clin Endocrinol Metab.* 1998;83(10):3411-3418.

Beauregard C, Truong U, Hardy J, Serri O. Long-term outcome and mortality after transsphenoidal adenomectomy for acromegaly. *Clin Endocrinol.* 2003;58(1):86-91.

Ben-Shlomo A, Melmed S. Acromegaly. *Endocrinol Metab Clin North Am.* 2008;37(1):565-583.

Biermasz NR, Dulken HV, Roelfsema F. Postoperative radiotherapy in acromegaly is effective in reducing GH concentration to safe levels. *Clin Endocrinol (Oxf).* 2000;53(3):321-327.

Buhk JH, Jung S, Psychogios MK, et al. Tumor volume of growth hormone–secreting pituitary adenomas during treatment with pegvisomant: a prospective multicenter study. *J Clin Endocrinol Metab.* 2010;95(2):552-558.

Chanson P, Salenave S, Kamenicky P, et al. Acromegaly. *Best Pract Res Clin Endocrinol Metab.* 2009;23:555-574.

Cohen-Gadol AA, Liu JK, Laws Jr ER. Cushing's first case of transsphenoidal surgery: the launch of the pituitary surgery era. *J Neurosurg.* 2005;103:570-574.

Colao A, Ferone D, Marzullo P, et al. Long-term effects of depot long-acting somatostatin analog octreotide on hormone levels and tumor mass in acromegaly. *J Clin Endocrinol Metab.* 2001;86(6):2779-2786.

Feenststra J, de Herder WW, ten Have SM, et al. Combined therapy with somatostatin analogues and weekly pegvisomant in active acromegaly. *Lancet.* 2005;365(9471):1644-1646.

Freda PU, Katznelson L, van der Lely AJ, et al. Long-acting somatostatin analog therapy of acromegaly: a meta-analysis. *J Clin Endocrinol Metab.* 2005;90(8):4465-4473.

Giustina A, Chanson P, Bronstein MD, et al. A consensus on criteria for cure of acromegaly. *J Clin Endocrinol Metab.* 2010;95(7):3141-3148.

Gutt B, Hatzack C, Morrison K, et al. Conventional pituitary irradiation is effective in normalising plasma IGF-I in patients with acromegaly. *Eur J Endocrinol.* 2001;144(2):109-116.

Jho HD, Alfieri A. Endoscopic endonasal pituitary surgery: E: evolution of surgical technique and equipment in 150 operations. *Minim Invasive Neurosurg.* 2001;44:1-12.

Laws ER, Vance ML, Thapar K. Pituitary surgery for the management of acromegaly. *Horm Res.* 2000;53(Suppl 3):71-75.

Melmed S. Medical progress: Acromegaly. *N Engl J Med.* 2006;355(24):2558-2573.

Melmed S, Casanueva F, Cavagnini F, et al. Consensus statement: medical management of acromegaly. *Eur J Endocrinol.* 2005;153(6):737-740.

Nachtigall L, Delgado A, Swearingen B, et al. Changing patterns in diagnosis and therapy of acromegaly over two decades. *J Clin Endocrinol Metab.* 2008;93(6):2035-2041.

Parkinson C, Trainer PJ. Pegvisomant: a growth hormone receptor antagonist for the treatment of acromegaly. *Growth Horm IGF Res.* 2000;10:S119-S123.

Powell JS, Wardlaw SL, Post KD, Freda PU. Outcome of radiotherapy for acromegaly using normalization of insulin-like growth factor I to define cure. *J Clin Endocrinol Metab.* 2000;85(5):2068-2071.

Racine MS, Barkan AL. Medical management of growth hormone-secreting pituitary adenomas. *Pituitary.* 2002;5:67-76.

Roberts BK, Ouyang DL, Lad SP, et al. Efficacy and safety of CyberKnife radiosurgery for acromegaly. *Pituitary* 2007;10(1):19–25.

Swearingen B, Barker FG, Kaznelson L, et al. Long-term mortality after transsphenoidal surgery and adjunctive therapy for acromegaly. *J Clin Endocrinol Metab.* 1998;83(10):3419-3426.

Zada G, Kelly DF, Cohan P, et al. Endonasal transsphenoidal approach for pituitary adenomas and other sellar lesions: an assessment of efficacy, safety, and patient impressions. *J Neurosurg.* 2003;98:350-358.

Zhang N, Pan L, Wang EM, et al. Radiosurgery for growth hormone-producing pituitary adenomas. *J Neurosurg.* 2000;93(suppl 3):6-9.

Numbered references appear on Expert Consult.

CHAPTER 19

Prolactinomas

JAMES K. LIU • MARK D. KRIEGER • ARUN P. AMAR • WILLIAM T. COULDWELL • MARTIN H. WEISS

Prolactinomas are the most common type of functioning pituitary tumors, accounting for approximately 50% to 60% of functioning pituitary adenomas.[1,2] These prolactin-secreting adenomas are the second most common type of pituitary tumor overall after nonfunctioning adenomas and represent 30% to 40% of all pituitary tumors.[3,4] Their prevalence is generally thought to be up to 100 cases per 1 million people,[5] and one meta-analysis of the literature estimated a much higher prevalence rate of approximately 17% of the population, with a third of tumors staining positive for prolactin.[6]

The objectives for treatment of hyperprolactinemia due to prolactinomas are normalization of the hyperprolactinemic state, preservation of residual pituitary function, reduction of tumor mass, and prevention of disease recurrence. Pharmacologic therapy with dopamine agonists remains the mainstay of treatment;[7-10] however, surgical removal of prolactinomas remains an important treatment in those patients who cannot tolerate or are resistant to medical therapy. Surgery may play a curative role in some cases of microprolactinomas.[1,11,12] The current surgical management strategies for patients with prolactinoma are discussed in this chapter.

Clinical Presentation

Patients with prolactinomas can present with clinical manifestations of hyperprolactinemia, endocrine dysfunction, local mass effect, or pituitary apoplexy (Table 19-1). The biologic effects of hyperprolactinemia predominantly affect the gonadal axis and breast tissue. The primary effects of prolactin are to stimulate lactation, but this hormone can also promote deleterious effects on the gonadal axis. Excessive prolactin centrally inhibits hypothalamic production of gonadotropin-releasing hormone and subsequently inhibits secretion of luteinizing hormone and follicle-stimulating hormone, resulting in infertility and hypogonadism.[13,14] Clinical presentation appears to differ between males and females.

In premenopausal women, the most common presentation includes galactorrhea, amenorrhea, and infertility. Although prolactinomas are equally distributed at autopsy, women are four times more likely to develop symptoms than men. Because of these readily identifiable symptoms, women generally present earlier in the course of the disease and have smaller tumors at the time of diagnosis. Hyperprolactinemia may not be detected until after discontinuation of an oral contraceptive.[15] Approximately 5% of women

with primary amenorrhea and 25% of women with secondary amenorrhea (excluding pregnancy) are found to have a prolactinoma,[16] and this incidence rises to 70% to 80% when galactorrhea accompanies amenorrhea.[17] Galactorrhea is present in 50% to 80% of women with hyperprolactinemia.[18-20] In men harboring prolactinomas, hypogonadal manifestations of decreased libido and impotence are often attributed to aging or functional causes rather than hyperprolactinemia, delaying detection until the tumor becomes large (mostly macroprolactinomas) and causes local mass effect on neighboring structures. Compression on the optic chiasm, cavernous sinus, and pituitary gland can result in symptoms of visual loss (visual acuity and/or visual field loss), cranial nerve dysfunction resulting in ophthalmoplegia, and/or hypopituitarism, respectively.[21] Galactorrhea and gynecomastia are extremely rare in men. About 2% of all men with impotence have a prolactinoma.[16] Low testosterone levels can result from either hyperprolactinemia or hypopituitarism secondary to mass effect on the normal pituitary gland.

In young individuals, prolactinomas are the most common type of pituitary adenoma overall, particularly in adolescents older than 12 years of age.[22,23] Prolactinomas are more common in girls and present with primary amenorrhea. Boys tend to have much larger tumors and higher preoperative prolactin levels than girls. They can also present with gynecomastia and hypogonadism and tend to have neurologic signs of mass effect.[23] Growth retardation and short stature can be common presentations because growth hormone is the first hormone to undergo hyposecretion in pituitary adenomas.[22] The signs and symptoms of hypogonadism in prepubescent children and postmenopausal patients, however, are clinically absent.[24-26] Adolescent children can present with delay or failure of sexual/reproductive development.[21,27-30]

Persistent gonadal dysfunction resulting in estrogen or testosterone deficiency from prolonged hyperprolactinemia that is left untreated can result in premature osteoporosis in patients of either sex.[17,31-34] These important but often overlooked effects of hyperprolactinemia are additional arguments for treating patients who may not be concerned about sexual dysfunction or fertility. Hyperprolactinemia-induced osteopenia is progressive and correlates with the duration of hypogonadism.[35] If treatment is undertaken, normalization of hyperprolactinemia can impede further bone loss; however, although bone density increases to a certain extent, it may not necessarily return to normal baseline values.[33,36-38]

Tumor compression on neighboring structures can result in symptoms from mass effect such as visual acuity and visual field deficits; cranial nerve palsies resulting in diplopia, ophthalmoplegia, and facial numbness; or impedance of cerebrospinal fluid flow resulting in obstructive hydrocephalus. Compression of the normal pituitary gland can result in hypopituitarism, namely hypocortisolism and hypothyroidism. Pituitary apoplexy from an acute hemorrhage and/or infarction into a prolactinoma can cause rapid enlargement of the tumor, resulting in hypopituitarism and acute compression of the sellar and parasellar structures.[39,40]

Diagnosis

The diagnosis of a prolactin-secreting adenoma is determined by elevation of serum prolactin with radiographic evidence of a pituitary adenoma on magnetic resonance (MR) imaging of the pituitary region with and without gadolinium enhancement.[41] Interpreting serum prolactin levels in conjunction with radiographic findings is important in making the correct diagnosis of a prolactinoma to ensure proper treatment. Serum prolactin levels generally correlate with tumor size: Levels from 100 to 250 ng/ml often signal a microprolactinoma (<10 mm), whereas levels greater than 250 ng/ml generally reflect a macroprolactinoma (>10 mm).[4,42] Extremely elevated serum prolactin levels that are greater than 1000 ng/ml may correlate with a macroprolactinoma that has invaded the cavernous sinus. Macroadenomas associated with a mildly elevated prolactin level, roughly 50 to 125 ng/ml, can be attributed to the stalk-section effect from a nonfunctioning pituitary adenoma. This is because prolactin is under tonic inhibition from the hypothalamus, and lesions or compression of the pituitary stalk may interfere with this inhibition, resulting in mild elevation of prolactin. However, it is important to rule out the "hook effect" in cases of giant and invasive macroprolactinomas in which the serum prolactin level is falsely low (25 to 150 ng/ml). This is due to excessive serum prolactin

saturating the binding sites of the two-site (monoclonal "sandwich") technique resulting in falsely normal levels of prolactin. Subsequent dilutional testing of prolactin samples can counteract this assay phenomenon and prevent incorrect diagnosis.[43-46]

The diagnosis of prolactinoma requires that other causes of hyperprolactinemic states (either physiologic or pathologic) and other mass lesions in the sellar and parasellar region are ruled out (Table 19-2).[13,14,42] Most cases of hyperprolactinemia can be ruled out on the basis of the history and physical examination, a pregnancy test, and thyroid and renal function tests. MR imaging with gadolinium enhancement should then be obtained to confirm the diagnosis of a prolactinoma. Other pituitary-related serum hormone levels (growth hormone, insulin-like growth factor-1, fasting AM cortisol, adrenocorticotrophic hormone, luteinizing hormone, follicular stimulating hormone, sex hormones, and thyroid function tests) can be used to test anterior pituitary function in all patients with a radiographically confirmed pituitary adenoma.

Medical Treatment

The primary goals of treatment for prolactinomas are to normalize hyperprolactinemia and its clinical sequelae, restore fertility, relieve tumor mass effect, preserve residual pituitary function, and prevent disease recurrence or progression.[41]

Table 19-1   Clinical Manifestations of Prolactinomas

Hyperprolactinemia
Amenorrhea (females)
Galactorrhea (females)
Gonadal dysfunction
Infertility
Decreased libido
Impotence (males)
Osteoporosis
Delayed puberty (adolescents)
Mass Effect
Headaches
Visual acuity and field loss
Diplopia
Ophthalmoplegia
Facial numbness
Facial pain
Hypothalamic impairment
Hydrocephalus
Hypopituitarism
Pituitary apoplexy

Table 19-2   Etiology of Hyperprolactinemia

Physiologic
Exercise
Stress
Pregnancy
Breast feeding (suckling reflex)
Pharmacologic
Antidepressants (tricyclic, MAO inhibitors, SSRIs)
Antihypertensives (a-methyldopa, reserpine, verapamil)
Neuroleptics (phenothiazines, haloperidol)
Metoclopramide
H-2 blockers
Sellar/Parasellar Lesions
Prolactinomas
Nonfunctioning pituitary macroadenomas with "stalk effect"
Craniopharyngiomas
Rathke cleft cysts
Meningiomas
Germinomas
Sarcoidosis
Lymphocytic hypophysitis
Histiocytosis X
Metastasis
Primary empty sella syndrome
Other Disease States
Ectopic secretion of prolactin
Primary hypothyroidism
Hypothalamic dysfunction
Chronic renal failure
Cirrhosis
Chest wall lesions (trauma, surgery, herpes zoster)
Seizures

For smaller tumors, such as microprolactinomas (tumors <10 mm), removal of tumor mass is less concerning since these are usually not large enough to produce symptoms related to mass effect. Studies have demonstrated a lack of tumor growth in the vast majority of patients with microprolactinomas, which may remain unchanged throughout the patient's life.[47-49] Thus, in a patient with a microprolactinoma with only mild elevation of prolactin who has normal anterior pituitary function and no desire for pregnancy, observation can be a reasonable option.[4]

The first-line of treatment for prolactinomas is pharmacological intervention with dopamine receptor agonists, which bind to D2 receptors on lactotrophs to inhibit prolactin synthesis and release and reduce tumor volume.[50,51] The agents that are currently approved for use in the United States are bromocriptine and cabergoline. Bromocriptine is very effective in normalizing prolactin levels in more than 90% of patients, significant reducing tumor mass in approximately 85% of patients,[7,52-54] and restoring gonadal and anterior pituitary functions in over 80% of patients. Most female patients resume menstruation within 6 months of initiating therapy. Tumor shrinkage can occur rapidly within several days, decompressing the

visual apparatus in patients with macroprolactinomas who present with visual deficits (Fig. 19-1).[16,52,55] About 5% to 10% of patients may not be able to tolerate side effects of bromocriptine, including dizziness, nausea, arrhythmias, gastrointestinal discomfort, and orthostatic hypotension. About 10% to 25% patients are partially or totally resistant to bromocriptine.[56-58]

More recently, cabergoline has become the preferred first-line agent.[59] Cabergoline is associated with less frequent and less severe side effects and is easier to administer than bromocriptine, although it is more expensive.[60] In one study, cabergoline normalized serum prolactin in 84% of bromocriptine-intolerant patients and in 70% of bromocriptine-resistant patients.[61] Cabergoline has been shown to be more effective in shrinking macroprolactinomas in naive patients than in patients pretreated with other dopamine agonists.[62]

After normalization of serum prolactin levels has been sustained for at least 2 years with adequate reduction and stabilization of tumor size, dopamine agonist therapy can be tapered to lower doses that continue to control hyperprolactinemia and tumor growth. In general, dopamine agonist therapy must be continued for life, and cessation of therapy usually results in recurrent hyperprolactinemia and

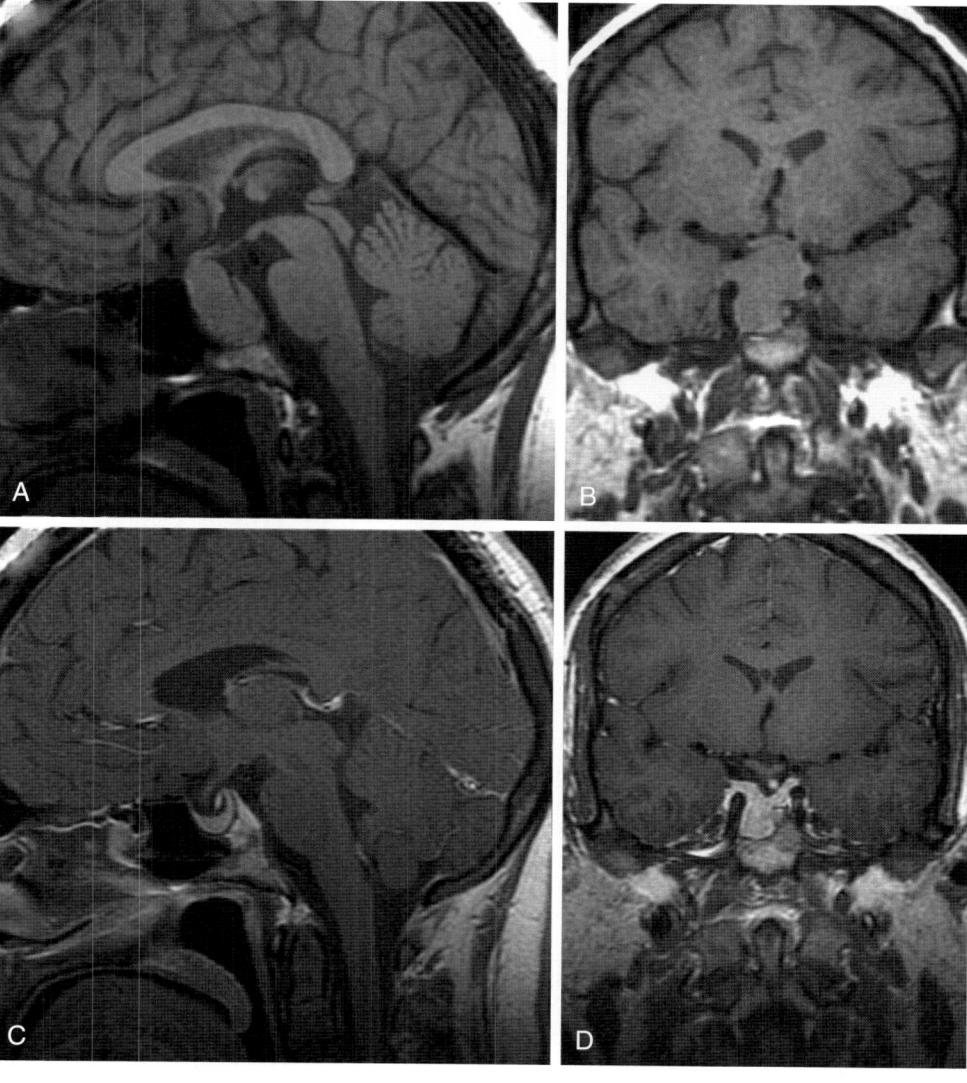

FIGURE 19-1 Initial T1-weighted MRI, sagittal (A) and coronal (B) views of a pregnant 27-year-old (26 weeks gestation) who presented with worsening headaches, right retro-orbital pain and right ptosis from a macroprolactinoma invading the right cavernous sinus and compressing the optic chiasm, with a serum prolactin of 1367 ng/ml. She was initially placed on bromocriptine about 1.5 years prior when her tumor was first diagnosed, and stopped bromocriptine when she became pregnant about 6 months prior. Bromocriptine therapy was restarted and her headaches and ptosis resolved within 24 hours. Her serum prolactin level 3 months later was 7.7 ng/ml. She went on to deliver a normal and healthy baby at term. Post-gadolinium MRI (C, sagittal; D, coronal) at 4 months after restarting bromocriptine showed significant tumor reduction with decompression of the optic chiasm. The pituitary stalk and gland were then visible.

tumor enlargement.[63-65] However, in one study, Colao et al.[5] reported sustained normalization of prolactin levels in 69% of patients with microprolactinomas and in 64% of macroprolactinomas without evidence of new tumor growth. Although there was no evidence of tumor recurrence in the face of recurrent hyperprolactinemia, the follow-up was relatively short and probably insufficient to detect delayed tumor recurrence.[66] Given the above data, we currently continue all patients on cabergoline for 2 to 3 years. If there is documentation of tumor disappearance and normalization of prolactin levels, we will discontinue medication and monitor the patient with twice-yearly review of prolactin levels and annual MR imaging scans. Recurrence detected by increasing prolactin levels would then indicate the need for repeat treatment with dopamine agonists.

It should be emphasized that primary resistance to dopamine agonist therapy occurs in 10% to 15% of prolactinomas[67] and secondary resistance may also rarely occur.[68] Thus, all patients treated with dopamine agonists should undergo serial prolactin measurements and yearly MR imaging surveillance studies.

In patients desiring pregnancy, bromocriptine is the drug of choice because of its safety record.[69,70] The experience with cabergoline is more limited, and it is not used as a primary therapy for infertility, although some reports state that it does not increase the risk of teratogenesis.[71,72] Once menses is restored, normal conception and pregnancy may follow. If a menstrual cycle has been missed, a pregnancy test should be obtained and bromocriptine or cabergoline use should be discontinued immediately.[18] If the patient develops symptomatic tumor enlargement during pregnancy, bromocriptine can be safely initiated (Fig. 19-1).[73-76] There does not appear to be an increased risk of congenital anomalies or spontaneous abortions with use of bromocriptine in this manner.[77] Alternatively, surgical debulking compression may also be an option if the patient does not respond to medical therapy. Patients with pre-existing macroprolactinomas tend to have a higher risk of symptomatic tumor enlargement (15%–35%)[77] than those with microprolactinomas (0.5%–1%).[3,55]

Surgical Treatment

INDICATIONS

The efficacy and success of dopamine agonist therapy has limited the indications of surgical therapy for prolactinomas. Furthermore, surgery is rarely curative in patients with macroprolactinomas and so should be reserved for patients who cannot tolerate the side effects of dopamine agonists or for whom medical therapy is ineffective (those with persistent hyperprolactinemia, progressive tumor enlargement, and persistent tumor mass effect despite maximal medical therapy) (Fig. 19-2).[11,78-80] Surgery may also be an option for treatment of microprolactinomas in patients who do not wish or cannot afford to be on life-long medical therapy (Fig. 19-3).[1,12,66,81,82] For patients whose tumors are more likely to be cured surgically (microprolactinomas or tumors with preoperative prolactin <200 ng/ml) and who desire fertility, surgery can be considered to limit the need for long-term medical therapy, and in some instances may be less costly.[66] Surgery may also be indicated in patients

who are dependent on anti-psychotic medications, because dopamine agonists can precipitate psychotic episodes.[83] Surgical resection should also be considered if impaired visual function or cranial nerve palsies are not immediately responsive to medical treatment, especially in cases of pituitary apoplexy, and in patients who present with a spontaneous cerebrospinal fluid leak after tumor shrinkage with dopamine agonist therapy.[4]

SURGICAL APPROACHES AND OUTCOMES

The trans-sphenoidal approach, either microscopic or endoscopic, is the preferred surgical route and is associated with low rates of morbidity and mortality.[84,85] The extended trans-sphenoidal approach may be used in some cases where the tumor is located beyond the confines of the sella.[86-89] Even in giant prolactinomas, a trans-sphenoidal approach should be considered first; however, a transcranial approach should be considered if there is extensive tumor extension lateral into the sylvian fissure.[80,89] The details of the trans-sphenoidal and transcranial approaches are well described elsewhere.[89-91]

Surgical outcomes appear to be correlated with tumor size and preoperative serum prolactin level.[4,11] In a large series of 489 prolactinomas surgically removed using the trans-sphenoidal approach, the overall remission rate was 42%.[4] For microadenomas, the remission rate was 82% if the preoperative prolactin level was less than 200 ng/ml and 50% if the level was greater than 200 ng/ml. For macroadenomas, the remission rate ranged from 15% to 52% and was 0% for giant adenomas. In the series by Amar et al.,[11] the immediate postoperative biochemical remission rate for microadenomas was 91%, which remained stable at 5 years after surgery. For macroadenomas, the remission rate immediately after surgery was 69%, which dropped to 33% at 5 years. The remission rates were also higher in patients with preoperative prolactin levels less than 200 ng/ml (86%) than in those with levels above 200 ng/ml (45%). Given this fact, we are reluctant to offer surgical treatment for microprolactinomas associated with a prolactin level of greater than 200 ng/ml in the absence of another indication (failure of medical therapy, intolerance to medical therapy, etc.).

Immediate postoperative serum prolactin levels have been used as potential predictors of biochemical cure. In a series of 222 patients who underwent trans-sphenoidal surgery for prolactinomas, fasting morning serum prolactin levels obtained on the first postoperative day that were less than 10 ng/ml predicted a 100% cure rate in microprolactinomas and a 93% cure rate in macroprolactinomas. In patients who had a postoperative level between 10 and 20 ng/ml, 100% of microprolactinomas and 0% of macroprolactinomas achieved biochemical remission.[11]

Although surgery may not be curative in most macroprolactinomas, surgical debulking has been used as a cytoreductive strategy to lower the dosage and increase the responsiveness of dopamine agonist therapy.[3,55] In patients with giant and invasive prolactinomas, pretreatment with bromocriptine resulting in significant tumor reduction may improve the cure rate with subsequent surgery.[53] However, Landolt[92] has reported that prior long-term treatment with dopamine agonists alters the tumor consistency by making the tumor more fibrous, preventing complete resection. We do not offer surgery to patients with

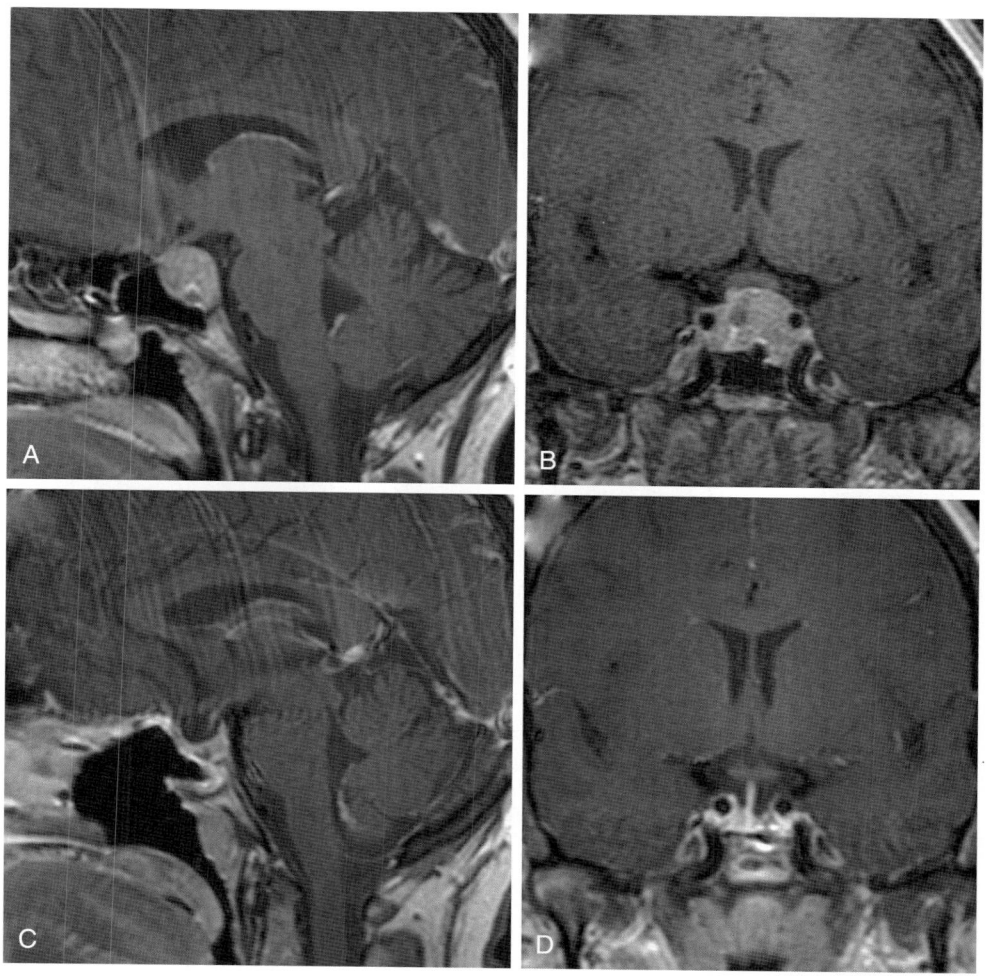

FIGURE 19-2 This 41-year-old woman presented with a recurrent prolactinoma that was not responsive to dopamine agonist therapy. She had undergone prior trans-sphenoidal resection by another surgeon 5 years ago and was continued on bromocriptine postoperatively. Her preoperative MRI (A, sagittal; B, coronal views) demonstrated a 1.5-cm enhancing pituitary adenoma with a persistently elevated serum prolactin of 70.9 ng/ml. An endoscopic trans-sphenoidal resection of the tumor was performed with gross total removal. Serum prolactin level on postoperative day 1 dropped to 5.2 ng/ml, indicating a surgical cure. The histopathology demonstrated pituitary adenoma cells that stained strongly positive for prolactin. Postoperative MRI (C, sagittal; D, coronal views) at 3 months demonstrated complete removal of the tumor with preservation of the pituitary gland and stalk.

macroprolactinomas who have not already tried medical therapy. The current indications used for surgery in these cases include lack of response to medication, development of resistance to medical therapy, intolerance to medical therapy, or cerebrospinal fluid leak after shrinkage of large tumor.

SURGERY FOR MICROPROLACTINOMAS

Trans-sphenoidal removal of microprolactinomas by an experienced pituitary surgeon can be considered in patients who do not wish to be on life-long medical therapy (Fig. 19-3).[1,11,12,81] The choice of trans-sphenoidal surgery for microprolactinomas should take into account the size and location of the tumor, the preoperative serum prolactin level, the age of the patient, the desire for restoration of fertility, the efficacy and tolerability of the dopamine agonists, the patient's desire to be free of long-term medical therapy, and the experience of the surgeon. Surgery should not be considered unless a complete removal with biochemical cure of the microprolactinoma is an expected outcome. The presence of a symptomatic microprolactinoma, especially in a young patient, should remain an indication for microsurgical or endoscopic trans-sphenoidal resection.

In patients with microprolactinomas with serum prolactin levels below 200 ng/ml, trans-sphenoidal surgery

performed by experienced pituitary surgeons at high-volume centers offers over a 90% chance of biochemical and oncologic cure[11,12,93,94] with minimal risks of morbidity and mortality of less than 1%.[85,88] Amar et al.[11] achieved a cure rate of 91% in patients with microprolactinomas. Similarly, although Tyrrell et al.[78] found that women with preoperative prolactin levels above 200 ng/ml and larger, more invasive prolactinomas had poorer outcomes (37%–41% cure rate), long-term remission was achieved in patients with microadenomas and noninvasive macroadenomas (moderate suprasellar extension and focal sphenoid sinus invasion). The continued evolution of endoscopic approaches for tumor resection, which are somewhat less invasive, may reduce the morbidity rate of the surgical approach even further.[95] The financial cost of treatment over a 10-year period is similar in uncomplicated surgical cases to that of long-term dopamine agonist therapy.[96]

PITUITARY APOPLEXY

Although most surgeons recommend emergent trans-sphenoidal decompression and administration of glucocorticoids for patients who present with pituitary apoplexy,[39,40,97-100] some have reported excellent results with dopamine agonist therapy in patients with pituitary apoplexy in prolactinomas.[39,101] In the absence of visual deficits, an initial trial of dopamine agonist therapy in

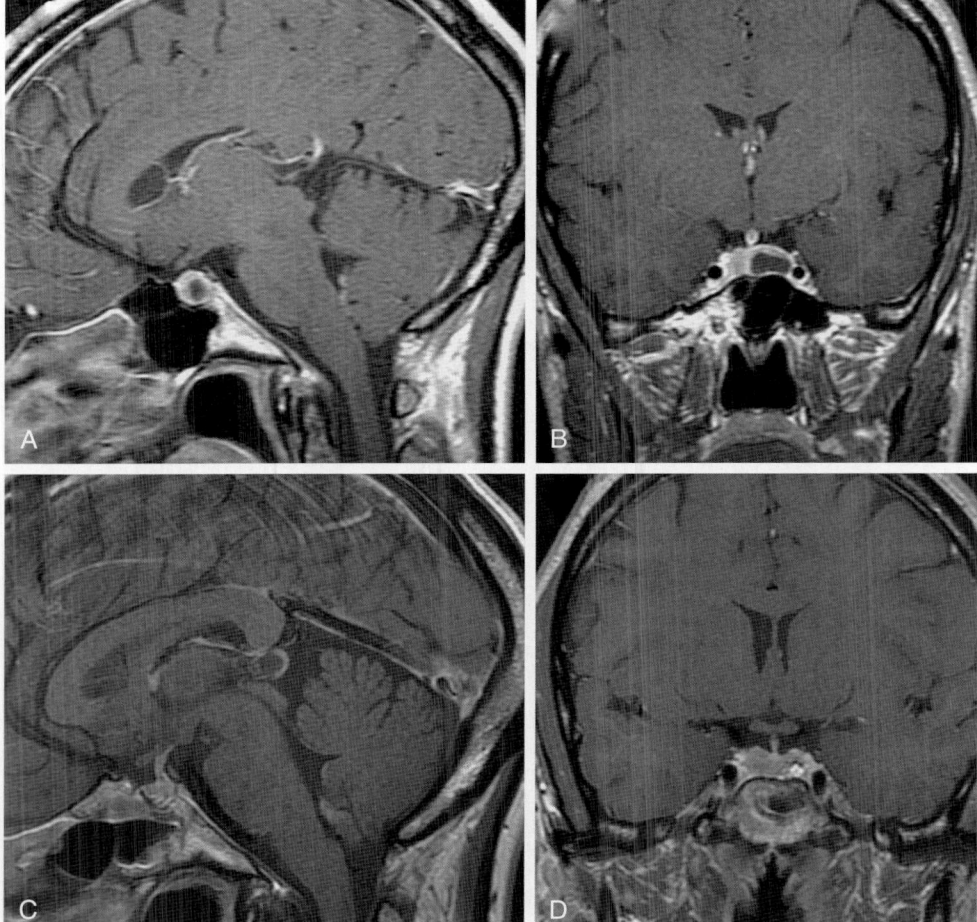

FIGURE 19-3 T1-weighted, post-gadolinium MRI (A, sagittal; B, coronal views) of a 31-year-old woman who presented with amenorrhea and galactorrhea secondary to a microprolactinoma in the left aspect of the sella. The initial serum prolactin level was 83.5 ng/ml. She underwent a complete microsurgical trans-sphenoidal resection of the tumor. The morning fasting serum prolactin level obtained on postoperative day 1 was 2.2 ng/ml, suggesting a biochemical cure. The histopathology demonstrated pituitary adenoma cells that stained strongly positive for prolactin. Postoperative MRI (C, sagittal; D, coronal views) at 3 months demonstrated complete removal of the tumor with preservation of the pituitary gland and stalk.

conjunction with glucocorticoids may be considered. However, the clinician should be prepared for urgent or emergent trans-sphenoidal surgery if visual loss is severe at presentation or if visual loss does not improve after dopamine agonist therapy.

STEREOTACTIC RADIOSURGERY

Stereotactic radiosurgery is an important modality in the armamentarium of treatment for prolactinomas as a secondary treatment after failed trans-sphenoidal surgery or failed medical therapy or as a primary treatment for prolactinomas in patients who are reluctant to undergo surgical resection but cannot tolerate medical therapy.[102-109] Current technology allows high-resolution targeting and dose planning with excellent accuracy. The preliminary data regarding tumor control and normalization of functioning pituitary adenomas after radiosurgery appear favorable. The proximity of the pituitary gland to the region of radiosurgical treatment, however, may carry the risk of hypopituitarism. Longer follow-up is necessary to assess the likelihood of this complication.

Landolt and Lomax[107] reported a 25% rate of normalization of hyperprolactinemia after gamma knife radiosurgery for residual prolactinoma after failed medical or surgical therapy. Eleven patients experienced improvement of prolactin levels decreased by at least 20%, while the treatment failed in four patients who were receiving dopamine agonist therapy at the time of radiosurgical treatment. Pollock et al.,[110] showed that absence of hormone-suppressive medications at the time of radiosurgery correlated with an endocrine cure, supporting the theory by Landolt and Lomax that dopamine agonist therapy may offer some radioprotective effect.[107] Pan et al.[109] reported that tumor growth was controlled in all but two of 128 patients with greater than 2-year follow-up. Biochemical cure was achieved in 52% of patients and improvement in 28%.

Castinetti et al.[111] reported a 46.6% normalization rate of hyperprolactinemia after radiosurgery in 15 patients with a mean follow-up of 96 months. Mean time to remission was approximately 24 to 28 months. Those that achieved remission had a smaller mean tumor volume and lower mean initial prolactin level than those that remained uncured. This raises the possible role of surgical or chemical debulking prior to radiosurgery to decrease the target size to achieve better radiosurgical results. Radiation-induced hypopituitarism was observed in 23% after a mean time of 48 to 96 months.

In another study of 35 prolactinomas treated with gamma knife radiosurgery, normoprolactinemia was achieved in 37.1% who discontinued dopamine agonists after radiosurgery, and in 42.9% who continued medical therapy after radiosurgery.[112] Median time to normalization was 96 months which suggests that the effects of treatment acts slowly and requires long-term follow-up.

PITUITARY TRANSPOSITION (HYPOPHYSOPEXY)

Surgical debulking with postoperative stereotactic radio-surgery of residual cavernous sinus tumor may provide another treatment option in patients with macroprolacti-nomas with cavernous sinus invasion that are refractory to medical therapy. To protect the pituitary gland during stereotactic radiosurgery, we perform a technique for pituitary gland transposition (hypophysopexy) after the tumor is adequately debulked.[113,114] This technique involves transposing the normal pituitary gland away from the cavernous sinus tumor and interposing a fat graft between the normal gland and the tumor in the cavernous sinus to increase the distance between the normal pituitary gland and residual tumor to facilitate radiosurgical treatment of the tumor, thereby reducing the effective biological dose to the normal pituitary gland. The goal of this reduction is to decrease the likelihood of the patient developing hypopituitarism.[113,114] Long-term results indicate a very low incidence of new hypopituitarism following the use of this technique (WT Couldwell, in prep.).

Summary

The management of prolactinomas requires proper diagnosis. The objectives of treatment are to normalize hyperprolactinemia and its clinical sequelae, restore fertility, relieve tumor mass effect, preserve residual pituitary function, and prevent disease recurrence or progression. Medical treatment with dopamine agonists remains the first line of therapy and is effective in normalizing hyperprolactinemia and shrinking tumor size in most cases. Surgical resection remains an important role in patients who fail or cannot tolerate medical therapy. It is also an option in patients with microprolactinomas who wish to avoid long-term medical therapy and in whom complete removal with biochemical cure is an expected outcome. Stereotactic radiosurgery is an option for those who fail medical and surgical treatments and may be considered as a primary treatment in those who do not wish to undergo medical or surgical treatment.

KEY REFERENCES

Amar AP, Couldwell WT, Chen JC, et al. Predictive value of serum prolactin levels measured immediately after transsphenoidal surgery. *J Neurosurg.* 2002;97:307-314.

Barkan AL, Chandler WF. Giant pituitary prolactinoma with falsely low serum prolactin: the pitfall of the "high-dose hook effect": Case report. *Neurosurgery.* 1998;42:913-915:discussion 915–916.

Colao A, Annunziato L, Lombardi G. Treatment of prolactinomas. *Ann Med.* 1998;30:452-459.

Colao A, Di Sarno A, Cappabianca P, et al. Withdrawal of long-term cabergoline therapy for tumoral and nontumoral hyperprolactinemia. *N Engl J Med.* 2003;349:2023-2033.

Colao A, Di Sarno A, Landi ML, et al. Macroprolactinoma shrinkage during cabergoline treatment is greater in naive patients than in patients pretreated with other dopamine agonists: a prospective study in 110 patients. *J Clin Endocrinol Metab.* 2000;85:2247-2252.

Colao A, Di Sarno A, Sarnacchiaro F, et al. Prolactinomas resistant to standard dopamine agonists respond to chronic cabergoline treatment. *J Clin Endocrinol Metab.* 1997;82:876-883.

Colao A, Loche S, Cappa M, et al. Prolactinomas in children and adolescents. Clinical presentation and long-term follow-up. *J Clin Endocrinol Metab.* 1998;83:2777-2780.

Comtois R, Robert F, Hardy J. Immunoradiometric assays may miss high prolactin levels. *Ann Intern Med.* 1993;119:173.

Couldwell WT, Rovit RL, Weiss MH. Role of surgery in the treatment of microprolactinomas. *Neurosurg Clin North Am.* 2003;14:89-92:vii.

Couldwell WT, Weiss MH. Medical and surgical management of microprolactinoma. *Pituitary.* 2004;7:31-32.

Landolt AM, Lomax N. Gamma knife radiosurgery for prolactinomas. *J Neurosurg.* 2000;93(suppl 3):14-18.

Liu JK, Couldwell WT. Contemporary management of prolactinomas. *Neurosurg Focus.* 2004;16:E2.

Molitch ME. Medical management of prolactin-secreting pituitary adenomas. *Pituitary.* 2002;5:55-65.

Molitch ME. Management of prolactinomas during pregnancy. *J Reprod Med.* 1999;44:1121-1126.

Molitch ME. Diagnosis and treatment of prolactinomas. *Adv Intern Med.* 1999;44:117-153.

Nomikos P, Buchfelder M, Fahlbusch R. Current management of prolactinomas. *J Neurooncol.* 2001;54:139-150.

Schlechte JA. Clinical practice. Prolactinoma. *N Engl J Med.* 2003;349:2035-2041.

Shrivastava RK, Arginteanu MS, King WA, et al. Giant prolactinomas: Clinical management and long-term follow-up. *J Neurosurg.* 2002;97: 299-306.

Thorner MO, Perryman RL, Rogol AD, et al. Rapid changes of prolactinoma volume after withdrawal and reinstitution of bromocriptine. *J Clin Endocrinol Metab.* 1981;53:480-483.

Turner THE, Adams CB, Wass JA. Trans-sphenoidal surgery for microprolactinoma: an acceptable alternative to dopamine agonists? *Eur J Endocrinol.* 1999;140:43-47.

Tyrrell JB, Lamborn KR, Hannegan LT, et al. Transsphenoidal microsurgical therapy of prolactinomas: initial outcomes and long-term results. *Neurosurgery.* 1999;44:254-261:discussion 261–263.

Vance ML, Thorner MO. Prolactinomas. *Endocrinol Metab Clin North Am.* 1987;16:731-753.

Wang MY, Weiss MH. Is there a role for surgery for microprolactinomas? *Semin Neurosurg.* 2001;12:289-294.

Weiss MH, Teal J, Gott P, et al. Natural history of microprolactinomas: six-year follow-up. *Neurosurgery.* 1983;12:180-183.

Weiss MH, Wycoff RR, Yadley R, et al. Bromocriptine treatment of prolactin-secreting tumors: Surgical implications. *Neurosurgery.* 1983;12:640-642.

Numbered references appear on Expert Consult.

CHAPTER 20

Cushing's Disease

JOSEPH WATSON • EDWARD H. OLDFIELD

Cushing's disease (CD), named for neurosurgery's influential forefather, Harvey Cushing, is best treated by surgery. With proper preoperative evaluation and careful surgical technique, most affected patients can be cured while preserving normal pituitary function. If surgery alone is unsuccessful, nearly all patients can be cured of hypercortisolism with irradiation therapy or bilateral adrenalectomy. On the other hand, without treatment, or in the case of treatment failure, the patient's quality of life is impaired and their lifespan is shortened.

Pathophysiology

Cushing's syndrome, the syndrome produced by chronic exposure to excess glucocorticoids, has several etiologies (Table 20-1). The most common cause of Cushing's syndrome is iatrogenic—that is, prescribed glucocorticoids for patients with chronic obstructive pulmonary disease, autoimmune disorders, and transplant patients requiring chronic immunosuppression, among others. Excluding iatrogenic causes, the most common cause of Cushing's syndrome is an ACTH-secreting pituitary adenoma, defined as CD, which affects 60% to 80% of patients with spontaneous (noniatrogenic) Cushing's syndrome (Table 20-1).[1] The other common causes of Cushing's syndrome, which must be distinguished from CD, are adrenal tumors and adrenal cortical hyperplasia, and ectopic ACTH secretion from a nonpituitary tumor, most commonly small-cell–lung cancer or bronchial carcinoid. Secretion of ACTH by lung carcinoma is not rare, but the ACTH is usually inactive, termed "big ACTH."[2] A rare cause of Cushing's syndrome is ectopic secretion of corticotropin-releasing hormone causing corticotroph hyperplasia.

Pathology

The typical pituitary adenoma causing CD is a microadenoma (<1 cm greatest diameter) that stains for ACTH by immunohistochemistry. Larger adenomas are occasionally seen and may even present with apoplexy. These tumors are monoclonal.[3] They disrupt the normal acinar pattern of the gland most clearly seen when stained for reticulin. They are typically basophilic by hematoxylin and eosin staining, but this terminology is no longer used, as immunohistochemistry for ACTH is more specific.

Occasionally Cushing's syndrome is attributed to corticotroph hyperplasia. When no definite tumor is identified at surgery and partial or total hypophysectomy is performed, the specimen must be meticulously and thoroughly examined with serial slices at closely spaced intervals, because tumors as small as 1 mm diameter, or less, may cause endocrinopathy from excess ACTH secretion. Corticotroph hyperplasia, which is usually a diagnosis of exclusion (i.e., only after no tumor can be found in the specimen from pituitary surgery), should be considered only after a careful search of the gland has ruled out a discrete adenoma. In our experience, hyperplasia is exceedingly rare (only two suspected, but unproven, cases from over 1200 operations for CD). A unique cytoplasmic staining pattern, known as Crooke's hyaline change, occurs in corticotrophs of the normal pituitary—cells from which ACTH production has been shut down by chronic exposure to hypercortisolemia. The "hyaline" is comprised of intracytoplasmic microfilaments, which do not stain for ACTH. Crooke's changes may also be found in the cells of the adenoma itself.

Mechanism of Hypercortisolemia in ACTH-Secreting Pituitary Adenomas

The basic endocrine disorder of the adenomas causing CD is that the sensitive negative feedback of cortisol on the production and release of ACTH is impaired (Fig. 20-1). However, ACTH-secreting pituitary adenomas are well-differentiated tumors derived from pituitary corticotrophs; thus, they typically retain negative feedback to glucocorticoids, it is just set at a higher threshold for suppression, as inhibition of ACTH release is retained in response to high doses of glucocorticoid. These well-differentiated tumor cells also retain their expression of CRH receptors and the cellular machinery necessary to respond to CRH. It is these features that underlie the typical diagnostic responses with provocative endocrine tests used for the differential diagnosis of Cushing's syndrome (see below). Excessive production of ACTH leads to hyperplasia and overproduction of cortisol by the adrenal cortex, loss of normal diurnal plasma cortisol rhythm, and sustained hypercortisolemia. It is the excessive cortisol, rather than ACTH per se that causes the clinical manifestations of CD.

Table 20-1	Etiology of Cushing's Syndrome	
ACTH-Dependent		**85%**
Cushing's disease		80–85%
Ectopic ACTH-secreting tumor		15–20%
Ectopic CRH-secreting tumor		Rare (<1%)
ACTH-Independent		**15%**
Adrenal adenoma		7%
Adrenocortical carcinoma		7%
Bilateral micronodular adrenocortical hyperplasia		Rare (1%)
Bilateral macronodular adrenocortical hyperplasia		Rare (<1%)

Table 20-2	Symptoms and Signs of Cushing's Syndrome
Fat Distribution	**Skin Manifestations**
Centripetal obesity	Purple striae
Moon facies	Plethora
"Buffalo hump"	Hirsutism
Supraclavicular fat pads	Acne
Epidural lipomatosis	Bruising
Musculoskeletal	**Metabolic/Circulatory**
Osteoporosis; fractures	Hypertension
Proximal muscle weakness	Glucose intolerance
Pituitary Dysfunction	Hypokalemic alkalosis
Amenorrhea	**Mental Changes**
Decreased libido, impotence	Irritability
Hypothyroidism	Psychosis
Dwarfism (children)	

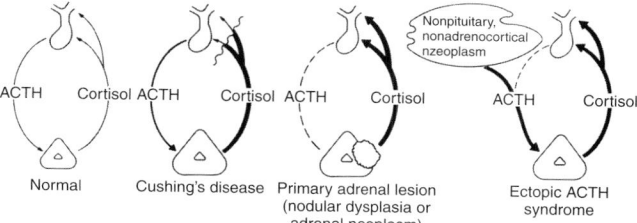

FIGURE 20-1 Normal physiology of the hypothalamic-pituitary-adrenal axis and pathophysiology of hypercortisolism. Left, Hypothalamic corticotropin-releasing hormone (CRH) stimulates production of and secretion of adrenocorticotropic hormone (ACTH) from the corticotrophs of the anterior pituitary. ACTH in turn regulates cortisol production and secretion by the adrenals. Cortisol potently exerts negative feedback on the pituitary and the hypothalamus. *(From Loriaux DL, Cutler GB Jr. Diseases of the adrenal glands. In: Kohler PO, ed. Clinical Endocrinology. New York: Wiley; 1986:167-238, with permission.)*[60]

Clinical Manifestations

The typical patient with Cushing's syndrome has truncal obesity with associated moon facies, enlarged dorsal fat pads ("buffalo hump"), and abdominal fat deposition with associated purple striae or "stretch marks" (Table 20-2). Hirsutism, especially noticeable on the face of women, is a common component, as are thin skin and easy bruisability, especially of the hands and forearms. Along with the outward appearance, mood or psychiatric disturbances are common, especially depression. A reversible form of brain atrophy is frequently displayed on imaging studies[4] and may be a clue to the presence of Cushing's syndrome in pediatric patients. Other signs include hypertension and hyperglycemia, often with frank diabetes mellitus. A hypercoagulable state has been described with Cushing's syndrome, so prophylaxis for deep venous thrombosis in high-risk situations has been encouraged.[5] Patients also may have complications related to immunosuppression, such as fungal or opportunistic infections. Spinal epidural lipomatosis may be symptomatic.[6] Osteoporosis is common; related complications include vertebral compression fractures and susceptibility to traumatic long-bone fractures with minor trauma. Pediatric patients with CD stop growing linearly and gain weight, often producing morbid obesity.[7] This "crossing of the weight and height curves" is so common in childhood Cushing's syndrome that many consider it diagnostic of the condition. Affected children often appear cherubic. Symptoms caused by tumor growth and pressure on the optic nerves and chiasm are rare with CD, as the tumors are usually microadenomas.

Life expectancy is greatly foreshortened by untreated CD. If left untreated, most patients succumb early to complications of the disease (diabetes, hypertension, myocardial infarction, stroke, or complications associated with immunosuppression).[8]

Diagnosis

The diagnosis of Cushing's syndrome, and its differential diagnosis, must be established with a high degree of certainty to avoid unnecessary surgery and treatment failure. Provocative endocrine testing is important in patients with Cushing's syndrome, as hypercortisolism may come from causes other than a pituitary tumor, and ectopic ACTH-secreting tumors (typically lung neoplasia) and the pituitary adenomas causing CD are often too small to be detected with radiographic techniques.

ESTABLISHING HYPERCORTISOLISM

Cushing's syndrome, when suspected clinically, is confirmed by demonstrating hypercortisolism or characteristics of its effects on the normal functioning of the hypothalamic-pituitary-adrenal axis. Confirmation of excess cortisol production is made by one or more standard testing procedures. Most commonly today these tests include one or more of the following: serial 24-hour urine-free cortisol measurements, diurnal plasma cortisol levels, evening salivary cortisol levels to detect loss of diurnal rhythm of cortisol secretion, or the overnight dexamethasone suppression test.

Urine-free cortisol (UFC) measurements are assayed using a variety of techniques. The normal upper levels vary with the technique used and with the laboratory performing the assay (Fig. 20-2). Hypercortisolism is associated with loss of normal diurnal variation in cortisol secretion, which is demonstrated by obtaining morning (8 to 9 a.m.) and evening (11 to 12 p.m.) plasma cortisol levels (Fig. 20-3). Salivary cortisol levels are also reliably used for this and are well suited for outpatient screening of adult and pediatric patients for hypercortisolism.[9] A study of more than 140 patients demonstrated a sensitivity of 93%

and a specificity of 100% using this test to determine the presence of Cushing's syndrome (Fig. 20-4).[10] Because of its simplicity, the overnight low-dose (1 mg) dexamethasone suppression test is commonly used to screen patients for hypercortisolism (Fig. 20-5). In persons with a normal hypothalamic-pituitary-adrenal axis, AM cortisol levels are suppressed by the overnight low-dose dexamethasone suppression test (1.0 mg given the night before a morning [7 to 8 a.m.] cortisol measurement). A morning plasma cortisol level greater than 1.8 μg/dl after the bedtime (11 p.m.) administration of 1 mg of dexamethasone detects most patients with Cushing's syndrome and justifies further diagnostic evaluation.[11]

DIFFERENTIAL DIAGNOSIS OF HYPERCORTISOLISM

Once excess cortisol production has been established, plasma ACTH levels are measured to distinguish between an ACTH-dependent and ACTH-independent etiology (Fig. 20-6; see also Fig. 20-1). With CD or ectopic ACTH secretion, the ACTH levels will be normal or elevated relative to the degree of glucocorticoid secretion. For this reason, these two entities are categorized as "ACTH-dependent" Cushing's syndrome (see Table 20-1), in contrast to adrenal disease, in which plasma ACTH is low (<5 pg/ml) or undetectable ("ACTH-independent" Cushing's syndrome, as the adrenal cortical cortisol secretion is autonomous).

At one time, the presence of Cushing's syndrome and then differentiating CD from adrenal disease or ectopic ACTH secretion were examined with the 6-day dexamethasone suppression test, as described by Liddle.[12,13] The first 2 days of the test were used for measurement of basal cortisol secretion. In most patients with CD, cortisol secretion, an indirect measure of ACTH secretion by the pituitary gland or the tumor, is not suppressed during the 2 days of low-dose dexamethasone (0.5 mg every 6 hours for 48 hours),

but 24-hour urinary cortisol secretion is suppressed to less than 10% of baseline values by 2 days of high-dose dexamethasone (2 mg every 6 hours for 48 hours). In contrast, high-dose dexamethasone fails to suppress cortisol secretion in most cases of ectopic ACTH secretion. Because of the difficulty in successfully completing this test today, it is now rarely used, but has been replaced with the high-dose overnight dexamethasone suppression test. For this test, 8 mg of dexamethasone is administered orally at 11 p.m. and a morning (7 to 8 a.m.) plasma cortisol measurement is obtained;[14] for greatest diagnostic accuracy, suppression of morning serum cortisol of greater than 68% is required to assign a diagnosis of CD (Fig. 20-7).[14,15]

Another test available today to distinguish ectopic ACTH secretion from an ACTH-secreting pituitary tumor is the CRH stimulation test.[16-18] Since they are well-differentiated tumors derived from pituitary corticotrophs, most ACTH-secreting pituitary adenomas retain receptors for, and response to, CRH, whereas most ectopic tumors, tumors that are not derived from pituitary tissue, do not express receptors for CRH and do not respond to it (Fig. 20-8). The sensitivity and specificity of the test are optimal using ≥35% for the maximum ACTH response from the 15- or 30-minute samples to indicate CD (see Fig. 20-8B).[18]

If ACTH-dependent hypercortisolism is established, a sella MRI with and without contrast is obtained (see below). In many patients with CD, a high-resolution sella MRI will demonstrate the presence and location of a pituitary tumor. However, a negative sella MRI does not rule out an adenoma, as the false-negative rate using the standard T1-weighted spin echo after contrast enhancement in CD is as high as 50% at some centers.

If the results of the high-dose dexamethasone suppression test and the CRH stimulation test are consistent with CD and the pituitary MRI reveals a definite adenoma, no further diagnostic testing is necessary. However, if either of these provocative endocrine tests is inconsistent with CD, inferior petrosal sinus sampling is performed.

The test with the greatest diagnostic accuracy for the differential diagnosis of CD versus ectopic ACTH syndrome is bilateral simultaneous inferior petrosal sinus sampling performed with and without intravenous CRH administration.[19] The test is performed by placement of catheters with their tips in the inferior petrosal sinuses and in a peripheral vein (Fig. 20-9A), and then obtaining serial, simultaneous samples for central and peripheral plasma ACTH concentrations at 2 and 0 minutes before and at 3, 5, and 10 minutes after intravenous CRH administration (1 μg/kg body weight). IPSS is only used in patients with confirmed hypercortisolism, as the test cannot discriminate between normal subjects and patients with CD. Further, since this is an invasive procedure with rare but serious associated risks,[20] it is generally used in patients in whom the results of provocative endocrine testing to distinguish ectopic ACTH secretion from CD are conflicting or equivocal and in instances in which the sella MRI is negative. In this test the levels of ACTH in the primary venous drainage of the pituitary, the inferior petrosal sinuses, are compared to simultaneous ACTH measurements in the peripheral blood. A peak ratio of 2:1 petrosal:peripheral during baseline (before CRH) or 3:1 before or after CRH indicates a pituitary source of the excess ACTH, that is, CD.[19] The sensitivity of the test is

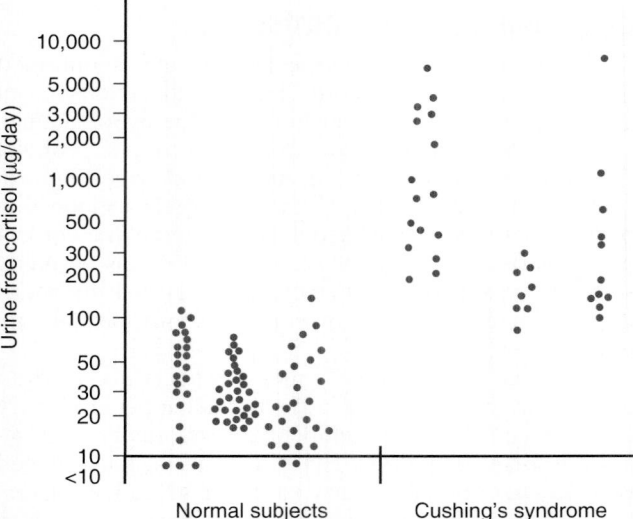

FIGURE 20-2 Twenty-four–hour excretion of urine-free cortisol to screen patients for Cushing's syndrome. Comparison of 24-hour excretion of urine-free cortisol value in normal subjects and patients with confirmed Cushing's syndrome. *(Modified from Loriaux DL, Cutler GB Jr. Diseases of the adrenal glands. In: Kohler PO, ed. Clinical Endocrinology. New York: Wiley; 1986:167-238, with permission.)*[60]

increased by sampling after administration of CRH, which, because it stimulates a pituitary adenoma to secrete ACTH, enhances the ACTH concentration differential between the central (inferior petrosal sinus) and the peripheral blood (Fig. 20-9B).[19] It originally seemed that the procedure had a diagnostic accuracy 100%. However, reports of diagnostic errors, almost all false negative, have appeared, although in our experience the diagnostic accuracy approaches 100%. The accuracy of the test also relies upon successful placement of the catheter tips in the petrosal sinus bilaterally, since a false negative result may arise if the blood from both inferior petrosal sinuses cannot be catheterized successfully. Thus, venography is performed to ensure correct catheter placement and to evaluate the venous anatomy.

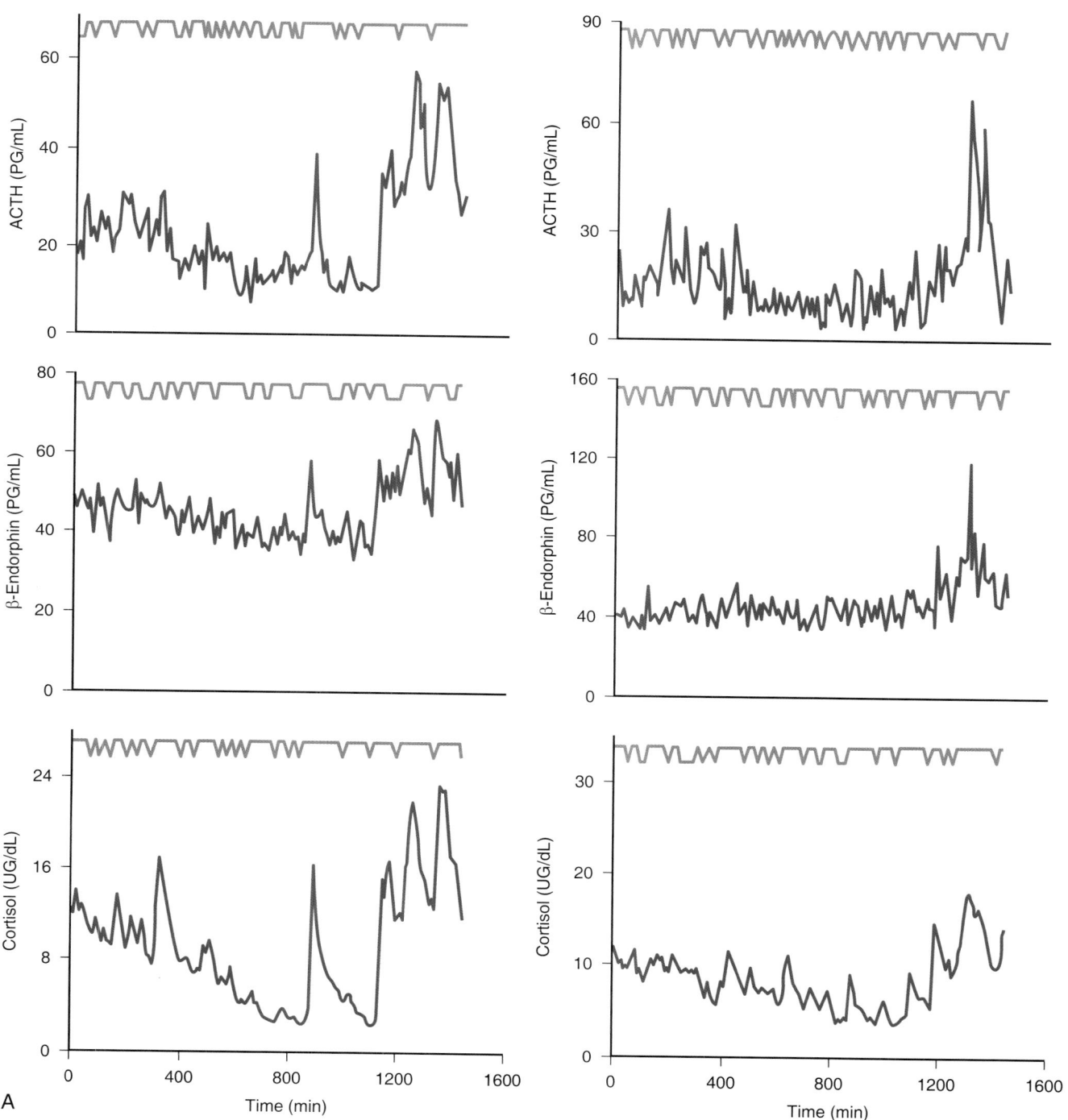

FIGURE 20-3 A. Diurnal rhythms of ACTH, β-endorphin, and cortisol in normal subjects. Plasma ACTH, β-endorphin, and cortisol concentrations in each of two (A and B) normal men who received blood sampling every 10 minutes for 24 hours. (Modified from Veldhuis JD, Iranmanesh A, Johnson ML, Lizarralde G. Amplitude, but not frequency, modulation of adrenocorticotropin secretory bursts gives rise to the nyctohemeral rhythm of the corticotropic axis in man. J Clin Endocrinol Metab. 1990;71:452-463.)

Continued

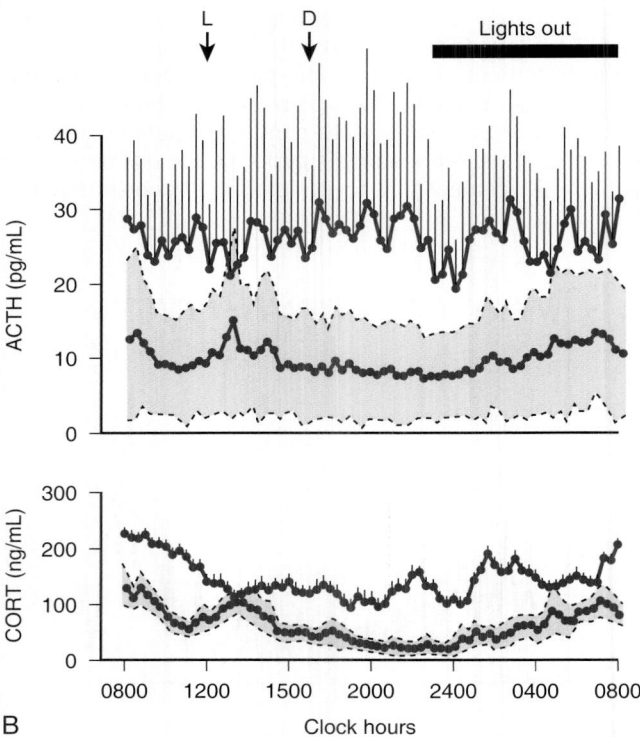

FIGURE 20-3, cont'd B, Diurnal rhythms of plasma ACTH and cortisol levels in nine normal women (shaded area; ±95% confidence limits) and in five women with CD (mean ± standard deviation). L, lunch; D, dinner. *(Modified from Liu JH, Kazer RR, Rasmussen DD. Characterization of the twenty-four hour secretion patterns of adrenocorticotropin and cortisol in normal women and patients with Cushing's disease. J Clin Endocrinol Metab. 1987;64:1027-1035.)*

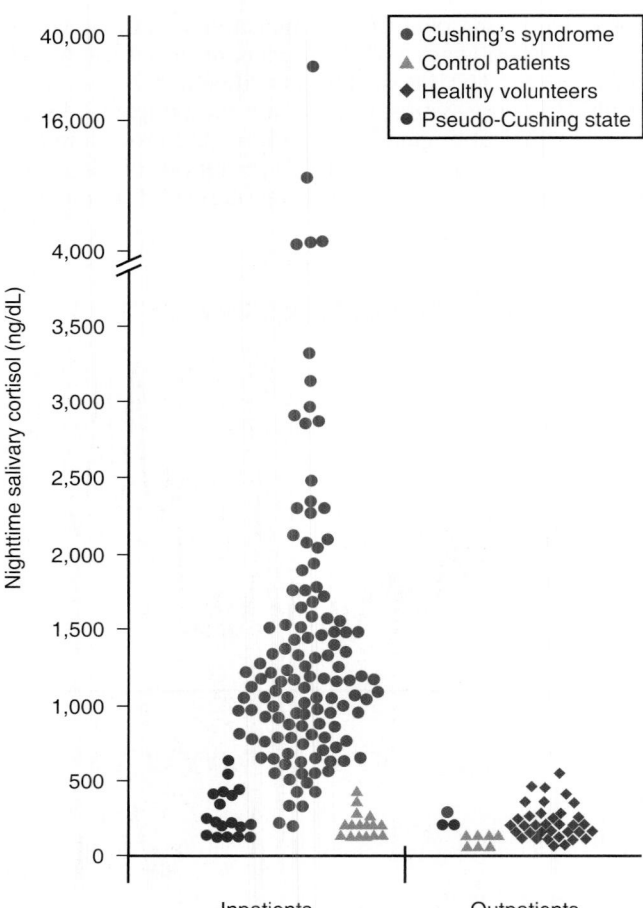

FIGURE 20-4 Salivary cortisols. Nighttime salivary cortisol values in healthy volunteers ◆, patient controls ▲, pseudo-Cushing patients ●, and patients with Cushing's syndrome ●. Samples were collected at 12 midnight from inpatients and at bedtime (11 p.m. to 2 a.m.) from outpatients. To convert salivary cortisol nanograms per deciliter to nanomoles per liter, multiply by 0.0276. *(Modified from Papanicolaou DA, Mullen N, Kyrou I, et al. Nighttime salivary cortisol: a useful test for the diagnosis of Cushing's syndrome. J Clin Endocrinol Metab. 2002;87:4515-4521.)*

A hypoplastic or anomalous inferior petrosal sinus in 0.8% of 501 patients was associated with false-negative results in patients with proven CD.[21] It was briefly thought that comparison of petrosal sinus ACTH from the right to left sides would accurately indicate the side of the pituitary in which a small pituitary tumor was located, permitting a more focused search for it at surgery, or permitting removal of the half of the pituitary containing an adenoma that was too small to identify despite a thorough search of the gland during surgery.[22] However, more experience with the technique for lateralization indicated that the lateralization accuracy is only about 70%, and even less so in pediatric patients,[23] compromising its usefulness as a localizing measure during surgery.[19]

IMAGING

Sella magnetic resonance imaging (MRI) is the imaging procedure of choice for detecting and localizing the pituitary adenoma in patients with CD. MRI should be performed with and without contrast, as the adenomas typically have decreased enhancement compared to the normal gland (Fig. 20-10). The resolution of a 1.5-T magnet may reveal tumors as small as 3 mm in diameter. MRI provides other important anatomical information for the surgeon: aeration of the sphenoid, parasellar anatomy, location of the carotid arteries or coexisting aneurysms, extent of supra- or parasellar extension of an adenoma, and ectopic parasellar tumors. Recently the spoiled gradient recalled acquisition

(SPGR) technique, used with 1-mm nonoverlapping slices was shown to be more sensitive than the conventional spin echo approach (sensitivity 80% vs. 49%), a finding also true in pediatric CD.[24,25] However, the incidence of false positives was also higher (4% vs. 2%). Since the sensitivity of the conventional MRI techniques (spin echo) for CD is only 50% to 75%,[26-29] many patients have a negative MRI. Furthermore, MRI is not always available or possible, as in patients with an MRI incompatible cardiac pacemaker or a morbidly obese patient who cannot be accommodated by the scanner. In these patients, a sella computerized tomography image (CT) with and without contrast may demonstrate a tumor, but CT is less sensitive than MRI. Furthermore, since the specificity of MRI is not 100% (MRI abnormalities consistent with adenomas occur in the pituitary gland in 10% of normal volunteers[30] and incidental adenomas are found in the pituitary gland in about 5% to 20% of subjects in unselected autopsy studies[31,32]), the results of MRI scanning must be confirmed by endocrinologic testing before surgery. In general, CD endocrine testing provides the

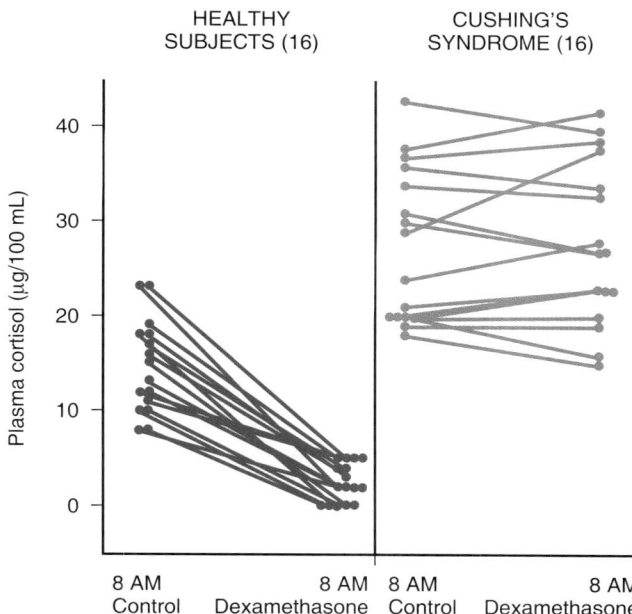

HEALTHY
SUBJECTS (16)

CUSHING'S
SYNDROME (16)

8 AM
Control

8 AM
Dexamethasone

8 AM
Control

8 AM
Dexamethasone

FIGURE 20-5 Detection of Cushing's syndrome with the low-dose overnight dexamethasone suppression test. Plasma cortisol levels at 8 a.m. on successive days before and after 1 mg dexamethasone given orally at 11:00 p.m. in healthy subjects and patients with Cushing's syndrome. *(Modified from Melby JC. Assessment of adrenocortical function. N Engl J Med. 1971;285:735-739.)*

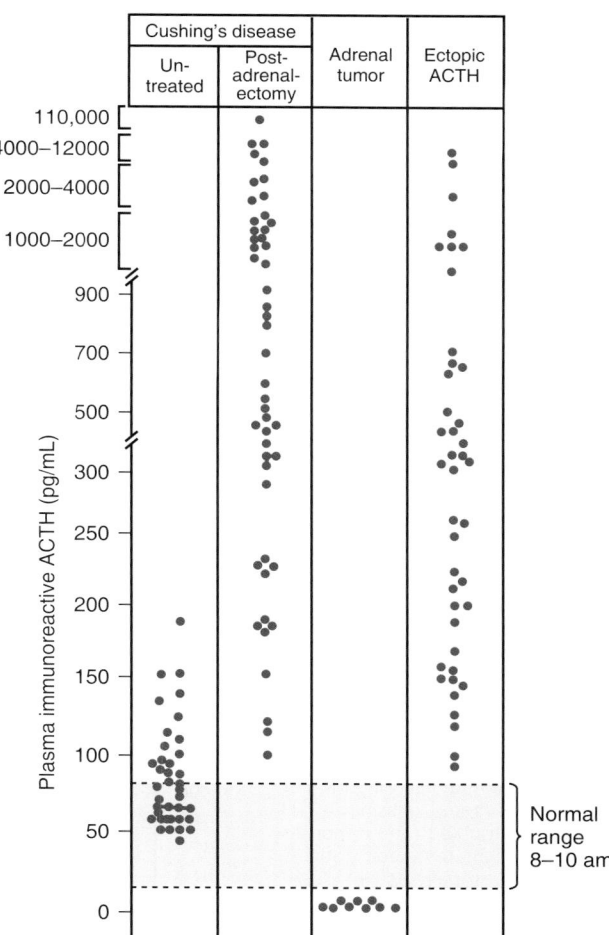

FIGURE 20-6 Plasma ACTH levels distinguish patients with ACTH-independent (primary adrenal disease) and ACTH-dependent forms of Cushing's syndrome. Plasma ACTH levels in 137 patients with Cushing's syndrome. *(From Besser GM, Edwards CRW. Cushing's syndrome. Clin Endocrinol Metab. 1972;1:451-490, with permission.)*[64]

diagnosis and CT localizes the adenoma within the pituitary and defines the anatomy in its vicinity.

Treatment

SURGERY

Trans-sphenoidal microsurgery is the treatment of choice for CD. Identification of the adenoma and selective adenomectomy provides remission of hypercortisolism in most patients with an adenoma that is contained within the anterior lobe and that is large enough to be detected by MRI. Surgery for these tumors is similar to the procedures that have been described for pituitary tumors in general.

However, many tumors that cause CD are small, frequently so small that they are not identified on the preoperative MRI. In these patients the first task for the surgeon is to locate the adenoma. A wide exposure of the pituitary gland permits visualization of the anterior lobe from one edge to the other. This requires removal of the bone of the anterior face of the sella until the medial portion of the cavernous sinus is visible bilaterally. The pseudocapsule of a microadenoma is almost always a grey-white or gray-yellow color. Because coagulation of the dura will discolor a circumscribed area of the pituitary surface, producing a local white region that can mimic an adenoma just beneath the site of dural coagulation, bipolar cautery of the dura is avoided. A wide cruciate dural opening extending to the lateral corners of the exposure, to the junction of the circular sinus with the cavernous sinus superiorly and to the medial wall of the cavernous sinus inferiorly, while avoiding entry into the capsule of the pituitary gland, allows visualization of most of the anterior surface of the anterior lobe. In many

cases, an adenoma will be seen during careful inspection of the gland's surface while using the operating microscope to look for a focal mass or discoloration on the surface of the gland. Localization of adenomas with intraoperative ultrasound, using a specially designed probe, has also proven useful in patients with negative MRI scans.[33] When it is used, intraoperative ultrasound is obtained after the bone removal is complete, but before the dura is opened, and with a bloodless field. However, in our experience the most reliable clue to the identification of a microadenoma is visualization of its pseudocapsule. This is especially important for the small tumors that are buried in the gland.

When the location of an adenoma is identified by inspection of the surface of the gland, the pituitary capsule is sharply incised just beyond the visible margin of the tumor pseudocapsule, which is a margin of compressed normal gland surrounding the adenoma (Fig. 20-11). If the adenoma is not identified by examining the pituitary capsule anteriorly and inspecting the lateral surfaces of the anterior lobe, a series of incisions is made vertically in the gland at intervals of 1.5 to 2 mm, each carried deeper in increments until either the pseudocapsule of the tumor is identified or the

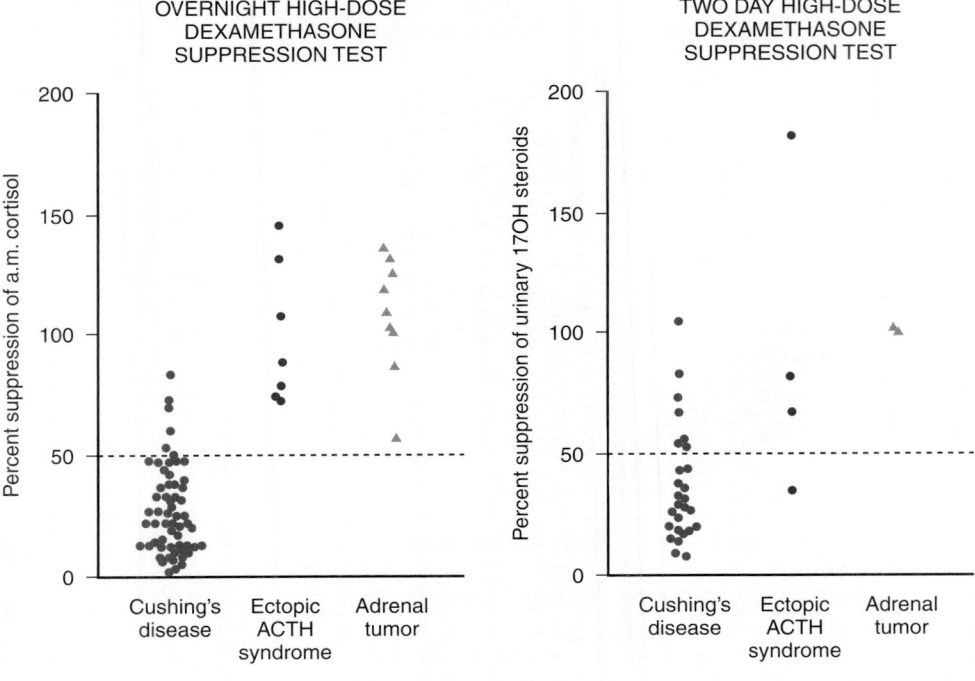

FIGURE 20-7 High-dose (8 mg) overnight dexamethasone suppression test for the differential diagnosis of Cushing's syndrome. Comparison of the high-dose overnight dexamethasone suppression test with the high-dose portion of the standard 6-day dexamethasone suppression test. *(Data from Tyrrell JB, Findling JW, Aron DC, Fitzgerald PA, Forsham PH. An overnight high-dose dexamethasone suppression test for rapid differential diagnosis of Cushing's syndrome. Ann Intern Med. 1986;104:180-186.)*

FIGURE 20-8 A, CRH stimulation test for the differential diagnosis of Cushing's syndrome. Plasma ACTH (top) and cortisol (bottom) responses to CRH in eight untreated patients with CD ●, six patients with Cushing's syndrome due to ectopic ACTH secretion ▲, and 10 human controls ●. *(Modified from Chrousos GP, Schulte HM, Oldfield EH, Gold PW, Cutler GB Jr, Loriaux DL. The corticotropin-releasing factor stimulation test. An aid in the evaluation of patients with Cushing's syndrome. N Engl J Med. 1984;310:622-626.)*

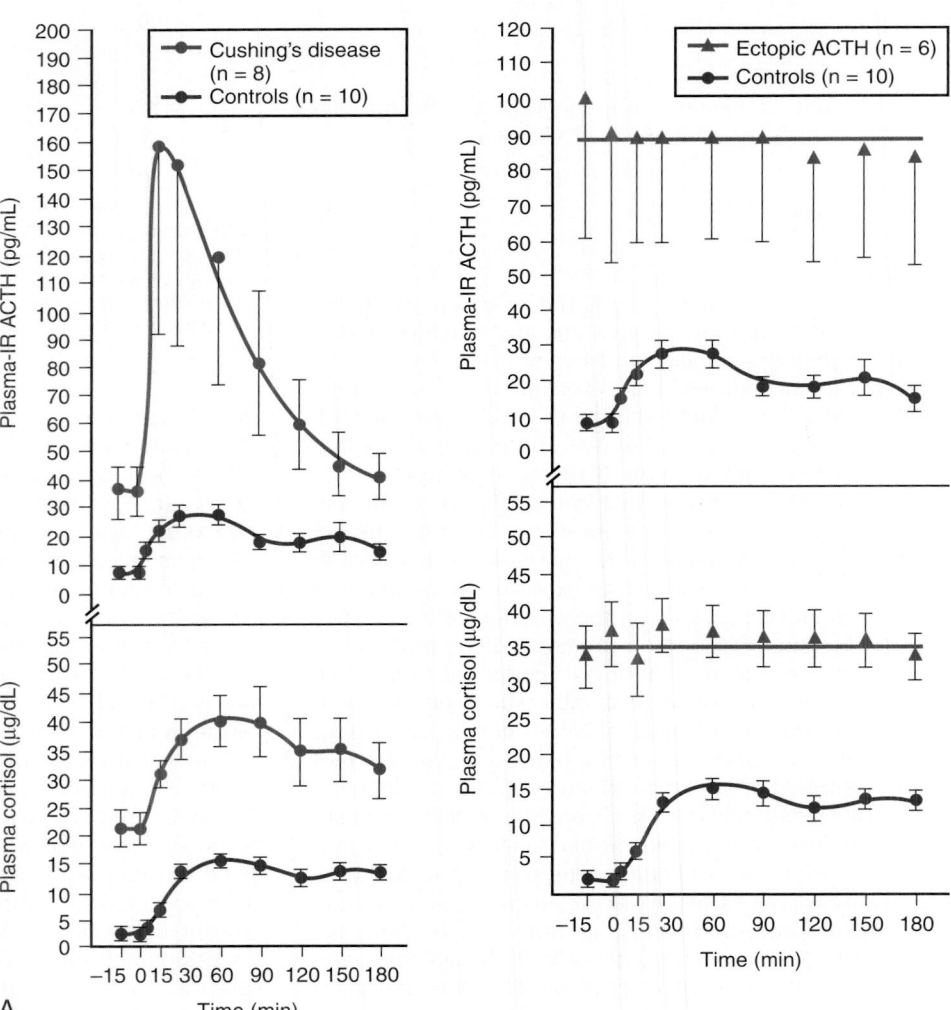

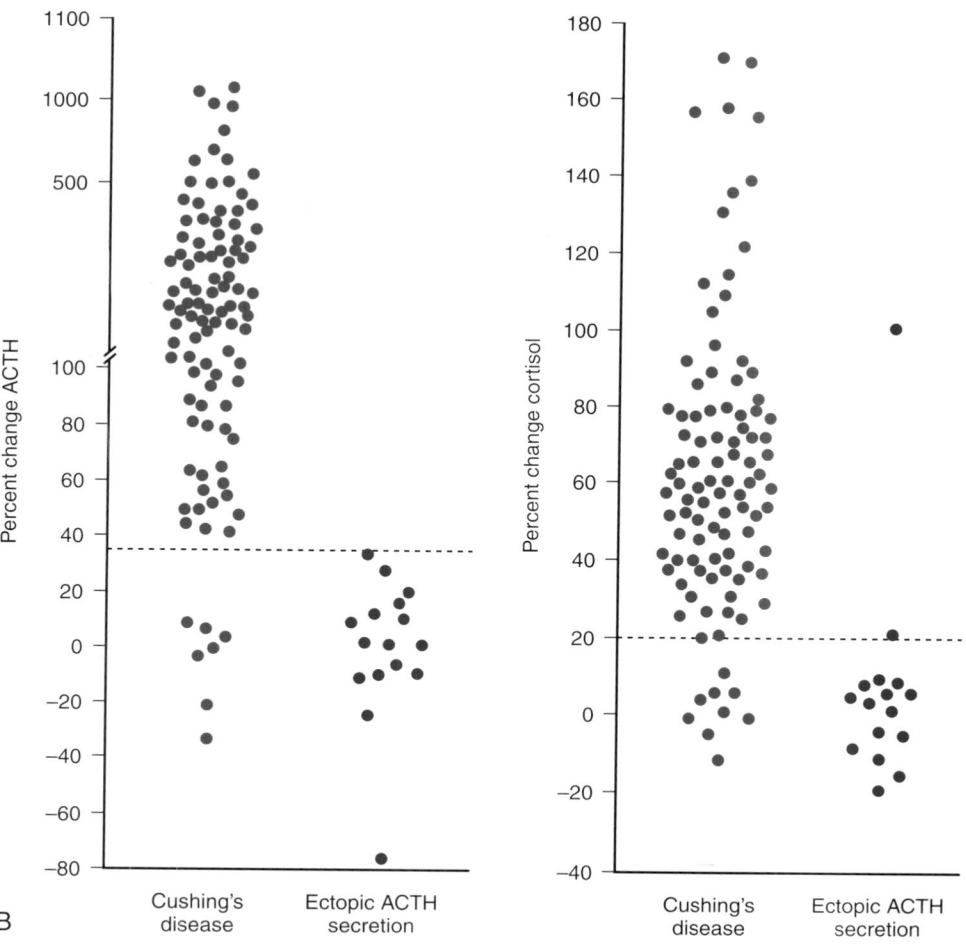

FIGURE 20-8, cont'd B, Responses of plasma ACTH and cortisol to intravenous administration of ovine CRH in patients with CD and ectopic ACTH secretion. ACTH responses are expressed as the percent change in mean ACTH concentration 15 and 30 min after CRH from the basal value 1 and 5 min before the injection. Dashed line indicates a response of 35%. Cortisol responses are expressed as the percent change in mean cortisol concentration 30 and 45 min after CRH from the basal value 1 and 5 min before the injection. Dashed line indicates a response of 20%. *(Modified from Nieman LK, Oldfield EH, Wesley R, et al. A simplified morning ovine corticotropin-releasing hormone stimulation test for the differential diagnosis of adrenocorticotropin-dependent Cushing's syndrome. J Clin Endocrinol Metab. 1993;77:1308-1312.)*

juncture of the anterior and posterior lobes is reached (Fig. 20-12). By identification of the interface between the pseudocapsule of the adenoma and the surrounding normal gland, the adenoma is discretely dissected from the normal pituitary, ideally without entering the soft body of the adenoma. In this way, total resection is commonly performed and lasting remission is achieved.[34] If the tumor breaches the capsule of the pituitary gland, careful inspection of the contiguous dura is performed to ensure that dural invasion by the tumor is not overlooked. This is particularly important laterally along the medial wall of the cavernous sinus, where even small tumors may spread into the adjacent dura and cavernous sinus.

ACTH-producing tumors may also be found in the posterior lobe,[35] so careful inspection of the gland back to the neurohypophysis should be preformed when no tumor is encountered anteriorly.

In the rare instance when the ACTH-secreting adenoma is located outside of the adenohypophysis, such as in a suprasellar (Fig. 20-13) or parasellar location,[36] special techniques are required. For tumors of the pituitary stalk in the suprasellar cistern, an extended trans-sphenoidal approach may be used.[37] With this technique, during the standard transseptal approach, bone removal is extended rostrally over the planum sphenoidale. The dura anterior to the gland is opened in the midline to expose the suprasellar cistern (Fig. 20-14). Bleeding from the opened circular sinus is stopped by packing it with small pieces of Gelfoam or with bipolar coagulation. Direct visual access of the pituitary stalk is thus provided.

Endonasal or endoscopic approaches to the sella are being examined, although their utility for resection of endocrine-active adenomas, such as CD, remains to be established.

POSTOPERATIVE ASSESSMENT

The chronic hypercortisolism associated with CD suppresses the hypothalamic CRH-producing cells and the secretion of ACTH by the normal corticotrophs, but does not fully suppress ACTH secretion by the tumor. In most patients who are cured by surgery it takes several months for the hypothalamic-pituitary-adrenal axis to recover and the patient suffers from hypocortisolism and requires glucocorticoid replacement therapy for the 6 to 24 months required for recovery of the hypothalamic neuron, the normal pituitary corticotroph, and the adrenal cortex and return of normal endogenous circadian cortisol secretion (Fig. 20-15). Therefore, complete removal of the abnormal source of ACTH should produce hypocortisolism in the immediate postoperative interval and for several months.[38] Thus, in almost all instances of successful surgery for CD, the patient will be hypocortisolemic (a morning cortisol of less than 5 µg/dl and 24-hour urine-free cortisol secretion of less than 20 µg). Because of this, postoperative cortisol replacement must be provided. There are several

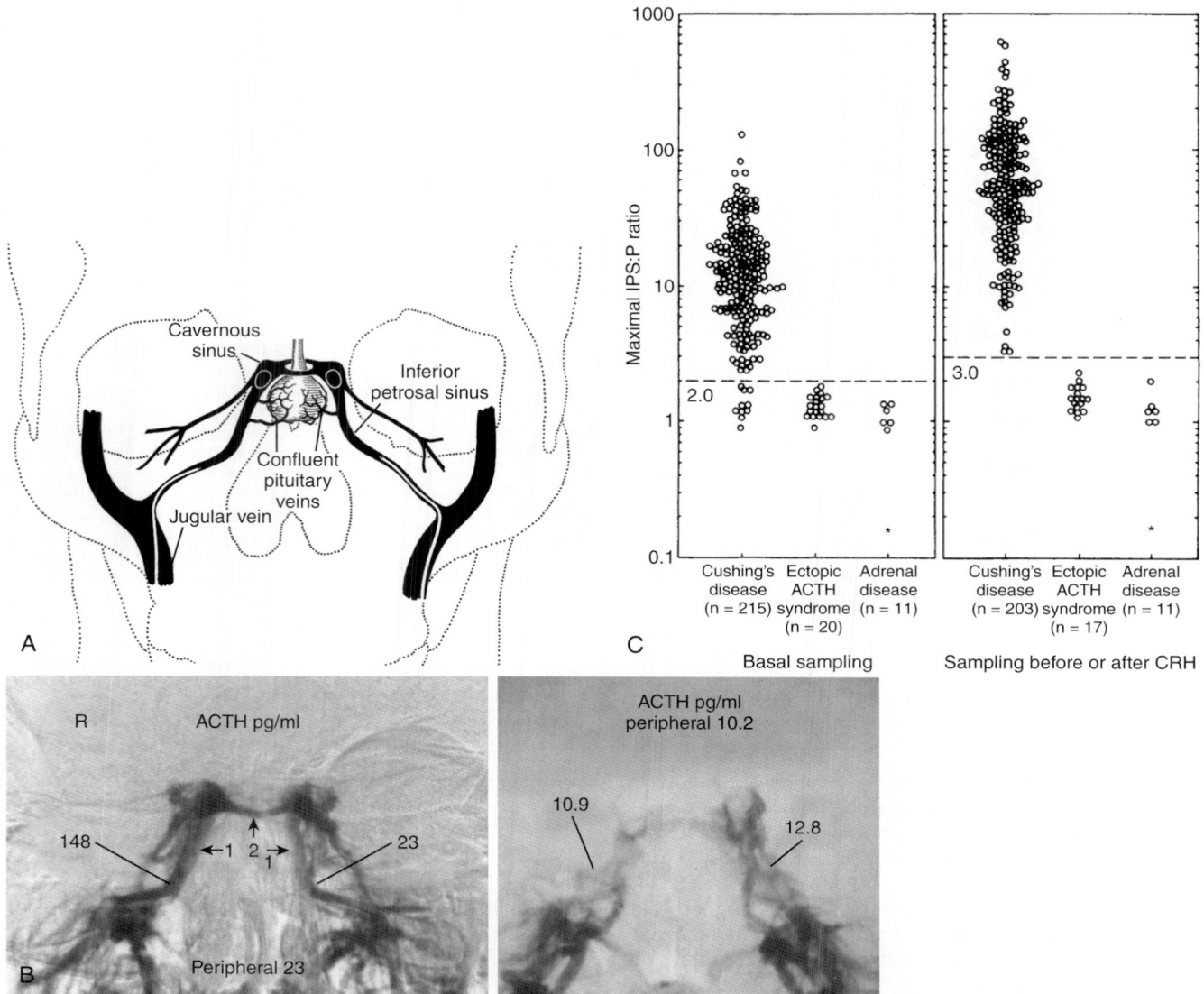

FIGURE 20-9 A, Anatomy and catheter placement in bilateral simultaneous blood sampling of the inferior petrosal sinuses. Confluent pituitary veins empty laterally into the cavernous sinuses, which drain into the inferior petrosal sinuses. B, Venous sampling during inferior petrosal venous sampling with ACTH levels from a patient with CD (left) and a patient with a bronchial carcinoid and ectopic ACTH secretion (right). C, Bilateral inferior petrosal vein sampling in the differential diagnosis of Cushing's syndrome. Maximum ratio of ACTH concentration from one of the inferior petrosal sinuses to the simultaneous peripheral venous ACTH concentration in patients with Cushing's syndrome in basal samples (left), and in basal and CRH-stimulated samples (right). During basal sampling, the maximum IPS:P ACTH ratio was ≥2.0 in 205 of 215 patients with confirmed CD, but was <2.0 in all patients with ectopic ACTH syndrome or primary adrenal disease. All patients with CD who received CRH had maximum IPS:P ACTH ratios of ≥3.0, whereas all patients with ectopic ACTH syndrome had IPS:P ratios of <3.0. The asterisks represent five patients with primary adrenal disease in whom ACTH was undetectable in the peripheral blood before and after CRH administration. *(A and C from Oldfield EH, Doppman JL, Nieman LK, et al. Bilateral inferior petrosal sinus sampling with and without corticotropin-releasing hormone for the differential diagnosis of Cushing's syndrome. N Engl J Med. 1991;325:897-905.)*

protocols for postoperative cortisol replacement therapy. One approach used in our practices is to administer 0.5 mg of dexamethasone every 6 hours for 36 hours. The dexamethasone is then discontinued and daily AM cortisol and 24-hour urine cortisol are obtained for 3 consecutive days. This permits immediate determination if surgery has been successful in eliminating hypercortisolism and provides the potential for immediate early reoperation, if indicated, which is successful in many patients.[39] Others use postoperative low-dose dexamethasone suppression testing as follows: on the first postoperative day, the patient receives 50 mg of hydrocortisone intravenously in the morning and 25 mg in the evening. On the second day, they are given 50 mg of hydrocortisone in the morning and 1 mg of dexamethasone in the evening at 10 p.m. Blood is withdrawn from the patient at 8 a.m. on the third postoperative morning and a fasting serum cortisol level is measured. With this approach patients with a morning plasma cortisol greater than 2 μg/dl will have a high likelihood of having recurrent disease: 100% of patients in the report by Arnott et al.[40] and in the larger experience of Chen et al.[41] On the other hand, 93% of patients with an AM cortisol value of

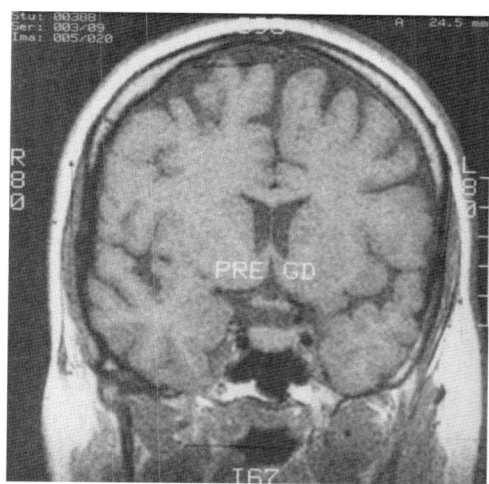 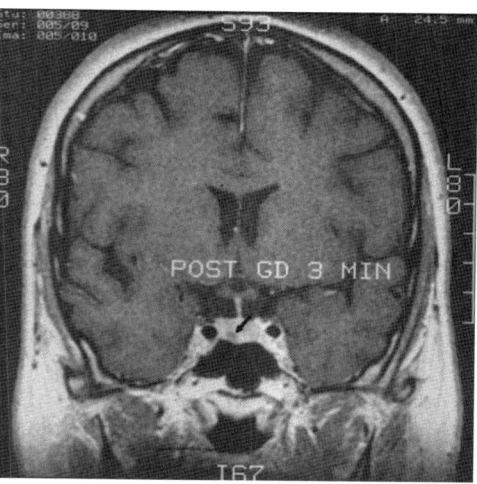

FIGURE 20-10 Magnetic resonance imaging of the pituitary in a patient with a 4-mm adenoma in the right half of the anterior lobe. This image was acquired before (left) and immediately after (right) infusion of gadolinium-DTPA (T1-weighted MRI, TR 500, TE 20). *(From Doppman JL, Frank JA, Dwyer AJ, et al. Gadolinium DTPA enhanced imaging of ACTH-secreting microadenomas of the pituitary gland. Correlation of MR appearance with surgical findings. J Comput Assist Tomogr. 1988;12:728-735.)*

2 µg/dl or less still had sustained remission of CD at 5 years (Fig. 20-16).[41] Many authors prefer either to provide cortisol replacement therapy and to test the patient's cortisol secretion several weeks after hospital discharge, or to provide no cortisol replacement and sample serum cortisol levels every 6 hours after surgery.[42-44] Most cured patients have serum cortisol drop below 2 µg/dl within the first 48 hours after surgery.

Without glucocorticoid replacement, the patient may be symptomatic from an Addisonian state and will typically complain of symptoms of lethargy, anorexia, and abdominal discomfort or nausea. As the patient's blood pressure will be normal or even low postoperatively, preoperative medications used to treat hypertension are withheld until it is determined that they are required after surgery. Similarly, since glycemic control may be restored after surgery, preoperative diabetic medications are withheld, and blood glucose is carefully monitored in the immediate postoperative interval. After discharge twice daily physiologic cortisol replacement is provided (cortisol, 15 to 20 mg in the morning and 5 mg in the evening) until normal function of the hypothalamic-pituitary-adrenal axis is re-established, which usually does not occur until 6 to 24 months after surgery.

In patients with eucortisolism immediately or within a few weeks of surgery, clinical remission is still likely, though CD is more likely to recur than in patients with postoperative hypocortisolism (Fig. 20-17).[45,46]

EARLY REPEAT SURGERY

If results of cortisol measurement shortly after surgery indicate persistent hypercortisolism, immediate repeat surgery should be considered in certain circumstances.[39] Early reoperation (within 1 to 6 weeks) can induce remission in the majority of patients, although with a risk of hypopituitarism. Surgical or pathologic confirmation of an ACTH-positive adenoma that is incompletely resected during the initial pituitary exploration is the most significant predictor of success with early re-exploration, in terms of both remission and avoidance of hypopituitarism. Patients who have undergone limited exploration of the pituitary and selective excision of an area that at surgery appears to be, but proves not to have been, a corticotroph adenoma, also are

likely to benefit from repeat surgery. On the other hand, patients who undergo an extensive initial exploration and partial resection of the anterior lobe are unlikely to benefit from a repeat operation if there is no ACTH-positive adenoma in the excised specimen.[39] With appropriate patient selection early repeat surgery deserves consideration, especially when prompt control of hypercortisolism is required.

SURGICAL MANAGEMENT OF RECURRENT CUSHING'S DISEASE

Patients who have remission of hypercortisolism following surgery occasionally develop recurrent CD. What should be done for the patient with recurrent CD after previous surgery? In a report detailing the results of trans-sphenoidal surgery in 31 patients who had previously undergone a trans-sphenoidal operation and two patients who had had previous pituitary irradiation only, in 24 (73%) of the 33 patients, remission of hypercortisolism was achieved by surgery.[47] Although CT identified an adenoma in only three of the 33 patients, in 20 patients a discrete adenoma was identified at pituitary exploration. The incidence of remission of hypercortisolism was greatest if an adenoma was identified at surgery and the patient received selective adenomectomy (19, or 95% of 20 patients), if there was evidence at surgery or by preoperative imaging that the previous surgical exposure of the pituitary was incomplete (seven, or 78% of nine patients), if an adenoma was seen on preoperative imaging (three of three patients), or if the patient had had prior pituitary irradiation without surgery (two of two patients). In contrast, only five (42%) of 12 patients who received subtotal or total hypophysectomy had remission of hypercortisolism. Surgically induced hypopituitarism occurred in six (50%) of these 12 patients, but in only one (5%) of the 20 patients who underwent selective adenomectomy. Three (13%) of the 24 patients who were in remission from hypercortisolism following repeat surgery developed recurrent hypercortisolism 10 to 47 months postoperatively.

More recent reports have established that the recurrent adenoma is always at, or immediately contiguous to, the site of the adenoma at the original surgery.[48,49] Furthermore, the recurrent tumor usually is invading the dura, usually the cavernous sinus wall contiguous to the former

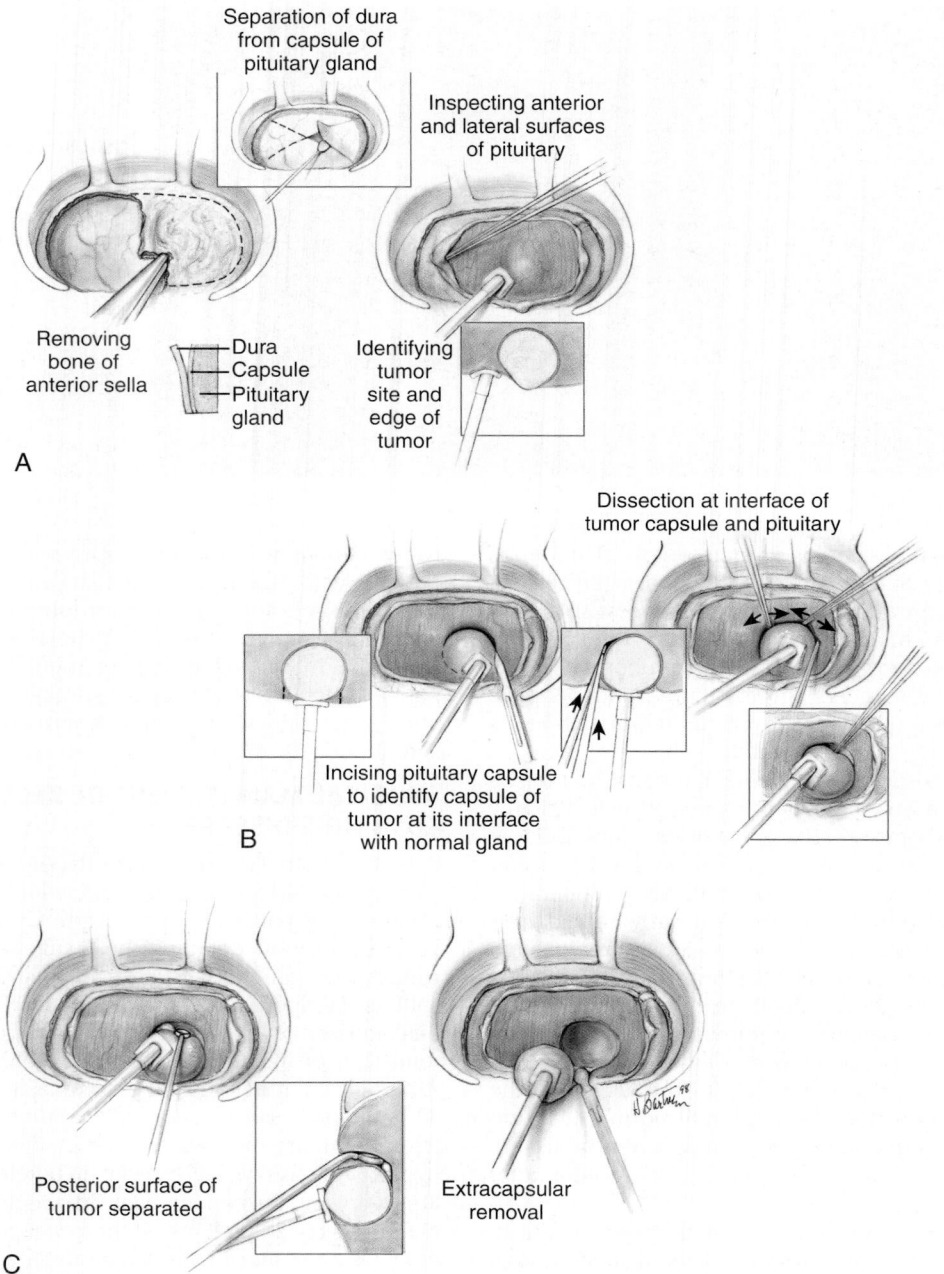

A

Separation of dura from capsule of pituitary gland

Inspecting anterior and lateral surfaces of pituitary

Removing bone of anterior sella

Dura
Capsule
Pituitary gland

Identifying tumor site and edge of tumor

B

Dissection at interface of tumor capsule and pituitary

Incising pituitary capsule to identify capsule of tumor at its interface with normal gland

C

Posterior surface of tumor separated

Extracapsular removal

location of the adenoma. In the Dickerman and Oldfield series, at repeat surgery (44 ± 35 months after the initial surgery), in all 43 patients in whom an adenoma had been identified at the initial surgery, the tumor was found at the same site or contiguous to the same site,[48] indicating that recurrence of CD is from growth of residual cells left in situ at the original surgery and that at repeat exploration the site occupied by the original tumor should be the focus of the exploration. Dural invasion by an ACTH-producing tumor was identified during repeated surgery in 42 (62%) of the 68 patients re-explored after prior surgery and recurrent or persistent CD. In addition, 39 (93%) of these 42 invasive adenomas were located laterally and involved the cavernous sinus. Adenoma invasion of the dura mater

was found in 31 (54%) of 57 microadenomas and in all 11 macroadenomas at repeated surgery. The presence of tumor was not detected in 28 of the 59 patients studied with MRI and in none of these 59 patients was dural invasion evident on MRI. The results of this study thus established that recurrent and persistent CD consistently results from residual tumor. At repeated surgery the residual tumor can be found at, or immediately contiguous to, the site at which the tumor was originally found. Unappreciated dural invasion with growth of residual tumor within the cavernous sinus dura, which frequently occurs without residual tumor or dural invasion being evident on MR images or to the surgeon during surgery, is the basis of surgical failure in many patients with CD.

FIGURE 20-11 A, Schematic drawings showing exposure of the pituitary. The initial opening of the anterior face of the sella turcica is performed using a drill with a 3- to 4-mm burr. A 2-mm Kerrison ronguer with a thin distal lip (0.75 mm) is used to remove the remaining thin layer of bone of the anterior sella face in small increments. These small pieces of bone can be flushed away with a brief pulse of saline irrigation, which is performed by the assistant, and suctioned away, permitting removal of the pieces without removing instruments from the working region. The bone is removed laterally until at least 2 mm of the most medial aspect of each cavernous sinus is visible. Superiorly bone removal extends to the tuberculum sellae. Inferiorly, a disc dissector is used to separate gently the dura from the bone of the sella floor after the anterior face of the sella has been removed. The sella floor is then removed with a small pituitary rongeur. Oozing bone margins are covered with a thin layer of bone wax and compressed into the bone interstices by using manipulation of a cotton pledget with the forceps tips. Because of the very low pressure in the cavernous sinus and the smaller dural veins draining into it, the same technique, or placement of small pieces of Gelfoam soaked in thrombin, can be used successfully for any site that slowly oozes blood from the layer between the dura and bone at the margins of the bone removal. At this stage the operative field should be bloodless and should expose the entire anterior sella dura and most of the inferior dura covering the pituitary. Much of the success of the surgery depends on achieving a wide and completely bloodless exposure. Inspection of the dura reveals any region of invasion of the anterior or inferior dura and, in cases of small tumors that reach the anterior surface of the pituitary gland, careful examination of the dural surface may provide clues to the site of the tumor, such as a slight local protuberance or a focal region of dark or light color. Because coagulation of the dura tends to glue it to the underlying pituitary capsule (impeding the capacity to open the dura sharply while leaving the pituitary capsule intact) and because it produces a region of white discoloration of the pituitary capsule and the contiguous region of the pituitary gland immediately beneath it (discoloration that may be misleading when searching for a small microadenoma), coagulation of the anterior or inferior dura is avoided during the exposure. All suction from this point is through a 0.5-inch square cotton pledget onto which the suction tip is placed close to the margin. The dura is opened using a No. 15 scalpel with care to take the incision completely through the dura, but not to enter the capsule of the pituitary gland. To achieve the widest available exposure, the superior margins of the incisions are extended laterally to reach the interface of the circular sinus and the medial margin of the cavernous sinus (upper inset). The cavernous sinus is often intentionally entered along the superior and lateral margin of the exposure, where the lateral aspect of the circular sinus meets the medial aspect of the superior portion of the cavernous sinus. Low-pressure venous bleeding from this opening is controlled by simply plugging the opening with a small piece of Gelfoam moistened in thrombin. To achieve a wide exposure laterally and inferiorly, the medial inferior region of the cavernous sinus is frequently opened during the lateral most extent of the incision and bleeding is controlled in a similar fashion. The dura is gently and cleanly separated from the pituitary capsule by using a disc dissector in the tissue plane between these layers. This exposes the entire anterior surface of the pituitary gland with an intact pituitary capsule in a bloodless field. Similar to the pia mater, the capsule of the pituitary gland (lower inset) is a strong layer despite its translucent nature and, even though it is visible histologically, like the pia mater, the capsule is invisible to the surgeon. It must always be cut sharply; blunt dissection will not open it and will only transfer pressure to the interior of the gland and to the tumor, potentially spilling the partially liquefied center of the tumor prematurely. B and C, The use of the surgical capsule for selective excision of small adenomas that are visible on MR imaging. When dealing with tumors within the gland that are visible on MR images, a curvilinear incision is made through the pituitary capsule just beyond the point at which the most superficial dome of the tumor reaches, or comes closest to reaching, the surface of the gland (B, left). Thus, this initial incision is not made directly into the tumor, as is common practice. This permits a thin layer of normal gland to be passed through before reaching the surgical capsule of the adenoma (left inset), allowing easy identification of the surgical capsule and the creation of a surgical plane of dissection at the margin of the tumor, at the interface of the normal gland and the surgical capsule of the adenoma. This interface between the adenoma and gland is further defined using the tips of the bipolar forceps in a series of movements parallel to the surface of the adenoma and in the crevice between the gland and adenoma (B, right and center and right insets). If the correct tissue plane is used, the dissection is unimpeded and the gray–white surface of the adenoma is spherical and smooth. After this interface has been clearly defined, gentle dissection of the interface between the adenoma and gland is continued following the curvilinear margin of the adenoma, and with further incisions in the capsule of the pituitary gland just beyond the tumor margin to release tension on the tumor as the dissection proceeds. A small Hardy sucker (2-mm tip) on the margin of a cotton pad is used to provide separation of the interface between the gland and the adenoma for dissection and for sponging the small amount of bleeding out of the field of view. Small pieces of Gelfoam soaked in thrombin help preserve the surgical space along the dissected margins while dissection takes place at other sites around the tumor margin (not shown here). After the most superficial portion of the tumor has been defined circumferentially, the deeper adenoma margins are defined and dissected in a similar fashion (C); the posterior margin of the adenoma often requires dissection using a disc dissector and a small and/or medium ring curette (C, left and center inset). This is performed gently; very little pressure is required if the correct tissue plane is being used, and most of the limited pressure that is applied is directed more toward the gland than the adenoma. After the margins of the tumor have been completely dissected, to prevent rupture of the tumor the last remaining connection between the pseudocapsule of the specimen and the pituitary capsule is grasped with a small cup forceps and the tumor is removed (C, right). In cases of tumors 8 to 10 mm or less in diameter, the entire tumor can usually be shelled out of its bed in the anterior lobe as an intact specimen. Successful and complete removal leaves a smoothly lined hemispherical tissue void in the anterior lobe. *(From Oldfield EH, Vortmeyer AO. Development of a histological pseudocapsule and its use as a surgical capsule in the excision of pituitary tumors. J Neurosurg. 2006;104:7-19.)*

Thus, repeat trans-sphenoidal exploration of the pituitary and treatment limited to selective adenomectomy should be considered in patients with hypercortisolism despite previous pituitary treatment. If an adenoma is identified during surgery, the chance of remission of CD is high and the risk of hypopituitarism is low; however, if no adenoma can be found and partial or complete hypophysectomy is performed, remission of hypercortisolism is less likely and the risk of hypopituitarism is about 50%.

RADIATION THERAPY

Fractionated radiation of the sella after failed trans-sphenoidal surgery achieves biochemical remission in most patients (80% at 4 years; Fig. 20-18).[50] Because remission is delayed 6 months to several years after radiation therapy, medical therapy is used to block adrenal[45] production of glucocorticoids permitting remission of the clinical syndrome of hypercortisolism until the effects of irradiation occur. Hypopituitarism is an expected side effect, but usually occurs 5 to 10 years after treatment. Other risks of sellar irradiation include, in decreasing likelihood, optic neuropathy, oculomotor neuropathy, and secondary neoplasia. Stereotactic radiosurgery may produce an earlier response than fractionated conventional radiation therapy, but whether it will reduce or increase the risk of radiation-induced complications has not been established. Radiosurgery of the sella, or of the focus of known residual tumor, is an option for treatment of CD after unsuccessful surgery,

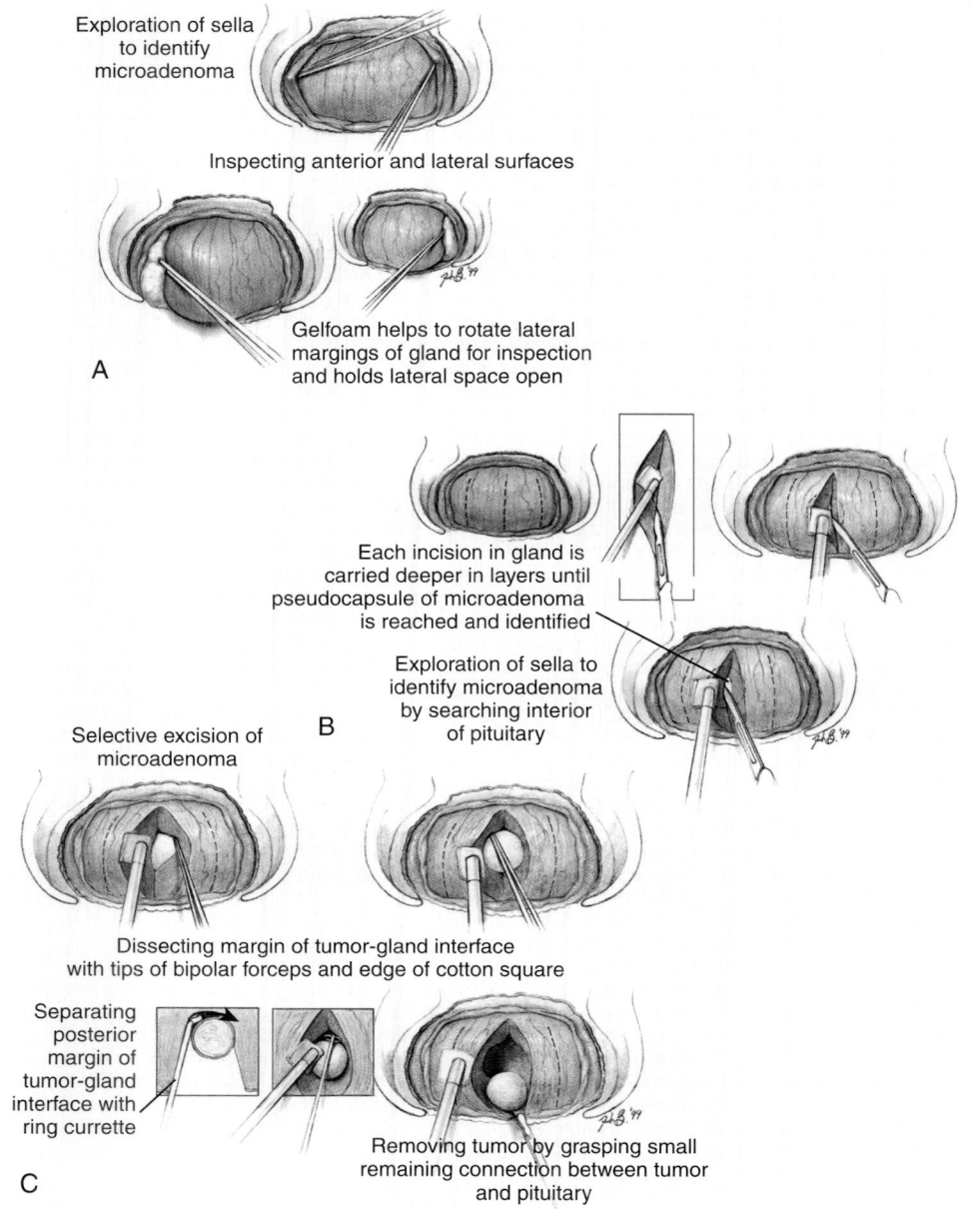

FIGURE 20-12 Exploration of the pituitary gland in patients with an endocrine-active adenoma whose imaging studies appear normal. The goal of the exploration is to find and identify the distinct encapsulated margin of the adenoma. Success depends on beginning with a widely exposed, bloodless surgical field (A). Coagulation of the anterior and inferior sella dura is avoided during the exposure and dural opening because it would produce a white area on the surface of the underlying gland that may falsely suggest the site of the adenoma. After widely opening the dura, which provides exposure of an intact pituitary capsule covering the anterior surface of the gland, and after exposure of the extreme lateral margins of the anterior surface, the surfaces are carefully inspected for regions of focal discoloration. The adenoma usually appears to be gray-blue or yellow-white, and can be identified against the background of the anterior lobe surface whose color is orange-pink. B, If no tumor is seen, the lateral surfaces of the anterior lobe are then inspected. For this the lateral dural wall of the sella (the medial wall of the cavernous sinus) is separated from the pituitary capsule by gently passing a disc dissector between these two layers from top to bottom. The space produced provides room for dissection of the interface between the lateral pituitary capsule and the dural wall with the closed tips of a fine-tipped bipolar forceps (B). Dissection is initially superficial and then progresses in stages to deeper levels until the posterior sella has been reached. After these two tissues have been separated, small pieces of Gelfoam are packed into the intervening space to rotate the lateral surface anteriorly and to gently displace it medially into the surgeon's direct view. After both lateral surfaces are exposed and examined in this fashion, the inferior surface of the gland is separated from the dura. (This is the site at which these two layers—the surface of the pituitary and the dura mater—are most tenaciously attached to each other.) If a tumor can be identified from inspection of the surface, it is removed as described in the text and the legend to Fig. 20-11. If no tumor is identified on inspection of the superficial gland, a series of vertical incisions is then made (B), each of which begins 1 to 2 mm below the superior edge of the pituitary exposure and is directed downward, initially to a depth of only approximately 1 mm, and then in stages deeper through the anterior lobe until either the intermediate lobe or the glistening white anterior surface of the posterior lobe is reached. Because the pituitary blood supply and the delivery of hypothalamic trophic factors to the pituitary is oriented vertically, vertical incisions should be less likely to cause an infarction in a portion of the pituitary or to isolate the gland from its hypothalamic regulation. A distinct tissue capsule is the primary object of the search, with the intent to identify the margin of the tumor before entering it and spilling its contents, by using the surgical capsule of the adenoma (B and C). When the surgical capsule of the adenoma is identified, the tumor is removed using dissection along the interface of the adenoma and the normal gland, as described in Fig. 20-11 (A and B). In cases of tumors lying in the posterior portion of the anterior lobe, a 2-mm-wide slice of the anterior lobe may be removed to provide space for dissection and removal of the deep microadenoma (not shown). *(From Oldfield EH, Vortmeyer AO. Development of a histological pseudocapsule and its use as a surgical capsule in the excision of pituitary tumors. J Neurosurg. 2006;104:7-19.)*

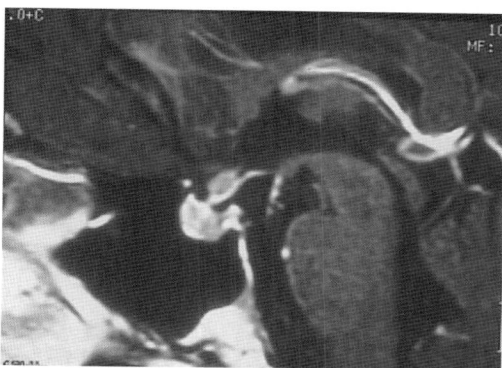
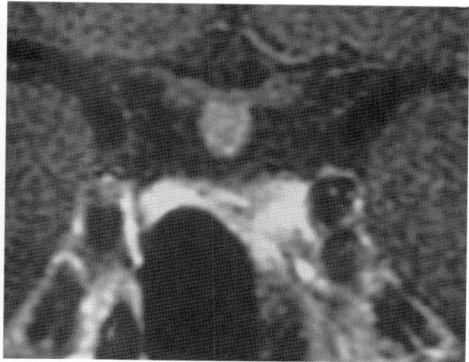

FIGURE 20-13 Adenoma in pituitary stalk. Magnetic resonance T1-weighted images revealing a 7-mm adenoma arising high in the pituitary stalk, just beneath the optic chiasm (left, sagittal view; right, coronal view) after contrast enhancement with gadolinium DTPA. Note enhancement of the anterior lobe and stalk, but not the tumor. *(From Mason RB, Nieman LK, Doppman JL, et al. Selective excision of adenomas originating in or extending into the pituitary stalk with preservation of pituitary function. J Neurosurg. 1997;87:343-351.)*

but, as in fractionated therapy remission of hypercortisolism, biochemical remission is delayed 1 to 3 years and the incidence of permanent hypopituitarism is expected to be similar to the incidence with fractionated irradiation therapy, and with new deficiencies being seen as long as 10 years after treatment.[51-53] In patients who have failed microsurgery, gamma knife radiosurgery provides remission in 40% to 80% of patients.[51-53]

MEDICAL THERAPY

"Chemical adrenalectomy," by medically blocking production of biologically active cortisol by the adrenal cortex, eliminates hypercortisolism and induces remission from the signs and symptoms of CD while awaiting transsphenoidal surgery or, more commonly, while awaiting the effects of pituitary irradiation. For this, ketoconazole, which blocks steroidogenesis, is used.[54,55] Its use is limited primarily by hepatic toxicity. Other side effects include reduced androgen production and gynecomastia in men, and a disulfiram reaction. Recent experience using a combination therapy using a new somatostatin analogue, pasireotide, with a dopamine agonist, cabergoline, prior to ketoconazole, proved effective in normalizing urine-free cortisol in 15 of 17 patients with CD.[56] Yet another option is metyrapone, which inhibits glucocorticoid and mineralocorticoid production, but its clinical usefulness is also limited by toxicity.

ADRENALECTOMY

Although, adrenalectomy was the treatment for CD in the mid-20th century, the current use of bilateral adrenalectomy is limited to patients in whom other treatments have failed.

Adrenalectomy may be used in lieu of irradiation to avoid hypopituitarism in young patients with CD refractory to surgery or it may be combined with irradiation to reduce the risk of development of Nelson's syndrome, which occurs in 10% to 20% of patients after adrenalectomy for CD.[57]

NELSON'S SYNDROME

As the adenomas of CD are under negative feedback, albeit incomplete negative feedback, by high circulating levels of glucocorticoids, plasma ACTH levels increase greatly after adrenalectomy for CD and some ACTH-secreting pituitary tumors aggressively enlarge after correction of hypercortisolism. Nelson's syndrome, hyperpigmentation (Fig. 20-19) associated with unbridled production of proopiomelanocortin and very high levels of plasma ACTH and α-melatonin–stimulating hormone and the appearance of a rapidly growing pituitary macroadenoma after bilateral adrenalectomy for CD, was identified in the era before microneurosurgery, when bilateral adrenalectomy was the treatment of choice for CD. The risk of Nelson's syndrome after adrenalectomy is 10% to 20% in most series, but is as high as 30% in others, and it may present 1 to 29 years after adrenalectomy.[58] It is a serious complication that is characterized by uncontrolled tumor growth and parasellar invasion and compression syndromes that are otherwise atypical of CD. The success of surgical treatment Nelson's syndrome is limited by the large size and invasiveness of these tumors; the incidence of remission from surgery is in the range of 20%,[59] but is higher if the tumors are detected before parasellar spread. Surgery followed by irradiation is the preferred treatment,[58] although many of these tumors are refractory to surgical and/or radiation therapy.

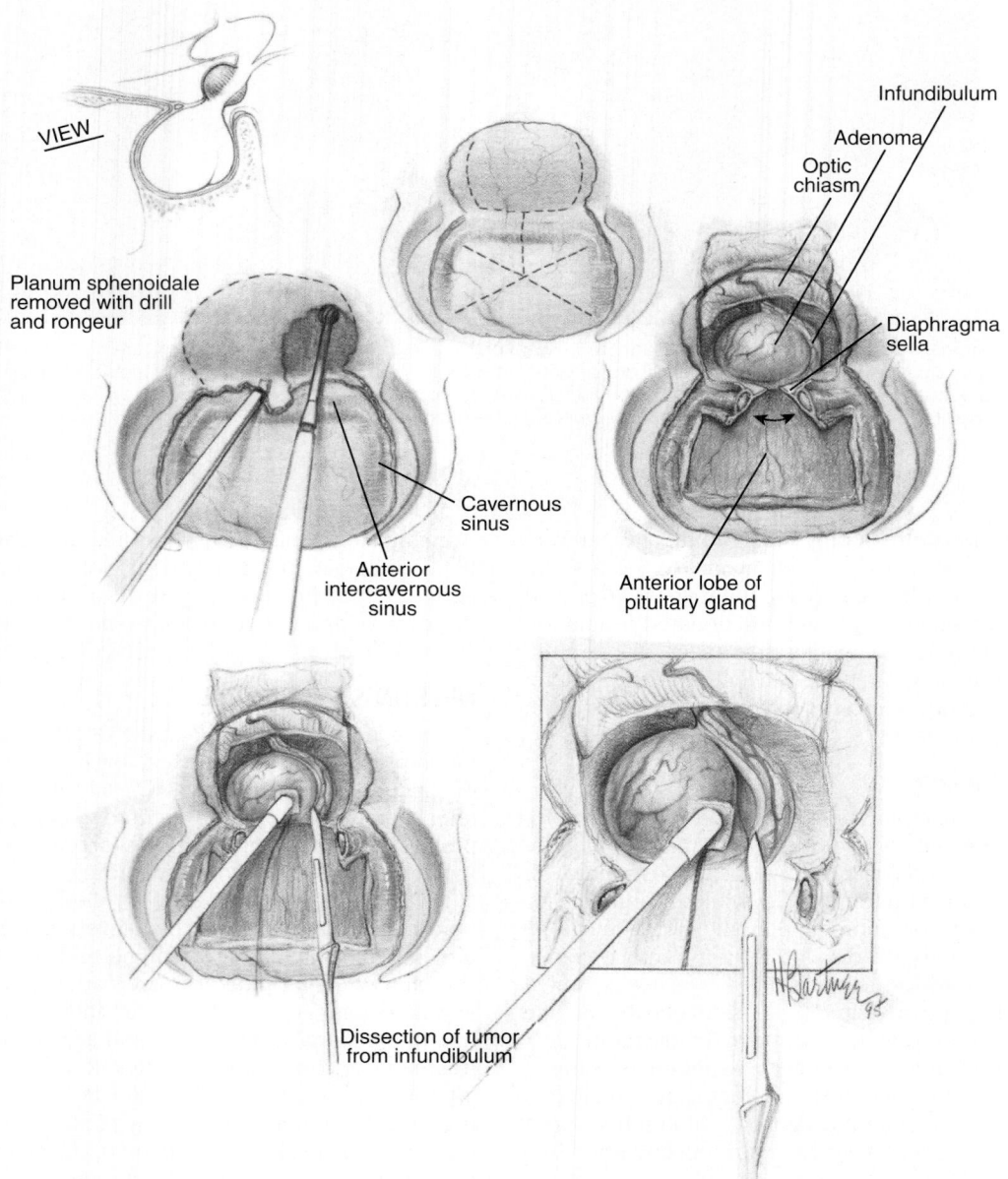

FIGURE 20-14 Extended trans-sphenoidal technique for removing suprasellar tumor of the pituitary stalk. Drawings depict the routine wide exposure of the anterior surface of the sella and bone removal to expose the medial portion of the cavernous sinus bilaterally. The posterior portion of the planum sphenoidale (the posterior 4–6 mm) is removed by first drilling with a rough diamond burr until the plate of bone was paper thin, and then using a 2-mm-thin–footplate cervical Kerrison rongeur. Removal of the planum sphenoidale aids access to the suprasellar cistern, the pituitary stalk, and the superior surface of the gland. The dura mater covering the anterior pituitary surface is opened widely. Bilateral parasagittal incisions are made 8 to 10 mm apart in the dura overlying the planum sphenoidale. A transverse incision just above the anterior portion of the circular sinus is then used to connect the parasagittal incisions. The resulting dural flap is opened posteriorly while, initially, preserving the intact arachnoid. After entering the suprasellar cistern, the superior hypophyseal artery is identified and care is taken not to injure it. The exposed diaphragma sella is incised in the midline, in an anteroposterior direction, to reach the stalk and the supradiaphragmatic tumor. A small piece of Gelfoam or cottonoid is placed superiorly in the subarachnoid space to prevent passage of blood into the cerebrospinal fluid. Characteristic vertical striations produced by the vertical course of the surface blood vessels permit identification of the stalk. A sharp incision is made in the pia with a No. 15 scalpel at the junction of the capsule of the tumor with the pituitary stalk and, when appropriate, in the superior surface of the anterior lobe at the margin of the adenoma. The adenoma is then resected using standard microsurgical technique. *(From Mason RB, Nieman LK, Doppman JL, et al. Selective excision of adenomas originating in or extending into the pituitary stalk with preservation of pituitary function. J Neurosurg. 1997;87:343-351.)*

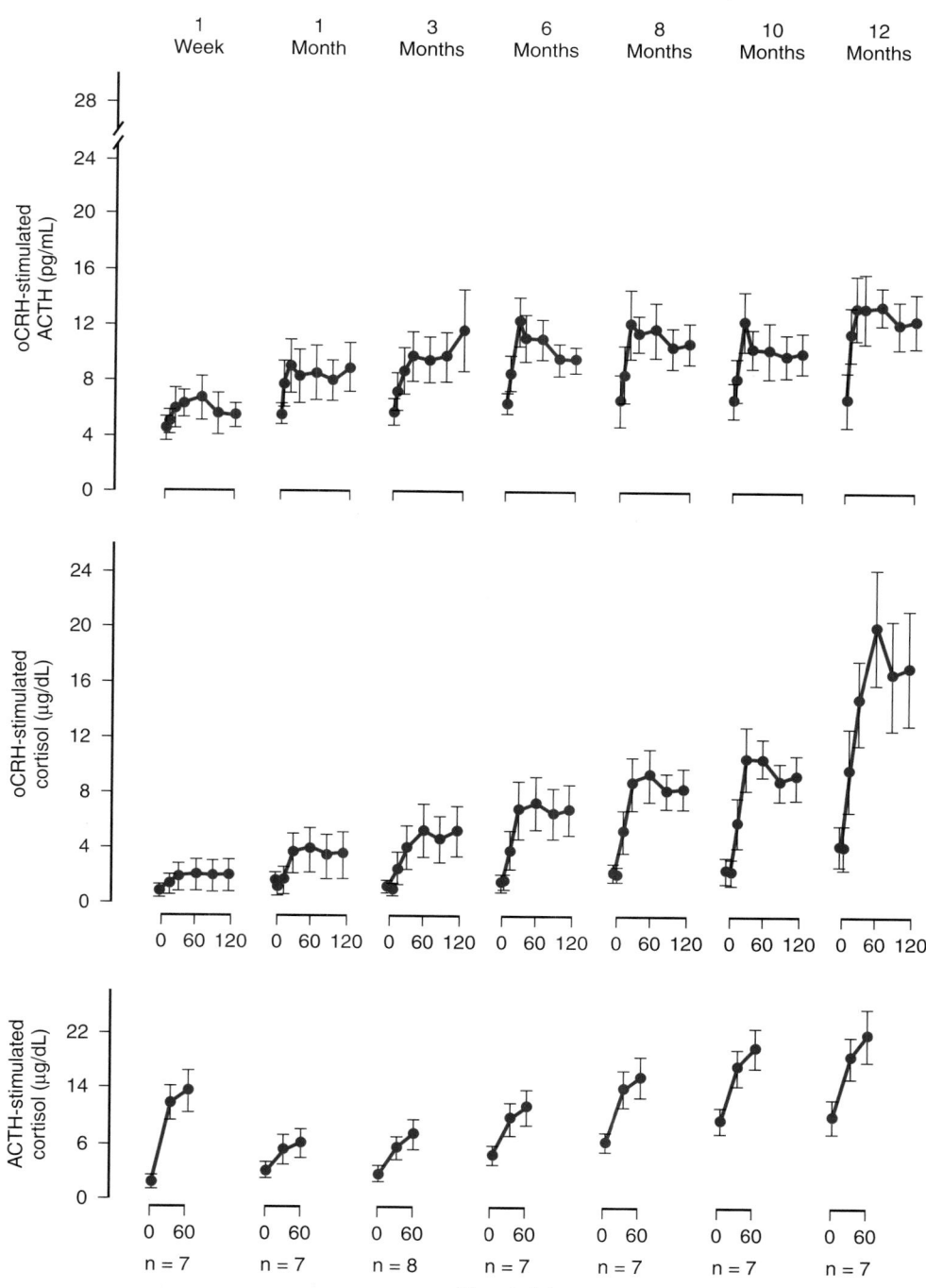

FIGURE 20-15 Recovery of the hypothalamic-pituitary-adrenal axis from chronic hypercortisolism. Nine patients with Cushing's syndrome (six patients with CD, two with adrenal adenomas, and one with ectopic ACTH syndrome) were tested longitudinally for 12 months after surgical correction of Cushing's syndrome with the 1-hour ACTH test (lower panel) and the oCRH test (upper and middle panels). The times at the top of the figure indicate the interval between the testing and surgery and the number of patients studied at each time point is shown at the bottom. The shaded areas represent the mean (± standard deviation) responses in normal subjects. *(From Avgerinos PC, Chrousos GP, Nieman LK, Oldfield EH, Loriaux DL, Cutler GB Jr. The corticotropin-releasing hormone test in the postoperative evaluation of patients with Cushing's syndrome. J Clin Endocrinol Metab. 1987;65:906-913.)*

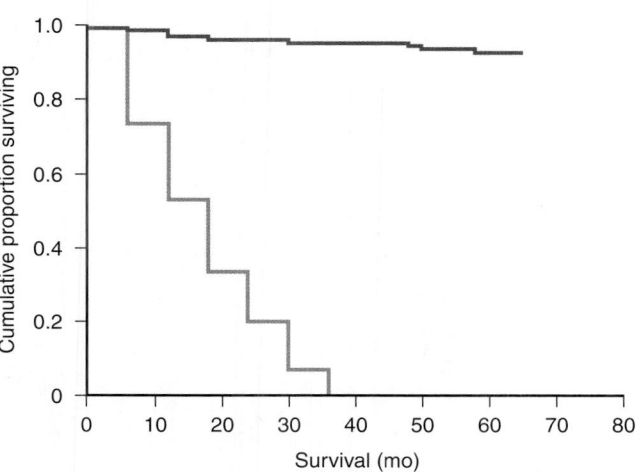

FIGURE 20-16 Postoperative remission of CD predicted by the overnight low dose dexamethasone suppression test. Kaplan-Meier graph compares recurrence-free survival for patients with AM plasma cortisol levels lower than 3 µg/dl (solid line) or 3 to 8 µg/dl (broken line) on the third postoperative day after receiving 1 mg of dexamethasone at 10 to 11 p.m. the previous evening. *(Modified from Chen JCT, Amar AP, Choi SH, et al. Trans-sphenoidal microsurgical treatment of Cushing's disease: postoperative assessment of surgical efficacy using overnight low-dose dexamethasone suppression test. J Neurosurg. 2003; 88:34-37.)*

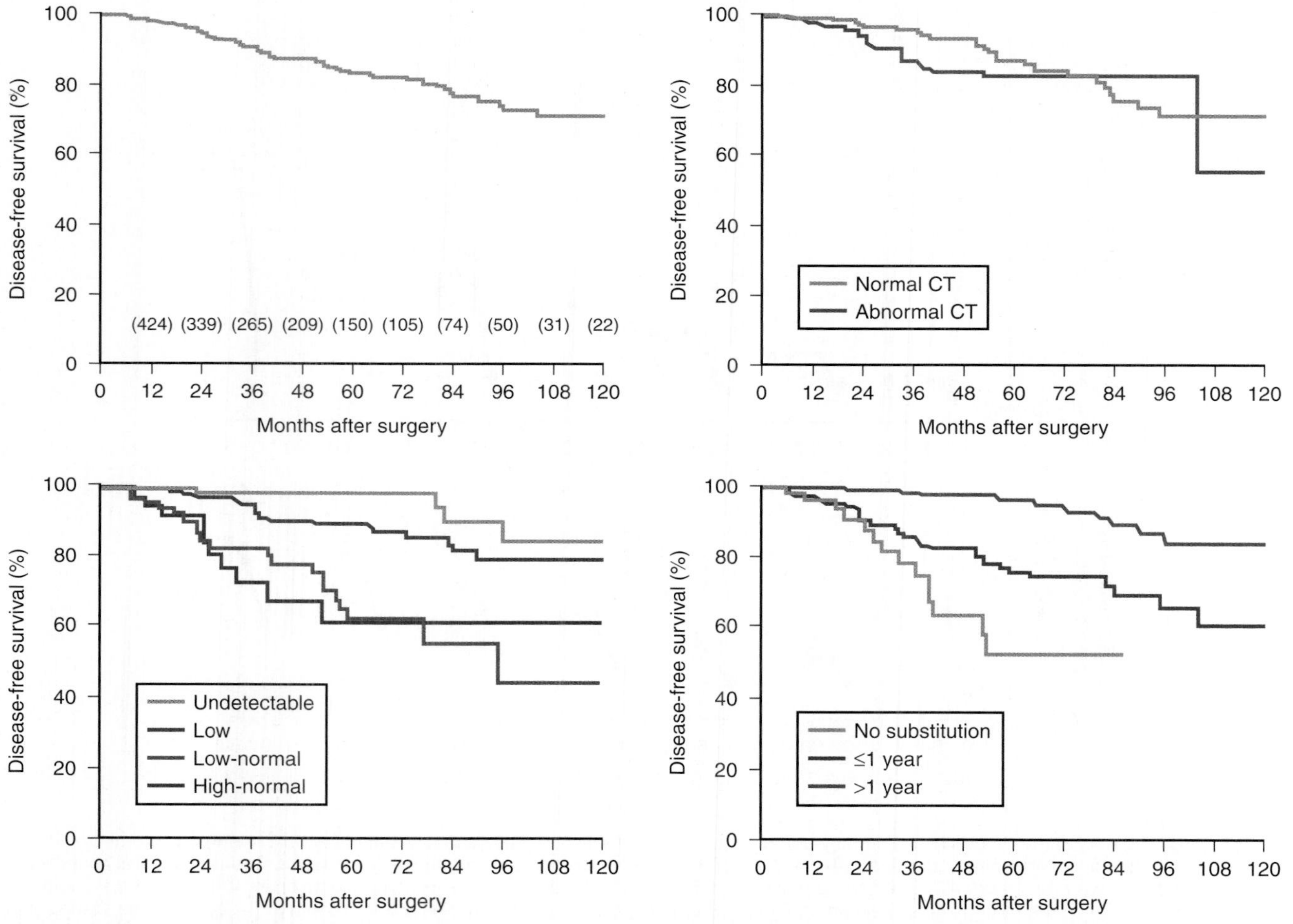

FIGURE 20-17 Analysis of the recurrence of CD in patients in remission after trans-sphenoidal operation. In the upper left, the disease-free survival in the whole group is shown (numbers in brackets represent patients at risk at the end of each year). In the upper right, the disease-free survival according to the presence of a normal (n = 220) or abnormal (n = 239) pituitary CT scan among the 459 patients who were examined before surgery is shown. Patients with an abnormal preoperative CT scan had a higher risk of recurrence, but the difference was of borderline significance (p = 0.053). In the lower left, the disease-free survival according to the early postoperative morning cortisol level is shown for the 482 patients for whom the result was available. Patients with undetectable (n = 94) and low (n = 250) cortisol levels had fewer recurrences during follow-up than did patients with low-normal (n = 97) and high-normal (n = 41) cortisol levels. The overall difference among the four groups was highly significant (p < 0.0001). In the lower right, the disease-free survival according to the length of glucocorticoid substitution therapy is reported for all of the 510 patients who had successful operations. Patients who did not need any substitution therapy (n = 821) and those who required glucocorticoid replacement for less than 1 year (n = 248) showed a higher risk of recurrence than did patients treated for more than 1 year (n = 180). The overall difference among the three groups was highly significant (p < 0.0001). *(Modified from Bochicchio D, Losa M, Buchfelder M. Factors influencing the immediate and late outcome of Cushing's disease treated by trans-sphenoidal surgery: a retrospective study by the European Cushing's Disease Survey Group. J Clin Endocrinol Metab. 1995;80:3114-3120.)*

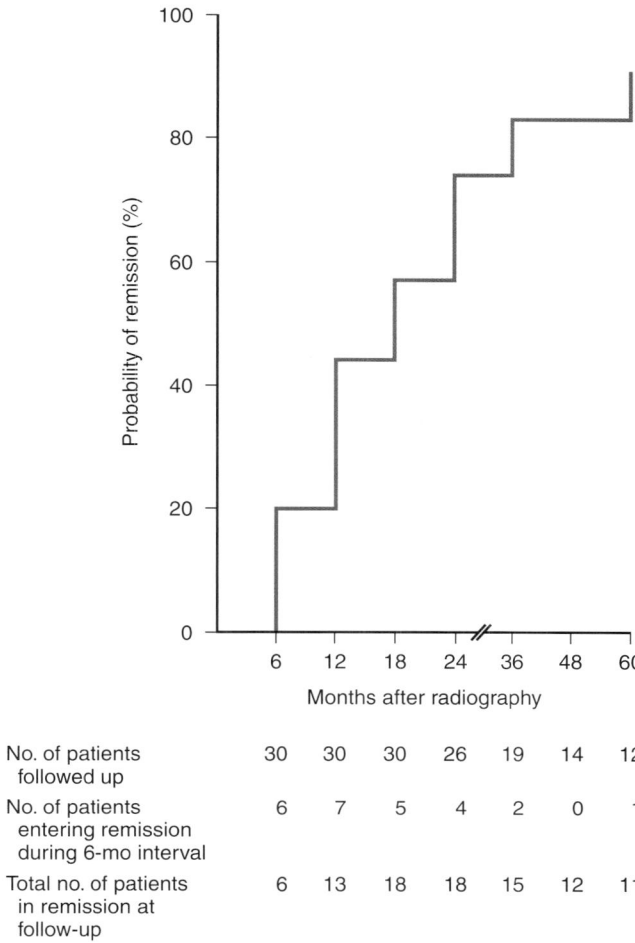

	6	12	18	24	36	48	60
No. of patients followed up	30	30	30	26	19	14	12
No. of patients entering remission during 6-mo interval	6	7	5	4	2	0	1
Total no. of patients in remission at follow-up	6	13	18	18	15	12	11

FIGURE 20-18 Probability of remission of CD in 30 patients treated with pituitary irradiation after unsuccessful transsphenoidal surgery. Response to XRT. *(Modified from Estrada J, Boronat M, Mielgo M, et al. The long-term outcome of pituitary irradiation after unsuccessful transsphenoidal surgery in Cushing's disease. N Engl J Med. 1997;336: 172-177.)*

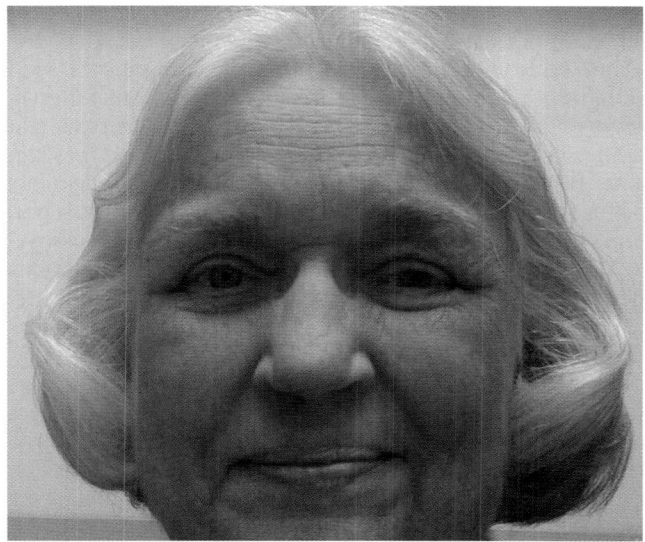

FIGURE 20-19 Nelson's syndrome. Photograph demonstrates the hyperpigmentation associated with excessive ACTH levels, made more noticeable by the patients light eyes and hair (with permission from the patient).

KEY REFERENCES

Bochicchio D, Losa M, Buchfelder M. Factors influencing the immediate and late outcome of Cushing's disease treated by transsphenoidal surgery: a retrospective study by the European Cushing's Disease Survey Group. *J Clin Endocrinol Metab.* 1995;80:3114-3120.

Chen JC, et al. Transsphenoidal microsurgical treatment of Cushing disease: postoperative assessment of surgical efficacy by application of an overnight low-dose dexamethasone suppression test. *J Neurosurg.* 2003;98:967-973.

Dichek HL, et al. A comparison of the standard high dose dexamethasone suppression test and the overnight 8-mg dexamethasone suppression test for the differential diagnosis of adrenocorticotropin-dependent Cushing's syndrome. *J Clin Endocrinol Metab.* 1994;78:418-422.

Dickerman RD, Oldfield EH. Basis of persistent and recurrent Cushing disease: an analysis of findings at repeated pituitary surgery. *J Neurosurg.* 2002;97:1343-1349.

Estrada J, et al. The long-term outcome of pituitary irradiation after unsuccessful transsphenoidal surgery in Cushing's disease. *N Engl J Med.* 1997;336:172-177.

Hall WA, Luciano MG, Doppman JL, et al. Pituitary magnetic resonance imaging in normal human volunteers: occult adenomas in the general population. *Ann Intern Med.* 1994;120:817-820.

Jagannathan J, et al. Outcome of using the histological pseudocapsule as a surgical capsule in Cushing disease. *J Neurosurg.* 2009;111:531-539.

Krikorian A, Abdelmannan D, Selman WR, Arafah BM. Cushing disease: use of perioperative serum cortisol measurements in early determination of success following pituitary surgery. *Neurosurg Focus.* 2007;23:E6.

Liddle GW. Pathogenesis of glucocorticoid disorders. *Am J Med.* 1972;53: 638-648.

Liddle GW. Tests of pituitary-adrenal suppressibility in the diagnosis of Cushing's syndrome. *J Clin Endocrinol Metab.* 1960;12:1539.

Losa M, Picozzi P, Redaelli MG, et al. Pituitary radiotherapy for Cushing's disease. *Neuroendocrinology.* 2010;92(Suppl 1):107-110.

Magiakou MA, Mastorakos G, Chrousos GP. Final stature in patients with endogenous Cushing's syndrome. *J Clin Endocrinol Metab.* 1994;79: 1082-1085.

Nieman LK. Diagnostic tests for Cushing's syndrome. *Ann N Y Acad Sci.* 2002;970:112-118.

Oldfield EH, et al. Petrosal sinus sampling with and without corticotropin-releasing hormone for the differential diagnosis of Cushing's syndrome. *N Engl J Med.* 1991;325:897-905.

Papanicolaou DA, Mullen N, Kyrou I, Nieman LK. Nighttime salivary cortisol: a useful test for the diagnosis of Cushing's syndrome. *J Clin Endocrinol Metab.* 2002;87:4515-4521.

Patronas N, et al. Spoiled gradient recalled acquisition in the steady state technique is superior to conventional postcontrast spin echo technique for magnetic resonance imaging detection of adrenocorticotropin-secreting pituitary tumors. *J Clin Endocrinol Metab.* 2003; 88:1565-1569.

Ram Z, et al. Early repeat surgery for persistent Cushing's disease. *J Neurosurg.* 1994;80:37-45.

Tyrrell JB, Findling JW, Aron DC, et al. An overnight high-dose dexamethasone suppression test for rapid differential diagnosis of Cushing's syndrome. *Ann Intern Med.* 1986;104:180-186.

Wilson CB, Tyrrell JB, Fitzgerald PA, Pitts LH. Cushing's disease and Nelson's syndrome. *Clin Neurosurg.* 1980;27:19-30.

Numbered references appear on Expert Consult.

CHAPTER 21

Endocrinologically Silent Pituitary Tumors

PAOLO CAPPABIANCA • FELICE ESPOSITO • LUIGI M. CAVALLO • ANNAMARIA COLAO

Epidemiology and Nomenclature

Accounting for approximately 15% to 20% of all intracranial neoplasms and being found in up to 27% of hypophyseal glands in autopsy studies and 22.5% of radiologic studies, pituitary adenomas are among the most frequent intracranial tumors. Most are pituitary incidentalomas and only a relatively small portion of such tumors become clinically evident.[1-6]

Once primarily classified according to their maximum diameter (microadenomas, <1 cm; macroadenomas, ≥1 cm), these tumors are further classified according to immunohistochemistry and functional status, since they display an array of hormonal and proliferative activity. Clinically silent pituitary adenomas (nonfunctioning, silent, or endocrine-inactive adenomas), which constitute the most frequent subtype of such pathologic entities, are pituitary adenomas that are not associated with syndromes of hormonal excess. They should not be preoperatively classified as nonsecretory adenomas, as it is known that after immunocytochemical studies, most produce one or more molecules, such as the α- or the β-subunits of the pituitary sexual glycoproteins (luteinizing hormone [LH], follicle-stimulating hormone [FSH]), in addition to the intact hormone; however, serum hormone levels may be not elevated, given that the secretion of such adenomas is often insufficient, incomplete, or inefficient.[7-14] Such gonadotroph adenomas account for 40% to 50% of all macroadenomas and up to 80% of clinically endocrinologically silent pituitary tumors (Fig. 21-1). The rest of these tumors is constituted by the true nonsecreting adenomas ("null-cell adenomas" in immunohistochemical and ultrastructural classifications) (Fig. 21-2) and adenomas that secrete an incomplete or mutated form of other pituitary hormones ("silent ACTH-omas," "silent GH-omas," and so on according to immunohistochemical and ultrastructural classifications).

We will not consider in this chapter the other sellar masses, whether tumoral and nontumoral, such as Rathke's cleft cysts, meningiomas (from the tuberculum sellae, diaphragma sellae, cavernous sinus, clivus), chordomas, germinomas, and so on, which are not adenomas originating from the pituitary gland. These other lesions may be misdiagnosed as nonfunctioning pituitary adenomas and require an accurate preoperative differential diagnosis.

Clinical and Anatomic Features

By definition, endocrinologically silent pituitary tumors do not cause symptoms related to hormone hypersecretion. Rather, their clinical presentation is dominated by mass effect symptoms. Consequently, the vast majority of them are not recognized until they become sizable macroadenomas. As a matter of fact, according to recent reports,[15,16] almost all such tumors are macroadenomas (96.5%) and the main presenting symptoms are visual defects (67.8%) and headache (41.4%), and the most frequent pituitary deficit is hypogonadism (43.3%).

VISUAL SYMPTOMS

Among the most common of such symptoms are the visual deficits, either qualitative and/or quantitative. Such symptoms are related to the suprasellar expansion of the pituitary tumor, with compression and distortion of the optic chiasm and consequent chiasmatic syndrome. That is characterized by visual field defect (classically, incomplete to complete bitemporal hemianopia) due to the compression of the nasal retinal fibers (Fig. 21-3). The deficit of one or of both the temporal hemi-fields begins in such a subdolous manner that it is not appraisable by the patient, in the superior temporal quadrants, progressing towards the bottom in a counterclockwise direction, for the left eye and in a clockwise sense for the right eye. Other perimetric defects are seldom present, such as binasal perimetric defects, resulting from a lateral compression of the chiasm; bilateral altitudinal hemianopia, from a lesion to the superior fibers or to the inferior ones, the latter being involved with greater frequency; homonymous hemianopia, because of the involvement of the posterior portion of the chiasm; and monocular perimetric defects.

Besides the visual field deficits, loss of vision of various degrees, even to blindness, may be present. The visus, especially in the initial stages, when the tumor does not compress the fibers originating from the macula (which are situated in the posterior-median portion of the chiasm), may be preserved. The reduction of visual acuity is often unilateral or is not the same in both eyes. More rare is palsy of the eye musculature, palpebral ptosis, ophthalmoplegia, and diplopia due to the adenomatous mass growing laterally, compressing and/or invading the cavernous sinus and therefore the oculomotor nerves. Another impairment of the ocular motility that could be encountered is a dissociated vertical-pendular nystagmus (see-saw nystagmus), sometimes associated with

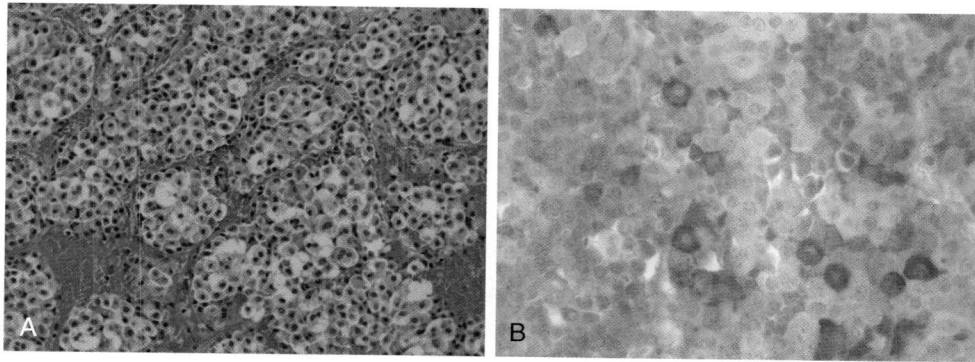

FIGURE 21-1 A, Histology of null cell adenoma: The tumor is characterized by trabecular architecture and is composed of moderated-sized cells, with slightly pleomorphic nuclei and with schromophobic cytoplasm (H/E, 20×). B, Some tumor cells immunoreactive for β-LH (40×).

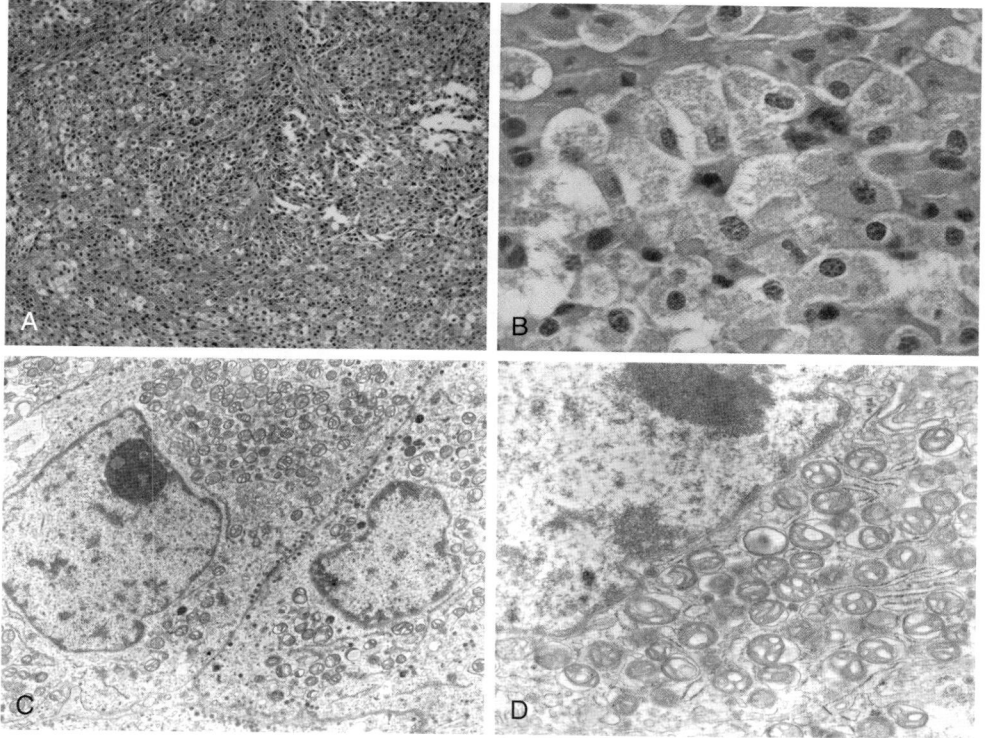

FIGURE 21-2 A, Histology of oncocytoma: The tumor is composed entirely of solid nests and sheets of epithelial cells (H/E, 10×). B, Histology of oncocytoma: The epithelial cells have abundant eosinophilic granular cytoplasm (H/E, 63×). C, Ultrastructure of oncocytoma: mitochondria occupy up to 50% of the cytoplasmic area. The cytoplasm contains scattered small secretory granules (E.M, 4400×). D, Ultrastructure of oncocytoma: The cytoplasm is almost entirely filled with mitochondria; other subcellular organelles are sparse (E.M, 12000×).

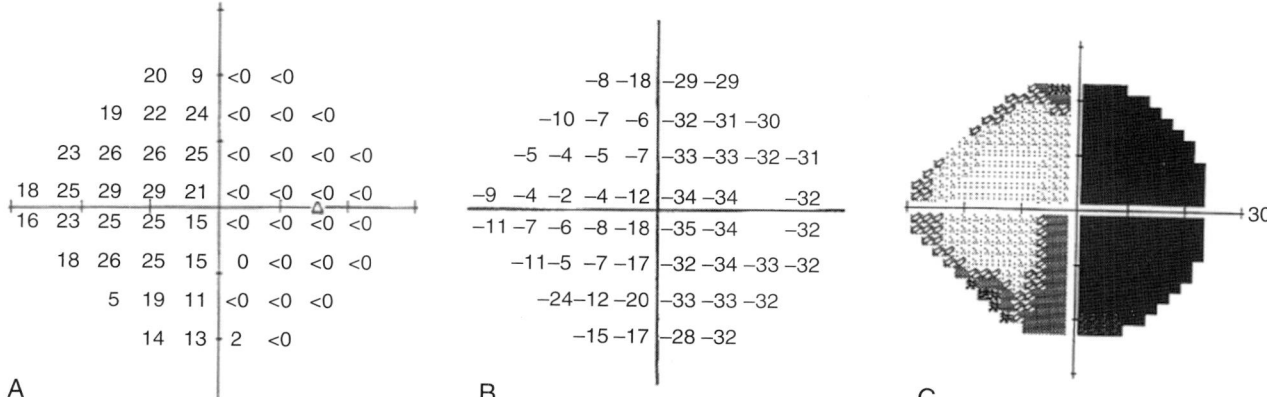

FIGURE 21-3 Graphical representation of an automatic static perimetric exam in a patient with bitemporal hemianopia (right eye). A, Numerical map (in Db): in every retinic point examined the levels of the light threshold are shown. B, "Total deviation" chart that shows the difference between the threshold value recorded for the patient and the computerized value statistically normal per age. C, Representation by means of a scale of grays.

bitemporal hemianopia, and thought to be related to a lesion of Cajal's interstitial nucleus. A splitting of the images could also be present in the absence of any muscular palsy, and this symptom is due to the fact that for the patient with bitemporal hemianopia, vision is missing in the outer (temporal or lateral) half of both the right and left visual fields.

HEADACHE

Another common symptom caused by endocrinologically silent pituitary tumors is headache, which does not seem to be correlated with the size of the adenoma.[17] Such symptom is due to the stretching of the diaphragma sellae and/or the medial wall of the cavernous sinuses, caused by an even mild or moderate intrasellar hypertension.[18]

ENDOCRINOLOGIC SYMPTOMS

Due to their usually large size, endocrinologically silent pituitary tumors can cause, indeed, endocrinologic symptoms. These are related with pituitary insufficiency caused by the compression on the residual gland and the stalk by the tumor mass and are most of the times subtle. As a matter of facts, patients harboring such tumors may present different symptoms of hormonal hyposecretion, such as secondary hypogonadism, oligo/amenorrhea in females (due to either hypogonadism and/or functional hyperprolactinemia), decreased libido, hypothyroidism, adrenal insufficiency, GH-insufficiency, etc. Such deficits can lead, ultimately, to complete pituitary insufficiency or panhypopituitarism.

Pretty common in case of macroadenomas is the functional hyperprolactinemia (AKA stalk effect) due to the compression/deviation of the pituitary stalk with consequent encroachment of the vessels of the pituitary portal system. This causes an insufficiency in the tuberoinfundibular pathway of the dopamine—an inhibitor of the prolactine production—with consequent disinhibition of the production of such hormone. Anyway, the increased serum levels of the HPRL are usually mild to moderate.

Diabetes insipidus is not a usual presenting symptom of nonfunctioning adenomas and, when present, should suggest reconsidering the diagnosis.

CRANIAL NERVE AND BRAIN SYMPTOMS

Although uncommon, deficits of one or more cranial nerves running inside the cavernous sinus may be present, depending on the grade of the involvement, in the event of compression of its medial wall or in the presence of a frank invasion of the sinus.

Exceptionally big tumors may cause psychiatric or other neurologic symptoms, such as personality changes and anosmia, due to the involvement of the frontal lobes, when the suprasellar expansion grows over the planum sphenoidale with shifting up the brain. Also, symptoms related with temporal lobe involvement, such as uncinate seizures, may be present, although rare.

PITUITARY APOPLEXY

Pituitary apoplexy is a relatively rare condition presenting with sudden headache, acute visual loss, ophthalmoplegia, altered level of consciousness, lethargy, and even collapse from acute adrenal insufficiency. It is caused by a hemorrhage into the tumor and/or its acute necrosis, with subsequent swelling and frequent spreading into the subarachnoid space, leading to other signs of meningeal irritation (Fig. 21-4). Clinical conditions or precipitating factors that are associated with an increased risk for such occurrence are coronary artery surgery and other major surgery, pregnancy, anticoagulant or antiaggregant therapy, and coagulopathies.[19] The related acute and severe clinical syndrome demands glucocorticoid replacement and surgical decompression, usually trans-sphenoidal, if visual loss is severe and progressive. These patients typically require a full hormonal replacement therapy in the perioperative period. If the patient has a subclinical or a mild form of apoplexy and is clinically stable, it is prudent to measure the serum prolactin, since some patients with prolactinoma present in this fashion and may be successfully treated with medical therapy.

PITUITARY INCIDENTALOMAS

The incidental discovery of a nonfunctioning pituitary adenoma is a fairly common occurrence. It usually happens when brain imaging studies are done for other reasons, such as motor vehicle accidents or head traumas. In such cases a more elaborate neuroradiologic work-up may be required, with the obtaining of a contrast-enhanced sellar MRI.

Preoperative Evaluation

Global management of pituitary masses usually involves a multidisciplinary team. Thus, an accurate, complete, balanced, and global preoperative evaluation of these patients

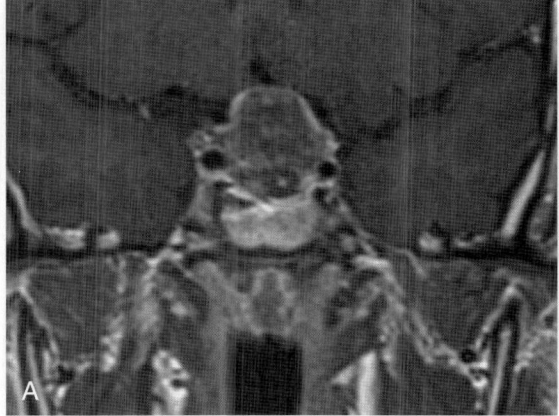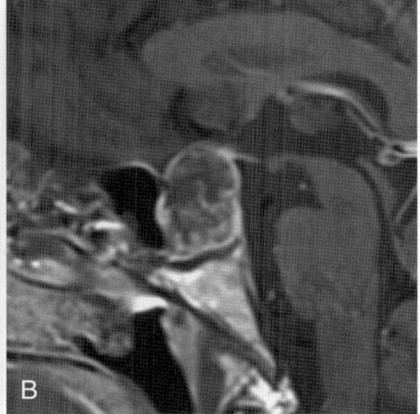

FIGURE 21-4 Preoperative coronal (A) and sagittal (B) contrast-enhanced sellar MRI showing a pituitary apoplexy. The mass compresses the optic apparatus, superiorly, and both the cavernous sinuses, laterally.

is critical, including diagnostic and clinical tests and laboratory investigations, to minimize surgical risks and optimize the outcome.

NEURORADIOLOGIC EVALUATION

A correct neuroradiologic evaluation of a patient with a nonfunctioning pituitary mass is mandatory. The aim of the neuroradiologic study of a suspected pituitary mass is mainly based on the evaluation of the characteristics of the lesion (origin, structure, extension, and relationships) and the shape and location of the residual pituitary gland. Its purposes follow:

- Identify the lesion, excluding various differential diagnoses
- Control effects of medical therapy
- Define spatial situation of the lesion (presurgical planning)
- Verify removal of the lesion (postsurgical follow-up)

The gold standard among the radiologic studies available is the magnetic resonance imaging. A complete MR protocol should include, at least T1- and T2-weighted images and T1-weighted postcontrast (postgadolinium) images (Fig. 21-5) in the three orthogonal planes and 3-mm thick sections.[20] Complementary MR sequences are also useful, such as dynamic sequences; MR angiography, namely when one suspects the vascular nature of a lesion; diffusion-weighted and/or perfusion-weighted MRI; and MR spectroscopy (Fig. 21-6).

Fibrous adenomas are encountered in approximately 10% of cases[21] and can be difficult to remove via the conventional trans-sphenoidal approach. In such cases, preoperative MRI may be useful in anticipating tumor consistency and allow planning of the surgical strategy correctly. Tumors with a hypo- or iso-intense appearance on T2-weighted MRI may be indicative of greater collagen content[21-23] and a more fibrous tumor consistency. In contrast, softer tumors are hyperintense on T2 (Fig. 21-7).

When a trans-sphenoidal approach is foreseen—especially the endonasal variant—axial and coronal CT scanning may be helpful in addition to an accurate assessment of the anatomy of the nasal cavities and the paranasal sinuses and for the definition of the best route from the nasal cavity toward the sella, since MR imaging alone does not provide the necessary detail of bone anatomy.[20] Axial and coronal CT scanning allows the neurosurgeon to more easily assess the three-dimensional (3D) aspects of the nasal and paranasal cavities, particularly the sphenoid bone, and the relationships with the sellar floor and carotid canals. CT study is essential in order to reveal the presence of eventual anatomic variations or pathologic changes of the cavities. Moreover, CT remains the diagnostic imaging study of choice in patients who are unable to undergo an MR study.

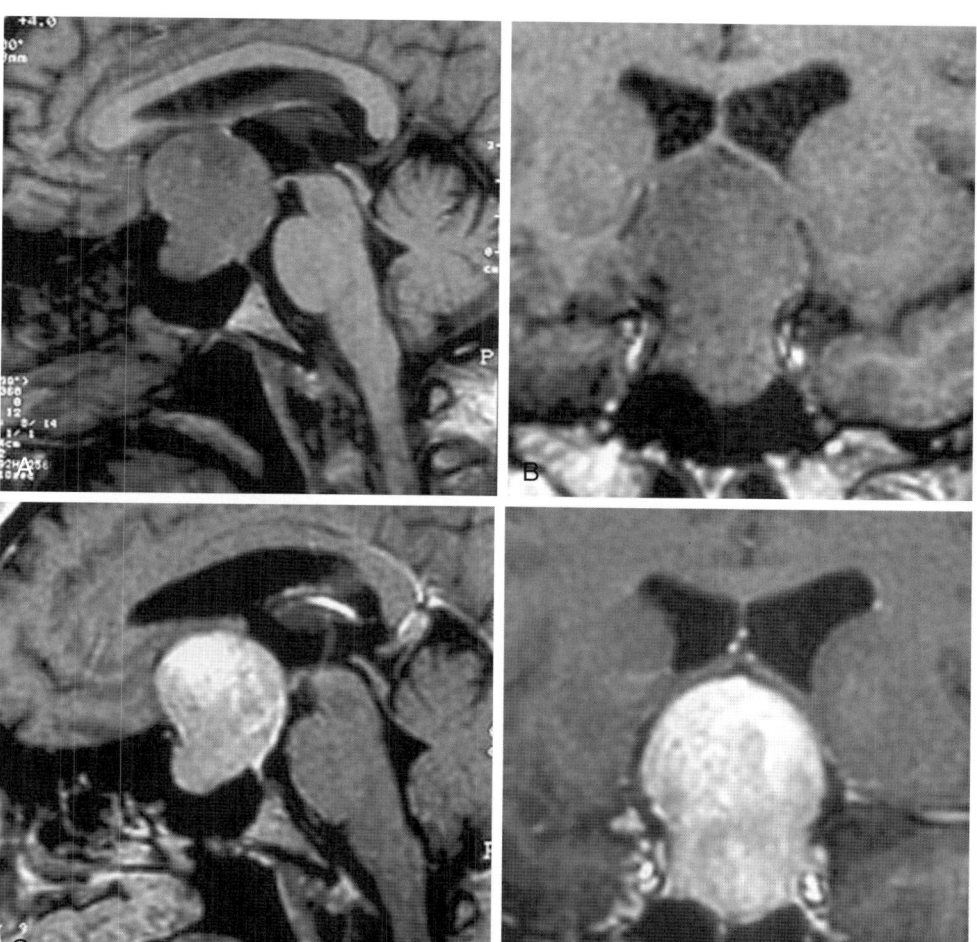

FIGURE 21-5 Preoperative sagittal (A) and coronal (B) and preoperative contrast-enhanced sagittal (C) and coronal (D) sellar MRI showing a large intra- and supra-sellar macroadenoma, strongly enhancing after contrast medium injection.

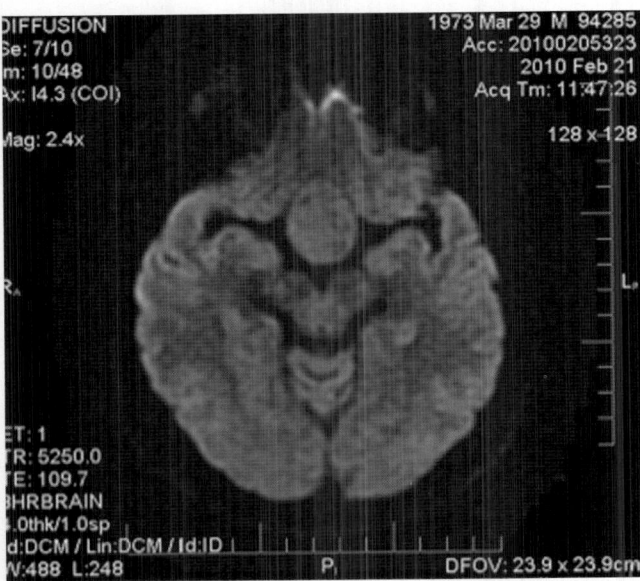

FIGURE 21-6 Preoperative axial MRI, diffusion-weighted sequence, of clinically nonfunctioning pituitary macroadenoma.

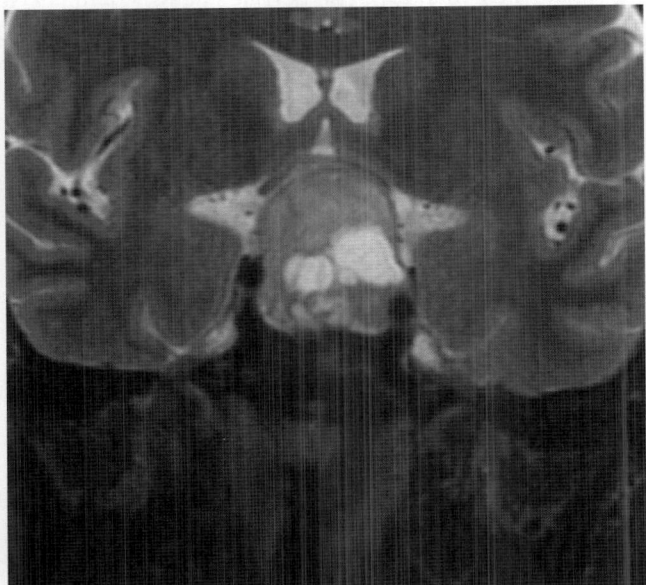

FIGURE 21-7 Preoperative coronal MRI, T2-weighted sequence, of a clinically nonfunctioning pituitary macroadenoma. The tumor mass is hyperintense with cystic areas within it, predicting a soft consistence of the tissue.

Although analysis of axial and coronal scans gives a detailed true depiction of rhino-sinusal anatomy, the 3D virtual endoscopy yields images similar to those provided by actual endoscopy, giving the surgeon a view before the operation and avoiding the complex task of mental reconstruction in the space of images obtained on traditional scan planes[20,24] (Fig. 21-8).

OPHTHALMOLOGIC EVALUATION

The ophthalmologist's evaluation is of utmost importance when a suprasellar lesion is suspected, in all the stages of the disease from the diagnosis to the pre- and post-operative evaluation.[25] The visual field evaluation, by means of either the manual kinetic technique or the computerized threshold static perimetry (Fig. 21-3) and the study of visual evoked potentials (VEPs) are the most suitable exams to show eventual functional deficits due to chiasmatic involvement, as well as to monitor the preservation or vision recovery after surgery. VEPs are useful in the evaluation of the pharmacologic or surgical treatment, rather than for routine diagnostic purposes, where the basic test was and still remains the field exam. The examination of chromatic sensibility is not considered a routine investigation, but it should be performed in cases where the field evaluation and VEPs are normal, but there is still suspicion of chiasmatic compression based on neuroradiologic studies.

ENDOCRINOLOGIC EVALUATION

The role of the endocrinologist in the preoperative settings of patients with endocrinologically silent pituitary tumors is of utmost importance. For such patients, a complete evaluation of the serum levels of the pituitary hormones together with the basal and functionality tests of the target organs of such tumors—including growth hormone, IGF-1, prolactin, TSH, T3, T4, FSH, LH, ACTH, and cortisol—is important to check for possible clinical or subclinical pituitary hypofunctions and to provide an adequate hormonal replacement therapy, if applicable. The correction of any eventual pituitary deficiency greatly helps improving the global outcome of these patients.

A full preoperative endocrinologic investigation is also conducted to ascertain the baseline pituitary gland function and to use its results to be compared with the postoperative ones, in order to demonstrate any postoperative pituitary function improvement or recovery or, conversely, any new hormonal deficit, also for medical legal purposes.

Management

MEDICAL MANAGEMENT

The medical approach to clinically silent pituitary adenomas has improved in recent years due to the availability of effective, well tolerated and safe molecules able to reduce, in some instances, the tumor mass.

It is now verified, by immunocytochemistry and ultrastructural studies, that the majority of such tumors are glycoprotein-producing, followed by nonfunctioning somatotroph, lactotroph, or corticotroph adenomas.[16] As a matter of facts, a large proportion of nonfunctioning adenomas (up to 90%) is shown to secrete low amounts of either intact FSH and LH and/or their α- and β-subunits and the vast majority of nonfunctioning adenomas also express on cell membranes different subtypes of somatostatin and dopamine receptors (respectively, sst_1-sst_5 and D_1-D_5) in a variable amount. Based on this feature, both dopamine agonists and somatostatin analogues have a rationale in the treatment of such tumors and such fact has opened a new perspective of medical treatment for these lesions.

SOMATOSTATIN RECEPTORS AND THEIR ROLE

Somatostatin (growth hormone-inhibiting hormone [GHIH] or somatotropin release–inhibiting factor [SRIF]) is a peptide hormone that regulates the endocrine system

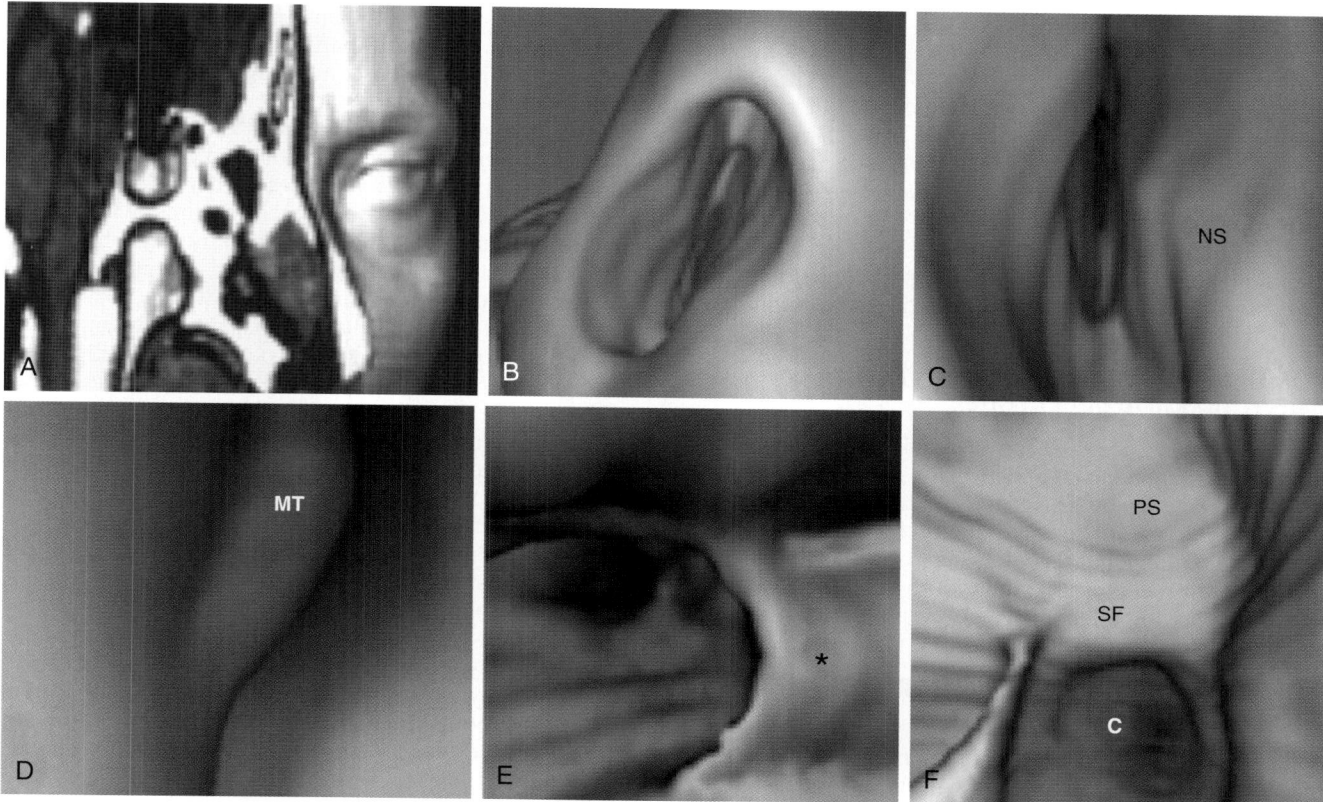

FIGURE 21-8 A, Three-dimensional surface CT reconstruction. B, Virtual endoscopy. Approach to the right nasal cavity. C, Virtual endoscopy. Entry into the right nasal cavity between the lateral wall and the septum. D, Virtual endoscopy. Identification of the middle turbinate. E, Virtual endoscopy. Entry into the sphenoid sinus with the intersinusal septum. F, Virtual endoscopy. Visualization of the sellar floor. NS, nasal septum; MT, middle turbinate; *, intrasphenoid septum; SF, sellar floor; PS, planum sphenoidale; C, clivus.

and affects neurotransmission and cell proliferation via interaction with G-protein–coupled somatostatin receptors and inhibition of the release of numerous secondary hormones. It is classified as an inhibitory hormone. Somatostatin analogs (SSAs) have been used in clinical practice over the past 20 years. They act through the somatostatin receptors, which have been demonstrated to be highly expressed in all pituitary adenomas with a predominance of sst_2 and sst_5 and infrequent expression of sst_4.[16,26-28] Another analogue, the slow-release lanreotide (LAN), showing a similar receptor affinity for sst to that of OCT, was made available for intramuscular injections every 7 to 14 days. More recently, OCT and LAN have been made available for injections either intramuscular or subcutaneous every 28 to 56 days, respectively. The response to octreotide and lanreotide is predicted by the expression of sst_2.[16,29] In nonfunctioning adenomas the receptor subtype expressed in a higher amount was found to be the sst_3 followed by the sst_2, also correlated with sst_5 expression.[30] The expression of sst_2 and sst_5 in nonfunctioning adenomas has been found to be associated with reduced cell viability by 20% to 80% (in 8 of 13 sst_2-positive tumors) and by 15% to 80% (in 10 of 13 tumors, all but three sst_5 positive).[31] More recently, pasireotide (SOM230), a somatostatin analogue binding sst_{1-3} and sst_5, completely abrogated the promoting effects of vascular endothelial growth factor (VEGF) on nonfunctioning adenoma cell viability.[32]

Only few clinical trials have been conducted to evaluate potential effects of SSA in patients with nonfunctioning adenomas. However, a meta-analysis of such data revealed that tumor reduction was reported only in 12% of cases, while the vast majority of patients had stable remnant tumors.[16] A still unexplained finding reported by some authors[33,34] is that OCT treatment was followed by a rapid improvement in headache and visual disturbances, without any change in tumor volume. This effect was likely not owing to a direct effect on tumor size but more likely to a direct effect on the retina and the optic nerve.[35] However, approximately in one third of the patients there was an improvement in visual field defects.[16]

DOPAMINE RECEPTORS AND THEIR ROLE

Dopamine receptors, namely the D_2 subtype, in the normal pituitary mediate the tonic inhibitory control of PRL secretion[36] by dopamine.[37] A meta-analysis of several studies[16] has shown the presence of dopamine binding sites (most likely D_2) in nonfunctioning adenomas. Furthermore, in gonadotropin-immunopositive adenomas, the D_2 were mainly localized in LH- and FSH-immunopositive cells.[38] Anyway, the D_2 receptor is not the only dopamine receptor expressed in the pituitary gland. Indeed, the D_4 receptor, in particular its $D_{4.4}$ variant, is also expressed, although its role in the physiology of the pituitary gland is not known.[39] Cabergoline is the actual most commonly used dopamine agonist, able to inhibit in vitro the α-subunit concentration in 56% of cases and such result was associated with D_2 expression,[40] while the tumor shrinkage after DA therapy is 27.6%.[16]

A recent study of our group[40] demonstrated that 1-year treatment with cabergoline at the dose of 3 mg/wk induced a more than 25% tumor shrinkage in 56% of patients with histologically proven nonfunctioning adenomas and such shrinkage was significantly correlated with the expression of the D_2 isoform. The counterpart of such evidence was the finding of tumor regrowth after stopping the dopamine-agonist treatment,[41] thus supporting the use of such treatment in these subjects.

CUMULATIVE ROLE OF SOMATOSTATIN AND DOPAMINE RECEPTORS

It is known that D_2 and sst_5 physically interact through hetero-oligomerization to create novel receptor with enhanced functional activity.[16,42] This fact constitutes the rationale of whether the combination treatment with selective ligands of these two individual receptors, as well as new molecules binding both receptors simultaneously, could be effective in nonfunctioning adenomas.[16] Anyway, such approach is still under investigation.[43]

GONADOTROPIN-RELEASING HORMONE ANALOGUES AND THEIR ROLE

Since a large percentage of nonfunctioning pituitary adenomas produce intact gonadotropins or, at least, the α-subunit, attempts were made to inhibit gonadotropin secretion by using GnRH analogues.[16] Unfortunately, the results of the different attempts were not conclusive and no data are available concerning the tumor shrinkage or the visual effects. Though, such treatment is not anymore proposed in patients with nonfunctioning adenomas.

OTHER MEDICAL APPROACHES

Type I interferon (IFN) molecules routinely used in the treatment of chronic hepatitis B and C, multiple sclerosis, and a few tumors[44] have been investigated in recent years for their possible regulatory role in the hypothalamic-pituitary axis. As a matter of facts, incubation with IFN-α resulted in 24% to 62% inhibition of the secretion of gonadotropins and/or alpha-subunit in a recent study of Hofland et al.[45] However, in healthy volunteers or in treated patients for hepatitis or multiple sclerosis, changes of testosterone or gonadotropin levels were found to be temporary.[44]

Ongoing experimental studies for other possible medical approaches concern the folate receptor (FR-α), which is significantly overexpressed in clinically nonfunctional adenomas but not in functional adenomas.[46,47] Such evidence may hold significant promise for medical treatment by enabling novel molecular imaging and targeted therapy.

SURGICAL MANAGEMENT

Surgical management of pituitary masses and, therefore, endocrinologically silent pituitary tumors, remains a distinct subspecialty of neurosurgery. It requires a precise knowledge and skills of basic neurosurgical techniques, together with specific knowledge, interest, and appreciation of pituitary-hypothalamic pathophysiology, allowing the surgeon to choose among different approaches based upon the specific features of the patient. The neurosurgeon must know the detailed surgical anatomy, must be experienced in neuroimaging, must know pathophysiology and the natural history of pituitary disease, and must be familiar with the various therapeutic options and the related pros and cons. Furthermore, surgery of the pituitary tumors yields the best outcomes when performed in dedicated centers where the entire range of pituitary specialties is offered in an environment of effective teamwork, which requires a "teamwork attitude" that is not just the addition of the expertise of the single contributors, but rather a cultural and psychological attitude, with the single units working with a goal of true exchange and sincere collaboration, thus allowing cooperative effort for the benefit of the patient and positive feedback for physicians and surgeons.[48] Pituitary surgery is not only choosing the correct surgical route and performing and uneventful operation but, rather, it also requires careful and specific postoperative management and long-term patient follow-up, with a continuous information exchange among the different specialists of the teamwork, i.e., the pathologist, the ophthalmologist, the neuroradiologist, the endocrinologist, the radiation oncologist and, of course, the neurosurgeon.

Therapy for pituitary adenomas is targeted to achieve multiple goals, such as normalization of excess of hormone secretion, if any; preservation or even restoration of normal pituitary function; elimination of mass effect; preservation or restoration of visual acuity and/or visual field; prevention of tumor recurrence; and achievement of a complete pathologic diagnosis.

Clinically silent pituitary tumors are primarily managed surgically, since such treatment modality is the sole that currently is able to achieve all the previously mentioned goals. As a general indication, surgery for such lesions should be especially indicated in the following conditions: pituitary apoplexy and progressive mass effect, producing compression of the surrounding neurovascular structures and usually causing visual deficits or cranial nerve palsy.

Large invasive pituitary tumors and those with a frank cavernous sinus invasion are thought to be difficult to cure regardless of the approach because the gross total removal of the tumor is often not achievable. Recently introduced extended trans-sphenoidal approaches sometimes can represent a valid alternative to transcranial options.[49]

The surgical approach, with respect to the basic principles for resecting pituitary adenomas, can be performed by two main approaches, each of them with several subcategories (Table 21-1). This chapter will focus on the

Table 21-1 Surgical Approaches for Pituitary Tumors
Trans-Sphenoidal Approach
Microscopic
Sublabial
Trans-septal
Endonasal
Endoscopic
Combined or endoscope-assisted microsurgery
Transcranial Approach
Pterional or frontolateral
Subfrontal unilateral
Subfrontal bilateral interhemispheric

trans-sphenoidal approaches only. Transcranial approaches will be described in a chapter dedicated to this issue.

TRANS-SPHENOIDAL APPROACHES

The statement that trans-sphenoidal route should be preferred among the other surgical options is based on the following simple but solid considerations:

1. It is the least traumatic route to the sella.
2. It does not leave visible scars.
3. It provides excellent visualization of the surgical field.
4. It offers excellent outcomes with a lower morbidity and mortality rate compared with transcranial procedures.
5. The hospitalization is usually shorter.

Indications for trans-sphenoidal surgery today include more than 95% of the surgical indications in the sellar area and approximately 96% of all pituitary adenomas.[50,51] Furthermore, absolute indications for such approaches include any condition that poses an elevated surgical risk via the transcranial route; the elderly patient; longstanding compression of the chiasm, and thus inability to tolerate additional trauma; acute endosellar hypertension, such as in pituitary apoplexy; paninvasive and not otherwise radically removable adenomas; adenomas with downward growth (into the sphenoid sinus); and microadenomas.

In case of exceptionally big adenomas or paninvasive tumors, an intentionally two-staged trans-sphenoidal operation may be scheduled. Such option is designed to encourage the descent of a suprasellar remnant of the adenoma incompletely removed in the first step, to limit the risks of a brisk decompression of huge lesions, and to manage the residual mass with a second surgery.[52]

The trans-sphenoidal approach represents a midline extracranial approach that has been performed since the 1960s by means of the *operating microscope* as visualizing tool, through transnasal trans-septal, sublabial trans-septal, or endonasal procedures (microsurgical trans-sphenoidal procedures) (Fig. 21-9A, B, and C). The trans-sphenoidal approach also can be performed by means of the *endoscope* as the sole visualizing tool during the entire surgical procedure, realizing a "pure" endoscopic endonasal trans-sphenoidal approach. The combined use of the microscope and the endoscope during the same approach defines the condition of *endoscope-assisted microsurgery*[48] (see Table 21-1).

Microsurgical Trans-Sphenoidal Approaches

Although many different trans-sphenoidal procedures and variations have been described, currently there are three basic microsurgical trans-sphenoidal approaches to pituitary tumors: the transnasal trans-septal trans-sphenoidal approach, the sublabial trans-septal trans-sphenoidal approach, and the endonasal trans-sphenoidal approach (Table 21-1). The procedure is performed with an operating microscope for visualization, illumination, and magnification of the surgical field. Intermittent fluoroscopy is used for trajectory guidance, or, more recently, neuronavigational systems permit the surgeon to gather information about the current position of anatomic structures or instruments during the procedure iself.[49,53-57] Intraoperative MRI (iMRI) may provide additional knowledge about the completeness of lesion removal.[58-60] The three main microscopic transsphenoidal methods differ slightly primarily in the initial phase up to the exposure of the sphenoid sinus; they then follow the same surgical sphenoidal and sellar steps.

Endoscopic Endonasal Trans-Sphenoidal Approach

Endoscopic endonasal trans-sphenoidal surgery is a more recent, minimally invasive trans-sphenoidal approach performed by means of the endoscope as a stand-alone visualizing and operating instrument, without the need of the trans-sphenoidal retractor[48,49,61,62] (Fig. 21-9D). It has the same indications as the conventional microsurgical technique and since the 1990s has enjoyed progressive acceptance among surgeons and patients for its minimal invasiveness and for the excellent surgical view it provides.[63-70] Based on these advantages of trans-sphenoidal surgery in combination with the continuous search for less invasive procedures and the development of endoscopic equipment, endoscopic endonasal trans-sphenoidal surgery has slowly and inexorably become an accepted technique in the field of pituitary surgery during the last decade of the 20th century.[62,63,71,72]

It requires detailed knowledge of the sinonasal anatomy and specific endoscopic skills, both favored by a close cooperation with an ENT/otolaryngologist with specific competences in endoscopy, and is based on a different concept because the endoscopic view that the surgeon receives on the video monitor is not the transposition of the real image, as it would be looking through the eyepiece of a microscope, but is the result of a microprocessor's elaboration.[48] Nevertheless, other factors have contributed to determine the success of the endoscopic skull base and pituitary surgery. As a matter of facts, if the operation itself has become increasingly simply, safe and elegant, that is unimaginable without an appropriate instrumentation.[73] Every operation and even every technique for each type of operation, requires a dedicated set of instruments—endoscope, camera, light source, monitor, video-recording systems, drills, and so on—which should be of the best quality possible and be dedicated to this type of operation. The instruments form a sort of chain, where each link must to be strong enough to perform its role in the operation otherwise the chain will break and the surgery will not be successful.[49,73,74]

As for other techniques of skull base surgery, the endoscopic endonasal procedure consists of three main aspects: exposure of the lesion, management of the relevant pathology, and reconstruction of the sella.[49]

Because trans-sphenoidal endoscopy is a more recent contribution to pituitary surgery, some advantages, pitfalls, and peculiar aspects related to this technique must be highlighted. The main advantages of the endoscopic procedure compared with the microsurgical procedures are related to the properties of the endoscope itself and to the absence of the nasal speculum.[62,68] As a matter of facts, the nasal speculum creates a "fixed tunnel" and an almost coaxial restriction of the microinstruments and, with its absence, the endoscope discloses its superior properties, permitting a wider vision of the surgical field, with a close-up "look" inside the anatomy. The angled lens endoscopes enable the surgeon to work on tumors located in suprasellar and parasellar regions under direct visual control. The endoscopic endonasal procedure seems to be less traumatic, and the percentage of many complications is reduced compared with the traditional microsurgical approach.[75] Since

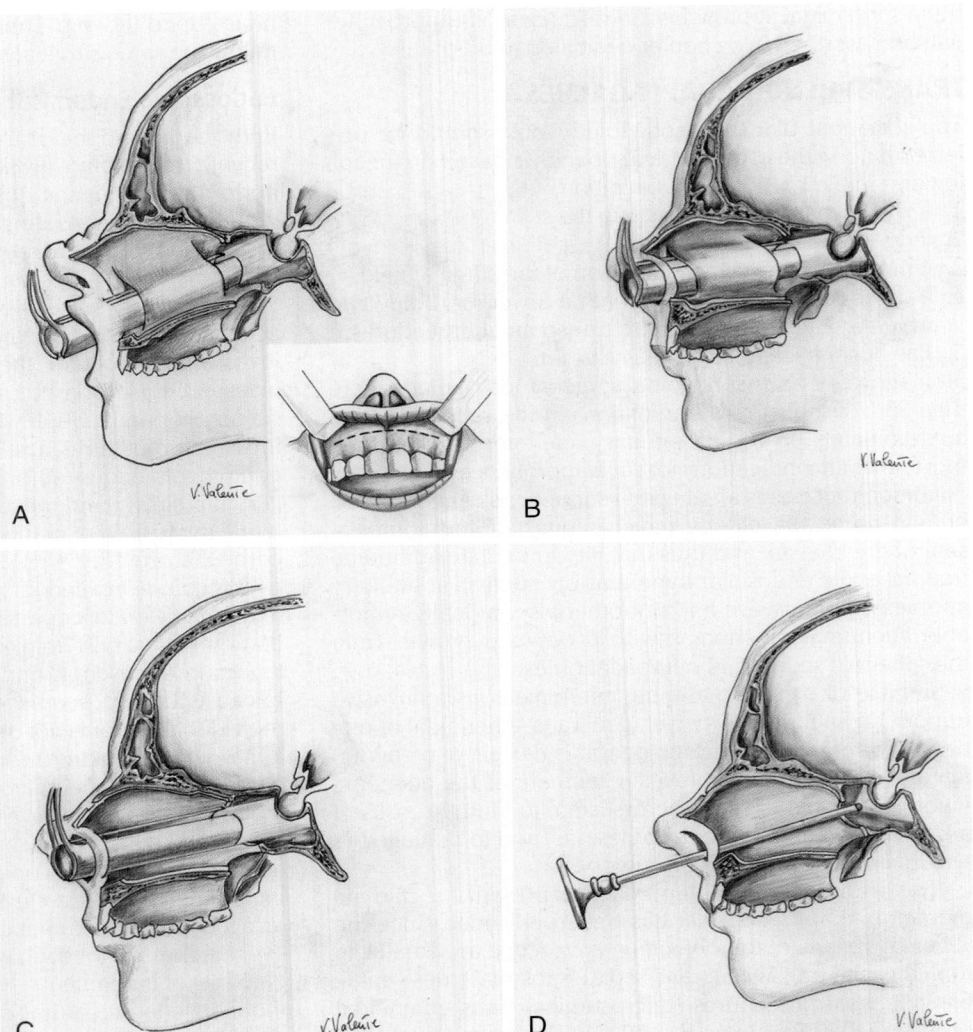

A

B

C

D

FIGURE 21-9 Schematic drawings illustrating the different variants of the trans-sphenoidal approach. A, Sublabial technique. B, Trans-septal technique. C, Endonasal microscopic technique. D, Endonasal endoscopic technique. (From Cappabianca P, et al. Pituitary surgery. In: Jameson JL, De Groot LJ, eds. Endocrinology: Adult and Pediatric, 6th ed. Philadelphia: Saunders-Elsevier; 2010: 358-376.)

the actual procedure starts from the natural ostium of the sphenoid sinus and the submucosal nasal phase is almost avoided, damage to the nasal spine and orodental complications due to the incision in the buccogingival junction are prevented. As a consequence, in almost all cases, no nasal packing is employed, and postoperative breathing difficulties are reduced. So, the endoscopic endonasal approach can be employed in cases of intentionally two-staged trans-sphenoidal operations[52] because of its excellent ability in reaching the sellar region during the second operation.

Furthermore, the endoscopic approach is particularly advantageous in the case of recurrent or sresidual tumors already treated with a trans-sphenoidal operation,[76] in which the surgeon usually finds distorted anatomy and may encounter nasal synechiae, septal perforations, mucoceles, and intrasellar scarring. With the endoscopic procedure, thanks to the avoidance of the submucosal nasal phase of the microsurgical operation, the real beginning of the operation is at the sphenoid sinus, already enlarged by the former approach, rendering the procedure faster and more straightforward, compared with the microsurgical trans-sphenoidal method. The wide anatomic view of the surgical field the endoscope offers in the sphenoid and sellar area

minimizes the chance of a misdirected orientation, when the midline anatomic landmarks are not recognizable or absent, reducing the possibility of injury to the intrasellar and parasellar structures, particularly if a neuronavigation system is used.

Disadvantages of the endoscopic approach include a learning curve to become confident with the unfamiliar anatomy of the nasal cavities and with the specific endoscopic dexterity. Nevertheless, after adequate experience, the operating time becomes the same or shorter than that required for trans-sphenoidal microsurgery, especially in case of recurrences. The endoscope offers only bidimensional vision on the video monitor. The sense of depth can be gained with the surgeon's experience, making the endoscope execute in and out movements, looking for many useful different anatomic landmarks and referring to the many protuberances and depressions in the sphenoid sinus, representing reflections and shadows corresponding to different structures. Dedicated microsurgical endoscopic instruments with secure grip, straight and not bayonet shaped, provided with different and variably angled tips are necessary to reach the surgical targets, particularly the targets that the angled endoscopes are able to show.[74,77]

Extended Endoscopic Endonasal Approach to the Suprasellar Area

For clinically silent pituitary tumors, indications for extended endoscopic endonasal approaches, such as to the suprasellar space or to the cavernous sinus, may be indicated when the lesion occupies such structures and one would avoid various extensive transcranial and/or nasofacial approaches, such as anterior and anterolateral.

First introduced by Weiss in 1987,[78] the *extended transsphenoidal approach is* a trans-sphenoidal approach with the removal of additional bone along the tuberculum sellae and the posterior planum sphenoidale between the optic canals. As a matter of fact, the dural opening was completely above the diaphragma sellae. More recently, the widespread use of the endoscope in trans-sphenoidal surgery has shed new interest on this surgical technique, affording the extension of the trans-sphenoidal approach.[49,79-86] Today, pituitary macroadenomas with suprasellar symmetric and/or asymmetric extension even inside the cavernous sinus, once considered all amenable to open transcranial surgery only are successfully treated by means of such approaches.[49,81,87]

The extended endoscopic approach to the suprasellar area requires the use of additional tools that could be useful to render the procedure safer and more effective:
- Detailed, complete preoperative planning, integrated by 3D reconstructions, in order to tailor the skull base opening with the 3D volume of the lesion
- An image-guided system (neuronavigator) to intraoperatively identify the limits of the lesion, the midline, and the trajectory, offering more precision in defining the boundaries of the bone removal and neurovascular relationships
- Dedicated instruments—that is, high-speed, low-profile microdrills, micro-Doppler probes (especially when approaching the cavernous sinus), bipolar forceps with angled tips, low-profile ultrasonic aspirator or radiofrequency cavitron-like coagulation—to properly manage lesions in such a delicate environment

It is interesting to note that with the endoscopic extended approaches, the surgeon could proceed performing a bimanual dissection while a "tuned" coworker holds the endoscope moving it dynamically and, as requested, insert another surgical instrument. This so-called "3-4 hands technique" requires a good collaboration between two surgeons that should be perfectly tuned, one holding the endoscope and another handling two surgical instruments inside the surgical field.[88] The two surgeons have therefore the possibility to continuously pass between the close-up view, as during the dissecting maneuvers, and a panoramic view of the neurovascular structures. However, it is possible to fix the endoscope to an autostatic holder that can be handled by a single surgeon.

Due to the conspicuous intraoperative cerebrospinal fluid (CSF) leakage resulting from the usually large osteodural opening required to approach the suprasellar area, an accurate reconstruction of the skull base defect is needed after lesion removal. The reconstruction has to be watertight in order to prevent postoperative CSF leak, which could occur even more frequently large openings of the arachnoid cisterns or of the third ventricle.[89,90] The

reconstruction is performed using various techniques, including intradural, extradural, and intra-extradural, and the recent adoption of the pedicled nasoseptal flap,[91-93] even though the most effective seems to be the extradural one.[90] No lumbar drainage is used by our group at the end of the procedure; nevertheless, we advise our patients to have bed rest for 3 to 5 days, depending also on the grade of the pneumoencephalus, while medical therapy with acetazolamyde, laxatives, and broad-spectrum antibiotics is administered.

When compared to the transcranial routes, the extended trans-sphenoidal approach provides a direct view of the neurovascular structures of the suprasellar region from below and no brain and optic nerve manipulation is required, with reduced risk of postoperative vision worsening.[94]

On the other hand, it should be minded that the extended endoscopic endonasal approach to the suprasellar area is more technically demanding and requires some additional skills, both related to the endoscope itself and the opposite anatomic point of view.[84] Besides, it is crucial to focus on some parameters, concerning either the lesion and the anatomy, that could affect lesion management via such a route.[6] Indeed, a well-pneumatized sphenoid sinus allows better visualization of all important landmarks in the posterior wall that, again, are necessary for maintaining surgical orientation while performing the bone removal.[49] On the contrary, a conchal-type sphenoid sinus could hinder the extended endonasal approach, whilst a small sella, with two close intracavernous carotids, could determine a narrower approach.

Transcranial Approaches

There are conditions that limit and sometimes contraindicate the choice of the trans-sphenoidal approach in favor of the transcranial, either related to the anatomy of the surgical pathway or to the morphology and consistency of the lesion. The size of the sella, the size and pneumatization of the sphenoid sinus, and the position and tortuosity of the carotid arteries can increase remarkably the difficulty of the trans-sphenoidal procedure and the final surgical result and may determine the opportunity or even the necessity for the transcranial alternative.

When such selected indications make a transcranial approach required, there are several options (see Table 21-1).

Postoperative Evaluation and Management After Uncomplicated Trans-Sphenoidal Operation

The patient is awakened from anesthesia and transferred to the PACU (postoperative care unit) for 1 to 3 hours; he/she then proceeds to the regular ward, and if the operation was uneventful (no intraoperative CSF leak nor major bleeding), will leave the bed, walk a few hours later, and have a light dinner.

Regarding the antibiotic therapy, it is our policy to adopt a short-term prophylaxis with intravenous third-generation cephalosporins (ceftriaxone or ceftazidime): 30 minutes before starting the procedure and 6 hours after the first injection, with no increased risk for infectious complication. Only in the case of intraoperative CSF leak, where a large communication exists with the subarachnoid compartment, we use prophylaxis for 3 days after the operation.

Since we are dealing with endocrinologically silent pituitary tumors, it is not obligatory to follow our policy as in case of hormonally active adenomas, where we advise checking hormone levels on postoperative days 1 and 2. In fact, as demonstrated by previous studies, if the operation is successful, the pituitary hormones fall into the normal ranges, or even in the subnormal ranges.[100,101] The patient is observed for developing diabetes insipidus by checking the fluid balance.[102]

The patient is usually discharged from the hospital on postoperative day 2 or 3, and is expected to contact the endocrinologist for hormonal follow-up. Furthermore, the patient will be instructed to have serum sodium checked on postoperative days 4 to 6 in order to control for incipient hyponatremia[17] that may be caused by a SIADH (syndrome of inappropriate antidiuretic hormone secretion). (Such hyponatremia is typically subclinical, although on occasion it is severe enough to require rehospitalization.) The patient will then be seen in the outpatient clinic 3 months later for a postoperative sellar-contrast–enhanced MRI. If grade-2 or -3 CSF has occurred during the operation, or in the case of large lesions, the patient is scheduled as an outpatient for an endoscopic evaluation of the nasal and sphenoid sinus cavities to ensure that the mucosa is healing well and that CSF leakage is not present.

Radiotherapy

As part of the armamentarium for managing pituitary tumors, radiotherapy/radiosurgery should be mentioned. Such approaches will be described more in detail in a chapter completely dedicated to this issue.

KEY REFERENCES

Black PM, Hsu DW, Klibanski A, et al. Hormone production in clinically nonfunctioning pituitary adenomas. *J Neurosurg.* 1987;66(2):244-250.

Cappabianca P, Cavallo LM, de Divitiis E. Endoscopic endonasal transsphenoidal surgery. *Neurosurgery.* 2004;55(4):933-940:discussion 940-931.

Cappabianca P, Cavallo LM, de Divitiis O. Pituitary surgery. In: DeGroot L, Jameson JL, eds. *Endocrinology.* 5th ed. vol 1. Philadelphia: Elsevier; 2006:511-535.

Cappabianca P, Cavallo LM, Esposito F, de Divitiis E. Endonasal approaches to the Cavernous sinus. In: Anand VK, Schwartz TH, eds. *Practical endoscopic skull base surgery.* San Diego, Oxford, Brisbane: Plural Publishing; 2007:187-199.

Cappabianca P, Esposito F, Cavallo LM, Corriero OV. Instruments. In: Cappabianca P, Califano L, Iaconetta G, eds. *Cranial, Craniofacial and Skull Base Surgery.* New York: Springer-Verlag; 2010:7-16.

Cavallo LM, Messina A, Esposito F, et al. Skull base reconstruction in the extended endoscopic transsphenoidal approach for suprasellar lesions. *J Neurosurg.* 2007;107(4):713-720.

Colao A, Di Somma C, Pivonello R, et al. Medical therapy for clinically non-functioning pituitary adenomas. *Endocr Relat Cancer.* 2008; 15(4):905-915.

de Bruin TW, Kwekkeboom DJ, Van't Verlaat JW, et al. Clinically nonfunctioning pituitary adenoma and octreotide response to long term high dose treatment, and studies in vitro. *J Clin Endocrinol Metab.* 1992;75(5):1310-1317.

Elias WJ, Chadduck JB, Alden TD, Laws Jr ER. Frameless stereotaxy for transsphenoidal surgery. *Neurosurgery.* 1999;45(2):271-275:discussion 275–277.

Esposito F, Dusick JR, Cohan P, et al. Clinical review: early morning cortisol levels as a predictor of remission after transsphenoidal surgery for Cushing's disease. *J Clin Endocrinol Metab.* 2006;91(1):7-13.

Ezzat S, Asa SL, Couldwell WT, et al. The prevalence of pituitary adenomas: a systematic review. *Cancer.* 2004;101(3):613-619:1.

Frank G, Pasquini E. Endoscopic endonasal cavernous sinus surgery, with special reference to pituitary adenomas. *Front Horm Res.* 2006;34:64-82.

Hofland LJ, Lamberts SW. Somatostatin receptor subtype expression in human tumors. *Ann Oncol.* 2001;12(suppl 2):S31-S36.

Iuchi T, Saeki N, Tanaka M, et al. MRI prediction of fibrous pituitary adenomas. *Acta Neurochir (Wien).* 1998;140(8):779-786.

Kassam A, Snyderman CH, Mintz A, et al. Expanded endonasal approach: the rostrocaudal axis. Part I. Crista galli to the sella turcica. *Neurosurg Focus.* 2005;19(1):E3:15.

Laws ERJ. Foreword. In: De Divitiis E, Cappabianca P, eds. *Endoscopic endonasal transsphenoidal surgery.* Wien, New York: Springer; 2003:v-vii.

Levy MJ, Jager HR, Powell M, et al. Pituitary volume and headache: size is not everything. *Arch Neurol.* 2004;61(5):721-725.

Minniti G, Gilbert DC, Brada M. Modern techniques for pituitary radiotherapy. *Rev Endocr Metab Disord.* 2009;10(2):135-144.

Pivonello R, Matrone C, Filippella M, et al. Dopamine receptor expression and function in clinically nonfunctioning pituitary tumors: comparison with the effectiveness of cabergoline treatment. *J Clin Endocrinol Metab.* 2004;89(4):1674-1683.

Prevedello DM, Doglietto F, Jane Jr JA, et al. History of endoscopic skull base surgery: its evolution and current reality. *J Neurosurg.* 2007;107(1):206-213.

Semple PL, Jane Jr JA, Laws Jr ER. Clinical relevance of precipitating factors in pituitary apoplexy. *Neurosurgery.* 2007;61(5):956-961: discussion 961–952.

Shirodkar M, Jabbour SA. Endocrine incidentalomas. *Int J Clin Pract.* 2008;62(9):1423-1431.

Snyder PJ. Gonadotroph and other clinically nonfunctioning pituitary adenomas. In: DeGroot L, Jameson JL, eds. *Endocrinology.* 5th ed. vol 1. Philadelphia: Elsevier; 2006:465-484.

Visot A, Pencalet P, Boulin A, Gaillard S. Surgical management of endocrinologically silent pituitary tumors. In: Schmideck HH, Sweet DW, eds. *Operative Neurosurgical Techniques. Indications, Methods and Results.* 5th ed. vol 1. Philadelphia: Elsevier; 2006:355-373.

Numbered references appear on Expert Consult.

CHAPTER 22

Endoscopic Endonasal Pituitary and Skull Base Surgery

DAVID H. JHO • DIANA H. JHO • HAE-DONG JHO

Neuroendoscopy was first implemented almost a century ago for choroid plexus surgery in a patient with hydrocephalus. General enthusiasm for ventricular endoscopy experienced an initial decline with the advent of ventricular shunt systems but was later revived for third ventriculostomies in selected patients. The first reported use of the endoscope specifically for trans-sphenoidal surgery was in a sublabial approach by Guiot and colleagues in 1963.[1] However, the general advancement of intracranial and spinal neuroendoscopy continued to be limited, in part trumped by historical developments in neuroimaging and microneurosurgery. Yet in the past three decades, a few pioneering endoscopic neurosurgeons continued to expand and refine the use of neuroendoscopy in endoscope-assisted microsurgery, endonasal trans-sphenoidal surgery, ventricular tumor surgery, extra-axial intracranial surgery, intra-axial brain surgery with stereotactic guidance, and spinal surgery. These advances were accompanied by concurrent technological developments in endoscopic optics, video-imaging systems, endoscopic accessory attachments for neurosurgical applications, specialized neuroendoscopic surgical instruments, radiologic imaging, and compatible frameless stereotactic image-guided systems. As neuroendoscopic surgical techniques and equipment have co-evolved, the addition of neuroendoscopy to the repertoire of the modern neurosurgeon has become increasingly practical. Of note, general interest has noticeably grown for the use of neuroendoscopy in endonasal trans-sphenoidal pituitary surgery, and the common use of neuroendoscopy in pituitary surgery became truly practical in recent years with the development of commercially-available neuroendoscopic equipment.

Although the removal of pituitary tumors completely through endoscopic visualization via an endonasal route has been a relatively recent development, the use of the endonasal pathway itself was initially reported in 1909 by Hirsch who performed his first pituitary surgery in Vienna by approaching the sella through an endonasal route using multiple-staged sinonasal operations with naked-eye visualization. Despite his first endonasal trans-sphenoidal surgery having reported success, Hirsch subsequently converted to a trans-septal submucosal approach, possibly due to fear of surgical infection through such a wide communication made between the nasal and the cranial cavity. Griffith and Veerapen revisited the endonasal approach in 1987, with insertion of a trans-sphenoidal retractor through

the natural nasal airway to the sphenoid rostrum for microscopic pituitary surgery.[2] In 1994, Cooke and Jones reported the lack of sinonasal and dental complications when an endonasal route was adopted for microscopic pituitary surgery.[3] But the most significant progression of the traditional sublabial and transfixional-trans-septal approaches to the direct endonasal route was highly facilitated by the neuroendoscope, with the initial use of sinonasal endoscopy in Europe four decades ago. In the field of Otolaryngology, the introduction of endoscopic sinus surgery to the United States kindled an evolution in surgical techniques such that endoscopic sinus surgery rapidly replaced many forms of conventional sinus surgery, with radical changes in concepts of sinonasal pathophysiology and associated treatments aided by endoscopic exploration. Rather than stripping the infected sinus mucosa as was done in conventional sinus surgery, endoscopic sinus surgery aimed to restore physiologic mucous drainage merely by eliminating obstructive pathoanatomy at sinus ostia via the endonasal route and became popularized as functional endoscopic sinus surgery (FESS). Successful advances in sinonasal endoscopy then enhanced interest in the use of endoscopy for trans-sphenoidal surgery. Endoscopic trans-sphenoidal surgery started with guidance during simple biopsy of a sellar lesion, and then evolved to assist visualization during insertion of trans-sphenoidal retractors or during microscopic removal of pituitary adenomas, and eventually the pure form of endoscopic endonasal pituitary tumor surgery emerged.[4-12]

This chapter describes endoscopic endonasal trans-sphenoidal surgery (EE-TS) along with related endoscopic endonasal approaches to the midline skull base such as the anterior cranial fossa (EE-ACF), optic nerve or cavernous sinus (EE-CS), pterygoid fossa or petrous apex (EE-Pterygoid or EE-Petrous), clivus or posterior fossa (EE-PFossa), and craniocervical junction (EE-CC junction). EE-TS is not merely endoscope-assisted microscopic surgery but is rather an operation done completely with an endoscope without any trans-sphenoidal retractor or nasal speculum, eliminating the need for postoperative nasal packing or other adjuncts. The physical nature of an endoscope with its optics at the tip and slender shaft allows simple access to the sella through the natural nasal air pathway via a nostril. EE-TS uses an endonasal route to the rostrum of the sphenoid sinus with an anterior sphenoidotomy about 1 to 1.5 cm in diameter.

The wide-angled panoramic view, angled-lens views, and a close-up zoom-in view provide optical advantages with distinct visualization at the surgical target site. The application of principles and anatomy in EE-TS was extended to the surgical treatment of midline skull base pathologies (from the anterior cranial fossa to the clivus and posterior fossa along with the craniocervical junction) and paramedian skull base pathologies (from the optic nerve and cavernous sinus regions to the pterygoid fossa and petrous tip). Endoscopic endonasal techniques can potentially be applied to nearly any lesion within approximately 2-cm width of the midline skull base from the crista galli at the anterior-superior skull base to the foramen magnum and atlantoaxial region at the posterior-inferior skull base.[13-23]

Preoperative Management and Surgical Indications

As with microscopic pituitary surgery, all patients with pituitary adenomas undergo formal endocrine evaluations preoperatively and postoperatively. Hypopituitarism is among the important endocrine conditions requiring treatment starting preoperatively, particularly for hypocortisolism and hypothyroidism. For patients with preoperative visual symptoms or tumors impinging on the optic apparatus on magnetic resonance imaging (MRI), formal neuro-ophthalmologic evaluation is obtained preoperatively with follow-up visual examinations postoperatively. MRI of the brain with and without contrast enhancement (ideally with a pituitary focused protocol and optionally with dynamic contrast imaging) is the diagnostic imaging modality of choice with best resolution for most pituitary adenomas. Patients who are unable to undergo MRI for various reasons can undergo the lesser alternative of computed tomography (CT) of the brain with pituitary focus and dynamic contrast protocol. Usually, the basic anatomy of the paranasal sinuses and any variations of an individual can be appreciated sufficiently on MRI for the purposes of trans-sphenoidal surgery. However, bone windowed CT scans with fine-cut axial and coronal views can disclose the bony anatomy of the paranasal sinuses in detail and may be obtained depending on surgeon's preference or for patients who have had previous paranasal sinus or trans-sphenoidal surgery. Image-guided systems (IGS) are not routinely required for EE-TS, but imaging protocol compatible with frameless stereotaxy may also be used for complex skull base lesions if desired.

Surgical indications for patients with pituitary adenomas to undergo endoscopic trans-sphenoidal surgery are essentially comparable to indications for conventional microscopic trans-sphenoidal surgery. Patients with hormonally inactive or nonfunctional pituitary adenomas are operated upon when the tumors cause symptomatic compression of the optic apparatus, hypopituitarism, pituitary apoplexy, or severe intractable frontotemporal headaches. Patients with hormonally active or functional pituitary adenomas causing acromegaly, Cushing's disease, or hyperthyroidism undergo trans-sphenoidal surgery as the primary mode of treatment. Patients with prolactinomas are operated upon only when they fail to respond appropriately to dopaminergic medications, develop intolerable side effects to the medications, or choose against the use of dopaminergic medications. Other symptomatic mass lesions or tumors at the pituitary fossa generally undergo surgery if needed for biopsy or resection. In contrast to conventional microscopic surgery, a large pituitary tumor with suprasellar extension can be directly visualized in EE-TS and bony exposure can be extended rostrally if further exploration at the planum sphenoidale is required. EE-TS can thus enhance the chance for total pituitary tumor resection and potentially reduce the need of a supplemental transcranial approach.

Following hundreds of EE-TS cases with the youngest patient being a teenager, we have yet to encounter a patient whose nasal passage was too small or narrow to undergo standard EE-TS. Notably, patients with acromegaly usually have hypertrophic turbinates and nasal-oral soft tissues such that the endonasal space can be disproportionately small. In addition, patients with Cushing's disease often have narrow nasal airways due to swollen hypertrophic mucosa, which also tends to bleed easily. Among our patients who have undergone EE-TS, two patients with Cushing's disease required a two-nostril technique with an endoscope inserted through one nostril and the surgical instruments inserted through the other. Reoperation by EE-TS for patients who have undergone previous conventional trans-sphenoidal surgery is not difficult if an appropriate anterior sphenoidotomy was previously performed, although reoperation can be challenging if bony sellar structures were excessively eliminated, complications were encountered at previous surgery, or distorting extensive reconstruction was performed.

Pertinent Sinonasal Anatomy

To perform endoscopic pituitary surgery, the functional physiology and anatomy of the sinonasal cavity must be understood. In the paranasal sinuses (that include the sphenoid, ethmoid, maxillary, and frontal sinuses), mucociliary movement is orchestrated by the delivery of mucus flow to the sinus ostia. From the sinus ostia, nasal mucosal ciliary movement is directed to establish the physiologic flow of mucus towards the nasopharynx. When the path of physiologic mucus flow is interrupted mechanically or functionally, the paranasal sinuses can retain stagnant mucus, which can subsequently become infected and result in sinusitis. The confluence of the draining mucus from the frontal sinus, anterior ethmoidal sinus, and maxillary sinus is located at the middle meatus. Mucosal drainage of the posterior ethmoidal sinus occurs at the superior meatus, and drainage of the sphenoid sinus is at the sphenoethmoidal recess, which is located between the posterolateral aspect of the middle turbinate, superior turbinate, and the rostrum of the sphenoid sinus.

The nasal cavity itself is bordered medially by the nasal septum (comprised of the septal cartilage, perpendicular plate of the ethmoid bone, and the vomer); superiorly by the cribriform plate of the ethmoid bone and bridge of the nose (consisting of the nasal portion of the frontal bone, nasal bone, and frontal process of the maxilla); inferiorly by the floor of the nasal cavity (involving the palatine process of the maxilla and the horizontal plate of the palatine bone); and conchae or turbinates laterally (inferior, middle, superior, and sometimes supreme turbinates). The superior and middle conchae (along with the occasional supreme concha) are components of the ethmoid bone, whereas the inferior concha is a separate bone. The EE-TS procedure traverses the region medial to the middle turbinate, between the middle turbinate and the nasal septum, on the way to the sphenoid sinus then the pituitary fossa at the sella turcica. Nasal septal deviation is not an uncommon phenomenon, such that often the larger nasal cavity is selected as the route for EE-TS based on preoperative imaging and intraoperative visualization.

The lateral wall of the endonasal route (with numerous projections of the ethmoid bone and individual anatomic variability) is more complex in anatomy than the medial wall, which consists of the nasal septum. From both a surgical and anatomic embryology standpoint, the ethmoid at the lateral wall of the nasal cavity has been divided into five sequential lamella from anterior to posterior consisting of the uncinate process, ethmoid bulla, basal lamella of the middle turbinate, basal lamella of the superior turbinate, and occasionally the basal lamella of the supreme turbinate (if present). The basal lamella of the middle turbinate divides the ethmoid sinuses into anterior and posterior air cells, and the middle turbinate attachments lie in three different planes with the anterior segment oriented along a sagittal plane (attached to the lateral portion of the cribriform plate superiorly), middle segment oriented along a coronal plane (attached to the lamina papyracea), and the posterior segment oriented nearly along an axial plane (attached to the medial wall of the maxillary sinus and perpendicular plate of the palatine bone). The normal sinonasal anatomy located laterally to the middle turbinate is referred to as the osteomeatal complex (OMC) and comprises a key set of structures for sinonasal function, forming the basis of FESS treatments for paranasal sinus pathologies.

The OMC consists of the middle turbinate, uncinate process, hiatus semilunaris, ethmoid infundibulum, and ethmoid bulla. Anterolateral to the middle turbinate is the uncinate process of the ethmoid bone, behind which lies a cleft between the uncinate and ethmoid bulla called the hiatus semilunaris, which is contiguous with the ethmoid infundibulum. The hiatus semilunaris is essentially a two-dimensional crescent-shaped opening leading from the middle meatus into the three-dimensional funnel-shaped ethmoid infundibulum to which the frontal sinus, anterior ethmoid sinus, and maxillary sinus usually drain. The frontal sinus drains anteriorly at the ethmoid infundibulum (via the hourglass-shaped frontonasal recess), anterior ethmoid sinus drains into the mid-portion, and the maxillary sinus drains through its ostium posteriorly at the maxillary infundibulum. Along the posterior-superior bank of the hiatus semilunaris is the ethmoid bulla, which is considered one of the most constant and largest of the anterior ethmoid air cells. The ethmoid bulla is bordered medially by the lamina papyracea of the medial orbit and projects medially in the middle meatus, and the posterior-superior portion of the hiatus semilunaris connects the middle meatus with the suprabullar and retrobullar recesses (collectively called the sinus lateralis), which are defined in relation to the ethmoid bulla. There are variations and debated nuances in the anatomic terminology of paranasal sinus anatomy, including the precise borders of the ethmoid infundibulum in relation to the hiatus semilunaris. Regardless, the more important point is that there are individual structural variations, which

can affect paranasal sinus physiology and surgical anatomy. For instance, there are three major variations to the superior attachment of the crescent-shaped uncinate process with the most common type attaching laterally to the lamina papyracea (~70% in cadaveric studies) resulting in frontal sinus outflow medial to the uncinate process at the middle meatus. The two other major patterns of uncinate superior insertions include medial attachment to the base of the middle turbinate at the cribriform plate (<20%) and superior attachment to the roof of the ethmoid at the skull base (<10%) that both result in natural frontal sinus outflow lateral to the uncinate at the ethmoid infundibulum. There are other unmentioned variations of uncinate insertions, and these variations may be considered a continuous spectrum of lateral-to-medial insertions rather than merely categorical entities. Anatomic variations may also include a pneumatized or aerated turbinate, most frequently the middle turbinate, which is referred to as concha bullosa and can be enlarged. There can also be variations of a paradoxical middle turbinate with the convexity of the turbinate curve oriented laterally instead of medially, which can alter the expected configuration of the OMC. Regardless of these variations or the presence of any nasal polyps, the main point is that structures of the OMC should not be significantly disturbed *en route* to the sphenoid sinus during EE-TS. The sphenoid sinus mucosa should also be minimally disrupted by limiting the mucosal removal only to the region required at the anterior sphenoidotomy site and the anterior wall of the sella.

As mentioned, there can be significant variability in the structure of the ethmoid sinus, which is sometimes termed the ethmoid labyrinth, with the ethmoid air cells having some surgically pertinent variations for EE-TS. The agger nasi is a mound or prominence on the anterior-lateral aspect of the nasal cavity formed by mucous membrane covering the ethmoidal crest of the maxilla near the anterior aspect of the middle turbinate. The agger nasi cells are the most anterior ethmoidal cells located just anterior and lateral to the nasofrontal recess and can sometimes be involved in frontal sinus outflow obstruction. For EE-TS, the surgeon should be aware that a hyperpneumatized agger nasi cell can occasionally present as a bulge that mimics the anterior view of a turbinate. Haller cells (infraorbital ethmoid air cells or maxilloethmoidal cells) are closely related to the ethmoid infundibulum along the medial roof of the maxillary sinus, inferior-lateral to the ethmoid bulla, and extend into the inferomedial orbital floor at the inferior margin of the lamina papyracea. Since Haller cells are quite lateral, these usually do not present a problem during EE-TS, although their proximity to the ethmoid infundibulum can result in inadvertent orbital entry during FESS if not recognized. Onodi cells (sphenoethmoidal cells) are posterior ethmoidal air cells that can project superiorly into the sphenoid sinus towards the lateral side and can potentially be confused with a septated region of the sphenoid sinus. The optic nerve and/or internal carotid artery can bulge into Onodi cells instead of the sphenoid sinus proper, or occasionally may have either partial or complete bony dehiscence at the sphenoid sinus, presenting risk for injury during surgery. It is also possible to have extensive pneumatization of the anterior clinoid process at the optico-carotid recess (OCR), which can also expose the optic nerve and internal carotid artery to additional risk. It is also possible for patients who have undergone previous trans-sphenoidal surgery to have a mucocele at the region of the sphenoid sinus, which can also potentially lead to intra-operative confusion, although this is usually recognizable on the preoperative MRI with the mucocele usually having a spherical type of shape and bright T2 signal such that it can be anticipated intraoperatively.

The rostrum of the sphenoid sinus is usually a relatively constant midline landmark regardless of any bowing or lateral deviation of the nasal septum and can be used as a reference for drilling. However, the sphenoid sinuses internally are divided by a highly variable intersinus septum (or configuration of septae) that can be oblique, multiple, or incomplete, and usually does not strictly respect the sagittal midline. Sphenoid sinus septations are generally oriented in a vertical direction and may attach to the regions of the optic canal or carotid artery; septations that are horizontally oriented are usually boundaries between the posterior ethmoid sinus and the sphenoid sinus, which can include Onodi cells (sphenoethmoid air cells). Variations in the pneumatization of the sphenoid sinus, asymmetries, and septal divisions along with the relationship of the optic nerve and internal carotid arteries should be studied on the preoperative MRI and/or CT to serve as a roadmap to the sella. The thickness and position of the sella turcica, plus anatomy of the presellar and retrosellar recesses, and tumor extension in the suprasellar region and laterally to the region of the cavernous sinuses should be noted preoperatively to allow anticipatory maneuvers intraoperatively.

When the sphenoid sinus is entered with an endoscope, the complex anatomy is visualized in a panoramic fashion. The clival indentation is seen at the bottom midline, the bony protuberances covering the internal carotid arteries are lateral to the clival indentation, the sella is at the center, the cavernous sinuses are seen lateral to the sella, the tuberculum sella is at the top, and the bony protuberances of the optic nerves are seen laterally. Surgical landmarks for endoscopic endonasal pituitary surgery consist of the choanae and nasopharynx along with the inferior margin of the

middle turbinate. The choana at the anterior-superior entry of the nasopharynx is always a useful landmark in order to confirm the middle turbinate. The extended line along the inferior margin of the middle turbinate leads to the region approximately 1 cm inferior to the sellar floor. Although the sphenoid sinus ostium at the sphenoethmoidal recess may also be visible under the endoscope, it may not always be easily identifiable or precisely consistent in its relationship to the sella. Thus, the sphenoid sinus ostium can be regarded as an inconsistent surgical landmark, whereas the choana and inferior margin of the middle turbinate tend to be quite consistent. Anterior sphenoidotomy measuring approximately 1.5 cm in diameter is performed at the rostrum of the sphenoid sinus at a location rostral to an extended line from the inferior margin of the middle turbinate (Fig. 22-1A and B).

Following pituitary tumor removal, the thin flaps of sellar bone are placed back into position to provide reconstruction at the anterior wall of the sella turcica. The sphenoid sinus is preserved as a natural air-filled cavity, and we routinely do not use any foreign surgical material at the sphenoid sinus (although reconstruction can be done with various materials or methods if absolutely needed for cerebrospinal fluid leaks or complex lesions involving significant bony defects). When an anterior sphenoidotomy is made, attention must be paid not to significantly disrupt the normal posterior mucus drainage channel at the sphenoid ostium of the sphenoethmoidal recess. Towards the conclusion of EE-TS, the middle turbinate is gently medialized back to its original position in order to avoid blockage of mucus drainage at the OMC.

The nasal mucosa is predominantly supplied by the sphenopalatine artery, with contributions from the greater palatine artery, branches of the facial artery, and the anterior and posterior ethmoidal arteries. The posterior septal artery arises from the sphenopalatine branch of the internal maxillary artery and passes to the posterior nasal septum at the inferior-medial aspect of the middle turbinate posterior

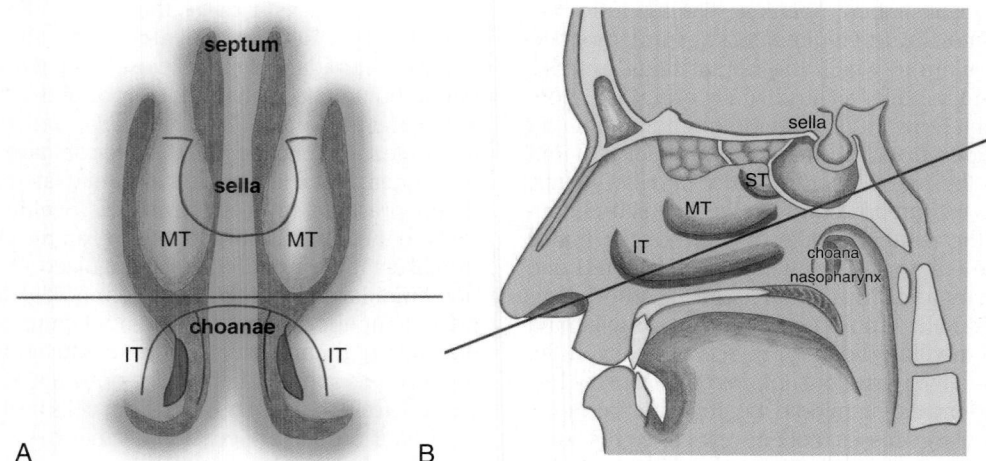

FIGURE 22-1 Schematic drawings of the sinonasal cavity, coronal (A) and sagittal views (B), demonstrate the anatomic landmarks leading to the sella. The inferior turbinate (IT) and middle turbinate (MT) are initially encountered along the endonasal route. A plane followed along the inferior margin of the middle turbinate leads to the clivus approximately 1 cm inferior to the floor of the sella, and just inferiorly lies the upper margin of the choana with view of the nasopharynx that serves as a key surgical landmark. Confirmation of the middle turbinate in relation to the nasopharynx prevents any confusion of the middle turbinate with the superior turbinate (ST), which is especially important in occasional cases of an anatomic supreme turbinate. Fluoroscopic C-arm imaging is not necessary because of the consistency of these surgical landmarks.

margin. When surgical access is obtained between the middle turbinate and nasal septum for an anterior sphenoidotomy, the posterior septal artery often requires coagulation and division to prevent unwanted intraoperative or postoperative nasal bleeding. Delayed copious nasal bleeding after trans-sphenoidal surgery usually arises from rebleeding of the posterior septal artery.

For endoscopic endonasal approach to the anterior cranial fossa (EE-ACF), the region of the ethmoid roof with the cribriform plate and the fovea ethmoidalis should be studied on preoperative imaging. Keros categorized three types of skull base conformations along a spectrum depending on the depth of the olfactory sulcus and corresponding height of the lateral lamella, with Type 1 having 1-3 mm depth, Type 2 having 3-7 mm depth, and Type 3 having 7-16 mm depth such that the ethmoid roof is significantly higher than the cribriform plate.[24] The Keros classification is more pertinent for ethmoid sinus surgery to avoid inadvertent entry through the thin lateral lamella of the cribriform plate, especially for a deep olfactory sulcus. However, for EE-ACF or EE-CS (via the middle meatal approach with posterior ethmoidectomy), one should be aware of the potential individual variations in depth of the olfactory sulcus and the specific anatomic configuration should be noted preoperatively to assist with optimal intraoperative maneuvering. In the same region, the ethmoidal sulcus is the groove in the lateral lamella for the anterior ethmoidal artery, which branches from the ophthalmic artery and enters from the orbit in a bony canal in the ethmoid roof (anterior ethmoidal canal) or just below the level of the ethmoid roof to course anteromedially with the anterior ethmoidal nerve and to penetrate the lateral lamellae to supply the dura in the region of the olfactory sulcus. The posterior ethmoidal artery traverses the posterior ethmoidal canal within a 3 mm planar region above the cribriform plate. The anterior and posterior ethmoidal arteries usually provide the major blood supply for olfactory groove or planum sphenoidale meningiomas at the skull base.

Optical Advantages of an Endoscope
WIDE-ANGLED PANORAMIC VIEW

As trans-sphenoidal pituitary surgery began its evolvement in the 19th century, one major advance was the adoption of the operating microscope in the 1960's. The use of the endoscope for pituitary tumor resection represents another significant advancement. Whereas the operating microscope provides a magnified view of a limited portion of the sella through a narrow corridor revealed by the trans-sphenoidal retractor, an endoscope can physically enter into the sphenoid sinus and provide a wide-angled panoramic view with zooming capability. An operating microscope renders a tubular parallel beam view, but an endoscope shows a diverging flask-shaped wide-angled view (Fig. 22-2A to D). This wide-angled panoramic view is particularly useful for pituitary tumor surgery because it allows excellent anatomical visualization at the posterior wall of the sphenoid sinus.

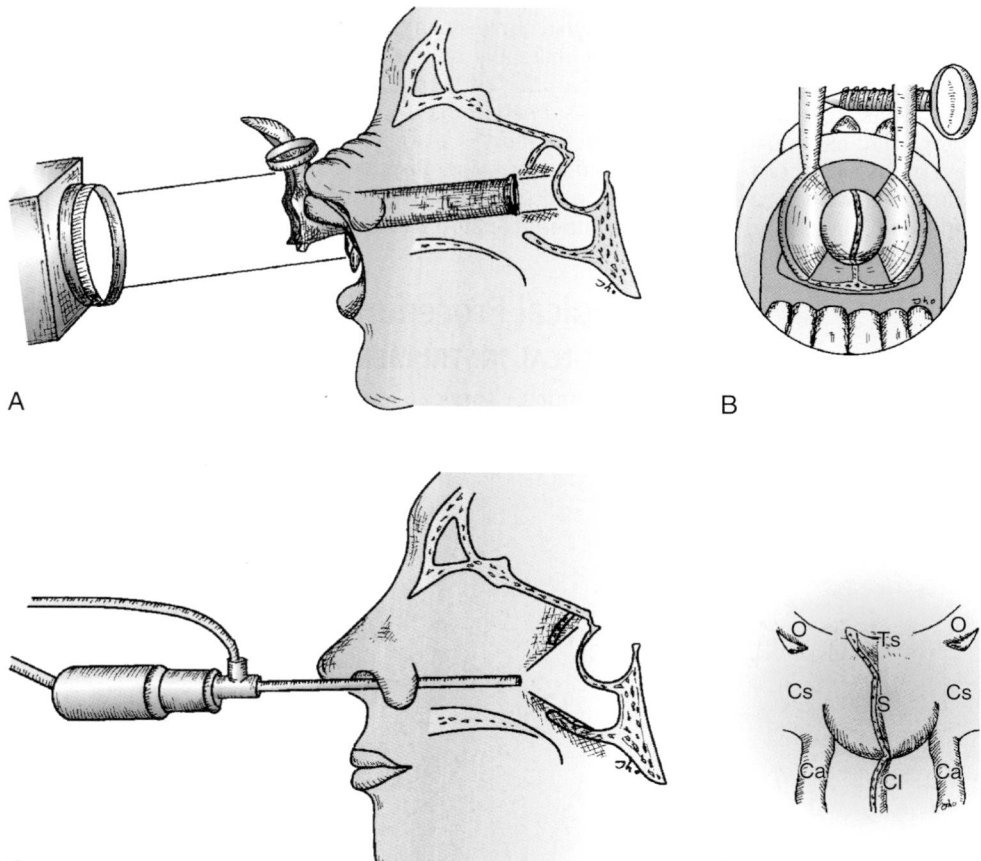

FIGURE 22-2 Schematic drawings demonstrate comparison views between microscopic and endoscopic exposure at the posterior wall of the sphenoid sinus during trans-sphenoidal pituitary surgery. The microscope view is stereoscopic but can be confined by the narrow tubular corridor for light projection to a central limited area of the sella (A, B). The endoscope view is monoscopic but reveals a wide region of the sphenoid sinus posterior wall due to the panoramic nature of endoscopic optics (C, D). The endoscope also has capabilities for dynamic visualization using freedom of endoscope movement at the surgical site and extra options for angled lenses. However, the endoscope lens does produce a degree of fish-eye effect with the center being maximally magnified and the periphery somewhat contracted. Endoscopic view demonstrates the sella (S) at the center, cavernous sinuses (Cs) laterally, the cavernous carotid arteries (Ca) inferolaterally, clivus (Cl) inferiorly, tuberculum sella (Ts) superiorly, and optic nerves (O) superolaterally.

However, it must be recognized that the endoscopic view renders a fish-eye effect with maximum magnification at the center and relative contraction at the periphery with visualization of a wide anatomical area. In the well-pneumatized sphenoid sinus, the sella is readily recognizable at the center of the surgical view, and a panoramic image of the surrounding anatomy at the posterior wall of the sphenoid sinus is revealed under direct endoscopic view. Unless the region of the sella is not pneumatized or the patient is a complicated reoperation case, the use of fluoroscopic roentgenogram is not necessary since endoscopic visualization can adequately reveal the distinct surgical anatomy.

ANGLED-LENS VIEW

The angled-lens endoscopic view provides direct visualization of the anatomical corners such as the suprasellar area or towards the cavernous sinus. These views can be of great assistance even if an endoscope is only used as an adjunctive tool during conventional microscopic surgery. Operating under an angled-lens endoscopic view requires specially designed surgical tools and advanced endoscopic surgical skills, particularly for the 70-degree-lens endoscope. As an angled-lens endoscope is rotated towards the surgical target, various anatomical corners can be visualized from the floor of the sella to the medial wall of the cavernous sinus and towards the suprasellar region. A fiberoptic endoscope can sometimes be used to inspect anatomical corners involving curved routes. This angled view is advantageous when large suprasellar macroadenomas are to be removed. It also allows clear visualization at the medial wall of the cavernous sinus when the lateral margin of a sellar tumor abutting the cavernous sinus is dissected away or when tumor tissue invading the cavernous sinus is to be removed under direct visualization. Although pituitary adenomas with significant invasion of the cavernous sinus were once generally regarded as inoperable, EE-TS allows safe access to the cavernous sinus for tumor removal. Angled views allow for direct surgical access to the pterygoid fossa, anterior cranial fossa, clivus, and posterior cranial fossa in addition to the cavernous sinus (Fig. 22-3A and B).

CLOSE-UP INTERNAL VIEW

When tumor resection is accomplished, an endoscope can be advanced into the sella or suprasellar area close to the surgical target. This close-up view in liaison with zooming of the camera enhances the magnification of the surgical site.

For microadenoma removal, the close-up view is utilized to confirm that the normal margin of the pituitary tissue is well-exposed at the tumor resection site. For macroadenomas, an endoscope can be advanced into the tumor resection cavity to visualize the internal anatomy at the resection cavity. When a 30-degree angled endoscope is inserted into the cavity and rotated through a full revolution, it can visualize the entire circumference of the cavity. Often a minute amount of tumor residue is revealed at the hidden corners for completion of removal. These close-up magnified views thus enhance complete tumor removal in microadenomas as well as macroadenomas.

PHYSICAL ADVANTAGES OF AN ENDOSCOPE

Endoscopes can be subdivided into two categories: fiberoptic flexible endoscopes and rod-lens rigid endoscopes. The number of fiberoptic fibers in most flexible endoscopes is approximately 10,000 although new flexible endoscopes carrying up to 50,000 fibers are being developed. Thus, the image quality of the flexible endoscope is still inadequate for pituitary surgery, and its use is limited to occasional inspection at deep curved anatomical regions. Three-mm or 4-mm rod-lens endoscopes can be used for primary visualization during pituitary surgery since they provide clear video images. Four-mm rod-lens endoscopes provide full-screen, high-quality images in contrast to the smaller, inferior quality images provided by 3-mm rod-lens endoscopes. The basic endoscopes used by the authors are 4-mm rod-lens endoscopes with 0-, 30-, or 70-degree lenses. As previously mentioned, the slender physical shape of the endoscope shaft with the visualizing lens at the tip allows navigation through a narrow anatomical space and eliminates the need to traumatically retract a straight tubular surgical corridor. Surgical incision, septal mucosal dissection, or removal of the nasal septum is unnecessary. Therefore, postoperative nasal packing is also not necessary. The occurrence or amount of postoperative bloody nasal discharge is very minimal, and postoperative comfort of the patient is related to the minimal anatomical disruption during surgery.

Surgical Procedure

SURGICAL INSTRUMENTS

Appropriate surgical equipment is necessary to perform optimal endoscopic pituitary surgery. Attempting an endoscopic operation of this nature with a borrowed

FIGURE 22-3 Schematic drawings show angled views with the 30-degree-lens endoscope directed towards the suprasellar region (A, B). The 30-degree-lens endoscopic view discloses the anterior cerebral artery, optic chiasm (C), diaphragma sella (D), left optic nerve (LtO), right optic nerve (RtO), and pituitary stalk (S).

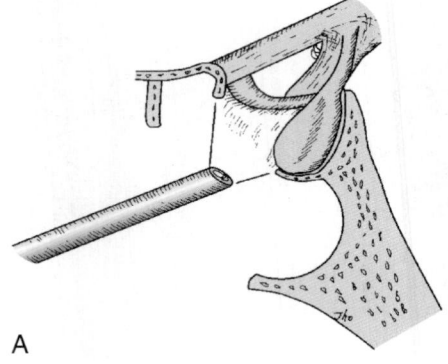

A

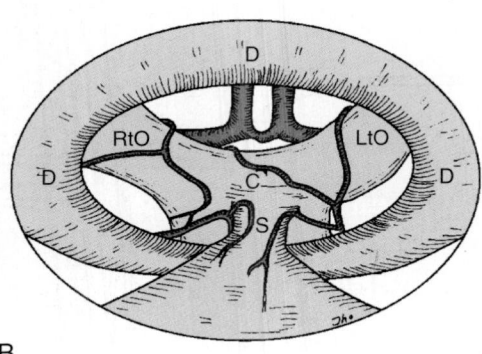

B

otolaryngologic endoscope can potentially result in frustration. Endoscopic surgical techniques are quite different from those of microscopic surgery. Being well-trained in microscopic surgery does not preclude the need for practice in endoscopy. The required surgical instruments are endoscopes with 0-, 30-, and 70-degree lenses (Fig. 22-4A) and their appendages, including a video-imaging system and light source connections, an endoscope lens-cleansing device, a rigid endoscope holder, and various other surgical instruments specifically designed for endoscopic pituitary surgery. The length of an endoscope must be 18 cm or longer. When an 18 cm-long endoscope was used for removal of a posterior fossa tumor through an endonasal transclival approach, it proved to be marginally short and restricted the surgeon's operating space between the endoscopic appendages and the patient's face. Fluoroscopic guidance, which was used in earlier patients, is no longer used in routine pituitary surgery. It is rarely but occasionally used for anterior or posterior cranial fossa surgery, and for pituitary tumor patients in which complexity of the sinonasal anatomy is anticipated.

An endoscopic lens-cleansing device is required to cleanse the lens so that the surgeon can operate without interruption (Fig. 22-4B). The device consists of a disposable irrigation tube, which has a loop of tubing passed through a battery-powered rotary device. The irrigation tube is connected into a warmed saline bag (the temperature prevents lens fogging), which is hung on a pole, and the motor-powered irrigation device is controlled by a foot pedal to flush saline forward. When the foot pedal is released, the motor reverses its rotary direction and draws the saline back for 1 to 2 seconds. The forward flow of irrigation saline cleans the lens, and the reverse flow clears water bubbles at the tip of the endoscope. Although this device is not yet perfect, it helps the surgeon significantly in the task of keeping the endoscope lens clean in order to preserve the optimal technical continuity and flow of the procedure.

Appropriate endoscope holders help provide stability of the visual image and bimanual instrument use during portions of the case during which this is optimal, such as drilling and the majority of tumor removal (Fig. 22-5). Although there are portions of surgery during which dynamic visualization is important, such as the initial approach to the sphenoid sinus rostrum and final visualization of any tumor remnants at anatomic corners of the sella, endoscope holders provide camera stability akin to a video camera tripod during appropriate segments of surgery and does not require the presence of a trained assistant to constantly drive or hold the endoscope camera. The endoscope holder should also provide rigid fixation of the endoscope while also allowing easy transition between stable fixation and manual dynamic steering. The holding terminal is necessarily compact and slender so as to render adequate operating space around the endoscope shaft for the surgeon to maneuver surgical instruments. We routinely use a customized manual endoscope holder specifically designed for EE-TS, in contrast to a nitrogen-powered holder called the Mitaka Point Setter (Mitaka USA; Park City, Utah) for our endoscopic transcranial approaches, and a nitrogen-powered holder called Unitrac (Aesculap; Tuttlingen, Germany) for our endoscopic spine surgery. Manual holders have multiple joints that are tightened by hand to set the final position, but only a single joint has to be loosened during a case to transition from endoscope fixation to manual driving or back. Manual holders are highly stable without significant constraints in range-of-motion or disadvantage of the settling phenomenon, but the configuration can purposefully be set such that the range-of-motion of the final joint is constrained to maintain the trajectory of the endonasal route for EE-TS and depth adjustments only require the simple untightening of a single joint. Nitrogen-powered holders are more expensive but conveniently provide release and tightening using a single button. The Mitaka Point Setter provides excellent stability and minimal settling phenomenon but is limited by the constrained range-of-motion to cases that require only minor maneuvering of the endoscope holder. The Unitrac is stable and highly maneuverable but displays significant settling phenomenon

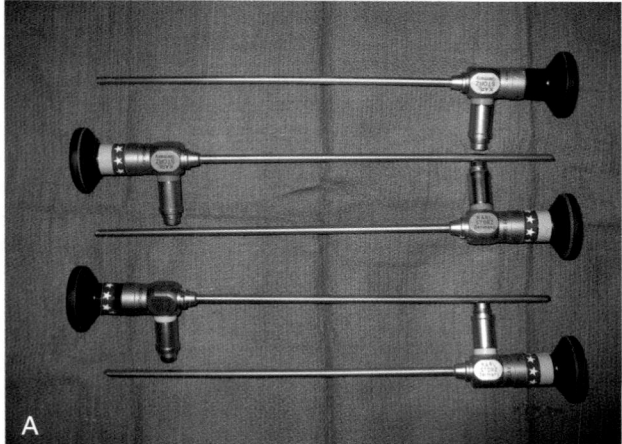 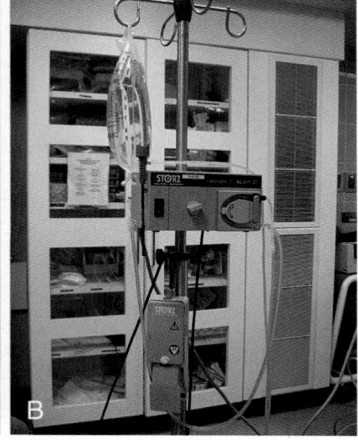

FIGURE 22-4 The sinonasal endoscopes used for endonasal pituitary surgery are 4 mm in diameter and 18 cm in length with 0-degree, 30-degree angled-up or angled-down, and 70-degree angled-up or angled-down lenses (A). The tube with green top and black tip is the sheath of the Endoscope Lens Cleansing Device (Endoscrub®, Xomed-Treace, Bristol-Myers Squibb, Jacksonville, FL). The base of the battery-powered lens cleansing device (Endovision®, Karl Storz, Tuttlingen, Germany) is connected to the endoscope sheath and serves as a tool for cleaning the lens using foot pedal control (for forward irrigation of warm saline solution at the lens followed by brief reverse flow) without removing the endoscope from the surgical field (B).

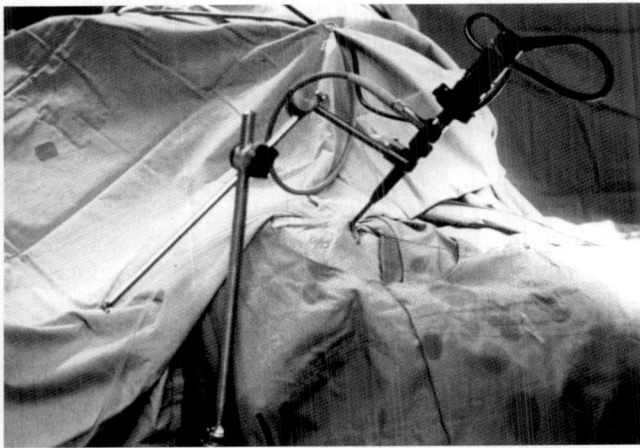

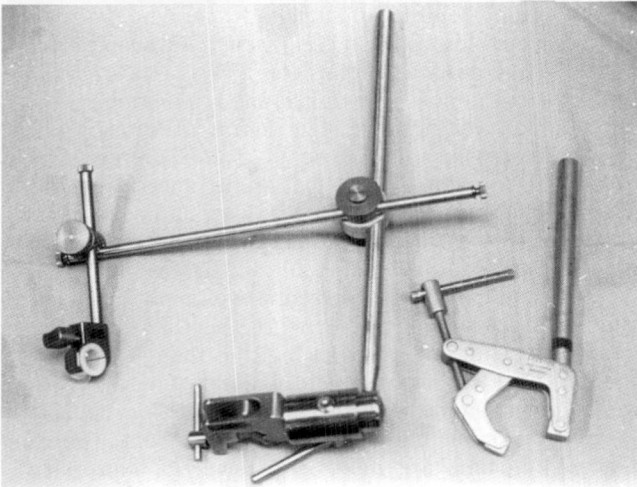

FIGURE 22-5 The customized manual endoscope holder consists of a custom-made distal joint in combination with a Greenberg retractor mounting system. The holder provides rigid fixation of the endoscope (akin to a video camera tripod) during specific portions of surgery such as drilling or tumor removal, to provide stable video images as well as bimanual capabilities for a lone surgeon to use surgical instruments. The holder is setup along a parallel trajectory with the surgical route to allow a smooth range of endoscope depth changes. The ergonomics of the customized holder also allows easy alternation between endoscope stabilization in the holder and single-handed endoscope steering as needed for dynamic surgical visualization or view adjustments during the operation.

such that the final endoscope position sinks somewhat with gravity before locking in final position. Other endoscope holders are still in development to attempt to maximize the strengths and minimize the weaknesses of the various endoscope holders.

Among various surgical instruments, a monopolar suction coagulator (No. 8 or 9 French cannula), a bipolar suction coagulator (No. 8 or 9 French cannula), and a single-bladed bipolar coagulator are useful tools for hemostasis. These are all disposable, and the monopolar suction coagulator is malleable and insulated. The malleable monopolar is useful in bloodless preparation of the nasal cavity for anterior sphenoidotomy. The bipolar suction coagulator and single-bladed bipolar coagulator have two cables for producing bipolar functioning, the single-bladed bipolar has one electrode at the core and the other at the shell. These bipolar instruments are used for dural or intradural hemostasis.

Suction cannulas with variously curved tips (No. 5 and 7 French cannulas) are used for sellar operations. Titanium microclips have been used as a dural suturing device and nitinol U-clips are also commercially available, but further evolvement would be ideal for endoscopic dural suturing. Other instruments used include a micropituitary rongeur, pituitary rongeur, ethmoid rongeurs, high-speed drill, micro-Kerrison rongeurs, pituitary ring curettes, Jannetta 45-degree microdissector, single-bladed Kurze scissors, and a specially-designed septal breaker. A slender high-speed drill is useful when the sphenoid sinus is small and not well-pneumatized.

MYTHS IN SINONASAL SURGERY

In early patients, topical application of a vasoconstrictor and local infiltration of lidocaine with epinephrine were used with the belief that intraoperative and postoperative bleeding would be reduced. Sometimes a piece of polytetrafluoroethylene (Teflon) or Gelfoam sponge was also left at the middle meatus in the hope that it would minimize postoperative bleeding and mucosal adhesions. However, these ineffective practices were gradually eliminated from our technique as experience accumulated. When the topical use of a vasoconstrictor and local injection of lidocaine with epinephrine were completely eliminated, delayed postoperative nasal bleeding markedly decreased. The use of vasoconstrictors may lessen bleeding intraoperatively, but postoperative nasal bleeding was increased presumably due to inadequate intraoperative hemostasis during the active vasoconstriction phase and rebound vasodilatation when the vasoconstrictor effects wore off postoperatively. Meticulous hemostasis using monopolar coagulation (and bipolar coagulation if needed) at the rostrum of the sphenoid sinus without the masking effect of intraoperative vasoconstrictors is the key to minimizing the incidence of postoperative nasal bleeding. When we performed careful hemostasis at the rostrum mucosa and anterior sphenoidotomy site, the placement of a Teflon or Gelfoam sponge was also unnecessary.

When an anterior sphenoidotomy was performed, care is taken not to strip the mucosa at the sphenoid sinus. When the sphenoidal mucosa is stripped unnecessarily from the sinus cavity, not only can the resultant excessive bone bleeding interfere with surgery, but the healing of the sinus is nonphysiologic. When the bony opening of an anterior sphenoidotomy is made, only the focal corresponding mucosa at the anterior sphenoidotomy site is opened to enter the sphenoid sinus. Minimal mucosa at the anterior wall of the sella is removed using electrocoagulation with the remaining mucosa of the sphenoid sinus preserved. When pituitary tumor removal is completed, the anterior wall of the sella is reconstructed by folding the flaps of thin sellar bone back in place. The sphenoid sinus is left intact without any packing, and these precautions allow physiologic healing of the open sphenoid sinus with normal mucosal lining.

Since the nasal cavity cannot truly be conventionally prepared with extensive antiseptic solutions, we prescribed postoperative oral antibiotic regimens empirically for 5 days in our early patients. Subsequently, postoperative antibiotic treatment has been completely abandoned without any evidence of increased infection. We still swab the nasal cavity with an antiseptic solution during surgical preparation, but even this practice may not be clearly necessary.

POSITIONING

The patient is positioned supine with the torso elevated about 15 to 20 degrees, and the head is positioned with the forehead-chin line set horizontally. The level of the head is placed a little higher than that of the heart with the intent that the cavernous sinus venous pressure stays low to minimize venous bleeding. The horizontally leveled head positioning allows the surgeon to access the region of the middle turbinate easily and naturally for EE-TS when the endoscope is inserted at approximately 25 degrees cephalad.[11] When the anterior cranial fossa is to be explored as in EE-ACF, the head is extended approximately 15 degrees.[19] Conversely, the head is flexed by 15 degrees when the clival or posterior fossa region is to be explored in EE-PFossa.[22] The head is rotated toward the surgeon at 10 to 20 degrees. A head pin fixation device can optionally be used but is not necessary. The hip and knee joints are gently flexed for patient comfort, and a soft pillow is placed underneath the knee joints. A Foley catheter is not routinely used but is inserted occasionally in selective patients who are expected to undergo longer operating hours or for the possible anticipated occurrence of diabetes insipidus. Fluoroscopic C-arm imaging is not used except in patients with anterior fossa or posterior fossa tumors or in patients with complex sinonasal anatomy. Ophthalmic eye ointment is placed on the cornea and conjunctiva, and the eyelids are taped closed with double-layers of soft vinyl adhesives to prevent corneal abrasions and infiltration by prep solutions. The oropharynx is packed with a 2-inch gauze roll to prevent the accumulation of blood at the perilaryngeal area during surgery, which may cause aspiration at the time of extubation.

The video monitor is placed a few feet away from the patient's head to face the surgeon directly. The lens-cleansing motor is placed next to the video monitor, and the scrub nurse is positioned adjacent to the surgeon. The entire face, nasal cavity, and abdominal wall are prepared and draped in an aseptic manner. When fat graft material is required to fill the tumor resection cavity, an appropriate amount of the abdominal fat tissue is obtained through a 1- to 2-cm infraumbilical transverse skin incision. Clindamycin is mixed with the endoscope's irrigation fluid. For the intraoperative antibiotic regimen, 2 g cefazolin is given intravenously in the operating suite before the start of the operation.

SURGICAL APPROACHES

An endoscopic endonasal approach to the sella can be made by a paraseptal, middle meatal, or middle turbinectomy approach.[10,19] The paraseptal approach is the least invasive and basic workhorse among these three approaches, and the surgical technique described here for EE-TS involves the paraseptal approach. The paraseptal approach is made between the nasal septum and the middle turbinate with temporary displacement of the middle turbinate laterally and contralateral displacement of the posterior nasal septum by fracturing at the sphenoid rostrum. The fractured nasal septum is pushed away by submucosal dissection at the contralateral side of the sphenoid rostrum.

For endoscopic endonasal access to the anterior cranial fossa (EE-ACF), the paraseptal approach can be used

between the nasal septum and middle turbinate with trajectory confirmed using fluoroscopic C-arm guidance or image-guidance systems. The middle meatal approach involves trajectory lateral to the middle turbinate and provides access to the ipsilateral anterior cranial fossa by an anterior ethmoidectomy or direct access to the anterior aspect of the cavernous sinus and optic nerve by a posterior ethmoidectomy. When a larger operating space is required, the middle turbinectomy approach can be used by resection of the middle turbinate. Although a wider corridor is provided to the sella, lack of the middle turbinate structure can be problematic when a supportive structure is required for skull base reconstruction.

SURGICAL TECHNIQUE OF ENDOSCOPIC ENDONASAL TRANS-SPHENOIDAL SURGERY

Positioning is done as previously mentioned with the patient's head resting such that the forehead and chin make a straight line parallel to the floor. The head may also be turned and angled slightly such that endonasal access is in a comfortable positioning for the operating surgeon who stands on one side of the patient during surgery. Optionally, approximately 15-degree bends can also be made at the level of the waist and knees to allow a comfortable degree of flexion at the hip and knee joints. The ipsilateral arm on the side of the operating surgeon is tucked, and the contralateral arm may be on an armboard. The nasal cavities, face, and a small region on the abdomen in case a fat graft is needed (usually the infraumbilical area is used for cosmesis) are prepped and draped in an aseptic manner. Double-layer eye protection is used to shield from prep solution, with the nose left exposed in a triangular fashion. Multiple long-handled disposable cotton swabs (routinely a total of 10 with 5 per side) are used to prepare the nasal passages.

The base of the endoscope holder is attached to the head of the bed, then there are two holder arms that are attached at appropriate angles (such that the attachment is in parallel with the course expected through the nasal passage) before the distal portion of the holder is attached that directly affixes the endoscope. The patient's head should be close to the top of the operating table but not so close that the endoscope holder runs into the head. As the nasal cavity is being prepared with the cotton swabs, the size of the nasal airway can be assessed to determine which nostril is to be used. The nasal septum is usually somewhat deviated to one side, and thus the nostril with the wider nasal airway can usually be selected for the surgical approach. The size of the nasal airway is also anticipated in advance by reviewing the axial view that includes the nasal cavity on preoperative MRI. When both nasal cavities are comparable in size, the nostril contralateral to the lesion is used in patients with microadenomas that are located laterally. Since the endonasal approach is a few degrees off from the midline, it is relatively easy to visualize the contralateral side of the sella and the cavernous sinus in the standard paraseptal approach.

The endoscopic endonasal trans-sphenoidal (EE-TS) procedure can now be thought of as four basic steps: manual endoscope navigation to the sphenoid sinus, opening of sphenoid and sella, tumor removal, and closure. As an overview, the initial step of endonasal navigation to the rostrum of the sphenoid sinus uses the pathway between the nasal septum medially and the middle turbinate laterally while steering the endoscope with one hand and using a suction in the other hand to help lead the endoscope under direct visualization (Fig. 22-6A). Once the target site of the sphenoid sinus rostrum is exposed, the endoscope can be placed in its holder and the drill is used in one hand with the suction in the other to make the anterior sphenoidotomy and to access the sellar target (Fig. 22-6B). When the anterior sphenoidotomy is complete, the endoscope can be adjusted to an optimal surgical position in the endoscope holder for sellar entry and tumor removal. Finally, after tumor removal, the sellar bone is replaced and the middle turbinate pushed back into position during closure of the operation.

The first part of EE-TS is done with the endoscope usually in the nondominant hand used to directly visualize a 7-French suction in the dominant hand that leads the endoscope into the nasal cavity. The inferior turbinate is often initially visualized, and then the inferior margin of the middle turbinate is followed to the posterior nasal cavity where the ipsilateral choana with the nasopharynx transition is located. Through the choana, the vertically-oriented ridges and valleys of the pharyngeal tonsils can be seen along with the auditory tube opening laterally. The endoscope and suction are backed out after confirming this relation between the middle turbinate and the choana, then the space between the middle turbinate and nasal septum is followed posteriorly to the sphenoid target.

When the endoscope is held in the hand, the palm and last three digits are generally used to stabilize the endoscope shaft, and the index finger and thumb are used to steer the video camera to maintain anatomic orientation of the video image. This endoscope grip will naturally keep the endoscope at a 25-degree incline and allows for continuous steering of the video camera for maintaining correct orientation of the video image. When the patient's head is positioned horizontally with the forehead-chin line parallel to the floor, the middle turbinate is easily visualized at the tip of the endoscope when it is inserted into the nasal cavity. If the space between the nasal septum and middle turbinate is limited, several half- by three-inch cotton patties are inserted between the septum and middle turbinate to gently widen the space with minimal trauma (Fig. 22-7A and B). The cotton patties are pushed down to the rostrum of the sphenoid sinus. Care must be taken not to traumatize the mucosa in the nasal cavity while surgical instruments are being inserted and removed. The degree of surgical trauma to the nasal mucosa is a crucial factor in determining the amount of postoperative nasal bleeding. When a sharp-edged surgical instrument is inserted, the instrument tip must be guided by direct endoscopic visualization. The insertion of the surgical instrument should ideally be impelled by the gravity of the surgical instrument itself rather than surgeon's mechanical push. If cotton patties are required to develop the middle turbinate-septal space, the cotton patties are removed after a

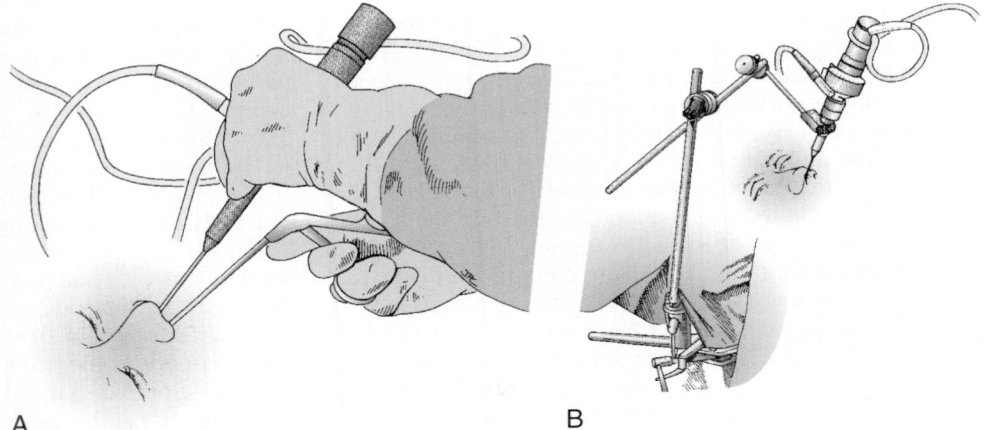

FIGURE 22-6 Schematic drawing shows manual endoscopic navigation into the nasal cavity with one hand holding the endoscope and the other hand, a suction cannula or other surgical instrument (A). When bimanual surgical maneuvering is required, the endoscope is anchored to the endoscope holder (B).

A   B

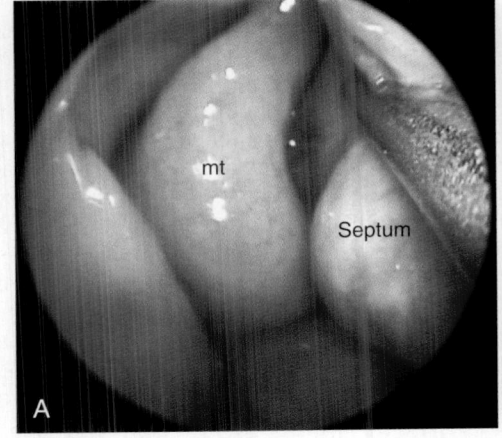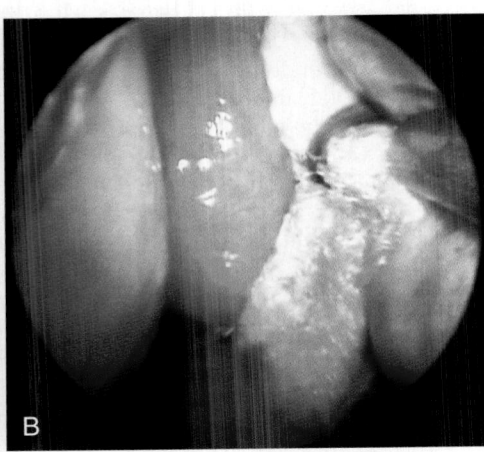

FIGURE 22-7 Under the 0-degree endoscope, the right-sided middle turbinate is exposed at the center of the surgical field (A). When the space between the nasal septum and middle turbinate (mt) is limited, several 0.5-by-3-inch cotton patties are inserted between the middle turbinate and the nasal septum anterior to the rostrum of the sphenoid sinus (B).

mt

Septum

A   B

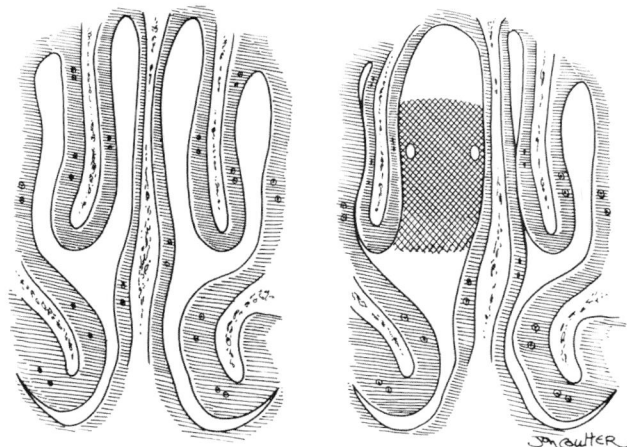

FIGURE 22-8 Schematic drawings demonstrate the target area for the anterior sphenoidotomy. The inferior margin of the middle turbinate follows a trajectory leading posteriorly to an area approximately 1 cm inferior to the sellar floor, useful as a consistent surgical landmark.

few minutes and the developed space will remain, although there may be some mild mucosal bleeding. Mucosal bleeding from the rostrum of the sphenoid sinus in the middle turbinate-septal space is controlled with electrocoagulation using the malleable monopolar suction coagulator. The mucosa at the rostrum of the sphenoid sinus is visualized with the manual-driven endoscope and completely coagulated before being divided vertically approximately 1.5 cm in length rostrally from the level of the inferior margin of the middle turbinate. The posterior septal artery arises from the sphenopalatine artery and passes at the inferolateral corner of the sphenoethmoidal recess, which is approximately the posteromedial corner of the inferior margin of the middle turbinate. The posterior septal artery must often be coagulated and divided to prevent intraoperative and postoperative nasal bleeding. The site for an anterior sphenoidotomy is again confirmed with reference to the surgical landmarks, which are the inferior margin of the middle turbinate and the choana of the nasopharynx (Fig. 22-8).

The second part of EE-TS involves use of the customized endoscope holder, which is an L-shaped connection from the operating table that connects to a reverse L-shaped segment running parallel to the trajectory of the endonasal pathway and a distal clamp that holds the endoscope itself. The endoscope is placed back into the nasal cavity following the same originally established trajectory along the endoscope holder with the coagulated sphenoid rostrum target reidentified at the sphenoid sinus and vomer interface. The endoscope is fixed in the endoscope holder, and a 4 mm diamond drill bit is used to drill the posterior nasal septum at the vomer and sphenoid rostrum to allow displacement towards the contralateral side. The floor of the sphenoid sinus is drilled along with only the underlying focal portion of mucosa (with the remaining sphenoid sinus mucosa left intact). The floor of the sella turcica presents as a bulge or mound with the prominences of the carotid arteries and cavernous sinuses bilaterally visualized and correlated with any anticipated anatomic variations from the preoperative MRI. The prominences of the optic nerves, the opticocarotid recess (OCR), and the tuberculum sella are often anterior to the pituitary target location and may not necessarily need to be exposed. The malleable coated suction monopolar is turned down to a setting of 10V (from 25V used for mucosal coagulation at the outer face of the sphenoid sinus during the first part of EE-TS) and the bipolar is routinely set at 35V (with adjustment as needed for any intradural use). The anterior sphenoidotomy to be made ranges from the inferior margin of the middle turbinate to the sphenoid sinus ostia, which is typically about 1 to 1.5 cm rostral from the inferior margin of the middle turbinate. However, the plane of the inferior margin of the middle turbinate is the consistent anatomic landmark. Although the sphenoid sinus ostia may be visualized directly (Fig. 22-9A), its identification is not necessary for performing an anterior sphenoidotomy. When the sphenoid sinus is entered near the level of the inferior margin of the middle turbinate, any further rostral exposure can be easily made relative to the exposed sellar floor. When an anterior sphenoidotomy is first attempted rostrally, the surgeon may erroneously enter the anterior cranial fossa because the superior turbinate can sometimes mimic the

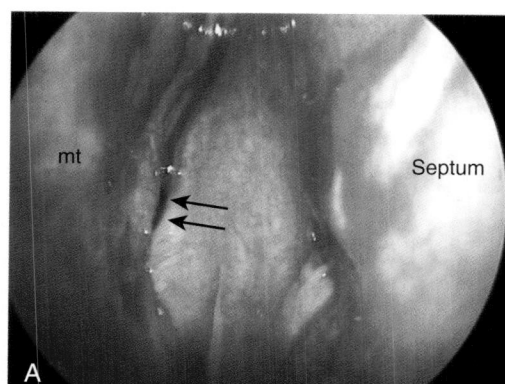
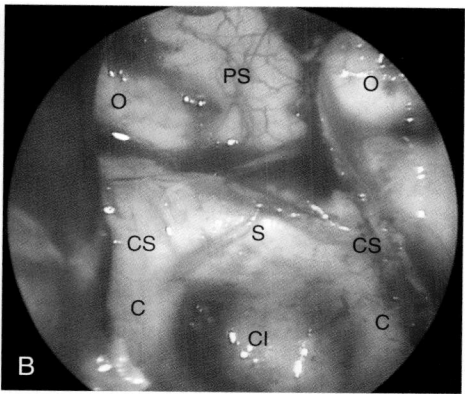

FIGURE 22-9 Cotton patties can be placed to create gentle expansion of the space between the middle turbinate and nasal septum, with the rostrum of the sphenoid sinus visualized upon removal of the patties. When mucosal bleeding is encountered, selective electrocoagulation is performed with monopolar suction cannula at the focal bleeding points. Sometimes the sphenoid ostium may be visible (double arrows), but can be a variable landmark (A). An anterior sphenoidotomy measuring approximately 1.5 to 2 cm in diameter is made using a high-speed drill or Kerrison and ethmoidal rongeurs. When the endoscope is advanced into the sphenoid sinus, a panoramic view (B) demonstrates the clival indentation (CI), internal carotid arteries (C), sella (S), cavernous sinuses (CS), planum sphenoidale (PS), and optic protuberances (O).

middle turbinate. Therefore, the middle turbinate must be confirmed in reference to the choana of the nasopharynx. The inferior margin of the middle turbinate is located just rostral to roof of the choana at the nasopharynx in a sagittal plane. Following the inferior margin of the middle turbinate posteriorly then leads to the clival indentation at approximately 1 cm inferior to the level of the sellar floor.

Anterior sphenoidotomy can be made with either of two different surgical techniques: power-drilling or rongeuring with fracture. In the first technique, use of a power-drill creates a clean opening at the anterior wall of the sphenoid sinus. The endoscope is placed on the endoscope holder, and the power-drill is inserted along with a suction cannula next to the endoscope shaft. The vomer is drilled first, and then the nasal septum is pushed to the contralateral side when it loosens. At the contralateral rostrum of the sphenoid sinus, submucosal dissection is carried-out to expose the bilateral rostrum of the sphenoid sinus. Then the exposure at the rostrum of the sphenoid sinus is very much similar to the exposure through a conventional trans-septal approach. Drilling is performed along the lateral gutter at the anterior wall of the sphenoid sinus, and the sphenoidal mucosa is exposed bilaterally. Using Kurze scissors, an opening is made at the sphenoid sinus mucosa. Then the posterior wall of the sphenoid sinus can be directly visualized demonstrating the tuberculum sella, clivus, cavernous sinus, and optic system. The second technique involves rongeuring after mechanical fracture of the nasal septum and vomer from the rostrum of the sphenoid sinuses using the septal breaker, which is a special instrument designed for this endoscopic operation. The rostral nasal septum is relatively easy to break; however, the caudally located vomer is often too thick to break without using the specially made septal breaker. The fractured nasal septum is pushed contralaterally, and the contralateral rostrum of the sphenoid sinus is dissected submucosally. The anterior aspect of the sphenoid rostrum is exposed bilaterally. With Kerrison rongeurs, the anterior wall of the sphenoid sinus is first opened along the lateral gutter. Then the bony opening of an anterior sphenoidotomy is completed using Kerrison rongeurs. The sinus mucosa is opened in the same manner as previously mentioned. Attention is paid not to strip the sphenoid sinus mucosa since inadvertent stripping can cause unwanted oozing of blood from the bony sinus wall. The anterior wall of the sphenoid sinus is removed performing an anterior sphenoidotomy about 1 to 1.5 cm in size. The sphenoid sinus septum is trimmed with a power-drill or rongeurs. Further rostral extension of the anterior sphenoidotomy is performed accordingly relative to the sella. Often the sella is exposed from the tuberculum sella to the clival indentation in the vertical dimension and from one cavernous sinus to the other cavernous sinus in the transverse dimension. At this point, endoscopic view demonstrates the tuberculum sella rostrally, optic protuberances at 11- and 1-o'clock positions, the bony wall covering the cavernous sinus and carotid artery laterally, clival indentation caudally, and the internal carotid arteries at 7- and 5-o'clock locations (Fig. 22-9B). The endoscope is adjusted in the endoscope holder as the endoscope tip is advanced for a close-up view of the sella.

Using a bipolar suction coagulator, the sphenoidal mucosa at the anterior wall of the sella is coagulated and removed. The suction is used to nudge the sellar floor and discern the thickness of the sellar bone via tactile feedback. A small entry hole is made at the inferolateral corner of the anterior bony wall of the sella by using either the drill for thick sella or a 1-mm Kerrison rongeur to gently punch through thin sella. The anterior bony wall of the sella is then removed with a 1-mm Kerrison punch circumferentially, from one cavernous sinus to the other cavernous sinus, and from the sellar floor to the tuberculum sella. When the sellar bone has adequate thickness, the anterior bone wall can be opened like a door with the hinge attached at the sellar floor or tuberculum sella. The sellar bone may be opened in an H-shaped flap with superior and inferior halves or as a single inverted-U flap. At the end of operation, the bony door can simply be closed for sellar reconstruction. The dura mater is coagulated along the periphery circumferentially with a single-bladed bipolar coagulator. The dural opening is made along the inferior margin at the floor of the sella using a Jannetta 45-degree microdissector. The anterior dural wall is incised and removed circumferentially for biopsy. Alternative option is an X- or cross-shaped incision of the dura mater.

The third part of EE-TS involves tumor removal with the identification of tumor tissue versus normal pituitary, and ring curettes are used to remove tumor along with pituitary forceps used to send specimens for frozen pathology sections as needed. Once all of the tumor tissue is removed, a very thin rim of normal pituitary gland is removed for margin. Tumor tissue is often soft and white, in contrast to firm orange-yellow anterior pituitary gland and firm white posterior pituitary gland. For larger pituitary tumors, classically the posterior portion of the tumor is removed first, followed by both lateral borders, and then the anterior portion of the tumor is allowed to fall down into the center of the field by gravity assistance if amenable. Otherwise ring curettes can simply be used to remove tumor tissue appropriate for the individual tumor configuration as needed.

In the case of a microadenoma covered by normal pituitary tissue, the pituitary tissue is sliced or split with a Jannetta 45-degree microdissector to locate the tumor tissue. The identified tumor tissue is removed by curettage; a thin layer of the normal pituitary tissue is then shaved-off at the margin of the resection site, especially to optimize the chance of endocrine cure for functional microadenomas. For macroadenomas, the tumor tissue often spills out when the dura mater is opened. Care has to be taken not to lose the tumor specimen by suctioning since the tumor tissue should be sampled for pathologic examination. Once enough of the tumor specimen is collected, the tumor is removed with a suction cannula at the central portion of the sella for debulking. A pituitary ring curette in one hand with suction in the other hand or dual suction cannulas (No. 5 or 7 French) can be used for soft tumor removal. When the tumor is fibrotic, either from previous medical and surgical treatments or by its intrinsic nature, the tumor tissue is gently curetted with a pituitary ring curette held in one hand, in addition to being suctioned with a suction cannula held in the other hand. When the tumor resection cavity is created at the central portion of the pituitary fossa, a 45-degree angled curette is first used followed by a 90-degree angled curette to remove the lower portion of the tumor from the floor of the sella. An inferiorly angled pituitary ring curette is used in one hand and an inferiorly curved suction cannula in the other hand for removal of the lower portion of the tumor. The dura mater at the floor of the sella is exposed directly when the lower portion of the tumor is removed. Next the lateral portion of the tumor is removed with a superiorly angled suction cannula and a superiorly angled pituitary ring curette, 45-degrees as well as 90-degrees. The medial wall of the cavernous sinus is directly exposed when the lateral portion of the tumor is removed. The rostral portion of the tumor is removed circumferentially with various superiorly curved and angled suction cannulas and pituitary ring curettes. When normal pituitary gland tissue is identified, it is preserved as much as possible. When the diaphragm sella is identified along the peripheral edge of the rostral portion of the tumor, the tumor is continuously removed circumferentially. When the tumor is removed along the edge of the diaphragma sella, the suprasellar portion of the tumor progressively descends through the central opening of the diaphragma sella. The suprasellar portion of the tumor that progressively descends is continuously removed with either two superiorly curved suction cannulas or a suction cannula and a pituitary ring curette, both angled superiorly.

Thinned pituitary tissue is often identifiable rostrally when the suprasellar portion of the tumor has been removed. When the pituitary tissue is severely stretched-out, the rostrally located pituitary tissue appears to be a transparent membrane similar to the arachnoid membrane. When this rostral tissue is penetrated, the arachnoid membrane may rupture, resulting in a cerebrospinal fluid (CSF) leak. Sometimes the arachnoid membrane bulges down along the anterior edge of the diaphragma sella in front of the thinned pituitary tissue. The last piece of the pituitary tumor is often located at the insertion point of the pituitary stalk. When this last piece of the tumor is removed at the reversed dimple of the pituitary stalk, the transparent and thinned pituitary tissue descends down, looking much like a lily with a dimple at the center. It continuously bulges downward with pulsation towards the floor of the sella. When the tumor resection cavity in the sella is large and the remaining tissue is very thin, the tumor resection cavity may have to be filled and supported with an abdominal fat graft in order to prevent postoperative CSF leak due to delayed rupture of this thin membrane. Delayed CSF leak can occur from unintentional Valsalva maneuvers produced by repeated coughs, bearing-down during extubation, or at anytime postoperatively.

When the tumor is so solid and fibrotic that the suprasellar portion of the tumor does not descend spontaneously, the suprasellar portion can be exposed directly using a 30-degree lens endoscope or by further removal of the bone at the planum sphenoidale or tuberculum sella. When the arachnoid membrane is ruptured, the optic nerves and chiasm, anterior cerebral artery system, and inferior aspect of the hypothalamus are under direct view with a 30-degree lens endoscope. When CSF leakage does not occur intraoperatively and the tumor is a microadenoma, an abdominal fat graft is unnecessary. After removal of a large macroadenoma, the tumor resection cavity is supported with an abdominal fat graft (Fig. 22-10A to F). Occasionally a piece of Gelfoam sponge is used instead of an abdominal fat graft when a sufficient amount of the pituitary tissue still remains

rostrally. An abdominal fat graft is harvested using a 1- to 2-cm transverse skin incision just inferior to the umbilicus. The anterior wall of the sella is reconstructed using autogenous bone saved at the time of the anterior sphenoidotomy (Fig. 22-11A). When autogenous bone is not available, a piece of thin titanium mesh is placed (Fig. 22-11B). No foreign material is placed in the sphenoid sinus or nasal cavity.

So the fourth and final part of EE-TS consists of closure and cleanup. The reconstruction of the sella in routine EE-TS involves replacement of the sellar bone flaps as previously mentioned. The endoscope is removed from the holder to be manipulated by hand again, the nasopharynx and nasal cavity are inspected and cleaned, and any stagnant blood is removed with a suction cannula. The middle turbinate is placed back to its normal position using a Cottle dissector-elevator. If a fat graft was used, the abdominal incision is closed in subcuticular fashion and covered with a small bandage to complete the operation.

ENDOSCOPIC ENDONASAL APPROACH TO THE ANTERIOR CRANIAL FOSSA

For meningiomas located in the olfactory groove, planum sphenoidale, or tuberculum sella and for repair of CSF leakage at the anterior cranial fossa, the endoscopic endonasal approach to the anterior cranial fossa skull base (EE-ACF) has been employed (Fig. 22-12A).[16,17,19] This approach is also useful for suprasellar craniopharyngiomas or large suprasellar pituitary tumors with fibrotic solid consistency. For tumor removal, a paraseptal approach is used (Fig. 22-12B). For CSF leak repair, either a paraseptal or a middle meatal approach can be used. Fluoroscopic C-arm imaging or frameless stereotactic image-guidance system can be used for optimizing the trajectory to the target lesion during EE-ACF.

The head is positioned in 15-degree extension of the forehead-chin line to maintain the endoscope insertion angle at about 25 degrees, which is naturally comfortable for the surgeon and follows the basic endonasal pathway. Otherwise the patient is prepared in the same manner as described earlier for EE-TS pituitary surgery. For the middle meatal approach, the middle turbinate is pushed medially and an ethmoidectomy is performed to reach the anterior skull base. Any CSF leak is often directly visible. The mucosa is dissected around the skull base defect, and an abdominal fat graft is inserted into the cranial cavity. After the entire fat graft is inserted into the cranial cavity, a portion of the fat is grabbed and pulled gently to wedge it into the skull defect in a dumbbell-shaped or snowman-shaped configuration. A piece of thin titanium mesh is then placed at the skull defect. The middle turbinate is placed back gently in its normal position.

For EE-ACF tumor surgery, a paraseptal approach is often used. For tumors located at the olfactory groove, planum sphenoidale, or tuberculum sella, the surgical approach is similar to the aforementioned EE-TS pituitary operation except that further rostral exposure is required. The middle turbinate is laterally displaced, and the nasal septum is fractured contralaterally. A rostral anterior sphenoidotomy is performed to enter the sphenoid sinuses, and then the sella and tuberculum sella are identified. Under fluoroscopic guidance, further rostral exposure is made at the anterior skull base removing the posterior ethmoid sinuses. This approach itself interrupts anterior or posterior ethmoidal

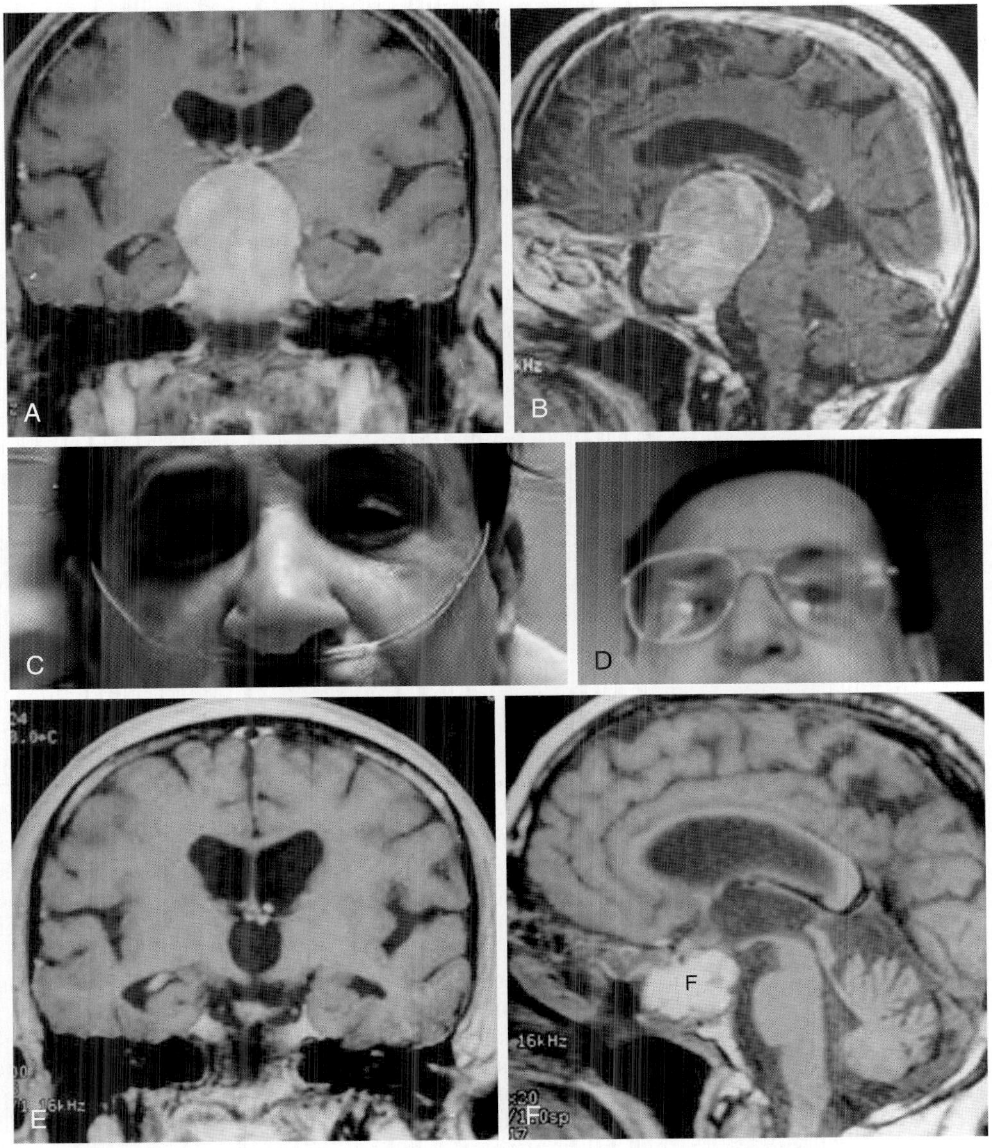

FIGURE 22-10 A 53-year-old man presented with visual deficits and panhypopituitarism associated with a large nonfunctioning pituitary adenoma demonstrated on T1-weighted MRI with contrast, coronal and sagittal views (A, B). Postoperative photos of the patient at the recovery room (C) and following morning just before his discharge from the hospital (D) reflect his uncomplicated recovery from EE-TS surgery. Postoperative T1-weighted MRI with contrast, coronal and sagittal views (E, F), demonstrate total tumor removal with fat graft (F) at the sella.

FIGURE 22-11 A small piece of abdominal fat graft is placed at the tumor resection cavity when the void is relatively large or cerebrospinal fluid leakage is encountered intraoperatively. The anterior wall of the sella is reconstructed with autogenous bone (A) or titanium mesh (B).

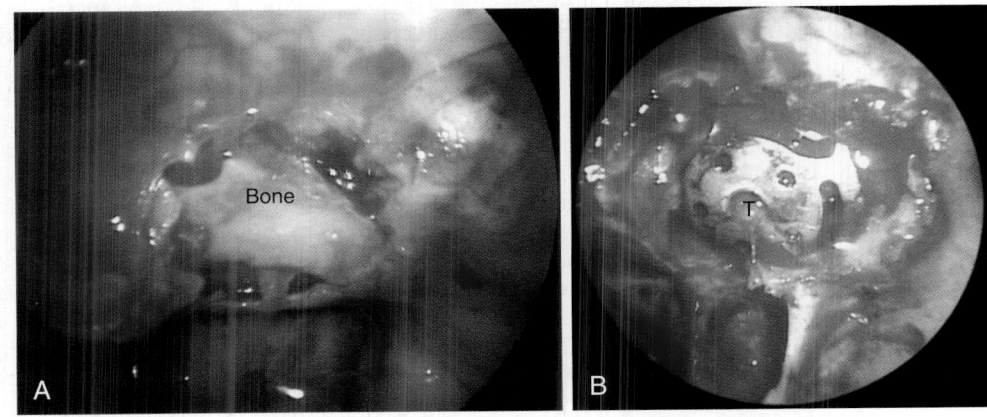

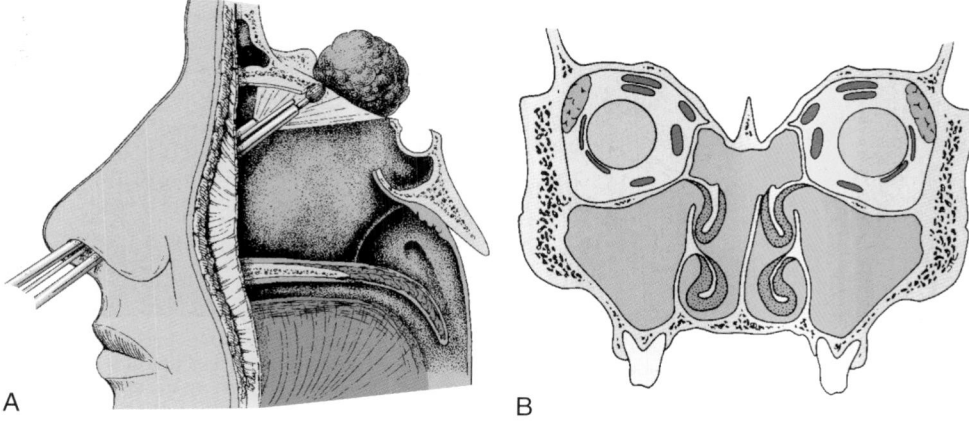

FIGURE 22-12 Schematic drawing (A) demonstrates an endoscopic approach to the anterior skull base. The paraseptal approach is the routine technique, although this can be extended to a middle turbinectomy approach to provide wider surgical space in selected cases as necessary (B).

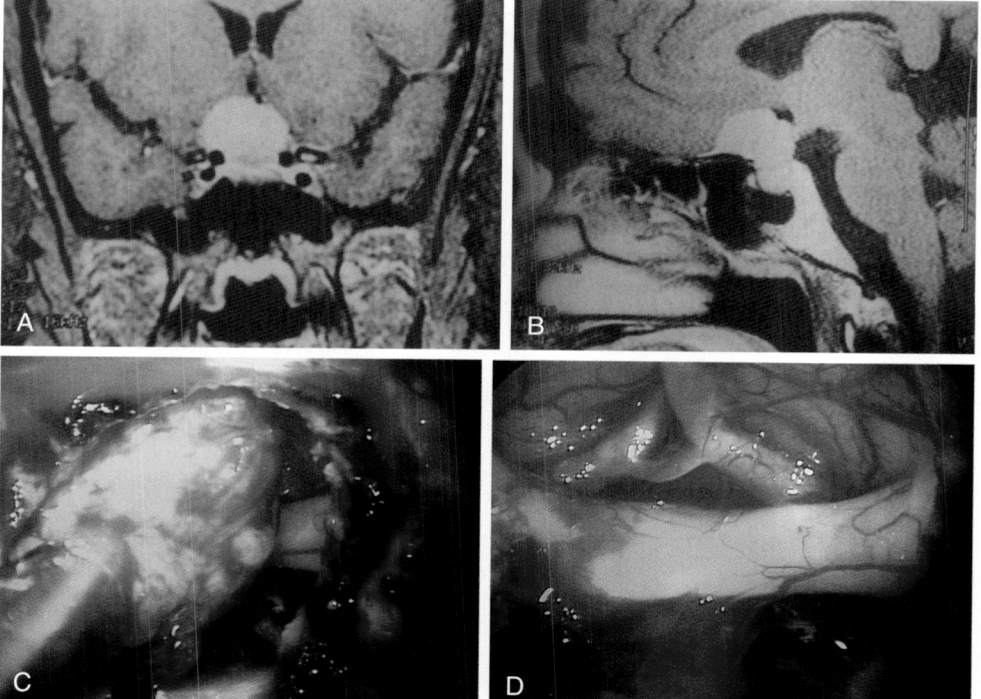

FIGURE 22-13 T1-weighted MRI with contrast, coronal and sagittal views (A, B), shows an anterior cranial fossa meningioma involving the planum sphenoidale and tuberculum sella in a 34-year-old woman. Intraoperative endoscopic photos demonstrate the meningioma, which was dissected and gently rotated towards the patient's right side in order to visualize the posterior anatomy, with the left optic nerve revealed (C). The anterior cerebral arterial complex, optic system, and pituitary stalk are displayed by view through a 0-degree-lens endoscope following tumor removal (D).

arteries during exposure, resulting in major devascularization of the meningioma. Approximately a 2-cm wide portion of the midline anterior skull base can be exposed with this technique. Bone of the skull base can be removed with a high-speed drill or Kerrison punch. The dura mater is opened, and the tumor is removed with central debulking followed by peripheral dissection. When the central portion of the tumor is excised, peripheral dissection is carried out to inspect the posterior aspect of the tumor. The remaining tumor is gradually flipped, and dissection along the posterior wall of the tumor is carried out until the remaining tumor is excised (Fig. 22-13A to D). Prudent selection of meningiomas should be considered for EE-ACF approaches versus transcranial approaches (whether minimally invasive endoscopic or open microscopic) because the inability to achieve at least a Simpson grade 2 resection due to inadequate exposure may result in suboptimal recurrence rates.

The main potential problem related to this surgery is postoperative CSF leak and subsequent meningitis. Therefore adequate skull base reconstruction is essential. When active CSF leak is noted at the time of surgery, a small piece of fat graft is inserted at the various corners intracranially in order to obstruct the active CSF inflow. Then a large dural graft is placed intradurally with enough margin overlapping, dural suture is performed with titanium clips, and another layer of dural graft is laid extradurally. There are other similar methods of dural graft reconstruction described such as composing the double-layer graft with a central suture prior to placement at the skull base defect or using alternative methods of dural suturing such as nitinol U-clips. The skull base defect reconstruction is then supported with autogenous bone graft or titanium mesh placement. Abdominal fat grafts are used at the ethmoidectomy site as additional support (Fig. 22-14A to C). When fat graft material is placed at the tumor resection cavity, care must be given not to cause

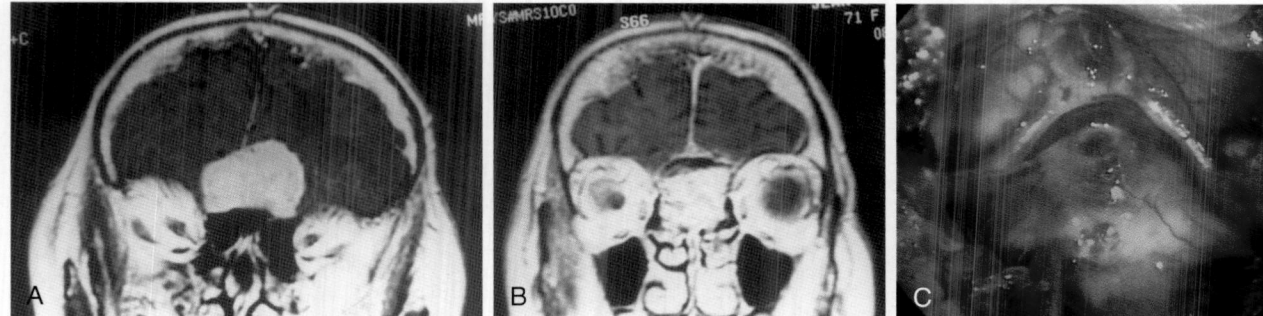

FIGURE 22-14 T1-weighted MRI with contrast, coronal views, preoperatively illustrates an olfactory groove meningioma (A), which was removed with an endoscopic endonasal approach, and postoperatively shows appearance of the skull base reconstruction (B). The skull defect is most commonly reconstructed with double-layered dural graft supported by titanium mesh, followed by abdominal fat graft placement at the ethmoidectomy area. Endoscopic view under a 0-degree-lens demonstrates the anterior cerebral arterial complex, lamina terminalis, and optic system (C).

unintended compression to the optic nerve system. Nasoseptal flaps have been reported but may not be routinely necessary depending on the skull base defect. The middle turbinate is placed back in its normal position to complete the operation.

ENDOSCOPIC ENDONASAL APPROACH TO THE OPTIC NERVE OR CAVERNOUS SINUS

Although surgical indication for decompression of the optic nerve is a controversial issue, the optic nerve at the optic canal can be easily exposed using this endoscopic endonasal approach.[13] The surgical approach to the cavernous sinus is similar to that of the optic nerve.[14,15,20,21] This endoscopic approach to the cavernous sinus is best suited for pituitary adenomas invading the cavernous sinus. Biopsy for the histologic diagnosis of cavernous sinus lesions can be performed with this technique. Tough fibrotic tumors in this region, such as some types of meningiomas, can be challenging to remove using endoscopic technique. The endoscopic endonasal cavernous sinus (EE-CS) procedure is an anteromedial approach, and the fact that cavernous cranial nerves are located towards the lateral wall of the cavernous sinus makes this approach advantageous.

Pituitary adenomas can involve the cavernous sinus by mechanical compression with lateral tumor bulging, by direct extension via dural infiltration, or by intrusion into the cavernous sinus through a defect of the medial wall of the cavernous sinus. A laterally bulged tumor can be removed by the pituitary approach described earlier and does not need any further particular maneuvering. The 30-degree lens endoscope discloses the medial wall of the cavernous sinus well when the lateral portion of the tumor is completely removed. Tumors that have intruded into the cavernous sinus by a defect of the medial wall can be removed completely under direct endoscopic visualization. The cavernous carotid artery is exposed during this procedure. Invasive pituitary adenomas of an infiltrating nature may not be completely resectable; however, they can be debulked to reduce the size of the tumor so that focused beam radiation treatment can be performed for the residual portion of the tumor postoperatively.

The optic nerves or cavernous sinuses can generally be approached through a paraseptal approach, with increasing exposure as needed by creating a middle meatal approach or even further exposure by using a middle turbinectomy

approach.[15] In the paraseptal approach, the endoscope visualizes the contralateral optic nerve or cavernous sinus better than it does the ipsilateral one, and this technique exposes the anteromedial aspect of the cavernous sinus (Fig. 22-15A). The anteromedial exposure of the optic nerve or cavernous sinus through the contralateral nostril using the paraseptal approach is similar to that of the previously described EE-TS for pituitary adenomas except that the trajectory is adjusted by entry through the contralateral nasal passage from the lesion. The middle meatal approach with a posterior ethmoidectomy provides a straight anterior approach to the cavernous sinus (Fig. 22-15B). The largest corridor to the optic nerve or cavernous sinus is provided by the middle turbinectomy approach, but overall the paraseptal approach is generally sufficient for approaching the optic nerve or cavernous sinus for the majority of lesions.

During the anterior sphenoidotomy, submucosal dissection at the contralateral side of the sphenoid rostrum is extended further laterally, and the anterior sphenoidotomy can be performed generously at the contralateral side of the sphenoid sinus. This exposes the contralateral cavernous sinus laterally up to the medial anterior temporal fossa. The bone is removed from the anterior aspect of the sella as well as from the cavernous sinus, and unroofing the internal carotid artery may be completed if necessary. The sellar portion of the pituitary tumor is removed first before attacking the portion of tumor in the cavernous sinus. For an isolated cavernous sinus tumor, the tumor is approached directly by opening the dura mater medial to the carotid siphon (Fig. 22-16A and B). The tumor is removed with various pituitary ring curettes and suction cannulas. Attention must be taken during tumor removal not to traumatize the lateral wall of the cavernous sinus since this can cause ocular cranial nerve dysfunction. The carotid artery pulsation is directly visible, and tumor resection is performed medially and posteriorly to the carotid siphon, which arcs in a C-shape for the patient's right carotid artery or a reverse C-shape for the left carotid artery with the convexity directed anterolaterally. When the tumor is completely removed, the lateral wall of the cavernous sinus can be completely visualized (Fig. 22-17A to C). The cavernous carotid artery is surrounded using an abdominal fat graft to protect the artery postoperatively. If necessary, the sphenoid sinus can additionally be filled with an abdominal fat graft for further protection of the exposed carotid artery. In

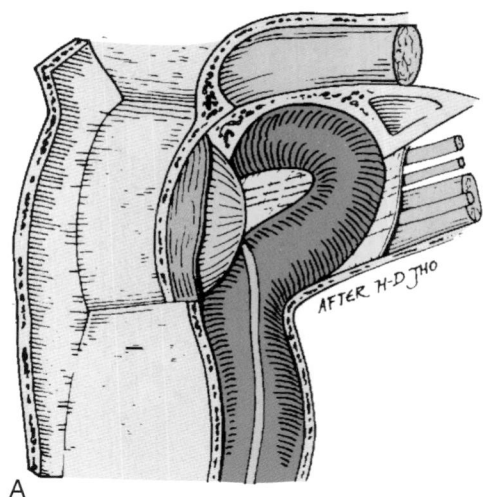
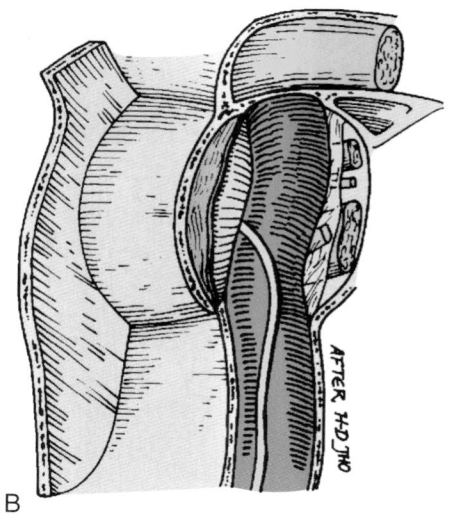

FIGURE 22-15 Schematic drawing indicates surgical exposure at the medial aspect of the cavernous sinus when surgical approach is made via a paraseptal approach through the contralateral nostril (A). However, when a middle meatal approach is made to the cavernous sinus through the ipsilateral nostril, a straight anterior view will be noted at the cavernous sinus with the possibility of access lateral to the cavernous carotid artery using an appropriate trajectory (B).

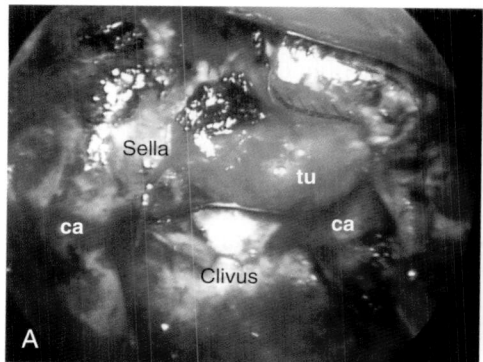
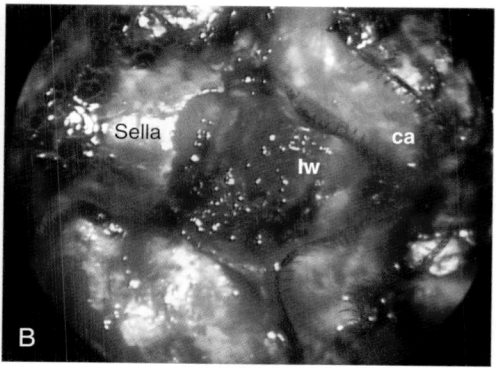

FIGURE 22-16 Endoscopic view under a 0-degree lens via the right-sided nostril discloses a pituitary adenoma (tu) at the left-sided cavernous sinus in a patient with acromegaly (A). After total tumor removal, the lateral wall (lw) of the cavernous sinus and carotid artery (ca) are exposed (B). The patient normalized IGF-1 levels postoperatively.

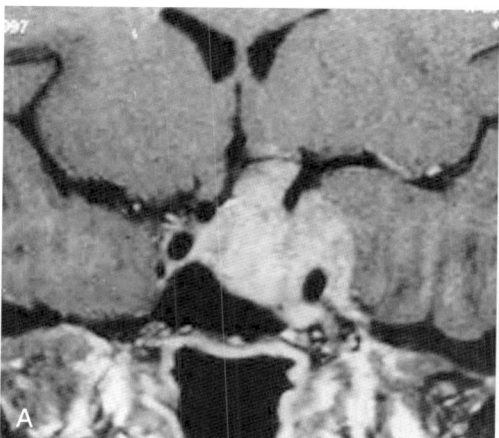
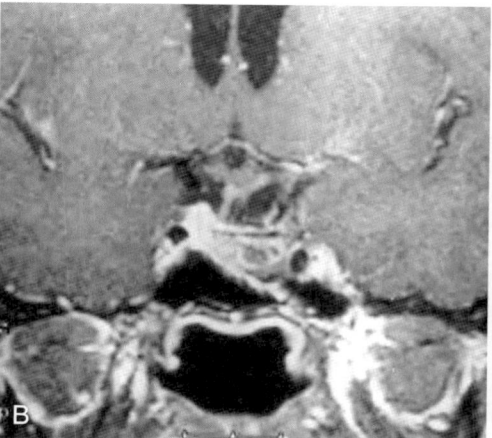
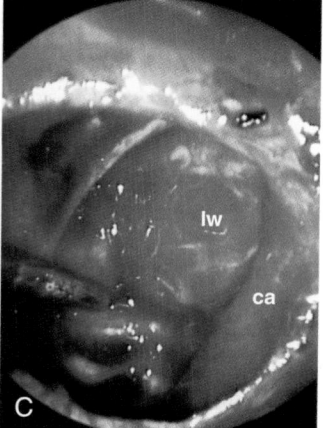

FIGURE 22-17 Preoperative T1-weighted MRI with contrast, coronal view, shows a recurrent nonfunctioning pituitary adenoma with extension to the left cavernous sinus (A). Postoperative T1-weighted MRI with contrast, coronal view, demonstrates total tumor removal via EE-TS (B). Intraoperative photo demonstrates a 30-degree-lens endoscopic view at the lateral wall of the left-sided cavernous sinus after total tumor removal (C). CA, carotid artery; LW, lateral wall of the cavernous sinus.

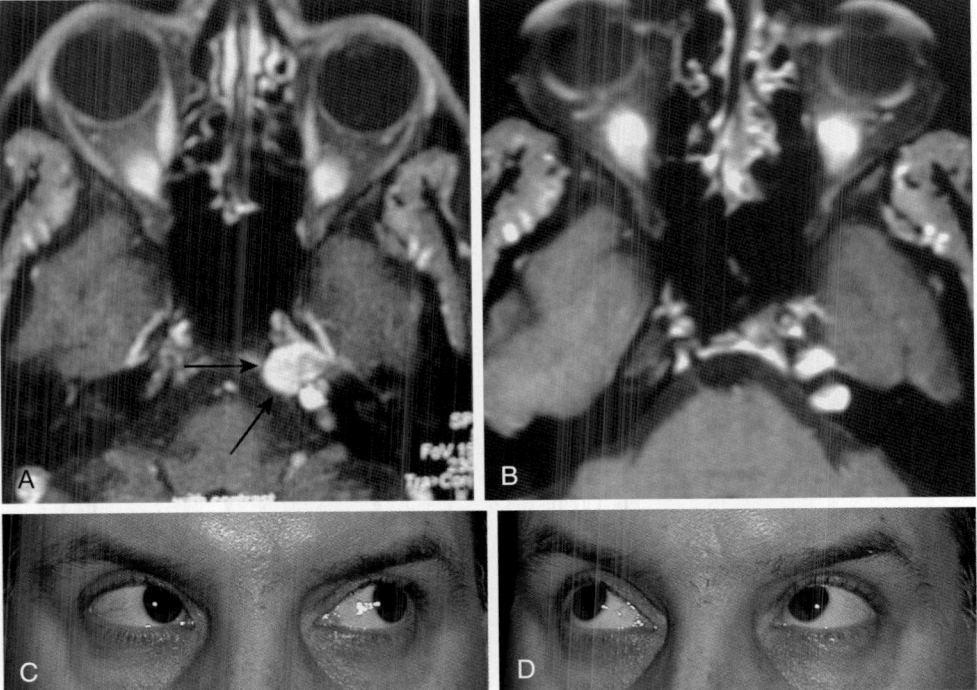

FIGURE 22-18 T1-weighted MRI with contrast, axial view, reveals a cholesterol granuloma at the left petrous tip in a 47-year-old man with 1-year history of left-sided partial sixth cranial nerve palsy (A). EE-Petrous approach was performed with drainage of the lesion, and T1-weighted MRI with contrast, axial view, demonstrates reduction of the cholesterol granuloma (B). Postoperative photographs demonstrate complete recovery of the left sixth cranial nerve palsy (C, D), and no recrudescence of the cholesterol granuloma has occurred in 7 years of follow-up.

contrast with pituitary surgery, the sphenoid sinus mucosa should be removed completely before the fat graft is placed in this case.

ENDOSCOPIC ENDONASAL APPROACH TO THE PTERYGOID FOSSA OR PETROUS APEX

Tumors involving the pterygoid fossa can be approached with a middle meatal or middle turbinectomy approach. The posteromedial wall of the maxillary sinus can be removed if necessary, and then the pterygoid fossa is fully exposed. The vidian nerve or sphenopalatine ganglion in the pterygoid fossa can also be approached with this technique. The petrous apex can be approached with a paraseptal approach. This endoscopic endonasal approach is particularly useful for drainage of cholesterol granulomas. Approach through the contralateral nostril gives a bit more lateral angulation in the trajectory to the petrous apex. When the sphenoid sinus is entered, the sellar floor and carotid artery protuberance provide anatomical orientation, and a stereotactic image-guidance device may assist with further anatomical orientation. The internal carotid artery is exposed at the medial margin, and the petrous apex is approached through the clivus inferior to the sellar floor and medial to the paraclival segment of the cavernous carotid. When the cholesterol granuloma is entered, xanthochromic fluid and material can be drained (Fig. 22-18A to D). Placement of fat graft material over the carotid artery for arterial protection is not necessary unless the aforementioned segment of the carotid artery is fully exposed by the exposure. Once the cholesterol granuloma is drained, the operation is complete.

ENDOSCOPIC ENDONASAL APPROACH TO THE CLIVUS OR POSTERIOR FOSSA

The advantage of the endoscopic technique in the endonasal surgical approach to the clivus and posterior fossa (EE-PFossa) is the flexibility and range of endoscopic visualization, which spans from the crista galli at the anterior cranial fossa to the foramen magnum at the posterior cranial fossa.[22,23] This endoscopic approach exposes the entire clivus from the floor of the sella to the foramen magnum at a midline width of approximately 2 cm (Fig. 22-19), with the internal carotid arteries serving as the lateral limits of this exposure. This technique has been used for the radical resection of clival chordomas and midline clival meningiomas. A paraseptal approach is most commonly used, but the middle turbinectomy approach can be used when a larger surgical corridor is required. Fluoroscopic C-arm imaging or frameless stereotactic system is used

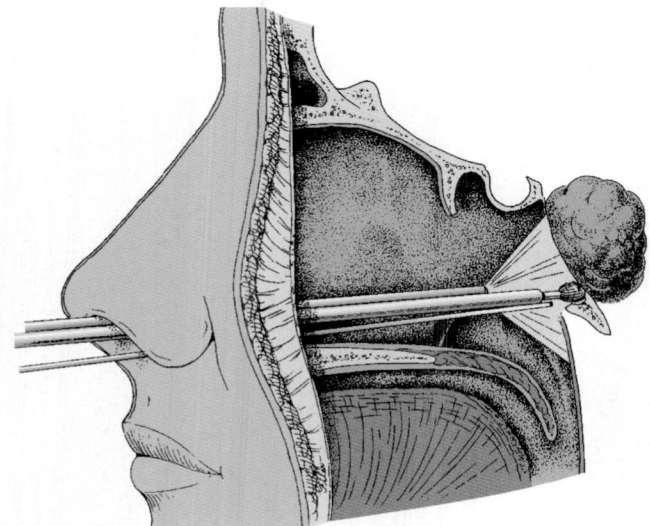

FIGURE 22-19 Schematic drawing demonstrates endoscopic approach to the clivus and craniocervical junction. Approximately a 2-cm midline window between the carotid arteries can be opened. Clival tumors or midline posterior fossa lesions can be approached with this technique.

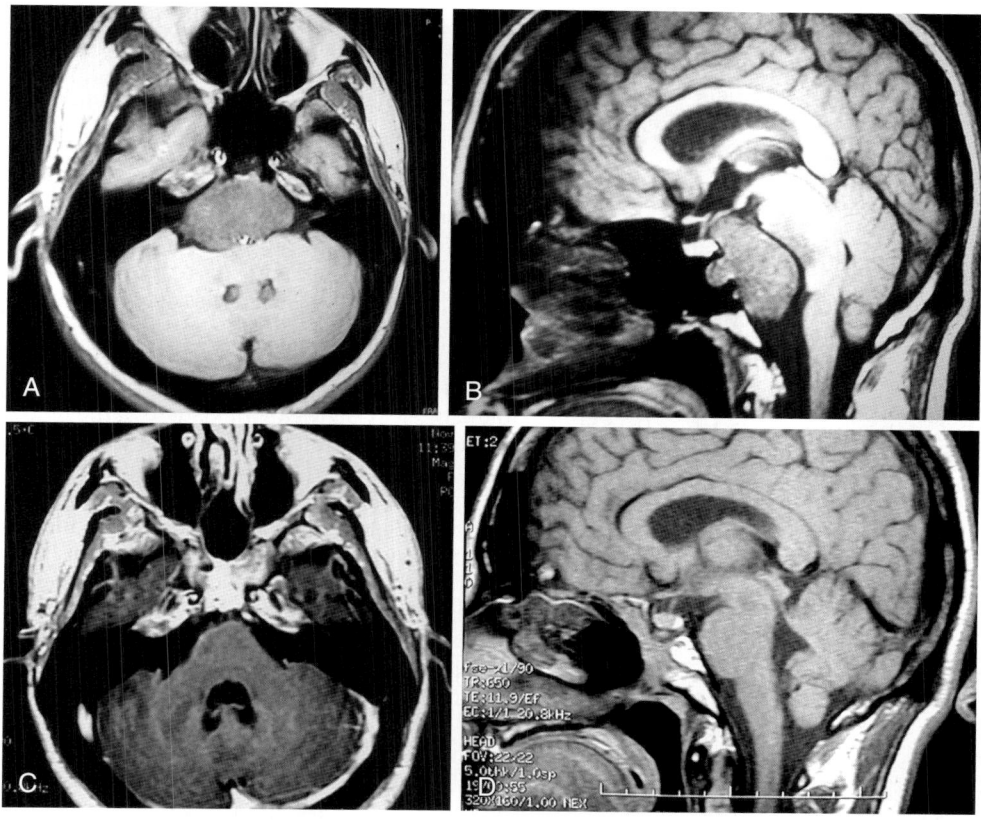

FIGURE 22-20 Preoperative T1-weighted MRI with contrast, axial and sagittal views, displays a large clival tumor with brainstem compression in a 28-year-old man with bilateral partial sixth cranial nerve palsies (A, B). Postoperative T1-weighted MRI with contrast, axial and sagittal views, shows total tumor removal of the clival chordoma by endoscopic endonasal approach (C, D).

for guidance to the vertical dimension. The clival bone is removed with a high-speed drill between the internal carotid arteries in the transverse dimension and from the floor of the sella to the foramen magnum or to the lower clival level as needed. The chordoma is then removed with suction cannulas and pituitary rongeurs. Bone is shaved at the tumor resection margin until normal bone is clearly documented. Intradural tumor is then resected, during which the pons and medulla can be visualized (Fig. 22-20A to D and Fig. 22-21A to C). A 30- or 70-degree lens endoscope visualizes the further rostral aspect of the brain stem or cranial nerves laterally (Fig. 22-22A and B). Dural defects are repaired with an abdominal fat graft, but once appropriate surgical instruments are fully developed, direct repair by a dural graft will be the ideal method for reconstruction. The dural titanium microclip applicator is currently available but is too short to be used effectively for this purpose.

ENDOSCOPIC ENDONASAL APPROACH TO THE CRANIOCERVICAL JUNCTION (EE-CC JUNCTION)

This endoscopic endonasal approach provides simple access to the craniocervical junction and the C1–C2 (atlanto-axial) area.[18] Pathologies such as chordoma, os odontoi-dum, basilar impression or invagination, rheumatoid basilar settling, or anterior lesions compressing the ventral aspect of the cervicomedullary junction can be approached with these techniques. Lateral fluoroscopic guidance or stereotactic image guidance can assist to access the surgical target. It can be done through one nostril or two nostrils. Under the endoscopic visualization, the nasopharyngeal mucosa and posterior pharyngeal muscles are incised at the midline

with electrocoagulation. The clivus at the ventral foramen magnum and the C1–C2 area can be exposed as indicated, and the clivus at the ventral foramen magnum, anterior rim of the C1, and odontoid can be drilled to the tectorial membrane. The dura mater can be exposed by incising the tectorial membrane. Lateral image using fluoroscopic guidance or frameless stereotactic image-guidance can help indicate the extent of surgical exposure. Additional posterior fusion surgery is necessary when stabilizing structures such as the C1 anterior arch and the transverse ligament are traversed to access the lesion. When the odontoid tip protrudes rostrally beyond the upper edge of C1 anterior arch, the protruding portion of the odontoid can sometimes be removed without removing the ventral C1 rim. In that case, C1–C2 stability can be preserved.

POSTOPERATIVE MANAGEMENT

Patients are kept in a regular hospital room overnight and are discharged home the next day if they do well. Postoperative discomfort is minimal and often does not require any strong analgesics. Postoperative nasal bleeding has also been very minimal since the techniques of meticulous hemostasis and eliminating intraoperative use of vasoconstrictors were adopted. Patients may note a few drops of bloody discharge for a day or two when they get up early in the morning or from a prolonged lying position. This minimal nasal drainage is usually accumulated bloody discharge at the sellar area in the sphenoid sinus during a recumbent position. Watery nasal discharge may indicate a postoperative CSF leakage, which is a potential complication that can delay hospital discharge. A few drops of fluid leakage are often benign, usually stopping in a day or so.

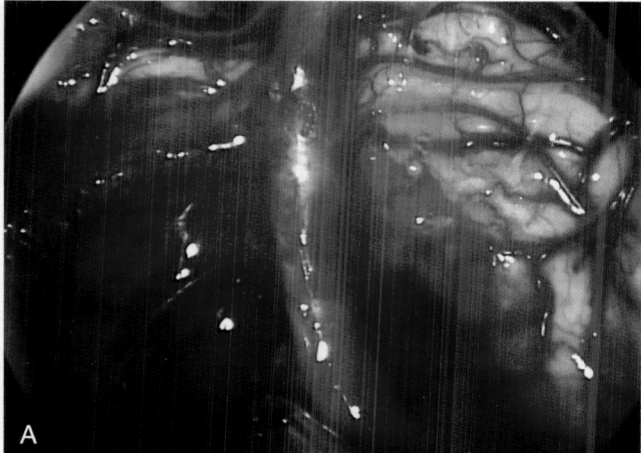

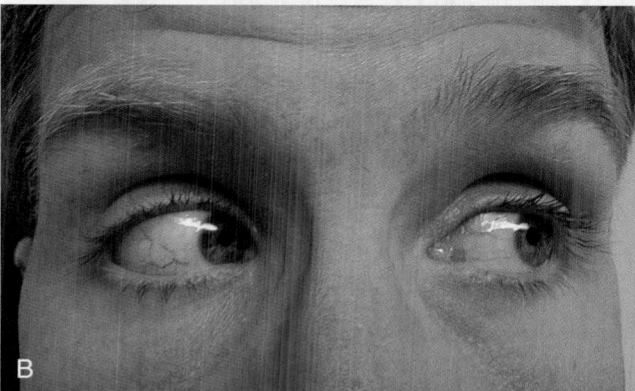

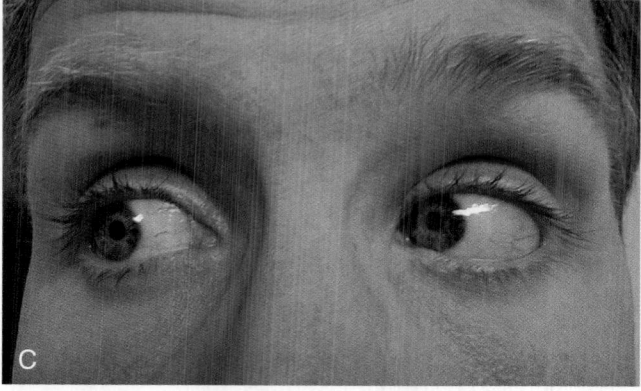

FIGURE 22-21 Intraoperative photo displays the appearance of the basilar artery and brain stem after removal of the clival chordoma shown on MRI in Fig. 22-20A. The 28-year-old male patient recovered bilateral sixth cranial nerve palsies completely within 1 year (B, C).

Although stress doses of corticosteroids were used intraoperatively and postoperatively in the earliest patients, routine intraoperative or postoperative corticosteroids are no longer used when the patient's preoperative hypothalamic-pituitary-adrenal (HPA) axis function is normal. Instead, a morning cortisol level is measured the day after surgery to confirm that it is higher than 15 μg/dl. If the morning cortisol level is less than 15 μg/dl, postoperative treatment is instituted with oral hydrocortisone, 20 mg every morning and 10 mg every night, until the HPA axis is proven to be normal. Target hormone levels for functioning adenomas are measured on the first postoperative day, such as prolactin

for prolactinomas, growth hormone for acromegaly, TSH for TSH-secreting adenomas, and cortisol for Cushing's disease. When target hormone levels are not within the expected normal ranges, they are measured again the following day. If the levels do not normalize by the third postoperative day, re-exploration is considered. For patients with Cushing's disease, dexamethasone is administered postoperatively 1 mg orally once or twice a day. Serum cortisol and 24-hour urinary free cortisol levels can be measured to judge the postoperative outcome of Cushing's disease when dexamethasone is used instead of hydrocortisone. Once serum cortisol and 24-hour urinary cortisol levels are confirmed to be normal postoperatively, dexamethasone medications can be changed to hydrocortisone.

Serum sodium or electrolytes are measured at the recovery room after surgery, on the first postoperative day, and 1 week postoperatively. During the hospital stay, urine specific gravity is measured each time patients urinate, and fluid intake and output are measured. In our early patients, postoperative diuresis was an annoying problem that often prolonged hospital stays to more than one night. However, we found that excessive intraoperative intravenous fluid administration was commonly responsible for this postoperative diuresis, and this stopped occurring when the intraoperative intravenous fluid volume was judiciously administered or limited. Vasopressin (Pitressin) is used when diabetes insipidus is confirmed by exhibition of the classic symptoms of polyuria and polydipsia, dilute urine with low urinary specific gravity, and increased serum osmolarity and sodium concentration. When patients develop diabetes insipidus, 1 μg of DDAVP is usually given intravenously. The intranasal form of DDAVP is instituted in the evening if patients experience a breakthrough of diabetes insipidus with increased urine volume. Patients who develop diabetes insipidus after surgery usually only require one or two doses of DDAVP because their diabetes insipidus is transient. Development of diabetes insipidus may delay hospital discharge by one or two nights.

In our early cases, we gave oral antibiotics (clarithromycin 500 mg twice a day) prophylactically for 5 days postoperatively because the endonasal approach traverses the presumed semi-contaminated sinonasal cavity. However, the use of postoperative antibiotics was found to be unnecessary, and we have not observed any increased incidence of infection in the absence of prophylactic antibiotics. A single dose of intravenous antibiotics is given intraoperatively in all patients, either as 2 g of cefazolin or a combination of 1 g vancomycin and 80 mg gentamycin. Formal endocrine evaluation, visual examination (if necessary), nasal examination, and postoperative MR scans are performed a few weeks postoperatively. Then patient follow-ups are made with interval endocrine evaluations and annual MR scans as needed.

Surgical Results

Among the 200 patients in our early series, 160 had pituitary adenomas, 10 had anterior skull base meningiomas, eight had clival chordomas, and 22 had other skull base pathologies. Fifty-five patients had undergone previous surgical and/or radiation treatments. Among the 160 patients with pituitary adenomas, 37 (23%) patients had microadenomas and 123 (77%) patients had macroadenomas. Among the

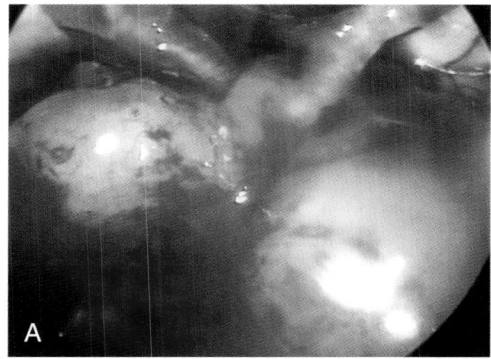
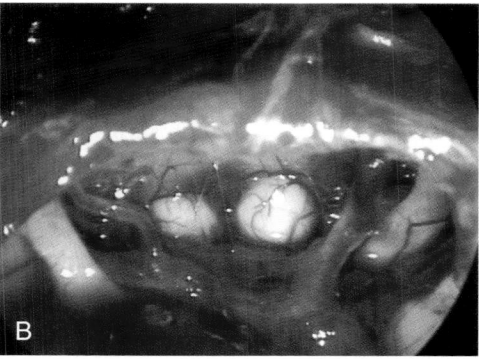

FIGURE 22-22 A 70-degree-lens endoscope discloses a chordoma encasing the basilar artery in another patient with a large clival chordoma (A). When the tumor was removed, the basilar bifurcation, III nerves, and mamillary bodies are visualized (B).

90 patients with nonfunctioning adenomas, 71 (79%) patients had gross total removal. Among the 38 patients with prolactinomas, 25 (66%) patients normalized their postoperative prolactin levels. Thirteen (72%) out of 18 patients with Cushing's disease had normal postoperative cortisol levels. Among the 13 patients with acromegaly, 11 (85%) had normalized postoperative IGF-1 levels. The length of hospital stay was less than 1 day in 75% of patients. One night of hospital stay has been routine for uncomplicated cases, although same-day surgery has occasionally been performed upon specific request and discussion with appropriate patients. Although our early surgical results are comparable to those reported with microscopic trans-sphenoidal surgery, we have continued to improve our surgical outcome with further increasing EE-TS experience. Of note, Tabaee et al. reported in a meta-analysis combining nine studies (totaling 821 patients) undergoing endoscopic pituitary surgery, including one of our early series of patients, gross total tumor removal in 78% and resolution of various hormone-secreting tumors ranging 81%-84%, along with complication rates of 2% CSF leak and 1% diabetes insipidus.[25]

Potential Complications and their Avoidance

CSF leakage is a potential complication in EE-TS, which can occur intraoperatively or in a delayed fashion postoperatively. There are two approaches for potential CSF leak with one approach being replacement of the sellar bone flaps without any further reconstruction required for routine EE-TS (and only placing a fat graft in a delayed fashion if uncommonly a CSF leak develops), and another approach is to perform abdominal fat graft and bone or titanium mesh reconstruction prophylactically. For routine EE-TS, we prefer the former method, but when the tumor resection cavity is large or if an intraoperative CSF leak is noted, an abdominal fat graft is placed and the anterior sellar wall is reconstructed with autogenous bone or a piece of titanium mesh. Fibrin glue or other adhesives are not routinely used but have been reported as supplements. The earliest postoperative leakage may be noted if patients are extubated with excessive coughing, which can result in rupture of thin arachnoid membranes at the surgical site. In our various patient series, the CSF leaks that do occasionally occur are usually delayed presentations within the first day of surgery. When patients merely leak a few drops of clear fluid from the nasal cavity, the leak usually stops quickly in a spontaneous fashion. However, if patients leak clear fluid continually when they sit with the head positioned leaning forwards, the leak must be repaired endoscopically without delay in order to prevent potential for meningitis. The challenging case in which to repair a CSF leak is in a patient following tumor removal from the tuberculum sella because excessive fat graft can cause compression to the optic system. The optic nerves located laterally at the tuberculum sella and the optic chiasm posteriorly can limit the adequate placement of fat graft material to seal the CSF leak. Reconstruction at the olfactory groove or clivus is much simpler than at the tuberculum sella. The use of a lumbar drain is reserved for rare occasions such as in patients with CSF leakage despite complete mechanical reconstruction. Although meningitis is an extremely rare occurrence, CSF leakage must be promptly repaired with administration of intravenous antibiotics if meningitis is confirmed, and CSF from a spinal tap can provide microbiologic information for antibiotic guidance.

Diabetes insipidus is another complication that can prolong hospital stay, but diabetes insipidus can be readily managed using the aforementioned remedies. However, the importance of corticosteroids in the postoperative management of patients with Cushing's disease cannot be overemphasized. When patients with Cushing's disease display the anticipated hypocortisolism postoperatively, they must take corticosteroid medications until they recover normal HPA axis function, which may take a few weeks to a year. Hypocortisolism with the lack of a cortisol stress response may be fatal if they fail to comply with their corticosteroid medications. In addition, postoperative hyponatremia can occur several days to a few weeks after surgery. Hyponatremic patients may need to be treated accordingly as inpatients as they may become symptomatic with nausea, vomiting, malaise, and altered consciousness.

There is a risk of delayed massive epistaxis occurring a few days to 2 weeks postoperatively. When patients go to an emergency room with significant epistaxis following EE-TS, intraoperative internal carotid artery injury with delayed pseudoaneurysm rupture is a diagnosis that emergency physicians may contemplate. However, the most common cause of such delayed nasal hemorrhage after trans-sphenoidal surgery is bleeding from the stump of the posterior septal artery, which can often be controlled acutely with direct pressure and can be addressed definitively with endoscopic electrocoagulation. But despite precautions, there is also rare risk of potential internal carotid artery injury with any technique of trans-sphenoidal surgery, and its occurrence requires tamponade with packing followed by endovascular intervention.

Advantages and Disadvantages of the Endonasal Endoscopic Technique

In our description of technique, we already outlined many of the advantages associated with EE-TS, but we will add a few additional comments. The endoscopic endonasal approach results in minimal postoperative discomfort or pain while obviating the need for postoperative nasal packing, and we have observed that avoidance of nasal packing offers a significant advantage for patient comfort and rapid recovery with early release from the hospital. Despite the naturally narrow nasal passages in pediatric patients (the youngest patient in our series was 13 years old) and in people of East Asian ethnicity, we have yet to encounter a patient who has nostrils too narrow for endoscopic endonasal surgery. This endonasal technique does not require sublabial or nasal transfixion incisions and subsequently minimizes the chance of dental, gingival, or sinonasal complications. The normal sinonasal physiologic anatomy is also well-maintained since the endoscopic endonasal technique is minimally traumatic. In addition, previously described optical advantages of an endoscope may improve overall surgical outcomes.

There are three major disadvantages of endoscopic pituitary surgery in comparison with conventional microscopic surgery: the inferior quality of two-dimensional monitor-generated flat images, inadequate development of commercially available surgical instruments, and the lack of formalized endoscopic training of pituitary neurosurgeons. Endoscopic two-dimensional video images may not quite reach the level of resolution of the stereotypic images generated by three-dimensional direct microscopic visualization, even though the endoscope allows close-up direct views unable to be achieved by the microscope and are enhanced by projection on a large high-definition monitor. A digitally enhanced camera has improved the picture quality to some degree, and high-definition cameras and monitors can further improve the quality of endoscopic views. Three-dimensional endoscopes with advanced video image such as super-definition camera and monitor may further enhance the visual quality of endoscopic surgery in the future. Second, commercially available instruments for endoscopic neurosurgery are still being optimized and may not be easily obtainable. Third, there is a steep learning curve for neurosurgeons who are already well-trained in conventional microscopic surgery. Maneuvering skills involved in endoscopic neurosurgery are quite different from conventional microsurgery techniques and may be compared to using a pair of chopsticks in each hand. Despite a neurosurgeon's painstaking training in microsurgery, most are not used to endoscopic surgical maneuvering and will need to spend considerable time getting accustomed to new endoscopic surgical skills. In addition, the neurosurgeon must adapt to operating with the endoscope shaft occupying the central portion of the surgical corridor. A major concern expressed by microscopic pituitary surgeons has been regarding the ability to control unexpectedly significant bleeding within a limited exposure. Although tumors involving high vascularity can bleed significantly as in microscopic pituitary surgery, the endoscopic endonasal technique has not proven to be a handicap for these types of tumors. Cavernous sinus bleeding may occasionally become cumbersome, but there has not been a single case that had to be aborted. Finally, the operating time for endoscopic surgery may initially be longer than that for microscopic surgery due to the intrinsic learning curve, but the operating time becomes comparable or shorter once the surgeon masters the technique.

Conclusions

As described, endoscopic endonasal trans-sphenoidal surgery is useful for the neurosurgical treatment of pituitary adenomas as well as for other skull base lesions located at the midline anterior cranial skull base, cavernous sinus, optic nerve, pterygoid fossa, petrous apex, and the midline clivus or posterior fossa.

ACKNOWLEDGMENTS

The authors thank Mi-Ja Jho and Robin A. Coret for their assistance in the preparation of this manuscript.

KEY REFERENCES

Alfieri A, Jho HD, Tschabitscher M. Endoscopic endonasal approach to the ventral cranio-cervical juncture: anatomical study. *Acta Neurochir (Wien)*. 2002;144:219-225.

Alfieri A, Jho HD. Endoscopic endonasal approach to the cavernous sinus. An anatomic study. *Neurosurgery*. 2001;48:827-837.

Alfieri A, Jho HD. Endoscopic endonasal approach to the cavernous sinus. Surgical approaches. *Neurosurgery*. 2001;49:354-362.

Carrau RL, Jho HD, Ko Y. Transnasal-transsphenoidal endoscopic surgery of the pituitary gland. *Laryngoscope*. 1996;106:914-918.

Ceylan S, Koc K, Anik I. Endoscopic endonasal transsphenoidal approach for pituitary adenomas invading the cavernous sinus. Clinical article. *J Neurosurg*. 2010;112:99-107.

Cooke RS, Jones RAC. Experience with the direct transnasal transsphenoidal approach to the pituitary fossa. *Br J Neurosurg*. 1994;8: 193-196.

de Divitiis E, Cavallo LM, Cappabianca P, Esposito F. Extended endoscopic endonasal transsphenoidal approach for the removal of suprasellar tumor: part 2. *Neurosurgery*. 2007;60:46-59.

Griffith HB, Veerapen R. A direct transnasal approach to the sphenoid sinus: technical note. *J Neurosurg*. 1987;66:140-142.

Guiot G, Rougerie J, Fourestier A, et al. Une nouvelle technique endoscopique: exploration endoscopiques intracraniennes. *Presse Med*. 1963;71:1225-1228.

Jho HD, Carrau RL, Ko Y, Daly M. Endoscopic pituitary surgery: an early experience. *Surg Neurol*. 1997;47:213-223.

Jankowski R, Auque J, Simon C, et al. Endoscopic pituitary tumor surgery. *Laryngoscope*. 1992;102:198-202.

Jho HD. Endoscopic transsphenoidal surgery. *J Neuro-oncology*. 2001;54:187-195.

Jho HD. Endoscopic endonasal approach to the optic nerve: a technical note. *Minim Invas Neurosurg*. 2001;44:190-193.

Jho HD, Alfieri A. Endoscopic endonasal pituitary surgery: evolution of surgical technique and equipment in 150 operations. *Minim Invas Neurosurg*. 2001;44:1-12.

Jho HD, Alfieri A. Endoscopic transsphenoidal pituitary surgery: various surgical techniques and recommended steps for procedural transition. *Br J Neurosurg*. 2000;14:424-432.

Jho HD, Carrau RL. Endoscopic endonasal transsphenoidal surgery: experience with 50 patients. *J Neurosurg*. 1997;87:44-51.

Jho HD, Carrau RL. Endoscopy assisted transsphenoidal surgery for pituitary adenoma: technical note. *Acta Neurochir (Wien)*. 1996;138: 1416-1425.

Jho HD, Carrau RL, Ko Y. Endoscopic pituitary surgery. In: Wilkins RH, Rengachary SS, eds. *Neurosurgical Operative Atlas.* vol 5. Baltimore: Williams & Wilkins; 1996:1-12.

Jho HD, Carrau RL, Mclaughlin ML, Somaza SC. Endoscopic transsphenoidal resection of a large chordoma in the posterior fossa. *Acta Neurochir (Wien).* 1997;139:343-348.

Jho HD, Ha HG. Endoscopic endonasal skull base surgery: part 1—The midline anterior fossa skull base. *Minim Invas Neurosurg.* 2004;47:1-8.

Jho HD, Ha HG. Endoscopic endonasal skull base surgery: part 2—The cavernous sinus. *Minim Invas Neurosurg.* 2004;47:9-15.

Jho HD, Ha HG. Endoscopic endonasal skull base surgery: part 3—The clivus and posterior fossa. *Minim Invas Neurosurg.* 2004;47:16-23.

Keros P. Uber die praktische beteudung der Niveau-Unterschiede der lamina cribosa des ethmoids. In: Naumann HH, ed. *Head and neck surgery,* vol 1. *Face and facial skull.* Philadelphia: WB Saunders; 1980:392.

Laufer I, Anand VK, Schwartz TH. Endoscopic endonasal extended transsphenoidal transplanum transtuberculum approach for resection of suprasellar lesions. *J Neurosurg.* 2007;106:400-406.

Tabaee A, Anand VK, Barron Y, et al. Endoscopic pituitary surgery: a systemic review and meta-analysis. *J Neurosurg.* 2009;111:545-554.

Numbered references appear on Expert Consult.

CHAPTER 23

Transcranial Surgery for Pituitary Macroadenomas

PABLO F. RECINOS • C. RORY GOODWIN • HENRY BREM
• ALFREDO QUIÑONES-HINOJOSA

The most common tumors affecting the suprasellar, intrasellar, or parasellar region include pituitary adenomas, craniopharyngiomas, meningiomas, germ cell tumors, and gliomas involving the hypothalamus or optic chiasm. Management is dictated according to each specific diagnosis. While medical therapies can be utilized in a subset of patients, many lesions require surgical management, which is most commonly carried out using a trans-sphenoidal approach. Sellar and suprasellar tumors are characteristically treated via a trans-sphenoidal approach because these operations are less invasive, provide direct access to the tumor with preservation of normal pituitary tissue, and have a quicker recovery of vision and visual field defects due to minimal manipulation of the optic nerves and chiasm. Despite the advantages of the trans-sphenoidal approach, certain pituitary tumors cannot be completely resected via the trans-sphenoidal approach and require transcranial surgery.

Transcranial approaches are used in approximately 1% to 4% of pituitary tumors that require surgical management.[1,2] The most common indications for transcranial surgery for pituitary tumors are large extrasellar tumor extension without sellar enlargement, marked frontal, middle fossa, or clival extension of tumors (particularly dumbbell shaped), very fibrous tumors not amenable to trans-sphenoidal resection (meningiomas), a persistent visual field deficit after incomplete decompression via the trans-sphenoidal approach, a coexistent aneurysm, loss of oculomotor function, ectatic midline carotid arteries, or sphenoid sinusitis.[1-3] Treatment selection depends on the tumor characteristics and its associated findings. A thorough understanding of the advantages and disadvantages of each transcranial approach is critical when choosing the most appropriate surgical option.

History

In 1893, Caton and Paul recorded the first attempted, but unsuccessful, pituitary tumor resection using a two-stage lateral subtemporal decompression in a patient with acromegaly.[4] This approach was suggested by Sir Victor Horsley, who from 1904 to 1906, used a subfrontal approach and a lateral middle fossa approach to operate on 10 patients with pituitary tumors.[5] In comparison to the 50% to 80% mortality rate of his colleagues, Horsley reported a mortality

rate of 20% using this approach. In 1904, Kilani showed an extensive bifrontal intradural approach using cadavers.[6] In 1905, Krause demonstrated that it was possible to reach the sella turcica via a frontal transcranial approach in a living patient.[7] In 1912, McArthur described an extradural approach via resection of the supraorbital ridge and orbital plate.[8] These approaches formed the basic foundation upon which subsequent neurosurgeons improved and modified surgical treatment of these pathologies.[8,9]

Harvey Cushing played a central role in standardizing the preference for transcranial surgery over the trans-sphenoidal approach. Cushing's initial experience with transcranial approaches to sellar neoplasms was very discouraging and as such, he adopted the trans-sphenoidal approach that was undergoing marked improvement at the time.[10] Cushing had a mortality rate of 5.6% in his series of 231 patients from 1910 to 1925 who had undergone surgical resection via the trans-sphenoidal approach.[11] The morbidity and mortality associated with the trans-sphenoidal approach at the time were primarily attributed to infection, most often associated with postoperative cerebrospinal fluid (CSF) leak, postoperative edema, and hemorrhage.[9] These complications coupled with Cushing's extreme interest in intracranial surgery prompted the development of a novel transcranial approach to sellar-based neoplasms. Cushing's increased experience with transcranial procedures, and subsequently the reduced mortality he experienced utilizing these approaches, led to a preferential treatment of sellar tumors using an intracranial approach.[9] The transfrontal craniotomy, performed via a direct midline approach, allowed Cushing to attain a more extensive resection, better visualization and decompression of the optic nerve and chiasm, lower recurrence rates, and better recovery of vision.[9,12] The transfrontal approach also avoided the potentially fatal complication of infection seen with the trans-sphenoidal approach. For these reasons, Cushing discarded the trans-sphenoidal operation, and with his prominence in American neurosurgery, he helped to usher in a strong preference for the transfrontal approach.[11,13,14]

From the 1930s to the 1950s, transcranial approaches to the pituitary dominated neurosurgical practice and teaching. In the late 1950s and 1960s, the trans-sphenoidal procedure received renewed interest as many technological and surgical advances improved this surgical approach including: (1) development of a lighted speculum retractor by Dott in 1956,[15] (2) enhanced surgical accuracy with the intraoperative radiofluoroscopy to define nasal passage anatomy and control the position of the instruments by Guiot,[16] (3) development of antibiotics in the 1950s to reduce the surgical mortality associated with this approach,[17] and (4) introduction of corticosteroids allowing safer surgeries to be performed on the pituitary gland.[12] Some of these advances were utilized by Hardy in 1971 in his landmark paper that demonstrated the trans-sphenoidal operation on over 300 patients undergoing hypophysectomy.[18] In his paper, he described the technical aspects of the trans-sphenoidal hypophysectomy and also reported a morbidity and mortality rate that was less than with transcranial approaches. Specifically, the risk of CSF leak was markedly reduced when the arachnoid was left intact. Since then, trans-sphenoidal surgery has dominated neurosurgical treatment of sellar-based lesions.

Specific Indications

While the trans-sphenoidal approach is standard for resection of sellar/parasellar region tumors, there are specific indications for transcranial approaches. The usual reason for using a transcranial approach is doubt about the diagnosis.[19] For instance, if the lesion is not a pituitary adenoma, but instead perhaps a meningioma or craniopharyngioma, a craniotomy is advised because these lesions are more safely removed transcranially.[19] For tumors with a wide extension on the cranial base, craniotomy remains a superior approach. Craniotomy is more effective in a variety of other surgical cases as well because it increases access to tumors, facilitates preservation of the surrounding neurovascular structures, improves visualization at the dural edge, and allows earlier identification of the cranial nerves and the feeding vessels.[20]

FAILED TRANS-SPHENOIDAL SURGERY

A major indication for a transcranial procedure is a failed trans-sphenoidal surgery. Failure can occur for multiple different reasons. Any intrinsic tumor characteristic that does not allow it to fall into the sella compromises the efficacy of trans-sphenoidal surgery. For instance, if a pituitary adenoma is too fibrous, a trans-sphenoidal approach will fail. In those circumstances, it is advisable to take no more than a biopsy specimen and obliterate the sphenoid sinus. The latter action may seem unnecessary with a large tough tumor between the nasal cavity and the CSF. The consistency of the tumor, not the size, limits the effectiveness of trans-sphenoidal surgery.[19]

Failure of the suprasellar extension to descend is another reason for failed trans-sphenoidal surgery. The usual cause is that a component of the tumor is extending superiorly, laterally, or anteriorly. If the suprasellar extension has pushed vertically, it usually falls into the tumor cavity created by the trans-sphenoidal surgeon. If an extension of tumor hooks around the optic nerve or carotid artery, this extension prevents descent of the tumor, and the tumor extension above the carotid artery or chiasm is inaccessible.[19] The anterior extension is particularly troublesome for the trans-sphenoidal surgeon because it is at the wrong angle for the line of

approach.[19] In addition, recurrent pituitary adenomas may not fall down satisfactorily because of adhesions between the tumor and the surrounding brain. In these circumstances, the combined transcranial/trans-sphenoidal approach may be the best method to completely remove the tumor. Thus, it may be justified if the tumor has recurred despite previous irradiation. Radical surgery is also indicated for hormone-secreting adenomas such as those that occur in patients with acromegaly (or Cushing syndrome), in which hormonal cure depends on total removal of the tumor.[19] A trans-sphenoidal procedure is also insufficient when the surgery fails to remove adequate amounts of tumor, particularly enough to decompress the optic chiasm.[19,21] The failure often manifests after incomplete decompression as a persistent visual field deficit or persistent loss of vision.

PARA/EXTRASELLAR EXTENSION

In cases with large extrasellar tumor extension without sellar enlargement, the pituitary gland may be vulnerable to a trans-sphenoidal approach. Usually in this case, the suprasellar component either encases optic nerves or intracranial arteries or it spreads over the surface of the planum sphenoidale.[21]

Also, pituitary adenomas can invade one or both cavernous sinuses. While the trans-sphenoidal approach is limited to the compartment of the cavernous sinus medial to the C4 segment of the internal carotid artery, this approach can be used in patients with non-secreting adenomas in which tumor debulking and neurovascular decompression is sufficient.[21] Transcranial approaches are warranted, however, if the adenoma is secretory, or if the parasellar extension ventures beyond the cavernous sinus into the middle fossa.[21] Transcranial approaches are also indicated when restoration of oculomotor function is the goal.

Dumbbell-shaped pituitary adenomas that have a 'narrow' waist created by a thick diaphragm sellae and a small pituitary stalk opening warrant a transcranial approach over a trans-sphenoidal. One can predict the failure of trans-sphenoidal surgery for a dumbbell shaped lesion based on tumor compression into the sella by intraoperative lumbar intrathecal injection of sterile saline and endoscopic navigation of the opening in the diaphragm sellae.[21]

OTHER

Co-existent aneurysms, ectatic carotid arteries, and severe sinus infection are indications for transcranial surgery. Aneurysms are found concomitantly in approximately 1.1% of all pituitary adenoma cases.[21,22] If an aneurysm adjacent to a pituitary adenoma (i.e. an aneurysm of the anterior cerebral artery) is detected preoperatively, both lesions can be potentially treated in the same operation. Co-treatment of these lesions is more applicable when an aneurysm will be affected by manipulation of the regional anatomy.[21] Alternative treatment strategies include a staged-procedure, surveillance of either lesion or nonsurgical treatments such as endovascular coiling for the aneurysm and radiotherapy for the pituitary adenoma.[21] In terms of ectatic vessels, the tumor's relationship to the intercavernous carotid arteries should be taken into account when deciding on an appropriate approach. There is commonly a 1 to 3 mm separation between the medial margin of the internal cerebral arteries and the lateral surface of the pituitary gland.[23]

Ectatic carotid arteries can veer into the midline trajectory preventing a trans-sphenoidal approach.[9] Also, if a sinus infection is severe and surgical delay will pose a threat of acute neurological deterioration, a transcranial approach is warranted.[20,21]

Diagnosis and Workup

The preoperative work-up for patients with signs or symptoms of a sellar neoplasm should include formal testing of the patient's visual fields and pituitary function. A T1-weighted magnetic resonance imaging (MRI) scan with and without gadolinium in the sagittal and coronal planes should also be performed to allow proper visualization of the optic nerves, optic chiasm, carotid arteries, cavernous sinuses and surrounding soft tissue.[19,24] A T2-weighted scan may be useful in determining the fibrotic nature of a tumor in this region to aid in surgical planning. Although no reliable predictor exists, evidence suggests that pituitary adenomas with a homogeneously isointense, as opposed to hypertense, signal on T2-weighted MRI are predicted to be firm and fibrotic, although this is not routinely used radiologic criteria.[20,21,25]

The position of the optic chiasm can be predicted on the sagittal MRI scan by finding the anterior communicating artery.[19] While the length of the intracranial optic nerves varies from patient to patient, tumor extension influences the distance of the optic nerves to the tuberculum sella. If the suprasellar extension is thrust between the optic nerves, it pushes the chiasm upward and backward, allowing good surgical access. On occasion the suprasellar extension pushes the chiasm upward and forward, severely limiting surgical access.[19] This is called a "prefixed chiasm."

Craniotomy for tumors in this region carries the same general risks as any operation (i.e., deep vein thrombosis, bleeding, infection, anesthetic risks), however there are specific risks associated such as damage to the optic nerves (resulting in impaired vision or visual fields), damage to the internal carotid artery or anterior cerebral artery, and damage to the pituitary stalk (resulting in hypopituitarism and diabetes insipidus).[19] The transcranial approach almost inevitably causes hypopituitarism because the normal pituitary tissue is pushed superiorly under the diaphragm sella, and this tissue is specifically coagulated and cut by the surgeon en route to the tumor.[19] The potential for harm to the vascular structures in this area necessitates cross-matching of 2 pints of blood. Anticonvulsants should be started preoperatively because epilepsy is possible after transcranial surgery. Cerebrospinal fluid rhinorrhea or anosmia can occasionally occur, especially if excessive retraction of the frontal lobe is indicated.[19]

AIMS OF SURGERY

The aims of pituitary surgery are ultimately to cure the patient of the tumor, without damage to the pituitary; to relieve the symptoms and the signs that have been caused by the tumor; and to achieve this relief without damage to the patient. When the tumor is secreting hormone, total extirpation of the tumor is necessary to achieve a cure. A nonfunctioning tumor does not necessarily require total removal, especially if the risks of such an attempt are

significant. In these circumstances, the aims should be an adequate debulking of the tumor to produce chiasmal and optic nerve decompression before radiotherapy or radiosurgery.

Pterional

The frontosphenotemporal or pterional craniotomy is the most commonly used transcranial approach to pituitary tumors (Fig. 23-1). It was popularized by Yaşargil as an approach to intracranial aneurysms and is now the most widely used transcranial approach in neurosurgery.[26-28] It provides a direct path to the sella turcica and allows removal of large pituitary tumors with minimal brain retraction. It should also be the transcranial approach of choice for tumors when a prefixed chiasm is present as the tumor can be resected safely underneath the optic chiasm.[27]

TECHNIQUE

A curvilinear incision is marked out. The caudal extent should start just below to the root of the zygomatic arch and 1 cm anterior to the tragus. The cranial extent depends on the patient's hairline and should end either at the midline or at the contralateral mid-pupillary line. The scalp is dissected in two layers with the fascia of the superficial temporalis muscle left intact. The superficial temporal artery should be left intact to maintain the vascular supply of the flap and to serve as a possible bypass donor artery. The superficial scalp flap should be reflected until the superficial temporal fat pad is seen. A curvilinear incision is made in the temporalis fascia posterior to the fat pad. The fascia is dissected sharply from the temporalis muscle, which protects the frontalis branch of the facial nerve. Usage of the monopolar cautery should be avoided because it can result in thermal injury to the frontalis branch of the facial nerve. The superficial temporal fat pad and fascia are elevated by dissecting the insertion of the fascia from the superior aspect of the zygomatic body and frontozygomatic process. The fat pad is then reflected along with the superficial skin flap.

After reflecting the skin flap and fat pad, the temporalis muscle is elevated. An incision is made in the temporalis fascia 1.5 cm posterior to the frontozygomatic process and continued posteriorly along the linea temporalis. A 1- to 2-cm cuff is left attached to the linea temporalis for reattachment of the temporalis flap during closure.[29] Using subperiosteal dissection, the temporalis myofascial flap is elevated off of the skull.[30] Once the myofascial flap is completely reflected anteriorly and inferiorly, it is held in place using fish hooks.

The frontosphenotemporal craniotomy may be created using varying numbers of burr holes and either a standard router with the footplate attachment or with the Gigli saw. We prefer to make our craniotomy using two burr holes: (1) in the squamous portion of the temporal bone just superior to the root of zygoma and (2) at the MacCarty keyhole. The ideal location for the MacCarty keyhole burr hole is to create it on the frontosphenoid suture approximately 5 to 6 mm posterior to the junction of the frontozygomatic, the sphenozygomatic, and the frontosphenoid sutures.[31] A Penfield #3 dissector is used to dissect the dura from the inner table. A standard router with footplate on a pneumatic drill

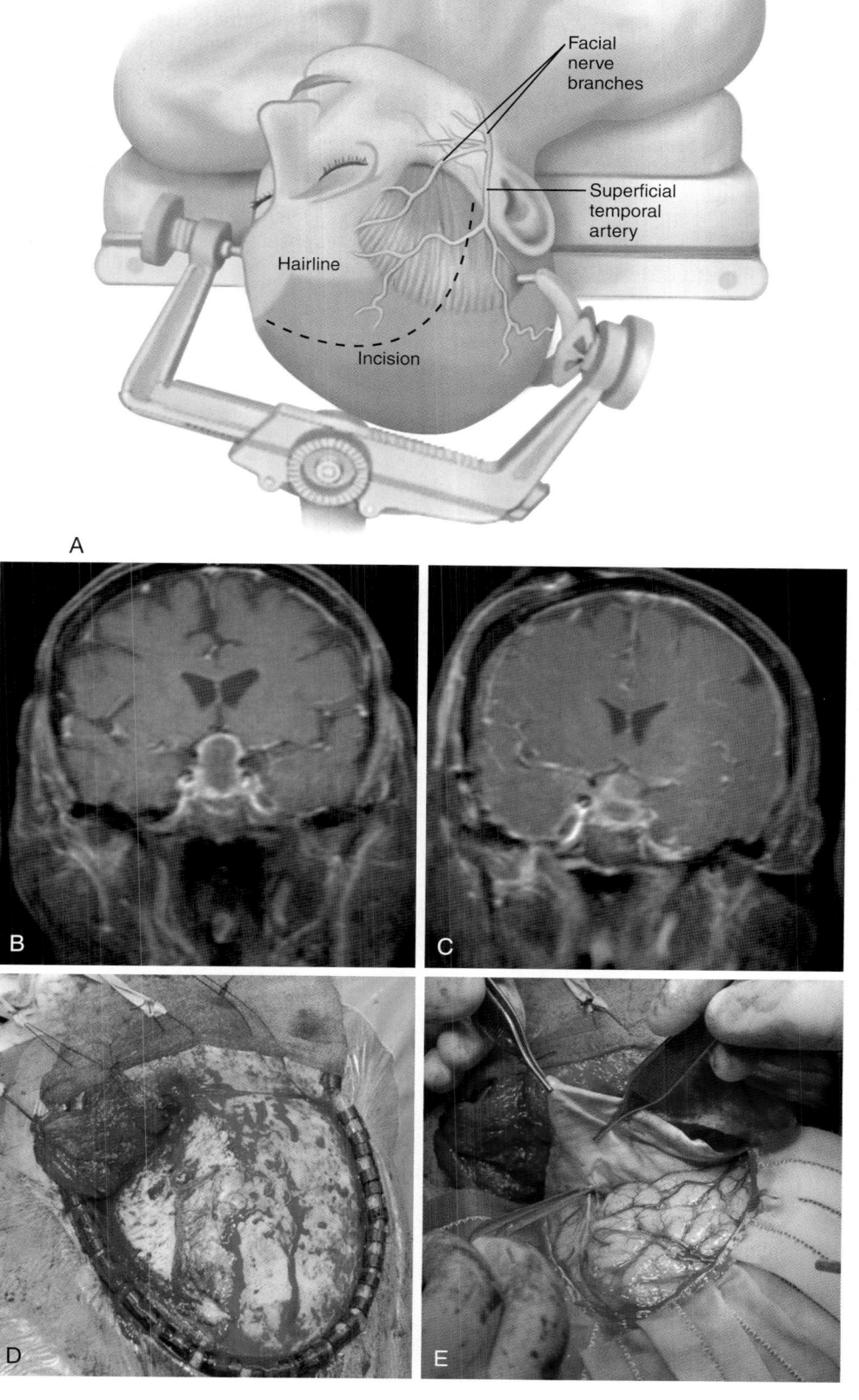

FIGURE 23-1 Pterionial approach. A, Artist representation of patient positioning and skin incision. B, Preoperative coronal T1-magnetic resonance image of a multicystic pituitary adenoma with lateral extension. C, Postoperative MRI demonstrating total tumor removal via a left pterional approach. D, Intraoperative photo of the myofascial flap reflected anteriorly and inferiorly. E, Intraoperative photo of a semicircular dural flap reflected anteriorly with dissection of arachnoid adhesions anchored to the dura. (Adapted from Brotchi J, Pirotte B. Sphenoid wing meningiomas. In: Sekhar LN, Fessler RG, eds. *Atlas of Neurosurgical Techniques, Brain*. New York: Thieme Medical Publishers; 2006:628.)

is utilized to turn the craniotomy. The supraorbital foramen serves as the medial border of the craniotomy. Once the bone flap it ready to be elevated, it is important to free the dura that remains attached to the inner table with a Penfield #3 dissector.

After the bone flap is removed, extradural bony removal continues prior to opening the dura. The frontal and temporal dura are dissected off of the ridge of the sphenoid bone with a Penfield #1 dissector. The bony sphenoid ridge is removed using rongeurs. The sharp edges of bone may be smoothed out with a pneumatic drill with a #2 or #3 diamond bit. It is important to constantly irrigate the drill to prevent thermal injury to the dura and underlying optic nerve. The optic canal is skeletonized and the anterior clinoid process completely removed. The underlying clinoidal segment of the internal carotid artery is then visualized. When approaching tumors with wide parasellar extension or that encroach the cavernous sinus, uncovering the foramen rotundum and foramen ovale gives additional needed exposure to minimize temporal retraction.[26]

Prior to opening the dura, cottonoids are then placed around the dural edges to wick the blood from the operative field. A semicircular dural flap is created and reflected anteriorly. Special care must be taken to dissect bridging veins and other adhesions anchored to the dura. Sutures are placed at the base of the dural flap and tied to the fish hooks retracting the temporalis flap to keep the dural flap under tension and out of the operative field.

The Sylvian fissure is split using a Nauta knife (18-gauge needle attached to 1cc tuberculin syringe). The extent of the dissection will be dependent on the size and extent of the tumor. Self-retractors may be placed on the frontal and temporal lobes with care to avoid excessive temporal lobe retraction. Placing moist telfa strips underneath the retractors provides an additional protective layer to the brain. Once the tumor is exposed, it is resected in a piece-meal fashion. The Cavitron ultrasonic aspirator is useful in coring out large, firm tumors. The tumor edges and capsule should be resected using bipolar cautery, microscissors, and suction in order to maintain direct visualization of critical adjacent structures.

Reconstruction of the one-piece bone flap is done using titanium burr-hole covers and plates to reattach the bone flap to the skull. The bone flap is preferentially situated as anterior as for an improved cosmetic result. Bone gaps that result from the osteotomies can be filled in with bone cement (such as CranioFix2®) or covered with molded titanium plates. After the bony reconstruction is completed, the temporalis muscle is reapproximated to the myofascial cuff. The galea and skin flap are then closed in standard fashion.

Orbitozygomatic Craniotomy

The orbitozygomatic craniotomy is a second option in the treatment of sellar masses that have significant extension (Fig. 23-2). It arose from the supraorbital craniotomy first described by Jane et al. and evolved into an approach incorporating the orbitozygomatic and pterional cranial segments as described by Pellerin et al. and Hakuba and colleagues.[32-34] This approach provides a greater degree of exposure with reduced brain retraction compared to the pterional approach. It is especially useful in approaching

lesions with considerable superior extension, those that extend laterally into the cavernous sinus, and those with significant parasellar and interpeduncular involvement.[26] However, given that it is less commonly used than the pterional approach, familiarity with the technical nuances of the orbitozygomatic approach is critical to minimize the increased risks associated with removal of the orbital rim.

TECHNIQUE

Planning, positioning, and initial flap creation are done according to the previous description for the pterional craniotomy. The temporalis dissection differs due to the need for inferior reflection of the temporalis muscle flap in order to gain additional bony exposure to perform the orbitozytomatic osteotomies. The incision in the temporalis muscle is made starting 2 cm posterior to the frontozygomatic process and carried posterior 1 cm below the superior temporal line. The incision is angled inferiorly and terminates at the root of the zygoma. The myofascial temporalis flap is then dissected using a fan periosteal elevator. The temporalis flap is then reflected inferiorly underneath the zygomatic process until the inferior orbital fissure is visualized. It is critical to have adequate exposure of the inferior orbital fissure since two of the osteotomies pass through it. The masseter can be detached from the inferior portion of the zygomatic process. Alternatively, the masseter can be left attached and simply reflected inferiorly after the osteotomies are made in order to reduce the risk of postoperative trismus.[35]

Dissection of the orbital rim and periorbita is performed with a #1 Penfield elevator. The supraorbital nerve is dissected out easily if it runs through a notch or chipped out carefully with an osteotome if it runs through a foramen. Upon dissection of the periorbita, the anesthesiologist should be warned about the possible production of vagal responses. Care must be taken not to violate the periorbita in order to minimize postoperative swelling. Dissection continues until the inferior orbital fissure is completely exposed.

The first step is to create a frontosphenotemporal craniotomy as described above. The second step is to create the orbitozygomatic osteotomies to release the superior orbital roof, lateral orbital wall, and zygoma. These have been described using varying number of cuts and instruments (e.g., oscillating saw). We accomplish this by making five osteotomies and prefer to use a long router bit with footplate for all of the cuts. The footplate provides a protective barrier that protects the soft tissues of the orbit. The first cut separates zygomatic arch from the root of zygoma. Placement of a dog-bone plate on the zygomatic arch that incorporates the location of the first osteotomy prior to making such cut will facilitate the reconstruction. The second cut separates the frontozygomatic process from the body of the zygoma. To accomplish this, a small retractor is placed gently on the periorbita, exposing the inferior orbital fissure. The footplate is then placed in the anterolateral portion of the inferior orbital fissure to initiate the cut. The third cut separates the temporal process of the zygoma from the zygomatic body. The footplate is placed on the inferior portion of the temporal process of the zygoma and directed obliquely to meet the second cut. The fourth osteotomy cuts through the superior orbital rim and orbital roof. Retractors are again used to protect the orbital contents and

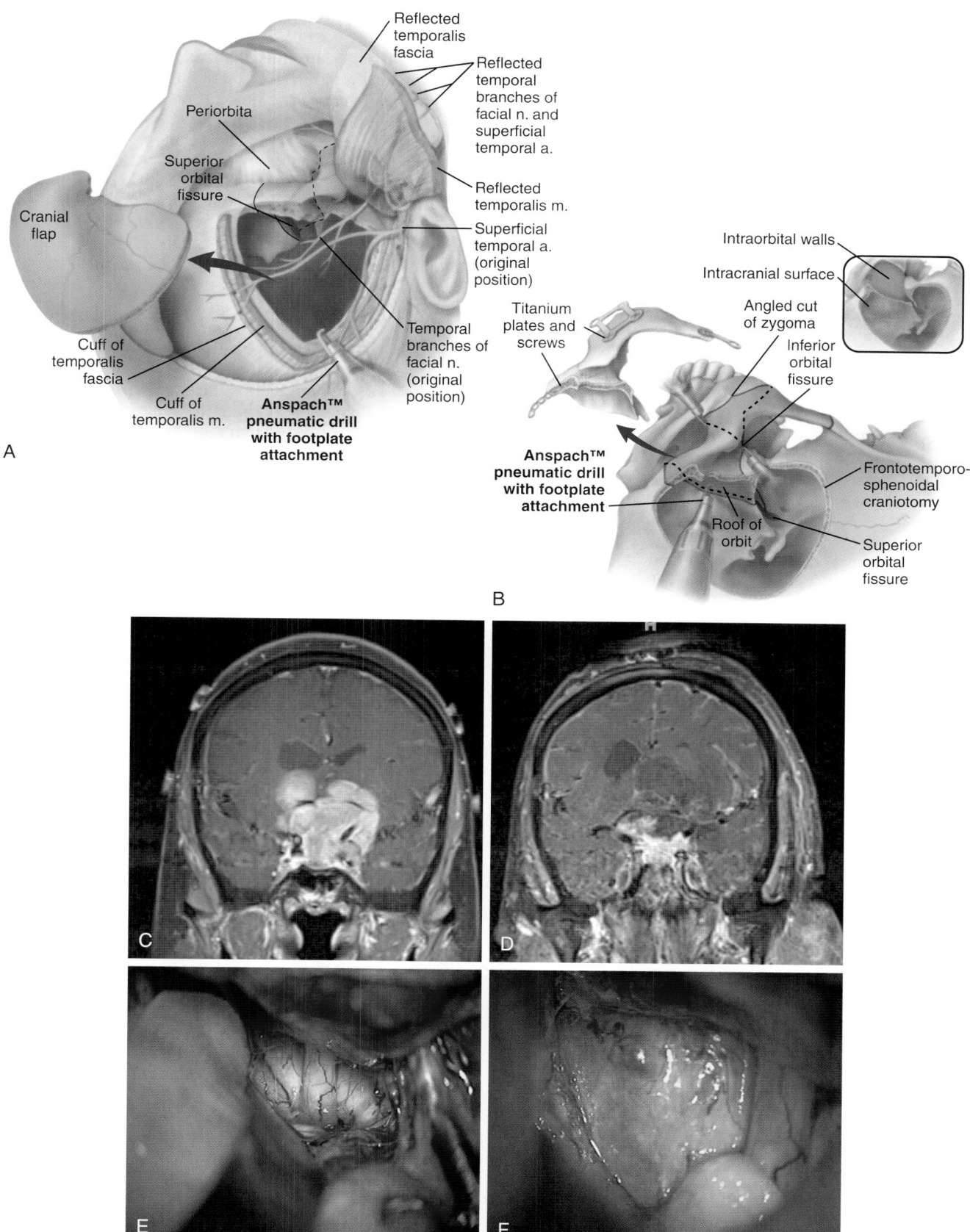

FIGURE 23-2 Orbitozygomatic approach. A, Artist rendering of anatomical dissection and frontosphenotemporal craniotomy. B, Artist rendering of orbitozygomatic osteotomies to release the superior orbital roof, lateral orbital wall, and zygoma. The bone flap is plated prior to making the cuts to ensure appropriate fit during reconstruction. C, Preoperative coronal T1-magnetic resonance with gadolinium demonstrating a pituitary tumor with significant superior extension and compression of the optic chiasm and third ventricle. D, Postoperative T1-MRI with gadolinium demonstrating tumor removal via an orbitozygomatic approach. E, Intraoperative photo with the tumor seen pushing up on the optic chiasm. F, Magnification of the intrachiasmatic space demonstrating the relationship of tumor to optic chiasm. (A and B, redrawn from Conway JE, Raza SM, Li K, McDermott MW, Quiñones-Hinojosa A. A surgical modification for performing orbitozygomatic osteotomies: technical note. Neurosurg Rev. 2010;33(4):491-500. Epub 2010 Jul 27.)

the frontal dura. The footplate is placed inside the orbit and directed immediately lateral to the superior orbital notch, over the supraorbital rim, and guided toward the superior orbital fissure. At the posterior orbital rim, the craniotome is directed laterally until reaching the junction of the superior and lateral orbital walls. It is then guided down the lateral wall of the orbit. The fifth osteotomy connects the fourth cut with the posterolateral portion of the inferior orbital fissure. The footplate is placed in the inferior orbital fissure in the infratemporal fossa and directed superiorly to complete second portion of the orbitozygomatic craniotomy.

Violation of the frontal sinus can occur during the orbitozygomatic craniotomy. The frontal sinus size and relationship to the relevant anatomy on preoperative MRI and/or computed tomography (CT) can help predict this event. If violation of the frontal sinus occurs and the nasofrontal duct is present, the frontal sinus mucosa does not have to be exenterated. In this case, large pieces of Gelfoam soaked in antibiotic solution can be used to pack the sinus. Alternatively, the mucosa of the sinus can be exenterated by monopolar cauterization followed by drilling the inner bony surfaces with a diamond burr. A pericranial flap is then used to tack down to the dura inferiorly to serve as a protective barrier to prevent CSF leak.

Reconstruction of the two-piece craniotomy is done by attaching titanium plates to reattach the bone flaps. The bone flap is preferentially approximated anteriorly in order to prevent a CSF leak from the frontal sinus (if violation occurred) and for an improved cosmetic result. Bone gaps that result from the osteotomies can be filled in with bone cement (such as CranioFix2®) or covered with molded titanium plates. After the bony reconstruction is completed, the temporalis muscle is reapproximated to the myofascial cuff. The galea and skin flap are then closed in standard fashion.

Bifrontal and Extended Bifrontal

The bifrontal and extended bifrontal are third-line transcranial options to approach pituitary tumors. The original concept of a bifrontal craniotomy was described by Frazier in 1913 and subsequently applied and developed to correction of craniofacial abnormalities by Tessier and to approaching skull base tumors by Derome.[36-38] These approaches are useful for tumors with significant superior and two-sided lateral extension and for those tumors that involve the medial orbits, clivus, upper air sinuses, and third ventricle. Removal of the orbital bar in the extended bifrontal craniotomy provides wide exposure of the anterior skull base and allows extensive inferior-superior viewing with minimal brain retraction.

TECHNIQUE

The bifrontal and bifrontal-extended approaches are options that can be used when a suprasellar tumor has significant superior, inferior, and/or lateral extension (Fig. 23-3). In the bifrontal extended approach the orbital bar is removed, which increases the inferior-to-superior mobility and allows generous bilateral exposure to the cavernous sinuses. Specifically, the orbital contents can be mobilized to widen the path of exposure. With the additional exposure afforded by removal of the orbital rim, the amount of retraction on the frontal lobes is minimized. However,

these approaches are considered as secondary alternatives to the more commonly used pterional and orbitozygomatic approaches because the amount of exposure attained is rarely needed for resection of pituitary macroadenomas.

The patient is positioned supine and placed in the Mayfield head clap. The pins are positioned posterior to the ears in the mastoid bone. The two-pin side should be rotated in a cranial-caudal direction so that it does not interfere with the opening or closing. The neck should be translated superiorly and flexed toward the chest without compressing the jugular veins. Care must be taken while draping to not place towels right above the eyebrow that cause compression on the orbit when the flap is rotated forward.

A standard bicoronal incision is planned and the hair is minimally shaved. The application of bupivicaine with epinephrine after the prep is applied is very useful for hemostasis during the opening. During the opening, great care must be taken to dissect the scalp in the subgaleal plane and to avoid damaging the pericranium. The scalp is reflected forward and retracted with fish hooks. A pericranial flap is elevated off of the superior temporal lines and based anteriorly on the supraorbital rim. The supraorbital nerves are then dissected out if they run through a groove or chipped out with an osteotome if they travel through a notch. The periorbita is dissected off the orbital rim and the pericranial flap is reflected past the nasofrontal suture. The temporalis muscles are dissected off of the superior temporal line bilaterally and reflected inferiorly.

The craniotomy is planned by marking eight burr hole drill points. Burr holes should be placed on each side of the superior sagittal sinus at the anterior and posterior extent of the bone flap, on the MacCarty keyholes bilaterally, and 2 cm below the superior temporal line at the posterior extent of the flap. Using the craniotome, the craniotomy is made saving the cuts across the sinus for last. During elevation of the bone flap, the dura mater is separated from the orbits but should not be dissected past the crista galli to avoid injury to the olfactory nerves.

In the extended bifrontal craniotomy, the orbital bar is removed by making five cuts. The long router bit with footplate attachment is used to make all cuts. The first cut is made at the frontozygomatic suture in a cranial to orbital direction. Using a malleable retractor to protect the orbit, the second cut extends from the lateral orbit to the nasion in a horizontal plane. This is repeated on the contralateral side. The final cut is made across the nasion connecting the medial extent of the second cuts on both sides. The orbital bar is then removed in one piece. The frontal sinus mucosa should be completely removed from the frontal sinus recesses to avoid the possibility of future mucocele development.

Depending on the extent of the tumor, a primarily intradural or extradural approach may be taken. Tumors with a large suprasellar extent and limited intrasellar/parasellar extension can be resected using a primarily intradural approach. However, tumors with significant parasellar and/or intrasellar extension may require a wider exposure by removing the additional bone of the skull base.

The superior sagittal sinus is suture ligated next to the crista galli and the falx is cut until its deep edge. Further dissection beginning with the olfactory tracts is performed under the microscope. The olfactory nerves should be

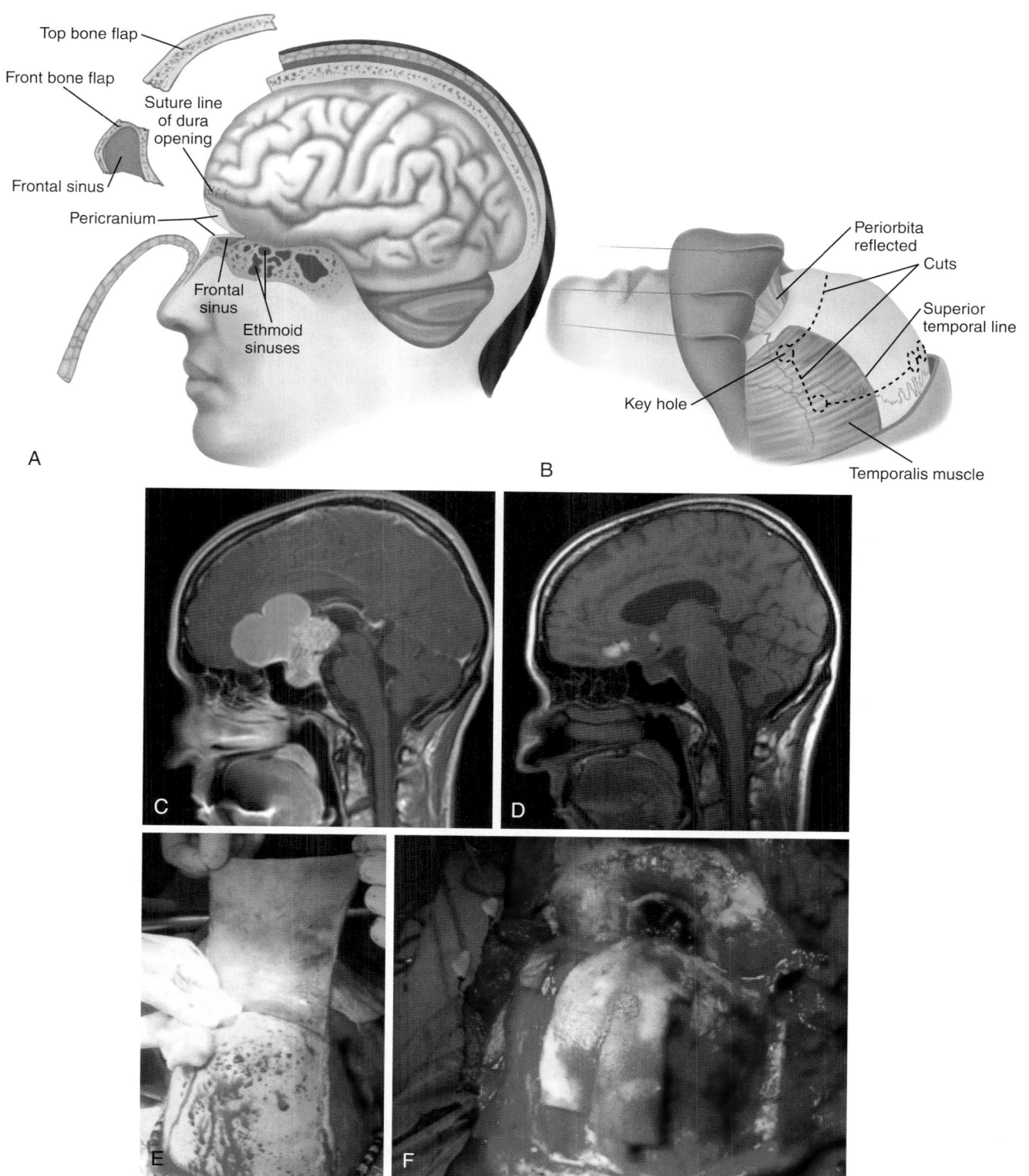

FIGURE 23-3 Bifrontal and extended bifrontal approaches. A, Artist representation of bifrontal and extended bifrontal approaches with removal of frontal bone flap and orbital bar, respectively. B, Artist representation demonstrating scalp reflection forward, and anatomical location of burr holes and craniotomy cuts. C, Preoperative sagittal nonenhanced T1-magnetic resonance image of a pituitary tumor with anterior extension. D, Postoperative MRI demonstrating total tumor removal via a bifrontal approach. E, Intraoperative photo of a pericranial flap elevated off of the superior temporal lines and based anteriorly on the supraorbital rim. F, Intraoperative photo of the extended bifrontal craniotomy with the orbital bar removed. (A and B, redrawn and modified from images by Michael McDermott, MD.)

covered during dissection to prevent dessication. They are then dissected from the pia-arachnoid surface of the frontal lobes. If additional removal of bone from the skull base is required, the olfactory nerves cannot be preserved. Sacrifice of the olfactory nerves allows separation of the dura from the cribriform plate and the crista galli. During dissection, a single silicon-covered brain retractor is utilized to minimize unnecessary, prolonged retraction.

Once the tumor is identified, any feeding vessels in the periphery may be coagulated. Debulking of the tumor helps to dissect the periphery of the tumor without placing significant retraction pressure on the frontal lobes. In cases of extensive skull base bone removal, the sphenoid is removed to expose the sphenoid sinus and superior turbinate. For tumors with significant inferior extension, the clivus may be drilled down while those with extension into the cavernous sinus may be approached by drilling the anterior clinoid process. For large tumors with significant mass effect posteriorly, the posterior margin must be dissected carefully off of the anterior cerebral arteries and anterior communicating artery.

After completion of the tumor resection, the dura is closed with 4-0 Nurolon sutures. The frontal sinus is packed with moist Gelfoam and fibrin glue applied. The pericranial flap is then reflected down over the frontal sinus to create an additional vascularized barrier to prevent CSF leak. The orbital rim is reconstructed by placing small, dog-bone titanium plates laterally, connecting the orbital rim and the zygoma, and medially, reattaching the orbital rim across the nasion. Burr-hole covers are applied over each burr hole and the frontal craniotomy flap reconstructed. The galea and skin flap are then closed in standard fashion.

Supraorbital (Keyhole)

The supraorbital (keyhole) craniotomy has been previously described to approach anterior and middle fossa lesions, and specifically sellar lesions[39-43] (Fig. 23-4). The advantages of this approach are that it requires a smaller incision, a single burr hole, carries a lower risk of injury to neurovascular structures that supply the temporalis muscle, minimizes the need for excessive brain retraction, and results in excellent cosmetic outcomes.[40,41] Pituitary macroadenomas that are confined to the sellar or region or those with minimal parasellar extension can be approached using the supraorbital (keyhole) approach. A supraorbital approach is not appropriate for pituitary tumors with extreme parasellar extension as the exposure is too limited for these tumors.[40,44] The presence of a large frontal sinus on preoperative imaging should discourage the use of this approach as well.[40] Overall, the selection of this approach will depend on the individual tumors and the surgeon's comfort level given that it is not the standard craniotomy for pituitary macroadenomas.[40,41] See Chapter 35 for the technical description of the supraorbital (keyhole) craniotomy.

Radical Combined Transcranial and Trans-Sphenoidal Approach

Occasionally, it is necessary to aim for a complete radical removal of the tumor (e.g., when a tumor has recurred despite radiotherapy). In these circumstances,

following complete removal of the suprasellar component, the tuberculum sella is drilled off between the optic nerves and the optic foramina. The sphenoid sinus is entered, allowing the mucosa to be displaced and the anterior wall of the pituitary fossa to be removed. Removal of the sellar component can be achieved under direct vision except for the ipsilateral intrasellar tumor, which is less visible. Alternatively, a separate trans-sphenoidal approach can be carried out; that has the advantage of better bilateral tumor exposure, but it also has the disadvantage of possibly failing to see remaining tumor superiorly. Whichever method the surgeon uses, particular care must be taken to achieve a tight CSF closure with obliteration of the sphenoid sinus.

The first is if a previous trans-sphenoidal operation has been performed and an inadequate obliteration of the sphenoid sinus has been achieved. Previous sections have alluded to the necessity to obliterate the sphenoid sinus during a trans-sphenoidal approach when a transcranial procedure is clearly going to be necessary in the future. This necessity exists even when no CSF is seen. Failure to do so means that CSF rhinorrhea is extremely likely to occur after the transcranial approach, because the dural lining of the pituitary fossa has been penetrated during the trans-sphenoidal approach. In these circumstances, fascia and fat may be introduced into the pituitary fossa transcranially, but it is not easy to obtain a watertight closure this way. The second circumstance in which CSF rhinorrhea may be seen is when bone is drilled away from the skull base, thus entering an extension of the sphenoid sinus. If recognized, a fat and fascia repair is necessary. Rhinorrhea usually ensues when such an occurrence has not been recognized.

Complications

FRONTAL LOBE DAMAGE

Frontal lobe damage is perhaps the most common complication, although it is often unappreciated because its manifestations may be subtle. Frontal lobe damage is particularly likely to occur in the elderly, and is caused by excessive frontal lobe retraction. The elderly take longer to recover from this surgery than from trans-sphenoidal surgery. There may be subtle changes of memory, judgment (on a social or professional level), concentration, and personality. These changes can be minimized by gentle surgical technique and, especially, by minimal brain retraction. A pattie or cotton strip should always be placed between the brain and the retractor. The retractor should be moved often, and should be removed when it is not needed. Splitting the sylvian fissure to separate the frontal and temporal lobes also minimizes the amount of retraction. If there is evidence of an area of soft, blue brain at the end of the operation, the surgeon should beware: this area may represent hemorrhagic infarction, which often causes postoperative bleeding and deterioration. Such areas should be removed surgically before closing the dura.

FRONTAL LOBE CYST FORMATION

Cystic enlargement of an area of frontal lobe damage, sufficient to act as a space-occupying lesion, may occur. Adams described one such case and speculated on the causal mechanism.[19,45]

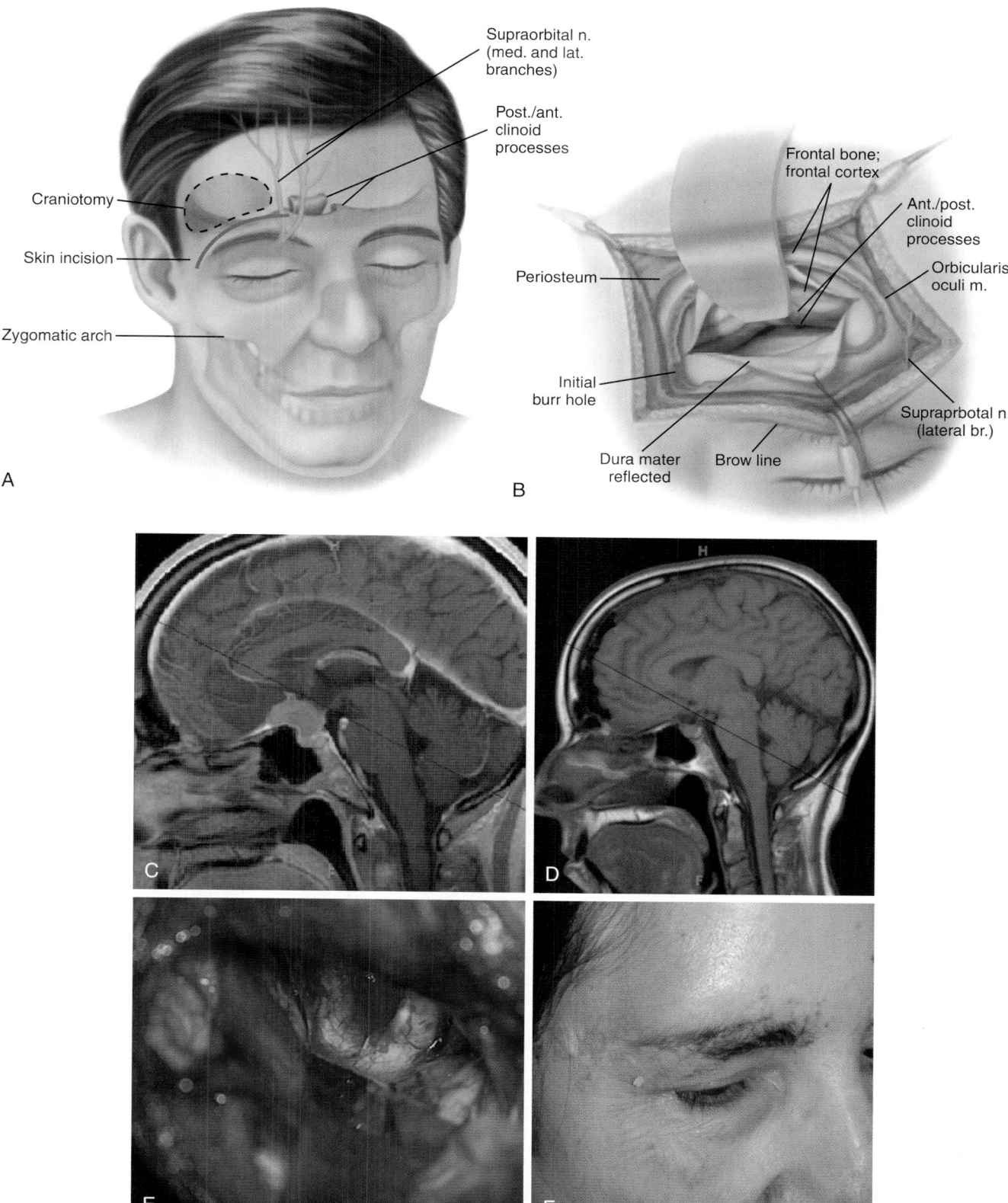

FIGURE 23-4 Supraorbital (keyhole) approach. A, Artist rendering of the skin incision and craniotomy. B, Anatomic dissection and exposure with single brain retractor placed under the frontal lobe C, Preoperative sagittal T1-magnetic resonance image of a pituitary tumor with minimal supra-sellar extension. D, Postoperative MRI demonstrating tumor removal via a supraorbital approach. E, Intraoperative view of the optic chiasm F, Skin closure following surgery. (A and B, redrawn from Jallo GI, Bognár L. Eyebrow surgery: the supraciliary craniotomy: technical note. Neurosurgery. 2006;59[Suppl 1]:ONSE157-158.)

ANOSMIA

Unilateral or bilateral anosmia often reflects the vigor of frontal lobe retraction. If there is a significant subfrontal extension of the pituitary tumor, anosmia is inevitable.

PERIOPERATIVE OPTIC NERVE DAMAGE

If an eye is blind preoperatively, it will not recover postoperatively. If vision is severely impaired preoperatively, it is also unlikely to recover. If an already-damaged optic nerve is manipulated at all, vision is likely to be lost altogether postoperatively. The patient should be thus warned.

The most vulnerable nerve is the ipsilateral optic nerve. The rule is not to touch or manipulate it, but this is rarely possible to achieve. Before teasing tumor away, the tumor should be debulked as much as possible; only at the last stage, when space has been created, should the remaining tumor be rolled away from the optic nerve. Meningiomas creep down the optic foramen, but in the authors' experience, pituitary tumors do not behave in that fashion.

The blood supply of the optic nerves and chiasm varies. The chiasm is supplied by small vessels from the anterior communicating artery, and these must be preserved. The rule is not to coagulate or cut any significant-looking vessel running to the chiasm or optic nerves. In general, however, it is suspected that manipulation of these structures, rather than ischemia, that usually causes the damage.

DAMAGE TO INTERNAL CAROTID, ANTERIOR CEREBRAL, OR ANTERIOR COMMUNICATING ARTERIES

The previous author of this chapter described the unpleasant occasion of cutting an internal carotid artery.[19] The patient was elderly, had undergone two previous craniotomies and radiotherapy for the pituitary tumor, and the artery was embedded in scar tissue. Although the artery was not visible, it should have been traced proximally from the middle cerebral artery. This tracing can be extremely difficult. On another occasion, he described damaging both anterior cerebral arteries. The tumor was firmly adherent to these vessels, and in hindsight the author stated he should have stopped the operation, leaving tumor behind around the vessels.

The literature describes such vascular damage repaired by fine sutures. Placing aneurysm clips so as to occlude the hole in the vessel without occluding the vessel has occasionally worked; usually, however, the vessel has to be occluded to stop the bleeding.

Occasionally a small vessel is pulled out of the side of a larger vessel. It can be difficult to stop the bleeding, but by placing the finest bipolar forceps on either side of the hole and using low bipolar coagulation, the hole is sealed without occluding the main vessel.

HYPOTHALAMIC DAMAGE

Hypothalamic damage is rare after removal of a pituitary adenoma, but it is easily caused by overenthusiastic removal of a craniopharyngioma. With hypothalamic damage, the patient loses the senses of thirst and hunger. Fluid control can be achieved only by weighing the patient, and excessive weight gain is usual. Hypothalamic wasting or precocious puberty occurs in the presence of tumors (usually hypothalamic gliomas) and not after surgical trauma. To remove or not to remove a craniopharyngioma intimately involved in the hypothalamus demands the finest surgical judgment to balance the desire to achieve a total removal with the need to avoid devastating hypothalamic damage.

PITUITARY DAMAGE, INCLUDING DIABETES INSIPIDUS

Damage to anterior pituitary function is common after transfrontal surgery because the normal pituitary gland is usually pushed superiorly against the diaphragma sella, rather like a rind around the tumor. The diaphragma is the first thing to be coagulated and cut when removing such tumor transcranially, hence destroying normal function. Pituitary hormone replacement therapy maintains reasonable health, but the patient never returns to normal. The patient seems sluggish, both physically and mentally, and gains weight. The standard hormone replacement therapy does not include growth hormone or other hormones given in the physiologically pulsatile fashion.

Fluids should be restricted to 2 l/day for 48 hours postoperatively. A postoperative diuresis is normal, especially in patients cured of acromegaly. If the urinary output is more than 200 ml/hr for 3 hours, plasma and urinary osmolalities are measured. If the former is increased and the latter is less than 295 mOsm/kg, desmopressin should be administered. The osmolality measurements should be repeated in 24 hours.

SALT-WASTING SYNDROME

Salt-wasting syndrome is rare. The syndrome is also alarming, and usually occurs 1 to 2 weeks after the operation.[4-7] Surgeons have described their patients developing a headache, rapidly lapsing into a coma, and on admission presenting with a low sodium value. The mechanism is unknown, but salt-wasting syndrome is assumed to be caused by inappropriate antidiuretic hormone secretion. It is difficult to measure antidiuretic hormone, and so not enough is known about this rare condition. It is advisable to place a central venous line to determine if the problem is primarily low sodium (low venous pressure) or water overload (high venous pressure). Patients should be treated empirically with rapid infusions of fluids and salt, then restricted fluids to increase the serum sodium. Until more is known about this mysterious condition, it can be treated only empirically. Kelly and colleagues[46] recommend using urea for salt-wasting syndrome, pointing out that urea enhances sodium reabsorption at the kidney.

POSTOPERATIVE VISUAL DETERIORATION

Acute visual deterioration within hours of surgery is usually caused by a postoperative hematoma in the tumor cavity. The best way to avoid this situation is to be sure to remove the tumor in its entirety. If, however, the tumor invades the clivus, bleeding from the cancellous bone can be difficult to stop, although bone wax, Surgicel, and patience are usually sufficient. Reoperation is necessary.

Olson and co-workers[47] have described acute deterioration after trans-sphenoidal surgery resulting from herniation of a chiasm into the pituitary fossa. This condition is amazingly rare, considering how, after trans-sphenoidal surgery, the diaphragma rapidly descends to the floor of the pituitary fossa on many occasions without visual impairment. The question can be asked if herniation per se (apart from the case reported by Olson and co-workers) can cause visual deterioration.

Occasionally, a unilateral loss of vision occurs about 8 days after surgery. Morello and Frera[48] describe a patient, and the author agrees with their conclusion that ischemic damage is the most likely explanation. Insidious visual deterioration is almost always caused by recurrent tumor, which usually reproduces the original visual field deficit (i.e., a bitemporal hemianopia). Another possibility is radiation damage to the optic nerves or chiasm after radiotherapy. This visual deterioration usually occurs 9 to 18 months after radiotherapy and is often sudden and unilateral. The mechanism is vascular damage and hence similar to stroke. Some improvement may occur. Guy and colleagues[49] suggest gadolinium-enhanced MRI scanning to confirm the diagnosis of radiation damage.

KEY REFERENCES

Couldwell WT. Transsphenoidal and transcranial surgery for pituitary adenomas. *J Neurooncol.* 2004;69:237-256.

Couldwell WT, Simard MF, Weiss MH, Norton JA. Pituitary and adrenal. In: Schwartz SI, Shires GT, Spencer FC, eds. *Principles of Surgery.* 7th ed. New York: McGraw-Hill; 1999:1613-1658.

Czirjak S, Szeifert GT. Surgical experience with frontolateral keyhole craniotomy through a superciliary skin incision. *Neurosurgery.* 2001;48:145-149:discussion 9-50.

Day JD. Surgical approaches to suprasellar and parasellar tumors. *Neurosurg Clin North Am.* 2003;14:109-122.

Derome P. Transbasal approach to tumors invading the skull base. In: Schmidek H, Sweet W, eds. *Operative Neurosurgical Techniques Indications, Methods, and Results.* 4th ed. Philadelphia: WB Saunders Company; 1993:427-441.

Frazier C. An approach to the hypophysis through the anterior cranial fossa. *Ann Surg.* 1913;7:145-150.

Hakuba A, Liu S, Nishimura S. The orbitozygomatic infratemporal approach: a new surgical technique. *Surgical Neurol.* 1986;26:271-276.

Hayashi N, Hirashima Y, Kurimoto M, et al. One-piece pedunculated frontotemporal orbitozygomatic craniotomy by creation of a subperiosteal tunnel beneath the temporal muscle: technical note. *Neurosurgery.* 2002;51:1520-1523:discussion 1523-1524.

Henderson WR. The pituitary adenomata. A follow-up study of the surgical results in 338 cases (Dr. Harvey Cushing's series). *Br J Surg.* 1939;26:811-921.

Jallo GI, Bognar L. Eyebrow surgery: the supraciliary craniotomy: technical note. *Neurosurgery.* 2006;59:ONSE157-ONSE158:discussion ONSE-8.

Jallo GI, Suk I, Bognar L. A superciliary approach for anterior cranial fossa lesions in children. Technical note. *J Neurosurg.* 2005;103:88-93.

Jane JA, Park TS, Pobereskin LH, Winn HR, Butler AB. The supraorbital approach: technical note. *Neurosurgery.* 1982;11:537-542.

Kadri PA, Al-Mefty O. The anatomical basis for surgical preservation of temporal muscle. *J Neurosurg.* 2004;100:517-522.

Kelly DF, Laws Jr ER, Fossett D. Delayed hyponatremia after transsphenoidal surgery for pituitary adenoma: report of nine cases. *J Neurosurg.* 1995;83:363-367.

Liu JK, Weiss MH, Couldwell WT. Surgical approaches to pituitary tumors. *Neurosurg Clin North Am.* 2003;14:93-107.

Musleh W, Sonabend AM, Lesniak MS. Role of craniotomy in the management of pituitary adenomas and sellar/parasellar tumors. *Expert Rev Anticancer Ther.* 2006;6(suppl 9):S79-S83.

Pellerin P, Lesoin F, Dhellemmes P, et al. Usefulness of the orbitofronto-malar approach associated with bone reconstruction for frontotemporosphenoid meningiomas. *Neurosurgery.* 1984;15:715-718.

Raza SM, Thai QA, Pradilla G, Tamargo RJ. Frontozygomatic titanium cranioplasty in frontosphenotemporal ("pterional") craniotomy. *Neurosurgery.* 2008;62:262-264:discussion 4-5.

Rhoton Jr AL, Hardy DG, Chambers SM. Microsurgical anatomy and dissection of the sphenoid bone, cavernous sinus and sellar region. *Surg Neurol.* 1979;12:63-104.

Sanchez-Vazquez MA, Barrera-Calatayud P, Mejia-Villela M, et al. Transciliary subfrontal craniotomy for anterior skull base lesions. Technical note. *J Neurosurg.* 1999;91:892-896.

Shimizu S, Tanriover N, Rhoton Jr AL, et al. MacCarty keyhole and inferior orbital fissure in orbitozygomatic craniotomy. *Neurosurgery.* 2005;57:152-159:discussion 159.

Tessier P, Guiot G, Derome P. Orbital hypertelorism. II. Definite treatment of orbital hypertelorism (OR.H.) by craniofacial or by extracranial osteotomies. *Scand J Plast Reconstr Surg.* 1973;7:39-58.

van Lindert E, Perneczky A, Fries G, Pierangeli E. The supraorbital keyhole approach to supratentorial aneurysms: concept and technique. *Surg Neurol.* 1998;49:481-489:discussion 489-490.

Vishteh A, Marciano F, David C, et al. The pterional approach. *Oper Tech Neurosurg.* 1998;1:39-49.

Youssef AS, Agazzi S, van Loveren HR. Transcranial surgery for pituitary adenomas. *Neurosurgery.* 2005;57:168-175:discussion 168-175.

Numbered references appear on Expert Consult.

CHAPTER 24

Craniopharyngiomas

PHILIP V. THEODOSOPOULOS • MICHAEL E. SUGHRUE •
MICHAEL W. McDERMOTT

Craniopharyngiomas are tumors of neuroepithelial origin that arise from squamous cell rests found along the path of the primitive craniopharyngeal duct. Their incidence ranges between 0.5 and 2.5 per 100,000 person years and does not vary by sex or race. Craniopharyngiomas account for 1.2% to 4.6% of all intracranial tumors (Central Brain Tumor Registry of the United States). They exhibit a bimodal distribution, first peaking during childhood (5–14 years) and later peaking in adults ranging from 50 to 74 years; they comprise 5% to 10% of pediatric brain tumors and 1% to 4% of adult brain tumors.[1-4] Craniopharyngiomas have a growth pattern that is often in close proximity to the pituitary infundibulum, and can occur within the sella, suprasellar space, or third ventricle, frequently spanning these spaces. These tumors tend to involve a number of neural structures, including the optic nerves, internal carotid arteries (ICAs), and pituitary gland, causing a variety of symptoms. Common clinical presentations include visual dysfunction with symptoms of chiasmatic as well as postchiasmatic compression, hypothalamic dysfunction with behavioral changes ranging from alterations in eating patterns, to apathy, and even obtundation and pituitary dysfunction, often manifesting as hypopituitarism.

During the past several years, treatment algorithms have evolved that now incorporate multiple modalities. Surgical resection remains the primary treatment whenever possible. However, the suprasellar space is replete with important neurovascular structures that include the perforator arteries supplying the optic chiasm, hypothalamus, and basal ganglia; their interruption results in permanent neurologic loss of function and disability. Proven therapies with low morbidities include nonradical surgical resection followed by fractionated radiation therapy, radiosurgery, cystic lesion aspiration with implantation of Ommaya reservoir for intracavitary radioisotope, or chemotherapy instillation. More recently, surgical resection via an expanded trans-sphenoidal resection has been advocated as the most direct route to the bulk of the lesion. Although the access provided through this corridor is unparalleled, this technique remains in development because of the lack of appropriate instrumentation to allow safe dissection and the difficulty in providing a watertight closure.

The natural history of craniopharyngiomas following treatment is one of recurrence. The need for re-treatment arises when these indolent lesions that exhibit slow growth in both their solid and cystic components become symptomatic at various times during a patient's lifetime.

Classification

Several authors who attempted to radiographically classify craniopharyngiomas include Rougerie, Pertuiset, Konovalov, Steno, Hoffman, Samii, and Kassam.[5-11] Although none have been universally adopted, these classifications all share the principle of subdividing lesions along the length of extension in the primary vertical axis; the resulting relationship is with the optic chiasm and the third ventricular floor immediately posterior to it.

Histologically, craniopharyngiomas are divided into adamantinomatous, papillary, and mixed. The most common form is adamantinomatous, which is often cystic and filled with dark fluid. Columnar or polygonal squamous cells with nuclear palisading arranged in broad bands, cords, and bridges with nodules of compact keratin and dystrophic calcifications are characteristic of the adamantinomatous type (World Health Organization). The wet keratin contrasts with the lamellar flaky keratin in epidermoid cysts. In contrast, papillary craniopharyngiomas consist of sheets of squamous cells that form papillae, lacking nuclear palisading, wet keratin, calcification, and cholesterol deposits.

Anatomy

Craniopharyngiomas arise in the parasellar space involving the sella, suprasellar space, and third ventricle. Unlike pituitary tumors, they often adhere to the neurovascular structures of the suprasellar space. Perforating vessels, arising from the anterior communicating artery as well as the proximal ICA, coat the tumor capsule anteriorly as they course toward the optic chiasm and anterior perforating substance. On their way to the basal ganglia and thalamus, laterally and posteriorly perforating vessels that originate from the posterior communicating artery and infrequently from the proximal posterior cerebral arteries are found adherent to the tumor capsule. This close anatomic relationship with vascular structures is an important factor that limits the extent of surgical respectability.

Another important limiting factor during surgical resection is the close apposition of craniopharyngiomas to the pituitary infundibulum. This opposition has led some to argue that gross total resection cannot be achieved without the section and removal of the involved part of the infundibulum. Although this point remains contested, the morbidity of sacrificing the infundibulum is significant, particularly in pediatric patients.[12-19] Diabetes insipidus and hypopituitarism after injury to the infundibulum can impact both the physical and mental growth of patients and limit their daily functional capacity.

Treatment Decision Making

The primary treatment of craniopharyngiomas remains surgical. The variability of the tumor extent make is imperative to tailor the surgical approach to the particular lesion. Of several different approaches described, no approach is overall preferred for the majority of the lesions. Adjuvant treatment with radiation therapy is often used; it is necessary in all cases when gross total resection is not achieved and in some tumor recurrences that appear after apparent gross total resection and are likely the result of microscopic residual disease.

Although most patients undergo both surgical and radiation treatments, a number of questions need to be addressed on an individual level. Choice of surgical approach depends primarily on the extent of the lesion along the vertical axis (Fig. 24-1). Lesions that are purely intrasellar are preferably approached through a trans-sphenoidal approach. Microscopic or endoscopic corridors have been well described and mimic the approach to pituitary adenomas. Because intrasellar lesions are often cystic, obliteration of the tumor cavity with fat may not be indicated unless a cerebrospinal fluid (CSF) leak is manifested intraoperatively, effectively allowing for a prolonged outlet that can delay or prevent future reaccumulation of fluid within the cavity. The trans-sphenoidal route can also be used successfully in the presence of significant suprasellar extension in mostly cystic lesions. The recent development of expanded endoscopic trans-sphenoidal approaches to the sella make the resection of the cyst wall possible when vascular adherence is not a significant issue.

Lesions with significant suprasellar extension, particularly when mostly solid, are preferably approached through intracranial corridors. Although expanded endoscopic trans-sphenoidal approaches can provide effective tumor resection, they are considered alternative approaches because of the dearth of appropriate instrumentation, which can cause difficulty in safely managing intraoperative bleeding. Additionally, the dural opening immediately inferior to the suprasellar cistern has proven to be difficult to seal effectively against CSF leaks. Finally, most lesions that are primarily suprasellar arise superior to the pituitary gland, displacing it inferiorly, making the mobilization of the gland itself a necessity for access to the lesion through a trans-sphenoidal route, a surgical maneuver that can result in hypopituitarism.

Transcranial routes to the suprasellar space range from a supraorbital corridor to the pterional approach (with or without an orbital or orbitozygomatic osteotomy) to the bifrontal craniotomy. Although each one of these approaches provides a similar exposure to lesions in the suprasellar space, they differ in several important ways. The supraorbital craniotomy, which minimizes soft-tissue morbidity and creates a shorter overall incision, is limited by the size of the frontal sinus. Violation of the frontal

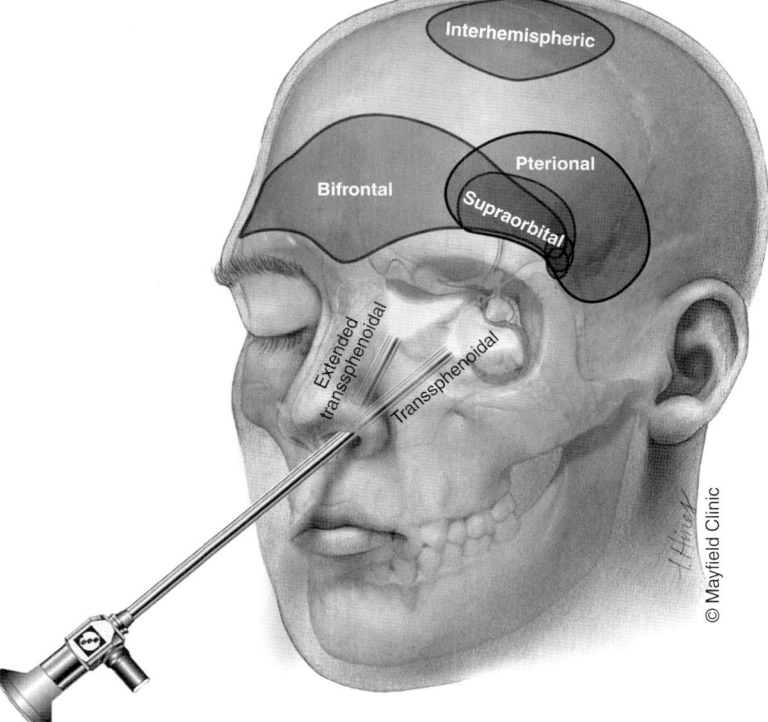

FIGURE 24-1 Approaches to the anterior fossa and sellar region include the trans-sphenoidal, extended trans-sphenoidal, bifrontal, interhemispheric, pterional, and supraorbital. *(From Mayfield Clinic, Cincinnati, OH.)*

sinus through the supraorbital approach can cause a CSF leak that is challenging to fix or a rotation periosteal flap is difficult. Additional limitations of the supraorbital craniotomy include the limited vertical exposure and difficulty with effective brain retraction.

The bifrontal subfrontal approach allows for a midline or medial exposure to the suprasellar space and can be the most effective in the presence of a post-fixed chiasm. Conversely, a prefixed chiasm is a limitation that may make access to the lesion all but impossible. Close study of preoperative imaging may give some indication to the location of the chiasm. Specifically, assessment can involve both direct visualization of the chiasm in the absence of severe distortion of normal anatomy and determination of the position of the anterior communicating artery as a surrogate for the location of the chiasm. Nonetheless, large lesions often make it difficult to ascertain the exact position of the chiasm preoperatively; in such cases, this approach can be limiting.

The pterional approach is the most versatile for accessing the majority of craniopharyngiomas. It allows for working channels in between the two optic nerves, between the optic nerve and ICA, and between the ICA and oculomotor nerve. The pterional approach is the one most often used for removal of the optic canal roof and anterior clinoid process, steps often necessary for safe mobilization of the optic nerve. The limitation of this approach relates to the location of the ipsilateral optic nerve in the direct line of sight; that is, resection of a significant part of the tumor deep to the nerve is difficult without substantial mobilization of the nerve itself.

Tumors that extend extensively into the third ventricle or infrequently arise primarily in the third ventricle pose the greatest surgical challenge, particularly when a significant cystic tumor component is absent. The two major corridors to such lesions are the translamina terminalis approach and the transventricular approach. The lamina terminalis forms the superior continuation of the optic chiasm; its fenestration allows for entry into the anterior third ventricle. It provides direct access to the anterior part of the lesion, yet is limited by the amount of retraction of the optic tracts and the anterior communicating artery necessary for visualization into the third ventricle. In large lesions, determination if a plane of safe dissection exists between the lateral walls of the tumor and hypothalamus can also be challenging. This determination is particularly difficult through a pterional approach that leads to blind dissection of the ipsilateral tumor margin.

Transventricular approaches are the most versatile to access large lesions within the third ventricle. A transfrontal or interhemispheric approach can be used to access the lateral ventricle. A transforaminal approach expanded through a subchoroidal extension provides wide access into the third ventricle and good visualization of the lateral margins of the lesion. Limitations of this approach are the significant depth at which the lesion is encountered, the thalamostriate vein that needs to be mobilized, and the potential for injury to the fornices.

Radiation therapy is often used as adjuvant therapy. However, a good indication for its use as primary treatment is the rare case of a solid third ventricular lesion with evidence of poor margins with the hypothalamus in an older patient. The radiation delivery method varies depending on the tumor's size and characteristics. The usual limitations for radiosurgical treatment, relating to both lesion size and proximity to the optic apparatus, hold true and often lead to the need for fractionated treatment.

For primarily cystic tumors, stereotactic- or endoscopic-transventricular cyst aspiration through an implanted catheter can allow for intracystic instillation of radioactive material or chemotherapy as well as subsequent percutaneous aspirations of fluid re-accumulation.

Surgical Techniques

TRANS-SPHENOIDAL/EXPANDED TRANS-SPHENOIDAL APPROACH

The patient is positioned supine; the head in the "sniffing" position allows for elevation above the level of the heart and drainage of bloody material inferiorly away from the surgical field. The traditional trans-sphenoidal approach through a microscopic or endoscopic approach can be used. Intrasellar tumors and mostly cystic craniopharyngiomas even with a significant suprasellar extension are excellent candidates for this approach (Fig. 24-2).

The expanded trans-sphenoidal approach requires significant bony removal superiorly past the tuberculum. Importantly, at the beginning of an expanded trans-sphenoidal approach, consideration should be given to raising a nasoseptal mucosal flap, which will be used during closure.[20] Visualization of the superior aspect of the lesion and its relationship to the undersurface of the optic chiasm is feasible with debulking of the tumor. The perforating vessels and the plane with the optic apparatus need to be sharply dissected under direct vision. However, present endoscopic instrumentation creates an obstacle to effective dissection in many patients.

Closure of a traditional or expanded trans-sphenoidal approach has important considerations. Intrasellar lesion resection can be associated with CSF leaks. Obliteration of the sella with abdominal fat grafting is our preferred reconstruction technique; it is reinforced by bone or cartilage obtained during the exposure and by tissue sealant onlay over the entire reconstruction. In the absence of a CSF leak, one may consider leaving the sella open to delay or obviate the re-accumulation of fluid within the cyst. Caution should be used in making this decision depending on the amount of arachnoid descent and herniation within the sella because a delayed CSF leak may ensue.

Although a watertight closure of expanded trans-sphenoidal approaches remains elusive, significant steps have been made during the past several years. Simple fat obliteration proves to be inadequate reconstruction. Multilayer reconstructions and the use of vascularized pedicled mucosal flaps have been promising as an effective reconstruction that can prevent leaks. Use of specialized clips that attempt direct dural reapproximation is an obvious improvement, yet technically very challenging. Deployment of inflatable balloons within the sphenoid sinus can augment the reconstruction. Lumbar subarachnoid drains for temporary CSF diversion offer mechanical advantages but must be balanced by their risk of potential complications,

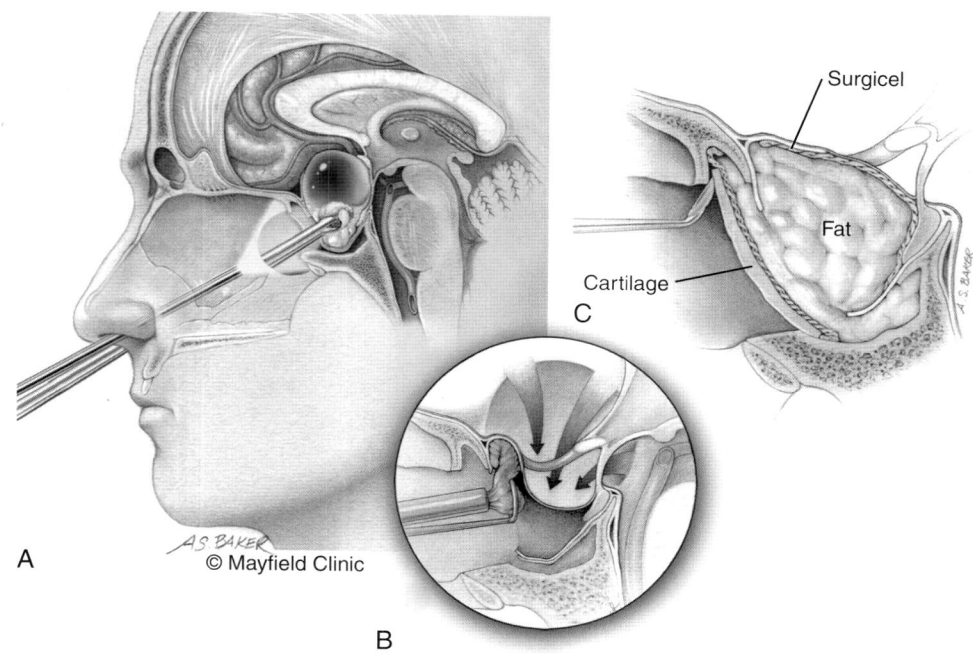

FIGURE 24-2 The trans-sphenoidal approach may be used for craniopharyngiomas that are primarily intrasellar or when the suprasellar component is cystic. A, An endoscope is inserted through one nostril and instruments are passed through the other nostril. A small portion of the posterior nasal septum is removed and the sphenoid sinus is opened. An opening is made in the sella to expose the tumor. Using curettes and suction, the surgeon debulks and removes the solid portion of the craniopharyngioma. B, Dissection into the cystic portion will release the fluid contents, then decompressing the optic nerves and vascular structures in the suprasellar space. C, The sella is lined with Surgicel and filled with fat harvested from the abdomen. Because the sella does not often support primary closure, the sphenoid sinus is obliterated with fat and closed with cartilage or cortical bone *(From Mayfield Clinic, Cincinnati, OH.)*

compression of neurovascular structures for the former, and development of pneumocephalus for the latter.

BIFRONTAL CRANIOTOMY

The patient is positioned supine with the head slightly extended in three-point pin fixation in the Mayfield clamp. Frameless stereotactic guidance is a useful adjunct for accurate localization of the lesion. A bifrontal incision is marked behind the hairline. Ensuring that the lateral limits are close to the zygomas bilaterally then limits the pressure on the skin flap and avoids flap ischemia. Burr holes are placed on either side of the superior sagittal sinus, approximately 5 cm above the nasion and laterally superior to the keyhole, just lateral to the superior insertion of the temporalis muscle, which is elevated in a limited fashion. The inferior bony cut is preferably made just superior to the frontal sinus; however, transgression of the sinus can be fixed easily with the use of a rotational pericranial flap. The dura is opened in a horizontal incision inferiorly and the superior sagittal sinus is divided with medium vascular clips. The falx is incised and the anterior interhemispheric space is explored (Fig. 24-3).

Once the lesion is localized, its relationship to the optic nerves and chiasm is assessed. A prefixed location of the chiasm is a limitation of this approach. In the absence of significant extension into the third ventricle, drilling the tuberculum often allows for increased exposure subchiasmatically. Although exposure is potentially adequate for resection of the lesion, this is a limited corridor for large lesions. Reconstruction of the skull base is crucial for a good outcome.

The anterior interhemispheric approach is perhaps the optimal approach for lesions with extension into the third ventricle. After exposing the chiasm, the surgeon identifies the lamina terminalis, dissects and gently retracts the anterior communicating artery superiorly, and a fenestration into the third ventricle. A midline fenestration at the thinnest area, as far superior to the chiasm as feasible, is most desirable. Correct identification of the optic nerves and optic tracts bilaterally is the safest way to avoid injury to the visual system.

Dissection of the tumor from the third ventricle can be safely achieved through the fenestration of the lamina terminalis. The principles that ensure safety and improved outcome are careful identification of the visual apparatus and careful dissection of the lateral margin of the tumor from the hypothalamus. In cases where the plane between the tumor and the lateral wall of third ventricle is not directly visible or absent, one needs to exercise caution to avoid hypothalamic dysfunction.

PTERIONAL CRANIOTOMY

The traditional frontotemporal or pterional craniotomy is perhaps the most widely used approach for the treatment of craniopharyngiomas. Reduction of the sphenoid wing is a standard part of this approach because it improves exposure superiorly. Once the basal cisterns are opened, there are two major corridors for lesion resection: the subchiasmatic corridor between the two optic nerves and the opticocarotid corridor between the lateral aspect of the ipsilateral optic nerve and ICA (Fig. 24-4).

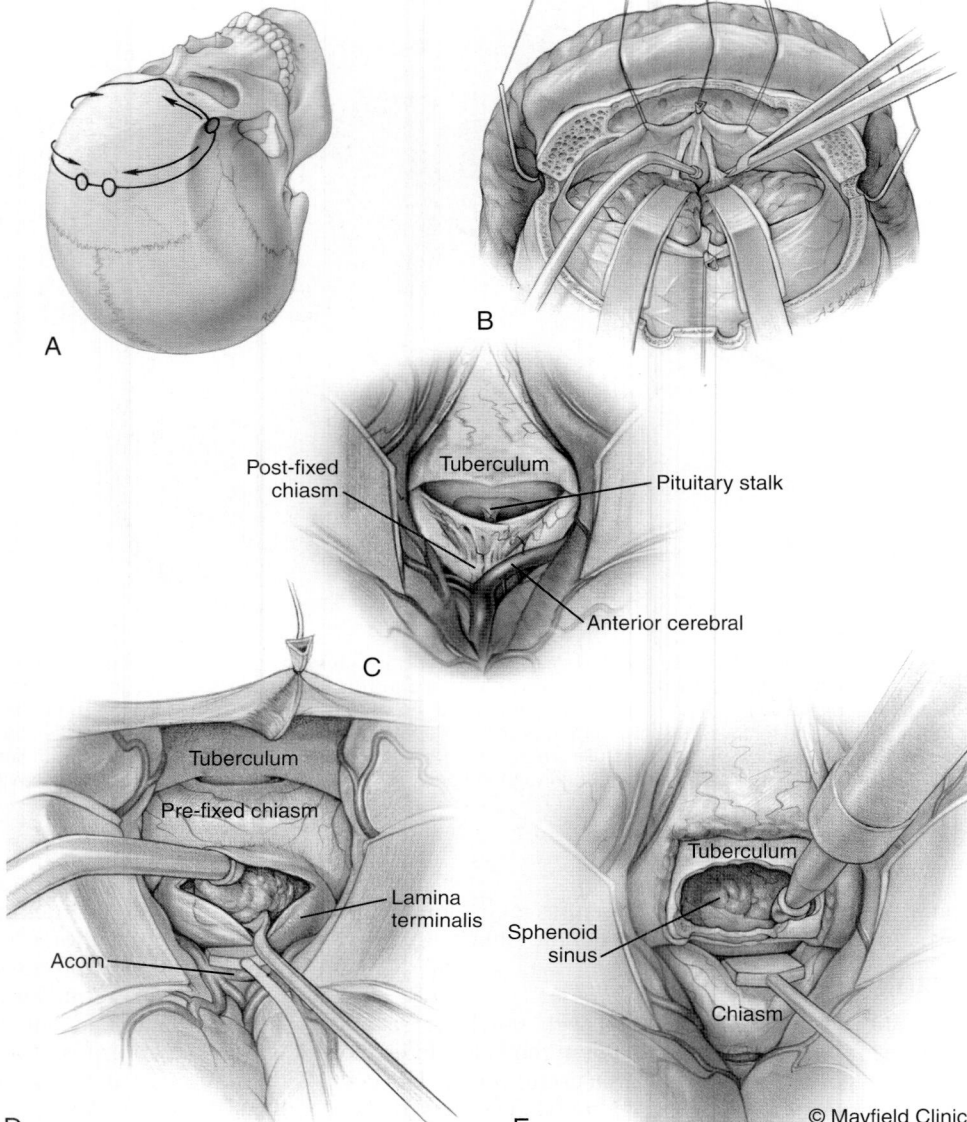

FIGURE 24-3 The bifrontal interhemispheric approach may be used for craniopharyngiomas in the suprasellar space and is most effective when a post-fixed chiasm is found. A, Bilateral burr holes are made at the pterion, and two additional burr holes are made on either side of the superior sagittal sinus. After a bone flap is cut to connect the burr holes, the posterior wall of the frontal sinus is down-fractured and the flap is removed. The dura is opened and the superior sagittal sinus is tied off and cut. The dural cut is extended down the falx until released. B, The frontal lobes are retracted and adhesions to the olfactory tracts separated. C, The anterior cerebral arteries and optic chiasm are identified and tumor is removed. D, If the tumor growth has prefixed the chiasm, entry into the lamina terminalis exposes tumor in the third ventricle. E, If the tumor growth extends inferiorly, the bone of the tuberculum sella can be drilled to access and remove tumor from the sphenoid sinus. *(From Mayfield Clinic, Cincinnati, OH.)*

This approach is familiar to most neurosurgeons, yet its relative limitation is that the lesion lies posterior to the ipsilateral optic nerve, which often is displaced anteriorly and superiorly as it is splayed over the tumor surface. Manipulation of the ipsilateral optic nerve is a maneuver that endangers visual function. Therefore, one needs to resist the temptation to mobilize the optic nerve for enhanced tumor exposure. Section of the falciform ligament and fenestration of the optic canal, and less often anterior clinoidectomy, are surgical adjuncts that minimize the risk to the ipsilateral vision.

The pterional approach allows for direct visualization of the microvasculature surrounding the lesion in the suprasellar cistern. Careful dissection of perforating vessels from the mesial wall of the ICA and the anterior cerebral artery prevents vascular injury to the anterior perforating substance, basal ganglia, hypothalamus, and visual system. The pterional approach is also a versatile one. An orbital osteotomy allows for wide access and improvement in the superior aspect of the surgical exposure. Dissection along the ipsilateral optic nerve and chiasm allows for fenestration of the lamina terminalis and access to the part of the lesion extending into the third ventricle. Care should be taken to correctly identify the location of the lamina terminalis. The 15- to 45-degree rotation off the vertical axis can disorient the surgeon with respect to midline, particularly at depth. Confirmation of midline anatomically is crucial with respect to the anterior communicating artery as well as with the use of frameless stereotactic guidance. Off-midline fenestration may result in both poor access to the lesion and injury to the visual system and hypothalamus.

The supraorbital craniotomy and its transorbital variant provide a similar degree of exposure with somewhat limited soft tissue dissection (Fig. 24-4B). The temporalis muscle is mobilized to a much lesser degree. With the incision is linear within the eyebrow, there is little need for subcutaneous dissection. The bone flap, which averages 3 × 2 cm, provides adequate access to most lesions in the

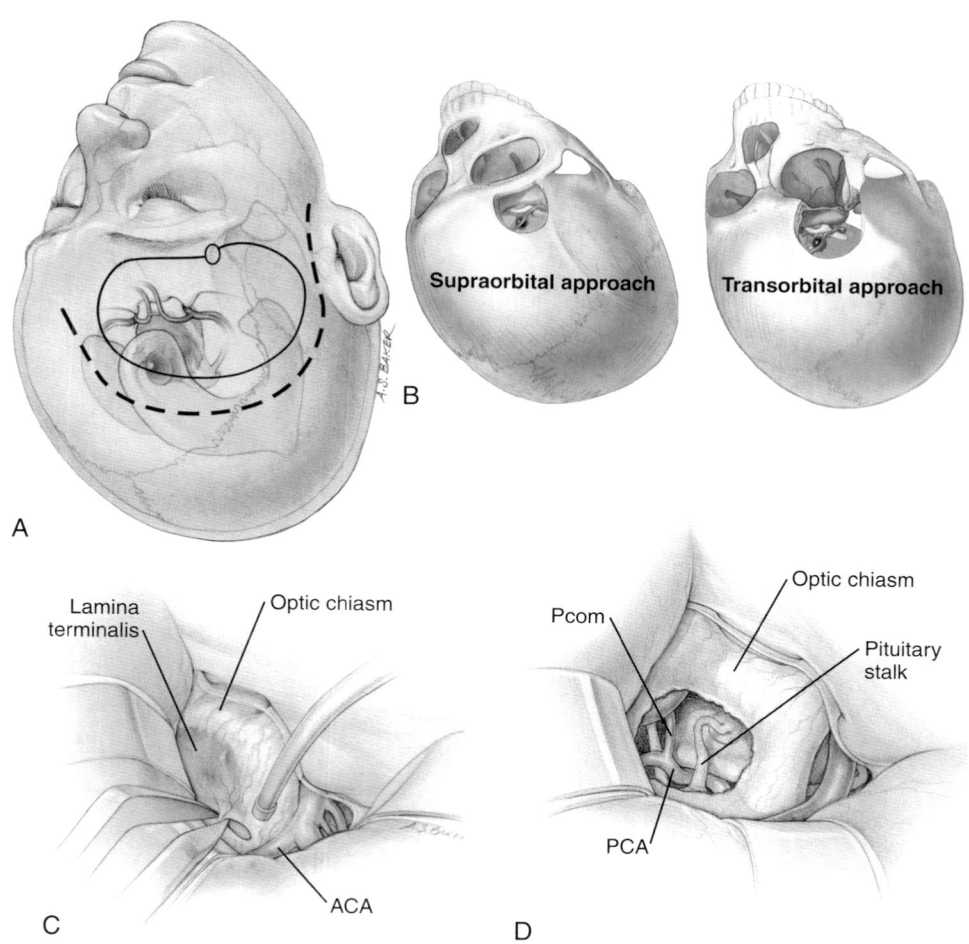

FIGURE 24-4 The pterional approach is the most versatile to access craniopharyngiomas by allowing the surgeon to work in between the two optic nerves, between the optic nerve and ICA, and between the ICA and oculomotor nerve. A, After a question-mark skin incision is made, a burr hole is placed at the anterior aspect of the superior temporal line. A bone flap is cut with a craniotome and removed. B, View of supraorbital and transorbital keyhole craniotomies. C, The dura is opened and retractors are used to access the optic nerve and chiasmatic cistern. A bipolar is used to coagulate tiny vessels and the lamina terminalis is opened. D, Tumor removal can be accomplished from the third ventricle and suprasellar space with preservation of the pituitary stalk. (From Mayfield Clinic, Cincinnati, OH.)

parasellar space. Care should be taken to avoid injury to the frontalis branch of the facial nerve along the lateral aspect of the incision. The use of frameless stereotactic guidance is recommended to prevent violation of the lateral recess of the frontal sinus. Reconstruction of the sinus from this approach is limited and may result in a transnasal CSF leak that can prove difficult to seal. In our practice, an extensive lateral recess of the frontal sinus is a contraindication for this approach.

TRANSVENTRICULAR APPROACH

The transventricular approach is an important surgical corridor for lesions that are primarily third ventricular in location. Although this can be used in most lesions that occupy the third ventricle, the presence of obstructive lateral ventriculomegaly makes this the preferred approach for such lesions. Access to the lateral ventricle can be achieved preferably in a transfrontal fashion in the presence of dilated lateral ventricles and in an interhemispheric fashion in the presence of normal or small-sized lateral ventricles. Our choice patient positions are the neutral supine for the transfrontal approach and the lateral side of access down with the head slightly tilted up for the interhemispheric approach (Fig. 24-5).

Once in the lateral ventricle, identification of the foramen of Monro and, in the absence of substantial dilatation

of the foramen, a subchoroidal dissection permits widening of the operative corridor into the third ventricle. This widening is a necessary maneuver for safe and effective surgery within the third ventricle. Retraction of the fornix as it forms the superior margin of the foramen of Monro, when necessary, should be done carefully to avoid injury to the structure with the potential result of memory dysfunction. Despite the depth at which dissection is performed in this approach, it remains the optimal corridor for exposure of third ventricular lesions. It allows for direct visual inspection of the lateral margins of the tumor and the relationship with the walls of the hypothalamus.

At the conclusion of the surgery, the placement of a ventricular catheter through the opening to the lateral ventricle is recommended in cases of symptomatic hydrocephalus preoperatively, an unusually bloody dissection, and the presence of residual tumor that may not relieve pre-existing hydrocephalus. We have found, however, that the need for CSF diversion usually becomes clinically apparent in a delayed fashion, when symptoms appear days to even several weeks postoperatively. The obvious exception to this is acute new-onset obstructive hydrocephalus that results from an immediate postoperative third ventricular hemorrhage. As a result, in our practice, the intraoperative placement of a ventricular catheter in this setting is infrequent.

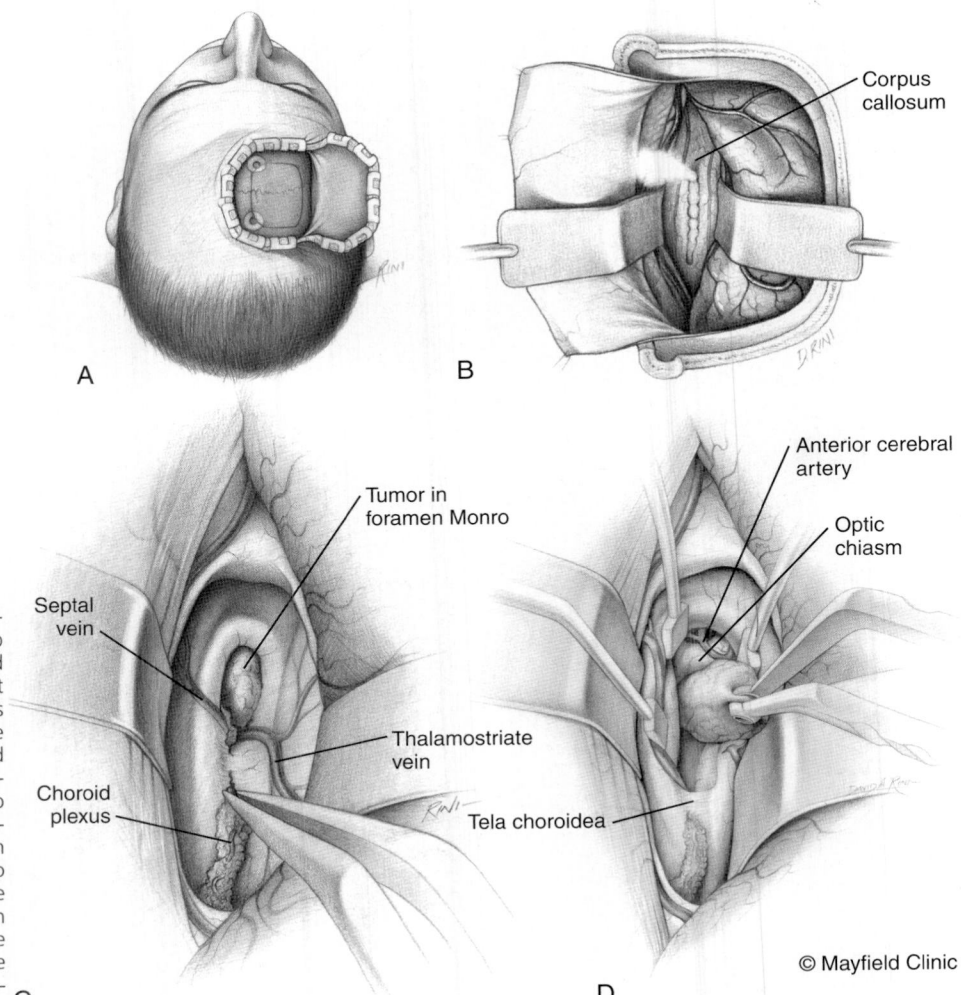

FIGURE 24-5 Interhemispheric trans-ventricular approach. A, A bone flap two thirds anterior and one third posterior to the coronal suture is cut with a craniotome. The frontal lobe is retracted from the falx and cingulate gyrus until the pericallosal arteries and corpus callosum are exposed. B, A 2- to 3-cm callosotomy is performed to enter the lateral ventricle. C, The choroid plexus and thalamostriate vein are followed to the foramen of Monro where the tumor is identified. The choroid plexus and thalamostriate vein are coagulated and sectioned. D, The choroidal fissure is opened to remove the tumor. (*From Mayfield Clinic, Cincinnati, OH.*)

CYST ASPIRATION

Cystic lesions at presentation or at recurrence may be safely treated with catheter drainage. With most symptoms arising from mechanical compression of the surrounding structures by the mass, symptom relief is often achieved by partial or complete collapse of the cystic lesion. Symptomatic resolution is often temporary because fluid tends to reaccumulate within the cyst. As a result, cyst aspiration is not a favored stand-alone treatment. However, the placement of an Ommaya reservoir that could allow for future re-aspiration is often an effective treatment for recurrent cystic craniopharyngiomas.

The placement of a catheter can be accomplished with stereotactic guidance or in an endoscope-assisted manner. Frameless stereotactic guidance is often accurate enough for safe catheterization of a large symptomatic cystic lesion and is recommended both in the case of simple aspiration, the placement of an Ommaya reservoir, or endoscope-assisted cyst fenestration (Fig. 24-6). In cases of hydrocephalus, an endoscope can safely navigate through the foramen of Monro, then allow for fenestration of a third ventricular cyst, and guide placement of a catheter within the deflated cyst under direct vision. However, it is a rare case of a craniopharyngioma that endoscopy can achieve more than fenestration and aspiration. Because most cyst walls have a close adherence of the third ventricle, endoscopic gross total resection is almost never possible.

RADIATION THERAPY

External Beam

The standard postoperative treatment for any residual or recurrent tumor is fractionated radiotherapy to a total dose of 60 Gy at 1.8 Gy per fraction. The total dose to the optic nerve ranges between 50 and 54 Gy, a dose generally well tolerated with no effects of vision. Intensity-modulated radiation therapy is the most recent evolution of the 3D-conformal radiation therapy delivery method and promises minimization of radiation dose to surrounding structures. Stereotactic radiosurgery and hypofractionated radiosurgical schemes have been used with good results. However, effective such treatments are limited to the treatment of lesions smaller than 3 cm.

Intracavitary Therapy

Intracavitary delivery of radiation therapy refers to the instillation of a radioisotope (90 yttrium, 32 phosphorus, or 186 rhenium) into a deflated tumor cyst cavity through an

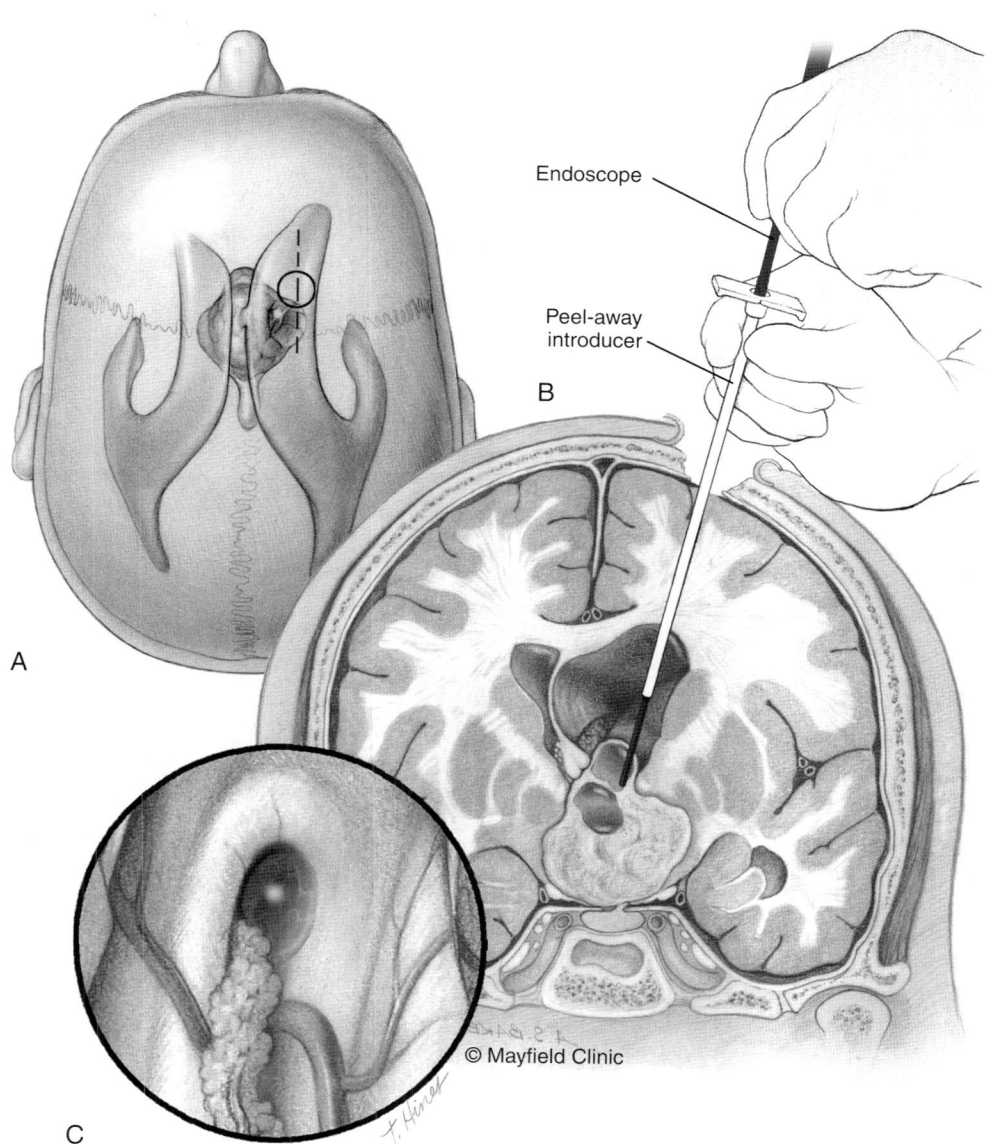

Endoscope

Peel-away
introducer

B

A

C

© Mayfield Clinic

FIGURE 24-6 The transventricular endoscopic approach. A, A 3-cm vertical incision, based on the coronal suture, is made 2.5 cm from the midline. A 1-cm burr hole is created slightly anterior to the coronal suture. B, A 12.5 French peel-away sheath introducer is used to cannulate the lateral ventricle. The flexible endoscope is inserted through the cannula to aspirate a large cyst blocking the foramen of Monro. C, Inset showing close-up view. *(From Mayfield Clinic, Cincinnati, OH.)*

indwelling catheter.[21,22] By this method, a high dose (about 150 Gy) can be delivered to the surrounding secretory epithelial layer that lines the cyst with good tumor control. In the literature, results with respect to vision and endocrine function vary widely, and are part of the reason that this technique has not been widely accepted.

Outcomes

The primary treatment of craniopharyngiomas remains surgical. The literature indicates rates of gross total resection range widely between 10% to 90%. Yet compilation of all surgical studies reviewed reveals a rough average of 58%—a number that is optimistic in our experience.[12,13,23-42] Estimates of gross total resection clearly depend on the postoperative imaging modality used; older studies in which CT was used reported lower rates of observed residuals.

Plenty of published evidence suggests that surgical resection is inadequate as the sole treatment for most craniopharyngiomas. Although it comes as no surprise that the rates of local tumor control after subtotal resection are generally low, rates after gross total resection are similar ranging between 6% and 57%.[25,29-31,34,38,39,43]

Operative morbidity includes postoperative visual dysfunction in 5.8% to 19% of patients and postoperative endocrinologic dysfunction in 50% to 100% of patients. Unlike most other brain tumors, an important consideration in the surgical treatment of craniopharyngiomas is perioperative mortality, which ranges between 1.1% to 10% in the early postoperative phase even in the most recent studies.[12,23-26,28-32,34,35,38,40,42-45] These rates undoubtedly are associated with the anatomic location of these lesions, and their infiltrative relationship with the hypothalamus and vascular structures. Evidence also exists on the association of improved perioperative outcomes with decreased degrees of surgical resection.[46-51]

Trans-sphenoidal approaches and their variants with extension to the parasellar region using either the

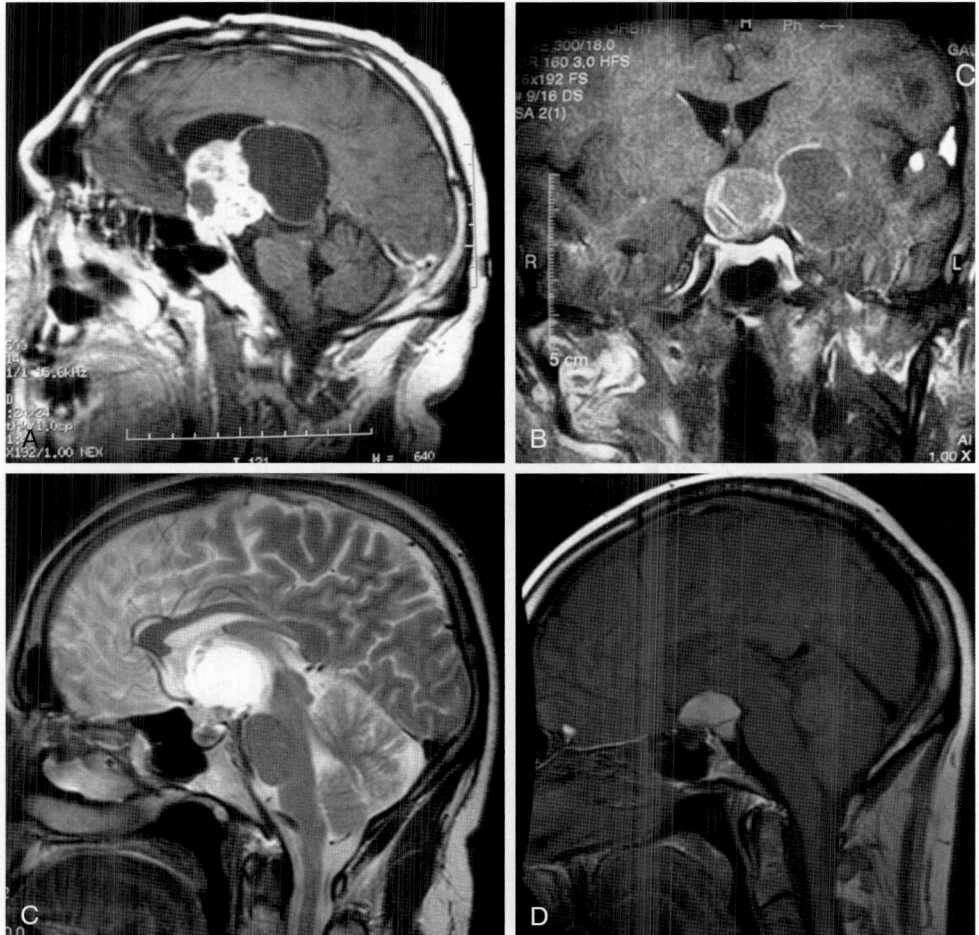

FIGURE 24-7 Examples of cranio-pharyngioma extension (and recommended approach). A, Large recurrent mostly third ventricular lesion (transcallosal). B, Multicystic lesion with lateral extension (pterional). C, Mostly cystic lesion with solid part filling the sella (transsphenoidal). D, Mostly cystic third-ventricular lesion separate from the sella (supraorbital, translamina terminalis).

microscope or endoscope are effective in the treatment of primarily cystic craniopharyngiomas.[11,20,52-67] Transventricular endoscopic approaches have a limited utility, primarily for fenestration of cystic lesions, followed by implantation of intracystic catheters under direct visualization.[68-71] Several other surgical approaches have been described but have limited clinical applicability and no proven significant benefit in operative outcomes.[72-75] A promising exception to this is the supraorbital craniotomy that has an increasing role, replacing the larger subfrontal and pterional approaches in less invasive and smaller tumors.[76] Examples of these tumors and recommended approaches are shown in Fig. 24-7 and an overall recommended management of these lesions is shown in Fig. 24-8.

The largest body of literature with respect to the radiation treatment of craniopharyngiomas deals with fractionated radiation therapy.[35,51,77-91] The majority of the studies include patients treated in the adjuvant setting either postoperatively or at recurrence. Local control ranged between 80% to 100% and follow-up was up to 12 years post-treatment. Morbidity is limited; no visual dysfunction in general is observed when doses less than 60 Gy are used. When compared with patients after gross total resection alone, patients after subtotal resection that was followed by adjuvant fXRT, particularly during the early postoperative period,

demonstrated improved tumor control rates and decreased morbidity.[31,44,86,92-97]

During the past decade, a number of publications on the treatment of craniopharyngiomas with stereotactic radiosurgery have reported that control rates range between 80% to 90% at 5 years post-treatment; response rates of 58% to 80% have been reported with median marginal dose of 9 to 16 Gy.[98-109] Morbidity of this approach appears to be low with visual dysfunction in 6.1% of patients.[100]

Given the cystic nature of many craniopharyngiomas, stereotactic aspiration of the cystic component with the instillation of radioactive material can be an effective minimally invasive route of treatment. Several types of beta-emitting isotopes have been used, including phosphorus 32, ytrium 90, and rhenium 186.[110-120] These colloid preparations can deliver high radiation doses of 100 to 200 Gy in the few surrounding millimeters, effectively treating the wall of cystic lesions, while depositing little radiation in the surrounding normal brain. Used as primary treatment after cyst aspiration or at recurrence, intracavitary radiation therapy has shown local tumor control rates of 70% to 96%.[111,112,115]

Stereotactic instillation of bleomycin has also shown 57% to 100% response rates.[121-126] Although peritumoral edema can be observed postprocedure, it is rarely clinically limiting.[121,122]

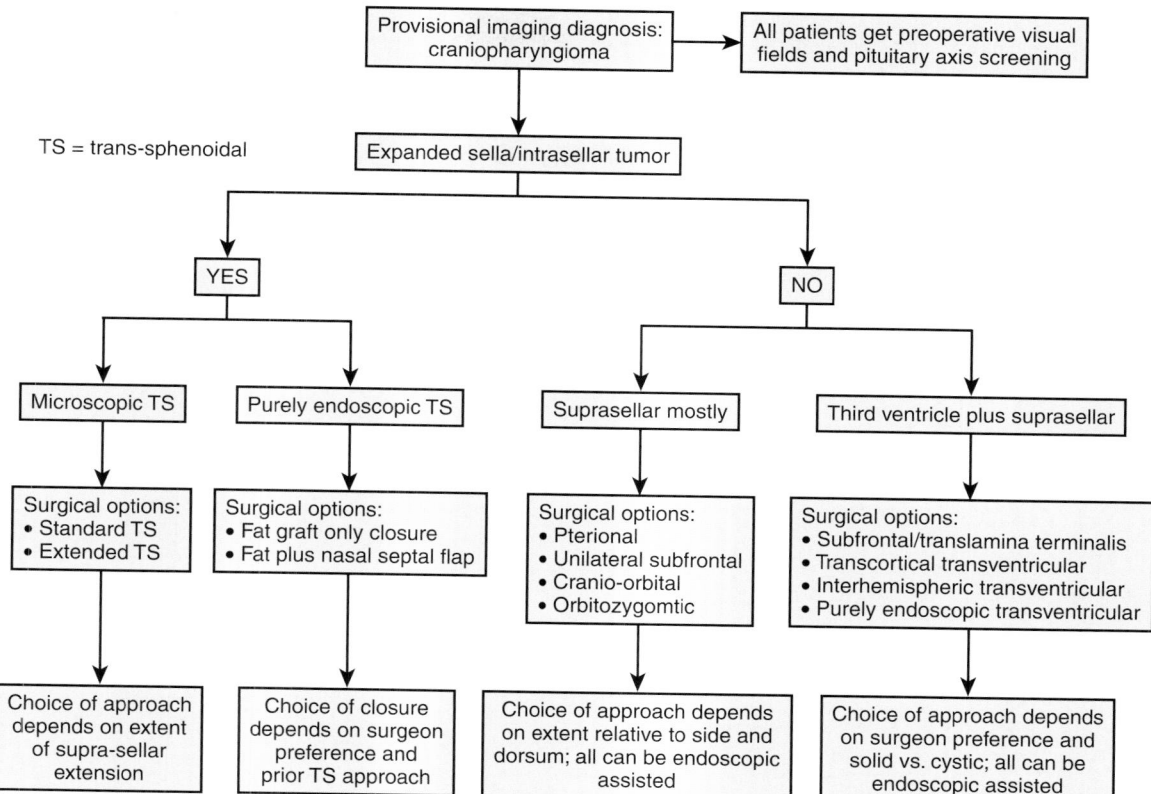

FIGURE 24-8 Diagram of recommended surgical management of craniopharyngiomas as per the authors' experience.

Conclusions

Despite technological advances in both surgical and radiation therapies, craniopharyngiomas remain especially challenging in achieving long-term tumor control at low levels of morbidity. These may be the single type of brain tumor whose surgical treatment even in the most modern series is associated with quantifiable mortality rates in the perioperative setting. The literature supports up front subtotal or near total resection. An effort is made to preserve neurovascular structures surrounding the lesion, including the pituitary stalk in most patients, except when a gross total resection appears clearly within reach. Regardless of the extent of resection, adjuvant radiation therapy should be considered in all patients. After gross total resection, patients should continue to undergo radiographic follow-up to ensure detection of a recurrence, which occurs more often than previously recognized. Considering recurrences are frequent, placement of Ommaya reservoirs for cyst aspiration and intracystic therapies are important parts of the treatment algorithm.

KEY REFERENCES

Albright AL, Hadjipanayis CG, Lunsford LD, et al. Individualized treatment of pediatric craniopharyngiomas. *Childs Nerv Syst.* 2005;21: 8–9:649-654.

Caldarelli M, Massimi L, Tamburrini G, et al. Long-term results of the surgical treatment of craniopharyngioma: the experience at the Policlinico Gemelli, Catholic University, Rome. *Childs Nerv Syst.* 2005;21: 8–9:747-757.

Cavallo LM, Prevedello DM, Solari D, et al. Extended endoscopic endonasal transsphenoidal approach for residual or recurrent craniopharyngiomas. *J Neurosurg.* 2009;111(3):578-589.

Chakrabarti I, Amar AP, Couldwell W, et al. Long-term neurological, visual, and endocrine outcomes following transnasal resection of craniopharyngioma. *J Neurosurg.* 2005;102(4):650-657.

Combs SE, Thilmann C, Huber PE, et al. Achievement of long-term local control in patients with craniopharyngiomas using high precision stereotactic radiotherapy. *Cancer.* 2007;109(11):2308-2314.

Derrey S, Blond S, Reyns N, et al. Management of cystic craniopharyngiomas with stereotactic endocavitary irradiation using colloidal 186Re: a retrospective study of 48 consecutive patients. *Neurosurgery.* 2008;63(6):1045-1053.

Dhellemmes P, Vinchon M. Radical resection for craniopharyngiomas in children: surgical technique and clinical results. *J Pediatr Endocrinol Metab.* 2006;19(suppl 1):329-335.

Di Rocco C, Caldarelli M, Tamburrini G, et al. Surgical management of craniopharyngiomas—experience with a pediatric series. *J Pediatr Endocrinol Metab.* 2006;19(suppl 1):355-366.

Fitzek MM, Linggood RM, Adams J, et al. Combined proton and photon irradiation for craniopharyngioma: long-term results of the early cohort of patients treated at Harvard Cyclotron Laboratory and Massachusetts General Hospital. *Int J Radiat Oncol Biol Phys.* 2006;64(5):1348-1354.

Gardner PA, Kassam AB, Snyderman CH, et al. Outcomes following endoscopic, expanded endonasal resection of suprasellar craniopharyngiomas: a case series. *J Neurosurg.* 2008;109(1):6-16.

Gardner PA, Prevedello DM, Kassam AB, et al. The evolution of the endonasal approach for craniopharyngiomas. *J Neurosurg.* 2008;108(5):1043-1047.

Gonc EN, Yordam N, Ozon A, et al. Endocrinological outcome of different treatment options in children with craniopharyngioma: a retrospective analysis of 66 cases. *Pediatr Neurosurg.* 2004;40(3):112-119.

Hukin J, Steinbok P, Lafay-Cousin L, et al. Intracystic bleomycin therapy for craniopharyngioma in children: the Canadian experience. *Cancer.* 2007;109(10):2124-2131.

Kassam AB, Gardner PA, Snyderman CH, et al. Expanded endonasal approach, a fully endoscopic transnasal approach for the resection of midline suprasellar craniopharyngiomas: a new classification based on the infundibulum. *J Neurosurg.* 2008;108(4):715-728.

Kim SD, Park JY, Park J, et al. Radiological findings following postsurgical intratumoral bleomycin injection for cystic craniopharyngioma. *Clin Neurol Neurosurg.* 2007;109(3):236-241.

Kobayashi T, Kida Y, Mori Y, et al. Long-term results of gamma knife surgery for the treatment of craniopharyngioma in 98 consecutive cases. *J Neurosurg.* 2005;103(suppl 6):482-488.

Lena G, Paz Paredes A, Scavarda D, et al. Craniopharyngioma in children: Marseille experience. *Childs Nerv Syst.* 2005;21:8-9:778-784.

Lin LL, El Naqa I, Leonard JR, et al. Long-term outcome in children treated for craniopharyngioma with and without radiotherapy. *J Neurosurg Pediatr.* 2008;1(2):126-130.

Maira G, Anile C, Albanese A, et al. The role of transsphenoidal surgery in the treatment of craniopharyngiomas. *J Neurosurg.* 2004;100(3):445-451.

Minniti G, Saran F, Traish D, et al. Fractionated stereotactic conformal radiotherapy following conservative surgery in the control of craniopharyngiomas. *Radiother Oncol.* 2007;82(1):90-95.

Mottolese C, Szathmari A, Berlier P, et al. Craniopharyngiomas: our experience in Lyon. *Childs Nerv Syst.* 2005;21:8-9:790-798.

Samii M, Samii A. Surgical management of craniopharyngiomas. In: Schmidek H, Roberts D, eds. *Operative Neurosurgical Techniques.* Philadelphia: WB Saunders; 2006:437-452.

Sosa IJ, Krieger MD, McComb JG. Craniopharyngiomas of childhood: the CHLA experience. *Childs Nerv Syst.* 2005;21:8-9:785-789.

Takahashi H, Yamaguchi F, Teramoto A. Long-term outcome and reconsideration of intracystic chemotherapy with bleomycin for craniopharyngioma in children. *Childs Nerv Syst.* 2005;21:8-9:701-704.

Numbered references appear on Expert Consult.

Endoscopic Endonasal Approach for Craniopharyngiomas

DANIEL M. PREVEDELLO • DOMENICO SOLARI •
RICARDO L. CARRAU • PAUL GARDNER • AMIN B. KASSAM

Craniopharyngiomas are benign tumors originating from squamous epithelial remnants of Rathke's pouch, and can arise from any area from nasopharynx to the hypothalamus.[1,2] Their consistency can be cystic, solid, or a combination of both; intralesional calcifications are a quite common finding (60% to 80% of cases). They are relatively infrequent, accounting for the 2% to 5% of all intracranial tumors, most frequently involving children (5–14 years) and older adults (50–74 years).[3,4] These features contribute to a somewhat unpredictable biological behavior; therefore, the correct management strategy is controversial.[5]

Surgical management is challenging, especially when complete removal has been advocated as the most effective treatment.[6-13] However, despite the benign nature of craniopharyngiomas, complete removal is not always possible due to their proximity and adhesions to vital neurovascular structures. Furthermore, craniopharyngiomas can recur even after radical resection and the surgical removal of recurrent craniopharyngiomas is even more complex due to the scarring and new adhesions.[6-12,14,15]

The surgical treatment of craniopharyngiomas has been historically performed using various microscopic transcranial approaches, such as the subfrontal, frontolateral, and pterional routes. Trans-sphenoidal approaches, either microsurgical or endoscopic, have been restricted to intrasellar or intrasuprasellar subdiaphragmatic tumors.[16,17] Nonetheless, in the last 20 years, the evolution of surgical techniques and technology have led to the progressive reduction of surgical invasiveness along with decreased morbidity. This has resulted in an increase of effectiveness for both transcranial and trans-sphenoidal approaches.[18-25]

The introduction and diffusion of the extended trans-sphenoidal approach, described by Weiss,[26] created a new paradigm in trans-sphenoidal surgery opening a new corridor to the suprasellar space. This extended route for the removal of craniopharyngiomas was successfully adopted by Edward Laws.[17,27]

The widespread use of the endoscope in sinus surgery was introduced to trans-sphenoidal surgery for the treatment of pituitary tumors.[28-30] The wider and panoramic view offered by the endoscope increased the versatility of the trans-sphenoidal approach and permitted its expansion to different parts of the skull base, thus allowing the removal of different "pure" supradiaphragmatic lesions.[18,31-45]

Furthermore, because craniopharyngiomas are infrachiasmatic midline tumors, the endonasal route provides the advantage of accessing the tumor without the need for brain or optic nerve retraction with a direct visualization through a linear surgical route.[46,47]

Since the approach has a caudal–cranial orientation, and the tumors are basically infrachiasmatic, the original classification of craniopharyngiomas in relation to the chiasm (pre or post fixed) is not practical. The infundibulum becomes the structure of reference; therefore, craniopharyngiomas have been recently classified accordingly[43] as type 1, preinfundibular; type 2, transinfundibular; type 3, post- or retro-infundibular, further subdivision is based on rostral or caudal extension, whether it is to the anterior third ventricular (infundibular recess, hypothalamic) and interpeduncular fossa; and type 4, isolated third ventricular (not well accessed via endonasal routes) (Fig. 25-1). Consequently, specific surgical variations are required for each modality.[43]

We present the surgical nuances based on our experience with the endoscopic endonasal approach for the treatment of craniopharyngiomas. We aimed to highlight the feasibility of this technique and evaluate its advantages and limitations as compared to the transcranial and trans-sphenoidal microscopic approaches.

Surgical Technique

TECHNICAL NUANCES IN CRANIOPHARYNGIOMA SURGERY

The endoscopic endonasal approach involves the team of two surgeons, using three- or four-hand technique using the visualization provided by rod lens endoscope (18 cm in 4-mm length in diameter; Karl Storz Endoscopy-America, Inc., Culver City, CA) of varying lens angulations (0 degrees and 45 degrees). The surgical team is usually composed of an otolaryngologist and a neurosurgeon experienced in endoscopic endonasal surgery. The otolaryngologist performs the sinonasal approach and then drives the endoscope to provide a dynamic view of the surgical field throughout the procedure, while the neurosurgeon performs a bimanual dissection of the intradural structures.[18]

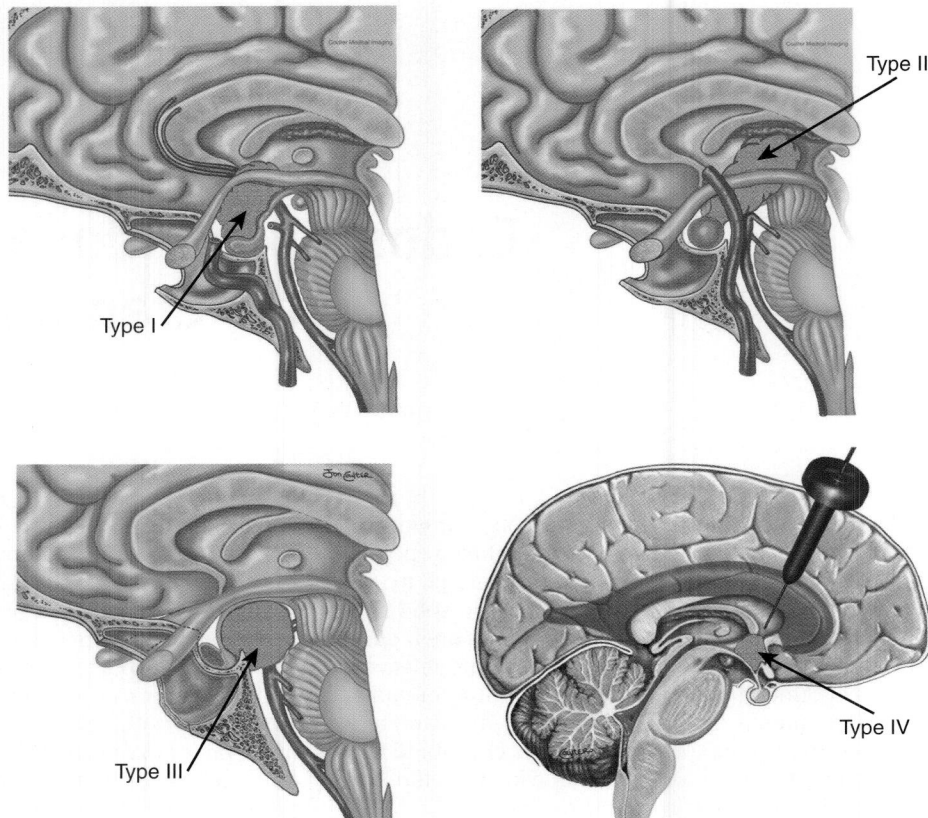

FIGURE 25-1 Types of craniopharyngiomas.

As in any other surgery, the EEA for the removal of craniopharyngiomas comprises three portions: exposure, tumor resection, and reconstruction.

EXPOSURE

Following the induction of general anesthesia the patient's head is placed in a three-point fixation system in a slightly extended position to optimize access to the anterior cranial base. The face is turned 5 degrees to 10 degrees toward the surgeons (the patient's right) and the neck is tilted to the left. Baseline somatosensory-evoked potentials and image guidance registration are obtained using a mask protocol (Stryker Navigation, Leibinger Corp., Kalamazoo, MI) preloaded with CTA and MRI. While the patient is being set-up the nose is decongested with topical 0.05% oxymetazoline applied with 0.5 × 3 inch cottonoids. The midface and the periumbilical area are prepped and draped and a third- or fourth-generation cephalosporin antibiotic is administered for perioperative prophylaxis.

We customarily initiate the procedure with removal of the inferior half of the right middle turbinate. Thereafter, the most posterior aspect of the posterior ethmoid sinuses is removed to expose the lamina papyracea bilaterally. A Hadad-Bassagasteguy (nasoseptal flap) is raised from the widest nasal cavity (usually the right in view of the middle turbinectomy) using a standard technique (see reconstruction section). At this point, the most posterior 2 cm of the nasal septum are removed and the left middle turbinate is displaced laterally (not resected). A wide sphenoidotomy is opened, enlarging the natural ostium until the lamina papyracea is in plane with the lateral wall of the orbit, the

roof of the sphenoid sinus is in plane with that of the nose, and the bottom of the sinus is in full view. All intrasinus septae are removed and, if the sinus is not well pneumatized, the bone is drilled until all surgical landmarks are well exposed. These include the optic nerves and intracranial carotid artery (ICA) canals as well as lateral and medial opticocarotid recesses (MOCR and LOCR, respectively), and the clival recess.[48,49] The LOCR lies at the junction of the optic nerve and ICA canals corresponding to the optic strut and the MOCR lies at the confluence of the optic canal and the paraclinoid carotid canal at the lateral portion of the tuberculum sellae. Image guidance is of assistance during these steps of the procedure. It should be remembered that continuous irrigation must be used to avoid thermal injury to the underlying optic nerve. Venous bleeding may be encountered in this region, which also represents the point of insertion of the SIS into the cavernous sinus. The bleeding can be controlled by packing microfibrillar collagen (Avitene, Ethicon, Inc.) or with the use of collagen (Surgifoam, Ethicon, Inc.) mixed with thrombin.

This opens an unobstructed corridor connecting the nasal cavities and the sphenoid sinus; thus, creating a single, large working cavity and bimanual access. The posterior ethmoidal arteries (PEA), encountered 4 to 7 mm anterior to the optic nerve and just anterior to the rostrum of the sphenoid, represent the anterior boundary of the exposure. Staying posterior to the PEAs prevents injury to the cribriform plate and the olfactory system associated with it. The surgical field extends from the posterior ethmoidal arteries rostrally to the clival recess caudally. Subsequently, the endoscope is kept in the patient's right nostril, slightly stretching it superiorly, over the 12 o'clock position, to create space for the suction tip that is introduced at the 6 o'clock position.

The bone over the sellar face is removed and the planum sphenoidale is removed anteriorly up to the anterior margin of the tumor, which is determined with image-guidance. Subsequently, a complete removal of the tuberculum sellae, including the MOCRs bilaterally, is mandatory to expose the subarachnoid opticocarotid cistern in order to allow adequate suprasellar exposure for tumor resection. At this point the dura can be opened.

As opposed to surgery for the resection of meningiomas, EEA for craniopharyngiomas have specific hallmarks due to the origin and spread of the tumor. Since the tumor has its origin on the pituitary stalk, it pushes the suprasellar arachnoid membrane with the superior hypophyseal artery (SHa) against the anterior dura of the tuberculum. This is very important since the SHa could be injured by a careless dural opening. A wide exposure, and the magnified view provided by the endoscope will facilitate the identification and preservation of the superior hypophyseal artery (SHa) and other subchiasmatic perforating vessels that are displaced over the lateral dome of the tumor; thus, preventing devascularization of the optic nerves, chiasm, and infundibulum.

Another difference with meningioma surgery is related to the management of the superior intercavernous sinus (SIS). In craniopharyngioma surgery, the common presence of both intrasellar disease and stalk involvement mandates the exposure of these areas; thus, the SIS should be transected for a craniopharyngioma surgery, whereas it is not necessary when dealing with a suprasellar meningioma.

Incisions above and below the SIS are undertaken to allow the insertion of a bipolar electrocautery with one blade on each side of the SIS to facilitate its coagulation. The incision is extended across the SIS posteriorly toward the pituitary stalk, which then will be completely exposed.

RESECTION

The endoscopic trans-sphenoidal approach to craniopharyngiomas follows the same principles and goals of the standardized microsurgical procedure: internal debulking of the solid part and/or cystic evacuation followed by fine and meticulous dissection of the tumor from the surrounding neurovascular structures. All dissection is performed under direct visual control shifting from a close-up to a wide panoramic view as needed.

Above all, it should be kept in mind that the concept of extracapsular dissection introduced by Laws[17] takes precedence over any other consideration. One highlight of the endoscopic technique is that it approaches the tumor at its ventral aspect and all of the critical neurovascular structures will lie on its dorsum and perimeter. Furthermore, the endonasal endoscopic technique provides direct visualization of the inferior aspect of the chiasm, the infundibulum, the third ventricle, and/or the retro and parasellar spaces, which can be dissected free from tumor. Debulking of the solid and/or cystic component is performed followed by capsule mobilization and extracapsular sharp dissection. Debulking can be effectively performed using the two-suction technique[43] or a combination of a suction and a cut-through instrument. It is important to mention that craniopharyngiomas are often adherent to the chiasm and/or

hypothalamus, particularly in cases of recurrence.[50] In these circumstances, we advise a partial resection in order to preserve critical neural tissue and its function.

In our experience, we have found that delicate "countertraction," with a controlled suction fine tip (4 or 6 French), can be very useful to facilitate the isolation of the arachnoid bands and/or the attachments to other neurovascular structures, which then can be sharply dissected,[43] as long there is no direct invasion.

RECONSTRUCTION

Due to the wide dural opening and the associated CSF leak, a reliable reconstruction of the skull base defect is mandatory. Our preferred method involves the use of vascularized tissue to prevent postoperative CSF leak. This is especially important during craniopharyngioma surgery as it often requires a large opening and dissection of the arachnoid cisterns and/or of the third ventricle.

The reconstruction starts with a subdural inlay collagen matrix graft (Duragen, Integra LifeSciences). This graft contains the flow of CSF and facilitates the placement and healing of the graft. Immediately after the inlay reconstruction, the nasoseptal flap is rotated to cover the skull base defect. It is important that osseous surfaces in contact with the flap are stripped of mucosa, which would otherwise prevent adherence and healing of the flap to the defect.[51,52] The flap is positioned to cover the defect overlapping its margins to allow contact with bone. In our experience this vascularized flap is superior to any other previously used technique. Its vascularity allows faster healing and an earlier, more resilient seal.

Finally, the flap is covered with Surgicel (Ethicon, Inc.) followed by Duraseal (Confluent Surgical, Inc., Waltham, MA) and Gelfoam. A 14-French Foley catheter balloon is then inflated in the posterior nasal cavity to buttress the reconstruction under direct endoscopic visualization. The catheter tip is placed into the nasopharynx and balloon inflation is monitored to avoid compression of intracranial or intraorbital structures. Sponge packings (Merocel Medtronic XOMED, Jacksonville, FL) are preferred when optic nerve canals were opened during the approach, or when the geometry of the defect and/or skull base is such that the round shape of the balloon would not conform to the area.

Lumbar drainage is performed only in cases in which the infundibular recess of the third ventricle has been opened for direct access into the ventricle, cases necessitating extensive arachnoid membrane dissection, or those in which perioperative high ventricular pressure is a concern.

SURGICAL CONSIDERATIONS BASED ON CRANIOPHARYNGIOMA TYPE

Type 1 craniopharyngiomas are preinfundibular and occupy the suprasellar cistern immediately anterior to the stalk. They tend to displace the chiasm superiorly and posteriorly. Concurrently, they displace the suprasellar arachnoid and the attached superior hypophyseal artery against the retrotubercular dura. These are the most accessible craniopharyngiomas via the endonasal route. Extreme care is critical during the dural opening to preserve the vascular supply for the optic nerves (SHa). Once the SHa are mobilized, the tumor can be debulked and this is followed by

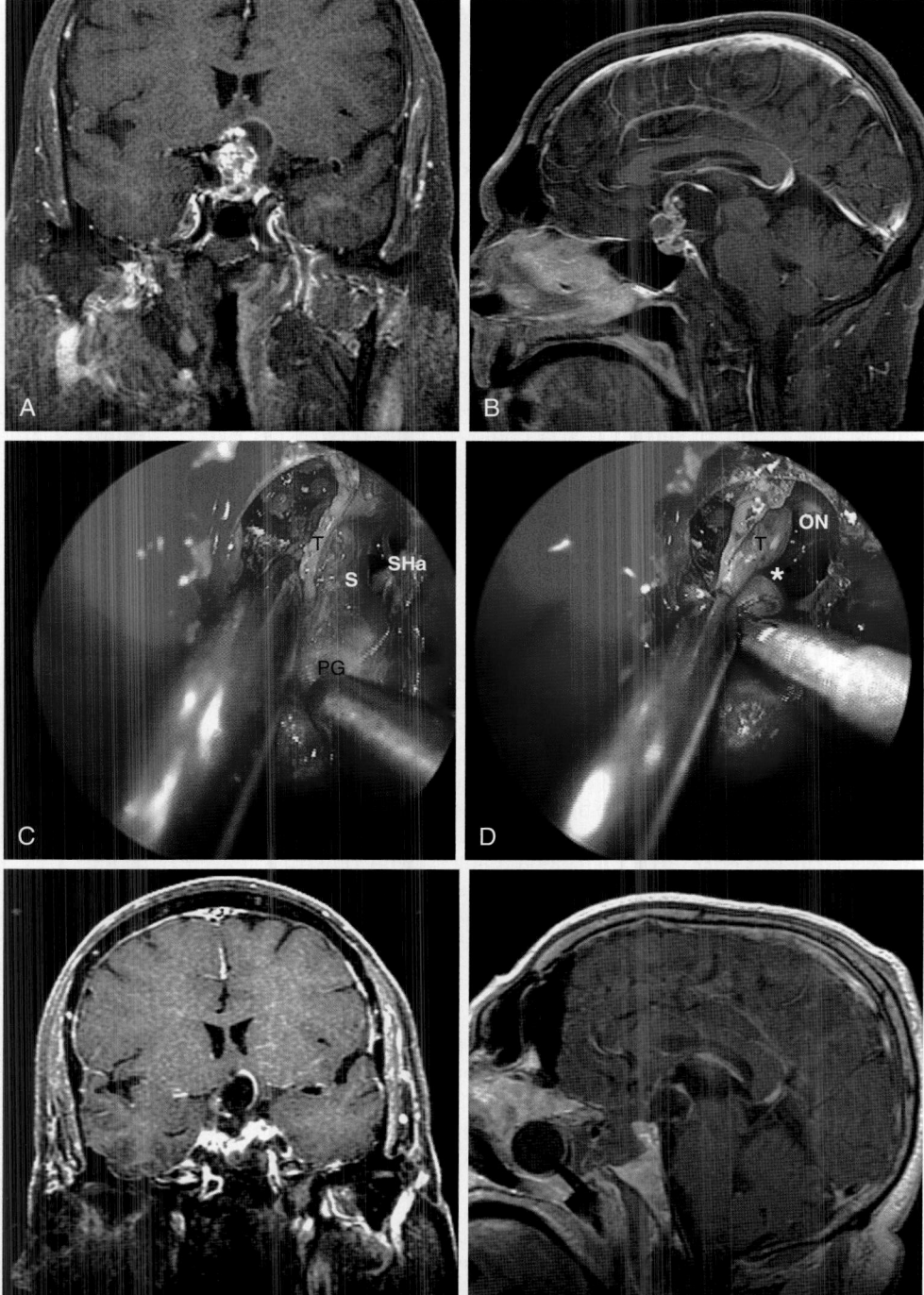

FIGURE 25-2 Preoperative (A) coronal and (B) sagittal: Preoperative post–contrast-enhanced T1-weighted MR images showing a case of a type 1 (preinfundibular) craniopharyngioma. Note that the tumor is entirely anterior to the pituitary stalk. C and D, Intraoperative endoscopic pictures confirming the tumor sitting in front of the pituitary stalk under the optic chiasm. Dissecting this type of tumor from a ventral route allows the surgeon to preserve the vascularization of the chiasm: indeed tiny vessels become visible in the close-up, wider endoscopic view. In addition, such a corridor allows for pituitary gland preservation. (E) Coronal and (F) sagittal early postoperative MRI demonstrate the removal of the lesion and residual capsule that was tightly adherent to chiasm and third ventricle floor. T, tumor; PG, pituitary gland; SHa, superior hypophyseal artery; S, pituitary stalk; *, pituitary stalk; ON, optic nerve.

extracapsular sharp dissection as described above. SIS ligation and sellar exposure helps in defining the possibility of stalk preservation once the tumor is grossly removed (Fig. 25-2).

Type 2 craniopharyngiomas comprise those in the infundibular area. They grow from the inner aspect of the stalk and they tend to expand it circumferentially. In these cases, the stalk forms the capsule of the tumor. Once the SIS and sella are exposed, the anterior tumor capsule (distended stalk) is visualized. The SHa are dissected away and the

capsule is entered. The center of the tumor is debulked and the capsule is dissected laterally and posteriorly. Unless there is a significant remaining stalk, the stalk/capsule should be sacrificed with a superior transection to avoid recurrence. This is the most difficult decision that has to be made in the operating room and becomes even more challenging when operating on children (Fig. 25-3).

Type 3 craniopharyngiomas are those that are retroinfundibular. They are posterior to the pituitary stalk, which is confirmed once the SIS and pituitary aperture are transected.

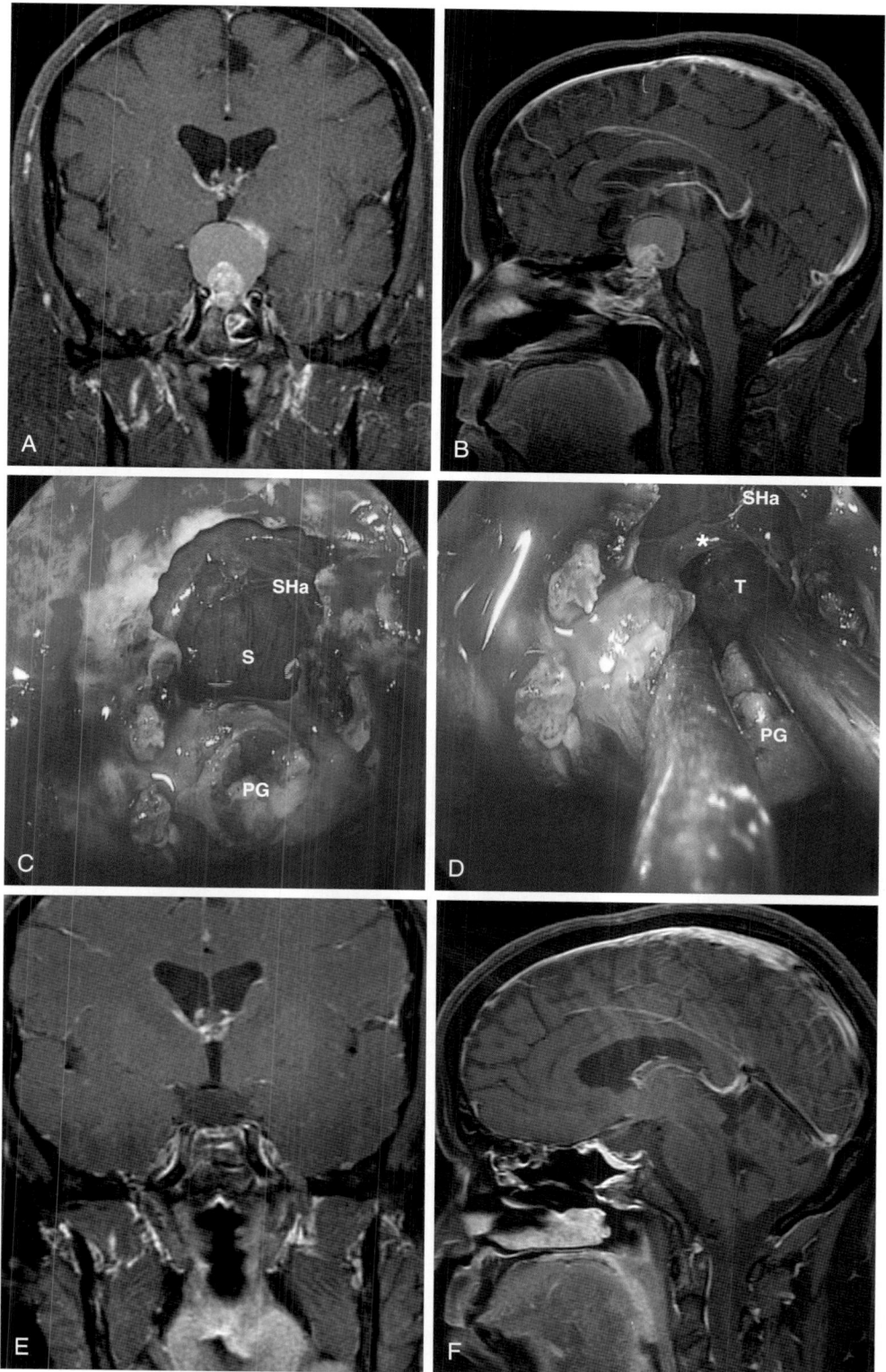

FIGURE 25-3 Preoperative (A) coronal and (B) sagittal MRI showing case of type 2 (infundibular) craniopharyngioma. The tumor seems to arise within the pituitary stalk, enlarging it in all directions expanding the infundibulum, which cannot be clearly visualized since it acts like tumor capsule. Intraoperative pictures showing (C) the presence, as soon as the dura of the planum has been opened, of the tumor completely inside the pituitary stalk that is thinned and stretched, encapsulating it; and (D) tumor dissection and removal maneuvers are performed with a two-suction technique that, once again, provides the surgeon with the possibility of sparing the vessels in close contact with the stalk and to work above the pituitary gland and thus respecting it. Coronal (E) and sagittal (F) postoperative MRI demonstrating total removal of the lesion. PG, pituitary gland; SHa, superior hypophyseal artery; S, pituitary stalk enlarged by the presence of the tumor; T, tumor; *, pituitary stalk.

The suprasellar cistern is going to be relaxed and looks like there is no tumor present, which is all hidden behind the infundibulum. In these cases, we advocate a pituitary transposition followed by a superior clivectomy with removal of the dorsum sellae in order to have a direct access to the interpeduncular cistern.[47] Once the transposition is done, a 45-degree endoscope is used to allow for a caudal–cranial orientation of dissection. The basilar artery is encountered initially with the Liliequist membrane. Craniopharyngiomas usually respect this membrane, displacing it downward. The tumor is debulked and the capsule is then dissected using microsurgical techniques with vascular proximal

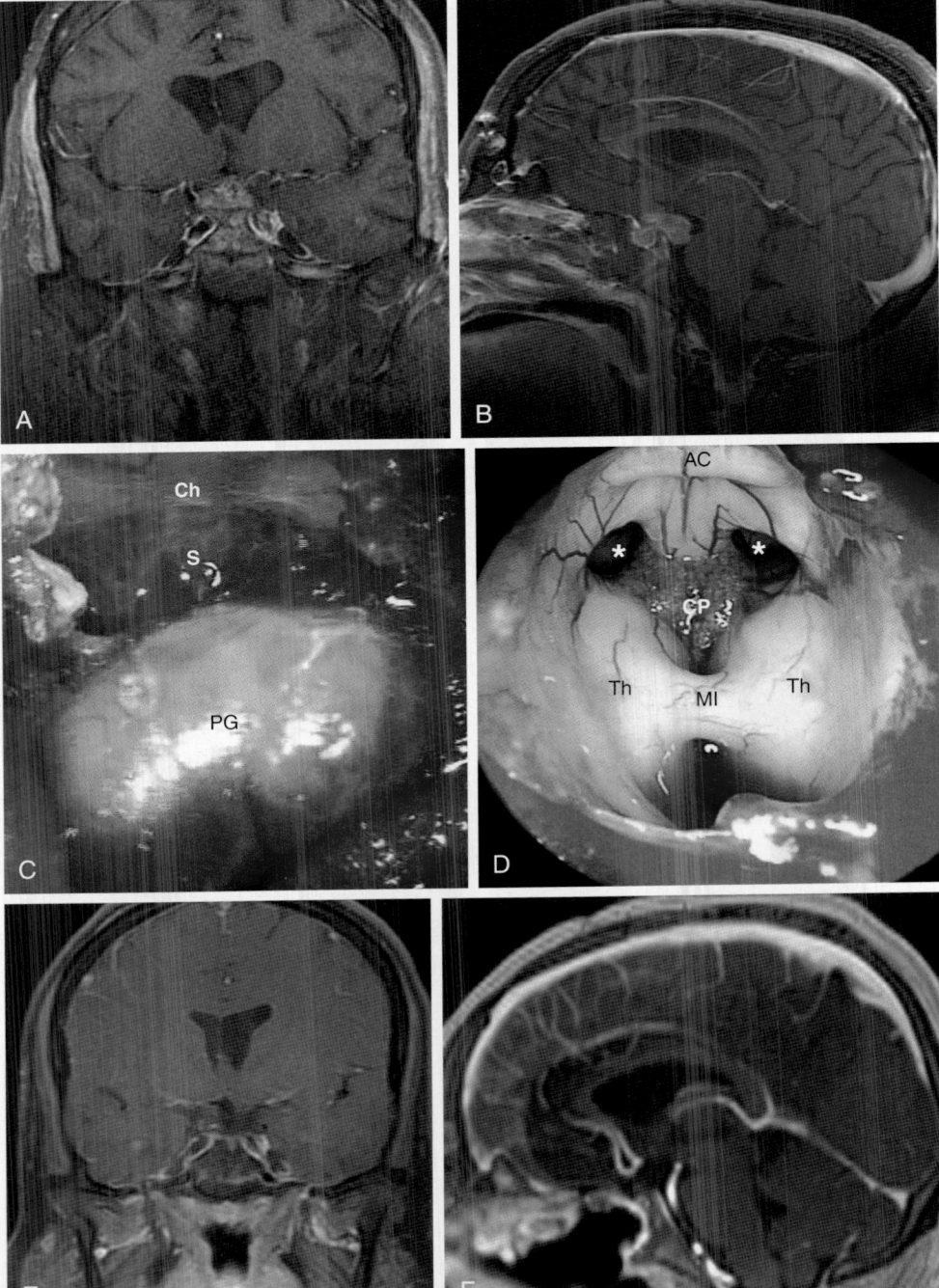

FIGURE 25-4 Preoperative (A) coronal and (B) sagittal MRI showing a case of a type 3 (retroinfundibular) craniopharyngioma. In this case, the tumor seems to extend into the retrosellar space compressing and displacing the stalk anteriorly. C, Intraoperative pictures showing the suprasellar space with the chiasm and the pituitary stalk, limiting access to the tumor. In such cases, pituitary transposition tremendously increases the corridor to the retrosellar area, providing enough room to dissect and remove this type of tumor once the dorsum sellae is removed. D, After removal of the lesion, the close-up endoscopic view with a 45-degree endoscope allows direct visualization of the third ventricle coronal (E) and sagittal (F) postoperative MRI demonstrating total removal of the lesion. (T, tumor; PG, pituitary gland; Ch, optic chiasm; S, pituitary stalk hiding the tumor; AC, anterior commissure; CP, choroidal plexus; Th, thalamus; *, foramen of Monro; MI, massa intermedia (interthalamic adhesion).

control on the basilar artery. The stalk is preserved anteriorly and the tumor is removed from its posterior surface. Often, the floor of the third ventricle is eroded by the tumor and this will allow a direct view at the end of the dissection (Fig. 25-4).

Type 4 craniopharyngiomas are pure intraventricular tumors and should be approached by a transcranial procedure. One alternative is a subfrontal approach with opening of the lamina terminalis. Another option is a transcortical or transcallosal approach followed by a transchoroidal approach to the third ventricle expanding the foramen of Monro. A potential alternative would be the interforniceal

approach; however, it adds the risk of loss of memory function; therefore, we do not advocate it.

Discussion

Craniopharyngiomas are challenging lesions with an extremely variable growth pattern. Their management is highly controversial.

Historically, transcranial microsurgical approaches have been advocated for the removal of craniopharyngiomas involving the suprasellar and ventricular areas. Transsphenoidal approach has been indicated for intrasuprasellar infradiaphragmatic lesions,[16,17] extending upward out of an enlarged sella turcica and only with partial involvement of the anterior inferior aspect of the third ventricle, such as craniopharyngiomas of grades 1 and 2, according to the Samii's classification.[53] Furthermore, patients with normal pituitary function were often considered as a contraindication for endonasal route. These indications have been recently revised since the introduction of extended transsphenoidal approaches.[54]

The concept of accessing median lesions via median approaches holds inherent appeal and many others have reported a successful experience with the use of such a technique.[26,32,36,40,45,55-59] Median approaches were boosted by the introduction of innovative tools such as the endoscope, high-definition cameras, and image guidance technology.

During the last decade multiple surgical centers around the world, already confident with the endoscopic endonasal management of pituitary tumors, began to perform "pure" extended endoscopic endonasal procedures for the removal of lesions involving different areas of the skull base.[18,31-34,36-38,41,42] This technique actually provides a median and two-sided access and direct visualization of the suprasellar space without brain manipulation. This technique provides a wider, close-up view of the surgical field that permits the identification of surgical landmarks, thereby allowing the safe dissection and removal of the tumor without brain or optic apparatus retraction, even with a normal-sized sella. Besides, the risk of postoperative visual loss, which is strictly related to the integrity of the blood supply of the optic chiasm, seems to be reduced.

In 2004, Kassam and coworkers[60] presented their initial experience with the treatment of craniopharyngiomas by mean of a fully endoscopic endonasal approach, describing an extension of the resection to the retrochiasmatic space and prepontine cisterns. Frank et al. in Bologna (Italy) reported a series of 10 patients with craniopharyngiomas who underwent a purely endoscopic endonasal approach.[37] Six were purely suprasellar tumors without

sellar enlargement. More recently, de Divitiis et al.[46] confirmed the feasibility of this approach for the treatment of craniopharyngiomas, describing the use of an EEA for the removal of 10 cases of craniopharyngiomas. Seven were classified as suprasellar (6 had intraventricular extension and one purely intraventricular).

Following these encouraging results, others adopted EEA as a surgical strategy for the removal of various skull base lesions including craniopharyngiomas.[46,50,61-64] The data from the main series of EEA for the removal of craniopharyngiomas is summarized in Table 25-1.

The analysis of data from these series, even though some included a small number of patients, confirmed the efficacy of the endoscopic endonasal technique for the treatment of craniopharyngiomas. In fact, it showed an overall gross-total/subtotal removal rate of 92.4% (residual tumor less then 25%) including a 60.4% of complete removal (no residual). These data seem to be at least equivalent to resection rates of the transcranial series[6,7,10-12,16] reported in the literature, where they range from 0% to 60% with the exception of the study by Yasargil et al.[12] (gross-total resection rate is of 90%). Notwithstanding the fact that the paramount aims of the surgery are the complete resection and cure at first attempt, we noted that with the direct subchiasmatic view offered by the endoscopic endonasal approach, there is no "blind" tumor dissection from hypothalamus, optic apparatus, and/or perforators resulting in a greater potential for preservation or even improvement of patient function, whether neurologic, ophthalmologic, or endocrinologic.

EEA has flourished thanks to the strict and systematic study of the anatomy of the skull base from the endoscopic perspective, the technological progress and the development and refinement of special instrumentation and the development of new approaches. Kassam et al. introduced the classification for craniopharyngiomas,[43] providing further understanding of the anatomy pertaining to craniopharyngiomas. Indeed, understanding a tumor's position relative to the stalk and other main vital surrounding

Table 25-1	Major Series Reporting the use of EEA for the Removal of Craniopharyngiomas					
Authors and Year	No. of Patients	Tumor Location	Tumor Removal	Post-Operative Endocrinology Outcome	Post-Operative Visual Outcome	Complications
Frank, 2006	10	4 Intra-suprasellar 6 Suprasellar	70% total 10% subtotal 20% partial	No improvement	70% improved 30% unchanged	CSF (33,3%) Permanent DI (33,3%)
de Divitiis, 2007	10	2 Intra-suprasellar 7 Suprasellar 1 Intraventricular	70% total 20% subtotal 10% partial	No improvement	90% improved 10% worsened	CSF (20%) Permanent DI (33,3%)
Laufer, 2007	4	4 Suprasellar	75% total 25% subtotal	100% Pan HP	100% improved	Permanent DI (100%)
Gardner, 2008	16	16 Suprasellar	50% total 31.2% subtotal 18.7% partial	82% unchanged 18% Pan HP	93% improved	CSF (58%) Permanent DI (8%)
Ceylan, 2009	2	2 Intra-suprasellar	100% total	N/A	N/A	N/A
Dehdashti, 2009	6	6 Suprasellar	17% total 83% subtotal	83% unchanged 17% Pan HP	84% improved 16% worsened	CSF (25%) Loss of vision (13%)
Cavallo, 2009*	22*	9 Intra-suprasellar 12 Suprasellar 1 Meckel's cave	40.9% total 54.6% subtotal 4.5% partial	91% unchanged 9% Pan HP	61% improved 22.2% normalized 4.5% worsened	CSF (13.6%) Permanent DI (9.1%) VI CN palsy (4.5%)

N/A: not available.
Subtotal: extent of resection > 70%.
*All cases were recurrent lesions; 9 of them were already present in the previous series.[16,28]

structures is critical for the surgical management of craniopharyngiomas. Accordingly, we approached type 1 lesions usually via a transplanum approach,[17,65] while for type 2 tumors, which generally extend intrasellar, SIS splitting[40] allows full resection with a more rostral trajectory.

For type 3 tumors, where the infundibulum blocks the direct access, we found very useful to mobilize the pituitary gland and stalk to gain direct retrosellar and retroinfundibular access without the manipulation of neurovascular structures.[47] Endoscope properties make safe removal of the posterior clinoid possible, which would be more difficult under a microscopic view. A skillful endoscopist is required to maintain the view in a narrow corridor while the clinoidectomy is performed. This latter maneuver is required to gain adequate access to retroinfundibular tumors, thus achieving a straight midline corridor to the interpeduncular cistern. It should be kept in mind that it is not always possible to determine the position of the infundibulum preoperatively and, above all, its relationships with the tumor, especially when dealing with large tumors. We learned that these relationships become clear after surgical exposure, so flaws in the preoperative planning can be accordingly modified.

Conversely, not all craniopharyngiomas are amenable to this kind of surgery, such as pure third ventricular tumors belonging to group 4.[43] Eccentric extensions of the tumor into the middle cranial fossa, out of the range of surgical instruments, or those encasing or adherent to critical neurovascular structures (ICA, AcomA, optic apparatus, hypothalamus) are clinical scenarios where the effectiveness of the surgery will be limited regardless of the approach. A more limited access to the suprachiasmatic areas is provided whether the chiasm is prefixed or anteriorly displaced.[18,33]

As the approach developed, its surgical limitations, ability to control catastrophic bleeding in a narrow space[31] and the higher risk of postoperative CSF leak[36] were significant concerns. Nevertheless, advances in the exposure techniques and improvements in reconstruction using vascularized flaps[51,66-68] have been developed and refined. These new strategies, combined with and the use of new haemostatic materials and customized instruments have significantly reduced such risks.[52,69,70]

Conclusion

Craniopharyngiomas represent a surgical challenge, whether they are resected via transcranial or transnasal approach or with microscopy or endoscopy. We learned that EEA should be part of the modern neurosurgical armamentarium. The extended endoscopic endonasal approach for suprasellar craniopharyngiomas avoids brain retraction; permits early exposure of the lesion; provides good visualization of the pituitary gland, stalk, and the main vascular structures; and minimizes optic apparatus manipulation. In our experience, it has permitted a better identification of the boundaries between the tumor and the normal tissue, and thus a safer and more radical excision. However, it must be emphasized that EEA cannot change the pathologic entity, its tendency to recurrence, or the fragility of invaded or associated structures.

Results have been promising in terms of tumor removal, preservation, or improvement of function and low complication rate. Definitive conclusions concerning disease control, however, will be drawn only after longer follow-up periods.

KEY REFERENCES

Caldarelli M, di Rocco C, Papacci F, Colosimo Jr C. Management of recurrent craniopharyngioma. *Acta Neurochir (Wien)*. 1998;140:447-454.

Cappabianca P, Cavallo LM, Esposito F, De Divitiis E. Craniopharyngiomas. *J Neurosurg*. 2008;109:1-3.

Cavallo LM, Prevedello DM, Solari D, et al. Extended endoscopic endonasal transsphenoidal approach for residual or recurrent craniopharyngiomas. *J Neurosurg*. 2009;111:578-589.

de Divitiis E, Cappabianca P, Cavallo LM, et al. Extended endoscopic transsphenoidal approach for extrasellar craniopharyngiomas. *Neurosurgery*. 2007;61:219-227:discussion 228.

Fahlbusch R, Honegger J, Paulus W, et al. Surgical treatment of craniopharyngiomas: experience with 168 patients. *J Neurosurg*. 1999; 90:237-250.

Fatemi N, Dusick JR. de Paiva Neto MA, et al: Endonasal versus supraorbital keyhole removal of craniopharyngiomas and tuberculum sellae meningiomas. *Neurosurgery*. 2009;64:269-284: discussion 284-286.

Frank G, Pasquini E, Doglietto F, et al. The endoscopic extended transsphenoidal approach for craniopharyngiomas. *Neurosurgery*. 2006; 59(suppl 1):ONS75-ONS83.

Gardner PA, Kassam AB, Snyderman CH, et al. Outcomes following endoscopic, expanded endonasal resection of suprasellar craniopharyngiomas: a case series. *J Neurosurg*. 2008;109:6-16.

Gardner PA, Prevedello DM, Kassam AB, et al. The evolution of the endonasal approach for craniopharyngiomas. *J Neurosurg*. 2008; 108:1043-1047.

Haupt R, Magnani C, Pavanello M, et al. Epidemiological aspects of craniopharyngioma. *J Pediatr Endocrinol Metab*. 2006;19(suppl 1):289-293.

Honegger J, Buchfelder M, Fahlbusch R, et al. Transsphenoidal microsurgery for craniopharyngioma. *Surg Neurol*. 1992;37:189-196.

Jane Jr JA, Laws ER. Craniopharyngioma. *Pituitary*. 2006;9:323-326.

Kassam AB, Gardner PA, Snyderman CH, et al. Expanded endonasal approach, a fully endoscopic transnasal approach for the resection of midline suprasellar craniopharyngiomas: a new classification based on the infundibulum. *J Neurosurg*. 2008;108:715-728.

Kassam AB, Prevedello DM, Thomas A, et al. Endoscopic endonasal pituitary transposition for a transdorsum sellae approach to the interpeduncular cistern. *Neurosurgery*. 2008;62:57-72:discussion 72-74.

Kassam AB, Thomas A, Carrau RL, et al. Endoscopic reconstruction of the cranial base using a pedicled nasoseptal flap. *Neurosurgery*. 2008;63:ONS44-52; ONS52-43:discussion 72-74.

Laws Jr ER. Transsphenoidal microsurgery in the management of craniopharyngioma. *J Neurosurg*. 1980;52:661-666.

Laws Jr ER. Transsphenoidal removal of craniopharyngioma. *Pediatr Neurosurg*. 1994;21(suppl 1):57-63.

Maira G, Anile C, Albanese A, et al. The role of transsphenoidal surgery in the treatment of craniopharyngiomas. *J Neurosurg*. 2004;100:445-451.

Minamida Y, Mikami T, Hashi K, Houkin K. Surgical management of the recurrence and regrowth of craniopharyngiomas. *J Neurosurg*. 2005;103:224-232.

Prevedello DM, Doglietto F, Jane Jr JA, et al. History of endoscopic skull base surgery: its evolution and current reality. *J Neurosurg*. 2007;107:206-213.

Samii M, Samii A. Surgical management of craniopharyngiomas. In: Schmidek HH, ed. *Schmidek and Sweet Operative Neurosurgical Techniques: Indications, Methods and Results*. vol 1. Philadelphia: WB Saunders; 2000:489-502.

Symon L, Sprich W. Radical excision of craniopharyngioma. Results in 20 patients. *J Neurosurg*. 1985;62:174-181.

Van Effenterre R, Boch AL. Craniopharyngioma in adults and children: a study of 122 surgical cases. *J Neurosurg*. 2002;97:3-11.

Wisoff JH. Surgical management of recurrent craniopharyngiomas. *Pediatr Neurosurg*. 1994;21(suppl 1):108-113.

Yasargil MG, Curcic M, Kis M, et al. Total removal of craniopharyngiomas. Approaches and long-term results in 144 patients. *J Neurosurg*. 1990;73:3-11.

Numbered references appear on Expert Consult.

CHAPTER 26

Arachnoid, Suprasellar, and Rathke's Cleft Cysts

DIETER HELLWIG • WUTTIPONG TIRAKOTAI • VINCENZO PATERNO • CHRISTOPH KAPPUS

Most of the intracranial cystic lesions are related to neoplasms, bacterial or parasitic infections, or loss of tissue due to malformation, infarction, or injury, including that resulting from surgical resection of brain tissue. These topics are discussed in other chapters of this book; however, an additional group of cystic intracranial lesions is encountered in neurosurgical practice, and three of these lesions are discussed in this chapter: the arachnoid, suprasellar, and Rathke's cleft cysts. Of particular interest is that the management of these lesions continues to evolve with the development of endoscopic neurosurgical techniques.[1-12]

Intracranial Arachnoid Cysts

Arachnoid cysts are intra-arachnoid benign cystic lesions filled with cerebrospinal fluid (CSF).[13] According to Cohen and Perneczky,[2] in 1831 Bright was the first to describe the intra-arachnoid location of intracranial arachnoid cysts. These lesions are probably developmental in origin and become symptomatic either because of their progressive enlargement or because of hemorrhage into the cyst. The enlargement of arachnoid cysts has been discussed controversially and is at this point in time a matter for discussion. There are various hypotheses to explain the growth of arachnoid cysts:

1. Active fluid secretion from the cyst wall[14,15]
2. Fluid accumulation caused by an osmotic pressure gradient[16]
3. Pumping of CSF through a persistent communication between the cyst and the arachnoid space due to vascular pulsation[17]
4. The so-called slit-valve mechanism, which is described later[1,18,19]

Arachnoid cysts occur throughout the neuraxis, and generally, no communication is demonstrable between the cyst and the subarachnoid space, although occasionally during surgery an arachnoid cyst is observed being filled through an apparent one-way valve.[20,21] Arachnoid cysts may be asymptomatic throughout life, and rarely, they may spontaneously regress;[22-24] however, if they do become symptomatic, the progression results from compression on the underlying brain, overlying bone, or both. There is an ongoing discussion whether space-occupying asymptomatic cysts should be operated on to prevent a hindrance to normal brain development and function.[25-27] Recently,

Di Rocco[28] commented on this. He discussed whether past failures in the management of this lesion have allowed to individuate reliable criteria to distinguish those subjects who may benefit of the surgical management from those who should be only observed. He emphasized that there are no clear-cut indications for operative treatment of Sylvian fissure arachnoid cysts, and the absence of defined criteria for postoperative success. In his conclusion, he argued that in many instances, surgical indications are offered based on preferences rather than objective evaluation of individual patients.

If the indication for surgery is questionable, intracranial pressure (ICP) monitoring should be performed to prove ICP elevation or pathologic pressure waves.[4,29] The clinical symptoms resulting from these arachnoid cysts depend greatly on their location—whether over the sylvian fissure; over the cerebral convexity; in the interhemispheric region; in the sella and suprasellar region; around the optic nerve, the quadrigeminal plate, or the cerebellopontine angle; in the region of the clivus; over the cerebellar vermis or cerebellar hemisphere; or within the lateral or fourth ventricle.[30-36] Arachnoid cysts have also been described extending across the region of the foramen magnum from the posterior cranial fossa into the upper cervical spine posterolateral to the spinal cord.[37-39] The midline lesions often lead to an obstruction of the CSF flow and result in focal symptoms and raised ICP.[40-43] There is a continuing discussion about whether intracranial arachnoid cysts are related to a specific seizure type and electroencephalographic focus.[44]

The arachnoid cyst wall is histologically indistinguishable from normal arachnoidal membrane. Moderate thickening of the arachnoid and an increase in connective tissue are common (Fig. 26-1).[45] Ultrastructural studies confirm the similarity of the cyst membrane with the normal meningeal counterpart, including the cell-cell connections and the occurrence of basal laminal structures. Quantitative differences in the contribution of the single components have been found both between different cysts and between cysts and normal arachnoid.

In a recently published microsurgical and endoscopic anatomical study, Inoue and colleagues[46] claimed that there are two types of arachnoid membranes: outer and inner. The outer arachnoidal membrane surrounds the whole brain, and the inner membranes divide the subarachnoid space into cisterns. Twelve inner arachnoid membranes

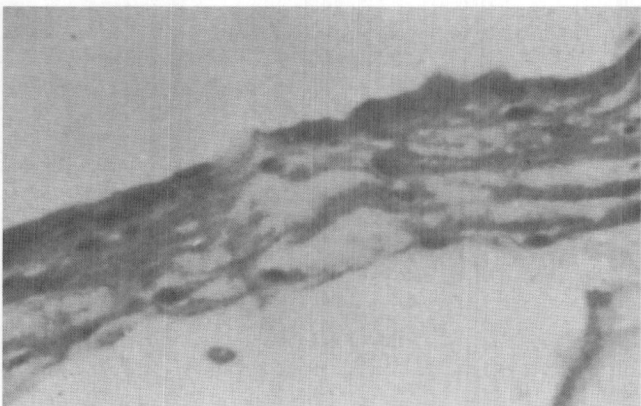

FIGURE 26-1 Lining of subarachnoid cysts consisting of a single layer of arachnoid and adjacent loose subarachnoid network and psammoma body. H&E stain. *(From Youmans JR. Neurological Surgery, 2nd ed, vol. 3. Philadelphia: WB Saunders; 1982:1437.)*

and 9 cisterns were identified in this study. A special kind of arachnoid cyst formation consists of a luminal epithelial layer connected with a glial sheet, followed peripherally by a thin connective tissue covering (Fig. 26-2.).

The glial nature of parts of the cyst lining can be shown by glial fibrillary acidic protein staining. Some authors have called these cysts "glioependymal."[47]

In many cases, arachnoidal cysts are incidental findings noted on CT scanning or MRI of the head performed for a reason unrelated to the cyst. Such patients are informed about the radiographic finding; provided with a copy of the study so they can present it to a physician at a later date, if necessary; and followed up annually. In approximately 15% of middle fossa arachnoid cysts, an asymptomatic lesion may become symptomatic as a result of bleeding in association with the cyst and raised ICP. This event may occur after minor head trauma.[48-50]

In a report of 6 cases of subdural hematoma occurring in 18 patients with previously asymptomatic middle cranial fossa arachnoid cysts, Rogers and colleagues[51] recommended a cystoperitoneal shunt to treat the cyst after evacuation of the hematoma. Auer and co-workers[52] also recommended evacuation of the hematoma and the cyst's wall in one procedure. Handa and associates[53] reported on the two-stage removal of bilateral cysts and hematomas. They recommend that the hematomas be drained initially through burr holes and that 3 months later the cyst wall be resected and a cystoperitoneal shunt inserted. Mori and colleagues as well propose a two-step procedure. Hematoma evacuation is adequate at first operation. If the preoperative symptoms persist, additional arachnoid cyst surgery should be considered.[54] Markakis and colleagues[55] also recommend a two-stage approach to the management of large arachnoidal cysts, beginning with a shunt procedure, which is followed several weeks later by the resection of the cyst wall and a ventriculostomy. Another treatment option is to evacuate the hematoma through an endoscopic burr hole approach and perform a cystostomy to the CSF space in one procedure.[56] Interestingly, successful treatment of middle fossa arachnoid, cysts, which means reduction of cyst size, may not reduce the risk of posttraumatic injury hemorrhage as demonstrated by Spacca and co-workers in

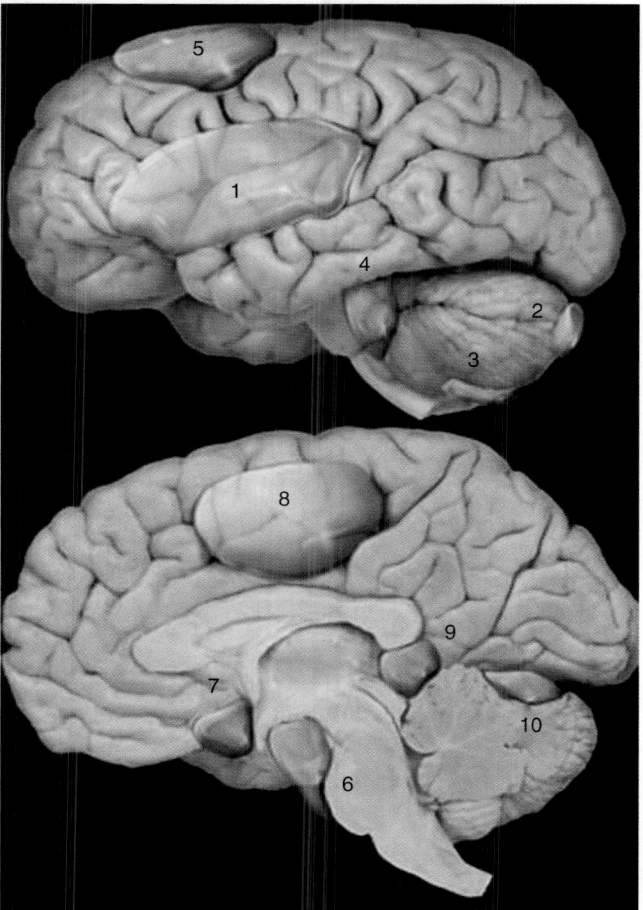

FIGURE 26-2 Typical localizations of intracranial arachnoid cysts. Supratentorial: sylvian fissure *(1)*, cerebral convexity *(5)*, interhemispheric fissure *(8)*, sellar and suprasellar *(7)*. Optic nerve: intraorbital, intracranial. Tentorial: quadrigeminal plate *(9)*. Infratentorial: clival *(6)*, cerebellopontine angle *(4)*, posterior midline *(10)*, vermis *(2)*, cisterna magna *(3)*.

a series of 40 patients operated with endoscopic fenestration. Four of these patients experienced a post-traumatic intracystic bleeding after surgery.[57]

Cerebral convexity cysts occurring in adults present as seizures, headache, raised ICP, and, sometimes, marked reactive thickening of the overlying skull with erosion of the inner table. These cases can be managed by the wide excision of the membranes and the establishment of communication between the cyst interior and the CSF of the subarachnoid space. The same approach has been used in the treatment of symptomatic interhemispheric arachnoid cysts and cysts in the region of the quadrigeminal plate that produce aqueductal obstruction that leads to hydrocephalus. Before the advent of MRI, arachnoid cysts of the cerebellopontine angle often presented a diagnostic dilemma that required differentiation from other mass lesions located in the cerebellopontine angle.[31] Cysts of the cerebellopontine angle may mimic other lesions in this location and may cause hearing loss and cerebellar signs. These cysts may present as intermittent downbeat nystagmus with an associated hydrocephalus or as vague symptoms, including hearing loss and disequilibrium, contralateral trigeminal neuralgia, or hemifacial spasm.[58-61]

Surgical options for the management of symptomatic arachnoid cysts include the endoscopic resection of the cyst wall with opening of the membranes, which establishes communication with the hemispheric or ventricular CSF pathways. Levy and co-workers described their results using the microsurgical keyhole approach for middle fossa arachnoid cysts.[62] This procedure can be performed with minimal morbidity via minicraniotomy. Compared with an endoscopic approach, better control of hemostasis can be obtained. The operative time and length of hospital stay were not excessively increased. Other options are stereotactic cyst aspiration,[63-65] shunt drainage or drainage of the lesion through a burr hole,[66] craniotomy with resection or marsupialization of the cyst walls,[67] and craniectomy and ventriculostomy of the cyst.[24,68] In a cooperative European study of the management of arachnoid cysts in children, total excision or marsupialization emerged as the first-choice surgical procedure, and shunting procedures were often applied to cysts located in deeper locations. Among the 285 patients, from birth to 15 years of age, there was a resultant reduction of the size of the cyst in approximately two thirds of the cases, and in 18%, the cyst had disappeared completely on follow-up CT scanning.[69] Another study of the relative merits of different approaches to the management of arachnoid cysts in children is based on an analysis of 40 children treated between 1978 and 1989 at the University of California, San Francisco. Of 15 patients with cysts that were treated initially by fenestration alone, 67% showed no clinical or radiographic improvement and subsequently required cyst-peritoneal or ventriculoperitoneal shunting. All of these patients improved postoperatively, although shunt revision was required in approximately one third of cases as a result of the recurrence of a cyst. These authors concluded that, irrespective of the location of the lesion, cyst-peritoneal or cyst-ventriculoperitoneal shunting is the treatment of choice.[25] However, there is considerable risk of overdrainage with posterior fossa overcrowding and acquired Chiari I malformation, or hindbrain herniation.[70]

Several groups reported about their results in neuroendoscopic treatment of arachnoid cysts. In a prospective study, Schroeder and coworkers[10] treated seven consecutive patients with symptomatic arachnoid cysts in different locations endoscopically. The authors performed cystocisternostomies and ventriculocystostomies via burr holes with the aid of a universal neuroendoscopic system. Symptoms were relieved in five patients and improved in one patient, whereas the size of the cyst decreased in six patients. Although the follow-up period was short (15 to 30 months), the authors recommend neuroendoscopic treatment of arachnoid cyst as the first therapy of choice. The second study was conducted by Hopf and co-workers.[6] They evaluated 24 patients with intracranial arachnoid cysts that were treated endoscopically. Their surgical strategy was to create broad communication between the cyst and the subarachnoid space. Various techniques were used: endoscopic fenestration (10 cases), endoscopic controlled microsurgery (5 cases), and endoscopy-assisted microsurgery (9 cases). In all patients sufficient fenestration of the cysts could be achieved, with a favorable outcome in 17 patients. Operative complications included infection (3 patients), bleeding into the cyst (1 patient), and subdural fluid collections

(4 patients). The authors conclude that different endoscopic techniques do provide sufficient treatment of selected arachnoid cysts. Recent advances in neurosurgical techniques and neuroendoscopy continue to favor cyst fenestration over shunt insertion as the method of choice for initial cyst decompression.[71]

CASE REPORT 1: ARACHNOID CYST

A 14-year-old boy was admitted with aggressive attitude, loss of motivation, headache, and nausea. The neurologic examination was normal. An electroencephalogram showed a left-sided reduction of activity in the frontotemporal region. Magnetic resonance imaging (MRI) demonstrated a large left, frontotemporal arachnoid cyst with a slight mass effect (Fig. 26-3). Epidural ICP measurement during a period of 24 hours revealed normal values (Fig. 26-4). We concluded that the cyst was not related to the patient's symptoms, and no further intervention was performed. Long-term follow-up examinations showed that the patient was in good neurologic condition with normal age-related capacity.

CASE REPORT 2: ARACHNOID CYST

A 72-year-old woman suffered from headache, stupor, and right hemiparesis. A large left hemispheric cystic process with a midline shift was diagnosed by computed tomography (CT) and MRI examination (Fig. 26-5A and B). Using three-dimensional (3D) stereotactic trajectory and target-point calculation, the cyst membrane was approached endoscopically through a right frontal burr hole. The gray membrane was opened by radiofrequency coagulation, and biopsies were taken (Fig. 26-5C). The cyst contained CSF-like fluid. There was no evidence of tumor or other pathology. The histopathologic diagnosis was that of an epithelial cyst. The cyst was opened endoscopically to the left lateral ventricle. After surgery, the CT scan showed that the midline shift was greatly reduced. The left frontal horn was enlarged again (Fig. 26-5D). A few days after the intervention, the patient was alert and she was discharged with only a slight hemiparesis.

CASE REPORT 3: ARACHNOID CYST AND CHRONIC SUBDURAL HEMATOMA

A 12-year-old boy had been hit on the head by a hockey stick. He suffered from headaches, and 2 weeks later his consciousness was impaired. MRI examination showed a left chronic subdural hematoma (Fig. 26-6A) related to a temporal arachnoid cyst (Fig. 26-6B). The subdural hematoma was drained through a silicone catheter. On CT examination, the subdural hematoma was greatly reduced with no signs of raised ICP or mass effect (Fig. 26-6C). We decided to leave the arachnoid cyst without further operative intervention. The patient did not develop complications during the postoperative course. Over a follow-up period of 9 years, the arachnoid cyst has remained.

CASE REPORT 4: ARACHNOID CYST AND POSTOPERATIVE CHRONIC SUBDURAL HEMATOMA

This female patient suffered from headache, vertigo, and partial oculomotor palsy. CT demonstrated a left-sided temporal arachnoid cyst (Fig. 26-7A). Endoscopic cystocisternostomy was performed. Postoperative CT examination

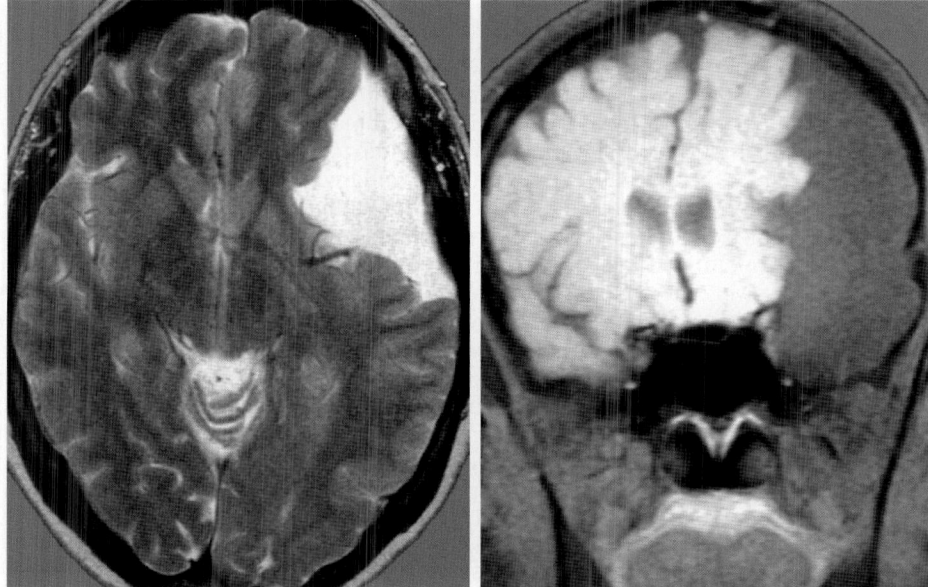

FIGURE 26-3 See Case Report 1: Arachnoid Cyst.

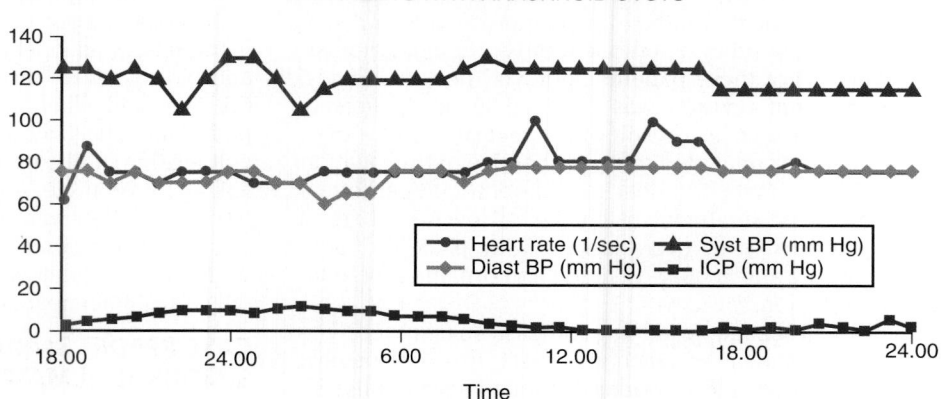

FIGURE 26-4 diastBP, diastolic blood pressure; ICP, intracranial pressure; syst BP, systolic blood pressure.

showed reduction of the cyst size (Fig. 26-7B), and symptoms improved. However, in the follow-up a subdural fluid collection with mass effect developed (Fig. 26-7C and D). This subdural hematoma was evacuated successfully via burr hole drainage as seen in control CT examination (Fig. 26-7E).

NEUROENDOSCOPIC INSTRUMENTATION AND OPERATIVE TECHNIQUE IN TREATMENT OF ARACHNOID CYSTS

Endoscopes

Various rigid and flexible endoscopes are available to perform cystostomy, cystoventriculostomy, or cystocisternoventriculostomy (Fig. 26-8A and B). The advantages of rigid-lens scopes are the brilliant and bright pictorial quality and the guidance via a predetermined direct trajectory. Angled rigid scopes are used together with microscopes and neuronavigational devices in endoscopy-assisted microsurgery.[72] They offer the possibility of looking around

corners. Flexible neuroscopes have the advantages of steerability and maneuverability, which make inspection and interventions on multifocal and multiseptated cystic lesions easier.[73]

Guidance

There are different methods to perform endoscopic interventions on arachnoid cysts. The easiest and most time-sparing technique is the "freehand method." The approach is a single burr hole, and during the intervention the surgeon orients on anatomic landmarks. The advantage is to be free from holding and guiding devices; however, the operative approach and the targeting could be inaccurate.

Frame-based stereotactic guidance provides high accuracy and ensures orientation but could be time consuming and restricts endoscope movements. Standard neuronavigation systems provide image guidance, which is interactive and precise.[74] These systems can be applied in a freehand

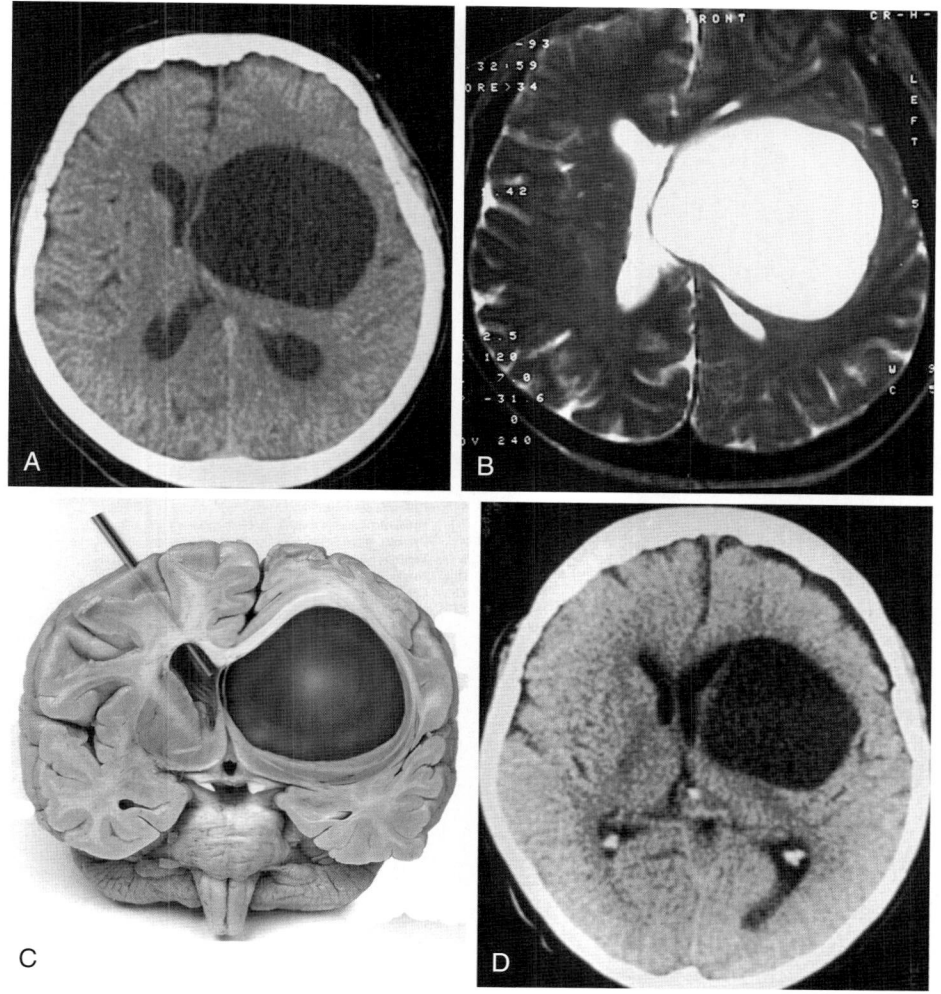

FIGURE 26-5 See Case Report 2: Arachnoid Cyst.

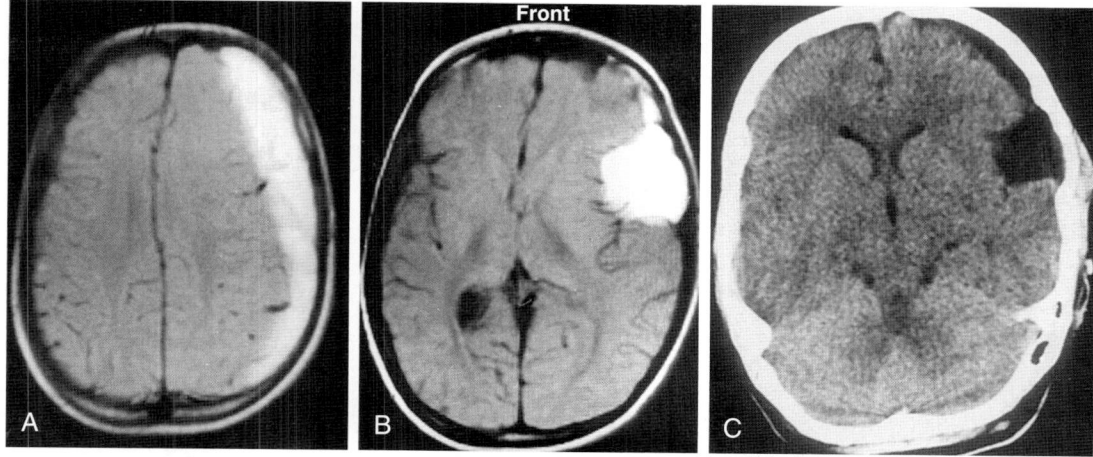

FIGURE 26-6 See Case Report 3: Arachnoid Cyst and Chronic Subdural Hematoma.

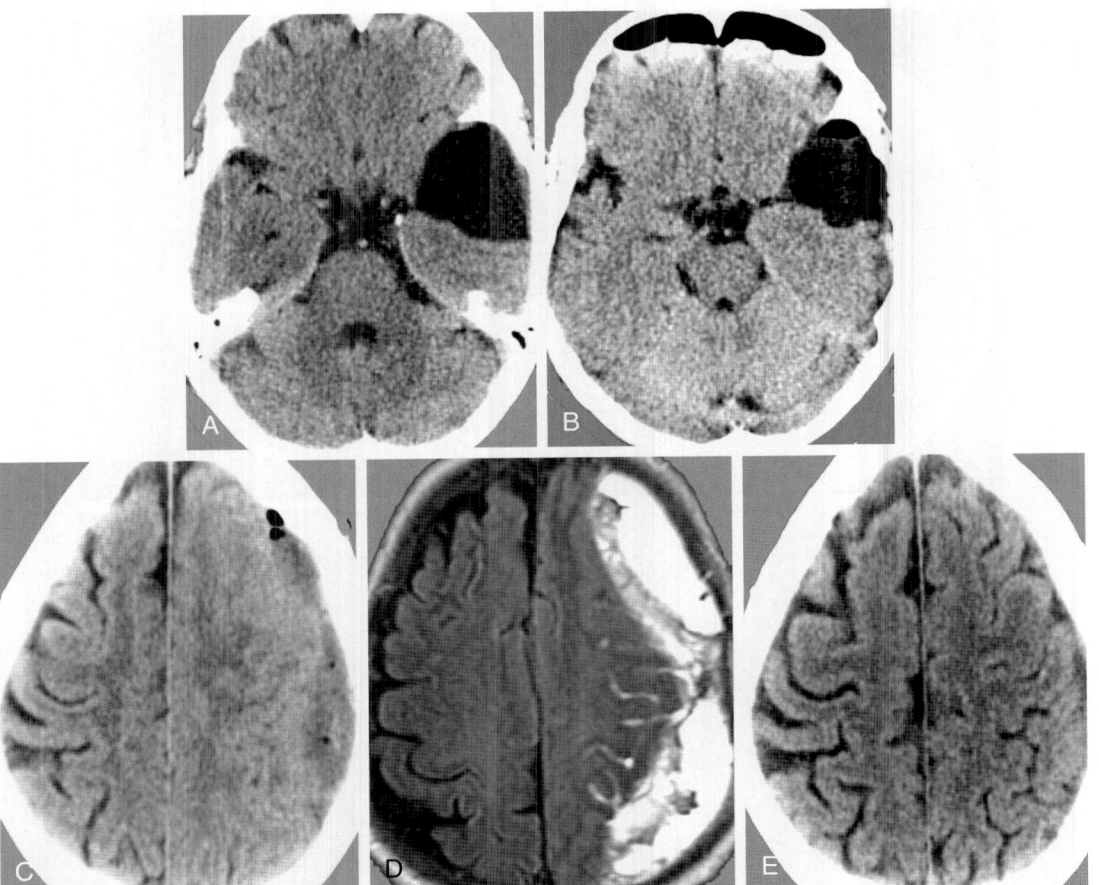

FIGURE 26-7 See Case Report 4: Arachnoid Cyst and Postoperative Chronic Subdural Hematoma.

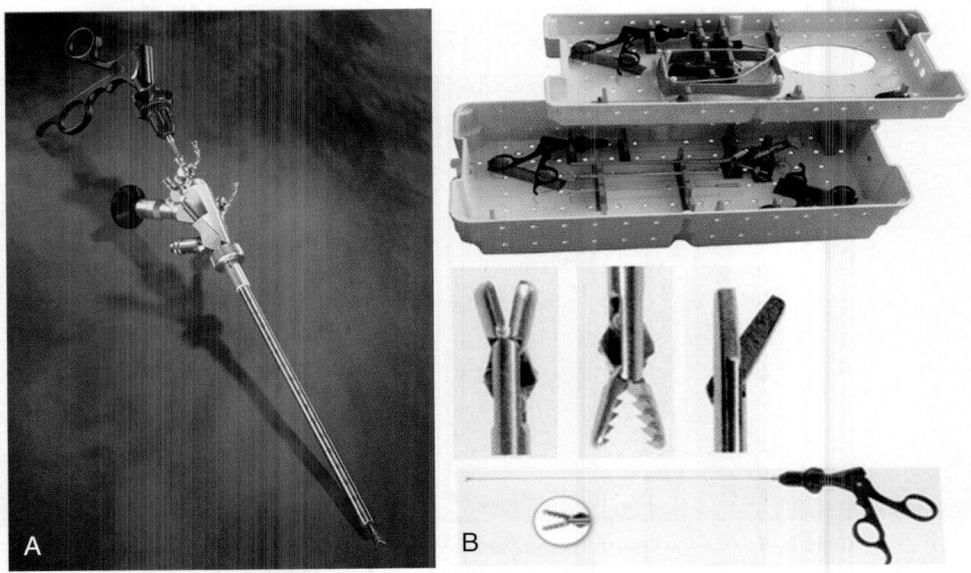

FIGURE 26-8 A, Rigid multipurpose endoscope: one working channel, one rinsing canal, one suction canal (outer diameter 6.5 mm, direction of view 5 degrees). B, Working instruments: biopsy forceps, grasping forceps, microscissors, diameter 1.6 mm for ETV, tumor biopsy and dissection of cyst walls. These instruments are detachable and rotatable. (A and B, Complete Set for Intraventricular Neuroendoscopy, Rudolf Medical Co., Tuttlingen, Germany.)

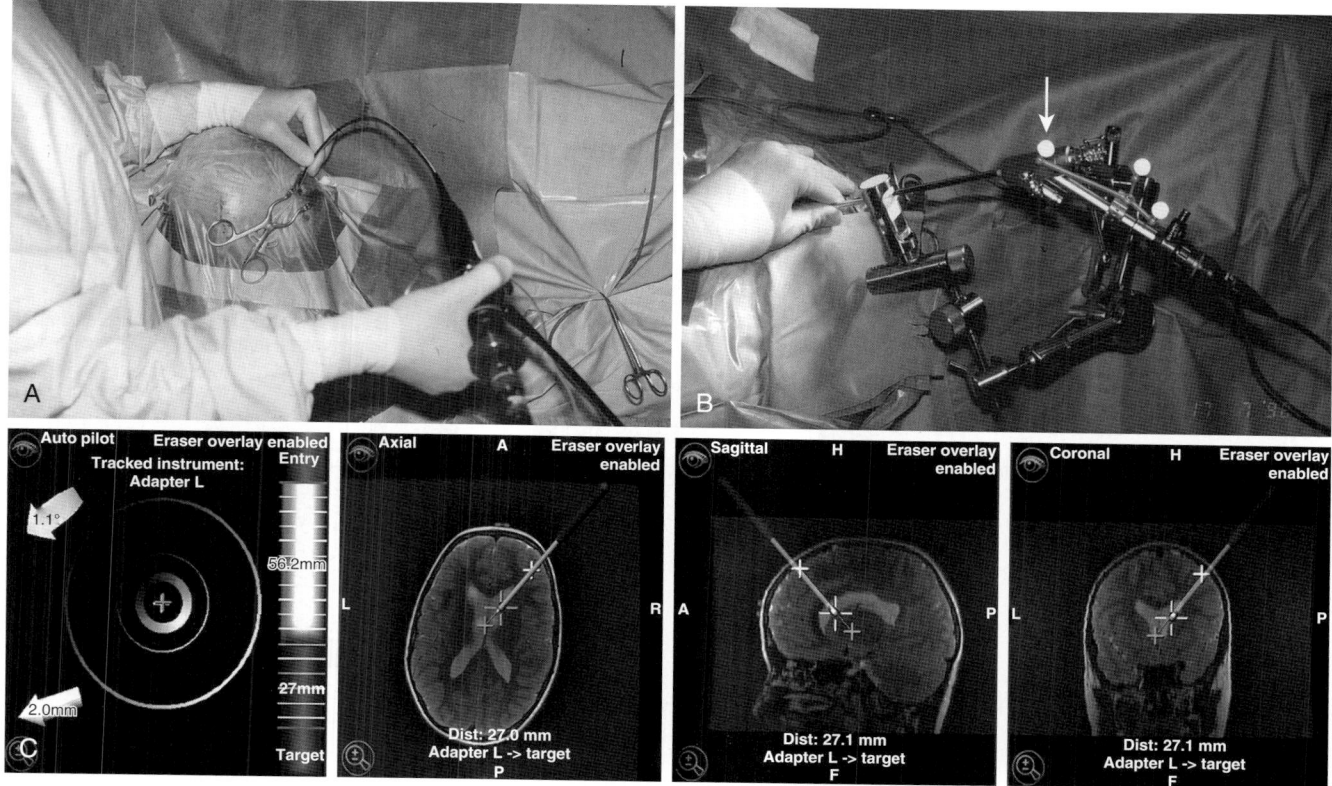

FIGURE 26-9 Various neuroendoscopy guiding techniques. A, Freehand technique with flexible steerable endoscope. B, Fixed technique with rigid endoscope (Zeppelin Co.) adjusted to a stereotaxy holding and guiding device in combination with neuronavigational guidance (*arrow*: see white star–shaped instrument adapters). C, Neuronavigation assembly for 3D calculation and real-time visualization of the endoscopic approach to ventricular cystic lesion.

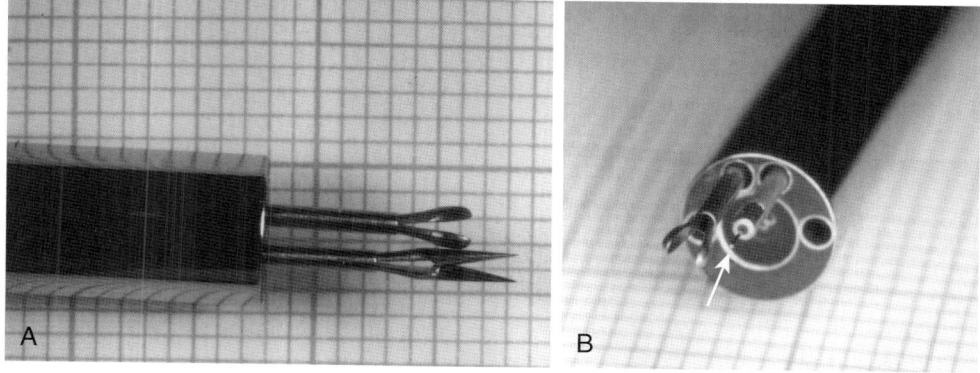

FIGURE 26-10 Supplementary endoscopy working instruments. A, Microscissors and grasping forceps guided through the rigid endoscope's working channel. B, Biopsy forceps and tip of bipolar coagulation and cutting microelectrode, which has a diameter of 0.9 mm (*arrow*) (Erbe Elektromedizin GmbH, Tübingen, Germany).

mode or in combination with holding and guiding devices (Fig. 26-9A to C).

Instruments

Moving neuroendoscopic working instruments within preformed or pathologic CNS cavities, as arachnoid cysts are, is not easy and requires training for several reasons: distances might be estimated incorrectly; the instrument may enter the viewing field from the side or is out of view; the surgeon controls the procedure at a video screen, and not directly as in microsurgery.

Various instruments are available for endoscopic interventions on arachnoid cysts. Microforceps and scissors are helpful to open and resect cyst membranes (Fig. 26-10A and B). Newly developed bipolar microforceps make it possible to dissect membranes and perform hemostasis using a single instrument (Fig. 26-11).[75]

In many cases, it is advisable to open the arachnoid cysts using electrosurgical devices. In cooperation with Erbe Company, we have developed a bipolar cutting and coagulation microprobe, which is controlled automatically by an electrosurgical unit. The regulated energy release avoids

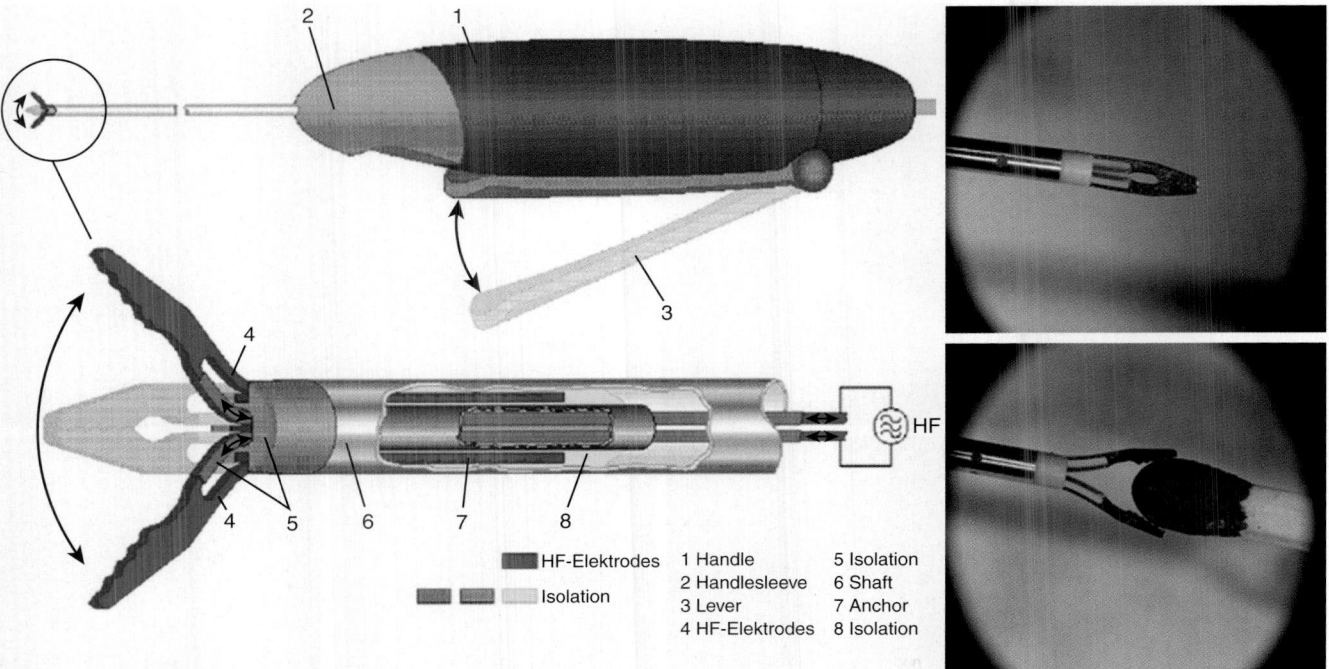

		1 Handle	5 Isolation
HF-Elektrodes		2 Handlesleeve	6 Shaft
Isolation		3 Lever	7 Anchor
		4 HF-Elektrodes	8 Isolation

FIGURE 26-11 Novel multipurpose bipolar instrument (Erbe Elektromedizin GmbH, Tübingen, Germany) for endoscopic neurosurgery (diameter 1.5 mm, length 360 mm). Branches can be opened smoothly to width of 6 mm, despite small diameter of instrument.

thermal damage to vulnerable structures. Safe hemostasis is ensured by pinpoint accuracy and effective coagulation of small vessels. The cutting depth is freely adjustable up to 3 mm. The cutting needle can be retracted into the endoscope's working channel. The probes are available for both rigid and flexible endoscopes with diameters of between 0.9 and 1.5 mm (Fig. 26-12).[76] Balloon catheters (Fogarty, double balloon) are very useful to enlarge the stomas in a nontraumatic fashion.

Imaging

Intraoperative digital dynamic subtraction cystography (cystoventriculography) is performed routinely to show the communication of the arachnoid cyst to the adjoining CSF compartments and the restoration of normal CSF flow. After the endoscopic intervention postoperative electrocardiogram-gated dynamic MRI examination demonstrates the normalized CSF flow under real-time conditions. In a recently published study Hoffmann and colleagues[77] could show 90% accuracy in diagnosis of communication between arachnoid cysts and neighboring CSF spaces using cine-mode MR imaging. Algin and coworkers[78] compared phase-contrast (PC) cine MRI versus MR cisternography to evaluate the communication between intraventricular arachnoid cysts and neighboring cerebrospinal fluid spaces. They found that PCMRI is an effective method for evaluating noncommunicating arachnoid cysts. The results should be confirmed with MR cisternography as suspected jet flow is depicted.

CASE REPORT 5: PINEAL CYST

A 38-year-old female suffered from vertigo, headache, and intermittent loss of consciousness. MRI revealed an obstructive hydrocephalus due to a sylvian aqueduct obstruction caused by a cystic lesion in the posterior part of the third ventricle (Fig. 26-13A). Cystoventriculostomy was performed using the flexible, steerable endoscope (Fig. 26-13B). Fluoroscopy was used for intraoperative control (Fig. 26-13C). Postoperative MRI shows a cyst-collapse and re-establishment of CSF flow through the aqueduct (Fig. 26-13D). Fig. 26-14 shows the intraoperative findings during the operative procedure. By moving the flexible endoscope nearly the whole dorsal part of the third ventricle can be explored, as shown in Fig. 26-14A.

Suprasellar Cysts

Suprasellar cysts are arachnoid cysts that occur in the sella region and become symptomatic as locally expanding lesions. Arachnoid cysts in relation to the sella turcica represent 10% of all cases.[79] The term *suprasellar cyst*, formerly a synonym for craniopharyngioma, designates a small group of lesions, usually congenital, with a thin, even transparent wall that is filled with clear, colorless, or light-yellow fluid. The congenital effect from these cysts, which constitute fewer than 1% of all intracranial mass lesions, was severe enough to cause symptoms in the first 2 decades in 46 of the 54 reports collected by Hoffman and co-workers.[80] The lesion evolves as a consequence of prevention of CSF circulation into the chiasmatic cistern or laterally from the interpeduncular cistern beneath the hypothalamus and behind the pituitary stalk and optic chiasm. The presence of CSF from below the pontine cistern then pushes the hypothalamic floor upward and thins it greatly, so that above the arachnoid dome are only at most a few glial and ependymal cells, as described by Harrison[81] in three of four cases. In many of the cases, thin, even transparent, connective tissue is the only lining to the cyst. As do arachnoid

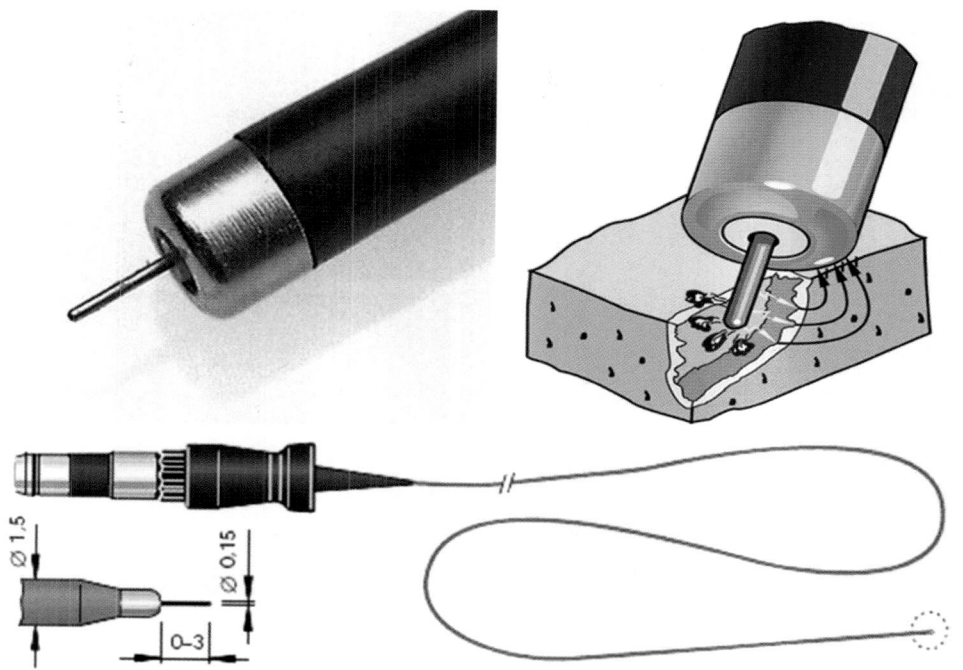

FIGURE 26-12 Flexible Marburg® cutting and coagulation probe. Specifications: diameter 0.9 mm, working length 600 mm, insulated, needle length adjustable from 0 to 3 mm, maximal operating voltage 500 Vp. (Erbe Elektromedizin GmbH, Tübingen, Germany.)

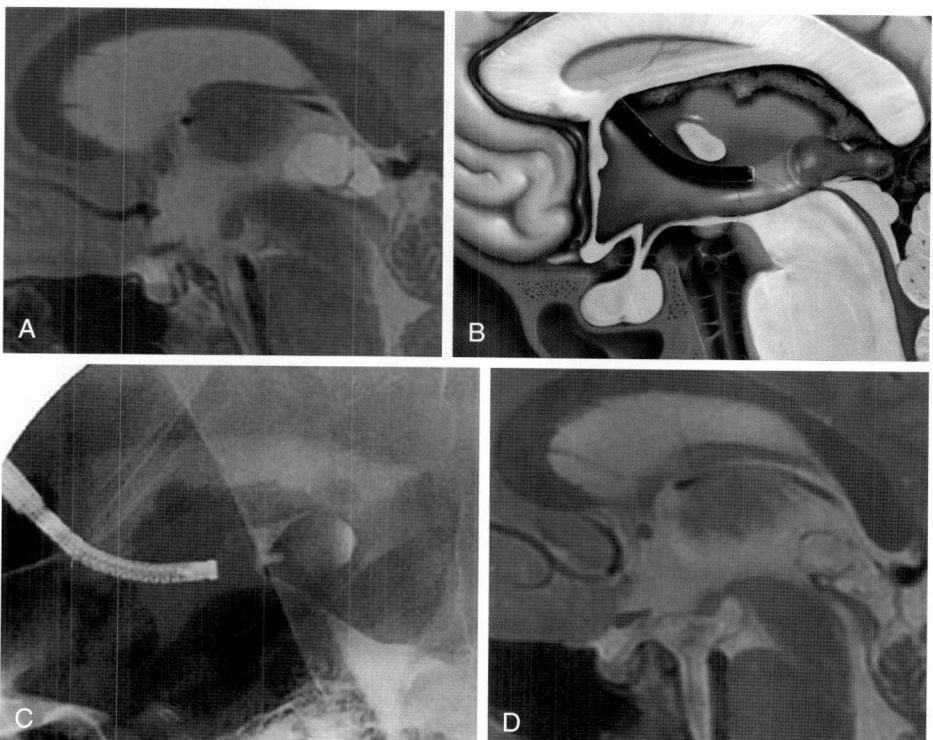

FIGURE 26-13 See Case Report 5: Pineal Cyst.

cysts in other locations, suprasellar arachnoid cysts may enlarge over time. This change could be effected by active secretion of the membrane[82] or from ectopic choroid-like structures[14] or osmotic pressure gradients.[16] Another theory for the enlargement of suprasellar arachnoid cysts is based on endoscopic and cine-mode evidence of a slit valve,[1,19,20] formed by an arachnoid membrane around the basilar artery. This valve is supposed to open and close with arterial pulsations and lead to an inflow of CSF into the cyst forced by a pressure gradient.

By the time that the diagnosis is made, much or all of the third ventricle is usually filled by the cyst, causing an obstruction of one or both foramina of Monro, lateral ventricular dilatation, and a huge head. Indeed, the dome of the

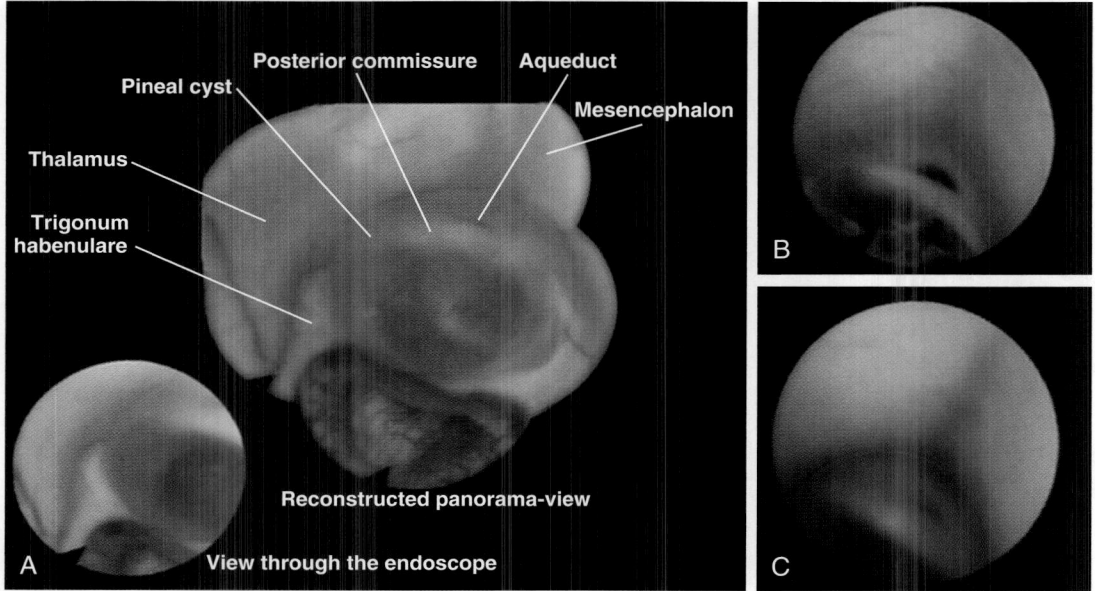

FIGURE 26-14 A, Demonstrates full range of endoscopic views during procedure for endoscopic orientation. B and C, Screenshots of aqueduct before and after fenestration of the cyst.

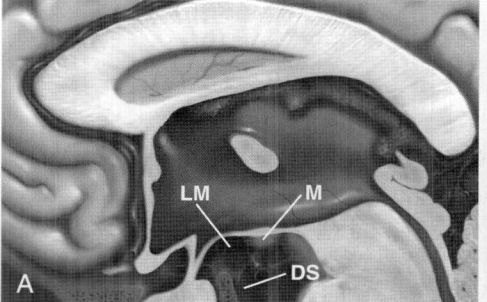
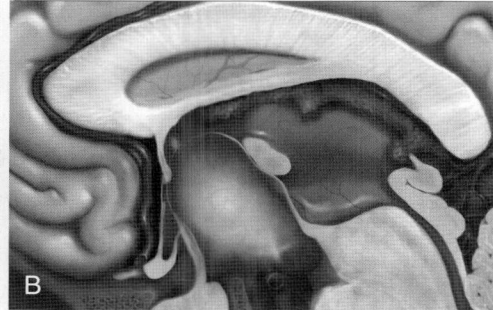

FIGURE 26-15 Anatomy of a suprasellar cyst. A, Artist's conception of sagittal section of normal brain and sellar region, looking to the right. M, mammillary body; LM, Lillequist's membrane; DS, dorsum sellae. B, The membrane of Lillequist has ballooned forward and backward, compressing the floor of the third ventricle to the level of the massa intermedia.

cyst is usually much higher than that shown in Fig. 26-15, lying just beneath the corpus callosum.

One possible mechanism for this block is excessive development of an arachnoidal curtain that extends from the posterior hypothalamus to the dorsum sellae below, originally described by Key and Retzius.[83] Its presence, confirmed by Lillequist[84] and by Fox and Al-Mefty,[85] becomes a menace when such curtain and the arachnoid lateral to it become imperforate. Another mechanism of pathogenesis, proposed by Starkman and coworkers,[86] is that intra-arachnoidal spaces in the embryo persist and expand exclusively within the arachnoid. This event was demonstrated incidentally at autopsy in a careful dissection of an intact suprasellar cyst by Krawchenko and Collins.[13] Most suprasellar arachnoid cysts occur in children, with a male prevalence.[2] The clinical picture often includes, in addition to hydrocephalus with a big head and ataxia, disturbed visual acuity and fields due to forward and upward displacement of the chiasm, and hypopituitarism due to pressure in the hypothalamus and pituitary stalk. These symptoms caused by a suprasellar cystic lesion had been first described by Pieter Pauw, a Dutch anatomist, in the 16th century.[87]

A constant forward and backward nodding of the head and neck, the bobble-head doll syndrome, is an inconstant sign.[88-90] Hagebeuck and coworkers[91] describe this syndrome in a 4-year-old boy, which resolved completely 3 years after endoscopic cystoventriculostomy. An unusual symptom is precocious puberty.[92] Headache may occur in older patients. On CT scans, the cyst has the density of CSF; its wall shows neither enhancement nor calcification and is often mistaken for a dilated third ventricle. According to Cohen and Perneczky,[2] suprasellar arachnoid cysts appear as midline round or oval hypodense lesions adjacent to the dilated frontal horns. They have a typical "Mickey Mouse" configuration on axial CT scans or MRI. Prenatal diagnosis is possible using antenatal ultrasound combined with antenatal MRI.[93] Effective surgical treatment, which would seem to require simply making a big opening between the cyst and a normal CSF compartment, proves to be surprisingly difficult. Various combinations have been tried, including the transfrontal removal of the lower anterior wall of the cyst beneath the chiasm, a transcorticoventricular or transcallosal approach to remove much of the dome, the insertion of catheters between the cyst and ventricle or chiasmatic cistern, and the insertion of shunts from the lateral ventricles. Any one of these operations alone has a poor chance of sustained success. Agreement seems to be converging on the insertion of a combination of shunts from the

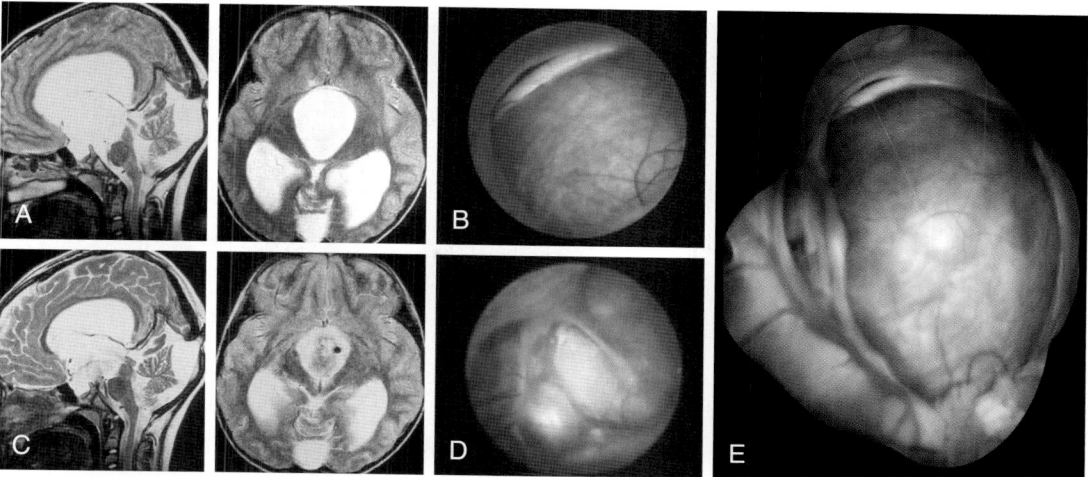

FIGURE 26-16 See Case Report 6: Suprasellar Arachnoid Cyst.

lateral ventricles to the peritoneal cavity, with either a transcallosal route to remove the cystic dome, which was used with sustained success by Hoffman and coworkers in five cases,[71] or subfrontal removal of the anterior cyst wall. This latter tactic was successful in two cases from Gonzalez and colleagues,[94] three cases from Raimondi and colleagues,[95] and two cases from Murali and Epstein.[96] However, the lower opening closed, and symptoms recurred in one case of each of the last two groups and in one of Hoffman and co-workers' cases. That shunts from the ventricles alone may not suffice was demonstrated in a case from Murali and Epstein, in a child in whom a neonatal shunt kept the ventricles small but who also required opening of a suprasellar cyst to control bilateral visual loss 9 years later. Ventriculoperitoneal shunting alone was satisfactory in Raimondi's fourth case. Each of the traditional approaches has been associated with a high rate of recurrence of cysts.[2]

Upcoming neuroendoscopic techniques seem to solve some of the major surgical problems in treatment of suprasellar arachnoid cysts. Pierre-Khan and associates[89] were the first to publish their results after performing endoscopic ventriculocystostomy of suprasellar arachnoid cysts. They used a monopolar electroprobe to create the wide stoma between the cyst and the ventricular cistern (ventriculocystostomy). In contrast to them, Caemaert and associates[1] prefer to use the neodymium:yttrium aluminum garnet (Nd:YAG) laser to open the cyst to the ventricular system and the basal cisterns (ventriculocystcisternostomy). None of the patients had postoperative complications or need for a secondary shunting procedure. Additional authors have published similar successful results.[2,19,97-100] Gangemi and associates[11] did an extensive literature review and described the postoperative follow-up of five patients with suprasellar arachnoid cysts at their own institution after endoscopic fenestration. They found among the reviewed cases, a rate of cure or improvement of 90% (92 of 102 patients including their own cases) after endoscopy and 81% (60 among 74 cases) after other surgical procedures. The results of this study suggest that endoscopic ventricle-cyst-cisternostomy is the best treatment for suprasellar arachnoid cysts, because it is less invasive, provides the best results, and avoids shunt dependency in most cases.

CASE REPORT 6: SUPRASELLAR ARACHNOID CYST

An 8-year-old girl presented with signs of raised ICP, ataxia, and a cognitive disorder. MRI showed a hydrocephalus caused by a large suprasellar cyst with brain stem compression (Fig. 26-16A). The girl was operated on with the neuroendoscopic technique using the frontal transventricular burr-hole approach. The cyst bulged into the foramen of Monro (Fig. 26-16B). After cystocisternostomy the pituitary stalk was clearly seen (Fig. 26-16D). Six days after the intervention, the girl's clinical condition was good and she was discharged. A control MRI, taken 1 year after the intervention, shows that the cystic lesion has reduced greatly in volume, and free CSF communication existed between the ventricular system and the basal cisterns, which is documented by a postoperative MRI scan with typical flow-void signal in T2-weighted sequences (Fig. 26-16C). The girl still has no neurologic signs.

Figure 26-16E was reconstructed from different endoscopic photographs to show the entire range of the endoscopic views while moving the endoscope during the procedure.

NEUROENDOSCOPIC TECHNIQUE IN TREATMENT OF SUPRASELLAR ARACHNOID CYSTS

Preoperatively, it is advisable to plan the operative approach whether stereotactically or by neuronavigation. Through a frontal precoronal burr-hole approach, the surgeon enters the frontal horn of the lateral ventricle with the endoscope.[74] The cyst dome is typically bulging through the foramen of Monro. Ventriculocystostomy is performed using microscissors and microforceps as well as the bipolar coagulation and cutting device. It is advisable to create a large stoma (10–15 mm in diameter). After inspection of the parasellar region, it is absolutely necessary to open the membrane of Lillequist (cystocisternostomy), which forms the inferior wall of the cyst toward the prepontine cistern, using the basilar artery as a landmark. Our bipolar coagulation and cutting electrodes prove to be the safe instruments to make bloodless openings and avoid thermal effects to the surrounding nerve tissue.[75,76]

Because many patients are severely impaired by the time of initial diagnosis, prompt aggressive effort and close

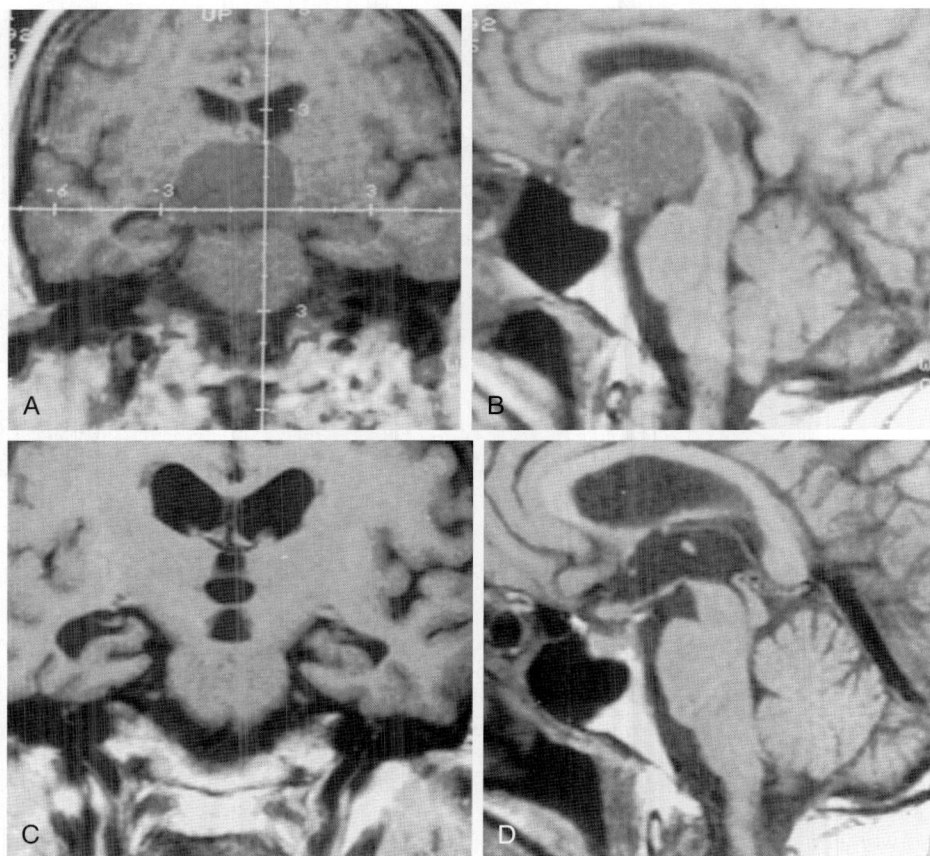

FIGURE 26-17 See Case Report 7: Low-Grade Astrocytoma.

follow-ups are required. In rare cases prepontine arachnoid cysts can disappear spontaneously as described by Dodd[101] and Thomas.[102]

CASE REPORT 7: LOW-GRADE ASTROCYTOMA

A 62-year-old woman was admitted with a progressive bitemporal hemianopia and agitated psychosis (Karnofsky score of 30%). On MRI, a large cystic suprasellar space-occupying lesion with a blockage of foramen of Monro (Fig. 26-17A and B) was noted. Endoscopic stereotactic cyst evacuation was performed as an emergency procedure. The cystic lesion was reached through a right frontal burr hole. The gray membrane that bulged into the foramen of Monro was coagulated and was opened by microscissors. The sticky yellow contents of the cyst were aspirated. The remaining cyst membrane was vaporized using a laser. The histopathologic diagnosis was of a low-grade astrocytoma. Visual loss and the psychological disturbances of the patient normalized immediately after the procedure. A postoperative MRI showed that the cystic process was totally evacuated (Figs. 26-17C and D). The patient was discharged 12 days after the procedure (Karnofsky score of 90%).

Rathke's Cleft Cysts

Rathke's pouch, the superiorly directed evagination from the stomodeum of the 4-week-old human embryo, becomes obliterated at all but its cranial portion by the seventh week of gestation. The anterior wall of the remaining small cavity, "the pituitary pouch," develops into the anterior lobe of the pituitary gland, and its posterior wall proliferates much less to become the pars intermedia of the gland. At autopsy, Shanklin[103] found that a residual lumen between a portion of these two structures persisted in 22 of 100 normal pituitary glands. Small asymptomatic, fluid-containing cysts were found in 13 of these 22 specimens. Such cysts of Rathke's cleft were recorded in 26% of routine autopsy series in five publications.[104-107] Infrequently, these cysts enlarge enough to produce symptoms. These residual clefts of Rathke's pouch are usually lined with cuboidal or columnar epithelial cells, which are often ciliated and include mucin-secreting goblet cells that stain positively by the periodic acid-Schiff method. Stratified or pseudostratified squamous epithelium may also be present and may rest on a collagenous connective tissue stroma.

By November 1989, Voelker and co-workers[108] had collected a total of 155 histologically confirmed symptomatic cases from the world literature, including their own 8 cases. The increased recognition of the disorder is evident from the total of only 35 cases found in the literature in 1977 by Yoshida and associates.[109] The Rathke's cleft cyst was both intrasellar and suprasellar in 90 patients, intrasellar in 22, suprasellar in 15, and intrasphenoidal in 1. The cyst capsule varies in thickness and can be any color. Common colors of the more watery fluids are yellow, blue, or green, at times with cholesterol crystals. The content of the cyst may vary from watery or serous (in 15 cases) to mucoid, gelatinous, caseous, or motor-oil-like consistency, to white and creamy. This last appearance may be suggestive of pus. The content of one of the cysts was so tough as to require a rongeur for

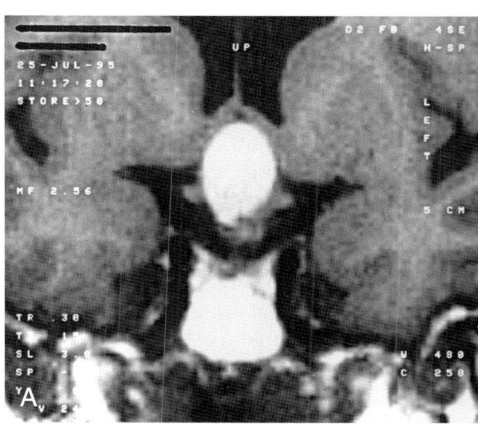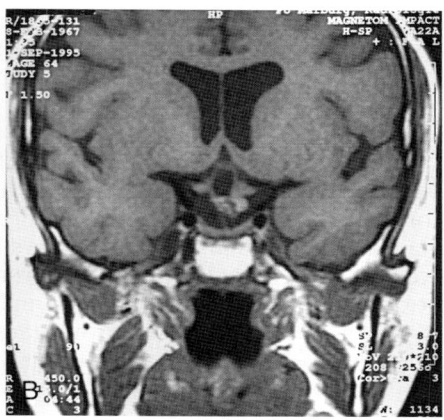

FIGURE 26-18 See Case Report 8: Rathke's Cleft Cyst.

removal. Although in these series reported with only a few patients and a limited range of abnormal appearances may be described in CT scans and MRI,[110] the extreme differences in the cystic content of protein and other chemicals are matched by similar variation in the scans, as pointed out by many authors.[111-117] However, the size and location of the lesion were delineated in approximately 100% of the MRI studies and 90% of the CT scans. Image features such as a sellar epicenter, smooth contour, absence of calcification, absence of internal enhancement, and homogeneous attenuation or signal intensity within the lesion suggest the diagnosis of a Rathke's cleft cyst.[118-120] Choi et al.[121] determined the differential magnetic resonance image (MRI) features of pituitary adenoma, craniopharyngioma and Rathke's cleft cyst involving both intrasellar and suprasellar regions in 64 patients. A snowman shape and solid characteristics, and homogeneous enhancement of the solid portion were more common in pituitary adenomas. A superior lobulated shape and third ventricle compression by superior tumor extension were more common in carniopharyngiomas. Finally, an ovoid shape, a small tumor volume, cystic characteristics, and no or thin cyst wall enhancement were typical in Rathke cleft cyst. The statistical accuracies of diagnosis were as follows: 92.1% in pituitary adenoma, 92.3% in craniopharyngioma, and 92.2% overall. Kunii et al.[122] described the value of single-shot, fast spin–echo, diffusion-weighted MR imaging to differentiate Rathke's cleft cysts from other cystic lesions. Several regions of interest (ROIs) for apparent diffusion coefficient (ADC) measurements were identified in the fluid component of the lesions.

Kleinschmidt and associates[123] proposed a new pathognomonic MR feature—the posterior ledge sign—of Rathke's cleft cysts. Ross and colleagues[111] stated that the diagnosis can be made at operation after the cystic cavity is irrigated. The lining of Rathke's cleft cyst is smooth and transparent; that of a craniopharyngiomatous or a pituitary adenomatous cyst is lined at least at some point by tumor.

CASE REPORT 8: RATHKE'S CLEFT CYST

A 28-year-old patient suffering from a secondary amenorrhea was admitted to our department. An MRI scan showed a cystic lesion growing up from the sellar region and bulging into the third ventricle (Fig. 26-18A). We decided to perform primarily an endoscopic cyst evacuation using the frontal transventricular burr hole approach. The cyst was totally evacuated, and the cyst membrane was partly resected

(Fig. 26-18B). The histopathologic diagnosis of the cyst membrane and its contents was ambiguous; some cells showed characteristics of craniopharyngioma cells, whereas others seemed to be of epithelial origin. Crystalloid and amorphic material was found in the contents of the cyst. The established histopathologic diagnosis was that of Rathke's cleft cyst; the differential diagnosis was a craniopharyngioma.

CLINICAL DATA OF RATHKE'S CLEFT CYST

Fager and Carter,[124] who had the earliest reported series of five living patients, found no solid abnormal tissue other than the thin wall in any of them. Visual fields and acuity, grossly abnormal in four of the patients preoperatively, improved greatly after the operation. The authors did not remove the cyst wall completely, but no symptoms recurred in any of the patients, who were followed up for as long as 9 years. They, therefore, regard total excision of the wall as unnecessary, concluding that a less radical approach suffices for these purely cystic intrapituitary or parapituitary lesions containing milky or mucoid fluid.

The following data are taken mainly from the reviews by Voelker and associates.[108] The female-to-male ratio was greater than 2:1, and patients ranged in age from 4 to 78 years, with a mean age of 38 years and the highest frequency in the sixth decade. The preoperative duration of symptoms was from 3 days to 18 years, with an average of 34.9 months. Clinical presentation of patients is characterized by the triad: pituitary dysfunction, visual impairment, and headache.[116,125] The most common symptoms were those caused by pituitary hypofunction. Dwarfism occurred in more than 70% of those younger than 18 years of age. Of the 37 patients with amenorrhea-galactorrhea, 14 had also a pituitary adenoma. Hyperprolactinemia might have occurred whether or not the amenorrhea-galactorrhea syndrome was present. Also precocious puberty in a 16-month-old child has been described by Acharya et al.[126] This child was suffering from breast enlargement, height increase, and an increase of growth velocity. Her vaginal mucosa was estrogenized. Treatment with leuprolide resulted in normalization of her growth rate and regression of the breast development; the vaginal mucosa became unestrogenized. Half of the patients had visual field defects, and about one fourth had decreased visual acuity. Almost half of the patients had headaches, which were often frontal headaches. Nausea and vomiting were noted in only 18 patients. Bouts of aseptic meningitis, though infrequent, should be recognized and are discussed later. A few patients described vertigo, diplopia, lethargy, or syncope. Intermittent episodes of fever in only six cases were, at least in the patient of Van Hilten and colleagues,[127] an unusual symptom of hypothalamic involvement. Attacks of fever at approximately 2-week intervals sometimes woke her at night or occurred randomly. They lasted for 6 hours, during which she had a rectal temperature of 39°C, followed by 3 hours of excessive sweating and a gradual return of temperature to normal. This picture proved to result from a 20 by 20 by 20 mm suprasellar cyst extending up to the foramina of Monro and causing dilatation of both lateral ventricles and increased ICP. After lasting drainage of the cyst (three operations), all symptoms virtually disappeared.

Surgical excision of the cyst (usually partial) was carried out in 137 of the 155 patients, the remaining 18 cysts having been found at necropsy. The approach was by craniotomy in 60 cysts and via the sphenoid sinus in 59 cysts. Ross and coworkers[111] used the trans-sphenoidal route in 40 of 43 patients. The three patients with suprasellar lesions involving the pituitary stalk had transcranial approaches. The 10 patients of Midha and coworkers[128] were all operated on trans-sphenoidally, as were the 28 patients of El Mahdy and Powell.[116] This route was selected in only three of Voelker and co-workers' eight patients, all of whom had suprasellar extensions from the main intrasellar mass.[108] Operative mortality was zero in each of these four series. The recurrence rate after a craniotomy is approximately twice as high as that following the trans-sphenoidal route. Furthermore, if the cyst wall is removed only partially at craniotomy, the material secreted by the remnant may provoke an aseptic meningeal reaction. However, headache is not satisfactorily controlled by the partial removal of cyst wall advocated by the neurosurgeon Ross and colleagues.[111] Of their 32 patients whose preoperative symptoms included headaches, 21 obtained relief. Of 14 patients in whom headache was the only preoperative symptom, the headache persisted after operation in 7 patients. No correlation existed between the size of the lesion and the incidence of headache or the likelihood of disappearance of the headache after operation. The two patients with the largest lesions (23 and 25 mm) did not have a headache. However, of the 17 patients who had preoperative hyperprolactinemia, only 3 have continued to have prolactin levels above normal after operation. No data have been collated on the results on these scores after craniotomies.

Ross and co-workers[111] advocate the extremely conservative simple drainage of the cyst trans-sphenoidally, "accompanied by biopsy of the cyst wall, when this is possible without entering the subarachnoid space or damaging normal structures." In fact, they took no operative pathologic specimen to confirm the diagnosis in 17 of their 40 patients. El Mahdy and Powell[116] performed a partial excision of the cyst wall and drainage of the contents into the sphenoid sinus. In seven patients with an intraoperative CSF leakage, they used fascia lata or fat grafts.

Midha and associates[128] obtained biopsies of the cyst wall in eight patients and removed all of it in two. The preoperative symptoms and signs in all 10 had disappeared, except those related to pituitary dysfunction and in 3 patients with visual problems. Although Ross and colleagues[111] followed up their patients for a mean of 68 months, with the longest follow-up at 126 months, they have seen only one symptomatic recurrence.

Totally benign behavior is far from invariable, however. One Japanese patient presented with acute adrenal insufficiency, which capped the hypopituitarism secondary to the intrasellar Rathke's cleft cyst.[129] There are two reports of an acute hemorrhage into a Rathke's cleft cyst.[130,131] Another report is of hemosiderin deposits in the calcified epithelium of a Rathke's cleft cyst,[132] which emerged with an abrupt onset of severe headache and gave rise to an enhancing intrasellar and suprasellar mass. The mass was successfully removed trans-sphenoidally. One of Yoshida and associates' patients had a small nodule on her cyst wall that was scraped out with a curet.[109] Only part of the cyst wall was removed, and a serious recurrence took place within 1 year. Raskind and coworkers' patient, whose cyst contained a clear, colorless fluid, experienced a recurrence requiring repeat surgery 26 years later.[133] The patient reported by Berry and Schlezinger[134] had only a fragment of the cyst wall removed at the first craniotomy. At a major recurrence 37 months later, the cyst was three times the original size but contained the same clear, colorless mucoid fluid. The recurrences described by Yoshida and colleagues,[109] Iraci and colleagues,[135] and Matsushima and colleagues[136] were in patients with solid components to their lesions that contained stratified epithelium. In Matsushima's case, although the cyst was filled with the typical mucinous, pus-like material and some of its lining comprised ciliated, mucin-containing columnar cells, most of it consisted of stratified squamous epithelium. This last component determined the outcome, namely death from recurrent tumor 20 months after its subtotal removal. Clearly, the solid portion of the tumor more than the appearance of the cystic fluid determines the prognosis. Two patients of Marcincin and Gennarelli[137] and one of Rout and colleagues[138] experienced recurrences in 4 months to 2 years after trans-sphenoidal evacuation of the cysts, even though the cyst fluid and wall were typical of pure Rathke's cleft lesions. A permanent visual loss ensued in one of the patients. The lesion was approached intracranially at recurrence in the second patient, and the entire cyst wall was removed. Two more recurrences after craniotomy have been reported by Yamamoto and co-workers[139] and by Leech and Olafson,[140] and four more have been reported after trans-sphenoidal approaches by Roux and co-workers,[141] Midha and co-workers,[128] Ross and coworkers,[111] and El Mahdy and Powell.[116] Surprisingly, Mukherjee and associates[142] describe a re-expansion rate of 33% in 12 patients with Rathke's cleft cysts during a follow-up time from 1 to 168 months (median of 30 months). They propose to evaluate the role of radiotherapy for recurrent symptomatic tumors. Raper and Besser[143] reported 5 recurrences out of 12 patients in an Australian population and conclude that the relatively high rate of recurrence may indicate a link between this pathology and craniopharyngioma. In a large series of patients with symptomatic Rathke cleft cysts (118 patients), who underwent trans-sphenoidal resection and participated in a long postoperative follow-up (1984–1995, at least 5 years), Aho and coworkers[144] found that recurrence was statistically associated with the use of a fat or fascial graft for closure and the presence of squamous metaplasia in the cyst wall. The extent of resection of the cyst wall was not associated with an increased rate of recurrence. They conclude, that the high recurrence rate (18%) supports the theory that a relationship exists between symptomatic Rathke cleft cysts and craniopharyngioma.

As the reports have accumulated, it has become clear that many patients have transitional lesions or even highly unusual accompanying lesions. Russell and Rubenstein[145] were among the first to point this out, describing in two patients dumbbell cysts, the intrasellar portion of which was lined by a single layer of ciliated epithelium that changed abruptly at the diaphragma sellae to the squamous epithelium characteristic of a craniopharyngioma for the suprasellar portion. In a case reported by Yoshida and associates,[109] there was a tumor nodule with an inner lining of columnar cells that covered many layers of stratified squamous epithelium. Tajika and coworkers[146] found some areas of stratified epithelium in two of their three patients with Rathke's cleft cysts; in one of the two patients, cholesterol crystals, calcification, and brown fluid were present. Conversely, some ciliated, combined with columnar, cell areas were found in two other patients with histologic findings otherwise typical of a craniopharyngioma. This underlines the assumption that Rathke's cleft cysts may originate from squamous cell rests along the craniopharyngeal canal, resulting in a spectrum of cystic lesions in this area ranging from simple Rathke's cleft cysts to complex craniopharyngiomas.[116,147]

Goodrich and coworkers[148] described a suprasellar soft necrotic tumor rather than a fluid-containing tumor that contained many ciliated cuboidal or columnar cells typical of the lesion under discussion; however, other parts of the tumor included masses of squamous epithelium. This assumption was underlined by a recently published case of Sato et al.[149] They suggest that the basal cells of Rathke cleft cyst transform to papillary type craniopharyngioma after squamous metaplasia, explaining the presence of cilia and goblet cells. Recently Okada and colleagues[150] described another case of ciliated craniopharyngioma developing from a Rathke cleft cyst.

Another Rathke's cleft cyst was reported that had characteristics of an epidermoid cyst.[151] Harrison and associates[152] suggested that Rathke's cleft cysts, epithelial cysts, epidermoid cysts, dermoid cysts, and craniopharyngiomas represent a continuum of ectodermally derived epithelial cystic epithelial lesions. Other groups described the association of pituitary adenomas with the typical histologic form of Rathke's cleft cyst.[153-159] The more solid tissue there is associated with the cyst, the more likely it is to include a chronic inflammatory process or the stratified epithelium of a craniopharyngioma or of the glandular tissue of a pituitary adenoma. These tissues are likely to show enhancement in a scan. In rare cases the association of a craniopharyngioma with a gonadotroph adenoma and of a Rathke cleft cyst with a corticotroph adenoma is possible.[160]

These lesions are also more likely to have a major or completely suprasellar portion. Yuge and coworkers[161] have added two more exclusively suprasellar Rathke's cleft cysts to the 15 cysts collected by Voelker and coworkers.[108] In the patients from Miyagi and co-workers,[155] the lesions extended into the third ventricle. The patients in each of two publications[161,162] actually presented with hypothalamic tumors, one as a noncystic hypothalamic mass. This patient had

an X, X, Y karyotype in all cells (Klinefelter's syndrome). These larger tumors were not totally removed. In the case from Itoh and Usui,[163] the subepithelial tissue consisted of normal pituitary gland. Wenger and colleagues added in 2001 another case of an entirely suprasellar Rathke's cleft cyst.[164] The Rathke's cleft cyst reported by Onda and colleagues[165] was associated with an arachnoid cyst; the cyst reported by Ikeda and colleagues[166] was associated with an eosinophil (acromegalic) adenoma. Arita and coworkers[167] described a case of Cushing's disease accompanied by Rathke's cleft cyst, and Ersahin and associates[168] presented a case of Rathke's cleft cyst with diabetes insipidus. Rathke's cleft cysts should be kept in mind as a potential cause for the syndrome of inappropriate secretion of antidiuretic hormone and adrenal insufficiency.[169] Two papers have reported chronic (granulomatous) hypophysitis related to Rathke's cleft cyst.[170,171]

Cannova and associates[172] found a granulomatous sarcoidotic lesion of the hypothalamic-pituitary region associated with a Rathke's cleft cyst. More distant accompanying lesions have been described by Koshiyama and colleagues[173] in the form of Hashimoto's thyroiditis with diabetes insipidus and by Kim and colleagues[174] as a maldevelopmental mass with absence of pituitary gland, a rudimentary prosencephalon, and two other cysts—one a pigmented epithelial cyst (possibly a rudimentary eye) and the other a dorsal ependymal cyst, plus several other congenital abnormalities.

A single case report was published of a large suprasellar tumor extending downward to attach to the anterior wall of the pituitary gland. The cyst wall of the tumor was consistent with Rathke's cleft cyst in many places, but both its immunohistochemical and ultrastructural features were indistinguishable from colloid cysts of the third ventricle.[175] The cyst wall was totally removed via a subfrontal approach, and the authors achieved an excellent clinical result. Graziani and associates[176] assumed a common embryologic origin of suprasellar neurenteric cysts, the Rathke's cleft cyst, and the colloid cyst.

The reports of recurrences after mere evacuation of cysts have provided support for those who, from the first, included readily removable cyst wall as part of the surgical objective. In a 1984 publication (when high-resolution CT scanning was available), Shimoji and coworkers[177] noted enhanced capsules around low-density cysts in all three of their patients. They, therefore, elected to remove "as much as possible of the capsule" in all three and achieved good clinical results. Specimens from all three patients showed a histologic pattern typical of Rathke's cleft cyst, with the addition of squamous epithelium in the third case. Swanson and coworkers[157] also used the presence of capsular enhancement at CT scanning of an intrasellar mass to guide them to a transfrontal excision of the cyst wall. Nonfunctional pituitary adenomatous cells constituted a part of that wall; therefore, they gave the patient a course of radiation therapy. This patient represented the sole reported case thus treated. The trans-sphenoidal route has been favored for most cases, especially when the suprasellar portion shows minimal enhancement. This approach offers an effective means of achieving complete cyst drainage for lesions requiring surgery. Fenestration and aspiration of the cyst are usually sufficient to achieve total resolution of symptoms and signs caused by RCC. Clinical symptoms such as headaches improve in the majority of patients after surgery, however hormonal disturbances can persist.[178] Madhoc and colleagues[179] favor the endoscopic endonasal approach for resection of Rathke cleft cysts. The authors retrospectively reviewed a series of 35 patients after endoscopic endonasal resection at the University of Pittsburgh between 1998 to 2008. Neither were there any intraoperative complications, postoperative CSF leaks, or new neurological deficits. The average hospital stay was 1.8 days. They concluded that the endoscopic endonasal approach is safe and effective in the treatment of Rathke cleft cysts. These positive results were confirmed by Cavallo and coworkers, who operated on a series of 76 consecutive patients with sellar lesions using the endoscopic endonasal approach. They performed endoscopic exploration of the sellar cavity during trans-sphenoidal surgery and recommended to use this technique to achieve maximal and safe tumor removal.[180]

In our experience with nontumorous cystic midline lesions, involving more than 100 patients, it is not necessary to resect the whole cyst membrane to prevent a recurrence. As an example, we have operated on 36 colloid cysts of the third ventricle in neuroendoscopic technique using the frontal burr hole approach. The cysts were evacuated and the membranes were resected subtotally. During a follow-up period from 6 months to 10 years, there were two recurrences which have been operated in a second endoscopic intervention.[181]

CASE REPORT 9: COLLOID CYST

For a 41-year-old woman had chronic headache and gait disturbances, CT and MRI including 3D reconstructions revealed a cystic lesion in the third ventricle with obstructive hydrocephalus (Fig. 26-19A to F). Through a right frontal burr hole, an endoscopic cyst perforation and evacuation of the colloidal material was performed (Fig. 26-19D). The histopathologic diagnosis was a colloid cyst. The cyst wall

was shrunk using the bipolar microelectrode. Membranous material adherent to the ventricular ependyma was left in situ. This was confirmed by a postoperative MRI examination (Fig. 26-19F). Seven days after the intervention, the patient was discharged without any new neurologic deficit. Five years after the operation, the patient showed no clinical or radiologic signs of cyst recurrence. Figures G and H show the typical endoscopic and illustrated macroscopic aspects of colloid cysts.

INTRASELLAR OR SUPRASELLAR ABSCESS

Gomez Perun and associates[182] stated in 1981 that 50 intrasellar abscesses had been reported; usually, the infection was propagated from a neighboring air or vascular sinus. The uninfected content of Rathke's cleft cyst may be a thick, white, or yellowish pus-like fluid that was mistaken for pus by the authors. Typically, the cellular reaction in the CSF is predominantly lymphocytic, and culture results of the "pus" and CSF are repeatedly negative. The patient is reacting to a "foreign body" that he himself has secreted, as described in the following section.[183]

Bouts of Chemical Meningitis: The Syndrome of the Toxin-Leaking Central Nervous System Cyst

An important point emerges from collation of the data from scattered individual case reports of patients with curious repeated febrile episodes, often with CSF pleocytosis. A culture was obtained from an organism in only one case. Attacks of recurrent chemical febrile meningitis in a craniopharyngioma, presumably from leakage of keratin or cholesterol, are a rare but well-authenticated occurrence.[184]

In the first such case of Rathke's cleft cyst, reported as an abscess by Obenchain and Becker,[185] the patient had five episodes in 3 years of severe headaches, nausea, vomiting, general malaise, and fever, all leading to hospital admissions but resolving spontaneously a few days later. Finally, blurring of vision in her inferior temporal

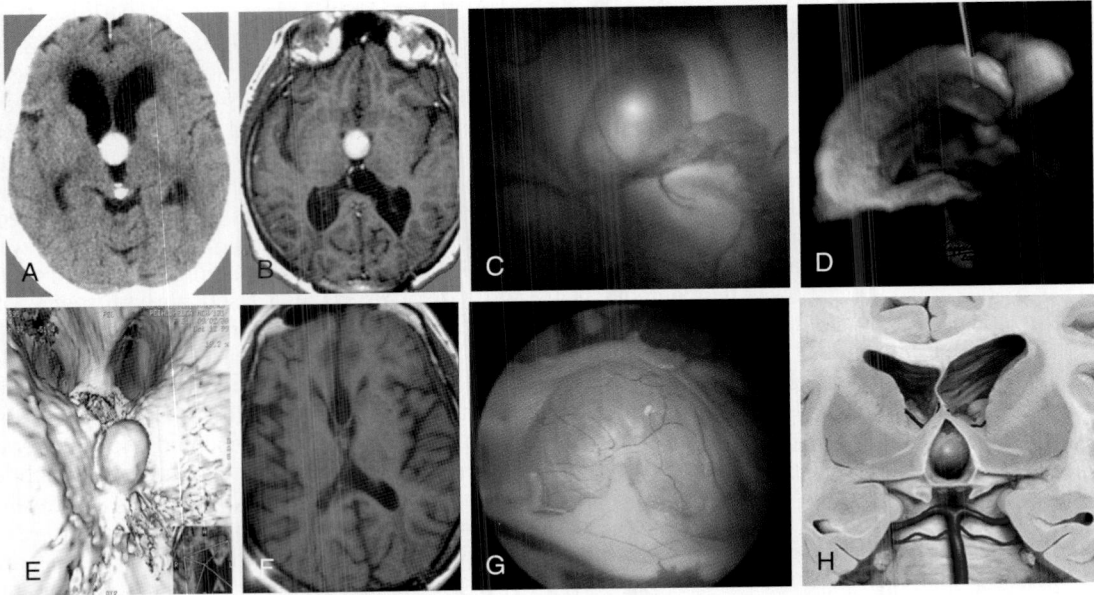

FIGURE 26-19 See Case Report 9: Colloid Cyst.

quadrants led to the diagnosis of her intrasellar and minimally suprasellar mass, from which, via a subfrontal route, 2 ml of "purulent" fluid was aspirated. *Staphylococcus epidermidis* was cultured from this fluid, and the patient was given penicillin, isoniazid, and ethambutol for 1 month. Then, via the trans-sphenoidal route, 3 ml of "pus" was aspirated, and the capsule was removed. Histologically, the wall was fibrous and lined by columnar epithelium with chronic inflammatory cells. The patient's recovery was excellent and sustained. The absence of acute inflammatory cells and the spontaneously subsiding brief attacks that had occurred for 3 years cast doubt on the role of the staphylococci.

In the next reported case,[186] similar recurrent brief episodes occurred. These episodes each lasted only 2 or 3 days and were characterized by intense supraorbital pain, fever to 39°C or 40°C, and about 50 clear-cut temporal lobe seizures a day. These seizures each lasted for several seconds and occurred mainly during the bouts of fever. These mysterious episodes continued for 10 years, during which time the patient's weight increased from 50 to 72 kg. Although the patient did not develop nuchal rigidity in the attacks, a lumbar puncture finally performed in 1977 revealed a largely lymphocytic pleocytosis and a normal protein level. Demonstration of an infratemporal quadrantanopia was followed by pneumography, which revealed a suprasellar mass. At a subfrontal exposure, thick, pus-like fluid was removed from a subchiasmatic cyst, the capsule of which was largely removed. The cyst wall was heavily vascularized and infiltrated with inflammatory cells but lined with the typical ciliated columnar and cuboidal epithelium. The patient had also developed the symptoms and laboratory findings of deficient thyroid-stimulating hormone, adrenocorticotropic hormone, and luteinizing hormone-releasing hormone. The febrile episodes involving a headache stopped at once after operation, and the patient gradually made a full recovery. The seizures continued to require phenobarbital and valproic acid for control.

The following year, Verkijk and Bots[151] described a patient in whom meningeal reactions developed after surgery on a cyst; these reactions resolved spontaneously in 9 months. In the case reported by Steinberg and coworkers,[187] the initial symptoms pointed to a pituitary origin because of defects in visual acuity and fields, but then over the next 2 years, the patient was in the hospital numerous times with bouts of severe headache, nausea, vomiting, confusion, stiff neck, decreased visual acuity, and ataxic gait. On different occasions, the CSF showed pleocytosis, an increased protein level, and elevated pressure. All culture results were always negative. The episodes either resolved spontaneously or disappeared promptly after increases in the dosage of dexamethasone. Decreases in this dosage were followed by a recurrence of the symptoms. The sella was found to be enlarged and to contain a mass without suprasellar extension; the sella was, however, partially empty, with its anterior portion filling with air. These findings were apparently considered to be incidental. The lateral and third ventricles became increasingly dilated, and egress of contrast was delayed through the aqueduct and out of the fourth ventricle. The hydrocephalus was treated by ventriculoatrial shunt in 1972. Intracranial obstruction of the shunt required

two revisions; each time, the symptoms promptly resolved. The patient died 1 year later of pneumonia. At autopsy, the Rathke's cleft cyst occupying the entire sella was filled with thick, yellow-green fluid. The cyst epithelium was largely ciliated and columnar, squamous in one area and keratinized in others. The leptomeninges adjacent to the chiasm and third ventricle were "moderately fibrotic with mild chronic inflammation."

Episodes of severe meningeal symptoms and signs, also with completely negative culture results, characterized a patient reported on by Gomez Perun and coworkers.[182] One episode in May 1977 was especially severe. When a suprasellar lesion was demonstrated and explored 6 months later, the cyst contained a thick, white fluid, which had an intense inflammatory reaction, and numerous vessels in the cyst wall, along with a lining of ciliated columnar epithelium. Also, an extensive frontal basal arachnoiditis was present that was not noted in the other cases. The "pus" was sterile, and the patient made a prompt recovery but soon regressed, with similar episodes of aseptic meningitis. Despite three more operations, he too died; no organism was ever grown.

The patient reported on by Sonntag and coworkers[188] had only two episodes of a lymphocytic aseptic meningeal reaction before his intrasellar-suprasellar mass was subfrontally exposed. Seven milliliters of "pus" were aspirated, and the cyst wall was subtotally removed. The aspirate was sterile, but rare gram-negative rods were seen, and chloramphenicol was administered for 1 week. The symptoms recurred in 1 month, leading to trans-sphenoidal drainage of 5 ml of "pus" and "extensive removal of its wall." Culture results from this fluid were also negative. Therapy with chloramphenicol was continued for 1 month, and the patient had remained well for almost 2 years as of this writing.

Shimoji and associates[177] described three clear-cut cases of chemical meningitis. In the first, brief episodes of headache, nausea, vomiting, and fever were accompanied by enough eye signs to point to the sellar region and its cyst. At craniotomy, the "abscess-like viscous fluid" was sterile. As much cyst wall as possible was removed, and an excellent result persisted 2 years later. In the second case, a 52-year-old woman, four episodes of aseptic meningitis were required before a trans-sphenoidal evacuation of "milky, abscess-like viscous fluid" occurred and "as much as possible" of the cyst wall was removed. She, too, made an excellent recovery, which continued at 2 years. Both patients were also given 3000 cGy of ^{60}Co radiation. In the third case, an intermittent fever to 38°C on hospitalization rose to 39°C after pneumoencephalography; the patient, a 42-year-old woman, had meningeal signs and a CSF pleocytosis of 456 neutrophils and 74 lymphocytes. No growth occurred on culture. A week of antibiotic therapy brought no change, but 30 mg/day of prednisolone given in addition to the antibiotics dropped the temperature to normal the next day. The yellowish white gelatinous cyst fluid and, "as far as possible," its capsule, were removed via craniotomy. The periodic acid-Schiff-positive stratified squamous epithelium was heavily infiltrated with inflammatory cells. Good recovery persisted at 28 months. Thick, yellow, pus-like material and a cyst wall accompanied by squamous epithelium and thick connective tissue infiltrated with inflammatory cells were described in two other reports.[138,189]

One more clear-cut case of a foreign body reaction to the content of Rathke's cleft cyst was reported by Albini and associates.[190] The 19-year-old woman developed headache, galactorrhea, and a few months later, amenorrhea. Bitemporal hemianopia and deficiencies in thyroid-stimulating hormone, adrenocorticotropic hormone, luteinizing hormone, and luteinizing hormone-releasing hormone were identified. There had never been any episodes of fever or other suggestion of an aseptic meningeal reaction. The sella was enlarged, and while in the hospital, the patient developed a partial right third nerve paresis along with polydipsia and polyuria. At right pterional craniotomy, a large cyst seen on CT scan arising from the sella turcica was emptied of its thick, white fluid, and the cyst wall was insofar as possible removed. An excellent clinical result was obtained. The cyst wall was lined by the ciliated columnar and squamous epithelium of a Rathke's cleft cyst. The rest of the specimen was infiltrated with lymphocytes, plasmacytes, and multinucleated giant cells among islands of preserved pituitary tissue. No organisms were ever demonstrated. Apparently, the cystic fluid never seeped into the subarachnoid space. At 3-year follow-up, the patient was free of headache and mass observed by CT. Bognàr and coworkers[191] reported on two more patients with symptomatic histologically typical Rathke's cleft cysts and no preoperative episodes, which suggested aseptic meningitis. In both of them, the cyst contents were removed via the sphenoid sinus. Inflammatory cells and bacteria were recognized in the operative specimen, but technical problems were said to have prevented identification of organisms. Antibiotics were used, and one patient recovered uneventfully. In the other patient, trans-sphenoidal partial removal was followed by worsening in 2 weeks, leading to a frontolateral craniotomy, which likewise did not eliminate all of the abnormal tissue. *Staphylococcus aureus* and *Streptococcus pyogenes* grown from the specimen at the second operation were treated by antibiotics, but they failed to avert death on the ninth postoperative day. This sequence suggests that the cyst content facilitated the bacterial growth seen only after the second operation. Because of the diagnosis of infection, neither of these patients was given large doses of corticosteroids. Both patients may have been reacting primarily to the chemicals in the cyst fluid. In 2008, Schittenhelm and colleagues[192] reported on a lymphocytic hypophysitis related to a ruptured Rathke's cleft cyst in a 45-year-old woman who initially presented with headache and temporary double vision followed by amenorrhea. The strongest inflammatory reaction was observed at the site of cyst integrity disrupture, suggesting that high protein levels from the rupture of Rathke's cleft cyst might have triggered a lymphocytic hypophisitis.

At least four reports have been published of spontaneous rupture of cystic craniopharyngiomas into the subarachnoid space that gave rise to a major but sterile meningeal reaction. This reaction was not different from those associated with Rathke's cleft cyst in that a predominantly neutrophilic, rather than lymphocytic, reaction occurred in severe cases.[177,193,194] Another case with spontaneous intraventricular rupture of a craniopharyngioma cyst was described in 2000 by Kulkarni and colleagues. The rupture resulted in an acute neurologic deterioration with consecutive bilateral optic nerve atrophy due to chemical meningitis. The patient was treated with ventricular drainage, steroids, and anticonvulsants. CSF showed high cholesterol and 1-lactate dehydrogenase levels. The diagnosis of craniopharyngioma was subsequently verified histologically.[195] Intracranial epidermoid tumors[196,197] and dermoid cysts[198,199] also rarely show this behavior as reported by several authors.

In conclusion, Rathke's cleft cysts tend to occur mainly within the sella; their precise extent can now be determined by modern CT and MRI scanning. Most of these cysts are best approached trans-sphenoidally; however, approximately 10% that are wholly suprasellar should be removed via craniotomy. Whether trans-sphenoidal aspiration of the cyst and biopsy suffice, as urged by Ross and colleagues,[111] the endoscopic transventricular approach with cyst opening and aspiration proposed by Hellwig and colleagues,[74] or whether removal of as much cyst wall as seems safe is preferable is currently unclear. The neurosurgeons who favor a more aggressive stance will need to show that they achieve better relief of symptoms such as significant headache as well as fewer recurrences. The suprasellar component may need to be removed to the full extent dictated by safety because a repeat craniotomy is probably more hazardous than a second trans-sphenoidal approach.

In patients suffering from Rathke's cleft cysts, recurrent episodes of systemic or usually meningeal febrile illness can occur. This finding suggests that some of these typically thin-walled cysts may contain a peculiar chemical irritant that can leak out enough to contaminate the CSF and possibly the bloodstream at intervals and produce these dangerous responses. In our experience, after endoscopic cyst evacuation (Rathke's cleft cyst, craniopharyngioma, colloid cyst), the contents that contact the CSF compartments lead to a temporary increase in body temperature as a result of aseptic meningitis, which lasts for almost 24 hours and recurs spontaneously.

CASE REPORT 10: CYSTIC CRANIOPHARYNGIOMA

A 44-year-old patient had two febrile episodes with headache and opisthotonos 2 years before admission. Repeated CSF punctures revealed a slight pleocytosis. The first MRI scan showed no evidence of an intracranial space-occupying lesion. Later, it was suggested that these symptoms were the result of aseptic meningitis after spontaneous perforation of a cystic craniopharyngioma. An MRI scan that was performed 3 months after the second febrile attack showed a cystic process in the anterior part of the third ventricle growing up from the suprasellar region (Fig. 26-20A and C). The cyst was approached by 3D stereotactic calculation under direct endoscopic control. The cyst wall was coagulated using bipolar radiofrequency, and the cyst was opened using microscissors. The cyst contained a thick yellow fluid. The cyst was emptied, and the capsule was coagulated. The postoperative follow-up was uneventful. On MRI, the residual tumor membrane was visible (Fig. 26-20B and D). The patient was discharged 12 days after the intervention without neurologic symptoms or psychological disorder (Karnofsky score of 100%). The patient decided to undergo gamma knife treatment for the remaining tumor capsule.

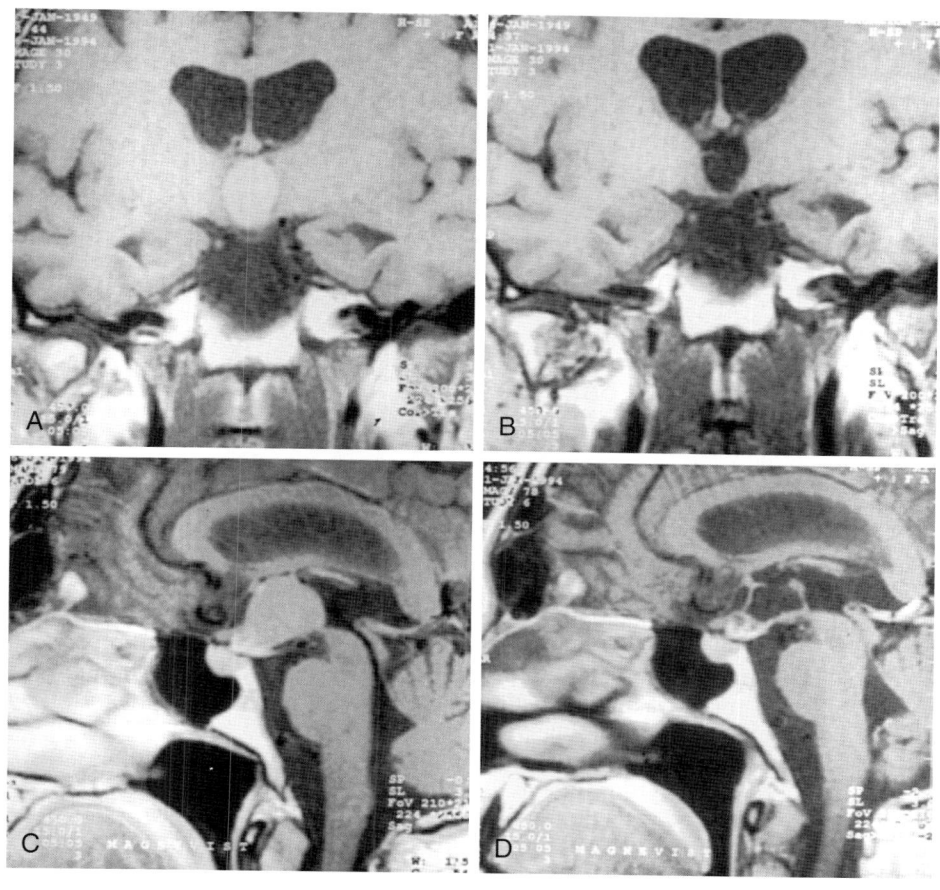

FIGURE 26-20 See Case Report 10: Cystic Craniopharyngioma.

ACKNOWLEDGMENT

In memory of Henry H. Schmidek and William H. Sweet, former authors of this chapter.

KEY REFERENCES

Aho CJ, Zelman V, Couldwell WR, et al. Surgical outcomes in 118 patients with Rathke cleft cyst. *J Neurosurg.* 2005;102(2):189-193.

Algin O, Hakyemez B, Gokalp G, et al. Phase-contrast cine MRI versus MR cisternography on the evaluation of the communication between intraventricular arachnoid cysts and neighbouring cerebrospinal fluid spaces. *Neuroradiology.* 2009;51(5):305-312.

Cavallo LM, Prevedello D, Esposito F, et al. The role of the endoscope in the transsphenoidal management of cystic lesions of the sellar region. *Neurosurg Rev.* 2008;31(1):55-64.

Choi SH, Kwon BJ, Na DG, et al. Pituitary adenoma, craniopharyngioma, and Rathke cleft cyst involving both intrasellar and suprasellar regions: differentiation using MRI. *Clin Radiol.* 2007;62(5):453-462.

Di Rocco C. Sylvian fissure arachnoid cysts: we do operate on them but should it be done? *Childs Nerv Syst.* 2010;26:173-175.

Ersahin Y, Kesikci H, Rüksen M, et al. Endoscopic treatment of suprasellar arachnoid cysts. *Childs Nerv Syst.* 2008;24(9):1013-1020.

Gangemi M, Coletta G, Magro F, et al. Suprasellar arachnoid cysts—endoscopy versus microsurgical cyst excision and shunting. *Br J Neurosurg.* 2007;21(3):276-280.

Grunert P, Gaab MR, Hellwig D, et al. German neuroendoscopy above the skull base. *Neurosurg Focus.* 2009;27(3):E7.

Hellwig D, Bauer BL, Schulte DM, et al. Neuroendoscopic treatment for colloid cysts of the third ventricle: the experience of a decade. *Neurosurgery.* 2008;62(6 Suppl 3):1101-1109.

Hellwig D, Haag R, Bartel V, et al. Application of new electrosurgical devices and probes in endoscopic neurosurgery. *Neurol Res.* 1999; 21:67-72.

Hellwig D, Riegel T. Stereotactic endoscopic treatment of brain abscess. In: Jimenez DF, ed. *Intracranial Endoscopic Neurosurgery.* Park Ridge, IL: AANS Publications Committee; 1998:199-207.

Hellwig D, Riegel T, Bertalanffy H. Neuroendoscopic techniques in treatment of intracranial lesions. *Minim Invasive Ther Allied Technol.* 1998;7:123-135.

Inoue K, Seker A, Osawa S, et al. Microsurgical and endoscopic anatomy of the supratentorial arachnoidal membranes and cistern. *Neurosurgery.* 2009;65(4):644-664.

Karavitaki N, Scheithauer BW, Watt J, et al. Collision lesions of the sella: co-existence of craniopharyngioma with gonadotroph adenoma and Rathke's cleft cyst with corticotroph adenoma. *Pituitary.* 2008; 11(3):317-323.

Martinez-Lage JF, Ruiz-Espejo AM, Almagro MJ, et al. CSF overdrainage in shunted intracranial arachnoid cysts: a series and review. *Childs Nerv Syst.* 2009;25(9):1061-1069.

Okada T, Fujitsu K, Miyahara K, et al. Ciliated craniopharyngioma-case report and pathological study. *Acta Neurochir.* 2009:(Epub ahead of print).

Pradilla G, Jallo G. Arachnoid cysts: case series and review of the literature. *Neurosurg Focus.* 2007;15:22(2):E7.

Raper DM, Besser M. Clinical features, management and recurrence of symptomatic Rathke's cleft cyst. *J Clin Neurosci.* 2009;16(3):385.9.

Riegel T, Freudenstein D, Alberti O, et al. Novel multipurpose instrument for endoscopic neurosurgery. *Neurosurgery.* 2002;51(1):270-274.

Tamburrini G, D'Angelo L, Paternoster G, et al. Endoscopic management of intra and periventricular CSF cysts. *Childs Nerv Syst.* 2007;23(6):645-651.

Thomas BP, Pearson MM, Wushensky CA. Active spontaneous decompression of a suprasellar-prepontine arachnoid cyst detected with routine magnetic resonance imaging. Case report. *J Neurosurg Pediatr.* 2009;3(1):70-72.

Tirakotai W, Bozinov O, Sure U, et al. The evolution of stereotactic guidance in neuroendoscopy. *Childs Nerv Syst.* 2004;20:790-795.

Tirakotai W, Hellwig D, Bertalanffy H, et al. The role of neuroendoscopy in the management of solid or solid-cystic intra- and periventricular tumours. *Childs Nerv Syst.* 2007;23(6):653-658.

Zada G, Ditty B, McNatt SA, et al. Surgical treatment of Rathke cleft cysts in children. *Neurosurgery.* 2009;64(6):1132-1137.

Numbered references appear on Expert Consult.

CHAPTER 27

Surgical Approaches to Lateral and Third Ventricular Tumors

TORAL R. PATEL • GRAHAME C. GOULD • JOACHIM M. BAEHRING •
JOSEPH M. PIEPMEIER

The majority of tumors of the lateral and third ventricles are benign or low-grade lesions. Because of their relatively slow growth rate, these lesions may reach several centimeters in size before they present to medical attention. The most common clinical manifestations of these tumors include headaches, memory loss, gait disorders, and cognitive changes.[1]

There are multiple surgical approaches to these tumors, all designed to minimally displace or disturb normal anatomy. Before embarking on an approach, the surgeon should be familiar with both the ventricular anatomy and the options for optimally accessing these lesions. The lateral and third ventricles can be reached by transcallosal, transcortical, and, in some cases, supracerebellar, subfrontal, pterional, and transtentorial approaches. Endoscopic techniques are a valuable addition to the surgeon's options for operative management.

Because intraventricular surgery requires manipulation deep within the hemispheres, proper patient positioning, adequate tumor exposure and brain relaxation are fundamental requirements for successful tumor removal. Intraoperative morbidity can be minimized by careful attention to presurgical planning and contingency strategies when required. Since cognitive deficits are the most commonly encountered preoperative sign of an intraventricular lesion, persistent postoperative cognitive liabilities and hydrocephalus merit close attention. There are several published alternative surgical approaches that have been utilized for accessing the ventricular system (interhemispheric-transcortical, trans-sylvian fissure) that this chapter will not present. While these alternative approaches may have some merit, the authors consider them to be of limited value for the vast majority of intraventricular tumors. This chapter will address proven and reliable methods to maximize tumor removal with minimal morbidity.

Lateral Ventricles

SURGICAL ANATOMY

The lateral ventricles are divided into five areas: frontal horns, bodies, atria, occipital horns, and temporal horns (Fig. 27-1).

The frontal horns are triangular extensions of the lateral ventricles anterior to the foramen of Monro and are bounded laterally by the head of the caudate, anteriorly and superiorly by the corpus callosum, and medially by the septum pellucidum. The foramen of Monro marks the posterior extent of the frontal horns, and the boundary consists of the forniceal columns that run just anterior to the foramen of Monro as they bend inferiorly to start their descent toward the mammillary bodies. The frontal horn contains no choroid plexus but has on its wall two important veins that help with surgical orientation. On its medial border, the septal vein leads into the medial foramen of Monro, where it enters the velum interpositum in the roof of the third ventricle to join the internal cerebral vein (ICV). Laterally, the anterior caudate vein runs medially to join the thalamostriate vein near the foramen of Monro.

The body of the lateral ventricles begins at the posterior edge of the foramen of Monro and extends posteriorly to the anterior border of the splenium of the corpus callosum. The body of the ventricle is covered superiorly by the corpus callosum and laterally by the body of the caudate. There are two sets of veins that travel on the lateral wall of the body: the more anterior thalamocaudate (the size of which is inversely proportional to the thalamostriate vein) and the posterior caudate vein, which drains either into the thalamostriate or directly into the ICV through the velum interpositum. Inferiorly, the junction of the lateral wall and floor of the body of the ventricle is demarcated by the striothalamic sulcus, which separates the caudate from the thalamus. In this sulcus, the thalamostriate vein courses anteriorly to the foramen of Monro to drain into the ICV. Separating the thalamus from the body of the fornix is the choroidal fissure. The medial posterior choroidal artery, which enters the ventricular system just lateral to the pineal and travels anteriorly in the roof of the third ventricle in the velum interpositum, can be seen in the lateral ventricle as it ascends through the foramen of Monro and bends posteriorly to run in the direction of the choroid plexus. Medially, the two leaves of the septum pellucidum separate the two ventricles.

The trigone or atrium of the lateral ventricles is a confluence of the body and temporal and occipital horns. The atrium begins as a continuation of the body at the posterior edge of the thalamus and ends further posteriorly as the corpus callosum blends into the occipital lobe. The splenium (superiorly) and the tapetum of the corpus callosum (more posteriorly) make up the roof of the atrium. Because the roof bends into the lateral wall posteriorly, the tapetum

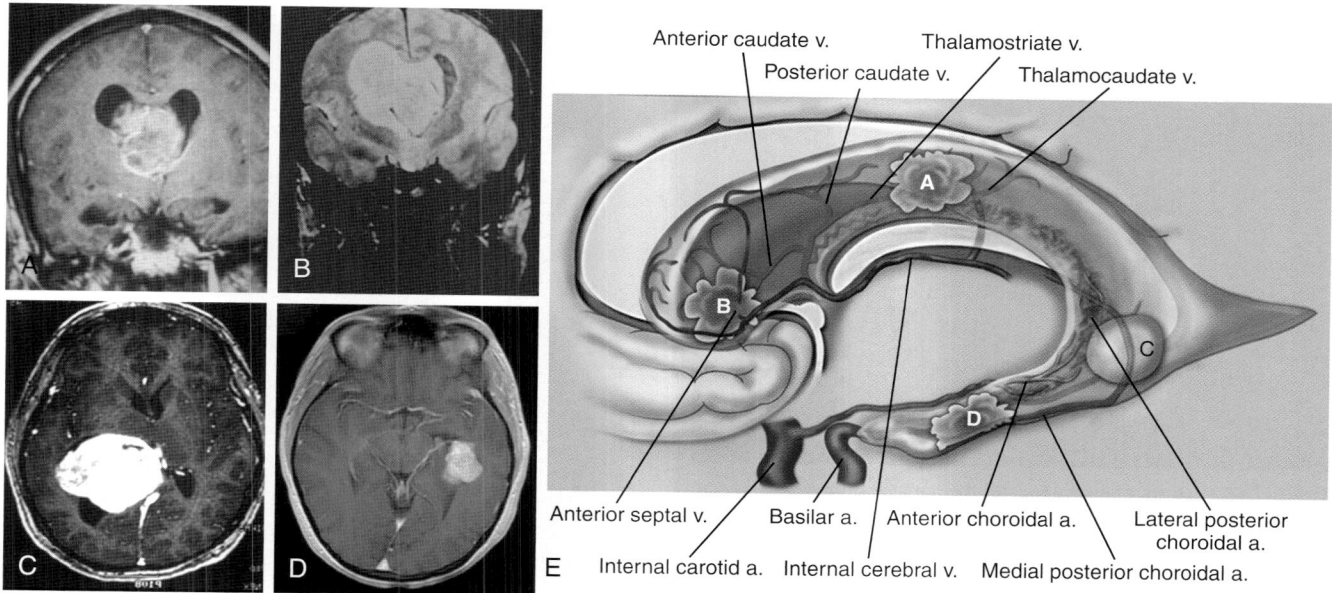

FIGURE 27-1 Enhanced magnetic resonance imaging of lateral ventricle tumors in common locations, with preferred surgical routes as denoted. A, Body, anterior transcallosal. B, Body and frontal horn, combined anterior transcallosal and anterior trans-sulcal. C, Atrium, posterior trans-sulcal/superior parietal lobule. D, Temporal horn, inferior temporal. E, Schematic representation highlighting common tumor locations (A, body; B, frontal horn; C, atrium; D, temporal horn) and relevant vascular anatomy of the lateral ventricle.

covers this lateral wall segment. More anteriorly, the caudate tail covers the lateral wall as it curves downward, on its way toward the temporal lobe. The anterior boundary of the atrium starts just medial to the caudate tail with the pulvinar eminence. Medial to the pulvinar, covered by choroid, is the crus of the fornix. At the atrial level of the choroid plexus, two choroidal arteries can often be seen, one curving with the choroid medially and the anterior choroidal artery, which can course into the body of the ventricle. More laterally, the lateral posterior choroidal artery, which may have several branches, runs to supply the atrium and body of the choroid. The triangular enlargement of the choroid plexus at the trigone is called the glomus. The medial wall of the atrium has two prominences. The upper prominence consists of the forceps major fibers and is called the bulb of the corpus callosum. The lower prominence is called the calcar avis and is simply the ventricular protrusion of the calcarine sulcus. The floor similarly consists of the upward protrusion of the collateral sulcus forming the collateral trigone.

The occipital horn is a posterior extension of the atrium and can vary in size. Medially, the wall consists of the same structures that make up the atrial medial wall, namely, the forceps major superiorly and, inferiorly, the calcar avis. Likewise, the collateral trigone forms the floor of the occipital horn. The roof and lateral wall blend into one and are both covered by the tapetum. There is no choroid in the occipital horn.

The temporal horn is an extension of the lateral ventricles into the medial temporal lobe. The floor displays two prominences: (1) laterally the collateral eminence formed by the underlying deep collateral sulcus and (2) medial to that, the hippocampus, which protrudes prominently into the floor. The lateral wall, which angles into the roof of the temporal horn, is lined by the tapetum. In the medial part of the roof, the tail of the caudate projects anteriorly toward the amygdaloid nucleus. Medial to the caudate tail, forming the medial wall of the temporal horn, is the thalamus and, inferior to it, the fimbria of the fornix. The choroid fissure separates the thalamus from the fornix. The choroid plexus is attached as it continues anteriorly to end just posterior to the amygdaloid nucleus at the inferior choroidal point. The anterior choroidal artery enters the choroidal fissure at approximately this point and courses posteriorly in the plexus. More posteriorly, the lateral posterior choroidal artery enters the fissure and is seen more laterally in the choroid plexus. The temporal horn ends in the amygdaloid nucleus.[2-5]

Surgical Options
ANTERIOR TRANSCALLOSAL APPROACH

The anterior transcallosal route is useful for lesions arising within the body of the lateral ventricle (Fig. 27-1A). Cortical veins draining into the sagittal sinus can be a significant obstacle to interhemispheric access and a preoperative cerebral angiogram or magnetic resonance venogram can be important for surgical planning. Furthermore, the ventricular venous and arterial structures can be distorted by the tumor and should be noted preoperatively. The patient is placed in a supine position, with the head slightly flexed. Alternatively, the patient's head is fixed in a lateral position with the affected hemisphere toward the floor to use gravity to assist with retraction. A bicoronal incision is made anterior to the coronal suture. The craniotomy is also centered anterior to the coronal suture. Midline exposure should extend up to the superior sagittal sinus. The dura is opened and reflected medially up to the sagittal sinus. Often, cortical draining veins enter the dura before reaching the midline. These veins may be preserved by opening the dura on all sides around the veins, leaving the dura covering the

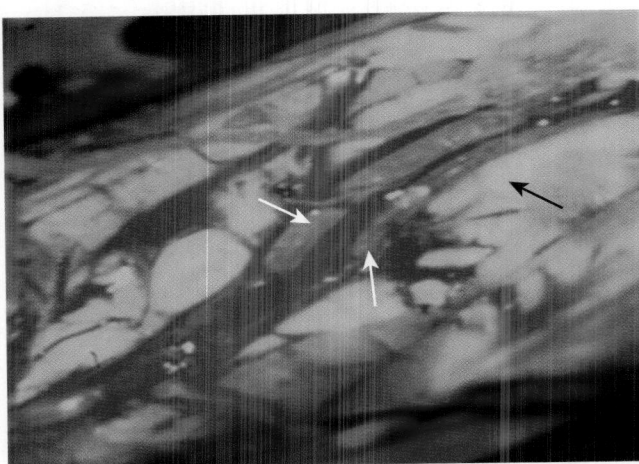

FIGURE 27-2 Intraoperative view of the pericallosal arteries (*white arrows*) over a distended corpus callosum (*black arrow*).

venous access to the sagittal sinus intact. If exuberant arachnoid granulations are encountered, they can be divided with sharp dissection and bipolar cautery. Once the midline is reached, the falx is followed to its depth. At this point, the operating microscope is used. The arachnoid below the falx may be adherent, and this must be carefully divided to avoid injury to the cingulate gyrus on either side. Once the corpus callosum is reached, the two pericallosal arteries are visualized (Fig. 27-2). Ventricular access between the two arteries helps to prevent vascular injury. The callosum midline is often demarcated by a very small callosal artery. The callosotomy can be started just posterior to the genu and developed 2 to 3 cm posteriorly to gain access to the lateral ventricle. By performing the callosotomy off midline and toward the ventricle of interest, opening the contralateral ventricle can be avoided. Proper orientation is confirmed by locating the choroid plexus and the thalamostriate vein entering into the foramen of Monro. If the vein is to the right of the choroid plexus, the surgeon is in the right ventricle, if the vein is to the left of the choroid, the surgeon is in the left ventricle (Fig. 27-3). Throughout the course of tumor resection, the interface between the tumor and the ependymal surface (Fig. 27-4) should be identified and preserved as this prevents losing the plane of dissection. Since many lateral ventricular tumors can reach a very large size, an internal decompression may be required prior to isolating the tumor capsule away from surrounding ventricular structures.[2,6-9]

The use of the operative microscope at this stage merits consideration. High magnification is helpful in identifying tumor anatomy and vascularity, but can diminish an appreciation of the volume of the lesion outside the field of view and its interface with regional anatomy. Expanding the operative field by zooming out to lower magnification can be helpful in reorienting the surgeon and in maintaining the interface with the ependymal surface.

ANTERIOR TRANS-SULCAL APPROACH

The anterior trans-sulcal approach (superior frontal sulcus) is used commonly for lesions in the anterior lateral ventricles, especially when associated with hydrocephalus. In addition, this approach is preferred over the transcallosal

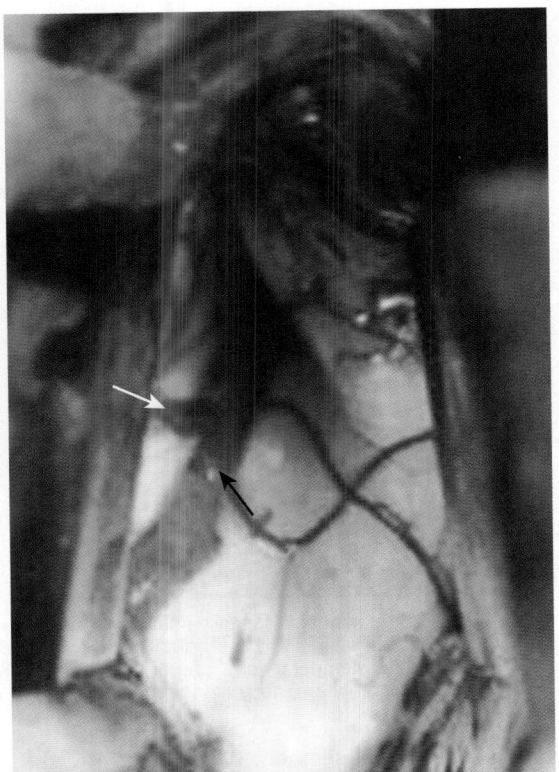

FIGURE 27-3 Intraoperative view of the left lateral ventricle showing the choroid plexus (*black arrow*), thalamostriate vein (*white arrow*), and septum pellucidum.

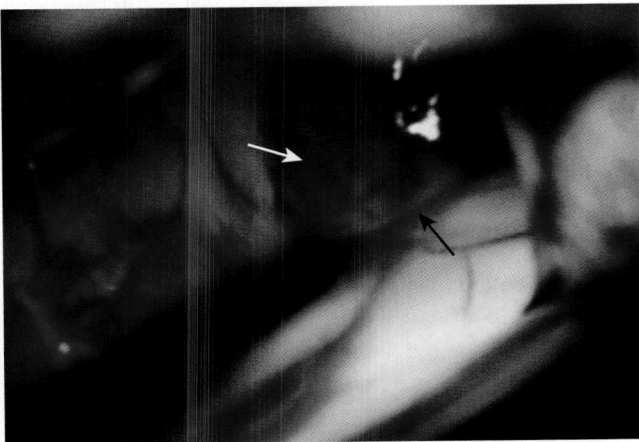

FIGURE 27-4 Intraoperative view of an intraventricular tumor (*white arrow*) and its interface (*black arrow*) with the ependymal surface.

route for large, midline-draining cortical veins. The craniotomy is similar to the one used for the transcallosal approach and uses a bicoronal incision lateral to the midline, measuring 4 to 6 cm in length. The superior and middle frontal gyri need to be exposed. Intraoperative ultrasound or stereotaxis can provide guidance for direct ventricular access. The sulcus is dissected open to its depths (or a 2 to 3 cm gyral incision is made) and developed down into the ventricle. The operative microscope is used after the ventricular chamber is opened. Tumor removal is achieved by delivering the lesion to the area of exposure while maintaining the tumor interface with the ependymal surface.

COMBINED APPROACHES

Very large tumors that extend into the frontal horn and body of the ventricle may require both a trans-sulcal and transcallosal approach (see Fig. 27-1B). This is necessitated by the limitations of each operative exposure. Entering the ventricle through the corpus callosum cannot provide access to the frontal horn without excessive retraction. Similarly, an anterior trans-sulcal exposure limits access to the posterior body of the ventricle. In those tumors that fill the lateral ventricle, an initial decompression through a trans-sulcal corridor can generate adequate relaxation of the hemisphere to permit interhemispheric dissection. Once this is achieved, the transcallosal corridor can be opened to complete the tumor resection without excessive retraction to either region.

POSTERIOR TRANS-SULCAL APPROACH

The interparietal sulcus approach (superior parietal lobule) is the preferred route to the atrium of the lateral ventricle and allows access to both medial and lateral segments of this part of the ventricle (see Fig. 27-1C). The patient is positioned in the three-quarter prone position with the parietal region at the highest point in the field. The craniotomy extends over the superior parietal lobule. A preoperative magnetic resonance venogram or cerebral angiogram is helpful in determining the position of major draining veins. The craniotomy does not cross midline. Once the cortex is exposed (or cortical incision is made), dissection proceeds along the interparietal sulcus. The atrium is more lateral at this location, and the dissection can be guided by ultrasound or stereotaxis. Once inside the atrium, the surgeon can visualize the thalamus anteriorly, the choroid plexus more medially, and the crus of the fornix. It should be remembered that the optic radiations define the lateral wall of the atrium, and the surgeon should avoid manipulation of that area. When tumors compress the lateral wall of the atrium, the tumor should be decompressed before separating it from this lateral ependymal surface. The vascular pedicle of the tumor should be identified and coagulated at the earliest possible time to avoid excessive bleeding.[2,10]

POSTERIOR TRANSCALLOSAL APPROACH

The posterior transcallosal approach gains access to the roof and medial part of the atrium of the lateral ventricles. This is achieved by splitting the splenium of the corpus callosum and is contraindicated for patients with a preoperative homonymous hemianopia contralateral to the dominant hemisphere due to a risk of alexia. Because the lateral ventricle extends laterally in this region, the lateral part of the atrium is not well visualized by this route. Preoperatively, as in the anterior approaches, a magnetic resonance venogram or cerebral angiogram helps to guide the placement of the craniotomy by visualizing the dominant cortical draining vessels. The patient is positioned in the three-quarter prone position, with the parietal area of the operated side in the dependent position. The craniotomy begins at the posterior edge of the postcentral gyrus and extends approximately 4 cm posteriorly. The craniotomy exposes the superior sagittal sinus and extends laterally

3 to 4 cm. The dura is reflected medially, and care is taken to maintain the large draining veins. The parietal lobe is gently retracted (approximately 2 cm) away from the falx. Once the arachnoid adhesions are opened, the distal pericallosal arteries and the splenium are identified. Below the splenium, the ICVs join Galen's vein, and these can be seen once the splenium is cut. The splenium is incised with a bipolar cautery, and this incision must be made lateral to the midline because the atrium of the lateral ventricle deviates laterally. Access into the atrium is now achieved; however, tumors not found in the medial part of the atrium will be hard to resect by this route, and the surgeon should consider the posterior transcortical route for lateral atrial tumors.[2,11,12]

POSTERIOR TEMPORAL APPROACH

The posterior temporal approach can be a useful route for lesions that are located laterally in the atrium. The patient is positioned either supine with the head tilted at least 60 degrees away from the craniotomy side or in the lateral position. The posterior temporal region is exposed just above the plane with the transverse sinus. Extreme care should be taken not to injure the vein of Labbe as it courses to the junction of the transverse and sigmoid sinus. Once the dura is exposed, on the nondominant side, an incision into the posterior middle or inferior temporal gyrus (middle temporal sulcus) will gain access to the atrium. The incision should be along the axis of the gyrus. Once the ventricle is accessed, the tumor is removed piecemeal and separated away from surrounding ependyma. In the dominant hemisphere, the approach can be varied to avoid impairment in language abilities. Specifically, the inferior temporal bone and mastoid air cells can be removed to gain access to the subtemporal area. The cortical incision is then made near the occipitotemporal gyrus. Although this avoids more of the optic radiations and is further removed from the speech cortex, this route requires more temporal lobe retraction. Care should be taken to avoid stretching or kinking the vein of Labbe. Furthermore, on closure of the subtemporal craniotomy, the mastoid air cells must be closed, and closure must be watertight to avoid postoperative CSF leakage. Lateral transcortical approaches to the atrium place the optic radiations at risk of injury minimizing the usefulness of this approach.

INFERIOR TEMPORAL APPROACH

This approach is used to gain access to temporal horn lesions (see Fig. 27-1D). The patient is placed supine, with the head tilted away by 45 degrees and extended. A reverse question mark incision is made starting at the level of the zygoma just anterior to the ear, then curving posteriorly over the ear and anteriorly toward the forehead. The temporalis muscle is mobilized anteriorly, and the craniotomy is extended inferiorly to the level of the zygoma. The dura is opened with its base positioned anteriorly. Access to the ventricle is achieved by making a cortical incision in the middle or inferior temporal gyrus or traversing the middle temporal sulcus. The more inferior temporal approaches are often used for lesions residing in the temporal horn or lateral atrium of the dominant hemisphere. Decompression of the tumor is followed by dissection away from surrounding ependyma.[2]

The Third Ventricle

SURGICAL ANATOMY

The third ventricle communicates with the lateral ventricles via the foramen of Monro and drains posteriorly into the aqueduct of Sylvius. Approximately one-third of the third ventricle is located anterior to the foramen of Monro and extends to the optic chiasm inferiorly. The anterior wall consists mainly of the lamina terminalis, a thin sheet of pia and gray matter that runs from the optic chiasm to the rostrum of the corpus callosum. The columns of the fornix are found at the superior lateral margins, and the anterior commissure crosses the anterior wall at its upper end. The lateral wall of the third ventricle is formed inferiorly by the hypothalamus and superiorly and posteriorly by the thalamus. In 75% of cases the massa intermedia, a thalamic projection, bridges the third ventricle at the superior-posterior end. The floor of the third ventricle starts at the optic chiasm at its anterior pole, dips into the infundibular recess before slanting superiorly and posteriorly over the tuber cinereum, the two mammillary bodies and the posterior perforated substance, located anterior to the cerebral peduncles. Posterior to the level of the peduncles is the aqueduct, which is surrounded by the tegmentum of the midbrain. The roof of the third ventricle starts anteriorly at the foramen of Monro and ends posteriorly in the suprapineal recess. The roof is separated from the lateral wall by the choroidal fissure, which runs in the cleft between the upper part of the thalamus and the fornix. Over the anterior part of the roof, the fornices run in parallel and are often attached into the body of the fornix, whereas over the posterior roof, the fornices separate into the forniceal crura, and the roof is draped in interforniceal-connecting white matter called the hippocampal commissure. However, the fornices and hippocampal commissure in the roof of the third ventricle are covered by a loose trabecular pial tissue that forms a double layer called the tela choroidea. Between these two layers of tela choroidea is a space, the velum interpositum, through which the internal cerebral veins (ICVs) and the medial posterior choroidal arteries course. The ICVs start at the posterior edge of the foramen of Monro and run posteriorly to exit the velum interpositum just above the pineal body. The third ventricular choroid plexus is attached to the roof by the tela choroidea, which communicates through the choroidal fissure with the lateral ventricular tela choroidea. The posterior wall of the third ventricle begins at Sylvius' aqueduct anteriorly and inferiorly. Proceeding in a posterior and superior direction, the posterior wall of the third ventricle contains the posterior commissure, the pineal body, the habenular commissure, and the suprapineal recess above.[13-15]

SURGICAL OPTIONS

The Anterior Third Ventricle

Transforaminal and Interforniceal Approaches

The transcallosal or trans-sulcal approaches to the third ventricle are a continuation of the approaches described for access into the lateral ventricles. The anterior transcallosal approach is the most commonly used for access to the third ventricle and affords an excellent, low morbidity pathway. This strategy provides several paths of dissection to open into the third ventricular chamber. The structures that are most at risk of injury with third ventricular tumors are the fornices and the vessels within the velum interpositum (the ICVs and the medial posterior choroidal arteries). These approaches are adequate for lesions extending to, or posterior to, the foramen of Monro. Lesions that are anterior to the foramen of Monro and inferior in the third ventricle may not be as readily accessible by this route.

Access to the anterior part of the third ventricle can be accomplished through an enlarged foramen of Monro. This transforaminal approach is particularly useful for tumors that dilate the foramen (Fig. 27-5A). Colloid cysts can be removed in this fashion with minimal manipulation of the foramen and the encircling fornix. The use of angled view endoscopes has allowed visualization of third ventricular structures. However, access to the third ventricle is limited by the size of the foramen of Monro, and when this limitation prohibits further removal of the tumor, alternative approaches to the third ventricle can be developed from this vantage point. The first method is enlargement of the foramen of Monro by unilateral transection of the fornix. This allows anterior access into the third ventricle. This approach, however, has been associated with potential significant morbidity in memory impairment. Thus it is not a recommended route.[16-20]

A second approach is the interforniceal route to the third ventricle, which gains access by splitting the fornices in the sagittal plane, along the direction of their fibers. In this approach, the septum pellucidum is opened and used as a guide to the midline. The great advantage of this approach is that posterior dissection can be carried out to expose the entire third ventricle. The ICVs have no reported branches between them and must be separated. The disadvantage of this method is the potential bilateral damage to the fornices. Consequently, the interforniceal approach is best used for patients who have a cavum septum pellucidum.[21-23]

Lateral Subfrontal Approach

This approach is useful for midline suprasellar and anterior third ventricular lesions (Fig. 27-5B). The patient is positioned supine and a bicoronal incision is used. The unilateral craniotomy starts laterally at the pterion and runs just above the orbital ridge. The brain is relaxed with mannitol and CSF drainage, while the frontal lobe is retracted gently. To reduce retraction and increase the upward angle of vision, the orbital ridges can be removed. Care should be taken to coagulate small draining veins because they may rupture during retraction. Past the planum sphenoidale, the optic nerves, the chiasm, and both internal carotid arteries are visualized. The tumor is generally evident at this stage. The A1 branches must be identified bilaterally to the level of the anterior communicating artery. If the tumor has a cystic component, such as in a craniopharyngioma, it is useful to decompress the cyst at this point. Care should be taken not to allow cystic contents to escape into the ventricle or subarachnoid space because they can cause aseptic meningitis. If the tumor does not contain a cystic component, then internal decompression is highly beneficial in reducing tension on the surrounding structures during dissection of the capsule. The resection can be performed through

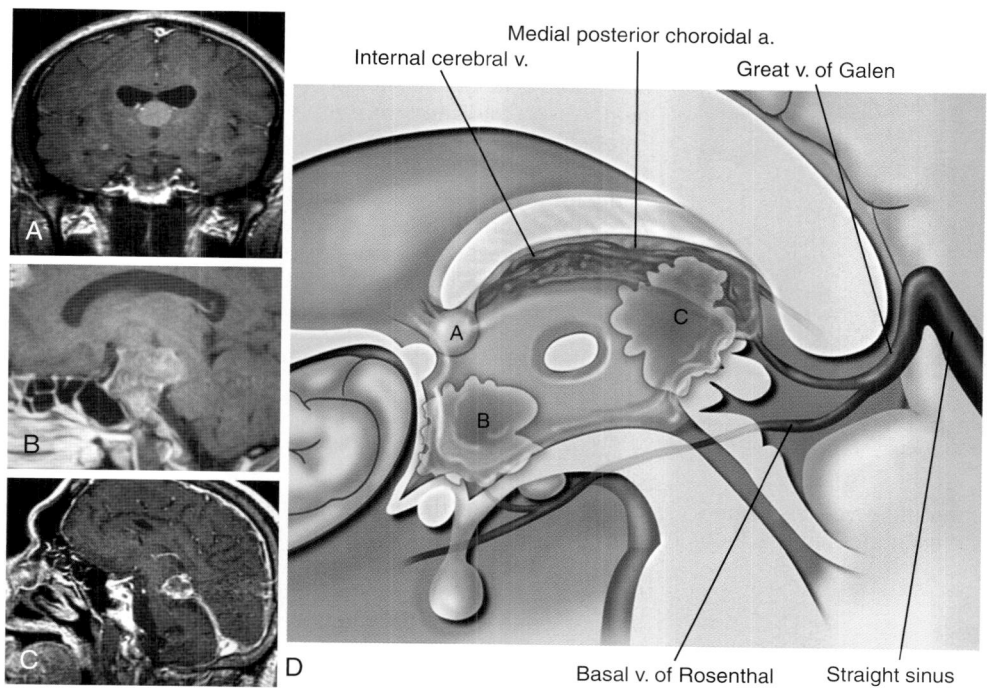

Medial posterior choroidal a.

Internal cerebral v.

Great v. of Galen

Basal v. of Rosenthal   Straight sinus

FIGURE 27-5 Enhanced magnetic resonance imaging of third ventricle tumors in common locations, with preferred surgical routes as denoted. A, Foramen of Monro, anterior transcallosal transforaminal or endoscopic. B, Anterior third ventricle, lateral subfrontal or pterional, C, Posterior third ventricle, occipital transtentorial or infratentorial supracerebellar. D, Schematic representation highlighting common tumor locations (A, foramen of Monro; B, anterior third ventricle; C, posterior third ventricle) and relevant vascular anatomy of the third ventricle.

the prechiasmatic space, the opticocarotid triangle, or the retrocarotid space. The latter two routes are the reasons for a wide craniotomy extending to the pterion. In patients with a prefixed chiasm, resection is particularly difficult to accomplish, and opening of the lamina terminalis may be required. The lamina is opened above the chiasm up to the anterior commissure. In suprasellar tumors that extend upward into the anterior third ventricle, the anterior floor of the third ventricle is pushed upward. Thus, on opening the lamina, the tumor is covered by a thin third ventricular floor, which every effort should be made to save. Occasionally, the tumor can be accessed and delivered through either the prechiasmatic space or the opticocarotid triangle.[24-27]

Pterional Approach

This approach is a common one to suprasellar tumors that extend into the anterior third ventricle (Fig. 27-5B). The weakness of this approach is the poor visualization of the ipsilateral third ventricular extension and contralateral opticocarotid and retrocarotid space. The positioning is supine, with the head tilted approximately 45 degrees to the left and in approximately 20 degrees of extension. The incision follows a hairline curve from the zygoma anterior to the ear to the frontal region. It is important to stay flush with the pterional base; alternatively, an orbital osteotomy maximizes the upward angle. The Sylvian fissure may need to be opened. Once CSF is released and brain relaxation is achieved, gentle retraction is applied to the frontal lobe. The tumor is accessed through the retrocarotid space, the opticocarotid triangle, and the prechiasmatic space. In addition, the lamina terminalis can be accessed and opened.[28]

Endoscopic Approaches

The endoscope offers a surgical approach that is useful for intraventricular tumor surgery (Fig. 27-5A). The improvement of endoscopic techniques and instruments has established

endoscopic approaches as an alternative to microsurgical techniques in selected cases.[29] The fluid-filled space of the ventricular system can be a very suitable region for endoscopy, including tumor biopsy under direct visualization and restoration of CSF flow by opening obstructed pathways.[30] The endoscope is also useful for inspecting regions not easily accessed with the operative microscope. The most commonly treated lesions using an endoscopic approach are colloid cysts of the third ventricle. Through a burr hole, a working sleeve is stereotactically inserted. A video unit is connected to a rigid endoscope with variable-degree angled optical systems. Endoscopic instruments and coagulation can be inserted through working ports and controlled in the visual field of the scope. This provides enough space and flexibility to separate tumor tissue or membranes and remove small intraventricular tumors, stereotactically aspirate the cyst contents, and relieve associated hydrocephalus by CSF diversion. The limitations of endoscopic techniques prohibit removal of tumors with high vascularity or fibrous consistency. Furthermore, the lesion can be engulfed by neural or vascular structures, such as the choroid plexus, or covered by large veins that cannot be mobilized during endoscopic surgery. In experienced hands, the endoscopic approach using optimal instrumentation may permit complete or near complete removal of the colloid cyst wall and should result in a low recurrence rate, mostly without the consequences described. Bleeding is a potential risk in endoscopic surgery. Since this problem may not be controlled without wide exposure, the surgeon should be prepared to perform a craniotomy when necessary.[31,32]

Endoscopy can be used in selected cases in ventricular surgery, but even in appropriate cases, the risks of incomplete tumor removal, bleeding, and a small operative corridor must be considered against the three-dimensional visualization of the operative microscope, wider operative field, greater chance of total resection, and better

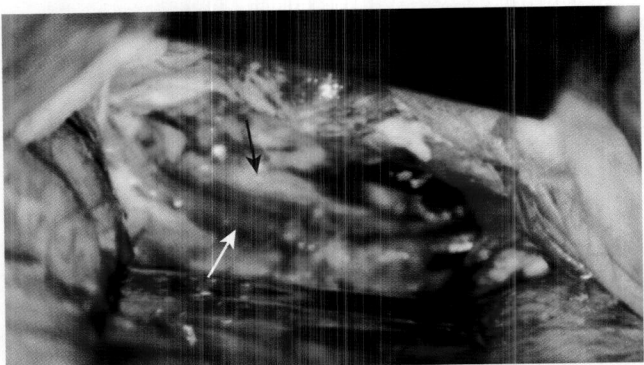

FIGURE 27-6 Intraoperative view of a transvelum interpositum approach to the third ventricle showing the internal cerebral vein (*white arrow*) and medial posterior choroidal artery (*black arrow*).

hemostasis. Additional expertise and improved instrumentation will continue to increase the usefulness of this technique in the future.

The Posterior Third Ventricle

Transcallosal Transvelum Interpositum Approaches

Following access to the lateral ventricle, the choroidal dissection is performed medial to the lateral ventricular choroid, through the tenia fornicis, separating the choroid from the body of the fornix. The choroid plexus is either removed or reflected laterally. This minimizes contact with the posterior choroidal artery and the superficial thalamic veins. Once the choroid is reflected laterally, the velum interpositum, the ICVs, and the medial posterior choroidal arteries are visualized (Fig. 27-6). At this point, the ICVs are separated and a plane is developed between them. Alternatively, the ICV is dissected from the ipsilateral fornix to expose the third ventricle. There are no reported bridging veins between these vessels; nevertheless, because they run closely together, they require manipulation and intermittent compression to gain access to the third ventricle. The last layer in this approach to be split is the third ventricular choroid plexus, which must also be separated in the midline. Finally, one should keep in mind that the anatomy is often distorted; in this case, the preoperative radiographic studies are particularly useful.[4,13,33,34]

Infratentorial Supracerebellar Approach

This approach is well suited for midline tumors in the pineal region and avoids retraction or manipulation of the cerebral hemispheres (Fig. 27-5C). The approach is not optimally suited if the tumor infiltrates laterally or superiorly above the tentorium. The patient can be placed in the sitting position, the three-quarter prone position, or the prone position. The sitting position is optimal for brain relaxation; the cerebellum falls away, while venous drainage is optimized. If this position is chosen, the patient is susceptible to air embolus; thus a central line, carbon dioxide monitor, PEEP, and compression stockings are advised. The incision is midline, and a wide suboccipital craniotomy is performed, thus exposing the transverse sinus and torculum. The dura is opened with its base superiorly. Retraction may be applied superiorly to the underside of the tentorium in the midline, while gentle inferior retraction can be placed on the vermis. Care

should be taken to coagulate and divide cerebellar bridging veins as they drain superiorly into the tentorium. The arachnoid is thick and should be divided before the parapineal vessels and the tumor are visualized. The precentral cerebellar vein, connecting the vermis to Galen's vein, can be sacrificed to gain access to the pineal region. Resection of the tumor proceeds inferior to Galen's vein, the ICVs, and Rosenthal's basal vein. The quadrigeminal plate should be well visualized. After tumor resection, communication of the posterior third ventricle can be confirmed by direct visualization.[35,36]

Occipital Transtentorial Approach

This approach is used for pineal and posterior third ventricular lesions with either supratentorial or infratentorial components (Fig. 27-5C). The patient can be placed in either the sitting or semiprone position. However, whereas the sitting position helps in the infratentorial approach by allowing the cerebellum to fall away, the three-quarter prone position helps the occipital lobe to fall away, thus reducing need for retraction. The trapdoor incision is made with its base inferiorly and across the midline. The occipital craniotomy can expose the midline and the transverse sinus. The dura is opened with its base on the sinuses. Minimal retraction on the occipital lobe is necessary with adequate CSF drainage and brain relaxation. There are rarely significant draining veins from the medial occipital lobe into the tentorium. The transection of the tentorium proceeds in a posterior to anterior direction by first making an incision proximally and then proceeding in a line approximately 1 cm off midline toward the tentorial edge. The tentorium is well vascularized, and hemostasis may require a bipolar cautery and clips. The thick arachnoid should be separated at the edge of the tentorium to avoid undue bleeding of small vessels. The deep veins around the pineal are surrounded in a thick arachnoid; this needs to be opened widely to expose the local anatomic landmarks. If necessary, the precentral cerebellar vein should be sacrificed to increase the working space. Tumor resection can proceed between the ICVs and Rosenthal's basal vein. The falx can be cut approximately 1 cm anterior to the insertion of the vein of Galen into the sinus, after coagulating or clipping the inferior sagittal sinus. Retraction on the falx allows further exposure. The splenium does not have to be cut but can be gently retracted upward to allow extra exposure.[37,38]

Complications

MORTALITY

Surgery of the lateral and third ventricle has carried an extremely high mortality rate in the past (as high as 75%). With advances in microsurgery and improved understanding of anatomic pathways, the 30-day postoperative mortality at present is 5% to 12%. Among the immediate causes of the mortality were cerebral hemorrhage, infarction, brain swelling, and pulmonary embolus.[11,39-42]

COGNITIVE DEFICITS

Intraventricular surgery can cause postoperative impairment of cognitive functions. Some of these symptoms are related to the corpus callosum disconnection and include disturbed consciousness, a transient state of mutism, memory impairment and apathy, contralateral leg weakness, incontinence, and disinhibition. The severity of these symptoms correlate with the length of the callosotomy and can be seen in as many as 75% of patients but tend to resolve within 3 weeks. Permanent changes in cognition are reported in 5% to 10%. Neuropsychological testing is useful in these cases. Persistent focal neurologic deficits such as impairment of motor function or a visual field cut are reported in 8% to 30% of cases.[9,11,41,42]

SEIZURES

Postoperative seizures are more common in patients who undergo transcortical procedures, and previous reports have indicated that approximately one-third of patients have seizures in the postoperative period. In patients undergoing transcallosal procedures, the incidence is unknown, although it is presumed to be lower. Although most approaches avoid transversing cortical tissue, retraction injuries to the brain may also cause postoperative seizures.[11,15,40]

HYDROCEPHALUS

It is common for lateral and third ventricular tumors to cause hydrocephalus. It should be remembered that following resection of the tumor, hydrocephalus persists in as many as 33% of patients. These patients require shunting. Furthermore, these shunts often (>20% of cases) malfunction, likely because of the higher protein content in the CSF of these postoperative patients, and there is also an increased risk of shunt infection. Overshunting can add to the problem of postoperative subdural hematoma collections, which are found in approximately 40% of patients. Only one fourth of these require surgery for drainage of the subdural collection; nevertheless, this implies that approximately 10% of patients who under-go ventricular surgery will require drainage of a subdural collection later on. The more pronounced the preoperative ventriculomegaly, the higher the risk of this complication.[43-45]

Multiple factors influence the successful outcome of surgery of the lateral and third ventricles. The approaches described have been developed to allow access to the ventricular system while minimizing manipulation of the surrounding brain. Among the numerous factors that are involved in choosing a particular surgical approach to these tumors are the location in the ventricles, size, vascularity, feeding blood supply, presumptive pathology, and the surgeon's comfort level with a particular approach. Although treatment of these lesions can be complex and often difficult, a good surgical outcome, which maximizes the patient's quality of life, can now be anticipated in most cases.

Conclusion

There are several general principles that guide successful intraventricular surgery. Each has an important role in providing the optimal conditions for tumor removal while minimizing morbidity. All surgery begins with patient positioning. Adequate exposure of the planned corridor of access, minimizing brain manipulation and utilization of gravity to assist in retraction are fundamental requirements.

Brain relaxation is mandatory to prevent further injury. Routine use of mannitol, hyperventilation and CSF drainage should be started early in the surgery to prevent injury from surgical manipulation of the brain. In patients with very large tumors filling the ventricle, these methods may be insufficient. Early access to the lesion (commonly by transcortical dissection) and decompressing the tumor may be the only method to achieve a relaxed hemisphere. Once this is achieved, microdissection of the margin between the tumor and the brain can proceed. Reliable identification and protection of the interface between the tumor and the ependymal surface can prevent dissection beyond the intended target lesion. Adjusting the field of magnification of the operating microscope to reorient to the surgical field can help to maintain this plane. Most operative approaches to intraventricular tumors create a corridor of exposure that is significantly smaller than the tumor. Consequently, the lesion must be removed in pieces and delivered into the field of view. This technique can result in significant blood loss since the vascular supply to the tumor (often the choroidal vessels) is not exposed early in the dissection. The surgeon must be prepared to attend to this issue and to approach the tumor's vascular supply as early as possible. Once the tumor has been removed, it is essential to remove blood and air from within the ventricles. This can prevent postoperative CSF obstruction and headache and cognitive impairment associated with pneumocephalus. Placing a cotton barrier over the foramen of Monro early in lateral ventricle tumor surgery can limit blood pooling within the third ventricle. Opening the septum pelucidum to inspect the contralateral ventricle can facilitate inspection for an accumulated hematoma as well as reducing the chances of a trapped ventricle. A postoperative ventricular catheter is commonly used for monitoring following this surgery. In patients with preoperative ventriculomegaly, the risk of an extra-axial hematoma is increased with rapid reduction in intracranial pressure and tumor volume. Consequently, any unexpected increase in intracranial pressure should be investigated with imaging before utilizing the catheter for removing CSF.

KEY REFERENCES

Asgari S, Engelhorn T, Brondics A, et al. Transcortical or transcallosal approach to ventricle-associated lesions: a clinical study on the prognostic role of surgical approach. *Neurosurg Rev.* 2003;26:192-197.

Bellotti C, Pappada G, Sani R, et al. The transcallosal approach for lesions affecting the lateral and third ventricles: surgical considerations and results in a series of 42 cases. *Acta Neurochir (Wien).* 1991;111:103-113.

Bruce DA. Complications of third ventricular surgery. *Pediatr Neurosurg.* 1991;17:325-330.

Bruce JN, Stein BM. Surgical management of pineal region tumors. *Acta Neurochir (Wien).* 1995;134:130-135.

Clark WK, Batjer HH. The occipital transtentorial approach. In: Apuzzo MLJ, ed. *Surgery of the Third Ventricle.* 2nd ed. Baltimore: Williams & Wilkins; 1998:721-741.

Dandy WE. Operative experience in cases of pineal tumor. *Arch Surg.* 1936;33:19-46.

Ehni G, Ehni BL. Considerations in transforaminal entry. In: Apuzzo MLJ, ed. *Surgery of the Third Ventricle.* 2nd ed. Baltimore: Williams & Wilkins; 1998:391-419.

Fuji K, Lenkey C, Rhoton Jr AL. Microsurgical anatomy of the choroidal arteries: lateral and third ventricle. *J Neurosurg.* 1980;52:165-188.

Hellwig D, Bauer BL, Schulte M, et al. Neuroendoscopic treatment for colloid cysts of the third ventricle: the experience of a decade. *Neurosurgery.* 2003;52:525-533.

Nagata S, Rhoton Jr AL, Barry M. Microsurgical anatomy of the choroidal fissure. *Surg Neurol.* 1988;30:3-59.

Ono M, Rhoton Jr AL, Peace D, et al. Microsurgical anatomy of the deep venous system of the brain. *Neurosurgery.* 1984;15:621-657.

Oppel F, Hoff HJ, Pannek HW. Endoscopy of the ventricular system: indications, operative procedure and technical aspects. In: Hellwig D, Bauer BL, eds. *Minimally Invasive Techniques for Neurosurgery.* Berlin: Springer; 1998:97-100.

Patterson RH. Jr: The subfrontal transsphenoidal and trans-lamina terminalis approaches. In: Apuzzo MLJ, ed. *Surgery of the Third Ventricle.* 2nd ed. Baltimore: Williams & Wilkins; 1998:471-487.

Piepmeier J, Spencer D, Sass K, et al. Lateral ventricular masses. In: Apuzzo MLJ, ed. *Brain Surgery: Complications Avoidance and Management.* New York: Churchill Livingstone; 1993:581-600.

Piepmeier JM, Sass KJ, et al. Surgical management of lateral ventricular tumors. In: Paoletti P, Takakura K, Walker M, eds. *Neurooncology.* Kluwer: Dordrecht; 1991:333-335.

Rhoton Jr AL, Yamamoto I, Pease DA. Microsurgery of the third ventricle. Part 2: Operative approaches. *Neurosurgery.* 1981;8:357-373.

Rhoton Jr AL. Microsurgical anatomy of the third ventricular region. In: Apuzzo MLJ, ed. *Surgery of the Third Ventricle.* 2nd ed. Baltimore: Williams & Wilkins; 1998:89-158.

Sass K, Novelly R, Spencer D, et al. Amnestic and attention impairments following corpus callosotomy section for epilepsy. *J Epilepsy.* 1988;1:61-66.

Stein BM, Bruce JN. Surgical management of pineal region tumors. *Clin Neurosurg.* 1992;39:509-532.

Sugita K, Kobayashi S, Yokoo A. Preservation of large bridging veins during brain retraction. *J Neurosurg.* 1982;57:856-860.

Timurkaynak E, Rhoton Jr AL, Barry M. Microsurgical anatomy and operative approaches to the lateral ventricles. *Neurosurgery.* 1986;19: 685-723.

Ture U, Yasargil MG, Al-Mefty O. The transcallosal-transforaminal approach to the third ventricle with regard to the venous variations in this region. *J Neurosurg (Wien).* 1997;87:706-715.

Wen WT, Rhoton Jr AL, de Oliveira E. Transchoroidal approach to the third ventricle: an anatomic study of the choroidal fissure and its clinical application. *Neurosurgery.* 1998;42:1205-1219.

Yasargil MG, Abdulrauf SI. Surgery of intraventricular tumors. *Neurosurgery.* 2008;62:1029-1040.

Yasargil MG, Curcic M, Kis M, et al. Total removal of craniopharyngiomas: approaches and long term results in 144 patients. *J Neurosurg.* 1990;73:3-11.

Numbered references appear on Expert Consult.

CHAPTER 28

Transcallosal Surgery of Lesions Affecting the Third Ventricle: Basic Principles

ALEXANDER TAGHVA • CHARLES Y. LIU • MICHAEL L.J. APUZZO

Intraventricular tumors represent a relatively small proportion of central nervous system lesions, accounting for approximately 10% of CNS neoplasms.[1] Despite this, they represent a diverse range of pathologic entities which pose technical challenges for neurosurgeons. Third ventricular lesions, in particular, are challenging in terms of surgical access and corridor, owing to their central location in the brain. As such, these lesions hold a special place in neurosurgical history and literature.

There is a wide differential diagnosis for third ventricular neoplasms, with the most common entities being colloid cysts, astrocytomas, and craniopharyngiomas. Other lesions include arachnoid cysts, pituitary adenomas, ependymomas, germinomas, metastasis, subependymoma, central neurocytoma, teratoma, dermoid, arteriovenous malformation, meningioma and choroid plexus papilloma (Table 28-1).[2,3] The differential can often be refined by location within the third ventricle; for example, astrocytomas and craniopharyngiomas tend to be located in the anterior third ventricle, meningioma and choroid plexus papilloma in the posterior third ventricle, and colloid cysts at the level of the foramen of Monro.[4]

Given that the majority of intraventricular lesions are benign, surgery is often the preferred, and potentially curative, option for tumors of this region.[5] However, owing to the relative rarity of these lesions, few surgeons have extensive experience with approaches to the ventricular system. Interhemispheric, transcallosal approaches to the third ventricle offer the advantage of potential avoidance of postoperative cortical hemispheric deficits or other long-term complications (e.g., seizures) as compared to transcortical approaches. Partial sectioning of the corpus callosum does not in general lead to significant neurologic impairment. In patients with crossed-dominance, where the hemisphere controlling the dominant hand is contralateral to the hemisphere controlling speech and language, callosal sectioning can lead to severe disability.[6-8] This condition can be present in patients with a history a childhood cerebral injury or other dysfunction forcing relocation of language function within the brain. Furthermore, sectioning the splenium of the corpus callosum in patients with a dominant hemisphere hemianopsia may also be contraindicated as this can lead to alexia.[8] In modern times, the complications related to transcallosal approaches are generally related to

manipulations in the floor of the third ventricle and not the approach.

Historical Notes

Dandy first described the transcallosal approach for accessing the ventricular system in 1922.[9] Before that time, localization of tumors of the third ventricle was limited by insufficient diagnostic methods, and the introduction of ventriculography by Dandy in 1918 helped in this regard.[10] Dandy accessed the third ventricle primarily through a posterior transcallosal approach. In 1944, Edward Busch described division of the midline forniceal raphe and entrance into the third ventricle by splitting of the plane between the two fornices.[11] Several series and reports detailing the use of transcallosal techniques began to appear in the 1950s and 1960s.[12-14] In the 1970s and 1980s, series reporting on psychometric and neuropsychological outcomes following transcallosal surgery further elucidated the then growing body of knowledge regarding the physiology of corpus callosum sectioning.[15-18]

Anatomic Considerations

The third ventricle is a narrow, funnel-shaped structure that lies in the center of the brain. It lies below the corpus callosum and body of the lateral ventricles, between the two thalami and walls of hypothalamus, and above the pituitary and midbrain (Fig. 28-1).[19] It is a unilocular cavity and communicates with the lateral ventricles at its anterosuperior margin via the foramen of Monro; posteriorly, it communicates with the fourth ventricle via the sylvian aqueduct.[19]

The roof of the third ventricle contains five layers and extends from the foramen of Monro anteriorly to the suprapineal recess posteriorly.[19,20] The fornices make up the upper, or neural, layer. The axons of the fornices arise in the temporal horns from the hippocampi and extend around the thalami to reach the mammillary bodies.[19] The inferior aspects, or fimbria, arise in the floor of the temporal horn and pass posteriorly to become the posterior portions, or crura of the fornices. These unite at the hippocampal commissure, which covers the posterior portion of the third ventricle; the bodies of the fornices cover the middle portion; the columns of the fornices, along with anterior

Table 28-1	Frequency of Tumors of the Third Ventricle	
Tumor	**Number**	**Percent**
Astrocytoma	5	21%
Craniopharyngioma	5	21%
Ependymoma	4	17%
Choroid plexus papilloma	3	13%
Cystercercosis	2	8.3%
Colloid cyst	1	4.2%
Epidermoid	1	4.2%
Dermoid	1	4.2%
Subependymoma	1	4.2%
Medulloblastoma	1	4.2%
Total	24	

Adapted from data in Morrison G, Sobel DF, Kelley WM, Norman D. Intraventricular mass lesions. Radiology. 1984;153:435-442.

commissure and lamina terminalis, cover the anterior portion of the third ventricle.[19] The second and fourth layers of the roof of the third ventricle are comprised of the superior and inferior layers of the tela choroidea. The superior and inferior layers of the tela choroidea form a space called the velum interpositum, which contains the third, and vascular, layer of the roof of the third ventricle.[20] In this vascular layer lie the internal cerebral vein (ICV) and posterior choroidal arteries (PChA). The fifth layer is the choroid plexus of the lateral ventricle, which extends from the foramen of Monro posterosuperolaterally toward the pineal gland.

The choroid plexus runs bilaterally in the choroidal fissures, which are incisuras between the lateral edge of the fornix and the superomedial surface of the thalamus.[21] The choroid plexus of the lateral ventricle has an ependymal attachment to the fornix and to the thalamus called the teniae fornicis and the teniae thalami, respectively.[22] The teniae fornicies contains no arteries or veins; however, tributaries of the internal cerebral vein, the superior and anterior thalamic veins and the thalamostriate vein, as well as the branches of the medial PChA traverse the teniae thalami.[23] Surgically, this is an important point, as opening the choroidal fissure along the teniae fornicis avoids these vascular structures.[24]

The floor of the third ventricle extends anteriorly from the optic chiasm to the sylvian aqueduct posteriorly.[19] The anterior half of the floor is formed by diencephalic structures and the posterior half is formed by those of the mesencephalon.[19] From anterior to posterior, structures encountered are the optic chiasm, the infundibular recess, the median eminence, the tuber cinereum, the pair of mammillary bodies, and the ventricular side corresponding to the posterior perforated substance, and part of the tegmentum of the midbrain.[19,25] The anterior wall of the third ventricle is formed from superior to inferiorly by the columns of the fornix, the foramina of Monro, the anterior commissure, lamina terminalis, optic recess, and optic chiasm. The posterior wall consists of, from superiorly to inferiorly, the suprapineal recess, the habenular commissure, and the sylvian aqueduct. The lateral walls are formed by the thalamus superiorly and hypothalamus interiorly, which are delineated by the hypothalamic sulcus extending from

the foramen of Monro to the sylvian aqueduct.[19] The massa intermedia connecting the two thalami is present in roughly three quarters of brains approximately 4 ml posterior to the foramen of Monro.[26]

Anatomy of the lateral ventricle and the relationship to the foramen of Monro is key in these approaches as well as these provide a corridor of access to the third ventricle. In the lateral ventricle, medial and lateral groups of veins converge at the level of the foramen of Monro to form the internal cerebral veins. The main medial vein is the septal vein, which crosses the septum pellucidum and the fornix. The lateral veins include the caudate veins, which run from posterolateral to anteromedial to cross the caudate nucleus and the thalamus, and the thalamostriate vein.[21] The thalamostriate vein is located in the body of the lateral ventricle. It is the largest tributary of the ICV and runs in the striothalamic sulcus between the caudate nucleus and the thalamus. At the posterior margin of the foramen of Monro, the thalamostriate vein curves medially around the anterior tubercle of the thalamus to form the ICV.[20] This U-shaped junction is termed the venous angle.[20,27,28]

Preoperative Radiographic Evaluation

Magnetic resonance imaging with and without contrast is the standard modality for imaging of neoplasms of the third ventricle. Surgical corridors should be planned to maximize visualization of the offending lesion with minimal possible disruption of normal anatomy. Posteriorly placed craniotomies will provide angulation toward the anterior portions of the third ventricle and vice versa for anteriorly placed craniotomies. Furthermore, as injury and sacrifice of parasagittal draining veins can lead to venous infarction and cortical deficits, magnetic resonance venography is often helpful for planning of the operative corridor. The advent of intraoperative navigation and stereotaxy makes it possible to plan approaches in corridors of relative venous paucity and should be considered, especially in cases of distorted or otherwise unusual anatomy.

Surgical Technique

After induction of general anesthesia with endotracheal intubation, we typically place the patient in Mayfield pin fixation with the patient supine and the head elevated 15-20 degrees above horizontal (Fig. 28-2). Some surgeons prefer a lateral head position with the head turned 90 degrees laterally with the vertex 30 to 40 degrees above horizontal. Usually in the lateral position, the nondominant hemisphere is placed inferiorly such that it falls away with gravity and opens up the midline corridor; however, based on anatomy of the offending lesion and the patient's venous drainage, it may be desirable to place the dominant hemisphere down. Advocates for lateral positioning cite that gravity may be used to allow the inferiorly placed hemisphere to fall away, giving midline access with minimal retraction and that lateral positioning of the head allows the surgeon to operate with hands side-by-side versus on top of one another. We have found in our experience that the main disadvantage of lateral positioning is the distortion of midline by displacement of the brain by gravity. This disadvantage is most significant in interforniceal approaches, as identification of the midline is crucial to the

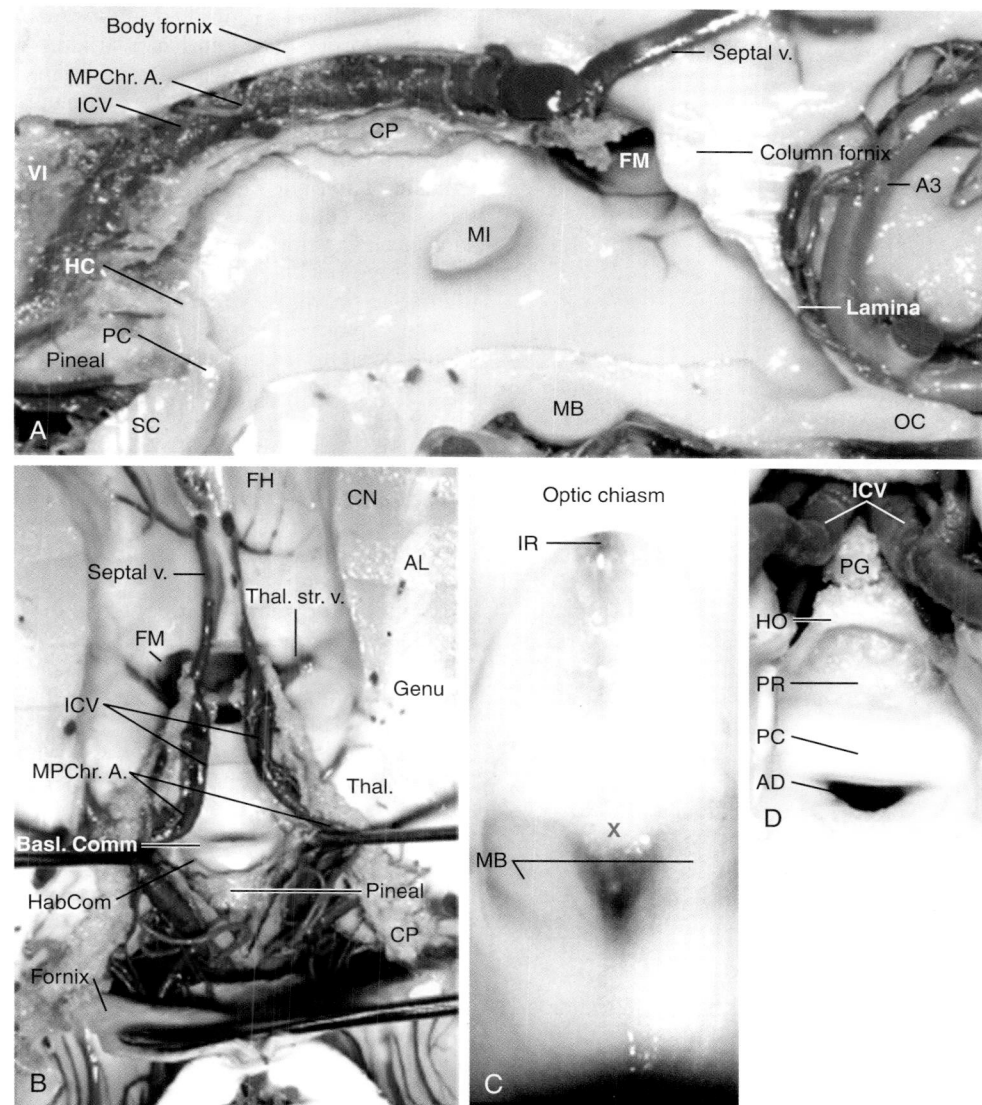

FIGURE 28-1 Photographs demonstrating the third ventricle. A, Mid-sagittal view of the third ventricle. B, View from above, looking into the third ventricle between the paired ICVs and paired distal branches of the medial PChAs. C, Close up view of the floor of the third ventricle. Prominent landmarks of the floor include (from anterior to posterior) the optic chiasm, infundibular recess, and paired mammillary bodies. The site for performing a third ventriculostomy lies just anterior to the mammillary bodies wherethe reddish color of the basilar apex can usually be seen through the transparent third ventricular floor. D, View of the posterior wall, which contains (from inferior to superior) the aqueduct, posterior commissure, pineal gland, pineal recess, and habenular commissure. A3, A3 segment; AD, aqueduct; AL, anterior limb of internal capsule; CN, caudate nucleus; CP, choroid plexus; FH, frontal horn; FM, foramen of Monro; Genu, genu of internal capsule; HC or HabCom, habenular commissure; IR, infundibular recess; Lamina Term., lamina terminalis; MB, mammillary body; MI, massa intermedia; MPChr. A., medial PChA; OC, optic chiasm; PC or Post. Comm, posterior commissure; PG or Pineal, pineal gland; PR, pineal recess; SC, superior colliculus; Septal V., septal vein; Thal., thalamus; Thal.Str.V., thalamostriate vein; VI, velum interpositum. *(From Ulm AJ, Russo A, Albanese E, et al. Limitations of the transcallosal transchoroidal approach to the third ventricle. J Neurosurg. 2009;111:600-609, with permission.)*

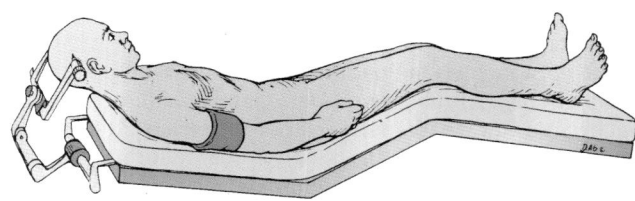

FIGURE 28-2 Patient in supine position with head flexed 15 to 20 degrees in Mayfield head fixation. *(From Apuzzo ML, Amar AP. Transcallosal interforniceal approach. In: Apuzzo ML, ed. Surgery of the Third Ventricle. Baltimore: Williams & Wilkins; 1998:421-452, with permission.)*

prevention of forniceal injury. Furthermore, we have found that by moving slightly to the patient's side, it is quite easy to operate with hands side-by-side in the supine position. For these reasons, we primarily utilize supine positioning.

Consideration is given to placement of preoperative ventriculostomy placement contralateral to the side of dissection. This assists in relaxation of the hemispheres for dissection and should be strongly considered in patients with preoperative ventriculomegaly. Typically, if preoperative ventriculostomy is not performed, we will leave behind a ventricular catheter at the time of closure. Furosemide and

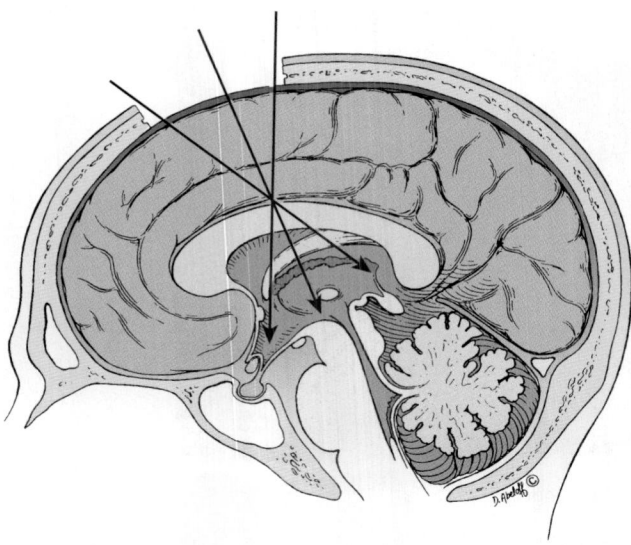

FIGURE 28-3 Craniotomy placement and the various viewlines into the anterior, middle, and posterior thirds of the third ventricle. *(From Apuzzo ML, Amar AP. Transcallosal interforniceal approach. In: Apuzzo ML, ed. Surgery of the Third Ventricle. Baltimore: Williams & Wilkins; 1998:421-452, with permission.)*

mannitol are also administered preoperatively to provide brain relaxation.

We typically use a two limbed curvilinear scalp flap or horseshoe flap, though other incisions can be tailored to achieve satisfactory cosmesis. A right-sided, 6 cm x 4 cm x 3 cm trapezoidal bone flap with the base at approximately 1 centimeter left of midline is most commonly used, with placement of burr holes at the vertices of the flap to obtain control of the sagittal sinus. For optimal access of the foramen of Monro, anatomy dictates that the bone flap should be placed such that it is bisected by the coronal suture.[29] However, the bone flap is classically placed two thirds in front of the coronal suture and one third behind it as generally there is a corridor of relative paucity of parasagittal draining veins at this location.[20,29] However, several factors influence craniotomy placement. A slightly more posterior bone flap with a more anteriorly angulated corridor will provide better access to the forniceal body and anterior third ventricle. More anteriorly placed bone flaps will provide better access to the posterior third ventricle (Fig. 28-3). Furthermore, with the advent of high-resolution MRI and frameless stereotaxy, parasagittal draining veins may be identified and a corridor chosen that provides access to the lesion without sacrifice of those veins.

Following craniotomy, a trapezoidal or curvilinear dural opening is made with the base toward the sagittal sinus (Fig. 28-4). Tack-up sutures are placed, and the addition sutures are placed to retract the dura toward the sagittal sinus to tamponade any bleeding from near the structure. Interhemispheric dissection is then undertaken until the corpus callosum is reached. Care should be taken to retract minimally on the exposed hemisphere. Progressively larger cotton balls can be placed at the anterior and posterior extents of the dissection to assist without use of retractor blades.[29,30] The cingulate gyri can be mistaken for the corpus callosum if the callosomarginal arteries are mistaken for the

pericallosal arteries running over the corpus callosum; however, the corpus callosum has a striking white appearance and is relatively hypovascular compared to the cortical pial color and vascularity of the cingulate (Fig. 28-5).[29] The number of A2, pericallosal arteries identified on the corpus callosum can range from one to three.[31,32] After the corpus callosum and pericallosal arteries are identified, incision of the corpus callosum is undertaken with a blunt dissector such as a Penfield 1 and 5 F suction. The incision is typically somewhere between 10 mm to 20 mm long, but should be tailored to provide optimal access to the lesion (Fig. 28-6).

After callosal incision, four possible entries into the ventricular system are possible: right lateral ventricle, left lateral ventricle, septum pellucidum with or without cavum, and forniceal body. In addition, three primary corridors for access to the third ventricle exist: through the foramen of Monro, through the choroidal fissure and velum interpositum, and interforniceal through the midline raphe. Choice of entry and approach taken depend primarily on the location, size, and texture of the lesion (Fig. 28-7). In addition, transcallosal entry into the ventricular system allows for emptying of the ventricular contents and brain relaxation. Furthermore, fenestration of the septum pellucidum will aid in this drainage.

A transforaminal approach is ideally-suited for cystic lesions in the anterior third ventricle and should be the first approach considered as it provides a natural aperture into the third ventricle without further dissection. Often times, the foramen is expanded secondary to the lesion, which allows decompression of the lesion without manipulation of critical structures.[8] Forniceal sacrifice is not necessary and should not be considered. From entry into the lateral ventricle, the septal vein medially, thalamostriate vein laterally, and choroid plexus can be identified and followed to the foramen of Monro. The choroid plexus is the most striking landmark leading to the foramen (Fig. 28-8). Again, at the posterior margin of the foramen, the thalamostriate vein joins the septal vein at a U-shaped junction forming the ICV, and this anatomy can be helpful in orienting the surgeon.

If the lesion is not accessible solely through the foramen of Monro, as with lesions in the middle or posterior portions of the third ventricle, other corridors of access should be considered. A detailed review of the three-dimensional radiographic anatomy will typically lend the surgeon the majority of the clues needed to plan an approach. One option as described by Yasargil and Abdulrauf is a combined transcallosal/trans-sylvian approach. This is an elegant approach and is now primarily used in a staged fashion for lesions with origins in the cranial base extending upward, such as craniopharyngiomas.[30] Therefore, the two other possible approach for lesions contained in the third ventricle are the transchoroidal approach and the interforniceal approach. The first approach we consider is the transchoroidal approach, as the choroidal fissure can be opened in a straightforward manner along a natural plane extending backward from the foramen of Monro. The choroid plexus of the lateral ventricle runs in the choroidal fissure, which is a C-shaped cleft between the fornix and thalamus extending from the foramen of Monro to the inferior choroidal point in the temporal horn.[20] The transchoroidal approach involves opening the choroidal fissure to expose the roof of the third ventricle by mobilization of the fornix to the contralateral

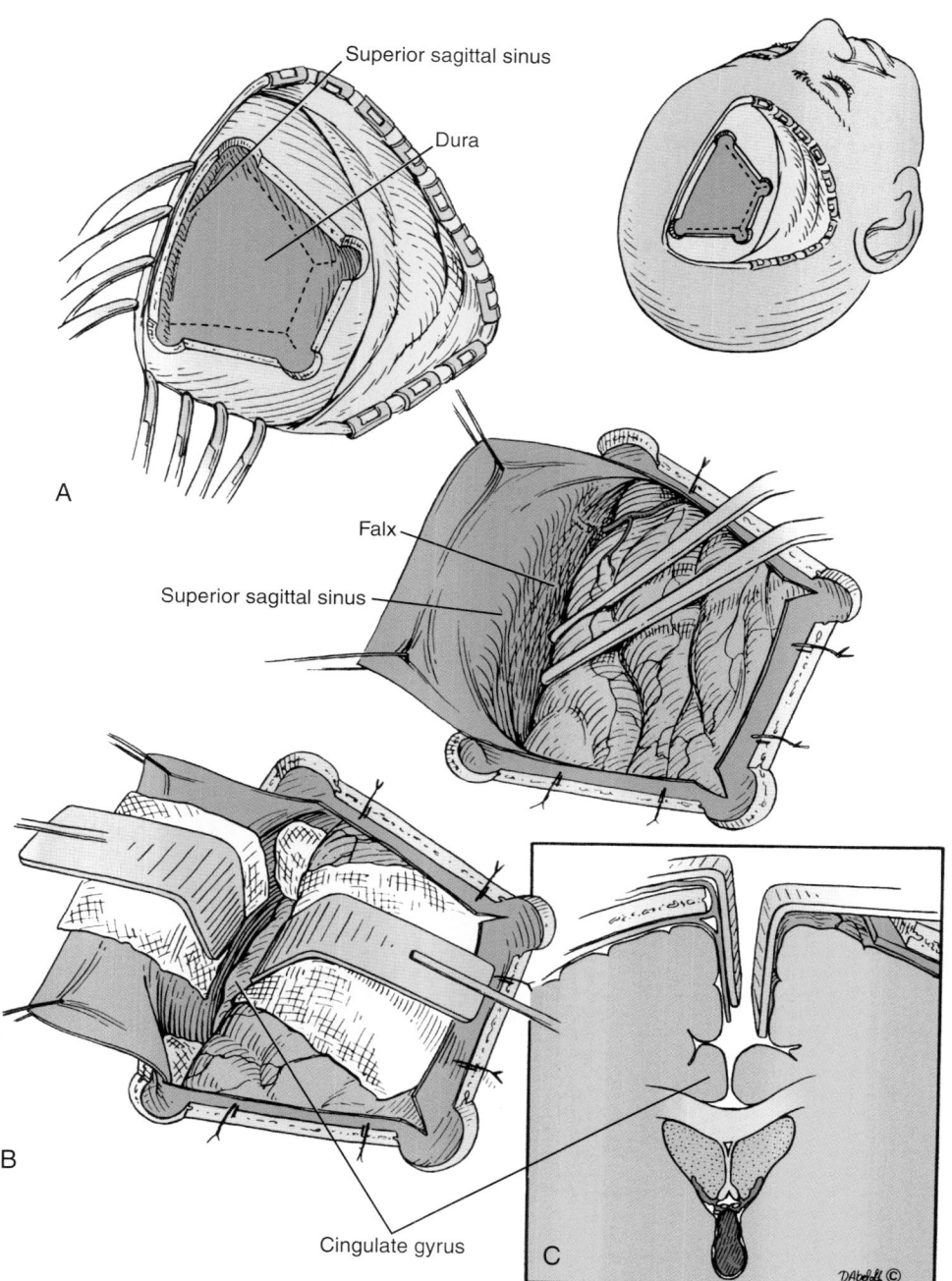

FIGURE 28-4 A, Dural incision takes advantage of the full extent of the bone flap with approximation of the midline and sagittal sinus. B, Initial development of the midline plane at the sagittal sinus with identification of the falx. C, Initial development of the exposure to the cingulate gyrus. Lateral retraction should not exceed 2 cm. *(From Apuzzo ML, Amar AP. Transcallosal interforniceal approach. In: Apuzzo ML, ed. Surgery of the Third Ventricle. Baltimore: Williams & Wilkins; 1998:421-452, with permission.)*

side.[30] This can be performed supra- or subchoroidally. Classically, in a subchoroidal approach, the taenia thalami is incised for access to the velum interpositum and third ventricle. In this approach, the ipsilateral thalamostriate vein may be injured due to manipulation of the fornix, and as described above, the superior and anterior thalamic veins, the thalamostriate vein, and the branches of the medial PChA pass through the taenia thalami, putting these structures at risk.[20,22,30] A suprachoroidal approach traverses the taenia fornicis, where no arteries or veins run, and also has a lesser risk of thalamostriate vein injury.[22] A recent anatomical analysis of the transchoroidal approach by Ulm et al.[20] found that the choroidal opening was limited to 1.5 cm

behind the foramen of Monro due to the expanding width of the fornix (Fig. 28-9). Furthermore, through this approach, they indicated that lesions in the middle third ventricle were most easily accessed, though anteriorly placed craniotomies and callosotomies were ideal for accessing posterior third ventricular pathology from an anterior to posterior angle. Access to the anterior third ventricle was limited by the columns of the fornix, and posteriorly placed craniotomies to achieve more anterior angulation was limited by the presence of parietal parasagittal draining veins.[20]

The interforniceal approach was originally described by Busch[6,11] in humans and studied in detail at our institution by Apuzzo et al. with the application of modern

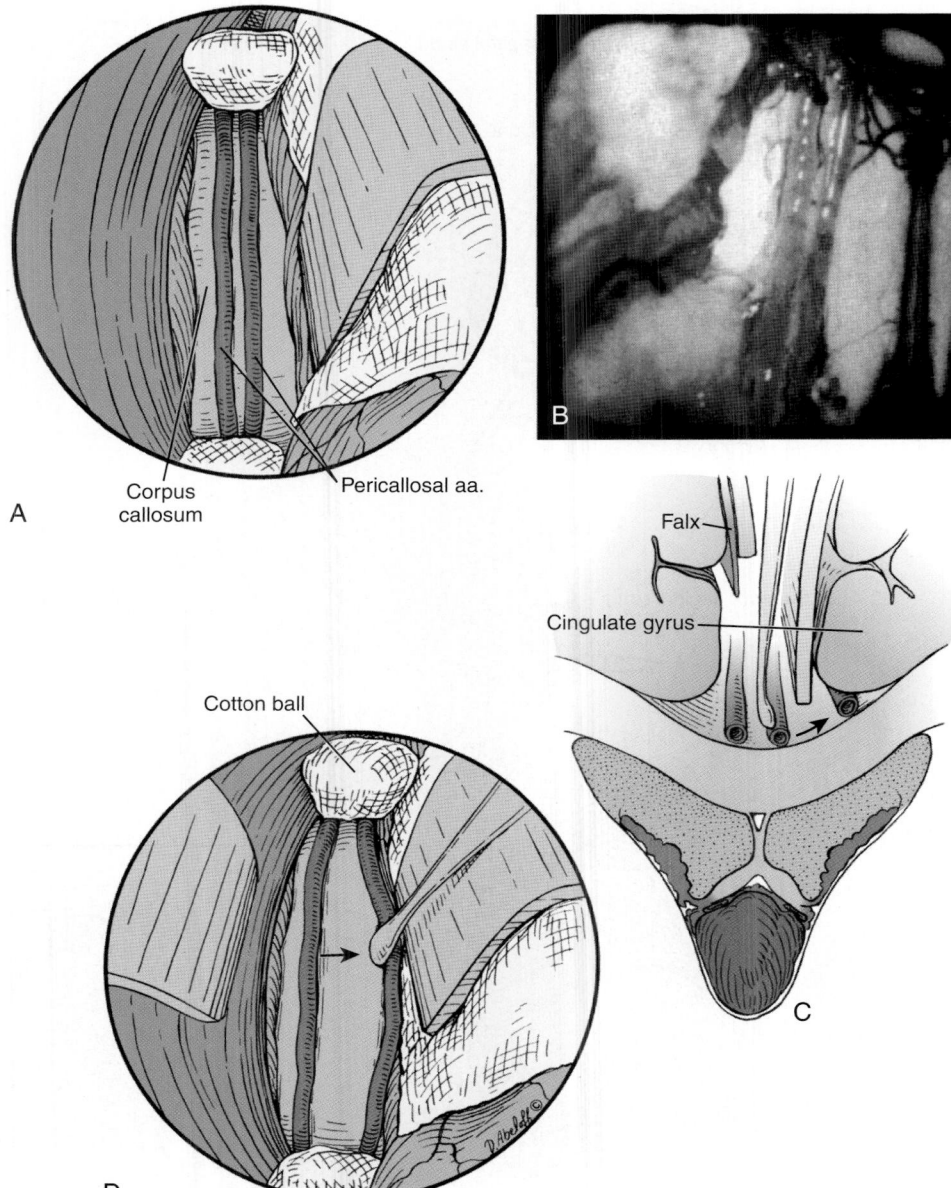

FIGURE 28-5 A, Initial exposure of the corpus callosum with the pericallosal arteries visualized. B, Photomicrograph of the callosal exposure with the anterior cerebral arteries in the midline. C, Coronal view. D, The anterior cerebral arteries are displaced toward the lateral callosal cistern. The falx gives a midline orientation for the incision. *(From Apuzzo ML, Amar AP. Transcallosal interforniceal approach. In: Apuzzo ML, ed. Surgery of the Third Ventricle. Baltimore: Williams & Wilkins; 1998:421-452, with permission.)*

microsurgical techniques.[15,29] In this approach, the midline raphe between the two fornices is opened at the roof of the third ventricle (Fig. 28-10). The interforniceal approach provides access to the anterior and middle third ventricle when the transforaminal approach inadequate and also provides a corridor to the related structures of the hypothalamus, infundibular recess, and mammillary bodies. One key advantage of this approach is that it allows the surgeon to work simultaneously through both foramina of Monro and the midline interforniceal plane. The midline raphe is opened from anterior to posterior beginning at the midpoint foramen of Monro and extending backward no more than two centimeters. Often, the lesion will splay open the plane between the fornices, which aids in dissection (Fig. 28-11). Beginning anterior to the midpoint of the foramen of Monro puts the anterior commissure at

risk[25,33] and injuries to this structure have been associated with deficits in visual retention.[34] Extending this incision beyond 2 cm puts the hippocampal commisure at risk and can lead to memory impairment.[29] In addition, injuries to the fornices are related to memory impairments; therefore, strict definition of the midline and natural cleavage planes is required. A variation of this approach, called the anterior interforniceal approach (AIF), has been described by Rosenfeld et al. (Fig. 28-12).[25,35] In this approach, a limited splitting of the fornices is performed anterior to the posterior border of the foramen of Monro using stereotactic navigation. This approach has been advocated for removal of hypothalamic hamartomas by Spetzler and Rosenfeld's groups.[25]

Closure is performed in the standard fashion, with careful attention to dural closure for the prevention of

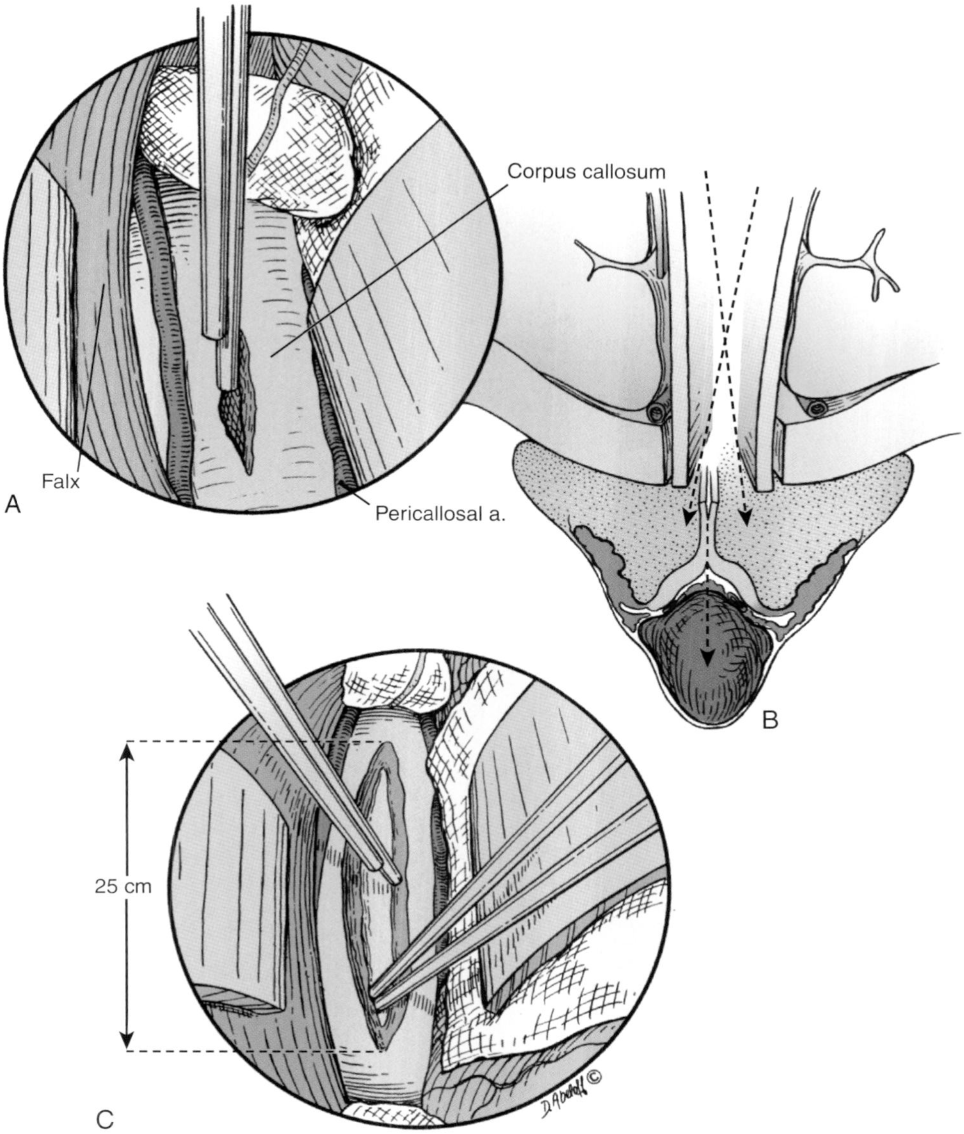

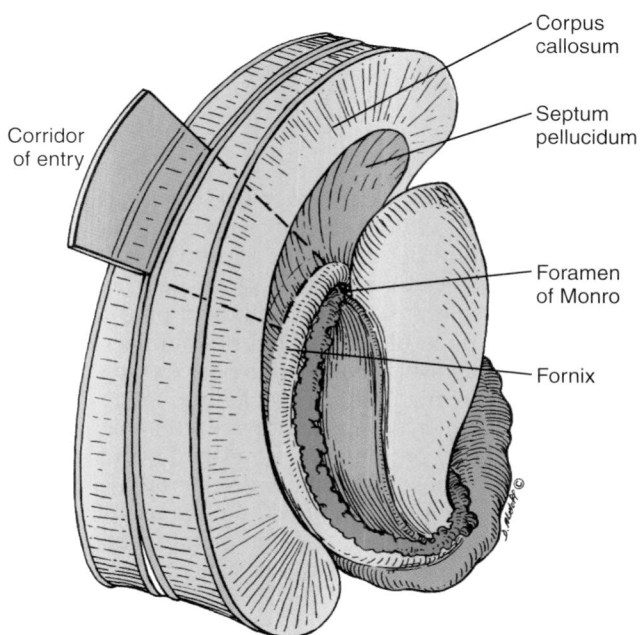

A

Falx

Corpus callosum

Pericallosal a.

B

25 cm

C

FIGURE 28-6 A, A suction device and bipolar forceps are used to incise the corpus callosum. Note in B the options for ventricular entry (left lateral ventricle, right lateral ventricle, midline interforniceal). C, Incision in the corpus callosum should not exceed 2.5 cm. *(From Apuzzo ML, Amar AP. Transcallosal interforniceal approach. In: Apuzzo ML, ed. Surgery of the Third Ventricle. Baltimore: Williams & Wilkins; 1998:421-452, with permission.)*

FIGURE 28-7 Angled anatomical schematic diagram demonstrating major incisions in midline neural structures to the third ventricular chamber. *(From Apuzzo ML, Amar AP. Transcallosal interforniceal approach. In: Apuzzo ML, ed. Surgery of the Third Ventricle. Baltimore: Williams & Wilkins; 1998:421-452, with permission.)*

Corpus callosum

Septum pellucidum

Foramen of Monro

Fornix

Corridor of entry

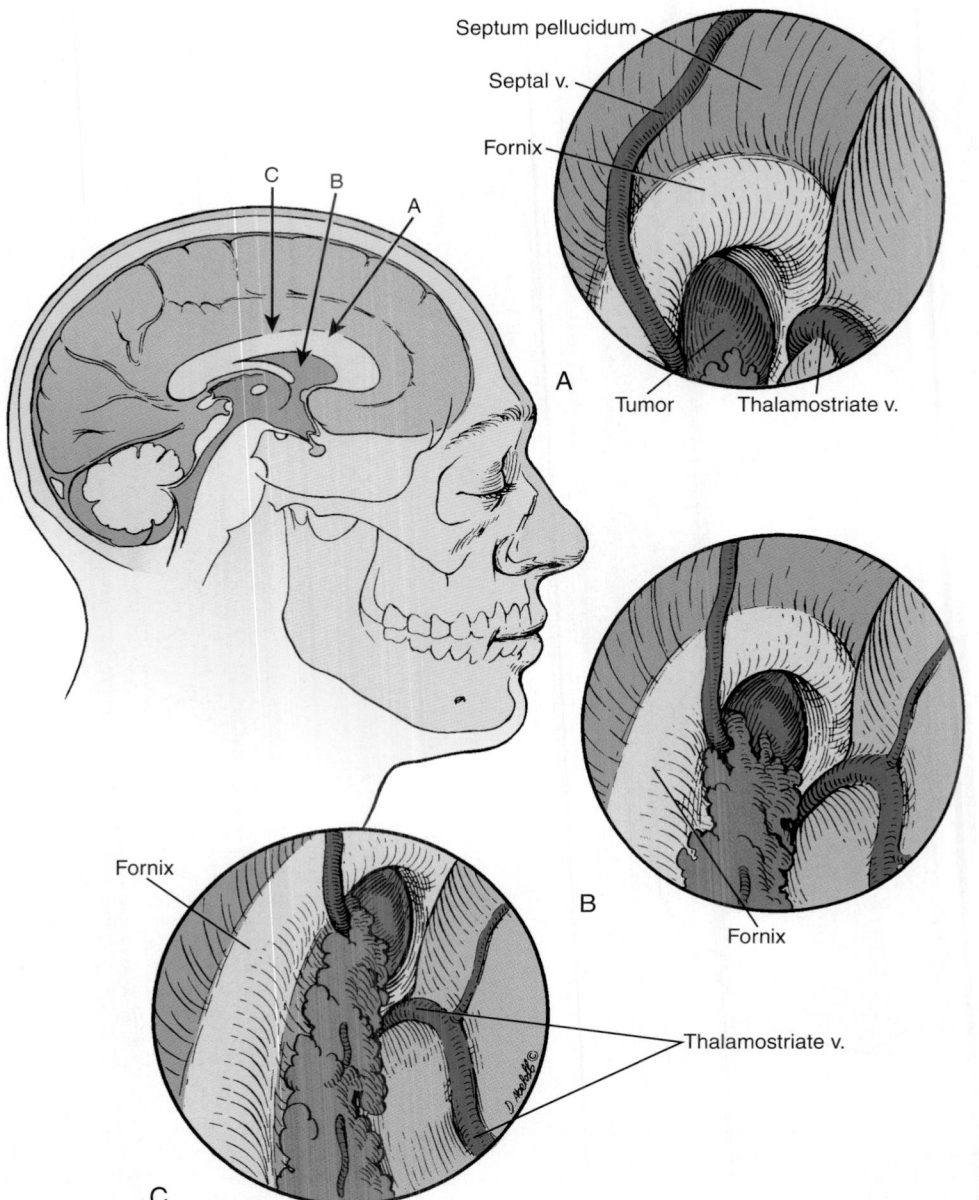

Septum pellucidum
Septal v.
Fornix
A
Tumor   Thalamostriate v.

B
Fornix

Fornix
Thalamostriate v.
C

FIGURE 28-8 Possibilities for field of view at the periforaminal region depending on sagittal entry angles. The angle of visualization will affect access to the raphe and the predominant perspective of the third ventricular chamber. A, Mid and posterior. B, Middle third. C, Mid and anterior. B is optimal for overall exposure. *(From Apuzzo ML, Amar AP. Transcallosal interforniceal approach. In: Apuzzo ML, ed. Surgery of the Third Ventricle. Baltimore: Williams & Wilkins; 1998:421-452, with permission.)*

pseudomeningocele. In cases where the dura cannot be closed to an acceptable degree of "water tightness," we generally use a dural substitute as an overlay or a suturable underlay. Ventriculostomy catheters are generally placed under direct visualization during closure if not placed preoperatively and either clamped for intracranial pressure monitoring or weaned slowly depending on the perceived risk of postoperative hydrocephalus.

Complications and Avoidance

Due to the delicate and eloquent anatomy traversed in approaching the center of the brain, transcallosal approaches carry a risk of postoperative deficits. However, most of these can be avoided if proper care is taken.

Craniotomy placement can lower risk to eloquent structures. Obviously, craniotomies placed primarily behind the coronal suture put the motor cortex at risk, and craniotomies on the dominant side place that hemisphere at risk. Furthermore, careful craniotomy placement can help avoid sacrifice of parasagittal draining veins. Sacrifice of parasagittal veins can lead to postoperative venous infarction and cortical deficits including hemiplegia. As described by Ulm et al.,[20] posteriorly placed craniotomies are limited by the presence of parasagittal veins related to the parietal lobes. In addition, preoperative magnetic resonance venography with or without the use of intraoperative navigation can be helpful in planning craniotomy placement and operative corridor so as to avoid major draining veins.

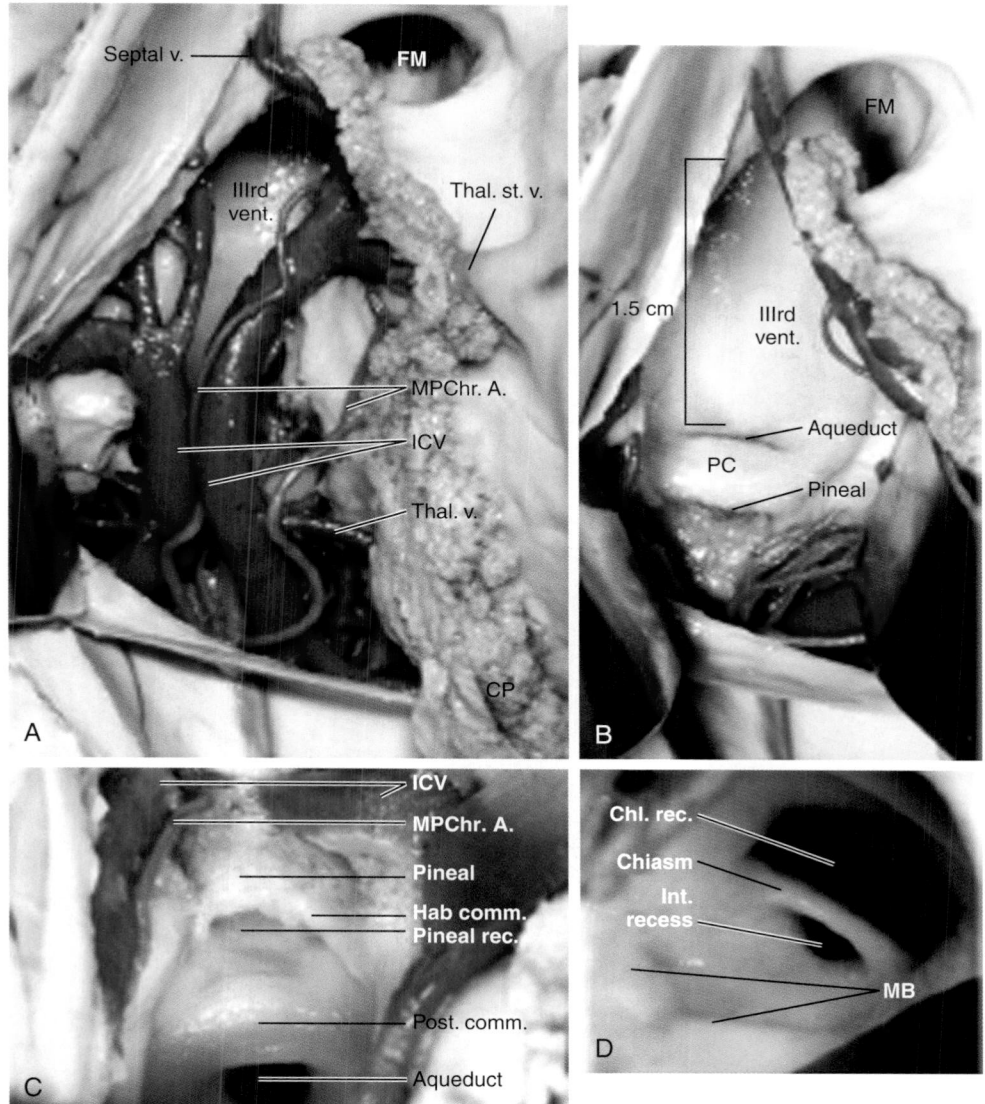

FIGURE 28-9 Photographs revealing various exposures seen during the transchoroidal approach. A, After the initial choroidal fissure opening, a dissection is performed between the ICVs to avoid damage to the draining veins of the thalamus, which enter the lateral side of the ICVs at varying sites along their course in the roof of the third ventricle. The paired medial PChAs course alongside the ICVs within the velum interpositum. The septal veins usually empty into the ICVs just behind the foramen. B, Exposure of the third ventricle after dissection through the layers of the ventricular roof. Exposed structures include the mammillary bodies just below the foramen, floor overlying the mesencephalic tegmentum, aqueduct, posterior commissure, and pineal gland. Note the amount of retraction and extension placed on the crus of the fornix needed to expose the structures posterior to the aqueduct directly from above. The bracketed black line denotes an opening limited to 1.5 cm behind the foramen of Monro. Through the more limited 1.5-cm opening, excessive stretch on the fornix is prevented. However, to access the posteriorly located landmarks, such as the aqueduct, through the limited choroidal opening, a more anterior-to-posterior approach must be taken; therefore, a more anterior incision through the corpus callosum is needed. C, Representative anterior-to-posterior view through a limited choroidal opening demonstrating exposure of the posterior third ventricle. Structures include the aqueduct, posterior commissure, pineal recess, habenular commissure, and pineal gland. D, Posterior to anterior view through the limited choroidal opening demonstrating the structures located in the anterior third ventricle, including the suprachiasmatic recess, optic chiasm, infundibular recess, and mammillary bodies. Chi.Rec, chiasmatic recess; Inf. Recess, infundibular recess; MB, mammillary bodies; PC, posterior commissure; Pineal Rec., pineal recess; Post. Comm., posterior commissure; SeptalV., septal vein; Thal. St. V., thalamostriate vein; Thal.V., thalamic vein; IIIrd Vent, third ventricle. *(From Ulm AJ, Russo A, Albanese E, et al. Limitations of the transcallosal transchoroidal approach to the third ventricle. J Neurosurg. 2009;111:600-609, with permission.)*

Care should also be taken to avoid other approach-specific complications. Complications related to the transchoroidal approach include infarction in the basal ganglia, mutism, and hemiparesis;[29] however, as discussed earlier, a suprachoroidal approach can avoid injury to the ipsilateral thalamostriate vein and fornix. Bilateral cingulate gyrus injuries can lead to akinetic mutism.[36] The main drawback to the interforniceal approach is that it puts both fornices at risk, and for that reason, some authors advocated limiting its use to cases where other approaches are inadequate.[8] These complications include transient memory loss and hemiparesis; however, definition of the anatomic midline and avoidance of parasagittal veins may mitigate this risk.[15]

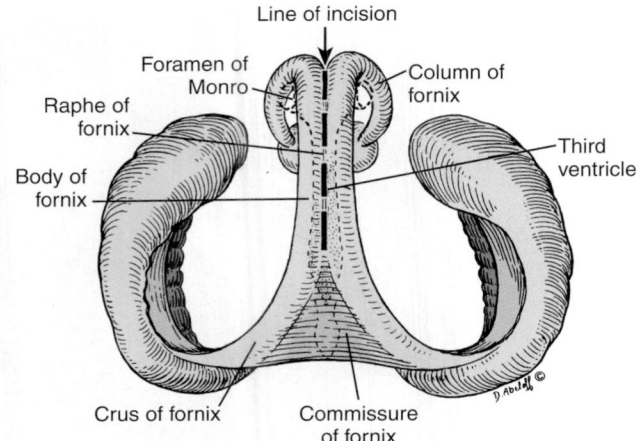

FIGURE 28-10 Dorsal fornix view with anatomical elements of structure, line of incision, and silhouette of the underlying third ventricle. *(From Apuzzo ML, Amar AP. Transcallosal interforniceal approach. In: Apuzzo ML, ed. Surgery of the Third Ventricle. Baltimore: Williams & Wilkins; 1998:421-452, with permission.)*

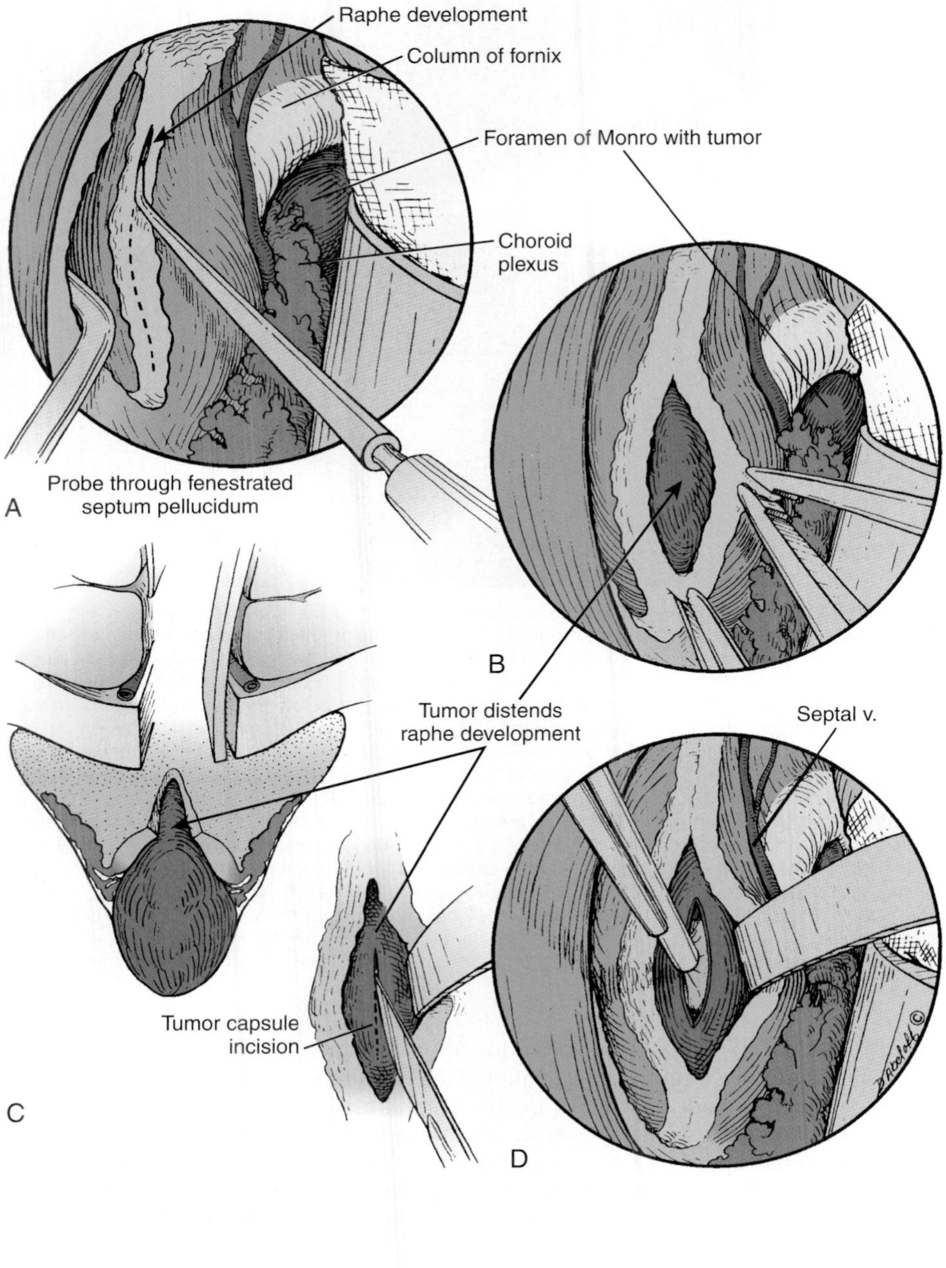

FIGURE 28-11 A, The junction of the septum and the fornix provides the landmark for the forniceal raphe, which may be established and developed. B and C, The mass lesion is identified and the raphe is developed over a 2-cm extent posteriorly from the foramen of Monro. D, The cystic lesion is incised and drained causing relaxation of the tens forniceal displacement and initiating the requirement for retraction on the forniceal body to maintain exposure. *(From Apuzzo ML, Amar AP. Transcallosal interforniceal approach. In: Apuzzo ML, ed. Surgery of the Third Ventricle. Baltimore: Williams & Wilkins; 1998:421-452, with permission.)*

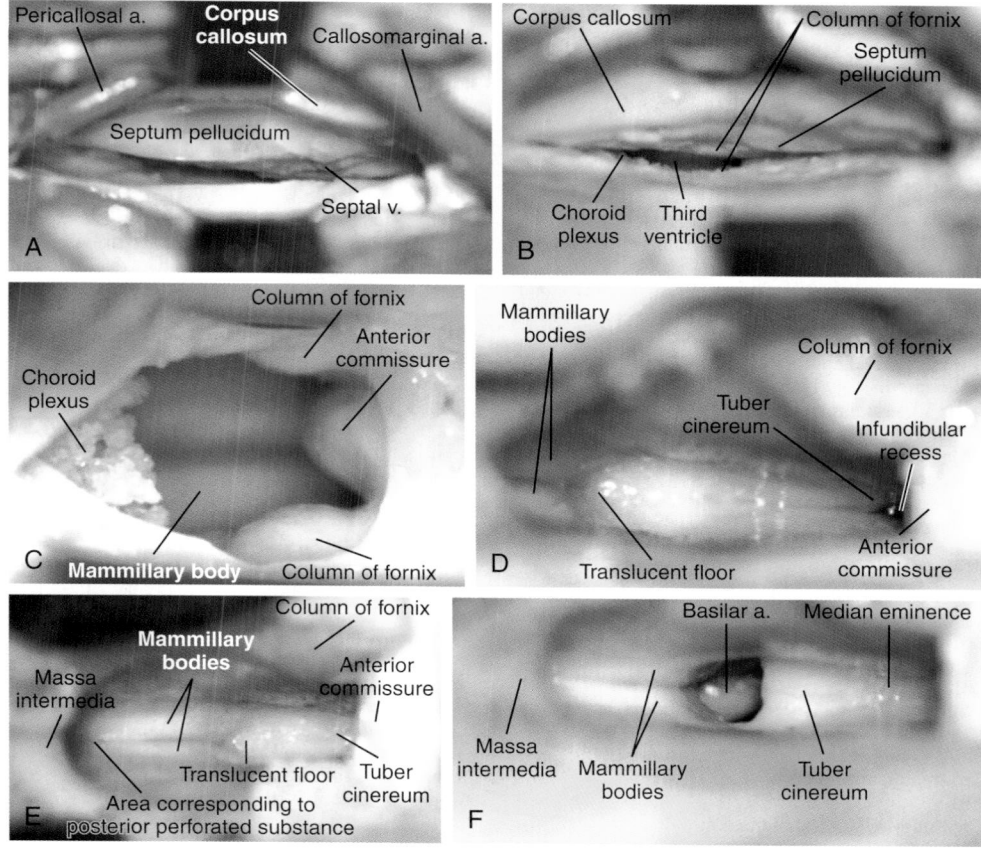

FIGURE 28-12 Stepwise dissection of the transcallosal anterior forniceal approach after callosotomy. A, The split septum pellucidum revealed the septal veins and their tributaries. B, The interforniceal plane and bilateral columns of the fornix. Note the transition from the thin septum pellucidum to the thick columns of the fornix. C, The third ventricle was accessed through the corridor bound anteriorly by the anterior commissure, laterally by the columns of the fornix, and posteriorly by the choroid plexus. D, Exposure of the structures at the floor of the third ventricle anteriorly to posteriorly: infundibular recess, tuber cinereum, translucent portion of the third ventricle, and mamillary bodies. The columns of the fornix on the lateral wall were also visible. E, Posterior view shows the posterior exposure bounded by the massa intermedia. An area posterior to the mamillary bodies corresponds to the posterior perforated substance. F, The third ventriculostomy performed through the translucent area anterior to the mamillary bodies exposed the basilar artery in the basal cistern. a., artery; v., vein. (*From Siwanuwatn R, Deshmukh P, Feiz-Erfan I, et al. Microsurgical anatomy of the transcallosal anterior interforniceal approach to the third ventricle. Neurosurgery. 2005;56:390-396; discussion 390-396, with permission.*)

Table 28-2   Advantages and Disadvantages of Transcallosal Approaches

Approach	Accessible Lesions	Advantages	Risks and Limitations
Transforaminal	Anterior to middle third ventricle	Requires least dissection and manipulation of critical anatomy. Can access tumors through enlarged foramen of Monro. Ideal for cystic lesions.	Limited primarily to tumors of the anterior third ventricle.
Trans/suprachoroidal	Middle to posterior third ventricle	Splitting of choroidal fissure provides a natural corridor of access to middle and posterior third ventricle.	Risk of ipsilateral thalamostriate vein injury, basal ganglia stroke, hemiparesis, mutism. These risks can be mitigated with suprachoroidal approach.
Interforniceal	Middle to anterior third ventricle, hypothalamus, mamillary bodies, infundibular recess	Versatile approach for lesions of the anterior, middle third ventricle and associated structures. Can work simultaneously through both foramina of Monro and midline raphe incision.	Risk of bilateral forniceal injury if midline structures not well-defined.

Conclusions

Surgery of the third ventricle represents in many ways one of the great frontiers in intracerebral surgery. The central location in the brain and anatomical and functional complexity of surrounding structures make the third ventricle a structure fitting for the rich history in attempts to reach it. Transcallosal approaches represent a set of highly refined corridors of entry into the third ventricle. The three primary variations of transcallosal approaches are the transforaminal, transchoroidal, and interforniceal approaches (Table 28-2). Preoperative planning is crucial for complication avoidance in these procedures. Venous anatomy should be elucidated with magnetic resonance venography in most cases and operative corridors planned to avoid venous sacrifice. Meticulous definition of critical structures intraoperatively also increases the safety of these procedures.

KEY REFERENCES

Apuzzo ML, Amar AP. Transcallosal interforniceal approach. In: Apuzzo ML, ed. *Surgery of the Third Ventricle.* Baltimore: Williams & Wilkins; 1998:421-452.

Apuzzo ML, Chikovani OK, Gott PS, et al. Transcallosal, interfornicial approaches for lesions affecting the third ventricle: surgical considerations and consequences. *Neurosurgery.* 1982;10:547-554.

Barris RW, Schuman HR. [Bilateral anterior cingulate gyrus lesions; syndrome of the anterior cingulate gyri.]. *Neurology.* 1953;3:44-52.

Botez-Marquard T, Botez MI. Visual memory deficits after damage to the anterior commissure and right fornix. *Arch Neurol.* 1992;49:321-324.

Busch E. A new approach for the removal of tumors of the third ventricle. *Acta Psychiatr Scand.* 1944;19:57-60.

Dandy WE. Diagnosis, localization and removal of tumors of the third ventricle. *Johns Hopkins Hosp Bull.* 1922;33:188-189.

Geschwind N. Disconnexion syndromes in animals and man. *I. Brain.* 1965;88:237-294.

Geschwind N. Disconnexion syndromes in animals and man. *II. Brain.* 1965;88:585-644.

Jeeves MA, Simpson DA, Geffen G. Functional consequences of the transcallosal removal of intraventricular tumours. *J Neurol Neurosurg Psychiatry.* 1979;42:134-142.

Ledoux JE, Risse GL, Springer SP, et al. Cognition and commissurotomy. *Brain 100 Pt.* 1977;1:87-104.

Milhorat TH, Baldwin M. A technique for surgical exposure of the cerebral midline: experimental transcallosal microdissection. *J Neurosurg.* 1966;24:687-691.

Morrison G, Sobel DF, Kelley WM, et al. Intraventricular mass lesions. *Radiology.* 1984;153:435-442.

Piepmeier JM, Spencer DD, Sass KJ. Lateral ventricular masses. In: Apuzzo MLJ, ed. *Brain surgery: complication avoidance and management.* New York: Churchill Livingstone; 1993:581-600.

Rhoton AL. *The lateral and third ventricles: Cranial Anatomy and Surgical Approaches.* Schaumburg, IL: Congress of Neurological Surgeons; 2003:235-298.

Rhoton ALJ. Microsurgical Anatomy of the Third Ventricular Region. In: Apuzzo ML, ed. *Surgery of the Third Ventricle.* Baltimore: Williams & Wilkins; 1998:421-452.

Shucart WA, Stein BM. Transcallosal approach to the anterior ventricular system. *Neurosurgery.* 1978;3:339-343.

Siwanuwatn R, Deshmukh P, Feiz-Erfan I, et al. Microsurgical anatomy of the transcallosal anterior interforniceal approach to the third ventricle. *Neurosurgery.* 2005;56:390-396:discussion 390-396.

Ture U, Yasargil MG, Al-Mefty O. The transcallosal-transforaminal approach to the third ventricle with regard to the venous variations in this region. *J Neurosurg.* 1997;87:706-715.

Ture U, Yasargil MG, Friedman AH, et al. Fiber dissection technique: lateral aspect of the brain. *Neurosurgery.* 2000;47:417-426:discussion 426-427.

Ture U, Yasargil MG, Krisht AF. The arteries of the corpus callosum: a microsurgical anatomic study. *Neurosurgery.* 1996;39:1075-1084: discussion 1084-1085.

Ulm AJ, Russo A, Albanese E, et al. Limitations of the transcallosal transchoroidal approach to the third ventricle. *J Neurosurg.* 2009;111: 600-609.

Wen HT, Rhoton Jr AL, de Oliveira E. Transchoroidal approach to the third ventricle: an anatomic study of the choroidal fissure and its clinical application. *Neurosurgery.* 1998;42:1205-1217:discussion 1217-1219.

Winkler PA, Ilmberger J, Krishnan KG, et al. Transcallosal interforniceal-transforaminal approach for removing lesions occupying the third ventricular space: clinical and neuropsychological results. *Neurosurgery.* 2000;46:879-888:discussion 888-890.

Yamamoto I, Rhoton Jr AL, Peace DA. Microsurgery of the third ventricle: Part I. Microsurgical anatomy. *Neurosurgery.* 1981;8:334-356.

Yasargil MG, Abdulrauf SI. Surgery of intraventricular tumors. *Neurosurgery.* 2008;62:1029-1040:discussion 1040-1041.

Numbered references appear on Expert Consult.

CHAPTER 29

Endoscopic Approach to Intraventricular Brain Tumors

JEFFREY P. GREENFIELD • MARK M. SOUWEIDANE •
THEODORE H. SCHWARTZ

Endoscopic surgery for intraventricular brain tumors is a logical application of endoscopic technology. Because of the central and deep location of intraventricular brain tumors, conventional neurosurgical approaches have a relative increase in potential morbidity. Auspiciously, the location of intraventricular tumors being within a cerebrospinal fluid (CSF) compartment affords excellent light and image transmission. The fact that most intraventricular tumors cause hydrocephalus makes endoscopic surgery particularly attractive since simultaneous procedures can be employed both for CSF diversion and tumor management. In addition, the inherent benefits of minimally invasive techniques including reduced surgical time, improved cosmetic results, shortened hospital stay, and reduced cost also factor into the appeal of neurosurgical endoscopy for managing intraventricular tumors.[1] Five commonly employed endoscopic procedures are highlighted including endoscopic fenestration, endoscopic tumor biopsy, simultaneous tumor biopsy with endoscopic third ventriculostomy (ETV), endoscopic removal of solid tumors and endoscopic removal of colloid cysts.

Patient Selection

Patient selection is critical in optimizing the desired surgical goal, avoiding unnecessary procedures, and minimizing surgical morbidity. The intended surgical goal must be carefully established prior to surgery. Many patients that can undergo endoscopic surgery may not be logical candidates since they will ultimately require conventional surgical tumor removal or no surgery. Examples that serve to highlight this point are the patient with a large intraventricular tumor of the ventricular atrium or the patient with a biochemically proven malignant germ cell tumor. In selecting patients, the less experienced surgeon should begin with less demanding cases (septal fenestration and endoscopic third ventriculostomy) and eventually incorporate more complex cases (colloid cyst and solid tumor resection). Although endoscopic surgery can be accomplished in patients with normal sized ventricles, concomitant hydrocephalus affords easier ventricular cannulation and intraventricular navigation.[2]

Equipment

Endoscopes vary in the type of optics (fiberoptic or solid lens), diameter of the scope, and the dimension and number of working portals. While the fiberoptic systems are appealing for their light weight and reduced cost, the greater image resolution with a sold lens system is preferred by the author for most endoscopic tumor surgery. For all procedures featured in this article, scopes should have at the very least one working channel, one irrigation port, and a dedicated egress channel. Navigational guidance is strongly encouraged not so much for ventricular cannulation, but for selecting an optimal trajectory (Figs. 29-1 and 29-2). This simple integration greatly reduces the tendency to torque once in the ventricular compartment thus reducing potential hemorrhage and neurological injury. Endoscopic courses are a useful means for becoming familiar with the requisite instrumentation and surgical techniques.

Endoscopic Tumor Procedures

ENDOSCOPIC FENESTRATION

Septal fenestration and tumor cyst fenestration are two of the simplest endoscopic procedures owing the relative avascular nature of these membranes. Fenestration of the septum pellucidum should be considered in any patient in which a tumor mass is situated in the anterior third ventricle or within the lateral ventricle at the foramen of Monro resulting in compartmentalized hydrocephalus (Fig. 29-3). Shunt burden can thus be reduced in the former situation or eliminated in the latter by simple endoscopic septal fenestration. Endoscopic fenestration of the septum pellucidum generally is performed via an entry site that lies more lateral than the conventional coronal burr hole. The entry site is thus positioned at least 4 cm from the midsagittal plane. It is recommended that the site of septal fenestration be positioned between the larger tributaries of the septal veins and as superior as possible from the fornix. Generous fenestrations are made with cautery and confirmation of effective communication is established with identification of contralateral ventricular landmarks including the choroid plexus and ependymal veins.

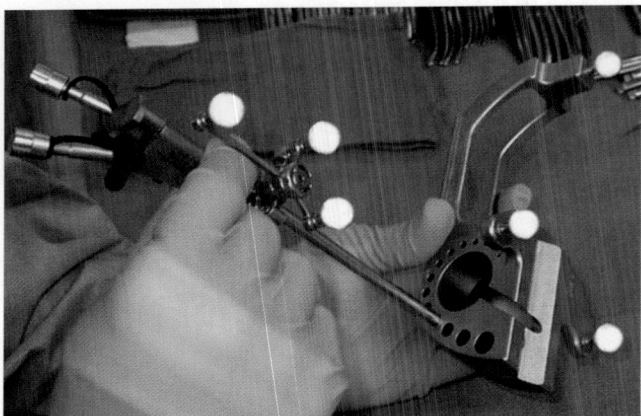

FIGURE 29-1 A solid lens endoscopic sheath integrated with an infrared navigational tracking device is being registered at the time of surgery.

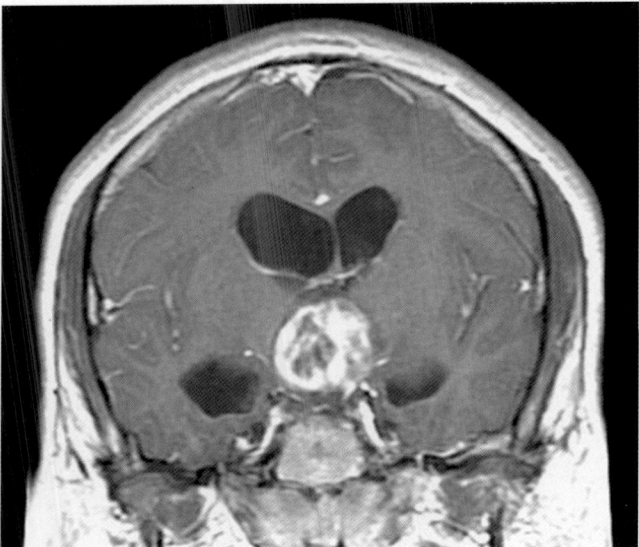

FIGURE 29-3 A coronal T1-weighted MRI obtained after gadolinium contrast administration shows a third ventricular tumor—pure geminoma—in a 12-year-old girl who presented with headache and polydipsia. A unilateral ventriculoperitoneal shunt was placed after endoscopic tumor biopsy and septal fenestration.

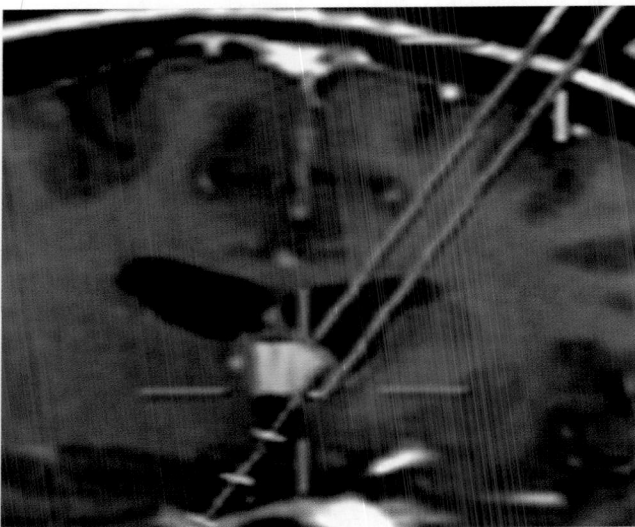

FIGURE 29-2 The endoscopic path is superimposed upon the preoperative MRI in selecting the ideal trajectory in a patient with a third ventricular tumor. The dimension of the endoscope is depicted so as to simulate the true size of the scope.

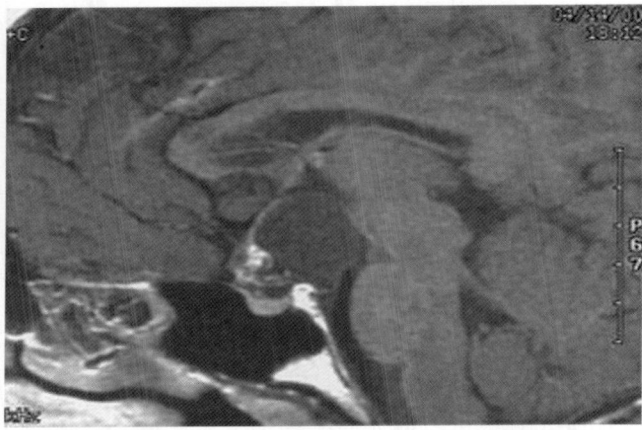

FIGURE 29-4 A sagittal T1-weighted MRI obtained after gadolinium contrast administration shows a presumed craniopharyngioma in a patient presenting with a bitemporal hemianopia. Visual fields normalized after a transventricular endoscopic cyst decompression. The residual mass was treated with fractionated stereotactic radiotherapy.

Tumor cyst fenestration is an appealing therapeutic option when a patient's symptoms can be relieved by cyst decompression and when aggressive tumor resection may be avoided (Fig. 29-4). Craniopharyngiomas, hypothalamic/chiasmatic astrocytomas, and suprasellar germ cell tumors are examples of such tumors.[3] Transventricular endoscopic cyst decompression is a minimally invasive method for temporarily or permanently alleviating obstructive hydrocephalus or visual loss. For most cystic tumors causing obstructive hydrocephalus at the level of the third ventricle, a standard coronal approach is an ideal trajectory. The transcavum interforniceal endoscopic approach[4] to the third ventricle is a further refinement of the technique for biopsy or fenestration of lesions within the third ventricle in those patients a large cavum vergae.

TUMOR BIOPSY

Endoscopic biopsy is a well-established method for sampling intraventricular brain tumors.[5-7] The procedure should always be considered in situations in which

surgical tumor removal may not be necessary or when the diagnosis would significantly alter the therapeutic approach. Primary examples of these situations include marker-negative germ cell tumors, Langerhans cell histiocytosis, and infiltrative hypothalamic gliomas. Candidates should have overt intraventricular extension of their tumor mass rather than a lesion that is entirely subependymal in location. The diagnostic yield is high and the risk is low.[8] In the authors' current series of 65 patients who have undergone endoscopic tumor biopsy the diagnostic yield was 98%. To maintain diagnostic accuracy it is imperative to avoid cauterizing the tumor prior to sampling. The samples are small and histologic interpretation can be challenging without superimposed artifact from cautery. If bleeding is encountered, continuous irrigation through

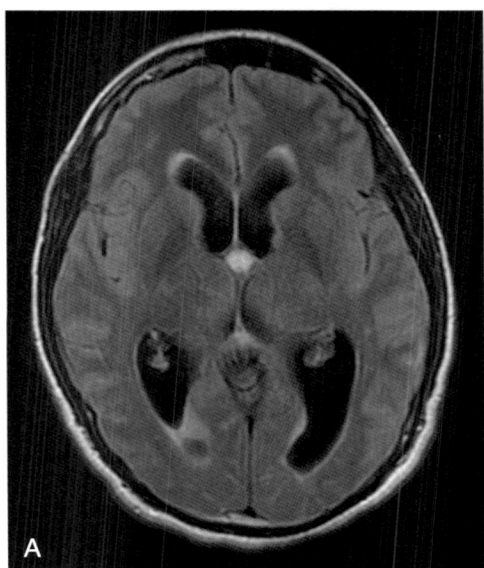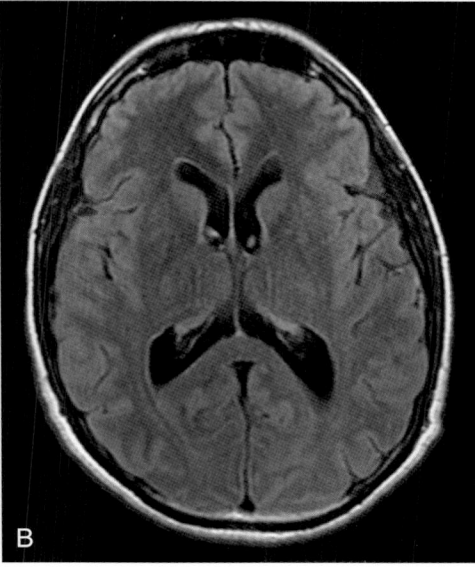

FIGURE 29-5 The colloid cyst of the third ventricle (A) is an ideal tumor for endoscopic removal. Postoperative imaging reveals resolution of preoperative hydrocephalus (B).

the endoscope or an external catheter is recommended until the efflux clears.

SIMULTANEOUS TUMOR BIOPSY AND ENDOSCOPIC THIRD VENTRICULOSTOMY

The prominence of pineal region tumors in children coupled with the high frequency of tumors that may not necessitate aggressive surgical resection converges nicely with endoscopic applications. Notably, primary central nervous system germ cell tumors (CNS GCT), both pure germinomas and nongerminomatous germ cell tumors, can be effectively treated without radical resection. Thus, children who present with noncommunicating hydrocephalus with a pineal region tumor should always be considered for primary endoscopic management by way of ETV and tumor biopsy. Serum biochemical analysis for alfafetoprotein (AFP) and human chorionic gonadotropin (HCG) should always precede endoscopic biopsy since marker-positive GCTs should be initially managed with neoadjuvant chemotherapy.[9-12] When performing simultaneous ETV and tumor biopsy, the CSF diversion should always be performed first. This recommendation is based on the fact that the patient's hydrocephalus is the more emergent clinical condition requiring treatment. Further, when tumor biopsy is performed some intraventricular hemorrhage is expected that may obscure vision. Given that the trajectory for ETV and pineal region tumor biopsy are different one must select between using one or two entry sites for performing these simultaneous procedures. The typical entry site for performing ETV is at the coronal suture 2 cm from midline while that for accomplishing a pineal region tumor biopsy is 4 to 6 cm precoronal. While two separate entry sites can be used one single entry site that is midway between these has been shown to be successful. It is the authors' preference to use a single precoronal approach that lies between the ideal entry sites for either separate procedure. This site is routinely dictated based upon stereotactic guidance. With the use of a 30-degree angled endoscope, it is rare that both procedures will not be possible simultaneously.

Solid Tumor Resection

Solid tumor removal, although a logical application of endoscopic techniques, is somewhat limited due to the inadequacy of compatible instrumentation and the small caliber of current endoscopic portals. Thus far, most descriptions for tumor removal have focused on the colloid cyst. The colloid cyst, unlike solid tumors, wonderfully lends itself to endoscopic removal given the primarily cystic nature of that mass. The success of endoscopic tumor removal is dependent upon the tumor characteristics including size, density, and vascularity. Tumors larger than 2 cm, those that have appreciable calcification on computed tomography (CT), and those that have significant subependymal infiltration are not currently amenable to endoscopic removal.[2,13] The resection of solid tumors is principally achieved through the use of aspiration with a variable, self-regulated suction catheter alternating with generous bipolar diathermy. It is critical to note that aspiration is only applied once the catheter tip is firmly and completely imbedded within the tumor tissue so as to avoid rapid evacuation of CSF. The feasibility of endoscopic removal of solid tumors within the ventricular system is expected to improve with the advent of compatible instrumentation designed for tissue ablation such as an ultrasonic aspirator.

Colloid Cyst Extirpation

PATIENT SELECTION

The colloid cyst of the third ventricle is an ideal tumor for endoscopic removal (Fig. 29-5A and B). This appeal is principally governed by the cystic nature of the mass. The deep central location within the ventricular compartment along with the associated complexity of standard microsurgical removal further enhances the desire for endoscopic management. Careful patient selection is critical given the frequency with which asymptomatic patients are diagnosed. Rationales for surgical intervention appropriately include symptoms of raised intracranial pressure, ventriculomegaly

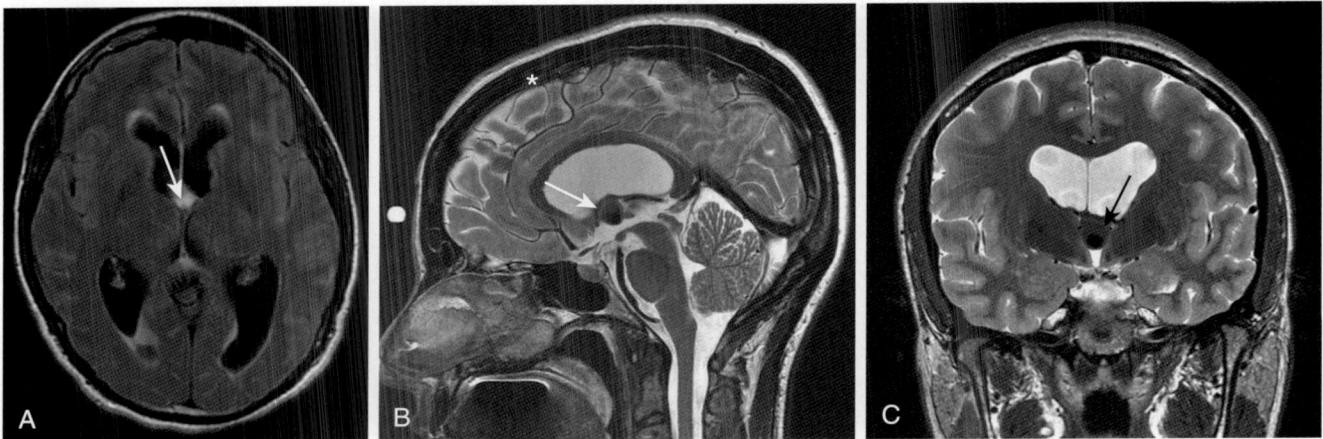

FIGURE 29-6 Integrated stereotatic navigation is critical for surgical planning and optimizing ventricular cannulation. Laterality should be determined based on a preoperative MRI with emphasis on the relative size of the frontal horns of the lateral ventricles and the dimensions of the foraminae of Monro when analyzed in the axial (A), sagittal (B), and coronal (C) planes.

in the absence of symptoms, and radiographic evidence of progression (ventricular size or tumor mass). Less-defined indicators include prophylaxis against clinical progression or sudden death and young age at the time of diagnosis. The ability to predict clinical progression is poorly defined. The natural history is not clear but is estimated that clinical or radiographic progression occurs in about 8% of patients over 10 years. The expectation of progression during a patient's lifetime is thus greater for younger patients. Variables that may precede clinical deterioration are ventriculomegaly, chronic headache, and cyst size (>1 cm diameter). Offering surgery to avoid the possibility of rapid deterioration must be balanced by a true estimation of operative risk to the patient, bearing in mind that many of the patients will have normal sized ventricles.

SURGICAL TECHNIQUE

It is strongly advised that familiarity and experience be obtained with intraventricular endoscopic surgery prior to treating colloid cysts or other intraventricular tumors. Pre-operative intravenous corticosteroids are administered to reduce the potential risk of chemical ventriculitis and subsequent hydrocephalus that may occur as a result of intraventricular spillage of colloid material. With familiarity it is not necessary to prepare the surgical site in anticipation of a craniotomy except when the cyst is large (>2 cm in diameter).

Because of variability in each patient's anatomy, surgical planning is critical in optimizing the surgical goal and reducing potential morbidity. Integrated stereotatic navigation is always used for surgical planning and optimizing ventricular cannulation (Fig. 29-6A through C). Laterality should be determined based on a preoperative MRI with emphasis on the relative size of the frontal horns of the lateral ventricles and the dimensions of the foraminae of Monro. Because the intent is to work below the ipsilateral column of the fornix, an entry site is used that is far forward of the coronal suture. In a sagittal dimension, the ideal trajectory passes just above the floor of the anterior horn, through the foramen of Monro, and below the roof of the third ventricle. In an axial and coronal plane, a trajectory is selected that passes between the head of the caudate and the column of

the fornix into the foramen of Monro. The entry site that is selected with stereotactic guidance is marked on the skin surface prior to the surgical prep. Regardless of the entry site, a curvilinear incision is planned on the hair line with a variable length depending upon the anterior location of the planned burr hole. A longer incision is needed to allow more anterior retraction of the scalp. In patients with a receding hairline the incision is alternatively placed within a forehead crease.

Once the frontal horn of the lateral ventricle is entered, the anatomical landmarks of the frontal horn are identified. Using a 30-degree angled lens the endoscopic is then rotated to offer a superiorly directed view toward the roof of the third ventricle; the site of attachment of the colloid cyst. The endoscope is then navigated toward the foramen of Monro where typically the wall of the colloid cyst is in clear sight obstructing the foramen of Monro (Fig. 29-7A and B). Generous bipolar coagulation of the choroid plexus is used to gain better visualization of the lateral cyst surface. Bipolar forceps are utilized to bluntly dissect the cyst wall away from the walls of the third ventricle. This coagulation device without current is used to push the cyst wall away from ependymal surfaces. When sufficient space exists between the cyst and the walls of the third ventricle power is then switched on to coagulate the cyst surface. Perforation of the cyst wall by either sharp dissection or electrocautery is utilized followed by aspiration of the cyst contents. A graduated 6-French endotracheal suction catheter that has had the distal fenestrations removed is preferred. This clear cannula allows direct visualization of the contents being suctioned. This ability is very helpful in gauging the strength of suction applied and in discontinuing aspiration if choroid plexus gets inadvertently aspirated. It is critical that aspiration only be applied once the tip of the device is placed within the cyst wall, thus avoiding rapid evacuation of CSF from the ventricular compartment. Utilizing suction aspiration the contents of the cyst can usually be fully evacuated. The viscosity of some contents may require repeated clearing of the cannula due to frequent clogging. With partial evacuation the cyst can commonly be drawn into the foramen with grasping forceps. This maneuver

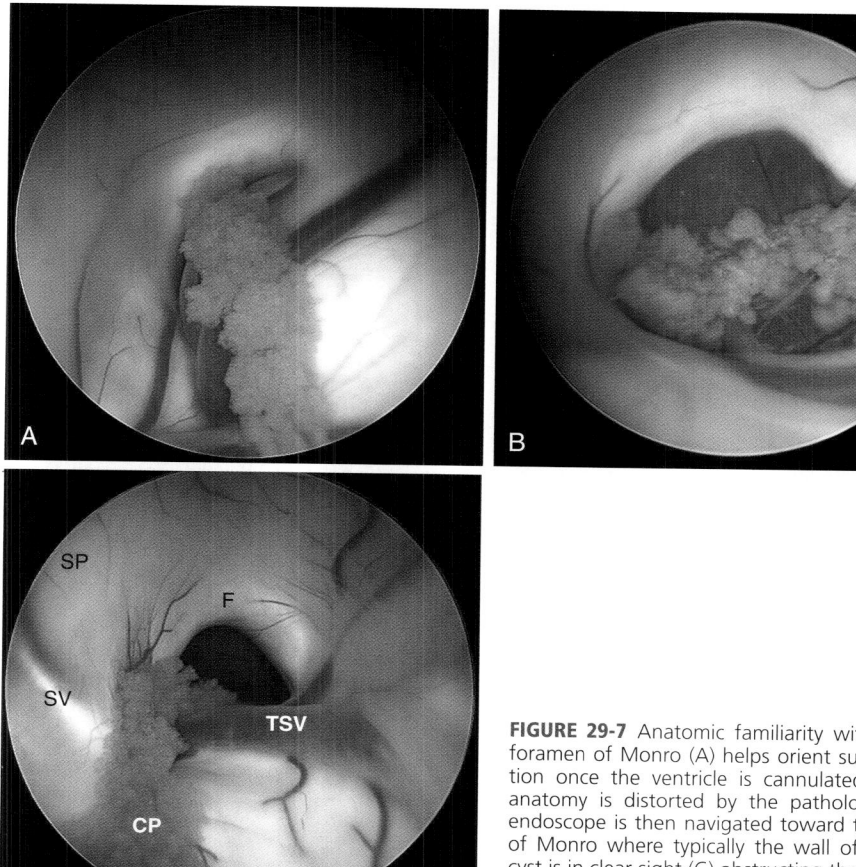

FIGURE 29-7 Anatomic familiarity with a normal foramen of Monro (A) helps orient surgical resection once the ventricle is cannulated when the anatomy is distorted by the pathology (B). The endoscope is then navigated toward the foramen of Monro where typically the wall of the colloid cyst is in clear sight (C) obstructing the foramen of Monro. SP, septum pellucidum; SV, septal vein; CP, choroid plexus; TSV, thalamostriate vein; F, fornix.

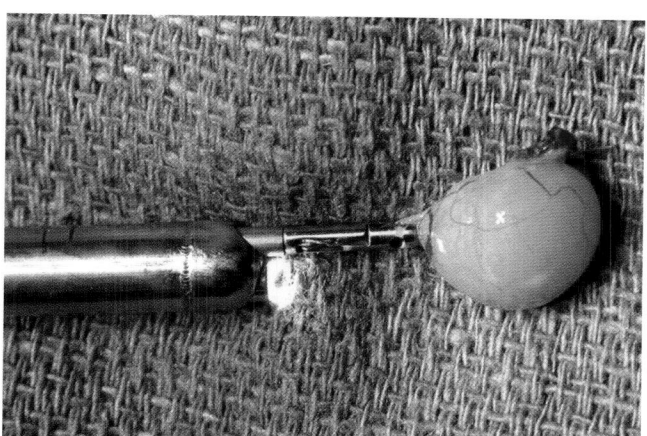

FIGURE 29-8 En bloc resection of colloid cyst is often possible with bimanual endoscopic manipulation, but requires removal of the entire endoscopic sheath with the cyst still adhered to the grasping forceps.

positions the lesion for continued aspiration and further coagulation. The superior aspect of the cyst can be dissected away from the roof of the third ventricle by using a rotary motion with grasping forceps in effect pulling the cyst in an inferior direction toward the floor of the ventricle. When visualized, adherent potions of choroid plexus should be coagulated and sharply divided.

Repeatedly using these techniques one of two situations usually occur. First, the cyst may freely separate from the confines of the third ventricular roof. If this situation occurs then the cyst should be removed by extracting the entire endoscope (Fig. 29-8). Because of the difference in size between the cyst and the working portal (1 to 2 mm) any attempt to extract the cyst through the sheath runs the risk of dislodging the cyst into the ventricular compartment. The second frequent scenario that occurs during endoscopic colloid cyst removal is that the cyst is entirely evacuated of contents leaving only adherent membrane. That membrane is then generously coagulated followed by sharp dissection. Some portions of the cyst wall may not be amenable to further removal due to adherence of venous structures. Any membrane remnants should be generously coagulated. Once the removal is complete, inspection of the third ventricle for residual clot is performed. If recognized small hematomas within the third ventricle are removed using aspiration applied directly to the clot. The placement of an externalized ventricular drain is advocated on an individual basis depending upon the degree of intraventricular hemorrhage. The overwhelming numbers of drains are discontinued the day after surgery based on intracranial pressures within a normal range and postoperative imaging failing to indicate any appreciable hematoma within the third ventricle.

Postoperative Management

Ventricular drainage for monitoring intracranial pressure is used on an individual basis depending on the degree of intraventricular hemorrhage and preoperative symptoms. If at the time of surgery moderate intraventricular hemorrhage is experienced, then an external drain is typically used for postoperative CSF egress until the CSF clears and the patient tolerates clamping of the drain during pressure monitoring. External drainage is also used in situations where the patient had significant preoperative symptoms of raised intracranial pressure. Preoperative obtundation, decreasing level of consciousness, or lethargy are all indicators that postoperative pressure monitoring is required, even when complete removal of the obstructing mass has been accomplished. The individual scenario gauges the duration of drainage or monitoring. If an externalized drain is to be used, consideration regarding the ultimate placement of a shunt should influence the site of externalization. A postoperative MRI or CT is routinely used during the early postoperative time period for assessing the extent of resection, evidence of intraventricular hemorrhage, or degree of hydrocephalus.

Summary

Endoscopic surgical management for intraventricular brain tumors has burgeoned over the past decade to a field with clearly defined surgical indications, dedicated instrumentation, and general acceptance by the neurosurgical community. Patient selection requires a thorough understanding of neuro-oncologic principles and the limitations of neuro-endoscopic methods. The appeal of endoscopic management is enhanced with the ability to simplify CSF diversion through endoscopic third ventriculostomy or septal fenestration. Endoscopic tumor biopsy and colloid cyst resection have been shown to be highly successful while affording significant advantages over conventional neurosurgical techniques. Endoscopic excision of solid intraventricular tumors, although feasible, remains challenging due to technical limitations. Intraoperative stereotactic guidance contributes greatly toward a safer and more efficacious procedure, and should be considered as an integral adjunct in patients undergoing endoscopic neurosurgery for third ventricular brain tumors or in patients without hydrocephalus. The potential of endoscopic surgery for intraventricular brain tumors is expected to expand with technological advancements in compatible instrumentation.

KEY REFERENCES

Cappabianca P, Cinalli G, Gangemi M, et al. Application of neuroendoscopy to intraventricular lesions. *Neurosurgery.* 2008;62(suppl 2): 575-597:discussion 597–598.

Delitala A, Brunori A, Chiappetta F. Purely neuroendoscopic transventricular management of cystic craniopharyngiomas. *Childs Nerv Syst.* 2004;20:858-862.

Depreitere B, Dasi N, Rutka J, et al. Endoscopic biopsy for intraventricular tumors in children. *J Neurosurg.* 2007;106:340-346.

Ellenbogen RG, Moores LE. Endoscopic management of a pineal and suprasellar germinoma with associated hydrocephalus: technical case report. *Minim Invasive Neurosurg.* 1997;40:13-15:discussion 16.

Luther N, Cohen A, Souweidane MM. Hemorrhagic sequelae from intracranial neuroendoscopic procedures for intraventricular tumors. *Neurosurg Focus.* 2005;19:E9.

Luther N, Edgar MA, Dunkel IJ, Souweidane MM. Correlation of endoscopic biopsy with tumor marker status in primary intracranial germ cell tumors. *J Neuro-Oncol.* 2006;79:45-50.

Pople IK, Athanasiou TC, Sandeman DR, Coakham HB. The role of endoscopic biopsy and third ventriculostomy in the management of pineal region tumours. *Br J Neurosurg.* 2001;15:305-311.

Schwartz TH, Ho B, Prestagiacomo CJ, et al. Ventricular volume following third ventriculostomy. *J Neurosurg.* 1999;91:20-25.

Shono T, Natori Y, Morioka T, et al. Results of a long-term follow-up after neuroendoscopic biopsy procedure and third ventriculostomy in patients with intracranial germinomas. *J Neurosurg.* 2007;107:193-198.

Souweidane MM. Endoscopic management of pediatric brain tumors. *Neurosurg Focus.* 2005;18:E1.

Souweidane MM. Endoscopic surgery for intraventricular brain tumors in patients without hydrocephalus. *Neurosurgery.* 2005;57:312-318:discussion 312-318.

Souweidane MM, Luther N. Endoscopic resection of solid intraventricular brain tumors. *J Neurosurg.* 2006;105:271-278.

Souweidane MM, Sandberg DI, Bilsky MH, Gutin PH. Endoscopic biopsy for tumors of the third ventricle. *Pediatr Neurosurg.* 2000;33:132-137.

Souweidane MM, Hoffman CE, Schwartz TH. Transcavum interforniceal endoscopic surgery of the third ventricle. *J Neurosurg Pediatr.* 2008 Oct;2(4):231-236:PubMed PMID: 18831654.

Numbered references appear on Expert Consult.

CHAPTER 30

Management of Pineal Region Tumors

JEFFREY N. BRUCE

Pineal region tumors encompass a diverse group of tumors that can arise from pineal parenchymal cells, supporting cells of the pineal gland, or glial cells from the midbrain and medial walls of the thalamus. These tumors occupy a central position that is equidistant from various cranial points traditionally used as routes of exposure. The deep central location places these tumors in intimate contact with important components of the deep venous system that lie dorsally, including the vein of Galen, the precentral cerebellar vein, and the internal cerebral veins.[1] In some instances, there may be a dense attachment to these structures and the tela choroidea. The tumor is often fed by small-caliber branches of the posterior choroidal arteries and branches of the quadrigeminal arteries that generally do not supply any clinically significant areas of the brain.

Although pineal region tumors affect a relatively small number of patients, their variable histology and difficult surgical challenge has generated a comparatively large volume of literature. This difficulty is underscored by Cushing's statement: "Personally, I have never succeeded in exposing a pineal tumor sufficiently well to justify an attempt to remove it."[2] Over the years, various supratentorial and infratentorial approaches have been developed by several prominent neurosurgeons including Dandy's interhemispheric approach,[3] Van Wagenen's transventricular approach,[4] and Poppen's occipital transtentorial approach.[5] The supracerebellar infratentorial approach was first described in 1926, when Krause reported three cases, each a different variety of tumor in the pineal or quadrigeminal region, which he approached through the posterior fossa, over the cerebellar hemispheres, and under the tentorium.[6]

In the 1970s, the increasing use of the operating microscope rekindled interest in direct surgical approaches to the pineal region.[7-9] This led to considerable debate over the best surgical route to the pineal region. More important than the route, however, was that debates stimulated interest in operating on these tumors to identify their nature and remove them whenever possible.[10,11] The more aggressive approach to pineal region tumors resulted in greater awareness of the histologic diversity of these tumors existing along an extensive continuum from benign to highly malignant.[12] Some of these tumors are mixed in nature, simultaneously containing benign as well as malignant elements or even glial and pineal cell constituents.[13] Despite advances in radiographic imaging and increased experience with tumor markers, preoperative diagnostic tests are insufficient and accurate determination of histologic typing requires operative intervention. With experience, the mortality and morbidity rates from the various surgical approaches dropped steadily and led to the current management philosophy for pineal tumors, which relies on an aggressive surgical approach for the removal of benign tumors and decompression and accurate histologic diagnosis of malignant tumors.[14]

Clinical Features

PATHOLOGY

The various cell types that comprise the mature pineal gland account for the diversity of histologic tumor subtypes that can occur in the pineal region. Lobules of pinealocytes surrounded by astrocytes form the pineal parenchyma with ependymal cells of the third ventricle lining the anterior border of the gland. Pineal tumors are grouped into four main categories:[1] germ cell tumors,[2] pineal cell tumors,[3] glial cell tumors, and[4] miscellaneous tumors (covering a wide range of histology). Each category contains tumors existing along a continuum from benign to malignant and can include mixed tumors of more than one cell type.[15] The term *pinealoma* was originally used by Krabbe and is a misnomer because it originally pertained to germ cell tumors.[16] Eventually this term was applied more generically to refer to any tumors of the pineal region. The term is now obsolete, in favor of *pineal region tumors* when a general reference is desired or an individual tumor's histology in that region when specificity is preferred (e.g., astrocytoma of the pineal region).

PRESENTATION

Tumors in the pineal region, regardless of their histology, generally become symptomatic by three mechanisms:[15]
1. Increased intracranial pressure from hydrocephalus.
2. Direct cerebellar or brain stem compression
3. Endocrine dysfunction

Headache, the most common presenting symptom, occurs after obstruction of the third ventricle outflow at the sylvian aqueduct. More advanced hydrocephalus can result in nausea, vomiting, papilledema, obtundation, and other cognitive deficits.

Direct brain stem compression may lead to disturbances of extraocular movements, classically known as Parinaud's syndrome.[17] Involvement of the superior cerebellar peduncles can lead to ataxia and dysmetria. Hearing disturbances can occasionally occur, probably from compression of the inferior colliculi.[18]

Endocrine dysfunction is rare and may be caused by direct tumor involvement in the hypothalamus or from secondary effects of hydrocephalus.[19] Diabetes insipidus and other neuroendocrine disturbances are often indicative of hypothalamic infiltration by tumor, even when not radiographically visualized.

LABORATORY DIAGNOSIS

α-Fetoprotein and β-hCG are markers of germ cell malignancy and should be measured in serum and cerebrospinal fluid, if possible, as part of the preoperative workup in all pineal region tumor patients.[14,20,21] Elevation of germ cell markers is pathognomonic for the presence of a malignant germ cell tumor, and under these circumstances, histologic verification is unnecessary as surgery does not improve the outcome with radiation and chemotherapy.[22] In patients with marker-positive germ cell tumors, measurement of marker levels can also be useful to monitor therapeutic response and as a sensitive early sign of tumor recurrence. The absence of germ cell markers should be interpreted cautiously because malignant germ cell tumors such as germinomas and embryonal cell carcinomas cannot be ruled out.

α-Fetoprotein, normally associated with fetal yolk sac elements, is markedly elevated with endodermal sinus tumors, whereas smaller elevations occur with embryonal cell carcinomas and immature teratomas. β-hCG, normally secreted by placental trophoblastic tissue, is markedly elevated with choriocarcinomas, with smaller elevations associated with embryonal cell carcinomas and those occasional germinomas containing syncytiotrophoblastic giant cells.[23] Most germinomas are nonsecretory and carry a better prognosis than β-hCG positive germinomas.[24]

IMAGING

The standard diagnostic workup includes magnetic resonance imaging (MRI), with and without contrast, which has proven to be the most accurate diagnostic examination. MRI provides information on type, size, and extent of the tumor, as well as anatomic features such as degree of invasion, vascularity and the anatomic relationships of the tumor with its surroundings (Fig. 30-1). Some tumors can be suspected from the appearance of the scans, particularly teratomas, which contain multiple germ layers (Fig. 30-2). Angiography is only performed if the MRI suggests a vascular lesion such as a vein of Galen aneurysm or arteriovenous malformation. Despite this broad diagnostic armamentarium, the exact histologic nature of the tumor cannot be reliably determined without surgery.[15]

The increasing use of MRI has revealed a large number of patients with lesions of the pineal gland that are mostly cystic but contain a small amount of solid tissue (Fig. 30-3).[25,26] In most cases, the aqueduct has not been compromised and the patients are not symptomatic from their lesion. Initially, they were considered to be low-grade cystic astrocytomas but, after surgical removal, were found to be composed of normal astrocytes and normal pineal cells. Histologically, these are pineal cysts and are normal anatomic variations of the pineal gland. As experience with pineal cysts has increased, it is clear that they should be managed conservatively with serial MRI scans and without surgery. Surgery is reserved for lesions that are symptomatic, progressing in size, or causing aqueductal obstruction.

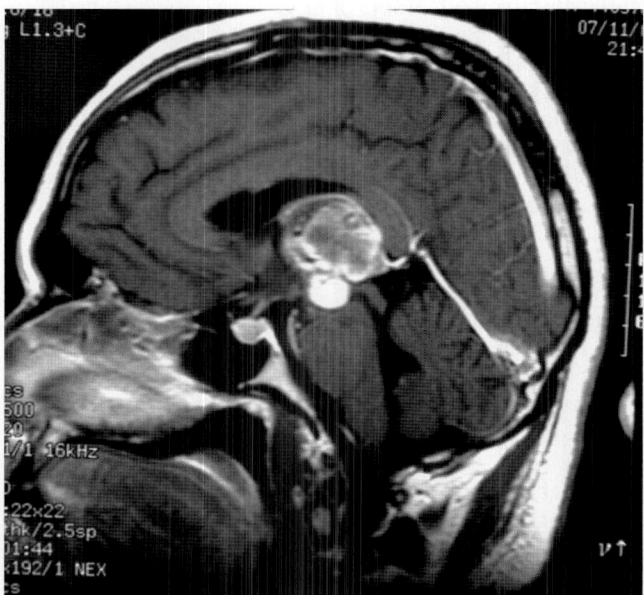

FIGURE 30-1 Sagittal magnetic resonance imaging with contrast shows a large pineal region tumor. The anatomic relationships of the tumor are well identified, including the third ventricle, aqueduct, and quadrigeminal plate.

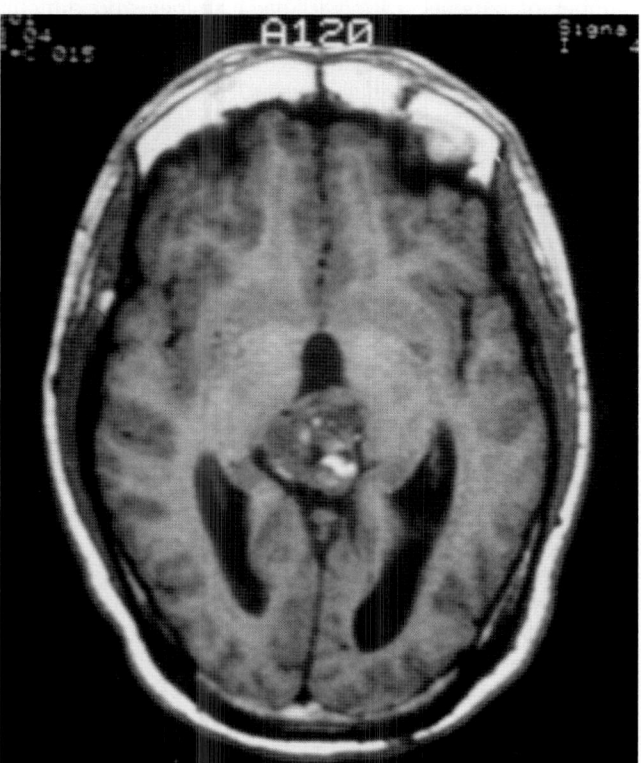

FIGURE 30-2 Magnetic resonance imaging with contrast (axial view) demonstrates the typical variegated pattern of a mixed germ cell tumor of the pineal region. The heterogeneity of lesions such as this in the pineal region can lead to misdiagnosis from sampling error.

Surgical Considerations

SURGICAL ANATOMY

Most tumors arise from and are attached to the undersurface of the velum interpositum, which includes the choroid plexus, deep venous system, and choroidal arteries. Depending on the degree of invasion of these important midline structures, the attachment may be minimal or comprehensive. Tumors rarely extend above the velum interpositum for any significant distance. Therefore, the blood supply comes from within the velum interpositum, mainly through the posterior medial and lateral choroidal arteries with anastomoses to the pericallosal arteries and quadrigeminal arteries.[1,27]

Some tumors extend to the foramen of Monro, but most are centered at the pineal gland, extending to the midportion of the third ventricle and posteriorly to compress the anterior portion of the cerebellum. In rare instances, the internal cerebral veins are ventral to the tumor. Mostly, however, vein of Galen, internal cerebral veins, Rosenthal's vein, and precentral cerebellar vein surround or cap the periphery of these tumors. The quadrigeminal plate may give rise to an exophytic astrocytoma or be infiltrated by the more malignant tumors of the pineal region, encompassing the aqueduct in the course of tumor growth. The most important aspects of the anatomy, which can be gleaned by radiographic imaging, are the relationship of the tumor to the third ventricle and quadrigeminal cistern, and the lateral and superior extent of the tumor. These features determine the route of the operation and the degree of difficulty likely to be encountered during surgery.[1]

MANAGEMENT OF HYDROCEPHALUS

Most patients present with obstructive hydrocephalus, a problem that may be managed in several ways.[14] When a complete tumor removal is anticipated and a permanent shunt may not be necessary, the hydrocephalus can be managed with a ventricular drain placed at the time of tumor surgery. The ventricular drain can be removed or converted

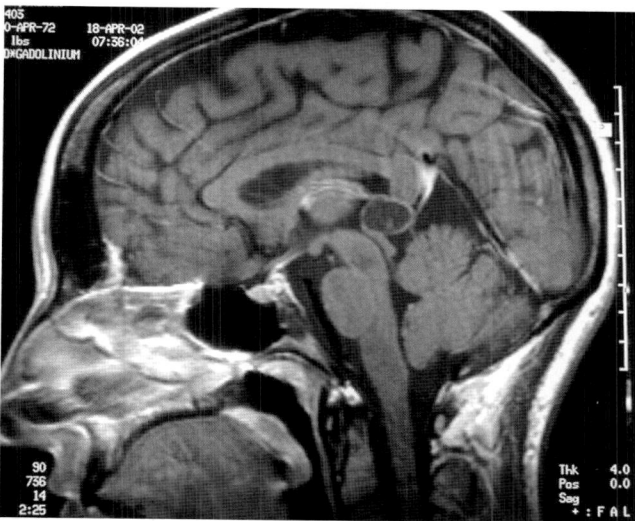

FIGURE 30-3 Sagittal magnetic resonance imaging with contrast shows an incidental pineal cyst discovered during the workup for unrelated headaches. The aqueduct is not compromised, and there is no hydrocephalus. Pineal cysts are anatomic variants and do not require treatment except in rare instances when they become symptomatic.

to a permanent shunt on postoperative day 2 or 3, depending on which circumstances prevail. Occasionally, no drain is necessary and the hydrocephalus resolves after complete tumor removal. The drain can be removed or converted to a shunt in the postoperative period as the circumstances dictate. Patients with more advanced symptomatology should be managed with an image-guided stereotactic endoscopic third ventriculostomy to allow a gradual reduction in intracranial pressure and resolution of symptoms.[28] This method is preferable to ventriculoperitoneal shunting as it eliminates potential complications such as infection, overshunting, and peritoneal seeding of malignant cells.

OPERATIVE APPROACHES: BIOPSY VERSUS OPEN RESECTION

The wide diversity of pathology that can occur in the pineal region makes histologic diagnosis a necessity to optimize patient management decisions.[14] Tissue histology has important implications for decisions concerning adjuvant therapy, metastatic workup, prognosis, and long-term follow-up. Cerebrospinal fluid cytology and radiographic examination are not sufficiently consistent to supplant the need for tissue diagnosis. The exception to mandatory histologic diagnosis is patients with elevated germ cell markers who can be treated with chemotherapy and radiation without a biopsy.[23,29] Some of these patients require a delayed surgical resection to remove residual radiographic abnormalities that may represent residual tumor.[30]

Specimens for tissue diagnosis can be obtained by either a stereotactic biopsy or an open operation. Passionate advocates for either approach can be found; however, it is important to recognize the relative advantages and disadvantages of each and use them in a complementary fashion for appropriate patients rather than having an inflexible dedication to one. The radiographic and clinical features of the tumor and the surgeon's experience will influence procedural decisions.

Experienced neurosurgeons using current microsurgical techniques can expect favorable results with open surgery.[14] Open procedures have the advantage of obtaining larger amounts of tissue to provide more extensive tissue sampling. This is particularly important for pineal region tumors where heterogeneity and mixed cell populations are common. This diversity is problematic for even experienced neuropathologists who can best resolve the subtleties of histologic diagnosis when free from the constraints of limited tissue sampling.[31-33] Additionally, open procedures provide a clinical advantage by facilitating tumor removal.[14,34,35] This is particularly important for the one third of patients with benign pineal tumors, in whom resection is usually complete but can also be useful for patients with malignant tumors in whom debulking may provide a more favorable response to adjuvant therapy and a better long-term prognosis. Additional advantages of aggressive tumor debulking include the potential to relieve hydrocephalus without additional procedures and the ability to control the risks of postoperative hemorrhage into an incompletely resected tumor bed. A disadvantage of open procedures is the relatively higher surgical morbidity compared with that of stereotactic biopsy, at least in the short term. This short-term disadvantage, however, may be a reasonable concession for the long-term advantage of better tumor control.

Any discussion about the relative risks and benefits of open procedures must recognize that the highly favorable outcome for patient with pineal tumor assumes an advanced level of experience, judgment, and expertise. These sophisticated surgical procedures are not recommended for novice surgeons as they can expect significantly less favorable outcomes. Stereotactic procedures, in contrast, can be appealing because of their ease of performance; however, the pineal region is among the most hazardous areas in the brain to safely biopsy, and careful forethought must be given to planning the target and trajectory to minimize hemorrhagic risks.[36] The potential for hemorrhage is increased because of several mechanisms including bleeding from any of several pial surfaces that must be traversed, bleeding in highly vascular tumors, damage to the deep venous system, and bleeding into the ventricle where the tissue turgor is insufficient to tamponade minor bleeding.[37,38] Despite this increased risk, several series have validated the effectiveness of stereotactic biopsy for these tumors.[36,39]

Stereotactic biopsy is ideally suited for patients with multiple lesions or clinical conditions that contraindicate open surgery and general anesthesia. Biopsy may also be preferable for tumors that are clearly invading the brain stem. However, the degree of invasion is not always easily discernible and tumors may have a surgically dissectible capsule that is not predicted on preoperative imaging studies.

STEREOTACTIC BIOPSY

Advances in radiographic imaging and software planning provide several alternatives for safely planning biopsy trajectories. Computed tomography-guided procedures are acceptable because of their high degree of accuracy and common availability. Although nearly any stereotactic frame system is sufficient, target-centered stereotactic frame systems such as the CRW (Cosman-Roberts-Wells) have the versatility to facilitate even complex biopsies. Local anesthesia with mild sedation is safe and usually sufficient to perform biopsies.

The most common surgical trajectory to the pineal region is via an anterolaterosuperior approach anterior to the coronal suture and lateral to the midpupillary line.[40] This trajectory passes through the frontal lobe and the internal capsule. The ependyma of the lateral ventricle and the internal cerebral vein should be avoided. An alternative approach is a posterolaterosuperior approach through the parieto-occipital junction, which is best suited for large tumors that have a lateral extension.

Whenever possible, multiple serial biopsy specimens should be obtained. Obviously, the risks of bleeding for each additional specimen must be considered, taking into account the size of the mass. A frozen section intraoperatively may be useful in verifying pathologic tissue; however, the high diversity of tissue types reduces the accuracy of a frozen tissue diagnosis.

ENDOSCOPY

Advances in endoscopic technique have led to investigations of biopsies via this method.[41,42] Endoscopy is sometimes performed in conjunction with an endoscopic third ventriculostomy to relieve hydrocephalus. Performing a ventriculostomy and biopsy simultaneously requires the use of a flexible endoscope because of the limited trajectory to the tumor through Monro's foramen. A rigid endoscope can be used but would necessitate a second burr hole and trajectory with a more inferior entry point on the forehead. The risks of an endoscopic biopsy are considerable due to the limited tissue sampling and difficulty achieving hemostasis within the ventricle. Even minor bleeding can obscure the operative field, making it difficult to identify the target. In general, given these limitations, a stereotactic biopsy is preferable to endoscopic biopsy in situations in which diagnostic tissue is desired.

Surgical Approaches

OPERATIVE CONSIDERATIONS

Common approaches to the pineal region include infratentorial supracerebellar, occipital transtentorial, and transcallosal interhemispheric (Fig. 30-4).[15] The best approach depends on the anatomic location as well as the degree of familiarity and confidence that the surgeon has with a given approach (Fig. 30-5).

Generally, the infratentorial supracerebellar approach is preferred for several reasons:

1. The approach is to the center of the tumor, which begins at the midline and grows eccentrically.
2. The approach is ventral to the velum interpositum and the deep venous system to which the tumor is often adherent. This minimizes the risk of damage to the vascular drainage of this critical region.
3. The exposure in the sitting position is comparable with that of other routes.
4. No normal tissue is violated on route to the tumor.

Either the transcallosal interhemispheric or occipital transtentorial approaches are used under the following circumstances:

1. Tumors that extend superiorly, involving or destroying the posterior aspect of the corpus callosum and deflecting the deep venous system in a dorsolateral direction
2. Tumors that extend laterally to the region of the trigone

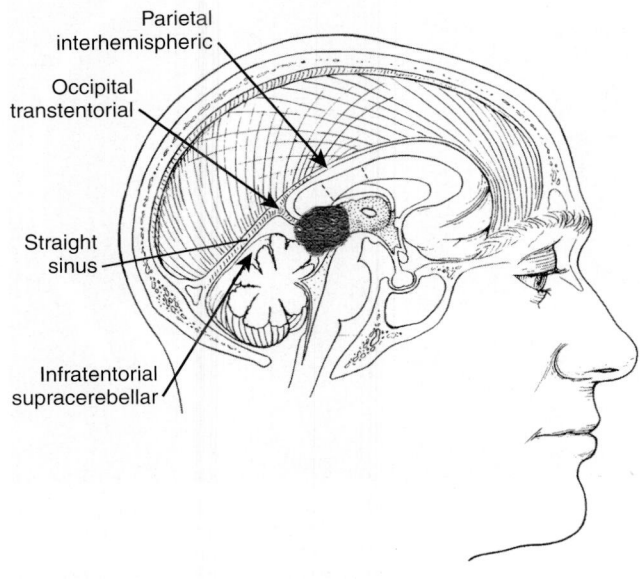

FIGURE 30-4 Surgical approaches to the pineal region.

3. Tumors that extend inferiorly into the quadrigeminal plate

4. In rare cases in which the tumor displaces the deep venous system in a ventral direction (often seen with meningiomas)

The transcallosal interhemispheric approach can provide extensive exposure, although the subtentorial portion of the tumor on the contralateral side of the approach is not easily visualized. This approach requires retraction of the parietal lobe and the disruption of bridging veins between parietal lobe and the sagittal sinus, creating the potential for venous infarct and retraction injury. Additionally, the veins of the deep venous system usually overlie the tumor, forcing the surgeon to work around them to avoid injury. Like the transcallosal approach, the occipital transtentorial approach has the disadvantage of encountering the deep venous system overlying the tumor. Once the tentorium is divided, however, this approach permits a wide view of the pineal region with particularly good visualization of the quadrigeminal plate. A major drawback is the high frequency of visual field deficits associated with this approach.[43]

PATIENT POSITIONING

Patient positioning is critical to successful pineal region surgery. There are three basic positions with variations and nuances of each that can be used somewhat interchangeably based on individual tumors and surgeon preferences. However, there are advantage and disadvantages to each. The three basic positions include sitting position, lateral position, and prone.

The sitting position is used most often for the infratentorial supracerebellar approach. This position enables gravity to work in the surgeon's favor by helping tumor dissection from the roof of the third ventricle and minimizing blood pooling in the operative field. It does carry the risk of air embolus or ventricular and cortical collapse with subsequent subdural hematoma or air. However, with proper precautions, these complications are infrequent. The occipital transtentorial approach often uses the three-quarter prone and lateral decubitus position, which, although avoiding many of the complications of the sitting position, does not allow gravity to work in the surgeon's favor. The Concorde position was developed to combine aspects of both the

prone and semisitting positions but still has the disadvantage of blood pooling in the operative field.[44]

The Sitting Position

The sitting position is accomplished by raising the back of the table to its maximal position. The patient's head, neck, and shoulders are brought forward by a pin vice head fixation device. The head must be strongly flexed so that optimal exposure of the tentorial notch can be achieved with the greatest comfort to the surgeon. The patient is tilted somewhat forward after being positioned on the operating table so that the surgeon actually works over the back of the patient's shoulders to the posterior fossa. A Doppler probe, central venous catheter, end tidal pCO_2 evaluation, and modest positive pressure ventilation are used to recognize and avoid air embolism which can occur during the bone opening or when large venous sinuses are exposed. A self-retaining retractor such as Greenberg's universal retractor is fixed via a bar to the operating table on the left side. The bars are then arranged in a rectangular configuration framing the operative field, facilitating placement of a retractor in the anterior position to depress the cerebellum. A cottonoid tray is fixed to the self-retaining retractor system and held by one of the retractor's arms.

Lateral Position

The lateral position and its variant the three-quarter prone position are generally preferred for the occipital transtentorial approaches. The lateral decubitus position is preferred with the dependent nondominant right hemisphere down. For the transcallosal approach, the head is raised approximately 30 degrees above the horizontal in the midsagittal plane, while with the occipital transtentorial approach, the patient's nose is rotated 30 degrees toward the floor.

The three quarter prone position is a useful variant of this approach. It is an extension of the lateral position with the head at an oblique 45-degree angle with a nondominant hemisphere dependent. It is particularly used for the occipital transtentorial approach as the nondominant hemisphere is retracted by gravity. Compared to the sitting position, the surgeon's hands are on a horizontal plane and less prone to fatigue. This position can be cumbersome to set up and it is important to avoid unnecessary pressure on the dependent axilla by placing in an axillary roll and supporting the right

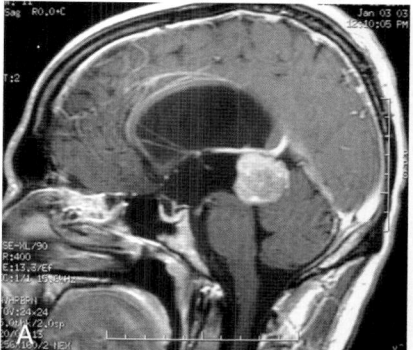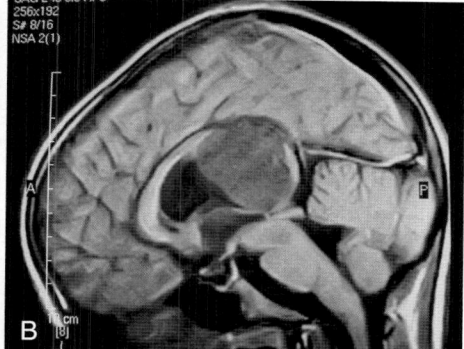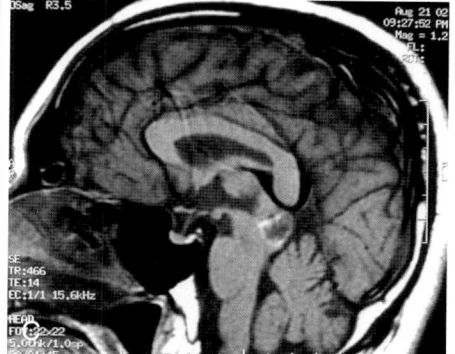

FIGURE 30-5 Midsagittal gadolinium enhanced magnetic resonance images illustrate the preferred surgical approaches. A, Meningioma of the velum interpositum with dorsal displacement of internal cerebral veins is best approached via the infratentorial supracerebellar corridor. B, Pilocytic astrocytoma arising from the corpus callosum with ventral displacement of the internal cerebral veins is best approach via the posterior-interhemispheric corridor. C, Tectal glioma is best approached via the occipital transtentorial corridor to facilitate access to the inferior portion of the tumor.

arm in a sling-like fashion. A supporting roll is placed under the left thorax and the head pin holder is used to support the head slightly extended and rotated to the left at a 45-degree oblique angle. The patient must be securely strapped at the table, which will facilitate rotation of the table as needed.

Prone Position

A simple prone position can be useful for the supratentorial approaches, particularly the transcallosal. The steep angle of the tentorium makes it difficult to use for the infratentorial approach. Without specialized operative tables, the head position can be considerably raised making it difficult for the surgeon to be seated during the surgery. A variant of the prone position known as the Concorde position has been advocated for infratentorial approaches particularly in the pediatric population. In the Concorde position, the position of the head is rotated 15 degrees away from the craniotomy side.

APPROACHES

Supracerebellar-Infratentorial Approach

Once the patient is optimal in the sitting position, a self-retaining retractor, such as Greenberg's Universal Retractor, is fixed via a bar to the operating table on the left side (Figs. 30-6 and 30-7). The bars are then arranged in a rectangular configuration framing the operative field, facilitating placement of a retractor in the inferior position to depress the cerebellum. A cottonoid tray is fixed to the self-retaining retractor system and held by one of the retractor's arms.

A long midline incision is used, extending approximately from the spinous process of the third vertebral body up into the occipital region, so that the pericranium and muscle attachments can be elevated on each side without disrupting their continuity. Freeing up the muscle layer facilitates closure later. A wide craniotomy is performed to include the lateral sinuses and torcula but without extending to the foramen magnum. Generally, using a high-speed air drill to perform a suboccipital craniotomy is preferred so that the

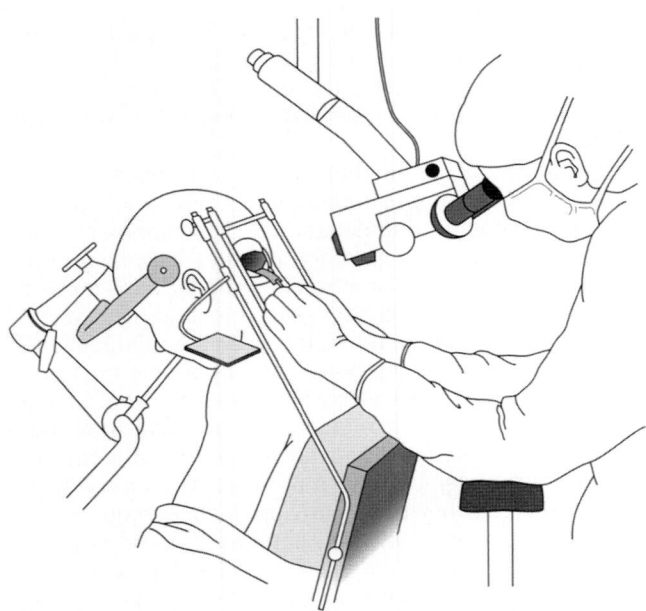

FIGURE 30-7 Diagram of the patient position and operative setup for the supracerebellar approach.

bone flap may be replaced at the end of the procedure. A craniotome is used to turn the flap after first exposing each of the dural sinuses to avoid tears. Brain relaxation and cerebellar retraction can be facilitated by mannitol, ventricular drainage, or removal of cerebrospinal from the cisterna magna. It is preferable to open the dura on either side of the midline so that the cerebellar falx and accompanying cerebellar sinus can be ligated and divided. The dural opening should extend bilaterally up to the lateral sinus (Fig. 30-8).

Once the dura is opened, all bridging veins over the dorsal surface of the cerebellum, including the hemispheres and vermis, can be sacrificed to free the cerebellum from the tentorium. The weight of cottonoids and a copper retractor, along with gravitational forces that are exerted in the sitting position, allow sufficient depression of the cerebellum

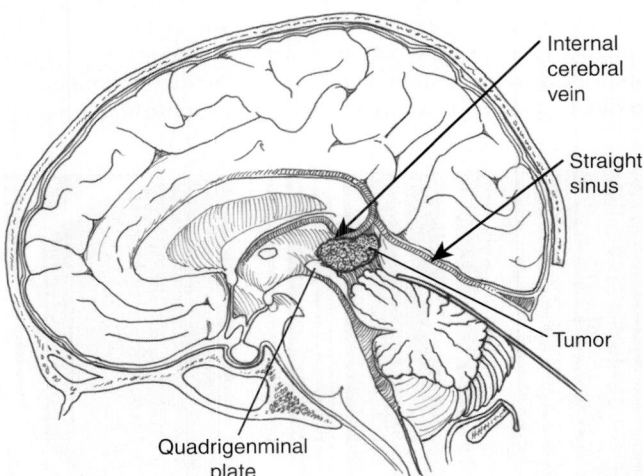

FIGURE 30-6 Drawing of the sagittal view shows the position of the pineal tumor with gravity facilitating retraction of the cerebellum to access the infratentorial supracerebellar corridor. (From Bruce JN. Tumors of the pineal region. In: Batjer HH, Loftus CM, eds. Textbook of Neurological Surgery, vol. 2. Philadelphia: Lippincott Williams and Wilkins; 2003:1365-1373.)

Internal cerebral vein

Straight sinus

Tumor

Quadrigenminal plate

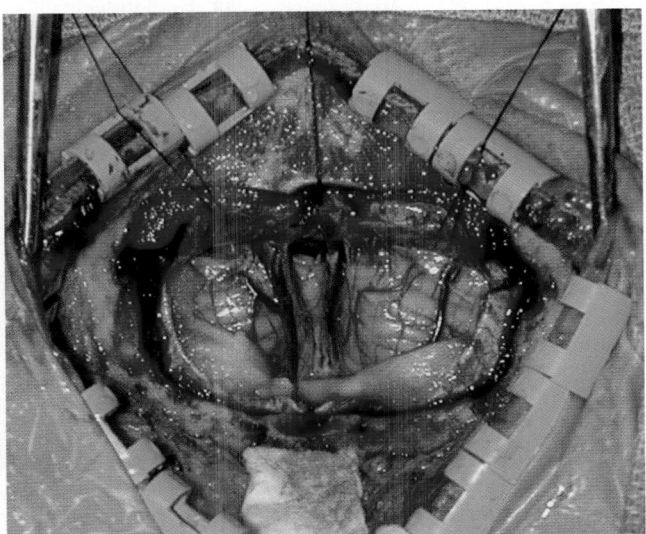

FIGURE 30-8 Dural opening prior to sacrifice of bridging veins.

to establish an unobstructed corridor to the pineal region under the tentorium. At this point, the operating microscope should be brought to the operating table. A microscope capable of varying the objective length from 275 to 400 mm is desirable because the operating distance for the surgeon changes throughout the operation, going from the dorsal surface of the cerebellum to the center of the third ventricle. The use of a freestanding armrest is also helpful in minimizing fatigue.

The arachnoid in the quadrigeminal region and around the incisura is usually thickened and opaque in the presence of tumors and must be opened by microdissection techniques to expose the surface of the tumor. The precentral cerebellar vein, which can be seen extending from the edge of the vermis to Galen's vein, should be cauterized and divided (Fig. 30-9). Galen's great vein and the internal cerebral veins are well above the tumor and are not encountered in these initial maneuvers. Laterally, the medial aspect of the temporal lobe and Rosenthal's veins can be seen as they course upward toward the confluence of veins in these regions. In general terms, the trajectory of the operation is toward the velum interpositum. This must be considered when attempting to remove segments of the tumor in the inferior portion of the third ventricle or directly over the quadrigeminal plate in relation to the anterior lobe of the cerebellum. The thickened arachnoid should be opened widely to appreciate the underlying anatomy. Using sharp dissection, the arachnoidal opening must be kept close to the anterior surface of the vermis and cerebellar hemisphere to avoid injuring the deep venous system, keeping in mind that the initial trajectory is toward Galen's vein. The anterior portion of the cerebellum is retracted by the inferior self-retaining retractor to expose the posterior surface of the tumor.

Because many of these tumors extend well into the third ventricle, even to the region of Monro's foramen, long instruments are required to reach the anterior margins of the tumor. With tumors of firm consistency, a Cavitron with a long, curved tip can be helpful for debulking. A long focal length is desirable to accommodate the large instrument

and maneuver into the operative field. The most difficult dissection involves the inferior portion of the tumor, where it is adherent to the collicular region of the dorsal midbrain. Small dental mirrors and angled instruments may be required to remove this portion of the tumor. Similarly, these techniques may be helpful for supratentorial tumor extensions. Further exposure can be gained by incising the tentorium if necessary. Tumors that are benign or encapsulated can usually be removed completely (Fig. 30-10). With tumors that are incompletely resected, particularly vascular ones such as pineal cell tumors, meticulous hemostasis is crucial. Surgicel is the preferred hemostatic agent, and it should be placed carefully so that it does not float and obstruct the aqueduct when the third ventricle fills with cerebrospinal fluid.

At the conclusion of the operation, after decompression of the tumor and the ventricular system, the dura can be closed to support the cerebellum. When a craniotomy has been performed, the bone flap is secured back in place with wires or miniplates. A greater degree of dural and bony closure seems to lower the incidence of postoperative aseptic meningitis.

Occipital-Transtentorial Approach

The occipital transtentorial approach uses an occipital craniotomy and by dividing the tentorium, it facilitates exposure of the quadrigeminal plate and tumors that have an inferior extension. A lateral or three-quarter prone position can be utilized. A spinal drain may be useful if the patient has not required a preoperative third ventriculostomy or shunt. The occipital transtentorial approach brings the surgeon at a slightly oblique angle which can be disorienting for a surgeon not familiar with the surgical anatomy since most tumors are midline.

A U-shaped right occipital scalp flap or a linear incision centered in the midline can be used. The craniotomy should extend across the sagittal sinus to the contralateral occipital lobe and should begin just above the torcula. Although some surgeons tried to avoid crossing the sagittal sinus, the bony overhang can limit the operative view. A burr hole is placed and slotted over the sagittal sinus just above the torcula and then a second burr hole slotted over the sagittal sinus 6-10 cm above this. The craniotomy is extended 1 to

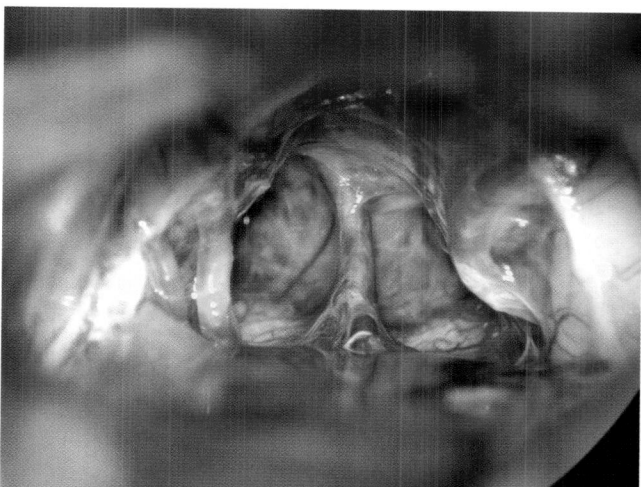

FIGURE 30-9 Operative view shows exposure of the posterior surface of a tumor in the pineal region before sacrificing the precentral cerebellar vein.

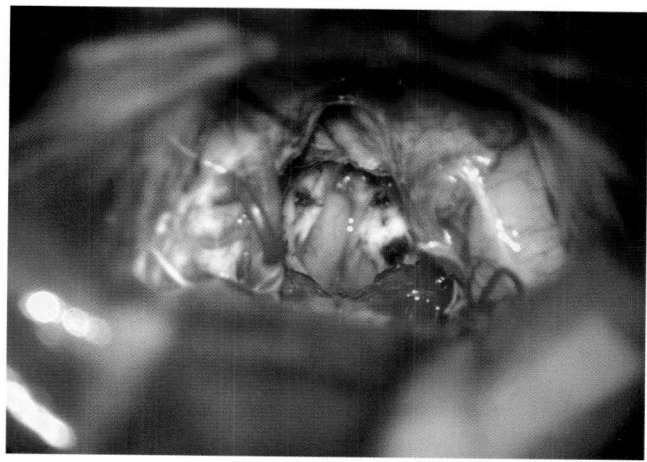

FIGURE 30-10 View into the third ventricle after pineal tumor removal.

2 cm left of midline providing an adequate exposure of the right occipital lobe. If the patient is positioned correctly, the nondominant occipital lobe will retract easily with gravity and brain relaxation. There are rarely any bridging veins near the occipital pole and minimal retraction is desirable to avoid hemianopsia. If the brain is tight, mannitol in ventricular drainage can be useful adjuncts.

The dura is opened in a U-shaped fashion and reflected towards the sagittal sinus. The interhemispheric fissure is accessed and the occipital lobe is gently retracted. Under the microscope, the straight sinus is identified and the tentorium can be divided adjacent and parallel to the straight sinus (Fig. 30-11). The tentorium can often be highly vascular and it is a CO_2 laser or unipolar cautery can facilitate the tentorial opening being careful to avoid damage to the underlying cerebellum and brain stem. If necessary, the falx can be retracted or even divided although this is rarely necessary. Once the tentorium is divided, the arachnoid overlying the tumor and the quadrigeminal cisterns can be seen and widely opened. Similar to what is described earlier in the supracerebellar approach, the tumor is entered dorsally, internally debulked, then gradually peeled away from the surrounding brain stem, deep venous system, and thalamus. Whenever possible, the plane between the tumor capsule and the surrounding structures should be developed.

Transcallosal, Interhemispheric Approach

The transcallosal interhemispheric approach (Fig. 30-12) provides a wide exposure between the falx and brain along the parietal occipital junction. One of the major drawbacks to this approach is the presence of bridging veins which can cause serious venous infarct if damaged or divided. Normally, one vein can be sacrificed if necessary. A generous craniotomy is desirable to provide some flexibility in the trajectory to the tumor if bridging veins are in the way. Although the sitting approach is often used for this approach, the lateral and prone positions can also be used.

Depending on where the tumor is located, the craniotomy is centered somewhere along the parietal lobe. Approximately 8 cm in length will provide the flexibility needed should bridging veins be in the way. It is desirable to extend the craniotomy across to the contralateral side

by slotting the boreholes over the sagittal sinus. If the sagittal sinus is not exposed, it can often be difficult to place retractors in the interhemispheric fissure and along the falx. Bleeding from the sagittal sinus can generally be controlled with routine hemostatic agents. In the sitting position, this bleeding is often less than another position.

The dura is opened in a U-shaped fashion and reflected towards the sagittal sinus. Although sacrifice of the bridging vein should be minimized to one, the operative angles mean that even a small opening at the superficial interhemispheric fissure can provide a wide angle of deep exposure. The hemisphere should be carefully protected and then gently retracted. If necessary, additional retraction can be placed on the falx which may be divided inferiorly if further retraction is necessary. The interhemispheric fissure should be easily opened without sacrificing any vessels that is a nonvascular corridor with a few adhesions between the falx and the cingulate gyrus. At the depth of the interhemispheric dissection, the corpus callosum is easily identified by its white appearance. The operating microscope is useful at this point to identify the pericallosal arteries as a paired structure running over the corpus callosum. Stereotactic guidance can be useful particularly for those uncomfortable with the surgical anatomy. The corpus callosum is opened over the maximal geometric center of the tumor. Corpus callosum is generally thin and easily opened with gentle suction and cautery. A two-centimeter opening is usually sufficient for most tumors and should not result in any disconnection syndromes or cognitive impairment. The deep venous system will be found in the midline just below the corpus callosum and deep to it and therefore, this should be looked for early on in the dissection to avoid damage to it. It is not safe to sacrifice the deep venous system. If necessary, even more posterior openings in the splenium can be safely performed. The tumors can often extent fore laterally and it is important to avoid damage to pericallosal arteries as the lateral aspects of the tumor are dissected.

Once through the corpus callosum, the deep venous system is identified and the tumor is internally debulked. As with the other approaches, once the tumor is internally debulked, it is helpful to work along the tumor capsule to avoid damage to the surrounding structures. There is considerable debate whether or not one internal cerebral vein

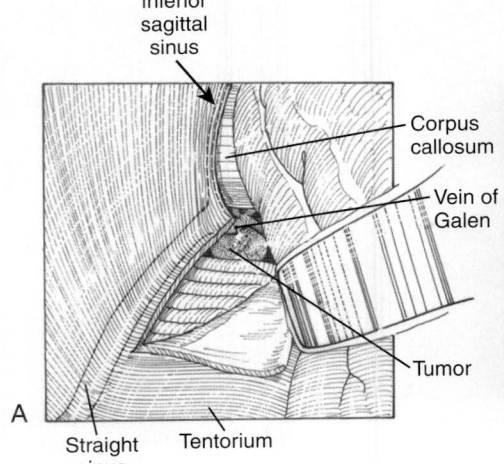
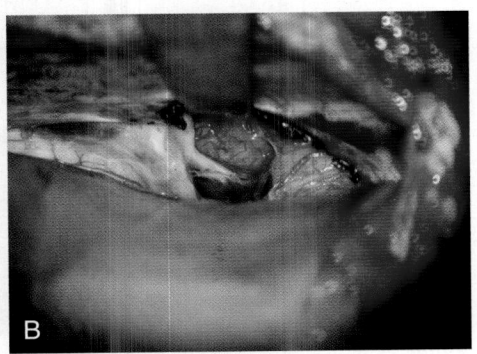

FIGURE 30-11 Diagram (A) and operative photo (B) of transtentorial approach. (From Bruce JN. Tumors of the pineal region. In: Batjer HH, Loftus CM, eds. Textbook of Neurological Surgery, vol. 2. Philadelphia: Lippincott Williams and Wilkins; 2003:1365-1373.)

Inferior sagittal sinus

Corpus callosum

Vein of Galen

Tumor

Straight sinus   Tentorium

can be safely dissected. Although there may be times when it is possible to get away with this, it is not desirable and should be avoided at all expenses.

Complications of Surgery

Serious complications of pineal tumor surgery, regardless of the route used, are related to the nature of the tumor and its potential for intra- or postoperative hemorrhage.[15] Hemorrhage has played a major role in most of the surgery-related deaths and can occur with a delay of as long as several postoperative days. This phenomenon is most prevalent with malignant pineal cell tumors (pineoblastomas), which tend to be soft and highly vascular. Hemorrhage can occur before surgery as a so-called pineal apoplexy or can be associated with stereotactic biopsy.

Complications of the sitting position, particularly with the posterior fossa approach, include air embolism, hypotension, and cortical collapse when hydrocephalus of significant degree is relieved by tumor removal. The incidence of cortical collapse can be reduced by preoperative shunting or third ventriculostomy to allow the ventricular system a chance to accommodate over several days before the major operation. This phenomenon can occur in varying degrees and, although striking on the postoperative computed tomography scan, gradually improves without major neurologic complications for the patient. Subdural shunting is rarely required to relieve chronic hygromas resulting from this complication.

The complications of the interhemispheric approach are related to retraction of the parietal lobe with transient sensory or stereognostic deficits on the opposite side. These have not been serious or permanent. Unlike the occipital transtentorial approach, the interhemispheric approach has not been associated with visual field defects.

Regardless of the operative approach used, various pupil abnormalities, difficulty focusing or accommodating, interocular palsies, and limitation of upward gaze can be expected whenever the tumor is dissected from the quadrigeminal region. These deficits improve gradually but may last for many months or as long as a year before normal function returns. Manipulation of the brain adjacent to the third ventricle can lead to impaired consciousness. The fourth cranial nerve is generally caudal to the tumor and is rarely identified or injured. Ataxia has been minimal and usually transient. The incidence and severity of deficits are increased with prior radiation therapy, presence of symptoms preoperatively, and a high degree of malignant and invasive characteristics. Shunt malfunction or blockage of a ventriculostomy can occur in as many as 20% of patients after surgery.

Surgical Results

Among large series of pineal region tumors in the microscopic era, operative mortality ranges from 0% to 8% and permanent morbidity from 0% to 25% (Table 30-1).[14] Pineal region tumors are among the most difficult surgical challenges, and outcome will vary significantly with the expertise and experience of the individual surgeon. For benign tumors, surgical resection is the treatment of choice with complete surgical removal likely to result in excellent long-term survival and likely cure (Table 30-2).[15] With malignant tumors, the impact of surgery is less delineated, although the degree of resection can correlate with improved prognosis.[14]

Adjuvant Therapy

POSTOPERATIVE STAGING

All patients with malignant pineal cell tumors, germ cell tumors, and ependymomas should have a postoperative staging consisting of a spinal MRI with contrast to look for spinal metastasis. Cerebrospinal fluid cytology is performed but is rarely helpful for guiding management decisions.

RADIATION THERAPY

Patients with malignant germ cell or pineal cell tumors require radiation therapy. The recommended radiation dose is 5500 cGy given in 180-cGy daily fractions with 4000 cGy to the ventricular system and an additional 1500 cGy to the tumor bed.[14,23,45-47] Recent studies suggest that using a

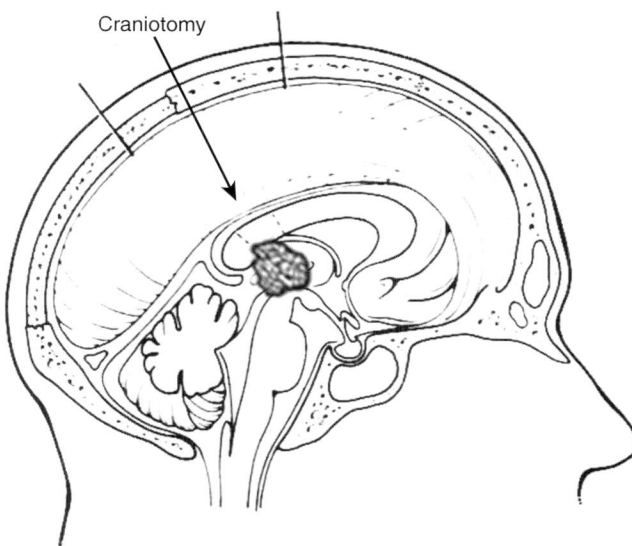

FIGURE 30-12 Transcallosal-interhemispheric approach. The arrow shows the operative trajectory and points to the potential opening in the corpus callosum.

Craniotomy

Table 30-1   Surgical Outcome for 128 Pineal Region Tumors at New York Neurological Institute, 1990–2009

Operative-related deaths, 2%
Permanent major morbidity, 1%
Transient major morbidity, 5%

Table 30-2   Extent of Resection for 128 Pineal Region Tumors at New York Neurological Institute, 1990–2009

Histology	Biopsy	Subtotal Resection	Radical Subtotal Resection	Gross Total Resection
Benign	2	5	11	37
Malignant	6	24	17	26
Total	8 (6%)	29 (23%)	28 (22%)	63 (49%)

more limited field of radiation that avoids the adverse side effects of ventricular exposure may be sufficiently efficacious; however, these studies lack long-term follow-up.[48]

Radiation therapy may be withheld for the rare, histologically benign pineocytoma or ependymoma that has been completely resected.[49] This distinction is based on the intraoperative observation of a well-circumscribed tumor that is well differentiated histologically. Surgical resection alone provides excellent long-term control in this group; however, careful follow-up is necessary so that radiation or radiosurgery can be offered at the first sign of recurrence. Pediatric patients are particularly vulnerable to adverse radiation effects.[50] In an effort to reduce the dose of radiation and minimize these effects, treatment strategies combining reduced radiation with chemotherapy are being investigated.[51]

Prophylactic spinal radiation is controversial and the current trend is to avoid spinal radiation unless there is documented evidence of spinal seeding or when pineoblastoma is present.[15] In patients with radiographic documentation of spinal seeding, a dose of 3500 cGy is recommended to the spine.

CHEMOTHERAPY

Patients with nongerminomatous malignant germ cell tumors have benefited most from advances in chemotherapy. Current chemotherapy regimens have resulted in reasonable expectations for long-term survival.[52] Additionally, patients with germinomas containing syncytiotrophoblastic giant cells have a less favorable prognosis and may benefit from more aggressive treatment with chemotherapy in addition to radiotherapy.[24]

Most of the germ cell chemotherapy regimens have been extrapolated from experience treating germ cell tumors of extracranial origin in which success has been remarkable.[23] Recent studies, using VP-16 (etoposide) in place of vinblastine and bleomycin to avoid the pulmonary toxicity have shown improved response rate with less morbidity. Currently a regimen of cisplatin or carboplatin with etoposide is among the most widely used.

Chemotherapy for pineal cell tumors has mostly been relegated to recurrent or disseminated pineal cell tumors.[45] Combined radiation and chemotherapy may be beneficial for pediatric patients with malignant pineal cell tumors.[53]

RADIOSURGERY

Radiosurgery has become more commonplace in the management of pineal tumors.[54,55] Several studies have clearly documented the relative safety of this method, although long-term follow-up results are currently lacking. Radiosurgery is generally limited to tumors less than 3 cm in diameter.

Distinct differences in radiobiologic effects between radiosurgery and conventional fractionated radiation must be considered when choosing optimal therapeutic strategies. Germinomas, for example, have excellent long-term response to fractionated radiation, and it is unlikely that radiosurgery will improve on these results. Additionally, because radiosurgery provides no therapeutic coverage to the ventricular system, tumors such as pineal cell and germ cell tumors are particularly vulnerable to ventricular recurrence. Radiosurgery may have its greatest benefit in providing a local boost to the tumor bed so that the radiation exposure to the ventricles and surrounding brain can be reduced.[56] It may also be useful for tumors that recur locally.

Conclusions

Advances in the treatment of pineal region tumors have led to significant improvements in survival as well as quality of life. The wide diversity of histologic subtypes in the pineal region necessitates a tissue diagnosis to optimally guide management decisions (the only exception being patients with elevated germ cell markers). A variety of operative approaches including stereotactic procedures can facilitate this with a reasonable risk. Surgical removal of benign or encapsulated tumors results in excellent long-term outcome. Most patients with malignant tumors will benefit from surgical removal as well, although successful surgical outcomes are dependent on advanced surgical expertise and experience. Adjuvant therapy with radiation and/or chemotherapy can be highly beneficial for most malignant pineal region tumors, with malignant germ cell tumors among the most responsive. Radiosurgery is a more recent addition to the armamentarium and may be most helpful for recurrent tumors.

KEY REFERENCES

Bruce JN, Ogden AT. Surgical strategies for treating patients with pineal region tumors. *J Neurooncol*. 2004;69:221-236.

Bruce JN, Stein BM. Surgical management pineal region tumors. *Acta Neurochir (Wien)*. 1995;134:130-135.

Chernov MF, Kamikawa S, Yamane F, et al. Neurofiberscopic biopsy of tumors of the pineal region and posterior third ventricle: indications, technique, complications, and results. *Neurosurgery*. 2006;59:267-277:discussion 267-277.

Edwards MS, Hudgins RJ, Wilson CB, et al. Pineal region tumors in children. *J Neurosurg*. 1988;68:689-697.

Jakacki RI, Zeltzer PM, Boyett JM, et al. Survival and prognostic factors following radiation and/or chemotherapy for primitive neuroectodermal tumors of the pineal region in infants and children: a report of the Childrens Cancer Group. *J Clin Oncol*. 1995;13:1377-1383.

Kobayashi T, Kida Y, Mori Y. Stereotactic gamma radiosurgery for pineal and related tumors. *J Neurooncol*. 2001;54:301-309.

Konovalov AN, Pitskhelauri DI. Principles of treatment of the pineal region tumors. *Surg Neurol*. 2003;59:250-268.

Kreth F, Schatz C, Pagenstecher A, et al. Stereotactic management of lesions of the pineal region. *Neurosurgery*. 1996;39:280-291.

Kyritsis AP. Management of primary intracranial germ cell tumors. *J Neurooncol*. 2010;96:143-149.

Lutterbach J, Fauchon F, Schild SE, et al. Malignant pineal parenchymal tumors in adult patients: patterns of care and prognostic factors. *Neurosurgery*. 2002;51:44-55:discussion 55-56.

Sands SA, Kellie SJ, Davidow AL, et al. Long-term quality of life and neuropsychologic functioning for patients with CNS germ-cell tumors: from the First International CNS Germ-Cell Tumor Study. *Neuro Oncol*. 2001;3:174-183.

Sawamura Y, de Tribolet N, Ishii N, Abe H. Management of primary intracranial germinomas: diagnostic surgery or radical resection? *J Neurosurg*. 1997;87:262-266.

Schild SE, Scheithauer BW, Haddock MG, et al. Histologically confirmed pineal tumors and other germ cell tumors of the brain. *Cancer*. 1996;78:2564-2571.

Stein BM. The infratentorial supracerebellar approach to pineal lesions. *J Neurosurg*. 1971;35:197-202.

Stein BM, Bruce JN. Surgical management of pineal region tumors. *Clin Neurosurg*. 1992;39:509-532.

Weiner HL, Lichtenbaum RA, Wisoff JH, et al. Delayed surgical resection of central nervous system germ cell tumors. *Neurosurgery*. 2002;50:727-733:discussion 733-734.

Yamini B, Refai D, Rubin CM, Frim DM. Initial endoscopic management of pineal region tumors and associated hydrocephalus: clinical series and literature review. *J Neurosurg*. 2004;100:437-441.

Numbered references appear on Expert Consult.

CHAPTER 31

Management of Tumors of the Fourth Ventricle

JONATHAN MILLER • ALIA HDEIB • ALAN COHEN

Tumors of the fourth ventricle offer a unique challenge to the neurosurgeon since they lie deep in the brain in close proximity to a number of vital structures. Although recent diagnostic and therapeutic advances have dramatically improved outcome for patients affected with these tumors, there are still many difficulties for which new solutions are always being offered. The purpose of this chapter is to provide a systematic and comprehensive review of tumors that occur in the region of the fourth ventricle. The first section reviews the relevant anatomy. The second section describes the surgical approach to fourth ventricular tumors and common complications associated with surgical resection. The third section describes in detail the epidemiology, clinical presentation, radiology, pathology, surgical techniques, and prognosis for specific fourth ventricular tumors.

Anatomy

The fourth ventricle is a broad tent-shaped cerebrospinal fluid (CSF) cavity located behind the brain stem and in front of the cerebellum in the center of the posterior fossa (Fig. 31-1). CSF enters through the cerebral aqueduct, which opens into the fourth ventricle at its rostral end. The ventricle widens caudally until its maximum width at the level of the lateral recesses, from which CSF exits through the two foramina of Luschka into the cerebellopontine cisterns on either side. The ventricle narrows again to its caudal terminus at the obliterated central canal of the spinal cord, called the *obex* from the Latin for "barrier." The foramen of Magendie is just posterior to the obex and allows CSF to exit into the cerebellomedullary cistern, which is continuous with the cisterna magna. There are no arteries or veins within the cavity of the fourth ventricle. All of the vessels associated with this region are in the fissures located just outside the fourth ventricular roof.

The glistening white floor of the fourth ventricle is the posterior surface of the brain stem (Fig. 31-2). The border between the pons and medulla occurs approximately at the level of the foramina of Luschka. The superior (pontine) part of the floor begins at the aqueduct and expands to the lower margin of the cerebellar peduncles. The inferior (medullary) part of the floor begins just below the lateral recesses at the attachment of the tela choroidea to the taenia choroidea and extends to the obex, limited laterally be the taeniae, which mark the inferolateral margins of the floor. Between these is the intermediate part, which extends into the lateral recesses on either side. There is a longitudinal midline sulcus in the fourth ventricular floor called the median sulcus. On either side of the median sulcus is the sulcus limitans, which also runs longitudinally parallel to the median sulcus. The sulcus limitans is an important landmark for functional anatomy of nuclei beneath the ventricular floor, as motor nuclei are medial and sensory nuclei lateral to the sulcus limitans. Medial to the sulcus limitans on either side of the median sulcus is the median eminence, a collection of four paired elevations in the fourth ventricular floor that are collectively referred to as the calamus scriptorius since they resemble the head of a fountain pen (Fig. 31-1). Rostral to caudal, the median eminence consists of the facial colliculus, which overlies the facial nucleus; the hypoglossal triangle, which overlies the hypoglossal nucleus; the vagal triangle, which overlies the dorsal nucleus of the vagus; and the area postrema, a tongue-shaped structure that is part of the brain-stem emetic center. Lateral to the sulcus limitans is the vestibular area, so named because is overlies the vestibular nuclei. This area is widest in the neighborhood of the lateral recess, where the striae medullaris cross transversely across the inferior cerebellar peduncles to disappear into the median sulcus. The auditory tubercle in the lateral part of the vestibular area overlies the dorsal cochlear nucleus and cochlear nerve.

The roof of the fourth ventricle is tent-shaped, rising to an apex called the fastigium that divides the superior roof from the inferior roof. The median part of the superior roof, called the superior medullary velum, consists of a thin lamina of white matter between the cerebellar peduncles. Just behind its outer surface is the lingula, the uppermost division of the vermis. The lateral walls of the superior roof are formed by the superior and inferior cerebellar peduncles, which lie between the fourth ventricle and the middle cerebellar peduncle. The rostral midline of the inferior roof is formed by the nodule, which lies directly in front of the uvula, the lower part of the vermis that hangs down between the tonsils (mimicking the appearance of the pharynx). Lateral to the nodule is the inferior medullary velum, a thin sheet of neural tissue that stretches over the fourth ventricle to connect the nodule to the flocculi on either side just superior to the outer extremity of the lateral recess. The inferior medullary velum is thus part of the primitive flocculonodular lobe of the cerebellum. The caudal inferior roof consists of the tela choroidea, two thin arachnoid-like membranes sandwiching a vascular layer of choroidal vessels to which the choroid plexus is attached. The junction between the tela choroidea and the nodule/inferior medullary velum

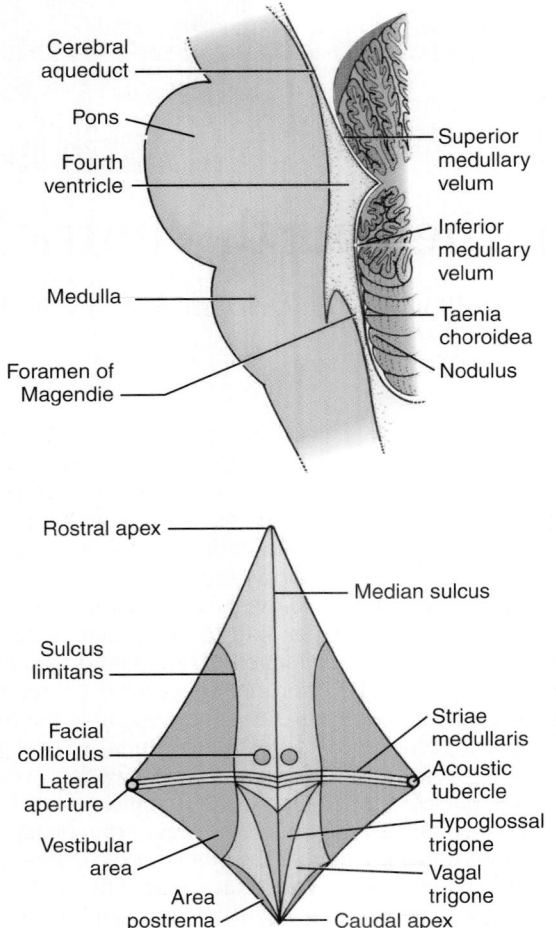

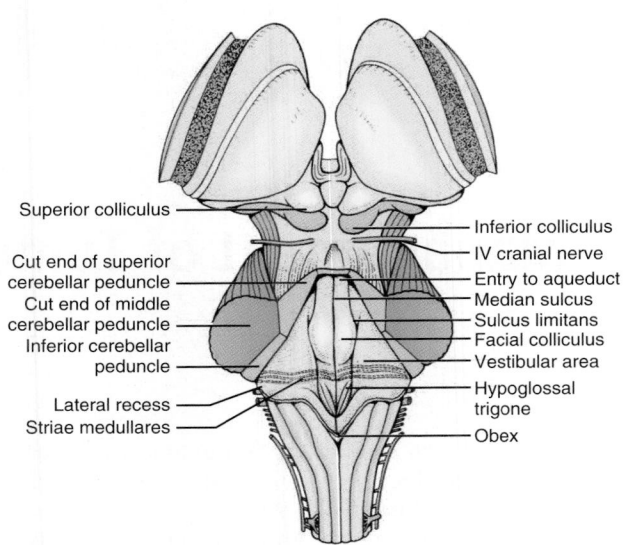

FIGURE 31-2 Fourth ventricle after removal of the cerebellum. *(Modified from Cohen AR. Surgical Disorders of the Fourth Ventricle. Cambridge, MA: Blackwell Science; 1996.)*

FIGURE 31-1 Fourth ventricle viewed from the side (A) and from behind (B). Landmarks such as the vertical median sulcus and oblique calamus scriptorius give the caudal floor the appearance of a fountain pen. *(Modified from Cohen AR. Surgical Disorders of the Fourth Ventricle. Cambridge, MA: Blackwell Science; 1996.)*

(telovelar junction) is at the level of the lateral recess. The tela choroidea is attached to the ventricular floor at narrow white ridges called taeniae choroidea, which meet at the obex and extend upward to turn laterally over the inferior cerebellar peduncles into each lateral recess, forming its lower border. As a result, the choroid plexus (extending from the ventricular surface of the tela) forms an upside-down L shape on either side of midline. There is a medial segment of choroid plexus that extends longitudinally from the foramen of Magendie up to the nodule and a lateral segment that extends transversely from the rostral ends of the medial segments out to the foramen of Luschka. The three fourth ventricular outlet foramina (Magendie and Luschka) are located in the tela choroidea itself, and frequently choroid plexus protrudes from these foramina.

External to the fourth ventricle are three deep V-shaped fissures between the cerebellum and brain stem that enclose subarachnoid cisterns and through which course the principle arteries and veins of the posterior fossa. These three fissures are intimately related to the structures of the posterior fossa. Located between the midbrain and cerebellum, the cerebellomesencephalic fissure (also called the

precentral cerebellar fissure) is the most rostral of the three and is intimately associated with the superior part of the fourth ventricular roof. This fissure is shaped like a V in the axial plain with the point facing posteriorly. The brain stem and fourth ventricle line the inner surface along with the lingula of the vermis, dorsal superior cerebellar peduncles, and rostral middle cerebellar peduncles. The outer surface of the V consists of the cerebellum, specifically the culmen and wings of the central lobule. The trochlear nerves run through the cerebellomesencephalic fissure, as do the superior cerebellar arteries (SCA). The SCAs leave the brain stem between cranial nerves IV and V to enter the fissure, and then after several sharp hairpin turns give rise to the precerebellar arteries that pass along the superior cerebellar peduncle to reach the superior fourth ventricle and dentate nucleus. Upon leaving the fissure the arteries supply end branches to the tentorial surface of the cerebellum. Venous drainage from the superior fourth ventricle occurs primarily through the vein of Galen. The vein of the cerebellomesencephalic fissure (also called the precentral cerebellar vein) is formed by the union of the paired veins of the superior cerebellar peduncle and ascends through the quadrigeminal cistern to drain into the vein of Galen either directly or through the superior vermian vein.

The cerebellopontine fissures are intimately related to the lateral recesses of the fourth ventricle. They are produced by the folding of the cerebellum laterally around the sides of the pons and middle cerebellar peduncles. Each cerebellopontine fissure is shaped like a V in the coronal plain with the point facing laterally. The outer surface of the V is made up of the petrosal surfaces of the cerebellum, and the inner surface is made up of the middle cerebellar peduncles. The lateral recess and foramen of Luschka open into the medial part of the inferior limb of the V near the flocculus. Several cranial nerves run through the cerebellopontine fissure, including the trigeminal (through the superior limb) and the facial, glossopharyngeal, and vagus (through the inferior limb). The anterior inferior cerebellar arteries (AICA) also run through these fissures. Each AICA courses posteriorly around the pons then sends branches to nerves of the acoustic meatus and choroid plexus protruding from the foramen of Luschka before passing around the flocculus on the middle cerebellar peduncle to supply the petrosal surface of the cerebellum. Venous blood from the cerebellopontine fissure and lateral recess primarily drains into the superior petrosal sinus. The vein of the cerebellopontine fissure is formed by the convergence of several veins on the apex of the fissure, including the vein of the middle cerebellar peduncle into which the vein of the inferior cerebellar peduncle drains. This vein courses near the superior limb of the fissure to drain into the superior petrosal sinus rostral to the facial and glossopharyngeal nerves.

The cerebellomedullary fissure is directly behind the inferior roof of the fourth ventricle. It is the most caudal of the three fissures and extends between the cerebellum and medulla. Like the cerebellomesencephalic fissure, it is shaped like a V in the axial plain with the point facing posteriorly. The ventral wall consists of the inferior roof of the fourth ventricle (inferior medullary velum and tela choroidea) and the posterior medulla. The dorsal wall consists of the uvula in the midline and the tonsils (paired ovoid structures attached to the cerebellar hemispheres along their superolateral borders) and biventral lobules laterally. The fissure communicates with the cisterna magna around the superior poles of the tonsils through the telovelotonsillar cleft (tonsils to tela/velum) and "supratonsillar cleft" (superior extension of this cleft over superior pole of tonsil). The posterior inferior cerebellar arteries (PICA) course around the medulla to reach the cerebellar tonsil and lower half of the floor of the fourth ventricle. They then loop superiorly at the caudal pole of the tonsil (caudal loop) to ascend in the fissure as far as the upper pole of the tonsil, and then loop again inferiorly over the inferior medullary velum (cranial loop). Branches of the artery radiate outward from the borders of the tonsils to supply the suboccipital surface of the cerebellum. Most of the venous blood from this region drains anteriorly into the superior petrosal sinus through the vein of the cerebellopontine fissure, although some drains posteriorly into the tentorial sinuses converging on the torcular Herophili. The vein of the cerebellomedullary fissure originates on the lateral edge of the nodule and uvula and courses laterally near the telovelar junction to reach the cerebellopontine angle.

Surgical Technique
SURGICAL APPROACH

The safest and most direct approach to the fourth ventricle is the midline suboccipital approach. The operative corridor to the fourth ventricle using this approach is somewhat superiorly directed. Preoperatively, all imaging and labs should be reviewed carefully. Antibiotics should be given with incision. Preoperative treatment with steroids can decrease vasogenic edema, alleviate headache and neck pain, decrease the incidence and severity of aseptic meningitis and the posterior fossa syndrome, and decrease nausea and vomiting allowing for better hydration and nutrition prior to surgery. It is helpful to have an automatic retractor system available.

Intraoperative monitoring may be helpful if there is danger of violating the brain stem or cranial nerves. The most sensitive measure of alteration of brain stem function is the pulse and blood pressure, since cardiovascular reflexes are mediated by structures near the fourth ventricle such as the nucleus tractus solitarius and dorsal motor nucleus of the vagus. Any alterations in vital signs while working near the floor of the fourth ventricle should be considered a serious warning sign to stop manipulation. The best option for direct monitoring of brain-stem function is brain-stem auditory-evoked potentials (BAEP), in which an auditory click is measured at earlobe and vertex electrodes. This produces five waves that correspond, respectively, to the proximal cochlear nerve, distal cochlear nerve, cochlear nucleus, superior olive, and lateral lemniscus/inferior colliculus. Evidence of pontomesencephalic transmission of the impulse implies that the brain stem has not been compromised. However, this pathway is fairly lateral and may be preserved in spite of serious damage to the central core of the brain stem. Another monitoring technique, somatosensory evoked potentials (SSEP), follows sensory signals through the medial lemniscus, but this is also some distance from the floor of the fourth ventricle, and SSEP is even less sensitive than BAEP. Finally, EMG with direct stimulation of the facial nerve or lateral rectus can be used to verify integrity of the cranial motor nerves if tumor abuts or envelops them.

There are three possibilities for positioning: prone, lateral oblique, or sitting. The prone position is optimal for very young children, but there is some controversy over which is the best position for older children and adults. Each of the positions requires the head to be pinned using a Mayfield or Sugita head holder as long as the patient is more than 2 years old. The pins are coated with an antibiotic ointment and placed two centimeters above the ear in the unshaven scalp. It is important to avoid the squamous temporal bone and shunt tubing if present. Use of pins in infants can lead to skull penetration producing depressed fracture, dural laceration, hematoma, or postoperative abscess. Therefore, rather than using pins, very young children should be placed face down with the head on a padded horseshoe, ensuring there is no pressure on the eyes. All three positions require a certain amount of neck flexion, so caution should be used if there is known preexisting neck pathology, especially a craniocervical anomaly, spinal instability, significant cervical spondylosis, or herniation of the cerebellar tonsils on preoperative imaging.

The most commonly used position for the midline suboccipital approach (especially in very young patients) is the prone position, in which the patient is rolled after induction of anesthesia so that the face is toward the floor (Fig. 31-3). There are many advantages to this position: the anatomy is clearly visualized, it is easy for two to work together since one operator can stand on either side, and the multiple complications of the sitting position do not occur. The most significant disadvantage of the prone position is venous congestion that can lead to more significant blood loss, pooling of blood in the operative field, and soft tissue swelling of the face. This congestion is much worse if the head is rotated and flexed, and is improved somewhat by elevating the head above the level of the heart. Also, nasotracheal rather than orotracheal intubation can minimize compression of the base of tongue and impairment of venous drainage of the tongue and pharynx. The weight is distributed to minimize pressure points that can lead to skin breakdown and neuropathy, especially at the ulnar nerve at the elbow, common peroneal nerve across fibular head, and lateral femoral cutaneous nerve at the iliac crest. Two longitudinal padded roles are placed under the patient, and the knees and ankles are padded. The neck is placed in the "military tuck position" with moderate flexion of the upper cervical spine (to open up the space between the foramen magnum and the arch of C1) and less flexion of the lower cervical spine (to bring the occiput parallel with the patient's back). The chin and chest at least two fingers apart. Finally, the table is positioned so that the neck is parallel to floor and the head is above the heart. The shoulders can be gently retracted toward the feet with some tape, and a strap under the buttocks is helpful to prevent sliding. The surgeon and assistant then operate from either side using the microscope, and the scrub nurse's Mayfield table can be placed over the patient's back.

The lateral oblique or lateral decubitus position is similar to the prone position, except that the patient is lying on his or her side. This allows superior visualization of pathology high in the fourth ventricle, in the lateral recesses, and in the cerebellopontine angle. The posterior fossa contents do not sink inward as they do in the prone position and the operative distance is more comfortable for the surgeon. The principle disadvantage of the lateral oblique position is that the anatomy is not centered so the surgeon must visualize all structures rotated. Also, it is constantly necessary to support the upper cerebellar hemisphere to maintain exposure, although the lower hemisphere naturally falls away. The patient is placed on the side with the dependent arm ventral on the table. A soft roll or IV bag wrapped in foam is placed in the axilla of the dependent arm to prevent brachial plexus injury or vascular compression, and

the dependent leg is padded with special attention paid to the fibular head of the upper leg to avoid peroneal palsy.

The third option for positioning is the sitting position, in which the patient is positioned sitting upright so that the operative corridor is parallel to the floor (Fig. 31-4). The sitting position offers a very clear operative field since blood and cerebrospinal fluid drain out of the operative site. However, there are many risks to the sitting position.[1] The most significant dangers are cardiovascular instability and hypotension, air embolism, and subdural hematoma. All patients should have an agitated saline echocardiogram to exclude right to left shunt through a patent foramen ovale that could complicate air embolism and presence of such a shunt is an absolute contraindication for the sitting position. Precordial Doppler ultrasonic flow and end-tidal CO_2 should be monitored throughout the case. The risk of subdural hematoma is greatly increased by presence of a shunt, and if possible the shunt should be occluded prior to attempting an operation in the sitting position. Other risks of the sitting position include tension pneumocephalus, cervical myelopathy, thermal loss (especially in children), surgeon fatigue, and sudden loss of CSF from enlarged lateral and third ventricles after removal of a fourth ventricle mass lesion. When applying the head holder, the pin sites must be covered with Vaseline gauze to minimize entry of air[2] and the head taped to the head-holder for extra support in case the pins become dislodged. The patient is elevated slowly into the sitting position so that the foramen magnum is at the surgeon's eye level with both of the patient's legs flexed at the knees to prevent postoperative sciatica. The instrument table is placed over the patient's head. Infants too young for pins may be taped to a padded headrest to support the forehead and chin, but it is probably safer to use the prone position. Throughout the case the patient should be carefully monitored for signs of hypotension or air embolism. If air embolism occurs, the wound should

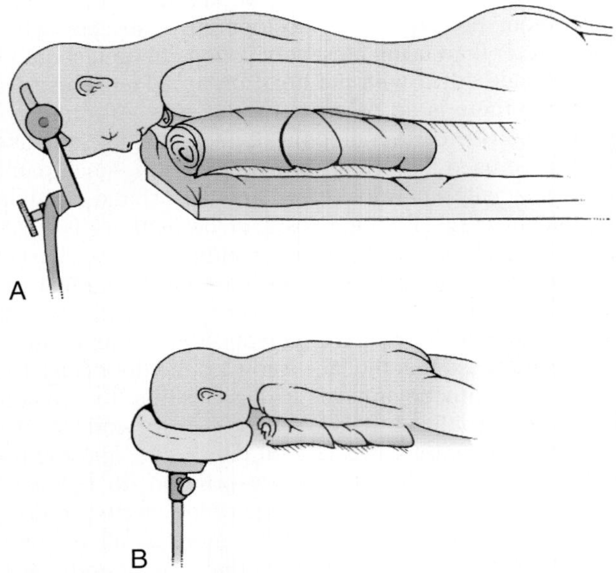

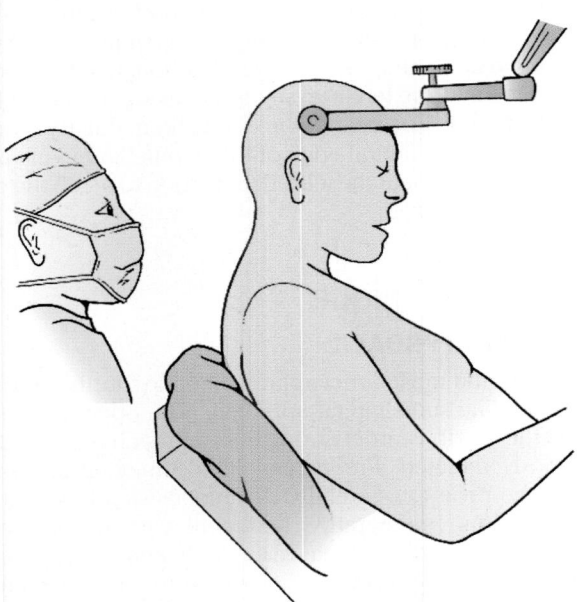

FIGURE 31-3 Prone position. The neck is in moderate flexion with the head higher than the heart. The surgeon and assistant stand on either side of the patient's neck. A, Skeletal fixation with a pin head holder. B, Padded horseshoe headrest for young patients. *(Modified from Cohen AR. Surgical Disorders of the Fourth Ventricle. Cambridge, MA: Blackwell Science; 1996.)*

FIGURE 31-4 Sitting position. Skeletal fixation is maintained using a pin head holder with the neck moderately flexed. *(Modified from Cohen AR. Surgical Disorders of the Fourth Ventricle. Cambridge, MA: Blackwell Science; 1996.)*

be packed with a saline-soaked sponge, and anesthesia should aspirate the atrial catheter to attempt to remove the embolus from the left atrium. If the embolus is severe, the patient should be placed in left decubitus position; otherwise, as soon as the patient is stable, the wound may be slowly exposed while covering the potential source of air with Gelfoam and Surgicel. If careful preparation is undertaken and complications dealt with promptly, the sitting position can be relatively safe.[3,4]

After positioning, the back of the head is shaved to expose the suboccipital region and the scalp degreased with acetone and alcohol then cleansed with a povidine iodine solution. A linear midline incision is outlined 1-2 cm above the external occipital protuberance down to the level of C4. The operative field is walled off with towels, draped with iodoform adhesive, and infiltrated with 0.25% lidocaine with 1/400,000 epinephrine (or 0.1% lidocaine with 1/1,000,000 epinephrine in infants less than 1 year old). If there is concern that it will be necessary to rapidly decompress the lateral ventricles intraoperatively or postoperatively, a burr hole may be drilled in the right posterior parietal region.

The incision is made with a number 10 blade applying firm digital compression, and bleeding points are coagulated (Fig. 31-5). The incision should be midline, but if the tumor is lateral, a hockey-stick incision can be used to allow for a wider craniectomy. The skin is undermined superficial to the fascia on both sides of the superior half of incision in preparation to create a fascial flap for closure (Fig. 31-6). The skin is then elevated with toothed forceps or a skin hook and a plane of dissection developed with knife or monopolar coagulation, sparing the occipital artery and nerve whenever possible. Even a slight deviation off midline will produce brisk bleeding from the muscles once deeper tissues are exposed. When anatomical landmarks are identified to confirm that the operative course is truly midline, cerebellar or Weitlaner retractors are placed to maintain

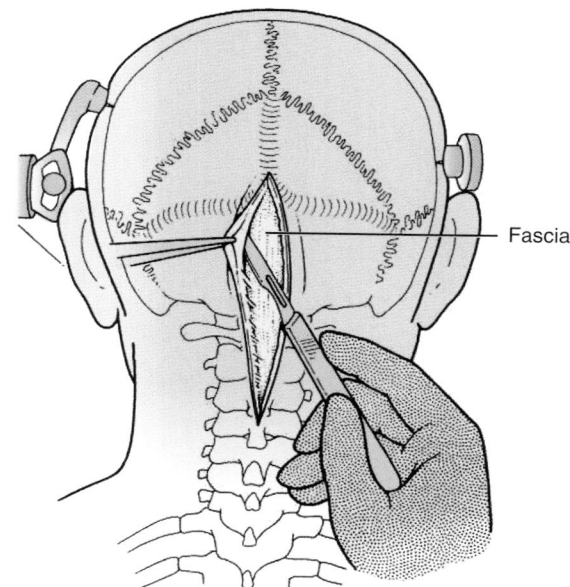

FIGURE 31-6 Fascial exposure. Skin flaps are mobilized by undermining the subcutaneous plane to prepare a fascial flap for closure. *(Modified from Cohen AR. Surgical Disorders of the Fourth Ventricle. Cambridge, MA: Blackwell Science; 1996.)*

exposure. As deeper layers are exposed, curved retractors may be used.

Next, the fascia is incised using a Y-shaped incision, keeping the lateral ends of the Y below the ligamentous insertion (Fig. 31-7). While a linear midline fascial incision without the upper limbs of the Y allows use of the avascular plane between the splenius capitus and semispinalis capitis muscles, it is often difficult to reapproximate such an incision tightly at the superior nuchal line. Muscle flaps

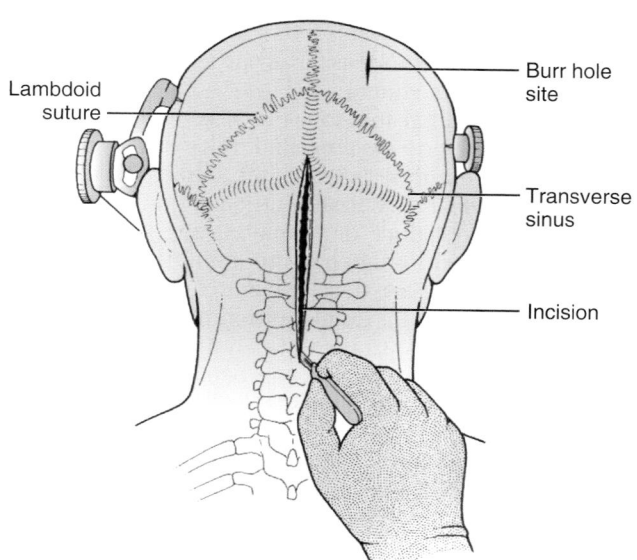

FIGURE 31-5 Skin Incision. The midline linear incision extends from just above the inion to the midcervical region. *(Modified from Cohen AR. Surgical Disorders of the Fourth Ventricle. Cambridge, MA: Blackwell Science; 1996.)*

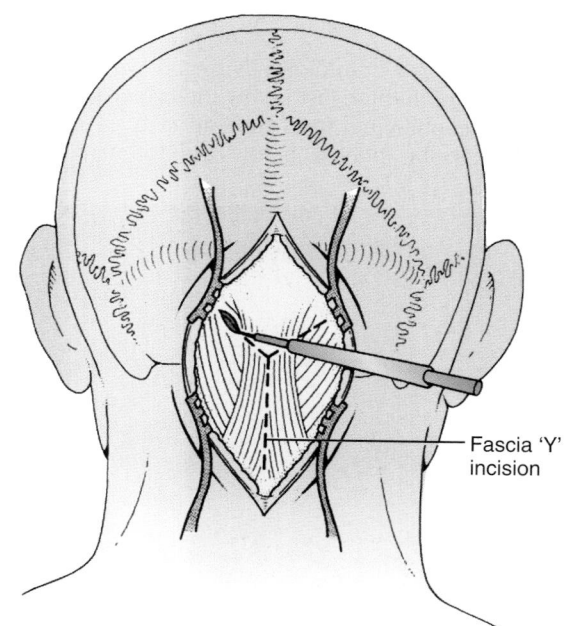

FIGURE 31-7 Fascial incision. The fascia and muscle are incised in the shape of a Y. The inferior limb of the Y passes through the avascular ligamentum nuchae. *(Modified from Cohen AR. Surgical Disorders of the Fourth Ventricle. Cambridge, MA: Blackwell Science; 1996.)*

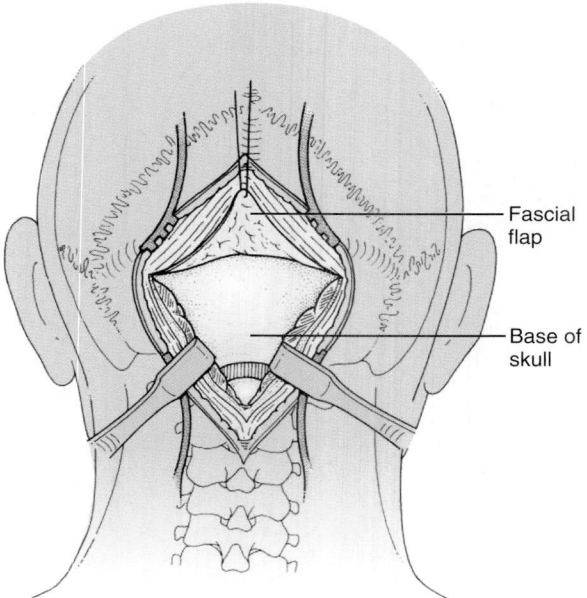

Fascial
flap

Base of
skull

FIGURE 31-8 Bony exposure. The occipital bone at the base of the skull is exposed widely using monopolar cautery and periosteal elevators. *(Modified from Cohen AR. Surgical Disorders of the Fourth Ventricle. Cambridge, MA: Blackwell Science; 1996.)*

are then developed with monopolar cautery and periosteal elevators, stripping the muscle from the bone as far as the mastoid emissary vein. This exposure is maintained with two curved cerebellar retractors and the rostral flap is placed under tension using a 3-0 silk suture to reflect it rostrally (Fig. 31-8). The muscle insertions are stripped off the spinous process and laminae of C2. Finally, the junction between the pericranium and dura at the foramen magnum is sharply dissected, and then the posterior fossa dura separated from the inner table of the occipital bone using a curette.

The suboccipital craniotomy is begun with burr holes on either side of midline just below the transverse sinuses, about three centimeters from midline (Fig. 31-9). A third burr hole can be placed below the torcular in older

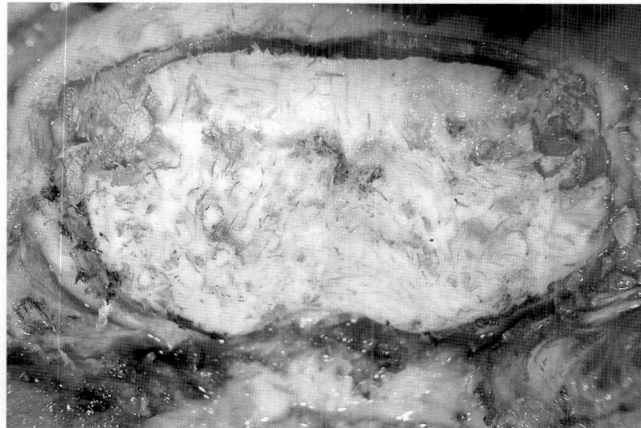

FIGURE 31-9 Suboccipital craniotomy. Burr holes are placed and a high speed drill is used to connect them. The bone flap is elevated after the dura is carefully stripped. *(Modified from Cohen AR. Surgical Disorders of the Fourth Ventricle. Cambridge, MA: Blackwell Science; 1996.)*

patients. In children, the dura is not firmly adherent to the skull so it is safe to drill close to or even on top of the sinuses, but more caution must be used with adults. The dura near the burr hole is then stripped using a Penfield and the bone removed using a high speed. The superior and lateral limits of the craniotomy are the transverse and sigmoid sinuses (Fig. 31-10). Inferiorly, the craniotomy should always include the posterior edge of the foramen magnum to prevent laceration of the brain against the closed bony rim when cerebellar elements are retracted downward and minimize damage from herniation if hematoma or swelling should occur postoperatively. The midline bone is removed last since it is often very vascular and contains a keel that can be quite deep. This keel must be stripped of dura with a Penfield, using extreme caution near the occipital sinus in the midline and the annular sinus near the foramen magnum. All exposed bone edges should be waxed, especially in the sitting position. Because of the irregular contour of the inner bone surface in adult patients, it is sometimes necessary perform a craniectomy rather than a craniotomy, removing the bone in a piecemeal fashion.

To expose the posterior arch of C1, the soft tissues overlying it are reflected laterally using a small periosteal elevator, stripping the inferior arch first since the vertebral artery is on its superior aspect. It is sometimes easier to do this after C2 has been exposed. The periosteum can sometimes be swept off the arch of C1 using an index finger covered with gauze. Monopolar cautery should be used with caution when dissecting the soft tissue over C1 (especially at the superolateral surface) to prevent injury to vertebral artery. It is important to remember that C1 can be bifid and is often cartilaginous in infants and young children. C1 laminectomy is helpful for lesions that herniate beneath the foramen magnum. To remove the lamina, small angled curettes can be used to strip the deep surface of the bone, and then the bone itself removed with an angled Kerrison punch or Leksell rongeur (Fig. 31-11). Because extending a laminectomy below C2 in young children increases the risk of swan neck deformity,[5] it is prudent to remove the smallest amount of bone possible. For most tumors, it is usually only necessary to remove as far as one level above the most caudal aspect of the tumor.

Prior to the dural incision, the wound should be irrigated and retractor systems and microscope prepared (Fig. 31-12). If the dura is tense, the intracranial pressure can be reduced with external ventricular drainage (if available), hyperventilation, or mannitol, although mannitol should be used with caution in the sitting position as it has been implicated in the development of subdural hematomas. All techniques for dural incision require crossing the occipital and annular sinuses, which may be very large in infants under age 2 years and can persist until 25 years of age. A Y-shaped incision allows wide visualization and can be extended if necessary (Fig. 31-13). One superior limb should be incised first with a number-15 blade. The incision should start just inferior to the transverse sinus and travel obliquely to the midline, stopping short of the occipital sinus. The other superior limb is incised next, and then they are connected over the midline. If there is significant bleeding from the midline occipital sinus, it should be controlled with obliquely placed hemostatic clips or suture ligatures (Fig. 31-14). Either way, both the superficial and deep layer

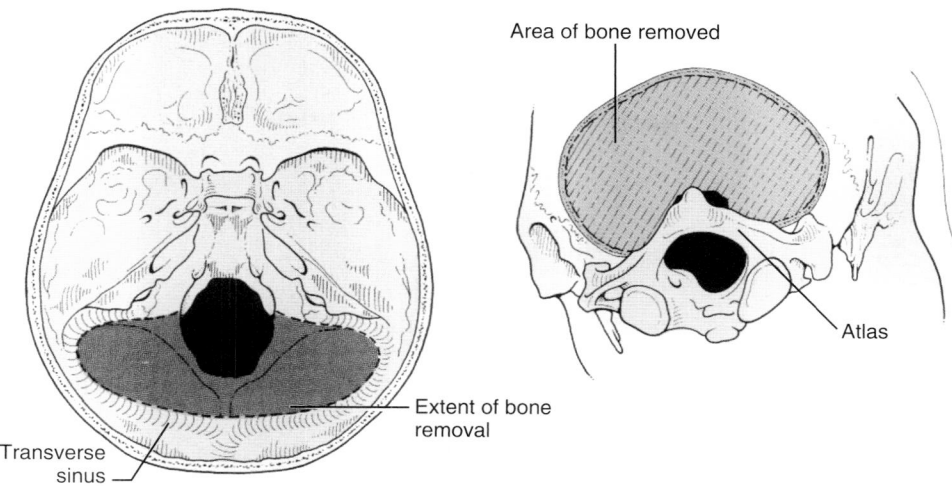

Area of bone removed

Extent of bone removal

Transverse sinus

Atlas

FIGURE 31-10 Suboccipital craniotomy. The craniotomy may be extended supriorly to the transverse sinus, laterally to the sigmoid sinuses, and inferiorly to the foramen magnum. *(Modified from Cohen AR. Surgical Disorders of the Fourth Ventricle. Cambridge, MA: Blackwell Science; 1996.)*

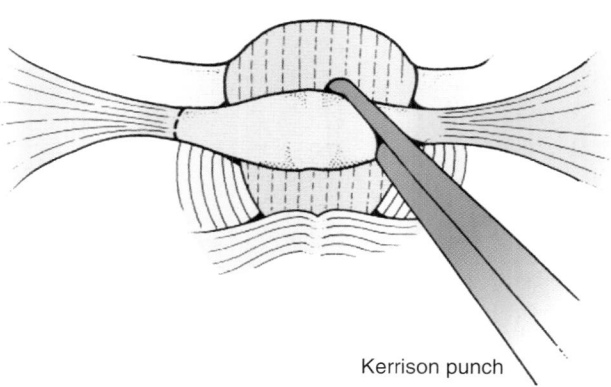

Kerrison punch

FIGURE 31-11 Removal of atlas (C1). This step may facilitate removal of some fourth ventricular tumors. To prevent injury to an aberrant vertebral artery, it is best to avoid use of monopolar cautery near the arches of C1 and C2. *(Modified from Cohen AR. Surgical Disorders of the Fourth Ventricle. Cambridge, MA: Blackwell Science; 1996.)*

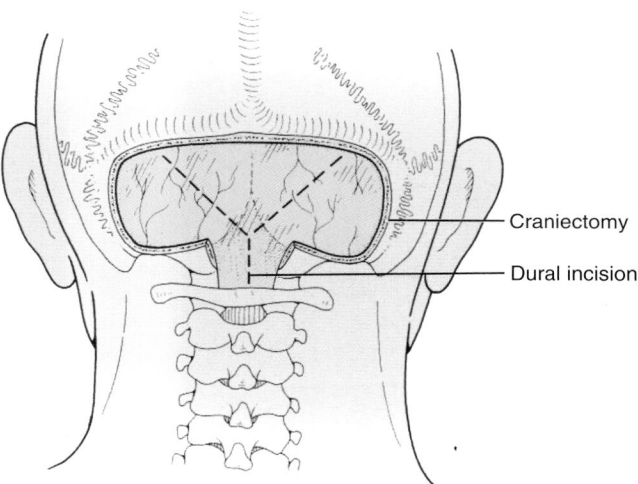

Craniectomy

Dural incision

FIGURE 31-13 Dural incision. The vertical limb of the Y-shaped incision, which overlies the occipital sinus, is opened last. *(Modified from Cohen AR. Surgical Disorders of the Fourth Ventricle. Cambridge, MA: Blackwell Science; 1996.)*

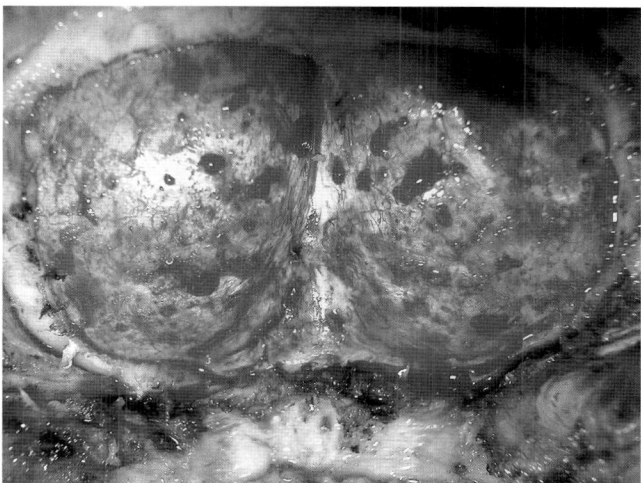

FIGURE 31-12 Dural exposure after removal of bone flap. The arch of C1 has been preserved in this patient.

of the dura must be incised or the sinus will be tented open. The vertical limb of the Y is opened last using scissors so that the dura can be tented if bleeding is seen. The vertical incision extends to the foramen magnum so that it will extend below the falx cerebelli, which is occasionally present in childhood. If bleeding is very troublesome, the dura can be opened paramidline. The dura is then covered with a moist collagen sponge or wet Gelfoam sandwich to prevent desiccation and anchored to the fascia with 4-0 neurolon suture. This allows wide exposure of the cerebellar vermis and hemispheres (Figs. 31-15 and 31-16). The arachnoid is opened next over the cisterna magna to allow drainage of CSF (Fig. 31-17). If the tumor is in the cerebellar hemisphere, another dural incision can be extended laterally to more fully expose the involved cerebellum.

Techniques for intradural exposure and resection of the tumor will vary depending upon the location and size of the tumor, and will be discussed in more detail for each individual tumor. Gentle separation of the cerebellar tonsils

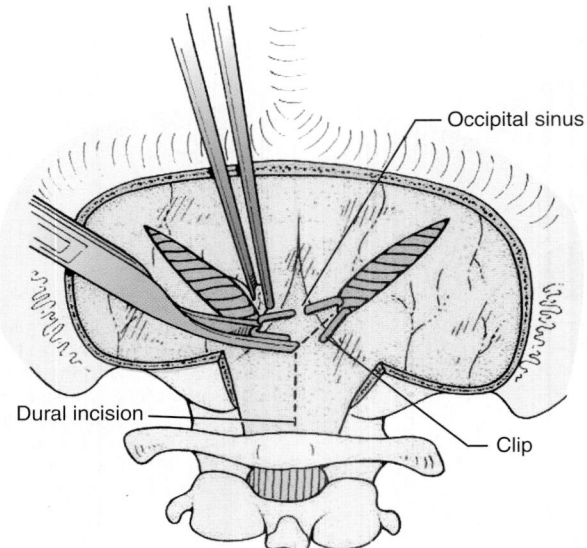

FIGURE 31-14 Control of bleeding from occipital sinus with clips. *(Modified from Cohen AR. Surgical Disorders of the Fourth Ventricle. Cambridge, MA: Blackwell Science; 1996.)*

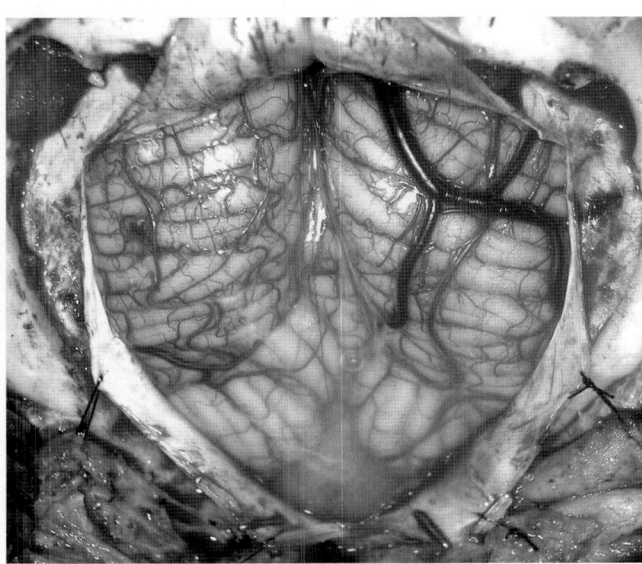

FIGURE 31-16 Exposure of cerebellar hemispheres and vermis. The tumor (in this case a medulloblastoma) can be seen between the hemispheric tonsils in the lower midline of the exposure.

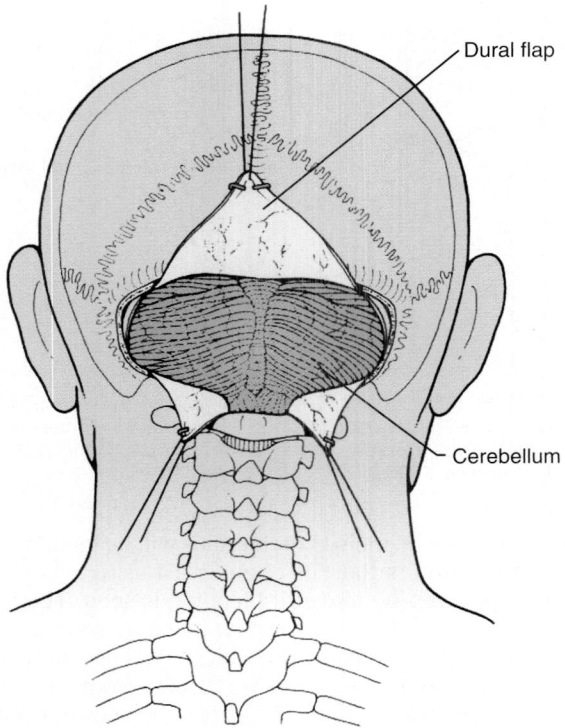

FIGURE 31-15 Exposure of cerebellar hemispheres and vermis. *(Modified from Cohen AR. Surgical Disorders of the Fourth Ventricle. Cambridge, MA: Blackwell Science; 1996.)*

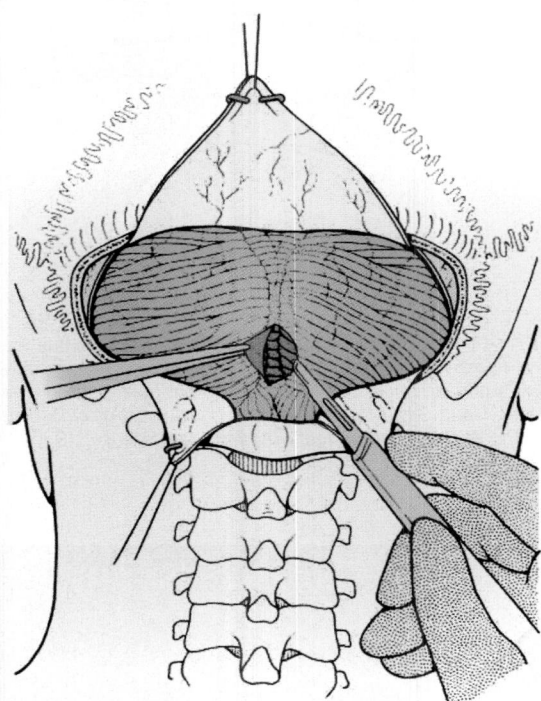

FIGURE 31-17 Opening the cisterna magna. This allows drainage of CSF and relaxes the posterior fossa. *(Modified from Cohen AR. Surgical Disorders of the Fourth Ventricle. Cambridge, MA: Blackwell Science; 1996.)*

will expose the cerebellomedullary fissure through the opened vallecula giving an unimpeded view of the inferior roof of the fourth ventricle (Fig. 31-18). Narrow malleable automatic retractors can be used to maintain separation of the tonsils; the retractor system should be kept close to the patient so as not to interfere with the subsequent operation. The operating microscope is brought into the field

and the anatomy is identified. In particular, the location of the caudal loops of PICA should be carefully noted since they are often tethered to the tonsils and the walls of the cerebellomedullary fissure by small perforating branches. The foramen of Magendie and the small tuft of choroid plexus protruding from it will be clearly seen, as well as any tumor that protrudes from the foramen. The thin layers forming the lower part of the roof can be opened to expose

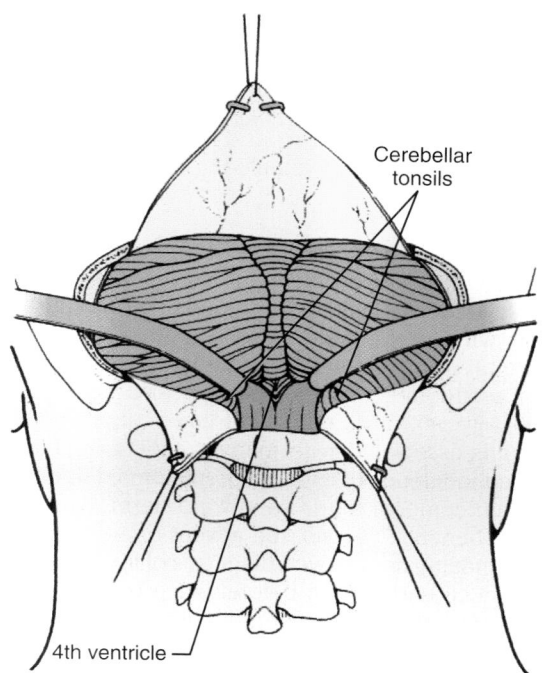

FIGURE 31-18 Exposure of the fourth ventricle. Retraction of the cerebellar tonsils widens the vallecula which allows visualization of the caudal fourth ventricle. Automatic retractors may be used to facilitate exposure. *(Modified from Cohen AR. Surgical Disorders of the Fourth Ventricle. Cambridge, MA: Blackwell Science; 1996.)*

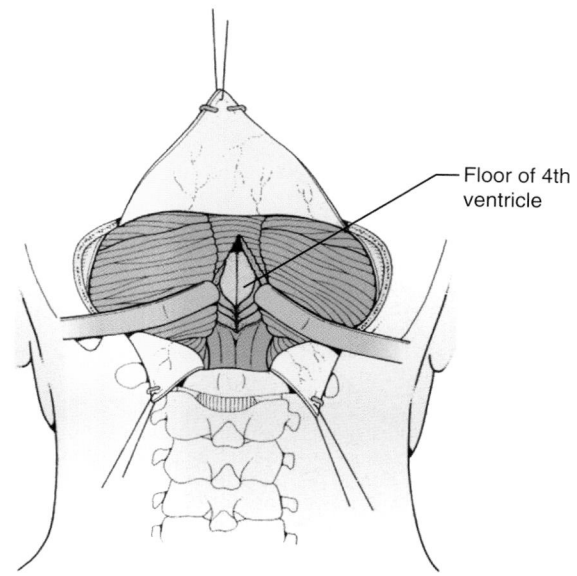

FIGURE 31-19 Splitting the vermis. Incision of the cerebellar vermis allows exposure of lesions situated more rostrally. Alternatively, some fourth ventricular tumors can be approached without splitting the vermis by opening the cerebromedullary fissure on each side. *(Modified from Cohen AR. Surgical Disorders of the Fourth Ventricle. Cambridge, MA: Blackwell Science; 1996. Reproduced with permission from Cohen AR., 1996.)*

the cavity of the fourth ventricle. Often this will provide sufficient exposure, but if not, it is sometimes helpful to retract the inferior vermis rostrally or incise the caudal vermis, avoiding the gutter between the vermis and the hemisphere to prevent injury to the inferior vermian veins there (Fig. 31-19). Lateral lesions may require removal of one tonsil by dividing the pedicle attaching the superolateral margin of the tonsil to the biventral lobule. To reach the lateral roof or lateral recess, part of the cerebellar hemisphere can be resected without significant morbidity as long as the dentate nuclei are not violated. If the tumor is not adherent to the floor of the fourth ventricle, cottonoid patties should be placed beneath the tumor to protect the delicate brain-stem structures just beneath the floor. These cottonoids should be placed under direct vision and never used as a tool to dissect the tumor from the floor of the fourth ventricle. After the tumor has been removed, the glistening white floor of the fourth ventricle should be clearly visible. The retractors are then removed and the cerebellar hemispheres allowed to fall back into place. If there is extension of the tumor through one of the foramina of Luschka into the cerebellopontine cistern, the ipsilateral tonsil and cerebellar hemisphere can be retracted medially to expose it. Sometimes it is necessary to do a secondary retromastoid approach to completely resect the tumor.

The dura is closed using a running 4-0 neurolon or polypropylene after approximating the dural edges with interrupted sutures (Fig. 31-20). A Valsalva maneuver will identify potentially dangerous venous bleeding. The dural closure should be watertight if possible, starting peripherally then working centrally to gradually overcome the tension. If the dura is not watertight, there is increased risk of

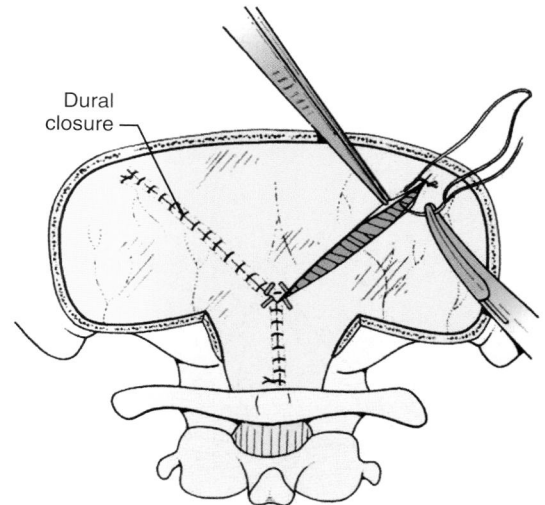

FIGURE 31-20 Dural closure. After the pathology is removed and hemostasis is obtained, the Y incision is closed with a running suture, starting peripherally. The lower midline limb is closed last. *(Modified from Cohen AR. Surgical Disorders of the Fourth Ventricle. Cambridge, MA: Blackwell Science; 1996.)*

pseudomeningocele due to a ball-valve effect or hydrocephalus from arachnoid adhesions produced by blood from the muscles. Sometimes the dura will be dried and shrunken by the end of the case, especially if measures have been taken to obliterate the occipital sinus. In this case, the remaining defect can be covered with a pericranial or fascial graft (Fig. 31-21). Freeze-dried bovine pericardium or human allograft dura can also be used, but use of autogenous material is less likely to produce postoperative aseptic meningitis.[6] If clips were used on the midline occipital sinus, they

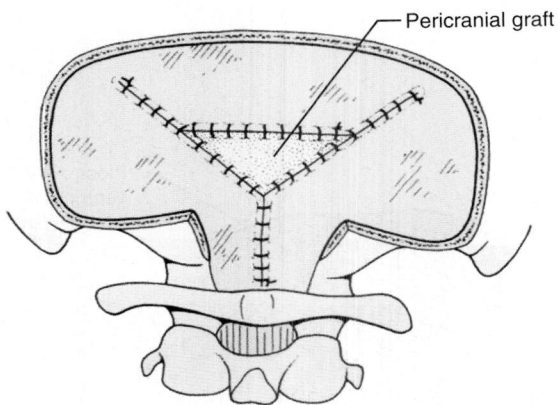

FIGURE 31-21 Use of a dural graft. If the dura cannot be easily brought together, a graft of pericranium or fascia can be used to complete the closure. (*Modified from Cohen AR. Surgical Disorders of the Fourth Ventricle. Cambridge, MA: Blackwell Science; 1996.*)

can be removed as the dura is sutured. The suture line may be covered with thrombin-soaked Gelfoam. If a craniotomy was performed, the bone flap can be secured with wires, plates and screws, or sutures. Alternatively, the defect can be covered with a titanium screen held in place by gently compressing the screen and allowing it to insert itself between the dura and inner margins of the bony defect. The fascia is closed with interrupted absorbable sutures to approximate the muscle and fascia (Fig. 31-22). If the fascia is dried and difficult to approximate, the skeletal fixation apparatus can be loosened and the neck extended to facilitate closure. An adequate amount of tissue must be left at the superior fascial flap to prevent buttonholes at superior nuchal line. The scalp is then closed in layers, ending with a subcutaneous

reapproximation using interrupted absorbable sutures with inverted knots. If in the sitting position, all layers should start from the caudal end of the wound so that the tails do not hang in the way. The wound is then closed with sutures or staples (Fig. 31-23). The wound is covered with a sterile dressing and the patient extubated in a supine position.

COMPLICATIONS

Hydrocephalus is common with fourth ventricular tumors, and is one of the most significant causes of morbidity and mortality associated with these tumors.[7,8] In the past, many patients with tumors and hydrocephalus underwent temporizing preoperative shunting to treat hydrocephalus and prevent pseudomeningocele, CSF leak, and meningitis from fistula. However, more recently it has been observed that shunting is associated with many complications, and the increased incidence of subdural hematoma, infection, and brain-stem compression from upward herniation may outweigh its benefits.[9-12] Also, the advent of advanced radiographic imaging has allowed diagnosis of fourth ventricular tumors much earlier than before, when patients were frequently moribund with dehydration and malnutrition from vomiting and hydrocephalus needed to be urgently treated. Today, only about 10% to 20% of patients with cerebellar and posterior fossa tumors require permanent shunting[7,8,13] and most of these have slow-growing tumors such as astrocytoma since more acute tumors distend the ventricles for a short period of time and do not allow outlet adhesions to form. Risk factors for shunt dependence include younger age, larger preoperative ventricle size, and more extensive tumors. In many cases, preoperative high dose steroids will produce satisfactory improvement in hydrocephalus. Otherwise, an appropriate alternative to shunting is perioperative

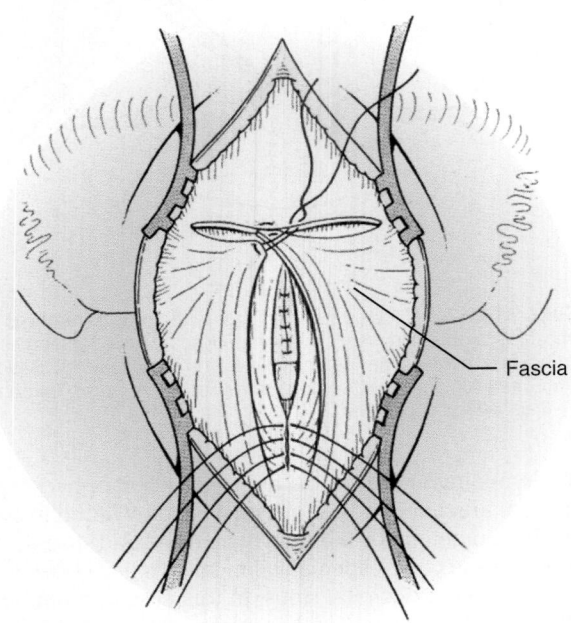

FIGURE 31-22 Fascial closure. The muscle and fascia are closed in layers using interrupted absorbable sutures. (*Modified from Cohen AR. Surgical Disorders of the Fourth Ventricle. Cambridge, MA: Blackwell Science; 1996.*)

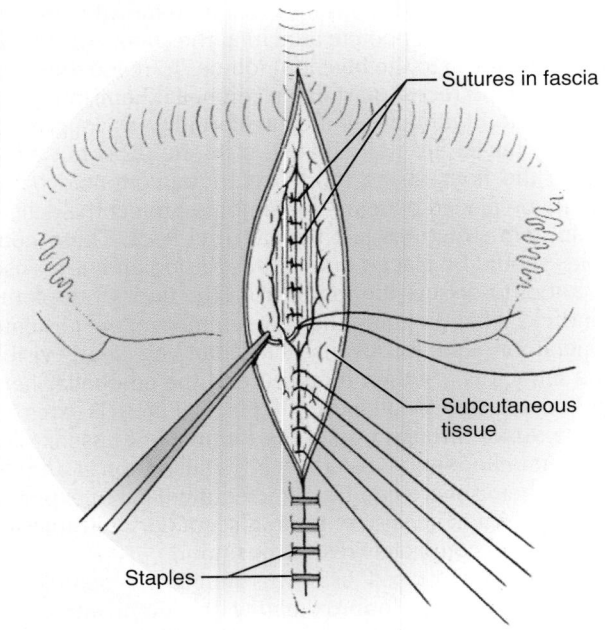

FIGURE 31-23 Skin closure. After closing the subcutaneous layer with interrupted inverted absorbable sutures, the skin is closed with staples or monofilament nylon suture material. (*Modified from Cohen AR. Surgical Disorders of the Fourth Ventricle. Cambridge, MA: Blackwell Science; 1996.*)

external ventricular drainage,[14] especially if a patient presents lethargic or obtunded. This allows for precise pressure monitoring and control of drainage rate to prevent upward herniation and, if continued postoperatively, clearance of debris, proteinaceous blood, and air from the operation. Although external ventricular drainage does reduce the necessity to use permanent shunts, the infection rate may be as high as 10%, so it should be used judiciously. If a shunt is required for a malignant tumor, there may be an increased risk of extraneural metastasis through the shunt tubing (especially to the peritoneum),[15] although some studies have suggested that such metastases may occur as often in patients without shunts.[16]

Pneumocephalus in the ventricles and subdural space is common after fourth ventricular surgery, especially when patients are operated in the sitting position,[17] although it also occurs after prone operations. It is much more common when patients have preoperative hydrocephalus, and frequently results from overzealous drainage of CSF through an external ventricular drain intraoperatively. Since nitrous oxide can diffuse into air filled spaces, it is possible that nitrous oxide contributes to tension pneumocephalus, although this is controversial. If tension pneumocephalus is recognized intraoperatively, the patient should be placed in Trendelenburg position and the operative bed irrigated to replace air with the irrigating fluid. Symptomatic postoperative tension pneumocephalus can be treated with a small frontal burr hole to relieve the pressure caused by the trapped air. Intraventricular air may cause ventriculoperitoneal shunt malfunction due to airlock.

Postoperative pseudomeningoceles affect 10% to 15% of all children with posterior fossa tumors. Normally, these are small collections of fluid that respond well to serial lumbar punctures. Occasionally they can put the closure under tension and eventually produce a leak, which carries a risk of meningitis. Pseudomeningocele may be a manifestation of hydrocephalus and in some cases may require a CSF diversion shunt to control.

Aseptic meningitis, also called posterior fossa fever, is a rare occurrence after posterior fossa surgery, especially for epidermoids or dermoids that rupture intraoperatively leaking cholesterol cyst fluid, although it also occurs after resection of astrocytoma or medulloblastoma. It may be a presenting symptom preoperatively but much more common as a postoperative complication.[18,19] Patients usually present about 1 week after surgery with fever, headache, irritability, and CSF pleocytosis. It can be difficult in some cases to differentiate aseptic meningitis from true bacterial meningitis, which should always be carefully excluded before treating for aseptic meningitis. The condition resolves with steroid or anti-inflammatory treatment and serial lumbar punctures to remove CSF.

Transient or permanent cranial nerve palsies sometimes occur after surgery of the fourth ventricle. These deficits are usually immediately evident in the recovery room. The most common deficit is cranial VI and VII palsy caused by disruption of the fourth ventricular floor along the facial colliculus where the intrapontine course of the facial nerve loops around the abducens nucleus. If this area is dissected or excavated, the deficit will often be permanent, but even gentle diathermy with low-current bipolar can produce a partial paralysis with total or near-total recovery. In most cases, patients with temporary facial weakness should be treated to prevent corneal desiccation with artificial tears, temporary tarsorrhaphy, or gold-weight implantation in the upper eyelid. Permanent weakness has been treated with facial-hypoglossal anastemosis, which can partially restore upper eyelid function. Abducens palsy is best treated with an eye patch to prevent diplopia (or amblyopia if the patient is under 5 years of age); if the condition persists beyond a few months, eye muscle surgery may be appropriate. Cranial nerve XII palsy can occur from injury to the hypoglossal trigone. While less common than facial palsy, this is a very serious complication since it is usually bilateral since the nuclei are close together by the median raphe. Patients present with dysarthria, swallowing apraxia, and continuous drooling. When combined with cranial nerve VII or IX/X deficits, even aggressive treatment with tracheostomy and feeding tubes may not prevent serious complications due to aspiration.

Skewed ocular deviation is a rare condition that is sometimes seen after fourth ventricular surgery during which the aqueductal opening is manipulated. This usually occurs with damage to the region of the cerebral aqueduct. It is thought to occur because vertical yoking of eye movements involves pathways that pass through the periaqueductal gray matter in the mesencephalic tegmentum. This condition usually resolves within weeks after surgery, and can be avoided by gentleness when working around the aqueduct.

The "posterior fossa syndrome," also called posterior fossa mutism or pseudobulbar palsy, is characterized by the delayed onset of mutism, emotional lability, and supranuclear lesions that occurs within a few days after midline posterior fossa operations.[20] The syndrome has been seen in as many as 15% of intraventricular approaches to lesions near the brain stem, but has also been described with supracerebellar infratentorial approach to the pineal region and retromastoid lateral cerebellar approach to the side or front of the brain stem. Patients present with global confusion, disorientation, combativeness, paranoia, or visual hallucinations. They are generally alert and will follow simple commands, but will sometimes refuse to speak or present scanning speech. Orofacial apraxia, drooling, dysphagia, pharyngeal dysfunction, and flat affect are common, but there is no actual weakness, hence the term pseudobulbar palsy. Because of the delay in onset, it has been suggested that edema from operative manipulation may play a role, for example through transmission of retractor pressure from the medial cerebellum through fiber pathways along the middle and superior cerebellar peduncles into the upper pons and midbrain. There are no consistent neuropathologic findings, and most patients have some improvement over several weeks to months.[20-22]

Generalized and focal seizures have been described after posterior fossa surgery. The incidence is higher in faster growing tumors and in the presence of ventricular drainage or shunting. Late-onset seizures may be related to remote hemorrhage, meningitis, or hydrocephalus.

Ipsilateral limb ataxia, dysmetria, dysdiadokinesis, and hypotonia usually results from damage to the cerebellar hemisphere, especially the dentate nucleus, which is located along the superolateral margin of the roof of the fourth ventricle adjacent to the upper pole of the tonsil. Most injuries to the dentate nucleus occur during dissection of a hemispheric tumor. Retraction during dissection of the superior vermis can injure the superior cerebellar peduncle (which) producing similar symptoms. Unless the dentate is completely ablated, most patients recover well within a few months with only minor residual intention tremor that does not interfere with motor development.

Since the superior and inferior cerebellar peduncles make up the lateral walls of the superior roof of the fourth ventricle, they are susceptible to damage during intraventricular procedures. The superior cerebellar peduncle contains pathways connecting the dentate nucleus to the red nucleus and thalamus, so damage to the superior cerebellar peduncle produces a similar clinical syndrome to damage of the dentate nucleus with ipsilateral ataxia and intention tremor. Injury to the inferior cerebellar peduncle produces a syndrome similar to ablation of the flocculonodular lobe with equilibrium disturbances, truncal ataxia, staggering gait, and oscillation of head and trunk on assuming erect position without ataxia of voluntary movement of the extremities. Injury to the middle cerebellar peduncle (which causes ataxia and dysmetria) is rare during intraventricular procedures, but can occur during an approach to the cerebellopontine cistern.

Postoperative dysarthria can result when resections extend into paravermian part of cerebellar hemisphere. This occurs more frequently from left hemisphere injury than from vermal or right hemisphere injury.

Acute urinary retention is an uncommon complication of dissection of the fourth ventricular floor near the striae medullaris, presumably due to injury to the pontine micturition center in the pontine tegmentum, the structure that integrates the cortex with sacral and pelvic sensory pathways that apprise bladder filling status.[23] Patients with this condition demonstrate inability to initiate voiding in spite of a full bladder with high intravesicular pressure. Since the pontine micturition center is deep in the pons near the reticular activating system, this symptom is usually associated with a disturbance in sensorium, but can occur in conscious patients. It is usually reversible but does not respond to detrusor augmenting agents or alpha-adrenergic blockers. Patients are best managed by intermittent catheterization.

Patients treated with radiation sometimes have significant learning disabilities,[24] and should undergo follow-up neuropsychiatric evaluation. Radiation treatment has also been associated with endocrine dysfunction, growth dysfunction, hypothyroidism, delayed or precocious puberty, and secondary malignancy.[25] Patients that have extensive laminectomies are predisposed to development of swan-neck deformity, and should be kept in a soft cervical collar for 6 to 8 weeks until the paraspinal muscles reattach and monitored with cervical spine x-rays every few months for a few years to check for spinal deformities.

Injury to major vessels is rare with fourth ventricular surgery. The most likely artery to be injured is PICA. Most patients with PICA injury present with postoperative flocculonodular dysfunction with nausea, vomiting, nystagmus, vertigo, and inability to stand or walk without appendicular dysmetria. Venous injury is extremely rare even if veins are sacrificed due to diffuse anastomosis in this region. Veins near the tonsils, vermis, and inferior roof can be safely sacrificed. Medial retraction of the cerebellar hemisphere to expose the lateral recess and cerebellopontine cistern can stretch bridging veins to the sigmoid sinus, but it is seldom necessary to sacrifice these. Most venous infarctions of the posterior fossa have followed sacrifice of the petrosal veins or veins of the cerebellomesencephalic fissure (including the precentral cerebellar vein).

Specific Tumors

MEDULLOBLASTOMA

The term "medulloblastoma" was initially introduced by Bailey and Cushing who noted the highly cellular architecture of small round basophilic cells that showed various degrees of differentiation along neuronal and glial lines. They assumed that the cell of origin (the "medulloblast") was a primitive cell capable of both neural and glial differentiation.[26] More recently, it has been theorized that these are related to tumors with similar histology in other locations, such as the pineal gland (pineoblastoma), ependyma (ependymoblastoma), retina (retinoblastoma), and elsewhere (neuroblastoma). The term "primitive neuroectodermal tumor" (PNET) was used to describe these tumors. A medulloblastoma would therefore be described as a PNET of the fourth ventricle.

Medulloblastoma is the most common malignant primary brain tumor in children, accounting for 20% to 25% of all childhood primary brain tumors and 40% of all childhood posterior fossa tumors.[27,28] Peak incidence is 3 to 5 years of age; half of all medulloblastoma patients are under 10 years of age at diagnosis, and three quarters are under age 15. Medulloblastoma is uncommon in infancy, and less than 5% of patients present under 1 year of age. There is a second peak between 20 and 40 years so that medulloblastoma accounts for 5% of all adult posterior fossa tumors and 1% of all adult brain tumors. Adult medulloblastomas are more likely to be hemispheric than midline, likely due to the lateral migration of cells of the granular layer of cerebellum from the inferior medullary velum. Adult medulloblastomas are also more likely to be cystic or necrotic, have poorly defined margins and less contrast enhancement.[29] They may even involve the cerebellar surface and resemble meningiomas. There is a slight male preponderance in most clinical series, and for reasons that are unclear, medulloblastomas have a significantly higher incidence in North America than elsewhere in the world.[30] Medulloblastomas frequently metastasize in the subarachnoid space, and some dissemination is evident in 20% to 30% of all patients and 50% of young patients at diagnosis.[31,32] Familial medulloblastoma has been reported.[33]

Medulloblastomas grow quickly, so onset of symptoms is usually fairly acute; most patients are symptomatic less than 2 months before the tumor is diagnosed, and very few report symptoms for longer than 6 months. Most patients initially experience symptoms of increased intracranial pressure from CSF obstruction. Symptoms typically begin with intermittent headache (often worst in the morning) followed by vomiting and eventually gait problems.[34] Gait difficulties include wide-based gait and inability to tandem walk; these findings are often subtle and not appreciated by the child or the parents but frequently alert the physician to the presence of a neurologic lesion. Clinical signs include ataxia for midline tumors or dysmetria/dysdiadokinesia for lateral tumors. Most patients have papilledema by the time they present for evaluation. Less common signs include diplopia from abducens palsy, facial paresis or lower cranial nerve palsy from tumor invasion, or head tilt from tumor extension into the upper spinal canal or impaction of the cerebellar tonsils at the foramen magnum against the first two cervical nerve roots. Since medulloblastomas can metastasize along the subarachnoid space, some patients present with cranial or spinal nerve root symptoms from distant metastases or even seizures from cortical metastases. Patients who present with signs of metastatic disease have a limited life expectancy.

Medulloblastomas usually appear as midline solid tumors on neuroimaging, although cystic change is sometimes observed. Eighty-five percent are midline vermian lesions, usually arising from the vermis or inferior medullary velum and growing into the fourth ventricle, sometimes appearing to be entirely intraventricular.[32] Adult lesions are much more likely to be in a lateral location. CT demonstrates a homogeneous hyperdense lesion that enhances intensely and diffusely after contrast administration with occasional heterogeneously enhancing regions due to necrosis, although rarely medulloblastomas do not enhance at all on CT.[35] Calcification will be apparent in 10% of medulloblastomas,[36] but presence of calcium or cystic change is more typical of ependymomas. On MRI, the lesion is hypointense to isointense to the brain on T1 and hyperintense or hypointense on T2 with heterogeneous signal due to microcysts, necrotic cavities, tumor vessels, or calcification (Fig. 31-24). The tumor displays irregular enhancement with MRI contrast material,[36,37] and enhanced MRI will disclose small cortical or basal metastases in 5% to 10% of cases. The sagittal MRI can help delineate the relationship of the tumor to the vermis, midbrain tectum, vein of Galen, and cervicomedullary junction. Additionally, sagittal MRI can differentiate true intraventricular tumors from extraventricular vermian tumors: intraventricular tumors will widen the aqueduct and displace the quadrigeminal plate posterosuperiorly, while dorsal lesions will kink the quadrigeminal plate giving it a C-shaped appearance.[38] Infrequently, the tumor will be seen to extend out of foramen of Luschka, but this is far more typical of ependymomas. In young children, medulloblastomas are often radiographically indistinguishable from ependymomas by radiographic appearance alone. Because of the frequency of craniospinal metastases, all patients should get a contrasted MRI of the entire craniospinal axis.

Grossly, medulloblastomas are discrete, soft tumors, although adult lesions tend to be firmer and more adherent to leptomeninges. Medulloblastomas can be divided into two broad histologic patterns: classical and desmoplastic. Classical medulloblastomas, which make up three quarters of the total, are seen to have dense, diffusely monotonous sheets of cells with intensely basophilic nuclei and scant cytoplasm ("small round blue cells"). There is regional variability in the size and shape of cells, number of mitoses, and appearance of nuclei, and necrosis is common. Desmoplastic medulloblastomas have a higher proportion of fibrous stroma associated with the perivascular collagen skeleton of tumor. Sometimes there are uniform compact lines of cells around islands of relative hypocellularity; when this is seen, the compact rims stain heavily with reticulin and the hypocellular areas stain for GFAP. Occasionally individual cells resembling oligodendrocytes are seen, having

perinuclear halos and staining with tubulin and synaptophysin. The desmoplastic variant is more common in older patients. In young patients location is not associated with histology, but older patients are more likely to have desmoplastic histology in more lateral tumors.[39] In both histologic patterns there are occasionally neuroblastic areas with histology similar to neuroblastomas with Homer-Wright rosettes (rings of nuclei surrounding a central zone of fibrillary processes) and perivascular pseudorosettes that resemble those in ependymomas except that they do not stain for GFAP. Mature ganglion cells are sometimes seen, although it is controversial whether these represent further neuronal differentiation or engulfing of deep cerebellar nuclei by the tumor. Also seen are islands of glial development characterized by clusters of GFAP-staining cells with pink cytoplasm commonly seen as circular whirls of cells with bipolar processes. These may represent entrapped or reactive astrocytes.

To resect a medulloblastoma, the posterior fossa is exposed as described above. Since most medulloblastomas arise from the vermis or inferior medullary velum, the tumor will often be immediately visible either protruding through the foramen of Magendie or immediately deep to the vermis. If the tumor protrudes through the foramen, it often will fill the cisterna magna and even extend into the upper cervical canal. If the tumor is deep to the vermis, the tonsils will usually be displaced backward, and it may be necessary to retract the cerebellar tonsils or biventricular lobules using self-retraining retractors to visualize the inferior vermis. By exposing the cerebellomedullary fissure on each side it is sometimes possible to resect the tumor without dividing the cerebellar vermis, although sometimes midline incision of the vermis is necessary to obtain adequate exposure. Gentle retraction of the cerebellar hemispheres will expose the intraventricular tumor, which generally appears purple-gray, friable, and quite vascular.

Even with a vermian incision, it is seldom possible to expose the entire tumor. Therefore, the next step is to debulk the central portion of the tumor using blunt or sharp dissectors with microscissors and microsuction aspiration. Desmoplastic tumors cannot be aspirated with microsuction, so ultrasonic aspiration can be used for these tumors, but this must be used with caution around the brain stem because of increased destruction of tissue. Bleeding is controlled with bipolar cautery. To expedite removal of the tumor and minimize blood loss, the tumor can be divided into four quadrants; as soon as bleeding becomes troublesome from one quadrant, a micropatty is placed there and attention turned to a different quadrant, and so on. By the time the dissection returns to the first quadrant the bleeding will have slowed enough to allow continued resection. After the tumor has been debulked, the shell of tumor is carefully stripped off the brain stem from inferior to superior using a small brain retractor and separated from the brain stem using cottonoid patties. Cottonoid patties should be placed along the fourth ventricular floor as early as possible to protect the brain stem, and it is important to constantly ensure that the trajectory is correct to prevent diving into the brain stem at an angle. When the brain stem is protected with a cottonoid patty, the inferior half of the tumor can then be safely removed. The tumor is rarely adherent or invasive into the brain stem, but when it is, gross total

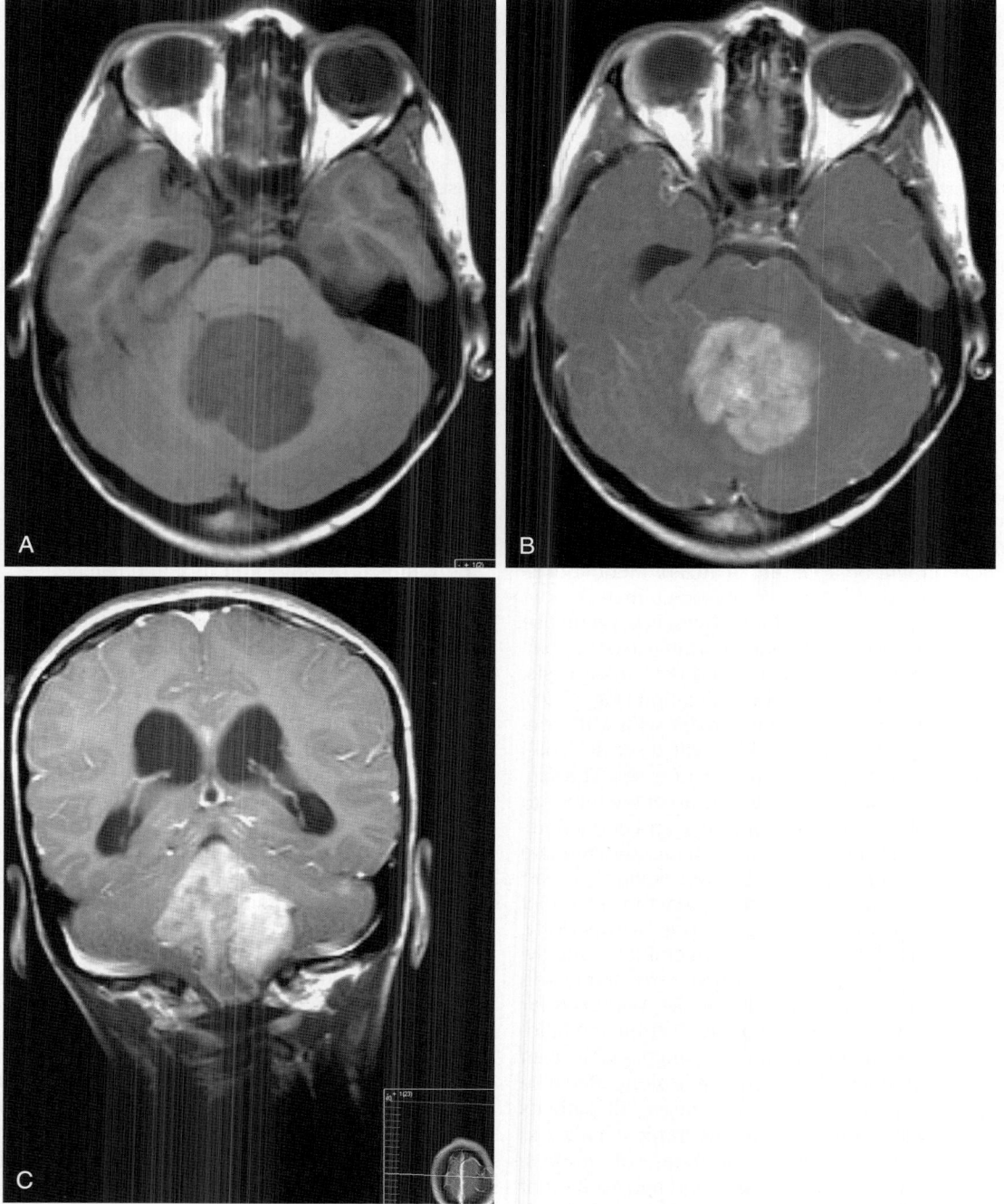

FIGURE 31-24 Medulloblastoma. A, T1 without contrast. The midline hypointense lesion usually arises from the inferior medullary velum. B, T1 with contrast. The lesion enhances brightly and heterogeneously. C, T1 with contrast, coronal section. The tumor is seen to fill the fourth ventricle and displace the cerebellar hemispheres laterally.

resection should not be attempted due to the risk of permanent cranial nerve defects. Rather, any focal areas of adhesion are separated using bipolar cautery and covered with a cottonoid. Later, when the tumor is entirely removed, the residual tumor tissue can be carefully aspirated parallel to the plane of the fourth ventricular floor until only a thin lining remains, and this lining can be coagulated with bipolar cautery to reduce the viability of remaining cells.

The next step is to resect the lateral and anterior portions of the tumor. The lateral and superior attachments of the

tumor usually blend with the paravermian brain so there is seldom a plane between tumor and normal brain. As a result, most residual tumor fragments are left in this area. Since there are minimal postoperative neurologic deficits that result from removing a thin rim of cerebellum, the dissection should be carried out on the brain side of the brain-tumor interface so that all tumor is resected and hemostasis is easier to obtain. At the end of the dissection there will be a bed of clean white brain. The lateral dissection is extended onto the ependymal surface, where the tumor attaches to the cerebellum, and this margin is defined upward and forward until the dilated caudal aqueduct is reached, producing a conical dissection field. Finally, the anterosuperior tumor pole is removed, leaving the tip of the tumor covering the opening of the caudal aqueduct until the end of the operation so that no blood from the dissection will enter the lateral or third ventricles.

If only a small amount of tumor extends laterally through the foramen of Luschka, it can usually be aspirated under direct vision from the ventricular side, since the tumor is not adherent to the ependyma. A large extraventricular segment that extends to the pons or mesencephalic peduncle may rarely require a secondary retromastoid approach after main tumor debulking with extension of the craniectomy and dural opening to lateral venous sinuses. The cerebellar hemisphere is retracted medially and dissection extended along the plane of the petrous bone to expose the lateral part of the tumor. It is important to identify the lower cranial nerves, since they are sometimes encapsulated by the tumor.

Since medulloblastoma often spreads through the subarachnoid space and the tumors are highly radiosensitive, radiotherapy to the entire neuraxis is considered standard even when there are no obvious lesions on postoperative imaging.[31] The best survival rates are obtained with 3600 to 4000 cGy to whole craniospinal axis supplemented to 5400 to 5600 cGy to the primary site and 1800 to 3000 cGy extra to any area of lump disease. Young children have a high incidence of postradiation neurocognitive deficits, so radiation should be delayed or eliminated in the very young; various studies have suggested lower dosage[40] or chemotherapy until the brain is mature enough to handle radiation.[28] Trials using various chemotherapy regimens have demonstrated improved survival with chemotherapy, especially for locally extensive or widely disseminated tumors.[28,41,42]

Prognosis for patients with medulloblastoma is related to size, invasiveness, and dissemination of tumor at diagnosis; age of the patient; and postoperative residual tumor. Large tumors have been shown to have a lower 5-year disease-free survival.[42] Brain-stem invasion also carries a poorer prognosis, and is problematic for preoperative staging because it cannot be predicted based on MRI.[42,43] Presence of dissemination through the neuraxis is the single most significant predictor of outcome for all histologic types of medulloblastoma. Even microscopic dissemination (determined by lumbar puncture performed at least 10 days postoperatively) carries a significantly lower 5-year survival.[28] Extraneural metastases to bone and even lymph nodes have been reported, but the incidence is too low to warrant screening all medulloblastoma patients.[44] Young patients are much more likely to have dissemination, but patients younger than 4 years of age have a worse prognosis out of proportion to the increased dissemination rates.[41] Finally, completeness of resection is thought to impact subsequent behavior of the tumor,[43,45] and presence of more than a cubic millimeter of residual tumor has been associated with worse survival. Histology has not been shown to impact prognosis except for rare tumor subtypes at the extreme ends of the histologic spectrum; specifically, medulloblastomas with extensive nodularity and large cell/anaplastic medulloblastomas are associated with better and worse clinical outcomes, respectively. However,

histologic features have not been shown to correlate with clinical outcome for the vast majority of medulloblastomas that lie between these extremes.[46]

Overall, with surgery and radiation, 5-year disease-free survival rates approach 80%.[28] Medulloblastomas have classically been said to follow Collin's law, which says that a cure has been obtained if there is no tumor recurrence over period equal to the age at diagnosis plus 9 months. However, one third of survivors at 5 years have recurrence, and one third of the recurrences are outside of the period predicted by Collin's law. Most recurrence occurs in the cerebellum or along CSF pathways. Surveillance imaging has been shown to improve survival.[32,47]

ATYPICAL TERATOID/RHABDOID TUMOR

Atypical teratoid/rhabdoid tumors share many clinical and pathologic features with medulloblastomas but appear to be unique entity with a more aggressive course and worse prognosis.[48] They may occur anywhere in the neuraxis but are most commonly found in the cerebellum, and clinical presentation is similar to that of medulloblastomas. Most patients are under 2 years of age at diagnosis. One third of patients have subarachnoid dissemination upon presentation. Histologically they are composed at least partly of rhabdoid cells but also have areas typical for medulloblastoma and malignant mesenchymal or epithelial tissue. They stain for epithelial membrane antigen, vimentin, and smooth muscle actin. They are associated with abnormalities of chromosome 22 whereas medulloblastomas typically have an i(17q) abnormality.[48] Prognosis is dismal, and most patients die within 1 year of diagnosis regardless of treatment.[49]

ASTROCYTOMA

In the pediatric population, astrocytomas account for about one fourth of all brain tumors, and one third of posterior fossa tumors. These tumors occur most often during the first 20 years of life, with peak incidence from 5 to 8 years of age, and very few patients are younger than 1 year or older than 40. Males and females are affected equally.[50,51] Unlike astrocytomas of the cerebrum, they are chronic and slowly progressive tumors that usually present subacutely and can be resected with minimal morbidity with a very high rate of cure.

Because they are slow-growing tumors, onset of symptoms is usually far more insidious than medulloblastomas and ependymomas. In 1931, Cushing remarked with amazement that "tumors of such high magnitude in such a critical situation and so certain to produce early hydrocephalus can be tolerated for so many years with no comparatively insignificant symptoms."[52] Most patients have had symptoms for many months by the time the tumor is diagnosed, and some undergo extensive gastrointestinal or neuropsychological investigation before the tumor is diagnosed. Although outside the lumen of the fourth ventricle, astrocytomas frequently disrupt the flow of CSF, so the most common presenting symptoms are those of increased intracranial pressure such as headache, vomiting, abducens palsy, and papilledema. Other common symptoms include altered gait, clumsiness, and head tilt. Common signs include papilledema, ataxia that is often unilateral, appendicular dysmetria, nystagmus, and macrocephaly that occasionally dates back several years even to infancy. Severe neck pain, opisthotonus, bradycardia, hypertension, and altered neurologic function are less common but require immediate attention, and rarely patients will present with signs of acute hydrocephalus such as stupor or coma, projectile vomiting, and oculomotor and facial palsies. Blindness was once a very common presenting symptom (present on presentation in 23 of the 76 patients reviewed by Cushing) but is rarely seen today.[50]

On imaging, astrocytomas are solid, cystic, or mixed lesions that arise from the medial hemisphere or vermis;[53,54]

one third are entirely in one cerebellar hemisphere (Fig. 31-25). When in the midline, they can be difficult to differentiate from medulloblastomas and ependymomas. MRI will usually disclose a round to oval mass with well-defined margins and of mixed intensity, hypointense to surrounding brain on T1 and hyperintense on T2. On CT the tumor is hypodense or isodense to surrounding brain. Unlike low-grade supratentorial astrocytomas, the tumor enhances brightly with CT and MRI contrast material. If the tumor is cystic, there may be an enhancing mural nodule and the cyst fluid will be slightly denser than CSF on T2-weighted images.

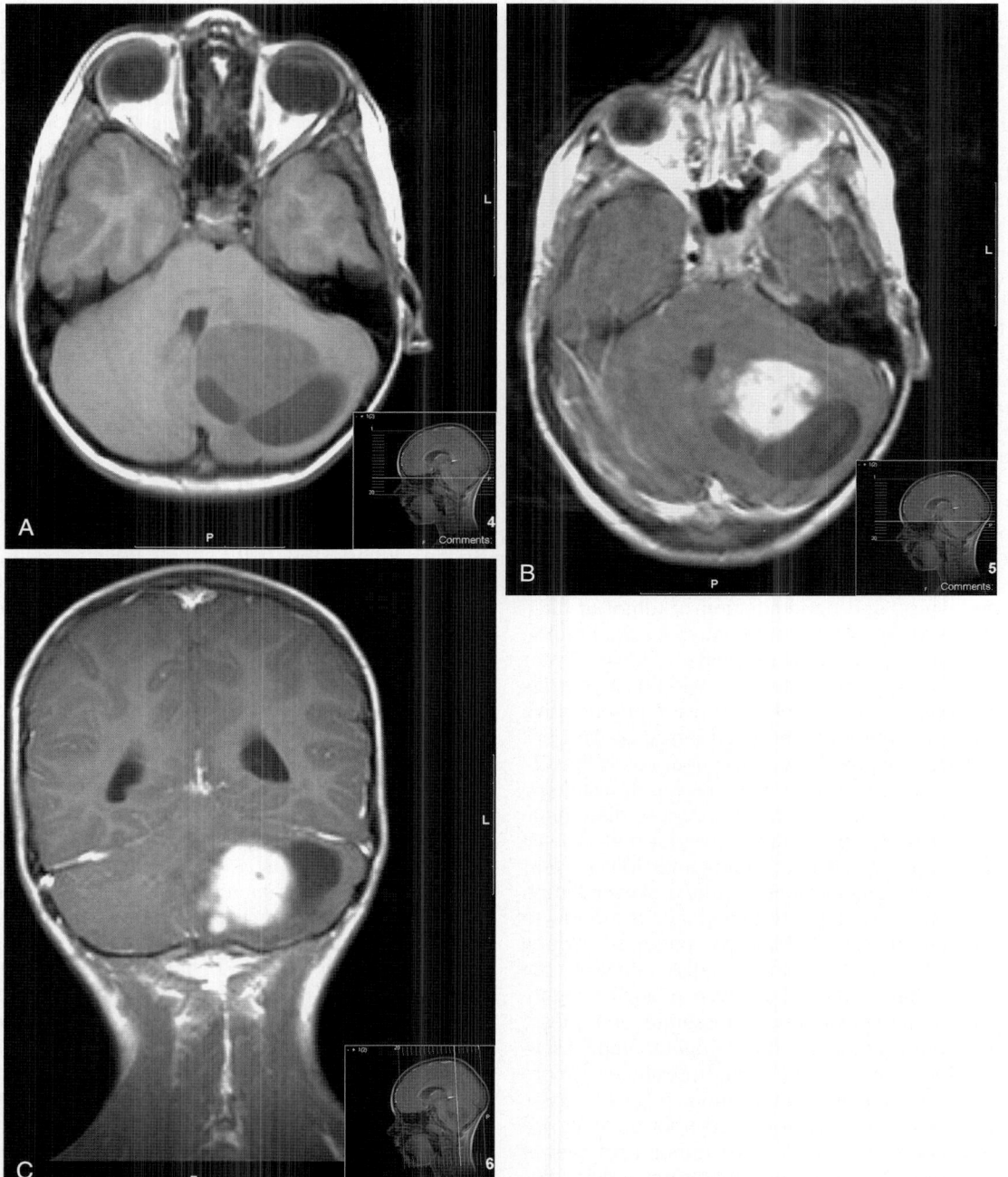

FIGURE 31-25 Astrocytoma. A, T1 without contrast. The hemispheric lesion is slightly hypodense to brain and has a cystic component. B, T1 with contrast. The solid portion of the tumor enhances irregularly. C, T1 with contrast, coronal section. These tumors are much more likely to involve the cerebellar hemisphere.

The cyst wall is sometimes denser than surrounding brain but does not contain tumor unless it enhances (Figs. 31-26, 31-27, and 31-28). Calcification and peritumoral edema are infrequently observed.[54] Skull x-rays are generally not helpful, although they may show signs of chronically increased intracranial pressure such as thinning or asymmetric bulging of occipital squama, chronic splitting of cranial sutures, or demineralization of sella turcica.

Grossly, astrocytomas are firm with discrete borders. About half will have some degree of cystic degeneration (compared with 80% of supratentorial astrocytomas). There is usually one cyst with a prominent mural nodule, although honeycombing of small cysts is also seen. The cyst wall is most commonly smooth and glistening, although sometimes there will be a coating of tumor or raised tumor nodules on the inner surface of the cyst (seen more often when there is enhancement of the cyst wall on neuroimaging). Histologically, areas of loose glial tissue resembling cerebral protoplasmic astrocytes with round or oval nuclei are intermixed with compact areas of fusiform, fibrillated cells that often have elongated eosinophilic bodies called Rosenthal fibers. When the cells conform to white matter tracts they have an elongated hair-like structure and are described as "pilocytic" (hair cell). The cells stain weakly for GFAP and have bundles of intermediate filaments in perikaryon and cell processes, both of which confirm their identity as astrocytes.

Some posterior fossa astrocytomas have histology and clinical behavior that deviates from the typical pilocytic astrocytoma described above. These tumors resemble low-grade astrocytomas of the cerebral hemispheres.[55-57] They have diffusely homogeneous histology, lack microcysts and Rosenthal fibers, and are characterized by pseudorosettes, high cell density, necrosis, mitoses, and calcification. Incidence of these tumors is much lower than pilocytic astrocytomas and they are more common in older patients, especially those who have previously received radiation.[55,58] They have a much higher rate of malignant degeneration,[51] and high-grade anaplastic astrocytomas and even glioblastomas have been reported in the posterior fossa.[59-61] Even when histologically low grade, they may infiltrate into cerebellar nuclei or peduncles and often lack clear tumor margins making gross tumor resection difficult. Survival rates with these tumors is lower than the typical astrocytomas,[59] and there are reports of diffuse leptomeningeal spread[55] and even spread to the muscles of the neck requiring several local surgical procedures to control.[62]

After exposing the posterior fossa, the tumor is usually immediately apparent as enlargement of the vermis or unilateral hemisphere with distended folia. The cerebellar tonsils may be pushed down on the side of the tumor. Intraoperative ultrasonography can be used transdurally to be certain bony exposure is adequate or after dura has been opened to demonstrate the closest location of tumor to cerebellar surface to minimize the amount of cerebellar tissue that must be removed to provide adequate exposure of the tumor. After incising the vermis or hemisphere, the tumor is removed with the ultrasonic aspirator until normal cerebellar tissue is seen. Very large tumors will cause the compressed cerebellum to relax inward after debulking so self-retaining retractors are helpful to keep the tumor bed open. If there is a cystic component to the tumor, the cyst is entered and cyst fluid quickly suctioned, supporting the hemisphere with self-retaining retractors to prevent collapse away from the tentorium with rupture of bridging veins. The mural nodule is then identified and removed using the ultrasonic aspirator. If the tumor is mixed or enhancement of the cyst wall is seen, the entire cyst wall should be removed and normal cerebellar tissue exposed; otherwise, simple removal of the mural nodule is curative. To prevent contamination of the CSF with blood and cyst fluid (which can produce chemical meningitis that increases the likelihood of postoperative communicating hydrocephalus), the

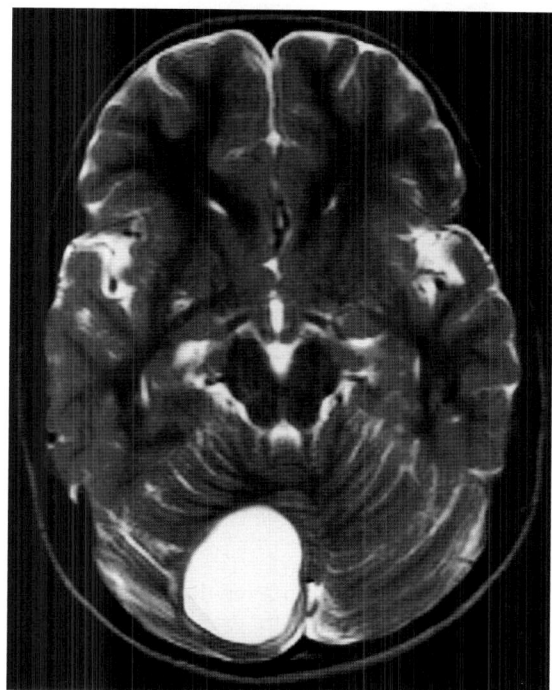

FIGURE 31-26 Astrocytoma, T2. The cyst associated with this tumor is often much larger than the mural nodule.

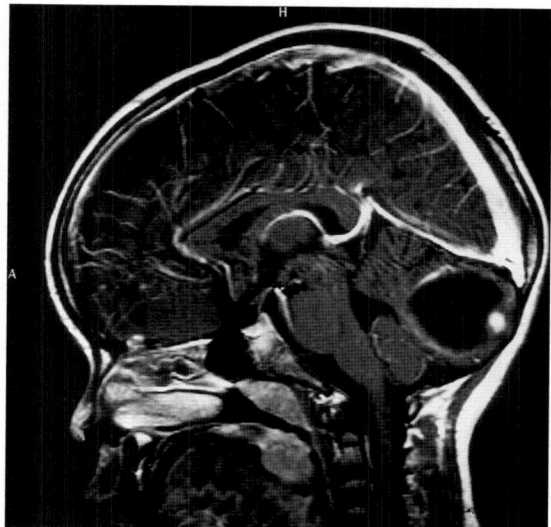

FIGURE 31-27 Astrocytoma, T1 with contrast, sagittal section. Note the small enhancing mural nodule posteriorly. If the cyst wall does not enhance, removal of the nodule is usually all that is necessary.

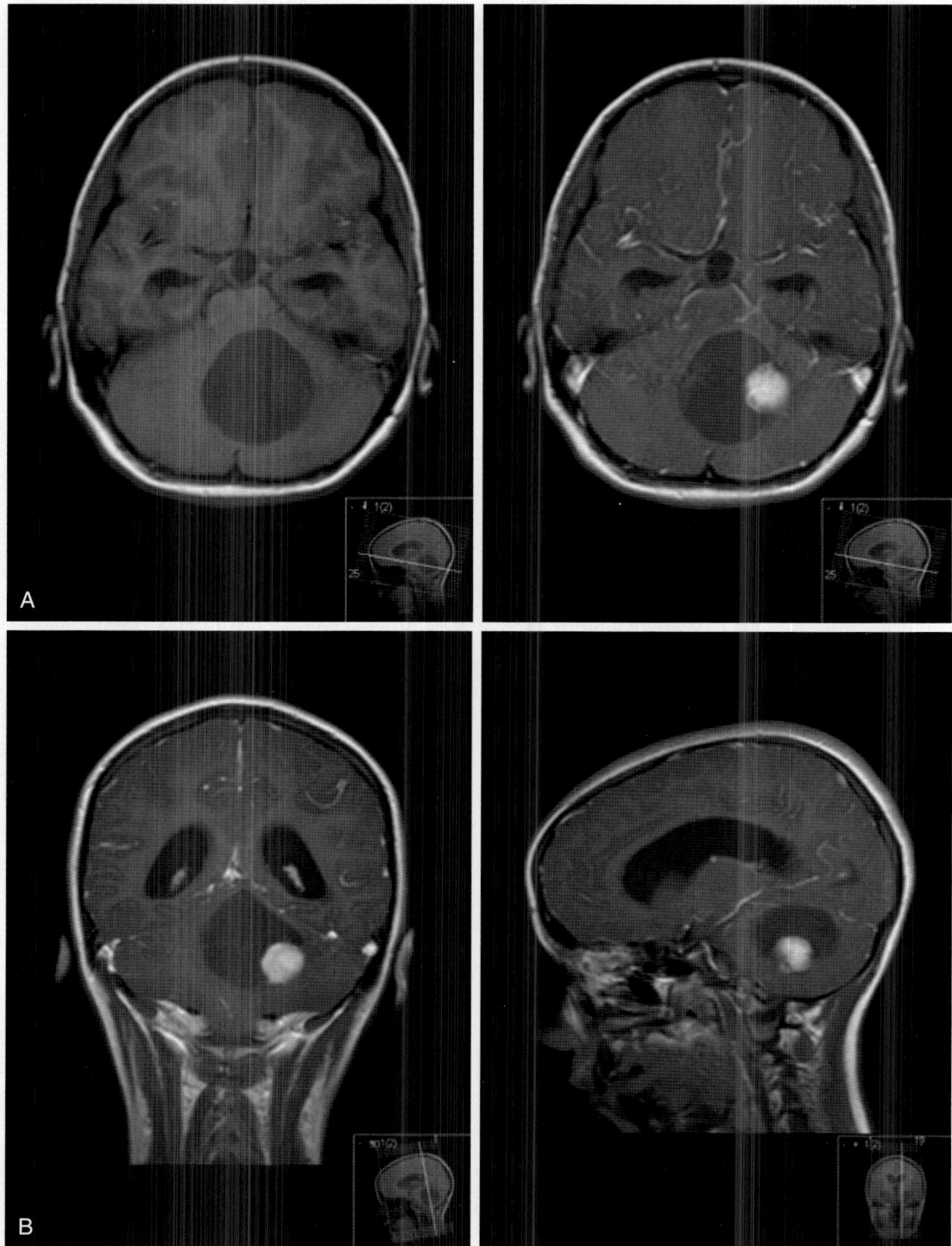

FIGURE 31-28 Pilocytic Astrocytoma. A, T1 without (*left*) and with contrast (*right*), axial section. Enhancing mural nodule and an associated cyst noted in a pilocytic astrocytoma in a 12-year-old patient. There is effacement of the fourth ventricle with hydrocephalus. B, T1 with contrast, coronal (*left*) and sagittal (*right*) sections demonstrating an enhancing mural nodule and an associated cyst in a pediatric patient with a pilocytic astrocytoma.

cisterna magna and fourth ventricle should not be opened unless it is necessary to do so to achieve gross total resection. All walls of the tumor bed are then carefully inspected to ensure there is no residual tumor. Finally, before closing, it is important to ensure that bridging tentorial veins are not stretched. These veins can be safely sacrificed but

tearing one later can lead to a life-threatening hematoma. All patients should get a postoperative contrast-enhanced scan within the first twenty-four hours to evaluate the extent of resection, provide a baseline if hydrocephalus should develop, and evaluate for cerebellar/brain-stem retraction edema or clinically silent hematomas. If more than one cubic centimeter has been left behind, early re-exploration to remove the residual tumor is indicated.

True pilocytic astrocytomas are almost always resectable by modern techniques and have excellent prognosis with no adjuvant therapy if gross total resection is possible.[53,56] Postoperative MRI is particularly poor at differentiating residual astrocytoma from postsurgical changes so early postoperative imaging to obtain a baseline is probably not helpful.[63] If there is a small amount of residual tumor, serial imaging can be used to follow its growth. Although there are several well-documented cases of low-grade astrocytoma undergoing malignant degeneration several years after surgical resection, this is probably quite rare and each of the documented cases had received radiation therapy. Radiation therapy has not been shown to be successful in the management of these tumors,[64] and is associated with significant side effects, although focused radiation may be helpful for surgically inaccessible or rapidly growing lesions.[65] Combined chemotherapy and radiotherapy for high-grade cortical astrocytomas has been shown to decrease rates of metastasis for children with high-grade astrocytomas. As with pilocytic astrocytomas, patients with more complete resections of infiltrative tumors fare better.

Recurrence of posterior fossa astrocytomas is related to the extent of resection, location, invasiveness, and histology of the original tumor.[51,67] Age of the patient does not appear to have any effect on outcome. Recurrence is most common at the primary site, and if any tumor is left behind, symptoms almost invariably recur. Cystic tumors can usually be totally extirpated, but solid tumors tend to regrow after prolonged remission even if grossly resected. Solid midline tumors are most likely to recur since they more often extend toward the cerebellar peduncles, aqueduct, or brain stem, which may prevent total excision. Invasion of the subarachnoid space often occurs but this does not indicate a poor prognosis as with most other tumors. Astrocytomas do not follow Collin's law for tumor recurrence and can have recurrences long after complete resection.[68] Overall 10-year survival for astrocytomas is close to 100% with complete resection, and 20-year survival is above 70%.[56,67]

EPENDYMOMA

Ependymoma is the third most common infratentorial tumor of childhood, representing 10% to 20% of all posterior fossa brain tumors, although in children under 3 years of age they represent 30% of all posterior fossa tumors. They occur very rarely in adults.[69] Since ependymomas arise from the cells lining the ventricles, they can appear in any of the ventricles or ependymal streaks (obliterated portions of ventricles). Sixty-five percent of these tumors are infratentorial, and the most common location is in the middle to lower fourth ventricle or at the junction of the lateral inferior medullary velum and foramen of Luschka. Males are affected about twice as often as females, and 60% of all patients are under 5 years old at diagnosis.[70] Recently, it has been suggested that ependymomas may have a viral etiology, since DNA sequences identical to segments of the SV40 virus have been identified in childhood ependymomas,[71,72] and ependymomas can be induced in rodents by intracerebral inoculation of SV40.[73] For unclear reasons, they are much more common in India than elsewhere in the world.[30]

Ependymomas are relatively fast growing tumors and present more acutely than astrocytomas but not as acutely as medulloblastomas. Median duration of symptoms is 2 to 3 months. The most common presenting symptoms are nausea and vomiting from increased intracranial pressure, ataxia, and nystagmus. Some patients have repeated vomiting in the absence of hydrocephalus due to direct stimulation of the brain-stem emetic center. At presentation, one third to one half of ependymomas will have grown through the foramen of Luschka or central canal with direct extension into the upper cervical spine, and this can produce nuchal rigidity, torticollis, posterior neck pain, or head tilt. Infiltration of the brain stem or direct tumor involvement within lateral brain-stem recesses can produce cranial nerve deficits, and this is associated with a particularly poor outcome.[70,74] Finally, ependymomas do metastasize (although not as often as medulloblastomas), and patients rarely present with signs of metastatic spinal cord or nerve root compression.[74,75]

Ependymomas usually appear isodense to brain on both MRI and CT, although they may be hypodense on CT, hypointense on T1-weighted MRI, and hyperintense on T2.[76] They are almost always seen on the floor of the fourth ventricle with the body of the ventricle expanded around the tumor, and are often quite large by the time they are discovered (Fig. 31-29). They frequently extend through the foramen of Luschka into the cerebropontine angle or through the foramen of Magendie occasionally compressing the upper cervical cord. This extraforaminal extension is an important diagnostic feature since other tumors in the differential (medulloblastoma, astrocytoma, and choroid plexus papilloma) almost never do this (Fig. 31-29B). Calcifications are seen in one quarter of ependymomas on CT, although a greater percentage of tumors have microcalcification;[77] these calcifications are usually soft and do not pose a problem during tumor removal, so preoperative CT is not necessary. MRI appearance is usually heterogeneous from calcification, cysts, blood products, necrotic foci, and tumor vascularity. Enhancement on both CT and MRI is more heterogeneous than most other tumors in this area, and peritumoral edema is often seen on T2-weighted images.[76]

Grossly, the tumor is gray, well-circumscribed, homogeneous or less often lobulated, and is seen to arise directly from the floor of the fourth ventricle. Microscopically, ependymomas are quite heterogeneous, and can have highly variable histology within a single tumor. The two most common ependymoma histologic patterns are cellular and epithelial. Cellular (or "glial") ependymomas consist of sheets of glial-appearing cells interrupted by perivascular pseudorosettes, in which fusiform cells with tapered fibrillary processes that stain for GFAP surround blood vessels. The pseudorosettes produce perivascular eosinophilic zones free of nuclei, giving the tumor a "leopard skin" appearance under low magnification. Epithelial ependymomas have cells with discernible boundaries that are arranged in canals and form true rosettes, reflecting the cell's origin as ventricular lining. As with normal ependyma, these cells have basal bodies that anchor cilia and intracytoplasmic spherical or rod-shaped structures called blepharoplasts. Other rare histologic variants include papillary in which tumor cells are seen to cover glial tissue, tanocytic with elongated cells that resemble astrocytes, and clear cell in which cell have perinuclear halos like oligodendrocytes. Regardless of histologic pattern, ependymomas frequently sometimes have small cystic areas, regions of necrosis, evidence of acute or chronic hemorrhage, and calcification. More than half of infratentorial ependymomas have evidence of microcalcification, which is important to differentiate the tumor from medulloblastoma,[77] and the chromatin is much denser than is seen with astrocytomas. Occasionally focal areas of anaplastic degeneration are seen with increased mitoses, cellular anaplasia, vascular proliferation, necrosis, and fewer

perivascular pseudorosettes, although this happens much more often with supratentorial ependymomas. Unlike astrocytomas and medulloblastomas, in which histologic grade and proliferative potential correlate with prognosis, it is controversial whether histologic grade affects prognosis; this is likely to be because of the diversity of pathology seen. High mitotic index and presence of focal areas of dense cellularity are associated with poor prognosis, but calcium and ependymal rosettes have no impact.

The so-called ependymoblastoma, which has been reclassified as an entirely separate embryonal PNET, usually

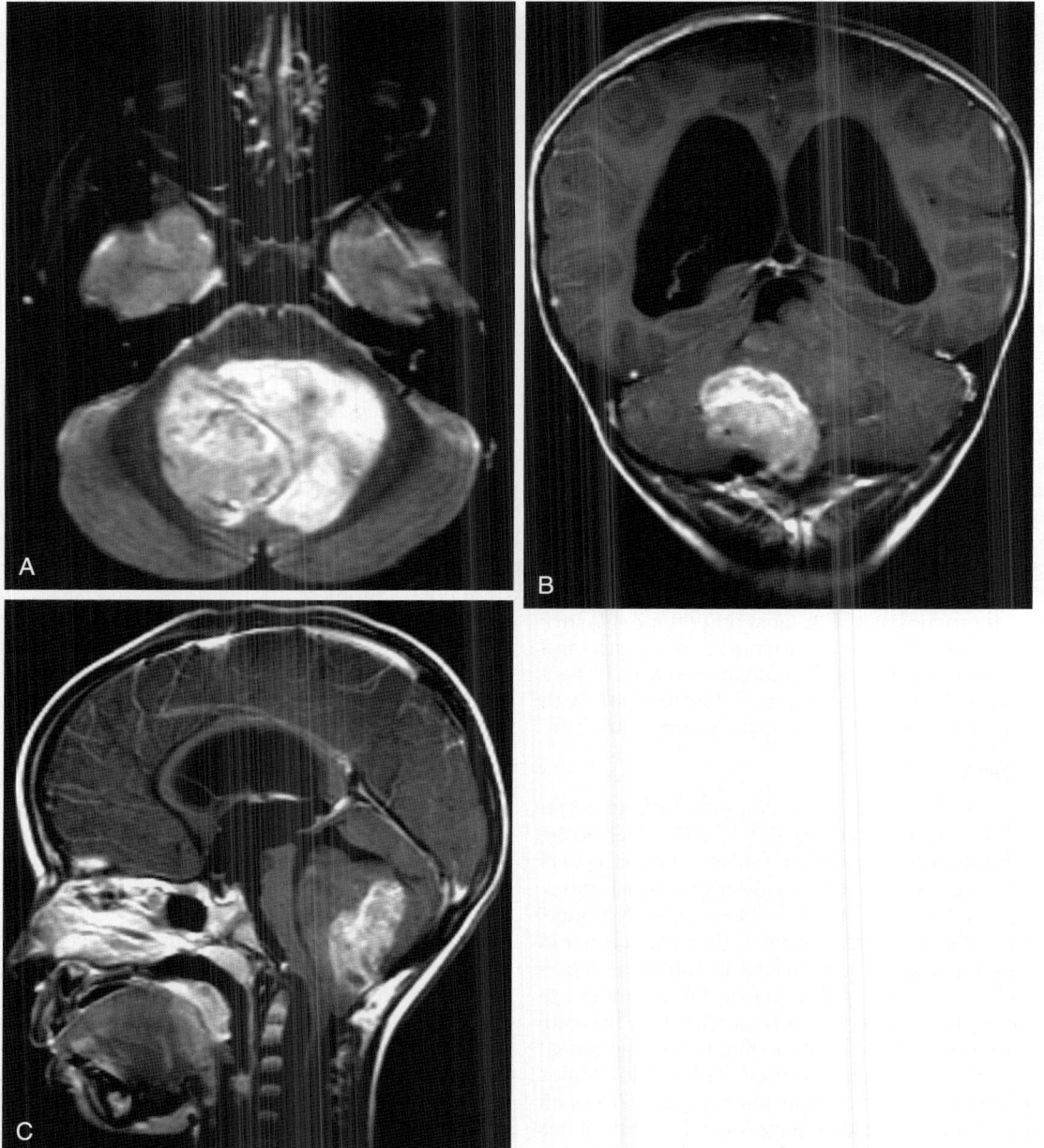

FIGURE 31-29 Ependymoma. A, T1 with contrast. The tumor arises from the floor of the fourth ventricle, is associated with marked peritumoral edema, enhances brightly and heterogeneously, and is often quite large by the time it is discovered. B, T1 with contrast, coronal section. The tumor is seen here to extend through the foramen of Magendie, a characteristic sign of ependymoma. Enhancement is more irregular than most other tumors in this area because of calcification, cysts, blood products, necrotic foci, and tumor vascularity. C, T1 with contrast, sagittal section. The tumor, which has extruded through the foramen of Magendie, is also causing herniation of the cerebellar tonsils with compression of the upper cervical cord.

occurs supratentorially in young children and consists of sheets of poorly differentiated cells with frequent mitoses and distinctive rosettes of pseudostratified cells surrounding a lumen and surrounded by terminal bars. Median survival for ependymoblastoma is a few months, and patients frequently have diffuse spread through the subarachnoid space by presentation.[79]

Since ependymomas usually arise from the floor of the fourth ventricle and are frequently adherent to the lower cranial nerves, it is often quite difficult to achieve gross total resection, and in the past surgery was limited to removing enough of the tumor to allow free flow of CSF. More recently, the benefits of total resection have been shown to outweigh the risks, as there is a significant difference in survival depending on extent of resection.[70,74] The posterior fossa is exposed by standard techniques. If there is extension of the tumor through the foramen of Magendie, it will be apparent in the cisterna magna immediately after the dura is opened. Any tumor tissue extending into the cervical canal is gently aspirated from the surface of the cord with suction or ultrasonic aspiration. This is usually easy to do since the tumor does not invade the pia. The cerebellar hemispheres are then retracted laterally and resection continued along the floor of the fourth ventricle until the point of origin is determined (usually caudal to the stria medullaris). Ependymomas rarely submerge deep into the brainstem, so a 1-mm thick carpet of tumor should be left at its point of attachment, and resection continued parallel to the floor of the fourth ventricle using the ultrasonic aspirator. It is vitally important to identify the glistening white fourth ventricular floor before attempting to remove tumor from its point of attachment. If the tumor extends through the foramen of Luschka, the area of origin will usually be found at the junction of the lateral medullary velum and the medial foramen of Luschka. In this case, the tumor should be resected from within the fourth ventricle as far laterally as possible and then the retractors removed from the fourth ventricle and placed underneath the cerebellar tonsil to expose the cerebellomedullary cistern where the rest of the tumor may be visualized and resected. Ependymomas are quite soft and can usually be safely aspirated off the lower cranial nerves, but it is important not to violate PICA and its lateral medullary branches, although the lateral medullary veins can be safely sacrificed if inadvertently entered. Any changes in cardiac rate or rhythm (more common when dissecting on the left side) can be abolished by soaking a micropatty in 1% lidocaine and placing it on the cranial nerve near the root entry zone for a few minutes. Removing tumors from deep within the cerebellopontine angle may require partial resection of the lateral cerebellar hemisphere to facilitate exposure. Occasionally the tumor arises from the roof rather than the floor of the fourth ventricle and will invade the roof and inferior vermis without attachment to the floor of the fourth ventricle. This often allows for complete tumor removal, but excessive resection of the inferior vermis or nodulus increases the risk of damage to the superior cerebellar peduncle producing postoperative ataxia or the posterior fossa syndrome. Recurrent ependymomas are usually invasive or adherent, so it is challenging to distinguish invasive disease from normal anatomy. As a result, resection of recurrent disease is almost always incomplete.[74]

Because recurrence is most common at the primary site, radiotherapy with 4500 to 5600 cGy to the primary site has shown to significantly improve overall rate and duration of disease-free survival in patients with incompletely resected ependymoma in several retrospective studies.[80,81] Most authors therefore recommend local radiotherapy even if gross total resection is confirmed by postoperative MRI and staging is negative for leptomeningeal spread,[80] although one recent study recommends withholding further treatment unless there is evidence for tumor recurrence.[74] If there are no radiographically evident metastases, craniospinal irradiation probably does not improve outcome, since only 3% of patients with low-grade tumors later develop have clinical evidence of metastatic disease (although one third have dissemination at autopsy). Also, most spinal seeding occurs only after recurrence at the primary site, and craniospinal irradiation has not been shown to prevent spinal metastases.[82] However, anaplastic ependymomas are much more likely to be disseminated and should be treated with craniospinal irradiation,[74] although it may not help.[83] If disseminated disease is confirmed, most authors recommend 3600 cGy to entire axis with an additional boost of 1980 cGy to the local site and areas of macroscopic dissemination.[80]

There is not much data concerning chemotherapy for ependymomas. Although chemotherapy does transiently reduce tumor bulk and stabilize tumor growth in patients with recurrent disease, no chemotherapeutic regimen has been shown to be effective after radiation at the time of initial diagnosis.[81,84]

Prognosis for patients with ependymoma is poor compared with medulloblastomas and astrocytomas, although survival studies are difficult to interpret because most include anaplastic histology and supratentorial tumors. Most studies show that long-term survival is strongly correlated to amount of residual tumor as judged by postoperative MRI. For example, 5-year disease-free survival approaches 70% to 90% if there is no evidence of residual tumor compared with 0% to 30% if residual tumor is untreated.[70,80,85] Other studies show no effect.[81] Because ependymomas tend to insinuate into crevices within and about the fourth ventricle, the surgeon's assessment overestimates completeness of resection as much as one third of the time, and so MRI should be used to determine completeness of resection. Therefore, any presence of residual enhancing tissue on imaging studies following completion of radiation should be explored and resected if possible. Overall 5-year survival is variously quoted at 15% to 50% for children and 50% to 75% for adults with fourth ventricle ependymomas.[70,85] Histology and age of the patient do not significantly impact survival,[70,74] although anaplastic ependymomas have a worse outcome,[68] and female patients do better.[80] Midline tumors have a better 5-year survival than lateral ependymomas out of proportion to their ease of resection.[86] Disseminated ependymomas, about 5% of low-grade and 15% of anaplastic tumors,[82] have a particularly poor prognosis, with 5-year survival rates near 12%.

BRAIN-STEM GLIOMA

Brain-stem gliomas are much more common in children than adults, and make up about 10% to 20% of intracranial pediatric tumors, and 15% to 30% of all posterior fossa tumors.[87,88] They are a heterogeneous group of tumors with many distinct clinical and pathologic varieties. Duration of symptoms prior to presentation varies widely but is generally 3 to 5 months with insidious onset. Unlike the tumors described above, increased intracranial pressure is infrequent except as very late manifestation. Most patients present with a triad of a cerebellar deficit, pyramidal tract deficit, and involvement of cranial nerve nuclei; more than half have clinically detectable facial weakness, pharyngeal weakness, trigeminal deficit, or paresis of conjugate gaze by admission. The vast majority of brain-stem gliomas are astrocytomas with gangliogliomas and oligodendrogliomas making up the remainder. Histologically, they resemble fibrillary or pilocytic astrocytomas of cerebellar hemispheres, although they can show anaplastic components and cytoarchitecture of glioblastoma multiforme. Brain-stem tumors can be classified into three general categories based on location: tumors of the midbrain (including tectal gliomas and focal midbrain tumors, not discussed here); dorsally exophytic brain-stem tumors; and cervicomedullary tumors.

Pontine tumors have the highest prevalence in the first decade but can present in adults as old as forty. They tend to be infiltrative with indistinct borders and are always malignant regardless of histology at diagnosis[89] and spread early through the leptomeningeal space[90] and even extraneurally.[91] Pontine tumors usually present with cranial nerve palsies followed by pyramidal tract signs, ataxia, and hydrocephalus in the most advanced stages. Imaging demonstrates diffuse pontine enlargement with hypodense signal to brain on CT, hypointense on T1-weighted MRI and hyperintense on T2-weighted MRI. Calcification and hemorrhagic foci are unusual. They are often seen to extend into the midbrain, medulla, or cerebellum, and can encircle the basilar artery.[92] They rarely enhance on CT (occasionally there are areas of focal enhancement) but do enhance with MRI (Fig. 31-30). These tumors are surgically inaccessible, and surgical intervention does not alter survival.[93,94] Radiation therapy is standard treatment, and many patients

initially exhibit a striking response in terms of alleviation of symptoms and even radiographic resolution of tumor. However, within 6 to 12 months of starting radiation, there is nearly always recurrence with diffuse leptomeningeal spread. Chemotherapy has not been shown to improve survival time. Most patients are dead within 2 years of diagnosis, and overall 5-year survival rates are less than 10%.[94]

A subset (about 20%) of patients with pontine gliomas will have dorsal exophytic growth in which the tumor has eroded the ependyma to produce a wide-based, lobulated intraventricular mass that does not involve the cerebellum.[95,96] These patients have more chronic and insidious symptoms such as failure to thrive, headaches, and loss of balance, but hydrocephalus is often an earlier finding. They have a lower rate of malignancy than diffuse pontine tumors and a much better prognosis. These tumors may be amenable to surgical resection using microsurgical techniques to achieve maximal subtotal removal.

Focal pontine astrocytomas have been described that are confined to half or part of half of the pons, sometimes extending into the fourth ventricle. These are more common in type one neurofibromatosis and have a variable natural history.[97-99] They are amenable to surgical debulking and may not require immediate intervention after surgery; some patients do well with an aggressive surgical approach.

Cervicomedullary tumors generally present in young children, with average age of onset at 6 to 7 years. They almost never extend above the pontomedullary junction because their superior growth is limited by crossing fibers in the lower medulla and pontomedullary junction.[100] They generally grow outward and extend into the fourth ventricle as a cystic or solid exophytic growth, and can eventually produce hydrocephalus from compression of the fourth ventricle or its outlet foramina. The symptoms are insidious and are often present for months or years. Most patients initially experience dysfunction of the lower cranial nerves manifested by difficulty swallowing, nasal speech, or recurrent aspiration. Sometimes they have torticollis or neck pain, and half will have some spinal cord dysfunction, usually insidious motor findings or paresthesias. MRI demonstrates the lesions quite well, but CT is of little utility because of the artifact created by the bones of the posterior fossa. These tumors are surgically accessible.[101]

Since most surgically accessible brain-stem gliomas extend to posterior aspect of brain stem or bulge into the fourth ventricle or cervicomedullary cistern, the standard fourth ventricle approach is useful to address them. For cervicomedullary tumors, intraoperative ultrasound should be used to identify the rostral and caudal poles of neoplasm prior to opening dura, and the initial myelotomy should initially be made in the middle of the tumor.[102] In all cases, the tumor should be carefully removed from the inside out using ultrasonic aspiration, laser, microsuction, or irrigating bipolar forceps. It is possible to work to the brain interface when resecting pontine or cervical lesions, but when resecting medullary tumors, it is prudent to stop after only half to three quarters of the tumor is removed so that there is no chance that normal medullary structures will be violated. In particular, the cranial nerve nuclei should be carefully avoided. Monitoring (especially SSEP) is helpful to ensure important structures are not inadvertently damaged. It is important to avoid excessive manipulation and to consider

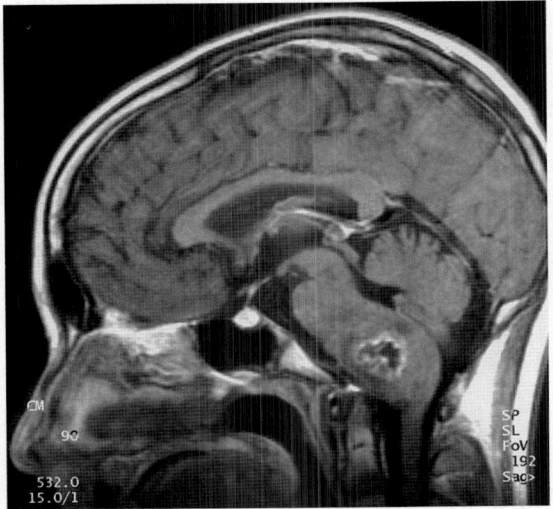

FIGURE 31-30 Brain stem glioma, T1 with contrast, sagittal section. The tumor is seen to enlarge the pons, which is a characteristic sign of brainstem glioma. Unless the tumor extends to the posterior aspect of the brainstem or bulges into the fourth ventricle or cervicomedullary cistern, it is not resectable.

every deviation in pulse or blood pressure to be a warning sign. Postoperatively, the most common threat to good recovery is respiratory difficulties, especially for medullary lesions. Therefore, patients should be monitored carefully and extubated only after fully awake. Postoperative radiation therapy may be helpful. If the tumor is focal and benign and gross total resection is obtained, many patients can have extended disease-free survival.

CHOROID PLEXUS PAPILLOMA

Choroid plexus papillomas are rare tumors, accounting for 2% to 3% of pediatric intracranial tumors and 0.5% of adult tumors.[103,104] Unlike most fourth ventricular brain tumors that are more common in the pediatric population, fourth ventricular papillomas are more common in adults and most pediatric choroid plexus papillomas are in the lateral ventricles. The third ventricle is an uncommon location at any age. Males slightly outnumber females in most clinical series. When in the fourth ventricle, they usually occur in the cavity, although rarely they are found in the lateral recess[105] or in the cerebellopontine angle arising from the small tuft of choroid plexus that extends through the foramen of Luschka.[106,107] Carcinomas of the choroid plexus account for about 20% of choroid plexus tumors and are usually found in the lateral ventricles,[103,108,109] but they occasionally involve the fourth ventricle. These malignant tumors almost invariably occur in young children, often during the first few days of life, and carry a grave prognosis with wide dissemination at or shortly after presentation.

Most choroid plexus papillomas present with symptoms of increased intracranial pressure such as headache, gait disturbances, and abducens palsy. Excessive formation of CSF is responsible for much of the hydrocephalus, although obstruction to CSF flow by the tumor or at the level of the arachnoid granulations due to hemorrhage is probably a more common cause. Because of CSF overproduction, affected infants often have papilledema in spite of an open fontanelle and macrocephaly disproportional to the size of the tumor. When in the cerebellopontine angle, dysfunction of lower cranial nerves and cerebellar ataxia are the main clinical findings.[106,107] In adults, these tumors usually do not produce excessive CSF and are sometimes discovered incidentally at autopsy.

On imaging, choroid plexus papillomas are usually seen as intraventricular masses. On CT they are hyperdense and enhance brightly and homogeneously with contrast.[110] Calcifications are common in childhood papillomas but are rare during infancy.[111] MRI demonstrates hypointensity on T1 and heterogeneous hyperintensity on T2. The tumor can be highly vascular, and angiography is useful for preoperative planning when faced with an extremely brightly enhancing tumor or one that demonstrates high vascularity on MRI to identify feeding vessels and develop a plan for early devascularization of the tumor. There is often hypertrophy of the feeding artery, which is usually PICA, although AICA supplies some tumors arising from choroid plexus far in the lateral recess. An important diagnostic clue is engulfing of the choroid glomus by tumor, which usually suggests choroid plexus papilloma.[112] Choroid plexus carcinomas are less homogeneous on neuroimaging due to necrosis, intratumoral hemorrhage, and cysts.[113]

Grossly, the papilloma is well-defined, lobulated, mulberry-like, and reddish purple, with a firm and vascular basal portion. Microscopically, these tumors strongly resemble normal choroid with a single layer of cuboidal epithelium that occasionally appears somewhat crowded and taller seated on a simple fibrovascular stroma with little or no abnormal mitotic activity. Calcification is common in these tumors and is extensive in 10%. Some atypical histologic features such as enlargement, irregularity, hyperchromasia, mitoses, and loss of papillary growth pattern is present in half of these tumors but have no prognostic significance. In infants there is occasionally evidence of ependymal differentiation with piling of ependymal cells or presence of cilia and blepharoplast. In these patients, it can be difficult to differentiate the tumor from papillary ependymomas. Rarely the tumors have a cystic portion within the tumor or in the brain parenchyma filled with CSF presumably secreted by the papilloma. The so-called "oncocytic variant of papilloma" resembles oncocytomas in other organs, with cytoplasm packed with mitochondria. Carcinoma of the choroid plexus is recognizable by heterogeneity, necrosis, invasiveness, cellular pleomorphism, and mitotic figures. The tumor has a tendency to form multilayered epithelium and invades the parenchyma.[111] This malignant tumor may be confused with metastatic adenocarcinoma, especially when it occurs in adults, and sometimes the only indication that it is a choroid tumor is the presence of cilia, microvilli, and zonula adherens on electron microscopy.

Complete surgical resection of fourth ventricular choroid plexus papillomas is frequently possible, since the tumor typically does not invade the parenchyma or floor of the fourth ventricle. Because they are very vascular tumors, it is important to prepare for significant blood loss. The fourth ventricle is exposed by standard techniques. Because of their extreme vascularity, it is important to identify feeding vessels during the resection. If the tumor is small, it may be possible to identify its point of attachment to normal choroid plexus and devascularize the tumor by coagulating and sectioning the tonsillar and vermian choroidal branches of PICA. Larger tumors may have feeding arteries embedded in the core of the tumor and occasionally envelope PICA, so the intraventricular papillary portion (which is less vascular than the core) is first shrunk with bipolar cautery or ultrasonic aspirator, and then the feeding branches identified and coagulated. Forceful retraction of the tumor should be avoided since there is sometimes a major draining vein on the dome of the papilloma and inferior vermian veins may be arterialized due to intratumoral shunting; these can produce significant hemorrhage if violated. It may be necessary to section the inferior vermis to reach the rostral end of the tumor. If there is extension through the foramen of Luschka into the cerebellopontine angle, the intraventricular part is resected first then the rest of the tumor is exposed by elevating the ipsilateral tonsil and hemisphere. There may be displacement of cranial nerves and brain stem but the papilloma can usually be easily be separated from these structures.[106]

At one time radiation therapy was commonly used for unresectable or recurrent papillomas, but it is controversial whether it is effective.[114-116] Since there are risks associated with radiation (especially in children), adjuvant radiotherapy is not warranted for these tumors, although some authors assert that radiotherapy may be effective in treating invasive benign tumors that could not be resected.[104] Choroid plexus carcinomas, on the other hand, should receive radiation to the entire craniospinal axis since these tumors often disseminate along CSF pathways; most long-term survivors of chroroid plexus carcinoma were treated with radiation.[109,115] Chemotherapy may be appropriate for young patients in which radiation is too risky.

Benign papillomas have a good prognosis. Total resection is usually curative without recurrence, and symptoms generally do not recur even following subtotal resection. Overall, 5-year survival rates for papillomas are nearly 100%.[103,104,114-116] Choroid plexus carcinomas have a much poorer prognosis because gross total resection is usually impossible due to frequent infiltration of brain stem and cerebellar peduncles and extreme vascularity, the tumor often disseminates through CSF pathways, and it usually occurs in very young children which limits use of adjuvant radiotherapy. While there are reports of gross total resection of choroid plexus carcinomas without recurrence,[103,109] they tend to recur even after total resection. Most authors agree that the degree of resection is the most important variable, followed by histology (cellular atypia, microscopic invasion, or mitosis).[116] Five-year survival rates vary significantly among reports, but are generally less than 50%, with carcinomas of the fourth ventricular choroid plexus having a worse prognosis than those in the lateral ventricles.[109,114]

HEMANGIOBLASTOMA

Hemangioblastomas are benign, slow-growing vascular tumors that are found exclusively in the neuraxis.[117] The most common location is the cerebellum, followed by the brain stem (usually on the floor of the fourth ventricle near the cervicomedullary junction) and spinal cord. They rarely occur supratentorially, but when they do and are dural based, it is difficult to distinguish them from angioblastic meningiomas. They account for 1% to 2% of all intracranial neoplasms, and 7% to 12% of adult postfossa tumors. Isolated sporadic hemangioblastomas are more common in middle-aged adults 30 to 40 years of age. Males slightly outnumber females.

Ten percent to 20% of hemangioblastomas occur as part of the von Hippel-Lindau syndrome. This syndrome was initially described in 1904 when von Hippel identified two patients with vascular retinal tumors. In 1926, Lindau noted an association with retinal tumors, cerebellar tumors, and visceral cysts.[118] It is now known that von Hippel-Lindau syndrome is an autosomal dominant condition with varying degrees of penetrance, similar to neurofibromatosis and other neurocutaneous syndromes.[119,120] In addition to multiple hemangioblastomas (which occur in 40% of patients with von Hippel-Lindau), there are multiple angiomatoses of the retina, visceral cysts and tumors especially of kidney and pancreas, pheochromocytoma, and papillary cystadenoma of epididymis or mesosalpinx (called "tubular adenomata" by Lindau). Recently the gene for von Hippel-Lindau has been mapped to a small region of chromosome 3p25-p26.[121] and a protein called pVHL identified that is a moderator of mRNA elongation and may be responsible for the syndrome. Whether associated with von Hippel-Lindau or not, hemangioblastomas are always benign tumors, and although there is occasional local subarachnoid seeding after surgery, distant metastases have never been reported.

As with most other tumors of the posterior fossa, the most common presenting symptoms are increased intracranial pressure and ataxia. Since the most common location is in the fourth ventricle at the level of the obex, some patients present with intractable nausea and vomiting from direct irritation of the area postrema in the fourth ventricular floor. The mass effect is usually due to cystic enlargement rather than the solid tumor itself.[122] In 10% of patients with hemangioblastoma, there will be a secondary polycythemia due to erythropoietin secreted by stromal tumor cells.[123,124] This is more common with solid tumors, but cyst fluid from hemangioblastomas often contains erythropoietin. Resection of the tumor usually improves this polycythemia. Any patient known to have retinal angioma and polycythemia should be scanned to rule out hemangioblastoma. If there is evidence of von Hippel-Lindau, it is necessary to image the entire neuraxis to search for multiple lesions. First degree relatives should also be screened since up to 20% will have the disease.

On CT and MRI, most fourth ventricular hemangioblastomas appear cystic with a mural nodule that is located next to the pial surface of the brain (usually inferior or lateral), but they can be solid or mixed (supratentorial and spinal lesions tend to be solid). The nodule (which contains the tumor) invariably enhances but the cyst wall does not. CT demonstrates an isodense tumor with hypodense cystic fluid. On MRI the solid portion of the tumor is hypointense to brain tissue on T1 and slightly hyperintense on T2, and the cyst fluid is isointense or hyperintense to CSF on T1 and hyperintense on T2 to CSF (Fig. 31-31). Most hemangioblastomas produce peritumoral edema visible on T2 and there are often flow voids that indicate enlarged draining veins (Fig. 31-32). There may be hemorrhage with a hemorrhagic fluid level within the tumor cyst or blood products such as hemosiderin within the solid tumor.[126] Tumors can be multiple with additional lesions in the brain stem and spinal cord; when in the spinal cord, they strongly resemble a syrinx except that they enhance dramatically with contrast.

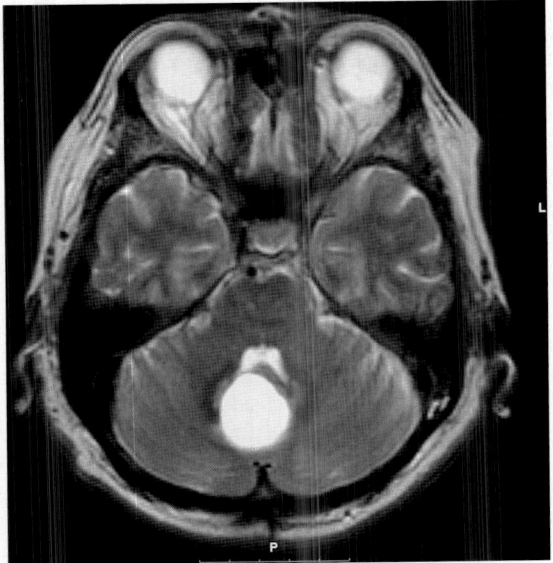

FIGURE 31-31 Cystic hemangioblastoma. T2. When in the posterior fossa, hemangioplastomas are usually cystic. This lesion had an enhancing subpial mural nodule that represented the tumor itself.

Leptomeningeal hemangioblastosis has been reported.[127] Because the tumors are extremely vascular, conventional or magnetic resonance angiography is essential in preoperative planning for successful removal of hemangioblastomas to identify the location of feeding vessels and develop a plan for early devascularization to avoid serious hemorrhage. For very large or vascular tumors, preoperative embolization of major feeding vessels may reduce intraoperative hemorrhage, although revascularization of the tumor occurs rapidly so the embolization should be carried out no more than 1 to 2 days prior to the operation. Patients with multiple small hemangioblastomas may be treated with embolization alone.

Grossly, hemangioblastomas are smooth orange tumors from high lipid content and the cut surface is beefy red from rich vascularity with multiple cysts. When cystic, there is always a mural nodule. The cyst fluid is golden yellow to brown and highly proteinaceous, and clots readily after aspiration. The inner surface of the cyst wall is smooth and made up of glial cells and compressed cerebellar tissue; the tumor itself never lines the cyst wall. Microscopically, the tumor consists of endothelial cells, pericytes, and stromal cells, but it is not known which of these cells participate in the neoplastic process or whether these cells interconvert. The most characteristic feature is the presence of numerous capillary channels that form an anastomosing plexiform pattern lined by a single layer of plump endothelial cells. This capillary network compartmentalizes larger, pale stromal cells with lipid vacuoles in the cytoplasm. Lindau thought these were endothelial cells that had ingested lipids that resulted from generation of myelin, but immunologic studies have shown that they do not originate from endovascular cells, and since they sometimes stain with GFAP and S100, it is possible that they are glial in origin. The nuclei are round, elongated, and sometimes multiple; this does not affect prognosis. There is no tumor capsule but the margin is well defined, and even if invasion occurs, complete resection is usually possible. There is often surrounding reactive astrocytosis. On frozen section, hemangioblastomas can be confused with cerebellar astrocytomas

or metastatic renal cell cancer (which coexists in 25% of patients with von Hippel-Lindau). Mast cells are common in hemangioblastomas and uncommon in other tumors, and negative staining for glycogen and epithelial membrane antigen should be able to differentiate hemangioblastoma from metastatic renal cancer.

Because hemangioblastomas are always benign and total removal is curative, surgical removal is the treatment of choice for fourth ventricle hemangioblastomas.[117] Perioperative steroids are helpful because of the extensive swelling, and sitting position may make hemorrhage easier to deal with intraoperatively. The fourth ventricle is exposed by standard techniques, and then different techniques are used to remove the tumor itself depending on whether it is cystic or solid. If the tumor is cystic, the cyst should be entered and the fluid drained. The mural nodule is then identified and dissected away from the cyst cavity using bipolar coagulating forceps. Occasionally the preoperative angiogram will identify a large feeding artery on the external surface of the cyst that must be divided prior to resecting the tumor; otherwise, the cyst wall should be left intact since it is not made up of tumor tissue but compressed gliotic cerebellum. If the tumor is solid, it is essential to avoid violating the tumor itself since this will lead to brisk hemorrhage. The dissection should be carried out between the external surface of the tumor and adjacent compressed gliotic cerebellum. Even after the major arterial supply has been controlled, there will frequently be many small perforating arteries or arterioles feeding the tumor that require coagulation. As soon as the dissection planes meet behind the tumor, it can be rolled out of the cerebellar bed and bleeding controlled. If the tumor tissue is violated prior to separation from the adjacent cerebellum, the tumor should be rapidly dissected from the cerebellar bed and hemorrhage controlled afterwards; attempting hemostasis within the center of tumor is futile and only leads to continued hemorrhage and delayed swelling.

All patients should get a postoperative enhanced MRI to determine if complete resection has been achieved. If no residual tumor remains, most patients have no recurrence, except in the case of von Hippel-Lindau. Partial resection usually leads to recurrence. Adjuvant radiotherapy is generally ineffective; although gamma knife can sometimes cause the solid portion of the tumor to stop growing or even to shrink, the cystic component does not respond and usually requires surgical treatment.[128]

EPITHELIAL CYSTS: EPIDERMOIDS AND DERMOIDS

Epidermoid and dermoid cysts occur intracranially as result of nests of epithelial cells remaining intracranially during embryogenesis probably due to failure of separation between neural and cutaneous ectoderm at the time of closure of the neural groove.[129] Epidermoids, also called pearly tumors or cholesteatomas, include only ectodermal elements. They are usually lateral in location; 50% are parapontine, and they frequently affect the cerebellopontine angle, suprasellar cistern, and cranial base.[130,131] By contrast, dermoid cysts include elements of all three germ layers and include skin appendages. They tend to be located along the central neuraxis anywhere from the pituitary to distal spinal cord, although the most common location is

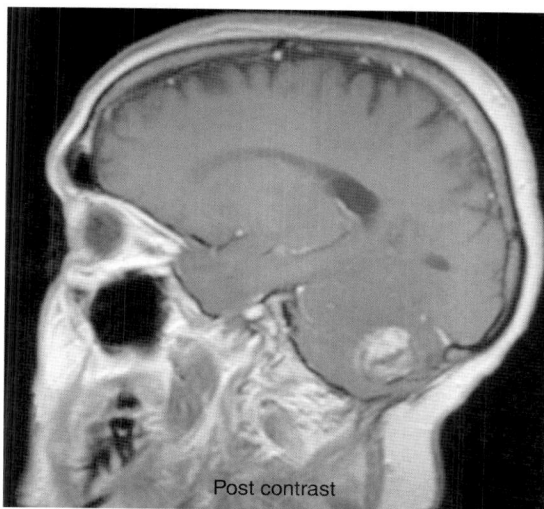

FIGURE 31-32 Solid hemangioblastoma, T1 with contrast, sagittal section. The tumor enhances brightly. Flow voids are seen that represent tumor vascularity.

in the posterior fossa, especially the fourth ventricle. Dermoids are sometimes associated with a dermal sinus tract that extends from the skin toward the tumor with an associated suboccipital skull defect,[132] and there will usually be a cutaneous marker such as hair, telangiectasia, pigmentation, or increased subcutaneous tissue. Together, epidermoids and dermoids account for 1% of intracranial masses, and epidermoids are somewhat more common in most clinical series. Males and females are affected equally.

Although congenital in origin, epidermoids and dermoids can become symptomatic at any age, although dermoids tend to manifest earlier, usually in childhood. Both tumors grow very slowly and by linear rather than exponential growth since they enlarge by deposition of stratified squamous epithelium and its products (such as keratin and cholesterol) into the center rather than mitotic proliferation as with true neoplasms. Dermoids grow somewhat faster since, in addition to growth by desquamation, they also fill with secretions of sebaceous glands, sweat glands, and hair follicles. Symptoms are related to site of the cyst and are not specific. Most become symptomatic due to mass effect, although epidermoids occasionally burrow into the brain stem. Epidermoids occasionally rupture causing sterile meningitis. Dermoids associated with a dermal sinus most often present with localized swelling, redness, tenderness, and purulent drainage from inflammation or infection of the dermal sinus. This often occurs several times before neurosurgical consult is obtained. Some patients present with meningitis or cerebellar abscess since the sinus tract can act as a portal for bacterial entry into the subarachnoid space,[133,134] and subsequent scarring can lead to hydrocephalus.

On CT, an epidermoid cyst appears as a nonenhancing hypodense mass with frond-like margins that interdigitate into normal brain structures. Dermoids have a similar appearance but are somewhat higher density and may also contain calcification or fat, and sometimes the cyst wall enhances with contrast. Both epidermoids and dermoids have well-defined margins and contain a central low-density area similar to CSF but with frequently nonhomogeneous contents ("dirty CSF"). On MRI, epidermoids appear homogeneous, hypointense to brain on T1-weighted images and hyperintense to CSF on T2. Dermoids appear more heterogeneous because of a greater variety of constituents (keratin debris has high attenuation and dermal elements have low attenuation), so their appearance varies considerably on different T-weighted images, but they are sometimes hyperintense to brain on T1 due to the presence of fatty tissue. Sometimes it is possible to see a dermal sinus tract. Both cyst types conform to adjacent anatomy but may produce some mass effect; they almost never produce edema.[135] Hydrocephalus can occur but is rarer than with other fourth ventricular tumors. Because the imaging appearance is so variable (especially for dermoids), the differential diagnosis can be extensive and includes abscess, cystic astrocytoma, hemangioblastoma, and even medulloblastoma or cystic ependymoma.

Grossly, epidermoids are pearly white from desquamated keratin, while dermoids are buttery yellow from pilosebaceous contents and sometimes contain hair. Because the connection between the dermal and neural ectoderm is small and there is minimal disturbance of mesoderm,

adjacent structures are usually not affected by the malformation. Epidermoids (but not dermoids) are sometimes seen to invaginate into adjacent brain, and the capsule of either can become adherent to surrounding neural structures, especially after infection or inflammation from fatty acids of degenerating material within the capsule. Microscopically, epidermoids are seen to be composed of stratified squamous epithelium, and dermoids also have skin appendages such as hair follicles, sebaceous glands, and sweat glands. Dermoids sometimes have areas of cystic degeneration. Malignant degeneration (squamous cell cancer) can occur, and is more common in epidermoids. Cysts of the fourth ventricle are almost invariably dermoids; if no skin appendages are seen on pathologic analysis, it is possible that the specimen does not include the whole tumor or dermal elements have been destroyed by inflammation.

Morbidity and degree of invasiveness of the tumor dictate decisions regarding surgical treatment. If surgically excised, these cysts must be totally removed since subtotal resection usually leads to recurrence. The capsule may separate easily or be densely adherent (especially if infected due to dermal sinus tract); either way, every effort should be made to keep the capsule intact to prevent spillage of cyst contents or purulent material into subarachnoid space, which can lead to severe chemical meningitis. If the cyst does rupture intraoperatively, the area should be copiously irrigated with corticosteroid irrigant and the patient should receive intravenous steroids postoperatively. Cysts that are densely adherent to the floor of the fourth ventricle or cervicomedullary junction can be gently coagulated with the bipolar forceps to minimize the risk of recurrence. If a dermal sinus tract is present, it must be explored even if imaging does not indicate any abnormality, although absence of bony defect on exploration excludes the possibility of intracranial extension. An elliptical incision is made around the opening of the dermal sinus tract and the bone is removed inferiorly since the tract always extends inferiorly below the torcular. The tract is then removed en toto. The sinus tract is often intimately related to torcula so it is important to be prepared for major venous bleeding. Postoperatively, all patients should receive an MRI scan with contrast to obtain a baseline; if residual cyst is seen immediate re-exploration is warranted. Overall, the long-term prognosis for patients with fourth ventricular dermoid or epidermoid cysts is quite good.[136]

In addition to epidermoids and dermoids, neuroepithelial and endodermal cysts can occur in the region of the fourth ventricle. Neuroepithelial cysts result from embryologic folding of primitive ventricular lining into or out of ventricles. These include ependymal cysts and colloid cysts that usually involve the anterior third ventricle but can rarely occur in the fourth ventricle.[137-139] They secrete solid or viscous exudate that results in gradual enlargement. Endodermal cysts are slow growing, endothelial-lined cysts that are most often located in the spinal canal but can occur in the fourth ventricle. They are likely due to an error in embryogenesis, probably early in gastrulation since their location tends to follow the location of the primitive notochord.[140,141] Each of these are very slow growing but can become symptomatic from mass effect due to local compression or obstruction of the ventricular system; many remain asymptomatic and are discovered only incidentally or at autopsy. Treatment options for symptomatic cysts include excision, fenestration, or shunting.

MENINGIOMA

Meningiomas can rarely produce a fourth ventricular mass. Overall, meningiomas are quite common and account for more than 15% of all primary intracranial tumors, but intraventricular meningiomas account for only 0.5% to 2% of all meningiomas, and most intraventricular meningiomas are in the trigone of the lateral ventricle. Fourth ventricular meningiomas without dural attachment are quite rare.[142-145] The first reported case of a fourth ventricular meningioma that was removed by Ernest Sachs in 1936 in a patient with diminished hearing, leading Cushing to suggest coexistent neurofibromatosis.[146] Since then, there have been only a few dozen additional cases reported. Meningiomas are believed to arise from arachnoid cap cells, which are specialized cells found on outer aspect of the arachnoid layer particularly at arachnoid granulations, because the distribution of location of meningiomas parallels the frequency of arachnoid cap cells in normal meninges.[147] It is possible that these cells are dragged into ventricles by vessels piercing the ependymal layer during choroid plexus development. Most fourth ventricular meningiomas arise from the choroid plexus or inferior tela choroidea, although they can extend into the posterior fossa from the posterior petrous ridge, clivus, tentorium, foramen magnum, or cerebellar hemisphere convexity. The blood supply is usually from PICA.

Meningiomas primary affect adults, and peak occurrence is during the fifth decade. Females are affected more often than males. Typically fourth ventricular meningiomas are asymptomatic until large enough to obstruct flow of CSF. The vast majority are larger than three centimeters by the time of presentation. The most common symptoms are headache, vomiting, nystagmus, cerebellar dysfunction such as ataxia and dysmetria, cranial nerve palsies, and behavioral change.[144]

Because they are so rare, there are few descriptions of radiologic appearance of fourth ventricular meningiomas. In general, meningiomas are isodense on CT and T1 MRI, bright on T2; they enhance brightly with contrast. There is usually no peritumoral edema. There is often calcification, and sometimes flow voids representing large blood vessels surround the tumor. Angiography can be used to identify tumor feeding vessels.

Grossly, meningiomas are firm, well-circumscribed, and globular or lobulated yellow to pink-gray tumors. They are usually homogeneous in consistency and can be cystic or gritty from calcification. Microscopically, meningiomas are divided into four categories: meningothelial, fibroblastic, transitional (between meningothelial and fibroblastic), and angioblastic. Meningothelial meningiomas have uniform sheets of cells with indistinct borders, occasional orientation into whorls, foamy yellow areas (call xanthomatous), and basophilic calcifications called psammoma ("sand") bodies. Fibroblastic meningiomas have spindle cells with elongated interwoven bundles of cell bodies with collagen and reticulin fibers. Angioblastic meningiomas have pathology very similar to hemangiopericytoma and hemangioblastoma, and some believe that they are not meningiomas at all. Among fourth ventricular meningiomas, pathologic

analysis has been roughly equally divided between meningothelial, fibroblastic, and transitional.[143] A few have been largely psamommatous, one osteoblastic,[148] one associated with Sturge-Weber syndrome,[149] and one with an associated inflammatory reaction.[150]

Because they are well circumscribed with distinct borders, fourth ventricular meningiomas can usually be completely resected. After exposing the fourth ventricle, the blood supply is identified (usually from the choroid plexus in lateral recess) and coagulated. The tumor is then resected in piecemeal fashion, progressively folding the capsule inward and using cottonoid patties to define the border between brain and tumor and protect the fourth ventricle. If the meningioma is very large, it may be necessary to debulk internally using suction or ultrasonic aspiration before identifying the attachment site to the choroid plexus. Alternatively, if very small, it is sometimes possible to remove the tumor en bloc. Most patients do quite well after complete resection with few recurrences.

SUBEPENDYMOMA

Fourth ventricular subependymomas are rare neoplasms that account for less than 1% of all tumors in adults.[151,152] Peak incidence is 40 to 60 years of age, and males are affected more often than females. They are usually found on the caudal fourth ventricular floor or roof of the fourth ventricle, but have also been described in the lateral recess of the fourth ventricle, the lateral ventricles, and rarely the third ventricle. They are frequently asymptomatic and usually found incidentally at autopsy, but can grow large enough to produce hydrocephalus or mass effect causing visual abnormalities, ataxia, or cranial nerve palsies.[153] They have been associated with the Chiari II malformation.[154]

On CT, subependymomas are assymmetric, lobulated, often calcified intraventricular masses that enhance moderately with contrast. MRI reveals a mass that is hypointense on T1 and hyperintense on T2 with little or no surrounding edema. Compared with lateral and third ventricular subependymomas, fourth ventricular subependymomas are more likely to have calcification and enhance (heterogeneously) with contrast[155] (Fig. 31-33). Grossly they can be firm or friable but are usually gray and soft with occasional cystic change and hemorrhage.[151] Small subependymomas often have a small area of attachment to the ventricular wall with sharp demarcation from the underlying brain, but larger tumors will often have several secondary sites of attachment.[151] Microscopically, subependymomas have a lobulated appearance with clusters of astrocytic nuclei in a dense fibrillary background of neuroglial fibers.[156] There are no cytologic features of malignancy such as mitoses but the tumor can infiltrate the brain.

It is controversial whether these tumors arise from subependymal glia, astrocytes of the subependymal plate, ependyma, a mixture of astrocytes and ependymal cells, or simply a non-neoplastic reaction to another process such as meningitis. Initially it was believed that the subependymomas originated from subependymal glia because microscopically the cells resemble fibrillary subependymal astrocytes. However, mixed ependymoma/subependymoma tumors have been described in which areas typical for subependymoma are adjacent to areas typical for ependymoma.[152] Also, electron microscopic analysis of

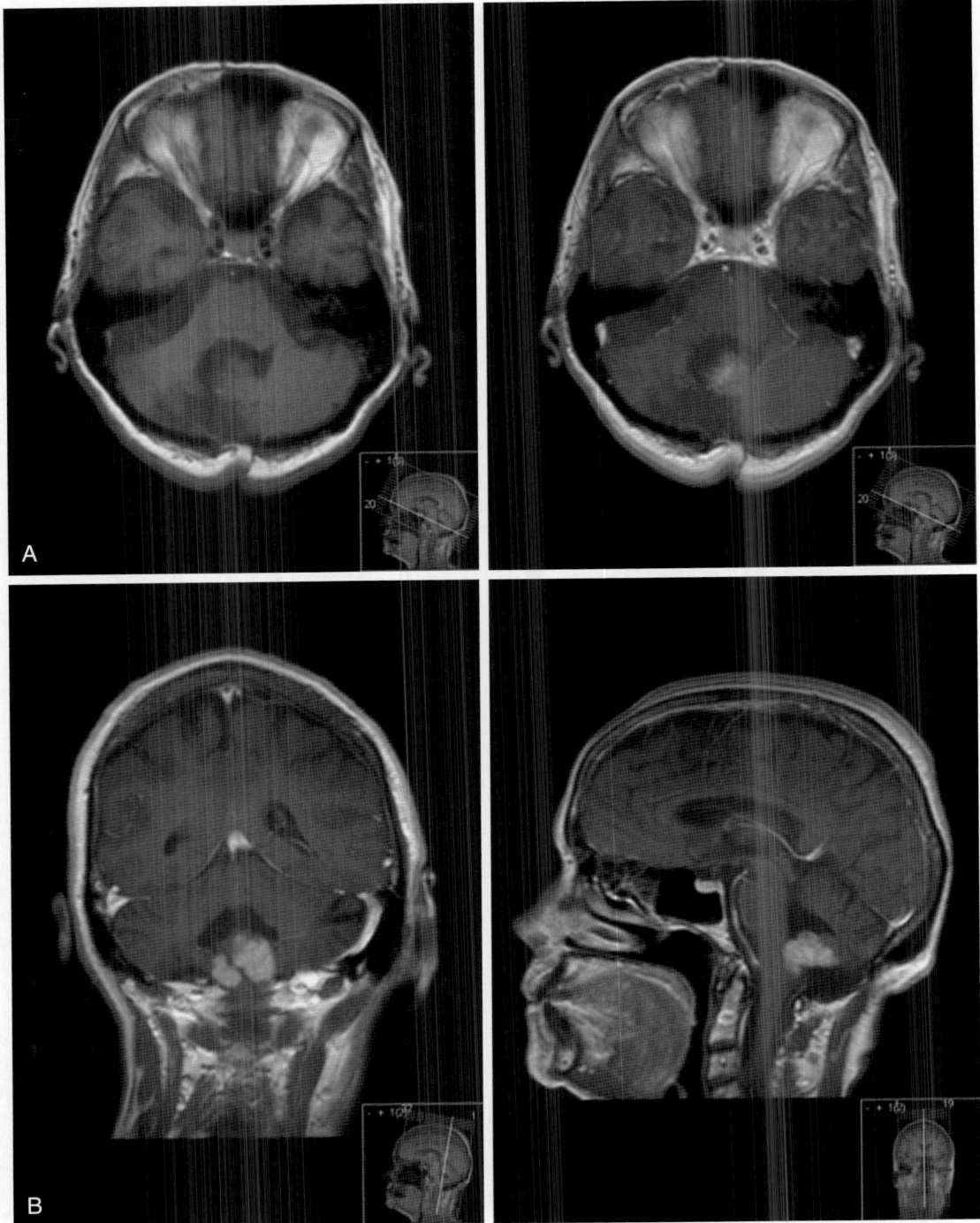

FIGURE 31-33 Subependymoma. A, T1 without (*left*) and with contrast (*right*), axial sections. Fourth ventricular subependymoma is noted in a 75-year-old patient. B, T1 with contrast, coronal (*left*) and sagittal (*right*) sections. Note enhancement present in this fourth ventricular subependymoma in an adult patient.

subependymoma reveals blepharoplasts, intermediate junctions, and microvilli that suggest ependyma, along with intermediate filaments that suggest astrocytoma.[157]

If the patient is asymptomatic and there is no sign of brain-stem compression, it is appropriate to follow with serial MRI scans to monitor growth of the tumor. Subependymomas occasionally become symptomatic and warrant surgical treatment. After internal debulking with ultrasonic

aspiration or laser, the tumor is gradually folded in on itself and dissected from the surrounding brain. There is usually a well-defined plane between the tumor and normal brain, but occasionally the tumor will be infiltrative and adherent, presumably due to an ependymal component of the tumor. In these cases, it is extremely important not to pull on the capsule attached to the fourth ventricle, since respiratory failure from brain-stem manipulation is the most common perioperative cause of death in patients with subependymoma.[152] If the patient is elderly and presents with obstructive hydrocephalus without brain-stem compression from a mass with radiologic appearance consistent with subependymoma, insertion of a ventriculoperitoneal shunt and observation with MRI may be a good alternative to removing the tumor surgically.

Most patients who survive surgery to completely resect a pure subependymoma do well with no recurrence,[151] although the natural history of incomplete resection is not known.[153] Presence of an ependymal component carries a worse prognosis and should be treated as a true ependymoma.

LHERMITTE-DUCLOS DISEASE

Lhermitte-Duclos disease is characterized by a cerebellar mass of abnormal ganglion cells producing circumscribed regions of enlarged cerebellar folia.[36,158] It is unclear whether it represents a congenital cerebellar malformation, hamartoma, phakomatosis, arrest of cell migration, graded hypertrophy of granular cell neurons, or true neoplasm. Immunohistochemical analysis confirms that the cells are derived from granule cells with a minor population of Purkinje cells, and they have no significant proliferative activity, which suggests that the disease is a non-neoplastic malformation predominantly derived from granule cells.[159] Because little is known about its pathogenesis, many names have been used to describe this lesion,[158] including dysplastic gangliocytoma, hamartoma, hamartoblastoma, neurocytic blastoma, diffuse ganglioneuroma, myelinated neurocytoma, granulomolecular cerebellar hypertrophy, gangliocytoma myelinicum diffusum, and purkinjeoma.

Most patients with Lhermitte-Duclos also have megencephaly. Other associated malformations include hydromyelia, cortical heterotopia, leontiasis ossea, neurofibromatosis, microgyria, hemihypertrophy, numerous hemangiomata, and polydactyly.[160] It is known to be familial in some cases,[161] and there is an association between Lhermitte-Duclos and Cowden disease,[162-165] an autosomal dominant condition characterized by multiple cutaneous trichilemmomas, oral papillomatosis, and increased incidence of breast, colon, adnexa malignancies. The association suggests that both conditions may represent a single disorder of cellular development, perhaps a phakomatosis involving all three germ layers with a tendency for malignant degeneration of lesions.[163]

Peak incidence is between 20 and 40 years of age,[158] but patients can present at any age, even at birth.[166] There is no sex predominance. In most cases, the lesion grows slowly and produces few symptoms until the abnormal bulk of the cerebellum becomes large enough to obstruct flow of CSF and produce brain-stem compression. Most patients have a history of several months of progressive headache, vomiting, gait disturbance, and cranial nerve dysfunction. The lesion almost always becomes progressively larger and is rarely an incidental finding at autopsy.

Imaging demonstrates unilateral cerebellar enlargement with a gyriform pattern within the lesion corresponding to the enlarged folia (Fig. 31-34). Most patients have hydrocephalus from fourth ventricular compression at the time of presentation. On CT, the mass is hypodense with ill-defined borders and no enhancement. There is sometimes thinning

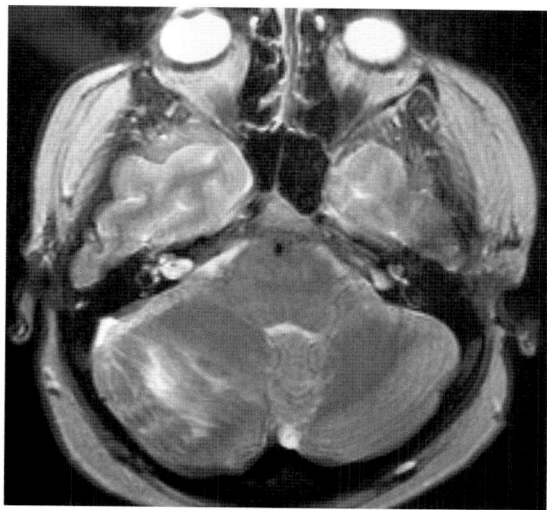

FIGURE 31-34 Lhermitte-Duclos disease. T2. Note the enlarged cerebellar folia on the right and mass effect on the fourth ventricle. This patient also had hydrocephalus.

of occipital squama and focal areas of calcification.[167-170] On MRI, the lesion is well defined, hypointense on T1 and hyperintense on T2. The lesion usually does not enhance on CT or MRI,[168,171] but there is occasionally peripheral enhancement due to proliferation of veins near the edge of the tumor in the molecular layer and leptomeninges.[172,173] Except for the lack of enhancement, the mass can closely resemble a low-grade astrocytoma.[170,174] The preserved folial pattern and lack of enhancement produces a striated "tiger-striped cerebellum" pattern that is characteristic of this tumor.[175,176]

Grossly, Lhermitte-Duclos appears as broad, pale cerebellar folia confined to one hemisphere or a portion of one hemisphere.[36,177] Microscopically, there is a thick outer layer of well-developed myelinated nerve fibers, encompassing an inner layer of abnormal densely packed neurons that superficially resemble Purkinje cells. There is no layering of Purkinje cells and granular neurons, the folia central white matter is often absent, and that transition between normal and abnormal areas is gradual.

As the lesion almost always continues to enlarge progressively, patients who become symptomatic from Lhermitte-Duclos invariably require surgery. Upon exposure of the cerebellum, the large pale broadened gyri should be immediately apparent. The affected tissue is usually hypovascular and easily removed with ultrasonic aspiration.[177] Since there is no clear plane between involved and normal cerebellum, the preoperative MRI should be used to determine the extent of resection. Recurrence years after initial resection have been reported,[159,178-180] so complete resection should be attempted and patients should get periodic follow-up MRI scans. Otherwise no adjuvant treatment is necessary.

METASTASIS

Brain metastases occur in about one quarter of all patients with metastatic cancer, so metastases outnumber all other brain tumors in adults. This is true in the posterior fossa as well, where 15% of metastases are located (equal to the proportional weight of brain tissue in the posterior fossa).[181,182]

In adults, the most common metastases to brain tissue are lung (30%), breast (20%), melanoma (10%), kidney (10%), and gastrointestinal tract (5%). Some cancers, like melanoma, metastasize to the brain very commonly, so melanoma brain metastases are often found even though it is a relatively rare tumor. Others, like gastrointestinal tumors, rarely metastasize to the brain but are so common that they are frequently found in the brain. Any tumor that metastasizes to the brain can be found in the posterior fossa, but gastrointestinal, bladder, and uterine tumors do so slightly more often than the others do, and lymphoma sometimes presents as a subependymal mass that extends into the ventricle. When they occur in the posterior fossa, metastatic tumors often become symptomatic from fourth ventricular compression, and most patients present with signs of increased intracranial pressure and hydrocephalus. In children, the most common metastatic tumors are neuroblastoma, rhabdomyosarcoma, Wilms' tumor, and ALL (chloromas).

The radiographic appearance of metastatic tumors is highly variable. CT may show hyperdensity (from dense cellularity of most metastatic tumors) or hypodensity, and MRI may be hyperintense, hypointense, or isointense on both T1 and T2. Metastases usually occur at the gray-white junction and are often multiple, although renal and gastrointestinal metastases tend to be solitary. Because they have no blood-brain barrier, virtually all metastatic tumors enhance on CT and MRI, either diffusely or at the tumor margins ("ring-enhancing"); there are sometimes nonenhancing central areas consistent with necrosis.[183,184] Hemorrhage is more characteristic of certain tumors, especially melanoma, choriocarcinoma, renal cell cancer, and lung cancer. Adjacent tissue usually has significant vasogenic edema that follows white matter tracts that is often so extensive that the tumor will be obscured on CT or T2-weighted MRI. The histology of metastases is similar to that of the tumor of origin. They differ from primary brain tumors in that they contain more collagen and have more distinct borders with adjacent normal brain.

Brain metastases are usually tertiary metastases from previously metastatic locations in the lung, liver, or lymph nodes; therefore, presence of metastases in the brain suggests advanced cancer, and the prognosis is very poor. Survival rates vary with different tumors, but few patients survive more than 1 year. Surgery for metastatic disease can prolong patients' survival and quality of life, especially if the metastasis is solitary, which is true in about 50%.[181] Radiation is often used as primary or adjunctive therapy.

OTHER TUMORS OF THE FOURTH VENTRICLE

Teratomas rarely occur in the fourth ventricle or cerebellar vermis, either along or in combination with the more common pineal location.[185-189] Clival chordomas, arising from the remnants of the primitive notochord, can spread along the floor of the posterior fossa to compress the brain stem and cranial nerves, and require adjuvant radiotherapy since complete surgical excision is rarely possible. Nerve root fibromas of the lower cranial nerves often affect the cerebellopontine angle, especially in neurofibromatosis type II, which includes bilateral vestibular schwannomas and silent fibromas of the vagus and trigeminal nerves. Gangliogliomas have been described in the cerebellum and brain stem.[190,191] Finally, single cases of fourth ventricular myxofibroxanthoma[192] and hemangioma calcificans[193] have been reported.

Molecular Biology and Cytogenetics

While some tumors of the fourth ventricle are benign and relatively curable by surgical resection alone, more malignant tumors pose a particular challenge for the neurosurgeon. With malignant subtypes, surgical cure is often not possible, and recurrence, prognosis, and novel treatment strategies become important in treatment paradigms. With advents in molecular biology and cytogenetics, our understanding of certain tumors of the fourth ventricle has become more robust. The goals are to use molecular advances to improve our current therapy regimens, develop new targeted treatments, and define markers for prognostic stratification.

MEDULLOBLASTOMA

Studies of the molecular biology and genetics of medulloblastomas have led to a better understanding of the disease, and to novel treatments. Medulloblastomas are difficult to cure, with some subtypes carrying a poorer prognosis. Various genetic alterations and molecular aberrations have been identified in these tumors, including mutations in the hedgehog (Hh), Wnt, and Notch pathways, which are active during embryogenesis as well as cellular proliferation and/or differentiation.[193-195] This understanding has led to important clinical translations. Other pathways are also implicated. More recently, several groups have tried to stratify medulloblastomas into molecular subgroups, currently four to five based on genetic profiles, each subgroup with predominant aberrations in the Wnt, Hh, and other pathways.[193,196-198] Though we are beginning to understand that some subgroups have a better prognosis and some a poorer one, more studies are needed to understand the clinical behavior of tumors with various molecular profiles active.[193]

In addition, understanding the molecular pathways active in medulloblastomas has led to novel treatments. Cyclophosphamide has been recognized as an Hh pathway inhibitor, with promising results in vitro and in vivo.[193-195] Small-molecule inhibitors have also been used to block the Hh pathway. ErbB pathway inhibition may also be a promising target, as well as HDAC inhibitors that act on histone deacetylases, which are involved in gene expression control.[193-195] New targets and pharmacologic agents are under investigation.

EPENDYMOMA

Ependymomas are common tumors encountered in the pediatric and adult population, and can occur in the posterior fossa, the spine, and the supratentorial regions. Though histologically they are often indistinguishable, current studies suggest that ependymomas from these different locations may have very distinct molecular and genetic profiles.[193] Frequent chromosomal abnormalities include losses of 6q, 17p, and 22q, and gains of 1q and 9q.[193] More recently amplifications of MYCN, EGFR, NOTCH1, NOTCH4, VAV1, YAP1, and deletion of CDKN2A and SULT4A1 have also been observed.[193] The search for driver genes involved in tumorigenesis is still ongoing. Despite our growing understanding of the molecular factors involved in the formation of these tumors, prognosis remains poor, and translation of genetic profiles into therapeutic targets is still needed.

PILOCYTIC ASTROCYTOMA

Though pilocytic astrocytomas in the posterior fossa can have a good outcome with complete surgical resection, those in locations near the brain stem can have a less favorable prognosis and outcome. Some chromosomal changes noted in pilocytic astrocytomas have been trisomy of 5 and 7, and gain of 7q.[193] More recently, smaller chromosomal aberrations have been identified, such as duplication of chromosome 7q34, containing the locus for the BRAF gene, which is beginning to be identified as an important oncogene in the development of these tumors.[193] Other gene alterations also have been noted. For instance, BRAF-KIAA1549 gene fusion but no mutation of IDH1 or IDH2 has been noted in up to 70% of pilocytic astrocytomas as compared to diffuse astrocytomas, further helping to stratify glial tumor subtypes occurring in this location as separate clinical entities for prognosis and treatment.[193]

Further studies of the molecular cytogenetics of fourth ventricular tumors remain promising. In addition, understanding alterations of epigenetic phenomena that govern tumorigenesis of these lesions can help further drive risk stratification, treatment, and perhaps prognosis.

Conclusion

Tumors that arise in the fourth ventricle present the neurosurgeon with a unique challenge since there are many vital neural structures in close proximity to the lesions. Most posterior fossa tumors occur in children, and medulloblastoma, astrocytoma, and ependymoma are the most common. In adults, the most common lesions are metastasis and hemangioblastoma. Improvements in surgical technique and instrumentation have resulted in better outcomes for patients with these tumors.

KEY REFERENCES

Albrecht S, Haber RM, Goodman JC, et al. Cowden syndrome and Lhermitte-Duclos disease. *Cancer.* 1991;70:869-876.

Bambakidis NC, Robinson S, Cohen M, et al. Atypical teratoid/rhabdoid tumors of the central nervous system: clinical, radiographic and pathologic features. *Pediatr Neurosurg.* 2002;37(2):64-70.

Berger MS, Wilson CB. Epidermoid cyst of the posterior fossa. *J Neurosurg.* 1985;62:214-219.

Bertolone SJ, Yates AJ, Boyett JM. Combined modality therapy for poorly differentiated gliomas of the posterior fossa in children: a Children's Cancer Group report. *J Neurooncol.* 2003;63(1):49-54.

Breslow N, Langholz B. Childhood cancer incidence: geographical and temporal variations. *Int J Cancer.* 1983;32:702-716.

Burkhard C, Di Patre PL, Schuler D, et al. A population-based study of the incidence and survival rates in patients with pilocytic astrocytoma. *J Neurosurg.* 2003;98(6):1170-1174.

Campbell JW, Pollack IF. Cerebellar astrocytomas in children. *J Neurooncol.* 1996;28(2):223-231:(3).

Carlotti CG, Smith C, Rutka JT, et al. The molecular genetics of medulloblastoma: an assessment of new therapeutic targets. *Neurosurg Rev.* 2008;31:359-369.

Desai KI, Nadkarni TD, Muzumdar DP, et al. Prognostic factors for cerebellar astrocytomas in children: a study of 102 cases. *Pediatr Neurosurg.* 2001;35(6):311-317.

Dubuc AM, Northcott PA, Mack S, et al. The genetics of pediatric brain tumors. *Curr Neurol Neurosci Rep.* 2010;10:215-223.

Duffner PK, Cohen ME, Thomas PRM, et al. The long-term effects of cranial irradiation in the central nervous system. *Cancer.* 1985;56:1841-1847.

Ellenbogen RG, Winston KR, Kupsky WJ. Tumors of the choroid plexus in children. *Neurosurgery.* 1989;25:327-335.

Epstein F, McCleary EL. Intrinsic brain-stem tumors of childhood: surgical indications. *J Neurosurg.* 1986;64:11-15.

Farmer JP, Montes JL, Freeman CR, et al. Brainstem gliomas. A 10-year institutional review. *Pediatr Neurosurg.* 2001;34(4):206-214.

Fernandez C, Figarella-Branger D, Girard N, et al. Pilocytic astrocytomas in children: prognostic factors—a retrospective study of 80 cases. *Neurosurgery.* 2003;53(3):544-553.

Guyotat J, Signorelli F, Desme S, et al. Intracranial ependymomas in adult patients: analyses of prognostic factors. *J Neurooncol.* 2002;60(3):255-268.

Northcott PA, Rutka JT, Taylor MD, et al. Genomics of medulloblastoma: from Giemsa-banding to next-generation sequencing in 20 years. *Neurosurg Focus.* 2010;28(1):E6.

Onvani S, Etame A, Smith CA, et al. Genetics of medulloblastoma: clues for novel therapies. *Exp Rev.* 2010;10(5):811-823.

Packer RJ, Sutton LN, D'Angio G, et al. Management of children with primitive neuroectodermal tumors of the posterior fossa/medulloblastoma. *Pediatr Neurosci.* 1985-86;12:272-282.

Smyth MD, Horn BN, Russo C, et al. Intracranial ependymomas of childhood: current management strategies. *Pediatr Neurosurg.* 2000;33(3):138-150.

Tarbell NJ, Loeffler JS. Recent trends in the radiotherapy of pediatric gliomas. *J Neurooncol.* 1996;28(2):233-244:(3).

Thompson MC, Fuller C, Hogg TL, et al. Genomics identifies medulloblastoma subgroups that are enriched for specific genetic alterations. *J Clin Oncol.* 2006;24(12):1924-1931.

van Veelen-Vincent ML, Pierre-Kahn A, Kalifa C, et al. Ependymoma in childhood: prognostic factors, extent of surgery, and adjuvant therapy. *J Neurosurg.* 2002;97(4):827-835.

Wanebo JE, Lonser RR, Glenn GM, et al. The natural history of hemangioblastomas of the central nervous system in patients with von Hippel-Lindau disease. *J Neurosurg.* 2003;98(1):82-94.

Weil RJ, Lonser RR, DeVroom HL, et al. Surgical management of brainstem hemangioblastomas in patients with von Hippel-Lindau disease. *J Neurosurg.* 2003;98(1):95-105.

Numbered references appear on Expert Consult.

CHAPTER 32

Surgical Management of Parasagittal and Convexity Meningiomas

ASHOK R. ASTHAGIRI • RUSSELL R. LONSER

There is today nothing in the whole realm of surgery more gratifying than the successful removal of a meningioma with subsequent perfect functional recovery…
—Harvey Cushing[1]

Epidemiology and Significance

Meningiomas are the most common primary brain and central nervous system tumor (incidence rate, 6.29 per 100,000 persons). Data from the 2004–2006 Central Brain Tumor Registry reveal that these tumors account for approximately 34% of all primary brain tumors. Meningiomas occur in females 2.25 times more frequently than males (incidence: 8.44 per 100,000 females vs. 3.76 per 100,000 males).[2] An increased incidence has been reported among Africans and black Americans.[3,4] The incidence rate increases with older age and peaks in persons over 85 years of age (incidence over age of 85 years of age: 36.9 cases per 100,000 persons).[2] Meningiomas occur most frequently on the convexity (19% to 34%) and parasagittal locations (18% to 25%), followed by the sphenoid wing and middle cranial fossa (17% to 25%), anterior skull base (10%), posterior fossa (9% to 15%), cerebellar convexity (5%) and clivus (<1%).[5-7] To optimize patient management and surgical outcome, understanding appropriate surgical objectives and technique based on the location and biology of these neoplasms is critical.

Etiology

SPORADIC

The etiology of the majority of meningiomas is unknown. Although head injury, viral infection, and cell phone use have been implicated in the development of intracranial meningiomas,[8,9] the data are inconclusive and conflicting for each of these potential etiologies. The strongest support for an etiologic role in the development and progression of sporadic meningiomas is hormonal. Specifically, studies have shown a potential progesterone influence in the development of meningiomas based on the propensity of these tumors to occur in females and the presence of progesterone receptors in the majority of meningiomas.[10-13] While few definitive etiologic correlations have been made for meningiomas, there are certain iatrogenic, environmental exposure and genetic causes that have been linked to their development. These tumorigenic etiologies have significant implications for the management of a meningioma patient who presents for treatment.

RADIATION INDUCED

Meningioma development is associated with irradiation exposure. This association was established by two large cohorts of individuals exposed to radiation that subsequently developed tumors, including meningiomas. Studies published on a group of nearly 11,000 Israeli children treated with low-dose (approximately 1.5 Gy) radiation for tinea capitis revealed a 9.5 times risk for development of meningioma compared to matched controls and untreated siblings.[14,15] Similarly, the incidence of meningioma formation among 68 survivors of the Hiroshima atomic bomb within a 2-km radius of the hypocenter identified a 2.9 times risk for the development of meningioma with higher risk for patients within a 1-km radius (6.7 times risk).[16] Other iatrogenic forms of ionizing radiation exposure have also been linked to the subsequent development of intracranial meningiomas, including higher-dose, full-mouth dental radiographs and radiotherapy provided for treatment of other cancers.[17-20] Generally, radiation-induced meningiomas have a dose dependent latency to development of 10 to over 30 years and have a higher propensity to recur after resection.[21]

Radiation-induced meningiomas tend to be a higher pathologic grade when compared to their sporadic counterparts, but even WHO grade I radiation–induced meningiomas exhibit more aggressive clinical behavior and have an increased proclivity to recur when compared to their sporadic counterparts.[19,22,23] Patients with radiation-induced meningiomas also have an increased incidence of multiple tumors, which must be accounted for when planning placement of the incison.[17,24,25] Further, atrophic changes in the scalp that commonly accompany cranial irradiation can require modification of standard multilayer scalp closure. Because radiation exposure can result in other delayed side effects, patients with radiation-induced meningiomas require close medical follow-up for other sequelae, including pituitary dysfunction, visual disturbances (optic atrophy), radiation necrosis, and development of other neoplasms (sarcoma, glioma).[26]

NEUROFIBROMATOSIS TYPE 2 (NF2)

NF2 is an autosomal dominant heritable tumor predisposition syndrome that leads to the development of central and peripheral nervous system tumors (meningiomas, schwannomas, ependymomas), ophthalmologic findings (cataracts, epiretinal membranes, retinal hamartomas) and cutaneous findings (skin plaques, subcutaneous tumors).[27] Intracranial meningiomas are identified in approximately half of NF2 patients and are a significant source of morbidity and mortality. NF2-associated intracranial meningiomas are frequently multiple and develop at a younger age than compared to sporadic cases of meningiomas.[28-31] Up to 20% of children presenting with a meningioma will have NF2, necessitating full clinical screening and longitudinal follow-up.[28,32] The presence of intracranial meningiomas is associated with a 2.5-fold rise in relative risk of mortality in patients with NF2.[33] Meningiomas associated with NF2 frequently have increased proliferative activity and a greater rate of atypical and anaplastic grades than do sporadic meningiomas.[34,35] Because of the frequent multiplicity of lesions, we perform resection of tumors based on the development of symptoms rather than radiographic tumor growth.

MULTIPLE MENINGIOMAS

Examination of a large series reporting on the presence of multiple meningiomas found that 1% to 10.5% of patients may present with multiple tumors.[34] Identification of patients with multiple meningiomas has increased significantly with the advent of improved imaging techniques. Both sporadic and familial forms of multiple meningiomas have been described in the literature, independent of NF2 or history of radiation exposure.[37-40] Familial forms of the disease follow an autosomal dominant inheritance pattern and are caused by a mutation independent of the *NF2* gene.[41,42] Tumors in patients with multiple sporadic meningiomas appear to originate from a single clone (suggesting metastatic spread), whereas others may develop these tumors independently, based on cytogenetic differences among tumors.[43-45] Patients with sporadic or familial forms of multiple meningiomas present dilemmas in management similar to patients with NF2, resection is often reserved until the development of symptoms rather radiographic tumor growth.

Classification

Meningiomas originate from arachnoid cap cells, which are distributed along the entire neuroaxis and reflect the wide spectrum of tumor localization. The preoperative classification of meningiomas is based on location of the tumor, primary dural attachment and relationship to neurovascular structures. In the Cavendish Lecture presented in 1922, Harvey Cushing coined the term "meningioma" and classified these tumors based on their site of origin.[1] Later, in 1938, Cushing and Eisenhardt used preoperative anatomic classification of meningiomas as a method to correlate clinical findings, help determine surgical approach and aide in developing a prognosis.[46] To this day, preoperative anatomic localization remains of critical importance, because it determines surgical positioning, placement of incision and risks involved with resection of the tumor.

CONVEXITY MENINGIOMAS

Convexity meningiomas refer to tumors of the supratentorial space that have their sole attachment to the dura covering the convexity of the cerebral hemispheres. The original classification of convexity meningiomas by Cushing included temporal, frontal, paracentral, parietal and occipital locations.[1] Several studies examining the distribution of convexity tumors reveal that the frontal region is the most common site of origin (over 50%), with the posterior locations least frequent (7% to 11%), and the remainder equally distributed between the temporal and paracentral locations.[47,48] Because of improvements in the ability to localize tumors and their relationship to functional cortices based on anatomic and functional imaging studies, it is possible to preoperatively classify convexity tumors, anticipate clinical symptoms and the specific risks associated with their management.

PARASAGITTAL MENINGIOMAS

Parasagittal meningiomas have an attachment to the dura forming the outer layer of the SSS and occupy the parasagittal angle displacing brain from this location (Fig. 32-1). Olivecrona first classified parasagittal meningiomas based on their anatomic location along the superior sagittal sinus (SSS). He divided the SSS into thirds anatomically (anterior, middle, posterior) because of the potential consequences of sinus occlusion during complete removal of meningiomas in each area.[49] The most common location for parasagittal meningiomas to arise is along the middle third of the SSS (from coronal suture to bregma). Tumors in this location account for 37% to 70% of parasagittal tumors. Fifteen to 42% of parasagittal meningiomas are located along the anterior third of the SSS (from the glabella to the coronal suture) and 9% to 16% of parasagittal tumors are located along the posterior third of the SSS (between the bregma and torcula).[50,51]

Differentiating parasagittal meningiomas from convexity and falcine meningiomas has significant implications for preoperative evaluation and surgical planning. In the instance where tumors of the convexity approach the SSS, they are distinguished from parasagittal tumors by the presence of brain tissue at the parasagittal angle and lack of attachment to the meninges that create the outer wall of the superior sagittal sinus itself. A similar distinction is made of falcine meningiomas, which are delineated from parasagittal tumors because their sole dural attachment is the falx cerebri. Parasagittal meningiomas vary in the amount of attachment to convexity dura and the falx cerebri, but they all have an attachment to the dura forming the outer layer of the SSS and occupy the parasagittal angle displacing brain tissue from this location (Fig. 32-1).

Clinical Presentation

Meningiomas are discovered incidentally or as a result of the development of related signs and/or symptoms. The increasing use of computed tomography (CT) and magnetic resonance (MR)-imaging has led to an increase in the number of incidentally discovered meningiomas over the last two decades. Currently, incidentally discovered meningiomas represent 10% to 20% of all meningiomas that are brought to clinical attention. Overall, clinical symptoms from meningiomas develop as a result of raised intracranial pressure, disruption of cortical electrophysiology or direct mass effect on adjacent neural structures.

CONVEXITY MENINGIOMAS

Similar to other mass-occupying lesion in the central nervous system, convexity meningiomas can present with a variety of signs and symptoms based on their anatomic location. Symptomatic convexity meningiomas most commonly are associated with headache (39% to 48%), seizures (20% to 34%), and/or hemiparesis (10% to 21%).[47,48,52] Other specific symptomatology, such as dysphasia, sensory changes, and visual disturbance occur less frequently but develop when tumors are located specifically over the respective eloquent cortices.

PARASAGITTAL MENINGIOMAS

Signs and symptoms associated with parasagittal meningiomas depend on their location along the SSS. Tumors of the anterior third of the SSS often cause headache and personality changes. Tumors of the middle third of the SSS often are associated with Jacksonian seizures, headache and progressive hemiparesis. Tumors of the posterior third of the SSS often cause headache, seizures and gradual hemianopsia.[50,51] Like convexity tumors, the most common symptoms associated with parasagittal meningiomas at the time of presentation are seizures (46% to 51%), headache (42% to 54%), and/or motor weakness (39% to 49%).

Indications for Surgery

INCIDENTAL MENINGIOMAS

Because they exhibit no growth or slow linear growth, the majority of asymptomatic, incidental meningiomas may be observed without surgical intervention.[53,54] Several studies reporting on the long-term natural history of these tumors also reveal that a smaller subset of tumors may demonstrate exponential growth or sigmoidal growth.[55,56] Variability in growth rates and patterns necessitate close surveillance until these properties can be established.[57] We perform follow-up MR-imaging 3 months after initial diagnosis for

incidentally discovered meningiomas. If the tumor demonstrates no growth or slow linear growth, we will monitor the tumor at 6 to 12 month intervals. Alternatively, we monitor tumors exhibiting exponential growth at 3 to 6 month intervals. Specific imaging and patient characteristics associated with more rapid meningioma growth rates have been identified. The likelihood of tumor growth is higher in young patients and tumors larger than 3 cm in size.[53,58,59] Tumors that lack calcification and are hyperintense on T2-weighted MR-imaging are also more likely to display an aggressive growth pattern.[55,57,60] For each clinical situation, the decision to recommend surgery should be evaluated on an individual basis, incorporating patient comorbidities, age, observed growth rate, and image-based predictive factors for growth.

CONVEXITY MENINGIOMAS

The indications for meningioma removal and timing of resection depend on several factors. Generally, the clearest indication for surgery is the development of neurologic symptoms attributable to the tumor. Rarely, tumors may present with significant hyperostosis or skin ulceration, necessitating surgical intervention for cosmesis and/or reducing the risk of infections. Meningiomas associated with significant peritumoral edema may also carry an increased epileptogenic potential and represent an indication for early removal, even if tumors are relatively small in size. Additionally, convexity tumors adjacent to important neurovascular structures (Sylvian veins, middle cerebral arteries, superficial anastomosing veins) and eloquent cortices may be resected before additional tumor growth places these structures at increased risk at the time of operation.

PARASAGITTAL MENINGIOMAS

In addition to the indications presented for convexity tumors, timing of parasagittal meningioma resection is influenced by the extent of SSS involvement. Because acute surgical obstruction of the patent SSS can cause significant cerebral edema and venous infarction, a tumor causing partial obstruction may be followed closely to observe for the development of complete occlusion, allowing that the intracranial component of the tumor does not greatly increase in size, cause symptoms, or encroach on large adjacent superficial

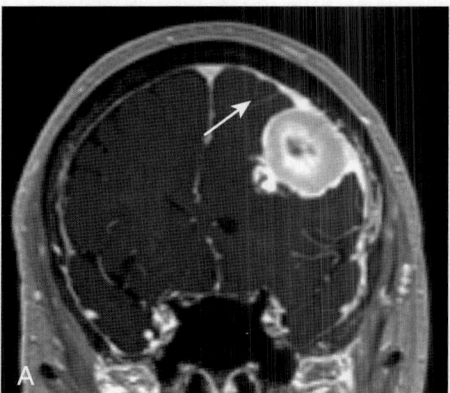 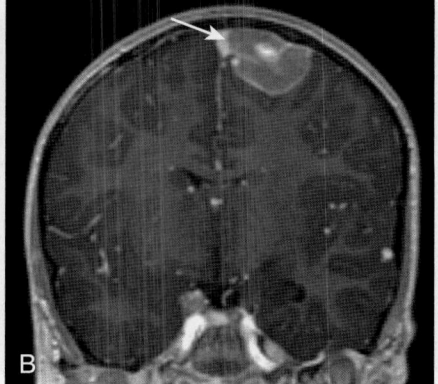 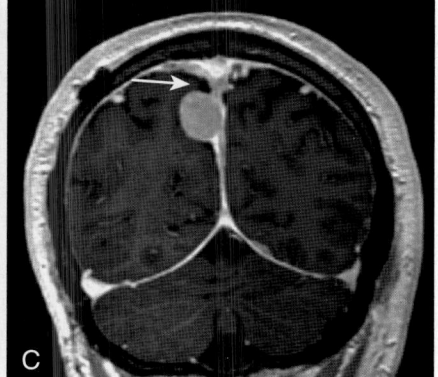

FIGURE 32-1 Anatomic differentiation of convexity, parasagittal and falcine meningiomas. A, Convexity meningiomas have no affiliation with the SSS and are separated from the SSS by intervening brain tissue that presents to the surface (arrow). B, Parasagittal meningiomas fill the angle between the convexity and falcine meningioma. They are at least attached to one wall (arrow) of the SSS and brain tissue at the angle is displaced laterally or deep. C, Falcine meningiomas primarily arise from the falx and are cloaked from the surface by convexity brain tissue (arrow).

anastomosing veins. Alternatively, an asymptomatic meningioma without evidence of invasion into the SSS may require intervention at the earliest sign of growth so that a complete resection can be performed without entering the SSS.

Preoperative Evaluation

After determining the necessity for tumor resection, a thorough preoperative evaluation minimizes the risk of perioperative morbidity and mortality, allows an appropriate estimation of the risks of surgery and identifies key points that will need to be addressed intraoperatively by the surgeon. There are three important tumor characteristics that can be assessed preoperatively that will significantly impact the objective and approach to resection of these tumors. These include the (1) involvement of the SSS and development of collateral veins, (2) the extent and type of bone involvement, and (3) the presence of edema and brain invasion in adjacent eloquent cortices.

SUPERIOR SAGITTAL SINUS INVOLVEMENT

With advancements in imaging and microsurgical techniques, reconstruction and bypass of the SSS have been used in an effort to enhance resection parasagittal meningiomas. Several large series have been published on the

complete removal of tumor with reconstruction or bypass of the SSS.[61] Despite performing more extensive resections (Simpson grade I, Table 32-1) with sinus reconstruction or bypass, which increased perioperative morbidity and mortality, the authors found that local recurrence remains a significant problem.[62] Subsequently, based on the potential morbidity with these cases, better understanding of the natural history of meningiomas and efficacy of adjuvant radiosurgery[63-65] in the management of residual and/or recurrent disease, many surgeons have adopted a more conservative approach to management of SSS invasion by meningioma.[62,63,66]

Derived from a surgical approach that does not include resection and repair/reconstruction of a patent or partially occluded SSS, a simple classification system can be used that permits stratification of parasagittal meningiomas based on preoperative imaging (Fig. 32-2). This classification scheme divides parasagittal tumors into three types that have direct surgical implications. Type I tumors are defined as tumors that attach to the external layer of dura forming the SSS. Type II tumors are identified as tumors that visibly invade the SSS and narrow its lumen, but do not cause complete obstruction. Grade III tumors are defined as tumors that invade the SSS and cause its complete obstruction. Each of the three types has surgical implications as defined below.

The evaluation of SSS patency, invasion and the development of collateral venous pathways are performed with contrast-enhanced MR-venography (CE-MRV). The sensitivity and specificity for these findings on CE-MRV is similar to that of digital subtraction angiography (DSA), with a reduction in risk and patient discomfort.[67,68] DSA is still performed if tumor embolization is considered or if arterial supply to the tumor needs to be better defined. In the setting of SSS obstruction, CE-MRV, and DSA may reveal significantly dilated scalp veins and diploic veins in addition to engorged cortical venous collaterals. These supplementary collateral venous pathways play a critical role in venous drainage, especially in the setting of parasagittal meningiomas causing occlusion of the middle or posterior third of the superior sagittal sinus. When possible, surgical

Table 32-1	Simpson Classification of Extent of Resection for Intracranial Meningiomas and Recurrence Rate	
Grade	**Extent of Resection**	**Recurrence Rate**
I	Gross total resection of tumor, dural attachments and abnormal bone	9%
II	Gross total resection of tumor, coagulation of dural attachments	19%
III	Gross total resection of tumor without resection or coagulation of dural attachment or its extradural extensions	29%
IV	Partial resection of tumor	44%
V	Simple decompression	

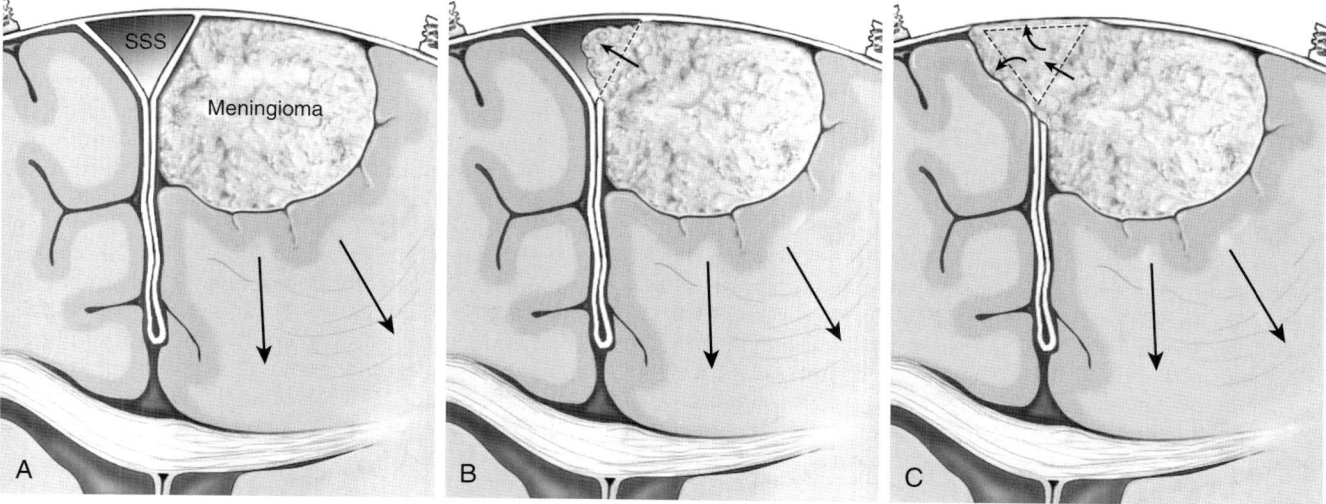

FIGURE 32-2 Clinical classification of parasagittal meningiomas. Parasagittal meningiomas may be classified based on their relationship with the superior sagittal sinus (SSS). A, Type I meningiomas are attached only to the outer surface of the SSS. B, Type II meningiomas invade the SSS but the lumen remains patent. C, Type III meningiomas invade the SSS and cause its occlusion.

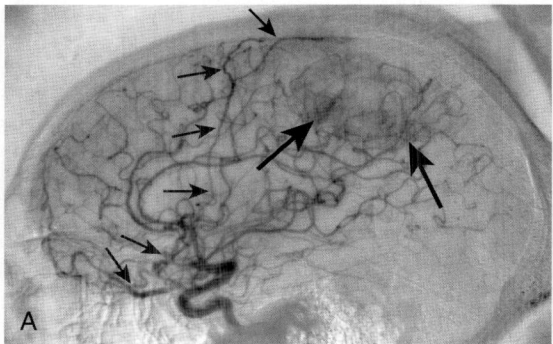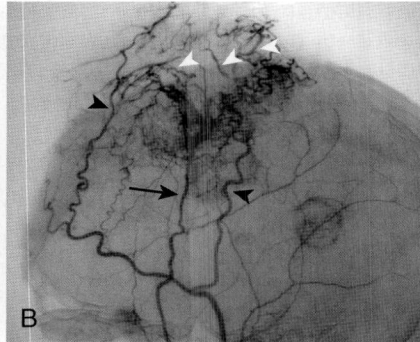

FIGURE 32-3 Arterial supply of meningiomas. Convexity and parasagittal meningiomas typically receive their primary blood supply from dilated meningeal arteries. A, Some tumors may develop feeding vessels from the internal carotid circulation (large arrows) with minimal contribution from meningeal vessels (small arrows). B, When tumors have significant bone involvement, arterial blood supply from scalp arteries (black arrowheads) may transgress the cranium (white arrowheads) to supply the intracranial portions of tumor. Also displayed is the middle meningeal feeding vessel (arrow). *(Images courtesy of Nicholas Patronas, National Institutes of Health.)*

approaches should avoid transgression of these structures with tailored scalp incisions and bone flaps.[62,69] Although convexity and parasagittal meningiomas typically receive their primary blood supply from dilated meningeal arteries, the surgeon should be aware that some tumors may develop additional blood supply through the internal carotid artery (pial parasitization) or dilated scalp arteries (Fig. 32-3).

BONY CHANGES

Preoperative evaluation of bone involvement is useful in assessing the need for bone removal and cranioplasty. Because MR imaging alone significantly underestimates bony changes associated with meningiomas, we routinely perform a cranial CT for evaluation of the extent of bony involvement of all parasagittal and convexity meningiomas.[70] Bony changes associated with meningiomas can be caused by hyperostotic changes or direct bone invasion by tumor. Hyperostotic changes are generally considered a benign form of inductive ossification caused by tumoral increases in alkaline phosphatase production.[71] In managing hyperostotic changes without bony invasion by tumor, we use the high-speed drill to remove the bulk of hyperostotic bone, at times just leaving the outer cortical table of bone intact. For tumors that present with significant bone destruction and replacement by tumor, removal of the invaded bone is necessary for complete tumor resection.

TUMOR AND BRAIN CHARACTERISTICS

The "gold standard" for evaluation of meningioma size, location, and impact on adjacent brain structures is MR-imaging performed with and without contrast. Meningiomas typically appear as isointense masses on pre-contrast T1-weighted imaging and enhance homogenously after the administration of contrast. Postcontrast MR imaging often reveals a trailing linear enhancing structure along its dural attachment referred to as the "dural tail."[72] The dural tail is not specific to the diagnosis of meningioma, but its management continues to be a point of controversy.[72,73] Although evidence suggests that most of the dural tail is an imaging correlate of dilated meningeal vessels and dural congestion,[74] many still advocate extensive resection of the dural tail believing that it can contain tumor. Generally, we resect at least a 1-cm margin of dura from its interface with the tumor.

T2-weighted MR-image sequences typically show more variability in tumoral intensity (50% isointense, 40% hyperintense, and 10% hypointense),[75] but may help predict clinical behavior of meningiomas. Identification of a T2-weighted hyperintense arachnoid cleft between tumor and brain is often indicative of a distinct anatomic plane (Fig. 32-4). Absence of an arachnoid cleft in combination with significant peritumoral edema may be indicative of pial vessel parasitization and/or brain invasion. Addressing brain invasion is a key aspect in the operative management of parasagittal and convexity meningiomas. Management balances preoperative expectations, age of the patient, and eloquence of the involved cortices. If extrapial resection is not possible in an area of eloquence, a small amount of tumor may be left attached to the cortical surface and observed postoperatively.[76] For tumors near eloquent areas with variable representation, such as Broca's and Wernicke's area, fMR imaging or awake surgery with mapping is valuable in elucidating their anatomic relationship and determining risks of resection.

Surgical Treatment

SURGICAL ADVANCES

In 1743, Lorenz Heister,[77] performed the first documented attempt of surgical treatment of a meningioma. During the operation, he applied a caustic of lime to the tumor of a 34-year-old Prussian soldier in an attempt to destroy the tumor tissue. Infection ensued shortly thereafter, leading to the death of the patient. In 1835, the first meningioma was successfully resected by Zanobi Pecchioli. The parietal convexity tumor, which had eroded through the calvarium, was excavated with a triangular craniectomy, and "a fine linen soaked in almond oil" was placed over the exposed brain. The open wound healed by granulation tissue formed over the course of 4 months. While wound healing occurred, the patient utilized a "skullcap of boiled leather with padded lining" to protect the brain.[78]

The development of monopolar cautery, in 1926, and then the widespread use of bipolar cautery, in the late 1950s, significantly improved meningioma resection results by reducing the significant blood loss that often occurred

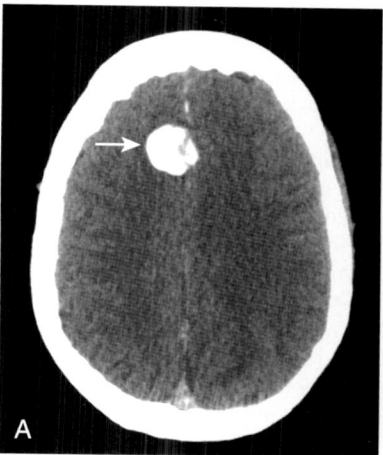 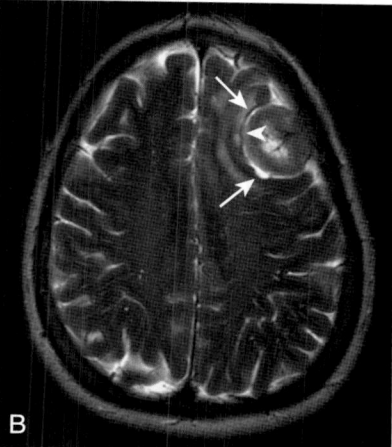 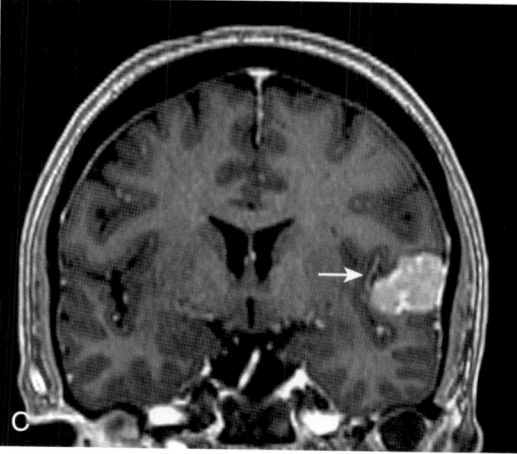

FIGURE 32-4 Important radiologic findings on preoperative imaging evaluation. A, Computed tomography scans may provide insight into tumor constituency and identification of bony changes. For tumors with significant tumoral calcification (arrow), the ultrasonic aspirator may be a less effective tool for central debulking. B, Identification of the arachnoidal cleft (arrows) is suggestive of a distinct anatomic plane and can be best visualized on T2-weighted imaging. Disappearance of the arachnoidal cleft (arrowhead) in combination with significant peritumoral edema may be indicative of pial vessel paratization or brain invasion. C, Resection of convexity meningiomas near the sylvian fissure requires meticulous extracapsular identification of feeding vessels and distinguishing middle cerebral native vessels of passage (arrow).

before their development.[79,80] The use of the operating microscope, beginning in the 1960s, enhanced the safe and complete resection of many meningiomas through improved visualization of the tumor–tissue plane, tumor associated vessels and other tumor-nervous system relationships. Recently, intraoperative image-guided surgical navigation systems have made it possible to more accurately localize these tumors before incision and craniotomy. This has enhanced the precision of incision placement and has led to minimization of the craniotomy size necessary for complete resection.

PREOPERATIVE CARE

For patients who present with seizure, antiepileptic medications are optimized to prevent complications that may result from intra- and peri-operative seizures including venous hypertension and brain swelling. For tumors with surrounding edema, preoperative steroids (dexamethasone) can be started 4 to 7 days before surgery to allow reduce peritumoral vasogenic edema and swelling. Concurrent administration of proton pump inhibitors for gastrointestinal ulcer prophylaxis is recommended.[81] Because most parasagittal and convexity tumors have a broad attachment to convexity dura, we prefer not to give diuretics such as Mannitol (osmotic diuretic) or Furosemide (loop diuretic). We typically reserve the use of these agents in the setting of a large parasagittal tumor with a primary falcine attachment to minimize the need for brain retraction. For deep venous thrombosis prophylaxis, all patients have graduated compression stockings and/or an intermittent pneumatic compression device applied before induction. According to guidelines, preoperative antibiotics (for appropriate grampositive coverage) are administered within 60 minutes of incision.[82]

EMBOLIZATION

Since embolization for preoperative management of meningiomas was introduced in 1971,[83] reports have indicated that it can be used to reduce intraoperative blood loss, which

can potentially reduce surgical complications and improve overall outcome.[84-86] Despite these theoretical advantages, the surgeon must balance the use of embolization against its known complications (6%), including ischemic stroke, hemorrhage, and acute cerebral edema.[87,88] While there is little benefit in performing preoperative embolization for small tumors,[89] the risks of angiography and embolization can be considered for treatment of larger tumors. In our experience, we have rarely found it necessary to embolize convexity or parasagittal meningiomas of any size, because the source of tumor bleeding is readily apparent at the working surface and can be controlled with meticulous hemostasis.

PARASAGITTAL MENINGIOMAS

Positioning

Positioning for resection of parasagittal meningiomas is determined by the anteroposterior location of the tumor along the SSS. For tumors located along the anterior third of the SSS, a supine position with the head and neck in a neutral or gently flexed position will permit direct access to the tumor. For tumors located along the middle third of the SSS, a supine semisitting position with slight head and neck flexion will often allow direct access to the tumor. Another positioning option for tumors in this location includes placing the patient lateral with their head elevated so that the scalp over the tumor is at the highest point in the field.[62] Finally, for parasagittal tumors located along the posterior third of the SSS, a prone position with the head and neck in neutral or slightly extended position can provide direct tumor access. Another positioning option for tumors in this location includes placing the patient three quarters prone with the tumor below the midline, allowing for the brain to fall away with minimal retraction.[76,90]

Incision

After patient positioning, frameless stereotaxic navigation is registered to patient. The use of frameless navigation facilitates the identification of the surface presentation of the underlying tumor with reference to the overlying scalp. Surgical navigation can be used to assist in determining the precise placement, shape and size of incision, as well as facilitate the planning and size of the craniotomy after incision and calvarial exposure.[91] During the course of resection (provided there is little shift of brain parenchyma), frameless neuronavigation is also helpful in affirming local relationships to major vascular structures (dural venous sinuses, superficial anastamotic veins and feeding arteries) and eloquent cortices. After the skin incision is marked, the incision site and surrounding region is sterilely prepared and draped. The skin of the incision site is then infiltrated with a local anesthetic with epinephrine (1:200,000).

Generally, parasagittal meningiomas of the anterior third of SSS are exposed via a bicoronal incision. Meningiomas of the middle and posterior third of the SSS can be exposed through a bicoronal, S-shaped or a U-shaped incision. Bicoronal or S-shaped incisions are centered over the tumor mass in the anteroposterior plane and should permit exposure of the uninvolved side of the SSS. Similarly, U-shaped incisions for parasagittal tumors should extend at least 2 cm past the midline to provide exposure to the uninvolved side of the SSS. U-shaped incisions should have a wide base that is 1.5 times the length of the pedunculated flap to ensure adequate perfusion to the distal portions. During incision, it is important to attempt to maintain large anastamotic collaterals that may have developed within the scalp and diploe to prevent venous congestion, brain swelling, and/or infarction.[69]

Exposure

Skin incision is made with a #10 scalpel through the skin, dermis, and galea to the level of the pericranium. After incision, hemostatic clips are applied to the scalp edges. Medium curved scissors or the back edge of the #10 scalpel are then used to separate the galea from the underlying the pericranium. Visualization of this tissue interface is enhanced by upward tension on the scalp flap at the point of dissection. Because the frontal sinuses may be entered during approach to tumors of the anterior third of the SSS, we maintain a vascularized pedicle for the pericranial graft. In this circumstance, we detach the pericranium laterally and posteriorly using bovie cautery, reflecting it anteriorly with the pericranial elevator over the scalp flap. For all other locations, a free pericranial graft is harvested and kept moist with saline until it is used to repair the dural defect.

Once the pericranium is dissected and the calvarium is exposed, bleeding of the bone surface can be visualized at times, representing a crude location of the tumor below, but does not necessarily represent direct invasion by tumor. The exposed cranium is examined closely for signs of bony invasion. The neuronavigation system and anatomical landmarks are utilized to outline the planned craniotomy. If bone invasion by tumor is present on preoperative imaging, this area of involved bone is marked with neuronavigation before performing the craniotomy. The craniotomy should be at least 1.5 to 2 cm away from the junction of the tumor mass and the dural tail. The craniotomy margins should be kept 1 cm within from the scalp edges. For parasagittal tumors, two burr holes are placed on the opposite side of the SSS, approximately 1 cm off

the midline and one burr hole is placed on the convexity ipsilateral to the tumor. A right-angle dural elevator or the Penfield-3 is used to separate the underlying dura along the craniotomy flap. It is imperative that the SSS is detached from the overlying cranium where the craniotome is to pass. Subsequently, the craniotome is used to connect the outside margin of the burr holes. Preferably under direct visualization, the craniotomy flap is separated from the underlying dura and the longitudinal section of the exposed SSS. If there is significant involvement of the bone by tumor, the intracranial tumor mass is sharply divided from the invaded bone to avoid avulsing the tumor from its bed. Hemostasis from the superficial bleeding edge of tumor and dural tears is obtained with bipolar cautery after the entirety of the bone flap is reflected. Bleeding from arachnoid granulations, venous lakes, or the area around the SSS is stopped with the application of woven oxidized cellulose polymer and Gelfoam. The bone flap is set aside for tumor resection. Removal of suspected areas of bony invasion and reshaping of hyperostotic bone is done at the time of closure. After the bone is removed, circumferential tack-up sutures are placed.

Resection

The major obstacles to a safe resection pertain to the management of the superior sagittal sinus and bridging superficial cortical vessels entering this structure. After craniotomy, intraoperative ultrasound or the neuronavigation can supplement the surgeon's observation and tactile tracing of the underlying tumor and adjacent neurovascular structures. A C-shaped dural opening, with its base towards the SSS is planned and small durotomy is made with the #15 blade over the ipsilateral brain convexity 1 cm from the tumor margin (Fig. 32-5). As the durotomy is extended along the "C" in both directions towards the SSS, great care is taken to examine cortical veins that may cross to bridge with the SSS. Because of the potential importance of these veins for critical drainage we prefer to alter the course of the durotomy than cause damage to these vessels.

Once the durotomy is completed, bipolar cautery applied to the center of the dural leaflet causes eversion of the cut margins and allows visualization of the intradural compartment. Initial separation of the tumor from the underlying cortex along arachnoid planes proceeds and the dura is reflected progressively over the contralateral hemisphere causing the tumor to evert. Cottonoid patties are placed in the tumor–brain arachnoid cleft. As this commences, we perform central debulking of the tumor to avoid avulsion or disruption of venous elements on the falcine side of the tumor and detachment of the convexity dura mater. Central debulking of the tumor is carried out with the use of the ultrasonic aspirator. For fibrous and heavily calcified tumors, the loop cautery device can sometimes be more effective than the ultrasonic aspirator. Care is taken never to breach the capsule of the tumor while internal debulking is performed. Alternating between extracapsular dissection and intratumoral debulking permits tumor dissection and removal, while minimizing brain tissue manipulation. The primary dural attachment at the convexity and/or falx is resected to within a few millimeters from the SSS, leaving a small portion attached to the SSS.

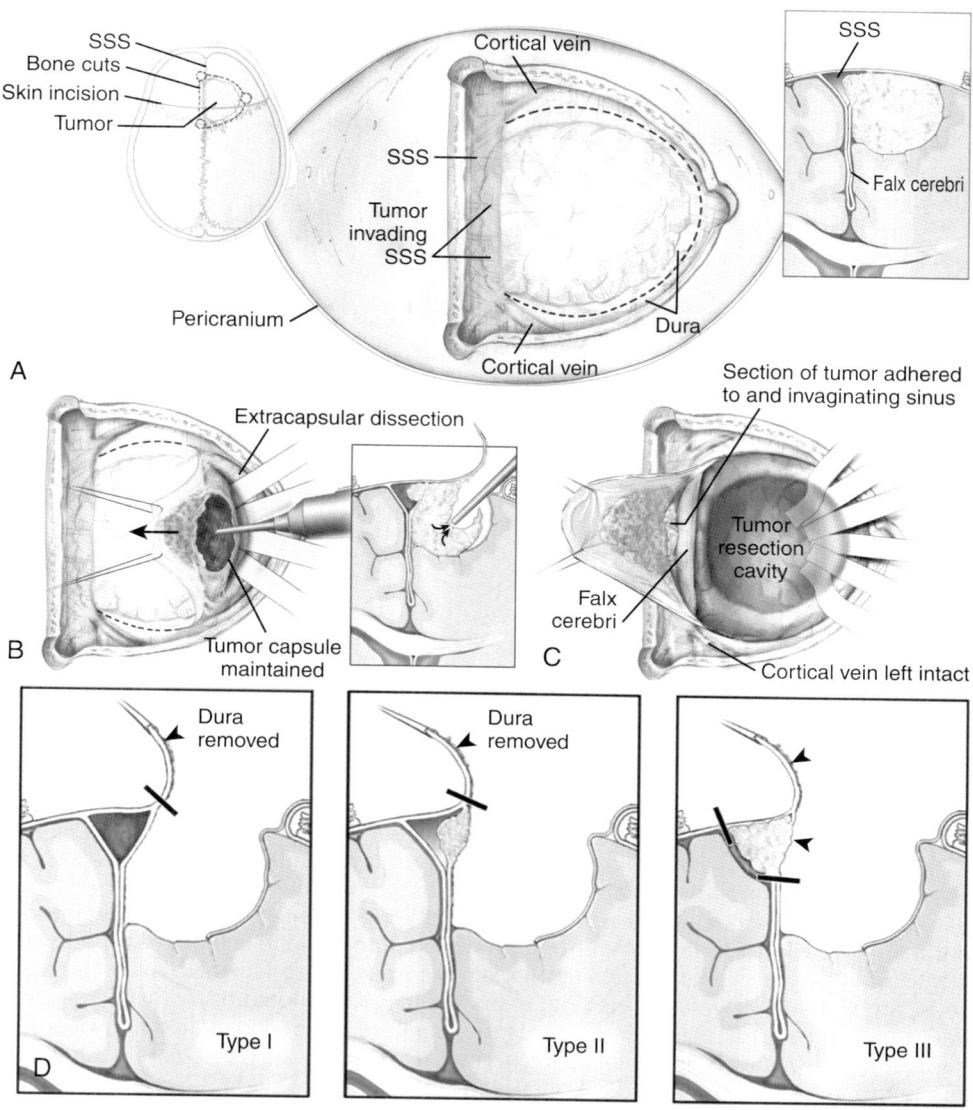

FIGURE 32-5 Surgical approach to parasagittal meningiomas. A, After pericranial graft harvest, two burr holes are placed on the opposite side of the superior sagittal sinus (SSS), approximately 1.5 cm off the midline and one burr hole is placed on the convexity ipsilateral to the tumor. B, The dura is opened and reflected contralaterally. Care is taken to avoid cortical veins that may cross to bridge with the SSS. Extracapsular dissection and intratumoral debulking is performed until the tumor is removed. C, After the principal mass is removed, areas of dural attachment to the convexity and/or falx are examined and extent of SSS involvement ascertained. D, For type I tumors, the tumor is peeled from the dura of the SSS and this area of attachment is cauterized (Simpson grade II resection). Areas of dural attachment can be resected (bold line) up to within a few millimeters of the SSS. For type II tumors, a layer of tumor residual invading the wall of the SSS is cauterized and left in situ. Areas of dural attachment can be resected (bold line) up to within a few millimeters of the SSS. Tumor within the sinus is not treated (Simpson grade III resection). For type III tumors, the occluded SSS is ligated and resected (bold line), along with involved convexity and/or falcine dura (arrowheads) (Simpson grade I resection).

SSS involvement

Type I tumors can be peeled from their attachment to the dura overlying the SSS (Fig. 32-5). After this is accomplished, the external layer of dura is cauterized to achieve a Simpson grade II resection. If preoperative assessment indicates tumor is present within the lumen of the SSS (type II), we perform a Simpson grade III resection. Tumor is debulked at its insertion through the wall of the superior sagittal sinus, but cannot completely be removed or peeled without entering the lumen of the SSS. Instead, this residual tumor is cauterized and the tumor residual within the lumen of the SSS left in situ. Type III tumors allow for ligation and resection of the SSS. Because immediately adjacent veins that enter the SSS just anterior or posterior to the obstruction represent important collaterals, it is imperative that these vessels not be compromised in an attempt for greater resection. In order to ligate the SSS, the dura over the contralateral hemisphere is opened approximately 1 cm from the SSS along the length of the planned SSS resection. At the anterior and posterior margins of the resection, 2-0 silk suture is passed through the falx under direct visualization, encircling the SSS. Once the SSS is ligated in this fashion, it may be transected and removed, achieving a Simpson grade I resection.

Closure

For all tumors, the pericranium is harvested at the time of exposure, kept moistened during resection and available for closure. Because shrinkage of dura is inevitable from management of meningeal feeding vessels, achieving a primary watertight dural closure is often not feasible. In cases with small convexity defects, portions of the pericranial graft may be placed as interposition grafts to gain a better seal. The pericranial graft can also be used to replace the entirety of large defects created by Simpson grade I resections (type III tumors) or resection of a large primary attachment to the convexity dura at the parasagittal angle (type I and II tumors). Several small, nonbraided, nonresorbable interrupted suture are used to tack the graft in position and augmented with a running suture. The dural closure is then completed with a running suture. The suture line is then

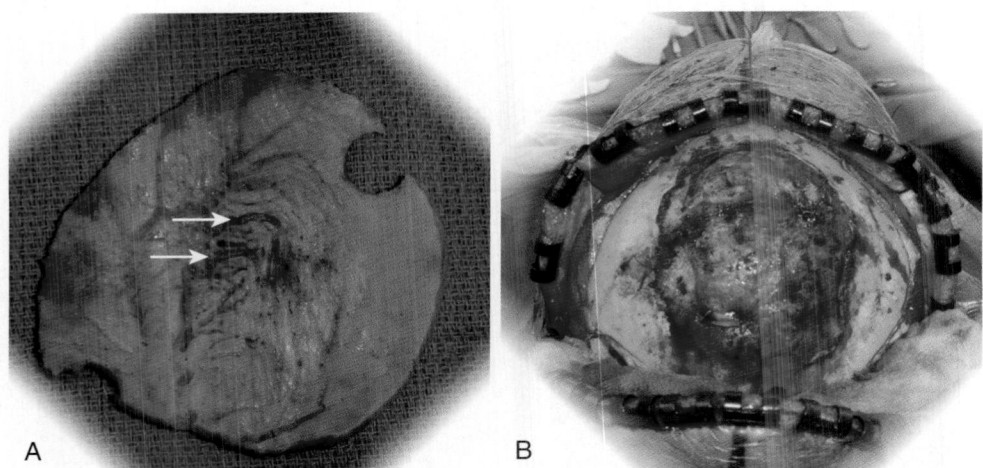

FIGURE 32-6 Bone involvement with convexity and parasagittal meningiomas. The preoperative extent of bony involvement is determined with computed tomography scanning. A, Markings on the inner table from dilated meningeal feeding vessels (arrows) or engorged emissary veins are not worrisome findings. The cranial flap is plated and returned to its native position. B, For tumors extensively involving the calvarium, we perform a resection of the involved bone with a margin of at least 1 cm of uninvolved bone and perform a complete cranioplasty for reconstruction. C, If meningiomas invade the calvarium focally, this portion of bone is outlined at the time of exposure using neuronavigation. After craniotomy, this area is removed and the defect bridged with either titanium mesh or methylmethacrylate.

augmented with a thin layer of fibrin sealant. Two to three central dural tack-up sutures are placed through the dura and bone flap at closure.

The bone flap is examined for evidence of bony changes (Fig. 32-6). Because direct tumor invasion can be identified with preoperative CT imaging, with co-register CT and MR-imaging in neuronavigation system to identify the extent of tumor involvement of bone before the craniotomy flap is elevated, as described previously. This allows accurate resection of the portion of the bone flap that is involved, instead of relying solely on visual inspection. Either titanium mesh or methylmethacrylate can be utilized to bridge the defect that is created in the craniotomy flap. If a craniectomy is needed because of extensive invasion of the bone by tumor, a cranioplasty is performed. A custom-designed cranioplasty for these larger defects can be included in the preoperative planning. Hyperostotic regions, without direct invasion by tumor, are removed with a high-speed cutting burr until the appropriate contour and thickness are achieved. The bone flap is then returned to its native position and aligned without gap in portions that are covered with thinned or nontrichogenic scalp. Titanium burr-hole cover plates and miniplates are held in place with titanium screws. Subsequently, the galea is reapproximated with inverted absorbable suture and the scalp reapproximated with staples.

CONVEXITY MENINGIOMAS

Positioning

During positioning, the head placed above the level of the heart and situated to present the tumor-bearing convexity parallel to the ceiling. This may require positioning the patient in a park-bench or prone position, especially for parietal and occipital tumors, depending on how mobile the neck and torso are in accommodating rotation. To simplify positioning, avoid the risk of venous air embolism,[92] and ideally place the tumor at the highest point of the

operative field so that brain retraction can be minimized, we generally avoid the sitting position for operation of convexity tumors.

Exposure

While smaller tumors of the convexity are approached via linear incision, larger tumors and those of the parietoccipital region are often approached via S-shaped or U-shaped incisions. For linear and S-shaped incisions, the diameter of the proposed cranial flap must be centered along the incision and should not exceed half the length of the proposed incision. U-shaped incisions should have a wide base that is 1.5 times the length of the pedunculated flap to ensure adequate perfusion to the distal portions. For tumors of the frontal convexity, a three quarters bicoronal incision or a pterional incision sparing the temporalis muscle and preserving the frontal branches of the facial nerve within the superficial fat pad, allows for great exposure with ideal cosmetic results. As with parasagittal tumors, a free pericranial graft is harvested and kept moist with saline on the back table.

Once the pericranium is dissected and the calvarium is exposed, we use neuronavigation and anatomic landmarks to outline the planned craniotomy and mark any area of tumor-invaded bone. Depending on the size of the tumor and age of the patient, anywhere from one to three burr holes may be placed circumferentially around the underlying tumor. More burr holes are placed in elderly patients because of the adherence of dura to the calvarium that increases with age. A right-angle dural elevator or the Penfield-3 is used to separate the underlying dura along the craniotomy flap. The craniotome is used to connect the outside margin of the burr holes. Preferably under direct visualization, the craniotomy flap is separated from the underlying dura. Tumor-invaded bone is detached sharply from the underlying intracranial mass. Bleeding from exposed tumor and dural tears are aggressively cauterized with the use of bipolar cautery once the craniotomy flap is completely elevated. Bleeding from arachnoid granulations and venous lakes near the superior sagittal sinus are stopped with the application of woven oxidized cellulose polymer and Gelfoam. The bone flap is set aside for tumor resection. Removal of suspected areas of bony invasion and reshaping of hyperostotic bone is done at the time of closure. After the bone is removed, circumferential tack-up sutures are placed.

Resection

The goal in surgery of convexity meningiomas is a Simpson grade I resection. After craniotomy, the junction of the tumor with dura is outlined circumferentially utilizing neuronavigation, intraoperative ultrasound, and visual inspection. An incision is made in the dura, at least 1 cm remote to the tumor mass attachment to the dural and is extended circumferentially around the tumor maintaining this margin. Care is taken to separate the underlying brain and directly visualize and avoid bridging veins to the dura. After encircling the tumor, bipolar cautery is applied to the center of the dural attachment, causing eversion of the cut margins. This allows clear visualization of the arachnoid margin. Alternatively, the dural attachment may be removed to expose the intracranial surface of the tumor. At this time, initial separation of the tumor capsule along these arachnoid planes is performed. Cottonoid patties are placed into the arachnoid cleft between tumor and brain to maintain dissected planes and avoid direct manipulation of cortical tissue. With small tumors, the tumor may completely be extirpated in this fashion.

Large tumors are centrally debulked for several reasons. First, this allows retraction on the tumor capsule into the tumor itself. Second, as tumors enlarge, they often begin to parasitize blood supply through the development of pial collateral feeding vessels. Careful identification, cautery, and sharp transection of these vessels allow minimal disruption of the underlying cortex. Lastly, debulking allows extracapsular differentiation between feeding vessels and vessels of passage, critical in removal of tumors near the Sylvian fissure (Fig. 32-4). If central debulking is planned, we generally acquire tissue for histologic evaluation at this time because subsequent cautery effect on the capsule causes significant histopathologic artifacts. Central debulking of the tumor is carried out with the use of the ultrasonic aspirator. For fibrous and heavily calcified tumors, the loop cautery device can be more effective than the ultrasonic aspirator. While proceeding during internal debulking of the tumor, it is useful to have hemostatic agents, such as thrombin-soaked Gelfoam available to place in the tumor cavity. With gentle application of pressure on top of thrombin-soaked Gelfoam, most intratumoral bleeding will stop. It is important to avoid breaching the capsule as internal debulking proceeds, making alternating internal debulking and subsequent extracapsular dissection an ideal way to proceed without significant lapses in time. Proceeding in this fashion, the tumor is gradually excavated from its bed.

Closure

For all convexity tumors, a free pericranial graft if obtained during exposure and preserved for use during closure. Because the graft is larger than the craniotomy flap that is created, it can easily replace the extent of dural resection performed with tumor resection. Several small, nonbraided, nonresorbable interrupted suture are used to tack the graft in position. The dural closure is then completed with a running suture. The suture line is then augmented with a thin layer of fibrin sealant. Two to three central dural tack-up sutures are placed through the dura and bone flap at closure. The bone flap is examined for evidence of invasion by tumor and significant hyperostosis. Hyperostotic regions are removed with a high-speed cutting burr and the bone flap is returned to its native position and aligned without gap in portions that are covered with thinned or nontrichogenic scalp. Titanium burr hole cover plates and miniplates are held in place with titanium screws.

The bone flap is examined for evidence of bony changes. Because direct tumor invasion can be identified with preoperative CT-imaging, we prefer to utilize CT/MRI registered neuronavigation to identify the extent of tumor involvement of bone before the craniotomy flap is elevated, as mentioned previously. This allows accurate resection of the portion of the bone flap that is involved, instead of relying solely on visual inspection. Either titanium mesh or methylmethacrylate can be utilized to bridge the defect that is created in the craniotomy flap. If a craniectomy is needed because of extensive invasion of the bone by tumor, a cranioplasty is performed. A custom-designed cranioplasty for these larger defects are generally included in the preoperative planning. Hyperostotic regions, without direct invasion by tumor, are removed with a high-speed cutting burr until the appropriate contour and thickness are achieved. The bone flap is then returned to its native position and aligned without gap in portions that are covered with thinned or nontrichogenic scalp. Titanium burr hole cover plates and miniplates are held in place with titanium screws. We do not utilize drains left in the operative bed, but rather emphasize obtaining adequate hemostasis during closure. Subsequently, the galea is reapproximated with inverted absorbable suture and the scalp reapproximated with staples. Meticulous attention to detail, at times difficult after a lengthy resection, is an absolute necessity during closure.

Postoperative Care and Complications

Immediately following placement of the dressing, patients are awoken from anesthesia and their neurologic status assessed. It is imperative that during awakening, pain and hypoxia be managed appropriately to prevent excessive agitation.[93] Coughing and valsalva maneuvers should be avoided during emergence and extubation. Once recovered from anesthesia, all patients are kept under neurologic observation with bedside examinations performed by nursing staff every 1 to 2 hours overnight. The head of bed is kept elevated at 30 degrees. Initiation of new antiepileptic drug therapy for postoperative seizure prophylaxis is not recommended.[94] Postoperatively, initiation of steroids is avoided and preoperative dosing is stopped (if patient on steroids less than 7 days before surgery) or systematically tapered over days. Strict assessment of fluid intake and outputs are recorded and euvolemia maintained.

For uncomplicated convexity surgeries that less than 3 hours, we routinely remove the Foley catheter before emergence and encourage increased activity as tolerated after the immediate postanesthetic recovery period. For patients undergoing longer operations or who have preoperative motor deficits, activity level is monitored and advanced as tolerated. Perioperative antibiotic prophylaxis is discontinued within 24 hours of surgery. Deep venous thrombosis prophylaxis with low-dose, unfractionated subcutaneous heparin or low-molecular-weight heparin is added to graduated compression stockings and/or an intermittent pneumatic compressive device on the first postoperative day and continued until patient discharge.[95]

With parasagittal tumors, any disruption of collateral veins warrants extended monitoring for the development of delayed sequelae (2 to 4 days after resection) such as venous infarction and seizures. Before increasing activity level and decreasing frequency of neurologic assessment, patients can be evaluated for occult complications with either CT or MR imaging. When early postoperative imaging is obtained, MR imaging is often preferred because it can serve as a baseline assessment of the resection. Dressings are removed on the second day after surgery and incisions are examined closely for signs of dehiscence or inflammation.

Despite standard implementation of extensive preoperative evaluations, medical morbidity still occurs in 2% to 5% of all convexity meningioma operations. While perioperative mortality from surgery of convexity meningiomas is very low, the morbidity remains at approximately 10%. These are equally divided between neurosurgical complications, including development of new neurological deficits (approximately 2%), wound infection (3%), cerebrospinal fluid leak (1%), postoperative hematoma (1%), seizure (1%), and delayed hydrocephalus (1%) and medical complications, including nonwound infections (1%), cardiac events (1%), deep venous thrombosis (3%), and pulmonary embolus (1%).[47,48]

Both medical and surgical complications are increased in patients undergoing resection of parasagittal meningiomas compared to convexity tumors. This is likely due to the increased complexity of surgical resection and management of the critical venous structures. Perioperative mortality, although significantly reduced in the microsurgical era, still occurs in 2% to 3% of cases.[51,61] Operations involving the SSS have the additional risk of air embolism (1%) and significant blood loss.[61] Permanent neurologic deficit and worsening of functional status (approximate 10%) occurs as a result of postoperative brain swelling and/or venous infarction, likely from acute occlusion of important collateral vessels.[51,61] Postoperative hematomas (3%) and wound infections (5%) are also more frequent in patients undergoing resection of parasagittal tumors and may be related to the increased time often required to remove meningiomas in this location compared to convexity tumors.

Outcomes and Follow-Up

The extent of surgical resection is the most important factor in the prevention of recurrence.[96,97] Simpson reviewed the recurrence rate among 265 patients who underwent operation for meningiomas and noted a proportional increase in recurrence that was associated with the amount of residual tumor remaining after surgery[97] (Table 32-1). Because convexity tumors are free of involvement of the major venous sinuses and are amenable to resection of involved dura, the 5-year recurrence rate of benign meningiomas in this location is 0% to 3%.[47,96] In contrast, the 5-year recurrence rate for parasagittal meningiomas is 2% to 18%.[50,51,61,96]

In addition to extent of surgical resection, the World Health Organization (WHO) histopathologic grading of meningiomas is the other major predictive factor of recurrence.[35,98] Eighty to 90% of meningiomas are benign tumors (WHO grade I), whose gross total resection results in recurrence rates of 7% to 25%.[99,100] Although some histologic variants of benign (WHO grade I) meningioma (secretory) are associated with increased findings of edema on preoperative imaging, no differential growth or recurrence rate has been identified between histologic subgroups of benign meningiomas.[101] Atypical meningiomas (WHO grade II) are associated with recurrence rates of 29% to 52% while anaplastic meningiomas (WHO grade III) recur in 50% to 94% of cases.[100] The WHO no longer classifies brain invasion as a feature of atypical (WHO grade II) meningiomas, although its clinical presence is an indicator of higher chance for recurrence.

ACKNOWLEDGMENT

The Intramural Research Program of the National Institute of Neurological Disorders and Stroke at the National Institutes of Health supported preparation of this manuscript.

KEY REFERENCES

Al-Mefty O. *Meningiomas.* New York: Raven Press; 1991.

Al-Mefty O, Kersh JE, Routh A, Smith RR. The long-term side effects of radiation therapy for benign brain tumors in adults. *J Neurosurg.* 1990;73(4):502-512.

Asthagiri AR, Parry DM, Butman JA, et al. Neurofibromatosis type 2. *Lancet.* 2009;373(9679):1974-1986.

Bratzler DW, Houck PM. Antimicrobial prophylaxis for surgery: an advisory statement from the National Surgical Infection Prevention Project. *Am J Surg.* 2005;189(4):395-404.

Claus EB, Bondy ML, Schildkraut JM, et al. Epidemiology of intracranial meningioma. *Neurosurgery.* 2005;57(6):1088-1094.

Cushing H, Eisenhardt L. *Meningiomas: their Classification, Regional Behavior, Life History, and Surgical End Results.* Springfield, IL: Charles C. Thomas; 1938.

Geerts WH, Bergqvist D, Pineo GF, et al. Prevention of venous thromboembolism: american College of Chest Physicians evidence-based clinical practice guidelines 8th ed. *Chest.* 2008(6 suppl. 6):133.

Hancq S, Baleriaux D, Brotchi J. Surgical treatment of parasagittal meningiomas. *Semin Neurosurg.* 2003;14(3):203-210.

Kondziolka D, Flickinger JC, Perez B. Judicious resection and/or radiosurgery for parasagittal meningiomas: outcomes from a multicenter review. *Neurosurgery.* 1998;43(3):405-413.

Kuijlen JMA, Teernstra OPM, Kessels AGH, et al. Effectiveness of antiepileptic prophylaxis used with supratentorial craniotomies: a meta-analysis. *Seizure.* 1996;5(4):291-298.

Larson JJ, Tew Jr JM, Simon M, Menon AG. Evidence for clonal spread in the development of multiple meningiomas. *J Neurosurg.* 1995;83(4):705-709.

Manelfe C, Lasjaunias P, Ruscalleda J. Preoperative embolization of intracranial meningiomas. *Am J Neuroradiol.* 1986;7(5):963-972.

Mirimanoff RO, Dosoretz DE, Linggood RM. Meningioma: analysis of recurrence and progression following neurosurgical resection. *J Neurosurg.* 1985;62(1):18-24.

Morokoff AP, Zauberman J, Black PM. Surgery for convexity meningiomas. *Neurosurgery.* 2008;63(3):427-433:discussion 433-434.

Nakamura M, Roser F, Michel J, et al. The natural history of incidental meningiomas. *Neurosurgery.* 2003;53(1):62-71.

Perry A, Louis DN, Cheithauer BW, et al. Meningiomas. In: Louis D, Ohgaki H, Wiestler OD, Cavenee WK, eds. *WHO Classification of Tumours of the Central Nervous System.* 3rd ed. Geneva: International Agency for Research on Cancer; 2007:164-172.

Ron E, Modan B, Boice Jr JD, et al. Tumors of the brain and nervous system after radiotherapy in childhood. *N Engl J Med.* 1988;319(16):1033-1039.

Sanai N, Sughrue ME, Shangari G, et al. Risk profile associated with convexity meningioma resection in the modern neurosurgical era. *J Neurosurg.* 2010;112(5):913-919.

Simpson D. The recurrence of intracranial meningiomas after surgical treatment. *J Neurol Neurosurg Psychiatry.* 1957;20(1):22-39.

Sindou MP, Alvernia JE. Results of attempted radical tumor removal and venous repair in 100 consecutive meningiomas involving the major dural sinuses. *J Neurosurg.* 2006;105(4):514-525.

Umansky F, Shoshan Y, Rosenthal G, et al. Radiation-induced meningioma. *Neurosurg Focus.* 2008;24(5).

Wen PY, Schiff D, Kesari S, et al. Medical management of patients with brain tumors. *J Neuro-Oncol.* 2006;80(3):313-332.

Wilkins R. Parasagittal meningiomas. In: Al-Mefty O, ed. *Meningiomas.* New York: Raven Press; 1991:329-343.

Yano S, Kuratsu JI. Indications for surgery in patients with asymptomatic meningiomas based on an extensive experience. *J Neurosurg.* 2006;105(4):538-543.

Numbered references appear on Expert Consult.

CHAPTER 33

Surgical Approach to Falcine Meningiomas

ERIC C. CHANG • FREDERICK G. BARKER II • WILLIAM T. CURRY

Falcine meningiomas arise from the falx cerebri and make up approximately 5% to 9% of all intracranial meningiomas.[1-2] Falcine meningiomas differ from parasagittal meningiomas in that parasagittal tumors originate from the dura mater enclosing the superior sagittal sinus and are up to 5 to 7 times more common that falcine lesions.[3-4] Cushing further distinguished falcine meningiomas from parasagittal tumors by how, from the surgeon's perspective, falcine tumors are often concealed by overlying cerebral cortex;[5] however, large falcine meningiomas can grow superiorly to secondarily invade the superior sagittal sinus.

For surgical considerations, like parasagittal tumors, falcine meningiomas can also be classified based on their relationship to the superior sagittal sinus. The anterior third of the superior sagittal sinus extends from the foramen cecum to the coronal suture, the middle third extends from the coronal suture to the lambdoid suture, and the posterior third extends from the lambdoid suture to the torcular herophili.

Symptoms and Presentation

Falcine meningiomas located at the level of the anterior third of the superior sagittal sinus often present somewhat insidiously and result in a frontal lobe syndrome (Fig. 33-1A to F). Slowly progressive symptoms include short attention span, poor short-term memory, personality changes, apathy, and emotional instability; often this complex is confused with age-related dementia, delaying diagnosis. Consequently, anterior third tumors are frequently larger in size at the time of presentation than tumors in other regions. In extreme cases, patients can also present with signs of increased intracranial pressure, including headache, papilledema, or optic atrophy. Of patients with anterior third falcine meningiomas, 25% have seizures, but they are less frequent and less localizing than when tumors abut motor cortex.[6]

Tumors along the middle third of the superior sagittal sinus are usually located adjacent to the motor and sensory regions and produce more focal and localizable symptoms that cause patients to seek earlier medical intervention. Earlier presentation of symptoms allows for earlier diagnosis, and, thus, tumors in this region rarely attain the same bulk as tumors in the anterior third. While symptoms of increased intracranial pressure are rare, tumors in this region are more likely to produce spastic weakness and focal seizures that involve the contralateral foot and leg.

Both motor cortices may be affected if the tumor extends bilaterally from the midline. Patients with meningiomas involving the posterior third of the sagittal sinus usually present with persistent headache and often are found on exam to have a hemianopsia (Fig. 33-2A to E). The degree of visual field involvement depends on the size and location of the tumor. Smaller tumors located above the calcarine fissure can cause anopia to the inferior quadrant. Smaller tumors along the tentorium cerebelli may involve the visual cortex below the calcarine fissure and only produce anopia in the upper quadrants. Larger tumors, on the other hand, can case homonymous hemianopsia with macular sparing. Some patients may present with reports of visual hallucinations. Tumors of the middle and posterior third can occasionally present with bilateral symptoms as the tumor extends across the falx.

Radiographic Findings

Magnetic resonance (MR) imaging is the gold standard for preoperative assessment of falcine meningiomas. Falcine meningiomas also frequently extend bilaterally, acquiring a dumbbell or bi-lobed shape with invagination into the medial aspects of both left and right hemispheres. Attempts to use MR imaging to differentiate histologic types of meningiomas have thus far been limited. Although efforts to differentiate benign from atypical meningiomas using MR spectroscopy (MRS) have been attempted, noninvasive measures have been unreliable.[7] The majority of tumors appear iso- or slightly hypo-intense relative to the cortex on noncontrast T1-weighted MR images. The T2-weighted characteristics can be variable and are believed to correlate best with histologic subtype, vascularity, and consistency.[8] Tumors that are hypo- to iso-intense on T2-weight imaging are found to be more firm and are histologically more fibroblastic or transitional (Fig. 33-1D and Fig. 33-2D). More malignant meningiomas, on the other hand, are more likely to exhibit greater brain edema that manifests as increased hyperintensity on T2-weight imaging and can be suggestive of pial invasion.[9-10]

For preoperative planning, multi-planar T1-weighted gadolinium enhanced MR images can provide coronal, sagittal and axial views that help in defining the tumor's anatomic location, size, and cortical involvement (Fig. 33-1A to C and Fig. 33-2A to C). Brain edema adjacent to the tumor can be a sign of pial invasion and can be assessed preoperatively using T2-weighted images and fluid-attenuated

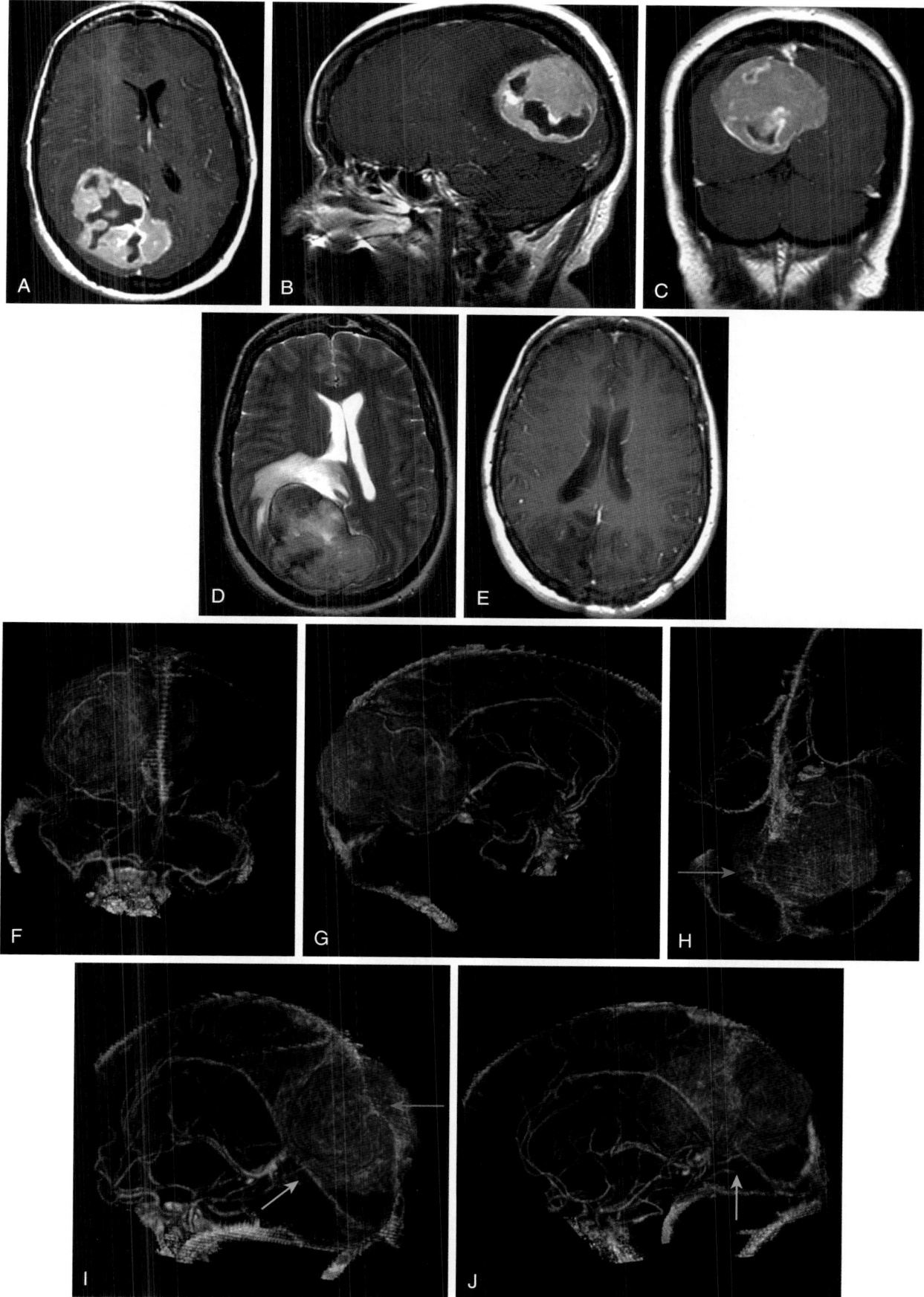

FIGURE 33-1 Fifty-two-year-old female presented with frontal headaches and found on workup to have a large right parietoccipital mass. On exam, patient was neurologically intact except for a slight left arm drift. A to C, T1-weighted images show a 7.5 cm × 7.0 cm × 6.0 cm heterogeneously enhancing cystic mass that extends across the posterior middle and posterior third of the falx. D, T2-weighted image shows a heterogeneous mass with increased hyperintensity along the anterior margin of the tumor. E, Four-year follow-up MRI after gross total resection. Patient continues to be neurologically intact with full visual fields. Histopathology showed atypical meningiomas. F to J, Preoperative CT angiography with Vitrea (Vital Images, Minnetonka, MN) 3D reconstructions. CTA shows compression and narrowing of the superior sagittal sinus (red arrows) and straight sinus (blue arrows). There is no radiographic evidence of sinus occlusion.

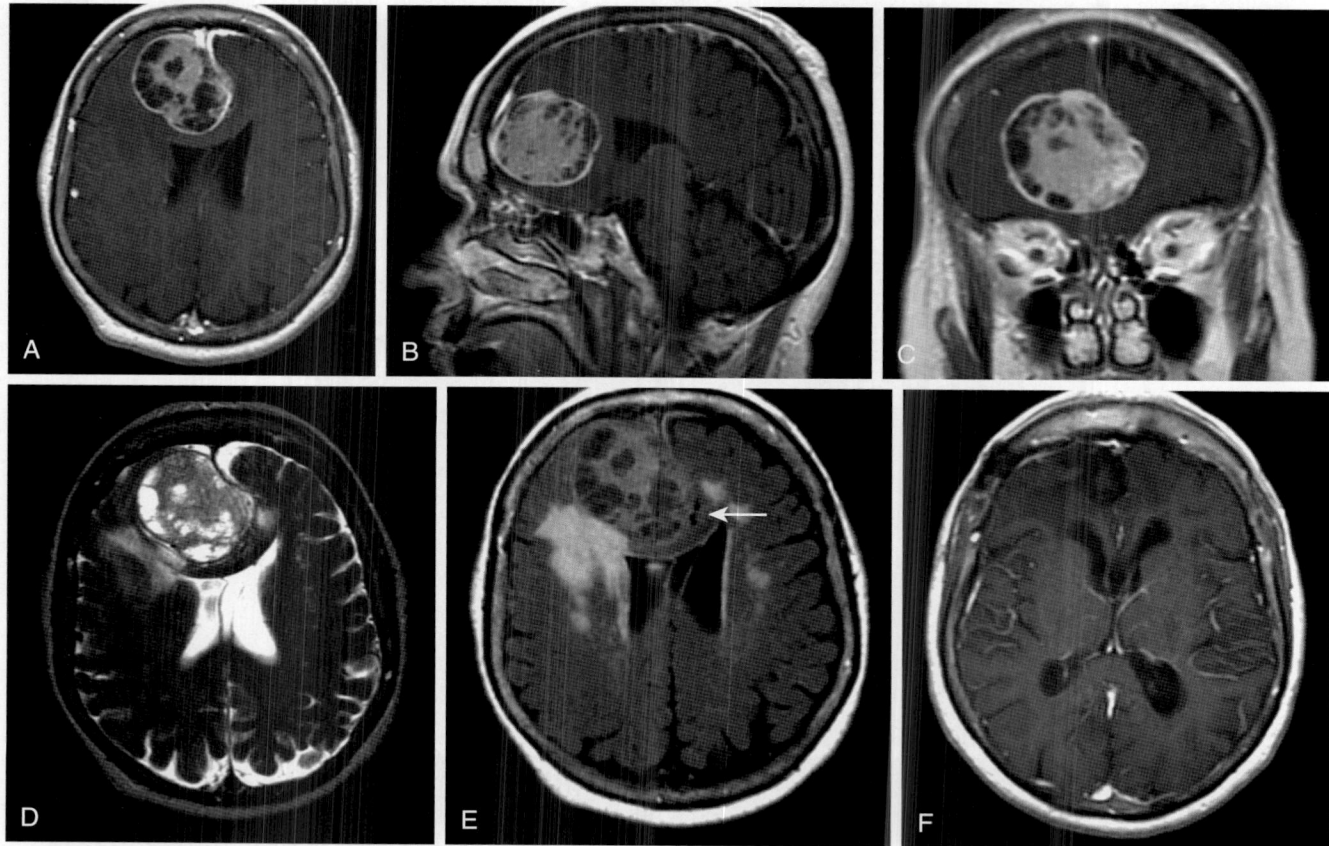

FIGURE 33-2 Seventy-seven-year-old female who presents with 1 month of worsening confusion, forgetfulness, and depressive symptoms. A to C, T1-weighted imaging showed a 4.7 cm × 4.6 cm × 4.3 cm heterogeneously enhancing cystic mass based along the anterior third of the falx and extending into the right frontal lobe. D, T2-weighted image shows a heterogeneous mass with minimal to moderate associated edema. E, FLAIR image shows the flow voids of both anterior cerebral arteries (arrow), which have been displaced posteriorly and to the left of the tumor. F, Two-year follow-up MRI that shows no evidence of tumor recurrence. Patient has persistent confusion, but is otherwise neurologically intact. Histopathology showed atypical meningiomas.

inversion recovery (FLAIR) sequences (Fig. 33-1E). Three-dimensional (3D) T1-weighted gadolinium enhanced multi-echo, magnetization-prepared, rapid gradient echo images can also be used with neuro-navigational tools to provide surgeons with intraoperative guidance.

Cerebral angiography can provide essential information delineating the tumor's arterial feeding pattern. Additionally, arterial phase of the angiography can provide crucial information on the course, displacement and possibly the encasement of the anterior cerebral arteries (ACA), pericallosal arteries, and callosomarginal arteries. The venous phase of the angiogram is also vital toward determining the patency of the superior sagittal sinus, understanding the anatomy of the draining cortical veins in relation to the tumor and the degree of collateral circulation.[11,12] If the sinus is occluded, the anatomy of the draining collateral vessels needs to be clearly identified during preoperative planning and meticulously preserved during surgery. Inadvertent occlusion of collateral vessels may result in severe postoperative complications such as venous infarct and cerebral edema.

The gold standard for cerebral angiography remains digital subtraction angiography (DSA). DSA provides a dynamic view of both the arterial and venous phases, better resolution of small vessel feeders, better accuracy in identifying sinus obstruction, and areas with reversal of normal venous flow. However, DSA is invasive and associated with a small, but not insignificant, risk for strokes, vessel injury, postdiagnostic hematoma, and possible renal injury from contrast use. Noninvasive means to evaluate the cerebral vasculature include MR angiography and CT angiography. MR angiography/venography capitalizes on its intrinsic sensitivity to flow to detect the patency of vessels. Vessels with high flow give rise to high signal intensity while the absence of flow is characterized by reduced signal intensity.[13,14] The technical limitations to MR-angiography include its susceptibility to flow-related artifacts such that patent but obstructed regions of the sinus may appear completely occluded due to decrease in flow and the ability for intracellular deoxyhemoglobin/methemoglobin found in clot can create false signals to suggest a patent vessel. Other practical limitations include longer image acquisition times, and sensitivity to patient movement. CT-angiography/venography (CTA/CTV) is acquired using thin 0.625-mm slices on a helical 64-channel multidetector scanner during the peak arterial and venous enhancements. The acquired images can be viewed using maximum intensity projection (MIP) images, multi-planar reconstruction (MPR) images, and Vitrea 3D reconstruction images (Vital Images,

Minnetonka, MN) to provide the surgeon a better sense of the tumor and its relationship to the vasculature (Fig. 33-2F to J). The faster image acquisition times as well as its ability to maintain high spatial resolution has made CTA/CTV the preferred method for routine preoperative vessel assessment at our institution. CTA/CTV has better small-vessel and sinus resolution and fewer motion and flow artifacts seen in MR venography.[15-16] In a study by Wetzel and colleagues, CTV was compared to digital subtraction angiography and CTV was found to have an overall sensitivity of 95% and 91% specificity while DSA had 90% sensitivity and 100% specificity.[17] Additionally, the shorter image acquisition times allow for less motion artifacts and makes CTA/CTV better suited for uncooperative or sick patients.

Operative Technique

ANESTHESIA AND PREPARATIONS

The patient is brought to the operating room and general anesthesia is administered via endotracheal intubation. A combination of intravenous furosemide, mannitol, and slight hyperventilation is used to reduce intracranial pressure. Preoperative antibiotics, stress dose steroids, and antiseizure prophylaxis, such as fosphenytoin, are also given prior to skin incision. If the preoperative plan involves resection or manipulation of the sagittal sinus, air emboli precautions are implemented. A precordial Doppler is securely placed over the right atrium to monitor for air emboli and an intra-atrial venous catheter is placed for aspirating the air bubbles if necessary. Intraoperative monitoring with somatosensory evoked potentials or direct cortical stimulation is often used when tumors are located adjacent to the motor or sensory areas, and attaching leads should be completed prior to incision.

POSITIONING

For tumors located in anterior third of the sagittal sinus, the patient is placed in a supine position with the head slightly elevated. Tumors around the middle third of the sagittal sinus can be approached with the patient supine with the head elevated and flexed, or, alternatively, a semiprone or lateral approach can be used, especially if the tumor is located more posteriorly. A semilateral, semisitting position with the head well elevated so that the scalp over the area of the tumor is at the highest point can also be considered for tumors in this area. For tumors involving the posterior third, the patient is placed in the lateral position and the head is elevated and turned to the opposite side so that the center of the tumor is uppermost.[18-19] The head is secured with the Mayfield 3-point fixation head rest and the patient's body is secured to table with tape. Foam padding and gel rolls are used to pad all pressure points.

NEURO-NAVIGATION

Advances in neuro-imaging and development of frameless neuro-navigational tools have been instrumental in improving surgical outcomes. After the patient's head and body are securely positioned, neuro-navigational tools are used to co-register the patient's head with a high resolution MRI.

Neuro-navigation can be helpful in planning out the skin incision and the borders of the craniotomy. The accuracy of the neuro-navigation needs to be considered after opening of the dura, as the degree of tumor resection and drainage of CSF can cause shifts in the anatomy.

SKIN INCISION

A bi-coronal incision is used to approach tumors along the anterior third of the sagittal sinus. Tumors at the level of the coronal suture and the middle third of the sagittal sinus are approached via a horseshoe/U-shaped incision that has its base laterally. For posterior-third tumors, a horseshoe/U-shaped incision that has its base toward the occiput provides the most flexibility and exposure. Care is taken to ensure that the base of all U-shaped incisions is broader than the length of the flap. The skin incision will extend across the midline for cases when the tumor involves both sides of the falx. For these cases, the skin incision is based off the side with the largest tumor burden. When possible, retraction on the dominant hemisphere is avoided.

CRANIOTOMY

The craniotomy should encompass the borders of the entire tumor by an addition of a 1- to 2-cm margin. The craniotomy for tumors that extend across the midline may be turned as a single piece or in two sections. Several burr holes are placed laterally along the superior sagittal sinus and the sinus is carefully stripped away from the bone before the bone is cut with the craniotome. If the sinus cannot be separated from the cranium easily, the ipsilateral bone flap may be turned first. Then, under direct tangential vision, the sinus can be stripped from the cranium before turning the second contralateral section of the bone flap. For tumors that extend to the surface, the bone flap may be adherent to the underlying tumor and care should be taken when dissecting the bone flap off over this region to avoid injury to underlying cortex and veins. Bone that has been invaded by tumor may be very thick and it may be necessary to drill the bone away in a piecemeal fashion to avoid injury and tearing underlying cortex. Once the bone flap is off, bleeding points along the sagittal sinus are controlled with a combination of bipolar cautery and use of Surgicel (oxidized cellulose), thrombin-soaked Gelfoam, and Cottonoid pads. Tears to the sinus need to be repaired using 5-0 or 6-0 prolene sutures. Bone bleeding can be controlled with bone wax and circumferential tenting sutures are used along the periphery to avoid further epidural bleeding.

DURAL OPENING

A U-shaped dura incision is made starting laterally with the hinge parallel to the falx. Care needs to be taken when elevating the dural flap medially to avoid tearing potentially important bridging veins. Adhesions and bridging veins need to be dissected and freed. If a large cortical vein enters a dural sinus prior to emptying into the superior sagittal sinus, the cortical vein, and the dural sinus need to be incised from the dural flap and be preserved as an attachment to the midline sinus. For bilateral tumors, the dura on the contralateral side is also incised and the free ends of the dura can be sutured together to help with retraction out of the surgical field.

TUMOR RESECTION

Once the midline cortex is exposed and the falx and superior sagittal sinus are visualized, steps are taken in preparation to retract the hemisphere out laterally. Again, before getting to the tumor, attention must be paid to the anatomy of the cortical veins emptying into the superior sagittal sinus and the falx, itself. While veins along the anterior third of the sinus can usually be ligated without neurologic consequences, the general principle is to preserve cortical veins since they may either directly drain eloquent areas or provide essential collateral drainage. If segments of the superior sagittal sinus are completely or partially occluded, preserving collateral drainage is vital to preventing venous infarcts and cerebral edema. Cortical veins traversing through the tumor and shown to be occluded by DSA can be resected or ligated. However, we re-emphasize that interruption of all other large draining cortical veins that drain toward the midline, particularly at the level of the middle and posterior thirds of the superior sagittal sinus, is fraught with risk. Veins that are encased by tumor need to be dissected free to the greatest extent possible and preserved.

For falcine meningiomas that are concealed beneath cortex, it is important to first establish the anterior and posterior limits of the tumor. From these limits, a corridor can be created by gently retracting the medial surface of the hemisphere. The cortex should not be retracted more than 2 cm away from the falx and the sinus. Overlying bridging veins that are within this corridor, again, need to be preserved and can be made slack by being dissected away from the superior sagittal sinus. If necessary, the bridging veins can also be freed from the cortex for a few millimeters to allow for the required retraction of the hemisphere without sacrificing the vessel. In rare cases where the tumor is exceedingly large or where the corridor is compromised by unyielding veins, the surgeon can create additional exposure by resecting some noneloquent cortex and white matter that is well anterior to the primary and supplementary motor areas. Resection of noneloquent cortex is preferable to taking cortical veins. Additionally, a contralateral interhemispheric approach to large deep-seated meningiomas has been reported.[20]

Once the corridor has been established, the blood supply to the tumor from the falcine arteries is sectioned by cauterizing and sectioning the falx in the inferior-to-superior direction approximately 1 cm anterior and 1 cm posterior to the margins of the tumor. The exposed tumor capsule is then entered using bipolar cautery. Intracapsular enucleation is used to debulk the tumor and this can be accomplished using a combination of bipolar cautery, aspiration, and/or sonic aspiration (e.g., CUSA). Once sufficiently debulked, the rest of the tumor can be delivered by invaginating the capsule into the hollowed tumor cavity. The capsule is peeled away from the cortex using gentle retraction and bipolar cautery. Only small vessels parasitized from the pia arachnoid that are entering the tumor from the brain can be divided. In areas where the capsule has been dissected from the cortex, the brain can be protected with either Gelfoam or Cottonoid pads. It should be noted that a cleavable pial–tumor plane is not always present. Sindou and Alaywan evaluated 150 patients with preoperative angiography.[21] Only 34.8% of meningiomas

with evidence of pial parasitization on angiogram were found to have a cleavable pial–tumor interface at surgery. Conversely, in meningiomas with primarily a dural supply, 83.6% had a cleavable plane. In addition, in cases where there is pial invasion in areas involving eloquent brain, total resection may result in significant and unacceptable postoperative deficits. In these conditions, it is advisable to leave a thin rim of tumor attached to the cortex rather than risk debilitating neurologic compromise.[22] As the tumor is resected, the surgeon should be mindful of the branches of the ACA, including the pericallosal and callosomarginal arteries. These relationships should be identified preoperatively. Smaller arteries directly feeding the tumor can be coagulated and divided; however, traversing branches that are adherent or encased by tumor should be dissected and freed. Once the tumor capsule has been separated from the cortex, the tumor attachment to the falx and sagittal sinus is excised and coagulated. Tumors that extend bilaterally will also require complete resection of the involved falx.

MANAGEMENT OF SINUS INVASION

Falcine meningiomas can grow and extend to involve the superior sagittal sinus. Although occurring less frequently than with parasagittal meningiomas, the surgical considerations for managing tumor infiltration into the sinus are essentially the same. When tumor extends into the sagittal sinus, surgeons are faced with the dilemma of leaving a fragment of invasive tumor and facing a higher rate of recurrence versus attempting to achieve a Simpson I resection but putting the venous circulation at greater risk. As is the case for all meningiomas, the likelihood of recurrence for falcine lesions depends on the Simpson grade at the time of initial resection.[3] Most pertinently, the falx and the encroached upon superior sagittal sinus are the dural attachments associated with these tumors. In a recent case review of 68 falcine meningiomas, Chung et al. found that those with Simpson grade I or II resections had a recurrence rate of 3.6% (2 cases out of 56) while those with a grade III or greater had a rate of 44% (4 cases out of 9).[3] The imperative for aggressive surgery needs to be tempered by the risks of unexpected and sudden occlusion of the middle or posterior thirds of the sagittal sinus. Such venous injury can lead to significant neurologic morbidity and mortality. Decisions regarding sinus management, therefore, should be tailored to individual patients based on their age, symptoms, tumor location, degree of sinus involvement, and the robustness of the cortical venous collaterals.

Three main surgical strategies can be employed in the management of sinus invasion. The first involves simple resection of the outer dural layer with the tumor and coagulation of the inner layer at the sites of tumor attachment. Simpson's series from 1957 demonstrated that complete tumor resection and coagulation of attached dura had a recurrence rate of 16% as compared to 29% recurrence rate when gross total resection was performed without dural coagulation.[23] Complete tumor resection with excision of attached dural attachments had the lowest rate of recurrence of 6%. The second technique for disease involving the superior sagittal sinus involves resecting the invaded sinus wall(s) and repairing the sinus by one of three techniques:[1] resection of the intraluminal tumor and suturing of the sinus edges primarily;[2] resection of the infiltrated wall(s) and repair with an autologous patch (e.g., venous or fascia temporalis); or[3] resection of the occluded portion with interposition of a bypass graft composed of either autologous vein (e.g., external jugular, internal saphenous vein) or a synthetic tube (e.g., Gore-Tex). The third option for management would be simple coagulation of residual tumor or resection of the involved sinus without venous reconstruction.[24]

Sindou and Alvernia propose a six-stage classification scheme for progressively tumor invasion into the sinuses.[25] Type I lesions involve just the outer surface of the sinus wall. Type II lesions have the tumor extending into the lateral recess of the superior sagittal sinus. Type III tumors infiltrate into the lateral sinus wall and when tumor invaded into the roof of the sinus, they are characterized as type IV lesions. Types V and VI tumors completely occlude the sinus, with and without wall invasion, respectively. For type I lesions, the tumor can be peeled off the wall of the sinus using bipolar cautery. Care is then taken to coagulate the areas of tumor attachment to prevent recurrence. Type II tumors that involve the lateral recess can be managed with opening the sinus edge, removing the residual plaque of tumor, and then progressively closing the edge of the sinus wall primarily with a continuous 5-0 or 6-0 prolene suture. Types III and IV tumors involve to the sinus walls to a greater extent and require more extensive sinus reconstruction. Details for this reconstruction are detailed elsewhere.[24,26-28] Type V and VI tumors can be approached on the basis of the location of sinus involvement: anterior, middle, and posterior. A partially or completely occluded superior sagittal sinus in the anterior third can usually be resected without risk of neurologic consequences. Traditionally, middle and posterior segments of the sinus that are found to be occluded on digital subtraction angiography can be resected without the need for venous reconstruction or bypass. Some author advocate testing with temporary occlusion prior to excision.[22] Sekhar temporarily occludes the sinus and measures proximal venous pressure for over 10 minutes.[22] If there is no change in sinus pressure and if there is evidence of brain swelling, the sinus can be resected. However, some authors warn that cerebral edema, venous infarction and subcutaneous cerebrospinal fluid collection can still occur and suggest the need for a venous reconstruction or sinus bypass. The 1955 study by Hoessly and Olivecrona evaluated 196 parasagittal meningiomas treated without venous reconstruction and reported perioperative morbidity of 12.3%, of which more than half was associated with venous drainage.[29] A more recent examination study of 108 cases of falcine or parasagittal meningiomas invading the superior sagittal sinus described 9 cases of severe cerebral edema, of which 3 involved en bloc resection without venous reconstruction.[30] However despite these risks, surgeons are still advised to consider each case individually and weigh the options which include adjuvant radiosurgery and radiotherapy for residual tumor.

CLOSURE

The dura can be closed primarily or if necessary, a duraplasty can be performed using a pericranial graft harvested from the undersurface of the skin flap or with allograft. The dura and/or graft are sewn in a water-tight fashion. The bone flap is re-evaluated for possible tumor invasion. If the bone flap has been invaded with tumor, the patient will require a bone reconstruction from titanium mesh, acrylic cranioplasty, or customized synthetic cranioplasty flap. The reconstruction can be done at the time of the original surgery, or can be done in a delayed fashion, especially if the brain appears swollen at the time of closure. Bone flaps that are free of tumor can be secured to the cranium with titanium miniplates and screws. The galea is closed with interrupted, inverted absorbable sutures and the skin is typically closed using a running nylon stitch.

Postoperative Care

The patient is emerged from general anesthesia and transported to the ICU for standard postoperative care. Postoperatively, the patient should be kept well hydrated to prevent the propensity for delayed venous thrombosis. Steroids that were started preoperatively are continued for a short course that typically last through the first 72 hours and then tapered rapidly. Antiepileptics should be continued for an additional 3 months in patients with no prior seizure history. Patients who present with seizure may require a longer course of antiepileptics and may be weaned off therapy if a sleep-deprived electroencephalogram shows no signs of further seizure activity. Postoperative imaging with noncontrast CT or MRI may be indicated if the patient has persistent or progressive lethargy or obtundation, or progressive focal neurologic deficits. CT or MR angiography/venography can be used to diagnose or follow evolving venous thrombosis. Patients who have undergone a venous graft need to be started on anticoagulation. For the first 24 to 48 hours these patients should be placed on titratable heparin drip. The goal PTT should be in the therapeutic range of 60 to 80 but each case should be evaluated to avoid postoperative hematomas. Once the patient has been stabilized, the patient can be transitioned to weight-based therapeutic doses of low-molecular weight heparin and Coumadin. The low-molecular-weight heparin can be discontinued when the patient's INR is between 2.0 to 3.0. Coumadin is then continued for at least 3 months postoperatively.

Summary

The surgical approach to falcine meningiomas is dictated by the tumor's location relative to the superior sagittal sinus. Preoperative and intraoperative high-resolution gadolinium-enhanced MR images can aide in understanding tumor size and location and can be helpful in planning patient positioning, skin incision, and the size of the bone flap craniotomy. Standard digital subtraction and noninvasive CT and MR cerebral angiography can provide critical insight on the course of the arterial feeders. Additionally, for cases where tumor infiltrates the superior sagittal sinus, cerebral angiography can reveal the degree of sinus occlusion and the anatomy of the collateral draining veins. Intraoperatively, the surgeon needs be judicious in the degree of cortex retraction and be meticulous in preserving surrounding cortical veins in order to avoid potentially devastating neurologic injuries. Occasionally falcine meningiomas can secondarily invade the superior sagittal sinus and in such cases, the surgeon needs to consider the patient's age, symptoms, degree of tumor infiltration, and the role of adjuvant radiosurgery and radiotherapy. The options for sinus repair and/or venous bypass should be discussed at length before pursuing tumor within the sinus. Intraoperative verification of completely occluded sinuses using manometry and temporary clipping is recommended prior to sinus resection. Finally, the surgeon needs to be aware of the risks for delayed sinus thrombosis and to keep patients well hydrated postoperatively.

KEY REFERENCES

Al-Mefty O, Origitano TC, Harkey HL, eds. *Controversies in Neurosurgery.* New York: Thieme; 1996.

Barajas Jr RF, Sughrue ME, McDermott MW. Large falcine meningioma fed by callosomarginal branch successfully removed following contralateral interhemispheric approach. *J Neurooncol.* 2009;97:127-131.

Casey SO, Alberico RA, Patel M, et al. Cerebral CT venography. *Radiology.* 1996;198:163-170.

Chung SB, Kim CY, Park CK, et al. Falx meningiomas: surgical results and lessons learned from 68 cases. *J Korean Neurosurg Soc.* 2007;42:276-280.

Demir MK, Iplikcioglu AC, Dincer A, et al. Single voxel proton MR spectroscopy findings of typical and atypical intracranial meningiomas. *Eur J Radiol.* 2006;60(1):48-55.

DiMeco F, Li KW, Casali C, et al. Meningiomas invading the superior sagittal sinus: surgical experience of 108 cases. *Neurosurgery.* 2004; 55:1263-1274.

Hoessly GF, Olivecrona H. Report on 280 cases of verified parasagittal meningioma. *J Neurosurg.* 1955;12:614-626.

Kim CY, Jung HW. Falcine meningiomas. In: Lee JH, ed. *Meningiomas: Diagnosis, Treatment, and Outcome.* London: Springer-Verlag; 2008.

Lawton MT, Golfinos JG, Spetzler RF. The contralateral transcallosal approach: experience with 32 patients. *Neurosurgery.* 1996;39(4): 729-735.

Liauw L, van Buchem MA, Split A, et al. MR angiography of the intracranial venous system. *Radiology.* 2000;214:678-682.

Longstreth WT, Dennis LK, McGuire VM. Epidemology of intracranial meningiomas. *Cancer.* 1993;72:639-648.

Maiuri F, Iaconetta G, de Divitiis O, et al. Intracranial meningiomas: correlations between MR imaging and histology. *Eur J Radiol.* 1999;31(1):69-75.

Ojemann RG. Management of cranial and spinal meningiomas. In: Selman W, ed. *Clinical Neurosurgery.* Baltimore: Williams and Wilkins; 1992.

Ojemann RG, Ogilvy CS. Convexity, parasagittal and parafalcine meningiomas. In: Apuzzo MLJ, ed. *Brain Surgery: Complication Avoidance and Managment.* New York: Churchill Livingstone; 1993.

Ozsvath RR, Casey SO, Lustrin ES, et al. Cerebral venography: comparison of CT and MR projection venography. *AJR Am J Roentgenol.* 1997;169:1699-1707.

Sekhar LN, de Oliveira E, Riedel CJ. Parasagittal, falx meningiomas. *Cranial Microsurgery: Approaches and Techniques.* New York: Thieme; 1997.

Simpson D. The recurrence of intracranial meningiomas after surgical treatment. *J Neurol Neurosurg Psychiatry.* 1957;20:22-39.

Sindou M. Meningiomas invading the sagittal or transverse sinuses, resection with venous reconstruction. *J Clin Neurosci.* 2001;8(suppl 1):8-11.

Sindou M, Alaywan M. Most intracranial meningiomas are not cleavable tumors: anatomic-surgical evidence and angiographic predictability. *Neurosurgery.* 1998;42:476-480.

Sindou M, Auque J. The intracranial venous system as a neurosurgeon's perspective. *Adv Tech Stan Neurosurg.* 2000;26:131-216.

Sindou M, Hallacq P. Venous reconstruction in surgery of meningiomas invading the sagittal and transverse sinuses. *Skull Base Surg.* 1998;8:57-64.

Sindou MP, Alvernia JE. Results of attempted radical tumor removal and venous repair in 100 consecutive meningiomas involving the major dural sinuses. *J Neurosurg.* 2006;105:514-525.

Sindou MP, Bokor J, Brunon J. Bilaeral thrombosis of the transverse sinuses: microsurgical revascularization with venous bypass. *Surg Neurol.* 1980;13:215-220.

Tamiya T, Ono Y, Matsumoto K, Ohmoto T. Peritumoral brain edema in intracranial meningiomas: effects of radiological and histological factors. *Neurosurgery.* 2001;49(5):1046-1051.

Wetzel SG, Kirsh E, Stock KW, et al. Cerebral veins: comparative study of CT venography with intraarterial digital subtraction angiography. *Am J Neuroradiol.* 1999;20:249-255.

Numbered references appear on Expert Consult.

CHAPTER 34

Surgical Management of Midline Anterior Skull Base Meningiomas

MATTHIAS KIRSCH • DIETMAR KREX • GABRIELE SCHACKERT

Surgical Anatomy

Meningiomas arising in the midline of the anterior fossa are generally separated in the more ventral olfactory groove meningiomas and the more dorsal planum sphenoidale and tuberculum sellae meningiomas. Olfactory groove meningiomas arise over the cribriform plate of the ethmoid bone and the area of the frontosphenoid suture. Those tumors may grow symmetrically around the crista galli and thus may involve any part of the planum of the sphenoid bone or extend predominantly to one side. They occurred with a frequency of less than 6% in our series of 1200 meningiomas. Of all anterior skull base meningiomas, 22% were pure olfactory groove meningiomas. Of these, 7% had at least one additional meningioma at a different location. Planum sphenoidale/tuberculum sellae meningiomas arise from the roof of the sphenoid sinus and the tuberculum sellae, which is an area between the optic nerves and the anterior clinoid processes belonging to the frontal part of the middle cranial fossa. The tuberculum sellae is located between the chiasmatic grooves and on either side at the optic foramen, which transmits the optic nerve and ophthalmic artery to the orbit. Behind the optic foramen, the anterior clinoid process is directed posteriorly and medially and attaches to the tentorium cerebelli. These structures are frequently overgrown by these types of meningiomas, as are the posteriorly located dural folds of the sella turcica and the lateral adjacent cavernous sinus (Fig. 34-1). Planum sphenoidale/tuberculum sellae meningiomas occurred at rates similar to those of olfactory groove meningiomas in our series: less than 6% of all intracranial meningiomas but 21% of anterior skull base meningiomas.

The planum sphenoidale and tuberculum sellae are part of the sphenoid bone. The former is a dorsal extension beyond the ethmoid bone and part of the anterior cranial base; the latter belongs to the middle cranial base. Whereas planum sphenoidale meningiomas usually push the optic nerves dorsally and caudally, tuberculum sellae meningiomas lead to an upward bulging of these structures. However, it is often difficult to clearly separate these tumors simply based on their bony covering. Rather, their relationship to the optic nerves and chiasm can distinguish these tumors as to their most likely origin. Both entities might grow between, around, and beyond the optic nerves. Depending on the exact extension, tuberculum sellae tumors are usually approached either frontolaterally or strictly laterally from the pterion using an angle that allows viewing posterior to the optic nerves.

Branches of the ethmoidal, meningeal, and ophthalmic arteries enter through the midline of the base of the skull and constitute the primary blood supply of those tumors. In smaller tumors, the A2 segments of the anterior cerebral arteries usually are not involved in the tumor capsule but rather are separated from the tumor by a rim of cerebral tissue and arachnoid. However, in large tumors, these and additional segments, e.g., the frontopolar or other small branches originating from the anterior cerebral arteries, may adhere to the posterior and superior tumor capsule. They should be meticulously coagulated and separated from the capsule to avoid postoperative bleeding.

The olfactory nerves either are displaced laterally on the lower surface of the tumor or are adherent, compressed, or even not visible while diffusely spread within the tumor capsule. Preservation of these nerves should be attempted in small tumors, resulting in displacement of one or both nerves. Once the olfactory nerves are compressed by large tumors or even tightly involved in the tumor capsule, it is difficult to preserve them, and this becomes almost impossible when the tumor has a broad attachment to the dura and infiltrates adjacent, often hypertrophic bone. In addition, in large tumors, the optic nerves and chiasm may be displaced downward and posteriorly, which is in contrast to tumors originating from the sella region.

Clinical Presentation

Olfactory groove meningiomas are on average larger than meningiomas at different locations in our series. This is most likely due to the relative lack of focal symptoms at the frontal base with smaller meningiomas. For large tumors, the slow growth rate allows surrounding tissues to adapt. Many symptoms are difficult to localize neurotopically, and the initial consultations of family and physicians often tend toward interpretation of these as functional personality changes rather than focal cerebral symptoms. Personality changes, such as apathy and akinesia, can be common when the tumors grow to larger size; in our series, this was found in up to 13% of patients. Onset of these symptoms is gradual, and they may not be observed early in their course. Other common symptoms include headache and

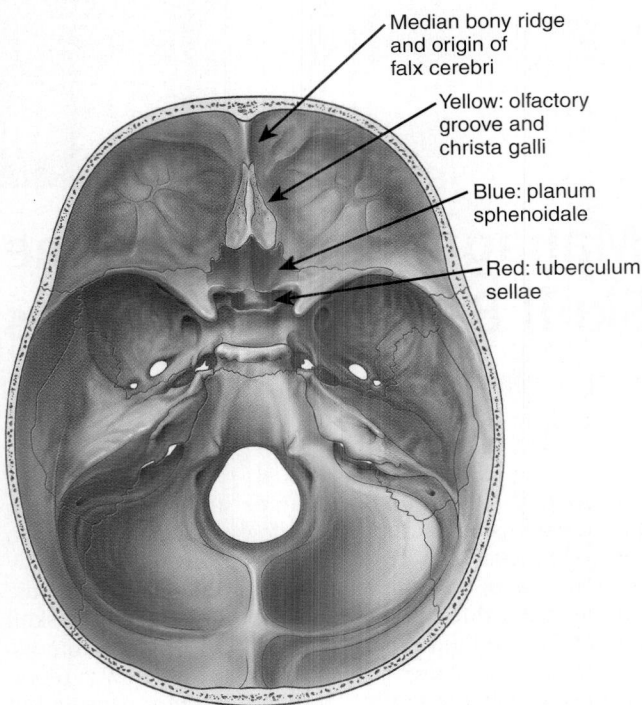

Median bony ridge and origin of falx cerebri

Yellow: olfactory groove and christa galli

Blue: planum sphenoidale

Red: tuberculum sellae

FIGURE 34-1 Anatomic skull base overview with the midline anterior skull base colored to show the most common origins of tumors: the cribriform plate, olfactory groove, and crista galli (yellow); the planum sphenoidale (blue); and the tuberculum sellae area (red), which reaches bilateral to the optic nerve canal. *(Adapted from Drake RL: Gray's Atlas of Anatomy, International Edition. Philadelphia: Churchill Livingstone, Elsevier, 2008.)*

visual deficits, both of which were more frequent in frontal meningiomas than in any other type of meningioma in our series. Because the optic nerves and chiasm are compressed superiorly by the tumor, an inferior visual defect was most common in up to one third of our patients. The Foster-Kennedy syndrome of unilateral optic atrophy and contralateral papilledema, although originally described in olfactory groove meningiomas,[1] occurred in only a small number of patients.

Double vision is a rare symptom, occurring in less than 6% of patients. In our series, smelling disorders up to anosmia were apparent in 64.5% of the patients that were diagnosed based purely on the routine preoperative workup. Only 7.1% were completely anosmic preoperatively. Interestingly, anosmia is not an important symptom for most patients, most likely because it develops slowly. In Cushing and Eisenhardt's series, the sense of smell was the primary symptom in only 3 of the 29 patients.[2] Bakay reported that even if anosmia was apparent, it was not the leading symptom.[3]

Epilepsy was less frequent, occurring in 12% of cases, compared to all other supratentorial sites and was only lower, occurring in 8% of cases, in medial sphenoid wing tumors. Planum sphenoidale and tuberculum sellae meningiomas encompassed a further 21% of frontobasal meningiomas in our series. They presented more frequently with visual pathway symptoms than did olfactory groove meningiomas and less frequently with disorders of smell. Symptomatic epilepsy was also rare in these more dorsal tumors and occurred only in very large lesions.

Evaluation of Radiologic Studies in Planning the Operation

The standard diagnostic means for evaluation of anterior midline meningiomas such is magnetic resonance imaging (MRI), because it can delineate the mass effect relationship to other important structures such as the optic nerves, the relationship to the anterior cerebral arteries, and the elevation of the frontal lobes. However, cranial computed tomography (CT) and angiography are important adjuncts if the destruction of the anterior skull base, the infiltration of the ethmoid bone, the relationship of the major vessels, and the vascular supply are of interest.

Noncontrast CT scanning classically demonstrates a dural-based, homogeneous tumor of increased density compared to the surrounding brain, with variable mass effect and surrounding edema. Hyperostosis of the adjacent skull base is a common feature. Contrast agent administration produces dramatic homogeneous enhancement of the tumor and often reveals a dural tumor tail.

For preoperative and diagnostic evaluation, MRI is essential and provides additional information and good soft-tissue differentiation. With T1-weighted MRI, the tumor is of equivalent signal intensity compared to the surrounding brain, and T2-weighted MRI reveals that the tumor signal is slightly increased compared to the normal brain but less than that of cerebrospinal fluid. Fluid-attenuated inversion recovery and T2-weighted MRI highlight surrounding edema. With administration of gadolinium contrast medium, MRI demonstrates homogeneous tumor enhancement. It is crucial to analyze the relationship of the optic nerves and anterior cerebral arteries to the tumor capsule. Magnetic resonance angiography may provide essential information about blood supply and displaced arteries or even arteries embedded within the tumor. In correlation with CT, the extension into the osseous structures, the underlying ethmoid and sphenoid sinuses, and the foramina yields additional information. Modern imaging tools easily facilitate the coregistration of many imaging modalities to visualize the tumor from any angle and to plan the operation virtually.

In recent years, angiography generally has not been indicated unless embolization is planned. The classic angiographic appearance of a meningioma is that of increasing hypervascular tumor blush throughout the arterial phase, persisting well into the late venous phase with slow washout. Hypervascularity may complicate and lengthen the operation. Therefore, embolization may be considered, which involves the devascularization of the tumor's blood supply through the placement of an embolic agent via a microcatheter into the feeding arteries. However, the surgeon should be aware of a considerable rate of hemorrhagic and ischemic complications when using small particles for embolization.[4-7]

General Aspects of Surgical Management

As the majority of meningiomas are benign, well-circumscribed extra-axial tumors, complete surgical removal should be the primary goal in most instances. The neurologic integrity has to be preserved as it would be in any other neurosurgical procedure. Due to the relation of anterior midline meningiomas to adjacent neurologic eloquent areas, complete tumor removal even with resection of infiltrated dura or removal of infiltrated bone might be achieved with low morbidity in most cases. However, when tumors are firmly attached to the anterior vessels or the optic chiasm, complete removal might constitute a high risk for damage of those structures. In these cases a small piece of adherent capsule might remain and is controlled by periodic MRI scans. Upon recurrence, reoperation and adjuvant radiation therapy may be considered.

The decision for surgery should not be based on age alone as long as the patient's general health condition is stable and the patient is increasingly hampered by neurologic symptoms. Because symptoms usually occur late and at larger tumor volumes that are often increased by surrounding edema, there are rarely alternatives to surgical treatment.

On examination, the sense of smell is often compromised; however, remaining function is difficult to test and a formal olfactogram should be requested. If unaltered, the patient should be warned about the loss of this function.

Preoperatively, steroids are only applied if significant edema is present. Intraoperatively, a steroid bolus, e.g., dexamethasone of up to 24 mg, is given and subsequently weaned over a period of 3 to 7 days postoperatively. When the patient arrives in the operating room, intravenous antibiotics are given once as a prophylaxis and for one week afterward if the frontal sinus was opened.

After induction of anesthesia, the application of intravenous glycerol or 15% mannitol might be considered in a case of extensive edema.

Bifrontal Approach

GENERAL CONSIDERATIONS

The bifrontal approach was first described by Horsley[8] and Cushing[9] and was later proposed by Tönnes,[10] who preserved the frontal brain tissue by a subfrontal approach.[11] Many others have used the bifrontal approach for large tumors of the frontal base, such as Al-Mefty,[12] Nakamura et al.,[13] and Ransohoff and Nockels.[14] A bifrontal craniotomy might be considered for patients with large tumors because this approach gives direct access to all sides of the tumor. Due to the wide exposure, retraction on the frontal lobes is minimal. It simultaneously allows interruption of the blood supply, preparation of the frontobasal matrix of the tumor, and concomitant decompression. There is usually no problem from the ligation of the anterior sagittal sinus. However, venous drainage should be evaluated by preoperative imaging to avoid venous congestion, and coagulation of draining veins from the anterior frontal lobe should be avoided of possible. A navigation system might be used to avoid opening the frontal sinus; however, if the frontal sinus is entered, meticulous closure of the defect should prevent any complications.

OPERATIVE TECHNIQUE

The patient is placed in the supine position with the knees slightly flexed and the head slightly elevated and extended. A three-point skeletal-fixation headrest system is used.

Usually, only a small area of hair needs to be shaved to prepare a coronal incision through the skin while preserving the pericranial tissue. The skin of the posterior aspect of the incision is elevated, and the pericranial tissue is incised below the skin. This step gives extra pericranial tissue, which might be used later to cover the floor of the anterior fossa and to patch the convex dura as needed. The skin flap and underlying tissue, including the pericranial tissue, are then turned down together using fishhooks. According to the size and extension of the tumor, bur holes are placed just below the end of the anterior temporal line or keyholes are placed above the pterion and on each side of the sagittal sinus anterior to the skin incision (Figs. 34-2 and 34-3).

After blunt dissection of the dura from the tabula interna of the skull bone, particularly in the midline area, the bone flap is usually cut in one piece. The bone is cut just above the supraorbital ridge from each side as far medially as possible. Usually, this process leaves about 1 cm of bone in the midline. Here, because of the irregular bone projecting from the inner table of the skull, sawing might be difficult. If complete cutting across the frontal sinus is not possible, the outer table is cut separately. The inner table is then broken as the bone is elevated, and the free bone flap is removed. A rarely necessary method is to cut a right frontal bone flap first, free the sagittal sinus, and then cut a second bone flap across the midline to the left side.

The frontal sinuses are entered frequently. Whether the mucosa needs to be completely removed remains controversial. A multilayered closure of the frontal sinus is prepared. First, a layer of bone wax is used to close the sinus during the intracerebral part of the operation. For final closure, a pericranial flap is formed (Fig. 34-3) that can be inserted once the tumor is removed. The pericranial flap should be sutured to the frontal edge of the dura and intradurally as far posterior as possible to cover any defects (Fig. 34-4). In addition, frontobasal dura gaps can be covered that occurred during tumor and dural matrix removal. In case of an opened ethmoid sinus, the pericranial tissue should cover this too. Sutures are placed along the edge of the craniotomy to control epidural bleeding.

A slightly curved dural incision is performed over each medial inferior frontal lobe adjacent to the edge of the craniotomy opening but leaving a sufficient rim for safe and convenient closure of the dura. Depending on the bony removal, the dural opening can be curved basally or upward. This incision can be tailored to the specific line of approach to the meningioma. If a lateral approach is needed, in addition to the midline approach, the dural opening is extended as needed. It is carried medially near the edge of the sagittal sinus, thereby allowing good exposure yet protecting most of both frontal lobes during the operation. Bridging veins from the anterior frontal lobe to the midline area might be coagulated and divided if necessary. To obtain better exposure of the sagittal sinus, the frontal lobes might be carefully retracted. Then the sagittal sinus is divided between two silk sutures, and the falx is cut (Fig. 34-3). The frontal lobes are gently retracted slightly laterally and posteriorly to open the view to the anterior and superior surface of the tumor, lying in the midline with attachments to the falx and crista galli.

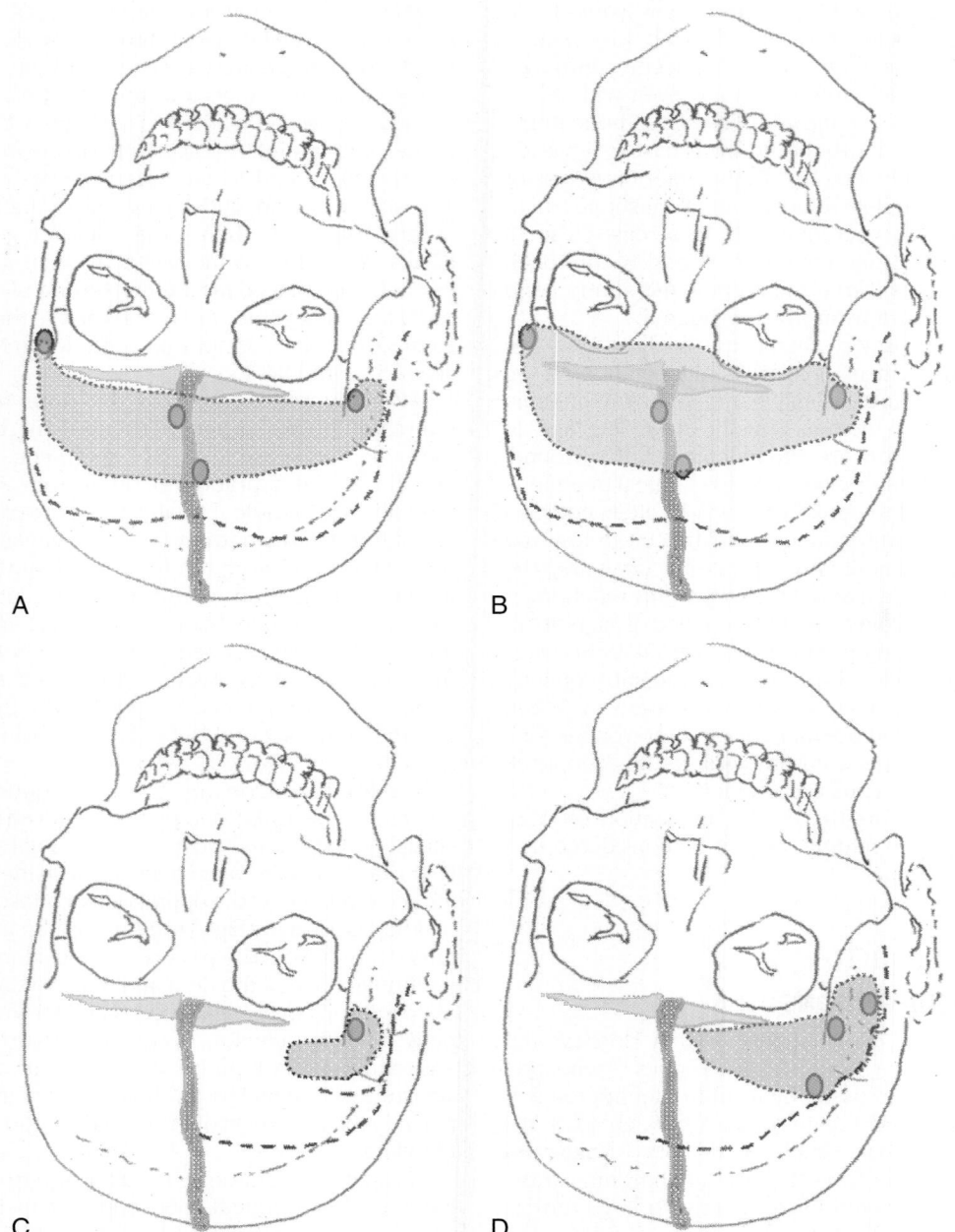

FIGURE 34-2 Skin incision (red dashed line), craniotomy (gray dotted line), frontal sinus (gray filled space) and burr holes (green ovals) for a bifrontal (A), extended bifrontal transbasal (B), limited right pterional/subfrontal (C), and extended subfrontal (D) approach that is sometimes used with an orbitozygomatic approach.

Generally, two alternative procedures are suggested. Particularly in large olfactory groove meningiomas, we prefer devascularization of the tumor as early as possible and only minor debulking for preparation along the base of the skull. This procedure seems to be associated with less blood loss and does not produce difficult angles for dissecting of the tumor capsule from the surrounding brain parenchyma. The dissection along the base is alternated with internal decompression of the tumor to gradually bring into view the base and to remove the bulk of the tumor. This brings down

the rim of the tumor and the brain tissue toward the skull base. The cerebral cortex is carefully separated from the tumor capsule by division of arachnoid and small vascular attachments. The self-retaining retractors are repositioned accordingly.

The alternative procedure is to remove the core of the tumor first. This leads to higher blood loss and poorer control of the blood supply during debulking. However, preparation of the skull base after debulking of the tumor is easier compared to the initial devascularization

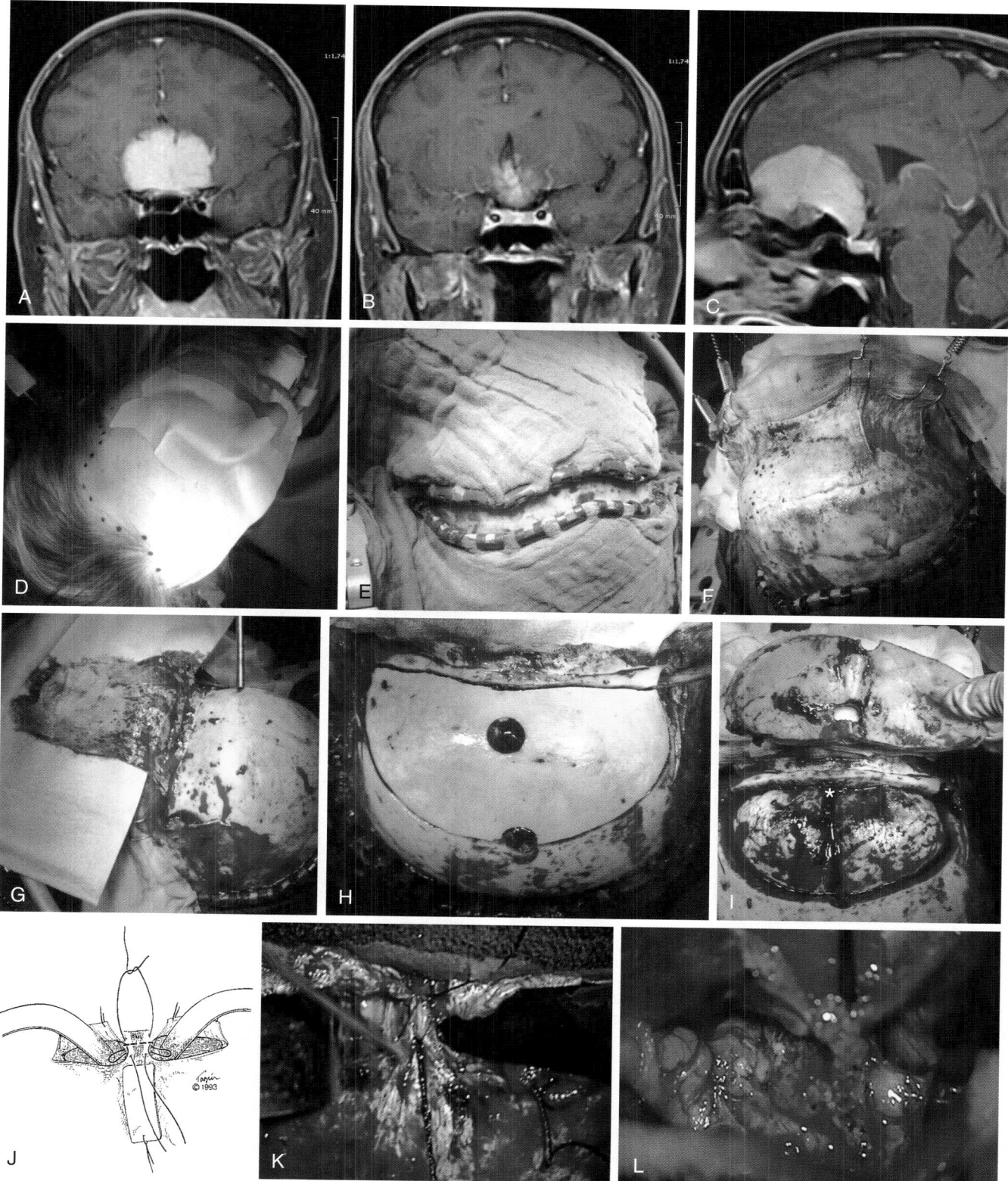

FIGURE 34-3 Craniotomy and dural opening for a typical large olfactory groove meningioma that is suited for a bifrontal approach. A-C, The fron-topolar artery branches and the A2 segments are engulfed in the tumor and the capsule; the anterior skull base midline structures are involved. C, Hyperostosis and concurrent growth into the ethmoid sinus are seen. D, A bicoronal incision is made 2 to 3 cm behind the hairline (dotted line). E-G, A vascularized galeal–periosteal flap is prepared. H and I, A bone flap is generated that can extend from the keyholes bilaterally on both sides to the frontal sinus (the opened frontal sinus is indicated by an asterisk) or might be limited to 3 cm bilateral of the midline. J-L, A slightly curved dural opening is made over both hemispheres, the anterior sagittal sinus is ligated, and the tumor is visualized growing around the falcine origin along the crista galli (L). (*J, © 1993 Edith Tagrin.*)

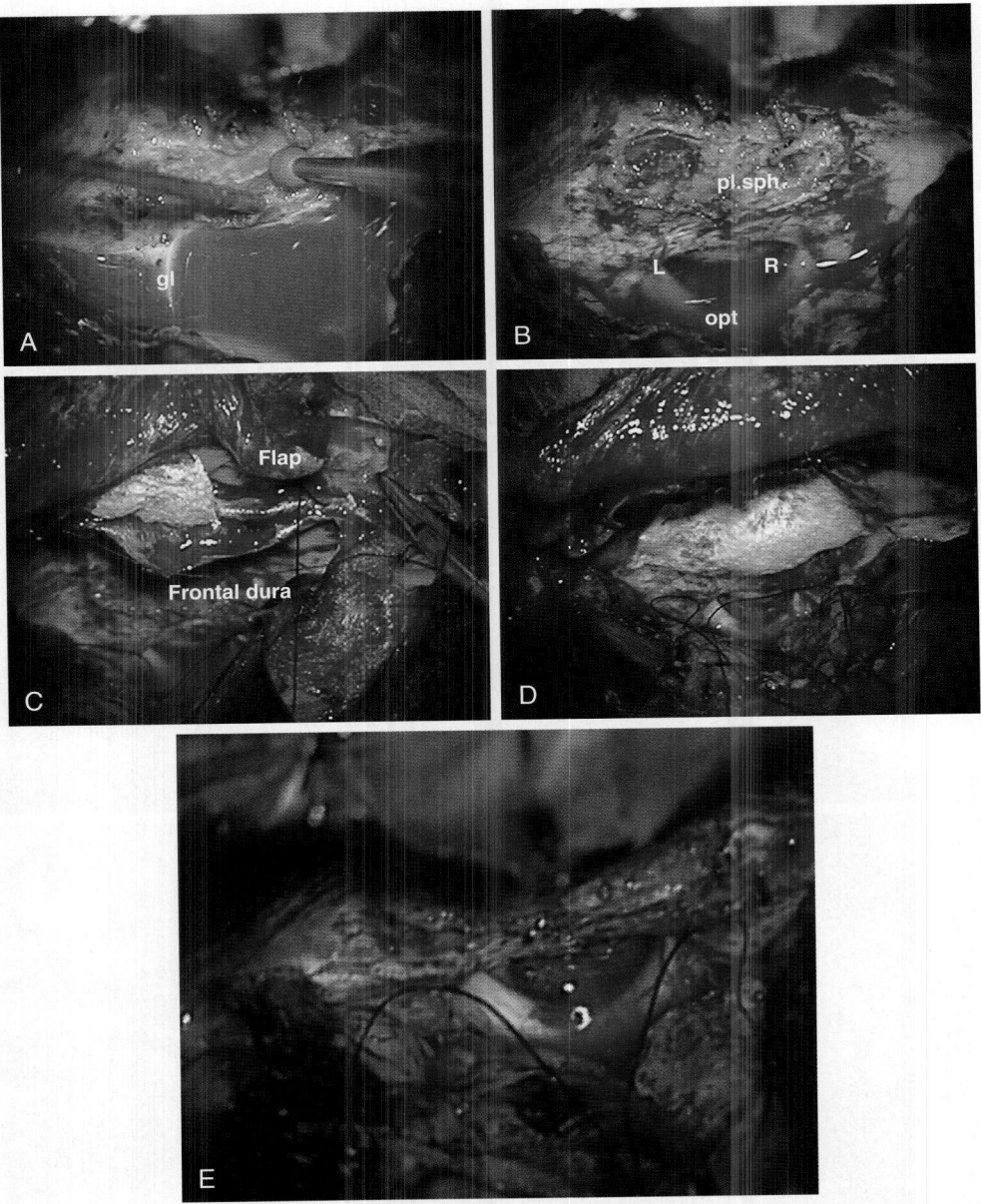

FIGURE 34-4 Closure of the bifrontal approach. The infiltrated part of the dura and osseous skull base is removed (A) until the dural fold before the tuberculum sellae (B). After opening the frontal sinus during craniotomy, a temporary closure with Gelfoam and bone wax was used during tumor removal. The definite two-layered covering is performed using TachoSil or a similar product and the vascularized periosteal flap (C), with a running suture along the frontal dural margin (C and D). The flap is inserted, and then it is necessary to fix the flap posteriorly (E) and laterally with sutures to the remaining basal dura; otherwise, the flap will contract and fold away over the next few days. In addition, fibrin glue is used to reinforce closure of any remaining holes. gl, protective piece of glove above the optic nerves; pl.sph., planum sphenoidale; opt, optic nerves and chiasm.

procedure. The initial step in that procedure is to open the anterior capsule of the tumor. If histology is in doubt, a biopsy might be taken now for frozen-section histology. Depending on the amount of bleeding, large parts of the anterior and midline portion of the tumor can be removed before the part of the tumor capsule that is attached at the anterior midline is divided. Numerous small blood vessels that penetrate the bone in the frontal fossa usually constitute the main blood supply for those tumors. Therefore, in cases of heavy bleeding after starting debulking the tumor, it might be necessary to switch strategies and do the basal

devascularization first. Those vessels are occluded by bipolar coagulation and, occasionally, bone wax or soft drilling with a diamond drill.

Devascularization of the tumor as early as possible is especially important in large olfactory groove meningiomas. As the debulking progresses, the remaining tumor is brought down away from the brain tissue toward the cribriform plate, where most of the work takes place. Thus, it is an alternating procedure of dissection along the base and internal decompression of the tumor, resulting in the exposure of the base and removal of the bulk of the tumor. For decompression,

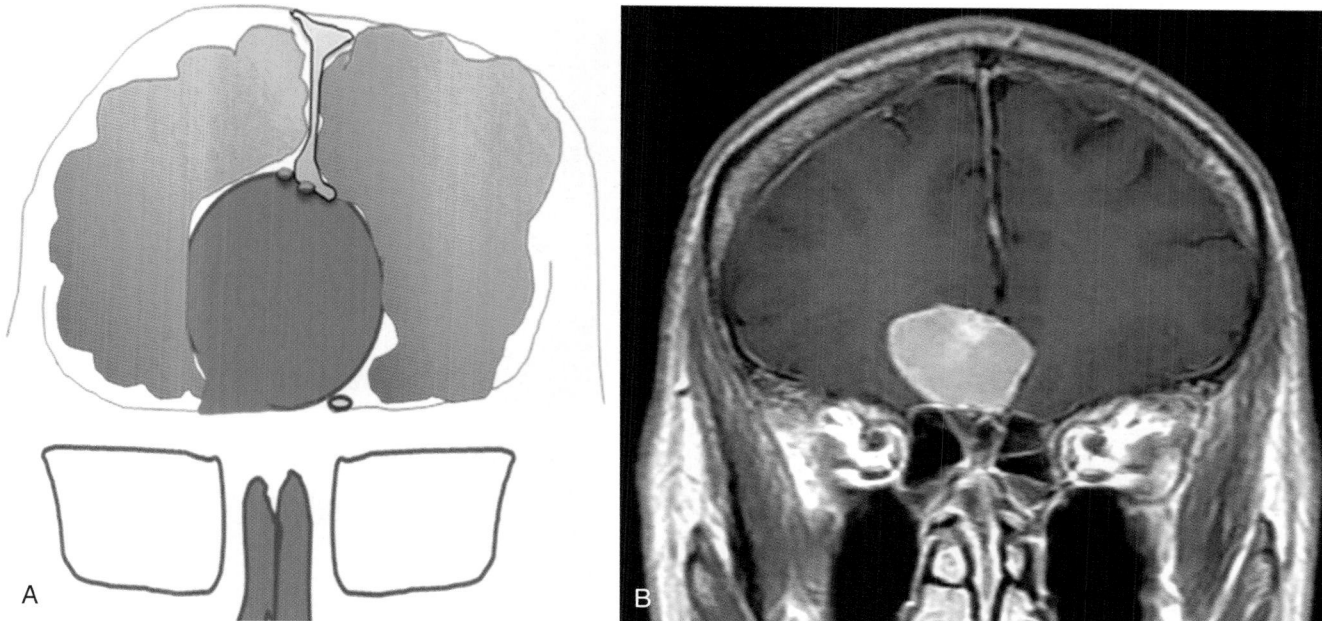

FIGURE 34-5 Schematic (A) and MRI (B) presentation for olfactory groove tumors eligible for one-sided removal, a right-sided approach in this case. The olfactory nerve and groove should be visible. The A2 segments should be approachable from this side.

an ultrasound surgical aspirator can be used that is effective even for tumors of firm consistency. By preventing the frontal lobes from falling into the decompression area by self-retaining retractors, there is enough space to dissect the tumor capsule from the adjacent frontal brain parenchyma. Care should be taken to avoid pressure on the frontal lobes and consecutive postoperative edema or even intraparenchymal hemorrhage. The preparation of the posterior tumor capsule is the most challenging step, because branches of the anterior artery complex might be adjacent to or even involved in the tumor capsule. In most cases, at least the larger vessels can be separated by a small rim of cerebral cortex and arachnoid between the adventitia and the outer tumor capsule. However, when those vessels are firmly embedded within the tumor capsule, a tumor remnant should be left in place. Smaller branches or the frontopolar artery being spread in the capsule might be considered to be occluded and divided if there is no alternative that may not cause a problem.[15]

The optic nerves and the anterior clinoid process can be visualized by preparing farther back to the sphenoid wing and then medially. If a large tumor has displaced the optic nerves posteriorly and inferiorly, localization might be more difficult because the displacement is frequently associated with arachnoid thickening.

After identification of the involved adjacent neurologic structures and removal of the bulk of the tumor, the area of dural attachment should be meticulously coagulated or preferentially excised. Infiltrated hyperostotic bone should be removed by a high-speed diamond drill. In our view, hyperostosis may contain remaining tumor cells, and the osseous and tumorous vascular supply usually originates from this area. Similarly, any tumor entering the ethmoid sinus should be resected. The region of the excised dura should be covered with a sheet of Tacho-seal, TachoSil,™ or something similar; with a vascularized galeal–periosteal patch or

fascia lata over the defect, the patch should be sutured to the remaining dura margin with single stitches and sealed along the border with fibrin glue (Fig. 34-4). Another layer of gelatin sponge is placed over the fascia. The layers might be augmented with fibrin glue.

The convexity dura is closed with another graft of pericranial tissue, and the bone flap is fixed by nonresorbable sutures or miniplates. The bur holes are filled with bone dust or cranioplasty material. A subcutaneous wound drain should be left in place before wound closure.

Unilateral Subfrontal Approach

GENERAL CONSIDERATIONS

The unilateral approach is preferred if the tumor grows prominently on one side and does not have an extensive basal dural attachment onto the contralateral side and if the contralateral olfactory nerve is expected to have a clear plane of dissection (Fig. 34-5A).

OPERATIVE TECHNIQUE

The patient's position depends on the involvement of the midline structures, the displacement and orientation of the A2 segments, and the optic nerve structures. In general, the head is slightly extended posteriorly to allow the frontal lobes to follow gravity. A regular frontal skin incision behind the hair line is used that might be extended over the midline, if anterior and medial visualization are considered. A pericranial flap is always prepared to cover potential dural tears or removed tumor matrix in case of anterior middle fossa involvement (Fig. 34-6). This is not necessary for isolated tuberculum sellae tumors. The craniotomy should aim to visualize the sylvian fissure if posterior retraction along the sphenoid wing is required, remain very low above the

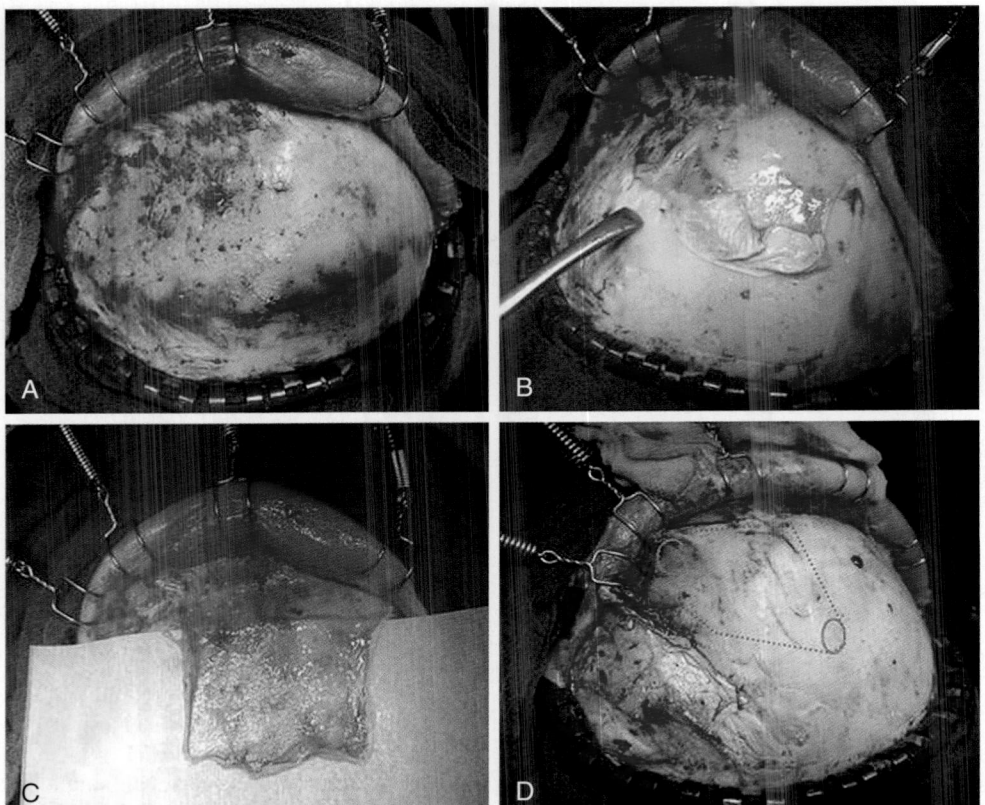

FIGURE 34-6 Left-sided unilateral approach for an anterior olfactory groove meningioma (A). The pericranial tissue (B) is scraped off the bone and maintained with vascular supply intact (C). The PCG is kept in a moistened pad. The temporal muscle is scraped off superiorly to expose the pterion, where the first burr hole is made. A second burr hole is made over the superior sagittal sinus (D, in light blue).

plane of the frontal skull base, and extend close to the midline as far as necessary. The craniotomy should be shaped according to the expected irregularities of the frontal skull base, which might otherwise hinder clear visualization along a one-sided trajectory.

For isolated tuberculum sellae tumors a regular pterional craniotomy suffices, whereas for very large tuberculum sellae tumors extending to the frontal base a modified frontal approach might be necessary.

DURAL OPENING

The dural opening is preceded by many sutures along the craniotomy edges. Depending on the bony removal, the dural opening can be curved basally or upward. If the frontal sinus is opened, a multilayered closure should be accomplished, including a pericranial flap that is sutured as far basally as possible. Dural closure is usually not difficult because the dura is lifted from the frontal skull base. However, the dura is lifted in a tentlike fashion, which can lead to epidural collection. If such an enlarged epidural space is created, the sinus covering should be double-checked prior to closure. If necessary, additional sutures secure the graft's attachment to the skull base.

TUMOR REMOVAL

Two principle approaches are feasible to begin tumor removal: (1) detach the tumor from its vascularization and dural matrix by dissecting the dural plane and then debulk the tumor safely without further blood loss or (2) enter the tumor directly and debulk before entering into the tumor–brain plane. Both approaches have their merits: we prefer initial dural detachment because the tumor can be rendered bloodless without increasing the compression of the surrounding structures. A narrow window is formed along the dural plane that devascularizes the tumor and makes it movable to a certain degree. Then, the interface of the tumor with the brain can be seen by gentle pulling of the tumor and continuous stepwise resection. With smaller lesions, the tumor can be extracted in toto at this time. The surgeon has to be aware that the arteries are pushed upward and are seen at a late stage of preparation. The contralateral olfactory nerve is the last structure to be identified along the frontal skull base clearly and often has a dense subarachnoid layer that should be preserved.

The alternative technique to initial devascularization is debulking, which was introduced as early as 1938 in the classic monograph by Cushing and Eisenhardt.[1] However, even central decompression rarely leads to shrinking of the tumor because these are usually rather stiff and attached to the surrounding brain. The preparation should aim to preserve the olfactory nerves and A2 segments. Therefore, these structures should be visualized as early as possible. Before approaching the dural matrix of the tumor, the olfactory nerve should be freed of the surrounding arachnoid scarring, which is easier from a lateral approach. Piecemeal

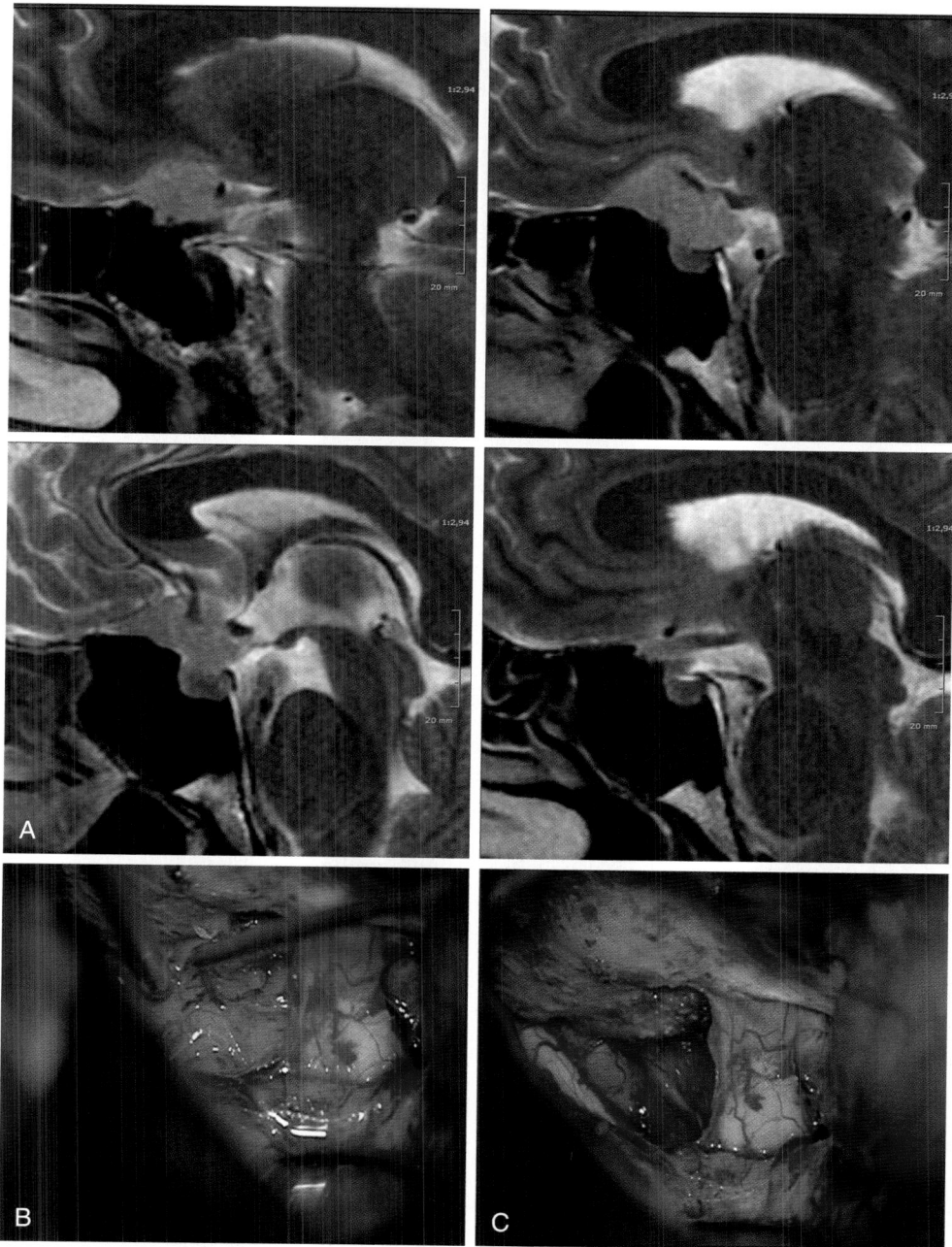

FIGURE 34-7 Tuberculum sellae meningioma: A, Sagittal T2-weighted MRI depicting the location and involvement of surrounding structures. B, A frontolateral right-sided craniotomy was performed, and a paramedian approach was chosen. After removal of the anterior skull base portion of the tumor, the reminder is gently pulled downward anteriorly. This is possible because there are only limited attachments to the medial and vascular structures. C, The tumor is removed, and the dura is coagulated and partially removed. The view from the anterior and lateral to the optic nerve, including the use of micromirrors, demonstrates complete macroscopic removal.

preparation might be necessary to maintain olfactory nerve integrity because this nerve is particularly vulnerable to bipolar cauterization and inadvertent suctioning. We prefer to protect the nerve with a nonadherent covering such as Bicol collagen sponges rather than using a Cottonoid. If the optic nerves are reached by the tumor, dissection should proceed in an arachnoid plane, which can be of varying thickness and clarity. If a thin layer of tumor is approaching the optic nerves and seems to enter the middle cranial fossa, careful inspection of this side using a bayonet mirror

or an endoscope should facilitate visualization of all tumor compartments and their removal using curettes and coagulation of the remaining matrix using an angled bipolar cautery.

Arteries are frequently embedded within thickened arachnoid layers of the tumor capsule. It is necessary to continuously reevaluate the correct plane of dissection because tumor feeding arteries are difficult to differentiate from frontal lobe branches. When the surgeon is in doubt, every vessel is prepared with its arachnoid covering.

Table 34-1 Results of Surgical Resection in Recent Series of Olfactory Groove Meningiomas*

Authors (Year)	Approach	Cases	Mean Size (Range)	Complete Resection	Anosmia/ Dysosmia Pre- > Postop	Mental Status Pre- > Postop	Vision/Visual Field Deficits/ Double Vision Pre- > Postop	Recurrence	Follow-Up Median (Range)
			(cm)	(%)	(%)	(%)	(%)	(%)	(time)
Mayfrank and Gilsbach (1996)[16]	Interhemispheric	18	1.5-7.0	100		NA	NA	NA	NA
Paterniti et al. (1999)[17]	Pterional	20	NA	100		NA	NA	0	1-21 yr
Tsikoudas and Martin-Hirsch (1999)[18]	Bifrontal	13	NA	NA		NA	NA	4	NA
Turazzi et al. (1999)[19]	Pterional	37	NA	100		100	100	0	4 yr (1-8)
Zevgaridis et al. (2001)[20]	Frontal	5	6.7 (5.5-8)	100		NA	80	NA	5 yr (2-8)
Hentschel and DeMonte (2003)[21]	Bifrontal, biorbital	13	5.6 (3.5-8)	85		85	83	0	2 yr (0-5)
Nakamura et al. (2007)[13]		82						5	63 mo
Romani et al. (2009)[22]	Lateral supraorbital	66		91				6	45 mo (2-128)
Present series 2011	Bifrontal, subfrontal, one sided	64	3.9	94	64 > 45	13 > 6	35 > 13	3	7 yr (1-16)

*Updated from Hentschel and DeMonte 2003.[21]
NA, not applicable.

Tuberculum sellae meningiomas that push the optic structures upward and do not extend anteriorly can be approached from a pterional craniotomy. Tuberculum sellae meningiomas extending anteriorly and pushing the optic nerves laterally should be considered for a modified frontal approach (Fig. 34-7). If the carotid artery is engulfed and the medial sphenoid wing or the cavernous sinus is involved, any combined approach that includes a pterional opening is recommended.

Olfactory groove meningiomas most frequently underwent radical removal (Simpson grade I and II in more than 94%), which was reflected in only two recurrences (3%) compared to 14% of recurrences/residual tumors for all intracranial meningiomas, in our series (Table 34-1).

SURGICAL MORBIDITY

Postoperative complications were significantly associated with tumor volume. The sense of smell improved in 10.3% of patients, and 25% worsened upon initial follow-up, although the olfactory nerves were only rarely severed macroscopically. The symptoms that were most likely to improve were associated with massive space-occupying lesions or massive surrounding edema; neuropsychologic symptoms and severe psychiatric symptoms improved for most patients. Also, symptomatic hemiparesis and motor dysphasia improved frequently. One patient suffered from extensive postoperative edema and peritumoral contusions displaying a significant thrombopathy and needed osteoclastic decompression. The most frequent postoperative nonneurologic morbidity was symptomatic deep venous leg thrombosis in 6% of cases, which in 3% was associated with pulmonary embolism despite routine postoperative antithrombotic treatment.

Surgical Outcome and Conclusions

Meningiomas of the anterior midline skull base have an excellent outcome compared to all other skull base meningiomas. They rarely recur, and the patients benefit from the removal of the space-occupying lesion.

Small tumors may be observed, whereas tumors with significant peritumoral edema or of large size should be removed. Rostral tumors should be exposed with an adequately sized craniotomy, whereas more dorsal tumors can easily be operated on using a unilateral approach. Recurring meningiomas are amendable to repeated surgical intervention. Stereotactic radiation represents an alternative to small residues or recurrences.

KEY REFERENCES

Al-Mefty O. Surgical technique for the juxtasellar area. In: Al-Mefty O, ed. *Surgery of the Cranial Base (Foundations of Neurological Surgery, 2 ed.).* Boston: Kluwer Academic Publishers; 2010:73-89.

Bakay L. Olfactory meningiomas. The missed diagnosis. *JAMA.* 1984;251:53-55.

Bendszus M, Monoranu CM, Schutz A, et al. Neurologic complications after particle embolization of intracranial meningiomas. *AJNR Am J Neuroradiol.* 2005;26:1413-1419.

Carli DF, Sluzewski M, Beute GN, et al. Complications of particle embolization of meningiomas: frequency, risk factors, and outcome. *AJNR Am J Neuroradiol.* 2010;31:152-154.

Cushing H, Eisenhardt L. *Meningiomas, Their Classification, Regional Behaviour, Life History and Surgical End Results.* Springfield, Illinois: Charles C. Thomas; 1938.

Hassler W, Zentner J. Pterional approach for surgical treatment of olfactory groove meningiomas. *Neurosurgery*. 1989;25:942-945.

Kallmes DF, Evans AJ, Kaptain GJ, et al. Hemorrhagic complications in embolization of a meningioma: case report and review of the literature. *Neuroradiology*. 1997;39:877-880.

Nakamura M, Struck M, Roser F, et al. Olfactory groove meningiomas: clinical outcome and recurrence rates after tumor removal through the frontolateral and bifrontal approach. *Neurosurgery*. 2007;60: 844-852.

Ransohoff J, Nockels RP. Olfactory groove and planum meningiomas. In: Apuzzo MLJ, ed. *Brain Surgery Complication Avoidance and Management*. New York: Churchill Livingstone; 1993:203-219.

Wakhloo AK, Juengling FD, Van Velthoven V, et al. Extended preoperative polyvinyl alcohol microembolization of intracranial meningiomas: assessment of two embolization techniques. *AJNR Am J Neuroradiol*. 1993;14:571-582.

Numbered references appear on Expert Consult.

CHAPTER 35

Supraorbital Approach Variants for Intracranial Tumors

RODRIGO RAMOS-ZÚÑIGA • SHAAN M. RAZA • ALFREDO QUIÑONES-HINOJOSA

The fundamental basis of "keyhole" neurosurgery lies in the fact that, if designed and tailored to the lesions, deep lesions can be approached via smaller incisions and craniotomies providing essentially the same anatomic visualization as the larger, more traditional cranial base approaches. The supraorbital craniotomy is the prime example of this trend in neurosurgery. With increased emphasis on maximizing cosmetic outcomes, minimizing tissue morbidity and reducing hospitalization stays, there is now increased importance in understanding minimally invasive approaches (i.e., supraorbital craniotomy, keyhole craniotomies in general, and endoscopic endonasal approaches).

Paramount to the success of these approaches is a thorough understanding of the anatomy, as they can be difficult for novice surgeons who do not have a solid grasp of microsurgical corridors and cranial base anatomy/compartments. Anatomically relevant is the orbital bone, since it forms the roof of the orbital cavity and a strategic part of the anterior floor of the skull base. The orbital ridge intersects with the zygomatic bone laterally and the ethmoid medially; the orbit is further contiguous with the anterior fossa and sphenoid bone. Consequently, it is an anatomic structure that is intimately associated with the orbital cavity and its structures, as well as with the intracranial region.[1-5]

The supraorbital craniotomy and its variants essentially provide a combined subfrontal–anterolateral microsurgical approach. Anatomic structures such as the anterior clinoid, sphenoidal plane, and sellar region are keys to this corridor extending toward the region of the sylvian fissure. Therefore, these anatomic structures are critical in planning any microsurgical trajectory to the anterior fossa floor, the middle fossa, the smaller wing of the sphenoid, and the sellar/parasellar region.[1,6,7]

Previous anatomic studies have critically evaluated anatomic corridors in this region and their utility in treating a variety of neurologic lesions; these studies have subsequently resulted in potential surgical alternatives. Such historical and fundamental contributions have been made by Durante, Krause, Frazier, Cushing, Heuer, Dandy, Yasargil, Brock and Dietz, Al-Mefty, Zabramski, and Perneczky. Although the supraorbital approach is not a new strategy (initially described by Frazier with his epidural approach described in 1913[8]), technological innovations have enhanced its applicability. The introduction of new tools (e.g., endoscopy) and new approaches (i.e., orbital ridge osteotomy) has improved access to and visualization of cranial base lesions. Ultimately, neurosurgical and technological innovations have aimed to reduce morbidity under the concept of minimally invasive neurosurgery.[9,10]

Orbital Anatomy

It is important to consider the orbital region as an anatomic compartment bound superiorly by the frontal bone, medially forming a close angle with the ethmoid bone, lacrimal bone, and lacrimal fossa. In addition, there are connections to the nasal region.[11-14]

In the inferior medial region we find the adjacent palatine bone and in the lower border the maxillary bone, where the infraorbital foramen is located. Going towards the midlateral inferior region, we find the area of the zygomatic bone which in turn extends through the zygomatic arch towards the posterolateral aspect, and going in an anterolateral location we find the facial zygomatic foramina. In the internal cavity of the orbital region the origin of the great wing of the sphenoid in its posterolateral portion is found—giving way to a virtual space between the small wing and the great wing of the sphenoid, known as the superior orbital fissure. Adjacent to the posterior medial portion are the optic canal located inferiorly and the inferior orbital fissure.[2,15]

The ethmoid bone represents a complicated component of the craniofacial skeleton with several critical components. Medially, the ethmoid presents a lamina to the nasal cavity while superiorly it presents the cribriform plate. In addition, the ethmoid bone articulates with the sphenoid bone and sphenoid sinus along several surfaces posteriorly and inferiorly. Furthermore, a majority of the volume of the ethmoid bone consists of trabeculated air spaces creating the ethmoid air cells.

The posterosuperior orbital cone is made of the superior margin of the orbital fissure and the extension of the small wing of the sphenoid. The intracavitary foramina are the lacrimal foramen, the optic canal, the superior orbital fissure, the inferior orbital fissure, and in the extracavitary portion we find the notch or foramen for the infraorbital nerve and the orbital zygomatic foramen (Fig. 35-1).[12]

The optic canal and the anterior clinoid process are closely located and associated with the origin of the small wing of the sphenoid bone; the superior orbital fissure is divided by a bone strut (optic strut) supporting the anterior clinoid process. The most important structures involved in this region looking above (from the intracranial frontal floor perspective) are the anterolateral floor or the platform and the orbital arch. Toward the anterior medial portion, the crista galli and the cribriform plate of the ethmoid bone are found. The sphenoid plane and the wing of the sphenoid that meets the optic foramen are located in the deep plane (Fig. 35-2).[16,17]

The anatomic intraorbital structures are basically represented by the extraocular muscles, predominantly the rectal and medial and lateralis muscles, such as the levator muscle for eye movement. We also find the periorbital fat or periorbit and the globe itself, the optic nerve, and other nerve structures from the ophthalmic branch of the trigeminal nerve, such as the frontal, nasociliary, and lacrimal nerves. The rest of the ocular motor nerves—III, IV, and VI—converge in a particular anatomic site after passing through the cavernous sinus (Fig 35-3).[16]

The most important arterial structures are the ophthalmic artery, its variants in the lacrimal artery and its connections to the ciliary artery, and the central retinal artery, whose venous return flows through the ophthalmic vein. The anterior ethmoidal artery is a significant vessel in the anteromedial region. It is closely related with the nasolacrimal region and the irrigation of the nasal mucosa, frequently managed in surgical procedures to control nose bleeds.[11,14,18-22]

This specific anatomy gives way to the possibility of removing the orbital roof to have wide access to all the orbital area and ocular contents, nerve structures, muscles and vessels,

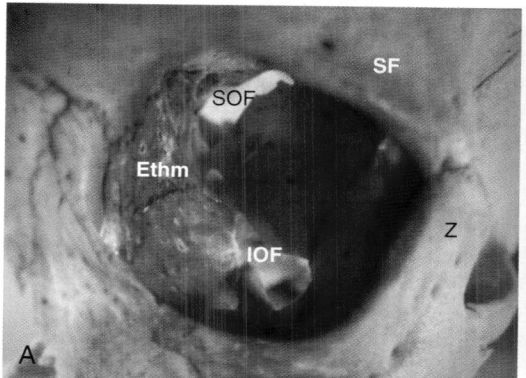
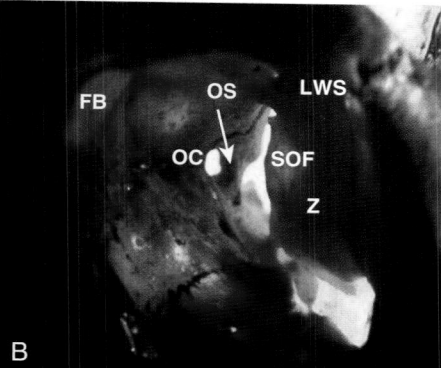

FIGURE 35-1 A and B, Overview of orbital anatomy. Ethm, ethmoidal bone; SF, supraorbital foramen; SOF, superior orbital fissure; IOF, inferior orbital fissure; GWS, greater wing of sphenoid; LWS, lesser wing of sphenoid; FB, frontal bone; OC, optic canal; OS, optic strut.

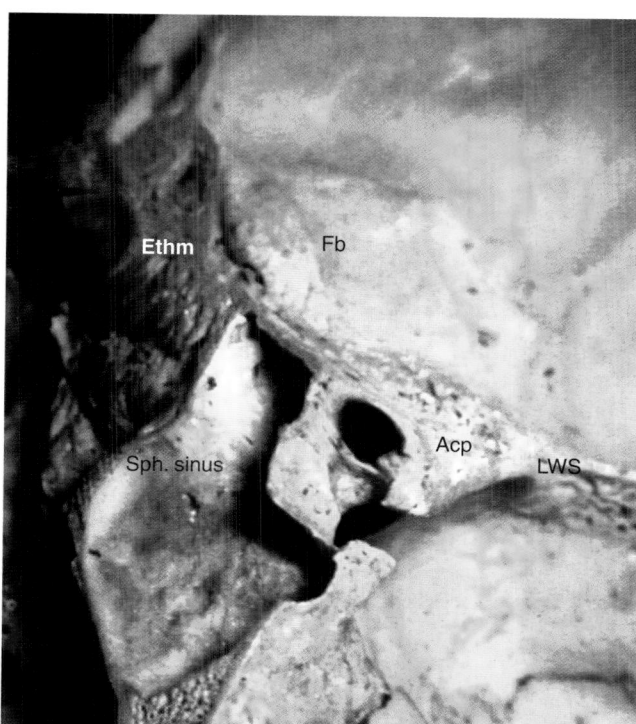

FIGURE 35-2 Sagital cut of skull and right side view. Ethm, ethmoidal bone; Fb, frontal bone; Sph sinus, sphenoidal sinus; Acp, anterior clinoid process; LWS, lesser wing of sphenoid.

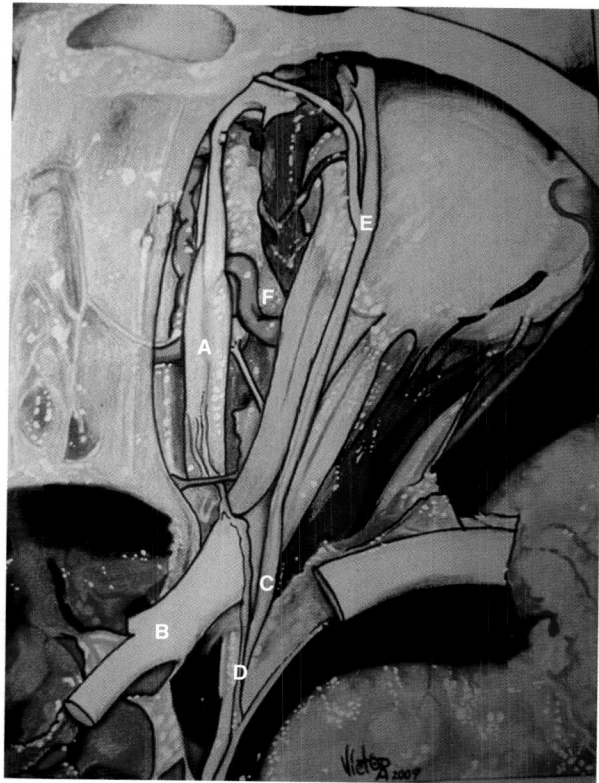

FIGURE 35-3 Overview of intraorbital anatomy. A, Superior oblique muscle. B, Optic nerve. C, Trochlear nerve. D, Oculomotor nerve. E, Supraorbital nerve. F, Ophtalmic artery. (Victor © 2009.)

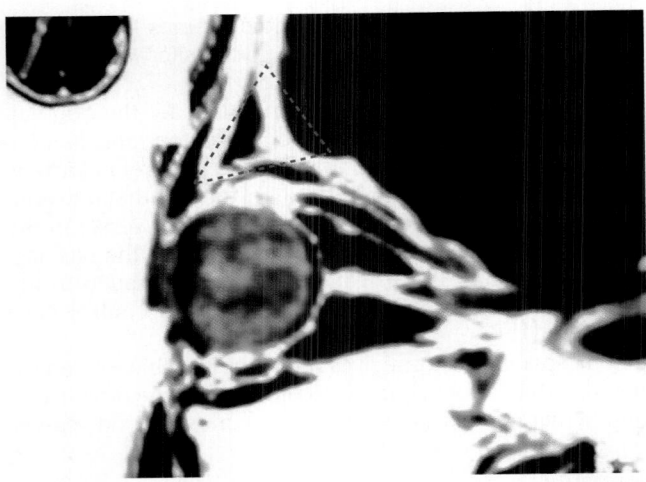

FIGURE 35-4 Operative corridor to deeper lesions via supraorbital approach.

and additionally have an intracranial access. An important anatomic structure from the surgical perspective is the lacrimal gland, located in the superior external area of the orbit. This is a region that can be compromised when using a surgical approach where the orbital roof is removed.[12]

From the surgical perspective as well, it is important to emphasize the orbital surgical triangle, represented by a geometric figure that, from its lateral projection, the base is the anterior part of the frontal bone and the orbital arch, the upper part is outlined by the base of the frontal lobe, and the inferior part is outlined by the periorbit.[13] This triangle, with an anterior base and a posterior vertex may offer several options for deep resection (also representing the angle of bone removal described in the trans-supraorbital approach; Fig. 35-4).[5,23]

Experimental Analysis of the Supraorbital Approach in Cadavers

A series of cadaver specimens were studied in order to assess the variations described for the supraorbital craniotomy in order to evaluate the extent of surgical access in identifying different anatomic landmarks. The conventional supraorbital keyhole approach was used to examine the optic nerve, ipsilateral anterior clinoid, sphenoidal plane, and the dorsum sellae. This approach, compared with the trans-supraorbital approach, showed some benefit with regard to accessibility and visualization.[24-28]

Subsequently, possible variants of this approach were analyzed in another experimental cadaveric study. In a series of 15 adult skulls, the differences between anatomic targets and the space around the sellar region were evaluated for these variants. Access to the following regions was assessed: the anterior clinoid process (ipsilateral), the chiasmatic sulcus, the optic canal, the center point of the sella turcica, and the dorsum sellae. Table 35-1 presents measurements for the classical supraorbital approach versus the supraorbital craniotomy combined with removal of the orbital arch.

Recognizing that the approach can be tailored, the craniotomy can be extended in different anatomic directions specific to the target pathology/region. For example, the supraorbital nerve can be mobilized in order to create a craniotomy more towards the midline. This modified approach facilitates a more comfortable and direct route to the prechiasmatic region, as well as other structures such as the crista galli, ethmoid lamina, olfactory bulb, sphenoidal plane, and anterior clinoid.[10,27-32]

On the other hand, lateral extension, as with the supraorbital-pterional approach, permits greater pterional access. This modification permits greater access to the lateral targets in the frontotemporal neurosurgical corridor and their neurovascular structures.[10,27,32]

Finally, if the principles of minimally invasive surgery and skull base surgery are combined, using the supraciliary incision, it is possible to remove the orbital arch in a block in the medial and lateral portion which provides an average of 1.5 cm more space to work in the craniotomy site, according to the anatomic studies of the trans-supraorbital approach.[22,33]

All of these variations of the supraorbital approach provide greater versatility and several possible adaptations to meet the surgical goal under the concept of supraselective craniotomy, which is the fundamental basis of the "keyhole" craniotomy. There are four basic variants of the supraorbital approach (Fig. 35-5):

1. Supraorbital medial
2. Supraorbital anterolateral (classical)
3. Supraorbital pterional
4. Trans-supraorbital

Intracranial Surgical Access and its Variants

The development of finer, more accurate, and angled instruments has been critical for success of the supraorbital approach and its variants. Likewise, a major breakthrough was the use of the surgical microscope complemented with endoscopy-assisted microneurosurgery. The concept of keyhole microsurgery set forth by Perneczky was based

Table 35-1	Volumetric Comparison of Exposure of Critical Structures (Mean ± Standard Deviation)				
Technique	Anterior Clinoid Process Ipsilateral	Chiasmatic Sulcus	Optic Canal	Pituitary Fossa	Dorsum Sellae
Classical supraorbital approach	5.57 ± 0.06	5.5 ± 0.09	5 ± 0.09	6.5 ± 0.09	6.97 ± 0.08
Supraorbital craniotomy with orbital ridge osteotomy	4.5 ± 0.09	4.5 ± 0.09	4 ± 0.12	5.4 ± 0.09	6 ± 0.12

on this new technology that contributed to providing several new options. Although seemingly contradictory, keyhole cranial base surgery advocates maximal resection through the use of current surgical technology and methodology taking into consideration the patient's condition and pathology. Thus, variations in the orbital approach itself have led to improved extension and use in various surgical spaces granting access to the most important accessible structures.[27,32-39]

Synonymous with the development of keyhole surgery has been the increasing acceptance of using smaller incisions, such as the eyebrow incision. The use of smaller incisions can have cosmetic, functional, and even psychological benefits for the patient. However, this fact should not limit the final surgical plan in view of the surgical goal. For example, a displaced frontal scalp flap/craniotomy can also be chosen to apply the principle of selective craniotomy. In other words, minimally invasive surgery does not simply mean a minimal incision or minicraniotomy; instead, the goal is to spare craniofacial and neurovascular structures using a tailored approach as broad as necessary and as selective as experience allows, with every possible manipulation of a conventional procedure.[36,40-48]

For example, disadvantages of the brow approach can include frontalis weakness that occurs as a result of damage to the frontal branch of the facial nerve or the potential posterior alopecia of the eyebrow. Another advantage of this approach is preservation of the temporalis muscle in comparison to other antero-lateral based approaches (i.e., pterional). Even with lateral extension of this approach, the soft tissue dissection only involves minimal mobilization of the superior and anterior most aspect of the temporalis—in this process the deep neurovascular supply is preserved.[40,47]

In order to truly benefit from minimally invasive strategies, cases must be carefully selected, upon consideration of the surgical objective, the patient's individual anatomic variations, and the experience and comfort level of the surgical team. This strategy allows proper evaluation and ultimately helps the surgeon to identify the most adequate and beneficial approach for the patient.

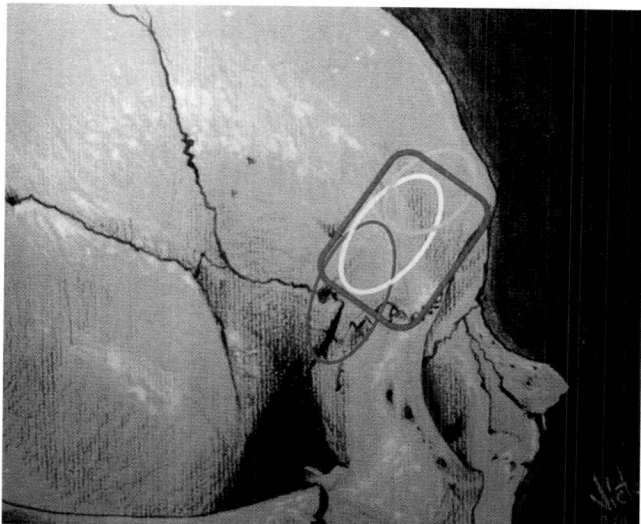

FIGURE 35-5 Supraorbital approach and its variants. *(Victor © 2009.)*

PATIENT POSITIONING

One of the most significant factors in supraselective approaches is patient positioning as part of the operative plan. It is crucial to consider not only the surgical plan, but also the general and neurovascular anatomy of the patient. The effect of gravity and potential brain shift as a result of positioning may provide patient benefits by creating comfortable and wide access.[11,45]

Consequently, is important to consider not only elevating the head above the chest in every case to facilitate the venous return but also retroflexing and rotating the head according to the surgical plan.[46,49] One of the goals is to have a three-dimensional view that gives full access to the surgical target with the least possible retraction, considering the conventional anatomic spaces promoted by cisternal drainage and subarachnoid dissection—fundamental microsurgical principles.[24]

SUPRAORBITAL VARIANTS

Basic Access through the Eyebrow

Meticulous planning places the incision lateral to the supraorbital foramen extending to the area of the fronto-zygomatic suture. The skin flaps are retracted with elastic holding sutures. After exposing the muscles of the area, the frontalis muscle is sectioned sharply parallel to the orbital rim after which dissection of the orbicularis and the fronto-temporal insertion of the temporalis muscle are also completed. Subsequently, the burr hole is made with high-speed drill, inferiorly to the temporal line, and use any of the variants described in the following.[36,41,50]

Medial Supraorbital Approach

In selected cases, this approach basically provides access to the subfrontal region, the medial gyrus rectus, the anterior interhemispheric portion, and medial bone annexa such as the cribriform region, olfactory sulcus, and nasolacrimal region.[11,15,21,24] This corridor gives access to several tumors in this area, including the basal interhemispheric region, the genu and rostrum of the corpus callosum, and the proximal pericallosal space. Direct access to the cribriform basal region and the olfactory nerves is provided (crista galli, olfactory groove, planum sphenoidale, tuberculum sellae, lamina terminalis, anterior third ventricle, pituitary stalk, anterior communicating artery, and dorsum sellae).[8,16,21,28,44,46,49-54]

An inconvenience of this approach is the decision to plan entry into the frontal sinus (unless the frontal sinus is reduced in size) and the potential external mobilization of the supraorbital nerve to obtain a totally medial access. Infection and fistula from the frontal sinus access should be seriously considered as risk factors for this procedure. Nevertheless, when closure of the dura is meticulous and careful, the frontal sinus is cleaned thoroughly, and specific antibiotics are used, the procedure can be done without any problem (Fig. 35-6).[14,24,45,53]

Classic Supraorbital Approach (Laterobasal)

The classic supraorbital approach—also called the fronto-lateral-basal approach—is the classic technique described by Perneczky. From this supraorbito-lateral corner, access is obtained to the frontobasal region, sylvian fissure, and

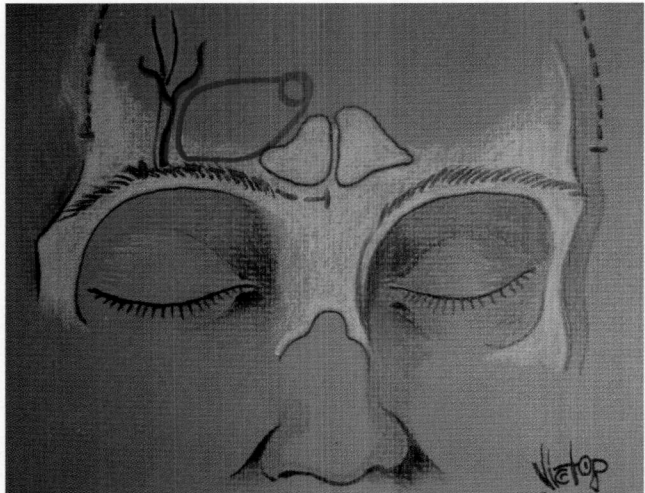

FIGURE 35-6 Relationship of frontal sinus to craniotomy. *(Victor © 2009.)*

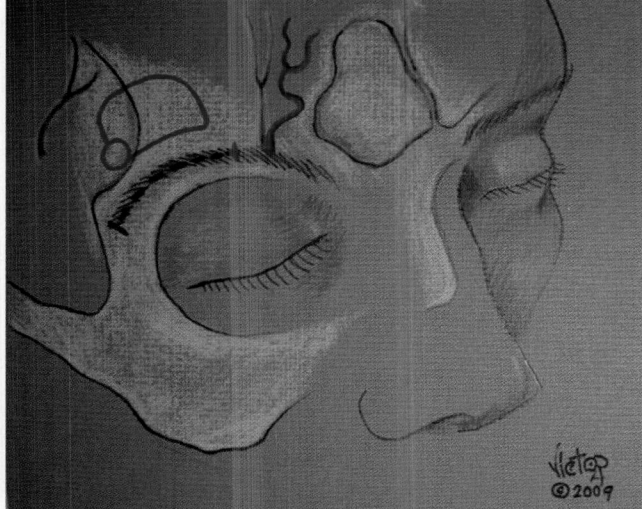

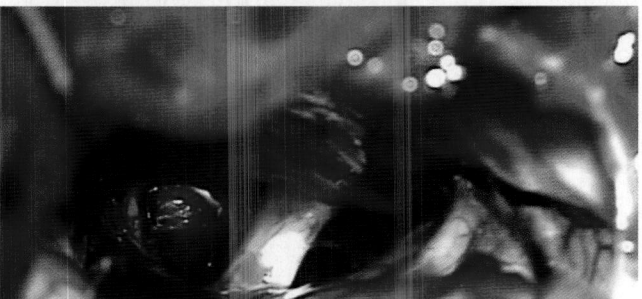

FIGURE 35-7 Right supraorbital approach surgical view after excision of pituitary adenoma in prechiasmatic region and optic-carotid cistern. *(Victor © 2009.)*

mesial temporal lobe. This approach provides such anatomic access due to the fundamental microsurgical principle of cerebrospinal fluid drainage via opening cisterns.[10,35]

This approach provides access to: the orbital roof, anterior clinoid process, posterior clinoid process, the roof and lateral wall of the cavernous sinus, the basal portion of the frontal lobe, gyrus rectus, sylvian fissure, temporal lobe, uncus, hippocampus, and cranial nerves of all this neurovascular corridor including CN1, CNII, CNIII, and CNIV; and extensions of the internal carotid artery, middle cerebral artery, and posterior cerebral artery in their proximal segments (ICA, Opht A, PCoA, AChA; perforators A1, A2, Mi, M2, P1, P2, SCA; and temporal vein) (Fig. 35-7).[10,12,21,51-53,55]

Supraorbito-Pterional Approach

This keyhole approach was created to achieve the angle of vision and advantages of the classic pterional approach. This surgical approach is based on the anatomic location of the sphenoid ridge and its relationship with the sylvian fissure and basal cisterns. The initial incision is made over the hairline behind the external border of the eye on the selected side, because the cosmetic outcome is better compared with an eyebrow incision. A skin and muscular flap is reflected anteriorly, and a small 3 × 3–cm craniotomy is completed around the external landmarks of the sphenoid ridge. Further extradural drilling is completed down to the anterior clinoid process. The dura is opened in a semilunar manner, and the sylvian fissure is opened completely to reach the sylvian and basal cisterns. Of course, if we consider that the actual microsurgical space is 20 mm, this approach gives the same benefits as the conventional pterional approach and the benefits of the access through the trans-sylvian corridor, for a well-outlined craniotomy at the usual extension of the dural opening (Fig. 35-8).[56]

Trans-Supraorbital Approach

With the conventional technique, a 3-cm incision is made through the eyebrow between the median line of the pupil and the external rim of the zygomatic-orbital joint.[25,26] In selected cases, the approach can be made through a fronto-temporal skin incision close to the hairline, to

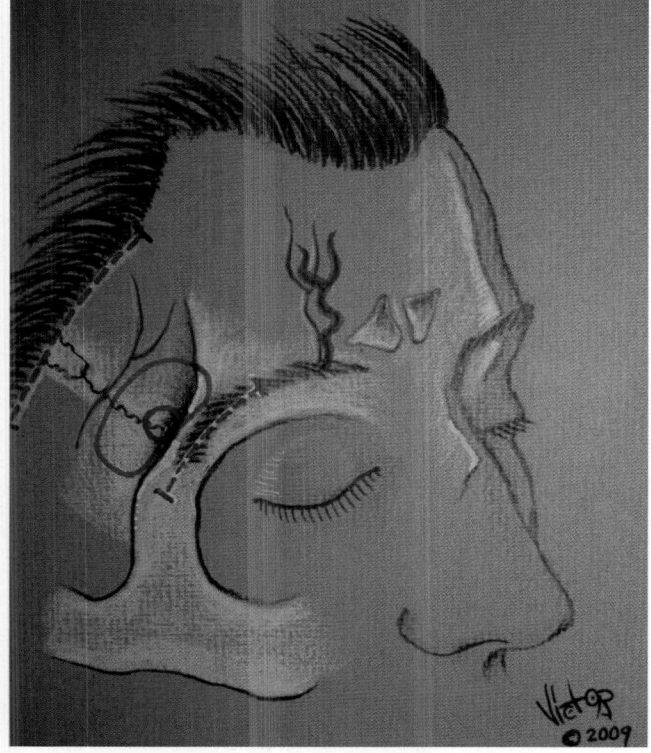

FIGURE 35-8 Supraorbital pterional approach. *(Victor © 2009.)*

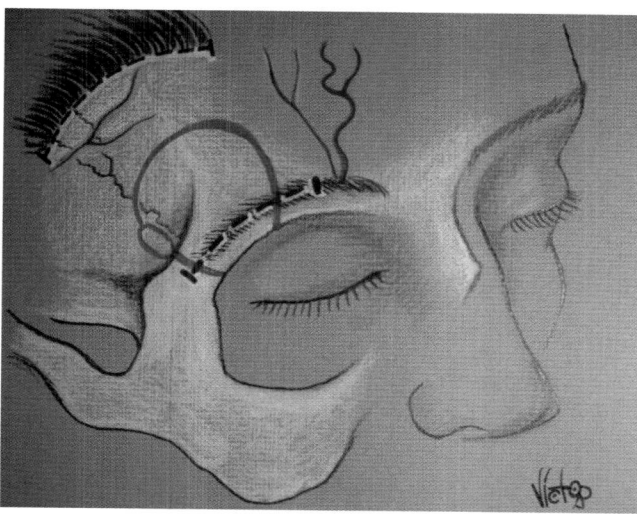

FIGURE 35-9 Trans-supraorbital approach. *(Victor © 2009.)*

prevent scarring in the eyebrow or a cosmetic compromise from weakness in the frontal branch of the facial nerve. After incision, the orbicularis muscle is dissected. Once the tissues are mobilized with elastic retraction, an en-bloc craniotomy is performed with the following borders: median line–supraorbital foramen; external line–the zygomatic-orbital joint; and in the lower border–the orbital arch and 1-cm extension into the depth of the orbital roof until the intracranial portion is found. An en-bloc resection is made at the superior margin of the frontal 1.5-cm craniotomy, after removing the periosteum and protecting the orbital fat. The orbital bone is drilled with different boundaries and choices according to the surgical target. This procedure allows us to work in the intraorbital space, the intracranial–extradural space, and the intracranial–subarachnoid space.[25,26]

Once the drilling of the inner edges of the craniotomy is completed, the dura mater is opened under the microscope and the appropriate microsurgical corridor is dissected. The trans-supraorbital approach provides access to the entire sellar region and its neurovascular structures, providing enough space for surgical manipulation in cases of pituitary tumors with extrasellar extension to the optic chiasm. In selected cases, endoscopy has been used[39-49] (Aesculap, Ventriculoscope, Tuttlingen, Germany, 0 and 30 degrees) to confirm patency of neighboring arteries, explore the intrasellar space and cavernous extension of the tumor, and finally, evaluate the pituitary stalk and sellar diaphragm (Fig. 35-9).[3,4,25,26,33,39,57]

Benefits and Limitations

One of the main advantages of the minimally invasive concept used in neurosurgery is that it involves a strategy that preserves the anatomic integrity of all structures, insofar as is possible, using a supraselective tailored approach. The latter should correlate specifically with the surgical target.[3,4,25-28,33,50] Therefore, the approach does not entail a reductionist or minimalist vision, but rather one based on experience to find the proper balance in the design and size of the craniotomy aimed at achieving the surgical goal

without subjecting the patient to unnecessary risk from tissue manipulation.

A practical example is shown by the historical progression from initially using large craniotomies to clip elective aneurysms to current use of tailored approaches. This progression is based on two basic principles. First, considering that microsurgery involves a 20-mm work space, it was concluded that resorting to greater exposure with the craniotomy was not strictly necessary (the evolution of a wide frontotemporal craniotomy to the pterional craniotomy). Second is inclusion anatomic integrity in the surgical plan, not only of cerebral structures with less retraction and manipulation, but also to preserve the craniofacial structures as well (avoiding atrophy of the temporal muscle, temporomandibular dysfunction, bone defects, fistula, flap necrosis, etc.).[5,10,36,47,48,58]

Thus, minimally invasive neurosurgery is not a discipline but a neurosurgical concept that may result in less morbidity due to the rational use and support of technology as part of the armamentarium and current multidisciplinary options used for the patient's benefit.[38] That is the reason why serious complications can result with a limited understanding of the principles of minimally invasive approaches and an overuse of technological support. Critical analysis of surgical experience accumulated thus far has demonstrated that major complications with minimally invasive approaches can occur if microsurgical principles are not properly followed. The key is to maintain a proper balance between overexposure and limited/reduced exposure. A crucial principle to obtain optimal outcome is that the selected approach must always allow performance of possible and necessary procedures, with conventional technology as support to facilitate the desired surgical goal with comfort and safety. Therefore, it is about correct planning—taking into account the patient's specific anatomy and disease as well as variables related to the availability and pertinent use of certain technologies, and finally the skills and ability of the neurosurgical team.

ACKNOWLEDGMENT

In memory of Axel Perneczky.

KEY REFERENCES

Brock M, Dietz H. The small frontolateral approach for the microsurgical treatment of intracranial aneurysms. *Neurochirurgia (Stuttg).* 1978;21:185-191.

Cohen AR, Perneczky A, Rodziewicz GS, Gingold SI. Endoscope-assisted craniotomy: approach to the rostral brain stem. *Neurosurgery.* 1995;36:1128-1129:discussion 1129-1130.

Davies HT, Neil-Dwyer G, Evans BT, Lees PD. The zygomatico-temporal approach to the skull base: a critical review of 11 patients. *Br J Neurosurg.* 1992;6:305-312.

Delashaw Jr JB, Tedeschi H, Rhoton AL. Modified supraorbital craniotomy: technical note. *Neurosurgery.* 1992;30:954-956.

Delfini R, Raco A, Artico M, et al. A two-step supraorbital approach to lesions of the orbital apex. Technical note. *J Neurosurg.* 1992;77:959-961.

Jane JA, Park TS, Pobereskin LH, et al. The supraorbital approach: technical note. *Neurosurgery.* 1982;11:537-542.

Jho HD. Orbital roof craniotomy via an eyebrow incision: a simplified anterior skull base approach. *Minim Invasive Neurosurg.* 1997;40: 91-97.

Noguchi A, Balasingam V, McMenomey SO, Delashaw Jr JB. Supraorbital craniotomy for parasellar lesions. Technical note. *J Neurosurg.* 2005;102:951-955.

Ramos-Zuniga R. The trans-supraorbital approach. *Minim Invasive Neurosurg.* 1999;42:133-136.

Ramos-Zuniga R, Velazquez H, Barajas MA, et al. Trans-supraorbital approach to supratentorial aneurysms. *Neurosurgery.* 2002;51:125-130: discussion 130-131.

Raza SM, Boahene KD, Quinones-Hinojosa A. The transpalpebral incision: its use in keyhole approaches to cranial base brain tumors. *Expert Rev Neurother.* 2010;10:1629-1632.

Raza SM, Garzon-Muvdi T, Boaehene K, et al. The supraorbital craniotomy for access to the skull base and intraaxial lesions: a technique in evolution. *Minim Invasive Neurosurg.* 2010;53:1-8.

Reisch R, Perneczky A. Ten-year experience with the supraorbital subfrontal approach through an eyebrow skin incision. *Neurosurgery.* 2005;57:242-255:discussion 242-255.

Numbered references appear on Expert Consult.

CHAPTER 36

Surgical Management of Sphenoid Wing Meningiomas

GERARDO GUINTO

Sphenoid wing meningiomas (SWMs) constitute about 14% to 20% of intracranial meningiomas.[1] Although they originate from arachnoid cells, they are usually attached to dural thickening or folding, where they receive their blood supply. Infiltration of the adjacent bone is not unusual; neither is growth around or inside the cranial base foramina.[2] Most SWMs are relatively easy to remove; however, they are sometimes challenging, especially when they invade the cavernous sinus, internal carotid artery (ICA), and visual pathway. In these cases, total excision is extremely difficult, resulting in high morbidity and a high rate of regrowth or recurrence.[3]

Anatomic Observations

The designation SWM refers to tumors that originate in any part of the bony crest formed by wings (lesser and greater) of the sphenoid bone, which represents the boundary between the anterior and the middle cranial floor.[4] This anatomic portion is also known as the sphenoid ridge, where the lesser wing constitutes its internal two thirds and the greater wing its external third. The lesser wing is the most complex area because of its relationship with the orbit, ICA, cavernous sinus, optic foramen, superior orbital fissure, sylvian fissure, middle cerebral artery (MCA), tip of the temporal lobe, and basal surface of the frontal lobe. In contrast, the greater wing is located in the external portion and is in relation to the frontal and temporal lobes (predominantly with their opercular areas) in its intracranial surface and with the orbit and zygomatic fossa in its extracranial surface, where it serves as insertion to the temporal muscle. It also forms the pterion when it articulates with the frontal squama, temporal, and parietal bones.[4]

Classification

In 1938, Cushing and Eisenhardt classified SWMs into two main varieties: en plaque and globoid (Fig. 36-1).

EN-PLAQUE MENINGIOMAS

Also known as spheno-orbital meningiomas or hyperostotic meningiomas of the sphenoid wing, en-plaque meningiomas refer to tumors with a carpet-like dural growth, which are associated with a reactive hyperostosis that, in most cases, is marked and principally responsible for clinical manifestations[5,6] (Fig. 36-1A). Sphenoid

wing hyperostosis has been reported as high as 42% of all meningiomas in this area.[7,8] Due to its extensive bone involvement, differential diagnosis should include fibrous dysplasia, osteoma, osteoblastic metastasis, Paget's disease, hyperostosis frontalis interna, erythroid hyperplasia, and sarcoidosis.[6,9,10] It frequently extends posteriorly toward the cavernous sinus and anteriorly toward the orbital apex, where it causes proptosis and oculomotor deficits, the primary clinical manifestations of these lesions.[5] Hyperostosis in meningiomas was initially described by Brissaud and Lereboullet in 1903.[11] Theories regarding the cause of hyperostosis include vascular disturbances, irritation of bone without actual invasion, previous trauma, bone production by tumor cells, or osteoblastic stimulation of normal bone. Currently, the most widely accepted theory is that this bone growth is actually bone invasion by tumor cells.[3,11,12]

GLOBOID MENINGIOMAS

Globoid meningiomas have traditionally been classified into three groups: (1) deep, inner, or clinoidal; (2) middle or alar; and (3) lateral, outer, or pterional (Fig. 36-1B). Middle or alar meningiomas have radiologic characteristics similar to lateral or pterional meningiomas. Surgical resection and clinical results of both types are almost identical. For this reason, some authors suggest that globoid meningiomas of the sphenoid wing can be classified into only two groups: deep, inner, or clinoidal and lateral, outer, or pterional, discharging the middle or alar variety.[13] Deep, inner, or clinoidal meningiomas represent the most complex variety of these tumors, whose resection, in most cases, implies increased morbidity and a high rate of recurrence.[14-17] In this region, the cavernous sinus is the most critical area; therefore, clinoidal meningiomas are subclassified into two groups: tumors without extradural growth and tumors with extradural growth into the cavernous sinus.[13,18]

There is a third and debatable variety of SWMs. These are tumors that grow within the diploë without an epidural, subdural, or subcutaneous component and are referred to as intraosseous or intradiploic meningiomas.[3,6] The origin of these tumors in the skull base is controversial. Arachnoid cells have been described, following the vessels and nerves in bone foramina or trapped within the sutures. However, some authors[19] doubt the existence of these tumors, proposing that they are really a variety of en-plaque meningiomas

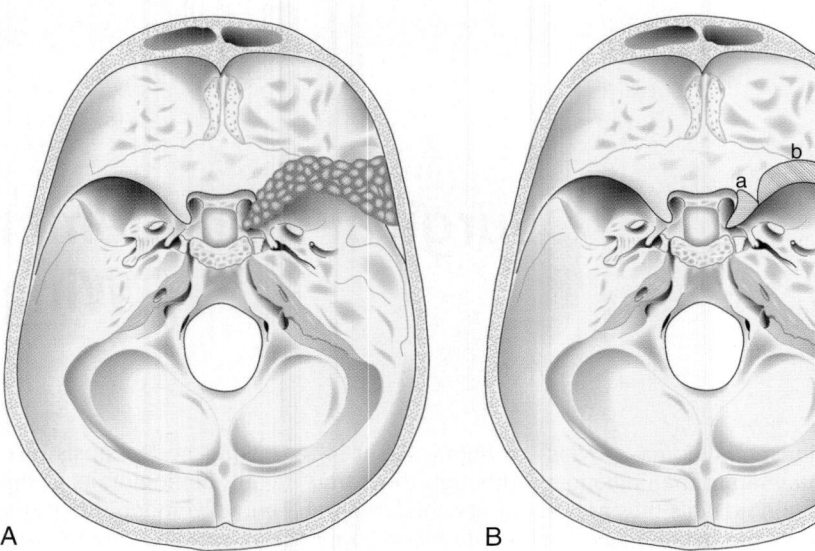

FIGURE 36-1 Classification. A, En plaque. Hyperostosis is the main finding, which is especially located on the sphenoid ridge and the orbital roof. B, Globoid. This variety has been subclassified into three types: (1) deep, inner, or clinoidal; (2) middle or alar; and (3) lateral, outer, or pterional.

in which the dural component of the tumor is not well identified on preoperative imaging studies, mostly considering that many of these tumors were described before the era of magnetic resonance imaging (MRI).

Clinical Course

The most common clinical sign of en-plaque meningiomas is proptosis, which usually is slowly evolving, unilateral, nonpulsatile, and irreducible.[11] Possible causes of this sign are hyperostosis of the orbital walls, periorbital tumor invasion, intraorbital tumor, and venous stasis caused by compression of the ophthalmic veins. Related symptoms include headache, orbital pain, visual deficit, ptosis, diplopia, ectropion, conjunctivitis, corneal ulceration, and scleral hemorrhages. Unilateral loss of vision is rare and is caused by a narrowing of the optic foramen.

In regard to clinoidal meningiomas, clinical manifestations are dominated by visual field problems presenting virtually any pattern. On the other hand, visual acuity deficits are only somewhat variable and are reported in between 39% and 92% of patients.[1,7] When these tumors invade the cavernous sinus, the most common symptoms are oculomotor deficit (especially on cranial nerve VI) and facial hypoesthesia.

Middle or alar meningiomas usually produce late symptoms and, when detected, generally have reached larger dimensions than inner third meningiomas. Clinically, these are characterized by headache and signs or symptoms suggesting increased intracranial pressure, such as nausea, vomiting, and papilledema. Due to frontotemporal compression, it is not uncommon for patients to begin with memory impairment, olfactory hallucinations, personality changes, seizures, and hemiparesis. Finally, pterional meningiomas frequently cause a silent hyperostosis but also may be associated with seizures, headache, intracranial hypertension, hemiparesis, and speech alterations, mostly when located on the dominant side.

Diagnosis

Although clinical manifestations may be strongly suggestive of the diagnosis, especially in spheno-orbital meningiomas, imaging studies are indispensable to establish the diagnosis and to propose the best therapeutic option (Fig. 36-2).

COMPUTED TOMOGRAPHY

Computed tomography (CT) is predominantly useful in en-plaque meningiomas because it provides more precise information regarding the extent of bone invasion, also allowing correct planning for reconstruction (Fig. 36-2A). The dural component of these tumors is typically found as an isodense image with contrast enhancement, being contiguous with the surrounding dura mater.[11] However, it is not always possible to observe this due to its carpet-like appearance. Also, it may be occulted by the high hyperdensity of the contiguous bone growth. There is no correlation between size of the hyperostosis and size of the meningeal tumor. In fact, small dural components are frequently found associated with large bone masses. A bone window algorithm is mandatory in terms of obtaining better definition of bone thickening. Performing axial and coronal projections, as well as three-dimensional (3D) reconstruction, also facilitates both complete resection and reconstruction. The most common locations of hyperostosis of en-plaque meningiomas are, in order of frequency, the lesser wing of the sphenoid bone, the greater wing of the sphenoid, the roof of the orbit, the inferior orbital fissure, the infratemporal fossa, and the orbital rim.

Globoid tumors appear on CT as well-defined isodense lesions that present an intense and homogeneous contrast enhancement. Even though they are usually slow-growing masses, it is not uncommon to find perilesional edema invading the temporal lobe and centrum semiovale, which is attributed to compression or occlusion in the superficial middle cerebral vein or sphenoparietal sinus; there is no direct relationship between the grade of edema and the size of the tumor. Clinoidal meningiomas usually show

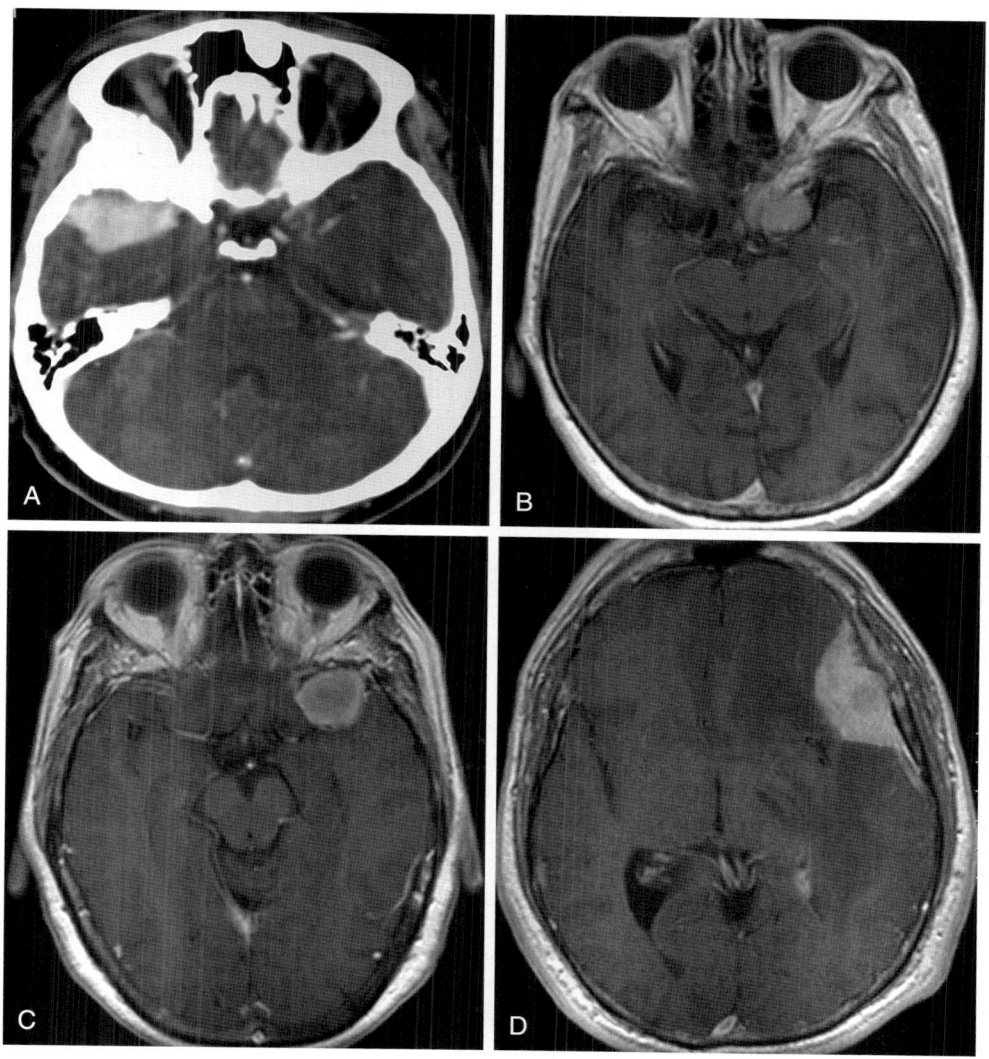

FIGURE 36-2 Radiologic findings. A, Contrast-enhanced CT axial view of a right en-plaque meningioma. Observe the hyperostosis on the entire sphenoid ridge, associated with a small dural component. The figure also shows a contrast-enhanced, T1-weighted axial MRI view of three left globoid SWMs: clinoidal (B), alar (C), and pterional (D).

hyperostosis of the anterior clinoid process (ACP), causing narrowing of the optic canal and the superior orbital fissure.[1] CT has some limitations when these tumors infiltrate the cavernous sinus; however, computed angiotomography (CAT) may help by providing more precise information about blood supply and vascular relations of the tumor.

MAGNETIC RESONANCE IMAGING

MRI is more useful in globoid meningiomas (Fig. 36-2B to D) and for the correct evaluation of the dural component of en-plaque meningiomas; however, this study's principal limitation is the osseous tissue. Globoid meningiomas show different appearances on MRI. When their vascularity is not so marked, they usually present as a homogeneous isointense lesion in both T1- and T2-weighted images;[20] on the other hand, when they are highly vascularized (angioblastic meningiomas), multiple hypointense images ("empty signals") can be seen in the interior of the tumor. Gadolinium enhancement is usually intense and uniform, and a T2-weighted image is particularly useful in demonstrating perilesional edema.

MRI is the ideal study for showing cavernous sinus invasion. MRI spectroscopy helps establish the differential diagnosis with other lesions; tractography, as well as functional MRI,

shows critical cerebral pathways and eloquent areas of the brain, information that is important when dealing with tumors on the dominant hemisphere. Finally, magnetic resonance angiography (MRA) demonstrates the pattern of displacement and permeability of the related neighboring vessels.

ANGIOGRAPHY

Considering the clear image of the vascular anatomy obtained with CAT and MRA, particularly with 3D reconstructions, angiography is indicated only in special SWM cases. Selective catheterization provides specific information about the blood supply of the tumor[1] and allows the possibility of preoperative embolization. Another indication for angiography is for performing carotid occlusion tests, especially in tumors invading the cavernous sinus and when arterial bypass is planned.

Treatment

Surgical management is, without doubt, the best therapeutic option for SWMs. This treatment is indicated considering the following factors: size of the lesion, presence of signs or symptoms, patient's condition, changes in the adjacent cerebral tissue (edema) on imaging studies, and surgeon's experience. In general, surgery is indicated in all patients who are in good health and have a tumor size greater than 2.5 cm. The goal of surgery in all cases should be radical excision of the tumor, which means resection of the lesion, along with the dural implant (1-cm margin) and all hyperostotic bone. This objective is accomplished in the large majority of SWMs except in some spheno-orbital and clinoidal meningiomas, particularly when they present invasion to the cavernous sinus. For these cases, most authors recommend excising the tumor, dura mater, and infiltrated bone on extracavernous areas but leaving the intracavernous portion for another adjuvant treatment, such as radiosurgery, because even in experienced hands, oculomotor morbidity is extremely high after a direct approach to this region.[1,2,4,18,21]

PREPARATION

Patients are operated under intravenous general anesthesia. Antiepileptic drugs, broad-spectrum antibiotics, and glucocorticoids are administrated when beginning the anesthesia. Neurophysiologic monitoring, especially electromyography of the extraocular muscles, is indicated only when the orbit contents, the cavernous sinus, or both will be manipulated.

POSITIONING

The patient is placed in the supine decubitus position with the head fixed in a three-pin headholder with slight extension and rotated toward the contralateral side of the tumor (Fig. 36-3). There are certain variations in this head rotation, depending on the exact location of the meningioma: for clinoidal tumors a lesser rotation (between 30 and 40 degrees) is preferred, whereas for alar and pterional lesions a major rotation (between 40 and 50 degrees) is indicated[2] (Fig. 36-3A and B).

SKIN INCISION

Most SWMs can be operated on through a frontotemporal (pterional) curvilinear skin incision starting at the root of the zygomatic arch, just 5 mm in front of the tragus, which

runs vertically upward. Once it passes the ear, it is curved rostrally and superiorly toward the ipsilateral frontal region until it reaches the midline or beyond, always keeping behind the hairline (Fig. 36-3C). The midportion of the incision can be extended backward, especially in cases of pterional meningiomas with large infiltration of the pterion. If an orbitozygomatic (OZ) approach is required, it is necessary to extend the incision vertically down to the level of the ear lobe.

DISSECTION OF EPICRANIAL PLANES

Beginning this dissection in the preauricular area of the incision is recommended for facilitating early identification of the superficial temporal artery, which must be preserved to maintain vascularity of the myocutaneous flap.[11] In this region, this vessel usually has a posterior branch that has to be coagulated and cut to allow anterior displacement of the main trunk, along with the skin flap. Dissection continues until the temporal fascia is identified in the entire area of the skin incision. It is important not to perform a wide separation between the temporal fascia and the skin flap because, in this manner, injury to the frontotemporal branch of the facial nerve is unavoidable. There are two forms to achieve the preservation of this branch of the facial nerve. The first consists of making the cut in a single plane from skin to bone, including the cut in the skin, temporal fascia, and muscle fibers. In this way, a single fasciomyocutaneous flap is created, which is detached from the bone and displaced forward. This is a simple and safe form to preserve facial function; however, it presents some problems. First, the fasciomyocutaneous flap created in this way is bulky and sometimes interferes with the surgeon's deep vision, especially when dealing with clinoidal tumors. Second, particularly in pterional meningiomas, there are some cases that present tumor infiltration to the temporal muscle that is not seen (and therefore not removed) because the muscle remains attached to the galea. For these reasons, there is another way to accomplish preservation of the facial branch, which consists of sectioning of the two layers

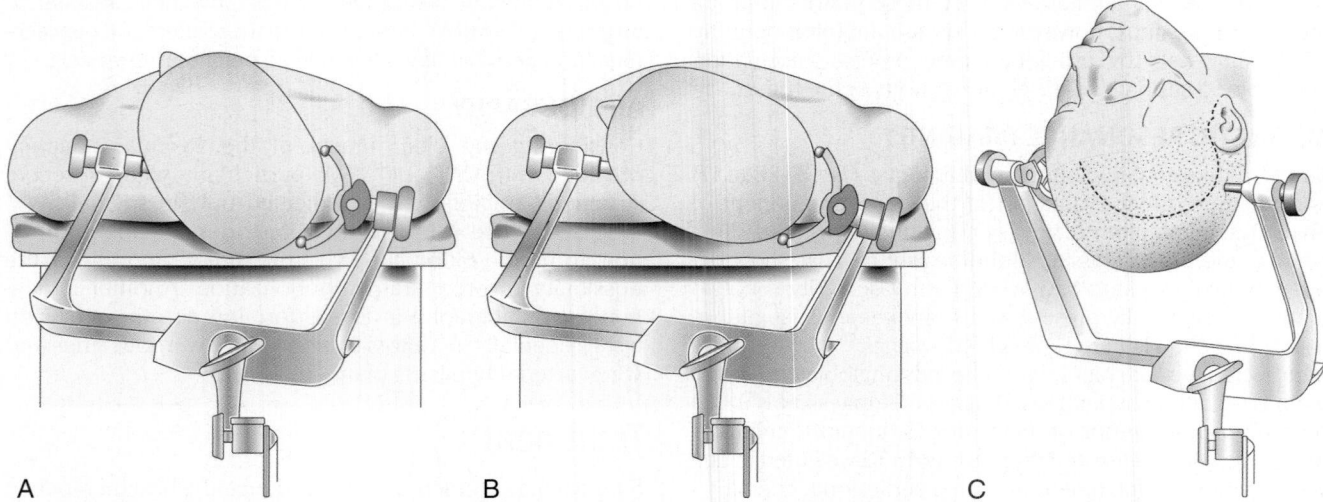

A   B   C

FIGURE 36-3 Positioning and skin incision. The patient is placed in a supine position with the head slightly extended and rotated toward the contralateral side of the tumor. A, For clinoidal meningiomas, a 30- to 40-degree rotation is preferred. B, For pterional meningiomas, the rotation recommended is 40 to 50 degrees. C, Skin incision.

(superficial and deep) of the temporal fascia in the same direction as the skin incision. In this way, the skin flap and the two layers of the temporal fascia (with the fat pad and the branch of the facial nerve lying between them) are separated from the temporal muscle fibers and reflected anteriorly.[11] Once this is completed, detachment and separation of the temporalis muscle is done. It is recommended to perform this dissection in a retrograde direction (from downward to upward) to preserve the epicranial surface of the temporal muscle and reduce its atrophy.[22] In this way, two epicranial planes are created: one composed by the skin and temporal fascia (fasciocutaneous flap) and the other formed by the temporal muscle alone (muscle flap). In this manner, the two flaps can be displaced in slightly different directions: the fasciocutaneous flap forward and the muscle flap downward, which facilitates exposure.[11]

CRANIOTOMY AND TUMOR RESECTION

The shape and size of the craniotomy and tumor resection technique specifically depend on the anatomic variety of the meningioma.

Pterional

In pterional tumors, hyperostosis is usually seen immediately in the pterion once the temporal muscle is detached. Craniotomy is then planned around the bone infiltration, forming a bone flap of about 5 cm around it; if the hyperostosis is not seen, a standard pterional craniotomy is performed (Fig. 36-4A). To raise and remove the bone flap, it is often necessary to section the tumor, leaving in situ the dural infiltration (Fig. 36-4B). This step must be done carefully because of risk of profuse bleeding that may be seen in some cases. Resection of the hyperostosis is done in the bone flap, being certain to remove at least a 1-cm free margin. The meningeal portion of the tumor is then removed, also being certain to include at least a 1-cm free margin of healthy dura mater[2] (Fig. 36-4C). However, in some cases of predominantly osseous tumors, its division is not possible during craniotomy. Under this condition, a craniectomy is then preferred, removing the bony tumor from the onset by using a high-speed drill until exposing the dural implant.

ALAR

In alar tumors, osseous infiltration is usually not seen from the beginning; therefore, a frontotemporal craniotomy is performed with standard dimensions of a 6- to 8-cm diameter centered on the pterion. Craniotomy is followed by extradural resection of the lesser wing of the sphenoid bone. This step is sometimes troublesome because of bleeding, which may be profuse, generated when performing dural detachment.[14,15] Bone removal is continued until complete exposure of the superior orbital fissure and base of the ACP. The dura mater is then opened following a curvilinear frontotemporal incision, reflecting the dural flap forward. Next, splitting of the sylvian fissure is done to gently separate the frontal and temporal lobes to expose the tumor. If the position is correct and cerebrospinal fluid (CSF) evacuation is adequate, it is usually not necessary to place automatic retractors. In these cases, "en bloc" resection is only possible in small tumors; therefore, initial debulking is preferred in the majority of these cases, leaving deeper portions and dural implant for the end of the procedure.

Clinoidal

In clinoidal tumors, a frontotemporal or standard pterional craniotomy is performed, as previously mentioned. Bone management is begun extradurally with resection of the sphenoid ridge from the pterion to the base of the ACP. The superior orbital fissure is also completely opened;[14] if there is an orbital component of the tumor, the posterolateral wall of the orbit is also removed.[14,16] In almost all clinoidal tumors, it is also necessary to perform an anterior clinoidectomy using a high-speed drill, being careful to irrigate profusely to avoid damage to the optic nerve due to heat generated by the drilling. This anterior clinoidectomy can also be performed by holding the ACP with a rongeur and applying a gentle "wiggle and jiggle" movement of the surgeon's wrist.[23] This maneuver may be difficult in cases with marked hyperostosis. Drilling is continued until the optic canal is completely unroofed, being careful not to open the sphenoid or ethmoid sinus when working

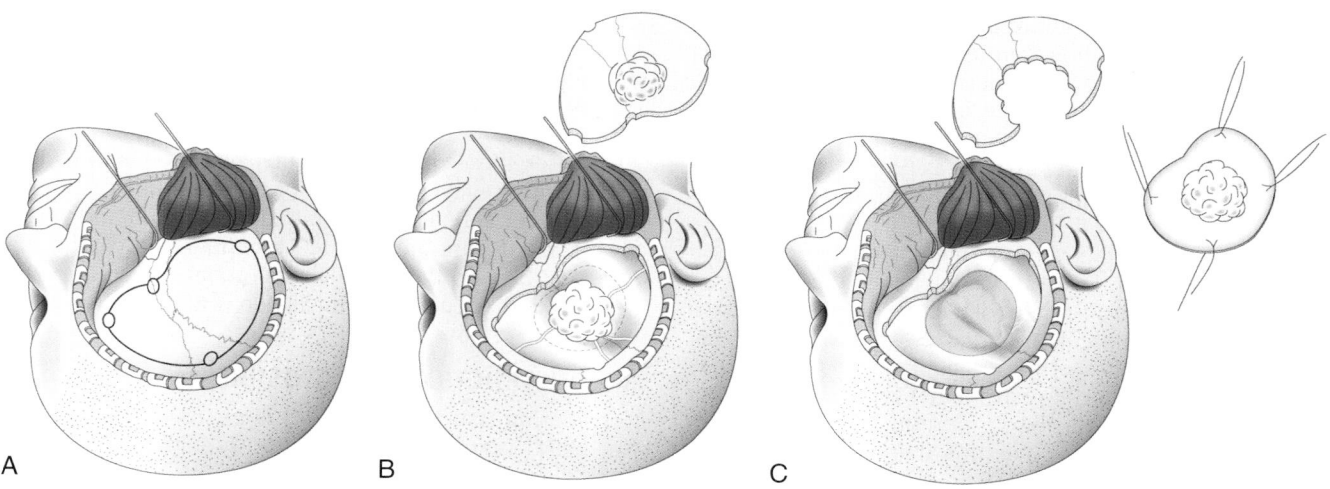

FIGURE 36-4 Craniotomy and tumor resection in pterional meningiomas. A, Standard pterional craniotomy planning. B, Cutting the tumor is usually necessary to elevate the bone flap. C, Tumor resection with a 1-cm free margin in the bone and the dura.

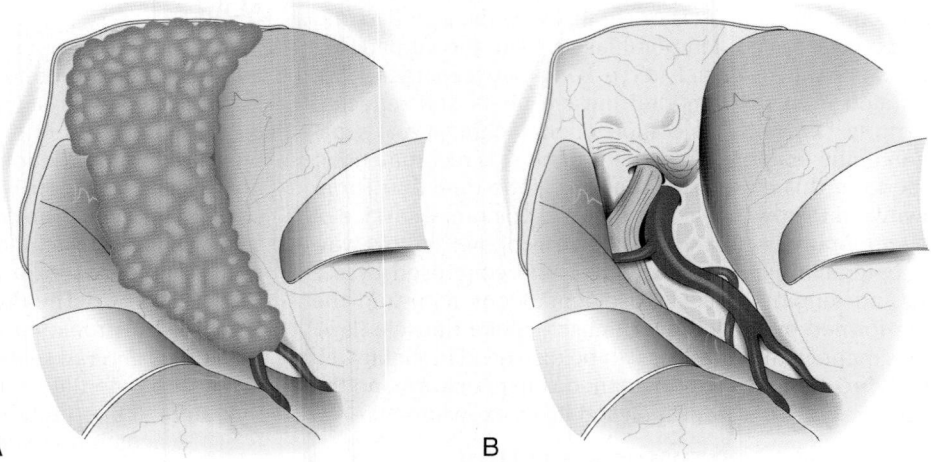

FIGURE 36-5 Surgical exposure and resection of clinoidal meningiomas. A, Exposing the tumor after a wide opening on the sylvian fissure. B, Surgical bed after resection. The ACP has to be drilled and removed, along with the dural implant.

A   B

in the superomedial portion of this channel. The curvilinear dural incision is the same as described earlier, and if the tumor is invading the optic nerve, it is recommended to make another incision following bisection of the dural flap toward the optic sheath and extending across the falciform ligament to the annulus of Zinn. This allows initial identification and free mobilization of the optic nerve before tumor removal.[15,16] Dural opening is followed by a wide splitting of the arachnoid membrane on the sylvian fissure and the free drainage of CSF (Fig. 36-5). Retractors are placed on the frontal and temporal lobes, more to protect their cortical surfaces than to actively retract them, and the lateral portion of the tumor is then identified (Fig. 36-5A). Initially, the dural implants in the frontal and temporal regions are coagulated, which reduces vascular supply of the tumor and facilitates its resection. The distal branches of the MCA and, if possible, the main trunk of this artery are then identified, focusing special attention on early identification and preservation of lenticulostriate branches. Dissection is followed in a distal to proximal direction, which in a large tumor necessarily implies an initial debulking. Arterial dissection is continued proximally to identify the carotid bifurcation and anterior cerebral, posterior communicating, and anterior choroidal arteries, reaching the ICA. The optic nerve is next referred intradurally and released from the tumor. Once macroscopic resection of the tumor is completed, extirpation of the dural implant is done, including margins as previously described (Fig. 36-5B). However, this is extremely difficult to achieve in the vicinity of the ACP.

Resection of intracavernous meningiomas deserves a special description. Due to its complexity, it is discussed in detail elsewhere in this book. This involves manipulation of the ICA and oculomotor nerves, as well as the first and second branches of the trigeminal nerve.[21] In these tumors, it is mandatory to have initial proximal control of the ICA, preferably in its petrous portion, which also serves as anatomic orientation. To do this, it is necessary to combine pterional craniotomy with an OZ approach. It is recommended to begin tumor resection extradurally by finely peeling the lateral wall of the cavernous sinus. If necessary,

it can be continued intradurally, entering through the different anatomic triangles. However, as has been previously mentioned, gross total resection is almost impossible when the tumor invades this region.

En Plaque

In en-plaque tumors, it is easier to expose the entire hyperostosis if pterional craniotomy is combined with an OZ osteotomy, particularly when the lesion extends into the inferior orbital fissure, infratemporal fossa, or orbit (Fig. 36-6). This osteotomy is performed with a reciprocating saw, beginning the cut in the orbital rim at the level of the supraorbital notch or slightly medial to this. The cut is directed backward over the orbital roof to a distance of about 1.5 to 2 cm, at which point the direction is changed and continues laterally to reach the inferior orbital fissure. The bone cut is then continued on the orbital surface from the inferior orbital fissure toward the malar bone. The cut on this bone is completed on its extracranial surface, making an inverted V shape to facilitate relocation. Finally, a diagonal cut is made at the root of the zygomatic arch (Fig. 36-6A). Once the OZ bar is extracted, it is easy to observe the totality of the hyperostosis from a lateral perspective and the drilling begins (Fig. 36-6B). Drilling should be systematic and must include all bony structures of the region invaded by hyperostosis. Occasionally, due to extensive bone invasion, opening the ethmoid and sphenoid sinuses is unavoidable; in such cases, these sinuses should be occluded with fat and fibrin adhesive. Once excision of the osseous component of the tumor is finalized, the intradural portion and, finally, all infiltrated dura are resected, attempting to extend this resection beyond the area of dural enhancement seen on imaging studies. This step is facilitated with the use of neuronavigation systems.

RECONSTRUCTION AND CLOSURE

Considering that in all SWMs it is necessary to resect a free dural margin, closure of the dura mater necessarily implies application of a graft. For this purpose, local tissue can be used, such as aponeurotic galea, pericranium, or temporal fascia. Distant tissues such as fascia

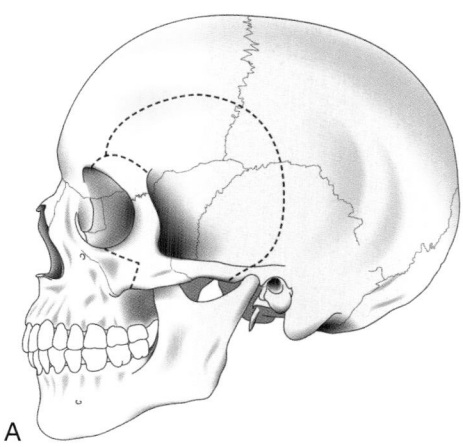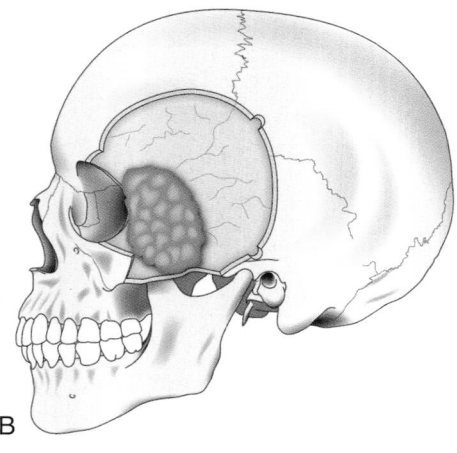

FIGURE 36-6 Craniotomy and OZ osteotomy for en-plaque meningiomas. A, Craniotomy and osteotomy planning. B, With a pterional OZ approach, the entire tumor is exposed.

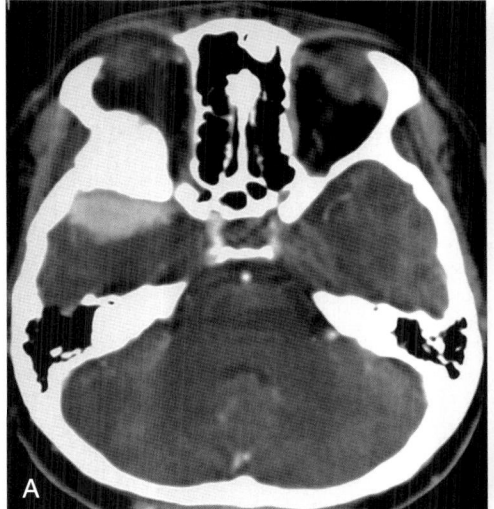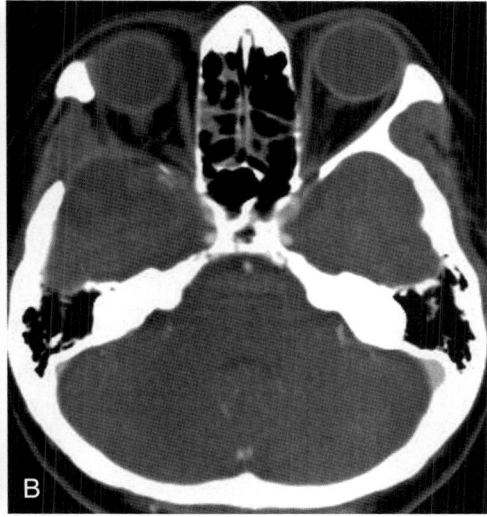

FIGURE 36-7 Contrast-enhanced CT axial view showing a radical removal of an en-plaque right SWM. A, Preoperative. B, Postoperative.

lata or abdominal fascia can also be used, as can synthetic and biologic materials, but with a slightly higher risk of infection. Watertight closure is mandatory and can be reinforced with the use of fibrin sealants. There is an ample variety of options for reconstruction of the pterional defect. Autologous materials such as split calvarial bone graft or ribs can be used, as well as synthetic materials such as methylmethacrylate and titanium, which have the advantage of offering a better cosmetic result. Reconstruction of the orbital walls is controversial. The only incontrovertible point regarding this issue is when the floor, the orbital rim, or both are removed; in these cases, all authors agree that reconstruction is required due to the high risk of orbital ptosis, postoperative diplopia, or cosmetic defect. The controversy focuses mainly on reconstruction of the superior and lateral walls of the orbit. Some authors mention that reconstruction is unnecessary when the roof is removed, as well as the greater and lesser wings of the sphenoid bone;[6] however, other authors have reported an increased risk of pulsatile enophthalmos or cosmetic deficit if this reconstruction is not performed.[5,11,24]

Complications and Results

Although surgery for an SWM has a high margin of safety, because in the majority of cases it is possible to get excellent surgical results (Figs. 36-7 to 36-9), there are some complications reported that must be considered. There is a risk of postoperative hematoma, especially epidural, due to the wide dural detachment done in some cases and the spaces created by resection of large bone formations. CSF leakage is another risk, which is secondary to wide resection of the dural implant. Possibility of seizures should also be considered because SWMs sometimes grow near potentially epileptogenic cortical areas. Finally, cosmetic results may be a problem after inadequate reconstruction. More serious complications are indeed rare. They are primarily associated with a lesion on functional areas of the brain, especially when they occur on the dominant side and are related to excessive manipulation of brain parenchyma, poor use of retractors, or vascular lesion in the MCA or its branches.

Risk of infection is also present, especially when prosthetic materials are used for reconstruction or when frontal,

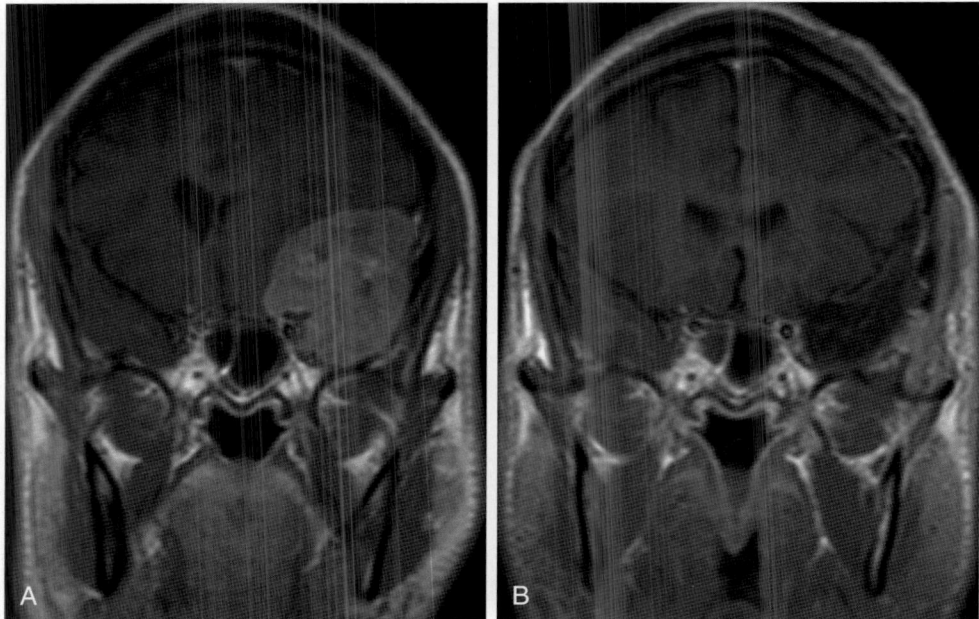

FIGURE 36-8 Contrast-enhanced, T1-weighted coronal MRI view showing a complete resection of a large left alar SWM. A, Preoperative. B, Postoperative.

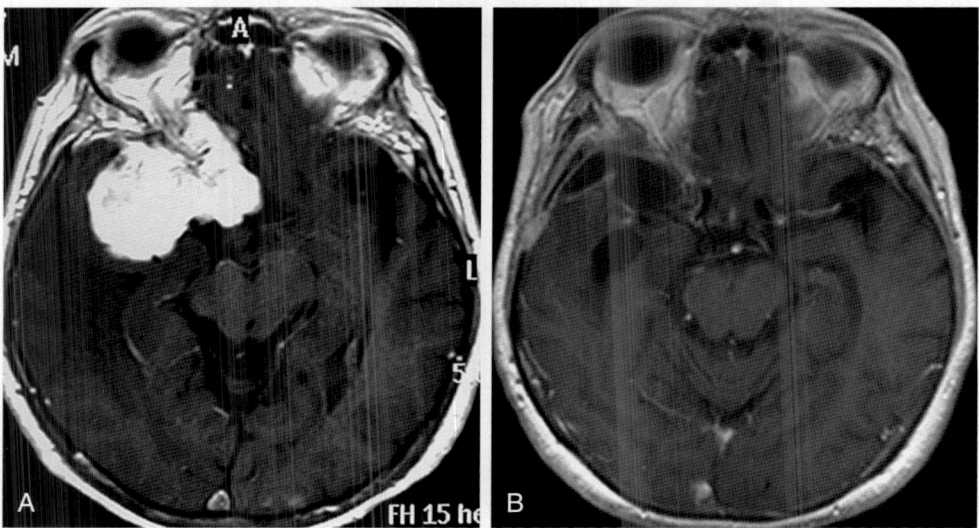

FIGURE 36-9 Contrast-enhanced, T1-weighted axial MRI view showing a total removal of a large right clinoidal meningioma. A, Preoperative. B, Postoperative.

ethmoid, or sphenoid sinuses are inadvertently opened. Finally, mortality after surgery for an SWM is very rare and, when this happens, is usually secondary to a concomitant preexisting problem.

In general, the short- and midterm follow-up results after SWM resection are excellent. In the majority of cases, gross total resection is accomplished with minimal morbidity. However, the critical point is in long-term follow-up because of the high risk of recurrence, which is inversely proportional to the degree of tumor resection.[11,18,19,25] Factors most commonly reported to be associated with incomplete resection of these tumors are extent of bone invasion, undervaluation of the dural component, and invasion of adjacent neurovascular structures. In addition, biologic behavior of the tumor must be considered because if anaplasia is demonstrated or if there is a high proliferative index or complex karyotype, recurrence risk significantly increases. In general, 10-year recurrence has been estimated to be between 9% and 15%, which increases to 19% in a 20-year follow-up. However, a 35% to 50% index of recurrence has been reported when associated with orbital extension.[6]

KEY REFERENCES

Abdel-Aziz KM, Froelich SC, Dagnew E, et al. Large sphenoid wing meningiomas involving the cavernous sinus: conservative surgical strategies for better functional outcomes. *Neurosurgery.* 2004;54: 1375-1384.

Bassiouni H, Asgari S, Sandalcioglu E, et al. Anterior clinoidal meningiomas: functional outcome after microsurgical resection in a consecutive series of 106 patients. *J Neurosurg.* 2009;111:1078-1090.

Basso A, Carrizo AG, Duma C. Sphenoid ridge meningiomas. In: Schmidek HH, ed. *Operative Neurosurgical Techniques. Indications, Methods and Results.* 4th ed Philadelphia: WB Saunders; 2000 pp. 316-324.

Bikmaz K, Mrak R, Al-Mefty O. Management of bone-invasive, hyperostotic sphenoid wing meningiomas. *J Neurosurg.* 2007;107:905-912.

Brotchi J, Pirotte B. Sphenoid wing meningiomas. In: Sekhar LN, Fessler RG, eds. *Atlas of Neurosurgical Techniques. Brain.* New York: Thieme; 2006 pp. 623-632.

Carvi y, Nievas MN. Volume assessment of intracranial large meningiomas and considerations about their microsurgical and clinical management. *Neurol Res.* 2007;29:787-797.

Chang DJ. The "no-drill" technique of anterior clinoidectomy: a cranial base approach to the paraclinoid and parasellar region. *Neurosurgery* 64 (suppl 3). 2009:ONS96-ONS106.

Cunha e Sa M, Quest DQ. Sphenoid wing meningiomas. In: Apuzzo MLJ, ed. *Brain Surgery. Complication Avoidance and Management.* New York: Churchill Livingstone; 1993 pp. 248-268.

Goel A, Gupta S, Desai K. New grading system to predict resectability of anterior clinoid meningiomas. *Neurol Med Chir (Tokyo).* 2000;40:610-617.

Guinto G, Abello J, Félix I, et al. Lesions confined to the sphenoid ridge. Differential diagnosis and surgical treatment. *Skull Base Surg.* 1997;7:115-121.

Honeybul S, Neil-Dwyer G, Lang DA, et al. Sphenoid wing meningiomas en plaque: a clinical review. *Acta Neurochir (Wien).* 2001;143:749-758.

Kim KS, Rogers LF, Goldblatt D. CT features of hyperostosing meningiomas en plaque. *AJR Am J Roentgenol.* 1987;149:1017-1023.

Leake D, Gunnlaugsson C, Urban J, et al. Reconstruction after resection of sphenoid wing meningiomas. *Arch Facial Plast Surg.* 2005;7:99-103.

Lee JH, Jeun SS, Evans J, et al. Surgical management of clinoidal meningiomas. *Neurosurgery.* 2001;48:1012-1021.

Lee JH, Sade B, Park BJ. A surgical technique for the removal of clinoidal meningiomas. *Neurosurgery.* 2006;59(1 Suppl 1):ONS108-ONS114.

Nakamura M, Roser F, Vorkapic P, et al. Medial sphenoid wing meningiomas: clinical outcome and recurrent rate. *Neurosurgery.* 2006;58:626-639.

Nakasu S, Nakasu Y, Nakajima M, et al. Preoperative identification of meningiomas that are highly likely to recur. *J Neurosurg.* 1999;90:455-462.

Oikawa S, Mizuno M, Muraoka S, et al. Retrograde dissection of the temporalis muscle preventing muscle atrophy for pterional craniotomy. *J Neurosurg.* 1996;84:297-299.

Pamir MN, Belirgen M, Özduman K, et al. Anterior clinoidal meningiomas: analysis of 43 consecutive surgically treated cases. *Acta Neurochir (Wien).* 2008;150:625-636.

Pieper DR, Al-Mefty O, Hanada Y, et al. Hyperostosis associated with meningiomas of the cranial base: secondary changes or tumor invasion. *Neurosurgery.* 1999;44:742-747.

Ringel F, Cedzich C, Schramm J. Microsurgical technique and results of a series of 63 spheno-orbital meningiomas. *Neurosurgery.* 2007;60(4 Suppl 2):ONS214-ONS222.

Russell SM, Benjamin V. Medial sphenoid ridge meningiomas: classification, microsurgical anatomy, operative nuances, and long-term surgical outcome in 35 consecutive patients. *Neurosurgery.* 2008;62(3 Suppl 1):38-50.

Schick U, Bleyen J, Bani A, et al. Management of meningiomas en plaque of the sphenoid wing. *J Neurosurg.* 2006;104:208-214.

Shrivastava RK, Sen C, Costantino PD, et al. Sphenoorbital meningiomas: surgical limitations and lessons learned in their long-term management. *J Neurosurg.* 2005;103:491-497.

Tobias S, Kim CH, Kosmorsky G, et al. Management of surgical clinoidal meningiomas. *Neurosurg Focus.* 2003;14:e5.

Numbered references appear on Expert Consult.

CHAPTER 37

Spheno-Orbital Meningioma

JOHN R. FLOYD • FRANCO DEMONTE

The original description of sphenoid ridge meningiomas by Cushing and Eisenhardt in 1938 defines a global type, which grows outward into the sylvian fissure from its attachment, and an en-plaque type, which has a carpet-like growth pattern and evokes hyperostotic changes in the adjacent bone.[1] Since the original description, myriad synonyms have been used in the literature to further describe hyperostosing meningiomas found along the sphenoid ridge, such as pterional tumors en plaque,[2] intraosseous meningiomas,[3] osteomeningiomas, hyperostosing lesions of the ala magna, hyperostosing meningiomas of the sphenoid wing,[4,5] invading meningiomas of the sphenoid wing,[6] and spheno-orbital meningiomas (SOMs).[7]

SOMs may be either globoid or en plaque; may invade the orbit, superior orbital fissure, or cavernous sinus; and may extend into the paranasal sinuses. Hyperostosis can occur regardless of lateralization on the sphenoid wing or invasion into the cavernous sinus.[8] Typically, SOMs exhibit hyperostosis of the squamosal temporal bone, greater sphenoid wing, lateral orbital wall and orbital roof, lesser sphenoid wing, anterior clinoid, and middle fossa floor. Structures involved may include the basal foramina, superior orbital fissure, optic canal, and ethmoid and sphenoid sinuses. The hyperostotic bone has been shown to be secondary to tumor invasion in the vast majority of cases.[9,10] The intradural component can be either globoid or carpet-like; can be attached to the convexity dura, basal sphenoid, and floor of the middle fossa dura; and can invade the cavernous sinus and superior orbital fissure. An intraorbital tumor can be extra- or intraperiorbital, can be extra- or intraconal, and can invade the orbital apex. Extracranial invasion of the temporalis muscle and the infratemporal fossa can occur.

Early management of these complex, hyperostosing meningiomas was conservative. In Castellano's early report in 1952, he discloses a mortality rate of 13.3% in 15 patients undergoing surgery for hyperostosing sphenoid wing meningiomas.[2] Based on this high perioperative mortality, the discomforts of severe proptosis and even unilateral vision loss were insufficient reasons to warrant surgical intervention.[2,11] It was not until the work of Derome[12] and others[6,13,14] in the 1970s that more complete resections were safely achieved with use of a coronal incision, pericranial grafting, and reconstruction of the anterior skull base with iliac bone or split calvarial bone grafts. Today, with greater understanding of surgical anatomy and the development of advanced skull base techniques,[15-19] the perioperative mortality has dropped from 20%[2,6,11,13] to

0% to 4%.[3,7,8,20-24] Even so, with efforts to preserve neurologic function,[25] residual tumors involving the cavernous sinus, orbital apex, and superior orbital fissure remain problematic surgical limitations. These areas are major sites for residual tumors, recurrence, and continued neurologic deterioration.[4-6,8,22-24,26] Adjuvant radiotherapy for residual tumors or recurrence commonly forms part of modern management plans,[27] but specific indications remain controversial.[22,26,28]

The most common presenting symptom of a SOM is by far unilateral eye bulging with the corresponding physical finding of proptosis.[2] Hyperostosis of the lateral orbital wall, orbital roof, and intraorbital tumor invasion contribute to proptosis. Other common symptoms include decreased vision, double vision, headache, temporal swelling, facial numbness, and seizures. Correlative neurologic findings include optic atrophy, decreased acuity and deficits of visual field, cranial nerve (CN) paresis, and trigeminal hypesthesia. CN III, IV, and VI paresis is the result of cavernous sinus, superior orbital fissure, or both types of invasion. However, diplopia can also result from rectus muscle compression and restricted movement from orbital invasion by tumor. Facial hypesthesia in the V1 distribution typically indicates superior orbital fissure invasion. Tumor invasion in the cavernous sinus or hyperostotic stricture of the basilar foramina can cause facial hypesthesia in the V2 or V3 distributions. Presenting symptoms and neurologic findings are summarized in Tables 37-1 and 37-2.

Data from the Central Brain Tumor Registry of the United States reveals that the most frequently reported primary brain tumors are meningiomas, at 33.4%. They are the most common type of tumor from age 35 on and occur more often in females than males, with a 2.2:1 (cbtrus.org). In Castellano's 1952 report of 608 cases of verified meningiomas,[2] 18.4% (n = 111) were located along the sphenoid ridge and 2.5% (n = 15) were associated with hyperostosis. Other series report a range of 4% to 9% for hyperostosis associated with sphenoid wing meningiomas.[5,29]

Presurgical Management
PHYSICAL EXAMINATION

Patients with hyperostosing sphenoid wing meningioma need to undergo a thorough physical evaluation. Due to the variable degree of hyperostosis, soft tissue invasion, and

Table 37-1	Symptoms in Patients with Hyperostosing SOMs
Symptom	**Percentage of Patients (mean)**
Eye bulging	36-100 (78)[2,5,8,10,21,24]
Decreased vision	16-60 (32)[2,5,8,10,24]
Double vision	5-21 (14)[5,10,21,24]
Headache	8-41 (25)[2,5,8,10,24]
Mass or swelling	7-61 (27)[2,5,21,24]
Facial numbness or pain	2-5 (3)[5,8,24]
Seizures	1-16 (8)[2,5,8,21,24]

Table 37-2	Findings in Patients with Hyperostosing SOMs
Neurologic Finding	**Percentage of Patients (mean)**
Proptosis	36-100 (79)[2,5,8,21,24]
Optic atrophy	16-29 (23)[2,5]
Decreased acuity	24-58 (43)[2,5,24]
Visual field deficit	10-32 (18)[2,5,24]
CN paresis	21-33 (26)[2,5,24]
Temporal swelling	7-61 (27)[2,5,21]
Trigeminal hypesthesia	3-8 (5)[2,5,24]

extracranial extension, a detailed neurologic examination is requisite. Patients may have deficits in CN II, III, IV, and V (V1, V2, and V3) and in CN VI. If a portion of the tumor is globoid, contralateral hemiparesis may exist, as may deficits of speech and language. Careful attention should be given to the patient's appearance, and proptosis and temporal bulging should be noted.

OPHTHALMOLOGIC EXAMINATION

A complete ophthalmologic examination should be performed on any patient with the diagnosis of a hyperostosing SOM. Proptosis can be quantified utilizing Hertel measurements. Visual acuity and visual field should be documented and followed. In addition, variable degrees of optic neuropathy should be fully evaluated: afferent pupillary defects, loss of color saturation, optic nerve atrophy and pallor, thinning of the retinal nerve fiber layer, and central field deficits. The degree of limitation of eye movement should be quantified, and attempts should be made to determine whether the limitation is due to neuropathy or extraocular muscle restriction.

NEUROLOGIC IMAGING

Neurologic imaging should begin with high-resolution thin section computed tomography (CT) scan of the head and skull base. Assessment of the bony windows identifies the affected hyperostotic bone. Structures commonly involved include the orbital roof and lateral wall, greater and lesser sphenoid wing, anterior clinoid, temporal squamosal bone, body of the sphenoid bone, and lateral wall of the sphenoid and ethmoid sinuses. Brain magnetic resonance imaging (MRI) with gadolinium enhancement gives greater detail of intradural and dural involvement. Fat-suppressed T1 sequences are essential when evaluating intraorbital invasion. Preoperative angiography is typically not necessary. Figure 37-1 demonstrates the variable radiologic presentations found with SOMs.

Operative Techniques

The surgical approach for SOMs is typically frontotemporal with possible modifications to include transzygomatic, orbitozygomatic, and orbital frontal approaches. The initial approach is extradural, which consistently enables access to the orbit and middle fossa for removal of hyperostotic bone and decompression of the optic canal. This also allows coagulation and control of extradural arterial blood supply and minimizes brain retraction during intradural tumor removal.[8,19] Accessing of the superior orbital fissure, cavernous sinus, and intraorbital compartment is facilitated by this approach as well. A coronal incision allows harvest of a vascularized pericranial graft for reconstruction purposes. The patient is typically positioned in the supine position. The head is rotated 30 degrees to the contralateral side and fixed. The patient's surgical position is then registered to the preoperative imaging data sets to allow intraoperative navigation. Preoperative high-resolution CT and MRI with gadolinium and fat suppression are coregistered. CT is utilized to assess intraoperative bone removal, and MRI with gadolinium and fat suppression is utilized to guide intradural and intraorbital tumor removal. An area of the abdomen is prepped for an autologous fat graft. The coronal incision is made, and the anterior branch of the superficial temporalis artery is preserved. Sharp dissection is utilized to elevate the scalp in the immediate subgaleal plane. The scalp is reflected anteriorly, leaving the periosteum and overlaying loose connective tissue layer attached to the calvarium. The posterior edge of the scalp is undermined 2 to 3 cm.

The temporalis fascia is incised 2 cm above the "keyhole" region and continued to the root of the zygoma (Fig. 37-2A). The periosteum is released posteriorly and then incised along the superior temporal line. Together, the periosteum and the superficial and deep layers of the temporalis fascia are elevated off the frontal bone, orbital rim, and zygoma while the frontalis branch of the facial nerve is protected. Subperiosteal dissection is utilized to elevate the temporalis muscle laterally and inferiorly, carefully preserving the blood supply and innervation. When infratemporal exposure is required, a zygomatic osteotomy is then performed, leaving the zygomatic arch attached to the masseter muscle (Fig. 37-2B and C). Tumor-infiltrated temporalis muscle is excised. Complete exposure of the frontal, temporal, and zygomatic bones is thus achieved (Fig. 37-2D). Intraoperative navigation is utilized to ensure sufficient exposure of involved bone, as well as underlying dural involvement.

The hyperostotic greater sphenoid wing, lateral orbital wall and rim, and temporal squamosal bone are then removed with a high-speed drill and rongeurs (Fig. 37-3A). Bony removal is performed as indicated clinically and by the preoperative evaluation of the CT scan, as well as intraoperative use of CT-guided neuronavigation. The superior orbital fissure and basilar foramina (foramen rotundum, vidian canal, foramen ovale, and foramen spinosum) all can be completely skeletonized (Fig. 37-3B). When the lesser wing of the sphenoid bone, anterior clinoid, orbital roof, or optic canal is involved, an orbital frontal craniotomy is performed. Removal of the lesser wing and anterior clinoid and wide opening of the optic canal is performed with a high-speed diamond burr under constant irrigation

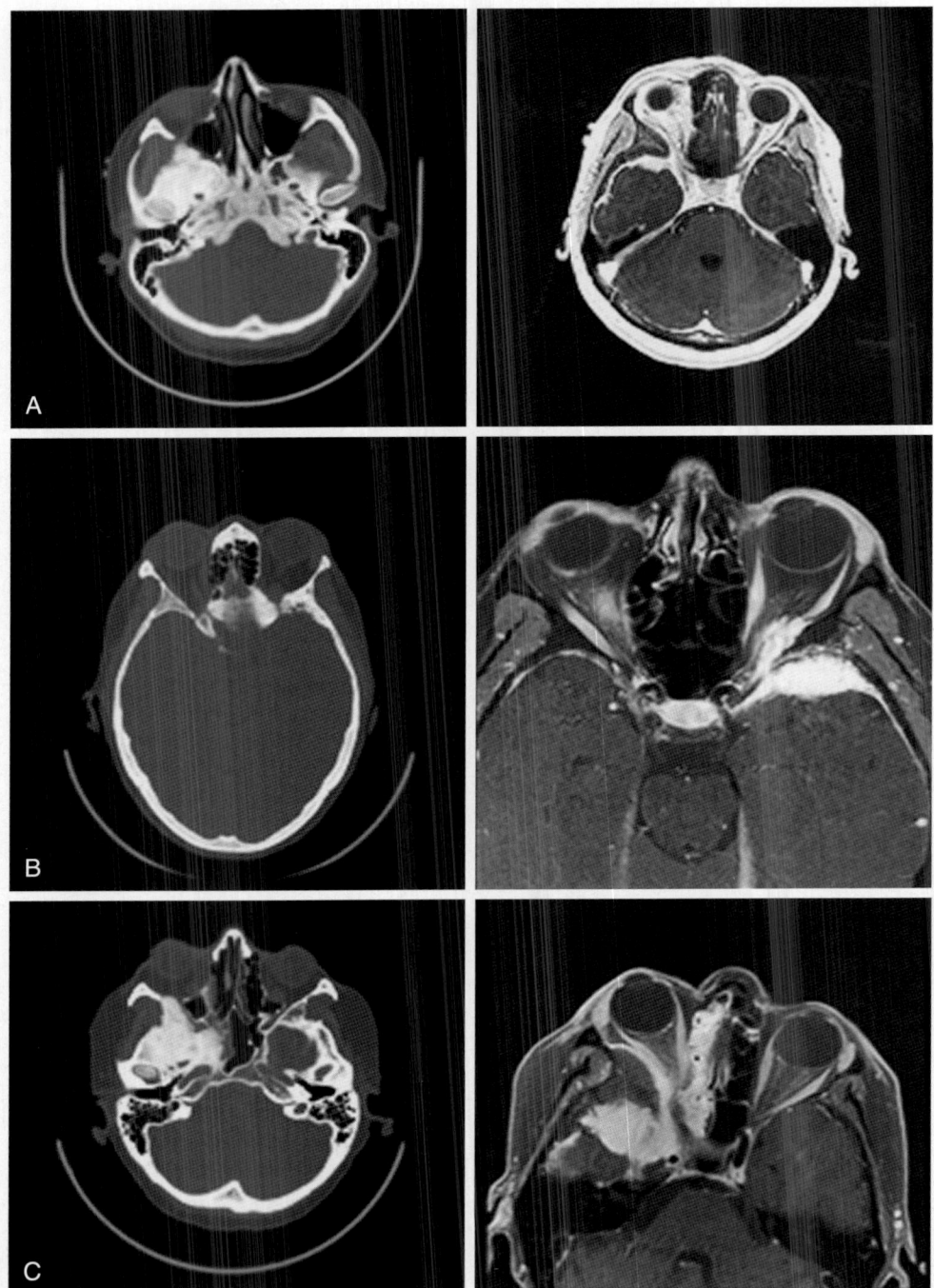

FIGURE 37-1 A, Axial noncontrast CT head and bone windows, showing hyperostosis of the right medial greater sphenoid wing to the foramen rotundum, ovale, and spinosum (left). Axial, gadolinium-enhanced MRI, showing a thin en-plaque intradural right anterior temporal pole meningioma (right). B, Axial noncontrast CT head and bone windows, showing hyperostosis of the left lateral greater sphenoid wing (left). Axial, gadolinium-enhanced, fat-suppressed, T1-weighted MRI of the orbits, demonstrating a left intradural temporal pole meningioma with extension to the superior orbital fissure and intraorbital extension (right). C, Axial noncontrast CT head and bone windows, showing hyperostosis of the right medial greater sphenoid wing medial to the foramen rotundum, ovale, and spinosum with involvement of the lateral sphenoid sinus (left). Axial, gadolinium-enhanced, fat-suppressed, T1-weighted MRI of the orbits demonstrating a right intradural temporal pole meningioma with cavernous sinus, orbital apex, and sinonasal extension (right).

and microscopic visualization. Involved dura is excised (Fig. 37-3C). Intradural or plaque-like tumor involvement is removed with sharp dissection and microsurgical techniques. When cavernous sinus invasion is noted, resection is carried forward to include the medial temporal dura of the

lateral cavernous sinus wall. Meningiomas within the cavernous sinus can directly invade the CNs and the connective tissue planes between them.[4,30] Thus, even with radical cavernous sinus resection, an oncologic cure is not possible and certainly not justified given the resultant morbidity.[31]

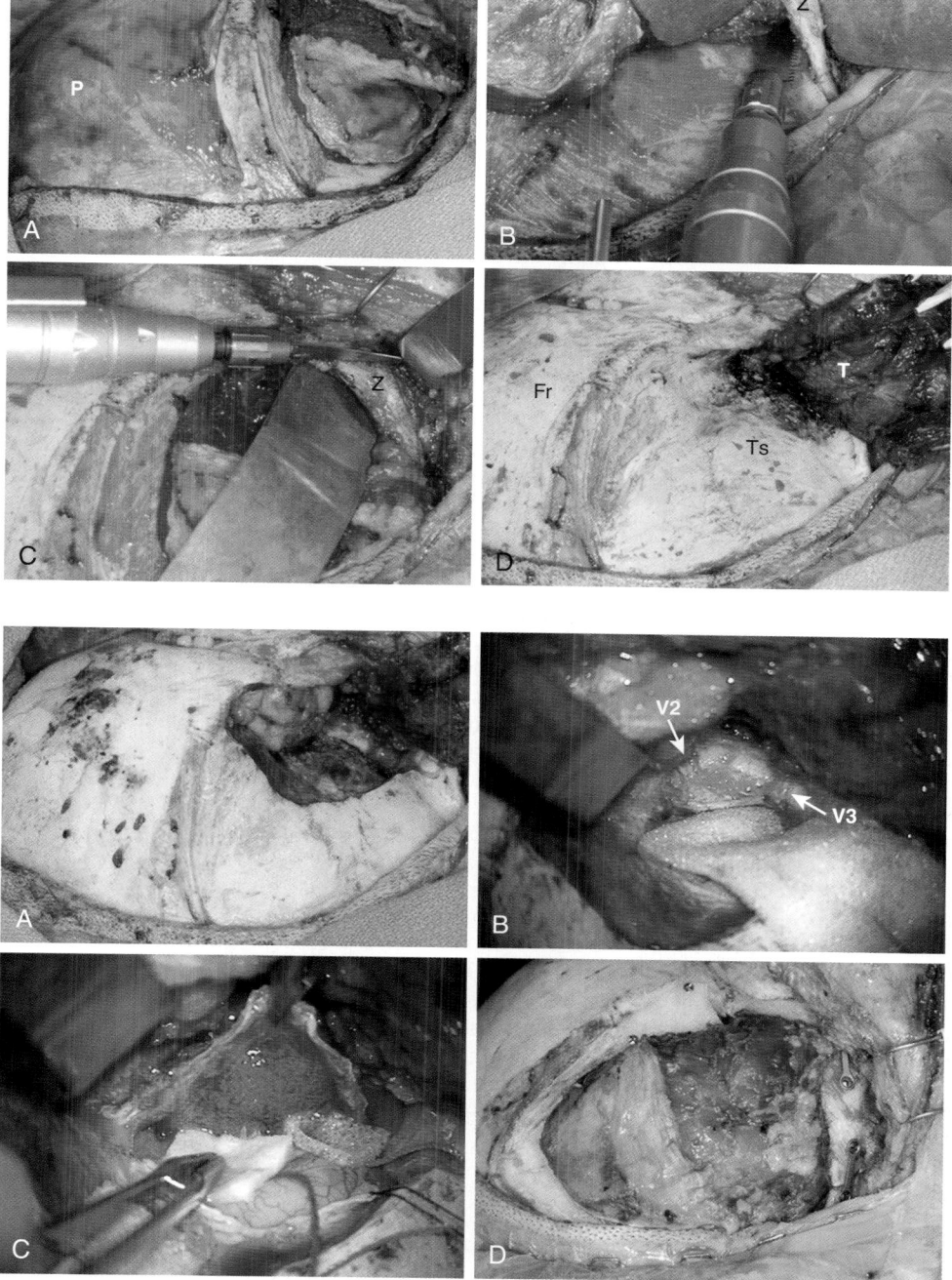

FIGURE 37-2 A, Exposure after performing coronal incision, elevation of the pericranial graft (P), and opening of the temporalis fascia (T). B and C, Zygomatic osteotomy, left attached to masseter muscle. D, Exposure of the frontal bone (Fr) and temporal squamosal bone (Ts) with inferior reflection of the temporalis muscle (T). Note the abnormal, hyperostotic bone.

FIGURE 37-3 A, Demonstration of complete removal of hyperostotic bone, including the lateral orbital wall, temporal squamosal bone, greater sphenoid wing, and temporal floor. B, Demonstration of the skeletonization of the second and third branches of the trigeminal nerve exiting through the foramina rotundum and ovale, respectively. C, Intradural tumor resection. D, Reconstruction consisting of pterional implant, plating of the zygoma, and suspension of temporalis muscle.

For these reasons, tumor within the cavernous sinus or superior orbital fissure is typically left in place to avoid neurologic complications. Once the intracranial portion has been excised, attention is turned to the intraorbital involvement. The dura is closed prior to the commencement of intraorbital tumor resection.

Often, tumor extension into the orbit is extraperiorbital. This tumor is typically removed when the bony lateral orbital wall is removed. When involved, the periorbita is resected and the intraorbital tumor invasion is removed. Intraoperative neuronavigation with fat-suppressed sequences is useful in identifying intraorbital meningioma. The lateral

rectus can be tagged through the conjunctiva with a nylon suture at the beginning of the case to help identify the muscle once tumor resection has started. All intraorbital and extraconal tumors can be removed. Invasion into the orbital apex, annulus of Zinn, or superior orbital fissure is left in place due to the high risk of injury to the CNs.

The dura is reconstructed with a portion of the pericranial graft, temporalis fascia, or allographic dural substitute. If the sphenoid or ethmoid sinuses are entered, these are obturated with autologous fat to prevent cerebrospinal fluid leak. If a periorbital defect is present, it is closed with locally harvested temporalis fascia. The pericranial graft is

Table 37-3   Perioperative Mortality in Hyperostosing SOMs

Series	Year	Patients	Mortality
Castellano et al.[2]	1952	15	3 (23%)
Columella et al.[14]	1974	3	0 (0%)
Bonnal et al.[6]	1980	21	3 (14%)
Pompili et al.[5]	1982	49	2 (4%)
McDermott et al.[18]	1990	8	0 (0%)
Carrizo and Basso[7]	1998	48	2 (4%)
Honeybul et al.[21]	2001	15	0 (0%)
Roser et al.[8]	2005	82	1 (1.4%)
Shrivastava et al.[4]	2005	25	0 (0%)
Sandalcioglu et al.[22]	2005	16	0 (0%)
Schick et al.[23]	2006	67	0 (0%)
Ringel et al.[24]	2007	63	1 (1.6%)
Bikmaz et al.[10]	2007	17	0 (0%)
Floyd and DeMonte	2012	20	0 (0%)

Table 37-4   Postoperative Outcomes: Proptosis and Vision

Symptom	Preoperative	POSTOPERATIVE	
		Improved	Worsened
Proptosis	233	185 (79%)	0
Vision	133	58 (44%)	3 (2%)

then rotated over the orbit. This helps compartmentalize the orbit from the intracranial space and avoid adhesion of the orbital tissues to the dura. Reconstruction of the orbital roof and lateral orbital wall is not necessary for a good cosmetic result[32] if the periorbita is intact or repaired. If the superior or lateral orbital rim is removed, it can be reconstructed with split calvarial bone grafts or commercially available orbital prostheses. The orbital and zygomatic osteotomies are fixated with low-profile cranial plating. Remaining dead space from hyperostotic bone removal can be filled with autologous fat. If a temporal fossa defect exists, a cranioplasty is performed. Options for cranioplasty include polymethylmethacrylate, various commercially available bone cements, or commercially available prostheses. Alternatively, prior to bone removal, titanium mesh can be molded to the calvarium and then utilized to cover the bony defect at the end of the case.[10] The temporalis muscle is reattached to a cuff of fascia, drill holes in the calvarium, or the reconstruction plates (Fig. 37-3D).

Outcomes

MORTALITY

In modern case series, perioperative mortality rates vary from 0% to 4% (Table 37-3). Since 2001, only two perioperative deaths have been reported, one from pulmonary embolus[8] and one from carotid laceration.[24]

MORBIDITY

Morbidity is inconsistently reported in the literature. Instances of subgaleal fluid collection, temporal hollowing, chemosis, meningitis, osteomyelitis, epidural hematoma, chronic subdural hematoma, retro-orbital hematoma, transient aphasia, brain edema, temporary hemiplegia, hemispheric stroke secondary to carotid injury, and blindness have all been reported.[4,5,7,21,22,24]

Specific outcomes related to the presenting clinical symptoms of proptosis, decreased vision, and cranial neuropathy have also been inconsistently detailed. Since 2001, 285 patients have been reported in case series.[4,8,10,21-24] With the addition of 20 patients from our series, 305 patients are considered.

PROPTOSIS

In the case series since 2001,[4,8,10,21-24] there have been 233 patients with proptosis identified, either by clinical inspection or by formal measurements. Of this number, 79% (n = 185) have been reported to have had significant cosmetic improvement postoperatively (Table 37-4). Methods used to evaluate the degree of proptosis varied; patient questionnaires, patient perception, clinical examinations, and formal Hertel measurements were all used. Five patients developed enophthalmos (2%) that required additional corrective surgery, and the remaining patients had stable degrees of proptosis. Maroon et al.[26] reported good cosmetic results without orbital reconstruction. However, no objective measurements or strict criteria were utilized in the evaluation of globe position. Subsequent reports that utilized objective measures emphasize that reconstruction of the orbit is necessary if more than one orbital wall is removed during surgery.[20,21] DeMonte et al.,[32] however, demonstrated that as long as the periorbita is intact, or has been primarily repaired, isolated bone defects of the medial or lateral orbital walls do not need to be reconstructed. Similarly, isolated defects of the orbital roof, or combined defects of the orbital roof and lateral wall, do not need reconstruction as long as the periorbita is intact or repaired. Large defects of the orbital floor always need reconstruction regardless of whether the periorbita is intact or repaired to prevent hypoglobus or enophthalmos.

VISION

In the literature reviewed,[4,8,10,21-24] 133 patients were reported to have decreased visual acuity at the time of diagnosis. Fifty-eight patients (44%) experienced an improvement in visual acuity postoperatively (see Table 37-4). Three patients (2%) were noted to have worsened visual acuity postoperatively.[23,24] One new case of transient decreased acuity and a permanent temporal hemianopsia occurred when a skull base fracture extended through the optic canal when elevating the bone flap.[21] The remaining patients retained stable vision after surgery. In Schick's series,[23] 7 patients had no useful vision; of those, 1 patient improved postoperatively. Another 28 patients had decreased vision, and 11 of those patients improved. In our series of 20 patients, 2 patients had light perception vision only and did not improve. Another 4 patients had vision loss that did not exceed 20/400, and 3 of these 4 patients improved after surgery. Complete optic nerve decompression is imperative

Table 37-5   Long-Term Outcomes

Series	Year	Follow-up Average (Months)	Patients	Incomplete Resections	Recurrence	Time to Recurrence (Months)	Average Time to Recurrence (Months)
Honeybul et al.[21]	2001	40	15	7 (47%)	2 (13%)	36, 96	66
Roser et al.[8]	2005	66	82	>51 (>62%)	25 (30%)	Not specified	32
Sandalcioglu et al.[22]	2005	68	16	5 (31%)	9 (60%)	16, 118, 13, 66, 47, 62, 9, 12, 17	40
Shrivastava et al.[4]	2005	60	25	7 (28%)	2 (8%)	12, 132	73
Schick et al.[23]	2006	46	67	27 (40%)	7 (10%)	29, 21, 47, 21, 14, 23, 13	24
Ringel et al.[24]	2007	54	63	42 (67%)	16 (25%)	Not specified	Not specified
Bikmaz et al.[10]	2007	36	17	3 (18%)	1 (6%)	72	72
Floyd and DeMonte	2012	42	20	12 (60%)	5 (25%)	96, 24, 18, 12, 9	32

in improving and stabilizing vision. When hyperostosis involves the orbital roof, lesser sphenoid wing, and clinoid process, extra attention must be given to avoid bone fractures into the optic canal. This is generally avoided by utilizing a two-piece approach to the orbital osteotomy when an orbital frontal approach is indicated. However, even with excellent surgical technique, once vision has deteriorated to greater than 20/400 or to light perception only, it is unlikely that acuity will improve.

CRANIAL NERVE FUNCTION

Ocular motility is often disturbed in SOMs secondary to either extraocular muscle restriction or CN dysfunction. Either can cause diplopia as a presenting symptom. When diplopia is secondary to extraocular muscle restriction, symptoms typically resolve after orbital decompression and reconstruction. In Shrivastava et al.'s series,[4] five patients presented with double vision, thought to be secondary to extraocular muscle restriction. All five patients eventually had significant improvement after surgery. In our series, nine patients presented with double vision. Five were secondary to extraocular muscle restriction and four due to CN dysfunction (CN III, IV, and IV palsies). Of the five patients with extraocular muscle restriction, four patients (80%) had improvement in double vision postoperatively. However, there was no improvement in patients who had preexisting CN palsies. Sandalcioglu et al.[22] reported nine transient CN deficits postoperatively, including ptosis and CN III palsy in seven patients and facial hypesthesia in two patients. One patient had a preexisting CN III palsy, and one patient had a new permanent CN III palsy following surgery. Ringel et al.[24] also reported eight transient CN III deficits, along with one CN VI and two CN IV deficits after surgery. In that series, there were eight additional permanent CN III palsies, one CN IV palsy, two CN VI palsies, and 10 cases of facial hypesthesia from CN V dysfunction. The number of CN deficits that may have been preexisting is unclear.

In summary, double vision when secondary to the restricted movement of the extraocular muscles improves with orbital decompression. When patients present with true CN III, IV, and VI deficits, these are unlikely to improve after decompression. True CN palsies are due to direct tumor invasion of the cavernous sinus, superior orbital fissure, or orbital apex and annulus of Zinn. Transient CN deficits occur most often with ptosis (CN III) and facial hypesthesia (CN V). New CN deficits are variably reported; however, it seems that CN III is most often reported.[22,23]

Long-Term Outcomes

The recurrence or progression rate for hyperostosing sphenoid wing meningiomas varies from 6% to 60%, with an average time to recurrence or progression of 24 to 73 months[4,8,10,21-23] (Table 37-5). Bonnal et al.[6] describe six early recurrences (within less than 2 years) in their series of 21 patients. Three areas attributed to the early recurrence, or more likely progression, are the cavernous sinus, sphenoid body, and annulus of Zinn. Shrivastava et al.[4] also reported one early recurrence (within less than 1 year) from direct extension from the superior orbital fissure. Maroon et al. in 1994 indicated that recurrences are multifactorial, including failure of early diagnosis, subtotal resection when tumor invades the cavernous sinus and superior orbital fissure, and incomplete removal of hyperostotic bone.[26] Today, it is clear that hyperostotic bone is tumor-invaded bone.[9,10] With advanced imaging by means of high-resolution CT scans and gadolinium-enhanced, fat-suppressed MRIs, corrected diagnosis is made earlier and more extensive resections are achieved. However, tumor invasion in the cavernous sinus, superior orbital fissure, and orbital apex remains problematic and is the main reason for tumor progression.[7,21,29] In our series of 20 patients followed for an average of 42 months, 5 patients developed tumor recurrence or progression at an average of 32 months. The areas of progression resulted from residual tumors in the cavernous sinus, superior orbital fissure, and intraorbital and intraconal locations.

Long-Term Management
POSTOPERATIVE FOLLOW-UP

Patients with hyperostosing SOMs need indefinite close and careful follow-up in the postoperative period, given the possibility for recurrence many years after the primary resection. Patients with recurrent hyperostosing SOMs most often present with progressive proptosis, followed by progressive vision loss and CN dysfunction.[23,26] For these reasons, serial ophthalmologic examinations should be part of the postsurgical evaluation of globe position, ocular motility, visual acuity, visual fields, and other signs of optic neuropathy. Early detection of a recurrent tumor can be made prior to clinical symptoms with high-resolution gadolinium-enhanced MRIs with fat-suppressed orbital sequences. This allows for the evaluation of intradural and intraorbital recurrences.

When faced with recurrence or progression of hyperostosing SOMs, the management goals are the same as with initial presentation: maximal tumor removal and reconstruction, preservation of ocular and CN function, and improvement in cosmesis with reduction of proptosis. The strategy varies according to the recurrence and symptomology. However, in most instances of recurrence, a second surgery for maximal tumor cytoreduction is indicated.[8] Excellent cosmetic results and vision preservation can be achieved with a second surgery.[26] Sandalcioglu et al. report that out of nine recurrences in their series, eight underwent reoperation; in three patients, a complete resection was achieved. In all eight patients, there were no additional neurologic deficits.[22] For these reasons, and because these are slow-growing tumors, Honeybul et al. advocate a second surgery unless additional surgery poses greater risk to the patient.[21] When this situation arises, either due to medical comorbidities or due to excessive neurologic risks, radiation treatment as primary therapy is a good option.

RADIATION TREATMENT

Radiation treatment has been shown to decrease the recurrence rate and increase the time to progression for benign meningioma.[28,33-35] Barbaro et al.[36] demonstrated that in subtotally resected meningiomas, 60% of patients had tumor recurrence at an average of 66 months if no additional radiation was given. In patients with subtotally resected meningiomas who received postoperative radiation, the recurrence rate was 32% at an average of 125 months. Later, Goldsmith et al. demonstrated a 5-year 98% progression–free survival rate in patients who had undergone a subtotally resected benign meningioma.[37] Soyuer et al.[28] also demonstrated that the 5-year progression-free survival is significantly improved in patients who have had adjuvant radiotherapy for subtotally resected meningiomas versus those patients who have had subtotal resections without additional treatment. However, there was no overall survival advantage when patients were receiving immediate postoperative radiation. This significant finding indicates that delaying adjuvant radiation therapy does not compromise the overall survival and may have the added benefit of delaying treatment-related toxicities. At the time of recurrence, most often a second surgery is advocated.

At that time, in most published clinical series, adjuvant radiation is given.[4,8,22,23,26]

Conclusions

Hyperostosing SOMs are rare tumors with complex presentations. Careful preoperative workup with formal ophthalmologic evaluations and neuroimaging is essential. The approach to hyperostosing SOMs has evolved from a nonsurgical stance, to a gross total tumor resection strategy, to a present-day patient outcome–oriented strategy. Excellent results in terms of reduction of proptosis and CN preservation can be achieved at both the primary surgical resection and the second surgery for recurrence. Radiation treatment decreases recurrence and increases progression-free survival in subtotally resected meningiomas.

KEY REFERENCES

Bikmaz K, Mrak R, Al-Mefty O. Management of bone-invasive, hyperostotic sphenoid wing meningiomas. *J Neurosurg.* 2007;107(5):905-912.

Carrizo A, Basso A. Current surgical treatment for sphenoorbital meningiomas. *Surg Neurol.* 1998;50(6):574-578.

De Jesus O, Toledo MM. Surgical management of meningioma en plaque of the sphenoid ridge. *Surg Neurol.* 2001;55(5):265-269.

DeMonte F, et al. Ophthalmological outcome following orbital resection in anterior and anterolateral skull base surgery. *Neurosurg Focus.* 2001;10(5):E4.

Derome P. [Spheno-ethmoidal tumors. Possibilities for exeresis and surgical repair]. *Neurochirurgie.* 1972;18(1):p. (suppl 1):1-164.

Honeybul S, et al. Sphenoid wing meningioma en plaque: a clinical review. *Acta Neurochir (Wien).* 2001;143(8):749-757:discussion 758.

Maroon JC, et al. Recurrent spheno-orbital meningioma. *J Neurosurg.* 1994;80(2):202-208.

Pieper DR. Hyperostosis associated with meningioma of the cranial base: secondary changes or tumor invasion. *Neurosurgery.* 1999;44(4):742-746:discussion 746-747.

Pompili A, et al. Hyperostosing meningiomas of the sphenoid ridge—clinical features, surgical therapy, and long-term observations: review of 49 cases. *Surg Neurol.* 1982;17(6):411-416.

Ringel F, Cedzich C, Schramm J. Microsurgical technique and results of a series of 63 spheno-orbital meningiomas. *Neurosurgery.* 2007;60 (4 suppl 2):214-221:discussion 221-222.

Roser F, et al. Sphenoid wing meningiomas with osseous involvement. *Surg Neurol.* 2005;64(1):37-43:discussion 43.

Sandalcioglu IE, et al. Spheno-orbital meningiomas: interdisciplinary surgical approach, resectability and long-term results. *J Craniomaxillofac Surg.* 2005;33(4):260-266.

Schick U, et al. Management of meningiomas en plaque of the sphenoid wing. *J Neurosurg.* 2006;104(2):208-214.

Shrivastava RK, et al. Sphenoorbital meningiomas: surgical limitations and lessons learned in their long-term management. *J Neurosurg.* 2005;103(3):491-497.

Soyuer S, et al. Radiotherapy after surgery for benign cerebral meningioma. *Radiother Oncol.* 2004;71(1):85-90.

Numbered references appear on Expert Consult.

CHAPTER 38

Tumors Involving the Cavernous Sinus

JOHN DIAZ DAY • DONG XIA FENG • TAKANORI FUKUSHIMA

Until 1965, when Parkinson's landmark article describing the direct surgical approach to carotid-cavernous fistulas was published, little reference was made in the neurosurgical literature to direct operative attack on lesions of the cavernous sinus.[1] This lack of information was largely a result of the inability in the premicrosurgical era to address effectively the extreme risks of significant hemorrhage and damage to the cranial nerves in the region. This anatomic locale has long been considered a true "no man's land" for direct surgical approaches. The modern era of microneurosurgery has realized expanded capabilities in microsurgical technique and has fostered the work of several neurosurgeons who have made great strides in effectively approaching this region with reduced morbidity.[2-20] In particular, the work of Dolenc should be recognized for the development of his combined epidural and subdural approach, which has become the standard method used to directly access lesions in this region.[6]

More recently, within the last decade, endonasal endoscopic approaches to the cavernous sinus region have been developed as an alternative to an open craniotomy.[21-24] These approaches are not commonly utilized, but the current trend in anterior and middle cranial base surgery is to incorporate these strategies as a minimally invasive alternative. These techniques are mentioned as they are becoming an important element of the armamentarium in dealing with these lesions. However, they are complex enough to warrant a separate and entire chapter themselves. Here we will focus on the transcranial techniques in detail.

Another contemporary development has gained increased importance in the general management paradigm of cavernous sinus lesions as an adjunct to surgical treatment, namely stereotactic radiosurgery. Radiosurgery has become an integral management option for these lesions, either as an adjunct to surgery, or as a stand-alone treatment. This modality must be considered in the discussion of surgical treatment of cavernous sinus lesions.

Indications

The indications for direct operative attack on neoplastic lesions arising in or involving the cavernous sinus have been a matter of debate. New forms of therapy, such as stereotactic radiosurgery, are providing alternatives in our armamentarium for treating these difficult tumors.[25-27] A more restrictive set of indications for operative intervention has evolved within the past decade. We briefly consider the presently acceptable indications for a direct operation on these lesions.

The presence of a mass in the cavernous sinus, of course, does not itself constitute an indication for a direct operation. Many variables must be taken into account, including the age and medical condition of the patient, imaging characteristics, adjacent structures involved, time course of the process, and functional severity of symptoms. Many patients, because of poor medical condition or refusal to undergo surgery, may not be candidates for intracavernous microsurgery under any circumstances. The primary indications for surgery in most cases at present depend upon whether radiosurgery can be done safely as the primary treatment or not. Patients that have direct involvement, for example, of the optic apparatus by extension of tumor, cannot have radiosurgical treatment without significant risk of radiation delivery over acceptable minimums to these structures. In such case, an expert debulking of the lesion with creation of sufficient space between residual tumor and the optic apparatus is indicated. Patients with symptoms such as severe retro-orbital pain are also considered candidates for a debulking procedure, in order to relieve them of symptoms. Reports have demonstrated that stereotactic radiosurgery presents a viable alternative in patients with most intracavernous meningiomas.[27] At present, most patients who harbor lesions of the cavernous sinus are considered for radiosurgical treatment as primary treatment, with the possibility of surgery as an adjunct to their overall treatment. In some cases, patients with benign, well-circumscribed tumors in the cavernous sinus are candidates for a primary surgical approach for resection of the lesion. Most of these patients have lesions that are consistent with benign tumors of the region (e.g., neurinomas, cavernous hemangiomas, pituitary adenomas, dermoids, chordomas, and chondrosarcomas). These tumors tend to be well-encapsulated masses that are dissectible from the surrounding structures.

Patients with apparent meningiomas of the cavernous sinus, although their tumors are benign, are considered for surgery only in select circumstances. Patients who are able to undergo surgery who have debilitating symptoms, such as rapid visual loss or painful ophthalmoplegia, are offered an operation with the goal of decreasing the mass of the tumor and providing space for the tumor to expand via decompression at the skull base. The goal of such an operation is decompression of the involved structures, with a total resection attempted only when circumstances are very favorable. Patients with asymptomatic, small meningiomas are followed up with serial scans until they show enlargement of the mass or neurologic symptoms. A select few patients with tumors that are located at the lateral wall of the cavernous sinus and involve the temporal dura propria without cavernous invasion may be offered surgery. This is reasonable in such situations as the tumor can be completely removed with a minimum of risk of permanent neurologic deficits. These decisions rely on the judgment of the surgeon experienced with tumors in this area.

Difficult decisions are made in cases in which cavernous sinus involvement occurs by extensions of malignant processes from the paranasal sinuses and pharynx. Procedures treating such disorders are palliative because of the characteristically aggressive nature of these tumors, such as squamous cell carcinoma. En bloc resection of the cavernous sinus and adjacent areas may represent merely a heroic effort on the patient's behalf, with little realistic chance of long-term survival. Localized malignancies are an entirely different prospect in most cases. Local invasion by chordomas or chondrosarcomas can be effectively resected almost totally in many cases, with long-term recurrence-free survival, even though these tumors are incurable.[13]

Regardless of the process, surgery for these lesions is a formidable undertaking. As experience with these lesions advances, the indications will change according to technological developments and growing surgical capabilities. This discussion outlines the methods for operative intervention when such an approach is deemed appropriate.

Surgical Anatomy

Work focusing on the microsurgical anatomy of the cavernous sinus and its adjacent structures has made a critical contribution to our understanding and capabilities in dealing with neoplasms involving the cavernous sinus.[7,28-32] The individual surgeon's facility with the anatomic details of this complex region cannot be overemphasized as a basis for successful surgical therapy. The anatomy as presented in conventional texts, although an important initial basis, provides insufficient knowledge for the neurosurgeon operating in this region. An intimate comprehension of the multiple entry corridors and their specific anatomic substrates and boundaries is critical to the safe implementation of these procedures. Adequate preparation, including judicious use of the cadaver dissection laboratory, enhances the chances for a successful approach to these lesions. This has become especially important with the introduction of advanced endonasal endoscopic techniques. These techniques introduce an entirely separate skill set that requires development in the laboratory to gain comfort and facility with the endoscope and the special instruments.

The cavernous sinus is a tetrahedron-shaped space that is bounded on all sides by dura mater. It is located on either side of the sella turcica at the convergence of the anterior fossa, middle fossa, sphenoid ridge, and petroclival ridge. The contents of the sinus are contained within a membranous structure. Inferiorly and medially, this membrane consists of a periosteal layer of dura that covers the middle fossa and sella turcica. The superior and lateral portion of this outer cavernous membrane is contiguous with the connective tissue sheaths of cranial nerves III, IV, and V. This "true," or outer, cavernous membrane contains the structures within the cavernous sinus. A heavy venous plexus with connections to the ophthalmic veins, the pterygoid plexus, the superior and inferior petrosal sinuses, the basilar venous plexus, and the superficial middle cerebral veins via the sphenoparietal sinus is contained in the space. The internal carotid artery (ICA) and its branches, accompanied by a sympathetic plexus of nerves, pass through the sinus. Also, the cranial nerve VI travels through the cavernous sinus to enter the superior orbital fissure under the ophthalmic division of cranial nerve V.

The anatomy of the intracavernous carotid artery deserves special attention. The artery enters the cavernous sinus, piercing the true cavernous membrane, at the foramen lacerum. It is surrounded here by a thickening of this connective tissue, which forms a fibrous ring around the artery. The artery then bends anterosuperiorly toward the superior orbital fissure. Just distal to this bend, the meningohypophyseal trunk typically arises on the superomedial side. This trunk has three branches: (1) the tentorial (Bernasconi-Cassinari), (2) the dorsal meningeal, and (3) the inferior hypophyseal arteries, all of which display some variability. The carotid artery usually gives rise to the artery of the inferior cavernous sinus on its lateral side as it courses anteriorly. This vessel traverses the sinus, usually crossing over cranial nerve VI, and anastomoses with several branches of the internal maxillary artery. These anastomoses include: (1) the recurrent meningeal artery at the superior orbital fissure, (2) the artery of the foramen rotundum, (3) the accessory meningeal artery at the foramen ovale, and (4) the middle meningeal artery at the foramen spinosum. The tentorial artery is absent from the meningohypophyseal trunk in some cases, and in these situations, a marginal tentorial artery is typically found arising from the artery of the inferior cavernous sinus.[29] In a few patients (~10%), branches off the medial side of this segment (known as McConnell's capsular arteries) supply the capsule of the pituitary gland.[29]

The artery makes another bend in the anterior portion of the cavernous sinus superomedially. This segment of the artery exits the cavernous sinus and pierces the enveloping membrane. The membrane in this region is called the carotico-oculomotor membrane, because it spans the gap between the oculomotor nerve in the medial wall of the cavernous sinus and the carotid artery.[29,33] This loop is then completed in the extracavernous, extradural space under the anterior clinoid process. This loop has been designated the siphon segment, or clinoidal segment, and continues posteriorly a short distance before piercing the dura. Here, it is surrounded by a fibrous ring of dura, and the ophthalmic artery typically originates just inside this fibrous dural ring.[33-35]

The ICA has been assigned nomenclature that divides it into several segments by different authors. We have been using the system described by Fischer in 1938, which numbers the segments beginning from the carotid bifurcation.[36] We make a small modification to the original system with regard to numbering the petrous carotid segment (Fig. 38-1).

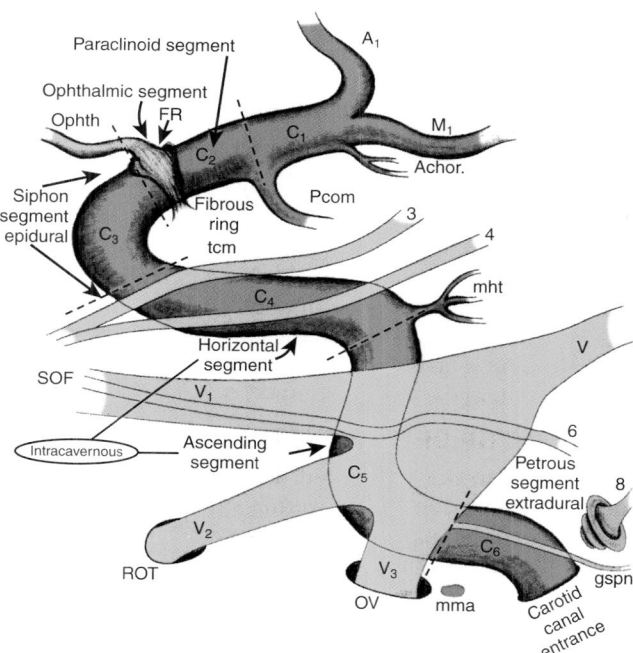

FIGURE 38-1 Illustration of the segmental nomenclature of the intracranial internal carotid artery. The divisions are indicated by the *dashed lines.* C1 begins at the bifurcation and extends to the origin of the posterior communicating artery (Pcom). C2 extends to the fibrous dural ring, making C1 and C2 the two intradural segments of the vessel. C3 corresponds to the extradural, extracavernous carotid siphon segment, which is delimited by the fibrous dural ring and the carotico-oculomotor membrane. C4 is truly intracavernous and extends to the origin of the meningohypophyseal trunk (mht). The C5 segment is mainly inferior to the trigeminal complex and extends from the meningohypophyseal trunk to the posterolateral fibrous ring, at which point the carotid artery becomes extracavernous. The C6 segment is the horizontal intrapetrous carotid artery. gspn, greater superficial petrosal nerve; mma, middle meningeal artery; SOF, superior orbital fissure; V2, mandibular division of trigeminal complex; V3, maxillary division of trigeminal complex. *(Modified from Fischer E. Die Lagabweichrugan der vorderen Hirnarterie in Gefassbild. Zentralb Neurochir. 1938;3:300-312.)*

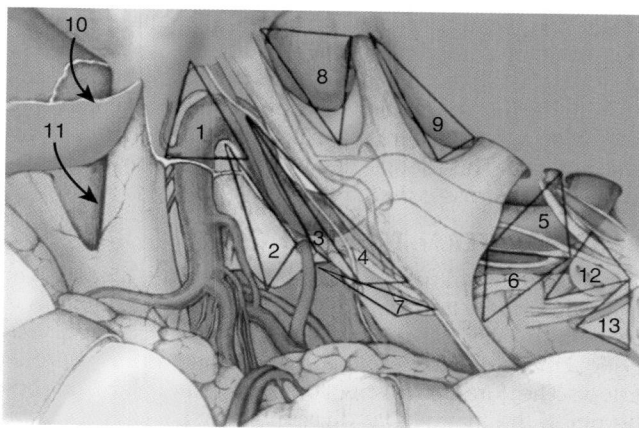

FIGURE 38-2 A geometric construct of the entry corridors to the cavernous sinus region. 1, anterior triangle; 2, medial triangle; 3, superior triangle; 4, lateral triangle; 5, posterolateral triangle; 6, posteromedial triangle; 7, posteroinferior triangle; 8, anterolateral triangle; 9, far lateral triangle; 10, anterior tip of the cavernous sinus route; 11, extended transsphenoidal route; 12, premeatal triangle; 13, postmeatal triangle.

The C1 segment begins at the carotid bifurcation and extends to the origin of the posterior communicating artery. C2 is the ophthalmic segment described by Day, stretching from the posterior communicating artery to the fibrous dural ring.[33] The extradural, extracavernous clinoid segment is given the designation of C3. C4 is the true intracavernous segment of the artery and is delimited by the carotico-oculomotor membrane anteriorly and the origin of the meningohypophyseal trunk posteriorly. From the meningohypophyseal trunk, the artery is designated as C5 until it has passed under the trigeminal nerve. The intrapetrous portion begins at the point at which V3 crosses over the artery and extends to its entrance into the carotid canal in the infratemporal fossa. This segment is designated as C6.

Crucial to the surgeon's understanding of the relevant surgical anatomy of the cavernous sinus is a thorough working knowledge of the multiple triangular entry corridors into the region. The various entry points have been described by various authors and were brought together into a unified geometric construct of the region in 1986 by Fukushima.[7] This scheme is illustrated in Fig. 38-2. Surgical facility with cavernous sinus lesions requires intimate knowledge of the entry spaces into the cavernous sinus in order to minimize morbidity. The anatomy as encountered from the endonasal endoscopic approaches is an important additional consideration. Understanding of the cavernous sinus from this additional perspective is an absolute prerequisite to such procedures.

A thorough working knowledge of the following entry corridors is a reasonable prerequisite to operating in the region. Because of the complicated anatomy and the potential for difficult hemostasis, this construct organizes the region in such a way that provides an anatomic foundation for the operative principles outlined herein.

ANTERIOR TRIANGLE

The anterior triangle describes an epidural space that contains the C3 portion of the ICA. It is exposed by removal of the anterior clinoid process, either intradurally or extradurally. The boundaries of the triangle are the extradural optic nerve, the fibrous dural ring, and the medial wall of the superior orbital fissure.[4-6,37] The C3 carotid segment enters this space by piercing the carotico-oculomotor membrane. It is important to bear in mind the proximity of the oculomotor nerve, which runs in the medial wall of the superior orbital fissure, thus in apposition to the lateral boundary of this space.

MEDIAL TRIANGLE

The medial triangle is delimited by the intradural carotid artery, the posterior clinoid process, the porus oculomotorius, and the siphon angle of the carotid artery.[9] This space is the primary corridor of access to the C4 portion of the carotid and thus is used for the direct approach to most intracavernous aneurysms. This space is also critical in terms of exposure for most intracavernous tumors.

SUPERIOR TRIANGLE

The medial and lateral boundaries of the superior triangle are cranial nerves III and IV, respectively.[7] The posterior margin is the edge of the dura along the petrous ridge. This triangle is the entry corridor used to locate the meningohypophyseal trunk.

LATERAL TRIANGLE

Described by Parkinson in 1965, the lateral triangle is a very narrow space that is delimited by the trochlear nerve medially and by the ophthalmic division of the trigeminal nerve laterally.[1] Again, the dura of the petrous ridge forms the posterior margin. This triangle can be opened to expose cranial nerve VI as it crosses the C5 segment of the carotid artery.

POSTEROLATERAL TRIANGLE

The posterolateral triangle, first described by Glasscock in 1968, describes the location of the horizontal intrapetrous carotid artery.[38] Exposure of the artery in this space is a critical maneuver in gaining proximal control of the carotid artery. The foramen ovale, foramen spinosum, posterior border of the mandibular division of the trigeminal nerve, and cochlear apex define this space. Removal of the bone of this triangle exposes approximately 10 mm of the C6 segment of the carotid artery.[39,40]

POSTEROMEDIAL TRIANGLE

The posteromedial triangle describes the anterior petrous projection of a volume of bone that can be removed to make a window in the petrous apex to the posterior fossa. First described by Kawase and colleagues, this space is delimited by the cochlea, the porus trigeminus, and the posterior border of V3 at the posterior apex of the posterolateral triangle.[41,42] If this triangle is used to make a window in the petrous bone, the anterior brain stem and root of the trigeminal nerve can be reached without encountering neural or vascular structures in the bone.

POSTEROINFERIOR TRIANGLE

The porus trigeminus, posterior clinoid, and entrance to Dorello's canal define this triangle. An incision in this area exposes the petrosphenoidal ligament (Gruber's ligament), which forms the roof of Dorello's canal. Cranial nerve VI can be observed in this space making the first of its two bends, the second occurring as it crosses the intracavernous carotid artery.

ANTEROLATERAL TRIANGLE

The anterolateral triangle is defined by the area between the first and second divisions of the trigeminal nerve as they exit the middle cranial fossa. The anterior border of the triangle is an imaginary line drawn from the lateral edge of the superior orbital fissure to the medial lip of the foramen rotundum. This space is the entry point for exposure of the superior orbital vein and cranial nerve VI and is used to gain access to carotid-cavernous fistulas.[43]

LATERALMOST TRIANGLE (LATERAL LOOP)

Analogous to the anterolateral triangle, this space is bounded by V2, V3, and an imaginary line from the foramen rotundum to the foramen ovale. Lateral extensions of cavernous sinus tumors are also reached through this route. In some patients, the sphenoidal emissary foramen and vein are found here, communicating the cavernous sinus with the pterygoid venous plexus.[29]

PREMEATAL TRIANGLE

The premeatal triangle is used to help define the location of the cochlea from the middle fossa angle of view. The boundaries are the medial lip of the internal acoustic meatus, the intrapetrous carotid genu, and the geniculate ganglion. The cochlea is located in the basal portion of this triangle. This triangle is important in cases in which the petrous apex is removed through the extradural middle fossa approach.[39,40]

POSTMEATAL TRIANGLE

The postmeatal triangle delimits the volume of bone located between the internal auditory canal (IAC) and the superior semicircular canal and is used to maximize bone removal of the petrous apex through an extradural middle fossa approach.[39] The boundaries are the geniculate ganglion, the lateral lip of the internal acoustic meatus, and the posterior end of the arcuate eminence.

ANTERIOR TIP OF THE CAVERNOUS SINUS

This entry corridor is affected through either an anterior transbasal approach to the cavernous sinus or an endonasal trans-sphenoidal approach, which exposes the apical portion of the region. Bilateral exposure of the carotid siphon and the C4 segment is obtained through this strategy.

BACK OF THE CAVERNOUS SINUS

Through an extended endonasal trans-sphenoidal approach, the posteroinferior aspect of the cavernous sinus is appreciated from the underside. The bilateral C4 segments are seen after wide removal of the sellar floor toward the carotid eminence. This exposure is useful in cases of large pituitary adenomas that extend into the cavernous sinus.

Anesthetic and Monitoring Techniques

The ability of modern neuroanesthesia to facilitate operative procedures by providing increased relaxation of neural tissue and pharmacologic protection against ischemia has realized great improvements over the past forty years. Several maneuvers are used in transcranial cases to help maximize exposure while minimizing retraction of the brain. Administration of osmotic diuretic agents is routine at the beginning of each surgery. We infuse 20% mannitol solution (0.5 mg/kg) along with furosemide (20–40 mg) at the time of skin incision. Further relaxation is attained by maintenance of end-tidal carbon dioxide in the range of 25 to 30 mm Hg. In some cases, these maneuvers alone may not be adequate to provide adequate relaxation, necessitating the use of cerebrospinal fluid (CSF) drainage. This procedure is performed either through a ventricular catheter or a lumbar drain. We rarely use lumbar drainage of CSF in our transcranial cases, mainly because of personal preference. Patients with significant elevation of intracranial pressure are not well served by insertion of a lumbar drain at the beginning of the operation. If necessary, the safest and least complicated method is insertion of a catheter into the frontal horn of the lateral ventricle; this provides ample and accurate drainage of CSF throughout the operation. Administration of osmotic diuretic agents is not on the whole necessary in endonasal endoscopic trans-sphenoidal approaches to the cavernous sinus. In some cases, the pressure gradient between the intracranial compartment and the sphenoid sinus works to the advantage of the surgeon in terms of delivery of tumor into the field for removal. In general, lumbar drains are inserted in these cases when diversion of cerebrospinal fluid is necessary for help in closure of dural defects.

Neurophysiologic monitoring is routinely used in all cases. The specific configuration is tailored to each case, taking into consideration the operative approach and the neural and vascular structures likely to be compromised. Somatosensory-evoked potentials and electroencephalographic data are always recorded when there is a potential for temporary occlusion of the carotid artery. When the operative approach involves exposure of any part of the facial nerve, facial nerve monitoring is employed.[44] Visual and brain-stem auditory-evoked potentials have not found much application in our cases of tumors involving primarily the cavernous sinus. But certainly in cases of posterior fossa skull base tumors with cavernous sinus extension, facial nerve monitoring is mandatory.

Before planned occlusion of the carotid artery, a suppressive agent (e.g., propofol) is administered to the point of electroencephalographic burst suppression. Burst suppression is then maintained for the entire period of occlusion. Even with burst suppression, the best results are obtained when occlusion time is minimal. Any attenuation of response is an indicator that tolerance to occlusion may be limited, and preservation of the evoked potentials predicts tolerance to ischemia induced by occlusion. However, this is not always the case.

Surgical Approaches

The cavernous sinus region may be approached through several different corridors. The appropriate choice of surgical approach is dictated mainly by the extent and character of involvement of adjacent structures. Some lesions are fairly well confined within the bounds of the cavernous sinus and require only a straightforward dissection of the region. Other lesions require the combination of two or more standard approaches to gain adequate access to the lesion. Others are best handled by some variation of one of the standard approaches, and this is a point that we wish to emphasize. Because of the high potential for morbidity associated with these operations, we approach each lesion individually, tailoring our approach according to the exposure expected to be necessary. Maneuvers that put particular structures at unnecessary risk and lengthen operating time are not used.

Mainly the specific entry corridors to the cavernous sinus expected to be used to resect the lesion dictate surgical strategy. The cavernous sinus can be divided into four separate quadrants. Lesions involving the anteromedial region are approached via the anteromedial and anterolateral triangles. Because these two triangles are exposed extradurally, in selected cases (e.g., neurinoma of V2), opening the dura might not be necessary in resecting such a lesion. This concept similarly applies to lesions located in the anterolateral quadrant, approached via the lateral loop and posterolateral triangles (Fig. 38-3A). This location of tumor also invites consideration of an endonasal endoscopic extended transsphenoidal approach. More posterior lesions, involving the posteromedial and posterolateral regions of the cavernous sinus, usually require exposure through the medial, superior, and lateral triangles (see Fig. 38-3B). These triangles, although possible to open through an extradural route, are typically entered intradurally. Posteromedial lesions without extension lateral to the cavernous carotid artery may also be considered for an endonasal endoscopic approach.

Masses confined mainly to the posterolateral quadrant of the region are best approached in our opinion laterally through the middle fossa (see Fig. 38-3C). Lesions involving more than one of these four areas, for example, a mass with extensive posterior cavernous involvement with extension into the posterior fossa, may require a combined approach for adequate exposure (see Fig. 38-3D). This type of lesion requires a combined strategy via an anterolateral and middle fossa transpetrosal approach. Many lesions require more than one of the standard approaches for satisfactory exposure, and the experience and judgment of the surgeon are necessary to adequately plan the procedure. We outline the standard approaches to intracavernous neoplasms used in our practice and discuss the general indications for their use.

FRONTOTEMPORAL EPIDURAL AND SUBDURAL APPROACH TO THE CAVERNOUS SINUS

Dolenc is credited with the initial development and use of the combined epidural and subdural frontotemporal approach (anteromedial transcavernous approach), originally used to directly approach intracavernous aneurysms.[4,6] This technique has become the standard by which lesions within the cavernous sinus are approached. This strategy effectively exposes lesions confined to the cavernous sinus and those with extension to the supratentorial compartment. Lesions with extension into the petroclival area and the posterior fossa are not well exposed by this approach. The method is, however, easily combined with a more lateral approach (e.g., middle fossa transpetrosal) to gain access to such posterior extensions of tumor. Dolenc's combined epidural and subdural strategy has been modified in several ways.[37,47-49] These modifications largely center around the bone flap used and the extent of extradural bone removal at the skull base. The following discussion presents these modifications as alternatives to the basic approach; the modifications are selected on the basis of the exposure expected to be necessary.

Positioning

After induction of general endotracheal anesthesia, the patient is placed in the supine position on the operating table. The table is flexed approximately 30 degrees, and the patient's legs are propped up on one or two pillows. The Mayfield pin headrest is applied with the two-pin arm on the dependent side. We place the posteriormost pin at the inion and rotate the arm such that the anterior pin comes to rest on the body of the mastoid. The single pin is placed inside the hairline, lateral to the contralateral mid-pupillary line. The head position is rotated approximately 30 degrees, with the vertex neutral. When in the proper orientation with respect to rotation, the malar eminence is the highest point of the head. The back of the table is then tilted such that the head is at, or slightly above, the level of the heart. The patient is now ready for the final skin preparation and draping.

Incision and Flap Elevation

We use three different methods of initial scalp incision and elevation, the choice of which depends mainly on the amount of inferior-to-superior exposure desired. Also, three different methods of craniotomy are used, again depending on the degree of inferior-to-superior exposure necessary.

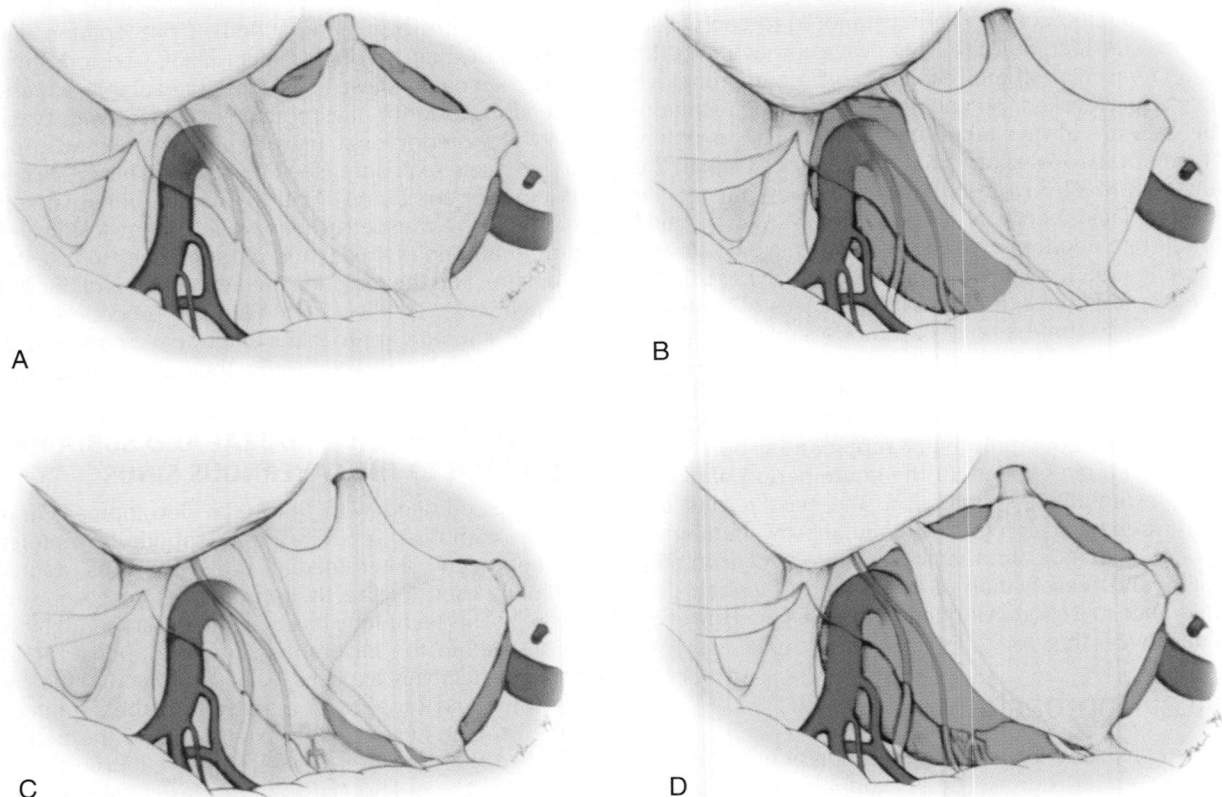

FIGURE 38-3 A, Tumors with their primary component located in the anterolateral quadrant of the cavernous sinus can often be approached exclusively through an extradural route to open the anterolateral and far lateral triangles. The mass illustrated may also require exposure via the posterolateral or posteromedial triangles but still remain extradural. B, This tumor is located in the posteromedial and anteromedial quadrants, which would require intradural exposure and dissection via the medial, superior, and lateral cavernous triangles. The anteromedial component could be resected via an extradural exposure of the anterior triangle. C, Masses with their greatest bulk in the posterolateral quadrant of the cavernous sinus are best handled via a lateral approach, again entirely extradural. D, Extensive lesions that involve all quadrants of the cavernous sinus and extend to the posterior fossa or the para/suprasellar regions require a combined approach for adequate exposure.

Single-Layer Technique

The standard one-layer technique is used when the requirement for extradural bone removal is minimal, and a limited inferior-to-superior viewing angle will be necessary. Also, this technique does not include the creation of a vascularized pericranial flap for use at closure. We begin the incision just anterior to the tragus at the level of the zygoma root and proceed superiorly, inside the hairline. The incision curves gently forward, ending in the midline. The temporalis muscle and fascia are incised. Particular attention is paid to the area around the zygoma root. The temporalis muscle is freed from its attachment to the zygoma root, which yields increased elevation of the muscle anteriorly. Use of monopolar cautery in this area should be restrained because of the proximity of the frontalis branch of the facial nerve. The pericranium medial to the superior temporal line is elevated with the temporalis muscle and fascia. This myocutaneous flap is elevated anteriorly to expose the frontozygomatic recess and is held in place with large hooks.

Half-and-Half Technique

The half-and-half method is used when a vascularized pericranial flap is desired and obtaining a high degree of inferior-to-superior exposure is not necessary. After the skin incision has been made, the flap is elevated medial to the superior temporal line in two layers by sharp dissection of the areolar connective tissue layer between the pericranium and the galea. Care must be exercised to avoid damaging the supraorbital nerve, which lies adherent to the galea and can be mistakenly included in the pericranial layer. At the superior temporal line, the pericranium is incised. The temporalis muscle and fascia are then elevated with the scalp and reflected anteriorly, just as in the single-layer technique. The pericranium is then elevated from the bone to the supraorbital rim and reflected anteriorly. We protect this flap by wrapping it in wet gauze, and we keep it moist during the operation.

Two-Layer Technique

The two-layer technique is used when increased inferior-to-superior trajectory is necessary, because this technique results in reflection of the temporalis muscle inferiorly and laterally. This method rotates the muscle away from the orbital rim and frontozygomatic recess, thus preventing the muscle mass from creating an obstruction when the microscope is radically rotated to obtain a more rostral view. The skin incision is typically started slightly more inferiorly, exposing the entire zygomatic root. Beginning medially, the galeal layer is elevated from the pericranium, and the areolar bands, which span the two layers, are sharply divided. Again, the supraorbital and supratrochlear nerves must be preserved with the galeal layer. As the superior temporal line is reached, the areolar connective tissue that is continuous with the pericranial layer is elevated with the galea, which exposes bare temporalis fascia. The critical step in this maneuver is handling the temporal fat pad. This fat pad consists of superficial and deep components. The superficial fat pad is surrounded by the loose areolar connective tissue overlying the temporalis fascia and contains the frontalis branches of the facial nerve. The fat pad is elevated with the areolar tissue and the galeal layer. The galeal layer is elevated to expose the supraorbital rim, lateral orbital rim, and entire zygomatic process, which is covered by fascia. The deep fat pad is situated over the inferior portion of the temporalis muscle as it passes under the zygomatic arch and is covered by fascia. This pad of fat is left in place and retracted with the muscle (Fig. 38-4).

The temporalis muscle is now elevated. This elevation is begun anteriorly at the lateral orbital rim, and the periosteum is incised so as to leave a cuff for reattachment of the fascia. The muscle is elevated without any incision being made in this structure and is reflected inferiorly and posteriorly. Elevation of the temporalis muscle is always done via subperiosteal dissection, avoiding the use of cautery. This helps to preserve the vascular supply and innervation of the muscle, leading to a decreased chance of postoperative atrophy. The vascularized pericranial flap is next elevated and reflected anteriorly as described earlier for the half-and-half technique.

CRANIOTOMY AND EXTRADURAL BONE REMOVAL

As with the elevation of the skin flap, the degree of inferior-to-superior exposure and the posterior limits of the expected dissection determine the type of bone flap to be used. A routine pterional bone flap is sufficient for masses limited to the anterior and anterolateral cavernous sinus. Tumors with much more extensive involvement posteriorly and those that escape the confines of the region require a more generous cranial opening for adequate exposure.

Frontotemporal Craniotomy

This is the most frequently used bone flap and provides satisfactory exposure in most cases. Two or three burr holes are made, preferably with the pediatric-sized burr hole drill bit. The first hole is placed in the keyhole area in an attempt to straddle the sphenoid ridge. The second hole is placed directly posterior, just below the superior temporal line, at the posterior limit of the exposed bone. The third hole is optional and is placed inferiorly, in the temporal squama, just above the floor of the middle fossa. Typically, the flap is made with a more generous frontal exposure than that typically used for an anterior circulation aneurysm. The dimensions are usually approximately 7 to 8 cm by 5 cm, centered one third above and two thirds below the superior temporal line. The temporal squama remaining inferiorly is removed, resulting in a flat angle of view along the middle fossa floor. The dura is then tacked to the posterosuperior bone margin with fine suture through obliquely drilled wire-pass holes.

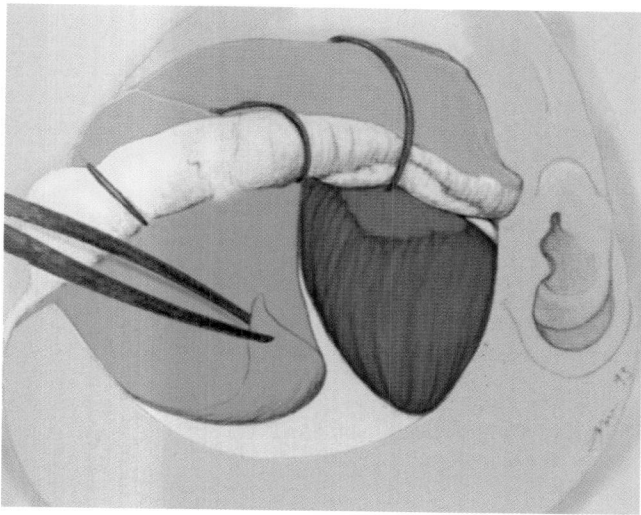

FIGURE 38-4 The two-layer scalp flap technique is illustrated, preserving the frontalis branches of the facial nerve by splitting the superficial and deep temporal fat pads. This technique preserves a vascularized periosteal flap, which is used in closure of the skull base. Note the preservation of the supraorbital nerve.

With a generous frontal extension toward the midline, the frontal sinus is frequently encountered. An open frontal sinus must be handled properly to avoid an annoying complication from a CSF leak or postoperative infection. It is not necessary to completely exenterate the mucosa of the sinus. Rather, the most important element of preventing a mucocele is to maintain patency of the nasofrontal duct. Incomplete or inadequate closure of the nasofrontal duct can lead to inadequate drainage from any remaining mucosa and result in a mucocele in a delayed fashion. The opening to the sinus is probably best handled by covering the opening with vascularized tissue, such as the pericranial flap, such that the opening is sealed.

Transzygomatic Craniotomy

This craniotomy method is infrequently employed. It is probably best suited for lesions with a large middle fossa extension where expanded access to the middle fossa is necessary. After the galeal layer is reflected by use of the two-layer technique, the periosteum of the zygomatic process and the lateral orbital rim is incised and elevated. We make this incision in such a way that leaves a cuff of tissue for later reapproximation. The temporalis muscle is freed from the temporal squama and of its attachment to the inner surface of the zygoma. The zygoma is now cut with a sagittal or reciprocating saw (Fig. 38-5). The anterior cut is made parallel to the lateral orbital rim, beginning at the frontozygomatic suture, leaving as little bone overhanging the frontozygomatic recess as possible. The posterior cut is made roughly parallel to the surface of the temporal squama through the root of the temporal zygomatic process, and care is taken to avoid invasion of the temporomandibular joint. This technique results in what we call a "T-bone" cut and maximizes inferior temporalis muscle retraction, resulting in an increased ability to gain an inferior-to-superior view. A frontotemporal craniotomy is now made as described earlier. The remaining temporal squama is removed to obtain a flat viewing angle along the middle cranial fossa floor.

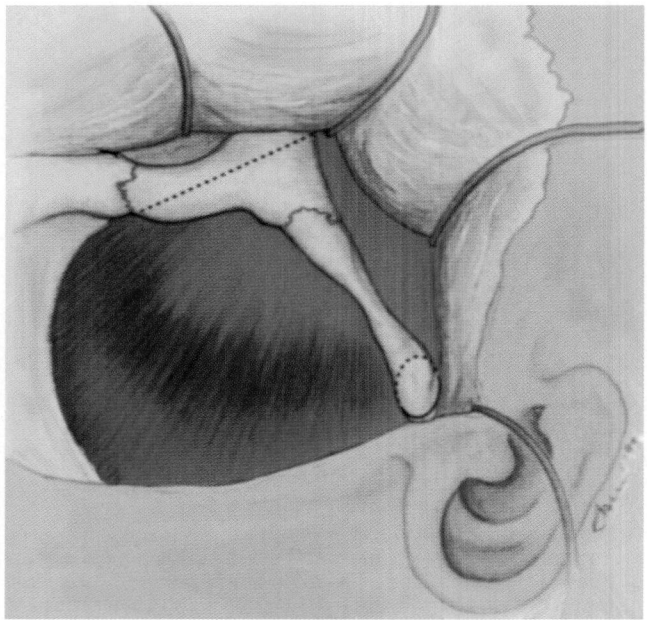

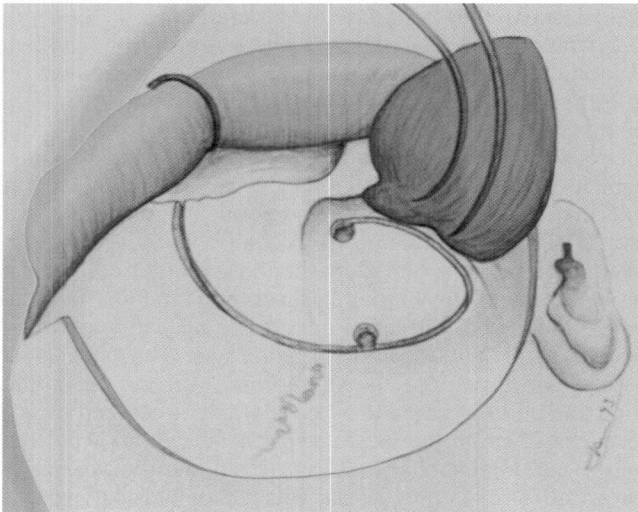

FIGURE 38-6 The initial craniotome osteotomy is illustrated, extending through the medial orbital rim.

FIGURE 38-5 The osteotomies used for the transzygomatic craniotomy are demonstrated. This method results in what is called a T-bone cut, maximizing inferior temporalis retraction.

Orbitozygomatic Craniotomy

This craniotomy technique results in maximal inferior-to-superior trajectory and allows the widest access to the cavernous sinus up toward the brain base. This technique is the most common craniotomy utilized for transcranial approaches to the cavernous sinus. The scalp flap must be made in two layers, and elevation of the pericranium is extended to include the periorbital fascia. The periorbital fascia is elevated from the midline superiorly to the inferolateral aspect of the orbit. This tissue must be freed to a depth of approximately 1.5 cm inside the orbit. If the supraorbital nerve travels through a supraorbital foramen, freeing the nerve is necessary. By use of a small osteotome, the bone of the foramen is removed in a wedge to free the nerve and allow forward reflection with the pericranium.

Two burr holes are then made, one in the keyhole area and the second about 5 cm posteriorly, inferior to the superior temporal line. Next, the thick bore that connects the anterior temporal base to the orbital wall is drilled away. Then, a cut is made with the craniotome beginning at the posterior burr hole, proceeding inferiorly toward the middle fossa floor, and then curving upward over the temporal line to meet the pterional burr hole (Fig. 38-6). A sagittal or reciprocating saw is now used to cut the zygoma root parallel to the squamosal surface, as described earlier (Fig. 38-7). The next cut is made roughly parallel to, and several millimeters above, the zygomaticomaxillary suture, cutting into the lateral wall of the orbit. The medial supraorbital rim is cut and continued posteriorly several millimeters into the orbital roof. The orbital wall is next incised, either with the sagittal saw or a small osteotome, from medial to lateral, thus freeing the supraorbital and lateral orbital rims (Fig. 38-8). The final cut made is through the articulation of the zygomatic and sphenoid bones from posterior. These bone incisions free the flap as a single unit. Sometimes the

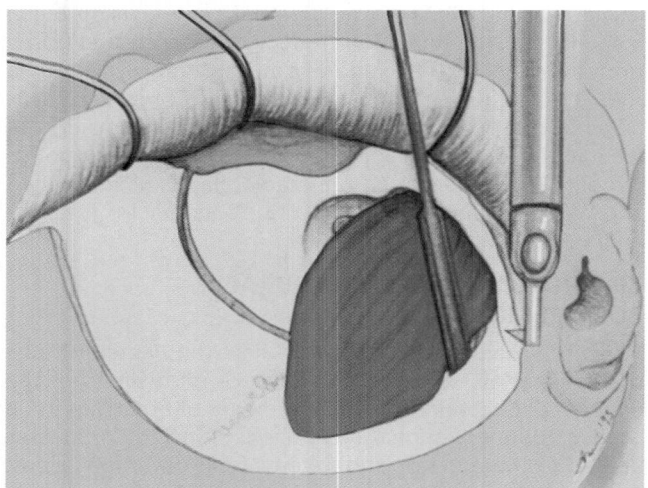

FIGURE 38-7 The root of the zygomatic process is cut parallel to the surface of the temporal squama to prevent any obstructing process to maximal inferior temporalis retraction.

flap needs to be freed from some remaining attachment of the sphenoid wing; this is easily accomplished via fracturing of that remaining attachment.

Extradural Bone Removal

Extradural removal of bone at the cranial base provides several advantages. Primarily, reduction of cranial base bone volume reduces the degree of necessary retraction of neural structures. Second, removal of bone surrounding neural structures as they pass through bone canals results in mobility of these structures without impingement against bone surfaces, which may result in pressure-induced ischemia. Third, transposition of neural and vascular structures from their bone canals results in wider corridors of access. In this chapter, we describe the technique for maximal removal of the anterolateral base; however, the extent of removal of the cranial base is individualized for each case. Risk is associated with every degree of bone removal at the

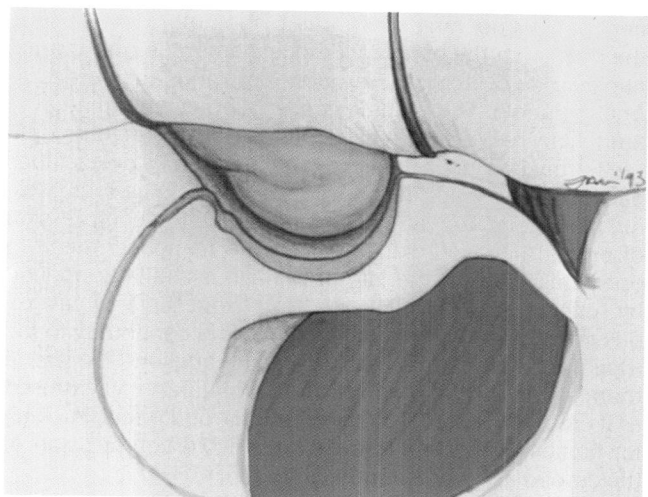

FIGURE 38-8 Intraorbitally, the osteotomy is made at a depth of approximately 10 to 15 mm. The zygoma is incised just superior to the zygomaticofrontal foramen (shown) and the zygomaticomaxillary suture.

skull base, and for this reason, determination of the exposure for each particular case is an important step in surgical planning.

The initial step in this procedure is reduction of the sphenoid wing. The dura is elevated and retracted with 4-mm tapered retractors. Under constant irrigation, the sphenoid wing is reduced with a high-speed drill. Initially, the wing is flattened down to the level of the meningo-orbital artery as it joins the dura at the superior orbital fissure apex. Bone irregularities of the frontal floor are reduced with a diamond burr, resulting in a smooth contour of the orbital roof. The superior orbital fissure is skeletonized to expose approximately 10 mm of periorbital fascia, and the foramen rotundum is unroofed to the infratemporal peripheral branches to expose 5 to 8 mm of V2. When lateral cavernous exposure is desired, the foramen ovale is similarly unroofed to mobilize V3. The orbit may now be skeletonized, leaving only a thin shell of bone adherent to the periorbital fascia. The meningo-orbital artery, typically at the superior orbital fissure apex, is coagulated and divided. The adhesion of the dura at the superior orbital fissure apex is divided approximately 4 to 5 mm. This goal can be achieved without risk to cranial nerves III and IV.

The next stage of extradural bone removal, optic canal unroofing, is the most technically demanding. It is helpful to first locate the exit point of the nerve from the optic canal. A very short segment (about 1 mm) can be identified as it spans the gap between bone and dura. On the medial side, care must be taken to avoid entering the sphenoid sinus, which lies just medial to the optic canal. If the sinus is opened, it must be carefully exenterated of its mucosa and packed with either muscle or fat. The sinus may likewise be entered on the lateral side when the surgeon drills between the optic canal and anterior clinoid, while reducing the optic strut.

The anterior clinoid process is next removed on the lateral side of the optic canal. Optimal technique is critical because the anterior clinoid process is surrounded by the optic nerve, ICA, and contents of the superior orbital fissure.

Under constant cooling from irrigation, the anterior clinoid process is hollowed out with the diamond drill. This structure must never be removed in a single piece. The sides are thinned to the point at which the sides can be lightly fractured and dissected free from the dura. The very tip of the anterior clinoid is usually removed with the aid of small alligator forceps, and the small (1 to 2 mm) tip is gently twisted free after careful dural dissection. When the anterior clinoid is hollowed out, the surgeon must be ever cognizant of the relative positions of the optic nerve, the carotid artery, and the superior orbital fissure contents. The optic nerve is medial; the carotid artery, anterior and inferior; and cranial nerve III, lateral in the medial superior orbital fissure wall. At times, this removal is complicated by the presence of a bridge between the anterior and posterior clinoid processes, forming a caroticoclinoidal foramen. Under such circumstances, completing the resection of this structure intradurally may be necessary. Occasionally, with final removal of the anterior clinoid, bleeding from the cavernous sinus occurs, typically from disruption from the carotico-oculomotor membrane. This bleeding is controlled by packing one or two small pieces of Surgicel in the defect. Bipolar cautery should not be used because it is ineffective, and current may spread to the oculomotor nerve.

Next, the full anterolateral cranial base is skeletonized, and the neural structures become capable of being mobilized, after being freed from the constraints of their respective bone foramina (Fig. 38-9). Hemostasis is attained with the use of bone wax and monopolar cautery. Monopolar cautery should be used only in areas that do not have underlying sensitive structures. A typical example is in the middle fossa in the region of the tegmen tympani. Heat transfer through bone here can damage cranial nerve VII or the hearing apparatus.

When extradural exposure of the intrapetrous carotid artery is desired, it is appropriately exposed in the posterolateral triangle (Fig. 38-9). The dura must be elevated from the middle cranial fossa to expose the greater superficial petrosal nerve running in the major petrosal groove. The middle meningeal artery must be coagulated and divided as it exits the foramen spinosum. This vessel is usually surrounded by a plexus of veins, which must be effectively coagulated. With the greater superficial petrosal nerve exposed, the landmarks delineating the position of the carotid artery are apparent because the artery lies under the nerve and is running parallel, toward V3. Drilling is begun posterior to V3, just medial to the foramen spinosum. The greater superficial petrosal nerve is typically divided near V3 and reflected posteriorly for greater exposure of the ICA. Bone over the artery is removed from the tensor tympani muscle lateral to bone that lies under V3. The greatest danger in this procedure is violation of the cochlea, which lies 1 to 2 mm from the carotid genu. Excessive bone removal posterior to the carotid genu carries significant risk for cochlear violation.

Intradural Transcavernous Dissection

Neoplastic lesions that escape the bounds of the cavernous sinus typically require intradural exposure of adjacent regions. In these cases, the cavernous sinus may be opened through the medial, superior, and lateral triangles via an intradural dissection. This intradural approach to the

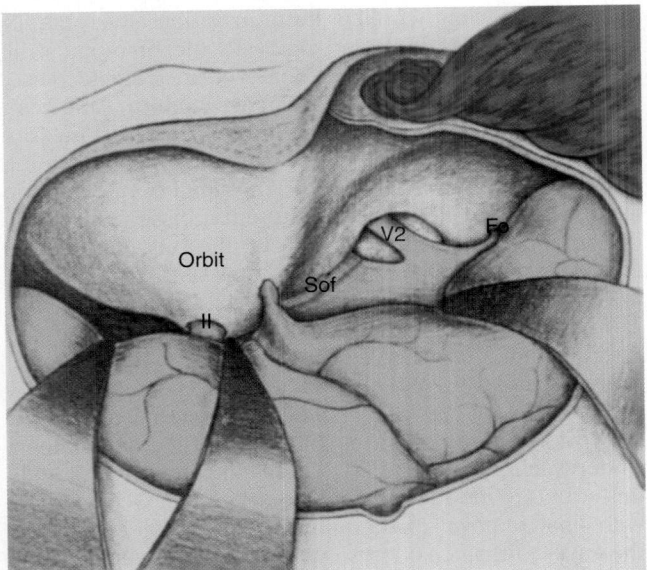

FIGURE 38-9 This figure illustrates the view of the anterior and middle cranial base at the completion of the extradural bone dissection to unroof the maxillary division of the trigeminal (V2), the superior orbital fissure (sof), and the optic nerve (II). fo, foramen ovale.

cavernous sinus begins with opening of the dura using a T-shaped incision. The incision starts at the anterior frontal corner of the exposure and curves downward, close to the posterior bone margin, toward the anterior temporal corner. A cut is then made along the dura that covers the sylvian fissure and proceeds toward the optic nerve dura, completing the T. The dural flaps are retracted forward and tacked down with fine suture.

Arachnoid dissection usually begins with splitting of the sylvian fissure. Dividing the anterior 3 to 4 cm is sufficient in most cases and provides adequate retraction of the frontal and temporal lobes while minimizing retractor pressure. It is often necessary to coagulate and divide the bridging veins of the temporal tip to mobilize the temporal lobe satisfactorily. The arachnoid surrounding the optic nerve and intradural carotid artery is then sharply divided, and damage to small perforating arteries is carefully avoided. Arachnoid division continues posteriorly to the tentorial edge, dividing the membrane of Lilequist to expose the oculomotor nerve as it enters the porus oculomotorius. The lateral dural wall of the cavernous sinus is now visible at this point of the dissection from the anterior margin of the middle fossa to the tentorial edge posteriorly.

The medial triangle of the cavernous sinus is readily opened at its apex after the carotid artery has been sharply liberated of its attachment at the fibrous dural ring. The dura over the triangle can then be incised toward the posterior clinoid, a procedure that produces a tremendous amount of bleeding, except when the region is filled with tumor. Bleeding is controlled by judicious packing with Surgicel. Medial and posterior packing can be fairly generous to close off the connections to the basilar venous plexus and inferior petrosal sinus. Lateral packing must be more modest to avoid compression of cranial nerve III.

Dissection of the superior triangle is best performed after opening of the medial triangle and liberation of cranial

nerve III by opening the porus oculomotorius, reflecting the dura from the outer cavernous membrane over cranial nerve III, and incising the outer cavernous membrane to free the nerve. The triangle can then be entered medial to cranial nerve IV. This triangle contains the meningohypophyseal trunk, which is subject to compression by overzealous packing of the space to control hemorrhage. Vigorous packing posteriorly and laterally can also result in compression of cranial nerve VI. Analogous to the maneuver made to open this triangle, the lateral triangle is similarly opened by reflecting the middle fossa dura from the true cavernous membrane over cranial nerve IV and continuing to the trigeminal first branch and semilunar ganglion. The lateral triangle can then be entered and cranial nerve VI exposed as it crosses over the intracavernous carotid artery. Packing for hemostasis in this triangle must avoid compression of the carotid artery and cranial nerve VI.

At the completion of the dissection, the anteromedial, anterolateral, and posteromedial quadrants of the cavernous sinus are exposed. The posterolateral portion is usually incompletely exposed via this dissection because of obstruction by the trigeminal complex. Intradurally, cranial nerve III is visible from the interpeduncular fossa to its entrance into the superior orbital fissure. Cranial nerve IV is seen from near its entrance into the incisural edge, crossing the cavernous sinus to enter the superior orbital fissure on top of cranial nerve III. Lateral to the trochlear nerve, in the lateral triangle, deflection of the ophthalmic division of the trigeminal nerve exposes cranial nerve VI crossing the intracavernous carotid artery. Incision of the incisural edge between the porus trochlearis and the porus trigeminus widely opens the posteroinferior triangle and Dorello's canal. Tumor is resected by use of the techniques outlined in the subsequent section, Special Techniques of Intracavernous Surgery.

Closure

Closure in these procedures is at times complicated. The goal of closure at the skull base is complete separation of the intradural compartment from extradural structures. A watertight dural closure is critical to the successful avoidance of postoperative complications secondary to CSF leakage and contamination, and fascial patch grafts are used as necessary to meet this goal. Even the most meticulous closure has the potential for small leaks. Therefore, all potential routes of communication should be closed off with autologous fat grafts and fascial barriers. As discussed earlier, opened paranasal sinuses must be exenterated of mucosa to avoid mucocele formation. Then, any ostia are obliterated and the sinus is occluded with muscle or fat. The fat or muscle graft is then best sealed from the dural closure by covering with an additional vascularized pericranial flap, and strategically placing tacking sutures prevents migration. We use titanium plates for securing the bone flap because of the superior cosmetic results obtained.

Anterolateral Temporopolar Transcavernous Approach

This approach provides access to the cavernous sinus from a more lateral trajectory than the standard frontotemporal method.[47] The technique makes use of extradural retraction of the frontal and temporal lobes, both to protect the cortical surface and to preserve the venous drainage of the temporal tip. The extensive extradural dissection provides a very wide corridor of access to the cavernous sinus region, as well as wide access to the infrachiasmatic and upper clival areas.

In contrast to the standard frontotemporal approach, the cavernous sinus triangles are opened from an extradural route, using minimal intradural dissection. Integral to the basis of this technique is an understanding of the anatomy of the lateral wall and roof of the cavernous sinus. The dura covering the cavernous sinus, on the undersurface of the temporal lobe, is adherent to the outer cavernous membrane. The outer (or "true") cavernous membrane is formed by the connective tissue sheaths of cranial nerves III, IV, and V and is continuous with periosteum at the bone margins. This membrane envelops the structures in the cavernous sinus. Thus the dura can be elevated from the outer cavernous membrane with minimal hemorrhage if no large tears are created in this membrane. The ability to expose the cavernous sinus in this way is the key element of this approach.

Closure typically requires a vascularized pericranial flap; therefore, the two-layer scalp flap technique is necessary. The incision is a generous frontotemporal incision, beginning at, or just below, the root of the zygomatic process. Any of the three bone flaps described earlier may be used for this approach. Again, the degree of inferior-to-superior trajectory that will be required dictates the use of the transzygomatic or orbitozygomatic flaps. Extradural bone removal proceeds as outlined earlier. The novel aspects of the approach begin when extradural bone removal is complete and the dura is ready to be opened.

Beginning at the superior orbital fissure apex, the meningo-orbital fibrous band is coagulated and divided. The temporal dura is retracted posteriorly. Elevation of the dural margin begins at the superior orbital fissure and extends laterally to the foramen ovale. At the junction of the periorbital fascia and dura, the cleavage plane is sharply developed, and the connective tissue fibrils bridging the dura and the outer cavernous membrane are divided, as the dura is retracted posteriorly. In this way, the dura is reflected from the outer cavernous membrane toward the petrous ridge (see Fig. 38-10). If this maneuver is performed properly, little bleeding occurs from the cavernous sinus. Cavernous sinus bleeding from small tears in the outer cavernous membrane is stopped by packing small pieces of Surgicel into the openings. The anteromedial limit in dural elevation is the tentorial edge, which is handled after the dura is opened.

The dura is now ready to be opened. An L-shaped incision is made beginning along the dura covering the sylvian fissure, approximately 5 cm from its attachment to the carotid artery. The incision is extended through optic nerve sheath dura and is then carried medially across the tuberculum sellae for 2 to 3 cm (Fig. 38-11). The retractors are replaced to provide posterior retraction on both the frontal and temporal lobes, and the fibrous dural ring surrounding the carotid artery is sharply freed from the vessel. The lateral portion of this fibrous ring is met by the tentorial edge, formed by a fold in the dura. The two layers composing this fold are then split. This maneuver elevates the temporal

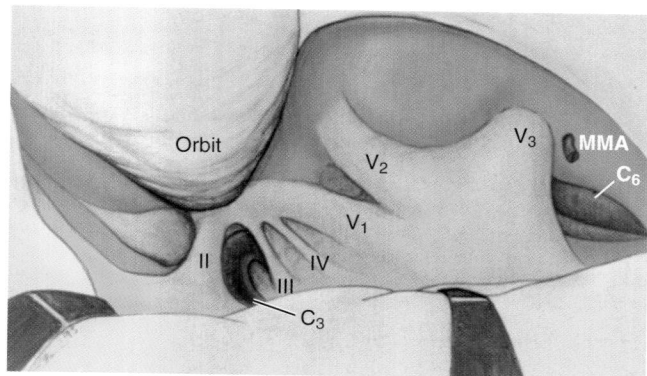

FIGURE 38-10 The dura propria is reflected from the outer cavernous membrane to expose the trigeminal complex (V1–V3), the trochlear, and the oculomotor nerves. With extradural resection of the anterior clinoid process, the carotid siphon is well exposed (C3). The extradural exposure of the intrapetrous carotid artery (C6) exposes approximately 10 mm of the vessel in the middle fossa. MMA, middle meningeal artery.

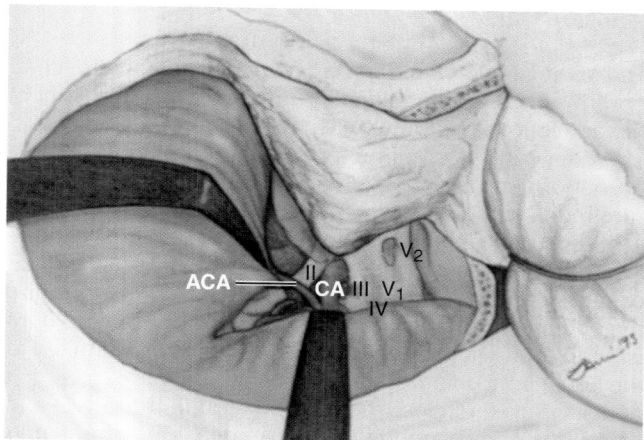

FIGURE 38-11 The dura is opened in an L-shaped incision to expose the sylvian fissure and intradural internal carotid artery. The sylvian fissure is split approximately 2 cm for additional retraction. ACA, anterior cerbral artery; CA, carotid artery.

dura from the outer cavernous membrane over the medial triangle and effectively frees the medial margin of temporal dura, resulting in full lateral and posterior retraction. Some arachnoidal dissection around the porus oculomotorius is typically a prerequisite to this move. At this juncture, the structures of the lateral wall of the cavernous sinus should be plainly visible through the thin veil of the outer cavernous membrane, from the sella to the trigeminal third division. The medial, superior, and lateral triangles are well delineated (Fig. 38-12).

The sylvian fissure is usually split to decrease the required retractor pressure, even though the degree of frontal and temporal lobe retraction is somewhat lessened with this approach. No more than the anterior 1 to 2 cm of the fissure need be split in most cases. During the dissection, it will be clear that the temporal tip bridging veins need not be sacrificed with this approach because the temporal dura is retracted with the temporal lobe, obviating sacrifice of these vessels. The arachnoid is opened over the optic nerve and chiasm, as well as the carotid artery to expose the A1

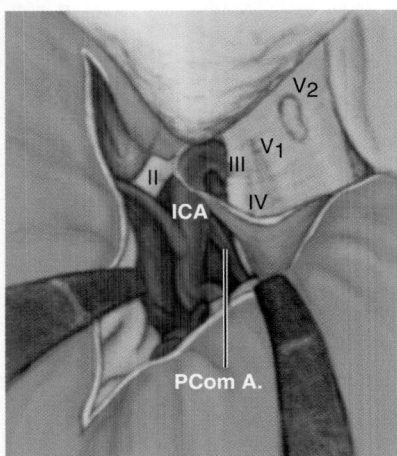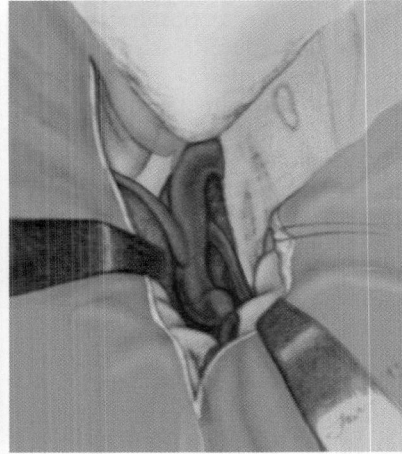

FIGURE 38-12 The opening of the fibrous dural ring and the porus oculomotorius with splitting of dural leaves composing the tentorial edge are shown. This maneuver allows lateral retraction of this dural edge and opening of the medial triangle. This also leads into the opening of the superior triangle in similar fashion. PCom A, posterior communicating artery; ICA, internal carotid artery.

and M1 segments (Fig. 38-13). The medial and anterolateral portions of the cavernous sinus are exposed at this point of the dissection, and tumor resection may proceed.

At the conclusion of the procedure, dural closure must be performed in as complete a manner as possible. Closure requires the use of a pericranial or fascial graft, and if any bone sinuses were opened during the extradural bone removal, these must be exenterated and packed with a fat or muscle graft. A problem area of closure is that around the optic nerve. The incision in the optic nerve sheath dura is not closed with suture because of the risk of damage to the nerve from compression or direct trauma. Fascial patch grafts are used to close the incision around the nerve, and then fat is placed around the nerve area. The fascial graft is tacked such that it will prevent migration of the fat graft, and the area is finally sealed with fibrin glue. For superior cosmetic results, the bone flaps are secured with one of the titanium plating systems.

LATERAL APPROACH TO THE POSTERIOR CAVERNOUS SINUS REGION (ANTERIOR TRANSPETROSAL APPROACH)

Although the posterior cavernous sinus region may be reached strictly through an anterior trajectory, the exposure is narrow, and cranial nerve V is an obstacle to adequate vision. This narrow corridor provides limited access to the posteroinferior triangle and region surrounding the porus trigeminus. For this reason, a more lateral and posterior approach is indicated, either subtemporal or transpetrosal, that provides a wider operative corridor and access inferolateral to the trigeminal complex. The extradural middle fossa anterior transpetrosal approach provides such exposure through a subtemporal route and is easily combined with the frontotemporal approach.[39-42,50,51] When bone removal through this approach is maximized, near-total resection of the petrous apex results.[39]

Avoidance of complications from this technique depends mainly on an intimate knowledge of the internal anatomy

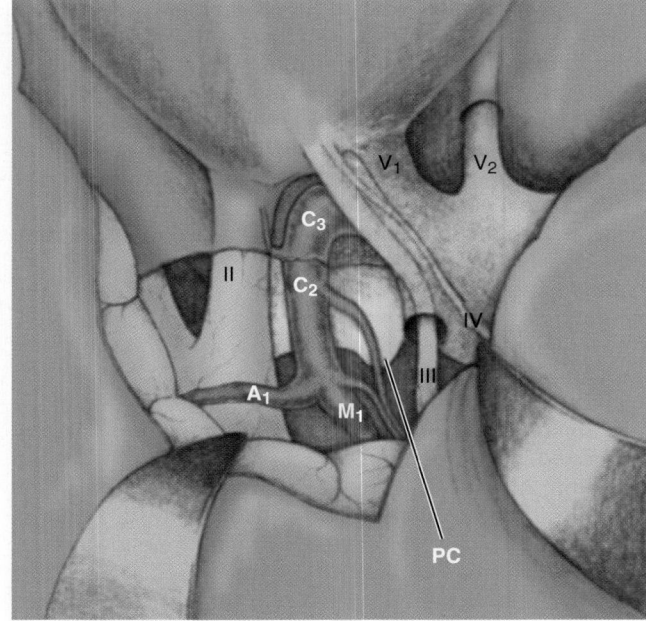

FIGURE 38-13 The final exposure of the anteromedial and posteromedial cavernous sinus via the temporopolar approach.

of the petrous bone and the relationships between internal structures and surface landmarks. The major potential complications of the procedure are hearing loss resulting from cochlear or bone labyrinth violation and compromise of facial nerve integrity and function. In an attempt to simplify the technique, we have devised a geometric construct of key middle fossa landmarks that delineates the volume of bone to be resected. This construct helps to locate, and thus avoid, internal structures of the petrous pyramid.[39]

The approach is performed with the head in the 90-degree lateral position, through a 4-cm by 4-cm temporal craniotomy centered two thirds anterior and one third

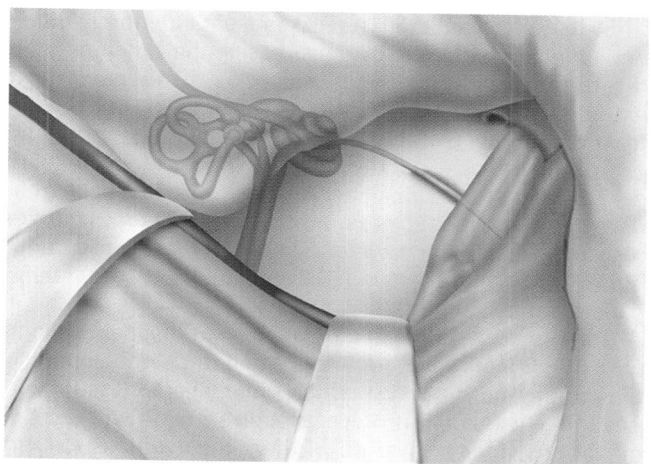

FIGURE 38-14 This middle fossa floor is exposed via the extended middle fossa approach, seen on the left side in this figure. The landmarks to begin the extradural bone removal are visible at this point in the procedure.

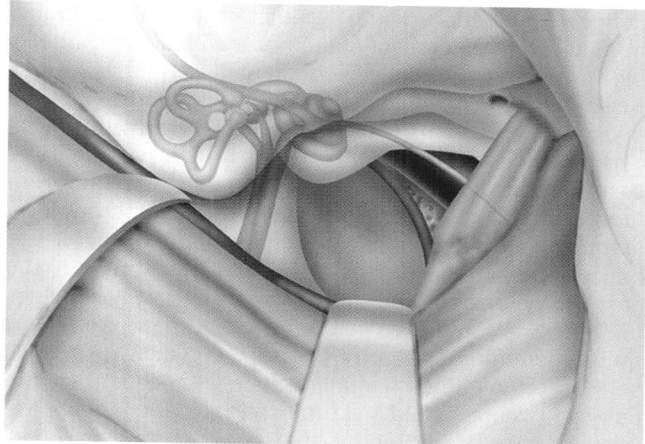

FIGURE 38-15 After the extradural bone resection is completed, the posterior fossa dura to the level of the inferior petrosal sinus (IPS) is exposed. The internal auditory canal (IAC) is skeletonized approximately 270 degrees. The posterior cavernous sinus is exposed via this route by elevating and medially translocating the trigeminal complex, opening the outer cavernous membrane inferior to the trigeminal ganglion.

posterior over the external auditory meatus. When performed in combination with a frontotemporal approach, a more generous temporal extension of the craniotomy must be made that reaches posterior to the root of the zygomatic process. Middle fossa dural elevation begins posteriorly and laterally, over the petrous ridge, and continues anteromedially to the foramen ovale. Dura is elevated in this manner to avoid traction on the greater superficial petrosal nerve (GSPN), which may result in facial nerve compromise. The GSPN lies in the major petrosal groove of the middle fossa floor and is covered by a thin layer of periosteum. The middle meningeal artery and surrounding venous plexus are coagulated and divided near the artery's exit from the foramen spinosum. The dura is then separated from the trigeminal complex at the foramen ovale, continuing posteriorly toward the porus trigeminus. Tapered retractors are used to retract the dura medially and posteriorly to expose the entire middle fossa floor (Fig. 38-14).

At this juncture, the landmarks necessary to begin the bone dissection are identifiable. The volume of bone that will be resected corresponds to a rhomboid-shaped complex of landmarks of the middle fossa floor. This geometric construct is defined by: (1) the intersection of the GSPN and V3, (2) the intersection of lines projected along the axes of the GSPN and the arcuate eminence, (3) the intersection with the petrous ridge, and (4) the porus trigeminus. Obliquely projecting this construct through the petrous bone to the inferior petrosal sinus delimits the volume of petrous bone that has no neural or vascular structures.

Bony resection begins with the exposure of the IAC. By use of a high-speed diamond drill, the IAC is found 3 to 4 mm deep to the middle fossa floor along the bisection axis between lines projected along the GSPN and the arcuate eminence. The entire length of the IAC is exposed. Next, the GSPN is uncovered lateral to the facial hiatus, until the geniculate ganglion is exposed. A thin shell of bone is left over the ganglion for protection. The GSPN is preserved if possible. In some cases, however, it must be sectioned and reflected lateral for exposure needs. The carotid is exposed in the posterolateral triangle from V3 to the tensor tympani

muscle. Then, the bone between the IAC and carotid can be safely removed to expose posterior fossa dura (Fig. 38-15). Great care must be taken to avoid the cochlea during this portion of bone dissection.

The cochlea is located in the base of the premeatal triangle, which is defined by the carotid genu, the geniculate ganglion, and the medial lip of the internal auditory meatus.[39] Resection of apical petrous bone is continued inferiorly to the level of the inferior petrosal sinus. The apical bone inferior to the trigeminal ganglion can be removed by coring out of the petrous apex. The wedge of bone remaining that lies lateral to the IAC can be removed, to result in an almost 270-degree exposure of the IAC. This lateral wedge of bone is defined by the postmeatal triangle, which is bounded by the geniculate ganglion, the arcuate eminence, and the lateral lip of the internal auditory meatus. It is often helpful to blue-line the superior semicircular canal during removal of this bone to avoid entering the vestibule.

With the bone dissection complete, the posterior and inferolateral cavernous sinus can be widely reached. The limits of this exposure are the foramen of Dorello medially and the inferior petrosal sinus below. The trigeminal complex can be completely freed of dura and then elevated or retracted medially. This exposure provides visualization of the C5 and C6 portions of the carotid artery. A prerequisite to this maneuver for increasing the exposure of the posterior cavernous sinus is extradural liberation of the V2 and V3 divisions in their respective bone canals. Elevation of the trigeminal complex in this way allows full exposure of the posterior cavernous sinus and complete petrous apex resection extradurally under direct vision.[40]

The dura is opened at the porus trigeminus above the superior petrosal sinus. This incision is carried laterally as far as the arcuate eminence and exposes the superior surface of the tentorium. A parallel incision is then made inferior to the superior petrosal sinus. The superior petrosal sinus is ligated and divided at its medial aspect. The retractors can then be placed on the undersurface of the tentorium, and the temporal lobe is retracted more superiorly under its protection. The trigeminal root is also liberated from its dural attachment at the porus trigeminus. Mobilizing the trigeminal complex medially and superiorly provides a corridor to the posterior cavernous sinus and the entrance of cranial nerve VI into Dorello's canal. To expose the intracavernous carotid artery, it is necessary to open the outer cavernous membrane between the trigeminal ganglion and the posterolateral fibrous ring surrounding the carotid's entrance to the cavernous sinus at the foramen lacerum. In this way, the intracavernous carotid can be exposed to the crossing point of cranial nerve VI. This strategy provides full access to the posterolateral quadrant of the cavernous sinus, and tumor resection may proceed. The main venous connections of the posterolateral cavernous sinus are to the pterygoid venous plexus via the sphenoidal emissary, the inferior petrosal sinus, and the basilar venous plexus. Effective hemostasis is obtained via packing oxidized cellulose in the direction of these venous connections.

Closure requires the use of an adipose graft placed into the bony defect in the petrous apex and floor of the middle fossa. We find it best to place the adipose tissue into the defect in strips and any open air cells are carefully covered.

SPECIAL TECHNIQUES OF INTRACAVERNOUS SURGERY

Intracavernous Tumor Resection

Proper instrumentation is one of the major assets to successful resection of cavernous sinus neoplasms. A full array of dissectors, including micro-ring curettes, is useful. A wide selection of Cottonoids is also necessary for protection of neural and vascular structures and dissection of tumor. An extremely useful tool is a pressure-attenuable suction tip that is invaluable for working around delicate structures to prevent damage induced by traction. The pressure-adjustable sucker is used for retraction and dissection as well as suction of blood and CSF. Proper instrumentation is key to application of the technical principles of tumor resection in this region.

The techniques used for resection of these tumors vary, depending on the degree of invasiveness and adherence to neural and vascular structures. Tumors such as trigeminal neurinomas that are well encapsulated and nonadherent can be relatively uncomplicated to remove. After exposure of tumor capsule through one of the triangular entry corridors, tumor debulking is performed with suction, ring curettes, and alligator biopsy forceps. Developing a plane between tumor capsule and the neural and vascular structures is usually possible within the confines of the cavernous sinus. This dissection is typically performed by use of a combination of fine dissectors and long, thin Cottonoids. The capsule is dissected free, continually collapsing solid tumor at the periphery into the center. Adjacent entry corridors may need to be utilized to completely free the tumor capsule. Usually, tumor is primarily resected from one or two triangular spaces, and adjacent portals are entered to dissect tumor and to push or sweep the mass toward the primary route of resection. When the capsule is freed, it is removed from the cavernous sinus, and hemostasis is attained with judicious use of Surgicel packing. This same general technique is used for any well-encapsulated, nonadherent tumor.

Invasive and adherent tumors present an entirely different surgical challenge. In these cases, the outcome with regard to morbidity depends mainly on the judgment and experience of the surgeon. Attempts at dissection of tumor from cranial nerves often result in damage either directly or from interruption of the nerves' blood supply. In some cases, when the cranial nerves have already been rendered nonfunctional by tumor invasion, the nerves can be resected with tumor to gain a more complete resection. This possibility is always considered and discussed with the patient before surgery.

Tumors such as meningiomas are approached initially with the primary intent of interrupting the blood supply to the tumor. These tumors can be quite tenacious and invasive, qualities that can prevent total resection without significant morbidity. Invasion of the intracavernous carotid artery may require a bypass procedure for total tumor resection. The dural origin and surrounding margin are resected in cases in which a complete resection is performed.

Invasive, malignant processes, such as squamous cell cancer, involve a very extensive procedure for removal. In these cases, the affected cavernous sinus and adjacent structures are removed en bloc. This procedure requires wide exposure of the cavernous sinus and adjacent regions as well as a bypass procedure to permit resection of the affected carotid artery.

TECHNIQUES OF HEMOSTASIS

Complete hemostasis throughout the surgical procedure is one of the primary determinants of the success or failure of any direct approach to the cavernous sinus. The potential for tremendous bleeding from the cavernous sinus requires familiarity and practice with certain techniques before such a surgical undertaking. A complete understanding of the anatomy and the elements of the triangular entry corridors is requisite to maintaining a dry operative field. Compulsive hemostasis begins with the skin incision and is maintained until final skin closure.

Preparation for the maintenance of hemostasis begins with the selection of instruments and the arrangement of materials by the scrub nurse. Bipolar cautery forceps should be available in a wide range of lengths and tip sizes. We prefer to use high settings during the initial phases of the operation to treat bleeding from scalp and muscle more effectively. As structures vulnerable to damage from the spread of heat or current are neared, the settings are reduced. Monopolar cautery is used frequently during the initial phases of these operations and is very useful to stop bleeding from bone at the skull base. When the bone of the middle fossa floor and sphenoid ridge is drilled, hemostasis is attained by several methods. Bone wax is judiciously used to seal off bleeding from porous bone. In addition to monopolar cautery, a high-speed drill, fitted with a diamond burr, cauterizes bone when used without irrigation. Bone bleeding at the skull base can often be persistent; therefore, patience and effective use of these techniques are necessary.

As the foramina of the cranial nerves are approached, the technical strategy changes. Heat and current from the monopolar cautery can spread for several millimeters through bone and can damage the nerves. Bone bleeding around neural foramina is controlled more with bone wax than with cautery or the diamond drill. Bleeding from the cavernous sinus also occurs via tiny rents in the cavernous membrane when the dura is separated from the margins of the foramina. This bleeding can be controlled by packing tiny pieces of Surgicel into the open cavernous membrane and covering for 1 or 2 minutes with a small Cottonoid. Coagulating the Surgicel for 1 to 2 seconds with the bipolar after it is packed in the hole is sometimes helpful. Bleeding can occur from a tear in the cavernous membrane during the final stages of removal of the anterior clinoid process. Although possible to remove without bleeding, more frequently, the carotico-oculomotor membrane develops a small tear that can bleed profusely. A small piece of Surgicel suffices when packed into the opening and covered with a Cottonoid for 1 to 2 minutes. An important principle in hemostatic technique in the cavernous sinus is patience. Much is gained by packing an area, moving to another area to work, then coming back later to the original bleeding site.

The geometric construct describing the entry corridors to the cavernous sinus region serves as a foundation for effective hemostasis. Knowledge of the nature and communications of the venous plexus residing within each triangle, as well as the proximity of anatomic structures, is critical. In cases of tumor resection, the tumor mass often tamponades the cavernous venous plexus. Surgicel packing for hemostasis then begins after the tumor mass is removed from the area. In the anterior triangle, lateral and medial packing must be conservative because of the position of cranial nerve III and the optic nerve. Anteroinferior packing is less constrained; however, constriction of the carotid siphon must obviously be avoided. The anterolateral triangle typically contains the anastomosis of the superior orbital vein with the cavernous venous plexus and, therefore, can produce brisk bleeding when opened. The main concern in this triangle is avoidance of overpacking in the direction of cranial nerve VI, because the abducens nerve is entering the superior orbital fissure on its underside. The lateralmost triangle can also produce significant bleeding if a sphenoid emissary vein is present beside the mandibular branch that exits the foramen ovale. This sphenoid emissary is seen only in a few patients; however, when present, it can be quite large.

The medial cavernous triangle can bleed tremendously when opened. Packing must be conservative laterally, in the direction of cranial nerve III; however, inferomedial packing can be quite generous. Here, the cavernous sinus communicates with the basilar venous plexus along the clivus and the inferior petrosal sinus. Therefore, a large amount of Surgicel may be packed in their direction without compromise of any vital structures. The superior triangle does not have such an area that may be so generously packed. The meningohypophyseal trunk is found in this triangle and is vulnerable to overzealous packing. The lateral triangle is the space entered to expose cranial nerve VI as it crosses over the C4 segment of the carotid artery. Surgicel placement must be modest, except in the inferomedial direction toward the clivus.

Exposure of the intrapetrous carotid artery in the posterolateral triangle does not usually produce significant bleeding. This segment of the carotid is, however, often covered by a venous plexus that is an extension of the cavernous venous plexus. This plexus must be coagulated with bipolar cautery before work with this segment begins. The

posteromedial triangle similarly is not a major concern for significant hemorrhage. When bone deep in this space is removed, the inferior petrosal sinus is encountered and must be occluded. Also, deep drilling to the clivus usually results in encountering the basilar venous plexus, which must be packed and coagulated. The posteroinferior triangle can also produce a fair amount of hemorrhage from connections with the basilar venous plexus and inferior petrosal sinus. In the floor of this space runs Dorello's canal and cranial nerve VI. Hemostasis in this space must be performed carefully to avoid compression of this structure.

CLOSURE TECHNIQUES

Avoidance of complications in these procedures includes meticulous attention to dural closure to prevent CSF leakage and subsequent contamination. Judicious use of fascial grafts is important in meeting this goal. Typically, abdominal fat and rectus fascia are harvested in these cases for dural closure and sealing of opened paranasal sinuses. In areas of difficult dural closure, such as around the optic nerve, fat grafts are placed and secured with fine sutures tamponading them against the open area. This arrangement is then covered with a layer of fibrin glue to hasten the fibrotic process. Muscle or fat is also tacked to areas where it is impossible to attain tight apposition of dural edges. Also, at the corner areas of complex dural incisions, fat or muscle is used to completely plug any small holes. Fibrin glue is applied to the entire dural surface at the completion of dural closure.

As discussed, open paranasal sinuses commonly result from extensive removal of bone at the skull base. Any open sinus must be meticulously exenterated of any mucosa. We prefer to use a high-speed drill fitted with a diamond burr for this purpose. The heat generated by the drill provides extra assurance of destroying any mucus-producing epithelial cells. Ostia are then occluded with muscle or bone wax to prevent communication with bacteria-laden adjacent sinus cavities. The sinus is then packed with autologous fat. We then cover the opening to the packed sinus with a vascularized pericranial flap and carefully tack the edges to adjacent surfaces to prevent migration.

The ultimate cosmetic result of these procedures is partially dependent on the proper reattachment of the bone flap, especially in cases in which a transzygomatic or orbitozygomatic flap has been used. One of the titanium plating systems now available provides superior cosmetic results over those obtained with wire or suture. We prefer to use one of the low-profile systems, especially at points where only skin is covering the bone surface to be approximated.

Another cosmetic consideration relates to the reattachment of the temporalis muscle. If the muscle is not supported in some manner along the superior temporal line, it tends to sink into the temporal fossa, resulting in a poor appearance. To combat this, oblique wire-pass holes are made along the superior temporal line before the bone flap is replaced. The superior edge of the muscle can then be sutured to the superior temporal line, maintaining its position during the healing process.

Skull Base Carotid Bypass Procedures

Invasive tumors often require sacrifice of the ICA if they are to be completely removed. Balloon test occlusion is performed before surgery to determine tolerance to occlusion of the involved ICA.[41] Patients who tolerate occlusion without incident may be treated without bypass, thus avoiding the potential major complications of thromboembolic sequelae and anticoagulation associated with these procedures. In cases in which occlusion is not tolerated, the carotid flow can be preserved by performing a bypass procedure.[8,28,30,53,54] This procedure was first performed in 1986 by Fukushima to treat a giant intracavernous aneurysm.[7,8,55] Over time, the procedure has evolved to include three variations. The most common form is a bypass between the C3 and C6 segments of the carotid. The second important variation is an anastomosis from the high cervical portion of the ICA to the C3 segment.[8,56]

The C3-to-C6 bypass procedure requires exposure of those two segments in sufficient length to perform the anastomosis procedure. The C3 portion is exposed in the anterior triangle through removal of the anterior clinoid process and detachment of the fibrous dural ring. The C6 segment is exposed in the posterolateral triangle.[57] It is usually helpful to free the dura from the posterior trigeminal complex, as discussed earlier, to gain several additional millimeters of exposure. Clips can then be placed to trap the intracavernous carotid segments. A saphenous vein graft is harvested from the upper thigh and prepared for anastomosis. Any loose adventitia is stripped from the vein, and tributaries are ligated with fine suture. The graft is flushed with heparinized saline solution, and proper orientation is maintained by marking either end of the graft. The distal anastomosis is then performed, either end to end or end to side, with 8-0, 9-0, or 10-0 suture. Suture selection depends on the wall thickness of both the graft and the carotid artery. Control of carotid flow is maintained either by a temporary clip near the genu or by exposure in the neck. The proximal anastomosis is performed between the origins of the ophthalmic artery and the posterior communicating artery. In some cases, the anastomosis may be performed in an end-to-end fashion if the tumor resection leaves a carotid stump including the ophthalmic origin or the ophthalmic artery is taken with tumor resection in the orbit. The anastomosis is performed under electroencephalographic burst suppression induced by barbiturates. Patients are given low-dose heparin therapy for several days postoperatively, and they are then given aspirin or warfarin (Coumadin) for approximately 3 months.

In cases of en bloc cavernous sinus resection, resecting carotid artery well into the infratemporal fossa and petrous bone may be necessary. In this case, the carotid is bypassed from the high cervical segment, near the origin at the carotid bifurcation. Saphenous vein is again harvested from the upper thigh in an appropriate length. The graft is anastomosed in end-to-end fashion and tunneled through the infratemporal fossa to enter the cranial vault subtemporally. The proximal end is then anastomosed to the C3 segment as outlined earlier.

Summary

Direct operative treatment of intracavernous neoplasms has realized great strides in the past decade. Several experienced centers have had success with treating these patients more aggressively, while limiting morbidity. Advances in microsurgical technique, neuroanesthesia, imaging techniques, neurovascular reconstruction, and microanatomic knowledge have all provided significant contributions to the successful surgery of these lesions. However, the therapeutic approach to these difficult tumors is still debated. The appropriate role of surgery in the overall management of these patients is still evolving as we continue to refine our management strategies.

We anticipate that direct surgery will continue to figure prominently in the treatment of these tumors, although it is increasingly combined with adjuvant therapies that present less risk to the cranial nerves while increasing the effectiveness of treatment. The indications for these procedures are still evolving as different centers gain wider experience with direct surgery, stereotactic radiosurgery, and endonasal endoscopic techniques. Clearly, much room for improvement remains in the overall results of treating these difficult lesions.

KEY REFERENCES

Al-Mefty O, Smith RR. Surgery of tumors invading the cavernous sinus. *Surg Neurol.* 1988;30:370-381.

Ceylan S, Koc K, Anik I. Endoscopic endonasal transsphenoidal approach for pituitary adenomas invading the cavernous sinus. *J Neurosurg.* 2010;112:99-107.

Day JD. Surgical approaches to suprasellar and parasellar tumors. *Neurosurg Clin North Am.* 2003;54(2):391-395.

Day JD. Cranial base surgical techniques for large sphenocavernous meningiomas: technical note. *Neurosurgery.* 2000;46(3):754-759.

Dolenc VV, Kregar R, Ferluga M, et al. Treatment of tumors invading the cavernous sinus. In: Dolenc VV, ed. *The Cavernous Sinus: Multidisciplinary Approach to Vascular and Tumorous Lesions.* Wien: Springer-Verlag; 1987:377-391.

Duma CM, Lunsford LD, Kondziolka D, et al. Stereotactic radiosurgery of cavernous sinus meningiomas as an addition or alternative to microsurgery. *Neurosurgery.* 1993;32:699-705.

Fraser JF, Mass AY, Brown S, et al. Transnasal endoscopic resection of a cavernous sinus hemangioma: technical note and review of the literature. *Skull Base.* 2008;18:309-315.

Fukushima T, Day JD, Tung H. Intracavernous carotid artery aneurysms. In: Apuzzo MLJ, ed. *Brain Surgery: complication Avoidance and Management.* New York: Churchill Livingstone; 1993:925-944.

Glasscock ME. Exposure of the intra-petrous portion of the carotid artery. In: Hamberger CA, Wersall J, eds. *Disorders of the Skull Base Region: Proceedings of the Tenth Nobel Symposium, Stockholm, 1968.* Stockholm: Almqvist & Wicksell; 1969:135-143.

Hakuba A, Suzuki T, Jin TB, Komiyama M. Surgical approaches to the cavernous sinus: report of 52 cases. In: Dolenc VV, ed. *The Cavernous Sinus.* Wien: Springer-Verlag; 1987:302-327.

Harris FS, Rhoton AL. Anatomy of the cavernous sinus: a microsurgical study. *J Neurosurg.* 1976;44:169-180.

House WF, Hitselberger WE, Horn KL. The middle fossa transpetrous approach to the anterior-superior cerebellopontine angle. *Am J Otol.* 1986;7:1-4.

Kassam AB, Gardner P, Snyderman C, et al. Expanded endonasal approach: fully endoscopic, completely transnasal approach to the middle third of the clivus, petrous bone, middle cranial fossa, and infratemporal fossa. *Neurosurg Focus.* 2005;19(1):E6.

Kawase T, Toya S, Shiobara R, Mine T. Transpetrosal approach for aneurysms of the lower basilar artery. *J Neurosurg.* 1985;63:857-861.

Kitano M, Taneda M, Shimono T, Nakao Y. Extended transsphenoidal approach for surgical management of pituitary adenomas invading the cavernous sinus. *J Neurosurg.* 2008;108:26-36.

Perneczky A, Knosp E, Czech T. Para- and infraclinoidal aneurysms. Anatomy, surgical technique and report on 22 cases. In: Dolenc VV, ed. *The Cavernous Sinus.* Wien: Springer-Verlag; 1987:252-271.

Pichierri A, Santoro A, Raco A, et al. Cavernous sinus meningiomas: retrospective analysis and proposal of a treatment algorithm. *Neurosurgery.* 2009;64:1090-1101.

Sekhar LN, Ross DA, Sen C. Cavernous sinus and sphenocavernous neoplasms. In: Sekhar LN, Janecka IP, eds. *Surgery of Cranial Base Tumors.* New York: Raven Press; 1993:521-604.

Spetzler RF, Fukushima T, Martin N, Zabramski JM. Petrous carotidto-intradural carotid saphenous vein graft for intracavernous giant aneurysm, tumor, and occlusive cerebrovascular disease. *J Neurosurg.* 1990;73:496-501.

Umansky F, Elidan J, Valarezo A. Dorello's canal: a microanatomical study. *J Neurosurg.* 1991;75:294-298.

Walsh MT, Couldwell WT. Management options for cavernous sinus meningiomas. *J Neurooncol.* 2009;92:307-316.

Zada G, Day JD, Giannotta SL. The extradural temporopolar approach: a review of indications and operative technique. *Neurosurg Focus.* 2008;25(6):E3.

Numbered references appear on Expert Consult.

CHAPTER 39

Surgery for Trigeminal Neurinomas

TAKESHI KAWASE

Anatomy

The trigeminal nerve courses in three compartments: middle cranial fossa, posterior fossa, and extracranial space. Therefore, tumors extending into multiple fossae are common (58%)[1] (Table 39-1). The most common origin is around the Gasserian ganglion (GG), showing a dumbbell-shaped tumor extending both middle and posterior fossae (MP type, 38.6%) through Meckel's cave (MC). MC is a subarachnoid space depressed from the posterior fossa, separated from the cavernous sinus by a thin meningeal dura (dura propria), and opened freely to the posterior fossa containing loose trigeminal nerve bundles without perineural covering.[2] However, the trigeminal nerves peripheral to the GG course in the interdural space, are wrapped with a so-called inner reticular layer (perineurium), and are easily separated from the lateral wall of the cavernous sinus by a cleavage plane[3] (Fig. 39-1A).

Therefore, the dumbbell-shaped tumor is spreading over the two anatomically different spaces: the interdural space anteriorly and the subarachnoid space posteriorly. The anterior part of the tumor can be removed through the interdural space by Dolenc's approach.[4] A small posterior fossa tumor can be removed through the orifice of MC; however, resection of the petrous apex, which obstructs the surgical field, is commonly necessary to observe the posterior fossa sufficiently. If the posterior fossa tumor is larger than 1 cm, the bone resection of the petrous apex plus detachment of the tentorium by the anterior petrosal approach (APA) is necessary.

Resection of the petrous apex may offer a surgical effect to widen the surgical space, as well as to decrease the tension of the trigeminal bundle bent by the petrous apex (Fig. 39-1B). The posterior fossa (P) type of tumor commonly attaches on the trigeminal nerve bundle alone, and it can be removed by the APA,[5] even when the tumor is large.

Selection of Surgical Approaches

Every type of trigeminal neurinoma can be removed safely by the following two approaches, plus their combination. The authors do not use the suboccipital approach to spare injury to the facial and auditory nerves.

- The subtemporal interdural approach (SIA) without zygomatic osteotomy is indicated for tumors of the middle fossa (M) or middle fossa and extracranial (ME) type (with infratemporal extension).
- The APA is indicated for MP-type (dumbbell-shaped) and P-type tumors.
- The zygomatic petrosal approach (ZPA), combining SIA and APA is indicated for large MP-type tumors or extension into three middle, posterior, and infratemporal fossae (MPE)–type tumors.

SIA WITH OR WITHOUT ZYGOMATIC OSTEOMY

The SIA is indicated for an M-type tumor with or without extracranial extension (Fig. 39-2). The zygomatic osteotomy is not always necessary but is effective to spare retraction damage to the temporal lobe by turnover of the temporal muscle inferiorly, especially for a large tumor extending higher than the tentorial fold. In the supine position, the patient's head is rotated 60 degrees with a downward axis. A curved hemicoronal incision along the auricle is followed by exposure of the zygomatic arch, which is cut in two points by a surgical saw. The craniotomy is created along the middle fossa base to expose the foramen rotundum and ovale epidurally. The middle meningeal artery is coagulated and cut at the foramen spinosum. The periosteal side of the dura mater is incised above the foramen rotundum, and the incision is extended above the foramen ovale and toward the superior orbital fissure.

The lower part of the tumor appears by this point, and the upper part can be exposed by tacking the parasellar dura superiorly (Fig. 39-3). The tumor is commonly covered by a thin semitransparent membrane, the so-called inner reticular layer, showing the course of the trigeminal nerves through it (Fig. 39-3A and B).

The nerves are clearly identified and separated from the tumor by removal of the membrane (Fig. 39-3C). In large tumors, the nerve fascicule is lost and the tumor is

Table 39-1	Location and Type of Tumor (MPE Classification)
Tumor Type	**Patients**
M	8 (14.0%)
P	12 (21.1%)
E	4 (7.0%)
MP	22 (38.6%)
ME	7 (12.3%)
MPE	4 (7.0%)
Total patients	57 (100.0%)
Compartment	
Single	24 (47.3%)
Multiple	33 (57.9%)

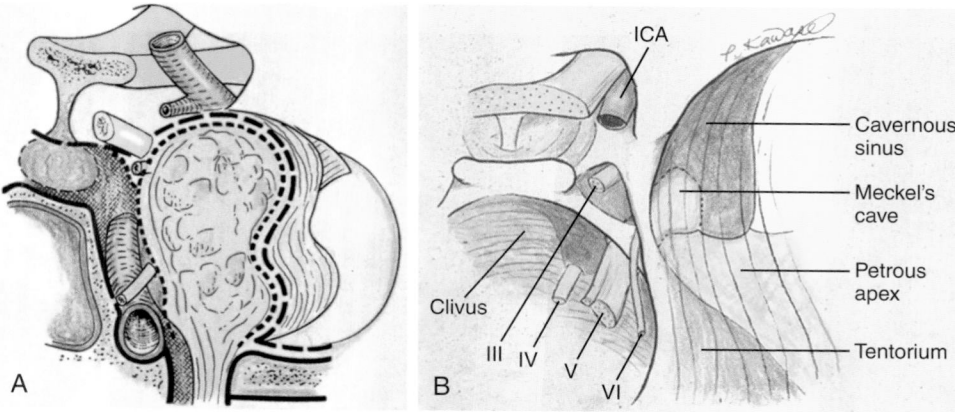

FIGURE 39-1 A, Parasellar trigeminal neurinoma based on the meningeal anatomy. The tumor is located between the meningeal dura (break line) and the cavernous sinus, wrapped with inner reticular layer (dotted line). Incision of the periosteal dura (broad line) on the foramen rotundum and ovale (arrow) offers tumor exposure without exposing the temporal lobe. B, An illustrative anatomy of MC. The orifice is covered by two meningeal folds: the petroclinoid fold (tentorium) and the petroclival fold. The inferolateral margin is surrounded by the petrous apex.

commonly wrapped by numerous isolated trigeminal nerve fibers. The surgical windows for tumor removal are created by mobilizing the nerve fibers.

The cavernous sinus is separated from the tumor by the medial wall of the inner reticular layer, and it does not open by careful preservation of the membrane. After tumor removal, the widened orifice of MC can be confirmed by cerebrospinal fluid discharge. The anterolateral aspect of the pons can be seen through MC (Fig. 39-3C). The opened MC is packed by the fascial flap at closure. The zygomatic arch is replaced and fixed by titanium plates.

There are two options:

1. In the case of tumor extension into the infratemporal fossa (MPE type), the middle fossa base is drilled off until the penetrating tumor is exposed. Venous bleeding from pterygoid plexus must be cared for.
2. In the case of tumor extension into the orbit (ME type 1), the surgical method is the same as Dolenc's approach.[4] Orbital unroofing, removal of the anterior clinoid process, and interdural dissection on the superior orbital fissure offer a total view from the orbit to the parasellar space. The orbital wall is reconstructed by an inner layer of the cranial flap or by a titanium plate.

ANTERIOR PETROSAL APPROACH

The technical details of the APA were described earlier. This approach is indicated for dumbbell-shaped MP-type tumors (Fig. 39-4) or P-type tumors (Fig. 39-5). A fishhook-shaped scalp incision is followed by dissecting a fascial flap of the temporal muscle available for tight dural closure. The temporal muscle is reflected anteriorly without incision. The craniotomy size is almost the same as that of the squamous suture. After elevation of the middle fossa dura from the skull base, the middle meningeal artery is cauterized and cut. The petrous apex medial to the greater petrosal nerve is commonly eroded by the tumor; thus, the petrous resection is easier. In a P-type tumor, the petrous apex must be resected completely. The middle fossa dura is cut into a T shape along the superior petrosal sinus (SPS), which is ligated and cut with the tentorium thereafter.

The posterior fossa part of the tumor is observed later. The orifice of MC, which the tumor occupies, is a thick dural ring formed by the petroclival fold; it is incised anteriorly along the tumor. The trigeminal nerves caging the tumor are fragile and are not covered with "inner reticular

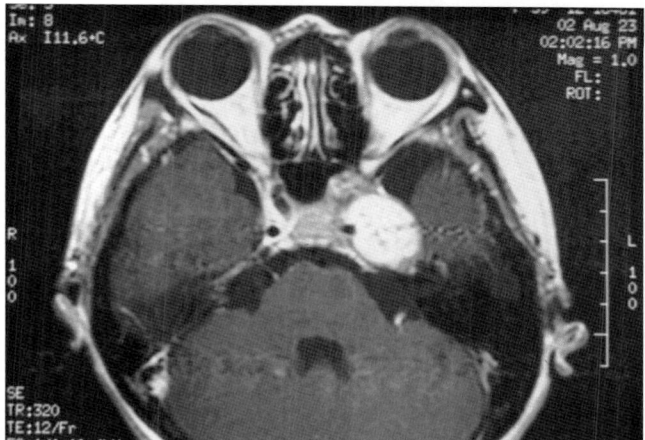

FIGURE 39-2 Parasellar type of trigeminal neurinoma. Note the compressed cavernous sinus medial to the tumor.

layer" because they are in the subarachnoid space. The GG is not clear in a large tumor. The tumor is removed from among the nerve fibers, and the nerve of the tumor origin must be amputated. A larger posterior fossa tumor can be removed through the petrous keyhole by retraction of the tumor margin toward the tumor attachment using a hooked tumor retractor. An advantage of this approach is visualization of the entry zone of the trigeminal nerve to which the tumor adheres. The course of the abducens nerve must be cared for in the inferomedial aspect of the tumor. The superior cerebellar artery and trochlear nerve course along the superior aspect of the tumor.

The facial–auditory nerve complex is not seen before tumor removal because it is pushed back by the tumor. Injury to the seventh to eighth nerves is very rare by this approach because these nerves are separated from the tumor by the cerebellopontine angle arachnoid and protected by the fan-like extended trigeminal nerve.

The complex can be confirmed by neuroendoscope after tumor removal. Also after tumor removal, the medial wall of MC, anterolateral aspect of the pons, and basilar artery complex are seen. For closure, a piece of abdominal fat is placed on the air cells of the petrous apex and rim of the craniotomy and is fixed with fibrin glue. Moreover, the cells are wrapped with a temporal fascia, which is sutured with

V neurinoma

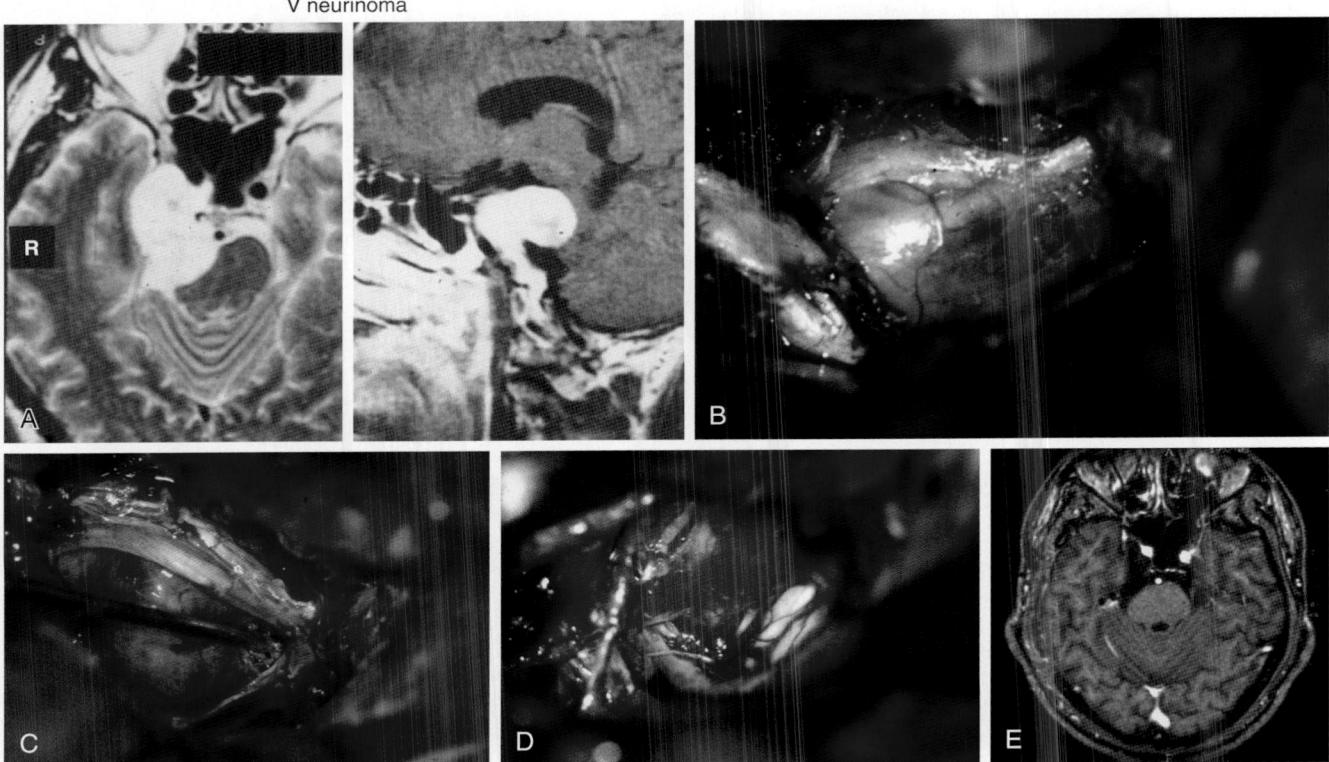

FIGURE 39-3 A 53-year-old male patient. A, Magnetic resonance imaging (MRI) with T2 weighting (left) and gadolinium enhancement in a parasellar tumor with a small bulge into the posterior fossa. B, A surgical photo after tacking the parasellar meningeal dura. The tumor is covered with a transparent membrane, the so-called inner reticular layer. C, After removal of this inner layer, the trigeminal nerves become clear. D, Pons and basilar artery observing through a widened MC. E, Postoperative MRI showing the intact temporal lobe and the cavernous sinus.

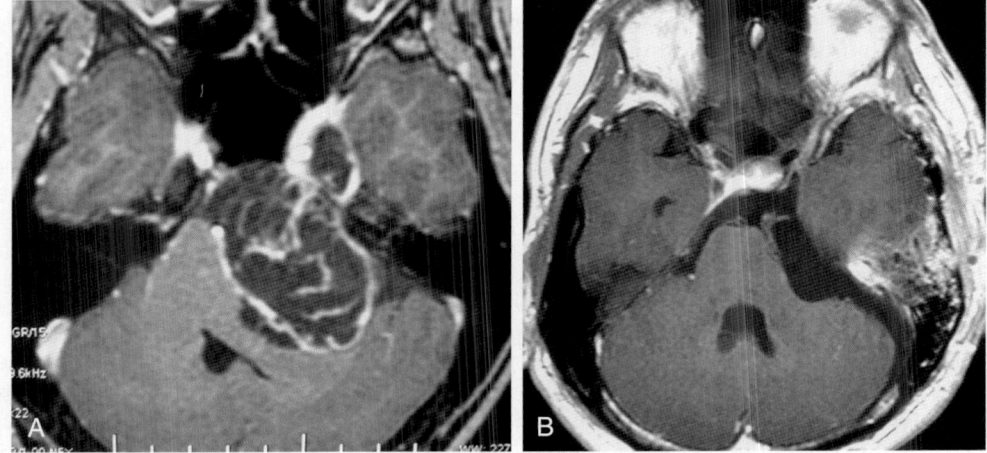

FIGURE 39-4 Large dumbbell-shaped (MP) neurinoma in a 26-year-old male before (A) and after (B) by the APA.

dura thereafter. The double-layer closure seldom causes complication of cerebrospinal fluid leakage or subcutaneous cerebrospinal fluid accumulation.

ZYGOMATIC PETROSAL APPROACH

The ZPA is a combination of SIA with zygomatic osteotomy and APA, indicated for a large MP-type tumor (Fig. 39-6) or a tumor extending into three fossae (middle, posterior, and infratemporal fossae); that is, a tumor of the MPE type. The operation has five steps. A question mark–shaped skin incision, zygomatic osteotomy, and basal craniotomy exposing the superior orbital fissure, foramen rotundum, foramen ovale, and petrous apex comprise the first step of operation. Skull base resection along the infratemporal tumor extension and resection of the petrous apex comprise the second step. The third step is removal of the tumor from the middle and infratemporal fossae. The fourth step consists of a dural incision along the SPS, a tentorial incision, and the opening of MC. The last step consists of removal of the posterior fossa tumor and closure. After tumor removal, the three fossae can

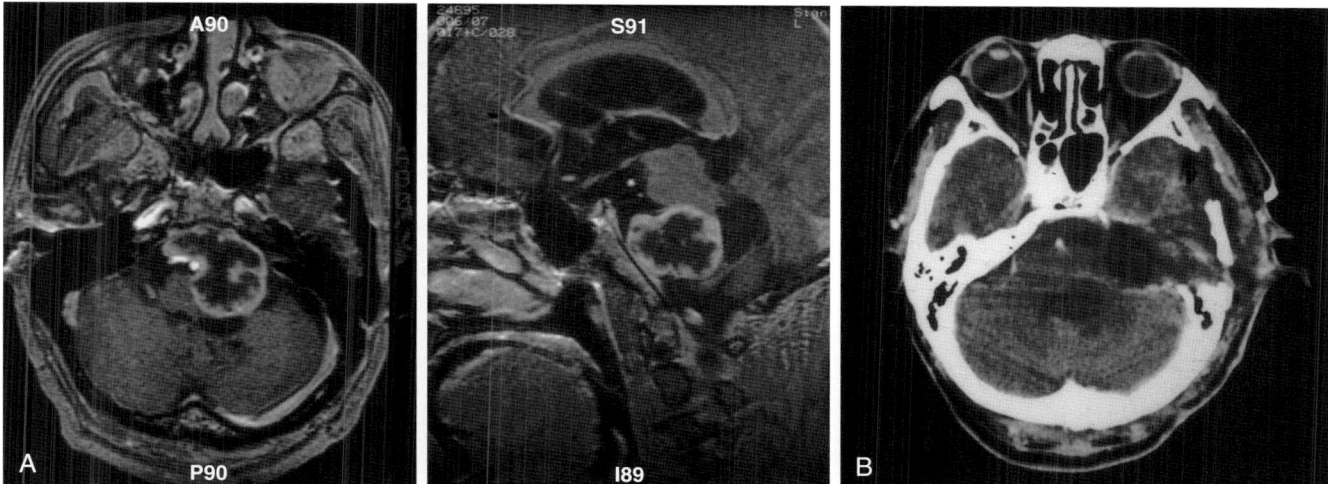

FIGURE 39-5 A 61-year-old male patient with a P-type tumor and a history of partial resection by the suboccipital approach. A, Magnetic resonance imaging with gadolinium enhancement before surgery. B, A contrast CT scan after surgery by the APA.

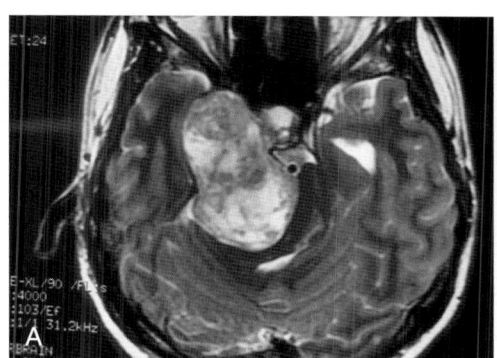 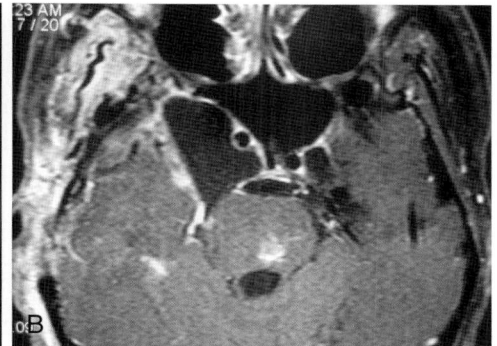

FIGURE 39-6 A 21-year-old male patient with a huge dumbbell-shaped (MP) tumor. A, Magnetic resonance imaging (MRI) with T2 weighting. The brain stem is severely compressed by the tumor. B, MRI with gadolinium enhancement after surgery. Note the intact temporal lobe and the cavernous sinus, operated by the ZPA. The brain stem is recovered to the normal configuration.

Table 39-2	Extent of Resection Using a Skull Base Approach
Extent	**Patients**
Total resection	43 (91.5%)
Nearly total resection	3 (6.4%)
Partial resection	1 (2.1%)
Total patients	47 (100.0%)

be observed from a single craniotomy along the trigeminal nerve. Retraction damage to the temporal lobe is uncommon because exposure of the brain is minimal.

Surgical Results

Among 57 patients with trigeminal neurinoma at our university, 47 have undergone skull base surgery since 1990. The most common method was APA, performed in 29 patients (61.7%). Another 12 patients (21.3%) underwent SIA, and zygomatic osteotomy was combined in 6 of them. A further group of 7 patients (14.8%) underwent ZPA. One patient was treated by the supraorbital approach for the tumor location in the orbit. The tumor was gross totally resected in 43 patients (91.5%) and nearly totally resected in 3 patients

(6.4%); partial resection was made only in 1 patient who had a history of surgery and gamma knife treatment (Table 39-2). Two patients with a small residue were treated by gamma knife, and a single patient underwent reoperation due to tumor regrowth. Patients did not present temporal lobe symptoms or long tract signs. No mortality occurred in this series. The major surgical complication was facial hypesthesia, which occurred in the territory of tumor origin. However, the patients' symptoms did not significantly affect their daily life because branches were preserved when possible. Only 1 patient with an M-type tumor complained of paresthesia. Permanent abducens palsy occurred in 3 patients, and hearing disturbance occurred in a single patient with a large tumor. Incomplete facial palsy, which might have resulted from retraction of the greater superficial petrosal nerve, occurred in 2 patients; however, the incidence might be lower compared to another reports.[6,7]

We concluded that the surgery was very safe with low morbidity. The surgical risk of facial palsy or hearing disturbance may be more optimistic in comparison with acoustic neurinoma surgery. Therefore, surgical treatment should be the first choice because complete removal after radiosurgery is difficult due to severe adhesion to the brain stem and cranial nerves.

KEY REFERENCES

Al-Mefty O, Ayoubi S, Gaber E: Trigeminal schwannomas: removal of dumbbell-shaped tumors through the expanded Meckel cave and outcome of cranial nerve function. *J Neurosurg.* 2002; 96:453-463 .

Dolenc VV. Frontotemporal epidural approach to trigeminal neurinomas. *Acta Neurochir (Wien).* 1994;130:55-65.

Kawase T, Shiobara R, Toya S. Anterior transpetrosal–transtentorial approach for sphenopetroclival meningiomas: surgical method and results in 10 patients. *Neurosurgery.* 1991;28:869-875:discussion 875-876.

Kawase T, van Loveren H, Kellar JT, Tew JM. Meningeal architecture of the cavernous sinus: clinical implications. *Neurosurgery.* 1996;39:527-534:discussion 534-536.

Muto J, Kawase T, Yoshida K. Meckel's cave tumors, relation to meninges and minimally invasive approaches for surgery—anatomical and clinical studies. *Neurosurgery.* 2010 Sep(suppl operative 3):67: 291-298; discussion 298-299.

Sami M, Tatagiba M, Carvalho GA. Retrosigmoid intradural suprameatal approach to Meckel's cave and the middle fossa: surgical technique and outcome. *J Neurosurg.* 2000;92:235-241.

Yoshida K, Kawase T. Trigeminal neurinomas extending into multiple fossae; surgical methods and review of the literature. *J Neurosurg.* 1999;91:202-211.

Numbered references appear on Expert Consult.

Surgical Management of Petroclival Meningiomas

KHALED M. AZIZ • SEBASTIEN FROELICH • SANJAY BHATIA • ALEXANDER K. YU •
ALBINO BRICOLO • TODD HILLMAN • RAYMOND F. SEKULA, JR.

Posterior fossa meningiomas comprise 10% of intracranial meningiomas. Clival and petroclival meningiomas comprise only 3% to 10% of the posterior fossa meningiomas. Petroclival meningiomas arise from the petroclival junction, above the jugular tubercle, medial to the trigeminal nerve, and anteromedial to the facial–vestibulocochlear nerve complex.[1-5] Petroclival meningiomas arise in the area surrounding the spheno-occipital synchondrosis. Tumors can involve the anterior portion of the tentorial incisura, Meckel's cave, middle cranial fossa floor, and parasellar region and cavernous sinuses (sphenopetroclival meningioma). Petroclival meningiomas can displace the brain stem and encase the surrounding critical neurovascular structures. Meningiomas arising posterolateral to the internal auditory canal (IAC) are defined as cerebellopontine angle meningiomas. The position of cranial nerves VII and VIII is the critical landmark to differentiate petroclival meningiomas from cerebellopontine angle meningiomas. Petroclival meningiomas originate anterior to the IAC and displace cranial nerves VII and VIII posteriorly. In contrast, cerebellopontine angle meningiomas originate posterior to the IAC and displace cranial nerves VII and VIII anteriorly. Foramen magnum meningiomas arise inferior to the jugular tubercles.[1,2,4-7]

Petroclival meningiomas are located in an anatomically demanding region. Despite a better understanding of the microsurgical anatomy and the great advances in standard operative technique, the surgical resection of petroclival meningiomas remains a substantial challenge. The emergence of cranial base surgery as a discipline has resulted in the revival, revision, and expansion of the surgical approaches that expose the petroclival region.

History

In 1874, "a 50-year-old woman developed paralysis of the arms, followed by the legs, then of respiration…and died after a few months. The autopsy revealed a nut-sized tumor of the inferior basilar gutter." This case, presented by Hallopeau,[8] may represent the first report of a petroclival meningioma in the literature. In the past, petroclival meningiomas were described only in postmortem studies.[9,10] In 1922, Cushing[11] acknowledged the difficulties in treating meningiomas of the clival region. He concluded his Cavendish lecture by saying, "The difficulties are admittedly great, sometimes insurmountable, and though the disappointments still are many, another generation of neurologic surgeons will unquestionably see them largely overcome." The petroclival clival region is an anatomically complex area. It has an irregular bony topography and contains complex collection of blood vessels, cranial nerves, and related brain stem. Despite Cushing's optimism, petroclival meningiomas remain the most demanding and formidable meningiomas to treat.

In 1927, Olivecrona[12] started his surgical exploration of clival meningiomas. He deemed them inoperable after an unacceptable experience with six patients. Early surgical experience with petroclival meningiomas was depressing. The reported surgical mortality exceeded 50%.[10,13,14] With the introduction of microsurgical techniques, Yasargil et al.[5] reported more promising results in 1980, with a mortality rate of 10%. With improved three-dimensional understanding of microsurgical anatomy and advancement and refinement of skull base techniques and approaches, management of petroclival meningiomas has been accomplished with much lower morbidity and mortality rates according to the recent literature.

Natural History

The incidence of petroclival meningiomas is low compared to that of other skull base meningiomas. Petroclival meningiomas are known to be slowly growing. However, the literature on the growth rates and natural history of petroclival meningiomas is insufficient. Jääskeläinen et al.[15] reported the growth rates of intracranial meningiomas among tumors with the same histologic grade. In 2003, Van Havenbergh et al.[16] reported the results of a long-term clinical and radiologic follow-up study of 21 patients with petroclival meningiomas treated conservatively. The follow-up period was from 48 to 120 months (mean 82 months, median 85 months). During follow-up, radiologic tumor growth was documented in 76% of the patients, and clinical deterioration occurred in 63% of these patients. The mean growth rates were 1.16 mm/yr in diameter and 1.10 cm^3/yr in volume. Rapid growth spurts were documented in small and medium-sized tumors. Small to medium-sized tumors tended to grow more than larger tumors. Therefore, active treatment was recommended for symptomatic patients with small or medium-sized tumors. The authors recommended surgical resection for younger and healthy patients and focused beam radiation therapy (stereotactic radiosurgery or radiotherapy) for elderly patients or unhealthy patients who cannot undergo surgery. The authors have the same recommendations for large growing asymptomatic tumors.

Recurrence Rate

It is difficult to compare the recurrence and regrowth rates in the published series due to the variation in the follow-up duration and the definition of the degree of resection. Recurrence rate depends on location, cavernous sinus involvement, brain stem infiltration, grade of resection, and histopathologic result.[17] Mathiesen et al.[18] provide comprehensive long-term results of resected skull base meningiomas. Recurrence rate after 5 years for Simpson grade I resection was 3.5%, for grade II resection was 4%, for grade III resection was 25%, and for grade IV to V resection 36% to 45%. After 15 years, recurrence rate for Simpson grade I resection was 7% to 10%, for grade II resection was 11% to 15%, for grade III resection was 37% to 43%, and for grade IV to V resection was 63% to 100%. Recurrence rate after 25 years for Simpson grade I resection was 13% to 16%, for grade II resection was 15% to 20%, and for grade III resection was 39% to 76%.

Recurrence rates for petroclival meningiomas in the published literature ranged from 0% to 42%[2,3,5,7,17,19-24, 26,30,31,65,66] (Table 40-1). Jung et al. followed 38 patients after subtotal resection of petroclival meningiomas for a mean period of 47.5 months. Radiographic evidence of tumor progression and recurrence occurred in 16 patients (42%). Among the previously mentioned factors, there were correlations among growth rate, old age, and occurrence of menopause.[19]

Clinical Picture

Clinical findings in patients with petroclival meningiomas can be related to four major etiologies: (1) involvement of cranial nerves, (2) cerebellar compression, (3) brain stem compression, and (4) increased intracranial pressure.[2,5,14] Presenting symptoms in petroclival meningiomas are nearly the same in all series reported in the literature. Cranial nerves affected, in order of greatest incidence, are V, VIII, VI, VII, IX, and X. Cranial nerves are affected by compression, stretching, incorporation into the tumor, or less frequently, invasion by the tumor. Other common neurologic findings include gait ataxia and motor and sensory deficits due to cerebellar and brain stem compression. Increased intracranial pressure, dementia, and change in visual acuity were frequently associated with hydrocephalus, secondary to aqueduct compression.

Based on the location of the tumor's dural attachment, Ichimura et al.[22] created four subtypes of petroclival meningiomas: the upper clivus type, the cavernous sinus type, the tentorial type, and the petrous apex type. Trigeminal neuropathy was the most commonly found symptom (45%); there was no significant difference in the frequency of trigeminal neuropathy among the four types. The upper clivus type comprises tumors medial to the trigeminal nerve with the primary presentation of ataxia. The cavernous sinus type comprises tumors originating from the posterior cavernous sinus medial to the trigeminal nerve and extends

Table 40-1	Outcomes Following Resection of Petroclival Meningiomas						
Series	Patients	Total Excision (%)	Mortality (%)	Major Morbidity (%)	New CN Deficits (%)	Average Follow-up (Months)	Recurrence/Regrowth (%)
Yasargil et al. (1980)[5]	20	35	10	30	50	NR	15
Mayberg and Symon (1986)[3]	35	26	9	34	54	34	11
Al-Mefty et al. (1988)[2]	13	85	NR	8	31	26	8
Hakuba et al. (1988)[31]	8	75	12	38	100	42	NR
Samii et al. (1989)[21]	24	71	NR	17	46	NR	NR
Bricolo et al. (1992)[7]	33	79	9	18	76	53	9
Kawase et al. (1994)[24]	42	76	NR	12	36	54	7
Sekhar et al. (1994)[26]	75	60	3	16	60	NR	3
Couldwell et al. (1996)[20]	109	69	3.7	15	33	73	13
Abdel Aziz et al. (2000)[23]	35	37	0	9	31	50	3
Little et al. (2005)[17]	137	55	0.8	26	23	29.8	17.6
Natarajan et al. (2007)[65]	150	32	0	20.3	20	102	5
Bambakidis et al. (2007)[66]	46	43	0	15	30	42	15

CN, cranial nerve; NR, not reported.

into the posterior fossa, with the characteristic symptom being abducens nerve palsy. The tentorial type originates from the tentorium and the petroclival junction; it displaces the trigeminal nerve inferomedially. The petrous apex type of tumor attaches to the petrous apex lateral to the trigeminal nerve and pushes it superomedially. Trigeminal neuralgia was common in patients with the petrous apex and tentorial types.

Neuroradiologic Evaluation

Thorough evaluation of preoperative neuroimaging studies is of utmost importance in the management of petroclival meningiomas. Multimodality imaging methods are utilized to assess the tumor's size, consistency, vascularity, location "zone" and extension of dural attachment, tumor–brain stem interface, degree of brain stem displacement encasement, displacement of the vertebrobasilar arterial system, and tumor extension into the cavernous sinus.[23]

Computed tomography of the temporal bone is valuable in evaluating the anatomy of the inner ear, its relation to the jugular bulb, the "height of the jugular bulb," and the degree of pneumatization of the mastoid bone. These data are helpful when transpetrosal approaches are contemplated. Tumor location zone can be identified from the temporal bone computed tomography.

Magnetic resonance imaging (MRI) T1-weighted images with and without contrast delineates the tumor and its relationships to the surrounding structures. MRI T2-weighted images are useful for assessment of the arachnoid cleavage plane, brain stem edema, and infiltration. Flow voids on MRI T2-weighted images can reveal the location of major vertebrobasilar vessels. The absence of a definite arachnoid cleavage plane between the tumor and the brain stem can make resection extremely challenging. This is one of the main obstacles preventing safe total resection of petroclival meningiomas. The lack of a definite arachnoid cleavage plane can be associated with brain stem pial infiltration. This can be predicted from preoperative MRI studies (Fig. 40-1) and has been associated with postoperative

morbidity.[4,24-27] Understanding the venous anatomy can reduce related complications during surgical approaches for petroclival meningiomas. Magnetic resonance venogram can illustrate the variations of the torcula and the relative sizes and patency of the transverse and sigmoid sinuses on either side. In addition, the vein of Labbé (posterior temporal venous drainage) and its drainage area are often visualized. This information may be useful if a sigmoid sinus needs to be divided (lateral to the temporal venous drainage) during surgery.

Cerebral angiography should be considered during the preoperative evaluation of petroclival meningiomas. Not only does it show the tumor's blood supply, it also can indirectly demonstrate the tumor causing mass effect on the vertebrobasilar system and its branches. Petroclival meningiomas are supplied by the meningohypophysial trunk of the internal carotid artery, the posterior branch of the middle meningeal artery, the meningeal branch of the vertebral artery, the clivus artery from the carotid siphon, the petrosal branches of the meningeal arteries, and the ascending pharyngeal branches of the external carotid artery.[28] Angiography can also be used for preoperative tumor embolization to reduce surgical blood loss.

Anesthetic Considerations

Neuroanesthesia continues to evolve with recent advances in neurosurgical procedures and intraoperative monitoring. The goals of modern neuroanesthesia are to provide a stable hemodynamic condition, maintain cerebral perfusion pressure, allow optimum intraoperative monitoring, and leave no residual anesthetic effects to facilitate the postoperative assessment of patient's neurologic condition.

Patient positioning may require maximal rotation of the patient's head and neck. A reinforced (armored) endotracheal tube is preferred to prevent kinking of the endotracheal tube to maintain the airway.

Brain relaxation can be provided by the judicious use of mannitol (0.25 to 1.0 mg/kg) and furosemide (10 to 20 mg), hypertonic saline (NaCl 3%), and a lumbar drain. It is

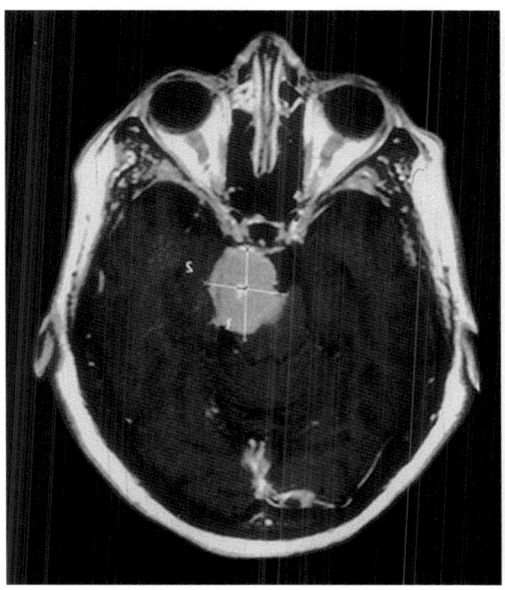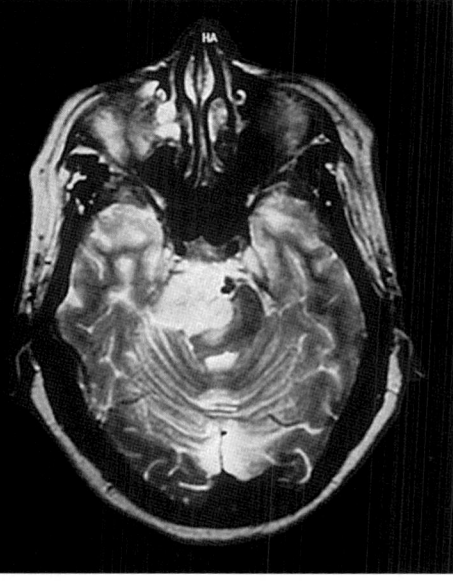

FIGURE 40-1 T1- and T2-weighted MRI images revealing brain stem infiltration by a petroclival meningioma. (From Abdel Aziz KM, Sanan A, van Loveren HR, et al. Petroclival meningiomas: predictive parameters for transpetrosal approaches. *Neurosurgery.* 2000;47(1):139-152.)

preferred to keep the patient normocapnic with maintained euvolemia. The ability to maintain and manipulate blood pressure in response to changes in monitoring parameters and surgical needs is crucial. Muscle relaxation is not utilized because of cranial nerve and motor tract monitoring. Most anesthesiologists use a narcotic-based technique, a remifentanil or sufentanil infusion for analgesia, and a low-solubility inhalational agent such as sevoflurane or an intravenous agent such as propofol for hypnosis. The hypnotic agents can be titrated based on bispectral index monitoring. This is especially useful when propofol is being used for long cases, because the context-sensitive half-life of propofol increases with the duration of use. Nitrous is not utilized with such a regimen. A phenylephrine drip is used to titrate the blood pressure to desired levels. Burst suppression can also be provided in conjunction with electroencephalogram monitoring.

Intraoperative Neurophysiologic Monitoring

Intraoperative neurophysiologic monitoring has been utilized to minimize neurologic morbidity from operative manipulations. Intraoperative monitoring has been effective in localizing cranial nerves, which helps guide the neurosurgeon during dissection. This facilitates safe tumor resection with cranial nerve preservation.

The following modalities are generally used:

- *Somatosensory evoked potentials (SSEPs).* SSEPs are recorded by electric stimulation of peripheral afferent nerves and recorded with the assistance of scalp electrodes. The sensory system is monitored from the peripheral nerves in upper and lower extremities via plexi, tracts, fasciculi, thalami, and the sensory cortex. The median nerve at the wrist is the most common stimulation site for upper extremity monitoring, and the posterior tibial nerve, just posterior to the medial malleolus, is most commonly used for lower extremity monitoring.
- *Motor evoked potentials (MEPs).* The motor system is monitored by transcranial stimulation of the motor cortex bilaterally and recording electromyogram activity in the muscles. Muscle relaxants cannot be used during MEP monitoring. MEPs can be difficult to detect at baseline, especially in older patients, and are very sensitive to the depth of anesthesia.
- *Brain stem auditory evoked potentials (BSAEPs).* BSAEPs record cortical responses to auditory stimuli. This allows monitoring of the function of the entire auditory pathway, including the acoustic nerve, brain stem, and cerebral cortex. Positive deflections are termed waves I to VII. Waves I, III, and V are the waves most consistently seen in healthy subjects (obligate waves). Wave V is the most reliably seen wave. A shift in latency of 1 msec or a drop in amplitude of 50% could be significant and should be reported to the neurosurgeon. Auditory evoked potential monitoring is crucial during dissection and retraction around cranial nerve VIII.
- *Electroencephalography.* This is generally used to monitor burst suppression. It may also detect ischemia with unilateral slowing.

Monitoring of cranial nerves III to VII and IX to XII is performed by recording electromyogram activity from the appropriately innervated muscles via an intraoperative stimulation probe. Again, muscle relaxants cannot be utilized during cranial nerve monitoring.

Goals of Surgical Management

Neurosurgeons must weigh the increased morbidity produced by aggressive surgery against the natural history of residual tumor, particularly in older patients. The optimal therapeutic strategy for each patient involves various considerations. These include prognostic factors, applicability of other options such as radiosurgery, and consequences of the outcome on the patient's quality of life. Evaluating the surgical results of petroclival meningioma removal requires special considerations. Grading schemes used for convexity meningiomas cannot be used to evaluate the excision of petroclival meningiomas. It is extremely difficult to achieve total excision of a petroclival meningioma, including excision of its dural attachment, its dural tail, and the involved bone. Therefore, it is impractical to apply the Simpson grading system to assess the degree of resection of petroclival meningiomas.[29]

Untreated petroclival meningiomas produce morbidity from the continuous brain stem compression (Fig. 40-2). Therefore, our primary goal is brain stem decompression to restore clinical function with either total or subtotal excision. We have developed a grading scale that evaluates the extent of resection and the degree of brain stem reexpansion. The extent of resection is considered maximal if the tumor is grossly removed. Brain stem reexpansion is maximal if the brain stem regains its normal contour and position (Table 40-2).

Petroclival meningiomas grow very slowly, and they may have a tendency to invade the brain stem, cranial nerves, and the basilar artery and its perforators. For tumors with neurovascular invasion, we prefer performing an excision of the tumor that leaves the parts infiltrating the neurovascular structures undisturbed, rather than attempting total excision of the tumor, which may leave the patient with a major neurologic deficit. Devascularization of the residual capsule of a petroclival meningioma may result in limited growth for a long period.[3,30]

The ideal goal of surgery is complete resection of the tumor without causing additional deficits to the patient. Preoperative imaging shows the extent of the tumor, its relationship to adjoining nerves and major blood vessels, and the lack or presence of an arachnoid cleavage plane. For petroclival meningiomas, the surgeon must constantly weigh the benefits of complete resection, the risk of morbidity by injury to vital structures and the natural history of potentially residual tumor. To keep morbidity to a minimum, other alternatives to surgery include safe debulking (incomplete, subtotal resection) and stereotactic radiosurgery or stereotactic radiotherapy.

Surgical Approaches

Petroclival meningiomas have been mainly exposed through the petrous portion of the temporal bone. Petrosal approaches have a distinctive advantage for exposure of the petroclival region compared to the other conventional approaches.[1,2,24,31-37] The variety of names for the petrosal approaches fall into one of two categories: anterior or

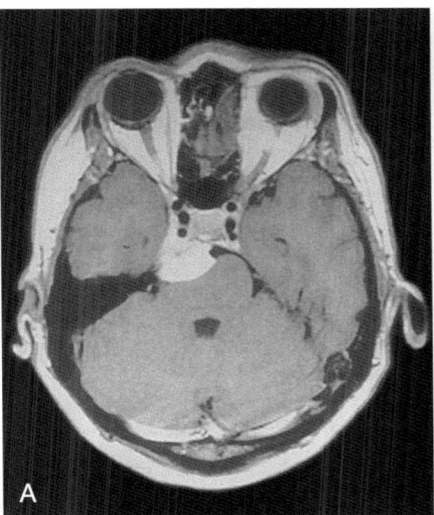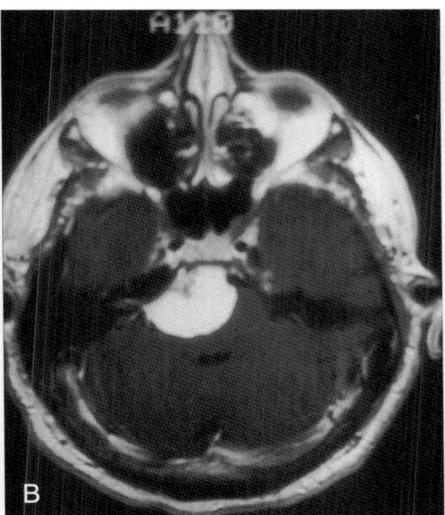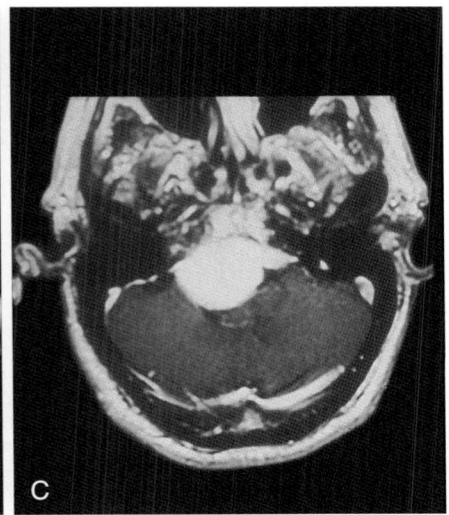

FIGURE 40-2 MRI revealing brain stem compression. A, Less than 25% compression. B, From 25% to 50% compression. C, More than 50% compression. (From Abdel Aziz KM, Sanan A, van Loveren HR, et al. Petroclival meningiomas: predictive parameters for transpetrosal approaches. *Neurosurgery.* 2000;47(1):139-152.)

Table 40-2	Grading Scale for Excision of Petroclival Meningiomas
Grade I	Total resection with coagulation of the dural attachment
Grade II	Total resection without coagulation of the dural attachment
Grade II	<10% residual tumor
Grade IV	10%-50% residual tumor
	A: Complete brain stem expansion
	B: >75% brain stem reexpansion
	C: <75% brain stem reexpansion
Grade V	>50% residual tumor
	A: Complete brain stem expansion
	B: >75% brain stem reexpansion
	C: <75% brain stem reexpansion

posterior petrosectomy.[33] The two approaches can be combined (i.e., combined petrosal approach), or they can be used as part of a more elaborate surgical exposure. We prefer to collaborate with the neuro-otologists to perform the temporal bone drilling. However, some neurosurgeons prefer to perform the whole approach in either one or two stages without a neuro-otologist. On the basis of surgical experience and anatomic dissections, we have designed an algorithm to predict the extent of resection possible via transpetrosal approaches.[23] The extent of exposure achieved via the anterior petrosal approach is from cranial nerve III down to the IAC (Fig. 40-3A). The extent of exposure achieved via the posterior petrosal (retrolabyrinthine) approach was from cranial nerve IV to the upper border of the jugular tubercle (Fig. 40-3B). Some pioneers achieved successful results through the lateral suboccipital "retrosigmoid" approach.[38-40]

Tumors that extend anteriorly to the cavernous sinus and the interpeduncular fossa need an additional frontotemporal approach with or without orbitozygomatic osteotomy for more exposure. Tumors extending into the foramen magnum require an additional suboccipital–transcondylar approach.

CLIVUS AND PETROCLIVAL ZONES

Based on the extent of surgical exposure achieved by surgical approaches, the clivus and petroclival region is divided into three zones (I, II, and III)[23] (Fig. 40-4). Petroclival meningiomas involving multiple zones require combined approaches.

Zone I (upper zone) extends from the dorsum sellae to the upper border of the IAC. This involves the retrosellar region and the region medial to the trigeminal impression (Meckel's cave) down to the IAC. Zone I can be exposed utilizing the Kawase approach,[32] also known as the anterior petrosal approach.[23,33] Zygomatic osteotomy can be added to the anterior petrosectomy to enhance the angle of exposure.[41] If the tumor only involves the retrosellar region of zone I, exposure can be via a trans-sylvian transcavernous approach, which involves mobilization of the oculomotor nerve and drilling of the posterior clinoid process and the dorsum sellae.[42] With endoscopic assistance, zone I of the petroclival region can be exposed via a subtemporal keyhole approach.[43]

Zone II (middle zone) extends from the IAC to the upper border of the jugular tubercle, representing the exposure provided via the posterior petrosal approach. The posterior petrosal approach achieves exposure from the trigeminal impression (in zone I) to the jugular tubercle. Tumors involving both zone I and zone II require a combined petrosal approach.[44] This is a combination of anterior and posterior petrosal approaches (Fig. 40-5).

Horgan et al. described the "transcrusal" approach, which adds drilling of the posterior and superior semicircular canals, while preserving hearing, to enhance the exposure of the petroclival region.[45]

Zone III (lower zone) extends from the jugular tubercle to the lower edge of the clivus. This is essentially the foramen magnum. Lateral suboccipital–transcondylar approaches provide exposure for zone III.

The angle between the petrous bone and the clivus (the petroclival angle) at the level of the IAC varies between patients.[23] There is no direct access to the small irregular volume of space bounded by the midline medially, the intermeatal plane superiorly, and the jugular tubercle inferiorly

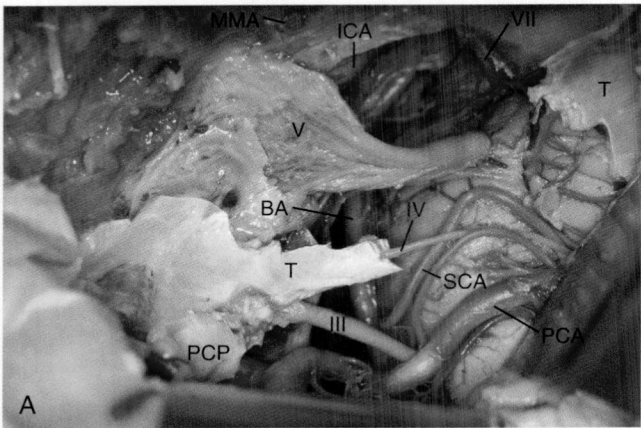

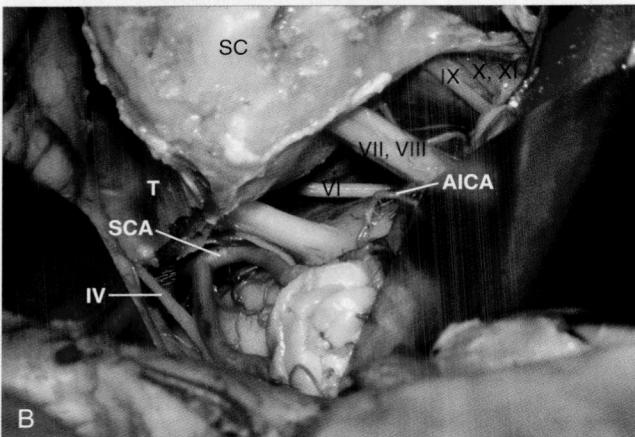

FIGURE 40-3 A, Cadaveric dissection showing the extent of exposure achieved via the anterior petrosal approach. B, Cadaveric dissection showing the extent of exposure achieved via the posterior petrosal approach. AICA, anteroinferior cerebellar artery; BA, basilar artery; MMA, middle meningeal artery; SCA, superior cerebellar artery; SC, semicircular canal; T, tentorium; ICA, internal carotid artery; PCA, posterior cerebellar artery; PCP, posterior clinoid process; III, oculomotor nerve; IV, trochlear nerve; V, trigeminal nerve; VI, abducent nerve; VII, facial nerve; VIII, superior vestibular nerve; IX, glossopharyngeal nerve; X, vagus nerve; XI, accessory nerve. (From Abdel Aziz KM, Sanan A, van Loveren HR, et al. Petroclival meningiomas: predictive parameters for transpetrosal approaches. *Neurosurgery.* 2000;47(1):139-152.)

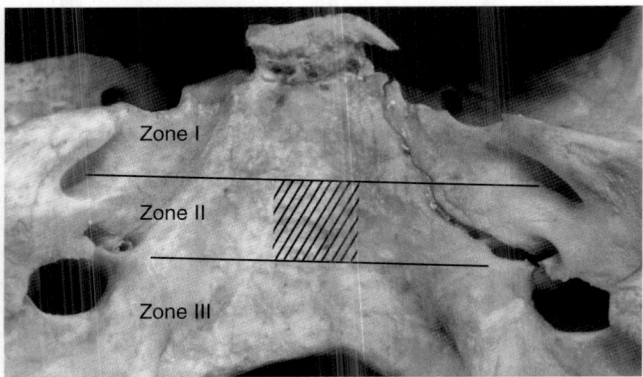

FIGURE 40-4 Photograph of a dry human skull showing the three clival zones separated by blue lines. Zone I (upper zone) extends from the dorsum sellae to the upper border of the IAC. Zone II (middle zone) extends from the upper border of the IAC to the upper border of the jugular tubercle. The central clival depression is shown by the hatched area. Zone III (lower zone) extends from the upper border of the jugular tubercle to the lower edge of the clivus. (From Abdel Aziz KM, Sanan A, van Loveren HR, et al. Petroclival meningiomas: predictive parameters for transpetrosal approaches. *Neurosurgery.* 2000;47(1):139-152.)

between the pregeniculate and the postgeniculate portions of the facial nerve, manipulation around the geniculate ganglion leads to ischemic injury of the facial nerve.[46-50] Posterior mobilization of the facial nerve results in complete postoperative nerve paralysis in 100% of patients. Facial nerve paralysis improves in about one third of patients to House-Brackmann grade III within 1 year.[51] In 1994, Cass et al.[52] reported the use of total petrosectomy (the translabyrinthine/transcochlear approach) for large petroclival meningiomas. Despite the sacrifice of hearing and a significant rate of facial nerve paralysis, only 55% of lesions were totally excised.

ANTERIOR PETROSAL APPROACH

The anterior petrosal approach[32] (Fig. 40-9) allows exposure of the middle fossa floor, the petrous bone apex, and zone I of the petroclival region. The anterior petrosal approach includes a subtemporal or frontotemporal craniotomy and anterior petrosectomy. The anterior petrosal approach can be combined with the posterior petrosal approach to expand the exposure down to the jugular tubercle (zone II). Patient positioning is the most crucial step of all operative procedures. For the subtemporal/anterior petrosal approach, we prefer placement of a lumbar drain prior to positioning. The patient is placed in a supine position with the head fixed in a three-point skull fixation device and rotated 90 degrees (the sagittal suture is parallel to the floor). The ipsilateral shoulder is elevated with a gelatin roll to prevent kinking and occlusion of the jugular vein and stretching of the brachial plexus. The head is tilted 15 degrees downward; this places the zygoma in the highest point of the surgical field, and the gravity effect minimizes the extent of temporal lobe retraction during surgery. The patient's upper back is elevated 25-30 degrees to facilitate venous drainage. The arms are securely padded to avoid pressure on the ulnar and radial nerves. Slight flexion of the knees prevents joint tension from hyperextension. Thromboembolic deterrent hose and compression stockings are placed around the legs to reduce venous stasis.

(Fig. 40-6). This is a relatively difficult-to-access or an inaccessible space called the "central clival depression."[23] The less obtuse the petroclival angle, the more difficult the exposure of the central clival depression (Figs. 40-7 and 40-8).

With posterior petrosectomy (retrolabyrinthine), our line of sight could not reach portions of tumor attached to the central clival region between the IAC and the upper border of the jugular tubercle. Exposure of the central clival depression necessitates the posterior petrosal translabyrinthine/transcochlear approach with posterior mobilization of the facial nerve. Resection of the labyrinth results in hearing loss, and posterior mobilization of the facial nerve to drill the cochlea results in a facial palsy, with limited expectation of facial recovery. To achieve posterior mobilization of the facial nerve, the nerve is unroofed from the IAC back to the stylomastoid foramen. The chorda tympani and the greater superficial petrosal nerve (GSPN) are cut, and the facial nerve is mobilized from the geniculate ganglion posteriorly. As there are few anastomotic arteries

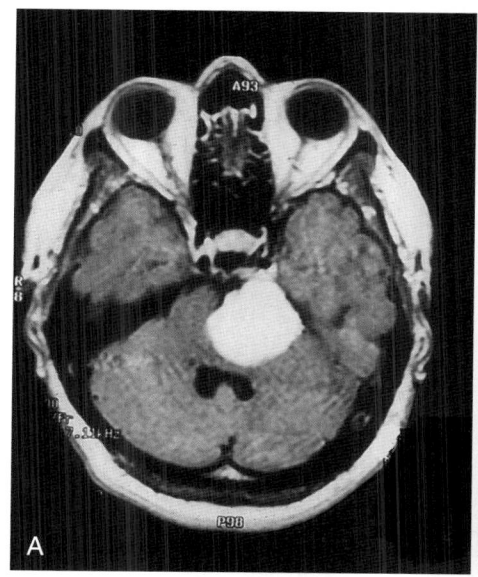
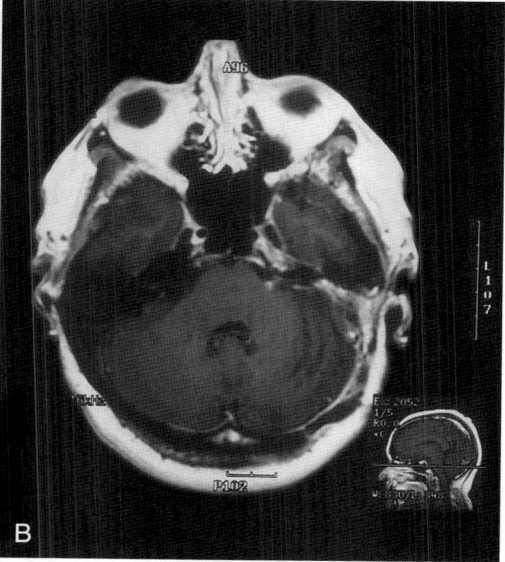

FIGURE 40-5 A, Preoperative MRI scan showing zone I and II petroclival meningiomas. B, Postoperative MRI scan showing grade II resection (combined petrosal approach). (From Abdel Aziz KM, Sanan A, van Loveren HR, et al. Petroclival meningiomas: predictive parameters for transpetrosal approaches. *Neurosurgery.* 2000; 47(1):139-152.)

A skin flap initiated posterior to the midpoint of the mastoid process extends superiorly and anteriorly, traversing the superior temporal line and ending at the middle of the zygomatic arch for a subtemporal anterior petrosal approach. The skin incision is extended anteriorly along the superior temporal line, ending just behind the hairline if a frontotemporal craniotomy is planned.

In the subtemporal approach, the temporalis muscle is reflected inferiorly with the skin flap as a myocutaneous flap. A rectangular craniotomy is designed along the squamosal suture (posterior third behind the external auditory canal and anterior two thirds in front of the external auditory canal). Zygomatic osteotomy allows more caudal displacement of the temporalis muscle and more inferior to superior trajectory with minimal temporal lobe manipulation. The bony edges are drilled flush to the floor of the middle cranial fossa. The key in the initial steps of this approach is to preserve the dura and remain extradural.

If the petroclival meningioma extends anteriorly beyond zone I into the interpeduncular fossa and the cavernous sinus, a frontotemporal craniotomy is designed. The previously mentioned skin flap is extended anteriorly, and a mycutaneous flap is reflected anteroinferiorly. The sphenoid wing is totally exposed and completely drilled; our craniotomy extends anteriorly to allow more exposure. The sphenoid wing is completely drilled (flush to the roof and lateral wall of the orbit). Extradural partial anterior clinoidectomy can be added. This allows exposure of the frontotemporal junction of the basal dura and facilitates extradural dissection and mobilization of the lateral wall of the cavernous sinus using the Hakuba technique[53] (directed from anterolateral to posteromedial). The dura is elevated from the middle fossa floor, and petrous bone via a posterior to anterior approach; elevation starts at the arcuate eminence and proceeds anteriorly. The middle meningeal artery is controlled with bipolar cautery and sectioned, and the foramen spinosum is packed with mixed bone wax–Oxycel. The GSPN is identified and kept intact; we always leave a thin dural layer covering the nerve. Geniculate ganglion location is confirmed with facial nerve monitoring. The GSPN is

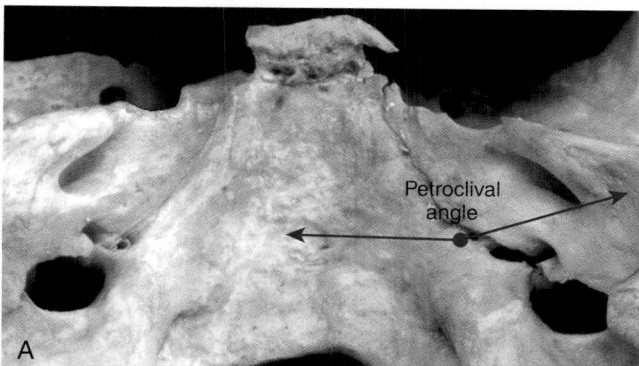
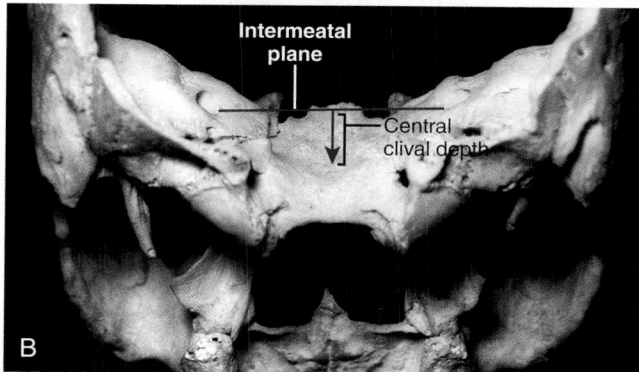

FIGURE 40-6 A, Photograph of the petroclival region in a dry human skull showing the petroclival angle (blue arrows). B, Photograph of the petroclival region in dry human skull demonstrating the intermeatal plane and the depth of the central clival depression (central clival depth). (From Abdel Aziz KM, Sanan A, van Loveren HR, et al. Petroclival meningiomas: predictive parameters for transpetrosal approaches. *Neurosurgery.* 2000;47(1):139-152.)

preserved, and dissection follows the GSPN from posterior to anterior until it courses under the third division of the trigeminal nerve (V3). More anteriorly, the mandibular division (V2) is identified at the foramen rotundum. Occasionally, the petrous segment of the internal carotid artery is visualized

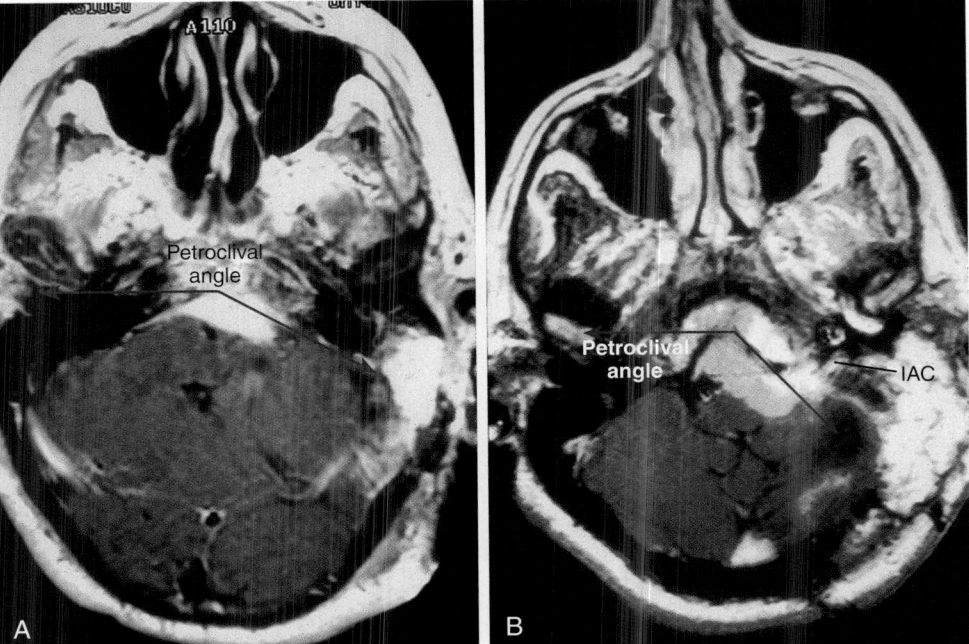

FIGURE 40-7 Postoperative MRI scans of residual tumor in the central clival depression with correlation to the petroclival angle (blue dashed lines). A, More obtuse petroclival angle with less residual tumor. B, Less obtuse petroclival angle with more residual tumor. (From Abdel Aziz KM, Sanan A, van Loveren HR, et al. Petroclival meningiomas: predictive parameters for transpetrosal approaches. *Neurosurgery.* 2000;47(1):139-152.)

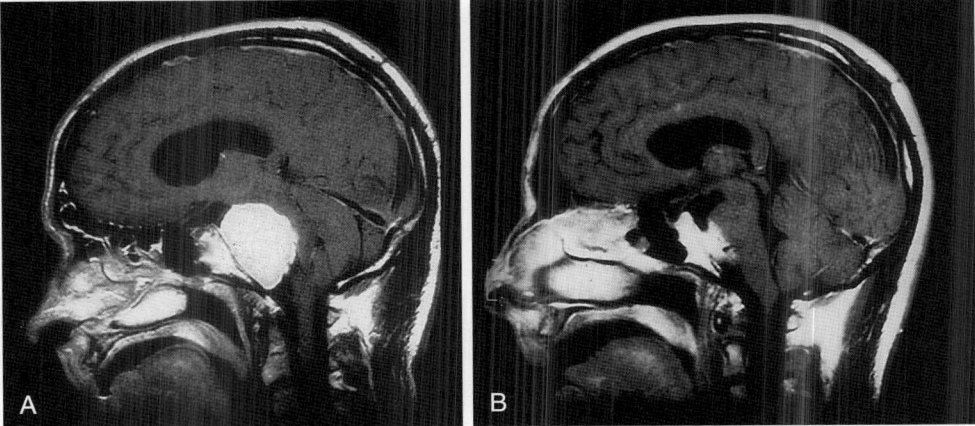

FIGURE 40-8 A, Preoperative MRI (sagittal section) showing zone I, II, and III petroclival meningiomas. B, Postoperative MRI scan showing grade III resection with complete brain stem reexpansion and residual tumor in the central clival depression and in the infiltrated brain stem. (From Abdel Aziz KM, Sanan A, van Loveren HR, et al. Petroclival meningiomas: predictive parameters for transpetrosal approaches. *Neurosurgery.* 2000;47(1):139-152.)

through a bony dehiscence in the petrous apex. Dissection continues medially to the petrous ridge indenting the superior petrosal sinus. Separation of the dura propria continues until the connective tissue sheath over V2, V3, and the Gasserian ganglion is visible (Meckel's cave). Kawase's quadrilateral is drilled under the microscope starting medially at the petrous ridge to identify the IAC. The arcuate eminence forms a 120-degree angle to the GSPN (or the internal carotid artery), and the IAC bisects this angle. Another, less commonly used, method to identify the IAC is to follow the geniculate ganglion to the labyrinthine segment of the facial nerve marking the IAC. This is associated with a high incidence of facial nerve injury. Drilling of the IAC continues to the bone crest dividing the facial nerve and the superior vestibular nerve (Bill's bar). The bone overlying the cochlea is drilled until the cochlea appears as a blue line. After identification of the dura covering the IAC posteriorly, the Kawase's

quadrilateral is drilled to the GSPN (preserved) laterally, the petrous segment of the internal carotid artery anterolaterally, V3 anteriorly, the superior petrosal sinus medially, and the posterior fossa dura and inferior petrosal sinus inferiorly. the inferior temporal lobe dura is open above and parallel to the superior petrosal sinus. The dura is reflected inferiorly; the superior petrosal sinus is secured with titanium hemoclips and is split. The tentorium is cut medially toward the tentorial incisura posterior to the dural entry of the trochlear nerve. The posterior fossa dura is further split inferiorly. This allows panoramic exposure from the oculomotor nerve superiorly, to the vestibulocochlear nerve inferiorly, to the nerve inferiorly (see Fig. 40-3A).

After completion of surgical resection, watertight dural closure is demanding. The IAC bony opening is plugged with a small piece of fat or muscle. The dura is approximated utilizing a synthetic dural graft and is sprayed with fibrin glue.

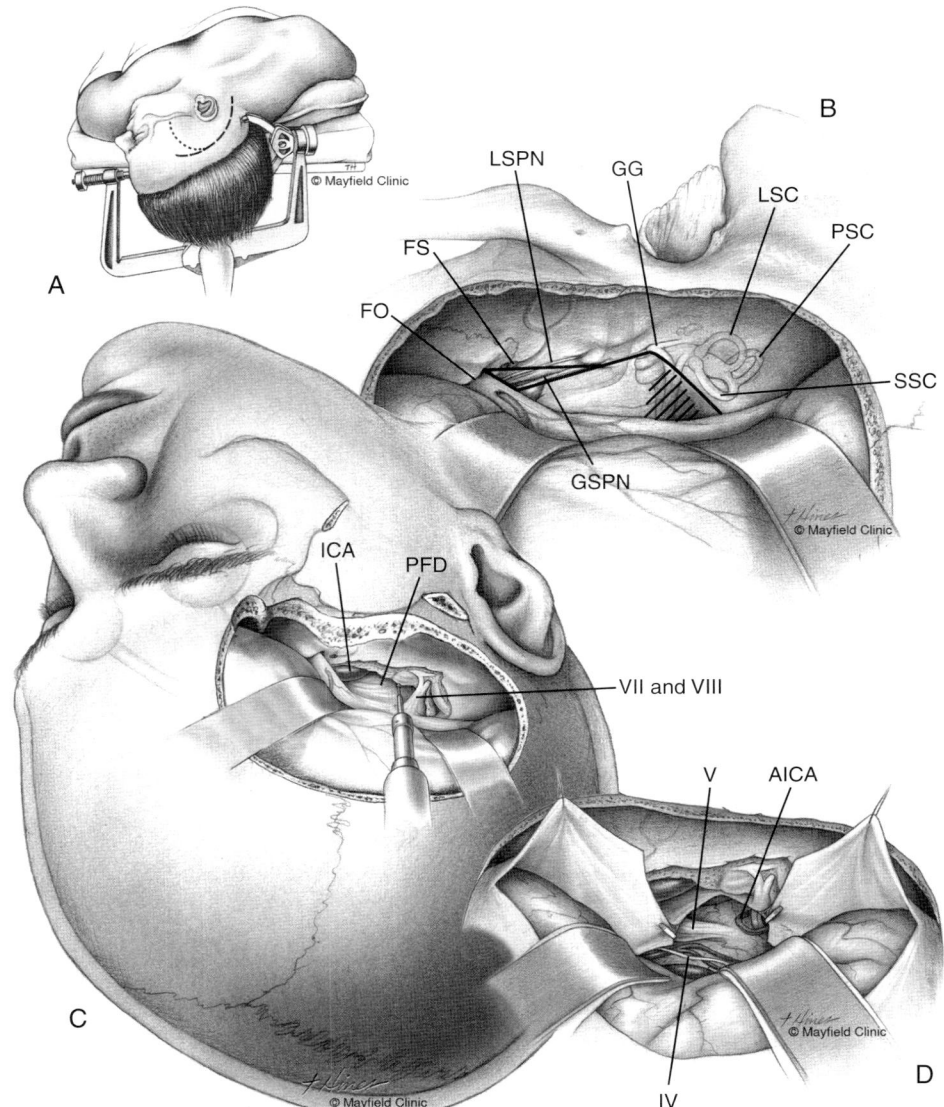

FIGURE 40-9 Diagram of the anterior petrosal approach. A, Patient position and skin incisions for anterior petrosal and posterior petrosal (dotted line) approaches. The approach (dashed line) if we plane to perform a frontotemporal craniotomy. B, Extradural exposure of the floor of the middle cranial fossa after a subtemporal craniotomy. Glasscock's and Kawase's triangles are outlined on the middle fossa floor. The boundaries of Glasscock's triangle are as follows: laterally, a line from the foramen spinosum to the facial hiatus; medially, the GSPN; and at the base, V3. The boundaries of Kawase's triangle are as follows: laterally, the GSPN; medially, the petrous ridge; and at the base, the arcuate eminence. The hatched area represents the meatal plane overlying the IAC. C, "Blue lining" of the cortical bone of the basal turn of the cochlea, with a diamond bur for maximum exposure while preserving hearing. The internal carotid artery is exposed in Glasscock's triangle. The posterior fossa dura is exposed down to the level of the inferior petrosal sinus by resection of the bone of Kawase's triangle. D, Intradural exposure achieved with anterior petrosectomy when coupled with a temporal craniotomy, section of the inferior temporal lobe dura, elevation of the temporal lobe, sacrifice of the superior petrosal sinus (shown with two titanium clips applied), section of tentorium cerebelli, and opening of the posterior fossa dura. LSPN, lesser superficial petrosal nerve; GG, geniculate ganglion; LSC, lateral semicircular canal; PSC, posterior semicircular canal; SSC, superior semicircular canal; FO, foramen ovale; FS, foramen spinosum; ICA, internal carotid artery; PFD, posterior fossa dura; VII, facial nerve; VIII, superior vestibular nerve; V, trigeminal nerve; AICA, anteroinferior cerebellar artery; IV, trochlear nerve. (©*Mayfield Clinic.*)

If there is a big filling defect, it can be judiciously obliterated with pieces of fat graft to prevent postoperative fluid collection and cerebrospinal fluid (CSF) leak. Bone flaps are connected and fixed with titanium plates and secures. Bony defects are filled with bone cement for cosmetic reconstruction and prevention of CSF leak. We prefer to keep the lumbar drain in place for 48 hours after obtaining an immediate postoperative computed tomography scan.

POSTERIOR PETROSAL APPROACH

The posterior petrosal approach (Fig. 40-10) consists of a temporal craniotomy combined with a presigmoid craniectomy and a small lateral retrosigmoid craniectomy. Depending on the preoperative hearing status, either retrolabyrinthine or translabyrinthine bony temporal bone drilling is added. The addition of a retrosigmoid craniotomy, sectioning of the superior petrosal sinus and tentorium, and

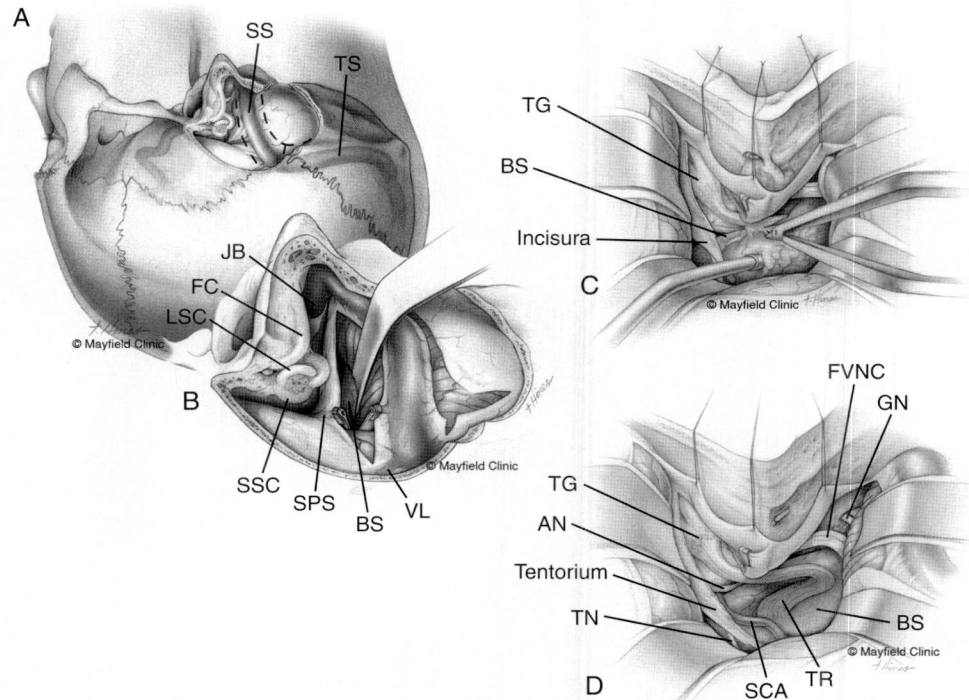

FIGURE 40-10 Diagram of the posterior petrosal approach. A, Posterior petrosectomy (mastoidectomy) with preservation of the labyrinth (semicircular canals) and skeletonization of the fallopian canal. The posterior petrosectomy is expanded to expose the temporal lobe to facilitate sacrifice of the superior petrosal sinus, section of the tentorium cerebelli, and placement of a relaxing incision above the transverse sinus, along with a small suboccipital (retrosigmoid) craniotomy. These maneuvers facilitate posterior displacement of the transverse–sigmoid sinus junction and sigmoid sinus. Dashed lines represent the dural incision. B, Initial intradural exposure achieved with the extended posterior petrosal approach. The superior petrosal sinus is sacrificed between two titanium clips. Also shown is a possible opening of the retrosigmoid dura for exploration from a conventional suboccipital approach, especially of lesions extending caudal to the jugular bulb. C, The tumor-involved dura overlying Meckel's cave is resected. The surgeon rolls the tumor posteriorly while sharply dissecting the adhesions and arachnoid of the trigeminal root to expose the brain stem. D, Caudal tumor remnants are removed from the dura adjacent to the cranial nerves of the jugular foramen TS, transverse sinus; SS, sigmoid sinus; SPS, superior petrosal sinus; JB, jugular bulb; LSC, lateral semicircular canal; SSC, superior semicircular canal; FC, facial nerve in the fallopian canal; VL, vein of Labbé; BS, brain stem. TG, trigeminal ganglion; AN, abducens nerve; TN, trigeminal nerve; SCA, superior cerebellar artery; TR, trigeminal root; FVNC, facial–vestibulocochlear nerve complex; GN, glossopharyngeal nerve. (©Mayfield Clinic.)

a relaxing incision in the dura above the lateral transverse sinus frees the sigmoid sinus and allows mobilization of the sigmoid sinus posteriorly to expand the presigmoid space. These steps are crucial to improving the presigmoid exposure of posterior fossa contents.

Head positioning is similar to that in the anterior petrosal approach. The lateral oblique position is an alternative if more posterior fossa exposure is required and to avoid venous congestion or if the patient is not tolerating neck rotation. Skin incision is marked three fingerbreadths circumferentially around the edge of the ear pinna, starting below the tip of the mastoid process. The skin flap is reflected inferiorly, and the temporalis muscle is reflected anteroinferiorly.

A temporal craniotomy is performed anterior to the transverse sinus, and a presigmoid and retrosigmoid craniectomy is performed using a drill. Drilling the bone overlying the dural sinuses prevents injury to the transverse and sigmoid sinuses. Other neurosurgeons prefer temporal and occipital craniotomy saddling the dural sinuses; however, our technique can be safer if performed in two or three pieces. The first set of bur holes is placed at the most anterior mastoid point and below the asterion, which puts the holes above and below the transverse sigmoid junction.

A second set of bur holes is placed above and below the superior nuchal line, which puts these holes above and below the transverse sinus. The drill footplate is utilized to connect the bur holes for a temporal and retrosigmoid craniotomy. The transverse sinus and the transverse–sigmoid junction are dissected from the overlying bone, and the initial bur holes are crossed using the drill footplate. If the dural sinuses are impeded in an inner table bony groove, the overlying bone is thinned with a drill bur and the final bone cut is made using a bone punch to allow safe bone flap elevation.

Retrolabyrinthine mastoidectomy is performed by a neuro-otologist. The spine of Henle is a landmark to the antrum. The mastoid bone is drilled, and the middle fossa and meatal bone plates are dissected until the antrum is identified. The floor of the antrum is the cortical bone of the lateral semicircular canal. After drilling the bone over the sinodural angle, the sigmoid sinus, superior petrosal sinus, and posterior semicircular canal are exposed. Following the lateral semicircular canal until it bisects the posterior semicircular canal is another technique to expose the posterior semicircular canal. The posterior semicircular canal is followed superiorly to expose the superior semicircular canal. The air cells of the mastoid tip are removed to expose the digastric ridge, which is a landmark to the stylomastoid foramen and the beginning of the fallopian canal. Preservation of the cortical bone of the fallopian canal avoids injury to the facial nerve. The combination of a temporal and suboccipital craniotomy with petrosectomy allows mobilization of the sigmoid sinus so that the surgeon can operate presigmoidally through the petrosectomy and retrosigmoidally through the suboccipital craniotomy.

The dural opening is made as follows: (1) the Dura is incised along the undersurface of the temporal lobe parallel to the superior petrosal sinus, taking care to preserve the vein of Labbé, which generally enters the transverse sinus within 1 cm of the transverse–sigmoid junction. (2) The posterior fossa dura in the presigmoid space is incised longitudinally between the superior petrosal sinus and the jugular bulb. (3) With gentle traction on the temporal lobe and cerebellum, the superior petrosal sinus is sectioned between two titanium hemoclips. (4) A relaxing dural incision is made along the upper border of the transverse sinus. (5) The tentorium is sectioned into the incisura at a point posterior to entrance of the trochlear nerve; the vein of Labbé on the surface of the temporal lobe is protected during the final dural cut. This wide dural opening allows panoramic posterior fossa exposure between the trigeminal nerve (cranial nerve V) and the upper border of the jugular tubercle (see Fig. 40-3B). If additional exposure caudal to the jugular tubercle (zone III) is required, a retrosigmoid craniectomy is expanded with partial condylar resection and C1 laminectomy to expose the foramen magnum (transcondylar approach) (Fig. 40-11; see also Fig. 40-8).

Watertight dural closure at the area of mastoidectomy is unachievable. The dural and edges are approximated. Pericranium or a synthetic dural graft is utilized to reinforce the dural closure. Open mastoid air cells are closed with wax. The antrum is plugged with a piece of muscle to close the middle ear cavity. The mastoidectomy defect is covered with an abdominal fat graft and sprayed with fibrin glue. Bone flaps are connected and fixed with titanium plates and secures. Bony defects are filled with bone cement for cosmetic reconstruction and prevention of CSF leak. The temporalis muscle is split to cover the mastoid defect and then firmly reattached to a fascial cuff. We prefer to keep the lumbar drain in place for 48 hours after obtaining an immediate postoperative computed tomography scan.

LATERAL SUBOCCIPITAL APPROACH

For petroclival meningiomas involving zones I, II, and III, the lower lateral suboccipital (retrosigmoid) approach is a viable alternative.[54,55] This provides exposure of the posterior surface of the petrous bone, the anterolateral brain stem, and the craniocervical junction. Intradural drilling of the petrous apex allows exposure of the tumor portion extending to the middle cranial fossa through Meckel's cave.[56]

The lateral oblique position is preferred for the lateral suboccipital approach. However, some surgeons prefer the supine position for lateral suboccipital approaches. This is applicable in slim patients with flexible necks. The lateral oblique position avoids excessive neck rotation and facilitates exposure of the posterior fossa and the upper cervical spine. The head is secured with a three-point skull fixation

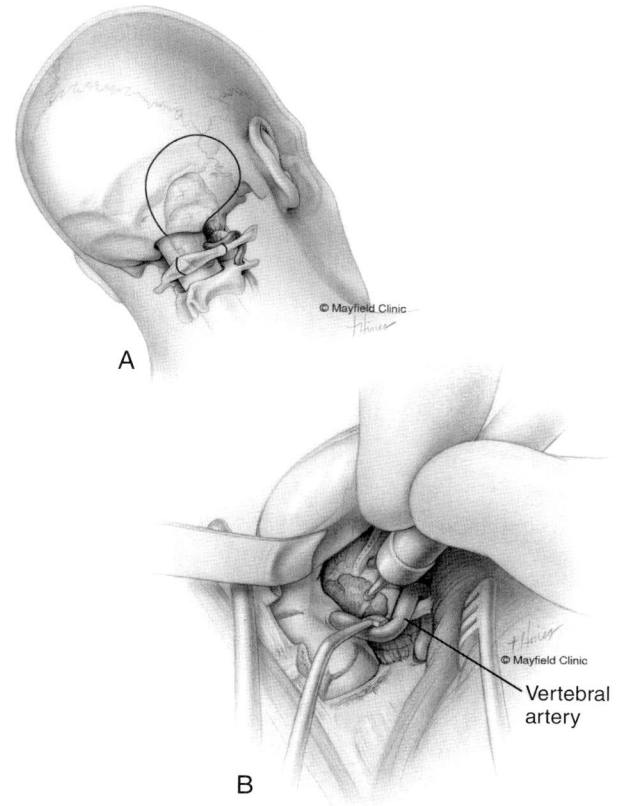

Vertebral artery

FIGURE 40-11 A, Petroclival meningioma involving zones I, II, and III. The surgical approach is a lateral suboccipital approach with opening of the foramen magnum, C1 hemilaminectomy, and upper transcondylar approach (partial resection of the posteromedial one third of the condyle without mobilization of the vertebral artery from the foramen transversarium of C1). The ghosted head depicts a lower lateral suboccipital craniotomy and C1 hemilaminectomy, and the relationship between the tumor and the regional anatomy. B, The vertebral artery can be retracted with a microretractor while the posteromedial one third of the occipital condyle is removed with a high-speed drill. (©Mayfield Clinic.)

while the patient is in the lateral position. An axillary roll is placed under the axilla to prevent brachial plexus compression. The lower extremities are flexed and separated with a pillow. Pressure points are padded; this includes the head of the fibula with the overlying peroneal nerve. The body is secured to the table with adhesive tape and safety belts. The patient's upper back is elevated 15 degrees to allow venous drainage. The head is maintained in a neutral position. The neck is flexed and tilted slightly downward so that three fingerbreadths can be easily placed between the chin and the manubrium. After the skin incision and subperiosteal muscle separation, craniotomy or craniectomy is designed. A keyhole bur hole is placed inferomedial to the asterion to avoid injury of the transverse sigmoid junction. The craniotomy flap does not extend beyond three to four fingerbreadths lateral to the external auditory canal. Mastoid bone is drilled to expose the medial edge of the sigmoid sinus and the inferior edge of the transverse sinus. We always prefer to open the foramen magnum. For a tumor that extends to zone III, C1 laminectomy and drilling of the posteromedial third of the occipital condyle and lateral mass of C1 allow lateral extension of the dural opening and better exposure to tumor portion anterior to the brain stem (see Fig. 40-11). The V3 segment of the vertebral artery is easily identified at the groove of the C1 lamina. This step can be achieved by following the periosteum covering the C1 lamina laterally; this usually keeps the neurosurgeon on top of the prevertebral venous plexus. If venous bleeding is encountered, it is controlled with Oxycel and bipolar cautery. The dural incision starts at C1, extends superiorly through the foramen magnum, and extends superolaterally to the top of craniotomy edge. After tumor resection, the dura is closed watertight. An autologous pericranial graft or a synthetic graft is usually required during closure, and the suture line is sprayed with fibrin glue. A craniotomy flap is placed using titanium plates and screws, and bony defects are filled with bone cement to minimize postoperative headache.

Radiosurgery

Stereotactic radiosurgery can be applied as a primary treatment modality for small petroclival meningiomas of less than 3 cm in diameter.[57] It can be utilized as an adjuvant treatment to prevent tumor regrowth and recurrence after maximal safe surgical resection. Subach et al.[58] retrospectively reviewed a heterogeneous group of 62 patients with a petroclival meningioma treated by gamma knife radiosurgery. During a median follow-up period of 37 months, tumor control was obtained in 92% of cases. Neurologic status improved in 21%, remained stable in 66%, and declined in 13%. Park et al.[59] reported on 12 patients who underwent stereotactic radiosurgery treatment with a median follow-up period of 52 months. These patients refused surgical treatment, suffered multiple medical problems, had a tumor that was asymptomatic and incidentally diagnosed, or in elderly patients, had a tumor that was small. The authors reported no clinical deterioration except in one patient, and two patients showed radiologic evidence of tumor progression during the follow-up period. The two patients with tumor progression underwent surgical treatment. Flannery et al.[60] reported the largest series in the literature of 168 patients with petroclival meningiomas treated with stereotactic radiosurgery as a primary or an adjuvant treatment with a median follow-up period of 72 months. The median tumor volume was 6.1 cm^3, and the median radiation dose to the tumor margin was 13 Gy. During the follow-up period, status improved in 44 patients (26%) who showed neurological improvement, 98 patients (58%) remained stable, and 26 patients (15%) showed neurologic deterioration. Tumor volume decreased in 78 patients (46%), remained stable in 74 patients (44%), and increased in 16 patients (10%). Major risk factors for tumor progression were tumor volume of 8 cm^3 and male sex.

In 2007, Couldwell et al.[61] report 13 patients with benign (World Health Organization grade I) skull base meningiomas who demonstrated tumor progression after stereotactic radiosurgery treatment. Radiosurgery was the primary or an adjuvant treatment. Tumor progression occurred within 6 months to 8 years after treatment in 10 patients and was between 8 and 14 years in 3 patients. With these recent data, it is strongly recommended to follow patients for longer durations after stereotactic radiosurgery treatment.

Outcomes

Preoperative neurologic deficits (diminished Karnofsky Performance Scale score), tumor size of 2.5 cm or more, multiple cranial fossae involvement and cavernous sinus infiltration, absence of arachnoid cleavage plane, brain stem compression and invasion, brain stem edema, adhesions to and encasement of vascular structures, high vascularity and direct tumor blood supply from the basilar artery, and firm tumor consistency affecting the extent of tumor resection have been associated with increased postoperative morbidity.

Various authors have reported gross total resection rates of 20% to 85%. Mortality varies from 0% to 10%, cranial nerve deficits range from 29% to 76%, and major morbidity is reportedly 8% to 45%.[2,3,5,7,17,23,24,26,30,31,62-66] The published series on petroclival meningiomas is summarized in Table 40-1.

Conclusions

As stated by Cushing in 1922, "There is today nothing in the whole realm of surgery more gratifying than the successful removal of a meningioma with a subsequent perfect functional recovery."[11] Despite the major attempts to perform total resection of petroclival meningiomas, there are microscopic nests of cells on the involved basal dura; dural attachment cannot be completely excised in the majority of cases. Ultimately, for meningiomas attached to the dura at the central clival depression in zone II, the surgical morbidity associated with total removal becomes prohibitive, and the chance of total removal, even with excellent exposure, remains poor.

The goal of surgical resection of petroclival meningiomas should be the avoidance of permanent neurologic dysfunction with maximum tumor removal. With classification of the petroclival region into three zones, it is clear that achieving total resection without permanent neurologic dysfunction is possible in either extreme of the clivus, but it becomes extremely demanding in certain areas. The difficulty arises from tumors that extend into the central clival depression and infiltrate neurovascular structures. Therefore, the art of resection of petroclival meningiomas should be simultaneously aggressive and judicious. Incomplete resection is not necessarily a failure, and for some tumors, brain stem decompression after subtotal resection is the most appropriate course of action. Residual tumors can be successfully followed or treated with focused beam radiation therapy. Stereotactic radiosurgery or stereotactic radiotherapy can be a viable primary treatment option for some patients.

KEY REFERENCES

Abdel Aziz KM, Sanan A, van Loveren HR, et al. Petroclival meningiomas: predictive parameters for transpetrosal approaches. *Neurosurgery.* 2000;47(1):139-152.

Al-Mefty O, Fox JL, Smith RR. Petrosal approach for petroclival meningiomas. *Neurosurgery.* 1988;22:510-517.

Bambakidis NC, Kakarla UK, Kim LJ, et al. Evolution of surgical approaches in the treatment of petroclival meningiomas: a retrospective review. *Neurosurg.* 2007;61(ONS suppl 2):202-211.

Couldwell WT, Weiss MH. Surgical approaches to petroclival meningiomas. I: upper and midclival approaches. *Contemp Neurosurg.* 1994;16:1-6.

Flannery TJ, Kano H, Lunsford LD, et al. Long-term control of petroclival meningiomas through radiosurgery. *J Neurosurg.* September 4, 2009.

Kawase T, Shiobara R, Toya S. Anterior transpetrosal–transtentorial approach for sphenopetroclival meningiomas: surgical method and results in 10 patients. *Neurosurgery.* 1991;28:869-876.

Kawase T, Shiobara R, Toya S. Middle fossa transpetrosal–transtentorial approaches for petroclival meningiomas: selective pyramid resection and radicality. *Acta Neurochir (Wien).* 1994;129:113-120.

Little KM, Friedman AH, Sampson JH, et al. Surgical management of petroclival meningiomas: defining resection goals based on risk of neurological morbidity and tumor recurrence rates in 137 patients. *Neurosurgery.* 2005;56(3):546-559.

Natarajan SK, Sekhar LN, Schessel D, Morita A. Petroclival meningiomas: multimodality treatment and outcomes at long term follow-up. *Neurosurg.* 2007;60:965-981.

Samii M, Tatagiba M. Experience with 36 surgical cases of petroclival meningiomas. *Acta Neurochir (Wien).* 1992;118:27-32.

Numbered references appear on Expert Consult.

CHAPTER 41

Surgical Management of Lesions of the Clivus

GIULIO MAIRA • FRANCESCO DOGLIETTO • ROBERTO PALLINI

The clivus is localized at the center of the skull base, and its deep location renders surgical access a challenge. Tumors that arise purely from the clivus are rare, but this region can be involved with numerous processes extending from the structures near the clivus, mainly from the petrous–clival line. Tumors may be limited to a part of the clivus, or they may involve the entire clivus; they may also extend superiorly to the suprasellar region, inferiorly to the foramen magnum and cervical spine, and laterally to the cavernous sinus, subtemporal region, or cerebellopontine angle.

Different pathologic lesions can develop in this region.[1] Histologically, clival lesions can be benign (e.g., meningiomas, epidermoid cyst, cholesterol granuloma, or glomus jugulare tumors with major petroclival involvement), of low-grade malignancy (e.g., chordomas and chondrosarcomas), or of high-grade malignancy (e.g., squamous cell cancer, adenocarcinoma, basal cell carcinoma, osteogenic sarcoma, or metastases). Some of these tumors have an intradural location, whereas others are extradural.

The lesions that most often involve this region are meningiomas (commonly intradural), followed (much less commonly) by chordomas, which are often extradural. The former grow from the dura that covers the clivus or the passage from the clivus and the petrous bone (petroclivus fold),[2] whereas the latter originate directly from embryonic residues enclosed in the bone of the clivus.[3-6]

Tumors in the region of the clivus may involve the lowest seven cranial nerves. The sixth cranial nerve can be within the tumor itself, where it runs through Dorello's canal in the lateral region of the clivus. The brain stem can be displaced dorsally or laterally. The basilar artery is usually displaced contralaterally; however, occasionally it is shifted dorsally or encased by the tumor.

Major advances in imaging modalities over the last two decades have allowed a more precise delineation of the anatomic extension of these tumors. In most cases, the nature of the lesion can be predicted.

Tumors in the region of the clivus are difficult to treat using conventional neurosurgical approaches. Until a few decades ago, because of the relative inaccessibility of the clivus and its proximity to the brain stem and surrounding neurovascular structures, the results of surgical treatment were so dismal that these tumors were often considered incurable.[1]

Advances in microsurgery of the skull base have resulted in the development and refinement of approaches to petroclival and clival lesions,[7-57] better methods for tumor removal, and innovative techniques[44,45,58-62] to minimize injury to neural and vascular structures during tumor removal. These factors enable the surgeon to treat these tumors more effectively, aiming at a radical excision with an acceptable morbidity and mortality.

In some cases, the combined effort of the neurosurgeon with those in other disciplines interested in skull base surgery (e.g., otolaryngology or maxillofacial surgery) constitutes real progress in the realization of special approaches that aim at improving the exposure of the tumor and reducing trauma to the brain during surgery. Endoscopic skull base surgery is the most recent result of this multidisciplinary concept.[63]

In general, surgical approaches to the clival region have followed two main strategies. The first strategy utilizes conventional approaches, which are technically simple and are characterized by a low approach-related morbidity. The disadvantages of these approaches include the limited surgical field, long working distance, and need for brain retraction, all of which make tumor dissection difficult. The second strategy implies the use of complex approaches, which require specific anatomic knowledge on cadaveric dissections; they are time consuming because of the extensive bone removal and are themselves related to some morbidity in terms of hearing loss, facial nerve dysfunction, and postoperative cerebrospinal fluid (CSF) leak. These approaches facilitate tumor dissection as a result of the wide surgical field and short working distance.

A third option implies that simple conventional approaches, such as the retrosigmoid or subtemporal routes, may be combined with conservative petrosectomies to create key openings to the tumor area, while preserving hearing and providing adequate exposure to the petroclival and prepontine regions. Such approaches appear suited for treating petroclival meningiomas. In clival chordomas, however, the extensive bony involvement by the tumor forces the surgeon to choose between a partial removal through a simple anterior approach (e.g., the trans-sphenoidal approach or Le Fort I maxillotomy) and an attempt for total tumor resection using more complex anterior or anterolateral approaches. Nevertheless, surgeons who have extensive experience with the trans-sphenoidal route for pituitary tumors have shown that gross total removal of clival chordomas can be achieved in up to 70% of cases with low morbidity and excellent long-term survival.

In recent years, the introduction of the endoscope in trans-sphenoidal surgery and the use of extended endoscopic approaches have allowed resection of chordomas involving the lower clivus, and even the odontoid, with good short-term results and low surgical morbidity.[64-72]

Surgical Anatomy

The clivus is located at the midline, in the deepest part of the skull base. It constitutes the inclined anteroinferior surface of the posterior cranial fossa and extends from the dorsum sellae to the foramen magnum (Fig. 41-1). It is formed by a sphenoidal part (corresponding to the superior third) that extends from the dorsum sellae to the spheno-occipital synchondrosis and by an occipital part (corresponding to the inferior two thirds) that reaches the anterior intraoccipital synchondroses.[3,73]

Surgical access to the clivus is complicated by the presence of osseous barriers corresponding to the sphenoid and facial bones (anteriorly and inferiorly) and to the petrous bones (laterally). Posteriorly and laterally, there are critical structures, including the basilar artery, brain stem, cavernous sinus, petrous carotid arteries, temporal lobes, and cranial nerves.

Because of the complexity of the clivus and its surrounding structures, knowledge of their anatomy is essential to planning a correct surgical approach in this region.

The clivus is usually divided into the upper, middle, and lower clivus[25] (see Fig. 41-1) or into superior and inferior halves of the clivus.[74]

The upper clivus is the part above the crossing of the trigeminal and the abducens nerves from the posterior to the middle cranial fossa; this part includes the dorsum sellae and the posterior clinoid processes. This area is bounded anteriorly by the sella turcica and sphenoid sinus, posteriorly by the basilar artery and midbrain, and laterally by the cavernous sinus, temporal lobes, and (from superior to inferior) cranial nerves III through VI.

The middle clivus is the part between the exits of the trigeminal and the glossopharyngeal nerves; it is bounded anteriorly by the upper nasopharynx and retropharyngeal tissues, posteriorly by the basilar artery and pons, and laterally by the petrous apices and cranial nerves VII and VIII.

The lower clivus is the part from the glossopharyngeal nerve to the foramen magnum. This part is bounded anteriorly by the lower nasopharynx and retropharyngeal tissues, posteriorly by the vertebral artery and medulla, and laterally by the sigmoid sinus, jugular bulb, and cranial nerves IX to XII.

The superior and inferior halves of the clivus extend, respectively, above the internal auditory canal and below it.

The topographic anatomy of the clivus makes several surgical approaches feasible.[1,11,34,35,37,41,75,76] The choice of an approach to remove a tumor from this region must take into account the nature and location of the lesion (i.e., whether the lesion is intradural or extradural, its position in respect to the clivus, and its lateral extension).

The surgical approaches to the clivus are divided into three general groups: (1) anterior, (2) anterolateral, and (3) posterolateral. Anterior approaches are mainly used for extradural lesions that primarily involve the clivus and

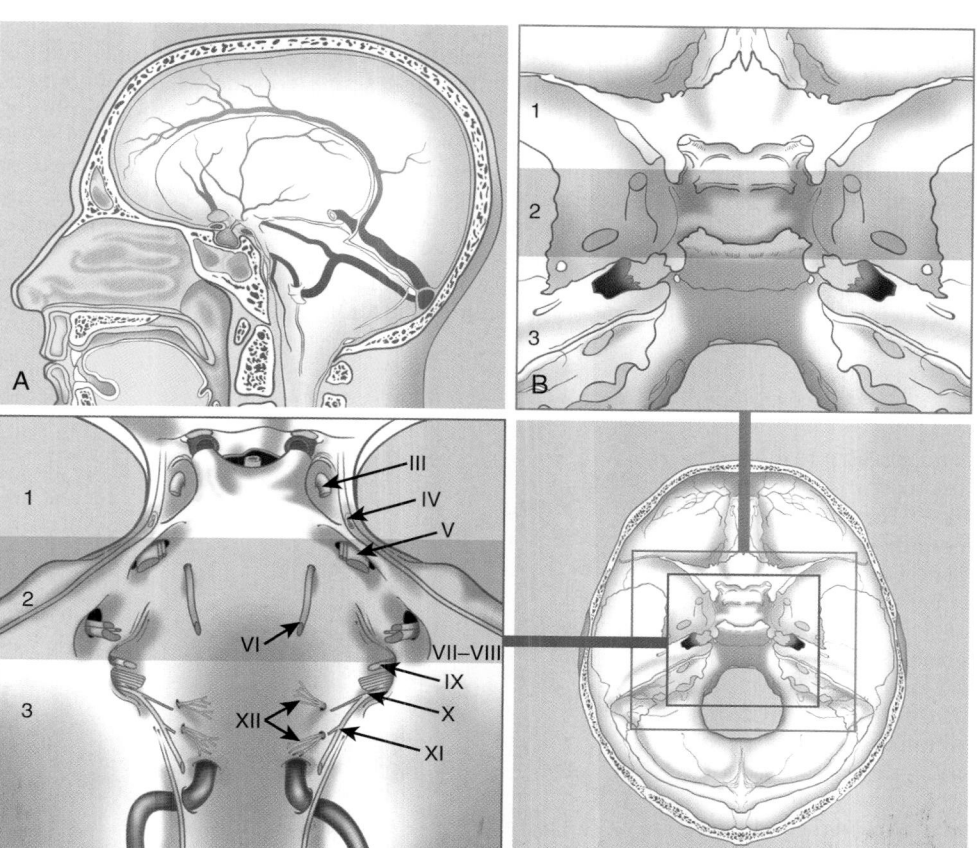

FIGURE 41-1 A, Anatomy of the clivus and adjacent structures. B, Anatomic division of the clivus in upper (1), middle (2), and lower (3) regions. C, The clivus and cranial nerves III and V to XII.

extend extracranially (e.g., chordoma and chondrosarcoma). For these tumors, the anterior approaches are usually extradural and include the trans-sphenoidal, transethmoidal, transoral–transpalatal, transmaxillary, and transcervical. A subfrontal transbasal extraintradural anterior approach can also be indicated for huge tumors with maximal involvement of the clival area and surrounding structures (e.g., chordoma, pituitary tumors, and craniopharyngiomas).

Anterolateral approaches are mainly utilized for intradural tumors that involve the upper and middle clivus and extend into the surrounding regions. The frontotemporal trans-sylvian approach exposes lesions of the upper clivus with extension in the suprasellar region. The subtemporal transtentorial approach exposes lesions of the upper and midclival region, with extension in the middle fossa and tentorial edge (a zygomatic osteotomy and anterior petrosectomy increase the exposure inferiorly and toward the clivus).

Posterolateral approaches are mainly utilized for tumors involving the medial and lower part of the clivus with extension to the petrous bone, cerebellopontine angle, foramen magnum, or upper cervical region. These approaches include the combined subtemporal suboccipital presigmoid with posterior petrosectomy (retrolabyrinthine, translabyrinthine, transcochlear, and total petrosectomy), the retrosigmoid, and the extreme lateral transcondylar approach.

Extradural Lesions: Chordomas

Chordomas are the most common extradural tumors of the clivus; they arise from remnants of the embryonic notochord and are located in all areas where the notochord existed (i.e., the entire clivus, sella turcica, foramen magnum, C1, and nasopharynx).[3,5] From there, they may spread to the upper cervical region, petrous bone, posterior fossa, cavernous sinus, middle fossa, nasopharynx, and sphenoid sinus.[3,5] Chordomas grow slowly but may present the characteristics of a malignant tumor in that they are locally aggressive with a tendency for regrowth.[77] About 20% of chordomas recur as early as 1 year after surgery despite extensive surgical resection.[48,78] Ten percent of chordomas show histologic signs of malignancy.[5] Although it is considered difficult to identify histologic features indicative of aggressiveness,[79,80] recent studies indicate that some molecular features of these tumors are associated with an aggressive biologic behavior.[47,48,78,81,82] Metastases are relatively rare.[78,80]

Chordomas infiltrate the bone and spread into the epidural space, seeding the dura with microscopic deposits well beyond the limits of the tumor bulk.[5,83] For this reason, they may invade the dura and become adherent to the arachnoid and pia mater. The tumor is often gelatinous and soft, with a jelly-like consistency, but it may also appear as a firm cartilaginous mass.

Chordomas are usually classified according to the portion of clivus involved by the tumor and by the extension to surrounding structures (e.g., upper clivus, middle clivus, lower clivus, and craniocervical junction tumors, with or without invasion of sphenoid, cavernous sinus, and petrous bone).[1,3]

Computed tomography (CT) scan and magnetic resonance imaging (MRI) are the most important radiologic tools for diagnosis. The CT scan reveals the destruction of bone, whereas MRI shows the extension of the tumor, which appears nonhomogenously hyperintense on T2-weighted images and with a variable contrast enhancement after gadolinium.[4]

The most commonly involved cranial nerve is the sixth, and diplopia is the most common presenting symptom, particularly in the midclivus chordomas. Other symptoms include headache, pituitary dysfunction, visual field defects, cerebellar syndrome, torticollis, and brain stem syndrome.[84]

SURGICAL TREATMENT

Its deep position (at the central base of the skull) and its tendency to infiltrate the bone make total removal of the clivus chordoma difficult. Total resection leads to a significant improvement in survival at 5 years, with 90% and 52% with complete and partial resection, respectively;[85] at 10 years, the recurrence-free survival rate in a large series for primarily operated patients (with a complete resection of 83%) was 42%; for reoperation cases (complete resection achieved in 30% of patients), it was 26%.[86]

In recent years, because of the development of innovative and complex approaches to the clival area[29,30,34,35,37,41,42,67,68,86-91] and the extensive application of standard procedures to this area,[12,13,16,36,38,84,92-100] many possibilities are at the disposal of the surgeon attempting radical removal of these tumors.

Because chordomas are basically extradural and midline tumors, they displace the neuraxis dorsally or dorsolaterally. Anterior midline extradural approaches are generally preferred (Fig. 41-2).[20,46,52,83,92,101-105] These approaches allow a midline exposure of the clivus and a short working distance, avoiding any retraction of the brain.

The choice of surgical approach depends on the location and extension of the tumor. Even when only anterior extracranial approaches are considered, many options exist. These include the transbasal,[13] extended subfrontal,[104] microscopic trans-septal trans-sphenoidal,[16,84,93-94] modified microsurgical endoscope-assisted sublabial or endonasal trans-sphenoidal,[98,99] endoscopic endonasal trans-sphenoidal,[64,67-71] trans-sphenoethmoidal,[92] transmaxillary transnasal,[106] transfacial,[107] facial translocation,[108] transmaxillary,[109-110] midfacial degloving,[103] transoral,[12] mandible-splitting transoral,[94] transcervical transclival,[111]

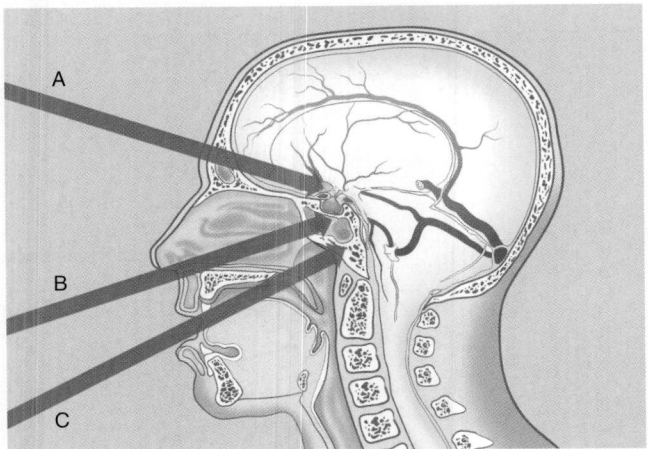

FIGURE 41-2 Anterior approaches to the clivus: subfrontal transbasal approach (A), transsphenoidal approach (B), and transoral approach (C).

and anterior cervical[112] approaches; Le Fort I osteotomy;[113] unilateral Le Fort I osteotomy;[114] total rhinotomy; and pedicled rhinotomy.[115]

All of these approaches are devoted to removing all clival lesions localized on the midline without important lateral extent. In the case of massive lateral extension, in which a midline approach is insufficient for the removal of the entire tumor, complex lateral approaches can be utilized as a primary or secondary procedure.[1,5] These include, for lesions of the upper clivus, the subtemporal, transcavernous, and transpetrous apex approaches; for lesions of the midclivus, subtemporal and infratemporal approaches; and for lesions of the lower clivus with lateral extension to the occipital condyle, jugular foramen, and cervical area, the extreme lateral transcondylar ("far lateral") approach.[26,43,86,116]

According to the level of the clival lesion, the approaches that we often utilize include the following:

- For chordomas located in the upper and middle clivus, the trans-sphenoidal approach is favored.
- For lesions of the lower clivus that involve the foramen magnum, C1, and C2, the transoral approach is preferred, with or without splitting of the palate.
- For tumors in the lower clivus, foramen magnum, and first cervical spinal bodies, with important lateral extension, the Le Fort I osteotomy can be used with a midline incision of the hard and soft palate and lateral swinging of the two flaps of the hard palate.
- For huge tumors involving the entire clival area, the sphenoid, and the sellar region and extending anteriorly to the optic nerves, the transbasal or extended subfrontal route is utilized.
- For lesions that involve the lower clivus and the upper cervical region and that extend laterally into the occipital condyle and the jugular bulb on one side, the extreme lateral approach with partial condylectomy seems particularly well suited.

Other anterior approaches can be utilized, including the following:

- The trans-sphenoethmoidal approach[92] provides access to the entire sphenoid sinus, prepontine space, and superior clivus; a limited medial maxillectomy improves access to the inferior clivus.
- The transfacial approach[107] is indicated for extradural tumors confined on the midline and extending from the level of the sellar floor to the foramen magnum. This approach offers direct access to the clivus along its rostrocaudal extent up to the anterior arch of C1; with depression of the palate, the odontoid can also be visualized. The main advantage is to add, by this single facial route, the possibilities of the trans-sphenoidal and transoral routes, avoiding any injury to the hard and soft palate. The disadvantages are a facial scar and osteotomy of the facial skeleton.
- The recent application of the endoscope to trans-sphenoidal surgery, in either endoscope-assisted or pure endoscopic approaches, provides wider visualization of lesions extending from the upper clivus to the odontoid process; in the future, they will probably be substituted for most transfacial routes, even for tumors extending inferiorly to the odontoid and laterally to the petrous apex.[64-72,117]

TRANS-SPHENOIDAL APPROACH

The trans-sphenoidal approach provides excellent exposure to chordomas of the sphenoid sinus, sella turcica, and upper and middle clivus (see Fig. 41-2), minimizing the morbidity of more complex surgical approaches[13,16,84,96] with a route that, where necessary, can easily be repeated. The technique utilized for the sublabial trans-septal trans-sphenoidal procedure has already been described.[118] Extensive experience obtained with pituitary tumors[119-120] and with craniopharyngiomas[121] has made this route safe and effective, even for other pathologies (Figs. 41-3 to 41-6). Several papers have reported that gross total tumor removal can be achieved in up to 70% of cases using the trans-sphenoidal approach, with excellent long-term survival and no evidence of disease at a mean of 38.6 months after surgery.[84,94,95,98,99]

The main disadvantages of this approach are represented by the limited lateral exposure and the deep and narrow field. Nevertheless, the correct use of long and angled curettes can allow a skillful surgeon to remove even large tumors (greater than 4 cm) that are not strictly confined to the midline.[78] Application of endoscopy to the trans-sphenoidal route may increase the surgical field and allow even extensive tumors to be removed.[45,64,67-71]

When the tumor is found to be located intradurally, an opening of the dura mater can be realized to remove the intradural tumor. Afterward, an accurate reconstruction must be realized. We usually use a dural patch and fibrin glue. When a major intraoperative CSF leak (grade 3[122]) is evident, a lumbar drain is kept in place for 48 to 72 hours postoperatively.

TRANSORAL APPROACH

The transoral route is indicated for extradural lesions of the inferior clivus that are confined to the midline, protrude into the posterior pharyngeal region, and extend to C1 to C2 (see Fig. 41-2). The approach provides good exposure with limited surgical trauma.[75,123] This route has been used for many years for epidural tumors of the cervical spine.[124] Several reports have described the utilization of this surgical route to treat clivus chordomas.[125-127]

A modified transoral version has been described for chordomas.[110,113] It combines the Le Fort I osteotomy with a midline incision of the hard and soft palate and allows lateral swinging of the two flaps of the hard palate based on their own palatine artery and nerves. The advantage is extensive exposure of the region, inferiorly and laterally (Fig. 41-7); the wound must be closed carefully to preserve occlusion and functioning of the palate. A unilateral Le Fort I osteotomy can be realized for laterally growing tumors.[114] Neuronavigation in transoral approach has been found to be a useful tool for planning and checking the limits of resection and for reducing morbidity in chordoma surgery.[44]

THE ENDOSCOPE: A SURGICAL ADJUNCT FOR WIDER VISION AND EXPOSURE

As a result of technological progress and collaboration between neurosurgeons and otolaryngologists,[63] the endoscope has been applied to trans-sphenoidal and transoral surgery to get visualization in these deep surgical corridors that is wider than the microsurgical vision. The use of

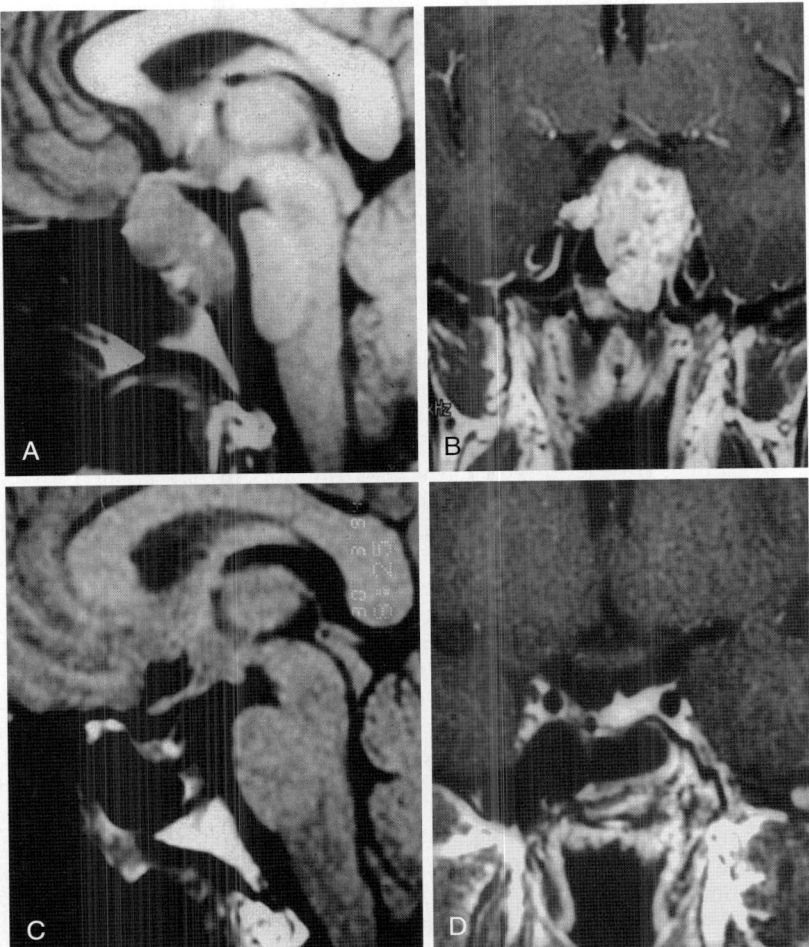

FIGURE 41-3 Transsphenoidal approach, showing an upper and middle clivus chordoma with prepontine extension and brain stem compression. Contrast-enhanced MRI is used. A, Preoperative sagittal image. B, Preoperative coronal image. C, Postoperative sagittal image. D, Postoperative coronal image.

the endoscopes in microsurgical approaches has allowed a view behind the corner achieved by angled (30 and 45 degrees) scopes.[98,99] The main limit of endoscope-assisted microsurgery remains though the narrow surgical corridor in which the endoscope is positioned; this reduces the endoscope to a complex mirror to visualize tumor remnants, as tumor removal under an endoscopic view may be not possible because of the space limitation created by the self-retractor.

In recent years, "pure" endoscopic trans-sphenoidal approaches have been developed[63] that use only the endoscope as a visualization tool. The approaches are performed through both nostrils to allow for a bimanual technique and a wide range of free motion. The major limit of pure endoscopic skull base surgery is the loss of the binocular vision provided by the microscopic technique. When the wider visualization achieved by the endoscope is coupled with wider exposure, the full advantage of the endoscopic technique is achieved, extending the realm of trans-sphenoidal surgery to the cavernous sinus,[128] petrous apex,[117] lower clivus, and odontoid process.[65,72]

Results of the endoscopic series in the treatment of clival chordomas are at least comparable to the microsurgical trans-sphenoidal series,[64,67,68,71] though the small number of patients and the short follow-up preclude definitive conclusions in terms of survival and recurrence rate.

The endoscope has also been applied to the transoral approach to the anterior craniovertebral junction in limited series.[129] A pure endonasal endoscopic approach to C1 and the odontoid process has also been described.[72,130] The main advantage of this approach, as compared to the transoral, is the visualization of the whole clivus and the avoidance of the soft palate splitting; its major limitation is the lowest extension of the surgical field, which is usually 9 mm above the base of the C2 body. The application of the endoscope to the transoral approach may reduce the need for splitting the soft palate yet maintain a satisfactory surgical maneuverability.[131]

SUBFRONTAL TRANSBASAL OR EXTENDED FRONTAL APPROACH

The subfrontal transbasal or extended frontal route can be utilized for chordomas with both intradural and extradural extension and with extensive involvement of the clivus and surrounding structures.[5] The approach is a modification of the "transbasal approach" of Derome.[13,132,133] After a bifrontal craniotomy (including the orbital roof and nasal bones), the anterior skull base is exposed extradurally on both sides (Fig. 41-8; see also Fig. 41-2). The planum sphenoidale and part of the anterior wall of the sella are removed. The clivus is reached anterior to the sella and exposed up to the rim of the foramen magnum (see Fig. 41-2). If the lesion presents

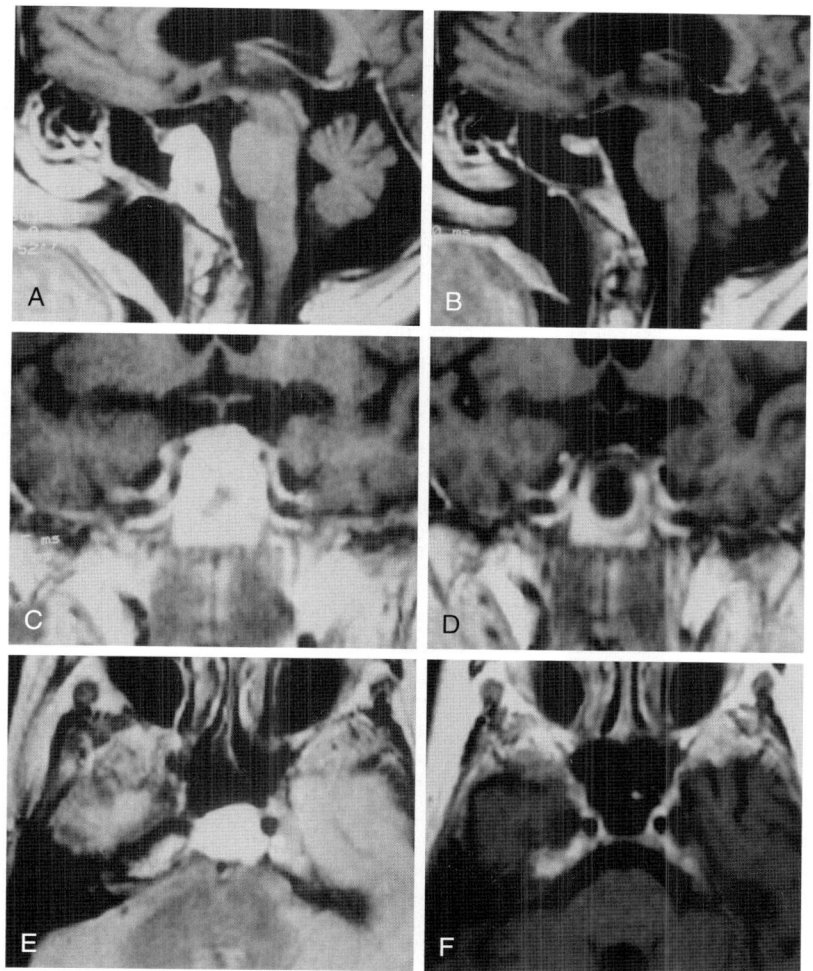

FIGURE 41-4 Transsphenoidal approach, showing an upper and middle clivus chordoma with a retroclival intradural extension (E). Contrast-enhanced MRI is used. A, Preoperative sagittal image. B, Postoperative sagittal image. C, Preoperative coronal image. D, Post-operative coronal image. E, Preoperative axial image. F, Postoperative axial image.

an intradural extension, the frontal dura is opened. It also allows for the removal of tumors that extend near to the clivus (i.e., the frontal suprasellar region, orbits, paranasal sinuses, and temporal fossa). This approach has been used for different tumors such as craniopharyngiomas (Fig. 41-9), meningiomas, or pituitary tumors.

EXTREME LATERAL TRANSCONDYLAR APPROACH

The extreme lateral transcondylar approach is useful for the management of both intradural and extradural lesions that involve the lower clival and foramen magnum regions (Figs. 41-10 and 41-11), with extension into the occipital condyles, jugular bulb, and upper cervical spine.[15,26,134,135] The technical steps of the approach have been described by many authors.[8,26,43,76,118,133] The main advantage of this route is the direct view that it offers to the ventral aspect of the foramen magnum without requiring brain stem retraction.

The patient is placed in a full lateral decubitus position, with the head in the neutral position. After skin incision and muscle dissection, the lateral mass of C1 is exposed and the vertebral artery is unroofed in the foramen transversarium of C1. The anatomic relationship of the vertebral artery with the foramen transversarium of C1 or C2 must be defined preoperatively by angiography or three-dimensional CT angiography. Then, a C1 laminotomy and suboccipital craniotomy are performed. The occipital condyle and the lateral

mass of C1 are partly removed. The vertebral artery can be transposed during the dural opening, when necessary.

POSTOPERATIVE ADJUNCTIVE RADIOTHERAPY

Although the definitive modality for treating clival chordomas is surgical resection, an adjunctive treatment can be considered in selected cases. A correlation between radiation dose and length of the disease-free interval has been indicated;[136] however, some authors remain somewhat skeptical as to the actual efficacy of postoperative radiotherapy in the management of chordomas.[86,137-139] Conventional external beam radiotherapy, after partial or subtotal removal, does not seem to affect the regrowth of the tumor.[140] Nevertheless, a better prognosis for small remnants is achieved with proton beam therapy.[141] Although used in small series, stereotactic radiosurgery, carbon ion radiotherapy, and radiofrequency ablation appear promising options for adjunctive treatment of chordoma tumors.[142-149]

Intradural Lesions: Meningiomas

Meningiomas of the clivus and apical petrous bone are the most common intradural neoplasms of this region. Their natural history is characterized by a slow but progressive growth that eventually leads these tumors to achieve an

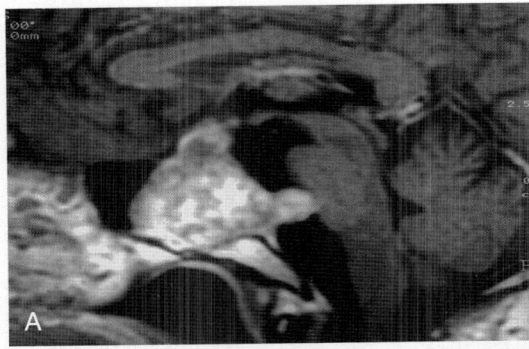
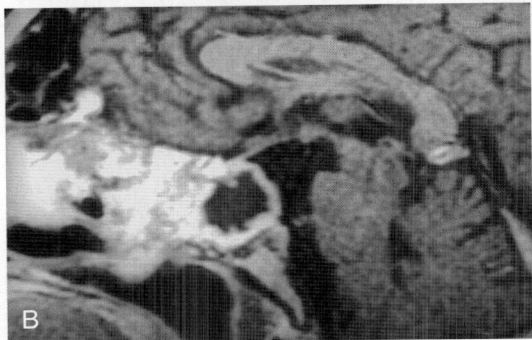

FIGURE 41-5 Transsphenoidal approach, showing an upper and middle clivus chordoma with an intradural retroclival nodule compressing the brain stem. Contrast-enhanced MRI is used. A, Preoperative sagittal image. B, Early postoperative sagittal image (1 month after surgery).

enormous size before manifesting neurologic symptoms related to distortion of the brain stem or cranial nerves III to XII. The growth pattern of these tumors may be unpredictable, and the major factors that influence their growth remain unknown.[150]

According to Yasargil et al.,[2] these meningiomas may be attached "at any of the lateral sites along the petroclival borderline, where the sphenoidal, petrous and clival bones meet." These authors suggested that such basal tumors can be divided into clival, petroclival, and sphenopetroclival, according to their points of insertion and extent.

Clival meningiomas originate from the clival dura. They are rare and commonly encase the basilar artery and its branches. Petroclival meningiomas are tumors that originate in the upper two thirds of the clivus at the petroclival junction, medial to the entry of the trigeminal root in Meckel's cave.[2,151,152] These meningiomas often displace the basilar artery and the brain stem on the opposite side; however, in up to 25% of patients, there is encasement of the artery.[153] Sphenopetroclival meningiomas are the most extensive of these lesions, involving the clivus and the petrous apex. These meningiomas invade the posterior cavernous sinus and the sphenoid sinus and grow into the middle and posterior fossae.[152]

The classification of meningiomas of this area can also be based on the anatomic location of the tumor with reference to the clivus (i.e., upper, middle, or lower) and to the size and volume of the tumor (i.e., medium, up to 2.5 cm in average diameter; large, 2.5 to 4.5 cm; and giant, more than 4.5 cm).[154]

Structures that are close to the clivus often may be involved by the tumor's growth. Meningiomas of the upper clivus may involve the cavernous sinus, sella turcica, Meckel's cave, and tentorial notch; from the middle clivus, they may extend into the cerebellopontine angle; and meningiomas of the lower clivus may involve the jugular bulb, hypoglossal foramina, and upper cervical region.

The location and volume of the tumor, its consistency and vascularity, the presence or absence of a subarachnoid plane between the meningioma and the brain stem, arterial and nervous displacement or encasement, and the correct choice of surgical approach are the factors that, ultimately, decide the extent of the surgical resection and the quality of the results.

SURGICAL TREATMENT

For safe excision of these deep tumors, an adequate exposure (with a low or basal approach to limit or avoid brain retraction) is necessary. The combined supratentorial and infratentorial approach, which Malis[20] called the petrosal approach,[9,155] was the first progress in the surgical exposure of the petroclival region. Thereafter, several surgical approaches were suggested to reach tumors in this region.[12,66,156-158] In these, the petrous part of the temporal bone is often removed to reduce retraction of the temporal lobe and cerebellum and to provide better exposure of the clivus and ventral surface of the brain stem.

Surgical removal of the petrous bone was first used by King in 1970.[159] A limited anterior resection (anterior transpetrosal approach), with preservation of hearing, was reported by Kawase et al. in 1985.[160] Since then, the transpetrosal approach has received many modifications and has become a relevant part of the surgical approaches to the clivus and brain stem.* As suggested by Miller et al.,[165] transpetrosal approaches can be divided basically into two types: (1) anterior petrosectomy, for lesions of the petrous apex and superior half of the clivus, and (2) posterior petrosectomy, for lesions of the petroclival area and cerebellopontine angle.

Meningiomas of the petroclival region can be reached through several routes that pass through the middle or posterior fossa (Fig. 41-12 and Table 41-1):

- Anterolateral route: frontotemporal trans-sylvian approach (usually combined with an orbitozygomatic osteotomy) for tumors of the upper clivus and tentorial notch
- Lateral route: anterior subtemporal approach with zygomatic osteotomy and anterior petrosectomy, for tumors of the petrous apex and upper half of the clivus (Fig. 41-13)
- Posterolateral route:
  - Posterior subtemporal suboccipital presigmoid approach with posterior petrosectomy for centrolateral midclival and petrous apex lesions (in the case of extensive meningiomas, this route can be combined with the anterior subtemporal approach)
  - Retrosigmoid approach for lateral, small, and medium-sized tumors of the midclivus (which are eventually combined with the previous approach)
  - Extreme lateral transcondylar approach for tumors of the lower clivus, foramen magnum, and cervical spine

---

*References 14, 18, 22, 23, 29-32, 34, 35, 37, 38, 40-42, 90, and 161-164.

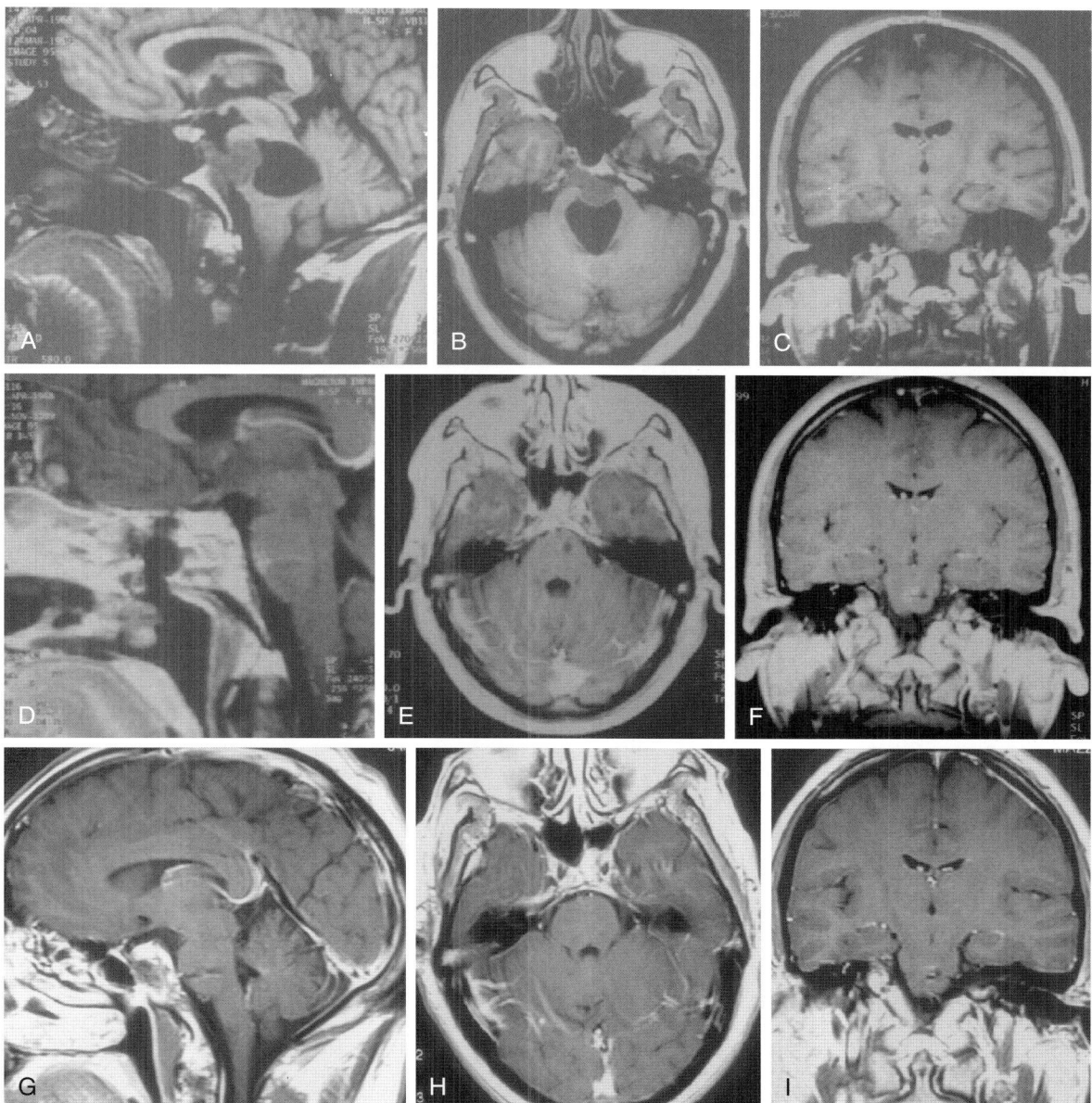

FIGURE 41-6 Transsphenoidal approach, showing a chordoma of the middle clivus with intradural retroclival extension causing an unusual intra-axial CSF cystic dilation. Contrast-enhanced, T1-weighted MRI is used. A, Preoperative sagittal image. B, Preoperative axial image. C, Preoperative coronal image. D, Postoperative sagittal image (6 months after surgery). E, Postoperative axial image (6 months after surgery). F, Postoperative coronal image (6 months after surgery). G, Postoperative sagittal image (5 years after surgery). H, Postoperative axial image (5 years after surgery). I, Postoperative coronal image (5 years after surgery).

FRONTOTEMPORAL TRANS-SYLVIAN APPROACH

The frontotemporal trans-sylvian approach provides enough exposure for the removal of small tumors in the upper clivus and tentorial notch. If necessary, the floor of the middle fossa can also be exposed by performing a zygomatic or orbitozygomatic osteotomy with inferior displacement of the temporalis muscle.[17,166,167]

ANTERIOR SUBTEMPORAL APPROACH WITH ANTERIOR PETROSECTOMY

The anterior subtemporal approach with anterior petrosectomy is indicated for lesions of the tip of the petrous bone or for those involving the middle upper clival area that do

not extend behind and below the internal auditory canal.[19] This approach is also indicated when the greater part of the tumor is in the middle fossa, involving the cavernous sinus.[25,41,154]

An anterior temporal craniotomy is performed, followed by an orbitozygomatic osteotomy to extend the exposure of the conventional craniotomy anteriorly or inferiorly. The superior orbital fissure and the foramen ovale are exposed. To increase exposure at the petrous apex and midclivus, part of the petrous bone is removed. Kawase et al.[19] described a triangle in the petrous bone (lateral to the trigeminal nerve and medial to the internal auditory meatus) that can be drilled, thus providing a route toward the lesions located

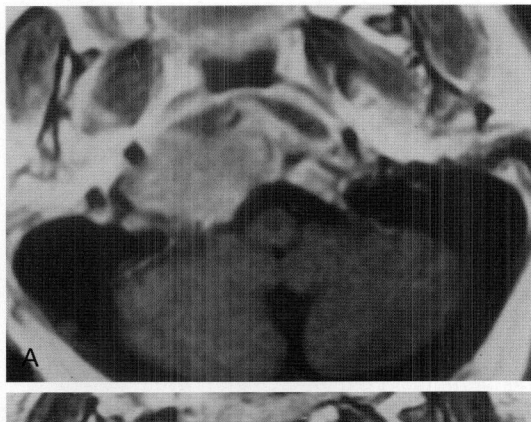

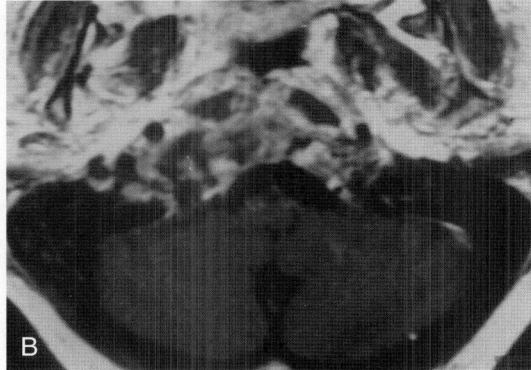

FIGURE 41-7 Modified transoral approach. Le Fort I osteotomy with a midline incision of the hard and soft palate. The middle and lower clivus chordoma are shown with left lateral extension. Contrast-enhanced MRI is used. A, Preoperative axial image. B, Postoperative axial image.

in the region of the midclivus (see Fig. 41-12). Anteroinferior to this area is the horizontal segment of the petrous carotid artery. The petrous apex can be drilled at the Glasscock triangle (demarcated laterally by a line from the foramen spinosum toward the arcuate eminence ending at the facial hiatus, medially by the greater petrosal nerve, and at the base by the third trigeminal nerve division).[165] The exposure can be further increased by anterior displacement of the carotid artery or by drilling the region of the cochlea and thus sacrificing hearing. During this procedure, care should be taken not to damage the abducens nerve that runs through Dorello's canal just medial to this area.

The approach to the clivus can be obtained by simple fenestration of the petrous bone and attached tentorium[19] or with an intradural transtentorial approach.[74,163] In the latter case, intradural and extradural subtemporal approaches are combined with division of the tentorium and with intradural removal of the petrous bone from its apex to the cochlea.

Taniguchi and Perneczky[164] suggested the application of the keyhole concept during surgery of petroclival lesions; this involves reduction of the conventional approach to its essential parts. The concept of restricting petrous bone removal to obtain the exposure necessary in individual cases has also been applied by several neurosurgeons.[29,34,42,56,62]

SUBTEMPORO–SUBOCCIPITAL PRESIGMOID APPROACH WITH POSTERIOR PETROSECTOMY

In 1992, Spetzler et al.[27] summarized neurosurgical approaches that required a posterior petrosectomy into three groups:
1. Approach that preserves hearing
2. Approaches involving sacrifice of hearing
3. Approaches involving mobilization of the facial nerve

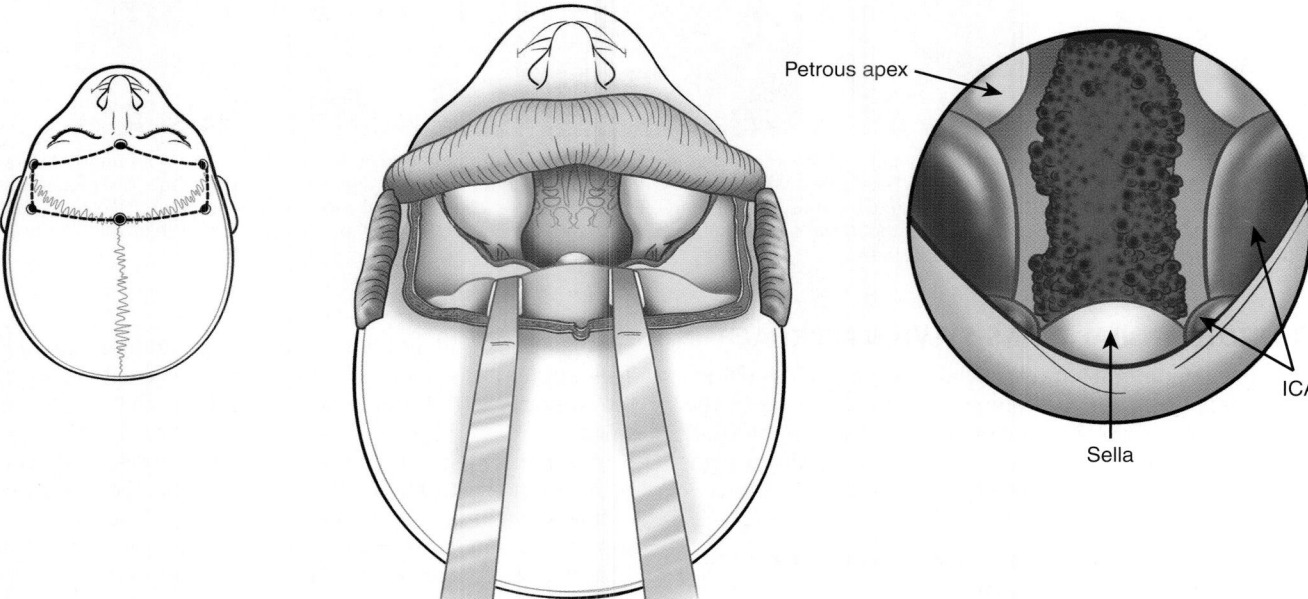

FIGURE 41-8 Artist's rendering of a subfrontal transbasal approach using a bifrontal craniotomy, including the orbital roof and nasal bones. Once the roof of the sphenoid sinus is opened, the intrasphenoidal protuberances are visible, including the sella, the ICA, and the petrous apex.

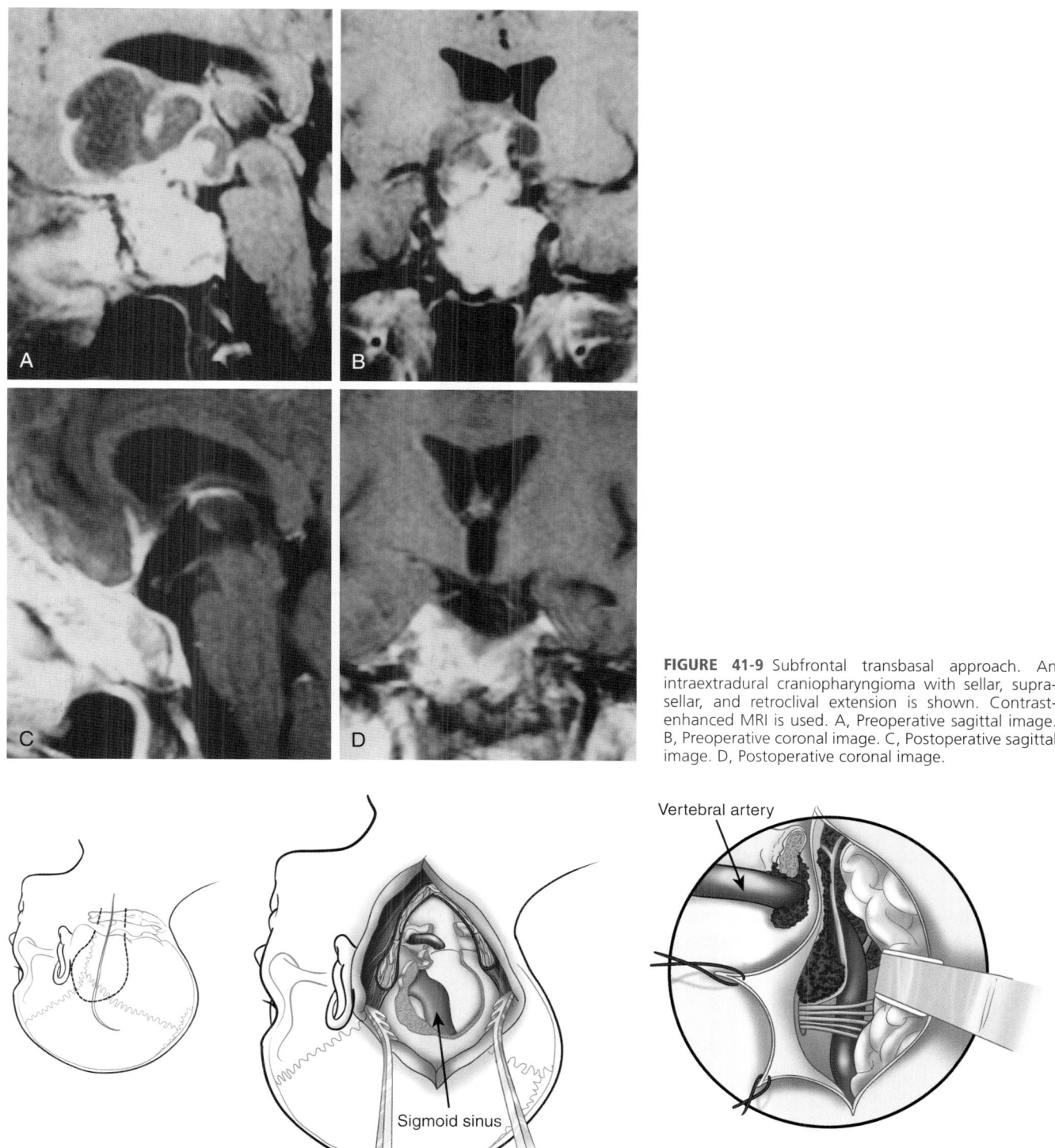

FIGURE 41-9 Subfrontal transbasal approach. An intraextradural craniopharyngioma with sellar, suprasellar, and retroclival extension is shown. Contrast-enhanced MRI is used. A, Preoperative sagittal image. B, Preoperative coronal image. C, Postoperative sagittal image. D, Postoperative coronal image.

FIGURE 41-10 Artist' rendering of the extreme lateral approach. Once the C1 hemilaminectomy, retrosigmoid craniotomy, and mastoidectomy are performed, the lowest portion of the cerebellopontine angle is widely exposed.

Approach That Preserves Hearing

The presigmoid retrolabyrinthine transmastoid approach is most suitable for tumors of the clivus with extension in the middle and posterior fossa. This approach provides excellent exposure of the region ventral to the midbrain and pons. Described by Hakuba et al.[168] in 1977 and refined by Al-Mefty and associates,[7,30] this approach requires a low posterior temporal craniotomy and a lateral retrosigmoid craniotomy.[161] A mastoidectomy is performed to expose the

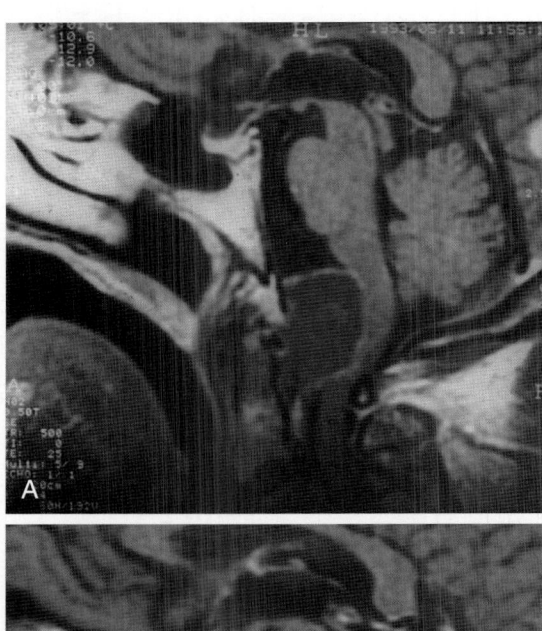

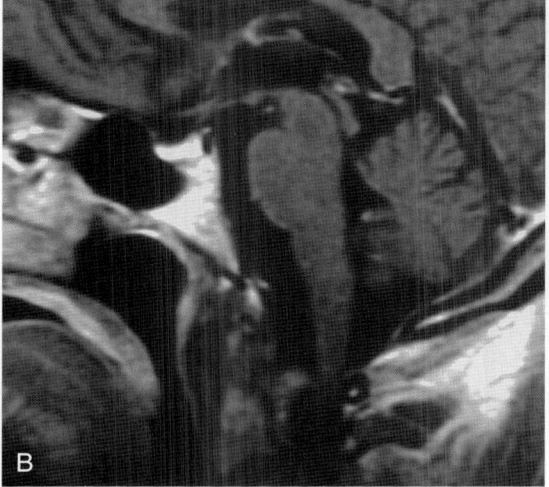

FIGURE 41-11 Extreme lateral transcondylar approach, showing the lower clivus and upper cervical chordoma. Contrast-enhanced MRI is used. A, Preoperative sagittal image. B, Postoperative sagittal image.

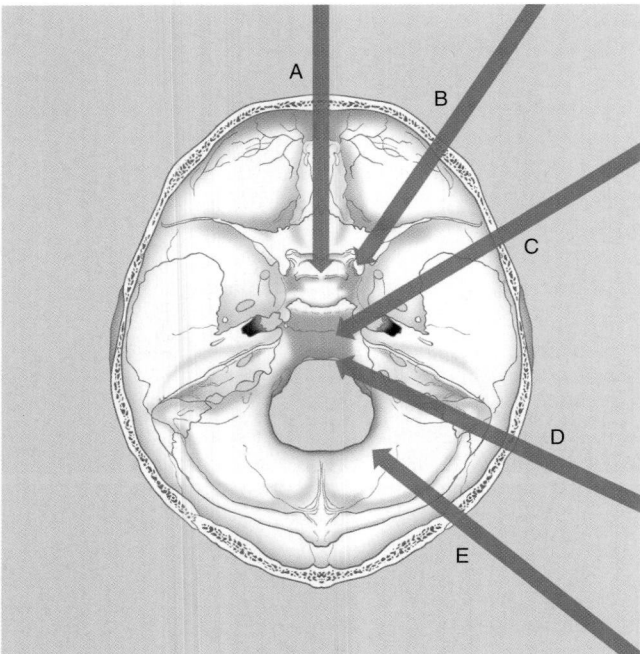

FIGURE 41-12 Approaches to the clivus. A, Anterior approaches. B, Frontotemporal approach. C, Anterior subtemporal approach with an anterior petrosectomy. D, Presigmoid retrolabyrinthine approach with a posterior petrosectomy. E, Extreme lateral transcondylar approach.

sigmoid sinus, the dura mater of the posterior cranial fossa situated anteriorly to the sinus, and the labyrinth. The sinus must be unroofed along its entire course to provide adequate length for mobilization, and the labyrinthine complex must be skeletonized completely from the mastoid cells to gain as much space as possible (Fig. 41-14). A labyrinthectomy improves access to the posterior fossa minimally: its use should be avoided unless hearing has been irreversibly lost. Some authors have suggested the use of a partial labyrinthectomy to widen exposure from the presigmoid route without affecting hearing.[34,169]

The dura mater of the posterior cranial fossa is incised anteriorly to the sigmoid sinus, and this incision is joined to that of the dura mater of the middle cranial fossa, thus preserving the sigmoid sinus, as described by Al-Mefty.[161] The superior petrosal sinus is then resected, and the tentorium is incised (see Fig. 41-14). The fourth nerve is identified by moving the edge of the tentorium. A crucial step in the petrosal approach is the identification and preservation of the venous drainage of the posterior temporal lobe (i.e., the vein of Labbé and other basal veins). The transverse sinus may be divided to obtain improved exposure of

structures below the auditory canal; this can be performed for patients who have good patency of the contralateral venous sinuses.

The advantages of this approach include minimal cerebellar and temporal lobe retraction and shortening of the operative distance to the tumor by 3 cm, when compared with the retrosigmoid approach. The surgeon has surgical access more anteriorly and closer to the clivus, which is important for the removal of lesions with a central location anterior to the brain stem (Figs. 41-15 and 41-16). Disadvantages are temporal lobe retraction and the possibility of injury to the vein of Labbé. Furthermore, paralysis of the lower cranial nerves constitutes one of the major sources of morbidity. Exposure of the lower clivus is limited by the jugular bulb, especially when it is high.

Access to the foramen magnum and inferior clivus can be improved by adding a retrosigmoid dural opening with anterolateral retraction of the sinus. If the lesion extends forward, the surgeon has to consider combining this approach with an anterior subtemporal zygomatic approach. Variants include the partial labyrinthectomy petrous apicectomy approach,[41,56] extended lateral subtemporal approach,[38] and anterior subtemporal medial transpetrosal approach.[42]

Approaches Involving Sacrifice of Hearing

The presigmoid translabyrinthine approach is an anterior extension of the presigmoid retrolabyrinthine approach. The approach involves the removal of the semicircular canals, thus enhancing the exposure. The transcochlear approach involves the anterior extension of the translabyrinthine approach.[32,170]

A combination of the transcochlear approach with extensive bone removal and anterior mobilization of the

Table 41-1   Choice of Surgical Approach in Relation to the Location of the Tumor

Location of Lesion (Sagittal Axis)	Surgical Approach	Location of Lesion (Coronal Axis)
Upper clivus	1. Frontotemporal approach with orbitozygomatic osteotomy	Lateral to Dorello's canal
	2. Subtemporal approach with a zygomatic osteotomy and an anterior petrosectomy	
	3. Trans-sphenoidal approach*	Medial to III-VI CNs
Upper and middle third of the clivus	1. Subtemporal craniotomy with an anterior petrosectomy	Anterior to V3
	2. Subtemporal–suboccipital craniotomy with a posterior petrosectomy	Posterior to V3
	3. Trans-sphenoidal approach*	Medial to V-VI CNs
Lower third of the clivus	1. Extreme lateral transcondylar approach	
	2. Trans-sphenoidal approach*	Medial to XII CN, no vascular involvement
Middle and lower third of the clivus	1. Combined posterior petrosectomy with an extreme lateral approach	
	2. Trans-sphenoidal approach*	Medial to XII CN, no vascular involvement
Entire clivus through the level of the foramen magnum	Far lateral–combined supratentorial and infratentorial approach (including posterior petrosectomy or total petrosectomy)	

*Endoscope assisted or purely endoscopic.
CN, cranial nerve.

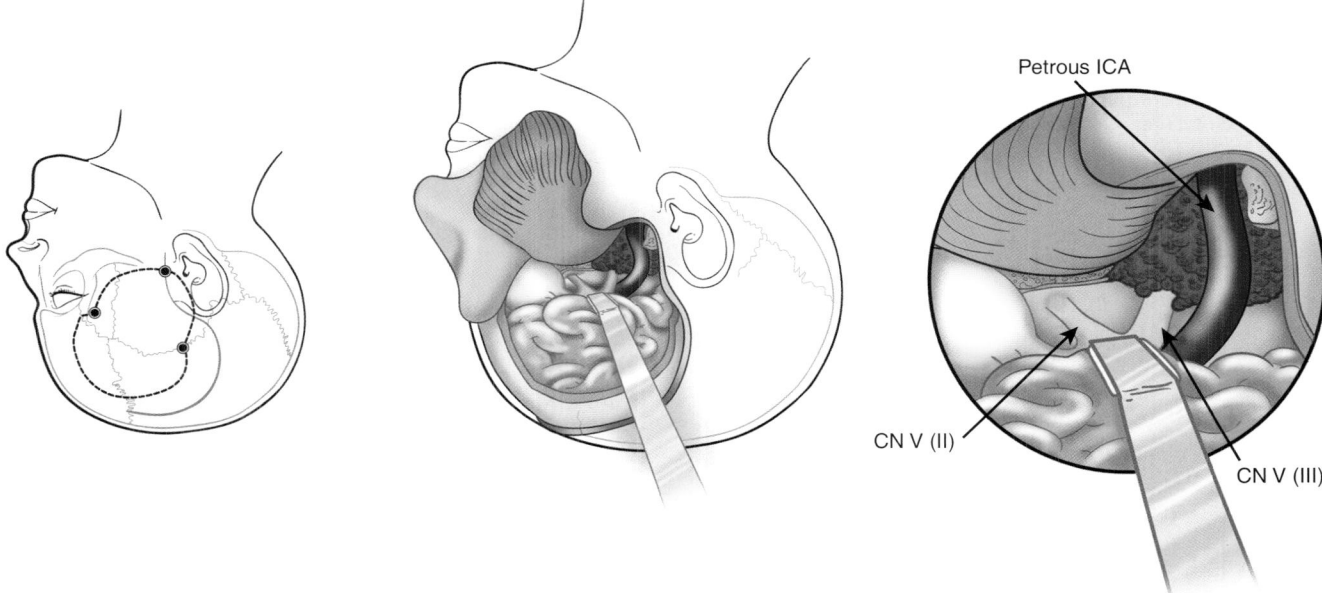

FIGURE 41-13 Artist's rendering of the anterior subtemporal approach with anterior petrosectomy. After a fronto-orbitozygomatic approach is performed, the intradural portion of the tumor, dislocating the ICA, is visible at the level of the clivus. The second and third division of the trigeminal nerve (cranial nerves V to II and III) are important landmarks.

petrous internal carotid artery (ICA) is called a total petrosectomy approach.[76]

Approaches Involving Mobilization of the Facial Nerve

Various elaborate transpetrous approaches have been described, some of which involve mobilization of the facial nerve. A total petrosectomy approach has been described by Sekhar et al.[154,163] The approach requires unroofing of the entire facial nerve and its posterior mobilization and anterior displacement of the petrous carotid artery.

RETROSIGMOID APPROACH

A retrosigmoid approach is generally indicated for lateral, small, and medium-sized tumors of the midclivus. The approach is easy, but it requires the surgeon to work between the cranial nerves and the blood vessels in the cerebellopontine angle and does not provide adequate exposure of more medial or contralateral extensions of the lesion.[171] Samii et al., who advocate the simple retrosigmoid route even for large petroclival meningiomas,[36] recently described an elegant variant, the retrosigmoid intradural suprameatal approach in which the suprameatus petrous

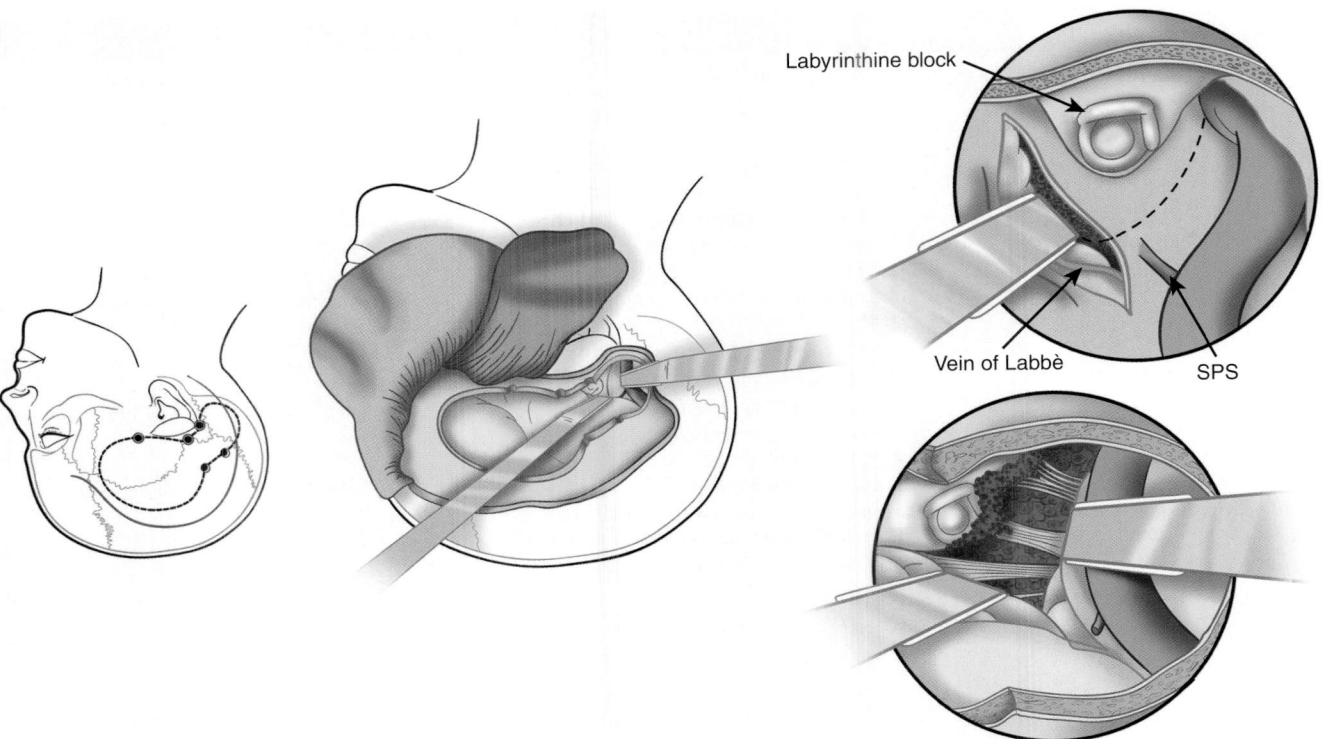

FIGURE 41-14 Artist's rendering of the presigmoid retrolabyrinthine approach. A temporal craniotomy, retrolabyrinthine craniectomy, and petrosectomy are performed. The tentorium is incised after opening of the presigmoid and temporal dura, taking care to preserve vein of Labbé. Once the superior petrosal sinus is ligated and cut and the tentorium is incised, the cerebellopontine angle and ambient cistern are visible.

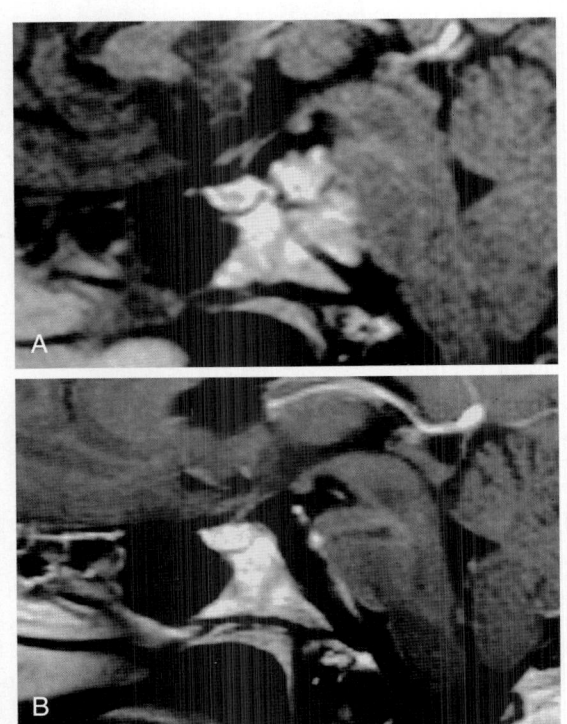

FIGURE 41-15 Presigmoid retrolabyrinthine approach, showing a central meningioma of the upper and middle clivus. Contrast-enhanced MRI is used. A, Preoperative sagittal image. B, Postoperative sagittal image.

bone is drilled, thus providing access to Meckel's cave and the middle fossa.[37] Samii's school is going to develop surgical "corridors" along the dural structures of the sphenopetroclival area to reach the lateral sellar compartment via the posterior fossa.[55]

EXTREME LATERAL TRANSCONDYLAR APPROACH

The extreme lateral transcondylar approach was already described among the approaches for extradural lesions.

FAR LATERAL–COMBINED APPROACH

The far lateral–combined approach combines the far lateral approach with subtemporal and transpetrosal exposures to gain an extensive view of the entire petroclival region for tumors involving the entire clivus and extending to the craniocervical region.[172,173] The approach incorporates a subtemporal craniotomy and posterior petrous bone resection into the far lateral approach to obtain an unobstructed view of the entire clivus and ventral brain stem.

SURGICAL ADJUVANTS

- Vascular embolization: Preoperative embolization of the external carotid artery feeders can be helpful in reducing intraoperative bleeding.
- Intraoperative lumbar drainage of CSF: Drainage of CSF is an important adjuvant to facilitate brain relaxation.
- Intraoperative monitoring of the brain and cranial nerve functions: This monitoring includes somatosensory and motor evoked potentials, auditory brain stem evoked potential, and cranial nerves III, IV, VI, VII, X, XI, and XII.

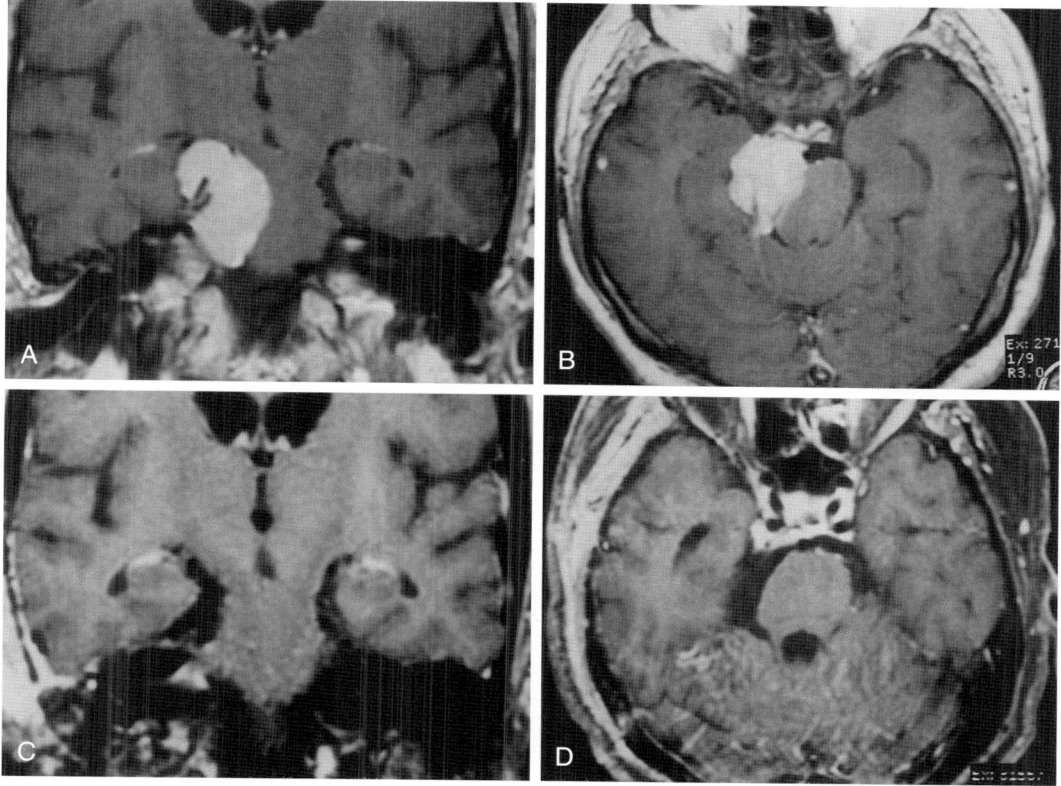

FIGURE 41-16 Presigmoid retrolabyrinthine approach, showing petroclival meningiomas. Contrast-enhanced, T1-weighted MRI is used. A, Preoperative coronal image. B, Preoperative axial image. C, Postoperative coronal image. D, Postoperative axial image.

- Frameless stereotactic navigation: This navigation aids surgical orientation, thus optimizing exposure and reducing risks, especially in complex approaches.
- Contact neodymium:yttrium–aluminum–garnet laser: This tool increases the chances of total removal, which can be achieved faster and with less bleeding.[58]
- Arterial bypass: When the tumor encases the petrous or cavernous carotid artery, if the patient fails the balloon occlusion test and vascular ligation is necessary, a vascular reconstruction is mandatory using a saphenous vein graft bypass or using an extracranial–intracranial arterial bypass.[174]
- Adequate reconstruction of the skull base to prevent CSF leakage: Reconstruction is done by placing a pericranial flap or autologous fat and biologic glue.
- Radiosurgery: Such surgery can be helpful for treating small remnants in critical areas.
- Postoperative hydroxyurea therapy: This therapy has been shown to stabilize and even reduce the size of residual petroclival meningiomas.[175,176]

KEY REFERENCES

Abdel Aziz KM, Sanan A, van Loveren HR, et al. Petroclival meningiomas: Predictive parameters for transpetrosal approaches. *Neurosurgery.* 2000;47:139-150.

Al-Mefty O, Kadri PA, Hasan DM, et al. Anterior clivectomy: surgical technique and clinical applications. *J Neurosurg.* 2008;109(5): 783-793.

Crockard HA, Steel T, Plowman N, et al. A multidisciplinary team approach to skull base chordomas. *J Neurosurg.* 2001;95:175-183.

Dassoulas K, Schlesinger D, Yen CP, Sheehan J. The role of Gamma Knife surgery in the treatment of skull base chordomas. *J Neurooncol.* 2009;94(2):243-248.

Dehdashti AR, Karabatsou K, Ganna A, et al. Expanded endoscopic endonasal approach for treatment of clival chordomas: early results in 12 patients. *Neurosurgery.* 2008;63(2):299-307.

Fatemi N, Dusick JR, Gorgulho AA, et al. Endonasal microscopic removal of clival chordomas. *Surg Neurol.* 2008;69(4):331-338.

Frank G, Sciarretta V, Calbucci F, et al. The endoscopic transnasal transsphenoidal approach for the treatment of cranial base chordomas and chondrosarcomas. *Neurosurgery.* 2006;59(1 suppl 1):ONS50-ONS57.

Fraser JF, Nyquist GG, Moore N, et al. Endoscopic endonasal transclival resection of chordomas: operative technique, clinical outcome, and review of the literature. *J Neurosurg Aug 21[Epub ahead of print].* 2009.

Hasegawa T, Ishii D, Kida Y, et al. Gamma Knife surgery for skull base chordomas and chondrosarcomas. *J Neurosurg.* 2007;107(4): 752-757.

Kassam AB, Snyderman C, Gardner P, et al. The expanded endonasal approach: a fully endoscopic transnasal approach and resection of the odontoid process: technical case report. *Neurosurgery.* 2005;57(suppl 1):E213.

Lang J. *Skull Base Related Structures: Atlas of Clinical Anatomy.* New York: Schattauer; 1995:85-86.

Maira G, Pallini R, Anile C, et al. Surgical treatment of clival chordomas: the transsphenoidal approach revisited. *J Neurosurg.* 1996; 85:784-792.

Martin JJ, Niranjan A, Kondziolka D, et al. Radiosurgery for chordomas and chondrosarcomas of the skull base. *J Neurosurg.* 2007; 107(4):758-764.

Pallini R, Maira G, Pierconti F, et al. Chordoma of the skull base: predictors of tumor recurrence. *J Neurosurg.* 2003;98:812-822.

Pallini R, Patel S, Salvinelli F, et al. Petroclival tumors. Anterolateral Approaches. In: Salvinelli F, De La Cruz A, eds. *Otoneurosurgery and Lateral Skull Base Surgery.* Philadelphia: Saunders; 1996:457-472.

Pillai P, Baig MN, Karas CS, Ammirati M. Endoscopic image-guided transoral approach to the craniovertebral junction: an anatomic study comparing surgical exposure and surgical freedom obtained with the endoscope and the operating microscope. *Neurosurgery.* 2009;64(5 suppl 2):437-442.

Samii A, Gerganov VM, Herold C, et al. Chordomas of the skull base: surgical management and outcome.*J Neurosurg.* 2007;107(2):319-324.

Samii M, Tatagiba M, Carvalho GA. Resection of large petroclival meningiomas by the simple retrosigmoid route. *J Clin Neurosci.* 1999;6:27-30.

Sekhar LN, Schessel DA, Bucur SD, et al. Partial labyrinthectomy petrous apicectomy approach to neoplastic and vascular lesions of the petroclival area.*Neurosurgery.* 1999;44:537-550.

Sen C, Triana AI, Berglind N, et al. Clival chordomas: clinical management, results, and complications in 71 patients.*J Neurosurg, Nov 20 [Epub ahead of print].* 2009.

Stippler M, Gardner PA, Snyderman CH, et al. Endoscopic endonasal approach for clival chordomas.*Neurosurgery.* 2009;64(2):268-277.

Tzortzidis F, Elahi F, Wright D, et al. Patient outcome at long-term follow-up after aggressive microsurgical resection of cranial base chordomas.*Neurosurgery.* 2006;59(2):230-237.

Van Havenbergh T, Carvalho G, Tatagiba M, et al. Natural history of petroclival meningiomas.*Neurosurgery.* 2003;52:55-62.

Vougioukas VI, Hubbe U, Schipper J, et al. Navigated transoral approach to the cranial base and the craniocervical junction: technical note. *Neurosurgery.* 2003;52:247-250.

Yoneoka Y, Tsumanuma I, Fukuda M, et al. Cranial base chordoma—long term outcome and review of the literature. *Acta Neurochir.* 2008;150(8):773-778.

Numbered references appear on Expert Consult.

CHAPTER 42

Surgical Management of Posterior Fossa Meningiomas

BEEJAL Y. AMIN • SAMUEL RYU • JACK P. ROCK

Posterior fossa meningiomas are uncommon lesions that are most often slow-growing neoplasms manifesting in clinically indolent fashion. Based on clinical and radiographic information, the differential diagnosis is relatively straightforward; however, the range of management options can be considerable, including observation, surgery, and radiation in various forms and combinations. Although chemotherapeutic agents have been and continue to be investigated, this form of therapy is generally considered only for intractable, atypical, and malignant tumors and is not part of the general armamentarium in the majority of patients. Although the surgical management of meningiomas located in the posterior fossa may be challenging, patient-based outcomes studies suggest that long-term results can be encouraging.[1]

Posterior fossa meningiomas can be found anywhere in the posterior fossa, and individualized management recommendations depend primarily on size, growth rate, clinical presentation, and location (i.e., surgical accessibility). Tumors are primarily classified by their anatomic origin along the suboccipital surface of the cerebellum, lateral (i.e., lateral to the internal auditory meatus) petrous bone, cerebellopontine angle (CPA), petroclival region and clivus, jugular foramen, foramen magnum, pineal region, fourth ventricle, or tentorium (Table 42-1). Surgical accessibility varies based on location, with the most straightforward originating on the suboccipital surface of the cerebellum and lateral petrous bone; the more difficult originating on the tentorial surface, in the fourth ventricle, and at the CPA; and the most difficult originating at the petroclival junction. Each location is associated with different clinical implications regarding presentation and treatment strategy. Contemporary radiation therapy and radiosurgical decisions also depend on tumor location and the proximity of the tumor to critical neural elements. This chapter reviews the topic of posterior fossa meningioma from diagnosis though management and follow-up, in terms of both general and specific approaches relative to the various anatomic sites.

General Clinical Presentation and Diagnosis

The clinical presentation of posterior fossa meningiomas varies according to the location and size of the tumor, but because meningiomas are mostly slow-growing tumors, size plays less of a role in presentation and more of a role in choice of treatment strategy. Anatomically, the presenting clinical symptoms most often are related to involvement of cranial nerves and to a lesser degree the cerebellum, brain stem (i.e., long tracts), and fourth ventricle (i.e., hydrocephalus). Headaches are a common but nonspecific symptom. More specific clinical features based on location are discussed in the individual sections (see Table 42-1).

The diagnosis of meningioma is generally made radiographically, and most tumors share certain imaging characteristics. Plain radiographs, although no longer commonly utilized, often demonstrate bony hyperostosis, bony erosion, calcification, and occasionally, evidence of enlarged vascular channels. Transaxial computed tomography (CT) most often shows a hyperdense tumor signal (75% of cases) that intensely and homogeneously enhances after contrast administration. Cystic regions within the tumor can be seen but are uncommon, and peritumoral low-density suggestive of edema is noted in up to 60% of tumors.[2] Calcification can also be noted on CT, but hemorrhage is distinctly uncommon. Three-dimensional computed tomography angiography (3D CTA) is useful in patients with skull base meningiomas. 3D CTA provides images that clearly depict the anatomic relationship between the meningioma and the bony structures of the skull base, as well as the relationship between the tumor and the neighboring vessels.[3] Magnetic resonance imaging (MRI) most often reveals an isointense or hyperintense lesion on T1-weighted imaging, which is heterogeneous on T2-weighted imaging. These tumors almost always intensely enhance after gadolinium administration. The dural tail sign is one of the most revealing characteristics of meningioma, even though it is not pathognomonic (Fig. 42-1). A high-intensity signal noted on T2-weighted imaging is typical of peritumoral edema.[2] While unproven in a large series of patients, diffusion-weighted MR imaging has been noted to correlate with the histopathologic features of certain meningiomas before resection.[4] Cerebral angiography commonly (but not invariably) reveals an intense vascular supply, primarily from the dural arteries; a prolonged stain in the late venous phase of the angiogram is also common. Given the efficacy of magnetic resonance angiography (MRA), magnetic resonance venography (MRV), and 3D CTA for diagnosis and surgical planning, conventional angiography is used less frequently today. Nevertheless, it is still required for preoperative embolization.

Table 42-1	Posterior Fossa Meningiomas		
Location	**Incidence**	**Symptoms**	**Common Surgical Approaches**
Occipital surface	10%	Headaches, cerebellar syndrome, increased intracranial pressure, hemianopsia, visual hallucinations	Suboccipital craniotomy ± occipital craniotomy
Lateral petrous surface	8%-10%	V, VII, and VIII cranial neuropathies; brain stem and cerebellar compression syndromes	Retrosigmoid craniotomy
CPA	10%-15%	V, VII, and VIII cranial neuropathies; brain stem and cerebellar compression syndromes	Retrosigmoid craniotomy, translabyrinthine craniotomy
Petroclival region	10%-38%	III, IV, V, VI, VII, VIII, IX, X, and XI cranial neuropathies; brain stem and cerebellar compression syndromes; spasticity; headaches	Petrosal craniotomy variants ± anterior petrosectomy
Jugular foramen	Rare	IX, X, and XI cranial neuropathies; brain stem and cerebellar compression syndromes	Retrosigmoid craniotomy, transjugular variants
Foramen magnum	4%-20%	Increased intracranial pressure; IX, X, XI, and XII cranial neuropathies; brain stem and spinal cord compression syndromes	Suboccipital craniotomy ± C1 laminectomy, transoral; far lateral approach
Pineal region	6%-8%	Increased intracranial pressure; visual symptoms; cerebellar dysfunction	Infratentorial–supracerebellar craniotomy, occipital–transtentorial craniotomy, supra/infratentorial–transsinus approach
Fourth ventricle	Rare	Headaches, increased intracranial pressure	Midline suboccipital craniotomy
Tentorial surface	30%	III, V, VI, VII, and VIII cranial neuropathies; headaches; increased intracranial pressure; brain stem and cerebellar compression syndromes; psychomotor epilepsy	Subtemporal craniotomy, petrosal craniotomy variants, retrosigmoid craniotomy

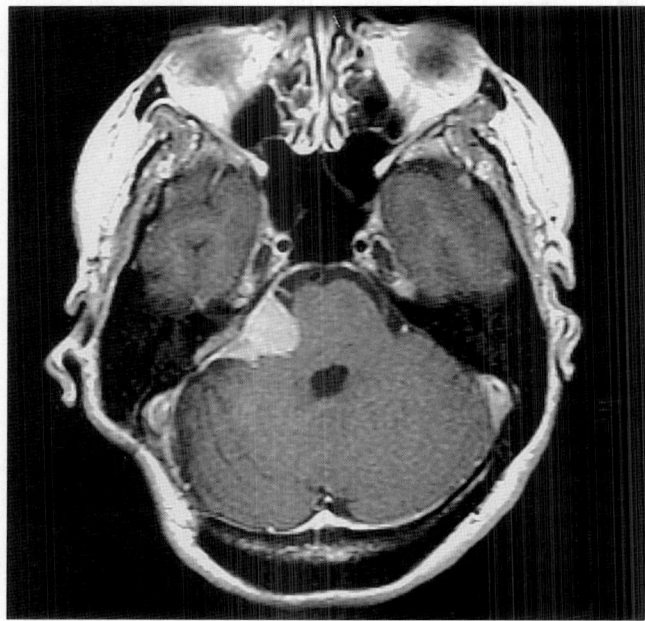

FIGURE 42-1 The thin layer of enhancement extending posterior to this CPA tumor is referred to as the dural tail. Although commonly noted with meningiomas, it may also be seen with other tumor types.

Although the differential diagnosis of posterior fossa tumors is extensive, the common radiographic features of meningioma usually establish the diagnosis from among the more common lesions. The most common tumors encountered along the dural margins of the posterior fossa include schwannomas, epidermoids, and metastases. Ependymomas and choroid plexus papillomas (in the fourth ventricle) and primary pineal tumors and germ cell tumors (in the pineal region) must also be considered.

PREOPERATIVE EVALUATION

Most posterior fossa meningiomas are radiologically evaluated in a similar fashion, although smaller tumors may not require extensive testing. The standard diagnostic workup includes MRI with and without contrast administration, MRA, MRV, and CTA. For lesions involving the petrous bone, a thin-cut temporal bone CT scan may be useful. Tumor extensions are best appreciated on contrast-enhanced MRI, and MRA and/or CTA generally demonstrates the degree of tumor vascularity. When optimally performed, MRV demonstrates (although in not as detailed a fashion as angiography) the venous anatomy, including the dominance of the transverse and sigmoid sinuses, the size of the jugular bulb, the superior and inferior petrosal sinuses, and the temporal lobe drainage pattern. Temporal bone CT indicates the extent of hyperostosis or erosion and demonstrates the relationship between the size of the jugular bulb and the surrounding bony anatomy.

CEREBRAL ANGIOGRAPHY AND EMBOLIZATION

The need for preoperative cerebral angiography as a diagnostic and surgical planning tool has largely been supplanted by CTA, MRA, and MRV. In most cases, the vascular supply to the tumor comes from arteries related to meningeal tumor origins. In the posterior fossa, arterial branches from the petrous and cavernous segments of the carotid, as well as branches from the vertebrobasilar and external carotid systems, constitute the main supply.

Given the limited space in the posterior fossa, the surgical removal of a highly vascular lesion can be fraught with difficulty (e.g., persistent bleeding obscures the operative field, requiring greater patience on the part of the surgeon to avoid increased morbidity), and although ideally the surgeon will select an approach that allows eradication of the tumor's vascular supply early in the operation, this is not always possible or sufficient. In these instances, preoperative arterial

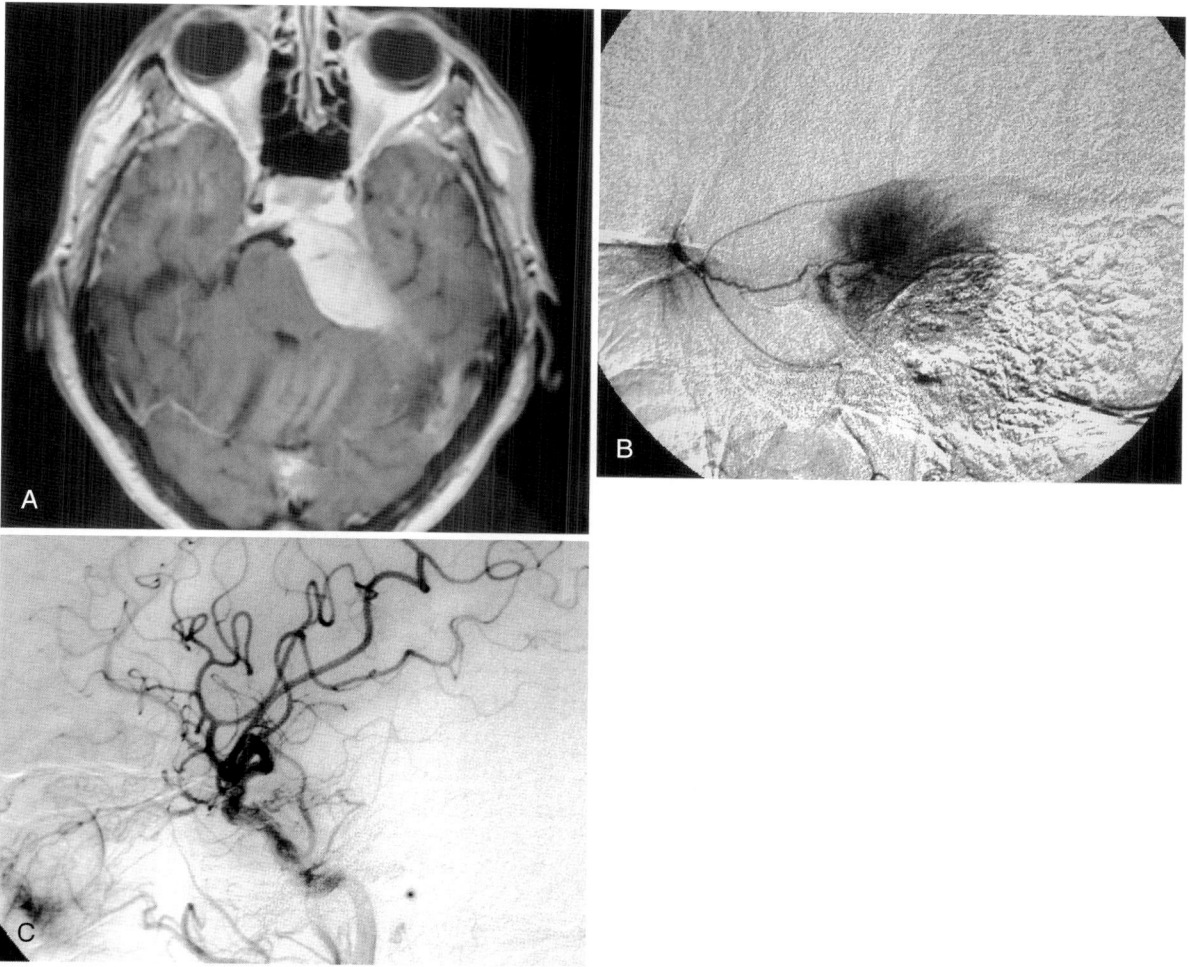

FIGURE 42-2 A, Petroclival meningioma. B, Preoperative angiogram with prominent vascular supply through the tentorial arteries. C, Angiogram postembolization. The patient was operated on 72 hours after embolization, and the tumor was significantly necrotic and removable by standard suction.

embolization can be helpful, especially for selected tumors in the posterior fossa[5] (Fig. 42-2). The primary reservations regarding embolization generally include risk of stroke, retroperitoneal hematoma, and secondary tumor necrosis and swelling (possibly leading to clinical deterioration). In addition, because the vascular supply is commonly made up of internal and external vessels, external carotid embolization may shift vascular supply to more-difficult-to-control internal carotid branches. Nevertheless, our experiences and those of others suggest that embolization can be helpful.[6,7] Most authors conclude that to be most helpful, embolization must achieve complete or near-complete eradication of the vascular supply to the tumor: partial interruption of the blood supply may leave the surgeon with a significant intraoperative bleeding challenge.

An additional issue relates to the timing of the surgical procedure relative to embolization. After an investigation of 50 patients, Chun and colleagues observed that more favorable results of embolization were noted with delays of longer than 24 hours, although the optimal delay was not specified.[8] It has become the practice with all posterior fossa tumors at Henry Ford Hospital to delay the surgical procedure 48 to 72 hours from the time of embolization;

because of the potential risk (albeit rare) of clinical deterioration from tumor swelling, the patient is admitted to the hospital until surgery.

GENERAL TREATMENT CONSIDERATIONS

The general management considerations surrounding meningiomas located in the posterior fossa run parallel to those for treating these lesions located in other regions of the brain. Because meningiomas are mostly slow-growing neoplasms, urgent and emergent management decisions are seldom required. Recent reports on residual disease after surgical resection of petroclival tumors indicate that the average growth rate is 0.37 cm/yr; this is associated with a median time to progression of 36 months, a median progression-free survival of 66 months, and a 5-year progression-free survival rate of 60%.[9] Older age, menopause, and previous radiation therapy can be associated with slower growth. In addition, we found that meningiomas with evidence of calcification on CT scan have longer doubling times. Despite this indolent nature, the neoplasms seem to grow relentlessly, often by en-plaque growth along tissue planes, along the dura, and through the basal cranial foramina, thereby making accurate growth assessment by

CT or MRI a challenge. For practical purposes, four management options are available: (1) observation alone, (2) surgical resection, (3) radiation therapy or radiosurgery, and (4) some combination of surgery and radiation.

OBSERVATION

Observation is usually selected when the patient is neurologically intact, the lesion is small, and especially, the patient is elderly or has significant comorbidities. Observation remains reasonable even when the diagnosis is histologically unproven, because these lesions usually can be correctly diagnosed with MRI. Given the known natural history, when a lesion grows more than a couple of millimeters in a 6-month period, either the accuracy of the diagnosis will be questionable or the tumor growth will be more aggressive; in either case, surgical treatment would be the most judicious recommendation. Another consideration leading to a decision to observe rather than treat in an asymptomatic patient would be the surgeon's experience and the consequent risks of resection, in addition to the risks of possible postoperative radiation therapy for lesions nestled tightly amid important neurologic structures in the posterior fossa. Whatever the reasons for choosing observation as a management strategy, when this form of management is selected, relatively frequent MRI (i.e., 6- to 12-month intervals) is recommended because, although the lesions are generally slow growing, occasionally rapid growth can occur.

Intervention as Opposed to Observation

Although it is difficult to set absolute standards for intervention, examples include the young patient without, or especially with, neurologic symptoms and signs; a large tumor (generally greater than 3 cm); the asymptomatic patient's preference for removal; and documented neurologic and/or radiographic progression. The recommendation to intervene then leads to selection of a treatment alternative that seems most reasonable from both the physician's and the patient's points of view.

SURGERY

Realistically, most surgeons focus primarily on the removal of the significant bulk (i.e., Simpson grade III) of the tumor and "decompression" of neurologic structures, including the brain stem and cranial nerves.[10] Although it is known that recurrence often follows when the tumor is not entirely removed, the morbidity associated with attempts at total resection is clearly higher. However, in the modern era, and in the hands of experienced surgeons, the extent of resection has dramatically improved and has been associated with a marked decrease in morbidity.[11] This decrease in morbidity largely relates to the use of skull base surgical approaches that rely on bone removal as opposed to brain retraction to create tumor exposure.

General concepts are important for the successful removal of most meningiomas; these include adequate bony exposure, early eradication of vascular supply, debulking of tumor mass, and maintenance of the arachnoid plane. A sufficient bony exposure greatly facilitates surgical manipulation and allows the surgeon an opportunity to move from one section of the tumor to another. Although it is preferable to internally debulk most tumors so that the

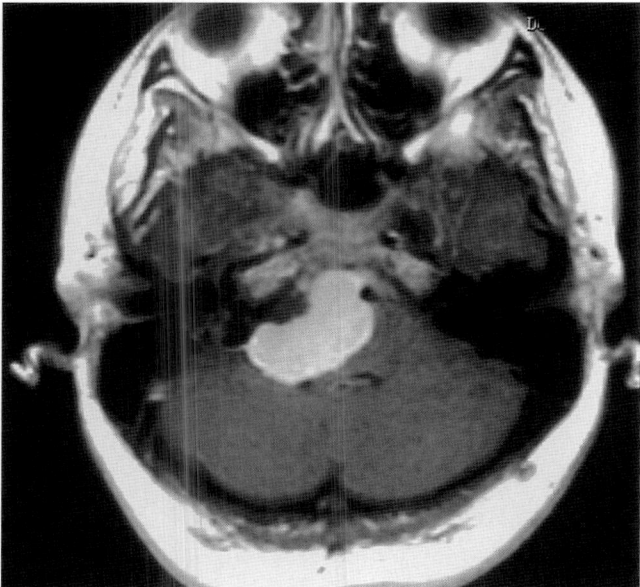

FIGURE 42-3 Petroclival tumor extending into the CPA. Although the lesion can be reached through a retrosigmoid exposure, the petrosal approach allowed ready access to and eradication of the feeding arteries. On the axial image, the basilar artery is displaced but not narrowed. The tumor readily separated from the artery in this case, and perforating vessels were preserved.

tumor capsule can be more easily separated from adjacent normal structures, for many vascular lesions, an approach that provides access to and early elimination of the vascular supply is desirable (Fig. 42-3). Once the vascular supply is eliminated, a far less challenging resection may be possible.

Although not essential, image guidance can facilitate tumor resections, especially those along the petrous bone and in the petroclival region. For the experienced surgeon, the surgical anatomy is so familiar that simply by maintaining the arachnoid planes the surgeon can appreciate the boundaries of the lesion; however, for those with less experience, image guidance can help with orientation, save considerable time by providing a map around petrous bone and clival structures, and indicate the extent of the residual lesion as the resection proceeds. Brain shift is a less significant problem for skull base tumors.

Caused partially by the location of the cells of origin of meningiomas, these tumors are commonly situated next to cerebral venous structures, the preservation of which is often critical. Generally, acute occlusion of major draining veins or sinuses as a result of surgical approach and/or dissection is likely to lead to cerebral edema and significant neurologic deficit, and it should be avoided. Despite this, instances of resection of the tumor-infiltrated walls of a patent sagittal sinus with successful repair, complete tumor resection, and maintenance of sinus patency have been reported.[12] In addition, division of the sigmoid and transverse sinuses during petrosal and pineal approaches, respectively, have been reported.[13,14] In principle, however, it is safest to avoid division of major veins and sinuses. It is quite reasonable to consider radical subtotal resections, leaving patent venous structures intact and following the patient to monitor growth of the residual tumor with consideration of delayed radiation.

RADIATION

Conventional Radiation Therapy

Meningiomas are best managed with total excision, if that is achievable with acceptable morbidity. However, about one third of meningiomas are not fully resectable because of tumor location, size, and proximity to adjacent tissue and vascular structures. The posterior fossa is also a common site of residual postoperative disease.[15] Because subtotal resection is associated with a higher chance of clinically significant recurrence than is total resection, postoperative radiotherapy has been common practice and is associated with improved local tumor control and low morbidity.[16,17] The goals of radiotherapy are to prevent tumor progression, prolong the interval to recurrence, and improve survival whether administered as adjuvant or primary therapy.

As primary therapy, radiation therapy has been shown to be efficacious for tumor control and long-term relapse-free survival.[18-21] The standard recommendation for external beam radiotherapy is a dose of 5400 to 6000 cGy in fractionated doses of 180 to 200 cGy to the entire tumor plus a 2-cm margin. Histologically benign meningiomas have most often been treated with a lower dose of about 5400 cGy, and malignant meningiomas have been treated with 6000 cGy. To these dosing standards, the recent addition of intensity modulated radiation therapy (IMRT) has significantly improved the delivery process. IMRT allows multiple and highly conformal radiation beams to be delivered to the tumor volume while significantly decreasing the dose to immediately adjacent tissue (e.g., the optic tracts, acoustic and facial nerves, and brain stem). Three-dimensional radiography, coupled with CT- or MRI-assisted computerized treatment planning, and precise tumor localization and patient immobilization techniques have all served to improve progression-free survival as compared with the techniques used previously.[22]

Radiotherapy has been used primarily as an adjuvant treatment after subtotal resection, for infiltrating tumor into the adjacent brain parenchyma or pathologic finding of atypia, and after multiple recurrences. Although postoperative radiotherapy has never been evaluated in a randomized trial, there have been large retrospective analyses, and the results of these strongly support its role following subtotal resection.[17,18] Recurrence rates of 60% after subtotal resection versus 32% after subtotal resection plus radiotherapy at mean follow-up of 78 months, and 5-year freedom from recurrence of 59% after subtotal resection alone versus 77% after postoperative radiation therapy, have been noted.[16] These studies also found that median time to recurrence was doubled by radiotherapy (i.e., 66 vs. 125 months), and this analysis was notable in that many of the irradiated patients had more adverse factors such as surgically unfavorable sites (e.g., posterior fossa) than did patients treated with surgery alone.

In another report, findings for skull base meningiomas (including those in the posterior fossa) did not differ significantly in terms of progression-free survival from similar findings for other, more favorable sites.[15] An interesting observation suggests that the progression-free survival rate at 5 years for those patients treated before 1980 was 77% versus 98% for those treated after 1980, when CT and MRI became available for tumor localization and treatment

planning.[22] The Royal Marsden Hospital experience also supported the role for postoperative radiotherapy, particularly following subtotal resection.[21] All patients were treated to a total dose of 5000 to 5500 cGy over 6 to 6.5 weeks. Interestingly, there was no significant difference in disease-free survival of minimum postoperative residual versus bulky residual; with actuarial disease-free survivals at 5, 10, and 15 years, patients with minimum residual tumor had survival rates of 78%, 67%, and 56%, respectively, whereas patients with bulky residual tumor had survival rates of 81%, 68%, and 61%, respectively.

As salvage therapy for patients with recurrent or progressive disease, radiotherapy may be used either alone or as an adjuvant to surgical resection. In these cases, local control with the radiotherapy appears equal or superior to that seen with resection alone.[17,23,24] With a total dose of 4500 to 5500 cGy using older megavoltage radiation, the crude salvage rate was 50% as compared with 37% for reoperation alone.[23] More recent reports showed 10-year tumor control rates in the range of 80% with adjuvant radiotherapy following reoperation, as opposed to 10% to 30% for surgery alone.[24] Although the local control rate following salvage radiotherapy compares favorably with rates seen with immediate postoperative radiotherapy, these data should not be interpreted as sole justification for withholding radiation in the early postoperative period. Given the natural history of many meningiomas, progression, although common, is often extremely slow, and the decision as to when to radiate (i.e., immediate postoperative period vs. time of recurrence) is a matter for the treating physician and patient. In our practice, radiation is generally postponed to the time of demonstrable radiographic or clinical progression.

Much of the available literature consists of retrospective studies. Currently, a prospective follow-up study is available. The Radiation Therapy Oncology Group 0539 clinical trial uses the most common treatment recommendations for radiotherapy for various clinical scenarios. This study groups three categories of clinical scenarios and treatments:

- Group I (low risk) includes gross total resection (Simpson grade I-III) and subtotal resection with World Health Organization (WHO) grade I. These patients will be closely observed.
- Group II (intermediate risk) includes gross total resection with WHO grade II and recurrent WHO grade I meningioma, irrespective of resection extent. These patients will undergo radiotherapy (54 Gy/30 Fr) by 3D CTA or IMRT.
- Group III (high risk) includes newly diagnosed or recurrent WHO grade III of any resection extent, recurrent WHO grade II of any resection extent, and newly diagnosed WHO grade II subtotal resection. These patients will be treated with radiotherapy (60 Gy/30 Fr) by IMRT.

Stereotactic Radiation Therapy and Radiosurgery

Despite the favorable results obtained with conventional fractionated radiotherapy for subtotally resected, unresectable, and "inoperable" meningiomas, the use of radiosurgery has evolved as both adjuvant and primary therapy. Controversy still exists, however, regarding the use and efficacy of radiosurgery. The arguments against the routine use of radiosurgery are largely based on the lack of long-term radiosurgical data and on the fear of potential delayed radiation injury to

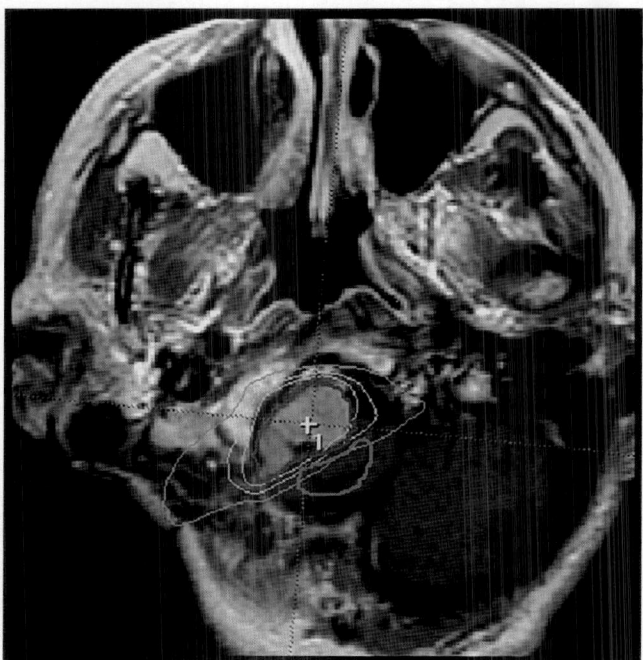

FIGURE 42-4 Fractionated radiosurgical treatment plan for a foramen magnum meningioma.

the brain tissue. However, considering the encapsulation of most benign meningiomas, the relatively low risk of infiltration into the adjacent brain tissue, the steep dose gradient characteristics, and the low reported morbidity (albeit after relatively short-term follow-up), the use of radiosurgery has become firmly established and is readily applied to meningiomas in the posterior fossa. Another significant concern has been the likelihood that secondary tumors will develop in the wake of radiosurgery, although few reports have appeared in the literature to date.[25] Fractionated radiosurgery has also become readily available (Fig. 42-4), largely as a result of noninvasive patient immobilization methods, including "head mask" frame (i.e., noninvasive) and frameless image-guidance systems.

A recent report evaluating fractionated stereotactic radiotherapy showed survival rates of 97% for 5 years and 96% for 10 years after treatment, with local failure seen in only 3 out of 189 patients with WHO grade I meningiomas (22.5% located in the posterior fossa).[26] These researchers noted tumor shrinkage (i.e., more than 50% reduction) in 14% of patients and resolution of preexisting cranial nerve symptoms in 28% of patients. Clinically significant treatment-related toxicity was seen in 1.6% of the patients.[26] Outcomes data for radiosurgery are available for intracranial meningiomas generally, as well as for those located in the posterior fossa. Engenhart et al. reported an experience of radiosurgery in 17 patients with histologically proven benign meningiomas. Using a linear accelerator radiosurgery system, a maximum single dose of 10 to 50 Gy was used, with mean dose of 29 Gy prescribed to the 80% isodose line matching the tumor volume.[27] The dose was chosen based on tumor volume, tumor location, and radiosensitivity of the adjacent brain tissue. Freedom from tumor progression was noted in 80% of patients, and late complications included transient neurologic deficits with perifocal brain edema and one case of visual loss.

Relating to intracranial meningiomas in general, Kondziolka et al. reported 2-year radiosurgical tumor control rates of 96% in 50 patients.[28,29] The radiosurgery dose was 10 to 25 Gy (mean 17 Gy) to the tumor margin using a gamma knife unit; the doses were chosen based on tumor volume, location, previous radiotherapy dose, and adjacent critical normal tissue (e.g., optic chiasm). Tumors greater than 35 mm in diameter and located within 5 mm from the optic chiasm were excluded for radiosurgery. Three patients experienced delayed neurologic complications, thought to be consistent with radiation injury at 3 to 12 months following radiosurgery.[28-30] In another report from the Mayo Clinic on radiosurgical results for meningioma (in which 77% of 206 tumors were located at the cranial base), the median tumor margin dose was 16 Gy and survival rates at 5 and 7 years were 94% and 92%, respectively.[31] The overall tumor control rate was 89% at 5 years, with 56% of tumors decreasing in size. Taken together, the available data relating intracranial meningiomas (with the endpoint being freedom from progression after radiosurgery) indicate that tumor control appears to be in the range of 90%, with tumor shrinkage noted in approximately one third of radiosurgical patients.

Meningiomas in the posterior fossa often require radiation as either adjuvant or primary therapy. The radiosurgical experiences for acoustic and other schwannomas, as well as those for various benign and malignant tumors, have provided an important database regarding the responses of the cranial nerves and brain stem. For practical purposes, most cranial nerves are tolerant to radiosurgical doses up to 16 Gy, whereas the optic nerves, chiasm, and tracts seem more sensitive; for these, lower doses up to 10 Gy seem reasonable.[32] The radiosurgical response may vary depending on the length of nerve irradiated; the microenvironment of the nerve (e.g., ischemia), the degree of compression by the tumor, prior surgery and radiotherapy effects, retreatment and treatment intervals, and additional host factors[33,34] (Fig. 42-5). Motor morbidity rates appear to be less than 5%. However, the assessment of sensory nerve function poses more difficult problems, depending on the tumor type and location. For example, whereas the radiosurgical impact on cochlear nerve function may be less significant when dealing with meningiomas, radiosurgical dosing for acoustic neuroma has undergone a gradual decrease, possibly as a result of the intimate relation of tumor to nerve. One recent report on 55 patients with skull base meningiomas (including three of the petrous apex, four of the tentorium, two of the clivus, five of the CPA, and three of the jugular foramen), with average follow-up of 48.4 months, noted tumor stabilization in 69%, shrinkage in 29%, and enlargement in 2%.[35] Mean tumor volume was 7.33 cm³, and doses ranged from 12 to 25 Gy. All complications were transient, including seven trigeminal pareses and three patients with diplopia. Radiosurgical data on 62 patients with petroclival meningiomas treated with tumor margin doses of 11 to 20 Gy documented tumor shrinkage in 23%, stabilization in 68%, and growth in 8%.[36] Median follow-up was 37 months.

For tumor residuals intimately attached to the dural sinuses, similar principles apply. Based on the current literature, it is reasonable to use radiosurgery for a tumor located adjacent to or inside a dural sinus. There does not appear to be increased risk of weakening of the walls of the sinus, venous infarction, or other vascular-related complications,

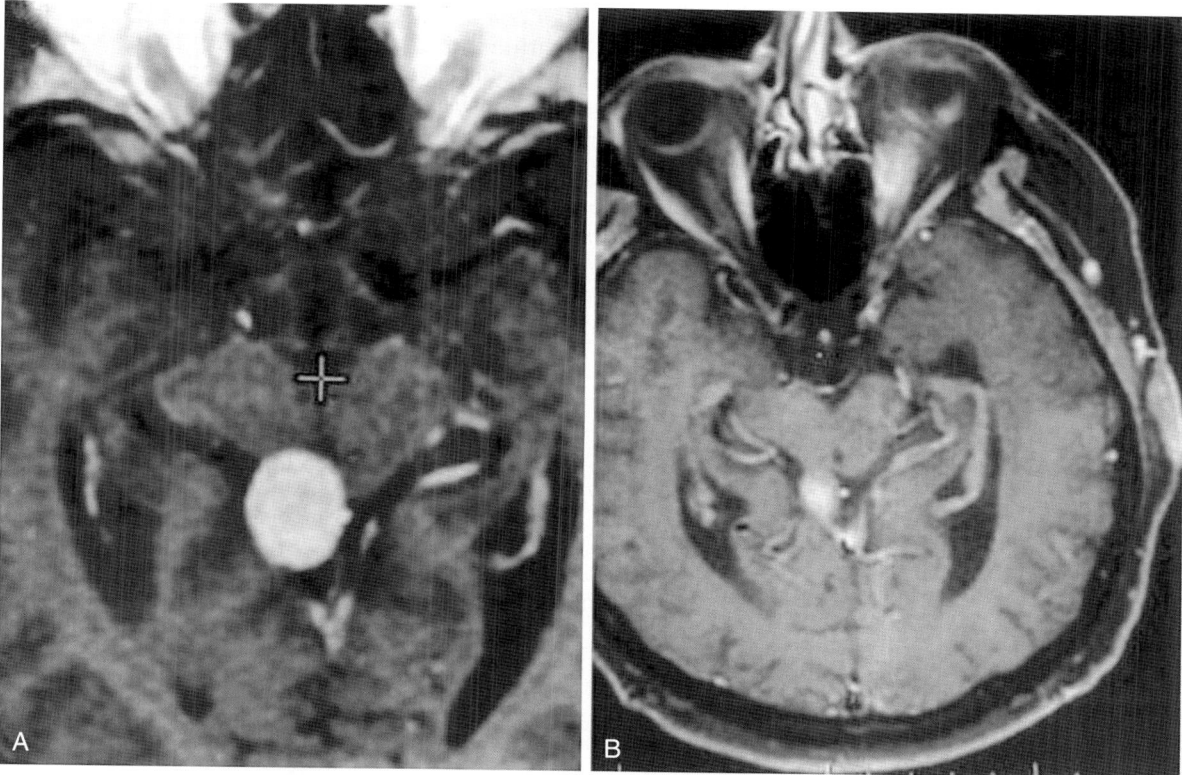

FIGURE 42-5 A, Axial contrast-enhanced MRI showing tentorial meningioma at the time of radiosurgery in 1992. B, Tumor regression 10 years later. *(From Kondziolka D, Nathoo N, Flickinger JC, et al: Long-term results after radiosurgery for benign intracranial tumors. Neurosurgery 53(4):815-822, 2003.)*

and it seems unlikely that radiosurgery will lead to progressive sinus occlusion. Larger experience and longer-term follow-up are needed to confirm these findings.

COMBINED SURGERY AND RADIATION

Ultimately, it seems logical to consider a combination of surgical resection and postoperative radiation treatment for the management of many meningioma patients. Many published reports have supported a planned, staged, microsurgery followed by stereotactic radiosurgery for selected patients with meningioma when indicated.[37,38] In these situations, microsurgical cytoreduction of a portion of the tumor can be achieved with minimal morbidity, as well as creation of adequate margins of space between the residual tumor surface and the differentially radiosensitive surrounding structures.

The optimal timing of the two stages remains a matter for debate. Delay of 12 to 18 months between stages allows for maximal recovery of any partial cranial neuropathy that occurs as a result of microsurgery before exposing the cranial nerves to an additional pathologic stress with radiation. However, delay between stages increases the likelihood of interval tumor growth and leads to loss of safety space achieved with surgery, because the previously compressed and displaced normal surrounding tissue returns to its natural position. If a delay between stages is contemplated, regular neuroimaging at 3-month intervals is recommended to detect and react to any unexpected circumstances.[39] This allows the surgeon to accelerate the radiation treatment to respond to the changing situation.

Perioperative Issues

Several issues, although not exclusively related to meningiomas, are commonly encountered in their management.

PREOPERATIVE EDEMA AND POSTOPERATIVE SWELLING

Many patients present with meningiomas that have significant associated peritumoral edema. The edema appears as a low-intensity signal on T1-weighted MRI and as a high-intensity signal on T2-weighted MRI. Unlike that seen with gliomas, with meningiomas this signal does not represent tumor infiltration but rather increased water concentration. Increased water content may lead to significant mass effect and must be considered in preparation for tumor removal. Edema can complicate the initial and postoperative stages of the operation. In the former, edematous brain forces its way out as the dura is opened; this can lead to unnecessary frustration and cortical resection in the early stages of the operation. In the postoperative stage, inadequate attention to peritumoral edema can lead to greatly increased pressure in the posterior fossa, herniation, and death. Significant preoperative edema is best managed by the administration of steroids; this should begin several days prior to the operation. When steroids (typically, Decadron at 4 mg every 8 hours) are begun several days prior to the operation, the likelihood of difficulty in the initial phases of the operation is low, even though the peritumoral T2 signal remains unchanged.

The postoperative problems secondary to edema are best dealt with during the operation by ensuring sufficient bony exposure, thereby limiting the extent of cerebellar retraction, which can aggravate the edema. A difficult tumor dissection may distract the surgeon, and when tumor removal requires ever-greater retraction, it is often best to resect the portion of the commonly contused cerebellum underlying the retractor rather than leave it alone, because this area can further swell and create significant, if not fatal, postoperative problems. Steroids are continued into the postoperative period and osmotic diuretics (i.e., mannitol and/or hypertonic saline solutions) may also be useful. Standard skull base approaches specifically for petroclival tumors now substitute bony removal for cerebellar retraction as the primary means to achieve the necessary exposure for safe tumor resection.

LARGE TUMOR WITHOUT PREOPERATIVE EDEMA AND POSTOPERATIVE SWELLING

An uncommon but important observation relates to large tumors without surrounding edema on preoperative MRI. Often after uneventful tumor resection (i.e., slack brain after total resection and no apparent venous injury), the patient does well for the first 24 to 48 hours and then becomes progressively sleepier, after which CT demonstrates extensive brain edema that has filled the resection cavity. The reason for this observation is not entirely clear, but aggressive management of elevated intracranial pressure with osmotic diuretics and possibly reintubation is required; reoperation for dural grafting and brain resection may be necessary.

TUMOR EN-PLAQUE EXTENSION BEYOND TYPICAL CRANIOTOMY

Meningiomas grow along the meninges, and a bony resection that closely conforms to the overtly contrast-enhancing mass of the tumor may often be insufficient. Because the tumor extends along the meninges, it is best to make a larger bony opening and therefore have the opportunity to remove the lateral en-plaque extensions of the tumor. In these instances, image guidance can be helpful.

HYPEROSTOSIS

Although still somewhat controversial, the hypertrophic bony changes often noted adjacent to meningiomas are known in most instances to be secondary to tumor invasion. Previous theories have suggested that these bony changes were related to vascular disturbances, "irritation" of the bone, osteoblastic stimulation by tumor, and direct tumor-derived bone formation.[40] Our experience, as well as the plentiful evidence in the literature, demonstrates that in many cases these changes are secondary to tumor invasion. The practical issue then relates to the potential for tumor recurrence, and it is well known that the best chance of cure follows radical tumor resection including the involved dura and bone (i.e., Simpson grade I).

VENOUS OBSTRUCTION AND INFARCTION

Although more obvious with supratentorial tumors, venous infarction can complicate surgery in the posterior fossa. Adequate exposure and internal debulking (when possible) of the tumor are the best means of avoiding this complication. After debulking, the tumor falls away or can be more easily separated from the adjacent vein. The effects of disrupting the venous sinuses (deep and superficial draining veins) are

not completely predictable. The veins near the roof of the fourth ventricle (i.e., around the cerebellar vermis and tonsils, petrosal veins, and veins of the cerebellomedullary fissure) can usually be sacrificed without major consequences. However, sacrificing the Galen vein, torcula, dominant lateral, or sigmoid sinuses is considered high risk.[13,14] Resection of a meningioma involving unilateral transverse sinus is feasible when the contralateral traverse sinus is open and close to the size of involved sinus. If a significant size discrepancy exists, prior to division of the involved transverse sinus, temporary sinus occlusion and pressure measurement should be considered.[14] When present, significant changes in manometric pressures during temporary occlusion and acute but temporary brain swelling indicate high risk.

When a dural sinus is partially occluded, the surgeon usually decides to radically remove the tumor mass but leave the patent sinus intact. Eventually, with continued tumor growth, the sinus occludes, and if adjuvant therapy is either not recommended or is ineffective, total resection can be considered at that time.

TUMOR–BRAIN INTERFACE

In most situations, the tumor does not adhere significantly to the brain surface. Although limited adhesions do exist, these are easily divided, and the tumor separates by simply advancing a cotton patty along the tumor–brain interface. The surgeon must pay attention so that small veins and arteries along this plane are not unnecessarily disrupted. On the other hand, invasive tumors (i.e., generally atypical and malignant subtypes) do invade the pial and brain surface, and great care must be exercised during dissection (especially along the brain stem) to remain on the tumor's immediate surface.

HYDROCEPHALUS

Hydrocephalus is one of the common presenting symptoms of posterior fossa meningiomas, particularly those located in the fourth ventricle. Although not all cases of hydrocephalus associated with posterior fossa meningiomas are obstructive, careful consideration must be given prior to recommending lumbar puncture, which can have serious ramifications. When surgical resection is delayed, it may be appropriate to relieve the hydrocephalus by temporary ventriculostomy, ventriculoperitoneal shunt, or third ventriculostomy. On many occasions, removal of the tumor with temporary postoperative ventricular drainage adequately manages hydrocephalus. At our center, external ventriculostomy is the preferred method for managing hydrocephalus because intracranial pressure can be better monitored after resection of the tumor and, ultimately, if there is no longer need for a shunt, it can be removed easily.

Specific Locations in the Posterior Fossa

OCCIPITAL AND LATERAL PETROUS SURFACE OF THE POSTERIOR FOSSA

Tumors located along the midline and lateral aspect of the occipital surface and lateral petrous bone (i.e., lateral to the internal auditory meatus) are, surgically, the least problematic (Fig. 42-6). Meningiomas in this region often present with

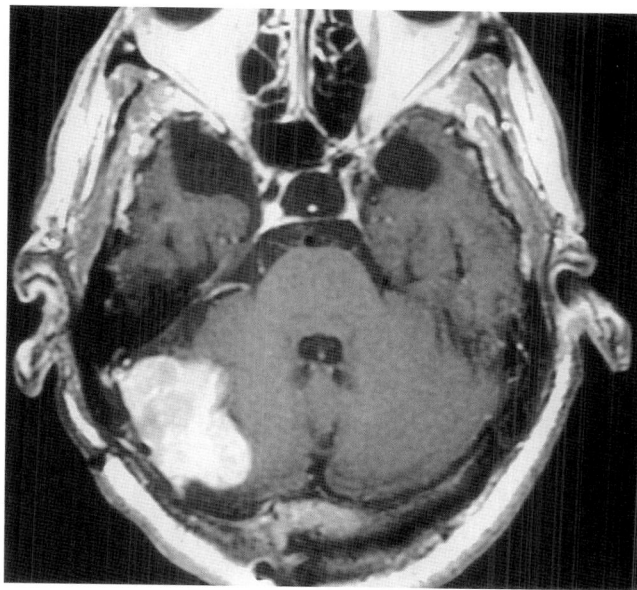

FIGURE 42-6 Preoperative MRI of a laterally based meningioma that originated from the suboccipital surface and was easily removed through a retrosigmoid incision and laterally oriented craniotomy without morbidity. Although the tumor separated from the transverse sinus, infiltration was apparent; radiation was not administered, and frequent follow-up is required.

symptoms of cerebellar dysfunction and headache, but they may also present as an incidental finding during workup for unrelated central nervous system symptoms. Occasionally, these tumors present with signs of elevated intracranial pressure. A suboccipital craniectomy/craniotomy is generally sufficient, and standard surgical techniques are employed to remove the tumor. The main surgical challenge is not to inadvertently open a patent dural sinus, although a simple suture or graft generally suffices as closure. The surgeon must realize that collateral venous drainage around an occluded sinus may be critical and should be protected. For those lesions located on the petrous bone lateral to the CPA, careful attention to the nerves coursing into the internal auditory meatus is required, and electrophysiologic monitoring of both the facial and the acoustic nerves is recommended. Although these lateral petrous tumors may be seen on MRI (T2-weighted images are usually best for this purpose) to be adjacent but lateral to the facial and acoustic nerve complex, the ability to stimulate the facial nerve, especially because it is located behind the tumor (i.e., in the surgeon's view), can be reassuring. It is important after the resection is complete to assess whether the adjacent cerebellum has been too heavily retracted or contused. In either case, resection of the injured brain may be prudent to avoid the postoperative risks associated with swelling.

TENTORIAL SURFACE

The clinical presentation of patients with tentorial meningioma is generally nonspecific. When the tumor originates in the anterior region of the tentorium, compression of the trigeminal and abducens nerves may lead to tic doloreaux and oculomotor paresis, but trochlear nerve signs are uncommon. Tumors originating from the posterior region of the tentorium rarely present with other than headache and,

perhaps, mild cerebellar signs. Occasionally, as a result of occlusion of the dural sinuses, a meningioma may present with signs of elevated intracranial pressure and visual loss (Fig. 42-7).

An additional but rare clinical presentation involves that of trigeminal neuralgia and hemifacial spasm secondary to a tumor that arises on the posterior portion of the tentorium but not involving the CPA.[41] In this case, the presumed cause of the neurologic symptoms and signs was rotation of the brain stem secondary to the large size of the tumor such that the cranial nerves were brought in contact with an ectatic vertebral artery. All symptoms and signs resolved after tumor removal.

Tumors originating from the posterior portion of the tentorium and extending into the posterior fossa are easily resected via standard suboccipital or retrosigmoid approaches. The tumor rarely invades the underlying cerebellum, and standard surgical techniques, as just noted for tumors located on the suboccipital and lateral petrosal surfaces, are sufficient. For those lesions extending toward the CPA, care must be taken to determine the location of the seventh and eighth cranial nerves, but generally this is not a significant obstacle to total resection. Every effort to preserve and even improve hearing should be made, because this is a more realistic goal with meningiomas (as opposed to acoustic schwannomas). Small lesions arising more anteriorly along the tentorium are usually adequately managed with a standard subtemporal approach, but for larger tumors, some variation on the transpetrosal approaches described later in the petroclival section may be necessary.

Although not a unique feature of tentorial meningiomas, an interesting surgical challenge concerns the handling of the dural venous sinuses. Generally, resection of these sinuses is not recommended if there is any indication of patency on CTA, angiography, or MRV or by direct intraoperative observation. When the sinus is completely occluded, it can be resected, but attention to the collateral venous drainage is critical because disruption of significant collateral drainage can be fatal.[42] Collignon et al. recently reported a case of occlusion of the torcula and bilateral transverse sinuses with hemangiopericytoma[43] (Fig. 42-8). The patient presented with visual blurring and bilateral papilledema, which was managed by bilateral occipital and suboccipital craniotomy. The tumor was noted to be filling the sinuses without extension beyond the walls of the sinuses. Total resection was achieved, and control of venous bleeding was accomplished with cotton balls, after which the sinus was repaired with bovine pericardial graft. Radiation therapy was used adjunctively, and 4 months after surgery the sinus remained patent, the patient was well, and papilledema had resolved. Although this unique case and others demonstrates the feasibility of sinus resection, it should not be undertaken lightly.

CEREBELLOPONTINE ANGLE

The CPA is the most common location for posterior fossa meningiomas, which are thought to originate from arachnoid cap cells in this region. The primary differential diagnostic consideration is acoustic neuroma, which arises from Schwann cells on the vestibular division of the statoacoustic nerve. Patients generally present in their fourth and fifth decades of life.[44] The clinical presentation, as

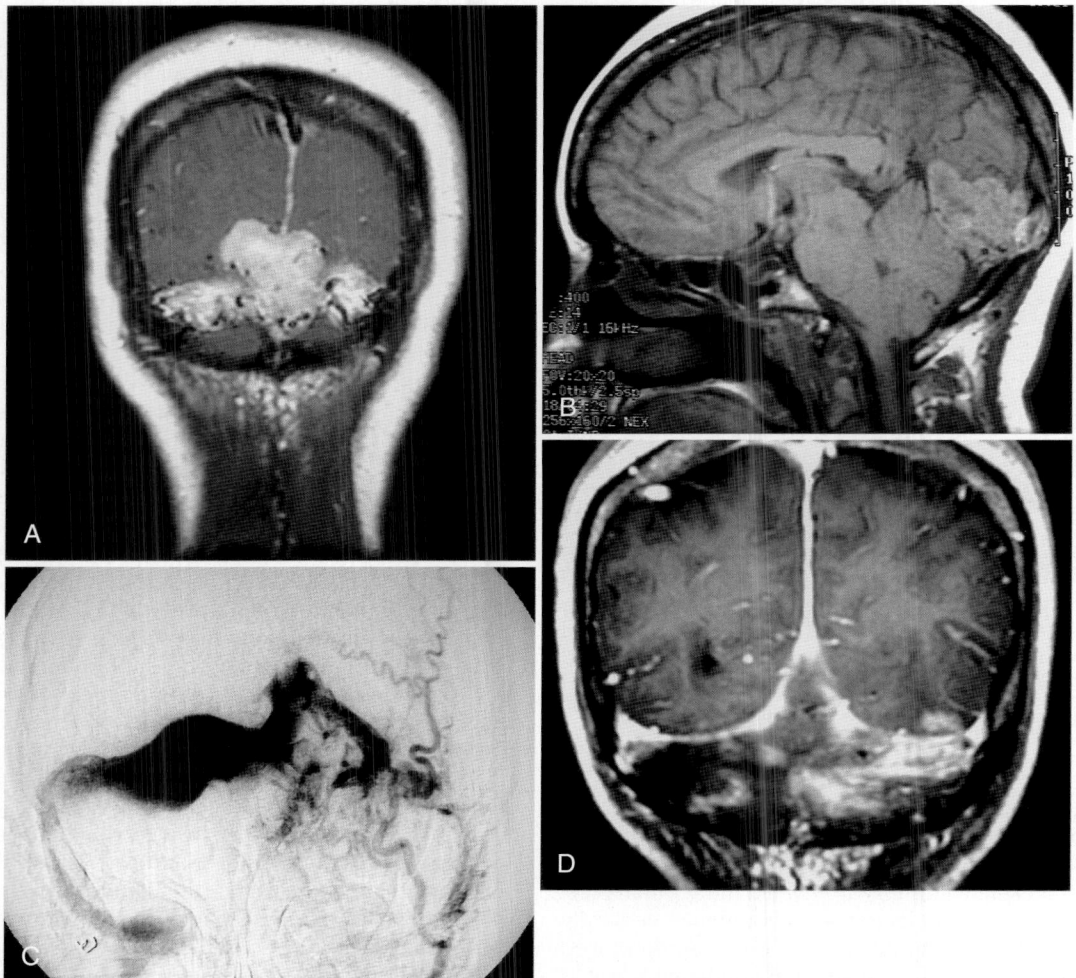

FIGURE 42-7 A, Coronal enhanced image of tentorial meningioma. B, Sagittal image of the same lesion. C, Pretreatment angiogram depicting the intense tumor stain and extensive collateral drainage. D, Coronal image 9 months after radiation treatment with 60 Gy.

for meningiomas as a whole, depends on the site of origin and direction of growth. Tumors growing superior to the internal auditory meatus commonly present with trigeminal symptoms (notably numbness and/or neuralgia), whereas those growing alongside the meatus may present with auditory and facial nerve dysfunction, the latter being distinctly uncommon with vestibular schwannoma. Those tumors growing inferior to the meatus may present with dysfunction of the lower cranial nerves (i.e., IX through XII). Symptoms and signs secondary to brain stem and cerebellar compression, because of the slow growth of the typical meningioma, are a late occurrence and often are not apparent even with very large tumors. CPA meningiomas cannot be distinguished from other tumor types based on clinical presentation alone, even though hearing loss and vestibular dysfunction are far less common with meningioma than with acoustic schwannoma.

MRI is the study of choice, although various auditory tests (e.g., pure-tone audiometry, speech discrimination, acoustic reflex, and brain stem auditory evoked responses) are commonly performed in neuro-otology practice, where many patients presenting with hearing loss are first evaluated. MRI findings (i.e., extra-axial CPA mass) can include

an enlarged CPA cistern, gray–white distortion of the adjacent cerebellum, and an indication of contrast enhancement extending along the skull base beyond the main tumor mass (i.e., dural tail) (Fig. 42-9). Calcification and cystic change are more common and less common, respectively, with meningiomas, whereas expansion of the porus acousticus is uncommon for the meningiomas. Although a typical acoustic schwannoma has the appearance of an ice cream cone, with sharply demarcated and rounded borders along the CPA portion with tumor extension filling the fundus of the internal auditory canal (IAC), meningiomas most often fill the CPA cistern with lateral extensions, irregular borders, and distinctly less notable growth into the IAC.

Because the epicenter of the tumor is the IAC, a standard lateral suboccipital approach generally provides sufficient exposure for complete tumor removal.[45] The patient is placed in a "park bench" position with the head slightly flexed and tilted toward the floor, after which the nose is rotated toward the floor. Mannitol and spinal drainage may facilitate the exposure and help to maintain this exposure, especially with larger tumors and longer dissections. The facial and acoustic nerves are routinely monitored. Given that the cranial nerves do not generally adhere to the tumor

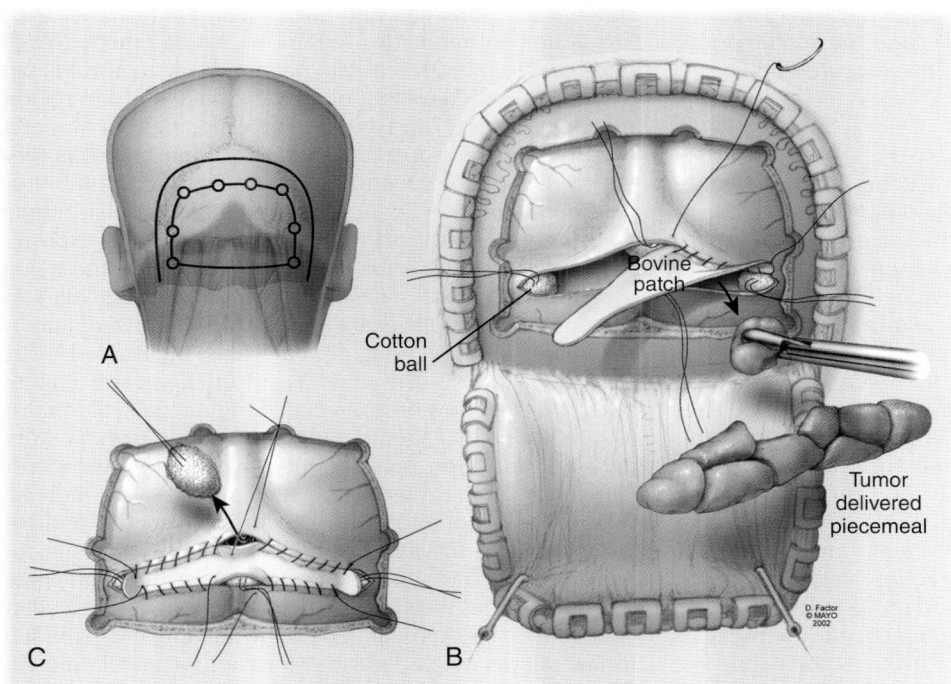

FIGURE 42-8 Illustration of the surgical steps. A, Exposure of the confluence of sinuses, bilateral transverse sinuses, and distal superior sagittal sinus via a bilateral occipital and suboccipital craniotomy. B, The transverse sinuses are opened and the tumor is removed piecemeal. Cotton balls control sinus bleeding while the venous sinuses are repaired with the aid of a bovine patch. C, Completion of the sinus repair after sequential removal of the cotton balls. *(From Collignon FP, Cohen-Gadol AA, Piepgras DG: Hemangiopericytoma of the confluence of sinuses and the transverse sinuses. J Neurosurg 99:1085-1088, 2003.)*

capsule, hearing preservation and even improvement should be reasonable expectations.

The craniotomy is centered about 1 cm behind the mastoid process, and partial exposure of the sigmoid sinus allows decreased retraction and about 0.5 to 1 cm of additional exposure anterior to the cerebellum. After durotomy and throughout subsequent dissection, attention must always be directed to brain stem auditory responses that will act as guides to the impact of cerebellar retraction on hearing function, which may easily be lost by direct medial retraction. The microscopic tumor dissection begins by assessment of tumor–cerebellar, tumor–brain stem, and tumor–cranial nerve relationships (when the nerves are lying on the surgeon's side). Constant attention to the maintenance of the arachnoid planes greatly facilitates subsequent resection and preservation of neural structures. The vascular supply to these tumors generally originates from vessels traversing the petrous bone and tentorium and commonly is difficult to interrupt early in the dissection, because the trajectories of the facial and acoustic nerves must be clearly defined before coagulating across the base of the tumor. With smaller tumors, interruption of the vascular supply greatly facilitates the subsequent dissection. With large tumors, internal debulking may be required to create "space" around tumor boundaries. As a rule, safe removal of posterior fossa tumors requires extensive internal debulking. As the tumor is debulked, small cotton patties are placed in the now-relaxed planes between tumor and neural structures. After the majority of the tumor has been removed from the CPA and the facial, acoustic, and trigeminal nerves are isolated, the portion located in the fundus of the IAC can be removed. The limits to bony removal along the IAC (i.e., generally less than 10 mm, but these may be precisely determined on preoperative temporal bone CT) are set by the location of the common crus of

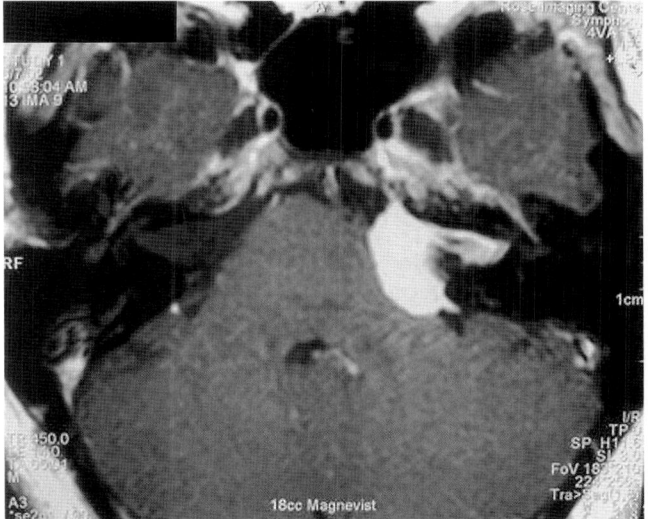

FIGURE 42-9 The extension of this CPA meningioma into the IAC is a relatively uncommon feature. Note also the normal diameter of the canal, an uncommon feature for acoustic schwannoma.

the posterior and superior semicircular canals. Disruption of this structure leads to deafness. At this point, the surgical resection is usually terminated (Simpson grade II). When possible, the surrounding dura that is invaded by tumor should be removed, but the resection generally will not be absolutely complete, and careful MRI follow-up over the next 5 to 10 years is required.

Other surgical approaches can be considered, but these have limitations. The translabyrinthine approach may be suitable when hearing is absent and may allow for early devascularization and identification of the facial and statoacoustic nerves, but the bony drilling is time consuming.

The standard petrosal approach is generally too extensive for most lesions limited to the CPA, and the subtemporal approach does not provide complete exposure to the CPA for most of these tumors.

PETROCLIVAL REGION

Anatomically, the petroclival region extends along the midline from the level of the posterior clinoid process to the jugular foramen and laterally to the CPA, incorporating cranial nerves III through XI and the brain stem. In a recent publication, Cho and Al-Mefty described hearing loss, facial and trigeminal pareses, gait disturbance, dysarthria, spasticity, and headache as the predominant clinical findings in patients with petroclival meningiomas prior to surgery.[46]

Surgically, meningiomas centered in the petroclival region are among the most challenging lesions to manage. Although there are many feasible surgical approaches to this region (e.g., transbasal, transoral, frontotemporal, subtemporal–transtentorial, combined subtemporal–suboccipital, transpetrous variations, and transsphenoidal), all except the transpetrous approaches have limitations in that they access only a small portion of the tumor. For lesions straddling a significant portion of the petroclival region, the most useful approach involves an exposure around and/or through the petrous bone.

Pioneered by Malis, transpetrous approaches provide exposure above and behind the petrous bone into the middle and posterior fossa, respectively.[47] Subsequent modifications of this approach provided additional exposure by incorporating various extents of petrous bone resection (i.e., retrolabyrinthine), which in keeping with standard skull base techniques, markedly decreases the need for temporal lobe, cerebellar, and brain stem retraction, thereby minimizing morbidity and allowing for total to near-total tumor resection.[48] This approach follows a route anterior to the sigmoid sinus and shortens the distance from the operator to the tumor. The approach also increases the risk to hearing loss by inadvertent drilling into the posterior semicircular canal; however, even this approach cannot easily visualize the most anteromedial portion of tumors extending along the midline clivus.

The anterior transpetrous approach is well suited for smaller lesions centered medial and superior to the internal auditory meatus and is based on the original description of the extended middle fossa approach.[46,49,50] In 1992, Spetzler et al. reported the results of various extents of petrous bone resection (i.e., retrolabyrinthine, translabyrinthine, and transcochlear) for 46 lesions including 18 petroclival meningiomas.[13] A recent report describes the addition of an anterior transpetrous bony removal (i.e., anteromedial to the cochlea, posteromedial to the petrous carotid, and inferior and medial to the gasserian ganglion) to a standard petrosal approach.[46] The authors report that in five of seven tumors, total resection was accomplished with neither mortality nor decrease in performance status, and only one patient lost hearing.

In the combined approach, the patient is placed in a supine position with a bolster under the shoulder and head turned about 30 to 45 degrees to the contralateral side.[46] The supra- and infratentorial craniotomy utilizes four bur holes placed above and below the transverse–sigmoid junction, plus one hole immediately above the zygoma, another at the superior temporal line, and one hole in the posterior fossa. The plate can frequently be removed as one piece. Next, a mastoidectomy with retrolabyrinthine bony removal is performed. The middle fossa dura is elevated, and the middle meningeal artery and greater superficial petrosal nerve are divided. The horizontal portion of the carotid is then exposed, and after identification and elevation of the third division of the trigeminal nerve, the anteromedial petrous apex (i.e., anteromedial to the cochlea) is removed, exposing the upper clivus. The dura is then opened above and below the superior petrosal sinus (SPS). The SPS is divided after the surgeon has carefully examined the MRV to ensure that no significant temporal bridging vein will be interrupted.[51] This maneuver exposes the middle and inferior clival regions. The tumor can now be appreciated, and piecemeal removal follows with initial attention to the vascular supply. By working back and forth between the inferior and the superior extremes of this exposure, the surgeon often can radically remove the tumor and safely work around vascular and nervous elements. The initial phases of the dissection may be facilitated by image guidance, especially regarding the anterior transpetrous resection. The approach provides excellent exposure for lesions centered on the midline and extending ipsilaterally, as well as for extensions across the midline. The most anteromedial portions of the tumor may occasionally be better visualized through the retrosigmoid portion of the exposure toward the end of the dissection (see Fig. 42-3). If hearing is to be preserved, this combined approach is generally required (especially for larger tumors); however, when hearing is not an issue, the translabyrinthine and transcochlear bony variations add considerably to the exposure.

JUGULAR FORAMEN

The jugular foramen region is a relatively uncommon origin for meningiomas.

Symptoms and signs reflect the local anatomy with involvement of cranial nerves IX to XI (and occasionally V and VIII), and larger tumors may be associated with brain stem compression.[52] Because of the nature of the preoperative neurologic deficits, otolaryngology evaluation should be performed to establish a preoperative baseline, but postoperative testing is also required and is more critical. Although most often temporary, postoperative swallowing deficits can be debilitating and require gastrostomy and tracheostomy.

Monitoring of cranial nerves VII, VIII, IX, XI, and XII should be performed because these nerves may be hidden (especially IX, X, and XI) by the tumor capsule. Arnautovic et al. describe a suprajugular, retrojugular, and transjugular approach for tumors in this region, with the patency and dominance of the jugular bulb dictating the choice.[53] The infralabyrinthine suprajugular approach requires a mastoidectomy, followed by skeletonization of the superior petrosal and sigmoid sinuses and jugular bulb, after which the tumor is dissected from the cranial nerves (Fig. 42-10). In the retrojugular approach, a lateral suboccipital craniotomy and mastoidectomy with skeletonization of the sigmoid sinus and jugular bulb are followed by removal of a portion of the occipital condyle and jugular tubercle. A durotomy posterior to the sigmoid sinus provides the exposure for tumor removal. In the transjugular variation, a mastoidectomy that exposes the sigmoid sinus, jugular bulb, and jugular vein

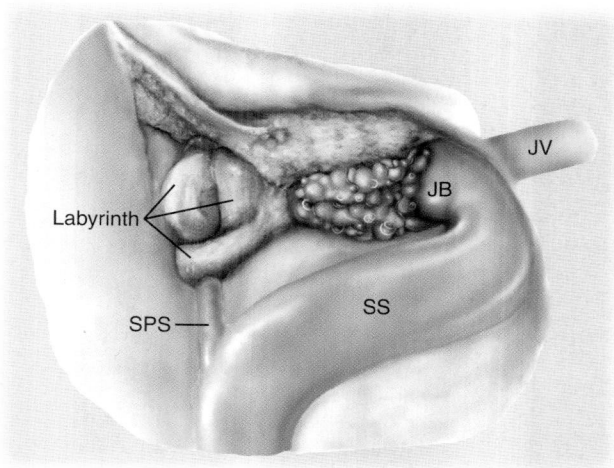

FIGURE 42-10 Drawing of the suprajugular approach. Note the infralabyrinthine position of the tumor; the sagittal sinus; the jugular bulb, which is patent; the jugular vein; the SPS; and the labyrinth (right side is shown). *(From Arnautovic KI, Al-Mefty O: Primary meningiomas of the jugular fossa. J Neurosurg 97:12-20, 2002.)*

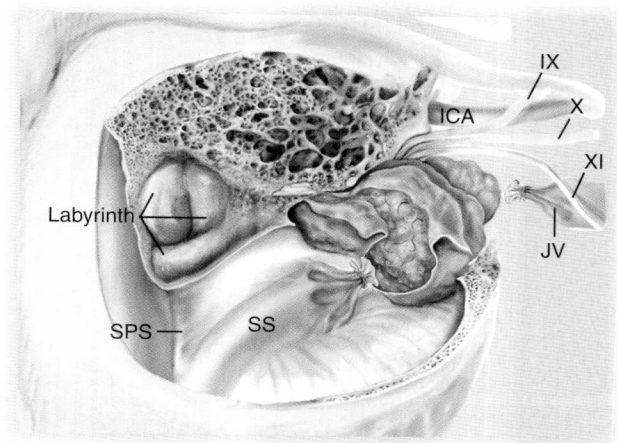

FIGURE 42-11 Drawing of the transjugular approach. Note the tumor occluding the jugular bulb, which is open; the sagittal sinus and jugular vein, both of which are ligated; the SPS; the internal carotid artery; the lower cranial nerves (ninth through eleventh nerves) extracranially; and the labyrinth (right side is shown). *(From Arnautovic KI, Al-Mefty O: Primary meningiomas of the jugular fossa. J Neurosurg 97:12-20, 2002.)*

and suboccipital craniotomy is performed. The posterior belly of the digastric muscle and the stylohyoid muscle are divided, after which the styloid process is removed. The sigmoid sinus and jugular vein are ligated above and below the tumor, respectively, and the tumor is dissected from the cranial nerves and carotid artery (Fig. 42-11). In this series of eight patients (nine surgeries), worsened or new deficits in three patients were reported, and some degree of recovery or stabilization was noted in all eight patients.[52]

FORAMEN MAGNUM

Meningiomas at the foramen magnum arise from the dura of the craniocervical junction; they account for 4.2% to 20% of posterior fossa meningiomas, depending on the referral status of the reporting institution[47] (Fig. 42-12). These tumors

tend to go undiagnosed or misdiagnosed for long periods because of the variety of presenting symptoms. Tumors can present with cerebellar signs, evidence of increased intracranial pressure, lower cranial nerve deficits, and brain stem or spinal cord signs mimicking cervical myelopathy with radicular signs and dysesthesias. In addition, symptoms of suboccipital pain may be seen.

As with all meningiomas, MRI is the study of choice and is complemented by CTA, MRA, and MRV, although thin-section CT better defines bony involvement. Selective angiography can be used to determine the blood supply and the utility of preoperative embolization. The vascular supply to these tumors is predominantly from the ascending pharyngeal artery and the middle meningeal artery, whereas the dura posterior to foramen magnum is supplied by the occipital artery and the posterior meningeal branch of the vertebral artery. Those tumors located ventral to the dentate ligaments should be differentiated from those arising dorsally because of significant differences in the clinical presentation, in the degree of operative difficulty, and in the likelihood of postoperative morbidity. The primary difference lies in truly ventral tumors originating anterior to the lower cranial (i.e., IX-XII), upper cervical nerves, posterior inferior cerebellar artery, and brain stem, all of which make surgical removal far more challenging.

Surgical approaches have included the standard posterior midline suboccipital approach with C1 laminectomy, the transoral approach, and the transcondylar approach.[54-56] For true ventral lesions, the posterior midline approach is insufficient for anything better than a Simpson grade IV removal, and it can be associated with significant morbidity because the spinal cord and lower brain stem will be interposed between the surgeon and the pathology. However, for lesions arising more laterally and dorsal to the dentate ligaments and displacing the spinal cord and brain stem medially, standard midline approaches may well be sufficient, although removal of the most medial extents of the tumor can be difficult in the final phases of the operation when the brain stem and spinal cord expand into the operative field. Theoretically reasonable from an anatomic viewpoint, the transoral approach provides limited exposure, carries the serious risk of postoperative cerebrospinal fluid leak through the oropharyngeal mucosa, and is best left to surgeons experienced with transoral techniques.[55] The transcondylar approach has been detailed by Sen and others[56-58] and is most suitable for practically all meningiomas in this location.

Preoperative considerations include the precise origin of the tumor, the relationship of the vertebral artery to the tumor, the relative sizes (i.e., contribution to stability) of the occipital–C1 joint, the vascular anatomy, the patency of the vertebral arteries (i.e., noted with CTA, MRA, and MRV), and the status of lower cranial nerve function (especially swallowing). Patients are placed in a park-bench position and are monitored for somatosensory and possibly auditory brain stem function, along with cranial nerves X through XII. The transcondylar approach for ventrally situated tumors generally requires transposition of the vertebral artery, which must be carefully rotated such that thrombosis will not occur during the commonly lengthy procedure. The microvascular Doppler can be helpful in locating the vertebral

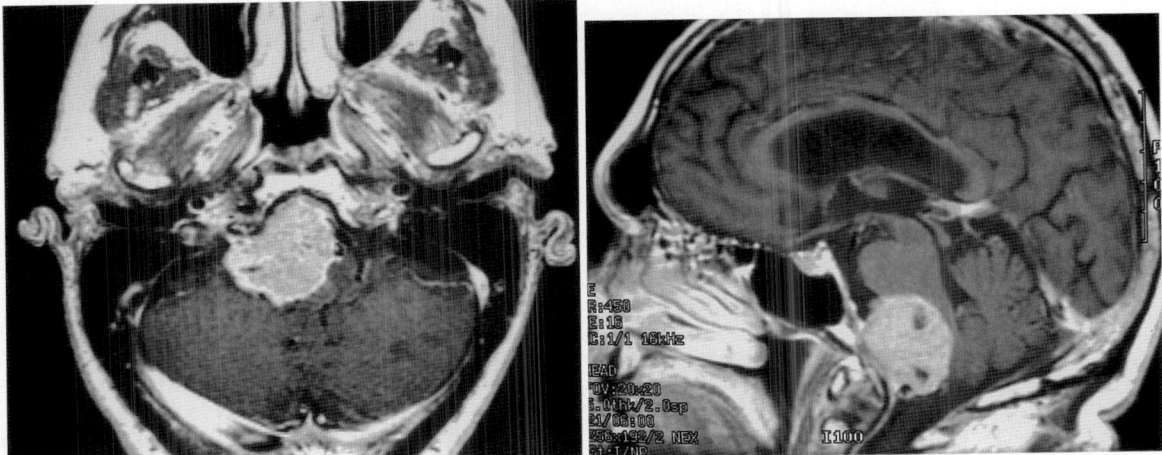

FIGURE 42-12 Enhanced T1-weighted MRI of a foramen magnum meningioma. Although the tumor has created space along the lateral aspect of the brain stem, a more lateral approach provides ample exposure for removal of the midline portion of the tumor toward the end of the procedure.

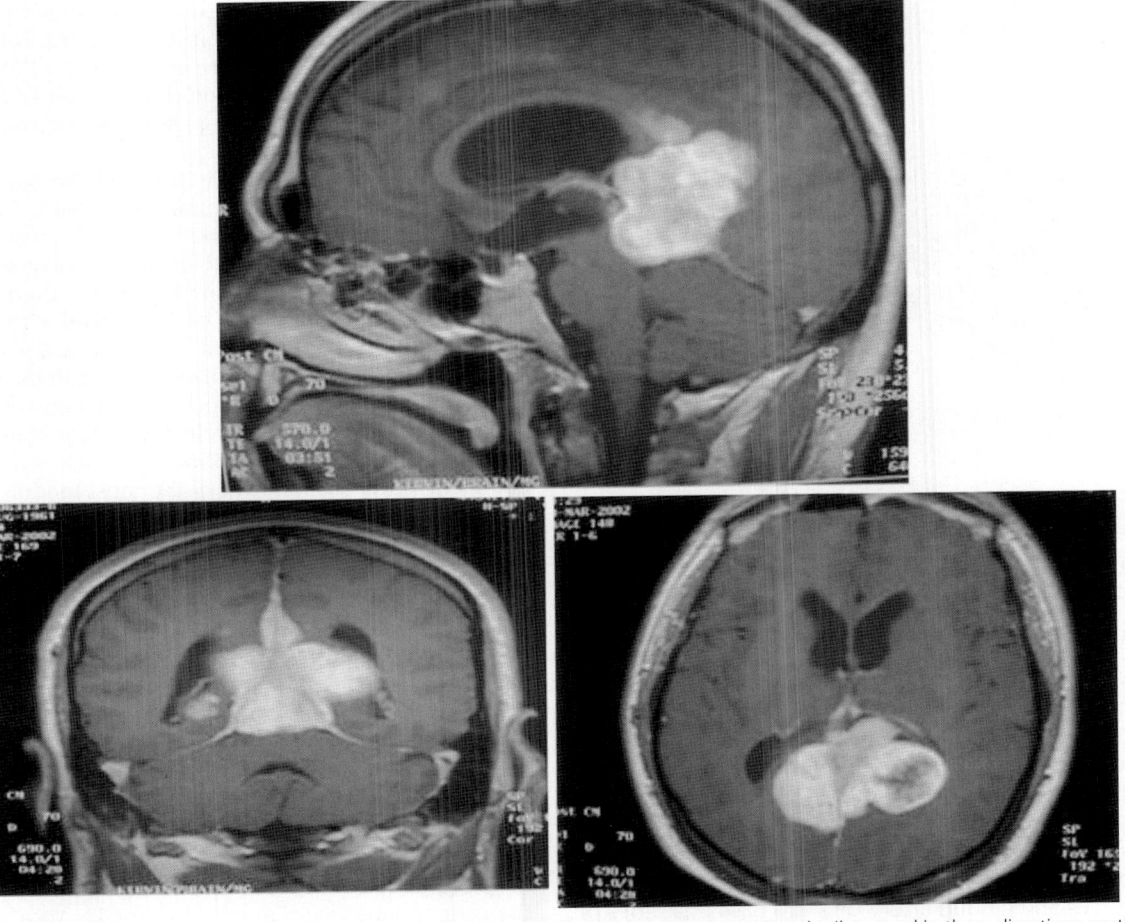

FIGURE 42-13 Sagittal, axial, and coronal T1-weighted MRI of a large pineal region meningioma. Dural tails extend in three directions on the coronal image. This tumor was resected (i.e., Simpson grade III) via an occipital–transtentorial approach.

artery in the early stages of the operation. To create the greatest extent of exposure, especially for tumors with extension across the midline, one half to two thirds of the condyle may be removed. Only rarely does this require surgical stabilization. The final element in the initial exposure involves the extent of venous engorgement in the so-called suboccipital

cavernous sinus, as detailed by Caruso et al., which can complicate the dissection.[59] From this point, careful attention to the cranial nerves traversing the tumor capsule is required while the tumor is debulked and dissected. In a review of 18 patients with ventral foramen magnum tumors followed for a mean of 40 months after first-time surgery, Arnautovic

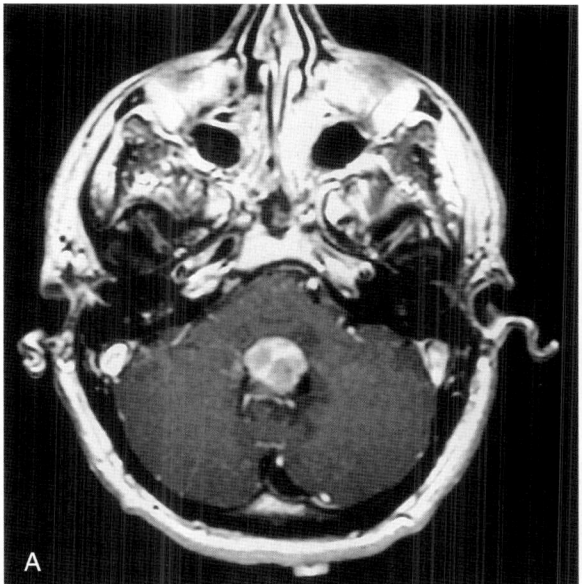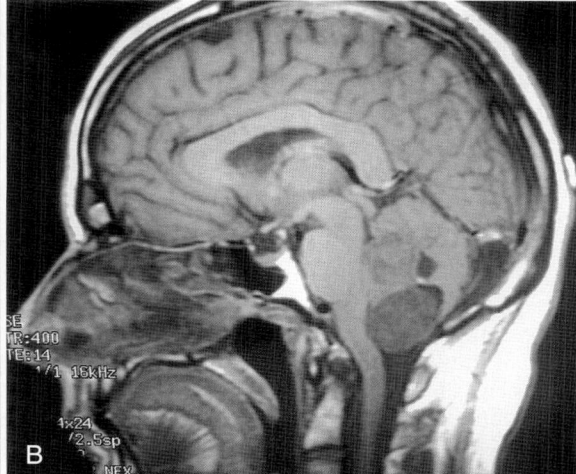

FIGURE 42-14 This fourth ventricular meningioma was totally resected by splitting the cerebellar vermis. A, Axial enhanced image. B, Sagittal non-enhanced image.

et al. described 75% with gross total resection (Simpson I-II), 12.5% with near-total resection (Simpson III), and 12.5% with subtotal excision (Simpson IV).[53] Ninth and tenth cranial nerve deficits were the most common consequence, and there was no 30-day operative mortality.

PINEAL REGION

Meningiomas in the pineal region are a rare entity constituting approximately 6% to 8% of neoplasms.[60] Most meningiomas arise from the tentorial edge or from the junction of tentorium and falx, although some instances of lesions with no dural attachment have been reported, in which case the tumor is believed to arise from the telachoroidea in the roof of the third ventricle.[61,62] Presenting symptoms are quite variable, partly reflecting the local anatomy. Common presenting symptoms are related to increased intracranial pressure (i.e., secondary to either tumor size or deep venous occlusion) and/or the visual system.[63] As with many meningiomas in various locations, headache is a common but nonspecific finding. Involvement of the tectal region may manifest as various degrees of upgaze paresis, pupillary, and convergence abnormalities culminating occasionally in a complete Parinaud syndrome. Symptoms and signs of cerebellar dysfunction may also occur but are uncommon. When the tumor compresses the cerebral aqueduct, hydrocephalus may develop.

The imaging study of choice is contrast-enhanced MRI with MRA and MRV, although with larger tumors cerebral angiography may be more useful for arterial and venous delineation (i.e., internal cerebral veins, basal Rosenthal vein, Galen vein, sinuses, and superficial venous system). Preoperative embolization, although rare, may also be considered (Fig. 42-13). Feeding vessels are commonly the medial and lateral posterior choroidal arteries, as well as the tentorial arteries. Given the usual operative choices (i.e., infratentorial–supracerebellar and occipital–transtentorial approaches), a clear understanding of the arterial and venous anatomy

may be important because early arterial occlusion during the surgical procedure is not always possible.

In the past, surgical treatment of pineal region meningiomas was associated with significant morbidity and mortality; however, as with meningiomas in all other locations, recent subspecialization and improvements in surgical techniques have markedly reduced these morbidities.[64] The main surgical approaches currently used are infratentorial–supracerebellar and occipital–transtentorial, with a supra/infratentorial–transsinus approach recently reported.[14] When significant obstructive hydrocephalus is detected preoperatively, insertion of a ventriculoperitoneal shunt may be considered; however, endoscopically guided third ventriculostomy is becoming the procedure of choice.

With the occipital–transtentorial approach, it is preferable to approach the tumor from the nondominant side, but tumor shape and vascular anatomy primarily determine this orientation. The patient may be sitting or semisitting, but we prefer a three quarter–prone position with the operated side down, which diminishes the degree of occipital lobe retraction.[65] The occipital lobe is gently retracted laterally, with attention paid to the bridging veins because their injury can lead to hemianopsia. After a paramedian tentorial incision, the tumor should come into view. The advantage of this approach is surgeon comfort (i.e., for those unfamiliar with the sitting position); disadvantages include limited space, potential for retraction injury to occipital lobe, off-midline anatomic orientation, and venous anatomy oriented between the surgeon and the tumor.

The advantages of the infratentorial–supracerebellar approach are the midline orientation, excellent tumor visibility below the venous system, and minimal cerebellar retraction. The main disadvantages of this approach, done with the patient in the sitting position, are limited exposure of tumors extending above the deep venous complex and fatigue in the surgeon's arm and hand, although with appropriate flexion of the patient's head and back such fatigue can be minimized.[66] As for any operation with the patient in a sitting position, air embolism is a possibility.[63]

For large tumors in the pineal region, a combined supra/infratentorial–transsinus approach has been described.[14] A craniotomy in three pieces is made over the torcula and transverse sinuses, with subsequent section of transverse sinus and tentorium. This approach provides a wide surgical corridor and large exposure with access to the tumor extending into the third ventricle, minimal retraction of cerebellum and occipital lobes, and a comfortable position for the surgeon.[14]

FOURTH VENTRICLE

Meningiomas located in the fourth ventricle are rare and usually present with signs of obstructive hydrocephalus; rarely, they present with cranial neuropathies secondary to compression of cranial nerves and nuclei in the floor of the ventricle (Fig. 42-14). The surgical approach generally requires a midline suboccipital craniotomy with vermian split and early devascularization of the tumor. Care to limit iatrogenic compression of the structures in the floor and not to intrude through the floor of the ventricle is paramount. With larger tumors, it is generally recommended to monitor somatosensory and brain stem auditory evoked responses along with lower cranial nerves (i.e., VI to XII).

Conclusions

Management strategies for patients with meningiomas in the posterior fossa have undergone considerable evolution during the past 25 years. For meningiomas (in general, as well as for those located in the posterior fossa), complete surgical resection remains the treatment of choice. For those tumors located at the petroclival junction, the jugular foramen, the CPA, or the pineal region, resection is best accomplished in centers with subspecialized and frequent experience. However, given the indolent natural history of these tumors, the diagnostic accuracy of radiography when combined with clinical data, the surgical challenges associated with posterior fossa tumors, and the modern refinements in radiation delivery methods, along with the extensive literature documenting tumor control and limited morbidity, it has become reasonable to consider radical subtotal resection combined with some form of adjuvant radiation therapy for many tumors and, for smaller tumors, radiosurgery alone as a primary therapy.

KEY REFERENCES

Akagami R, Napolitano M, Sekhar LN. Patient-evaluated outcome after surgery for basal meningiomas. *Neurosurgery*. 2002;50:941-949.

Ausman JI, Malik GM, Dujovny M. Three-quarter prone approach to the pineal–tentorial region. *Surg Neurol*. 1988;29:298-306.

Barbaro NM, Gutin PH, Wilson CB, et al. Radiation therapy in the treatment of partially resected meningiomas. *Neurosurgery*. 1987;20:525-528.

Bendszus M, Rao G, Burger R, et al. Is there a benefit to preoperative meningioma embolization. *Neurosurgery*. 2000;47:1306-1312.

Bonnal J, Brotchi J. Reconstruction of the superior sagittal sinus in parasagittal meningiomas. In: Schmidek HH, ed. *Meningiomas and their Surgical Management*. Philadelphia: WB Saunders; 1991:221-229.

Carella RJ, Ransohoff J, Newall J. Role of radiation therapy in the management of meningioma. *Neurosurgery*. 1982;10:332-339.

Cho CW, Al-Mefty O. Combined petrosal approach to petroclival meningiomas. *Neurosurgery*. 2002;51:708-716.

Chun JY, McDermott MW, Lamborn KR, et al. Delayed surgical resection reduces intraoperative blood loss for embolized meningiomas. *Neurosurgery*. 2002;50:1231-1237.

Elster AD, Challa VR, Gilbert GH, et al. Meningiomas: MR and histopathologic features. *Radiology*. 1989;170:857-862.

Forbes AR, Goldberg ID. Radiation therapy in the treatment of meningioma: The Joint Center for Radiation Therapy experience. *J Clin Oncol*. 1984;2:1139-1143.

House WF, Hitselberger WE, Horn KL. The middle fossa transpetrous approach to the anterior–superior cerebellopontine angle. *Am J Otol*. 1986;7:1-4.

Kinjo T, Al-Mefty O, Imad K: Grade zero removal of supratentorial convexity meningiomas: clinical study. *Neurosurgery*. 1993;33:394-399.

Kondziolka D, Lunsford LD. Radiosurgery of meningioma. *Neurosurg Clin N Am*. 1992;3:219-230.

Kondziolka D, Lundsford LD, Flickinger JC. Stereotactic radiosurgery of meningiomas. In: Lundsford LD, Kondziolka D, Flickinger JD, eds. *Gamma Knife Brain Surgery*. Vol. 14. Basel: Karger; 1998:104-113.

Kondziolka D, Nathoo N, Flickinger JC, et al. Long-term results after radiosurgery for benign intracranial tumors. *Neurosurgery*. 2003;53(4):815-822.

Mirabell R, Linggood RM, de la Monte S, et al. The role of radiotherapy in the treatment of subtotally resected meningiomas. *J Neurooncol*. 1992;13:157.

Rock JP, Monsell EM, Schmidek HH. Meningiomas of the cerebellopontine angle. In: Schmidek HH, ed. *Meningiomas and Their Surgical Management*. Philadelphia: WB Saunders; 1991: Harcourt Brace Jovanovich, 417-425.

Sekhar LN, Janetta PJ. Cerebellopontine angle meningiomas. *J Neurosurg*. 1984;60:500.

Sen CN, Sekhar LN. An extreme lateral approach to intradural lesions of the cervical spine and foramen magnum. *Neurosurgery*. 1990;27:197-204.

Simpson D. The recurrence of intracranial meningioma after surgical treatment. *J Neurol Neurosurg Psychiatry*. 1957;20:22.

Spetzler RF, Daspit P, Pappas CT. The combined supra- and infratentorial approach for lesions of the petrous and clival regions: Experience with 46 cases. *J Neurosurg*. 1992;76:588-599.

Stafford SL, Pollock BE, Foote RL, et al. Meningioma radiosurgery: tumor control, outcomes, and complications among 190 consecutive patients. *Neurosurg*. 2001;49:1029-1038.

Tishler RB, Loeffler JS, Lundsford LD, et al. Tolerance of cranial nerves of the cavernous sinus to radiosurgery. *Int J Radiat Oncol Biol Phys*. 1993;27:215-221.

Yasargil MG, Mortara RW, Curcic M. Meningiomas of basal posterior cranial fossa. *Adv Tech Stand Neurosurg*. 1980;7:1-15.

Ziyal IM, Sekhar LN, Salas E, Olan WJ. Combined supra/infratentorial–transsinus approach to large pineal region tumors. *J Neurosurg*. 1998;88:1050-1057.

Numbered references appear on Expert Consult.

CHAPTER 43

Surgical Management of Tumors of the Foramen Magnum

JOSE ALBERTO LANDEIRO • ROBERTO LEAL SILVEIRA
• CASSIUS VINÍCIUS CORRÊA DOS REIS

The foramen magnum (FM) comprises a bony channel formed anteriorly by the lower third of the clivus, the anterior arch of the atlas, and the odontoid process. The lateral limits are the jugular tubercle (JT), the occipital condyle (OC), and the lateral mass of the atlas. Lastly, the FM is limited posteriorly by the lower part of the occipital bone, the posterior arch of the atlas, and the two first intervertebral spaces.[1-3]

The FM encloses the vertebral arteries (VAs) and their meningeal branches, the anterior and posterior spinal arteries, the lower cranial nerves (IX, X, and XI), and the roots of the C1 and C2 vertebrae. The neural structures located at the FM are the cervicomedullary junction, the cerebellar tonsils, the inferior vermis, and the fourth ventricle.[1-3] It is surrounded by veins, venous sinuses, and the jugular bulb. Hence, when approaching this region, surgeons must avoid manipulation and retraction of those neurovascular structures and, consequently, preserve anatomy and function.

There is a broad spectrum of intra- and extradural surgical pathologies of the FM. Tumors represent almost 5% of spinal and 1% of intracranial neoplasms,[1] which consist mostly of meningiomas, neurinomas, and chordomas.[1-5]

In the past, these lesions were approached posteriorly and eventually via the transoral route; however, the results of these techniques were disappointing.[6] The introduction of computed tomography (CT) scan and magnetic resonance imaging (MRI) allowed the improvement of anatomic knowledge and the development of microsurgical techniques and skull base approaches. Therefore, treatment of these tumors has evolved and remarkable improvement in surgical results has been achieved. Nevertheless, despite these advances, surgery of FM tumors is still associated with a high rate of morbidity.

Clinical Presentation

The clinical presentation associated with FM tumors is insidious. Because of their slow-growing pattern, their indolent behavior, and the wide subarachnoid space at this level, the mean length of symptoms before diagnosis is 30.8 months.[3,7] In early stages, patients complain of occipital headache and cervical pain. This pain is described as deep and is aggravated by neck motion, coughing, and straining. As the tumor grows, sensory and motor deficits develop. The classic syndrome of FM tumors, mainly of meningiomas

placed anteriorly, is an asymmetrical deficit defined by weakness, paresthesis, and spasticity, first in the ipsilateral arm and progressing to the ipsilateral leg, then to the contralateral leg, and finally to the contralateral arm. Long tract signs characteristic of upper-motor lesions are the presence of atrophy in the intrinsic muscles of the hands. Later findings include spastic quadriparesis, respiratory dysfunction, and lower cranial nerve deficits.[6,7] In extradural tumors, especially in cranial base chordomas, diplopia is the symptom most commonly reported and headache is the second-most-common symptom.[5]

Classification of the Tumors

Tumors of the FM are classified according to their origin. They can arise in the FM itself or secondarily from surrounding areas. Most classifications focus on meningiomas and usually do not regard bone tumors. Among the many classifications of meningiomas of the FM,[6-8] the one most frequently used by neurosurgeons is the classification from Bruneau and George.[3] The main objective of this system is to define the surgical strategy preoperatively. Based on this classification, meningiomas of the FM are classified as intradural, extradural, or intra- and extradural. According to their insertion on the dura, meningiomas are anterior if insertion happens on both sides of the anterior midline, anterolateral if insertion occurs between the midline and the dentate ligament, or posterior if insertion is posterior to the dentate ligament. The other landmark used for classification is the relation to the VAs, because meningiomas of the FM can develop above, below, or on both sides of the VAs. Intradural meningiomas are the most common type, and most of them arise anterolaterally;[4-8] these are followed in frequency by posterolateral tumors. Tumors that arise purely posteriorly and anteriorly are rare.[7]

The surgical approach to extradural tumors is based on their relationship with the C1 lateral mass, OC, clivus, intradural extension, cavernous sinus, jugular foramen, retropharynge, VAs, and carotid artery. Although there are various kinds of tumors, they present a similar surgical aspect. A position in front of, or lateral to, the cervicomedullary junction; a closer relationship with the VAs and their branches; lower cranial nerves; and complex articulation between the occipital bone and the C1 and C2 vertebrae are some of these surgical aspects. The size, position, and nature of the tumors define the surgical approach and steps, such as drilling the lateral wall of the FM and transposing the VAs. The definition of the space between the cervicomedullary junction and the lateral wall of the FM, the so-called surgical corridor,[7] is also an important consideration. Large tumors, either anterior or anterolateral, push the cervicomedullary junction posteriorly, creating a surgical avenue for tumor removal. In contrast, small tumors and an elongated FM may require additional space, which can be obtained via the condyle or the lateral mass of C1, with transposition of the VAs.[5]

Preoperative Imaging

The preoperative workup includes MRI and CT scan. With the availability of CT angiography and magnetic resonance angiography, conventional angiography is rarely indicated unless embolization is planned in highly vascularized tumors. Preoperative imaging studies allow for planning of the surgery; for this, the following information must be retrieved from the images: the nature of the tumor (intra- and/or extradural), its location and attachment, its relationship with the cervicomedullary junction, its caudal and rostral extension, the position and possible involvement of the VAs and their branches, the shape of the FM, the dominance of the VAs, the venous drainage patterns and dominance, and bony involvement. T1-weighted MRI with contrast enhancement clearly defines the tumor and the dural attachment site and discriminates between the tumor and the brain stem. T2-weighted MRI provides information on the arachnoid plane between the tumor and the cervicomedullary junction. CT using sagittal, coronal, and axial viewing and bone window remains the tool of choice for the study of bone involvement, the shape of the FM, and the surgical corridor.[1-3,6,7]

Choosing the Best Approach

The principal factors that determine access to the lesions placed at the craniovertebral junction are the nature, position, and size of the tumors and the shape of the FM.[5] Tumors located posteriorly or posterolaterally to the cervicomedullary junction can be approached from the posterior midline, which allows an extensive sagittal view from the skull base to the entire cervical spine; however, this approach does not work well for tumors located anterolaterally. This midline route does not allow control of the VAs when the bone needs to be removed ventrolaterally. Anterior approaches via transcervical or transoral routes have been used but are not accepted widely. The transoral approach is essentially a midline and extradural approach to the inferior clivus and upper cervical spine that, combined with maxillotomy or labiomandibulotomy and glossotomy, can provide access from the superior clivus to the middle cervical spine. Nevertheless, this approach is limited laterally from both carotid arteries and VAs at the clival and spinal levels. Removal of an intradural pathology carries a high risk of cerebrospinal fluid (CSF) leakage. The dura is difficult to repair, because it comprises a limited amount of soft tissue and the subarachnoid space is exposed to the contaminated field.[9] Anterior approaches are suitable for small extradural and bony lesions without VAs and carotid artery involvement.[4,6,7,10]

However, minimization of the cervicomedullary retraction and of risk of CSF leakage, a firm watertight closure, and management of the OC and of the VAs are the main factors considered when choosing the approach. Among the approaches available to the FM, the so-called far lateral approach, the extreme transcondylar approach, and its variants of the lateral suboccipital approach meet these criteria. These approaches can be combined with petrosal, retrosigmoid, transtuberculum, transfacetal, and infratemporal approaches, according to the rostrocaudal extension and nature of the tumor.[6,11]

Extradural tumors located frontal to the cervicomedullary junction that present with or without involvement of the VAs and the lower cranial nerves, that invade the dura, and that invade and/or destroy the OC and the articulation among OC, C1, and C2 can be approached via the same route; however, these tumors often require combined approaches.[6,9-11]

Far Lateral Approach

POSITIONING

Surgical results depend on the positioning of the patient. Malpositioning may result in a narrow microsurgical view, cerebral edema, increased bleeding because of impairment of venous return, and lesions of the eye, peripheral nerves, and spinal cord.[12] At our institution, we adopt the three quarter–prone position to perform lateral approaches.[6] The side of the approach is ipsilateral to the lesion. If the lesion is placed midline, the side of the approach is usually the side of the nondominant VAs and the nondominant jugular bulb. The body is placed in a lateral position, falling to the side of the craniotomy, and the arm contralateral to the operating side is placed out of the operating table and toward the floor and is padded with an axillary roll to avoid peripheral nerve damage. The knees and other pressure points are also padded to avoid damage to the peripheral nerves, and the legs are flexed to protect the femoral nerves. To avoid displacement of the patient's body during operating table movements, adhesive tape is attached to the operating table and then applied at the hip and shoulder. The position of the head is crucial, as the surgeon needs good exposure of the occipitocervical region for a good angle of view of the contents of the posterior fossa. A three-point head holder is placed so that the mastoid bone is at the highest point of the approach. The neck should be slightly flexed and the vertex angled down, up to 30 degrees, with the face rotated slightly ventrally. The head should not be flexed more than two to three fingers from the thyroid and should not be rotated more than 45 degrees to prevent impairment of venous drainage. The results of this positioning are the cerebellum falling away from the operating field and the contents of the lateral aspect of the FM and posterior fossa being placed right under the surgeon's view. Intraoperative monitoring is composed of somatosensory evoked potentials, auditory evoked responses, facial nerve monitoring, and monitoring of the X, XI, and XII cranial nerves, although their use is based on surgeon preference and acceptance.[4,5,7,10]

SKIN INCISION AND MUSCULAR DISSECTION

An inverted hockey stick–shaped incision is made, as it provides good exposure of the muscular layers, brings the surgeon closer to the surgical field, and requires lesser retraction of the soft tissues of the head and neck. A linear incision can also be used. The incision starts at the midline of the neck 5 cm below the inion and extends superiorly toward this reference. At the level of the inion, the incision is moved laterally right above the superior nuchal line and ends at the top level of the ear, about 2 to 3 cm medial to the pinna in the sagittal plane. From the last point, the incision extends down toward the mastoid and straight down over the posterior border of the sternocleidomastoid muscle. Knowledge of the muscular layers and of the neurovascular structures of the posterior neck is essential for the performance of the posterolateral approach and its variants. Dissection of each muscle is not recommended, as it creates extra dead space, increases the risk of infection, and causes muscle ischemia, which leads to wound dehiscence. We can summarize the muscular stage in three main steps: (1) elevation of the superficial muscles to expose the suboccipital triangle, (2) dissection of the suboccipital triangle to expose the VAs, and (3) transposition of the VAs if needed. At our institution, we avoid the use of cauterization to dissect the musculature, as it can damage the VAs with an abnormal loop out of the suboccipital triangle and disrupt the boundaries of the muscular layers, which damage the venous plexuses of the posterior neck, increasing bleeding and the risk of air embolism.

The skin flap is usually composed of the incised skin and galea, which are first elevated to expose the underlying pericranium. This structure, in addition to the superficial fascia of the neck, is elevated to expose the musculature of the posterior neck. The pericranium should be preserved to make a fascial graft for dural closure at the end of the operation. The first muscular layer that is exposed using this maneuver is composed by the sternocleidomastoid and trapezius muscles. They are incised near their insertion at the superior nuchal line and mastoid, leaving a cuff of tissue that is used later for closure of the incision. The underlying muscular layer (second or middle layer) is composed by the splenius capitis, longissimus capitis, and semispinalis capitis muscles. They are also incised and reflected as a single layer to expose the third layer, which forms the suboccipital triangle. The triangle is formed medially by the rectus capitis posterior major muscle, inferiorly by the inferior oblique muscle, and superolaterally by the superior oblique muscle; the VAs and its venous plexus are located in its center. Anatomic knowledge of the suboccipital triangle muscles and their insertions is essential to provide the best and safest exposure of the VAs. The rectus capitis major muscle inserts onto the inferior nuchal line and the spinous process of C2 and should be detached from the inferior nuchal line and reflected posteriorly. The inferior oblique muscle inserts onto the transverse process of C1 and onto the spinous process of C2 and the superior oblique muscle inserts at the inferior nuchal line and onto the transverse process of C1. Both muscles should be detached from the transverse process of C1 and reflected posteriorly. This maneuver exposes the C1 lamina, the VAs, the VAs venous plexus, and the C1 root.[13]

Knowledge of the muscular layers of the posterior neck is useful to prevent bleeding from the vascular structures of this region. Each muscular layer covers a vascular layer composed by a venous plexus and muscular arterial branches. Arterial blood supply for the muscles is provided by the occipital artery and by the muscular branches of the VAs. As the muscular branches of the VAs pass through the suboccipital triangle to reach the muscles, this is a crucial point for homeostasis. The main source of bleeding and air embolism in this region is the venous network. The venous system of the posterior neck is divided into two connected plexuses: (1) the suboccipital venous plexus and (2) the plexus around the VAs. The suboccipital venous plexus is superficial and is located in a space formed by the splenius capitis muscle superiorly and the longissimus capitis semispinalis capitis muscles inferiorly. The suboccipital plexus reaches the suboccipital triangle via the muscular cleft between the latter muscles and drains it into the plexus, thus surrounding the VAs through the anterior vertebral vein.[14] Using the scalpel blade to cut through the muscles allows easier identification of these vascular layers and enables coagulation before bleeding and air embolism to occur.

EXPOSURE OF THE EXTRADURAL VAs

The VAs is divided into four segments. V1 is the segment that runs from the origin of the artery at the subclavian artery and ends at the vertebral foramen of C6. V2 runs within the vertebral foramina from C6 through C1. V3, which is the horizontal segment of the vessel, begins at the transverse foramen of the atlas, runs through a groove on the upper surface of the posterior arch of the atlas, and ends by piercing the dura of the posterior fossa, medial and to the right of the OC. V4 is the intradural segment of the VAs and joins the opposite side vessel to form the basilar artery[13] (Fig. 43-1).

Exposure and transposition of the VAs is not needed in the basic far lateral approach, in which drilling of the OC is not required.[15,16] To transpose the vessel in the other variations of the far lateral approach, dissection and manipulation of the venous plexus around the VAs, which is sometimes referred to as the suboccipital cavernous sinus, is needed. The suboccipital cavernous plexus is connected to the suboccipital plexus through the suboccipital triangle and via the anterior vertebral vein.[4] It is also connected to the internal vertebral venous plexus, posterior and anterior condylar veins, and occipital marginal sinus. To avoid intense bleeding from the plexuses, subperiosteal detachment of the VAs from its groove in C1 is recommended. To transpose the VAs, unroofing of the C1 transverse process is also mandatory. After detachment of the VAs and plexus, laminectomy of the C1 arch as laterally as possible can be performed to expose the OC for drilling.[1,2,4,5,10]

The V3 segment of the VAs has some branches that need to be coagulated during the approach. The first and largest is the anterior VAs, which passes through the suboccipital triangle to reach the muscles of the posterior neck. The posterior meningeal artery is another branch that can be coagulated. Care should be taken not to coagulate a posteroinferior cerebellar artery (PICA) or a posterior spinal artery that arises extradurally from the V3.

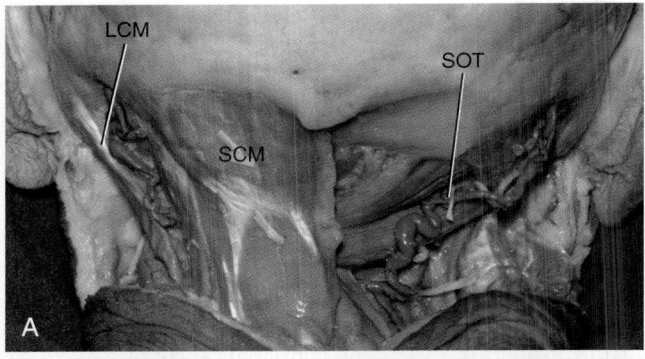

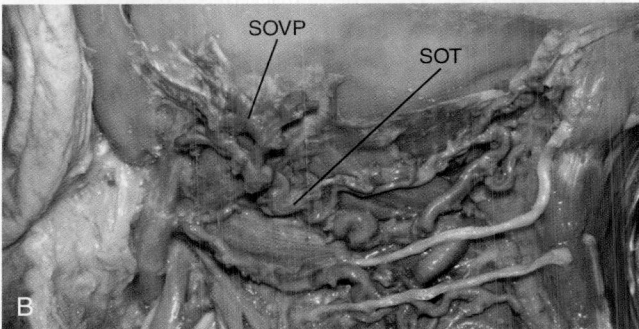

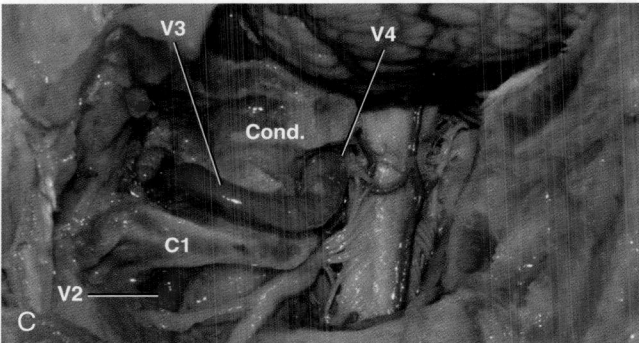

FIGURE 43-1 A, Muscular layers of the posterior neck dissected in a cadaver specimen. B, Venous plexus of the posterior neck. C, Segments of the VAs and their relation to the OC and the arch of C1. LCM, longissimus capitis muscle; SCM, semispinalis capitis muscle; SOVT, suboccipital venous plexus; SOT, suboccipital triangle; Cond., occipital condyle.

Osseous Stage: Suboccipital Craniectomy and Hemilaminectomy

The target points of the osseous stage of the approach are (1) exposure of the borders of the sigmoid and transverse sinuses, (2) resection of the ipsilateral margin of the FM, (3) resection of the squama of the occipital bone to the midline, and (4) resection of the ipsilateral border of the posterior arch of C1. If additional lateral space is needed, the OC can be removed in a subsequent step.

The landmarks for orientation of the craniotomy are (1) the asterion, (2) the midline, (3) the posterior border of the mastoid, (4) the inion, and (5) the superior nuchal line. The asterion is closely related to the lateral portion of the sulcus of the transverse sinus, especially with its inferior margin. To expose the lateral angle of the junction between the transverse and the sigmoid sinuses, a bur hole is placed immediately posterior and inferior to the asterion. This retrosigmoid point is the keyhole to the lateral suboccipital

approach and exposes the posterolateral border of the cerebellar hemisphere.[17] The inferior margin of the transverse sinus is located over a 50-mm line beginning at the inion and running across the superior nuchal line. This is the upper limit of the lateral suboccipital approach.

A high-speed drill is used to thin the squama of the occipital bone, and rongeurs are used to perform an occipital craniectomy. Another option is to perform a craniotomy of the posterior fossa. The mastoid air cells are the lateral limit of the suboccipital approach and are drilled until the borders of the sigmoid sinus and jugular bulb are exposed. The ipsilateral border of the FM is removed, and the occipital bone is removed to the point where it joins the OC.

To improve the inferior dural exposure, a hemilaminectomy of C1 is performed after detachment of the VAs and its plexus from its groove in C1. If additional exposure is needed, the C2 and C3 laminas can be removed.

Small tumors without rostral extension require small craniectomy; however, craniotomy is preferred for tumors with rostral extension, as replacing the bone protects the dura and limits the postoperative occipital pain.

Condylar Stage

The OC, which is an oval-shaped osseous structure located at the base of the occipital bone, articulates the skull in relation to the cervical spine. The anterior portion of the condyle is directed anteriorly and medially toward the basion. The posterior portion ends at the level of the middle portion of the FM and blocks the angle of view to an anterior portion of the FM and of the craniovertebral junction. The resection of the posterior aspect of the condyle increases the angle of exposure, reduces brain stem retraction, and increases the working area of the posterior fossa.[4-8,10,18,19] The presence of small anterior tumors, an elongated FM, a short distance between the foramen and the brain stem, and relatively large OCs represent the ideal conditions for resection of the condyle.[20]

A high-speed drill is used to remove the posterior portion of the condyle after displacement of the VAs to avoid injury of the vessel. The amount of condyle that can be safely removed is controversial; however, biomechanical studies showed that the removal of more than 50% of the condyle leads to considerable hypermobility of the craniocervical junction, in which case fusion is indicated.[5,21] The removal of the cortical bone (which forms the external capsule of the condyle) exposes cancellous bone (which forms the core of the condyle). Drilling of this bone exposes the lateral aspect of the intracranial portion of the hypoglossal canal; this landmark is approximately at the limit of the posterior third of the condyle. Another maneuver that can be used to achieve a better view of the anterior portion of the clivus is the removal of the JT, a bony prominence situated above the hypoglossal canal, in cranial and medial extensions of the tumor.[8,11]

Many variants of the far lateral approach have been proposed, according to the amount of bony resection at the condylar region.[4,5,10,18] The basic far lateral approach comprises the steps described earlier, without condylar drilling. An occipitoatlantal transarticular transcondilar approach is performed after the condyle and the C1 superior articular facet are removed. The occipital–transcondylar approach exposes the clivus and the lower medulla and is performed after drilling the atlanto-occipital joint, condyle, and lower border of the hypoglossal canal. A supracondylar variant increases the exposure of the lateral aspect of the clivus and is directed above the condyle. During the transtubercular approach, the JT above the hypoglossal canal is removed to expose the area in front of the lower cranial nerves. The paracondylar approach is achieved via drilling of the area lateral to the condyle to resect lesions of the jugular process and of the posterior aspect of the mastoid.[5,11,13]

INTRADURAL EXPOSURE

The dura is opened parallel to the sigmoid sinus, crossing the circular sinus at the FM. Extreme care must be taken when opening the circular sinus, as the large venous plexus renders homeostasis more difficult and the risk of embolism increases.

All procedures performed after opening of the dura are carried out under the microscope. The arachnoid is opened and kept in place to facilitate the dissection or identification of the following neurovascular structures: the VAs and PICA (identification and dissection), the anterior spinal artery, and the cranial nerves (spinal division of the XI, IX, X, and XII cranial nerves, as well as identification and dissection, if possible, although sometimes the lower cranial nerves and the VAs are encased by the tumor). In general, tumors that encase the VAs can be removed via an arachnoid plane. In tumors located below the VAs, the lower cranial nerves may be identified in the superior part of the tumor. In contrast, the position of these nerves cannot be anticipated in tumors with superior extension.

The tumor is approached first via the side of the main vasculature at the dural attachment. The tumor is devascularized and removed piecemeal using an ultrasonic aspirator, with protection of the neurovascular structures involved. The bone and the dura involved by the meningioma attachment are also removed, if possible, to avoid recurrence. A meticulous homeostasis is performed, and the dura is closed in a watertight manner with the aid of patches from the pericranium or of dural substitutes. The mastoid bone, if open, is filled with bone wax, pieces of muscle, and fibrin glue. To avoid dead space, the posterior part of the aponeurotic-muscle flap is made and is sutured onto the dura.

Immediate Postoperative Measures

The lower cranial nerves are often encapsulated by the tumors, and surgical manipulations may lead to permanent or transitory deficits, such as swallowing and airway protection. Patients must remain intubated after surgery, and removal of the tube is performed only after functional studies of the larynge and pharynge are completed. Tracheostomy is indicated in cases that exhibit several lower cranial nerve deficits.

Instability can occur in cases with bone tumors that require extensive bone removal; in these instances, functional studies should be performed as soon as possible.

Illustrative Cases

PATIENT 1

A 63-year-old woman presented with chronic upper neck pain, headaches, and neck stiffness. She also complained of weakness of the limbs. Thorough neurologic examination revealed hypotrophy of the tongue, tetra-hyperreflexia, bilateral paresis of the trapezium, hypophonia, and left-palate deviation during phonation. MRI revealed the presence of a right anterolateral extramedullary tumor of the FM, with superior extension toward the jugular foramen and along the right hypoglossal canal, and development on both sides of the VAs. The tumor was hypointense on T1-weighted MRI and hyperintense on fluid-attenuated inversion recovery and T2-weighted MRI, with homogenous enhancement after the infusion of gadolinium. CT angiography was performed to obtain relevant information on the VAs and the sigmoid sinus. CT with bone windows was also performed to assess the shape of the FM. Stereotactic image guidance was used. The surgical procedures were planned using an imaging database that included stereotactic CT and MRI scans (Fig. 43-2).

The tumor was resected using a far lateral suboccipital approach. The patient was placed in the three quarter–prone position, with the head fixed with a three-pin head holder (Fig. 43-3). Excessive superior shoulder traction was avoided. The head of the patient was tilted slightly downward to open the space between the mastoid and the neck. The incision ran laterally in an inverted hockey stick–shaped fashion, from the right mastoid process to the occipital protuberance, and then curved medially to the spinous process of C4. After exposure of the VAs (V2 to V3), a right far lateral suboccipital craniectomy was performed that included the rim of the FM. The JT was drilled because of the upward extension of the tumor. A right C1 hemilaminectomy without condyle resection was tailored. The dura was opened in a linear shape over the cerebellum, after identification of the VAs entry point. The next step consisted of draining the CSF by opening the cisterna magna. The procedure led to the spontaneous sinking of the cerebellum, which rendered significant retraction unnecessary. The dentate ligament was sectioned before the initiation of tumor removal and widening of the surgical corridor. A small portion of the V4 was identified before tumor involvement, and the dissection was performed by following the artery inside the tumor along an arachnoid plane. Microsurgical resection of a firm, consistent, and hypervascularized lesion with dural attachment was performed. The bulk of the tumor was removed using microscissors, cupped forceps, and an ultrasonic aspirator and was continued piecemeal. The tumor matrix was then coagulated, the basal dura was partially resected, and Simpson grade II resection was achieved. The only nerve that was identified initially was the spinal portion of cranial nerve XI and the posterior rootlets of the first cervical nerve. All of them were preserved. The other nerves and the VAs branches were identified during tumor removal. Control MRI and CT scan showed complete resection of the tumor (Figs. 43-4 and 43-5). After surgery, in the immediate postoperative period, videolaryngoscopy showed that paresis of the lower cranial nerves worsened, providing evidence that a tracheostomy and gastrostomy were needed. The patient's symptoms resolved, with the exception of some mild facial paresis and transient right brachial paresis (brachial plexus neuropraxis). Histopathologic analysis revealed the presence of a transitional meningioma.

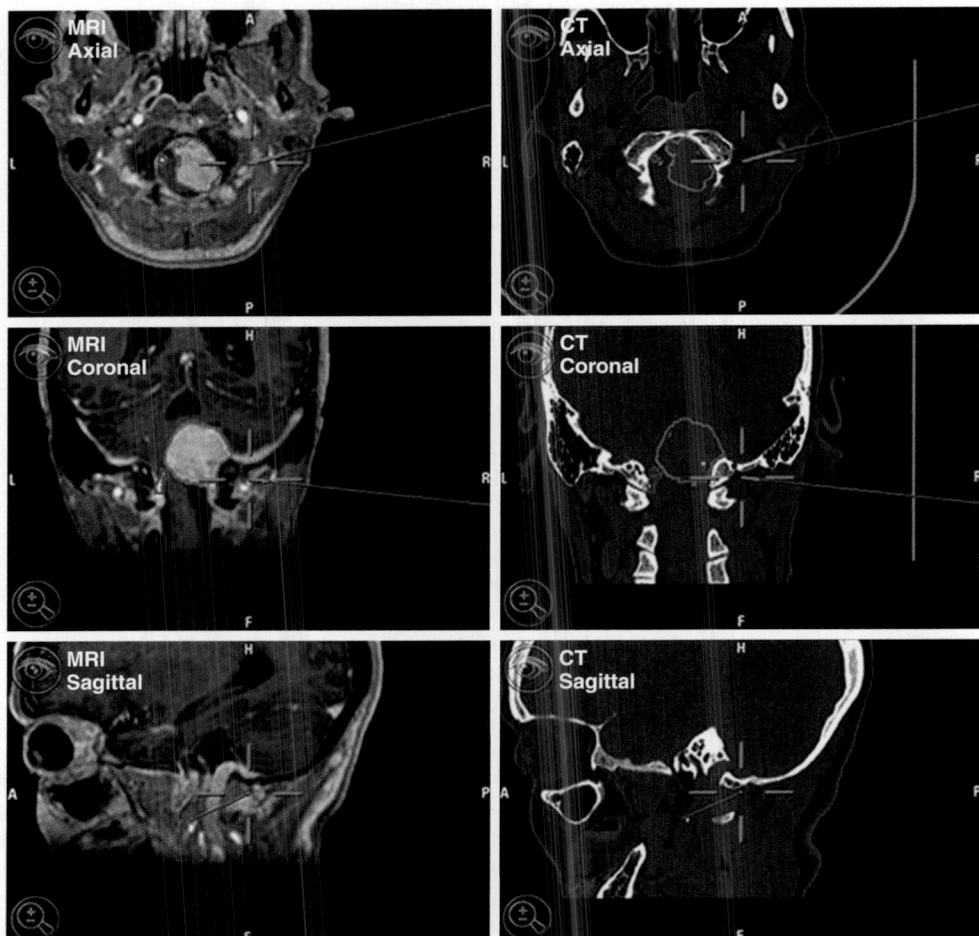

FIGURE 43-2 Image-guided tumor resection. Three-dimensional reconstructions were obtained by CT and MRI through automated segmentation processes. During surgery, the neuronavigation displays the position of the VAs (red dots) and the location of the tumor in relation to the OC (green circle).

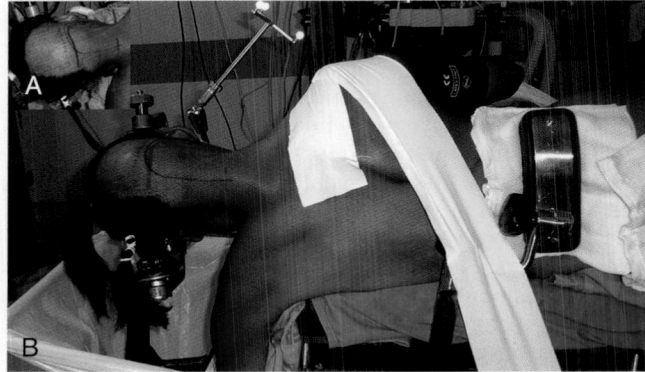

FIGURE 43-3 Patient in a lateral position, with the lesion side facing up, head on a three-point head holder, and a cushion placed below the dependent axilla. A, Green line, inverted J-shaped incision; red line, transversal, and sigmoid sinus outlined previously and guided by neuronavigation.

PATIENT 2

A 44-year-old male patient was admitted for the first time in 2003. At that time, he complained of progressive weakness of the legs and arms (mainly of the left arm) for a few months prior to admission. At neurologic examination, he exhibited mild tetraparesis and hyperreflexia. Imaging demonstrated the presence of a vast lesion based on the anterolateral portion of the FM, which was suggestive of a meningioma that compressed the medulla. He was operated on in 2003 via a suboccipital extreme lateral approach and the lesion was partially removed. The surgery was stopped when the resection caused transitory cardiac arrhythmia.

The patient was supposed to undergo follow-up; however, he did not comply in full, as he was afraid of a second surgery, which was recommended and necessary. Five years later, the patient returned because his symptoms had worsened. He was tetraparetic, in a wheelchair, and unable to stand up. In addition, he had dysphonia, dysphagia, and nocturnal apnea, with paralysis of the IX, X, XI, and XII cranial nerves, suggesting the presence of pyramidal-tract deficits and brain stem compression. Imaging revealed that the lesion had grown considerably and had infiltrated the medulla, engulfing the VAs. At that time, he finally accepted the second operation, as he had no other options. We started by performing a traqueostomy, as a fibroendoscopy examination showed that he had pulmonary microaspiration. He was reoperated on with complete monitorization of the affected neurologic functions and by using the same approach; however, we extended the surgery laterally and extradurally, as the tumor infiltrated the extradural portion of the VAs. The tumor was radically removed after we found an irregular and incomplete plane between the tumor and the brain stem. The postoperative period was uneventful. He recovered partially from his

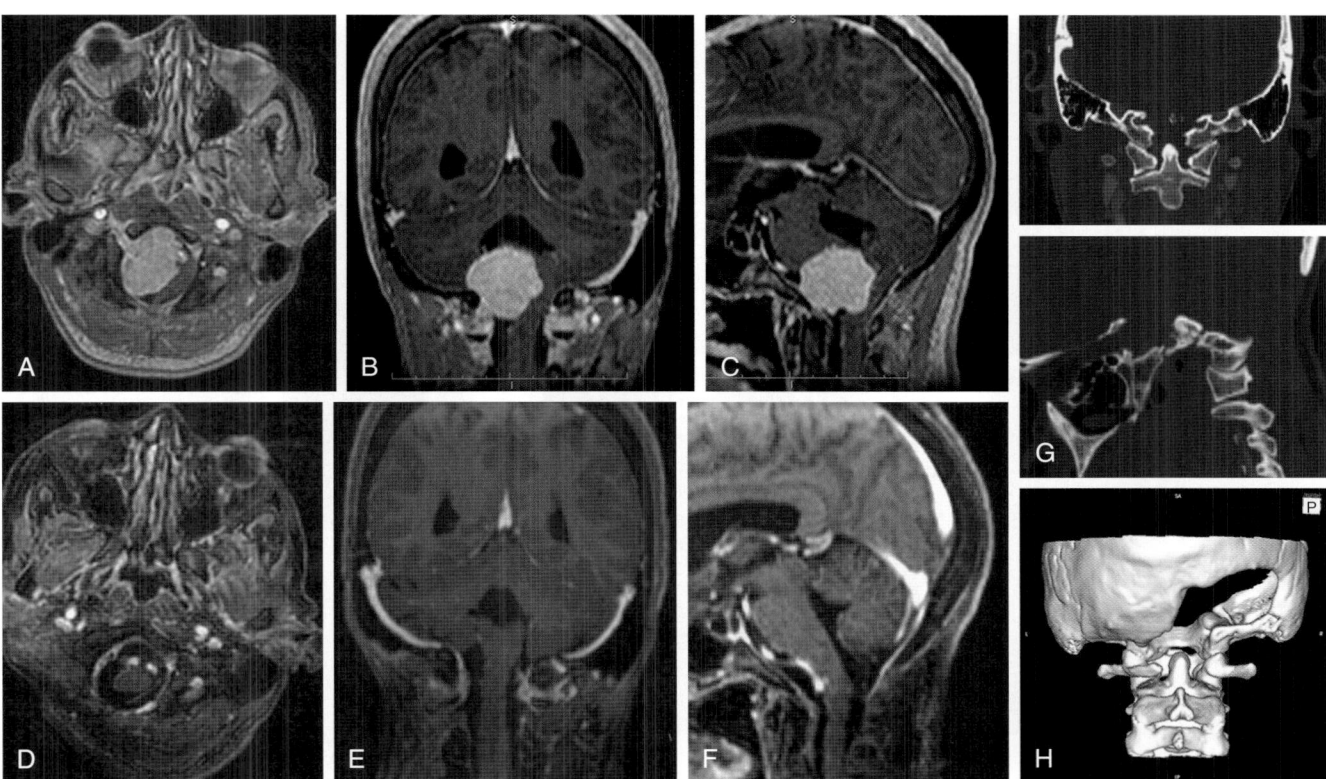

FIGURE 43-4 A, B, and C, Preoperative contrast-enhanced T1-weighted MRI showed the presence of a hyperintense lesion located at the antero-lateral surface of the FM and that compressed the brain stem. D, E, and F, Postoperative contrast-enhanced T1-weighted MRI confirmed the gross total resection of the tumor. G, Coronal and sagittal CT showing complete preservation of the OC. H, Three-dimensional CT reconstruction showing the suboccipital approach.

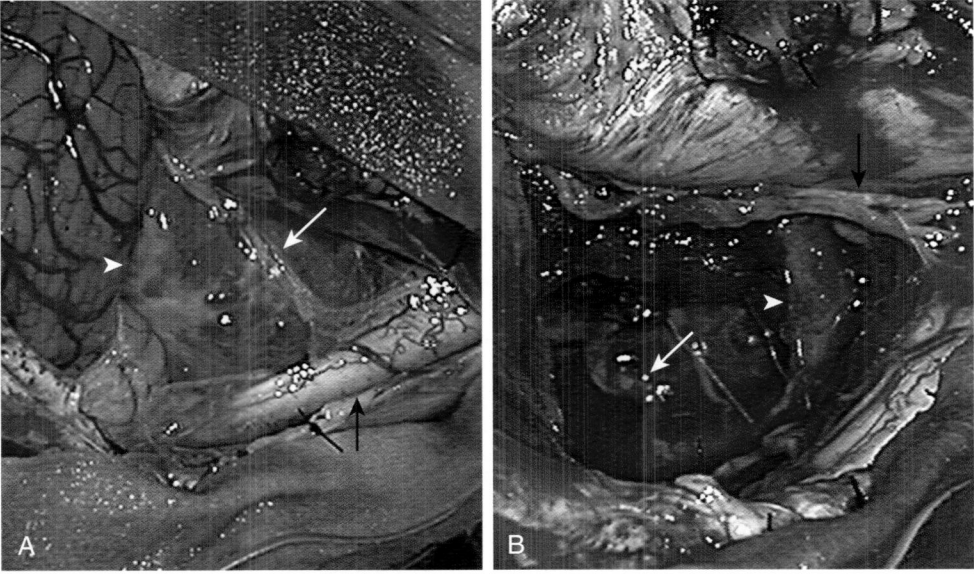

FIGURE 43-5 A, Intraoperative view before tumor excision: tumor (white arrowhead), cranial nerve XI out-stretched by the lesion (white arrow), and brain stem (black arrow). B, Intra-operative view after tumor excision: VAs (white arrowhead), cranial nerve XI after decompression (white arrow), and cranial nerve XII (black arrow).

deficits, and at the last follow-up, he was able to stand up and walk, with the only remaining symptom being cranial nerve XII paresis (Fig. 43-6).

PATIENT 3

A 13-year-old girl presented with difficulty in swallowing and a severe occipital headache that was aggravated by physical activity. The symptoms started 15 months before

examination. Neurologic examination was normal. MRI showed the presence of a widespread retropharyngeal tumor. The tumor involved both carotid arteries, displaced both VAs, and extended caudally to C3. The tumor seemed to replace the OCs bilaterally, as well as the arch of C1 and the inferior border of the clivus, from whence it invaded the subarachnoid space posterolaterally and ventrolaterally. CT showed intense bone involvement.

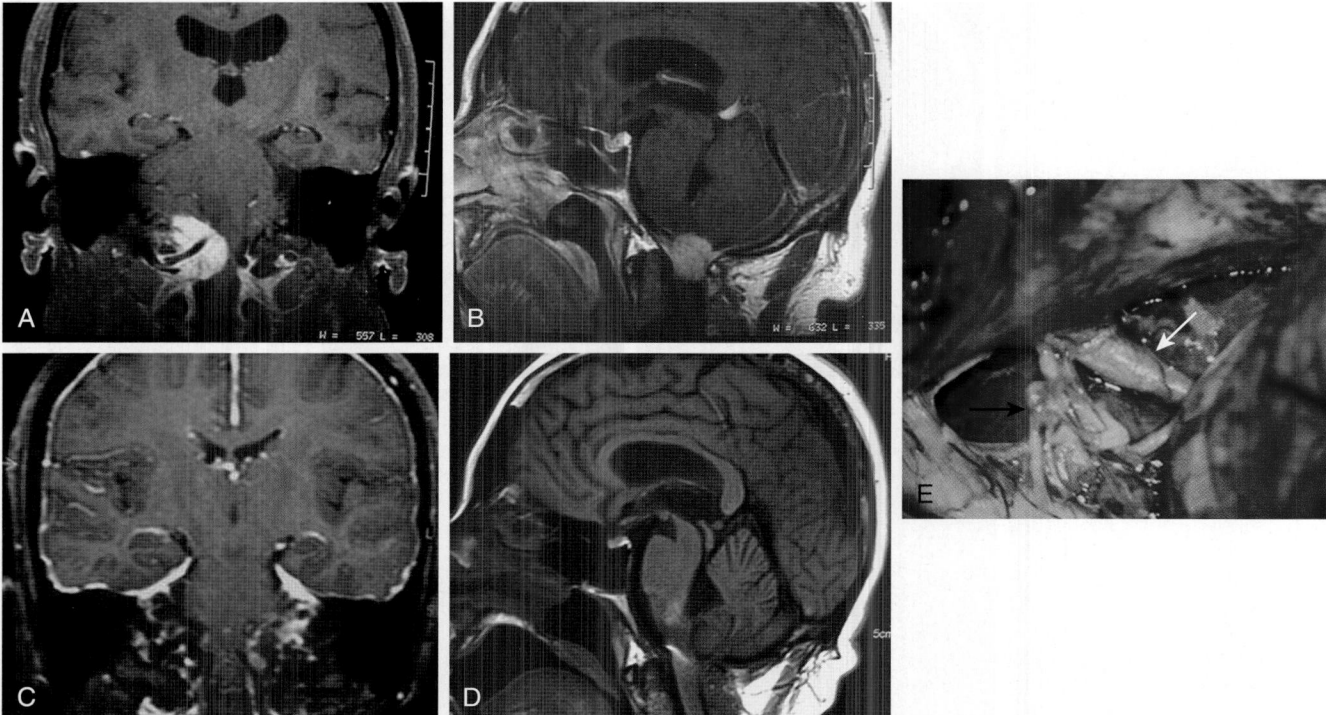

FIGURE 43-6 A, B, Preoperative T1-weighted MRI shows a hyperintense lesion located at lateral wall of the FM compressing the brain stem. C, Postoperative coronal postcontrast T1-weighted MRI demonstrates complete resection of the lesion. D, Postoperative sagittal T1-weighted MRI reveals complete resection of the lesion. E, Intraoperative view before tumor excision: white arrow, VAs; black arrow, lower cranial nerves.

Because the symptoms were the result of the retropharyngeal location of the tumor, we thought that midline anterior and posterolateral exposure was required. First, we felt that the midline anterior approach would be the best for the removal of the anterior mass. Thus, an extended transoral–transpalatopharyngeal approach was performed. After retraction of the pharyngeal mucosa and of the longus colli and longus capitis muscles, a gelatinous yellow mass was found that did not have a capsule. The tumor, which was suckable and firm, was removed piecemeal using a drill and an ultrasonic aspirator under microscopic view. The anterior arch of the atlas was resected, as were the inferior border of the clivus, which is limited bilaterally by the JT and the lateral mass of C1 and C2. The midline dura was infiltrated. Careful closure was performed, during which the longus colli and the longus capitis muscles were covered with the pharyngeal mucosa. The palatal layers were closed, and a nasogastric feeding tube was placed under direct vision. A postoperative MRI scan showed a decompression of the retropharyngeal mass; however, marked ventral and posterolateral compression of the cervicomedullary junction remained.

The second stage of the tumor resection was performed using the far lateral approach. A midline incision was performed because the tumor invaded the spinal canal bilaterally. Gross tumor resection was achieved that included part of the OC (on the right side) and the JT, with bilateral transposition of the VAs. The tumor that invaded the subarachnoid space was removed after careful dissection from the lower cranial nerves. A dorsal occipitocervical fusion was performed that spanned C1 and C2 and reached the fusion at the C3 or C4 level. Postoperatively, the patient exhibited

swallowing deterioration; thus, gastrostomy and traqueostomy were performed. The traqueostomy was discontinued after the end of the third week after surgery, and the gastrostomy was discontinued after 3 months. Histopathologic examination revealed the presence of a chordoma. Postoperative MRI showed the presence of a residual mass, without compression (Fig. 43-7). The patient was able to return to her normal life and underwent MRI-based follow-up periodically.

Results

Our group of authors treated 22 patients with FM tumors. The mean age of the 14 women and eight men was 57.3 years. There were 12 meningiomas, all of them located intradurally and 10 arising from the anterior or anterolateral rim. One tumor was located in the posterior midline, and another had a posterolateral origin. One hypoglossal schwannoma had intradural and extradural components, and a C1 neurofibroma completed the intradural tumors in this series. Chordomas were the most common type of extradural tumors. The most common symptom was suboccipital neck pain and/or headache. Other symptoms included motor weakness, gait imbalance, myelopathy, and numbness. Table 43-1 lists the types of tumors, and Table 43-2 shows the clinical presentations of the patients in our cohort.

The posterior midline approach was performed in 2 patients with posterior and posterolateral meningioma, respectively. The far lateral approach was used in the other 10 patients. The rostrocaudal extension tailored the size of the craniotomy. For tumors with upward extension or located above the intracranial VAs, a combined retrosigmoid approach was performed in four cases and a petrosal

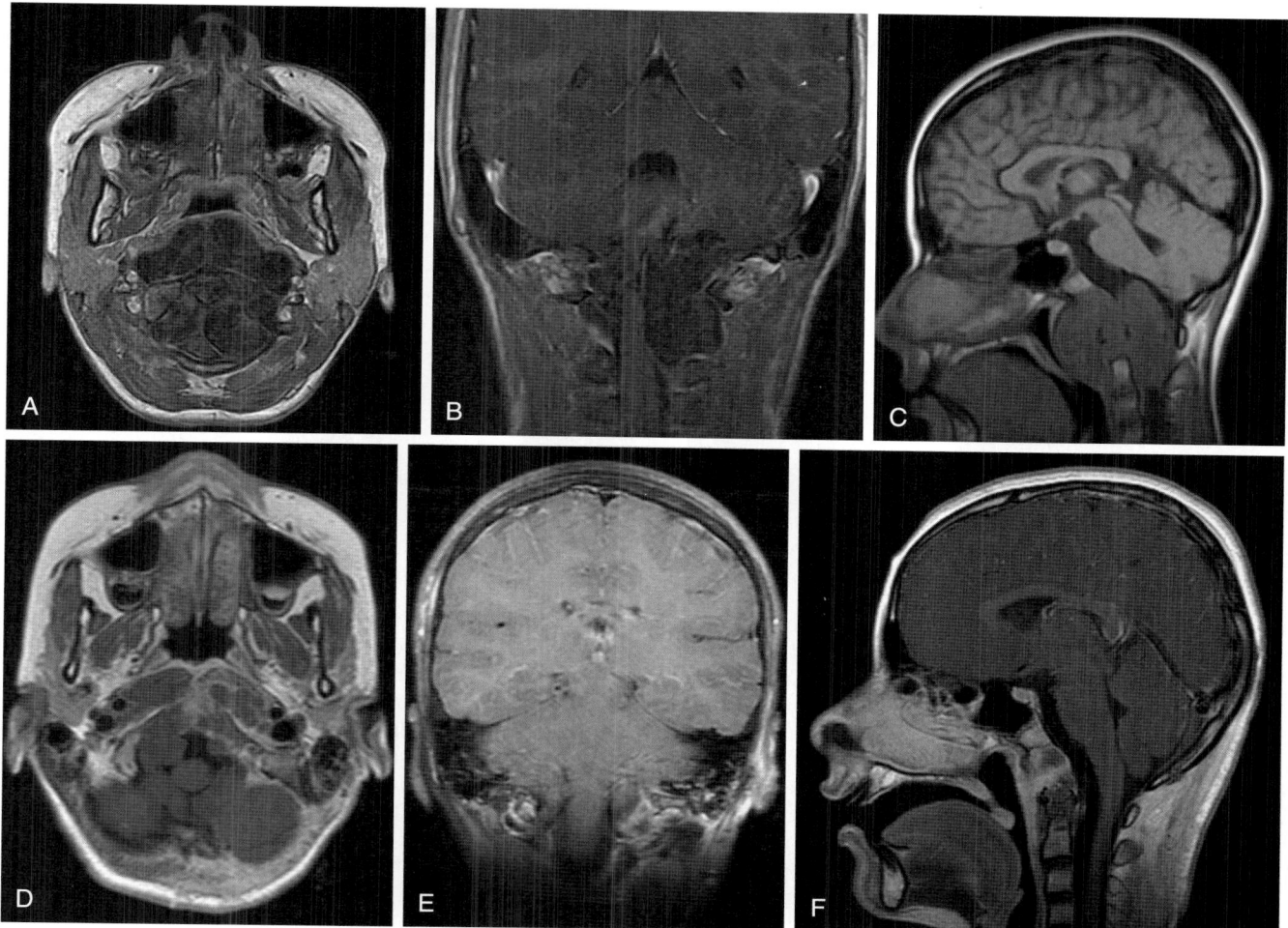

FIGURE 43-7 MRI of a patient with a large chordoma involving the clivus superiorly and extending to the level of C2 inferiorly. The tumor was partially removed via two steps: an extended transoral–transpalatopharyngeal approach and a far lateral transcondylar approach. Preoperative (A) sagittal, (B) coronal, and (C) axial and postoperative (D) sagittal, (E) coronal, and (F) axial T1-weighted MRI with gadolinium.

Table 43-1	Distribution of Pathology
Tumor Type	**Patients**
Meningioma	12
Schwannoma	1
Neurofibroma	1
Chordoma	5
Glomus tumor	1
Chondrosarcoma	1
Metastatic kidney carcinoma	1
Total patients	22

Table 43-2	Clinical Presentation of Patients with FM Tumors
Signs and Symptoms	**Cases by Presented Symptom (Confirmed after Examination)**
Suboccipital neck pain	12
Headache	8
Motor weakness	9 (5)
Gait imbalance and myelopathy	5 (2)
Numbness	5 (6)
Cranial nerves	
Swallowing difficulty	7 (5)
Tongue atrophy	3 (2)
Speech problems	3 (2)
Diplopia	1 (2)
Hearing deficit	1 (2)
Hand deficit	1 (1)
Vomiting	1 (1)

approach was used in three cases, all of which had predominantly extradural tumors. An extended transoral–transpalatopharyngeal approach was used in two patients, both with chordomas. These patients required additional petrosal and far lateral transcondylar access. Drilling of the JT was performed in four cases that had FM meningiomas with cephalad extension. Partial resection of the lateral mass of C1 was performed in one patient with a C1 neurofibroma. The OC was partially resected in three patients with meningioma and in one patient with hypoglossal schwannoma (Table 43-3).

For intradural tumors, the VAs was mobilized in five cases, although it was encased or displaced in all cases. This maneuver was performed at the dural entry of the artery at the FM. For extradural tumors, the VAs was encased in four patients with chordomas, and it was

Table 43-3 Patients with Intradural Tumors

Patient No.	Tumor Type/Pathology	MRI Feature	Condyle/JT Drilling	VAs Mobilization	Tumor Resection Grade (Simpson)
1	M/meningothelial	A	Yes/yes	FM	II
2	M/meningothelial	AL	No/yes	No	I
3	M/fibroblastic	AL	No/no	No	I
4	M/psammomatous	PL	No/no	C1	I
5	M/meningothelial	A	Yes/no	C3	III
6	M/psammomatous	AL	No/yes	No	I
7	M/meningothelial	AL	No/no	No	II
8	M/fibroblastic	P	No/no	No	I
9	M/meningothelial	AL	Yes/yes	FM	I
10	M/meningothelial	AL	Yes/no	C3	I
11	M/fibroblastic	PL	No/no	No	III
12	M/psammomatous	AL	No/no	No	I
13	Neurofibroma	PL	No/no	C3	Total
14	Hypoglossal schwannoma	AL	Yes/no	V3	Total

A, anterior; AL, anterolateral; M, meningioma; P, posterior; PL, posterolateral.

displaced in another four patients. In extradural tumors, the VAs was mobilized in all cases, either for dissection or for improved exposure. In these cases, the VAs was transposed at the C1 transverse foramen and mobilized medially. There were no injuries in the VAs, neither in extradural nor in intradural tumor cases.

Seven patients with extradural tumors had some degree of condylar resection. The resection of the condyle performed in these patients was done because of the invasive nature of the tumors and/or direct involvement by the tumors in five patients with a chordoma. A complete condylar resection was performed in one patient with metastatic kidney carcinoma. One chordoma patient underwent a partial condylar resection because of extensive bone invasion; the purpose of the surgery was decompression. In the case of a glomus tumor, the lesion was approached more anteriorly and required partial condylectomy and resection of the JT.

Occipitocervical fusion was performed in four chordoma patients and in one patient with metastatic kidney carcinoma who had complete resection of the condyle. These surgeries were performed after the removal of their tumors using an elective fusion procedure.

The grade of tumor resection for intradural tumors was based on Simpson's classification.[21] For nonmeningiomas, the degree of resection was divided into three categories: (1) total resection, in which the entire tumor was removed; (2) subtotal resection, in which a small fragment of the tumor remained on vital structures, such as the VAs, cranial nerves, or the brain stem; (3) partial resection, in which the bulk of the tumor remained.[5]

For meningiomas, radical excision (Simpson grades I and II) was achieved in 10 cases (83.3%). In most cases, the dura insertion was coagulated or removed. Two patients had Simpson grade III resection. The incomplete resection performed in one patient was attributable to a firm adhesion of the lower cranial nerves to the VAs and poor dissection planes; in another patient, intentional decompression was planed because of the clinical condition. Other patients underwent two surgeries (see the illustrative case of patient 2). The patient

with hypoglossal schwannoma had a total resection, and the patient with a dumbbell-shaped neurofibroma of C1 had total tumor removal via a transfacetal approach (Fig. 43-8).

Total resection was achieved in two cases of chordoma tumors; the remaining three patients had a partial removal because of the extensive nature of the tumor, which occupied multiple compartments, invaded the jugular foramen and the cavernous sinus, and encased the carotid arteries. The patient with chondrosarcoma also had partial tumor removal because of the firm adherence to the lower cranial nerves (Table 43-4).

There was no surgical mortality in this series. The patient with metastatic kidney carcinoma died because of multiple metastases. The second death was a chordoma patient who was in poor condition and in whom tumor removal was intentionally partial.

A postoperative CSF leak occurred in four patients and required surgical repair in one case. A new deficit of the accessory nerve was observed in one patient, and a deficit of the hypoglossal nerve occurred in another individual who underwent partial recovery. Dysphagia developed in four patients; however, their recovery was complete. Transient hoarseness occurred in two patients, and abducens nerve palsy occurred in two subjects (one of whom developed a permanent deficit). Three patients required postoperative traqueostomy, and two underwent gastrostomy. After 6 months, these problems were resolved completely. Periodical clinical examination and MRI scans were performed for all patients. The mean Karnofsky performance scale score improved in 13 cases (63.6%), was kept stable in 8 cases (36.3%), and worsened in 1 case.

Comments

Surgical treatment is the best approach to treat tumors of the FM, especially meningiomas, schwannomas, neurofibromas, and chordomas. Most lesions can be removed using posterior approaches; however, when the tumors are located anteriorly or anterolaterally, resection using traditional approaches becomes more difficult. Some authors

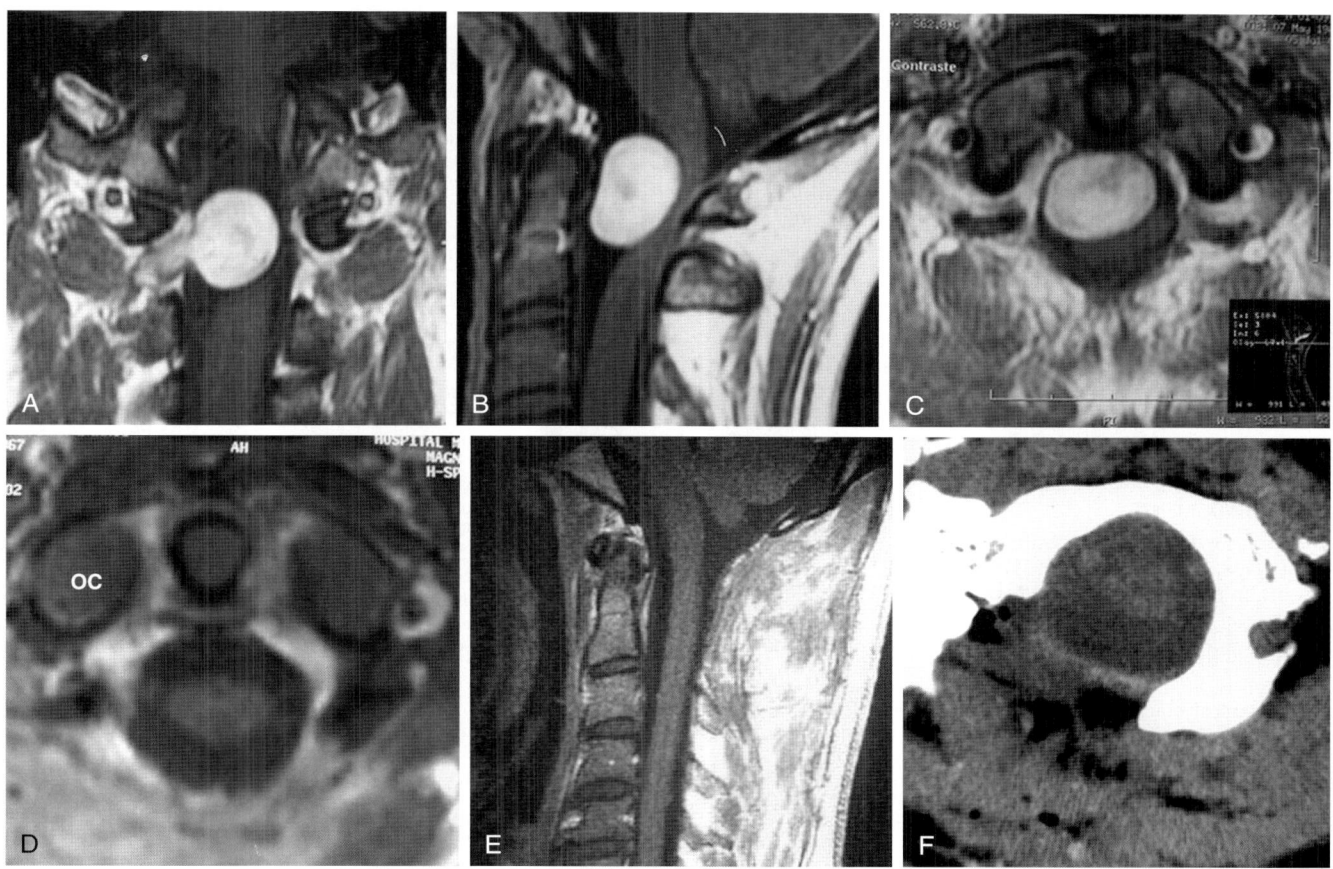

FIGURE 43-8 Preoperative coronal (A), sagittal (B), and axial (C) T1-weighted MRI shows a right C1 neurofibroma. D, In postoperative axial T1-weighted MRI, the OC was left intact. E, Postoperative sagittal T1-weighted MRI after total resection. F, Postoperative CT scan at the level of the OC.

Table 43-4 Degree of Resection in Patients with Nonmeningioma Tumors

Tumor Type	RESECTION CATEGORY			Total Patients
	Total	Subtotal	Partial	
Chordoma	2	2	1	5
Schwannoma	1			1
Neurofibroma	1			1
Glomus tumor		1		1
Chondrosarcoma		1		1
Metastatic kidney carcinoma		1		1
Total patients	4	5	1	10

used posterior approaches to reach posterolateral and anterolateral tumors located at the FM,[22,23] as large tumors provide a working space that is sufficient for resection of the tumor. However, there is not enough space to control the VAs between C2 and C3 and to reach essential anterior midline and small tumors.

Intradural extramedullary tumors, which are located anterolaterally or ventrally and are mostly meningiomas, generally tend to extend cranially and caudally. For this reason, and to obtain sufficient exposure of the cervicomedullary junction, tumor interface, rostrocaudal extension, and attachment at the dura, as well as to achieve dissection of the lower cranial nerves and control of the VAs and their branches, approaches that are more lateral are required. Among them, the far lateral approach and its variants, such as the transcondylar, transtubercle, and transfacetal methods, met the criteria. Resection or drilling of the condyle posterior to and below the hypoglossal canal provides an enhanced view of the target area. The extreme lateral transcondylar approach, which implies drilling the condyle, was used by some neurosurgeons.[4-6,8,9,24] This procedure is not required for most intracranial tumors because there is risk of vertebral artery injury.[16]

Transposition of the VAs is another controversial point. Injury of this vessel or transposition of atherosclerotic VAs may result in permanent or transient neurologic deficit.[16] For intradural tumors in patients with a normal VAs, the artery can be mobilized at the dural entry but not transposed posteromedially, because this implies drilling the condyle and unroofing the transverse foramen of C1. For patients with extradural tumors, resection of the condyle is not as controversial; in such patients, drilling the bone is part of the surgical treatment.[5,10]

Incomplete resection is a challenge for neurosurgeons. The size and the rostral extension from the tumor to the midline of the clivus are factors that influence morbidity.[24] Remnants of tumors with strong adherence to the brain stem or to the VAs and their branches should not be resected. We prefer to follow the patient periodically instead of sending the patient to radiation therapy because of the risk of complications and because a second procedure would be more difficult.[5,16,25]

Nowadays, the entire circumference of the FM can be accessed. Anterior extradural lesions located on the midline can be exposed and removed from transoral approaches combined with mandibular splitting and maxillotomy.

The far lateral approach with or without condylar resection has the advantage of being combinable with the petrosal, retrosigmoid, and infratemporal approaches. It also allows the removal of most of tumors, either intradural or extradural lesions.

ACKNOWLEDGMENTS

We acknowledge the contribution of Mariangela Barbi Gonçalves, MD, and Cristian Ferrareze, MD (Rio de Janeiro, Brazil), in the preparation and completion of this chapter.

KEY REFERENCES

Bassiouni H, Ntoukas V, Asgari S, et al. Foramen magnum meningiomas: clinical outcome after microsurgical resection via a posterolateral suboccipital retrocondylar approach. *Neurosurgery.* 2006;59: 1177-1187.

Boulton MR, Cusimano M. Foramen magnum meningiomas: concepts, classifications, and nuances. *Neurosurg Focus.* 2003;14(6):10.

Bruneau M, George B. Foramen magnum meningiomas: detailed surgical approaches and technical aspects at Lariboisiére Hospital and review of the literature. *Neurosurg Rev.* 2008;31:19-33.

George B. Foramen magnum tumors. In: Shmidek HH, Roberts DW, eds. *Schmidek and Sweet. Operative Neurosurgical Techniques: Indications, Methods, and Results.* 5th ed. Philadelphia: WB Saunders; 2005.

Gupta SK, Khosla VK, Chhabra R, et al. Posterior midline approach for large anterior/anterolateral foramen magnum tumors. *B J Neurosurg.* 2004;18(2):164-167.

Margalit NS, Lesser JB, Singer BA, Sen C. Lateral approach to anterolateral tumors at the foramen magnum: factor determining surgical procedure. *Neurosurgery.* 2005;56(ONS suppl 2):ONS-324-ONS-326: pp. 324-336.

Menezes AH. Surgical approaches: postoperative care and complications "posterolateral–far lateral transcondilar approach to the ventral foramen magnum and upper cervical spinal canal". *Childs Nerv System.* 2008;24:1203-1207.

Rhoton Jr AL. The posterior cranial fossa: microsurgical anatomy & surgical approaches. *Neurosurgery.* 2000;47(suppl 3):S131-S153.

Roberti F, Sekhar LN, Kalavaconda C, et al. Posterior fossa meningiomas: surgical experience in 161 cases. *Surg Neurol.* 2001;56:8-21.

Salas E, Sekhar LN, Ziyal IM, et al. variations of extreme-lateral craniocervical approach: anatomical study and clinical analysis of 69 patients. *J Neurosurg (Spine 2).* 1999;90:206-219.

Wanebo JE, Chicoine MR. Quantitative analysis of the transcondylar approach to the foramen magnum. *Neurosurgery.* 2001;49:934-943.

Numbered references appear on Expert Consult.

CHAPTER 44

Surgical Management of Tumors of the Jugular Foramen

JAMES K. LIU • GAURAV GUPTA • LANA D. CHRISTIANO • TAKANORI FUKUSHIMA

The management of jugular foramen tumors remains challenging for the skull base surgeon. They are formidable lesions because of their difficult location, their proximity to cranial nerves and critical neurovascular structures, and their tumor vascularity. These tumors may involve adjacent structures such as the jugular bulb, carotid artery, middle ear, petrous apex, clivus, infratemporal fossa, and posterior fossa. Advances in neuroimaging, endovascular embolization techniques, neuromonitoring, microneurosurgery, and modern skull base surgery have allowed safe resection of these tumors with lower rates of morbidity and mortality. In this chapter, we discuss the surgical management of jugular foramen tumors, primarily glomus jugulare tumors, schwannomas, and meningiomas.

Historical Background

In 1840, Valentin[1] observed a small cellular formation near the origin of the tympanic nerve that he identified as ganglionic tissue and termed "ganglionium tympanicum" or "intumescentia gangliosa." In 1878, Krause[2] further demonstrated highly vascular glomus tissue along the tympanic branch of the glossopharyngeal nerve ("glandula tympanica") that was histologically similar to the carotid body, as reported by Von Lushka in 1862.[3] This work received little attention until 1941, when Guild[4,5] described glomus tissue as a flattened ovoid body in the adventitia of the dome of the jugular bulb and coined the term "glomus jugularis" to describe paraganglionic tissue composed of capillary or precapillary vessels interspersed with numerous epithelioid cells found along the jugular bulb. In sectioning human temporal bones, Guild found that 50% of this tissue occurred in the jugular bulb, approximately 25% occurred along the course of the tympanic branch of the glossopharyngeal nerve (Jacobson's nerve), and 25% occurred along the auricular branch of vagus nerve (Arnold's nerve). This observation explained the existence of "glomus tumors" that occurred both in the middle ear (glomus tympanicum tumors) and in the region of the jugular bulb (glomus jugulare tumors). Rosenwasser[6] in 1952, was the first to suggest a possible relationship between the "glomus jugularis" and the "carotid body–like" tumors in the temporal bone. The designation "tumors of the glomus jugulare" was first mentioned by Lattes and Waltner in 1949.[7]

Management of jugular foramen tumors has evolved over the years. The inaccessibility of the jugular foramen because of its relatively deep location, high vascularity, and proximity to cranial nerves made tumor management extremely challenging; surgery in this region was often associated with a poor outcome. Surgery in the 1930s was primarily performed using a suboccipital approach with removal of bone around the jugular foramen to avoid excessive bleeding.[8] A subtotal resection followed by radiation therapy was generally performed.[9-12] Most patients had resultant postoperative lower cranial palsies. Mobilization of the facial nerve to better access the jugular foramen was first described by Capps[13,14] in 1952 and later by others.[15,16] Capps combined this with proximal and distal control of the sigmoid sinus and the jugular vein; however, attempts to remove the jugular bulb were met with excessive bleeding and poor outcomes.

In the 1960s and 1970s, the advent of better surgical technology resulted in better surgical outcomes. These innovations included the operating microscope, microneurosurgery dissection techniques, bipolar electrocautery, safer neuroanesthesia, arteriography,[17,18] polytomography,[19] retrograde jugular venography,[16,20] computed tomography (CT),[21] and magnetic resonance imaging (MRI).[22] Hearing preservation surgeries were advocated by House and Glasscock[23] and Farrior[24] (modified endaural postauricular hypotympanotomy). In 1969, McCabe and Fletcher[25] proposed that the size and extent of the tumor were the determining factors for selecting the most appropriate surgical approach. Soon after, new classification schemes were proposed by Fisch[26] and by Jackson et al.[27] based on tumor size, intracranial extension, and surgical operability. The 1970s saw the emergence of multidisciplinary skull base approaches,[27] including the combined lateral skull base approach (suboccipital craniectomy with mastoidectomy),[28-30] and infratemporal fossa approaches by Fisch[31] (modified after Farrior's hypotympanic approach). Other modifications to access the jugular foramen using skull base approaches were further advocated by Al-Mefty and colleagues,[32-34] Bordi et al.,[35] Patel et al.,[36] and Liu et al.[37]

Despite the improvements in surgical exposure, extreme vascularity of the tumor was still a major challenge during surgery. The introduction of preoperative superselective transarterial embolization[38-41] of jugular foramen tumors significantly reduced the vascularity of the tumor, making surgery safer.

Anatomic Considerations of the Jugular Foramen

The jugular foramen, also called the posterior foramen lacerum, is situated in the posterior fossa lateral to the carotid canal. The walls of the jugular foramen are formed anterolaterally by the petrous bone and posteromedially by the occipital bone.[42,43] The foramen is directed in an anterior, lateral, and inferior direction. According to morphometric studies, the jugular foramen can be more accurately described as a triangular canal with an endocranial (~14.5 × 7 mm) and an exocranial opening (~9 × 17 mm). It lies about 23 mm medial to the apex of the mastoid tip, 15 mm medial to the tympanomastoid suture, and 5 mm above the intracranial orifice of the hypoglossal canal.[44-47]

The pars venosa (or pars vascularis) is situated in the posterolateral aspect of the jugular foramen and contains the internal jugular vein (IJV), the jugular bulb, the posterior meningeal branch of the ascending pharyngeal artery, the vagus nerve (cranial nerve X), the auricular branch of the vagus nerve (Arnold's nerve), and the spinal accessory nerve (cranial nerve XI). A smaller pars nervosa is located in the anteromedial portion of the jugular foramen and contains the glossopharyngeal nerve, the tympanic branch of the glossopharyngeal nerve (Jacobsen's nerve), and the inferior petrosal sinus. This nomenclature can be somewhat misleading, because both structures contain neural, as well as vascular, structures.[44]

The important structures surrounding the jugular foramen include the mastoid segment of the facial nerve laterally, the petrous segment of the internal carotid artery (ICA) anteromedially, the vertebral artery inferiorly, and the hypoglossal nerve medially. Access to the jugular foramen from a lateral trajectory is obstructed by the mastoid and styloid processes, the transverse process of C1, and the mandibular ramus.[42] The deep potential spaces along the foramen include the middle layer of the deep cervical fascia (buccopharyngeal fascia) anteromedially, the deep layer of the deep cervical fascia (prevertebral fascia) posterolaterally, and the superficial layer of the deep cervical fascia laterally.[44] These potential spaces are important in understanding the spread of tumors in this region.

The cranial nerves run anteromedially to the jugular bulb and maintain a multifascicular histoarchitecture, especially cranial nerve X, which is formed by multiple fascicles, in contrast to cranial nerves IX and XI, which are formed of only one or two fascicles. The tympanic branch of the glossopharyngeal nerve (Jacobson's nerve) and the auricular branch of the vagus nerve (Arnold's nerve) cross the jugular foramen. A dural septum separates cranial nerve IX from the fascicles of cranial nerves X and XI.[45,46,48] The only intradural site at which the glossopharyngeal nerve is consistently distinguishable from the vagus nerve is just proximal to this dural septum. In about 23% to 30% cases,[44] a bony partition of the jugular foramen may be seen. The facial nerve exits the stylomastoid foramen approximately 5 mm lateral to the lateral edge of the jugular foramen. The hypoglossal nerve does not traverse the jugular foramen; however, it joins the nerves exiting the jugular foramen

just below the skull base and runs with them in the carotid sheath.[42] Tumors in this area can cause Vernet syndrome (jugular foramen syndrome),[49] which is characterized by paralysis of cranial nerves IX, X, and XI caused by tumor expansion within the jugular foramen.

The muscular relationships encountered during surgery at the jugular foramen include the sternocleidomastoid (SCM), situated superficially in the lateral neck, and the splenius capitis, longissimus capitis, levator scapulae, and scalenus medius muscles in a deeper muscular layer. Anteriorly, the posterior belly of the digastric muscle is encountered. Immediately laterally, the styloid process and its attached musculature (stylopharyngeus, stylohyoid, and styloglossus muscles) appear in a triangular zone bounded by the posterior belly of digastrics muscle, the external auditory canal, and the mandibular ramus. Displacement of the digastric muscles exposes the transverse process of C1 (where the superior and inferior oblique muscles attach). The rectus capitis lateralis is the muscle most intimately related to the jugular formen.[42]

Specific Pathologic Conditions
GLOMUS JUGULARE TUMORS

Glomus jugulare tumors are rare lesions with an annual incidence of approximately 1 in 1.3 million people per year.[50,51] Women are affected more often than men (6:1 ratio).[52,53] Glomus tumors have also been referred to as paragangliomas, chemodectomas, nonchromaffin tumors, glomerocytomas, and receptomas. Glomus jugulare tumors arise from paraganglia in the adventitia of the jugular vein. In contrast, glomus tympanicum tumors arise from paraganglia associated with Arnold's and Jacobson's nerves within the middle ear. Tumors occur most frequently in patients between 40 and 70 years of age, but some have been reported in patients as young as 6 months and as old as 88 years. Although they are histologically benign and only rarely metastatize[54] or display malignant features,[55] these tumors may locally invade neighboring structures, such as bone, dura, carotid artery, and cranial nerves.[48] Jansen et al.[56] estimated the doubling time of the size of head and neck paragangliomas to be 13.8 years, with an annual growth rate of 0.79 mm/yr. The incidence of multicentric glomus tumors is 3.7% to 10% in sporadic cases[57,58] and up to 55% in familial cases.[59] For familial glomus tumors, the mean age of patients at presentation is younger, almost 50% of patients have multicentric tumors, and a higher proportion have bilateral tumors.[60,61] Four hereditary paraganglioma syndromes have been described, referred as PGL 1 to 4.[62]

The most common presenting symptoms include conductive hearing loss and pulsatile tinnitus, which is due to the highly vascular nature of these tumors. Pain in the ear and temporal region associated with progressive cranial neuropathies should raise suspicion for malignancy. These tumors are locally invasive with erosion of the neighboring bone and dura. Larger tumors have the potential to cause progressive lower cranial nerve palsies, facial nerve palsy, and symptomatic brain stem and cerebellar compression.

Pathologically, glomus tumors appear as highly vascular nonencapsulated masses (Figs. 44-1 and 44-2). Histologically, they are indistinguishable from glomus tympanicum, glomus vagale, and carotid body tumors. These tumors are characterized by large groups of polyhedral epithelioid cells (chief cells) with centrally located uniformly hyperchromatic nuclei and finely granular cytoplasm.[63] There is an extensive thin-walled capillary and reticulin network surrounding the nests of chief cells, creating the characteristic *Zellballen* appearance.[48] Immunohistochemical analysis of chief cells demonstrates positivity for chromogranin, synaptophysin, neuron-specific enolase, and neurofilament. Malignant glomus tumors demonstrate immunoreactivity to *MIB-1, p53, Bcl-2,* and *CD34.* The extreme vascularity of these tumors is due to angiogenesis from vascular endothelial growth factor and platelet-derived endothelial cell growth factor.[64] Ultrastructurally, secretory granules containing norepinephrine, epinephrine, and dopamine may

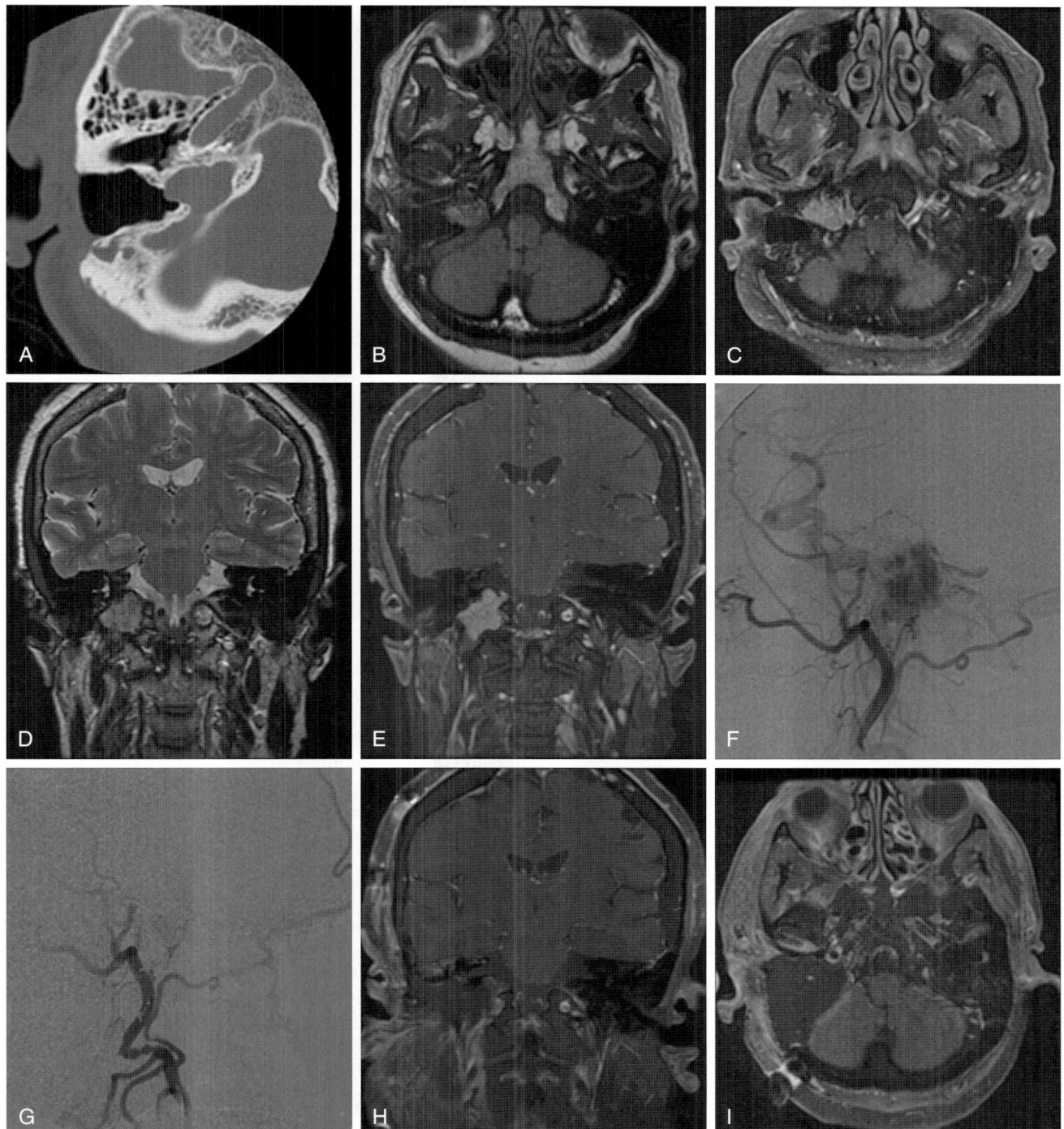

FIGURE 44-1 A, Preoperative axial CT shows enlargement of the right jugular foramen from a glomus jugulare tumor. Preoperative MRI—fluid-attenuated inversion recovery (B) and axial T1-weighted (C), coronal T2-weighted (D), and coronal T1-weighted (E) postgadolinium enhancement—demonstrates a right-sided glomus jugulare tumor in a patient who presented with lower cranial nerve palsies. F, Preoperative angiogram demonstrates a hypervascular tumor fed by the ascending pharyngeal and posterior auricular arteries. G, Postembolization angiogram shows significant reduction of the tumor blood supply. Postoperative coronal (H) and axial (I) T1-weighted postgadolinium enhancement MRI shows gross total resection of the glomus jugulare tumor using the transjugular posterior infratemporal fossa approach.

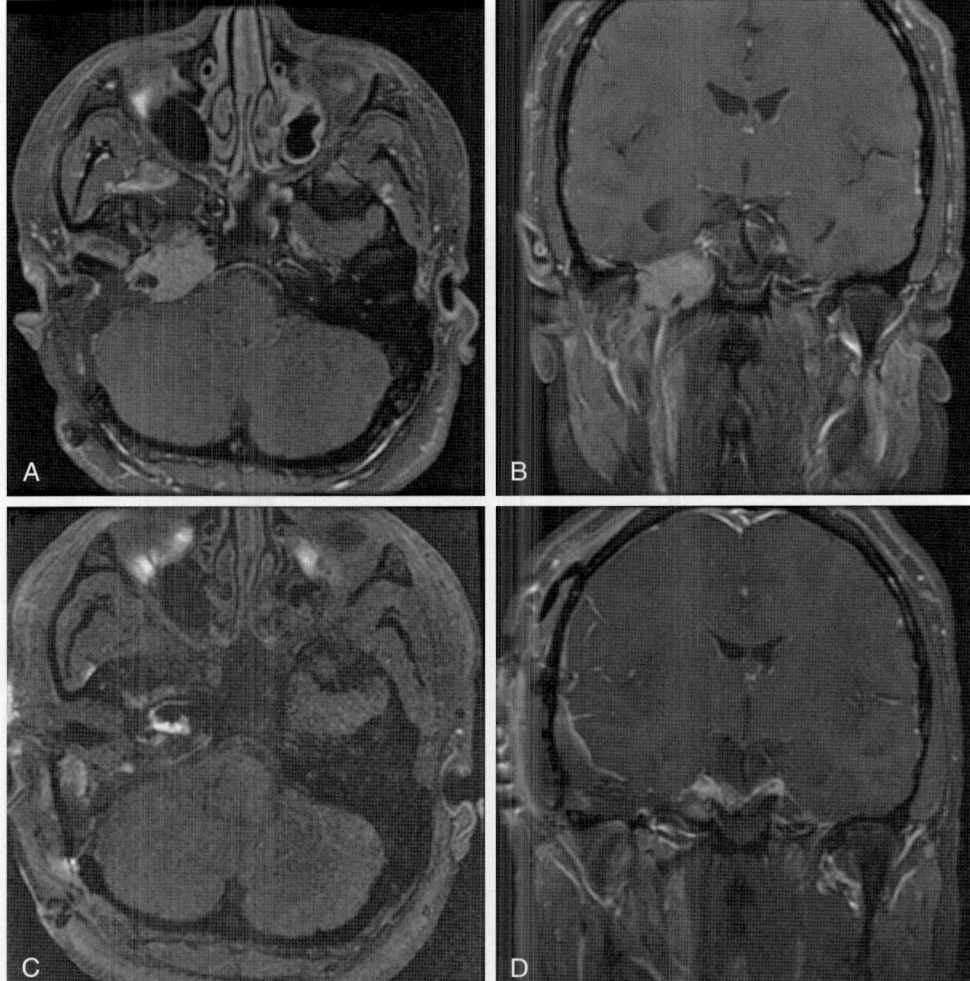

FIGURE 44-2 Preoperative axial (A) and coronal (B) T1-weighted post-gadolinium enhancement MRI demonstrates a recurrent glomus tumor in the petrous apex encasing the petrous ICA. The patient tolerated a BTO with hypotensive challenge, and endovascular embolization and sacrifice of the petrous ICA were subsequently performed. A combined extended middle fossa and infratemporal fossa approach was performed to remove the tumor and involved carotid artery without bypass. Postoperative axial (C) and coronal (D) MRI shows complete removal of the tumor. The patient had no postoperative neurologic deficits.

be seen. Because of the presence of catecholamines and neuropeptides, they are included in the amine precursor uptake and decarboxylase system[65] or the diffuse neuroendocrine system.

SCHWANNOMAS

Schwannomas are the second largest group of tumors at the jugular foramen (Figs. 44-3 to 44-5).[66] Ninety percent of jugular foramen schwannomas originate from cranial nerve IX or X.[67,68] Samii et al.[69] classified these tumors into four subtypes based on location. Type A tumors are those that primarily occupy the cerebellopontine angle with minimal enlargement of the jugular foramen. Type B tumors are primarily located in the jugular foramen with intracranial extension. Type C consists of primarily extracranial tumors with extension into the jugular foramen. Type D consists of dumbbell-shaped tumors with both intra- and extracranial components.

On unenhanced CT scans,[70] schwannomas appear isodense to the brain and enhance brightly as well-demarcated tumors after contrast administration. As opposed to glomus tumors, the bony remodeling of the jugular foramen appears smoothly scalloped and well corticated. On T1-weighted MRI,[71] schwannomas are isointense to brain and markedly enhance after gadolinium administration. On T2-weighted imaging, they are hyperintense to brain. On angiography, schwannomas do not appear very vascular and often compress the jugular bulb, in contrast to glomus tumors, which are highly vascular and invade the jugular bulb.[71]

At surgery, jugular foramen schwannomas appear as well-circumscribed, firm or rubbery, tan–white masses. Histologically, they comprise alternating patterns of compact spindle cells called Antoni A areas, interspersed with loose, hypocellular regions called Antoni B areas. Whorling or palisading formation of the nuclei may be seen. The hyperchromatic nucleus is elongated and twisted with indistinct cytoplasmic borders. These tumors often demonstrate retrogressive changes in the form of cystic degeneration, hyalinization, necrosis, calcification, and hemorrhage. Immunohistochemically, they demonstrate a uniformly intense S-100 protein positivity.[72] Malignant transformation of these benign lesions is rarely seen.[49]

MENINGIOMAS

Although basal posterior fossa meningiomas often extend into the jugular fossa, primary jugular foramen meningiomas are rare, with fewer than 100 cases reported in the literature.[73-76] The jugular foramen as a location for primary meningiomas accounts for only 4% of all posterior fossa

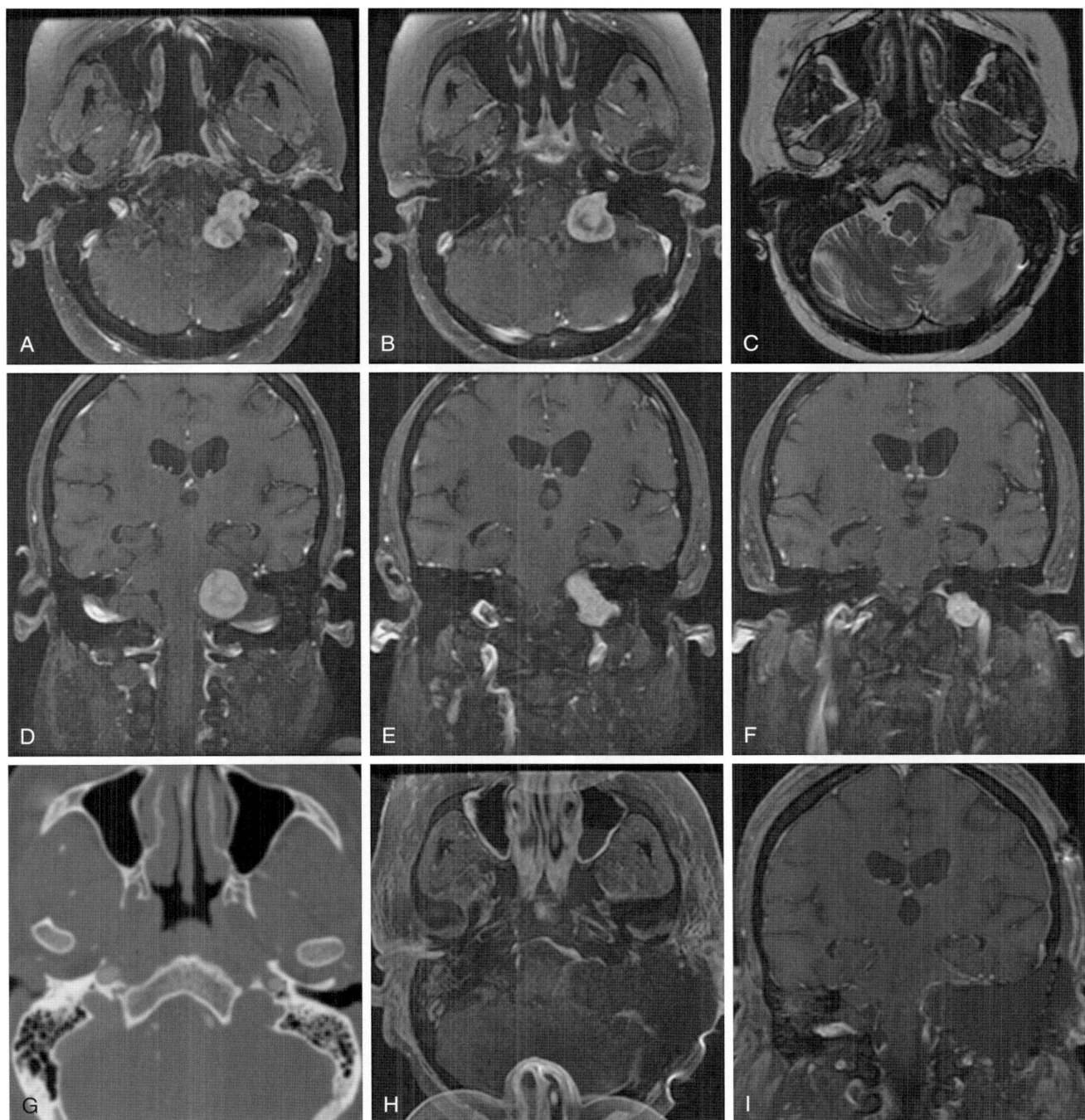

FIGURE 44-3 Preoperative MRI—axial T1-weighted (A and B), axial T2-weighted (C), and coronal T1-weighted (D to F) postgadolinium enhancement—demonstrates a left-sided, enhancing, dumbbell-shaped, type D jugular foramen schwannoma with cerebellar edema. G, Preoperative axial CT scan shows enlargement of the left jugular foramen with smoothly scalloped edges. Postoperative axial (H) and coronal (I) T1-weighted postgadolinium enhancement MRI shows gross total resection of jugular foramen schwannoma using the transjugular posterior infratemporal fossa approach.

meningiomas.[77] Primary jugular foramen meningiomas presumably arise from the arachnoid cap lining the jugular bulb and are more common in women (2:1).[78] These meningiomas tend to exhibit an invasive growth pattern with extensive skull base infiltration, differentiating them from the meningiomas that are centered in the posterior fossa and secondarily extend into the jugular foramen.[44,79] These lesions infiltrate surrounding temporal bone and

neurovascular structures and require wide margins of excision to minimize risk of recurrence. A centrifugal pattern of spread, a permeative-sclerotic appearance of the bone margins of the jugular foramen, the presence of dural tails, and an absence of flow voids are particularly important features that assist in differentiating these from more common jugular foramen tumors. On CT scans, they appear isodense to the brain and show marked enhancement with contrast

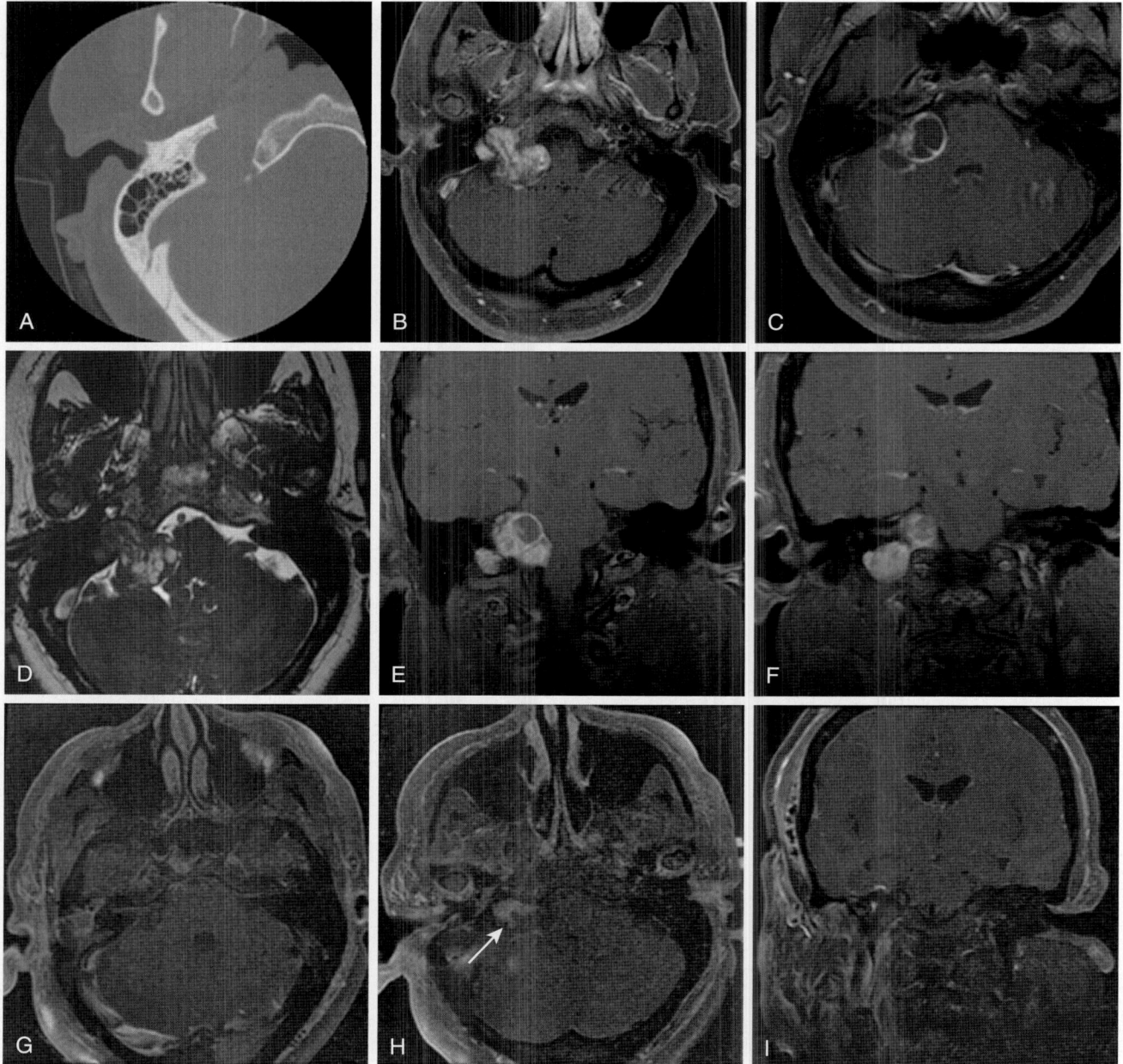

FIGURE 44-4 A, Preoperative axial CT shows enlargement of the right jugular foramen with smoothly scalloped edges from bony remodeling by the tumor. Preoperative MRI—axial T1-weighted (B and C), axial T2-weighted (D), and coronal T1-weighted (E and F) postgadolinium enhancement—demonstrates a right-sided, cystic, dumbbell-shaped, type D jugular foramen schwannoma with brain stem compression. Postoperative axial (G and H) and coronal (I) T1-weighted postgadolinium enhancement MRI shows subtotal resection of jugular foramen schwannoma using the transjugular posterior infratemporal fossa approach. The small extracranial residual tumor (arrow, H) was later treated with stereotactic radiosurgery.

administration; there is occasional calcification and infiltration of the skull base with a characteristic hyperostosis.[75]

At surgery, they are solid, well-circumscribed extra-axial masses and are usually sessile with a broad dural base. On MRI studies, they are typically isointense to hypointense on T1-weighted imaging and enhance markedly after gadolinium administration. Moreover, the angiographic blush time is significantly longer than that of a glomus tumor. As compared with surgical intervention for glomus tumors or schwannomas, surgery on primary jugular foramen meningiomas often has a worse cranial nerve outcome[76] (approximately 60% for meningiomas, 30% for glomus jugulare

tumors, and 15% for schwannomas).[80] There is also a higher recurrence rate of up to 25% at 5 years after resection.[79]

Classification

The main pathways of direct tumor spread are important in understanding the clinical and neurologic manifestations, operative strategies, and risk assessment. Glomus tumors tend to expand within the temporal bone via the pathways of least resistance, that is, air cells, vascular lumens, skull base foramen, and the Eustachian tube.[81,82] According to Spector et al.,[83] glomus tumors can spread through the

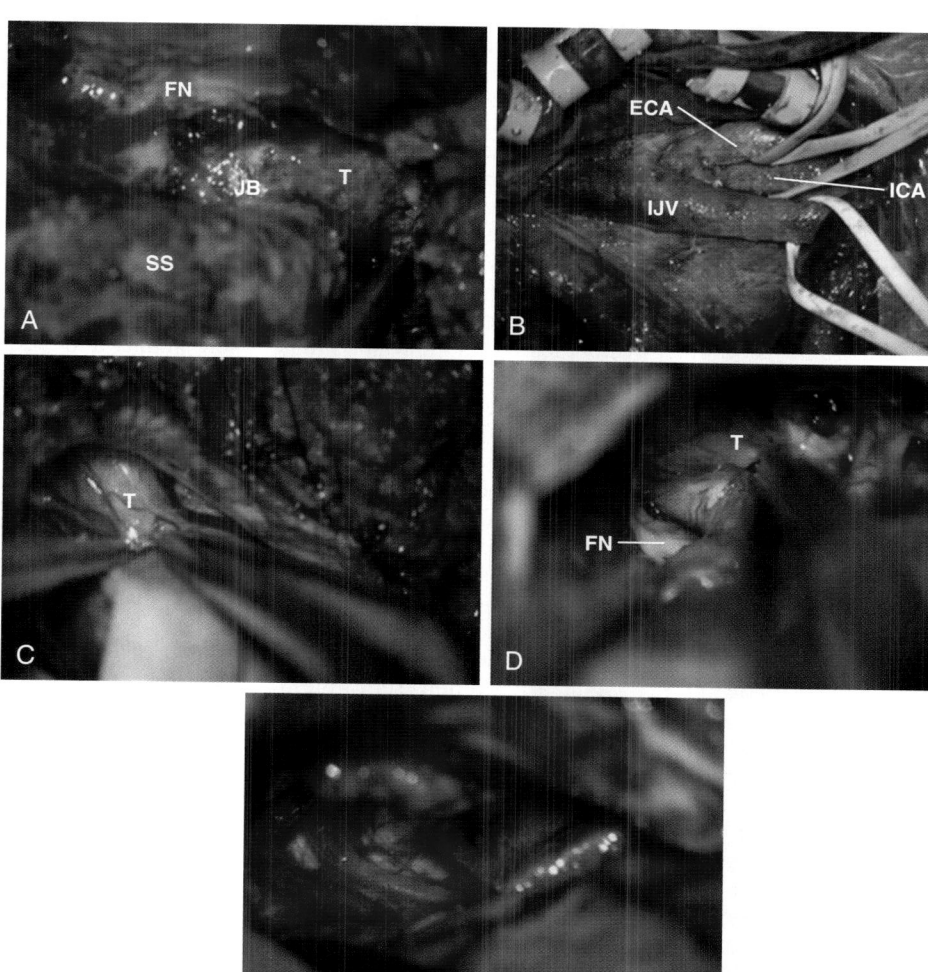

FIGURE 44-5 Intraoperative photographs of a right-sided transjugular posterior infratemporal fossa approach for removal of a jugular foramen schwannoma. A, Infralabyrinthine mastoidectomy has been performed, and the sigmoid sinus and jugular bulb have been skeletonized to expose the tumor at the jugular foramen. B, High cervical exposure of the IJV (white vessel loop) and internal and external carotid arteries (blue vessel loops). C, Retrosigmoid exposure of the intradural portion of the tumor in the cerebellopontine angle. D, The tumor capsule is dissected off of the root of the facial nerve. E, The brain stem is decompressed after removal of the intradural portion of the tumor. FN, facial nerve; JB, jugular bulb; SS, sigmoid sinus; T, tumor; ECA, external carotid artery.

Table 44-1	Fisch Classification
Fisch Grade	**Extent of Tumor**
A	Middle ear cleft (glomus tympanicum)
B	Tympanomastoid area with no infralabyrinthine compartment involvement
C	Infralabyrinthine compartment of the temporal bone and extending into the petrous apex
C1	Limited involvement of the vertical portion of the carotid canal
C2	Invasion of the vertical portion of the carotid canal
C3	Invasion of the horizontal portion of the carotid canal
D1	Intracranial extension <2 cm in diameter
D2	Intracranial extension >2 cm in diameter

Table 44-2	Glasscock-Jackson Classification
Glasscock-Jackson Grade	**Extent of Tumor**
I	Involves the jugular bulb, middle ear, and mastoid; generally small in size
II	Extends under the internal auditory canal; intracranial canal extension possible
III	Extends into the petrous apex; intracranial canal extension possible
IV	Extends beyond the petrous apex into the clivus or intratemporal fossa; intracranial canal extension possible

following pathways once they have locally invaded into the temporal bone and middle ear: (1) down the Eustachian tube into the nasopharynx and then through the skull base foramina, (2) along the carotid artery into the middle fossa, (3) along the jugular vein or hypoglossal canal toward the posterior fossa, (4) through the tegmen tympani to the middle fossa floor, or (5) through the round window, with extension via the internal auditory canal into the cerebellopontine angle.[83,84] Extension within the sigmoid and inferior petrosal sinus may be present as well. Although glomus tumors are usually considered benign and locally invasive, distant metastases to cervical lymph nodes, lung, and bone have been reported in about 4% to 19% of cases.[84,85]

The two most commonly used classifications of glomus tumors are those proposed by Fisch and colleagues[26,86] and Jackson et al.[27] (Tables 44-1 and 44-2). These systems are based primarily on tumor location and size. In 2002, Al-Mefty and Teixeira[32] defined a subgroup of complex glomus jugulare tumors as those having one or more of the following criteria: giant size, multiple paragangliomas (bilateral or ipsilateral), malignancy, catecholamine secretion, association with other lesions such as dural arteriovenous malformations or adrenal tumors, or previous treatment with adverse outcome (prior surgery, radiation, or embolization).

Clinical Presentation and Diagnosis

Patients with jugular foramen tumors often present with initial symptoms of hearing loss and swallowing difficulty, as well as pulsatile tinnitus with glomus tumors. Invasion of the middle ear results in conductive hearing loss. The glomus tumor may erode through the floor of the hypotympanum, presenting as a middle ear mass; if there is erosion of the tympanic membrane, it may present as an aural polyp. Extension of the tumor through the facial recess results in facial nerve encasement and a deficit of the facial nerve.[87,88]

Glomus tumors, meningiomas, and schwannomas of the jugular foramen can each present with lower cranial nerve deficits. Only a small subset of patients exhibits the pathognomonic Vernet syndrome, characterized by paresis of cranial nerves IX, X, and XI with or without XII. However, most patients present with at least one of the following symptoms: vertigo, hoarseness, dysphagia, tongue weakness, or paresis of the SCM and trapezius muscles. If there is extensive intracranial involvement, brain stem and cerebellar compression may result in gait ataxia, nystagmus, and hemiparesis. Mass effect on the fourth ventricle may result in obstructive hydrocephalus. Large tumors with sigmoid sinus occlusion may present with venous hypertension.

A thorough history and physical examination, including a detailed neurologic and otologic assessment, is essential. Specifically, each cranial nerve should be tested and documented preoperatively. There may be a characteristic pulsatile, reddish-blue tumor behind the tympanic membrane. A loud intracranial bruit may be audible over the mastoid or temporal bone. A formal audiogram should be performed to assess hearing function, because this facilitates risk assessment and guides surgical planning.

Glomus tumors have been associated with multiple endocrine neoplasia type 2, neurofibromatosis type 1, and Von Hippel–Lindau syndrome.[87] Familial paragangliomas, in contrast to sporadic cases, are commonly multiple and bilateral, present at an earlier age, and are inherited almost exclusively via the paternal allele.[53,89] Genetic mapping has identified loci *11q13* and *q23* as sites likely responsible for tumorogenesis.[90]

Although the incidence of catecholamine secretion is approximately 4%,[52,91] complications of blood pressure and pulse fluctuations intraoperatively can occur during surgical manipulation.[32] Therefore, preoperative assessment for catecholamine secretion should be performed, including urinary vanillylmandelic acid and metanephrines.[92,93] An abdominal CT or MRI should be obtained in all such patients to rule out a pheochromocytoma as an adrenal tumor source of catecholamine secretion.[32] In patients with catecholamine-secreting tumors, pretreatment with alpha- or beta-blockers is warranted. Epinephrine release during surgical manipulation can provoke a hypertensive crisis, whereas histamine and bradykinin release can cause severe hypotension.[94]

Radiologic Imaging

On thin-section axial CT, glomus jugulare tumors produce a characteristic "moth-eaten" pattern of destruction of the temporal bone and adjacent structures, particularly the jugular spine and the carotid crest (the bone separating the petrous carotid artery from the jugular bulb). These tumors can also cause dehiscence of the floor of the tympanic cavity, with extension into the middle ear and destruction of the bony labyrinth. The tendency of glomus jugulare tumors to erode bone helps distinguish them from glomus tympanicum tumors, which are generally smaller and arise from the cochlear promontory, enveloping but not usually destroying the ossicular chain.[44] In some cases, however, the differentiation cannot be made between the two tumors; therefore, they are called glomus jugulotympanicum tumors. On T1-weighted MRI, glomus tumors demonstrate a characteristic "salt and pepper" pattern caused by flow voids within the highly vascular tumor.[95] They enhance heterogeneously after gadolinium administration.[96] More recently, [111]indium octreotide, a radiologic somatostatin analogue, has been used to selectively identify paragangliomas, especially for detecting multicentricity, recurrence, and metastatic disease.[97]

Jugular foramen schwannomas, on the other hand, enlarge the jugular foramen with widened smooth, scalloped, sclerotic margins seen on CT scans. Unlike meningiomas, there is a lack bony invasion in schwannomas.[95,98] Meningiomas frequently invade bone, particularly the jugular spine and jugular tubercle, resulting in hyperostosis.[96] Schwannomas are usually solid and well circumscribed but occasionally demonstrate cystic degeneration. On MRI, they appear hypointense on T1-weighted images and hyperintense on T2-weighted images; they also brightly enhance, though the enhancement can be heterogeneous if there is associated necrosis or cystic degeneration.[95] When there are intra- and extracranial components, a pathognomonic dumbbell-shaped tumor can be seen best on coronal or sagittal views. Meningiomas typically appear isointense to hypointense on T1-weighted images and enhance considerably after gadolinium administration. A pathognomonic "dural tail" is usually seen.

On diagnostic cerebral angiography, glomus jugulare tumors demonstrate an intense tumor blush because of their hypervascularity.[95] Large feeding vessels and early draining veins are commonly associated with glomus tumors. The main blood supply of glomus tumors comes from the external carotid artery via the inferior tympanic branch of the ascending pharyngeal artery.[89] Large tumors may also parasitize their blood supply from meningeal branches of the occipital artery, the posterior auricular artery, caroticotympanic branches from the petrous ICA, ascending cervical branches from the thyrocervical trunk, the posterior inferior cerebellar artery, and the vertebral artery.[87,96] Narrowing and irregularities of the ICA may indicate tumor infiltration of the carotid wall. In comparison with glomus tumors, meningiomas and schwannomas are only mild to moderately vascular. Meningiomas of the jugular foramen do not necessarily demonstrate the early, prominent, and prolonged tumor blush that is frequently seen with supratentorial meningiomas.[96] Cerebral angiography is also useful in demonstrating the patency of the sigmoid sinus and jugular vein to assess the venous outflow of the tumor during preoperative planning.

Treatment

In 1934, Seiffert performed the first reported exploration of the jugular bulb.[9] Since then, several techniques and modalities have been tried to find the optimal approach to facilitate complete removal of paragangliomas. Early treatment options were extremely limited because of the inaccessibility and the relatively deep location of the jugular foramen,[99] as well as the proximity to and involvement of the cranial nerves and the very high vascularity.[100] With the advancements in the field of neuroimaging, endovascular techniques, anesthesia, microsurgical techniques, and radiosurgery, the treatment of even large jugular foramen tumors has become safer with good outcome.

For catecholamine-secreting tumors, pretreatment is required. Alpha- and beta-blockers are used for catecholamine-secreting tumors and are given 2 to 3 weeks before surgery or embolization to avoid potentially lethal intraoperative blood pressure lability and arrhythmias. Beta-blockers should never be started before full alpha-blockade, because unopposed alpha-agonism in the setting of beta-blockade can lead to severe vasoconstriction and a hypertensive crisis; the beta-blocked heart may not be able to compensate for the increased systemic vascular resistance, leading to myocardial ischemia, infarction, and heart failure.[94] The recommended regimen includes phenoxybenzamine administered 1 to 2 weeks before elective surgery (initial dosage of 10 mg twice daily gradually increasing to final dosages of 40 to 100 mg/day). This drug blocks postsynaptic $alpha_1$-receptor and presynaptic $alpha_2$-receptors, stimulation of which causes increased catecholamine secretion and symptoms thereof. In emergent cases, 3 days of treatment is adequate. Prazosin, a selective $alpha_2$-blocker, can also be used (1 mg three times a day gradually increasing to a final dosage of 8 to 12 mg/day). This has the advantage of causing less tachycardia and is shorter acting, therefore resulting in less prolonged postoperative hypotension. Labetelol (combined alpha- and beta-adrenergic blocker) can also be used. For serotonin-producing tumors, a combination of somatostatin and octreotide is used.[94]

PREOPERATIVE CONSIDERATIONS

Patient Considerations

Small, asymptomatic tumors in patients without a family history can be monitored radiographically with serial imaging. The growth rate of glomus tumors has been estimated at 0.79 mm/yr, with a doubling time of 13.8 years.[56] Surgical removal should be considered in younger patients with symptomatic tumors, in patients with intracranial extension, in those with neural compression, and in patients with tumors demonstrating progressive growth.[101] In patients with bilateral glomus tumors, the larger and more symptomatic side should be treated first. If the resection does not result in significant cranial nerve palsies, then surgery on the remaining contralateral side can be considered. If the patient already has significant postoperative cranial neuropathies, then radiation therapy should be considered on the contralateral side.[32,61] Radiation therapy should also be considered in patients of advanced age with significant medical comorbidities who cannot tolerate the surgical risk,

although other studies have shown that the patient's age is not correlated with the postoperative surgical outcome.[69]

Endocrine Secretion

Paragangliomas are capable of secreting catecholamines and may produce symptoms similar to those of pheochromocytomas. Although the incidence of catecholamine secretion is approximately 4%,[52,91] complications of wide blood pressure and pulse fluctuations intraoperatively can occur during surgical manipulation.[32] Therefore, preoperative assessment for catecholamine secretion is done in all patients.[92,93] This includes measuring plasma catecholamines, metanephrines/normetanephrines and urinary metanephrines/normetanephrines, and/or vanillylmandelic acid. Preoperative hypertension, arrhythmias, palpitations, headaches, or nausea are indicative of a norepinephrine-secreting tumor.[89] An abdominal CT or MRI scan should be obtained in all patients with elevated levels of catecholamines to rule out an adrenal source of secretion.[32]

The endocrine secretion capabilities of paragangliomas are not limited to norepinephrine. Paragangliomas can also secrete 5-hydroxytryptamine (serotonin), kallikrein, and 5-hydroxytryptophan, which are precursors of serotonin and histamine, producing a carcinoid-like syndrome.[94] Clinical symptoms of bronchoconstriction, tricuspid regurgitation, pulmonary stenosis, abdominal pain, explosive diarrhea, violent headaches, cutaneous flushing, hypertension, hepatomegaly, and hyperglycemia are all consistent with carcinoid syndrome. Serotonin-secreting tumors are even less common than norepinephrine-secreting tumors; therefore, preoperative screening is needed only if there are clinical symptoms of concern.

Preoperative Endovascular Treatment

Extreme vascularity of the tumor is another preoperative consideration. Preoperative embolization of the paragangliomas is performed for highly vascular lesions and is useful to reduce bleeding, surgical time, and intraoperative blood transfusion.[41] The various endovascular embolization agents described are Gelfoam, polyvinyl alcohol particles, cyanoacrylate glue,[102] and Onyx.[103] Not all paragangliomas need preoperative embolization (e.g., tympanic paragangliomas confined to the middle ear cavity do not). Balloon test occlusion (BTO) can be helpful in assessing the degree of collateral flow if the ICA were to be sacrificed. If there is poor collateral flow, a superficial temporal artery–middle cerebral artery[104] or saphenous vein reconstruction and high-flow bypass of the carotid artery may be necessary.[105,106] The risk of permanent carotid artery occlusion is high even in patients who pass a preoperative BTO test,[33,107] which carries an inherent risk of 3.7%.[108] Sanna et al.[104] advocate ICA stent placement preoperatively in cases with extensive ICA involvement. They suggest that this maneuver also decreases the intraoperative risk of carotid artery injury; however, if a stent is placed, the patient must be continued on prolonged antiplatelet therapy until the stent has endothelialized.

Intraoperative Neurophysiologic Monitoring

Real-time intraoperative neurophysiologic monitoring is critical not only in preventing inadvertent intraoperative injury to neural elements but also in mitigating further nerve injury after injury is first detected intraoperatively.[109] Baseline curves for brain stem auditory evoked potentials, somatosensory evoked potentials, motor evoked potentials, and facial nerve monitoring are obtained before starting surgery, monitoring is continued intraoperatively, and final runs are obtained at the conclusion of surgery. Electrodes are placed into the SCM muscle and tongue for monitoring cranial nerves XI and XII, and an electromyographic endotracheal tube (Medtronic Xomed Inc., Jacksonville, FL) is used for cranial nerve X monitoring. Cranial nerves at risk during surgery at the jugular foramen include cranial nerves IX, X, XI, and XII (and V, VI, VII, and VIII in the case of large tumors).[37]

SURGICAL PROCEDURE

Choice of Approach

The location, size, and presence of vascular encasement dictate the choice of approach. Access to the jugular foramen is blocked laterally by mastoid and styloid processes, the transverse process of the atlas, and the mandibular ramus.[42] Tumors of the jugular foramen can be typically accessed through a transjugular posterior infratemporal fossa approach. This generally involves mastoid–neck approach that includes a retrolabyrinthine mastoidectomy, upper cervical neck exposure, and skeletonization of the sigmoid sinus and jugular bulb with or without anterior translocation of the facial nerve.[110] For resection of large paragangliomas (Fisch types C and D), several lateral infratemporal fossa approaches have been described by Fisch.[111] These involve transection and blind sac closure of the external ear canal with permanent routing of the facial nerve and anterior displacement of the mandible to expose the vertical segment of the ICA (C7). This procedure has inherent limitations, including conductive hearing loss, facial nerve palsy, and problems with mastication because of the displacement of mandible. For Fisch type D2 (greater than 2-cm intracranial extension), a combined two-stage resection has also been described.[112-115]

We previously described a one-stage transjugular posterior infratemporal fossa approach that allows radical resection of tumors that are located around the jugular foramen, lower clivus, and high cervical region from an anterolateral direction.[37] Transection of the external ear canal, permanent rerouting of the facial nerve, and mandibular displacement are not required as in the Fisch approach. Instead, slight anterior transposition of the facial nerve, in select cases, allows exposure of the vertical C7 segment of the petrous ICA. Both intracranial and extracranial components of tumor can be removed in one stage with total exposure of the jugular foramen. Additional exposure of the lower clivus can be achieved by translocating the vertical infratemporal ICA anteriorly and translocating the lower cranial nerves in the pars nervosa inferiorly. If, however, the patient has nonserviceable hearing and the tumor extends into the middle ear (as in glomus jugulotympanicum tumors), transection of the external ear canal with blind sac closure may be necessary to achieve better tumor exposure and removal.

One-Stage Transjugular Posterior Infratemporal Fossa Approach

The one-stage transjugular posterior infratemporal fossa approach is a combination of the transmastoid, retro- and infralabyrinthine, transjugular, extreme lateral infrajugular–transcondylar–transtubercular, and high-cervical approaches.[116] Multidirectional working corridors to the jugular foramen can be achieved including suprajugular/infralabyrinthine, transjugular, and infrajugular (retrosigmoid–transcondylar) exposures. The main steps of this approach are: (1) postauricular infratemporal incision; (2) retrolabyrinthine mastoidectomy; (3) high cervical exposure; (4) skeletonization and anterior translocation of the facial nerve; (5) lateral suboccipital craniotomy and transcondylar–transtubercular exposure; (6) removal of the IJV, jugular bulb, and sigmoid sinus; and (7) intradural exposure. This approach is versatile and can be used to remove a variety of jugular foramen tumors, including glomus tumors, schwannomas, meningiomas, chordomas, and chondrosarcomas.

Patient Positioning

The patient is placed in the supine position, and the head is held in a three-point Mayfield pin fixation system and turned laterally away from the side of the lesion. A shoulder roll is used to elevate the shoulder ipsilateral to the lesion, and all bony prominences and pressure points are carefully padded with foam and gel pads. The patient is secured to the operating table with adhesive tape to allow safe tilting during the operation. Intravenous corticosteroids and antibiotics are given at the time of skin incision. The abdomen is prepared in anticipation of a need for harvesting an abdominal fat and fascia graft. If facial nerve reconstruction and grafting are anticipated, the sural nerve or greater auricular nerve region is prepped for harvesting.

Postauricular Infratemporal Incision

A curvilinear C-shaped combined retroauricular–high cervical skin incision is made starting 2 to 3 cm posterior to the upper border of the ear and continuing inferiorly toward the neck over the anterior border of the SCM muscle (Fig. 44-6). After the galeal layer/temporoparietal fascia is undermined, the skin flap is reflected anteriorly and the posterior auricular muscle is identified behind the external ear canal. At this point, we must identify and preserve the greater auricular nerve, which runs obliquely 2 to 3 cm below the mastoid across the anterior border of the SCM. If facial nerve reconstruction is planned, the nerve is harvested now. As noted earlier, the sural nerve is another alternative for reconstruction. The muscular attachments at the mastoid tip are then carefully dissected in layers. First the superficial layer (including the SCM and splenius capitis) and then the middle layer (longissimus capitis and semispinalis capitis) are reflected posteriorly, exposing the deep layer muscles of the suboccipital triangle. Next, the deep layer, including the rectus capitis posterior major and obliquus capitis superior and obliquus capitis inferior (suboccipital triangle), is dissected. The styloid diaphragm, a membranous structure covering the posterior belly of the digastrics muscle, is also identified. The occipital artery runs under the styloid diaphragm and the posterior belly of the digastric muscle.

Retrolabyrinthine Mastoidectomy

A retrolabyrinthine mastoidectomy with skeletonization of the sigmoid sinus and jugular bulb is performed, and the mastoid air cells are totally removed until the presigmoid dura, the superior petrosal sinus, the middle fossa dura,

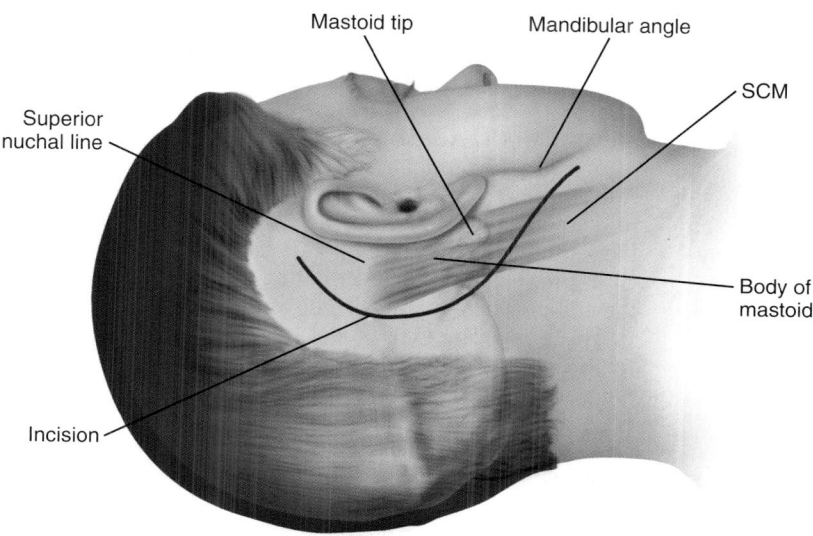

Mastoid tip

Mandibular angle

SCM

Superior
nuchal line

Body of
mastoid

Incision

FIGURE 44-6 Right-sided retroauricular high cervical skin incision for transjugular posterior infratemporal fossa approach. *(From Fukushima T, Manual of Skull Base Dissection, 2nd ed., AF-Neurovideo Inc.)*

the sinodural angle, and the retrosigmoid dura are identified (Fig. 44-7). The digastric ridge, which marks the exit of cranial nerve VII from the fallopian canal through the stylomastoid foramen, is then identified. The fallopian canal is located 12 to 15 mm deep to the outer cortical surface of the mastoid and 1 to 3 mm anterior and parallel to the posterior semicircular canal. The facial nerve is carefully skeletonized using a high-speed drill under constant copious irrigation to prevent thermal injury to the facial nerve. The retrofacial air cells are removed to further skeletonize the jugular bulb.

High Cervical Exposure

The goal of the high cervical exposure part of the procedure is identification of the extracranial portions of the lower cranial nerves, the ICA, and the IJV (Fig. 44-8).[117] The anterior limit of the approach is defined by the posterior border of the angle of the mandible, and the posterior limit is defined by the mastoid tip. The subcutaneous tissue and the platysma are divided, and blunt dissection is used to demarcate the posterior angle of the mandible, along with the anterior border of the SCM. The anterior part of the SCM

is retracted posteriorly to achieve adequate exposure of the posterior belly of the digastric muscle. Next, the stylomastoid diaphragm is removed and the underlying occipital artery coagulated. The posterior belly of the digastric muscle is reflected superoanteriorly to cover and protect the facial nerve. For identification of the accessory nerve, the transverse process of C1 is palpated.[118] The lateral point located 3 to 15 mm inferolaterally to the anterior edge of the C1 transverse process is an important landmark for identifying the accessory nerve, which runs in a posteroinferior direction between the posterior belly of digastric and the IJV. The hypoglossal nerve is identified running over the IJV on the lateral surface of the carotid sheath. After the carotid sheath is opened, the vagus nerve is identified in the dorsal aspect of the ICA. The stylohyoid muscle is identified lying anterior to the ICA and attached posteriorly to the styloid process at the cranial base. The stylopharyngeus and styloglossus are also attached to the styloid process, which can be subsequently removed from its insertion at the skull base to increase the exposure of the ICA where it enters the cranial base. The glossopharyngeal nerve can be seen

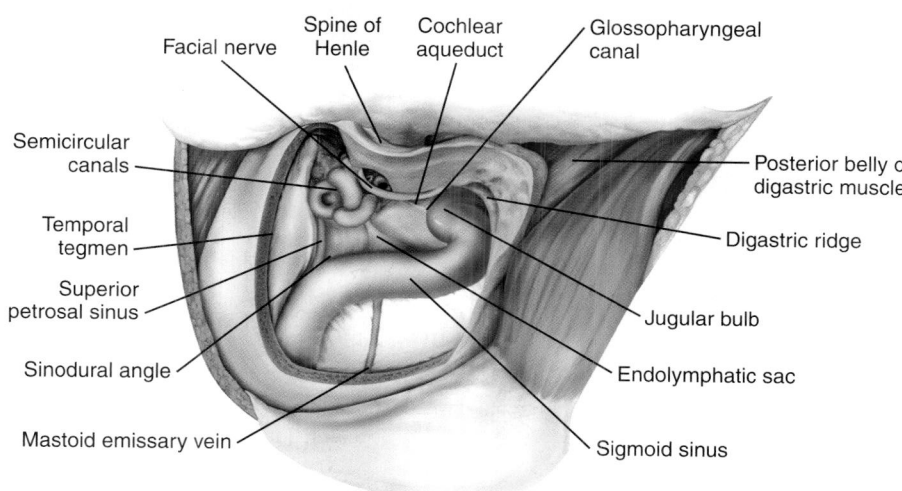

Facial nerve

Spine of
Henle

Cochlear
aqueduct

Glossopharyngeal
canal

Semicircular
canals

Temporal
tegmen

Superior
petrosal sinus

Sinodural angle

Mastoid emissary vein

Posterior belly of
digastric muscle

Digastric ridge

Jugular bulb

Endolymphatic sac

Sigmoid sinus

FIGURE 44-7 Retro- and infralabyrinthine mastoidectomy is performed to skeletonize the sigmoid sinus, jugular bulb, and facial nerve. *(From Fukushima T, Manual of Skull Base Dissection, 2nd ed., AF-Neurovideo Inc.)*

crossing the ICA 1 to 2 cm inferior to this point, and posterior retraction of the IJV helps expose the carotid branch of the glossopharyngeal nerve (the carotid sinus nerve). The pharyngeal branch of the vagus nerve is identified inferior to the glossopharyngeal nerve.

Anterior Translocation of the Facial Nerve

The mastoid segment of the facial nerve in the fallopian canal is skeletonized from the second genu to the stylomastoid foramen. The mastoid tip is removed with care to preserve the periosteum surrounding the facial nerve because this protects stylomastoid artery, which provides blood supply to the facial nerve. This maneuver allows better exposure of the jugular bulb where it meets the superior aspect of the IJV at the level of the jugular foramen. The vertical C7 segment (infratemporal) of the ICA is exposed by detaching the styloid process, as mentioned earlier. If additional exposure of the ICA is necessary, anterior translocation of the mastoid segment of the facial nerve can be performed. This maneuver is used selectively and produces decreased risk of facial nerve palsy postoperatively, in contrast with permanent facial nerve rerouting. Further drilling of the petrous carotid canal is performed to expose the petrous ICA. The glossopharyngeal nerve is identified exiting dorsal to the ICA and behind the IJV. Jacobson's nerve (tympanic nerve) diverges from the glossopharyngeal nerve and exits between the C7 segment of the ICA and the jugular bulb.

Retrosigmoid and Transcondylar–Transtubercular Exposure

A retrosigmoid craniectomy is performed and carried down to include the lip of the foramen magnum. Extradural reduction of the occipital condyle and jugular tubercle allows exposure of the hypoglossal canal and the posterior condyle and opens up the posterior rim of the jugular foramen (Fig. 44-9). Care is taken to identify and protect the vertebral artery, which lies in the C1 vertebral sulcus on the arch of C1. A safe way to identify the vertebral sulcus is to follow the lamina of C1 toward the transverse process. A J-shaped groove can be identified where the vertebral artery, which is encased by a venous plexus, courses from the foramen transversarium of C1 behind the lateral mass of C1 in the vertebral sulcus and then turns medially to pierce the atlanto-occipital membrane and dura.

The posteromedial aspect of the occipital condyle is removed with a high-speed diamond drill while protecting the vertebral artery. Venous bleeding from the condylar emissary vein can be controlled with bone wax and Surgicel. Further drilling exposes the extradural hypoglossal canal, which is situated superior to the occipital condyle and inferior to the jugular tubercle. The canal contains the hypoglossal nerve, a meningeal branch of the ascending pharyngeal artery and the venous plexus of the hypoglossal canal, which communicates the basilar venous plexus with the marginal sinus that encircles the foramen magnum. Identification of the medial aspect of the hypoglossal canal usually indicates that approximately one third of the posterior condyle has been removed. Because the hypoglossal canal is directed anteriorly and laterally at a 45-degree angle with the sagittal plane, further skeletonization of the canal to its lateral extent usually results in approximate removal of the lateral aspect of the posterior two thirds of the condyle. Skeletonization of the entire hypoglossal canal should not result in occipitocervical instability as long as care is taken not to drill the occipital condyle inferior to the hypoglossal canal and violate the articulation to the lateral mass of C1. Further drilling of

FIGURE 44-8 High cervical exposure is performed to expose the lower cranial nerves and the ICA and IJV. The mastoid tip is removed to expose the jugular foramen. *(From Fukushima T, Manual of Skull Base Dissection, 2nd ed., AF-Neurovideo Inc.)*

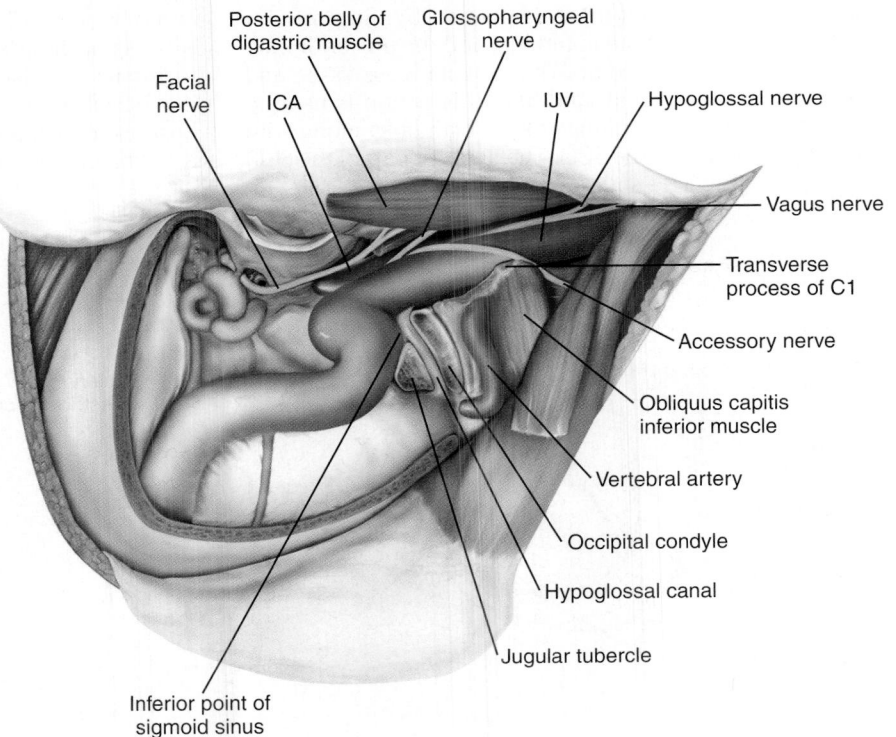

Posterior belly of digastric muscle
Glossopharyngeal nerve
Facial nerve
ICA
IJV
Hypoglossal nerve
Vagus nerve
Transverse process of C1
Accessory nerve
Obliquus capitis inferior muscle
Vertebral artery
Occipital condyle
Hypoglossal canal
Jugular tubercle
Inferior point of sigmoid sinus

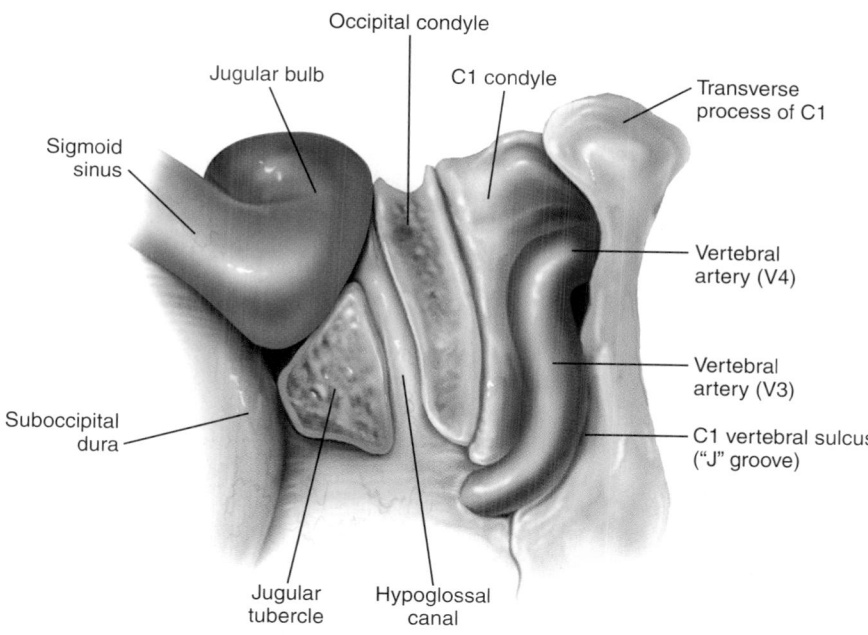

Occipital condyle

Jugular bulb   C1 condyle

Sigmoid sinus

Transverse process of C1

Vertebral artery (V4)

Vertebral artery (V3)

Suboccipital dura

C1 vertebral sulcus ("J" groove)

Jugular tubercle   Hypoglossal canal

FIGURE 44-9 The medial third of the occipital condyle and jugular tubercle is removed. The extradural hypoglossal canal is skeletonized. Care is taken to preserve the joint articulation between the occipital condyle and the C1 lateral mass. *(From Fukushima T, Manual of Skull Base Dissection, 2nd ed., AF-Neurovideo Inc.)*

the jugular tubercle can facilitate an unobstructed view of the basal cistern and clivus anterior to the lower cranial nerves.

Removal of IJV, Jugular Bulb, and Sigmoid Sinus

In glomus jugulare tumors, the tumor situated within the IJV, jugular bulb, and sigmoid sinus can now be palpated. The jugular bulb is the connective link between the sigmoid sinus and the IJV and varies in both height and position. The average bulb has a width of approximately 15 mm

and a height of about 20 mm.[32] The hypervascularity of the tumor contributes to the prominence of the vasa vasorum of the IJV. All arterial feeders to the tumor are then meticulously coagulated. The tumor mass is isolated by ligating the IJV inferior to the tumor mass and ligating the sigmoid sinus superior to the tumor mass (Figs. 44-10 and 44-11). The lateral wall of the IJV is then opened with a No. 11 blade, and the tumor is removed from within. Brisk venous bleeding arising from the inferior petrosal sinus can be readily controlled with Surgiflo (Ethicon Inc.), followed by

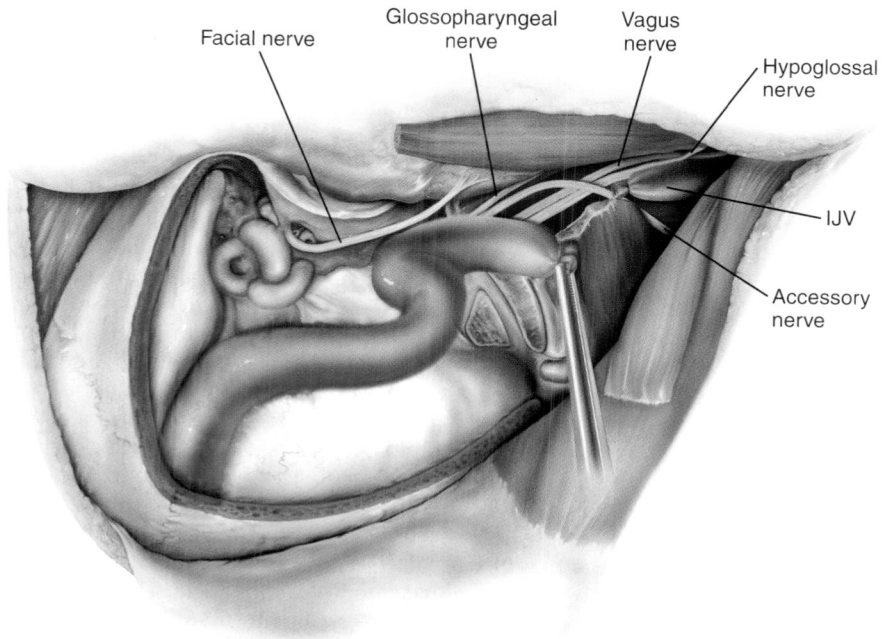

Facial nerve

Glossopharyngeal nerve

Vagus nerve

Hypoglossal nerve

IJV

Accessory nerve

FIGURE 44-10 The IJV is ligated and divided just inferior to the tumor mass. *(From Fukushima T, Manual of Skull Base Dissection, 2nd ed., AF-Neurovideo Inc.)*

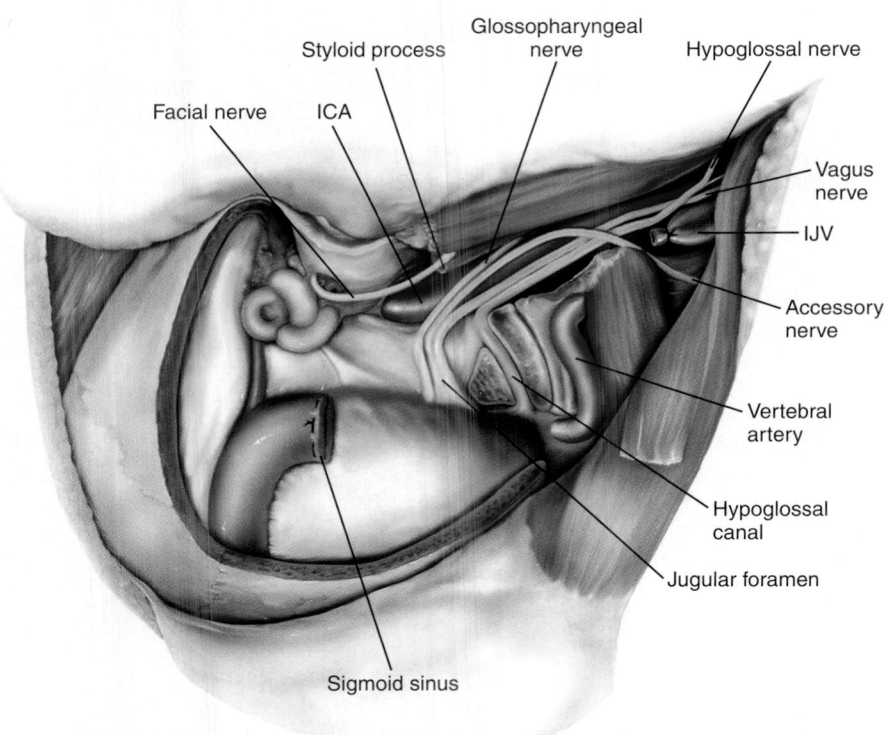

FIGURE 44-11 The sigmoid sinus is ligated and divided just superior to the tumor mass. The medial wall of the jugular foramen is left intact to better preserve the lower cranial nerves. *(From Fukushima T, Manual of Skull Base Dissection, 2nd ed., AF-Neurovideo Inc.)*

gentle packing with cottonoid patties. The tumor is coagulated with a bipolar cautery and carefully dissected from the pars nervosa while preserving the plane of dissection between the tumor and the medial wall of the jugular bulb. By preserving the medial wall of the jugular bulb, the lower cranial nerves at the jugular foramen are protected and are at less risk for injury. This technique can only be performed as long as the tumor has not invaded the medial wall of the jugular bulb or infiltrated the lower cranial nerves. The lower cranial nerves in the pars nervosa can be translocated inferiorly, and the vertical C7 segment of the ICA can be translocated anteriorly to establish an operative corridor to the lower clivus if necessary. For functional preservation of the lower cranial nerves, we must preserve the dural sleeve covering of the nerves. For schwannomas and meningiomas extending through the jugular foramen, ligation of the IJV and sigmoid sinus and opening of the IJV and jugular bulb can be useful in removing these tumors situated at the jugular bulb.

Retrosigmoid Intradural Exposure

Intradural exposure provides access to the ventral craniovertebral junction, including the inferior part of the cerebellopontine angle and the cerebellomedullary angle, and allows removal of the intradural part of the tumor, including careful dissection of the tumor off the lower cranial nerves (Figs. 44-12 and 44-13). A curvilinear incision of the dura is made 3 to 4 mm posterior to the sigmoid sinus all the way inferiorly to meet the point where the vertebral artery enters the dura. Additional exposure of the cerebellopontine angle is achieved by extending this incision superiorly to the transverse–sigmoid junction. An adequate reduction

of the occipital condyle and jugular tubercle, as explained in the previous section, is key for providing a good surgical corridor to the ventral craniovertebral junction and the inferior part of the cerebellopontine angle, including the cerebellomedullary angle. This gives an excellent view of cranial nerves V through XII, the vertebral artery, the vertebrobasilar junction, the basilar artery, the posterior inferior cerebellar artery, and the anterior inferior cerebellar artery. The next step is inspection of the intradural part of the jugular foramen for any tumor invasion and dissecting the tumor carefully off the lower cranial nerves.

Reconstruction of Skull Base after Tumor Removal

Cranial base reconstruction and excellent watertight dural closure are key to prevention of cerebrospinal fluid (CSF) leakage. A watertight dural closure should be the goal if possible. Autologous fascia lata or a dural substitute can be used to close dural defects primarily. If a primary closure is not attainable, then an autologous fat graft is used to plug the remaining dural defect. For larger defects, an autologous fascial graft or pericranial flap can be used followed by fibrin glue. Care is taken to seal off any entrance to the middle ear with autologous muscle, bone wax, or bone cement to prevent CSF fistula to the middle ear. Additional fat is used to plug the mastoid defect and any remaining anatomic dead space. The mastoid and suboccipital cranial defect can be repaired with a sheet of malleable titanium embedded in polyethylene (Medpor Titan) that is easy to shape and secure to the skull with titanium screws. Multilayer soft tissue wound closure is performed. Temporary lumbar drainage can be used to facilitate healing of the dural closure.

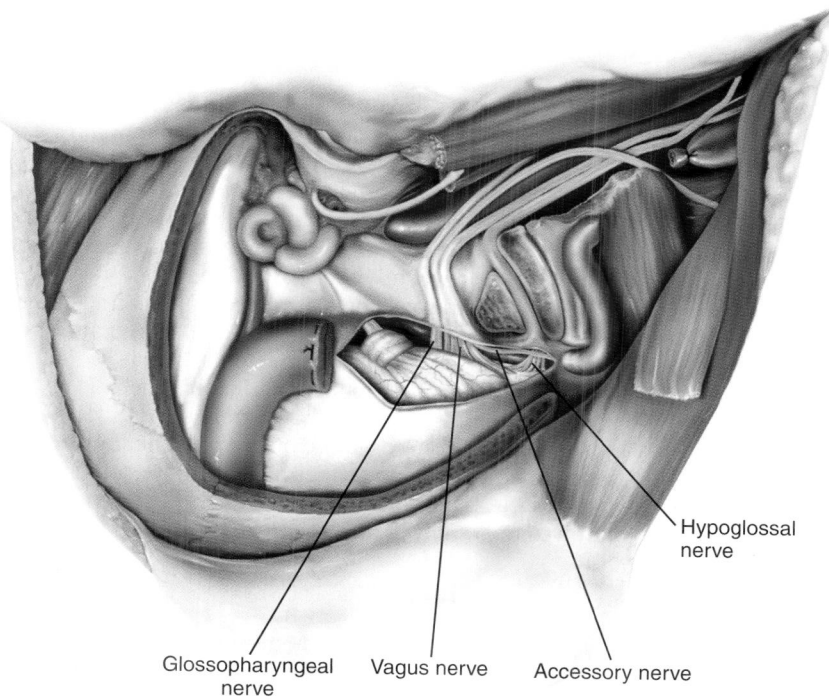

Glossopharyngeal nerve   Vagus nerve   Accessory nerve   Hypoglossal nerve

FIGURE 44-12 Intradural exposure is performed to inspect for intracranial extension of tumor through the jugular foramen. *(From Fukushima T, Manual of Skull Base Dissection, 2nd ed., AF-Neurovideo Inc.)*

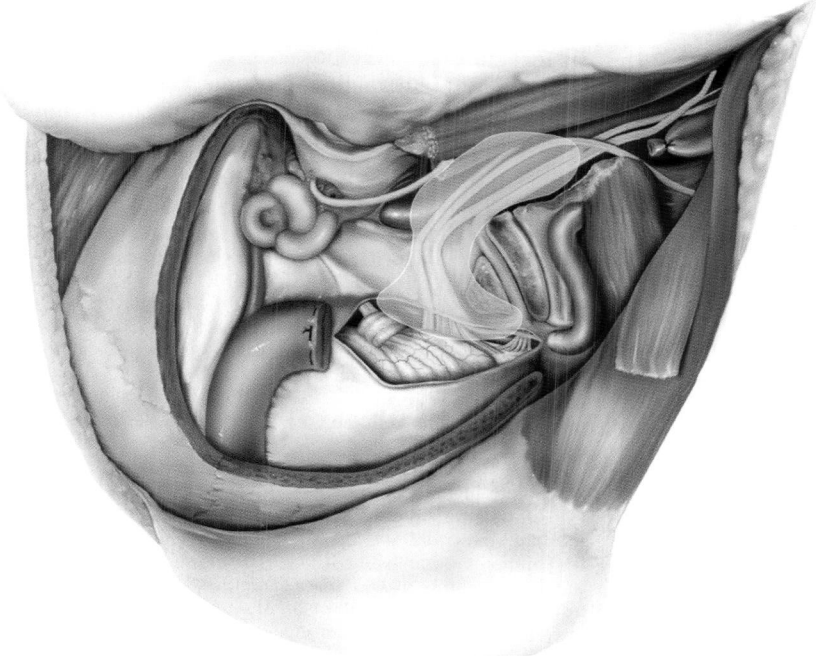

FIGURE 44-13 Final view after the tumor has been removed. The yellow shadow represents the tumor's previous location in the jugular foramen. *(From Fukushima T, Manual of Skull Base Dissection, 2nd ed., AF-Neurovideo Inc.)*

Complication Avoidance

Complications from surgical removal of jugular foramen tumors include new cranial nerve deficits, vascular injury, CSF leakage, and meningitis. Postoperative morbidity can be considerable, largely from permanent cranial nerve palsies.[119] Although patients with larger tumors can present with preexisting cranial nerve palsies, it is important not to incur new and permanent cranial nerve palsies. Anatomic preservation of cranial nerves and intraoperative cranial nerve monitoring are useful in minimizing these complications. Anterior translocation of the facial nerve should be used judiciously, because this can increase the risk of transient facial nerve palsy. Preservation of the medial wall of the jugular bulb is helpful in preserving lower cranial nerve integrity and function, as long as there is no tumor invasion of the medial wall or cranial nerves. In a report by

Green et al.,[57] 29% of patients had postoperative dysphagia, 29% had persistent hoarseness, 19% were treated for vocal cord paralysis (medialization laryngoplasty), 8% required primary thyroplasty, 8% required prolonged nasogastric feedings, and 2% to 6% experienced additional complications, including pneumonia, pulmonary embolism, wound infection, aspiration, and meningitis. Patients with facial nerve palsy and incomplete eye closure may require a tarsorrhaphy or upper lid gold weight to protect the eye until facial nerve function improves. In cases of intraoperative carotid injury, attempts should be made at repairing the ICA primarily. Alternatively, ICA sacrifice with or without a bypass can be performed, depending on the results of the preoperative BTO study.[111,120,121]

TREATMENT OF RESIDUAL AND RECURRENT LESIONS

Although gross total resection is the goal of surgery, residual tumor may be left behind in some cases to preserve lower cranial nerve function. Treatment options of residual tumor include conservative management with periodic reimaging (every 3 to 6 months), reoperation, stereotactic radiosurgery, or conventional fractionated external beam radiation.[122] Repeat surgery for tumor recurrence, sometimes even in cases of failed radiation, is technically more difficult because of tissue fibrosis, loss of surgical planes, and previous irradiation.

RADIOSURGERY

The use of stereotactic radiosurgery as a primary and a secondary treatment modality for jugular foramen tumors has been increasing in frequency.[123] Radiosurgery is effective in controlling growth while minimizing permanent disability in patients with jugular foramen tumors.[124] It involves a shorter treatment time than conventional fractionated external beam radiation and offers precise stereotactic localization. Some have recommended radiosurgery for tumors of less than 2 to 3 cm, with documentation of growth on serial MRI and for patients with other relative contraindications to surgery, such as patient age, significant comorbidities, or simply patient preference.[125] The main goal of radiosurgery is tumor control. The main indications of primary radiosurgery are (1) age greater than 60 years; (2) medical or surgical contraindications to surgery; (3) unresectable or bilaterally large tumors; (4) major vascular risk, including failed BTO; (5) patient preference; and (6) absence of neurologic deficits.[126-128] Radiosurgery should not be considered primary therapy in patients with large tumors resulting in mass effect and brain stem compression.

The primary effects of radiation therapy occur from direct injury to the cells by damaging cellular deoxyribonucleic acid and by radiation-induced vascular injury.[129] There is no association between radiation dose and clinical outcome,[130] tumor control,[130,131] or toxicity.[132,133] Although paragangliomas treated primarily with radiation have shown excellent tumor control,[134] there is no effect of radiation on the catecholamine secretion of the tumor.[125,135]

Stereotactic radiosurgery can be used in the treatment of jugular foramen tumors as a primary therapy,[136] in conjunction with surgery[137] for unresectable or subtotally resected tumors, or when the patient may not be a candidate for surgery based on age,[138] medical problems, tumor size, or

prior treatment failure. A multicenter study[139] involving 66 patients with paragangliomas treated with gamma knife radiosurgery demonstrated that 95% had clinical improvement or remained stable, 60% had no change in tumor size on follow-up CT or MRI, and 40% had reduction in the size of their tumor. For jugular foramen schwannomas, stereotactic radiosurgery showed 5- and 10-year control rates of 97% and 94%, respectively.[140]

Radiation-induced neoplasms,[136,141] hearing loss, alopecia, facial weakness, imbalance, and vocal cord dysfunction[125,129,141] have all been described after radiotherapy for benign paragangliomas. Acute complications of radiosurgery include mucositis and nausea. Late complications include hair loss, xerostomia,[142] otitis media, vertigo, secondary tumor development, radiation necrosis of brain, bone, and muscle,[133] radiation-induced cranial neuropathies,[143] ICA thrombosis, and poor wound healing. Although excellent tumor control rates have been reported over relatively short periods, only a few studies have reported long-term tumor control rates.[133,143,144]

Conclusions

The surgical management of jugular foramen tumors remains a formidable challenge in cranial base surgery. Knowledge of surgical anatomy and microsurgical skull base approaches to the jugular foramen are critical for successful removal of these lesions. The primary goals of surgical removal are to preserve neurologic function while treating the underlying pathology. The ultimate goal is gross total resection, if safely possible, with minimal morbidity and mortality. Stereotactic radiosurgery remains an important part of the armamentarium in the overall multimodal treatment of complex jugular foramen tumors.

KEY REFERENCES

Al-Mefty O, Fox JL, Rifai A, et al. A combined infratemporal and posterior fossa approach for the removal of giant glomus tumors and chondrosarcomas. *Surg Neurol.* 1987;28(6):423-431.

Al-Mefty O, Teixeira A. Complex tumors of the glomus jugulare: criteria, treatment, and outcome. *J Neurosurg.* 2002;97(6):1356-1366.

Arnautovic KI, Al-Mefty O. Primary meningiomas of the jugular fossa. *J Neurosurg.* 2002;97(1):12-20.

Brackmann DE, Fayad JN, Owens RM. Paragangliomas and schwannomas of the jugular foramen. In: Sekhar LN, Fessler RG, eds. *Atlas of Neurosurgical Techniques: Brain.* New York: Thieme; 2006:752-758.

Fayad JN, Schwartz MS, Brackmann DE. Treatment of recurrent and residual glomus jugulare tumors. *Skull Base.* 2009;19(1):92-98.

Fisch U. Infratemporal fossa approach for glomus tumors of the temporal bone. *Ann Otol Rhinol Laryngol.* 1982;91(5 Pt 1):474-479.

Fisch U. Infratemporal fossa approach to tumours of the temporal bone and base of the skull. *J Laryngol Otol.* 1978;92(11):949-967.

Gardner G, Cocke Jr EW, Robertson JT, et al. Combined approach surgery for removal of glomus jugulare tumors. *Laryngoscope.* 1977; 87(5 Pt 1):665-688.

Gottfried ON, Liu JK, Couldwell WT. Comparison of radiosurgery and conventional surgery for the treatment of glomus jugulare tumors. *Neurosurg Focus.* 2004;17(2):E4.

Graham MD, Larouere MJ, Kartush JM. Jugular foramen schwannomas: diagnosis and suggestions for surgical management. *Skull Base Surg.* 1991;1(1):34-38.

Green Jr JD, Brackmann DE, Nguyen CD, et al. Surgical management of previously untreated glomus jugulare tumors. *Laryngoscope.* 1994;104(8 Pt 1):917-921.

Jackson CG, Glasscock 3rd ME, Harris PF. Glomus Tumors. Diagnosis, classification, and management of large lesions. *Arch Otolaryngol.* 1982;108(7):401-410.

Katsuta T, Rhoton Jr AL, Matsushima T. The jugular foramen: microsurgical anatomy and operative approaches. *Neurosurgery.* 1997;41(1):149-201:discussion 201-202.

Liu JK, Sameshima T, Gottfried ON, et al. The combined transmastoid retro- and infralabyrinthine transjugular transcondylar transtubercular high cervical approach for resection of glomus jugulare tumors. *Neurosurgery.* 2006;59(1 suppl 1):ONS115-ONS125.

Patel SJ, Sekhar LN, Cass SP, et al. Combined approaches for resection of extensive glomus jugulare tumors. A review of 12 cases. *J Neurosurg.* 1994;80(6):1026-1038.

Ramina R, Maniglia JJ, Fernandes YB, et al. Tumors of the jugular foramen: diagnosis and management. *Neurosurgery.* 2005;57(suppl 1): 59-68.

Ramina R, Neto MC, Fernandes YB, et al. Meningiomas of the jugular foramen. *Neurosurg Rev.* 2006;29(1):55-60.

Samii M, Babu R, Tatgiba M, et al. Surgical treatment of jugular foramen schwannomas. *J Neurosurg.* 1995;82:924-932.

Sheehan J, Kondziolka D, Flickinger J, et al. Gamma knife surgery for glomus jugulare tumors: an intermediate report on efficacy and safety. *J Neurosurg.* 2005;102(suppl):241-246.

Varma A, Nathoo N, Neyman G, et al. Gamma knife radiosurgery for glomus jugulare tumors: volumetric analysis in 17 patients. *Neurosurgery.* 2006;59(5):1030-1036:discussion 1036.

Numbered references appear on Expert Consult.

Suboccipital Retrosigmoid Surgical Approach for Vestibular Schwannoma (Acoustic Neuroma)

ROBERT L. MARTUZA

For the surgery of vestibular schwannoma (acoustic neuroma), refinements of microsurgical techniques, combined with improvements in intraoperative monitoring of facial and cochlear nerve function and advances in neuroimaging, have resulted in the shift of focus from reduction of mortality to optimizing facial nerve function,[1-4] hearing preservation,[1,2,5] and preservation of other cranial nerves.[6] Facial nerve dysfunction is a major concern among patients undergoing unilateral vestibular schwannoma surgery, and loss of useful hearing can be debilitating.[7] Patients with vestibular schwannoma have many options, including watchful waiting, radiosurgery, fractionated radiation, and surgery through one of several routes: translabyrinthine, middle fossa, or suboccipital retrosigmoid. The ideal treatment strategy depends on several factors, including the age, medical condition, and hearing status of the patient and the anatomy of the tumor as seen on imaging studies. Surgeons generally try to save hearing if the speech discrimination is above 50% and the average pure tone loss is less than 50 dB.[8,9] However, even worse hearing is worth saving in some circumstances, such as when poor hearing is present on the contralateral side or in a patient with neurofibromatosis type 2 (NF2), where bilateral hearing loss could later occur. Moreover, these various treatments are not mutually exclusive; in some patients, a combination of subtotal surgical tumor removal followed by radiosurgery of the residual may prove appropriate.

Preoperatively, whenever appropriate, we have the patient see not only the neurosurgeon but also an otologist and a radiosurgeon or radiation oncologist to explore the various options. If surgery is the chosen option, the various risks and complications are explained, the patient is tested with the neck in the position of surgery to assure that no symptoms are produced from spinal cord compression due to a secondary cervical lesion, and preoperative laboratory studies are performed. An audiogram with speech discrimination and magnetic resonance imaging (MRI) with gadolinium and fine cuts through the posterior fossa are routinely performed. We do not routinely perform a computed tomography (CT) scan or combined CT and magnetic resonance angiogram or CT and magnetic resonance venogram; these are only done if indicated by the initial MRI. If the patient has NF2, cervical MRI with gadolinium is performed to detect possible cervical spinal cord and nerve tumors.

The patient is started on dexamethasone (8 mg twice daily) for 48 hours prior to surgery, along with a gastric proton blocking agent such as pantoprazole (40 mg twice daily) or a related pharmaceutical. The patient is admitted the day of surgery, and the side and site of surgery are confirmed with the patient and marked on the skin. The surgical team reviews the plans for the procedure. The anesthesiologist places an intravenous line, and general anesthesia is administered. Care must be taken not to use paralytic agents that will last into the procedure and interfere with monitoring of facial or other cranial nerve function. An arterial line and embolism-prevention airboots are placed. Antibiotics are administered, and a urinary catheter and nasogastric tube are placed. Dexamethasone (10 mg) and furosemide (10 mg) are administered intravenously. An infusion of mannitol is begun (250 to 500 cc of a 20% solution). If hearing is to be saved and if there is no medical contraindication, nimodipine (60 mg) is given via the nasogastric tube.

The patient is positioned supine with one or two folded soft cotton blankets beneath the ipsilateral shoulder and padding beneath the knees and is secured with one or two belts to allow the table to be rolled if necessary during surgery. For patients with a cervical tumor (as in NF2) or elderly patients with cervical spondylosis or limitations in neck movement, additional blankets are used to further turn the upper body of the patient and thereby require less turning of the neck. However, too much turning of the body can place the shoulder in a position that interferes with surgery. To prevent peripheral neural compression, the surgeon must ensure the contralateral ulnar and fibular head areas will not be under pressure if the bed is rolled and pad them appropriately. The head is gently turned toward the contralateral side. Hair is shaved from about 7 cm behind the ipsilateral ear, and the patient is fixed in a three-pin headrest (Fig. 45-1A). The surgeon must assure that there is adequate space between the chin and the clavicle and that contralateral jugular compression is avoided. Physiologic monitoring equipment is placed. Bipolar facial monitoring electrodes are routinely placed in the orbicularis oculi and orbicularis oris. If trigeminal nerve function is of concern, an additional electrode is placed in the masseter. For hearing monitoring, the ear canal is inspected and cleaned if necessary; an electronic clicker is placed in the ipsilateral ear and the contralateral ear, with electrodes in the scalp to record a brain stem auditory evoked response (BAER) during surgery. If lower cranial nerves are involved, we use an endotracheal tube with an embedded electrode.

The self-retaining retractor post is secured to the side of the headrest away from the surgical site. A metal triangle is used to protect the face and allow both the anesthesiologist and the neurophysiologist or audiologist visualization of the airway and of facial movement. The endotracheal tube exits the mouth on the contralateral side to avoid distortion of the ipsilateral lip and cheek. A fiberoptic tube delivers a cool but bright light to the area under the drapes and assures that the small TV camera also under the drapes has a well-illuminated view of the patient's ipsilateral face (Fig. 45-1B). Stimulation of the facial nerve in the operative field causes a clearly visible "smile" reaction, which can be seen on the external TV monitors. In contrast, electric activity that causes stimulation of the motor branch of the trigeminal nerve in turn causes jaw movements due to activation of the masseter muscle. An audiologist or neurophysiologist monitors facial movements, electromyogram (EMG), and BAER throughout the procedure.

The area behind the operative ear and an area on the ipsilateral abdomen are sterilely prepared and draped for surgery. A linear incision is made approximately 3 cm

behind the insertion of the pinna and going from approximately 1 cm above the tip of the pinna to 1 cm below the ear lobe. Superiorly, a 3-cm piece of pericranium is removed and placed in sterile solution during the procedure for later use in closing the dural defect. The muscles are then divided inferiorly, hemostasis is obtained, and two muscle self-retaining retractors are placed. They are angled such that the medial skin area is free from these muscle retractors, because that is where the cerebellar retractors will later be situated (Fig. 45-2A).

The transverse sinus and sigmoid sinus generally curve around the asterion. Therefore, a bur hole is placed inferomedial to the asterion. A high-speed drill with irrigation, as well as rongeurs, is used to define the inferior edge of the transverse sinus and the medial edge of the sigmoid sinus. The medial dura is then stripped from the bone using a No. 3 Penfield dissector, and a craniotome is used to remove a free bone flap, which is placed with the pericranial graft for later insertion. The bone edges are waxed, paying particular attention to the areas of the mastoid where nonsecured air cells can be a cause of postoperative cerebrospinal fluid (CSF) leakage.

The incisional area is surrounded with antibiotic-soaked sponges and towels in preparation for dural opening. The dura is opened with a linear vertical incision approximately

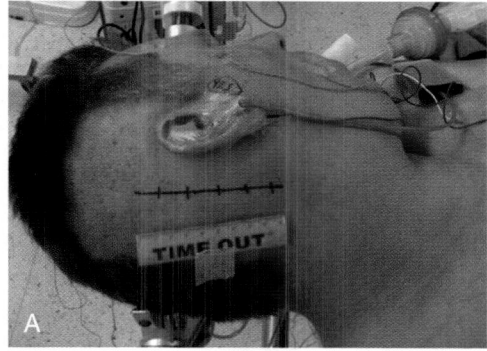
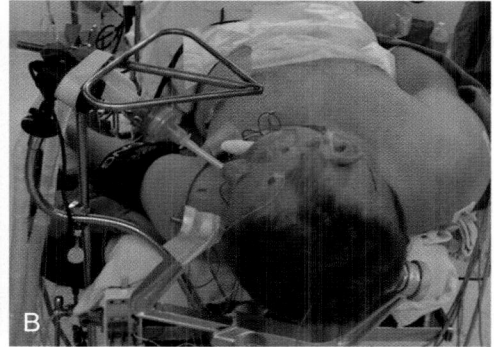

FIGURE 45-1 Positioning. A, The patient is positioned supine, with the head gently turned toward the contralateral side and fixed in a three-pin headrest. A timeout is taken for the surgical team to assure the correct patient, correct site, and correct procedure. The incision and the monitoring apparatus are demonstrated. B, The supine position of the patient is seen from the vertex. The endotracheal tube exits the mouth on the contralateral side to avoid distortion of the ipsilateral lip and cheek. The small TV camera (secured with yellow tape) has a well-illuminated view of the patient's ipsilateral face beneath a triangular metallic protector that will hold the operative drapes upward.

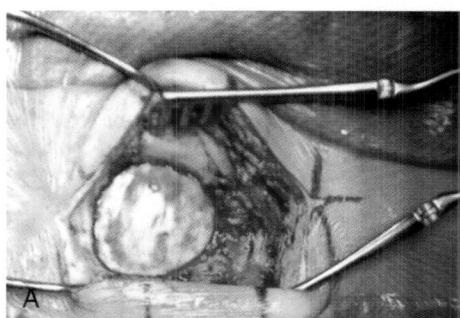
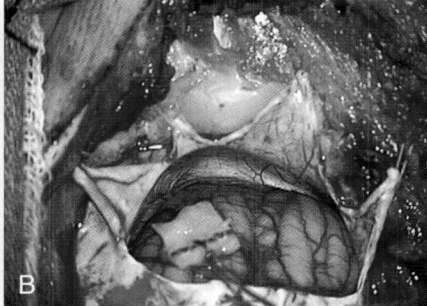
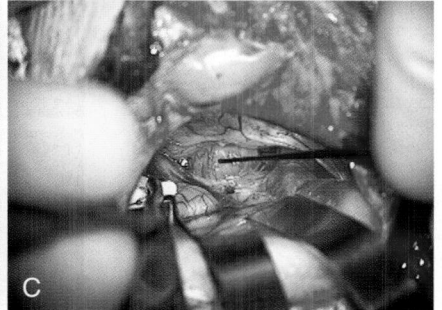

FIGURE 45-2 Opening and tumor exposure. A, The skin, muscle, and bone opening exposing the dura. (Cranial is to the left. Lateral is upward.) The superior limit of the exposure is the inferior edge of the transverse sinus. The lateral limit of the exposure is the medial edge of the sigmoid sinus. The retractors are angled such that the medial skin area is free to make room for the cerebellar retractors. B, The dural opening. CSF has been removed, and the cerebellum falls away from the cerebellopontine angle because of gravity in this supine position. A ½-inch cottonoid patty gives a reference as to the size of the exposure. C, Three ¼-inch retractors are placed on Telfa and a rubber dam is placed on the cerebellum and positioned to spare the very large vein located superiorly (left side of the photo). The tumor is being stimulated with a monopolar facial nerve stimulator.

2 cm medial to the edge of the sigmoid sinus. The medial dura is left intact to protect the cerebellum. Additional dural incisions are made laterally toward the edge of the venous sinuses. The resulting triangular-shaped dural leaves are sutured to the surrounding tissue with 4-0 Vicryl sutures. An adjustable bar is attached to the retractor bar that previously had been affixed to the headrest, and a long flexible arm and long narrow retractor are attached. The inferior cerebellum is gently elevated with the retractor, and the arachnoid of the cistern is opened sharply to release CSF and provide for cerebellar relaxation. For larger tumors, a ventriculostomy catheter is put into the cistern, secured to the inferomedial dura with a 4-0 Vicryl suture, cut off at the dural edge, left in place for continuous CSF drainage throughout the procedure, and removed during closure. For smaller tumors, this is often unnecessary. At the time of initial dural opening, if the cerebellum is under a lot of pressure, it is often beneficial to open initially the most inferior triangular dural flap only and then release a small amount of CSF to allow the remainder of the dural opening to be performed under more controlled conditions. The surgeon must, however, be cautious not to remove too much CSF when the dura is not fully opened; doing so can be associated with too much cerebellar relaxation, causing a venous tear near the tentorium or in the area of the petrosal sinus. This can be difficult to control and forces a more rapid dural opening than might be desired.

Once the dura is opened and CSF removed, the cerebellum is generally relaxed and, in this position, falls away from the cerebellopontine angle because of gravity (Fig. 45-2B). A piece of moistened rubber dam covered with Telfa is placed on the cerebellum. Three long flexible arms and three long, ¼-inch-wide self-retaining retractors are used. The retractors are placed on the Telfa with the tips on the cerebellum 1 or 2 mm proximal to the tumor edge. Care must be taken to be sure the retractors do not occlude

important vascular structures or impinge on or stretch cranial nerves. They should be formed to sit securely on the skin edge to prevent unwanted movement. Occasionally, with a large tumor and an operculum of cerebellum overhanging the tumor, it is safer to resect the lateral cerebellar operculum than to retract it for long periods.

The operating microscope is engaged. At this point, stimulation of the posterior capsule of the tumor is necessary (Fig. 45-2C). I use a monopolar stimulator and first check it at 3 mA on the exposed neck muscles to be sure the stimulator is working and the patient is not pharmacologically paralyzed. If muscle stimulation occurs, the stimulator is turned down to 1 mA and the posterior capsule is stimulated at all points to exclude a posteriorly placed facial nerve. If no stimulation is encountered, the tumor may be entered. In more than 80% of patients, the facial nerve is anterior or inferior. However, if stimulation occurs, the surgeon must determine whether this is due to transmission to a distant facial nerve or whether the nerve is indeed on the posterior tumor surface. To determine this, the posterior capsule is mapped out at sequentially lower milliampere levels to determine the course of the facial nerve. The surgeon must define an entry point into the tumor that is devoid of facial nerve fibers.

The surgeon must pay close attention to the arachnoid over the tumor. If this can be stripped away without coagulation, it provides not only the best plane for dissection but also a protective barrier for the cranial nerves and their small feeding vessels. After peeling away the arachnoid, a nonstimulating area on the posterior tumor is coagulated with bipolar cautery and opened with microscissors and specimens are sent for pathologic study. The internal portion of the tumor is then decompressed using an ultrasonic aspirator (Fig. 45-3A). Hemostasis is obtained, and the tumor capsule is dissected from the arachnoid plane and rolled inward. Depending on the size of the tumor, this process of

FIGURE 45-3 Tumor removal. A, Internal decompression of the tumor is performed with an ultrasonic aspirator in one hand and No. 16 suction in the other. B, The internal auditory canal is being exposed using a high-speed drill in one hand and a continuous suction-irrigator in the other. C, The dura of the internal auditory canal is exposed. Superiorly (to the left) within the canal is a large mastoid air cell. D, The microdissector and No. 16 suction are being used to dissect the tumor off the vestibular–cochlear and facial nerves. The tumor is rolled from medial to lateral. Some bleeding over the facial nerve, as seen in this photo, is best stopped with irrigation.

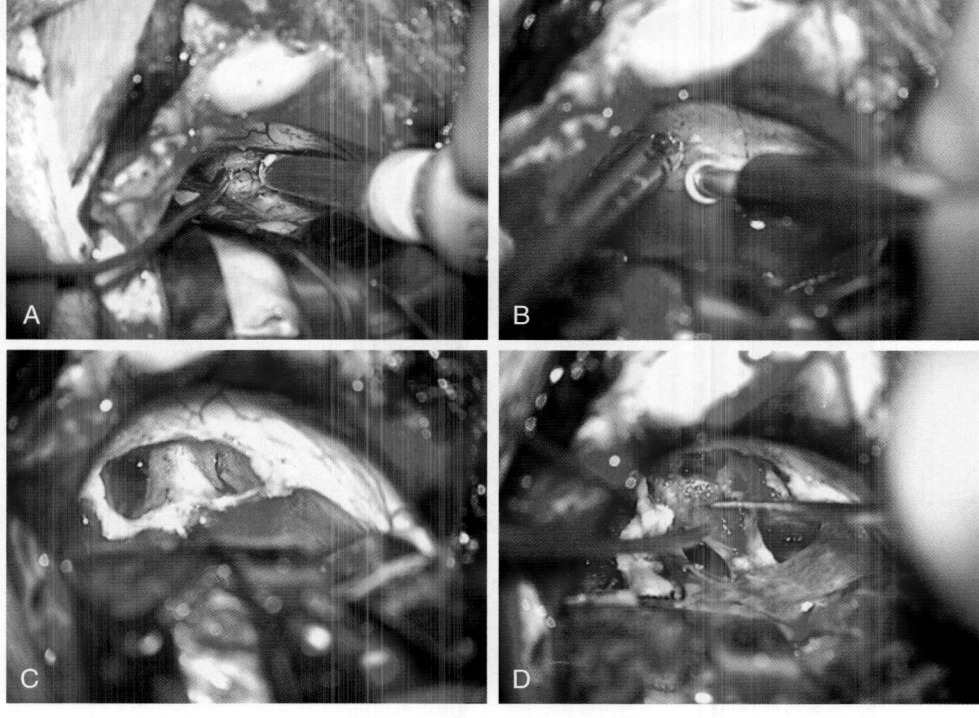

internal decompression followed by dissection and inward rolling the capsule may need to be repeated several times. Each time, some of the capsule is also cut away but always leaving a visible portion to make the next round of microdissection easier. The retractors may need to be moved, but the surgeon must always keep them low profile, affixed to the skin, and with the tips on the cerebellum, not the cerebellar peduncle, brain stem, or critical blood vessels.

At some point, the limiting factor becomes the entry of the tumor into the internal auditory canal and its attachments at the medial edge of the canal. It then becomes necessary to open the canal. I usually work with an otologist to do this part. However, in some circumstances, the neurosurgeon may do this portion of the procedure. The superior and inferior lips of the internal auditory canal are defined. If there are open CSF cisterns, they are occluded with moistened gelfoam pledgets to prevent entry of bone dust. However, all patties with strings on them must be removed from the field prior to using a drill. The dura over the canal is coagulated and flapped medially. Using a suction-irrigator and high-speed diamond drill (Fig. 45-3B), the canal is opened to expose the dura of the canal (Fig. 45-3C). Attention is paid to air cells that will later need to be secured (Fig. 45-3C) and to a high jugular bulb if present. If hearing is being spared, the drilling of the canal should be limited to 10 mm or less and must not include the vestibular apparatus. Once drilling is completed, the entire operative field is washed clear of bone dust, the temporary gelfoam pledgets are removed, and the CSF spaces are irrigated with saline. The dura of the canal is then opened sharply.

For a case in which hearing is being spared, we do not necessarily define the facial nerve at this point in the canal; rather, because these are smaller tumors, we proceed to define the facial nerve medially as it enters the brain stem. The tumor can then be rolled medially to laterally, sparing both the facial and the cochlear nerves (Fig. 45-3D). There is often a nice arachnoid plane, and as the tumor is rolled into the canal, parts of the tumor may need to be removed to decrease the bulk. During the dissection of tumor off the facial nerve or cochlear nerves, the surgeon must minimize the use of bipolar cautery. If bleeding starts between the tumor and the facial nerve, it can often be stopped with irrigation or temporary application of Surgicel. Even using bipolar cautery at low levels can cause facial or cochlear nerve damage. Ultimately, the most lateral portion of the tumor can be removed with microdissectors. Ideally, the surgeon desires not only that the facial nerve be anatomically intact but also to stimulate at low milliamperes at the brain stem level and that a good wave V remains on the BAER.

In the case of larger tumors and patients for whom hearing cannot be saved, once the dura of the canal is opened, using the stimulator initially on 1 mA but then gradually lowering to 0.1 mA, the facial nerve is identified in the distal canal as distinct from the tumor and from the other nerves. The vestibular and cochlear nerves are cut, and the tumor is rolled out of the canal from distal to proximal, with the facial nerve preserved under direct view. The tumor is invariably tightly attached at the proximal edge of the internal auditory canal. These attachments must be isolated. Stimulation is used to exclude the presence of the facial nerve; the attachments are then bipolar coagulated and sharply divided. At this point, the surgeon can start to roll

the tumor in on its internally decompressed self and away from the facial nerve. The petrosal vein may hinder dissection at the superior part of the tumor. For large tumors, the petrosal vein is usually coagulated and divided. For smaller tumors, this may not be necessary. Occasionally, the petrosal vein is particularly large and may be the only major draining vein in this area. In such instances, it is wise to preserve it if possible to minimize the possibility of cerebellar venous infarction.

If the tumor is being dissected from lateral to medial, the facial nerve most commonly adheres to the tumor just medial to the internal auditory canal. This often limits the lateral to medial dissection, and the surgeon must start dissection in a different direction. If the superior tumor capsule is rolled in on the main bulk of the tumor, the trochlear nerve (cranial nerve IV) becomes visible parallel to the tentorial edge. Deeper and slightly inferiorly, the fibers of the trigeminal nerve (cranial nerve V) are encountered. At times, there appears to be a nice plane between the trigeminal nerve and the tumor; however, do not be tempted by this, as it is often a different plane from the plane between the facial nerve and the tumor and, if followed, may lead to transection of a thinned-out facial nerve tightly attached to the tumor capsule.

In contrast, if the surgeon goes to the inferomedial part of the tumor, the facial nerve and vestibular–cochlear nerves can be seen as separate from the tumor as they enter the brain stem. The vestibular–cochlear nerves do not stimulate and can be divided (provided hearing is not being spared), and the tumor can then be rolled from medial to lateral away from the facial nerve and from inferior to superior away from the glossopharyngeal (cranial nerve IX), vagus (cranial nerve X), and accessory (cranial nerve XI) nerves. Deep in the cavity of the dissection may be the abducens (cranial nerve VI) nerve.

The arachnoid plane must be retained between the facial nerve and the tumor; however, as the surgeon comes to the area near the internal auditory meatus, where the facial nerve can be more tightly attached to the tumor, it may be necessary to sharply cut the tumor away from the facial nerve if blunt dissection is not adequate. Even if the facial nerve is tightly stretched and has the appearance of wet tissue paper such that the surgeon can see through it, the nerve can still be functional. I have found that if it stimulates at 0.3 mA or less at the brain stem level after tumor removal, good facial function will likely ensue.

Although much of the focus is on removing the tumor while sparing the important cranial nerves, blood vessels may also be encountered, including the anterior inferior cerebellar artery, which may loop near the internal auditory canal or be displaced in various other locations, including near the facial nerve. Superiorly, the surgeon may encounter the superior cerebellar artery; deep to the tumor, the larger vertebral–basilar trunk may be seen. These must be preserved and with microdissection can usually be dissected away from the tumor. In cases for hearing preservation, it must be remembered that the internal auditory artery is the only blood supply to the cochlea and must be saved if hearing is to be saved.

Once the tumor is removed and hemostasis is obtained, the internal auditory canal that has been drilled must be secured to prevent CSF leakage postoperatively. A 1-inch incision is made in the skin of the abdomen that had been previously prepared sterilely. A piece of subcutaneous adipose tissue is removed, hemostasis is obtained, and the incision is closed with 3-0 Vicryl sutures in the subcutaneous tissue plus a 4-0 Vicryl subcuticular closure and Steri-Strips. If large air cells are visible where the internal auditory canal had been drilled, some Tisseel or fibrin glue is placed within (Fig. 45-4A) and then packed with one or a few small pieces of adipose tissue covered with bone wax. The drilled surface of the canal is secured with bone wax, and a larger piece or multiple pieces of adipose tissue are then placed over the bone wax. This is covered with one piece of moistened surgicel to secure it to the surrounding dura (Fig. 45-4B). This is then further sealed and secured to the surrounding dura with Tisseel or fibrin glue.

The retractors are removed, along with the Telfa, rubber dam, and temporary CSF drainage tube that was placed in the cistern. All cottonoid patties and rubber dams are accounted for. The cerebellum should appear relaxed and away from the dura. The extra space is filled with sterile saline. The dura is then repaired using the previously removed pericranial graft and 4-0 Vicryl sutures (Fig. 45-4C), with two tenting sutures in the middle. The bone defect is then repaired with a construct consisting of the removed bone plus a preformed titanium mesh cranioplasty plate (Fig. 45-4D). The two dural tenting sutures of 4-0 Vicryl are threaded through this construct, and it is secured to the surrounding bone with a combination of miniplates and screws, taking care not to put any screws in an area of possible mastoid air cells. The tenting sutures are secured. The muscle retractors are removed, hemostasis is obtained, and the layers of muscle and the galea are reapproximated with 2-0 and 3-0 Vicryl. The skin is closed with running 3-0 monofilament nylon, and a sterile dry dressing is applied to this incision and the one on the abdomen.

The patient is awakened, extubated, examined, and taken to the postanesthesia care unit and/or the neuroscience intensive care unit overnight. The next day, the patient is usually ambulatory and moved to a regular room. Antibiotics are stopped after 24 hours. Steroids are generally tapered off over 4 to 7 days, and the gastric proton inhibitor is then stopped. Most patients leave the hospital on the third to fifth postoperative day and return for suture removal around the 10th postoperative day. Walking is encouraged, but strenuous activities are discouraged for 1 month postoperatively.

Outcomes and The Importance of Cranial Nerve Monitoring

The importance of adequate cranial nerve monitoring must be emphasized. I had the opportunity to operate on 200 sequential patients in two centers where different monitoring techniques were used: center 1 (Massachusetts General Hospital, 1982 to 1991 and 2000 to 2001) and center 2 (Georgetown University Hospital, 1991 to 2000) using (1) only facial monitoring electrodes versus (2) electrodes

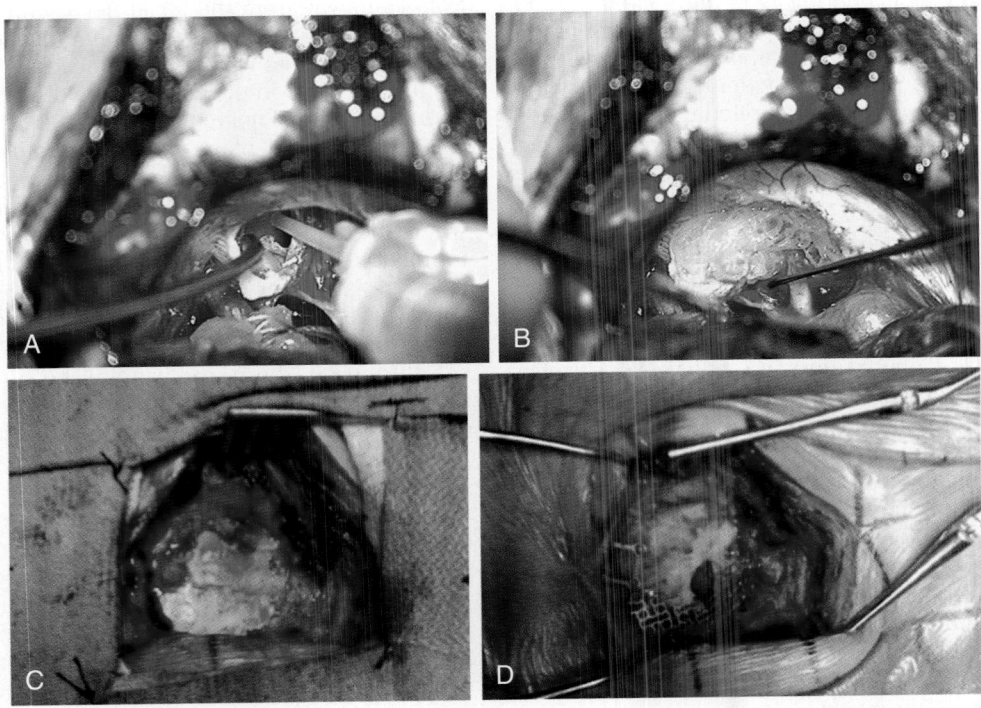

FIGURE 45-4 Closure. A, The tumor has been removed, but the facial and cochlear nerves have been spared. The large air cell is filled with some Tisseel via a syringe. A few small pieces of adipose tissue removed from a small incision in the abdomen will then be placed within the air cell. B, The drilled bone of the internal auditory canal has been waxed, and the entire canal is filled with a larger piece of adipose tissue, which is then further secured to the surrounding dural with Surgicel and Tisseel. C, The previously removed pericranial tissue is used to repair the dural defect in a watertight manner using a running suture of 4-0 Vicryl. Two central dural tenting sutures are placed. D, The previously removed craniotomy bone plate is reinserted in the superior–lateral portion of the defect and held in place with a superiorly placed miniplate and screws to avoid placing screws into mastoid air cells. Medially, a preformed titanium cranioplasty plate is secured both to the surrounding bone and to the craniotomy bone plate to obtain a firm construct to which the dural tenting sutures are then secured.

plus mechanical means of verifying facial nerve stimulation or damage. Because the surgeries at center 2 occurred between the two surgical periods at center 1, changes that might occur with a later period are negated. In all, 164 patients (82%) underwent the suboccipital approach using the techniques noted earlier. (The others were done via the middle fossa or translabyrinthine approaches but are not the subject of this chapter.) Outcomes of vestibular schwannoma surgery, including facial nerve function, hearing preservation, neurologic function (other cranial nerves, cerebellar function, and gait) and postoperative complications, were evaluated.

All patients who had NF2, intentional partial removal, prior vestibular schwannoma surgery, significant preoperative facial nerve dysfunction, or inadequate follow-up and 21 patients whose complete medical records could not be retrieved were excluded from this series.

Hearing function preoperatively and postoperatively was classified using the Hanover classification.[5] In cases where the speech discrimination score and pure tone average differed, the lower of the two was used to determine the patients' hearing grade. The correlation between tumor size and hearing preservation, as well as preoperative hearing class and hearing preservation, were assessed. Regression and analysis of variance were performed utilizing the Minitab statistical software.

Facial nerve function was determined at multiple time points whenever possible using the House-Brackmann facial nerve outcome scale.[10] Tumors were classified as large (more than 3 cm), medium (2.1 to 3 cm), and small (no more than 2 cm),[8] as measured from maximal diameter on MRI or CT image. Neurologic function of cranial nerves V, VI, IX, X, and XII; cerebellar function; and gait were assessed. The postoperative improvement is reported as a percentage of preoperative symptomatic patients who experienced improvement or resolution of their symptoms. Postoperative complications are reported as a percentage of that patient subgroup, as categorized by tumor size.

INTRAOPERATIVE MONITORING TECHNOLOGIES

Hearing Assessment

In both centers, BAERs were measured in response to click stimuli to the ipsilateral ear. In center 1 only, the response to clicks of the auditory nerve was also measured via electrocochleogram (EcochG) using a transtympanic needle electrode resting in the bony prominence or, more recently, an extratympanic electrode (a cotton wick) resting on the exterior surface of the tympanic membrane.[9] The standard methodology is to apply clicks to the ipsilateral ear via a special earphone (tube insert) and a low-level (60 dB typically) white noise via a similar earphone to the contralateral ear. Responses to the click stimuli are added, averaged, and noted in the BAER. If EcochG is available, the primary response (N1) corresponding to the auditory significance is the amplitude and latency of wave V in the BAER if present and the amplitude of N1 in the EcochG. Irreversible loss of N1 is often associated with an irreversible postoperative hearing loss (deafness). The status of wave V in the BAER is not perfect in predicting hearing status but we have found that if it is unchanged at the end of surgery, hearing is usually good.

Facial Nerve Monitoring

In both centers, standard EMG measurements were continually assessed from selected muscles in the face that are innervated by the ipsilateral facial nerve (orbicularis oculi and orbicularis oris). Intraoperative nerve stimulation was performed with a monopolar handheld probe. At center 1, in addition to EMG, I monitored facial nerve function mechanically with either a closed-circuit camera alone or such a camera in conjunction with a midface motion sensor.

HEARING PRESERVATION

Hearing preservation was analyzed in patients who underwent the suboccipital approach for large, medium, and small tumors. Tumor size was negatively correlated with postoperative hearing preservation ($p \leq 0.003$) (Table 45-1). Preoperative hearing class was positively correlated with postoperative hearing preservation ($p \leq 0.001$). Important to the patient in situations of daily living is preservation of hearing with 40% or greater speech discrimination (H1 to H3). Patients with medium and small tumors who presented with preoperative hearing ranging from class H1 to class H3 and were operated on by the suboccipital approach had a 6/13 (46%) and 31/38 (82%) chance, respectively, that their hearing would be maintained within hearing classes H1 to H3. Comparison of patients with small tumors and preoperative hearing ranging from class H1 to class H3 who were operated on by the suboccipital approach revealed no difference in hearing preservation between center 1 (11/13 = 85%) and center 2 (20/24 = 83%). In evaluable patients with small tumors operated on with the middle fossa approach ($n = 9$) during this same period, 78% had hearing preservation, which was not statistically different from the result of small tumors using the suboccipital approach (82%). However, all "small" tumors operated by the middle fossa approach were strictly intrameatal tumors, whereas those operated by the suboccipital approach included larger tumors up to a maximal diameter of 2 cm.

FACIAL NERVE PRESERVATION

Of the 164 patients operated by the suboccipital route, tumor size was negatively correlated with favorable facial nerve outcome or positively correlated with House-Brackmann facial nerve grade; that is, large tumors were associated with worse House-Brackmann grades immediately postoperatively ($p \leq 0.04$), at 2 to 3 months postoperatively ($p \leq 0.02$), and at 2 to 3 years postoperatively ($p \leq 0.02$). The impact of size of the vestibular schwannoma on facial nerve preservation employing the suboccipital approach assessed at three time points is seen in Table 45-1. In general, with a smaller tumor size, the facial nerve outcome is better.

DIFFERENCE IN FACIAL NERVE OUTCOMES BETWEEN VESTIBULAR SCHWANNOMAS OPERATED ON AT THE TWO CENTERS USING DIFFERING FACIAL MONITORING TECHNIQUES

Facial nerve outcomes for patients who underwent unilateral vestibular schwannoma surgery via the suboccipital approach by me were assessed at various time points. Compared to patients with large tumors operated on at center 2, a significantly higher proportion of patients with large tumors operated on at center 1 had grade I facial nerve outcomes

Table 45-1	Facial Nerve Grade Following Vestibular Schwannoma Surgery by Suboccipital Approach at Center 1											
	POSTOPERATIVE				**2-3 MONTHS**				**2-3 YEARS**			
	Grade I	Grade II	Grade III-IV	Grade V-VI	Grade I	Grade II	Grade III-IV	Grade V-VI	Grade I	Grade II	Grade III-IV	Grade V-VI
Tumor Size												
Large	14 (50%)	6 (21%)	4 (14%)	4 (14%)	16 (55%)	5 (17%)	4 (14%)	4 (14%)	17 (77%)	1 (5%)	4 (18%)	0
Medium	15 (65%)	3 (13%)	1 (4%)	4 (17%)	13 (72%)	2 (11%)	3 (17%)	0	13 (93%)	1 (7%)	0	0
Small	19 (86%)	1 (5%)	1 (5%)	1 (5%)	17 (89%)	1 (5%)	1 (5%)	0	12 (100%)	0	0	0

immediately postoperatively (50% vs. 31%) ($p = 0.03$), 2 to 3 months postoperatively (55% vs. 35%) ($p = 0.02$), and 2 to 3 years postoperatively (77% vs. 53%) ($p = 0.01$). A higher proportion of patients with medium-sized tumors operated on at center 1 had grade I facial nerve outcomes at 2 to 3 years postoperatively compared to patients with medium-sized tumors operated on at center 2 (93% vs. 73%) ($p = 0.03$). For small tumors, there was no significant difference in facial nerve outcome at any time point between the two centers.

Outcomes for Cranial Nerves, Cerebellar Function, and Gait following Vestibular Schwannoma Surgery

Outcomes for cranial nerves V, VI, IX, X, and XII; cerebellar function; and gait were assessed following vestibular schwannoma surgery, as demonstrated in Table 45-2. In patients operated on by the suboccipital approach, preoperative trigeminal nerve symptoms of decreased facial and corneal sensation were most frequent among patients with large tumors. Postoperative resolution of symptoms was observed in the majority of patients. Diplopia from abducens nerve dysfunction (diplopia) was observed preoperatively in two patients with large tumors, and these resolved following surgery. However, one patient with a large tumor and normal preoperative abducens nerve function developed diplopia postoperatively. Lower cranial nerve dysfunction as manifested by decreased gag reflex and dysphagia was observed preoperatively in one patient harboring a large tumor, and this resolved following resection via the suboccipital approach. One patient with a large tumor and normal preoperative lower cranial nerve function developed postoperative symptoms. Hypoglossal nerve dysfunction manifested by tongue deviation was also observed in only one patient preoperatively who harbored a large tumor, and this resolved postoperatively following resection via the suboccipital route.

Cerebellar and/or vestibular dysfunction, as manifested by ataxia and an abnormal Romberg test, was directly related to tumor size. Preoperative cerebellar and/or vestibular dysfunction was observed in 37% of patients harboring a large tumor, 24% of patients harboring a medium tumor, and 6% of patients harboring a small tumor operated on by the suboccipital approach. Postoperative improvement following resection via the suboccipital approach was demonstrated in 55% of patients with large tumors, 73% of

patients with medium tumors, and 100% of patients with small tumors. Preoperative gait dysfunction was directly correlated to tumor size. Preoperative gait dysfunction was observed in 37% of patients with large tumors, 20% of patients with medium tumors, and 2% of patients with small tumors operated on by the suboccipital approach. Postoperative improvement was observed in the majority of patients.

Other Complications

Overall, as noted in Table 45-3, the incidence of postoperative CSF leak for patients who underwent the suboccipital approach was 5.5% (large tumors 7.4%, medium tumors 2.2%, and small tumors 6.2%). Of the patients who underwent the suboccipital approach and developed CSF leaks, only one patient required repeat surgery with obliteration of the mastoid air cells with an adipose graft; the rest of the patients were treated with lumbar subarachnoid drains, which led to resolution of the leak.

The other significant complications occurred exclusively in patients with large tumors. Wound infection occurred in one patient with a large tumor who suffered from *Staphylococcal meningitis* and was successfully treated with nafcillin and metronidazole. A posterior fossa cyst occurred postoperatively in one patient with a large tumor who also developed hydrocephalus. The hydrocephalus in this patient was successfully treated with a ventriculoperitoneal shunt; the cyst was then asymptomatic.

Postoperative cerebellar hematoma occurred in one patient with a large tumor. This was managed by posterior fossa reexploration for decompression and hematoma removal with good recovery.

One intraoperative technical complication was documented for a patient with a large tumor and with an aberrant extracranial vertebral artery that was entered during the muscle dissection of surgical opening. The vertebral artery was ligated and the operation stopped. There were no adverse effects postoperatively. The tumor resection was done several weeks later without incident.

There were no deaths in this series.

Conclusions

We are now in an era where multiple alternatives for the treatment of vestibular schwannomas exist. These include three surgical approaches, fractionated radiotherapy, and three single-fraction radiosurgery techniques (gamma knife, linear accelerator, and proton beam). If surgery is

Table 45-2 Preoperative Deficits and Postoperative Status of Trigeminal, Abducens, and Glossopharyngeal Cranial Nerves; Cerebellar or Vestibular Function; and Gait*

Tumor Size	CN V Preop.	CN V Postop. Improved	CN V Postop. Worse	CN VI Preop.	CN VI Postop. Improved	CN VI Postop. Worse	CN IX and X Preop.	CN IX and X Postop. Improved	CN IX and X Postop. Worse	CN XII Preop. Deviation	CN XII Postop. Improved	CN XII Postop. Worse	Cerebellar/Vestibular Function Preop.	Cerebellar/Vestibular Function Postop. Improved	Cerebellar/Vestibular Function Postop. Worse	Gait Preop.	Gait Postop. Improved	Gait Postop. Worse
Large	27 (50%)	21 (78%)	0	2 (4%)	2 (100%)	1 (2%)	1 (2%)	1 (100%)	1 (2%)	1 (2%)	1 (100%)	0	20 (37%)	11 (55%)	1 (2%)	20 (37%)	12 (60%)	0
Medium	9 (20%)	5 (56%)	0	0	0	0	0	0	0	0	0	0	11 (24%)	8 (73%)	0	9 (20%)	5 (56%)	0
Small	3 (4.6%)	2 (67%)	0	0	0	0	0	0	0	0	0	0	4 (6%)	4 (100%)	0	1 (2%)	1 (100%)	0
Total SOC	39 (24%)	28 (72%)	0	2 (1%)	2 (100%)	1 (1%)	1 (1%)	1 (100%)	1 (1%)	1 (1%)	1 (100%)	0	35 (21%)	23 (66%)	1 (1%)	30 (18%)	18 (60%)	0

*Preoperative deficits are presented as a percentage of the entire suboccipital subgroup. Postoperative percentages of improvement are presented as percentages of the preoperative symptomatic patients in this subgroup. Postoperative new deficits are presented as percentages of the total subgroup.
CN V, trigeminal nerve (functions tested: facial and corneal sensation); CN VI, abducens (functions assessed: diplopia and ocular movement abnormality); CN IX and X, glossopharyngeal and vagus (functions assessed: dysphagia, hoarseness, or decreased gag reflex); CN XII, hypoglossal (functions tested: tongue protrudes midline or deviation on right–left movement); SOC, suboccipital craniotomy.

Table 45-3 Complications Other Than Cranial Nerve Dysfunction in 164 Cases Following Vestibular Schwannoma Surgery by the Suboccipital Route

Tumor Size	CSF Leak	Wound Infection	Posterior Fossa Cyst	Hematoma	Hydrocephalus	Technical	Death
Large	4 (7.4%)	1 (1.9%)	1 (1.9%)	1 (1.9%)	1 (1.9%)	1 (1.9%)	0
Medium	1 (2.2%)	0	0	0	0	0	0
Small	4 (6.2%)	0	0	0	0	0	0
Total	9 (5.5%)	1 (0.6%)	1 (0.6%)	1 (0.6%)	1 (0.6%)	1 (0.6%)	0

the chosen method of treatment, the operative approach should be dictated by tumor size and location and the preoperative hearing status of patients. I have used the suboccipital approach for large and medium-sized tumors and even for small tumors in patients with preserved hearing. I considered the translabyrinthine approach for certain medium and small tumors in patients with loss of hearing. Some surgeons use the translabyrinthine approach even for large tumors when hearing is absent. However, I feel there are several benefits to employing the suboccipital approach: it affords the ability to remove a tumor of any size, to preserve cranial nerve function, and to better visualize the brain stem and its vascular supply. I find that the middle fossa approach is best suited when hearing preservation is desired and the tumor is strictly intracanalicular, especially for those with lateral extension.

Hearing preservation is inversely related to tumor size[1,4,8,11-19] and is most likely in patients with small tumors (less than or equal to 2 cm) and with good preoperative hearing. I have found no statistical difference in hearing preservation whether or not an EcochG is used. Therefore, I currently use only a BAER and no longer use a transtympanic electrode.

Functional preservation of the facial nerve is inversely correlated to tumor size. Over the follow-up period, improvement was observed in patients with all three tumor sizes, emphasizing that if anatomic preservation of the facial nerve is achieved and care is taken to minimize intraoperative injury, excellent long-term outcomes can be achieved even with large tumors. Normal facial nerve outcomes were achieved in a significantly higher proportion of large tumors at all periods and in medium tumors at 2 to 3 years at center 1, where both a mechanical and an electric means of monitoring were utilized. These results stress the importance of intraoperative facial nerve monitoring techniques, which significantly affect facial nerve outcome. Although electrode monitoring of facial nerve function is sensitive and essential to this operation, in multiple cases I noted that the mechanical methods could detect facial movement in the absence of detection by the electrodes. In addition, electrode monitors can be ineffective during use of bipolar cautery, although this does not affect the mechanical systems. For this reason, I routinely use a video monitor, in addition to electric monitoring on all cases.

ACKNOWLEDGMENTS

The author thanks Saad A. Khan, MD, and Asad Khan, PhD, for their help with preparation of the data used in this manuscript and Joseph B. Nadol, MD, and Michael J. McKenna, MD, for their assistance with some surgical procedures and the development of some surgical concepts and monitoring techniques. The author particularly thanks Robert G. Ojemann[20] for his initial instruction in these operative techniques.

KEY REFERENCES

Arriaga MA, Chen DA, Fukushima T. Individualizing hearing preservation in acoustic neuroma surgery. *Laryngoscope.* 1997;107:1043-1047.

Delgado TE, Bucheit WA, Rosenholtz HR, Chrissian S. Intraoperative monitoring of facial muscle evoked responses obtained by intracranial stimulation of the facial nerve: a more accurate technique for facial nerve dissection. *Neurosurgery.* 1979;4(5):418-421.

Ebersold MJ, Harner SG, Beatty CW, et al. Current results of the retrosigmoid approach to acoustic neuroma. *J Neurosurg.* 1992;76(6): 901-909.

Fischer G, Fischer C, Remond J. Hearing preservation in acoustic neuroma surgery. *J Neurosurg.* 1992;76:910-917.

Gardner G, Robertson JH. Hearing preservation in unilateral acoustic neuroma surgery. Annals of Otology. *Rhinology & Laryngology.* 1988;97(1):55-66.

House JW. Brackmann DE. Facial nerve grading system. *Otolaryngology—Head & Neck Surgery.* 1985;93(2):146-147.

Levine RA, Ronner SF, Ojemann RG. Auditory evoked potentials and other neurophysiological monitoring techniques during tumor surgery in the cerebellopontine angle. In: Lotus CM, Traynelis VC, eds. *Intraoperative Monitoring Technique During Tumor Surgery in the Cerebellopontine Angle.* New York: McGraw-Hill; 1994:175-192.

Moffat DA, da Cruz MJ, Baguley DM, et al. Hearing preservation in solitary vestibular schwannoma surgery using the retrosigmoid approach. *Otolaryngol Head Neck Surg.* 1999;121(6):781-788.

Nadol Jr JB, Chiong CM, Ojemann RG, et al. Preservation of hearing and facial nerve function in resection of acoustic neuroma. *Laryngoscope.* 1992;102(10):1153-1158.

Ojemann RG. Management of acoustic neuromas (vestibular schwannomas). *Clinical Neurosurgery.* 1993;40:498-535.

Ojemann RG, Martuza RL. Acoustic neuroma. In: Youmans J, ed. *Neurological Surgery.* 3rd ed. Philadelphia. Ch: WB Saunders Co. 1990; 113: 3316-3350.

Rand AW, Kurze T. Facial nerve preservation by posterior fossa transmeatal microdissection in total removal of acoustic neuroma. *J Neurolo Neurosurg Psychiatry.* 1965;28:311-316.

Rhoton Jr AL. Microsurgical removal of acoustic neuromas. *Surgical Neurology.* 1976;6(4):211-219.

Samii M. Microneurosurgery of acoustic neuromas with emphasis on preservation of seventh and eighth nerves and scope of facial nerve grafting. In: Rand RW, ed. *Microsurgery.* St. Louis: CV. Mosby Co.; 1985:366-388.

Samii M, Matthies C. Management of 1000 vestibular schwannomas (acoustic neuromas): the facial nerve—preservation and restitution of function. *Neurosurg.* 1997;40(4):684-694.

Samii M, Matthies C. Management of 1000 vestibular schwannomas (acoustic neuromas): hearing function in 1000 tumor resections. *Neurosurg.* 1997;40(2):248-260.

Sampath P, Holliday MJ, Brem H, et al. Facial nerve injury in acoustic neuroma (vestibular schwannoma) surgery: etiology and prevention. *J Neurosurg.* 1997;87(1):60-66.

Sterkers JM, Morrison GA, Sterkers O, El-Dine MM. Preservation of facial, cochlear, and other nerve functions in acoustic neuroma treatment. *Otolaryngology—Head & Neck Surgery.* 1994;110(2):146-155.

Strauss C, Fahlbusch R, Berg M, Haid T. Function saving microsurgery in suboccipital removal of large acoustic neuromas. *HNO.* 1989;37(7):281-286:[German].

Tatagiba M, Samii M, Matthies C, et al. The significance for postoperative hearing of preserving the labyrinth in acoustic neurinoma surgery. *J Neurosurg.* 1992;77(5):677-684.

Wiegand DA, Fickel V. Acoustic neuroma—the patient's perspective: subjective assessment of symptoms, diagnosis, therapy, and outcome in 541 patients. *Laryngoscope.* 1989;99(2):179-187.

Numbered references appear on Expert Consult.

CHAPTER 46

Translabyrinthine Approach to Vestibular Schwannomas

LARS POULSGAARD

Vestibular schwannomas can be surgically accessed via a subtemporal, a translabyrinthine, or a suboccipital and retrosigmoid approach.[1,2] The number of centers that have mastered all approaches has increased. The translabyrinthine approach was reintroduced approximately 35 years ago[3] and is successfully used by several otologic specialist centers.[4-6] After developments in skull base surgery, neurosurgeons have become aware of the advantages of the translabyrinthine approach for vestibular schwannomas and for other skull base lesions.

Advantages of the Translabyrinthine Approach

The most obvious advantages of the translabyrinthine route that it offers a direct approach to the cerebellopontine angle and that the cerebellum requires a minimum of retraction. The tumor is lifted away from the brain stem, avoiding pressure on the brain stem and cerebellum.

It has been stated that the usefulness of the translabyrinthine approach is limited to small tumors. In fact, no tumor is too large to be approached by the translabyrinthine route.[7-9] In large and giant tumors, it is a significant advantage to be able to go directly to the center of the tumor; after debulking the center of the tumor, the neoplasm collapses and is displaced toward the opening by the surrounding brain structure.

The procedure offers excellent exposure of the lateral end of the internal auditory meatus and allows identification of the facial nerve as it enters the fallopian canal. This identification ensures complete tumor removal from that area and the best chance to preserve the facial nerve.

I find it convenient that two surgeons may help each other in the removal of the tumor. As pointed out later, this approach offers two surgeons comfortable placement during a lengthy procedure.

Disadvantages of the Translabyrinthine Approach

The translabyrinthine procedure destroys the labyrinth and, as a consequence, hearing. This approach is not used if preservation of hearing is attempted. Only a limited number of patients with vestibular schwannomas have hearing worth preserving, however. If the tumor exceeds 2 cm in size, the chances of preserving hearing are known to be poor.[10]

If the patient has had active otitis media in the past, the approach involves crossing a potentially infected field, and alternative exposure should be considered. In the case of a mastoid cavity, a total obliteration with blind sac closure of the external auditory canal should be performed and healed before the translabyrinthine approach can be done. Finally, the procedure is generally more time consuming than the suboccipital or middle fossa approach, which must be considered if a limited duration of the operation is desirable.

Surgical Anatomy

The bone opening for the translabyrinthine approach is done in the mastoid part of the temporal bone (Fig. 46-1). The mastoid is filled with air cells, and the air cells are connected to the middle ear through the tympanic antrum. In the translabyrinthine approach, the bone is removed between the sigmoid sinus and the external ear canal. The sigmoid sinus is located in the sigmoid sulcus in the temporal bone. From the posterior aspect of the sigmoid sinus, emissary veins run through the mastoid foramen to subgaleal veins.[11-13]

Removing the air cells creates a space that is bounded posteriorly by the wall of the sigmoid sulcus, superiorly by the tegmen tympani, and anteriorly by the prominence of the lateral semicircular canal. Above the prominence of the lateral semicircular canal, the antrum communicates with the tympanic cavity. The facial canal runs close to the mastoid wall of the tympanic cavity. The genu of the facial canal is just inferior to the lateral semicircular canal, and it continues inferiorly to emerge below the skull base at the stylomastoid foramen (Fig. 46-2). The sigmoid sulcus meets the roof of the cavity at a sharp sinodural angle from which the superior petrosal sulcus runs anteriorly. When removing the bone in the sinodural angle, the superior petrosal sinus is exposed in a dural duplex.

The lateral semicircular canal is an important landmark for the location of the entire labyrinth. After removing all three semicircular canals, the vestibule is open. The vestibule is the bone cavity that harbors the soft-tissue part of

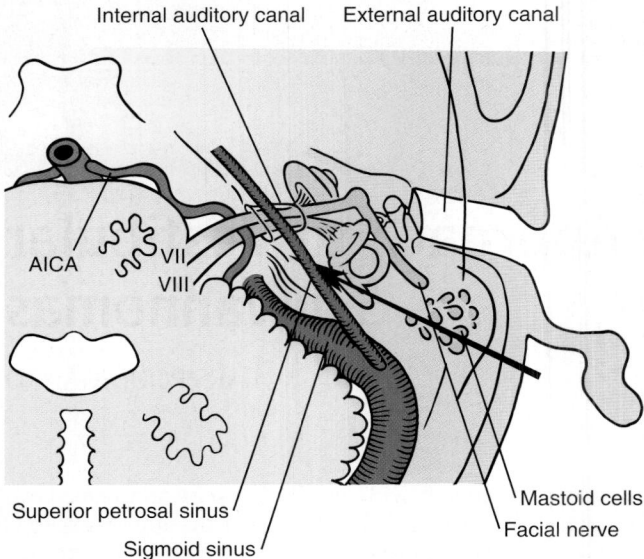

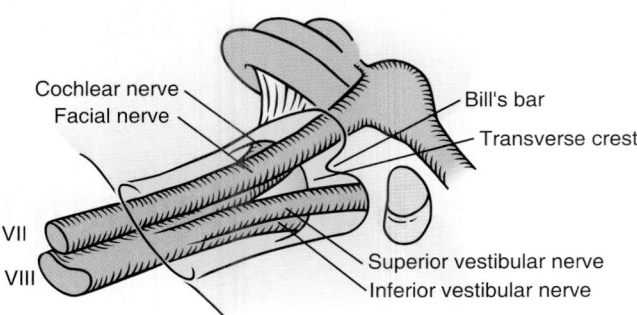

FIGURE 46-3 Contents of the internal acoustic canal, which shows the relation of the facial nerve to Bill's bar.

FIGURE 46-1 Approach to the cerebellopontine angle through the mastoid and labyrinth. The arrow indicates the surgical view after an extended mastoidectomy.

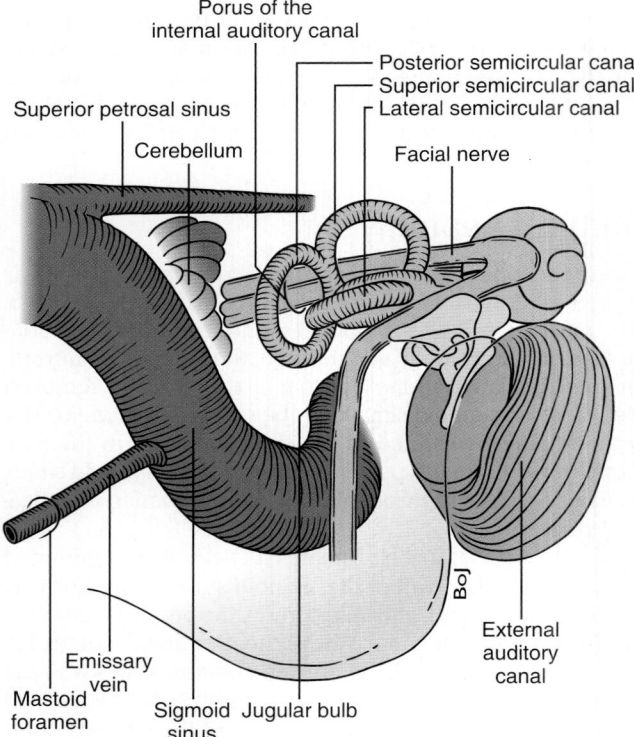

FIGURE 46-2 Relationship of the labyrinth, the internal acoustic canal, the facial nerve, and the sigmoid sinus.

the labyrinth utricle and saccule. Through the aperture of the vestibular aqueduct runs the endolymphatic duct that connects the utricle to the endolymphatic sac. The internal auditory canal contains four separate nerves: two vestibular nerves, the facial nerve, and the cochlear nerve. Located laterally are the superior and inferior vestibular nerves separated at the fundus by a bony crest called the transverse crest. Anterior to the superior vestibular nerve, the facial nerve enters the fallopian canal. Laterally, the facial nerve is separated from the superior vestibular nerve by a small vertical bony septum called the vertical crest or Bill's bar (Fig. 46-3).

Most vestibular schwannomas arise from one of the vestibular nerves in the internal auditory canal. The facial nerve is often displaced in the internal auditory canal, and its location may vary. The nerve can always be identified laterally in the internal auditory canal.

After maximal translabyrinthine bone removal and opening of the dura, the cerebellopontine angle with its nerves and vessels is seen. Superiorly, the exit of cranial nerve V is seen on the pontine surface near the cerebellum. The exits of cranial nerves VI, VII, and VIII are located on a vertical line on the medulla oblongata near the crossing to the pons. The exit of the cranial nerve VIII is just anterior and superior to the flocculus. The entry zone for the abducens nerve is anteriorly on the medulla oblongata. It runs in a superior direction anteriorly on the pons to enter the Dorello canal.

The blood vessels in the cerebellopontine angle display greater variability than do the nerves. The posterior–inferior cerebellar artery emerges from the vertebral artery. Loop formations of this artery are often seen to extend cranially to the level of cranial nerves VIII and IX, and in these cases, it may be seen using the translabyrinthine approach. The anterior–inferior cerebellar artery extends from the basilar artery, and in most cases, it forms a loop that protrudes against or into the internal auditory canal. From the loop of the anterior–inferior cerebellar artery, the labyrinthine and the subarcuate arteries extend.

Preparation for Surgery

A cephalosporin is given intravenously just before surgery and repeated every 3 hours. The patient is placed in a supine position on the operating table. The patient's head is turned toward the opposite side and maintained in position with a Sugita head frame. Excessive rotation of the head should be avoided because it may cause venous obstruction in the neck. Decreased mobility of the neck in elderly patients may make sufficient rotation of the head difficult to achieve. This problem may be solved by lifting the ipsilateral shoulder with a pillow and by rotating the whole table.

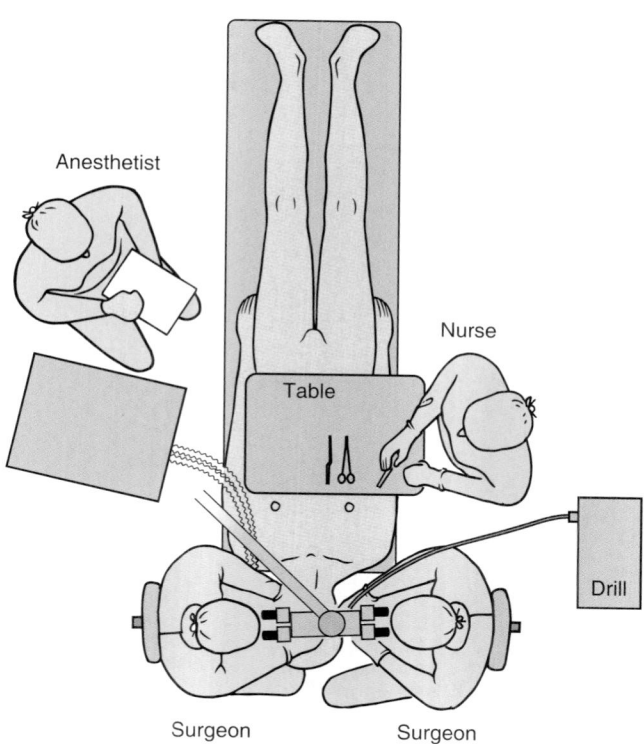

FIGURE 46-4 Room arrangement for the translabyrinthine approach. Note the positions of the two surgeons. Both have comfortable access to the microscope.

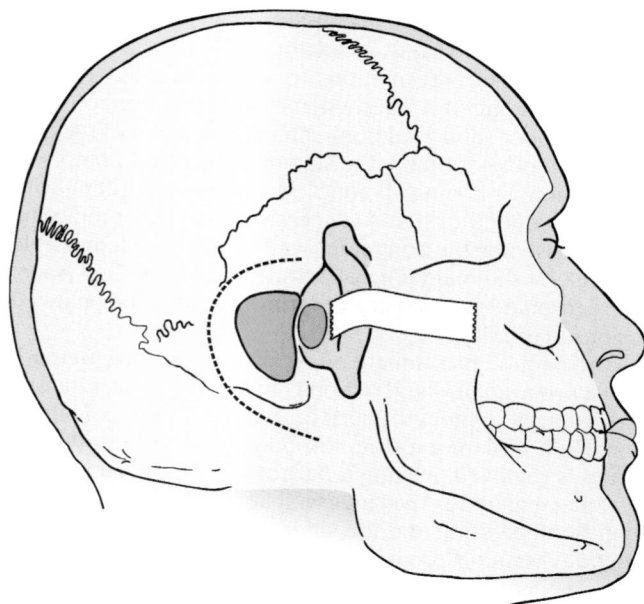

FIGURE 46-5 Skin incision behind the right ear. The area planned for a mastoidectomy is indicated.

Continuous electrophysiologic monitoring of facial nerve function is performed during the operation.[14-16] This monitoring has become an established procedure and is mandatory in my operations. To accomplish this, electrodes are placed in the frontal and oral orbicular muscles. We use a floor-standing operating microscope with the two surgeons sitting opposite each other on each side of the patient's head. This setup enables both surgeons to be in a comfortable sitting position with a direct view in the microscope. The lead surgeon sits on the same side as the tumor. In left-sided tumors, the drill is placed between the two surgeons, and in right-sided tumors, the drill is placed between the scrub nurse and the surgeon on the right side (Fig. 46-4). The anesthesiologist is placed at the lower left side of the table at the level of the hip of the patient.

The surgical view of the cerebellopontine angle occurs along the posterior fossa dura. It is limited posteriorly by the sigmoid sinus and anteriorly by the horizontal part of the facial nerve. The operating microscope can be moved in all directions, and the table can be tilted in all directions, which ensures visualization of all surgical planes.

Surgical Procedure

Although some surgeons advocate routine cannulation of the lateral ventricle to relieve hydrocephalus or prevent surgically induced hydrocephalus, I do not find this necessary because, even in large tumors, it is easy to access the cistern magna beneath the tumor, open the arachnoid, and allow cerebrospinal fluid (CSF) to drain. The skin incision is made using the cutting cautery to decrease the amount of bleeding from the skin. The incision starts at the upper edge

of the helix, superior to the linea temporalis; it continues 4 to 5 cm posteriorly, turns inferiorly, and ends near the tip of the mastoid process (Fig. 46-5).

The incision is made first only through the skin. Second, a curved incision is made in the muscle fascia and pericranium. This incision is made similar to but with a smaller radius than the skin incision. This procedure enables a watertight closure of the muscle fascia and pericranium layer. The skin and muscle/pericranium layer is elevated and turned anteriorly over the auricle, where it is covered with a piece of moist gauze and fixed with hooks attached to the Sugita head frame. Because of the size of the skin incision, it is not necessary to retract the skin at the superior, posterior, or inferior margin.

MASTOIDECTOMY

An extended mastoidectomy is performed with removal of bone over the sigmoid sinus and the middle cranial fossa (Fig. 46-5). In cases with an anteriorly placed sigmoid sinus or large tumors, I also remove bone over the posterior cranial fossa behind the sigmoid sinus.[17,18] The extended bone removal ensures good visualization of the entire surgical field. The power drill, driven by either an electric motor or an air turbine, is an essential tool in the translabyrinthine procedure. The cortical bone covering the mastoid region is removed by a large cutting drill. In cases with pronounced pneumatization, a large hole can be made quickly and safely. The anterior margin for cortical bone removal is just behind the external ear canal. The opening is gradually widened backward to the sigmoid sinus and upward to the dura in the middle cranial fossa. Removal of bone over the sigmoid sinus must be done carefully. If the cutting drill tears the sigmoid sinus, profuse bleeding ensues, requiring packing with Surgicel or direct suture of the sinus wall. Large emissary veins often drain into the posterior aspect of the sigmoid sinus. They can be identified through the bone as it is removed. The emissary veins must be controlled with bipolar coagulation and are filled with bone wax. With a drill, the sigmoid sinus is skeletonized.

There are several methods to skeletonize the sigmoid sinus, including the eggshell method, creation of Bill's island of bone, and total bone removal. The aim of the eggshell method is to make the sigmoid sinus wall compressible without removing all bone. By continuous drilling with a large diamond drill and successive pressing of the bone with a dissector, the bony sinus wall becomes compressible because of the many microfractures in the eggshell bone. The preserved periosteum covering the sinus helps avoid lesions in the sinus.

The method recommended by House and Hitselberger[19] is to leave a small island of bone (Bill's island) over the sigmoid sinus to protect the surface from the trauma of retraction. With a diamond drill, the bone around the outlined island is removed, leaving a part of the sinus wall with an oval piece of bone. The sinus wall and the bony island can then be depressed, and the sinus wall that corresponds to the bony island is protected. I find this method less appropriate because of the risk of lesions in the sinus wall that may be produced by the sharp edge of the bony island.

I prefer total bone removal. This method is initiated by carefully drilling away all bone covering a small part of the sinus. Through this hole, the adjacent sinus wall can be depressed with a Freer elevator, and the edge of the bone can safely be removed with Kerrison bone punches without damage of the sinus wall. This method ensures an easily compressible sinus wall.

With blunt dissection, the adjacent dura in the middle and posterior cranial fossa is loosened, and the remaining bone may be removed by either bone punches or drilling.

LABYRINTHECTOMY

As soon as the mastoid cortical bone has been removed and the sigmoid sinus and the middle fossa dura have been outlined, the operating microscope is used. The facial nerve is an important landmark, and its position must be established early in the surgical dissection. After skeletonizing the middle fossa dura, the antrum is opened, and the compact bone of the labyrinth is visualized.

It is essential to open the antrum and to identify the lateral semicircular canal (Fig. 46-6). This canal is a main landmark, and once the positions of this canal and of the antrum are known, the three-dimensional anatomy of the facial nerve is known. After identification of the facial nerve, the labyrinthectomy is performed. The bone in the sinodural angle is removed, followed by opening along the superior petrosal sinus until the labyrinthine bone is encountered. The lateral semicircular canal is drilled away until the ampulla is reached anteriorly. Then the posterior and superior semicircular canals are identified and removed to their entrance in the vestibule. After opening of the vestibule, the facial nerve is skeletonized from the genu inferiorly to near the stylomastoid foramen. It is not necessary to remove all bone around the nerve. I always make a small window in the fallopian canal near the second genu to ensure the position of the nerve and to ensure correct function of the facial nerve monitoring device. To avoid injury to the facial nerve, a thin, eggshell bone is left on the nerve. Only posteriorly, where access is needed to approach the cerebellopontine angle, is the nerve exposed.

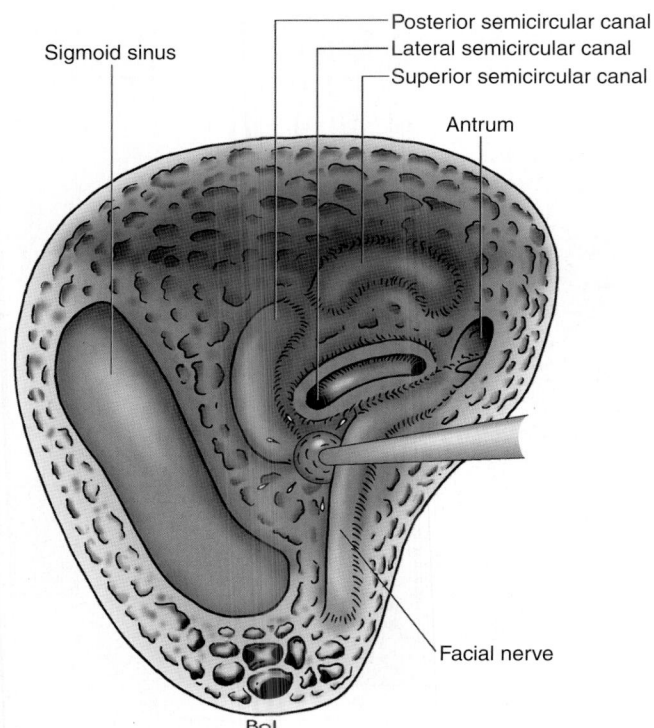

FIGURE 46-6 The facial nerve and the sigmoid sinus have been skeletonized. The lateral semicircular canal is opened.

After removal of all semicircular canals, the labyrinthectomy is completed, and the vestibule is opened. The endolymphatic duct must be excised from the endolymphatic sac on the posterior fossa dura. The vestibule is removed, and the cribriform area in the saccule marks the most lateral extent of the internal auditory meatus. In the center of the labyrinth, the subarcuate artery is located, and it is usually bleeding when it is opened by the drill.

INTERNAL AUDITORY CANAL DISSECTION

The dura of the internal auditory canal is identified posteriorly, where it continues as the dura of the posterior cranial fossa. The dura at the opening of the canal can be loosened from the bone with slightly bent sharp dissectors. The bone around the canal is gently removed with a diamond drill. A more than 180-degree arc of bone around the canal is removed. At this point, the surgeon must remove as much bone as possible on both sides below and above the meatus, because this helps in accessing the superior and inferior borders of the tumor. Care is taken not to open the dura covering the nerves and tumor in the canal. If the dura is accidentally damaged, the facial nerve should be identified by stimulation.

All bone between the internal meatus and the jugular bulb is removed. The location of the jugular bulb is extremely variable. When its position is low, all bone removal necessary for tumor removal can be performed without seeing the jugular bulb. In other cases, its position is high and occurs as a bluish spot in the bone after removing the ampulla of the posterior semicircular canal. The surgeon should always be aware of the blue color of the jugular bulb when drilling medial to the facial nerve and inferior to the posterior semicircular canal. All bone covering the jugular bulb must be removed in cases with a high-positioned jugular bulb, in which the bulb is an obstacle to proper bone removal from the inferior aspect of the internal acoustic meatus.

The technique of bone removal from the jugular bulb is the same as described for the sigmoid sinus. With the egg-shell method, the bone can be thinned so much that the jugular bulb can be compressed and allow further removal of bone from the inferior part of the porus. Bone is removed until the cochlear aqueduct is identified. The cochlear aqueduct enters the posterior fossa directly inferior to the midportion of the internal auditory canal above the jugular bulb. It is an important landmark because it identifies the location of cranial nerves IX, X, and XI in the neural compartment of the jugular foramen. Bone dissection should be confined to the area superior to the cochlear aqueduct to avoid injury to these nerves. After removal of bone on the inferior part of the internal auditory canal, the dissection is carried out on the superior and anterior parts.

The facial nerve often underlies the dura along the anterior–superior aspect of the internal auditory canal, and extreme care must be taken not to allow the bur to slip into the canal. The facial nerve is especially vulnerable at this point. The lateral end of the internal auditory canal is divided by the transverse crest in an inferior and a superior compartment (Fig. 46-7). The bone around the inferior compartment can be drilled away to the most lateral extent of the canal without risk of facial nerve injury. In the superior compartment, bone removal allows identification of a bar of bone (Bill's bar), which separates the superior vestibular nerve from the facial nerve. The bone is removed at the porus and the medial part of the internal auditory canal first; the more difficult lateral part is left until last, when most of the bone removal has been completed.

All bone between the middle fossa dura and the internal auditory canal must be removed. With the visualization of the most lateral end of the internal auditory canal, the bone work is completed. Up to this point, all dissection has been extradural and the morbidity of the approach consequently low.

DURAL OPENING

The dural incision is started superiorly in the sinodural angle near the sigmoid sinus continuing down to the porus (see Fig. 46-7). Care is taken to avoid vessels on the surface of the tumor. Posteriorly, the petrosal vein lies just beneath the dura. This vein originates in the cerebellum and drains into the superior petrosal sinus near the level of the internal auditory canal. If the dura is pulled laterally with a small hook, the space between the cerebellum and the dura is enlarged, and injury to the vessels may be avoided. At the porus, a small incision is made on both sides of the porus. Around the porus, the dura often forms a distinct constriction ring that usually adheres to the surface of the tumor, and there are small vessels going from the dura to the tumor. The dural ring must be divided, and a further incision is made over the dura in the meatus. In the meatus, the dura is often extremely thin, and sometimes it is opened while removing the bone around the meatus. The small vessels in the thickened dura at the porus can be coagulated with bipolar coagulation. Cottonoids are advanced into the

plane between the tumor and the cerebellum. The surgeon must develop this plane accurately, because doing so separates the major vessels of the cerebellopontine angle from the tumor. To widen the opening, retractors are attached to the Sugita head frame and placed on the dura of the middle fossa and on a cottonoid on the cerebellum and the sigmoid sinus.

TUMOR REMOVAL

After opening the dura, the posterior part of the tumor is exposed. Rarely, the facial nerve may lie on the posterior surface of the tumor, and this surface must be carefully inspected for nerve bundles. In large tumors, it is essential to begin tumor removal with intracapsular debulking to reduce tumor size and subsequently develop the extracapsular dissection planes. In small tumors, the surgeon can readily identify the inferior and superior extracapsular dissection planes of the tumor. An ultrasonic aspirator is useful for debulking and removing intracapsular tumor.

IDENTIFICATION OF THE FACIAL NERVE IN THE FUNDUS OF THE INTERNAL AUDITORY CANAL

In approximately 15% of vestibular schwannomas, the fundus of the internal auditory canal is empty, and all four nerves are visible and easily recognizable. In these cases, bone work in the internal auditory canal does not need to be as extensive as described. The identification of the vertical crest (Bill's bar) is not necessary. Exact determination of the facial nerve is done with stimulation.

In the remaining cases, the fundus of the internal auditory canal is filled with tumor, and identification of the facial nerve is more difficult. During bone removal, the medial part of the fallopian canal is opened, which uncovers a labyrinthine segment of the facial nerve. Bill's bar separates the facial nerve anteriorly from the superior vestibular nerve. A fine hook is inserted lateral to Bill's bar and gently placed beneath the superior vestibular nerve and Bill's bar. The superior vestibular nerve can then be pulled out from its canal. Likewise, the two nerves inferior to the transverse crest (the inferior vestibular nerve and the cochlear nerve) are pulled out from their canals, along with the tumor (Fig. 46-8). Positive identification of the facial nerve at the lateral end of the internal auditory canal is one of the principal advantages of the translabyrinthine approach.

FREEING THE TUMOR FROM THE FACIAL NERVE IN THE INTERNAL AUDITORY CANAL

The arachnoid sheath completely surrounds the tumor, nerves, and vessels in the meatus, and the arachnoid strands that attach the facial nerve to the tumor must be divided. The meatal part of the tumor is gently retracted backward. Small hooks or fine microscissors are used to free the facial nerve from the arachnoid fibers that bind the nerve to the tumor. Because cutting of the arachnoid occurs along the facial nerve, the surgeon must have identified the inferior and the superior edges of the nerve accurately. Usually, it is relatively easy to develop the dissection plane between the facial nerve and the tumor in the internal auditory canal, but difficulties often arise at the porus. Around the entire circumference of the porus, dural adhesions to the tumor make dissection of the facial nerve from the tumor difficult. The exact position of the facial nerve in the porus

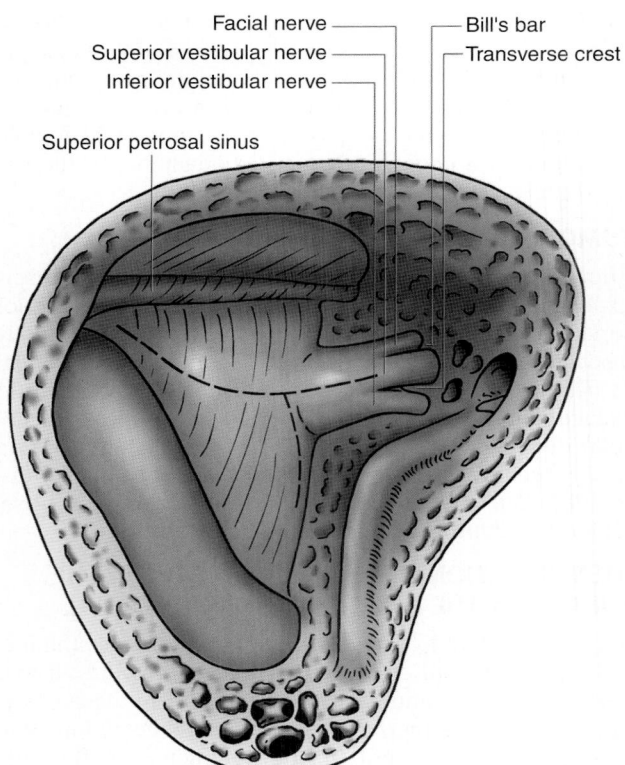

Facial nerve — Bill's bar
Superior vestibular nerve — Transverse crest
Inferior vestibular nerve —

Superior petrosal sinus

FIGURE 46-7 The mastoidectomy has been completed. The internal auditory canal is opened and allows the facial nerve to be identified. The broken lines indicate the dural incisions.

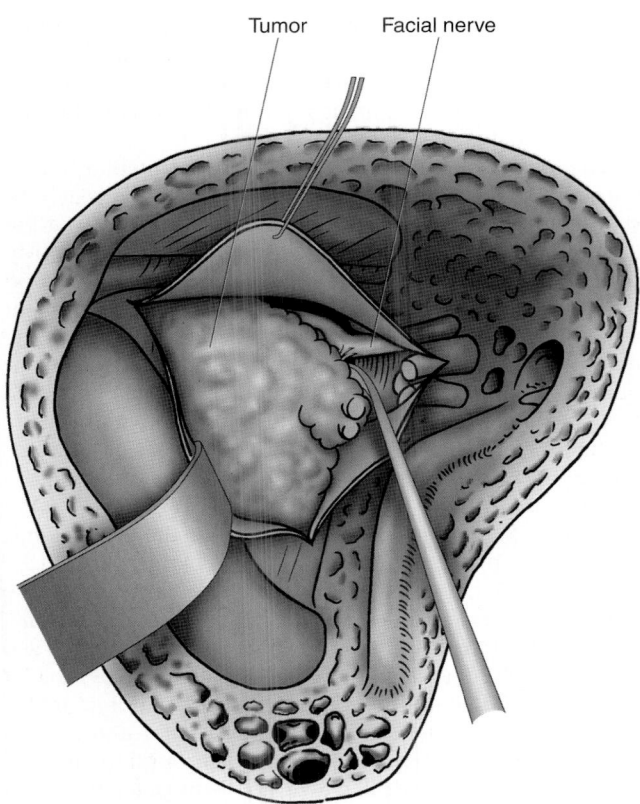

Tumor   Facial nerve

FIGURE 46-8 After the dural opening, the tumor can be separated from the facial nerve in the internal auditory canal. The vestibular nerves and the cochlear nerve are divided laterally in the internal auditory canal.

must be established before the adhesions between the dura and the tumor are removed. Inferiorly, freeing of the tumor from the porus is simpler because damage to the cochlear nerve is insignificant. Superiorly, the facial nerve may be at risk. At times, it is difficult to isolate the facial nerve at the porus. In these cases, it is wise to carry out a partial tumor removal, identify the facial nerve medially, and follow the nerve laterally until the porus is reached. During this work, the surgeon must be careful not to push the tumor forward or medially, because stretching the facial nerve, especially at the porus level, can damage the nerve. Early mobilization of the tumor from the internal auditory canal has the advantage that the landmarks are well defined and are not obscured with blood, as tends to happen later in the surgical dissection.

REDUCING TUMOR SIZE

In large tumors, there is inadequate space in the cerebellopontine angle to mobilize the tumor in the superior, inferior, and lateral directions, which is necessary to identify and free the facial nerve. In these cases, the posterior surface of the tumor capsule is incised in a superior–inferior direction, and an intracapsular removal is gently performed with the ultrasonic aspirator.

ISOLATION OF THE TUMOR

With tumors of all sizes, the surgeon must work in the proper cleavage plane between the tumor and the arachnoid. Tumor growth pushes the arachnoid membrane of the pontocerebellar cistern and causes it to double in the distal

part of the internal auditory canal and in the cerebellopontine angle. In large tumors, there is duplication of the cerebellar cistern and the cerebellomedullary cistern, causing formation of the third and fourth arachnoid layers. Through these layers, cranial nerves IX, X, and XI run at the inferior aspect of the tumor. The petrosal veins run through the layers of cisterna cerebelli at the superior–posterior aspect of the tumor.

TUMOR REMOVAL

The principle method for removal of large tumors is intracapsular gutting to reduce tumor bulk, followed by mobilization and removal of the adjacent capsule segment. The point of attack must be changed progressively, and as the limits of mobilization are reached at one point, the surgeon moves to another. Once the interior part of the tumor has been extensively removed, the capsule is displaced into the tumor space. Opening of the arachnoid layers and dissecting within these layers facilitates the isolation of the tumor. Semisharp dissectors and sometimes small cottonoids are used in the proper dissection plane to separate the tumor from the surrounding structures. The dissection is made from four directions: inferior, superior, medial, and lateral.

Inferior Dissection

Dissection at the inferior aspect of the tumor usually leads into the large cerebellomedullary cistern, which allows CSF to escape. This step improves the operative condition, and if any difficulties are encountered because of lack of room

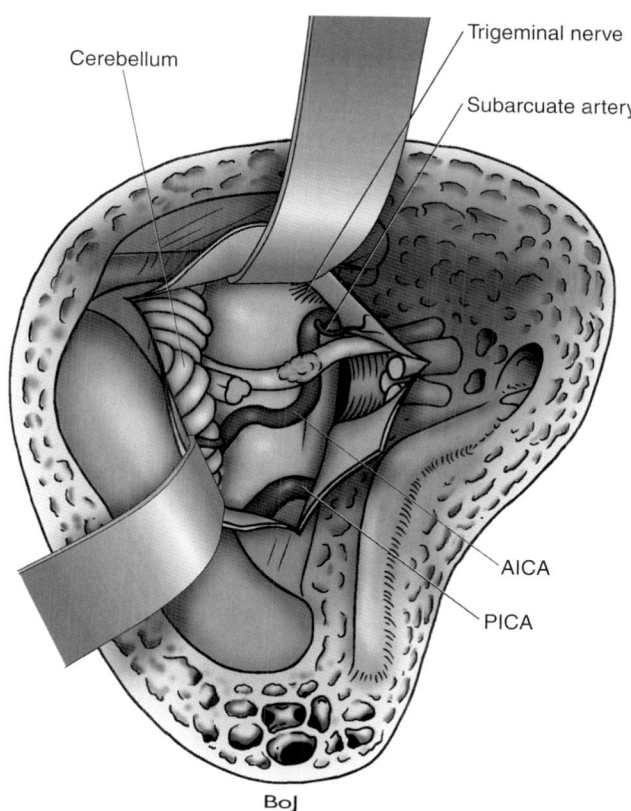

Cerebellum

Trigeminal nerve

Subarcuate artery

AICA

PICA

BoJ

FIGURE 46-9 The tumor has been removed. A small tumor remnant is left on the facial nerve.

in the posterior fossa, draining the cerebellomedullary cistern as soon as possible is valuable.

On the inferior aspect of the tumor, it is possible to localize cranial nerves IX and X, which are best identified near the jugular foramen medial to the jugular bulb. These nerves must be freed from the tumor and isolated. Sometimes they are not well seen because they tend to lie around the corner of the opening. During manipulation of cranial nerves IX and X, changes in the pulse rate may occur. Stopping the manipulation restores the pulse rate.

The posterior–inferior cerebellar artery is at the inferior aspect of the tumor and must be carefully separated from the tumor capsule and preserved. The labyrinthine artery supplies branches to the facial nerve and should be preserved. Dissection inferior to the tumor continues until the brain stem is reached and is completed with removal of that portion of the capsule.

Superior Dissection

The facial nerve is normally located anteriorly to the tumor, but it is not unusual to find the facial nerve over the top of the tumor. If the precise location of the facial nerve is unknown, when starting the dissection at the superior aspect of the tumor, it is imperative to inspect the tumor surface carefully and to use the nerve stimulator to identify the nerve and avoid injury.

The petrosal vein and cranial nerve V are located in the superior aspect of the tumor. These structures must be identified and carefully separated from the tumor. The trigeminal nerve is a broad white structure running in the

inferior–posterior direction. Near the brain, the nerve lies in close contact with the tumor capsule but is usually easy to separate from the tumor. Handling of the nerve must be avoided if recovery of sensory loss in the face is to be achieved. The petrosal vein and vein branches are stretched over the tumor and enter the superior petrosal sinus. To stay in the proper cleavage plane, it is better to separate the vein from the tumor rather than coagulate the vessels. The coagulation seals the layers together and makes later separation difficult. The superior dissection is continued until the pons is reached and the attachment of the trigeminal nerve to the brain stem is visualized.

Medial Dissection

The medial dissection is the most difficult part of the tumor removal because of the risk of damaging the facial nerve or the pons. After the posterior part of the tumor is debulked, a small portion of tumor capsule is left attached to the cerebellum and the pons. The tumor capsule is lifted, and the proper cleavage plane is identified. In large tumors, the posterior pole may protrude far under the cerebellum and deep into the brain stem. This protrusion requires maximal rotation of the operating table toward the surgeon to visualize the dissection plane. The vessels are dissected away, and the branches that extend into the capsule are coagulated and divided. The capsule and tumor remnant are pushed anteriorly, and arachnoid and veins are dissected from the capsule. When the brain stem has been reached from all directions and the tumor has gradually been removed, the remaining small portion of tumor covers a part of the brain stem, facial nerve, and cochlear nerve.

Anterior Dissection and Final Tumor Removal

In small tumors, the main approach is from the anterior aspect. In these cases, the facial nerve can easily be located at the brain stem, and the precise position of the nerve is easy to ascertain early. Separating the tumor from the facial nerve is done from the porus and against the brain stem.

In large tumors, the dissection of the facial nerve is done in an anterior–posterior direction. The small portion of tumor that covers the facial nerve from the brain stem to the porus is the most difficult to remove (Fig. 46-9). The anterior part of the tumor capsule usually contains a number of small vessels from arteries and vein, and dissection can easily provoke bleeding. Veins are often present around the facial nerve's entry zone from the brain stem. Coagulation of the bleeding vessels is dangerous and must be precise to avoid facial nerve injury.

For several reasons, dissection on the anterior aspect of the tumor is troublesome and time consuming:
- The facial nerve is often stretched and spread out over the largest prominence of the tumor, which sometimes makes the nerve nearly invisible.
- The facial nerve is not protected by an epineurium and is vulnerable to injury.
- At the porus, the facial nerve is often embedded in the tumor capsule, causing problems when loosening the tumor.

Care must be taken not to leave fragments of tumor on the nerve, because the dissection continues inside the tumor and obscures the location of the nerve, which may be lost.

Once the facial nerve has been separated from the tumor, the last bit of tumor is removed from the brain stem. The adhesions between the tumor and the brain stem are not usually dense, but if they are, clearing the brain stem of tumor demands particularly careful dissection. Once the tumor has been removed, the field is inspected and the facial nerve is examined with the stimulator. If a signal can be obtained by stimulating the nerve at the brain stem, it is likely that the patient will have normal facial nerve function. The wound is then irrigated with saline, and all bleeding points are controlled. Absolute hemostasis is required and may be time consuming.

FACIAL NERVE REPAIR

If the nerve has been divided during operation, the surgeon may get an acceptable level of function by anastomosing the nerve ends, provided that the central stump can be found and isolated. If the nerve ends can reach each other, they are anastomosed end to end and fixed with a suture and fibrin glue.[20-22] If a gap exists, a great auricular nerve or sural nerve graft is used to bridge the gap between the nerve ends.

CLOSURE

An essential part of wound closure involves preventing rhinorrhea. CSF may escape through the middle ear and the eustachian tube. The middle ear is entered through the antrum, and the incus is removed with a small hook. The eustachian tube can be reached below the malleus and is occluded with muscle. The middle ear is packed with a small piece of fat. The dural opening and the mastoid cavity are filled with large pieces of adipose tissue taken from the abdomen. Fibrin glue is injected around the adipose tissue. The muscle fascia/pericranium flap is closed watertight with absorbable sutures. The postauricular skin incision is closed in two layers with absorbable subcutaneous suture and nylon suture in the skin. I do not use a subgaleal drain but make a solid compression of the wound by gauze supported by a solid elastic bandage.

Postoperative Management and Complications

Surgery on large tumors in the posterior fossa is not without risks.[23-25] Large tumors sometimes adhere strongly to the surface of the cerebellum and the brain stem. Dissection of the tumor from the surroundings may elicit cerebellar edema and infarction. Veins can often be coagulated, but sometimes packing is necessary, especially of the bulb of the sigmoid sinus and the petrosal vein. Hematomas or reactive edema of the cerebellum may necessitate immediate response. Close observation of the patient is necessary in the initial postoperative phase by trained nurses in the intensive care unit. Acute hydrocephalus resulting from obstruction of CSF drainage from the ventricles may occur because of edema or hematoma at the level of the fourth ventricle.

HEMATOMA

Postoperative hematoma after a translabyrinthine approach is a rare but serious complication. This complication is the cause of most of the mortality seen after translabyrinthine removal of vestibular schwannomas. Even when excellent hemostasis appears to have been achieved, however, postoperative hemorrhage may occur,[26] and it seems most likely among elderly patients and patients with large tumors. The hematoma is most likely to occur shortly after the operation but may be seen days after surgery.

The clinical course is often insidious. If the patient does not regain consciousness after surgery or if the patient after a period with normal sensorium develops decreasing consciousness, a hematoma must be suspected. If the symptoms develop quickly, it may be necessary to open the wound immediately in the intensive care unit. If the symptoms develop more slowly, computed tomography can confirm the diagnosis. I always perform a control computed tomography scan the day after surgery to avoid clinical deterioration or death because of slowly progressive hematomas.

ACUTE HYDROCEPHALUS

Acute dilatation of the cerebral ventricles may be observed immediately postoperatively or in the following days. Failure to wake up or decreasing consciousness should arouse suspicion, and a computed tomography scan should be obtained. If the complication is diagnosed soon after surgery, ventricular drainage is undertaken. If the complication arises slowly and later after surgery, a permanent CSF shunt may be considered.

FACIAL PARALYSIS

Facial paralysis is often difficult to detect immediately postoperatively, when full wakefulness and cooperation are absent and, for unknown reasons, eye closure may be present. If the face is paralyzed, eye care is of great importance. In the first days after surgery, the eye is covered with a protective shield and viscous eyedrops are used. Shortly thereafter, a tarsorrhaphy is performed. The patient is warned to protect the eye and to wear protective spectacles. An ophthalmologist should be consulted.

Even though the nerve seems anatomically intact at the end of the operation, some patients exhibit postoperative facial paralysis. These patients still have a good chance for some function of the facial nerve. At least 6 months of observation should be allowed before any further treatment is considered. If permanent facial paralysis exists, a faciohypoglossal anastomosis is carried out after a delay of approximately 1 year.[27]

CSF LEAKAGE

CSF leakage is a common complication after vestibular schwannoma surgery,[28] and it is seen in 5% to 15% of the cases. The leakage may occur either through the skin at the wound site or through the nose. Rhinorrhea is more common than leakage through the wound. The diagnosis of postoperative CSF rhinorrhea is often obvious within a few days of surgery, but its recognition may be delayed. Some patients report only a sensation of postnasal dripping or a salty taste in the mouth. In these cases, the diagnosis may be subtle. The patient should be tested in a head-down position for watery escape from the nose before discharge.

When rhinorrhea is diagnosed, a lumbar drain is inserted for 3 to 5 days; however, the success with CSF drainage is not as high as in the wound leakage, probably because the defect is located in the bone, which is not as easily overgrown as is a defect in soft tissue. If the lumbar drainage fails to close the defect, reoperation and resealing the communication to the middle ear and eustachian tube with muscle graft and bone wax in the communicating air cells is necessary.

CSF escape through the postauricular wound may be prevented by meticulous closure of the wound followed by a tight head bandage. If wound leakage occurs, spinal drainage is often sufficient to solve the problem, and reoperation is rarely necessary.

MENINGITIS

Because the translabyrinthine approach is time consuming and involves opening of an air-filled cavity, meningitis is among the more common complications, occurring in up to 5% of cases. The peak incidence is seen from the third to the fifth postoperative day. Delayed meningitis is often caused by an undiagnosed otorhinorrhea. Early recognition of meningitis with demonstration of high polymorphonuclear cell count in the CSF usually ensures rapid resolution.

A high or persistent fever, combined with severe headache or signs of altered mental status, is likely to be caused by meningitis. Because postoperative fever and headache are common after the translabyrinthine procedure, the clinician should have a low threshold for performing a lumbar puncture when suspicion of meningitis arises.

A large proportion of postoperative meningitis after vestibular schwannoma surgery is aseptic.[29] It is not always clear from the CSF findings whether an infection is present. If there is any doubt, the patient should be treated with intravenous antibiotics.

Conclusions

The results from translabyrinthine and retrosigmoid approaches are comparable, with less than 1% mortality, 97% total removal, anatomic preservation of facial nerve in 90% to 95% of cases, and a functioning facial nerve in more than 70% of cases 1 year after surgery.[4,30-32] Except for hearing preservation, the published results do not favor one method over the other, and preference of one method should be based mostly on personal experience.

No comparison exists regarding the clinical outcome of the two approaches in vestibular schwannomas larger than 3.5 cm. In such cases, hearing preservation is seldom an issue. The standard retrosigmoid approach, as used in most neurosurgical departments for other pathologies in the cerebellopontine angle, does not, in my opinion, offer the same control of the tumor surfaces, especially the relation to the brain stem, as that achieved by a large, translabyrinthine exposure.

Summary

Three different surgical approaches can be used for vestibular schwannoma surgery: subtemporal, suboccipital, and translabyrinthine.

In patients with nonserviceable hearing, the translabyrinthine approach offers the most direct route to the cerebellopontine angle and can be used for removal of tumors regardless of the size.

The patient is placed in a supine position with the head turned toward the opposite side. Intraoperative facial nerve monitoring is mandatory. A curved skin incision is made behind the ear, and the skin and muscle/pericranium layer are retracted anteriorly.

An extended mastoidectomy is performed. The facial nerve is identified close to the lateral semicircular canal. The nerve is exposed by making a small window in the fallopian canal. After complete removal of the labyrinth, a more than 180-degree arc of bone around the internal auditory canal is removed. The dura is open from the internal auditory canal to the sinodural angle near the sigmoid sinus.

After opening the dura, the posterior part of the tumor is exposed. Small tumors can be removed en bloc after careful dissection of the facial nerve away from the tumor. In large tumors, it is essential to begin removal with intracapsular debulking to reduce the tumor size and subsequently develop the extracapsular dissection planes. Around the entire circumference of the porus, dural adhesions to the tumor make dissection of the facial nerve difficult.

When tumor removal has been accomplished, absolute hemostasis must be obtained.

To prevent rhinorrhea, the eustachian tube is packed with a small piece of muscle, the middle ear is packed with abdominal fat, and the dural opening and the mastoid cavity are filled with large pieces of abdominal fat. Fibrin glue is injected around the adipose tissue. The muscle fascia/pericranium flap is closed watertight, and the skin incision is closed in two layers.

Complications after using the translabyrinthine approach may be serious or even fatal. Close observation of the patient is necessary in the initial postoperative phase by trained nurses in the intensive care unit. Hematomas may necessitate immediate response.

ACKNOWLEDGMENT

The author is indebted to Bo Jespersen, MD, who provided all illustrations for this chapter.

KEY REFERENCES

Anson BJ, Donaldson JA. *Surgical Anatomy of the Temporal Bone and Ear.* 2nd ed. Philadelphia: WB Saunders; 1973.

Barrs DM, Brackmann DE, Hitzelberger WE. Facial nerve anastomosis in the cerebellopontine angle: a review of 24 cases. *Am J Otol.* 1984;5:269-272.

Benecke JE. Complications of acoustic tumor surgery and their management. *Semin Hear.* 1989;10:341-345.

Briggs RJ, Luxford WM, Atkins Jr JS, Hitselberger WE. Trans-labyrinthine removal of large acoustic neuromas. *Neurosurgery.* 1994;34:785-790.

Briggs RJS, Fabinyi G, Kaye AH. Current management of acoustic neuromas: review of surgical approaches and outcomes. *J Clin Neurosci.* 2000;7:521-526.

Day JD, Chen DA, Arriaga M. Translabyrinthine approach for acoustic neuroma. *Neurosurgery.* 2004;54:391-395.

Ebersold MJ, Harner SG, Beatty CW, et al. Current results of the retrosigmoid approach to acoustic neurinoma. *J Neurosurg.* 1992;76:901-909.

Helms J. Indications for the suboccipital, translabyrinthine, and transtemporal approaches in acoustic neuroma surgery. In: Tos M, Thomsen J, eds. *Proceedings of the First International Conference on Acoustic Neuroma.* Amsterdam: Kugler; 1992:501-502.

House WF, Hitselberger WE. Fatalities in acoustic tumor surgery. In: House WF, Leutje CM, eds. *Acoustic Tumors.* Baltimore: University Park Press; 1979:235-264.

House WF, Hitselberger WE. Translabyrinthine approach. In: House WF, Leutje CM, eds. *Acoustic Tumors.* Baltimore: University Park Press; 1979:43-87.

House WF (ed). Monograph. Transtemporal microsurgical removal of acoustic neuromas. *Arch Otolaryngol Head Neck Surg.* 1964; 80: 597–756.

Jackler RK, Pitts LH. Selection of surgical approach to acoustic neuroma. *Otolaryngol Clin North Am.* 1992;25:361-387.

King TT, Morrison AW. Translabyrinthine and transtentorial removal of acoustic tumours: results of 150 cases. *J Neurosurg.* 1980;52:210-216.

Mamikoglu B, Wiet RJ, Esquivel CR. Translabyrinthine approach for the management of large and giant vestibular schwannomas. *Otol Neurotol.* 2002;23:224-227.

Mass SC, Wiet RJ, Dinces E. Complications of the translabyrinthine approach for the removal of acoustic neuromas. *Arch Otolaryngol Head Neck Surg.* 1999;125:801-804.

Rhoton Jr AL. Microsurgical anatomy of the brainstem surface facing an acoustic neuroma. *Surg Neurol.* 1986;25:326-339.

Rhoton Jr AL, Tedeschi H. Microsurgical anatomy of acoustic neuroma. *Otolaryngol Clin North Am.* 1992;25:257-294.

Selesnick SH, Liu JC, Jen A, Newman J. The incidence of cerebrospinal fluid leak after vestibular schwannoma surgery. *Otol Neurotol.* 2004;25:387-393.

Slattery III WH, Francis S, House KC. Perioperative morbidity of acoustic neuroma surgery. *Otol Neurotol.* 2001;22:895-902.

Sterkers JM. Life-threatening complications and severe neurologic sequelae in surgery of acoustic neurinoma. *Ann Otolaryngol Chir Cervicofac.* 1989;106:245-250.

Sterkers JM, Corlieu C, Sterkers O. Acoustic neuroma surgery (1300 cases), the translabyrinthine method. In: Tos M, Thomsen J, eds. *Acoustic Neuroma.* Amsterdam: Kugler; 1992:377-378.

Thomsen J, Tos M, Børgesen SE, Møller H. Surgical results after removal of 504 acoustic neuromas. In: Tos M, Thomsen J, eds. *Proceedings of the First International Conference on Acoustic Neuroma.* Amsterdam: Kugler; 1992:331-335.

Tos M, Thomsen J, Harmsen A. Results of translabyrinthine removal of 300 acoustic neuromas related to tumour size. *Acta Otolaryngol Suppl (Stockh).* 1988;452:38-51.

Tos M, Thomsen J, eds. *Translabyrinthine Acoustic Neuroma Surgery: A Surgical Manual.* Stuttgart: Georg Thieme; 1991.

Yates PD, Jackler RK, Satar B, et al. Is it worthwhile to attempt hearing preservation in larger acoustic neuromas? *Otol Neurotol.* 2003;24: 460-464.

Numbered references appear on Expert Consult.

Transtemporal Approaches to Posterior Cranial Fossa

FRANK D. VRIONIS • KAMRAN V. AGHAYEV • GALE GARDNER • JON H. ROBERTSON • JASON A. BRODKEY

Traditional approaches to the posterior cranial fossa do not permit direct access to complex lesions of the lateral skull base, cerebellopontine angle (CPA), or clivus. To circumvent brain retraction and allow for complete resection, approaches have been developed that position the dissection both lateral and anterior to the brain stem and cerebellum. All of these skull base approaches are combinations and variations of transtemporal bone routes (Table 47-1 and Fig. 47-1). Unlike craniotomies performed elsewhere, entry to the posterior fossa through the temporal bone poses special problems for the surgeon if the internal carotid artery (ICA), sigmoid sinus (SS), cranial nerves VII and VIII, and specialized structures for hearing and balance are to be preserved. Despite the widely varied nomenclature, often only subtle differences exist among these approaches. It is imperative that the location, type, and extent of the lesion dictate the type of the approach. Tailored approaches to the lesion instead of standard ones are recommended for minimal disruption of normal structures. In this respect, transtemporal approaches represent an anatomic continuum of temporal bone dissection, with frequent overlaps and minor discrepancies or differences among the various approaches. The complicated nomenclature has arisen because skull base tumors tend to extend into different anatomic compartments, often necessitating combined approaches. Because of the overlap of neurosurgery and otology in this area, collaboration of neurosurgeons and otologists is mandatory.

This chapter is divided into three sections: anterior transpetrosal approaches, describing anterior approaches within the temporal bone through the middle cranial fossa; posterior transpetrosal approaches, for those that are situated more posteriorly through the mastoid process; and combined approaches. We define the external auditory canal (EAC) as the dividing structure between the anterior and the posterior approaches. We divide each approach into sections, giving a brief historical perspective, indications, surgical approach, and complications and disadvantages.

Anterior Transpetrosal Approaches

Anterior transpetrosal approaches are based on a standard subtemporal extradural middle fossa approach. We divide the anterior approaches into three types: (1) middle fossa approach, (2) extended middle fossa approach (anterior petrosectomy), and (3) middle fossa transtentorial approach. The middle fossa approach provides a subtemporal extradural exposure of the middle fossa floor designed for removing acoustic neuromas situated laterally within the internal auditory canal (IAC). For more extensive tumors, the extended middle fossa approach provides additional exposure of the petrous apex and supraclival region. With the addition of division of the tentorium, the middle fossa transtentorial approach provides access to the middle clival region and posterior fossa, as well as the posterior cavernous sinus.

MIDDLE FOSSA APPROACH

House developed the middle fossa access to the IAC and adjacent structures in 1961 in an effort to remove foci of labyrinthine otosclerosis.[1-3] Although he used this approach briefly for the removal of acoustic tumors, he soon directed his efforts to a translabyrinthine approach. Fisch and Mattox further refined the middle fossa approach.[4,5]

Several techniques for localization of the IAC have been described. House's technique identifies the greater superficial petrosal nerve (GSPN), follows it to the geniculate ganglion (GG), and then proceeds along the labyrinthine segment of the facial nerve to the IAC.[2] Another popular method described by Fisch and Mattox uses the superior semicircular canal (SSC) as the primary landmark.[5] Using this method, once the SSC is identified, the meatal plane overlying the IAC is located in a 60-degree plane centered over the SSC ampulla. Garcia-Ibanez and Garcia-Ibanez[6] advocate a technique beginning at the bisection of the angle between the GSPN and the arcuate eminence. Lan and Shiao, in a cadaveric study, described the technique of finding the IAC by drilling a point that is 9.9 mm medial from the GG on a line angled with the GSPN by 96 degrees.[7] Because the medially IAC dura enlarges threefold, and there are no neural structures anterior to it, the medial or proximal "safe" part of the IAC is first identified and is followed laterally: once the IAC dura is exposed, it can be distinguished from the posterior fossa dura by its "pinkish" color in contrast to the "white" posterior fossa dura.[8] Other techniques involve drilling to expose the semicircular canals and exposure of the ossicles in the middle ear as

Table 47-1	Temporal Bone Approaches

Anterior Approaches
Middle cranial fossa
Extended middle cranial fossa
Middle cranial fossa transtentorial
Posterior Approaches
Retrolabyrinthine—presigmoid
Retrolabyrinthine—trans-sigmoid
Retrolabyrinthine—retrosigmoid
Translabyrinthine
Transotic
Transcochlear
Infralabyrinthine
Transcanal–infracochlear
Combined Approaches
Petrosal
Infratemporal fossa
Endoscopic Approaches
Endonasal endoscopic approach

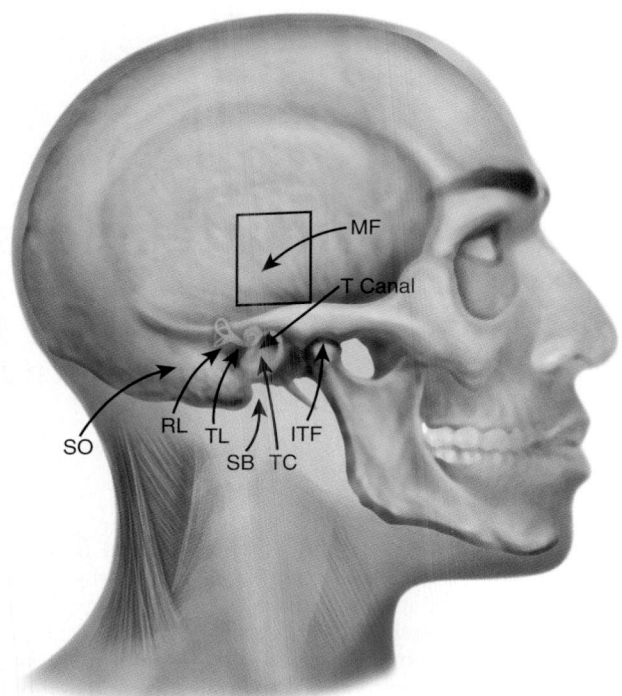

FIGURE 47-1 Multiple approach routes through the temporal bone to the posterior fossa. ITF, infratemporal fossa; MF, middle fossa; RL, retrolabyrinthine; SB, skull base; SO, suboccipital; TC, transcochlear; T Canal, transcanal; TL, translabyrinthine.

a reference point.[9] Because of the wide variations in anatomy[4,6] and small working space, no single technique can ensure avoidance of injury to important structures. Careful dissection and a detailed understanding of the regional anatomy are important for success. Image-guided navigation through the temporal bone has been introduced as an accurate alternative method to localize the IAC without the need to expose the GG or the SSC.[10,11]

Indications

The middle fossa approach is best suited for lesions situated lateral within the IAC that have limited extension into the CPA (less than 1 cm) and where hearing preservation is the goal.[2,12] It is especially useful when preoperative computed tomography (CT) of the temporal bone demonstrates the proximity of the posterior semicircular canal (PSC), common crus, or vestibule to the posterior lip of the IAC. In those circumstances, retrosigmoid approaches are less preferable and the middle fossa approach becomes the hearing-preservation approach of choice. Tumors that are medial in position and do not extend to the fundus of the IAC are best approached by posterior approaches (e.g., retrosigmoid approach).

The middle fossa approach provides access to the labyrinthine segment of the facial nerve without sacrificing hearing. Thus, decompression of the facial nerve in trauma or Bell's palsy, or resection of facial nerve tumors can be accomplished. During vestibular schwannoma removal, early identification of the facial nerve allows better functional preservation. In a recent retrospective literature review that included 296 studies and more than 25,000 patients, facial nerve preservation was highest in patients treated with middle fossa (85%) approach compared to translabyrinthine (81%) and retrosigmoid (78%) approaches.[13] However, the main factor contributing to the facial nerve preservation was found to be tumor size, which is consistent with other studies.[14] Therefore, bias can be a contributing factor, because most schwannomas treated with the middle fossa approach are small or medium sized. This approach also permits selective sectioning of the

vestibular nerve fibers for Ménière's disease. In theory, it could also be used to expose the horizontal portion of the ICA, eustachian tube, and temporomandibular joint (TMJ). Other indications include advanced otosclerosis, nerve section for tinnitus, facial nerve repair and facial nerve neuroma, repair of middle fossa encephaloceles, and cerebrospinal fluid (CSF) leakage through the tegmen.[2]

Surgical Approach

The patient is positioned supine on the operating table with the head turned opposite the side of the tumor.[2,4,6,12,15] Facial and auditory nerve monitoring is used. An incision is planned that begins at the level of the zygoma just anterior to the tragus and extends superiorly to approximately the superior temporal line. We prefer an S-shaped incision curving first anteriorly and then posteriorly to allow for greater spreading of the soft tissues.

The temporalis muscle is divided and reflected anteriorly. A 4- by 5-cm bone flap is planned approximately two thirds anterior and one third posterior to the EAC. The inferior margin should be placed as close to the middle fossa floor as possible. A subtemporal craniectomy is performed. The dura is then elevated from the middle fossa floor in a posterior to anterior direction. This direction of dissection helps avoid inadvertent elevation of the GSPN and subsequent traction injury to the GG and facial nerve. Injury to the GSPN can produce a dry eye secondary to loss of lacrimal gland innervation. In approximately 16% of cases, the GG is not covered by bone and inadvertent injury can occur.[4] To maintain a visible plane of dissection, a self-retaining brain retractor is used. Some retractors are limited to only 4 to

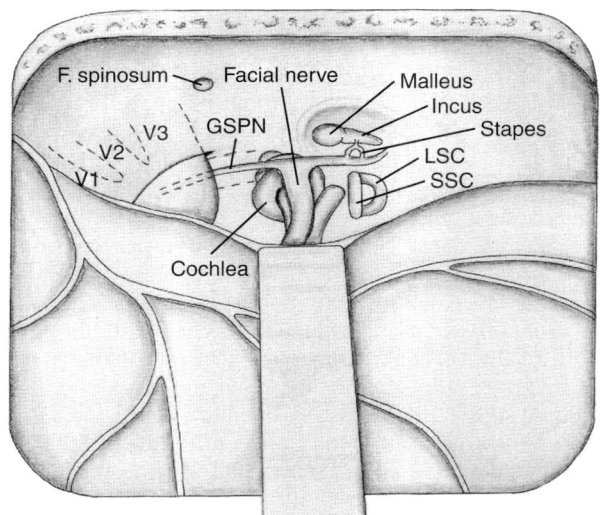

FIGURE 47-2 Middle fossa approach to the IAC. The illustration depicts the facial nerve, GG, and GSPN. The petrous carotid artery is shown as a dotted structure under the GSPN. The tegmen is opened, and the head of the malleus, the incus, and the stapes are seen. Anteriorly, the branches of the trigeminal nerve (V1, V2, and V3) are depicted.

5 cm of spread; thus, too wide a craniotomy can impair the capability of the retractor to elevate the dura adequately.

Several landmarks must be identified before bone removal can begin over the IAC: (1) the middle meningeal artery, (2) the arcuate eminence, (3) the GSPN, and (4) the facial hiatus (Fig. 47-2). The first landmark is typically the middle meningeal artery at the foramen spinosum. This can be obliterated and divided if necessary. The foramen may be, albeit rarely, duplicated or absent. It marks the anterior limit of the dural elevation. As dural elevation continues, the arcuate eminence, a rounded elevation of the petrous bone, can be identified. It is usually produced by the underlying SSC. Lateral to the arcuate eminence is the tegmen tympani, a thin lamina of bone that forms the roof of the tympanic cavity. The GSPN originates from the GG, exits through the petrous bone at the facial hiatus, and runs extradurally in an anteromedial direction toward the trigeminal ganglion. The GSPN serves as a landmark for the lateral margin of the horizontal segment of the petrous carotid artery. Care should be taken at this stage not to apply force to the floor of the middle fossa, because the bone over the carotid artery and the area of the tegmen can be quite thin and even dehiscent in up to 20% of cases.[4] The arcuate eminence is drilled until the dense bone of the SSC is encountered. The SSC is visualized with a bluish hue through the bone, the so-called blue line. In approximately 15% of cases, however, the arcuate eminence is absent; in 50% of cases where it is present, it is rotated in relationship to the SSC.[16]

Once the key landmarks have been identified, the IAC can be localized using two key angles. Traditionally, the GSPN-SSC angle (120 degrees)[6] and the SSC-IAC angle (60 degrees)[17] have been used. Unfortunately, these angles have been shown to be quite variable,[15] and in one study the GSPN-SSC angle ranged from 90 to 135 degrees and the SSC-IAC angle from 34 to 75 degrees.[4] Thus, simply relying on angles can lead to inadvertent injury to the SSC and hence loss of hearing. House's technique places the facial nerve at risk, because this structure is first identified and then followed

to the IAC.[2] Fisch's technique places the SSC at risk. Orientation can be aided by removal of the tegmen and identification of the head of the malleus.[9] This can help predict the location of the GG and IAC because these structures are usually collinear, at the expense of risking a CSF leak through the middle ear.[2] None of these techniques is failsafe, and the best method of localizing the IAC is what the surgeon finds most comfortable in his or her own experience.

Once the IAC has been identified, exposure proceeds from lateral to medial until the entire IAC has been exposed along its superior surface. A safer technique is to begin medially, expose the porus acousticus first, and then work laterally, taking advantage of the larger margin for error in the region of the porus.[8,12,15] At the fundus of the IAC, the vertical crest (Bill's bar), a bone spicule that separates the superior vestibular nerve from the facial nerve, is identified. Finally, the dura over the IAC is opened, first posteriorly over the superior vestibular nerve to avoid facial nerve injury.

In the case of vestibular schwannomas, the tumor can be removed by separating the superior vestibular nerve and tumor from the facial nerve. The tumor is usually delivered posteriorly away from the facial nerve. Small hooks are necessary to palpate the limits of the IAC and gently free the tumor, particularly from its inferolateral portion, where the view is especially obscured. The approach carries a higher risk to the facial and cochlear nerves when the tumor less commonly arises from the inferior vestibular nerve. A rigid 0- or 30-degree endoscope can be used at the end of the procedure to inspect for residual tumor, facial and cochlear nerve integrity, and opened air cells.[18] Closure of the IAC defect is accomplished with a small free graft or temporalis muscle.

Complications and Disadvantages

The middle fossa approach requires retraction of the temporal lobe;[19] therefore, injury can potentially occur (e.g., aphasia, hemiparesis, or seizure). There is potential for CSF leakage through unwaxed air cells or through the middle ear, if the tegmen is opened. Careful hemostasis and tenting sutures can lessen the risk of postoperative hematoma (e.g., epidural hematoma).

As with any temporal bone approach, high-speed drilling can potentially cause injury to the underlying neurovascular structures as a result of the vibration and heat from the drill. Using a diamond bur with continuous-suction irrigation lessens this risk.

Specifically, with the middle fossa approach, during drilling of bone over the facial nerve there is a small margin for error. Inadvertent injury to the nerve, which is in the most superficial plane of the surgical field, can occur. The SSC, cochlea, and petrous portion of the carotid artery are obvious structures at risk with this approach. Also, the working zone is quite restricted, making this a somewhat technically demanding approach. If major bleeding occurs in the posterior fossa, control may necessitate conversion to a middle fossa transtentorial or a translabyrinthine approach.

EXTENDED MIDDLE FOSSA APPROACH (ANTERIOR PETROSECTOMY)

The traditional middle fossa approach works well for lesions in the IAC;[2,3] however, the exposure is limited. For that reason, extensions of the middle fossa approach have been developed to permit wider access to the petrous apex, clivus, and posterior fossa. The extended middle fossa approach involves a petrous apex resection, in addition to the temporal craniotomy described for the middle fossa approach.[20] The horizontal segment of the carotid artery and the cochlea limit the inferior exposure to the level of the inferior petrosal sinus. The TMJ, ossicles, and petrous carotid artery laterally; the trigeminal ganglion anteriorly; and the SSC and vestibule posteriorly represent the limits of the extended middle fossa approach.

Indications

The anterior petrosectomy provides access to the petrous apex and superior clival region. It provides access to the posterior fossa past the carotid artery and trigeminal and facial nerves. Although the extended middle fossa approach is considered a hearing-preservation approach, it can provide additional exposure in the posterior fossa by sacrificing the SSC and labyrinth—and thus hearing.[20,21] Sacrifice of the cochlea improves visualization of the lateral extreme of the IAC, the medial wall of the tympanic cavity, and the jugular foramen if needed.

The extended middle fossa approach permits resection of vestibular schwannomas that extend more medially in the CPA. Meningiomas and chordomas of the anterior CPA and clivus can be resected through this approach, as well as lesions of the petrous apex (i.e., cholesteatomas and petrositis). The middle fossa approach is not recommended for cholesterol granulomas because of the absence of permanent aeration and the need for temporal lobe retraction.[22] Large lesions may be difficult to resect by this approach, and the angled endoscope can be used to deal with blind spots.[23] Lesions of the posterior cavernous sinus, basilar artery, and anterior brain stem up to the level of pontobulbar junction can also be approached.[24] The petrous carotid artery can be also approached for bypass anastomosis.[25]

Surgical Approach

A temporal craniotomy is performed, similar to the middle fossa approach. Occasionally, a zygomatic osteotomy is added for exposure of the middle fossa floor. The middle meningeal artery, foramen ovale, GSPN, and arcuate eminence are identified. The dural sheath of the trigeminal ganglion and its continuation as V3 forms the superior limit of this approach.[24] The petrous carotid artery can be exposed at this point by drilling bone along the course of the GSPN (see Fig. 47-2). This area is also known as the posterolateral or Glasscock's triangle.[26] The boundaries of Glasscock's triangle are a line extending from the foramen spinosum to the arcuate eminence laterally, the GSPN medially, and the third division of the trigeminal nerve (V3) at the base. Medial to this triangle is Kawase's, or the posteromedial, triangle, which consists of the bone in the area of the petrous apex. Drilling this bone provides access to the clivus and the infratentorial compartment.[27] Kawase's triangle is defined laterally by the GSPN, medially by the petrous ridge, and at the base by the arcuate eminence. Usually the GSPN is sacrificed to avoid traction to the GG and subsequent facial paralysis. Arcuate eminence is absent in significant number of the patients. Therefore, foramen ovale and spinosum can

be used alternatively as landmarks to start drilling.[24] The cochlea represents the posterolateral limit of exposure within Kawase's triangle. Infracochlear lesions are hard to access with the conventional approach, and an endoscope can be helpful.[23]

The IAC is identified by one of the means described in the previous section. Once the IAC is identified, bone is removed, exposing the canal widely and the dura of the posterior fossa. The otic capsule bone is particularly dense and lighter in color than the remaining bone of the petrous apex. To identify the cochlea, Miller et al.[28] advocate drilling bone along an imaginary line extending from the tip of the vertical crest to the junction of the petrous carotid artery and cranial nerve V3 until the cochlea is identified. With this exposure, the dura along the medial temporal lobe and infratentorially to the level of the inferior petrosal sinus can be exposed. The superior petrosal sinus (SPS) can be clipped and divided. A dural incision can be extended across the SPS and then inferiorly into the posterior fossa. Occasionally, the dura over Meckel's cave is divided to mobilize the trigeminal nerve anteriorly and increase exposure of the petroclival region.

The approach can be extended into the infratemporal fossa by removing the bone from lateral to medial toward the foramen ovale. This maneuver eventually connects the temporal and infratemporal fossae, allowing tumor removal, especially in the case of trigeminal schwannomas, with extension along V3.[19]

Complications and Disadvantages

Complications of the extended middle fossa approach are similar to those with the standard middle fossa approach. Because of the additional bone removal at the petrous apex, potential injury to the carotid artery and trigeminal nerve are possible. The main advantage of the extended middle fossa approach compared with posteriorly based approaches (e.g., translabyrinthine and transcochlear), when used to remove petrous apex lesions, is hearing preservation. One of the disadvantages is the time spent for the exposure of the posterior fossa. Usually the approach requires several hours to accomplish. In comparison, a retrosigmoid approach is more straightforward from a surgical point of view and requires significantly less time to finish. Another major disadvantage is that in the majority of cases (such as petroclival meningiomas) the pathology is encountered first, whereas the cranial nerves are typically compressed medially and encountered last. Again, posterior approaches are more advantageous from this point of view, because early identification of neurovascular structures allows better control.

MIDDLE FOSSA TRANSTENTORIAL APPROACH

The middle fossa transtentorial approach was first reported by Kawase et al.[27] in 1985 for approaching aneurysms of the midbasilar artery through the petrous pyramid. In 1991, Kawase et al.[29] applied this approach for resection of petroclival meningiomas that extended into the parasellar region (sphenopetroclival meningiomas). This approach uses a combination of the extended middle fossa approach with the addition of intradural resection of the tentorium to allow wider posterior fossa exposure. It is in many ways similar to the subtemporal transtentorial approach, with the added advantage of drilling the anterior petrous ridge.

Indications

The middle fossa transtentorial exposure can be accomplished with an anterior or posterior petrosectomy or a combined petrosal approach.[20,29-31] It is suitable for meningiomas extending along the superior and middle clivus or along the posterior wall of the petrous ridge, which can have long dural attachments. Hearing is preserved with this approach, as with all middle fossa approaches. It also permits resection of tumors that extend to the parasellar region and posterior cavernous sinus. It is particularly attractive for small tumors in the petroclival region, laterally located pontine lesions (cavernous malformations and gliomas), or basilar trunk aneurysms. Compared with the extended middle fossa approach, it provides wider posterior fossa exposure because of sectioning of the tentorium.

Surgical Approach

The extent of petrous pyramid resection is similar to that obtained by the extended middle fossa approach. The dura is opened above and below the SPS. Cranial nerves IV and V are identified. The SPS is clipped between cranial nerves V and VII, with care taken to avoid sacrificing the petrosal vein. Alternatively, the SPS can be embolized preoperatively.[24] The tentorium is cut until the tentorial notch is seen. The tentorium can then be tented open with retention sutures, exposing the petroclival region from cranial nerves III through VII.[30] The inferomedial triangle of the cavernous sinus can be visualized, mobilization of the trigeminal nerve can be accomplished by opening Meckel's cave, and Dorello's canal can be seen through this exposure.

Complications and Disadvantages

The middle fossa transtentorial approach carries the additional risk of injury to cranial nerve IV as a result of the tentorial incision. Furthermore, the degree of retraction and thus the risk of possible injury to the temporal lobe may be slightly higher than in the middle fossa or extended middle fossa approaches.

Posterior Transpetrosal Approaches

Most posterior transpetrosal approaches involve a certain degree of mastoid resection, positioning the surgical corridor inferior to the middle fossa approaches. There are wide variations among these approaches, although often portions of approaches are used in combination to create more extensive exposure (e.g., the presigmoid approach as part of the petrosal approach).

RETROLABYRINTHINE APPROACHES
Presigmoid Approach

The retrolabyrinthine presigmoid approach was first described by Hitselberger and Pulec[32] in 1972, and was popularized by Norrell and Silverstein[33] in 1977 and by House et al.[34] in 1984. It is performed through the mastoid air cells, with elevation of a dural flap between the labyrinth and the SS. The concept of this procedure is based on its allowing entry into the CPA anterior to the SS, thus lessening the need for cerebellar retraction. It was originally described as being useful for partial sectioning of the fibers of the sensory roots of cranial nerve V for trigeminal neuralgia. It has been used for selective sectioning of the vestibular division of cranial nerve VIII for treatment of vertigo and for endolymphatic duct surgery. It can occasionally be used to remove small acoustic tumors when preservation of hearing is desirable. The major advantage of this approach is that it provides direct access to the CPA without sacrificing hearing and without extensive cerebellar retraction. Its major disadvantage is the limited exposure, which can be compromised even further by a large dominant SS or when the mastoid air space is contracted ("crowded mastoid").

Trans-sigmoid Approach

The trans-sigmoid approach can be used as part of any posterior transpetrosal approach. Exposure is increased by ligating the SS, usually between the superior and the inferior petrosal sinuses or between the inferior anastomotic vein (vein of Labbé) and the SPS. Thus, the inferior anastomotic vein drains into the transverse sinus and retrogradely into the opposite jugular system. A preoperative angiogram or magnetic resonance venogram is essential to ensure patency of the torcular. A nondominant sinus in the presence of a patent torcular can be sacrificed in selected cases. Temporary clipping across the SS is recommended to assess for the presence of temporal lobe or cerebellar swelling. The SS can be opened and packed with Surgicel and its lumen sutured, or it can be ligated and clipped. Uyar et al.[35] described an original technique for sinus closure without opening the dura or the sinus itself. Posterior fossa and presigmoid dura are exposed first, and parallel suture is passed in front and back of the sinus. The muscle graft is placed between and sutures are tied, resulting in bending and obliteration or the lumen. Cadaver and angiographic studies show that the incidence of unilateral transverse sinus is rather infrequent (2.5%) and absence of any communication at the torcular is even rarer.[36,37] Despite this, given the catastrophic results of ligating a unilateral SS, a preoperative arteriogram or magnetic resonance venogram is recommended. This approach is advantageous in cases of tumor growth into the SS with spontaneous obstruction. Jugular foramen tumors spreading into the jugular bulb and SS can be managed by ligation of the internal jugular vein in the neck followed by opening the SS, packing, and tumor removal.[38]

Retrosigmoid (Suboccipital) Approach

The retrosigmoid approach, also known as the lateral suboccipital approach, is not a true transtemporal approach. This approach is most familiar to neurosurgeons and has been the traditional exposure used for resection of tumors of the CPA.[39,40] This approach provides wide entry into the posterior fossa, with maximal exposure for tumors such as vestibular schwannomas. Using this approach, the neurovascular structures of the temporal bone are avoided at the expense of cerebellar retraction. The development of monitoring techniques using evoked response methods has greatly increased the practicality of this approach.

Indications

Most tumors in the CPA can be approached through a suboccipital craniotomy (i.e., vestibular schwannomas, meningiomas, and epidermoids). Cranial nerves V to XI can be visualized with this exposure. Tumors with extension into the petroclival region or with significant spread anterior to the brain stem are not optimally treated with this exposure because of the need for increased cerebellar retraction and a long surgical corridor. This exposure can be combined with other transpetrosal approaches to provide maximal supratentorial and infratentorial exposure for extensive lesions of the CPA.

Surgical Approach

The retrosigmoid approach can be done with the patient sitting, lateral, or three fourths prone. The head position is carefully adapted to the procedure type that is performed. With upper complex exposure (cranial nerve V and SCA) the vertex should be tilted downward. If the procedure involves the middle complex (cranial nerves VII and VIII, anteroinferior cerebellar artery) or the lower complex (cranial nerves IX-XI, posteroinferior cerebellar artery), the degree of tilt decreases or is reversed. An incision is made approximately 2 cm posterior to the mastoid tip, extending cephalad to slightly above the transverse sinus and caudally into the suboccipital musculature. The asterion has been used as a useful landmark for the junction of the transverse sinus and SS. However, a study showed that it is a quite unreliable landmark and that placing a bur hole over it can potentially lead to sinus damage.[41] Neuronavigation alternatively has been shown to locate the position of the transverse sinus–SS junction more accurately.[42] Craniectomy or "silver dollar" craniotomy can be performed such that the edges of the transverse sinus and SS and their junction are clearly identified. In difficult reoperative cases, a line drawn from the root of the zygoma to the inion can reliably locate the course of the transverse sinus.[43] Bone removal can include the posterior lip of the foramen magnum, as well as the upper cervical lamina. The arachnoid at the foramen magnum should be opened first to permit CSF egress and facilitate cerebellar retraction.

The "extended retrosigmoid approach" involves removing of the bone over the SS to expose its entire length from the transverse sinus to the jugular bulb. This allows some degree of sinus retraction when the dura is reflected anteriorly, lessening the degree of cerebellar retraction.[44,45] However, venous flow can be impaired intra- or postoperatively. so frequent reassessment should be performed.[44]

In the case of vestibular schwannoma resection, the tumor is immediately visualized. It can be explored initially with a rigid endoscope to verify the position of neurovascular structures to the tumor and extent of the tumor to the IAC.[18] The facial nerve usually lies anterior to the tumor. For tumors that extend into the IAC, the porus is drilled until the dura over the IAC is seen. In a cadaver study, the amount of posterior IAC that can be safely unroofed averaged 5.9 mm (range 4-8 mm). The best available way to avoid critical labyrinthine structures during the suboccipital approach is to use preoperative high-resolution CT. A line is drawn on axial CT images from the medial aspect of the SS to the fundus of the IAC. If this line crosses any labyrinthine structures, the risk of injury and hearing loss during drilling of the IAC significantly increases.[46] In addition, air cells can be encountered during drilling with possibility of postoperative CSF leakage. Alternatively to drilling of the IAC a 70-degree rigid endoscope can be used to visualize the canal and remove tumor remnants.[47]

Complications and Disadvantages

This exposure requires a certain amount of cerebellar retraction; thus, cerebellar edema or hematoma can occur. This is especially true for large tumors requiring lengthy surgery. If the surgeon maintains gentle retraction (1-2 cm), these types of complications can usually be avoided. In cases of small or medium-sized tumors, an endoscope alone can be used for tumor removal to reduce the amount of cerebellar retraction.[48] The extended retrosigmoid approach also reduces the degree of cerebellar retraction. However, there is risk of postoperative sinus thrombosis.[44] The facial nerve lies on the anterior surface of the tumor somewhere between the superior and the inferior poles. Therefore, some amount of tumor removal is required to visualize the nerve. This is one of the disadvantages, because manipulation alone can cause nerve traction injury. A possible way to avoid injury to the facial nerve is to start medial to the tumor close to the brain stem or lateral in the region of IAC, where the nerve relation to tumor is relatively constant. After identification of the nerve, tumor removal can be performed safely. Other complications include CSF leakage and postoperative incisional pain attributed to adherence of the suboccipital muscles to the dura. The incisional pain can be lessened by either replacing the bone flap, in the case of a craniotomy, or performing a cranioplasty to fill the bone defect. The incidence of CSF leakage may be lessened by identifying and waxing small air cells in the IAC with the use of an endoscope. In 9% of cases, a high jugular bulb may make drilling of the meatus through the retrosigmoid approach impossible and is associated with increased risk of bleeding and air embolism.[49] As previously mentioned, loss of hearing can occur during drilling of the posterior aspect of the IAC.

TRANSLABYRINTHINE APPROACH

The first report of a translabyrinthine approach was in 1904 by Panse,[50] who advocated this approach for its shortest distance to the CPA. In 1961, House[3] described the middle fossa approach for resection of vestibular schwannomas located laterally in the IAC with minimal CPA extension. Because of limited exposure, incidence of facial paresis, need for temporal lobe retraction, and limited control of vascular structures, House and Hitselberger[51] introduced the translabyrinthine approach for resection of vestibular schwannomas. This was a more lateral approach and gave direct control of the facial nerve by drilling through the labyrinth. They emphasized the vertical crest at the lateral end of the IAC as a landmark. Differentiation between the superior and the inferior vestibular nerves was more readily apparent with this approach.

Variations of the translabyrinthine approach have been described for more extensive exposure of the SS, with mobilization of the jugular bulb, as well as drilling out of the infralabyrinthine air cells to increase access for large tumors.[52] Furthermore, there is evidence that in rare cases hearing preservation may be possible with the translabyrinthine approach, such that in one case ablation of all three semicircular canals with preservation of the cochlea and saccule left the patient with useful, though decreased, hearing.[53] Another variation of the translabyrinthine approach is the addition of a suboccipital approach with a partial labyrinthectomy, such that only those elements that are required for visualization of the vertical crest and the lateral IAC are removed.[54]

One advantage of the translabyrinthine compared with the middle fossa approach is that after drilling the labyrinth, the tumor is encountered, together with the superior and inferior vestibular nerves. Thus, the facial nerve, being anterior, is well protected. This is in contrast to the middle fossa approach, where the facial nerve is immediately beneath the dura, and the retrosigmoid approach, where the facial nerve is anterior to the tumor. The advantage of the translabyrinthine approach over the suboccipital approach is the lack of cerebellar retraction. Thus, for large tumors when surgery is expected to be long, this approach minimizes the chance of postoperative cerebellar edema, hematoma, or infarction. Its main disadvantages are the added surgical time for the labyrinthectomy, need for sacrificing hearing, and limited exposure in comparison with the retrosigmoid approach.

Indications

The objective of the translabyrinthine approach is to expose the IAC and CPA through the labyrinth without entering the middle ear. Larger tumors occupying the IAC and CPA can be approached. Hearing and vestibular function are sacrificed by definition. Therefore, it is indicated only in those vestibular schwannomas with nonserviceable hearing (i.e., speech reception threshold of more than 50 dB and speech discrimination score of less than 50%). It is an ideal approach for vestibular neurectomy for intractable vertigo when hearing is lost. For patients with normal hearing, this approach is contraindicated.

Surgical Approach

The patient is positioned supine with the head turned opposite to the side of the tumor. A retroauricular C-shaped skin incision is made, and an anteriorly based periosteal flap is elevated and preserved.[55]

A simple mastoidectomy is first accomplished by removing the mastoid cortex from the mastoid tip inferiorly, to the supramastoid crest superiorly, and to the posterior wall of the EAC anteriorly. The SS is visualized and skeletonized to the level of the jugular bulb. The angle formed by the middle fossa dura above, the posterior fossa dura below, and the SS is called the sinodural angle. After exposure of the sinodural angle, the SS, the transverse sinus, and SPS are identified.

The mastoid antrum is then entered, and the short process of the incus in the fossa incudis is identified. This provides a useful landmark for the lateral semicircular canal (LSC), which is found immediately below. The solid angle is located medial to the mastoid antrum and houses the three semicircular canals (Fig. 47-3). The air cells are then removed inferiorly to the level of the digastric groove. The air cells posterior to the LSC are removed, and the PSC, located between the LSC and the posterior fossa plate, is exposed. The vertical segment of the facial nerve is then located within the fallopian canal by removing the

remaining inferior mastoid and retrofacial air cells. The facial nerve passes from the external genu at the inferior surface of the LSC to the stylomastoid foramen, located just anterior to the digastric ridge. The facial nerve is skeletonized only to facilitate exposure of the jugular bulb and foramen; it is otherwise left within the dense bone of the fallopian canal. It is important to stay parallel to the facial nerve course during drilling of the bone around the fallopian canal. This technique avoids inadvertent penetration of the canal if the direction of drilling is perpendicular to the facial nerve.[56] The SSC is identified by following the sinodural angle through the supralabyrinthine air cells. The final area of posterior exposure is removal of the middle, posterior, and sigmoid plates, completing the subtotal petrosectomy. The roughly triangular area of bone bounded by the SS, SPS, and bony labyrinth (i.e., solid angle) is known as Trautmann's triangle. This bone is drilled to expose the presigmoid posterior fossa dura.

After the retrofacial air cells, the jugular bulb is exposed. At this point in the exposure, the tympanic and mastoid segments of the facial nerve mark the anterior limit, the jugular bulb the inferior limit, the SS the inferior limit, and the middle cranial fossa the superior limit of the dissection.

The LSC, PSC, and SSC are removed, as well as the bone over the posterior fossa, revealing the endolymphatic sac. Next, the vestibule is opened and completely exposed beneath the facial nerve. Bone is removed over the medial and posterior vestibule until the nerves to the superior, lateral, and inferior ampullas are exposed. These nerves define the superior and inferior limits of the IAC. Bone removal continues over the IAC until a transparent shell remains. The transverse crest separating the superior and inferior division of the vestibular nerves can be seen through the thinned bone.

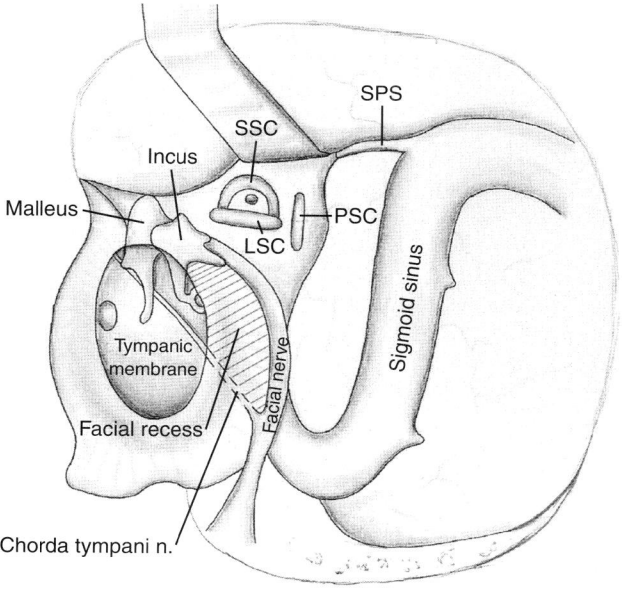

FIGURE 47-3 Critical structures of the temporal bone as seen by posterior transmastoid approaches. The solid angle, housing the three semicircular canals, is shown. The facial recess anterior to the facial nerve (hatched area) is illustrated. Opening the facial recess provides access to the middle ear structures, ossicles, and round and oval windows.

The facial nerve is then identified by palpation of the vertical crest. Care should be taken when removing bone from the superior wall of the IAC, because the facial nerve is superficial under the dura and can be injured. Once the facial nerve has been skeletonized, the remaining bone over the IAC is removed. The dura over the IAC can then be opened for tumor removal or vestibular neurectomy.

Because this approach is limited in comparison with the retrosigmoid approach for large vestibular schwannomas, several modifications have been added to House's classic description. Sanna introduced the enlarged translabyrinthine approach in 2003 with transapical extension as an extension for dealing with vestibular schwannomas greater than 4 cm.[57-60] The principle of transapical extension is to increase bone removal anterior and posterior to SS, along the middle fossa, and around IAC up to 320 degrees (type I) or 360 degrees (type II). To increase vertical extension of the exposure in cases with a high jugular bulb (which is one of the limitations of the classic translabyrinthine approach), the bulb is depressed inferiorly with Surgicel and bone wax.[57]

The wound is closed by placing a free muscle graft over the malleus, incus, and attic. To gain access to the middle ear, the facial recess is sometimes opened. The facial recess is a triangular area defined superiorly by the fossa incudis, medially by the facial nerve, and inferiorly by the chorda tympani (see Fig. 47-3). In this situation, a muscle plug is placed to close the opening of the eustachian tube. The cavity is filled with fat graft, and the periosteal flap is closed. The skin is closed tightly, and a pressure dressing is applied.

Complications and Disadvantages

The main disadvantage of the translabyrinthine approach is inadequate exposure of the tentorium, petroclival area, and foramen magnum. Thus, for large posterior fossa tumors, especially meningiomas with broad-based tentorial attachment, the translabyrinthine approach by itself is inadequate, requiring expansion of the approach. Also, it may be difficult to control vascular structures (e.g., the anterior inferior cerebellar artery) if inadvertent injury occurs.

The main complication with this approach seems to be a high incidence of CSF leakage (up to 30% in some series but usually in the 10% to 20% range).[61] Access to the eustachian tube through the middle ear (facial recess) or the epitympanum can lessen the risk of CSF leakage but involves additional exposure and drilling. Placing a free muscle graft over the attic, filling the operative cavity with fat graft, and closing with a periosteal graft decrease the chance of CSF leakage. In a series of 110 patients treated with the expanded translabyrinthine approach closed with abdominal fat, the rate of CSF leakage was 1.8%.[57] Other complications include posterior fossa subdural hematoma, brain stem hematoma, cerebellar and cerebral swelling, and lower cranial nerve palsies. In cases of highly pneumatized temporal bone, preventive closure of the eustachian tube can be performed. This is accomplished by "cul de sac" closure of the EAC, removal of the ossicular chain, and additional drilling of hypotympanic air cells with exposure of eustachian tube, which is plugged with a piece of muscle.[62]

TRANSOTIC APPROACH

The transotic approach was developed by Fisch and Mattox[61] in response to the limitations of the translabyrinthine approach. Unlike the posteriorly directed translabyrinthine approach, the transotic approach permits more extensive temporal bone resection and positions the dissection both anterior and posterior to the facial nerve, giving excellent visualization of the anterior CPA and petrous apex. The early description included transposition of the facial nerve and had similarities with the transcochlear approach of House and Hitselberger.[63] Unfortunately, the rate of facial nerve paralysis was unacceptable, and modifications followed such that the facial nerve is not transposed but left in situ in the fallopian canal.[61,64]

Indications

The indication for the transotic approach is essentially identical to that for the translabyrinthine approach. It was designed for vestibular schwannomas of up to 2.5 cm,[61,65] although it can certainly be used for larger schwannomas and other lesions, such as meningiomas, hemangiomas, arachnoid cysts, and mucosal cysts, involving the IAC.[66] In contrast to the translabyrinthine approach, the transotic approach circumvents the problem of a high jugular bulb because of the anterior exposure obtained. Because of additional anterior exposure, this approach can be used for treating some petrous apex cholesteatomas.[67]

This approach may be useful for large vestibular schwannomas, because it provides an additional corridor anterior to the facial nerve compared with the translabyrinthine approach. Less extensive petrosectomies (e.g., translabyrinthine) are probably adequate for most vestibular schwannomas. Its other main advantage is the obliteration of the eustachian tube, resulting in a decreased chance for CSF leakage.

Surgical Approach

The surgical approach for the transotic approach is similar to that for the transcochlear approach, with the important difference that the facial nerve is not mobilized (Fig. 47-4). It involves blind sac closure of the EAC, exenteration of the otic capsule including the cochlea, and exposure of the jugular bulb by drilling infralabyrinthine air cells and petrous carotid artery. The additional exposure is obtained by drilling the bone anterior to the tympanic and mastoid segments of the facial nerve. By the end of the exposure, the facial nerve from its entrance into the IAC to its exit at the stylomastoid foramen is exposed in the middle of approach yet remains within bone, thus reducing the potential risk for injury.[61,66,68]

Complications and Disadvantages

The original transotic approach was associated with a high incidence of facial nerve paralysis secondary to transposition of the facial nerve.[65] The modification of leaving the facial nerve within the fallopian canal reduced this risk.[64] In Fisch and Mattox's[61] series of 73 patients, for tumors less than 1.4 cm, all patients had normal facial nerve function at 2 years after surgery. For tumors measuring 1.5 to 2.5 cm, facial nerve function was normal in 61% at 2 years. CSF leakage was contained subcutaneously in 4% and was transient in 3%, and no patient required revision. Removal of all of the middle ear mucosa and pneumatic air cells related to the middle ear space and obliteration of the eustachian tube orifice, combined with dural closure and filling of the defect with fat, lessen the chances for CSF leakage.[66] In

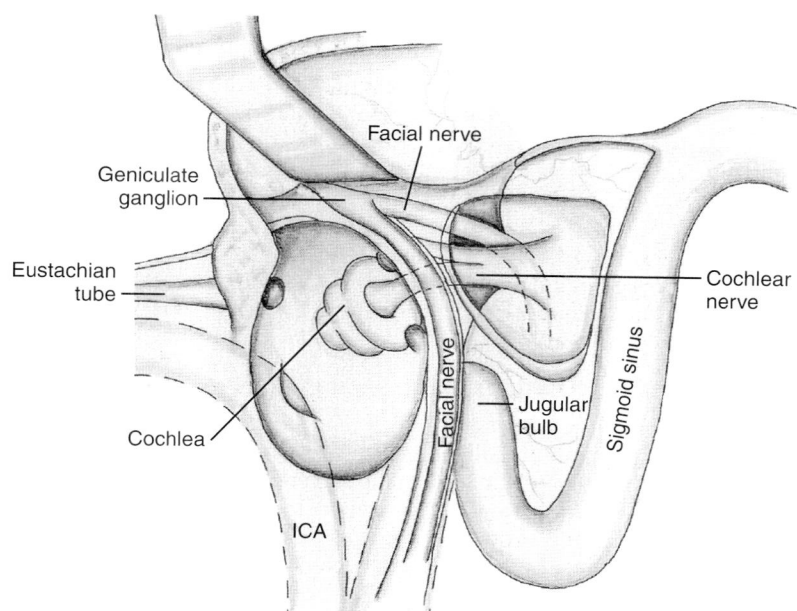

FIGURE 47-4 Exposure of the temporal bone as seen during a transcochlear approach. The cochlea is shown. The ICA is shown anterior and inferior to the cochlea. The facial nerve lies in its canal (not transposed).

their series, meningitis occurred in 1%, and death occurred in 1%. Disadvantages of this approach are that it adds operative time compared with other procedures (e.g., translabyrinthine approach) and that the presence of facial nerve in the middle of approach not only limits surgeon maneuverability but also exposes the nerve to inadvertent injury.[69]

TRANSCOCHLEAR APPROACH

In 1976, House and Hitselberger[63] described the transcochlear approach. This approach is a forward extension of the translabyrinthine approach in which the facial nerve is mobilized and the cochlea removed. This exposure essentially removes the entire petrous bone, giving maximal transpetrosal exposure. The transcochlear approach involves the same extent of petrous bone drilling as the transotic approach, but during a transcochlear approach the facial nerve is mobilized posteriorly, giving the surgeon additional working space and maneuverability. Both approaches give access to the CPA anterior to the IAC, but the transotic approach can be converted to a transcochlear approach if wider exposure is required.[70]

The operative field given by the transcochlear approach is limited by the EAC wall and middle ear and, although more anterior than the translabyrinthine approach, remains posteriorly directed. The modified transcochlear approach was developed to give additional anterior exposure by removing the EAC and the tympanic membrane.[65] It also offered more extensive exposure and circumferential control of the petrous ICA.[71-75] Some authors also include resection of the glenoid fossa, joint capsule, and meniscus and partial resection of the posterior aspect of the zygomatic arch.[74] Others combine it with a neck dissection,[76] and some describe extended exposures, including tentorial section for supratentorial exposure.[77]

Indications

The transcochlear approach was designed for large tumors in the CPA extending anterior to the IAC along the superior two thirds of the clivus, as well as for aneurysms of the middle and lower basilar artery. It is also suitable for complex petrous apex cholesteatomas encasing vital structures.[78] Its main advantage is the broadness of the exposure, giving the surgeon a parallel triangular view of the middle clivus. In addition, contralateral cranial nerves and the CPA are exposed.[70] The addition of the modified transcochlear approach gives the surgeon a more direct and most laterally directed approach to the CPA, as well as circumferential exposure of the petrous ICA. This is important for selected cases in which a carotid bypass is required. It can be combined with resection of the mandibular condyle, closure of the EAC, zygomatic osteotomy, and drilling of the floor of the middle cranial fossa for tumors extending into the infratemporal fossa and nasopharynx.

Surgical Approach

The initial exposure for the transcochlear approach is similar to that for the translabyrinthine approach. A curvilinear C-shaped retroauricular skin incision is made, and the skin of the cartilaginous EAC is everted and sewn shut (see Fig. 47-4). A musculoperiosteal flap from the mastoid process is used medially as a second layer of closure.[74] The skin of the bony EAC and tympanic membrane were initially left in place, but removal of this bone improves access to the midline without increasing morbidity. The entire osseous EAC can be removed without affecting the function of the mandibular condyle in the glenoid fossa.

A mastoidectomy is performed exposing the canal wall inferiorly. The middle and posterior fossa plates, along with the SS, are then skeletonized. The facial nerve is skeletonized from its entrance into the IAC to its exit from the stylomastoid foramen. The facial recess is opened. The middle ear space and epitympanum are entered, and the ossicles can then be removed. The chorda tympani is then sectioned inferiorly at its origin from the descending portion of the facial nerve. Drilling is continued into the retrofacial air cells. The GSPN is then divided just anterior to its origin at the GG. The facial nerve can then be mobilized from its bony canal and transposed posteriorly. This invariably results in facial nerve paralysis, because it disrupts the blood supply to the GG. It is best to leave the facial nerve within the canal, if possible. If transposition is necessary, then anterior transposition by mobilizing the mastoid segment and the nerve exiting at the stylomastoid foramen is safer.

Next, the cochlea is removed, including the bony septum between the basal turn and the ICA (see Fig. 47-6). The jugular bulb is also exposed completely. Care should be taken not to injure the underlying neurovascular structures, namely, cranial nerves IX through XI near the jugular bulb and foramen, as well as the facial nerve in the dura of the IAC.

The complete petrosectomy gives exposure from the SPS superiorly to Meckel's cave and inferiorly to the inferior petrosal sinus and jugular bulb. The osseous removal extends anteriorly to the petrous carotid artery and TMJ and medially to the clivus. The dura is opened triangularly parallel to the SPS, inferior petrosal sinus, SS, and IAC. It can also be opened on both sides of the IAC. This exposes the CPA widely.

Complications and Disadvantage

The main disadvantage of the transcochlear approach is that hearing is sacrificed. The extensive mobilization of the facial nerve places it at risk, and all patients have significant facial nerve paralysis.[79] Although it usually improves after surgery, facial nerve function infrequently exceeds grade III on the House-Brackmann grading scale,[80] and the nerve often is permanently impaired. Section of the GSPN can result in an ipsilateral dry eye. There is also a risk of CSF leakage and meningitis. Resection of the mandibular condyle can result in TMJ dysfunction.

Given the high frequency of facial nerve paralysis and time-consuming exposure, some groups advocated the use of relatively simple retrosigmoid approach in combination with an orbitozygomatic approach for petroclival meningiomas.[79]

INFRALABYRINTHINE APPROACH
Indications

In 1985, Gherini et al.[81] advocated the infralabyrinthine approach for the surgical management of cholesterol granulomas of the petrous apex and CPA. The purpose of this approach is to permit access to that portion of the petrous apex that is inferior to the labyrinth. As such, it is valuable in decompression of a cholesterol granuloma of the petrous apex.[82] The advantages of this approach for cholesterol granulomas include absence of ossicular chain work and risk of ICA injury, as well as easiness of revision surgery. It can also be useful in conjunction with the suboccipital approach for resection of meningiomas of the petrous ridge with extension into the temporal bone, but without involvement of the labyrinth[76,83] and jugular paragangliomas.[84]

Surgical Approach

In the infralabyrinthine approach, a simple mastoidectomy is first performed. The middle and posterior fossa plates, along with the SS, are then skeletonized. At this point, the PSC and LSC can be identified and protected. The facial nerve is identified and skeletonized along its

mastoid segment and left in its bony canal. Communication between the labyrinth superiorly and the jugular bulb inferiorly is then developed until the petrous apex is entered. The bulb can be skeletonized, and its superior portion is carefully dissected to free it of its adjacent bony covering. It is then packed inferiorly with bone wax so that additional exposure is obtained. In the case of a cholesterol granuloma, drainage of dark, thick fluid, sometimes under pressure, occurs on opening the cavity. Cultures are obtained, the opening into the cavity is widened to approximately 0.5 to 1 cm to provide permanent drainage, and a catheter is placed from the granuloma cavity into the mastoid cells.

Complications and Disadvantages

If the jugular bulb is in a high position, access below the labyrinth and above the bulb can be limited. A careful preoperative evaluation using high-resolution CT is useful.[46,49] Measuring the distance between the labyrinth and the jugular bulb on coronal images can be particularly useful; a distance of less than 1 cm was found to be inadequate for satisfactory drainage of cholesterol granulomas.[85] In those instances, another approach is recommended (e.g., the transcanal–infracochlear approach, described later).

Other complications include injury to the facial nerve, carotid artery, jugular bulb, and labyrinth. The opening made for drainage of the cholesterol granuloma may scar, and the granuloma may recur.

TRANSCANAL–INFRACOCHLEAR APPROACH

The transcanal part of the transcanal–infracochlear approach was first described by Farrior[85,86] in 1984.

Indications

The transcanal–infracochlear approach is used for access to the petrous apex cholesterol granulomas when hearing preservation is a goal and the jugular bulb is positioned high, limiting exposure through an infralabyrinthine approach. Because this approach is directed cephalad, it provides dependent drainage for cholesterol granulomas of the petrous apex. Additional advantages are drainage to a well-aerated region near the eustachian tube and easy reexploration through an inferior myringotomy.[22] Because of these advantages over other approaches, the transcanal–infracochlear approach is considered the approach of choice for cholesterol granulomas of the petrous apex.[22,85,87]

Surgical Approach

The transcanal–infracochlear approach uses a C-shaped retroauricular skin incision similar to that used for the translabyrinthine and infralabyrinthine approaches. The soft tissues are reflected forward, and the ear canal is transected just medial to the bony cartilaginous junction. The anterior, inferior, and posterior portions of the ear canal skin are lifted superiorly to the level of the umbo. Bone is removed from over the anterior, inferior, and posterior portions of the bony canal wall, effectively achieving near-total removal of the tympanic bone and enlargement of the canal. The thin bone over the TMJ is preserved. The carotid artery is then skeletonized anterior and inferior to the eustachian tube orifice. Bone is then removed between the ICA and the internal jugular vein without actually exposing the jugular bulb. The region of the facial nerve is identified using continuous electrical monitoring, but the nerve is not exposed. Inferiorly, the cholesterol granuloma sac is identified, opened for drainage, and irrigated. Essentially, the silicone catheter should be positioned to maintain the patency of fenestration.[22] Finally, the tympanomeatal flap is repositioned and the resultant bone defect is filled with bone plate.

Complications and Disadvantages

The complications of the transcanal–infracochlear approach are similar to those with the translabyrinthine approach except that injury to the cochlea, carotid artery, and jugular bulb is possible. This approach provides only limited exposure of the petrous apex and therefore is useful only in the specific indications of drainage of a cholesterol granuloma or petrous apicitis. Mattox reported use of a combination of microscope and endoscope for cholesterol granulomas and cholesteatomas.[88] An endoscope facilitates the exposure of cystic cavity and allows the surgeon to clean any sediment, as well as fenestrate all cysts into a single cavity.[89,90]

Combined Approaches
PETROSAL APPROACH

The petrosal approach is also referred to as the combined suprainfratentorial approach because it combines both supratentorial and infratentorial exposures to give wide anterior access to the CPA and ventral brain stem. The first reported transtentorial exposure was in 1896 by Stieglitz et al.,[91] in which a CPA tumor was approached through a supramastoid–suboccipital exposure. Several authors followed with modifications of the occipital flap with a suboccipital craniectomy, including ligation of the SS for wider exposure,[92] combined occipitotemporal craniotomy with or without ligation of the lateral sinus,[93] and reapproximation of the lateral sinus,[94] as well as other approaches,[95,96] including the addition of a mastoidectomy.[97,98]

The petrosal approach was popularized by Malis,[98] who described ligation of the SS between its junction with the superior anastomotic vein and the SPS for increased exposure. Spetzler et al.[99] operated on 83 patients with the petrosal approach and sacrificed the SS in 50% of cases. Al-Mefty et al.[100] described the petrosal approach in detail, emphasizing an extensive petrous resection and directing the approach more laterally, thus lessening the operative distance to the clivus. They also stressed the importance of preserving the venous sinuses.

Indications

The petrosal approach includes a combined temporal craniotomy with a posterior fossa craniectomy–craniotomy for supratentorial and infratentorial exposure. Crucial to this approach is sectioning of the tentorium. With the addition of an extensive petrous resection, the anterior surface of the brain stem can be approached to the level of the inferior one third of the clivus. The lowest portion of the clivus is often obscured by the jugular tubercle. The petrosal approach provides access to lesions in the CPA and petroclival junction (upper two thirds of the clivus), such as meningiomas, trigeminal schwannomas, epidermoids, or chondrosarcomas. Vascular pathologies such as aneurysms of the middle

third of the basilar artery can be accessed.[101] For lesions of the lower third of the clivus and the foramen magnum, the far lateral transcondylar approach provides better access.

Not only the posterior fossa structures but also the supratentorial ventrolateral brain stem can be exposed through this approach. Hakuba et al.[102] first used this route for retrochiasmatic craniopharyngiomas. The main advantage of this approach in comparison with pterional or orbitozygomatic approaches is the ability to attack the tumor from an inferior to a superior direction. This is especially important for tumors with significant superior extension.[103,104]

Surgical Approach

The patient is placed in a lateral position. The incision begins approximately 1 cm anterior to the ear and is directed posteriorly in a gentle curve to the postauricular area approximately 2 cm posterior to the mastoid process. The temporalis fascia and muscle are elevated and reflected anteriorly on a pedicle.

A mastoidectomy is first accomplished with preservation of the labyrinth and exposure of the mastoid segment of the facial nerve. A combined temporo-occipital bone flap is then raised (Fig. 47-5). The transverse sinus and SS were previously identified during the mastoidectomy. This gives exposure along the middle fossa floor, transverse sinus, SS, and suboccipital dura. The dura can then be opened on the inferior aspect of the temporal lobe and anterior or posterior to the SS. After opening the dura over the temporal lobe and the presigmoid dura, the SPS is clipped and divided. The tentorium can be divided in three directions (Fig. 47-6). The first cut is done posteriorly along the transverse sinus to allow for retraction of the transverse sinus–SS junction posteriorly, thus enlarging the presigmoid corridor. The second cut is aimed medially toward the free edge to identify and protect the trochlear nerve. The third cut is parallel to the petrous pyramid and the SPS. This allows resection of the lateral tentorial leaflet and a view of the supratentorial and infratentorial compartments. Ipsilateral cranial nerves IV through X are well visualized (Fig. 47-7). A retractor can be placed to retract the temporal lobe superiorly, and another one can be placed to retract the transverse sinus and SS posteriorly. If the surgeon decides to work through the retrosigmoid corridor, a cerebellar retractor can be placed. Care

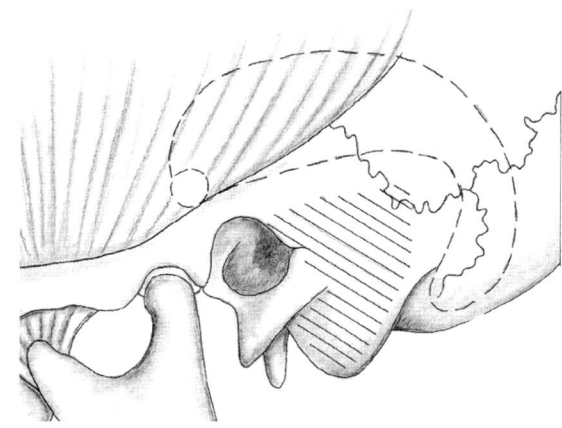

FIGURE 47-5 Petrosal approach. Outline of the craniotomy (interrupted line) and mastoidectomy (hatched area). The asterion and EAC are shown.

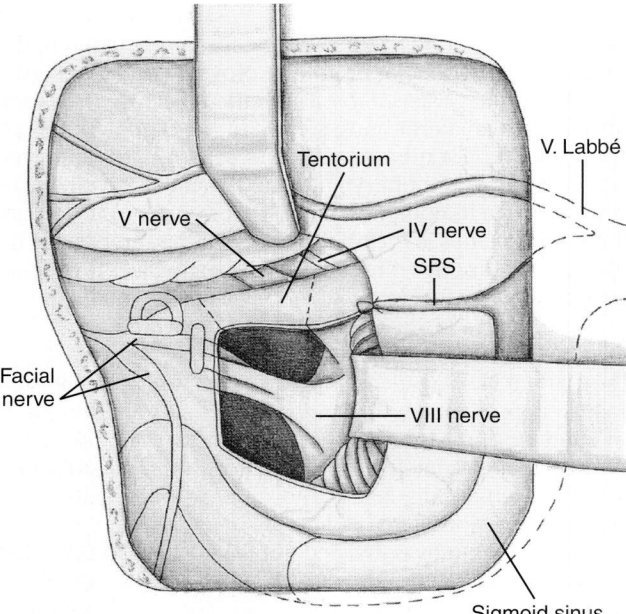

FIGURE 47-6 Exposure obtained by the petrosal approach. Two retractors, one superiorly and another posteriorly, elevate the temporal lobe and the cerebellum, respectively. The SPS is ligated. The vestibulocochlear nerve bundle and the facial nerve are shown as they course toward the internal auditory nerve. The semicircular canals are also shown. The tentorium is cut in three directions—one anteriorly parallel to the petrous pyramid, another medially toward the free edge (cranial nerves IV and V are shown medially), and one posteriorly along the transverse sinus (not shown here).

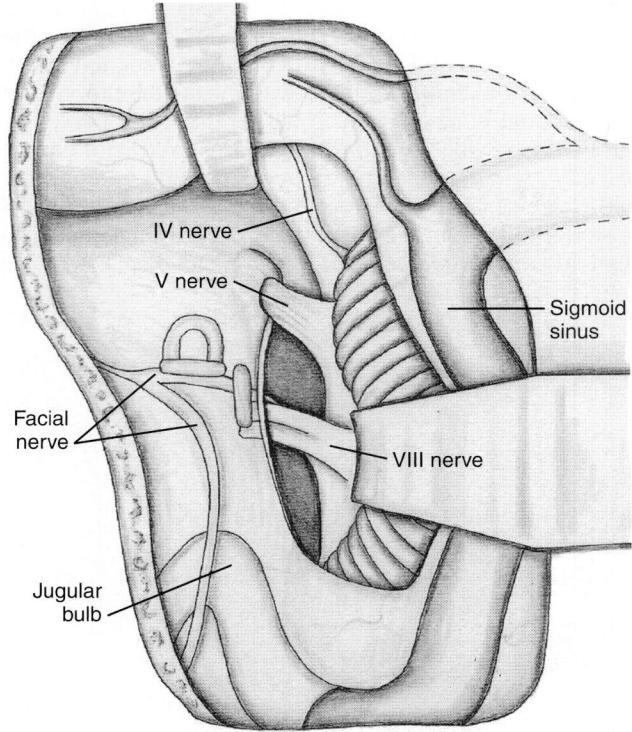

FIGURE 47-7 Petrosal approach. The presigmoid retrolabyrinthine corridor is shown. Exposure is obtained after sectioning the tentorium. The trochlear, trigeminal, facial, and vestibulocochlear nerves are seen.

must be taken to avoid injury to the inferior anastomotic vein. In certain cases, the presigmoid avenue is limited and ligation and division of the SS can provide maximum anterior exposure of the CPA.

The surgical technique for resection of retrochiasmatic craniopharyngiomas with the petrosal approach has several nuances.[102-105] Exposure is performed as described earlier, except that the presigmoid dura is exposed only enough for opening and closure. The temporal dura is opened along the floor of the middle fossa, the SPS is clipped and cut, and the incision is carried along the SS. Care is taken to avoid damage to the vein of Labbé. The tentorium is cut to the free edge, which enables retraction of the SS posteriorly, creating a presigmoid working corridor. The approach is then directed toward the crural and ambient cisterns. Opening the arachnoid exposes the tumor anterior and superior to the basilar artery, inferior to chiasm, and medial to cranial nerves III and IV. As mentioned previously, this approach allows retrochiasmatic tumor resection with minimal brain retraction.

Wound closure begins with reapproximation of the dura. A dural defect usually remains after suturing. Any opened air cells are waxed. The mastoid antrum is sealed with fascia or muscle, and an autologous fat graft is used to fill the petrosectomy defect. Alternatively or additionally, the posterior temporalis vascularized flap can be used to cover the petrosectomy defect and prevent CSF leakage. The inner table from the craniotomy can be shaped and anchored with miniplates for a more cosmetic mastoid appearance. Spinal drainage can be used for several days after surgery, depending on preference.

Complications and Disadvantages

Typical complications as described earlier for any intracranial approach may be encountered with the petrosal approach. In addition, there is potential for injury to the sinuses and for significant blood loss and air embolism if that occurs. Specific to this approach is the potential for injury to the inferior anastomotic vein, which provides significant venous drainage to the temporal lobe. Hence, edema and venous infarction are a possibility. During drilling of the petrous apex, injury to the semicircular canals (especially the posterior one) and facial nerve may occur.

INFRATEMPORAL FOSSA APPROACH

The infratemporal fossa approach, developed by Fisch[106] in 1977, is a craniotemporocervical approach for exposure of the lateral inferior skull base. This approach is divided into three exposures, types A, B, and C, depending on the amount of anterior exposure required. The type A approach is similar to the combined lateral skull base approach reported by Gardner et al.[107] in 1977. With the type A exposure, a subtotal petrosectomy with transposition of the facial nerve is accomplished for exposure of the apical and infralabyrinthine temporal bone, as well as the mandibular fossa and posterior infratemporal fossa. The type B exposure gives additional anterior exposure of the clivus and horizontal segment of the ICA. The anterioposterior limits are from the foramen ovale to the SS. The type C approach is an anterior extension of the type B approach, giving exposure of the infratemporal fossa, pterygopalatine fossa, parasellar region, and nasopharynx. The exposure is obtained by removal of middle cranial fossa bone. With most indications for the type C approach, the surgeon can use a more anterior, preauricular pterional type of incision with a zygomatic osteotomy and subtemporal craniectomy.[108]

Indications

According to Fisch,[106] the type A infratemporal fossa approach is useful for lesions involving the jugular foramen (e.g., class C and D glomus jugulare tumors), lesions of the petrous apex, lower cranial nerve schwannomas, high cervical and petrous carotid artery lesions, and certain infratemporal fossa lesions. Modifications of the approach can be made according to the therapeutic goal. Deveze et al.[109] reported a modified type A approach for vascular lesions of high cervical and petrous carotid artery with subsequent reconstruction of EAC and ossicular chain. Despite the aggressiveness of the approach, patients had satisfactory facial and hearing preservation.

The type B approach is indicated for lesions of the petrous apex and clivus. The type C approach is best for lesions such as juvenile nasopharyngeal angiofibroma and nasopharyngeal carcinoma or for those involving the pterygopalatine fossa, cavernous sinus, and nasopharynx.

Surgical Approach

The details of the types of infratemporal fossa approaches were well described by Fisch and Mattox[5] and are summarized here. The skin incision is an extension of the standard C-shaped retroauricular incision. The skin and periosteal flap is reflected anteriorly, with transection and closure of the EAC. Facial nerve is exposed distal to the stylomastoid foramen in the parotid gland. Next, the great vessels

(carotid artery and jugular vein) and nerves of the neck (glossopharyngeal, vagus, spinal accessory, and hypoglossal) are exposed (Fig. 47-8). The posterior belly of the digastric muscle is divided near its insertion at the mastoid process. The external carotid artery and its branches are ligated and transected above the lingual artery. The ICA is followed to the carotid foramen. Next, a subtotal petrosectomy is done by exposing the temporal bone and reflecting the sternocleidomastoid muscle away from the mastoid tip. The operation proceeds with removal of the EAC, mastoidectomy with complete mobilization of the facial nerve for anterior transposition, exposure and possible ligation of the SS, removal of the styloid process for exposure of the ICA, obliteration of the eustachian tube, and exposure of the infratemporal fossa. This includes anterior translocation of the mandible. The exposure obtained with this approach spans from the middle ear to the mastoid and upper neck, exposing the posterior portion of the infratemporal fossa.

The type B approach includes exposure of the ICA from the neck to the cavernous sinus posterior to the foramen ovale. To expose the horizontal segment of the ICA, the middle meningeal artery is divided and the eustachian tube is sacrificed. By sacrificing the eustachian tube at this point and preserving the middle ear cleft, hearing can be preserved. The approach to the clivus requires division of cranial nerve V3 and complete removal of the bony eustachian tube.

The type C approach adds anterior exposure to the type B approach. The nasopharynx can be entered by removing the lateral pharyngeal wall behind the medial pterygoid process. Exposure here gives visualization of the vomer, opposite inferior turbinate, and pharyngeal end of the opposite

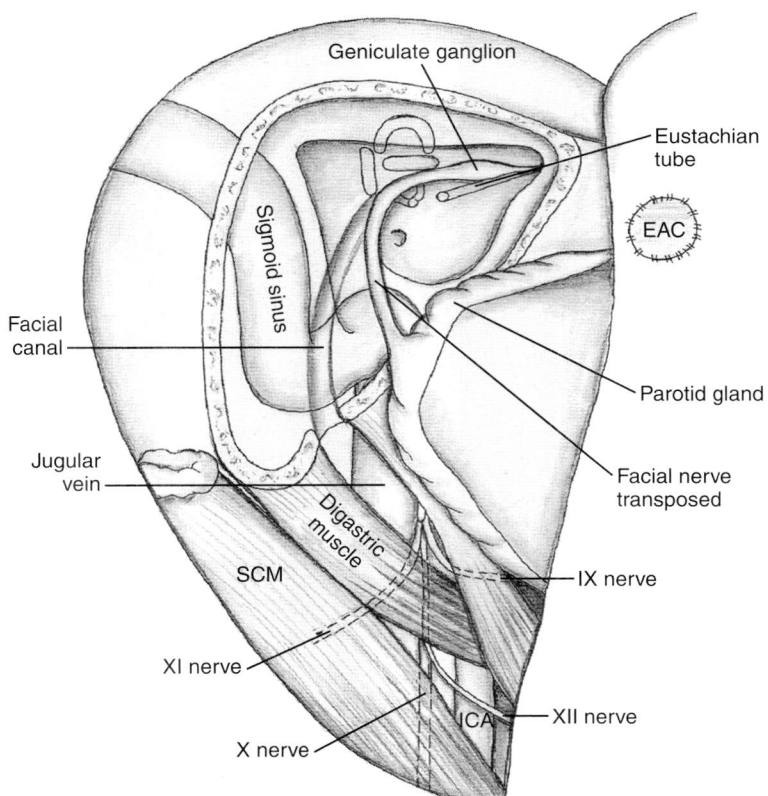

FIGURE 47-8 Exposure is obtained by a type A infratemporal fossa approach. The sternocleidomastoid muscle (SCM) and posterior belly of the digastric muscle are shown. Cranial nerves IX, X, XI, and XII are shown in the neck. The EAC, malleus, and incus have been removed. The facial nerve has been transposed anteriorly.

eustachian tube. The pterygopalatine fossa is exposed by removing the pterygoid process. To expose the parasellar region, the zygoma and basal portion of the sphenoid are removed. The ipsilateral sphenoid and maxillary sinus are opened. For complete exposure of the cavernous sinus, the maxillary nerve is divided and the bone at the floor of the middle fossa is removed for extradural elevation of the temporal lobe.

We have used a combination of middle fossa and infratemporal fossa approaches for treating en plaque meningiomas of the temporal bone (Fig. 47-9). This particular combination of approaches is a logical extension of either individual approach when both areas are involved pathologically. This approach could be of value in providing wider access to the petrous carotid artery.

Complications and Disadvantages

According to Fisch and Mattox,[5] transposition of the facial nerve always results in some paresis, but the average recovery of function (to House-Brackmann grade II) was 80%. A conductive hearing loss is common in all infratemporal fossa approaches because of removal of the tympanic membrane and ossicles. Tachycardia can occur after removal of glomus jugulare tumors. Preoperative laboratory evaluation of suspected glomus tumors should include blood vanillylmandelic acid levels and possible use of alpha-adrenergic blockers. With the additional exposure of the eustachian tube, ascending infection can occur even with subsequent primary closure of the eustachian tube. CSF leakage and meningitis can obviously occur. Fisch and Mattox[5] recommend obliteration of the wound with muscle rather than free fat graft to aid in closure of the eustachian tube. For the type C approach, the major risks include hearing loss,

which occurs in most, and loss of mandibular function as a result of translocation of the mandibular condyle and resection of the articular disc and glenoid fossa during exposure. Initially, there may be limitation in jaw opening, but this eventually resolves if the mandibular condyle is preserved. Resection of cranial nerves V2 and V3 usually results in facial and tongue anesthesia; this generally improves over 9 months.[5]

ENDONASAL ENDOSCOPIC APPROACH

The endoscopic approach to the cranial base is not truly a transtemporal approach. The first report of a transsphenoidal approach was reported by Montgomery,[110] who used an open access through the medial canthus. Fucci et al.[111] first used an endoscope to drain a giant cholesterol granuloma of the petrous apex. However, it was not until recently that technological advances popularized endoscopic skull base surgery. The advantages of this approach are less invasiveness, better cosmetic results, hearing and vestibular function preservation, and shorter operative time.[112,113] In addition, as in the case of cholesterol granuloma, stent patency can be easily assessed and the stent can be removed during office follow-up.[114] The endonasal endoscopic approach is considered appropriate for patients with benign cystic lesions abutting, prolapsing, or invading the sphenoid sinus, such as cholesterol granulomas or cholesteatomas,[112,115,116] yet solid lesions can also be resected.[114]

Indications

The endoscopic endonasal approach provides excellent visualization of midline structures from the dorsum sella to C2. Therefore, it is suitable for midline and paramedian lesions, such as chordomas, chondrosarcomas, osteosarcomas,

FIGURE 47-9 Combined middle fossa–infratemporal fossa approach. Adjacent structures are shown. The facial nerve is displaced, and the ICA is exposed. *(From Gardner G, Robertson JH, Clark C: Transtemporal approaches to the cranial cavity. Am J Otol 6(Suppl):118, 1985.)*

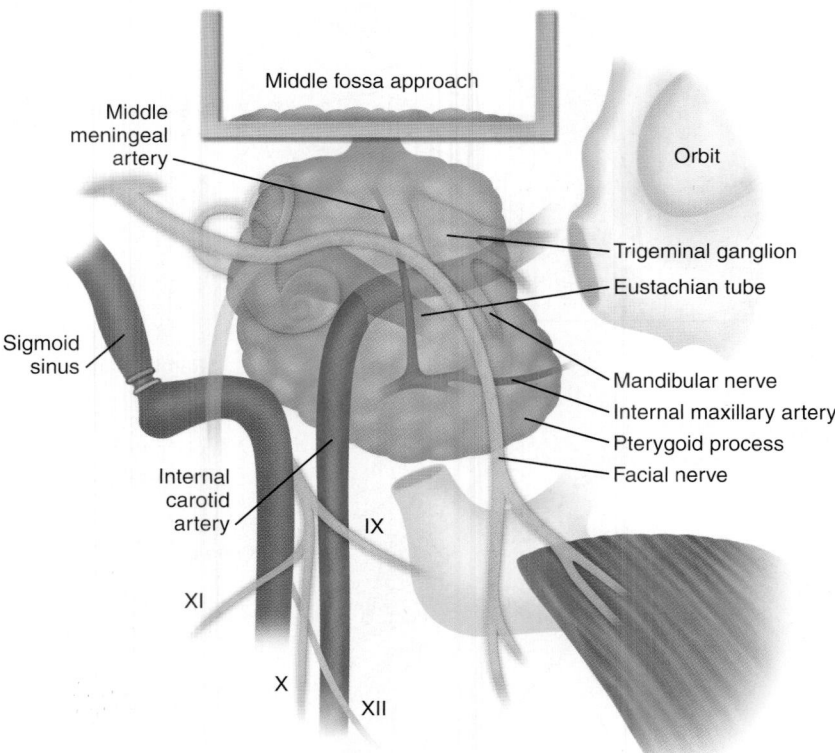

cholesterol granulomas, and cholesteatomas. The carotid arteries laterally are the main limitation of the exposure. Therefore, petrous apex lesions lying medial to the carotid artery can be exposed. An additional advantage for treating a cholesterol granuloma is the presence of the sphenoid sinus, which can be used for aeration of the cavity. Unique to the endoscopic approach is the ability to visualize blind spots with angled rigid 30- and 70-degree scopes. This allows the surgeon to reexplore the surgical field for tumor remnants. Image guidance systems allow early identification of the carotid arteries, as well as an entry point into the petrous apex.[117,118] One of the advantages of image guidance in skull base surgery is the absence of the shift seen during intracranial procedures. Generally, intradural lesions are not considered for endoscopic treatment because of the high risk of postoperative CSF leakage and meningitis.

Surgical Approach

The endoscopic endonasal approach is centered over the sphenoid sinus. Usually a right-sided approach is preferred for right-handed surgeons. However, for paramedian structures, a contralateral approach allows a slightly oblique view—more in line with the axis of the lesion. Depending on the lesion size, a unilateral or bilateral approach can be selected. For lesions requiring less manipulation, a unilateral approach through an enlarged sphenoid ostium can be performed. We prefer to use an anterior trans-sphenoidal approach with lateralization of the posterior nasal septum and opening of both sphenoid ostia, because this method provides better visualization of the sinus cavity. Septations in the sinus are removed carefully to avoid injury to the carotid arteries. Usually both carotid and optic protuberances can be visualized. If not visualized adequately, the position of carotid artery can be identified with a Doppler probe[119] or image guidance.[117,118] Midline tumors are identified in the clival recess. Paramedian lesions protruding into the sinus—so-called sphenopetroid cholesterol granulomas are visualized at this stage. In those cases, marsupialization can be done.[113,114] Usually the petrous apex is entered from a point halfway between the medial surface of the ICA and the midline of the sphenoid sinus at a horizontal level one third of the way up from the posteroinferior aspect of the sphenoid sinus wall. Additional exposure can be done by mobilizing of the carotid artery as described by Zanation et al.[114]

Complications and Disadvantages

The absence of three-dimensional perception is one of the main handicaps of endoscopic surgery. The exposure is limited by the carotid arteries laterally, giving the surgeon relatively narrow working space. Because watertight dural closure is problematic, the approach is currently used to address extradural lesions.

Early experience with the endoscopic approach for petrous apex cholesterol granulomas showed subsequent stenosis.[120] However, subsequent studies showed satisfactory results, broadening the applications.[114] The main risk during surgery is carotid artery injury. It can be avoided by intraoperative visualization of anatomic landmarks or image guidance. Optic nerves, the vidian nerve, and intercavernous and cavernous sinus structures are also at risk during exposure.

Conclusions

The ability to approach the posterior cranial fossa in a variety of ways is advantageous, because it allows the neurosurgeon more options to reach and treat tumors in this area. The ability to drill away selected segments of the temporal bone, without major sacrifice of function, and thus achieve access for surgical procedures presents a continuing and exciting challenge to both neurosurgeons and their otologic colleagues.

ACKNOWLEDGMENT

Portions of this chapter are reproduced with permission from Brodkey J, Vrionis FD: Surgical approaches through the temporal bone. In Robertson JT, Coakham H, Robertson JH (eds): Cranial Base Surgery: Management, Complications and Outcome. Edinburgh, Churchill Livingstone, 2000.

KEY REFERENCES

Al-Mefty O, Ayoubi S, et al. The petrosal approach: indications, technique, and results. *Acta Neurochir Suppl (Wien).* 1991;53:166-170.

Brackmann DE, Toh EH. Surgical management of petrous apex cholesterol granulomas. *Otol Neurotol.* 2002;23(4):529-533.

Deveze A, Alimi Y, et al. Surgical management of lesions of the internal carotid artery using a modified Fisch type A infratemporal approach. *Otol Neurotol.* 2007;28(1):94-99.

Fisch U, Mattox DE. Infratemporal fossa approach type B. In: Fisch U, Mattox DE, eds. *Microsurgery of the skull base.* New York: Stuttgart; 1988:286-343.

Fisch U, Mattox DE. Translabyrinthine approach. In: Fisch U, Mattox DE, eds. *Microsurgery of the Skull Base.* New York: Stuttgart; 1988:546-576.

Fisch U, Mattox DE. Transotic approach to the cerebellopontine angle. In: Fisch U, Mattox DE, eds. *Microsurgery of the Skull Base.* New York: Stuttgart; 1988:74-127.

Fisch U, Mattox DE. Transtemporal supralabyrinthine approach. In: Fisch U, Mattox DE, eds. *Microsurgery of the Skull Base.* New York: Stuttgart; 1988:418-454.

Horn KL, Hankinson HL, et al. The modified transcochlear approach to the cerebellopontine angle. *Otolaryngol Head Neck Surg.* 1991;104(1):37-41.

House W. Surgical exposure of the internal auditory canal and its contents through the middle, cranial fossa. *The Laryngoscope.* 1961;71(11):1363-1385.

House WF. Middle Cranial Fossa Approach to the Petrous Pyramid. Report of 50 Cases. *Arch Otolaryngol.* 1963;78:460-469.

Kabil MS, Shahinian HK. A series of 112 fully endoscopic resections of vestibular schwannomas. *Minim Invasive Neurosurg.* 2006;49(6): 362-368.

Kawase T, Shiobara R, et al. Middle fossa transpetrosal–transtentorial approaches for petroclival meningiomas. Selective pyramid resection and radicality. *Acta Neurochir (Wien).* 1994;129(3-4):113-120.

Mann WJ, Amedee RG, et al. Transsigmoid approach for tumors of the jugular foramen. *Skull Base Surg.* 1991;1(3):137-141.

Mattox DE. Endoscopy-assisted surgery of the petrous apex. *Otolaryngol Head Neck Surg.* 2004;130(2):229-241.

Oyama K, Ikezono T, et al. Petrous apex cholesterol granuloma treated via the endoscopic transsphenoidal approach. *Acta Neurochir (Wien).* 2007;149(3):299-302:discussion 302.

Quinones-Hinojosa A, Chang EF, et al. The extended retrosigmoid approach: an alternative to radical cranial base approaches for posterior fossa lesions. *Neurosurgery.* 2006;58(4 suppl 2):ONS-208-214: discussion ONS-214.

Sanna M. *Lateral Skull Base Surgery. Atlas of Temporal Bone and Lateral Skull Base Surgery.* New York: Stuttgart; 1995:37-50.

Sanna M. Transotic approach. *The Temporal Bone: A Manual for Dissection and Surgical Approaches.* New York; 2006:98-105.

Sanna M. *The Translabyrinthine Approaches.* In: Sanna M, et al, eds. *Atlas of Microsurgery of the Lateral Skull Base.* New York: Thieme; 2008:34-77.

Sanna M, Dispenza F, et al. Otoneurological management of petrous apex cholesterol granuloma. *Am J Otolaryngol.* 2009;30(6):407-414.

Shiobara R, Ohira T, et al. A modified extended middle cranial fossa approach for acoustic nerve tumors. Results of 125 operations. *J Neurosurg.* 1988;68(3):358-365.

Vrionis FD, Cano WG, et al. Microsurgical anatomy of the infratemporal fossa as viewed laterally and superiorly. *Neurosurgery.* 1996;39(4):777-785:discussion 785–776.

Vrionis FD, Foley KT, et al. Use of cranial surface anatomic fiducials for interactive image-guided navigation in the temporal bone: a cadaveric study. *Neurosurgery.* 1997;40(4):755-763:discussion 763–754.

Vrionis FD, Robertson JH, et al. Image-interactive orientation in the middle cranial fossa approach to the internal auditory canal: an experimental study. *Comput Aided Surg.* 1997;2(1):34-41.

Vrionis FD, Robertson JH, et al. Asterion meningiomas. *Skull Base Surg.* 1998;8(3):153-161.

Numbered references appear on Expert Consult.

CHAPTER 48

Surgical Management of Neurofibromatosis Types 1 and 2

JAMES H. TONSGARD • BAKHTIAR YAMINI • DAVID M. FRIM

Neurofibromatosis types 1 and 2 (NF1 and NF2) are genetic diseases that commonly affect the brain, peripheral nerves, spinal roots, spinal cord, and dura. While the type of neurologic complications in NF1 and NF2 are also found in patients without NF, management frequently is different. It is important for the neurosurgeon to be aware of not only the range of neurologic complications that occur in NF but also their clinical course in NF patients. This chapter covers the neurologic complications, the indications for surgery, and the surgical approach to the tumor types found in NF1 and NF2. The details of the techniques of tumor removal are similar to those used for removal of the same tumors in patients without NF. Because NF1 and NF2 have very different complications, the two diseases are presented separately.

Neurofibromatosis Type 1

NF1 is an autosomal dominant genetic disorder caused by a mutation or deletion of the neurofibromin gene on the long arm of chromosome 17.[1] The diagnosis of NF1 requires the presence of two or more major criteria: six or more café-au-lait spots, two cutaneous neurofibromas, one plexiform neurofibroma, certain bony abnormalities, an optic glioma, iris Lisch nodules, or a first-degree relative with NF1.[2] Diagnosis has primarily been clinical, but genetic testing identifies at least 95% of patients who meet the clinical criteria. While there are no silent carriers of NF, clinical manifestations are variable, even within the same family.[3] Because NF1 may affect virtually any organ system and some complications such as plexiform neurofibromas commonly involve adjacent organs, a multidisciplinary team is essential for management. Such a team should include a pediatrician, neurologist, geneticist, ophthalmologist, neurosurgeon, orthopedist, plastic surgeon, and oncologist. NF1 is a progressive disorder. Some complications worsen with age. Moreover, complications of NF1 are usually age specific. Plexiform neurofibromas can be considered congenital, although they may not require surgical intervention until later in life. Optic gliomas usually present between 18 months and 7 years of age.[4] Iris Lisch nodules usually appear between 10 and 21 years of age. Cutaneous neurofibromas commonly occur in teenagers or young adults, and malignant peripheral nerve sheath tumors (MPNSTs) are a complication of young adults.[5]

NEUROLOGIC COMPLICATIONS OF NF1 AND INDICATIONS FOR NEUROSURGICAL INTERVENTION

The neurologic complications of NF1 include headaches, learning disabilities, seizures, peripheral nerve tumors, spinal nerve root tumors, dural ectasias, deafness, optic gliomas, areas of high-intensity signal on magnetic resonance imaging (MRI), tumors of the brain parenchyma, and aqueductal stenosis.[6] Migraine headaches are a common feature.[7] Learning disabilities and hyperactivity occur in at least 50% of patients.[8] Deafness occurs in 10% of NF1 patients and is not caused by tumors.[9] Brain tumors and optic gliomas occur in a small percentage of patients. The incidence is increased compared with the normal population.[10] All patients with NF1 develop peripheral nerve tumors.

Peripheral Nerve Tumors

Five types of peripheral nerve tumors occur in NF1: schwannomas, discrete neurofibromas (sometimes called cutaneous or dermal neurofibromas), diffuse neurofibromas, plexiform neurofibromas, and MPNSTs. Schwannomas are infrequently found in patients with NF1. This tumor is more typical of NF2 and is discussed in the section on NF2. Diffuse neurofibromas most commonly present as boggy caplike lesions of the scalp that involve the subcutaneous tissue, stopping at the fascia.[11] Diffuse neurofibromas of the scalp do not progress beyond the hairline and are best left alone unless there is evidence of rapid growth.

Discrete neurofibromas and plexiform neurofibromas involve a proliferation of fibroblasts, Schwann cells, perineural cells, mast cells, extracellular matrix, axons, and blood vessels.[12] These two tumors differ histologically, primarily in the extent of extracellular matrix. Plexiform neurofibromas have more extracellular matrix. Both tumors cause expansion of the nerve. Nerve fibers run through the tumor. Plexiform neurofibromas may involve small peripheral nerves, large peripheral nerves, nerve trunks, plexus, or spinal roots. Motor nerves, sensory nerves, or both are affected. Plexiform neurofibromas may be associated with markedly dilated veins. Plexiform neurofibromas involve the skin with or without involvement of underlying muscle, or they may be confined to deeper tissues. Plexiform tumors are felt to be congenital or to appear within the first year of life. Growth is highly variable. Some tumors remain static, others relentlessly increase, and still others undergo spurts of growth and periods of quiescence. Plexiform neurofibromas may appear discrete and isolated, diffuse and infiltrative, or nodular with multiple grapelike clusters.[13] Plexiform neurofibromas commonly infiltrate adjacent muscle and sometimes infiltrate adjacent organs, such as the bladder or esophagus. Plexiform neurofibromas occur in at least 50% of all patients.[14] Large areas of hyperpigmentation with fine hair may overlie plexiform neurofibromas.

Discrete or cutaneous neurofibromas occur in all patients with NF1. These tumors usually appear in teenagers or adults.[15] Early appearance of large numbers of neurofibromas is associated with complete deletion of the NF1 gene.[16] Isolated neurofibromas may involve both motor and sensory nerves in the epidermis and/or dermis.

MPNSTs occur in 4% to 10% of all patients with NF1. These tumors arise within plexiform neurofibromas usually between 15 and 50 years of age.[5] Earlier onset is uncommon but occurs. MPNSTs may be multifocal in some patients. MPNSTs are highly malignant, with rapid hematogenous dissemination. Outcome for patients with MPNSTs is poor. The best outcome is associated with radical resection.[17]

Indications for Removal of Peripheral Nerve Tumors

Neurofibromas, either discrete or plexiform, should be removed or resected only if they are symptomatic. Discrete neurofibromas may be associated with some discomfort and/or itching as they grow. Rarely, isolated neurofibromas cause compression of a motor nerve with distal weakness. Discrete neurofibromas should be removed if they produce significant discomfort or are located in exposed areas that are stigmatizing. Discrete neurofibromas may recur near the site of removal but usually not for several years if removal is complete. Resection of plexiform neurofibromas is more difficult. Plexiform neurofibromas frequently have diffuse projections that make complete removal impossible. Moreover, plexiform neurofibromas sometimes involve large nerves or nerve roots, so complete resection results in disability. Nevertheless, resection of plexiform neurofibromas should be considered if they cause cosmetic disfigurement, pain, or compromise of function. No successful chemotherapy has been identified for plexiform neurofibromas, although there are ongoing experimental trials of medication. Growth of plexiform neurofibromas is sometimes stimulated by radiation therapy. Histologic identification is not an indication for surgery unless the tumor is suspected to be malignant.

MPNSTs are commonly associated with pain. There are no reliable radiologic characteristics to distinguish MPNSTs from plexiform neurofibromas.[12] While MPNSTs commonly enhance with contrast and lack a homogeneous appearance, the same is true of some benign plexiform tumors. A helpful distinguishing feature is that MPNSTs commonly take up gallium in radioisotope scans.[18,19] Positron-emission tomography scans may also be useful in diagnosis.[20] Because MPNSTs arise within plexiform neurofibromas, in which only a small portion of the tumor is malignant, biopsies can be negative. Computed tomography (CT)–directed needle biopsy is preferred when an MPNST is suspected. MPNSTs do not respond well to chemotherapy or radiation therapy.[20]

Spinal Nerve Root Tumors and Dural Ectasias

Tumors of spinal roots are plexiform neurofibromas. One nerve root or multiple roots may be affected. Nerve root involvement is associated with enlargement of the neural foramen on MRI or scalloping of vertebral bodies on radiography. Virtually any nerve root may be affected, but the high cervical and lower lumbar spine are the most common sites. There is a subset of patients who show involvement of virtually all spinal roots. Nerve root tumors may extend through the neural foramen and expand and compress the cord, or they may remain static. Surgery is indicated if there is pain or compression of the spinal cord.

Dural ectasias are a weakening or expansion of the dural covering of a spinal root that is independent of a nerve root tumor. Dural ectasias commonly erode the vertebral body and may produce large dilated pockets anterior to the vertebral body (so-called anterior meningoceles). This is associated with pain, scoliosis, and sometimes vertebral instability.[21] Dural ectasias increase in size or remain static. They can be seen in early childhood, suggesting that they may be congenital defects. Surgery is indicated if there is intractable pain or vertebral instability.

Brain Tumors, MRI Abnormalities, and Hydrocephalus

High-intensity signals are present on T2 images in MRI of the brain in roughly 50% of all patients with NF1. Common locations are the basal ganglia, cerebellum, midbrain, and pons. The lesions do not enhance and are less easily visible on T1 images. They are not visible on CT scans. These areas of increased signal are sometimes referred to as unidentified bright objects, heterotopias, or hamartomas. The latter terms are misleading, because the etiology of the lesions is unclear.[22] They may be more common in children with learning disabilities but also occur in children without any cognitive difficulties. Areas of hyperintensity depend on age. They are less common after age 20.[23] In younger patients, the hyperintense signals may increase or decrease over time. They are not tumors and do not require radiologic follow-up or biopsy.

Optic gliomas or visual pathway tumors occur in 15% of patients with NF1.[24] Optic gliomas are pilocytic astrocytomas (World Health Organization grade I).[25] They commonly affect the chiasm, as well as one or both optic nerves. The tumors may extend into the hypothalamus or along the optic radiations.[4] Impairment of vision occurs in only 20% to 30% of patients with optic gliomas.[26] If treatment is required, chemotherapy is preferred.[27] The tumors do not require biopsy. The age of onset is between 16 months and 8 years of age. Screening is done with regular eye exams rather than imaging. Optic gliomas are almost never symptomatic after age 8,[4] but progression of tumors after treatment may occur. Not all optic gliomas respond to current chemotherapy regimes.

Tumors of the brain parenchyma (not including optic pathway tumors) occur in 2% to 3% of patients with NF1.[28] The cerebellum and brain stem are the most common locations.[29] Brain stem tumors involve the midbrain, pons, or medulla. They commonly have an exophytic component. Some enhancement with contrast may be seen. The natural history of brain stem tumors is usually benign.[30] Almost all are grade I astrocytomas. They may be associated with recurrent coughing, intermittent difficulty swallowing, or choking, but they are not associated with any weakness or persistent cranial nerve palsies. Rarely, they produce obstructive hydrocephalus. Once a brain stem tumor has been identified, it is prudent to obtain imaging at intervals for a few years to prove that the lesion is stable.[31] Brain tumors in other locations can vary from grade I to grade IV astrocytomas. In general, brain tumors in patients with NF1 are more indolent than in normal individuals. Some tumors even regress over time. Highly malignant gliomas also occur in patients with NF1. Tumors should not be biopsied unless they are clearly symptomatic or show progression over time.

Aqueductal stenosis is a rare complication of NF1. Symptoms include headache, vomiting, progressive gait disturbance, incontinence, and cognitive difficulties.[32] The onset may be insidious and recognition delayed. Surgical intervention usually results in significant improvement, even when the symptoms appear to be long-standing.

SURGICAL APPROACH TO THE LESIONS OF NEUROFIBROMATOSIS TYPE 1

Peripheral Nerve Lesions

Tumors of small peripheral nerves are usually discrete neurofibromas. The surgical approach is a direct linear incision along the length of the nerve. Care must be taken to dissect down to the expanded nerve sheath, incise it, and deliver the lesion through the incision. Electric nerve stimulation is useful to ensure that motor function is identified and preserved. In the absence of any motor function, nerve sectioning above and below the lesion with complete removal is appropriate. The cut nerve endings should be sewn into a nearby muscle to reduce the likelihood of painful postresection neuroma. When motor function is identified in the nerve entering the neurofibroma, we advocate intracapsular removal, incising the tumor sheath to deliver the intracapsular portion and remove it in its entirety but leaving the residual nerve in continuity. Often the bulk of the functional nerve is expanded and external to the tumor capsule. Function can be preserved by leaving the capsule in continuity with the nerve. After resection, the wound is closed in layers.

Large Nerves and Plexus

Neurofibromas of large peripheral nerves, such as the sciatic, common peroneal, or divisions of the brachial and lumbosacral plexus, are more complicated to approach than tumors of small cutaneous nerves. Tumors of large nerves are invariably plexiform tumors. The anatomic structures entering and leaving the area of the tumor must be carefully identified and dissected before tumor resection is attempted. The approach to the brachial plexus and lumbosacral plexus is similar to that of any lesion in those areas. However, plexiform neurofibromas often adhere to and follow the nerve trunks as an axis of growth. The tumors often envelop the entire plexus and adjacent tissue. Maximal debulking should be attempted while preserving function. The dissection must proceed along the anatomic plane of the nerve, and electric stimulation and monitoring of all involved nerves in the plexus

is mandatory. Some success has been reported with a more radical approach to plexiform neurofibromas of the plexus with postresection nerve grafting. We do not advocate that approach because of the potential for disability, the long recovery period, and the likelihood of recurrence.

Spinal Nerve Root Tumors

Spinal nerve root tumors are plexiform neurofibromas that grow from the nerve root into the intraspinal space either intradurally or epidurally and exit through the neural foramen, producing a dumbbell appearance. The tumors may occur at any level of the spine. Because some patients have enlargement of multiple nerve roots, care must be taken to identify tumors that are symptomatic. Only those lesions that are symptomatic or threaten to become symptomatic should be approached. Spinal cord compression or canal compromise is the most reliable indication for surgery.

In the cervical spine, spinal root tumors are usually approached posteriorly to relieve spinal cord compression. A laminectomy is performed through a midline incision. In young adults and children, an osteoplastic laminoplasty provides stability to the spine. In addition, the presence of bony lamina provides a landmark for dissection if patients require reoperation for recurrent tumor.

Intradural tumors without any extradural component are approached similarly to any nerve sheath tumor in the intradural space. They are usually dorsal or dorsolateral to the spinal cord but occasionally occur more ventrally. A midline or paramedian durotomy is performed once adequate exposure has been achieved by bony decompression. The nerve root involved is identified and stimulated. If it is a sensory root, which is usually the case, the root is sectioned proximal to the tumor. The tumor bulk is removed as the tumor is followed into the neural foramen. When there is minimal extension of the tumor beyond the neural foramen, the bulk of the tumor is removed from the intraspinal space. Residual tumor in the foramen is left to ensure adequate cerebrospinal fluid (CSF) closure. The dura is closed either primarily or with an expansile duraplasty patch graft, and the lamina is replaced where appropriate. This approach presumes that tumor regrowth, though likely, will be slow and easily monitored. We do not resect a small residual epidural tumor. Radical excision does not enhance symptomatic relief. An epidural tumor is highly vascular, and radical resection may cause significant bleeding. Radical resection entails removal of the lateral or ventral dura, resulting in CSF leakage. Moreover, recurrence from small amounts of a residual tumor is rare.

When the plexiform neurofibroma is primarily extradural, the approach is posterior with wide unilateral or bilateral bony decompression. The tumor is dissected in the epidural space. The epidural venous structures above and below are cauterized and divided. The tumor capsule is entered sharply and removed intracapsularly. We recommend the intracapsular approach to epidural tumors to preserve nerve root function. Removal of the tumor with its capsule and dural sheath interrupt both sensory and motor nerve function. In the thoracic region, radical removal can be performed, but radical removal in the cervical and lumbar region would cause significant morbidity.

Spinal Nerve Root Tumors with Large Extra-axial Components

Spinal nerve root tumors with significant extra-axial extension are particularly challenging. In the cervical spine, extension of the tumor may compress the trachea or invade the esophagus. In the lumbosacral region, extra-axial tumor commonly compresses the rectum or invades the bladder.[14] An interdisciplinary surgical team is essential for resection of these tumors. The intraspinal portion of the procedure is performed identically to the procedure for purely spinal tumors, whether they be intradural or epidural. However, patient position and the incisions are dictated by the extra-axial portion of the tumor.

In the cervical spine, where all nerve roots carry significant function, the tumor is removed intracapsularly. Upon decompression of the intraspinal space, the posterior incision is closed and a separate incision is made for resection of the extra-axial extension into the neck. The diffuse nature of plexiform neurofibromas frequently results in poorly defined margins of adjacent organs. Care must be taken to avoid entry into the trachea, esophagus, and great vessels. The goal of tumor resection in the neck is usually decompression of the airway. Plexiform neurofibromas almost never compromise the great vessels. Preservation of function of adjacent structures limits the extent of removal of the tumor.

In the thoracic region, when the extra-axial extent of the tumor is large, tumor removal is accomplished in the lateral position using either a single or two adjacent incisions—one for thoracotomy and a second (or an extension of the first) for laminectomy. The patient is positioned for a thoracotomy, and the approach to the intrapleural space is performed by a thoracic surgeon. The neural foramina are identified in the pleural space. The extra-axial portion of the tumor is removed, along with its pleural investment, with dissection along major vascular structures. The enlarged spinal foramina can be approached from the front by the neurosurgeon. When the foramina are wide and the intraspinal tumor is small, the resection can be completed from the anterolateral approach by foraminotomy and partial vertebrectomy. When the intraspinal extent is large or difficult to reach through the neural foramina from the front, we enlarge the incision or make a separate midline posterior incision. The lateral position for laminectomy (or osteoplastic laminoplasty) permits a standard approach to the epidural or intradural components of the tumor. In general, plexiform neurofibromas in the thoracic space requiring a transthoracic approach can be resected in their entirety, if there is no intradural extension, by sectioning the nerve root as it exits the dural sac. An intraspinal tumor can be delivered through the widened foramen, along with a portion of the extraspinal intraforaminal tumor, achieving a near-complete resection. This is one of the few situations in which removal of the involved neural structure causes minimal residual functional loss.

Tumors in the lumbosacral region with large extra-axial extensions are best approached in the lateral position through a large flank incision. The tumor is dissected through the retroperitoneum, and the lumbosacral plexus is identified. The extra-axial portion of the tumor is followed to the neural foramen and removed. If the tumor cannot be adequately removed from the lateral approach, the intraspinal portion of the tumor is approached posteriorly. This can be accomplished during the same procedure through a laminectomy, either by lengthening the flank incision or by creating a separate midline lumbar incision. Occasionally, the flank incision is closed and the patient is repositioned for a posterior approach. If the retroperitoneal surgery is extensive, the spinal portion of the tumor can be removed at a later date in the prone position. Because the lumbar and sacral nerves are functionally important, tumors of these nerves must be approached intracapsularly. Resection should be limited to decompression and debulking. Recurrence is unusual.

Lesions of the Cranial Vault and Brain

Patients with NF1 may have a variety of parenchymal abnormalities on MRI. Of the parenchymal brain lesions in NF1, only symptomatic tumors with radiologic characteristics of malignancy or progression require surgical intervention. Treatment of these lesions entails biopsy and aggressive resection, where possible, followed by adjunctive chemotherapy and radiotherapy. The treatment protocols are identical to high-grade astrocytomas in normal individuals. Treatment of the optic pathway tumors is not surgical. Diagnostic biopsy is not required. When optic pathway tumors progress, chemotherapy may be indicated.[27]

The aqueductal stenosis that is associated with NF1 is treated as any congenital aqueductal stenosis lesion. Endoscopic third ventriculocisternostomy is the approach of choice. If that procedure is not available or a large optic glioma limits access to the floor of the third ventricle, standard lateral ventricular shunting adequately treats this problem.

Neurofibromatosis Type 2

NF2 is an autosomal dominantly inherited disease due to a mutation or deletion in the long arm of chromosome 22 of the merlin gene.[33] The diagnosis depends on the presence of bilateral eighth-nerve tumors or the presence of a unilateral eighth-nerve tumor before 30 years of age in an individual with a first-degree relative with NF2 or two of the following: neurofibroma, meningioma, glioma, schwannoma, or juvenile posterior cataract.[9] Genetic testing is also available and may identify as many as 95% of patients with germline mutations. NF2 is characterized by the presence of multiple central nervous system (CNS) tumors. The clinical hallmark is bilateral vestibular nerve schwannomas. Patients may have multiple supratentorial meningiomas and schwannomas of the cranial nerves, in addition to vestibular tumors. Meningiomas occur along the spine, and schwannomas may develop along spinal nerve roots.[34] Roughly 33% of NF2 patients have intramedullary tumors of the spinal cord or brain stem that are either ependymomas or astrocytomas.[35] Juvenile posterior subcapsular cataracts and retinal hamartomas occur in 80% of patients.[36] Skin tumors occur in patients with NF2 but are not particularly prominent.

The clinical presentation of NF2 in adults is usually unilateral deafness. Facial weakness, visual impairment, dizziness, or painful peripheral nerve lesions may also be presenting complaints.[37] Spinal cord compression or seizures are late symptoms. Children with NF2 more commonly present because of a cataract or signs and symptoms related to cranial meningiomas, brain stem tumors, or spinal cord tumors.[38] The spectrum of severity of NF2 is variable. Early studies suggested two clinical phenotypes: the Gardner phenotype with milder disease, fewer tumors, and later onset and the Wishart phenotype with more tumors, earlier onset, and rapid progression.[37] Molecular studies demonstrate that more severe disease is seen in patients with frameshift or nonsense mutations. These patients are also more likely to have intramedullary spinal tumors. A milder phenotype is seen in patients with missense mutations, in-frame deletions, or large deletions.[38] A mild phenotype, particularly in patients with a unilateral vestibular schwannoma with no family history of NF2, may also be due to somatic mosaicism of the NF2 gene. Somatic mosaicism is found in one third of patients with no family history of NF2 and has a lower rate of transmission of the disease than germline mutations.[39]

NF2 is completely distinct from NF1, although rare patients may have features of both diseases. Two additional disorders must be distinguished from NF2: Schwannomatosis is characterized by multiple schwannomas of the peripheral, spinal, or cranial nerves without evidence of a vestibular schwannoma.[40] Schwannomatosis can be familial, although most cases are sporadic.[41] Meningiomatosis is an autosomal dominant disorder characterized by multiple meningiomas along the spinal cord, as well as supratentorially.[42]

TUMORS ASSOCIATED WITH NF2

Schwannomas

Schwannomas are typically nodular masses surrounded by a fibrous capsule consisting of epineurium and some nerve fibers. The tumors consist predominantly of Schwann cells with alternating patterns of cellularity.[43] Glandular or cystic areas sometimes occur. Schwannomas are virtually never malignant. Unlike neurofibromas, in which axons run through the tumor, schwannomas are usually extrinsic to the nerve and separate from the majority of the axons. However, when schwannomas involve small nerves, the tumor frequently engulfs the nerve, making separation from the nerve difficult. Schwannomas of the vestibular nerves are histologically similar to schwannomas of other nerves. Frequently, vestibular schwannomas in NF2 are multinodular and less vascular than sporadic tumors.[44] Although these tumors were originally called acoustic neuromas, they arise from the vestibular nerve. They usually impair hearing, but vestibular symptoms may also be prominent at the time of presentation. Schwannomas of the other cranial nerves are found in at least 25% of patients, particularly the third and fifth cranial nerves.[9] Schwannomas of the spinal nerves are present in the majority of patients.[35,37]

Meningiomas

Meningiomas arise from arachnoid cells of the leptomeninges. Meningiomas in patients with NF2 are predominantly fibrous, but meningothelial tumors also occur.[45] Meningiomas infrequently show evidence of pleomorphism or malignancy and act more aggressively, invading bone. Orbital meningiomas may occur in childhood and must be distinguished from optic gliomas. Meningiomas of the cerebellar pontine angle are occasionally confused with vestibular

schwannomas. Meningiomas of the skull base produce brain stem compression and are an important cause of mortality in NF2. An en plaque meningioma occurs in some patients with NF2 late in their disease.

Astrocytomas, Ependymomas, and Hamartomas

Astrocytomas and ependymomas occur in as many as a third of NF2 patients.[35] The most common site is the brain stem or cervical cord.[46,47] Syrinx formation is not uncommon. These tumors are typically indolent in NF2. A more malignant profile in spinal cord tumors is rare and usually related to prior radiation therapy. Evidence of rapid growth or symptoms related to the tumors is an indication for surgery, but radiation and chemotherapy are usually not indicated. Hamartomas of the brain are frequently found in patients with NF2. They are a mixture of Schwann cells, glia, and meningeal cells.[47]

INDICATIONS FOR NEUROSURGERY

NF2 is not a surgically curable disease. Lesions recur and progress. The entire CNS can be involved. The tumors of NF2 do not respond to conventional chemotherapy. However, molecular studies are beginning to suggest alternative chemotherapeutic approaches.[48] Radiation therapy can be considered for lesions that are not surgically accessible. Lesions are usually addressed surgically when they are symptomatic. Special considerations involved in the surgery of the vestibular schwannomas are discussed later. In patients with the more benign phenotype, with few and slow-growing tumors, surgical intervention is reserved for prevention of impending symptoms or for symptomatic tumors. In its most aggressive form, however, the disease can progress rapidly and cause severe disability that leads to death. In that situation, surgical intervention is palliative to improve quality of life.

A variety of approaches with different goals and complications are available for vestibular schwannomas. Single or multiple fraction stereotactic radiosurgery (i.e., gamma knife, as well as other types) is advocated in some centers.[49,50] Studies of NF2 patients with vestibular schwannomas treated with these techniques suggest good local disease control and a relatively low incidence of side effects that is at least comparable to results with microsurgery techniques.[51,53] However, both single dose and multiple fraction radiotherapy are not without potential complications for NF2 patients.[38,49,50,54] Radiotherapy may have limited usefulness and limit the options for recurrent or new vestibular tumors. We prefer a microsurgery approach to vestibular schwannomas. Regardless of the approach, all centers agree that intervention should only occur when there is documentation of tumor growth or progressive hearing loss. Because of the variety of approaches available, it is important to discuss the risks and benefits of each with the patient. For those opting for a microsurgery approach, it is important to discuss goals for surgery and define the degree of aggressiveness of the surgical approach with the patient before surgery. Aggressive removal of vestibular schwannomas may cause facial nerve injury. Facial nerve injury may be extremely distressing to patients and predisposes them to ocular injury. These complications should be discussed with patients. Consideration of cochlear implantation may also influence surgical decisions.[55] Surgical removal of intramedullary spinal cord tumors is indicated only when there are signs of spinal cord compression. Because multiple tumors may develop over time along the length of the spine, the number of surgical interventions is limited. Schwannomas of the spinal nerves rarely cause problems. Surgery on these tumors should be avoided.

SURGICAL APPROACH TO THE LESIONS OF NF2
Vestibular Schwannoma (Acoustic Neuroma)

The technical approach to a vestibular schwannoma in an NF2 patient is identical to sporadic tumors. However, surgical decisions in NF2 patients are affected by the presence of bilateral disease and the knowledge that the disease is not surgically curable. Surgical approaches include radical resection, partial removal, and decompression. Suboccipital retrosigmoid, translabyrinthine, or middle cranial fossa approaches can all be appropriately used for tumor removal. The arguments for these various approaches are outlined elsewhere in this text. The translabyrinthine approach permits greater exposure of the tumor but results in deafness. The middle cranial fossa approach is used primarily for decompression. We prefer the suboccipital retrosigmoid approach, with the goal of sparing hearing.[52] This operation entails drilling open the posterior aspect of the internal auditory meatus, followed by subtotal resection of the tumor, preserving facial nerve function at all costs. Electrophysiologic monitoring of the eighth cranial nerve helps to preserve hearing.

We advocate early surgery on one side if one of the vestibular tumors is less than 1.5 cm in diameter. When the tumor is small, early surgery reduces the size of the tumor and preserves hearing and facial nerve function. If the tumors are greater than 1.5 cm, we prefer to wait until there is significant motor dysfunction due to brain stem compression. When motor dysfunction is present in patients with large bilateral tumors, we recommend subtotal resection of one of the tumors. If brain stem compression is predominantly unilateral, subtotal resection of the larger tumor relieves brain stem compression and preserves facial nerve function and hearing. However, when patients have very large bilateral tumors and bilateral brain stem compression, the appropriate operation may be a radical subtotal resection on one side, sacrificing hearing and preserving facial nerve function. In the latter situation, aggressive tumor removal may compromise facial nerve function. Chemotherapy with bevacizumab may also be an option.[48]

In patients with large vestibular tumors, the presence of additional CNS tumors may affect the surgical approach to a vestibular tumor. If there are multiple large CNS tumors and the vestibular schwannoma is causing brain stem compression, subtotal resection of the vestibular tumor for brain stem decompression alone may be more appropriate than radical resection. Because vestibular schwannomas may remain stable for prolonged periods, simple decompressive subtotal resection can provide symptomatic relief for several years.

In children and young adults, the vestibular tumors may be small. If one of the tumors is less than 1.5 cm in size, we recommend operating on the smaller tumor. Resection is performed with the goal of preserving hearing on that side. Successful resection of the smaller tumor, with preservation of hearing on that side, permits radical resection of the contralateral tumor at a later time, when hearing loss on that side will not affect quality of life.

Other Intracranial Tumors

The technical surgical approach to the removal of brain tumors in patients with NF2 is identical to the same tumor in normal individuals. However, the potential for multiple recurrent CNS tumors and multiple surgeries must be considered before deciding on surgery. Tumors are only removed when they are symptomatic. Meningiomas in NF2 are removed for cortical compression causing neurologic deficit or for seizure generation. En plaque meningiomas, even when very large and diffusely compressive, should be watched in patients with NF2, especially if there is a large additional tumor burden. Meningiomas invading the bone require an aggressive surgical approach with wide margins and demand the participation of a cranial facial surgeon.

Spinal Cord Lesions

The surgical approach to intramedullary spinal tumors of NF2 is identical to intramedullary spinal tumor in normal individuals. The levels of interest are exposed by generous bony removal, the dura is opened and retracted, a midline myelotomy is performed, and pial retraction stitches are placed after the tumor has been reached by gentle dissection under the microscope. Ependymomas in NF2 are usually well circumscribed. They can be debulked and dissected from normal spinal cord tissue with care. Although the spinal cord may appear thinned and compressed, recovery from a first surgery is generally good.

Hydrocephalus

Hydrocephalus can occur either from tumor obstruction of CSF pathways or from tumor protein production within the CSF, causing reduced CSF absorption. Hydrocephalus is treated with tumor removal or ventriculoperitoneal shunting. Frequently, hydrocephalus is observed postoperatively after removal of an intraventricular or subarachnoid tumor (e.g., vestibular schwannoma). Despite treatment with anti-inflammatory glucocorticoids, the malabsorption of CSF, presumed to be from inflammatory insult at the villus absorptive surface, rarely resolves. Knowledge of the type of hydrocephalus, obstructive versus absorptive, as well as consideration of the presumed elevated CSF protein in the presence of multiple CNS tumors, may affect the choice of shunting valve system.

Conclusions

The NFs are not surgically curable diseases. Unfortunately, the limited usefulness of adjuvant therapy leaves surgery as the primary treatment to alleviate symptoms. While surgery provides symptomatic relief, it may not alter the course of disease. Surgery should be limited to the removal of tumors that are symptomatic or that threaten to cause symptoms. The technical surgical approach to the tumors of NF1 and NF2 is generally similar to the approach of the same tumor in patients without NF. However, the decision of when to operate and to what level of aggressiveness is often affected by the disease and is of critical importance in NF. Even though the relentless progression of disease may at times be discouraging, the ability of neurosurgery to alleviate symptoms and improve longevity and quality of life is significant.

KEY REFERENCES

Aoki S, Barkovich AJ, Nishimura K, et al. Neurofibromatosis types 1 and 2: cranial MR findings. *Radiology.* 1989;172:527-534.

Balasubramniam A, Shannon P, Hodaie M, et al. Glioblastoma multiforme after stereotactic radiotherapy for acoustic neuroma: case report and review of the literature. *Neuro Oncol.* 2007;9:447-453.

Chan AW, Black P, Ojemann RG, et al. Stereotactic radiotherapy for vestibular schwannomas: favorable outcome with minimal toxicity. *Neurosurgery.* 2005;57:60-70.

Cohen BH, Rothner AD. Incidence, types, and management of cancer in patients with neurofibromatosis. *Oncology.* 1989;3:23-38.

Duffner PK, Cohen ME, Seidel FG, et al. The significance of MRI abnormalities in children with neurofibromatosis. *Neurology.* 1989;39: 373-378.

Evans DGR, Baser ME, O'Reilly B, et al. Management of the patient and family with neurofibromatosis 2: a consensus conference statement. *Br J Neurosurg.* 2005;19:5-12.

Friedrich RE, Korf B, Funsturer C, et al. Growth type of plexiform neurofibromas in NF1 determined on magnetic resonance images. *Anticancer Res.* 2003;23:949-952.

Huson SM, Harper PS, Compston DAS. Von Recklingausen neurofibromatosis: a clinical and population study in southeast Wales. *Brain.* 1988;111:1355-1381.

Ilgren EB, Kinnier-Wilson LM, Stiller CA. Gliomas in neurofibromatosis: a series of 89 cases with evidence for enhanced malignancy in associated cerebellar astrocytomas. *Pathol Ann.* 1985;20:331-358.

Listernick R, Charrow J, Greenwald MJ, et al. Natural history of optic pathway tumors in children with neurofibromatosis type 1: a longitudinal study. *J Pediatr.* 1994;125:63-66.

Louis DN, Ramesh V, Gusella J. Neuropathology and molecular genetics of neurofibromatosis 2 and related tumors. *Brain Pathol.* 1995;5: 163-172.

Mathieu D, Kondziolka D, Flickinger JC, et al. Stereotactic radiosurgery for vestibular schwannomas in patients with neurofibromatosis type 2: an analysis of tumor control, complications, and hearing preservation rates. *Neurosurgery.* 2007;60:460-470.

Mautner VF, Tatagiba M, Lindenau M, et al. Spinal tumors in patients with neurofibromatosis type 2: MR imaging study of frequency, multiplicity, and variety. *Am J Roentgenol.* 1995;165:951-955.

McCormick P, Torres R, Post K, et al. Intramedullary ependymoma of the spinal cord. *J Neurosurg.* 1990;72:523-532.

McKenna M, Halpin C, Ojemann R, et al. Long-term hearing results in patients after surgical removal of acoustic tumors with hearing preservation. *Am J Otolaryngol.* 1992;13:134-136.

Mulvihill JJ, Parry DM, Sherman JL. NIH Conference. Neurofibromatosis 1 (Recklinghausen disease) and neurofibromatosis 2 (bilateral acoustic neurofibromatosis): an update. *Ann Intern Med.* 1990;113:39-52.

Neff B, Wiet RM, Lasak JM, et al. Cochlear implantation in the neurofibromatosis type 2 patient: long-term follow-up. *Laryngoscope.* 2009;117:1069-1072.

Packer RJ, Ater J, Allen J, et al. Carboplatin and vincristine chemotherapy for children with newly diagnosed progressive low-grade gliomas. *J Neurosurg.* 1997;86:747-754.

Plotkin SR, Stemmer-Rachamimov AO, Barker 2nd FG, et al. Hearing improvement after bevacizumab in patients with neurofibromatosis type 2. *N Eng J Med.* 2009;361:358-367.

Pollack IF, Shultz B, Mulvihill JJ. The management of brainstem gliomas in patients with neurofibromatosis 1. *Neurology.* 1996;46:1652-1660.

Samii M, Gerganov V, Samii A. Microsurgery management of vestibular schwannomas in neurofibromatosis type 2: indications and results. *Prog Neurol Surg.* 2008;21:169-175.

Sordillo PP, Helson L, Hajdu SI. Malignant schwannoma: clinical characteristics, survival, and response to therapy. *Cancer.* 1981;47:2503-2509.

Sorensen SA, Mulvihill JJ, Nielsen A. Long-term follow-up of von Recklinghausen neurofibromatosis: survival and malignant neoplasms. *N Engl J Med.* 1986;314:1010-1015.

Tonsgard JH, Kwak SM, Short MP, et al. CT imaging in adults with neurofibromatosis-1: frequent asymptomatic plexiform lesions. *Neurology.* 1998;50:1755-1760.

Warbey VS, Ferner RE, Dunn JT, et al. [18F]FDG PET/CT in the diagnosis of malignant peripheral nerve sheath tumors in neurofibromatosis type-1. *Eur J Nucl Med Mol Imaging.* 2009;36:751-757.

Numbered references appear on Expert Consult.

CHAPTER 49

Hearing Prosthetics: Surgical Techniques

WADE W. CHIEN • HOWARD FRANCIS • JOHN K. NIPARKO

Tumors in the cerebellopontine angle and internal auditory canal can result in hearing loss. In addition, surgical resection of these tumors often leads to hearing impairment due to manipulation and/or sacrifice of the cochlear nerve. This chapter examines the current technologies that enable a restored perception of sound and the clinical application of implantable hearing technologies. We describe the application of an osseointegrated implant, cochlear implant, and auditory brain stem implant to the solution of hearing loss in the neurosurgical patient.

Hearing Loss

Hearing loss can be divided into two broad categories: conductive and sensorineural. In conductive hearing loss, the sound conduction mechanism in the outer and middle ear is impaired. This results in a decrease in the perception of air-conducted sound delivered through the external auditory canal. If the transduction of sound to neural signals continues normally in the inner ear, the perception of sound transmitted to the cochlea through the skull (bone conduction) is not disturbed. In sensorineural hearing loss, the inner ear, cochlear nerve, or central auditory pathway are affected, disturbing the perception of sound delivered through both air and bone conduction. Both conductive and sensorineural hearing loss are present in patients with mixed hearing loss.

Hearing loss is usually evaluated through audiologic testing. A typical audiogram has two parts: pure tone audiometry and speech audiometry. In pure tone audiometry, air- and bone-conduction thresholds are tested at different frequencies (Fig. 49-1). In conductive hearing loss, the disparity between air- and bone-conduction thresholds results in an air–bone gap. In sensorineural hearing loss, both air- and bone-conduction thresholds are elevated. In speech audiometry, the ability to perceive and discriminate words and sentences is tested. The speech reception threshold is a measure in decibels (dB) of the speech perception threshold, whereas the speech discrimination score (SDS) is a measure as a percentage of words from a standardized list presented at suprathreshold levels that are recognized and repeated by the patient.

Some patients may have mild hearing loss on pure tone audiometry but significant impairment in speech audiometry. Therefore, sound awareness does not guarantee the presence of useful hearing. It is always important to consider both types of audiometry when evaluating patients with hearing loss. Furthermore, the presence of normal

hearing in one ear underestimates the negative impact of acquired unilateral hearing loss on the ability to comprehend speech and access information in the presence of background noise.

The rehabilitation challenges posed by hearing loss are modest when threshold elevation is the primary deficit but become increasingly complex as speech perception is impaired. Referral to and close collaboration with specialists in otolaryngology–head and neck surgery and audiology provides comprehensive consideration and delivery of options that meet the specific needs of the patient. Threshold deficits in the setting of normal or near-normal speech discrimination can be overcome by a conventional hearing aid through a combination of amplification and sound filtering. In patients with lower SDS, more complex filtering, other speech processing strategies, and a directional microphone are required to overcome speech perception challenges, particularly in background noise. If the hearing loss is primarily conductive and the ear canal has been surgically altered so that it cannot accommodate a conventional hearing aid, a bone-conduction hearing aid can be used to deliver sound transcutaneously or via an osseointegrated implant. When the loss of acuity and speech discrimination is too advanced for conventional hearing aids to provide benefit, a normal contralateral ear may serve as the conduit for sound input from the deaf side using wireless transmission from an ear-level microphone to a receiver by the contralateral routing of sound (CROS) hearing aid or using bone transmission across the skull using osseointegrated technology. The presence of significant sensorineural hearing loss and speech perception deficits in both ears poses the greatest challenge. In this scenario, the delivery of relevant neural codes to the central nervous system can be accomplished by electrical stimulation of the cochlear nerve or the auditory brain stem using implantable prostheses.

Bone-Anchored Osseointegrated Implants

Osseointegrated implants were first introduced into clinical practice in Scandinavia in the late 1960s, ostensibly for intraoral rehabilitation.[1] Since then, osseointegrated implants have gained widespread acceptance in the fields of dental, oral/maxillofacial, craniofacial, and orthopedic surgery. Application of this technology to bone-anchored hearing devices represents a refinement of conventional bone-conduction hearing aids. In bone-conduction hearing

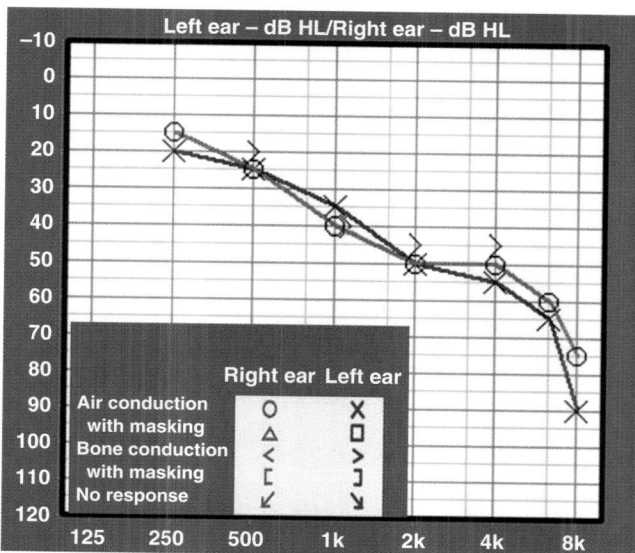

FIGURE 49-1 Pure tone audiometry in a patient with bilateral sensorineural hearing loss. Frequency (in hertz) is plotted on the x-axis, and loudness of sound (in the decibel hearing level) is plotted on the y-axis. The air- and bone-conduction thresholds are elevated in both ears (right ear in red, left ear in blue), particularly at higher frequencies.

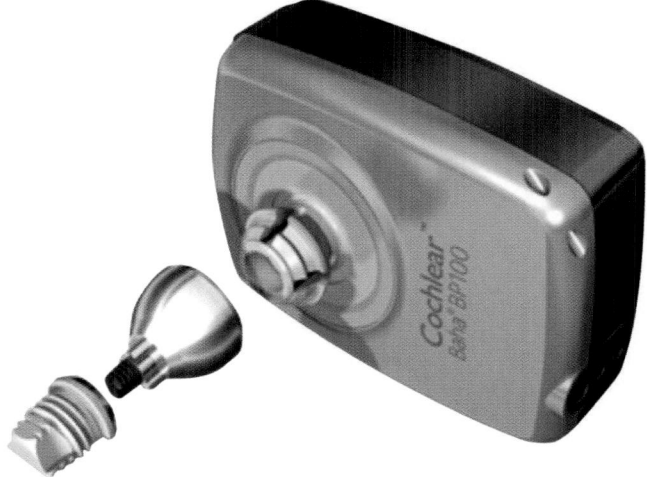

FIGURE 49-2 Baha osseointegrated implant. It consists of three parts: the sound processor, the connecting abutment, and the titanium implant. *(Courtesy of Cochlear Corporation, Englewood, CO.)*

aids, sound is transmitted through vibration of the skull to the cochlea. However, the utility of conventional bone-conduction devices is now considered limited due to patient discomfort and limited sound fidelity secondary to soft tissue attenuation. Coupling the bone vibrator to an osseointegrated implant, as originally performed by Tjellström and his team at the Institute of Applied Biotechnology in Sweden in 1977, averts many of these limitations of conventional bone conducting devices.[2]

The success of this technology relies on two basic principles: the creation of a permanent percutaneous connection and the placement of an osseointegrated titanium abutment upon which a transducer is coupled. The cutaneous-implant interface as originally conceived by Brånemark[3] is based on biologic principles observed throughout nature. Teeth and nails (as well as talons, tusks, or claws as found in other species) all interface with a thin, firmly attached cutaneous or mucosal border with little to no hair. This tissue architecture limits tissue mobility and preserves stability of tissue planes while inhibiting the penetration of microbes and subsequent inflammation or infection.[4,5] By mimicking these attributes in the skull, the surgeon creates a permanent cutaneous-implant border that the patient may easily maintain.

Advances in metallic biomaterials facilitate the creation of permanent, well-tolerated implant fixtures upon which the transducer is placed. Titanium is the most notable among several materials that have found clinical application in anchoring dental prostheses. This is because of its ability to create a corrosion-resistant oxide layer on the surface of the implant that confers osseointegration potential.[6,7] Because the implant may be worn for several decades or longer, the toxicity and carcinogenicity of the oxide coating takes on particular importance.[8] Reports have shown that titanium is superior to stainless steel, lacking steel's high potential for corrosion or the toxicity of its components.[9,10]

To date, pure titanium appears free of the adverse sequelae seen with other metals and thus continues to represent an ideal implant material.[7]

Currently, the most widely used osseointegrated hearing device is the Baha implant (Cochlear Corporation, Englewood, CO), shown in Fig. 49-2. The Baha consists of a pure titanium implant and a sound processor. The processor couples directly to the titanium implant via a skin penetrating abutment, utilizing a force-fit, plastic coupling.

INDICATIONS

Baha implants were first developed for patients with conductive hearing loss and chronically draining ears, those with discomfort from the sound levels required from a traditional hearing aid, and patients unable to tolerate a hearing aid because of a large mastoid bowl or meatoplasty following chronic ear surgery. Patients with aural atresia are also candidates for Baha implants. Patients who have undergone external auditory canal closure following extensive skull base surgery with preserved inner ear function are also not amenable to traditional hearing aids. This group of patients may benefit from a device that offers bone-anchored hearing.[11] Baha implants are also approved for patients with single-sided deafness, for example, due to the effects of a tumor in the cerebellopontine angle or its treatment. In this instance, sound is delivered to the skull on the side lacking sensorineural function and transmitted by bone conduction to the normal contralateral ear, where it is perceived (Fig. 49-3).

SURGICAL TECHNIQUE

The postauricular area is cleaned and shaved, and the site of the abutment placement is marked. The abutment is typically placed 50 to 55 mm posterior to the ear canal along the temporal line. A dermatome is used to raise an anteriorly based skin flap. The underlying and surrounding soft tissues are removed, leaving the periosteum intact. A small circle of the periosteum (about 6 mm^2) is removed, exposing the underlying bony cortex. A 4-mm hole is drilled at the center of the exposed bony cortex. A countersink is then used to

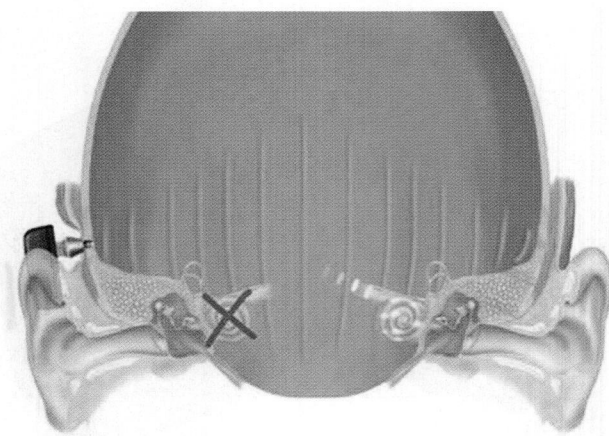

FIGURE 49-3 The osseointegrated implant can be used for single-sided deafness, because it relies on bone conduction, which stimulates both cochleae simultaneously. As sound comes in from the deaf side, it is picked up by the sound processor, which activates the contralateral cochlea by bone conduction, achieving sound transmission. *(Courtesy of Cochlear Corporation, Englewood, CO.)*

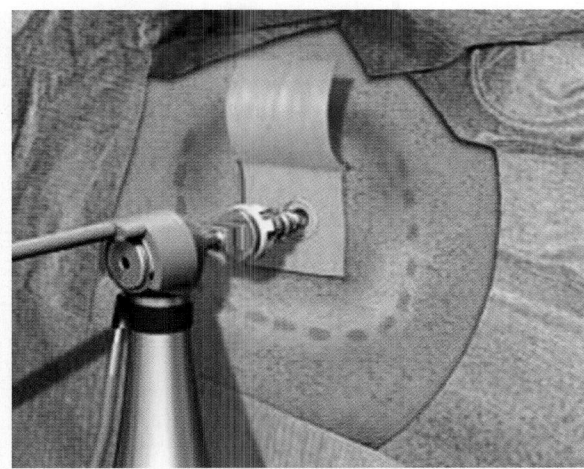

FIGURE 49-4 Surgical placement of the Baha implant. The connecting abutment and the titanium implant are placed securely into a previously drilled hole in the skull. *(Courtesy of Cochlear Corporation, Englewood, CO.)*

enlarge the hole. The abutment is slowly threaded into the previously prepared hole using the abutment inserter (Fig. 49-4). The skin flap is reflected back to its original position, with a central opening to accommodate the abutment. The edges of the skin flap are then sutured to the surrounding periosteum and skin. The abutment is left undisturbed for 3 to 4 months, which allows osseointegration to occur. Once the abutment is osseointegrated, it is ready for coupling to the sound processor.

COMPLICATIONS

In a study looking at postoperative complications of Baha implant in 149 patients, House and Kutz[12] found that the most common complication is skin growth over the abutment (7.4%). This is managed by either steroid application or skin flap revision with removal of the underlying scar tissues. In some cases, a split-thickness skin graft may be needed. Other complications include implant extrusion (3.4%), wound infection (1.3%), and flap necrosis (0.7%). Implant extrusion is more likely to occur in radiated bone and in the pediatric population. Pretreatment with hyperbaric oxygen is suggested in radiated patients. The delay to use is extended in this population and in children by 2 to 3 months to allow for optimal osseointegration.

OUTCOMES

In one of the largest series to date studying the Baha implant, Håkansson et al.[13] reported results from 147 patients over 10 years. Patients were divided into three groups based on their pure tone average (PTA) bone-conduction thresholds: 0 to 45 dB, 46 to 60 dB, and more than 60 dB hearing level. The authors noted a strong relationship between PTA and successful rehabilitation. In the group with the best cochlear reserve (PTA of up to 45 dB), 89% of patients said their hearing was subjectively improved by the implant, while 8% felt their hearing was worse. Conversely, in the groups with progressively less cochlear function (the 46 to 60 dB and the more than 60 dB groups), 61% and 22% of patients reported subjective hearing improvement,

respectively. Furthermore, SDSs improved on average from 14% unaided and 67% with a traditional hearing aid to 81% with the Baha. This number increased to 85% if people with a sensorineural loss greater than the 60 dB hearing level were excluded and to 89% if subjects with a PTA worse than 45 dB were excluded. Based on these results, the authors recommended that to be in consideration for a "high success rate" with the Baha, patients should have a PTA by bone conduction that is less than the 45 dB hearing level, though improvements in hearing should still be expected for a PTA of up to 60 dB.

Lustig et al.[14] performed a review of experience with the Baha in the United States. The most common indications for implantation included chronic otitis media and external auditory canal stenosis and/or aural atresia. Patients who had undergone skull base surgery and had complete closure of the external auditory canal were also included. Overall, each patient had an average improvement of 32 ± 19 dB with the use of the Baha. Complications were limited to local infection and inflammation at the implant site in 3 of 40 patients and failure to osseointegrate in 1 patient. Patient response to the implant was uniformly satisfactory.

In addition to implantation for purely conductive or mixed hearing losses, emerging data indicate the value of Baha amplification for patients with unilateral profound sensorineural hearing loss. The Baha on the deafened ear effectively expanded the sound field for the patient and improved the patient's speech understanding in noise, much like a CROS hearing aid or transcranial CROS system.[15,16] However, in contrast to CROS, the Baha does not require the placement of an ear mold in the better-hearing ear. As the better-hearing ear functions normally, the acoustic "head shadow" can be used to isolate sounds incident to the deafened side but heard in the better ear through transcranial bone conduction from the Baha. This avoids the potential discomfort and perceptual costs of wearing an ear mold on the better-hearing ear. Preliminary results show subjective improvement in both sound quality and speech understanding in noise.[17]

Cochlear Implants

Cochlear implants are neural prostheses that convey sound information to the auditory cortex via electrical stimulation of the auditory nerve, bypassing the dysfunctional cochlea in individuals with bilateral severe to profound sensorineural deafness. A typical cochlear implant consists of an external component, which includes the microphone and the speech processor, and an internal component, which includes the receiver-stimulator and the stimulating electrodes. The speech processor is battery powered and is housed in a behind-the-ear unit similar to a hearing aid or in a "body" style encasement worn at the waist, carried in a pocket, or otherwise harnessed to the body. A microphone captures acoustic input and delivers it to the speech processor that, in turn, converts it into electrical signals. An external antenna magnetically retained behind the ear transmits the encoded signals across the scalp via radiofrequency to the antenna of the internal device. The signals are then sorted tonotopically and are delivered to different auditory nerve fibers along the cochlear spiral. An example of a cochlear implant is shown in Fig. 49-5.

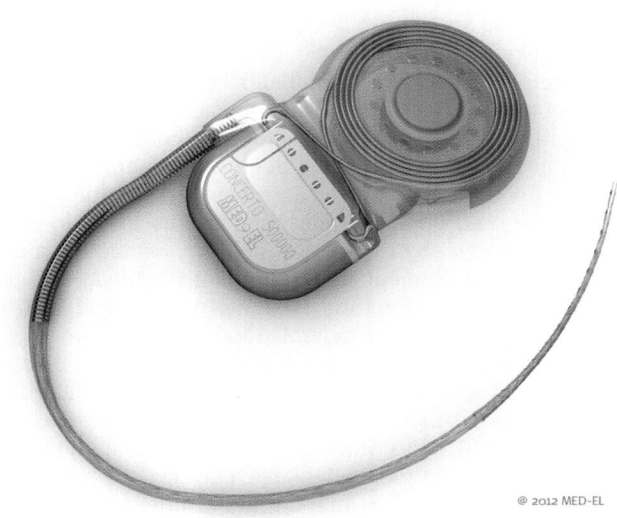

FIGURE 49-5 Cochlear implant. The electrode array and the ground lead are connected to the internal processor. *(Courtesy of Med El.)*

INDICATIONS

Severe to profound impairment of cochlear function in both ears and anatomic preservation of the auditory nerve in the implanted ear are requirements for cochlear implantation. Currently, criteria vary somewhat but generally include an upper threshold of 40% to 50% speech discrimination with a hearing aid for the poorer hearing ear, with up to 60% in the better-hearing ear, and PTA hearing loss (the average threshold for 500, 1000, and 2000 Hz) of 70 dB or greater in both ears. As experience with cochlear implants grows, outcomes have continued to improve and candidacy criteria based on speech discrimination have continued to evolve toward higher levels of function over the past 25 years.[18,19] Mean recognition scores for words in isolation after implantation now far exceed the 40% level, and individuals with some preserved speech-recognition ability preoperatively often score substantially higher postoperatively than prior to implantation.[20,21] Residual hearing as reflected in aided speech-recognition levels is an important predictor of implant success.[22,23] When combined with duration of deafness, preoperative scores on tests of sentence recognition provide a predictive composite that accounts for approximately 80% of the variance in postoperative word recognition.[19]

Cochlear implants have been widely used for the management of cochlear dysfunction due to congenital or acquired causes, including genetic, ototoxic, infectious, and autoimmune etiologies. In these instances, the auditory nerve is rarely affected and remains viable for electrical stimulation by an electrode array inserted within the cochlea and adjacent to spiral ganglion (auditory nerve) cell bodies. Cochlear implants may also be useful for cases in which radiation therapy or the surgical removal of a posterior fossa tumor threatens function in the only-hearing ear. If the contralateral ear was previously deafened by cochlear disease and had no retrocochlear lesion or surgery, it would be an excellent candidate for cochlear implantation if tumor removal could lead to profound hearing loss in the only hearing ear. In such an instance, appropriate consultation and discussion of cochlear implant rehabilitation should be included in the preoperative planning and counseling process.

Preservation of auditory nerve integrity should be strongly considered in all neurofibromatosis type 2 (NF2) cases—whether or not the contralateral ear has already demonstrated hearing loss—because it provides an opportunity for future benefit from prosthetic hearing at the cochlea. If the contralateral tumor ear continues to benefit from a hearing aid but is undergoing measurable decline in function, early implantation of the resected side provides an opportunity for the patient to transfer to electrical hearing as acoustic hearing diminishes. Lustig et al. reported on audiologic results in seven patients with NF2 who were implanted following surgical resection with nerve preservation or stereotactic radiation of vestibular schwannomas.[24] Whereas hearing acuity and awareness of environmental sound was achieved in all cases, the variability in speech understanding exceeded what is typical for cochlear implantation for cochlear disease. Three patients acquired open-set speech perception in auditory-only testing conditions. In most cases, even when speech understanding was poor, lipreading was enhanced by improved sound awareness, as was sound localization in cases with some residual hearing in the contralateral ear. Trotter and Briggs[25] observed favorable communication results in three NF2 patients with cochlear implants in ears whose tumors were treated with stereotactic radiation. Subtotal removal of vestibular schwannoma in two patients and stereotactic radiation therapy in a third were associated with high open-set function in all patients.[26] Neff et al. reported sustained open- and closed-set speech perception benefit during an average of 7.9 years.[27] They emphasized the utility of promontory electrical stimulation as a predictor of favorable outcome.

Comprehensive assessment of candidacy is essential to minimize risks and realize benefits of cochlear implantation. To ensure complete assessment of candidacy, clinicians should consider the many factors likely to affect performance with a cochlear implant, including audiologic, medical, surgical, developmental, cognitive, and psychosocial factors. Candidates should understand that the cochlear implant is a communication tool and is not a cure for deafness, because expectations largely shape postoperative satisfaction with any form of auditory rehabilitation.[28]

Candidacy should be considered in the context of current functional status and likely outcome with and without cochlear implantation. Patient age, etiology of hearing loss, unaided and aided hearing, duration of deafness, and circumstances of social support surrounding the candidate carry predictive value. Environments that enrich and promote spoken language are likely to exert a favorable influence over use of the device and contribute to maximal benefit from it. Tyler and Summerfield[29] observed evidence of the influence of auditory plasticity in adults with postlingual hearing loss. They found that speech perception ability and the duration of profound/total deafness before implantation were significantly correlated with postimplantation hearing outcome. Performance improved over time after implantation. For adult patients, the level of performance measured shortly after implantation was about half the level measured eventually. Performance tended to reach an asymptote after approximately 3 years of implant use. Such observations suggest that an established pathway for auditory processing is present even in profound sensorineural hearing loss and that refined processing develops over time. Although there are additional negative correlations between duration of deafness and performance,[20,22,23,29] such correlations do not apply to every case. Even a prolonged period of deafness does not rule out prospects for speech understanding with a cochlear implant, provided that basic foundations of communicating through audition (e.g., prior hearing aid use, use of lipreading, and production of speech) are in place.

A thorough preoperative medical examination should be performed to determine suitability for general anesthesia. An otologic evaluation, including history and physical examination, is essential to identifying structural changes in the temporal bone that may affect surgical approach and feasibility. Clinical evaluation of the vestibular system may help guide the choice of which ear is implanted and may help predict whether implantation will produce vestibular sequelae.

Optimal performance with a cochlear implant requires continued long-term use of the device. Observations that speech-recognition performance asymptotes only after at least 3 years of use underscore the importance of patient engagement with the intervention.

Consideration should be given to conditions for which a patient may need future assessment with magnetic resonance imaging (MRI). Implantation of a magnet in the internal device may be contraindicated in these patients.

A nonmagnetic modification of commercially available devices is available for patients whose medical or neurologic condition mandates future MRI studies.[30] However, Baumgartner et al.[31] found that MRI applied to cochlear implant patients using different devices with indwelling magnets did not cause implant malfunction or patient injury when imaged at 1 tesla (T). Our own experience (unpublished) suggests that MRI with a 1.5-T magnet poses no significant threats if the device is immobilized using externally applied molding material and is firmly bound.

IMAGING STUDIES

High-resolution computed tomography (CT) scans of the temporal bone define surgical anatomy and provide information about cochlear abnormalities that can aid the surgeon in surgical planning and patient counseling. Temporal bone CT scans should be obtained and reviewed for evaluation of temporal bone anatomy, with particular attention paid to mastoid pneumatization, ossicular anatomy, position of great vessels, position of the facial nerve, caliber of the internal auditory canal, and labyrinthine anatomy.[32] Scans are examined for evidence of cochlear malformation and ossification, enlarged vestibular aqueduct, and other inner ear and skull base anomalies that can affect implant surgery. CT findings of cochlear patency generally correlate with surgical findings,[33] but significant discrepancies can occur as a result of volume averaging.[34,35]

MRI may be a useful adjunct to CT for assessment of implant candidacy.[36-38] Whereas CT is the procedure of choice for detailing bony anatomy, MRI is ideal for imaging soft tissues such as the membranous labyrinth, nerves in the internal auditory canal, and soft tissue within a cochlea en route to cochlear ossification after meningitis. High-resolution T2-weighted MRI is especially helpful for determining cochlear patency (by revealing the presence or absence of fluid within the scalae) and the presence or absence of nerves within the internal auditory canal.

SURGICAL TECHNIQUE

Contemporary cochlear implantation surgery represents modifications of surgical procedures historically employed in managing chronic infections of the mastoid and middle ear. Prophylactic antibiotics are routinely administered to provide coverage for the placement of a prosthetic device; however, the necessity for this measure has not been established. General anesthesia is employed, paralytic agents are avoided, and a facial nerve monitor is often used. An extended postauricular incision is made, and the mastoid cortex and surrounding squamous portion of the temporal bone are exposed by raising a "flap" of mastoid periosteum pedicled anteroinferiorly. Soft tissue flaps should accommodate stable placement of the implant at a safe margin from overlying incisions and enable internal device placement sufficiently away from the pinna to leave room for an ear-level external processor.

A simple mastoidectomy is performed, preserving a slight overhang at the superior and posterior cortical margins. This provides protection for the connecting leads. The facial recess is opened to maximize visualization of the incudostapedial joint and cochlear promontory after adequate thinning of the bony canal wall, opening of the antrum, and removal of adequate air cells to enable systematic exposure of the horizontal semicircular canal, fossa incudus, and chordafacial angle. Before insertion of the electrode array, a well is created behind the mastoid to accommodate the receiver-stimulator portion of the internal device.

Thinning of the bone anterior to the vertical segment of the facial nerve maximizes visualization of the round window niche via the facial recess. The round window niche should be exposed, and the round window membrane should be identified.[39] Inspection of the posterior promontory allows for identification of the round window niche if it is bridged with bone; the niche is never more than 2 mm from the inferior margin of the oval window. A cochleostomy is created in the scala tympani, either directly through the round window membrane or indirectly through the promontory anteroinferior to the center of the round window niche. The preferred approach is debatable, but the priority should be to access the scala tympani without inducing direct injury to the basilar membrane yet while providing adequate space for unimpeded insertion of the electrode array.[40] This array is advanced under direct visualization along a trajectory tangential to the basal turn of the scala tympani (Fig. 49-6). Resistance to array insertion suggests the risk of buckling of the carrier. Because buckling of the implant can injure the spiral ligament, basilar membrane, or cochlear nerve endings, aggressive insertion is avoided. Full insertion of the array within the basal turn of the cochlea requires an insertion depth of 25 to 30 mm, depending on array length. After insertion of the array, the cochleostomy should be sealed gently with a small piece of fascia. The connecting lead should be stabilized within the facial recess to reduce the likelihood of the array extruding from the cochlea. Drilling a notch in the bridge of bone that defines the superior end of the facial recess provides a convenient slot in which the array lead can be stabilized. Once the electrode array is in place, the receiver-stimulator is stabilized with sutures to the bony cortex or by a tight-fit pocket subjacent to the pericranium and deep fascia of the temporalis muscle. As the incision is closed, the implanted device is covered completely with the scalp. Initial activation of the cochlear implant typically takes place 3 to 6 weeks after implantation to allow sufficient time for healing

of the surgical incision and resolution of the accompanying edema.

COMPLICATIONS

The risks for cochlear implantation include the risks inherent in extended mastoid surgery and those associated with the implanted device. Cohen et al.[41] characterized implant-related complications as *major* if they required revision surgery and *minor* if they resolved with minimal or no treatment. A survey of 459 cochlear implant operations reported 55 major (12%) and 32 minor (7%) complications. Webb et al.,[42] reporting on their experience with 153 patients, found 13.7% major complications and 13.7% minor complications. Hoffman and Cohen[43] noted that in later follow-up, 220 (8%) major and 119 (4.3%) minor complications occurred among 2751 implantations. Direct comparisons of complication rates between reports fail to include information on duration of device use, and studies vary in length and frequency of follow-up. Notwithstanding these limitations, longitudinal tracking indicates a substantial reduction in the incidence of major complications in the past 10 years.[43]

Major complications include facial nerve paralysis and implant exposure due to flap loss. Facial nerve injury is uncommon and, when recognized promptly, is unlikely to produce permanent, complete paralysis. Loss of flap viability can lead to wound infection and device extrusion, necessitating scalp flap revision. When intractable infection is present, device removal with or without replacement may be necessary.

Major complications that are strictly device-related involve partial or complete device failure. As the materials used to fabricate the internal device are expected to maintain a hermetic seal for beyond 100 years, use-related failure per se is not expected. Device failure is attributed to either flaws in manufacturing or trauma. Device failure as a result of loss of electrical function in the external processor commonly produces a sudden loss of function and therefore hearing. Intermittent hearing loss and "popping" sensations occur before processor failure. External processor function may be lost with direct trauma, exposure to water, and most frequently, normal wear and tear of connecting lead wires linking the processor unit with the magnetically retained antenna that relays information to the internal device.

Although much less prevalent, device failure as a result of loss of electrical function in the internal device is of considerably greater concern. An internal device failure typically presents as either immediate cessation of hearing or intermittent hearing loss associated with reduced quality of sound and a period of diminishing function over days to weeks. Reports of painful stimulation have been noted but are rare. A review of experiences at Johns Hopkins University reveals a 1.3% annual risk of revision surgery, including reimplantation, in adults.[44] Device failure (65%) was the most common indication of reimplantation, of which about one third presented with complete cessation of device function and two thirds experienced less dramatic declines in function. Other indications included infection (12%), electrode extrusion (15%), and facial nerve stimulation (8%). Cochlear implants have maintained a historical reliability of 99% at 1 year. Reported trends suggest that device reliability has improved over the past 30 years.[45] For example, the

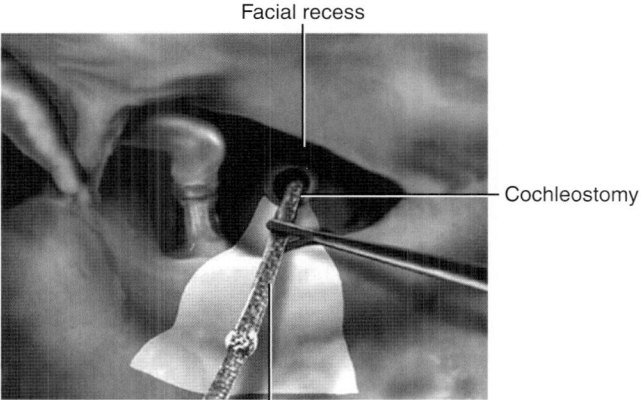

FIGURE 49-6 Surgical placement of cochlear implant electrode. The facial recess is opened, and a cochleostomy is created to allow for implant electrode insertion. *(Courtesy of Med-El Corporation, Durham, NC.)*

failure rate for the third-generation Cochlear Corporation (Lane Cove, New South Wales, Australia) device released in 2001 (0.3% per year) is approximately one third of that associated with the company's first-generation device (0.8% per year) used from 1985 to 1998.

Prevention of device failure begins with proper securing of the implant, particularly the connecting lead between the receiver-stimulator and the electrode array, where the device is vulnerable to shearing. Surgeons should secure the device by embedding it in a well drilled in bone and fixing it in place with permanent suture material. While the evolution of implant design has diminished the rate of device failure, these precautions may help to shield the device from traumatic events.

The risk of bacterial infection of an implanted device producing labyrinthitis or meningitis and associated reactive fibrosis and destruction of neural elements appears to be low. Franz et al.[46] inoculated the bullae of implanted cats with streptococci to evaluate the risk of infection spreading from the middle ear into the implanted cochlea. Despite resulting inflammation of the round window niche, cochlear inflammation was absent. This finding was attributed to a seal that had formed around the electrode at the entrance to either the round window or the cochleostomy, thus forming a protective barrier against implant-surface colonization and bacterial biofilm.[47]

In 2002, an increase in the number of postimplantation meningitis cases was noted anecdotally. Initial reports suggested a higher risk of meningitis in patients implanted with a particular device design—especially when placed with an intracochlear shim (electrode positioner)—and the manufacturer ultimately recalled unimplanted devices utilizing the positioner. The level of risk did not suggest the need for positioner removal unless repeated infections occurred. Since then, continued studies have revealed a higher risk for the disease in patients with all cochlear implants compared to the general population. Children appear to be particularly affected: of the 52 cases originally reported by the U.S. Food and Drug Administration, 33 (63%) were under the age of 7.[48]

Reefhuis et al.[49] conducted a study of 4264 children implanted between 1997 and 2002 and found 29 cases of bacterial meningitis in 26 children. This rate of meningitis (caused by *Streptococcus pneumoniae*) was 30 times the incidence in the general population. While the use of a positioner increased the likelihood of contracting meningitis, even children implanted without a positioner had rates of meningitis 16 times higher than the general population. Case-control analysis found the following risk factors: a history of placement of a ventriculoperitoneal cerebrospinal fluid (CSF) shunt, a history of otitis media prior to implantation, the presence of CSF leakage alone or inner ear malformations with CSF leakage, the use of a positioner, incomplete insertion of the electrode, signs of middle ear inflammation at the time of implantation, and exposure to smoking in the household. While the incidence of meningitis decreased considerably after the perioperative period, cases still appeared even 2 years after implantation.

The design of the study conducted by Reefhuis et al.,[47] as noted by the authors, did not permit the comparison of meningitis risk between deaf children with and without a cochlear implant. That is, there is no comprehensive epidemiologic analysis of the risk of meningitis in deaf children in general. It is biologically plausible that deafness itself poses a greater risk of meningitis given the strong association of deafness with skull base anomalies that predispose individuals to the disease. It is also possible that any surgical implant placed in or near the skull base of toddlers and young children (e.g., CSF shunts) carries a prolonged risk of meningitis.

OUTCOMES

Clinical observations in adult patients with current processors indicate that for patients with implant experience beyond 6 months, mean scores on word recognition approximate 40%, with a range of 0% to 100%.[22] Results achieved with the most recently developed speech processing strategies reveal mean scores above 75% correct on words-in-sentence testing, again with a range of scores from 0% to 100%.

BILATERAL COCHLEAR IMPLANTATION

In an effort to expand the benefits obtained with unilateral cochlear implantation, bilateral implantation has been offered to increasing numbers of patients. Implantation of the second ear some time after implantation of the first ear and bilateral, simultaneous implantations have been described. The potential benefit of bilateral implantation relies on the capacity for patients to integrate bilateral electrical stimulation within the central auditory system. Laboratory trials have focused on an examination of whether the advantages of binaural acoustic hearing extend to those with bilateral implants. Binaural advantages are (1) increased auditory sensitivity (i.e., improved pure tone thresholds) as a result of summation effects, (2) improved sound source localization, and (3) improved speech recognition in noise. The latter can occur through acoustic effects when the second ear is away from the noise or by neurologic effects when the second ear is closer to the noise source. In the first scenario, distance and head shadow establish a favorable signal-to-noise ratio for the ear farthest from the noise. In the second, neural integration of bilateral inputs results in "binaural squelch," whereby suppression of the noise enhances speech perception.

Tyler et al.[50] noted that bilateral cochlear implantation generally enables head shadow effects in discerning speech in noise. However, only some patients benefit from summation and squelch effects. Most adult bilateral recipients have shown improved horizontal plane localization. Similarly, Litovsky et al.[51] and Schoen et al.[52] have observed general trends toward additional benefit with the use of a second implant. However, different binaural benefits were obtained in different subjects, and these studies document cases wherein no additional benefit with bilateral implantation was achieved.

Although the "era of bilateral implantation" has been introduced, there are few controlled trials to date. Preliminary results show promise in enabling the use of the head shadow, an expanded sound field, and some sound localization ability to the majority of bilateral recipients.[53,54] Moreover, some observed benefits are attributable to improved summation and squelch. These findings have demonstrated that the brain can integrate electrical stimulation from the two ears. However, systems that enable integrated, bilateral sound field processing have not yet been introduced clinically, possibly limiting the potential benefits of bilateral implantation.

Auditory Brain Stem Implants

Patients with bilateral hearing loss due to bilateral vestibular schwannomas (e.g., in NF2) experience devastation of their spoken communication abilities. In such patients, auditory nerve damage due to tumor progression or tumor removal may render cochlear implantation ineffective. Instead, electrical hearing can be achieved with an electrode device placed on the cochlear nucleus of the pontomedullary brain stem. The first single-channel auditory brain stem implant (ABI) was placed by House and Hitselberger.[55] Since then, significant technical advancement and modifications have taken place. The current ABI device (Fig. 49-7) consists of an electrode array with 21 channels (Cochlear Corporation, Englewood, CO). Newer designs employing multitined penetrating microelectrodes may permit access to deeper and more discrete populations of cochlear nucleus neurons and may offer improved spectral and dynamic range.[56]

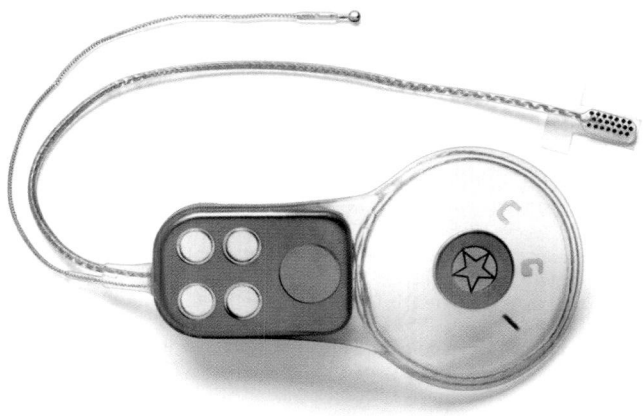

FIGURE 49-7 Auditory brain stem implant. *(Courtesy of Cochlear Corporation, Englewood, CO.)*

INDICATIONS

In the United States, ABIs are only approved for patients with NF2 manifesting bilateral vestibular schwannomas. The criteria for implantation are (1) evidence of bilateral cranial nerve VII and VIII tumors involving the internal auditory canal or cerebellopontine angle, (2) language competency, (3) age 12 years or older, (4) psychologic suitability, and (5) realistic expectations. An ABI can be placed during the surgical resection of the first- or second-side vestibular schwannoma. The advantage of implantation during the first-side tumor resection is that it allows the patients to have early exposure to the device before total deafness after the second-side tumor resection.

More recently in Europe, ABIs have been placed in non-NF2 patients.[57-58] These patients have conditions that preclude cochlear implant placement: severe cochlear malformations, cochlear nerve dysplasia/hypoplasia, cranial nerve VIII avulsion, or cochlear ossification.

SURGICAL TECHNIQUE

ABIs can be placed via the translabyrinthine or the retrosigmoid approaches, often in the same setting as tumor resection. The details of these two surgical approaches are discussed elsewhere in the text. A well is created in the bony cortex posterior to mastoidectomy cavity or the retrosigmoid craniotomy site to allow for placement of the receiver-stimulator, similar to cochlear implantation. Once the receiver-stimulator is secured in place, the cochlear nucleus is located. The anatomic landmarks for locating the cochlear nucleus include the choroids plexus, which marks the entrance to the foramen of Luschka (lateral opening of the fourth ventricle) and lateral recess.[55] Cranial nerves V and VII through X and the anterior inferior cerebellar artery are identified and used to locate the area in which the cochlear nuclei reside in the superolateral aspect of the floor of the fourth ventricle (Fig. 49-8). Anatomic landmarks may be obscured by choroids plexus and displaced by effects of tumor growth. The electrode array is placed on the surface of the brain stem overlying the ventral cochlear nuclei, in the anterosuperolateral aspect of the lateral recess. Placement is adjusted based on intraoperative

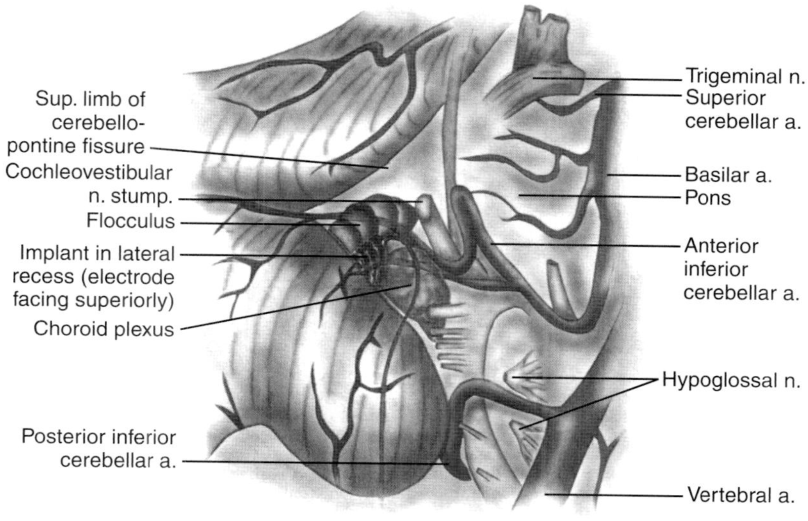

FIGURE 49-8 Surgical placement of an ABI. The implant electrode is placed in the lateral recess in the proximity of the cochlear nuclei. *(Salvinelli F, De la Cruz, A. Otoneurosurgery and Lateral Skull Base Surgery. Philadelphia, WB Saunders, 1996.)*

Sup. limb of cerebello-
pontine fissure
Cochleovestibular
n. stump.
Flocculus
Implant in lateral
recess (electrode
facing superiorly)
Choroid plexus

Posterior inferior
cerebellar a.

Trigeminal n.
Superior
cerebellar a.

Basilar a.
Pons

Anterior
inferior
cerebellar a.

Hypoglossal n.

Vertebral a.

auditory brain stem response waveforms elicited by stimulation via the implant, and then the implant is stabilized. The surgical site is then closed as in translabyrinthine and retrosigmoid approaches for tumor resection, taking every precaution to prevent CSF leakage.

COMPLICATIONS

The main complication with ABIs is CSF leakage. Such leakage associated with an ABI often presents as fluid collection under the skin flap. CSF leakage can be prevented by meticulous dural closure, as well as packing the eustachian tube and mastoid cavity or air cells with various materials. Meningitis is also a complication after an ABI. It can arise either on its own or as a result of CSF leakage.

OUTCOMES

The ABI is usually activated within 4 to 6 weeks after surgery. Otto et al. reviewed the ABI experience at the House Ear Institute.[59] This study included 61 patients who underwent placement of an ABI. In this cohort, 6 patients report no useful auditory sensation after the ABI. Patients with the ABI scored well above chance for closed-set speech tests (Monosyllable Trochee Spondee, or MTS, test and Northwestern University Children's Perception of Speech test), but significant open-set word recognition was rare. Otto et al. found that for most patients with an ABI, the benefit in communication occurs when sound is used in conjunction with lipreading. There were 2 patients who experienced CSF leakage that resolved with pressure dressing and lumbar drain placement.

In a study by Nevison et al., the results of an ABI in 27 patients were reviewed.[60] All but 1 patient received useful auditory sensation after implantation. In the study, 16 patients were tested using a closed-set MTS word test. Of the 16 patients, 15 scored close to 100% in the auditory–visual condition. In the auditory-only condition, scores were lower but were well above chance. Seventeen patients underwent open-set sentence-recognition tests. Eight patients scored at or greater than 50% in auditory–visual condition. One patient even scored 68% in the auditory-only condition. Two patients experienced facial nerve stimulation, which resulted in nonuse. One patient experienced a gradual increase in epileptic seizures after ABI. No CSF leak was reported in this study.

As mentioned earlier, ABI has been placed more recently in non-NF2 patients with deafness, which precludes cochlear implant placement. In a study comparing the ABI hearing outcomes in NF2 patients versus non-NF2 patients, Colletti et al. found that the average open-set speech-recognition score for non-NF2 patients was 59%, whereas the average score for NF2 patients was 10%.[58] Colletti et al. postulated that the poorer performance seen in NF2 patients is secondary to damage to the cochlear nucleus by tumor; thus, the central auditory system never receives sufficient information from the auditory periphery.

Conclusion

There are multiple rehabilitative options for patients who have lost their hearing from presbycusis, experienced sudden sensorineural hearing loss, or lost their hearing as a result of lateral skull base tumor progression or resection.

An osseointegrated implant offers patients with conductive hearing loss a way of bypassing the external and middle ear by using bone conduction for sound transmission. It is also beneficial for patients with single-sided deafness. A cochlear implant offers favorable hearing outcomes in many patients, with the possibility of achieving open-set speech recognition. Even though the hearing outcome for an ABI is not as good as that for a cochlear implant, it can be used for patients who are not candidates for cochlear implant and offers access to speech for lipreading and environmental sounds for improved safety.

KEY REFERENCES

Brackmann DE, Hitselberger WE, Nelson RA, et al. Auditory brainstem implant: I. Issues in surgical implantation. *Otolaryngol Head Neck Surg.* 1993;108:624-633.

Cohen NL, Hoffman RA, Stroschein M. Medical or surgical complications related to the nucleus multichannel cochlear implant. *Ann Otol Rhinol Laryngol Suppl.* 1988;135:8-13.

Colletti V, Shannon R, Carner M, et al. Outcomes in nontumor adults fitted with the auditory brainstem implant: 10 years' experience. *Otol Neurotol.* 2009;30(5):614-618.

Friedland DR, Venick HS, Niparko JK. Choice of ear for cochlear implantation: the effect of history and residual hearing on predicted postoperative performance. *Otol Neurotol.* 2003;24(4):582-589.

Håkansson B, Liden G, Tjellström A, et al. Ten years of experience with the Swedish bone-anchored hearing system. *Ann Otol Rhinol Laryngol Suppl.* 1990;151:1-16.

House JW, Kutz Jr JW. Bone-anchored hearing aids: incidence and management of postoperative complications. *Otol Neurotol.* 2007;28(2):213-217.

Lustig LR, Arts HA, Brackmann DE, et al. Hearing rehabilitation using the BAHA bone-anchored hearing aid: results in 40 patients. *Otol Neurotol.* 2001;22(3):328-334.

Lustig L, Niparko J. Osseointegrated implants in otology. *Adv Otolaryngol Head Neck Surg.* 1999;13:105-126.

Lustig LR, Yeagle J, Driscoll CLW, et al. Cochlear implantation in patients with neurofibromatosis type 2 and bilateral vestibular schwannoma. *Otol Neurotol.* 2006;27:512-518.

NIH Consensus Conference. Cochlear implants in adults and children. *JAMA.* 1995;274(24):1955-1961.

NIH Consensus Development Statement. Cochlear Implants. *NIH Consensus Statement.* 1988;7(2):1-25.

Niparko JK, Cox KM, Lustig LR. Comparison of the bone anchored hearing aid implantable hearing device with contralateral routing of offside signal amplification in the rehabilitation of unilateral deafness. *Otol Neurotol.* 2003;24(1):73-78.

Otto SR, Brackmann DE, Hitselberger WE, et al. Multichannel auditory brainstem implant: update on performance in 61 patients. *J Neurosurg.* 2002;96(6):1063-1071.

Rauschecker JP, Shannon RV. Sending sound to the brain. *Science.* 2002;295(5557):1025-1029.

Reefhuis J, Honein MA, Whitney CG, et al. Risk of bacterial meningitis in children with cochlear implants. *N Engl J Med.* 2003;349:435-445.

Rivas A, Marlowe AL, Chinnici JE, et al. Revision cochlear implant surgery in adults: indications and results. *Otol Neurotol.* 2008;29(5):639-648.

Rubinstein JT, Parkinson WS, Tyler RS, et al. Residual speech recognition and cochlear implant performance: effects of implantation criteria. *Am J Otol.* 1999;20(4):445-452.

Tjellström A, Lindstrom J, Hallen O, et al. Osseointegrated titanium implants in the temporal bone. A clinical study on bone-anchored hearing aids. *Am J Otol.* 1981;4:304-310.

Waltzman SB, Fisher SG, Niparko JK, et al. Predictors of postoperative performance with cochlear implants. *Ann Otol Rhinol Laryngol Suppl.* 1995;165:15-18.

Webb RL, Lehnhardt E, Clark GM, et al. Surgical complications with the cochlear multiple-channel intracochlear implant: experience at Hannover and Melbourne. *Ann Otol Rhinol Laryngol.* 1991;100(2):131-136.

Numbered references appear on Expert Consult.

Multimodal Treatment of Orbital Tumors

SHAAN M. RAZA • ALFREDO QUIÑONES-HINOJOSA • PREM S. SUBRAMANIAN

The surgical management of intraorbital tumors requires a thorough understanding of not only orbital anatomy but also the objectives of surgical intervention. The orbital contents abut the skull base, paranasal sinuses, and intracranial compartment or anterior cranial fossa. The orbit is a quadrangular compartment that can be approached through a variety of trajectories along one of its four walls or posteriorly from its apex. From the surgical standpoint, the orbit represents an anatomic compartment that is encountered by several specialties—neurosurgery, ophthalmology and otolaryngology—with their own approaches derived from the pathologic processes they usually encounter.

From the neurosurgical perspective, the orbit is exposed in the surgical management of pathologic processes involving the orbit, in addition to the skull base or intracranial cavity. The neurosurgeon often becomes involved in orbital disease cases when tumors or vascular lesions are present. Orbital tumors are often benign (i.e., meningioma, cavernous hemangioma, and schwannoma) but may be locally invasive or infiltrative. Malignant lesions (i.e., cranial base sarcomas, esthesioneuroblastomas, and squamous cell carcinomas) are even more likely to require a multidisciplinary approach because of their spread across multiple anatomic compartments. Primary orbital tumors are often discrete from normal orbital structures and may engulf, although not necessarily invade, the extraocular muscles and/or optic nerve; secondary tumors extend into the orbit along normal anatomic structures (often nerves) or by bony destruction. As such, the surgical objectives for processes involving the orbit range from the need for negative margins or aggressive resection to purely orbital decompression.

Selecting the most appropriate surgical treatment for orbital disease processes requires an understanding of the various open and endoscopic surgical approaches and their advantages, indications, and limitations. The primary considerations are the location and size of the tumor, including its relationship to crucial orbital structures, the site of origin, the other extraorbital anatomic compartments involved, and histologic diagnosis.

Orbital Anatomy

ORBITAL BONY ANATOMY

The bony orbit not only lies close to other compartments in the facial skeleton but also contains several foramina through which critical neurovascular structures pass[1]

(Fig. 50-1). The orbital roof is formed by the frontal bone and lesser wing of sphenoid; its superior surface is the floor of the anterior cranial fossa. The roof also lies below the frontal sinus. The orbital plate of the maxillary bone forms most of the orbital floor, in addition to the roof of the maxillary sinus; the palatine and zygomatic bones also contribute to the floor. Medially, the medial wall, also known as the lamina papyracea, forms a thin wall separating the orbit from the ethmoid sinus anteriorly and the sphenoid sinus more posteriorly, a structure through which most endoscopic approaches to the orbit can be directed. It is comprised of four bones: the maxillary, lacrimal, ethmoid, and lesser wing of sphenoid. The medial wall of the orbit also contains the foramina through which the anterior and posterior ethmoidal arteries pass. The lateral orbital wall is covered externally by the temporalis muscle and formed by the frontosphenoid process of the zygomatic bone, in addition to the greater wing of the sphenoid. The apex of the orbit is directed in a medial oblique direction and contains three critical foramina: optic canal, superior orbital fissure, and inferior orbital fissure. The optic canal bridges the intracranial space and orbit inferomedial to the anterior clinoid process while it is bordered laterally by the lesser wing of the sphenoid. The superior orbital fissure is bordered laterally by the greater wing of the sphenoid.

MUSCLE CONE AND ANNULUS OF ZINN

The annulus of Zinn serves as the origin of six of the seven extraocular muscles (Fig. 50-2). Superiorly, the superior rectus arises from the annulus, which at this point is fused with the dura of the optic nerve. The levator palpebrae arises medial and superior to the superior rectus muscle but remains intimately associated with it. More medial and inferior to this are the origins of the medial rectus and superior oblique muscles. Although it is firmly fused to the optic nerve dorsally, the annulus of Zinn loops widely around the nerve laterally and inferiorly, giving rise to the lateral rectus muscle, in addition to the inferior rectus. The space between the insertion sites of these two muscles is known as the oculomotor foramen. Based on this arrangement, there are evident portals of entry of neurovascular structures into the orbit: the optic canal and the superior orbital fissure.

OPTIC NERVE AND ORBITAL NERVES

The optic nerve, throughout its entire course from the chiasm to sclera, is covered with a pial membrane (providing vascular supply) and associated subarachnoid space (Fig. 50-3).

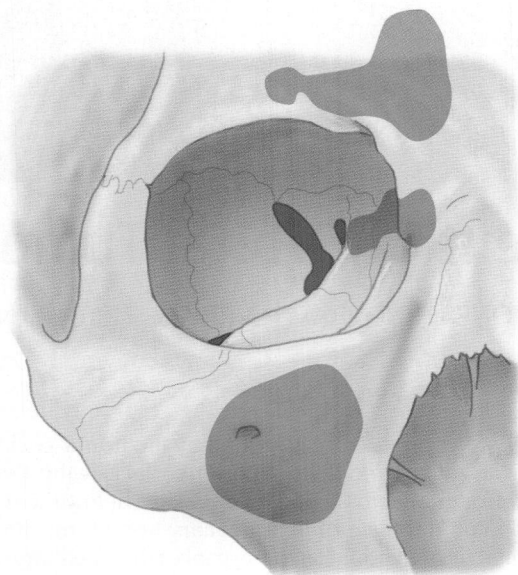

FIGURE 50-1 Integrity of the bony orbit and the size and shape of its fissures and foramina can be defined by plain skull radiographs and CT bone windows. The frontal, ethmoidal, and maxillary sinuses are shown diagrammatically. Attention is directed to one of the two roots of the lesser wing of the sphenoid, which lies beneath the anterior clinoid and forms the lateral margin of the optic canal in the medial margin of the superior orbital fissure.

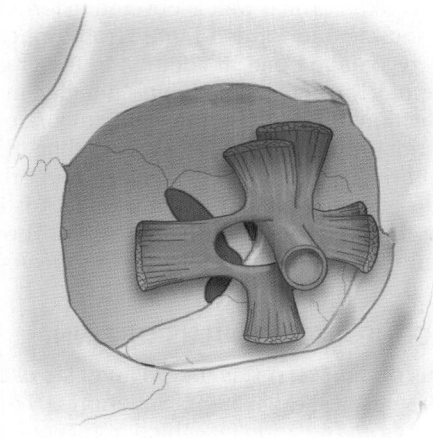

FIGURE 50-2 The anulus of Zinn is a fibrous band giving rise to the origins of six of the seven extraocular muscles. This fibrous tissue is in continuity with the dural sheath of the optic nerve. The two heads of the lateral rectus loop around that portion of the superior orbital fissure known as the oculomotor foramen.

As the optic nerve enters the optic canal, the intracranial dura splits, with the outer leaf forming the orbital periosteum and the inner leaf remaining with the optic nerve. The superior orbital fissure contains the remaining cranial nerves that enter the orbital compartment. The trochlear nerve and the frontal and lacrimal branches of the trigeminal nerve enter through the superior orbital fissure above the extraocular muscles and annulus of Zinn. The remaining nerves—the oculomotor nerve (superior and inferior divisions) and the abducens nerve—pass through the superior orbital fissure and annulus of Zinn.

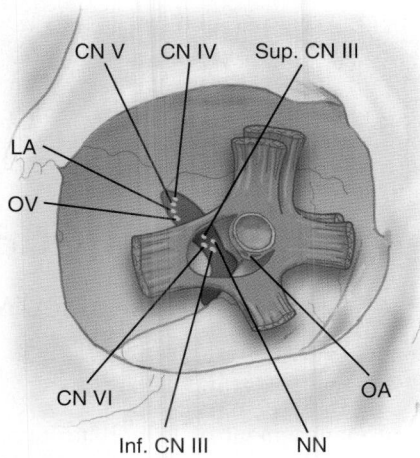

FIGURE 50-3 Partial obliteration of the subarachnoid space of the optic nerve at the anulus of Zinn is shown, and the medial origin of the levator muscle is evident. The ophthalmic artery (OA) enters the orbit through the optic canal. The trochlear (CN IV), frontalis (CN V), and lacrimal (LA) nerves and the ophthalmic vein (OV) enter through the superior orbital fissure and thus lie within the periorbita but outside the muscle cone, whereas the superior division of the oculomotor nerve (Sup. CN III), the abducens nerve (CN VI), the nasociliary nerve (NN), and the inferior division of the oculomotor nerve (Inf. CN III) enter the muscle cone through the oculomotor foramen and lie within the muscle cone.

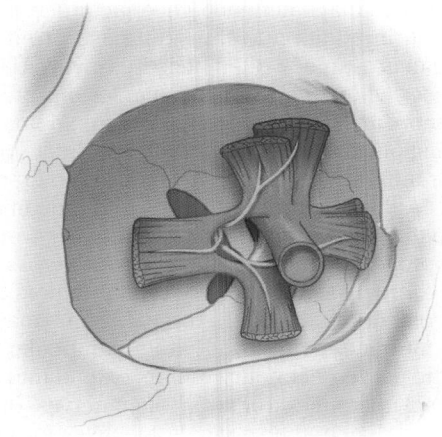

FIGURE 50-4 The nerve supply to the extraocular muscles is shown entering through the oculomotor foramen. A medial superior approach to the optic nerve between the lateral and the medial rectus muscles provides direct access, with minimal chance of injury to this nerve supply to the extraocular muscles.

Because of this arrangement, it is evident that the optic nerve can be approached directly through the medial compartment, between the medial rectus and the levator muscles, without fear of injury to the nerve supply of any extraocular muscle (Fig. 50-4).

Case Selection

The treatment strategy for orbital lesions is primarily determined by the nature of the lesion. An overview of the types of orbital lesions is provided in Table 50-1.[2] While medical management is best suited for infectious and inflammatory

Table 50-1	Overview of Orbital Lesions
Category	**Lesions**
Vascular	Capillary hemangioma
	Cavernous hemangioma
	Hamartoma
	Hemangiopericytoma
	Lymphangioma
Nerve sheath	Neurilemomas
	Neurofibroma (plexiform and solitary)
Osseous and cartilaginous	Osteoma
	Osteogenic sarcoma
	Chondroma
	Fibrous dysplasia
	Aneurysmal bone cyst
Neuroepithelial	Optic nerve glioma
Meningioma	
Mesenchymal	Rhabdomyosarcoma
	Lipoma
	Liposarcoma
Inflammatory	Nonvasculitic
	Vasculitic, nongranulomatous
Carcinoma	
Cystic	
Other	

processes involving the orbit, definitive surgical treatment remains the mainstay for a majority of symptomatic orbital tumors and dysthyroid orbitopathy.

The diagnostic workup proceeds logically after clinical examination and primarily consists of imaging. Magnetic resonance imaging (MRI) with fat suppression provides excellent definition of orbital pathology.[3,4] Fat suppression eliminates the T1 bright signal associated with orbital fat that can obscure intraorbital pathology. Contrast-enhanced MRI provides excellent soft tissue resolution and is the best modality to determine intracranial extension of orbital pathology.[5,6] Computed tomography (CT) imaging provides excellent definition of orbital pathologic process and regional bone anatomy. An adequate study includes thin cuts through the orbits and shows normal orbital anatomy, including the size and position of the globe, optic nerve, and extraocular muscles. CT is superior to MRI in surgical planning because of its ability to show bony anatomy, but MRI is preferred when optic nerve involvement by the tumor or disease process must be examined.

Once a thoughtful sequential diagnostic workup has been completed, the location and extent of the pathologic process must be defined and following questions considered:

- Is a tumor present?
- Is it likely benign or malignant?
- Is it confined to the muscle cone?
- Does it arise from the optic nerve, or is it medial or lateral to the optic nerve?
- Is the bony integrity of the orbit violated?
- Is the optic canal or any of the foramina or fissures enlarged or hyperostotic?
- Is the process destructive?

- Does the process extend from or enter the cranial cavity?
- Does the process extent from or enter the paranasal sinuses?

Surgical Approaches

Anatomically, orbital tumors can be divided into intraconal, extraconal, and intracanalicular. This distinction is made on the basis of the tumor's relationship with the muscle cone, with intracanalicular tumors at least partially extending into the optic canal. There are two primary types of surgical approaches to the orbit: transorbital approaches (performed primarily by ophthalmologists) and extraorbital approaches (often performed by a team that includes a neurosurgeon or head and neck surgeon, as well as an ophthalmologist).[7,8] This chapter focuses on the intra- and extraorbital approaches not discussed in other sections of this book. Extraorbital approaches typically employed by neurosurgeons include extended bifrontal craniotomy, orbitozygomatic craniotomy, subcranial craniotomy, and unilateral maxillectomy. As a general paradigm, lesions based anteriorly can be approached via transorbital approaches while lesions in the posterior third of the orbit are often managed by extraorbital approaches (open or endoscopic). There are instances in which a combination of approaches may be necessary.

Ultimately, there are four primary transorbital routes: anterior orbitotomy (superior or inferior), medial orbitotomy, lateral orbitotomy, and a combination of medial and lateral orbitotomies. These approaches are discussed here, in addition to endoscopic approaches to the medial orbit.

APPROACHES TO THE ANTERIOR ORBIT

The anterior approach is typically employed for lesions in the anterior third of the orbit. For superior-based approaches, an incision is typically made through the eyelid crease or a parallel curvilinear fashion superior to it. Such an incision provides excellent access and postoperative cosmesis. A direct sub-brow incision also may be used if eyelid anatomy is unfavorable. For inferior orbital lesions, the incision is usually placed in the conjunctival fornix. The skin and subdermal tissue are retracted after incision, at which point the periosteum (periorbita) is identified. Depending on the location of the lesion, the periorbita may be elevated and incised or the orbital septum may be entered directly. After incision and dissection of the periorbita or septum, the lesion is typically visible, and the remainder dissection proceeds according to the lesion. The periorbita can then be closed with interrupted 5-0 polygalactin sutures, although the orbital septum should not be closed to avoid eyelid retraction. The skin incision is closed with a running 8-0 nylon suture.

For larger lesions located in the anterior superior orbit, a superior osteotomy may be necessary. For this modification, a longer incision is made in the eyebrow, with the surgeon taking care to visualize and preserve the supratrochlear and supraorbital neurovascular bundles. The superior orbital rim can be removed with a sagittal saw or osteotomes, after which the remainder of the dissection proceeds as described earlier. The use of fine osteotomes ultimately results in thinner bone cuts (with minimal resultant bone loss) and improved cosmetic outcomes.

APPROACHES TO THE MEDIAL ORBIT (OPEN)

From a neurosurgical standpoint, medial approaches to the orbit are typically preferred when dealing with meningioma or optic glioma. They are also effective in the management of small tumors, such as cavernous hemangiomas and isolated neurofibromas. The medial orbitotomy can be performed via a transconjunctival approach, where a medial peritomy is performed in which relaxing incisions are angled superiorly and inferiorly to expose the insertion of the medial rectus onto the globe. The medial rectus is subsequently freed from its intramuscular septum and ligaments and retracted medially. At this point, a medial orbital retractor is employed and a malleable retractor is used to retract the globe laterally. Dissection through the deeper orbital fat is often necessary before the tumor is identified within the cone. After tumor resection, the medial rectus is then reattached to its insertion site and the conjunctiva is closed with interrupted sutures. A transcaruncular approach is also effective in accessing extraconal tumors in the medial space. An incision is placed directly through the caruncle, and Stevens scissors are used to palpate the posterior lacrimal crest. Blunt dissection reveals the periorbita, which is opened sharply. Access to the medial orbit back to the apex can then be achieved, with ligation of the anterior and posterior ethmoidal arteries as needed to allow for adequate exposure.

APPROACHES TO THE LATERAL ORBIT

The lateral orbitotomy is useful for retrobulbar lesions and more posterior lesions. The technique removes the lateral wall of the orbit to visualize lateral, superolateral, and inferolateral tumors; such lesions include cavernous hemangiomas. After induction of general anesthesia, the patient is positioned supine with the head turned contralaterally. A curvilinear incision is made starting in the eyelid crease and extending inferolaterally in a lazy S shape (modified Kronlein incision). The incision follows natural skin tension lines and is lateral to the lateral canthus. As an alternative, an incision is made from the lateral canthus alone and directed posteriorly, dividing the canthus sharply with scissors. This Burke-type incision permits better access to the inferolateral orbit.

After incision and subcutaneous dissection, the periorbita is incised along the orbital rim in a T shape. With blunt dissection, the lateral periorbita is distracted posteriorly to the posterior one fourth of the orbit to expose the lateral wall of the orbit. The periosteum and temporalis muscle are

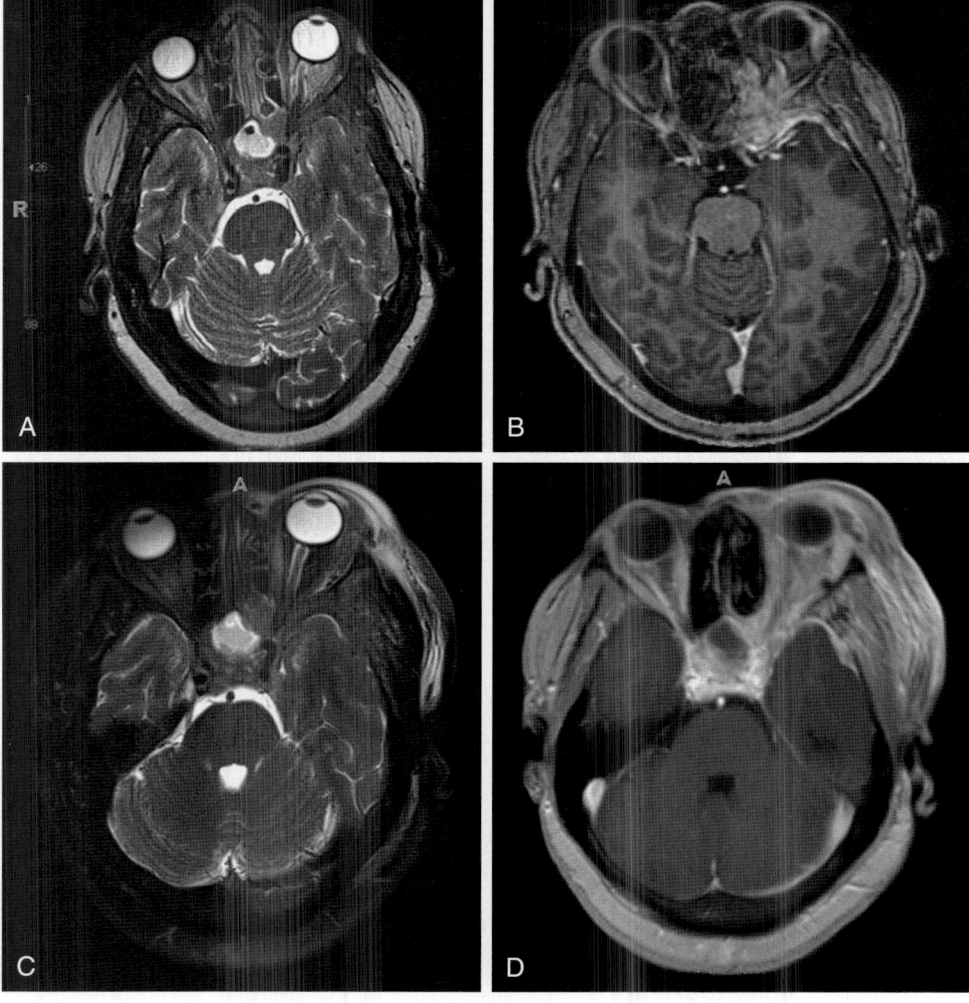

FIGURE 50-5 Patient with a metastatic breast cancer lesion at the orbital apex presenting with visual decline and diminished extraocular movements. A, Preoperative T2-weighted image demonstrating compression of the left optic nerve at the orbital apex. B, Preoperative T1-weighted axial image with contrast demonstrating an enhancing lesion at the orbital apex involving the anterior cranial fossa, orbit, and middle cranial fossa. C, Postoperative T2-weighted image demonstrating decompression of left optic nerve. D, Postoperative T1-weighted axial image with contrast demonstrating the debulking of the lesion.

similarly freed from the bone. To perform the lateral orbital wall osteotomy, initial angled cuts are made along the lateral aspects of the superior and inferior orbital rims. These cuts are directed toward one another to result in a keystone-shaped portion of bone that is removed from the lateral wall. After this initial osteotomy, further posterior visualization is made through removal of bone with a series of rongeurs and drills. Exposure can be extended posteriorly all the way to the orbital apex. Once bone removal has been completed, an incision is made in the periorbita—avoiding the lateral rectus muscle. After entry, the lateral rectus may be retracted superiorly or inferiorly, based on the location of the lesion.

At the completion of the resection, hemostasis is achieved and the integrity of the lateral rectus is verified. The periorbita need not be closed with sutures but merely smoothed into place. The bone is placed back and reconstructed with low-profile craniofacial fixation plates. The periosteum should be closed over these plates to enhance healing and cosmesis. A subcuticular suture is then used to close the skin incision.

ENDONASAL ENDOSCOPIC APPROACHES TO THE MEDIAL ORBIT

With the introduction of endoscopic sinus surgery in the 1980s, endoscopic techniques and approaches have developed to various compartments of the cranial base. The endoscope provides excellent illumination, magnification, a panoramic view, and the capacity for angled vision. With increasing understanding of the advantages and limitations of endoscopic skull base surgery, this technique has also been applied to the management of orbital lesions. Endoscopic visualization ultimately has provided surgeons with the possibility to reach medial and inferior orbital structures and the orbital apex with no facial incisions and minimal soft tissue disruption. In addition, endoscopic approaches limit globe retraction. Endoscopic approaches have been approached for a variety of situations, ranging from optic canal decompression (in situations of displaced bone fractures) to resection of tumors in the medial orbit.

After positioning the patient supine, the endoscope is introduced into the ipsilateral nostril. After identification of key landmarks (inferior turbinate, middle turbinate, and nasal septum), the middle turbinate is retracted medially to expose the uncinate process and ethmoid bullae. The middle turbinate is subsequently removed with caution to avoid injuring the ethmoidal roof. In addition, a posterior septectomy is performed after identification of the sphenoid ostium.

To enter the medial orbital wall, an anterior and posterior ethmoidectomy must be performed. After the nasal steps of the surgery, a unicinacetomy and maxillary antrostomy is performed and the bulla ethmoidalis is entered. The maxillary antrostomy allows definition of the medial wall of the orbit, which lies in the same vertical plane as the maxillary ostium. The inferoanterior wall of the ethmoid bulla is opened, and the anterior ethmoid cells are entered and resected. Recognizing the posterior ethmoid air cells can be entered safely through the horizontal portion of the middle turbinate lamella, the posterior ethmoidectomy proceeds until facing the sphenoid sinus. Throughout the anterior and posterior ethmoidectomy, the surgeon must recognize that the lateral wall of the ethmoid bullae is the lamina papyracea, which is the medial orbital wall.

Prior to the medial orbitotomy, the anterior and posterior ethmoidal arteries must be identified. If the artery is injured prematurely, it may retract into the orbit and cause a dangerous retrobulbar hematoma. After complete resection of the medial orbital wall, the orbital periosteum and underlying periorbital fat tissue are exposed. The fat tissue can be removed and medial rectus identified, after which dissection proceeds according to the tumor.

Ultimately, this technique provides sufficient exposure for particular benign lesions with minimal neurovascular retraction. During dissection, potential complications can be related to globe perforation, optic nerve injury (during canal decompression), and vascular injury (damage to the anterior and posterior ethmoidal arteries).

Conclusions

There are two major types of surgical approaches for the removal of orbital tumors: transorbital and extraorbital approaches. The extraorbital approaches employed typically include extended bifrontal craniotomy, orbitozygomatic craniotomy, and craniofacial approaches (such as unilateral maxillectomy). Transorbital approaches primarily include open approaches (anterior, lateral, and medial orbitotomies) that can be done via cosmetically appealing incisions in the conjunctiva. With the growing understanding of the advantages and limitations of endoscopy, minimally invasive approaches to the medial orbit can now be done for benign pathology. Ultimately, the selection of surgical approach and goals of surgery are dictated by the location (primarily orbital vs. involvement of the intracranial space and paranasal sinuses) and goals of resection (i.e., need for negative margins with malignancies).

CASE EXAMPLE

The patient is a 50-year-old female, status postmastectomy and postchemotherapy for breast cancer, who presented to our service with vision loss and motility abnormalities in her left eye. The patient was at neurologic baseline until 2 months prior to presentation, when she noted dull color perception in her left eye associated with blurring of vision. Several days after onset of her symptoms, the patient also experienced difficulty in abduction of her left eye, which prompted further workup by her oncologist. MRI (Fig. 50-5A and B) demonstrated an extra-axial enhancing mass along the floor of the anterior fossa extending into the left orbit and middle cranial fossa with encasement of the left optic nerve. On initial neuro-ophthalmologic evaluation, the patient's exam was notable for the following: no light perception in the left eye, a left pupil that was amaurotic, and extraocular movements in the left 95% of abduction, 60% of normal elevation, 60% of normal depression, and 10% of abduction past midline. Furthermore, numbness in the left V2 distribution was noted. On orbital echography, enlargement of the left periophthalmic vein was noted.

The patient was taken to the operating room for tissue diagnosis and decompression. Via an eyebrow incision, a left-sided orbitozygomatic craniotomy was performed. Extradurally, the remaining diseased bone was drilled to decompress the superior orbital fissure and optic canal.

Postoperatively, the patient was monitored in the neurocritical care unit and discharged home postoperative day 1. Postoperative MRI demonstrated adequate debulking (Fig. 50-5C and D); final pathology indicated metastatic poorly differentiated adenocarcinoma, consistent with the patient's history of breast cancer.

At 1-month follow-up, the patient exhibited improvement with her extraocular movements, but her vision demonstrated no improvement. In light of the diagnosis of metastatic disease and the low-probability of visual improvement, she was referred for radiation therapy.

KEY REFERENCES

Bejjani GK, Cockerham KP, Kennerdel JS, Maroon JC. A reappraisal of surgery for orbital tumors. Part I: extraorbital approaches. *Neurosurg Focus*. 2001;10:E2.

Cockerham KP, Bejjani GK, Kennerdell JS, Maroon JC. Surgery for orbital tumors. Part II: transorbital approaches. *Neurosurg Focus*. 2001;10:E3.

Darsaut TE, Lanzino G, Lopes MB, Newman S. An introductory overview of orbital tumors. *Neurosurg Focus*. 2001;10:E1.

Haik BG, Saint Louis L, Bierly J, et al. Magnetic resonance imaging in the evaluation of optic nerve gliomas. *Ophthalmology*. 1987;94:709-717.

Housepian EM. Microsurgical anatomy of the orbital apex and principles of transcranial orbital exploration. *Clin Neurosurg*. 1978;25:556-573.

Jakobiec FA, Depot MJ, Kennerdell JS, et al. Combined clinical and computed tomographic diagnosis of orbital glioma and meningioma. *Ophthalmology*. 1984;91:137-155.

Jakobiec FA, Yeo JH, Trokel SL, et al. Combined clinical and computed tomographic diagnosis of primary lacrimal fossa lesions. *Am J Ophthalmol*. 1982;94:785-807.

Rhoton Jr AL. The orbit. *Neurosurgery*. 2002;51:S303-S334.

Numbered references appear on Expert Consult.

CHAPTER 51

Surgical Approaches to the Orbit

UTA SCHICK • ANDREAS UNTERBERG

The surgical treatment of orbital processes presents a border area between different surgical specialties, including otorhinolaryngology, oral/maxillofacial surgery, ophthalmology, and neurosurgery. Neurosurgeons encounter more neural tumors such as meningiomas and optic pathway gliomas in contrast to ear, nose, and throat (ENT) or head and neck surgeons, who more often deal with secondary lesions such as mucoceles and paranasal sinus neoplasms. Patients treated by ophthalmologists have a greater incidence of thyroid-related orbitopathy and inflammatory pseudotumor. [1]

The spectrum of pathologies is broad and the potential operative approaches are numerous. A better understanding of the variety of disease processes in the orbit and of the available interdisciplinary approaches is needed to determine the optimal mode of treatment. Only specialized centers are able to overview the broad variety of these rare lesions and possible minimal invasive surgical approaches.

History

The history of orbital approaches begins in the 19th century. Krönlein performed the first extracranial orbitotomy in 1889 and Berke in 1954. [2,3] Kennerdell and Maroon picked up this approach in 1988. [4] Niho [5] chose a transethmoidal approach in 1970, Colohan [6] a frontal trans-sinusoidal path in 1985, and Hassler [7] a transconjunctival approach in 1994.

Regarding the transcranial approaches, the subfrontal approaches published by Dandy [8] in 1941 and Housepian [9] in 1978 are well recognized. Naffziger [10] chose a frontolateral pterional approach in 1948. In 1964 and 1975, Yasargil [11] reported about experiences with the same approach. Kennerdell and Maroon [4] also operated via this frontolateral approach. Seeger and Hassler used a pterional extradural approach in 1983 and 1985. [12] Dolenc [13,14] opened the orbit by unroofing it while operating on parasellar lesions and tracing them through the orbital roof directly or through the superior orbital fissure in 1983. Hassler [15] described a contralateral pterional approach in 1994.

Choice of Surgical Approach

The choice of surgical approach is largely determined by the location, extension, and type of the lesion. The goals of the surgery such as biopsy, debulking, or gross-total resection have to be considered. The general guidelines recommend choosing the most direct approach, not to cross the optic nerve, and to avoid or hide skin incisions. In anterior locations, bone removal should be avoided. Today, there is a tendency towards less invasive approaches. Thus, the transcranial approaches are performed less frequently in favor of minimally invasive extracranial approaches. In most cases, the lateral orbitotomy and increasingly also the supraorbital orbitotomy are used to treat orbital pathologies. Anterior approaches without osteotomy such as superior or lower-eyelid incisions, sub-brow incision or inferior transconjunctival or subciliary incisions may be used for smaller anterior lesions. [16]

One of the more recently developed approaches, such as the transconjunctival, pterional (frontotemporal) contralateral, or pterional extradural approach, can be used as an alternative to a classic extracranial approach (lateral orbitotomy) or a more extensive transcranial approach. [7,12,17,18] Some specialists may choose to operate through the neighboring paranasal sinuses (transethmoidal or transmaxillary approach).

TOPOGRAPHIC DISTRIBUTION

Certain types of lesions occur at certain locations (Table 51-1). Thus, the most common intraconal processes affecting the optic nerve are optic nerve glioma, optic sheath meningioma, and lymphoma. Other intraconal processes include cavernoma, neurinoma, and metastases. The intraconal space is delimited by the conus, which connects the four rectus muscles to each other. The extraconal compartment takes up only a small amount of space within the orbit, surrounding the muscular conus like a tube. The most common extraconal processes are dermoid tumor (dermoid cyst) and pleomorphic adenoma of the lacrimal gland. The subperiosteal compartment is defined as the potential space between the periosteum and the bony orbit. Mucoceles are the most common processes affecting this compartment. The bony orbit and the sphenoid wing can be the site of an osteoma, a malignant tumor, or fibrous dysplasia, but the most common process affecting these structures is a sphenoid wing meningioma. Meningiomas are often found at the orbital apex, the superior orbital fissure, and the cavernous sinus. The intracranial periorbital dura mater heading toward the optic nerve may be infiltrated by an optic sheath meningioma or by other types of meningioma of variable size and extent. Pleomorphic adenomas and carcinomas arise within the lacrimal gland and duct system. Lymphomas and infections can affect the preseptal segment or the lids.

Table 51-1 Topographical Distribution

Intraconal (optic nerve)	Optic nerve glioma, optic nerve sheath meningioma
Intraconal	Cavernoma, schwannoma, metastases, lymphoma, lymphangioma
Extraconal	Dermoid cyst, pleomorphic adenoma of the lacrimal gland, pseudotumor
Subperiosteal	Mucocele
Sphenoid wing, bony orbit	Meningioma, osteoma, malignant tumor, fibrous dysplasia
Orbital apex, superior orbital fissure, cavernous sinus	Meningioma, cavernoma
Lacrimal gland, duct system	Pleomorphic adenoma, carcinoma
Muscles	Endocrine orbitopathy, rhabdomyosarcoma
Preseptal, lid	Lymphomas, infections, lipoma

Surgical Techniques

SUPRAORBITAL ORBITOTOMY

The more lateralized supraorbital approach has been used by neurosurgeons for vascular lesions of the anterior segment of the Circle of Willis and some tumorous lesions from the intradural side during the last two decades (Fig. 51-1).[19]

Eyebrow incision may also be used for a transperiostal approach to the superior orbit (Table 51-2) (Fig. 51-1A).[20,21] Lesions are approached by simple skin incisions of 4 cm along the orbital rim (Fig. 51-1A). After detachment of the periosteum, the supraorbital nerve is dissected and the periorbita is exposed. An osteotomy of the middle part of the supraorbital rim is performed using a reciprocating saw. Miniplates are fitted on both sides of the orbital rim (Fig. 51-1C to G). A small 2 × 3 cm frontobasal osteoclastic trepanation is carried out respecting the lateral border of the frontal sinus (Fig. 51-1C to E). In case of accidental opening of the frontal sinus, the mucous tissue is removed and the tear is closed with subcutaneous fat and fibrin glue. The basal dura of the frontal lobe is pushed away and the orbital roof is removed (Fig. 51-1F). The periorbita is opened and the levator palpebrae and superior rectus muscles are identified (Fig. 51-1E). In deeper intraconal lesions, three self-retaining retractors are positioned in the orbital fat; the tumor is exposed and removed. In extraconal tumors no spatula are necessary. There is no limitation of size of the tumor. The angle of approach allows tumor removal far behind the globe with minimal manipulation of brain and orbit. The surgical corridor is quite broad (3 to 3.5 cm). Finally, the periorbita is closed with sutures in intraconal lesions. In extraconal lesions the periorbita is partially resected and replaced by a dural patch, fixed with fibrin glue. The orbital rim is replaced and fixed by miniosteosynthesis (Fig. 51-1G). The frontobasal trepanation is filled with polymethyl-methacrylate. The orbital roof is not reconstructed. The muscular and subcutaneous layers are closed with interrupted sutures. A small suction drain is placed for 1 day and the skin is closed with a reabsorbable 6-0 suture. Two weeks postoperatively, the cosmetic result is good.

The supraorbital approach can be used in all kinds of intra- and extraconal pathologies that are located cranially

to the optic nerve (Fig. 51-1B). It combines the extracranial approach in the eyebrow with the advantages of a frontobasal craniotomy. Thus, it is a mixed approach between the purely extracranial and transcranial approaches. The main advantages are only minimal orbital and brain retraction and it also is not limited by the size of the lesion. The only drawback consists in temporary hypaesthesia in the territory of the supraorbital nerve.

The eyelid crease approach (Fig. 51-1A) is useful for biopsies of lacrimal gland lesions, such as lymphoma, sarcoidosis, or pseudotumor.[22] Superior extraconal lesions can be reached via a supraorbital or sub-brow incision. Larger extra- and intra-conal lesions require a superior supraorbital approach with an osteotomy as described above.

LATERAL ORBITOTOMY

Lateral orbitotomy provides excellent exposure of the temporal compartment of the orbit and it is indicated for well defined periorbital and intraconal tumors which are located lateral, dorsal and basal to the optic nerve (Table 51-2) (Fig. 51-2B).[20] It is useful for lacrimal gland tumors, retrobulbar lesions, such as cavernomas, and can be extended for posterior lesions.

In the past, the skin incision started superiorly and laterally in the eyebrow and was extended posteriorly along the zygomatic bone (Fig. 51-2A). Nowadays, the incision is usually smaller and runs along the lid crease towards the corner of the eye to the lateral canthus or even lateral to it (Fig. 51-2A). Then the temporalis fascia is incised, beginning at the midportion of the frontozygomatic bone and extending posteriorly the length of the skin incision. A reciprocating saw is used to incise the lateral rim of the orbit above the zygomaticofrontal suture line and inferiorly at the superior margin of the zygomatic arch (Fig. 51-2C and E). During the osteotomy the globe is protected with a retractor. The anterior edge of the greater wing of the sphenoid bone may be further reduced with rongeurs (Fig. 51-2D and F). The lateral orbit can be approached between the superior and lateral rectus muscles. Finally, a patch of artificial dura is placed to avoid a prolapse of the temporalis muscle into the orbit. Then the frontozygomatic bone is closed using plate and screw fixation. Alternatively, the bone may be held in position by nonabsorbable 4-0 nylon sutures. The periorbita and the slip of the temporalis muscle and periosteum are attached to the lateral orbital margin with 4-0 vicryl sutures.

There are numerous modifications of this lateral approach. The lateral canthothomy (Fig. 51-2A) presents the approach with the smallest incision, sufficient for lateral decompression in endocrine orbitopathy. An osteotomy is not required in all cases. Several anterior approaches through an eyelid crease incision, supraorbital or sub-brow incision are available to approach the anterior third of the orbit.[22]

TRANSCONJUNCTIVAL APPROACHES

The inferior transconjunctival approach[17,23] is restricted to basal and medial intra- and extraconal tumors (Fig. 51-3A and B) (Table 51-2). Following antiseptic preparation, the eyelids held apart, the conjunctiva is incised inferiorly along the corneal edge and the flap created thereby is opened in a caudal direction (Fig. 51-3A and C). The inferior rectus muscle is hooked with a suture and retracted laterally, and the inferior oblique muscle is hooked and retracted caudally.

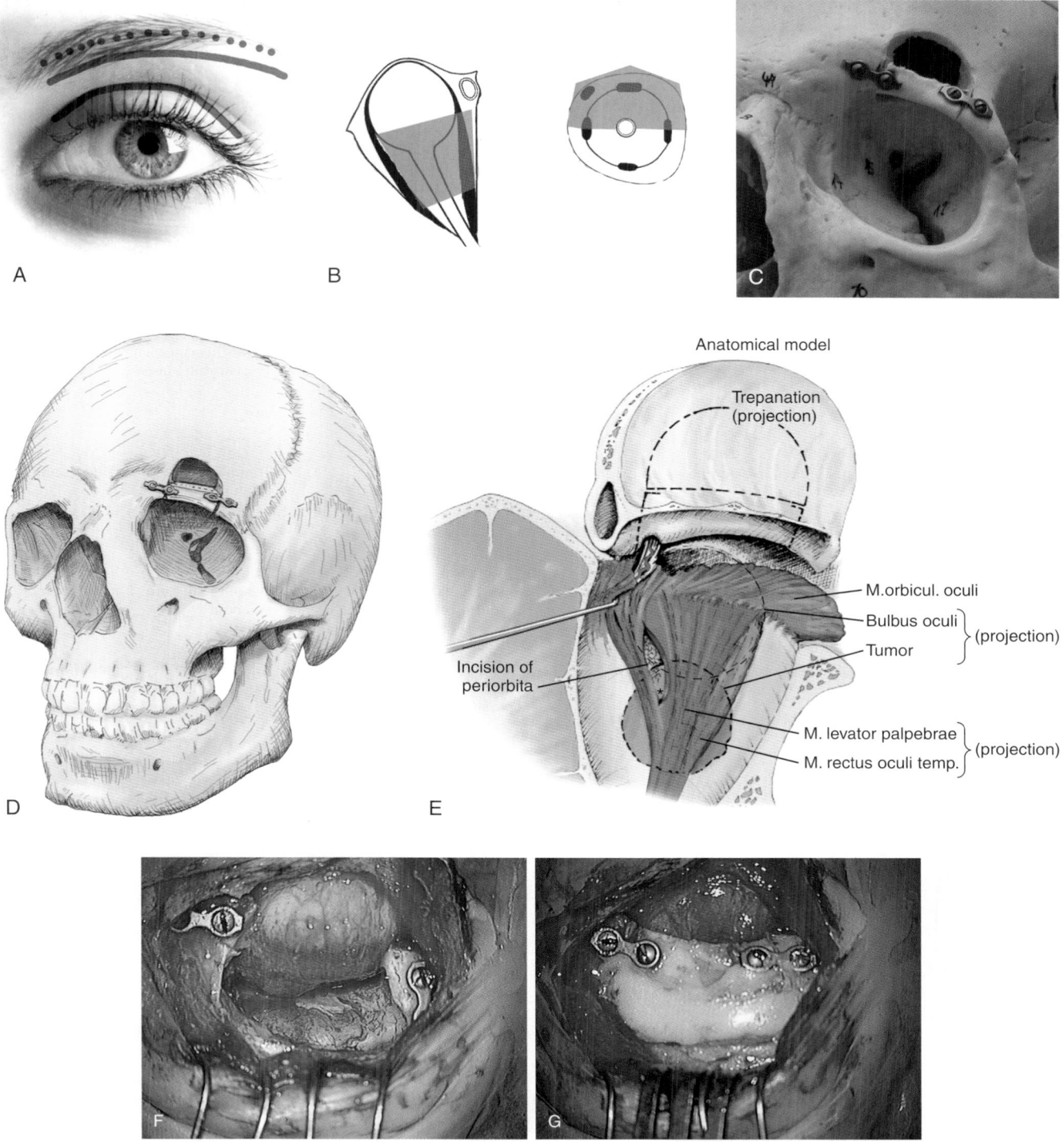

FIGURE 51-1 A, Scin incisions for eyebrow, sub-brow, and trans-septal upper eyelid crease approaches. B, Schematic drawing demonstrating the surgical area accessible by the supraorbital orbitotomy. C and D, Skull and drawing showing the frontobasal trepanation, removed orbital roof, and orbital rim with screw fixation. E, View from above on the partially incised periorbita, overlying the levator palpebrae and rectus superior muscles. The orbital roof is removed. (Courtesy of Dr. W. Seeger, Linden-Forst, Germany.) F, Removal of the orbital rim and view on the frontobasal dura and periorbita. G, Refixation of the orbital rim with plates and screw and reconstruction of the frontobasal bony defect with methyl-methacrylat.

After a superficial preparation and dissection of the layers of connective tissue and orbital fat, the lesion surface can be seen and approached. Due to the small access the tumor is removed piecemeal. After hemostasis, the inferior rectus muscle is released and the conjunctiva is closed with 8 to 10/0 suture (Fig. 51-3D). Limits of the transconjunctival approach are inability to deal with deep intraconal lesions and lesions of the apex (Fig. 51-3B). The advantage is that even masses larger than the eyeball can be removed transconjunctivally without bone destruction and without scars.

Table 51-2   Approaches to the Orbit

Approach	Indications	Advantages	Disadvantages
Extracranial Approaches to Orbit			
Lateral orbitotomy	Intra- and extra-conal tumors, lateral and basal to optic nerve; orbital apex, lacrimal gland tumors	Good exposure, well-tolerated procedure	Visible but minimal scar
Transethmoidal	Extraconal tumors medial to optic nerve, traumatic injury of optic canal	Well tolerated, usually used by ENT surgeons, no brain retraction	Limited exposure, approach through unsterile sinuses, more bleeding
Frontal trans-sinusoidal	Tumors or trauma of frontal sinus, retention cysts, extraconal processes	Minimally invasive, particularly for retention cysts	Visible scar, risk of infection, limited indications
Transmaxillary	Basal lesions, intra- or (preferably) extraconal, close by the maxillary sinus	Well tolerated, performed in collaboration with ENT surgeons	Limited exposure, hemorrhage, approach through unsterile sinuses
Transconjunctival	Basal, medial intra- and extraconal tumors, biopsy of intra-conal processes	Minimally invasive, ideal for cavernomas, excellent cosmetic result	Only for highly experienced surgeons (collaboration with ophthalmologists is recommended)
Combined Extra- and Intra-Cranial Approach			
Supraorbital via eyebrow incision	Well-circumscribed intra- and extra-conal processes above optic nerve	Minimally invasive extradural approach with minimal manipulation of orbital structures and brain, no limitation by size, excellent cosmetic result	Hypesthesia for 8 months (supraorbital nerve)
Transcranial Approaches to Orbit			
Subfrontal	Intraorbital optic nerve glioma, growing into cranial cavity, lateral tumors of optic nerve	Good general exposure	Traumatizing approach, requiring brain retraction
Fronto-lateral, pterional	Ideal approach for tumors of superior orbital fissure, optic canal, orbital apex, and intraorbital optic nerve; tumors located dorsal to optic nerve; and lateral extra- and intraconal tumors	Broad exposure, minimal brain retraction, good access to extra- and intradural and intraorbital compartments	No disadvantages
Pterional-extradural	Ideal for decompression of optic nerve in optic canal, suitable for periorbital tumors and for tumors near superior and inferior orbital fissures and cavernous sinus	Well tolerated, no brain retraction, clear exposure	Detailed anatomic knowledge is essential
Pterional-contralateral	Tumors of medial orbital apex, aneurysms of ophthalmic artery	Direct approach to medial processes medial and below optic nerve	Difficult without navigation, injury to olfactorian nerves is possible, may involve extensive brain retraction

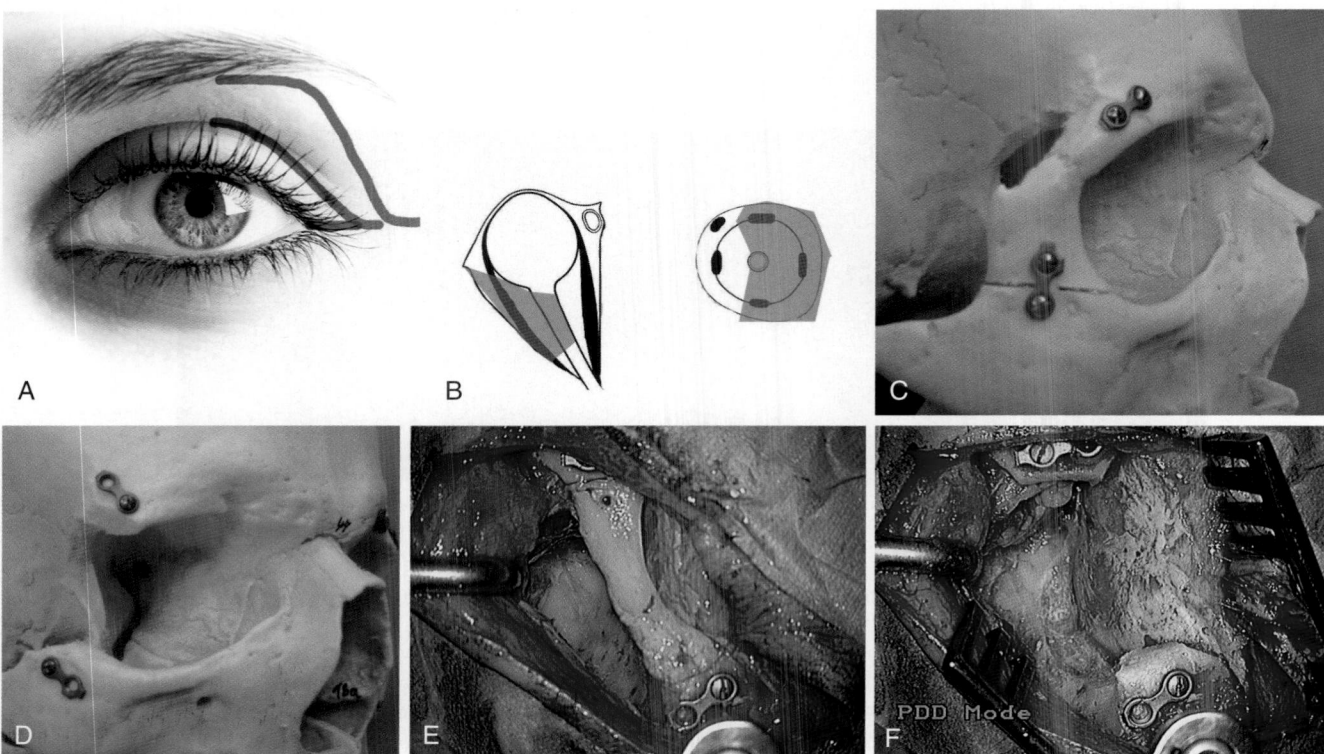

FIGURE 51-2 A, Scin incisions for eyebrow, lid crease, and lateral canthal approach. B, Schematic drawing demonstrating the surgical area accessible by the lateral orbitotomy. C and D, Skull showing the lateral orbitotomy with screw fixation, removed lateral rim and wall. E, Intraoperative view from above on the exposed lateral rim with screws. F, Intraoperative view from above on the periorbita with removed lateral orbital wall.

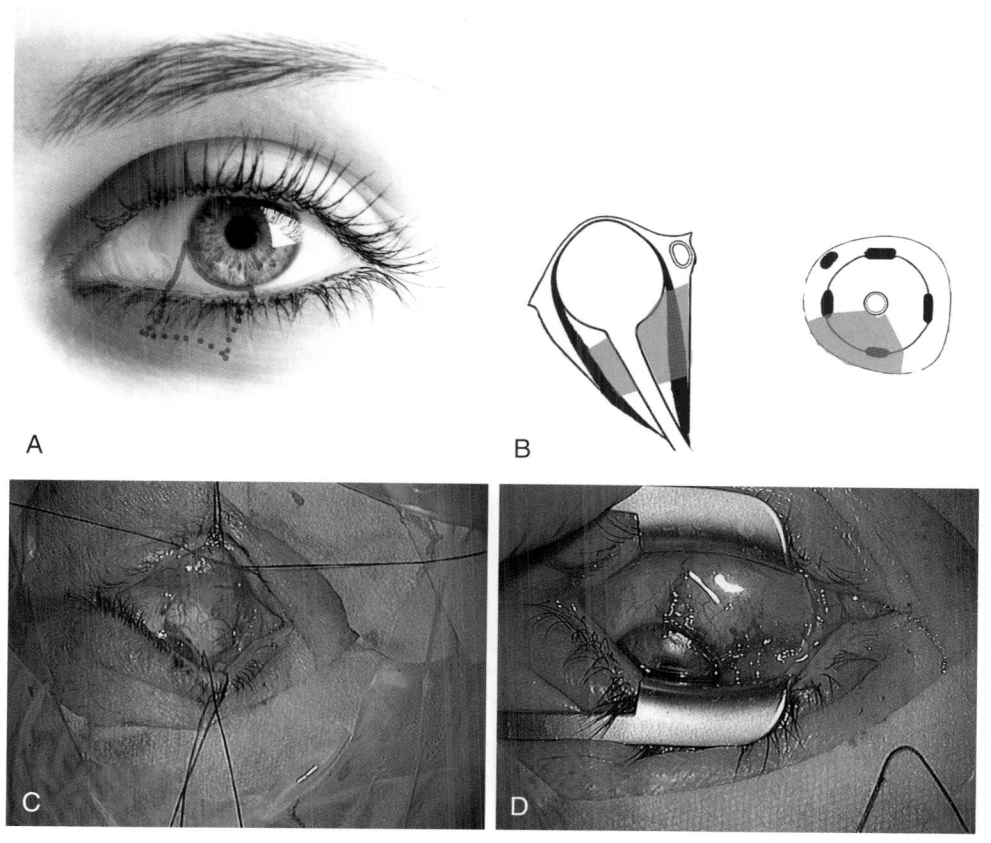

A

B

C

D

FIGURE 51-3 A, Lower transconjunctival incision line. B, Schematic drawing demonstrating the surgical area accessible by the transconjunctival approach. C, Intraoperative view creating a conjunctival flap. D, Intraoperative view with repositioning of the conjunctival flap with 8/0 suture.

A lower transconjunctival preseptal approach to the orbital floor is used to repair orbital blowout fractures, and in the maxilla in cases of congenital malformation. However, this lower approach carries the risk of ectropion, entropion, and tearing of the lid margin. In combination with a lateral cantothomy, this dissection may cause facial scarring, partially erasing the aesthetic advantage of the conjunctival approach. Therefore, the incision should be positioned between the lower border of the tarsus and the lowest point in the fornix, to avoid ectropion as well as injury of the inferior oblique muscle.

Subciliary and transcutaneous lower lid incisions are alternatives to access the inferior orbital rim and floor (Fig. 51-4). The medial transconjunctival approach with release of the insertion of the medial rectus muscle and readaption at its ends is used by our ophthalmologists to access the medial anterior orbit for biopsy or fenestration of the optic nerve sheath in pseudotumor cerebri. The transcaruncular approach is an alternative to reach the extraconal medial orbital wall and may be combined with the transconjunctival approach for repair of large medial orbital wall fractures.[24]

TRANSANTRAL APPROACH

The transantral approach[18] is performed by ENT surgeons to deal with basal intra- and extra-conal lesions in direct contact to the sinus (Table 51-2). The canine fossa is infiltrated for hemostasis and incised. The mucosa of the mouth is elevated from the anterior wall of the maxillary sinus. An osteotomy is made into the anterior wall with an osteotome and mallet. Using a Kerrison punch, the anterior wall is

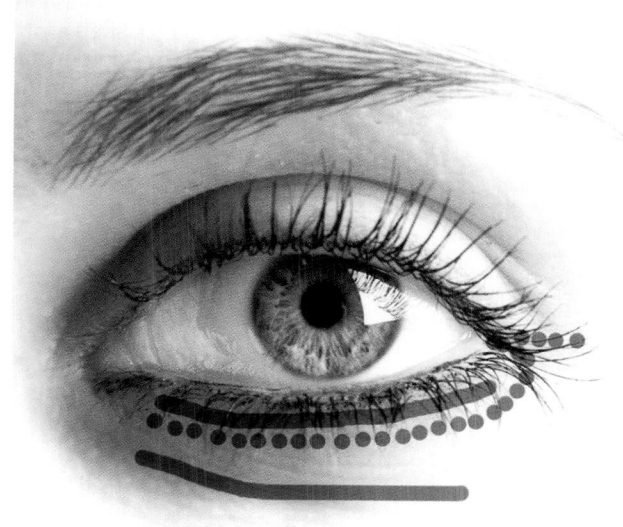

FIGURE 51-4 Subciliary, transconjunctival preseptal and transcutaneous lower eyelid incision lines.

removed. Any manipulation of the infraorbital neurovascular bundle should be avoided. The bone can be removed up to the orbital rim to provide visualization. The medial orbital floor is removed under preservation of the infraorbital nerve. Then the medial wall and the inferior aspect of the orbital apex are removed. A longitudinal incision of the periorbita is made. Today, endoscopic endonasal approaches are used to approach the medial and inferomedial orbit.[25]

TRANSCRANIAL APPROACHES

Pterional Approach
The pterional approach is a standard operation well described in the literature.[26] This approach provides an excellent view of the superior and lateral aspects of the posterior orbit and the optic canal as well as the superior orbital fissure and the anterior temporal fossa (Fig. 51-5A) (Table 51-2). The upper part of the medial orbit can also be exposed. If necessary, the ipsilateral orbital canal can be opened (Fig. 51-5B).

Extradural Pterional Approach
The extradural pterional approach[12,27] is an excellent approach to tumors near the superior and inferior orbital fissure and the cavernous sinus (Fig. 51-5B).

Example: Endocrine Orbitopathy, Neurosurgical Approach
The head is turned to the opposite side about 45 degrees and overstretched about 20 degrees and fixed with a Mayfield clamp. This position causes the frontal lobe to drop back from the orbital roof. The skin is incised in a curvilinear fashion from the top of the head along the hairline down to a point in front of the tragus. The skin-muscle flap is retracted downward. All steps of the operation are extradural. The pterional craniotomy is performed via three burr holes (frontal above the frontozygomatic suture, parietal at the temporal line, and temporal). The craniotomy is extended to the middle of the orbital rim and the dura is pushed away frontobasal and temporal while the orbital rim is left intact. Then the lesser wing of the sphenoid bone is drilled down

to the superior orbital fissure. The superior orbital fissure is first decompressed laterally and the bone of the lateral orbital wall (greater wing of the sphenoid bone) is drilled away down to the foramen rotundum and the beginning of the inferior orbital fissure is exposed. Finally, the orbital roof is removed up to the orbital rim, which is left intact. In endocrine orbitopathy, the periorbita is incised vertically parallel to the muscles (three to four incisions). Lyophilized dura with tissue glue is inserted around the decompressed periorbita to prevent ingrowths of the temporalis muscle into the orbit. The bone flap is repositioned and the basal defects of the sphenoid wing and the lateral expanded orbital wall are reconstructed with polymethyl-methacrylate. The temporalis muscle is reattached to the temporal line with good aesthetic results.

This approach provides good access to the superior and lateral walls, facilitates adequate proptosis reduction without induction of double vision, relieves the pressure at the orbital apex, allows decompression of the superior orbital fissure and optic canal, and leaves only scars behind the hair line. This approach is an alternative to other two- or three-wall decompressions and should be taken into consideration in patients with severe ophthalmopathy at greatest risk for permanent visual disability if left untreated.[27]

Example: Spheno-Orbital Meningioma
The hyperostotic bone is drilled away until the normal shape of the bone (compared with the contralateral side) is remodeled.[28] The craniotomy is usually extended to the middle of the orbital rim and the dura mater is dissected from the sphenoid bone. The first steps of the operation are entirely extradural and involve drilling the lesser wing of the sphenoid bone down to the superior orbital fissure (Fig. 51-5C and D) and the bone of the lateral orbital wall down to the

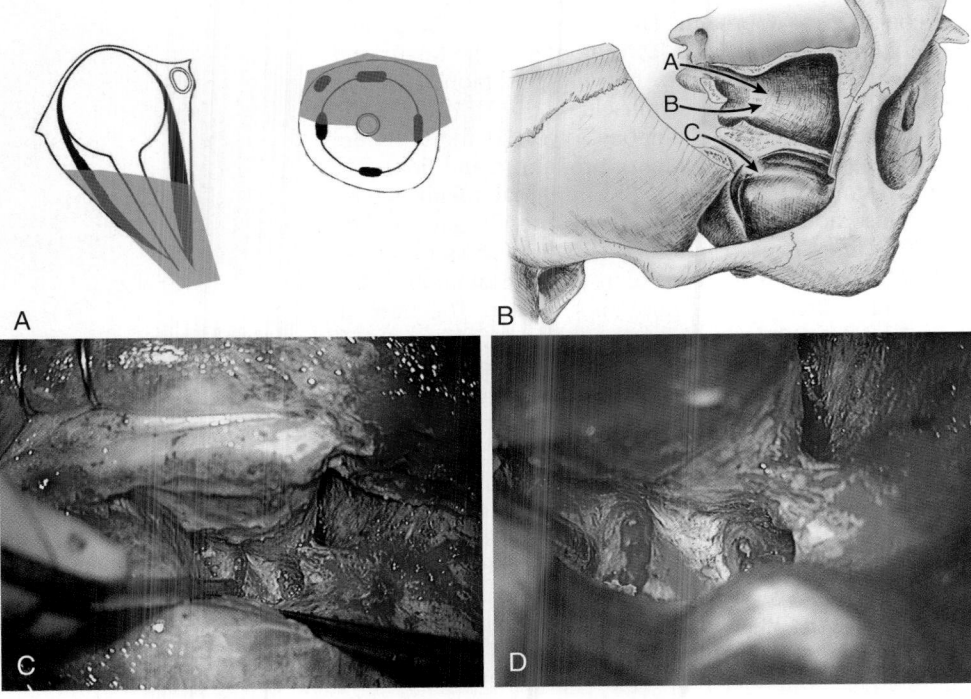

FIGURE 51-5 A, Schematic drawing demonstrating the surgical area accessible by the pterional extradural craniotomy. B, View of the right lateral orbit following removal of bone by an extradural pterional approach. The optic canal (upper arrow), superior orbital fissure (center arrow), and foramen rotundum (lower arrow) are indicated. (Courtesy of Dr. W. Seeger, Linden-Forst, Germany.) C and D, Intraoperative overview and close-up of the orbital apex, unroofed optic canal, and exposed superior orbital fissure.

foramen rotundum until the beginning of the inferior orbital fissure is exposed. Then a partial anterior clinoidectomy is performed, and the optic canal is unroofed extradurally (Fig. 51-5C and D) whenever tumor involvement is present. The extent of orbital access is tailored for each individual patient. The periorbita is only opened if there is tumor infiltration of intraorbital structures. The lateral periorbital tumor is dissected from the beginning of the superior orbital fissure to the annulus of Zinn and intraorbitally to the superior rectus and levator muscles or the lateral rectus muscle. In cases of infiltration of the ocular muscles, only the exophytic tumor is removed and muscles are not resected. Usually, the tumor is located only in the lateral and/or superior region. Following resection of the anterior temporal bone, the intracranial tumor is removed. Opening of the dura over the cavernous sinus is not recommended in patients without cranial neuropathy. The basal dura is excised as far as possible up to the superior orbital fissure and the optic canal.

Lyophilized dura with tissue glue is inserted around the resected dura and the periorbita to prevent ingrowth of the temporal muscle into the orbit. The bone flap is denatured in boiling water for 10 minutes and is repositioned. Before 1999, an autoclave was available in the operating room and this was used to clean the bone flap. Only the basal defects of the sphenoid wing and the lateral orbital wall are reconstructed using methylmethacrylate. Further reconstruction of the orbital roof is not required.

Intradural Pterional Approach
Example: Optic Nerve Sheath Meningioma

For intradural procedures, the sylvian fissure is routinely opened (Fig. 51-6A and B).[29] The basal cisterns are incised to drain cerebrospinal fluid (CSF). The ipsilateral optic nerve and carotid artery are identified and the intracranial tumor is first coagulated and resected along the dura around the optic canal. Preservation of the small feeding vessels between the carotid artery and the optic nerve is important and can be reached by sucking the tumor within the arachnoidal plane. At this step mainly irrigation instead of coagulation should be used. The ipsilateral optic canal should always be opened (Fig. 51-6C). We favor early lateral opening of the dural part of the optic canal to avoid narrowing of the optic nerve through this band. The dura is resected around the optic canal and the bony optic canal is decompressed. The drilling should begin laterally until the floor of the optic canal is reached to prevent any contact to the nerve. Finally, the optic canal is unroofed. In case of lacerating the medially located sphenoid sinus or ethmoidal cells, subcutaneous tissue with fibrin glue is inserted. The tumor around the optic nerve and the dura is carefully removed (Fig. 51-6C). In tumors infiltrating the nerve, resection is limited to the exophytic part. In blind patients with disfiguring painful proptosis, a prechiasmatic trans-section of the optic nerve is performed intradurally and the intraorbital part is removed as well. The intraorbital optic nerve is trans-sected just behind the globe and deep in the apex.

During the last years we changed our technique of decompression and performed an extradural pterional decompression of the optic canal in the last 20 patients. This extradural drilling is much easier, more extensive, and safer for the optic nerve avoiding any damage. The second step remains intradurally with tumor removal.

Contralateral Pterional Approach

The contralateral pterional approach is required for lesions of the posterior medial portion of the orbit, located inferior and medial to the optic nerve (Fig. 51-7A).[7,20] A standard pterional approach is performed. The proximal sylvian fissure is opened. The sphenoid plane is reached intradurally

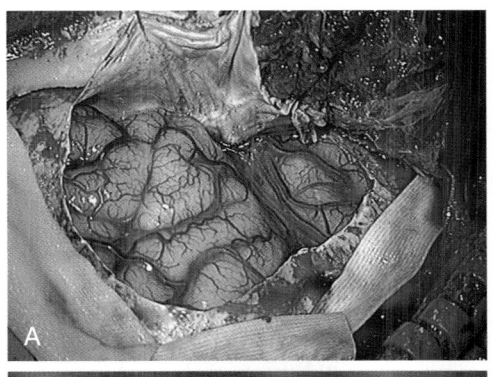

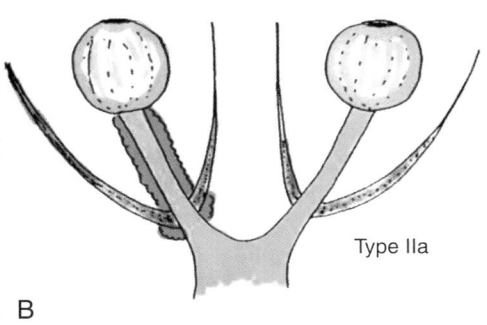

Type IIa

FIGURE 51-6 A, Intraoperative view of a frontalized pterional approach (two thirds frontal, one third temporal) with exposed sylvian fissure, downflected dura and temporalis muscle. B, Type IIa of an optic nerve sheath meningioma with extension via the optic canal into the cranial cavity. (From Schick U, Dott U, Hassler W. Surgical management of meningiomas involving the optic nerve sheath. J Neurosurg 2004;101:951-959.) C, Exposed optic nerve following tumor removal and intradural decompression of the optic canal.

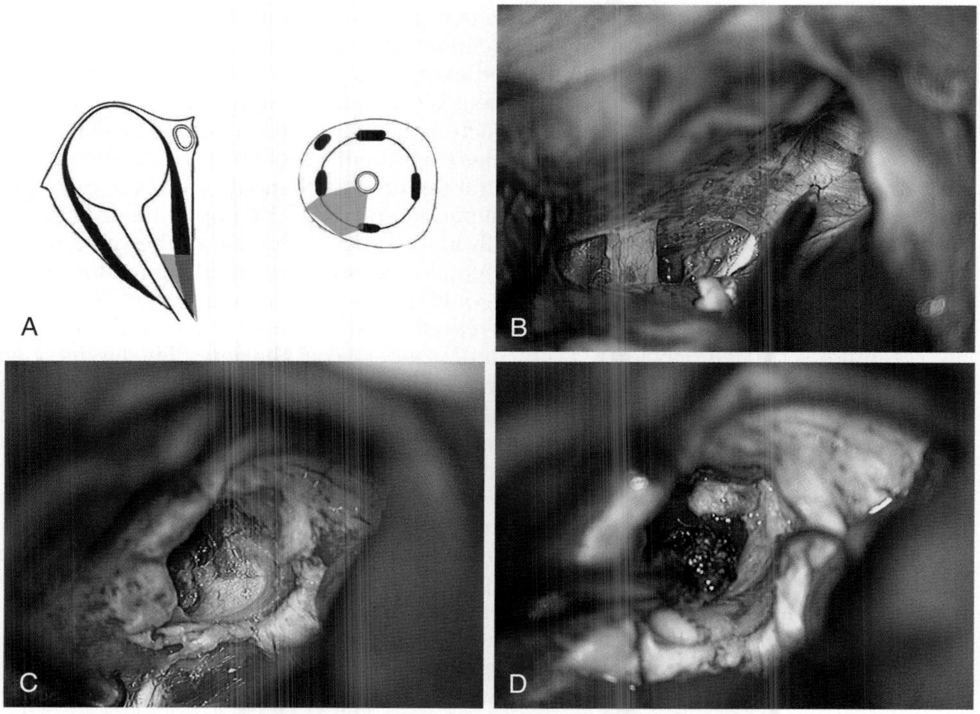

FIGURE 51-7 A, Schematic drawing demonstrating the surgical area accessible by the contralateral pterional craniotomy. B, Intraoperative view of the intradural contralateral pterional approach with exposed right optic nerve, carotid artery, partially visible left optic nerve, and tip of the neuronavigational pointer at the planned entrance point at the planum sphenoidale on the left. C, Intraoperative view of the dural flap, ethmoidal cells on the left, and intraorbital medial rectus muscle and optic nerve on the right below the dural plane. D, Removal of the cavernoma between the medial rectus muscle and the optic nerve.

subfrontally, and both optic nerves and the optic chiasm are visualized. Neuronavigation should be used to define the entrance point at the sphenoid plane and a rectangular patch of dura is removed over this area (Fig. 51-7B). Using a diamond drill, the sphenoid sinus and posterior ethmoidal cells are unroofed and its mucous membrane is exposed (Fig. 51-7C). Care must be taken not to injure the membrane, but rather to dissect it from the bone and to push it anteriorly into the ethmoidal sinus. The posterior medial wall of the contralateral orbit is then exposed with a diamond drill. The periorbita is incised. Between the superior oblique and medial rectus muscles, the lesion can be identified, and dissected carefully from the optic nerve (Fig. 51-7D). Therefore, the axis of the optic nerve should be visualized in extension from the contralateral intradural entrance point to the intraorbital course. After resection, abdominal fat is packed into the sinuses with fibrin glue. The sphenoid sinus is then sealed with a patch of lyophilized dura.

The potential problems of this approach consist of injury to the frontal lobe by extensive retraction, damage of the olfactorian nerves, and cerebrospinal fluid leak after rupture of the mucous membranes of the sinuses.

Orbitozygomatic Approach

The combined pterional and orbitozygomatic approach may be useful in selected cases to access extensive tumors of the lateral and laterobasal orbit and orbital apex and tumors extending from the orbit to the superior orbital fissure and temporal fossa.[30]

The variation from the standard pterional technique is the skin incision extending to the mandible. The lesser wing of the sphenoid bone is drilled down to the superior orbital fissure. The anterior clinoid process and roof of the optic canal are removed if necessary. The zygomatic arch,

zygomatic process of the frontal bone and zygomatic bone above the zygomatico-orbital foramen are trans-sected with the oscillating saw. The temporalis muscle is reflected downward. Direct access to the lateral basal orbit, the superior and inferior orbital fissure, the optic canal, and the anterior temporal fossa with foramina rotundum and ovale is possible. Finally, the zygomatic bone flap is repositioned and fixed with microplates. The temporalis muscle is reattached to the temporal line for restoration of mastication.

There is an ongoing discussion about one-piece versus two-piece orbitozygomatic craniotomy.[31] The two-piece orbitozygomatic craniotomy allows for more extensive orbital roof removal and better visualization of the basal frontal lobe.

Surgical Adjuvants

Neuronavigation became a standard procedure in neurosurgery. Accuracy improved due to improved software and registration processes, as well as framework became less complicated. Neuronavigation and more recent modalities at our center in Heidelberg such as intraoperative CT and MR imaging have helped us in the surgical management of difficult orbital apical tumors and are recommended in the contralateral pterional approach to localize small lesions in the apex in an operative distance about 11 to 13 cm from the entrance at the skull to the lesion. Neuronavigation in other intraconal lesions sometimes offers little advantage due to the dissection and dislocation of the orbital fat. However, neuronavigation is useful in defining the dural opening in small lesions within the superior orbital fissure approached via an ipsilateral extradural pterional way. Instruments such as drills and suction may be used as localizing wands with neuronavigation. More than one image localizer can be used at a time. Neuronavigation is often used in endoscopic cases. Endoscopic techniques have evolved dramatically and are effective in approaching the ethmoidal or maxillary sinuses. In the past, endoscopic use in orbital surgery was limited to optic canal decompression and thyroid decompression. This minimally invasive endoscopic surgery has progressed to a "maximally invasive endoscopic" surgery of the skull base in some centers.

Discussion

OPERATIVE APPROACHES

The choice of approach depends on the location, size, demarcation, and histologic type of the lesion. The least traumatic approach should be chosen. The procedures that can be performed range from open biopsies for confirmation of a diagnosis to the subtotal resection of diffusely infiltrating processes with preservation of function and the complete excision of well-circumscribed lesions. Very extensive surgery, with wide excision of bone followed by complicated reconstructive techniques, is rarely necessary. In general, open operations in the orbit are performed by one of two types of approach: transcranial or direct extracranial (Table 51-2).[1,18,32-37]

A transcranial approach is preferable for processes extending behind the orbit into the cranial cavity or located in the optic canal or the superior orbital fissure.[20,28] A classic pterional approach is a standard technique and is also used by the authors for orbital apex tumors.[38] An exclusively extradural pterional approach can be used to decompress the optic nerve in the optic canal and superior orbital fissure, as well as for tumor biopsy or resection.[12] Usually, a subfrontal approach with significant brain retraction is not necessary for intraorbital tumors. However, there is an indication for this approach in large periorbital tumors with secondary orbital involvement.

Processes located exclusively within the orbit can be reached by a wide variety of relatively noninvasive extracranial approaches, including lateral orbitotomy,[2,39] the transethmoidal[40-42] and transconjunctival approaches,[7,17,23,43] and the frontal-sinusoidal approach.[1,44]

LATERAL ORBITOTOMY

The basic approach to tumors lateral to the optic nerve is the lateral orbitotomy. This approach is useful for well-circumscribed periorbital and intraconal tumors and for tumors located dorsally, basally, and laterally to the optic nerve, as well as for tumors of the lacrimal gland. Tumors of the orbital apex or located medial to the optic nerve should not be operated on via this approach. Shields and Shields[36] describe a less extensive superolateral orbitotomy as an alternative to this lateral orbitotomy to remove tumors located laterally in the orbit. Carta et al.[39] advocated a posterolateral orbitotomy for the orbital apex. This approach, through a small opening on the orbital and temporal portions of the greater wing of the sphenoid, allowed adequate exposure of the orbital apex. Goldberg et al.[45] presented a deep transorbital approach to the apex and cavernous sinus. By enlarging the bony incision of a classic lateral orbitotomy to include a generous marginotomy and removing the deep sphenoid wing up to the superior orbital fissure, they obtained good exposure of the lateral orbital apex. We recommend a standard pterional approach to orbital apex tumors.

TRANSCONJUNCTIVAL APPROACH

The authors favor a transconjunctival approach for basal, medial intra- and extra-conal tumors, and particularly for biopsies of intraconal processes. Even masses larger than the eyeball can be removed transconjunctivally without bone destruction and an excellent cosmetic result.[23] Gdal-On and Gelfand[43] also favor a transconjunctival extraction for intraconal cavernoma. About 10% of the patients had to undergo secondary lateral orbitotomy, because the tumor could not be identified via the transconjunctival approach. For small lesions, image guidance is required.[23] The transcaruncular approach is available for medial orbital fracture repair.[24]

TRANSANTRAL APPROACH

Basal lesions in direct contact to the sinus may be approached transantrally. Kennerdell et al.[44] used a posterior inferior orbitotomy through the maxillary sinus to treat patients with orbital apex tumors between the optic nerve and inferior rectus. Mir-Salim and Berghaus[42] performed an endonasal microsurgical transethmoidal access to remove an intraconal hemangioma. However, this is a long operative distance with limited view. Herman et al.[40] reported on a transnasal endoscopic approach in a case of inferomedial and posterior intraconal cavernoma. Endoscopic endonasal techniques became more frequent to approach the medial and inferomedial orbit.[25,46]

SUPRAORBITAL APPROACH

Our new supraorbital approach[21] occupies an intermediate position between the extra- and trans-cranial approaches. Well-circumscribed processes superior to the optic nerve can be reached either intra- or extra-conally through an eyebrow incision. The supraorbital approach is particularly useful for the removal of cavernomas and schwannomas.[20] The earliest technical note of a supraorbital approach via a bicoronal flap, Jane et al. described a burr hole behind the zygomatic process with detached temporal muscle in 1982.[47] Maus and Goldman[48] used a transorbital craniotomy through a suprabrow approach to remove a cavernoma of the orbital apex. Our supraorbital approach is comparable to this approach but less invasive considering the extent of bone removal. The major advantage is that only a small transient resection of the upper supraorbital rim is necessary to create a focused surgical corridor. Brain and orbital manipulations are minimized. The size of the lesion is not a limiting factor. This extradural approach is also well tolerated in elderly patients. The hypaesthesic area in the territory of the supraorbital nerve usually recovers within 7 months. The cosmetic result compared to the lateral orbitotomy is much better, hiding the scar completely within the eyebrow. This new approach presents quite a useful addition to the variety of currently utilized operative techniques.

PTERIONAL APPROACHES

The ipsilateral pterional approach is our standard neurosurgical approach to tumors of the superior orbital fissure, optic canal, and orbital apex. Tumors located dorsal to the optic nerve, lateral, extra- and intra-conal tumors can be easily reached. Only tumors medial and basal to the optic nerve should not be operated on via this approach. These lesions in the posterior intraconal space can also be approached by a pterional contralateral way.[7] This route leads from the contralateral side through the sphenoid and ethmoidal sinus without opening the mucous membrane. This approach provides excellent exposure and straight access to the lesion. A transethmoidal operation has more limited space and an unfavorable angle for dissection.

Tumors of the superior orbital fissure such as cavernomas or neurofibromas are best approached extradurally. Detailed anatomic knowledge is essential to perform a lateral-to-medial dissection and incise the periorbital between the lateral and superior rectus muscle.[12,16]

The authors' classification scheme[38] distinguishes intraorbital (type 1) from intracanalicular (type 2) optic sheath meningiomas and from those that are both intraorbital and intracanalicular (type 3). When an intraorbital tumor (type 1) begins to affect visual acuity, it should be treated with radiation at first,[49-51] and any large exophytic tumor mass should be resected. For type 2 tumors, surgical decompression of the optic canal can stave off the impending loss of vision. Type 3 tumors growing toward the intracranial compartment are best treated with extradural decompression of the optic canal, intracranial tumor resection, and postoperative irradiation of the intraorbital portion.[38]

Conclusions

The optimal surgical approach to the orbit is determined by the lesion's type and location. Surgical planning and the chosen approach should allow tumor removal without significant morbidity. Transcranial approaches are chosen for lesions with retro-orbital, intracranial extension and for lesions involving the optic canal or superior orbital fissure. Purely intraorbital lesions can be reached via numerous less invasive extracranial approaches. Of these, the lateral orbitotomy is still the most practiced, followed by transconjunctival approaches and the supraorbital approach.

KEY REFERENCES

Al-Mefty O, Fox JL. Superolateral orbital exposure and reconstruction. *Surg Neurol.* 1985;23:609-613.

Bejjani GK, Cockerham KP, Kennerdell JS, Maroon JC. A reappraisal of surgery for orbital tumors. Part I: extraorbital approaches. *Neurosurg Focus.* 2001;10(5):E2.

Berke RN. Modified Krönlein operation. *AMA Arch Ophth.* 1954;51: 609-632.

Cockerham KP, Bejjani GK, Kennerdell JS, Maroon JC. Surgery for orbital tumors. Part II: transorbital approaches. *Neurosurg Focus.* 2001;10(5):E3.

Dandy W. Results following the transcranial operative attack on orbital tumors. *Arch Ophthalmol.* 1941;25:191-216.

Dolenc VV. Direct microsurgical repair of intracavernous vascular lesions. *J Neurosurg.* 1983;58:824-831.

Hassler WE, Eggert H. Extradural and intradural microsurgical approaches to lesions of the optic canal and the superior orbital fissure. *Acta Neurochir (Wien).* 1985;74:87-93.

Hassler WE, Meyer B, Rohde V, Unsöld R. Pterional approach to the contralateral orbit. *Neurosurgery.* 1994;34:552-554.

Hassler W, Schick U. The supraorbital approach—a minimally invasive approach to the superior orbit. *Acta Neurochir.* 2009;151:605-612.

Hejazi N, Hassler W, Farghaly F. Transconjunctival microsurgical approach to the orbit: a retrospective preliminary review and analysis of experience with the first 15 operative cases. *Neurosurg Q.* 1999;9:197-208.

Housepian EM. Microsurgical anatomy of the orbital apex and principles of transcranial orbital exploration. *Clin Neurosurg.* 1978;25:556-573.

Jane AJ, Sung Park T, Pobereskin LH, et al. The supraorbital approach: technical note. *Neurosurgery.* 1982;11:537-542.

Kennerdell JS, Maroon JC, Malton ML. Surgical approaches to orbital tumors. *Clin Plast Surg.* 1988;15:237-282.

Krönlein R. Zur Pathologie und operativen Behandlung der Dermoidzysten der Orbita. *Beitr Klin Chir.* 1889;4:149-163:(German).

Mauriello JA, Flanagan JC. Surgical approaches to the orbit. In: Mauriello JA, Flanagan JC, eds. *Management of orbital and ocular adnexal tumors and inflammations.* Berlin, Heidelberg, New York: Springer; 1990:149-169.

Naffziger HC. Exophthalmos. Some principles of surgical management from the neurosurgical aspect. *Am J Surg.* 1948;75:25-41.

Rhoton AL, Natori Y. Microsurgical Anatomy and Operative Approaches. *The Orbit and Sellar Region.* New York and Stuttgart: Thieme; 1996:208-308.

Rohde V, Schaller K, Hassler W. The combined pterional and orbitocygomatic approach to extensive tumours of the lateral and latero-basal orbit and orbital apex. *Acta Neurochir (Wien).* 1995;132:127-130.

Schick U, Bleyen J, Bani A, Hassler W. Management of meningiomas en plaque of the sphenoid wing. *J Neurosurg.* 2006;104:208-214.

Schick U, Dott U, Hassler W. Surgical management of meningiomas involving the optic nerve sheath. *J Neurosurg.* 2004;101:951-959.

Shields JA, Shields CL, Scartozzi R. Survey of 1264 patients with orbital tumors and simulating lesions: The 2002 Montgomery Lecture, part 1. *Ophthalmology.* 2004;111:997-1008.

Turbin RE, Pokorny K. Diagnosis and treatment of optic nerve sheath meningioma. *Cancer Control.* 2004;11:334-341.

Yasargil MG, Fox JL. The microsurgical approach to intracranial aneurysms. *Surg Neurol.* 1975;3:7-14.

Numbered references appear on Expert Consult.

CHAPTER 52

Anterior Midline Approaches to the Skull Base

IVO P. JANECKA • SILLOO B. KAPADIA

Comprehensive oncologic management of neoplasms involving the cranial base is an expanding field. Surgery has emerged as the primary modality of treatment for most tumors in this region, either as a single modality (for benign tumors) or in combination with irradiation and chemotherapy (for most malignant tumors). As with most tumors, the control of the primary site is one of the most important determinants of the ultimate outcome of treated patients, and thus a three-dimensional (3D) tumor resection with histologically clear margins is the primary goal of cranial base oncologic surgery. Extensive resections must be balanced with an acceptable functional and esthetic morbidity. Gross central nervous system involvement or internal carotid encasement in a patient with poor collateral cerebral circulation is considered a relative contraindication to oncologic surgery.

Neoplastic growth affecting the anterolateral skull base often originates from central and paracentral craniofacial anatomic structures (dura, orbit, ethmoid, sphenoid and maxillary sinus, pterygoids, infratemporal fossa, clivus, etc.). Histologically this group of tumors includes a great diversity of cell origin.

The surgical approach to such tumors should accommodate the following features: (1) tumor-specific predilectional neoplastic growth; (2) when feasible, protection of key anatomic structures such as the internal carotid artery (ICA), the optic nerves, and the content of the cavernous sinus and the superior orbital fissure; (3) the best cosmetic result; and (4) the stability of the craniovertebral junction.

The principal goal of an anterolateral approach to the skull base is to achieve an unobstructed view of the midline and paramedian skull base region. Strictly midline lesions of the anterior cranial fossa are treated with craniofacial resection using a low (basal) subfrontal approach combined with a midfacial translocation approach. For small clival (central) skull base lesions, a transoral approach may be satisfactory. For larger lesions, we have combined that with midfacial translocation. Midline lesions extending laterally can be resected through various units of the facial translocation system of approaches.

Anatomic Considerations

The intimate relationship of the skull base to the cranial as well as facial structures requires tissue displacement of one or both of these compartments to reach the desired section of the skull base. It is important to consider the effects of surgery on the normal but surgically manipulated tissues so as to select the most optimal approach. Any operative tissue displacement produces alterations in the anatomy and physiology of affected structures. Such changes have variable consequences when they occur in the neurocranium or the facial viscero-cranium. For example, facial swelling is usually self-limiting, with minimal long-term consequences for the patient. Similar edema, however, may be very deleterious when it involves the neurocranium.

The anterolateral skull base constitutes the floor of the anterior and middle cranial fossa. The proximate paranasal sinuses (ethmoid, sphenoid) with the nasal cavity and the orbits are intimate components of this skull base section.

The proximity of the face to the anterior cranial base gives this region a unique significance. The craniofacial skeleton gives protection to the organs of olfaction and vision and provides support for the configuration of the soft-tissue facial anatomy. This arrangement, however, hinders a direct surgical approach to the cranial base for tumors and requires planning of incisions and osteotomies that respect not only function but esthetics as well.

Anterolateral skull base approaches permit visualization of the surgical anatomy of the skull base that may extend from the ipsilateral temporomandibular joint and geniculate ganglion through trigeminal nerve branches of V3 and V2 as well as the ICA to the cavernous sinus, inferior and superior orbital fissures, and both anterior clinoids with corresponding optic nerves.

Diagnostic Evaluation

Several essential issues guide our evaluation of cranial base neoplasms: (1) tumor biology and its extent, (2) tumor composition, and (3) relationship of the tumor to the ICA and its importance to cerebral circulation (Fig. 52-1).

Tumor biology is best determined by preoperative histologic evaluation obtained after biopsy. New endoscopic instrumentation permits access to many skull base sites for direct visualization and tissue biopsy, or an open biopsy can be performed. The tumor extent determines the potential for surgical resection of the neoplasm. This is currently best determined by multiplanar CT as well as MRI. Both tests are also very useful in assessing the character of the lesion in terms of its vascular, bony, or soft-tissue content.

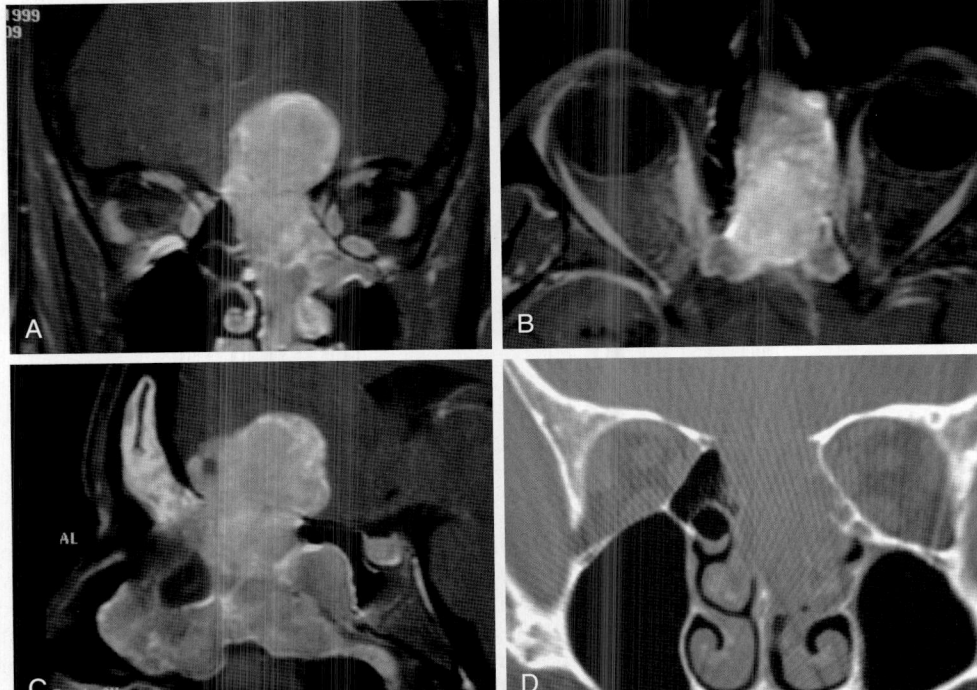

FIGURE 52-1 Diagnostic evaluation with imaging. A, Coronal MR with contrast, demonstrating an enhancing midline and paramedian transcranial mass (esthesioneuroblastoma). B, Axial MR with contrast showing involvement of interorbital space. C, Sagittal MR with contrast, outlining the tumor extent into the anterior cranial fossa and its subcranial penetration. D, Coronal CT, bone algorithm, delineating bone destruction of the anterior cranial base and subcranial nasal structures.

The location of the ICA, and its contribution to the tumor vascularity as well as the relationship of this vessel to the tumor perimeter, are assessed by MRI, MR angiography, or invasive angiography. The tolerance of the patient to temporary occlusion of the ICA can be evaluated with a series of tests known as temporary balloon occlusion test and xenon blood flow studies.[1] These tests permit us to estimate the risk of neurologic deficit with a permanent occlusion in the ICA.

For orbital or periorbital tumors, a detailed neuro-ophthalmologic evaluation is valuable. Not only must the precise level of visual acuity, extent of visual fields, and ocular mobility be ascertained, but the completeness of function or the degree of dysfunction of the superior orbital fissure structures, optic nerve, and lacrimal apparatus should be known as well.

Endocrinologic evaluation is necessary preoperatively and in the follow-up period for tumors of the sellar or parasellar region.

Selected Tumors

CARCINOMA

Carcinoma that involves the anterior cranial base originates primarily in the paranasal sinuses, the nose and nasopharynx, or occasionally as a metastatic disease. Carcinoma of the nose and sinuses makes up less than 1% of all malignancies. It carries an overall 30% 5-year survival rate. In general, the prognosis of a patient with a carcinoma is very much related to the histologic type. Anaplastic carcinoma must be differentiated from lymphoma and melanoma with leukocyte common antigen and S-100 protein. Anaplastic carcinoma appears to be a separate entity from poorly differentiated squamous cell carcinoma, which still exhibits some squamous differentiation. It is found more often in women, with occurrence on the left side predominant. Among these patients, 33% develop cervical metastases, but only 70% of these have obvious evidence of bone destruction on radiographs. The survival of patients with anaplastic carcinoma varies with the site of origin. If it occurs in the nose, the 5-year survival rate is 40%. If it originates in the sinuses, the 5-year survival rate decreases to 15% (see Thorup et al.[2]).

The signs and symptoms common to most malignancies in the sinus–nose region include nasal obstruction, discharge, epistaxis, facial pain, as well as swelling, proptosis, or cervical node metastases.

The nasal passages and the sinuses are intimately related, permitting tumor to spread easily from one cavity to the other. Therefore, ethmoid sinuses are often involved secondarily by tumor spread from the nasal cavity or the maxillary sinus. This is reflected in the fact that isolated ethmoid carcinomas compose no more than 5% to 20% of all carcinomas involving the ethmoid sinus. The initial symptoms are usually insidious and trivial, accounting for a significant delay of diagnosis from the onset of symptoms. Sixty to 75% of patients with malignant tumors of the ethmoid sinuses do not survive for 5 years. The ethmoid sinus is closely related to the orbit. Both the orbit and the ethmoid sinus are simultaneously involved in 60% of malignant sinus neoplasms, and 45% of the patients are likely to require orbital exenteration. Most sinus tumors arise from the mucous membrane lining that is in continuity with the mucosa of the remaining sinuses, nasopharynx, and lacrimal draining system. The respiratory mucosa of the ethmoid sinus gives rise to two types of neoplasm. The first is squamous cell carcinoma, arising from the metaplastic epithelium. Of all malignant neoplasms of the sinuses, 75% to 95% will be squamous cell carcinomas, and the ethmoid sinus is the second most common site for this neoplasm. The second is a glandular tumor, arising from mucous glands. The submucosal glands give rise to adenocarcinomas or adenoid cystic carcinomas. Adenocarcinoma occurs most frequently in the ethmoid sinus, and its behavior is similar to that of squamous cell carcinoma. There is some suggestion that this tumor is found more frequently among workers in woodworking industries than in the population in general.[3] The lymphatic drainage from the ethmoid sinus is into the superior cervical chain and the retropharyngeal nodes. The incidence of metastases at the time of diagnosis is low, but 25% to 35% of patients will eventually develop metastatic disease. Distant metastases may occur in up to 18% of the cases.[4]

ESTHESIONEUROBLASTOMA

This is a rare tumor originating from the olfactory epithelium and represents 3% of all intranasal neoplasms. It was originally described by Berger and Luc.[5] This tumor has been identified under different terms, including olfactory neuroblastoma, esthesioneurocytoma, and olfactory esthesioneuroblastoma. It arises from cells of neural crest origin and resembles childhood neuroblastoma. The tumor does contain neurosecretory granules and is linked to other neural crest tumors, such as carcinoid, chemodectoma, and pheochromocytoma. It occurs most frequently in the third decade of life and is more common in males. Unilateral nasal obstruction and epistaxis are the most common symptoms. The tumor may fill the nose and paranasal sinuses and involve the cribriform plate.

A staging system has been proposed by Kadish and colleagues that recognizes three stages[6]:
Stage A: Tumor involves only nasal cavity
Stage B: Tumor extends also to sinuses
Stage C: Tumor extends beyond stage B
However, correlation of tumor extent with prognosis has not been as accurate as the relationship of clear surgical margins.

Esthesioneuroblastoma is known to have a slow but insidious malignant course, and death comes from local recurrence, intracranial invasion, and/or metastatic disease. Differential diagnosis must exclude lymphoma, melanoma, and metastatic neuroblastoma. The characteristic histologic picture includes a fibrillary intercytoplasmic background that on electron microscopy is identified as representing neuronal cell processes. The 5-year survival rate is approximately 50%, with a median survival of 58 months. When the cranial base is invaded, the survival rate drops to about 40%. Long-term recurrence has also been observed 10 to 20 years after the original diagnosis. This tumor is characterized by local persistence and recurrence. There is a 20% to 40% potential that this tumor will metastasize into cervical lymph nodes, lungs, and bones. The current modality of treatment includes a radical resection of the area involved that includes the cribriform plate with or without the attached dura followed by a full course of irradiation and possibly chemotherapy as well.

NASOPHARYNGEAL CARCINOMA

Nasopharyngeal carcinoma is a rare tumor among non-Chinese patients, with an incidence of 1 in 100,000 among the North American population as compared with 2 in 100,000 among Chinese, especially those living in the Canton province of the People's Republic of China. Several

etiologic factors have been implicated in the development of nasopharyngeal carcinoma, for example, the Epstein-Barr virus and numerous external inhalation as well as dietary carcinogens. The male-to-female ratio heavily favors male patients (3:1), with an average age of onset of 45 years.

Clinically, the tumor appears to arise primarily at the superior or lateral aspect of the nasopharynx. The symptomatology often includes epistaxis, nasal and Eustachian tube obstruction, and eventual cranial nerve neuropathies (the fifth cranial nerve is most commonly involved). Histologically, these tumors are predominantly poorly differentiated carcinomas with a high propensity for metastatic regional spread, so that at the time of diagnosis, 50% of patients are expected to have regional disease. In the diagnostic evaluation, direct nasopharyngoscopy and biopsy, as well as a CT scan and MRI, provide for full assessment of the primary site. Irradiation is still considered a primary therapeutic modality for the nonkeratinizing squamous cell carcinoma of the primary site and the regional lymph node draining area.[7] The cure rate, however, varies tremendously depending on the histologic type of the tumor, stage of the disease, and subsequent therapy. The most frequent recurrence of nasopharyngeal carcinoma is in the neck.[8] Reirradiation of recurrent nasopharyngeal carcinoma gives a 5-year cure rate of only 14%, with a high chance of radiation-induced complications. It is important prognostically to separate patients with metastatic nasopharyngeal carcinoma in the neck on the basis of their response to the primary irradiation. If metastatic neck nodes disappeared completely following irradiation, the recurrence rate was only 13%. If nodes persisted throughout the course of irradiation, the recurrence rate was 91%.

With the advent of new approaches to the nasopharynx, surgery is becoming a therapeutic option for the treatment of resectable recurrent nasopharyngeal cancer with expected survival of over 50% (5 years). For tumors with very poor response to the primary radiotherapy (e.g., keratinizing squamous cell carcinoma, adenoid cystic carcinoma), surgery should be considered as the initial treatment.

FIBROUS DYSPLASIA

Fibrous dysplasia is a progressive benign fibro-osseous lesion. Its natural growth is one of gradual expansion beyond its bony margins with concomitant displacement of surrounding soft tissue. It was first described by Lichtenstein in 1938.[9] It may be placed into three categories on the basis of its clinical presentation. The monostotic form represents a localized disease to one osseous structure and is the most frequent form (up to 70%). A polyostotic form involves several bones but usually on the same side of the body. Here the frequency ranges from 30% to 50%. The third form is disseminated, in which numerous bones are involved, along with the possibility of extraskeletal developments such as skin pigmentation and precocious puberty. The incidence ranges from 3% to 30%. These individual clinical forms retain their categorization during the course of the disease and do not seem to change from, for example, the monostotic to the polyostotic form. Fibrous dysplasia is more common in females. In the head and neck region (0.5% of all head and neck tumors), it is the maxilla, frontal bone, mandible, and parietal and temporal bones that are most frequently involved. It is of interest that the progression of the disease is often limited after completion of skeletal maturation.[10]

The clinical symptomatology usually includes swelling at the tumor site with displacement of surrounding soft tissues. For example, diplopia, when present, is usually caused by mechanical displacement of the globe. If the cribriform plate is directly involved, alteration in olfaction can be perceived. Histologic verification can be considered in addition to the clinical and radiographic examination. In the differential histologic diagnosis, fibrous dysplasia may mimic meningioma, and sarcoma is also a possibility. Radiographically, a sclerotic form manifests itself with dense bone. The cystic and pagetoid forms are distinguished radiographically from each other by the greater amount of fibrous component in the former.

Fibrous dysplasia can be treated by surgical resection when functional or esthetic deformity warrants it.[11] Full preoperative evaluation should include CT scan, with and without contrast, in the axial and coronal planes with bone algorithms.

Osseous reconstruction of the surgical defect is necessary only when the tumor involves key aspects of the craniofacial skeleton. Autogenous bone graft or alloplastic materials can be used. In the orbital region, most of the fibro-osseous lesions involve the orbital roof. Prolonged ocular displacement by the tumor often produces a secondary concavity in the orbital floor. This must be taken into account, since after orbital tumor removal superiorly, the globe may not return to the expected normal level. Secondary bone grafting of the deformed orbital floor may have to be considered.

JUVENILE ANGIOFIBROMA

Juvenile angiofibroma is a relatively rare tumor occurring primarily in adolescent boys. The site of origin of the tumor is thought to be the medial pterygoid region. Clinically, the tumor has the potential to involve the nasopharynx, nose, infratemporal fossa, sphenoid, orbit, middle cranial fossa, and cavernous sinus. There is a preferential growth through preformed anatomic fissures and foramina. The symptomatology is one of nasal obstruction with episodes of nasal hemorrhage that can be profound. The diagnostic evaluation usually consists of CT scan and MRI as well as angiography. The CT scan demonstrates classical widening of the pterygopalatine fossa. MRI is assuming a greater importance in the diagnosis of this tumor, its extent, as well as the degree of its vascularity. Angiography determines the blood supply to this lesion, which originates primarily in the external carotid system, usually the internal maxillary or the ascending pharyngeal artery. There may be additional blood supply from the internal carotid system. In the differential diagnosis, angiomatous polyp, pyogenic granuloma, and hemangioma are included in the benign group. Carcinoma, rhabdomyosarcoma, and chordoma should be considered among the malignant tumors.[12]

The primary treatment has been surgical through a trans-facial or transpalatal approach, or, for extensive cases, craniofacial resection. Because of its vascularity and potential for a recurrence, a complete removal of this tumor should be attempted. The need for preoperative embolization can be determined at the time of the diagnostic angiography as well as from the appearance of tumor vascularity

on the MRI scan. However, the potential complications from embolization must be considered and its advantage weighed against the potential risks. Recurrent tumors are usually treated again with surgery (if accessible) or irradiation. Hormonal therapy, originally thought to be beneficial, has not proved to be of significant value. Histologically, this tumor is composed of fibrous stroma and multiple vascular channels without a definite layer of muscularis in the vessel walls.[13]

Careful postoperative and long-term evaluation of patients with juvenile angiofibromas is important. MRI provides the best modality of clinical assessment. Harrison published a personal series of 44 patients treated by surgical removal in whom there was a 23% incidence of recurrence.[14] These 10 patients with recurrent tumor received another operation. Of these 10 patients, 3 developed a second recurrence that was subsequently treated successfully with irradiation.

CHORDOMAS

Chordomas are tumors that are thought to arise from remnants of the notochord, which is the embryonic precursor of the axial skeleton. Chordomas constitute only 1% of all intracranial tumors, and 30% to 40% of all chordomas arise in the skull base area. Chordomas may involve the sphenoethmoidal area, the petrosphenoid synchondrosis, and the cavernous sinus region, the upper, middle, or lower clivus. The symptoms produced depend on the location of the tumor. Patients may develop cranial nerve palsies, brain stem compression, or merely a nasal or nasopharyngeal mass with nasal airway obstruction.

There are two histologic types of chordoma. The chondroid variety demonstrates a cartilaginous matrix histologically and is associated with much better long-term survival. Patients with chondroid chordoma may live as long as 20 to 30 years. The regular variety of chordoma is associated with a poorer prognosis (5-year survival rate of 30% to 50%). Death is usually caused by local recurrence of tumor. Metastasis to distant sites occurs in about 10% of patients and is more common with longer survival periods. Chordomas are relatively radioresistant to standard radiotherapy and do not respond to chemotherapy.

During the last 15 years, two new developments in the treatment of chordomas have occurred that may change the prognosis for cranial base chordomas. First, the advances in cranial base surgery have allowed a more complete resection of chordomas from difficult regions such as the clivus, the petrous apex, and the cavernous sinus. Second, irradiation with high-energy particles, such as proton beams (Bragg peak) or helium ions, has permitted the delivery of large amounts of radiation to a restricted area. The effects of both of these advances will require many years to evaluate, since chordomas are slow-growing tumors. The current management principle consists of surgical removal and postoperative irradiation.[15-17]

CHONDROSARCOMA

Since the bones of the cranial base are derived from a cartilaginous matrix through endochondral ossification, 60% to 70% of chondrosarcomas involve the cranial base skeleton. Such tumors may involve any area of the cranial base but have a predilection for the petrosphenoid synchondrosis.

The prognosis of chondrosarcomas in general depends on the histologic grade, which is worse in patients with a poorly differentiated tumor. The majority of cranial base chondrosarcomas are low grade, locally confined for many years. They recur repeatedly after local resection and metastasize rarely.

Similar to the management of skull base chordomas, our present management consists of tumor resection. Irradiation is administered to patients with residual tumor or high-grade chondrosarcoma.

OSSEOUS MENINGIOMAS

Meningiomas of the cranial base area are often associated with hyperostosis of the cranium. In 30% to 50% of cases, such hyperostosis is due to actual tumor invasion into the bone. In the others, it occurs as a reaction to the tumor resulting from increased vascularity. A patient with a hyperostotic bony reaction or tumor may have either a carpet-like "meningioma en plaque" or a globular "meningioma en masse" involving the dura, the periorbita, and the paranasal sinuses. Osseous meningiomas may be discovered when a patient presents with signs and symptoms caused by a globular tumor. With the en plaque variety, such osseous involvement is often the reason for neurologic symptoms, commonly proptosis, extraocular muscle palsies, and visual loss.

Failure to remove the osseous portion of the tumor will result in eventual progression of symptoms. Regrowth of osseous tumor is often slow, permitting conservative surgery in many patients.

Surgery

Several basic principles, well utilized in other surgical areas, are applicable to cranial base tumor surgery. One is simplicity. Even in complex cranial base surgery, the simplicity and thus the proper sequential logic of the procedural steps should be high on the priority list. The second principle is exposure. It is essential that adequate surgical access to the tumor be achieved with good visualization to allow its complete removal and preservation of uninvolved anatomic structures. In particular, the blood supply to the overlying skin and surrounding muscles must be respected during exposure and tumor resection, so as to have adequate and viable soft tissue available for reconstruction. The cranial nerves, if free of neoplastic growth, are preserved or reconstructed following tumor removal.

CRANIOFACIAL RESECTION

This procedure is performed for neoplasms involving the midline anterior cranial base. For example, tumors involving the ethmoid sinuses and cribriform plate would be encompassed by this procedure.

A bicoronal incision is used with removal of the craniofacial skeleton (Fig. 52-2). This incision outlines the distal end of the fronto-parietal scalp flap used for the exposure of the cranium. It is based inferiorly on supraorbital and supratrochlear vessels and laterally on branches of the superficial temporal arteries. It is a broad-based flap. It can include all the layers of the scalp, including the underlying pericranium, or it can be raised at the galeopericranial plane. Anterolateral extensions of this bicoronal incision, in front of each ear, permit reflection of the flap over the face (a greater rotational arch was achieved) and thus unhindered exposure to the cranium, the roof of the orbit, and both zygomatic arches. The frontalis branch of the facial nerve is preserved and reflected inferiorly in a fascial layer with the overlying scalp flap. The supraorbital neurovascular pedicle can be dissected out of its foramen or groove on each side and preserved. The nasion is well exposed, permitting access to both medial orbital walls. Loss of the sense of smell is always a consequence of this approach.

In addition to the bicoronal scalp flap for superior exposure, inferior facial incisions are made (see Fig. 52-2). Several options are available, from a purely midline "face-splitting" incision (from the nasion through the upper lip) to a paramedian incision, a modification of a lateral rhinotomy incision. It is also possible to avoid direct facial skin incisions by performing what is referred to as a "degloving" procedure (a horizontal mucosal incision from one maxillary tuberosity to the other in the gingivolabial sulcus with elevation of all the soft tissues of the face including the nose). This approach, however, provides wide surgical access only at the level of the incision and significantly narrows at the skull base. Optimal visualization at the skull base is not achieved in the majority of cases. Also, reconstruction of the skull base, if needed, is difficult with this approach.

The "exposure osteotomies," done in a zigzagging fashion, are performed with the intent to remove, as a free graft, the supraorbital bar, usually from one supraorbital nerve to the other. The facial bony segments are displaced following osteotomies, with the attached soft tissues. They may extend from one medial orbit across the nasion to the opposite

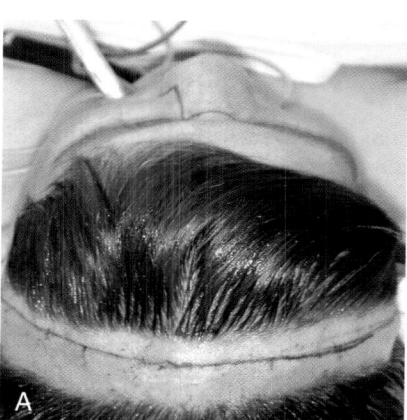
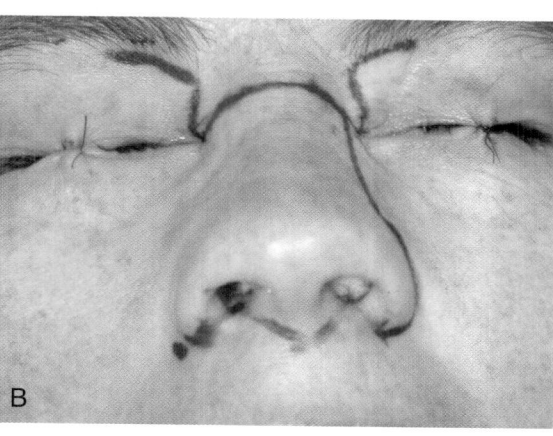

FIGURE 52-2 Incisions. A, Markings for bicoronal incision. B, Outline of midfacial and subcranial incisions.

orbit (usually to the level of the superior orbital nerve on the opposite side). If the orbital content is involved with the tumor, then it becomes part of the specimen. Before tumor extirpation, when needed, the ICA is isolated in the neck. The craniotomy used in this approach is a bifrontal craniotomy. After dural elevation from the anterior cranial fossa, tumor extent is appropriately assessed with preservation of as many uninvolved anatomic structures as possible including cranial nerves and the carotid artery.

The planning for 3D tumor resection should include the natural anatomic boundaries to tumor progression. These include dura, one or both medial walls of the orbit, the cribriform plate, and the nasal septum. A portion of the frontal bone, corresponding to the upper boundary of the interorbital space, is usually removed with the specimen. If the frontal sinus is not involved by the tumor, it is possible to replace the most anterior portion of this bone.

MIDFACIAL SPLIT AND MIDFACIAL TRANSLOCATION

Midfacial split provides a direct access and a unified surgical field at the central cranial base. It is performed utilizing bilateral facial osteotomies and soft-tissue mobilization. It extends in the sagittal plane from the anterior cranial fossa floor and sphenoid sinus to the level of C1. In the axial plane, the surgical reach extends between medial orbits superiorly, through the plane between V2 to the level of the palate. If the tumor demands wider exposure, an extended facial translocation with palatal split can be utilized.[18]

Incision consists of either a midline or a paramedian nasal incision with supraorbital extensions. If needed, it may continue inferiorly through the upper lip. The uninvolved nasal septum is reflected with one of the lateral composite tissue components. Facial soft tissues are elevated from the nasomaxillary bones to both infraorbital foramina.

The upper end of the nasal incision is extended laterally below the medial eyebrows, exposing the superior and medial orbital rims. Elevation of the periorbita reveals the anterior and posterior ethmoid foramina; cauterization of the ethmoid vascular pedicles is performed. Inferiorly, the nasolacrimal duct is identified and preserved (or repositioned for subsequent dacryocystorhinostomy).

Bone cuts are made from the medial orbit on one side to the other, through the nasion followed by LeFort I osteotomy. Vertical maxillary cuts are made just medial to the infraorbital nerves. The osteotomies in the medial and inferior orbit are then connected. A midline nasal osteotomy completes bony disassembly if a central nasal incision is used; if a paramedian nasal incision is selected, the entire nasal-midfacial complex is rotated laterally as a composite flap on a single soft-tissue pedicle. Nasal cavities and maxillary sinuses are now widely exposed, allowing resection of the medial maxillary walls. Nonessential nasal septum and vomer can be removed or dislocated to one side, providing direct access to the nasopharynx, sphenoid sinus, and clivus.

For more inferior exposure, the procedure is modified (by omitting the LeFort I osteotomy and separating the maxillary segment from the pterygoid plates posteriorly) and splitting the hard palate in the midline. Each hemipalate (still attached to its vascular pedicle and the rest of the maxilla) is then rotated laterally and retracted. The soft palate can also be divided in the midline, giving access to the entire orona-sopharynx and C1–C4 area.

If further inferior exposure is needed, a tranoral-transmandibular approach can be selected.[19] For more lateral access, an extended facial translocation[18,20] can be added.

FACIAL TRANSLOCATION

This approach to the skull base has undergone a significant evolution since its original description in 1989 and now comprises a system of approaches based on a principle of facial disassembly along embryonic planes of fusion.[18,20,21] Due to its modular design, it permits great versatility of design and accommodates the surgical needs for limited as well as complex procedures at the skull base. The operative manipulation of cranial base anatomy and pathology, crucial for oncologic surgery, can be tailored with this system of approaches very precisely to a specific skull base tumor. Maximum preservation and functional and esthetic reconstruction of craniofacial anatomy is an integral part of this procedure.

The current underlying principle of skull base approaches is to minimize brain retraction while maximizing skull base visualization reflected in disassembly and displacement of craniofacial bony and soft-tissue anatomy while preserving the intactness of the brain. This concept facilitates 3D tumor resection, tumor margin verification, and functional reconstruction with appropriate esthetic concerns. Facial translocation approach to the skull base through its great versatility contributes to this goal.

In general, surgical treatment of lesions located anterior to the neuroaxis should be done through an anterior approach. This requires selection of a transfacial approach because of the anteroinferior anatomic relationship of the facial viscerocranium to the cranial base.

The advantages of the facial translocation system of approaches include the following:

1. Facial anatomy has developed through the embryonic fusion of nasofrontal, maxillary, and mandibular processes. Normally, the fusion takes place in the midline or in the paramedian region, thus logically presenting optimal lines of "separation" of facial units for a surgical approach, permitting the least consequential displacement.
2. The primary blood supply to the "facial units" is through the external carotid system, which also has a lateral-to-medial direction of flow, thus ensuring viability of displaced surgical units.
3. The midface contains multiple "hollow" anatomic spaces (oronasal cavity, nasopharynx, paranasal sinuses) that facilitate the relative ease of surgical access to the central skull base.
4. Displacement of facial units for an approach to the cranial base offers much greater tolerance to postoperative surgical swelling, as opposed to similar displacement of the content of the neurocranium.
5. Reestablishment of the normal anatomy, following repositioning of the facial units during the reconstructive phase of surgery, has a high degree of functional as well as aesthetic achievement.

However, there are some disadvantages:

1. Contamination of the surgical wound with oropharyngeal bacterial flora.

2. The need for facial incisions with subsequent scar development.
3. Emotional considerations for the patient related to "surgical facial disassembly."
4. The potential need for supplementary airway management (postoperative endotracheal intubation, temporary tracheostomy).

The listed disadvantages are of much lesser consequence to the patient when viewed from the perspective of the procedure's overall safety, tumor control potential, and the facilitation of excellent reconstructive options.

In the past, several surgeons worked on achieving additional oncologic exposure of the facial viscerocranium. Barbosa[22] expanded exposure for the treatment of maxillary sinus cancer and Altemir[23] did the same for the nasomaxillary area access.

OPERATIVE TECHNIQUE

Modular craniofacial disassembly is the principle of the facial translocation approach to the skull base. It is based on the creation of composite facial units that are designed along key neurovascular anatomy and esthetic lines. The individual units merge into larger composites without compromising their function. It is possible to attach eponyms to the technical variations of facial translocation for ease of communication and comparison. Thus we can recognize "mini," "standard," "expanded" (vertically, medially, posteriorly), and "bilateral" facial translocation procedures.[24] Complementary craniotomies or craniectomies are added to these approaches as necessary to assist with 3D tumor resection.

Minifacial translocation-central is designed to reach the medial orbit, sphenoid and ethmoid sinuses, and the inferior clivus. The port of entry is through the displaced ipsilateral nasal bone, the nasal process of the maxilla, and the medial orbital rim (with an attached medial canthal ligament, the lacrimal duct, and the skin). The skin incision is made along the lateral aspect of the nose and the inferior aspect of the medial eyebrow with a triangular design at the level of the medial canthal ligament to limit potential scar contracture. Osteotomies create a rectangular window with a lateral extent being just medial to the inferior orbital nerve. The entire unit is displaced laterally for surgical exposure. Closure is accomplished with replacement of this composite unit (skin, bone, mucosa). Rigid fixation of the bone is accomplished with microplating. The perimeter of this approach can be further augmented with endoscopic instrumentation.

Minifacial translocation-lateral opens the infratemporal fossa. The incisions run from the inner canthus horizontally in the inferior fornix of the lower eyelid through the lateral canthus to the preauricular area. Here, it joins vertical temporal and preauricular incisions. The frontal branches of the facial nerve are temporarily disconnected through entubulation (see later). The temporalis muscle is reflected inferiorly after displacement of the zygomatic arch/malar eminence. The head of the mandible, when needed, may be either displaced or resected.

Standard facial translocation achieves surgical access to the anterolateral skull base. The ipsilateral facial skin (including the lower eyelid) is displaced laterally and inferiorly with the attached underlying maxilla (with or without the hard palate). The nasal incision may extend inferiorly to include an upper lip split. Superior incision continues from the nose to the inferior fornix of the lower eyelid, and again through the lateral canthus horizontally to the preauricular area. In some cases (more anterior tumors), it is possible to conclude the horizontal canthal incision about 1.5 cm beyond the lateral orbital rim after identifying and preserving the most anterior frontal branch of the facial nerve. This point then serves as the point of rotation of the displaced composite unit, providing sufficient surgical space for some paracentral tumors. When the entire extent of the horizontal temple incision is needed, the frontal branches of the facial nerve are identified with a nerve stimulator, placed in silicone tubings, and transected (entubulation). During the reconstruction, only these transected tubings are reconnected, approximating the facial nerve branches, and providing a stable, enclosed milieu for nerve regeneration. Osteotomies correlate to LeFort I or II or the midpalatal lines when the entire maxilla is being displaced. The inferior orbital nerve is electively sectioned along the floor of the orbit, tagged, and repaired at the end of the procedure. Rigid fixation is achieved with mini- and microplates. With this technique of facial translocation, good exposure of the anterolateral skull base is achieved, especially when the infratemporal fossa is involved as well.

Extended facial translocation-medial incorporates the standard translocation unit plus the nose and the medial one half of the opposite face (up to the infraorbital nerve). It can be rotated at the LeFort I level or include the ipsilateral palate and upper lip split. The skin incisions are similar to the standard technique, except that the paranasal incision is made on the contralateral side. The surgical exposure includes the ipsilateral infratemporal fossa and the central and paracentral skull base bilaterally. The entire clivus is accessible, as are the optic nerves, both precavernous ICAs, and the nasopharynx. The wide communication with the infratemporal fossa allows the placement of the temporalis muscle flap for vascularized reconstruction of any skull base defect. Bony fixation of craniofacial osteotomies is done with miniplates and a lag screw for the palate. The occlusal plane is reestablished with the help of an orthognathic splint prefabricated preoperatively. In addition, a full palatal splint is attached to the contralateral stable palate for additional stability and protection of the palatal incision. Temporary silicone intranasal stents are inserted, as are bilateral lacrimal stents.

Extended facial translocation-medial and inferior includes the aforementioned procedure with an inferior extension via mandibular split. The lower lip split incision is performed in a zigzagging fashion to conform to the tension lines of the skin with a horizontal extension into the upper neck. Mandibular osteotomy is performed just medial to the mental foramen. Usually an interdental space is found wide enough to permit placement of a reciprocating saw for the osteotomy. This is performed in a step fashion, which then permits more stable reconstructive reapproximation of the bone. Before performing the osteotomy, it is wise to select an appropriate miniplate for eventual fixation, contour it to the mandible, and create drill holes. This maneuver assists in the reestablishment of a normal occlusion during reconstruction. This extended translocation procedure adds a significant inferior as well as upper cervical surgical access.

Bilateral facial translocation combines complete right and left basic translocation units with or without palatal split. The exposure incorporates both infratemporal fossae, central and the entire paracentral skull base. Both distal cervical ICAs are in view, as is the full clivus. The palatal split permits a reach to the level of C2–C3. If further inferior extension is needed, a mandibular split can be added so a vertical reach to C3–C4 is accomplished. A single temporalis muscle flap is sufficient for the coverage of the surgical defect at the skull base.

RECONSTRUCTION

The repair of any dural defect is performed with a pericranial graft harvested posterior to the bicoronal incision. In addition, a pericranial flap, based on supraorbital vessels, is utilized to enclose the cranial cavity and complete the separation of the cranial cavity from the extracranium. The reestablishment of external craniofacial bony continuity is done by replacing any skeleton displaced for exposure. Any surgical defect can be augmented with a split cranial bone graft or a titanium mesh. The most inferior portion of cranial base defects (floor of cranial fossae) is usually not bone grafted (Fig. 52-3). Further soft-tissue repair may include regional muscle transposition (temporalis) or free muscle–skin flap transfer (rectus abdominis or latissimus dorsi myocutaneous flaps).

Complications

Complications of a craniofacial resection can be categorized into fatal and nonfatal groups. Terz and colleagues reported an 11% fatal complication rate in their group of 28 patients. The three deaths in this series resulted from pulmonary embolus, brain injury, and tracheal abscess. In the nonfatal complication group, reported by the same investigators, there were several CSF leaks, meningitis, and osteomyelitis of the bone flap, for a 35% nonfatal complication rate.[25]

Careful attention to even minor details during the preoperative evaluation, the operation, and the postoperative period can often prevent major complications. For instance, when severe lower cranial nerve dysfunction is expected, a temporary tracheostomy and gastrostomy can prevent aspiration pneumonia and malnutrition. Since many of the initial postoperative problems are neurologic, cardiac, or respiratory, the patient should be observed in a unit with facilities for neurologic and cardiorespiratory intensive care. Because of the close collaboration among neurosurgery, otolaryngology, and plastic surgery, the incidence of postoperative problems following extensive cranial base surgery has been greatly reduced.[26]

Adjuvant Therapy

External beam irradiation is usually administered as an adjuvant treatment to patients with malignant cranial base neoplasms. The value of such combined therapy (surgery and irradiation) for extensive skull base tumors is unproven at this time in the absence of prospective controlled trials. However, such combined modalities have become a standard in head and neck surgery for extensive neoplasms (T3–T4).

High-energy–focused radiation, with proton beams or helium ions, has been used to treat cranial base chordomas and chondrosarcomas with encouraging results.[17]

Although benign tumors such as meningiomas and neurilemmomas have been considered radioresistant, recent reports suggest that recurrent or residual tumors can be treated with external beam irradiation, reducing their

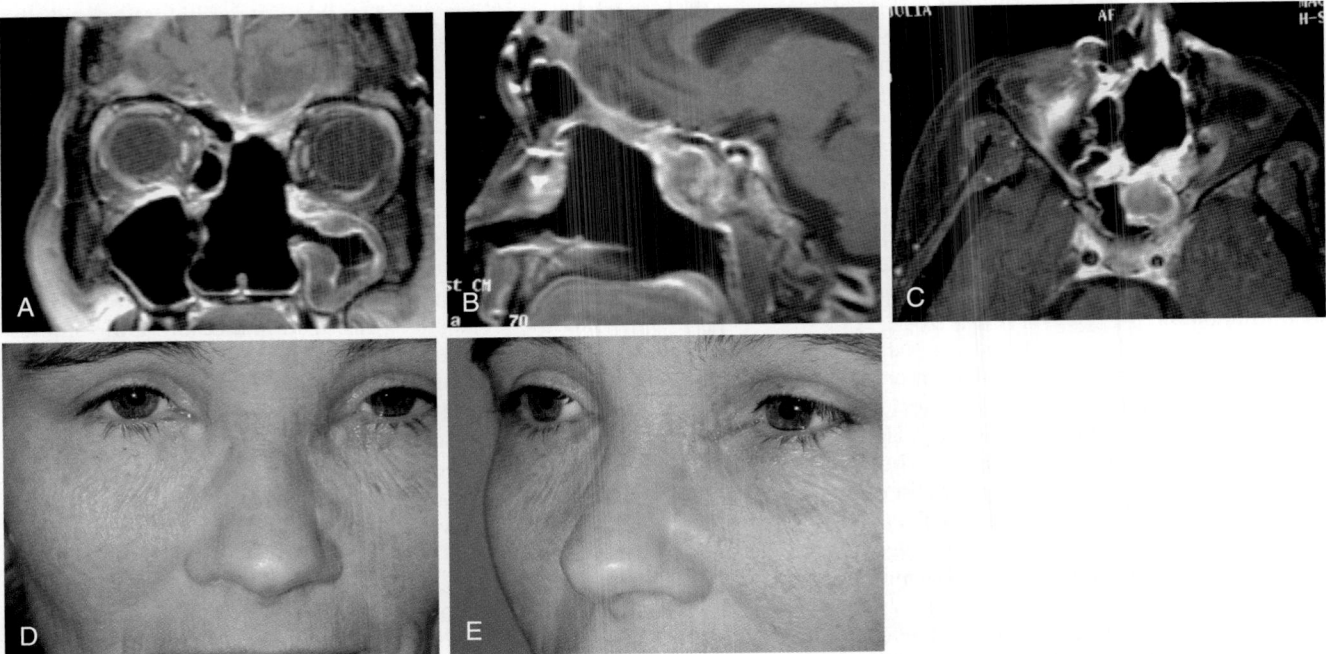

FIGURE 52-3 Postoperative scans. A, Coronal MR with contrast, showing total removal of midline transcranial tumor and soft-tissue–only reconstruction of the anterior cranial fossa. B and C, Sagittal and axial MR revealing the same as A. D and E, Postoperative facial appearance with well-healed incisions.

growth rates.[27] However, the deleterious effects of irradiation (carcinogenesis, normal tissue growth retardation) must be kept in mind.

For small benign lesions (<2.5 cm), such as meningiomas or acoustic neurilemmomas, stereotactically focused cobalt radiation has been used. Such "gamma knife" treatments appear to be effective in arresting the growth of tumors in many cases and offer an alternative to surgical treatment.[28]

In general, chemotherapy for cranial base tumors has not been successful. Tissue assay, performed on a sample of a removed tumor, may offer a potential for finding a more specific chemotherapy drug for each patient. In vitro drug testing on tumor cells is in its infancy and still not a perfect predictor of clinical response. However, treatment with assay "positive" drugs is reported to be more strongly associated with clinical response than is treatment with assay "negative" drugs (Weisenthal Cancer Group, "Functional Tumor Cell Profiling," Huntington Beach, CA, http://www.weisenthal cancer.com/). We have obtained assays on several skull base tumors. Clinical conclusions cannot be drawn yet at this early stage; these findings could be used only as guidance to planning when chemotherapy option needs be considered.

Case 1: Chordoma of clivus. The tumor assay showed sensitivity to Cisplatin and Ifosfamide.

Case 2: Myxoid fibrosarcoma. The tumor assay showed sensitivity to Gemcitabine+Cisplatin, Gemcitabine+Melphan, Gemcitabine+Melphan+High dose of Tamoxifin.

Case 3: Meningioma, middle and infratemporal fossa. The tumor assay showed sensitivity to Taxol.

Case 4: Chordom of clivus. The tumor assay showed sensitivity to Docetaxel, Gemcitabine+Cisplatin, Gemcitabine+CP+High dose of Tamoxifin, Gemcitabine+Melphan+High dose of Tamoxifin, Vinorelbine+High dose of Tamoxifin.

Case 5: Synovial cell sarcoma of upper neck. The tumor assay showed sensitivity to Doxyrubicin, Gemcitabine+Melphan+High dose of Tamoxifin, Isosfamide.

Case 6: Squamous cell carcinoma, maxilla. The tumor assay showed sensitivity to Bleomycin, Cisplatin, Gemcitabine, Gemcitabine+Cisplatin, Docetaxel, Irinotecan+Cisplatin, Irinotecan+Cisplatin+High dose Tamoxifin, Topotecan+Cisplatin.

Case 5: Neuroendocrine carcinoma, ethmoid sinuses. The tumor assay showed sensitivity to Trimetrexate.

Case 6: Meningioma, orbit, middle, and infratemporal fossae. The tumor assay showed sensitivity to Extramusine, Decarbazine, and Taxanes.

Case 7: Myxoid fibrosarcoma, orbit, infratemporal fossa, skull base. Tumor assay showed sensitivity to Doxil, Doxorubicin, Epirubicin, Gemcittabine, Gemcitabine+Cisplatin, Gemcitabine(+Doxil+High dose of Tamoxifin, Gemcitabine+Isofosfamice(4HI), Gemcitabine+Melphan.

Conclusions

The management of complex cranial base neoplasms by a team approach, combined with other therapeutic advances, has greatly improved the outlook for these patients in the past 15 years. The next decade will witness the consolidation of such advances and the conduction of cooperative and prospective clinical trials to assess further the efficacy of such aggressive approaches in controlling neoplastic disease at the skull base. Patients with extensive cranial base neoplasms often need considerable help with psychological, social, and financial problems. Such problems are best handled with the assistance of psychology, nursing, and social service departments.

The oncologic benefit of cranial base surgery is continuously being assessed. The percentage of patients living disease free after cranial base surgery for malignant disease has increased to 60% to 65% at 5 years. This "overall" percentage (all histologies, all sites) reflects not only the slow biologic aggressiveness of some tumors (e.g., chondrosarcomas, adenoid cystic carcinomas), but also the high aggressiveness of others (e.g., squamous cell and anaplastic carcinomas). Most encouraging is that primary cranial base surgery (done as the initial treatment) has a significantly greater chance of oncologic success than "salvage" procedures following failure of other therapeutic modalities (e.g., non–skull base surgery, radiotherapy).

For most benign tumors, cranial base surgery is the only therapeutic modality and has a high degree of effectiveness.

KEY REFERENCES

Choussy O, Ferron C, Védrine PO, et al. Adenocarcinoma of ethmoid: a GETTEC retrospective multicenter study of 418 cases. *Laryngoscope.* 2008;118(3):437-443.

Chung WY, Pan DH, Lee CC, et al. Large vestibular schwannomas treated by gamma knife surgery: long-term outcomes. *J Neurosurg.* 2010;113(suppl):112-121.

Durante M, Loeffler JS. Charged particles in radiation oncology. *Nat Rev Clin Oncol.* 2010;7(1):37-43.

Ganly I, Patel SG, Singh B, et al. Complications of craniofacial resection for malignant tumors of the skull base. Report of an International Collaborative Study. *Head Neck.* 2005;27(6):445-r51.

Ganly I, Snehal G, Patel SG, et al. Craniofacial resection for malignant paranasal sinus tumors: report of an International Collaborative Study. *Head Neck.* 2005;27(7):575-584.

Holzmann D, Reisch R, Krayenbühl N, et al. The transnasal transclival approach for clivus chordoma. *Minim Invasive Neurosurg.* 2010;53(5):211-217.

Janecka IP. New reconstructive technologies in skull base surgery. Role of titanium mesh and porous polyethylene. *Arch Otolaryngol.* 2000;126:396-401.

Janecka IP, Tiedemann K, eds. *Skull base surgery.* Philadelphia: Lippincott-Raven; 1998.

Kadish S, Goodman M, Wang CC. Olfactory neuroblastoma: a clinical analysis of 17 cases. *Cancer.* 1976;37:1571-1576.

Patel SG, Singh B, Polluri A, et al. Craniofacial surgery for malignant skull base tumors: report of an international collaborative study. *Cancer.* 2003;98(6):1179-1187.

Roos DE, Brophy BP, Taylor J. Lessons from a 17-year radiosurgery experience at the Royal Adelaide Hospital. *Int J Radiat Oncol Biol Phys.* 2010 Oct 30:[Epub ahead of print].

Sen C, Triana AI, Berglind N, et al. Clival chordomas: clinical management, results, and complications in 71 patients. *J Neurosurg.* 2010;113(5):1059-1071.

Suárez C, Rodrigo JP, Rinaldo A, et al. Current treatment options for recurrent nasopharyngeal cancer. *Eur Arch Otorhinolaryngol.* 2010;267(12):1811-1824.

Numbered references appear on Expert Consult.

CHAPTER 53

Orbitozygomatic Infratemporal Approach to Parasellar Meningiomas

KENJI OHATA • TAKEO GOTO

Lesions located high in the parasellar region and the interpeduncular fossa are challenging and often difficult to approach, as a result of both the deep position and the surrounding vital structures that obscure the view. In 1977, we developed a new surgical approach, the orbitozygomatic infratemporal approach,[1] consisting of an orbitozygomatic osteotomy, a fronto-temporo-orbital craniotomy, and removal of the posterolateral wall of the orbital bone and major sphenoid wing lateral to the foramen spinosum. This approach provides a good exposure of the infratemporal fossa, permits access obliquely upward to the parasellar region and the interpeduncular fossa, and permits safe manipulation of parasellar and interpeduncular lesions via the shortest distance.[2-4]

Operative Technique

The patient is placed in the supine position with the thorax elevated 30 degrees to facilitate venous drainage. By using a three-pin head-holder, the head is rotated to the side opposite the lesion without creating excessive torsion of the neck, so that the right pterion is the highest in the surgical field.

A bicoronal scalp incision is made to gain sufficient exposure of the zygomatic arch and superior and lateral orbital margins, starting at the inferior end of the base of the earlobe, running along the anterior margin of the ear cartilage, extending upward and forward, and running within the hairline to a level 3 cm above the upper margin of the contralateral zygomatic arch. The superficial layer of deep temporal fascia is incised and reflected with the skin flap to avoid the injury of the frontal branch of the facial nerve. The skin flap is reflected farther anteriorly with the frontal pericranium to expose the orbitozygomatic complex, cutting the supraorbital notch for the preservation of the right supraorbital nerve.[5,6] To preserve the temporal and zygomatic branches of the facial nerve, the fascia covering the temporomandibular joint capsule is carefully pulled away, and the periosteum covering the outer surface of the zygomatic arch is incised vertically just in front of the tuberculum articulare. The entire outer surface of the zygomatic arch from its frontal process to its pedicle is then fully exposed subperiosteally. The superior and lateral orbital margins are then exposed, maintaining continuity of the pericranium and the periorbita. The superior and lateral periorbita are separated from the superior and lateral posterior walls of the orbit.

Multiple burr holes are made, the first of which, in the lateral frontal bone just behind the frontal process of the zygomatic bone, is the key burr hole. The second burr hole is at the pterion, the third in the temporal bone just above the pedicle of the zygomatic process, the fourth in the squamous suture about 3 cm above the zygomatic arch, the fifth in the coronal suture about 6 cm above the zygomatic arch, and the sixth in the frontal bone 3 cm above the orbital ridge (Fig. 53-1). The anterior and posterior ends of the zygomatic arch are then cut using a sagittal saw, and it is retracted downward hinged on the masseter muscle.

The second, third, fourth, fifth, and sixth burr holes are then connected with a craniotome (see Fig. 53-1). Using a reciprocating saw, osteotomy of the lateral and superior walls of the orbit is performed from the inferior orbital fissure. The orbital content is protected by a spatula during this osteotomy. The frontotemporal bone flap and the orbitozygomatic flap are kept in saline solution containing an antibiotic. While protecting the periorbita and the dura mater with self-retaining retractors with spatulas, the remaining major sphenoid wing lateral to the foramen spinosum, forming the posterolateral orbital wall and the anterolateral part of the middle fossa, and the posterior portion of the orbital roof lateral to the superior orbital fissure, are divided, using either a sagittal saw or small chisel (see Fig. 53-1). The remaining medial part of the minor sphenoid wing is then partially removed with an air drill and a bone rongeur. The bone fragments are kept in the saline solution to be replaced at the end of the procedure.

The exposed frontotemporal dura mater is opened in semicircular fashion, from the medial superior orbital margin to the midportion of the inferior temporal region. Alternatively, in a combined orbitozygomatic epidural and subdural approach,[7-9] an inverted T-shaped dural incision is made along the sylvian fissure to the superior surface of the optic nerve sheath forward with a short vertical incision at the distal sylvian fissure. The orbital contents are retracted medially downward by retracting the anterior dural fringe forward.

The operative microscope is now introduced, and either a trans-sylvian approach or a subtemporal approach can be taken with minimal retraction of the brain. In the trans-sylvian approach, the sylvian fissure is widely opened, with

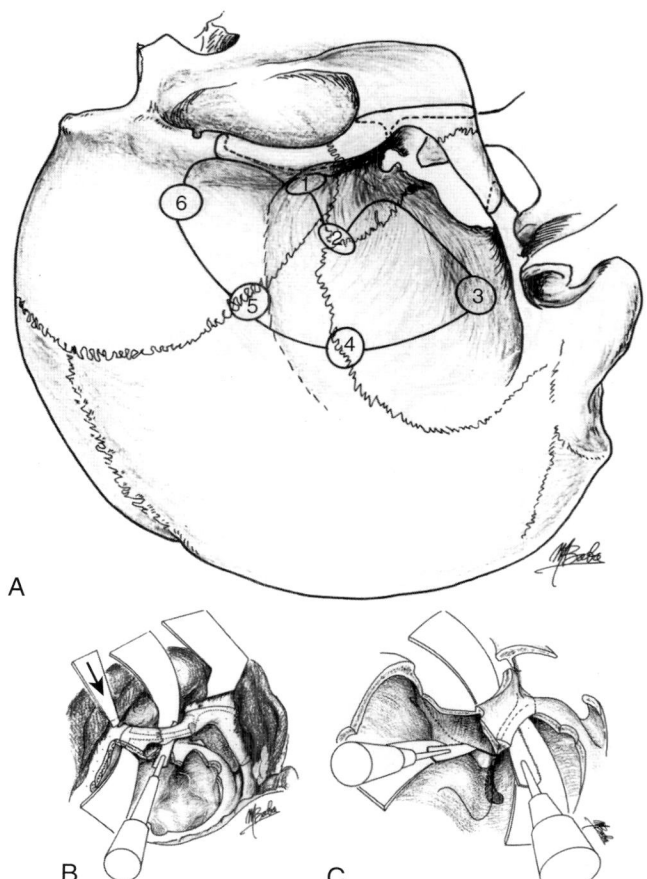

FIGURE 53-1 A, Location of the burr holes and the extent of craniotomy. The first burr hole, made at the frontal bone just behind its zygomatic process, is the "key burr hole." The second burr hole is made at the pterion, the third on the temporal bone just above the pedicle of the zygomatic arch, the fourth in the squamous suture, the fifth in the coronal suture, and the sixth in the frontal bone 3 cm above the orbital ridge. B, An orbitozygomatic osteotomy. The zygoma has been well exposed down to the zygomaticofacial canal. The supraorbital canal has been opened by a chisel to prevent its nerve from stretching. The osteotomy of the lateral and superior wall of the orbit is done from the inferior orbital fissure using a reciprocal saw. The orbital content is protected with a spatula during this procedure (the temporal muscle is not drawn). C, Osteotomy of the greater sphenoid wing. The dura mater of the frontal base and temporal pole are retracted to expose the greater and lesser sphenoid wings. The line of osteotomy passes 5 to 10 mm lateral to the lateral margin of the superior orbital fissure. *(From Ohata K, Baba M. Orbitozygomatic infratemporal approach. In: Hakuba A, ed. Surgical Anatomy of the Skull Base. Tokyo: Miwa Shoten; 1996:1-35.)*

preservation of the bridging veins coming from the tip of the temporal lobe. The parasellar region as well as the interpeduncular fossa can be reached at a short distance through the space formed via this approach.

When the tumor is invading the cavernous sinus (CS),[5] the CS is explored by a combined orbitozygomatic infratemporal epidural and subdural approach, which has been described elsewhere.[7-9] The periosteal reflection, which is continuous with the periorbita, is divided at the superior and inferior margins of the superior orbital fissure by sharp dissection using either microscissors or a knife; then the temporal dura propria, forming the superficial layer of the CS, can be separated from the content of the superior orbital fissure (Fig. 53-2A). The lateral part of the

anterior clinoid process is shelled out, leaving a thin layer of its cortical bone. The optic canal is then opened along its length. The cortical bone of the anterior clinoid process and the optic strut are removed by a bone-cutting forceps and a small diamond drill (Fig. 53-2B). The dural incision passes along the sylvian fissure to the superior surface of the optic nerve sheath forward, and then turns laterally at a right angle (Fig. 53-2C). It passes backward at a right angle and runs along the medial part of the distal carotid ring, then along the carotid artery 2 mm away from the artery (Fig. 53-2D). Opening of the medial triangle (Hakuba's triangle, which is a triangle in the subdural space) starts from the distal ring along the medial side of the triangle to the posterior clinoid process and turns laterally at a right angle along the posterior side of this triangle to the dural entrance of the third cranial nerve. The lateral dural fringe of the medial triangle is elevated. Then the remaining outer layer of the CS is separated farther backward from the inner layer of the lateral wall of the CS consisting of the nerve sheaths of the third through fifth cranial nerves (Fig. 53-2E), and the entire CS is unveiled (Fig. 53-2F). Bleeding from the CS is easily controlled by elevating the head side of the table, and the opened venous pathway in the CS is immediately sealed off by insertion of either a fibrinogen-soaked oxidized cellulose sponge or a collagen sponge into the CS, and a bipolar coagulation. Because the intracavernous internal carotid artery (ICA) has its own dural sheath,[10] the plane between the ICA and the tumor is usually found relatively easily, and the tumor is freed from the ICA if it is not invasive. When the artery is torn during dissection, 8-0 monofilament nylon interrupted sutures are applied while trapping this segment of the artery between two temporary clips at both C3 and either C5 or the intrapetrous portions of the ICA, with intravenous administration of barbiturates for brain protection[8] (pentobarbital 4 mg/kg as the initial dose, followed by 2 mg/kg/hr).

Closure of the Opened Paranasal Sinus and Dural Defect

If laceration of the paranasal sinus mucosa is large, it is better to open this sinus wall maximally, and the mucosa of the opened sinus should be removed entirely to prevent postoperative sinusitis and empyema. The opened sinus is closed with a piece of the abdominal fat fixed with fibrin glue. If the laceration of the sinus mucosa is small, the defect is closed by application of a small piece of the temporal muscle. If the mucosa is intact, the bony defect is closed simply with insertion of either a sheet of the temporal fascia or the fascia lata in the epidural space. The dural defect developed by tumor removal is closed by a free pericranial graft. For watertight closure of the dura mater, fibrin glue is applied after approximation of the margins of the graft to the edges of the dura mater using interrupted 6-0 monofilament nylon sutures. Miniplates are used for adequate bone closure to fix the bone flaps to bone edges.

SUMMARY OF CASES

Between 1977 and 2009, 181 cases were treated using the orbitozygomatic approach either alone or combined with other approaches, such as the oticocondylar approach[11]

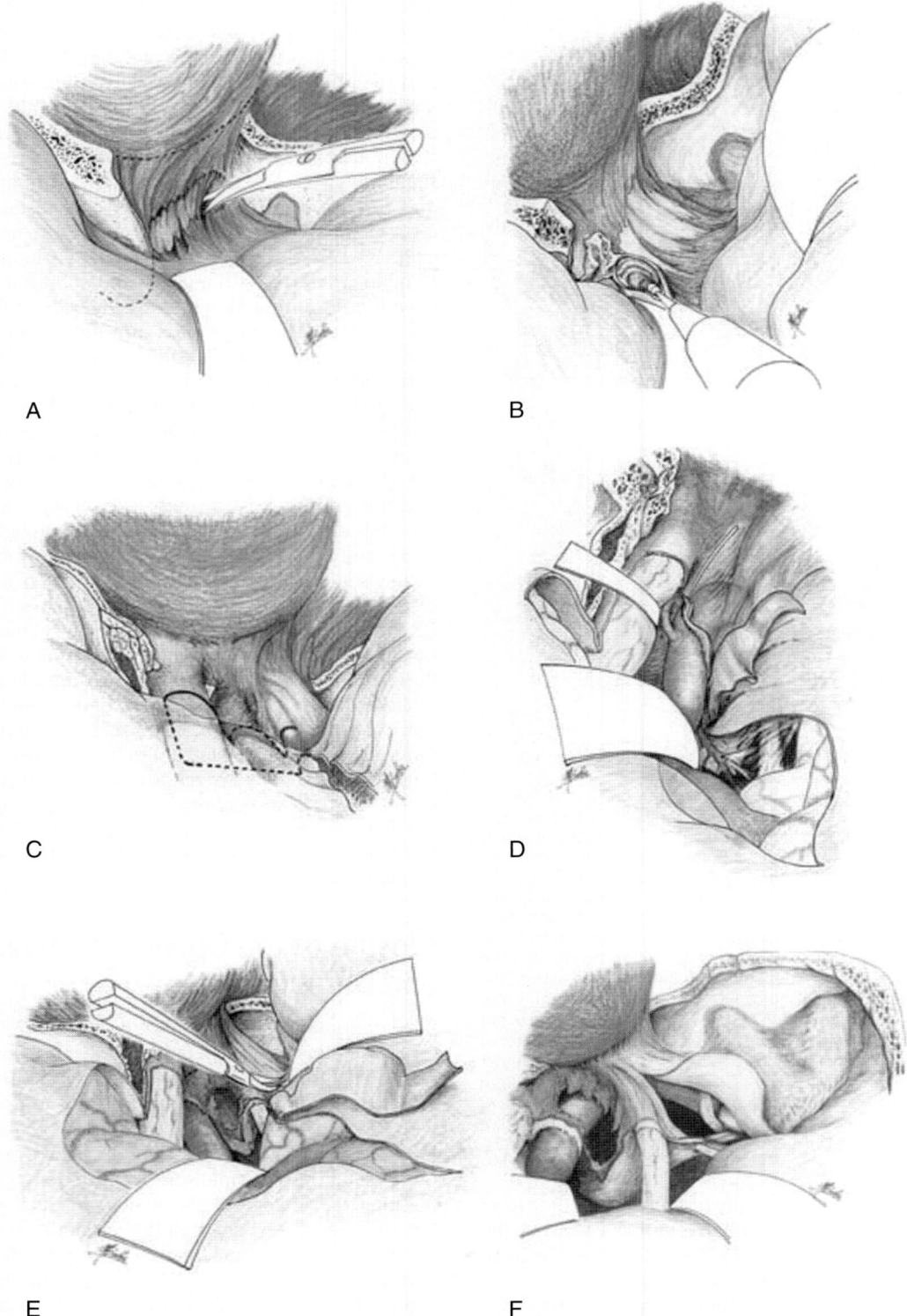

A

B

C

D

E

F

FIGURE 53-2 Combined orbitozygomatic infratemporal epidural and subdural approach. A, The periosteal reflection, which is continuous with the periorbita, is divided at the superior and inferior margins of the superior orbital fissure. Then the temporal dura propria, forming the superficial layer of the cavernous sinus (CS), can be separated from the content of the superior orbital fissure. B, The cortical bone of the anterior clinoid process and the optic strut are being removed by a bone curette and a small diamond drill, respectively. C, Dural opening around the paracavernous region. The dotted line shows the dural incision that passes along the sylvian fissure to the superior surface of the optic nerve sheath forward and is then turned laterally at a right angle. D, Dural incision passes backward at a right angle and runs along the medial part of the distal carotid ring and then along the carotid artery. E, Peeling off the temporal dura propria, the dural incision runs along the medial side to the posterior clinoid process and finally along the posterior side of the medial triangle (Hakuba's triangle) to the dural entrance of the oculomotor nerve. F, Finally, the CS is opened so as to expose the internal carotid artery. *(From Ohata K, Baba M. Orbitozygomatic infratemporal approach. In: Hakuba A, ed. Surgical Anatomy of the Skull Base. Tokyo: Miwa Shoten; 1996:1-35.)*

or transpetrosal approach.[7] These cases included 44 parasellar meningiomas, 24 pituitary adenomas, 26 basilar tip aneurysms, 12 trigeminal neurinomas, 19 chordomas, 11 internal carotid aneurysms, 21 craniopharyngiomas, 3 CS cavernomas, and 21 other lesions (Table 53-1). Of 44 parasellar meningiomas, 19 patients were men and 25 women. Ages ranged from 35 to 76 years (mean of 57.2 years). Total removal of the tumor was accomplished in 32 cases, subtotal removal in 8, and partial removal in 4. Postoperative bacterial meningitis and either an epidural or a subdural hematoma was seen in three cases, wound infection in two, and pneumonia in one. In the cases of the tumors involving the CS, impairment of extraocular movement was seen postoperatively in five cases, trigeminal nerve injury in four, and ipsilateral blindness in two. There was no mortality, but four patients developed disturbance of their conscious level (severely disabled in one case and moderately disabled in three). The operative results were classified as follows: excellent, when the patients have no neurologic deficit; good, when the patients have normal activity in daily life with minor neurologic dysfunction; fair, when the patients are moderately disabled but independent with major neurologic deficit; and poor, when the patients are severely disabled and totally dependent. The operative results were excellent in 23 patients and good in 17 patients (Table 53-2). Three of the remaining four patients were fair postoperatively as a result of bacterial meningitis in one; hypothalamic damage, which had been seen preoperatively, in one; and a combined epidural and subdural hematoma in one. The last one was poor because of a postoperative epidural hematoma. Two representative cases are described briefly.

TABLE 53-1 Summary of Cases Accessed with Orbitozygomatic Approach

Pathology	No. of Cases
Parasellar meningioma	44
Pituitary adenoma	24
Basilar tip aneurysm	26
Trigeminal neurinoma	12
Chordoma	19
Craniopharyngioma	21
IC aneurysm	11
CS cavernoma	3
Others	21
Total	181

CS, cavernous sinus; *IC*, internal carotid.

TABLE 53-2 Surgical Outcome of 44 Parasellar Meningiomas Removed by Orbitozygomatic Approach

Grade	No. of Cases
Excellent	23
Good	17
Fair	3
Poor	1

Case Report 1

The right orbitozygomatic infratemporal approach with a combined epidural and subdural (medial triangle) approach was used on a 57-year-old, right-handed man with a large right parasellar meningioma who had total ophthalmoplegia after partial removal of the tumor in the past (Fig. 53-3). A large tumor occupied the entire CS with encasement of the intracavernous segment of the right ICA. The tumor extended backward subdurally behind the upper clivus with marked compression of the pons and extended inferiorly into the right sphenoid sinus. All the cranial nerves were encased and invaded by the tumor in the CS and had to be sacrificed and removed with the tumor. The intracavernous ICA was carefully dissected out and preserved. The upper basilar artery and its tributaries, which were displaced backward and partially encased, were also well preserved, with total removal of the tumor (Fig. 53-4). The patient had moderate left hemiparesis, which lasted 2 weeks postoperatively; he was neurologically intact except for permanent total ophthalmoplegia at 4 months.

Case Report 2

A 57-year-old woman presented with progressive visual deterioration of the left eye. Radiologic study showed a large left parasellar meningioma (Fig. 53-5). A left orbitozygomatic

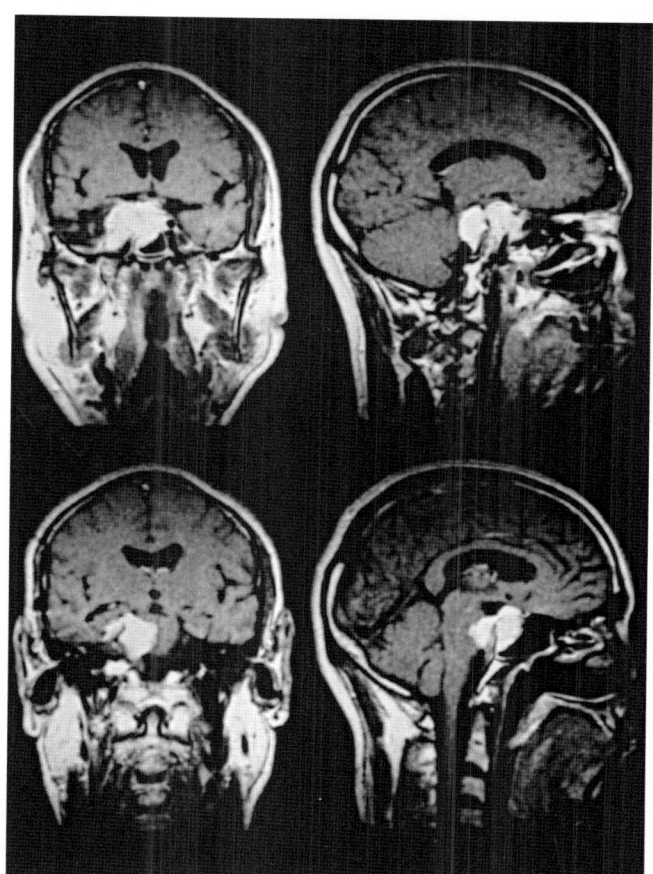

FIGURE 53-3 Preoperative T1-weighted magnetic resonance imaging scan with contrast of a right parasellar meningioma that was partially removed previously. The tumor is encasing the right internal carotid artery and extending to the sphenoid sinus anteriorly. It also extends posteriorly, compressing the pons.

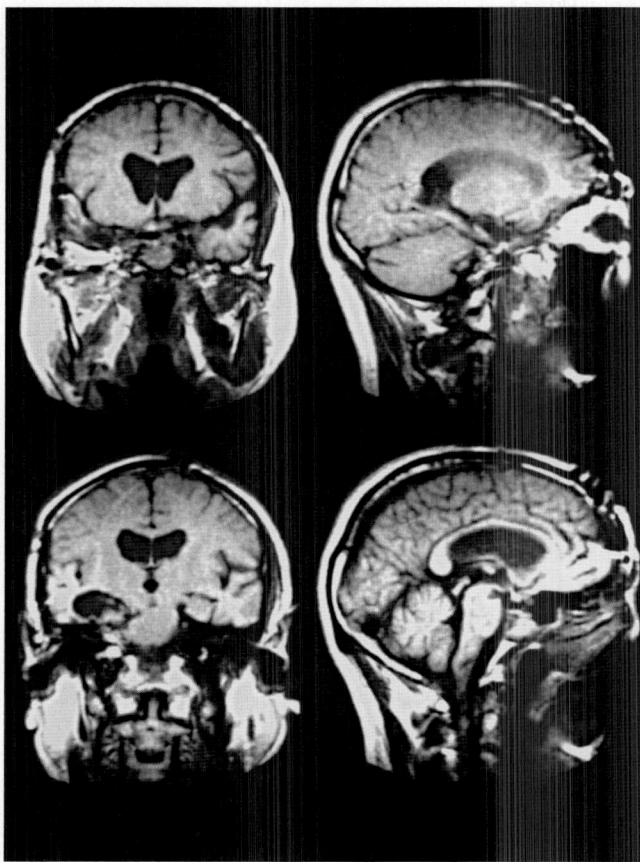

FIGURE 53-4 Postoperative study showing the complete removal of the tumor. The sphenoid sinus is repaired with a vascularized temporal musculofascial flap.

FIGURE 53-5 Preoperative study of coronal and axial T1-weighted magnetic resonance imaging scan with contrast injection showing the parasellar meningioma encasing the internal carotid artery and extending to the interpeduncular cistern (*top*). Postoperative study after total excision of the meningioma (*bottom*).

approach was used for total removal of the tumor. The tumor was engulfing the ICA, but it could be easily separated from it because of the presence of arachnoid space between the artery and the tumor. The tumor extended into the left optic canal and compressed the optic nerve. The canal was opened for excision of that part of the tumor. The anterior part of the lateral wall of the CS was invaded by the tumor, but intracavernous structures were not involved by the tumor. The pituitary stalk was shifted and flattened by the tumor. All these structures were preserved, and total removal of the tumor was achieved (Fig. 53-6 see also Fig. 53-5). Postoperatively the patient showed mild left oculomotor palsy, which improved gradually.

Discussion

Radical removal of parasellar meningiomas usually involves difficult surgical procedures.[12] With the orbitozygomatic infratemporal approach, the working distance to the lesions in the parasellar region and the interpeduncular fossa is about 3 cm shorter and the angle to the lesions about 1 to 3 cm lower than with either the pterional or the subtemporal approach. With the combined orbitozygomatic infratemporal epidural and medial triangle approach, the intracanalicular portion of the optic nerve is well exposed, so that much more space can be obtained between the optic nerve and the carotid artery. With this combined approach, the parasellar region, including the CS, and the interpeduncular fossa can be accessed in the shortest possible distance with minimal retraction of the temporal lobe.[2-4] Manipulation of the vital structures is much easier and safer, even with large parasellar meningiomas, than with the conventional operative approaches.

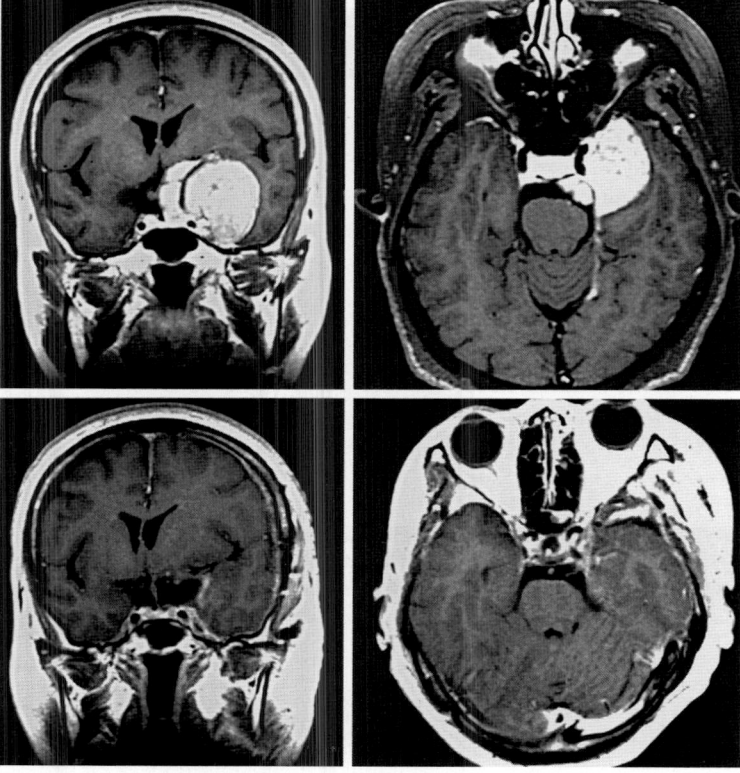

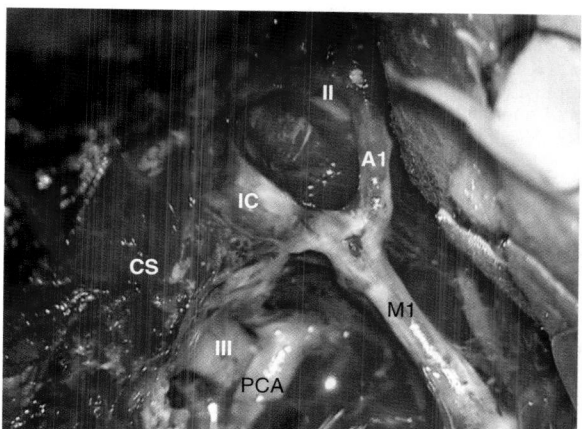

FIGURE 53-6 Operative photograph after total excision of the tumor via the orbitozygomatic infratemporal approach with resection of the anterior clinoid process and opening the medial triangle to remove the tumor, involving the lateral wall of the cavernous sinus (*CS*). *A1,* anterior cerebral artery; *M1,* middle cerebral artery; *IC,* internal carotid artery; *PCA,* posterior cerebellar artery II and III, second and third cranial nerves; *sca,* superior cerebellar artery.

In the orbitozygomatic infratemporal approach, wide exposure of the parasellar lesions can be obtained exclusively by aggressive posterior temporal lobe retraction, which may be at risk of temporal lobe contusion. Surgical strategy should consider the preoperative imaging study of the venous system. The contusion is avoidable by preservation of temporal venous drainage. In the cases of parasellar meningiomas invading the medial sphenoid ridge, the sphenoparietal sinus is usually occluded by tumor and collateral flow via cortical veins is well developed, so that safe posterior temporal lobe retraction is possible after transecting the sylvian vein at its orifice to the sphenoparietal sinus. If the sphenoparietal sinus is patent, an extradural orbitozygomatic approach should be taken for preservation of the venous drainage of the sylvian vein to the pterygoid venous plexus. Peeling off of the temporal dura propria from the inner layer of medial wall of the cavernous sinus is feasible down to the dural entrance of the trochlear nerve.[13] In cases of retrochiasmatic parasellar meningioma in which either the superficial or deep sylvian vein is draining directly into the CS without efficient transcortical collateral circulation, the orbitozygomatic approach risks its damage. In such cases, we select the combined anterior and posterior transpetrosal approach.

The petrosal portion of the ICA, 1 cm long, is epidurally exposed with removal of the petrosal apex at the posterior portion of the trigeminal impression medial to the great petrosal nerve groove by using an air drill. Therefore, when parasellar tumors extend into the CS, the intracavernous portion of the procedure is performed relatively safely while trapping the intracavernous portion of the ICA between its petrosal and C3 portions if necessary.[14] Because the petrosal bone is removed, both medial to the petrosal ICA and anterior to the internal auditory meatus and cochlea, a transzygomatic preauricular transpetrosal approach[9] can be readily carried out. Therefore, parasellar tumors extending into the posterior fossa can be totally removed at one stage with this combined epidural and subdural approach.

If the sphenoparietal sinus is not involved by the parasellar meningiomas, the venous drainage from the sylvian vein should be preserved. Sphenoparietal sinus runs within the dura propria of the temporal lobe and drains usually into the pterygoid venous plexus through the foramen ovale. Preservation of the venous drainage can be done by using the described combined orbitozygomatic epidural and subdural approach, in which the dura propria of the temporal lobe forming the outer layer of the lateral wall of the CS medial to the foramen rotundum and ovale is separated from the inner layer consisting of the dural sheaths of the third and fourth cranial nerves and the first and second branches of the fifth cranial nerve. This dura propria is elevated and retracted backward together with the lateral leaf of the medial triangle opened along its medial and posterior sides. By this means, the infratemporal approach to the interpeduncular fossa can be taken via the temporopolar epidural space without cutting the temporopolar bridging veins.

To preserve the peripheral facial nerve in such low craniotomies, it is necessary to know its topographic anatomy.[15] After exiting from the stylomastoid foramen, the facial nerve crosses the posterior margin of the mandible about 2 cm below the inferior base of the earlobe and enters the parotid gland from behind, where it is situated between the superficial and deep portions of the gland. The branches leave the gland at its superior, anterior, and inferior borders, forming a pattern of rami located superficial to Bichat's fat pad and underneath the facial muscles, entering them from their deep surface. The temporal and zygomatic rami cross the zygomatic arch about 2 cm anterior to the anterior margin of the external auditory canal. Therefore, it is safe to make the skin incision along the anterior margin of the ear cartilage. The temporal and zygomatic rami of the ipsilateral facial nerve are usually well preserved by elevating the superficial temporal fascia together with the skin flap and subperiosteally dissecting the zygomatic arch and zygomatic bone.

Conclusions

An orbitozygomatic infratemporal approach to the parasellar region, including the CS, and interpeduncular fossa has been presented and evaluated. We believe that an orbitozygomatic infratemporal approach may provide a better anatomic assessment of the lesions in the parasellar region and interpeduncular fossa and their surrounding structures than the conventional approach. This operation, however, is technically more demanding because familiarity with the use of chisels and sagittal saw, in addition to microsurgical techniques, is essential to its execution.

KEY REFERENCES

Ammirati M, Spallone A, Ma J, et al. An anatomical study of the temporal branch of the facial nerve. *Neurosurgery.* 1993;33:1038-1043.

Bruder N, Ravussin P, Young WL, et al. Anesthesia for surgery of intracranial aneurysms. *Ann Fr Anesth Reanim.* 1994;13:209-220.

Chanda A, Nanda A. Anatomical study of the orbitozygomatic transsellar-transcavernous-transclinoidal approach to the basilar artery bifurcation. *J Neurosurg.* 2002;97:151-160.

Day JD. Cranial base surgical techniques for large sphenocavernous meningiomas [technical note]. *Neurosurgery.* 2000;46:754-759.

Hakuba A. Surgical approaches to the cavernous sinus via the medial triangle: report of an aneurysm at the C4–C5 junction of the internal carotid artery [Japanese]. *Geka Shinryo.* 1965;26:1385-1390.

Hakuba A, Liu SS, Nishimura S. The orbitozygomatic infratemporal approach: a new surgical technique. *Surg Neurol.* 1986;26:271-276.

Hakuba A, Matsuoka Y, Suzuki T, et al. Direct approaches to vascular lesions in the cavernous sinus via the medial triangle. In: Dolenc VV, ed. *The Cavernous Sinus.* New York: Springer-Verlag; 1987:272-284.

Hakuba A, Tanaka K, Suzuki T, et al. A combined orbitozygomatic infratemporal epidural and subdural approach for lesions involving the entire cavernous sinus. *J Neurosurg.* 1989;71:699-704.

Lemole Jr GM, Henn JS, Zabramski JM, et al. Modifications to the orbitozygomatic approach [technical note]. *J Neurosurg.* 2003;99:924-930.

Millesi H. Extratemporal surgery of the facial nerve—palliative surgery. In: Krayenbuhl H, et al. ed. *Advances and Technical Standards in Neurosurgery.* Vol 8. Vienna: Springer-Verlag; 1980:180-308.

Ohata K, Baba M. Orbitozygomatic infratemporal approach. In: Hakuba A, ed. *Surgical Anatomy of the Skull Base.* Tokyo: Miwa Shoten; 1996:1-35.

Ohata K, Baba M. Otico-condylar approach. In: Hakuba A, ed. *Surgical Anatomy of the Skull Base.* Tokyo: Miwa Shoten; 1996:37-75.

Ohata K, Hakuba A, Branco SJ. Development of the meninges: Application to microneurosurgery [Japanese]. In: Ishii R, ed. *Surgical Anatomy for Microneurosurgery.* Tokyo: SIMED Publications; 1997:58-64.

Sindou MP. Working area and angle of attack in three cranial base approaches: pterional, orbitozygomatic, and maxillary extension of the orbitozygomatic approach. *Neurosurgery.* 2002;51:1526-1527.

Takami T, Ohata K, Nishikawa M, et al. Transposition of the oculomotor nerve for resection of a midbrain cavernoma [technical note]. *J Neurosurg.* 2003;98:913-916.

Numbered references appear on Expert Consult.

Section Two

OPERATIVE TECHNIQUES IN PEDIATRIC NEUROSURGERY

KURTIS AUGUSTE

Methods for Cerebrospinal Fluid Diversion in Pediatric Hydrocephalus: From Shunt to Scope

AABIR CHAKRABORTY • JAMES M. DRAKE • BENJAMIN C. WARF

Introduction

DEFINITION AND EPIDEMIOLOGY OF HYDROCEPHALUS

Hydrocephalus is one of the more common neurologic sequelae following insult to the central nervous system. It can be congenital or acquired. The incidence of congenital hydrocephalus has been estimated to be 0.48 cases per 1000 live births,[1] whereas the incidence of neonatal hydrocephalus is 3 to 5 cases per 1000 live births.[2] Table 54-1 lists common causes of pediatric hydrocephalus.[3] Acquired causes of hydrocephalus include postintraventricular hemorrhage hydrocephalus, brain tumors, infections, and head injury.[3] An estimated 33,000 shunts are placed in patients of all ages annually in the United States, with an estimated shunt prevalence of more than 56,000 in children younger than 18 years.[4] In the United States, shunt placement accounts for 38,200 to 39,900 hospital admissions and 3.1% of all pediatric hospital charges ($1.4 billion to $2.0 billion).[5] Hydrocephalus has not been clearly defined but represents a disparity between production and absorption of cerebrospinal fluid (CSF), resulting in raised intracranial pressure with or without ventricular dilatation.

CLINICAL AND RADIOLOGIC FEATURES

The diagnosis of hydrocephalus is based on clinical features, radiologic appearances, and occasionally invasive intracranial pressure recordings. As seen in Table 54-2,[3] children most commonly present with symptoms of irritability, delayed development, and vomiting. For infants, examination often reveals an increasing head circumference and a bulging fontanelle. Seizures are an uncommon presentation. Papilledema, when present, is highly suggestive of raised intracranial pressure. Papilledema is not particularly sensitive for acute raised intracranial pressure but is specific. If seen, it is highly suggestive of raised intracranial pressure; however, it has been shown to be absent in 86% of patient with shunt blockage.[6] Sixth nerve palsy or loss of upward gaze may be a false localizing sign indicative of raised intracranial pressure.

Imaging that is commonly used in the primary assessment of a child with suspected hydrocephalus includes ultrasound, computed tomography (CT), and magnetic resonance imaging (MRI). The aim of imaging is to assist in the diagnosis and the etiology of hydrocephalus. MRI provides superior resolution to other imaging modalities and thus is useful when assessing the etiology of hydrocephalus. In addition, T2-weighted sequences such as fast imaging employing steady-state acquisition (FIESTA) and time-spatial labeling inversion pulse sequences[7] provide information of fluid movement within the ventricles.

Ultrasound through the open anterior fontanelle is quite practical in critically ill premature infants with intraventricular hemorrhage or in patients with myelomeningocele in whom the cause is not in doubt. In patients with mild ventricular enlargement, evidence of transependymal flow of CSF usually suggests that the process is more acute. Other signs of progressive hydrocephalus—enlargement of the temporal horns, dilation of the third ventricle, and effacement of the sulci—are not absolutely specific. In cases in which there is doubt, careful observation with serial images, rather than subjecting the patient to the known risks of shunt failure, is prudent.

The risk of radiation from CT has prompted increased interest in limited-sequence or "quick" MRI.[8] When evaluating patients with potential shunt dysfunction, brain imaging

Table 54-1 Common Causes of Hydrocephalus in 344 Pediatric Patients[3]	
Cause	**Patients**
Intraventricular hemorrhage	24.1%
Myelomeningocele	21.2%
Tumor	9.0%
Aqueduct stenosis	7.0%
CSF infection	5.2%
Head injury	1.5%
Other	11.3%
Unknown	11.0%
Two or more causes	8.7%
Total patients	99.0% (344)

Table 54-2 Presenting Clinical Features of Hydrocephalus in Pediatric Patients[3]

Symptoms	Children
Irritability	26.6%
Delayed developmental milestone	19.8%
Nausea or vomiting	19.0%
Headache	17.5%
Lethargy	17.5%
New seizures or change in seizure pattern	6.6%
Diplopia	5.8%
Worsening school performance	4.2%
Fever	2.6%
Signs	**Infants**
Increasing head circumference	81.3%
Bulging fontanelle	70.6%
Delayed developmental milestones	20.9%
Loss of upward gaze	15.8%
Decreased level of consciousness	12.6%
Other focal neurologic deficit	12.4%
Papilledema	12.0%
Sixth nerve palsy	4.6%
Hemiparesis	3.8%
Nuchal rigidity	1.8%

in conjunction with radiographs of the shunt tubing, known as a shunt series, should be obtained. A shunt series consists of two views of the head, neck, chest, and abdomen so that the whole shunt system is imaged. The current ventricular size in a patient with a possible shunt blockage based on contemporary imaging is not necessarily a good indicator of shunt blockage. Comparison to a previous scan when the patient was well with the same valve in place is far more reliable in terms of diagnosis of shunt blockage.

PHYSIOLOGY AND PATHOPHYSIOLOGY OF CSF CIRCULATION

Historically, it has been suggested that CSF is produced by the choroid plexus in the lateral and fourth ventricles, flows out through the foramina of Luschka and Magendie, and is absorbed by the arachnoid granulations near the venous sinuses. This model has been called into question for two main reasons:

- CSF radionuclide cisternography and MRI have not shown flow of CSF through the arachnoid granulations.[9]
- There is growing evidence in animal models (and human cadavers) that the nasal lymphatics may be the primary absorptive mechanism at normal pressure.[10]

Recently, there has been a different approach to the pathology of hydrocephalus.[9,11] The CSF can be seen as extracellular fluid. The choroid plexus is the driving force for circulating the CSF along the pathway described earlier, but the absorption and, to a lesser extent, the production occur in the subarachnoid spaces and Virchow-Robin spaces. Regional changes in capillary bed caliber and permeability may affect this absorptive mechanism. When an obstruction develops, be it at the level of the aqueduct, the fourth ventricle, or the arachnoid on the brain surface, the absorptive capacity is reduced; therefore, a higher hydrostatic pressure is required to reach equilibrium between

absorption and production. More research is required to substantiate these theories.

Treatment with Cerebrospinal Shunts
HISTORY OF SHUNTS

The history of hydrocephalus is a fascinating one and dates back to the dawn of civilization. A good summary of the history is presented by McCullough.[12] Early 20th-century attempts at achieving closed ventricular drainage included gold, glass, silver, and rubber tubes, as well as catgut and linen threads passed from the ventricle to the subdural space.[12-15] Similar techniques were used to connect the lumbar thecal sac to the peritoneum or renal pelvis.[16-18] After attempts at third ventriculostomy by Dandy[19] and by Mixter[20] and choroid plexectomy by Dandy,[21] shunts from the lateral ventricle to cisterna magna (Torkildsen shunts[22]) and shunts from the lumbar spine to the ureter came into more widespread use.

The treatment of hydrocephalus was revolutionized when Nulsen and Spitz[23] reported in 1952 the successful use of a ventriculojugular shunt using a spring and stainless-steel ball valves. The two valves were housed in rubber intravenous tubing, which acted as a flushing device, and connected to polyethylene tubing at either end. Unfortunately, occlusion of the venous catheter by blood clot was a frequent problem.

Holter's shunt was the first to use silicone, and he designed a multislit valve out of silicone for use in his son, who had developed hydrocephalus.[24] About the same time, Pudenz[25] concluded that silicone was the best material and designed two valves to use as ventriculoatrial (VA) shunts.

Surgical Technique: Initial Shunt Insertion

Shunt surgery is one of the most unforgiving types of surgery undertaken by the neurosurgeon. The vast majority of shunt complications are due to either blockage or infection. The incidence of these complications is largely related to factors that the surgeon can influence. Meticulous attention to detail and thorough planning of the procedure prior to surgery are likely to reduce shunt-related complications. There are many techniques for shunt insertion.

In essence, a shunt consists of a ventricular catheter, a valve, and a distal catheter, the purpose of which is to divert CSF from the ventricle to the another site capable of absorbing the extra fluid load. The most common locations for distal catheter insertion include the peritoneum (ventriculoperitoneal, or VP, shunts), the pleura (ventriculopleural shunts), and the right atrium (VA shunts).

This section details some principles of shunt surgery and then discusses in detail the steps involved in insertion of VP, ventriculopleural, and VA shunts.

PRINCIPLES

Once the decision to implant or revise a shunt is made, the surgeon should begin planning the procedure. Informed consent discussing the rationale for the procedure, the potential complications, and the potential outcome should be sought in a timely fashion prior to surgery. The surgeon should pick out the shunt hardware prior to surgery. The following are important patient factors to consider when planning:

1. The most appropriate site for insertion of the ventricular catheter. The scan should be inspected, and the most appropriate site should be determined. In general, most ventricular catheters are inserted via a parieto-occipital or frontal bur hole on either the right or the left side. The most appropriate choice out of these four sites is often related to the underlying pathology driving the hydrocephalus. For example, it would not be appropriate to insert a VP shunt into the contralateral side of a tumor causing mass effect and midline shift, because this may exacerbate the midline shift. For patients who have had a recent shunt infection, it is optimal to use an uninfected bur hole site.

2. The most appropriate site for insertion of the distal catheter. In general, the preferred location for the distal catheter is the peritoneum, followed by the pleura or right atrium. The latter two choices should only be entertained when there is clear evidence that use of the peritoneum is highly likely to result in malabsorption, infection, or abdominal content damage.

3. The most appropriate valve to implant. A valve is required to maintain one-way flow and prevent reflux. Avoiding overdrainage of CSF and gravity-dependent swings in intracranial pressure, the effects of which include low-pressure headache and subdural hematoma,[26-28] may also be accomplished to some degree. The most appropriate valve depends on a number of factors, including the age of the patient, what valve was used previously, the symptoms the patient exhibits, the number of previous shunt revisions, and whether having flexibility in the opening pressure is important. A more detailed account of the types of valve and the evidence pertaining to outcome based on valve choice is given in the next section. In general, patients should have the same valve reinserted if there were no clinical or radiologic problems before shunt dysfunction. For new shunts, the age of the patient is important. Neonates and young infants with open fontanelles have relatively low intracranial pressure compared to patients with a closed fontanelle. Hence, the valve inserted should allow drainage at lower pressures. We tend to implant medium-pressure valves in older children. Variable pressure valves are reserved for patients with complex shunt problems in whom the likely optimal intraventricular pressure based on history, examination, and investigations remains unclear.

4. Inspection of the site of the insertion of the ventricular and peritoneal catheter, as well as the proposed peritoneal catheter trajectory. Specific issues to consider include the site of previous incisions (avoid tunneling under scar tissue), the quality of skin (patients with multiple shunt revisions with large amounts of scar tissue and patients who have undergone radiotherapy are likely to be at higher risk of wound complications), the skin thickness (very young children with thin skin may require a low-profile valve and reservoir), and the presence of other devices such as central venous catheters, gastrostomies, Mitrofanoff devices, pacemakers, and other implanted devices may impede safe tunneling. The underlying pathology may also affect the bur hole site.

5. Evidence of concurrent illness. It is preferable to avoid inserting a VP shunt in the presence of infection elsewhere. In critically ill patients, even if their illness has been attributed to shunt malfunction, it may be more appropriate to insert an external ventricular drain (EVD). This gives the clinician a means for intracranial pressure measurement, allows intracranial pressure modulation by altering CSF drainage, and eliminates uncertainty whether the newly inserted shunt has failed if the patient fails to improve neurologically.

6. Past shunt history in patients who require a VP shunt revision. It is important to know what valve and shunt tubing were inserted previously, what difficulties were faced intraoperatively, and whether redundant shunt tubing was left in place and why. The last operation note, previous scans, and discharge summaries are invaluable pieces of information.

7. Need for assistance. If there has been a past history of bowel surgery, difficulty entering the peritoneum, or adhesions, consideration of performing the procedure with the assistance of a general surgical colleague is important.

VP SHUNTS

For a parieto-occipital VP shunt insertion, positioning is important. Once the patient is under general anesthesia and following administration of antibiotics on induction of anesthesia, we use the horseshoe headrest with a bolster placed under the shoulder ipsilateral to the ventricular catheter insertion site for positioning. The head is tilted such that the cranial incision site is accessible. This is usually achieved by rotation and lateral flexion of the neck to the contralateral side (Fig. 54-1A). This position is optimal for tunneling because it keeps the skin around the neck under some traction, provides a straight line from the cranial incision to the abdominal incision, and allows good access to the both abdominal and cranial incisions.

For patients in whom a laparoscopic peritoneal insertion with an abdominal trocar is being used, the bladder should be emptied. Hair is clipped (not shaved) in the operating room to prevent hair from becoming tangled within the wound. The site of the bur hole and abdominal incisions should be selected and marked before draping.

Many techniques have been described to determine the appropriate location for the bur hole.[29] For example many people measure distances from either the ear or the midline to approximate the site of the bur hole. Whichever method is chosen, it is important to correlate the projected bur hole location with the optimal location on the preoperative imaging. Measurements made from CT scan are probably more accurate than choosing the site of the bur hole based on arbitrary surface landmarks. It is important to obtain localization in two planes. The use of neuronavigation removes all guesswork in localization of the optimal bur hole location but may increase cost and time. Furthermore, rigid cranial fixation is usually required, and this can hamper tunneling. Newer neuronavigation techniques such as electromagnetic-based systems eliminate the requirement for head fixation in pins, thus allowing easier tunneling.[30]

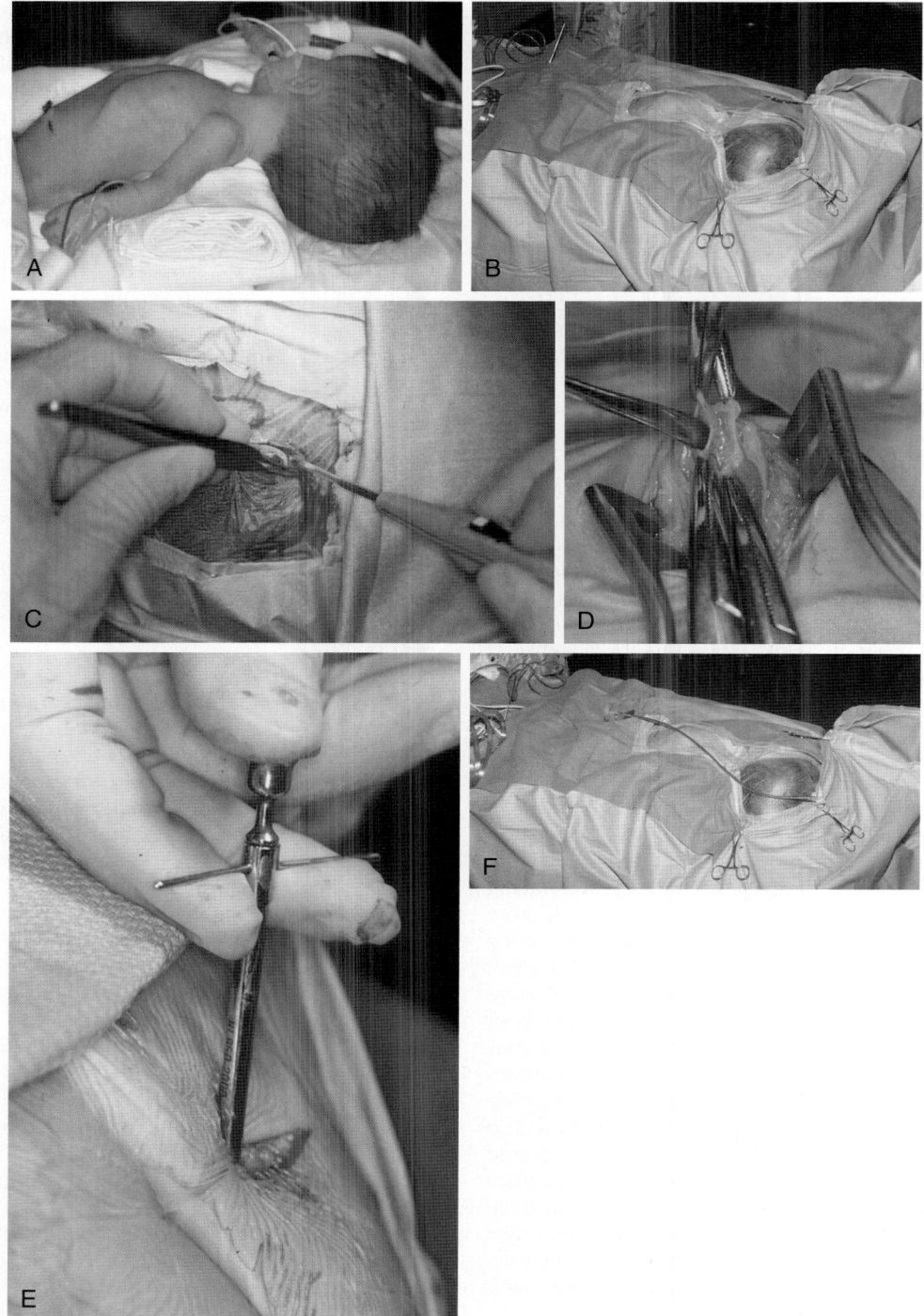

FIGURE 54-1 Sequential steps on shunt insertion. A, Patient positioning and marking of incisions. B, Draping. C, Making a small incision that will not cross over shunt equipment. D, Passing a blunt dissector into the peritoneal cavity. E, Using an abdominal trocar. F, A tunneling device.

Continued.

For frontal bur hole placement, the patient is usually positioned supine with the head tilted to the contralateral side. The bur hole site is usually just anterior to the coronal suture 2 to 3 cm from the midline (the midpupillary line is a good estimation). Preparation of a small intervening incision just posterior to the ear is important because it is usually required to tunnel through the subcutaneous tissue plane from the frontal region to the abdomen.

The skin is meticulously prepared with an antiseptic solution such as povidine–iodine or chlorhexidine. We use disposable, adhesive drapes to cover the patient and the operating table entirely, except for a small band of skin from the bur hole site to the abdomen (Fig. 54-1B). We use iodine-impregnated transparent adhesive drapes, although there is no evidence to suggest that shunt infection rates are reduced with this technique.

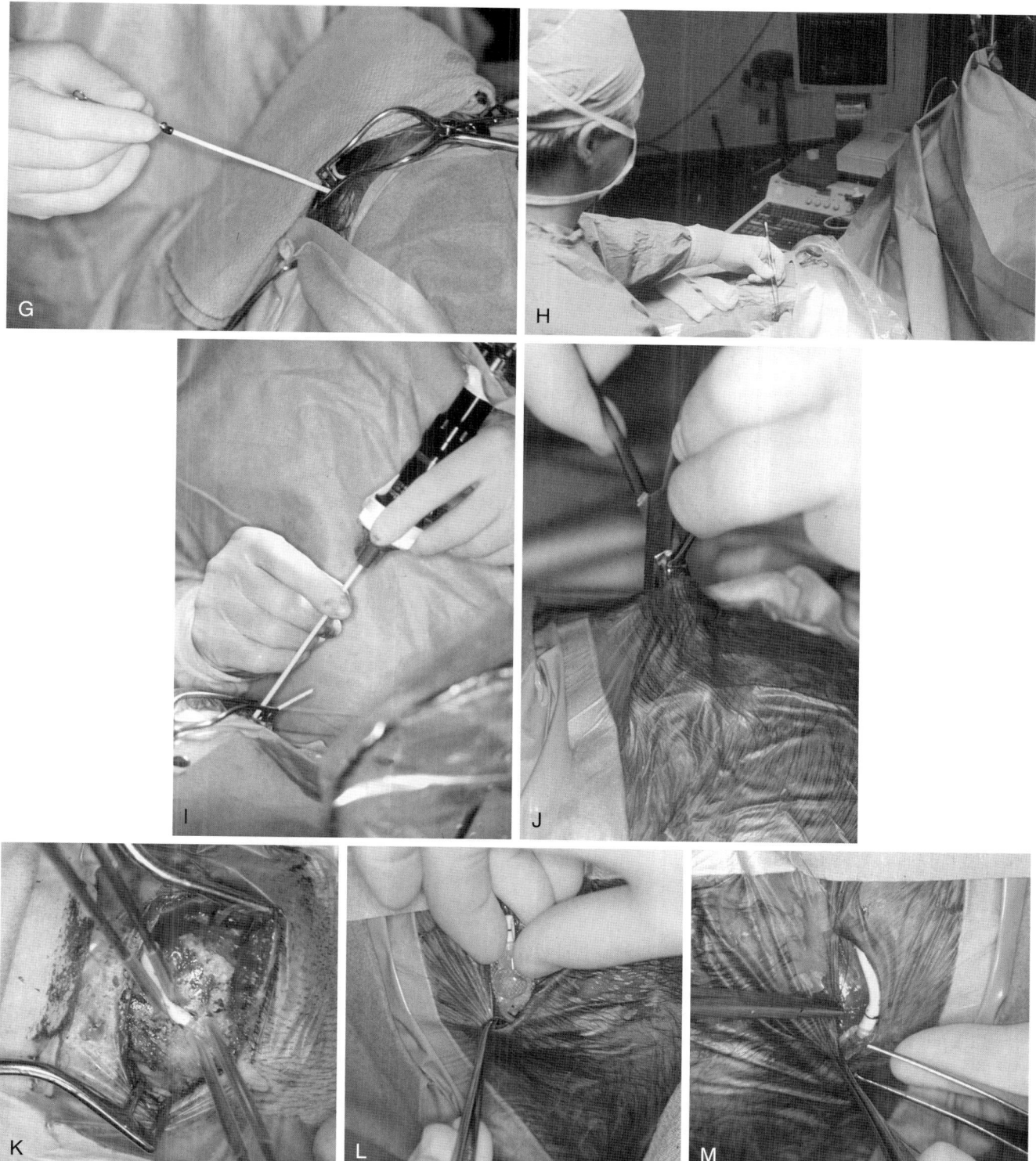

FIGURE 54-1, cont'd G, Cannulating the ventricle according to landmarks. H, Using ultrasound guidance to place the ventricular catheter. I, Using a shunt scope to place the ventricular catheter. J, Making the subcutaneous pocket for the valve. K, Silastic-sleeved forceps coaxing the tubing onto the connector. L, Placing the valve into its pocket. M, Suturing the valve to the pericranium.

During the "time out," we ensure that an appropriate dose of prophylactic antibiotics has been administered to achieve desired tissue concentrations and that we are operating on the correct patient, are operating on the correct side, and have the scans and equipment available. We do

not infiltrate the wound with local anesthetic mixed with adrenaline, because this has the potential to increase the number of punctures of the skin and reduce blood supply to the wound. We use a horseshoe incision (Fig. 54-1C) that has its pedicle based on the direction the shunt will initially be tunneled. It is important to keep this pedicle wide and large so that no shunt equipment lies under the incision and blood supply to the flap is not restricted. For frontal bur holes, this may mean an obliquely oriented pedicle.

The size of the bur hole should be adequate to insert the ventricular catheter. We insert all our ventricular catheters under direct, real-time ultrasound guidance so that the bur hole required is quite large and allows access to the probe and the ventricular catheter simultaneously.[31] In infants, particularly if premature, an opening between the splayed sutures at either frontal or occipital sites is often all that is required for dural access. A small dural incision just large enough to allow passage of the ventricular catheter is optimal, because this may reduce the risk of CSF extravasation into the subgaleal space. This is especially true in patients with thinned cortical mantle. The brain pia is cauterized and opened.

The abdominal incision is simultaneously opened by the second operator. There is no evidence that any specific location on the abdomen results in reduced complications. We avoid umbilical incisions because it is difficult to clean the umbilicus. The peritoneum should be approached by dissection in layers. It is vital to confirm that the peritoneum has been entered, for example, by observation of intraperitoneal contents such as bowel and liver, by flooding the field and watching fluid drain into the peritoneum, or by passing a blunt dissector into the abdominal cavity (Fig. 54-1D). The use of abdominal trocars to enter the peritoneum is a safe and acceptable technique, although we tend to ask our general surgical colleagues to assist when performing this maneuver (Fig. 54-1E).

Tunneling is a potentially dangerous maneuver. The aim is to ensure the tunneling device is subcutaneous throughout its course. There is no evidence that the direction of tunneling, be it cranial to caudal or caudal to cranial, affects complications. A preassembled valve and tubing may not pass in the direction required because you have tunneled in an incorrect direction; hence, planning is important. Potential errant entries while tunneling include the skin, the peritoneum and its contents, the pleural space and lung, the heart and the great vessels of the neck, and the skull base, including the foramen magnum. As a rule, the tip of the trocar should be palpable below the skin at all times and the tip should pass superficial to the ribs and the clavicle. A common site of resistance to tunneling is at the deep cervical fascia of the neck (Fig. 54-1F). If you feel excessive force is required to pass the tunneler, a separate incision should be made and retunneling should commence from that location. If passing to a frontal bur hole, an intervening incision is usually required behind the ear. When tunneling along the chest wall, especially in neonates, there is potential to affect ventilation. The anesthetist should be made aware when tunneling, and the time during which the tunneler is subcutaneous should be kept to a minimum. The peritoneal tubing, with the attached valve, is then passed along the tube, attaching suction to the distal end and irrigating. The valve should then be irrigated to fill it with fluid. It is important to connect the valve in the correct direction (according to manufacturer's instructions). We make a subcutaneous pocket to seat the valve (Fig. 54-1J).

The ventricular catheter trajectory is then determined according to external landmarks or using some form of image guidance, be it ultrasound or neuronavigation (Fig. 54-1G and H). From a frontal bur hole, traditional landmarks for the foramen of Monro are the intersection of the planes through the midline and just anterior to the external auditory meatus (or simply perpendicular to the skull). If the patient's head is tilted, these landmarks can be difficult to appreciate, so palpable electrocardiogram electrodes placed at these points prior to draping may be of assistance. From the occipital location, a target at the midpoint of the forehead just at the normal hairline ensures that the catheter proceeds into the frontal horn instead of the temporal horn. For frontal bur holes it is generally accepted that the optimal position of the ventricular catheter tip is just anterior to the foramen of Monro, whereas for occipital bur holes the optimal position is the atrium of the lateral ventricle. In both cases, it is optimal to have the tip of the catheter away from the ventricular walls or choroid plexus. Endoscopic insertion allows visualization of the ventricular catheter in real time (Fig. 54-1I).

The ventricular catheter can often be felt to "pop" once the ependyma is breached with a concomitant "gush" of CSF. This "gush and pop" can be visualized on ultrasound. Gently irrigating the catheter may show pulsatile CSF flow into and out of the catheter. Withdrawing vigorously may draw brain tissue into the catheter and plug the shunt and thus is not recommended. There is no evidence that multiple catheter passes affect outcome; however, making fewer passes is likely to result in having fewer complications. We believe that ultrasound guidance in real time may reduce the number of passes required, thus optimizing catheter position and potentially reducing operating time.

Iatrogenic intraventricular hemorrhage is an uncommon complication that usually occurs as a result of choroid plexus hemorrhage. If the CSF is quite blood stained, it may be more appropriate to convert the operation to an EVD and obtain an urgent CT scan postoperatively.

The ventricular catheter is then connected to the valve and ties are placed along any connections (Fig. 54-1K and M). The valve system is then positioned into the subcutaneous pocket that had been created (Fig. 54-1L). Once in place, the peritoneal catheter should be checked for spontaneous CSF flow. The surgeon should not close until it is clear that the shunt is working. If there is any doubt, the system should be disconnected to verify that both ends are patent.

The distal catheter is then inserted into the peritoneum, with the surgeon making sure that it enters easily and there is enough length to account for patient growth. If the catheter keeps backing out of the abdomen, it may be coiling up in the preperitoneal space or there may be abdominal adhesions. The abdomen is closed in layers, as is the cranial incision. We do not advocate closure of the peritoneum because this layer is often thin and does not contribute to preventing a hernia.

Skin closure is critical. Any CSF leak predisposes to wound breakdown or infection. The rate of shunt infection has been shown to be as high as 57.1% in the presence of perioperative CSF leakage.[32] We place an occlusive dressing on the wounds, particularly on young children, who may irritate or pick at their incisions.

Positioning in the postoperative period can be important. Premature infants may be particularly prone to skin ulceration if positioned with the full weight of the head on the valve hardware. In patients with large ventricles, early ambulation may predispose the patient to a subdural hemorrhage. In patients with high-resistance valves, placing them in an upright posture may promote CSF drainage and prevent accumulation under the skin. We allow patients to eat on completion of their surgery and clearance of anesthetics.

The postoperative hospital stay is typically 2 to 3 days. Intravenous prophylactic antibiotics are normally given preoperatively and sometimes postoperatively for two doses only. Shunted patients typically have rapid resolution of acute symptoms. In infants, a sunken fontanelle with standard valves is typical. Low-pressure headache can occur in older patients, particularly if the hydrocephalus is longstanding. Low-pressure headaches can be managed with bed rest, hydration, and simple analgesia. A postoperative scan is important to obtain as a baseline; however, the timing is up to the individual surgeon. Some evidence shows the ventricles do not reach their final size on average until 1 year of age.[33] We tend to scan immediately postoperatively, after 1 year, and then approximately every 5 years in asymptomatic patients.

VENTRICULOPLEURAL SHUNTS

Ventriculopleural shunts are an additional option for distal catheter placement. Contraindications include previous chest surgery and adhesions, active pulmonary disease including infection, and borderline pulmonary function in patients in whom a significant pleural effusion might push them into respiratory failure. Infants are more likely to develop a significant effusion temporarily. We recommend a preoperative chest x-ray and pulmonary function testing.

The pleural space can be entered at a variety of sites. A common site is along the anterior axillary line, in the fourth to sixth intercostal space on the right. A muscle-splitting approach along the upper border of the rib (to avoid the neurovascular bundle) reveals the translucent pleura and the lung moving with ventilation.

The pleura is opened sharply. There is no need to ask the anesthetist to collapse the lung; it moves away slightly because it usually is at subatmospheric pressure during inspiration and thus retracts slightly from the chest wall once the pleural space is opened. The distal catheter is then introduced gently and is carefully guided along the chest wall and away from the lung parenchyma. The catheter may need to be cut to avoid putting excess tubing, even allowing for growth, into the chest. A Valsalva maneuver by the anesthetist inflates the lung adequately. At that point, the site should be closed in three layers. Rapidly closing the muscles with a few sutures avoids further air entry into the chest.

A small pneumothorax is usually seen postoperatively on chest x-ray. It resolves over the next few days, whereas the CSF usually accumulates as a small pleural effusion. These patients must be monitored for any evidence of respiratory distress, with serial chest films and continuous oxygen saturation monitoring.[34,35] Usually, the intrapleural fluid disappears over the next several weeks. In patients in whom the pleural fluid progressively accumulates, leading to respiratory distress with significant shift of the mediastinum, percutaneous drainage of the fluid and accessing another site for the tubing are required.

VA SHUNTS

The right atrium is another alternative to the peritoneum for distal catheter placement. The aim is to place the distal catheter just above the right atrium. Atrial catheters have a slit valve to prevent reflux of blood up the tubing. The patient is placed in the supine position with the head slightly down to avoid air embolus. The anesthetist should be involved throughout the procedure because ventricular ectopic beats are commonly encountered. The ventricular catheter inserted as described in the preceding section. The distal catheter is tunneled to the neck area in the proximity of the site of insertion of the atrial catheter.

There are broadly two methods for performing the distal portion of the procedure: open or percutaneous. For an open procedure, a right-sided neck incision is made to expose the common facial vein, which is tied proximally and held with a stay suture distal to the venotomy site. The catheter is then advanced down the jugular vein into the superior vena cava. Fluoroscopy is used to identify the final position of the tip of the catheter.

The percutaneous method involves cannulating the subclavian vein under color flow Doppler ultrasound guidance. A Seldinger wire is then passed into the vein and progressed to the entrance to the right atrium. A dilator expands the entrance to the subclavian vein. Following this, a peel-away ventricular catheter is inserted. Under fluoroscopic guidance, the tip of the catheter is positioned just above the right atrium.[36] The atrial catheter is then connected with a straight connector to the distal catheter, and all incisions are closed in two layers.

OTHER SITES OF INSERTION

Other options include reinsertion into the peritoneum, insertion into the gallbladder,[37] insertion into the superior sagittal sinus retrograde to the direction of flow,[38] and use of the vascular surgeons to assist in insertion into another peripheral vein. We have limited experience in any of these techniques.

Evidence-Based Approach to Complication Prediction and Avoidance During Shunt Surgery

VP shunt surgery has a considerable long-term complication rate. The rate of shunt complications 1 month following insertion is 15%, rising to 25% after 1 year and reaching 34% after 5 years[39] (Fig. 54-2). This figure does not appear to have improved with time.[40] Failure rates in pediatric studies are even higher: 38% shunt failure rate at 1 year, going up to 48% at 2 years.[41] By far, the two most common complications are shunt blockage and infection. Much of the neurosurgical literature pertaining to shunt complications relates to these two complications.

A number of factors affect the shunt complication rate. These have been categorized as follows:

- Hardware issues
- Patient factors
- Surgical environment and surgical technique

The following sections discuss these three issues in greater depth, highlighting the current evidence on shunt-related complications.

ALL PATIENTS

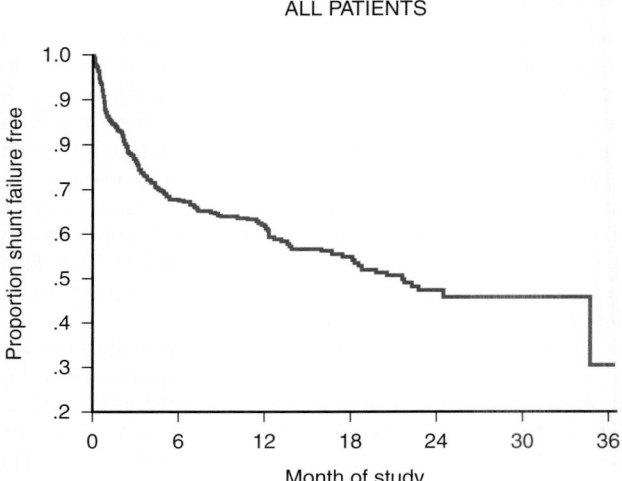

FIGURE 54-2 Pediatric shunt failure from the time of the first shunt insertion. Most failures occur within 6 months. The 2-year failure rate is 50%. *(From Drake JM, Kestle J, Milner R, et al. Randomized trial of cerebrospinal fluid shunt valve design in pediatric hydrocephalus. Neurosurgery 43:294-305, 1998.)*

HARDWARE ISSUES

The primary components of a VP shunt include a ventricular catheter, a valve, and a distal catheter.

Valve Selection

There are many shunt valves available on the market.[42] They can broadly be categorized into either pressure- or flow-regulated systems. Pressure-regulated valves are either open or closed to CSF flow, depending on the pressure across them (Fig. 54-3A and B). Pressure-regulated valves can be grouped into four design categories:

- Slit valves, where slits within tubing open when the pressure is high enough. This type of valve is commonly used when inserting lumboperitoneal shunts, such as the Spetzler lumbar peritoneal shunt system (Integra NeuroSciences, Plainsboro, NJ).
- Miter valves, where two opposing leaflets are in the closed or open position depending on the pressure differential. Examples include the Mischler Dual chamber valve (Integra NeuroSciences) and the UltraVS cylindrical in-line valve system (Integra NeuroSciences).
- Diaphragm valves, where a mobile flexible membrane moves in response to pressure changes. Examples include the Heyer-Schulte Pudenz flushing valve (Integra NeuroSciences).
- Metallic spring ball valves,[28] where a spring moves up and down depending on the pressure. Examples include the Miethke ProGrav valve (BBraun, Melsungen, Germany) and Polaris valve (Sophysa, Orsay Cedex, France).

The pressure at which valves open is termed the opening pressure and is fixed. Typically, there are low, medium, and high designations, which generally correspond to 5, 10, and 15 cm H_2O pressure, respectively, although there are no universal standards.

Flow-regulated valves work by reducing the caliber of the tube through which CSF flows when pressure increases but ensuring that some flow is maintained at all times.[43]

An example is the OSV II Orbis Sigma valve (Integra NeuroSciences) (Fig. 54-3C). This valve has a variable-diameter pin that partially occludes a ring whose position depends on the pressure. This alters the cross-sectional area through which CSF can flow. Thus, increased pressure would reduce the cross-sectional area; conversely, low pressure would increase it. The result is that, in an idealized system, the flow is constant irrespective of the pressure.

Measures to limit large changes in intracranial pressure based on the patient's position include siphon-reducing devices. Antisiphon devices have a mobile membrane that moves to narrow an orifice in response to a negative pressure inside the shunt system when the patient is vertical (Fig. 54-3B).[44,45] Examples are the antisiphon device and PS Medical Delta valve (Medtronic, Goleta, CA). Other valves try to reduce the effects of gravity by changing their configuration according to how they are positioned (Fig. 54-3D). In some designs, metallic balls rest on top of a standard spring ball valve to increase the opening pressure when the valve (and patient) is vertical. In another, a single metallic ball rests in an asymmetrical valve seat in upright position, increasing the resistance.

Programmable valves allow the opening pressure to be altered using an externally applied device. Examples include the Miethke ProGrav valve (BBraun), the Polaris valve (Sophysa), the PS Medical Strata valve (Medtronic), and the Codman Hakim valve (DePuy, Raynham, MA). Some factors that are important when evaluating these devices include the ease of assessing the pressure at which the valve is set and ease of altering the pressure. Many of these systems rely on a magnet to alter the setting, so the setting may need to be checked following an MRI (see individual manufacturer guides for details). The newer valves are MRI compatible, with a trade-off of increased difficulty in changing the setting.

Does the Chosen Valve Affect Patient Outcome?

It is generally accepted that a valveless shunt with the diameter of tubing commonly available can cause siphoning, leading to intracranial hypotension with the attendant risk of subdural hematomas. However, there is some evidence that the use of a valveless system with a small internal diameter of tubing and a longer length of tubing may act as a flow-controlled system that prevents overdrainage.[46] This mechanism by which overdrainage is prevented is similar to the mechanism by which a flow-regulated valve prevents overdrainage. This system exploits the Hagen-Poiseuille equation that states that the flow through a tube is inversely proportional to the radius of the tube,[3] the length of the tubing, and the viscosity of the fluid.

There is much debate about the efficacy of flow-controlled valves compared to pressure-controlled valves. Kan et al.[47] suggested that the incidence of slit ventricle syndrome (described in a later section) is lower in patients who have had a flow-controlled valve inserted compared to differential- and fixed-pressure valves; however, the diagnosis of slit ventricle syndrome was based on radiology, and clinical correlation was not performed. There is no compelling evidence that the shunt obstruction rate is related to whether a flow- or a pressure-controlled system is used.[3]

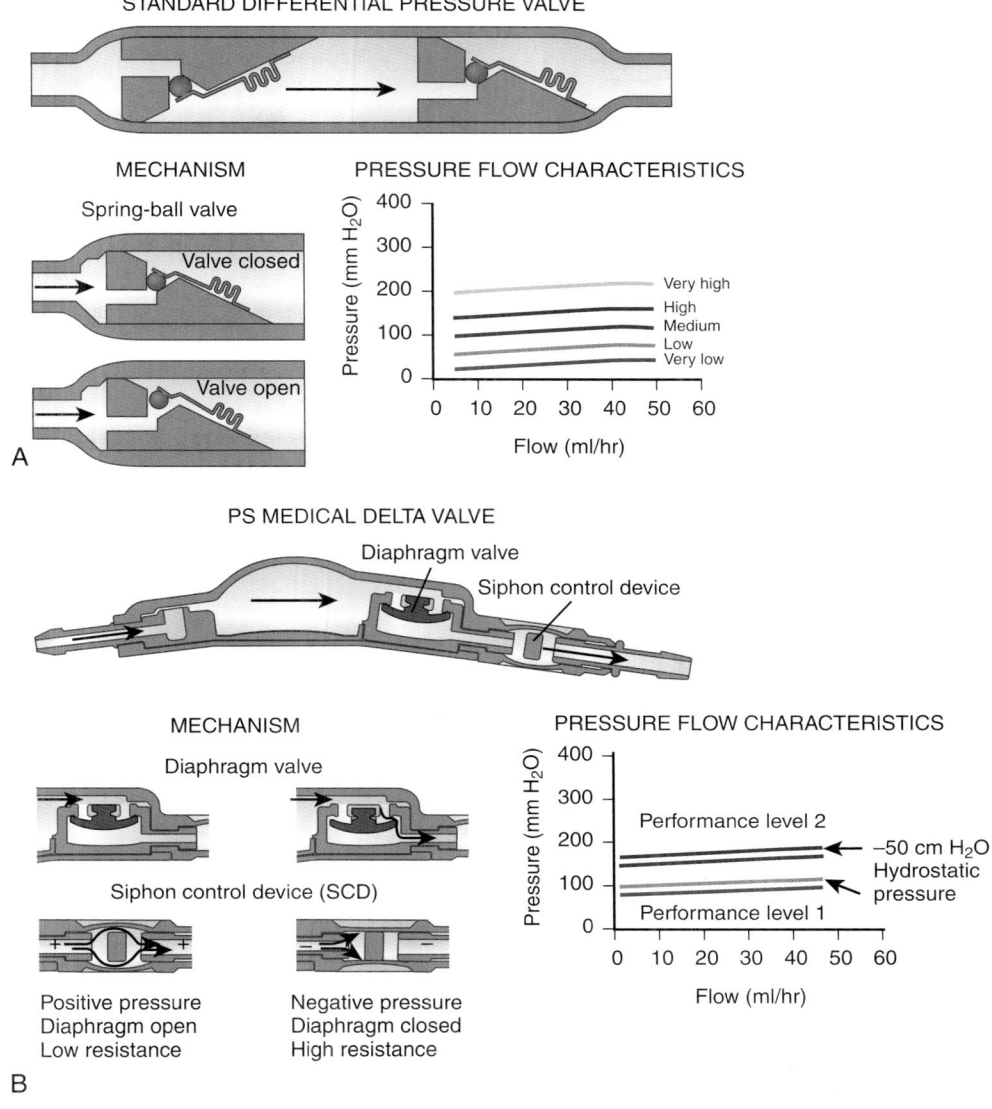

FIGURE 54-3 Shunt valve designs. A, Standard differential-pressure shunt, spring valve. Flow increases rapidly once opening pressure is exceeded. B, Siphon-reducing device distal to a standard differential-pressure valve, diaphragm type. The effects of gravity are reduced in the upright position.

Continued.

Ventricular and Distal Catheter Material Selection

The majority of shunt catheters are made from silicone rubber. During the manufacturing process, it is now possible to impregnate the catheter with other materials. The Codman Bactiseal catheter (DePuy) is a silicone rubber catheter impregnated with the antibiotics clindamycin and rifampin. Silver-impregnated polyurethane catheters (Silverline, Spiegelberg, Hamburg, Germany) are also available. In vitro testing of silver-impregnated catheters suggests that the silver prevents formation of bacterial colonies on the tubing, whereas antibiotic-impregnated catheters form a zone of inhibition of bacterial growth. It is thought that antibiotic-impregnated catheters prevent a bacterial biofilm from developing on the shunt tubing, thus preventing shunt infection.[48]

There are a number of ways of connecting the ventricular catheter to the distal system, including bur hole reservoirs, right-angle connectors, right-angle guides, and preshaped catheters. There are systems with a completely and partially unitized ventricular catheter, valve, and peritoneal catheter.

Does the Type of Catheter Affect Complications?

Numerous studies have investigated the efficacy of these catheters in prevention of infection. Table 54-3 lists many of the studies looking into the infection rate when different catheters are used. The results suggest that there may be a reduction in shunt infection rate when antibiotic-impregnated catheters are used; however, further studies are warranted to confirm this finding.

PATIENT FACTORS

Age appears to be a strong predictor of shunt-related complications. Table 54-4 shows the hazard ratio of shunt-related complications based on age in a cohort of 19,284 patients of all ages. The incidence of shunt-related complications in

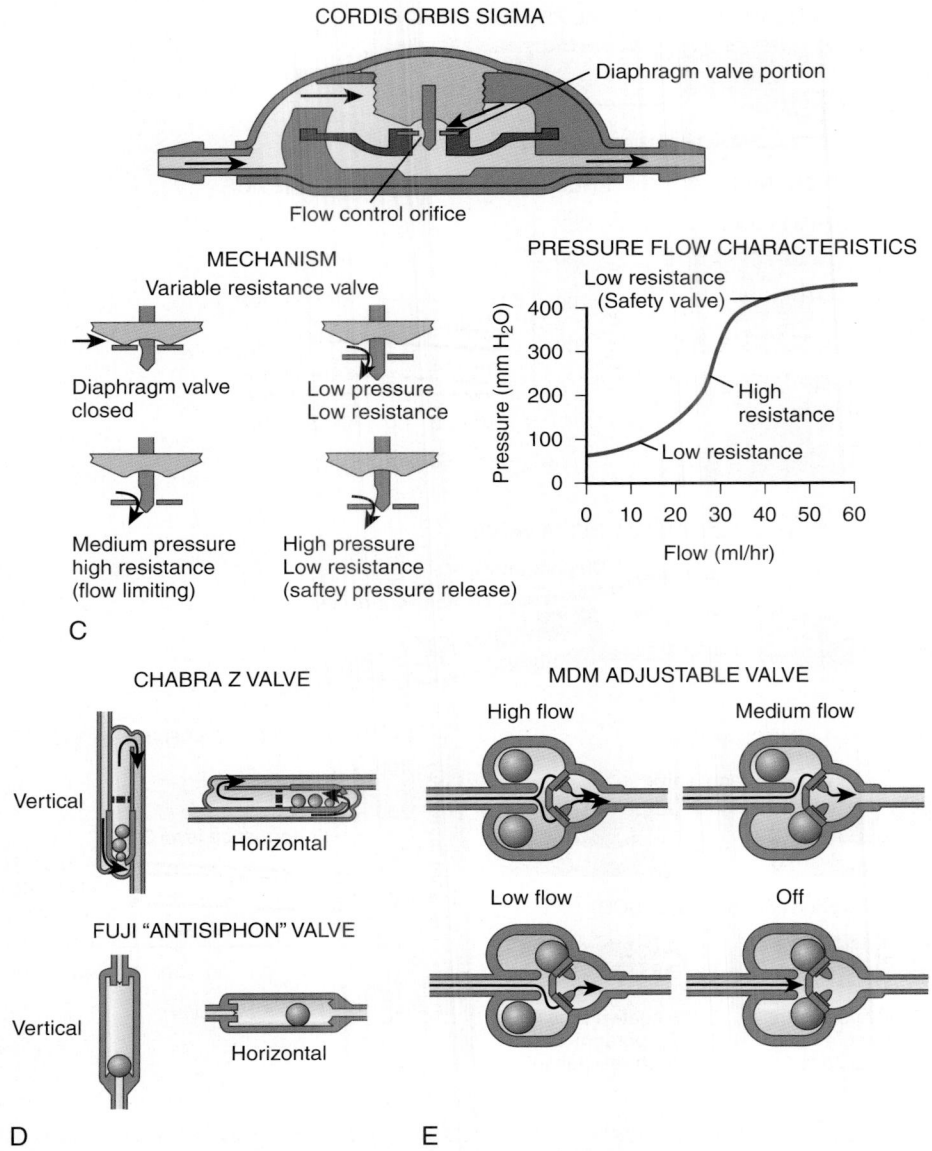

FIGURE 54-3, cont'd C, Flow-limiting valve with a variable-resistance orifice leading to flow limit, as seen in the flow–pressure curve. D, Two gravity-actuated devices that increase the opening pressure (above) or the resistance (below) in the vertical position. E, Percutaneous adjustable valve that can be completely occluded. (A to C, Drake JM, Kestle J. Determining the best CSF shunt valve design: The pediatric valve design trial. Neurosurgery 38:604-607, 1996. D and E, Drake JM, Sainte-Rose C. The Shunt Book. New York, Blackwell Scientific, 1995, p 1.)

children in this cohort was in the region of 48%, compared to 27% in adults.[39] Tuli et al. also found age to be a significant factor in shunt failure.[58]

The underlying etiology of hydrocephalus is also an important predictor of shunt-related complications. Common causes of hydrocephalus in the pediatric population include aqueduct stenosis, Dandy-Walker malformations, obstruction by tumor, postintraventricular hemorrhage of prematurity, and hydrocephalus associated with myelomeningocele.[59] Table 54-5 shows the incidence of shunt-related complications based on the condition warranting shunt insertion.

It has also been shown that the incidence of shunt failure is greater if multiple shunt revisions have been performed.

Shunts are also more likely to fail within 6 months of implantation.[33] The majority of patient risk factors for shunt failure are not alterable, so it is important for the surgeon to be aware of these risk factors when consenting patients.

SURGICAL ENVIRONMENT AND SURGICAL TECHNIQUE

The surgical environment has a great potential effect on the outcome of shunt surgery.

Surgeon and Surgical Experience

The number of shunt-related cases performed by the surgeon affects the incidence of complications. Smith et al.[60] studied the in-hospital mortality rates for patients undergoing

Table 54-3   Shunt Infection Rates of Standard Catheters versus Antibiotic-Impregnated Catheters

Study	Study Design (device tested, patient population)	Patients with Non-Antibiotic-Impregnated Catheter	Infection Rate	Patients with Antibiotic-Impregnated Catheter	Infection Rate	p Value
Zabramski et al. (2003)[49]	Randomized, controlled study in six centers (EVDs, adults)	139	36.7%	149	13.9%	<0.0012
Govender et al. (2003)[50]	Randomized controlled, study in one center (VP shunts, adults and children)	60	10%	50	3%	0.038
Sciubba et al. (2005)[51]	Retrospective, historically matched controls (VP shunts, children)	208	12%	145	1.4%	<0.01
Kan and Kestle (2007)[52]	Retrospective, historically matched controls (VP shunts, children)	80	8.8%	80	5%	0.534
Ritz et al. (2007)[53]	Retrospective, surgeon's preference (VP shunts, children and adults)	172	8.7%	86	9.6%	1.0
Hayhurst et al. (2008)[54]	Retrospective, historically matched controls (VP shunts, children)	77	10.4%	214	9.8%	0.884
Eymann et al. (2008)[55]	Retrospective, historically matched controls (VP shunts, adults and children)	120	5.8%	197	1.1%	0.01
Richards et al. (2009)[56]	National registry, matched control analysis (VP shunts and EVDs, adults and children)	1139	4.7%	1139	3.0%	0.048
Parker et al. (2009)[57]	Retrospective, historically matched controls (VP shunts, children)	570	11.2%	502	3.2%	<0.01

*Study design and infection rates from selected trials. The p value is in boldface if <0.05.

Table 54-4   Hazard Ratio for Shunt-Related Complications Based on Age on a Cohort of 19,284 Patients[39]

Age Group	Hazard Ratio	95% Confidence Interval	p Value
Adult	Reference	Reference	
Neonate	1.4	1.1-1.7	0.002
Infant	1.3	1.2-1.5	<0.001
Child	1.7	1.5-1.8	<0.001

VP shunt insertion or revision in the United States between 1998 and 2000. They observed that high-volume institutions (more than 121 admissions per year) had a lower in-hospital mortality rate compared to low-volume institutions (fewer than 28 admissions per year).

A number of studies have looked into the seniority of the surgical staff. Cochrane and colleagues demonstrated that the surgeon's experience significantly correlates to the survival of a VP shunt.[5,61,62] The so-called July effect, looking

Table 54-5   Shunt-Related Complications Based on the Etiology[5]

Condition	Shunt-Related Complication
Aqueduct stenosis	6.7%
Myelomeningocele	22.8%
Postintraventricular hemorrhage of prematurity	13.6%
Posterior fossa tumor	22.6%
Postinfection	4.8%
Congenital condition	10.8%
Post-trauma	2.3%

at whether the start of new residents and fellows within a particular unit affects shunt complications, has also been reviewed. Kestle et al.[63] showed a small detrimental effect in terms of shunt-related complications when new residents arrive to service.

Preoperative Prophylactic Antibiotics

There is some evidence that the routine use of perioperative antibiotic prophylaxis reduces the shunt infection rate. Haines and Walters[64] performed a meta-analysis demonstrating a 50% reduction in shunt infection when antibiotic prophylaxis was used. There is no evidence on which antibiotic is most appropriate; however, most units have a local policy.

Skin Preparation

There is no evidence that any particular skin preparation results in a lower shunt infection rate; however, Darouiche et al.[65] recently published a multicenter prospective, randomized, controlled study demonstrating reduced infection rates in clean, uncontaminated surgery (not including shunt surgery) when using chlorhexidine–alcohol compared to povidone–iodine.

Hair Shave

There is little evidence that shaving hair at the site of the procedure reduces infection rates.[66-68] Our policy is to clip hair minimally at the site of incision and to ensure that hair does not enter the sterile field, thus avoiding hair becoming tangled within the wound when closing.

Double-Gloving

The use of two pairs of gloves or a new pair of gloves when handling shunt hardware has not been proved in the literature to reduce shunt infection.[69] However, double-gloving is likely to reduce the incidence of glove perforations. Many surgeons elect to double-glove or change gloves, because this is an inexpensive maneuver that has the potential for reducing shunt infection.

Length and Position of the Ventricular Catheter

There is some evidence that the position of the ventricular catheter affects shunt survival. Tuli et al.[33] demonstrated that a ventricular catheter surrounded by CSF on a postoperative image had a significantly lower risk of blockage compared to a catheter tip touching the brain or completely embedded in parenchyma. Many surgeons suggest that the optimal position for a ventricular catheter placed from a parieto-occipital bur hole is in the atrium of the lateral ventricle and placed from a frontal bur hole is just above and in front of the foramen of Monro; however, individual factors such as the ventricular morphology should be accounted for. The optimal length of the ventricular catheter for frontally placed shunts has been said to be in the region of 5 to 5.5 cm, whereas the length for occipitally placed shunts is 5.5 to 6 cm. Again, however, the ventricular anatomy based on preoperative imaging should dictate the length of the catheter. There is little evidence that the incidence of shunt blockage is different when comparing a frontal to a parietal insertion.[70,71]

The site of the incision and the trajectory for cannulation of the ventricle have historically been based on surface landmarks. More recently, neuronavigation techniques have been increasingly applied, especially in the context of the patient with small ventricles.[72] Ultrasound is becoming more popular intraoperatively during shunt placement. Bur hole probes are commercially available, allowing for real-time insertion of ventricular catheters.[31] We hope that image guidance will improve catheter placement and thus reduce the shunt failure rate.

Placement of the Distal Catheter

A number of sites can be chosen for distal catheter placement, as mentioned previously, including the peritoneum, pleura, right atrium, and subgaleal space. Other sites rarely used include the superior sagittal sinus, gallbladder, and ureter.

The peritoneum over the right atrium has been the preferred site for distal catheter placement for a number of years. Borgberg et al.[73] demonstrated that the shunt revision rate was 51% for VA shunts, compared to 38.5% for VP shunts. Furthermore, the mortality rate of VA shunts has been quoted to be as high as 3%.[74,75] Complications specific for VA shunts include right-sided heart failure, venous thrombosis, chronic septicemia and shunt infection, intraoperative air embolus, and cardiac arrhythmias.

The pleural space is occasionally used for distal catheter placement; however, the absorptive capacity of the space is variable; thus, symptomatic pleural effusion is not an uncommon complication.

Ventriculosubgaleal shunts have recently had a resurgence in the context of posthemorrhagic intraventricular hemorrhage of prematurity with associated hydrocephalus.[76] Small studies suggest that the complication rate may be lower compared to the intermittent use of a ventricular access device.

Management of Shunt Complications

SHUNT BLOCKAGE

No data demonstrate a reliable relationship between the duration of shunt blockage and the speed of clinical deterioration of the patient. Some patients may have clinical symptoms for long before becoming unwell, whereas other patients become unwell quickly. The Birmingham, Alabama, group has analyzed their experience of shunt-related death.[77] Symptoms of raised intracranial pressure longer than 24 hours prior to death were present in at least 10 of the 28 patients who died. Of these, 5 patients had symptoms for 1 to 4 weeks. They also found that 8 patients died prior to arriving at the hospital. We find that, given that the duration of symptoms prior to a catastrophic event is variable in shunted patients, the safest approach is to review the patient as soon as possible. The Birmingham, Alabama, group's follow-up study also emphasizes the importance of patient education to prevent such events.[78]

The principles underlying the management of shunt blockage are to make the diagnosis, aim to identify where the blockage is likely to be, and then plan surgery to relieve the blockage by replacing the faulty components. Any obtunded patient with a shunt in situ requires careful evaluation for shunt blockage followed by clear objective evidence that a shunt blockage is not the cause for the reduced level of consciousness.

The diagnosis of shunt blockage is usually made on clinical evaluation combined with a CT/MRI scan and a shunt series (Fig. 54-4). Clinical history in a patient with shunt blockage may reveal symptoms suggestive of raised intracranial pressure. However, subtle deterioration in intellectual performance may be the only symptom of shunt dysfunction. Examination of the site of the shunt may provide some evidence of shunt dysfunction. Fluid around the ventricular site is indicative of proximal shunt blockage or of fracture/disconnection of the shunt apparatus, whereas fluid around the distal catheter and/or ascites is indicative of a CSF malabsorption process.

Although pumping of the shunt reservoir is a time-honored technique, this is often misleading.[79] Shunts whose reservoirs remain depressed for a long time raise the possibility of proximal shunt obstruction. However, this may simply represent a small ventricular size. A reservoir that is difficult to depress or refills apparently instantaneously frequently indicates a distal obstruction. Some shunt reservoirs contain proximal and distal occluders. By occluding the distal reservoir and depressing and allowing the reservoir to refill, we can infer that the proximal catheter is patent. Similarly, by occluding the proximal reservoir and flushing distally, we can confirm patency of the distal catheter.

Another commonly used preoperative method of shunt interrogation is tapping of the reservoir. Placing a small gauge butterfly needle connected to a manometer provides an evaluation of the pressure required for CSF to flow distal to the reservoir. The valve is usually distal to the reservoir, so we are, in effect, interrogating the valve and the distal tubing. Evaluation of the proximal catheter is more difficult and subjective and requires gentle aspiration of CSF from the butterfly needle. If flow is "easy," then the probability of a proximal shunt blockage is low. CSF can also be sent for

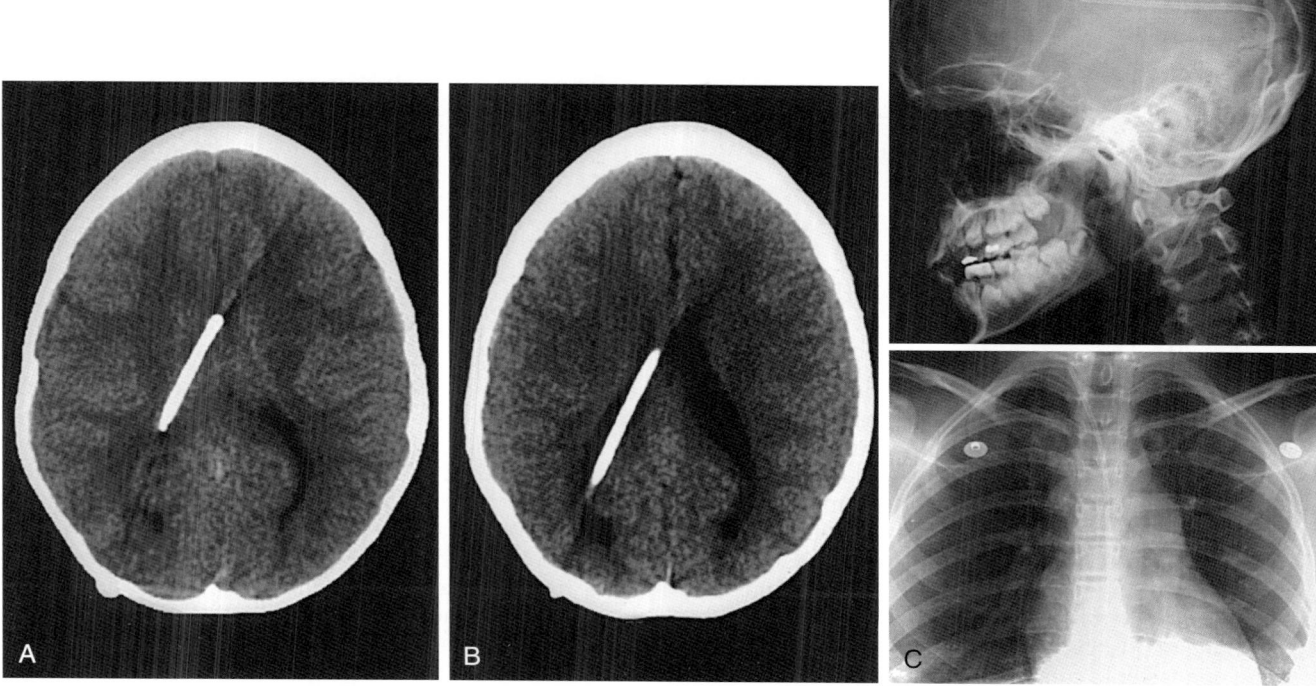

FIGURE 54-4 Diagnosis of shunt failure. A CT scan before (A) and after (B) shunt obstruction from a disconnection. The size of the ventricles in the scan in panel B appears normal, indicating the importance of a control CT scan when the patient is well. C, Plain films of the same patient showing a disconnection in the neck, which is a common site for this occurrence.

microbiologic examination in the process. The risks of this bedside procedure include introducing infection.

When operating on patients with shunt blockage, it is important to prepare and drape the abdomen, as well as the head, because the only definitive method for diagnosing shunt blockage is operation with the proximal catheter, valve, and distal catheter visible. For this reason, we usually open the cranial incision in the first instance. Careful dissection with the monopolar cautery onto the shunt tubing is an effective method for exposing the tubing without damage (Fig. 54-5A). The components are then systematically disconnected and interrogated. If there is no spontaneous flow from the proximal catheter, then a proximal blockage is diagnosed and the proximal catheter needs revision. It is preferable to remove the catheter and replace it with a new catheter. Often, especially when shunts have been in place for a long time, the ventricular catheter is quite stuck. The catheter should not be pulled out because this is likely to result in intraventricular hemorrhage. It may be possible to free the catheter by placing a stylet through the catheter and using the monopolar cautery to coagulate any choroid plexus occluding the holes at the tip while twisting the catheter (Fig. 54-5B). If this is not possible, the catheter should remain. If the ventricular catheter inadvertently slips into the ventricular system, an endoscopic approach is usually indicated to "fish" the catheter out. CSF should always be

obtained and sent for microbiologic examination for all shunt procedures.

For valve and distal catheter blockages, the component or components that are not functioning should be replaced. If the valve is to be replaced and the distal catheter is to remain, the wound needs to be extended to expose a length equivalent to the new valve to avoid kinking and coiling of the distal catheter. For distal revisions, great care must be taken if the same incision site in the abdomen is used because localized adhesions may be present, increasing the risk of bowel perforation.

VP SHUNT INFECTION

Shunt infection is a common complication of shunt surgery. A proportion of patients with shunt infection will have a blocked shunt; hence, it is important to consider shunt infection in anyone who presents with shunt blockage relatively early following VP shunt insertion. The majority of shunt infections occur within 3 months of the shunt surgery. The spectrum of clinical manifestations include the following:

- Wound infection: an incision or shunt tract with signs of inflammation, purulent discharge, and organisms seen on Gram stain or culture. Wound breakdown with shunt tubing exposed should be treated as a shunt infection.
- Meningitis: fever, meningismus, CSF leukocytosis, and organisms seen on Gram stain or culture.

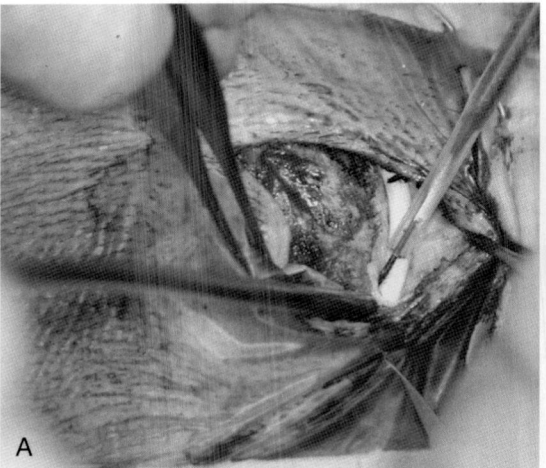 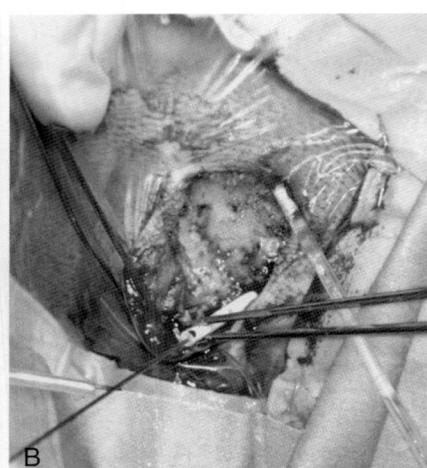

FIGURE 54-5 A, Dissecting the shunt apparatus during a shunt revision with a cutting cautery, which will not harm the Silastic material. B, Applying cautery to the ventricular catheter stylet to free a stuck ventricular catheter.

- Peritonitis: fever, abdominal tenderness (abdominal pseudocyst and abdominal abscess may present with mass with or without fever), and organisms seen on Gram stain or culture. For vascular shunts, findings are fever, leukocytosis, and positive blood culture, with or without evidence of shunt nephritis or cor pulmonale.
- Infected shunt apparatus: minimal signs of CSF contamination with bacteria recovered from purulent exudate in or on shunt material, Gram stain of CSF withdrawn from the shunt, or positive culture on fluid aspirated from the shunt under sterile conditions.[80]

One of the more common and difficult clinical situations to manage is the patient with a VP shunt who has a temperature. If the child is well, other more common causes of a temperature such as a urinary tract infection and upper respiratory tract infection should be excluded. Routine blood tests may reveal a polymorphonuclear leukocytosis and a raised C-reactive protein. Culture of the urine or other obvious sites of infections, for example, the wound, should also be taken. In the absence of another source or in an unwell child, it is prudent to perform a shunt tap as described earlier to diagnose whether the shunt reservoir can be performed preoperatively or by obtaining CSF intraoperatively. In most cases, CSF should be sent for cell count, Gram stain, culture and sensitivity, glucose, and protein. Shunt aspiration should be done using an aseptic technique so as not to iatrogenically contaminate a shunt system. Shunt aspiration provides a high diagnostic yield of shunt infection of approximately 95% and is quite safe.

The most common organisms infecting CSF shunts are staphylococci. Approximately 40% of shunt infections are caused by *Staphylococcus epidermidis* infections and 20% by *S. aureus*.[81-83] Other species isolated from infected shunts include the coryneforms, streptococci, enterococci, aerobic gram-negative rods, and yeasts. *Propionobacteria acnes* is a relatively common organism causing shunt infection but requires prolonged culture to diagnose.[84] We recommend anaerobic culture with prolonged incubation. Because these organisms are commonly part of the normal skin flora, and shunt infection usually occurs within 2 months of surgery, endogenous spread from the patient or surgical staff is the logical route of infection. Most surgeons would agree that a relatively early shunt infection (i.e., within 6 months of insertion) is seen as a surgical complication.

Bacteria colonize the shunt in the form of a continuous biofilm. This biofilm is composed of bacterial cells, either singly or in microcolonies, all embedded in an anionic matrix of bacterial exopolymers and trapped macromolecules.[85] The biofilm offers protection against many common antibacterial agents, including antibodies, white blood cells, surfactants, and antibiotics. For this reason, treatment of shunt infections by the exclusive use of systemic or intraventricular antibiotics[82,86] has been generally ineffective, although a recent report in patients without *S. aureus* infections had reasonable resolution if infections with intraventricular antibiotics were injected into a separate CSF reservoir.[87]

It has been shown that shunt removal with interval antibiotic treatment (usually with EVD) carries the highest shunt infection cure rate and the lowest mortality rate.[88] CSF shunt removal with immediate replacement carries an almost equal shunt infection cure rate and a higher morbidity and mortality rate. Antibiotic treatment alone has the lowest cure rate and the highest mortality rate. Continuous discussion with the microbiology/infectious disease team members throughout treatment is important. They should advise on isolation of the organism, the appropriate antibiotic based on sensitivity testing, the duration of antibiotic treatment, and when it is appropriate to internalize the shunt. Intrathecal administration is commonly instituted in many units. It is important to ensure that the person administering the antibiotics has been appropriately trained.

When reinserting a VP shunt following shunt infection, we tend to prefer inserting the ventricular catheter in a site that has not been operated on.

INTRA-ABDOMINAL PATHOLOGY

Contamination of the shunt can occur from other general surgical procedures,[82] such as insertion of a gastrostomy with peritoneal shunts. If a patient presents with obvious peritoneal sepsis (e.g., ruptured appendicitis or perforated bowel), it is generally accepted practice to externalize the shunt by making an incision over the chest wall (i.e., distal to the valve) and connecting the catheter to an external ventricular drainage system. When performing this procedure, the level the drain should be placed at is 0 cm above the foramen of Monro because the valve will still be functioning. Reinternalization should be performed only when the intra-abdominal sepsis has been eradicated. If there is a high chance of bowel adhesions, it may be more prudent to convert to a ventriculopleural or VA shunt. When reinternalizing a distal catheter, it is important to retunnel from an area proximal to the exit site, usually the valve, and to use new catheter tubing. This approach can be applied for the unusual complication where the shunt migrates through the bowel wall and out through the anus.

Patients with VP shunts occasionally present with abdominal swelling. Ultrasound and/or CT may demonstrate intra-abdominal pseudocysts. In this scenario, there is a high chance that a low-grade pseudocyst infection is present. The principles of management include making the diagnosis and treating the infection. The shunt can be externalized over the chest wall and the pseudocyst drained by aspirating from the distal catheter. The fluid should be sent for microbiologic examination, and antibiotic therapy should be initiated. Once the sepsis has been treated, reinsertion at another site, including another part of the abdomen, is appropriate.

SHUNT OVERDRAINAGE

CSF overdrainage occurs relatively commonly following shunt insertion. Patients with shunt overdrainage may complain of postural headache, lack of energy, and "feeling washed out." Causes of overdrainage include valve dysfunction or selection of a valve that is inappropriate for that patient. The complication of subdural hematoma is often associated with overdrainage. Treatment involves increasing the pressure in a programmable valve or upgrading to a higher pressure valve. Large subdural hematomas should be treated surgically in the appropriate fashion, in combination with a valve change.

SLIT VENTRICLE SYNDROME

A consequence of chronic overdrainage is slit ventricle syndrome. Nomenclature in the literature is confusing. Some authors define the condition as small ventricular size associated with symptoms of intermittent shunt blockage. When the ventricles are very small, the shunt blocks. As the ventricles expand, the shunt unblocks, thus creating a cycle of intermittent shunt blockage.[89] A product is noncompliant ventricles. There are three theories as to the pathogenesis of noncompliant ventricles; however, it is likely that the true pathophysiology involves more than one mechanism. The first is that ventricular pressure is intimately related to intracranial venous pressure and when CSF pressure drops, uncoupling occurs. This leads to increased venous congestion and increases brain elasticity. The second is that increased pressure with subependymal flow can cause subependymal gliosis and periventricular gliosis with increased ventricular wall stiffness. If this happens, intraventricular pressure would need to be higher than usual to obtain ventricular dilatation. The third proposed mechanism is that low-pressure valves in neonates lead to overshunting with radiologic slit ventricles, the development of microcephaly, and synostosis. This in turn predisposes the ventricular catheter to obstruction and prevents the ventricles expanding in response to obstruction.

This group of patients is among the most difficult to manage. They can be difficult to diagnose because their ventricles do not change significantly in size when the intraventricular pressure is high. The principles of management of a patient with slit ventricles and possible features of shunt blockage include accurate characterization of the intracranial pressure. Careful evaluation of the CT scan may demonstrate subtle changes suggestive of raised pressure, such as reduced CSF over the hemispheres. Intracranial pressure (ICP) monitoring, although invasive, is often required and is the gold standard investigation in the assessment for potential shunt malfunction in the context of complex hydrocephalus. Another recognized technique is to externalize the VP shunt and modulate the pressure according to symptoms. ICP monitoring, if performed, should be continued for 24 to 48 hours, in conjunction with a headache and activity diary, and should be maintained during sleep.

Treatment usually involves shunt revision. Variable pressure valves are often used in this instance so that the pressure can be altered with ease. CSF flow-limiting valves, such as the Orbis Sigma, may also normalize intracranial pressure, possibly by improving intracranial compliance. Intraoperative image guidance is important because the ventricular size is often so small. In cases where multiple shunt revisions have been performed, subtemporal decompression has been shown to be effective. By removing bone (in effect creating a new fontanelle), the defect can act as an alternative pressure relief valve to the shunt, thus increasing intracranial compliance. Endoscopic third ventriculostomy (ETV) and cranial vault expansions have also been attempted.

MANAGEMENT OF PATIENTS WITH ISOLATED VENTRICLES

An additional challenge to managing a patient with hydrocephalus occurs when the ventricular system is not one contiguous fluid compartment. This situation occasionally occurs following treatment of ventriculitis or meningitis, but similar principles apply to the management of arachnoid cysts compressing specific parts of the ventricular system. We tend to manage these patients with a combination of endoscopic fenestration of cysts and VP shunting. The aim is to drain as many cysts with as few ventricular catheters as possible. Endoscopic fenestration of the septum pellucidum is a useful method for allowing communication between the two lateral ventricles in the presence of obstruction at the foramen of Monro.

COMATOSE PATIENTS WITH FIXED, DILATED PUPILS

Patients presenting in coma are fortunately a rare occurrence; however, when seen, management must be prompt. A large bore spinal needle can be placed through the bur hole along the presumed trajectory of the ventricular catheter if the patient is in extremis. Patients presenting in coma should have an EVD inserted, rather than a shunt revision, because if the patient has a VP shunt revision and does not come out of coma immediately, it is difficult to ascertain whether the prolonged coma is caused by blockage of the new shunt or the neurologic damage from the initial presentation was so severe to keep the patient in a comatose condition.

HEADACHES IN PATIENTS WITH VP SHUNTS

Headaches are common in patients with VP shunts. There are numerous causes for headaches, and not all headaches are related to the shunt. A detailed history and examination are often necessary. Options for investigation to exclude shunt malfunction include CT, MRI, shunt series, shunt tapping and manometry, altering the valve setting, headache diaries, and ICP monitoring. In the absence of any objective evidence of shunt dysfunction, it is appropriate to refer the patient to your neurology and pain services.

Endoscopic Third Ventriculostomy

HISTORY

The earliest endoscopic treatment for hydrocephalus was choroid plexus fulguration performed by Lespinasse in 1910.[91] Dandy[92] subsequently described an open technique for third ventriculostomy for the treatment of noncommunicating hydrocephalus. A percutaneous ventriculostomy technique using an endoscope was first described by Mixter in 1923.[20] Fay and Grant[93] published the first intraventricular photographs that same year, providing the first visual record of endoscopic anatomy. Because of the limited illumination and large size of early endoscopes, open ventriculostomy procedures, as well as percutaneous fluoroscopic and later CT-guided techniques, remained popular for many years. Johns Hopkins provided the technical advances necessary for the revival of neuroendoscopy.[94] Hopkins' innovative solid-rod lens and coherent quartz fiber lens systems underlie the basic design of all modern rigid and flexible endoscopic systems. The improved optics and illumination and reduced size of modern endoscopes have greatly increased their utility and reduced their associated morbidity and mortality.

PATIENT SELECTION

ETV has been intended to treat noncommunicating hydrocephalus with patent subarachnoid spaces and adequate CSF absorption. Results of ETV have been related to the cause of hydrocephalus encountered, as well as clinical and radiographic features of the individual patient. Table 54-6 lists causes of obstructive hydrocephalus classified according to reported success rates of ETV (see the later section on outcome). Patients with acquired aqueductal stenosis or tumors obstructing third or fourth ventricular outflow have demonstrated the highest success rates, exceeding 75% in carefully selected series of patients.[95-98] Previously shunted patients with or without myelomeningocele and patients with congenital aqueductal stenosis or cystic abnormalities leading to obstruction (i.e., arachnoid cyst or Dandy-Walker malformations) have shown intermediate responses.[96,97,99-101] Infants presenting with hydrocephalus associated with myelomeningocele, hemorrhage or infection have generally demonstrated poor response to ventriculostomy,[94,102,103] and despite limited reports of success in such patients,[97,99,100,104-107] they have been more controversial candidates for this procedure. The procedure is not advisable in patients who have undergone prior radiation therapy because of the extremely poor response rates, altered anatomy (i.e., thickened third ventricular floor), and increased risk of bleeding.[97,99,103]

Table 54-6   Ventriculostomy Success Rates by Hydrocephalus Cause

High Success Rates (≥75%)
Acquired aqueductal stenosis
Tumor obstructing ventricular outflow
· Tectal
· Pineal
· Thalamic
· Intraventricular

Intermediate Success Rates (50%-70%)
Myelomeningocele (previously shunted, older patients)
Congenital aqueductal stenosis
Cystic abnormalities obstructing CSF flow
Arachnoid cysts
Dandy-Walker malformation
Previously shunted patients with difficulties
Slit ventricle syndrome
Recurrent or intractable shunt infections
Recurrent or intractable shunt malfunctions

Low Success Rates (<50%)
Myelomeningocele (previously unshunted, neonatal patients)
Posthemorrhagic hydrocephalus
Postinfectious hydrocephalus (excluding aqueductal stenosis of infectious origin)

Several clinical features influence the outcome of ETV (Table 54-7). There appears to be a significant association between increasing patient age and a more favorable outcome.[96,97,99,108] Evidence suggests that this association applies to the age at which hydrocephalus initially developed, as well as the age at the time of ventriculostomy.[97,108] Several studies show success rates of approximately 50% in patients younger than 2 years, regardless of cause.[96,97,100] Results have been reported as even poorer in patients younger than 6 months.[108]

In recent years, the value of endoscopic treatment for hydrocephalus in the developing world has been demonstrated.[109-115] Given the obstacles to urgent access for treatment of shunt malfunction in this environment, shunt dependence is more dangerous in the context of the developing world.[109] However, the low success rate for treatment of infant hydrocephalus by ETV alone has been problematic. The addition of bilateral lateral ventricle choroid plexus cauterization (CPC) to the ETV procedure has significantly increased the likelihood of success for endoscopic treatment of infant hydrocephalus regardless of etiology, thus expanding the applicability of endoscopic treatment for infants in this setting.[110-112] In the extensive experience from Uganda, combined ETV/CPC has been successful in treating hydrocephalus among infants younger than 1 year with postinfectious hydrocephalus (62% success), hydrocephalus associated with myelomeningocele (76% success), and other hydrocephalus of noninfectious origin (72% success). The role of ETV/CPC in treating posthemorrhagic hydrocephalus of prematurity is not apparent from the East African experience, but this is currently under investigation in the United States where, unlike Africa, this is a common cause of infant hydrocephalus.

Many studies had demonstrated a trend toward more successful ventriculostomy outcome in patients with

Table 54-7 Favorable Clinical and Radiographic Features for ETV

Clinical

Cause of hydrocephalus in high or intermediate success group (see Table 54-6)

Age >6 months at time of hydrocephalus diagnosis

Age >6 months at time of procedure

No prior radiation therapy

No history of hemorrhage or meningitis

Patient previously shunted

Radiographic

Clear evidence of ventricular noncommunication

Obstructive pattern of hydrocephalus

Aqueductal anatomic obstruction

Lack of aqueductal flow void on T2-weighted MRI

Favorable third ventricular anatomy

Width and foramen of Monro sufficient to accommodate endoscope

Rigid >7 mm

Flexible >4 mm

Thinned floor of third ventricle

Downward bulging floor draped over clivus

Basilar posterior to mammillary bodies

Absence of structural anomalies impeding procedure

AVM or tumor obscuring third ventricular floor

Enlarged massa intermedia

Insufficient space between mammillary bodies, the basilar, and the clivus

Basilar artery ectasia

AVM, arteriovenous malformation.

existing shunt systems.[96,100,108] Indeed, ETV has been found to be useful in the treatment of intractable shunt infections and malfunctions and even slit ventricle syndrome refractory to other treatments.[95,99,116-120] However, other series of ventriculostomy in previously shunted patients have been less promising.[101,113] These contradictory results may reflect the mix of patients in small series. An improved outcome in previously shunted patients was attributed by some to increased CSF absorptive capacity; however, the effect of the shunt itself on CSF absorption is difficult to distinguish from the effect of increased age in these patients. More recently, a history of prior shunt dependence was found to be an independent risk factor for ETV failure in the analysis of a large database from developed countries.[114]

Formalized methods for predicting the likelihood of ETV success, and thus for improved patient selection, have been recently reported.[114,115,122] An ETV success score based on a large database from developed countries incorporates the parameters of age, etiology, and previous shunt.[114] Another success score developed from the Ugandan experience is based on age, etiology, and the extent of CPC as variables that independently influence outcome.[115] The presence of scarring in the prepontine cistern has been shown to independently double the risk of ETV failure, whereas an open aqueduct has been shown to increase the risk of failure by 50%.[123] Where available, MRI FIESTA (constructive interference in steady state) imaging may prove useful in defining the status of the cistern and of the cerebral aqueduct preoperatively.

Table 54-7 also depicts preoperative radiographic criteria that have been frequently cited for improving outcome and limiting morbidity of ETV. Preoperative MRI optimally demonstrates all relevant anatomic features and should be obtained for all proposed ETV patients. Initially, confirmation of noncommunicating hydrocephalus of favorable cause should be established by the pattern of ventricular dilatation. Anatomic obstruction of CSF pathways between the aqueduct and the fourth ventricular outflow foramina may be visible on T2- or T1-weighted images. Additionally, T2-weighted images may reveal absence of the aqueductal CSF flow void frequently present in normal individuals. Extraventricular sites of obstruction, such as posterior fossa arachnoid scarring, may also cause noncommunicating hydrocephalus.[124] In addition, ETV has been reported to successfully treat cases in which ventricular outlet obstruction is not apparent, such as idiopathic normal pressure hydrocephalus, as well as communicating hydrocephalus secondary to trauma, hypertensive intracranial hemorrhage, tuberculous meningitis, and subarachnoid hemorrhage.[125-129] Given the significant risk of ETV failure in the face of prepontine cistern scarring,[123] preoperative MRI with FIESTA sequences may prove useful in refining patient selection.

Once the patient's suitability for the procedure has been established, the neurosurgeon must clarify the details of third ventricular anatomy that are likely to affect morbidity. First, the width of the third ventricle and diameter of the foramen of Monro must be sufficient to accommodate the endoscope of choice (see the later section on technique). Additionally, the thickness of the third ventricular floor and the anatomy of the proposed puncture site in relationship to vital structures, particularly the basilar artery and its branches, must be assessed. A downward-bulging third ventricular floor draped over the clivus has been cited as a prerequisite for this procedure in the past, but others have not found this to be necessary.[97,103] Ultimately, the surgeon must be satisfied that there is no structural lesion (i.e., tumor or arteriovenous malformation) or anatomic variation that would render the procedure unduly difficult or hazardous. In cases of doubt, it is reasonable to visualize the floor of the third ventricle and abandon the procedure if the floor is unsuitable.

TECHNIQUE

An ever-increasing variety of endoscopic equipment is available for neuroendoscopic procedures. For uncomplicated ETV, a 0- or 30-degree rigid scope is most commonly used. This offers superior optics and anatomic orientation. The Gaab endoscope (Johnson & Johnson, Randolph, MA), inserted through a 7-mm rigid cannula, provides the advantage of two working ports with a third for continuous irrigation. A 3.7-mm flexible steerable endoscope (Karl Storz, Tuttlingen, Germany) introduced through a No. 12 French peel-away sheath allows improved maneuverability within the ventricular system, at the expense of some image quality. Alternatively, this endoscope can be passed directly into the lateral ventricle without the use of a sheath in infants with a thin cortical mantle. In addition to performing the ETV, flexible scopes are useful for accessing more remote portions of the ventricular system (i.e., pineal recess or aqueduct), as well as for bilateral cauterization of the lateral ventricular choroid plexus. Several miniature fiberoptic endoscopes are also now available. These scopes can be inserted through a standard ventricular catheter; however, their inferior optics and lack of an irrigating or working channel limit their potential applications (i.e., ventricular catheter placement).

A miniature video camera is attached to the endoscope, and orientation is adjusted before insertion. The monitor should be placed at a comfortable distance and height for viewing throughout the case. Use of the camera allows the senior surgeon, trainee, and operating room staff to view the entire procedure, greatly enhancing the opportunities for learning without added morbidity. Newer cameras have digital filters that can be used to "clean up" the picture when flexible fiberoptic scopes are being used.

Adequate continuous or intermittent irrigation is imperative for proper visualization, particularly if bleeding is encountered. This irrigation is provided by body temperature Ringer's lactate solution. An uninterrupted release pathway for irrigation fluid is essential to avoid dangerous elevations of intracranial pressure. A separate channel for fluid release can be intermittently or partially blocked to provide transient pressure tamponade for control of bleeding. Direct, gentle pressure using the scope cannula itself, the tip of an instrument such as a Bugby wire, or a balloon compression catheter can also be useful for hemostasis.

ETV can be performed with either a flexible or a rigid endoscope. The patient is positioned supine in a horseshoe headrest with the neck flexed 15 to 20 degrees. A bur hole is made over the right coronal suture, along the midpupillary line. Optimal positioning of the bur hole varies slightly depending on the proposed trajectory, as determined from preoperative MRI. The bur hole is placed more anteriorly to provide access to the posterior third ventricle if desired. The dura is opened in cruciate fashion, and the pial surface is coagulated and incised. A 3-mm-diameter, blunt-tipped

brain needle is inserted into the right frontal horn, directed toward the foramen of Monro. After CSF sampling and intracranial pressure assessment, the needle is withdrawn, and the same tract is used for insertion of the endoscope sheath or cannula. This technique allows blunt separation of the ependymal layer and progressive enlargement of this opening, minimizing ependymal bleeding, a common cause of poor intraventricular visualization. In infants, an approach is easily made from the right lateral corner of the anterior fontanel without any bone removal. This allows for formal dural incision and primary closure of the durotomy at the end of the procedure, which minimize the risk of postoperative CSF leakage. Use of this technique is especially important for infants with severe ventriculomegaly and a thin cortical mantle. Infants can be conveniently positioned, prepped, and draped as for a right frontal VP shunt placement in the event that technical failure necessitates shunt placement.

Once insertion of the endoscope into the lateral ventricle has been achieved, the foramen of Monro is located by identification of the choroid plexus and septal and thalamostriate veins (Figs. 54-6A and B and 54-7A). After passage of the endoscope through the foramen of Monro, the optic chiasm, infundibulum, mammillary bodies, massa intermedia, and aqueduct can all be observed along the floor of the third ventricle from anterior to posterior, depending on trajectory (Figs. 54-6C and D and Figs. 54-7B and G). A flexible scope is generally necessary to view the lamina terminalis, suprapineal recess, or third ventricular roof. In cases of obstructive hydrocephalus, a diamond-shaped transparent membrane is commonly seen between the mammillary bodies and the infundibulum. The dorsum sellae, clivus, and basilar artery are often visible through this membrane (Fig. 54-7B). This area of the third ventricular floor between the clivus and the basilar artery is the ideal site for ETV.

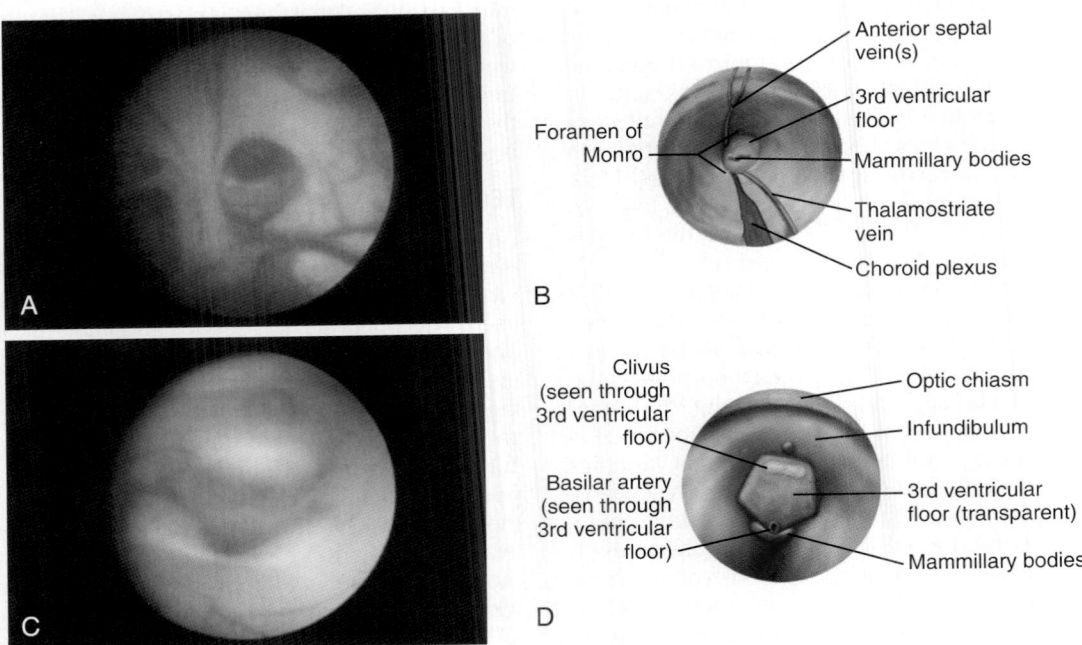

FIGURE 54-6 Anatomy of the foramen of Monro as viewed from the lateral ventricle: operative photograph (A) and diagram (B). Close-up view of anatomy of the third ventricular floor: operative photograph (C) and schematic diagram (D).

Numerous methods of perforating the third ventricular floor have been described that use the scope itself, a cautery unit, laser, or endoscopic instrument.[96,99,103,130-132] We advise never penetrating the third ventricular floor with cautery or laser because of increased risk of damage to underlying structures, such as the basilar artery. A closed blunt biopsy forceps for initial fenestration can be used, followed by dilation of the stoma with a No. 4 French Fogarty balloon catheter (Fig. 54-7C through E). Care is taken to inflate the balloon with sterile irrigation fluid only under direct vision within the opening, because blindly withdrawing an inflated balloon from the basal cisterns carries a significant risk of injury to perforating vessels. Alternatively, if using a flexible endoscope, the floor can be penetrated with the tip of a Bugby wire, using no electrocautery, and the opening subsequently widened by gentle stretching at the margins of the developing stoma. This is easily accomplished by flexing the steerable tip of the endoscope. After adequate enlargement of the ventriculostomy, the scope can be advanced to inspect the prepontine and interpeduncular cisterns (Fig. 54-7F). The flexible endoscope also allows access to the lamina terminalis, which can be used as an alternative ETV site if technical or anatomic issues preclude use of the third ventricle floor.

Postoperative management of patients after ETV must be individualized to address the unique preoperative and intraoperative details of each case. Infants or patients presenting with subacute hydrocephalus and uneventful procedures may require only short-term postoperative observation, whereas patients with acute presentations, prior shunt dependence, or significant intraoperative bleeding often require an EVD with continuous ICP monitoring in an intensive care unit setting. Patients undergoing

a simultaneous endoscopic tumor biopsy or removal of a prior existing shunt system require particularly close observation and monitoring.

In the past, postoperative CSF shunting was recommended to promote expansion of pericerebral CSF spaces and improve absorption.[104,106,113] Compelling evidence suggests, however, that CSF flow through the ventriculostomy maintains its patency, and shunts can lead to closure of the opening.[95,113] We do not recommend a coexisting CSF shunt and ETV.

CHOROID PLEXUS CAUTERIZATION

Bilateral lateral ventricle CPC, when performed in combination with ETV, has been demonstrated to be significantly more successful than ETV alone in infants younger than 1 year.[110-112] The combined procedure (ETV/CPC) can be performed with a flexible steerable ventriculoscope via a single approach through the right lateral corner of the anterior fontanel in the midpupillary line, as described earlier. After completing the ETV, attention is turned to the choroid plexus of the right lateral ventricle. Beginning at the right foramen of Monro, the plexus is cauterized with the tip of the Bugby wire (Fig. 54-8A). A monopolar current is used at its lowest effective setting. The tip of the wire is not buried in the substance of the plexus but rather is used to work along its surface, keeping the tip in view. It is imperative to avoid transgressing the ependyma or the choroidal fissure. The plexus is cauterized along its axis back to and including the glomus choroidea (Fig. 54-8B). The superior choroidal vein is typically in view, running along the surface of the plexus, and this is coagulated completely. Care must be taken to avoid injury to the thalamostriate and internal cerebral veins. Once at the atrium, the flexible

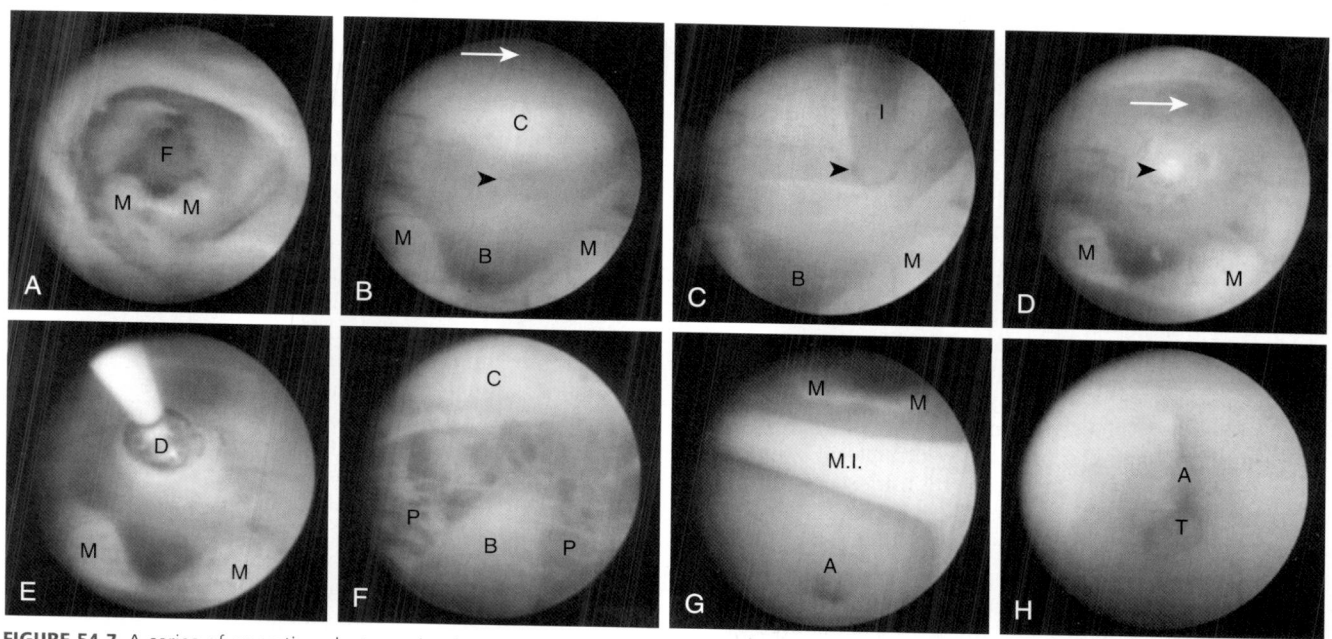

FIGURE 54-7 A series of operative photographs demonstrating the ETV procedure. A, Entrance is through the foramen of Monro from the right lateral ventricle. B, Close-up of the third ventricular floor, with the proposed ventriculostomy site indicated (*arrowhead*). C, Blunt forceps piercing the third ventricular floor. D, View of the initial ventriculostomy opening. E, Dilatation of the ventriculostomy using a Fogarty balloon catheter. F, View of basal cisterns through the ventriculostomy opening. G, View of the middle third ventricular floor. H, View of the aqueduct, demonstrating an obstruction by a tectal tumor (black arrowhead). Ventriculostomy site (*white arrow*); infundibular recess. A, aqueduct; B, basilar artery; C, clivus; D, Fogarty balloon; F, floor of third ventricle; I, blunt forceps; M, mammillary bodies; MI, massa intermedia; P, basilar perforators; T, tectal tumor.

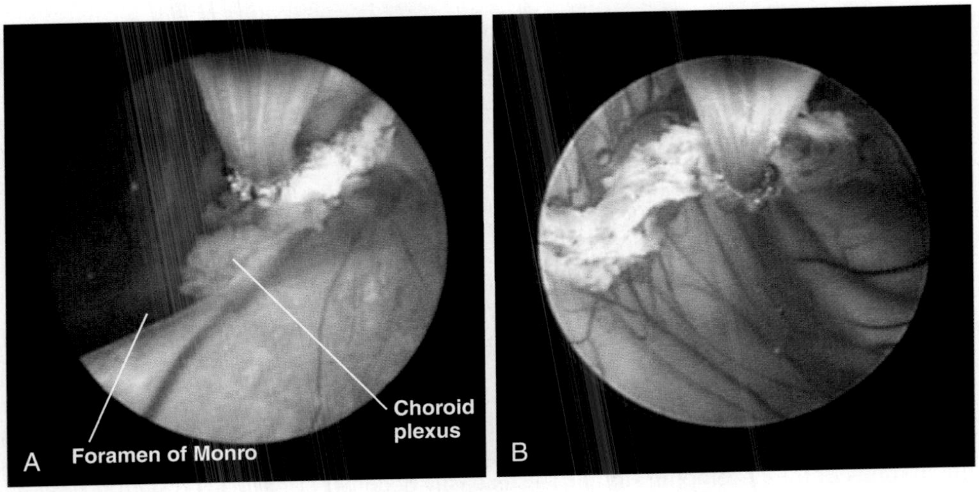

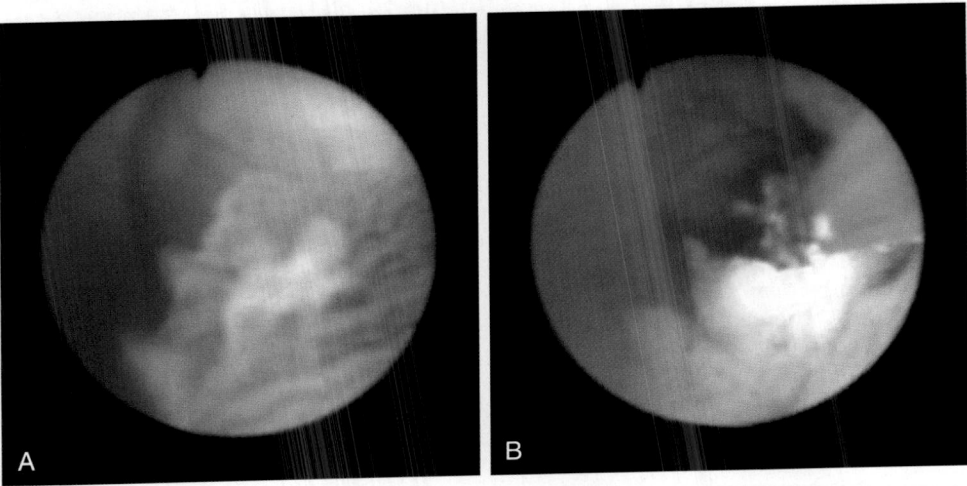

FIGURE 54-8 A, Bugby wire cauterizing the choroid plexus at the right foramen of Monro; B, Bugby wire cauterizing the choroid plexus just anterior to the glomus choroidea in the atrium of the right lateral ventricle.

FIGURE 54-9 A, Choroid plexus adjacent to the hippocampus within the temporal horn of the right lateral ventricle; B, Bugby wire cauterizing the choroid plexus within the temporal horn of the right lateral ventricle.

scope is advanced slightly into the occipital horn posterior to the thalamus, where the tip is flexed and the scope slightly torqued to direct the procedure along the plexus within the temporal horn to its anterior extremity (Fig. 54-9A and B). Once all accessible plexus in the right lateral ventricle has been coagulated and shriveled, the left lateral ventricle is accessed. This requires a septostomy if the septum pellucidum is competent. The point for septostomy is chosen superior to the posterior margin of the foramen of Monro in an avascular region, avoiding the septal vein and its branches. A small circular area is cauterized and then penetrated with the Bugby wire. A cavum septum pellucidum requires deliberate fenestration of each distinct leaf. The scope is passed into the contralateral lateral ventricle, avoiding any contact with the underlying forniceal columns. The contralateral choroid plexus is then easily accessed and cauterized in the same fashion (Fig. 54-9B).

OUTCOME

The goal of ETV and, to date, the best objectively quantifiable measure of a successful outcome is shunt independence. ETV has yielded a higher success rate with lower morbidity and mortality than earlier methods of third ventriculostomy. Mortality rates for open ventriculostomy procedures varied between 5% and 27%, with success rates

of 37% to 75%.[19,95,103,105,113,133] Percutaneous radiographic and later CT-guided techniques reduced this mortality rate to 2% to 7%, with a 44% to 75% rate of shunt independence.[95,102,103,106,113,134] Studies using modern endoscopic techniques and equipment, with or without stereotactic CT or MRI guidance, have reported low morbidity (3% to 12%) and essentially no mortality, with success rates greater than 75% for carefully selected patient groups. Table 54-8 depicts the results of earlier ETV studies with success rates by cause where this information is available. The new success prediction scores cited previously have helped define appropriate indications and predict the likelihood of success in an individual patient. Objective measures for postoperative assessment of these patients need to be refined.

One of the most confusing aspects of outcome evaluation in ETV patients is the failure of the ventricles to return to normal size. Most studies report a gradual decrease in the ventricular size over months to years postoperatively, with resolution of periventricular edema and increased extracerebral spaces, coinciding with clinical improvement.[95-98,113,135] One series of patients treated with either CSF shunts or ETV showed no difference in intellectual outcome despite enlarged ventricles in the ETV group.[135] A more recent study of infants with myelomeningocele and hydrocephalus demonstrated no difference between patients

Table 54-8 Summary of ETV Trials

Author (Year)	Procedure	Patients (n)	Overall Success (%)	Morbidity (%)	Procedure Abort Rate (%)	Follow-up (Mean)	SUCCESS (SHUNT INDEPENDENCE) (%) BY CAUSE (N)						
							AS	M	Tumor	SVS	Shunt	PHH	Other
Hirsch et al. (1986)[145]	ETV	114	70	—	—	—	70 (114)	—	—	—	—	—	—
Jones et al. (1990)[99]	ETV	24	50	8	16	NS	57 (14)	40 (5)	67 (3)	—	—	—	0 (2)
Kelly (1991)[95]	SETV	16	94	0	0	1-5 yr (3.5 yr)	94 (16)	—	—	—	—	—	—
Dalrymple and Kelly (1992)[146]	SETV	85	87	—	—	1-66 mo	65 (31)	40 (10)	86 (7)	—	—	—	—
Jones et al. (1992)[96]	ETV	54	60	7	9	3 mo-7 yr (27 mo)	—	—	—	—	75 (4)	0 (2)	—
Goodman (1993)[147]	MRETV	3	100	0	0	6-14 mo (10 mo)	100 (3)	—	—	—	—	—	—
Jones et al. (1994)[97]	ETV	101	61	5	6	NS	78 (9)	52 (21)	81 (16)	—	—	—	—
Sainte-Rose and Chumas (1996)[98]	ETV	82	81	NS	NS	(1.8 yr)	67 (111)	—	—	—	—	—	—
	RTV and STV	104	68	—	—	(5.7 yr)	—	—	>80 (53)	—	—	—	—
Teo and Jones (1996)[100]	ETV	69	72	3	9	1-17 yr (32 mo)	—	72 (69)	—	—	—	—	—
Goumnerova and Frim (1997)[139]	ETV	23	73	9	—	7-44 mo (17 mo)	69 (13)	—	71 (7)	—	—	0 (1)	100 (2)
Baskin et al. (1998)[116]	ETV	16	63	12	—	(18.8 mo)	—	—	—	63 (16)	—	—	—
Brockmeyer et al. (1998)[101]	ETV	97	49	6	26	15-69 mo (24.2 mo)	56 (16)	50 (16)	61 (18)	50 (4)	—	0 (4)	38 (13)

AS, aqueductal stenosis; ETV, endoscopic third ventriculostomy; MMC, myelomeningocele; MRETV, stereotactic (MR-guided) endoscopic third ventriculostomy; MS, not significant; PHH, posthemorrhegic hydrocephalus; RTV, radiography-guided third ventriculostomy; SETV, stereotactic (CT-guided) endoscopic third ventriculostomy; STV, stereotactic (CT-guided) third ventriculostomy; shunt, intractable shunt infection of malfunction; SVS, slit-ventricle syndrome.

treated by shunting or those treated by combined ETV/CPC in regard to early developmental outcomes.[113] In that study, there was little difference among shunted patients, patients treated by ETV/CPC, and patients who required no hydrocephalus treatment in regard to ventricular size. Furthermore, no association was demonstrated between ventricle size and developmental outcome. Multiple authors have reported late failures, in which the ventriculostomy closes sometimes years postoperatively.[97,109,136] However, late ETV failure appears to be rare. Importantly, in contrast to the ongoing lifetime risk of shunt failure, the majority of ETV failures have been shown to become apparent within 6 months of the procedure.[112,115,135] Radiographic evaluation of suspected closure is confounded by the presence of persistently enlarged ventricles, and closure must often be suspected solely on the basis of clinical evidence.

Studies detailing the serial measurements of multiple radiographic indices of ventricular size postoperatively show that the third ventricular size responds more quickly (usually within 3 months) than the lateral ventricular size (2 years).[135,137] Additionally, third ventricular size appears to correlate most closely with outcome in these patients.[98,135,137] Several newer modalities appear promising as potential objective measures of ventriculostomy function. MRI detection of T2-weighted flow void around the ventriculostomy has been correlated with clinical outcome in ETV.[138-140] This observation has proved most helpful in confirming ventriculostomy patency postoperatively, particularly in patients with persistent ventriculomegaly.[139,140] Actual quantification of flow velocity through ventriculostomies has also been demonstrated by phase-contrast MRI and Doppler ultrasonography.[141,142] Intraventricular pressure has been observed to return to normal over 3 months in a patient after third ventriculostomy who underwent concurrent implantation of a telemetric ICP monitor.[143] For patients in whom an EVD is placed postoperatively, such as those undergoing ETV in the face of shunt failure, ICP may take several days to normalize, and serial lumbar puncture has been reported to facilitate this process.[144] We hope that methods of quantifying ventriculostomy function will allow neurosurgeons to refine further the techniques necessary to improve outcome. Radiographic confirmation may also help define indications with more subjective outcomes, for example, the observation of less fulminant shunt malfunctions in patients after ventriculostomy.[99]

COMPLICATIONS

Several series of ETVs report no mortality and low morbidity (Table 54-8).[95-101,109-112,116,139,145-147] The most common serious complications are related to structures in and around the floor of the third ventricle. In patients with aqueductal obstruction, the third ventricular floor is usually thinned out and transparent and the hypothalamic nuclei displaced laterally. When the floor is not thinned or the ventriculostomy is not performed at the preferred midline site, injury to the hypothalamus or bleeding can result. These complications have been attributed to direct pressure from the perforating instrument, elevated CSF temperature from cautery or the light source, or distention of the third ventricle from continuous irrigation without adequate drainage.[98] Reported complications from injury to this area include the syndrome of inappropriate secretion of antidiuretic hormone,

diabetes insipidus, loss of thirst, amenorrhea, and trance-like states.[136,148] These complications are usually transient. Bradycardia is also observed occasionally, when perforating a thickened third ventricular floor, and a near-fatal cardiac arrest has been reported.[149] Transient postoperative fevers, which frequently occur in these patients, are commonly attributed to irritation of the ependyma from blood or manipulation of the hypothalamus.[131]

Other structures at risk in this area include the third and sixth cranial nerves, fornix, and caudate. Injuries to all of these structures, usually transient or clinically silent, have been reported.[136,148] The major life-threatening risk during the procedure is injury to the basilar artery and its branches. The basilar bifurcation is usually visible through the thinned third ventricular floor. Extreme caution should be taken to avoid injuring these vessels, particularly when preoperative imaging suggests a thickened ventricular floor or aberrant location (i.e., anterior to the mammillary bodies) of these vessels. We perform the initial fenestration with a blunt instrument rather than the cautery or laser to minimize the risk of arterial damage. Injury to these vessels can result in catastrophic hemorrhage, stroke, or pseudoaneurysm formation.[150] Other routine complications, associated with most neurosurgical procedures, have also been observed. Superficial wound infections, meningitis and ventriculitis, subdural hematomas, and CSF leaks have all been described.[98,136,148]

Other Endoscopic Applications

Endoscopic techniques, with and without the addition of stereotactic assistance, are increasingly used for treating a variety of conditions and complications related to hydrocephalus. In stereotactic-guided techniques, the scope target can be selected and intervening structures (i.e., the foramen of Monro) can be chosen as part of the trajectory.[95,151] CT- or MRI-based frame systems have commonly been supplanted by newer frameless stereotactic systems. These can be easily adapted for use with a rigid endoscope. These systems are particularly useful when planning the trajectory in patients with small ventricles, distorted anatomy as a result of prior shunting procedures or infection, or approaching intraventricular lesions. They are also helpful when operating in large ventricles where the light is diffused, in loculated ventricles where there is essentially no recognizable anatomy, and in CSF turbid from debris or blood when scope image quality is poor. Collapse of the ventricular system or cystic cavities can rapidly render the preoperative imaging data useless.

Intracranial cysts and loculated regions of the ventricular system have been successfully treated with these techniques.[130,152,153] Endoscopic procedures for colloid cysts and suprasellar arachnoid cysts have been particularly successful.[154-156] Several studies have examined the role of ventriculoscopic shunt catheter placement.[157,158] However, a prospective, randomized study of the usefulness of this procedure failed to demonstrate any significant benefit in regard to shunt survival.[159] Likewise, treatment of intraventricular tumors and their associated hydrocephalus with endoscopic techniques requires further study, particularly in midline posterior fossa tumors.[98,160-164] Ventriculoscopic procedures for pineal, suprasellar, and tectal lesions have proved most useful to date.[165-168] Further study and technical refinements will lead to many more potential uses for these procedures in the treatment of hydrocephalus and its associated causes. The challenge for neurosurgeons is to continue defining the indications and outcomes and refining the techniques for safely performing these useful procedures.

KEY REFERENCES

Drake JM. Ventriculostomy for treatment of hydrocephalus. *Neurosurg Clin N Am.* 1993;4:657-666.

Drake J, Chumas P, Kestle J, et al. Late rapid deterioration after endoscopic third ventriculostomy: additional cases and review of the literature. *J Neurosurg.* 2006 Aug;105(2 suppl):118-126.

Greenfield JP, Hoffman C, Kuo E, Christos PJ, Souweidane MM. Intraoperative assessment of endoscopic third ventriculostomy success. *JNS Peds.* 2008;2:298-303.

Kulkarni AV, Drake JM, Mallucci CL, et al. Canadian Pediatric Neurosurgery Study Group Endoscopic third ventriculostomy in the treatment of childhood hydrocephalus. *J Pediatr.* 2009;155:254-259.

Warf BC. Comparison of endoscopic third ventriculostomy alone and combined with choroid plexus cauterization in infants younger than 1 year of age: a prospective study in 550 African children. *J Neurosurg.* 2005 Dec;103(6 suppl):475-481.

Warf BC. Hydrocephalus in Uganda: the predominance of infectious origin and primary management with endoscopic third ventriculostomy. *J Neurosurg.* 2005 Jan;102(1 suppl):1-15.

Warf BC, Campbell JW. Combined endoscopic third ventriculostomy and choroid plexus cauterization as primary treatment of hydrocephalus for infants with myelomeningocele: long-term results of a prospective intent-to-treat study in 115 East African infants. *J Neurosurg Pediatr.* 2008 Nov;2(5):310-316.

Warf BC, Kulkarni A. Endoscopic third ventriculostomy in the treatment of childhood hydrocephalus in Uganda: report of a scoring system that predicts success. *J Neurosurg Pediatrics.* 2010;5:143-148.

Warf BC, Kulkarni A. Intraoperative assessment of cerebral aqueduct patency and cisternal scarring: impact on success of endoscopic third ventriculostomy in 403 African children. *J Neurosurg Pediatrics.* 2010;5:204-209.

Numbered references appear on Expert Consult.

CHAPTER 55

Posterior Fossa Tumors in the Pediatric Population: Multidisciplinary Management

TAE-YOUNG JUNG • JAMES T. RUTKA

Primary brain tumors are the most common solid tumors in the pediatric population, comprising 20% to 25% of all childhood cancers. About 60% to 70% of all pediatric brain tumors originate in the posterior fossa.[1-4] The reason that pediatric brain tumors have a propensity to occur in the posterior fossa has not yet been elucidated. By far, the most common posterior fossa tumors of childhood are medulloblastomas, ependymomas, and astrocytomas. As for uncommon tumors, these include atypical teratoid/rhabdoid tumors (AT/RTs), teratoma, hemangioblastoma, dermoid, and epidermoid. Each tumor may have a vastly different prognosis and response to treatment depending on the pathologies. Recent advancements have increased our knowledge of the cell biology, facilitated earlier diagnosis and improved neurosurgical resections and adjuvant treatment. These in turn have not only improved the survival of children but also their quality of life. Although much progress has been made in the diagnosis and treatment of posterior fossa tumors, they still cause the most cancer-related deaths in this age group.[5,6] This review focuses on the multidisciplinary management of the major types of pediatric posterior fossa tumors. Current advances in tumor diagnosis and surgery, along with adjuvant therapeutic modalities, will be discussed.

Symptoms and Signs

The signs and symptoms of posterior fossa tumors are typically not specific for pathology subtype. Rather, children with these tumors may present with a variety of signs and symptoms. The diagnosis is often difficult to establish in a child because many of the signs and symptoms may mimic those of more common childhood illnesses.

Posterior fossa tumors often cause hydrocephalus by blocking cerebrospinal (CSF) outflow pathways, with resulting signs and symptoms of raised intracranial pressure (ICP).[7] Symptoms typically begin with intermittent headache, often worse in the morning followed by vomiting and eventually gait disturbance. Funduscopy must be performed in children with suspected posterior fossa or supratentorial tumors because papilledema is a common finding. Sixth nerve palsies resulting from intracranial hypertension and ataxia from a combination of cerebellar compression and hydrocephalus are also common.

The presenting signs and symptoms are dependent on the growth rate of tumors, the age of the patient and the location of the tumor. Most children with medulloblastomas present with a short clinical history, for less than 1.5 months in approximately 50% of patients and less than 3 months in approximately 75% of patients.[7] Ependymomas are relatively fast-growing tumors and the median duration of symptoms is 2 to 3 months.[8] As for cerebellar astrocytoma, the symptomatic period ranges from 5 to 9 months and is usually significantly longer than other posterior fossa tumors.[9] Rapid, sudden deterioration in neurologic status may result from acute obstructive hydrocephalus or hemorrhage into either the tumor or the subarachnoid space.[10-13] Older children may complain of headache, neck stiffness, dizziness or diplopia. On neurologic examination, they will demonstrate truncal or appendicular ataxia, dysmetria, nystagmus, or cranial nerve palsies. In comparison with older children, the presentation in infants and young children is often more insidious, with gradual progression.[14] The diagnosis is suspected in the setting of irritability, loss of appetite, weight loss and failure to thrive. In addition, they may display signs of increased ICP, including lethargy, drowsiness, vomiting, sun-setting, a full fontanelle, or an increasing head circumference. Midline tumors of the cerebellum usually cause truncal ataxia, whereas hemispheric lesions cause ipsilateral dysmetria. Tumor in the obex and area postrema causes vomiting even if the tumor is small and there is no hydrocephalus. Cranial neuropathies such as facial weakness, hearing loss and swallowing dysfunction may present in tumors that exit the foramen of Luschka from the cerebellopontine angle or in tumors demonstrating brain stem invasion.

Head-tilt, signifying descent of the cerebellar tonsils into the foramen magnum with compression of the C1 or C2 nerve roots, may be observed. Development of a stiff neck or head tilt usually suggests tonsillar involvement by the tumor or signs of impending herniation.[15-17] Rarely, children initially present with symptoms of spinal dissemination, such as back and leg pain or paraparesis.[18] The transmission of increased pressure to the upper cervical spinal cord may cause syringomyelia and related symptoms in patients with cerebellar astrocytomas.[19]

Radiologic Findings

MEDULLOBLASTOMA

Approximately two thirds of medulloblastomas are located in the midline arising from the vermis or inferior medullary velum and widening the space between the cerebellar tonsils. Isolated involvement of the hemisphere is seen in older children and young adults.[20,21]

Due to the increased nuclear to cytoplasmic ratio of the tumor cells, medulloblastoma typically appears as a homogenous iso- to hyper-dense midline mass within the posterior fossa on non-contrast CT scan (Fig. 55-1A), with variable amounts of peritumoral edema and hydrocephalus whereas the solid portion of cerebellar astrocytomas are hypodense on precontrast studies.[22] By CT, medulloblastoma can also contain calcification, necrosis, cystic degeneration, and hemorrhage and can invade the brain stem. Following contrast administration, this tumor demonstrates homogenous enhancement (Fig. 55-1B).

On MRI, medulloblastoma typically appears as a hypo- to iso-intense mass on T1-weighted images (T1WI), and iso- to hyper-intense on T2-weighted images (T2WI)[22,23] (Fig. 55-1C). Diffusion-weighted images (DWI) demonstrate restricted diffusion.[24] The enhancement pattern is variable: enhancement may be uniform or patchy[22,23] (Fig. 55-1D). The heterogeneity probably results from cysts and calcification. Intracranial subarachnoid or intraventricular dissemination should be carefully identified because the perimesencephalic cisterns, tentorial surface and suprasellar cisterns are frequent sites for dissemination at the time of tumor diagnosis.

EPENDYMOMA

On CT scan, a posterior fossa ependymoma is an iso- or hyper-dense midline cerebellar mass with calcifications, small cysts, and heterogeneous enhancement after intravenous contrast administration[25] (Fig. 55-2A). Hemorrhage is present in up to 13% and calcifications are frequent in 25% to 50%. MR imaging shows marked heterogeneity of the tumor due to small cysts as well as areas of old hemorrhage. Precontrast T1- and T2-weighted images commonly reveal an iso- to hyper-intense signal intensity. Most tumors show heterogeneous and irregular enhancement following gadolinium administration[26] (Fig. 55-2B).

The most characteristic appearance supporting the diagnosis of ependymoma is of a mass arising from the lower brain stem and projecting into the fourth ventricle; in half or more tumors, extension through the foramen of Luschka

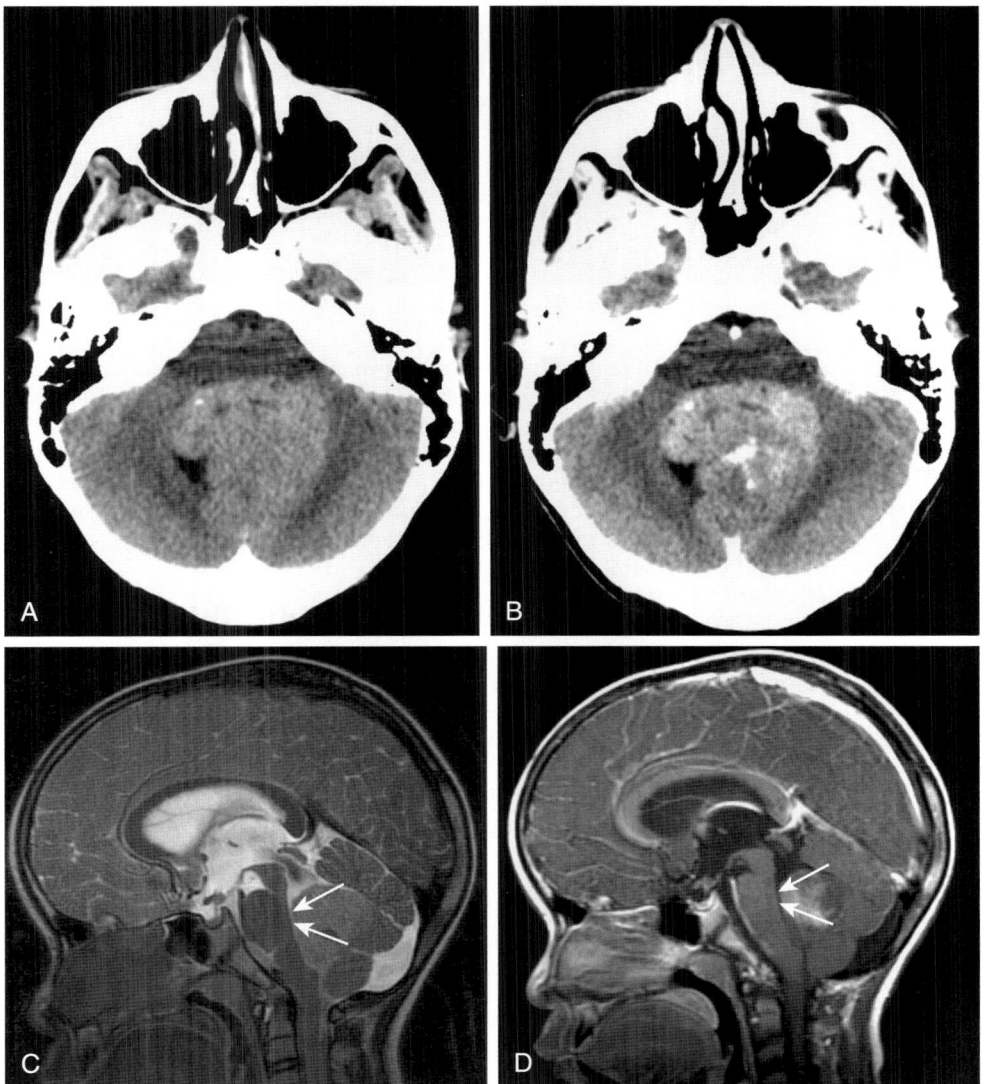

FIGURE 55-1 Radiologic findings of medulloblastoma. A, Noncontrast axial CT shows a hyperdense mass in the cerebellar vermis and foci of calcification. B, On postcontrast CT, the tumor enhances heterogeneously. C, T2-weighted sagittal MRI shows a hyperintense mass projecting into the fourth ventricle and compressing the brain stem caudally. D, Postcontrast sagittal MRI following gadolinium administration shows the tumor with heterogeneous enhancement. On these MR midsagittal images (C, D), a cerebrospinal fluid space between the tumor and the floor of the fourth ventricle (*black arrows*) is seen, which suggests that there is no invasion of the floor of the fourth ventricle.

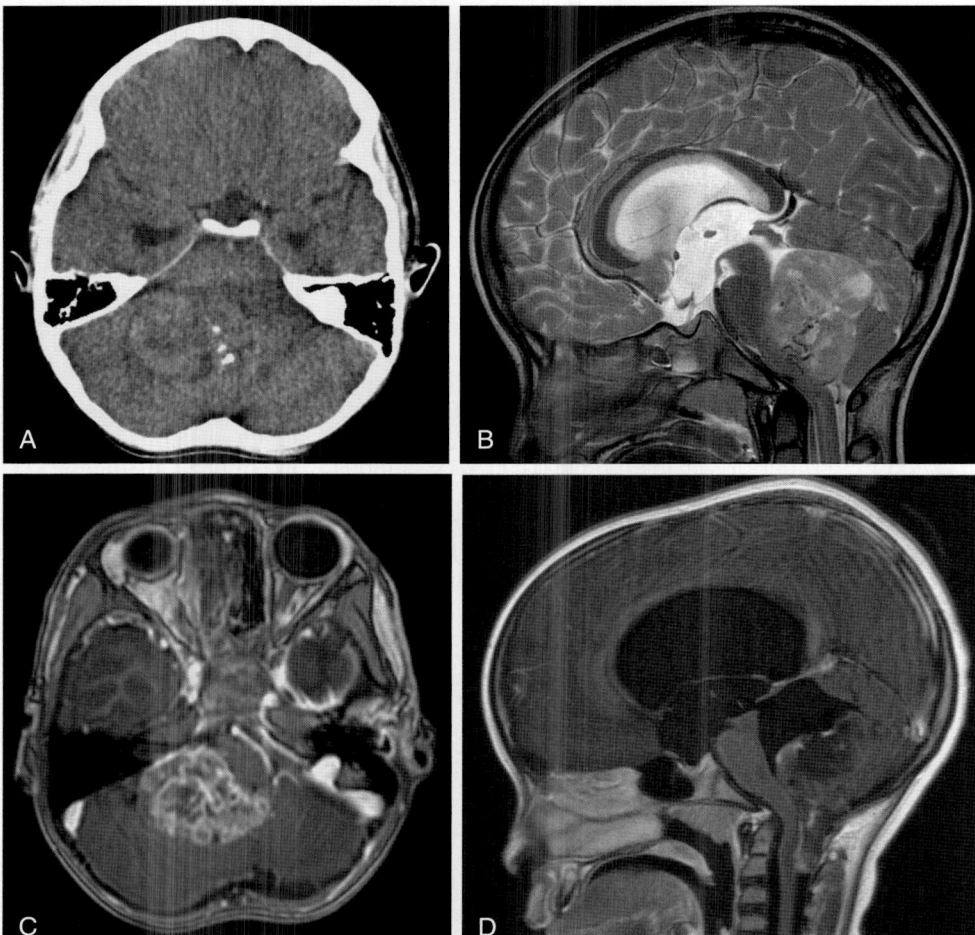

FIGURE 55-2 Radiologic findings of ependymoma. A, Precontrast axial CT shows an isodense midline cerebellar mass with calcifications. B, On T2-weighted sagittal MRI, there is a fourth ventricular mass showing compression of the surrounding cerebellum and brain stem. C, Postcontrast axial MRI shows a heterogeneously enhancing mass extending through left foramen of Luschka into the cerebellopontine angle. D, Postcontrast sagittal MRI showing an ependymoma extending through the foramen magnum.

into the cerebellopontine angle or through the foramen magnum into the cervical spinal canal is found (Fig. 55-2C and D). The vertebral arteries and posterior inferior cerebellar arteries may be displaced or encased.

CEREBELLAR ASTROCYTOMA

Cerebellar astrocytomas can be either vermian or hemispheric in location. They can be predominantly cystic with a solid mass, the so-called mural nodule, in 30% of cases; they can be, solid with cystic areas in 40% to 50%; and wholly solid in 20% to 30%.[9,27,28] Cystic tumors tend to be located within the hemispheres and solid tumors in the midline alone or in combination with extension into one or both hemispheres.[29,30]

On noncontrast CT, the solid portion of the tumor is usually iso- to hypodense and the cyst is hypodense but denser than CSF because of the high protein concentration (Fig. 55-3A and C). Calcification can be seen in up to 20%, and cysts in 70%.[31,32] On MRI, solid parts of the tumor are generally iso- or hypo-intense signal intensity masses on T1-weighted sequences and hyperintense masses on T2-weighted and FLAIR sequences.[33] Contrast enhancement is usually irregular caused by cysts and tumor necrosis[22] (Fig. 55-3B and D). Tumors of pilocytic pathology show intense enhancement of their solid portions.[34] Nonenhancing tumors are almost never of pilocytic histology.

Frequently, the infiltrative fibrillary astrocytomas do not show much gadolinium enhancement.[35] Both pathologies can invade the cerebellar peduncle and brain stem.

A mural nodule in a nonenhancing cyst in child is almost pathognomonic for a benign cerebellar astrocytoma. Similarly, cystic hemangioblastoma in the cerebellum mimics this appearance, but hemangioblastoma rarely occurs in children.

ATYPICAL TERATOID/RHABDOID TUMORS

AT/RTs usually originate in the cerebellar hemispheres instead of the midline and have a predilection for the cerebello-pontine angle.[36,37] Their pattern of growth is aggressive with significant mass effect on the adjacent fourth ventricle and brain stem, and early CSF dissemination. AT/RTs may also arise in the spinal cord, pineal gland and suprasellar region.[38,39]

On noncontrast CT, the solid portions of the tumor demonstrate hyperdensity, presumably due to the high cellularity of the tumor[36,38] (Fig. 55-4A). On MRI, solid portions of the tumor are low signal intensity on T1-weighted images and isointense or decreased signal on T2-weighted images.[36,38,40] In addition, frequent necrosis, cysts, and sometimes hemorrhage are identified, giving an appearance of striking heterogeneity.[36,37,41] Enhancement can be variable (Fig. 55-4B to D).

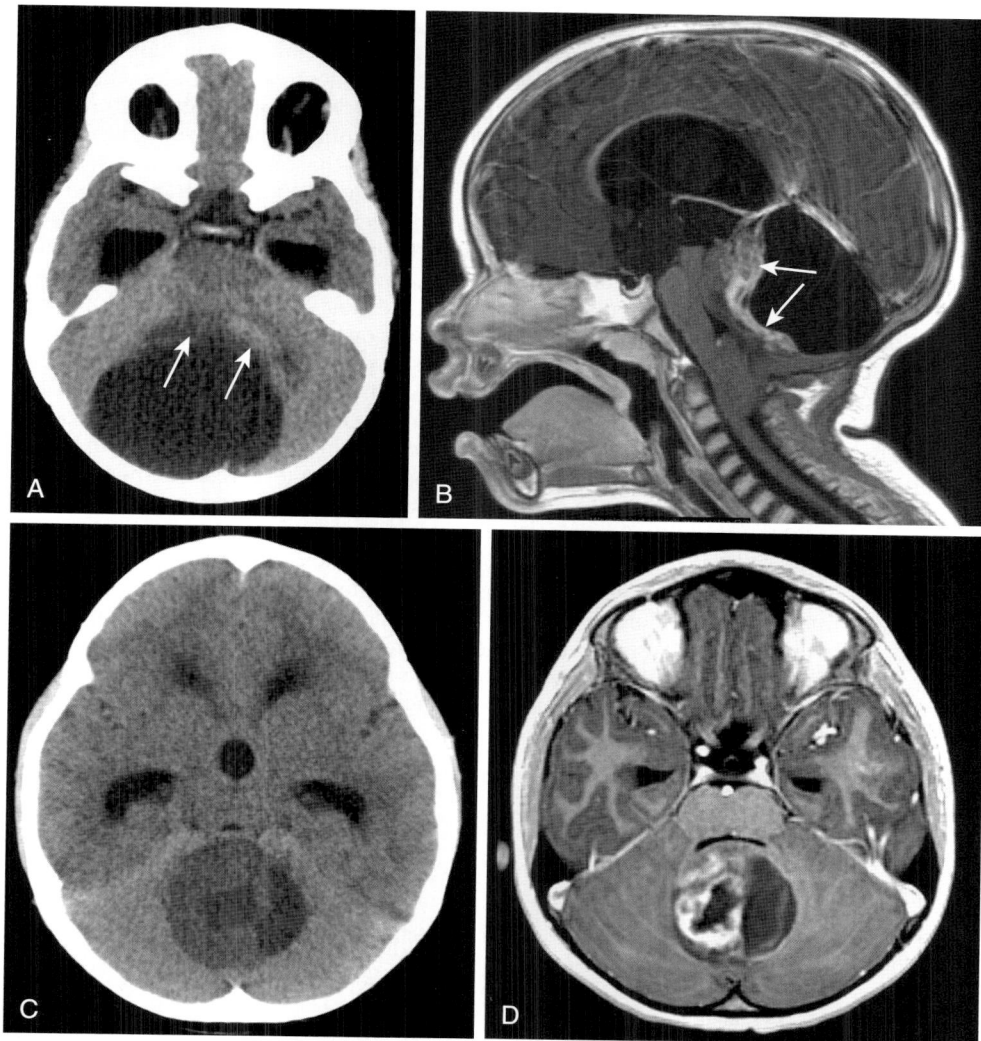

FIGURE 55-3 Radiologic findings of cerebellar astrocytoma. Predominantly cystic cerebellar astrocytoma with mural mass lesion. A, On precontrast CT, the solid portion of the tumor (*white arrows*) is iso- and hypo-dense and the cyst is hypodense. B, Sagittal T1-weighted image shows a large posterior fossa tumor cyst associated with a contrast-enhancing mural mass lesion (*white arrows*). C, Predominantly solid cerebellar astrocytoma with small cystic area: Precontrast CT shows a hypodense vermian mass. D, Postcontrast MRI with contrast shows an irregularly enhancing mass lesion.

INVASION OF THE BRAIN STEM AND CEREBELLAR PEDUNCLE

Invasion of the brain stem and cerebellar peduncle is found in up to 40% of newly diagnosed medulloblastoma.[4,42] In another study, brain stem or peduncle involvement is identified in 34% of cerebellar pilocytic and diffuse astrocytomas.[43] Cerebellar peduncle involvement is suggested by an ill-defined border on the affected side on postcontrast MRI (Fig. 55-5). On MR midsagittal images without/with contrast infusion, a cerebrospinal fluid space between the tumor and the floor of the fourth ventricle may be found, which can indicate that there is no invasion of the floor of the fourth ventricle (Fig. 55-1C and D). However, absence of a cerebrospinal fluid space does not always indicate the invasion of tumor. As such, it is difficult to affirm unequivocally that the tumor is compressing or invading the floor of the fourth ventricle by imaging studies alone.

Work-Up for Tumor Dissemination

At diagnosis, patients rarely present with symptoms of tumor dissemination. However, spinal metastases can be found in about 20% to 50% of medulloblastoma, 11% to 17% of ependymoma, 25% to 34% of AT/RT at the time of diagnosis.[38,39,44-49] The current standard of care should be to obtain pre- and post-contrast scans of the brain and spine when the presumptive diagnosis of a malignant posterior fossa tumor is made. In the first few weeks after posterior fossa surgery, artifacts from blood products can be very difficult to differentiate from CSF spread of tumor.[50,51] These problems are avoided by performing preoperative staging MR studies of the spine. Postsurgical MRI should be performed within 48 to 72 hours of surgery or at least 2 weeks later to avoid the difficulty of distinguishing between postoperative changes and tumor dissemination or residual tumor. By MRI scans, leptomeningeal dissemination appears as diffuse enhancement of the meninges and/or enhancing clumps along the spinal cord and cauda equina on T1-weighted images (Fig. 55-6).

In addition to spinal MRI, CSF cytologic examination for malignant cells has been used for the diagnosis of leptomeningeal disease pre- or post-operatively. However, spinal MR imaging has a greater diagnostic accuracy than CSF cytology in the early detection of disseminated disease.[52,53] CSF cytologic analysis performed more than 2 to 3 weeks after surgery can reduce false-positive results. Negative

CSF cytologic results do not always exclude the tumor dissemination.[54,55]

Surgery

MANAGEMENT OF HYDROCEPHALUS

Obstructive hydrocephalus is reported in 70% to 80% of children with posterior fossa tumors and is frequently the cause of clinical deterioration at the time of diagnosis.[56,57] Depending on the patient's symptoms and the severity of the associated hydrocephalus, a decision must be made whether to treat the hydrocephalus up front or at the time of tumor resection. In the 1960s, when a child presented in a poor clinical state as a result of a delayed diagnosis, the routine placement of a preoperative shunt significantly reduced the overall morbidity and mortality rate.[58,59] However, neurosurgeons have questioned the need for a routine shunt because only 15% to 30% of patients ultimately require permanent CSF diversion following resection of the tumor.[57,60] In addition to the usual complications associated with ventriculoperitoneal (VP) shunts such as infection and blockage, rare complications such as upward herniation, tumor hemorrhage, and peritoneal seeding of the intracranial tumor may occur.[61] Accordingly, most centers are using a combination of corticosteroids, early surgery, and external ventricular drainage rather than VP shunting.[62,63]

In the majority of cases, patients with symptomatic hydrocephalus may be managed with preoperative intravenous corticosteroids alone, with surgical resection performed on a semi-urgent basis. Dexamethasone alleviates headaches, nausea, and vomiting within 12 to 24 hours after administration and allows for better hydration and nutrition before surgery. This effect usually lasts several days. If a patient is lethargic or obtunded, emergent insertion of an external ventricular drain (EVD) is the most common strategy employed. The gradual decompression of the ventricular system over 12 to 24 hours with slow drainage at initially high (20 to 30 cm H_2O) and subsequently, normal outflow pressures. It is maintained in the early postoperative period, followed by gradual weaning and discontinuation. Difficulty weaning off an EVD, or the development of a tense pseudomeningocele should raise the question of whether permanent CSF diversion is required because of continued hydrocephalus.

Postoperative hydrocephalus occurs within the first few days to months after surgery. Rarely, it will develop several months or years after surgery, or at the time of a local recurrence or of subarachnoid spread.[64,65] Factors requiring placement of postoperative shunt include more severe hydrocephalus at diagnosis, young age, large preoperative

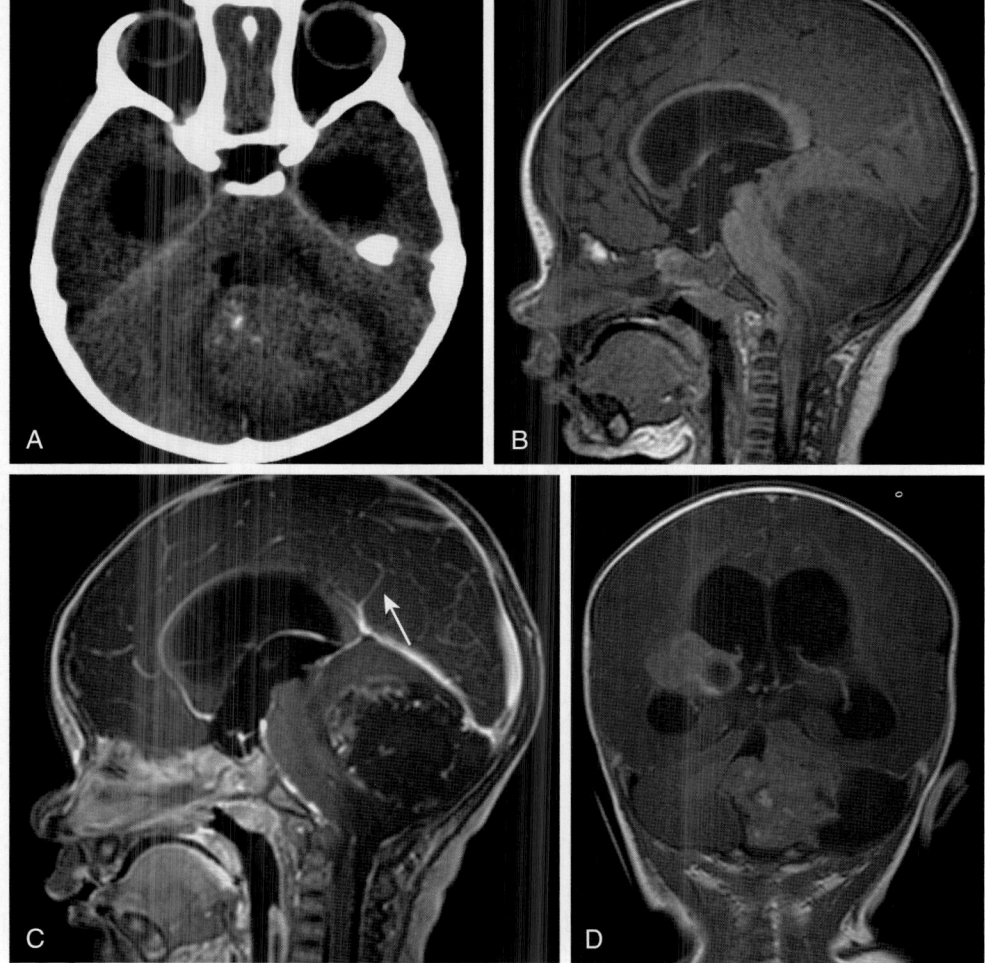

FIGURE 55-4 Radiologic findings of AT/RT. A, On noncontrast axial CT, the solid portion of the tumor is hyperdense. B and C, T1-weighted sagittal MRI without and with gadolinium enhancement, shows a hypointense lesion in the cerebellar vermis that enhances heterogeneously and is associated with perilesional edema. D, Postcontrast coronal MRI showing a metastatic ATRT with a lesion in the posterior fossa and one in the right lateral ventricle.

tumor size, midline localization and incomplete tumor removal.[56,60,66,67] Patients with medulloblastoma, as opposed to other posterior fossa tumors, also appear to be at higher risk for postoperative hydrocephalus requiring a VP shunt.[56,68]

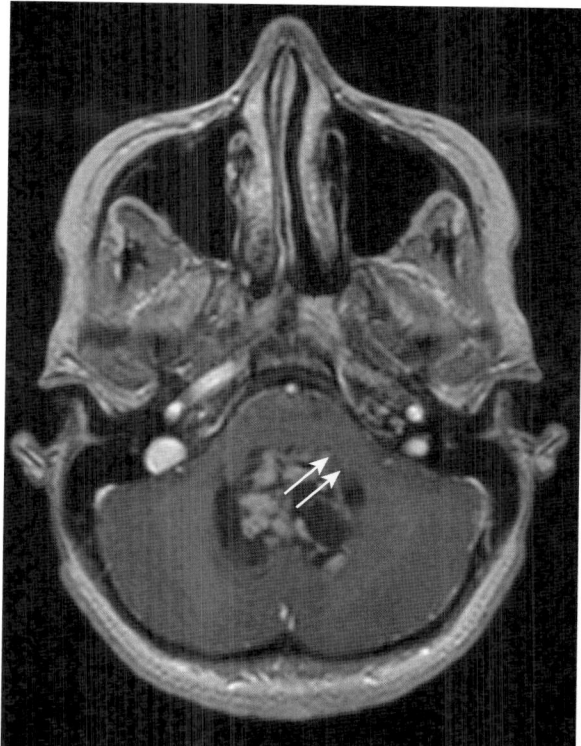

FIGURE 55-5 Radiologic finding of invasion of the cerebellar peduncle. Postcontrast axial MRI of an ependymoma showing an ill-defined border of the left middle cerebellar peduncle, which suggests tumor infiltration at this location (*arrows*).

The effectiveness of endoscopic third ventriculostomy (ETV) has been evaluated in the management of pre-operative and postoperative hydrocephalus. ETV, when performed prior to posterior fossa surgery, reduces the incidence of hydrocephalus because preoperative normalization of CSF hydrodynamics decreases the risk of permanent postoperative impairment of the CSF circulation.[67] However, the routine application of preoperative ETV is not indicated because of the small number of patients requiring definitive treatment for hydrocephalus.[57,68] ETV may be used for persistent or progressive hydrocephalus following tumor removal.[57]

NEUROSURGICAL APPROACHES

The neurosurgical goals of posterior fossa tumor removal include obtaining a tissue diagnosis, achieving maximal safe tumor resection, relieving critical structures from mass effect and addressing associated hydrocephalus. Operative adjuncts that may be employed during surgery include frameless stereotaxy, ultrasonography, and evoked potential and/or cranial nerve monitoring.

PATIENT POSITIONING

Several options for patient positioning are available for patients with posterior fossa tumors: prone, Concorde, lateral decubitus, "park-bench" and the sitting position. Pediatric patients are typically placed in the prone position. For lesions extending superiorly through the aqueduct, the head is tilted slightly to the patient's right, away from the surgeon and flexed far forward (Concorde position) so that the rostral extent of the tumor can be removed with the surgeon sitting behind the patient's shoulder. The lateral decubitus positioning can be used for tumors that occur in the cerebellopontine angle or lateral cerebellum. The sitting position has several distinct advantages including limited use of retraction, and a clear operative field. However, it is difficult to position infants and young children in the sitting

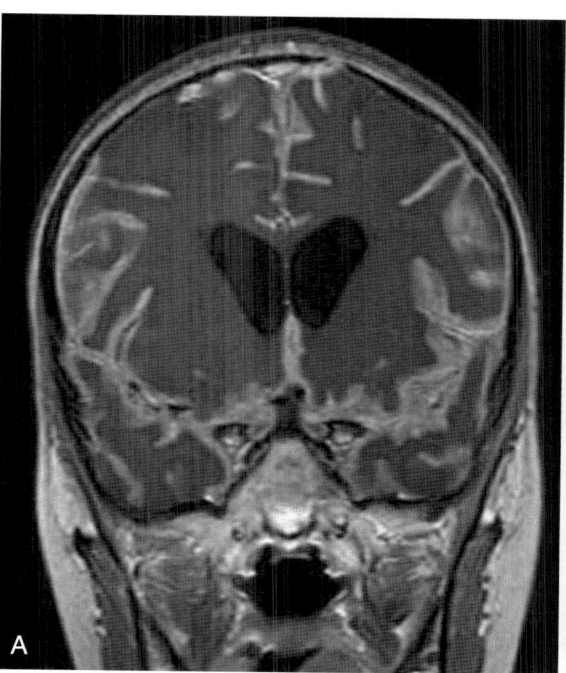

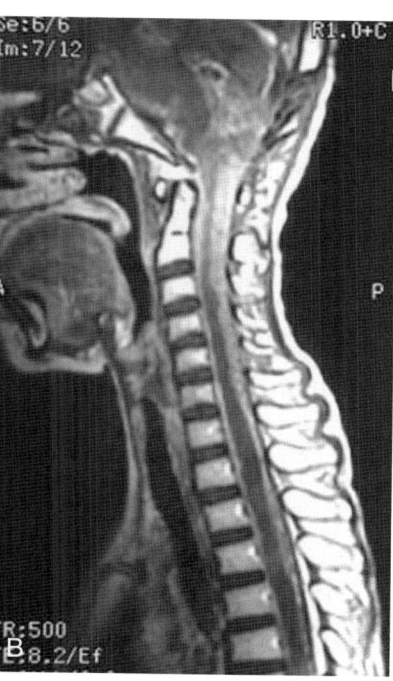

FIGURE 55-6 Radiologic findings of leptomeningeal dissemination. A, Postcontrast T1-weighted coronal MRI shows diffuse leptomeningeal enhancement in the subarachnoid space. B, Coating of the spinal cord with tumor is seen on postcontrast T1-weighted sagittal image.

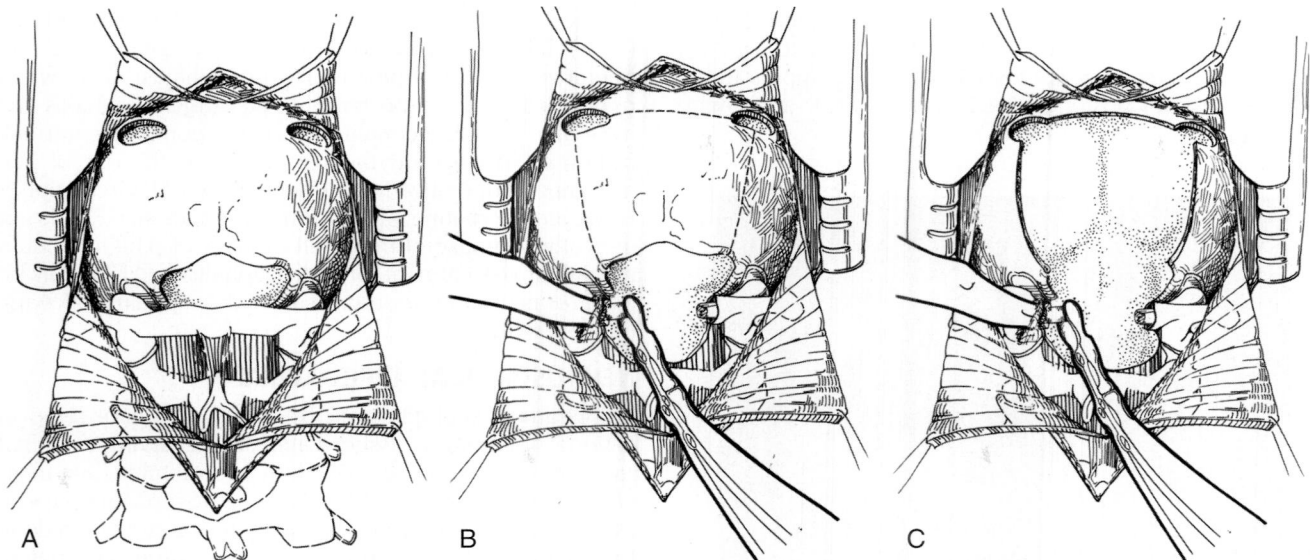

FIGURE 55-7 Posterior fossa craniotomy. A, Bilateral burr holes are made just below the transverse sinus. B, The dura is separated from the inner table of the skull, and if the tumor extends into the upper cervical spinal canal, a laminectomy of the upper cervical vertebrae is performed. C, Craniotomy inferiorly includes the posterior edge of the foramen magnum.

position. Dangers include cardiovascular instability, hypotension, air embolism, pneumocephalus, subdural hematoma, and the rapid escape of cerebrospinal fluid from the ventricular system.

In the prone position, and likewise in the Concorde position, the neurosurgeon works comfortably, looking onto the operative field. The most significant disadvantage of the prone position is venous congestion that can lead to blood loss, pooling of blood in the operative field, and soft-tissue swelling of the face. An armored tube or nasotracheal intubation may lessen the risk of the occlusion of the endotracheal tube. The head of the operating table is elevated until the patient's head is parallel to or just above the heart, which decreases venous pressure of the sinuses. A moderate degree of neck flexion is important to prevent these disadvantages and to access the occipitoatlantal junction. The chin and chest are at least two finger-breadths apart. Pin fixation can be used readily in children over age 3 years. Under age 3, a padded horseshoe headrest is used. The use of a satellite parietal burr hole for CSF drainage is optional depending on patient age, ventricular size, and type of tumor encountered.

OPENING AND CLOSURE

If the lesion is located in the vermis or paravermian region, a midline skin incision suffices. If the lesion occupies one hemisphere without a contiguous attachment to the midline, a paramedian incision is preferred and a hockey stick incision can be used to allow for a wider craniectomy. In the midline posterior fossa exposure, the incision is extended from slightly rostral to the inion down to the C1–C2 spinal process. Skin flaps are mobilized by undermining the subcutaneous plane to prepare a fascial flap for closure and the fascia is incised using a Y- or T-shaped incision for reapproximating tightly at the superior nuchal line. The cervical musculature is mobilized laterally off the occiput and cervical laminae in the midline avascular plane. The foramen

magnum is exposed, and the dura is identified up to the posterior arch of C1. A posterior fossa craniotomy is then performed (Fig. 55-7). Bilateral burr holes are made just below the transverse sinus from the midline. The dura is separated from the inner table of the skull, which is typically not adherent in children. At the foramen magnum, the junction of the pericranium and the dura is sharply dissected with caution because of the occipital sinus in the midline near the foramen magnum. If the tumor extends into the upper cervical spinal canal, a laminectomy of the upper vertebrae may be performed. Monopolar cautery should be used carefully when dissecting the superolateral surface of C1 to prevent injury to an aberrant vertebral artery. C1 can be bifid and is often cartilaginous in infants and young children. After extending a laminectomy below C2, young children have an increased risk of swan neck deformity.[69] Therefore, it is prudent to remove the smallest amount of bone possible.

The dura is then opened in a Y-fashion with care taken to obtain hemostasis of the occipital sinuses (Fig. 55-8A). When the vertical incision extends to the foramen magnum, it may extend below the falx cerebella. If there is significant bleeding from the midline occipital sinus and circular dural sinuses, it should be controlled with obliquely placed hemostatic clips or suture ligatures. If clips are used, they can be removed as the dura is sutured because metal clips may result in artifact on postoperative MRI studies. Intraoperative ultrasonography and neuronavigation may be used to define the location of tumors. The surgeon should inspect the surface of the exposed cerebellum and spinal cord for evidence of leptomeningeal seeding. After the cisterna magna has been exposed, cerebrospinal fluid is aspirated for cytology and drained to decrease ICP.

After tumor removal, meticulous hemostasis is achieved with judicious use of bipolar coagulation and gentle pressure, and may be confirmed with a Valsalva maneuver. The dura is always closed in a watertight fashion, followed by

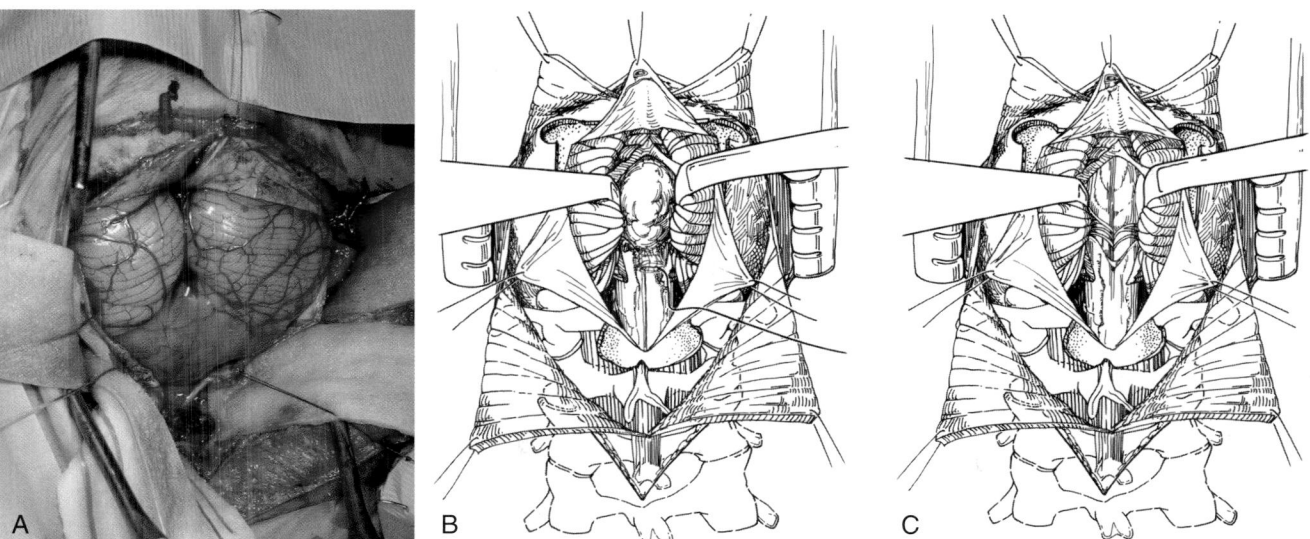

FIGURE 55-8 Tumor exposure and removal. A, Intraoperative photograph after opening the dura. An ependymoma is seen in the midline beneath the cerebellar hemispheres. B, The distal portion of the vermis is divided to expose the dorsal surface of tumor. C, After the removal of tumor, the floor of the fourth ventricle is identified.

replacement of the bone flap and multilayer closure of the superficial tissues. It is important to close the fascial layer tightly near the inion to prevent postoperative leak of cerebrospinal fluid and the formation of a pseudomeningocele.

TUMOR REMOVAL

Transvermian and Telovelar Approaches to Midline Cerebellar Tumors

The two most common surgical approaches to midline cerebellar tumors adjacent to the fourth ventricle are the transvermian and telovelar approaches. The transvermian approach involves incising the inferior vermis of the cerebellum and retracting the two halves of the vermis in opposite lateral directions to remove the tumor. The telovelar approach uses the dissection of the cerebellomedullary fissure, which is a natural cleft between the cerebellum and medulla oblongata, and the dissection of the tela choroidea and inferior medullary velum along the natural avascular planes.[70-74] The greatest advantage of the telovelar approach is the superolateral exposure of the fourth ventricle and the complete exposure of the foramen of Luschka, which can be accessed without removal of cerebellum or adjustment of the retractors.[75,76] However, a limitation of this exposure can be expected when approaching the rostral portion of the fourth ventricle. The transvermian approach provides a greater working angle in this area and a better visualization of the midline inferior portion of the superior medullary velum and fastigium. Nevertheless, the main disadvantages of this approach are a limited lateral exposure and the potential for complications due to iatrogenic injury from excessive vermian dissection and retraction.

In the transvermian approach, the cerebellar tonsils are separated in the midline and it is sometimes helpful to retract the inferior vermis rostrally or incise the caudal vermis to prevent injury to the inferior vermian veins. The posterior inferior cerebellar arteries are usually displaced laterally. The distal portion of the vermis is divided to expose the dorsal surface of tumor (Fig. 55-8B). Cottonoid patties are used

to help to protect the normal neural structures and to dissect along the tumor–cerebellar interface. Once planes around the tumor are developed, the tumor is internally debulked, with suction or with the Cavitron. Specimens are now taken for pathologic assessment and tumor banking. As the tumor is debulked, the lateral tumor–cerebellum interface continues to be developed. The uninvolved side of the cerebellar peduncle is first dissected from the surrounding cerebellar tissue, the floor of the fourth ventricle and the aqueduct are then identified, and tumor invading the involved cerebellar peduncle is resected (Fig. 55-8C). The dentate nucleus is located just above the ipsilateral tonsil, and one should take meticulous care to avoid trauma to it during resection of the tumor from the upper pole of the tonsil.

The telovelar approach is performed by opening the cerebellomedullary fissure, which includes dissection of the tonsillomedullary and uvulotonsillar space. The two cerebellar tonsils are then retracted laterally to expose the floor of the fissure, which includes the inferior medullary velum and tela choroidea. The tela choroidea, which forms the caudal part of the roof of the fourth ventricle, is incised from the foramen of Magendie and then followed laterally to the foramen of Luschka on both sides. In large tumors, the uvulotonsillar cleft is stretched, and the anatomy may be distorted. Aggressive dissection in this area before decompression can result in breaching the pial plane and entering either the vermis or tonsil leading to neurologic deficit, such as ataxia and cerebellar mutism. Placing the retractor on the superomedial part of the tonsil to visualize the superolateral corner of the fourth ventricle can injure the dentate nucleus. Dissection and decompression should be done simultaneously to minimize retraction and reduce associated injuries in large-sized tumors.[77,78]

Techniques When Operating Near the Brain Stem

Care must be taken to identify areas where tumor may invade the floor of the fourth ventricle. One of the most important factors of successful tumor resection is the identification of the floor of the fourth ventricle. If the tumor is not adherent to the floor of the fourth ventricle, one can place Cottonoid patties along the ventricular floor as the dissection proceeds. If the tumor adheres to or invades the floor of the fourth ventricle, the intact floor of the fourth ventricle next to the invasive tumor is identified and the last portion of the tumor is resected at the plane of the floor of the fourth ventricle. The sylvian aqueduct should be covered with Cottonoid patties to prevent blood from entering the third ventricle. The tumor should not be chased into the brain stem as this will lead to serious neurologic morbidity. Hemorrhage from the floor of the fourth ventricle should not be cauterized, because this may result in unexpected cranial nerve damage. Placement of a Gelfoam pack and gentle compression should result in the hemostasis needed.

Cerebellar Hemispheric Tumors

If the lesion occupies one hemisphere, a linear incision should be made through the cerebellar cortex as the shortest distance from the tumor. In the case of a cerebellar astrocytoma with a mural nodule, the non-enhancing cyst wall does not need to be resected. If any portion of the cyst demonstrates contrast enhancement on the preoperative imaging study, it should be removed.

INTRAOPERATIVE NEUROMONITORING

Intraoperative monitoring of the cranial nerves and the brain stem is frequently used for posterior fossa tumors. Monitoring may be helpful to decrease morbidity and to allow a more aggressive resection. Brain stem auditory-evoked potentials (BAEPs) are resistant to most anesthetic agents. Somatosensory-evoked potentials (SSEPs) are affected by the inhalation anesthetics, although the effects to nitrous oxide are minimal.[79] Intravenous anesthetics affect SSEPs significantly less than do inhalation anesthetics. Propofol with nitrous oxide has minimal latency shift and amplitude reduction effects on SSEPs and offers promise as an effective adjunct to neuroanesthesia.[80,81]

The best option for direct monitoring of brain stem function is BAEPs; and median nerve SSEPs can be used simultaneously. The short-latency auditory-evoked potentials are generated from the cochlea, eighth nerve, and the brain stem, while the somatosensory-evoked potential is generated in the median lemniscus. The SSEPs are less sensitive than the BAEPs. If there is a 50% amplitude reduction, a greater than 10% latency increase, a loss of waveform or any alterations in vital signs, these should be considered warning signs to stop tumor manipulation, to relax on brain retractors, and to allow vital signs to normalize. Intraoperative electromyography can be recorded from directed stimulation of the following: The masseter or temporalis muscle (CN V), the lateral rectrus (CN VI), both orbicularis oculi and the oricularis muscles (CN VII), the soft palate (CN IX), the trapezius muscle (CN XI), the anterior third of the tongue (CN XII), and the posterior vocalis muscle or cricothyroid muscles (CN X).

OPERATIVE COMPLICATIONS

The most common complication is cerebellar ataxia. This may be transient and often rapidly resolves over several weeks. The portion of the tumor involving the unilateral cerebellar peduncle can be aggressively resected, and

gross total resection is possible with minimal neurologic deficits.[82] However, if bilateral cerebellar peduncles are involved, radical surgical manipulation should be avoided and may result in severe permanent cerebellar ataxia. When the dentate nucleus is damaged, the disequilibrium and intentional tremor during voluntary movement of the extremities may be found.

Cerebellar mutism is a unique postoperative complication seen in 5% to 30% of children following the resection of a posterior fossa mass lesion.[71,83,84] Vermian incision and lateral retraction of the dentate nuclei may explain the development of the cerebellar mutism syndrome particularly in children. Cerebellar mutism is a transient complication that may appear after removal of midline cerebellar tumors involving the vermis in children. It typically arises 1 to 2 days following surgery with patients initially displaying diminished speech progressing to mutism and typically resolves during the ensuing weeks to months. Cerebellar mutism is characterized by a lack of speech output in awake patients with intact speech comprehension, and is sometimes associated with oropharyngeal apraxia.

Cranial nerve dysfunction, such as abducens palsy and facial weakness, internuclear ophthalmoplegia, horizontal gaze palsy, swallowing difficulty, and vocal cord palsy are related to irritation of the brain stem or lower cranial nerve. Deficits with vocal cord apposition and swallowing may cause complications such as aspiration pneumonia and respiratory distress. Swallowing problems related to lower cranial nerve manipulation can generally be expected to recover function over time.[3,85,86] On the contrary, the symptoms with nuclear involvement of the brain stem may take longer to recover or may never recover completely.

Postoperative pseudomeningoceles or subsequent CSF leak affect 23% to 28% of all children with posterior fossa tumors.[87,88] The mechanisms leading to pseudomeningocele formation are unclear, but probably include inadequate dural and wound closures. Small pseudomeningoceles may respond well to pressure bandages, needle aspiration, and lumbar CSF drainage. However, pseudomeningoceles may be a manifestation of hydrocephalus and in some cases may require CSF diversion to control.

Aseptic meningitis is related hemorrhage into the subarachnoid space during tumor resection. It manifests with postoperative headaches, fever, irritability, photophobia, neck stiffness, and CSF pleocytosis at approximately 1 week after surgery. This complication is rare if appropriate hemostasis is achieved. Before treating for aseptic meningitis, true bacterial meningitis should be carefully excluded. A low-dose steroid or anti-inflammatory therapy may be helpful.

Specific Tumors

MEDULLOBLASTOMA
Epidemiology and Genetics

Medulloblastomas are the most common malignant brain tumor in children comprising 20% to 25% of all pediatric brain tumors and are usually found in the posterior fossa.[89] The majority (85%) arise from the cerebellar vermis and in the minority, they arise laterally from the cerebellar hemisphere. The median age at diagnosis is approximately 6 to 9 years.[20,90] There is a slight male predominance (male:female ratio 2:1).[91,92] Up to 30% of cases occur in adulthood.[93]

Several cancer predisposition syndromes are associated with medulloblastoma including Gorlin's syndrome, Turcot's syndrome, Li-Fraumeni syndrome, and Rubenstein-Taybi syndrome.[94] A frequent genetic abnormality is amplification of the MYC family of oncogenes, which is seen in up to 10% of cases.[95-97] Molecular subgroups, characterized by Wnt/wingless signaling, sonic hedgehog signaling (SHH), expression of neuronal differentiation genes or photoreceptor genes have been identified.[97-99] Based on these signaling pathways, targeted therapies have been suggested using agents such as cyclopamine and HhAnTag (small molecule inhibitor of the SHH).[100-102] Common chromosomal copy number changes include gain of chromosomes 1q and 7, as well as loss of chromosomes 22, 11, 10q, and 17p.[95,103,104] Loss of 17p is observed in up to 50% of cases, and may occur in the context of an isochromosome 17q.[95,103]

Pathology

Medulloblastomas are considered WHO grade IV tumors.[104] Histologic variants include the classic, desmoplastic/nodular, medulloblastoma with extensive nodularity, anaplastic, and large-cell subtypes. The classic medulloblastomas (70% to 80% of cases) appear as a dense sheet of small, basophilic cells with little cytoplasm, round-to-oval hyperchromatic nuclei and frequent mitoses (Fig. 55-9A). Homer-Wright rosettes are commonly seen.[104] Evidence of differentiation along neuronal or glial lineage is seen in up to 50% of cases.[105] The desmoplastic/nodular subtype accounts for approximately 15% to 20% of cases and is characterized by pale, reticulin-free nodules surrounded by reticulin-positive collagen fibers.[106] These nodules represent regions of more advanced neuronal differentiation. The large-cell and anaplastic subtypes have a greater percentage of poorly differentiated, anaplastic cellular regions. Medulloblastoma with extensive nodularity typically occurs in patients under 3 years of age, and shows the presence of lobular, grapelike nodules as a result of expansion of the reticulin-free zones.

Staging and Prognostic Factors

Careful pre- and postoperative staging is crucial in order to direct therapy and provide an estimate of patient prognosis. The staging system proposed by Chang et al. classified patient lesions based on two parameters: tumor and metastasis stage.[107] Currently, high-risk patients are defined as children with more than 1.5 cm² postoperative tumor residual, presenting at 3 years old or younger and/or the presence of metastases. All other patients are considered standard or average-risk.

One of the factors most consistently associated with prognosis is age at diagnosis.[44,108] Poor outcomes in younger patients may be a reflection of differences in treatment patterns, such as the delay or avoidance of adjuvant radiotherapy. Absence of metastatic disease at diagnosis and maximal safe surgical resection have been associated with improved survival. With respect to histologic subtypes, medulloblastoma with extensive nodularity has a very good prognosis and the desmoplastic subtype may have a better prognosis.[109-113] The large-cell and anaplastic subtypes demonstrate the worst prognosis.[114,115]

As for molecular markers, over-expression of TrkC (neurotrophin-3 receptor) and nuclear positivity for β-catenin (a marker of Wnt pathway activation) have been associated with a better prognosis.[116-119] High expression of the oncogenes erbB2 and myc are associated with worse outcomes.[120-122] Metastatic medulloblastoma has been associated with increased expression of genes involved with mitogen signaling including platelet-derived growth factor-alpha (PDFGR-α) and RAS/MAPK signaling components.[123]

Treatment

Medulloblastoma is frequently a radiosensitive and chemosensitive tumor. The current treatment protocol starts with maximal surgical resection followed by adjuvant craniospinal irradiation and chemotherapy.

Radiation Therapy

Craniospinal radiation (CSI) is an essential adjuvant treatment because medulloblastomas have a propensity for leptomeningeal spread. The standard postoperative CSI regimen is 36 Gy to the entire neuraxis, with a boost to the posterior fossa to a total dose of 54 Gy.[124,125] In recent years, a risk-adapted therapeutic strategy has been employed due to adverse sequelae of full dose radiation. High-risk patients older than age 3 years typically receive the standard-dose CSI plus adjuvant chemotherapy. In average-risk patients, reduced-dose CSI has been examined. The average-risk patients receiving reduced-dose CSI without adjuvant chemotherapy demonstrated a worse outcome compared with conventional dose CSI.[126-128] However, the reduced-dose CSI (23.4 Gy) in combined with adjuvant chemotherapy offered survival and disease control rates comparable to those achieved with standard dose CSI.[129-131] In a phase III study, the 5-year overall survival and event-free survival rates were 86% and 81%, respectively.[130] Another method being investigated for maximizing target radiation dose and reducing toxicity to adjacent normal brain includes the use of conformal boost radiotherapy limited to the tumor bed alone. The limited radiotherapy boost to the tumor bed produced disease control rates comparable to studies in which the entire posterior fossa is targeted.[131-134] For average-risk patients, 5-year disease-free survival and posterior fossa control rate were 86% and 94%, respectively.[134]

CSI can be associated with long-term CNS toxicities. Acute postradiation effects occur in the first week and consist of temporary drowsiness, nausea, and headaches. Subacute effects occur after 6 to 10 weeks and are reversible lethargy and fatigue. Late changes include cognitive impairment, growth abnormalities, hypopituitarism, severe sensorineural hearing loss, moyamoya syndrome, and secondary neoplasms (gliomas, meningiomas).[135]

Chemotherapy

Chemotherapy regimens have been developed for high-risk patients, those with progressive disease, and very young patients to avoid or delay radiation therapy, as well as average-risk patients. Current investigations attempt to determine the optimal timing and dosage of adjuvant therapies to maximize efficacy and minimize toxicity. As a result, multiagent chemotherapy has now become commonplace.

Several studies reported a survival benefit for average and high-risk patients treated with adjuvant chemotherapy

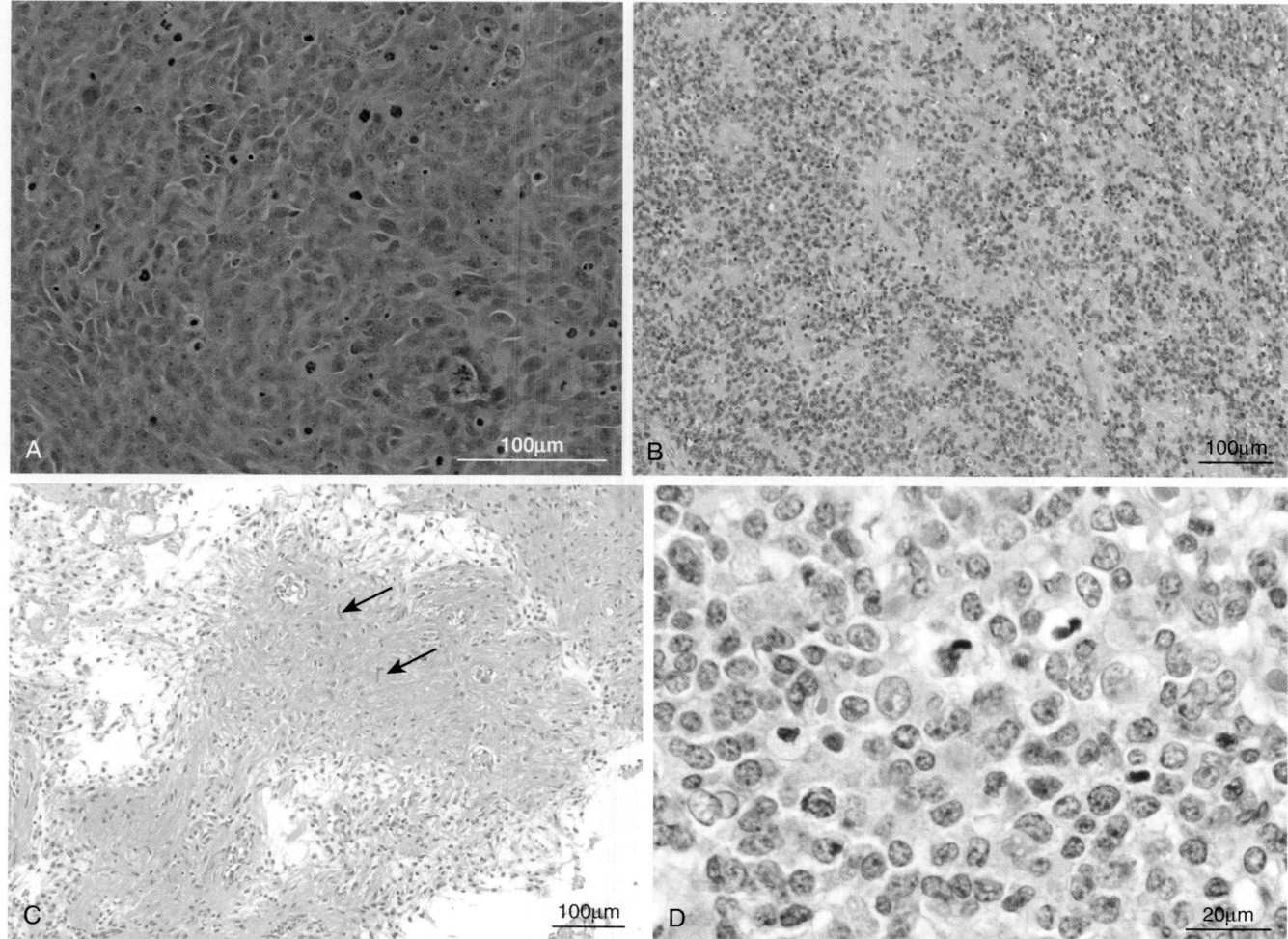

FIGURE 55-9 Histopathologic features of childhood posterior fossa tumors. A, Classic medulloblastoma is composed of a dense sheet of undifferentiated tumor cells with little cytoplasm and round-to-oval hyperchromatic nuclei (H&E). B, In ependymoma, the cells are uniform, cuboidal to elongated with oval or round nucleus, and perivascular pseudorosettes are seen (H&E). C, Pilocytic astrocytomas exhibit a biphasic appearance of compact, fiber-rich areas and hypocellular areas with microcysts (*black arrows:* Rosenthal fiber, H&E). D, Typical rhabdoid cells have an eccentric round nucleus with a prominent nucleolus and a plump cell body (H&E).

following surgical resection and CSI.[52,129,136,137] After CSI plus adjuvant chemotherapy, the 5-year, progression-free survival rate was 67% for patients with metastatic disease at the time of diagnosis.[52] Neoadjuvant chemotherapy has received attention but showed no clear benefit over conventional therapeutic strategies.[127,138-140] In the CCG921 trial, high-risk patients treated with postradiation chemotherapy had better 5-year progression-free survival (63%) compared with a neoadjuvant chemotherapy plus postradiation chemotherapy (45%).[140] Neoadjuvant chemotherapy was also associated with subsequent radiotherapy-induced myelotoxicity, leading to higher rates of treatment interruptions.[139] The strategy of high-dose, myeloablative chemotherapy followed by hematopoietic stem cell rescue has been tried as an option for recurrent disease, high-risk patients, disseminated disease, or children less than 36 months of age, in the avoidance of radiotherapy.[136,141-145] Overall, treatment-related mortality rates between 10% to 20% are seen with this strategy. For children less than 3 years old without metastasis, the 5-year event-free and overall survival rates for patients with gross total resection and residual resection

were 64% and 79%, and 29% and 57%, respectively.[144] In average- and high-risk patients, 5-year overall survival rates of 85% and 70% have been reported following postoperative risk-adapted CSI followed by high-dose chemotherapy and stem cell rescue, respectively.[136]

Chemotherapy has been associated with a variety of adverse events such as fatigue, nausea, vomiting, loss of appetite, stomatitis, myelosuppression, and infection. Some studies have found greater hematologic toxicity when chemotherapy was combined with radiation therapy compared with radiotherapy alone.[139] Less common side effects include nephrotoxicity, hepatotoxicity, cardiomyopathy, urinary bladder, sensorineural hearing loss, acute myelogenous leukemia, or pulmonary fibrosis depending on the agent used.

Follow-up and Recurrence

Long-term follow-up imaging has become the standard of care for medulloblastoma patients, with most receiving repeat brain and spine MRI every 3 to 6 months in the first 2 years following treatment.

Collin's law states that tumor relapse should occur within a period equal to the patient's age at diagnosis plus 9 months. This usually holds true for medulloblastoma in spite of several exceptions. The most common site of recurrent disease is the primary tumor site. However, up to 60% of patients will display evidence of disseminated disease at relapse.[90,146] Metastasis outside the nervous system is uncommon.[146] Bone lesions are the most common and lymph nodes are the second most common site. Early detection of recurrence offers the opportunity to test novel therapies in the setting of minimal disease burden. However, there is a controversy to the proven benefit because of the high percentage of dissemination at recurrence.

EPENDYMOMA

Epidemiology and Genetics

Ependymomas account for 5% to 10% of pediatric CNS tumors and can be located throughout the CNS.[147] They are the third most common brain tumors in children, following astrocytoma and medulloblastoma. More than 70% of ependymomas occur in the posterior fossa.[148] The mean age at the time of diagnosis is between 3 and 6 years, with more than 25% found in children under the age of 3 years. Males are 1.4 times more likely to develop ependymomas than females are.

The genetic alterations observed are loss of heterozygosity in chromosome 22q, monosomy 17, and loss of a region on 6q.[149-151] The 22q region is of special interest because it contains the neurofibromatosis type 2 (NF-2) tumor suppressor gene and an increased incidence of ependymomas is seen in NF-2. The intriguing finding of SV40-like DNA sequences raises the question of a possible viral role in tumor pathogenesis.[152] Although ependymomas from the supratentorial space, posterior fossa, and spinal cord have very similar histology, they are biologically distinct diseases with their own transcriptional profiles and distinct sets of genetic abnormalities.[153]

Pathology

Ependymomas are glial neoplasms arising from ependymal cell layers adjacent to the ventricular system or central spinal canal.[154] According to the WHO criteria, the two-tiered classification of ependymoma (ependymoma as grade II and anaplastic ependymoma as grade III) has been used. The cells are usually uniform, cuboidal to elongated with oval or round nuclei. The key pathologic feature is perivascular pseudorosettes, in which tumor cells are arranged radially around vessels (Fig. 55-9B). True ependymal rosettes may be present in a minority of cases. The histological differences between ependymoma and anaplastic ependymoma include the presence of nuclear atypia, marked mitotic activity, high cellularity, and often prominent vascular proliferation. Numerous studies concerning the correlation between histopathologic features and clinical outcome have yielded conflicting, inconsistent results.[46,47,155,156]

Prognostic Factors

Surgical resection is the best prognostic factor. A number of studies have shown that complete surgical resection offers the best hope of cure.[47,48,157,158] Surgery and radiation therapy yield 5-year progression-free survival ranging from 60% to 87% after complete resection to 0% to 33%

after incomplete surgical resection.[47,148,159-165] Postoperative imaging is essential. In patients where postoperative imaging shows residual disease that is surgically accessible, there may be a role for early second look surgery or perhaps delayed surgery for resection of residual disease after chemotherapy and radiation. These tumors are relatively well-demarcated and distinct from adjacent brain parenchyma. However, depending on location, tumors arising from the roof of the fourth ventricle are the easiest to totally remove. Lateral tumors with a large cerebellopontine angle component are the most difficult to totally remove as they are often adherent to cranial nerves and vascular structures.[166] Morbidity remains high secondary to brain stem and cranial nerve injury. The complete removal rates of the mid-floor type (origin of fourth ventricular floor), lateral type (extension to cerebellopontine angle), and roof type (origin of fourth ventricular roof) tumors are approximately 23%, 0%, and 100%, respectively.[167]

The incidence of dissemination of ependymoma is only 11% to 17%.[47,48] Nonetheless, it is important to demonstrate its presence or absence, because disseminated disease is a strong adverse prognostic factor. Perioperative disease staging with craniospinal MRI and CSF cytology is recommended. Controversial results have been published regarding the efficacy of age, histologic composition, radiotherapy, and chemotherapy on progression-free survival.[147,165,168]

Treatment

Intracranial ependymomas are relatively radiosensitive and chemoresistant. This further supports the need to completely extirpate primary ependymoma when feasible. Radiation therapy is the adjuvant therapy of choice. It is generally recommended that even after a gross total tumor resection, patients with localized disease undergo local tumor bed irradiation. The dose of radiation for the treatment of ependymoma has traditionally been in the range of 4500 to 5600 cGy. Craniospinal irradiation (CSI) is indicated for patients with disseminated disease and anaplastic histology does not appear to be an indication for CSI because most of subtypes are prone to local treatment failure. There was no difference in the distant failure rate for those receiving CSI versus posterior fossa only, for ependymoma (5%) versus anaplastic ependymoma (8.7%).[156,169-171] With the advent of stereotactic conformal radiotherapy, treatment can be highly focused on the tumor bed while sparing adjacent normal brain or brain stem in order to minimize radiation-associated toxicity.[172]

Adjuvant chemotherapy combined with radiation therapy has not yielded a significant improvement in survival for pediatric infratentorial ependymoma.[170,173,174] However, chemotherapy is efficacious to defer irradiation at the time of relapse and provide improved survivals in very young patients.[161,175-178] High-dose chemotherapy followed by autologous bone marrow transplantation has been tried for recurrent disease, but ependymoma does not appear to be as sensitive as medulloblastoma.[179,180] These data are not sufficient to justify the use of chemotherapy except in younger children to substitute for or delay radiation therapy, or patients in whom surgery and radiation therapy have failed to control tumor growth.

Tumors recur predominantly at the primary tumor site, suggesting that they arise from residual ependymoma cells.[46,160,162,181,182] Most instances of spinal metastases follow failure in the posterior fossa. It is very unusual to see isolated recurrence in the spine. After recurrence, repeated surgeries can be performed. Because the primary problem with ependymomas is local tumor control, brachytherapy with [125]iodine and radiosurgery have been reported to be an option in patients with recurrent disease. In current treatment paradigms, brachytherapy has been replaced with radiosurgery.[165,170,183]

CEREBELLAR ASTROCYTOMA

Epidemiology

The cerebellar astrocytoma represents over 10% of pediatric brain tumors and over 25% of posterior fossa tumors, making it one of the most common intracranial neoplasms of childhood. Over 70% of cerebellar astrocytomas are seen in children.[184] A mean age at presentation of 6 to 8 years is found, and these tumors are rarely found in children under 1 year of age or in adults over the age of 40.[9] There is no gender predilection.

Pathology

Most cerebellar astrocytomas are low grade neoplasms, especially in childhood. These are divided into two pathologic entities. Pilocytic astrocytomas are WHO grade I lesions and account for 65% to 85% of cerebellar astrocytoma.[9,27,28] Diffuse astrocytomas are considered as WHO grade II and account for 15% to 35%. Pilocytic astrocytomas exhibit a biphasic appearance, with compact areas composed mainly of bipolar cells with hair-like projections alternating with areas of loosely aggregated astrocytes containing stellate astrocytes and microcysts (Fig. 55-9C). In this pathology, the presence of endothelial proliferation does not imply a higher grade. Diffuse astrocytomas are composed of fibrillary neoplastic astrocytes on the background of loosely structured tumor matrix. Malignant tumors account for less than 5% of all pediatric cerebellar astrocytomas.[185]

Prognostic Factors

Long-term prognosis is dependent on the extent of resection, presence of brain stem invasion and histological features of malignancy.[9,27,28,185-188] Total resection is associated with considerably better outcome than is subtotal or partial resection. Total resection overall carries a 5-year survival of 90%, compared to subtotal resection with 48.5%.[27] There is no difference between diffuse and pilocytic astrocytoma in outcome for totally resected tumors. The diffuse type has been considered more prone to recurrence but the histologic type is not as definitive a predictor of recurrence as is extent of removal. Brain stem involvement is a significant adverse prognostic factor for cerebellar astrocytoma and the poor prognosis of solid tumors is related with the increased likelihood of brain stem involvement. There is a tendency for some tumors to invade the subarachnoid space and grow along the surface of the cerebellum, but this is not ominous and does not usually portend a negative prognosis. However, patients with malignant pathology will have poor clinical courses.

Treatment

The surgical goal is gross total resection of all contrast-enhancing tumor tissue, which virtually guarantees the patient a cure. Total tumor resection is limited by attachment or invasion of the tumor into the brain stem and both pilocytic and diffuse astrocytomas can invade the brain stem. Tumors of the cyst-mural nodule form are more often amenable to total gross removal because of their discrete margins and lateral placement. Tumors of the solid form may also be clearly demarcated from the surrounding cerebellum. However, with or without visible cysts, these may show an increased involvement of the brain stem, which in turn may make complete neurosurgical resection more difficult to achieve.[27,32,189]

All patients should have postoperative brain imaging with and without contrast enhancement to evaluate the extent of resection. The postoperative imaging is more accurate than the surgeon's assessment in determining whether a total removal has been accomplished.[28] If surgically accessible, bulky disease is seen on the postoperative images, early second-look surgery and resection of tumor may be advisable in some cases. If there is unexpected postoperative enhancement (with small residual tumor) in the patients in whom a total resection was thought to have been accomplished, the neurosurgeon can safely follow these patients with serial imaging studies rather than pursue a second operation. The growth potential of these tumors is low and the dedifferentiation to a more malignant type is rare.

There is no role for adjuvant radiation or chemotherapy once a cerebellar astrocytoma has been completely removed with confirmation by postoperative imaging. The value of postoperative radiotherapy as initial adjuvant treatment following subtotal removal has been debated and does not significantly improve survival.[27,190] However, it may be useful for the treatment of progression following a subtotal surgical excision where there is obvious infiltration of the brain stem or cerebellar peduncles.[191] These tumors may violate Collins' law by recurring late.[192]

ATYPICAL TERATOID/RHABDOID TUMORS

Epidemiology and Genetics

AT/RTs of the CNS in infants and children are unique histologic entities with an extremely aggressive natural history. AT/RTs form 1% to 2% of all brain tumors in the pediatric population.[38,39,49,193,194] Two thirds of AT/RTs will take origin in the posterior fossa. Three quarters of patients are age 3 years or younger at the time of diagnosis and the median age at diagnosis ranges from 16 to 32 months. There is a 3:2 male predominance.

Monosomy 22 is the principal cytogenetic abnormality, and was initially demonstrated in 1990.[195] Subsequently, truncating mutations of *hSNF5/INI1* on chromosome 22q11 were found in a series of cell lines derived from renal rhabdoid tumors. Somatic mutations of *hSNF5/INI1* were then identified in a series of CNS AT/RT.[196,197] These studies suggest that mutations in the tumor suppressor gene *INI1* predispose children to the development of AT/RTs.

Pathology

Histologically, AT/RTs resemble the more common and less aggressive primitive neuroectodermal tumor/medulloblastoma (PNET/MB) with which they have been misdiagnosed in the past. It is important to distinguish AT/RTs from PNET/MBs because AT/RTs are aggressive and usually fatal malignancies, whereas PNET/MBs have well-defined treatment protocols leading to decent 5-year survival rates.

The microscopic characteristics of AT/RT may be variable, but they almost always contain visible rhabdoid cells. The typical rhabdoid cells have an eccentric round nucleus with a prominent nucleolus and a plump cell body (Fig. 55-9D). Careful study of these tumors disclosed fields of rhabdoid cells with or without areas of primitive neuroepithelial cells, which are composed entirely (13%) or partly (77%) of rhabdoid cells.[38] In a quarter to a third of tumors, mesenchymal and/or epithelial elements are seen as well. Mitotic figures are typically abundant, and necrosis and hemorrhage are also common. In immunohistochemical studies, there are three antibodies whose epitopes are almost always expressed: epithelial membrane antigen (EMA), vimentin, and smooth-muscle actin. Today, immunohistochemistry for INI1 protein typically shows absence of expression in AT/RTs, but not in PNET/MBs.

Treatment

The initial treatment for most children with AT/RT is maximal safe neurosurgical resection of tumor. The interface of the AT/RT and cerebellum may be infiltrative and ill-defined, and tumors primarily in the cerebello-pontine angle may incorporate cranial nerve roots in the vicinity.[39] Total or near total resection of the tumor is feasible in about 30% of patients.[38] Postoperative cranio-spinal imaging is essential. Spinal imaging at initial presentation reveals evidence of disease in 25% to 34% patients.[38,39,49] Patterns of relapse show local disease alone in 31%, leptomeningeal dissemination alone in 11% and both in 58%.[38] The prognosis for children with AT/RT remains poor. The median time to progression is 4.5 months and the median reported survivals range from 6 to 11 months.[38,39,49] The few patients who underwent surgery with our without radiation therapy but had no chemotherapy experienced a median survival of 2.5 months.

As children with AT/RT frequently present with leptomeningeal dissemination, or develop it at the time of relapse, it is desirable to administer CSI after primary tumor resection for children greater than age 3 years and chemotherapy. While radiation therapy does not seem to alter the progression of disease in children with AT/RT, most children will receive radiation at some point in the course of their disease.[38,39] Patients with AT/RT respond poorly to chemotherapy with or without radiation therapy, and only 6 in 36 children had a greater than 50% reduction in tumor mass. The longest lasting response to chemotherapy was 10 months.[38] However, there are a few reports with prolonged survival after intensified chemotherapy. One study showed that after intensive therapy including intrathecal chemotherapy, two of three children were alive without evidence of disease 36 and 89 months after diagnosis.[194] Three of four children in another study treated with high dose chemotherapy with stem cell rescue survived more than 12 months and one is alive with no evidence of disease 46 months from diagnosis.[49]

Conclusions

Surgery is the mainstay of treatment for the child with a posterior fossa tumor. Surgery alone can guarantee a cure in the case of cerebellar astrocytoma, and complete neurosurgical resection promises extended survival in children

with posterior fossa ependymoma. While in and of itself insufficient to guarantee prolonged survival in medulloblastoma, gross total resection or near gross total resection has been shown to provide children with a survival advantage over those with bulk residual disease. As such, the neurosurgeon has a significant role to play in the management of posterior fossa tumors in children.

Recently, progress has been made in the design of clinical trials using enhanced adjuvant therapies such as intensity modulated radiation therapy (IMRT), and novel chemotherapeutic agents. However, many challenges persist with tumor types such as AT/RT and anaplastic ependymoma or anaplastic astrocytoma. Children with these tumors typically have a very poor prognosis. At the present time, the collaborative efforts of interdepartmental and multiinstitutional groups are crucial to delivering appropriate and timely multimodality therapy. In the future, we envision the use of new biological therapies targeting known aberrant molecular pathways to improve the survival of children with these more aggressive neoplasms.

ACKNOWLEDGMENT

This work was supported by the Laurie Berman and Wiley Funds at the Hospital for Sick Children. T-Y Jung is a visiting neurosurgical fellow from Chonnam National University Medical School, Gwangju, South Korea.

KEY REFERENCES

Abdollahzadeh M, Hoffman HJ, Blazer SI, et al. Benign cerebellar astrocytoma in childhood: experience at the Hospital for Sick Children 1980-1992. *Childs Nerv Syst*. 1994;10:380-383.
Culley DJ, Berger MS, Shaw D, et al. An analysis of factors determining the need for ventriculoperitoneal shunts after posterior fossa tumor surgery in children. *Neurosurgery*. 1994;34:402-407.
David KM, Casey AT, Hayward RD, et al. Medulloblastoma: is the 5-year survival rate improving? A review of 80 cases from a single institution. *J Neurosurg*. 1997;86:13-21.
Hayostek CJ, Shaw EG, Scheithauer B, et al. Astrocytomas of the cerebellum: a comparative clinicopathologic study of pilocytic and diffuse astrocytomas. *Cancer*. 1993;72:856-869.
Koral K, Gargan L, Bowers DC, et al. Imaging characteristics of atypical teratoid-rhabdoid tumor in children compared with medulloblastoma. *AJR Am J Roentgenol*. 2008;190:809-814.
Lee YY, Van Tassel P, Bruner JM, et al. Juvenile pilocytic astrocytomas: CT and MR characteristics. *AJR Am J Roentgenol*. 1989;152:1263-1270.
Louis DN, Ohgaki H, Wiestler OD, Cavenee WK. *World Health Organization Classification of Tumours of the Central Nervous System*. Lyon: IARC; 2007.
Meyers SP, Kemp SS, Tarr RW. MR imaging features of medulloblastomas. *AJR Am J Roentgenol*. 1992;158:859-865.
Meyers SP, Wildenhain SL, Chang JK, et al. Postoperative evaluation for disseminated medulloblastoma involving the spine: contrast-enhanced MR findings, CSF cytologic analysis, timing of disease occurrence, and patient outcomes. *AJNR Am J Neuroradiol*. 2000;21:1757-1765.
Miller JP, Cohen AR. Surgical management of tumors of the fourth ventricle. In: Schmidek HH, Roberts DW, eds. *Schmidek and Sweet operative neurosurgical techniques: indications, methods, and results*. 5th ed. Philadelphia: Elsevier; 2006:881-909.
Mussi AC, Rhoton Jr AL. Telovelar approach to the fourth ventricle: microsurgical anatomy. *J Neurosurg*. 2000;92:812-823.
Nazar GB, Hoffman HJ, Becker JE, et al. Infratentorial ependymomas in childhood: prognostic factors and treatment. *J Neurosurg*. 1990;72:408-417.
Nejat F, El Khashab M, Rutka JT. Initial management of childhood brain tumors: neurosurgical considerations. *J Child Neurol*. 2008;23:1136-1148.
Park TS, Hoffman HJ, Hendrick EB, et al. Medulloblastoma: clinical presentation and management. Experience at the hospital for sick children, Toronto, 1950-1980. *J Neurosurg*. 1983;58:543-552.

Rorke LB, Packer RJ, Biegel JA. Central nervous system atypical teratoid/rhabdoid tumors of infancy and childhood: definition of an entity. *J Neurosurg.* 1996;85:56-65.

Rutka JT. *Medulloblastoma. Clin Neurosurg.* 1997;44:571-585.

Rutka JT, Kuo JS. Pediatric surgical neuro-oncology: current best care practices and strategies. *J Neurooncol.* 2004;69:139-150.

Rutka JT, Kuo JS, Carter M, et al. Advances in the treatment of pediatric brain tumors. *Expert Rev Neurother.* 2004;4:879-893.

Sainte-Rose C, Cinalli G, Roux FE, et al. Management of hydrocephalus in pediatric patients with posterior fossa tumors: the role of endoscopic third ventriculostomy. *J Neurosurg.* 2001;95:791-797.

Schneider Jr JH, Raffel C, McComb JG. Benign cerebellar astrocytomas of childhood. *Neurosurgery.* 1992;30:58-62.

Shemie S, Jay V, Rutka J, et al. Acute obstructive hydrocephalus and sudden death in children. *Ann Emerg Med.* 1997;29:524-528.

Tanriover N, Ulm AJ, Rhoton Jr AL, et al. Comparison of the transvermian and telovelar approaches to the fourth ventricle. *J Neurosurg.* 2004;101:484-498.

Taylor MD, Mainprize TG, Rutka JT. Molecular insight into medulloblastoma and central nervous system primitive neuroectodermal tumor biology from hereditary syndromes: a review. *Neurosurgery.* 2000;47:888-901.

Tortori-Donati P, Fondelli MP, Cama A, et al. Ependymomas of the posterior cranial fossa: CT and MRI findings. *Neuroradiology.* 1995;37:238-243.

Undjian S, Marinov M, Georgiev K. Long-term follow-up after surgical treatment of cerebellar astrocytomas in 100 children. *Childs Nerv Syst.* 1989;5:99-101.

Numbered references appear on Expert Consult.

Supratentorial Tumors in the Pediatric Population: Multidisciplinary Management

CHETAN BETTEGOWDA • LINDA C. CHEN • VIVEK A. MEHTA • GEORGE I. JALLO • JAMES T. RUTKA

Epidemiology

In the pediatric population, primary central nervous system (CNS) malignancies are the most common solid organ tumor, totaling approximately 20% of cancers in children ages 1 to 4 years and approximately 30% in children ages 5 to 9 years. In the United States, there are more than 3700 newly diagnosed cases of CNS tumors per year in children below 19 years of age. With a 66% 5-year survival rate for this age group, it is estimated that 26,000 children in the United States have a CNS tumor. The incidence rate for CNS tumors is higher in males than in females (29.9 vs. 25.1 per million) and is greatest in Caucasian individuals (29.4 per million). Based on the World Health Organization (WHO) classification system, 75% of all primary childhood CNS tumors are of neuroepithelial origin (gliomas). These include astrocytic tumors, embryonal CNS tumors, neuronal and mixed neuronal–glial tumors, and ependymomas. Ependymomas account for 15% of nonastrocytic neoplasms in the pediatric supratentorial space. Supratentorial tumors constitute 31% of pediatric CNS tumors (Table 56-1).[1,2]

Clinical Presentation

The clinical presentation is often determined by the tumor type and location, because symptoms are produced by local invasion, compression of adjacent structures, and increased intracranial pressure. More than 50% of patients have had symptoms for 6 months or longer at the time of diagnosis.[3] They can be broadly categorized into generalizing and localizing symptoms. Generalizing symptoms are due to increased intracranial pressure, often a result of blockage of normal cerebrospinal fluid (CSF) flow. The most common generalizing symptoms for childhood CNS tumors include headache, nausea and vomiting, and lethargy.[4] Localizing symptoms result from direct irritation, destruction, or impairment of neuronal function caused by the tumor. These include seizures, endocrinopathies, hemiparesis, cranial nerve deficits, and visual field defects[5] (Table 56-2).

When considering the youngest pediatric patients, the constellation of symptoms differs because children are often unable to articulate their complaints. In this case, a thorough history with the caregiver and a physical exam are essential to uncover subtle and nonspecific signs. For children under the age of 4, the most commonly found symptoms include macrocephaly, nausea, vomiting, irritability, and lethargy.[4]

In the case of supratentorial tumors, symptoms are generally nonspecific and children typically have a delayed diagnosis when compared to those with infratentorial tumors. However, seizures are often seen in low-grade supratentorial lesions, either as an isolated finding (30% of patients) or with other symptoms, such as changes in personality, cognition, and development.[2]

Though headache is the most common manifestation of CNS tumors in children, its character is nonspecific and can vary from focal to diffuse. Thus, headaches in pediatric and adolescent patients are often attributed to benign causes, including migraines or tension headaches. However, on closer examination, these patients often present with other neurologic symptoms. Therefore, children with headaches in the setting of another neurologic deficit require further evaluation with neuroimaging. The options for imaging children include ultrasound if the fontanelle is open; x-ray, which can be of limited use in select cases; computed tomography (CT); magnetic resonance imaging (MRI); and if vascular abnormalities are suspected, angiography. The use of CT scans should be limited in the pediatric population, given the increasing evidence for radiation-induced malignancies that occur many years after image acquisition.[6] If neuroimaging does confirm the presence of a mass, tissue diagnosis is often necessary to determine the appropriate treatment regimen.[4]

The most common pediatric supratentorial tumors include low-grade glioma, high-grade glioma, pineal region tumors, germ cell tumors, and intraventricular tumors. In this chapter, we examine the epidemiology, diagnosis, treatment, and relevant operative approaches for these lesions.

Low-Grade Glioma

BACKGROUND

Pediatric low-grade gliomas, consisting of WHO grade I to II tumors, are a heterogeneous group of lesions that include pilocytic astrocytomas, oligodendrogliomas, and mixed neuroglial tumors, with pilocytic astrocytomas predominating. The overall prognosis is favorable with an indolent course and a remote risk of malignant transformation.[5] While rare, there have even been case reports of spontaneous

Table 56-1 Breakdown of the Anatomic Location of Pediatric Supratentorial Tumors

Supratentorial Brain Lesions	Patients
Temporal lobe	7%
Frontal lobe	6%
Multilobar	6%
Ventricle	6%
Parietal lobe	4%
Occipital lobe	2%
Total patients	31%

Matula C. Tumors of the pineal region. In Rengachary SS and Ellenbogen RG (eds), Principles of Neurosurgery, 2nd ed. Philadelphia, Elsevier, 2005.

Table 56-2 Breakdown of the Most Common Presenting Symptoms for Pediatric Supratentorial Tumors

Presenting Symptom	Frequency	Presenting Symptom	Frequency
Headache	33%	Declining academic performance	7%
Nausea and vomiting	32%	Macrocephaly	7%
Abnormal gait or coordination	27%	Cranial nerve palsies	7%
Papilledema	13%	Lethargy	6%
Seizures	13%	Abnormal eye movement	6%
Intracranial pressure symptoms	10%	Hemiplegia	6%
Squinting	7%	Weight loss	5%

Matula C. Tumors of the pineal region. In Rengachary SS and Ellenbogen RG (eds), Principles of Neurosurgery, 2nd ed. Philadelphia, Elsevier, 2005.

regression of low-grade astrocytomas.[7,8] Low-grade astrocytomas account for 30% to 50% of all pediatric CNS tumors,[9] with hemispheric (10%-15%), deep midline (10%-15%), and optic pathways (5%) being the most common locations.

The two most common pediatric low-grade gliomas are pilocytic astrocytomas (WHO grade I) and diffuse fibrillary astrocytoma (FA) (WHO grade II). Pilocytic astrocytomas typically occur in children between the ages of 5 to 19, whereas only 10% of FAs occur before the age of 20.[5] Other less common pathologies include pilomyxoid astrocytoma, pleomorphic xanthoastrocytoma (PXA), ganglioglioma, subependymal giant cell astrocytoma, and oligodendroglioma. Pilomyxoid astrocytomas (WHO grade II) were first introduced in 1999; tend to occur early in life, with a median age of 18 months; and typically occur in the hypothalamus.[10] Gangliogliomas and PXAs, both WHO grade II, typically occur in the temporal lobe and can present with seizures. Subependymal giant cell astrocytomas are WHO grade I lesions that occur almost exclusively in patients with tuberous sclerosis. Oligodendrogliomas (WHO grade II) are rare and account for less than 5% of brain tumors in children. When they do occur, they typically are found in the frontal lobe.[5]

The molecular triggers that lead to formation of low-grade gliomas are poorly understood. Few recurrent genetic changes have been described. Karyotype analysis has only revealed gain of chromosome 7 in a minority of tumors.[11,12] Recently, groups have identified recurrent duplications in 7q34 in a large fraction of pilocytic astrocytomas, implicating BRAF and the RAS/RAF/MEK pathway in the pathogenesis.[13,14]

Pilocytic astrocytomas are the most common glial tumor in the pediatric patient and can occur anywhere in the CNS. The most common supratentorial location is the optic pathway, contributing to approximately 60% of optic pathway gliomas.[5] These lesions are typically diagnosed early, with 75% of optic pathway gliomas being diagnosed before 10 years of age. More than 70% of children with optic pathway gliomas have neurofibromatosis type 1 (NF1), and many of those with NF1 develop bilateral optic nerve lesions.[15]

Optic Pathway Gliomas

EPIDEMIOLOGY

Optic nerve gliomas comprise approximately 1% of all intracranial tumors, are most commonly unilateral, and occur more frequently in females.[16,17] While they can present at any age, 75% become symptomatic in the first decade of life and 90% become symptomatic before age 20.[18] Rush et al. reported that in their series of 33 patients that the median age at diagnosis was 6.5 years and the mean age was 10.9 years, with a range of 2 to 46 years.[19] The signs and symptoms of optic nerve gliomas typically consist of decreased visual function, proptosis, optic disc swelling, and strabismus.[17] Patients can have vascular compromise of the optic apparatus from chronic compression of the central retinal vein, leading to occlusion, venous stasis retinopathy, optociliary shunt vessels, or neovascular glaucoma.[17] In rare cases, acute loss of vision can occur in the setting of tumor hemorrhage. Patients typically do not present with orbital or ocular pain.[17]

A firm link has been established between NF1 and optic pathway gliomas. The incidence of NF1 among patients with optic nerve or chiasmal gliomas has ranged from 10% to 70% based on the series, while the incidence of optic nerve glioma in patients with NF1 varies from 8% to 31%.[17,20]

DIAGNOSIS

The diagnosis of an optic nerve glioma can largely be made by either CT or MRI. The radiographic appearance varies depending on whether the person has NF1. In patients without NF1, the optic nerve is almost always enlarged in a fusiform manner with a clear-cut margin produced by the intact dural sheath. In patients with NF1, the nerve is irregular, with kinking and buckling secondary to the mass.[17] On MRI, the tumor is typically hypo- to isointense on T1-weighted imaging and hyperintense on T2-weighted imaging. After intravenous administration of gadolinium-based contrast agents, the glioma may not enhance, have patchy enhancement, or demonstrate avid enhancement (Fig. 56-1).[21] Additionally, MRI imaging may demonstrate abnormalities that extend beyond the optic nerve into the chiasm.[17] Patients may have an enlarged optic canal ipsilateral to the side of the lesion, but this does not always indicate extension of the tumor intracranially. Arachnoid hyperplasia may be sufficient by itself to cause canal enlargement. Conversely, a normal caliber optic canal does not rule out the possibility of tumor extension beyond the orbit.[17]

The natural history of optic nerve gliomas is usually benign, with most growing slowly in a self-limited manner

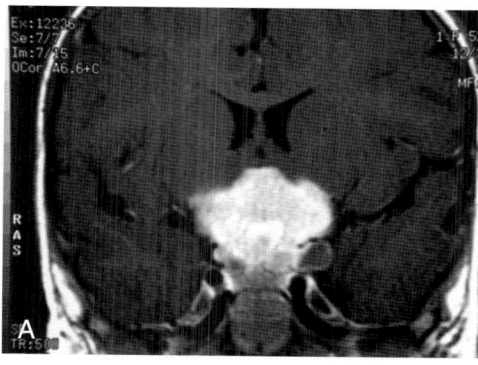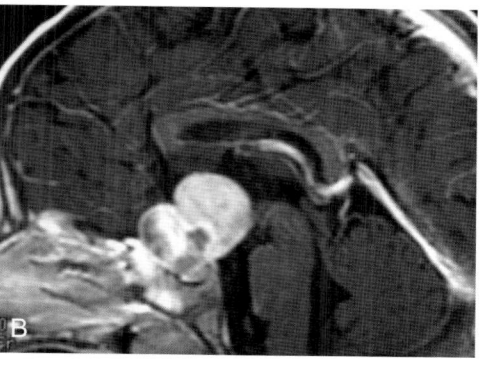

FIGURE 56-1 Coronal (A) and sagittal (B) postcontrast MRI demonstrating a large enhancing optic pathway pilocytic astrocytoma.

or, in extremely rare cases, spontaneously regressing.[8] As a result, many patients retain excellent or maintain existing visual function without treatment. Rarely, WHO grade III and IV lesions arise from the optic nerve and result in rapid visual loss, neurologic deficit, and eventual death. These high-grade lesions almost always occur in adults.[22]

PATHOLOGY

The gross appearance of an optic nerve glioma often causes diffuse expansion of the nerve that may extend the entire length of the nerve or affect only a portion. The expanded portion can be solid or gelatinous, with hemorrhagic and necrotic regions. In children with NF1, the tumor not only expands the nerve but often breaks through pia mater and enters the subdural space.[17,23] However, as long as the glioma lies within the confines of the orbit or optic canal, the tumors are typically limited to within the optic dural sheath. If the glioma extends intracranially, it can remain intraneural or become an expansile mass that can compress adjacent structures, including the chiasm or contralateral optic nerve.[17]

The most common type of optic nerve tumor is the pilocytic astrocytoma, which has three predominant histologic patterns: (1) coarsely reticulated, (2) finely reticulated, and (3) coarsely fibrillated or spindle cell.[21] The most common pattern is coarsely reticulated, with a biphasic pattern histologically of coarse bipolar astrocytes that are either tightly compacted around blood vessels or loosely associated around microcystic spaces. These tumors frequently have Rosenthal fibers and eosinophilic granular bodies. Finely reticulated pilocytic astrocytomas can be confused with WHO grade II diffuse low-grade astrocytomas and demonstrate an expansion of the indigenous neuroglia of the optic nerve. Within the finely reticulated tumors, a delicate reticulated syncytium of neuroglia fibers is embedded among multiple, small, round or ovoid nuclei. The coarsely fibrillated variant consists of coarse neuroglial fibrils and spindle cells arranged in bundles and is more often seen in adults.[21]

MANAGEMENT

Treatment for pilocytic astrocytoma of the optic pathway continues to evolve. Management is highly variable, depending on the patient's age, location of tumor, degree of infiltration of the optic chiasm, visual function in both eyes, and whether the patient is comorbid with NF1. In pediatric patients who do not display symptoms, close observation with serial MRI scans and visual function assessment is recommended until there is a change in tumor size or clinical status. While no universally accepted criteria have

been developed regarding when to treat optic gliomas, most would agree that intervention is indicated if there is (1) cosmetically unacceptable proptosis, (2) progressive deterioration of visual function, (3) MRI findings of definite tumor enlargement or extension, or (4) progressive neurologic deficit attributable to the tumor.

The three major treatment modalities are surgery, chemotherapy, and radiation therapy. Surgery still plays a role in the management of optic pathway gliomas, especially in individuals without NF1 for whom MRI findings are not compelling and tissue diagnosis is required.[24-26] Often in those cases, stereotactic or open biopsies can be safely performed. However, in cases where a large tumor creates mass effect or hydrocephalus, recurrent tumors refractory to chemo- or radiotherapy or cystic lesions with compression of the optic pathway can benefit from more radical surgery.[25,26] Advocates of aggressive surgical resection argue that radical tumor excision allows long-term remission, given the slow-growing nature of pilocytic astrocytomas. Additionally, it could delay the initiation of radiation therapy, which has significant long-term sequelae in children. While some studies have demonstrated that aggressive resection can be safely performed if done carefully,[27,28] the outcomes after surgery remain variable. For example, Sawamura et al. reported on the visual outcomes after 26 cases treated surgically with the intent to debulk as much tumor as possible.[25] Of this group, 20 patients underwent radical resection with greater than 90% tumor removal, and the remaining 6 patients had partial resection. Of the 26 children, only 2 had visual improvement, 2 remained static, 10 remained blind, and 12 worsened.

Given the unclear role for each of the treatment modalities and that overall survival rate for pilocytic optic gliomas is greater than 90%, each patient should be treated case by case in a multidisciplinary fashion that involves pediatricians, neurologists, neurosurgeons, medical oncologists, and radiation oncologists. Preserving overall quality of life and vision should be key endpoints during the decision-making process.

Thalamic Glioma

Pediatric thalamic gliomas arise as primary gliomas or secondary gliomas from adjacent structures, including the cerebral hemispheres, caudate nuclei, brain stem, or pineal gland. The deep, central location of the thalamus makes surgical treatment of these tumors difficult without significant patient morbidity and mortality. Even though thalamic gliomas are rare and account for 1% to 1.5% of all CNS tumors, both low-grade, well-circumscribed lesions and high-grade, diffuse, infiltrating gliomas have been described.[29] Although pilocytic astrocytomas classically occur in the hypothalamic/optic pathway, they can also occur as unilateral thalamic masses. Higher-grade FAs also occur in this region and are typically unilateral, with little involvement of the visual pathways. Finally, bilateral infiltrating astrocytomas, a rare variant of FAs, are lesions in bilateral thalami that have a poor outcome due to their intrinsic aggressive biology and the difficulty in attaining adequate surgical debulking of the tumor, resulting in mass effect on the thalamus.[30,31] Treatment considerations concerning the necessity, feasibility, and safety of surgery in children with these lesions are varied.

EPIDEMIOLOGY

Thalamic gliomas are rare and account for 0.84% to 5.2% of pediatric intracranial tumors.[29] This discrepancy in incidence is due to difficulty in differentiating primary thalamic tumors from secondary lesions that grow to involve thalamic structures. In a retrospective analysis of 69 children with thalamic tumors, 32 had low-grade thalamic tumors and 22 had high-grade tumors; the remaining 15 had 9 bilateral thalamic and 6 thalamopeduncular tumors. It was found that low-grade lesions had statistically improved survival rates, particularly when patients had symptom duration longer than 2 months and tumor excision greater than 90%.[32]

PATHOLOGY

Primary thalamic gliomas include pilocytic astrocytomas, FAs, and bilateral infiltrating astrocytomas. Pilocytic astrocytomas are low-grade gliomas, with histologic grade I. FAs are a heterogeneous group of astrocytic cells and are graded by the WHO from grade II to grade IV. They are prone to malignant progression. Bilateral infiltrating astrocytomas are a rare variant of FAs histologically that are highly infiltrating but well-differentiated grade II tumors.[30] They are extremely rare, and though benign and well differentiated, patients have

a poor prognosis due to thalamic nuclei involvement and inadequate surgical resection.[31] It is unknown whether these bilateral tumors arise from one side of thalamic nuclei and cross the midline to the other or arise independently from tumors in the subependymal region of the third ventricle.

DIAGNOSIS

Clinical signs and symptoms include weakness, increased intracranial pressure, motor deficits, seizures, ophthalmologic abnormalities, and in some cases, mental deterioration and personality change. It has been reported that the majority of patients have symptoms of increased intracranial pressure, headache, and vomiting.[33] Though the thalamus plays an important functional role in movement, only 12% of patients have movement disorders such as tremors and dystonia. More commonly, 30% of patients present with epilepsy, despite the tumor's deep-seated location. Another common finding in thalamic lesions includes contralateral paresis that affects one or both extremities.[34] In addition, clinical presentation is correlated with tumor location. Specifically, tumors of the anterolateral thalamus are associated with sensation deficits and paresis, while those of the posteromedial thalamus are associated with early hydrocephalus.[35] The presentation can also include deficits in vision such as hemianopia, a mitotic poorly reactive pupil, and ipsilateral oculomotor palsy.[34]

Patients typically undergo MRI prior to treatment and during follow-up. Thalamic lesions are heterogeneous and often cystic, with calcification, edema, and contrast enhancement on T1- and T2-weighted MRI[32] (Fig. 56-2). The most common neuroimaging finding is hydrocephalus. Imaging is helpful in distinguishing between pilocytic astrocytomas and more infiltrative FAs. Pilocytic astrocytomas are characteristically well circumscribed, solid, and contrast enhancing. Grade II FAs are diffuse and hyperintense on T2-weighted and fluid-attenuated inversion recovery (FLAIR) sequences, and grade IV FAs enhance with contrast. Bithalamic infiltrating astrocytomas present as symmetrical T2 signal hyperintensity in both thalami.[36]

FIGURE 56-2 Axial (A) and coronal (B) postcontrast MRI scan depicting a thalamic pilocytic astrocytoma with heterogenous enhancement and a small cystic component.

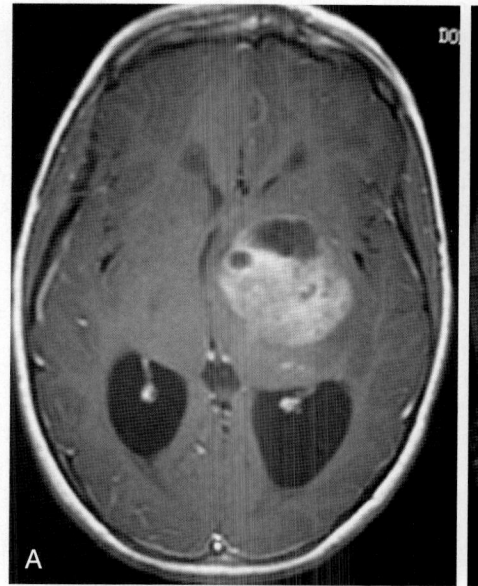
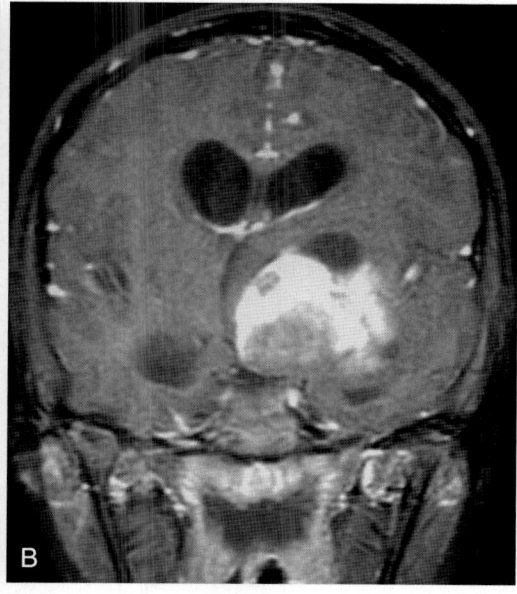

MANAGEMENT

Overall surgical management of pediatric thalamic tumors is individualized and largely depends on the pathologic grade of the tumor, location, and neuroimaging characteristics such as vascular involvement and enhancement. These characteristics are needed when considering surgical course.

The correlation between extent of resection and prognosis of a particular tumor type is of considerable importance. Historically, biopsy with irradiation was the standard of treatment due to patient morbidity and mortality with surgery. However, in low-grade thalamic tumors, radical resection can be curative. Consensus within the literature for low-grade astrocytomas includes stereotactic biopsy to verify histology, followed by surgery for curative intent. In a study examining the mortality rate of complete resection of benign thalamic astrocytomas in 26 children, the procedure was found to be associated with improved prognosis when postoperative MRI showed no residual tumor but was associated with a 7.7% mortality rate.[37] Surgical resection of bilateral infiltrating astrocytomas of the thalamus is difficult to achieve, and biopsy for histologic diagnosis is preferred. These patients have a poor outcome despite adjuvant radiation and chemotherapy.

Anatomic considerations are important because the thalamus is adjacent to critical structures. The thalamus is bound anteriorly by the foramen of Monro and posteriorly by the posterior commissure. It also is bound superiorly by the stria medullaris and inferiorly by the hypothalamic sulcus. Finally, the thalamus is medially bound by the third ventricle and laterally bound by the internal capsule. The terminal vein lies in the groove between the thalamus and the caudate and serves as a landmark for the position of the internal capsule.[34] Factors that must be considered by neurosurgeons include MRI appearance of the tumor, extent of tumor involvement, regions of enhancement, evidence of hydrocephalus, and relationship of the tumor to vital vascular structures.[34] Surgical approaches that have been used with endoscopic or stereotactic guidance include transcallosal–interhemispheric, infratentorial–supracerebellar, and trans-sylvian transinsular approaches.[34] Surgical resections can be performed while minimizing morbidity using concomitant neuronavigation and intraoperative neuromonitoring of the corticospinal tracts.

If the patient is in extremis because of elevated intracranial pressure secondary to hydrocephalus, the surgeon should perform emergent CSF drainage. The most rapid method is to place an extraventricular drain (EVD). If surgery for gross total resection is planned, the surgeon can attempt to wean the EVD postoperatively because the normal CSF flow is sometimes restored. If only biopsy is planned or a CSF blockade persists, the surgeon can perform an endoscopic third ventriculostomy or place a ventriculoperitoneal shunt.[38]

Postoperative imaging is obtained to evaluate the extent of resection and residual tumor. Adjuvant radiation and chemotherapy for high-grade gliomas are required. In a study of 57 patients, despite surgical resection and multimodal therapy, the median survival length remained 73 weeks.[33] In contrast, children who have low-grade gliomas that have been resected in their entirety can be observed serially for tumor recurrence. Upward of 90% 10-year survival rates have been reported for low-grade thalamic gliomas. For partially resected or unresectable low-grade thalamic tumors, the timing of additional therapy is controversial. Most surgeons advocate a "wait and see" approach. Often adjuvant therapy can be delayed until signs of clinical worsening or radiographic growth. In one series looking at 128 children with subtotal resection of low-grade gliomas, 58% had no evidence of tumor progression 7 years after diagnosis despite undergoing no additional therapy. Furthermore, there was no difference in survival in those children that did receive immediate postoperative radiotherapy and those that not.[39]

Given the increasing data regarding the detrimental effects of radiation on children, many centers recommend chemotherapy as frontline adjuvant therapy in children with progressive low-grade gliomas. One combination that has shown promise is a combination of carboplatin and vincristine, which has been shown to generate a 68% 3-year progression-free survival rate.[40] Unfortunately, 40% of children experience hypersensitivity reactions with carboplatin. These patients are often started on a regimen of 6-thioguanine, procarbazine, lomustine, dibromodulcitol, and vincristine, which has shown a 45% 3-year progression-free survival rate.[40]

Pediatric Glioblastoma

Glioblastoma multiforme (GBM) are WHO grade IV gliomas, which are rarely diagnosed in the pediatric population but cause significant morbidity and mortality. While GBMs are primarily an adult-age tumor, pediatric GBMs are also classified as high-grade gliomas, along with anaplastic astrocytomas and intrinsic pontine gliomas.[41,42] Anatomically, the majority of these tumors are located supratentorially, but GBMs also occur in the brain stem.[43] The current treatment recommendations include aggressive surgery, radiotherapy, and chemotherapy.

EPIDEMIOLOGY AND PROGNOSIS

Pediatric GBMs compose 3% of childhood primary brain tumors and are rarely diagnosed among children and adolescents. Overall, the prognosis of glioblastoma is better in children than in adults.[44] The majority of patients experience recurrence after surgical resection within 2 years of diagnosis, with the overall survival rate at 67% 1 year, 52% 2 years, and 40% 5 years after diagnosis.[44,45] The median overall survival length is 43 months, with a median progression-free survival length of 12 months.[44] Survival is correlated with tumor location, and patients with superficially located GBM had a median survival length of 52 months, while those with deeply located tumors had a median survival length of 7 months.[44] Furthermore, there is no significant relationship between patient age and survival.[45] Histologic features, while prognostically significant in adults, have been found to have no association with survival in pediatric patients.[45] Extent of resection was found to be a significant predictor of outcome. Radical tumor resection, defined as resection of greater than 90% of the tumor by postoperative imaging, was found to have a survival advantage when compared to partial resection in pediatric patients.[42] Specifically, the median survival length for patients with completely resected tumors was 106 months, while those with incompletely resected tumors had a median survival length of 11 months.[44]

PATHOLOGY

GBMs are classified as WHO grade IV infiltrating astrocytomas. Pathologic diagnosis is based on histologic features that include pleomorphism, mitotic figures, endothelial proliferation, and tumor necrosis.[46] Unlike adults, histologic grading has not been found to have a strong prognostic significance for children, as the difference in overall progression-free survival of pediatric glioblastoma and anaplastic astrocytoma is not statistically significant.[47] Individual genetic alterations such as epithelial growth factor receptor (EGFR) amplification, p53 mutations, retinoblastoma loss, IDH1 mutations, and deletion of phosphatase and tensin homology (PTEN) are common in adults; however, such alterations are distinctly different in pediatric GBMs.[46] In pediatric GBMs examined in the Children's Cancer Group cohort of 945 patients, EGFR, PTEN, and IDH1 gene expression aberrance were rare in pediatrics, while p53 alterations were more frequent.[47,48] In addition, overexpression of O-6-methylguanine-DNA methyltransferase, which is an important mechanism of resistance to temozolomide, is limited in pediatric glioblastomas and has driven investigation of the use of temozolomide in children.[49] Pediatric GBMs are molecularly distinct from their adult counterparts and warrant therapies specifically directed toward these molecular targets.

DIAGNOSIS

Presenting signs and symptoms vary by location and age. The history may include a short evolution of symptoms on the order of days and weeks to months.[42] Cortical lesions may be manifested through seizures, hemiparesis, visual deficits, and headaches. Indications of obstructed CSF leading to hydrocephalus include morning headaches, vomiting, and papilledema.[42] Infants commonly present with nonspecific symptoms, including irritability, lethargy, vomiting, failure to thrive, and macrocephaly. Nonspecific symptoms coupled with a neurologic deficit are particularly suspicious for a brain lesion in young children.

MRI is the preferred diagnostic imaging modality to determine whether symptoms are consistent with high-grade glioma. Imaging including axial, sagittal, and coronal planes pre- and postgadolinium should be obtained. T1 sequence characteristics include irregular margins, enhancement with contrast, invasion of surrounding brain parenchyma, heterogeneous enhancement patterns, and areas of cystic necrosis with a rim of enhancement (Fig. 56-3). Edema is commonly evidenced on FLAIR or T2. When imaging is consistent with high-grade glioma, biopsy—at a minimum—is indicated for tissue diagnosis. Stereotactic biopsy is appropriate for deep-seated tumors in functionally important areas.[42] Further surgical management, including open resection, is dictated by tumor location.

MANAGEMENT

Therapy for pediatric GBMs consists of surgery, radiotherapy, and chemotherapy. Complete or near-complete surgical resection is recommended when operative risks are acceptable, because gross total resection of the tumor significantly improves prognosis compared to subtotal resection.[42] In 131 children with GBM treated with surgery, as well as chemotherapy and radiation, patients undergoing gross total resection had a 5-year progression-free survival rate of 26% compared to a rate of 4% in patients with subtotal resection.[50] Because of the survival advantage for radical tumor resection, surgery with the intent of providing maximal safe resection while preserving normal or near-normal neurologic function should be attempted. However, in diencephalic tumors, more conservative management is warranted.

Postoperative imaging is needed to objectively assess the volume of residual tumor. Postoperative MRI should be obtained within 48 hours of surgery to minimize postoperative changes, such as surgery-related enhancement and encephalomalacia, which may complicate image interpretation.

Focal radiotherapy is commonly utilized, because progression in the majority of patients occurs locally.[45] Specifically, doses between 54 and 60 gray is delivered to a target volume of the tumor bed and additional margin for tumor infiltration.[51] Use of fractionated radiotherapy, brachytherapy, stereotactic radiosurgery, and gamma knife radiosurgery allows for sparing of uninvolved surrounding tissues. Irradiation of the entire neuraxis is reserved for leptomeningeal spread, which occurs in 10% to 31% of patients at the time of progression.[45] Radiation

FIGURE 56-3 Axial (A) and sagittal (B) postcontrast MRI demonstrating a large left frontal enhancing pediatric GBM with an associated mass effect.

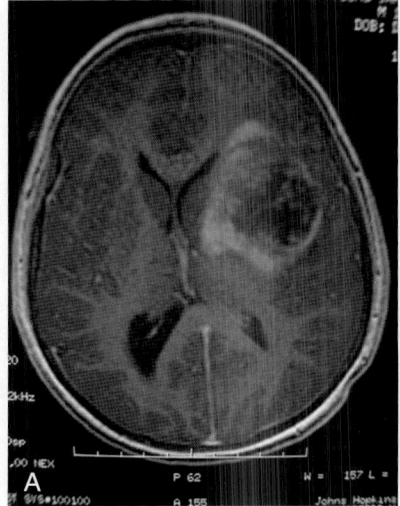
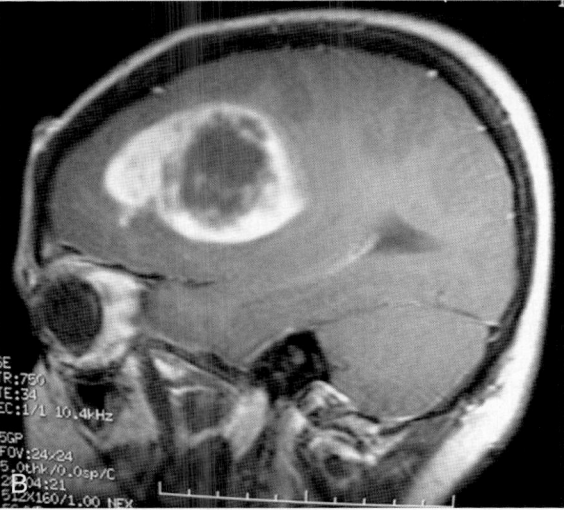

therapy is primarily indicated for pediatric brain tumors in patients older than 3 years. For children younger than 3 years, multiagent chemotherapy is recommended to delay radiation therapy.[52] In the Children's Cancer Group study, 299 enrolled infants with malignant brain tumors were found to have a high response rate (42%) to intensified induction therapy, but unfortunately the 5-year event-free survival rate was only 27%.[52]

The role of multimodal therapy for pediatric GBM with chemotherapy is less clear, with one study demonstrating a long-term survival rate of less than 20% in a study of 58 pediatric patients, despite the addition of chemotherapy.[51] The improvement in outcome with temozolomide in adult GBMs has spurred interest in its use in the pediatric population. The efficacy of temozolomide in children with high-grade gliomas has been found to vary, and in a phase II trial with temozolomide the median progression-free survival was found to be 3 months in 24 patients.[53,54] New therapies, as well as clear data on chemotherapy, are needed to achieve improved outcome in children.

Pineal Region Tumors

Tumors of the pineal region make up 0.4% to 2% of all primary CNS tumors in children.[55] Germ cell tumors, pineal parenchymal tumors, and astrocytomas make up the vast majority of lesions in this area. When considering all CNS germ cell tumors, two thirds occur in the pineal region.[56,57]

PRESENTING SIGNS AND SYMPTOMS

The development of signs and symptoms of pineal region tumors relates to the aggressiveness of the tumor based on its histology, normal pineal gland anatomy, and the confines of adjacent structures. The signs and symptoms of pineal region tumors develop due to three major reasons: (1) tumor-induced hydrocephalus producing increased intracranial pressure, (2) direct compression of the brain stem or cerebellum, and (3) tumor-induced endocrine dysfunction. However, the asymptomatic patient with a small, incidental lesion found on MRI is likely to be an increasingly common presentation as a result of increasing of frequency and resolution of MRI and CT scanning.

The most common symptoms of pineal region tumors are those related to hydrocephalus due to obstruction of the outflow of the third ventricle at the sylvian aqueduct.[58,59] The symptoms of headache, lethargy, increasing head circumference, seizures, nausea, and vomiting are common in the early symptomatic period, but papilledema, subacute cognitive deficits, and obtundation can develop with worsening hydrocephalus. The pathognomonic constellation of signs known as Parinaud's syndrome occurs in 50% to 75% of patients and refers to the triad of paralysis of upward gaze, retraction nystagmus, and near-light papillary dissociation occurring as a result of compression of the superior colliculus in the pretectal region.[60,61] As the tumor involves greater ventral midbrain, there is a greater impairment of downward gaze.

Less common presentations occur in patients presenting late in their disease with large tumors and relate to infiltration or compression of adjacent structures. Compression of the periaqueductal gray region can cause mydriasis, convergence spasm, papillary inequality, and convergence of

refractory nystagmus. Compression or infiltration of the cerebellar efferent fibers within the superior cerebellar peduncle can cause motor impairments such as ataxia and dysmetria. Infiltration of the thalamus or internal capsule can occur with large, invasive tumors and cause contralateral hemihypesthesia, paresthesia, and typical thalamic pain syndromes.[62] Exceedingly rare signs include compression of the inferior colliculus, causing hearing deficits; compression of elevatory inhibitory fibers in the posterior commissure, causing lid retraction (Collier's sign); and fourth nerve palsy, causing double vision.[63,64] While rare in children, drop metastasis from CSF or extracranial metastasis can occur and present with radiculopathy; myelopathy, which is more commonly observed in pineoblastomas; and germ cell tumors.[65,66]

Children with tumors of the pineal gland can present with symptoms of endocrine dysfunction, including diabetes insipidus and pseudoprecocious puberty either primarily due to tumor involvement of the hypothalamus or secondarily as a consequence of hydrocephalus.[67] Precocious puberty has historically been reported to occur in approximately 10% of males, but reexamination suggests true precocious puberty is rare and may be a uncommon finding. This occurs due to ectopic secretion of beta-human chorionic gonadotropin (β-hCG) by choriocarcinomas and germinomas. Alternatively, mass effect on the posterior diencephalon augments secretion of gonadotropins by blocking the inhibitory effect on the median eminence of the hypothalamus or by decreasing secretion of a substance in the pineal gland with antigonadotropic effect.[62] This is termed pseudopuberty because the mechanism is secondary stimulation of the Leydig cell to secrete androgen, resulting in the development of secondary sexual traits prematurely.

A rare but potentially lethal initial presentation is the acute onset of Parinaud's syndrome and hydrocephalus due to pineal apoplexy. The highly vascularized pineal gland is at greater risk for hemorrhage, particularly with primary pineal cell tumors and choriocarcinoma. An acute decline in mental status with extraocular movement dysfunction in a child with a known or suspected pineal region lesion should raise concern for this phenomenon. Hemorrhage into a partially resected pineal lesion is a significant concern and can present in a similar manner.

DIAGNOSIS

The preoperative diagnostic workup consists of high-resolution MRI of the brain and entire spine, measurement of tumor makers in the serum and CSF, and biopsy to confirm diagnosis and guide subsequent management.

High-resolution MRI with and without gadolinium is important to appreciate tumor size, lateral and superior extension, contrast enhancement, marginal irregularities, and relationships with surrounding structures. Particularly important are the degree of involvement and position of the tumor within the third ventricle, extension into or above the corpus callosum, superolateral extension into the region of the ventricular trigone, involvement or compression of the quadrigeminal region, relation to the anterior cerebellar vermis, and location of the deep venous system. Angiography is not routinely recommended unless the MRI suggests potential vascular involvement with the Galen vein or an arteriovenous malformation. While imaging is not predictably diagnostic, radiologic patterns that are associated with specific tumor histology types can provide valuable information for preoperative planning and postoperative adjuvant management (Table 56-3).

As a rule, malignant gliomas and germ cell tumors invade through the wall of the third ventricle, while pineal parenchymal tumors, meningiomas, and low-grade astrocytomas are more likely to cause expansive compression.[68] Pineocytomas and pineoblastomas are typically hypointense to isointense on T1-weighted MRI, display increased T2 signal, and enhance homogenously after gadolinium administration. Pineoblastomas (Fig. 56-4) are larger (>4 cm) and have an irregular shape compared to pineocytomas. Astrocytomas are hypointense on T1-weight MRI and hyperintense on T2-weighted MRI. These lesions enhance in variable patterns because they can arise from either the glial stroma of the pineal gland or the surrounding tissue. Calcium may be present in either pineal cell tumors or astrocytomas. Meningiomas display smooth, distinct borders and often have a homogenously enhancing dural tail. A lesion fitting this pattern located dorsal relative to the deep venous system should raise suspicion for a tentorial meningioma. Germinomas are isointense on T1 and slightly hyperintense on T2 MRI. They enhance strongly in a homogenous pattern (Fig. 56-5) and can display a peripheral calcification that surrounds the pineal gland. By contrast, the calcification in pineocytomas can be differentiated from germinomas in that there is primarily intratumoral calcium; they may also have intratumoral cysts. Teratomas have a heterogeneous appearance on MRI, are multilocular, and enhance in an irregular pattern. These lesions are often well circumscribed and can be distinguished from other pineal region tumors by the low attenuation from the adipose tissue. Other malignant nongerminomatous germ cell tumors have a mixture of benign and malignant germ cell components and a heterogeneous appearance. Choriocarcinoma, a specific subtype, is characterized by areas of intratumoral hemorrhage. Incidental findings of a mostly cystic pineal gland, known as pineal cysts, are becoming more common with the increasing use of MRI scans. These lesions do not require surgery unless they are progressing in size or cause symptomatic obstruction of the aqueduct and may be followed with serial MRI scans.

LABORATORY DATA

The measurements of markers specific for tumors of the pineal gland are important to establish a diagnosis and to follow post-treatment response and recurrence (Table 56-4).

Table 56-3 Clinical and Radiographic Overview of Pediatric Pineal Region Tumors

	Germinoma	Teratoma	Pineoblastoma	Glioma	Pineocytoma	Meningioma
Age	Child	Child	Child	Child	Adult	Adult
Sex predilection	Male	Male	None	None	None	None
Pineal vs. parapineal	Pineal	Pineal	Pineal	Parapineal (usually)	Pineal	Parapineal (usually)
Signal intensity (heterogenous vs. homogenous)	Homogenous (but often hemorrhagic)	Strikingly heterogenous	Homogenous (unless hemorrhagic)	Homogenous (usually)	Homogenous	Homogenous
Hemorrhage	Common	Typical	Common	Rare	Common	Rare
Calcification	Rare	Typical	Common	Uncommon	Common	Common
Brain edema or invasion	Common	Variable	Common	Primarily mid-brain neoplasm	Uncommon	Occasional
Tendency to metastasize	Yes	Variable	Yes	Variable	No	No
Enhancement	Dense	Variable	Dense	Variable	Dense	Dense
Prognosis	Excellent (83%)	Variable (33%)	Poor	Variable	Variable	Excellent

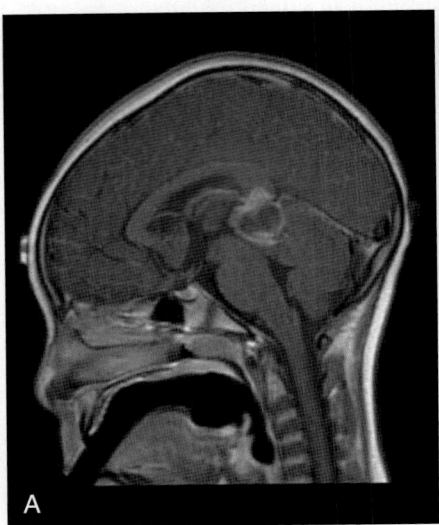
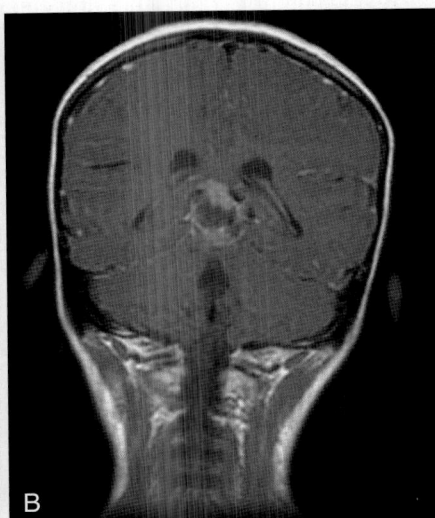
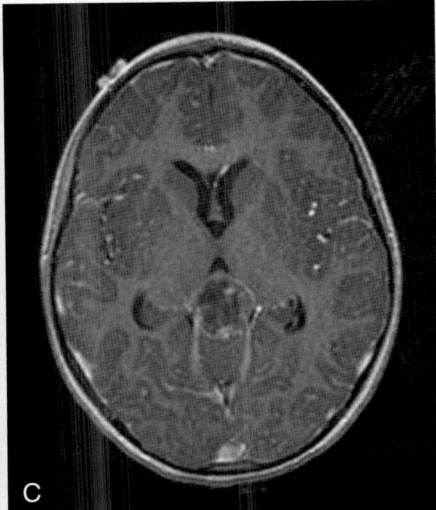

FIGURE 56-4 Sagittal (A), coronal (B), and axial (C) postcontrast MRI demonstrating a heterogeneously enhancing pineoblastoma.

Alpha-fetoprotein (AFP) and β-hCG are the most specific makers for malignant germ cell tumors, and these levels are important to ascertain as the treatment of these lesions is nonoperative.[58] AFP is greatly elevated with endodermal sinus tumors, but smaller elevations occur with immature teratomas and embryonal cell carcinomas.[58] β-hCG is elevated in choriocarcinomas and germinomas containing a syncytiotrophoblastic giant cell, which is associated with a worse prognosis.[69] Lactate dehydrogenase and placental alkaline phosphate are less specific than AFP and β-hCG but are also often used to follow response to therapy. The candidate tumor makers for pineal parenchymal cell tumors are melatonin and the S antigen, but neither has proved valuable for establishing diagnosis or for following recurrence. Theoretically, undetectable levels of melatonin in the serum following surgery suggest a gross-total resection. A combination of tumor-maker evaluation and neuroimaging should be a routine part of the preoperative evaluation; it provides the greatest diagnostic accuracy and plays an important in optimal surgical and medical management.

SURGICAL INDICATION

The surgical indications for children with tumors of the pineal region must take into consideration the presence and severity of hydrocephalus, results of CSF sampling to

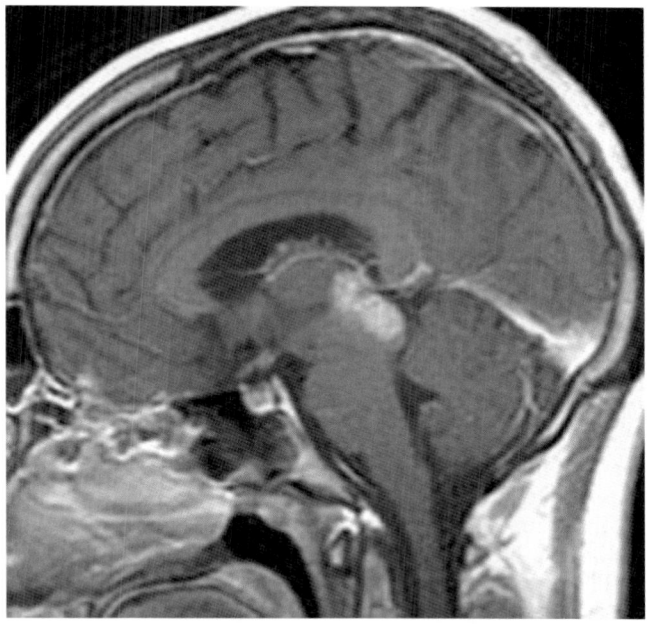

FIGURE 56-5 Sagittal T2 postcontrast MRI showing a homogenously enhancing germ cell tumor without evidence of hydrocephalus.

diagnose nonoperative germ cell tumors, imaging findings, presence of local or regional metastasis, and results of biopsy.

Any patient presenting acutely with hydrocephalus should have an immediate CSF diversion procedure, either by external ventricular drainage or by endoscopic third ventriculostomy. The decision for more definitive CSF diversion can be made at the time of surgical resection. If surgical resection is not likely to occur soon and there is a concern for worsening hydrocephalus, the primary concern should be interval CSF diversion. Often, surgical or nonsurgical treatment of the tumor results in decreased tumor size with restoration of normal CSF flow.[70] In cases of nonacute hydrocephalus, definitive CSF diversion can take place at the time of biopsy with endoscopic third ventriculostomy or with a ventriculoperitoneal shunt or temporary ventricular drain. Ultimately, the decision of CSF diversion must be based on the degree of normalization of CSF flow at the end of treatment. While extremely rare, metastasis of pineal cell tumors from CSF diversion has been reported.[71,72]

CSF-Based Management

The finding of elevated serum or CSF AFP or β-hCG suggests a germ cell tumor with malignant components and may obviate the need for further direct surgical intervention, including biopsy or resection. In these children, surgical resection combined with adjuvant therapy has not been shown to have any advantage over radiation therapy and chemotherapy alone. However, many of these children may require delayed neurosurgical resection for a residual focal mass after radiation and chemotherapy.

Biopsy

In cases of nondiagnostic CSF findings, the decision must be made to attempt stereotactic biopsy or open biopsy with planned resection. The advancement of neuroendoscopic and image-guided stereotactic techniques has played an important role in the diagnosis of these lesions. Large retrospective series of both adults and children report mortality rates of less than 1.5%, and morbidity rates ranging from 2% to 10%, with diagnosis made in greater than 90% of cases.[73] To ensure safety, consider variation in anatomy due to the tumor, including displacement of vasculature. Some tumors, such as pineoblastoma or choriocarcinoma, are also known to be highly vascular. In cases of a clearly nonresectable lesion, evidence of metastatic disease, or a patient who is a poor surgical candidate, histologic diagnosis is still crucial for adjuvant management with chemotherapy and radiation therapy. The primary drawback of endoscopic or sterotactic biopsy is the inability to obtain sufficient tissue for definitive diagnosis, particularly in tumors with mixed

Table 56-4	Laboratory Values Used in Diagnostic Workup of Patients with Pineal Region Tumors			
	α-Fetoprotein (<5 ng/ml)	β-hCG (<5 IU/ml)	Placental Alkaline Phosphatase	Melatonin
Germinoma	–	+ (<770 IU/ml)	++	–
Teratoma	+ (<1000 ng/ml)	–	–	–
Yolk sac tumor	+++	–	±	–
Embryonal carcinoma	++ (<1000 ng/ml)	++ (<770 IU/ml)	+	–
Choriocarcinoma	–	+++ (>2000 IU/ml)	±	–
Pineocytoma	–	–	–	+
Pineoblastoma	–	–	–	++

components, such as teratomas. In cases of clearly resectable tumors, the risks of biopsy should be avoided and the preferred approach is open biopsy with resection at the same time.

SURGICAL APPROACHES

The decision to attempt surgical resection should be based on results of CSF findings, biopsy results, location and appearance of the lesion on MRI, and severity and progression of the clinical presentation.

Anatomic Considerations

The anatomic considerations of surgical resection of pineal region tumors have been well described by prior authors, notably Bruce et al.[59] In their large experience, among the most important considerations are the location and degree of attachment of these lesions to the undersurface of the velum interpositium, including the choroid plexus, deep venous system, and choroidal arteries. Because tumors rarely extend above the velum interpositium, the major vascular supply occurs from within the velum interpositium, mainly through the posterior medial and lateral choroidal arteries and with anastomoses to the quadrigeminal and pericallosal arteries.[59] The majority of these lesions are centered on the pineal gland, and they may extend to the midportion of the third ventricle and compress the anterior portion of the cerebellum with posterior extension. Important vascular structures, including the Galen vein, internal cerebral veins, basal Rosenthal veins, and precentral cerebellar veins, commonly encapsulate these tumors. Rarely, the internal cerebral veins can be found ventral to the tumor. Essential information that must be taken into account includes knowing the tumor's position within the third ventricle, its lateral and supratentorial extension, its position relative do the deep venous system, and the degree of brain stem involvement.

Approaches

At least five distinct approaches have been developed for lesions of the pineal gland because of its location in the geometric center of the intracranial cavity.[62] The two most common approaches are the infratentorial–supracerebellar and the occipital–transtentorial approaches; in certain cases, the parietal/transcallosal–interhemispheric approach is also used. The midline sagittal MRI with gadolinium is often the best sequence with which to make a decision regarding the approach.

The infratentorial–supracerebellar approach is generally preferred for three distinct reasons: (1) it provides the most direct route to the center of the tumor; (2) it provides a corridor ventral to the velum interpositium and deep venous system, minimizing the risk of damage to this venous drainage; and (3) there is minimal injury to normal tissue by this approach. The major disadvantages of this approach are limited lateral exposure and limited exposure and access above the deep venous complex and anteriorly into the third ventricle. The transcallosal–interhemispheric or occipital–transtentorial approaches are the preferred approaches with tumors that require extensive exposure, such as tumors that extend superiorly to involve the posterior aspects of the corpus callosum and deflect the deep venous system dorsolaterally, tumors that extend laterally to

the trigone, and tumors that cause ventral displacement of the deep venous system.

The primary advantage of the occipital–transtentorial approach is the excellent view provided above and below the tentorium. The major disadvantages of the transcallosal–interhemispheric approach are the extensive reaction required on the parietal lobe, the potential risk of venous infarction if disruption of the bridging veins between the sagittal sinus and the parietal lobe occurs, and the need to work around the veins of the deep venous system that overlie the tumor.[59,62] The major disadvantages of the occipital–transtentorial approach also include the need to work around the deep venous system around the tumor and the high frequency of visual deficits due to retraction of the occipital lobe and damage to the calcarine cortex.[59]

Positions

Patient positioning is an important part of the preoperative plan and is largely dictated by the approach selected. In the transcallosal–interhemispheric and infratentorial–supracerebellar approaches, the sitting slouch position can be used. The major advantages of this position include minimal blood pooling in the operative field and the cerebellum falling away because of gravity to improve exposure. The major disadvantages include air embolus, pneumocephalus, and epidural or subdural hematoma from ventricular and cortical collapse, though these are rare occurrences.[59] This position is contraindicated in children younger than 2 years with severe hydrocephalus, in which case the three quarter prone, lateral decubitus, and Concorde position are appropriate alternatives. In the occipital–transtentorial approach, the three quarter prone position or lateral decubitus position can be used. This position reduces the risk of complications of the sitting slouch position but does not allow gravity to work in the surgeon's favor.[59] The Concorde position was designed specifically for tumors of the pineal region and combines aspects of both the prone and the semisitting positions. While this position is more comfortable for the surgeon and reduces the risk of air embolism, a major disadvantage is the pooling of blood in the operative field.[59] Ultimately, the approach and position selected depend on the presence and degree of hydrocephalus, whether the tumor is more anterior or posterior in location, and surgeon experience and preference.

The infratentorial–supracerebellar approach was first described by Karuse in 1913 and popularized by Stein in 1979.[74] This is the preferred approach for tumors of the pineal region because of the wide lateral exposure obtained and because it provides an intuitive orientation for the surgeon.[59] The primary anatomic structures exposed are the cerebellum, cerebellar veins, cerebellar vermian veins, internal cerebellar veins, basal Rosenthal veins, Galen vein, pineal body, posterior commissure, quadrigeminal plate, splecinum of corpus callosum, and posterior third ventricle. The skin incision is made along the midline from the occipital region down to the spinous process of the third vertebral body. A wide craniotomy is performed to include the transverse sinuses and torcula. After the dura is opened, the arachnoid is dissected and the superomedial cerebellar bridging veins are divided to allow for inferior retraction on the cerebellar hemispheres. Alternatively, some degree of upward retraction on the sinus complex decreases the degree of downward retraction on the cerebellum. An operating microscope is then brought in and the arachnoid spanning the interval between the cerebellar vermis and the central posterior incisura is opened with microdissection to exposure the pineal gland. Several vascular structures are important to consider. The precentral cerebellar vein, which can be seen extending from the edge of the cerebellar vermis to the Galen vein, can be cauterized and divided. In the lateral aspects of the exposure, the Rosenthal veins can be seen coursing upward toward the confluence of veins. Branches of the choroidal arteries often supply these tumors. The tumor may be removed with a combination of tumor forceps, curets, suction, cautery, or ultrasonic aspiration based on its consistency.[59]

Occipital–Transtentorial Approach

Compared to the infratentorial–supracerebellar approach, the occipital–transtentorial approach is more laterally directed and the primary anatomic structures exposed include the splenium of the corpus callosum, internal cerebral veins, basal Rosenthal veins, Galen vein, precentral cerebellar vermian vein, pineal body, posterior commissure, and quadrigeminal plate. An inverted L-shaped skin incision is made to clearly expose the inion. The superior margin of the bone flap is 1 to 2 cm below the lambdoid suture, and the inferior margin is below the inion. The dura is opened in an H shape. Retraction of the occipital lobe laterally exposures the posterior edge of the incisura, where it is attached to the falx cerebri. The tentorium is incised, and sharp dissection of the arachnoid brings the Galen vein and the ipsilateral basal Rosenthal vein into view. The pineal gland is visible inferior to this venous complex.[59]

POSTOPERATIVE MANAGEMENT AND ADJUVANT THERAPY

Immediate Postoperative Management

The most common postoperative complications following pineal region surgery are extraocular movement dysfunction, ataxia, and altered mental status. These findings are particularly pronounced in patients with invasive and malignant tumors, prior radiation therapy, and severe preoperative neurologic deficits.[59] A potential lethal complication is postoperative hemorrhage in a subtotally resected lesion, particularly vascular lesions such as primary pineal cell tumors. Acute worsening of symptoms up to 1 week following surgery or hydrocephalus should raise concern for this phenomenon. Less common postoperative complications include venous infarction, hemorrhage related to third ventriculostomy if performed, aseptic meningitis, and in the case of supratentorial approaches, seizures, hemianopsia, and hemiparesis. An MRI should be obtained 24 to 48 hours following surgery to assess the extent of resection and as a baseline for future studies.[59]

Chemotherapy

Primary chemotherapy or adjuvant chemotherapy plays an important role in the management of children with tumors of the pineal region. Germinomas and nongerminomatous germ cell tumors are primarily treated with radiation, but their chemosensitivity has been demonstrated and chemotherapy is now routinely used to improve the efficacy and reduce the dose of subsequent radiation therapy.[75]

Common agents used with germinomas include cyclophosphamide, ifosfamide, etoposide, cisplatin, carboplatin, and bleomycin. Common agents used in nongerminomatous germ cell tumors include platinum-based regimens, often used in combination with vinblastine, etoposide, and/or bleomycin.[76] Children with pineoblastomas receive the same chemotherapy regimen for medulloblastomas, particularly infants to delay the age at first radiation treatment.[76] There are limited data regarding the use of chemotherapy in children with pineocytoma because they are treated primarily with surgical resection and radiation therapy.

Radiation Therapy

While radiation therapy also plays an important role in the management of children with pineal region tumors, there is greater concern given the effects of radiation on cognitive development, particularly because these children are often long-term survivors. Germinomas are among the most radiosensitive tumors, with greater than 90% disease control with radiation therapy alone. The addition of chemotherapy reduces the dose of radiation required and is particularly effective in children presenting prior to puberty.[76] There is great ongoing debate as to the type, dose, volume, and regions that should be irradiated. Though the data are limited, it appears that postoperative radiation therapy improves the outcome in children with pineoblastoma and pineocytoma, particularly in those with subtotal resection or with progressive disease.[77] For pineoblastoma, the use of craniospinal irradiation is frequently recommended depending on patient age.

Long-Time Follow-Up

Children with tumors of the pineal region require lifelong follow-up for primary recurrence, which can occur as late as 5 years after diagnosis, and secondary lesions induced by treatment. MRI should be performed routinely, the exact interval dictated by histology, extent of resection, and adjuvant treatment. In the case of germ cell tumors, evaluation of serum and CSF for tumor makers should be done routinely, even if the levels of these makers were normal at the time of diagnosis.

Second-look surgery is considered in relapse germ cell tumors, particularly when nongerminomatous germ cell tumors do not have complete radiographic response to adjuvant chemotherapy. The differential for residual on neuroimaging may be necrosis and fibrosis or residual malignant elements. In some rare instances, growing teratoma syndrome is a pathophysiologic phenomena in mature teratoma, where tumor masses enlarge during chemotherapy in the presence of normal or declining tumor markers.[78] Second-look surgery is also considered when patients have persistently positive tumor markers in CSF and/or serum, which require histologic evaluation and confirmation.[79]

Intraventricular Masses

Intraventricular tumors are rare masses that are found more commonly in the pediatric population. These tumors are a heterogeneous group of histologically varying tumors that can be divided into primary and secondary intraventricular tumors. Primary tumors are considered those that develop from the ependyma and subependymal glia of the ventricular lining, the epithelium of the choroid plexus, and the arachnoid supporting tissue.[80] Secondary, paraventricular

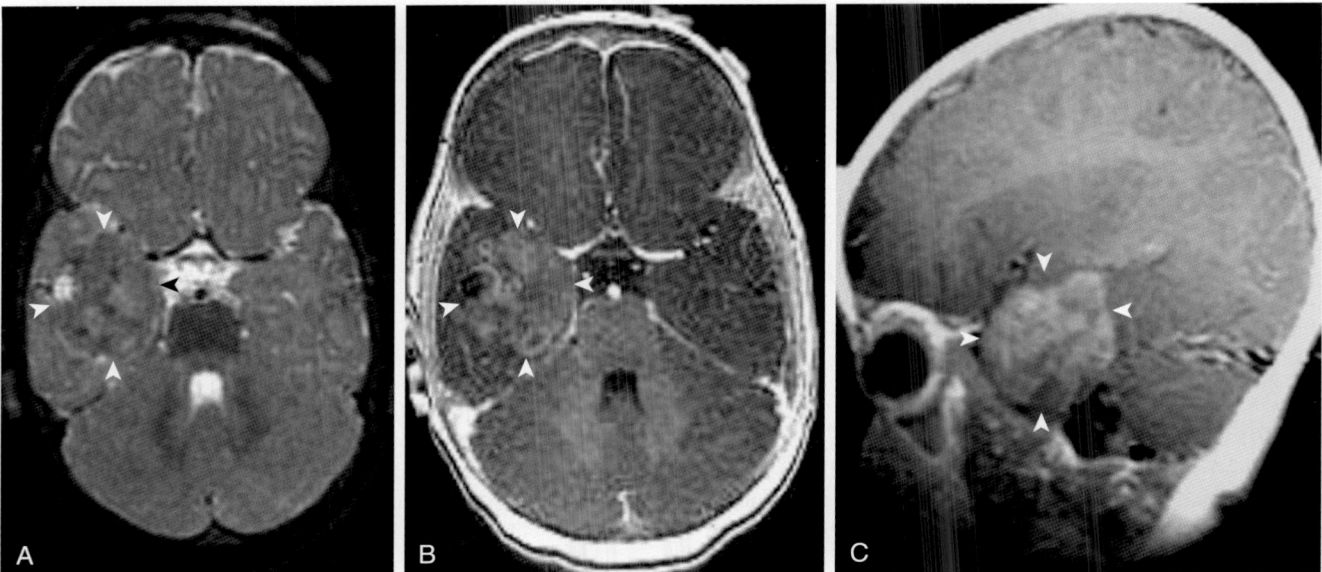

FIGURE 56-6 Axial T2 (A), axial T1 (B), and sagittal T1 postcontrast (c) MRI, demonstrating a large right temporal ependymoma.

tumors are masses that develop within the brain parenchyma, rather than the ventricular wall. They are defined as secondary intraventricular masses when more than two thirds of the tumor's surface bulges into the ventricle.[80] For example, third ventricular tumors tend to be germ cell tumors, pineal cell tumors, and glial cell tumors from the pineal gland that occupy this ventricular space.

Though extremely heterogenous, intraventricular tumors are grouped together due to their commonalities in clinical development, management, and difficulty in surgical resection due to their deep-seated location. The most common pediatric intraventricular tumors include ependymomas, choroid plexus papillomas (CPPs), and astrocytomas that frequently occur in the lateral and frontal horn.[81-83] Less common intraventricular tumors include subependymal giant cell astrocytomas, oligodendrogliomas, subependymomas, pilocytic astrocytomas, neurocytoma, and choroid plexus carcinomas.[82] The vast majority of intraventricular tumors are benign, and these rare intraventricular tumors make up 0.8% to 1.6% of all CNS tumors. These tumors occupy a nonfunctional space and are often able to grow into a considerable size before clinical manifestations. Given their benign nature, these masses are treated surgically but pose a significant challenge to neurosurgeons.

EPIDEMIOLOGY

Intraventricular tumors are more common in children than adults and comprise 16% of childhood and adolescent intracranial tumors. In a retrospective study of 112 pediatric patients with intraventricular tumors within the lateral ventricles, it was found that 42.8% of tumors occurred in the frontal horn and foramen of Monro, 22.3% in the body of the ventricle and septum pellucidum, 19.7% in the atrium or trigone, 8.9% in the temporal horn, and 6.3% in the occipital horn.[81,84] Tumor type varies with age. Younger children with lateral ventricular neoplasms most commonly have CPPs or choroid plexus carcinomas, while in older children low-grade gliomas such as subependymal giant cell

astrocytomas, pilocytic astrocytomas, and ependymomas are more frequent.[83,85]

Ependymomas

Ependymomas are uncommon, slow-growing, glial tumors that arise either within or adjacent to the ependymal lining of the ventricular system. Within pediatric patients, the median age of diagnosis is 5 years. These patients commonly present with seizures and focal neurologic defects when the tumors are in the supratentorial space.[86] On pathologic exam, they are commonly characterized by calcification, hemorrhage, and cysts. Upon neuroimaging, ependymomas are hypointense on T1-weighted and hyperintense on T2-weighted MRI, and they enhance prominently with gadolinium contrast (Fig. 56-6). Their diagnosis requires biopsy and histologic confirmation. Due to the favorable outcome of gross resection of these benign tumors, open resection is recommended over stereotactic biopsy.[87] Gross total resection followed by adjuvant radiation is recommended for children older than 3 years, and adjuvant chemotherapy is advisable for those younger than 3 years old to avoid radiation. Management also includes MRI of the entire neuraxes, as well as CSF cytology to exclude metastatic disease.[88]

Choroid Plexus Papillomas

CPPs arise from the endogenous neuroepithelial tissue of the choroid plexus.[89] CPPs are distributed according to ventricular surface area, where 50% of these tumors occur in the lateral ventricle, 40% in the fourth ventricle, and 5% in the third ventricle. These tumors make up 10% to 20% of intracranial tumors in pediatric patients younger than 1 year. CPPs are benign WHO grade I tumors that histologically resemble normal neuroepithelium of the choroid plexus.[90] CT and MRI are recommended imaging modalities. CPPs are often calcified and can be difficult to distinguish from ependymomas. On MRI, CPPs are hypo- to isointense on T1, are hyperintense on T2, and enhance with contrast (Fig. 56-7). The vascular nature of these tumors, which commonly obtain blood supply from the choroidal arteries, may lead to flow voids visible on MRI.

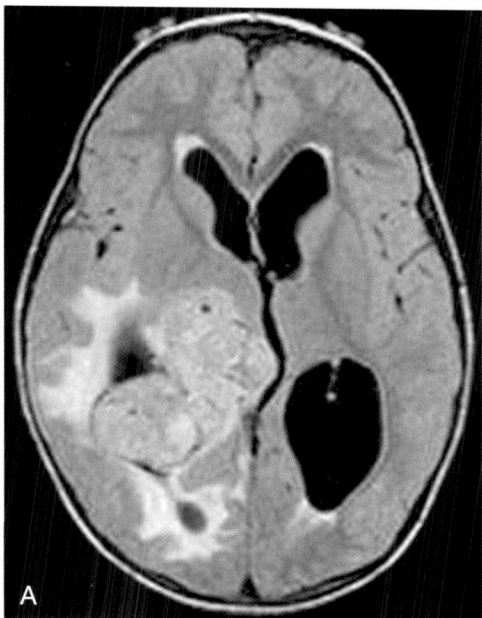
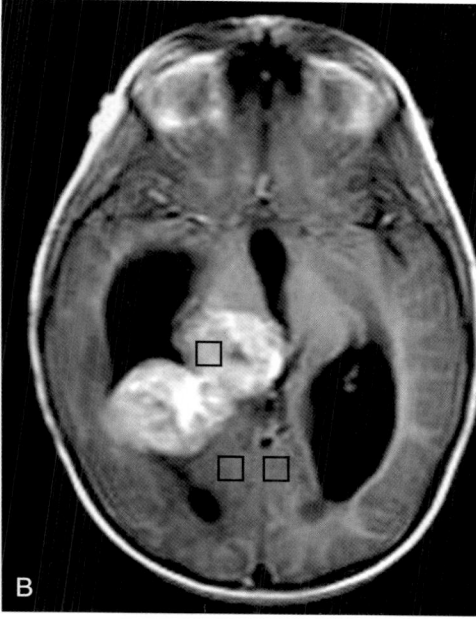

FIGURE 56-7 Axial FLAIR (A) and T1 postcontrast (B) MRI depicting a CPP with associated edema and contrast enhancement.

Management includes complete surgical resection, with adjuvant radiotherapy reserved for recurrent tumors.[91] Malignant transformation into a choroid plexus carcinoma rarely occurs, and the majority of incompletely resected CPPs remain benign.

CLINICAL PRESENTATION

The range of pathologies that arise within the ventricles, as well as the diversity in location of intraventricular tumors, does not lend to a stereotypic neurologic or behavioral pattern of signs and symptoms. However, the majority of clinical manifestations result from either obstructed CSF flow or hydrocephalus secondary to an overproduction of CSF.[83] Common symptoms include papilledema, headache, motor disturbance, sensory disturbance, nausea and vomiting, visual field defects, low vision, and mental status changes.[82] Memory loss secondary to mass effect on the fornix from direct compression or hydrocephalus is also known to occur. Finally, in rare instances, spontaneous bleeding and acute clinical deterioration have been reported.[80]

SURGICAL MANAGEMENT

Treatment of intraventricular tumors is controversial due to the challenges presented by their location, size, association with hydrocephalus, and surrounding functional anatomy. Imaging with MRI is the preferred modality for preoperative evaluation. Important considerations include tumor size, tumor vascular supply and drainage, hydrocephalus, and surrounding neural structures.[80] Finally, in instances where intraventricular tumors are inaccessible, intraventricular endoscopy can be utilized to achieve diagnosis. Such minimally invasive procedures are attractive and successful for smaller lesions or radiosensitive tumors that require biopsy for pathologic diagnosis, followed by definitive treatment with radiation or chemotherapy.[92]

Relevant Anatomy

During surgical resection, visible landmarks within the lateral ventricle should be identified to orient the surgeon. In particular, the veins that line the white ependymal surface are significant. The thalamostriate vein lies in the groove separating the caudate nucleus from the thalamus. This vein joins the septal vein, and together the two form the internal cerebral vein that lies proximal to the foramen of Monro, beneath the choroid plexus. The choroidal fissure serves as another important intraventricular landmark, because the choroid plexus lies within it, and the fissure divides the fornix and thalamus. The choroid plexus itself is within the medial aspect of the body, atrium, and temporal horns of the lateral ventricles. It courses through the foramen of Monro to the roof of the third ventricle.[80] Additional important functional structures adjacent to the ventricles include the Rolandic area, language areas on the dominant hemisphere, fornices, internal cerebral veins, and the Galen vein.[82]

Surgical Approach

The ideal surgical exposure allows sufficient exposure for removal of the tumor, rapid identification of supplying vessels, and minimal brain retraction and damage to functional cortex.[80] The most direct trajectory between the surgeon and the lesion is often the most appropriate, but the choice is variable and depends on experience (Table 56-5). The tumor location within the ventricle, hydrocephalus, hemispherical dominance, tumor size, tumor blood vessel supply, and histopathologic features are all significant factors. Stereotactic guidance systems are helpful in choosing tailored approaches that allow for safe and aggressive tumor removal. Historically, neurosurgeons have used a transcortical approach to the lateral ventricle. More recently, transcallosal–interhemispheric approaches are more frequently used due to the provision of direct access to the ventricles without damaging cortical brain tissue.[93-95] For third and posterior intraventricular tumors, transcortical temporal, superior parietal lobule, and transcallosal–interhemispheric approaches are the most common.[96]

The most common surgical approaches to lateral ventricle tumors are anterior, temporal, and parietal transcortical approaches, followed by anterior and posterior

Table 56-5   Operative Approaches to Intraventricular Tumors*

Tumor Location	Advantages	Disadvantages	Approach	Complications
• Frontal horn and anterior body of the lateral ventricles • Anterior third ventricle	• Access to large tumors • Facilitated by hydrocephalus or enlarged ventricle	• Difficult to expose the lateral ventricle on the opposite side • Contraindicated for tumors of the midventricular body due to lesions in motor and sensory cortex	Frontal transcortical–middle frontal gyrus	• High incidence of epilepsy • Transient hemiparesis • Speech difficulties
• Choroidal tumors • Temporal horn and trigonal regions	• Early identification of anterior choroidal vessels • Facilitated by hydrocephalus or enlarged ventricle	• Poor visualization of the posterior choroidal artery	Temporal transcortical–middle temporal gyrus	• Visual field loss secondary to optic radiation injury • Speech dysfunction
• Trigonal region • Posterior body	• Exposure of large masses • Facilitated by hydrocephalus or enlarged ventricle • Reduced incidence of language impairment	• Delayed visualization of afferent vessels	Parietal transcortical–superior parietal lobule	• Visual field impairment • Apraxia • Acalcula • Gerstmann syndrome
• Midbody or anterior horn of the lateral ventricle	• Access to both lateral ventricles • Absence of cortical incision • Reduced incidence of postoperative seizures	• Injury to bridging veins • Venous hypertension, infarction of basal ganglia, and internal capsule	Anterior transcallosal	• Hemiparesis • Aphasia, mutism, and confabulation • Memory deficits • Astereognosis • Alexia without agraphia
• Medial tumors with blood supply from posterior choroidal arteries	• Avoidance of primary motor and sensory gyri, which preclude the transcortical approach	• Not appropriate for large trigone region tumors	Posterior transcallosal	• Alexia • Verbal–visual disconnection

*Data from references 78, 80-82, 92, 93, 96-98.

interhemispheric approaches.[80] Anterior approaches include anterior transcallosal, transcortical, and frontal. Posterior approaches include posterior transcallosal, transcortical, and occipital. Inferior approaches include temporal and posterior frontotemporal.

Intraoperative Considerations

Highly vascular intraventricular tumors necessitate division and coagulation of arterial supply prior to resection of the tumor. Once hemostasis is achieved, it is recommended that the ventricle be filled with saline and emptied to identify leaking vessels. The tumor resection cavity should also be filled with saline to prevent collapse of brain parenchyma once retractors are removed. Lining the cavity with hemostatic agents should be done cautiously, given the possibility of dislodging and obstructing CSF flow. Septal fenestration and placement of a ventricular drain is also recommended to avoid postoperative hydrocephalus by diversion of blood, debris, and CSF.[80]

POSTOPERATIVE MANAGEMENT

Patients require intensive care unit monitoring postoperatively. Medications include 24 hours of antibiotics and a 10- to 14-day corticosteroid taper. If a transcortical approach was utilized, antiepileptic prophylaxis should be considered. Postoperative MRI is also needed to confirm the extent of tumor resection. If an external ventricular drain was placed, this can be weaned over 3 to 5 days. Patients need close monitoring because complication rates of intraventricular tumors can approach 20%.[82] The

most common complications include severe brain edema, intraventricular hemorrhage, subdural hematoma, and epidural hematoma. Severe memory difficulties can also occur because tumors of the lateral ventricles can lead to forniceal injury.[80,95,97]

Conclusion

Pediatric supratentorial tumors are composed of a diverse spectrum of lesions that range from benign to uniformly lethal malignancies. The workup of a child found to have a supratentorial mass should take into consideration several factors including age, presentation, and imaging characteristics. In nearly all cases, the treatment plan should be developed in a multidisciplinary fashion that includes neurosurgeons, radiation oncologists, medical oncologists, and pediatricians. The surgical indications, as well as the risks and benefits of any proposed procedure, should be explained in great detail to the family. The goals of surgery should be consonant with the tumor type, prognosis, family wishes, and availability of adjuvant therapies. Ultimately, an individualized treatment plan for each child needs to be developed to provide the best possible care.

KEY REFERENCES

Ahn Y, et al. Optic pathway glioma: outcome and prognostic factors in a surgical series. *Childs Nerv Syst.* 2006;22(9):1136-1142.

Albright AL. Feasibility and advisability of resections of thalamic tumors in pediatric patients. *J Neurosurg.* 2004;100(5 suppl Pediatrics):468-472.

Apuzzo ML, et al. Transcallosal, interfornicial approaches for lesions affecting the third ventricle: surgical considerations and consequences. *Neurosurgery.* 1982;10(5):547-554.

Bhattacharjee MB, et al. Cytogenetic analysis of 120 primary pediatric brain tumors and literature review. *Cancer Genet Cytogenet.* 1997;97(1):39-53.

Bruce J, ed. Pineal region masses: clinical features and management. In: R.D. Schmidek H. ed. *Schmidek and Sweet's Operative Neurosurgical Techniques: Indications, Methods, and Results,* 5th ed. Vol. 2. Saunders; 2005:786-797.

Bruce JN. Pineal tumors. In: Winn HR, ed. *Youman's Neurological Surgery.* WB Saunders; 2004:1011-1029.

Cuccia V, Monges J. Thalamic tumors in children. *Childs Nerv Syst.* 1997;13(10):514-520:discussion 521.

Dutton JJ. Gliomas of the anterior visual pathway. *Surv Ophthalmol.* 1994;38(5):427-452.

Fisher PG, et al. Outcome analysis of childhood low-grade astrocytomas. *Pediatr Blood Cancer.* 2008;51(2):245-250.

Heideman RL, et al. Supratentorial malignant gliomas in childhood: a single institution perspective. *Cancer.* 1997;80(3):497-504.

Jennings MT, Gelman R, Hochberg F. Intracranial germ-cell tumors: natural history and pathogenesis. *J Neurosurg.* 1985;63(2):155-167.

Lau C, Teo W-Y. Clinical manifestations and diagnosis of central nervous system tumors in children. *UpToDate Online.* 2009;17.2:May 26, 2009 [cited 2009 August 18].

Listernick R, et al. Optic pathway gliomas in children with neurofibromatosis 1: consensus statement from the NF1 Optic Pathway Glioma Task Force. *Ann Neurol.* 1997;41(2):143-149.

Lozier AP, Bruce JN. Surgical approaches to posterior third ventricular tumors. *Neurosurg Clin N Am.* 2003;14(4):527-545.

Miller NR. Primary tumours of the optic nerve and its sheath. *Eye (Lond).* 2004;18(11):1026-1037.

Perkins SM, et al. Glioblastoma in children: a single-institution experience. *Int J Radiat Oncol Biol Phys.*

Pollack IF, et al. Rarity of PTEN deletions and EGFR amplification in malignant gliomas of childhood: results from the Children's Cancer Group 945 cohort. *J Neurosurg.* 2006;105(suppl 5):418-424.

Pytel P. Spectrum of pediatric gliomas: implications for the development of future therapies. *Expert Rev Anticancer Ther.* 2007; 7(suppl 12):S51-S60.

Ruggiero A, et al. Phase II trial of temozolomide in children with recurrent high-grade glioma. *J Neurooncol.* 2006;77(1):89-94.

Sawamura Y, et al. Role of surgery for optic pathway/hypothalamic astrocytomas in children. *Neuro Oncol.* 2008;10(5):725-733.

Sievert AJ, Fisher MJ. Pediatric low-grade gliomas. *J Child Neurol.* 2009;24(11):1397-1408.

Song KS, et al. Long-term outcomes in children with glioblastoma. *J Neurosurg Pediatr.* 6(2):145–9.

Souweidane MM, Hoffman HJ. Current treatment of thalamic gliomas in children. *J Neurooncol.* 1996;28(2-3):157-166.

Stein BM. Supracerebellar–infratentorial approach to pineal tumors. *Surg Neurol.* 1979;11(5):331-337.

Stoiber EM, et al. Long term outcome of adolescent and adult patients with pineal parenchymal tumors treated with fractionated radiotherapy between 1982 and 2003—a single institution's experience. *Radiat Oncol.* 5:122.

Winkler PA, et al. The transcallosal interforniceal approach to the third ventricle: anatomic and microsurgical aspects. *Neurosurgery.* 1997;40(5):973-981:discussion 981-2.

Numbered references appear on Expert Consult.

CHAPTER 57

Mapping, Disconnection, and Resective Surgery in Pediatric Epilepsy

BRENT O'NEILL • JEFFREY G. OJEMANN • MATTHEW SMYTH • JOHANNES SCHRAMM

Children present many unique challenges to the epilepsy surgeon necessitating the use of special techniques and equipment. A large portion of adult epilepsy surgery treats mesial temporal sclerosis, while in children, extratemporal epilepsy is more common and developmental lesions are frequently encountered. The scope of surgical treatment of pediatric epilepsy may involve mapping the site of seizure onset and surrounding essential brain functions, resection of a seizure focus, or disconnection of the majority or even the entirety of a hemisphere.

The incidence of epilepsy is higher in children than adults with about 5% of children experiencing a seizure before the age of 20.[1,2] The majority of these (80%) will never have another seizure, and therefore not meet the diagnosis of epilepsy.[2] Among children with epilepsy, 20% will be refractory to medical therapy even with the numerous new medications available.[3] Epilepsy surgery provides a powerful treatment modality for the subgroup of children with refractory epilepsy who are candidates. Determining appropriate surgical candidates requires a team specialists and a number of diagnostic modalities.

Another important distinction from adult epilepsy is the dynamic, developing nervous system of children. Repetitive seizures and anticonvulsive medications present noxious stimuli that may inhibit brain development.[4] Seizures may additionally hamper socialization and school integration, causing deleterious impacts beyond the physiologic.[5,6] However, brain plasticity could also benefit the child in recovering from resective or disconnective surgery. While these factors weigh significantly in the decision to pursue surgical treatment and the timing of such treatment, each child and family must assess their particular situation with the advice of the epilepsy team to help them weigh the risks of ongoing epilepsy, the risks of surgery, and the likelihood of seizure control with surgery.

Mapping

All evaluations for resective epilepsy surgery focus on identifying a localized source of seizure onset. Noninvasive tools used to accomplish such localization include seizure semiology, neurologic exam (including neuropsychology), scalp electroencephalogram (EEG), and imaging. In the most straightforward of cases, all modalities of localization identify a single, safely-resectable source of seizure onset. In such cases, invasive mapping is unnecessary. In some cases, many of the nonoperative localization modalities give equivocal results or discordant localization. In these cases, operative mapping can reveal an otherwise obscure epileptic focus.

In addition to identifying a seizure focus, mapping can define the extent of a subtle or diffuse epileptic focus such as cortical dysplasia. Such mapping guides the extent of surgical resection.

Finally, mapping can localize neurologic function, defining the relationship between functional brain tissue and an epileptic focus. Such information predicts what if any neurologic deficit will be induced by resection, vital information for a family and care team in deciding whether to proceed with resection. Advances in functional imaging are increasingly able to localize neurologic function, often supplanting or supplementing invasive mapping.

NONOPERATIVE LOCALIZATION

Attempts at nonoperative localization of an epilepsy focus include an array of specialized testing and a team of trained personnel to administer and interpret them. History (particularly of seizure semiology), neurologic exam (including neuropsychology to elucidate subtle cognitive deficits), prolonged video electroencephalography, and advanced imaging are all vital elements of the epilepsy surgery workup.

Semiology

The clinical semiology of a seizure provides the first clue to localizing its onset. Penfield described an assortment of mental, sensory, and physical aspects of seizures specific to various brain regions.[7] These range from mental phenomena such as déjà vu and ill-defined epigastric rising to olfactory and gustatory auras to motor convulsions. The first manifestation of a given seizure most accurately reflects the area of onset, whereas seizure spread can lead to later involvement of other areas outside to true site of seizure onset.

Seizures of temporal lobe origin are the most likely to have auras. Those originating in the mesial temporal structures classically begin with an ill-defined epigastric sensation accompanied with panic or autonomic disturbance. Neocortical temporal seizures commonly have auditory, visual, or perceptual hallucinations. Head turning, posturing, automatisms, and behavioral arrest are common accompaniments of temporal seizures.

Frontal lobe seizures are often brief, occur in clusters, and may include complex motor posturing, versive eye movements, or vocalization. They can rapidly spread yielding early generalization, drop attacks, or early signs of temporal lobe activation.

Parietal lobe seizures often present with somatosensory symptoms but may have abdominal symptoms such as nausea or a gustatory sensation. Occipital seizures may be heralded by visual phenomena including scotoma.[8]

Neuropsychology

The classic neuropsychology workup of an epilepsy patient consists of a variety of standardized tests and questionnaires that establish a profile of the patient's cognitive, emotional, and behavioral abilities. This testing quantifies the patient's abilities, deficits, and coping strategies. Such information can localize areas of dysfunctional cortex, which may be the site of seizure onset. Neuropsychology also predicts the deficits likely to be incurred by resection of a given focus and the impact that such deficits will have on the individual's life.[9]

In many emerging technologies such as functional magnetic resonance imaging (fMRI), the neuropsychologist plays a vital role in administering verbal and functional tasks and assessing the patient's cooperation with such tests. As these tests are very dependent on cooperation from the child while in the MRI machine, the neuropsychologist plays a vital role in extracting and interpreting information from an otherwise uncooperative patient.[9,10]

Electroencephalography

Electrophysiologic data are acquired by placing electrodes on the scalp and recording electrical differences between them. Interictal EEG can reveal epileptiform discharges such as spike and sharp waves, providing clues to the lateralization and localization of seizure onset, but prolonged video EEG provides an electrophysiologic picture of the seizures themselves. Video EEG data can confirm that spells are seizures (as opposed to breath-holding or other nonepileptic spells) and in many instances begin to localize the onset of the seizure. Most centers want to record several typical seizures and will continue monitoring until this is accomplished.[11]

Ictal video EEG will precisely localize the seizure focus in about a third of patients with temporal lobe epilepsy.[12] Precise localization is even less common in those with extratemporal epilepsy where seizures tend to spread rapidly. Rapid spread from the orbitofrontal or posterior parietal cortex can falsely localize to the temporal lobe.[13]

Dense-array EEG is a newer technology that holds promise for more precise seizure localization. The dense array consists of 256 electrodes held to the head by an elastic mesh, giving substantially more information and spatial resolution than the standard 32-electrode array.[14]

Imaging

Surgical epilepsy cases are sometimes divided into lesional and nonlesional. Classically lesional cases from well-circumscribed pathologies such as cavernoma,

dysembryoplastic neuroectodermal tumors (DNETs), and ganglioglioma have a significantly better prognosis than nonlesional cases. The identification of a structural abnormality on MRI is a strong predictor of localization.[15] When the scalp EEG confirms seizure onset from the lesion, localization is strongly suggested, and resection often proceeds without invasive mapping.

The distinction between lesional and nonlesional epilepsies has blurred a bit as improved imaging has revealed cortical dysplasias, focal sclerosis, or other pathologies previously noted only by histology. Higher-field MRI, diffusion tensor imaging, and other MRI methods (e.g., MR spectroscopy and fMRI) may also show abnormalities. Voxel-based MRI postprocessing has been recently shown to help visualize blurred gray–white matter junctions or abnormal extension of cortical bands otherwise not recognizable on MRI.[16] A negative MRI may still allow for further surgical planning. In a recent series of pediatric temporal lobectomies, half of those eventually shown to have histologically confirmed mesial temporal sclerosis had normal hippocampus on MRI.[17] In such cases, other imaging such as positron emission tomography (PET), single-photon emission computed tomography (SPECT), and magnetoencephalography (MEG) can help to further define the extent of the epileptic-onset zone and the functionality within and surrounding the malformation.

PET provides a tomographic image of brain glucose utilization, while SPECT images blood flow. Both can reveal areas of metabolic derangement (hypometabolism interictally and hypermetabolism during a seizure) that can represent a seizure focus.[18,19] MEG collects minute magnetic potentials generated by bands of synchronized neural currents, a technique that can reveal epileptic foci as well as functional circuits (e.g., motor units).[20] The specific role for these various modalities is not determined and considerable variability exists across programs.[21]

INVASIVE MONITORING

Invasive mapping can identify a focus of seizure onset, define the extent of an epileptic zone, or localize neurologic functions. The intraoperative mapping needed is determined by the preoperative workup and must be determined on an individualized basis.

In some patients, no definitive focus can be identified on preoperative studies, and invasive monitoring is needed to lateralize. This may occur in a child with classic temporal lobe epilepsy but evidence for bilateral onset on scalp EEG recordings. In this setting, bilateral strip or depth electrodes may reveal lateralized onset with rapid spread and allow the child to be a candidate for temporal lobectomy.

In the setting of infiltrative low-grade tumors or focal cortical dysplasia, invasive EEG recording may be used to define the relationship of epilepsy onset to the lesion. This may guide the surgeon to resect epileptogenic tissue beyond the bounds of the imaging abnormality. Such infiltrative tumors and cortical dysplasias can have functional neurologic tissue within them. If these lesions are anatomically near motor or speech cortex, mapping of these functions can further define this relationship. It may be found that a lesion has displaced the motor fibers in such a way that resection can be accomplished while preserving function or an aberrant localization of speech function may be present precluding violation of a typically ineloquent area of cortex.

Direct cortical recording and stimulation mapping can be accomplished via intraoperative electrocorticography (ECoG) or via implantation of grid, strip, and/or depth electrodes for extraoperative study. The choice of technique depends on the information needed and the familiarity of the epilepsy team with the various techniques.

Some centers approach poorly defined lesions and occult lesions on MRI with MEG, PET, and ECoG alone, avoiding grid placement entirely.[22] While good results from this approach[22] have been published, it is difficult to directly compare it to the liberal use of prolonged grid monitoring. At our center, both ECoG and extraoperative grid monitoring are a part of the armamentarium. The approach used is determined on a case-by-case basis depending on the information from the preoperative workup and what vital questions remain.

Electrocorticography

A significant amount of information about the epileptogenicity and function of an area of tissue can be obtained from intraoperative electrical monitoring. ECoG data are obtained by placing electrodes on the exposed brain and observing the EEG record for epileptiform discharges (spike and sharp waves).[23,24] Anesthetic considerations are important to avoid suppressing or altering the EEG record. Benzodiazepenes should be avoided except at induction or after ECoG. Inhalational agents above 0.5 MAC will dampen the record beyond interpretation. A combination of sevoflourane and dexmetomidate is preferred at our (BO and JGO) institution, but a total intravenous anesthetic is also possible.[25]

Some functional information can be obtained in the anesthetized patient. A distinct pattern of cortical activity (phase reversal) of evoked-somatosensory responses can localize the central sulcus. Direct stimulation of motor cortex can elicit motor responses that are visualized or recorded on EMG. Awake craniotomy in cooperative older children (sometimes as young as 10) can be used to map language cortex.[25] Current is passed through a hand-held bipolar stimulator (Ojemann stimulator) to inhibit an area of cortex while the patient is performing speech tasks. Speech arrest induced during this procedure reflects an area of vital speech function.[24]

ECoG guidance adds little risk to an epilepsy resection, and can avoid the second operation and likely some morbidity of implanted electrode monitoring. The information gained, however, is limited to the anesthetized, interictal state. Time constraints also limit electrophysiologic data.

Implanted Electrodes (Grids, Strips, Depths)

Implanted electrodes allow for EEG monitoring and stimulation mapping outside of the operating room. Recordings include the awake, drowsy, and sleep states and ideally will include several of the patient's seizures. Monitoring typically continues for 5 to 7 days but can be extended if additional information is needed. Very brief intracranial monitoring (24 or 48 hours) can be a useful technique in toddlers who would not tolerate prolonged implantation.

Intracranial monitoring electrodes are typically placed in the subdural space but epidural placement is employed at times, and yields comparable information.[26,27] Placement below the skull dramatically increases the amplitude of cortical electrical signals collected and diminishes muscle artifact, the main source of noise. Implanted electrodes also greatly increase the spatial resolution of the EEG. A typical grid consists of 64 electrodes on an 8×8 cm array, whereas scalp EEG typically employs 32 electrodes to cover the entire head.

Effective definition of an epileptic focus relies on placement of electrodes as close to the region of interest as possible while electrodes covering distant sites, including the opposite hemisphere can exclude multifocal onset of seizures.

Implanting electrodes additionally allows for prolonged functional mapping outside the operating room by stimulating through the same electrodes.[2] By applying current across two neighboring electrodes, the intervening area of cortex (about a centimeter of tissue) is inhibited. Deficits observed can identify the function of the cortex and the deficits likely to be incurred by resection. Lower stimulation of motor cortex may produce muscle contraction rather than inhibition. Many children who cannot tolerate with awake intraoperative mapping will cooperate with extraoperative mapping.[30] Additionally, the mapping can take place during complex activities such as drawing, writing, or playing a musical instrument potentially identifying important integrative functions.

Cortical stimulation for mapping can induce seizure activity, causing inhibition beyond the intended stimulation both temporally and spatially. The EEG must be monitored for after-discharges reflective of stimulation induced seizure.

Grid electrodes consist of a broad array of contacts that can cover a large area of cortex. They can be particularly helpful in defining an epileptic zone within a lobe or defining the relationship of a lesion to seizure onset. Convexity sites are particularly amenable to grid placement.[31] Extraoperative language and motor mapping are typically performed through grids as they give ample coverage of the hand and face motor area as well as the typical language sites.

Strip electrodes consist of a single or double row of electrodes spaced along a flexible strip that can be safely passed along the subdural space. Coverage of the interhemispheric cortex, orbitofrontal cortex, and mesial temporal lobe can be achieved by passing strip electrodes, all locations poorly monitored by scalp recordings.[28,32] A strip passed along the undersurface of the temporal lobe will typically place the distal electrode just at the parahippocampal gyrus, providing good monitoring of the mesial temporal structures.[33] Placement of strip electrodes requires only a burr hole, allowing for limited monitoring of distant sites, including the contralateral hemisphere without requiring a craniotomy.

Distant and mesial temporal recordings can also be obtained with depth electrodes. These electrodes line a narrow probe that passes directly into the region of interest. Some centers also place depth electrodes directly within or along the deep margins of a lesion infiltrating the white matter (e.g., cortical dysplasia) to evaluate the depth of resection necessary.[28,34] These various electrodes are often used in combination to monitor all areas of interest.

Complications

Electrode implantation procedures require two separate operations (occasionally more) with a prolonged hospitalization between. The most common complications are cerebrospinal fluid (CSF) leakage, fever, and infection. Minor CSF leak is common while electrodes are in place, but rarely problematic. While low-grade fevers are common and wound infection much less so, suspicion should remain high in order to recognize and treat infections promptly.[35]

Cerebral edema combined with the mass effect of the implants can cause elevated intracranial pressure. This occurs more commonly with more electrodes implanted. Mannitol and steroids typically will control intracranial pressure, but on rare occasions, grids may need to be removed.

Strip electrodes have fewer complications than grids, 1% overall compared to 3% to 4%. Strips also appear to be safer than depths. Isolated cases of permanent neurologic deficit and death have been reported.[35-39] The risk of complications, as well as the additional hospitalization time, need to be balanced against the information gained by invasive monitoring.

Disconnection

Disconnective operations include hemispherotomy, the modern iteration of hemispherectomy, to isolate a diffusely pathologic, epileptogenic hemisphere and lobar or multilobar disconnection, for pathology that affects multiple lobes (Fig. 57-1).

TRANS-SYLVIAN HEMISPHERIC DISCONNECTION OR FUNCTIONAL HEMISPHERECTOMY

Hemispheric deafferentation, hemispheric disconnection, hemispherotomy, or functional hemispherectomy are synonyms for surgical procedures that aim to disconnect all cortical structures of one hemisphere from the deeper lying structures of the brain, i.e., the basal ganglia by combination of disconnective steps and additional more or less extensive resective steps. The various terms mirror the development in the last 20 years away from classic anatomic hemispherectomy to procedures that combine more and more disconnective steps with less and less resective steps. In the last 15 years, several procedures have been described[40-44] that step by step have replaced anatomic hemispherectomy and Rasmussen's functional hemispherectomy technique.

Indication

These procedures are primarily indicated in patients with pre-existing unihemispherical damage and typical neurologic deficits such as hemianopia and hemiparesis combined with drug resistant epilepsy. If these cases occur in early infancy, are combined with holohemispheric dysplasias or extensive damage and severe drug resistant seizures they are frequently called "catastrophic epilepsy." Other typical diagnoses seen in these patients include hemimegalencephaly, multilobar cortical dysplasia, and various disorders of gyration such as polymicrogyria or lisencephaly. Hemimegalencephaly (HME) is a quite rare malformation of the cortical development arising from an abnormal proliferation of anomalous neuronal and glial cells that leads to the hypertrophy of the whole affected cerebral hemisphere. Epilepsy typically presents in infancy with severe, drug-resistant seizures. Many infants with HME undergo hemispherotomy before 2 years of age. HME patients have more operative complications and worse seizure outcomes than other hemispherotomy patients.[45,46]

Frequently hemispheric damage is due to perinatally acquired brain defects or intrauterine hemorrhagic damage. Perinatal stroke is in many ways an ideal pathology for hemispherotomy as patients typically have little function stored in the affected hemisphere and rarely incur new deficits from the operation. Development and cognition often improve when seizures are controlled and epilepsy

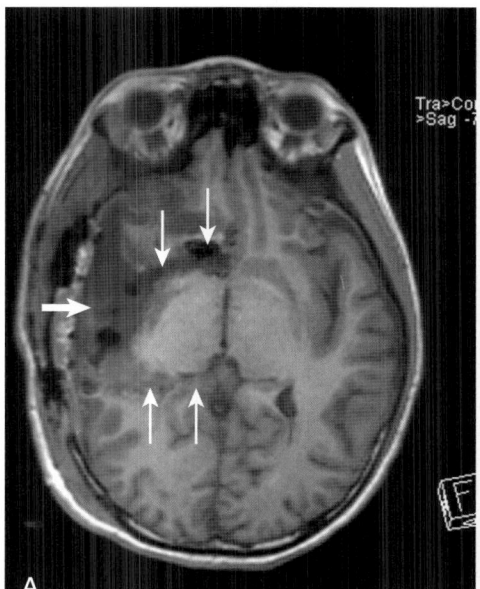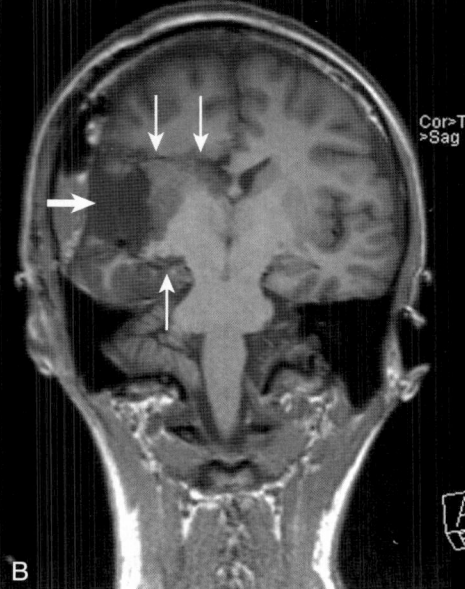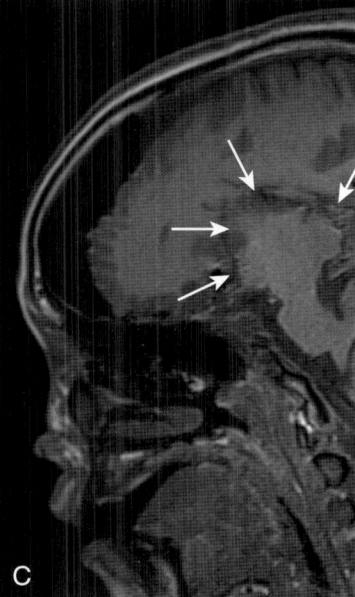

FIGURE 57-1 Hemispherectomy. Axial (A), coronal (B), and sagittal (C) images of a 13-year-old patient 1 day after peri-insular hemisphereotomy. The thick white arrows show the area of central resection, while the smaller arrows demonstrate the disconnecting cuts.

medicines are decreased or discontinued. Many of these children have cystic encephalomalacia in continuity with the ventricular system or separated by a thin membrane. This expanded space gives additional surgical access and easier visualization of the deep anatomy that needs to be disconnected, but this anatomy can be distorted. Care must be taken to maintain orientation.

Hemispherotomy may also be considered in diseases such as Sturge-Weber syndrome, a sporadically occurring phakomatosis consisting of unilateral facial port-wine stain in the V1 distribution, glaucoma, and unilateral leptomeningeal angioma. The intracranial angioma causes progressive cortical atrophy and calcification. Epilepsy occurs in 75% to 90% of Sturge-Weber patients, usually presenting in infancy. In some patients, the angioma is focal enough to be resected, but most are candidates for hemispherotomy.[47,48]

Other pathologies potentially amenable to hemispherotomy include Rasmussen's encephalitis, and postencephalitic and post-traumatic hemispheric damage. Rasmussen's encephalitis or chronic focal encephalitis is a chronic T-lymphocyte inflammation that remains localized to one hemisphere. Presentation is usually between 5 and 10 years of age with acute, drastic onset of focal seizures and progressive loss of hemispheric function. Anticonvulsants typically have little success in controlling seizures. Medical treatments to control inflammation, including steroids, intravenous immunoglobulin (IVIG), tacrolimus, and plasmapheresis are the first line of therapy, although their efficacy is limited.[49,50]

Timing of hemispherotomy has been debated in Rasmussen's patients particularly. Permanent loss of hemispheric function eventually occurs in a large majority from the disease, prompting recent recommendations for early hemispherotomy. Some evidence supports improved cognitive outcomes with early surgery,[46,51] but this must be balanced against the acute loss of hemispheric function from surgery performed before hemispheric dysfunction is fully actualized.

As hemispherotomy disconnects the motor and visual cortices, hemiparesis and visual field defects are inevitable consequences of the operation. The procedure is more appealing if these deficits are already present or if they are an inevitable outcome of the underlying pathology. Postoperative hemiparesis affects the upper extremity more than the lower. Ability to walk is almost always maintained.[52,53] Improved development and cognition commonly follow hemispherotomy in cases where seizures stop and anticonvulsants can be weaned.[52,54-56]

Diagnostics

The most important presurgical diagnostics include MRI and EEG recording of ictal events. MRI may show larger defects, frequently in the distribution of the middle cerebral artery, and malformations of cortical development. MRI findings include gross malformations of the hemisphere, ectopic gray matter, disorders of gyration, extensive postencephalitic damage, or holohemispheric atrophy. In the ideal case all ictal activity can be localized to the affected hemisphere. However, hemispherectomy may be indicated even in the setting of contralateral EEG or even MRI abnormalities. MRI abnormalities on the opposite hemisphere are particularly concerning for predicting poor success.[57,58]

If the disease has started after the fourth year it is important to demonstrate transfer of language to the other hemisphere for which the intracarotid amobarbital test, or possibly functional MRI,[10] is useful. However, the association between speech outcome and hemispherectomy is multifactoral with congenital etiologies having a more favorable outcome, even with age considered.[59]

Choice of Approach

It has become clear that the disconnective procedures carry the same success rate, may be even higher success rates as those procedures that involve larger resective steps.[60,61] In the 10 to 15 years of available follow-up for these disconnective procedures the complications known from anatomic hemispherectomy have not been reported thus far, and in particular no cases of cerebral hemosiderosis, which was reported for earlier procedures. The availability of CT and MRI-scanning has also minimized the potential problem of shunt malfunctions. However, postoperative hydrocephalus is also much rarer in disconnective procedures such as trans-sylvian keyhole deafferentation or trans-sylvian keyhole disconnection, or the alternatives described by others.[40,43,44] Other advantages of the trans-sylvian keyhole disconnection procedure favored by us have been confirmed by other series.[43,60,62] The keyhole procedures are less well suited for cases with extensive hemispheric malformation such as hemimegalencephaly. In these cases we combine the trans-sylvian approach with a perisylvian window technique such as has been described by Villemure and Mascott.[44]

Surgical Technique

Preoperatively, anticonvulsive medication is not discontinued. Dexamethasone is given in cases with normal brain volume or hemimegalencephaly, not in cases with large central cysts and huge ventricles. Testing of clotting mechanisms and blood typing should be done and before skin incision a prophylactic antibiotic is given. The placement of an arterial line is important as well as a central venous line in small babies. As always in pediatric neurosurgery, keeping the patient warm during surgery is important.

The patient's head is brought into a horizontal and slightly downward pointed position. The skin incision starts right before the tragus and can be linear or slightly curvilinear to allow for a craniotomy flap of 4×4 or 5×6 cm, depending on the size of the cranium. This small craniotomy size is possible because one just has to reach in front and behind the corpus callosum, which in children is no longer than 7 cm. Neuronavigation may be helpful to place the craniotomy in an ideal position, that is, the upper border at the level of the corpus callosum and the lower about 1 cm below the level of the M1. The sylvian fissure is opened and the temporal and frontal opercula are dissected away from the insular cortex (if those opercula still exists) and thus the insular cortex is exposed. Due to atrophic processes or postinfarction cyst built-up orientation may be more difficult. The tree of the M2–M3 branches is a good guide, although one should keep in mind that in cases with perinatal infarction, the M2 and M3 branches are smaller in diameter. In some cases the block of basal ganglia, thalamus, and insular cortex is considerably smaller than in healthy brains. If multiple cysts are present, these vascular structures inside the ventricle the choroid plexus are helpful as guides to orientate the surgeon.

Once the insular cortex has been exposed, the temporal horn is opened from its anterior tip to the trigone, approaching it through the inferior circular sulcus of the insular cistern. As the next step, the cella media and the frontal horn are also exposed by a transcortical incision along the circular sulcus following the outline of the circular sulcus to its superior part underneath the frontal operculum. In that way finally the whole ventricular system is exposed through a U-shaped incision along the circular sulcus from the temporal horn tip through the trigone and forward again to the tip of the frontal horn.

At this stage the basal ganglia bloc is disconnected from its cortical input but the four lobes are still connected through their mesial and basal structures to the deeper lying brain structures.

The mesial disconnection begins with removal of the uncus, transecting mesially through the amygdala to the choroidal fissure in the temporal horn and then taking the hippocampus/parahippocampus en bloc for accurate histology. Using the tentorial rim as a guideline the mesial disconnection is then carried backward around the trigone through the mesial brain structures. Always leaving the mesial arachnoid intact one exposes step by step the falcotentorial edge, works upward through the trigone to the inferior rim of the falx, to the cella media. Now working very close to the midline one in fact does a paramesial callosotomy all the way anteriorly to the frontal horn. The frontal and parietal opercula are reflected with self retraining retractors, looking through the exposed ventricle one can easily disconnect the callosal fibers close to the mesial ventricular roof or wall.

The most difficult step considering orientation is the fronto-basal disconnection. This is facilitated by creating a disconnection line through the basal part of the frontal lobe. A dissecting plane through the fronto-basal cortex and white matter along the M1 branch is created starting on the surface of the brain always aiming for the major M1 branch and following it down toward the midline. After a short distance the carotid bifurcation is reached and exactly in the same direction as the outward bound M1, one then follows the inward bound A1 to the interhemispheric fissure. Leaving the basal and mesial arachnoid intact one disconnects the fronto-basal brain tissue. After reaching the midline, the A1 turns into the A2 and now one is following the ascending pericallosal artery around the anterior bend of the corpus callosum. In this way one will finally reach the posterior disconnection line which originally went from the trigone to the anterior aspect of the frontal horn.

Important guide structures for the temporo-mesial, occipital, and parietal disconnection are the rim of the tentorium, and later the falco-tentorial margin and finally the inferior rim of the falx. In the frontal part of the brain the guide structure for the surgeon are the M1, the A1, and then the pericallosal artery. The two transection lines will meet at the roof of the anterior horn where the surgeon, following the pericallosal artery from the fronto-basal area will meet the transection line that was created when following the inferior rim of the falx from the trigonal area.

In the event of preserved insular cortex, we prefer its routine removal by CUSA, since postoperatively there will be no discussion about the importance of persisting insular cortex if case persisting seizures are observed.

Postoperative Care

Patients spend one or two nights on intensive care, particularly very small babies, and patients with hemimegalencephaly stay one night more. Wakefulness, verbal response, and motor response are classically monitored, as are pulse frequency, blood pressure, and temperature. In cases with more than expected blood loss, especially in hemimegalencephaly patients with larger blood loss, replacement of erythrocytes and coagulation factors will have been done during surgery and should be completed on intensive care. We have seen the occasional case with electrolyte disorder, so these also need to be followed. Postoperative anticonvulsive medication remains the same as preoperative. In case postoperative seizures are observed they need to be recorded and described carefully. In some patients deterioration of motor function of the leg makes postoperative treatment in a rehabilitation unit mandatory. An early postoperative MRI nicely demonstrates completeness of transection because fresh blood acts like a contrast medium.

Complications may be similar to all craniotomies, that is, subdural hemorrhage, epidural hemorrhage, or infection of ventricular space and bone flap. Dreaded complications would occur if the midline is transgressed, particularly in the area of the septum pellucidum where the contralateral fornix is close. Patients frequently develop pyrexia, which may last for a few days or for more than a week and they are usually noninfectious.[63] An elevated cell count may also be caused by contamination of CSF with blood.

As with all intraventricular surgeries a certain rate of patients needing a shunt or developing intraventricular cysts or adhesions appears to be unavoidable. Large series of hemispherotomy (20 to 83 patients) report rates of hydrocephalus ranging from 2% to 16%, commonly presenting months after the operation. Hemimegalencephaly and widespread cortical dysplasia patients are more likely to develop hydrocephalus than others. Infections and hemorrhages have also been reported, at times as often as 5% for each.[42,53,64,65]

In the Bonn groups pediatric series, one of us (JS) has reviewed 93 children with a minimum follow-up of 1 year (mean 100 months, range 12–265 months) with five shunts required (5.4%) and a few cases with hygromas and meningitis. Severe blood loss, not infrequently seen in anatomic hemispherectomy or with Rasmussen's functional hemispherectomy technique was never seen with the trans-sylvian technique. There was one death in the total series, a hemimegalencephalic 5-year-old boy was found dead in his bed on day 6 without recognizable intracranial complications.

A certain degree of deterioration in motor function, especially of the affected hand pincer movement and sometimes in movement of the leg, is unavoidable, whereby ability to walk is typically regained after rehabilitation in those few cases where significantly deterioration in walking ability occurred.[52,53]

Outcome

Cognitive and developmental outcomes have garnered significant attention recently with quite positive results. An increasing number of studies show improved postoperative development following hemispherotomy as fewer seizures and anticonvulsant medications improve cognitive abilities and social integration.[52,54-56] Early surgery has been increasingly recommended to avoid seizures during the critical periods of brain and social development. These points must be balanced against the increased anesthetic and blood loss risks of young children[66] and the potential for ongoing development or radiologic revelation of a pathology (as with cortical dysplasia or Sturge-Weber syndrome) that would have argued against hemispherectomy.

Good seizure outcomes have been demonstrated from all forms of hemispheric surgery, with more than two thirds of patients seizure-free. Rasmussen's encephalitis, Sturge-Weber, and perinatal stroke patients consistently have better seizure outcomes, with reported rates ranging from 73% to 93% seizure-free. Case series of cortical dysplasia and hemimegencephaly are seizure-free between 63% and 80% of the time.[53,64,65]

In Schramm's series (mentioned above) of 93 pediatric and juvenile patients with a minimum follow-up of 1 year, Engel class 1 outcome was 88%. Other all-pediatric series have reported similar results.[67] Thus, hemispherotomies continue to be a successful type of epilepsy surgery.

PALLIATIVE DISCONNECTION—CALLOSOTOMY

For children with generalized seizures, and drop attacks in particular, corpus callosotomy is a palliative disconnection consideration. The disconnection will, in theory, prevent the spread and generalization of a seizure. Callostomy has been considered for drop attacks, primary and secondary generalized seizures, and medically refractory mixed seizure types like Lennox-Gastaut.[68-72] Traditionally, anterior callosotomy has been the preferred option to avoid disconnection syndromes, but recent reports in the literature suggest that a one-stage complete callosotomy may be a better choice for initial surgical treatment in some patients.[73-75]

The surgical approach for both anterior two thirds or complete callosotomy can be done through the same incision placed over the coronal suture with the patient in the supine position in a head holder. Brain relaxation may be used to minimize the degree of frontal retraction. Frameless stereotactic navigation can optimize flap location, trajectory, and avoidance of large midline venous complexes. A midline craniotomy, biased to the right, is performed. The dura is opened based medially until the interhemispheric fissure is visualized. Cortical veins are respected and the frontal lobe retracted until pericallosal vessels found. Azygous vessels must be considered as the dissection proceeds to find the avascular midline. The pearly white callsoum is then exposed and divided. In an anterior two-thirds procedure, the anterior genu is disconnected to just before the splenium. The callosum is sectioned staying within the leaves of the septum and ideally preserving the ependymal lining of the ventricles. In complete callosotomies, the resection is taken more posteriorly and the internal cerebral vein and vein of Galen that lie just anterior to the splenial reflection of the callosum are preserved by remaining inside the adjacent pial membrane.

When analyzed by seizure type, atonic spells, myoclonic seizures, and absence seizures appear to be the seizure types most affected by a corpus callosotomy.[75-78] Cognitive and psychosocial outcomes have been demonstrated by family surveys and other assessments administered following surgery.[79,80] Operative complications of callosotomy can include hydrocephalus, aseptic meningitis, and cerebral edema.[75]

Resections

Resective operations for pediatric epilepsy include a diverse array of underlying pathologies and diverse prognoses. Resection of circumscribed lesions in ineloquent cortex can have low risk, good prognosis, and straightforward decision making, while other cases may require an involved search for the seizure focus and difficult decision making about whether to proceed with surgery.

TEMPORAL LOBE RESECTIONS

The results of pediatric temporal lobe resections are less consistent than adult series and the pathologies more varied. Structural lesions are present in as many as half of pediatric temporal lobectomy candidates.[15,81] Hippocampal sclerosis does occur in pediatric patients, but often in association with other neocortical pathology.[82] The presence of such dual pathology alters the surgical approach, and the suspicion of such will at times mandate invasive monitoring.

Common temporal lobe pathologies in children include tumors, vascular lesions, and dysplasias. In the subset of patients with a well-circumscribed, neocortical lesion such as DNET, ganglioglioma, or cavernous malformation, the decision must be made whether to resect mesial temporal structures. Lesionectomy alone can yield seizure freedom, but often mesial structures are also involved and may need to be included[83-85] typically this is a consideration in the case of a prolonged seizure history. Dysplasia in the anterior temporal lobe can often be seen in the setting of hippocampal changes in the young patient (Fig. 57-2).

Technique

Many different terms are applied to temporal lobectomies. An "aggressive" temporal lobectomy would typically be employed only when extensive dual pathology is present. In what historically might be considered a standard anterior temporal lobectomy, the lateral cortex is resected back 4 cm on the dominant side and 6 cm on the nondominant side.[86] Compared to selective procedures, this "standard" temporal lobectomy would be less desirable for cases of isolated medial temporal pathology.[87]

So-called "selective" approaches cover a variety of strategies. When the lateral temporal lobe is suspected to be pathologic, the resection can be tailored to address the specific imaging or electrophysiologic abnormalities.[88,89] Such a "tailored-selective" approach may use ECoG or prolonged monitoring through grids and strips to identify the extent of the epileptic zone when a diffuse lesion is present. In children old enough for consideration of language preservation, functional MRI, invasive mapping, or in some adolescents, awake language mapping may be necessary to identify and preserve speech cortex[90] and such considerations may also modify the surgical approach.

In any access to mesial structures, the temporal horn must be accessed, this may be through middle temporal,[91] inferior temporal, or basal temporal[92,93] in the various "anatomic-selective" approaches that address isolated mesial temporal pathology. Approaches through sylvian

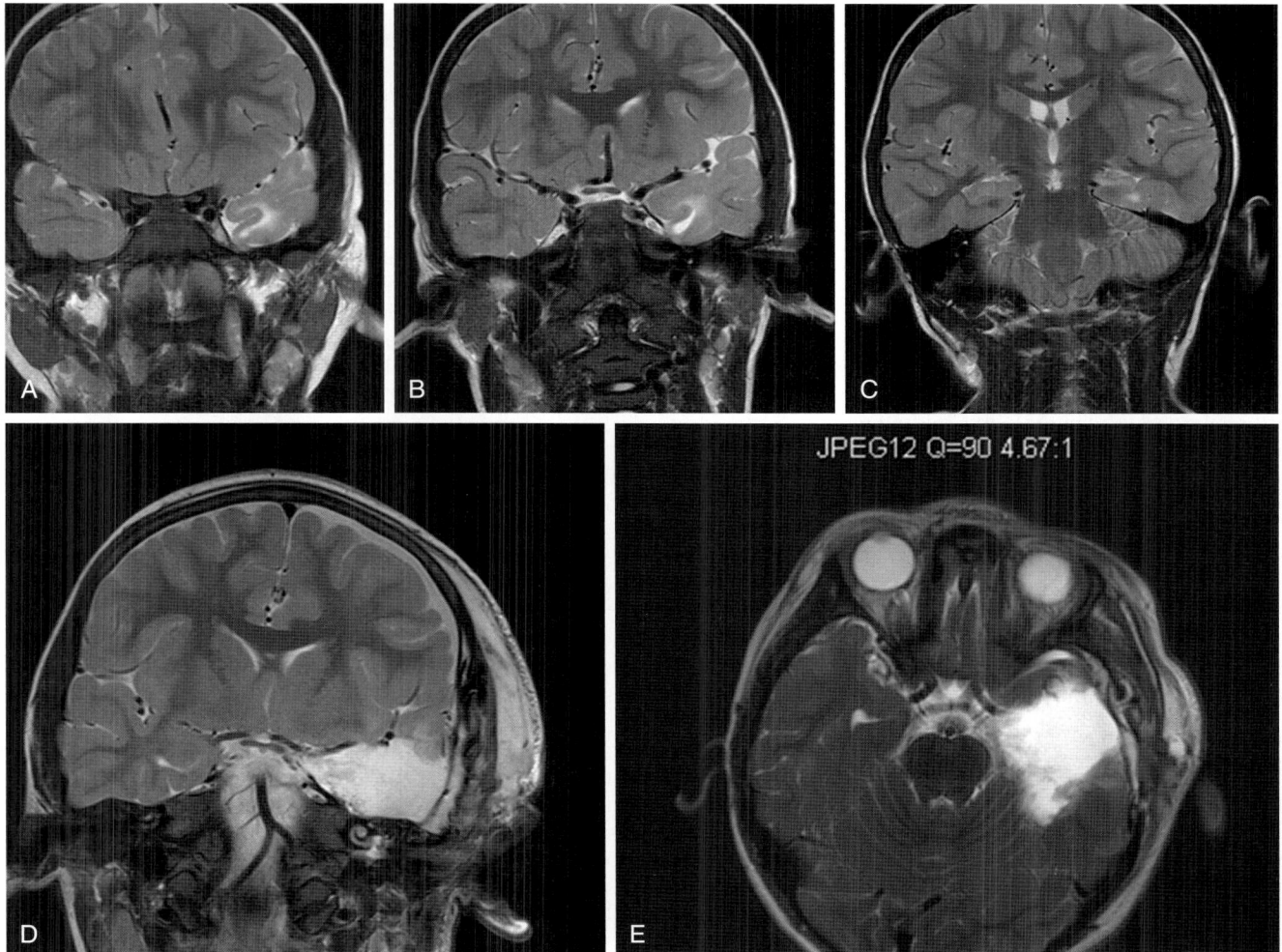

FIGURE 57-2 Temporal lobe pathology with hippocampal involvement. Preoperative (A to C) and postoperative (D and E) T2 images of 9-year-old boy with intractable epilepsy due to temporal lobe cortical dysplasia. Electrocorticography revealed epileptiform spikes extending to much of the posterior hippocampus. An extensive temporal lobe resection was performed.

fissure access to the hippocampus are also described primarily in adult populations.[94,95] The amygdalohippocampectomy can then be performed. While these approaches are often appropriate in adult patients where hippocampal sclerosis is usually isolated and evident on imaging, they are applicable to only the pediatric case that displays these clear preoperative criteria for isolated mesial temporal sclerosis.[17] More tailored resections may be indicated, varying the amount of lateral resection, depending on preoperative imaging and other evaluations.

The hippocampal resection is carried back beyond the choroidal point between 1.5 to 3 cm, or until the lateral brain stem is visualized beyond the arachnoid. Direct hippocampal recording has been described to further tailor the operation.[96] Care must be taken to maintain a subpial resection as the oculomotor nerve, carotid artery, optic nerves, and brain stem lie medial to the hippocampus.

Complications

Some degree of superior quadrant visual field defect is expected from interruption of Meyer's loop pathways running through the temporal lobe, even for many selective approaches,[93,97,98] but small deficits typically goes unnoticed by the patient and on bedside exam. Dominant temporal lobectomies in rare instances cause severe anomia and more commonly cause a variable decline in verbal ability on neuropsychology testing and difficulty with naming specific proper nouns.[99] Good verbal memory preoperatively and a normal MRI are risk factors for decline in language function in adults,[100] but the effects in children are less studied. "Selective" procedures appear to have better cognitive outcomes than "standard" temporal lobectomy, but an anatomic-selective versus a tailored-selective approach have not been directly compared. Damage to medial structures can occur, including the brain stem, cranial nerves, or major vessels. Respect for the pial boundary between the temporal lobe and these structures helps to prevent such complications. CSF leak, infection, and hemorrhage complicate temporal lobectomy at similar rates as other craniotomy procedures.[101]

Outcomes

Outcomes in pediatric patients undergoing temporal lobe surgery for intractable epilepsy are difficult to compare for several reasons. Temporal lobe pathology is less common in pediatric epilepsy series than adult, and the pathologies vary between different series, with some institutions reserving surgery for lesional resections while others take a more aggressive approach. The outcome measures also vary among the reported series. The inclusion of adolescents, who more commonly have mesial temporal sclerosis, can also affect the outcome of a series.

In three recent series of pediatric temporal lobe operations for epilepsy, the rate of Engel class 1 or 2 outcome has varied from 63% to 88.5%.[17,102,103] Cortical tumors have the best seizure outcome in most series.[103]

Mesial temporal sclerosis (MTS) confirmed on pathology also bore a favorable prognosis in a recent multi-institution study.[17] MTS was identified histologically in 53% of their series of children younger than 14 years with nontumor temporal lobe pathology. Children with MTS had Engle class 1 or 2 outcome 77% of the time as compared to 57% in those without MTS, a group consisting mostly of cortical dysplasia and gliosis.

Despite the added complexity of dual pathology cases, some series report similar outcomes in cases with preoperatively recognized dual pathology to other children undergoing temporal lobe epilepsy surgery.[103] Negative predictors of seizure outcome include developmental delay, multifocal EEG, and multiple seizure types. All of these factors point to diffuse seizure onset.[17,103]

EXTRATEMPORAL RESECTIONS

Extratemporal epilepsy foci are far more common in children than in adults where mesial temporal sclerosis dominates. Many authors group lateral temporal sources of seizure with extratemporal sources under the category of neocortical epilepsy as distinct form MTS. This taxonomy better reflects the underlying pathology and more starkly divides pediatric from adult epilepsy populations, but when planning a surgical approach we find the geographical categorization of temporal versus extratemporal epilepsy more useful (particularly with the possibility of dual pathology). Extratemporal epilepsy foci occur most commonly in the frontal lobe followed by the parieto-occipital regions.[104]

Search for a lesion with brain imaging is a key component to any epilepsy evaluation. MRI is the mainstay of this evaluation. Particularly with higher resolution MRIs, subtle areas of cortical dysplasia or migrational disorders can be identified to focus the further evaluation. Common lesions seen in surgical pediatric epilepsy include low-grade tumors, malformations of cortical development, and less commonly, vascular lesions and acquired gliosis (from trauma, infection, or other cause).

Developmental tumors such as gangioglioma, ganglocytoma, and dysembryoplastic neuroectodermal tumor (DNET) most commonly present with seizure. Epilepsy from such lesions has a very high likelihood of intractability, reaching 90% by 10 years after diagnosis.[105] Resection of a low-grade tumor provides very good seizure control, with Engle class 1 or 2 in as many as 95% in some series.[103] Often after scalp EEG confirmation of the involvement of the lesion in seizures, lesionectomy is undertaken with or without electrocorticography guidance.[106,107] Complete resection of the lesion is an independent predictor of good outcome.[108]

Malformations of cortical development appear on imaging as variations in the depth of sulci, distribution of sulci, thickness of the cortex, or presence of gray matter in the depths of white matter. Focal cortical dysplasia is the most common of these amenable to epilepsy surgery.[109] It histologically consists of disorganization of lamellar structure, large neurons, neuronal heterotopias extending into the deep white matter, usually tailing toward the lateral ventricle, and balloon cells with focal gliosis. Cortical dysplasias are most commonly located at extratemporal sites.[110] High-resolution MRI or PET may reveal lesions that are otherwise occult.

Vascular malformations including cavernous malformation and arteriovenous malformation (AVM) are a less common cause of pediatric epilepsy. Cavernous malformations are well circumscribed lesions surrounded by an area of hemosiderin-stained brain. For either, lesionectomy outcome resembles that of low-grade tumor resection.[111]

Technique

When a diffuse lesion such as FCD is identified, the extent of the epileptogenic zone often requires better characterization. Type 2 dysplasias are typically visible on MRI, but PET or MEG may show areas of abnormal metabolism that are more extensive than the visualized malformation. Functional imaging may also reveal type 1 cortical dysplasia which is occult on MRI.[112] Several approaches have been taken for cortical dysplasia. Tuberous sclerosis in particular is managed differently across institutions.

Invasive seizure monitoring and cortical mapping are often employed to tailor the resection of diffuse lesions to include the full seizure focus and avoid important functional tissue (Fig. 57-3). In a two stage approach to mapping such a lesion, a grid is typically placed over the lesion to precisely localize seizure onset. Strip electrodes are useful in monitoring otherwise hard to sample areas such as the interhemispheric fissure, the orbitofrontal cortex, or at times, the contralateral hemisphere. Depth electrodes can define the epileptogenicity of a tail of gray matter extending toward the ventricle from a cortical dysplasia. In some cases, a replacement of the subdural electrodes immediately after an initial resection.

Other groups rely on the preoperative evaluation, including MRI, PET, and/or MEG to identify candidates who undergo a single stage approach. ECoG will give feedback on the presence of epileptiform spikes in given brain areas and the effect of resection on these.[113] Outcomes from both strategies are quite similar, although patient selection processes are not the same.

Limiting functional impairment is often a challenge in diffuse lesions. Generally, resection of motor and language cortices are avoided in focal resections because the morbidity of hemiparesis or aphasia exceeds the benefit of seizure control offered, although in some instances, the epilepsy is so disabling that a family is willing to consider such a trade-off. Mapping of such functions is often a critical step in resective epilepsy surgery and pathology is known to potentially contain function.

When an epileptic focus is within an area of critical function, multiple subpial transections (MSTs) can offer some reduction of seizures without functional impairment. In this technique, the surface of the cortex is transected along the width of the gyrus. This is thought to disrupt seizure spread while preserving cortical output through descending fibers.[114,115]

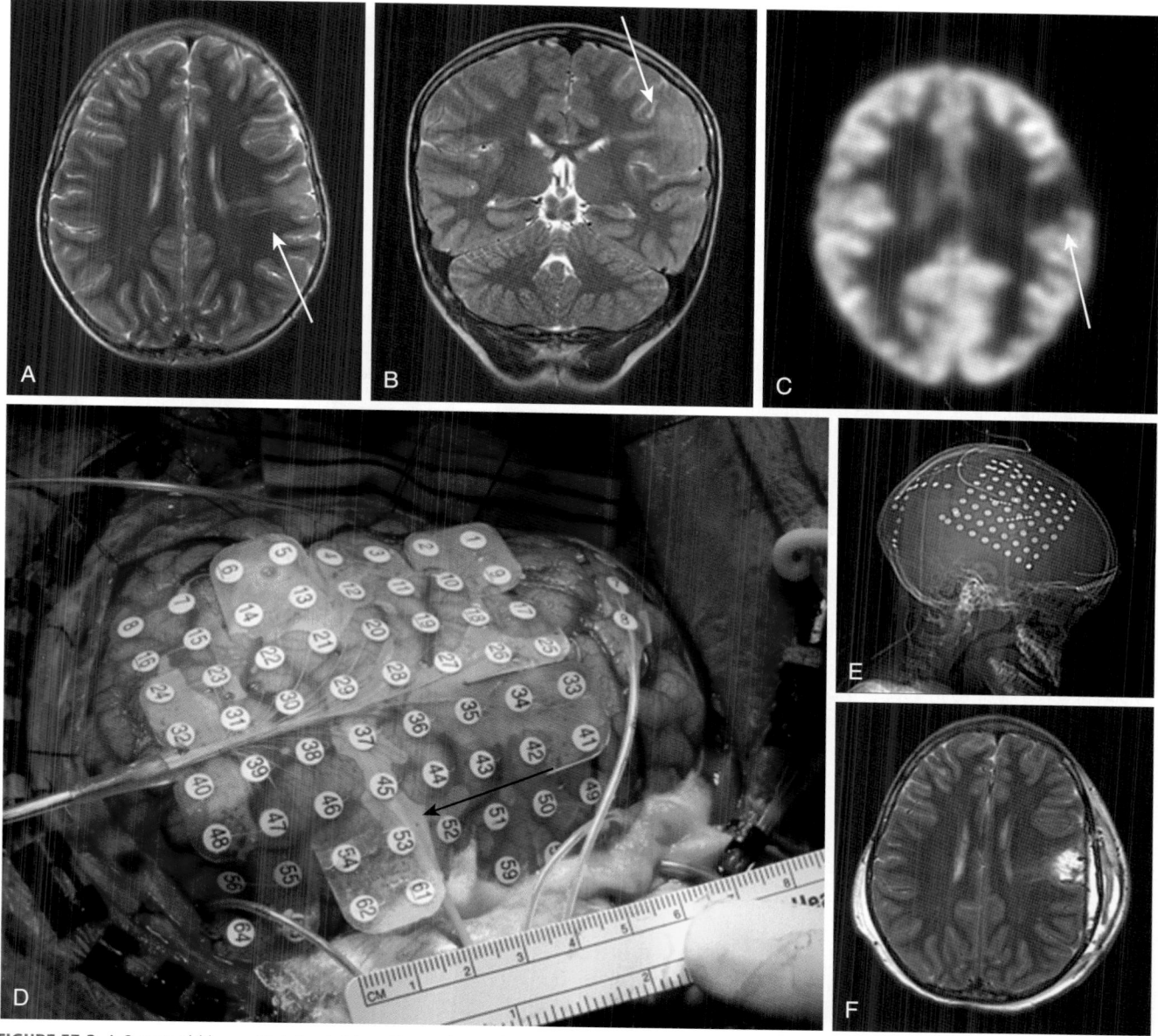

FIGURE 57-3 A 9-year-old boy with intractable epilepsy due to focal cortical dysplasia. Preoperative axial (A) and coronal (B) T2 MRI showed thickened cortex in the parietal lobe with a tail of dysplasia extending to the ventricle (arrows). C, PET showed corresponding hypometabolism (arrow) in dysplastic focus. D, Grids, strips, and depth electrodes were implanted to more precisely localize seizure onset and map motor and language functions. Arrow shows insertion site of depth electrode under grid. E, X-ray of final electrode arrangement. All recorded seizures began superficially in the dysplastic area. Language and motor function were sufficiently removed to allow for a focused, superficial resection of the dysplasia as shown by the postoperative MRI. F, Representative axial T2 image.

Outcome

Extratemporal resections overall carry a poorer prognosis than temporal lobe resections. As in temporal lobe epilepsy, lesional resection has a better prognosis than cortical dysplasia or nonlesional resections where the boundaries of the epileptogenic zone are poorly defined.[116] Many different approaches report similar outcomes and are typically center-specific. Complete resection of MRI-evident lesions is one emerging predictor of outcome.

Multiple subpial transections have shown some benefit, but poorer outcomes than resection. In cases where most of a seizure focus can be resected, MST can be a useful adjunct in nearby functional tissue that is epileptic.[117]

Conclusion

The pathologies encountered in pediatric epilepsy and the surgical techniques used often differ from adult epilepsy. Mapping is a key component to many pediatric epilepsy cases as children often have diffuse congenital epileptic foci. The resection of such foci is often safe when guided by modern techniques. Technological advances, particularly in imaging, are rapidly changing the field and improving the care of epileptic children. The improved technique of hemispherotomy allows a chance for safe treatment of diffuse hemispheric pathologies not amenable to other approaches.

KEY REFERENCES

Boshuisen K, van Schooneveld MM, Leijten FS, et al. Contralateral MRI abnormalities affect seizure and cognitive outcome after hemispherectomy. *Neurology.* 2010;75:1623-1630.

Clarke DB, Oliver A, Anderman F, et al. Surgical treatment of epilepsy: the problem of lesion/focus incongruence. *Surg Neurol.* 1996;46:246-585.

Commission on Classification and Terminology of the International League against Epilepsy: proposal for revised clinical and electroencephalographic classification of epileptic seizures. *Epilepsia.* 1981;22:489-501.

Di Rocco C, Tamburrini G. Sturge-Weber syndrome. *Childs Nerv Syst.* 2006;22:909-921.

Hallbook T, Ruggieri P, Adina C, et al. Contralateral MRI abnormalities in candidates for hemispherectomy for refractory epilepsy. *Epilepsia.* 2010;51:556-563.

Hemb M, Velasco TR, Parnes MS, et al. Improved outcomes in pediatric epilepsy surgery: the UCLA experience, 1986-2008. *Neurology.* 2010;74:1786–75.

Jonas R, Nguyen S, Hu B, et al. Cerebral hemispherectomy: hospital course, seizure, developmental, language, and motor outcomes. *Neurology.* 2004;62:1712-1721.

Mathern GW. Challenges in the surgical treatment of epilepsy patients with cortical dysplasia. *Epilepsia.* 2009;50(suppl 9):45-50.

Mohamed A, Wyllie E, Ruggieri P, et al. Temporal lobe epilepsy due to hippocampal sclerosis in pediatric candidates for epilepsy surgery. *Neurology.* 2001;56:1643-1649.

Morrell F, Whisler WW, Bleck TP. Multiple subpial transections: a new approach to the surgical treatment of focal epilepsy. *J Neurosurg.* 1989;70:231-239.

Morrison G, Duchowny M, Resnick T, et al. Epilepsy surgery in children: a report of 79 patients. *Pediatr Neurosurg.* 1992;18:291-297.

Paolicchi JM, Jayakar P, Dean P, et al. Predictors of outcome in pediatric epilepsy surgery. *Neurology.* 2000;54:642-647.

Schramm J. Temporal lobe epilepsy surgery and the quest for optimal extent of resection: a review. *Epilepsia.* 2008;49:1296-1307.

Schramm J, Behrens E, Entzian W. Hemispherical deafferentation: an alternative to functional hemispherectomy. *Neurosurgery.* 1995;36:509-515.

Schramm J, Kral T, Clusmann H. Transsylvian keyhole functional hemispherectomy. *Neurosurgery.* 2001;49:891-901.

Shields WD, Peacock WJ, Roper SN. Surgery for epilepsy: special pediatric considerations. *Neurosurg Clin North Am.* 1993;4:301-310.

Sillanpaa M, Falava M, Kaleva O, et al. Long-term prognosis of seizures with onset in childhood. *N Engl J Med.* 1998;338:1715-1722.

Smyth MD, Limbrick DD, Ojemann JG, et al. Outcome following surgery for temporal lobe epilepsy with hippocampal involvement in preadolescent children: emphasis on mesial temporal sclerosis. *J Neurosurg.* 2007;106(suppl 3 Pediatrics):205-210.

Spencer SS, Schramm J, Wyler A, et al. Multiple subpial transection for intractable partial epilepsy: an international meta-analysis. *Epilepsia.* 2002;43:141-145.

Spooner CG, Berkovic SF, Mitchell LA, et al. New-onset temporal lobe epilepsy in children: lesion on MRI predicts poor seizure outcome. *Neurology.* 2006;67:2147-2153.

Tanriverdi T, Olivier A, Poulin N, et al. Long-term seizure outcome after corpus callosotomy: a retrospective analysis of 95 patients. *J Neurosurg.* 2009;110:332-342.

Villemure JG, Daniel RT. Peri-insular hemispherotomy in paediatric epilepsy. *Childs Nerv Syst.* 2006;22:967-981.

Wyler AR, Ojemann GA, Lettich E, et al. Subdural strip electrodes for localizing seizure foci in children. *J Neurosurg.* 1984;60:1195-1200.

Wyllie E. Surgical treatment of epilepsy in pediatric patients. *Can J Neurol Sci.* 2000;27:106-110.

Wyllie E, Comair YG, Kotagal P, et al. Seizure outcome after epilepsy surgery in children and adolescents. *Ann Neurol.* 1998;44:740-748.

Numbered references appear on Expert Consult.

CHAPTER 58

Surgical Decision-Making and Treatment Options for Chiari Malformations in Children

TODD C. HANKINSON • R. SHANE TUBBS • W. JERRY OAKES

Significant herniation of the cerebellar tonsils through the foramen magnum is termed the Chiari malformation, type I (CMI). Individuals with CMI may present with symptoms, or this entity may be found incidentally. Headache is the most common presenting symptom, but hydrocephalus is found less than 10% of patients. One common presentation is scoliosis, which is found in 10% to 20% of these patients. Syringomyelia, which may or may not be the underlying etiology of the scoliosis, is present in 12% to 85% of patients.[1-3] Currently, surgical treatment of the CMI is the only available treatment for symptomatic patients.

This chapter discusses the current literature regarding two aspects of surgical decision-making for children with CMI. The first is the current opinion regarding when surgery is indicated. The second is the decision regarding what operation to perform. In the absence of hydrocephalus, the first-line surgical management for CMI is a posterior fossa decompression (PFD) through a midline suboccipital craniectomy and removal of the posterior arch of the atlas with or without dural opening. If hydrocephalus is present, appropriate cerebrospinal fluid (CSF) diversion should be undertaken prior to any other surgical intervention. This may be accomplished through the insertion of a ventriculoperitoneal shunt or performance of an endoscopic third ventriculostomy.[4] These points are widely accepted; however, there is controversy regarding the role of opening the dura as a component of PFD. This chapter discusses the merits and shortcomings of PFD with and without dural opening. When a dural opening is chosen, the surgeon may elect to perform further maneuvers, such as cerebellar tonsillar reduction or resection. Few studies directly compare dural opening with and without additional intradural maneuvers. This chapter therefore does not specifically address decision-making with regard to the completion of further intradural maneuvers after dural opening.

Treatment algorithms regarding patients with Chiari malformation, type II (CMII) differ significantly from those used in patients with CMI and are not discussed here. Treatment algorithms for patients with the more recently described Chiari 0 (syringohydromyelia in the absence of cerebellar tonsillar herniation) and Chiari 1.5 (tonsillar herniation with associated brain stem herniation) are based on the principles that are discussed here in the context of CMI.

Decision-Making Regarding When to Operate

Recent publications regarding operative intervention for CMI demonstrate the varying opinions regarding both when and how to intervene.[5-7,9-21] The availability of magnetic resonance imaging (MRI) has resulted in an increased number of asymptomatic patients being diagnosed with CMI.[1] In addition to tonsillar herniation, these patients may present with asymptomatic syringomyelia and/or scoliosis. Similarly, patients may present with symptoms referable to any of these three structural lesions. Alden et al. used their experience to design a straightforward algorithm to help guide surgical decision-making.[6] Our surgical decision-making tree is shown in Fig. 58-1.

SURGICAL INTERVENTION FOR CMI

First-line surgical therapy for patients with CMI in the absence of hydrocephalus is PFD via midline suboccipital craniectomy, with appropriate removal of the posterior arch of the atlas with or without dural opening (Figs. 58-2 through 58-4). PFD attempts to reestablish bidirectional CSF flow across the craniocervical junction. This is accomplished through the expansion of the posterior fossa subarachnoid space, thus decompressing the cerebellar tonsils and brain stem. PFD may also eliminate the craniospinal CSF pressure differential that is postulated to contribute to syrinx formation.[5] For the remainder of this discussion, the acronym PFD, when used alone, refers to bony suboccipital decompression with dural scoring or splitting but without frank opening of both layers of the dura mater. Most commonly, PFD is undertaken with duraplasty (PFDD) with or without cerebellar tonsil coagulation or resection. Other intradural interventions, such as fourth ventricular stenting and syrinx shunting, have been largely abandoned or are reserved for second- or third-line therapies.[6-9]

Asymptomatic Patients

With regard to asymptomatic patients, survey data collected from the American Association of Neurological Surgeons/Congress of Neurological Surgeons section on pediatric neurosurgery in 1998[7] demonstrated that 83% of pediatric neurosurgeons would not operate on an asymptomatic child with CMI with or without syringomyelia. However, if

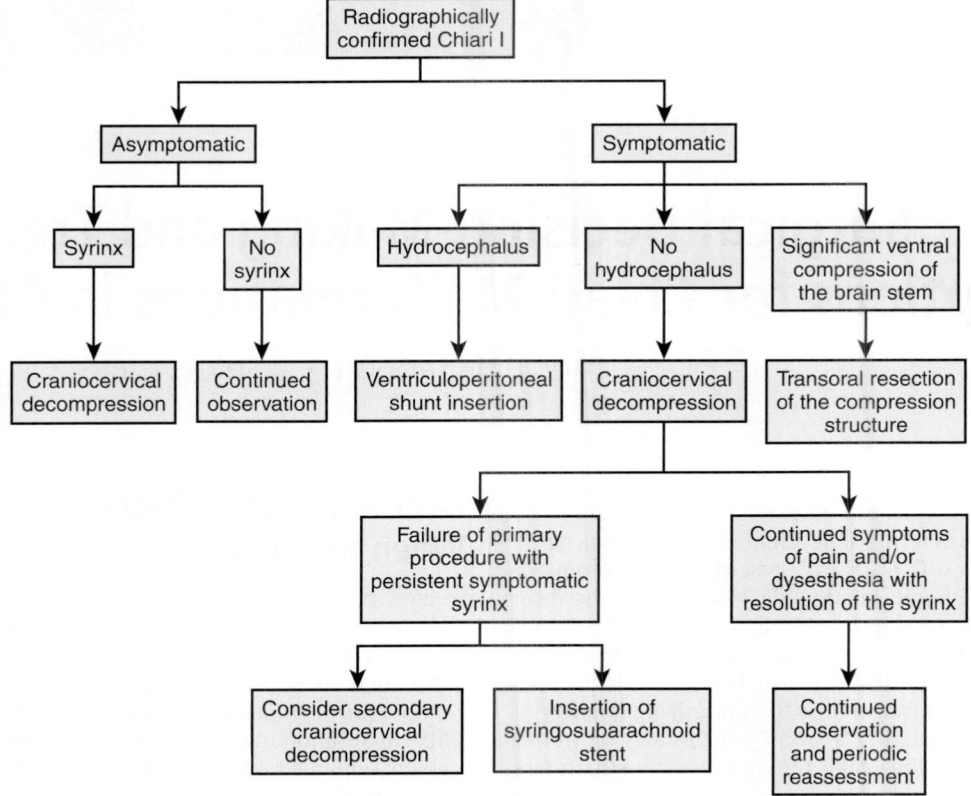

FIGURE 58-1 Surgical decision-making.

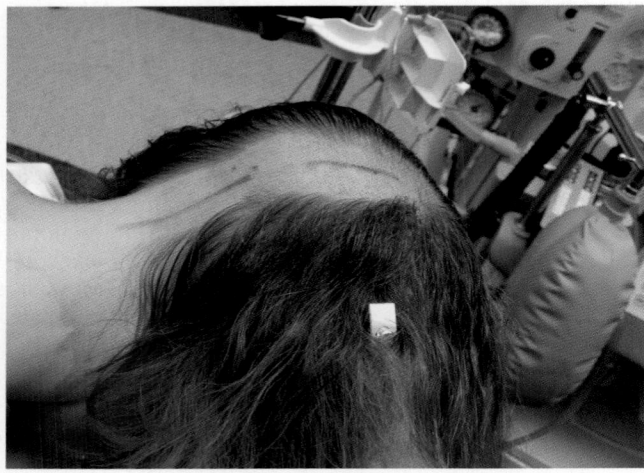

FIGURE 58-2 Positioning of the patient.

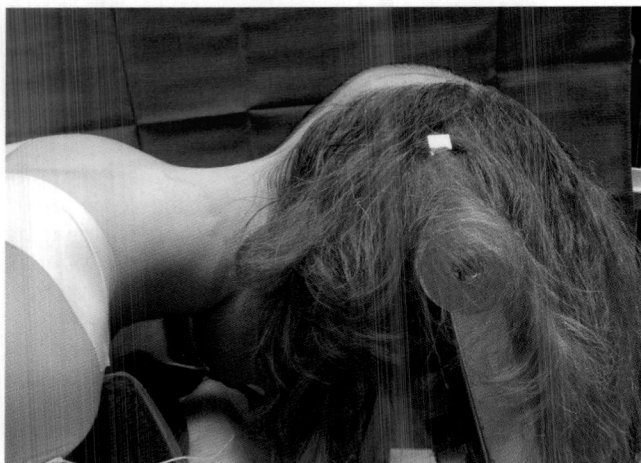

FIGURE 58-3 Skin incisions for PFD. The upper incision is used to harvest a periosteal graft for duraplasty.

the patient subsequently demonstrated asymptomatic syrinx progression, 61% of respondents would intervene. More recent international survey data[9] similarly demonstrated that only a small minority (8%) of pediatric neurosurgeons would intervene for a patient with an asymptomatic CMI without syringomyelia. Rates of surgical treatment increased to 28% and 75% when the same patient presented with a thoracic syrinx of 2 and 8 mm in diameter, respectively. Novegno et al.[20] conservatively managed 22 asymptomatic or minimally symptomatic children with CMI, 1 of whom had syringomyelia. Over a 5.9-year follow-up period, 17 children (77.3%) remained asymptomatic or had symptom improvement (including the patient with syringomyelia), 2 children (9%) had mild worsening of symptoms, and 3 children (13.6%) required surgical intervention. In our institution, children with asymptomatic CMI without syringomyelia do not undergo operative intervention, while those with a syrinx generally receive treatment. Asymptomatic CMI patients with scoliosis in the absence of syringomyelia are rare and should be evaluated individually.

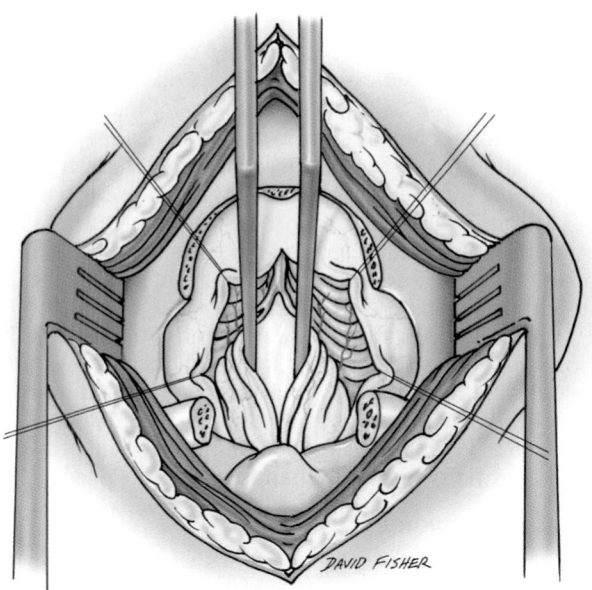

FIGURE 58-4 Schematic drawing of the PFD. Sutures are shown retracting the dura, and the forceps are shown spreading apart the left and right cerebellar tonsils for identification of the floor of the fourth ventricle.

Symptomatic Patients

There is a consensus that patients with symptomatic CMI merit surgical decompression under most circumstances. The most common presenting symptom of a child with CMI is headache. The subjective and nonspecific nature of this symptom requires neurosurgeons to apply strict criteria for a headache to be attributed to CMI. In most cases, the headache must be posteriorly located, must be of short duration, and should be exacerbated or reproduced with a Valsalva maneuver. Surgical treatment of CMI in children with other headache patterns and no additional symptoms referable to the condition may not achieve satisfactory results. Other common symptoms include neck, shoulder, and back pain; motor and sensory changes in the extremities; and sleep apnea and/or feeding difficulty in younger patients.[22]

In cases of progressive syringomyelia, Schijman and Steinbok[9] reported that 97% of respondents would intervene and that 58% would do so in cases of CMI with progressive scoliosis in the absence of syringomyelia, although such cases are not common. McGirt et al.[23] attempted to identify which patients would be most likely to have improvement in symptoms following PFD or PFDD. The authors retrospectively reviewed the clinical response of symptomatic patients who underwent preoperative cine phase-contrast MRI. They concluded that patients with preoperative CSF flow abnormalities, both ventral and dorsal to the caudal brain stem, were less likely to suffer from recurrent symptoms than were patients who lacked such evidence of preoperative CSF flow obstruction.

Decision-Making Regarding Surgical Technique

As previously discussed, once the decision to operate has been made, the surgeon must determine the extent of decompression that will be performed. The goals of surgery in the CMI population include improvement/resolution of symptoms, stabilization/improvement of scoliosis (when present), and radiologic decrease in the extent of syringomyelia (when present). With the postoperative assessment of syringomyelia, there is some debate regarding the extent of diminution that is necessary to demonstrate effective treatment.[11,24] This section describes the current evidence regarding PFD with and without dural opening.

STUDIES DIRECTLY COMPARING SURGICAL TECHNIQUES

Despite significant literature describing the treatment of CMI, no randomized trials comparing PFD against PFDD have been completed. Among the studies that directly compare the two techniques, only one meta-analysis and two surveys have been completed.[7,9,13]

Durham and Fjeld-Olenec[13] published a meta-analysis of studies that directly compare cohorts of pediatric patients who underwent PFD with cohorts who were treated with PFDD. A total of seven studies met their inclusion criteria.[18,19,25-29] The authors concluded that patients who undergo duraplasty are less likely to require reoperation (2.1% vs. 12.6%) for persistent or recurrent symptoms but are more likely to suffer CSF-related complications (18.5% vs. 1.8%). There was no statistical difference in clinical outcomes between the two groups, specifically with regard to symptom improvement and syringomyelia. In summary, rates of clinical improvement were 65% in the PFD patients and 79% in the PFDD patients. Rates of radiologic syrinx improvement were influenced by small numbers in some studies but were 56% in the PFD patients and 87% in those undergoing PFDD. The authors appropriately acknowledged that their conclusions were limited by the patient selection methods of the studies they examined. Among the seven papers, five studies used intraoperative ultrasound to help determine whether or not to perform a dural opening.[18,19,26,28,29] The inherent subjectivity of this technique limits the degree to which the findings of each work may be generalized. Additionally, no study included a randomization or blinding process.

Using expert opinion as an indicator of current practice, Haroun et al.[7] reported that 25% of survey respondents would perform PFD for children with symptomatic CMI, 32% recommended PFDD, and 55% recommended further intradural manipulations (some respondents chose more than one intervention). International survey data published by Schijman and Steinbok[9] demonstrated that 76% of pediatric neurosurgeons always open the dura mater for treating CMI.

STUDIES OF PFD WITHOUT DURAL OPENING

There is significant literature retrospectively examining the results of PFD and PFDD. With regard to outcomes, three general categories can be assessed: clinical improvement, syrinx resolution, and scoliosis progression.

Electrophysiologic evidence suggests that neurologic improvement can be achieved without a dural opening. Groups from Columbia University and Ohio State University found that improved conduction of nerve impulses through the brain stem occurs after bony decompression rather than after dural opening.[30-32] As mentioned previously, multiple groups have used intraoperative ultrasound findings to aid their decision-making with regard to dural opening in children with CM-I.[10,19,29,33] Yeh et al.[29] found that factors that were associated with adequate decompression without duraplasty included age of less than 1 year. Factors that were more likely to be associated with the need for duraplasty included spinal symptoms (motor, sensory, or scoliosis) and a greater magnitude of tonsillar descent.

Clinical Outcome

The majority of studies that report rates of clinical and radiologic improvement following PFD also include patients who were treated with PFDD and have therefore been referenced in the preceding section. Two Italian reports demonstrated excellent results in series of patients who underwent PFD alone.[11,34] Genitori et al.[34] reported the results of their experience using PFD in 26 patients. Among 16 patients (61.5%) without syringomyelia, 13 (81.3%) had complete symptom resolution and the remaining 3 (18.8%) had partial resolution. Among 10 patients with syringomyelia, symptoms improved or resolved in all cases with the exception of one of three cases of scoliosis (33.3%) and one of five cases of sensory loss (20%). Rates of complete symptom resolution, however, ranged from 25% (sensory loss) to 100% (vertigo). Two patients (7.7%) required reoperation. The authors acknowledged that it is difficult to draw definitive conclusions from their study due to the small numbers in each group.

Caldarelli et al.[11] reviewed their experience with PFD in 30 children. After a mean follow-up period of 4.7 years, 28 patients (93.3%) demonstrated a "significant improvement in their clinical condition."

Syrinx Resolution

In the PFD groups of the studies included in their meta-analysis, Durham and Fjeld-Olenec[13] reported an aggregate 56.3% (9 of 16 patients) rate of syrinx reduction, which was not statistically different from the 87.0% (40 of 46 patients)

rate calculated for the PFDD group. As previously mentioned, in the series of Genitori et al.,[34] 10 of 26 patients (38.5%) patients presented with syringomyelia. Following PFD, the syrinx disappeared in 8 (80%). The remaining 2 children (7.7%) had initial clinical improvement but required further surgery, with duraplasty, for persistent syringomyelia. Syringomyelia was present preoperatively in 12 of 30 patients (40%) in Caldarelli et al.'s report.[11] Postoperatively, half of these patients (6) had a decrease in the size of the syrinx. Two patients (6.7%) demonstrated recurrent symptoms and postoperative syrinx growth (one *de novo* and another who had a syrinx preoperatively) and required reoperation. The authors argued that, in the context of clinical improvement, radiologic change (either in syrinx size or in posterior fossa subarachnoid volume) was not mandatory for a successful result. Wetjen et al.[24] also argued that the absence of syrinx distention is more important than complete collapse.

Scoliosis Improvement

In two studies that describe outcomes with regard to scoliosis following PFD without duraplasty, Genitori et al.[34] reported improvement in 2 of 3 patients and Caldarelli et al.[11] reported mild improvement in 2 of 2 patients. In their series of 21 patients with CMI, syringomyelia, and scoliosis, Attenello et al.[35] described a single patient who underwent PFD. This patient had progression of scoliosis and underwent PFDD reoperation.

STUDIES OF PFD WITH DURAL OPENING

Clinical Outcome

In a series of PFDD in 130 patients, Tubbs et al.[3] reported relief of preoperative symptoms in 83% of patients. Headache did not resolve in 12%, and perioperative complications occurred in 2.3%. Smaller series using PFDD (with or without further intradural manipulation) reported clinical improvement rates of 92% to 100% and complication rates of 0% to 16.7%.[12,14,15,17,30,31,36-38] In the context of a comparison

Table 58-1 Rates of Symptom/Syrinx Improvement and Reoperation in Studies Including Both Techniques

Author (year)	Points	Dural Opening	Clinical Improvement (%)	Syrinx Improvement (%)	Scoliosis Stable/ Improvement (%)
Galarza et al. (2007)[25]	20	N	4 (33.3, $n = 12$)	2 (40, $n = 5$)	NR
	21	Y	11 (73.3, $n = 15$)	0 (0, $n = 2$)	NR
	19	Y*	8 (88.9, $n = 9$)	7 (100, $n = 7$)	NR
Yeh et al. (2006)[29]	40	N	36 (90.0)	4 (66.7)	1 (100)
	85	Y	83 (97.6)	17 (85)	9 (100)
Limonadi and Selden (2004)[18]	12	N	1.67†	NR	NR
	12	Y	1.53†	7 (70, $n = 10$)	NR
Navarro et al. (2004)[19]	56‡	N	40‡ (72.2)	NR	NR
	24‡	Y	16‡ (68.4)	NR	NR
	29‡	Y*	17‡ (60.8)	NR	NR
Ventureyra et al. (2003)[28]	6	N	4 (66.7)	0 (0, $n = 2$)	NR
	10	Y	10 (100)	5 (100, $n = 5$)	NR
Munshi et al. (2000)[27]	11	N	8 (72.7)	3 (50.0, $n = 6$)	NR
	21§	Y	18 (85.7)	7 (63.6, $n = 11$)	NR

*With intradural maneuvers.
†Aggregate scoring system with a range from −1 to 2, with 2 = all preoperative symptoms resolved.
‡Extrapolated from percentages.
§Dural opening as the initial procedure.
NR = not reported.

of duraplasty materials (autograft vs. synthetic allograft), Attenello et al.[39] demonstrated mild to moderate symptom recurrence at 16 months follow-up in 14 of 67 patients (20.9%), with 4 of these (6.0%) requiring revision decompression. A pseudomeningocele observed on imaging was identified in 10 patients (17%), but only 1 of these became symptomatic. A total of 5 patients (7%) suffered CSF-related complications: 2 (3%) with CSF leakage and 2 (3%) with aseptic meningitis.

Syrinx Resolution

Reported rates of syrinx improvement in children following PFDD range from 55% to 100%.[3,10,14,17,30,31,36-39] The variability in these results may stem partly from the small sample size of some studies and additionally from the absence of a standard definition of "improvement" when considering syrinx size (Table 58-1). As previously mentioned, Durham and Fjeld-Olenec[13] found an overall rate of 87% syrinx reduction in the PFDD arms of studies that directly compared PFD with PFDD.

Following initial PFDD, Tubbs et al.[3] found that only 8 of 75 syringes (10.7%) did not improve. Of these, 7 syringes (87.5%) improved with repeat PFDD[40] (Fig. 58-5). No radiographic parameters predicted failure of syrinx response. As such, we maintain a policy of repeat PFDD in cases of persistent syringomyelia. Attenello et al.[10] retrospectively examined the syrinx response rate following hindbrain decompression in 49 consecutive children with CMI, 46 of whom underwent PFDD and 3 of whom underwent PFD alone. They reported a 55% overall syrinx improvement rate at 14 months, with 26 of the 46 (56.5%) in the PFDD group improving. Of 5 patients (10.2%) who underwent repeat decompression, 1 (2.0%) was due to syrinx expansion at 5 months after PFDD. Of the 49 patients, 39 (79.6%)

had preoperative symptoms attributable to syringomyelia. Of these, 21 patients (54%) experienced symptom resolution. Complications included aseptic meningitis and wound breakdown in 2 patients (4%) and pseudomeningocele in 1 (2%). None of these complications required reoperation. In the PFD group, 2 of the 3 did not have syrinx improvement. One required reoperation with PFDD, and another underwent spinal fusion for scoliosis.

The expected time to and magnitude of syrinx improvement following PFDD remain incompletely understood. Although a subjectively significant decrease in the syrinx size on the first postoperative imaging examination is reassuring to the surgeon, complete resolution of the fluid collection is likely unnecessary[11,24] and syringes may dissipate after a prolonged interval.[41]

Scoliosis Progression

In the vast majority of cases, scoliosis in the context of CMI is associated with syringomyelia.[42] Although the exact mechanism through which the syrinx produces scoliosis remains unknown, it is believed that lower motor neuron injury imbalances innervation to the trunk musculature, predisposing the patient to scoliosis.[43-45] Consistent with this theory, multiple authors have reported scoliosis improvement following PFDD in children with CMI. Reported rates of scoliosis improvement are 0% to 73%, and rates of progression are 18% to 72%,[3,8,46-53] demonstrating that PFDD may slow or halt scoliosis progression in some cases—although there remains a considerable risk of progression. In some series, younger children (younger than 8-10 years) have been less likely to suffer from scoliosis progression.[8,46,47,52,53] Female gender and a smaller presenting Cobb angle have also been associated with improved outcomes; however, Brockmeyer et al.[46] found that a decrease in syrinx size did not

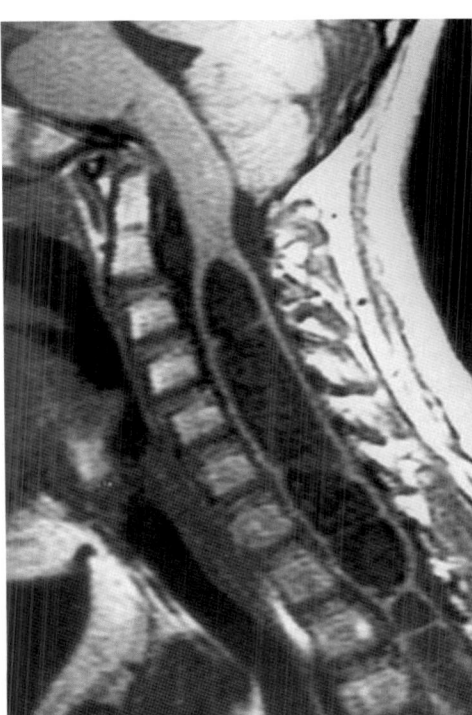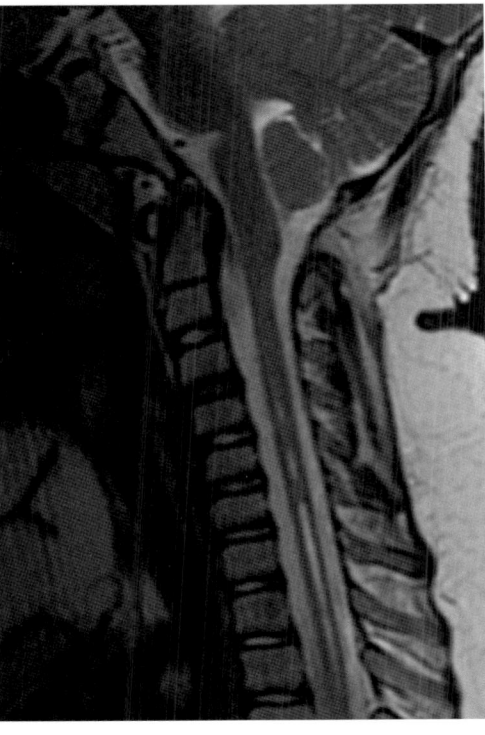

FIGURE 58-5 Preoperative and postoperative sagittal MRI demonstrating significant improvement of holocord syringomyelia in a child with CMI who was treated with PFDD.

necessarily correlate with scoliosis improvement. In 20 pediatric patients with CMI-associated scoliosis treated by PFDD, Attenello et al.[35] reported that 8 (40%) demonstrated a postoperative improvement of their scoliosis and 9 (45%) progressed. The authors reported that an increased magnitude of the scoliosis curve at presentation was predictive of scoliosis progression, as were thoracolumbar junction scoliosis and a lack of postoperative radiologic syrinx response.

Summary

THE CASE FOR PFD

Electrophysiologic data support the assertion that effective PFD occurs with bony decompression and dural scoring, not necessarily requiring dural opening.[30-32] Although rates of reoperation for persistent or recurrent symptoms are higher with PFD, the technique is attractive because it minimizes potential surgical complications. Theoretical complications that are avoided with PFD include pseudomeningocele, chemical meningitis, bacterial meningitis, arterial injury, venous sinus bleeding, stroke, and hydrocephalus. Multiple studies have demonstrated that CSF-related complication rates are lower for PFD than for PFDD.[18,19,27,29] Additionally, nondural opening PFD is likely to require less operative time.[18] The case for PFD is also strengthened because no study directly comparing PFD and PFDD has demonstrated a statistically significant difference in clinical outcomes between the two techniques. Furthermore, while many studies have demonstrated a trend toward a greater pace and magnitude of syrinx collapse following PFDD, the clinical significance of this result has yet to be clearly defined,[11,24] making syrinx resolution a questionable measure of efficacy regarding hindbrain decompression for CMI. Lastly, the use of PFD does not preclude patients from undergoing further decompression should this become necessary (Table 58-2).

THE CASE FOR PFDD

Although direct comparisons have not demonstrated a statistically significant difference in clinical outcomes, the large majority of studies reporting the clinical efficacy of PFDD for the most common presentations have demonstrated rates of improvement superior to those of PFD.[26-29] Durham and Fjeld-Olenec[13] demonstrated a significantly lower rate of reoperation following PFDD versus PFD (2.1% vs. 12.6%). Although their meta-analysis also demonstrated a higher complication rate with PFDD, it must be acknowledged that multiple groups have reported very low complication rates with PFDD.[3,15,17] Additionally, at least 12% of patients with CMI and syringomyelia who undergo PFD are likely to require reoperation, because without opening the dura, it is not possible to release arachnoid veils that have been described at the foramen of Magendie in some patients.[40] Lastly, in some circumstances, such as rapidly progressive neurologic decline or scoliosis, there is little debate that PFDD is necessary.[54] As such, PFDD is the treatment that offers the greatest likelihood of improving the presenting signs and symptoms in any given child.

Table 58-2   Relative Advantages of PFD and PFDD

PFD	PFDD
Lower CSF-related complication rate	Lower reoperation rate
Shorter operative time	Better radiological outcomes
Optional shorter incision	Inspection possible of arachnoid veils/scarring
± adequate syrinx decompression	± better clinical outcomes

Conclusions

Surgical decision-making for children with CMI may be considered in two steps: when to operate and what operation to perform. With the growth of MRI availability, neurosurgeons are asked to evaluate many asymptomatic and minimally symptomatic children with tonsillar herniation. In this population, a characteristic finding such as syringomyelia or scoliosis is generally required for surgical intervention to be indicated. In a patient with a symptom complex that is consistent with posterior fossa compression, surgical decompression is likely to improve the condition. Similarly, children with CMI and syringomyelia should be considered for surgical intervention regardless of their presenting symptoms.

Selection of the most appropriate surgical technique for CMI is not yet guided by type I or II evidence. Although most authors agree that the combination of hindbrain decompression through suboccipital craniectomy and removal of the posterior arch of the atlas is the best first-line treatment for CMI, the use of duraplasty remains debated. Current data leave the treating surgeon to choose between a procedure that is more likely to require reoperation (PFD) and one that is more likely to result in perioperative CSF-related complications (PFDD). The frequency of these suboptimal outcomes (12.6% and 18.5%, respectively, in Durham and Fjeld-Olenec's meta-analysis[13]) does little to clarify which approach is most appropriate for a given patient. Furthermore, wide ranges of clinical efficacy and complications have been reported. Lastly, the spectrum of presentation in children with CMI extends from asymptomatic to potentially life-threatening symptomatology. It is therefore not surprising that no single surgical approach is universally recommended. As such, if a particular neurosurgeon has significant problems with dural opening, then PFD is an attractive option. If, however, PFDD is associated with hospital discharge in fewer than 3 days and very low reoperation rate (<1%), then adding the additional steps of opening the dura, looking for IV ventricular outlet obstruction, and grafting the dura to prevent chemical meningitis has great appeal.

KEY REFERENCES

Anderson RC, Dowling KC, Feldstein NA, Emerson RG. Chiari I malformation: potential role for intraoperative electrophysiologic monitoring. *J Clin Neurophysiol.* 2000;20:65-72.

Durham SR, Fjeld-Olenec K. Comparison of posterior fossa decompression with and without duraplasty for the surgical treatment of Chiari malformation type I in pediatric patients: a meta-analysis. *J Neurosurg Pediatr.* 2008;2:42-49.

Haroun RI, Guarnieri M, Meadow JJ, et al. Current opinions for the treatment of syringomyelia and Chiari malformations: survey of the Pediatric Section of the American Association of Neurological Surgeons. *Pediatr Neurosurg.* 2000;33:311-317.

Hayhurst C, Osman-Farah J, Das K, Mallucci C. Initial management of hydrocephalus associated with Chiari malformation type I—syringomyelia complex via endoscopic third ventriculostomy: an outcome analysis. *J Neurosurg.* 2008;108:1211-1214.

Oldfield EH, Muraszko K, Shawker TH, Patronas NJ. Pathophysiology of syringomyelia associated with Chiari I malformation of the cerebellar tonsils. Implications for diagnosis and treatment. *J Neurosurg.* 1994;80:3-15.

Schijman E, Steinbok P. International survey on the management of Chiari I malformation and syringomyelia. *Childs Nerv Syst.* 2004;20: 341-348.

Tubbs RS, McGirt MJ, Oakes WJ. Surgical experience in 130 pediatric patients with Chiari I malformations. *J Neurosurg.* 2003;99:291-296.

Numbered references appear on Expert Consult.

CHAPTER 59

Fetal Surgery for Open Neural Tube Defects

NALIN GUPTA

The goal of fetal surgery is to prevent or reduce the adverse consequences of a congenital disorder without increasing the risks for the fetus and mother. A number of diseases, such as congenital diaphragmatic hernia and sacrococcygeal teratoma, can be treated by surgical procedures performed directly on the fetus prior to the anticipated delivery date.[1] An open neural tube defect, or myelomeningocele, is different in that it is not a fatal disease and fetuses with this condition will usually complete a normal gestation.[2] This is an ethical challenge for the treating physicians because the potential benefits must be balanced by a well-defined risk to the fetus, and also to the mother who is a "bystander" with respect to the perceived benefits.

The development of fetal surgery for a specific condition has usually moved in a series of steps starting from the development of an animal model, definition of the natural history, refinement of techniques in test cases, and finally, evaluation of efficacy in prospective clinical trial. The reported benefits of fetal surgery for myelomeningocele as determined from retrospective case series include a reduction in shunt insertion rates and improvement in the hindbrain abnormality.[3-5] To obtain more conclusive data, the potential benefit of fetal surgery for myelomeningoceles is being examined in a clinical trial directly comparing patients randomized into prenatal and postnatal treatment groups.

Rationale for Fetal Repair

Although there is large spectrum of abnormalities observed in children with myelomeningoceles, it is useful to separate the neurologic deficits into two groups: primary and secondary. The primary neurologic deficits are those directly caused by the arrested development of the neural placode, which usually occurs in the lumbosacral region.[6] Because neural tube closure occurs during the third and fourth weeks of gestation, the spinal cord in this region is very immature at the stage when a myelomeningocele develops. Although the structure of the spinal cord is severely disrupted at the involved level, it is unknown whether the placode is capable of further development.[7] The functional neurologic level is either at the same level as the vertebral anomaly, or actually higher than the vertebral level, resulting in worse neurologic function, in more than 80% of patients with open forms of spina bifida.[8]

The secondary neurologic deficits in patients with spina bifida include delayed loss of motor function, worsening bowel and bladder control, and scoliosis. These symptoms and signs are typically attributed to a symptomatic tethered spinal cord, although other conditions, such as a Chiari II malformation, syrinx, and hydrocephalus, all worsen neurologic function. Magnetic resonance imaging (MRI) studies of most myelomeningocele lesions following repair show a dysplastic spinal cord terminating in the overlying soft tissues at the site of the repaired defect. For this reason, virtually all patients with myelomeningocele have a tethered spinal cord by radiological criteria. It is not clear, however, why some patients with a myelomeningocele have either minor or no symptoms of a tethered spinal cord.

The theoretical advantage of fetal repair for myelomeningoceles is that the neural tube is covered and protected many months before the expected delivery date. The basis for expecting improved neurologic function is that restoration of the dysplastic neural placode within the spinal canal isolates it from the amniotic fluid and prevents ongoing injury.[9,10] Mueli and others surgically created a spinal-cord lesion in fetal sheep at 75 days of gestation that simulated a spina bifida lesion.[11] After delivery at term, the gross and microscopic appearance of the exposed spinal cord resembled a human spina bifida lesion and the animals were incontinent and had loss of sensation and motor function below the lesion level. One group of animals with surgically created spina bifida lesions were then treated using a myocutaneous flap at 100 days of gestation. These animals were then carried to full-term gestation and had near-normal motor function and normal bowel and bladder control. The results of these experiments suggested that early repair of an exposed spinal cord may preserve neurologic function and may allow improvement through plasticity.[12] Although provocative, these large animal experiments clearly rely on a model system that has distinct differences with the human disease.

Timing for Fetal Surgery

If closure of an open neural tube defect reduces secondary injury occurring to the placode, then surgical intervention should be performed as early as possible. In practice, surgical timing is determined by diagnosis and technical limitations of the actual procedure. Most myelomeningoceles are detected during the second trimester, either during an investigation of a positive maternal screening test, or during a routine ultrasound study. The quality of current ultrasonography allows detection of most fetuses with myelomeningoceles by the mid-portion of the second trimester.[13] From a practical viewpoint, this means that a diagnosis is made between 18 and 22 weeks of gestation. Taking into consideration current obstetrical practice, it is unlikely that detection of fetuses with spina bifida will occur any earlier unless new, more sensitive screening tests are discovered.

Preoperative fetal imaging studies usually begin with a detailed ultrasonogram (Fig. 59-1A). This study is able to determine some anatomic features with great precision. These include size of the overlying sac, the level of the defect, the position of the cerebellar tonsils, and the presence of lower-extremity deformities. Limitations include difficulty determining some associated brain anomalies, other intraspinal anomalies, and at times, the exact dysraphic level. Most patients being considered for fetal surgery will undergo a fetal MRI study (Fig. 59-1B). Because of motion, images in sagittal, axial, and coronal planes are obtained randomly by repeatedly imaging the fetus over time. The preferred MRI technique is a single-shot, fast spin-echo T2-weighted sequence. There is some evidence that MRI may improve the ability to detect coexisting spinal and brain anomalies that may not be apparent on ultrasound studies.[14,15]

Hysterotomy and Exposure

Several technical hurdles needed to be overcome before fetal surgery could be performed safely. These include: (1) the ability to open the uterus and prevent separation of the chorioamniotic membranes, (2) achieve watertight uterine closure, and (3) prevent the onsent of preterm labor in the post-operative period.[1] The ability of the mother to carry and deliver subsequent pregnancies does not appear to be jeopardized by fetal surgery.

The patient is anesthetized with a halogenated agent and an epidural catheter is used for pain control. The fetus is monitored using pulse oximetry, radiotelemetry, and intraoperative ultrasound. A low transverse incision is made and ultrasound is used to localize the position of the placenta and fetus. An anterior or posterior hysterotomy is performed using an absorbable uterine stapler device that provides hemostasis and seals the membranes to the myometrium. In general, the uterine incision should be made directly over the back of the fetus and as small as possible. The fetus is rarely removed from the uterus in order to avoid unnecessary manipulation and torsion of the umbilical cord. A narcotic and paralytic agent is administered to the fetus intramuscularly. Warm lactated Ringer solution is continuously infused around the fetus and open uterus to maintain fetal body temperature.

After the hysterotomy is completed, the edges of the uterine wall are inspected carefully to stop any significant bleeding and prevent separation of the amniotic membranes. Catheters are placed into the uterus to allow continual irrigation to maintain the level of amniotic fluid. The fetus floats in the uterine cavity and this will tend to push the torso up against the hysterotomy. This is preferred since the fetus will tend to move or drift during the surgery, which can make the actual repair quite difficult. After repair of the defect, the fetus is returned to the womb and amniotic fluid is restored with warm saline containing an antibiotic such as nafcillin. The uterine incision is closed with in two layers, and fibrin glue is used to help seal the uterine incision.

Surgical Repair of the Defect

The overall steps used during fetal surgery are similar to those of the postnatal procedure: (1) identification of the neural placode, (2) separation of the placode from the surrounding epithelium, (3) identification and closure of the dura, and (4) elevation of the surrounding soft tissues and closure of the skin. The major difference between the pre- and post-natal procedures is the tenuous nature of the fetal tissues. The neural placode is extremely fragile and even limited manipulation leads to loss of tissue integrity. Although the nerve roots are able to withstand some handling, excessive tension will cause avulsion from the placode. The dura is often insubstantial, transparent when mobilized, and has the characteristics of arachnoid in older children. The skin is able to handle surgical dissection but excessive tension leads to tearing.

The neural placode is usually more visible in the fetus than in the term infant. The arachnoid is extremely thin and

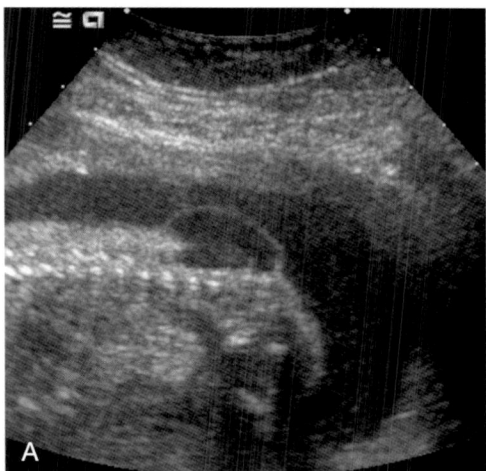
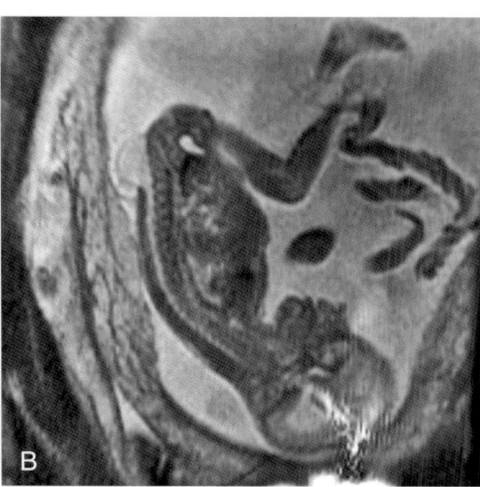

FIGURE 59-1 A, Prenatal ultrasound performed at approximately 20 weeks gestational age shows a typical lumbar myelomeningocele in patient who underwent fetal surgery. B, Fetal MRI of the same patient. The resolution of the T2-weighted image is low, but the spinal cord can be seen terminating in the placode. The myelomeningocele sac is clearly visible above the defect in the soft tissue.

FIGURE 59-2 A, Fetal myelomeningocele exposed through a hysterotomy. The placode is oriented in a horizontal direction and is surrounded by a moderate-sized sac. The arachnoid at the margins of the sac is extremely thin and translucent. Uterine staples can be seen at the edge of hysterotomy. B, The same lesion following repair showing a single-layer closure of the skin. C, A different patient with a flat placode with no sac. The arachnoid is transparent and the surrounding skin is several millimeters from the edge of the open spinal canal. D, The width of the skin defect precluded primary closure of the skin. Excessive tension on the skin leads to tearing. An acellular dermis patch was used to close the skin.

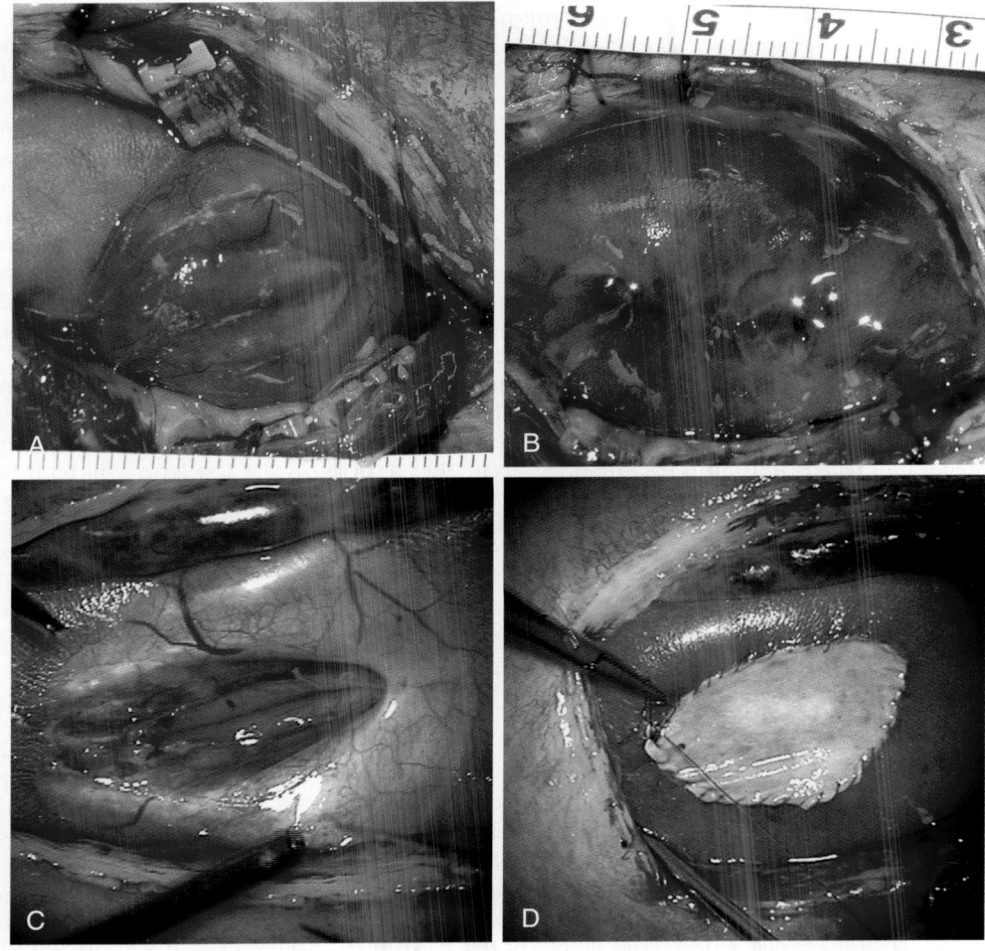

translucent and the junction between it and the placode is readily apparent. If the myelomeningocele sac is intact, the placode is usually lifted upward away from the surface of the back (Fig. 59-2A). In other situations, the placode is flat and at the same level as the surrounding skin (Fig. 59-2C). The epithelium of the skin does not usually reach the edge of the placode. The clear identification of the intervening arachnoid usually allows the placode to be divided from its attachments with sharp dissection. Depending on the consistency of the placode, the neural tube can be retubularized; however, if the placode is particularly fragile, this step may not be possible.

The dura is loosely attached to the underlying subcutaneous tissues just lateral to the spinal canal. After incising the dura at its lateral junction with the dermis, gentle instillation of saline into the epidural plane with a small angiocatheter lifts the dura away from the underlying tissues, which minimizes trauma. Between 18 to 20 weeks of gestation, the dura can be very thin and difficult to handle. After 22 weeks of gestation, the dura becomes more substantial and can be handled more easily. Once the dura is circumferentially detached from the dermis and separated from the underlying lumbar fascia, it can be closed using a running suture. If the amount of dura is insufficient, then a patch is used to close the opening. The use of acellular human dermis to repair the dura may contribute to the

formation of intracellular dermoid cysts.[16] For this reason, a synthetic collagen matrix (DuraGen, Integra Life Sciences, Plainsboro, NJ) can be used to create a dural barrier.

Following dural closure, the skin is closed as a single layer incorporating the superficial and deeper tissues (Fig. 59-2B). In general, dissection of the underlying muscle and fascia is not attempted because excessive fetal blood loss must be avoided and the duration of the procedure minimized. Elevation of the skin and separation from the underlying subcutaneous tissues is relatively easy, although increased tension on the skin inevitably leads to tearing. Small openings in the skin caused by handling with forceps or tension from suture points generally close rapidly. If the skin can be brought together, the final postnatal appearance is often excellent. For situations where insufficient skin is available to close the lesion, either skin flaps, relaxing incisions, or acellular dermis can be used as a patch (Fig. 59–2D). In most cases, this patch becomes incorporated into the healing scar tissue.

Results

Experimental evidence suggested that early closure of myelomeningoceles should improve neurologic function by preventing the secondary injury to the exposed nervous tissue.[9,11] Early clinical results, however, from fetal repair

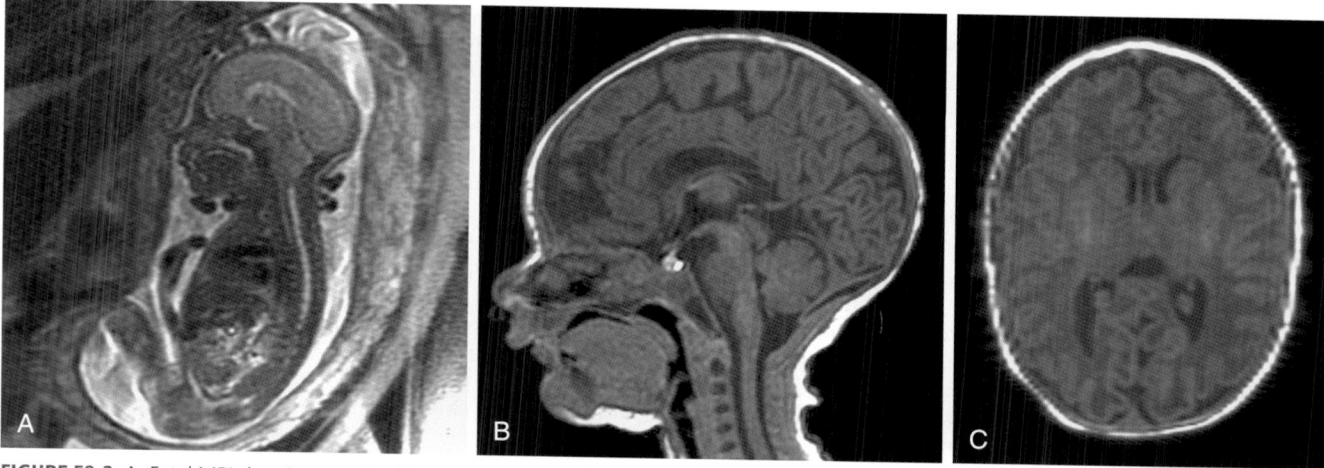

FIGURE 59-3 A, Fetal MRI showing a sagittal image of the craniocervical junction and upper spine. Although the resolution is low due to the size of the fetus, the cerebellum appears displaced downwards. B, After fetal repair, the cerebellum appears to be in the normal position and the secondary changes normally seen in the brain stem are markedly improved. C, The axial brain image shows normal ventricular size without hydrocephalus.

of human myelomeningoceles have been disappointing. Tubbs and colleagues examined a cohort of patients ($n = 37$) who had undergone fetal repair between 20 and 28 weeks of gestation and compared their neurologic function to a cohort ($n = 40$) of patients who underwent postnatal procedures.[17] No statistical difference was observed in lower extremity function between the two groups. This study, along with others, has limitations inherent with any retrospective analysis, such as an unmatched control group, lack of standardization of surgical technique, and lack of randomization to treatment arms. Nevertheless, the lack of clear improvement in neurologic function with fetal surgery suggests that the animal models used to study this disorder do not recapitulate the human disease.

The incidence of delayed signs and symptoms such as lower-extremity weakness, worsening of bladder and bowel control, and/or pain in patients who have had fetal surgery is unknown. Based on a few cases, re-exploration in patients who have had previous fetal repair appears to be more difficult because tissue planes in the area of the placode are poorly defined. Urodynamics performed on a small group of children who had undergone fetal surgery showed clear abnormalities such as vesicoureteral reflux and a significant postvoid residual urine volume. These results were indistinguishable from those of patients who had undergone postnatal repair.[18] This is not unexpected since urologic function should be strongly related to sacral spinal cord function.

Data from centers performing fetal surgery for myelomeningocele have indicated that the benefits of surgery are a reduction in the rate of CSF shunt insertion, and improvement in the appearance of the Chiari II malformation on imaging studies (Fig. 59-3).[5,19] The shunt rate in a cohort of 116 children treated with fetal surgery and followed in the postnatal period for at least 12 months was 54%.[20] The strongest predictor for postnatal shunt placement was the upper level of the spinal lesion, with those above L3 showing the highest rates of shunt insertion. This trend is similar to a historical series where lesion level affected shunt

rates.[8] The overall percentage of patients requiring shunt placement, based on retrospective series, is usually in the range of 80% to 95%. By this measure, the reduction in shunt insertion rates reported in the fetal surgery group is encouraging. However, it is possible that selection bias alone may account for this benefit. In order to measure this presumed reduction in shunt insertion rates and to accurately assess maternal and fetal risks, a randomized, prospective clinical trial sponsored by the National Institutes of Health is underway (see Addendum).

Conclusion

Fetal surgery for myelomeningocele can be performed safely with acceptable maternal and fetal risks. Whether these risks are balanced by a benefit to the child over many years of follow-up is unknown. Initial reports do not indicate that fetal surgery improves neurologic or urological function, although it may reduce the need for shunt insertion. The impact on other long-term disabilities such as tethered cord syndrome remains unknown and will only be determined as groups of patients are followed over time.

KEY REFERENCES

Bruner JP, Tulipan N, Paschall RL, et al. Fetal surgery for myelomeningocele and the incidence of shunt-dependent hydrocephalus. *JAMA.* 1999;282(19):1819-1825.

Bruner JP, Tulipan N, Reed G, et al. Intrauterine repair of spina bifida: preoperative predictors of shunt-dependent hydrocephalus. *Am J Obstet Gynecol.* 2004;190(5):1305-1312.

Meuli M, Meuli-Simmen C, Hutchins GM, et al. In utero surgery rescues neurological function at birth in sheep with spina bifida. *Nat Med.* 1995;1(4):342-347.

Tulipan N, Hernanz-Schulman M, Lowe LH, et al. Intrauterine myelomeningocele repair reverses preexisting hindbrain herniation. *Pediatr Neurosurg.* 1999;31(3):137-142.

Adzick NS, Thom EA, Spong CY, et al. A randomized trial of prenatal versus postnatal repair of myelomeningocele. *NEJM.* 2011;364:993-1004.

Numbered references appear on Expert Consult.

Addendum

The Management of Myelomeningocele Study (MOMS), a prospective randomized clinical trial, was stopped for efficacy in early 2011 after 183 of a planned 200 patients were recruited. Mothers with a singleton pregnancy, and a fetus with a myelomeningocele between T1 and S1 were randomized between prenatal surgery and standard postnatal repair. The fetal repairs were carried out between 19 and 26 weeks gestational age. Baseline characteristics were the same between the two treatment groups; although the lesion level was more severe in the prenatal surgery group.

The children with spina bifida were evaluated at 12 and 30 months. Two primary outcomes were measured: a) the first, at 12 months of age, was a composite of fetal or neonatal death, or the need for placement of a cerebrospinal fluid shunt, and b) was a composite of mental development and motor function. Secondary outcomes included fetal and maternal complications, radiographic features, the time to first shunt placement, locomotion, and developmental progress as measured by several validated instruments.

The data and safety monitoring committee evaluated the results of the study on an ongoing basis. Of the 183 women who underwent randomization, 158 had children who were evaluated at 12 months. The first primary outcome, shunt placement, occurred in 68% of the infants in the prenatal surgery group and in 98% of those in the postnatal surgery group (relative risk, 0.70; 97.7% confidence interval [CI], 0.58 to 0.84; P<0.001). An independent group of neurosurgeons evaluated patients' medical records and imaging studies, and according to pre-determined criteria, determined if the primary outcome was met. Because patients were being followed in their own communities, actual rates of shunt placement were 40% in the prenatal-surgery group and 82% in the postnatal surgery group (relative risk, 0.48; 97.7% CI, 0.36 to 0.64; P<0.001). Of note, the proportion of children who had no evidence of a hindbrain herniation (Chiari II malformation) was higher in the prenatal surgery group (36%) than the postnatal surgery group.

The second primary outcome, a score derived from the Bayley Mental Development Indez and the difference between the functional and anatomical level, was determined in 134 patients whose children had reached 30 months of age. The outcomes in the prenatal surgery group were significantly better (p=0.007) than the postnatal group. There was also an improvement in several secondary outcomes, such as ambulation by 30 months. Parent-reported self-care and mobility was significantly better in the prenatal surgery group. However, prenatal surgery was associated with an increased risk of preterm delivery and uterine dehiscence at delivery.

Prospective, randomized clinical trials are difficult to conduct for surgical procedures. Based on 12 and 30 month outcomes, prenatal repair of myelomeningocele results in better neurologic function than repair deferred until after delivery. This successful conclusion of this study demonstrates the efficacy of prenatal surgery, and supports the hypothesis that at least some of the disability caused by myelomeningocele is reversible.

CHAPTER 60

Surgical Management of Spinal Dysraphism

JAMES B. MITCHELL • DACHLING PANG

The term "spinal dysraphism" describes many different forms of congenital malformations of the neural tube.* Table 60-1 classifies dysraphic malformations according to accepted theories of embryogenesis and conveniently divides most of them into primary and secondary neurulation lesions, plus an additional class of preneurulation malformations whose basic error of embryogenesis probably occurred before primary neurulation. The surgical repair of these malformations varies as widely as their morbid anatomy. The "surgical" classification in Table 60-2 therefore has less to do with embryogenesis, structural characteristics, neurology, or region of involvement within the neuraxis, than with whether the lesion is "open" or "closed" in its external boundary, a factor that strongly influences the timing and urgency of surgery. A transitional class incorporates lesions that may have "limited" exposure to the outside, although their main features are mostly enclosed. Each class consists of malformations that have radically dissimilar features. The difference in surgical techniques necessitates individual description under the appropriate lesion heading.

Open Spinal Dysraphism

An open spinal dysraphism, synonymous with open myelomeningocele or open neural tube defect (ONTD), refers to a cerebrospinal fluid (CSF) filled, membrane-bound sac with an unclosed segment of the neural plate (the neural placode) floating on top. It is the most severe form of spinal neurulation failure.

EMBRYOLOGY AND MORBID ANATOMY

Normal development of the spinal cord begins around postovulatory day (POD) 22 to 23, when the neural groove deepens and the neural folds meet in the dorsal midline to form the *primary neural tube* (eFigs. 60-1 and 60-2).* The dorsal midline fusion of the neural folds proceeds in a "zipper-fashion" both caudally and rostrally beginning near the sixth cervical somite. This phase of development, called *primary neurulation,* ends with the formation of the lower lumbar cord segments opposite somites 30/31 around POD 28. As the primitive streak shortens to almost nothing with elongation of the primary neural tube, the caudal cell mass, a cluster of pluripotent primitive stem cells appearing around POD 27 to 28 (O'Rahilly and Muller's stage 12),[2] begins

forming (among other caudal embryonic tissues) a solid cord of future neural cells called the medullary cord.[2] This connects with the primary neural tube, and then undergoes central vacuolization (cavitation) to form a secondary neural canal. This second phase of development, called *secondary neurulation*, culminates in the conus from somites 30/31 downward. A final process of degeneration involving extensive apoptosis of the coccygeal segments of the medullary cord occurs resulting in the filum terminalis.[3-5]

Most ONTDs contain a *terminal* neural placode with no recognizable neural tube caudal to the flattened neural plate.[6] It appears that in most cases, the complete failure of dorsal folding and fusion of the primary neural plate inhibits secondary neurulation so that no conus is formed and the placode ends abruptly. In some cases, remains of an abnormal secondary medullary cord can be found in the form of a filum-like band attached to the lower margin of the neural placode. The dorsal surface of the terminal placode corresponds to what would have been the ependymal lining of the cord if neurulation had taken place, and its ventral surface corresponds to the outer surface of the "would-be" neural tube. The sensory and motor roots from the neural placode therefore project from its ventral surface only, the more lateral sensory roots issuing from the alar plates and the medial motor roots from the basal plates. The cutaneous ectoderm from each side of the embryo normally destined to fuse in the midline is kept widely apart by the unneurulated placode. The dorsal surface of the placode is therefore either "naked," or covered by an

Table 60-1 Classification of Spinal Dysraphic Malformations According to Theories of Embryogenesis

Primary Neurulation Malformations
Open neural tube defect, terminal and segmental
Spinal cord lipomas (dorsal and transitional)
Limited dorsal myeloschisis (LDM)
Dermal sinus tract (cyst)
Secondary Neurulation Malformation
Caudal agenesis (caudal cell mass abnormalities)
Thickened or fatty filum
Spinal cord lipomas (terminal, chaotic?)
Terminal myelocystocele
Retained medullary cord
Malformation of Gastrulation
Split cord malformations, types I and II

---

*e-Figures are located on Expert Consult.

Table 60-2   Classification of Spinal Dysraphic Malformations According to Surgical Significance

Open Dysraphism
Open neural tube defect with terminal neural placode
Open neural tube defect with segmental neural placode
Closed Dysraphism
Spinal cord lipomas
   Dorsal
   Transitional
   Chaotic
   Terminal
Thickened filum
Split cord malformations, types I and II
Caudal agenesis and associated caudal spinal cord malformations
Terminal myelocystocele
Retained medullary cord
Transitional Forms of Dysraphism
Limited dorsal myeloschisis
Dermal sinus tract (cyst)

epithelial membrane of variable thickness grown in from the surrounding pia-arachnoid layer (eFig. 60-3A). The placode also effectively prevents dorsomedial migration of the mesenchyme, and thus the completion of the posterior neural arch (hence the term spina bifida), dorsal paraspinous muscles, and lumbodorsal fascia.

Because the meninges develop adjacent to the basal surface of the neuroepithelium, only the ventral (basal) surface of the unneurulated placode receives meningeal investment.[7,8] As CSF accumulates between the ventral surface of the placode and underlying leptomeninges, the flat placode is subjected to increasing dorsally directed forces and, lacking dorsal integumentary and myofascial support, is ultimately pushed out dorsally to ride on the dome of the distended cyst (eFig. 60-3B). The remaining dorsal wall of the sac on each side of the placode is composed of leptomeninges that were also ballooned out by the CSF and stretched between the lateral edge of the placode and the margin of abnormal skin. Intact dura lines the ventral portion of the sac, being also prevented from dorsal midline fusion and instead fuses with the margin of the unclosed skin, dorsal musculature, fascia, and periosteum of the incomplete neural arch on both sides of the myelomeningocele sac.[8]

PREPARATION FOR SURGERY

The goals of surgical management of ONTD are (1) preservation of functional neural tissues, (2) reconstruction of the dural tube, (3) securing sound myofascial and skin closure, and (4) minimizing the chances of future retethering of the cord. Most open lesions are closed within 24 hours after birth. If the child is initially unstable, closure may be safely delayed for up to 72 hours without an increase in complications. Performing surgery after that time carries a substantial risk of meningitis, wound abscess,[9,10] and neurologic deterioration.

Preoperative chest and spine films are obtained to exclude obvious cardiac anomalies and a severe kyphosis. A quick neurologic assessment suffices to document the sensorimotor level as well as whether gross hydrocephalus

necessitates simultaneous external ventricular drainage. About 10% of infants with ONTD are born with severe macrocephaly, tense fontanels, and cardiorespiratory instability. The infant should also be checked for pulmonary insufficiency and for coexisting life-threatening anomalies such as renal agenesis and irreparable cardiac defects with ultrasound studies. Lethal chromosomal abnormalities such as trisomy 18 must be verified with an emergency karyotype. Presence of any such untreatable lesions incompatible with a decent quality of life should prompt a realistic discussion with the parents and recommendation of no intervention.

While awaiting surgery, the infant is placed prone, and the placode is protected by a warm, sterile, saline-soaked, nonadherent dressing, reinforced with a plastic wrap to minimize rapid desiccation. An intravenous line is started and antibiotics are given if there is a history of premature rupture of membranes.

SURGICAL TECHNIQUE

Positioning and Sterile Preparation

The operating room must be kept warm to avoid hypothermia. All prep solutions are warmed to body temperature. The infant is intubated in the lateral position or supine with a doughnut-sponge on the back to accommodate the sac. The pelvis is propped up with a horizontal roll to render the lumbar spine hyperlordotic and give maximum relaxation of the skin and soft tissues. The membranous portion of the sac, containing the exposed neural placode, is irrigated profusely with antibiotic-reinforced saline (betadine compounds have been shown to be neurotoxic), and the surrounding skin scrubbed with the usual antiseptic agents.

Opening the Sac

Magnification is used from the very beginning. The sac is entered through the diaphanous leptomeningeal membrane halfway between the margin of healthy skin and the edge of the placode (eFig. 60-4). Neural tissue of the placode is recognizable by its pink, felty surface, transverse wrinkles, and a straight, longitudinal median raphe (Fig. 60-1A) and since the epithelialized membrane itself is relatively avascular, any substantial bleeding from the cut edges signifies breaching of the neural tissue (Fig. 60-1B). Bleeding is controlled with a pair of ultrafine irrigating bipolar cautery forceps. After the initial gush of CSF and collapse of the cyst, the edge of the neural placode is gently flipped up to identify the ventral nerve roots. Several crossing blood vessels may have to be coagulated to free the placode margins. The pearly epithelium must be meticulously trimmed circumferentially from the placode to avoid later occurrence of inclusion dermoid cyst. At the caudal extreme of a terminal placode, the epithelial membrane may remain thin, or one may encounter a band-like thickening probably representing remnant of the medullary cord that must be divided to free the tip. At the rostral extreme of the placode, careful incision of the epithelium–neural tissue junction on both sides exposes the delicate bevel-shaped transition between the neurulated cylindrical spinal cord and the un-neurulated, flat placode (eFig. 60-5). At the apex of the bevel, the central canal of the normal cord can be seen unfurling into the median raphe of the placode, from which CSF sometimes slowly oozes.

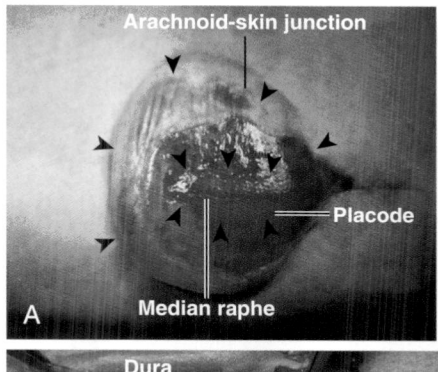
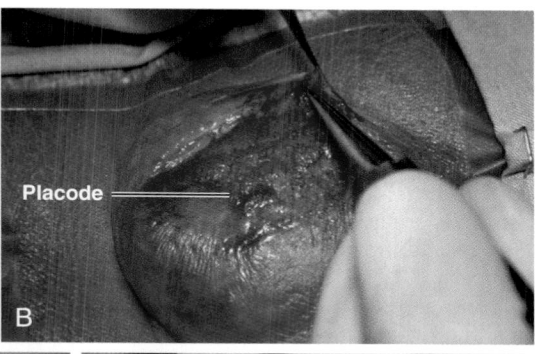
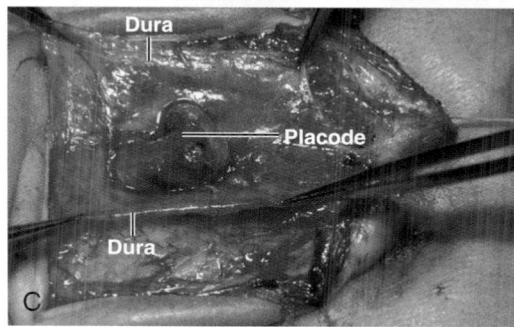
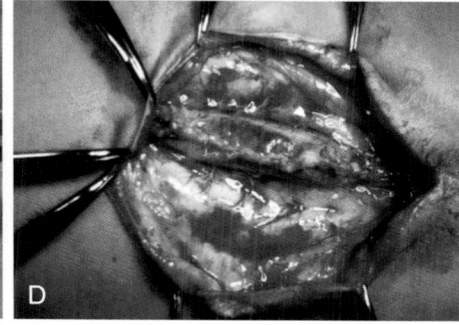

FIGURE 60-1 A, Open myelomeningocele with a terminal neural placode. Note longitudinal median raphe on the neural placode. Small arrowheads outline margin of placode. Glistening leptomeningeal membrane stretches between placode and skin. Large arrowheads outline skin edge. Triangular end of the sac is toward the anus. B, Cutting into the leptomeningeal membrane just outside the margin of the placode. C, Neural placode after dural edges from all sides have been defined and dissected free, ready for dural closure. D, Closed dural tube. Paraspinous muscles and periosteum of bifid neural arch are exposed on each side of the closed dural tube. Anus to the right of picture.

Handling the Neural Placode

The neural placode is always handled gently with jeweler's micro-forceps. If the placode is pliable and thin enough, it is rolled on itself and sewn up with 8-0 nylon sutures through the delicate pial edges (eFig. 60-6). There is no evidence that this improves neurologic function, but it reduces the "sticky" surface from a flat plate to a seam and theoretically lessens the chances of later tethering. If the placode is too thick or too stiff, it should not be forced to roll up for fear of strangulation. Also, tugging too hard on the proximal spinal cord will cause ascension of the neurologic level. In addition, the caudal end of the placode must be checked for the presence of a *neurulated cord* in the rare case of a *segmental* placode (see below).

Paradoxically, small and compact neural placodes are likely functional and therefore should be treated with extreme care, whereas large, thin, and "spread-out" placodes commonly found in middle to high thoracic lesions are usually nonfunctional. It is sometimes advisable to cordectomize these large placodes, for whilst they do not convey volitional movements, the decentralized neuronal pools within them can produce pathologically hyperactive local reflexes underlying high-pressured, spastic bladders and prominent ureteral reflux. Reflux is less prevalent when the bladder is rendered flaccid following elimination of this type of placode.

Dural Closure

The margins of the dural flaps are created by sharply incising the ventral dura from the lumbosacral fascia and periosteum (Fig. 60-1C and eFig 60-7; see also eFig. 60-4A and B), and a new dural tube is reconstructed in the midline (Fig. 60-1D). One aims to obtain as capacious a dural sac as possible commensurate with the size of the placode, the theory being if the placode passively flops freely within a large CSF space, it is less likely to adhere to the dorsal dura. This is almost always achievable with the patient's own dura, even if some of the periosteum overlying the bifid neural arches have to be mobilized with the dura proper to enlarge the sac. In the rare event of insufficient dura, bovine pericardium can be used as a graft because its texture is compatible with newborn dura and because it seldom has suture-hole leakage of CSF. At the end of closure, the suture line is tested with a Valsalva maneuver held at a pressure of 30 to 35 cm of H_2O for 10 seconds.

Skin and Myofascial Closure

The true size of the skin defect is only apparent after completely excising the epithelialized membrane back to full thickness skin. Defects up to 5 or 6 cm diameter can usually be closed primarily after the subcutaneous layer is mobilized a short distance centrifugally, just enough to reduce the tension on the skin edges. The subdermal layer is closed with interrupted absorbable sutures, and the skin with fine nylon sutures. A number of surgical techniques have been developed to minimize suture line tension in large defects. Lateral relaxing incisions with bipedicle flap closure in the midline have been effective,[11] but the relaxing incisions themselves then require skin grafting at the same time or at a later date. Complex multiple rotation skin flaps have also been tried, but this necessitates extensive skin undermining and still does not altogether eliminate all tension spots. For impossibly large defects, I favor using composite skin--muscle (myocutaneous) flaps. There are three advantages to this technique. Cadaver vaso-latex studies show that a rich vascular anastomosis exists in the skin overlying the gluteus maximus and the latissimus dorsi muscles on each side and across the midline; the muscles themselves are supplied by the gluteal and thoracodorsal arteries, respectively. As long as these arterial pedicles are preserved, blood supply to the lumbosacral skin is well maintained when the four muscles are apposed in the midline, even if the short paraspinous arterial perforators deep to the muscle are taken.[12] Secondly, because there is no undermining of the subcutaneous tissues, the skin tension is mostly absorbed by the muscle closure. Finally, this method results in a triple-layered (muscle, subcutaneous tissue, and skin) closure with extra insurance against CSF leak. The flaps survival rate even for enormous defects is greater than 92% with this technique, and the blood loss and extra anesthetic time are quite acceptable.[12]

It is important to avoid large wound seroma or hematoma, which increases skin tension and prevents flap adherence to the underlying tissue from which revascularization for the flap must be derived. If the flaps are large and "wet," a small drain without negative suction may be left in for 24 hours. Suction drains may perpetuate a CSF fistula and are best avoided.

POSTOPERATIVE MANAGEMENT

The immediate postoperative concern is wound healing. The wound should be kept moist with a generous spread of bacitracin ointment and covered with a light nonsticking dressing (e.g., Telfa), fashioned so that it can be easily lifted up for inspection several times daily. The infant is nursed prone at all times for the first 7 to 10 days, and the hips should be hyperextended by a horizontal roll under the anterior iliac crests to allow maximum relaxation of the back skin. Even though temporary hypothermia may be problematic, a heat lamp is forbidden because direct radiated heat on the wound may induce relative ischemia to the flaps from hypermetabolism.

Hydrocephalus normally does not pose a problem until at least 5 to 7 days after closure of the sac, which hitherto acted as a pressure reservoir. It is preferable to await insertion of a CSF shunt until the back wound shows initial healing without signs of breakdown, CSF leak, or infection. On the other hand, high CSF pressure may cause a leak, and often precipitates early signs of brain stem compression due to the Chiari malformation. If there is any question with the integrity of the wound and more time is needed, the ventricles can be decompressed by serial ventricular taps.

An indwelling bladder catheter is usually left in for as long as the infant is prone. Intermittent catheterization is difficult in this position. Male infants are recommended to have circumcision before hospital discharge for ease of clean catheterization by the parents at home. The infant can usually be nursed in the lateral and supine positions after 5 to 7 days, depending on the strength of the skin closure, and at this time urodynamics and renal ultrasound scan are performed to assess intravesicular pressure, bladder capacity, and ureteral reflux. Clean intermittent catheterization (CIC) is recommended if the leak point pressure on cystometry is over 20 cm H_2O, or if there is demonstrable reflux.

Early Complications (First Postoperative Week)

The operative mortality for children undergoing repair of an ONTD should be close to 0.[13-15] The most common cause of postoperative death is related to hindbrain dysfunction (73%),[10,16] but this seldom occurs acutely in the first week of life. Most of the immediate complications pertain to the wound itself.

Wound Dehiscence

A study of the nutritional status of newborn infants who have had myelomeningocele surgery using body weight, nitrogen balance, serum protein, and total lymphocyte count as parameters, showed that these neonates undergo an initial period of severe catabolic changes that do not readjust themselves for as long as 1 month after surgery. This nonspecific catabolic response is caused by rises in circulating levels of ACTH, cortisol, thyroxin, growth hormone, and antidiuretic hormone, stimulated by the extreme stress of surgery, general anesthesia, and blood transfusion.[8] During this period, the resistance to infection is lowered, and all anabolic processes, including wound healing, are temporarily slowed. This metabolically unstable time also coincides with feeding difficulties caused by hydrocephalus, postoperative ileus, neurogenic dysphagia (due to brainstem compression), and prematurity. It is no surprise that wound dehiscence is the single most common complication during the first postoperative week.[8]

Local factors, mostly avoidable, also contribute to this problem. A large sac means higher wound tension and precarious blood supply. An untreated kyphus adds stretching to the suture line and aggravates the local ischemia. Any additional external pressure caused by a tight dressing or improper patient positioning also interferes with healing.

It is common to see erythema along an 8- to 10-mm strip on either side of the suture line, particularly in areas of high tension. Sometimes the skin flaps may even look deep red to dusky as a result of venous stasis. These color changes often pass after a few days. When there is necrosis, the intensely dark red skin edges will turn black, but the necrosis may be limited to the epidermis, and the dermis and subdermis may survive, which should make adequate coverage. If full-thickness necrosis occurs, the blackness extends farther laterally. The junction between dead and viable skin demarcates, and the surrounding skin becomes erythematous and edematous. The sloughing skin edge also begins to pull away from the sutures, and serous exudate from subjacent fat necrosis seeps from the exposed subcutaneous tissues. Demarcation and sloughing are usually complete by the 7th or 10th day.

Sloughing of only the epidermis in small areas requires only simple dressing changes because the wound eventually epithelializes over the underlying dermal and subdermal layers. Skin grafting is unnecessary. If the skin necrosis is full thickness but there is healthy muscle underneath, the wound edges should be carefully debrided back to bleeding skin. It may then be dressed for second intention healing from below, but this will take some time and delay CSF shunting. A faster way would be partial-thickness skin grafting, which should take well over a well vascularized bed. If full thickness necrosis exposes the dural tube, some measure of immediate coverage must be instituted to prevent desiccation and meningitis. This usually means a more radical and extensive flap rotation or even pediculated full thickness skin flap grafting.[17]

Finally, parenteral or enteral hyperalimentation should be set up to ensure adequate nutrition.

Wound Infection

Considering how badly the exposed neural placode is contaminated during and shortly after birth, it is surprising how rarely wound (extradural) infections occur after closure of an ONTD. The wound infection rate is about 1.5% to 2.5%, which is only moderately higher than *clean* neurosurgical procedures.[8] However, if one counts the intradural infections, the infection rate rises to 7% to 10% even for early closure.[15,18]

The initial period of obligatory catabolism in these infants lowers both their cellular and humoral defenses. In as much as the infant must depend on transplacentally acquired maternal antibodies during the first 3 months of life, and IgA does not cross the placenta well, infections from enteric bacteria are particularly common. Chief among local predisposing factors to infection is a large sac with redundant, folded membranes. It is virtually impossible to sterilize all the creases and folds of the wobbly sac and the placode is therefore recontaminated during surgery. During closure, the contaminated placode is put inside a closed intradural space, which explains why intradural infection is more common than extradural infection.

Systemic signs of sepsis due to gram-negative meningitis are usually present 1 to 3 days after closure. In neonates, these early signs tend to be nonspecific, such as poor feeding, lethargy, or an ashen complexion. It is more common to see hypothermia than pyrexia, and the systemic white blood cell count often drops below 4000/mm.[3] If the dural sac is well invested with a myocutaneous coverage, an intradural abscess may eventually form without any external signs. It is important to obtain CSF for culture from a ventricular tap if there is clinical suspicion of sepsis, for the long-term prognosis of gram-negative ventriculitis in the newborn depends almost solely on the promptness of diagnosis and treatment.

If the infection is confined to the extradural space, the wound will become red and fluctuant on day 5 to 7. The surrounding skin will also appear edematous but, unlike CSF infection, there is often no systemic signs of sepsis and the infant may continue to feed and move normally. A red, fluctuant wound should be diagnostically aspirated for purulent material. An abscessed wound must be opened immediately, widely debrided, irrigated with antibiotic solution, and reclosed over suction drains. Associated vascular occlusion and myonecrosis may require refashioning of a new myocutaneous closure. Depending on whether the CSF indices indicate intradural infection, the dura may have to be opened to rule out an intradural abscess. The patient is then put on broad spectrum, CSF-penetrating antibiotics.

Cerebrospinal Fluid Leak

The dura nearest its lateral margin may be severely attenuated in large myelomeningocele defects. This plus the often tense and precarious myocutaneous closure makes large lesions particularly prone to leak CSF. Also, the timing of the slowly climbing CSF pressure happens to coincide with weakening of the tenuous suture line, around the 5th to 8th postoperative day. A small amount of transdural CSF leak probably occurs through the suture holes in most cases, considering the thinness of the newborn dura. The appearance of slight fluctuance under the skin flaps during the first few postoperative days is likely due to a combination of CSF and blood. As long as the skin closure holds, and there is no *outward* leak of CSF, there is no risk of infection. This small amount of seepage is self limiting. A large transdural leak causes a tense subcutaneous accumulation that will eventually threaten the viability of the suture line. When CSF actually breaks through the skin barrier, the risk for gram-negative infection rapidly rises, and treatment must be promptly initiated.

A shunt is effective in *preventing* CSF leak but is not recommended *after* the leak has sprung, especially if the leak has already breached the skin closure. Even a low pressure shunt maintains a constant lumbar CSF pressure of 5 to 6 cm H_2O, still considerably higher than that in the subcutaneous pocket, which is near atmospheric. The preferential passage of CSF is still out through the back wound and not through the shunt. If a CSF leak persists in the presence of a shunt, the latter becomes infected sooner or later. The external ventricular drain (EVD) is a much better means of decompression after a substantial leak has already existed. The drainage chamber can be lowered to subzero pressure to siphon CSF away from the back wound. With elimination of outward leak, the probability of infection is mitigated. The skin edges can now be oversewn, and the infant may have to be sedated to minimize the milking action of muscles overlying the thecal sac. Many leaks can be successfully managed by such measures without a reoperation. If the leak persists post-EVD, the wound needs to be explored to close the dural defect.

ONTD WITH SEGMENTAL PLACODE

The term segmental placode describes a portion of open neural plate bounded both rostrally and caudally by perfectly neurulated spinal cord (eFig. 60-8). It is found in approximately 4% of all open neural tube defects. The exact mechanism of its genesis is unknown, but somehow it must involve a "square-pulse" type teratogenic insult to the process of primary neurulation; that is, normal neurulation resumes post facto to an isolated failure of neural plate fusion, both in space and time. Or, it could be a manifestation of "collision site" failure from two adjacent neurulation sites proceeding in opposite directions, although no proof of the multisite closure hypothesis yet exists.[19] The most common site for the segmental placode seems to be midthoracic to thoracolumbar. It is unclear why the teratogenic insult in these cases, unlike in terminal placodes, does not disrupt secondary neurulation, and allows for normal closure of the posterior neuropore and formation of the conus.

It is important to recognize the placode as segmental *before* surgical closure because the surgeon should be mentally prepared to handle the distal end of the placode delicately. One reliable clinical clue is the preservation of distal lower extremity movements while the open defect is located high up in the thoracic region. A preoperative MR should be obtained, not only to visualize the distal spinal cord beyond the placode, but to spot other associated paradysraphic malformations such as a split cord malformation (SCM),[20,21] a lipoma,[22] or a thickened filum. It is even possible the segmental placode represents a hemimyelomeningocele in that the other hemicord of the SCM is fully neurulated and stays uninvolved in the open defect itself.[23,24]

The technique of closure of the segmental placode is the same as for the terminal one. Every bit of neural tissue must be preserved during trimming of the extraneural membrane, and every effort should be made to reconstruct the tube (eFig. 60-9). The critical decision is whether to deal with the other associated malformation at the same time or at a later date. I recommend the latter since one wants to inflict as little stress to the newborn infant as possible and the immediate goals of infection prevention and neural conservation have been met by the mere closure of the open sac. The definitive procedure of "complete" untethering usually involves more extensive bone and soft tissue dissection, and should be left till 2 to 3 months later when the infant can better withstand a longer anesthesia and larger blood loss, when hydrocephalus is no longer an issue, and after thorough neuroimaging studies have been obtained.

ONTD AND KYPHECTOMY

A prominent kyphus is almost exclusively found with large, thoracic myelomeningoceles when the neurologic deficits are profound and at a high level. Presumably, the lack of lumbosacral paraspinous muscle action allows overpull by the thoracic cord, that is, innervated anterior abdominal and intercostal muscles, which causes dorsal buckling of the thoracolumbar spine and secondary wedging of the vertebral bodies at the apex of the kyphosis. A sharp and prominent kyphus exerts enormous tension on the skin flaps and compromises their vascularity. Resection of a bad kyphus not only rids this perpendicular tension but also in effect shortens the spine and helps in relaxing the surrounding soft tissues. However, kyphectomy should only be attempted if there is no other way to achieve adequate soft tissue closure. When kyphectomy is unavoidable at the time of sac closure, it should be approached with painstaking regard to details because the procedure is fraught with potential mishaps.

Before kyphectomy, the thin, nonfunctional placode is resected, and the dural tube is sewn up as a blind stump rostral to the designated upper cut of the kyphectomy. The vertebral bodies intended for resection are now cleared of its surrounding musculotendinous attachment with careful subperiosteal dissection using the monopolar cautery. Considerable bleeding from the epidural veins may be expected because their thin walls are adherent to the relatively unyielding posterior longitudinal ligament, which prevents the veins from collapsing with the bipolar cautery. The monopolar cautery needle must stay close to bone, particularly while separating the ventral muscles off the bodies. The inferior vena cava, aorta, iliac arteries, and kidneys are all retroperitoneal structures that could be injured by the heat of the cautery or by injudicious action of the periosteal elevator.

The apex of the kyphus is resected through the intervertebral discs with the monopolar cautery. The extent of resection must take into account the feasibility of apposing the remaining ends of the spine to fill the gap. The two ends of the stump are then cleared of cartilaginous endplates, and brought together using two parallel wires forced through the bony part of the vertebral bodies with sharp cutting needles. A certain amount of downward pressure must be exerted on the bodies during the apposition and twisting of the wires. During twisting of the wires, the fusion surfaces and the wire loops are subjected to tremendous distracting and persistent dorsal-pointing stresses. The wires should never pass through any cartilaginous part of the body or the intervertebral disc. The infant is immediately immobilized in a fitted thermoplastic body brace for a minimum of 3 months and up to 2 years. Nonunion is a serious problem because discarding one or two crumbled and defunct vertebral bodies essentially means widening the gap even more and an even greater stress for the new construct.[8,25]

Spinal Cord Lipomas

We advocate strongly for total resection of spinal cord lipomas and radical reconstruction of the neural placode over partial resection because aggressive surgery, contrary to traditional view, is safe and gives far better long-term progression-free survival.[26] The rationale for total lipoma resection is based on three hypotheses: (1) the high rate of symptomatic recurrence after partial resection is due to retethering; (2) retethering is promoted by three factors: a tight content-container relationship between spinal cord and dural sac, a large "sticky" raw surface of residual fat, and incomplete detachment of the terminal neural placode from residual lipoma; and (3) total resection can eliminate the factors conducive to retethering and thus reduces the probability of symptomatic recurrence.

The object of surgery is therefore to create conditions that will minimize retethering. The first condition relates to the fact that the normal spinal cord exhibits intradural motions to gravity and postural changes on ultrasonography and dynamic imaging.[27,28] Reducing the content-container ratio and amplifying the degree of freedom of the cord within the dural sac must lessen resticking by limiting sustained contact between cord and dura, this sustained contact being intuitively a necessary condition preceding the formation of fibrous adhesions. To do this, the cord bulk must be drastically reduced. For large rambling "virgin" lipomas, this means resection of all or most of the fat down to the thin, supple neural placode. For redo lipomas, the hard, grasping cicatrix must also be removed. The aim is to render the thinnest, most pliant neural placode possible that can be atraumatically neurulated without distortion or strangulation to form a slender, round tube. The raw, sticky lipoma bed is simultaneously concealed within the tube and the sac is enlarged by a capacious dural graft. Finally, total resection also enhances the chances of terminal untethering.

ANATOMY AND CLASSIFICATION

In the literature, the nomenclature of spinal cord lipoma is imprecise and inconsistent. Here, we are defining the types of lipomas as follows, based loosely on Chapman's original classification.[29]

Dorsal Lipoma

The lipoma–cord interface is entirely on the dorsal surface of the lumbar spinal cord, sparing the distal conus (Fig. 60-2A). The junctional demarcation between lipoma, cord, and pia, the *fusion line*, can always be traced neatly along a roughly oval track, separating fat from the dorsal root entry zone (DREZ) and dorsal nerve roots laterally (Fig. 60-2B and eFig 60-10). The lipoma therefore never

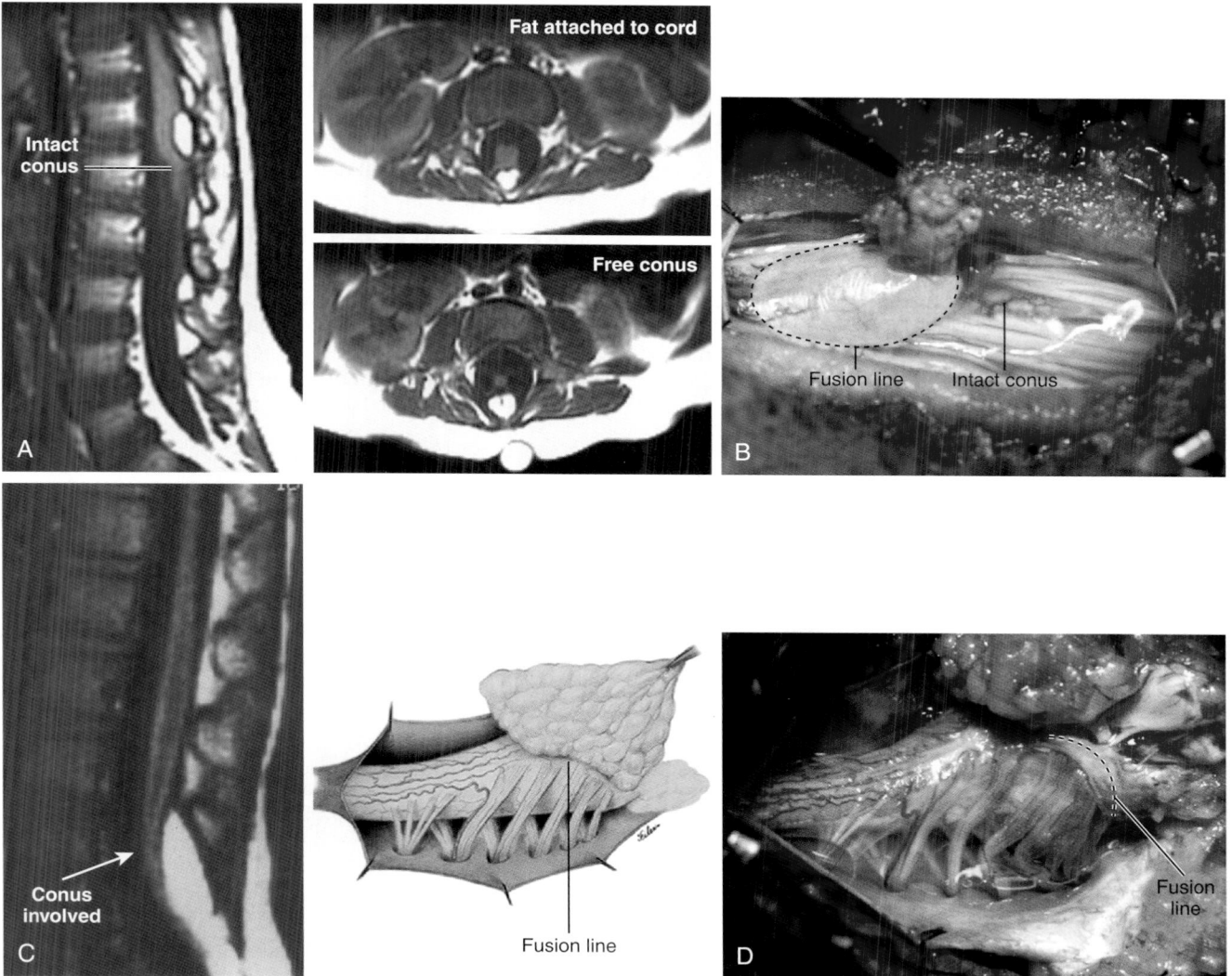

FIGURE 60-2 A, Dorsal lipoma on MRI. Sagittal image shows intact conus caudal to lipoma stalk. Axial images: upper shows site of lipoma attachment to cord; lower shows free conus just caudal to the level of lipoma attachment. B, Intraoperative picture shows neat oval fusion line around lipoma–cord interface on a horizontal plane. Note intact conus and caudal sacral roots. C, Transitional lipoma. *Left:* Sagittal MRI shows lipoma begins dorsally but involves entire conus. Ventral side of neural placode is free of fat. *Right:* Plane of the fusion line begins dorsally and then cuts obliquely toward the tip of the conus. The array of DREZ and dorsal roots is also forced to slant dorsoventrally. D, Transitional lipoma. Intraoperative picture showing massive lipoma but very distinct dorsoventral fusion line separating fat from the DREZ and dorsal roots, which always lie lateral and ventral to the fusion line. The ventral side of placode is always free of fat in a regular transitional lipoma. DREZ, dorsal root entry zone.

contains nerve roots. The lipomatous stalk runs through an equally discrete dorsal dural defect to blend with extradural fat. The uninvolved conus often ends in a thickened filum terminale.

Transitional Lipoma

The rostral portion of this type is identical to that of a dorsal lipoma, with a discrete fusion line and easily identifiable DREZ and dorsal roots. Unlike the dorsal type, however, which always spares the conus, the transitional lipoma then plunges caudally to involve the conus as the plane of the fusion line cuts ventrally and obliquely towards the tip of the conus likened to making a slanting, beveled cut on a stick (Fig. 60-2C). The lipoma–cord interface thus created may be undulating and tilted so that the neural placode is rotated to one side or even spun into a parasagittal edge-on orientation, but the neural tissue is always ventral to it and

the DREZ and the nerve roots are predictably localizable lateral and ventral to the fusion line and therefore do not course through the fat (Fig. 60-2D). There may or may not be a discrete filum. The dorsal dural defect extends to the caudal end of the thecal sac and may be much larger on the biased side.

Terminal Lipoma

Unlike the dorsal and transitional types, terminal lipomas insert into the caudal extremity of the conus without blending with the spinal cord or its root entry zones. All the sacral roots unmistakably leave the conus rostral to the lipoma, and in most cases the conus itself looks normal. The dural sac and the dorsal myofascial coverings are intact. The lipoma either replaces the filum entirely, or is separated from the conus tip by a short, thickened filum (Fig. 60-3A and B).

Chaotic Lipoma

This previously undescribed type is so named because it does not "follow the rules" of either the dorsal, transitional, or terminal lipoma. It begins dorsally in an orderly fashion as in a dorsal or transitional lipoma, but its caudal portion is *ventral* to the neural placode and does engulf neural tissue and nerve roots (eFig. 60-11). The fusion line may be distinct rostrally but quickly becomes blurred distally, and the location of the DREZ and nerve roots is less predictable. The moniker "chaotic" depicts the sometimes confusing blend of the ventral fat and neural placode, and the often impossible task of separating fat from neural tissue at surgery (Fig. 60-3C). Chaotic lipomas are uncommon but are characteristically seen with sacral agenesis.

The literature[30,31] describes one other lipoma type, the lipomyelomeningocele, in which part of the distal conus extends into the extraspinal compartment, dragging with it a small collar of dural sac (Fig. 60-3D). The basic structure is either that of a transitional or a dorsal lipoma. Accordingly, we choose to classify this type as either a transitional or dorsal lipoma with a descriptive qualifier of "extraspinal extension."

SURGICALLY RELEVANT EMBRYOLOGY

Embryogenesis of Dorsal and Transitional Lipomas

In the embryo, a progressive disparity exists between the spinal cord and vertebral column as a result of the faster growth rate of the latter.[32-35] The caudal end of the cord ascends gradually from opposite the coccyx in the 30-mm human embryo to the L_1–L_2 level at birth.[34-37] Proper ascent

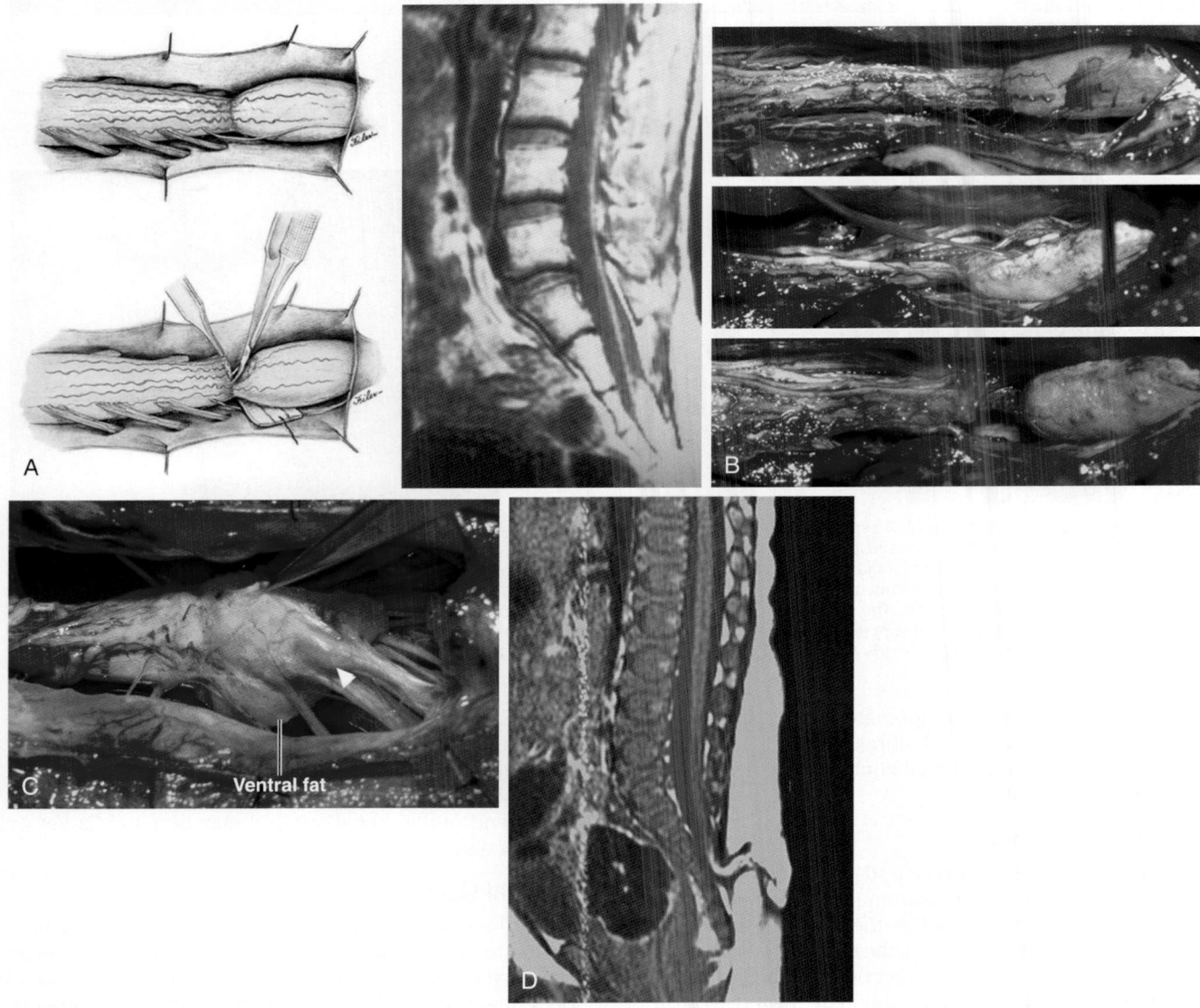

FIGURE 60-3 A, Terminal lipoma. Drawings showing insertion of fat directly on the end of the conus, which is itself intact. Resection plane is right through a clear transition plane. Typical MR appearance is shown at right. B, Intraoperative pictures for terminal lipoma. Top shows the typical terminal lipoma. Middle shows separation of "hitch-hiker" nerve roots from lipoma. Lower shows conus after transaction through separation plane. C, Choatic lipoma. Intraoperative picture showing fat ventral to placode and on one of the sacral roots (*arrow*). Note absence of discrete fusion line. D, Lipomyelomeningocele with the lipoma stalk, cerebrospinal fluid sac, and part of the conus extending out of the spinal canal through a dorsal defect.

of the cord requires a well-formed neural tube and a smooth pia-arachnoid covering. If during early development a dorsal defect exists in the dura (duraschisis) and neural tube (myeloschisis), mesodermal elements from the surrounding mesenchyme will enter the dural sac and form attachment with the sliding neural tube in the form of a fibro-fatty stalk, resulting in its entrapment. This theory features a fundamental defect in neural tube closure during primary neurulation (secondary neurulation does not involve dorsal neural fold closure), and thus applies only to the dorsal and transitional lipomas (see below). It is compatible with the observation that these two types of lipomas are always associated with neural arch defects.

The embryologic error leading to the mesodermal invasion of the neural tube probably lies in *premature disjunction* between the cutaneous and neural ectoderms[38-40]; that is, the separation of one from the other occurs *before* the converging neural folds fuse with each other. This allows the paraxial mesenchyme to roll over the still gaping neural folds and enter the central canal. Once contact between mesenchyme and ependymal neuroectoderm is made, further closure of the neural tube is permanently prevented and a segmental dorsal myeloschisis is created (eFig. 60-12A and B). Alternatively, the fault may lie in a delay in neural folds fusion secondary to an insufficiency of the paraxial mesoderm in impelling their dorsal convergence,[41-47] so that ectodermal disjunction again precedes neural folds fusion. Lastly, faulty fusion of the neural folds due to metabolic disturbance of the cell membrane-bound glycosaminoglycans, which are vital to cell–cell recognition and adhesion,[48-51] could likewise reverse the temporal relationship between disjunction and neural folds fusion.

Experimental studies show that the pluripotent mesenchyme forms derivatives according to the inductive properties of the adjacent neuroectoderm (eFig. 60-12C).[6,9] The ependymal side of the neural tube induces mesenchyme to form fat, muscles, collagen, and occasionally bone and cartilage, whereas the outer surface of the neural tube induces the formation of meninges.[52] However, no dura can now form over the dorsal opened portion of the neural tube, and the dural defect neatly surrounds the evolving lipomatous stalk, which tethers the neural tube to the subcutaneous adiposity. In like manner, deficiencies in the overlying myofascial layers (from myotomal mesoderm) and neural arches (from scleromesoderm) also neatly surround the lipomatous stalk (eFig. 60-12D).

Within the neural tube, the intramedullary fat and muscles fuse with the developing alar and basal plates. Since the dorsal root ganglions develop from neural crest cells at the outer aspect of the neural fold lateral to the site of failed fusion, the dorsal nerve roots grow outward ventrolateral to, *but never traverse*, the lipomatous stalk. The DREZ must correspondingly lie very near, *but always lateral to*, the exact junctional boundary between lipoma and spinal cord. This boundary, called *fusion line*, is of tremendous surgical significance[22,53,54] (eFig. 60-12D). Meanwhile, the cutaneous ectoderm, long detached from the neuroectoderm, heals over in the dorsal midline to form wholesome skin over the subcutaneous lipoma.

The genesis of a dorsal lipoma perfectly exemplifies mistimed disjunction during *primary* neurulation. Its fibro-fatty stalk always involves cord segments above the conus,

which mainly forms from secondary neurulation. Furthermore, failure of primary neural tube closure appears to be *segmental*, normal closure takes place "business-as-usual" immediately following the abnormal event. This "square pulse" nature is illustrated by the fact that the sharp fusion line between fat, spinal cord, and pia-arachnoid can be neatly traced circumferentially around the lipomatous stalk[53-55] (see Fig. 60-2B and eFig. 60-10). Dorsal lipomas therefore result from a segmental closure abnormality *involving only primary neurulation*. They are found in less than 15% of spinal cord lipomas in our series.[22,26]

In transitional lipoma, the myeloschisis involves much more than an isolated segment of the primary neural tube. Even though its rostral part resembles the dorsal lipoma, the involvement of the whole of the caudal spinal cord means that not only primary but also secondary neurulation have been profoundly disturbed by the mesodermal invasion. This is supported by the observations that in many transitional lipomas the filum is incorporated into the distal fat, and within the lipomas are often spaces resembling the vacuoles within the secondary neural tube. Also, while the rostral part of the transitional lipoma is always dorsal and aptly reflects premature disjunction of primary neurulation, the distal part sometimes involves both the dorsal and ventral aspects of the conus, a situation compatible with misguided mesenchymal inclusion during the much less orderly events of secondary neurulation. Intramedullary mesenchyme may migrate within the neural tube after invasion and travel caudally across the boundary from the primary to the secondary neural canal, since the two neural canals are in continuity.[56] In fact, the hypothesis that the rostral part of the transitional lipoma arises from aberrant primary neurulation (involving only the dorsal cord) and the caudal lipoma arises from abnormal condensation of the secondary neural cord (affecting more ventral aspects of the conus) furnishes at least one explanation for the dorsoventral obliquity of the lipoma–cord interface.

Embryogenesis of Chaotic Lipomas

Chaotic lipomas do not quite fit into either the dorsal or transitional schema. They often do not have a distinct dorsal part with the symmetry of a dorsal lipoma, and the lipoma–cord interface is irregular and ill-defined, with fat running through the neural placode to the ventral side in large and unruly measures. Even in the context of the less orderly transitional lipoma, the interplay between lipoma and cord in this type of lesion seems to be in constant chaos.

This degree of anatomic unpredictability in chaotic lipoma and its strong association with caudal agenesis (82% in our series[22]) suggest that the embryogenetic error occurs during the early stage of secondary neurulation as part of the general failure of the caudal cell mass (eFig. 60-13).[57,58] Secondary neurulation comprises three distinct stages: (1) condensation of neural material from the caudal cell mass to form the solid medullary cord, (2) intrachordal cavitation of the medullary cord[56,58,59] and its integration with the primary neural tube, and (3) partial degeneration of the cavitary medullary cord through massive apoptosis to result in the thin filum terminale.[34,56] It is possible that formation of the chaotic lipoma involves the entanglement of lipogenic mesenchymal stem cells with cells from the caudal cell mass during aberrant condensation of the medullary cord, forming an inseparable mixture of neural tissue and fat, with nerve roots projecting out haphazardly.[22]

Embryogenesis of Terminal Lipoma

Terminal lipomas result from abnormal *secondary* rather than primary neurulation, as evidenced by the unexcepted rule that the lumbar and upper sacral cord segments, products of primary neurulation, are never affected in a terminal lipoma. Furthermore, dorsal myeloschisis and duraschisis, both hallmarks of failed (primary) neural fold fusion, are never seen. Lastly, the terminal lipoma either replaces or forms part of a thickened filum, which temporally places the pathogenetic process at secondary neurulation. The fact that the distal conus in terminal lipomas always remains fat-free argues against an abnormal condensation phase during early secondary neurulation. On the other hand, the terminal lipoma often contains (disorganized) spinal cord elements and ependymal tubules,[60,61] which suggests rather an incomplete or ineffective degeneration phase at late secondary neurulation.

INTRAOPERATIVE ELECTROPHYSICOLOGIC MONITORING

Intraoperative monitoring has become *sine qua non* in lipoma surgery.[22,62,63] Electromyography (EMG) is routinely used to accurately identify the motor roots and to detect functional spinal cord within ambiguous tissues. The muscles commonly employed are sartorius (L_1), rectus femoris (L_2, L_3), anterior tibialis (L_4, L_5), extensor hallucis longus (L_5), gastrocnemius (S_1), and abductor hallucis (S_2). Half-inch long, 25- to 27-gauge–needle recording electrodes and input gains of 50 to 80 microvolts are selected to enable maximum capturing of far-field evoked action potentials of the indexed muscle without undue artifacts. Smaller needle electrodes are inserted directly through the anal verge to record activities of the external anal sphincter (S_2-S_4). All stimulations and recordings in our cases are done with the Cadwell Cascade Intraoperative Monitoring System (Cadwell Laboratories, Kennewick, WA) using the Cascade Software Version 2.0.

For nerve root and direct spinal cord stimulation, we use a concentric coaxial bipolar microprobe (Kartush Concentric Bipolar, Medtronic Xomed, www.xomed.com) (Fig. 60-4) capable of generating extremely focused and confined current spread at its 1.75-mm tip, and is thus best suited in precise localization of small functioning neuron-axonal units. Larger double-pronged bipolar electrodes, or worse, monopolar electrode, which in essence converts the spinal cord into a giant volume conductor, are undesirable because they cause unwanted recruitment of adjacent depolarizable tissues. Stimulating currents from 0.5 to 3.0 milliamperes are used depending on target impedance. The stimulation frequency is usually set at 10 per second. This allows spontaneous random firing due to nerve irritation from surgical manipulation to be distinguishable from the rhythmic evoked contractions.

For monitoring L_4 to S_1 spinal cord conduction we use standard somatosensory evoked potentials (SSEP) with stimulating needle electrodes placed near the posterior tibial nerve behind the medial malleolus and near the common peroneal nerve over the fibular neck. Pudendal SSEP for monitoring S_2-S_4 cord segments can be used with

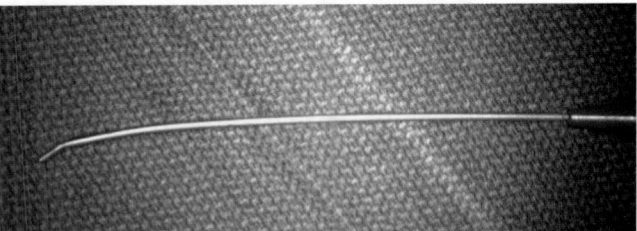
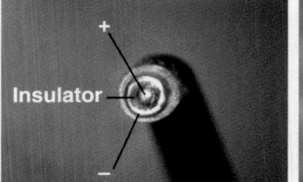
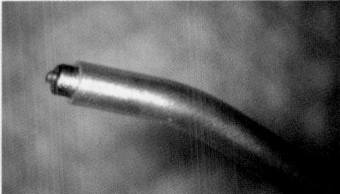

FIGURE 60-4 Concentric coaxial bipolar microprobe stimulator, in which the concentric cathode and anode are separated by a coaxial insulator. Tip diameter is approximately 1.75 mm.

disc electrodes affixed to the dorsum of the penis or on the periclitoral skin, but the evoked cortical tracings in infants tend to be disorganized, unstable, and extremely susceptible to inhalation anesthetics, which considerably limits the value of pudendal SSEP in children younger than 1 year.

SURGICAL TECHNIQUE OF TOTAL/NEAR-TOTAL RESECTION

Step 1. Exposure

The skin and soft tissue incision should go straight through the subcutaneous lipoma if one is present. Removing this will leave behind a large subdermal space into which CSF could collect under tension and consequently hinder wound healing. Frequently a discrete fatty stalk connects the subcutaneous with the intraspinal lipoma through a defect in the lumbodorsal fascia. This stalk is continuous with the spinal cord and should not be tugged on during fascial dissection.

The upper extent of the bony exposure should include one level above the rostral end of the lipoma. This reveals for proper orientation the "last" normal set of nerve roots and DREZ before starting lipoma resection. Wide laminectomy is essential to afford full access to the lateral edges of the dural sac (see below). Visualization of the normal dura rostral to any lipoma gives a depth perspective as to how far out neural tissue and CSF sac might have extruded beyond the plane of the dura. The heavy bulk of extradural fat could then be safely lopped off to give room for intradural dissection and lighten the tug on the conus.

Step 2. Detachment of Lipoma from Dura

The dura rostral to the lipoma is opened in the midline. For dorsal lipoma, the dural incision is carried circumferentially around the discrete lipoma stalk and then down the middle again to expose the conus (eFig. 60-10). For transitional lipoma, the dura is cut close to the lipoma edge on each side as far caudal as possible, though the two side incisions seldom could meet distally. The dural edges are then tautly and widely retracted with sutures. This is a crucial maneuver because full lateral exposure of the intradural span, made possible by the generous bone removal, reveals the "crotch" where the far lateral fringe of the lipoma attaches to the inner surface of the dura (see Fig. 60-6A).

Next, the *fusion line* is identified where pia, spinal cord, and lipoma join in a continuous furrowed border that travels from rostral to caudal outlining the entire attachment of the lipoma stalk to the cord. In a dorsal lipoma, the fusion line forms a neat *complete* oval or circle from side to side, usually upon a leveled horizontal plane, often bilaterally symmetrical, and always sparing the conus below (Fig. 60-2B and eFig 60-10). In a transitional lipoma, the rostral fusion line starts distinctly enough but then edges ventrally towards the tip of the conus and tends to wander laterally and asymmetrically, often becomes sheltered by the overhanging fat, and never meets its mate from the other side at the caudal end (see Fig. 60-2C and D).

True to the events of embryogenesis, the DREZ and dorsal roots are always lateral to the fusion line, and at the rostral end of the fatty stalk of both lipoma types, this orderly arrangement can be depended upon on both sides, thus presenting a convenient place to start the dissection. In most transitional lipomas, however, the more caudal nerve roots are quickly covered from view by the overflowing fat which tends to fuse with the dura at a far lateral point (Fig. 60-5A). Hence the term "crotch dissection," which depicts the key step of grasping the overhanging fat and pulling it medially under tension against the tagged dural edge, then sharply separating the fat-dura attachment with dissecting scissors (Fig. 60-5B and eFig. 60-14). It is absolutely requisite to lean the round curve of the scissors firmly against the inner lining of the dura while cutting this attachment to avoid blindly injuring the nerve roots, which project from the cord slightly medial to the "crotch" and lie just deep to the fat. The hidden roots should spring into view wherever the detached fat is pulled back, and can be gently coaxed away from the dura by blunt dissection toward the exit foramina (Fig. 60-6B). At the same time, the free CSF space ventral to the dorsal roots, and the fat-free, pia-covered ventral surface of the neural placode, hitherto hidden by the overhang, now "pop" into view (Fig. 60-6C).

It is clear from this description that in each successive axial slice, all lipomas big or small, dorsal or transitional, are roughly divided by a transverse line joining the points of the far lateral fat-dura attachment on each side, where the lipoma–cord assembly is in effect suspended like a hammock against two lateral hinges over an uncluttered ventral CSF pool. Dorsal to this transverse line is the visible but disorderly, massive, and unrevealing fat and ventral to this line is the orderly fusion line, DREZ, dorsal nerve roots, neural placode, and ventral CSF space but all initially rendered invisible to the surgeon by the overhanging fat (Fig. 60-5A). The purpose of the "crotch dissection" is therefore to release this suspension so that the hammock of neural placode and nerve roots can be folded inward enough to be identified and preserved during the next phase of lipoma resection (Fig. 60-5B).

This laborious but indispensable step of "crotch dissection" is carried all the way caudally (Fig. 60-6C) until all the "useful" nerve roots are identified and the entire neural placode, with a profusion of lipoma still attached, is completely unsuspended from the dura and has literally "fallen" to the basin of the dural trough (Fig. 60-6D).

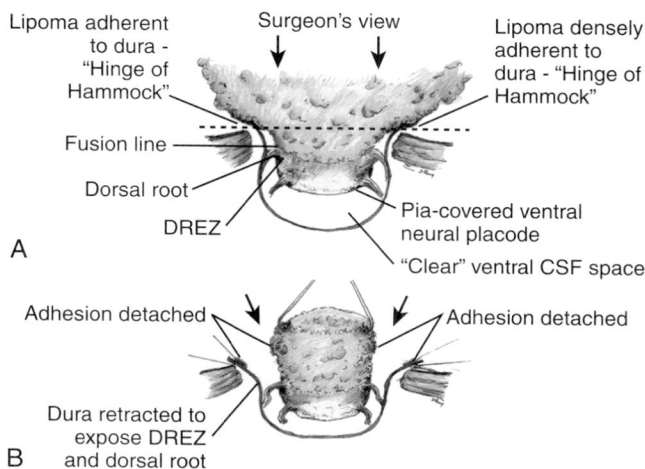

FIGURE 60-5 Drawing depicting relationship among lipoma, neural placode, nerve roots, and dural sac in an axial slice. A, The lipoma–cord assembly is suspended at the dural edge at far lateral adhesion points like a hammock against side hinges. The dotted transverse line that joins the two side hinges divides the assembly into a dorsal disorderly fibro-fatty half that completely blocks the surgeon's view to a much more orderly ventral half containing the important anatomic landmarks of fusion line, dorsal root entry zone, dorsal roots, fat-free ventral placode, and pristine, ventral cerebrospinal fluid space. B, After detaching the far lateral adhesion points (the hinges) by careful "crotch dissection," and folding-in the fatty mass, the ventral anatomic landmarks can now be visualized.

Step 3. Lipoma Resection

Resection of the lipoma begins at the rostral end where the anatomic relationships between fat, DREZ, and nerve roots are clearly decipherable (Fig. 60-7 and eFig. 60-15). Sharp dissection with microscissors is used to locate a thin but distinct silvery *white plane* between fat and cord at the demi-lune of the rostral fusion line (Fig. 60-8A). It takes some determination, for the initiate, to cut into this traditionally forbidden place, seemingly straight into the spinal cord right at the fusion line, but with experience, this white plane can be found in every case. We strongly discourage using the CO_2 laser because it chars the surface (no more white plane!) and negates the tactile feedback through the microscissors on which the surgeon depends to differentiate between cutting through the grittiness of fibrous fat and the formless softness of spinal cord. Bleeding on the white plane can be handled with the ultra-fine irrigating bipolar cautery (0.2-mm tips) and a very low current setting. The cold irrigation mitigates against sticking but more importantly it dissipates heat rapidly from the cord. Minimal cauterization is used on the DREZ to avoid postoperative dysesthesia.

As long as all the activities are rendered medial to the fusion line, thus also medial to the DREZ and nerve roots, dissection along the white plane can be conducted safely all the way to the end with no damage to the cord or nerve roots (eFigs. 60-16 and 60-17). In a dorsal lipoma, this is a simple feat because the white plane is basically horizontal and flat, the two banks are symmetrical, and the caudal end well defined rostral to the conus so that a completely circumscribed attack on the fat is possible from multiple angles (eFig. 60-18). In a large transitional lipoma, navigating the white plane is more difficult because it always

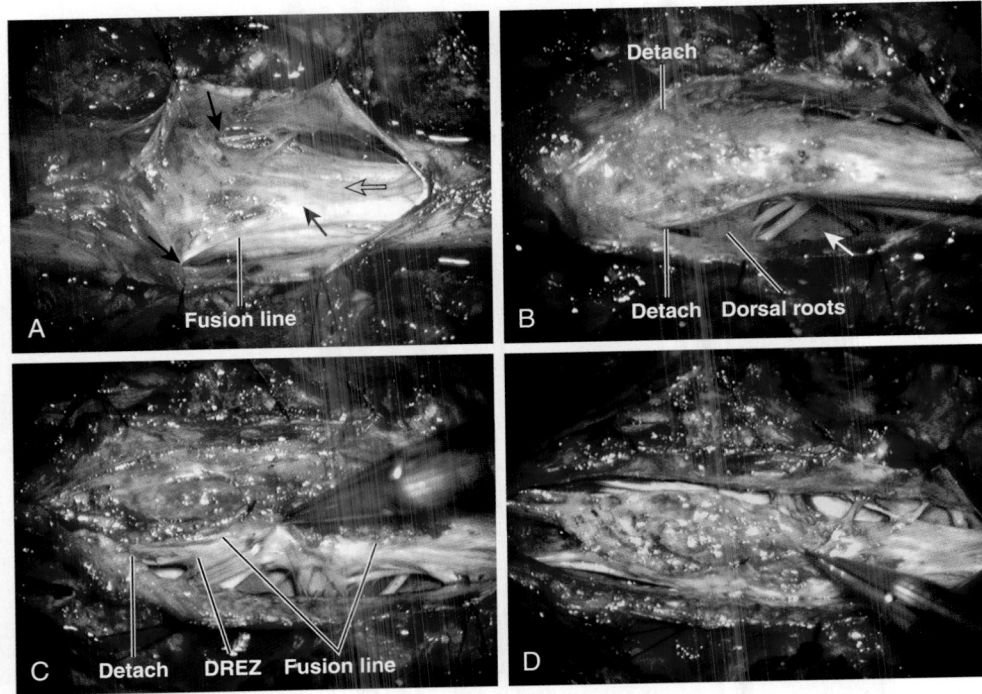

FIGURE 60-6 Transitional lipoma. A, Exposure of the rostral lipoma, showing the normal cord to the right and the swath of yellow fat indicating beginning of the lipoma (*small arrow*). The *large arrows* locate the far lateral adhesion points (the "crotches") between the flanges of the lipoma and the inner dura. The rostral starting point of the fusion line is also indicated (*open arrow*). B, Exposure of the pristine ventral CSF space (*arrow*), nerve roots, and fat-free ventral side of the neural placode. C, Exposure of all relevant anatomy vital to the next stage of the actual resection of the lipoma: the fusion line, dorsal root entry zone, dorsal roots, ventral side of placode and free CSF space, in dorsal-ventral order. D, Complete bilateral detachment of the adherent hinges and terminal untethering; the neural placode now "sinks" into the basin of the dural trough. CSF, cerebrospinal fluid.

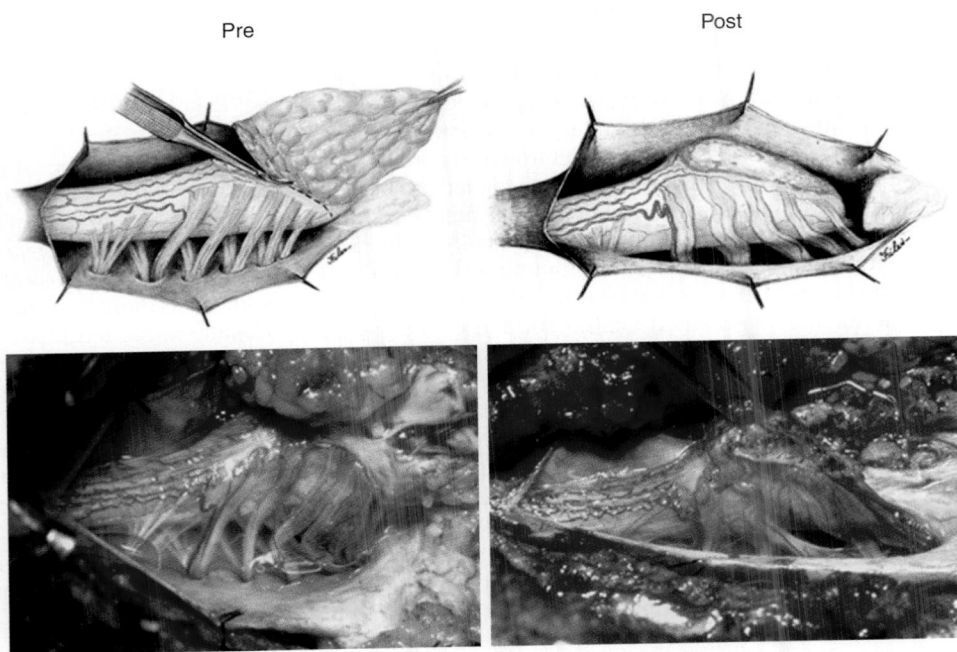

FIGURE 60-7 Basic technique for transitional lipoma resection: resection on an asymmetrical and oblique fusion line along an occasionally undulating lipoma–cord interface plane, showing pre- and post-operative pictures.

slopes ventrally, often undulates, and one side may be tilted so steeply that the corresponding DREZ and nerve roots are shifted ventrally and the placode so rotated that its ventral surface now faces the side. Such a white plane is almost turned vertically "on edge," its orientation confusing unless one remembers the transverse line concept dividing one "clean" ventral hemisphere from the "messy" dorsal one.

The white plane sometimes seems never-ending in large transitional lipomas and the caudal thecal sac is thronged with fat admixed with suspicious strands. This is when systematic stimulation and identification of the ventral nerve roots become invaluable in localizing the termination of the *functional* spinal cord. As soon as two to three pairs of sphincter-activating sacral roots are identified, any tissue distal to the last pair can be considered nonessential and be cleanly cut across to consummate the final liberation of the placode (eFig. 60-19). A good chunk of the now isolated distal fatty stump should be excised to prevent reconnection with the terminal placode.

In chaotic lipomas, electrophysiologic determination of the functional extent of the neural placode may be the only

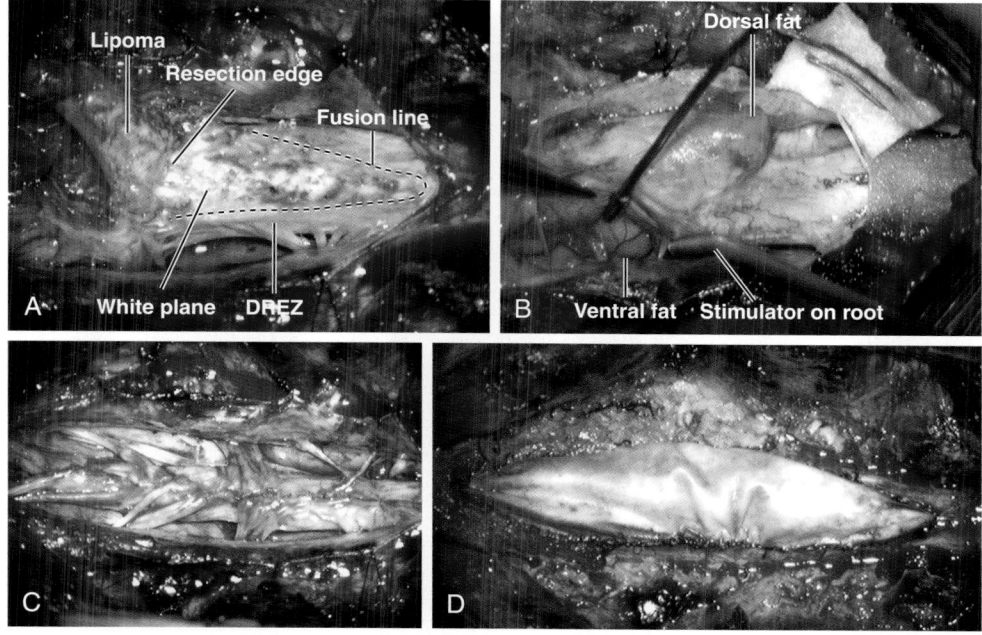

FIGURE 60-8 A, Transitional lipoma. The "white plane" of thin glistening fibrous netting separating fat from spinal cord, bounded always by the fusion line. Note detached rostral portion of the lipoma lifted away from the white plane to show the resection edge. B, Chaotic lipoma. Note ventral pia-covered fat medial to ventral nerve roots (being stimulated by concentric microprobe), and dorsal fat perched on the dorsal side of the placode. C, Transitional lipoma. Completed neurulation. D, Completed expansile graft duraplasty with bovine pericardium.

way to achieve final untethering; the caudal fat-cord-fibrous jumble can only be sorted out functionally and not anatomically by direct stimulation of the placode and the projecting nerve roots. The handling of the white plane on the dorsal side of a chaotic lipoma is the same as with the other lipoma types, but the billows of fat on the ventral side of the placode should be left alone and its smooth pial surface left unviolated (Fig. 60-8B and eFig. 60-20). It is always the dorsal and never the ventral part (unless iatrogenically invaded) of the lipoma that actually tethers the spinal cord.[22]

Step 4. Neurulation of the Neural Placode

Total resection of the dorsal fat and thorough unhinging of the placode convert a bulky, transfixed lipoma–cord complex into a free-floating, thin, supple, purely neural plate (eFig. 60-17), eminently suitable for pia-to-pia, midline, dorsal closure with interrupted 8-0 nylon sutures without strain or strangulation to the neural tissue (eFig. 60-21). It is helpful to leave a narrow cuff of pia along the cut edges of the white plane to accommodate the sutures, which are tied with inverted knots. Neurulation thus transforms a broad, wafery, sticky sheet into a trim, sturdy, pia-covered tube bearing a single seam, evocative of the natural neurulation process (Fig. 60-8C).

Step 5. Expansile Graft Duraplasty

The argument for a graft dural closure comes from the belief that if the neurulated placode could slosh about in ample CSF within a capacious sac, the likelihood of reattachment to the dura would be diminished. Thus we prefer a slightly full-bodied yet texturally compatible (to infant dura) material such as bovine pericardium that can maintain its shape, to a filmy-soft graft such as autologous fascia lata that may swell and ebb with respiration and body movements and thus collapse on the cord. The bovine graft is carefully measured and shaped to prevent inward folds. Running prolene sutures are used to achieve watertight closure, confirmed with Valsalva maneuvers (Fig. 60-8D).

TECHNICAL POINTS

Our data show that total or near-total resection of spinal cord lipomas can be done in more than 90% of cases[22] (Fig. 60-9A). In most instances, the small amount of residual fat is adherent to the DREZ and had been invaginated out of mischief during neurulation (Fig. 60-9B). In the 8% of patients with unusually large amount of residual fat, the fat belongs to the ventral component of a chaotic lipoma and has been intentionally left pia-covered and therefore harmless.

To assess the "looseness" or degree of freedom of the reconstructed placode within the newly formed dural sac, we created the cord–sac ratio, defined as the ratio of the diameter of the cord to the diameter of the sac on the postoperative axial MRI at the bulkiest portion of the reconstructed segment. The ratios are grouped into low, less than 30%, in the loosest sacs; medium, between 30% and 50%, in moderately loose sacs; and high, greater than 50%, in the tightest sacs (Fig. 60-9C). In the total group of 238 patients, 162 (68%) had low cord–sac ratios, 61 (25.6%) had medium ratios, and only 15 (6.3%) had high ratios.[22]

The size of the lipoma is not an important determinant of the completeness of resection. Much more relevant is the configuration of the lipoma–cord interface, which contains the "white plane." The white plane is a filmy netting of relatively compact collagen fibers. It may be extremely contorted and asymmetrical in some transitional lesions, and there is no better way than boldly cutting into the tongue of the rostral lipoma to find the glistening fibers beneath the first few globules of yellow fat. Once the plane is located, one can follow it with sharp dissection by feeling the grittiness through the microscissors and by spotting the glistening white stripes between yellow fat and pink spinal cord. With large dorsolateral transitional lipomas, the placode may be twisted 90 degrees and the lipoma–cord interface can look almost vertical. Access to the DREZ of the ventral (down) side can be awkward unless the "hammock" is first unhinged, and the placode is swung back to a more

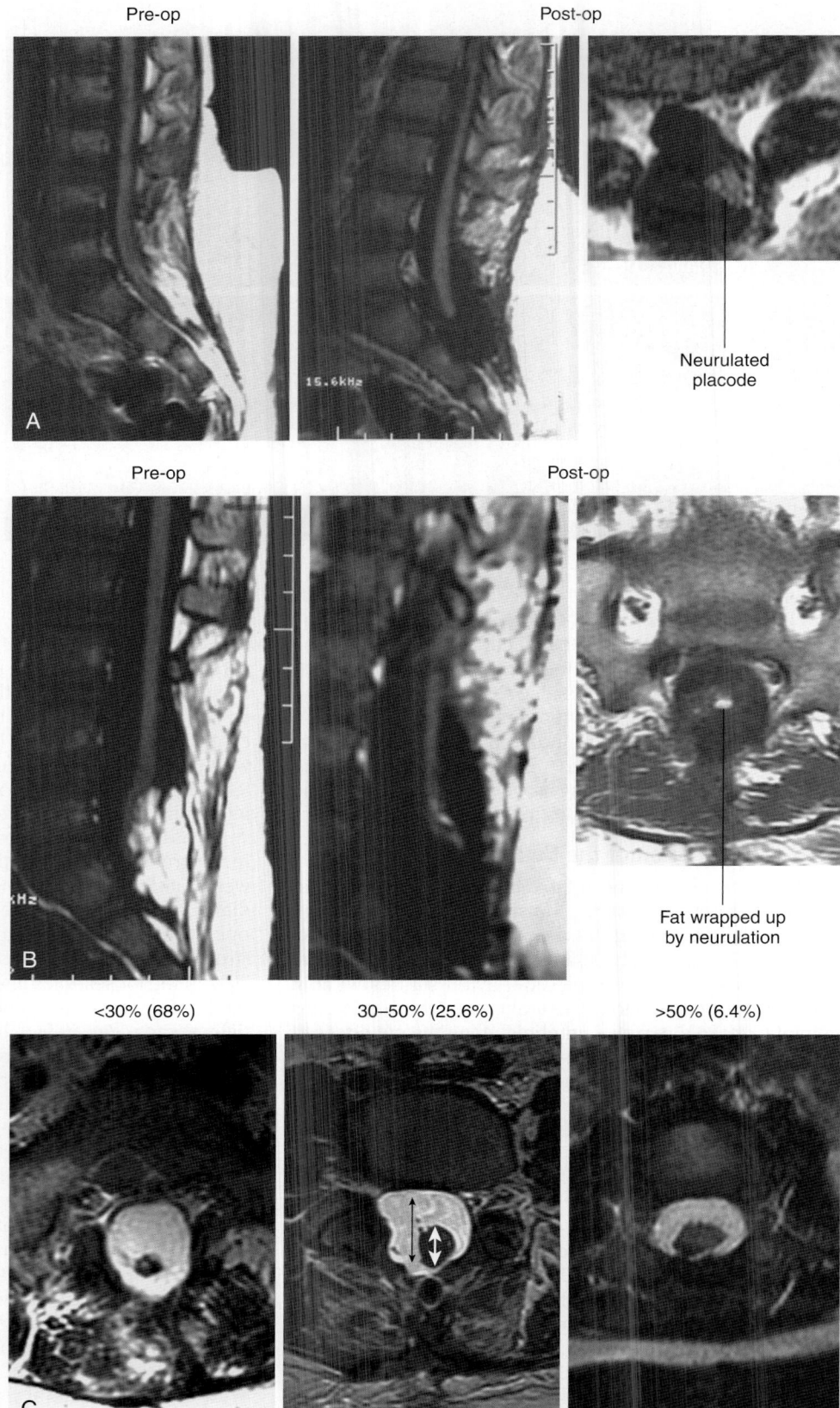

FIGURE 60-9 A, Preoperative and postoperative MRI of a case of transitional lipoma with no residual fat after total lipoma resection. Note neurulated oblong-shaped, fat-free, neural placode within a large dural sac. B, Preoperative and postoperative MRI of a case of complex transitional lipoma with a very small amount (<20 mm³) of residual fat after resection. Axial image shows the small round piece of fat is wrapped up within the roundly neurulated neural placode and therefore not exposed on the surface. C, Cord–sac ratios in the postoperative axial MRI after total/near-total resection of lipoma. This ratio is obtained by dividing the sagittal diameter of the most bulbous portion of the postneurulated neural placode by the sagittal diameter of the dural sac. Sixty-eight percent in our series have very loose sacs with cord–sac ratios <30%; 25.6% have intermediate ratios 30% to 50%; and 6.4% have ratios greater than 50% with the least commodious cord–sac relationship. Cord–sac ratio estimates the degree of freedom of motion of the postneurulated spinal cord within its container sac.

horizontal position. On the more involved side, festoons of overhanging fat may obscure the emergent dorsal roots to give the false impression that they *course through* and not underneath the lipoma. In fact, this overhang can be readily teased and lifted off the "knee-turn" of the dorsal rootlets to allow these to be traced under the verandah of fat into the true DREZ, at which site the white plane can once again be picked up. In general, a sinuous and severely rotated white plane makes it more likely to leave behind residual fat.

Redo lesions are associated with a higher rate of residual fat and a higher cord–sac ratio. When the fat layer is infiltrated by heavy cicatrix from previous surgery, the cementing hold to the surrounding dura is much more tenacious and harder to detach, and the bright yellow of "virgin" fat is lost to a gray dense concretion much harder to distinguish from the white plane. The dissection often stops short of the white plane for fear of cutting too deep, and the result is a stiffer slab of residual scar-studded fat that not only augments the bulk of the placode, but also makes it awkward to fold at neurulation. The presence of this unyielding fat-scar at the DREZ often leads to "gouging," which may well be the cause of postoperative dysesthetic pain in redo patients.[26]

Incomplete terminal untethering of the placode predictably ends in recurrence of symptoms.[64-66] We ascribe two explanations for the surgeon's hesitation to commit the final disconnecting cut. With very large transitional lipomas, the distal neural placode is buried in fat, and unless visualization is improved by substantial removal of fat, safe untethering cannot be done. Also, nerve twigs are sometimes seen issuing in pairs from the distal placode, making it seem impossible to complete the detachment without sacrificing functional cord. This assumption is spurious, for as long as two or three anal sphincter-activating roots, presumably S_2 to S_4, are identified and preserved, there should be no loss of function if the terminal cut is made just *caudal* to these roots. The small nerve twigs within the discarded stump that did not stimulate are probably coccygeal roots and therefore vestigial in human and have no essential function.[22,26,29]

Thus, thorough lipoma and scar resection and terminal untethering impart the optimal bulk, texture, and maneuverability to the neural placode for tensionless neurulation. A low postoperative cord–sac ratio has been shown to be the single most important factor in securing a long progression-free survival (PFS) in lipoma surgery.[26]

Finally, our experience unequivocally shows that chaotic lipomas are the most treacherous lesions. They can be recognized in the preoperative MRI by the presence of ventral fat medial to the ventral nerve roots and by their association with sacral agenesis (eFig. 60-13). Compared to other lipoma types, chaotic lipomas are more likely to show conspicuous residual fat and high cord–sac ratio on the postoperative MRI.[22,26] The strategy for chaotic lesion is knowing just when to stop excavating deeper after the dorsal portion of the lipoma has been removed to enable neurulation. If the ventral fat is judged not amenable to total excision and neurulation, then its pial surface that had hitherto laid freely against the adjacent ventral dura should be left unsullied to avoid creating new adhesions (eFig. 60-20).

COMPLICATIONS

Our combined neurologic-urologic deterioration rate following total/near-total resection is 4.2%, which compares favorably with rates in the literature ranging from 0.6% to 10%[30,31,66-80] and averaging 3% to 7%, associated with partial resection using more conservative techniques. Only 1.7% of patients had new weakness and approximately 4% had neuropathic pain, which, we suspect, is due to close encounters of the DREZ and dorsal roots with heat from the electrocautery. Most minor bleeding on the cord can be stopped with gentle tamponade and Gelfoam, and if electrocoagulation has to be applied, only the ultrafine microtipped irrigating bipolar cautery is used with very low current intensity.

The CSF leak rate (0.8%) and wound complication (1.3%) with total resection are much lower than almost all of the published series (of partial resection), which record CSF leak rates from 2% to 47%,[31,66,69,70,74-76,78,80] and wound dehiscence and infection rates of 2% to 26%.[31,66,70,73,74,76,78,80] Good results are owed to the following technical stipulations: (1) Enough bony exposure must be done caudally so that a cuff of healthy dura *past* the lowest extent of the lipoma can be made available for graft anastomosis. The graft should never be sewn to the web of fat at the remaining lipoma stump. (2) Absolute water-tight closure of the graft with Prolene must be achieved, and challenged by Valsalva maneuvers. (3) Synthetic or organic tissue glues are used if there is even a suggestion of a leak. (4) In large sacral lesions, there are often gaping muscle and fascial defects that cannot be primarily approximated. In these cases, paramedian relaxing incisions can be used on the flanking lumbodorsal fascia to facilitate sliding midline closure of the myofascial edges. (5) The large subcutaneous lipoma is never removed at the time of intraspinal surgery. The creation of this immense dead space will encourage collection of CSF which may turn into an enlarging pseudomeningocele and ultimately threaten skin flap viability.

RESULTS OF TOTAL RESECTION

When the outcome of total lipoma resection is analyzed against preoperative symptoms, the best result is seen with pain. Most of the sharp, dysesthetic leg and perineal pain will significantly diminish within 3 months, but not necessarily low back pain that is likely mechanical in origin.[81,82] Children also become more active and playful, and virtually never have chronic back complaints. Sensorimotor deficits also respond favorably with surgery. Although less than 20% of patients have actual normalization of motor function, the majority will substantially improve.[22,26] As with other forms of tethered cord, the milder and more recent deficits have better chance for good recovery. Bladder dysfunction responds favorably in about 20% to 30% of patients.[22] The subtype of neuropathic bladder with the best prognosis is the small capacity, spastic bladder with uninhibited detrusor contraction. Atonic bladders seldom improve with surgery, and intermittent catheterization usually needs to be continued indefinitely. The response of detrusor-sphincter dyssynergia to surgery is unpredictable. It is mandatory that cystometry and voiding cystourethrogram be repeated 3 to 6 months after surgery to determine what other urologic procedures such as bladder augmentation or ureteral conduits may be necessary to prevent reflux and frequent infections. Surgery has been known to arrest the rapid worsening of existing scoliosis in tethered cord. However, severe scoliosis still requires surgical realignment and fixation with instrumentation and fusion.

The immediate benefits of total lipoma resection are due to the abrupt cessation of spinal cord tethering and are thus comparable to those from partial resection.[22] However, the long-term benefits of total resection become very obvious if progression-free survival (PFS) of the two techniques are calculated for periods of 15 to 16 years. The total resection PFS for all lipoma types and clinical subgroups is 84% versus 34% for partial resection.[26] When the select group of young children without symptoms or prior lipoma surgery is considered, the PFSs for total versus partial resection are 98.9% and 43%, respectively.[26] Considering conservative management of lipoma without surgery carries a PFS of only 60%,[83] these robust statistics argue strongly for total resection, not only for symptomatic patients but also as prophylactic treatment for all comers.[26]

Terminal Lipoma

There is no controversy surrounding the technique of resecting terminal lipomas, and the surgical result is essentially that of filum surgery. The terminal lipoma inserts directly into the caudal extremity of the conus. The junction between lipoma and conus is usually readily identifiable by the yellow color of the fat, the sparse vasculature compared to the conus, and the lack of nerve roots exit. Roots may become adherent to the ventral surface of the lipoma. It is important to identify and preserve "hitch hiker" roots arising from the conus but become adherent to the pia over the lipoma (see Fig. 60-3B). The conus–lipoma junction is then cut across transversely.

Split Cord Malformations

EMBRYOGENESIS, MORBID ANATOMY, AND CLASSIFICATION

All double spinal cord malformations probably arise from a common embryogenetic error during gastrulation: a failure of prospective notochordal cells to achieve midline integration following their ingress through Hensen's node, allowing the simultaneously lengthening ectoderm and endoderm to form an adhesion across this central fenestration in the notochord[20,24,32,84] (eFig. 60-22). The subsequent incorporation of pluripotent mesenchyme into this adhesion constitutes the endomesenchymal tract, which not only permanently bisects the notochord but also forces each overlying hemineural plate to neurulate against its own heminotochord in a severely compromised manner. The basic malformation, therefore, consists of two heminotochords and two hemineural plates separated by a midline tract containing ectoderm, mesenchyme, and endoderm (eFig. 60-23). Further evolution of this basic form into the full-grown malformation depends on four factors: (1) the ability of the heminotochords and hemicords to achieve midline healing, (2) the interaction between each heminotochord and hemineural plate during neurulation, (3) persistence of the endomesenchymal tract, and (4) the developmental fates of the three germ elements.

Variable healing of the notochord results in the spectrum of associated vertebral anomalies ranging from bifid vertebral body (butterfly vertebra), to a widened body with a midline tract, to plain widened body. Partial healing of the hemineural plates results in the so-called cleft cord, a single cord with double central canals and a deeply indented midsection. Abnormal neurulation of the hemineural plate, hinged to the cutaneous ectoderm only on one side and receiving mechanical and inductive influence from only one (lateral) set of paraxial mesoderm, results in a misshapen hemicord with unpredictable internal cytoarchitecture varying from four healthy gray horns to a single rudimentary gray column. Complete inability of one or both hemineural plates to neurulate, perhaps due to an untenable relationship with the heminotochord(s) on whose sonic hedgehog protein neurulation depends, results in an associated hemimyelocele or "complete" myelomeningocele, respectively. Persistence of the dorsal (ectodermal) portion of the endomesenchymal tract causes a patent dermal sinus tract to maintain continuity with the midline septum; the tract sometimes encysts to form a dermoid between the hemicords. Persistence of the ventral (endodermal) portion of the mesenchymal tract and its connection with the embryonic gut explains the associations of split spinal cords with intestinal diverticulum and malrotation. Finally, and in some respects most importantly, the developmental fates of the germ elements within the midline endomesenchymal tract determine the state of the meningeal investment of the hemicords, the nature of the mature septum, the presence of ganglion cells and nerve roots bridging between a hemicord and the septum, the tethering of the hemicords to the dorsal dura by fibroneurovascular bands (myelomeningocele manqué), and the rare occurrence of an enterogenous (neurenteric) cyst in the midline cleft.

Classification of split cord malformations (SCM) into the well-known types I and II lesions depends on activities of specialized mesodermal cells destined to form dura and neural arch. These meninx primitive cells are normally found in the region between the notochord and neural tube around postovulation days 27 to 29 (eFigs. 60-2 and 60-23D), slightly later than the formation of the endomesenchymal tract. If they become incorporated into the endomesenchymal tract, a median dural layer forms next to the medial aspect of the hemicord and joins the dura that normally grows around the lateral aspect of the hemicord to complete a separate dural tube for each hemicord. Additionally, in accordance with their sclerogenic function, the meninx primitiva cells within the endomesenchymal tract facing away from the hemicords also form a midline bone spur between the two median dural walls, continuous with the bone of the developing vertebral centrum. This configuration, designated type I SCM, therefore consists of two hemicords each contained within its own dural tube, separated by a dura-sheathed rigid osseocartilaginous median septum (Fig. 60-1A). Inasmuch as the endomesenchymal tract frequently reaches the neural arches, the median bone spur bisects the spinal canal into two separate compartments. The spinal cord is transfixed solidly to the spinal canal by the bony and dural septum. The sclerogenic effect of the meninx primitiva cells when these admix with cells of the developing neural arches accounts for the often massively hypertrophic fusion of several adjacent laminae at the level of a type I SCM (Fig. 60-10A, lower right).

In contrast, the endomesenchymal tract in a type II SCM does not recruit meninx primitiva cells. A thin fibrous septum, texturally different from dura, will form from the "ordinary" mesenchyme in the space between the hemicords. Here also, no arachnoid, bone, or cartilage will form. Both hemicords will lie within a single arachnoid and dural tube inside a noncompartmentalized spinal canal, separated by a fibrous rather than a rigid osseocartilaginous median septum (Fig. 60-10B). However, this fibrous septum is always adherent to the medial aspect of the hemicords, and by virtue of its firm peripheral attachment to the ventral and/or dorsal dural wall, it is as real a tethering lesion as the bone spur of a type I SCM (Fig. 60-10B, lower right).

What causes some endomesenchymal tracts to entrap meninx cells while other tracts exclude them is unclear. Since gastrulation and therefore formation of the endomesenchymal tract occur round POD 18 to 22 in a rostrocaudal direction, an early tract would have completed its development long before the appearance of the meninx cells, whereas a later tract might be more likely to ensnare meninx cells during its evolution. This is consistent with the fact that the "earlier" cervical and high thoracic SCMs are almost exclusively type II SCMs whilst type I SCMs are mostly located in the lower thoracic and lumbar regions.

The determining features of this classification do not overlap between the two types; there is never a type I SCM with dual dural sacs that does not have a rigid midline bone or cartilage within the median dural cleft, nor is there ever a type II SCM with a single dural sac but a naked piece of bone or cartilage unlined by dura. Typing is thus easily made with preoperative MRI, an important step because the surgical techniques are different for the two types of SCM. The other commonly associated features of SCM such as paramedian nerve roots, myelomeningocele manqué, dermoids, dermal sinus tracts, centromedian blood vessels, thickened filums, and intestinal anomalies occur in both types of SCM in relatively similar frequencies.

SURGICAL INDICATION

There is no doubt both types of SCM are tethering lesions. As with all other tethering lesions, the mere presence of a SCM in a child is sufficient indication for surgical release of the cord because neurologic deterioration is very common in these children, and because lost function is seldom reclaimable when treatment is rendered late. In both types of SCM, the operation aims at removing the median septum and all other associated bands, dermoids, lipomas, or enterogenous cysts that might be attaching or otherwise anchoring the hemicords to the surrounding dura. Unlike the obvious bony-dural septum in a type I lesion, the thin fibrous septum in a type II SCM may not show up on preoperative neuroimaging studies. This should not deter an exploration because in every case of type II SCM the author has explored, a taut fibrous septum or fibroneural bands had been found to tether the hemicords. In addition, most SCMs located in the low thoracic or lumbosacral region have at least one associated lesion tethering the tip of the conus, which must also be removed during the same procedure.

In contrast to children with SCM, the evidence to support prophylactic surgery in asymptomatic adults with SCM is much less convincing, and most adults have been operated on for symptoms and/or progressive deficits. However, it is known that neurologic deterioration can be precipitous after a fall or strenuous exercise. I, therefore, recommend operating on asymptomatic adults who are otherwise healthy and lead a physically vigorous life, but managing conservatively those who are old or infirm, or have a sedentary lifestyle.

PREOPERATIVE NEUROIMAGING STUDIES

Magnetic resonance imaging (MRI) is an excellent screening test but will miss the details of structures within the median cleft. Computed tomographic myelography (CTM) with iohexol is more sensitive than MRI for displaying fine soft tissue bands and associated myelomeningocele manqué, and it also shows the bony anatomy (such as the neural arches) to great advantage. It is superior to MRI in providing important information for precise localization of the septum and for delineating the size, obliquity, and relationships of a type I median septum. CTM is recommended if there is remaining ambiguity after MRI.

OPERATIVE TECHNIQUE

Because the relationship between septum and hemicords is so drastically different between type I and type II SCMs, the surgical techniques for the two lesions are also very different.

Type I SCM

Planning the skin incision requires knowledge of the exact vertebral level of the median septum. A linear midline skin incision is made to span at least two laminar levels above and two below the septum. In a type I SCM, the bony septum is always extradural, being completely surrounded and excluded from CSF by the medial walls of the double dural tubes which form a complete sleeve for the bone in the sagittal midline. The septum itself is frequently fused with, and thus hidden under, the neural arches so that it is not immediately visible at exposure. Noting the adjacent bony anatomy on the preoperative scan such as a bifid or eccentric spinous process, exostoses, and abnormal fusion is helpful in localizing the level. Another useful hint is that the septum is often located where the spinal canal is widest, or where the neural arches and spinous processes are hypertrophic and fused with adjacent laminae.

The extent of the laminectomy should include at least one level rostral and one caudal to the septum-bearing laminae. The hypertrophic laminae are rongeured away piecemeal around the attachment of the septum until only a small island of lamina is left attached to the dorsal end of the septum (Fig. 60-11A, upper). This affords a circumferential view of the bone spur still within its dural sleeve so that its dural attachment can be safely dissected off the bone deep within the cleft. However, once the dorsal support of the septum (by the laminae) is eliminated, the septum is no longer held rigidly at both ends and could be pushed from side to side depending on how solidly it is anchored ventrally. Excessive lateral movement of the septum thus may injure the subjacent hemicords and must be avoided. A Woodson dental elevator with a thin, angulated, sharp

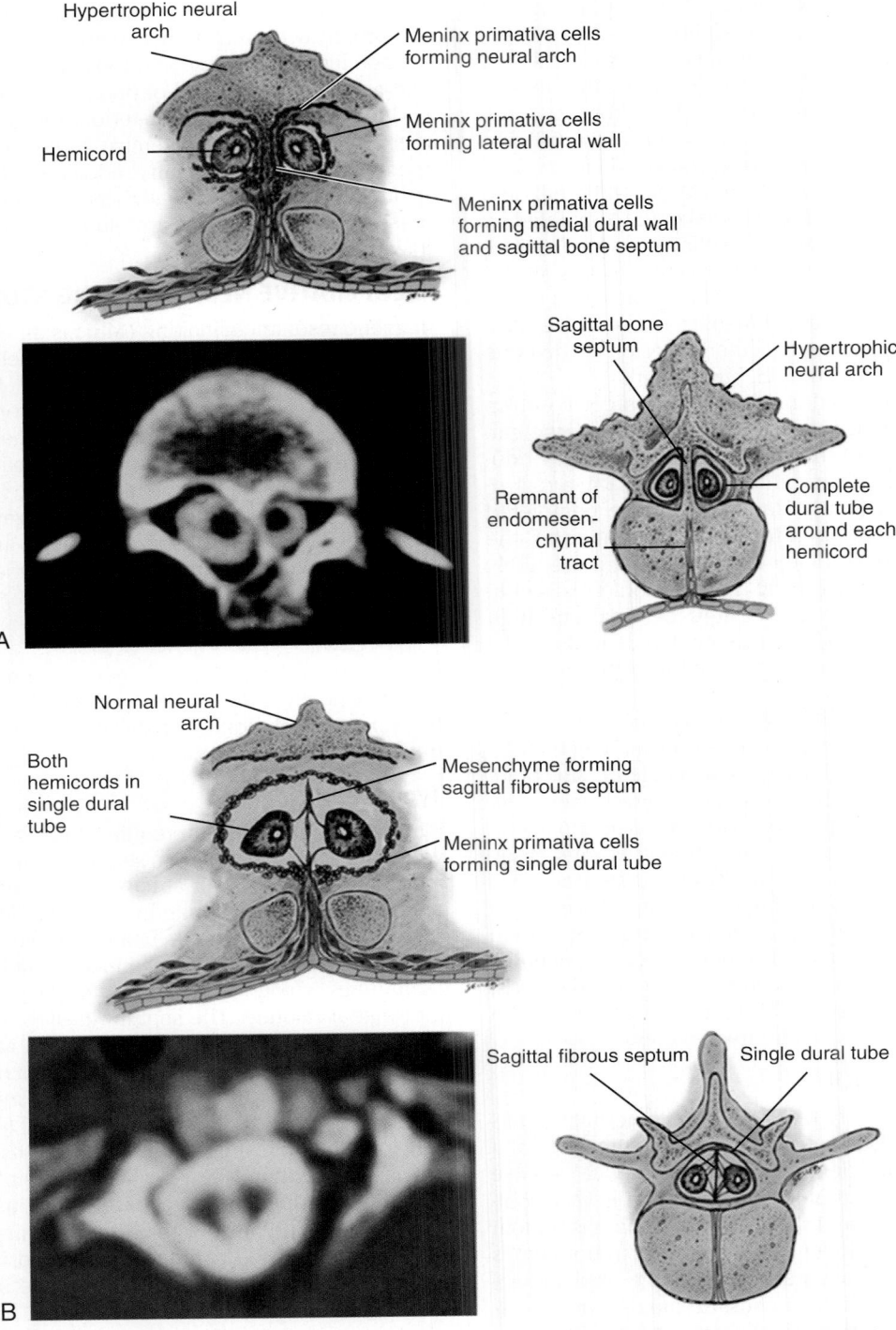

FIGURE 60-10 A, Formation of a type I SCM. *Upper left:* Meninx primitiva cells become admixed with the endomesenchymal tract and situate in the midline between the hemicords, where they form a medial dural wall that ultimately completes the dural sac that surrounds each hemicord. The sclerogenic potential of these specialized cells enables them to also form the median bone septum between the medial dural sleeve, as well as the hypertrophic neural arch attached to the dorsal end of the septum. *Lower left,* CT myelogram; and *right,* drawing of fully formed type I SCM, showing the double dural sacs, the median bone septum, and the hypertrophic neural arch. B, Formation of type II SCM. *Upper left:* Meninx primitiva cells are uninvolved in the endomesenchymal tract, and enclose only the outer aspect of each hemicord to form a single dural sac that surrounds both hemicords. The absence of these cells in the median cleft explains the absence of the sagittal bone septum, its investing dural sleeve, and possibly also the low incidence of hypertrophic neural arches in type II SCM. The mesenchyme from the endomesenchymal tract persists in the midline to form a sagittal fibrous septum, which is frequently adherent to the medial aspect of the hemicords. *Lower right:* Fully formed type II SCM, showing the single dural sac, the thin sagittal fibrous septum, and the adhesions between the septum and the medial surface of the hemicords. Such adhesions tether the hemicords to the adjacent dural tube. *Lower left:* Computed tomography myelogram of a type II SCM. SCM, split cord malformation.

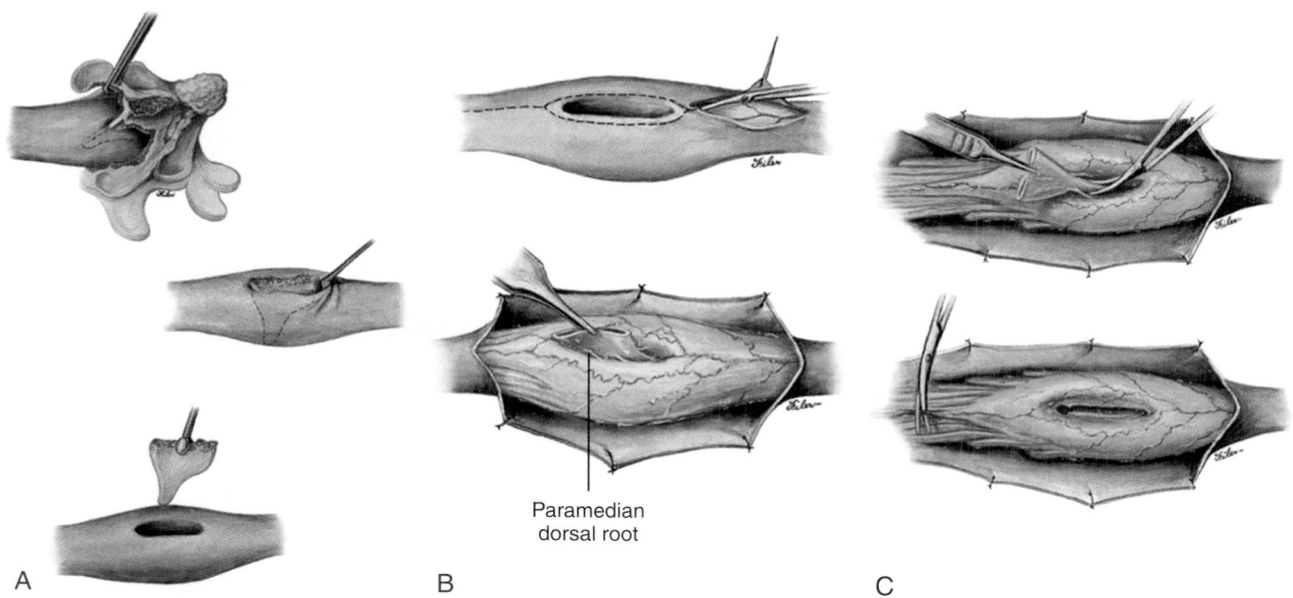

Paramedian
dorsal root

A   B   C

FIGURE 60-11 A, Exposure of a type I bony septum. *Upper:* After the laminae rostral and caudal to the midline septum are resected, the septum-bearing laminae are removed carefully around the dorsal "stump" of the septum where it is attached to the ventral surface of the hypertrophic neural arches. *Middle:* Surgeon then performs subperiosteal separation of the median dural sleeve from the bony septum with a small dental elevator. *Lower:* Bony septum is then avulsed from its ventral attachment, which is often slender. B, *Upper:* Dural opening is made from rostral to caudal along the medial edge of the median dural sleeve (*dashed line*). *Lower:* After lateral retraction of the dura, the median dural sleeve is isolated except ventrally. Note the paramedian dorsal roots attaching the medial aspect of each hemicord to the dural sleeve. C, *Upper:* Dural sleeve is resected flush with the ventral dural surface, proceeding from the rostral "free part" to the caudal end. Note the thickened filum terminale. *Lower:* Ventral dural defect is left after complete resection of the dural sleeve flush with the vertebral body. Note the sectioning of the thickened filum after it has been cauterized. The conus is now completely untethered.

edge is well suited to peel off the dura with minimal lateral "wedging" motions (Fig. 60-11A, middle).

For most type I septa, their dorsal attachment is broad but their ventral junction with the vertebral body is usually flimsy; they could thus be easily avulsed from the dural cleft (Fig. 60-11A, lower). If the ventral attachment happens to be stout and bony, the septum may be carefully chipped away using a small rongeur. Complete extradural removal of the bone spur at this stage greatly facilitates later resection of the dural sleeve. Also, most type I septa are either purely bony or partly cartilaginous. Purely cartilaginous septa are rare. Embedded in the septum is a fairly constant central artery which can bleed briskly on avulsion. A deft plunge with some bone wax on a cotton patty deep into the cleft should handle the bleeding.

The dura is opened on both sides of the now-empty dural cleft to isolate the median dural sleeve (Fig. 60-11B, upper). The medial aspect of each hemicord is often tightly adherent to the dural sleeve by fibrous bands that must be cut. Paramedian dorsal nerve roots, when present in a type I lesion, typically stretch from the dorsomedial aspect of the hemicords to end blindly within the median dural sleeve (Fig. 60-11B, lower). These are nonfunctional and must be cut prior to resection of the dural sleeve. The dural sleeve is always wedged against the caudal reunion site of the hemicords, and the split cord rostral to the septum is therefore a safe, relatively spacious area to begin resection of the dural sleeve. Proceeding caudally from the rostral edge of the sleeve where the hemicords are least adherent, the surgeon cauterizes the ventral attachment of the sleeve to seal the central vessels and then cuts it flush with

the ventral dural wall (Fig. 60-11C, upper). Not having the enclosed stump of the bone spur greatly simplifies the low resection of the sleeve. The most hazardous part of this undertaking is at the caudal end where the reunited "crotch" of the hemicords hugs tightly against the caudal end of the sleeve. The pressure on the crotch is readily felt here, and upward migration of the cord is often seen right after the sleeve resection.

Complete resection of the dural sleeve exposes the ventral extradural space in the sagittal midline (Fig. 60-11C, lower). Any remaining bony stump must now be trimmed down until it is no longer in contact with the ventral surface of the hemicords (Fig. 60-12). Closure of the anterior dural defect is unnecessary because of the abundant adhesions of the ventral dura to the posterior longitudinal ligament which would naturally prevent CSF leakage. Anterior dural closure is actually undesirable because the anterior suture line can potentially tether the hemicords.[84] Posterior dural closure ultimately converts the double dural tubes into a single sac.

Frequently, a fibroneurovascular stalk containing paramedian dorsal nerve roots, fibrous bands, and large blood vessels (myelomeningocele manqué) tautly tethers the hemicords to the dorsal dura. These bands always penetrate the dura at a level more caudal than their origin from the hemicords, and they often form an exuberant tuft of fibroadipose tissue which, unlike ordinary loose extradural fat, clings tenaciously to the outer surface of the dura, and marks the underlying myelomengocoele manqué. These bands must be cut flush with the hemicords to complete the untethering process.

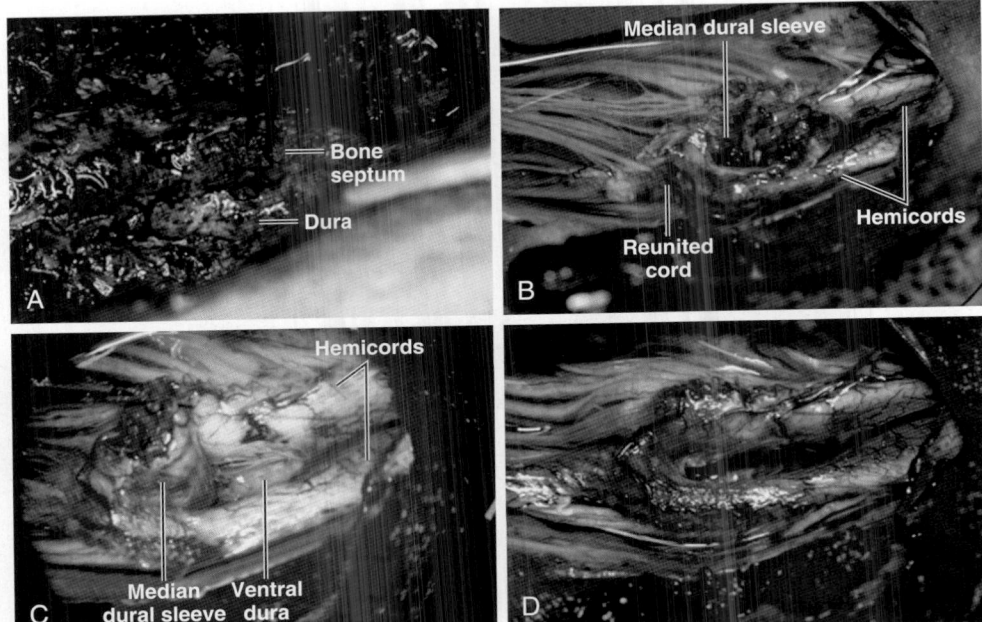

FIGURE 60-12 Resection of type I split cord malformation septum. A, Bone septum is isolated after laminectomy to expose the double dural sleeve. B, Bone septum has been removed and dura opened, exposing median dural sleeve and hemicords. C, Median dural sleeve is being pulled caudally to expose the rostral free space between the hemicords. D, Free hemicords and reunited cord after complete resection of median dural sleeve.

In 5% to 10% of type I SCMs, the bony septum is oblique. It arises from the midline posterior surface of the vertebral body but then cuts diagonally across the spinal canal to divide it into two asymmetrical compartments. Without exception, the hemicord contained within the larger compartment (major hemicord) is much larger than the hemicord in the smaller compartment (minor hemicord), sometimes by a factor of 2 or 3. Moreover, the larger hemicord frequently possesses one set of lateral ventral roots but two sets of dorsal roots, whereas the smaller hemicord only gives off a single set of ventral roots. In these unusual cases, the exposure of the minor hemicord is hampered because it is partly sheltered by the overhanging oblique bone spur as well as being ventrally rotated away from the surgeon's view. Moreover, the smaller hemicord is extremely delicate. It can thus be injured inadvertently during the removal of the bone spur. This unusual pattern of asymmetric splitting must be recognized through preoperative scan as a signature of heightened risk.

Type II SCM

In all cases of type II SCM, some form of fibrous (mesenchymal) septum or band is found within the midline cleft. Three patterns of such nonrigid median septa are encountered in type II lesions: (1) The least common is a complete fibrous septum stretching between the ventral and dorsal surfaces of the dural sac. Except for it being nonosseous, the complete fibrous septum transfixes the hemicords to the surrounding dura in the same manner as does the type I bony septum. (2) Slightly more common is the purely ventral fibrous septum. Its intimate adherence to the ventromedial aspects of the hemicords in effect anchors the cord ventrally where the septum arises from the ventral dura. (3) By far the most prevalent kind is the purely dorsal septum that attaches the dorsomedial aspects of the hemicords to the dorsal dura. A tuft of fibrovascular tissue in the extradural space is sometimes found connected to the septum through a small defect in the dorsal dura (Fig. 60-13B).

Hypertrophic and fused laminae, common in type I lesions, are seldom found in type II SCMs. In fact, the neural arches of type II lesions are often attenuated or even bifid. Laminectomy for these SCMs is technically easy and safe. A midline dural opening immediately exposes a dorsal or complete septum (Fig. 60-13) but a purely ventral septum has to be sought for either between the hemicords or by gently rotating the hemicords to one side (Fig. 60-14). Like the type I bony septa, all type II fibrous septa are found near the caudal end of the split. However, the length of the split in type II SCMs is, by comparison, much shorter than that of the type I SCM, and, because all fibrous septa are thin, the hemicords in type II SCM are apposed much closer together, with very little "free" part. Intracleft exploration is not recommended. Fortunately, the excessive width of the spinal canal should allow the hemicords to be rolled gently to one side for ventral inspection.

The point of attachment between hemicords and septum is invariably rostral to the point of attachment between dura and septum (Figs. 60-13 and 60-14). This is true of all three kinds of fibrous septa, giving testament to the fact that the fibrous septum was dragged upward by rostral movement of the cord after formation of the primordium of the septum. This upward dragging converts the incomplete (ventral or dorsal) septum into an oblique backward-pointing sheet and the complete septum into a V-shaped sheet with the apex pointing rostrally. Blood vessels often skirt the edge of the septum (Fig. 60-14C) or are loosely incorporated within the centromedian fibroneural bands. Very rarely, a true arteriovenous malformation is found within the median cleft. Unless these large vessels are contributing to the tethering of the hemicords, they should be left alone. Paramedian dorsal nerve roots and myelomeningocele manqués are commonly found in type II SCMs (Fig. 60-13), coursing dorsally from the dorsomedial aspect of the hemicords. The puny nerve roots usually end blindly in the septum but the more robust myelomeningocele manqués often penetrate the dorsal dura caudal to their hemicord origin (Fig. 60-13).

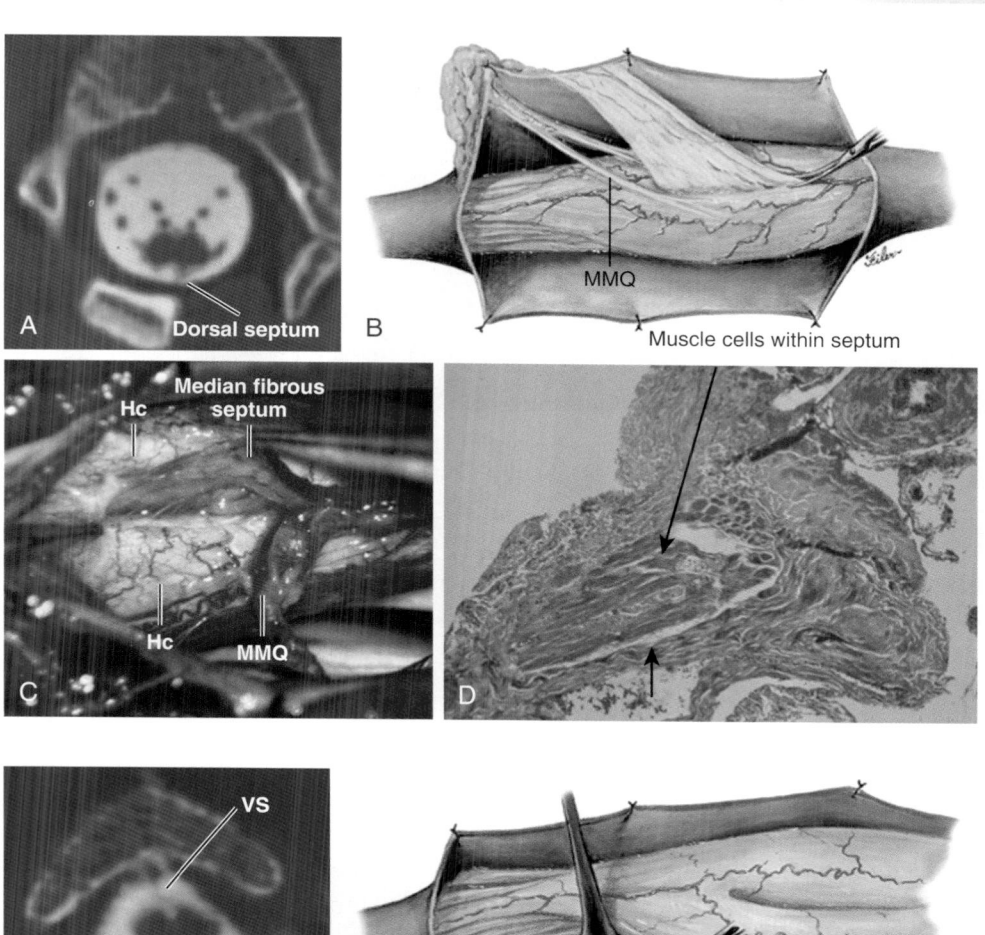

FIGURE 60-13 Resection of type II split cord malformation septum. A, Computed tomography myelogram shows dorsal septum. B, Drawing of the median septum and MMQ. C, Fibrous septum and a large blood vessel, and an MMQ. D, Muscles within fibrous septum. MMQ, myelomeningocele manqué.

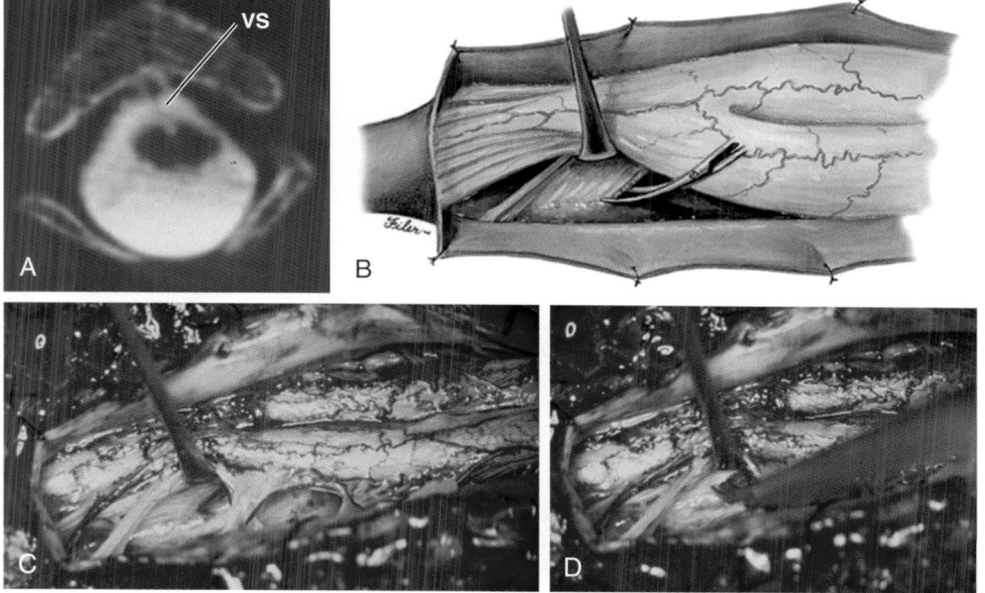

FIGURE 60-14 Type II split cord malformation with ventral fibrous septum. A, Computed tomography myelogram shows VS. B, Drawing of VS with a skirting artery being cut. C, VS with skirt blood vessel. D, VS being cut. VS, ventral septum.

These bands contribute to the tethering and must be cut. Untethering is completed by simply cauterizing the central vessels and excising the median fibrous septum. The ventral septum and bands come through a small defect in the ventral dura, presumably where the original endomesenchymal tract arose, but this small defect never leaks CSF and does not need to be repaired.

SPECIAL CIRCUMSTANCES
Composite SCMs and Multiple SCMs
A composite SCM consists of two or more SCMs of differing types occurring in tandem, with no normal cord in between. The most common constituents of a composite SCM are a type I–type II–type I combination (Fig. 60-15A). Each individual component is typical of its kind: the type I lesion has an extradural bone spur and a median dural sleeve, and the type II lesion has a median fibrous septum within a single dural tube. The three median elements are continuous, suggesting that the entire lesion results from a single (but very large) endomesenchymal tract in which meninx primitiva precursor cells have been included at both ends to cause the type I lesion, but not in the middle where the median septum remains fibrous. The total length of the septa can sometimes span as many as seven vertebral levels. The split cord is coextensive with the septa so that the rostral and caudal reunion sites of the hemicords hug tightly the rostral

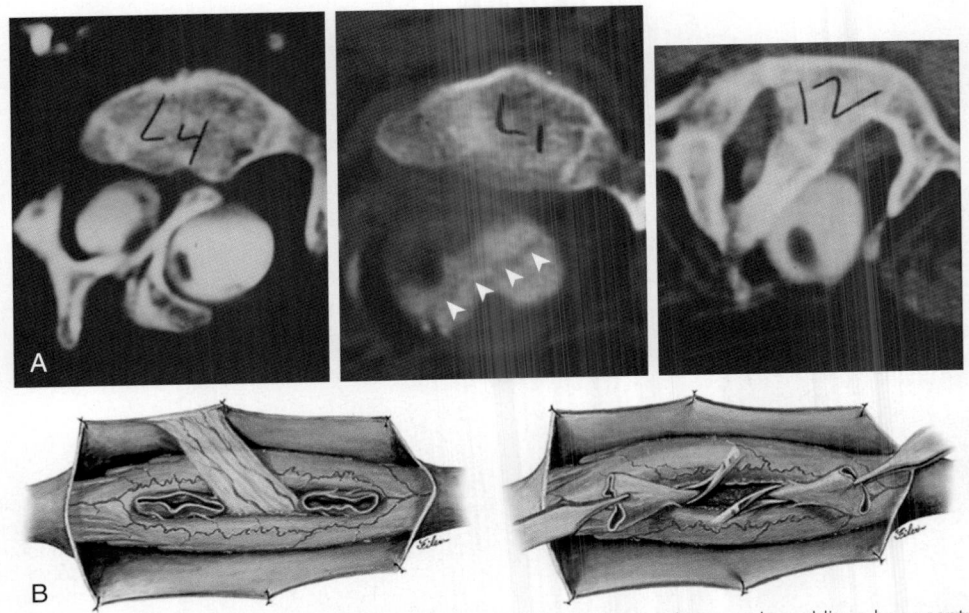

FIGURE 60-15 A, Composite SCM. Right: CTM at T12 shows a type I SCM with double dural sacs and an oblique bone septum dividing the cord into a small right hemicord and a large left hemicord. Middle: CTM at L1 shows a type II SCM with a single dural sac and an oblique fibrous septum (*small arrowheads*). Left: CTM at L4 shows a second type I SCM with an oblique bone septum. All three septi are oblique in the same plane. B, Intraoperative drawings of a composite SCM after the two type I bony septa have been removed. Upper: Midline type II fibrous septum fills the Interval between the median dural sleeves of the two type I lesions. Lower: Fibrous septum has been resected, which provides room in the middle; the dural sleeves now can be resected safely from a middle free space toward the respective "crotches" of the split cord. CTM, computed tomography myelogram; SCM, split cord malformation.

margin of the rostral bone spur and the caudal margin of the caudal bone spur, respectively.

The dural opening for composite SCMs begins rostral to the rostral dural sleeve, skirts around it, returns to the midline over the type II lesion, and finally skirts around the second dural sleeve (Fig. 60-15B, upper). Resection of the middle type II fibrous septum should then be done to gain a "free" area within the midportion of the median cleft. This will provide working room to begin resection of the type I dural sleeves above and below: for the rostral dural sleeve, resection goes from caudal to rostral, whereas resection goes from rostral to caudal for the caudal dural sleeve. This way, the manipulation of the dural sleeve is always directed *toward* and never *away from* the tight reunion site of the hemicords at either end (Fig. 60-15B, lower). Release of the cord is accomplished with total excision of all three septa (eFig. 60-24).

If two or more SCMs occur in the same patient but are separated by an interval of normal spinal cord, they are true multiple SCMs. These are rare because they result from multiple endomesenchymal tracts, that is, from multiple embryologic errors in the same neural tube. The individual SCMs may be all type I or type II, or of mixed types.[23] Their surgical treatment is as described.

Associated Dermal Sinus Tract and Dermoid Cyst

A dermal sinus tract is formed when the original connection between the endomesenchymal tract and the cutaneous ectoderm is retained (eFig. 60-25A). Because of this embryologic relationship, the deep end of the sinus tract is always in continuity with the mesenchymal median septum, but because the septum is either extra- or intrathecal depending on the SCM type, the clinical significance of the retained dermal sinus tract also varies with the SCM type.

For a type I lesion, the dermal sinus tract can be traced all the way from the skin pit through defects in the myofascial layers and neural arches to the bone spur (eFig. 60-25B). Thus, the tract is always extradural and usually does not contribute to the tethering. It is removed together with the bone spur (eFig. 60-25A). Even if the tract may occasionally encyst to form a dermoid cyst, it lies outside the dural sac and seldom becomes large enough to cause compression of the hemicords.

In a type II SCM, however, the dermal sinus tract is of necessity intradural where it retains connection with the median fibrous septum. In its intradural course, the sinus tract is often densely adherent to the hemicords, thereby exerting a separate tethering effect (eFig. 60-26). In addition, over 50% of dermal sinus tracts in a type II SCM will develop a dermoid cyst within the dura, often large enough to cause cord compression. The entire intradural sinus tract and cyst must be excised to prevent recurrence. The cyst is first collapsed by intracapsular evacuation of its cheesy content and the cyst wall is then carefully peeled off the pial surface of the cord. Its deep end is removed with resection of the fibrous median septum (Fig. 60-16).

Associated Myelomeningocele and Hemimyelocele

Approximately 25% to 35% of SCMs have an associated ONTD.[20,22,23] Depending on whether one or both hemicords are involved in the dysraphic sac, the lesion may contain a hemimyelocele or a full-blown myelomeningocele, respectively.

In most myelomeningoceles, the open neural placode is terminal and thus is caudal to the SCM. Less commonly, the open placode is segmental and may therefore be rostral

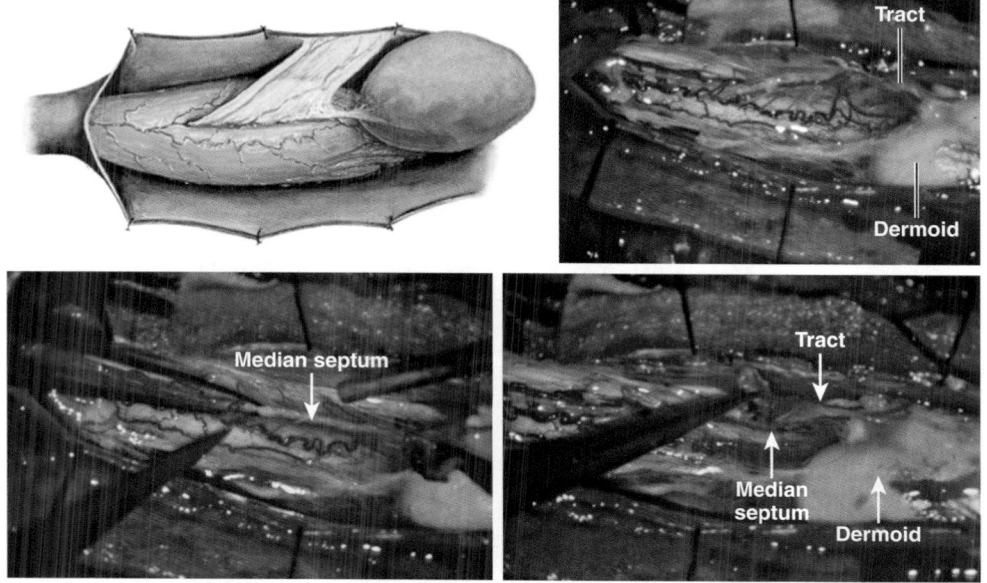

FIGURE 60-16 Intraoperative pictures of type II split cord malformation and associated dermoid cyst showing dermal sinus tract continuous with the median fibrous septum and tract.

to the SCM. Because the open dysraphic sac is usually treated at birth, by the time the SCM is diagnosed by later neuroimaging studies and explored via a second surgical procedure, the original neural placode would have already developed dense adhesions to the dorsal dura. Because the placode is always adjacent to the split cord and may well be contributing to the tethering, it is always freed from the dura when the SCM is being treated. Depending on whether the placode is rostral or caudal to the SCM, it is carefully detached from the dorsal dura by sharp dissection either before or after the median septum is excised.

Most hemimyeloceles are segmental (eFig. 60-27). The unaffected hemicord is usually hidden from view by the median septum during the original sac closure, when the hemiplacode is mistaken to be the whole lesion. During the definitive procedure for the SCM, the entire dural sac (double or single) must be exposed to give access to both hemicords (Fig. 60-17). This often requires cutting into dense scar tissue. Removing the adjacent normal laminae helps to define the full width of the dura rostral to the scar. After identifying and resecting the median septum, the hemiplacode is detached from the dorsal dura with sharp dissection.

Associated Neurenteric Cyst and Other Intestinal Anomalies

Since the ventral endomesenchymal tract is continuous with and partially composed of yolk sac endoderm, it is no surprise that enterogenous remnants and other intestinal anomalies coexist with SCMs. Neurenteric (enterogenous) cysts are rare (presumably because extrinsic induction of endodermal progenitor cells is fastidious) but have been found along the entire endomesenchymal tract, from subcutaneous layers to the prevertebral space in front of the split cord[84] (eFig. 60-28). These cysts can cause compression when found in between the hemicords (Fig. 60-18) or as intramedullary masses within the hemicords (Fig. 60-19). They must be resected in toto to avoid recurrence.

Intestinal malrotation results when the ventral endomesenchymal tract remains as a tethering band in the proximal

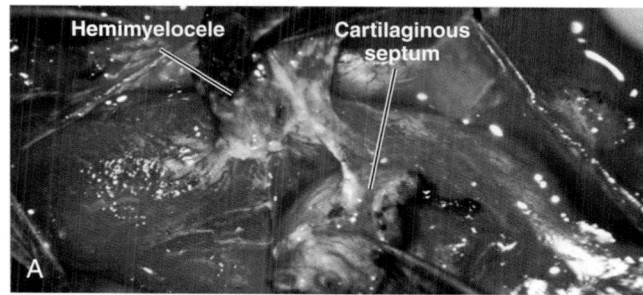

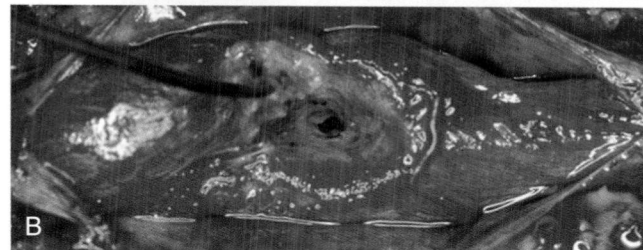

FIGURE 60-17 Intraoperative pictures of type I split cord malformation with associated hemimyelocele. A, 8-mm thick stalk of neural tissue arising from the right hemicord just rostral to the median dura-clad cartilaginous septum. B, Both hemimyelocele stalk and median septum have been removed.

intestine (Ladd's band) that prevents normal clockwise rotation of the primitive fore-gut (eFig. 60-29). If the portion of the endomesenchymal tract continuous with the yolk sac differentiates into mature bowel epithelium, a patent intestinal diverticulum linking small bowel with the prevertebral tissue may occur as an impressive mass lesion in the thoracic cavity (eFig. 60-30). This will require a combined thoracotomy and spinal exposure for complete resection.

COMPLICATIONS AND PRECAUTIONS

Neurologic Injury

Worsening of neurologic function occurs in less than 3% of patients following surgery for SCM. The surgical morbidity is higher with a type I SCM due to hemicord injury during

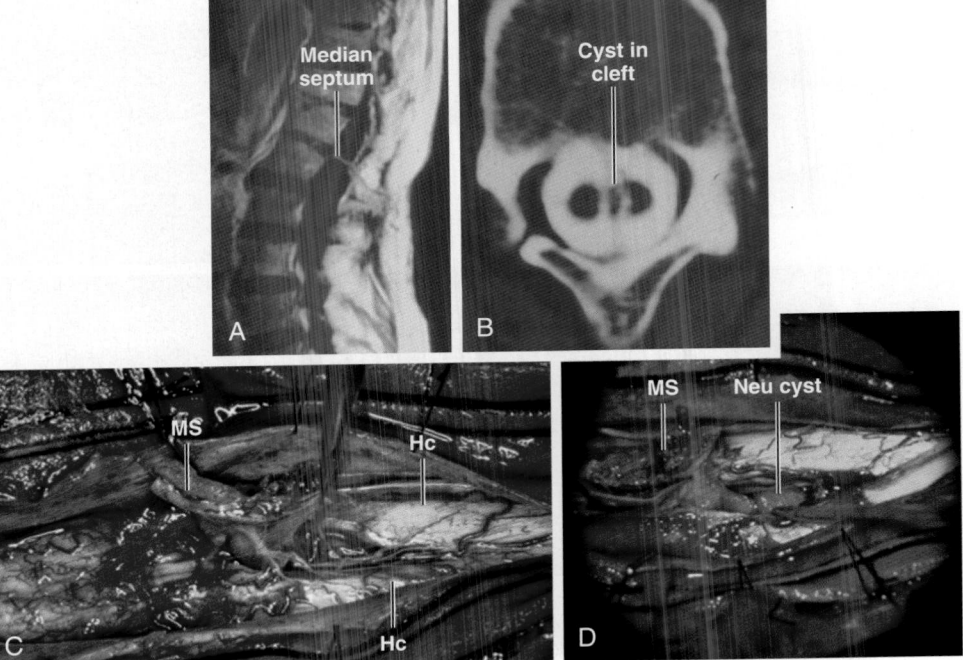

FIGURE 60-18 Intracleft neurenteric cyst in a type I split cord malformation. A, Sagittal magnetic resonance image shows the median septum. B, Computed tomography myelogram shows the cyst within the median cleft. C, Shows bony median septum (MS) within median dural sleeve. D, Shows neurenteric cyst (Neu cyst) rostral to the dura-clad bony median septum (MS) within the median cleft. Hc, hemicord.

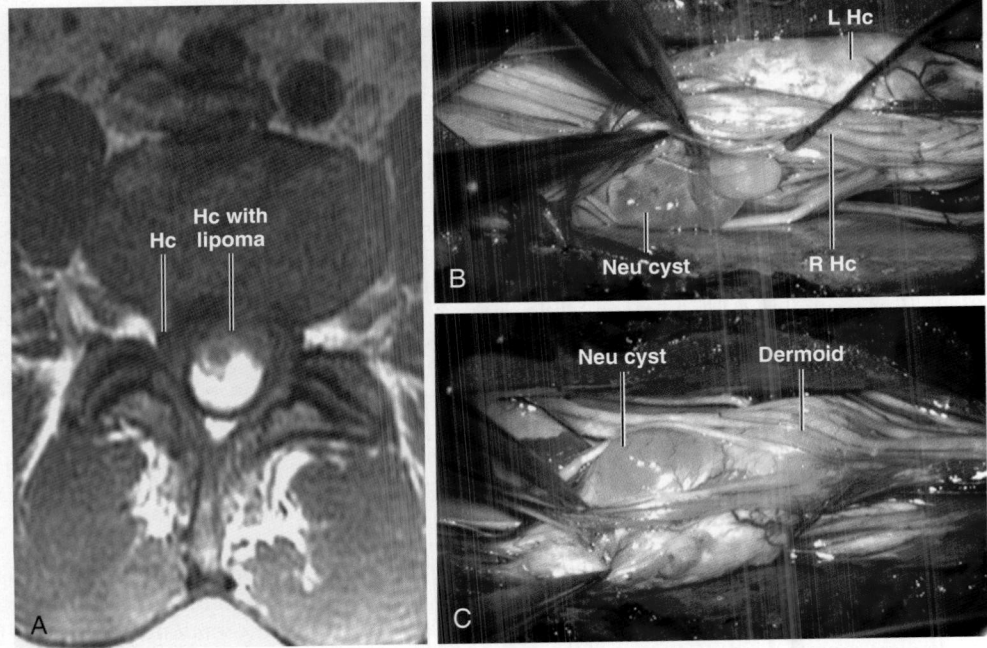

FIGURE 60-19 Intracleft neurenteric cyst and intramedullary neurenteric cyst in a patient with type II split cord malformation, who also has a lipoma in the left Hc. A, magnetic resonance imaging shows Hc's and lipoma in the L Hc. B, Shows intracleft neurenteric cyst (Neu cyst) after the R Hc is lifted up. C, Shows intramedullary neurenteric cyst with L Hc, adjacent to a dermoid cyst. Hc, hemicord; L Hc, left hemicord; R Hc, right hemicord.

removal of the bone spur. This is especially true when the bony septum is oblique and the delicate minor hemicord is tucked under the overhanging septum. The risk of hemicord injury is minimized by the following precautions:

1. Accurate preoperative depiction of the peculiar angulation of the bony septum and the relationship of the minor hemicord to the bony overhang.

2. Wide laminectomy at the site of the septum to improve exposure of both dural sacs. Without wide exposure, the oblique bone spur may be mistaken for the lateral wall of the spinal canal.

3. Extremely careful piecemeal resection of the dorsal end of the septum. As more of this end of the septum is bitten away, more of the minor dural tube is exposed.

Cerebrospinal Fluid Leakage

Wound complications are seldom encountered in patients with SCM except when there is a previously treated open neural tube defect adjacent to the split cord. These children often have poor myofascial coverage as well as tenuous, scar-ridden skin over the dural sac and may develop CSF leakage. This underscores the importance of a watertight dural closure. In addition, these children should be managed in the fully prone position for 5 to 7 days after surgery similar to the newborn with a newly repaired myelomeningocele. Heavy sedation may be necessary to prevent an infant from wiggling and pulling at the incision.

Postoperative Bladder Management

Transient detrusor weakness and urinary retention is not uncommon after the resection of a type I SCM. It can last from a few days to several months and tends to be more common in adults than in children. Permanent worsening in bladder function occurs in about 3% of patients.[20,23,24] A bladder catheter is left in the first two postoperative days when the patient is confined to complete bed rest. The catheter is removed on the third postoperative day as the patient is encouraged to ambulate and use bathroom facilities. If there is obvious difficulty in micturition or if a large postvoid residual urine volume is obtained repeatedly, the patient is given a cholinergic agent such as bethanechol chloride to strengthen detrusor contraction, or an α-sympathetic blocker such as prazosin hydrochloride to encourage relaxation of the internal urethral sphincter. If the postvoid residual urine volume remains high on medication, an intermittent catheterization program is started in the hospital and is continued on an outpatient basis. After 4 to 6 weeks, a cystometrogram is obtained to evaluate bladder function and to determine whether therapy can be discontinued.

Limited Dorsal Myeloschisis

This form of spinal dysraphism is called transitional because it is neither open, with a leaking sac, nor is it truly closed, with its obvious cutaneous signature and a potentially patent tract. The basic structure of a limited dorsal myeloschisis (LDM) consists of a fibroneurovascular stalk containing neurons, glia, and nerves emanating from the dorsal surface of the spinal cord and penetrating through a narrow dorsal dural opening to reach the surface of the skin. The presence of an LDM is always indicated on the overlying skin by one of two main types of cutaneous manifestations: (1) the flat or nonsaccular type, consisting of a prominent dimple or crater made of pearly, squamous epithelium without an underlying dermis, often surrounded by elevated skin edges, hemangioma, or hair tufts (eFig. 60-31), and (2) the saccular type consisting of either a fluid-filled, fluctuant mass with a skin-covered base capped by a thick, purplish, raw-looking squamous epithelial membrane (eFig. 60-32A), a skin sac with an unobtrusive epithelial crater at the dome (eFig. 60-32B), or a sac with a thin epithelial cap that is not full-thickness skin (eFig. 60-32C). LDMs are rare lesions found in all areas of the spine, but more commonly in the lumbar and thoracolumbar regions.[20,24] In the cervical region, LDMs are almost always of the sac type, particularly with the purplish lichenized squamous epithelial cap[21,85] forming an imposing protrusion in the back of the newborn's neck.

EMBRYOGENESIS

Embryogenetically, LDM is a defect of primary neurulation and thus never involves the conus. It probably differs from the open myelomeningocele only in the degree of the incompleteness of neurulation. In LDM, most of neurulation has occurred except for the final fusion of the opposed neural folds (hence *dorsal myeloschisis*). The basic configuration of the neural tube has taken shape but for a thin slip in the dorsal midline (hence *limited*). Here, disjunction between cutaneous ectoderm and neuroectoderm never truly happens, but the midline gap between the converging cutaneous ectoderm and dorsal scleromyotomes from opposite sides of the embryo remains very narrow (eFig. 60-33A). Further development of the full-thickness, dorsal myofascial tissues (except for a narrow strip in the midline) progressively sets the integument farther away from the neural tube, which ultimately retains its primarily intraspinal location. A dorsal median stalk of central nervous system tissue, however, remains as the original link between the *nearly* closed neural tube and the still slightly gaping cutaneous ectoderm (eFig. 60-33B). Underneath, normal meninges develop around the neural tube and extend around the midline neural stalk as a sleeve that projects to the surface (eFigs. 60-34 and 60-35). Superficially, the small dimple or pearly thin membrane belies the small unclosed gap of the cutaneous ectoderm. In the flat or nonsaccular LDM, thick squamous epithelium grows across and bridges this gap, even though this membrane lacks a full-thickness epidermis and dermis.[21] In the saccular LDM, the formation of the requisite fibroneural stalk linking cutaneous with neuroectoderm is the same as in the flat type, but in the sac type, CSF squeezes into the dorsal dural fistula around the neural stalk and ultimately distends the thinner, less well-supported squamous epithelial portion of the gap into a fluid-filled and mostly skin-covered sac (eFig. 60-36A). The crater, dimple, and otherwise "un-skin-like" cap of the dome always belie the original dorsal myeloschisis.

The internal structure of the saccular LDM dorsal to the fibroneural stalk can be of three forms. If there is an associated hydromyelia in the part of the cord bearing the dorsal myeloschisis, CSF may distend the center of the distal neural stalk dorsal to the myofascia into a large myelocystocele within the meningocele sac[21,86] (eFig. 60-36). If there is no hydromyelia, the neural stalk remains solid and narrow and fans out on the dome of the sac (eFig. 60-37). Or the CSF pressure within the sac may compress the neural stalk ventrally into a series of basal neural nodules lining the bottom of the sac (eFig. 60-38). In all 3 variants, the spinal cord underneath the sac is tethered to the myofascial tissue by way of the fibroneural stalk and its meningeal investment. Neurologic deficits develop because of this tethering effect and vary according to the location of the LDM.

SURGICAL TECHNIQUE

LDMs are frequently associated with other tethering lesions that should be simultaneously treated. For example, a thickened filum is invariably found in thoracolumbar and

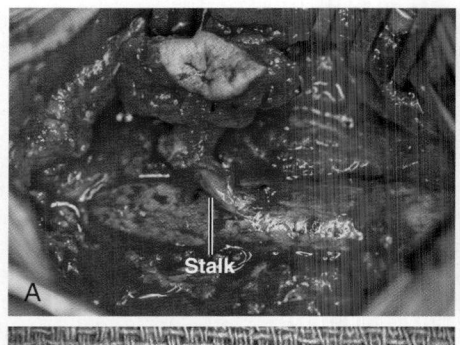

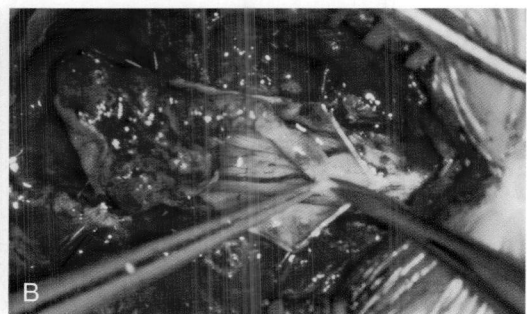

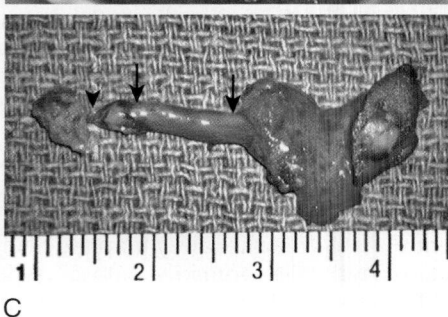

FIGURE 60-20 Surgical resection of a lumbar crater-type, flat (nonsaccular), limited dorsal myeloschisis. A, Extradural stalk and dural fistula. B, Resection of stalk flush with cord surface. C, En bloc specimen showing, from right to left, skin ellipse bearing pale epithelial crater, the subcutaneous portion bearing fat, the extradural portion of the stalk (between *arrows*), intradural stalk (between *arrow* and *arrowhead*), and an exuberant cuff of tissue on the cord.

lumbar LDMs and in some cervical LDMs; about 50% of cervical LDMs have coexisting Chiari II malformation[21,85] and hydrocephalus; and SCMs have also been reported.

The operation for the crater-type LDM is usually uncomplicated (Fig. 60-20). The superficial crater or pit is excised with an elliptical cuff of skin; the fibroneural stalk is followed through to the laminar defect and ultimately to the dorsal dura after laminectomy. The fibroneural stalk itself may be thin or thick, but the principle is always to resect it flush with the dorsal surface of the cord and leave as inconspicuous a scar as possible (Fig. 60-21 and eFigs. 60-39 and 60-40).

The operation for saccular LDMs is the same whether the internal structure of the sac contains a myelocystocele, a basal neural nodule, or a slender, simple fibroneural band. The skin incision incorporates an elliptical split around the base of the sac exposing at least one set of intact laminae both above and below the dural-neural stalk. The often thick subcutaneous tissues are carefully dissected to reveal the funnel of dura at the base of the sac where the discrete stalk penetrates the myofascial layer (Fig. 60-22A and eFig. 60-41A). Laminectomy is done to display the normal dural tube rostral and caudal to this dural fistula, which is thus seen in-continuity with the dorsal dural outpouching. The dura is opened in the midline to show the fibroneural stalk and the almost always discrete attachment of the stalk with the spinal cord (Fig. 60-22B). The stalk is simply cut flush with the surface of the cord (eFig. 60-41B), and the dura is closed primarily. The superficial sessile sac, now detached, can be resected *en masse*.

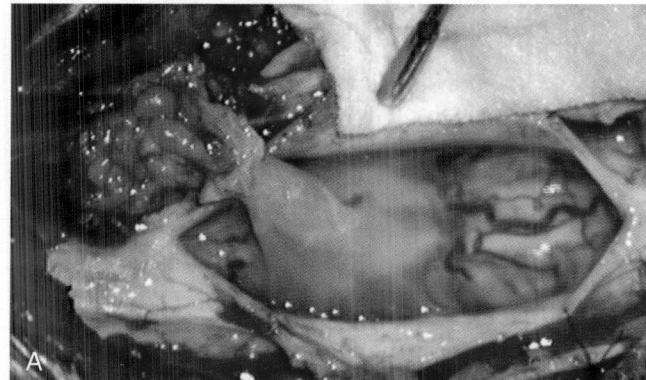

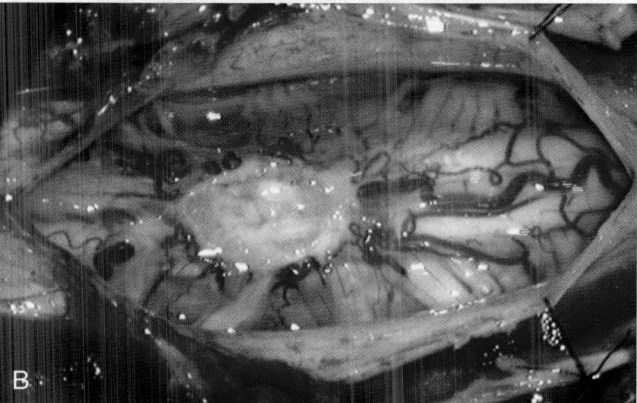

FIGURE 60-21 Moderate-sized limited dorsal myeloschisis stalk. A, Stalk has a flared-out cord attachment. B, Stalk resection leaves a fish-mouth–shaped scar.

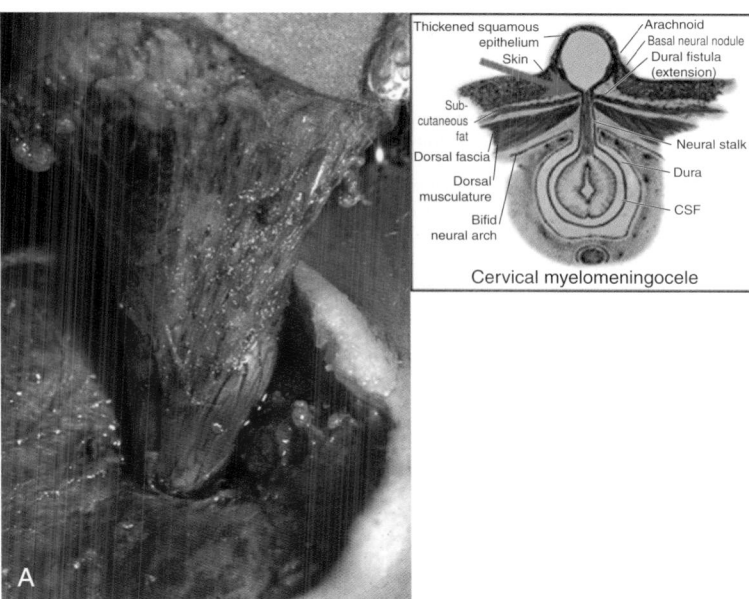

Thickened squamous epithelium
Skin
Sub-cutaneous fat
Dorsal fascia
Dorsal musculature
Bifid neural arch
Arachnoid
Basal neural nodule
Dural fistula (extension)
Neural stalk
Dura
CSF
Cervical myelomeningocele

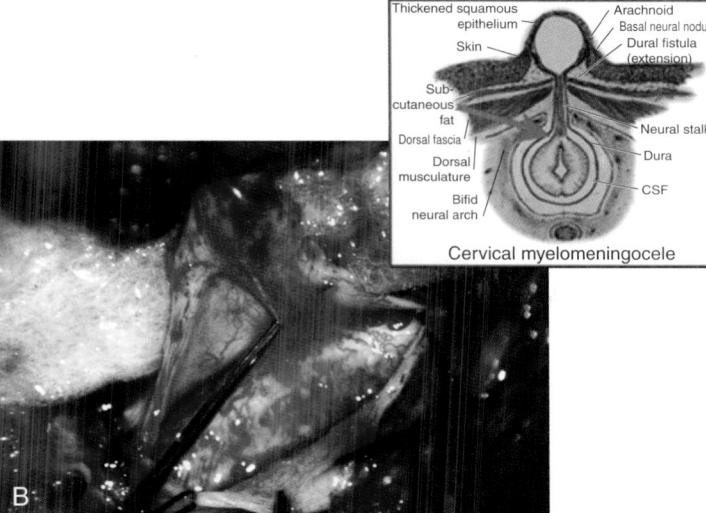

Thickened squamous epithelium
Skin
Sub-cutaneous fat
Dorsal fascia
Dorsal musculature
Bifid neural arch
Arachnoid
Basal neural nodule
Dural fistula (extension)
Neural stalk
Dura
CSF
Cervical myelomeningocele

FIGURE 60-22 Large cervical saccular limited dorsal myeloschisis. (*Arrows* in insets show direction of surgeon's vision.) A, Exposure of the dorsal fistula at the level of the nuchal fascial defect. B, Dural fistula opened into the main thecal sac, showing the thin fibroneural stalk inserting on to the dorsal spinal cord.

KEY REFERENCES

Chapman PH. Congenital intraspinal lipomas. Anatomic considerations and surgical treatment. *Child's Brain*. 1982;9:37-47.

Chapman PH, Davis KR. Surgical treatment of spinal lipomas in childhood. *Pediatr Neurosurg*. 1993;19:267-275.

Dias M, Pang D. Human neural embryogenesis: a description of neural morphogenesis and a review of embryonic mechanisms. In: Pang D, ed. *Disorders of the Pediatric Spine*. New York: Raven Press; 1994.

Kulkarni HV, Pierre-Kahn A, Zerah M. Conservative management of asymptomatic spinal lipomas of the conus. *Neurosurgery*. 2004;54:868-875.

La Marca F, Grant JA, Tomita T, McLone DG. Spinal lipomas in children: outcome of 270 procedures. *Pediatr Neurosurg*. 1997;26:8-16.

McLone DG, Naidich TP. Spinal dysraphism: experimental and clinical. In: Holtzman RN, Stein BM, eds. *The Tethered Spinal Cord*. New York: Thieme-Stratton; 1985.

McLone DG, Suwa J, Collins JA, et al. Neurulation: Biochemical and morphological studies on primary and secondary neural tube defects. Concepts Pediatr. *Neurosurg*. 1983;4:15-29.

Muller F, O'Rahilly R. The development of the human brain, the closure of the caudal neuropore, and the beginning of secondary neurulation at Stage 12. *Anat Embryol (Berl)*. 1974;176:413-430.

O'Rahilly R, Meyer DB. The timing and sequence of events in the development of the human vertebral column during the embryonic period proper. *Anat Embryol (Berl)*. 1973;157:167-176.

O'Rahilly R, Müller F. *Developmental Stages in Human Embryos, Including a Revision of Streeter's Horizons and a Survey of the Carnegie Collection*. Washington, DC: Carnegie Institution of Washington; 1987.

Pang D. Electrophysiological monitoring for tethered cord surgery. In: Yamada S, ed. *Tethered cord syndrome*. 2nd ed. New York and Stuttgart: Thieme; 2010.

Pang D. Split cord malformations, theories and practice. In: Batjer H, Loftus C, eds. *Textbook of Neurological Surgery*. Philadelphia: Lippincott, Williams & Wilkins; 2002:916-945.

Pang D. Ventral tethering in split cord malformation. *Neurosurg Focus*. 2001;0(1):e6.

Pang D. Surgical complications of open spinal dysraphism. *Neurosurg Clin North Am*. 1995:6243-6257.

Pang D. Cervical myelomeningoceles. *Neurosurgery*. 1993;33(3):363-373.

Pang D. Split cord malformation. Part II: the clinical syndrome. *Neurosurgery*. 1992;31:481-500.

Pang D, Dias M, Ahdab-Barmada M. Split cord malformation. Part I: A unified theory of embryogenesis for double spinal cord malformation. *Neurosurgery*. 1992(31):451-480.

Pang D, Zovickian JG, Oviedo A. Long term outcome of total and near total resection of spinal cord lipomas and radical reconstruction of neural placode. Part II: Outcome analysis and preoperative profiling. *Neurosurgery.* 2010;66(2):253-273.

Pang D, Zovickian JG, Ovieda A. Long-term outcome of total and near total resection of spinal cord lipomas and radical reconstruction of the neural placode. Part I: surgical technique. *Neurosurgery.* 2009;65:511-529.

Pierre-Kahn A, Lacombe J, Pichon J, et al. Intraspinal lipomas with spina bifida: prognosis and treatment in 73 cases. *J Neurosurg.* 1986;65:756-761.

Pierre-Kahn A, Zerah M, Renier D, et al. Congenital lumbosacral lipomas. *Childs Nerv Syst.* 1997;13:298-334.

Saitsu H, Yamada S, Uwabe C, et al. Development of the posterior neural tube in human embryos. *Anat Embryol (Berl).* 2004;209:107-117.

Schoenwolf GC. Histological and ultrastructural observations of tail bud formation in the chick embryo. *Anat Rec.* 1979;193:131-148.

Schoenwolf GC, Nichols DH. Histological and ultrastructural studies of secondary neurulation in mouse embryos. *Am J Anat.* 1984;169:361-376.

Steinbok P. Dysraphic lesions of the cervical spinal cord. *Neurosurg Clin North Am.* 1995;6:367-376.

Numbered references appear on Expert Consult.

CHAPTER 61

Revascularization Techniques in Pediatric Cerebrovascular Disorders

EDWARD SMITH • R. MICHAEL SCOTT

This chapter focuses on methods used to revascularize the brain in the setting of treating pediatric cerebrovascular disease. While there are many situations that might require some form of surgical revascularization, there are three conditions in particular—atherosclerotic carotid disease, intracranial aneurysms, and moyamoya syndrome—that are most commonly encountered by neurosurgeons. However, age-specific differences in disease presentation mean that the spectrum of cerebrovascular disease encountered by neurosurgeons who treat children is notably different than what is seen in adult patients. Atherosclerotic carotid disease is not present in the pediatric population and using revascularization techniques to treat the rare pediatric intracranial aneurysm is rarely feasible. Since these conditions are rare in children, the use of revascularization techniques in these diagnoses will not be discussed here and the reader is referred to the relevant descriptions elsewhere in this textbook. This chapter will thus primarily center on the surgical revascularization of children with moyamoya syndrome.

Moyamoya Syndrome

Moyamoya syndrome is an arteriopathy characterized by progressive stenosis of the distal internal carotid arteries as they enter the cranial vault.[1,2] With narrowing of the internal carotids, cerebral blood flow is reduced, cerebral ischemia develops, and collateral blood vessels develop in the region of the carotid bifurcation, on the cortical surface, and from branches of the external carotid artery (ECA). This alternative blood supply—comprised of maximally dilated pre-existing arteries and growth of new vessels—provides circulation to the region formerly supplied by the internal carotids. Although usually limited to the anterior circulation, this process may involve the posterior circulation as well; including the basilar and posterior cerebral arteries. The appearance of this basal collateral network on angiography has been compared to a hazy cloud or puff of smoke: the disease defined by the Japanese word "moyamoya." Because of the natural propensity in patients with moyamoya for collateral vessels to the brain to develop from branches of the external carotid and because these arteries and those on the surface of the brain are not involved by the moyamoya arteriopathy, most of the surgical revascularization techniques in this condition utilize the external carotid circulation as a donor source of new blood flow to the ischemic brain.

Surgical Treatment of Moyamoya

Two general methods are employed: direct and indirect. In direct revascularization, a branch of the ECA (usually the superficial temporal artery [STA]) is anastomosed end to side to a cortical artery (usually a distal branch of the middle cerebral artery [MCA]), the so-called "STA-MCA bypass." In contrast, indirect techniques involve mobilizing vascularized tissue supplied by the ECA (dura, muscle, pedicles of the STA) and placing it in contact with the brain to promote in-growth of new vessels to the cortex.

Historically, direct procedures have been used in adults, with immediate increase of blood flow to the ischemic brain cited as a major benefit of the procedure. Augmentation of cerebral blood flow usually does not occur for several weeks with indirect techniques. However, direct bypass is often technically difficult to perform in children because of the small size of donor and recipient vessels; making indirect techniques appealing. Nonetheless, direct operations have been successful in children as have indirect procedures in adults.[3-5] Considerable debate exists regarding the relative merits and shortcomings of the two approaches; in fact, some centers advocate combinations of both approaches.[5-7]

Numerous indirect revascularization procedures have been described: *encephaloduroarteriosynangiosis* (EDAS) whereby the STA is dissected free over a course of several inches and then sutured to the cut edges of the opened dura; *encephalomyosynangiosis* (EMS) in which the temporalis muscle is dissected and placed onto the surface of the brain to encourage collateral vessel development; the combination of both, *encephalo-myo-arterio-synangiosis* (EMAS), a variant of EDAS in which the STA is sutured to the brain; *pial synangiosis*, described in detail below; and the drilling of multiple burr holes without vessel synangiosis.[8-14] *Dural inversion*, carrying out a craniotomy, opening the dura, and turning the dural flaps inward over the surface of the brain has also been described as a revascularization technique.[13] Cervical sympathectomy and omental transposition or omental pedicle grafting have also been described.[2] We have found the technique of pial synangiosis particularly effective in the pediatric moyamoya population, and in a

Table 61-1 Perioperative Management Protocol Used at Our Institution for Patients with Moyamoya

At 1 Day Before Surgery

Continue aspirin therapy (usually 81 mg once a day orally if <70 kg, 325 mg once a day orally if ≥70 kg).

Admit patient to hospital for overnight intravenous hydration (isotonic fluids 1.25–1.5 × maintenance).

At Induction of Anesthesia

Institute electroencephalographic monitoring.

Maintain normotension during induction; also normothermia (especially with smaller children), normocarbia (avoid hyperventilation to minimize cerebral vasoconstriction, pCO_2 > 35 mm Hg), and normal pH.

Placement of additional intravenous lines, arterial line, Foley catheter, and pulse oximeter.

Place precordial Doppler to monitor for venous air emboli (relevant with thicker bone resulting from extramedullary hematopoiesis).

During Surgery

Maintain normotension, normocarbia, normal pH, adequate oxygenation, normothermia, and adequate hydration.

Electroencephalographic slowing may respond to incremental blood pressure increases or other maneuvers to improve cerebral blood flow.

Postoperatively

Avoid hyperventilation (relevant with crying in children); pain control is important.

Maintain aspirin therapy on postoperative day 1.

Maintain intravenous hydration at 1.25–1.5 × maintenance until child is fully recovered and drinking well (usually 48–72 hours).

Revised from Smith ER, McClain CD, Heeney M, et al. Pial synangiosis in patients with moyamoya syndrome and sickle cell anemia: perioperative management and surgical outcome. Neurosurg Focus. 2009;26:E10.

review of 143 patients treated with pial synangiosis, demonstrated marked reductions in stroke frequency following surgery.[14] Regardless of the revascularization procedure utilized, the perioperative strategies for complication avoidance are relevant to all moyamoya patients, regardless of surgical technique employed.

PIAL SYNANGIOSIS

We have recently published a specific perioperative protocol for patients with moyamoya[15] (Table 61-1). This protocol has been adapted from our practice for all patients with moyamoya and highlights general strategies we have found useful in the surgical management of this condition.

Indications for Surgery

In the setting of patients with radiographically confirmed moyamoya syndrome, surgery is indicated in the cases with (1) history of neurologic symptoms such as stroke, TIA, seizures, and so on, due to cerebral ischemia; and (2) progressive moyamoya changes detected on surveillance scans in susceptible populations (e.g., following radiation therapy for brain tumor). We use cerebral blood flow and metabolism studies, such as MRI perfusion sutides, PET, and SPECT, only in problematic cases where the indications for surgery are not as well-defined.

Surgery is relatively contraindicated in patients who are at significant operative risk (severe cardiac disease, advanced debilitation from stroke burden, or other severe comorbidities). In addition, patients with an unclear diagnosis or whose arteriopathy is very mild, with a low Suzuki grade (I or, rarely, II), are occasionally observed closely with serial imaging before we consider surgical revascularization.

Overall, we generally advocate surgical treatment for patients with radiographically confirmed moyamoya, even if asymptomatic, as the preponderance of evidence suggests that moyamoya is a relentless, progressive process in children. Surgical treatment, both direct and indirect, has been shown to be safe when performed by experienced surgeons and confers long-lasting, durable protection from stroke relative to medical therapy alone.

Preoperative Strategy and Imaging

Preoperative management of moyamoya patients is critical to the success of surgery. Strategy is based on the utilization of appropriate imaging for planning and the maintenance of hypervolemia, normocarbia, and prevention of thrombosis. A full five- or six-vessel (both ICAs, both ECAs, and one or both vertebrals as indicated) diagnostic angiogram is critical to the planning of the procedure for:

1. Accurate identification of disease status
2. Identification of transdural collaterals so that they may be preserved during surgery
3. Confirmation of the presence of a suitable donor scalp vessel (usually the parietal branch of the superficial temporal artery [STA])

Once the decision to operate has been made, we follow a standardized perioperative protocol. Dehydration is a significant risk given the hypoperfused intracranial circulation. To minimize shifts in blood pressure during the induction of anesthesia, we routinely admit patients to the hospital on the evening prior to surgery for intravenous hydration. If there are no underlying cardiac or renal limitations, isotonic fluids are run at 1.5 times maintenance rate. Barring medical contraindication, patients are treated with daily aspirin therapy from the time of their diagnosis of moyamoya in order to minimize the risk of thrombosis in the slow-flowing cortical vessels. Dosing is continued up to and including the day prior to surgery (and restarted the day after surgery). Pain and anxiety must be aggressively managed, especially with children since hyperventilation, as occurs with crying, can induce cerebral vasoconstriction; leading to stroke. Steroids, cerebral dehydrating agents such as mannitol and anticonvulsants are not administered on a routine basis.

Anesthetic Issues and Monitoring

An experienced team of anesthesiologists is critical to the success of the operation. Generally, premedication is useful to minimize crying in children to prevent cerebral vasoconstriction and possible ischemic events. Hypotension, hyperthermia, and hypercarbia are to be avoided at all times, especially during induction. Muscular blockade is established by a non-depolarizing muscle relaxant prior to intubation. Anesthesia is maintained with low-dose isoflurane (a cerebral vasodilator) and a balanced nitrous oxide/oxygen mixture with fentanyl. End-tidal CO_2 is usually kept on the high-normal side (35 to 40 mm Hg) to minimize cerebral vasoconstriction. Normotension is maintained. Diuretics (mannitol and Lasix) are usually avoided due to the possibility of hypotension.

We routinely supplement routine anesthetic monitoring with the use of intraoperative EEG. EEG is employed during surgery to identify focal slowing, indicative of compromised cerebral blood flow, so that immediate compensatory measures can be instituted by the operative team. EEG technicians must communicate changes in the EEG promptly to allow the team to respond immediately with appropriate titration of blood pressure, pCO_2, and anesthetic agents.

OPERATIVE TECHNIQUE AND SETUP

In cases with bilateral disease, we will commonly treat both sides in a single operative sitting in order to reduce total anesthetic time (the anesthesia set-up time for a young child may take up to 1.5 hours if EEG electrodes are to be placed and if IV access is difficult, and having these already in place shortens the anesthesia time for the second side) and to limit the number of inductions and wake-ups; always a critical period for these compromised patients. We will usually treat the most affected side first, as determined either by clinical history or radiographic studies. If both sides are comparable in Suzuki grade and clinical status, then we will often treat the dominant hemisphere first.

The technique involves the following steps, which are described in more detail in following sections: (1) a scalp donor artery (most commonly, the parietal branch of the superficial temporal artery) is identified by Doppler and dissected, using a microscope from the very beginning of the dissection, from distal to proximal along with a cuff of galea and surrounding soft tissue; (2) the temporalis muscle is incised into four quadrants and retracted, and the largest possible craniotomy flap is turned in the available bony exposure; (3) the dura is opened into at least six flaps in order to increase the surface area of dura exposed to the pial surface and thereby enhance formation of collateral vessels from the dural vascular supply; (4) the arachnoid is opened widely over the surface of brain exposed by the dural opening; and (5) the intact donor artery is sutured directly to the pial surface using four to six interrupted 10-0 nylon sutures placed through the donor vessel adventitia and the underlying superficial pia. The bone flap is replaced over a Gelfoam cover of the dura, which is left widely open; the flap carefully secured to avoid compression of the donor artery. The temporal muscle and skin edges are carefully closed with absorbable sutures to similarly avoid compression of the donor vessel. The rationale behind the synangiosis procedure is that opening the arachnoid removes a barrier to the in-growth of new blood vessels into the brain and provides greater access of growth factors from the spinal fluid and brain to the donor vessel; the suturing of the donor vessel's adventitia to the pial surface insures that the donor vessel will remain in contact with the brain in areas where the arachnoid has been cleared, again, to promote the rapid ingrowth of new blood supply to the underlying brain.

The specific equipment needed for the procedure includes:

- Hand-held "pencil" Doppler probes—necessary for mapping the STA.
- Intraoperative microscope
- Powered drill (including footplate attachment)
- Microdissection instruments (including jeweler's forceps, micro-tying instruments, Vanass ophthalmic scissors, and a disposable arachnoid knife)
- Colorado tip electrocautery (a very fine tip for the monopolar cautery)
- Multiple #15 blades (for STA dissection)
- Papaverine

The operating room is then set up in a standardized fashion. The EEG tech is in the room with EEG monitors available for viewing. The microscope set for an assistant on the right side of the surgeon (assuming a right-handed surgeon) and is draped and ready from the onset of the case. The scrub is also on the surgeon's right. Immediate equipment is placed on mayo stands over the patient's torso. The microscope is positioned with the base to the left of the surgeon. The anesthesia team is to the surgeon's left or at the foot of the table.

The patient is then positioned. EEG electrodes are affixed in a standard array and the scalp is shaved over the expected course of the STA based on the angiogram. The parietal branch of the STA is mapped out using the Doppler probe and the skin is carefully marked with fine scratches from a sterile 22-gauge needle to outline its course from the distal end near the vertex to the root of the zygoma. The head is placed in pin fixation and the patient is positioned supine with the head turned parallel to the floor such that the STA site is level. Rolls are used as needed to reduce tension on the neck and the head is translated superior to the torso to facilitate venous drainage. The STA site is prepped; usually leaving the ear and face out of the field.

OPERATIVE APPROACH

Prior to incision, intravenous antibiotics are given. The microscope is employed from the onset of the case. No infiltration of the scalp with local anesthetic or epinephrine is used in order to avoid injury to the vessel.

Vessel Dissection

Using high magnification, a #15 blade is used to score the dermis at the distal end of the STA. A thin, curved pediatric hemostat and toothed Adson pickups are used by the surgeon (with suction and a second pickup by the assistant) to identify the STA under the skin. Using a repeated technique of subcutaneous dissection with the hemostat over the STA followed by elevation of the skin by the hemostat and an incision over the hemostat by the assistant, the STA is dissected along its length down to the root of the zygoma. Care must be taken to avoid tearing the vessel; particularly at tortuous bends or side branches. Irrigating bipolar (usually set at 25 with fine tips) is employed for hemostasis of small scalp vessels. A 0.05×3 cm Cottonoid is often useful to cover the exposed vessel to gently tamponade scalp bleeding as proximal dissection continues; electrocautery is used sparingly to control bleeding points along the incision line. A longer length of STA dissection is preferable (10 cm is optimal, although not always possible, especially in smaller children) (Fig. 61-1).

Following dissection of the STA branch, the "Colorado needle" electrocautery device (at low settings, usually one half to one third of the standard skin setting) is used in conjunction with the bipolar and microscissors to divide the galea and soft tissue on either side of the STA down to the temporalis fascia; leaving 1 to 2 mm of cuff on either side of the vessel. Two self-retaining retractors are then placed: one proximal and one distal. Dissection often terminates at the take-off of the frontal branch which should be preserved, if possible. However, if the bifurcation is high enough to

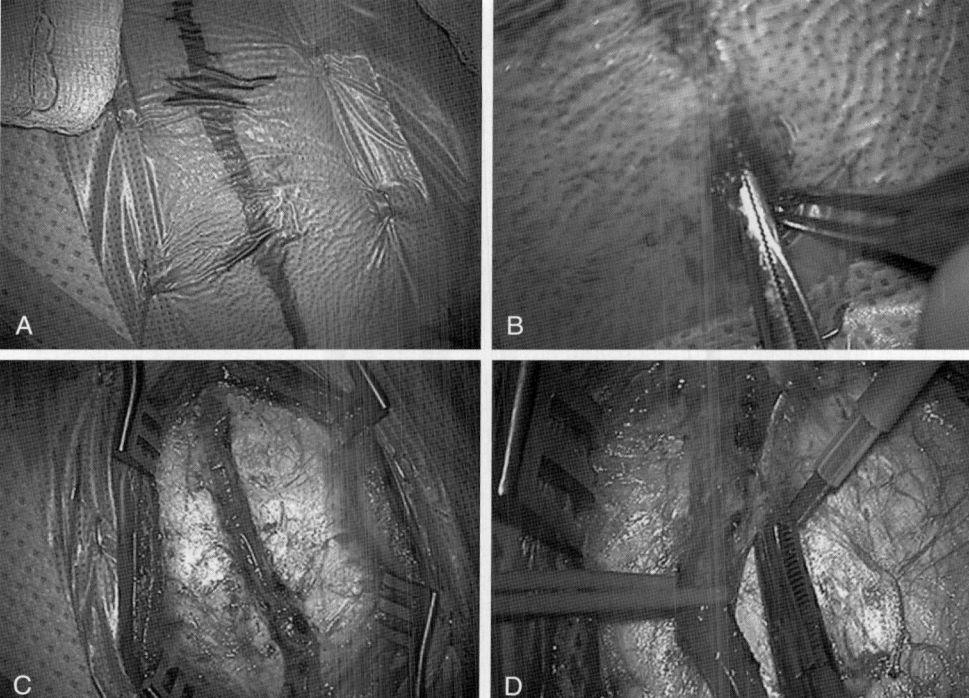

FIGURE 61-1 These images demonstrate the initial steps in performing a pial synangiosis. A, Course of the parietal branch of the STA marked out following Doppler mapping. B, Distal incision with subcutaneous dissection using a fine curved hemostat. C, Completed dissection of the STA branch prior to freeing up an adventitial cuff. D, Elevation of the STA with an associated adventitial cuff, using the monopolar cautery. Note that all of the surgery occurs under the microscope.

prohibit mobilization of the STA then the frontal branch of the STA often must be divided. The preoperative arteriogram will indicate whether the frontal branch provides any significant intracerebral collaterals that can be relevant to the decision to potentially sacrifice the branch. Following the dissection of the vessel, a vessel loop is placed under the distal end of the STA and used to elevate the dissected portion of the vessel from the temporalis muscle. Monopolar electrocautery is then used to free up connective tissue around and beneath the vascular pedicle.

Craniotomy

Once the STA is freed, the microscope is removed and scalp flaps are developed using the electrocautery to minimize bleeding: creating a subgaleal dissection plane anteriorly and posteriorly. The temporalis is then divided into quadrants with the electrocautery. The muscle is reflected from the bone (with use of the electrocautery) and held back with multiple Lone Star retractors (fish hooks). Two burr holes are made; one inferior and one superior, in the bony exposure at the proximal and distal sites of the STA over the exposed bone. Following dural dissection with a #3 Penfield, the footplate is then used to turn the widest possible craniotomy flap. Care must be taken to avoid injury to the vessel. This is usually best performed by the assistant protecting the vessel with retractor (Fig. 61-2).

Dural Opening

Review of the angiogram is helpful to attempt to avoid disrupting pre-existing dural collaterals. If the middle meningeal artery is providing an important source of collateral flow, it is kept intact and the dura is opened in two separate windows on either side. The dura is opened with a #15 blade; with the initial incision line along the axis of the donor vessel, with the opening extended into six

leaves of dura, three per side, retracted with 4-0 sutures. Small pieces of Gelfoam are placed between the retracted dura and craniotomy edge for hemostasis. Care is taken to minimize use of the bipolar on the dura in order to maximize collateral vessel development; although hemostasis is paramount in these patients. We avoid the use of thrombin after the dura is opened because of its demonstrated tendency to induce vasospasm in this patient population and all hemostatic substances such Gelfoam are from this point on in the operation moistened with saline solutions only.

Microsurgical Arachnoid Opening and Pial Synangiosis

Under the microscope, the arachnoid is opened widely; using the arachnoid knife, van Ness scissors, and jeweler's forceps. Bleeding is controlled with irrigation or small dots of Gelfoam. The donor vessel is laid on the brain surface in apposition to areas of open arachnoid. The adventitia of the donor vessel is sutured to the superficial pia of the subjacent cortex, using 10-0 nylon suture on a BV-75 needle using three knots per suture. Generally, at least three sutures are placed. Vasospasm, if seen, is treated with topical papaverine.

Closure

After synangiosis, the microscope is removed. The dural flaps are repositioned on the brain surface but not sutured. The entire craniotomy exposure is then covered with a large piece of Gelfoam soaked in saline. The burr holes on the bone flap are enlarged to facilitate entry and exit of the vessel (Fig. 61-3). The bone flap is replaced with small titanium plates (not over the burr holes) and the temporalis muscle is closed only vertically to prevent pressure on the entering and exiting STA. Galea is closed with interrupted 3-0 vicryls

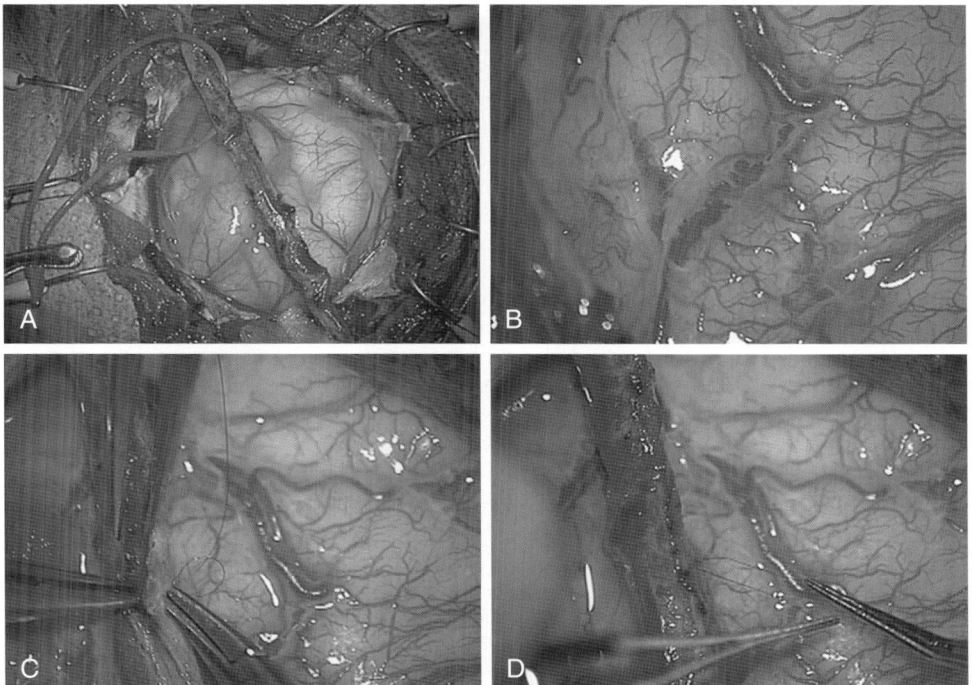

FIGURE 61-2 Intraoperative photographs documenting the steps of the craniotomy for pial synangiosis. A, Initial dural opening with stellate flaps and course of the STA. B, Arachnoidal opening, usually performed over vessels first, followed by subsequent opening over the cortex, if possible. C, Technique for placing 10-0 nylon stitch through pia and STA adventitial cuff. D, Completed suture, demonstrating good pial apposition to the vessel.

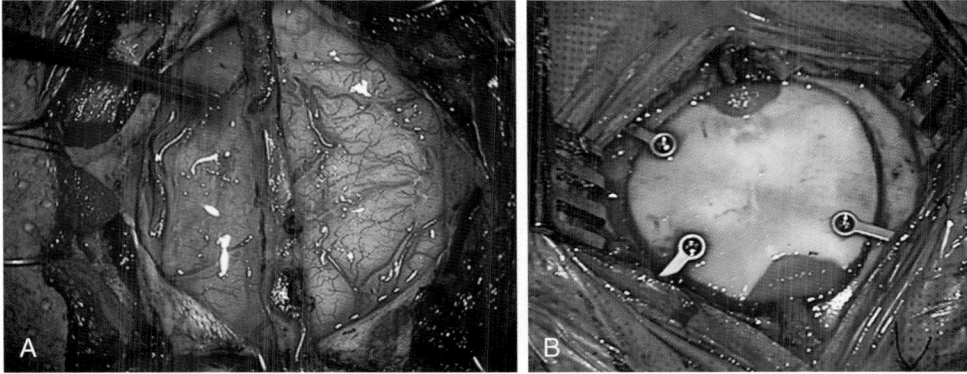

FIGURE 61-3 Images taken at the conclusion of pial synangiosis. A, Final view of syangiosis prior to folding dural flaps down and placing Gelfoam on site. Note the course of the artery, wide arachnoidal opening, and significant area of the brain exposed to facilitate collateral development. B, View following replacement of the craniotomy flap. It is important to leave tension-free entry and exit sites for the STA at the base and apex of the craniotomy.

(4-0 in smaller patients), taking care to avoid injuring the STA. Finally, the skin is closed with a running 4-0 rapide or other absorbable suture. Occasionally, EEG slowing will be noted with replacement of the bone flap. These usually resolve by adjusting anesthetic management or occasionally by briefly lifting the bone flap, followed by replacement of the bone.

Contralateral Side

If the EEG is stable and the contralateral side is affected, then the wound is dressed. The patient is repositioned and the same operation is performed on the contralateral side. Loss of CSF from the first operation may make arachnoid opening more difficult on the second side. As previously discussed, the dominant or most symptomatic side is generally done first so that if there are intraoperative events that preclude continuing with the second side; the most important hemisphere has been treated.

Complication Avoidance

The most significant postoperative complication in our series has been stroke, which in a series of 143 patients occurred at about 4% per operated hemisphere. Patients at the greatest risk appear to be those with neurologic instability around the time of surgery, those who have suffered a stroke within 1 month of the operation, or those with certain angiographic risk factors such as moyamoya disease in the posterior circulation. There have been two perioperative deaths related to ischemic stroke: one in a 5-year-old child operated on in the midst of a crescendo of strokes preoperatively and one in a 15-year-old boy with unusually fulminant disease with pre-existing basilar artery occlusion whose internal carotid artery—the sole supply of his posterior circulation—thrombosed following a unilateral operation. Other complications include four subdural hematomas requiring evacuation and two spinal fluid leaks.

Preoperative

As discussed in the preoperative section, careful management of moyamoya patients before they get to the OR can have a significant influence on complication avoidance. Patients, ideally, should be neurologically stable prior to surgery and at least 1 month out from any significant stroke. Patients must be medically optimized for surgery including prehydration, as described in our protocol (Table 61-1). Preoperative imaging is critical to planning vessel selection (the parietal branch of the STA may be small or absent, necessitating utilization of a frontal or retroauricular branch).

Intraoperative

Avoid hyperventilation and hypotension at all times, and remain aware of EEG slowing. Anesthetic efforts to restore normal physiology often improve EEG changes. Throughout the case, meticulous hemostasis is vital to prevent postoperative hemorrhage in the setting of ASA. Careful dissection of the STA is critical to avoid tears or avulsion of side branches. Cautery of side branches further out from the donor vessel helps to minimize risk of inadvertently injuring the graft. Attentive detail to the closure reduces the likelihood of a CSF leak.

Postoperative

Continue IV fluids at 1.5× maintenance for 48 to 72 hours until clearly taking enough liquids orally. Aggressive pain control is important to minimize blood pressure fluctuations and hyperventilation. Frequent and detailed neurologic examinations by nursing staff and physicians are critical to identify possible postoperative ischemia such that interventions can be instituted in an attempt to avoid progressing to a completed stroke.

Follow-Up

Careful follow-up of patients with moyamoya is warranted to monitor for disease progression and for response to therapy.[16,17] We routinely obtain MRI and MRA studies 6 months after surgery. Postoperative angiograms are usually obtained 12 months after surgery and typically demonstrate excellent MCA collateralization from both the donor STA and the meningeal arteries. A repeat MRI and MRA is done for comparison purposes and for a new baseline. For high-risk patients, MRI/A may be obtained in lieu of an angiogram if contrast from the angiogram presents a substantial risk to the kidneys. Generally, annual MRIs are obtained in all patients for 3 to 5 years after the initial 1-year angiogram and then spaced out subsequent to the 5-year time point. Particular attention must be paid to patients with unilateral moyamoya as the opposite side can progress in up to one third of patients, especially in children.[18] Patients are maintained on lifelong ASA therapy.

A review of 143 children with moyamoya syndrome treated with pial synangiosis had marked reductions in their stroke frequency after surgery especially after the first year postoperatively. In this group, 67% had strokes preoperatively and only 3.2% had strokes after at least 1 year of follow-up. The long-term results are excellent with a stroke rate of 4.3% (2 patients in 46) in patients with a minimum of 5 years of follow-up.[19] This work supports the premise that pial synangiosis provides a significant protective effect against new strokes in this patient population.

Conclusions

Moyamoya syndrome is an increasingly recognized entity associated with cerebral ischemia. Diagnosis is made on the basis of clinical and radiographic findings, including a characteristic stenosis of the internal carotid arteries in conjunction with abundant collateral vessel development. Treatment is predicated on revascularization of the ischemic brain which can be direct (STA-MCA bypass) or indirect (including pial synangiosis). The use of pial synangiosis is a safe, effective, and durable method of cerebral revascularization in moyamoya syndrome and should be considered as a primary treatment for moyamoya, especially in the pediatric population.

KEY REFERENCES

Dauser RC, Tuite GF, McCluggage CW. Dural inversion procedure for moyamoya disease. Technical note. *J Neurosurg.* 1997;86:719-723.

Fukui M. Guidelines for the diagnosis and treatment of spontaneous occlusion of the circle of Willis ("moyamoya" disease). Research Committee on Spontaneous Occlusion of the Circle of Willis (Moyamoya Disease) of the Ministry of Health and Welfare, Japan. *Clin Neurol Neurosurg.* 1997;99(suppl 2):S238-S240.

Fung LW, Thompson D, Ganesan V. Revascularisation surgery for paediatric moyamoya: a review of the literature. *Childs Nerv Syst.* 2005;21:358-364.

Houkin K, Kamiyama H, Abe H, et al. Surgical therapy for adult moyamoya disease. Can surgical revascularization prevent the recurrence of intracerebral hemorrhage? *Stroke.* 1996;27:1342-1346.

Houkin K, Kuroda S, Nakayama N. Cerebral revascularization for moyamoya disease in children. *Neurosurg Clin North Am.* 2001;12:575-584:ix.

Ikezaki K. Rational approach to treatment of moyamoya disease in childhood. *J Child Neurol.* 2000;15:350-356.

Isono M, Ishii K, Kobayashi H, et al. Effects of indirect bypass surgery for occlusive cerebrovascular diseases in adults. *J Clin Neurosci.* 2002;9:644-647.

Kawaguchi S, Okuno S, Sakaki T. Effect of direct arterial bypass on the prevention of future stroke in patients with the hemorrhagic variety of moyamoya disease. *J Neurosurg.* 2000;93:397-401.

Matsushima T, Inoue T, Ikezaki K, et al. Multiple combined indirect procedure for the surgical treatment of children with moyamoya disease. A comparison with single indirect anastomosis with direct anastomosis. *Neurosurgical Focus.* 1998;5:e4.

Matsushima T, Inoue T, Katsuta T, et al. An indirect revascularization method in the surgical treatment of moyamoya disease—various kinds of indirect procedures and a multiple combined indirect procedure. *Neurol Med Chir (Tokyo).* 1998;38(suppl):297-302.

Scott RM, Smith ER. Moyamoya disease and moyamoya syndrome. *N Engl J Med.* 2009;360:1226-1237.

Scott RM, Smith JL, Roberstson RL. Long-term outcome in children with moyamoya syndrome after cranial revascularization by pial synangiosis. *J Neurosurg Spine.* 2004;100:142-149.

Scott RM, Smith JL, Robertson RL, et al. Long-term outcome in children with moyamoya syndrome after cranial revascularization by pial synangiosis. *J Neurosurg.* 2004;100:142-149.

Sencer S, Poyanli A, Kiris T, et al. Recent experience with moyamoya disease in Turkey. *Eur Radiol.* 2000;10:569-572.

Smith ER, McClain CD, Heeney M, et al. Pial synangiosis in patients with moyamoya syndrome and sickle cell anemia: perioperative management and surgical outcome. *Neurosurg Focus.* 2009;26:E10.

Smith ER, Scott RM. Surgical management of moyamoya syndrome. *Skull Base.* 2005;15:15-26.

Smith ER, Scott RM. Progression of disease in unilateral moyamoya syndrome. *Neurosurg Focus.* 2008;24:E17.

Suzuki J, Takaku A. Cerebrovascular "moyamoya" disease: disease showing abnormal net-like vessels in base of brain. *Arch Neurol.* 1969;20:288-299.

Veeravagu A, Guzman R, Patil CG, et al. Moyamoya disease in pediatric patients: outcomes of neurosurgical interventions. *Neurosurg Focus.* 2008;24:E16.

Numbered references appear on Expert Consult.

CHAPTER 62

Management of Pediatric Severe Traumatic Brain Injury

JOTHAM MANWARING • P. DAVID ADELSON

Traumatic brain injury (TBI) still remains a leading cause of injury-related morbidity and mortality among the pediatric population of the United States. The impact on the individual child as well as the injured child's family provides a potent stimulus for improving management techniques within the neurosurgical community. While the exact financial cost of pediatric TBI to the family, society, and the medical system is not known, it has been estimated to be in excess of $35 billion annually in direct costs with additional indirect costs to the families of these children including lost wages, other nonmedical expenditures, and so on. It is known, however, that chronically disabled children require approximately four times the medical expenditures compared to their non-disabled cohorts.[1] This burden along with the relative lack of defined standards of care for pediatric TBI serves to create new methods for prevention and innovative intervention for pediatric neurotrauma.

Approximately 600,000 children in the United States visit the emergency department (ED) for TBI yearly and results in 60,000 hospitalizations and 7400 deaths per year. Children less than 4 years old visit the emergency department most frequently while adolescents more commonly are hospitalized and have the highest death rate of 24.3 per 100,000 secondary to TBI.[2,3] In those areas where it has been instituted, regionalization of pediatric trauma centers has taken a large step in reducing the morbidity and mortality of TBI among this population.[4] It has been demonstrated that injured children with moderate or severe TBI are more likely to undergo neurosurgical intervention and have improved outcomes when treated at a pediatric trauma center as opposed to adult trauma centers. With the likely future shortages in pediatric specialists, future steps to maintain and improve these outcomes may require regionalization to ensure volume and expertise.

This chapter will briefly review the past and present art of neurosurgical management of pediatric neurotrauma. Core topics will include diagnostic and management technologies, surgical guidelines and strategies, as well as adjuncts for optimization of care. The balance of the chapter will focus on the newest innovations in diagnosis, management, and surgical intervention as a means to stimulate forethought and creativity among the neurosurgical community toward optimizing outcomes among children who have incurred TBI.

Imaging in Pediatric Neurotrauma

Diagnostic imaging protocols and technology in the setting of acute pediatric TBI has received much attention in recent years. A general trend toward minimizing some imaging modalities, in particular the use of computed tomography (CT), has been due to concerns of potential delayed radiation injury.[4-6] In turn, the use of other modalities as well as the improvement in technology and further refinement of CT protocols have lessened the radiation exposure of these children yet still provide the requisite early, accurate, clinically significant information.

PLAIN RADIOGRAPHS

Plain skull films are rarely used today in pediatric trauma centers. While previously useful for evaluation of fractures, as well as for pneumocephalus, evaluation of bony fragments in depressed, comminuted fractures, and for evaluation of diastatic sutural fractures has been offset by CT, which provides soft tissue assessment as well as excellent cranial vault imaging especially with the more routine use of three-dimensional (3D) reconstruction algorithms. Today the role of the skull radiograph is used primarily as a map for identification of foreign bodies, or to document child abuse.[7] Plain films, however, still remain helpful to rule out spinal column injury while minimizing radiation exposure to the developing child that would come from a full-body, spine CT study. Since children more often suffer ligamentous injury, a screen with plain x-rays followed by magnetic resonance imaging (MRI) has provided an alternative to the radiation incurred with a full-body scan with mixed efficacy. If the child is awake and particularly uncomfortable due to either limitation to care in the intensive care unit setting or anxiety associated with wearing a rigid cervical collar, flexion/extension radiographs or dynamic fluoroscopic films may be used. Patients with diminished responsiveness are challenging, as actual clearance and collar removal requires radiologic in combination with clinical clearance, and thus there is little indication for cervical clearance in the early period in these patients. MRI for evaluation of ligamentous injury within the first 48 hours of the event can be performed if removal of the collar is necessary for the care of the patient, such as in operative intervention requiring manipulation of the neck. Unfortunately, MRI use has become increasingly popular as a screen, although it may be an unnecessary expense or risk due to frequent need for sedation and limited monitoring ability to obtain the requisite images. Based on extrapolation from recent studies in adult trauma patients, the risk of missing an occult unstable cervical injury in the teenage group with adequate prior static radiographs is less than 1%;[8-11] these data may not apply to the very young pediatric population. In pediatric spine injury, since there is a predominance of upper cervical and occipitocervical pathology in the younger pediatric population, we prefer imaging the cervical spine alone with CT including 3D reconstructions as necessary for initial radiologic clearance. Due to the low incidence of injury, the thoracic and lumbar spine can be imaged by plain radiograph unless a CT is desired for an area of pain or deformity, or the mechanism of injury is significantly violent, such as motor vehicle collision.

COMPUTED TOMOGRAPHY

For TBI, the noncontrasted axial head CT is the imaging modality of choice in pediatric neurotrauma. The scan can be performed very rapidly providing immediate information regarding cranial injury, intra- and extra-axial blood, fractures, ventriculomegaly associated with TBI, and to a less-specific degree, ischemia. The progression of intra- and extra-axial hemorrhagic lesions has been well documented. A repeat CT scan may be obtained within twelve hours if significant blood is present or there is a change in neurologic status. Data have failed to reconcile personal practice bias into standard protocols and practice regarding early repeat CT scanning. Repeat imaging should be conservatively considered given the "trauma" of transport and potential for worsening of hemodynamic instability. In adults, Oertel and colleagues evaluated 142 cases and described hemorrhagic progression by hematoma type as follows: 51% in parenchymal contusions, 22% in epidural hematomas, and 11% of subdural hematomas on 24-hour, follow-up CT scanning.[12] Unique to the pediatric population is the usual absence of anticoagulant use for comorbid conditions; this likely decreases the development of a delayed insult on CT from 85% to 31%.[13] These results can be applied to the pediatric TBI patient as a general guide in assessing the need for repeat CT evaluation.

Concern has been raised about the effect that ionizing radiation has on the immature central nervous system. Prediction models for the use of CT in mild TBI (Glasgow Coma Scale (GCS) 14 to 15) for the pediatric population have recently been investigated. The estimated rate of lethal malignancies from CT is 1 per 1000 to 1 per 5000 scans with increased risk with younger age.[4,5] Of 14,969 pediatric patients who underwent CT-scanning of the head for suspected TBI and met study parameters, 376 (0.9%) had clinically important TBI (defined as requiring acute intervention including neurosurgery), and only 60 (0.1%) underwent neurosurgery. The negative predictive value is 100% if the following criteria were met: (1) normal mental status, (2) no scalp hematoma except frontal, (3) no loss of consciousness or loss of consciousness for less than 5 seconds, (4) non-severe injury mechanism, (5) no palpable skull fracture, and (6) acting normally per parents. The negative predictive value is equivalent in children over 2 years of age with normal mental status, no loss of consciousness, no vomiting, no severe headache, no evidence of basilar skull fracture, and non-severe injury mechanism. It can be concluded from these data that CT scanning in the low risk TBI pediatric population may be avoided based on provider preference and likelihood of surgery.[6] Even in the higher risk categories, the authors' preference is not to repeat imaging unless there is consideration for a change in management strategy, that is, decision making for surgical intervention.

Recently there has been an increased utilization of the so-called "pan scan" including head, cervical spine, chest, abdomen, and pelvis. Tillou and colleagues reported on the effectiveness of the "pan CT scan" in an adult cohort indicating that if any study was omitted, from 311 CT scans, 17 injuries (5.4%) requiring immediate attention would have been missed.[14] We recommend caution and careful consideration of each patient's mechanism of injury, neurologic status, and age prior to undertaking a "pan scan" to limit the potential radiation exposure; however, this is determined in large part by trauma surgery. With the advent of "pediatric" protocols developed to lower the radiation load without compromising image quality, these studies, especially if limited to the head and cervical spine, can facilitate the care of the patient, reducing time in the radiology department and providing a wealth of information useful for clinical decision making.

MAGNETIC RESONANCE IMAGING

Magnetic resonance imaging in the pediatric trauma population is problematic primarily due to time constraints. The time for examination is significantly longer than the CT and frequently requires sedation in the young to ensure adequate image quality. If the patient is intubated in the field or on arrival to the ED, MRI becomes a more practical modality with extension of sedation, although the decision should be based on a specific question particularly as it relates to the cervical spine. In emergent and urgent settings, the potential benefits of subtler imaging seldom outweigh the screening achieved by CT alone for cranial trauma. This may differ in the cervical spine where bony abnormalities are less common and soft tissue injury may be better imaged by MR. Following the emergent acute phase, it must be recognized that certain implants such as intracranial pressure (ICP) sensors or cranial bolts have to be removed or disconnected to ensure safety from potential further injury or artifact,[15] such as inducible radio frequency heating, movement in the magnetic field leading to further parenchymal damage, or metallic artifact from skin staples, and thus, at this time MR in the acute setting has little efficacy.

In contrast, cervical spine or other spinal injury in a child is often best assessed by MR, although it is often impractical to image the entire spine in the acute setting. The initial screening of patients with clinical exam and CT usually provide a target area for more focused regional imaging. A patient with a spinal fracture and correlating neurologic findings can be better assessed for surgical pathology such as a hematoma or disc protrusion into the canal. As mentioned, since in children most often it is the extent of the ligamentous injury that is being evaluated, T2, FLAIR, or FIESTA sequences provide more information as to the extent of significant ligamentous injury, the potential for instability, and need for surgical intervention.

REMOTE IMAGING/TELEMEDICINE

With the advent of further regionalization for neurotrauma care, patients arriving with a variety of radiographic studies from the initial triage referring hospital is becoming more common. Often various proprietary image software packages for viewing the patient's studies can be encountered on a daily basis, leading to incompatibility and the need to repeat radiographic assessment in a vulnerable patient population. Teleradiology or the unification of systems under a single compatible program needs investigation to reduce costs and danger to the patient due to delayed intervention. Further, early communication from the primary emergency room to the trauma surgeon and neurosurgeon can commonly guide more appropriate selection of screening images and allow more expedient delivery of care upon arrival. Standardization in the "spokes and hub" model, where the receiving neurosurgeon has reviewed imaging studies remotely or from his office or home, can have substantial impact on timing from arrival to surgery for emergency craniotomies. Since shorter time from injury to surgery has been repeatedly shown to improve outcome dating back to the 1970s, efforts at broadening teleradiographic access along with regionalization of neurosurgical care/emergencies, particularly from rural areas, are likely to be more common in the near future.

Technology for Management of Intracranial Hypertension in Pediatric Head Trauma

The detection of intracranial hypertension and prompt treatment are typically the primary focus of the neurosurgeon. In those patients with moderate and severe TBI, the potential for intracranial hypertension or its evolution is sufficiently high enough that recommendations for monitoring have been established.[16] Despite these recommendations and algorithms for treatment as delineated in the pediatric guidelines, implementation and compliance in children remain modest except in tertiary academic and neurosurgical centers. While clearly ICP monitoring is not the optimal mode of understanding real-time neurophysiology, it is the most established and understood means of providing insight to the injured brain. Standard methods of ICP transduction are broadly available and frequently although inconsistently used, particularly in children. Keenan and Bratton[2] surprisingly reported in 2006 that only 33% of infants and young toddlers (<2 years of age) with severe TBI, defined as GCS score of less than 8, received ICP monitoring in the state of North Carolina. While newer monitoring systems, including efforts at noninvasive ICP monitoring, brain compliance monitoring, oximetry, local and regional cerebral blood flow, electroencephalography, and cerebrospinal fluid (CSF) biomarkers are emerging into protocols or research trials, their utilization is still infrequent and inconsistent from center to center. At a minimum, and despite the lack of a level I recommendation, the evaluation for increased ICP must be strongly considered in the setting of a GCS score ≤8. The overall assessment of the patient needs to be considered. As many patients arrive intubated, sedated, or with pharmacologic paralytics, careful examiner reassessment at post-CT scan screening and postresuscitation once medication has been metabolized, is essential to ensure that the data are consistent. Even in the setting of a "normal" CT, or in the infant with a normal head circumference and fontanel assessment, elevated ICP should still be considered in children. While a normal fontanelle does not indicate normal ICP, an elevated convex fontanelle most often does indicate ICP.

Three methods for monitoring ICP have been widely adopted:[1] the use of an inserted external ventricular drain (EVD) coupled with an adjustable drain bag and external saline column strain gauge;[2] parenchymal pressure sensors, which work by strain gauge or fiber optic methods; and[3] combination sensors integrating the transducer to the implanted EVD. Older technologies including epidural and subarachnoid sensors are rarely used due to concerns about accuracy. Among all of these, a key concern for accuracy rests on high-fidelity transduction of the ICP waveform with its systolic/diastolic peaks. If the waveform morphology cannot be discerned, accurate pressure transduction cannot be assumed. Further, the experienced neurosurgeon will observe in that waveform morphology features of risk for poor compliance, such as more vertical or rapid rise time or elevated P2 segment. Various commercial kits have been developed that simplify bedside placement of the EVD or ICP transducer. The authors use a combination of the EVD as a treatment modality with continuous CSF drainage and a concurrent strain gauge catheter for continuous monitoring of ICP (Fig. 62-1).

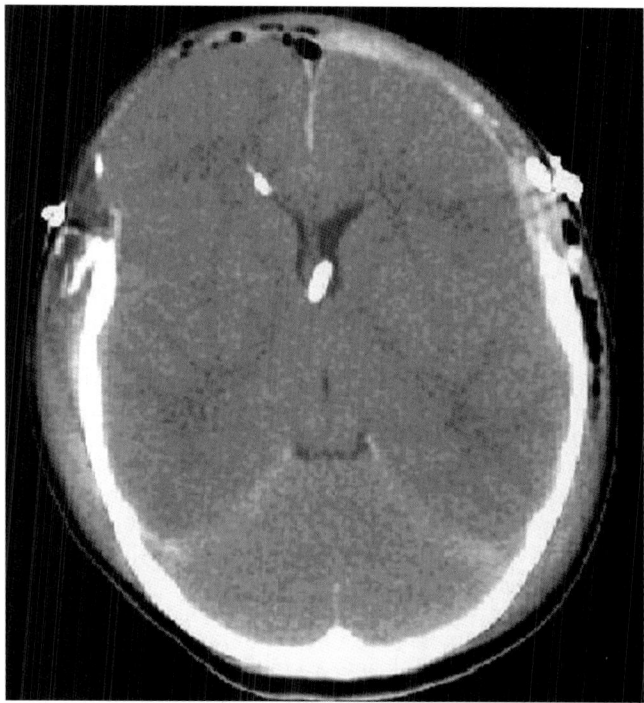

FIGURE 62-1 Five-year-old female as pedestrian hit by a motor vehicle with presenting GCS 3. EVD placement is noted at the left foramen of Monroe with ICP sensor placement in the deep white matter of the right frontal lobe. Decompressive bifrontal craniectomy with duraplasty was performed 12 hours post trauma due to rapid failure of medical management. Craniectomy led to immediate resolution of intractable ICP.

EXTERNAL VENTRICULAR DRAIN PLACEMENT

Many institutions have developed protocols to be followed when an EVD is inserted. The major potential risks of ventriculostomy placement are ventriculostomy-related infection (VRI) or insertional hemorrhage. A recent review of VRI indicated that a body of retrospective studies was limited by nonuniform definitions of infection versus colonization versus contamination. It lists, however, the rate of VRI from 0% to 22% among 23 studies with 5733 EVD insertions. The cumulative rate of positive cultures was 8.08% per EVD placed. With an earlier, more stringent definition of VRI in 1988, the incidence of VRI among the 5733 EVD insertions dropped to 6.1%.[17] Most studies have defined VRI as a single positive CSF culture obtained from the ventricular catheter or from CSF drawn via lumbar puncture. To limit this potential complication, prophylactic intravenous antibiotics or antibiotic impregnated catheters have been used. A controlled multicenter, prospective, randomized trial performed by Zabramski et al., showed striking results when antibiotic-impregnated catheters were used. In adult patients randomized to minocycline and rifampin-impregnated versus nonimpregnated drains, the rate of positive CSF cultures dropped from 9.4% to 1.3%, and the colonization rate of the drain dropped from 37% to 18%.[18] In contrast, another prospective, randomized, controlled trial in a single institution established equivalent infection rates among 116 patients comparing antibiotic-impregnated catheters to that of nonimpregnated drains with systemic antibiotics. These investigators concluded that impregnated catheters may diminish the cutaneous opportunistic infections associated with systemic antibiotics without tradeoff of VRI.[19] Technical aspects of insertion have been investigated; it has been showed that extended tunneling of the catheter has no effect on infection rate.[20] Risk factors for VRI development have been established in multiple reports, including subarachnoid hemorrhage (SAH), intraventricular hemorrhage (IVH), craniotomy, cranial fracture with CSF leak, ventriculostomy irrigation, concomitant systemic infection, and duration of placement.[21,22] Factors not associated with VRI include hydrocephalus, closed head trauma, tumor, CSF drainage, multiple catheters, and concomitant ICP sensors.[22] Most agree that sterile placement with some prophylactic antibiotic coverage whether impregnated or systemic can reduce the potential for VRI.

Less frequent risks of placement include malposition, hemorrhage, and neurologic injury. Almost all of the above studies were performed in the adult population. Generalization to the pediatric population seems appropriate but warrants further study. A recent retrospective study of 96 EVD placements in pediatric patients reported complication rates of infection (9.4%), malposition (6.3%), hemorrhage (4.2%), and obstruction (3.1%).[23] The senior author in a database of 147 consecutive EVD placements using nonantibiotic-impregnated catheters has had zero culture positive infections utilizing a culture screening protocol while the EVD was in place and prophylactic antibiotics with a second- or third-generation cephalosporin in each case (PD Adelson, unpublished data). As studies proceed in the future, we can expect that an optimal catheter, the ideal tunneling distance, the use of periprocedural antibiotics, and catheter indwelling time may be clarified.

MULTIMODALITY AND OTHER SENSOR TYPES

While there has been a lack of adjunct neuromonitoring use, advancing neurocritical care management is likely to have a multimodal approach to better understand the real time environment of the injured brain in the recovery phase. It is likely that no single modality will be the penultimate monitor to identify brain tissue at risk; meanwhile, the employment of numerous technologies in a multimodal approach may provide a broader understanding of brain function and risk in real time. Various multimodality EVDs and parenchymal sensors measuring blood flow, brain oxygenation, and so on have been developed as part of these new initiatives. Presently, the most utilized sensors and catheters are invasive and require operative placement. In general, while transduction from an EVD is considered the "gold standard," parenchymal sensing in the frontal white matter in the same trajectory appears equivalent. The advantage of the EVD, of course, is the ability to drain or divert CSF for control of intracranial hypertension as needed, either intermittently or continuously. The search for noninvasive ICP or compliance monitoring is ongoing. Various noninvasive pressure-monitoring methods are in preclinical and clinical trials and include tympanic-membrane displacement monitoring, retinal elevation and vascular change measurement, as well as transcranial acoustic transmission assessment. The most attractive aspect is its noninvasive nature and the ability to institute monitoring of brain function and physiology in the field and in triage. These devices must be shown to be as useful and as accurate as the inserted pressure sensor and EVD catheter, however.

In addition, indwelling sensors which incorporate temperature, pH, and pO2 measurements have become commercially available. Local tissue intraparenchymal oxygen sensors (LICOX, Integra Neuroscience) and regional noninvasive brain oxygen sensors using near-infrared technology (Foresite, CASmed, INVOS, Somanetics) are available and can be integrated into various monitoring protocols in an effort to further refine clinical decision making toward a better outcome. The LICOX oxygen sensor is placed through a bolt into the cranium, although free catheter placement is also possible (Fig. 62-2). Concerns as to its value have been raised due to the limited sensing of the surrounding area and the known regional effects of evolving brain edema, contusion, or traumatic infarction. Recent literature on both adult[24] and pediatric[25] patients, however, has shown the potential efficacy of this type of modality in conjunction with ICP/cerebral perfusion pressure (CPP)-directed therapy. While the transcutaneous near-infrared monitoring of frontal lobe oxygenation may be of limited benefit depending on the distribution of the regional insult, children more commonly suffer diffuse types of injuries, and at present, the potential to monitor one region with adequate generalizability is preferable to no monitoring. Preliminary data coupled with ICP monitoring is emerging. Although it is unclear at this time whether focal oxygenation is representative of global oxygenation in the damaged cerebrum, it is believed that it assists in the avoidance of second insults and further secondary injury. Similarly, the use of microdialysis and cerebral blood flow measurement may contribute in the future, although presently they are minimally utilized in only limited settings and have not been shown to be efficacious.

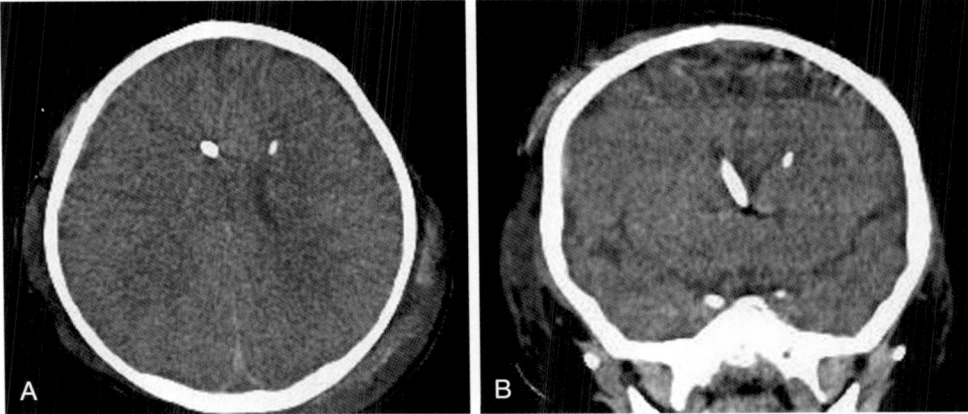

FIGURE 62-2 Placement of right frontal external ventricular drain and left frontal LICOX monitor in the setting of diffuse cerebral edema.

CURRENT PEDIATRIC ICP MANAGEMENT GUIDELINES

As mentioned earlier, the mainstay of evaluation for acute TBI is the neurologic examination and assignment of a GCS score, preferably reassessed during initial hours by the same clinician. After initial evaluation, the recommended "standard" management of acute severe TBI is at a minimum, ICP and CPP-based. If the GCS score is 8 or less, intubation and ventilation are warranted followed by emergency CT. Even if there is no recognized mass effect on CT or obvious injury at that time, the patient has the potential for elevated ICP or its emergence, and therefore ICP monitoring is undertaken. If an acceptable coagulation/platelet profile is present, and no other clear reason for the observed exam (e.g., intoxication or seizure) exists, an ICP sensor and/or EVD is placed preferentially on the nondominant side.

Once an ICP monitor is in place and there is an ICP elevation, first steps may include analgesia and sedation, head of bed elevation, and if an EVD has not yet been placed, insertion and CSF diversion. Within the first-tier therapies, further steps would then include paralytic agents, that is, vecuronium or cisatracurium. While a definitive time frame for paralysis duration has not been delineated, ICP normalization remains the goal of management. The next level of first-tier therapies for refractory ICP is hyperosmolar treatment with either hypertonic saline or mannitol, although these agents are and can be frequently used earlier in the introduction of therapy. Once continuous mild hyperventilation is required to temporize elevated ICP, first-tier therapy has failed and then second-tier therapy warrants consideration.

Repeat CT imaging may help to guide second-tier management and is dependent on the findings on the first scan and risk benefit of transporting a critically ill child to the scanner. The increasing use of portable CT scanners may help to obviate this concern. Focal mass lesions, especially with documented expansion, should be evacuated if deemed appropriate. If parenchymal swelling is unilateral or diffuse, the unilateral decompressive craniectomy (DC) or bifrontal craniectomy may be performed, respectively, and is discussed in more detail below. The addition of barbiturate therapy with escalation to 90% burst suppression, or moderate (32–34°C) hypothermia may also prove beneficial if all other measures fail[16] (Figs. 62-3 and 62-4).

Surgical Management of Pediatric Neurotrauma

Pediatric head trauma differs from adult brain injury in that the pediatric brain less often has an acute significant surgical lesion (i.e., epidural hematoma). In contrast, the pediatric brain post-TBI more frequently results in a diffuse type of response with resultant cytotoxic and vasogenic cerebral edema. This difference impacts surgical management of the pathophysiology in that acute unilateral evacuation of hematomas and decompression are infrequent especially relative to adult patients. As a result, most management to date has been medical with surgical interventions for hematomas less common. Similarly, in children decompressive craniectomy has not been as widely utilized as compared to adults. DC, a useful, albeit controversial intervention, has been shown to decrease mortality,[26-31] but is only at a class III level through a number of small case series and will likely have a more prominent role in the next edition of the Pediatric Guidelines.

One question is the timing (early vs. delayed) of surgical intervention after failed medical therapy as it relates to controlling elevated ICP. Survival benefit in many retrospective series of DC in children has been well-documented.[26-31] The results of a 10-year, single-institution retrospective study appear encouraging, in that survivors benefited from immediate postoperative ICP control (83%) with a 30% perioperative mortality rate. Eventually, 81% returned to school and 18% were dependent on a caregiver.[31] Further studies and particularly randomized controlled trials regarding early versus delayed treatment will hopefully refine indications and timing in the future.

While some have advocated early DC for certain subgroups without an acute surgical lesion, the literature currently supports instituting medical therapy first and only if secondary swelling due to regionalized cerebral edema with contusion, should a unilateral decompression be considered, especially if the source of swelling is not within the temporal lobes. As frontotemporal brain trauma is so common in the adult population, unilateral hemicraniectomy with emphasis on sufficiently low decompression of the temporal lobe is most frequently employed. In children, however, diffuse global cerebral edema is more commonly managed with bifrontal decompression. The Pediatric Guidelines provide

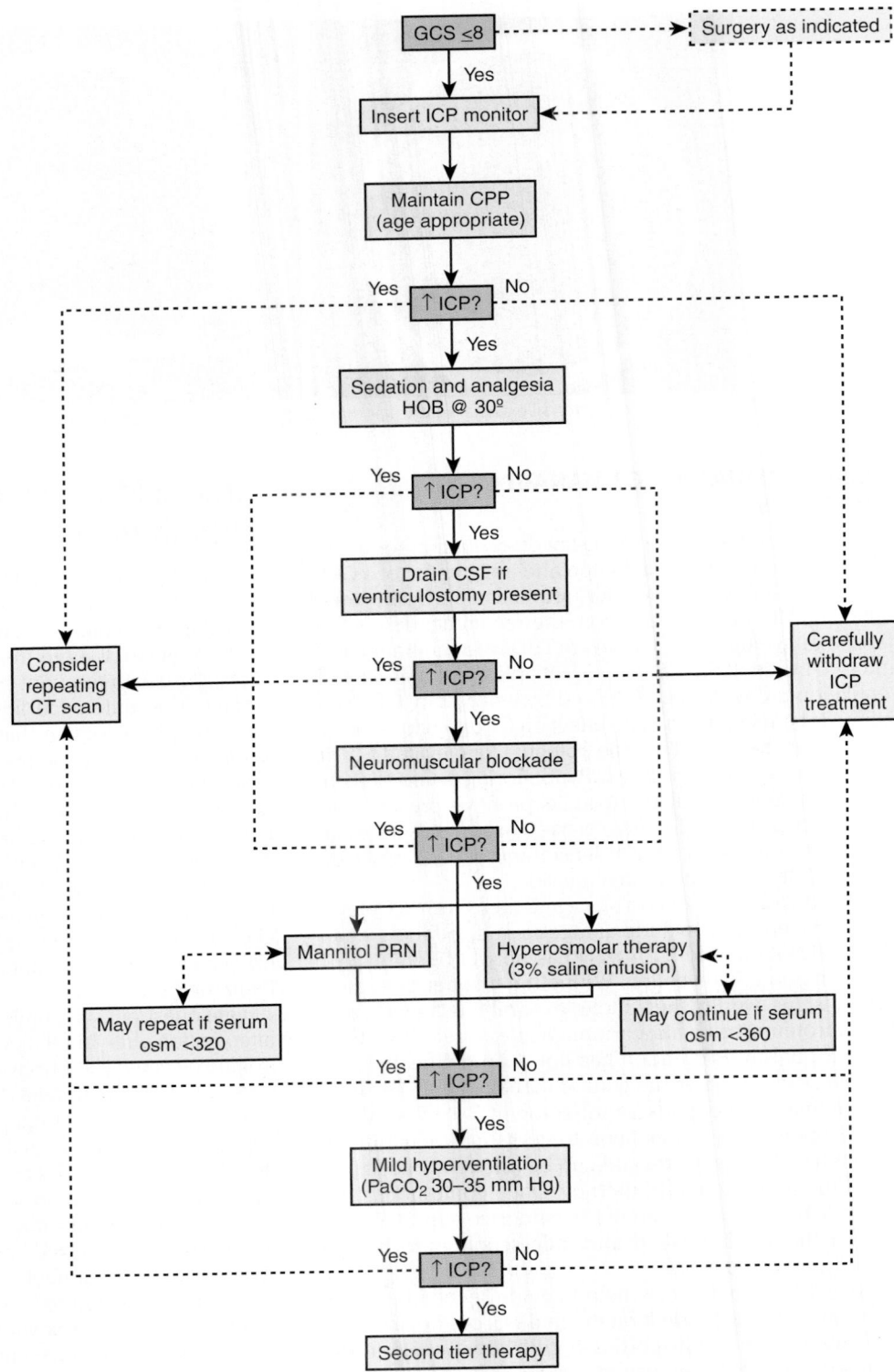

FIGURE 62-3 Clinical algorithm for first-tier therapy as a level-III recommendation from the Pediatric Guidelines. *(From Lozier AP, Sciacca RR, Romagnoli MF. Ventriculostomy-related infections: a critical review of the literature. Neurosurgery. 2002;51:170-182.)*

upper limits of utilization of medical therapy, that is, serum osmolality of 360 osm/ml when utilizing hypertonic saline, and burst suppression with pentobarbital. In the setting of rapidly failing first-tier and even second-tier therapy or the drift toward higher levels of therapies with diminishing efficacy, a DC should be considered as a next approach.

There are various techniques of hemicraniectomy and bifrontal craniectomy as described in an evolving, small literature, which for the most part, would seem fairly standard. If the patient presents with a surgical lesion requiring immediate surgical intervention for evacuation or hemostasis, the decision to leave the bone flap out is dependent on clinical judgment secondary to the intraoperative findings. The extent of damage, tightness of the dura/brain, etc. represents the degree of swelling, the physiologic state, and the expectation of secondary injury development. While

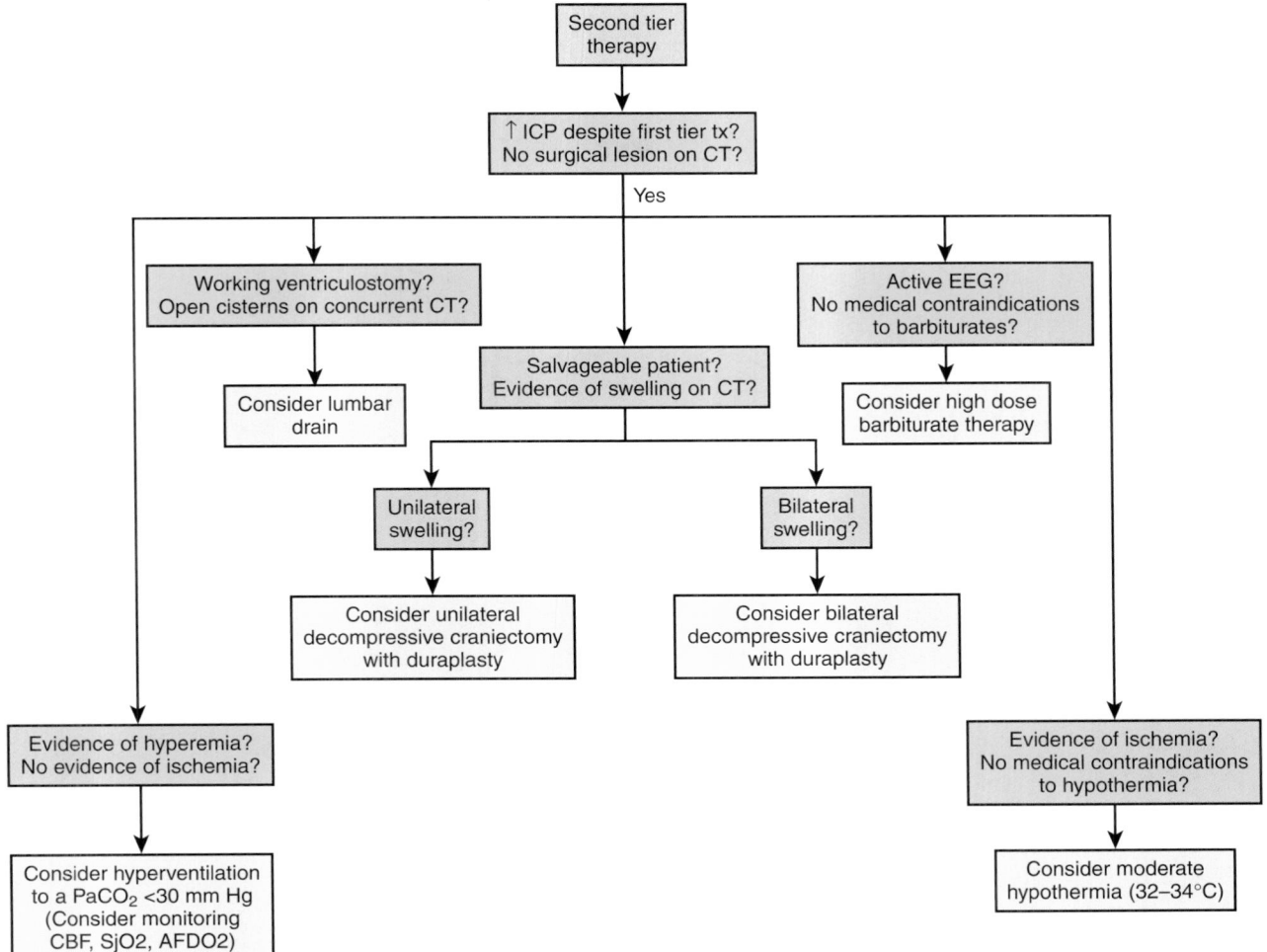

FIGURE 62-4 Clinical algorithm for second-tier therapy as a level-III recommendation from the Pediatric Guidelines. *(From Lozier AP, Sciacca RR, Romagnoli MF. Ventriculostomy-related infections: a critical review of the literature. Neurosurgery. 2002;51:170-182.)*

most techniques for DC emphasize width and breadth of decompression including low temporal exposure to allow for adequate swelling of the brain and avoidance of herniation, differences in technique include leaving midline bony and/or dural bridges, opening of the dura, inclusion of dural substitutes, dural substitutes and closure, incising across the superior and inferior sagittal sinuses and take down of the falx, storing or not of the bone flap, various types of storage (i.e., abdominal vs. freezer), and various methods for cranial reconstruction such as autologous graft, titanium mesh, or customized implants.

TECHNIQUE: DECOMPRESSIVE BIFRONTAL CRANIECTOMY

A curvilinear myocutaneous flap is created from the tragus of one ear to that of the contralateral ear with careful planning to remain behind the hairline, generally overlying the coronal sutures. The scalp is then incised to the level of the galea and reflected anteriorly carefully in an attempt to preserve continuity of the intact pericranium as a possible dural substitute. In children, burr holes can most easily be placed straddling the sagittal sinus, immediately posterior to the coronal suture at the bregma and paramedian supraglabellar. The cranial flap is then created with the foot-plate

craniotome as a bifrontal bone flap including generous margins into the temporal cranium, usually approximately 10 mm above the orbital rim, to adequately decompress the anterior and middle fossa. Extreme care should be taken when crossing the area of the superior sagittal sinus and bridging veins so as to avoid potentially catastrophic bleeding as well as taking bridging veins that then compromise adequate venous drainage of already compromised brain. Similarly, the frontal sinus needs to be taken into consideration in older children, as they usually become aerated beginning at 6 years of age.

Once the dura is exposed, preemptive planning is important in regard to brain swelling as well as risk of bleeding. The patient should likely have received maximal medical therapy with mannitol or hypertonic saline, and brief hyperventilation to ensure the lowest possible ICP when the durotomy is made. The senior author creates the durotomy along the frontal polar region and then carries the incisions posteriorly parallel along the lateral bone incisions creating a U-shaped dural flap hinged medially by the superior sagittal sinus. The most anterior midline incision includes suture and coagulation ligation of the superior sagittal sinus at its anterior origin from the ethmoidal emissary vein, and division of the falx to release the dura and accommodate greater frontal swelling.

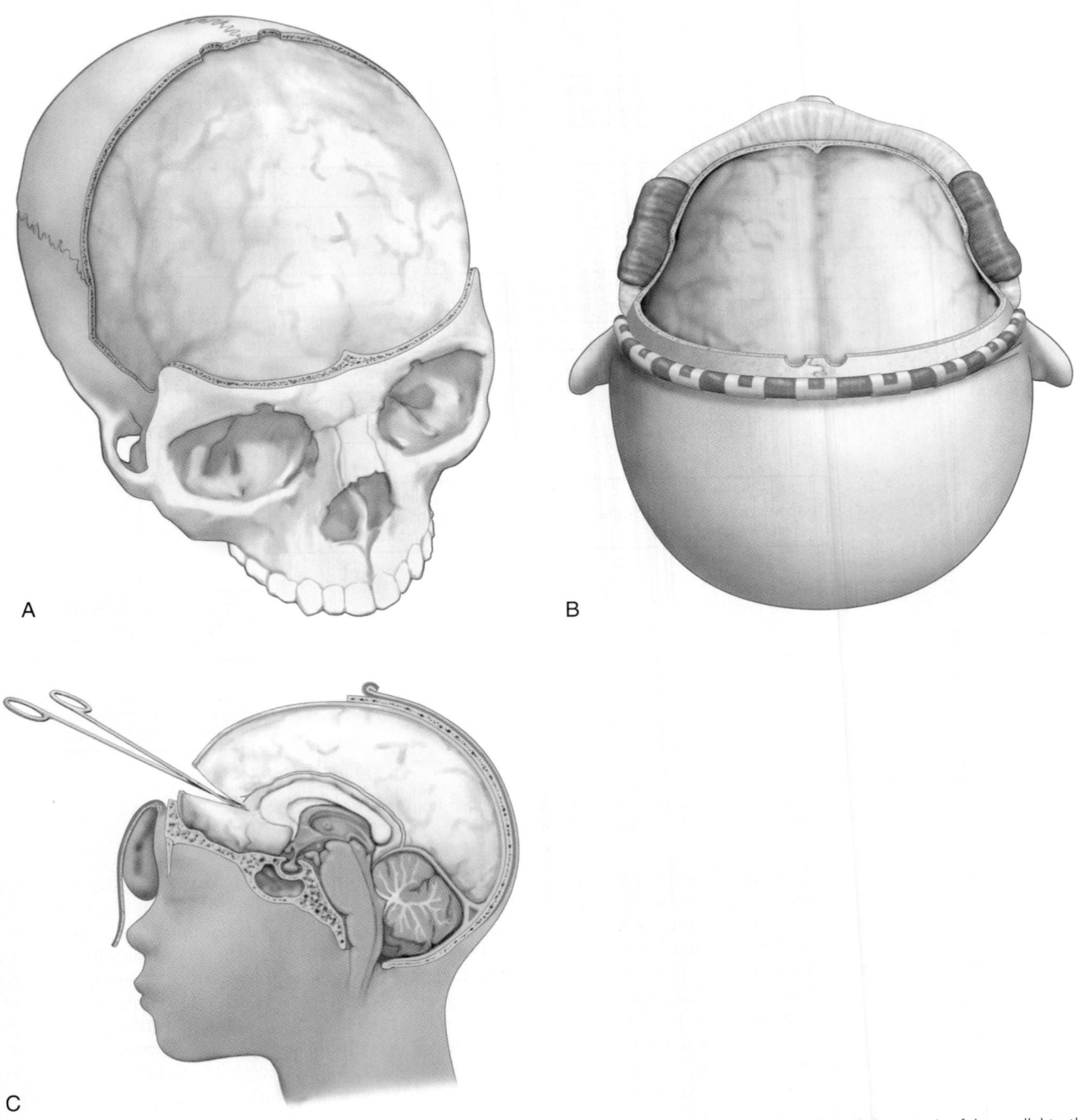

A

B

C

FIGURE 62-5 Depiction of bifrontal decompressive craniectomy with ligation of proximal sagital sinus and cutting of the anterior falx parallel to the frontal fossa base.

The flow volume at the origin of the sagittal sinus is minimal. The falx is incised parallel to the frontal fossa base and does not necessarily include the inferior sagittal sinus (Fig. 62-5). As mentioned, care should be exercised when handling bridging veins in this region to prevent stretching or tearing of the veins and resultant bleeding directly from the sinus. The pericranium can be harvested, trimmed into lenticular form, and grafted into the dural decompression site in watertight fashion or left as vascularized flap sutured in multiple locations for brain coverage. Alternatively, dural collagen substitutes can be cut to size and sutured to the dural margins for a watertight or coverage-only closure. Deep galeal stitches are followed by skin closure. A subgaleal drain may be employed as scalp serum and CSF leakage across the dural closure can contribute to constrictive tightness despite wide decompression, although the senior author does not use a drain to avoid creating a CSF fistula, preferring to drain CSF through an EVD. If an EVD is still necessary after the decompression has been performed, this can be placed easily with the use of ultrasound and then tunneled posteriorly over the bone edge.

The decision of how to store the flap depends on provider preference, facility limitations, the patient's infection status, and whether additional injury to the abdominal cavity occurred in the trauma. For bone that is to be stored, it is doubly packaged and labeled and stored in the hospital freezer. Another option, equally supported, is placement of the bone flap in the subcutaneous tissue of the abdomen in the epifascial plane above musculature, although this may be difficult in young children due to size constraints and whether abdominal injuries exist. In a setting of polytrauma that may necessitate laparotomy, storage in the subcutaneous abdominal tissue may create unnecessary difficulty and risk of infection secondary to repeated manipulation. In the absence of abdominal trauma, it may be preferable to divide the frontal cranium symmetrically into two portions through the metopic suture to avoid a curvilinear constraint in the abdominal wall.

TECHNIQUE: DECOMPRESSIVE HEMICRANIECTOMY

For the unilateral decompressive hemicraniectomy, the question mark incision or a large T-shaped incision can be employed with the goal of broad hemicranial exposure from anterior frontal cranium to posterior parietal cranium. The temporalis muscle must be elevated to allow low decompression of the temporal lobe and outward relief from uncal compression on the brain stem. The extent of the hemicraniectomy is important in that it is truly hemicranial as early literature highlighted frequent herniation/mushrooming of swollen brain at the craniotomy margin resulting in constriction of either venous outflow or arterial inflow extending parenchymal damage and furthering cerebral swelling. Once the craniectomy has been completed, the dura can be opened in a stellate fashion although any method can be used to allow broad swelling. Harvested pericranium or dural substitute can be sutured in place in watertight fashion or, at a minimum, for coverage. The bone is banked in similar fashion to the bilateral DC.

REPLACEMENT OF BONE FLAP

The bone is not replaced until the brain relaxation is sufficient. This allows replacement without exerting pressure upon the brain surface and is typically 4 to 6 weeks after head injury. This time frame also allows for adequate skin healing, improved nutrition, and freedom from systemic infection as well as assurance that there is no evidence of delayed post-traumatic hydrocephalus. Protective head gear may be necessary to shield the brain until replacement if the patient has recovered well and has begun the rehabilitation process. If only a few months have passed, banked bone can commonly be replaced utilizing sutures or permanent or absorbable plates (Fig. 62-6). In the latter instance, it is essential to obtain a follow-up CT scan 6 months later to ensure the expected healing and fixation. If banked bone is not suitable or was discarded, an excellent alternative material is titanium mesh, which can be shaped to an acceptable conforming calvarial contour on the surgical field and may be coated with a bone substitute as a matrix for bone reconstitution if desired (Fig. 62-7). In the instance of extensive replacement or reconstruction of a cosmetically sensitive area, computer-generated, customized synthetic materials or titanium are available.

POTENTIAL COMPLICATIONS OF CRANIAL DEFECT REPAIR

Complications of cranial defect repair can include infection, poor fit or contour matching, dislodgement, excessive constraint upon the underlying dura and brain, and CSF leak across a durotomy. In the setting of autologous bone flap replacement, bone resorption is an additional, undesirable outcome. Each is generally avoidable by careful planning and attention to detail at the time of replacement. Given the generally less than optimal medical condition of the post trauma patient, ensuring optimal timing, absence of systemic infection, well-healed incision, and adequate nutritional state is crucial. Furthermore, it is sometimes beneficial to involve plastic surgery, especially when scalp viability is tenuous.

Considerations for Temperature Regulation in Optimizing Outcome

HYPERPYREXIA

Cerebral metabolism is known to increase in the setting of fever. It is also known that the autoregulatory capacity of the prearteriolar sphincter is overcome in TBI causing mismatch of cerebral blood flow and the oxygen requirement of brain. In order to prevent secondary insults and further secondary injury due to this mismatch, fever should be aggressively treated with antipyretics and cooling blankets. Most studies of temperature regulation in TBI were performed in adults and have established that fever is a negative predictor of outcome.[32] Attempts at therapeutic intervention for fever include newer methods of localized cooling, specifically to the head. One such device delivers vaporized substances to the nasal cavity creating a cerebral cooling effect. Intravenous cooling devices are likewise in use and provide very reliable cooling but are plagued by complications (e.g., deep vein thrombosis) and not likely efficacious in young children due to the large bore size of the catheters placed in the femoral vein. It should be stressed that, prior to initiating any treatment modalities aimed at cooling, a febrile patient must be worked up for potential infectious etiologies and treated appropriately.

HYPOTHERMIA

Hypothermia for neurotrauma has been considered as a therapeutic option for quite some time. One of the first TBI studies in the modern era focused on moderate hypothermia as a neuroprotective management strategy in TBI[33] and showed initial positive results in a single-institution trial. Nevertheless, these results were not substantiated by a multicenter, prospective, randomized, controlled trial performed by Clifton et al.[34] Despite inconsistent results, it appears that with early cooling, younger patients did trend toward better outcomes than adults. Still, the level III recommendations in Adult Guidelines for the use of hypothermia in adults with TBI was based on a meta-analysis of eight randomized controlled trials ($n = 781$) that showed a deceased mortality and improved global function (relative risk [RR] = 0.51) with hypothermia at the possible expense of increased risk for pneumonia (RR = 2.37). They also concluded that the neurologic outcome was more likely to be

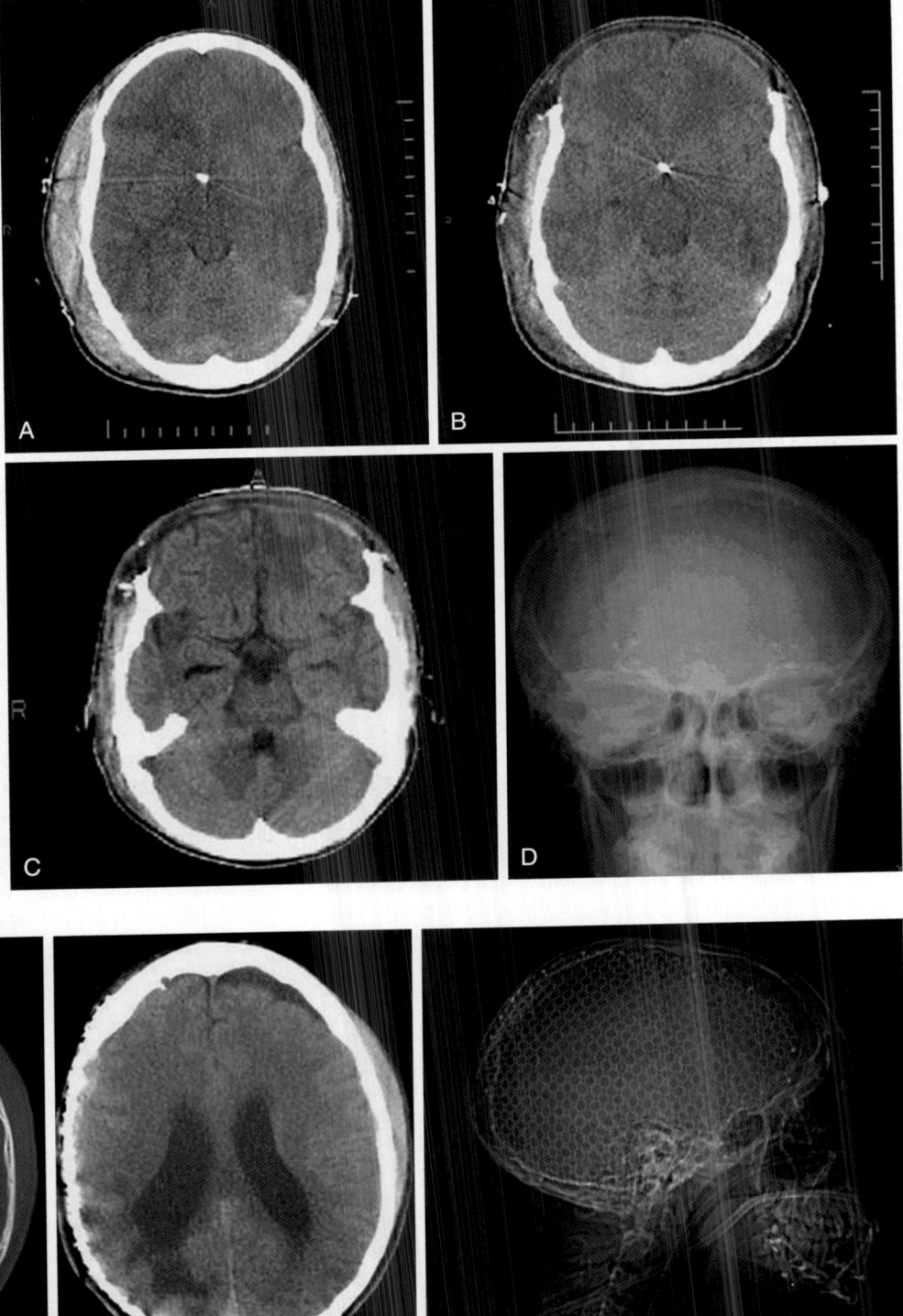

FIGURE 62-6 A, Fourteen-year-old male victim of auto-versus-pedestrian accident. Intracranial pressure became recalcitrant to medical therapy over the first 12 to 18 hours after admission. Given the absence of any localizing lesion, the patient was taken to the operating room for a bifrontal decompressive craniectomy. B, Postoperative image showing adequate frontal decompression and diffuse swelling. Patient's ICP was well controlled and medical therapy was successfully weaned. C, Screening CT in advance of reconstruction. The child was doing well in rehabilitation beginning to regain function. D, Postoperative x-ray showing replacement of bone flap 6 weeks following operative decompression.

FIGURE 62-7 CT and x-ray imaging of preformed titanium mesh cranioplasty after decompressive hemicraniectomy. The bone flap was discarded due to multiple comminuted fractures.

favorable (RR = 1.91) if hypothermia was maintained for at least 48 hours.[35] The best times for initiation and total duration of treatment have not been established.

In the 2003 Pediatric TBI Guidelines, Adelson et al.[16] again highlighted a lack of clinical trials specifically addressing hypothermia in children but there was a level III recommendation for the use of hypothermia as a second-tier therapy. Biswas et al. noted in a single-institution, randomized study that moderate hypothermia significantly decreased intracranial hypertension.[37] More recently, a phase II clinical trial of moderate hypothermia after severe TBI by the senior author (PDA) showed no significant increase in complications including arrhythmias, infection, or coagulopathy[36] and preliminarily showed improved mortality and global functional outcome. A phase-III, multicenter, international randomized controlled trial of a moderate hypothermia protocol (32.5 ± 0.5°C) initiated within 8 hours and continued for 24 hours among children and adolescents actually showed a trend toward worsened mortality at 6 months and possibly increased morbidity. There has been some criticism of the study due to issues with the screening process that may have included sicker patients in the hypothermia treatment arm (higher number of GCS 3)[38,39] as well as increased hypotension and hypoxia in the hypothermia study arm, lack of uniform clinical management (ICP monitoring was not required), variability of time to initiation of cooling, and a significant number of children lost to follow-up. The protocol also included rapid rewarming of 0.5°C every 2 hours paralleled by significant increases in ICP. These results substantiated the findings of Adelson et al., (2005) who found a significant decrease in ICP during cooling but rebound intracranial hypertension with rewarming.[36] Recognizing the potential for worsened secondary injury with rapid rewarming, more recent methodology includes a much slower rewarming of 0.5°C to 1.0°C every 12 to 24 hours. Using this methodology, the Pediatric Traumatic Brain Injury Consortium: Hypothermia or the "CoolKids Trial," was initiated as a phase-III trial investigating moderate hypothermia (32°C to 33°C) beginning within 6 hours of injury and maintained for 48 hours with a slow rewarm for children to evaluate efficacy versus mortality. This trial includes the less than 18-year-old age group with postresuscitation GCS scores of 4 to 8, who appeared to derive improved mortality benefits from moderate hypothermia.

Treatment strategies using hypothermia among the pediatric TBI population are being developed as further clinical trials proceed. Multiple methods for whole-body versus localized cerebral cooling have been developed and continue in experimental phases. These include widely varying methods such as intranasal selective cooling, transarterial or transvenous endovascular cooling, extraluminal vascular cooling, epidural cerebral cooling, and surface cooling.

Conclusion

The pediatric brain in the acute setting, similar although different from the adult, undergoes a multitude of complex pathophysiologic processes following TBI. The present-day goal of management is to provide an environment for recovery that includes lessening secondary insults and minimizing the impact of the secondary injury. At present, the armamentarium for treatment of acute TBI in children is limited, although the Pediatric Guidelines have spawned a number of studies that the revised edition now in preparation will hopefully begin to address. Most important is the development of a clinical algorithm that helps to improve communication and consistent management within a given critical care unit based on the Pediatric Guidelines. While there are a number

of recommendations in the guidelines, a well-defined clinical pathway can be developed that provides a clear communication amongst the critical care team as to the necessity and timing of these approaches. Once maximal medical therapy has been reached or medical therapy is failing, surgical intervention should be considered that is initially focused on the acute evacuation of intracranial mass lesions, and then secondarily on management of intracranial hypertension as there is growing evidence as to the potential efficacy of decompression. The timing of early versus late decompression is being investigated but aggressive use still needs to be addressed, and the risk benefit needs to be considered.

ACKNOWLEDGMENT

Medical illustrations were drafted and refined by Dr. Shih Liu, USF Department of Neurosurgery.

KEY REFERENCES

Adelson PD, Ragheb J, Kanev P, et al. Phase II clinical trial of moderate hypothermia after severe traumatic brain injury in children. *Neurosurgery.* 2005;56:740-754:discussion 740–754.

Adelson PD, Bratton SL, Carney NA, et al. Chapter 17. Critical pathway for the treatment of established intracranial hypertension in pediatric traumatic brain injury. *Pediatr Crit Care Med.* 2003;4(Suppl 3):S65-S67.

Biswas AK, Bruce DA, Sklar FH, et al. Treatment of acute traumatic brain injury in children with moderate hypothermia improves intracranial hypertension. *Crit Care Med.* 2002;30:2742-2751.

Bota DP, Lefranc F, Vilallobos HR, et al. Ventriculostomy-related infections in critically ill patients: a 6-year experience. *J Neurosurg.* 2005;103:468-472.

Brenner DJ. Estimating cancer risks from pediatric CT: going from the qualitative to the quantitative. *Pediatr Radiol.* 2002;32:228-231.

Clifton GL, Miller ER, Choi SC, et al. Lack of effect of induction of hypothermia after acute brain injury. *N Engl J Med.* 2001;344:556-563.

Figaji AA, Fieggen AG, Argent AC. Intracranial pressure and cerebral oxygenation changes after decompressive craniectomy in children with severe traumatic brain injury. *Acta Neurochir Suppl.* 2008;102:77-80.

Figaji A A, Fieggen AG, Peter JC. Early decompressive craniotomy in children with severe traumatic brain injury. *Childs Nerv Syst.* 2003;19:666-673.

Harris OA, Moure FC, Chappell ET. Use of modified EAST practice parameters in clearing the cervical spine in the obtunded trauma patient: a prospective study. *J Neurosurg.* 2001;94:413A-414A.

Hutchinson PJ, Kirkpatrick PJ. Decompressive craniectomy in head injury. *Curr Opin Crit Care.* 2004;10:101-104.

Hutchison JS, Ward R, Lacroix J, et al. Hypothermia therapy after traumatic brain injury in children. *N Engl J Med.* 2008;358:2447-2456.

Jagannathan J, Okonkwo DO, Dumont AS. Outcome following decompressive craniectomy in children with severe traumatic brain injury: a 10-year single-center experience with long-term follow-up. *J Neurosurg Pediatr.* 2007;106(4):268-275.

Keenan HT, Bratton SL. Epidemiology and outcomes of pediatric traumatic brain injury. *Dev Neurosci.* 2006;28(4-5):256-263.

Lozier AP, Sciacca RR, Romagnoli MF. Ventriculostomy-related infections: a critical review of the literature. *Neurosurgery.* 2002;51:170-182.

Lozier AP, Sciacca RR, Romagnoli MF, et al. Ventriculostomy-related infections: a critical review of the literature. *Neurosurgery.* 2002;51(1):170-181:discussion 181–182.

Marciano FF, Apostolides PJ, Vishteh AG, et al. Cervical spine management in severe, nonpenetrating closed head injury: a prospective study. *Neurosurgery.* 1997;41:740-741.

Ngo QN, Ranger A, Singh RN, et al. External ventricular drains in pediatric patients. *Pediatr Crit Care Med.* 2009;10(3):346-351.

Oertel M, Kelly DF, McArthur D, et al. Progressive hemorrhage after head trauma: predictors and consequences of the evolving injury. *J Neurosurg.* 1980;96:109-116.

Peterson K, Carson S, Carney N. Hypothermia treatment for traumatic brain injury: a systematic review and meta-analysis. *J Neurotrauma.* 2008;25:62-71.

Ruf B, Heckmann M, Schroth I, et al. Early decompressive craniectomy and duraplasty for refractory intracranial hypertension in children: results of a pilot study. *Crit Care.* 2003;7:133-138.

Rutigliano D, Egnor MR, Priebe CJ, et al. Decompressive craniectomy in pediatric patients with traumatic brain injury with intractable elevated intracranial pressure. *J Pediatr Surg.* 2006;41:83-87.

Stiefel MF, Spiotta A, Gracias VH, et al. Reduced mortality rate in patients with severe traumatic brain injury treated with brain tissue oxygen monitoring. *J Neurosurg.* 2005;103(5):805-811.

Tillou A, Gupta M, Baraff LJ, et al. Is the use of pan-computed tomography for blunt trauma justified? A prospective evaluation. *J Trauma.* 2009;67(4):779-787.

Wong GK, Poon WS, Ng SC, et al. The impact of ventricular catheter impregnated with antimicrobial agents on infections in patients with ventricular catheter: interim report. *Acta Neurochir Suppl.* 2008; 102:53-55.

Zabramski JM, Whiting D, Darouiche RO, et al. Efficacy of antimicrobial-impregnated external ventricular drain catheters: a prospective, randomized, controlled trial. *J Neurosurg.* 2003;98(4):725-730.

Numbered references appear on Expert Consult.

CHAPTER 63

Contemporary Dorsal Rhizotomy Surgery for the Treatment of Spasticity in Childhood

DONIEL DRAZIN • KURTIS AUGUSTE • MOISE DANIELPOUR

Cerebral palsy is a movement disorder resulting from an insult to the immature brain. As a result of the cerebral lesion, there are peripheral motor manifestations such as muscle contractures and joint deformities. Traditionally the contractures and joint abnormalities have been dealt with by physical therapists and orthopedic surgeons. Yet, their success has been limited as they have not addressed the primary pathology. Because the primary pathology is within the nervous system, neurosurgeons have attempted to treat the disorder closer to its source. Although there are many abnormal features associated with cerebral palsy, spasticity has been the only one accessible to neurosurgical techniques. As survival rates have improved among very low birth-weight infants, the incidence of cerebral palsy has increased to 1 in every 500 live births. Currently, cerebral palsy is estimated to affect 500,000 people in the United States alone.[1]

Spasticity is characterized by a velocity-dependent increase in tonic stretch reflexes with exaggerated tendon jerks resulting from hyperexcitability of the stretch reflex.[2] It is recognized by its characteristic "clasp-knife" quality during passive limb motion. Although over the past several decades, a variety of treatments have been developed for reduction of spasticity, more recently selective dorsal rhizotomy has been widely and successfully used in treatment of spastic cerebral palsy. Here we describe the operative technique for selective dorsal root rhizotomy.

History of Selective Posterior Rhizotomy

Sherrington in his classic studies on the neurophysiologic basis of muscle tone and spasticity, divided the brain stem from the spinal cord in cats and found that they became spastic. He then opened the spinal canal, cut the posterior rootlets and the spasticity was abolished.[3]

This work was applied to humans by Foerster in 1905, when he first performed the dorsal (sensory) rhizotomy in four patients. Subsequently, in 1913, he expanded his use of the dorsal rhizotomy to 159 patients.[4] Foerster used electrical stimulation during the surgery to identify the level of the nerve roots. He described division of whole posterior nerve roots from L2 to S2, with sparing of L4 and L3 sensory roots to preserve sensation and quadriceps tone for standing.

Although he was able to relieve spasticity, the dorsal rhizotomy was not widely used for the next 60 years.

In 1967, Gros[5] modified the technique to a partial posterior rhizotomy by saving one or two rootlets in each root to safeguard proprioception. Gros demonstrated that his more conservative procedure resulted in the same beneficial reduction of spasticity. Gros's "partial cutting" procedure, however, did not adequately predict and target which muscles would be affected by the surgery. To improve the outcomes, Gros's associates subsequently made adjustments to the rhizotomy procedure.

In 1972, Sindou published anatomic documentation of the location of the 1A sensory fibers of nerve roots (believed to be responsible for spasticity) where they entered the spinal cord.[6] In 1975, based on the Sindou thesis, Fraioli and Guidetti further modified the rhizotomy to sever these 1A sensory fibers and preserve other sensory fibers.[7] In 1977, Fraioli and Guidetti[7] modified the technique to a hemisection of nerve rootlets.

Fasano and colleagues published a method of selective posterior rhizotomy based on electromyographic responses to electrical stimulation.[10,11] Working at the level of the conus, they stimulated the dorsal spinal rootlets at increasing frequencies while recording the responses in corresponding anterior roots and muscles. This intervention, the "functional dorsal rhizotomy," widened understanding of abnormal responses and identified which rootlets should be cut. This system of identification and selective cutting to preserve proprioceptive sensation remains the basis of current surgical rhizotomy procedures.

Operation at the level of the conus medullaris made identification of the lower sacral rootlets involved in bowel and bladder function difficult. In 1981, Peacock modified the procedure by shifting the site of surgery from the conus medullaris region used by Fasano to the cauda equina region.[12,13] This shift allowed for easier identification and preservation of both the S3 and S4 nerve roots, as well as separation of individual rootlets of the ventral and dorsal roots. In a consecutive series of 105 children with spastic cerebral palsy who underwent selective dorsal rhizotomy, wound infection, cerebrospinal fluid leak, hemorrhage, and bowel or bladder disturbance were absent.[14] In a 20-year follow-up of his original series from Cape Town, 60 patients were shown to have maintained a decrease in muscle tone, increased range of motion, and improved function, including gait.[15]

Selective dorsal rhizotomy has proven to be a safe and effective procedure for treatment of spasticity, with long lasting results when performed in a methodical and careful fashion.[14,15]

Patient Selection

Proper patient selection is critical to the desired reduction of spasticity from selective dorsal rhizotomy. First, spasticity must be confirmed and differentiated from other abnormal movement patterns or dystonia.[16] Next all of the factors affecting the child's motor function should be identified and the role of spasticity considered in the overall motor disability. A team approach to evaluation and treatment is used involving a pediatric neurosurgeon, physical therapist, orthopedic surgeon, physiatrist, pediatric neurologist, and developmental pediatrician.

Patients are first screened to rule out those with dystonic disorders. The majority of children with cerebral palsy who are purely spastic have a history of prematurity with or without intraventricular hemorrhage. Those who suffered a traumatic or anoxic injury at a later stage are more likely rigid and therefore less likely to benefit from rhizotomy. Progressive and degenerative disorders, such as a progressive encephalopathy should also be ruled out. Development milestones are documented, as are the child's current motor function, equipment needs, therapy program, and orthopedic deformities. The goals of the patient and family are discussed and realistic expectations are set.

The neurologic examination begins with evaluation of muscle tone and range of motion. Velocity-dependent resistance to passive motion, brisk tendon reflexes, clonus, and clasp-knife phenomenon are all hallmarks of spasticity. Some children with spastic cerebral palsy will have relatively normal tone at rest, but their tone increases with activity highlighting the importance of observing these patients in motion, especially walking, if possible.

Spasticity can also mask underlying motor weakness or poor control of trunk muscles. The child's unsupported sitting posture is observed. Inability to sit upright can indicate weakness of the trunk muscles. The child's reaction to disturbances of equilibrium while sitting are also noted. Only then is antigravity control of the trunk and lower extremities best evaluated. The child's ability to control body weight while standing upright and with unilateral standing is assessed. Evaluation of flexion and extension ability at the hip, knee, and ankle in unilateral standing is also a useful estimate of motor strength.[16]

Children with dystonia are relatively poor surgical candidates, unless spasticity is severe and only mild signs of dystonia are present. Because selective posterior rhizotomy does not address dystonia, it is important to differentiate it from true spasticity. More severe dystonia can be associated with rotatory movements around the axis of both upper and lower limbs, facial grimacing and dysarthria.

Orthopedic examination is performed and appropriate radiographs of the hip and spine are obtained. Range of motion is assessed and any limitations of hip abduction, the popliteal angle, and ankle dorsiflexion are documented. Hip and knee flexion contractures, increased hip internal rotation, and abnormal posture of the foot and ankle are common and need to be assessed. In instances where significant structural deformity is present, input from the orthopedic surgeon is used to determine whether corrective surgery is required before, after, or instead of rhizotomy.

In summary, the children who are appropriate candidates for selective dorsal rhizotomy fall into two groups, severely affected quadriplegic patients with little or no independent function and spastic diplegic children who are walking, with or without support. In the first group of children, the goals of surgery are improved comfort, positioning, and ease of positioning and transport by the caregiver. In spastic diplegics the goal of surgery is improving functional skills including gait and decreasing the risk of developing flexion contractures with the need for orthopedic intervention. Ambulatory patients who have poor trunk control, or poor lower extremity antigravity control, are poor surgical candidates. They are unlikely to have significant benefit from this procedure. The ideal candidates are spastic diplegic children between 4 to 6 years of age who walk independently but with an abnormal gait pattern (due to excessive hip adduction, a flexed hip and knee posture, limited range of hip and knee motion, and an equine posture of the foot and ankle). These children typically have good trunk control and antigravity muscle strength in the hip abductors which are crucial for stability in standing and walking.[16]

Procedure

Induction of general anesthesia may be performed with short-acting muscle relaxants. This allows easier intubation, positioning, and less need for retraction during surgical exposure. Nerve root stimulation is absolutely critical to ensuring the desired outcome with low associated morbidity. Neuromuscular paralysis must be reversed pharmacologically before nerve stimulation and recording. Adequate use of analgesics during and after the procedure are also very important to a successful outcome. Intravenous lines and an arterial line are established. A Foley catheter is placed. The child is then turned to the prone position with surgical bolsters under the hips and chest allowing the abdominal wall to move freely with respiration. Proper positioning is critical to prevent abdominal compression, secondary unwanted venous congestion and the risk of hemorrhage from epidural veins. All bony prominences are well padded with foam, and the head is turned to one side on a circular gel head rest. The patient's back is kept in a neutral position, and the hips are flexed. The legs are supported by pillows. The arms are bent at the shoulder and the elbow. The plane between the highest point on the iliac crests is used as the level of the interspace between the spines of the fourth and fifth lumbar vertebrae. The spinous processes are carefully counted up to the spine of L1 and down to that of S2 allowing a midline incision to be marked out.

The skin is prepped in the usual sterile fashion. Two screens are placed to allow the head and the lower extremities to be visible to the anesthesiologist and the physiologist, respectively, during the procedure. The lower portion of the drapes is placed over a Mayo table so that the physiologist will be able to see and feel for muscle contractions and clonus in the lower extremities during the procedure. Needle electrodes for electromyography are placed in five lower extremity muscle groups bilaterally: adductor, quadriceps, tibialis anterior, hamstrings, and gastrocnemius. Electrodes are also placed in the external anal sphincter so that reflex arcs involved in sphincter control can be detected.

The incision is infiltrated with 0.25% Marcaine with 1:400.000 epinephrine at a total of 1 ml/kg. The incision is made with a #15 blade and self-retaining retractors are placed at both ends. Hemostasis is maintained with bipolar cautery. The lumbodorsal fascia is cut on either side of the supraspinous ligament, which is kept intact, and subperiosteal dissection is carried out to retract the paraspinal muscles laterally from L1 to S1. This can all be done with minimal blood loss, or use of the cautery.

Using a #15 skin knife the ligamentum flavum is opened at the inferior margin of the L5 lamina, and entrance in the epidural space is confirmed by visualization of fat or dura. A Penfield #4 can be used to confirm entry into the epidural space as well, but care must be taken not to cause any bleeding from epidural veins. The footplate of a small craniotome is inserted and brought up against the inferior margin of the lamina of L5, halfway between the spinous process and the facet. Care is taken not to injure the facets. A multilevel laminotomy is performed from L5 up to L2 in one step (Fig. 63-1). The same process is replicated on the opposite side. The supraspinous and interspinous ligaments are divided between L5 and S1 and the inferior portion of the laminar plate is then gently lifted up towards the cephalad extent of the surgical incision (Fig. 63-2). First, drill holes are placed at the base of the spinous process on either side at each level. Then, drill holes are placed in the lateral portions of the lamina at each level and threaded with non-absorbable sutures, each of which is held out laterally with a small hemostat. Then the plate is secured with suture and mosquito hemostats to the drapes superiorly. The lamina of S1 is cut on either side of the spinous process using a thin angled bone rongeur, with the supraspinous ligament left intact (Fig. 63-3). A suture is placed through the spine, which is then reflected caudally to expose the upper portion of the sacral dura. Bone bleeding is controlled with a slurry made from fibrin and Avatin. Bone wax is used to stop any persistent bone bleeding. Use of bone wax is minimized, as it can interfere with bone healing. Bleeding from epidural veins is controlled with bipolar coagulation.

At this point the child is put in mild reverse Trendelenburg position to decrease the amount of cerebrospinal fluid loss during the procedure. After the dura has been cleared of epidural fat, it is opened in the midline with a sharp #15 skin knife and held by traction sutures to the muscular layer. The arachnoid layer is left intact initially. A patty is placed over the arachnoid before a small opening is made. Following gentle cerebrospinal fluid aspiration, the arachnoid is opened widely to expose the cauda equina (Fig. 63-4).

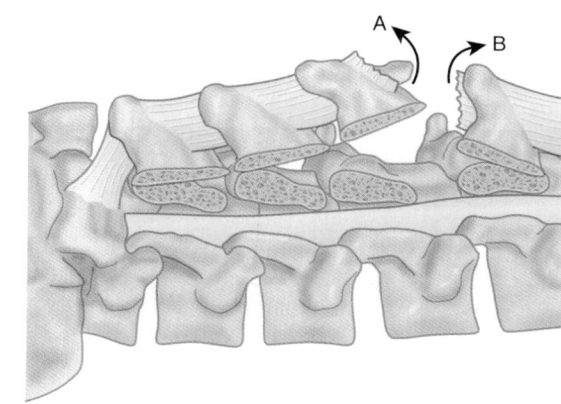

FIGURE 63-2 A, The inferior portion of the laminar plate is then gently lifted up towards the cephalad extent of the surgical incision. B, The lamina of S1 is cut on either side of the spinous process with a thin, angled bone rongeur, with the supraspinous ligament remaining intact.

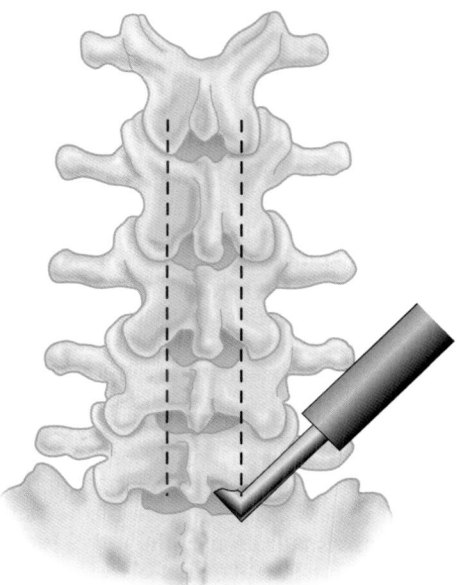

FIGURE 63-1 A multilevel laminotomy is performed from L5 up to L2 in one step.

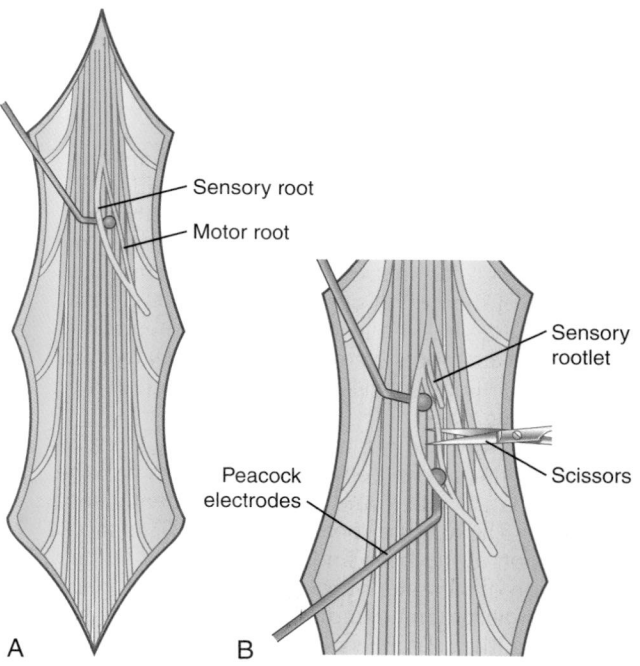

FIGURE 63-3 A, Using the rhizotomy electrodes, the groove between the posterior and the anterior roots is identified and the two are gently separated. B, The rootlet is elevated with rhizotomy electrodes and then sectioned with microscissors.

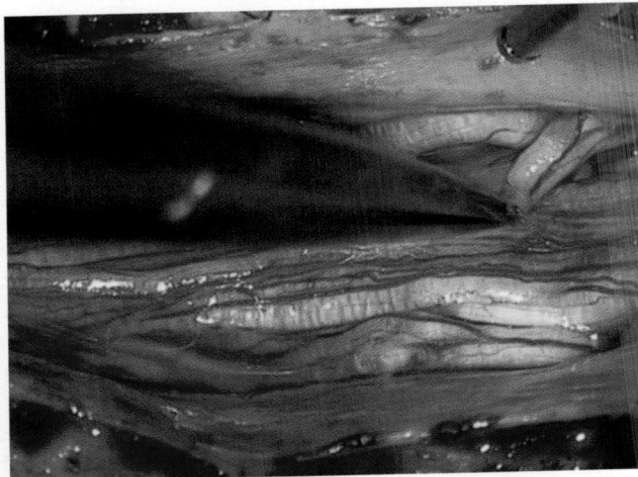

FIGURE 63-4 Intraoperative micrograph illustrating arachnoid dissection with microscissors to expose cauda equina.

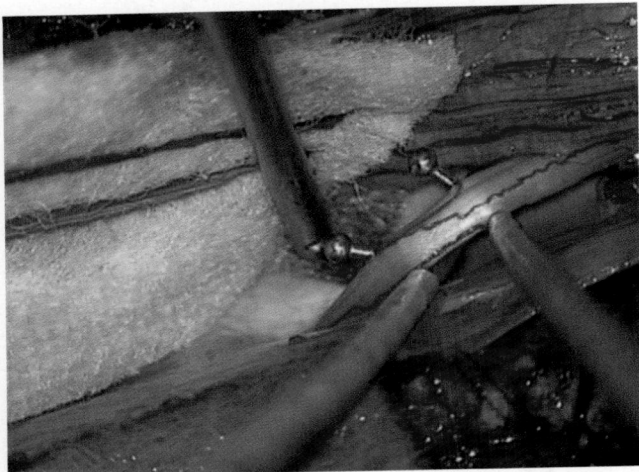

FIGURE 63-5 Intraoperative micrograph demonstrating the larger caliber and vascular tortuosity of a representative ventral nerve root.

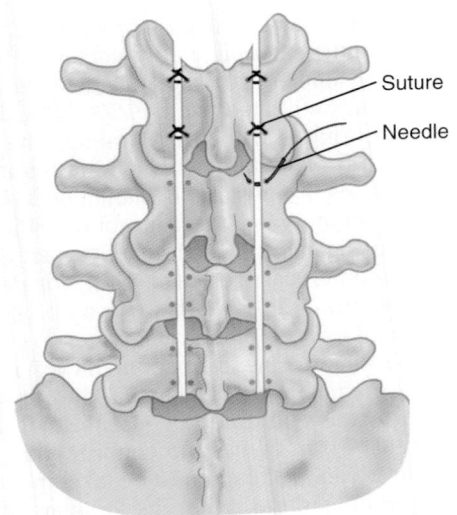

Suture

Needle

FIGURE 63-6 The laminar plate is secured back into position using the previously threaded sutures. The spinous process of L5 is also sutured to the spinous process of S1.

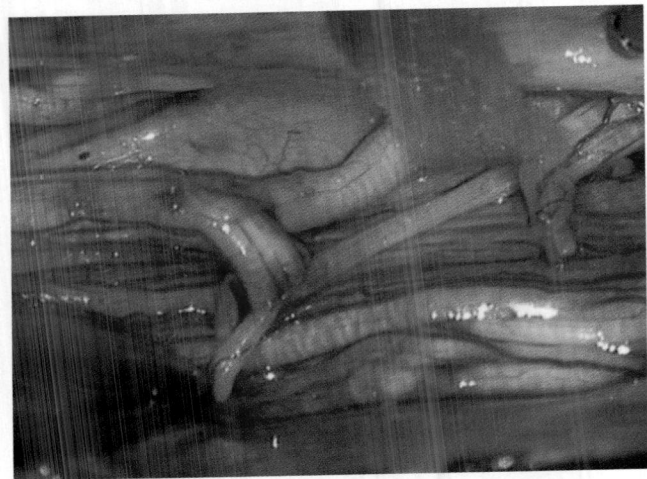

FIGURE 63-7 Intraoperative micrograph depicting multiple dorsal nerve roots after selective rhizotomy and sectioning.

Two insulated rhizotomy hook electrodes are connected by sterile cords to the electrical stimulator. Electric stimulation and recording are then used to identify root levels, and differentiate between motor and sensory bundles. The nerve roots are inspected at the exit foramina. At the dural exit of the nerve root, the motor root generally lies just slightly cephalad and anterior in the neural foramen. The motor nerve roots are generally slightly larger and have increased tortuosity of vasculature compared to the posterior roots (Fig. 63-5).

The largest nerve root is that of S1. Using the rhizotomy electrodes, the groove between the posterior and the anterior roots is identified and the two are gently separated (Fig. 63-6). The anterior root is stimulated. This should produce flexion at the knee and plantar flexion at the ankle. Stimulation of the anterior root of S2 should produce plantar flexion at the ankle and flexion of the toes. By counting upward, the L2 root is identified and separated into its anterior and posterior components. The posterior root of L2 is initially stimulated with a single 0.1-millisecond stimulus until the threshold for muscle contraction is reached. After a threshold to a single-pulse stimulus has been established,

a subthreshold tetanic stimulus at 50 Hz is applied, and the response is monitored. Abnormal responses are used to identify which rootlets should be divided. The selection of rootlets for division is discussed in more detail in the section on intraoperative monitoring. The stimulation and recording are done at each level, starting at L2 and continuing to S2 on the side opposite to the surgeon. There are normally two to four rootlets at the L2 level and an increasing number at each subsequent level down to S1, where there are approximately 8 to 11 rootlets. The S2 root is the first root that is smaller than the preceding root and usually contains two to six rootlets. The surgeon then moves to the opposite side of the operating room table and the process is repeated on the contralateral side of the patient. This allows for superb visualization of the nerve roots on each side while limiting the lateral extent of the laminotomy.

After those dorsal rootlets associated with an abnormal response have been sectioned (Fig. 63-7), the subarachnoid space is irrigated. Persistent bleeding is controlled with

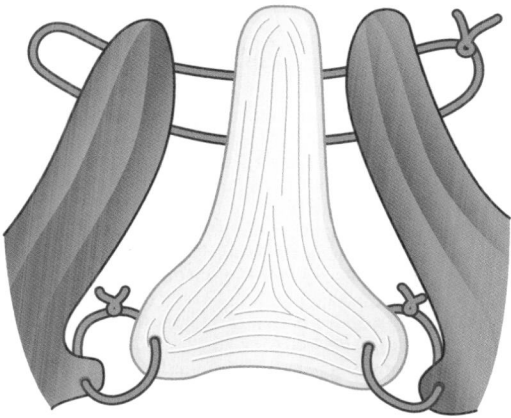

FIGURE 63-8 The paraspinal muscles are sutured to the interspinous ligament by suturing through the muscle on one side, then through the interspinous ligament into the muscle on the opposite side, and then back again through the interspinous ligament into the muscle on the original side before the suture is tied.

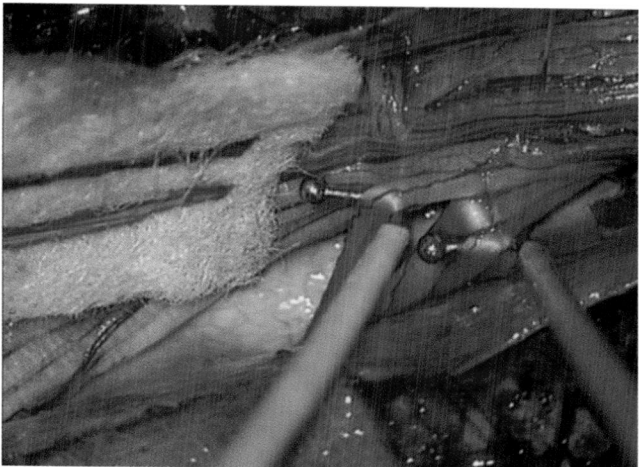

FIGURE 63-9 Intraoperative micrograph of nerve root dissection performed with gentle sweeping movements of insulated rhizotomy hook electrodes in line with nerve fibers.

bipolar cautery at low settings. The dura and arachnoid layers are then closed in a continuous locking watertight fashion. The child is taken out of reverse Trendelenburg and a tuberculin syringe and needle are used to inject intrathecal preservative free morphine. The dura is covered with fibrin glue. A brief Valsalva maneuver is applied to confirm watertight dural closure. The laminar plate is secured back into position using the previous partially threaded sutures. The spinous process of L5 is also sutured to the spinous process of S1 (Fig. 63-8). The paraspinal muscles are reattached to the interspinous ligament by suturing through the muscle on one side, then through the interspinous ligament into the muscle on the opposite side, and then back again through the interspinous ligament into the muscle on the original side before the suture is tied. This brings the muscles into tight apposition with the bone and ligaments, eliminating any surgical dead space. The supraspinous ligament is then sutured to the lumbosacral fascia covering the muscle before the skin closure. The skin is closed in two layers. The inner layer is closed with vicryl suture while the outer layer is closed with a continuous locking nylon suture. The wound is dressed, and the child is taken to the recovery room.

Intraoperative Monitoring

Responses to rootlet stimulation are evaluated by a neurologist with expertise in intraoperative neuromonitoring, and if possible a physical therapist or physiatrist who is familiar with the child's clinical picture. Rootlet selection for division is based on electromyographic response to dorsal rootlet stimulation, visual and palpable muscle contraction, and the child's clinical picture. Sacral-level rootlets associated with anal sphincter activity are spared.

Ten lower extremity muscle groups and the anal sphincter are evaluated with electromyography. The rootlets are stimulated using the rhizotomy electrode hooks with a constant-voltage electrical stimulator that allows delivery of single pulses and trains of stimuli. Recordings are made with pairs of noninsulated 2.5-cm needle electrodes and displayed on an 11-channel electroencephalography chart recorder.

Motor roots can be identified from sensory roots based on their lower threshold for inducing muscle contraction. The motor and sensory roots are identified and easily separated using the rhizotomy hook electrodes (Fig. 63-9). Because the threshold for muscle contraction is much lower for anterior roots (usually 100 mV to 1 V) than for whole posterior roots (usually 1 to 10 V), electrical stimulation can also be used to confirm separation of the posterior and anterior roots.

Stimulation of the anterior roots provides confirmation of spinal levels. Identifying root levels helps prevent injury to the lower sacral roots, thereby reducing the risk of developing bowel or bladder incontinence. First the S1 level is identified as the largest nerve root. Stimulation should produce flexion at the knee and plantar flexion at the ankle. Stimulation of the S2 nerve root should produce plantar flexion at the ankle and flexion at the toes. Stimulation of posterior rootlets is then carried at every level beginning at the L2 dorsal root. Rootlets producing contraction of the anal sphincter (S3–S4) can be identified using EMG.

Using gradual increases in the voltage of single square-wave pulses of 1-millisecond duration, threshold levels are established for simulation of the posterior root. This serves as a guideline to the stimulation threshold for the individual rootlets in that root. The root is then subdivided into its rootlets, which are stimulated in turn. The operator applies trains of stimulation, starting at about 50% of the single-pulse threshold and gradually increases the voltage until a small movement of the lower extremities is detected or a distinct electromyography recording is obtained.

The electromyographic response is analyzed in three ways: by duration, location, and pattern. The responses associated with rootlets that are to be spared have a duration no longer than that of the stimulus (1 second), are located in muscles innervated by that nerve root level, and have a decremental, squared-off wave pattern. Responses associated with rootlets that are to be divided may be associated with one or more of the following abnormalities: sustained duration (longer than 1 second), spread to muscles not innervated by that level, and an incremental, clonic, multiphasic or irregular waveform.

Suprathreshold stimulation should be avoided, as it may produce diffuse spread throughout the lower extremity, which may be misinterpreted as an abnormal response. Ongoing background activity may also be present and confuse the operator. If excessive background firing is present, or on the other hand responses are obtained only with higher voltages, small changes in the depth of anesthesia may alleviate the problem.

If there were not an appropriate number of rootlets at S1 associated with an abnormal response as would be expected in that child, S2 rootlets are evaluated for abnormal responses and sectioned only if stimulation did not result in contraction of the anal sphincter. If the patient does not have much spasticity in the quadriceps, but is in severe equinus, only the S1, L5, and L4 dorsal roots are sectioned.

Postoperative Care

Postoperatively, the patient is kept comfortable with appropriate analgesics. The Foley catheter is kept in place for 72 hours, given the risk of urinary retention with the use of intrathecal morphine. For the first three postoperative days, patients are kept flat in bed to help prevent cerebrospinal fluid leaks. On the third postoperative day, physical therapy is begun for positioning, range of motion, bed mobility, and family instruction. Sitting and maximally-assisted transfers are started on the fourth postoperative day. Flexor spasms, hypersensitivity of the lower extremities, and weakness are common in the patients in the early days after surgery and may last for several weeks. Continued physical therapy must be provided on an outpatient basis following discharge to help patients regain previous functional status and to improve skills and abilities beyond the preoperative levels.

KEY REFERENCES

Clark SL, Hankins GD. Temporal and demographic trends in cerebral palsy—fact and fiction. *Am J Obstet Gynecol.* 2003;188:628-633.

Decandia M, Provini L, Taborikova H. Mechanisms of the reflex discharge depression in the spinal motoneurone during repetitive orthodromic stimulation. *Brain Res.* 1967;4:2284-2291.

Fasano VA, Barolat-Romana G, Zeme S, et al. Electrophysiological assessment of spinal circuits in spasticity by direct dorsal root stimulation. *Neurosurgery.* 1979;4:2146-2151.

Fasano VA, Urciuoli R, Broggi G, et al. New aspects in the surgical treatment of cerebral palsy. *Acta Neurochir.* 1977;24(Suppl):53-57.

Foerster O. Resection of the posterior spinal nerve roots in the treatment of gastric crises and spastic paralysis. *Proc R Soc Med.* 1911;4:226-246.

Fraioli B, Guidetti B. Posterior partial rootlet section in the treatment of spasticity. *J Neurosurg.* 1977;46:618-626.

Lance JW. Symposium synopsis. In: Feldman RG, Young RR, Koella WP, eds. *Spasticity: Disorder of Motor Control.* Chicago: Year Book Medical Publishers; 1980:485-494.

Langerak NG, Lamberts RP, Fieggen AG, et al. A prospective gait analysis study in patients with diplegic cerebral palsy 20 years after selective dorsal rhizotomy. *J Neurosurg Pediatr.* 2008;1:3180-3186.

Peacock WJ, Arens LJ. Selective posterior rhizotomy for the relief of spasticity in cerebral palsy. *S Afr Med J.* 1982;62:119-124.

Peacock WJ, Arens LJ, Berman B. Cerebral palsy spasticity: selective posterior rhizotomy. *Pediatr Neurosci.* 1987;13:61-66.

Peacock WJ, Staudt LA. Functional outcomes following selective posterior rhizotomy in children with cerebral palsy. *J Neurosurg.* 1991;74: 380-385.

Sherrington CS. Decerebrate rigidity and reflex coordination of movements. *J Physiol. (London).* 1898;22:319-337.

Van de Wiele BM, Staudt LA, Rubinstien EH, Nuwer M, Peacock WJ. Perioperative complications in children undergoing selective posterior rhizotomy: a review of 105 cases. *Paediatr Anaesth.* 1996;6: 6479-6486.

Numbered references appear on Expert Consult.

CHAPTER 64

Instrumentation and Stabilization of the Pediatric Spine: Technical Nuances and Age-Specific Considerations

JOSHUA J. CHERN • KATHERINE RELYEA • ANDREW JEA

A wide variety of congenital, developmental, and acquired abnormalities may affect the pediatric spine. The decision for surgical intervention must be tailored to the disease pathology as well as each patient's clinical situation. Spinal instability may be iatrogenic or caused by the disease process, requiring installation of spinal instrumentation. Placing instrumentation in the pediatric spine is challenging given the small anatomy of a child, lack of "pediatric-specific" instrumentation, and at times, inability to adapt adult techniques to the pediatric patient.

This chapter discusses some posterior and anterior spinal instrumentation techniques used in the pediatric spine. Posterior instrumentation techniques are far more widely used than anterior techniques. Advantages and disadvantages of various biomaterials used in the pediatric spine are discussed. Lastly, we briefly discuss the effect of spinal instrumentation on a growing spine, a problem unique to the pediatric population.

Posterior Spinal Instrumentation in the Pediatric Age Group

CRANIOCERVICAL JUNCTION (O-C2)

Occipital Screws

Most of the limitations of occipitocervical fixation systems reside in the cranial part of the construct.[1,2] The occiput does not easily accommodate instrumentation.[2-4] The slope of the occipital bone and the angle it makes with the cervical spine impose unique geometric constraints. These limitations may lead to poor occipital screw purchase, screw loosening, pullout, breakage, and difficulties with screw insertion,[5] culminating in catastrophic hardware failure.

Numerous methods of obtaining occipitocervical stabilization have been described, including the use of methylmethacrylate,[6] onlay bone graft with wires,[7] contoured rods with wires,[8] and metal plates with wires or screws.[9-11] Internal fixation is advised to guarantee postoperative stability[11] and to enhance the rate of arthrodesis.[12]

In a biomechanical investigation of occipital screw pullout strength, the bicortical pullout strength was found to be 50% greater than unicortical; wire pullout strength was

not significantly different from that of unicortical screws,[13] although some authors find a posteriorly wired contoured rod less likely to provide a good fusion environment because of less stabilizing potential and greater potential and greater likelihood of loosening with fatigue.[14]

Although bicortical screw placement may result in superior holding strength secondary to greater cortical purchase,[15] caution is needed to avoid overpenetration and potential neurological injury.[16] Bicortical occipital screw insertion risks dural laceration, cerebrospinal fluid (CSF) leakage, dural venous sinus injury/thrombosis,[17] and subdural/epidural hematoma formation. CSF leakage and sinus bleeding can be stopped with placement of the occipital screws; if a screw cannot be placed, bone wax may be used to plug the drill hole in the bone.

Bicortical screw failure is directly related to screw length, and screw length is dictated by bone thickness.[4] Because the occiput is thickest in the region of the midline keel, multiple bicortical fixation points directed towards the midline have been advocated.

Like much of pediatric spine surgery, instrumentation techniques are adapted from the adult spine surgery experience. Careful preoperative study of a thin-cut CT including the occiput is mandatory to confirm enough midline bone thickness to accommodate the shortest 6-mm occipital screw inserted obliquely.

The basiocciput below the external occipital protuberance and posterior to the foramen magnum represents the squamous portion and is the site of occipitocervical fusion.[2] Screw fixation is more secure in the bone above the inferior nuchal line because bone below this landmark is thin. Screw purchase is improved closer to the superior nuchal line and external occipital protuberance. However, the superior nuchal line does not reflect the location of the transverse sinus accurately, ranging from 15 mm below the superior nuchal line and 17 mm above.[4] Unicortical screw purchase at and above the superior nuchal line may be warranted to decrease risk of dural venous sinus penetration.

Careful drilling with triangulation towards midline should be performed millimeter-by-millimeter until the inner table of the occiput is breached; the dura should be palpable with a ball-tipped probe. This "stop-drill" technique is routinely

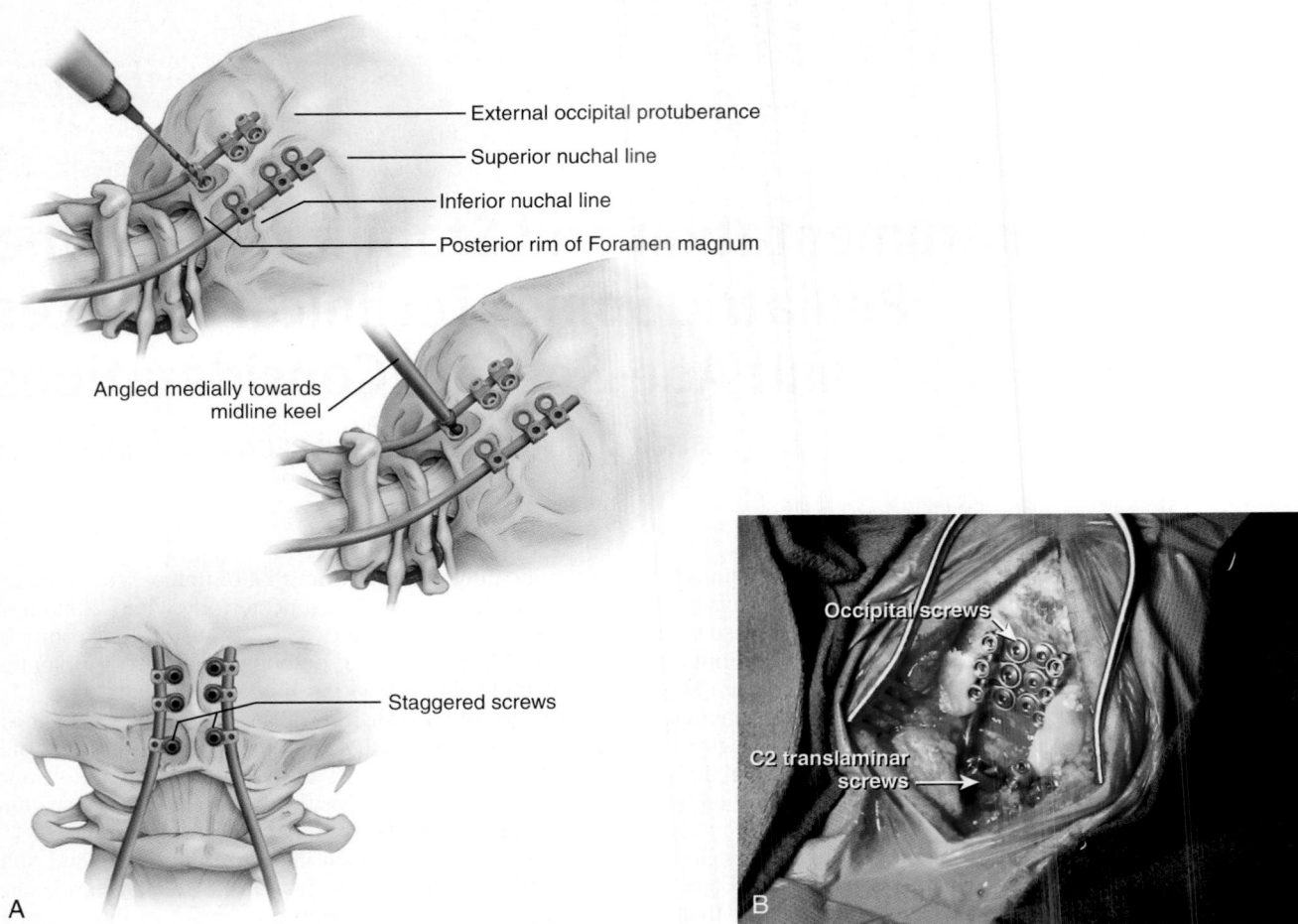

External occipital protuberance

Superior nuchal line

Inferior nuchal line

Posterior rim of Foramen magnum

Angled medially towards midline keel

Staggered screws

A

Occipital screws

C2 translaminar screws

B

FIGURE 64-1 A, Occipital screw technique. Prior to drilling, anatomic landmarks are identified. Four bony landmarks on the outer occipital cortex should be visible: the posterior rim of the foramen magnum, the superior nuchal line, the inferior nuchal line, and the external occipital protuberance. Safe placement of occipital instrumentation is placed between the inferior and superior nuchal line. 4.0–4.5-mm–diameter occipital screws may be placed in a bicortical fashion using the stop-drill or step-wise drill technique in 2-mm increments. Drill and screw trajectories should be angled medially toward the thick midline keel. Left and right occipital screws are staggered to avoid intersection of screw paths. B, Intraoperative picture. *(Illustrations by K. Relyea MS. Printed with permission from Baylor College of Medicine.)*

used. With left- and right-sided screws directed towards midline, screw paths may intersect causing even more unwanted difficulty with screw placement. It is useful to stagger the screws on each side of midline, being conscientious to direct the next screw trajectories slightly more cephalad or caudad away from the previous trajectory (Fig. 64-1).

C1 Lateral Mass Screws and C1–C2 Transarticular Screws

Transarticular C1–C2 screws as described by Magerl[13] provide a very rigid and biomechanically sound construct with the incorporation of four cortical surfaces, but the insertion procedure is technically demanding because of the danger of vertebral artery injury especially in cases were atlantoaxial subluxation remains irreducible preoperatively. Although successful transarticular screw fixation of the atlantoaxial complex has been extensively reported in adult series, there have been only a handful of reports in the pediatric population. Analysis of clinical experience in the largest series of pediatric patients[10,18,19] suggested a 4% rate of vertebral artery injury during screw placement; none of these injuries resulted in any long-term morbidity or mortality.

Because of the anatomical limitations complicating transarticular screw placement in adults and even more so in children, variations of C1–C2 screw fixation have been reported in adult patients in whom independent C1 lateral mass screws and C2 pars/pedicle screws were connected with either a plate[11] or a rod.[12] Atlantoaxial screw-rod fixation has been suggested as a safer procedure, and perhaps, as we have found, the technique is applicable in more patients despite anatomic variations, even in the smallest of pediatric patients. It is an ideal technique to fix and reduce occipitoatlantoaxial deformities that remain irreducible with closed reduction (Fig. 64-2).[21,22]

It is imperative that the entry point for the C1 lateral mass screw in the pediatric spine be placed at the confluence of the C1 lamina and the C1 lateral mass. The pediatric spine is unsuitable to accept a C1 lateral mass screw at alternative entry sites, such as the C1 lamina itself[14] because of the high risk of violating the superior wall of the lamina and injuring the vertebral artery in the sulcus arteriosus.[1]

It is also important to note how the pediatric atlas differs from the adult atlas. In the adult atlas, the medial side of the C1 lamina is typically flush with the medial C1 lateral mass. However, in the pediatric atlas, the medial aspect of the C1

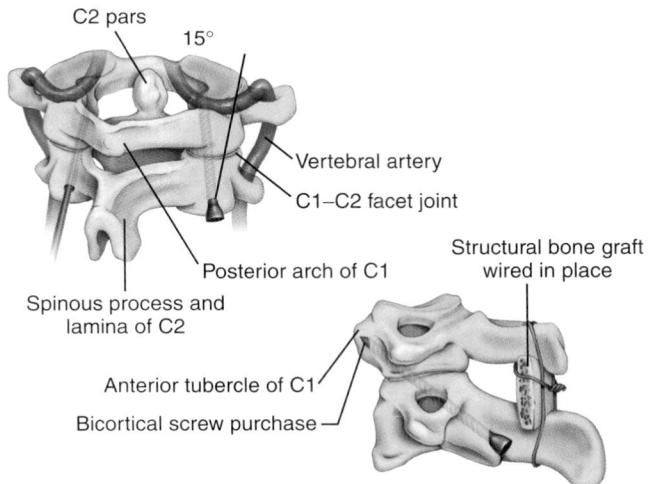

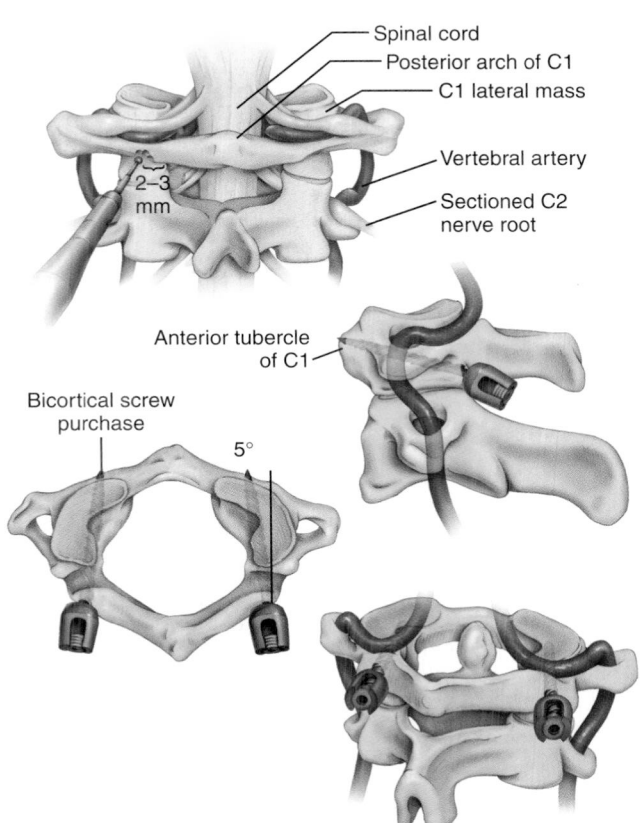

FIGURE 64-2 C1–C2 transarticular screw technique. A midline incision is made to expose the posterior elements from C1 to C3 with particular attention paid to C2–C3 facet joints. The superior and medial aspects of the C2 pars are exposed. There is no reason to expose the lateral aspect of the C2 pars; in fact, this may be a dangerous maneuver because of the proximity of the vertebral artery. The roof of the C2 pedicle is followed to the C1–C2 facet joint. The C2 entry point may be identified by first locating the medial edge of the C2–C3 facet joint. The C2 entry site is just lateral and rostral to this point, and may be estimated by visualizing the course of the medial pars (approximately 3 mm up and 3 mm out). The drill or K-wire, either through a stab incision lateral to the T1 spinous process or through an extended incision, is typically directed 15 degrees medial, with the superior angle visualized by fluoroscopy. The drill or K-wire is directed down the C2 pedicle and across the C1–C2 joint, aiming at the anterior tubercle of C1. The tip of the drill or K-wire is advanced to a point 4 mm short of the anterior C1 tubercle, attaining purchase of the anterior cortex of C1. After tapping, a fully threaded 3.5- or 4.0-mm–diameter cortical screw is used. The necessary screw length can be measured directly from the drill or the K-wire. Screws are typically 34 to 44 mm in length. The technique is repeated on the contralateral side. *(Illustrations by K. Relyea MS. Printed with permission from Baylor College of Medicine.)*

FIGURE 64-3 C1 lateral mass screw technique. The posterior arch of C1 is identified and followed laterally to visualize the lateral masses. Notably, there is a step-off between the medial aspect of the C1 lamina and the medial surface of the C1 lateral mass; this anatomic feature is different than in adults where the medial C1 lamina is flush with the medial C1 lateral mass. Subperiosteal dissection of the C2 nerve roots and associated venous plexi from the junction between the posterior arch of C1 and lateral masses was performed to minimize bleeding. Alternatively, the C2 nerve roots and venous plexi can be coagulated with bipolar electrocautery and divided with little clinical significance. After palpating the medial and lateral surfaces of the lateral mass, a pilot hole may be drilled in the center of the lateral mass, usually no more than 2 to 3 mm from the medial surface. The rest of the placement of the C1 lateral mass screws proceeds using the technique described by Harms and Melcher, using either 3.5-mm or 4.0-mm–diameter polyaxial screws. The drill and screw trajectory is angled 0 to 5 degrees medial, and is aimed at the superior half of the anterior arch of C1 on fluoroscopy. Bicortical purchase is usually achieved about 4 mm from the anterior cortex of the anterior arch. *(Illustrations by K. Relyea MS. Printed with permission from Baylor College of Medicine.)*

lamina is typically 2 to 3 mm laterally stepped-off from the medial surface of the C1 lateral mass. An entry point based on the medial aspect of the C1 lamina will place the entry of the C1 lateral mass screw dangerously lateral in extreme proximity to the vertebral artery. Instead, the medial surface of the C1 lateral mass itself must be used as a landmark for starting the C1 lateral mass screw[23,24] (Fig. 64-3).

Bleeding from the venous plexus around the C2 nerve root can be substantial as dissection down to the junction of the C1 lamina and C1 lateral mass is carried out. This blood loss can be life-threatening in small children without a large blood volume to begin with and may lead to unwanted blood transfusions. Bipolar coagulation of the venous plexus and division of the C2 nerve root may obviate much of this venous hemorrhaging while improving exposure without incurring any significant neurologic sequelae.

Although C1 lateral mass screw placement is still technically challenging and the potential risk of vertebral artery injury persists, our initial experience[22] is that it is a feasible and efficacious part of an occipitocervical or atlantoaxial screw-rod construct in young patients.

C2 Pars/Pedicle and Translaminar Screws

C1–C2 transarticular screw placement is technically demanding because of the close proximity of the vertebral artery to the screw path. Vertebral artery injury has been reported to occur in 2% to 8% in several large series.[25-27] Pars/pedicle screws may have a lower incidence of arterial injury,[28] but these screws still place the vertebral artery and spinal cord at risk.[29]

Wright[30,31] described a new technique for rigid screw fixation of the axis involving the insertion of polyaxial screws into the laminae of C2 in a bilateral crossing fashion and their feasibility for placement in the general adult population. Because the C2 translaminar screws are not in proximity to the vertebral artery, this technique allows rigid fixation of C2 through a safer technique. Recently, teams of authors[32,33] have reported their experience with this technique of crossing and noncrossing screws in small series of children (Fig. 64-4).

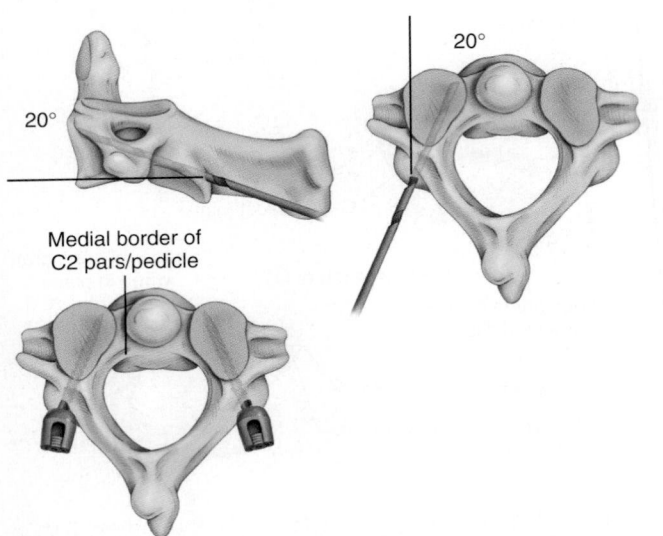

FIGURE 64-4 C2 pars/pedicle screw technique. The entry point of a C2 pars/pedicle screw is similar to that of C1–C2 transarticular screw placement. The medial, superior, and roof the C2 pars/pedicle should be exposed, dividing the C2 nerve root and venous plexus, if necessary. The medial trajectory of the C2 pars/pedicle screw parallels the medial border of the C2 pars/pedicle, and the superior trajectory guided by fluoroscopy aiming for the anterior tubercle of C1; however, the C2 pars/pedicle screw stops short of the C1–C2 joint. Screw length is typically one-half the screw length for a C1–C2 transarticular screw, measuring 16 to 22 mm in length. *(Illustrations by K. Relyea MS. Printed with permission from Baylor College of Medicine.)*

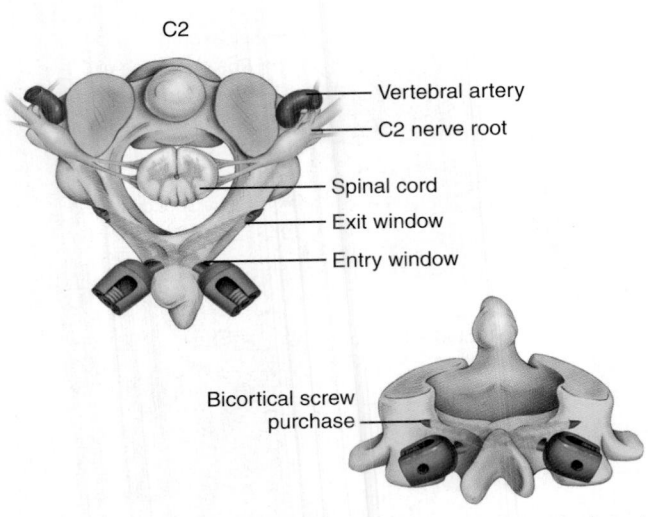

FIGURE 64-5 C3–C7 lateral mass screw technique. The entire lateral mass of the subaxial cervical spine is exposed from its medial junction with the lamina to the lateral step-off. The entry point is identified approximately 1 mm inferior and 1 mm medial to the center of the two-dimensional "square" posterior surface of the lateral mass. The drill and screw trajectory is directed superior and lateral (approximately 20 degrees up and 20 degrees out) to avoid the nerve root and vertebral artery, respectively, aiming for the superolateral "deep" corner of the 3D "cube" of the lateral mass in the mind's eye of the surgeon. Unicortical purchase is safe, but bicortical purchase may afford a biomechanical advantage. Fluoroscopy may be used, but is unnecessary. Boys usually tolerate 12–16-mm × 3.5-mm screws, and girls tolerate 10–14 mm × 3.5-mm screws. *(Illustrations by K. Relyea MS. Printed with permission from Baylor College of Medicine.)*

SUBAXIAL CERVICAL SPINE (C3–C7)

Lateral Mass Screws

Although lateral mass screw fixation in the cervical spine has been shown to provide excellent stability and high rates of fusion in adult patients,[34-36] little has been published about the use of subaxial lateral mass screws in the pediatric age group. Unlike the adult age group, there is limited cadaveric biomechanical analyses of these types of constructs. In addition, based on comparative biomechanical studies of the cervical fixation procedures, there is not much difference in stability between lateral mass screw fixation and conventional nonscrew fixation methods, such as sublaminar wiring.[37-41]

The two most popular techniques for lateral mass screws are the Roy-Camille and the Magerl techniques. However, nerve roots, vertebral arteries, facet joints, and the dura and spinal cord are at risk during the placement of lateral mass screws. A recent review of the literature[42] indicated that the youngest patient where subaxial lateral mass screws were successfully used was 8.2 years old. This correlates with the age at which most authorities agree that the developing spine takes on an "adult" configuration.[43,44] Despite this, the authors were only able to place 3.5 × 10 mm screws — the shortest screw length that is manufactured. Although a solid fusion was achieved in this case after 3 months of rigid immobilization, another study[36] of predominantly adult patients has suggested that a minimum subaxial lateral mass screw length of 14 mm is needed to confer any degree of biomechanical stability (Fig. 64-5).

Pedicle Screws

Pedicle screw fixation systems have been widely used for reconstruction of the thoracic and lumbar spine because of their biomechanical superiority. Abumi et al.[45,46] reported clinical results of pedicle screw fixation for reconstruction of traumatic and nontraumatic lesions of the middle and lower cervical spine. However, the procedure in the upper cervical spine has been criticized due to the potentially high risk to neurovascular structures, except at the C2 level.[47-49]

Translaminar Screws

Recently, translaminar screws have been promoted as a safe alternative to pedicle screws in the axis and in the upper thoracic spine, as they decrease the risk of violation of the transverse foramen and vertebral artery injury in the cervical spine and the risk of damage to the spinal cord and exiting nerve roots in the upper thoracic spine[50,51] without the need for image guidance. We now propose that translaminar screw fixation in the subaxial cervical spine is a consideration in highly selected cases, as an alternative to subaxial lateral mass screws in children with small lateral masses.

Translaminar screw placement in the subaxial pediatric cervical spine has numerous potential advantages compared with current instrumentation techniques. The entire length of the subaxial cervical lamina can be readily visualized. Important neurovascular structures can be avoided. A screw can be placed of much longer length than a lateral mass screw at the same level to confer a greater degree of biomechanical advantage.

Potential drawbacks of this technique must also be noted. Although the dorsal laminar surface is exposed during surgery, the surgeon must be careful to avoid penetration of the nonvisualized ventral laminar wall because penetration could lead to damage to the thecal sac or spinal cord. A modification of Wright's method of translaminar screw placement with an "exit" window in the dorsal lamina at the laminofacet line can help the surgeon avoid intracanicular violation of the translaminar screw.[52] Preoperative fine-cut CT scans with axial, sagittal, and coronal views should be used to estimate the screw length and to determine if the subaxial lamina can accept a minimum 3.5-mm diameter screw. We suggest that the acceptable width of the lamina should be at least 4.0 mm. Clearly, translaminar screws should not be used without intact posterior elements.

Although the biomechanics of lateral mass screw fixation of the subaxial cervical spine are well described, there is no report comparing construct stability or screw pullout strength of translaminar and lateral mass screws in this region. CT morphometric analysis for axial and subaxial translaminar screw placement in the pediatric cervical spine shows the anatomy in 30.4% of patients younger than 16 years of age could accept bilateral C2 translaminar screws; however, the anatomy of the subaxial cervical spine only rarely could accept translaminar screws.[53] Nonetheless, feasibility of translaminar screw placement in the subaxial cervical spine should be assessed on a case-by-case basis by careful study of preoperative thin-cut CT and sagittal and coronal reconstructions (Fig. 64-6).

THORACIC AND LUMBAR SPINE
Wires, Hooks, and Pedicle Screws

The history of spinal implants began in Kansas in 1887 when Dr. B.F. Wilkins reduced and fixed a T12–L1 dislocation with silver wires which he passed around the pedicles. Stainless steel wires were developed in the late 1930s. The surgical treatment of spinal deformity was transformed in the 1960s when the Harrington rod instrumentation system was introduced.[54] The next major advance in spinal instrumentation came in 1982, when Luque rods and sublaminar wires were introduced. The Luque instrumentation system provided segmental correction and fixation, allowing a more rigid construct that avoided mandatory postoperative external immobilization.[55] The Cotrel-Dubousset instrumentation system, developed in Europe in 1978 and introduced in the United States in 1984, has been described as a third-generation system that achieves three-dimensional correction of spinal deformity. The hallmark of this instrumentation system was the segmental nature of the hook attachment that allowed multiple forces to be applied on the same rod to correct the spinal deformity. Since then, other third-generation spinal systems combining the use of longitudinal members with different anchors including pedicle screws in variable positions have been developed.

In the surgical correction of spinal deformities, addition of internal fixation serves the dual function of improving solid arthrodesis by rigid immobilization of the instrumented segments and correcting preexisting deformities by facilitated application of the corrective forces. Since the introduction of spinal pedicle screws by Boucher[56] in the late 1950s and the Harrington instrument[57] in the early 1960s, spinal internal pedicle screw fixation has gained widespread use and popularity in the correction of spinal deformities.[58-61]

Noted advantages of pedicle screw fixation include three-column fixation; improved coronal, sagittal, and rotational correction; lower pseudoarthrosis rates, lower implant failures; and few postoperative external orthosis requirements when compared with hook and wire constructs.[62-65]

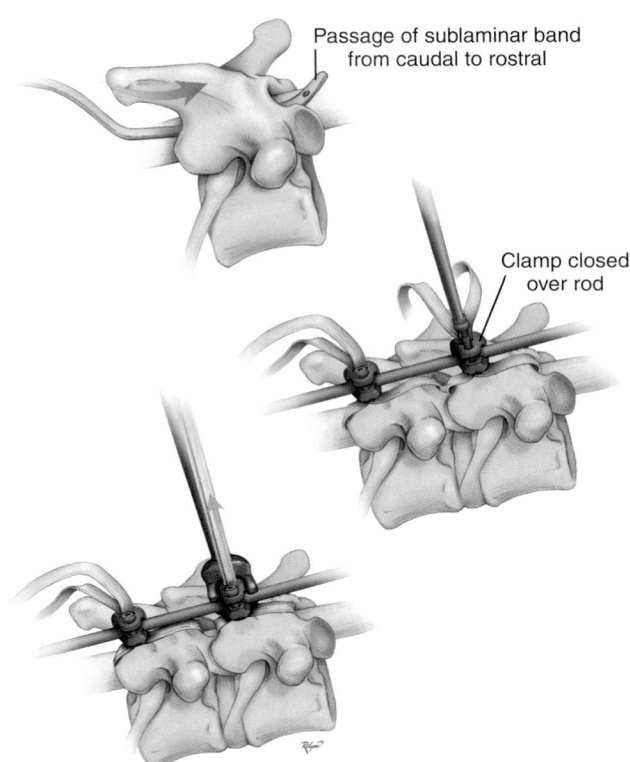

Passage of sublaminar band from caudal to rostral

Clamp closed over rod

FIGURE 64-6 Translaminar screw technique. A high-speed drill is used to open a small "entry" cortical window at the junction of the spinous process and lamina, close to the rostral margin of the lamina. Similarly, a high-speed drill is used to open a small "exit" cortical window at the junction of the facet and lamina, close to the rostral margin of the lamina. Using a hand drill as described by Wright, the contralateral lamina is carefully drilled along its length, with the drill visually aligned along the angle of the exposed contralateral laminar surface, aiming for the "exit" point. The drill tip should then be observed at the "exit" window. This gives confirmation that the drill did not violate the inner cortex of the lamina, allows bicortical screw purchase, and enables accurate measure of the appropriate screw length. Typically, a screw, 20 to 30 mm in length and 3.5 mm or 4.0 mm in diameter, could be placed. A small "entry" cortical window is then made at the junction of the spinous process and lamina, close to the caudal aspect of the lamina on the opposite side. The above technique is then repeated for this crossing translaminar screw. Fluoroscopy is not used during this technique. It neither guides screw trajectory nor confirms screw placement, as it is difficult to interpret on anteroposterior and lateral views where the screw lay in relation to the spinal canal. *(Illustrations by K. Relyea MS. Printed with permission from Baylor College of Medicine.)*

Despite their established role at the thoracolumbar, lumbar, and lumbosacral spine,[63,66-69] the use of pedicle screws in the thoracic spine (T1 through T10) had limited acceptance among earlier spine surgeons. This is due to concerns related to the small pedicle size and the tight proximity of vascular, nervous, and visceral structures in the thoracic cavity and the thoracic spine itself.[70-76] However, since the early 1990s, spine surgeons have been using pedicle screws for the management of thoracic deformities and have not observed any serious vascular or visceral complications[65,69,77-81] (Fig. 64-7).

Polyester Bands

Recently, polyester bands with a locking mechanism to provide rod coupling (Universal Clamp, Zimmer Spine, Warsaw, IN) were developed as an alternative to traditional anchors—wires, hooks, and screws. The material properties of polyester

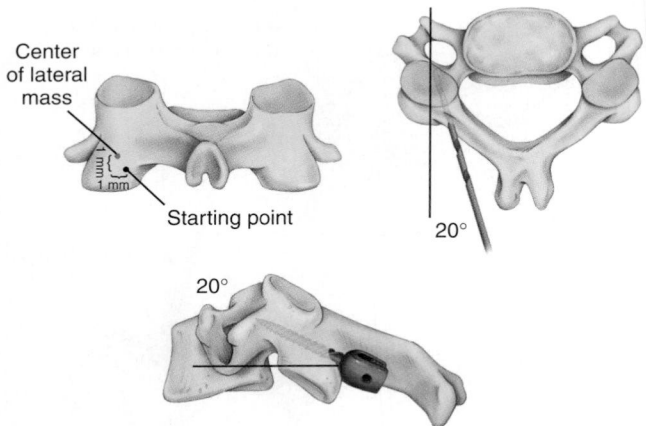

FIGURE 64-7 Thoracic and lumbar pedicle screw technique. The entry point for pedicle screw placement may be consistently found at the confluence between the pars interarticularis and transverse process. A thorough knowledge of pedicle anatomy and the sagittal and axial angulation of the individual pedicles is mandatory for safe screw placement. Angles for the pedicle finder, tap, and screw are best judged using preoperative CT or MRI of the thoracic or lumbar region. Intraoperative real-time guidance with fluoroscopy or direct palpation of the pedicle through a laminotomy may aid in screw placement, as an alternative to free-hand placement. *(Illustrations by K. Relyea MS. Printed with permission from Baylor College of Medicine.)*

are characterized by its high tensile strength, high resistance to stretch, wet or dry, and resistance to degradation.[82] Polyester is biocompatible without an exorbitant inflammatory reaction in surrounding tissue, including the dura. Polyester has been in use for more than 18 years in spinal implants in Europe (K. Mazda, personal communication, October 17, 2007).

Its woven fabric makes it gentle, and its flexibility make it an excellent alternative to implantation into the pediatric spine. This is most applicable when the anatomy is extraordinarily

small to accept hooks or screws, or when the anatomy is marked by significant congenital structural abnormalities where free-hand or fluoroscopic-guided hook or screw placement may lead to unacceptably high risk of neurologic injury. The polyester bands and locking mechanism to the rod may be placed at multiple levels, similar to wires, hooks, and screws, to effect segmental control, reduction, and fusion (Fig. 64-8).

With the passage of any sublaminar instrumentation into the spinal canal, there is a risk of neurological injury. Theoretically, a polyester band, compared to a metal cable, should conform safely to the undersurface of the lamina, which may lead to a decrease in neurological injury. However, as illustrated in the case above, neurological injury is still a risk with passage of sublaminar polyester bands.

Like sublaminar wires, sublaminar polyester bands can directly traumatize the spinal cord.[83-89] Meticulous technique can reduce the risk of injury, particularly in the thoracic and thoracolumbar spine.[90] Because the metal tip is not visible during the sublaminar passage of the polyester band, the surgeon is unable to appreciate the depth of tip penetration into the spinal canal. Important points to consider when using this technique include: (1) the radius of curvature of the malleable metal tip should be at least equal to the length of the lamina; (2) the bend of the tip should not be greater than 45 degrees; (3) lateral passage of sublaminar polyester bands should be avoided; (4) removal of additional bony lamina is not necessary because it does not significantly decrease the depth of band penetration but potentially weakens the lamina and increases the risk of instrumentation failure; (5) removal of the spinous process is recommended before direct midline passage of the sublaminar band; and (6) maintaining tension on the band throughout passage by using a push-pull technique to prevent bowing of the band into the spinal canal.

FIGURE 64-8 A, Sublaminar wire/band technique. Passing a metal wire or polyester band under the lamina does require a learning curve. The malleable metal end of the wire or polyester band is shaped into a gentle curve for passage around the lamina. The wire or band is always passed in a caudal-to-rostral direction. The tip of the wire or band is gripped with hemostats or forceps, and the rest of the passage follows a push-pull technique being mindful to keep tension so that a loop of band does not compress the thecal sac. After all of the sublaminar wires or bands have been passed, each of the wires or clamps is closed over the rods. The loop around the lamina is tightened with a tensioner. The final tension is primarily evaluated by the surgeon, taking into account the strength of the bone of the patient. B and C, Intraoperative pictures. *(Illustrations by K. Relyea MS. Printed with permission from Baylor College of Medicine.)*

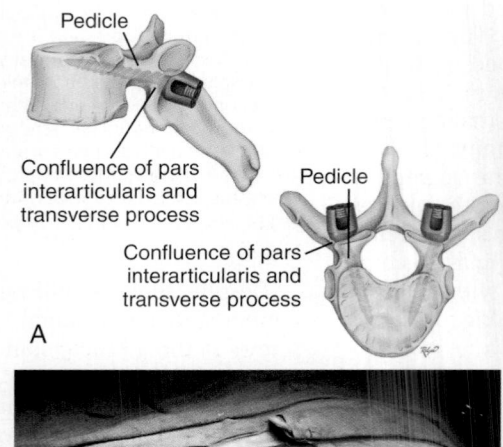

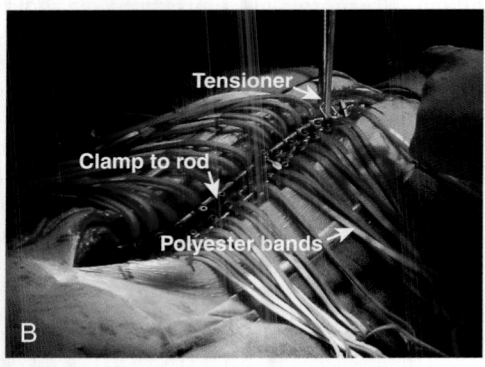

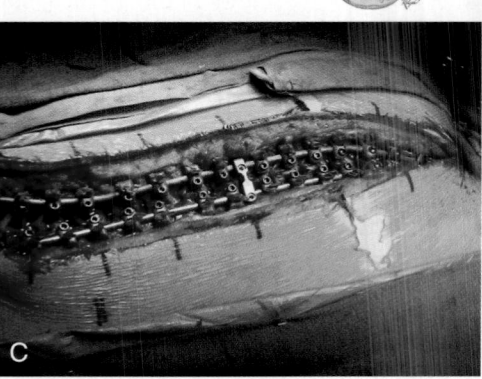

Care must be taken not to overtighten the bands, which can cause the bands to pull through or fracture a weak or skeletally immature lamina, as occurred in one of our cases. Excessive laminotomy in preparing for band passage may weaken the lamina; aggressive decortication in preparing the bony bed for arthrodesis may likewise decrease laminar strength[91] and increase the risk of laminar fracture in the follow-up period.

Anterior Spinal Instrumentation in the Pediatric Age Group

Anterior spinal instrumentation is used far less commonly than posterior spinal instrumentation. Still, surgical management of congenital deformities, such as kyphosis or scoliosis, may involve anterior instrumentation. Tumor, trauma, or inflammatory disorders of the spine may also occasionally require anterior instrumentation in children or adolescents as well.

ADVANTAGES OF ANTERIOR INSTRUMENTATION

Some advantages of anterior instrumentation compared to posterior instrumentation include preservation of motion segments and decreased blood loss with less muscle dissection.[92,93] Improved fusion rates and decreased operative times have also been proposed by some authors.[93,94] Anterior instrumentation also provides a reduced infection rate compared to posterior procedures.

For skeletally immature patients, circumferential fusion incorporating anterior instrumentation serves to arrest further anterior and posterior column growth and prevents the occurrence of "crankshaft" deformity.[95]

DISADVANTAGES OF ANTERIOR INSTRUMENTATION

The principle disadvantage of anterior approaches to the pediatric spine for placement of anterior hardware is that they may frequently require a second procedure for decompression of posterior pathology or placement of posterior spinal instrumentation. However, many current pediatric spine surgeons feel comfortable placing anterior spinal instrumentation through a posterior or posterolateral approach, gaining both anterior and posterior exposure of the spinal column through a single approach. A costotransversectomy or lateral extracavitary approach for the thoracic and lumbar spine will allow simultaneous placement of anterior spinal instrumentation with the installation of posterior spinal instrumentation.

As with posterior instrumentation, standard spinal instrumentation such as titanium or polyetheretherketone (PEEK) cages may have too large a profile for general pediatric use; careful study of preoperative CT is mandatory to determine if the anatomy of the patient will be able to accept anterior instrumentation. Other potential complications include the risk of nerve root injury; implant loosening and migration; injury to critical vascular structures such as the carotid artery, aorta, or inferior vena cava; injury to the spinal cord or its covering; visceral injury; adjacent level disease especially in the mobile cervical spine;[96] stenosis; and possible instability resulting from rigidity of the construct.[97]

Biomaterials

Autologous bone graft is widely used in the pediatric population. Sources of bone graft include iliac crest, fibula/tibia and rib grafts. Donor site morbidity is no different than what has been described in the adult population. However, iliac crest and rib graft may be cartilaginous in young children and lack sufficient rigidity. Alternative implants include calvarium and allograft which have both been used successfully.[98,99] Synthetic materials such as titanium mesh cages and PEEK cages are possible substitutes as well. Titanium mesh cages have been used mainly in the thoracolumbar and lumbar spine for adolescent idiopathic scoliosis correction[100] and less so for anterior column reconstruction after total spondylectomy for en bloc tumor resection.[101] Because of its size, the titanium cage is mainly used in older adolescents. While its effectiveness in maintaining spine alignment in the adult population has been shown,[102] there have been no reports on long-term follow-up in pediatric patients.

An additional problem associated with the titanium cage is its lack of radiolucency, which makes radiographic assessment of bony fusion difficult. A radiolucent alternative is the PEEK cage. PEEK biomaterial is strong, inert and biocompatible, and it is now broadly accepted as an alternative to metallic biomaterials in spine surgery.[103] Its use in the pediatric spine, however, remains undefined.

The biomechanical principle and advantages of using anterior cervical plating systems in the pediatric spine are no different than in the adult spine. An anterior plate may maintain cervical alignment, prevent graft extrusion, and kyphotic deformity. The latter may be of particular concern in the pediatric population, as a higher incidence of kyphosis had been noted in pediatric patients after cervical trauma.[104,105] Increased posterior ligamentous laxity and the relatively larger head are contributing factors. A particular problem facing the pediatric spine surgeon is that there is no commercially available anterior cervical plate small enough for some infants and young children. A cranial fixation miniplate is sometimes used.[106]

The bio-absorbable anterior plate is especially attractive in children. It eliminates the possibility of plate migration and imaging degradation associated with implants later in life. Its use in adult patients was first reported in the early 2000s with good clinical and radiographic results.[107,108] Use of resorbable material in the form of a macropore craniofacial miniplate was reported in an 18-month-old and a 2-year-old child, both undergoing circumferential fusion.[109,110] In these two case reports, both patients were placed in a halovest due to the gross instability of the cervical spine. It is not clear whether that is necessary if the pathology is purely anterior. Furthermore, a direct comparison between titanium and resorbable plates in terms of clinical outcome is not yet available either in the adult or pediatric population.

Long-Term Consequences of Fusion in a Growing Spine

A major consideration in pediatric spine fusion is the fact that the pediatric spine continues to grow from childhood into adolescence. For this reason, fusion and stabilization techniques have often been avoided in children and adolescents. Issues include range of motion, limitation on future growth, and development of secondary deformity.

After occipitocervical fusion, three studies had shown that the impact on growth potential and the incidence of secondary spinal malalignment were not significant at a minimum follow-up of 33 months.[111-113] Furthermore, vertebral remodeling may even improve sagittal postoperative malalignment to restore the straight, or even lordotic, position of the cervical spine.[113,114] With older children, the growth potential of the cervical spine after age 10 is very small, and that may limit the scope of the problem.[115] A study by Anderson et al.[116] reported on 17 patients aged 6 years or younger who underwent occipitocervical fusion and found no cases of sagittal malalignment or adjacent osteophyte formation or subluxation. In their estimation, based on comparison with radiographic studies of normal cervical spine growth,[117] vertical growth potential was not impaired.

To the best of our knowledge, there is no dedicated study on spinal alignment and growth in children after subaxial cervical fusion.

The consequence of thoracic and lumbar fusion for scoliosis correction is related to the etiology of the scoliosis and therefore the age at which the fusion is performed. In the largest published series of congenital scoliosis fused posteriorly (291 patients), the most common problem was bending of the fusion mass (crankshaft phenomenon, defined as more of 10 degrees of bending), which occurred in 14% of their patients.[118] Patients who were fused without instrumentation before 5 years of age did equally well in terms of maintaining sagittal balance.[119] With the addition of newer generation implants that are reduced in size, even better correction could be obtained while eliminating or shortening the periods of cast immobilization.[120] While all of these studies have emphasized generally favorable results in maintaining sagittal balance, the effect of long segment fusion at a young age on the overall body height, spine length, and torso-to-leg ratio is seldom reported.[121]

Anterior column growth after a posterior column fusion may result in the "crankshaft phenomenon".[122-124] Because of the posterior fusion, all longitudinal growth in the posterior elements ceased. The vertebral bodies continue to grow anteriorly and eventually start to pivot on the posterior fusion resulting in progressive angulation and rotation of the spine. It is more of a problem in patients 10 years of age and younger who are skeletally immature,[124] and in patients with idiopathic scoliosis than congenital scoliosis. This latter observation may be related to the "sick" anterior growth plate in congenital scoliosis, as healthy growth plates are necessary to produce the crankshaft effect.

One possible solution to crankshafting would be the addition of an anterior fusion.[125,126] Various authors have used age, Risser sign of 0, open triradiate cartilage, peak height velocity,[127] and a combination of these factors to help to identify those at risk. Others, however, question the indication and the efficacy of additional anterior fusion.[128] There are also authors who believe that the newer instrumentation systems that emphasize stiff segmental fixation (e.g., Cotrel-Dubousset, Texas Scottish Rite Hospital, Isola instrumentation) may better prevent this secondary deformity than the older Harrington, Luque or Harri-Luque instrumentation. This is currently an important and active area of research.

KEY REFERENCES

Abumi K, Ito H, Taneichi H, Kaneda K. Transpedicular screw fixation for traumatic lesions of the middle and lower cervical spine: description of the techniques and preliminary report. *J Spinal Disord.* 1994;17:19-28.

Akamaru T, Kawahara N, Tsuchiya H, et al. Healing of autologous bone in a titanium mesh cage used in anterior column reconstruction after total spondylectomy. *Spine.* 2002;27(13):E329-E333.

Anderson RC, Ragel BT, Mocco J, et al. Selection of a rigid internal fixation construct for stabilization at the craniovertebral junction in pediatric patients. *J Neurosurg.* 2007;107:36-42.

Anderson RCE, Kan P, Gluf WM, Brockmeyer DL. Long-term maintenance of cervical alignment after occipitocervical and atlantoaxial screw fixation in young children. *J Neurosurg.* 2006;105(1 Suppl Pediatrics):55-61.

Brockmeyer DL, York JE, Apfelbaum RI. Anatomical suitability of C1-2 transarticular screw placement in pediatric patients. *J Neurosurg (Spine 1).* 2000;92:7-11.

Chamoun RB, Relyea KM, Johnson KK, et al. Use of axial and subaxial translaminar screw fixation in the management of upper cervical spinal instability in a series of 7 children. *Neurosurgery.* 2009;64:734-739.

Dickerman RD, Morgan JT, Mittler M. Circumferential cervical spine surgery in an 18-month-old female with traumatic disruption of the odontoid and C3 vertebrae. *Pediatr Neurosurg.* 2005;41:88-92.

Dubousset J, Herring JA, Shufflebarger H. The crankshaft phenomenon. *J Pediatr Orthop.* 1989;9:541-545.

Ebraheim NA, Jabaly G, Xu R, Yeasting RA. Anatomic relations of the thoracic pedicle to the adjacent neural structures. *Spine.* 1997;22:1553-1556.

Farey ID, Nadkarni S, Smith N. Modified Gallie technique versus transarticular screw fixation in C1-C2 fusion. *Clin Orthop Relat Res.* 1999;359:126-135.

Gluf WM, Brockmeyer DL. Atlantoaxial transarticular screw fixation: a review of surgical indications, fusion rate, complications, and lessons learned in 67 pediatric patients. *J Neurosurg Spine.* 2005;2:164-169.

Goel A, Laheri V. Plate and screw fixation for atlanto-axial subluxation. *Acta Neurochir (Wien).* 1994;129:47-53.

Harms J, Melcher RP. Posterior C1-C2 fusion with polyaxial screw and rod fixation. *Spine.* 2001;26:2467-2471.

Harrington PR. Treatment of scoliosis: correction and internal fixation by spine instrumentation. *J Bone Joint Surg (Am).* 1962;44:591.

Jea A, Sheth RN, Vanni S, et al. Modification of Wright's technique for placement of bilateral crossing C2 translaminar screws: technical note. *Spine J.* 2008;8:656-660.

Jea A, Taylor MD, Dirks PB, et al. Incorporation of C1 lateral mass screws in occipitocervical and atlantoaxial fusions for children 8 years of age or less: technical note. *J Neurosurg.* 2007;107:178-183.

Jeanneret B, Magerl F. Primary posterior fusion C1/2 in odontoid fractures: indications, technique, and results of transarticular screw fixation. *J Spinal Disord.* 1992;5:464-475.

Kretzer RM, Sciubba DM, Bagley CA, et al. Translaminar screw fixation in the upper thoracic spine. *J Neurosurg Spine.* 2006;5:527-533.

Majid ME, Castro FP, Holt RT. Anterior fusion for idiopathic scoliosis. *Spine.* 2000;25:696-702.

Parisini P, Di Silvestre M, Greggi T, Bianchi G. C1-C2 posterior fusion in growing patients: long-term follow-up. *Spine.* 2003;28:566-572.

Roberts DA, et al. Quantitative anatomy of the occiput and the biomechanics of occipital screw fixation. *Spine.* 1998;23:1100-1107.

Roy-Camille R, Saillant G, Laville C, Benazet JP. Treatment of lower cervical spinal injuries—C3 to C7. *Spine.* 1992;17:S442-S446.

Roy-Camille R, Saillant G, Mazel C. Plating of thoracic, thoracolumbar, and lumbar injuries with pedicle screw plates. *Orthop Clin North Am.* 1986;17:147-159.

Sasso RC, et al. Occipitocervical fusion with posterior plate and screw instrumentation. A long-term follow-up study. *Spine.* 1994;19:2364-2368.

Seitz H, Marlovits S, Schwendenwein I, et al. Biocompatibility of polyethylene terephthalate (Trevira hochfest) augmentation device in repair of the anterior cruciate ligament. *Biomaterials.* 1998;19:189-196.

Shacked I, Ram Z, Hadani M. The anterior cervical approach for traumatic injuries to the cervical spine in children. *Clin Orthop Relat Res.* 1993;292:144-150.

Singh H, Rahimi SY, Yeh DJ, Floyd D. History of posterior thoracic instrumentation. *Neurosurg Focus 16:Article.* 2004;11.

Smith JL, Ackerman LL. Management of cervical spine injuries in young children: lesson learned. Report of 2 cases. *J Neurosurg Pediatrics.* 2009;4:64-73.

Suk S, Kim WJ, Lee SM, et al. Thoracic pedicle screw fixation in spinal deformities: are they really safe? *Spine.* 2001;26:2049-2057.

Vaccaro AR, Balderston RA. Anterior plate instrumentation for disorders of the subaxial cervical spine. *Clin Orthop Relat Res.* 1997;335: 112-121.

Winter RB, Moe JH, Lonstein JE. Posterior spinal arthrodesis for congenital scoliosis. An analysis of the cases of two hundred and ninety patients, five to nineteen years old. *J Bone Joint Surg Am.* 1984;66(8): 1188-1197.

Winter RB, Moe JH. The results of spinal arthrodesis for congenital spine deformity in patients younger than five years old. *J Bone Joint Surg Am.* 1982;64:419-432.

Wright NM. Posterior C2 fixation using bilateral, crossing C2 laminar screws: case series and technical note. *J Spinal Disord Tech.* 2004;17:158-162.

Numbered references appear on Expert Consult.

CHAPTER 65

Methods of Cranial Vault Reconstruction for Craniosynostosis

JOSE HINOJOSA

Cranial sutures are essential components in the development of the skull. Nonfunctional sutures during the evolution of the cranial vault and the skull base lead to evolving deformities that may end in neurologic sequel. Although the term *craniosynostosis* was first used by Bertolotti in 1914, referring to the premature closure of a cranial suture, it was Sommerring who described in 1791 the anatomy of the suture and postulated not only its role in normal skull growth but also the effects of early closure.[50] During the 19th century Otto, and later Virchow, asserted that premature closure of sutures *(craneostenosis)* prevented growth perpendicular to the suture and was accompanied by compensatory growth at others. Premature closure may affect a single suture, but several sutures may be involved and severe deformities can develop, including the orbits and anterior fossa in the process. This is even more evident in craniofacial syndromes, where the main difference between single-suture and nonsyndromic craniosynostosis is the alterations not only in *neurocranium* but also in *viscerocranium*, resulting in anomalies in the midface skeleton.

The true incidence of craniosynostosis is not known, but it is estimated to occur in 1 of 2500 newborns. Sagittal synostosis is the most frequent (40%-60% of all cases), followed by metopic, coronal, and lambdoid, which is unusual.[1,2] More than 150 associated syndromes have been described, but in most cases craniosynostosis is an isolated phenomenon. Several theories have been postulated to explain the appearance of premature synostosis and posterior deformities. Virchow was the first to suggest in 1852 that the premature closure of the suture was the primary event, while the vault deformity was a consequence of this closure.[71] In 1959, Moss suggested that the deformity in the cranial base was the primary event. For this author, dura mater is an important regulator in the activity of the sutures and vault development and the main factor for the alteration in the cranial growth and suture dysfunction. The abnormal mechanical strengths driven through dural structures from certain maldeveloped points at the skull base (crista galli, petrous pyramids, or sphenoidal wings) would be responsible for cranial deformities and suture dysfunction.[3] Park and Powers referred to mesenchymal abnormalities in bone structures, related to genetic anomalies, that would explain more thoroughly hypoplasia affecting the craniofacial region in syndromic cases.[67,68,70]

Mechanical restraint could explain a number of isolated craniosynostosis, such as in some cases of scaphocephaly, lambdoid synostosis, or trigonocephaly. However, genetic abnormalities are increasingly described as the cause of many instances of craniosynostosis. This is particularly true in craniofacial syndromes, in which mutations in six genes have been related to a constant presence of different syndromes. The identification of these mutations would lead to a new classification of craniofacial syndromes, based on molecular changes instead of phenotype. These genes are FGFR1, FGFR2, FGFR3, MSX2, TWIST, and EFNB1.

EFBN1 codes for a structural protein, fibrillin. TWIST and MSX2 are transcriptional factors that control and mediate the expression of other genes. TWIST codes for a transcriptional factor type II that joins as a heterodimer, representing the active functional factor joining deoxyribonucleic acid (DNA). Most mutations in this gene produce a lack of union to DNA, resulting in an abnormal expression of the gene and a loss of function in protein TWIST.

Fibroblast growth factor receptors (FGFRs) are a subgroup of the family of tyrosine kinase receptors. They consist of an extracellular domain (glycoside acidic box, immunoglobulin-like domain, and calmodulin-like domain), a transmembrane domain, and an intracellular tyrosine kinase domain. Its active form is the dimer that provokes phosphorylation of the tyrosine intracellular endings. This promotes activation of intracellular events that lead to Ca^{2+} release, protein kinase C activation, and kinase phosphorylation that ends with activation of transcription factors. FGFR1, FGFR2, and FGFR3 interact in the cell-to-cell signaling process. They have complex functions involving proliferation, the end of the cellular cycle, cellular migration, differentiation, and apoptosis. FGFR2 promotes proliferation, and FGFR1 acts in the differentiation of cranial sutures. A mutation in any of these genes promotes lengthening of the signal, which causes early maturation of bone cells in the developing embryo and premature fusion of sutures, hands, and feet. FGFR3 is an inhibitor of proliferation during chondrogenesis.

In the end, all of these mechanisms and changes produce a cosmetic deformity, as well as incompetence of the cranial and facial structures—unable to properly contain the organs inside the vault (brain and cerebellum) and the orbits (optic nerves and eyeballs)—and hypoplasia of the midface and oropharyngeal region. All of these factors are related, and depending on the affected region, there is a predominance of one abnormality. However, as explained later, in craniofacial syndromes the situation is more complicated. The presence of raised intracranial pressure (ICP) (multiple suture closure), hydrocephalus and cerebrospinal fluid (CSF) circulation anomalies, venous hypertension (skull base sutures closure affecting jugular foramina drainage, as well as genetic factors including endothelial proliferation in dural venous sinuses), chronic hypoxia and hypercapnia (obstructive airway in relation to midface retrusion and amygdalar hyperplasia), and chronic tonsillar herniation leads to a complex situation in which staged treatment has to be the rule, particularly after careful and proper understanding of the pathophysiology underlying these cases and always in a multidisciplinary team.

Scaphocephaly

Sagittal synostosis is the most common form of craniosynostosis. The premature closure of the sagittal synostosis has an estimated prevalence of 2 in 1000 births. Up to 80% of the cases are sporadic, and there is a male-to-female ratio of 3:1 to 4:1.[1] Sporadic cases are mainly related to intrauterine constraint, but some may have a heterogeneous cause. In particular cases, a dominant autosomal inheritance has been described, with 38% penetrance.[1] The frequency of twinning in a series was 4.8%, with only one monozygotic twin pair being concordant for sagittal synostosis.[4]

Histology usually shows synostotic ridging on the posterior part of the fused suture, which is consistent with the sagittal suture being thicker on the ectocranial cortex than on the endocranial side, and the bony edge of the suture becomes progressively thicker from anterior to posterior under normal conditions.[5] When the sagittal suture is the only involved suture, the head becomes long from front to back (Figs. 65-1 to 65-3). It is narrow from side to side, and frontal compensational bossing may occur when the anterior fontanel is patent. When both fontanels are closed and the posterior part of the suture is predominantly affected, there is a posterior deformity typically referred to as an occipital knob. It is usually accompanied by a thin forehead with severe pterional indentation (*leptoscaphocephaly*). In the severest forms of scaphocephaly, the head adopts the shape of a saddle, and it is named *bathrocephaly*. Accurate diagnosis of isolated sagittal synostosis can be made clinically, and operative correction can proceed without a need for radiologic investigations, unless the clinical features are not completely typical.[6] This could be the case in which Crouzon syndrome in some patients can resemble, early in evolution, an isolated scaphocephaly.

There is a plethora of techniques for the treatment of scaphocephaly[7-11] but most of them include the excision of the sagittal suture with different kinds of parietal and occipital osteotomies with or without frontal osteotomies and remodeling. Surgical correction, whatever the technique, when performed early in infancy, results in satisfactory and persisting reshaping of the skull (Figs. 65-1 to 65-3). Delays in diagnosis, as well as treatment, result in a small subset of patients with uncorrected craniosynostosis that require the development of more extensive calvarial reconstruction techniques (Fig. 65-4). Due to calvarial maturity, these more advanced cases would not be amenable to treatment using less aggressive

techniques. After 1 year of age the child's cranial vault has developed abnormally, resulting in a severe skull base deformity, as shown in the figure. Subsequently, the skull is significantly thicker and less pliable to reshaping. At this age, cranial defects due to aggressive surgical remodeling procedures may not reossify, and there is a lack of the driving mechanism that leads to closure of the sutures. For these patients, an approach with a more comprehensive calvarial reconstruction includes multiple interleaving osteotomies crossing the midline, leading to improvements in biparietal narrowing combined with a bifrontal reconstruction.

Trigonocephaly

Trigonocephaly is considered a fairly common type of craniosynostosis. The term was first coined by Welcker in 1862.[12] Formerly denoted as unusual,[12,13] it is now considered to represent about 10% of all patients with deformities related to craniofacial centers[12,14,15] and its frequency is increasing.[2] Its incidence is estimated to be 1 in 2500 births,[16] and there is a male predominance of 65% to 85%.[14]

Closure of the metopic suture starts under normal circumstances at the end of the first year and may last until the end of the second year.[12] When premature suture closure occurs, usually before birth, a typical craniofacial malformation develops. The premature arrest of growth of the metopic suture may present as a spectrum of manifestations, depending on the timing and extent of the suture closure. Its mildest form is a familial and ethnically inherited facial morphology.[17] Milder forms of metopic synostosis consist of only a somewhat prominent metopic ridge that does not need surgical intervention. In severe forms, a characteristic keel-shaped forehead can be observed, with absence of frontal eminences, retruded orbital rims, hypotelorism, and epicanthus giving a peculiar craniofacial appearance to these children. Different degrees of involvement of the anterior chondrocranial structures seem possible, such as presphenoid, mesoethmoid, and ectoethmoid structures.[18] Another explanation for the broad phenotype of affected children could be a nonspecific process acting at different evolutive ages. Trigonocephaly may appear either as an isolated anomaly or as part of syndromes involving prosencephalic or rhinencephalic structures (holoprosencephaly), such as Opitz syndrome,[19,20] Say-Meyer syndrome, or Frydman syndrome.[12] Recently a new fronto-ocular syndrome has been described with trigonocephaly.[21]

Several genetic defects also have been described associated with trigonocephaly. Abnormalities including deletions and duplications of chromosomes 3p, 9p, 1, 1q, and 13q have been published.[22-25] Isolated trigonocephaly has an unknown etiology. Autosomal dominant inheritance with very low penetrance has been proposed in 2% to 5% of the cases for familial cases.[15,26] The possible involvement of mutated FGFRs in newborns affected by trigonocephaly has recently been investigated by molecular screening in a search for mutations in FGFR2, which has been implicated in complex craniofacial syndromes. However, none of the cases studied carried mutations, except one that evolved later toward a Crouzon syndrome–like profile.[25]

Mental delay may occur in isolated trigonocephaly and has been observed in as many as 10% of these children.[12] Development delays may consist of subtle changes in the

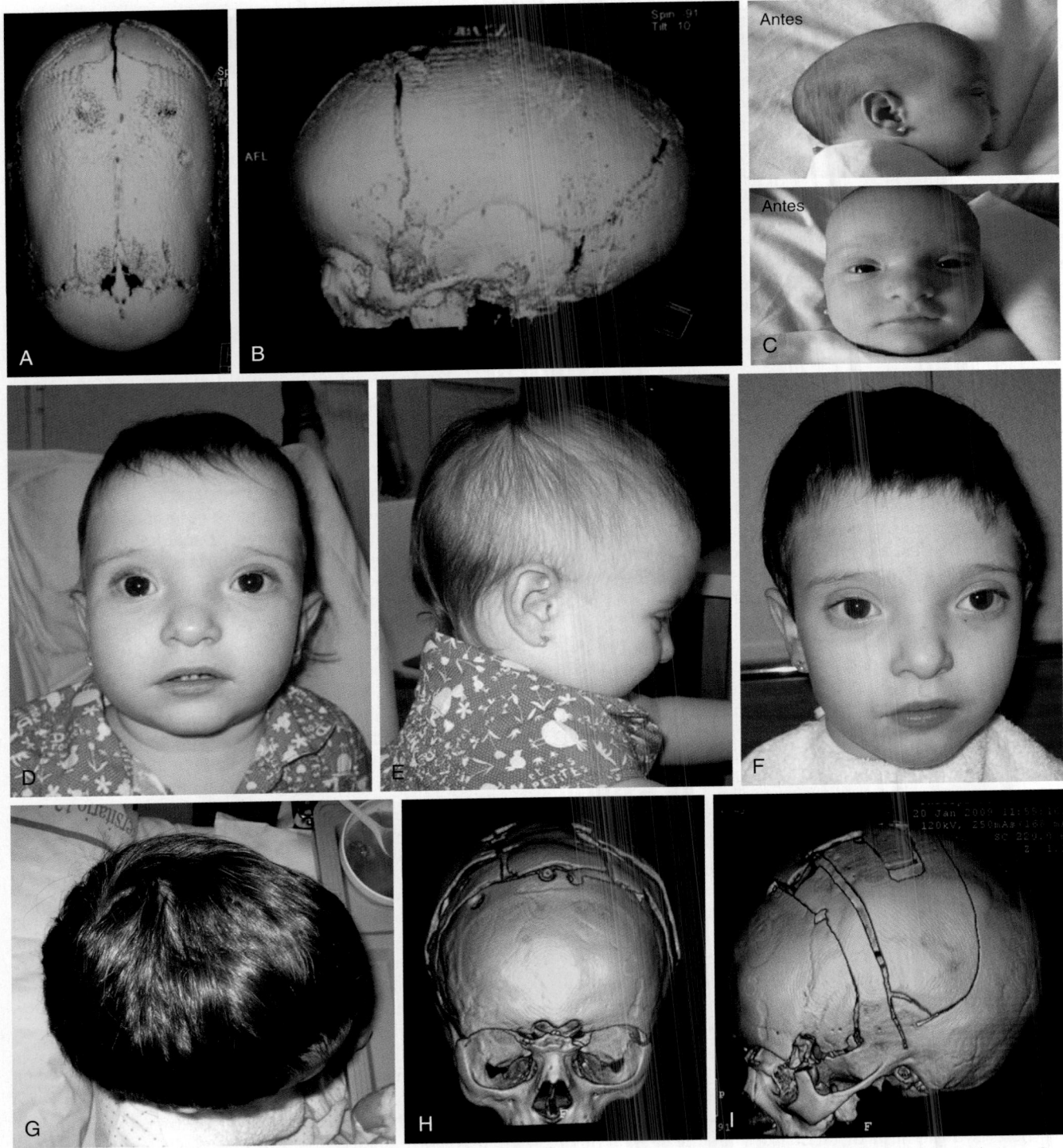

FIGURE 65-1 Scaphocephaly and differential diagnosis. Preoperative three-dimensional reconstructed CT in bird's eye (A) and lateral (B) views. Preoperative photographs are shown in side and front (C) views. The appearance 2 years after endoscopic correction is seen from front (D) and side (E) views. The patient later developed raised ICP despite excellent aesthetic outcome (frontal view, F; bird's eye view, G). Genetic studies revealed a mutation in FGFR2, compatible with Crouzon syndrome. CT showed pansynostosis with oxycephaly (not shown). Three-dimensional reconstructed CT after surgical correction is shown in frontal (H) and side (I) views. The patient's elevated ICP resolved with a favorable outcome.

time of acquisition of head control or sitting position or include more severe forms of mental retardation, with or without intracranial hypertension.

Di Rocco et al. proposed two subgroups on the basis of clinical and radiologic findings.[18] Group I presents with

bilateral frontal bone hypoplasia associated with extreme retrusion of the supraorbital margins. In this group, hypotelorism is associated with abnormally deep position of the cribriform plate, giving the ethmoidal region a hollow appearance. In these patients, the nasion–pterional

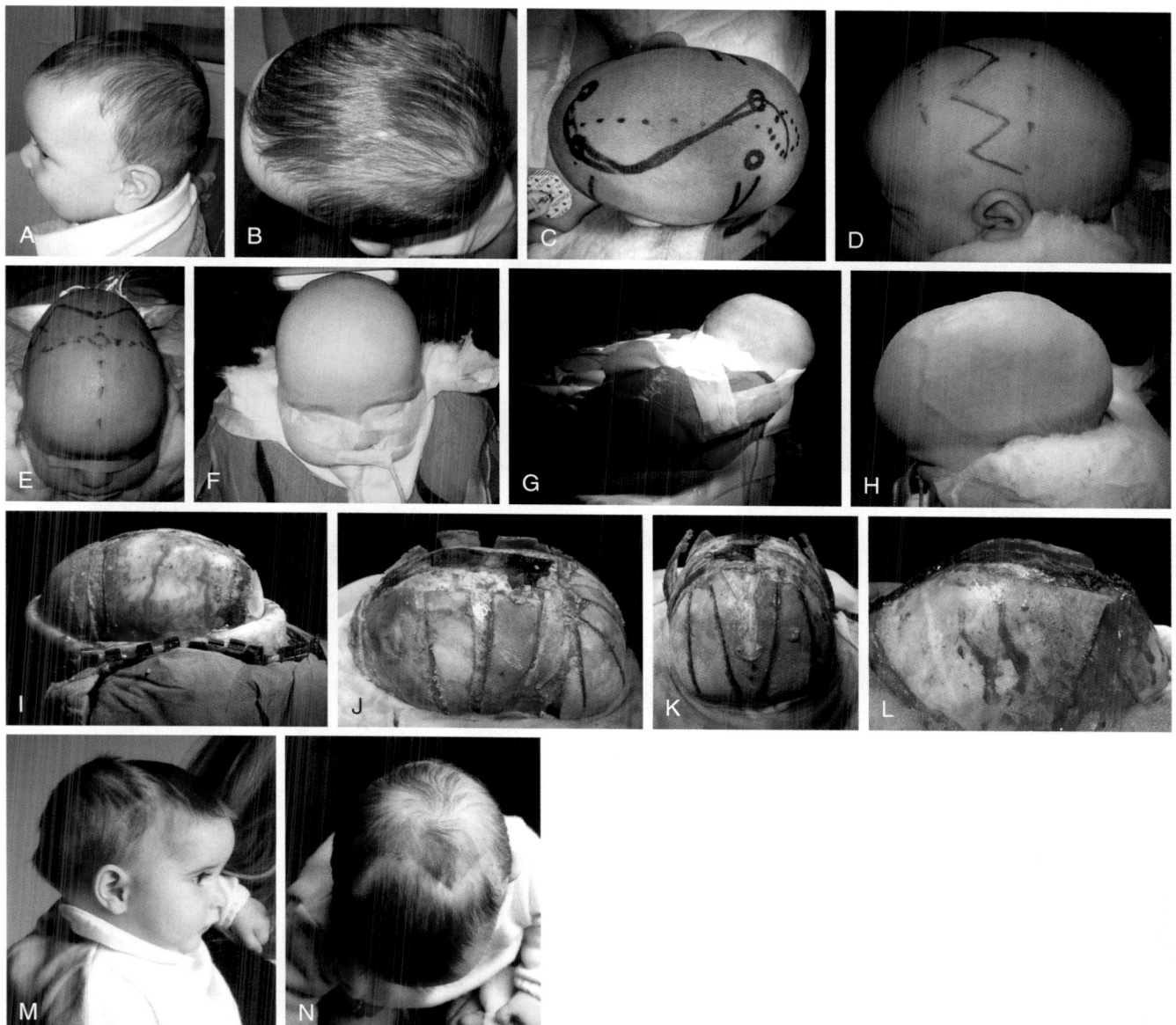

FIGURE 65-2 Open technique for surgical correction of scaphocephaly in side (A) and bird's eye (B) views. An S-type incision is seen from a bird's eye (C) view. Bicoronal modified incision is seen from side (D) and bird's eye (E) views. A modified prone position allows exposure of entire cranial vault from frontal (F), side (G), and higher-magnification side (H) views. Sagittal suturectomy (I) and osteotomies are seen from side (J) and frontal (K) views. A side (L) view details the lambda and the occipital isle. Postoperative side (M) and bird's eye (N) images demonstrate correction of scaphocephaly.

angle is severely restricted and the nasion–clinoidal distance significantly increased. Group II also shows bilateral frontal hypoplasia with hypotelorism, supraorbital retrusion, and a reduced nasopterional angle. However, the nasion–clinoidal distance is almost normal, and pterional evidence is scarcely evident.[18] Moreover, patients in group II showed a lesser degree of temporal compensatory expansion. The authors postulate that in some patients a compensatory elongation of the nasion–clinoidal distance and an incomplete synostosis of the frontoethmoidal sutures allows partial lateral expansion of the anterior cranial fossa, which could diminish the need for posterior calvarial expansion. On the other hand, children with more severe involvement of

the nasoethmoidal sutures, resulting in diminished lateral expansion of the anterior fossa, need compensatory changes in the temporal and parietal regions. Patients in group II accomplished good correction of associated hypotelorism, whereas patients in group I did not reach normal interorbital values when treated with the same surgical procedure, which did not include specific treatment of hypotelorism. Other authors have addressed the importance of the moment and degree of involvement of pathologic changes in the anterior chondrocranial structures.[14,27-31] Milder forms of trigonocephaly would affect only the upper metopic suture, whereas more severe forms include involvement of presphenoid, mesoethmoid, and ectoethmoid structures.

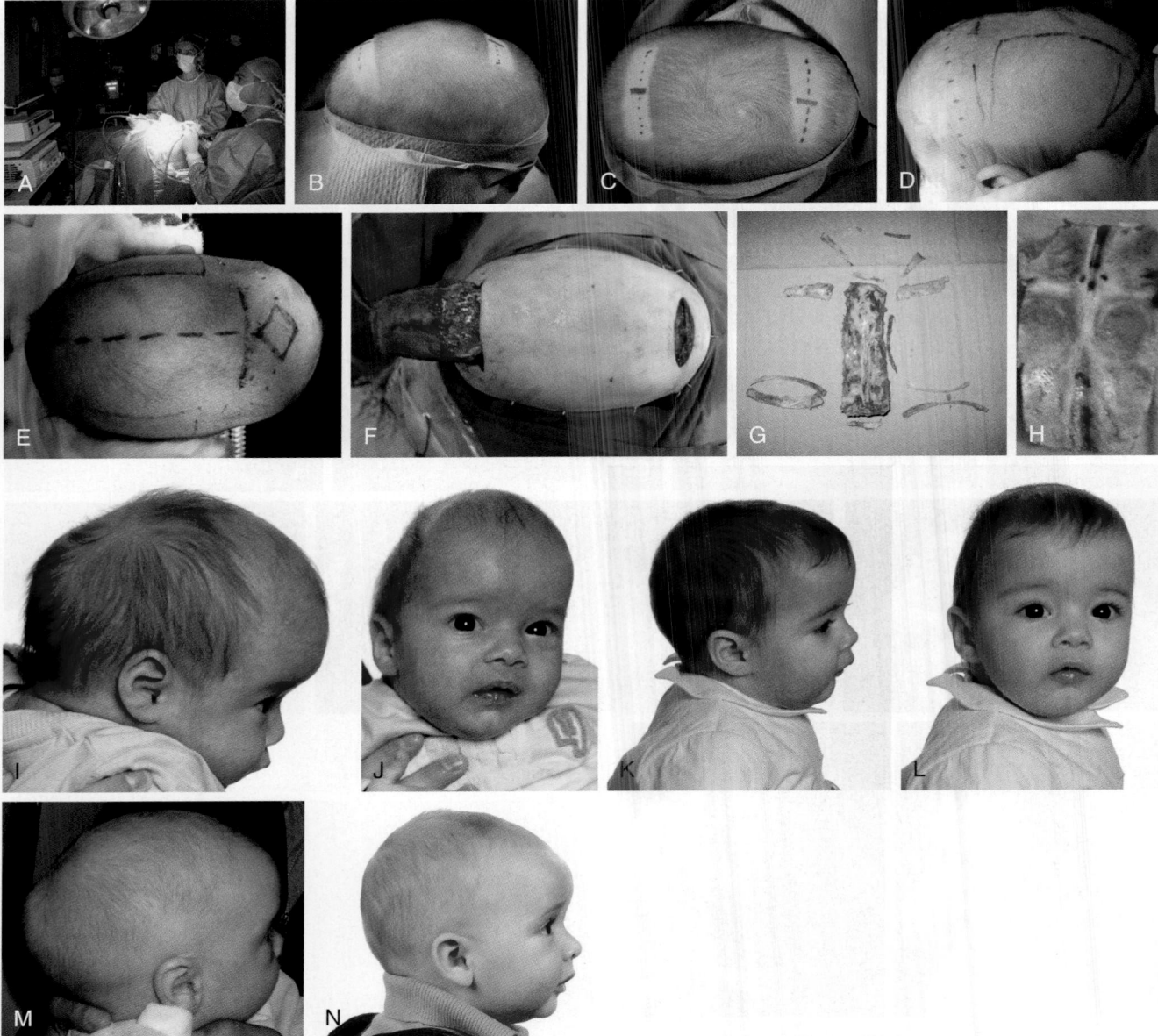

FIGURE 65-3 A, Endoscopically assisted surgical correction of scaphocephaly. Patient positioning is seen from side (B) and bird's eye (C) views. Surgical planning is also seen from side (D) and bird's eye (E) views. Sagittal suturectomy is seen from a bird's eye (F) view. Osteotomies are completed, as shown at low (G) and high (H) magnification: Observe emissary veins from the superior sagittal sinus. For patient 1, preoperative images are seen from side (I) and frontal (J) views, and postoperative images are seen from side (K) and frontal (L) views. For patient 2, preoperative side (M) and postoperative side (N) views are shown.

SURGICAL TECHNIQUE

The standard approach to surgical technique for trigonocephaly consists of bifrontal craniotomy, flap remodeling, and fronto-orbital advancement with recontouring. A standard bicoronal approach is scheduled with retroauricular incision and elevation of a bifrontal flap in the loose areolar plane between the periosteum and the galea pericrania. Frontal branches of the facial nerve run inside the external fascia of the temporalis muscle, so care must be taken to not damage them. However, these patients often show low implantation of the temporalis muscle, and dissection under the deep fascia of the muscle opens broad exposure of the pterion and lateral wall of the orbit. The periosteum is incised at this level, and dissection proceeds in the subperiosteal plane, exposing the frontal and pterional areas; the lateral walls of the orbit, with partial elevation of the temporalis muscle to expose the greater wing of the sphenoid; and the superior walls of the orbits up to the medial canthus, which is usually preserved.

Before starting osteotomies, the obliquity of frontal bones, retrusion of the lateral portions of the orbital bandeau, and pterional indentation are assessed. A bifrontal craniotomy is performed after a supraorbital bandeau is created. The marks are extended from the sphenosquamosal suture to its contralateral equivalent prepared for a tongue-in-groove advancement.[18] The bifrontal flap includes the

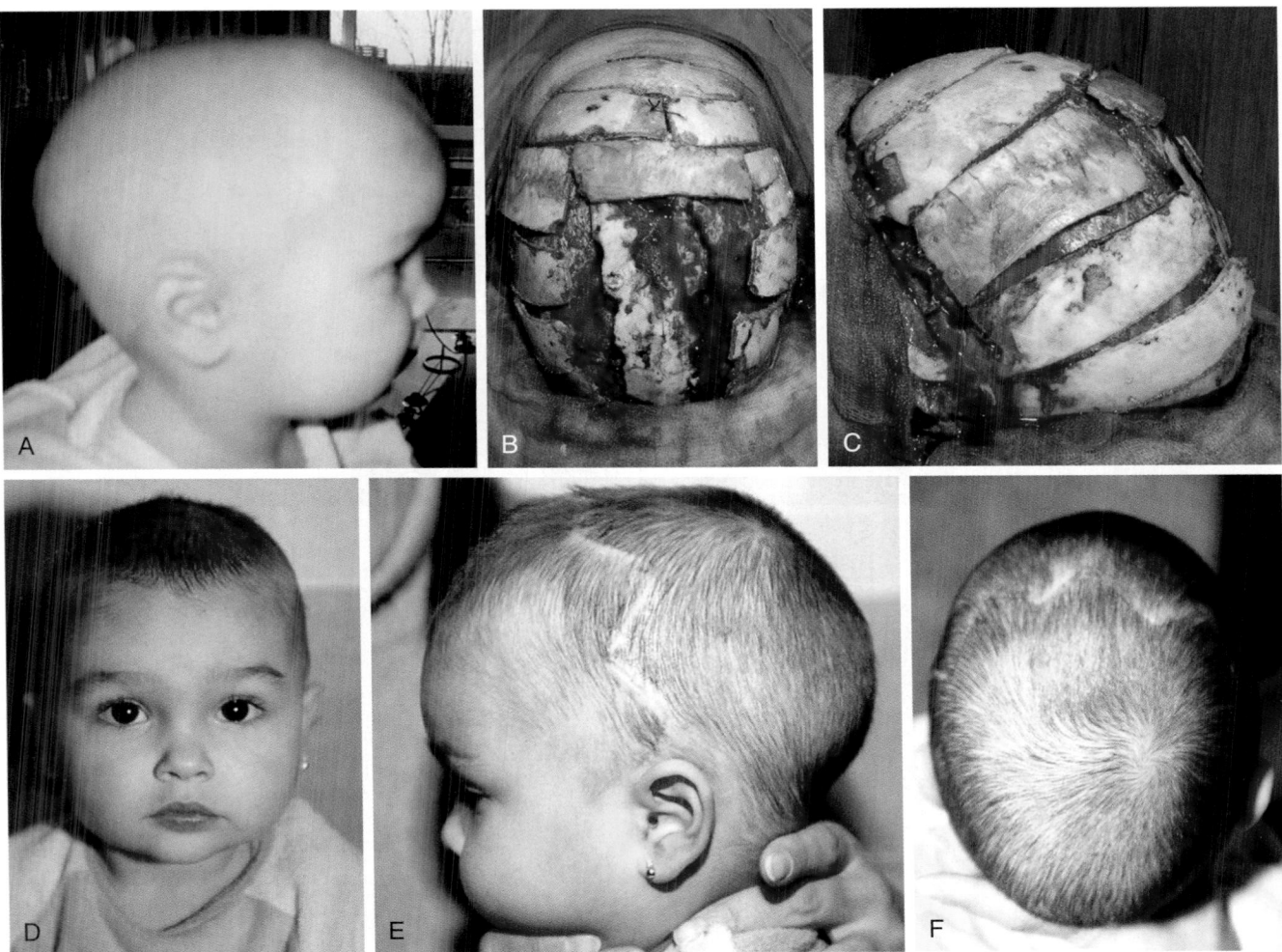

FIGURE 65-4 Holocranial dismantling in an older scaphocephaly patient. A, The preoperative side view demonstrates scaphocephaly. Intraoperative bird's eye (B) and side (C) views demonstrate osteotomies and synostectomy. Postoperative frontal (D), side (E), and bird's eye (F) views show correction of scaphocephaly.

anterior part of the bregmatic fontanelle and both coronal sutures. The anterior fossa is exposed extradurally with visualization of the anterior two thirds of the orbital roof.

Osteotomies on the orbitofrontal bandeau are now performed starting on the lateral orbital ridge over the fronto-zygomatic suture, and opening of the orbital roof includes the portion over the cribriform plate at the midline. There is commonly severe sphenoid thickening at the pterional level, where osteotomies are the last step to obtain a free orbital bandeau. Pterions are resected up to the level of the anterior fossa. The bandeau is anteriorly displaced, with rotation of the lateral extremes of the bandeau projecting forward, maintaining the medial aspect of the bandeau in place. Orbital roofs and supraorbital ridges are aligned in proper position and then fixed in place with absorbable miniplates. After recontouring of the frontal bone, closure proceeds in the standard way, with anterior rotation and elevation of the temporalis muscle bilaterally and covering of the field with the periosteum and galea.

There is not yet a consensus on hypotelorism correction. Several papers have addressed the importance of associated hypotelorism[17,28] and the need for direct surgical approach. Different authors[17,27,28,36,37] propose adding a nasofrontal osteotomy and an interpositional bone graft to the supraorbital bar and nasoethmoidal area to correct hypotelorism simultaneously with lateral orbitary wall expansion[17] or three quarter orbital wall osteotomies.[27] On the other hand, there are others[13,34] who do not advocate direct approach to the hypotelorism in the belief that internasalis grafting widens only nasal bones without increasing interorbital width, as far as osteotomies usually remain anterior and superior to nasoethmoidal complex.[36] I recommend a standard approach without grafting and thus consider the latter ineffective and unnecessary. Both techniques have achieved statistically significant improvement in hypotelorism, greater than that expected from normal growth curves. However, undercorrection of hypotelorism and persistence of abnormally low interorbitary distances occur frequently when orbital widening is not addressed.[18,27,35]

Anterior Plagiocephaly

Premature closure of a single coronal suture produces the most complex set of craniofacial deformities due to the peculiarities of the fronto-orbital region and the close relationship between the sutures of the anterior cranial base

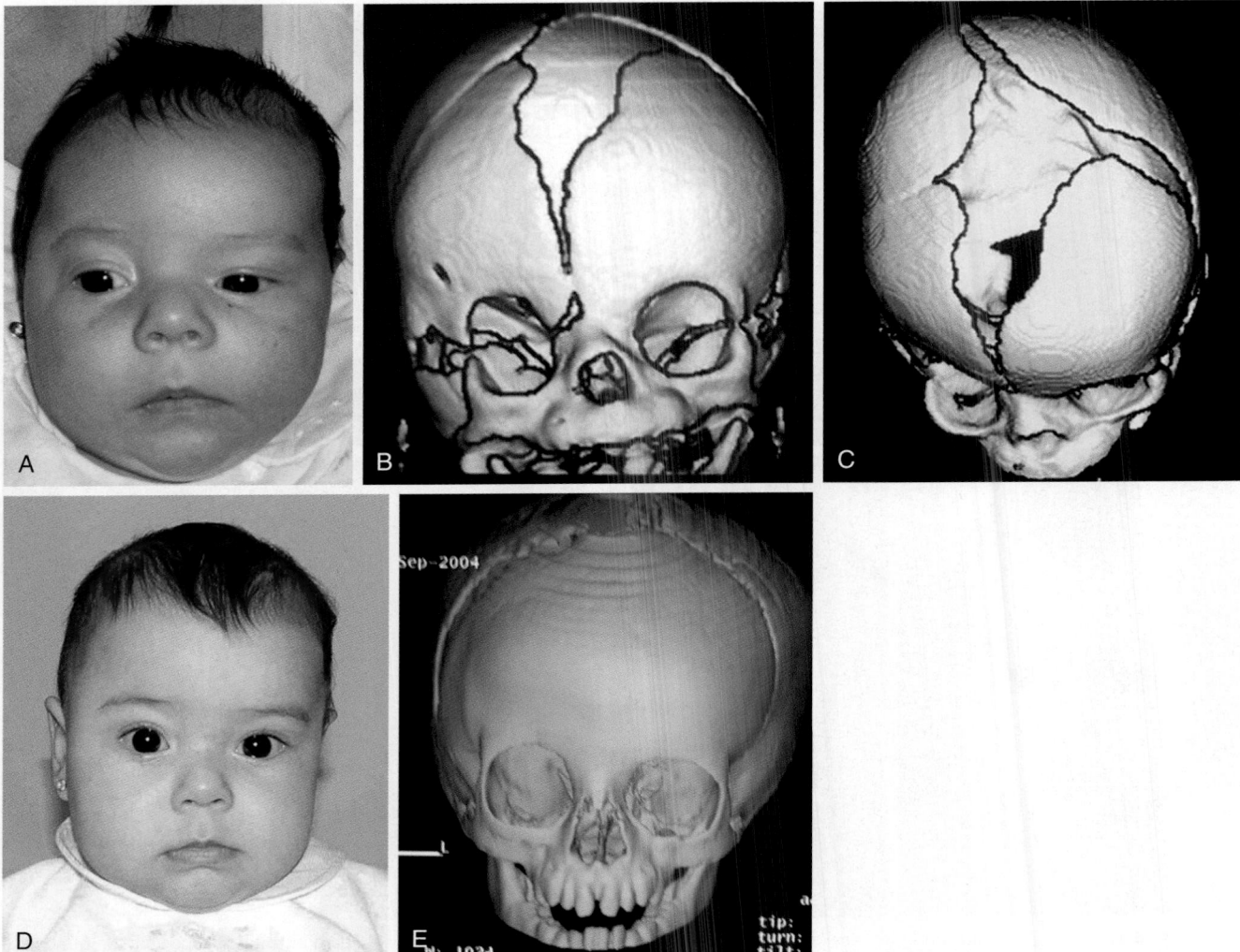

FIGURE 65-5 Endoscopically assisted correction of unilateral coronal suture synostosis. A, A preoperative image from a frontal view shows right forehead flattening and superior displacement of the right superior orbital ridge. A preoperative three-dimensional reconstructed CT demonstrates right coronal suture synostosis from frontal (B) and bird's eye (C) views. D, A postoperative image from a frontal view demonstrates improvement in facial asymmetry. E, A postoperative three-dimensional CT shows improvement in forehead shape and patency of the right coronal suture.

and the orbits and maxillary complex. The incidence of coronal craniosynostosis has been reported to be variable but can be approximated to be 0.4 per 1000.[40] Although most cases are sporadic, a familiar incidence of up to 8% in uncomplicated coronal synostosis has been reported.[40]

Frontal or anterior synostotic plagiocephaly has been described in association with unilateral coronal synostosis,[41-44] but it is known to occur with synostosis of other parts of the coronal ring, such as the frontosphenoidal or frontoethmoidal sutures.[41,45-47] In some rare cases, it has been reported to be the result of fusion of the frontosphenoidal[48] or the frontozygomatic sutures alone.[49] The deformity is manifest as a progressive cranial, orbital, and facial asymmetry of varying severity, with secondary deformities, considered to be compensatory, existing on the contralateral side (Figs. 65-5 and 65-6). Associated cranial anomalies affect the development of all facial bones and have been referred to as "the most complete presentation of craniofacial asymmetry."[50] There is a flat and retruded frontal bone in the affected side with a contralateral bossing. The orbital

rim on the synostotic side is also elevated and retruded, while the ipsilateral orbit is elevated and twisted. There is a variable degree of vertical orbital dystopia. The nasal root is deviated toward the closed sutured with an oblique nasal axis. The tip of the nose points to the nonsynostotic side. The zygoma and maxilla are hypoplastic on the affected side, and the ipsilateral temporal bone is malpositioned in an anterior and descended configuration.

Different reconstructive techniques have been described,[42,43,46,47,50-53] but most of them can be divided between unilateral and bilateral approaches. There is a long-standing controversy on the timing and type of surgical approach. Some authors have advocated early surgery (younger than 6 months),[40,54] whereas others support treating these patients later (between 9 and 10 months).[41,45,51] The former group uses the concept of rapid brain growth leading to advancement of the frontal bones and supraorbital rims.

Proponents of late surgery argue that delayed surgery allows for further maturation and growth of the craniofacial skeleton. There is less reliance on brain growth, and blood

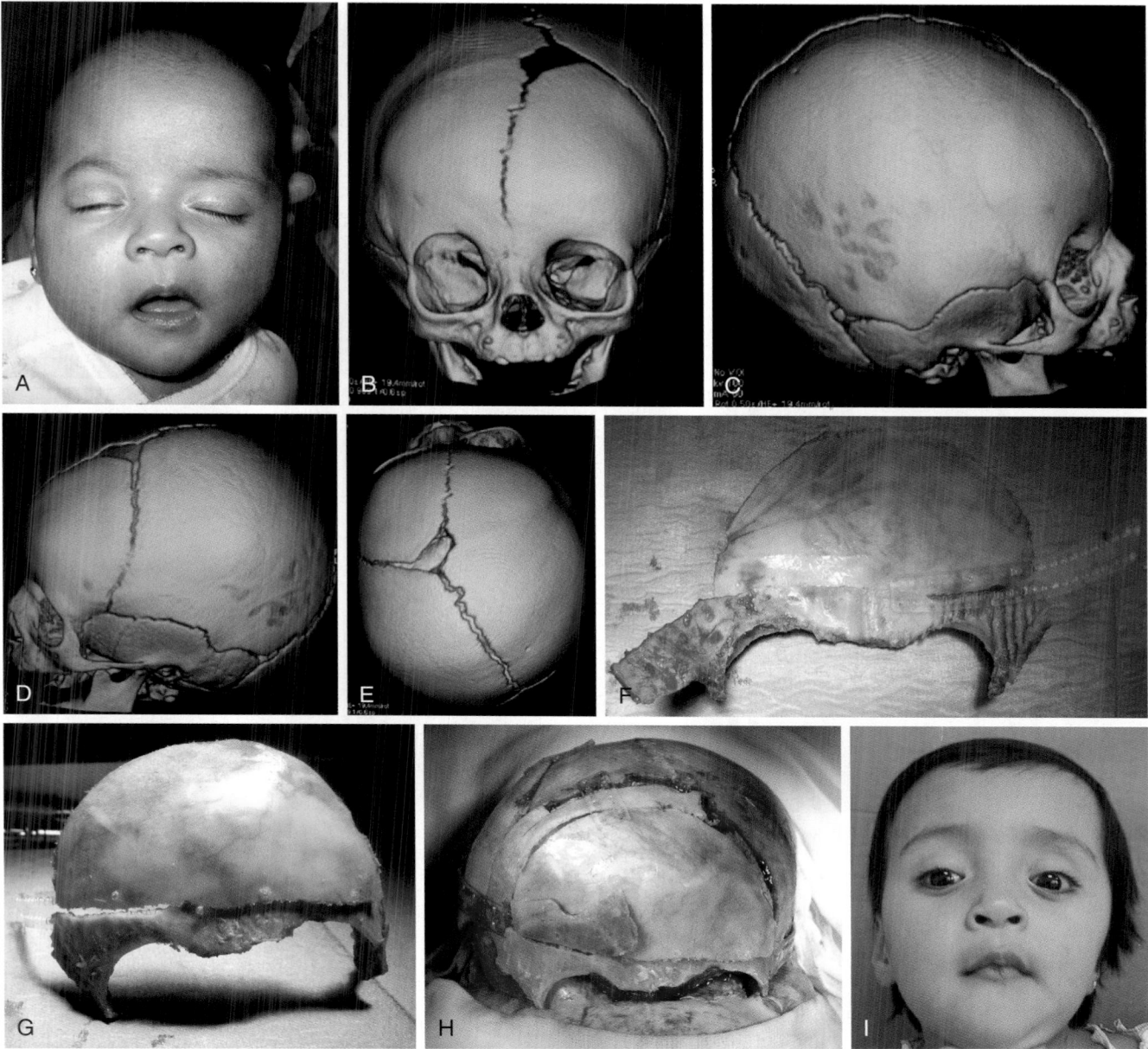

FIGURE 65-6 Standard fronto-orbital reconstruction for correction of unilateral coronal suture synostosis. A, A preoperative image from a frontal view shows right forehead flattening and superior displacement of the right superior orbital ridge. A preoperative three-dimensional reconstructed CT demonstrates right coronal suture synostosis from frontal (B), side (C), and bird's eye (D) views. E, In comparison, the contralateral coronal suture remains patent. The intraoperative technique is standard fronto-orbital reconstruction, as seen immediately after bony removal (F), during reconstruction (G), and at completion of reconstruction (H). I, A postoperative image is seen from a frontal view at 4 years of age.

loss is better tolerated. Also, there is immediate correction of the deformity. Surgical procedures have expanded from simple suturectomies (Fig. 65-5) to frontal–calvarial vault remodeling consisting of bifrontal craniotomes and orbital frontal bandeau advancement (Fig. 65-6). Aggressive surgical approaches have been supported by the theory of "coronal ring" synostosis, which states that there is an extension of the coronal synostosis into the cranial base.[55,56] However, in most cases of isolated, nonsyndromic, unilateral coronal synostosis, the sphenofrontal, sphenoethmoidal, ethmoidofrontal, and pterional sutures are patent. Furthermore, review of the literature of these patients who have undergone more extensive procedures indicate that the results

are inconsistent and mixed. Often, there is restriction of forward anterior skull base growth and advancement, and late correction (older than 9 months) fails to improve vertical dystopia, which persists into adulthood.[40] Most craniofacial centers use the classic fronto-orbital advancement with unilateral or bilateral correction. Undoubtedly, in cases with severe contralateral compensation (frontal and/or temporal bossing), a bilateral correction is preferred. The correction of orbital dystopia warrants careful preoperative evaluation. Orbital hypoplasia is a consequence of the elevated orbital roofs, frontal development of the greater sphenoidal wings, and descent of the ethmoidal position, secondary to early closure of the coronal sutures. Orbital axes are also

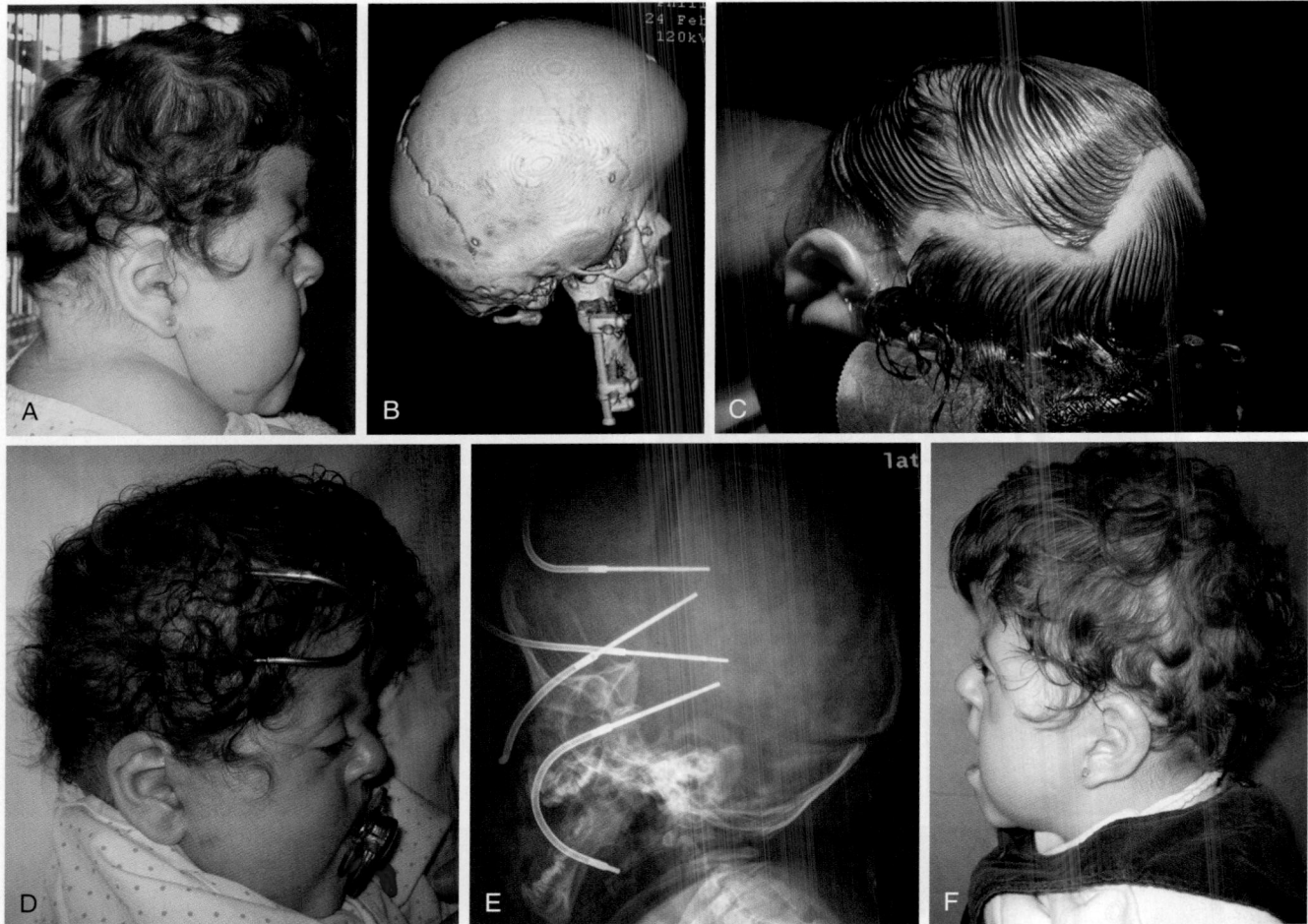

FIGURE 65-7 Occipital advancement by internal distraction in Apert syndrome. A preoperative side view (A) demonstrates the result of underlying pansynostosis, including squamosal region, bicoronal, and occipitotemporal sutures seen on side view three-dimensional reconstructed CT (B). Mandibular internal distraction avoided tracheostomy in this patient with severe mandibular hypoplasia. C, Surgical planning and positioning are prone with a horseshoe headholder and a bicoronal incision. Internal resorbable devices in place during distraction are seen from a side view in the immediate postoperative period (D) and on lateral postoperative x-ray images (E). F, A postoperative side view image shows successful occipital advancement. Fronto-orbital and midface advancement are pending as the next step of treatment.

altered and point downward and outward. In the severest cases, failure to achieve early treatment or undercorrection may lead to strabismus, amblyopia, and anomalies in the binocular vision.

Multiple Suture Craniosynostosis

BRACHYCEPHALY

Brachycephaly is most commonly the result of premature synostosis of both coronal sutures. The anterior fossa adopts a characteristic deformation, and there are retruded frontal bones and orbital rims with a vertical, broad, flat forehead and a high bregmatic point. Brachycephaly may appear as an isolated synostosis and has then a favorable prognosis. Often, it is the common final appearance of different syndromic craniosynostoses that share a premature closure of bicoronal sutures and similar phenotype (e.g., some cases of Saehtre-Chotzen or Pfeiffer type I). For this reason, every patient with brachycephaly should be assessed by a clinical geneticist (Figs. 65-7 and 65-8).

OXICEPHALY

The premature closure of both coronal sutures and metopic gives the head a pointed appearance (*oxis* is the Greek for "arrowhead"). The sagittal suture may be involved to a variable degree, resulting in a cone-shaped head with a high bregma. It is commonly associated with intracranial hypertension when left untreated.

CROUZON SYNDROME

Crouzon syndrome is an autosomal dominant disorder characterized by craniosynostosis that causes secondary alterations of the facial bones and facial structure. Common features include hypertelorism, exophthalmos and external strabismus, parrot-beaked nose, short upper lip, hypoplastic maxilla, and a relative mandibular prognathism. First described by Crouzon in 1912,[59] it was not until 1959 that Shiller observed an autosomal dominant transmission.[60] Crouzon syndrome represents approximately 4.8% of cases of craniosynostosis at birth, and the birth prevalence is estimated to be 16.5 per million births. Crouzon craniofacial dysostosis is

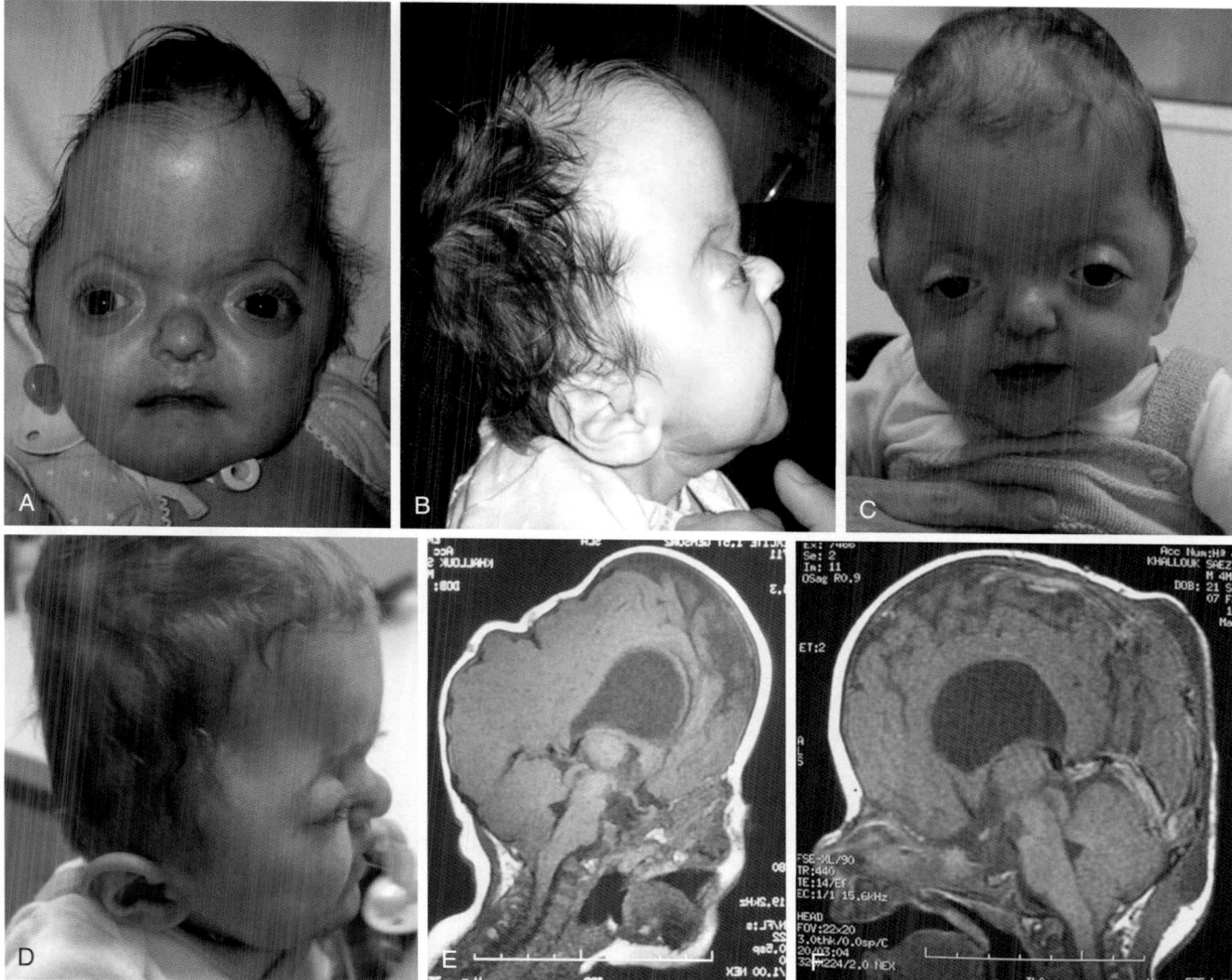

FIGURE 65-8 Kleeblattschädel deformity in Apert syndrome. Preoperative frontal (A) and side (B) views. Postoperative frontal (C) and side (D) views after occipital expansion (morselization of the parietal–occipital region). Note the improvement in the anterior (fronto-orbital and pterional) after posterior expansion by simply releasing the posterior two thirds of the cranial vault. Comparison of preoperative (E) and postoperative (F) MRI also demonstrates improvement.

linked to a high number of different mutations, but most of them are located on IgIII of FGFR2 (exons 7 and 9) on chromosome 10q. An association between Crouzon syndrome and acanthosis nigricans has been described and is related to an A391E mutation in the FGFR3 gene on chromosome 4p.

Crouzon syndrome is characterized by a premature synostosis of both coronal sutures, with a resultant brachycephalic shape of the skull. Sagittal, metopic, or lambdoid sutures may also be prematurely affected, isolated, or combined (Figs. 65-9 and 65-10). The cranial base and upper facial sutures are involved with a variable degree of midface hypoplasia and malocclusion. The orbits are hypoplastic, and the orbital floor is hollow, resulting in proptosis and additional orbital dystopia that may produce mild to moderate orbital hypertelorism and divergent strabismus. Maxillary hypoplasia results in pseudoprognatism. Nasal septum deviation, together with maxillary hypoplasia, may produce a chronic obstruction to respiratory flow and may be associated with choanal atresia, velopharyngeal incompetence,

and relative macroglossia. All of these malformations may lead to severe respiratory obstructions and apneas, which may cause a chronic raised ICP by an increase in venous pressure after hypercapnia and even contribute as an etiopathogenic mechanism in the development of hydrocephalus.

The initial treatment for Crouzon syndrome generally requires cranio-orbital decompression, including bicoronal suture release and osteotomies of the anterior cranial vault and upper orbits with reshaping and advancement. They are usually performed by the age of 8 to 11 months unless signs of increased ICP are found earlier. Sometimes, it is necessary to perform a combined approach, including midface advancement.[61] When Chiari malformation (CM) is identified precociously, an occipital–parietal calvarial decompression may be preferable to achieve a bigger expansion of the intracranial volume, with or without suboccipital decompression.[62] After proper release of the ICP, fronto-orbital remodeling can be achieved via an anterior approach.

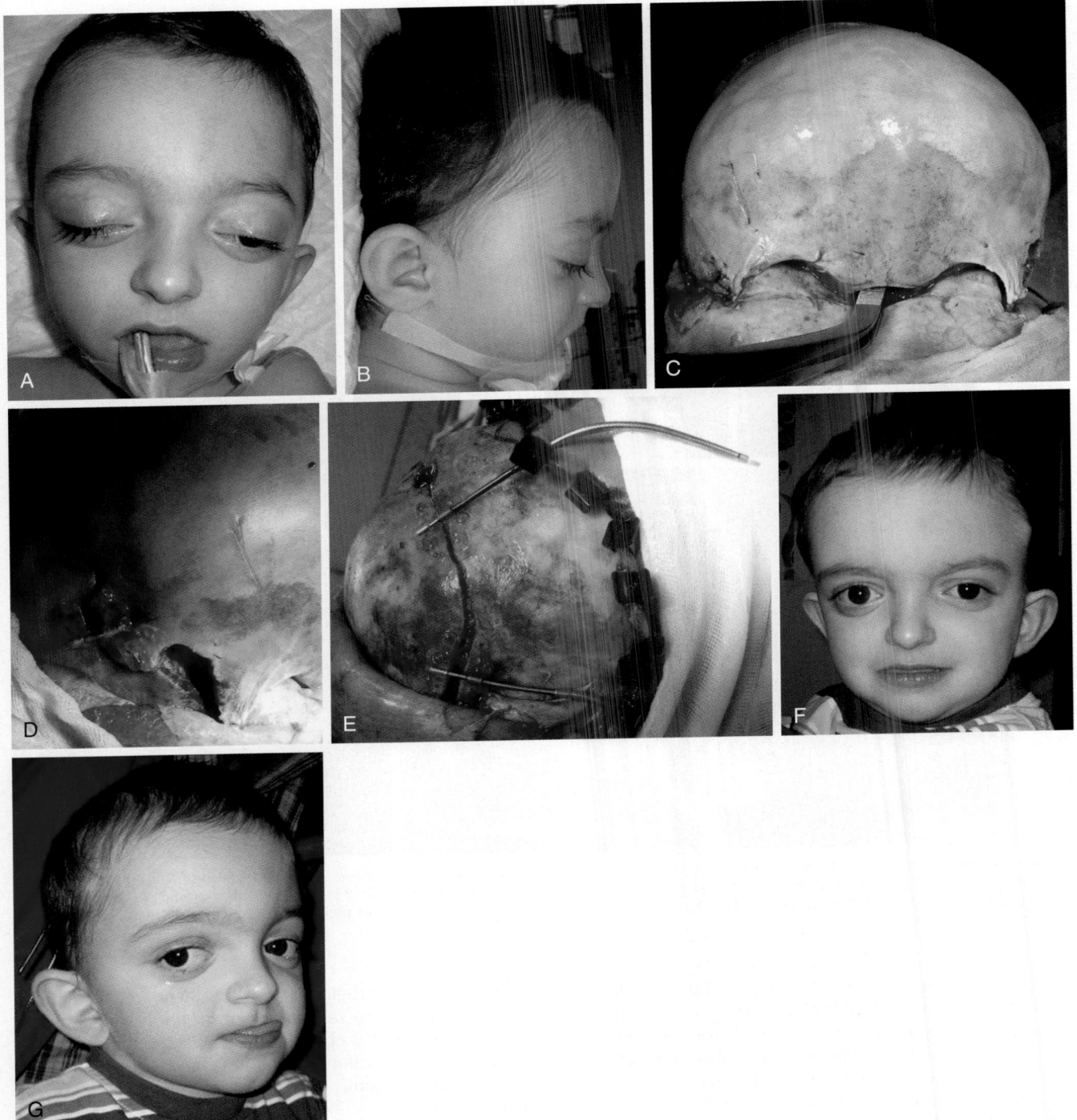

FIGURE 65-9 Fronto-orbital distraction with resorbable devices for anterior advancement. Predistraction frontal (A) and side (B) views show a harmonic Crouzon syndrome patient. In intraoperative frontal (C) and side (D) view images, observe pterional resection and osteotomy lines. E, Intraoperative high magnification of distraction devices. Postoperative frontal (F) and oblique (G) views are shown during distraction. Observe improvement in proptosis. Polysomnography also improved at the end of distraction in this patient with preoperative raised ICP and central apnea.

APERT SYNDROME

Apert syndrome, also known as acrocephalosyndactyly type I, is a congenital disorder characterized by multiple craniosynostoses, facial hypoplasia, and osseous syndactyly of the hands and feet. Approximately 1 in 65,000 to 165,000 of live births is affected. It is usually classified among a group of craniofacial syndromes with Crouzon, Pfeiffer,

and Saehtre-Chotzen syndromes, all of which are allelic disorders with similar clinic manifestations and common genetic background. Wheaton first noted the coincidence of craniosynostosis and syndactyly (1894), but it was Apert who fully characterized the syndrome in 1906.[63,64] Apert syndrome consists of a craniosynostosis in the shape of an acrocephaly or a brachycephaly due to the premature closure

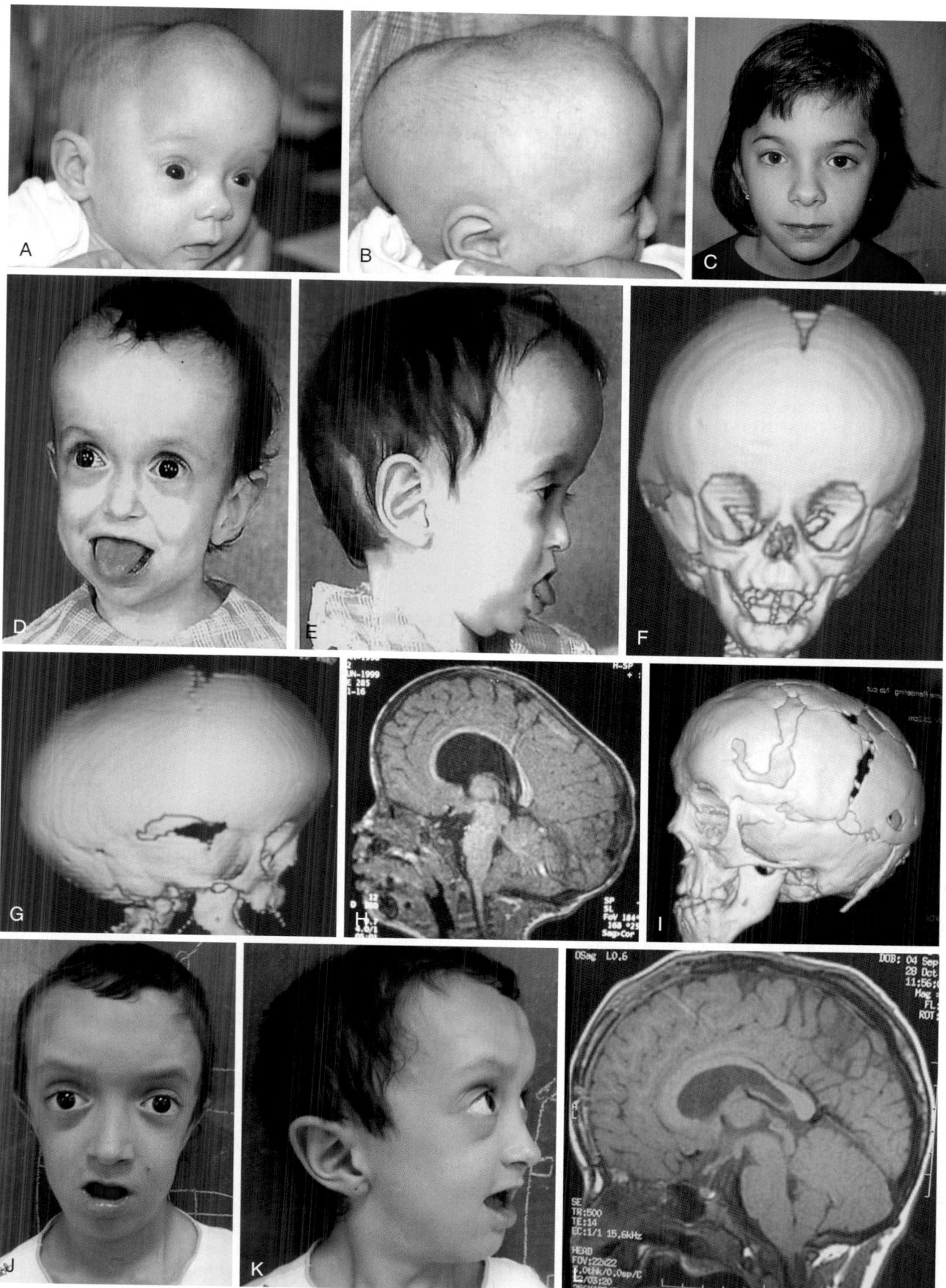

FIGURE 65-10 Holocranial dismantling in multiple sutures craniosynostosis. For patient 1, multiple suture nonsyndromic synostosis are seen in pre-operative oblique frontal (A) and side (B) views and postoperative frontal (C) views. Patient 2 had Crouzon syndrome. Preoperative images are seen in the frontal (D) and side (E) views, as well as preoperative three-dimensional reconstructed CT from frontal (F) and side (G) views and from sagittal view MRI (H). Postoperative frontal (I) and side (J) views of the same patient show marked improvement, as do side views from (K) three-dimensional reconstructed CT and from sagittal MRI (L).

of several cranial sutures, typically coronal sutures and later those of the anterior cranial base and posterior fossa. The sagittal suture is typically widened and opened. It is always accompanied by osseous syndactyly of hands and feet and by fusion of the distal phalanxes. There is usually severe hypoplasia of the midface with an ogival-fissured hard palate. The orbital rims are retruded and elevated, and the skin possesses a characteristic acneiform appearance, mostly over the nasal bridge, shoulders, and back. Midface anomalies and anterior fossa craniosynostoses produce a decrease in the orbital volume that may lead to proptosis, strabismus (V syndrome), hypermetropia, or astigmatism. Most of these patients present with central nervous system anomalies, including hypoplasia of the corpus callosum and limbic and mesial temporal structure malformations. Approximately 10% of these children develop hydrocephalus, but only 2% of them suffer from a CM, in contrast to Crouzon syndrome, where 75% of the patients develop a hindbrain herniation.[61] If left untreated, the incidence of raised ICP has previously been reported as 45%.[64,65] Untreated intracranial hypertension may result in insidious optic atrophy, visual loss, and possible developmental delay.

Antenatal diagnosis is possible, but most cases are diagnosed at the time of delivery. The possibility of a dominant autosomal inheritance has been described, but most cases are sporadic. Advanced paternal age has been reported to have a role in its pathogenesis. The genetic failure occurs over the long arm of chromosome 10 (10g26 region) due to a mutation of exon 7, which codifies for FGFR2. In most cases, a S252W or P253R mutation is present. Mutations in FGFR2 produce an increase in the number of precursor cells that take part in osteogenesis (preosteoblastic cells) and lead to an increase in subperiosteal osseous matrix formation, precocious ossification, and premature closure of the cranial vault during the fetal development.

Early cranial decompression with occipital expansion or fronto-orbital advancement is the treatment of choice, although some authors have advocated avoiding routine vault expansion in the first year of life. Instead, careful clinical, ophthalmologic, and respiratory monitoring would allow raised ICP to be treated in the most appropriate manner only when it occurs.[65] Midface hypoplasia accounts for the exorbitism, strabismus, and respiratory difficulties seen in this condition. In the absence of any clinical sequelae from this hypoplasia, midface advancement is usually postponed until an age of 4 to 6 years. In cases of functional or clinical compromise, it may be necessary to intervene earlier with different techniques, such as monobloc advancement, maxillotomies, and/or mandible distraction. Facial hypoplasia and ogival palate abnormalities are responsible for phonetic disorders, abnormal dental eruption, and malocclusion.

Apert syndrome patients present with a variable degree of mental retardation. Early treatment of the craniosynostosis has been related to better outcomes. Some authors have shown that up to 50% of patients with Apert syndrome have a normal or near-normal intelligence quotient (IQ), with the rest being moderately to severely retarded. Renier et al.[72] found an IQ greater than 70 in 50% of Apert syndrome patients when they were treated by cranial expansion in the first year of life but only in 7.1% of those who were treated later.

PFEIFFER SYNDROME

Initially described by Pfeiffer in 1964,[67,75] Pfeiffer syndrome is characterized by turribrachycephaly, maxillary hypoplasia, and antimongoloid slant of the orbits. There is hypertelorism and a marked degree of proptosis due to the bicoronal synostosis and subsequent recession of supraorbital rim and short anterior fossa. Extremities are notable for broad thumbs and large toes. There may be a variable degree and number of soft tissue syndactyly (most commonly between the second and the third digits), in comparison to Apert syndrome, where bony syndactyly is the hallmark. There may also be symphalangism (phalangeal fusion), ankylosis of the elbow joints, and cervical vertebral fusions (all of them also possible in Apert syndrome).

There are three clinical subtypes of Pfeiffer syndrome,[73] which have clinical and prognostic significance. Type I (classic) is a lesser craniosynostosis that has a typical appearance of brachycephaly but usually is associated with normal or near-normal intelligence. Children with this type of Pfeiffer syndrome can develop normally, but there is often increased ICP if the synostoses are left uncorrected. Type II is associated with cloverleaf deformity, and although compatible with life, prognosis is poor. Type III is characterized by striking proptosis, but kleeblattschädel is absent. Long-term prognosis is poor.

CLOVERLEAF SKULL (KLEEBLATTSCHÄDEL)

Kleeblattschädel syndrome is characterized by a trilobar skull caused by frontal and bitemporal bossing. The first description of a trilobar cranial malformation in a newborn was made by Vrolik in 1849,[77] but the term kleeblattschädel syndrome was not introduced until 1960 by Holtermuller and Wiederman.[77,78] These authors reported a series of children with a trilobar or "cloverleaf" cranium associated with multiple craniosynostoses. In 1965, Commings et al. published the first case in the United States and translated the term *kleeblattschädel syndrome* into *cloverleaf skull*.[78] This malformation has been described in children with Crouzon, Apert, Carpenter, Beare-Stevenson, or type II Pfeiffer syndrome, the latter being most frequently associated (up to 20% in some series).[75,77] The etiology of this syndrome is still unknown and has been attributed to abnormalities of both the calvarium and the skull base, probably due to the presence of a combination of prematurely fused cranial sutures and hydrocephalus.

The surgical management of cloverleaf skull remains one of the most formidable challenges for the craniofacial surgeon (Fig. 65-8). The natural history of this deformity without surgery was well described in the 1960s and 1970s. Just a few of these children survived beyond infancy, and those who did developed severe neurologic deficits. The first attempt at surgical correction was reported by Angle in 1967.[77] Since then, a number of surgical series have been reported, without a clear conclusion on prognosis and outcome. Review of the literature reveals a lack of consistent surgical strategies.[74-76] Postoperative data are sparse, and reoperation is the rule in these patients, with a consequent increased morbidity. In addition to the significant cosmetic deformity, the constant coexistence of intracranial hypertension, hydrocephalus, hindbrain herniation, severe skull base dysplasia, and anomaly in venous drainage (Fig. 65-11)

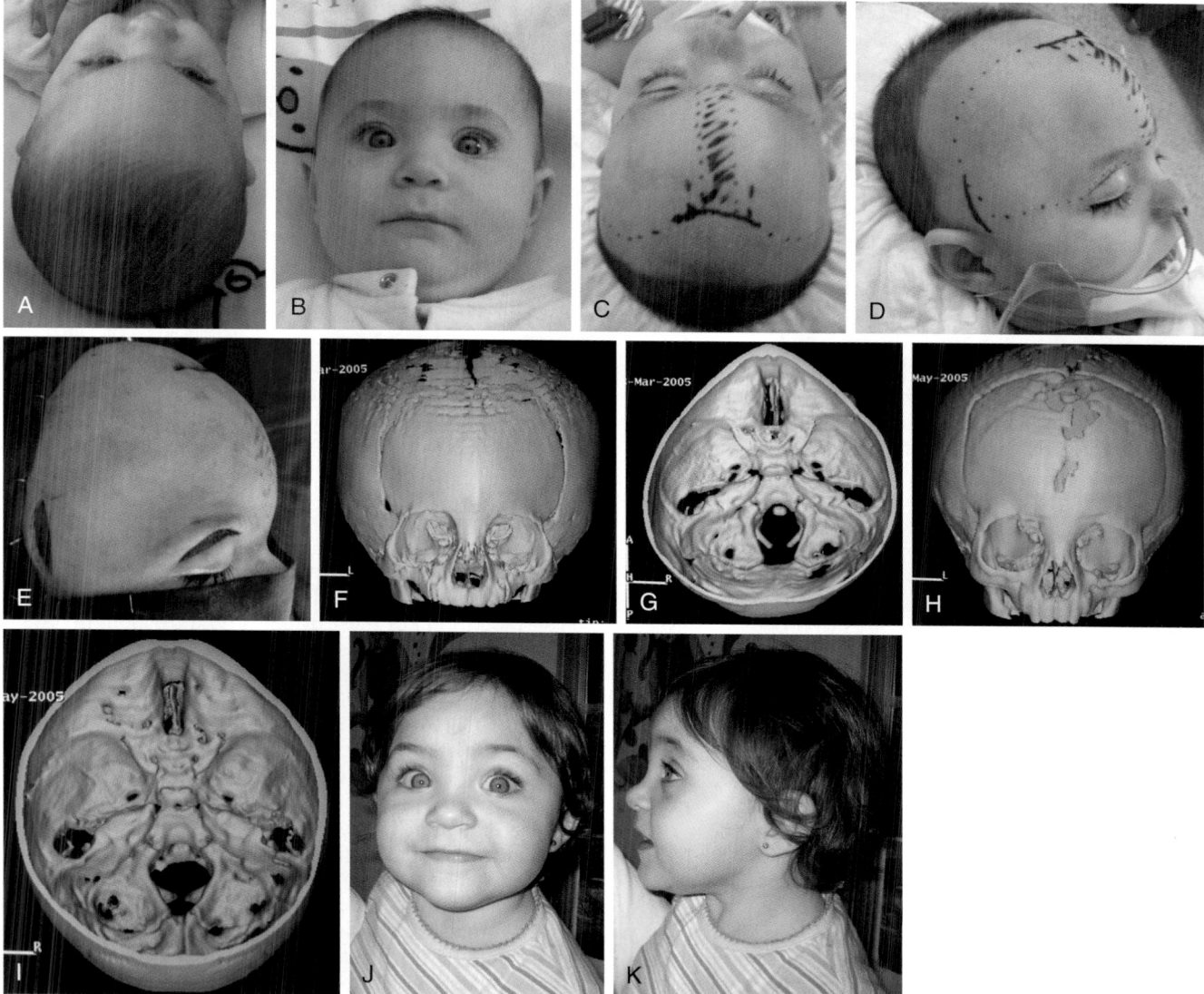

FIGURE 65-11 Endoscopically assisted surgical correction of trigonocephaly. Preoperative bird's eye (A) and frontal (B) views. Surgical planning from bird's eye (C) and oblique (D) views. E, Hairline and eyebrow incisions used for surgical access. Preoperative three-dimensional reconstructed CT from frontal (F) and bird's eye (G) views. Postoperative three-dimensional reconstructed CT from frontal (H) and bird's eye (I) views. Patient appearance 1 year after the operation from frontal (J) and side (K) views.

imposes important neurosurgical considerations throughout treatment.

Hydrocephalus in Craniosynostosis

Ventriculomegaly and ventricular asymmetry are frequent even in children with single-suture craniosynostosis, but they require treatment only in selected cases. Abnormal dilatations of the subarachnoid spaces are a common finding and may imply some disturbance in CSF absorption.[77] In sagittal synostosis, for example, the frequent encasing of the superior sagittal sinus in the bone groove formed by the fused suture may account for some impairment of CSF absorption. This may lead to mild ventricular dilatation and enlarged CSF subarachnoid spaces over the cerebral hemispheres. In comparison, hydrocephalus is a common feature in patients with complex craniosynostosis. Ventricular

dilatation has been reported in 30% to 70% of patients with Crouzon and Pfeiffer syndromes and in 40% to 90% of Apert syndrome patients.[66,77,78] With Apert syndrome, most cases of enlarged ventricles remain stable without a shunt, but with Crouzon syndrome and the severest Pfeiffer syndrome cases, shunting is frequently necessary at some stage of treatment. True hydrocephalus has seldom been reported in single-suture pathologies and can almost always be attributed to coincidental disorders independent of craniosynostosis, such as ventricular hemorrhage, meningitis, aqueductal stenosis, or neural tube defects.

Some patients develop rapidly evolving hydrocephalus before any surgical intervention, and this is expected mainly in kleeblattschädel or a severe Pfeiffer condition. In most of the remaining patients, ventricular dilatation only develops following decompressive surgery for craniosynostosis. In these patients, the indication for shunting is mainly based on progressive ventricular dilatation or evidence of persistent intracranial hypertension, which may need to be ascertained by direct pressure monitoring. After cranial surgery, the artificially created spaces are quite often accommodated by some enlargement of the intra- and extracerebral CSF spaces, and the possibility of a compensated or even slowly progressive hydrocephalic state should be taken into account.[77,79]

Two combined pathogenic factors have been offered as an explanation for the frequent association of hydrocephalus and complex craniosynostosis: a mechanical increase of the CSF outflow resistance due to constricted growth of the posterior fossa[62,80-82] and an impaired CSF absorption resulting from venous outflow obstruction.[82-84] Crowding of the posterior fossa appears to be an acquired disorder secondary to deficient occipital cranial expansion.[79,85] It has been related to the timing of fusion of the lambdoid suture, which in Crouzon and Pfeiffer syndromes is completed at an earlier age than in Apert syndrome. This would explain the delayed appearance of hydrocephalus in patients with Apert syndrome. The mechanical restriction to CSF outflow would worsen after the development of tonsillar herniation in a small posterior fossa. This theory alone fails to explain the incidence of hydrocephalus, because hindbrain herniation is missing in a number of cases of progressive hydrocephalus.[83,86] And while it is present in many other cases not affected by hydrocephalus, posterior fossa decompression has often failed to sufficiently restore normal CSF circulation.[80] Therefore, constriction of the posterior fossa may not be a single causative mechanism for hydrocephalus in craniosynostosis.

Venous hypertension has been accepted as another major pathogenic mechanism by several authors, with descriptions of venous sinus hypertension caused by a stenosis of the jugular foramen in hydrocephalic Crouzon syndrome patients.[84] The venous obstructions could be secondary to the abnormalities of bone growth that affect the base of the skull in children who have craniosynostosis, with early closure of lambdoid and petro-occipital sutures leading to decreased venous outflow through the jugular foramina.[79] Another possible explanation is that the disordered venous anatomy is primary rather than secondary and results from the same dysplastic processes that affect the cranial vault sutures, the basicranium, and the facial skeleton. The expression of FGFR gene products in the infant craniosynostotic sutures has been described; these products also have been localized by immunohistochemistry to the cranial vascular endothelia of patients with syndromic craniosynostosis.[79,86,87] Therefore, premature endothelial proliferation and subsequent differentiation in the sigmoid and jugular sinuses may result in the narrowed lumen.[86] Most patients with progressive hydrocephalus simultaneously exhibit signs of venous outflow obstruction and crowded posterior fossa, favoring a combined action of both mechanisms[77] by assuming that venous hypertension causes a CSF absorption deficit, as well as brain swelling resulting in tonsillar herniation,[82] or that it aggravates the preexistent cephalocranial disproportion by venous engorgement.[79,81-83]

Finally, the contribution of upper airway obstruction to raised ICP has long been recognized; in particular, an increase in ICP during episodes of respiratory obstruction has been documented, as has an improvement in the ophthalmologic signs of increased ICP after nasal airway dilation, nocturnal positive airway pressure, or maxillofacial advancement procedures. Possible underlying mechanisms include carbon dioxide retention during obstructive episodes in nocturnal apneas and cerebral flow changes during active sleep, particularly if they occur in the presence of reduced cerebral compliance.[82,86,88] All of these factors would lead in the end to a venous hypertension that would ultimately interfere with the CSF absorption.

Clinical evaluation is aimed at identifying progressive hydrocephalus. Diagnosis is sometimes difficult, and ventricular dilatation often becomes evident only after decompressive cranial surgery. As in other forms of hydrocephalus, subjective symptoms of intracranial hypertension like headaches, nausea, and vomiting may be missed, mostly in younger patients in whom classic clinical signs may be absent. Papilledema, however, was a rather common sign in my patients, and often the only sign of increased ICP. Mild ventriculomegaly may also exist with intracranial hypertension; therefore, careful monitoring of ICP and ventricular size in the pre- and postoperative period is a mainstay. My department has developed a strict protocol for the follow-up of complex craniosynostosis, which includes close monitoring of these patients with frequent neuroimaging, ophthalmologic survey (funduscopic examination and visual evoked potentials), polysomnography to detect sleep apnea, and invasive monitoring of ICP and cerebral blood flow when necessary to rule out a chronic increase in ICP.

A percentage of craniosynostosis patients goes on to require hydrocephalus treatment.[79] Improvement of ventricular dilatation has been anecdotally reported following removal of constricting bony ridges or decompressive craniectomies alone.[81,86] Some authors (Genitori, personal communication) have discussed the use of endoscopic third ventriculostomy for selected cases with the rationale that an acquired stenosis of the aqueduct may develop due to periaqueductal compression during progression of the multiple synostoses. In the presence of hindbrain herniation, there is certainly no place for lumbar peritoneal shunts. Therefore, despite other proposed treatment options, ventriculoperitoneal shunting is widely accepted as the most effective treatment for these patients. Overdrainage must be avoided when selecting the shunting system, because it may induce a pseudo–tumor-like state of venous origin, worsening the preexisting venous problem.[86]

When shunting is needed soon after cranial reconstruction, the stability of synostosis surgery may be endangered if the dural envelope does not rapidly expand because of artificial depletion of CSF spaces[86] and failure of cranial contents to support the bone plates. If shunting is addressed before cranial reconstruction, there is a real possibility of developing new suture closure due to sustained low ICP.

There is little evidence that dilated ventricles per se have an adverse effect on intelligence,[72,77] except that severe congenital hydrocephalus, as observed in the most complex craniofacial syndromes, carries an increased risk of a lower performance level. As in other hydrocephalic states, the prognosis mainly depends on coincidental cerebral abnormalities and on the detrimental effect of long-standing elevated CSF pressure.[77]

Chiari Malformation in Craniosynostosis

The association between CM and premature craniofacial synostosis was first noted by Saldino et al.[89] in 1972 in one patient with Pfeiffer syndrome. Since then, numerous authors have reported the incidence of chronic tonsillar herniation in multiple suture craniosynostosis,[62,81,90-92] and it is a frequent finding in syndromic and multisuture craniosynostosis, characterized by early fusion of lambdoid sutures and cranial base synchondroses. The incidence of CM has been reported as high as 70% in Crouzon syndrome,[90,92,94] 75% in nonsyndromic oxycephaly,[95] 50% in Pfeiffer syndrome, and 100% in kleeblattschädel deformity.[62] CM was found in other types of syndromic craniosynostosis, in some cases of nonsyndromic complex craniosynostosis involving the lambdoid suture, and in some rare cases of scaphocephaly.[85,92]

Downward herniation of neural tissue through the foramen magnum is usually an acquired malformation in craniosynostosis and may be secondary to a disproportion between the posterior fossa and the growing hindbrain structures.[96,97] In most cases of craniosynostosis, hindbrain herniation is not present at birth; rather, it develops in response to the changes in the skull base and posterior fossa secondary to premature closure of the lambdoid and cranial base sutures (usually between 3 and 6 months of age), supporting the pathogenetic hypothesis of overcrowding of the posterior fossa secondary to premature suture fusion.[90,97] The excellent review by Cinalli et al. gives a comprehensive overview on the pathogenic mechanisms involved in the development of hindbrain herniation in craniosynostosis.[97] The progressive fusion of the lambdoid suture produces alteration in the skull base and stenosis of the jugular foramina (if the petro-occipital synchondroses are primarily involved). The first result would be a small posterior fossa, with consequent herniation of the cerebellum into the cervical canal during the phase of rapid neural growth in the first months of life. The second result would be venous hypertension, induced both by jugular foramen stenosis (if the petro-occipital synchondroses are involved) and by crowding of the posterior fossa, with consequent compression of the sigmoid sinus. These factors can obstruct and alter CSF circulation at the level of the posterior fossa and impair CSF reabsorption at the level of the arachnoid granulations, with the overall final result of increased CSF outflow resistance. Severe crowding of the foramen magnum may result not only in hindbrain herniation but also in brain stem compression and deformation of the fourth ventricle. Thus, hindbrain herniation can be considered as a condition creating or aggravating a hydrocephalic state, not a consequence of hydrocephalus. This explains the cases of CM without hydrocephalus that are frequently observed in craniosynostosis without primary involvement of skull base synchondrosis (e.g., oxycephaly) or in the first stages of Crouzon syndrome, where CM is a frequent finding without hydrocephalus.

Under normal conditions, the posterior cranial fossa grows in length in early childhood along the intraoccipital, petro-occipital, and spheno-occipital synchondroses. Growth in the intraoccipital synchondrosis ceases in early childhood, whereas growth in the spheno-occipital synchondrosis continues after puberty.[98] In syndromic and complex multisutural craniosynostosis, unlike monosutural craniosynostosis, the facial skeleton and the cartilaginous cranial base are primarily involved.[98] In Crouzon and Apert syndromes, the degree of involvement of the skull base synchondroses and the timing of fusion are different. In Apert syndrome, the spheno-occipital, petro-occipital, and occipital synchondrosis are fused later, beginning after 12 to 48 months of life and ending at the age of 4 years, than in Crouzon syndrome, where they can be completely fused in the first year of life. All this could be conditioned by a different genetic pattern. In syndromic craniosynostosis, the genetic mutations responsible for the disease are located mainly in FGFR1 (Pfeiffer syndrome), FGFR2 (Crouzon, Apert, and Pfeiffer syndromes), and FGFR3 (Crouzon syndrome and acanthosis nigricans). Some authors have suggested a correlation between the mutation observed and the presence or absence of CM.[83,85] In Crouzon syndrome, the patients affected by CM and syringomyelia would present with a variety of mutations that spread over exons IIIa and IIIc of the FGFR2 gene.[92,98] This could explain the significant differences found in the final anatomy of the skull base and the posterior cranial fossa. The Apert basiocciput is larger than normal, whereas in Crouzon syndrome it is smaller.[99] According to Cinalli et al., Crouzon syndrome patients preferentially expand along a superoinferior axis, whereas little or no growth is allowed along an anteroposterior axis[97]; the foramen and the basion–opisthion area incur only small changes, whereas the more significant alterations are in the cranial base posterior to the foramen.[99] Previous conditions would result in altered dimensions of the posterior cranial fossa: normal or larger than normal in the Apert syndrome[99] and smaller, shortened in the anteroposterior axis, and elongated in the superoinferior and lateral axis in Crouzon syndrome.

If the petro-occipital synchondroses are involved, their premature closure may lead to stenosis or atresia of the jugular foramen. Venous hypertension, induced by jugular foramen stenosis,[100] increases the sagittal sinus pressure and results in a higher CSF pressure request to maintain CSF balance. In patients with closed sutures, ICP may rise to very high levels, overcoming the high sagittal sinus pressure and permitting absorption of CSF, with normal-sized or small ventricles, as seen in some cases of pseudotumor cerebri.[83,84] In contrast, in infants and children with open sutures (or following surgical cranial suture release), increased CSF pressure induces progressive head enlargement and dilatation of the ventricles and subarachnoid spaces.[83,84] This is usually followed by the development of collateral venous drainage, through the foramen magnum and/or through emissary veins and scalp veins. This venous pattern highlights a crucial point: In some cases, the main venous drainage occurs through emissary veins rather than through the usual jugular pathway, and the distortion of the previous could lead to a fatal outcome after surgery.[101] Enography should form part of the routine magnetic resonance imaging (MRI) protocol for diagnostic assessment of children with complex and syndromic craniosynostosis.[100] Quantification of venous hemodynamics may also have a role, allowing more accurate, noninvasive monitoring of change at follow-up studies.[102]

The rest of the sutures (lambdoid, sagittal, coronal, and metopic) could also play a role in the development of CM.

In the setting of in utero closure of sagittal and coronal sutures, a cephalocranial disproportion in the supratentorial compartment occurs early, forcing the neural growth to be directed posteriorly and inferiorly and pushing down the tentorium. This can induce a lower attachment of the tentorium (near the foramen magnum), reducing the size of the posterior fossa and increasing the risk of CM, especially if premature lambdoid synostosis is also involved. The precocity of coronal and sagittal suture synostosis does not seem to play a role in the pathophysiology of CM in Apert (where the sagittal suture is wide open) and Crouzon syndromes. The premature closure of the lambdoid suture reflects the primary closure of the spheno-occipital synchondrosis and could be a reliable radiologic indicator of synostosis of the posterior cranial base sutures. In Crouzon syndrome, the sagittal and lambdoid sutures close early (median 6 and 21 months, respectively), and they close significantly earlier in the cases of Crouzon syndrome associated with CM compared to in Crouzon syndrome patients without CM.[90] On the contrary, in Apert syndrome, where CM only occurs in approximately 2% to 5% of the cases, the cranial vault synostosis occurs early for the coronal suture (median 5 months) and significantly later for the sagittal and lambdoid sutures (median 51 and 60 months, respectively).

More than one third of patients with hindbrain herniation become symptomatic for CM or develop syringomyelic cavities. Usually, the onset of symptoms occurs late in life, but they may be dramatic—especially in very young children—with appearance of respiratory problems such as central apnea, bilateral vocal cord paralysis, bulbar palsy, ventilatory control abnormalities, persistent cyanosis, and breath-holding spells.[97] Careful radiologic and clinical follow-up is needed in patients with syndromic or complex craniosynostosis to assess the presence and evolution of CM. MRI with venous angiography is the gold standard for the evaluation of these patients.[100,103]

MANAGEMENT OF CM IN CRANIOSYNOSTOSIS

In cases of multiple suture synostosis—mainly in patients with a Crouzon syndrome or kleeblattschädel deformity, where cranial vault (bicoronal and both lambdoid) and skull base sutures are affected—the correction of a CM may need to be treated by a complete calvarial reconstruction. This may be performed as a one-step procedure, as described by Pollack et al.[104] The child is set in the "modified prone position," allowing exposure from the orbital ridge to the foramen magnum. This approach, however, requires marked hyperextension of the neck, and it is contraindicated for patients who present with anomalies of the craniovertebral junction, because hyperextension of the neck for several hours[104] may lead to prolonged severe compression on the spinal cord and medulla. I have used the same approach (described later in the section on type X holocranial dismantling) but in two steps: first fronto-orbital advancement with the child supine, and then, after closure of the skin incisions, occipital expansion with the patient prone in the same surgical session.

For patients with severe syndromes and marked flattening of the posterior vault and overcrowding of the posterior fossa, occipital expansion and suboccipital craniectomy may be indicated.[62] It is possible to perform occipital craniectomy and remodeling through a bicoronal incision. Dissection proceeds in the subperiosteal plane, elevating the occipital musculature over the external protuberance and exposing all suboccipital bone that can be removed and then reaching the posterior and lateral margins of the foramen magnum. The infratentorial compartment is left uncovered, and the occipitoparietal region is conformed, repositioning the bone. In cases such as cloverleaf malformation, a parietal craniectomy can only be performed piecemeal, and extreme care must be exercised when dissecting free the thin external layer of the superior sagittal sinus, which is often imbibed or pinched by bone spikes that enter the sinus.[75,76,94] In these cases, it is often not possible to perform an intradural approach, but even if some degree of tonsillar herniation remains after suboccipital craniectomy, crowding of the foramen magnum is reduced and more CSF can be observed around the medulla on postoperative MRI. Dural opening and cervical laminectomy may be indicated in cases of severe compression of the medulla, but this carries the risk of severe bleeding from the dural edges because of the abnormal anatomy of dural venous sinuses, which usually includes a prominent occipital longitudinal sinus over the suboccipital bone and a dominant marginal occipital sinus around the foramen magnum and frequently includes significant collateral circulation in the muscular plane. Computed tomography (CT) and/or magnetic resonance angiograms/venograms are mandatory studies in these patients to avoid catastrophic introperative bleeding.

SURGICAL TECHNIQUES

Type I. Endoscopically Assisted Suturectomies and Osteotomies

Different authors have proposed minimally invasive techniques[106] and endoscopic-assisted osteotomies[9,11,29,40,106] applied to younger patients using the concept of surgically created open sutures that take advantage of the rapid brain growth during the first months of life. Craniectomies and osteotomies (Figs. 65-1, 65-3, 65-5, and 65-12) are designed to mimic new cranial sutures and are followed by active head molding using custom-made helmets. These techniques are used for the treatment of single-suture premature synostosis, although good results have been reported when they are applied to multiple suture synostosis and syndromic involvement.[136] Small skin incisions (between 1.5 and 2 cm for anterior plagiocephaly and 3.5 and 4 cm for scaphocephaly) are placed over the suture to be resected.

In scaphocephaly (Fig. 65-3), the anterior incision is placed 2 cm behind the anterior fontanel, while a posterior incision is over the posterior fontanel. A solution with 0.25% bupivacaine and 1:100,000 epinephrine is injected over the area of dissection. The two small transverse incisions (approximately 2-3 cm length) are lengthened, and a subgaleal plane is developed over the pericranium with the assistance of a rigid endoscope (lens 0 degrees, 2.7 mm) and with electrocautery at a low setting. Bur holes at both sides of the sagittal suture are fashioned at each incision site. The dura is dissected, and bur holes are connected with epidural rongeuring. The sagittal sinus is then separated from the skull using the endoscope, suction, and a Penfield dissector. This moment is particularly helpful in the direct vision of the emissary veins, which can be coagulated with bipolar cautery. Bur holes are longitudinally connected with bone scissors to complete a sagittal suturectomy measuring

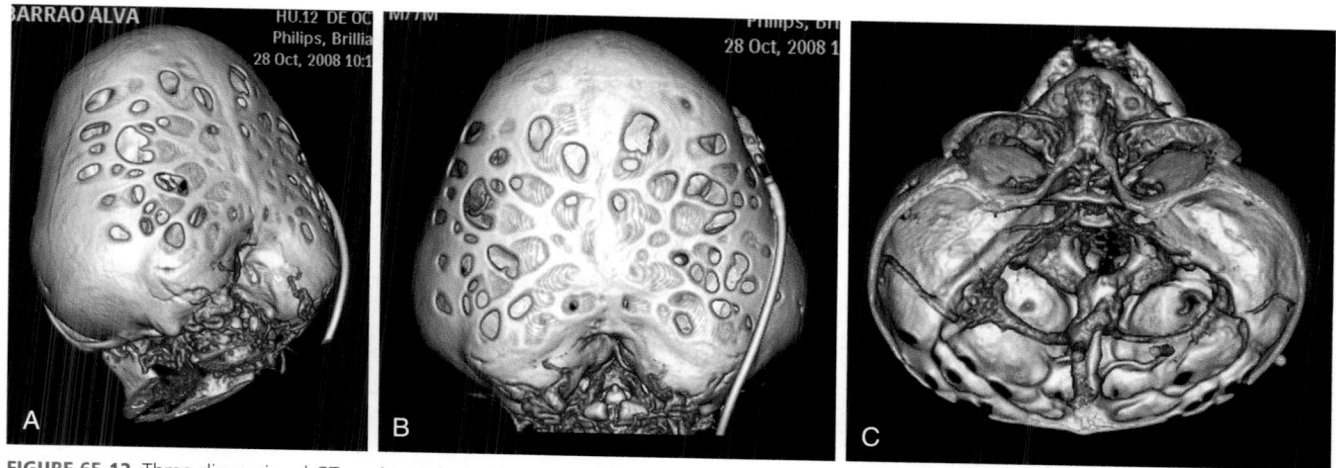

FIGURE 65-12 Three-dimensional CT angiography in cloverleaf deformity. Vascular studies are mandatory in surgical planning before craniotomies in complex craniosynostosis. Observe the vascular draining pattern and relationship between the torcular region and the emissary veins in oblique posterior (A), posterior (B), and bird's eye (C) views.

approximately 3 to 4 cm in width and between 6 and 11 cm in length. The sagittal bone plate is then freed and can be removed. Hemostasis is performed over the bone cuts with tip-insulated electrocautery and with oxidized cellulose and bipolar cautery over the superior sagittal sinus and dura mater. Further dissection is carried out under endoscopic assistance laterally over the parietal areas to achieve wedge osteotomies on both sides, immediately posterior to the coronal suture and immediately anterior to the lambdoid suture, reaching the squamosal sutures. Hemostasis is performed, and resorbable sutures are used for closure. No bandages are needed, and the patient is positioned in a strict supine position during the postoperative stay in the hospital.

For trigonocephaly (Fig. 65-4), the patient is placed supine on a horseshoe headrest. A 2- to 3-cm transverse incision is made just behind the hair line, approximately 3 cm in front of the anterior fontanelle. A subgaleal dissection over the metopic ridge is carried down to the nasion and frontonasal suture with endoscopic assistance and electrocautery. Two bur holes are placed along both sides of the metopic suture at the level of the skin incision and connected crossing the midline. Metopic suturectomy starts posterior to the bregmatic fontanelle. Then, with the aid of the rigid endoscope, epidural dissection under the fused metopic suture proceeds down to the nasofrontal suture. Suturectomy is completed with rongeurs or heavy bone scissors. At this point, some help with a high-speed drill may be needed to cross the thick glabella and may be used for smoothing the frontal bone edges. In some cases, I added frontal oblique-releasing osteotomies. For the severest cases, I advocated a variation of the technique previously published by Cohen et al.[107] The ultimate point of this approach is to achieve a complete fronto-orbitary osteotomy, including both orbital roofs and resection of the entire pterional region, together with metopic suturectomy.

For anterior plagiocephaly (Fig. 65-5), the patient is positioned supine in a neutral position. A 2.5-cm incision is placed halfway along the coronal suture, closer to the bregmatic fontanelle than to the ipsilateral pterion. A dissection plane is carried between the galea and the pericranium with electrocautery, exposing the whole affected coronal

suture under endoscopic vision with a rigid lens (0 or 30 degrees). A bur hole is created under the skin incision, and a 1- to 2-cm broad suturectomy is done with rongeurs or bone scissors up to the anterior fontanelle. Then, epidural dissection proceeds downward under endoscopic magnification, exposing the pterion and lesser wing of the sphenoid. Suturectomy is carried out behind the pterional region until the squamosal suture is reached. The osteotomy must be extended down to the pterion and allow the orbit to move forward.[9,40,108] Most patients undergoing endoscopic techniques are later sent for helmet molding therapy.

Type II. Scaphocephaly: Standard Technique

The standard scaphocephaly technique is applied in cases of scaphocephaly in children between 5 and 9 months of age, regardless of the presence of severe compensating frontal bossing (Fig. 65-2). It consists of a sagittal suturectomy with expanding green-stick parietotemporal and occipital osteotomies. The patient is placed in a beanbag horseshoe with the head extended in prone position. A modified retroauricular bicoronal incision (zigzag) is usually preferred for all craniofacial procedures for cosmetic purposes. This approach promotes healing without resulting in wide scars. A subperiosteal dissection separates the calvaria from the coronal sutures to the occipital knob. After sagittal suturectomy, I proceed with biparietal and temporo-occipital wedge osteotomies, expanding the biparietal diameter. In cases of severe occipital prominence, an "island" occipital craniectomy helps correct the posterior deformity (Fig. 65-2L).

Type III. Scaphocephaly: Standard Technique Plus Frontal Remodeling

In children older than 10 months with scaphocephaly and severe anterior bulging, a two thirds anterior cranial vault reconstruction is achieved by obtaining a new frontal bone from a parietal donor site and transposition or remodeling of the former frontal bone by midline split and repositioning. At the same time, bitemporal and parietal osteotomies and subsequent fixation are conducted to expand laterally the pterional indentation.

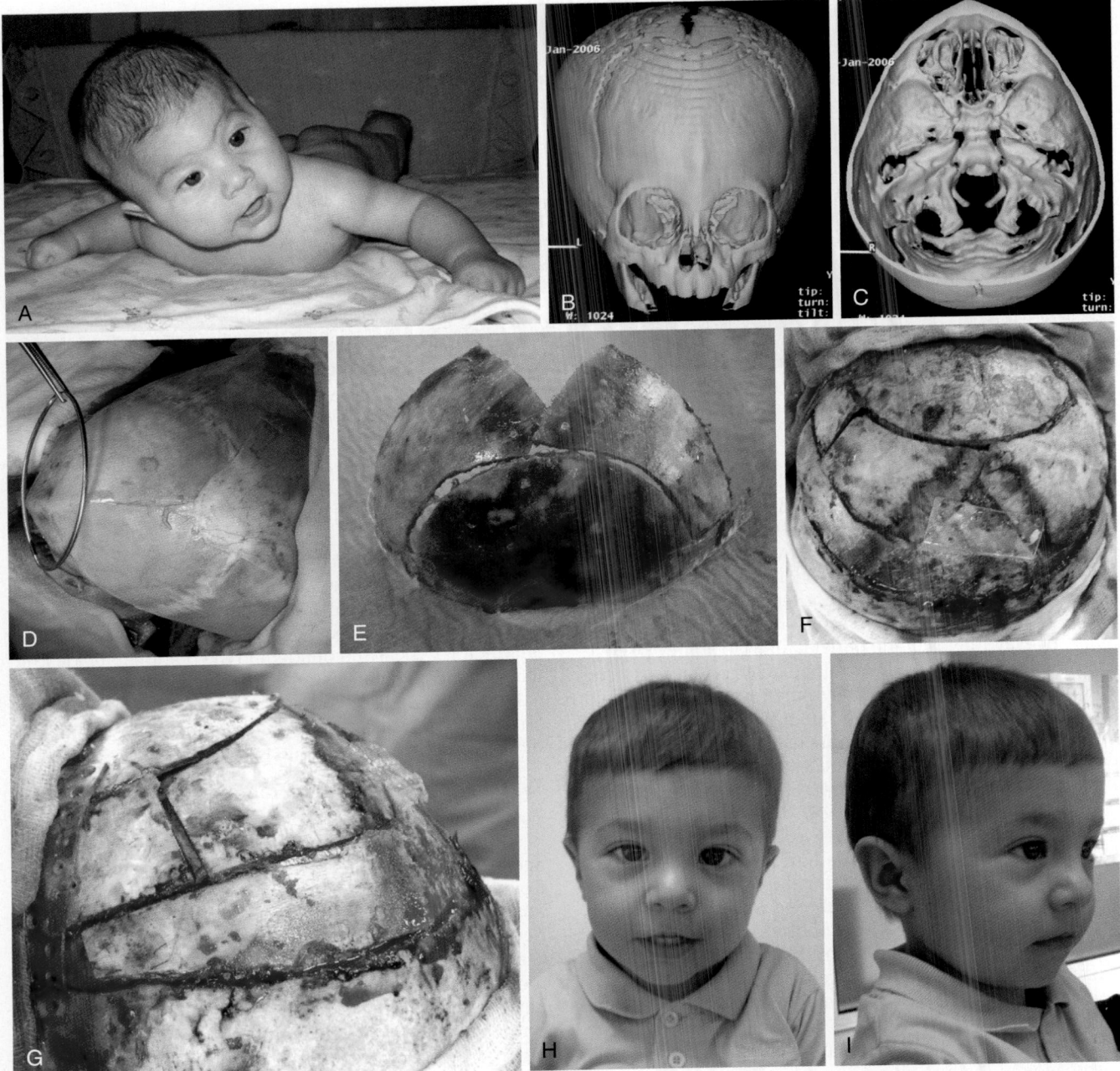

FIGURE 65-13 Standard fronto-orbital correction for trigonocephaly. A, Preoperative imaging demonstrates bitemporal narrowing and midline forehead ridging. Preoperative three-dimensional CT is seen from frontal (B) and bird's eye (C) views. Intraoperative images show metopic suture synostosis in situ (D) and after suturectomy (E); frontal (F) and oblique (G) views show detail of cranial vault reconstruction. Postoperative images from frontal (H) and oblique (I) views show correction of trigonocephaly.

Type IV. Scaphocephaly: Total Cranial Vault Remodeling (Holocranial Dismantling)

In children older than 12 to 14 months with scaphocephaly, a complete calvarial reconstruction is necessary to achieve an adequate cosmetic result (Fig. 65-4). Severe cranial base distortion and the necessity to change the three diameters (vertical, posterior–anterior, and biparietal) precludes the use of more aggressive techniques that include the dismantling and transposition of multiple bone fragments in the shape of arches (clamshell technique), crosses (holocranial

dismantling), or plates and posterior fixation with resorbable material.

Type V. Trigonocephaly: Frontal Remodeling without Fronto-Orbital Bandeau

For patients with trigonocephaly (Fig. 65-13), I routinely use a technique that has been previously reported from my department.[30,31] With the patient in a supine position and through the standard modified retroauricular bicoronal incision, the anterior two thirds of the calvaria; temporal region; both supraorbital margins, including the anterior roof of the orbita; and nasion are exposed subgaleally. A very low bilateral fronto-orbital craniotomy is performed, reaching the frontonasal junction, and pterional regions are rongeured away. Both supraorbital eminences and glabella are then drilled and contoured. Finally, a donor parietal bone is selected with the Marchac template, transposed and fixed with resorbable material.

Type VI. Anterior Plagiocephaly/Coronal Suture Synostosis: Frontal Remodeling without Fronto-Orbital Bandeau

The same technique of frontal remodeling without fronto-orbital bandeau that is used in trigonocephaly may be used in selected cases of anterior plagiocephaly, assuming that there is no severe orbital dystopia and retrusion of the affected coronal suture. A bifrontal craniotomy is performed to the level of the glabella and supraorbital region. Both pterional regions are thoroughly resected, including the lesser wing of the sphenoid on the affected side. The supraorbital region is then drilled away and contoured. A donor parietal bone is selected with the size and shape appropriate for new fronto-orbital remodeling and fixed with resorbable material. This technique is applied only in cases of plagiocephaly with very mild or no orbital dystopia and symmetric anterior fossa. For the majority of the plagiocephaly cases, a standard fronto-orbital bandeau with the classic tongue-in-groove advance (type VII) is preferable.

Type VII. Anterior Plagiocephaly/Coronal Suture Synostosis: Frontal Bilateral Remodeling with Fronto-Orbital Bandeau

Frontal bilateral remodeling with fronto-orbital bandeau is the technique that I select for most cases of anterior plagiocephaly, where vertical orbital dystopia, short and oblique anterior fossa, and compensating bossing in the contralateral side are consistent findings (Fig. 65-6).

A standard bicoronal approach is achieved with a retroauricular incision and elevation of a bifrontal flap in the loose areolar plane between the periosteum and the galea pericrania. Frontal branches of the facial nerve run inside the external fascia of the temporalis muscle, so care must be taken to not damage them. However, these patients often show low implantation of the temporalis muscle, and dissection under the deep fascia of the muscle opens a broad exposition of the pterion and lateral walls of the orbit. The periosteum is incised at this level, and dissection proceeds in the subperiosteal plane, exposing both the frontal and the pterional areas, the lateral walls of the orbit with partial elevation of the temporalis muscle to expose the greater wing of the sphenoid, and the superior wall of the orbits up to the internal canthus, which is preserved. Before initiating osteotomies, obliquity of the frontal bones, retrusion of the lateral portions of the orbital bandeau, and pterional deformation are assessed. A bifrontal craniotomy is performed after a supraorbital bandeau is created. The marks are extended from the sphenosquamosal suture to its contralateral equivalent prepared for a tongue-in-groove advancement. The bifrontal flap includes the anterior part of the bregmatic fontanelle and both coronal sutures. The anterior fossa is exposed extradurally, with visualization of the anterior two thirds of the orbital roof.

Osteotomies on the orbitofrontal bandeau are now performed, starting on the lateral orbital ridge over the frontozygomatic suture and opening the orbital roof anterior to the cribriform plate at the midline. There is commonly severe sphenoid thickening on the affected side over the pterion, where osteotomies are the last step to obtain a free orbital bandeau. The pterions are then thoroughly resected. The bandeau is anteriorly displaced, with rotation of the lateral extreme of the bandeau projecting forward in the side of synostosis, maintaining the medial aspect of the bandeau in place. The orbital roofs and supraorbital ridge are aligned in proper position, descending the affected side and elevating the nonsynostotic side as needed. Transposed new frontal bone is fixed on the orbital bandeau with absorbable miniplates. Closure proceeds in the standard way, with anterior rotation and elevation of the temporalis muscle bilaterally and covering of the field with the periosteum and the galea. I place two subgaleal drains and close the skin with subcutaneous absorbable sutures and an intradermal suture.

Type VIII. Occipital Remodeling: Occipital Advancement

Single synostosis of the lambdoid suture seldom happens, and surgical indication must be done only in cases of severe cosmetic deformation. In these cases, I performed a bilateral occipital craniotomy with complete posterior remodeling. In younger patients, an endoscopically assisted resection followed by helmet therapy may render good results.[11]

Posterior occipital advancement, however, is frequently used as the starting procedure for severe craniofacial syndromes, such as Pfeiffer syndrome, Crouzon syndrome, or kleeblattschädel with early elevated ICP when a vault expansion is needed (Fig. 65-7), or in cases of CM associated with multiple craniosynostoses when a single stage procedure for complete calvarial remodeling is not advisable due to elevated venous pressure.[62] Occipital advancement has been shown to be superior to fronto-orbital advancement in terms of total volume expansion[62,109] and has shown efficacy in correcting the fronto-orbital appearance, even prior to anterior advancement (Fig. 65-8).

Type IX. Standard Bilateral Fronto-Orbital Advancement with Expansive Osteotomies

A standard advancement technique is selected when bilateral anterior fossa advancement and bifrontal remodeling are the goals. The technique consists of standard bilateral fronto-orbital advancement with or without fronto-orbital bandeau plus expansive frontoparietal osteotomies. Characteristically, it allows only a short decrease in the vertical position of the bregma, as the posterior parietal region is not addressed. It is the technique selected in multisutural cases of syndromic (Crouzon, Apert, or Pfeiffer) and nonsyndromic (brachycephaly) involvement of the anterior fossa due to premature fusion of coronal, ethmoidosphenoidal, and frontosphenoidal sutures.

Type X. Holocranial Dismantling (Total Vault Remodeling) in Multiple Craniosynostosis

Holocranial dismantling in multiple craniosynostosis consists of a complete cranial vault remodeling for correction of multiple synostosis to achieve adjustment of the three skull diameters (vertical, interparietal, and posterior–anterior distances) (Fig. 65-10). It can be done in a single surgical step with the patient in a prone position (Persing's technique)[110] or in two steps in the same surgical session (first supine and then prone after closing the bicoronal incision). The two-step variation, commonly used in my department, is preferred over Persing's technique when venous hypertension, induced both by jugular foramen stenosis and crowding of the posterior fossa with subsequent compression of the sigmoid sinus, makes the hyperextended prone position unadvisable.

With the patient in a supine position, standard bilateral fronto-orbital advancement and frontoparietal remodeling are performed (type IX). A crossbar is designed over the bregmatic region, which allows decrease of the vertical diameter (Fig. 65-10C). After positioning the patient prone, occipital remodeling and advancement are completed (type VIII) (Fig. 65-8). These constitute an extensive procedure with higher morbidity rates that must be reserved for the complex cases in which multiple sutures are involved and early expansion of the whole cranial vault is needed.

Type XI. Fronto-Orbital Advancement by Distraction

The standard fronto-orbital advancement procedure requires elevation of both frontal and orbital bones (Fig. 65-9). This can result in partially resorbed advanced bone and convoluted dura mater that is herniated through the inner table of the skull. If a second operation is performed via the intracranial approach, the dura may be easily torn during calvarectomy and the bone that is advanced can be further resorbed and deformed. Distraction osteogenesis has been used in fronto-orbital advancement for patients with coronal synostosis (nonsyndromic brachycephaly)[111] or for those patients with a craniofacial syndrome in whom fronto-orbital advancement is needed at any moment. The main advantage of this technique is the possibility to avoid cranial vault defects, because separation between the dura mater and the bone flap is not necessary and therefore deterioration of the dura mater and resorption of the advanced fronto-orbital bone are minimized.[111,112] The concomitant expansion of the scalp prevents postoperative relapse and provides the advancement of soft tissues, thus helping in stability and the final postoperative result. In syndromic patients, "harmonic" Crouzon or Pfeiffer cases (those who present without severe frontal bossing or orbital dystopia) are best candidates. A small but nondisfigured fronto-orbital region may be advanced to avoid intracranial hypertension caused by closure of the anterior cranial fossa and to diminish typical proptosis. The whole fronto-orbital console is advanced to the new position without a change in the shape of the fronto-orbital bandeau. Apert patients usually present with severe retrusion of the supraorbital bar and a large lacunae over the metopic region, which makes them worse candidates for this technique. However, my colleagues and I use it in these patients when preliminary fronto-orbital advancement is needed and a second surgery is planned over the anterior region of the skull. This technique helps us prevent iatrogenic lacunae (Fig. 65-14) and pseudomeningoceles that occur through the standard osteotomies.

Among its disadvantages are the necessity for a second surgery to remove devices and the inability to reshape deformed fronto-orbital and temporosquamousal bones. For example,

the surgeon could not simultaneously reduce an increased bitemporal distance or lower a turricephaly as with the standard techniques. In addition, fronto-orbital advancement by distraction has the disadvantage of technical difficulty in the osteotomy at the anterior cranial base (orbital roof). When the surgical technique is not exquisite, orbital meningoceles resulting from intracranial hypertension have been described.[94,103]

The patient is in a supine position under general anesthesia. A zigzag coronal skin incision is made posterior to the planned coronal osteotomy line, and the dissection is performed in a subperiosteal plane down to the supraorbital rims. The anterior one third of the orbital roofs is exposed, carefully preserving the periorbita. The temporalis muscle is detached so that the bur holes can be placed at the middle cranial fossa just behind the sphenoid wing. The osteotomy lines are similar to those of conventional fronto-orbital advancement except for the nonexisting tongue-in-groove osteotomy. Bur holes are placed bilaterally at the pterion just behind the sphenoid wing. Two more bur holes are placed on the glabella at both sides of the end of the superior sagittal sinus. The pterion is then drilled away to expose the anterior fossa behind the wing of the sphenoid and the lateral wall of the orbit anterior to it. The thickened sphenoid ridge is also largely removed. Next, 2- to 3-mm-wide cuts are made in the bone at the lateral and medial orbital rims. The osteotomy is performed to connect the pterional bur holes with the bregma (anterior fontanel) as for standard bifrontal craniotomy. Using a groove director, a Gigli saw is passed from the bur hole at the pterion to the bur holes at the glabella. The Gigli saw is then guided into the cut at the medial orbital rim, and the osteotomy of the anterior cranial base is continued just posterior to the supraorbital rim, joining with the cut at the lateral orbital rim. After the osteotomy is complete, two to four internal distraction devices are placed bilaterally. The detached temporal muscles are sutured back to their original position. Finally, the distraction device rods are allowed to pierce the scalp. I used resorbable distractors to avoid a second operation to remove them. Distraction is initiated on postoperative day 3 or 4 and continued until the desired advancement is achieved. The distraction devices are activated twice daily, moved approximately 0.5 mm per activation, and left in place for an additional 3 weeks. They are then removed through the initial incision, with the patient under sedation, by simply screwing them backward.

Recurrences

As a rule, any craniosynostosis may recur, even after proper treatment, during development. This is particularly true in cases of multiple synostosis and craniofacial syndromes, where the dysplastic processes that affect the cranial vault sutures, the basicranium, and the facial skeleton by the expression of FGFR gene products remain as an underlying condition. This is also a consequence of the cranial base, which remains unchanged despite treatment, because most surgical procedures address the cranial vault but have little effect on the skull base. Recurrences consist mainly of a progressive vault deformation, but the presence of an evolving fracture or the appearance of a new hydrocephalic condition should alert the surgical team to the possibility of unresolved craniosynostosis. Secondary deformations and the appearance or progression of a new suture closure may also

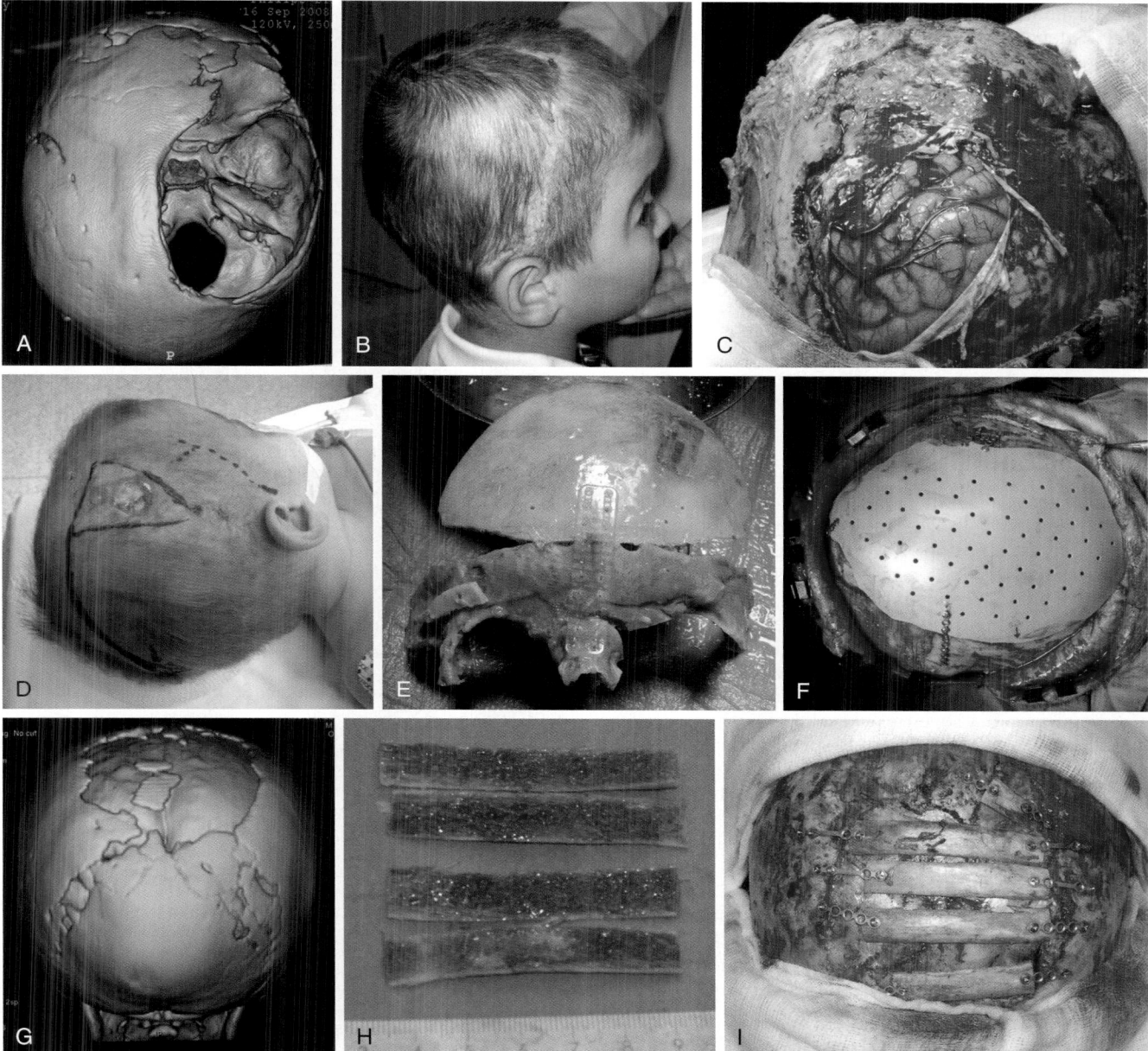

FIGURE 65-14 Complications. Craniolacunae are common complications after repeated surgeries (A and B), infection (C and D), or growing fractures (E). They can be treated with customized heterologous implants (F) or, preferably, with autologous bone implants (G-I).

indicate overdrainage and a pseudotumor state after shunting in a craniosynostosis patient with hydrocephalus.

Prognosis

Prognosis in craniofacial surgery depends mostly on the underlying condition. The majority of simple craniosynostosis patients with a single affected suture do not develop mental retardation, and surgical treatment on a proper schedule and with the right technique by an experienced team renders good results in terms of cosmetic and functional outcome. Although it has been stressed that the occurrence of raised ICP in single-suture synostosis is low,[109,110,113] up to 15% to 20% of patients with single-suture craniosynostosis have a documented increase in ICP.[86] This is particularly

true in patients with severe trigonocephaly,[117] and special attention must be paid to these children. The possibility of elevated ICP is higher as the number of affected sutures increases. The risk is very high in untreated patients with a craniofacial syndrome where craniosynostosis is an evolving condition that worsens during the first years of life and frequently leads to intracranial hypertension. Restricted skull volume contributes to this elevation in ICP, but it is not the only factor responsible. Venous congestion (sometimes with anomalous venous drainage), hydrocephalus, and/or upper airway obstruction are sometimes associated in these patients and are capable of increasing ICP.

Early detection of intracranial hypertension is important to reduce the risks for brain development and visual function. However, in children with craniosynostosis, the clinical manifestations of abnormally increased ICP are difficult to detect, as the majority of patients may have neither warning signs nor symptoms for a long period.[86] As a result, these children warrant extensive clinical surveillance.

The treatment of complex craniosynostosis and craniofacial syndromes requires the participation and coordination of a multidisciplinary team with profound knowledge of the underlying pathophysiogic mechanisms; the use of multiple diagnostic tools, surgical techniques, and staged approaches; and the management of multiple aspects of patient care. The collaboration of neurosurgeons; syndromologists; pediatricians; plastic and maxillofacial surgeons; ear, nose, and throat surgeons; psychologists; and occupational therapists in a multidisciplinary team is undoubtedly the best approach to treating this pathology. The support provided by specific parental associations with affected children is also a tremendous help for many of these families.

Complications

Mortality rates in craniofacial surgery literature are fortunately very low.[118,119] The most frequent complication in surgical series is postoperative hyperthermia (13.17%), possibly related to more extensive tissue dissection and a higher amount of blood component transfusion, followed by cranial infection (8.2%).[99] In the series of my department, infection was below 10%.[119-122] We also encountered subgaleal hematomas (6.0%), dural tears (5.1%), and CSF leaks (2.7%) with significantly lower incidence than that given in prior reports.[120]

Several issues have been related to infectious complications: type of craniosynostosis,[119] age and surgical timing,[120] number of surgeons and intensive care unit time,[123] and proportion of surgical reoperations.[121] My department found two important factors related not to just infections but to all complications: (1) surgical reoperations and (2) type of surgical procedure.

SURGICAL REOPERATIONS

The rate of relapse in the series of my department (12.8%) is similar to that of other authors.[124,125] In a pattern reminiscent of previous reports,[121] my department found that of the 8.2% rate of total infection for craniofacial surgery patients, 62.5% belonged to the group that underwent reoperations. There is an even stronger apparent relationship with dural tears (5.1%), of which 93% took place at the time of reintervention. Adhesions within the cleavage plane, mostly in the extradural space, make surgery more difficult and may predispose to a patient complications, including dural tears. The use of resorbable material may promote adherences in the epidural space, making reintervention more difficult and increasing the possibility of dural tears.

TYPE OF SURGICAL PROCEDURE

Fronto-orbital distraction by internal devices and combined fronto-orbital and midface advancement[126-129] are techniques most often associated with complications. Recently, Pelo et al.[130] performed an exhaustive literature review of 130 cases and added 8 personal patients. Complications included local infection, device breakage, and CSF leakage, though the patient's clinical condition is not mentioned in this paper. In the series of my department, complications were frequent in patients under distraction.[94,103] In the 26 patients treated, there were eight CSF leaks and three dural

tears, as well as eight local infections around the distracting devices. There was only one case of device breakage. This relatively high morbidity may be related to the role of distraction as a "rescue technique" in cases of relapses after the first standard fronto-orbital advancement. Dissection of the pterional and anterior fossa region is not easy without elevation of the frontal bones, and the possibility for dural tears is higher among reoperated patients, where multiple previous adherences and resorbing miniplates make dissection more hazardous. Leptomeningeal cysts,[131] encephalocele,[94] and growing fractures[132] have also been described.

KEY REFERENCES

Cinalli G, Chumas P, Arnaud E, et al. Occipital remodeling and suboccipital decompression in severe craniosynostosis associated with tonsillar herniation. *Neurosurg.* 1998;42:66-73.

Cinalli G, Sainte-Rose CH, Kollar EM, et al. Hydrocephalus and craniosynostosis. *J Neurosurg.* 1998;88:209-214.

Cinalli G, Spennato P, Sainte-Rose C, et al. Chiari malformation in craniosynostosis. *Childs Nerv Syst.* 2005;21:889-901.

Cohen M. Pfeiffer syndrome: update, clinical subtype and guidelines for differential diagnosis. *Am J Gen.* 1993;45:300-307.

Collman H, Sörensen N, Krauß J. Hydrocephalus in craniosynostosis: a review. *Childs Nerv Syst.* 2005;21:902-912.

Di Rocco C, Velardi F, Ferrario A, Marchese E. Metopic synostosis: in favour of a "simplified" surgical treatment. *Child's Nerv Syst.* 1996;12:654-663.

Esparza J, Hinojosa J. Complications in the surgical treatment of craniosynostosis and craniofacial syndromes: a propos of 306 transcranial procedures. *Child's Nerv Syst.* 2008;24:1421-1430.

Goodrich JT. Skull base growth in craniosynostosis. *Child's Nervs Syst.* 2005;21:871-879.

Hayward R. Venous hypertension and craniosynostosis. *Child's Nervs Syst.* 2005;21:880-888.

Hinojosa J, Esparza E, Muñoz MJ. Endoscopic-assisted osteotomies for the treatment of craniosynostosis. *Child's Nerv Syst.* 2007;23:1421-1430.

Hirabayashi S, Sugawara Y, Sakurai A, et al. Fronto-orbital advancement by distraction: the latest modification. *Ann Plast Surg.* 2002;49:447-451.

Jiménez DF, Barone CM, Cartwright CC, Baker L. Early management of craniosynostosis using endoscopic-assisted strip craniectomies and cranial othrotic molding therapy. *Pediatrics.* 2002;110:97-104.

Marucci DD, Dunaway DJ, Jones BM, Hayward RD. Raised intracranial pressure in Apert syndrome. *Plast and Reconstruct Surg.* 2008;122:1162-1168.

McCarthy JG, Glasberg SB, Cutting CB, et al. Twenty-year experience with early surgery for craniosynostosis: II. The craniofacial synostosis syndromes and pansynostosis—results and unsolved problems. *Plast Reconstr Surg.* 1995;96(2):284-295.

Pollack IF, Losken HW, Hurwitz DJ. A combined frontoorbital and occipital advancement technique for use in total calvarial reconstruction. *J Neurosurg.* 1996;84:424-429.

Posnick JC, Ruiz RL. The craniofacial dysostosis syndromes: current surgical thinking and future directions. *Cleft Palate Craniof J 37.* 2000;434(5):1-24.

Renier D, Arnaud E, Cinalli G, et al. Prognosis for mental function in Apert's syndrome. *J Neurosurg.* 1996;85:66-72.

Renier D, Cinalli G, Lajeunie E, et al. L'oxycéphalie, une craniosténose sévère. A propos d'une série de 129 cas. *Arch Pediatr.* 1997;4:722-729.

Sgouros S, Goldin JH, Hockley AD, Wake MJC. Posterior skull surgery in craniosynostosis. *Child's Nerv Syst.* 1996;12:727-733.

Sun PP, Persing JA. Craniosynostosis. In: Albright AL, Pollack IF, Adelson PD, eds. *Operative Techniques in Pediatric Neurosurgery.* New York: Thieme; 2001:51-64.

Tamburrini G, Caldarelli M, Massimi L, et al. Intracranial pressure monitoring in children with single suture and complex craniosynostosis: a review. *Childs Nerv Syst.* 2005;21:913-921.

Taylor WJ, Hayward RD, Lasjaunias P, et al. Enigma of raised intracranial pressure in patients with complex craniosynostosis: the role of abnormal intracranial venous drainage. *J Neurosurg.* 2001;94:377-385.

Thompson DN, Harkness W, Jones BM, Hayward RD. Aetiology of herniation of the hindbrain in craniosynostosis. *Pediatr Neurosurg.* 1997;26:288-295.

Numbered references appear on Expert Consult.

Section Three

VASCULAR DISEASES

CHRISTOPHER S. OGILVY

BRIAN L. HOH

Surgical Management of Extracranial Carotid Artery Disease

MARKUS BOOKLAND • CHRISTOPHER M. LOFTUS

Since the first description of a carotid endarterectomy (CEA) for the prevention of stroke,[1] the operation has been widely debated and often criticized; yet the numbers of end-arterectomy procedures performed annually have steadily increased.[2] Early studies suggested that medical management was superior to surgical intervention.[3,4] This is clearly no longer the case. Gratifying and unimpeachable results from recent multicenter trials have advocated surgical therapy over medical management in specific cases[5-7] of both asymptomatic and symptomatic carotid stenosis. The North American Symptomatic Carotid Endarterectomy Trial data indicate that CEA has benefit for all symptomatic patients with lesions of more than 70% linear stenosis and for specific subgroups of symptomatic patients with more than 50% stenosis. The Asymptomatic Carotid Atherosclerosis Study indicates that asymptomatic patients with more than 60% stenosis have a better outcome with CEA than with medical management.[8]

In this chapter, we describe our standard technique for CEA and discuss the various surgical options and different variations of the procedure. Although there are numerous ways to perform a CEA, one must adhere to several basic principles of carotid reconstruction. The surgeon must have complete preoperative knowledge of the patient's vascular anatomy, must maintain complete vascular control at all times, must have sufficient working anatomic knowledge to prevent harm to adjacent structures, and must assure the patient of a repair that is widely patent and free of technical errors.

Surgical Technique

SURGICAL MAGNIFICATION

We perform the operation with 3.5× loupe-magnified technique. Microscopic repair of the internal carotid artery (ICA), which we have also tried, allows a primary repair that is unquestionably finer than a loupe-magnified technique,[3,9-11] but which in our experience did not alter the overall patient outcome or incidence of restenosis or acute occlusion. In the ongoing effort to reduce morbidity, we have instead adopted universal patch grafting with collagen-impregnated Dacron (Hemashield graft), which has essentially eliminated the problem of acute postoperative thrombosis or rapid restenosis. In our opinion, the graft procedure is more easily and expeditiously accomplished with 3.5× magnification rather than the microscope. There is no doubt that the suture lines are not as fine with this method, but the added lumen diameter with patch angioplasty renders the microscopic technique unnecessary in our routine practice.

ANESTHETIC TECHNIQUE

General anesthesia and local anesthesia are both in common use for CEA. We routinely use general anesthesia with both full-channel electroencephalographic and concurrent somatosensory-evoked potential (SSEP) monitoring. Proponents of local anesthesia cite the advantages of patient response to questioning as a superior method of assessing the need for intraoperative shunting while minimizing anesthetic risks, reducing postoperative morbidity, and shortening length of stay. The patient has local anesthesia with light sedation, which allows the patient to perform a simple task with the contralateral hand during cross-clamping. The disadvantages include risk of contamination and patient movement during the procedure, along with the increased psychological stress of remaining awake. A recent review comparing our technique with that of an institutional vascular surgeon using local anesthesia showed a decreased incidence of electroencephalographic changes and intraoperative shunting with local anesthesia. However, there was no difference in stroke rate, complications, length of stay, or overall outcome.[12,13]

We prefer general anesthesia for a number of reasons, not the least of which is the controlled environment. Additionally, all commonly used inhalational anesthetic agents and intravenous barbiturates significantly reduce the cerebral metabolic rate of oxygen consumption,[14] giving a theoretical protective effect in the setting of cerebral ischemia. We keep our patients normocapnic. Although there has been much interest in arterial levels of carbon dioxide, nonphysiologic hypercapnia and hypocapnia provide no cerebral protection.[15-18] Gross and colleagues[19] found that there was a 40% decrease in electroencephalographic changes with cross-clamping in those patients receiving either one or two units of 6% hetastarch (500 to 1000 ml). They had acceptable outcomes with a postoperative stroke and mortality rate of 1.3%. We ourselves have not adopted this technique because of our policy of shunting quickly without hesitation for any hint of an EEG or SSEP change. Finally, blood pressure is maintained at normotensive levels with a tolerance of as high as a 20% increase in systolic pressure.[11] Although some surgeons prefer to induce hypertension at cross-clamping if there are electroencephalographic changes and then shunt if no improvement is seen in the electro-encephalographic recordings, we are not trying to avoid shunt use, and as mentioned we have a policy to shunt immediately if any monitoring changes are evident.

MONITORING TECHNIQUES

Monitoring techniques can be divided into two categories: (1) tests of vascular integrity, such as stump pressure measurements, xenon regional cerebral blood flow studies, transcranial Doppler and, to a lesser extent, intraoperative oculoplethysmography (OPG), Doppler/duplex scanning, and angiography; and (2) tests of cerebral function, such as electroencephalography, electroencephalographic derivatives, and/or SSEP monitoring. The newly described near-infrared spectroscopy technique bridges both categories. We use a full-channel electroencephalography interpreted by a neurologist. After completion of arteriotomy closure, an intraoperative Doppler examination is performed of the common carotid artery (CCA), the ICA, and the external carotid artery (ECA).[20,21]

INTRAOPERATIVE SHUNTING

Generally speaking, there are three schools of thought about intraoperative shunting.[22] Carotid surgeons shunt in every case, shunt when indicated by some form of intraoperative monitoring, or never place a shunt.[23] In our institution, we perform monitor-dependent shunting based on electroencephalographic criteria. We use a custom commercial shunt of our own design (Loftus shunt, Integra Neurocare, Plainfield, NJ).[24] In our experience, we shunt approximately 15% of CEAs. This increases to approximately 25% if the contralateral carotid is occluded. After the shunt is placed, the monitoring should return to baseline. If this does not occur, the shunt must be inspected for possible kinking, thrombosis, or misplacement. We always auscultate the shunt with a Doppler probe that confirms patency and shunt flow.

Proponents of universal shunting tout the benefits of the maximal degree of cerebral protection in every case while eliminating dependence on specialized intraoperative monitoring techniques. They assert that shunt placement is benign and allows extra time to ensure meticulous intimal dissection and arteriotomy repair.[25-30]

Proponents of nonshunting believe that shunt placement is not benign. In one series, there was a higher stroke rate with shunting compared with nonshunting,[31] indicating that embolization from shunt placement, especially by surgeons inexperienced in the procedure, is a real risk. Another documented concern is distal intimal damage leading to embolization or carotid artery dissection.[32]

Many surgeons, in part because of the concerns previously discussed, choose not to shunt. There have been multiple series that have good surgical results with no shunts being used.[33-40] These authors do not deny the existence of postoperative stroke, but they strongly believe that neurologic deficits from carotid artery surgery are invariably embolic rather than hemodynamic in nature and that intraoperative monitoring and/or shunt placement will not further reduce the already low morbidity in their series.[39]

As discussed previously, we prefer to shunt when there are changes in the EEG and/or SSEP with cross-clamping. This policy has been well supported by several reports of large series of patients.[41,42] Of note, there are also several authors who normally practice selective shunting but who advocate shunting all patients who have had recent strokes or reversible neurologic events (due to their belief that intraoperative monitoring is unreliable in the face of recent ischemic events).[43-45] Whereas we understand their concerns, this has not been our practice.

PATCH GRAFT ANGIOPLASTY

Almost all carotid surgeons perform patch angioplasty for recurrent carotid stenosis. Many will also use selective patching in cases in which the internal carotid is small, where the arteriotomy may have extended far up the ICA, or in any similar case in which compromise of the lumen and a high risk of thrombosis is anticipated. We have taken this policy one step further, and for a number of years have used a Hemashield patch graft primarily in all our patients. We have not encountered any restenosis or acute occlusions since using the patch universally. There are several other synthetic grafts available depending on surgeon preference, and of course autologous sapenous vein grafts can be used, but we prefer Hemashield, mindful of the real concern of central patch rupture with autologous vein, especially in women and patients with diabetes. Rupture risk can be reduced by harvesting the graft from a high femoral site rather than at the ankle.[46]

HEPARINIZATION

A single dose of intravenous heparin is given to the patient at some point before cross-clamping. This dose is between 2500 and 10,000 U of heparin, depending on the surgeon's preference. There are no published reports to support one dose versus another; however, Poisik and colleagues[38] recently reported their results using weight-based dosing of heparin at 85 U/kg. Although they did not see any statistically significant differences between fixed-dose heparinization (5000 U) and weight-based dosing, there were trends of decreased complications of hematoma formation and neuropsychometric testing differences. Some individuals reverse the heparinization with protamine after the operation.[39,40] We have not found any benefit in this practice. For those patients who come to the operating room on a continuous heparin drip, we continue the infusion until the arteriotomy closure is finished. With meticulous technique, bleeding in these cases has not been a problem.

TACKING SUTURES

Tandem sutures to secure the distal intima in the ICA after plaque removal are considered a great advance by some[26] and are deemed unnecessary by others.[27,39,40] The concern with tacking sutures is that they may narrow the lumen, but to us this risk seems small compared with the concern of intimal dissection from an unsecured intimal flap. Several authors[28,39,40] state that, if the arteriotomy is carried far enough to see normal intima distal to the plaque, the tacking sutures are unnecessary. We strongly agree with an arteriotomy that extends past the plaque, but we are not always satisfied with how the intimal plaque tapers at the distal endpoint. In recent years, because of negative experiences with plaque that does not feather cleanly when pulled down from the distal ICA, we have adopted the use of fine scissors to "trim" the plaque cleanly in the ICA as it is removed. When this is done, tacking sutures are rarely necessary. We estimate that we now selectively place tacking sutures in the distal ICA in approximately 10% of cases.

Surgery

We think that the meticulous anatomic dissection and identification of vital cervical structures needed to minimize postoperative complications can be achieved only with a bloodless field. Accordingly, we do not consider elapsed time to be a factor in the performance of carotid artery surgery. In our institution, CEA requires from 2 to 2.5 hours of operating time and the average cross-clamp time is between 30 and 40 minutes. No untoward effects from the length of the procedure have been observed in any patient, and we are convinced that the risk of cervical nerve injury or postoperative complications related to hurried closure of the suture line is significantly reduced by meticulous attention to detail.[47]

Two surgeons trained in the procedure are always present during carotid surgery. Both surgeons may stand on the operative side, the primary surgeon facing cephalad and the assistant facing the patient's feet, or the surgeons may stand on each side of the table. The operative nurse may stand either behind or across the table from the primary surgeon. The patient is positioned supine on the operating room table with the head extended and turned away from the side of operation. Several folded pillowcases are placed between the shoulder blades to facilitate extension of the neck, and the degree of rotation of the head is determined by the relationship of the ECA and the ICA on preoperative angiography or magnetic resonance angiography. The carotid vessels are customarily superimposed in the anteroposterior plane, and moderate rotation of the head will swing the ICA laterally into a more surgically accessible position. In those patients in whom the ICA can be seen angiographically to be laterally placed, the head rotation need not be as great. Conversely, occasional patients will demonstrate an ICA that is rotated medially under the ECA (sometimes called the "twisted" or "side-by-side" carotid configuration), and in such cases, no degree of head rotation will yield a satisfactory exposure. When faced with such a case, the surgeon must be prepared to mobilize the ECA more extensively and swing it medially to expose the underlying internal carotid (even tacking it up to medial soft tissues if necessary).

The position of the carotid bifurcation has been likewise determined before surgery from the angiogram and the skin incision is planned accordingly. We always use a linear incision along the anterior portion of the sternocleidomastoid muscle (Fig. 66-1). This may go as low as the suprasternal notch and as high as the retroaural region depending on the level of the bifurcation. The skin and subcutaneous tissues are divided sharply to the level of the platysma, which is always identified and divided sharply as well. Hemostasis often requires the generous use of bipolar electrocautery. If careful attention is paid to all bleeding points during the opening, there will be little or no bleeding when heparin is administered and the closure will be much simpler.

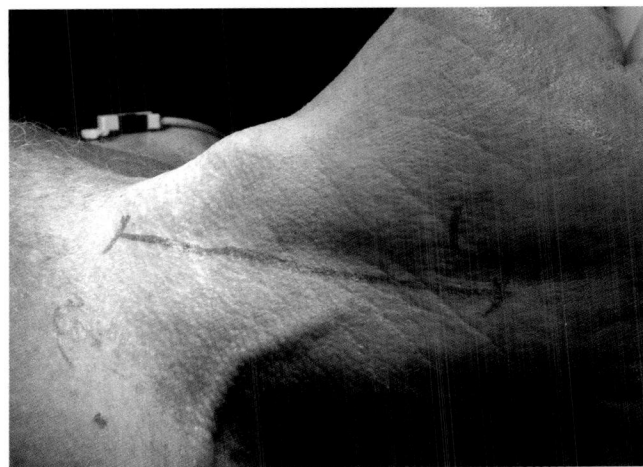

FIGURE 66-1 Positioning and surgical incision planning in a left carotid endarterectomy are shown. The incision parallels the anterior border of the sternomastoid muscle. The L-shaped mark indicates the angle of the mandible.

Self-retaining retractors are next placed and the underlying fat is dissected to identify the anterior edge of the sternocleidomastoid muscle. Retractors are left superficial at all times on the medial side to prevent retraction injury to the recurrent laryngeal nerve in the traceo-esophageal groove, but laterally they may be more deeply placed. Dissection proceeds in the midportion of the wound down the sternomastoid muscle until the jugular vein is identified. Care must be taken under the sternomastoid muscle, however, to prevent injury to the spinal accessory nerve, which can be inadvertently transected or stretched.

It is to be emphasized that the jugular vein is the key landmark in this exposure and complete dissection of the medial jugular border should always be carried out before proceeding to the deeper structures. In some corpulent individuals, the vein is not readily apparent and a layer of fat between it and the sternomastoid must be entered to locate the jugular itself. If this is not done, it is possible to fall into an incorrect plane lateral and deep to the jugular vein. As soon as the jugular is identified, dissection is shifted to come along the medial jugular border and the vein is held back with blunt retractors.[48] The importance of the blunt retractor in preventing vascular injury at this point cannot be overemphasized. In this process, several small veins and one large common facial vein are customarily crossing the field and need to be doubly ligated and divided (Fig. 66-2). The underlying carotid artery is soon identified once the jugular is retracted. Most often we come upon the CCA first, and at the point of first visualization, the anesthesiologist is instructed to give 5000 U of intravenous heparin, which, as discussed previously, is never reversed. Dissection of the carotid complex is then straightforward, and the CCA, ECA, and ICA are isolated with the gentlest possible dissection and encircled with 00 silk ties (or vessel loops, if preferred) passed with a right-angle clamp. We no longer routinely inject the carotid sinus; however, the anesthesiologist is notified when the bifurcation is being dissected, and if any changes in vital signs ensue, the sinus can be injected with 2 to 3 ml of 1% plain Xylocaine through a short 25-gauge needle (this has not been necessary for the past several years). Although the carotid complex is completely exposed, the CCA and ECA are not routinely dissected free from their underlying beds to prevent postoperative kinking and coiling of these vessels. These arteries are dissected circumferentially only in those areas where silk ties or clamps are placed around them. Posterior dissection is more extensive in the region of the ICA, where in an occasional case posterior tacking sutures may later be placed and tied.

The CCA 0 silk is passed through a wire loop that is then pulled through a rubber sleeve (Rummel tourniquet), thereby facilitating constriction of the vessel around an intraluminal shunt if this becomes necessary. The ECA and ICA ties or loops are merely secured with mosquito clamps. Particular attention is paid to the superior thyroid artery, which is dissected free and secured with a double loop 00 silk ligature (some prefer an aneurysm clip for this). A hanging mosquito clamp keeps tension on this occlusive Potts tie. Occasionally, multiple branches of this artery are identified on the preoperative angiogram and must be individually dealt with so that no troublesome back-bleeding will ensue during the procedure through ignorance of these vessels. It is also essential that the ECA silk tie (and subsequent cross-clamp) be placed proximal to any major external branches, lest unacceptable back-bleeding occur during the arteriotomy and repair.

Proper placement of the retractors facilitates the control of the carotid system. The hanging mosquitoes and silk ties are draped over these retractor handles to keep the field uncluttered. Of particular note is a blunt, hinged (modified Richards) retractor, which is invaluable in exposing the ICA when a far distal exposure is necessary. Dissection of the ICA must be complete and clearly beyond the distal extent of the plaque before cross-clamping is performed. A clear plane can be developed if the jugular vein is followed distally and dissection follows the plane between the lateral carotid wall and the medial jugular border. By following this plane, the hypoglossal nerve is readily identified as it swings down medial to the jugular and crosses toward the midline over the ICA. The nerve is mobilized along its lateral wall adjacent to the jugular vein, after which it can

be isolated with a vessel loop and gently retracted from the field. Hypoglossal paresis is rare and seems to result instead in cases in which the nerve is not visualized and is blindly retracted. On occasion, adequate mobilization of the hypoglossal nerve requires ligation of a small arterial branch of the ECA to the sternocleidomastoid muscle, which loops over the nerve. We have never seen inadvertent transection of the hypoglossal nerve.

There are several nerves that can be injured during carotid exposure and CEA. The spinal accessory and hypoglossal nerves have already been discussed. The vagus nerve lies deep to the carotid in the carotid sheath and can be inadvertently cross-clamped if not identified. The marginal mandibular branch of the facial nerve can be stretched by medial retraction in the high exposure of the ICA. The greater auricular nerve is at risk with a high incision, leaving the patient with a troublesome numb ear if it is transected. We have seen Horner's syndrome (always transient) from unrecognized injury to the pericarotid sympathetic chain. Cutaneous sensory nerves will always be transected with the skin incision, and we advise patients that the anterior triangle of their neck will be numb for approximately 6 months after endarterectomy, after which sensation customarily reverts to normal.

It is vital to have adequate exposure of the ICA and control distal to the plaque before opening the vessel. The extent of the plaque can be readily palpated with some experience by a moistened finger. There is also a visual cue when the vessel becomes pinker (instead of hard and yellow) and more normal appearing distal to the extent of the plaque. If high exposure is needed, the posterior belly of the digastric muscle can be cut with impunity, although this is necessary only in a small percentage of cases. When complete exposure is achieved, the final step in preparation for cross-clamping is to ensure that the shunt clamp can be fitted around the ICA to secure the shunt if one is used. We designed and use a custom commercial spring-loaded pinch clamp (Loftus carotid shunt clamp, Scanlan Instruments, St. Paul, MN), which is available in several angles and has a special head exactly sized to grasp the ICA and indwelling shunt without leakage from back-bleeding. The Loftus shunt clamp is illustrated in Fig. 66-3.

We also use a sterile marking pen to draw the proposed arteriotomy line along the vessel, which is helpful in preventing a jagged or curving suture line (Fig. 66-4). The

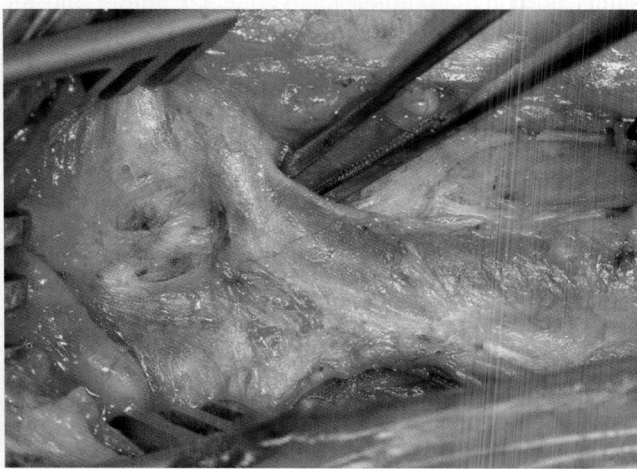

FIGURE 66-2 Intraoperative photograph shows the right jugular vein with a forcep behind the right common facial vein. The carotid cannot be visualized yet.

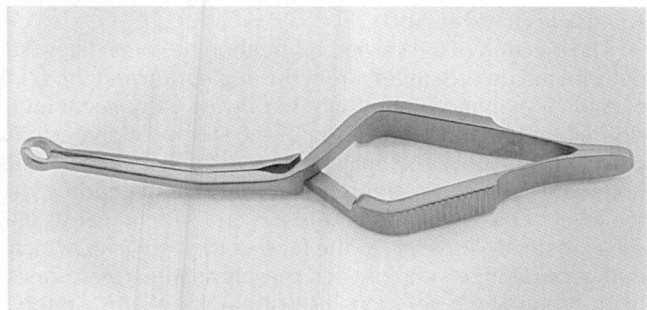

FIGURE 66-3 The Loftus shunt clamp. This customized spring-loaded clamp is slightly angled with an encircling atraumatic end. This clamp is used to secure the indwelling shunt in the internal carotid artery.

arteriotomy is made on the anterior surface of the ICA to facilitate the subsequent repair.

The monitoring systems (we use concurrently both EEG and SSEP now) are then rechecked, and the technicians are notified of impending cross-clamping. Once a suitable period of baseline has been recorded, the CCA is occluded with a large DeBakey vascular clamp and small, straight bulldog clamps or Yasargil aneurysm clips are used to occlude the ICA and ECA. We always occlude the ICA first in the belief that this approach has the lowest risk of embolization associated with clamping. A no. 11 blade is then used to begin the arteriotomy in the CCA and when the lumen is identified, a Potts scissors is used to cut straight up along the marked line into the region of the bifurcation and then up into the internal until normal ICA is entered (Fig. 66-5). In severely stenotic vessels with friable plaque, the lumen is not always easily discerned and false planes

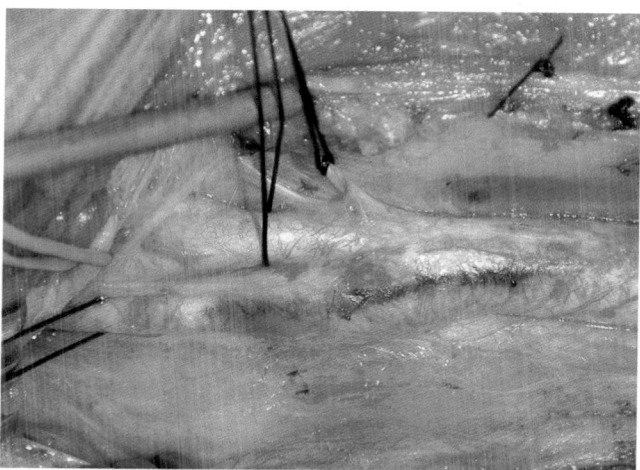

FIGURE 66-4 The carotid system has been cleanly dissected, and the arteriotomy site has been marked with a black marking pen. In the left upper quadrant, the hypoglossal nerve has been dissected and isolated with a vessel loop. The external carotid and superior thyroid arteries have silk ties around them. At the left edge, the internal carotid artery that is plaque free has a silk tie around it.

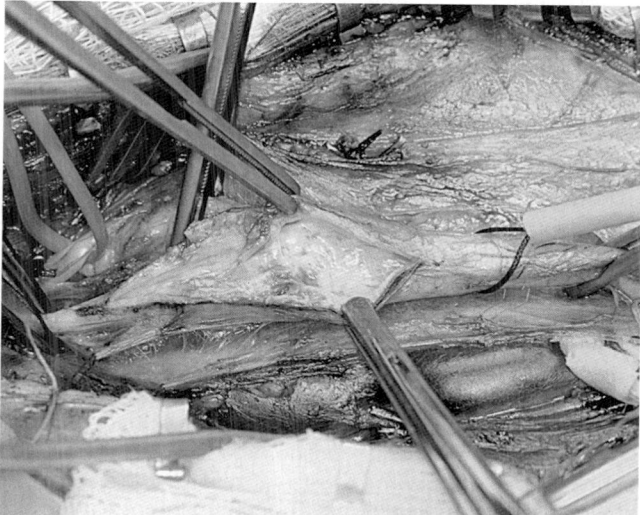

FIGURE 66-5 After the vessel has been opened, the plaque can best be seen by gently everting the edges of the artery with vascular forceps.

within the lesion are often encountered; great care must be taken to ensure that the back wall of the carotid is not lacerated and that the true lumen is identified before attempted shunt insertion.

Changes in the electroencephalogram mandate a rapid trial of induced hypertension for some surgeons, but for an intraluminal shunt is placed for any change on any monitor. The wisdom of shunt use is discussed elsewhere in the text. Numerous shunt types are available. We now use and recommend a customized indwelling shunt, the Loftus carotid endarterectomy shunt (Integra Neurocare, Plainsboro, NJ) (Fig. 66-6). This is a 15-cm straight silicone tube, singly packed in two diameters (10 Fr and 12 Fr), with tapered ends for easy insertion and a bulb at the proximal end to facilitate anchoring by the Rummel tourniquet. This shunt has a black marker band directly in the center of the shunt, so that cephalad shunt migration can be readily discerned and corrected. The shunt is first inserted into the CCA and secured by pulling up on the silk ties; a mosquito clamp then holds the rubber sleeve in place to snug the silk around both the vessel and the intraluminal shunt. The shunt tubing is held closed at its midportion with a heavy vascular forceps and then briefly opened to confirm blood flow and evacuate any debris in the shunt tubing. Suction is then used by the assistant to elucidate the lumen of the ICA, and the distal end of the shunt tubing is placed therein. After the shunt is again bled, flushing any debris from the ICA, the bulldog clamp is removed and the shunt is advanced up the ICA until the black dot lies in the center of the arteriotomy. The shunt, if properly placed, should slide easily into the ICA, and no undue force should be employed to prevent intimal damage and possible dissection. The Loftus shunt clamp is then used to secure the shunt distally in the ICA. Visualization of the dot in the center of the arteriotomy confirms constant correct positioning of the shunt (Fig. 66-7). A handheld Doppler probe can be applied to the shunt tubing to audibly confirm flow.

With or without the shunt, the plaque is next dissected from the arterial wall with a Freer elevator. A vascular pickup is used to hold the wall, and the Freer elevator is

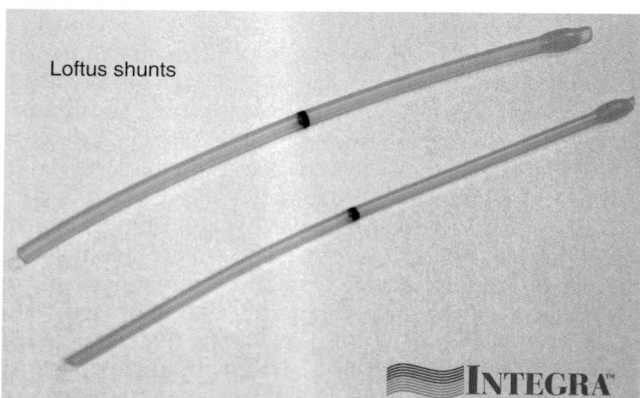

Loftus shunts

FIGURE 66-6 The Loftus shunt set. The set contains two shunts of differing diameters to allow for sizing preferences and a special scissors (disposable) to hook and cut the shunt cleanly for removal without damaging the back wall of the carotid. The shunt is a straight silicone tube beveled and rounded at both ends for safe insertion. A built-up bulb is present on the proximal (common carotid artery) end to anchor the shunt within the Rummel tourniquet.

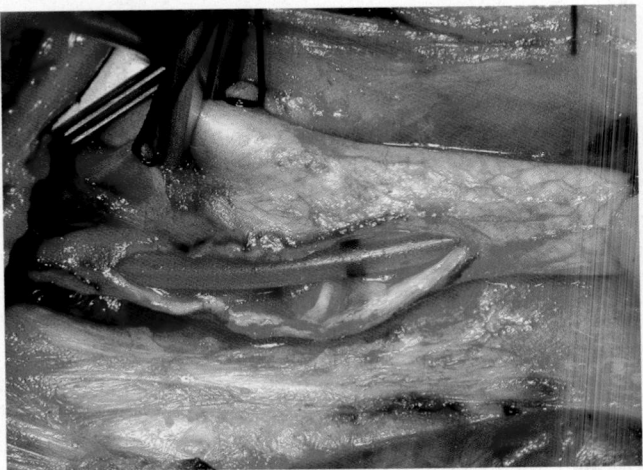

FIGURE 66-7 The Loftus shunt in place. The shunt is secured at the common carotid artery end by a Rummel tourniquet and in the internal carotid artery by the Loftus shunt clamp. The black band indicates the center of the shunt and helps prevent unrecognized shunt migration (which should also be prevented by the fat bulb on the common carotid artery end anchored by the Rummel tourniquet).

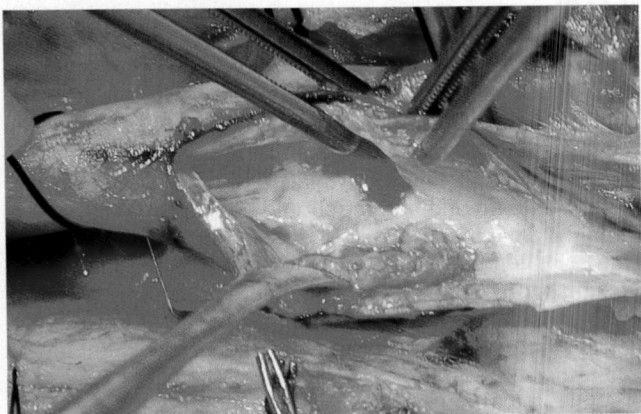

FIGURE 66-8 Plaque dissection is started by using a Freer elevator to develop a plane at the lateral edge of the arteriotomy. In this left carotid endarterectomy, the medial edge has already developed a plane, while the surgeon starts on the lateral edge.

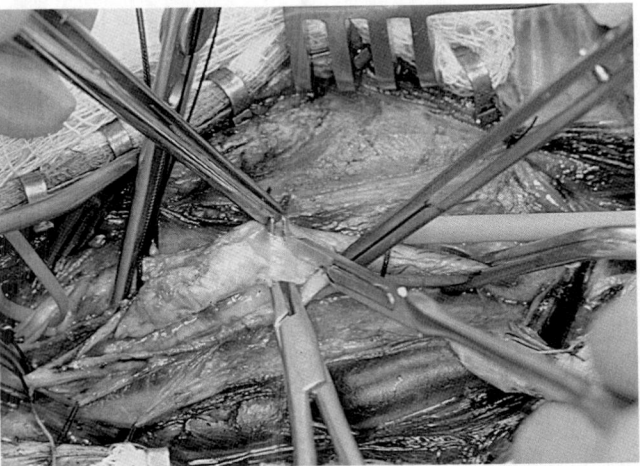

FIGURE 66-9 By using a right-angled clamp, the plaque can be incised in the common carotid artery by slipping the clamp under the plaque and then using a No. 15 knife to cut cleanly along the lower blade of the clamp.

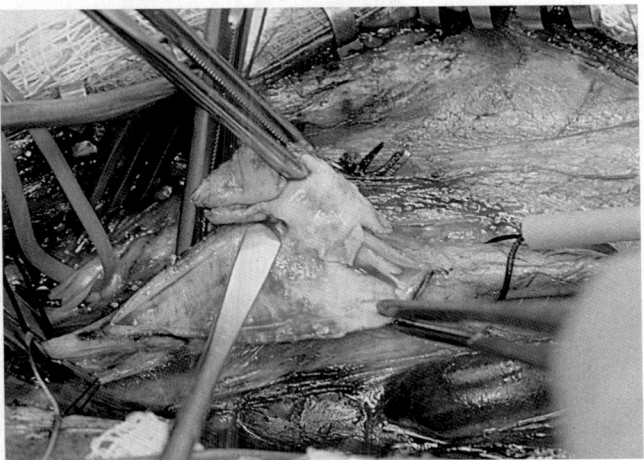

FIGURE 66-10 The dissection of the plaque is continued with the Freer elevator along the medial edge.

moved from side to side developing a plane first in the lateral wall of the arteriotomy (Fig. 66-8). The plaque is usually readily separated in a primary case, and we go approximately half way around the wall before proceeding to the other side. The plaque is then dissected on the medial side of the CCA and transected proximally with a Potts or Church scissors. A clean feathering away of the plaque is almost never possible in the CCA, and the goal here is to transect the plaque sharply, leaving a smooth transition zone. We like to pass a right-angle clamp between the plaque and the normal vessel and cut sharply along the clamp blade with the no. 15 knife (Fig. 66-9). It is important to note that, despite the direction of flow, the proximal end point can create a flap and the surgeon should ensure that the CCA end point is adherent. Attention is then directed to the ICA where likewise the plaque is dissected first laterally and then medially and then an attempt is made to feather the plaque down smoothly from the ICA (Fig. 66-10). However, we find that, in some cases no matter how far up the ICA

we go, a shelf of normal intima remains and tacking sutures are required. Attention is finally directed to the final point of plaque attachment at the orifice of the ECA. The vascular pickup is used to grip across the entire plaque at the ECA opening, and, with some traction on the plaque, the ECA can be everted such that the plaque can be dissected quite far up into that vessel (Fig. 66-11). The eversion of the external and thus optimal plaque removal can be facilitated by "pushing" the distal external artery proximally with the clamp or forceps. The plaque is often tethered in the ECA by the clamp and as long as the lumen is held closed with the heavy forceps, this clamp can be removed without untoward bleeding, allowing avulsion of the distal plaque. The clamp must be quickly reapplied to stem back-bleeding that occurs when the plaque is removed from the ECA. It should be stressed that if plaque removal is inadequate in the ECA, thrombosis may ensue, which can occlude the entire carotid tree with disastrous results. If there is any question of incomplete removal of the external plaque, we do not hesitate to extend the arteriotomy up the ECA itself and close it via a separate suture line.

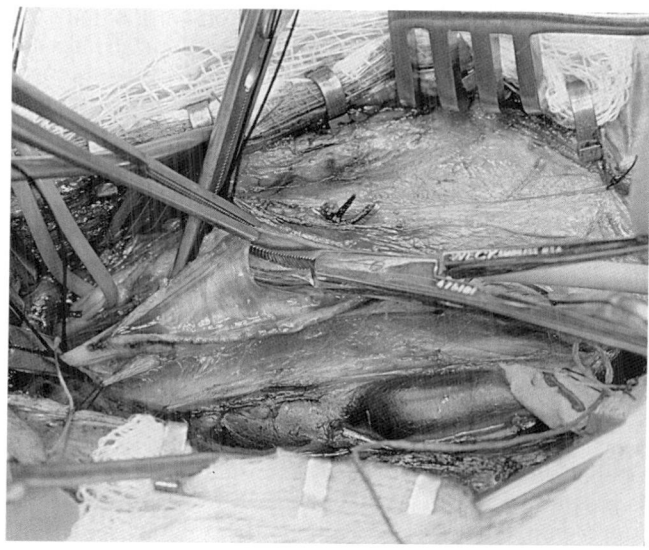

FIGURE 66-11 After plaque removal from the internal and common carotid arteries, attention is then turned to the external carotid artery. The plaque is gently removed from the external artery with a fine hemostat and gentle traction.

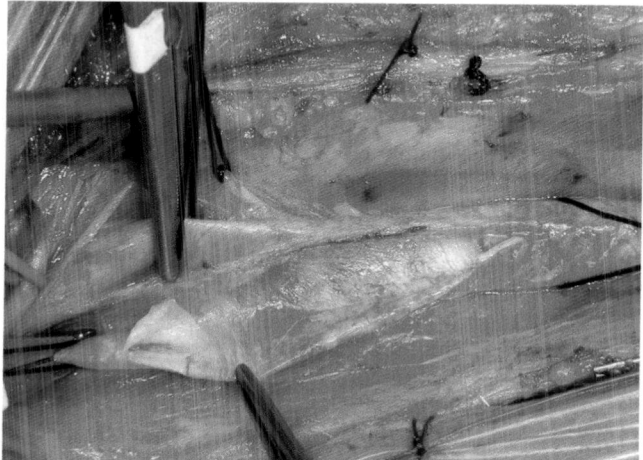

FIGURE 66-12 The lumen is then checked for any remaining fragments that are adherent to the wall.

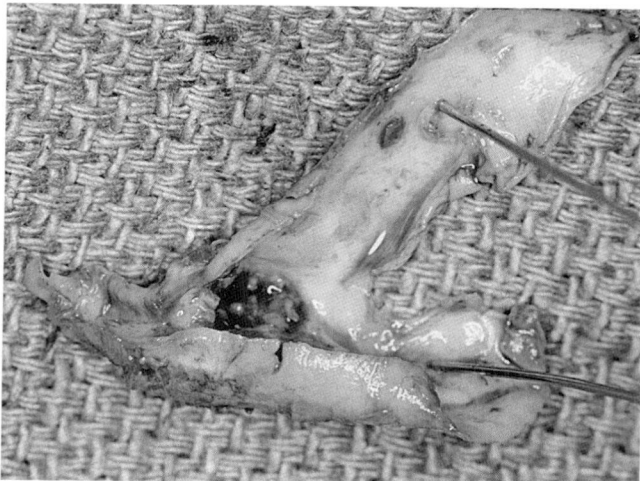

FIGURE 66-13 A soft, friable plaque with a small thrombus.

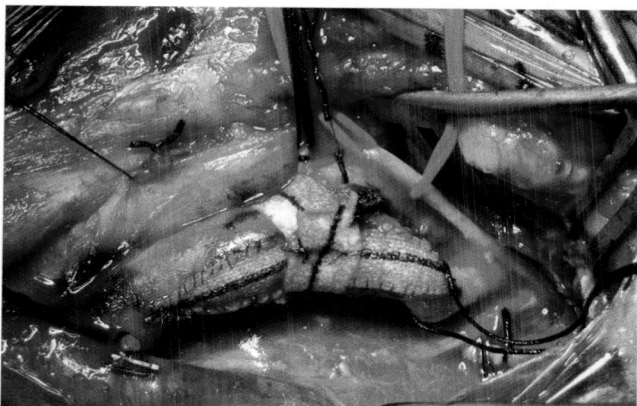

FIGURE 66-14 A Hemashield is wrapped around the carotid reconstruction to reinforce a tenuous back wall.

After gross plaque removal, a careful search is made for any remaining fragments adherent to the arterial wall (Fig. 66-12). Suspect areas are gently stroked with a peanut sponge, and every attempt is made to remove all loose fragments in a circumferential fashion, elevating them the complete width of the vessel until they break free at the arteriotomy edge. (The fine Scanlan Loftus micro-ring-tip forceps are ideal for this, as the fragments are often too fine to be grasped with conventional DeBakey forceps.) Although it is important to remove all loose fragments, no attempt is made to elevate firmly attached fragments, which pose no danger of elevating or breaking off.

Several special aspects of plaque removal need to be considered. The simplest plaque to remove is the soft, friable plaque with intraplaque hemorrhage and thrombus, which dissect quite readily and from which fragments are easily removed (Fig. 66-13). The more difficult is the severely stenotic, stony hard plaque in which a plane of dissection at

the lateral border of the carotid may not be readily apparent. This situation is analogous to the gross appearance in a case of recurrent carotid stenosis. In these instances, even the most gentle plaque removal results in areas of thinning, where only an adventitial layer is left in the posterior wall of the carotid. We have occasionally treated these thin spots by primary plication with one or two double-armed interrupted stitches of 6-0 Prolene placed in the same fashion as the tacking sutures, and no untoward consequences have ensued. Likewise, we have occasionally encountered an intraluminal thrombus emanating from a congenital web or shelf in the lumen of the vessel, and the shelf has been successfully tacked down with a posteriorly placed stitch of double-armed 6-0 Prolene. In all cases, the goal is to leave as smooth an arteriotomy bed as is possible with minimal areas of denudation or roughness available as sites of thrombus formation. Finally, at the completion of the repair, when the clamps are off, we sometimes reinforce thin back wall areas with an encircling "diaper" of Hemashield graft, loosely held together at the top by 6-0 sutures (Fig. 66-14).[49]

Attention is then directed to the arterial repair. If desired, the operating microscope can be brought into the field at this point or in some cases sooner to allow for removal of the small fragments under high magnification.[9-11,50] Our

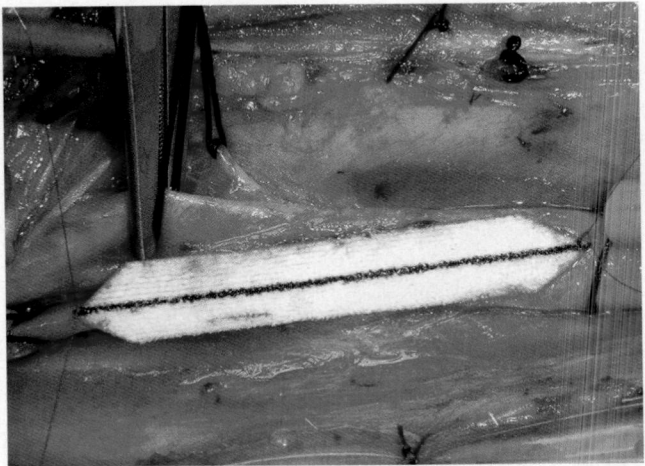

FIGURE 66-15 The Hemashield patch is attached to both ends of the arteriotomy with a double-armed 6-0 Prolene stitch. The needles are left attached to allow closure of the patch graft. Note that both ends of the patch are tapered.

personal preference is to continue with 3.5× loupe magnification. If tacking sutures are required, double-armed sutures of 6-0 Prolene are placed vertically from the inside of the vessel out such that they traverse the intimal edge and are tied outside the adventitial layer. Most often two such sutures are used, placed at the 4- and 8-o'clock positions.

The patch, whatever material is employed, is then fashioned, if the surgeon has chosen this option. The patch material (Hemashield for the purposes of this description and illustrations) is placed over the arteriotomy and cut to the exact length of the opening. After removal from the field, the ends are trimmed and tapered to a point with fine Metzenbaum scissors. Each end of the patch is then anchored to the arteriotomy with double-armed 6-0 Prolene sutures, and the needles are left on and secured with rubber-shod clamps (Fig. 66-15). The medial wall suture line is closed first, and a running, nonlocking stitch is brought from the ICA anchor to the CCA anchor where it is tied to a free end of the CCA anchor Prolene (Fig. 66-16). The lateral wall is then closed (with the remaining limb of the ICA anchor stitch) from the ICA to just below the level

of the carotid bulb. At this point, the second arm of the CCA anchor stitch is used to run up the CCA lateral wall to meet the ICA limb. Small bites are taken just at the arterial edge throughout (being certain, however, that all layers are included), and sutures are placed relatively close together to prevent leaks. Care is also taken so that no stray adventitial tags or suture ends are sewn into the lumen where they might induce thrombosis. Several millimeters of unsewn vessel are left on the lateral wall ensuring room to remove the shunt, if one has been used. After the EEG/SSEP teams are again notified, the shunt is double-clamped with two parallel straight mosquitoes and then cut between them and removed in two sections, one from each end. A common error at this point is to mistakenly entangle the suture material in the shunt clamps and thereby hamper smooth shunt removal. With or without shunt, the arteriotomy is completely closed as follows: all three vessels are first opened and closed sequentially to ensure that back-bleeding is present from the ICA, ECA, and CCA. The ICA is back-bled last to ensure that it is free of debris. The two stitches are then held taut by the surgeon while the assistant introduces a heparinized saline syringe with a blunt needle into the arterial lumen. The vessel is filled with heparinized saline, and in this process, all air is evacuated from the lumen. As the stitches are drawn up and a surgeon's knot is thrown, the blunt needle is withdrawn, allowing no air to enter. Ten more knots are then placed in this most crucial stitch (Fig. 66-17). The declamping sequence is first from the ECA, then from the CCA, and, finally, some 10 seconds later, from the ICA. In this fashion, all loose debris and remaining microbubbles of air are flushed into the ECA circulation. Meticulous attention is paid to evacuation of all debris and air before opening the ICA in every case. However, in the rare case in which there is a known ECA occlusion (although most of these can be reopened at surgery with an ECA endarterectomy), this technique is extremely crucial as there is no ECA safety valve and all intraluminal contents will be shunted directly into the intracranial circulation.

An alternative method for completing the repair involves removal of the ligature or clip from the superior thyroid artery or ECA before final closure, allowing back-bleeding from that vessel to fill the lumen and eliminate the air and debris while the final stitches are placed and tied. We do not use this because we find the bleeding to be annoying.

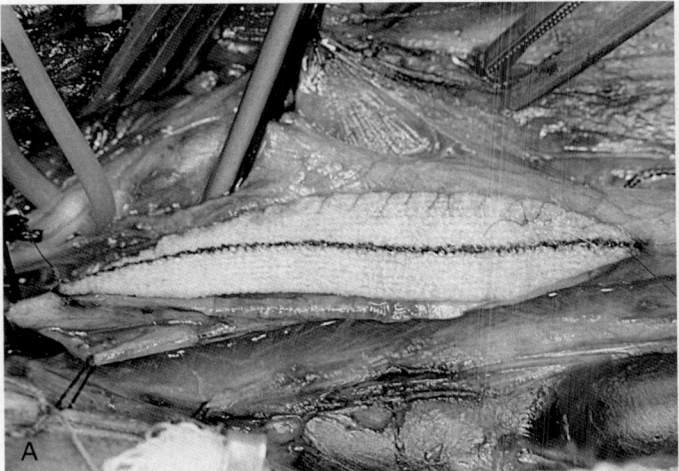
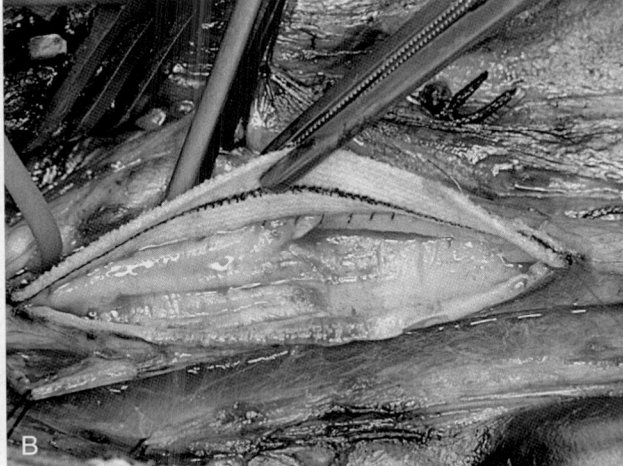

FIGURE 66-16 A, The medial wall is closed first from the internal to the common carotid arteries. B, The patch is lifted to show the sutures from the luminal side.

When the clamps have been removed, the suture lines are inspected for leaks, which are customarily controlled with pressure, patience, and Surgicel gauze. In occasional cases, a single throw of 6-0 Prolene is necessary to close a persistent arterial hemorrhage. Suture repairs of bleeding points are more likely if a patch graft has been placed. It is almost never necessary to reapply clamps to the artery if the repair has been properly performed. The repair is then lined with Surgicel, and the three vessels are tested with a handheld Doppler to ensure patency. The retractors are removed and hemostasis is confirmed both along the jugular vein and from the surrounding soft tissues. Persistent oozing is often encountered in these patients who have often received large doses of antiplatelet agents in addition to their intraoperative heparin. A final Doppler check is made, and the wound is closed in layers. The carotid sheath is first closed to provide a barrier against infection, and the platysma is then closed as a separate layer to ensure a good cosmetic result. Either running or interrupted subcuticular stitches may be used to close the skin edges. A Hemovac drain is left inside the carotid sheath. It is removed on the first postoperative day. Patients are continued on aspirin after surgery and are discharged in 1 to 2 days.[51-57]

We manage any postoperative neurologic deficit, including a transient ischemic attack alone, with immediate assessment of the technical adequacy of repair. If high-quality color duplex ultrasonography is available, this may allow quick documentation of patency and identify any partially obstructing defects. Computed tomography angiography is another excellent and rapid strategy, and these techniques have essentially replaced the rush to catheter angiography. Any occluded carotid artery postoperatively is re-explored and repatched immediately, although since adopting the primary Hemashield patch repair, the incidence of postoperative occlusion has been zero.[58]

Special Situations

COMPLETE OCCLUSION

Surgery is generally indicated for cases of acute carotid occlusion if the patient is not so debilitated as to make recovery untenable. Surgery is essentially always indicated for known acute postoperative occlusion, reflecting technical error in most cases. Surgery is sometimes indicated for cases of subacute carotid occlusion and in cases of chronic occlusion if the possibility of a "string sign" minimally patent vessel (which can usually be reopened) exists, justifying exploration. Our surgical technique for complete CCA/ICA occlusion involves opening (or reopening) of the CCA and ICA once the vessels have been controlled. The thrombus is usually seen at the carotid bulb and extending into the distal ICA; in our experience, the ECA is usually patent. Removal of thrombus and associated ICA plaque may establish back-bleeding; if not, the ICA can be explored with a no. 8 feeding tube cut to a 15-cm length and attached to a 10-ml syringe. The tube is advanced into the ICA, and the syringe is drawn back to establish suction, which often will pull down the distal thrombus as the tubing is withdrawn. If this fails, Fogarty catheters are passed into the ICA, but the risk of establishing a carotid-cavernous fistula with these must be considered. If back-bleeding cannot be established, we cleanly ligate the distal and proximal ICA stumps and perform a CCA/ECA endarterectomy and repair. If 6 hours or more have passed since occlusion, the likelihood of successful neurologic salvage is diminished, and the risk of intracerebral hemorrhage appears to increase.[59]

STUMP SYNDROME

The term "stump syndrome" describes the continuation of ipsilateral ischemic symptoms after ICA occlusion; the mechanism for this is the retrograde passage of emboli from the ICA intraluminal thrombus that gain entry to the intracranial circulation via the ECA and its collateral blood flow. After strict indications criteria are met,[60] surgical correction is undertaken via a standard common to external carotid CEA. After removal of the thrombus from the ICA stump, we attempt to reopen the ICA and establish back-bleeding. If this is not possible (it usually is not), the stump is obliterated with inside-out sutures or with external application of large Weck clips. We stress that the ICA lumen must be obliterated. A standard external CEA is then performed (we place a CCA to ECA patch graft), and the arteriotomy is closed in the usual fashion.

BILATERAL CAROTID ENDARTERECTOMY

Bilateral CEA runs the risk of extreme swings in blood pressure from concurrent denervation of both carotid sinuses[61] and from the risk of bilateral cranial nerve injury. For those patients who require bilateral endarterectomy, we recommend a staged procedure, with at least a 6-week window between the procedures. We customarily have laryngoscopy performed by an otolaryngologist to rule out recurrent laryngeal nerve palsy before the second procedure is undertaken. Unilateral nerve dysfunction in the cervical region is troublesome, but a bilateral one can be disabling. We have on occasion deferred the second surgery due to an occult vocal cord paralysis. When this happens, the patient is maintained on medical management until such time as cord function returns (as it usually does), after which the second side CEA is performed.

PLAQUE MORPHOLOGY

The correlation of plaque ulceration with ischemic neurologic symptoms and the need for surgery is difficult for several reasons. First, studies have shown poor interobserver variability, either on ultrasound or arteriographic

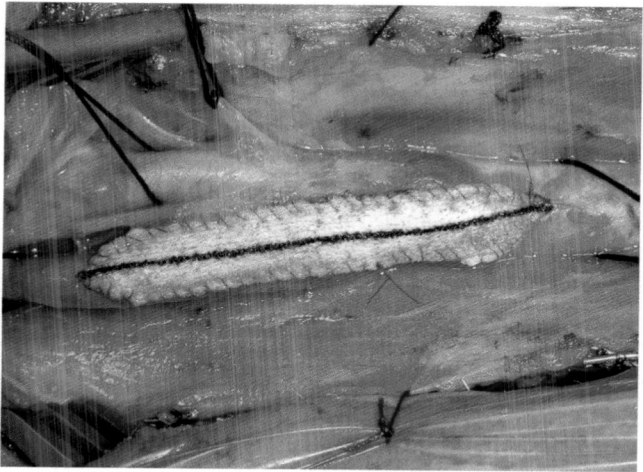

FIGURE 66-17 The lateral wall is then closed halfway down the internal carotid artery and then with the second stitch halfway up the common carotid artery.

examinations, and poor correlation between pathologic specimens and radiographically demonstrated ulceration. Second, in symptomatic patients, deep ulceration is most commonly found in conjunction with significant degrees of carotid stenosis, and it becomes difficult to separate clinical symptomatology between these two findings.[62,63] The most recent data from the North American Symptomatic Carotid Endarterectomy Trial[7] show that in medically treated patients with 50% to 99% stenosis (now proven to be unequivocal surgical candidates), the presence of plaque ulceration in conjunction with stenosis significantly increases the risk of stroke.[64] Whether the presence of ulceration in plaques of less than 50% linear stenosis significantly increases the risk of stroke remains an unanswered question that has not been addressed by cooperative trial data.

The significance of intraplaque hemorrhage as a predictor of ischemic symptoms is also unclear. Heterogeneous plaque morphology on duplex scanning (consistent with intraplaque hemorrhage) was a significant risk factor for subsequent neurologic events in one study if the underlying stenosis was more than 50%.[65] Although one recent review also suggested that intraplaque hemorrhage was found more commonly in patients with symptomatic carotid artery disease,[62] other studies suggest that there is a low correlation between ischemic symptoms and plaque hematoma in patients who undergo CEA.[66]

CONCURRENT CORONARY ARTERY DISEASE

Surgical intervention is the most effective treatment option for patients with carotid artery stenosis.[67] Alternate treatment modalities have arisen—the most notable being carotid artery stenting (CAS)—offering novel therapeutic options for extracranial carotid stenosis; but the preponderance of data continues to favor CEA as the therapeutic of choice.[68-72] Even so, there is a subset of high-risk patients with carotid artery stenosis and significant comorbidities such as poor cardiac function who, in the past, have justified consideration of alternative therapies and/or more measured approaches to CEA. For the most part, these patients still benefit greatly from CEA; but the timing of surgery and the spectrum of attendant risks can vary depending on the patient's comorbidities.[73]

Cardiac disease is probably the most common comorbidity that we deal with in planning strategy for carotid patients.[74,75] The basic dictum is—fix the offending lesion first.[76] In general, patients with symptomatic coronary artery disease (CAD) severe enough to warrant coronary artery bypass grafting (CABG), and surgical but asymptomatic carotid stenosis, should have their CEA delayed until they have had their CABG performed and been allowed adequate time to recover. While true that there appears to be some increase in stroke risk among CABG patients with synchronous carotid disease, the bulk of post-CABG cerebral infarctions (85%) occur in patients with little to no (<50% stenosis bilaterally) carotid disease.[77] Likewise, reviews of ischemic patterns in post-CABG patients with carotid artery disease and CVAs have found that 60% to 80% of their infarctions lie in either the posterior circulation or bilateral territories, making their ischemia difficult to attribute to unilateral carotid disease.[77,78] Particularly for those patients with unilateral, asymptomatic disease, the risk of post-CABG stroke appears to be exceedingly low (0%–2.9%).[79-81] Within this patient population, the risk of myocardial infarction in the perioperative period post-CEA appears to outweigh the potential risk of stroke post-CABG. It has therefore been recommended that surgeons consider delaying CEA for asymptomatic disease in patients with significant cardiac disease until after their cardiac issues have been adequately addressed.

Patients with symptomatic carotid disease are more aggressively managed even in the face of significant CAD. Naylor, et al. noted in a series of 4638 patients undergoing isolated CABG procedures that those with less than 50% carotid stenosis bilaterally had a 1.8% rate of CVAs, those with more than 50% unilateral stenoses had a rate of 3.2%, and those with unilateral carotid occlusions had a rate of 11.6%.[77] These data do not distinguish between symptomatic or asymptomatic patients, but imply that the risk of postprocedural cerebral infarction after a CABG becomes unacceptably high (>1%–2%) when carotid disease is compounded by tandem lesions or complete occlusion.[82,83] Similarly, some small studies have noted that coronary artery revascularization patients with pre-CABG complaints of strokes or TIAs ipsilateral to known carotid artery disease suffered a roughly sixfold increase in post-CABG strokes compared to patients with carotid artery disease who were asymptomatic or had discordant neurologic symptoms.[79] Taken together, these data argue for preemptive CEAs among cardiopaths with preoperative symptomatic carotid disease or marked bilateral stenoses/occlusions.[84]

ADVANCED AGE

Age over 70 years, is considered by many to be an independent risk factor for carotid reconstruction, and suggestions are made that elderly patients are better treated with CAS-P. Current data do not support this for two reasons: the risk of CEA is probably not significantly higher in the elderly; and the risk of CAS-P clearly is much higher with advancing age, because of the tortuosity of the great vessels and the difficulty of access for endovascular treatment. A review of 53 patients over 70 years old at the University of Iowa Hospital found no differences in CEA outcomes when compared to historic, younger controls.[85] Likewise, several prospective and retrospective studies have compared CEA and CAS in the elderly and found that age does not significantly alter CEA results. A meta-analysis of 8 CAS study groups and 33 CEA study groups that selected for patients over 80 years of age identified increased rates of postprocedure stroke among CAS patients, similar to those rates noted in past randomized controlled trials (RCTs). No other differences were seen in periprocedural or long term mortality and myocardial events in these studies.[86] Finally, the lead-in data from the credentialing phase of the CREST trial confirm that the risk of CAS-P in patients in their 70s and 80s is unacceptably high compared to routine CEA (stroke/death rate 5.3% for ages 70 to 79 and 12.1% for ages over 80).[87] As long as the predicted life expectancy of the patient exceeds 5 years, CEA should continue to be considered as the treatment of choice for extracranial carotid disease exceeding 50% to 60% among the elderly.[88,89]

COMPLICATED NECK ANATOMY

Patients with previous neck surgeries, high carotid bifurcations, irradiated cervical fields, and inextensible necks may be considered by some more efficaciously approached via an endovascular route. Although such anatomic challenges may make for a more difficult dissection, an experienced surgeon offers long-term benefits with CEA for such patients with significant carotid stenosis. A case-controlled trial in 2009 looking at 154 carotid artery stenosis patients prospectively followed and paired CEA and CAS patients. In the final analysis, no difference in periprocedural ischemic events or mortality was noted. A higher rate of postprocedural cranial nerve injuries (5 vs. 1, $p = 0.03$) did appear in the CEA group, although long-term outcomes did not vary.[90] These initial data would give credence to the thought that the "hostile neck" has little bearing on CEA outcomes when a skilled surgeon performs the procedure. In addition, the application of a NIMS endotracheal tube for vocal cord monitoring during the procedure was not reviewed in the above series and may resolve or at least minimize the issue of increased cranial nerve injuries among CEAs performed in "hostile neck" patients. We now use this method in every case.

INTRALUMINAL THROMBI

The problem of surgical timing in patients with angiographically demonstrated propagating intraluminal thrombus remains an open question among cerebrovascular experts.[74,75,91-98] In patients who present with a transient ischemic attack (which, in our experience, has always resolved with anticoagulation) and a long intraluminal thrombus (which goes too far up the internal carotid to be exposed and controlled), we have opted for delayed surgery (at 6 weeks after repeat angiography) in every case and have never seen a negative outcome from intercurrent embolization once heparin is instituted. The small "bullet-type" thrombus at the bifurcation, which can be isolated with cross-clamps, is operated without delay.

Likewise, there is a small subset of patients with postoperative neurologic events (most often transient ischemic attacks) after CEA who are found to have a fresh thrombus adherent to the suture line (by angiography), partially occluding the artery, and which is presumably the source of embolic phenomena. If there is no other angiographic evidence of technical inadequacy, we have chosen to manage these patients conservatively as well, with full anticoagulation and 6-week follow-up angiography. In every case, the thrombus has resolved, and there have been no negative neurologic outcomes in our series with this plan of management.[93] Despite the surgeon's natural inclination to fix a problem with bold action, we have found that a measured conservative approach yields good results in cases of fresh or propagating thrombus and in our experience is superior to undertaking a high-risk surgical procedure.

TANDEM LESIONS OF THE CAROTID SIPHON

In the North American Symptomatic Carotid Endarterectomy Trial, symptomatic patients were excluded if the degree of siphon stenosis exceeded that at the carotid bifurcation.[7] The presence of stenotic disease at the carotid siphon has been proposed as a contraindication to CEA because of both the inability to pinpoint the symptomatic source and the reputed increased possibilities of postoperative occlusion from decreased carotid flow velocity. This has not been our experience, and we do not hesitate to operate on patients with tandem lesions if we are convinced that an active plaque at the carotid bifurcation is the source of their embolic phenomena.

INTRACRANIAL ANEURYSM (SILENT)

There is always a concern that cervical carotid revascularization (for either symptomatic or asymptomatic carotid stenosis, especially high grade) will lead to rupture of a known intracranial aneurysm when both lesions are present. Although this is no doubt a small risk, several articles have shown that it is safe to proceed with a CEA with a silent intracranial aneurysm discovered on angiography.[94,95] Obviously, the symptomatic lesion should be treated first. We do not hesitate to operate in the light of an asymptomatic intracranial aneurysm, but we do customarily recommend subsequent craniotomy and aneurysm clipping as well.

RECURRENT STENOSIS

There is a quantifiable incidence of recurrent carotid stenosis after primary CEA. We have seen a decrease in our restenosis rate (to zero) after adopting patch graft angioplasty in all our cases. Piepgras and colleagues[96] show a symptomatic restenosis rate of 1% with an asymptomatic restenosis rate of 4% to 5% at 2-year follow-up using a patch graft. Aside from technical inadequacies, it has been difficult to identify risk factors associated with recurrent carotid stenosis, although continuation of smoking habits after endarterectomy has proved to be a significant risk factor in several studies,[97,98] whereas hypertension, diabetes mellitus, family history, lipid studies, aspirin use, and coronary disease may not be as important.

Reoperation for carotid stenosis, like the "hostile neck," is a technically difficult procedure. It is associated with significantly higher risks than primary endarterectomy. In our institution, the possibility of reoperation for carotid stenosis is entertained in patients who present with angiographically proven disease and classic neurologic symptoms referable to the appropriate artery or with documented progression to severe stenosis while being followed with annual serial duplex examinations.

CAROTID ENDARTERECTOMY VERSUS CAROTID ARTERY STENTING

There have been, to date, over 11 RCTs comparing CEA and CAS.[99-110] The results have roundly failed to validate CAS as a noninferior treatment for carotid artery stenosis. More to the point, several have found CAS to bear a much higher risk of subacute CVAs than carotid surgery. In 1998, the Leicester trial, although limited by a small sample size, found a 45% increase in periprocedure CVAs among CAS patients compared to CEA patients; and, in 2001, the WALLSTENT multicenter RCT demonstrated an alarming rate of ipsilateral strokes and deaths among CAS patients (CAS 12.1% vs. CEA 3.6%).[106,108] These results have been cause for much concern, but supporters of CAS have often only responded by citing the nascent understanding of CAS and lack of experience with the procedure during these early studies.

As such, a number of RCTs since WALLSTENT have attempted to reverse the stigma of 30-day and 1-year infarcts from carotid stenting. Largely, they failed. The SAPPHIRE trial, released in 2004, stands as the lone exception. It showed in a group of 334 randomized patients a 24.6% and 30.3% stroke rate between CAS and CEA. The difference was not statistically significant. We note, however, that there were an enormous number of patients (415 of the original 741 patients), nearly all stented, who were treated outside of the trial, which always introduces the specter of selection bias against surgery. In addition, the SAPPHIRE results claiming equipoise, unfortunately, have not been reproducible in subsequent, larger RCTs.[109,110]

The latest and most comprehensive RCT investigating the efficacy and safety of CAS and CEA in the treatment of carotid artery stenosis, as of this chapter's publication, is the Carotid Revascularization Endarterectomy versus Stenting Trial (CREST). This multicenter RCT attempted to address the numerous failings of past RCTs comparing CEA and CAS and so provide a convincing answer to the debate between the two treatments.

A total of 2,502 patients (1,262 CEA and 1,240 CAS) were enrolled in CREST. The study included both asymptomatic and symptomatic patients with either ≥60% or ≥50% stenosis of the carotid artery by angiography (other radiographic studies were permitted for diagnosis, though with higher cutoffs). Symptomatic patients needed to present within 6 months of randomization, and all surgeons and interventionalists had to be certified for their procedure in order to participate in the trial. Within the CAS arm of the study, an embolic protection device had to be employed wherever feasible. The primary endpoint for the study was all periprocedural stroke, myocardial infarction, and death, as well as any stroke or myocardial infarction ipsilateral to the diseased artery up to 4 years following.

In the final analysis, the authors of CREST noted no difference in primary endpoints between the two treatment arms (7.2% CAS versus 6.8% CEA; 95% CI, 0.81 to 1.51; $p = 0.51$). Though these results have been lifted as evidence of equipoise between CAS and CEA, the data underpinning these conglomerate endpoint data leads to a different interpretation. Looking at stroke and myocardial infarction independently, the two largest endpoints comprising CREST's general endpoint, the study found an elevated periprocedural stroke rate among CAS patients (4.1% CAS versus 2.3%, $p = 0.012$), on par with previous studies, and an elevated myocardial infarction rate among CEA patients (1.1 CAS versus 2.3%, $p = 0.032$). Looking at quality of life measures recorded over the study's 4-year follow-up (Medical Outcomes Study 36-Item Short-Form Health Survey (SF-36)), myocardial infarctions had no demonstrable effect on patients' quality of life, while periprocedural strokes did. Further, the rate of major ipsilateral stokes among CAS-treated patients, despite the use of an embolic protection device, ran nearly double that of the CEA patients (15.2% CAS versus 8.0% CEA).[111]

Taken in total, these subset data from CREST beg similar conclusions as previous trials. CREST seems to have reaffirmed that CAS bears an unacceptably high risk of periprocedural stroke compared to CEA and that this risk is not significantly rescued by the use of modern distal embolic protection devices. The failure of distal protection devices to limit CAS-related stroke likely derives from aortic arch disease concurrent with carotid stenosis. Such plaques must be traversed by endovascular interventionalists long before these embolic protection devices can even be deployed.

While CAS (with distal protective devices) has been an innovative new technique for the treatment of carotid stenosis, and no doubt has its place in the management of this disease. But the evidence to date is unequivocal, and strongly favors surgical repair. Numerous RCTs have demonstrated consistent and reproducible evidence for a lower 30-day stroke and death rate for patients randomized to CEA. In the absence of novel data to support CAS, however, current evidence-based medicine continues to confirm the superiority of CEA over CAS for the management of carotid stenosis patients.

Conclusions

Now that cooperative study data are available to support the clear superiority of surgery in the management of both asymptomatic (>60%) and symptomatic (>50%) carotid stenosis, carotid artery reconstruction will endure and flourish. The neurovascular principles are standard, but the indications for surgery are continually refined. Some conditions suggested to be unsuitable for CEA (such as contralateral occlusion, tandem stenosis, and fresh stroke) really do not prevent successful surgery in competent hands. In our opinion, the expanded acceptance of carotid surgery arises from more rigorous training and credentialing of surgeons, improved monitoring and anesthetic techniques, and the scientific application of cooperative trial methodology to the carotid problem.

The surgical methods presented here have been successful in producing superior postoperative results in patients who are candidates for CEA. Minor technical details, which may vary among surgeons, are probably of little significance. Conversely, subtleties of technique, which may add operative time to the routine CEA, assume greater importance when difficult lesions or high exposures are encountered or when the patient is unstable. The importance of a good outcome under these more difficult circumstances leads us to approach all carotid surgery, no matter how simple it may seem, with the same technical approach. Perhaps the most important factor in ensuring technically acceptable carotid surgery is the availability of a skilled cerebrovascular surgeon with demonstrable morbidity and mortality of less than 3% and a proper understanding of both vascular principles and cerebral physiology.

Summary

Multicenter trials have advocated surgical therapy over medical management in the cases of symptomatic patients with more than 50% stenosis, and asymptomatic patients with more than 60% stenosis. We perform the operation using a 3.5× loupe-magnified technique. Universal patch grafting has essentially eliminated the problem of acute postoperative thrombosis or rapid restenosis. We prefer general anesthesia with full-channel EEG and concurrent SSEP monitoring. We perform selective shunting based on monitoring criteria. This has resulted in an approximately 15% shunt placement rate in our experience. We do not reverse heparinization with protamine after the operation. We only place tacking sutures in approximately 10% of cases due to the use of fine scissors to trim the plaque cleanly in the ICA as it is removed. We emphasize meticulous hemostasis in our technique.

We recommend a staged procedure in those requiring bilateral CEA, with at least a 6-week window between procedures. In the case of intraluminal thrombi, we recommend full anticoagulation and repeat angiography in 6 weeks. We do not hesitate to operate on patients with tandem lesions if we are convinced that an active plaque at the carotid bifurcation is the source of their embolic phenomena. We do not hesitate to perform CEA in the setting of an asymptomatic intracranial aneurysm, but we do customarily recommend subsequent craniotomy and aneurysm clipping as well. In the setting of concurrent coronary and carotid disease, we recommend staged procedures with endarterectomy first in symptomatic patients. We do not believe that the presence of advanced age or hostile neck anatomy obviates endarterectomy's application in the treatment of carotid stenosis. Reoperation for carotid stenosis is proposed to patients who present with angiographically proven disease and classic neurologic symptoms referable to the appropriate artery or with documented progression to severe stenosis while being followed with annual serial duplex examinations, and with a somewhat greater filter, to asymptomatic recurrent stenosis as well.[121]

KEY REFERENCES

Alberts MJ, McCann R, Smith TP, et al. A randomized trial of carotid stenting versus endarterectomy in patients with symptomatic carotid stenosis: study design. *J Neurovasc Dis*. 1997;2:228-234.
Bailes J, Spetzler RF. *Microsurgical Carotid Endarterectomy*. New York: Lippincott-Raven; 1996.
Brooks WH, McClure RR, Jones MR, et al. Carotid angioplasty and stenting versus carotid endarterectomy: randomized trial in a community hospital. *J Am Coll Cardiol*. 2001;38:1589-1595.
Eliasziw M, Streifler JW, Fox AJ, et al. Significance of plaque ulceration in symptomatic patients with high-grade carotid stenosis. *Stroke*. 1994;25:304-308.
Executive Committee for the Asymptomatic Carotid Atherosclerosis Study. Endarterectomy for asymptomatic carotid stenosis. *JAMA*. 1995;273:1421-1428.
Fields WS, Maslenikov V, Meyer JS, et al. Joint study of extracranial arterial occlusion. V: progress report of prognosis following surgery or nonsurgical treatment for transient cerebral ischemic attacks and cervical carotid artery lesions. *JAMA*. 1970;211:1993-2003.
Heros RC. Carotid endarterectomy in patients with intraluminal thrombus. *Stroke*. 1990;19:667-668.

Honeycutt JH, Loftus CM. Carotid stump syndromes and external revascularization. In: Loftus CM, Kresowik TF, eds. *Textbook of Carotid Artery Surgery*. New York: Thieme; 2000:315-320.
Loftus CM. *Carotid Artery Surgery: Principles and Technique*. 2nd ed. New York: Informa Publishing; 2006.
Loftus CM. Carotid endarterectomy: the asymptomatic carotid. In: Batjer HH, ed. *Cerebrovascular Disease*. New York: Lippincott-Raven; 1996:409-420.
Loftus CM. *Carotid Endarterectomy: Principles and Technique*. St. Louis: Quality Medical Publishing; 1995.
Loftus CM. Concomitant carotid and coronary disease. *Patient Care*. 1992;15:49-66.
Loftus CM. Propagating intraluminal carotid thrombus: surgery or anticoagulation? In: Loftus CM, Kresowik TF, eds. *Carotid Artery Surgery*. New York: Thieme; 2000:321-327.
Loftus CM. Surgical management options to prevent ischemic stroke. *Neurosurg Q*. 1994;4:1-38.
Loftus CM. Technical aspects of carotid endarterectomy with hemashield patch graft. *Neurol Med Chir (Tokyo)*. 1997;37:805-818.
Loftus CM. Technical fundamentals, monitoring, and shunt use during carotid endarterectomy. *Tech Neurosurg*. 1997;3:16-24.
Loftus CM, Kresowik TF. Anatomic basis and technique of carotid endarterectomy. In: Loftus CM, Kresowik TF, eds. *Carotid Artery Surgery*. New York: Thieme Medical Publishers; 2000:245-256.
Naylor AR, Bolia A, Abbott RJ, et al. Randomized study of carotid angioplasty and stenting versus carotid endarterectomy: a stopped trial. *J Vasc Surg*. 1998;28:326-334.
Naylor AR, Mehta Z, Rothwell PM, Bell PRF. Stroke during coronary artery bypass surgery: a critical review of the role of carotid artery disease. *Eur J Vasc Endovasc Surg*. 2002;23:283-294.
North American Symptomatic Carotid Endarterectomy Trial Collaborators. Beneficial effect of carotid endarterectomy in symptomatic patients with high-grade carotid stenosis. *N Engl J Med*. 1991;325:445-453.
Schiro J, Mertz GH, Cannon JA, et al. Routine use of a shunt for carotid endarterectomy. *Am J Surg*. 1981;142:735-738.
Solomon RA, Loftus CM, Quest DO, et al. Incidence and etiology of intracerebral hemorrhage following carotid endarterectomy. *J Neurosurgery*. 1986;64:29-34.
Sundt TM. The ischemic tolerance of neural tissue and the need for monitoring and selective shunting during carotid endarterectomy. *Stroke*. 1983;14:93-98.
Yadav JS, Wholey MH, Kuntz RE, et al. Protected carotid-artery stenting versus endarterectomy in high-risk patients. *N Engl J Med*. 2004; 351:1493-1501.

Numbered references appear on Expert Consult.

CHAPTER 67

Management of Dissections of the Carotid and Vertebral Arteries

GREGORY J. VELAT • BRIAN L. HOH • CHRISTOPHER S. OGILVY

Arterial dissection is an important cause of stroke. The symptomatology, natural history, pathology, and management of extracranial and intracranial arterial dissections differ. The majority of dissections affect the extracranial carotid and vertebral arteries and result in ischemic strokes. Intracranial dissections mainly affect the vertebral and basilar arteries and present most commonly with subarachnoid hemorrhage. The treatment of carotid and vertebral artery dissections has evolved significantly since the early diagnosis and management descriptions by Fisher and colleagues in the 1970s.[1] Modern treatment of extracranial carotid and vertebral dissections is prolonged anticoagulation or antiplatelet therapy with surgical or endovascular intervention being reserved for refractory luminal irregularities or worsening neurologic status despite medical therapy. With recent innovations in neuroendovascular therapies, intracranial dissections are commonly treated with stents and/or coil embolization of associated pseudoaneurysms. This chapter reviews the presentation, treatment, and clinical outcomes for patients with extracranial and intracranial carotid and vertebral artery dissections.

Arterial Histology and Surrounding Milieu

Differences in arterial histology reflect the pathophysiologic dissimilarities between extracranial and intracranial arterial dissections. Craniocervical artery dissections (CAD) arise from a tear in the vessel lumen. Depending upon the extent of the tear, associated hemodynamic forces, and strength of the various arterial layers, a dissection may result in stenosis or aneurysmal dilatation of the artery. Subintimal dissections tend to cause stenosis of the parent artery, while subadventitial dissections may result in pseudoaneurysm formation and compression of surrounding soft tissue structures. Compared to extracranial arteries, intradural arteries have a thinner tunica media and adventitia with a relative paucity of elastic fibers making them more susceptible to subadventitial dissection resulting in pseudoaneurysm formation and potential subarachnoid hemorrhage.[2] Extradural arteries are more likely to have subintimal dissections presenting with arterial stenosis or thromboembolic complications.[1,3] The relatively weak milieu consisting of cerebrospinal fluid and brain parenchyma that surrounds the intracranial arteries predisposes patients to hemorrhagic complications in addition to potential thromboembolic phenomena.

Epidemiology

Craniocervical artery dissection accounts for approximately 2% of all ischemic strokes, but 10% to 25% of strokes in young and middle-aged patients.[3] Extracranial arterial dissection is more common than intracranial dissection. Specifically, the extracranial carotid artery is the most common site of arterial dissection, with an incidence estimated at 2.5 to 3.0 per 100,000 people.[3-5] Extracranial vertebral artery dissection occurs less frequently with an estimated incidence of 1.0 to 1.5 per 100,000 people.[3-7] Intracranial arterial dissection is relatively rare, with the intradural vertebral artery (V4 segment) being the most commonly affected vessel. In Yamaura's series of 338 patients with intracranial arterial dissections, 60% involved the intradural vertebral artery while only 9% affected the internal carotid artery.[8]

The etiology of CAD is multifactorial and appears to be linked to both environmental and genetic factors. Trauma has been proposed as an inciting factor of dissections, although in many cases there is no clear antecedent injury. The severity of trauma may range from a seemingly trivial injury (i.e., vigorous nose blowing or chiropractic maneuvers) to severe high-impact motor vehicle collisions resulting in blunt or direct injury to the craniocervical arteries.[9] Genetic factors have also been associated with CAD. In a population-based study by Schievink et al., approximately 5% of patients with CAD had a positive family history of spontaneous arterial dissections.[10] Patients with heritable connective tissue disorders such as Ehlers-Danlos syndrome type IV, Marfan's disease, autosomal dominant polycystic kidney disease, osteogenesis imperfecta type I, and α_1-antitrypsin deficiency have an increased risk of spontaneous extra- or intra-cranial artery dissection.[11-13] Recently, hyperhomocysteinemia has been linked to CAD. A significant reduction in methylenetetrahydrofolate reductase (MTHFRT) levels due to a mutation in the coding region of this gene results in increased serum levels of homocysteine.[14] Respiratory infections have also been associated with spontaneous CAD in a case-controlled study.[15]

Radiographic Diagnosis

Pathognomonic radiographic features of CAD include intramural hematoma, the presence of a double lumen, and/or intimal flap. Digital subtraction angiography (DSA) is the gold standard method for diagnosing CAD. The "string sign," a long arterial segment with a narrowed lumen, is the most common angiographic finding diagnostic of an arterial dissection. Intimal flaps and/or double lumens are appreciated in less than 10% of CAD cases diagnosed using DSA.[16] DSA is an invasive test with an estimated iatrogenic stroke rate of 0.5% to 1%.[17] Other risks of DSA include potential contrast-induced nephropathy and symptomatic hemorrhage at the arteriotomy site. Doppler ultrasonography (DUS) is a safe and effective method of diagnosing arterial dissections with reported sensitivity rates estimated at 90% when used in combination with hemodynamic signs and direct ultrasonic findings.[18] However, DUS is limited by bony regions that cannot be accurately insonated (i.e., skull base and/or carotid canal) and may overestimate the degree of stenosis.[19,20]

Magnetic resonance (MR) and computed tomographic (CT) angiography have replaced conventional angiography at many institutions as the primary diagnostic modalities for CAD. Advances in MR and CT angiography techniques have improved overall sensitivity and specificity rates at detecting CAD.[21] Intramural hematomas can be readily identified on T1-weighted MR series as hyperintense signals due to methemoglobin accumulation with a characteristic crescent shape adjacent to the arterial lumen. Fat suppression techniques may accurately differentiate small intramural hematomas from surrounding soft tissues in the acute period. MR angiography can accurately display luminal stenosis and/or occlusion. The temporal relationship between dissection occurrence and MRI/MRA imaging is a potential limitation to this diagnostic modality as the sensitivity is highest within the first 2 days following the dissection.

Multidetector row CT angiography provides improved spatial resolution of less than 1 mm sections with relatively short acquisition times and reduced doses of contrast material.[22] CT angiography may be superior to MR angiography at detecting acute intramural hematoma.[23] Complete hyperintense signal in the affected artery may be difficult to distinguish between intramural hematoma and vessel occlusion on MRI. In addition, CT angiography more accurately depicts near complete arterial occlusions and pseudoaneurysms than time-of-flight MR angiography, which is not as sensitive in slow flow arterial segments.[24] For these reasons, CT angiography is the primary diagnostic modality used at our institution in the rapid diagnosis of CAD. Recent public and governmental concerns regarding patient and healthcare worker radiation exposure during diagnostic testing have tempered our institutional use of CT angiography for interval follow-up imaging in favor of MRI/MRA especially in young patients.[25,26] Figs. 67-1 to 67-3 illustrate classic radiographic findings associated with extracranial carotid and vertebral artery dissections.

Extracranial Carotid Artery Dissection

The extracranial carotid artery is the most common site of CAD, with an estimated incidence of 2.5 to 3.0 cases per 100,000 people.[3-5] Cervical internal carotid artery dissection occurs approximately 2 cm distal to the artery's origin

and usually terminates proximal to its entry into the petrous bone.[1,27,28] The classic clinical triad for presentation of extracranial carotid dissection is ipsilateral pain in the head, face, or neck,[1] post-ganglionic partial Horner's syndrome characterized by ipsilateral miosis and ptosis without anhidrosis,[2] and cerebral or retinal ischemic symptoms.[3] All three components are found in less than one third of patients with extracranial carotid artery dissection.[3] Dissection-induced ischemia may manifest as transient ischemic attacks (TIAs) or cerebral infarctions. Fisher coined the term "carotid allegro" to describe dissection-associated TIAs as they tend to occur more frequently than ischemic episodes due to atherosclerotic disease.[1] Ipsilateral lower cranial nerve palsies may result from extracranial carotid artery dissection. In a retrospective series of 190 consecutive adult patients diagnosed with spontaneous dissection of the internal carotid artery, 23 (12%) presented with cranial nerve palsies.[29] The hypoglossal nerve was most frequently affected (5.2% of patients), with or without involvement of cranial nerves IX, X, and XI. Oculomotor and trigeminal nerve palsies were also observed in this series, possibly due to indirect interruption of nutrient vessels supplying the respective cranial nerves. Taste disturbance and tongue weakness are the most common manifestations of hypoglossal nerve compression due to its proximity to the carotid sheath. Pulsatile tinnitus may be experienced in up to one third of patients.[30]

Treatment of extracranial carotid artery dissections is medical, with neurointerventional and surgical procedures being reserved for dissections refractory to medical therapy and/or symptomatic associated pseudoaneurysms or flow-limiting stenosis. Anticoagulation with intravenous heparin followed by conversion to oral warfarin has been recommended as first-line treatment of patients with extracranial carotid artery dissections to prevent the risk of thromboembolic complications.[3,31,32] After 3 to 6 months of anticoagulation with a goal international normalized ratio of 2.0 to 3.0, patients should undergo reimaging to evaluate for dissection resolution. Arterial recanalization rates range from 50% to 70% with an estimated 10% of patients suffering a delayed thromboembolic event during medical therapy.[33-35] Patients should be reimaged following completion of anticoagulant therapy. No randomized controlled trial has investigated the optimal medical treatment of CAD. A 2003 Cochrane Database Review found no significant differences in mortality or clinical outcomes among 327 patients in 27 studies with carotid artery dissections who were treated with either anticoagulation or antiplatelet therapy.[36] A small, non–statistically significant increased incidence of intracranial hemorrhage was observed in patients treated with anticoagulation (0.5%). A prospective multicenter nonrandomized study conducted by the Canadian Stroke Consortium found a non–statistically significant increased risk of recurrent stroke in patients with CAD treated with aspirin (12.4%) versus anticoagulation (8.3%).[37] The Cervical Artery Dissection in Stroke Study (CADISS) is an ongoing multicenter, prospective study investigating the medical treatment of extracranial arterial dissections.[38] Patients diagnosed with acute extracranial carotid and/or vertebral artery dissection are randomized to antiplatelet or anticoagulation therapy. The primary end points are ipsilateral stroke or death within 3 months of randomization. The results of this trial should be available in the next several years.

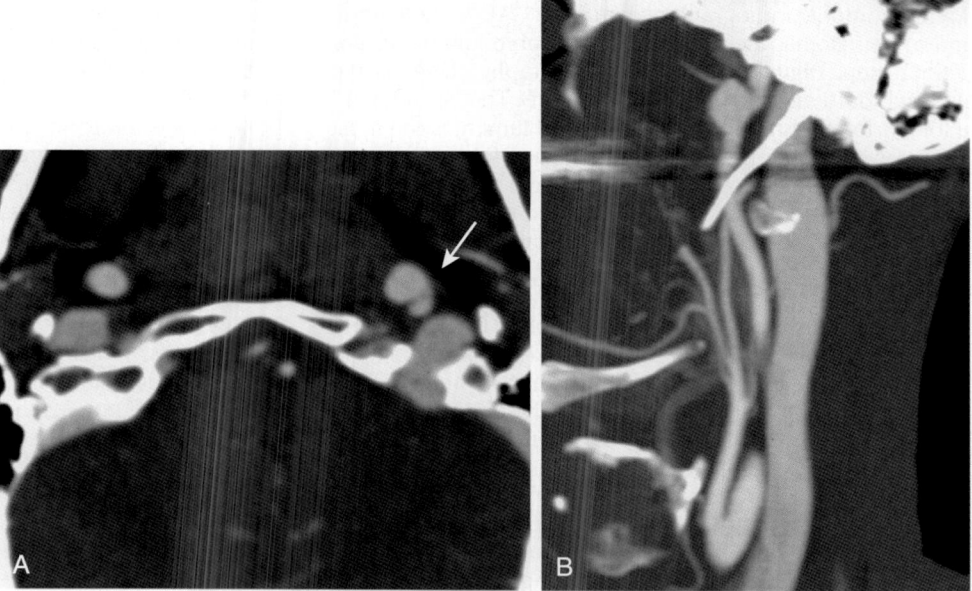

FIGURE 67-1 A, Axial CT angiogram revealing a left internal carotid artery extracranial dissection with intimal flap and associated pseudoaneurysm *(arrow).* B, Sagittal CT angiogram reconstruction illustrating the left internal carotid artery dissection with associated extracranial pseudoaneurysm.

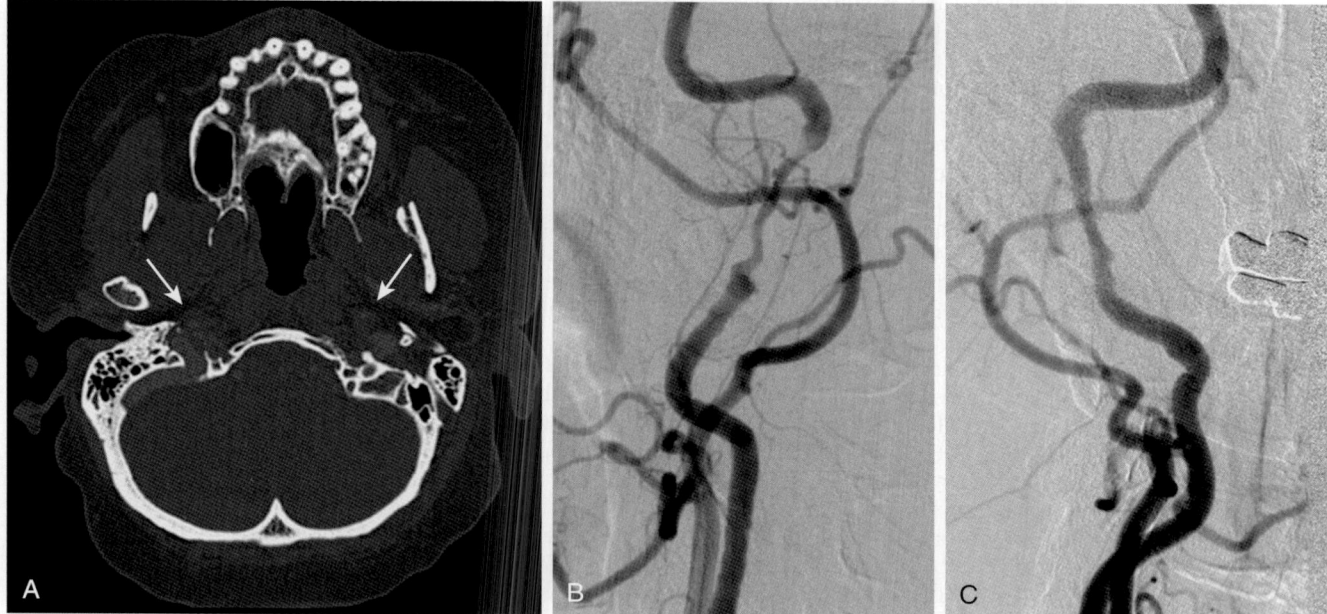

FIGURE 67-2 A, CT angiogram revealing bilateral extracranial carotid artery dissections following a high-speed motor vehicle collision *(arrows).* B, Left common carotid artery lateral digital subtraction angiogram revealing segmental narrowing (string sign) of the internal carotid artery with luminal reconstitution proximal to the skull base. C, Right common carotid artery lateral digital subtraction angiogram showing moderate stenosis of the internal carotid artery distal to the arterial dissection.

Endovascular and surgical treatments are typically reserved for cases of anticoagulation treatment failure defined by persistent luminal irregularities in the setting of recurrent thromboembolic disease and/or enlarging associated pseudoaneurysms. Endoluminal stenting and/or coil embolization of associated dissecting aneurysms are effective therapies for the treatment of extracranial carotid artery dissections.[39-44] Multiple stents may be deployed in a telescoping fashion for treatment of long segment arterial dissections.[40] In a 2008 review article that analyzed 13 clinical studies on 62 patients with 63 extracranial carotid artery dissections, endoluminal stents were successfully deployed in all patients with primary and 1-year stent patency rates of 100%.[45] Seven postprocedural strokes occurred (11%) without any mortalities within 30 days of treatment. One case of delayed asymptomatic in-stent stenosis occurred 22 months following initial treatment. Associated pseudoaneurysms may be effectively treated through coil embolization or deployment of covered stents. Yi et al. published a recent series of 10 patients

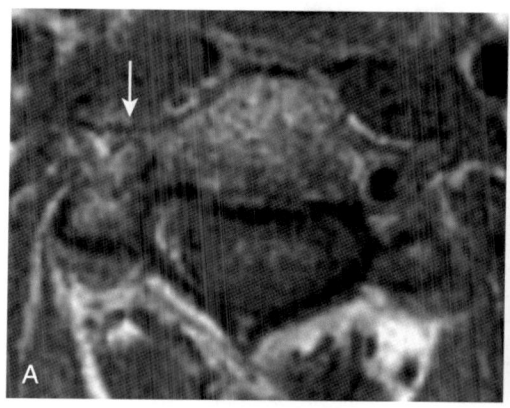
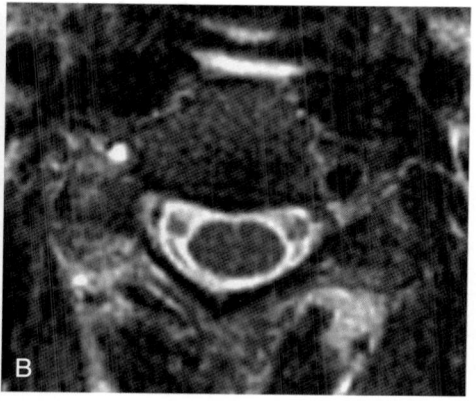

FIGURE 67-3 A, T1-weighted axial MRI of the neck revealing dissection of the right extracranial vertebral artery with associated isointense intramural hematoma *(arrow)*. B, T2-weighted axial MRI scan of the neck demonstrating loss of flow void in the dissected right extracranial vertebral artery.

with extracranial carotid ($n = 7$) or vertebral artery ($n = 1$) dissections and associated pseudoaneurysms successfully treated with covered stents.[46] Systemic intravenous and intra-arterial thrombolytic therapies have also shown promise in the treatment of dissection-induced extracranial carotid artery occlusion with a low incidence of intracranial hemorrhage.[31,47-49] Stent-assisted intra-arterial thrombolysis for the treatment of tandem carotid artery dissection or occlusion in the setting of acute stroke has been reported in several small case series.[50-52]

Surgical management of extracranial carotid artery dissections includes endarterectomy of the involved segment,[1] carotid ligation with or without external-to-internal carotid artery bypass contingent upon the patient's tolerance of balloon test occlusion,[2] and pseudoaneurysm wrapping or resection.[3] The major risks of surgical treatment include stroke and lower cranial nerve deficits. In Schievink's series of surgically treated extracranial carotid artery dissections, 9% of patients suffered a postoperative stroke within 30 days of surgery and nearly one third experienced transient lower cranial nerve palsies.[53]

Extracranial Vertebral Artery Dissection

Extracranial vertebral artery dissection incidence is estimated to be 1.0 to 1.5 per 100,000 people.[3,6,7] Traumatic injury is the main etiologic factor associated with extracranial vertebral artery dissection, with spontaneous dissections accounting for an estimated 4% of cases among middle-aged adults.[54] Chiropractic therapy of the cervical spine carries a risk of extracranial vertebral artery dissection and resultant stroke estimated at 1 in 20,000 manipulations.[55] The relative increased mobility of the extracranial vertebral artery at the atlanto-axial segments makes this region particular vulnerable to dissection.[9] Clinical manifestations of extracranial vertebral artery dissection include severe posterior cervical and occipital pain and stroke. More than 90% of patients with extracranial vertebral artery dissections present with ischemic symptoms of the brain stem, the thalamus, or the cerebral and/or cerebellar hemispheres.[56] Lateral medullary infarctions commonly result in dysarthria, dysphagia, ataxia, vertigo, diplopia, and sensory disturbances (Wallenberg's syndrome). TIAs occur less frequently than in extracranial internal carotid artery dissections.[9]

First-line treatment of extracranial vertebral artery dissections is anticoagulation with intravenous heparin

followed by conversion to oral warfarin with a goal international normalized ratio of 2.0 to 3.0 for 3 to 6 months.[3,31,32] Similar to extracranial carotid artery dissections, endovascular and surgical therapies are typically reserved for cases in which anticoagulation has failed due to persistent luminal irregularities with resulting thromboembolic events or hemodynamic insufficiency. Angioplasty and stent placement may effectively recanalize extracranial vertebral artery dissections.[42,57] Dissection-induced extracranial vertebral artery occlusions may be treated with intravenous or intra-arterial pharmacological thrombolysis with or without stent deployment to achieve vessel recanalization.[31,58,59] Vertebral artery sacrifice through endovascular obliteration or surgical ligation may be considered as tolerated in the setting of failed medical therapy. Extracranial-to-intracranial bypass procedures may be utilized prior to arterial sacrifice to improve symptomatic hemodynamic insufficiency related to dissection-induced arterial occlusion.[60]

Intracranial Arterial Dissection

The most common site of intracranial arterial dissections is the intradural vertebral artery (V4 segment). Although thromboembolic events may occur, the major risk of intracranial arterial dissections is subarachnoid hemorrhage due to the relatively thin arterial walls and weak surrounding milieu consisting of cerebrospinal fluid and brain parenchyma. Unruptured intracranial dissections typically follow a benign course, although the natural history of these lesions is poorly understood. Dissection appears to be a dynamic process with approximately 90% of stenoses resolving over time.[61,62] However, patients remain at risk of subsequent thromboembolic events and subarachnoid hemorrhage while the intracranial arterial dissection heals. In a review of 457 patients presenting with intradural vertebral artery dissection, 79% presented with subarachnoid hemorrhage and recurrent hemorrhage occurred in 37% of patients, particularly within the first 24 hours of the initial bleed.[63] Dissecting pseudoaneurysms of the vertebrobasilar arteries are estimated to account for 3% to 7% of all nontraumatic subarachnoid hemorrhage cases each year.[2] Treatment of ruptured dissecting intracranial aneurysms should be performed emergently due to the high rate of recurrent hemorrhage estimated at 30% to 70%[64,66] with mortality rates approaching 50%.[65,66]

Anticoagulation is not recommended for the treatment of intracranial arterial dissections due to the potential risk of

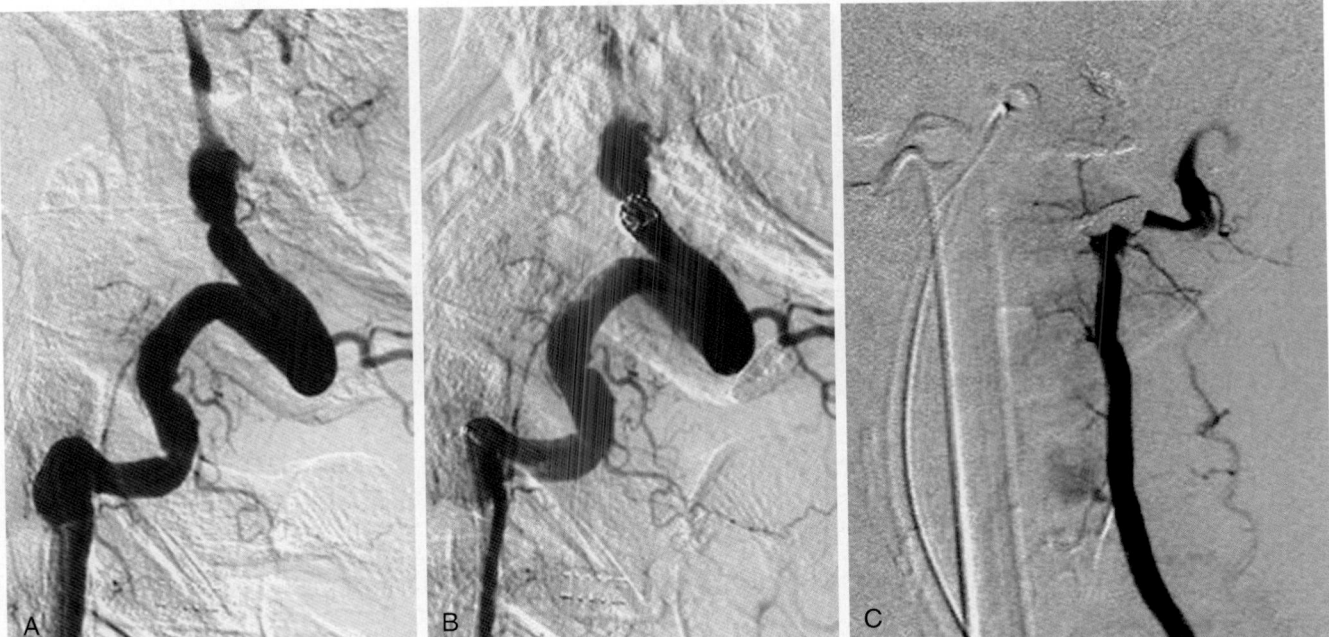

FIGURE 67-4 A, Left vertebral artery lateral digital subtraction angiogram revealing a dissection with associated intracranial pseudoaneurysm. This patient presented with diffuse subarachnoid hemorrhage and hydrocephalus. B, Left vertebral artery lateral digital subtraction angiogram following coil occlusion of the parent artery to treat the dissection and associated pseudoaneurysm. C, Post-coil embolization A/P digital subtraction angiogram illustrating occlusion of the distal left vertebral artery.

subarachnoid hemorrhage. Despite this recommendation, Metso et al. treated 81 consecutive adult patients with intracranial dissections using intravenous heparin followed by conversion to oral warfarin for 3 months without any reported cases of intracranial hemorrhage.[67] The mainstay treatment for intracranial dissections is surgical or endovascular therapy. At most institutions, surgical therapy is being replaced by neurointerventional techniques due to relatively high perioperative morbidity and mortality rates related mostly to lower cranial nerve deficits.[63,68] Surgical options include ligation of the affected artery without or with extracranial-to-intracranial bypass and direct clipping or wrapping of associated intracranial dissecting pseudoaneurysms.[63,68-73] Surgical procedures may be limited by the friable nature of the affected dissecting arteries and potential associated pseudoaneurysms.

Endovascular techniques include parent artery occlusion and coil embolization of associated pseudoaneurysms without or with stent deployment. The need for prolonged antiplatelet therapy to prevent parent artery re-stenosis is a relative contraindication to stent placement in the setting of subarachnoid hemorrhage. Our neurovascular group attempts to use balloon assistance, if required, during coil embolization of ruptured dissecting pseudoaneurysms. Fig 67-4 illustrates a ruptured dissecting intracranial vertebral artery pseudoaneurysm that was successfully treated with occlusion of the vertebral artery using coils. Several groups have successfully treated intracranial dissecting pseudoaneurysms via coil embolization alone.[74-81] Rabinov et al. treated 26 patients diagnosed with vertebrobasilar dissecting pseudoaneurysms utilizing endovascular parent artery occlusion (*n* = 14) or pseudoaneurysm coiling (*n* = 12).[72] Twenty patients (77%) presented with subarachnoid hemorrhage and 6 (23%) complained of headache or experienced stroke-like symptoms. The majority of patients (81%) had good clinical outcomes

(modified Rankin Scale score ≤2). Three patients (11.5%) died in the periprocedural period. Stent-assisted coiling followed by stent-within-a-stent technique has been recently reported for treatment of ruptured vertebrobasilar dissecting artery aneurysms. Suh et al. successfully treated 11 patients with dissecting aneurysms affecting either the basilar artery, the dominant vertebral artery in the setting or poor collateralization, or the segment bearing the origin of the dominant posterior inferior cerebellar artery using this technique.[82] Patients were not loaded with antiplatelet agents prior to the intervention, but were maintained on aspirin and clopidogrel for 3 months without any episodes of re-bleeding or stent re-stenosis. Only one patient died in the series due to complications from the initial subarachnoid hemorrhage. Stent deployment in combination with mechanical and/or chemical thrombolysis has been performed to successfully treat vertebrobasilar occlusion in patients presenting with acute stroke without significant hemorrhagic complications.[58]

KEY REFERENCES

Antiplatelet therapy vs. anticoagulation in cervical artery dissection: rationale and design of the Cervical Artery Dissection in Stroke Study (CADISS). *Int J Stroke.* 2007;2:292-296.

Beletsky V, Nadareishvili Z, Lynch J, et al. Cervical arterial dissection: time for a therapeutic trial? *Stroke.* 2003;34:2856-2860.

Donas KP, Mayer D, Guber I, et al. Endovascular repair of extracranial carotid artery dissection: current status and level of evidence. *J Vasc Interv Radiol.* 2008;19:1693-1698.

Dziewas R, Konrad C, Drager B, et al. Cervical artery dissection—clinical features, risk factors, therapy and outcome in 126 patients. *J Neurol.* 2003;250:1179-1184.

Fisher CM, Ojemann RG, Roberson GH. Spontaneous dissection of cervico-cerebral arteries. *Can J Neurol Sci.* 1978;5:9-19.

Kocaeli H, Chaalala C, Andaluz N, Zuccarello M. Spontaneous intradural vertebral artery dissection: a single-center experience and review of the literature. *Skull Base.* 2009;19:209-218.

Lyrer P, Engelter S. Antithrombotic drugs for carotid artery dissection. *Cochrane Database Syst Rev.* 2003:CD000255.

Metso TM, Metso AJ, Helenius J, et al. Prognosis and safety of anticoagulation in intracranial artery dissections in adults. *Stroke.* 2007;38:1837-1842.

Provenzale JM, Sarikaya B. Comparison of test performance characteristics of MRI, MR angiography, and CT angiography in the diagnosis of carotid and vertebral artery dissection: a review of the medical literature. *AJR Am J Roentgenol.* 2009;193:1167-1174.

Rabinov JD, Hellinger FR, Morris PP, et al. Endovascular management of vertebrobasilar dissecting aneurysms. *AJNR Am J Neuroradiol.* 2003;24:1421-1428.

Schievink WI. The treatment of spontaneous carotid and vertebral artery dissections. *Curr Opin Cardiol.* 2000;15:316-321.

Schievink WI. Spontaneous dissection of the carotid and vertebral arteries. *N Engl J Med.* 2001;344:898-906.

Schievink WI, Piepgras DG, McCaffrey TV, Mokri B. Surgical treatment of extracranial internal carotid artery dissecting aneurysms. *Neurosurgery.* 1994;35:809-815:discussion 815-806.

Thanvi B, Munshi SK, Dawson SL, Robinson TG. Carotid and vertebral artery dissection syndromes. *Postgrad Med J.* 2005;81:383-388.

Yamaura A. Nontraumatic intracranial arterial dissection: natural history, diagnosis, and treatment. *Contemp Neurosurg.* 1994;16:1-6.

Numbered references appear on Expert Consult.

CHAPTER 68

Management of Unruptured Intracranial Aneurysms

VIKRAM V. NAYAR • KAI FRERICHS • ARTHUR L. DAY

Subarachnoid hemorrhage, when caused by the rupture of an intracranial aneurysm, has a mortality rate near 50% at 30 days, and approximately half of the survivors sustain irreversible brain damage.[1] To avoid such a catastrophic event, it is important to identify and treat patients who harbor aneurysms that carry a significant risk of rupture. With the increased use of brain imaging in recent medical practice, including noninvasive tests like CT and MR angiography, a growing number of unruptured and usually asymptomatic intracranial aneurysms are being diagnosed. The decision of whether such lesions should be treated, and if so, whether by surgical or endovascular therapy, has been the subject of great controversy. This chapter evaluates the data available for making management decisions for unruptured aneurysms.

Natural History

Intracranial aneurysms are common, and may generally be classified as saccular (hemodynamic or "berry") and fusiform (dissecting, infectious, arteriosclerotic, or traumatic) types. The saccular type is by far the most common, and is the focus of this chapter.[2-7] Autopsy studies have shown that the overall prevalence of intracranial aneurysms in the general population ranges from 0.2% to 9.9%.[6-10] The population-based incidence of aneurysmal subarachnoid hemorrhage varies from 6 to 21.6 cases per 100,000 persons per year.[11-16]

The decision of whether to treat an unruptured aneurysm is based on the likelihood of its rupture during the patient's lifetime. The natural history study with the longest follow-up comes from Helsinki, Finland, where Juvela and colleagues reviewed a series of 142 patients with unruptured aneurysms followed without treatment from 1956 to 1978 (median follow-up of 19.7 years).[17] An advantage of the study is that it avoids treatment selection bias, because no unruptured aneurysms were treated in Helsinki before 1979. During 2575 person-years, 33 of the 142 patients (23%) had subarachnoid hemorrhage, resulting in an annual rupture rate of 1.3%. The cumulative rates of rupture were 10.5% at 10 years, 23% at 20 years, and 30.3% at 30 years.[17] Twenty-nine of 33 aneurysms that eventually ruptured were smaller than 10 mm in diameter at the time of the original diagnosis (18 were ≤6 mm).[8,17,18] Those aneurysms that ruptured were more likely to have increased in size (≥1 mm)

compared to those that did not rupture. Notably, the majority of the patients (131 of 142) had previous subarachnoid hemorrhage from another aneurysm, thus comprising a group of patients which may have had a higher rupture rate compared to those with no prior history of subarachnoid hemorrhage. Nevertheless, the study by Juvela and colleagues provided substantial long-term data on the natural history of unruptured aneurysms, and the annual rupture rate of 1.3% was similar to previously published reports (1% to 2.3%).[19-21]

Between 1976 and 1997, Tsutsumi and colleagues observed 62 patients who had noncalcified unruptured intradural aneurysms and no prior history of subarachnoid hemorrhage.[22] For small aneurysms (<10 mm), the 5- and 10-year rupture risks were 4.5% and 13.9%, respectively, an annual rupture rate similar to that reported by Juvela and colleagues.[8,17,18] For large aneurysms (>10 mm), the 5- and 10-year rupture risks were several-fold higher, 33.5% and 55.9%, respectively.

From 2003 to 2006, Ishibashi and colleagues elected to observe unruptured intracranial aneurysms at their institution. Of a total of 419 patients with 529 aneurysms, 19 aneurysms ruptured during the observation period, resulting in a 1.4% annual rupture rate.[23] Eight of the 19 aneurysms that ruptured were under 5 mm in size.

In 1998, a large retrospective international study, Phase I of the International Study of Unruptured Intracranial Aneurysms (ISUIA), evaluated the natural history of 1937 unruptured aneurysms in 1449 patients.[24] Patients harboring at least one unruptured aneurysm were divided into two groups: those with no history of subarachnoid hemorrhage (group 1) and those with a history of subarachnoid hemorrhage from another aneurysm (group 2). Patients in these two groups were not selected for surgical repair for various and often unknown reasons. The mean duration of follow-up was 8.3 years. As shown in Table 68-1, for aneurysms smaller than 10 mm, the annual rupture rate was 0.05% in group 1 (727 patients) and 0.5% in group 2 (722 patients). For aneurysms 10 to 24 mm in size, the annual rupture rate was approximately 1% in both groups. For giant aneurysms (25 mm or larger), the rupture rate was 6% in the first year, and declined thereafter. Aneurysms of the posterior circulation (the vertebrobasilar system) were significantly more likely to rupture than aneurysms of the anterior circulation, with basilar apex aneurysms carrying a relative risk

Table 68-1	Annual Rupture Risks as Reported in ISUIA I and II Studies				

	<10 mm		10–24 mm	≥25 mm	
ISUIA I	Group 1	Group 2			
	0.05%	0.5%	1%	6%	
ISUIA II	<7 mm		7–12 mm	13–24 mm	≥25 mm
	Group 1	Group 2			
Anterior circulation	0	0.3%	0.5%	2.9%	8%
Posterior circulation (including Pcom)	0.5%	0.7%	2.9%	3.7%	10%

Notes: Patients with unruptured aneurysms were separated into two cohorts: those with no history of subarachnoid hemorrhage (group 1), and those with a history of subarachnoid hemorrhage from another aneurysm (group 2). For larger aneurysms, the studies noted no significant differences in rupture rates between groups 1 and 2. Although the two studies stratified aneurysm size differently, ISUIA II reported rupture rates that were generally higher than ISUIA I.
ISUIA, International Study of Unruptured Intracranial Aneurysms; Pcom, posterior communicating.

of 13.8 compared to other locations. The study concluded that small unruptured aneurysms, particularly those in the anterior circulation with no history of prior aneurysmal subarachnoid hemorrhage, should be left untreated, especially when the morbidity and mortality rates of surgical repair were considered. This study generated significant controversy because its results were substantially different from previously published reports of a 1% to 2% annual rupture risk.[8,17-23]

In 2003, prospective data from the ISUIA was published as Phase II.[25] Aneurysms in this study were categorized by size into four groups: under 7 mm, 7 to 12 mm, 13 to 24 mm, and 25 mm or larger. Noncavernous anterior circulation aneurysms had 5-year cumulative rupture rates of 0% to 1.5%, 2.6%, 14.5%, and 40%, by size category, respectively. Posterior circulation aneurysms (including [Pcom] aneurysms, which are usually considered part of the anterior circulation) had cumulative 5-year rupture rates of 2.5%, 14%, 18.4%, and 50%. Although the two ISUIA studies stratified aneurysm size differently, ISUIA II reported rupture rates that were generally higher than ISUIA I (Table 68-1). For aneurysms in the 7-10-mm size range, ISUIA II suggested an annual rupture risk (0.5%–2.9%) that was several-fold greater than the rate of 0.05% to 0.5% purported by ISUIA I, which grouped together all aneurysms under 10 mm in size for the analysis.

Both ISUIA studies have been widely criticized for underestimating the true rupture risk of intracranial aneurysms, and certain limitations may have affected their results:

1. *Selection bias*: To be included in either study, a patient first had to be recommended for conservative management by a neurosurgeon. It is quite possible that those aneurysms included in the studies were judged to be very low risk, based on their benign morphology or location (i.e., intracavernous). In ISUIA I, internal carotid artery (ICA) aneurysms represented 42% of the total in group 1 and 27% in group 2; of these, cavernous-segment ICA aneurysms represented 16.9% in group 1 and 9.5% in group 2. In addition, a significant number of patients (32.7% in group 1 and 61.2% in group 2) had very small aneurysms (2–5 mm in size) which could also carry a lower rupture risk. Thus, the ISUIA I study population included large numbers of patients who harbored intracranial aneurysms considered to have little risk of rupture, at least during the study duration.

2. *Crossover*: In both ISUIA phases I and II, some patients who were initially chosen for observation were later advised to have treatment. In phase II, of the 1692 patients in the observation cohort, 534 patients were switched to therapeutic intervention. It is possible that the management strategy changed because of new symptoms or increased aneurysm size, both of which are risk factors for rupture. If those patients were left untreated, the observation cohort rupture rate may have been much higher.

3. *Incomplete follow-up*: Mean follow-up for the retrospective phase I study was 8.3 years, and for the prospective phase II study was 4.1 years. Of the 193 patients (11%) who died of causes other than subarachnoid hemorrhage, 52 patients died of intracranial hemorrhage. These patients were excluded from the analysis. It is unknown how these hemorrhages were determined to result from causes other than aneurysm rupture.

Given the disparity between the ISUIA data and other published reports, a population analysis based on prevalence of unruptured aneurysms and incidence of subarachnoid hemorrhage would be helpful. To estimate the prevalence of aneurysms, Winn and colleagues reviewed 3684 cerebral angiography studies performed at the University of Virginia between April 1969 and January 1980.[10] During the pre-CT era, the cerebral angiogram was a commonly performed neuroimaging test for a variety of indications. The authors found 24 asymptomatic unruptured aneurysms in 3684 patients, yielding a prevalence rate of 0.65%. Nearly 80% of the aneurysms were smaller than 10 mm. Because only 53% of the patients underwent a complete angiography study, the authors estimated that the true prevalence ranged from 0.65% to 1.3%. That would mean that in a population of 100,000, between 650 and 1300 people would have an unruptured intracranial aneurysm. Given an annual incidence of subarachnoid hemorrhage of 11 per 100,000 people,[26] a person with an unruptured aneurysm can be estimated to have a 0.85% to 1.7% yearly risk of rupture.

RISK FACTORS FOR RUPTURE
Aneurysm Size
It is now generally accepted that there is a strong correlation between aneurysm size and risk of rupture. ISUIA I used a historical classification scheme to separate aneurysms into small (<10 mm), large (10–24 mm), and giant (≥25 mm) categories (ISUIA 1998). ISUIA II separated nongiant aneurysms into three groups: <7 mm, 7 to 12 mm, and 13 to 24 mm (ISUIA 2003). Both studies demonstrated increased rupture rates with larger sizes. The exact size beyond which

an aneurysm becomes "dangerous," however, is unclear. In both clinical and autopsy series, aneurysms that present with hemorrhage are most commonly between 7 and 10 mm in size, and many are smaller than 7 mm.[27-29] Aneurysms smaller than 7 mm in size account for 55% of the aneurysms that ruptured in Juvela's series, 58% of the aneurysms that ruptured in the study by Ishibashi and colleagues, and 22% of the aneurysms that ruptured in ISUIA II.[18,23,25] Some aneurysms may enlarge prior to rupture, allowing for the premise that unruptured aneurysms can be followed until a change in size is noted.[30] Unfortunately, enlargement may more often occur near the time when the aneurysm ruptures, a quite unpredictable (and potentially fatal) moment.

Aneurysm Location

Both phase I and phase II ISUIA studies showed that posterior circulation aneurysms, especially basilar apex aneurysms, have a higher relative rupture rate compared to those at other sites.[24,25] A similar increased risk was also noted for lesions arising from the Pcom artery, a site traditionally considered to be within the anterior circulation. The distribution of aneurysms described in these series differs markedly from that encountered in ruptured aneurysm series. In the ISUIA studies, cavernous and small parasellar ICA aneurysms are highly represented, while in series dealing with ruptured aneurysms, anterior communicating (Acom) and Pcom aneurysm sites predominate.[27] In our personal experience, proximal (paraclinoid) ICA aneurysms are much more common than previously described, and may in fact be the most common aneurysm site, particularly in females. In series of ruptured aneurysms, however, lesions at this site are far less frequent, perhaps indicating that their relationship to and reinforcement by the parasellar dura provides some protection against subarachnoid hemorrhage.

Aneurysm Shape

Several reports suggest that aneurysms with irregular morphology, particularly those that are multilobed with daughter domes, have a significantly higher hemorrhage risk compared to smooth-walled, more spherical lesions.[20,31,32] In recent years, as aneurysm shapes and origins have become more important in determining "coilability," several quantifiable parameters have been evaluated for their contribution to rupture risk, including aspect ratio, ellipticity index, nonsphericity index, and undulation index. Of these parameters, aspect ratio (aneurysm height/neck width) has correlated best with rupture risk.[27,33] Several studies have shown that ruptured aneurysms have higher aspect ratios than unruptured aneurysms, but there is no consensus on a threshold value for increased risk.[34-38]

SYMPTOMS OTHER THAN RUPTURE

Unruptured aneurysms may present with cranial neuropathy (particularly oculomotor nerve or optic nerve/chiasmal deficits), ischemia, or other symptoms related to mass effect. New nonhemorrhagic symptoms suggest an acute change in the aneurysm (i.e., expansion), indicating a higher risk of imminent rupture compared to asymptomatic lesions. Data supporting this assertion is scant and retrospective, but in general, symptomatic aneurysms are treated with relative urgency, especially small Pcom aneurysms that cause oculomotor deficits.[27]

Significant Family History

In families that have multiple members with intracranial aneurysms, an aneurysm's risk of rupture is higher, and rupture may occur at an earlier age, compared to aneurysms that arise in individuals with no known family history.[39] Familial intracranial aneurysms are discussed later in this chapter.

Prior History of Aneurysmal Subarachnoid Hemorrhage

Phase I of ISUIA showed that a small unruptured aneurysm had a tenfold increase in rupture risk if it occurred in a patient with a history of subarachnoid hemorrhage from a different aneurysm, rather than in a patient with no history of subarachnoid hemorrhage.[24]

RISK FACTORS FOR ANEURYSM FORMATION

Age and Gender

Female gender seems to be a risk factor affecting both aneurysm formation and growth, with aneurysms 1.6 times more likely to occur in women than in men.[17,40] A series of 1230 autopsies showed two peaks in the prevalence of aneurysms in women, ages 40 to 49 and ages 60 to 69, which correlate with a peak incidence of subarachnoid hemorrhage between ages 40 and 60.[15] Interestingly, in this series, the prevalence of aneurysms in men was unchanged across the range of age groups.

Smoking

Cigarette smoking may hasten the growth of a preexisting aneurysm, and may contribute to an increased rupture rate, with hemorrhage occurring at smaller sizes.[17] In smokers, there is an increased ratio of elastase to alpha$_1$-antitrypsin in the walls of cerebral arteries, which may contribute to aneurysm formation or rupture.[18,41]

Genetic Conditions

In families in which two people have known intracranial aneurysms, first-degree relatives have a 9% to 11% chance of having an aneurysm in adulthood. Autosomal dominant polycystic kidney disease (ADPKD) is associated with a 15% prevalence of intracranial aneurysms.[40] Genetic conditions with at least some evidence of having an increased incidence of intracranial aneurysms are outlined in Table 68-2.

Aneurysm Detection

TRANSFEMORAL CEREBRAL ANGIOGRAPHY

Digital subtraction angiography (DSA), with selective injections of dye into the intracranial arteries, has long been the gold standard for imaging intracranial aneurysms. Since cerebral angiography is invasive (procedural stroke risk ranges from 0.07% to 0.5%) and requires a 2 to 6 hour hospital stay after the procedure, it is generally not advocated as a screening procedure.[42,43] A more recent innovation in angiography is three-dimensional reconstruction (3D-DSA). This technology permits rotation of the virtual image in any direction, allowing neurosurgeons and endovascular practitioners to evaluate specific anatomic characteristics of the

Table 68-2 Genetic Conditions Associated with Increased Incidence of Aneurysm Formation

Autosomal dominant polycystic kidney disease
Type IV Ehlers-Danlos syndrome
Hereditary hemorrhagic telangiectasia
Neurofibromatosis type 1
Alpha$_1$-antitrypsin deficiency
Klinefelter's syndrome
Tuberous sclerosis
Noonan's syndrome
Alpha-1,4-glucosidase deficiency

aneurysm, including the neck width and the relationship of the aneurysm to the parent artery and branch vessels. Both conventional and 3D-DSA reveal only the patent lumen of an aneurysm; heavy calcification or intraluminal thrombosis are not visualized, and CT and MRI provide useful complementary information.[44]

MAGNETIC RESONANCE ANGIOGRAPHY

The quality and the spatial resolution of noninvasive imaging have significantly improved in recent years, approaching that of DSA. Magnetic resonance angiography (MRA) is useful for screening and follow-up, and in some cases, it is sufficient for treatment planning.[45] Aneurysms with diameters as small as 2 mm and vessels as small as 1 mm can be detected.[46] Aneurysms 6 mm or more in diameter have been detected with 100% sensitivity. The sensitivity decreased to 87.5%, 68.2%, 60%, and 55.6% for aneurysms with a diameter of 5, 4, 3, and 2 mm, respectively. Three-dimensional reconstructions are valuable for anatomic evaluation; 3D contrast-enhanced MRA may be superior to 3D time-of-flight MRA in the detection of aneurysms.[44,47,48] Imaging of an aneurysm's morphology and relationship to branch vessels may be improved with 3-Tesla and 7-Tesla time-of-flight MRAs.[49,50] MRA does not expose a patient to radiation risks, and thus its utility is quite attractive in those patients with anticipated multiple studies during their follow-up, as long as the area of interest is seen in sufficient detail by this technology.

COMPUTED TOMOGRAPHY ANGIOGRAPHY

Multislice CT scanners allow simultaneous acquisition of as many as 64 slices by using multirow detector systems.[49] The concurrent acquisition of multiple slices results in a dramatic reduction of scan time. The major advantages of multislice CT are a longer scanning range, shorter scanning times, and a higher two-axis resolution.[51] The high scan speed of multislice helical CT permits scanning with a smaller slice thickness than is possible with conventional helical CT.[52] As a result, volumetric data with superior resolution in the z-axis can be obtained. Acquired data can be reformatted to provide 3D angiographic images, called CT angiography (CTA). Many physicians routinely use CTA in clinical practice. A recent review reported that the sensitivity of the CTA ranged from 53% for 2-mm aneurysms (Fig. 68-1) to 95% for 7-mm aneurysms. The overall specificity was 98.9%, but there was interstudy heterogeneity.[53] A meta-analysis comparing CTA with DSA in the diagnosis of cerebral aneurysms revealed that CTA had an overall sensitivity of 93.3% and a specificity of 87.8%.[54]

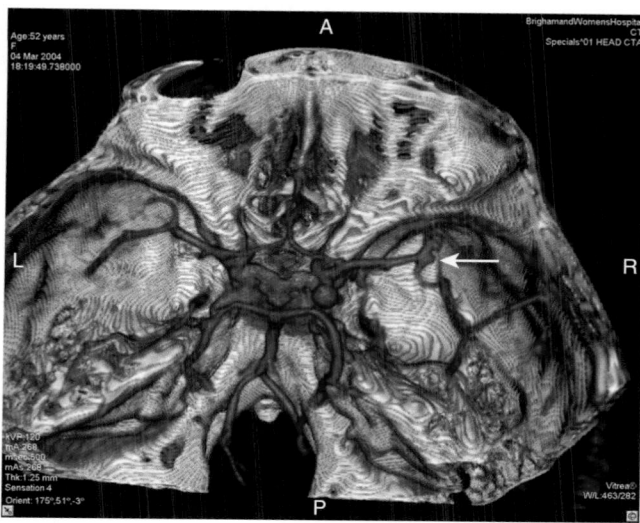

FIGURE 68-1 Three-dimensional reconstruction allows small intracranial aneurysms to be detected on CT angiography. The arrow points to a 2-mm aneurysm at the right middle cerebral artery bifurcation. An 8-mm right posterior communicating artery aneurysm is also seen.

The advantages of CTA over DSA are the following:
1. Data can be obtained more quickly and less expensively.
2. CTA provides additional anatomic information (information on surrounding bony structures and the presence of calcium or atheromas).
3. CTA can be used for the rapid planning of craniotomies for clip obliteration, and the preliminary determination of whether aneurysms are suitable for coil embolization.
4. CTA subjects patients to virtually no stroke risk and negligible discomfort.

The disadvantages of CTA are as follows:
1. Less sensitive and specific than the standard method, DSA, for the detection of cerebral aneurysms.
2. Difficulty detecting aneurysms at the skull base, such as those of clinoidal or cavernous segments of the ICA, due to the aneurysms' proximity to bone.
3. Sensitive to bolus timing, and opacified veins may be incorporated into the reconstructed image,[44] making interpretation of the arterial tree anatomy difficult.
4. May be inadequate in patients with left ventricular failure due to suboptimal opacification of the intracranial vasculature.[55]
5. Like standard CT, it is subject to motion artifact.
6. Provides no information regarding flow in all phases of the bolus transit in the cerebral vessels.
7. Has not been validated to detect vasospasm or other flow-limiting lesions with the same reliability as DSA.

At present, most cerebrovascular centers still use DSA to plan the surgical treatment of aneurysms. The use of DSA will likely diminish as CT and MR technology continues to improve. Endovascular intervention, which still depends on fluoroscopic technology, will remain closely linked to DSA.

Indications for Treatment

Aneurysmal subarachnoid hemorrhage carries a high fatality rate. In the retrospective part of ISUIA, 66% of the patients whose aneurysms ruptured died (83% in group 1 and 55% in group 2).[24] In the natural history study by Juvela and colleagues, 52% of patients whose aneurysms ruptured died.[8] Tsutsumi and colleagues reported a mortality rate of 86% after subarachnoid hemorrhage.[22] Thus, there are clear reasons to obliterate an unruptured aneurysm that has a significant risk of rupture.

Before deciding to treat an unruptured aneurysm, the cumulative risk of rupture over the patient's expected lifetime needs to be estimated and weighed against the risks of treatment.[56-60] Juvela advocated that all young and middle-aged patients with unruptured aneurysms should be surgically treated, regardless of the size of the aneurysm.[17] White and Wardlaw suggest that in patients under age 50 with no prior history of subarachnoid hemorrhage, all posterior circulation aneurysms and those anterior circulation aneurysms 7 mm or larger should be treated.[61] In patients over age 50 with no prior history of subarachnoid hemorrhage, they favor treatment for posterior circulation aneurysms larger than 7 mm and anterior circulation aneurysms larger than 12 mm.

In 2000, after the publication of phase I of ISUIA, the Stroke Council of the American Heart Association issued the following recommendations for the management of patients with unruptured intracranial aneurysms.[62]

The existing body of knowledge supports the following recommendations (options) regarding the treatment of UIAs:

1. The treatment of small incidental intracavernous ICA aneurysms is not generally indicated. For large symptomatic intracavernous aneurysms, treatment decisions should be individualized on the basis of patient age, severity, and progression of symptoms, and treatment alternatives. The higher risk of treatment and shorter life expectancy in older individuals must be considered in all patients and favors observation in older patients with asymptomatic aneurysms.

2. Symptomatic intradural aneurysms of all sizes should be considered for treatment, with relative urgency for the treatment of acutely symptomatic aneurysms. Symptomatic large or giant aneurysms carry higher surgical risks that require a careful analysis of individualized patient and aneurysmal risks and surgeon and center expertise.

3. Coexisting or remaining aneurysms of all sizes in patients with SAH due to another treated aneurysm carry a higher risk for future hemorrhage than do similar sized aneurysms without a prior SAH history and warrant consideration for treatment. Aneurysms located at the basilar apex carry a relatively high risk of rupture. Treatment decisions must take into account the patient's age, existing medical and neurologic condition, and relative risks of repair. If a decision is made for observation, re-evaluation on a periodic basis with CT/MRA or selective contrast angiography should be considered, with changes in aneurysmal size sought, although careful attention to technical factors will be required to optimize the reliability of these measures.

4. In consideration of the apparent low risk of hemorrhage from incidental small (<10 mm) aneurysms in patients without previous SAH, treatment rather than observation cannot be generally advocated. However, special consideration for treatment should be given to young patients in this group. Likewise, small aneurysms approaching the 10-mm diameter size, those with daughter sac formation

Table 68-3	Factors That Influence Management of Unruptured Intracranial Aneurysm	
Favoring Treatment	**Favoring Observation**
Patient Factors	
Age <70	Age >70
Prior SAH from another aneurysm	Significant medical comorbidities
Family history of intracranial aneurysms	Patient preference
Symptoms caused by aneurysm	
Size	
Size approaching ≥7 mm	Size much <7 mm
Location	
Within the subarachnoid space	Intracavernous or clinoidal segment
Posterior circulation aneurysm	Small superior hypophyseal aneurysm
Shape	
Irregular with bleb	Regular
Daughter dome	Unilobed
High aspect ratio	Low aspect ratio

SAH, subarachnoid hemorrhage.

and other unique hemodynamic features, and patients with a positive family history for aneurysms or aneurysmal SAH deserve special consideration for treatment. In those managed conservatively, periodic follow-up imaging evaluation should be considered and is necessary if a specific symptom should arise. If changes in aneurysm size or configuration are observed, this should lead to special consideration for treatment.

5. Asymptomatic aneurysms of ≥10 mm in diameter warrant strong consideration for treatment, taking into account patient age, existing medical and neurologic conditions, and relative risks for treatment.

After the above recommendations were issued, prospective results from phase II of ISUIA were published, which showed that 7- to 10-mm aneurysms had a higher rupture rate than was suggested by the phase I study. In light of those results, most neurosurgeons and endovascular practitioners give strong consideration to treating aneurysms ≥7 mm in diameter in patients who are not elderly. As stated in recommendation (4) above, treatment may be favored for some smaller aneurysms, with worrisome anatomic features, young patient age, or significant family history (Table 68-3).

Treatment Options

OBSERVATION

If intervention is not recommended for an unruptured intracranial aneurysm, periodic follow-up imaging with either CTA or MRA should be considered. In patients of advanced age or a limited life expectancy, no further imaging may be necessary for an asymptomatic aneurysm. A subsequent change in aneurysm size or morphology warrants consideration for treatment. In a retrospective series of 191 unruptured aneurysms with median follow-up of 47 months, 10% of aneurysms showed enlargement on serial MRAs.[30] In the time course of the study, aneurysms smaller than 8 mm had a 6.9% risk of growth, while those 8 mm or larger had a 44% chance of growth. The authors report that at least one aneurysm ruptured during the study, but they state that their follow-up information regarding aneurysm rupture was incomplete.

No noninvasive measures have been shown to prevent aneurysm rupture. However, since smoking has been associated with an increased rate of aneurysm growth and rupture, cessation is generally advocated. Among smokers, the number of cigarettes smoked daily seems to correlate with aneurysm growth more than the lifetime history of tobacco use. Patients who had quit smoking had no increased risk of aneurysm growth.[17,41]

Questions commonly arise about whether patients with unruptured aneurysms should be anticoagulated for other disorders (i.e., atrial fibrillation, pulmonary embolus), or whether they should take aspirin or NSAIDs. There is no evidence that anticoagulation increases the chance of subarachnoid hemorrhage in a patient with an unruptured aneurysm. However, should an aneurysm rupture occur, patients on anticoagulation have a twofold increase in mortality.[40] On the other hand, aspirin or NSAID use preceding aneurysmal subarachnoid hemorrhage does not significantly affect outcome.

SURGICAL TREATMENT

Since the operating microscope revolutionized neurosurgery over 40 years ago, the microsurgical clipping of aneurysms has been the mainstay of treatment, and is considered the time-tested way to obliterate aneurysms[63-65] (Fig. 68-2A and B). Over the years, microsurgical techniques have been developed and refined, and surgical instrumentation has been innovated and modified. Intraoperative angiography has been used to verify occlusion of the aneurysm, and preservation of the parent and branch arteries. Recently, fluorescence videoangiography has provided real-time intraoperative visualization of blood flow through small arteries that would not be visible on standard angiography.

The various innovations have been designed to reduce surgical risks. The decision to proceed with surgery requires an adequate assessment of these risks. High-volume centers and specialized neurosurgeons with cerebrovascular expertise offer better outcomes and fewer complications.[59]

Risks of Surgery

A meta-analysis of surgical treatment for unruptured aneurysms identified 61 studies published between 1966 and 1996, with a total of 2460 patients (57% female; mean age 50 years) and at least 2568 unruptured aneurysms.[56] Mean follow-up was 24 weeks, 27% of the aneurysms were over 25 mm in size, and 30% were located in the posterior circulation (vertebrobasilar system). Overall postoperative mortality and morbidity were 2.6% and 10.9%, respectively. Mortality and morbidity for nongiant aneurysms and anterior circulation aneurysms were significantly lower in more recent years; surgery for small anterior circulation aneurysms had a 0.8% mortality and 1.9% morbidity, whereas surgery for large posterior circulation aneurysms had a 9.6% mortality and 37.9% morbidity.

In a cohort of 1917 patients who underwent aneurysm surgery, ISUIA phase II reported surgical mortality to be 0.6% in patients who had a history of subarachnoid hemorrhage

from another aneurysm (group 2), and 2.7% in patients with no history of subarachnoid hemorrhage (group 1).[25] Neurologic outcome was graded at 1 year using the modified Rankin scale, and cognitive status was included in the assessment of morbidity, and the rates of morbidity were 9.8% and 9.9% for groups 1 and 2, respectively.

A review of the Nationwide Inpatient Sample hospital discharge database from 1996 to 2000 showed that surgical outcomes were better at high-volume hospitals (treating 20 or more cases per year) than at low-volume hospitals (treating less than four cases per year).[59] In recent years, specialized vascular neurosurgeons have reported low complication rates in appropriately selected patients. There are also various other predictors of surgical outcome besides hospital case volume and the expertise of surgeons, including patient age, aneurysm size, and aneurysm location.

Factors Associated with Surgical Outcome
Age

In ISUIA phase II, patients age 50 or older had an increased rate of adverse outcomes, with a relative risk of 2.4.[25] Takahashi found that patients age 80 or older had the worst surgical outcomes.[66] Khanna and colleagues report a that a 70-year-old patient has a sixfold higher risk of a poor outcome than a 30-year-old patient, keeping aneurysm size and location constant.[67] This increased complication incidence could be due to an increased frequency of atherosclerotic and/or calcified aneurysm necks in the elderly, as well as medical comorbidities in the older age group.

Aneurysm Size

Solomon and colleagues found that aneurysm size had an important influence on surgical outcome.[68] The combined morbidity and mortality of unruptured aneurysms was 0% for aneurysms 10 mm or smaller, 6% for aneurysms between 10 and 25 mm, and 20% for aneurysms greater than 25 mm. Drake reported 15% morbidity and mortality in nongiant posterior circulation aneurysms, compared with 39% for giant posterior circulation aneurysms, although ruptured aneurysms were also included in his series.[69] The ISUIA Phase II study showed a 2.6 relative risk of poor surgical outcome for an aneurysm greater than 12 mm in diameter.[25]

Aneurysm Location

In the ISUIA studies, posterior circulation aneurysms were associated with worse surgical outcomes.[25] Solomon and colleagues observed 50% morbidity and mortality after surgery for unruptured giant basilar aneurysms, compared with 13% for anterior circulation giant aneurysms.[68] Drake reported a 14.3% morbidity for unruptured asymptomatic posterior circulation aneurysms, compared with a 0% morbidity in the anterior circulation.[69]

Some anterior circulation aneurysms may have a higher morbidity and mortality compared to others, due to the technical challenges of surgical exposure and treatment. These include Acom aneurysms that project posterosuperiorly[70] and ICA aneurysms of the clinoidal and cavernous segments.[71,72]

Risk/Benefit Analysis

To determine the best course of treatment for an individual harboring an UIA, the risk of an adverse surgical outcome should be weighed against the cumulative risk of aneurysm rupture in the patient's lifetime. If a 50-year-old woman with a projected life expectancy of 80 years has an aneurysm with a 1% annual rupture risk, then she has a 30% lifetime risk of subarachnoid hemorrhage, with likely devastating consequences. If her surgical risk is under 5%, then after 5 years the cumulative risk of leaving the aneurysm untreated would outweigh the risk of having surgery up front. Sometimes, however, a high-risk natural history is weighed against a high surgical risk. For example, a giant basilar apex aneurysm may have a 5-year rupture risk of 50% to 60%, with a 40% to 50% risk of death or severe disability; the surgical morbidity and mortality could be in the same range. Endovascular treatment, if feasible, could be a safer alternative in that situation.

ENDOVASCULAR TREATMENT

In 1991, Guglielmi and colleagues introduced the detachable coil for treating intracranial aneurysms.[73,74] The coiling procedure involves passing a catheter through the arterial tree to the aneurysm, and then deploying platinum wire coils into the aneurysm to pack and occlude it (Fig. 68-2C to F). The Guglielmi detachable coil (GDC) system (Boston Scientific/Target) received U.S. Food and Drug Administration approval in 1995. Aneurysms considered unsuitable for surgery were the initial candidates for GDC coil embolization. In 1999, Guglielmi's group reported the coiling of 120 unruptured aneurysms, and in subsequent years, criteria for endovascular therapy have broadened to make it the first line of treatment at many centers.[75]

Experience with Ruptured Aneurysms

In 2002, the International Subarachnoid Aneurysm Trial (ISAT) Collaborative Group published the first prospective randomized trial comparing endovascular treatment with surgery for 2143 patients with ruptured intracranial aneurysms.[76] Inclusion in the trial was based on a pretreatment estimation that the ruptured aneurysm could be treated successfully by either coiling or clipping. At the 1-year follow-up, the combined rates of death and disability were 23.7% after endovascular therapy, and 30.6% after surgical clipping.

For ruptured aneurysms, ISAT achieved prominence as the only randomized trial comparing the two modalities of

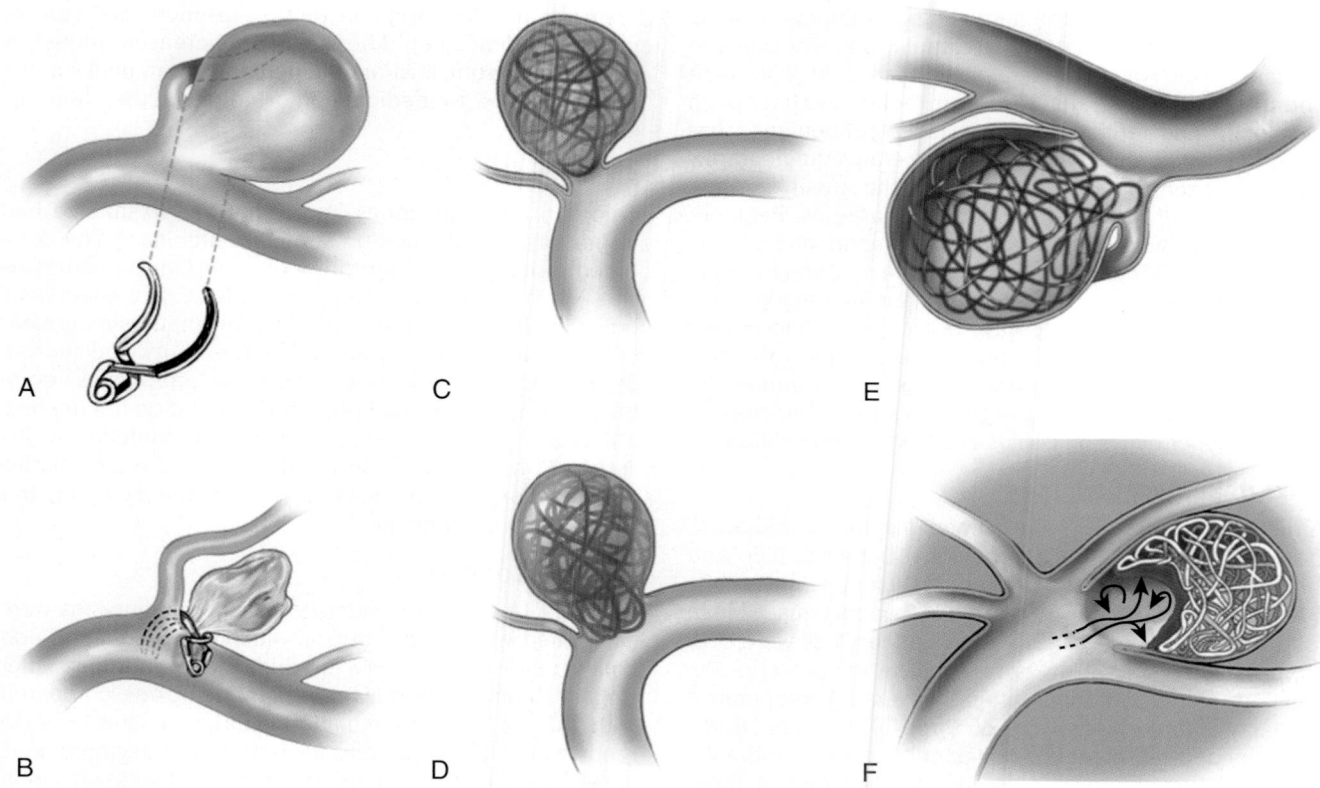

A

B

C

D

E

F

FIGURE 68-2 A and B, Microsurgical clipping of an aneurysm. Under an operating microscope, a titanium clip is placed across the neck of an aneurysm (A), and then closed (B). Multiple clips of various shapes and sizes may be used to exclude the aneurysm from the circulation, and preserve blood flow through the parent and branch artery. C to F, Coiling of an aneurysm, and some potential problems. Endovascular treatment involves passing a catheter through the arterial tree to the aneurysm. Platinum wire coils are placed in the dome, preventing blood flow into the aneurysm (C). When an aneurysm has a wide neck, coils may prolapse into the parent artery (D). Deploying a stent into the parent artery allows many wide-necked aneurysms to be coiled, but stenting carries higher risk. Coiling is generally not recommended when a branch vessel originates from the neck of an aneurysm, because blood flow into this artery would be obstructed (E). Recurrence of aneurysm after coiling is often due to coil compaction, when hemodynamic stress pushes coils deeper into the dome (F).

treatment. The study may have implications for the types of patients that were selected for randomization, and for neurosurgeons and endovascular practitioners with similar outcomes as the participating providers. Unfortunately, no information is provided on the level of expertise of the neurosurgeons who participated in the study, almost all of whom practiced in Europe. Furthermore, there is limited information about what constituted a randomizable aneurysm for the trial. The spectrum of aneurysms that was considered coilable at the time of the trial was much narrower than it is now. While newer techniques may allow the endovascular treatment of previously uncoilable aneurysms, these techniques would be associated with different morbidity and mortality rates than those represented in ISAT.

Certain aneurysm morphologies and locations favor surgical clipping over endovascular treatment. Younger patients with subarachnoid hemorrhage, and patients with good clinical status, could potentially benefit from the long-term aneurysm occlusion that clipping provides. Recognizing the conclusions and the limitations of ISAT, the Stroke Council of the American Heart Association issued the following recommendation in the 2009 *Guidelines for the Management of Aneurysmal Subarachnoid Hemorrhage*[77]:

> For patients with ruptured aneurysms judged by an experienced team of cerebrovascular surgeons and endovascular practitioners to be technically amenable to both endovascular coiling and neurosurgical clipping, endovascular coiling can be beneficial. Nevertheless, it is reasonable to consider individual characteristics of the patient and the aneurysm in deciding the best means of repair, and management of patients in centers offering both techniques is probably indicated.

For unruptured aneurysms, there are no randomized trials comparing surgical and endovascular therapy. Many cerebrovascular centers in the United States continue to favor surgical treatment for most unruptured aneurysms, particularly in younger individuals harboring lesions in the anterior circulation. Early results of the endovascular experience with these lesions are now allowing practitioners to evaluate the safety and efficacy of this alternative treatment.

Risks of Endovascular Treatment

In 2008, initial results were published for the first prospective multicenter study of the endovascular treatment of unruptured aneurysms (Analysis of Treatment by Endovascular approach of Non-ruptured Aneurysms [ATENA]).[78] During the 17-month study period, a total of 649 patients in Canada and France underwent coil embolization of 739 unruptured aneurysms, all less than 15 mm in size. Anterior circulation aneurysms accounted for 92% of the total, while 8% were in the posterior circulation. Balloon remodeling was employed in 37.3%, and stenting in 7.8%. The report describes the immediate clinical outcome of patients in the study. Endovascular treatment was attempted but aborted in 4.3% of aneurysms, because of anatomic and technical problems. Complications were encountered in 15.4% of patients, including infarction

(7.1% risk per procedure), intraprocedural aneurysm rupture (2.6% risk per procedure), device-related problems such as coil stretching and inappropriate coil detachment (2.9% risk per procedure), and nonspecific complications (2.3% risk per procedure). With intraprocedural rupture, there was 50% risk of death or disability. The 30-day mortality of the study population was 1.4%. The rate of infarction was higher in middle cerebral artery (MCA) (9.6%) and anterior communicating artery (ACA)/Acom (8.8%) aneurysms, and lower in ICA (4.6%) and posterior circulation lesions (3.3%). Intraprocedural rupture occurred in 4.1% of MCA aneurysms, 2.2% of ACA/Acom aneurysms, 1.9% of ICA aneurysms, and 0.0% of posterior circulation aneurysms.

The complication rates in the ATENA study are similar to those in a recent multicenter retrospective study.[79] Gallas and colleagues reported 321 unruptured aneurysms treated by coiling, with a treatment-related morbidity and mortality of 14.4% and 1.7%, respectively. Infarctions occurred in 9% of patients, and intraprocedural aneurysm rupture in 2.6%.

A few studies have used diffusion-weighted MRI to show that the true rate of ischemic complications after endovascular treatment may be higher than is clinically apparent. In a prospective evaluation of 66 patients who underwent coiling of their unruptured aneurysms, Soeda and colleagues found new hyperintense diffusion-weighted imaging (DWI) lesions in 61% of patients.[80] Grunwald and colleagues found a 42% incidence of new DWI lesions after coiling in their 68 patients.[81] Both series reported a much lower rate of permanent neurologic morbidity, similar to other studies of endovascular treatment. For comparison, there is very sparse prospective data from the microsurgical literature. In a prospective surgical series with preoperative and postoperative MRIs, Krayenbuhl and colleagues report a 9.8% occurrence of new DWI lesions after the clipping of 51 aneurysms, both unruptured and ruptured, with a 2% risk of symptomatic infarction.[82]

Efficacy of Coiling

The immediate and long-term efficacy of the endovascular treatment of unruptured aneurysms is an issue under investigation. Excluding those patients in whom coiling attempts failed, Gallas and colleagues report complete occlusion of unruptured aneurysms in 70% of 302 patients on initial post-treatment angiogram.[79] In aneurysms that were initially completely occluded, a 16.5% rate of recurrence or recanalization was observed at final follow-up, which ranged from 3 months to 2 years. Choi and colleagues report that 26.4% of completely occluded aneurysms recanalized after an average follow-up of 26.4 months, and noted that aneurysms with wide necks (4 mm or larger) had a higher rate of recanalization.[83] Secondary endovascular and surgical treatments of recanalized aneurysms have been described, but the success rate of re-treatment is unknown.[79,83,84] Clearly, longer follow-up is necessary to determine the durability of endovascular treatment. Proposed in 2008, the TEAM trial (Trial on Endovascular Aneurysm Management) plans to be a 14-year, large, randomized controlled trial comparing endovascular treatment to observation for unruptured aneurysms.[85] The ultimate results of that study may show whether, and under what conditions, coiling improves long-term outcome compared with the natural history of the disease.

Since the development of balloon-assisted and stent-assisted coiling, various technologies have emerged, designed to increase the efficacy of endovascular procedures. Self-expanding stents permit the coiling of wide-necked aneurysms that would otherwise be unsuitable for endovascular treatment. Recent studies show an increased morbidity of stent-assisted coiling. Use of the Neuroform stent (Boston Scientific) has been associated with a 5.8% risk of delayed in-stent thrombosis, and a 4.6% rate of delayed thromboembolic events, despite the combined use of antiplatelet agents and heparinization.[86,87] As a multicenter study of the newer Enterprise stent (Cordis) shows, there are also immediate procedural complications associated with this technique, including failed or inaccurate stent deployment, and a high mortality (12%) when used to treat ruptured aneurysms.[88]

Coils with a bioactive coating have been designed to induce thrombosis and reduce recanalization after the initial treatment. However, a study of 165 aneurysms treated exclusively with the bioactive Matrix coils (Boston Scientific) showed no better recanalization rates than those reported for bare platinum coils.[89] In addition, the authors noted a 3.3% rate of delayed infarction with the bioactive coils.

As newer techniques and materials are developed for endovascular treatment, careful analysis with standardized reporting will help determine their efficacy and safety.[90] Each new technology will add to the high device cost of coils. The endovascular treatment of unruptured aneurysms is associated with shorter hospitalization but higher hospital costs than surgical treatment, particularly because of the high cost of coils.[91]

A MULTIDISCIPLINARY APPROACH TO TREATING ANEURYSMS

A review of the Nationwide Inpatient Sample hospital discharge database from 1993 to 2003 showed that the number of endovascular procedures for ruptured and unruptured aneurysms doubled, while the number of surgeries for clipping remained the same.[92] In-hospital mortality rates for endovascular therapy showed no significant change during the 11-year period. In-hospital mortality rates for surgical clipping decreased by 30% throughout the study, reaching the mortality rates of endovascular therapy. Teaching hospitals were associated with better outcomes and lower mortality rates, especially in patients who underwent aneurysm clipping. From 1993 to 2003, the number of admissions for unruptured aneurysms doubled, while the in-hospital mortality for this group decreased by 50%.

It has become increasingly apparent that both surgical and endovascular options should be considered for each unruptured intracranial aneurysm, and treatment should be weighed against the natural history of the untreated disease. At centers that receive a high volume of cerebrovascular cases, specialized cerebrovascular surgeons and endovascular practitioners can work together to offer patients the optimal choice of treatment. The recommendation for either clipping or coiling depends on the characteristics of the aneurysm, the patient's clinical situation, and the expertise of the treatment team. The following factors guide that selection:

- Location of the aneurysm
- Relationship of the aneurysm to the parent or branch arteries
- Aneurysm dome-to-neck ratio
- Presence of mass effect or thrombus
- Accessibility of the aneurysm
- Patient's age and medical comorbidities

1. *Location:* Aneurysms in some locations are associated with a high surgical risk. During surgical repair of posteriorly projecting basilar apex aneurysms, thalamoperforating arteries may be injured. When these aneurysms warrant treatment, the endovascular alternative is generally safer.[93] The clipping of cavernous segment ICA aneurysms may result in cranial nerve palsies, while these aneurysms carry very little or no risk of rupture when left untreated. Paraclinoid aneurysms and posterosuperior-projecting ACA aneurysms have intermediate surgical risks.[70,94,95] MCA aneurysms are associated with a high endovascular failure and complication rate, and are usually more safely treated with surgical clipping.[96,97]

2. *Relationship to parent or branch arteries:* Aneurysms with branch vessels originating from the neck are not suitable for endovascular treatment. Surgical clip reconstruction generally allows the parent and branch vessels to be preserved while the aneurysm is obliterated (Fig. 68-3).

3. *Dome-to-neck ratio:* An aneurysm with a neck larger than 4 mm, or a dome-to-neck ratio of less than 2, is generally not amenable to simple coiling, and surgical clipping may be preferable.[98-100] The use of stents has made many wide-necked aneurysms coilable, but such treatment is associated with higher complication rates. Clipping may be the better alternative if the surgical risk is low.

4. *Presence of Mass Effect or Thrombus:* Aneurysms that are symptomatic from mass effect, such as those that present with vision loss or oculomotor palsy, can be decompressed with surgical clipping, but not with endovascular therapy. Partially thrombosed aneurysms are likely to recur after coiling, due to shifting and compaction of the coil mass. Surgical clipping offers definitive treatment, and the complete recovery of cranial nerve deficits is more often seen after clipping than after coiling.[101]

5. *Endovascular/surgical accessibility:* Tortuosity or occlusion anywhere along the arterial pathway to the aneurysm may prohibit endovascular treatment. It is not infrequent to find tortuosity of the aortic arch, carotid or vertebral arteries; or chronic occlusion of the carotid or vertebral arteries. In contrast, aneurysms of the midbasilar artery require an extensive and complex skull base approach for surgical treatment.

6. *Age and medical condition:* Elderly patients, and those who are at high risk for prolonged general anesthesia, are generally better candidates for endovascular treatment.[77] With very advanced age, the long-term durability of treatment is less of an issue. A few recent studies have reported good outcomes after the coiling of symptomatic unruptured aneurysms in septuagenarians and octogenarians.[102-104] Surgery may be preferable for patients with renal insufficiency who might not tolerate the significant dye load required for endovascular treatment.

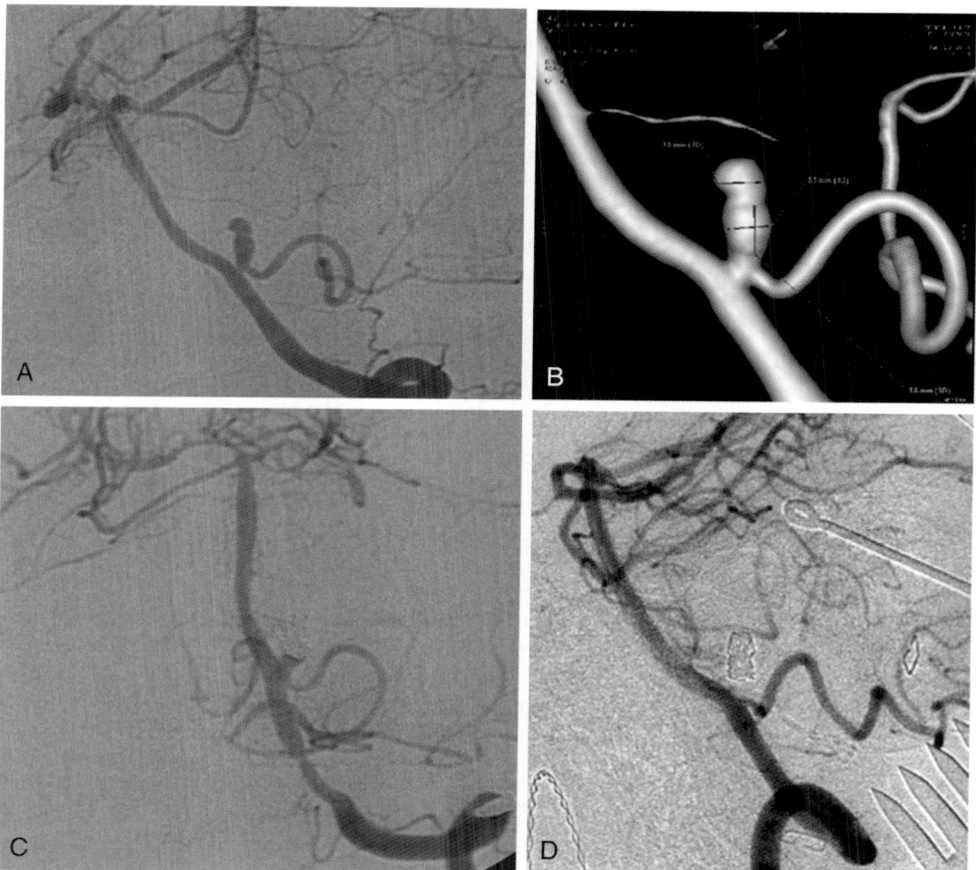

FIGURE 68-3 Digital subtraction angiography (A) with 3D reconstruction (B) showing a left vertebral artery aneurysm at the origin of the posterior inferior cerebellar artery (PICA). The aneurysm has a daughter dome and a high aspect ratio. The aneurysm was initially thought to be completely coiled; follow-up arteriography showed recanalization of the aneurysm base; recoiling to cure was thought hazardous because the PICA originates from the neck of the aneurysm (C). The patient subsequently underwent a far lateral suboccipital approach to clip the remaining aneurysm, after she recovered from her subarachnoid hemorrhage. Intraoperative angiography shows obliteration of the aneurysm and preservation of the PICA (D).

Follow-Up After Treatment

RISK OF ANEURYSM REGROWTH

In a surgical series with long-term angiographic follow-up, David and colleagues report 135 aneurysms that were clipped without residual. Of these aneurysms that were completely treated at surgery, two aneurysms (1.5%) recurred at long-term follow-up (2.6 to 9.6 years).[105] Of the 12 aneurysms in their series that were known to have residuals after clipping, 3 (25%) enlarged. In contrast, endovascular treatment is associated with a relatively high rate of aneurysm recanalization. In 145 aneurysms that were completely occluded by coiling, Raymond and colleagues found recurrences in 20%, which appeared on follow-up angiography at a mean of 12.3 months after treatment.[106] Of the 187 aneurysms in their series that had residual necks after coiling, enlargement occurred in 40%. Of the 47 aneurysms that had a dome residual after coiling, 51% enlarged. Of the recurrent aneurysms that underwent re-treatment with endovascular therapy, 48.6% showed a second recurrence. Data from a longer duration of follow-up is needed to determine the long-term recurrence rates after coiling.

Given these aneurysm recurrence rates, patients who undergo endovascular treatment require serial cerebrovascular imaging over an extended, sometimes indefinite period of time. Patients who undergo surgical clipping, and who have no evidence of residual on a postoperative angiogram, may not need further imaging. Delayed imaging after surgical clipping should be considered when there is concern for residual aneurysm. Delayed imaging may also be appropriate in young patients or those with multiple aneurysms, to evaluate for de novo aneurysms.

DE NOVO ANEURYSMS

In a series of 142 patients with unruptured aneurysms followed for 20 years, Juvela found that 19 new aneurysms developed in 15 patients, of which 2 caused subarachnoid hemorrhage.[17] The chance that an aneurysm would form de novo was 0.84% per year. A similar annual rate of 0.89% was reported by Tsutsumi and colleagues.[107] The annual risk of de novo aneurysm formation may be higher (1.8%) in patients with multiple aneurysms.[105]

Screening for Intracranial Aneurysms

PATIENTS WITH A FAMILY HISTORY OF INTRACRANIAL ANEURYSMS

Adults who have two first-degree family members with known intracranial aneurysms, or who have one first-degree and one second-degree affected family members, have a 9% to 11% chance of harboring an aneurysm.[56,57,108] In families with multiple affected individuals, first-degree relatives who have a history of smoking or hypertension have a 20.6% chance of harboring an unruptured intracranial aneurysm, according to early results from the Familial Intracranial Aneurysm Study.[39] This frequency is much higher than the prevalence in the general population. The rupture risk is also likely higher for familial aneurysms than for sporadic aneurysms of similar size. Subarachnoid hemorrhage may occur at younger ages in subsequent generations.[109] In siblings, aneurysm rupture tends to occur within the same decade of life.[110,111] It is therefore reasonable to screen individuals with multiple affected family members, with either MRA or CTA, beginning in early adulthood. The optimal age and subsequent frequency to screen these individuals is unknown.

AUTOSOMAL DOMINANT POLYCYSTIC KIDNEY DISEASE

Approximately 500,000 persons in the United States carry a genetic mutation for autosomal dominant polycystic kidney disease (ADPKD), making it one of the most common inherited disorders.[112] ADPKD is associated with an increased prevalence of intracranial aneurysms and an increased risk of subarachnoid hemorrhage. The prevalence of asymptomatic aneurysms in patients with ADPKD is 14% to 16% by autopsy and angiography studies.[113] When aneurysm rupture occurs in these patients, it happens at a mean age of 35 to 40 years,[114-116] which is 10 to 20 years earlier than the mean age for patients with sporadic intracranial aneurysms. Therefore, MRA screening is reasonable for young adults with this disease.

Conclusion

The issues regarding the management of unruptured intracranial aneurysms are complex and often multi-factorial. This chapter addresses whom to screen for asymptomatic lesions, and discusses the imaging tools used for diagnosis and evaluation. Once an aneurysm is identified, understanding the natural history and the risk factors for growth and rupture is essential for deciding whether or not to treat the lesion. With recent data on the efficacy and safety of surgical and endovascular therapy, a neurosurgeon can make informed recommendations regarding the optimal modality of treatment for an individual patient. Patients may benefit from referral to centers that offer specialized cerebrovascular care. A plan for follow-up should be determined, based on the modality and success of therapy. With appropriate, safe, and effective treatment of unruptured aneurysms, the burden of subarachnoid hemorrhage on society may eventually be reduced.

KEY REFERENCES

Andaluz N, Zuccarello M. Recent trends in the treatment of cerebral aneurysms: analysis of a nationwide inpatient database. *J Neurosurg.* 2008;108:1163-1169.

Bederson JB, Awad IA, Wiebers DO, et al. Recommendations for the management of patients with unruptured intracranial aneurysms: a statement for healthcare professionals from the Stroke Council of the American Heart Association. *Stroke.* 2000;31:2742-2750.

Bederson JB, Connolly ES, Batjer HH, et al. Guidelines for the management of aneurysmal subarachnoid hemorrhage: a statement for healthcare professionals from a Special Writing Group of the Stroke Council, American Heart Association. *Stroke.* 2009;40:994-1025.

Broderick JP, Brown RD, Sauerbeck L, et al. Greater rupture risk for familial as compared to sporadic unruptured intracranial aneurysms. *Stroke.* 2009;40:1952-1957.

Chappell ET, Moure FC, Good MC. Comparison of computed tomographic angiography with digital subtraction angiography in the diagnosis of cerebral aneurysms: a meta-analysis. *Neurosurgery.* 2003;52:624-631.

Choi DS, Kim MC, Lee SK, et al. Clinical and angiographic long-term follow-up of completely coiled intracranial aneurysms using endovascular technique. *J Neurosurg.* 2010;112(3):575-581, erratum 2010; 112(3):690.

Fiorella D, Albuquerque FC, Woo H, et al. Neuroform in-stent stenosis: incidence, natural history, and treatment strategies. *Neurosurgery.* 2006;59:34-42.

Gallas S, Drouineau J, Gabrillargues J, et al. Feasibility, procedural morbidity and mortality, and long-term follow-up of endovascular treatment of 321 unruptured aneurysms. *Am J Neuroradiol.* 2008;29:63-68.

Grunwald IQ, Papanagiotou P, Politi M, et al. Endovascular treatment of unruptured intracranial aneurysms: occurrence of thromboembolic events. *Neurosurgery.* 2006;58:612-618.

International Study of Unruptured Intracranial Aneurysms Investigators: Unruptured intracranial aneurysms—risk of rupture and risks of surgical intervention. *N Engl J Med.* 1998;339:1725-1733.

Ishibashi T, Murayama Y, Urashima M, et al. Unruptured intracranial aneurysms: incidence of rupture and risk factors. *Stroke.* 2009;40:313-316.

Juvela S. Natural history of unruptured intracranial aneurysms: risks for aneurysm formation, growth, and rupture. *Acta Neurochir Suppl.* 2002;82:27-30.

Juvela S, Porras M, Heiskanen O. Natural history of unruptured intracranial aneurysms: a long-term follow-up study. *J Neurosurg.* 1993;79: 174-182.

Krayenbuhl N, Erdem E, Oinas M, et al. Symptomatic and silent ischemia associated with microsurgical clipping of intracranial aneurysms: evaluation with diffusion-weighted MRI. *Stroke.* 2009;40:129-133.

Lall RR, Eddleman CS, Bendok BR, et al. Unruptured intracranial aneurysms and the assessment of rupture risk based on anatomical and morphological factors: sifting through the sands of data. *Neurosurg Focus.* 2009;26(E2):1-7.

Mocco J, Snyder KV, Albuquerque FC, et al. Treatment of intracranial aneurysms with the Enterprise stent: a multicenter registry. *J Neurosurg.* 2009;110:35-39.

Molyneux A, Kerr R, Stratton I, et al. International Subarachnoid Aneurysm Trial (ISAT) of neurosurgical clipping versus endovascular coiling in 2143 patients with ruptured intracranial aneurysms: a randomised trial. *Lancet.* 2002;360:1267-1274.

Pierot L, Spelle L, Vitry F, et al. Immediate clinical outcome of patients harboring unruptured intracranial aneurysms treated by endovascular approach: results of the ATENA study. *Stroke.* 2008;39:2497-2504.

Piotin M, Spelle L, Mounayer C, et al. Intracranial aneurysms coiling with Matrix: immediate results in 152 patients and midterm anatomic follow-up from 115 patients. *Stroke.* 2009;40:321-323.

Raaymakers TW, Rinkel GJ, Limburg M, Algra A. Mortality and morbidity of surgery for unruptured intracranial aneurysms: a meta-analysis. *Stroke.* 1998;29:1531-1538.

Raymond J, Guilbert F, Weill A, et al. Long-term angiographic recurrences after selective endovascular treatment of aneurysms with detachable coils. *Stroke.* 2003;34:1398-1403.

Soeda A, Sakai N, Sakai H, et al. Thromboembolic events associated with Guglielmi detachable coil embolization of asymptomatic cerebral aneurysms: evaluation of 66 consecutive cases with use of diffusion-weighted MR imaging. *Am J Neuroradiol.* 2003;24:127-132.

Tsutsumi K, Ueki K, Morita A, Kirino T. Risk of rupture from incidental cerebral aneurysms. *J Neurosurg.* 2000;93:50-53.

Wiebers DO, Whisnant JP, Huston 3rd J, et al. Unruptured intracranial aneurysms: natural history, clinical outcome, and risks of surgical and endovascular treatment. *Lancet.* 2003;362:103-110.

Yahia AM, Gordon V, Whapham J, et al. Complications of Neuroform stent in endovascular treatment of intracranial aneurysms. *Neurocrit Care.* 2008;8:19-30.

Numbered references appear on Expert Consult.

CHAPTER 69

Surgical Management of Intracerebral Hemorrhage

MANISH K. AGHI • CHRISTOPHER S. OGILVY • BOB S. CARTER

Epidemiology

Intracerebral hemorrhage (ICH), or hemorrhage within the brain parenchyma, occurs with an incidence estimated to range from 15 to 35 cases per 100,000 people per year. The incidence is up to twice that of subarachnoid hemorrhage by some estimates. Each year, approximately 37,000 to 52,000 people in the United States have an ICH. The rate is expected to double during the next 50 years as a result of the increasing age of the population and changes in racial demographics. A 1993 report found that only 38% of patients affected with ICH survive the first year,[1] while a 2009 report found improvement up to 51% for 3-year survival in ICH patients.[2]

Six risk factors for ICH have been identified—age, male sex, race, hypertension, high alcohol intake, and low serum cholesterol. Regarding other possible risks, current or past smoking and diabetes mellitus are weak risk factors, if at all.[3] The incidence of ICH increases significantly after age 55 and doubles with each decade of age until the age of 80, at which point the incidence increases 25-fold each decade.[4] ICH is more common in men than women. ICH also affects blacks and Japanese more than whites. During the 20-year period covered by the National Health and Nutrition Examination Survey Epidemiologic Follow-up Study, the incidence of ICH among blacks was 50 per 100,000, a little over twice the incidence among whites.[5] It has been hypothesized that hypertension and factors leading to limited access to health care result in the higher incidence of ICH within the African-American community. The higher incidence of ICH in Japan has been attributed to a higher incidence of hypertension in Japanese populations and diets leading to low serum cholesterol, another risk factor for ICH. The reversibility of the dietary factor may lead to reductions in ICH seen when Japanese people emigrate to the United States, while their persistent hypertension may explain why their rates never drop to the same level as whites even after they emigrate to the United States.

There have been 11 case-controlled studies on hypertension and risk of ICH, with all showing a positive association between hypertension and ICH. Hypertension is classified as high normal (systolic 130–139 or diastolic 85–89), stage I hypertension (systolic 140–159 or diastolic 90–99), stage II hypertension (systolic 160–179 or diastolic 100–109), or stage III hypertension (systolic $\geq$ 180 or diastolic > 110). Suh et al. found a relative risk of 2.2 for high normal, 5.3 for stage I

hypertension, 10.4 for stage II hypertension, and 33 for stage III hypertension.[6] Iribarren et al. found for each one standard-deviation increase in systolic blood pressure (18 mm Hg in men; 19 mm Hg in women) a relative risk of 1.14 in men and 1.17 in women.[7] Leppala et al. found a relative risk of 2.20 for systolic blood pressure 140 to 159 mm Hg and 3.78 for systolic blood pressure greater than 160 mm Hg compared with systolic blood pressure less than 139 mm Hg.[8] The correlation between blood pressure and ICH also leads to diurnal and seasonal variations in the onset of ICH. In general, ICH onset is usually during activity and rarely during sleep, which may be related to elevated blood pressure or increased cerebral blood flow. One study covering a decade of ICH cases in a Japanese city found that men 69 years of age and younger had a bimodal distribution of ICH-onset time, with an initial peak between 8:00 a.m. and 10:00 a.m., and a second, lower peak between 6:00 and 8:00 p.m. Men 70 years of age or older and women of all ages exhibited only a single evening peak, between 6:00 and 10:00 p.m.[9] Men exhibited peak ICH in winter and a trough in summer, while women had no seasonal patterns.[9] The incidence of ICH correlates with the daily times of blood pressure peaks in the sexes, and the ability of the autonomic nervous system to raise blood pressure during the winter may particularly affect men because they tend to work outdoors more often.

Alcohol consumption is a risk factor in both the short term and long term. During the 24 hours preceding an ICH, moderate alcohol consumption (41 to 120 g of ethanol, where one standard drink averages 12 g of ethanol) causes a 4.6 relative risk of ICH, while heavy alcohol consumption (>120 g of ethanol) causes an 11.3 relative risk of ICH. During the week preceding ICH, low (1–150 g of ethanol), moderate (151–300 g of ethanol), and heavy (>300 g of ethanol) alcohol consumption carry relative risks of 2.0, 4.3, and 6.5, respectively.[10] ICH in patients with high ethanol consumption tends to be lobar.[11] Ethanol promotes ICH by impairing coagulation and by directly affecting the integrity of cerebral vessels.[11]

A counterintuitive finding has been the identification of low serum cholesterol as a risk factor for ICH. Iribarren et al. found that for each one standard deviation increase in serum cholesterol (1.45 mmol/L in men and 1.24 mmol/L in women), there was a relative risk reduction of 0.84 in men and 0.92 in women.[7] One potential mechanism may be that patients with low serum cholesterol may exhibit reduced consumption of animal products, and such patients will have reduced concentrations of arachidonic acid in their cell membranes.[12] Arachidonic acid is a vital structural component of the cell membranes of vascular endothelium and its metabolites are involved in regulation of vascular tone and repair of injured vascular endothelium.[12] Defects in this pathway may increase the risk of ICH. However, hypercholesterolemia is a proven risk factor for morbidities such as myocardial infarction that are far more common than ICH and should therefore be avoided. Furthermore, patients taking cholesterol lowering statin drugs before experiencing an ICH have been shown to have lower hematoma volumes, although the difference has not been shown to impact clinical outcome after ICH.[13]

Etiology

Depending on the underlying cause of bleeding, ICH is classified as either primary or secondary. Primary ICH, accounting for nearly 80% of all ICH cases, originates from the spontaneous rupture of small vessels damaged by chronic hypertension or amyloid angiopathy, more commonly the former. Secondary ICH occurs in a minority of ICH patients in association with vascular abnormalities, tumors, cerebral infarction, or impaired coagulation. Although primary ICH from vessels damaged by chronic hypertension remains the most common etiology of ICH, secondary ICH from vascular abnormalities should always be investigated as a possible source because of the high risk of recurrent hemorrhage and the necessity of surgical or endovascular treatment to prevent recurrent hemorrhage. Underlying vascular abnormalities can be searched for using computed tomographic angiography (CTA) or digital subtraction angiography (DSA) when the combined opinion of the medical team and radiologist interpreting the CT deems it necessary.

In primary ICH, the hemorrhage arises from vessels damaged by chronic hypertension or amyloid angiopathy. Chronic hypertension causes degenerative changes in the walls of small penetrating arteries originating from the anterior, middle, or posterior cerebral arteries. These changes reduce vessel compliance and increase the likelihood of spontaneous rupture. Patients with chronic hypertension incur an annual risk of recurrent ICH of 2%, but this risk can be reduced by treatment of hypertension.[14] In 1868, Charcot and Bouchard attributed ICH to rupture at points of dilation in the walls of small arterioles that they called microaneurysms.[15] These microaneurysms were later found to be subadventitial hemorrhages or extravascular clots resulting from endothelial damage by the hematoma. Electron-microscopy studies have since suggested that most ICH occurs at or near the bifurcation of affected arteries, where prominent degeneration of the media presumably caused by chronic hypertension can be seen.

In amyloid angiopathy, β-amyloid protein, an acellular eosinophilic material, is deposited within the media of small- and medium-sized arteries in the cerebral cortex and leptomeninges, which causes primary ICH in the white matter of the cerebral lobes, particularly the parietal and occipital areas, in persons older than 70 years of age who exhibit no evidence of systemic amyloidosis. These patients face an annual risk of recurrent hemorrhage of 10.5%.[16] Cerebral amyloid angiopathy is present in the brains of 50% of people over the age of 70; however, most do not experience ICH. Amyloid angiopathy may be associated with genetic factors

including the apolipoprotein E allele and may be more prevalent in patients with Down's syndrome. O'Donnell et al. reported that the presence of the ε2 or ε4 alleles of the apolipoprotein E gene was associated with a tripling of the risk of recurrent ICH among survivors of primary lobar ICH attributable to amyloid angiopathy.[16] Among patients with lobar ICH, those with the apoE ε4 allele typically have their first ICH more than 5 years earlier than noncarriers (average age of 73 versus 79),[17] and experience a statistically independent decrease in survival.[18] Although they are distinct diseases, there is some overlap between amyloid angiopathy and Alzheimer's disease, in that the amyloid in amyloid angiopathy is identical to that found in the senile plaques of Alzheimer's disease and apolipoprotein-ε4 is associated with both the parenchymal plaque amyloid seen in Alzheimer's disease and the deposits of β-amyloid protein in cerebral vessel walls seen in amyloid angiopathy. Cerebral amyloid angiopathy may increase the risk of ICH by potentiating plasminogen, a finding that may be of some relevance to patients receiving tissue plasminogen activator (t-PA) to treat myocardial infarcts or cerebrovascular accidents. Amyloid angiopathy can be diagnosed suggestively on the basis of radiologic findings such as hemosiderin deposits from small cortical and subcortical petechial hemorrhages on gradient-echo magnetic resonance imaging (MRI). Histologic findings include deposits of acellular eosinophilic material in the media of vessels in the hematoma or in non-involved brain (Fig. 69-1). Perivascular microglia, thickened vessel walls, vessel dilatation, and microaneurysms are also seen in the vessels of patients with cerebral amyloid angiopathy. After staining with Congo red, the amyloid in the media of vessel walls exhibits apple-green birefringence under polarized light. A definitive diagnosis can be made on the basis of all three of the following findings: lobar, cortical, or corticosubcortical ICH; severe cerebral amyloid angiopathy on histopathologic exam; and absence of another diagnostic

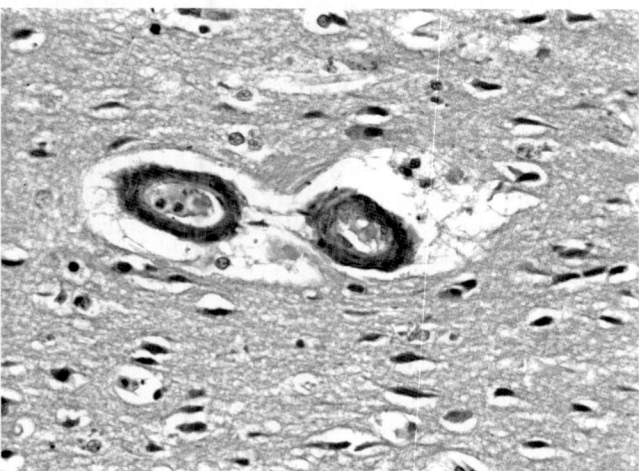

FIGURE 69-1 A pair of lobar intracerebral blood vessels from autopsy of a patient who experienced a lobar ICH with radiographic findings consistent with amyloid angiopathy. Shown here is peroxidase immunostaining using an antibody to the β-amyloid protein, an alternative to the Congo red staining that can also detect β-amyloid protein. Note that the β-amyloid protein localizes to the thickened media of both involved blood vessels, a typical finding in amyloid angiopathy. *(Courtesy of Matthew P. Frosch, MD, PhD, Massachusetts General Hospital, Department of Neuropathology.)*

lesion. A probable diagnosis with supporting pathologic evidence occurs with all three of the following findings: lobar, cortical, or corticosubcortical ICH; some degree of vascular amyloid deposition on histopathologic exam; and absence of another diagnostic lesion. Probable amyloid angiopathy without pathologic evidence occurs with all 3 of the following findings: age over 60 years; a history of multiple hemorrhages in the lobar, cortical, or subcortical regions; and absence of another cause of hemorrhage. A diagnosis of possible amyloid angiopathy occurs with age over 60 combined with either a single lobar, cortical, or cortico-subcortical hemorrhage without another cause or multiple hemorrhages with a possible but not a definitive cause.

Secondary ICH is far less common than primary ICH but because the etiologies of secondary ICH include tumors and vascular malformations that will need surgical intervention, or coagulopathies that need to be immediately corrected, attention must always be paid to secondary ICH as a possibility with any ICH. Tumors that produce ICH are usually malignant metastases. Hemorrhage is present in 3% to 14% of metastases and is most commonly seen in metastases from renal cell carcinoma, choriocarcinoma, melanoma, and renal cell carcinoma, with hemorrhage occurring in 70%, 50%, 40%, and 25% of the brain metastases from these respective primaries.[19] However, bronchogenic carcinoma represents the most common source of hemorrhagic cerebral metastases because, although only 9% of metastatic bronchogenic carcinomas undergo hemorrhage, it is a much more common metastasis than the other four tumor types. When ICH appears on an initial CT scan, the presence of nonhemorrhagic necrotic or hypodense tissue and pronounced surrounding vasogenic edema are radiologic clues to the underlying neoplasm and warrant an MRI with gadolinium to look for tumor. Vascular malformations that can give rise to secondary ICH are usually arteriovenous malformations (AVMs), with 81% of hemorrhages from AVMs having a significant intraparenchymal component. Cavernous malformations also tend to cause hemorrhage with a significant intraparenchymal component, but only represent 10% of central nervous system vascular malformations. The diagnosis is strongly suggested by finding a mixed signal core indicative of old hemorrhage and a T2 dark rim on an MRI. ICH is unusual from aneurysmal rupture, which usually causes subarachnoid hemorrhage. Aneurysms that become adherent to the brain surface due to fibrosis from inflammation or previous hemorrhage can sometimes produce ICH rather than subarachnoid hemorrhage when they rupture. Oral anticoagulant therapy is a known source of secondary ICH. The relative risk of ICH during oral anticoagulant therapy increases more than 10-fold in patients over the age of 50.[20] Bleeding is more protracted and hematomas larger in patients treated with anticoagulants than in those with spontaneous ICH.[21] The management of these patients requires rapid reversal of their coagulopathy. Vitamin K provides long-term reversal and stabilization of the international normalized ratio (INR), while fresh frozen plasma (FFP) provides faster reversal, although one study showed that 24 hours after administering 1000 ml of FFP, patients on coumadin with ICH dropped their INR from 3.35 to 1.40.[22] Slightly less than one third of these patients experienced radiographic hematoma enlargement within 24 hours of their initial CT scan,[22] suggesting that the time it takes FFP to reverse a coagulopathy may be too slow, particularly in elderly patients who cannot tolerate rapid administration of volume. A suggested alternative is prothrombin complex concentrate (PCC), which can counteract the effects of warfarin as early as 10 minutes in much smaller volumes than FFP.[22]

Pathophysiology

Edematous parenchyma, often discolored by degradation products of hemoglobin, is visible adjacent to the clot and correlates with areas of CT and MRI T1 hypodensity and MRI T2 hyperdensity. Histologic sections are characterized by edema, neuronal damage, macrophages, and neutrophils in the region surrounding the hematoma. The hemorrhage spreads between planes of white matter, causing varying degrees of tissue destruction, leaving nests of intact neural tissue within and surrounding the hematoma. This pattern of spread accounts for the presence of viable and salvageable neural tissue in the immediate vicinity of the hematoma.

The presence of hematoma initiates edema and neuronal damage in the surrounding parenchyma. Animal models of ICH have identified three phases of perihematoma edema—immediate (within 24 hours), intermediate (24 hours to 5 days), and late onset (from 5 days to several weeks after ICH). Immediate edema occurs within the first 24 hours and can often be seen at a histologic, but not radiographic level. This initial edema develops secondary to osmotically active plasma proteins accumulating in the extravascular space.[23] The blood–brain barrier is intact at this point, so the proteins most likely arise from the hematoma. After the initial hemorrhage, the clotting cascade activates thrombin, which disrupts the blood–brain barrier and activates the complement cascade, leading to lysis of red blood cells and other bystander cells. Vasogenic edema and cytotoxic edema subsequently follow owing to the disruption of the blood–brain barrier, the failure of the sodium pump, and the death of neurons.[24] This represents the intermediate edema seen at 24 hours to 5 days. This intermediate edema is noticeable radiographically and histologically. Red blood cell lysis releases hemoglobin and leads to formation of free radicals, which account for the late onset edema. The role of the coagulation cascade in intermediate perihematoma edema may explain why ICH related to thrombolysis or coagulopathy causes less perihematoma edema than spontaneous ICH.

Studies in animals and humans have refuted the notion that cerebral ischemia in areas of ICH occurs due to mechanical compression by the hematoma, and have suggested that secondary mediators may cause the delayed development of neuronal injury adjacent to a hematoma.[23] It is currently thought that blood products mediate most secondary processes initiated after ICH.[25] Recent evidence has suggested the presence of apoptosis or programmed cell death in neurons adjacent to ICH associated with nuclear factor-kB expression in neuronal nuclei.[26] Other studies have suggested that heme derived from erythrocytes extravasated during ICH is degraded into bilirubin and bilirubin oxidation products, which activate microglia, which secrete cytokines that recruit leukocytes into the brain, which contribute to the injury process.[27]

Presentation by Location

Intracerebral hemorrhage commonly occurs in the cerebral white matter (10%–20%); basal ganglia, usually the putamen but also including lenticular nucleus, internal capsule, and globus pallidus (50%); thalamus (15%); the pons (10%–15%); other brain-stem sites (1%–6%); and cerebellum (10%). Common arterial feeders of ICHs are the lenticulostriate branches of the anterior and middle cerebral arteries which form Charcot-Bouchard microaneurysms and are the source of putaminal ICH; thalamoperforators branching off the anterior and middle cerebral arteries which are the source of thalamic ICH; and paramedian branches of the basilar artery, which are the source of pontine and cerebellar ICH.

Intracerebral hemorrhage into the cerebral white matter includes ICH into the occipital, temporal, frontal, and parietal lobes, including ICH arising from the cortex and subcortical white matter, as opposed to ICH of deep structures such as the basal ganglia, thalamus, and infratentorial structures. Frontal lobe ICH causes frontal headache with contralateral hemiparesis, usually in the arm with mild leg and facial weakness. Parietal lobe ICH causes contralateral hemisensory deficit with mild hemiparesis. Occipital lobe ICH causes ipsilateral eye pain and contralateral homonymous hemianopsia, with some sparing of the superior quadrant. Temporal lobe ICH can be asymptomatic on the nondominant side, but, on the dominant side, produces fluent dysphasia with poor auditory comprehension but relatively good repetition. Lobar ICH is more likely to be associated with structural abnormalities such as AVMs or tumors than deep hemorrhages. Lobar ICH is also more common in patients with alcohol consumption. In one study, significant independent risk factors for lobar ICH included the presence of an apolipoprotein E ε2 or ε4 allele, frequent alcohol use, prior stroke, and first-degree relative with ICH, while significant independent risk factors for nonlobar ICH were hypertension, prior stroke, and first-degree relative with ICH,[28] suggesting different etiologies for lobar ICH than the other locations of ICH. Lobar ICH may also have a more benign outcome than basal ganglia and thalamic ICH.

In putaminal ICH, 62% of patients experience smooth gradual deterioration with only 30% exhibiting their maximal deficit at the onset. In some studies, the 30-day mortality rate has been 50%.[29] The clinical presentation of putaminal hemorrhage may vary from relatively minor pure motor hemiparesis to profound weakness, sensory loss, eye deviation, hemianopsia, aphasia, and depressed level of consciousness. Headache is a presenting symptom in only 14% of putaminal ICHs. In putaminal ICH, intraventricular extension portends a poor prognosis, because the hematoma must be quite large to track through the internal capsule and reach the ventricle.

Thalamic ICH usually causes contralateral hemisensory loss out of proportion to any weakness. Hemiparesis can ensue when the internal capsule becomes involved. Extension into the upper brain stem can cause vertical gaze palsy, retraction nystagmus, skew deviation, loss of convergence, ptosis, miosis, and anisocoria. Nearly 30% of patients with thalamic ICH present with headache. Hydrocephalus may result from obstruction of cerebrospinal fluid reabsorption pathways. In a series of 41 patients with thalamic ICH, all with hemorrhage diameter greater than 3.3 cm on CT died, with smaller hematomas causing permanent disability.

Patients with supratentorial ICH involving the putamen, caudate, or thalamus have contralateral sensory-motor deficits of varying severity due to involvement of the internal capsule. Higher-level cortical dysfunction, including neglect, gaze deviation, hemianopsia, and, for dominant hemisphere lesions, aphasia, can occur as a result of disruption of connecting fibers in the subcortical white matter and functional suppression of overlying cortex, known as diaschisis.[30]

Any deep, large hematoma can extend into the ventricles causing intraventricular hemorrhage (IVH). Common nonspecific initial symptoms include headache and vomiting due to increased intracranial pressure and meningismus resulting from blood in the ventricles. As any hematoma becomes larger, patients will exhibit a decreased level of consciousness due to increased intracranial pressure and direct compression or distortion of the thalamic and brain-stem reticular activating system. Small, deep lesions can occasionally impair consciousness due to decreased central benzodiazepine receptor binding on cortical neurons.[31]

Cerebellar ICH can cause patients' level of consciousness to progress from impaired to comatose due to direct compression of the brain stem, without any associated hemiparesis, unlike supratentorial ICH. Cerebellar ICH can present with the abrupt onset of vertigo, headache, vomiting, and inability to walk without any associated hemiparesis. Cranial nerve palsies are common, particularly an abducens palsy or a peripheral facial palsy. In one study, at least two of the three characteristic clinical signs—appendicular ataxia, ipsilateral gaze palsy, and peripheral facial palsy—were present in 73% of the cases of cerebellar ICH.[32]

Evaluation

Initial evaluation is typically through a CT scan, which is rapid and easily demonstrates ICH as high-density material within the brain parenchyma. Although mass effect on adjacent brain is common, the tendency for the hemorrhage to dissect through brain tissue often results in less mass effect than would be anticipated from the size of the clot. Clot volume can be estimated by computer programs that allow one to outline the hematoma on each slice and then model the hematoma in three dimensions and estimate a volume, or it can be approximated using the established practice of the modified ellipsoid volume, $(A \times B \times C)/2$, where A, B, and C are the diameters of the clot in each of three orthogonal dimensions, with one of the dimensions, C, being superoinferior such that C is equal to the number of slices with hematoma × slice thickness.[33] Clot volume carries significant prognostic significance. One study demonstrated a much steeper dependence of mortality on clot volume for deep ICH than lobar ICH, consistent with the fact that deep areas of the brain are less able to accommodate large volumes. Hematomas were divided into small (≤ 30 cm^3), medium (30–60 cm^3), and large (≥ 60 cm^3). The 30-day mortalities for small, medium, and large hematomas were 23%, 60%, and 71% for lobar ICH, compared to 7%, 64%, and 93% for deep ICH.[34] The overall 30-day mortality was 39% for lobar ICH and 48% for deep ICH. Hematoma volume also correlates with risk of rehemorrhage, with one retrospective study showing that 39% of ICH patients who experienced rehemorrhage had initial clot volumes greater than or equal to 25 cm³, compared to only 23% of ICH patients who did not experience rehemorrhage.[35]

Magnetic resonance imaging is not the initial study of choice, as it is more time consuming, makes it difficult to access a patient who may acutely deteriorate, and does not show blood well within the first few hours. MRI may, however, may be useful later once a patient stabilizes to identify cerebral amyloid angiopathy, cavernous malformations, or underlying tumors. Gradient-echo MRI is the most useful modality for identifying ICH of various ages. Gradient-echo MRI increases the amount of signal dropout from deposits of iron representing residual blood products as a result of past hemorrhage. This increases the potential for detecting two findings that are typical of patients with cerebral amyloid angiopathy: (1) small prior punctuate petechial hemorrhages; and (2) previous lobar ICH, as manifested by a dark hemosiderin ring around an area of lobar encephalomalacia (Fig. 69-2). MRI has improved to the point that gradient echo can now detect ICH as early as 2.5 hours with 99.5% sensitivity.[36] However, the specificity of MRI is limited in the hyperacute stage.[37] Overall, MRI remains a secondary study compared to CT, and is most useful when a CT scan has findings listed above that suggest an underlying lesion such as a tumor or cavernous malformation. In these cases, MRI with gadolinium can be used to search for enhancing areas consistent with tumor; MR spectroscopy can be used to identify areas with high choline peaks, an inverted lactate peak, and absence of creatinine and N-acetyl-aspartate peaks; or T2 MRI can show a central mixed density core suggesting old hemorrhages surrounded by a hypodense rim.

Cerebral aniography is used to identify arteriovenous malformations (AVMs) and aneurysms in patients with ICH. In a prospective study in which 206 ICH cases were investigated with CT and angiography, anigoraphic yield was significantly higher in patients (1) at or below the age of 45, and (2) without preexisting hypertension.[38] Analysis of angiographic yield of different sites of hemorrhage taken together with these two factors showed that (1) lobar ICH had a 10% angiographic yield in patients older than 45 with preexisting hypertension; (2) putaminal, thalamic, and posterior fossa hemorrhages in patients of all ages with preexisting hypertension had a 0% angiographic yield; (3) lobar ICH had a 65% angiographic yield in normotensive patients younger than 45; (4) putaminal, thalamic, and posterior fossa hemorrhages in normotensive patients younger than 45 had a 48% angiographic yield; and (5) putaminal, thalamic, and posterior fossa hemorrhages in normotensive patients older than 45 had a 7% angiographic yield. Isolated intraventricular hemorrhage (IVH) patients had 63% yield in the older and 67% yield in the younger groups. Taken together, these findings led the authors to recommend DSA in ICH patients except those older than 45 years who also have preexisting hypertension and thalamic, putaminal, or posterior fossa hemorrhages. More recently, the safer and more rapid technique of three-dimensional (3D) CTA has begun to replace DSA. CTA involves a head CT with thin 2.5-mm axial cuts occurring 5 seconds after administering a 45 mL contrast bolus at 7 cc/sec. Imaging software programs, which reformat the axial cuts and subtract out all but the contrast and adjacent brain tissue, are used to generate 3D images of the cerebral circulation. Preliminary studies have shown that CTA is 95% as sensitive and just as specific as DSA in the detection of cerebral aneurysms,[39] a gap that is expected to close as CTA technology improves.

Acute Rehemorrhage

Although it was initially believed that ICH was largely a monophasic event that stopped quickly as a result of clotting and tamponade by the surrounding regions, a number of investigators have shown that rehemorrhage is common, with one study of 627 ICH patients showing a 14.0% rehemorrhage rate within 24 hours of admission.[40] Brott et al. found that the hematoma expanded in 26% of ICH patients within 1 hour of the initial CT scan and in another 12% within 20 hours.[41] Expansion has been attributed to continued bleeding from the primary source and to the mechanical disruption of surrounding vessels from compression by the hematoma. Acute hypertension after the initial ICH, a local coagulation deficit, or both may be associated with expansion of hematoma.[35]

Factors associated with rehemorrhage in the initial 24-hour period include: (1) a previous history of brain infarction, (2) liver disease, (3) uncontrolled diabetes, (4) systolic blood pressure on admission greater than 195, (5) a history of alcohol abuse, (6) coagulation abnormalities, (7) a hematoma larger than 25 cm³ on the initial CT scan, (8) irregular hematoma shape because irregularly shaped hematomas seem to indicate active bleeding from multiple sources, (9) a large peripheral white cell count, and (10) elevated body temperature on admission.[40] CT angiography performed within 12 hours of the ICH revealing extravasation of contrast predicts

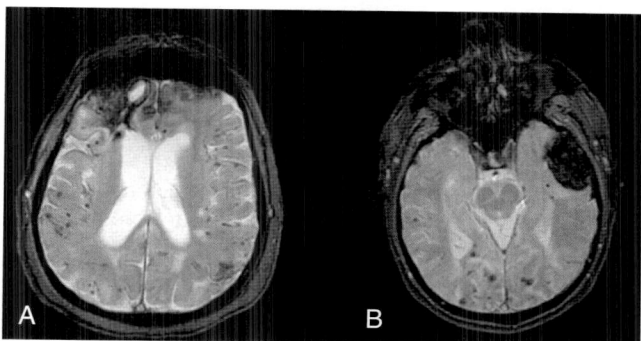

FIGURE 69-2 Axial MRI susceptibility pulse sequence images of the brain from patients showing findings consistent with amyloid angiopathy. A, This 74-year-old male presented with mental status changes. MRI susceptibility identified: (1) extensive areas of punctate darkness in both cerebral hemispheres, consistent with hemosiderin deposition from previous punctate petechial hemorrhages; and (2) cystic encephalomalacia with gliosis in right frontal lobe, consistent with a prior lobar ICH. The combination of these two findings is consistent with cerebral amyloid angiopathy. B, The susceptibility pulse sequences on this 82-year-old man with confusion, headache, and speech difficulty show (1) a 3×2×3 cm anterior left temporal hypodensity, which was also hypointense on T1 and T2 (not shown), consistent with acute lobar ICH; and (2) numerous punctate foci of abnormal signal dropout throughout the right and left cerebral hemispheres, concentrated in the occipital, parietal, and temporal lobes. The findings are consistent with hemosiderin deposits from multiple foci of chronic hemorrhage, likely secondary to amyloid angiopathy. (Courtesy of Stuart R. Pomerantz, MD, Massachusetts General Hospital, Department of Neuroradiology.)

rehemorrhage on a 24-hour post ICH CT scan with 60% specificity and 100% sensitivity.[42]

Systolic blood pressure control using an arterial line and intravenous drips of antihypertensives like nitroprusside remains the primary medical intervention designed to prevent rehemorrhage. Recommendations written by a panel of experts commissioned by the American Heart Association (AHA) in 1999 are to maintain the mean arterial blood pressure below 130 mm Hg (systolic BP < 180 and/or diastolic BP < 105) in patients with a history of chronic hypertension,[43] but therapeutic trials are needed. In patients with elevated ICP documented by an ICP monitor, cerebral perfusion pressure should be kept above 70 mm Hg.

Medical Management

Whether ICH is best managed medically or with a combination of surgery and medicines remains a subject of considerable debate. Regardless of which therapy is chosen, the goal is improvement in function, an objective that is based on the concept of a penumbra around ICH. There is now mounting evidence that there is a penumbra of functionally impaired, but potentially reversible, neuronal injury surrounding a hematoma. Adjacent brain tissue is displaced and compressed by extravasated blood. Animal models have shown that compression causes edema, ischemia, and hemorrhagic necrosis at the margin of the clot.[44] The volume of this penumbra may exceed the volume of the ICH several-fold. SPECT studies have confirmed that the penumbra tissue exhibits reversible ischemia.

We admit all ICH patients to the neurologic intensive care unit. An arterial line is placed and systolic blood pressure is kept between 100 and 140 mm Hg using intravenous antihypertensives. Traditional medical measures utilized in the treatment of ICH include therapies that directly or indirectly treat intracranial pressure such as mannitol, external ventricular drainage, and antiepileptics; therapies that protect the penumbra adjacent to the ICH such as maintaining normal blood sugars and body temperature; and administration of hemostatic agents to reduce the incidence of rehemorrhage.

Mannitol has been shown to improve mortality in ICH patients, primarily by acting as an osmotic agent that lowers intracranial pressure caused by the hematoma.[45] Because of issues of mannitol failure and rebound increases in ICP, new osmolar agents have been investigated, including hypertonic saline, which can be given in 30-ml boluses of 23.4% saline as needed for refractory intracranial pressure documented via an ICP monitor. Such treatments can lower ICP, with the effect lasting 15 hours in our hands. Randomized studies are needed for these alternative osmolar agents.

External ventricular drains (EVDs) are placed for ICH cases with associated IVH that has led to an obstructive hydrocephalus. Unfortunately, in the presence of a large amount of IVH, the EVD will fill with blood, which will clot and occlude the EVD frequently. For these cases, we administer 5 mg of intraventricular tissue plasminogen activator (tPA) twice a day for 5 days, in a fashion similar to previous reports.[46] After each administration, the EVD is clamped for 30 minutes if the intracranial pressure (ICP) transduced by the EVD does not elevate, in order to prevent the tPA from leaking out of the ventricles. We have experienced no complications from the use

of intraventricular tPA in treating EVDs occluded with blood products, although it is not our policy to use this therapy in the presence of an unsecured vascular lesion.

Convulsive seizures occur in 5% to 10% of patients with supratentorial ICH.[47] Because seizures increase intracranial pressure, prophylactic antiepileptic drugs (AEDs) have traditionally been given to patients with lobar ICH, the group of ICH patients with the largest seizure risk.[43] However, seizures have been shown to not be associated with poor outcome after ICH[47] and a recent retrospective analysis of 295 ICH patients found that AEDs were initiated on 8% of patients without documented seizure and that initiation of AEDs was robustly associated with poor outcome even after adjusting for other known predictors of outcome after ICH.[48] The mechanism by which AEDs impact outcome is unclear, but it may be related to sedation or cardiovascular side effects of AEDs. A randomized trial may therefore be warranted to determine whether prophylactic AEDs are indicated for lobar ICH patients, or if AED use is only appropriate when ICH patients have had a seizure but not as a prophylactic measure.

Fever of 37.5°C or higher is seen in over 90% of supratentorial ICH patients.[49] The incidence, duration, and magnitude of fever are even greater in patients with ventricular hemorrhage.[49] The duration of fever is associated with poor long-term outcome.[49] Therefore, we aggressively treat fever with acetaminophen and cooling blankets, targeting a temperature of ≤37.5°C.

Hyperglycemia in nondiabetic patients and worsening of baseline blood sugars in diabetic patients both occur after ICH.[50] Regardless of whether there is pre-existing diabetes, hyperglycemia is a predictor of poor outcome after supratentorial ICH.[50] We utilize intravenous insulin infusions titrated to maintain blood glucose between 80 and 110 mg/dl, rather than treating high blood glucose levels with subcutaneous insulin based on a sliding scale. Although this type of strict blood sugar control has been shown to reduce mortality, particularly due to septic end organ failure, in surgical intensive care units,[51] a study focusing on the outcomes associated with strict blood sugar control in neurosurgical patients is still needed.

Given the evidence that ongoing bleeding can occur for several hours after the onset of ICH, it is plausible that ultra-early hemostatic therapy may minimize hematoma volume and improve outcome by preventing early worsening related to hematoma growth, as well as late deterioration related to perihematoma edema and mass effect. Replacement therapies such as fresh frozen plasma, prothrombin complex concentrate, and factor IX concentrate are used to treat bleeding in coagulopathic ICH patients, such as those who take coumadin, but would not enhance hemostasis in patients with normal coagulation. Human and recombinant factors VIII and IX are used as replacement therapy for patients with hemophilia A or B, respectively, but, similarly, a strong procoagulant effect in patients with normal levels of these factors would not be expected. Cryoprecipitate enhances hemostasis in patients with hypofibrinogenemia, and desmopressin diacetate arginine vasopressin (ddAVP) is used in patients with primary or acquired platelet disorders.

In patients with normal coagulation, the most feasible hemostatic agents for ultraearly ICH therapy include the antifibrinolytic amino acids aminocaproic acid and tranexamic acid, aprotinin, and activated recombinant factor VII. The amino acids have a risk of cerebral ischemia, while aprotinin can cause hypersensitivity reactions and arterial or venous thrombosis, so attention in ICH patients has focused on factor VII. Factor VII, of which only 1% circulates in the active form, forms a complex with exposed tissue factor in the subendothelial layer of a damaged vessel wall, activating the hemostatic mechanism locally to form a hemostatic plug. In the randomized, phase-III fVIIa for Acute Hemorrhagic Stroke Treatment (FAST) trial, 841 ICH patients were randomized to receive placebo or intravenous recombinant activated factor VII administered within 4 hours of the onset of symptoms. Recombinant, activated factor VII reduced the growth in ICH volume at 24 hours from 26% in the placebo group to 11% in the group receiving the higher of two factor VII doses studied, but there was no significant difference among the groups in mortality or in the proportion of patients with poor clinical outcomes.[52]

There has been interest in neuroprotectant medications to protect the at-risk penumbra surrounding the ICH. A randomized phase III clinical trial of NXY-059, a free radical–trapping neuroprotectant, studied 607 patients and found that, while NXY-059 was associated with slightly less hematoma growth than placebo, the drug had no effect on long-term mortality or disability.[53] Neuroprotectants that have shown promise in the laboratory whose benefit remains to be proven clinically include the GABA antagonist muscimol and the NMDA receptor antagonists MK801 and D-(E)-4-(3-phodphonoprop-2-enyl)-piperazine-2-carboxylic acid (D-CPP-ene), which have been shown to increase tolerance of larger hematomas, reduce edema 24 hours after ICH, and protect adjacent white matter in animal models.[54]

There are other medical agents that some have suggested for ICH but have not proven to be beneficial. A randomized study following 93 patients with ICH showed no statistical difference in neurologic outcome in patients who received decadron, with the group receiving decadron exhibiting 11 times more complications than the control group, including hyperglycemia, septicemia, and gastrointestinal bleeding.[55]

Hyperventilation is not recommended for ICH patients, since homeostatic mechanisms adjust to the lowered pH rapidly and since the cerebral vasoconstriction causes increased ischemia and worse outcomes.

Parenchymal ICP monitors are infrequently used in our institutions for ICP monitoring in ICH patients, as we prefer to place ventricular catheters in ICH patients (particularly ICH associated with IVH) because the combination of ICP monitoring and ventricular drainage to reduce ICP can be useful. In addition, a focal parenchymal ICP monitor can lend a false sense of security, in that a hematoma typically causes a variety of focal pressure gradients, such that the pressure transduced in the right frontal lobe, where the monitor is typically placed, will not always reflect the pressure near the hematoma or in the brain stem.

Medical versus Surgical Management

There have been 10 randomized prospective clinical trials comparing medical versus surgical management of ICH. The number of patients enrolled in these trials has ranged from 20 to 1033. The results are summarized in Table 69-1. Three trials showed somewhat better outcomes with medical

treatment, with none achieving statistical significance in long-term outcomes, while seven trials showed somewhat better outcomes with surgical treatment, with two achieving statistical significance in long-term outcomes (Table 69-1). The largest trial by far was the International Surgical Trial in Intracerebral Hemorrhage (STICH), the results of which were released in January 2005.[56] The STICH trial showed that surgical intervention within 24 hours of randomization offered no benefit in survival or prognosis-based indices for patients with lobar, basal ganglia, or thalamic ICH measuring greater than 2 cm in diameter and a Glasgow Coma Score (GCS) of 5 or more.[56] Analysis of subgroups defined by age, GCS, ICH laterality, ICH location, ICH volume, distance from cortical surface, method of evacuation, motor and speech deficits, anticoagulation treatment, and country found that the only subgroups to show heterogeneity of outcome were those defined by distance of the ICH from the cortical surface, with a favorable outcome from early surgery more likely if the hematoma was 1 cm or less from the cortical surface (absolute benefit 8%; $p = 0.02$).[56] Of note, of patients randomized to initial conservative treatment, 26% went on to require surgery a few days after randomization due to clinical deterioration, and the outcome for this group was poorer than for patients who had early surgery or who were maintained on conservative management.[56] Thus the STICH trial suggests that a significant benefit for early operative intervention existed only for patients with superficial hematomas. These findings will be confirmed in the recently commenced STICH II trial, which will prospectively test the benefits of surgery in lobar ICH patients with hematomas extending to within 1 cm of the cortical surface without intraventricular extension. For deeper ICH, until factors are identified that can predict which patients will go on to experience clinical deterioration, the results of the STICH trial suggest that operative intervention should be reserved for patients who experience clinical deterioration, at which time surgery will improve outcomes relative to not operating but will unfortunately not restore outcomes to what they would have been had the deterioration not occurred.

Overall, considerable variability remains in ICH management among physicians worldwide. Recently reported operation rates for spontaneous supratentorial ICH spanned a wide range, including 2% in Hungary, 20% in the United States, 50% in Germany and Japan, and 74% in Lithuania.[57]

The choice of intervention is influenced by the location of the ICH. We routinely operate on lobar ICH associated with a structural lesion such as an AVM or tumor that is surgically accessible in noneloquent cortex. In stable patients, we avoid operating on dominant hemisphere lobar ICH near Broca's or Wernicke's. Operations are also performed on otherwise healthy patients with large lobar ICH who are clinically deteriorating.

The basal ganglia is the most common site of ICH, representing 60% of hypertensive ICH, and basal ganglia ICH is associated with a 50% mortality rate.[29] The majority of these basal ganglia hemorrhages occur in the putamen. In an early study by Kanaya and Kuuoda, patients who received medical treatment for basal ganglia hemorrhages less than 30 ml in volume fared better than those treated surgically.[58] A follow-up study by Tan et al. randomized 34 patients with basal ganglia hematomas greater in volume than 30 ml into surgical and nonsurgical treatment groups. No difference in

Table 69-1 Summary of Prospective Randomized Controlled Trials Comparing Surgery to Medical Treatment for Intracerebral Hemorrhage

| Author | Year | ICH Location | Surgery Method | Time Window from ICH to Surgery (hours) | NUMBER OF PATIENTS | | OUTCOME AT 6 MONTHS | | | | | | Odds Ratio for Death or Dependence with Surgery at End of Follow-up (95% CI; p-value) |
| | | | | | | | % OF PATIENTS INDEPENDENT | | % OF PATIENTS DEPENDENT | | % DEAD | | |
					M	S	M	S	M	S	M	S	
McKissock et al.[90]	1961	All	Craniotomy	72	91	89	34	20	15	15	51	65	0.49 (0.25–0.96; p = 0.2)
Juvela et al.[91]	1989	All	Craniotomy	48	26	26	19	4	42	50	39	46	5.68 (0.62–52.43; p = 0.2)
Auer et al.[60]	1989	All	Endoscopic	48	50	50	26	44	4	14	70	42	0.45 (0.19–1.04; p<0.05)
Batjer et al.[92]	1990	Putamen	Craniotomy	24	9	8	22	25	0	25	78	50	0.55 (0.06–4.91; p = 0.5)
Morgenstern et al.[67]	1998	Lobar and putamen	Craniotomy	12	17	17	41	35	35	47	24	18	0.52 (0.12–2.25; p = 0.5)
Zucarrello et al.[93]	1999	All	Craniotomy	24	11	9	36	56	36	22	18	22	0.46 (0.08–2.76; p>0.05)
Cheng et al.[94]	2001	All	Craniotomy	48	231	263	NS	NS	NS	NS	NS	NS	0.66 (0.46–0.95; p = 0.4)
Teernstra et al.[63]	2003	All	Stereotactic	72	33	36	10	11	88	75	59	56	1.52 (0.31–7.35; p = 0.4)
Hattori et al.[95]	2004	Putamen	Stereotactic	24	121	121	NS	NS	NS	NS	NS	NS	0.47 (0.28–0.78; p = 0.01)
Mendelow et al.[56]	2005	All	All	24	530	503	NS	NS	NS	NS	37	36	0.91 (0.65–1.25; p = 0.4)

Note: Dependence defined as Barthel index <60, score 3 to 5 on the Rankin scale, or 1 to 3 on the Glasgow Outcome Scale.
CI, confidence interval; ICH, intracerebral hemorrhage; M, medical treatment; NS, not stated; S, surgical treatment.

outcome was reported at 1-year follow-up.[59] Although stereotactic and endoscopic techniques minimize surgically morbidity from basal ganglia hematoma evacuation, Auer et al. failed to demonstrate any benefit from stereotactically guided endoscopic basal ganglia hematoma evacuation.[60] While recent studies[61-63] have shown that stereotactic aspiration of basal ganglia hematomas can aspirate over 80% of the hematoma, this volume reduction has not proven to be of benefit, perhaps due to the ability of residual blood products to trigger persistent and consequential perihematoma edema.

In the end, complete surgical clot evacuation through open craniotomy may prove beneficial if the proper patient group is selected and the surgery is performed by a group experienced in the surgical approach to the basal ganglia. A study by Kaya et al. 2 years after the study by Tan et al. compared conservative medical treatment to open craniotomy for putaminal hematomas greater than 30 mL volume.[61] The surgical group had 34% mortality at 6 months, compared to 63.1% in the medically treated group. When subdivided by initial neurologic grade, patients in stupor or semicoma without herniation signs fared better with nonsurgical treatment, while patients in semicoma with herniation signs fared better with surgical treatment. The more favorable results for surgery obtained by Kaya et al. compared to Tan et al. may reflect improved ability to evacuate basal ganglia hematomas safely through open craniotomies during the 2 years that transpired between the studies. Figure 69-3 illustrates results when we used an algorithm similar to that followed by Kaya et al. in the management of two different basal ganglia hematomas.

Thalamic ICH is almost always managed medically with external ventricular drain placement when third ventricular outlet obstruction is present. Anatomically, the thalamus is difficult to access safely. There is a high risk of causing neurologic deficits from the parietal lobe, internal capsule, or transcallosal transventricular dissection when approaching thalamic hematomas. Regardless of whether the approach is open craniotomy, stereotactic, or endoscopic, the risk of damaging adjacent functional thalamic tissue often precludes a surgical approach. The only study comparing surgical versus medical treatment for thalamic ICH showed no benefit to endoscopic evacuation compared to medical treatment.[60]

Most patients with pontine hematoma are managed conservatively due to the difficulty in achieving safe surgical access to the brain stem and the morbidity associated with the brain-stem manipulation that is required for hematoma evacuation. The mortality from pontine ICH is estimated to be around 18% during hospitalization[64] and 69% at 1 year.[65] Most mortality is associated with hypertensive pontine ICH and large paramedian pontine ICH, with pontine ICH from cavernous malformation and lateral tegmental pontine ICH having a better outcome.[64,65] Uncontrolled case series have documented successful stereotactic aspiration of pontine hematomas, but the effect on outcomes remains uncertain.

Cerebellar ICH is unique in that the posterior fossa is unable to tolerate large changes in volume without causing significant brain-stem compression, which can lead to rapid and often fatal deterioration. A second source of morbidity and mortality in these patients is hydrocephalus when the hematoma compresses the fourth ventricle. Although the use of external ventricular drainage would seem a reasonable, less invasive means of addressing the hydrocephalus, there is concern about upward cerebellar herniation and rostral brain-stem compression if surgical decompression of the posterior fossa is not performed simultaneously. Cohen et al. studied 37 patients with cerebellar ICH and found that patients with hematomas less than 3 cm in maximal diameter had 100% good outcomes, compared to 57% of these patients who underwent surgery.[66] On the other hand, patients with hematomas larger than 3 cm in maximal diameter who were not operated on immediately had a good outcome in only 33% of cases, compared to a good outcome in 50% of surgical patients with hematomas of this size.[66] Other studies have confirmed 3 cm in diameter as the recommended threshold for surgical intervention for cerebellar hematomas (Fig. 69-4), with an external ventricular drain placed if hydrocephalus is present.

Regarding the timing of surgery, Morgenstern et al. demonstrated improved neurologic function regardless of hematoma location if ICH patients were operated on within 12 hours of the onset of symptoms.[67] In a follow-up study evaluating ultraearly surgery at less than 4 hours after the onset of symptoms, they found an increased rehemorrhage rate associated with increased mortality, with rebleeding occurring in 40% of the patients operated on within 4 hours compared to 12% of the patients operated on at 12 hours.[68] These results suggest that the optimum timing for surgical clot evacuation may be within the 4- to 12-hour window after symptoms begin.

As a result of the paucity of data, guidelines for ICH management written in 1999 by a panel of experts commissioned by the American Heart Association (AHA) were largely limited to grade C recommendations based on case series and nonrandomized cohort studies.[43] The only grade A or B recommendations (based on randomized trials) were to use head CT for ICH diagnosis; to avoid corticosteroid therapy for ICH; to avoid surgical evacuation in patients with a Glasgow Coma Scale of 4 or less, or ICH volume below 10 cm^3; and to consider surgical evacuation in young patients with moderate or large lobar hemorrhages who are clinically deteriorating. Surgical evacuation was recommended for the following three categories of patients: (1) patients with cerebellar hemorrhages greater than 3 cm in diameter who have brain-stem compression and hydrocephalus or who are neurologically deteriorating (grade C recommendation); (2) ICH associated with a structural lesion such as an AVM or tumor that is surgically accessible (grade C recommendation); and (3) young patients with moderate or large lobar ICH who are clinically deteriorating (grade B recommendation). More recently, in 2006 and 2007, the American Stroke Association (ASA) Stroke Council[69] and the European Stroke Organization (EUSI)[70] released guidelines in which they did not recommend routine evacuation of supratentorial ICH by craniotomy within 96 hours of ictus. Both guidelines recommend surgery for patients presenting with lobar ICH within 1 cm of the surface, particularly for those with good neurologic status who are deteriorating clinically. Guidelines acknowledge that operative removal within 12 hours, particularly with minimally invasive methods, has the most evidence for beneficial effect and could be considered for deep ICH causing mass effect. Guidelines also noted that very early craniotomy might be associated with an increased risk of recurrent ICH.

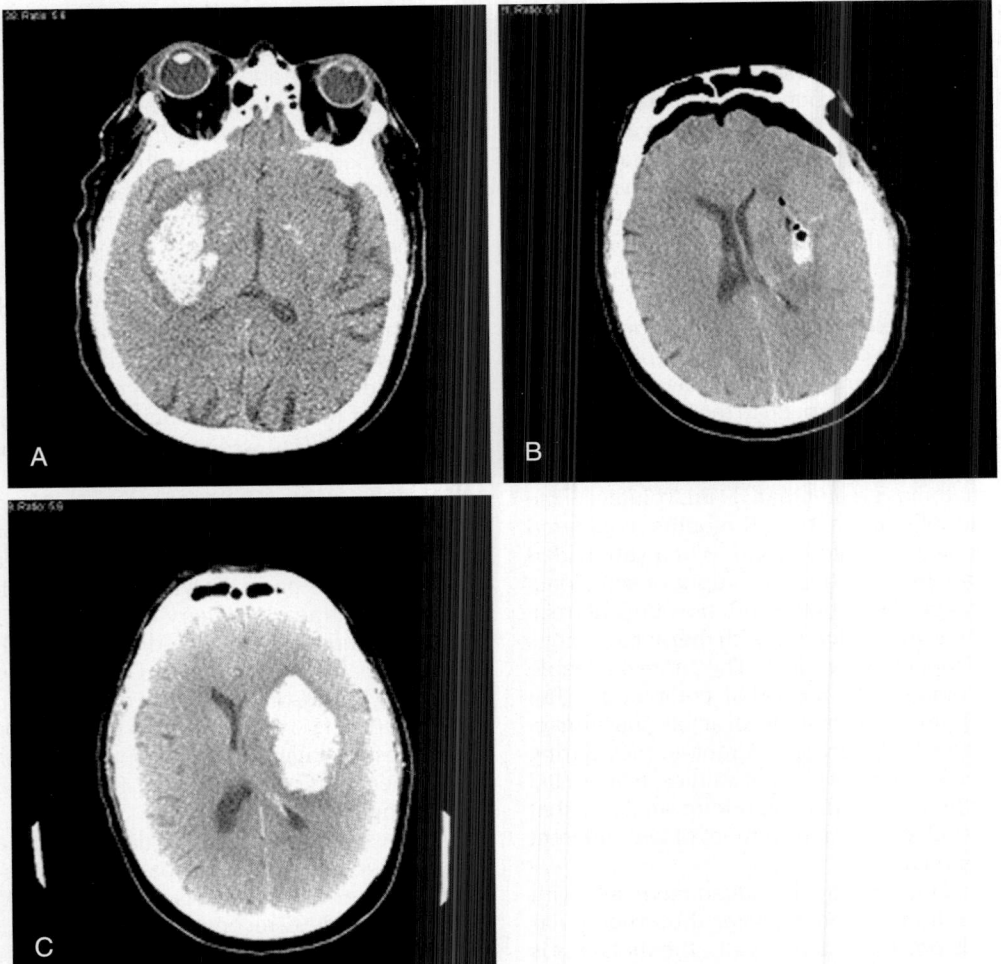

FIGURE 69-3 Management of hypertensive basal ganglia hemorrhages based on size of clot and other radiographic and clinical findings. Kaya et al.[61] suggest that patients with basal ganglia hematomas larger than 30 cm³ who exhibit diminished mental status and radiographic signs of herniation fare better with surgical rather than medical treatment. A and B, Sixty-two-year-old male with a history of hypertension presented with right hemiparesis and aphasia. CT scan (A) identified a left basal ganglia hemorrhage measuring 6 cm (AP) × 3 cm (LR) × 8 cuts (4 cm SI) = 144 cm³, causing 9-mm midline shift, and effacement of the cisterns. We went to the operating room and evacuated the hematoma through a left frontal craniotomy, eliminating much of the midline shift and herniation (B), consistent with recommendations of Kaya et al.[61] Unfortunately, the patient succumbed to an aspiration pneumonia 45 days after his surgery. (C) Sixty-nine-year-old male with a history of hypertension presented with left arm weakness but intact mental status. CT scan (C) identified a right basal ganglia hemorrhage measuring 5 cm (AP) × 2 cm (LR) × 7 cuts (3.5 cm SI) = 35 cm³ causing 2-mm midline shift with no cisternal effacement. He was managed conservatively, consistent with recommendations of Kaya et al.,[61] and remained awake and conversant with stable left arm weakness.

The degree of neurologic deterioration must also be considered before recommending surgery, as one study of lobar ICH evacuated in patients with a mental status of stupor or worse or midline shift greater than 1 cm with cisternal obliteration showed that 22% of operative patients regained independence afterward, 22% remained severely disabled, and 56% died.[71] All patients who had absent papillary, corneal, or oculocephalic reflexes combined with extensor posturing died, indicating a level of severity beyond salvage surgically.

Specific Surgical Techniques

CRANIOTOMY

Lobar hemorrhages are evacuated using craniotomies and corticectomies centered over the hematoma, with sparing of eloquent tissue. The head should be positioned so that the trajectory to the clot is as vertical as possible. Self-retaining brain retractors are attached to the Mayfield fixation device. After the corticectomy, superficial hematomas can be accessed by using a combination of bipolar cautery and small suction tips until the hematoma cavity is entered. Once in the hematoma, tumor forceps or a pituitary biter can be used to remove solid portions of the hematoma. Semisolid portions of the hematoma can be removed using suction tips. Hemostasis can then be achieved with a combination of topical hemostatic agents such as Avitene (microfibrillar collagen, Alcon, Humacao, PR), FloSeal (gelatin matrix thrombin sealant, Baxter Healthcare, Deerfield, IL), hydrogen peroxide–soaked cotton balls, thrombin-soaked Gelfoam (gelatin sponge, Baxter), and Surgicel (oxidized cellulose, Ethicon, Somerville, NJ). The systolic blood pressure can be raised 10 to 20 points before closure to identify any potential bleeding sources. The mass effect is typically

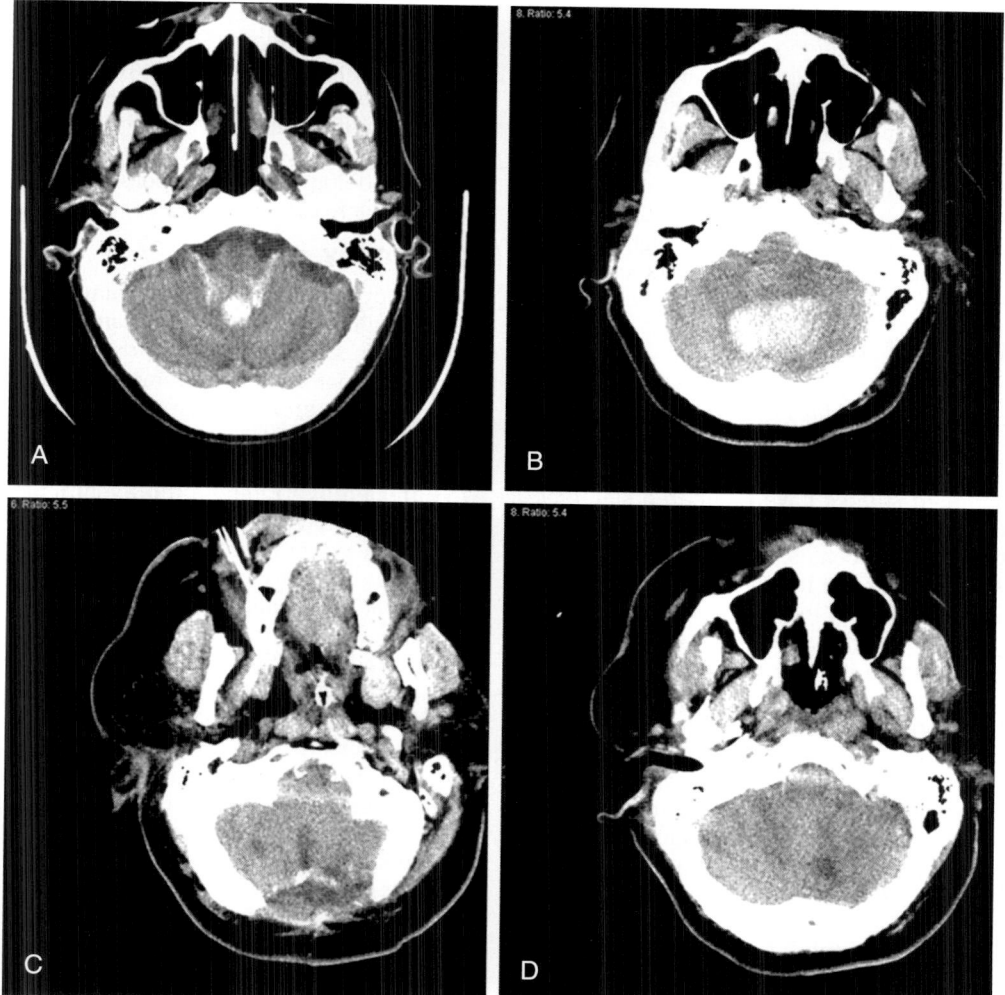

FIGURE 69-4 Management of cerebellar ICH depends on clinical status of patient and size of blood clot. A, A 75-year-old man with a history of hypertension presented with headache, nausea, vomiting, and syncope. Head CT identified a 1.7 cm (AP) × 1.5 cm (LR) × 2 cuts (1 cm SI) vermian cerebellar hemorrhage extending into the fourth ventricle, causing moderate hydrocephalus. Because of his intact mental status and because the hematoma was less than 3 cm in maximal diameter, he was managed medically with an admission to the intensive care unit and an external ventricular drain placed for the hydrocephalus. The hydrocephalus subsequently resolved, the drain was discontinued, and he was discharged from the hospital 10 days later. B to D, A 65-year-old woman with a history of hypertension collapsed. She was unresponsive to painful stimuli with intact brain-stem reflexes in the emergency room. Head CT (B) identified a 4.6 cm (AP) × 3.1 cm (LR) × 6 cuts (3 cm SI) cerebellar hematoma centered in the dentate nucleus, but favoring the left over the right cerebellar hemisphere, causing moderate hydrocephalus. Because of her clinical condition, she was brought emergently to the operating room, where a suboccipital craniectomy (C) and cerebellar hematoma evacuation (D) were performed. Unfortunately, she did not regain neurologic function and care was withdrawn by her family 1 week later. These two cases illustrate the finding documented before that 3 cm in maximal diameter is the cutoff after which cerebellar hematomas are likely to impair mental status and will likely require immediate surgery in order to have any chance for clinical improvement.[66]

relieved after hematoma removal, and the bone flap can be replaced. For deeper lobar hematomas, intraoperative ultrasound can be used for hematoma localization and to verify complete removal of the hematoma. Ultrasound can also be used to guide placement of a ventriculostomy catheter into the hematoma cavity. Self-retaining retractors can then be placed alongside the ventriculostomy and a 1-cm corticectomy can be opened down to the clot by following the ventriculostomy catheter, thereby minimizing damage to nearby cortex.

For putaminal hemorrhages, two approaches can be used: transtemporal or transsylvian. The transsylvian approach involves a pterional craniotomy, sylvian dissection under the microscope, and a 0.5- to 1-cm long corticectomy along the insular cortical surface in an area determined by

the largest and closest point of hematoma on the CT scan. This is followed by clot evacuation and hemostasis. In the hands of an experienced surgeon who can dissect the middle cerebral branches in the insular cortex, the trans-sylvian approach puts the smallest amount of brain at risk, since the insular cortical point of entry is closest to the putamen. For putaminal hematomas that extend significantly into the temporal lobe, the transtemporal approach can be used.

Thalamic and pontine hemorrhages are not evacuated with open craniotomies, due to the amount of intact cerebral tissue put at risk during such a procedure. The stereotactic or endoscopic procedures described below have been somewhat successful in evacuating pontine hemorrhages, but a benefit has yet to be shown in a large randomized trial.

Cerebellar hemorrhages are evacuated using a suboccipital craniotomy for medial hemorrhages, or a paramedian straight incision for unilateral cerebellar hemorrhage. Because the posterior fossa has less room to accommodate any postoperative bleeding than supratentorial sites after evacuating lobar ICH, we prefer doing a suboccipital craniectomy and not restoring the bone, which better accommodates posterior fossa bleeding and swelling than a bone flap craniotomy, an advantage that often outweighs the disadvantage of craniectomy headaches. A ventriculostomy is placed to relieve hydrocephalus.

STEREOTACTIC ASPIRATION

Benes et al. first reported the use of stereotactic hematoma drainage in 1965, with limited success.[72] With improvement in techniques, including administration of fibrinolytics, the success rate has improved. Although no randomized, prospective, controlled studies have compared stereotactic aspiration with craniotomy and conservative therapy, studies show favorable outcomes, especially with deep-seated lesions such as those in the basal ganglia or pons. Use of a stereotactic frame or the endoscopy and frameless stereotaxy approaches described below are less invasive procedures than open craniotomies, but still require that the patient be intubated if not already so, because ICH patients often have too tenuous a mental status to tolerate the sedation and lack of airway access associated with awake stereotactic procedures. Honda et al. retrospectively compared stereotactic aspiration and medical therapy for thalamic hemorrhages.[73] Patients with hematomas smaller than 2.5 cm in diameter had significantly higher activities of daily living (ADL) scores with aspiration. In another study, 71 ICH patients were randomized into a group that received stereotactic aspiration and administration of urokinase and another group that received systemic medical management only.[63] Although stereotactic aspiration reduced hematoma volume by 18 ml over 7 days, compared to 7 ml of reduction in the control group, no difference in morbidity or mortality was noted at 180 days.[63] The volume reduction achieved by stereotactic aspiration may be less beneficial than the more complete hematoma evacuation achieved by a craniotomy because residual hematoma can still cause considerable edema and mass effect. To make hematomas more amenable to stereotactic aspiration, various techniques have been incorporated into the stereotactic hematoma drainage, including (1) repeated injection of urokinase or recombinant tissue plasminogen activator into the hematoma to liquefy the clot and render it amenable to subsequent aspiration, and (2) equipment aimed at physical fragmentation of the clot like systems based on the Archimedes screw,[74] devices using high-pressure fluid irrigation,[75] ultrasonic aspirators,[76] or the Nucleotome probe.[77] The lack of direct visualization and the risk of rebleeding may still limit this technique to patients whose neurologic condition warrants drainage rather than medical treatment alone but whose hemorrhages are deep and whose overall medical condition precludes open craniotomy, especially during the hyperacute phase of hemorrhage. The stereotactic treatment of intracerebral hematoma by means of a plasminogen activator (SICHPA) multicenter randomized trial was published in 2003 and showed a slight but statistically insignificant benefit on survival and independence of

stereotactic hematoma removal after liquefaction by means of plasminogen activator.[63] These encouraging results have led to the ongoing minimally invasive surgery plus tissue plasminogen activator for intracerebral hemorrhage evacuation (MISTIE) trial, which will study different doses of recombinant tissue plasminogen activator to better refine the methodology and will hopefully enroll enough patients to achieve a result with statistical significance.[78]

ENDOSCOPY

Endoscopy represents another minimally invasive means of ICH draining, which, unlike stereotaxy, is not limited to the chronic stage of ICH. In a recent technical note, four pontine hematomas were removed using a 1.7-mm fiberscope placed through a burr hole 3 cm from the midline at the bregma.[79] After entering the third ventricle through the foramen of Monro, patients with acute hydrocephalus were treated by forming a third ventriculostomy, followed by slight dilation of the aqueduct of Sylvius. The guide tube was advanced into pontine areas found to have yellow discoloration. Hematoma was evacuated by repeated rinsing with physiologic saline. Hemostasis was achieved using a KTP laser. An external ventricular drain was left in place, and flushed with 6000 U of urokinase 3 hours after surgery. The urokinase must be administered because only liquid blood products could be washed out of the pons using the endoscope, and areas of clot had to be treated with intraventricular urokinase. The procedure typically took 1 hour. Advantages of endoscopic treatment over stereotaxy and open craniotomy were rapidity of the procedure and ability to treat associated hydrocephalus. Ability to anticoagulate is an additional advantage over stereotaxy.

FRAMELESS STEREOTAXY AND INTRAOPERATIVE MRI

Tyler and Mandbybur reported on 10 patients harboring intracerebral hematomas who were treated by frameless stereotactic means without fiducial markers.[80] Using an intraoperative MRI scanner, these patients underwent frameless stereotactic evacuation of 70% to 90% of each clot, with no complications or rehemorrhages. All patients showed some improvement. Similarly, Bernays et al. reported complete evacuation in 62% of their 13 ICH patients treated with a specially designed artifact-free aspiration cannula using intraoperative MRI.[81] No rebleeding was demonstrated and neurologic function improved in 11 of 12 patients.

Long-Term Outcome

Recently, Becker et al. pointed out that the most important variable predicting poor outcome in ICH patients is the level of provided medical support. Perception of futility of aggressive therapy leads to early withdrawal of medical support, which is less likely in ICH patients who are surgically treated.[82] It may be worth studying if ICH patients have better outcomes in high volume centers that frequently treat ICH patients medically and surgically, a phenomenon demonstrated in the operative management of unruptured aneurysms.[83]

Reported 30-day mortality for lobar, basal ganglia, thalamic, pontine, and cerebellar ICH have been 13%, 50%, 23%, 13%, and 16%, respectively.[84,85] Lobar ICH has consistently been shown to have the lowest mortality and best long-term outcomes, and basal ganglia ICH the worst. One of the sources of debate in long-term post-ICH management remains when it is safe to resume anticoagulation. In one study, epidemiologic data from the medical literature was used to generate a Markov-state transition decision model, in which effectiveness of therapy was measured in quality-adjusted life-years.[86] The authors found that, for patients with prior lobar ICH, withholding anticoagulation therapy indefinitely led to the best outcome regardless of the indication for anticoagulation, leading to an improvement of life expectancy by 1.9 quality-adjusted life-years. On the other hand, patients with deep interhemispheric ICH, because of a lower risk of recurrent ICH due to the lack of amyloid angiopathy in this group, should never receive anticoagulation for nonvalvular atrial fibrillation, but should resume anticoagulation with aspirin when the risk of thromboembolic event is moderately higher and with coumadin when

the risk of thromboembolic events is in the highest range. Both the ASA Stroke Council[69] and the EUSI guidelines[70] recommend that warfarin anticoagulation can be resumed in patients with a high risk of thromboembolism (artificial heart valve) 7 to 14 days after the onset of ICH.[87]

The overall long-term recurrence rate of ICH has been estimated to be 2.4% per year, and is 3.8-fold higher after lobar ICH caused by cerebral amyloid angiopathy (Fig. 69-5) than it is with hypertensive deep ICH.[88] Factors that are positive predictors of recurrent hemorrhage include age greater than 65 years and male sex.[89] Use of anticoagulation after ICH triples the risk of recurrent hemorrhage.[89]

Conclusion

Clinical evidence suggests the importance of achieving three goals in managing ICH patients: stop further bleeding, remove hematoma when appropriate, and controlling cerebral

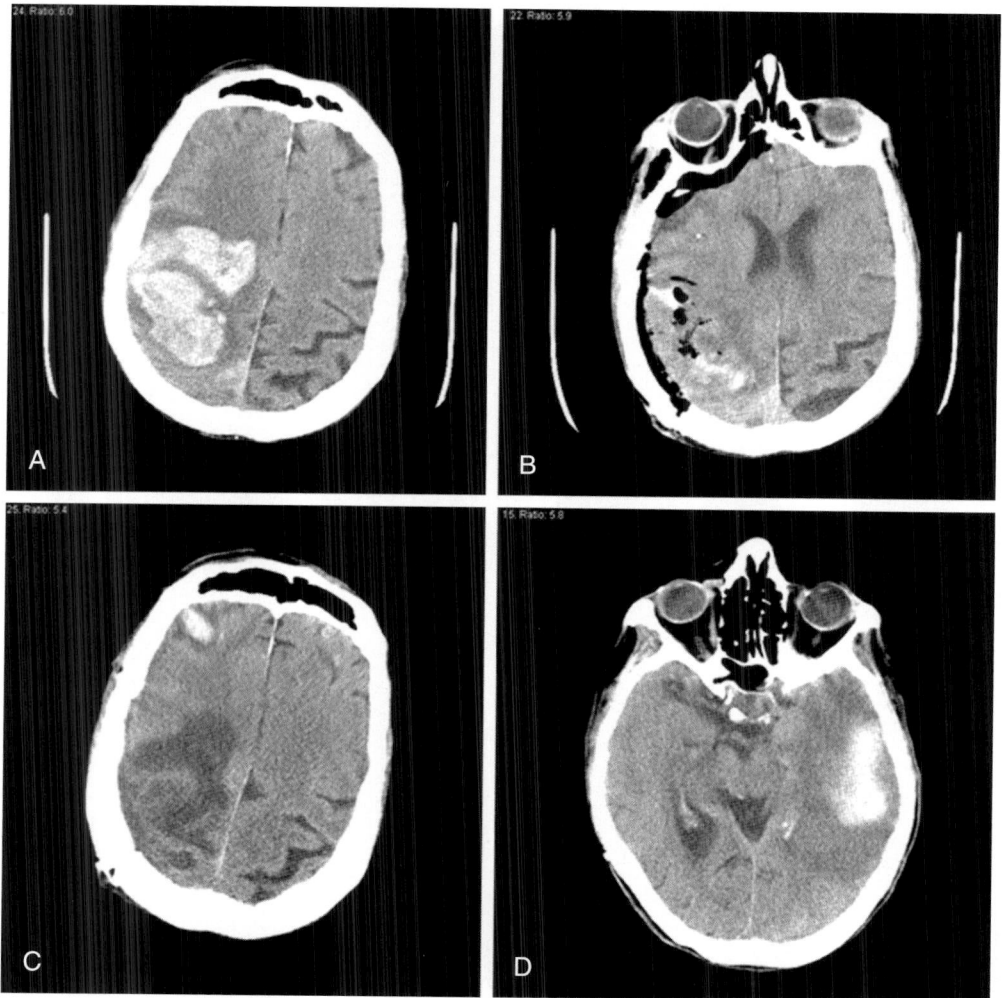

FIGURE 69-5 Amyloid angiopathy causes high risk of recurrent ICH. A 77-year-old woman presented to our institution with left hemiparesis. CT scan (A) showed 7 cm (AP) × 6 cm (LR) × 11 cuts (5.5 cm SI) = 231 cm³ right frontoparietal hematoma with surrounding edema, causing 8 mm of midline shift. She was brought to the operating room, where a right frontoparietal craniotomy enabled nearly complete hematoma evacuation and resolution of midline shift (B). Pathologic analysis of the clot confirmed the diagnosis of amyloid angiopathy. She was discharged from the hospital with some improvement in left-sided strength. Unfortunately, 1 month later, she was found unresponsive. CT scan showed encephalomalacia in the area of the evacuated right frontoparietal hematoma and two new hematomas—a 1.8 cm (AP) × 0.7 cm (LR) × 3 cuts (1.5 cm SI) = 2 cm³ right frontal hematoma (C) and a 4.9 cm (AP) × 1.9 cm (LR) × 7 cuts (3.5 cm SI) = 33 cm³ left temporal hematoma (D). She was managed medically because her history of prior ICH and the bilateral nature of her most recent ICH meant that surgery would have a high morbidity. She remained unresponsive, and was eventually discharged to a nursing home after a tracheostomy and gastrotomy tube were placed.

perfusion pressure. While several agents have been shown to slightly reduce hematoma expansion, none of these have shown clinical benefit. And the STICH trial raised questions about the role of early operative intervention in ICH patients. Because the outcome after ICH is still extremely poor, ongoing trials will be needed to identify agents capable of exerting a more powerful effect on preventing further bleeding or protecting the at-risk penumbra in a manner that leads to improved outcomes. Another key area of research will be determining which subset of ICH patients benefit from early operative intervention, an issue that will be addressed for lobar ICH patients during the upcoming STICH II trial.

KEY REFERENCES

Cheng XC, Wu JS, Zhou XP. The randomized multicentric prospective controlled trial in the standardized treatment of hypertensive intracerebral hematomas: the comparison of surgical therapeutic outcomes with conservative therapy. *Chin J Clin Neurosci.* 2001;9:365-368.

Hattori N, Katayama Y, Maya Y, Gatherer A. Impact of stereotactic hematoma evacuation on activities of daily living during the chronic period following spontaneous putaminal hemorrhage: a randomized study. *J Neurosurg.* 2004;101:417-420.

Kaya RA, Turkmenoglu O, Ziyal IM, et al. The effects on prognosis of surgical treatment of hypertensive putaminal hematomas through transsylvian transinsular approach. *Surg Neurol.* 2003;59:176-183: discussion 183.

Mayer SA, Brun NC, Begtrup K, et al. Efficacy and safety of recombinant activated factor VII for acute intracerebral hemorrhage. *N Engl J Med.* 2008;358:2127-2137.

Mendelow AD, Gregson BA, Fernandes HM, et al. Early surgery versus initial conservative treatment in patients with spontaneous supratentorial intracerebral haematomas in the International Surgical Trial in Intracerebral Haemorrhage (STICH): a randomised trial. *Lancet.* 2005;365:387-397.

Morgan T, Zuccarello M, Narayan R, et al. Preliminary findings of the minimally-invasive surgery plus rtPA for intracerebral hemorrhage evacuation (MISTIE) clinical trial. *Acta Neurochir Suppl.* 2008;105:147-151.

Morgenstern LB, Frankowski RF, Shedden P, et al. Surgical treatment for intracerebral hemorrhage (STICH): a single-center, randomized clinical trial. *Neurology.* 1998;51:1359-1363.

Salvati M, Cervoni L, Raco A, Delfini R. Spontaneous cerebellar hemorrhage: clinical remarks on 50 cases. *Surg Neurol.* 2001;55:156-161: discussion 161.

Tan SH, Ng PY, Yeo TT, et al. Hypertensive basal ganglia hemorrhage: a prospective study comparing surgical and nonsurgical management. *Surg Neurol.* 2001;56:287-292:discussion 292-293.

Teernstra OP, Evers SM, Lodder J, et al. Stereotactic treatment of intracerebral hematoma by means of a plasminogen activator: a multicenter randomized controlled trial (SICHPA). *Stroke.* 2003;34:968-974.

Zuccarello M, Brott T, Derex L, et al. Early surgical treatment for supratentorial intracerebral hemorrhage: a randomized feasibility study. *Stroke.* 1999;30:1833-1839.

Numbered references appear on Expert Consult.

CHAPTER 70

Surgical Management of Cerebellar Stroke—Hemorrhage and Infarction

VIKRAM V. NAYAR • ARTHUR L. DAY

Cerebellar stroke, either hemorrhage or infarction, often presents with poorly lateralizing symptoms, and its diagnosis is often delayed, especially when compared to strokes occurring in the supratentorial region. Both kinds can potentially compromise the already limited space within the rigid constraints of the posterior fossa, and increasing local mass effect can quickly lead to coma or death via direct compression of the brain stem and/or obstructive hydrocephalus with further increased intracranial pressure. Since patents with a cerebellar stroke and even a seemingly indolent course can abruptly decline via these mechanisms, an early evaluation and close follow-up by a neurosurgeon is a mainstay of management. Timely and appropriate surgical decompression saves lives, and such patients can often make a very good functional recovery, especially if the intervention is done earlier in the clinical course, before coma or vital sign changes are evident.

Relevant Anatomy

Composed of two hemispheres and a midline vermis, the cerebellum sits in the posterior fossa dorsal to the brain stem, in a space constrained by three surfaces: (1) the tentorium superiorly, (2) the skull base formed by the petrous bone and clivus ventrally, and (3) the suboccipital skull convexity surface dorsally and inferiorly (Fig. 70-1A). The posterior fossa communicates with the supratentorial space via the tentorial incisura, through which passes the upper brain stem (midbrain); and it communicates with the spinal canal via the foramen magnum, through which passes the lower brain stem (medulla) and upper cervical spinal cord.

The cerebellum modulates motor function, and corrects for differences between intended and actual movements. Because pathways to and from the hemispheres are mostly uncrossed or doubly crossed, hemispheric lesions cause coordination deficits in the ipsilateral limbs. Lesions of the vermis result in truncal ataxia and dysarthria, and lesions of the inferior cerebellum tend to cause vestibular dysfunction. When axial muscle groups are affected, deficits may not have an obvious laterality.

Blood is supplied to the cerebellum via three pairs of arteries from the vertebrobasilar system, each of which originates ventrally in the posterior fossa, and must encircle (and supply) the appropriate brain-stem region to reach the cerebellum (Fig. 70-2). These three trunks include: (1) the posterior inferior cerebellar artery (PICA), which originates from the vertebral artery 1 to 3 cm proximal to the vertebrobasilar junction and supplies the lateral medulla, inferior vermis, and posterior-inferior cerebellar surface, (2) the anterior inferior cerebellar artery (AICA), which usually originates from the inferior third of the basilar artery, and supplies the caudal pons and the petrosal surface of the cerebellum, and (3) the superior cerebellar artery (SCA), which supplies the caudal midbrain/rostral pons, the superior cerebellar peduncle and dentate nucleus, the superior vermis and the tentorial surface of the cerebellum.

Pathogenesis of Cerebellar Hemorrhage and Infarction

The infratentorial compartment, or posterior fossa, is approximately one-eighth of the entire intracranial space.[1] Based on MRI volumetric analysis, the volume of the posterior fossa is approximately 200 cc in men and slightly less in women.[2,3] The three components of that volume are brain parenchyma (80%), circulating blood (10%), and CSF (10%).[4] An expanded cerebellum associated with a clot or edema can directly compress the brain stem against the clivus, obliterating the subarachnoid cisterns. A mass lesion in the cerebellum, such as a hematoma or edematous infarct, can also cause effacement of either the fourth ventricle or the aqueduct, and lead to obstructive hydrocephalus.

If we estimate 18-20 cc of CSF in the posterior fossa, an infarct or hematoma adding 18 cc of mass to the posterior fossa is sufficient to displace the entire volume of CSF in this compartment. After the CSF reserve space is obliterated, any further enlargement of the hematoma or edema of the surrounding brain and/or infarction reduces the volume of circulating blood, and begins to force brain parenchyma out of the posterior fossa through the tentorial incisura or the foramen magnum (Fig. 70-1B). Given that the volume of a sphere is $4/3 \times \pi r^3$ (where r is the radius), an 18-cc spherical hematoma with a diameter of 3.2 cm (radius 1.6 cm) correlates with the popular assertion that a 3-cm cerebellar hematoma usually warrants urgent surgical evacuation. The causes of cerebellar infarction and hemorrhage are outlined in Table 70-1.

HEMORRHAGE

Hypertension is the most common identifiable risk factor for cerebellar hemorrhage, occurring in 36% to 89% of cases in various series.[5] Hematomas occur in the cerebellar hemisphere

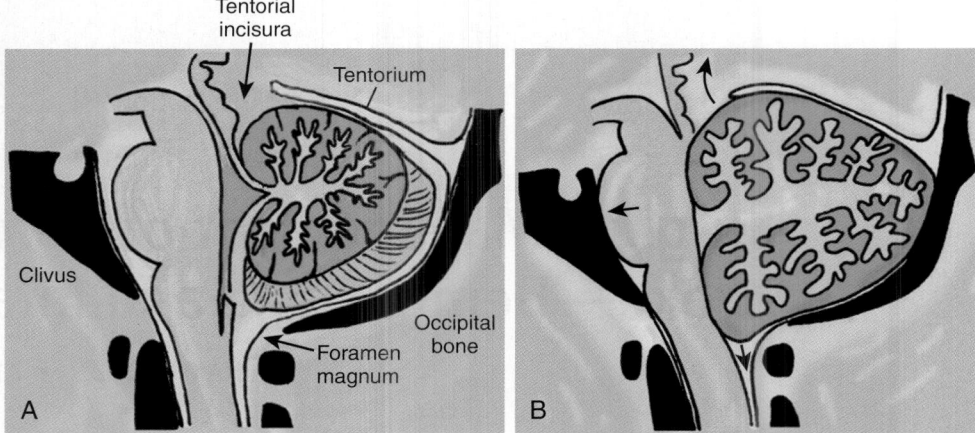

FIGURE 70-1 Posterior fossa. A, Anatomy (midsagittal view). Note the space constrained by three surfaces: (1) the tentorium superiorly, (2) the skull base formed by the petrous bone and clivus ventrally, and (3) the suboccipital skull convexity surface dorsally and inferiorly. Also note the communications with the supratentorial space via the tentorial incisura and with the spinal canal via the foramen magnum. B, Consequences of mass: cerebellar hemorrhage, or infarction with swelling, may cause effacement of the fourth ventricle, compression of the brainstem against the clivus, obstruction of CSF flow through the aqueduct, and herniation upward through the tentorial incisura and/or downward through the foramen magnum.

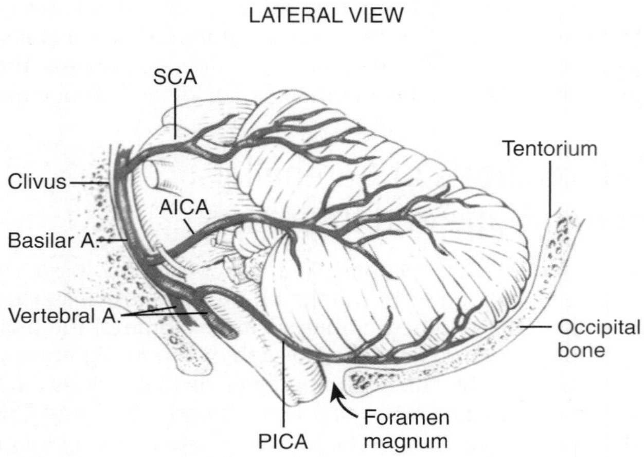

LATERAL VIEW

FIGURE 70-2 Blood supply of the posterior fossa. Three pairs of arteries originate from the vertebrobasilar system ventral to the brainstem, and then encircle and supply the appropriate brainstem region to reach the cerebellum. These trunks include the posterior inferior cerebellar artery (PICA), the anterior inferior cerebellar artery (AICA), and the superior cerebellar artery (SCA), which are seen on this lateral view. Most infarctions arise in the inferior-lateral cerebellum (PICA territory), while most hemorrhages arise near the deep cerebellar nuclei.

Table 70-1 Causes of Cerebellar Hemorrhage and Infarction	
Cerebellar Hemorrhage	**Cerebellar Infarction**
Hypertension	Vertebral artery atherosclerosis
Coagulopathy	Cardioembolism
Amyloid angiopathy	Artery to artery embolism
Hemorrhagic transformation of an infarct	Patent foramen ovale
Tumor	Vertebral artery dissection
Arteriovenous malformation	Hypercoagulable states
Cavernous malformation	Vasculitis
Supratentorial surgery with cerebral spinal fluid drainage	Venous sinus thrombosis
Spinal surgery with durotomy	Cocaine use

and vermis with roughly equal frequency, and may extend into the ventricular system. The SCA and AICA territories are more often involved, particularly in the region of the dentate nucleus, which is supplied by perforating arteries from the SCA.[6] A few cases of microaneurysms have been reported in histopathologic studies of perihemorrhagic tissue.[7]

Less frequent causes of cerebellar hemorrhage are coagulopathy (typically warfarin use), amyloid angiopathy, hemorrhagic transformation of an infarct, tumors, and vascular malformations.[8-10] Remote cerebellar hemorrhage related to the release of large volumes of CSF intra- or perioperatively has been well described in the literature as an unexpected outcome of supratentorial or spinal surgery.[11-14]

INFARCTION

The most common cause of cerebellar infarction in older patients is vertebral artery atherosclerosis, which may be intracranial, extracranial, or both. The PICA distribution is the most likely territory involved clinically. Cardiac and artery-to-artery embolization is also an important cause, and may explain "nonterritorial" infarcts that involve smaller regions of the cerebellum.[15] In patients under age 40, patent foramen ovale is an important consideration.[16] Vertebral artery dissection is another important cause, with or without a history of trauma, chiropractic manipulation, or prolonged neck hyperextension ("beauty parlor stroke"). Most infarcts caused by vertebral artery dissection also occur in the PICA territory.[17]

Less common disorders associated with cerebellar infarction include hypercoagulable states, vasculitis, venous sinus thrombosis, and cocaine use.[16] Such infarcts may involve the typical PICA, SCA, or AICA territories, watershed regions, or smaller, nonterritorial areas.[15]

Clinical Manifestations

While cerebellar stroke is the most worrisome cause of dizziness, nausea, and gait instability, the same constellation of symptoms may result from a peripheral disorder, such as vestibular neuritis or labyrinthitis. Furthermore, the clinical presentation of cerebellar hemorrhage is not reliably distinct from that of cerebellar infarction. In Raco's series

Table 70-2	Posterior Circulation Stroke Syndromes
Infarct Territory	**Clinical Features**
Posterior inferior cerebellar artery (lateral medullary syndrome or Wallenberg's syndrome)	Dysphagia Hoarseness Ipsilateral absent gag Hemifacial analgesia or pain Contralateral hemibody analgesia Horner's syndrome Hemiataxia Dysarthria Nystagmus
Anterior inferior cerebellar artery (Foville's syndrome)	Abducens palsy Hemifacial palsy Ipsilateral deafness Horner's syndrome Hemifacial analgesia Hemiataxia Dysarthria Nystagmus
Superior cerebellar artery (Mill's syndrome)	Ipsilateral tremor Hemiatonia Contralateral hemibody analgesia Hemiataxia Dysarthria
Cerebellar stroke with secondary brain-stem compression	Initially: Hemiataxia Dysarthria Nystagmus Delayed: Contralateral gaze deviation Hemifacial palsy Altered sensorium Abnormal respirations Coma

comparing 70 patients with cerebellar hemorrhage and 52 patients with cerebellar infarction, both entities commonly presented with the acute onset of nausea, vomiting, dizziness, and unsteady gait. Headache was more common as an initial symptom in cerebellar hemorrhage.[6] Dizziness may occur with or without vertigo.[16] On physical exam, dysarthria, ataxia, and nystagmus are common. Ataxia may be appendicular, axial or both, depending on the relative involvement of the cerebellar hemispheres and vermis. Nystagmus and/or hearing loss may be a sign of cerebellar stroke or of a peripheral vestibular disorder.[16]

Posterior circulation strokes, particularly infarction, often involve both the cerebellum and the brain stem. In such situations, various brain-stem stroke syndromes are evident in combination with the manifestations of cerebellar dysfunction. Depending on the level affected, these syndromes may include ipsilateral hemifacial analgesia, contralateral hemibody analgesia, Horner's syndrome, motor deficits, and cranial neuropathies (Table 70-2). The neurologic deficit often indicates the arterial territory affected by the infarct, but anatomic variations are common between AICA and PICA, and the territory affected can vary considerably.

Distinguishing the signs of primary brain-stem stroke from those of secondary brain-stem compression is extremely important. Direct brain-stem compression can manifest either as gaze restrictions, lower cranial nerve dysfunction, or altered sensorium from suppression of the reticular activating system. After the early symptoms and signs of the infarction are defined, delayed neurologic deterioration 1 to 7 days following symptom onset is often indicative of cerebellar swelling and impending upward (transtentorial) or downward (tonsilar) herniation.[18-23] Hydrocephalus may further contribute to the decline. Certainly, any change in sensorium warrants urgent surgical intervention, as the patient can quickly proceed through the later stages of brain-stem compression, which include coma, abnormal respirations, posturing, and death.

Radiologic Evaluation

CT scanning is the definitive diagnostic procedure of choice for cerebellar hemorrhage, and is also useful in defining subacute or chronic infarction. The initial CT may be normal for several hours following a cerebellar infarct, during which time a diffusion-weighted MRI can be diagnostic. Both types of studies (CT or MRI) provide information about any mass effect on surrounding structures, and shows hydrocephalus when present. Posterior fossa mass effect can be visualized as distortion or effacement of the fourth ventricle, compression of the brain stem, effacement of the basal cisterns, and cerebellar herniation through the tentorial incisura (vermis) or foramen magnum (tonsils). They can also identify primary brain-stem involvement in the stroke, which carries a worse prognosis.

Several CT criteria have been correlated with neurologic deterioration and the need for surgical intervention. The concept of a "tight posterior fossa" was described by Weisberg in a series of 14 patients with cerebellar hemorrhage, all of whom had effacement of the basal cisterns and obstructive hydrocephalus. Nonsurgical management resulted in 100% mortality; of the eight patients who underwent craniectomy and hematoma evacuation, all survived and six became ambulatory.[24] Taneda and colleagues correlated the degree of quadrigeminal cistern effacement with patient outcomes.[25] Many surgeons consider a hematoma diameter of greater than 3 cm to be an indication for surgery.[26-28] Another treatment algorithm stresses the importance of fourth ventricular compression over hematoma size.[5]

MRI scanning is preferable in defining an underlying tumor or vascular malformation. Vascular imaging (MRA or CTA) can often effectively define a parent vessel thrombosis, peripheral branch occlusion, or dissection of the vertebral artery. In questionable circumstances, four-vessel transfemoral arteriography is required to establish a final diagnosis and dictate future management. Echocardiography and laboratory tests can help identify cardiac and systemic risk factors.

Initial Management

An acute cerebellar hemorrhage or infarct requires neurosurgical evaluation. A patient with an acute cerebellar stroke without hydrocephalus or mass effect should be admitted for observation and continued evaluation, generally in a neurologic ICU. Serial neurologic exams and brain imaging are complementary. For ischemic stroke, antiplatelet and thrombolytic therapy may be given in accordance with American Heart Association guidelines, but should be avoided if surgical intervention is likely.[30]

In cerebellar hemorrhage, follow-up CT scans should be done daily (or more often in unstable patients) for the first several days following the ictal event, to evaluate for edema progression and/or rehemorrhage. Cerebellar infarction can be expected to increase in volume, with the first radiographic signs of mass effect developing 1 to 6 days after onset. Patients with progressive neurologic deterioration typically have characteristic findings over time on CT scanning, including fourth ventricular shift, basal cistern compression, brain-stem deformity, and hydrocephalus.[29]

Indications and Timing for Surgical Intervention

HEMORRHAGE

There is now general consensus that in cases of cerebellar hemorrhage with a tight posterior fossa, early surgery reduces mortality and can have good outcomes.[5,24,25,31-34] This group of patients has a high mortality when the hematoma is not evacuated, whether or not a ventriculostomy is performed.[31,35] While a hematoma diameter of 3 cm or larger is a popular indication for surgery, any cerebellar hemorrhage causing obstructive hydrocephalus, compression of the brain stem, or effacement of the cisterns should be a potential candidate for emergent surgical decompression and clot evacuation.

INFARCTION

The surgical management of cerebellar infarction has been the subject of debate. Cerebellar infarction, or "softening" as it was called, was first recognized as a neurosurgical emergency by Fairburn and Oliver in 1956.[36] It is now commonly agreed that surgical decompression can be lifesaving. Nevertheless, some surgeons favor a "gradual" approach to the treatment of massive infarction, beginning with ventriculostomy. If neurologic deficits progress despite this measure, these surgeons would proceed with craniectomy.[6,37] Several series describe a subgroup of patients with cerebellar infarcts who were treated with ventriculostomy alone.[38-40] Of those initially treated with ventriculostomy, 30% to 40% ultimately required a suboccipital craniectomy.

With cerebellar infarction causing brain-stem compression, it is well-established that suboccipital craniectomy reduces mortality.[19,41] In a series of 13 patients with cerebellar infarction and progressive deterioration of consciousness, all 7 who underwent craniectomy lived; the one patient treated with ventriculostomy alone died, and 4 of the 5 patients treated medically died.[31] With timely decompression, good functional outcomes are common.[18,42-44] One series reports that even comatose patients have a 38% chance of good recovery with decompressive surgery.[38]

When cerebellar infarction is massive enough to cause hydrocephalus, there are intuitive reasons that suboccipital surgery (often with ventriculostomy) is preferable to ventriculostomy alone. Hydrocephalus in this setting is caused by effacement of the fourth ventricle or the aqueduct, and it implies some degree of acute brain-stem compression, which would not be relieved by CSF drainage alone. Waiting to see if the brain-stem compression increases and causes progressive neurologic deterioration puts the patient at undue risk of acute decline and often catastrophic outcome. Other disadvantages of ventriculostomy without suboccipital craniectomy include the risk of upward transtentorial herniation and the prolonged need for catheter drainage, with associated rates of infection and shunt requirement.[18,45]

Surgical Intervention

Acute cerebellar stroke, whether ischemic or hemorrhagic, requires an initial clinical assessment to identify signs of hydrocephalus or brain-stem compression, and surgical decompression via a suboccipital craniectomy and a ventriculostomy should be considered an urgent decision in such patients. The neurosurgeon should be involved early in cases likely to need surgery.

Some patients have a very poor prognosis that may limit the treatment offered, particularly those in prolonged deep coma or those whose stroke primarily involves the brain stem. When a cerebellar hemorrhage or infarction does not initially warrant surgery, the patient should be admitted to an ICU or similar setting for serial neurologic exams and brain imaging.

After a decision is made to proceed with surgery, preparations for the procedure should be rapid, to optimize the patient's chances of a good recovery. Mannitol, head elevation, hyperventilation, and ventriculostomy can be temporizing measures to control increased intracranial pressure. The ventriculostomy is often placed frontally, and can be done while waiting for the operative theater to become available. Once the patient is in the operating room and asleep, the patient is positioned prone in three-point pin fixation with the head elevated above the heart. The neck and upper back are slightly flexed to open the craniocervical junction and allow a comfortable working angle to the posterior fossa, carefully avoiding excesses that can cause jugular venous obstruction or kinking of the endotracheal tube. Securing the patient with straps allows for axial rotation which makes the operative position more comfortable for the operating surgeon. The occipital and suboccipital regions are prepped and draped in the traditional fashion, with room to place an occipital burr hole and ventricular drain if needed.

A midline incision is preferable for the craniectomy, although occasionally a paramedian incision may be utilized. Bone removal is wide enough to decompress cerebellar swelling as well as to provide access to remove the offending pathology. The bone removal must extend inferiorly to access the cisterna magna and widely decompress the foramen magnum, and generally includes removal of the posterior arch of C1. The dura is opened to expose the midline and lateral cerebellar surface affected by the hematoma or infarct, and the incision is carried inferiorly below the foramen magnum so that the tips of the cerebellar tonsils are visualized and that adequate decompression of the brain stem has been accomplished.

Once the dura is opened, the operating microscope is used for the intradural portion of the procedure. With cerebellar hemorrhage, ultrasound can be helpful in localizing the hematoma and planning the incision in the cerebellar cortex. The entire clot does not need to be removed, but the evacuation should be aggressive enough to remove most of the mass effect caused by the hematoma; surrounding edematous tissue should be preserved. For cerebellar infarction, the clearly dead and necrotic tissue, which is more soft and suctionable than the surrounding normal cerebellum, should be removed, especially those portions in the lateral hemisphere and near the foramen magnum. No attempt should be made to define the ischemic penumbra; injury to the PICA, deep cerebellar nuclei, and brain stem must be avoided. After adequate decompression, the cerebellum and foramen magnum appear much more relaxed within the dural opening.

The dura is closed loosely, but in a watertight fashion, invariably using a patch graft. The suboccipital bone is not replaced; the muscle, fascia, and dermis are closed securely to minimize the chance of pseudomeningocele formation, CSF leak, and wound breakdown. Postoperatively, the ventriculostomy is opened to measure and control ICP and to keep CSF build-up from the recently closed wound. After several days of stability, the catheter is weaned as tolerated, and a ventriculoperitoneal shunt is later placed as necessary. Prior to feeding, the patient's risk of aspiration is evaluated, and early tracheostomy and feeding tubes are placed in high-risk patients.

Cases

CASE 1

A 51-year-old woman with a history of hypertension presented to the emergency room of another facility after the acute onset of headache, nausea, vomiting, and gait instability. She became comatose in the ER and was intubated.

After a CT showed a large right cerebellar hemorrhage with hydrocephalus, a right frontal ventriculostomy was placed, and the patient was transferred to our institution. Her CT showed a 5×3-cm hematoma in the right cerebellar hemisphere and vermis, causing deformity of the brain stem, effacement of the basal cisterns, compression of the fourth ventricle, and hydrocephalus (Fig. 70-3). She underwent an emergent suboccipital craniectomy and evacuation of the hematoma, and made a dramatic recovery postoperatively. At follow-up 4 months later, she was neurologically intact except for mild gait instability.

CASE 2

An 81-year-old man with a history of hypertension and atrial fibrillation presented after the acute onset of nausea and gait instability. His neurologic examination showed left dysmetria and gaze-paretic nystagmus. His initial CT was normal, and MRI showed diffusion restriction in the left PICA distribution (Fig. 70-4A and B). He was admitted to the neurologic intensive care unit, and found to have dysarthria 40 hours after the onset of symptoms. A CT showed the left cerebellar infarction with mass effect, causing transtentorial compression of the brain stem (Fig. 70-4C and D). He underwent an emergent suboccipital decompression, and recovered well after the surgery.

Conclusion

While the pathophysiology of cerebellar hemorrhage is distinct from that of cerebellar infarction, it is appropriate to consider these two entities together, because they have similar neurologic sequelae. Both conditions typically present acutely with symptoms and signs of cerebellar dysfunction, and may progress rapidly to coma from mass effect in the posterior fossa. When brain-stem compression and obstructive hydrocephalus occurs, urgent suboccipital decompression is warranted. Timely surgery can be life-saving, and patients often have a good functional outcome.

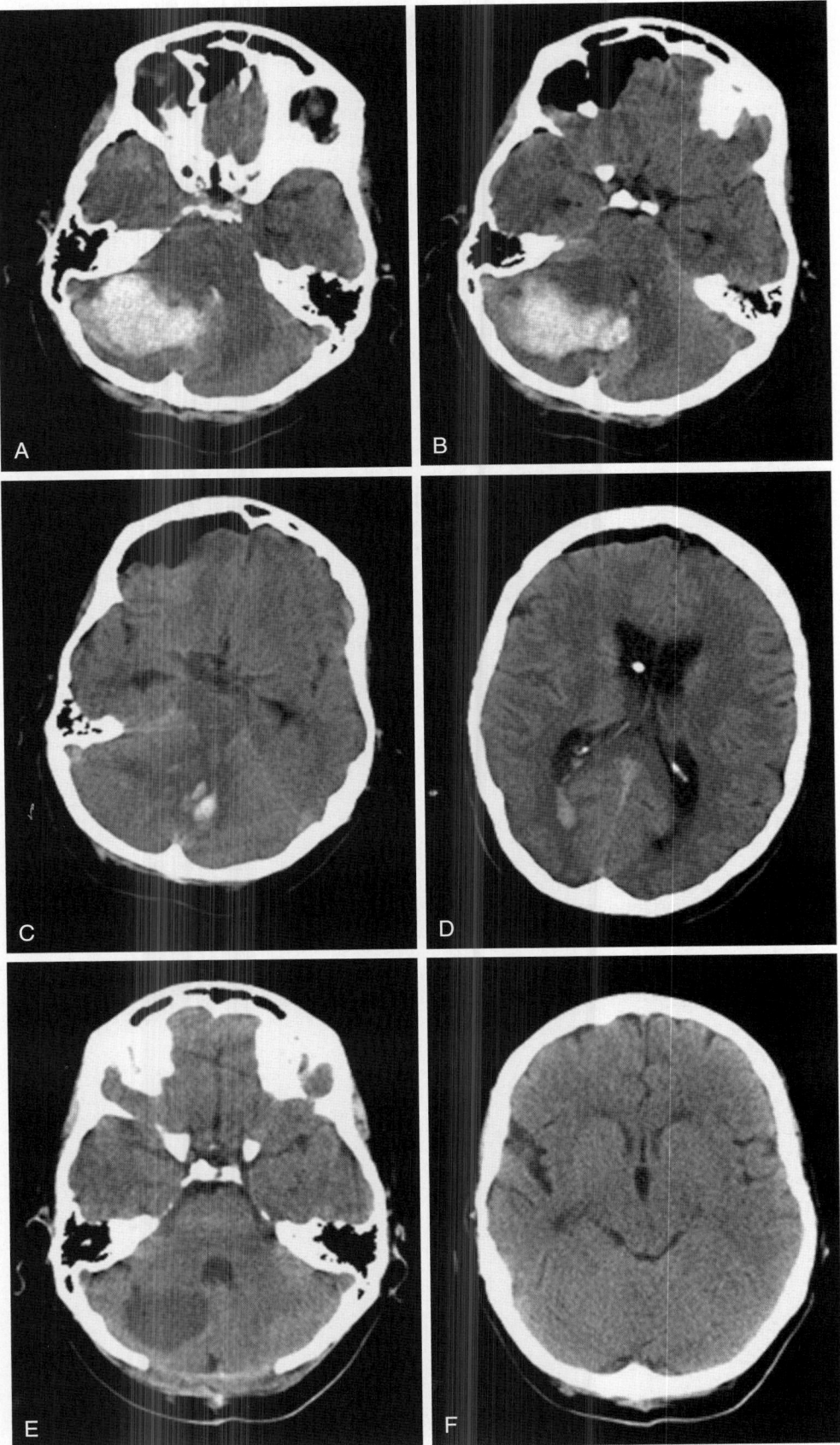

FIGURE 70-3 Cerebellar hemorrhage. A to D, Large right cerebellar hemorrhage, causing compression of the brainstem and basal cisterns. The upper fourth ventricle is effaced and there is obstructive hydrocephalus. Prior to the patient's transfer to our institution, a right frontal ventriculostomy catheter had been placed, with associated frontal pneumocephalus. E and F, CT 1 month after suboccipital craniectomy and evacuation of the hematoma. The brain stem is decompressed, the cisterns are open, and there is no hydrocephalus.

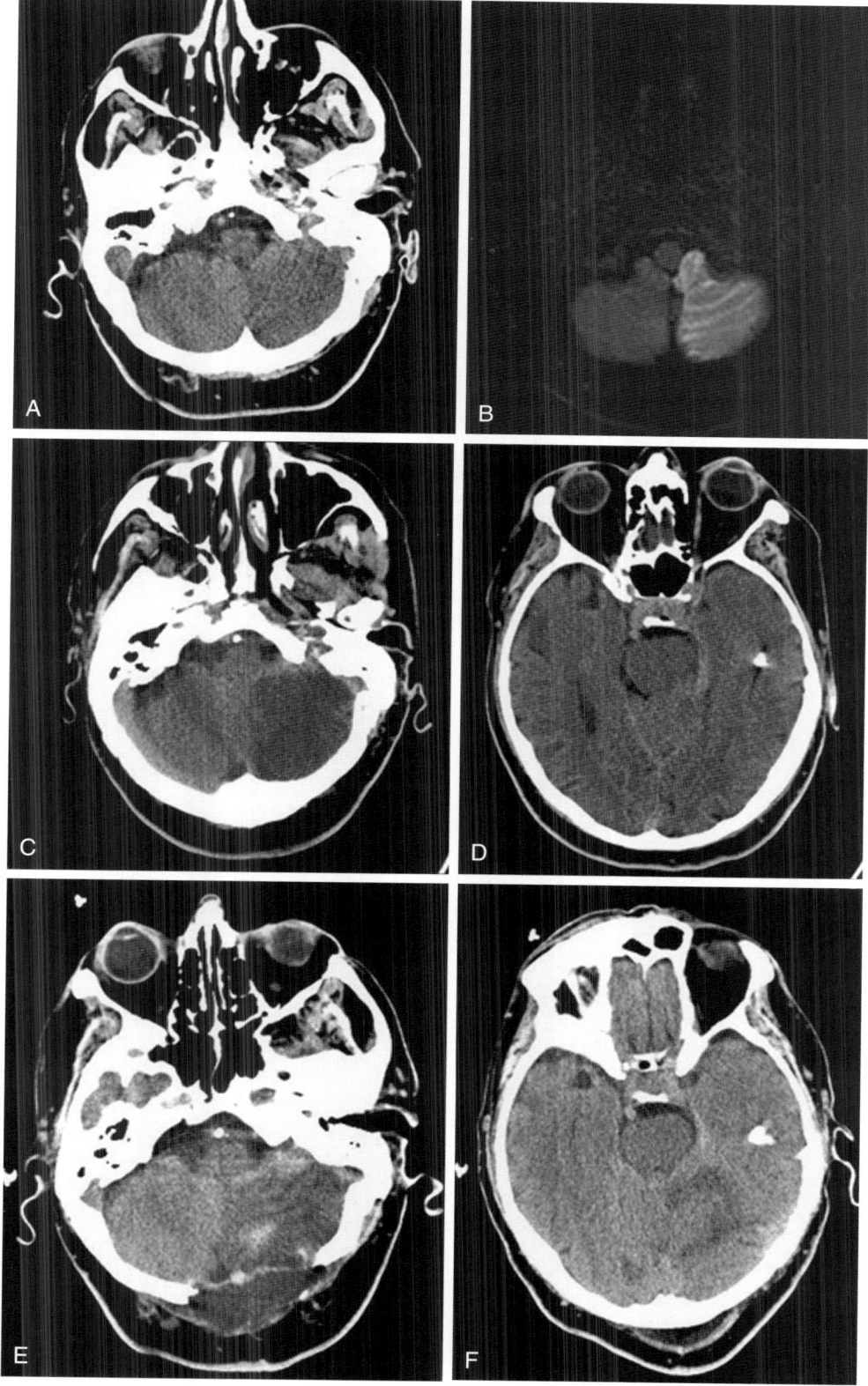

FIGURE 70-4 Cerebellar infarction. A, Normal initial CT in a patient with acute cerebellar symptoms. B, MRI shows diffusion restriction in the left PICA territory. C and D, Forty hours after the onset of symptoms, CT shows edematous left cerebellar infarction with transtentorial compression of the brainstem. E and F, CT 10 days after suboccipital craniectomy shows decompression of brain stem.

KEY REFERENCES

Adams HP, del Zoppo G, Alberts MJ, et al. Guidelines for the early management of adults with ischemic stroke. *Stroke.* 2007;38:1655-1711.

Amarenco P, Levy C, Cohen A, et al. Causes and mechanisms of territorial and nonterritorial cerebellar infarcts in 115 consecutive patients. *Stroke.* 1994;25:105-112.

Auer LM, Auer T, Sayama I. Indications for surgical treatment of cerebellar hemorrhage and infarction. *Acta Neurochir (Wien).* 1986;79:74-79.

Barinagarrementeria F, Amaya LE, Cantu C. Causes and mechanisms of cerebellar infarction in young patients. *Stroke.* 1997;28:2400-2404.

Chen HJ, Lee TC, Wei CP. Treatment of cerebellar infarction by decompressive suboccipital craniectomy. *Stroke.* 1992;23:957-961.

De Oliveira JG, Rassi-Neto A, Ferraz FAP, et al. Neurosurgical management of cerebellar cavernous malformations. *Neurosurg Focus.* 2006;21:1-8.

Duncan GW, Parker SW, Fisher CM. Acute cerebellar infarction in the PICA territory. *Arch Neurol.* 1975;32:364-368.

Edlow JA, Newman-Toker DE, Savitz SI. Diagnosis and initial management of cerebellar infarction. *Lancet Neurol.* 2008;7:951-964.

Fairburn B, Oliver LC. Cerebellar softening: a surgical emergency. *BMJ.* 1956;1:1335-1336.

Friedman JA, Piepgras DG, Duke DA, et al. Remote cerebellar hemorrhage after supratentorial surgery. *Neurosurg.* 2001;49:1327-1340.

Heros RC. Surgical treatment of cerebellar infarction. *Stroke.* 1992;23:937-938.

Hornig CR, Rust DS, Busse O, et al. Space-occupying cerebellar infarction: clinical course and prognosis. *Stroke.* 1994;25:372-373.

Juttler E, Schweickert S, Ringleb PA, et al. Long-term outcome after surgical treatment for space-occupying cerebellar infarction: experience in 56 patients. *Stroke.* 2009;40:3060-3066.

Kirollos RW, Tyagi AK, Ross SA, et al. Management of spontaneous cerebellar hematomas: a prospective treatment protocol. *Neurosurg.* 2001;49:1378-1387.

Kobayashi S, Sato A, Kageyama Y, et al. Treatment of hypertensive cerebellar hemorrhage: surgical or conservative management. *Neurosurgery.* 1994;34:246-251.

Koh MG, Phan TG, Atkinson JLD, et al. Neuroimaging in deteriorating patients with cerebellar infarcts and mass effect. *Stroke.* 2000;31:2062-2067.

Kudo H, Kawaguchi T, Minami H, et al. Controversy of surgical treatment for severe cerebellar infarction. *J Stroke Cerebrovasc Dis.* 2007;16:259-262.

Park JS, Hwang JH, Park J, et al. Remote cerebellar hemorrhage complicated after supratentorial surgery: retrospective study with review of articles. *J Korean Neurosurg Soc.* 2009;46:136-143.

Pfefferkorn T, Eppinger U, Linn J, et al. Long-term outcome after suboccipital decompressive craniectomy for malignant cerebellar infarction. *Stroke.* 2009;40:3045-3050.

Raco A, Caroli E, Isidori A, et al. Management of acute cerebellar infarction: one institution's experience. *Neurosurgery.* 2003;53:1061-1066.

Rhoton AL. Cerebellum and fourth ventricle. *Neurosurgery.* 2000;47:S7-27.

Salvati M, Cervoni L, Raco A, et al. Spontaneous cerebellar hemorrhage: clinical remarks on 50 cases. *Surg Neurol.* 2001;55:156-161.

Wakai S, Nagai M. Histological verification of microaneurysms as a cause of cerebral haemorrhage in surgical specimens. *J Neurol Neurosurg Psychiatry.* 1989;52:595-599.

Weisberg LA. Acute cerebellar hemorrhage and CT evidence of tight posterior fossa. *Neurology.* 1986;36:858-860.

Yanaka K, Meguro K, Fujita K, et al. Immediate surgery reduces mortality in deeply comatose patients with spontaneous cerebellar hemorrhage. *Neurol Med Chir (Tokyo).* 2000;40:295-300.

Numbered references appear on Expert Consult.

CHAPTER 71

Surgical Treatment of Moyamoya Disease in Adults

LEONIDAS M. QUINTANA

Moyamoya disease is a chronic, cerebrovascular occlusive disease, in which the terminal portions of the intracranial internal carotid arteries and the initial segments of the middle and anterior cerebral arteries progressively become narrowed or occluded. Due to this phenomenon, reduced blood flow to the brain is produced, and tiny collateral vessels at the base of the brain enlarge to become collateral pathways. These vessels are called "moyamoya vessels" because the angiographic appearance of these vessels resemble the "cloud" or "puff" of cigarette smoke, which is described as "moya-moya" in the Japanese language; also, "moya-moya" is the Japanese word to describe a hazy appearance or an unclear idea about something.[1]

In the 1950s, leading Japanese neurosurgeons began to notice a new clinical entity that came to be called moyamoya disease. Since its etiology was unknown, it was named in various ways. Takeuchi and Shimizu described it as a hypoplasia of bilateral internal carotid arteries.[2] Later, Suzuki and Takaku described in detail the angiographic appearance and development of this disease,[1] and gave it the name moyamoya disease. Kudo named it officially as the spontaneous occlusion of the circle of Willis[3] (Fig. 71-1).

Clinical Findings and Preoperative Assessment

Symptoms and signs of moyamoya disease include brain ischemia and hemorrhage. Initial symptoms in moyamoya disease, both juvenile (under age 15 years) and adult cases considered together, are most frequently motor disturbances. In the experience of Suzuki.[4] these were found in 36% of patients, followed by intracranial hemorrhage in 25%, headache in 20%, and convulsions in 6%. This is similar to the experience reported by Yamaguchi et al.,[5] who reported motor disturbances in 62.7% of males and 53.8% of females, disturbances of consciousness in 28.1% of males and 34.6% of females, signs of meningeal irritation in 10.3% of males and 20.5% of females, and speech disturbances 16.7% of males and 14% of females.

However, when these symptoms are studied with regard to age, large differences between juvenile and adult cases become apparent.

Among the juvenile cases, motor disturbances, including monoparesis, paraparesis, and hemiparesis are found in 60%,

and in these juvenile cases, some 20% show motor disturbances indicative of transient brain ischemia.[4]

If we also included other symptoms thought to be due to brain ischemia, such as sensory disturbances and mental and psychic disorders, then 85% of these juvenile cases show symptoms of brain ischemia. Intracranial hemorrhage was seen in only 4% of juvenile cases.[4]

In other Japanese reported experiences,[4,6,7] the onset of adult cases was accompanied by intracranial hemorrhage in 43% of patients, and symptoms due to brain ischemia,[8,9] including motor, mental, and psychic disturbances, were seen in 20% of these adult cases.

Moyamoya disease is basically diagnosed both by clinical symptoms and angiographic findings.

Neuroimaging

X-ray computed tomography (CT) is useful to differentiate brain ischemia from brain hemorrhage in the acute stage. However, CT is not definitely diagnostic for moyamoya disease. As a non-invasive mode of imaging, the following magnetic resonance and angiographic MRI imaging modalities are considered first line.

Catheter angiography is essentially required for the diagnosis of moyamoya disease and is the gold standard of the neuroimaging in this disease. However, catheter angiography has an inherent risk of cerebral infarction, drug allergy, etc, although the incidence is very low.

The widespread availability of magnetic resonance imaging (MRI) and magnetic resonance angiography (MRA) as useful and safe imaging methods has led to the increasing use of these methods for primary imaging in patients with symptoms suggestive of moyamoya.[10-12] An acute infarct is more likely to be detected with the use of diffusion-weighted imaging, whereas a chronic infarct is more likely to be seen with T1- and T2-weighted imaging. Diminished cortical blood flow due to moyamoya can be inferred from fluid-attenuated inversion recovery (FLAIR) sequences showing linear high signals that follow a sulcal pattern, which is called the "ivy sign."[13]

The finding most suggestive of moyamoya on MRI is reduced flow voids in the internal, middle, and anterior cerebral arteries coupled with prominent flow voids through the basal ganglia and thalamus from moyamoya-associated collateral vessels. These findings are virtually

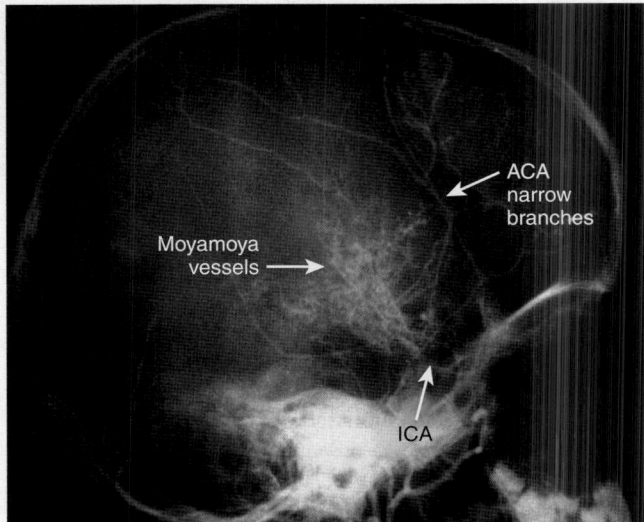

FIGURE 71-1 Lateral view, right carotid angiography showing moyamoya vessels. Supraclinoidal segment of ICA. MCA cannot be seen clearly. The ACA branches are extremely narrowed.

diagnostic of moyamoya,[14] and also called "the sign of termite nest."[15]

When we search for the classical findings of moyamoya disease, both studies, catheter angiography and MRA, show the terminal portions of the intracranial internal carotid arteries and the initial segments of the middle and anterior cerebral arteries progressively become narrowed or occluded. According to the report by Suzuki et al.[1] that named this disease, tiny collateral vessels at the base of the brain enlarge to become collateral pathways. These vessels are called "moyamoya vessels" because the angiographic appearance of these vessels resemble the "cloud" or "puff" of cigarette smoke, which is described as "moya-moya" in the Japanese language.

Suzuki and Takaku[1] classified the development of moyamoya disease into six stages. According to this classification, many patients fall into stage 3. Fukuyama and Umezu[16] then further divided stage 3 into three.

Stage 1: Narrowing of carotid fork.

Stage 2: Initiation of the "moyamoya vessels"; dilatation of the intracerebral main arteries.

Stage 3: Intensification of the "moyamoya vessels"; nonfilling of the anterior and middle cerebral arteries.

   3a: Partial nonfilling of the anterior and middle cerebral arteries.

   3b: Partial preservation of the anterior and middle cerebral arteries.

   3c: Complete lack of the anterior and middle cerebral arteries.

Stage 4: Minimization of the "moyamoya vessels"; disappearance of the posterior cerebral artery.

Stage 5: Reduction of the "moyamoya vessels"; the main arteries arising from the internal carotid artery disappear.

Stage 6: Disappearance of the "moyamoya vessels"; the original moyamoya vessels at the base of the brain are completely missing and only the collateral circulation from the external carotid artery is seen (Fig. 71-2).

Inconveniences of this classification are as follows: Many cases belong to stages 3 to 5, especially to stage 3. There are few cases in stages 1 and 6. Stages of moyamoya disease

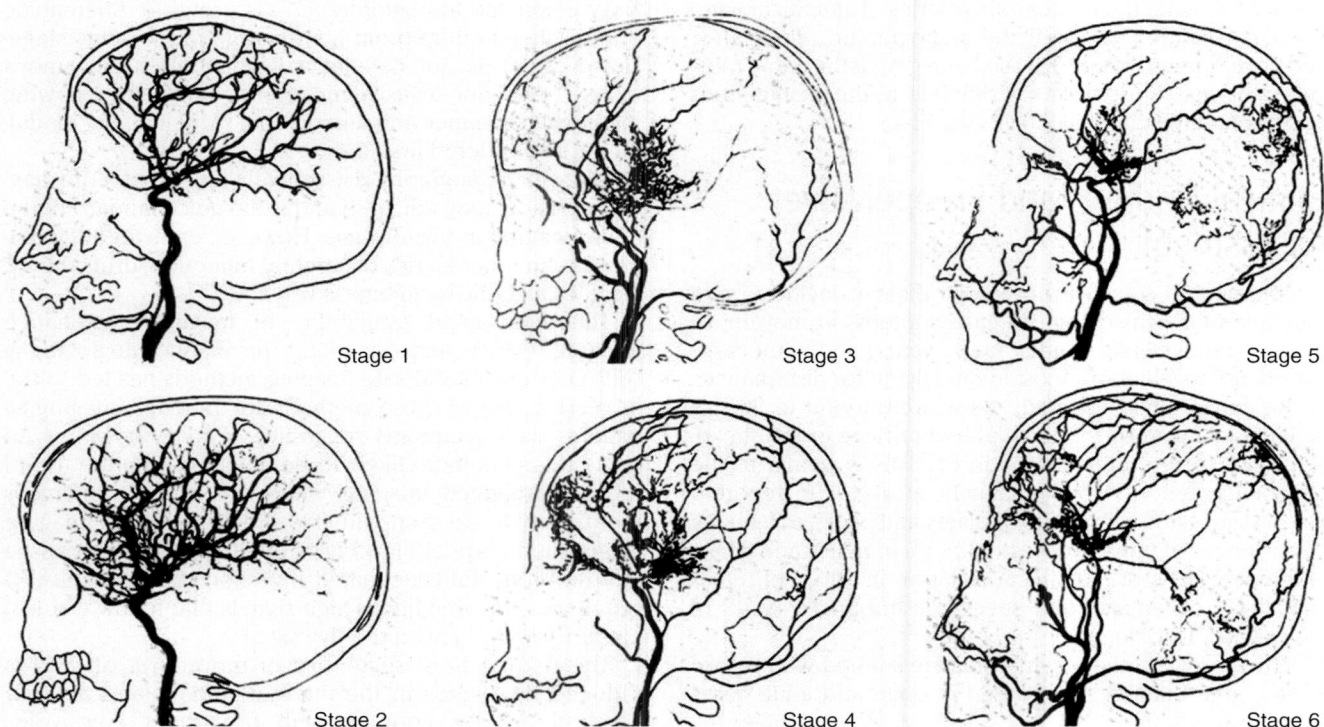

FIGURE 71-2 Angiographic staging of moyamoya disease. *(From Suzuki J, Takaku A. Cerebrovascular "moyamoya" disease showing abnormal net-like vessels in base of brain. Arch Neurol. 1969;20:288-299.)*

are not strongly related to clinical symptoms. In stages 1 and 6, there are no moyamoya vessels on cerebral angiography, which is not moyamoya disease by definition. There is some doubt that vascular dilatation in stage 2 really exists.

Progression of angiographic stages is commonly observed in children, but in adults many patients often remain in the same stages. However, when there is good correlation between the clinical picture and the imaging above presented, this angiographic classification is useful.

CBF, positron-emission CT or single-photon CT, or xenon inhalation CT are commonly used to obtain greater detail. Recently, perfusion x-ray CT and MRI with contrast materials have been used for this purpose.[17,18]

Emergency Treatment

In the acute stage, the treatment is the same as for brain infarction or spontaneous intracerebral hemorrhage due to other etiologies.[19] In the event of ventricular hemorrhage, an external ventricular drainage operation is performed if the patient presents in acute evolution with signs of intracranial hypertension.[20,21]

In the case of intracerebral hemorrhage (ICH), initial medical treatment is indicated if the hemorrhage totals less than 25 cc in volume. If the hemorrhagic volume totals more than 25 cc, is associated with a lobar topography, and demonstrates mass effect over the midline structures, then surgical evacuation is indicated.[20] In patients with ICH, infusion of osmotic agents is frequently used to control the intracerebral pressure and edema, as well as administration of anticonvulsants to control seizures, is also required.[21]

Bypass surgery in the acute stage of the disease is not indicated.[19]

Treatment in the Chronic Stage

PATIENTS WITH CEREBRAL ISCHEMIA

There is no consensus on medical treatment with aspirin, other antiplatelet agents, anticoagulants, vasodilators, or corticosteroids to prevent future ischemic attacks in patients with chronic disease.[22]

Surgical Anastomosis

In order to eliminate ischemic symptoms or to prevent recurrent ischemic stroke, bypass surgery is accepted as the treatment of choice. Site of the bypass is also determined occasionally by the results of the examination of cerebral blood flow (Xe[133]-CT scan, SPECT, PET scan).[22] The rationale to initiate some form of revascularization follows:

Clinical picture: As already described, there are mainly different forms of ischemic stroke in children (juvenile cases), and hemorrhagic and ischemic stroke in young adults.

Laboratory studies: The following studies may be indicated in patients with moyamoya disease: In a patient with stroke of unclear etiology, a hypercoagulability profile may be helpful. Significant abnormality in any of the following is a risk factor for ischemic stroke: protein C, protein S, antithrombin III, homocysteine, and factor V Leiden. Erythrocyte sedimentation rate (ESR) can be obtained as part of the initial workup

of a possible vasculitis. However, a normal ESR does not rule out vasculitis.

Imaging studies: Cerebral angiography is the criterion standard for diagnosis. The following findings support the diagnosis:

1. Stenosis or occlusion at the terminal portion of the internal carotid artery or the proximal portion of the anterior or middle cerebral arteries. Abnormal vascular networks in the vicinity of the occlusive or stenotic areas.

2. Bilaterality of the described findings (although some patients may present with unilateral involvement and then progress). Magnetic resonance angiography (MRA) can be performed. Any of these findings on MRA may preclude the need for conventional angiography.

3. One very important clinical finding is the presence of moyamoya vessels at the angiographic study or MRA, correlated with the previously described clinical picture. The moyamoya vessels only are present when the patient is suffering a chronic brain ischemia, and these vessels are representative of the development of collateral ways for the cerebral blood flow to the ischemic brain.[22]

Vascular anastomoses are classified as direct or indirect. In direct anastomosis, the superficial temporal artery (STA) in the scalp is dissected and anastomosed with the middle cerebral artery (MCA) on the brain surface under microsurgery. This surgical technique gives the patient a high cerebral blood flow (CBF) immediately after the surgery.[23-26] However, in this disease the diameters of the cortical arteries are very small, and the anastomotic technique requires for its proper implementation cortical arteries of at least 1 mm in diameter.

In the indirect anastomosis, the periosteum, dura mater, or a slice of the temporal muscle is placed over the brain surface, in anticipation of the development of new spontaneous anastomoses between extra and intracranial circulation. Some time is required to establish such anastomoses that also function with utility. Thus, the brain parenchyma is provided with collateral circulation through these structures, the STA, deep temporal artery, middle meningeal artery, and anterior meningeal artery. During the surgical technique (synangiosis), these arteries must be preserved. In some cases, and to ensure close contact between the STA and galea surrounding the cerebral cortex, the extirpation of the pia mater is done in zones or "windows," suturing the edges of the galea to the piamater.[27] While using these indirect techniques, a high increase of cerebral blood flow does not develop immediately; early revascularization is frequently observed between 3 to 6 months following the intervention, especially in cases that course with cerebral ischemia.

It is common to add an indirect bypass more or less when a direct bypass is scheduled.[23] In other situations, multiple burr-hole surgery is performed, in which multiple small holes are made on the skull bone, in anticipation of the development of spontaneous anastomoses.[28,29] Other less frequent surgeries are omental transplantation[30] and omental transposition.[31]

In moyamoya disease, usually both cerebral hemispheres are ischemic; thus bypass surgery is required bilaterally. First,

Table 71-1 Procedures Using Different Tissues for Indirect Anastomoses

1. Procedures using scalp artery
2. Procedures using galea
3. Procedures using dura mater
4. Procedures using temporal or other muscles
5. Procedures using omentum
6. Procedures using a combination of the above
7. Direct and indirect anastomoses combined

one-sided operation for the hemisphere that is more ischemic is performed, and then bypass surgery for the opposite side is scheduled 2 or 3 months later.

The indirect revascularization techniques most widely used are the encephalo-duro-arterio-synangiosis (EDAS) and the encephalo-myo-synangiosis (EMS).[32-34] There are many modes of indirect anastomoses. Such techniques reviewed by Matsushima et al.[35] are summarized in Table 71-1.

PATIENTS WITH INTRACEREBRAL HEMORRHAGE

It has been reported that the ICH occurs as a consequence of a hemodynamic overload over the small collateral arteries of neovascularization, the "moyamoya vessels," with terminal circulation in the deep zones of the brain in the vicinity of the ventricular wall. However, in these hemorrhagic cases, the advantages of the surgical treatment using direct or indirect bypass with the surgical techniques described here have yet to be proven. In these hemorrhagic cases, the patients suffering systemic hypertension must be treated with antihypertensive drugs, and platelet antiaggregants are not indicated.

We will describe the most common surgical techniques for this disease that have shown the best results, including one direct technique and six indirect techniques. In relation to general surgery, patients are positioned with the head above the heart atrium to reduce the cerebral venous congestion. Hyperventilation and alpha-adrenergic drugs are not recommended for their vasoconstrictor effect, but moderate hypothermia (32°–34°C) and barbiturates, or anesthetics like propofol, are used for cerebral protection during times of temporary arterial occlusion according to the local anesthesiologist's experience. Mean blood pressure should be maintained at normal or slightly elevated parameters (90–100 mm Hg), and plasma expanders should be used intraoperatively to prevent any ischemic event. Intraoperative monitoring with EEG and/or somatosensory-evoked potentials allows the detection of ischemic changes in early stages, using the drugs mentioned previously. The operating microscope and microsurgical instruments are used routinely in revascularization procedures.

Donor vessel (the STA) should be selected with an external diameter not less than 1 mm because vessels of smaller diameter have a high percentage of occlusion, deliver a low blood flow, are not useful, and are more difficult to anastomose.[23-26] To prevent mechanical vasospasm, it is useful to apply topical diluted papaverine or nimodipine.

The patient is placed on the operating table with the head rotated toward the contralateral side and the temporal bone is parallel to the floor, kept in position by the head holder with three points. After the scalp is shaved, the standard Doppler ultrasound is used over the donor artery and correlated

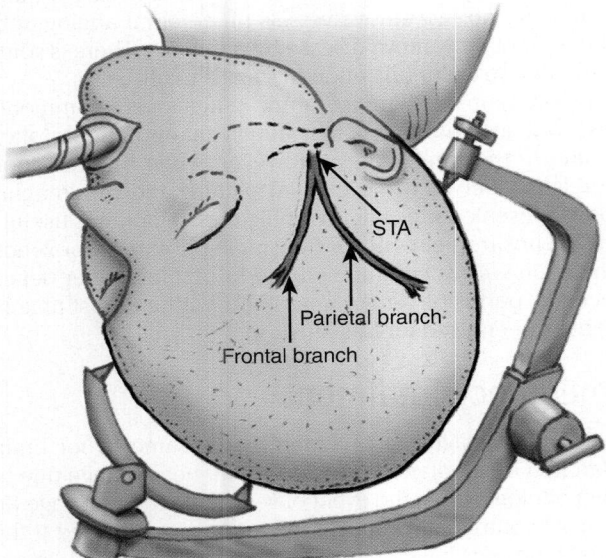

FIGURE 71-3 Position of patient's head. The patient is placed on the operating table with the head rotated toward the contralateral side, the temporal bone parallel to the floor, and kept in position by the head holder with three points.

with the preoperative angiography to locate the most suitable branch of the STA. The skin is painted with its branches using a marker pen. Usually there are two branches of the STA, the frontal and parietal. Both must be marked during the proceedings (Fig. 71-3).

Direct Bypass Surgery

Superficial Temporal Artery–Middle Cerebral Artery

The first bypass STA-MCA as treatment for moyamoya disease and other ischemic cerebrovascular pathologies, was performed in 1972 by Yasargil,[24] and since then, several clinical series have been reported showing good results in the immediate postoperative period with an isolated direct surgical technique[25,26] or combined with other indirect revascularization techniques.[23,35]

After sterile preparation, an incision is made beginning on the zygoma with a scalpel no.15; the STA is identified and skeletonized using smooth dissection, both with the scalpel and scissors tips. When necessary, a Doppler device is used to check the correct path of the STA. Either the frontal or parietal branch are used, depending on the diameter and length, preferably using the larger diameter branch, with the occasional exception of a wider frontal branch passing very low over the forehead. It is advisable to leave a sleeve of collagen tissue support around the artery to avoid injury, decreasing the mechanical vasospasm of the artery and allowing the surgeon to handle the vessel without damaging the artery walls. Small side branches are coagulated with bipolar and cut. The length of the artery required depends on the distance from the origin of the visible STA to the bypass site. The artery is separated and protected. Next a superomedial temporal craniotomy of least 4 cm in diameter is created crossing the anteroposterior projection of the sylvian fissure.

The dura mater is opened widely relative to the craniotomy, and the microscope is installed to select the recipient artery, which should ideally have an outer diameter of 1 mm or more. We must also take into account the orientation of the recipient artery and the location of the branch of the MCA in relation to the sylvian fissure. As closer branches allow better blood flow back to the internal carotid artery bifurcation, it is best to choose an M3 branch of the MCA emerging from the sylvian fissure. The exposure of the recipient vessel is performed with a meticulous dissection of the surrounding arachnoid membrane, over a segment from 6 to 10 mm in length, around the direction of the artery. Small collaterals that emerge from the recipient artery are coagulated and cut. It is preferable to place a small piece of plastic underneath the elected branch of the MCA, which increases visibility in the operating field.

A temporary clip is secured to the proximal segment of the STA and the distal end is cut; the blood flow of the STA can be evaluated by temporarily releasing the clip. Next, the lumen of the STA is irrigated with heparinized saline to prevent clot formation inside the lumen artery. The distal portion of the STA is confronted and adapted to the appropriate length to reach the recipient artery without tension. Next, the distal cuff of connective tissue around the artery is removed in a long, approximately 3- to 5-mm piece, preparing this segment for anastomosis. The distal end of the STA is cut in oblique form. Microclips are then installed on each side of the dissected segment of the recipient artery, and a diamond-shaped incision in the wall is made using microsurgical scissors.

Subsequently, under a microscope, the anastomosis is performed using 10-0 monofilament suture. Sutures are placed first at the corners of the diamond-shaped incision and then five interrupted sutures are placed over the distal wall edges. The procedure is repeated with five interrupted sutures over the nearest wall. The intima are always included in the suture to avoid any increased tension at the sutured site (Fig. 71-4).

We recommended using interrupted sutures.[23-25,36,37] but some authors prefer a continuous suture.[38] Proceed to remove the first distal clip and then the proximal clip of the recipient artery. Finally, the temporary clip on the STA is removed. Classically, it is recommended that the time of temporary clipping of the recipient artery should be no more than 30 minutes. After removing the clips, Cottonoids are applied with gentle pressure on the site of the anastomosis. If a higher rate of bleeding occurs at any time during the anastomosis with a higher rate of bleeding, then an additional suture must be placed. Minor oozing usually ceases with Surgicel (vegetal oxidized cellulose mesh, Ethicon®) and pressure on the anastomosed site. Once the anastomosis is complete, Doppler can be used to examine anastomotic patency.

Proceed to suture the dura mater carefully to avoid narrowing of the STA. The bone plate is replaced so as to prevent any pressure on the STA. Finally, the temporalis muscle, galea, and skin are sutured in the conventional manner.

In the immediate postoperative stage, hemodynamic monitoring is critical. The main complications of this procedure are intracranial hypertension and increased cerebral perfusion, which can cause leakage between nodes of the anastomosis and consequently a subdural hematoma at the site of the bypass. Conversely, hypotension may cause occlusion and ischemia, triggering a clinical complication that requires an emergency angiography and review of the

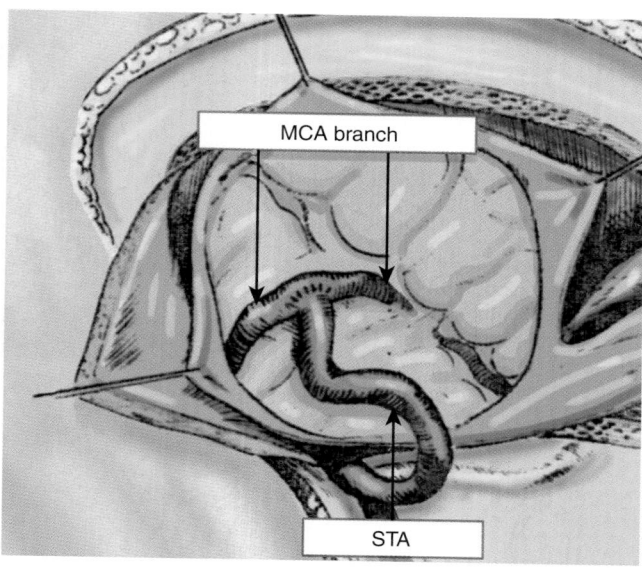

FIGURE 71-4 Classic anastomosis superficial temporal artery–middle cerebral artery branch.

bypass surgery. Another extremely rare but potential complication is cerebrospinal fluid fistula, which may occur if the dura is not closed under appropriate tension. On the first postoperative day, one may restart aspirin as a form of platelet antiaggregant therapy.

Indirect Bypass Surgery
Encephalo-Duro-Arterio-Synangiosis

The encephalo-duro-arterio-synangiosis (EDAS), described by Matsushima et al.,[32,33] is an alternative to the STA-MCA bypass. EDAS is an indirect way to increase collateral blood flow to the ischemic brain. This indirect technique does not increase cerebral blood flow immediately. Rather, indirect techniques are most often used in cases of cerebral ischemia and are associated with revascularization between 6 to 12 months following intervention, specially in cases that occur with cerebral ischemia.[15,23,32,33,35]

In this surgical technique, the STA is dissected, as in the technique described above, but the vessel is left in continuity, not sectioned. Then, an incision is made over the temporalis muscle. A diamond-shaped or biconvex craniotomy is performed with two holes using an automatic drill and with the directionality of the craniotomy site mirroring the direction of the underlying STA. Taking care to avoid damage to vessels of the extraintracranial collateral circulation, some authors advocate creating little windows[15,33] in the dura mater and pia-arachnoid to allow for greater, closer contact between the area of the STA and the cerebral cortex.

Next, the cuff of connective tissue surrounding the STA is sutured to the edges of the dura mater with monofilament 5-0 interrupted sutures. It is necessary to be careful that the path of the artery, sutured to the dura mater, is not curved on the edges of the craniotomy, which must be lowered to prevent this complication. Topical papaverine may be used to prevent mechanical vasospasm, and Doppler imaging can be used once the craniotomy has been repositioned to verify that there is adequate distal flow through the artery. After fixation of the craniotomy, the temporalis muscle, galea, and skin are sutured in a conventional manner (Figs. 71-5 and 71-6).

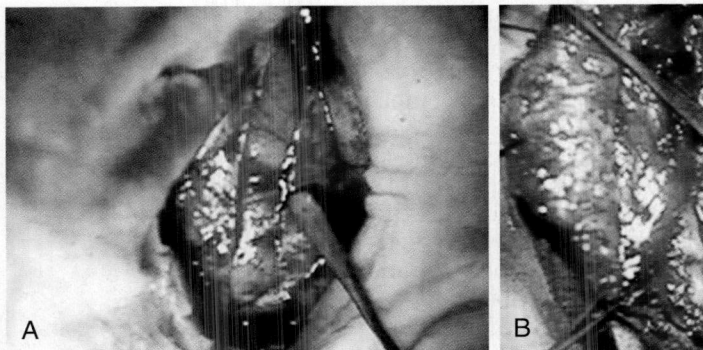

FIGURE 71-5 Encephalo-duro-arterio-synangiosis (EDAS). A, Dural opening. B, Suture of superficial temporal artery (STA) with galea edges to the edges of the dura.

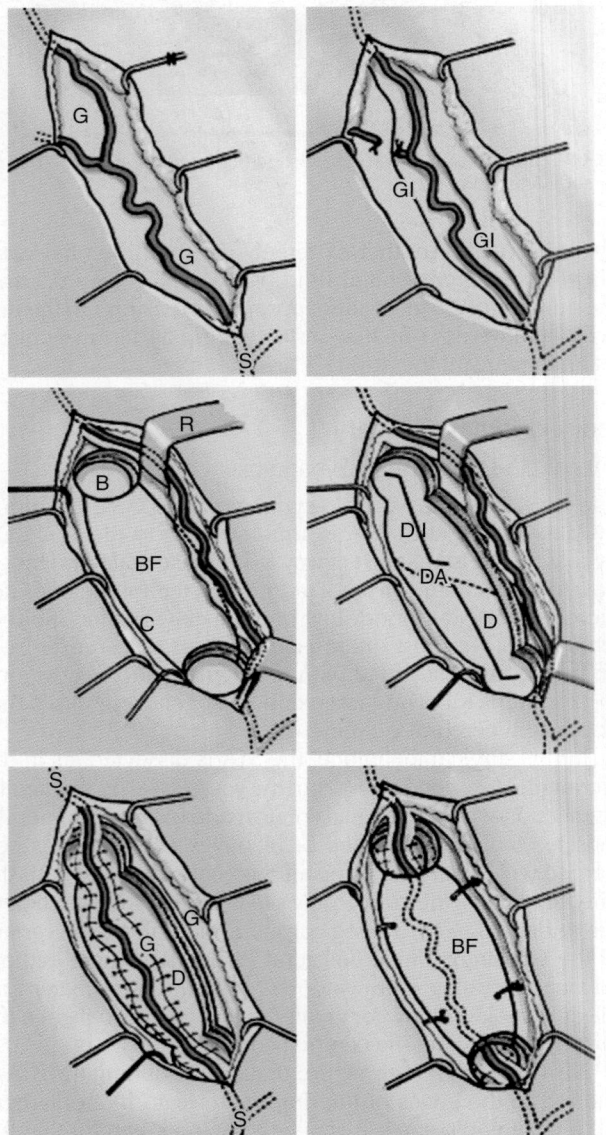

FIGURE 71-6 Shows the stages of encephalo-duro-arterio-synangiosis (EDAS), described by Matsushima et al. *(From Matsushima Y, Fukai M, Tanaka K, et al. A new surgical treatment of moyamoya disease in children: a preliminary report. Surg Neurol. 1981;15:313-320.)*

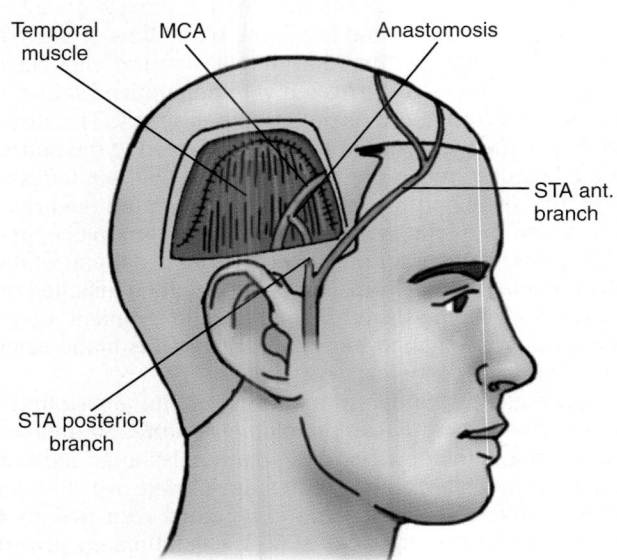

FIGURE 71-7 Encephalo-myo-synangiosis (EMS). Diagram shows the temporal muscle flap sutured to the edges of the dura and a superficial temporary artery/middle cerebral artery (STA-MCA) anastomosis. *(From Houkin K, Ishikawa T, Yoshimoto T, Abe H. Direct and indirect revascularization for moyamoya disease—surgical techniques and peri-operative complications. Clin Neurol Neurosurg. 1997;99:(Suppl 2):142-145.)*

The authors advocate that in the EDAS, temporary clipping over the branches of the MCA is not required. The extraintracranial spontaneous anastomoses that develop through the dura mater generally have good patency, and this procedure is technically much easier to perform than the STA-MCA procedure.[15,32,33] Furthermore, EDAS can be performed in cases where a donor or recipient artery of appropriate size is not available, which may occur as a function of the underlying disease.

Matsushima et al. reported their results treating moyamoya disease in 38 pediatric cases (70 hemispheres). In these cases, 100% of revascularization was obtained, with most patients showing improvement in symptoms due to cerebral ischemia.[32,33]

Encephalo-Myo-Synangiosis

In the encephalo-myo-synangiosis (EMS), a flap of the temporalis muscle is sutured to the edges of the dural surgical opening so that the muscle is positioned closer to the

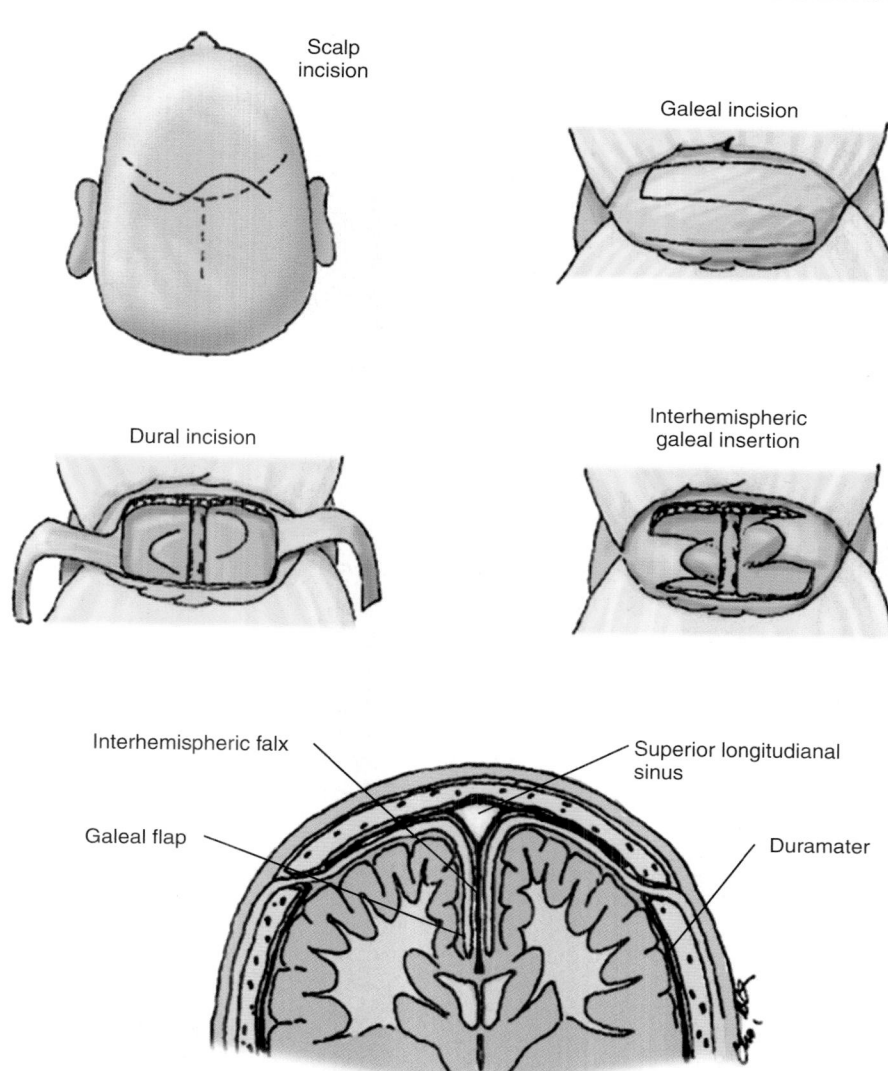

Scalp incision

Galeal incision

Dural incision

Interhemispheric galeal insertion

Interhemispheric falx

Superior longitudianal sinus

Galeal flap

Duramater

FIGURE 71-8 Encephalo-duro-arterio-synangiosis (EDAS) and encephalic galeo-sinangiosis. *(From Kim SK, Wang KC, Kim IO, et al. Combined encephaloduroarterio-synangiosis and bifrontal encephalogaleo (periostial) synangiosis in pediatric moyamoya disease. Neurosurgery. 2002;50:88-96.)*

brain surface. As in the EDAS, a frontotemporal craniotomy is performed and the arachnoid over the brain surface in question is opened as widely as possible. Next, the edges of the dura mater are sutured to the edges of the muscle flap.

Neovascularization occurs from muscle to the brain parenchyma, providing greater collateral blood flow to the brain. As in the EDAS, the EMS is technically simpler to perform than the direct STA-MCA bypass and does not require identification of a recipient artery. Additionally, the EMS can be combined with a direct STA-MCA bypass in some patients[23,34] (Fig. 71-7).

However, this procedure has been associated with an increased risk in some patients to developing an epileptogenic focus.[23,34,35] Yet, several series have shown that EMS improves the clinical condition of patients and promotes revascularization in the region of the MCA in 70% to 80% of all patients.[26,34]

EDAS plus Encephalo-Galeo-Synangiosis

The EDAS is performed according to the technique described by Matsushima and Inaba.[33] This surgery is performed in two stages, initially on the more hemodynamically affected cerebral hemisphere, with an average time between the first and second procedure being 6 to 8 months. To further increase collateral circulation in the territory of the anterior cerebral arteries, EDAS is performed with encephalo-galeo-synangiosis (EGS) in the bifrontal region as detailed below.[39]

The scalp is incised twice, once for the EDAS and again for the EGS. At the site of the EGS, an elongated S-shaped, 2-cm incision is made anterior to the coronal suture. Then, the galea and/or the periosteum are dissected and are incised in a Roman S-shape in the anteroposterior direction, like a zigzag.

A craniotomy is performed of approximately 4 to 8 cm in length, crossing the superior longitudinal sinus. Then, the dura mater is incised in both hemispheres, with two separate flaps down to the venous sinus. Next, the arachnoid surface is removed to expose the underlying brain. Galeal flaps and/or periosteum is overlaid on the cerebral cortex and inserted into the deepest possible interhemispheric fissure, suturing it to the dura mater.

Finally, the craniotomy is fixed, and the skin and galea are closed via a conventional technique[39] (Fig. 71-8).

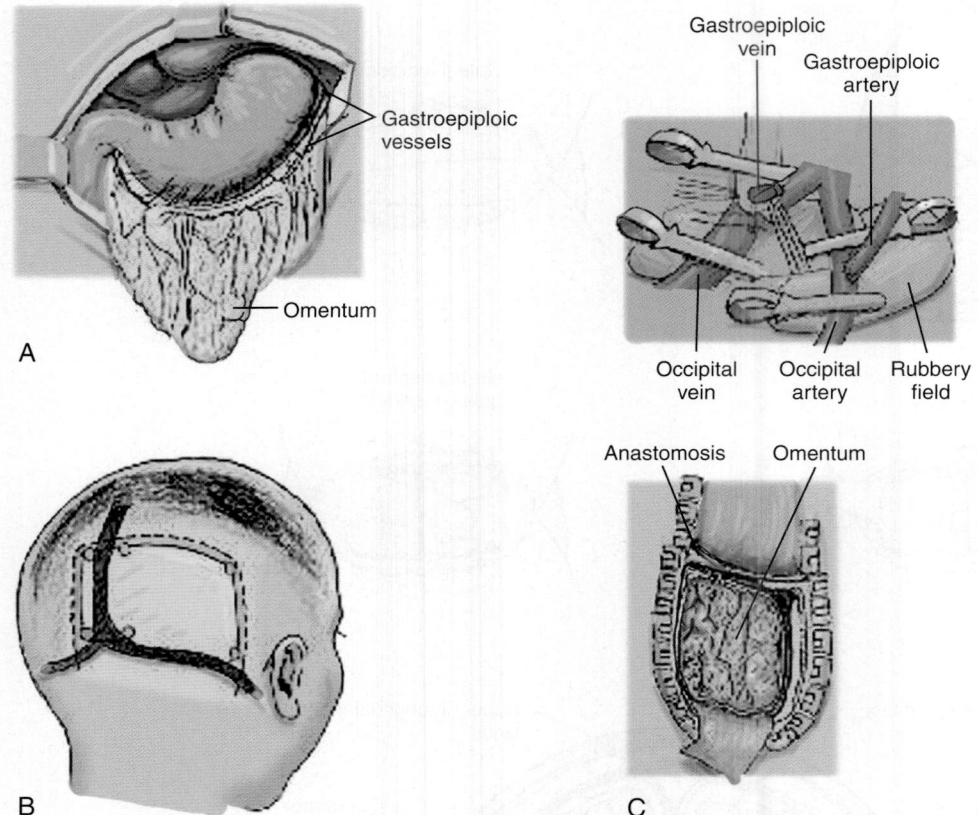

FIGURE 71-9 Omentum autograft. A, Piece of graft with omentum. B, Occipital craniotomy at right with region to be treated. C, Anastomosis of gastroepiploic artery and vein to occipital artery and vein. Details of the anastomosis are shown at top.

Revascularization Using Omentum

The omentum can be surgically used as a traditional flap nourished by the gastroepiploic vessels directly, or as a free flap, autotransplanted and vascularized from arteries and veins of the scalp. In both cases, the omentum is obtained through a median supraumbilical laparatomy.

Omental Transplantation

A median supraumbilical laparatomy with careful dissection and isolation of the gastroepiploic artery and vein exposes the omentum and preserves the vascular gastroepiploic pedicle. The omentum is separated from its vascular pedicle immediately before the autotransplantation to preserve omentumal perfusion as long as possible. The autograft is preserved wet. The gastroepiploic artery and vein are sectioned and irrigated with heparinized saline to prevent intraluminal thrombosis.

The STA (or the occipital artery) is dissected as described previously. For omentumal transplant, however, one must dissect the superficial temporal vein (STV) (or occipital vein). A craniotomy is performed over the region where the revascularization is desired.

Using microsurgical techniques, end-to-end anastomoses or end-to-side anastomoses between the STA (or occipital artery) and the gastroepiploic artery, as well as between the STV (or occipital vein) and the gastroepiploic vein are established, using 10-0 monofilament suture. First, arterial anastomosis is performed. Next, a temporary clip is placed

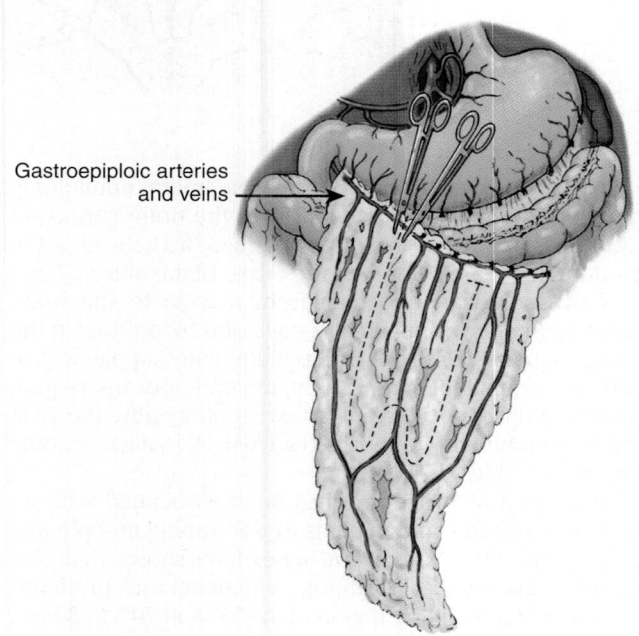

FIGURE 71-10 During the omentum transposition, the omentum is elongated by performing incisions in the form of an "L," preserving the lymphatic, venous, and arterial circulation.

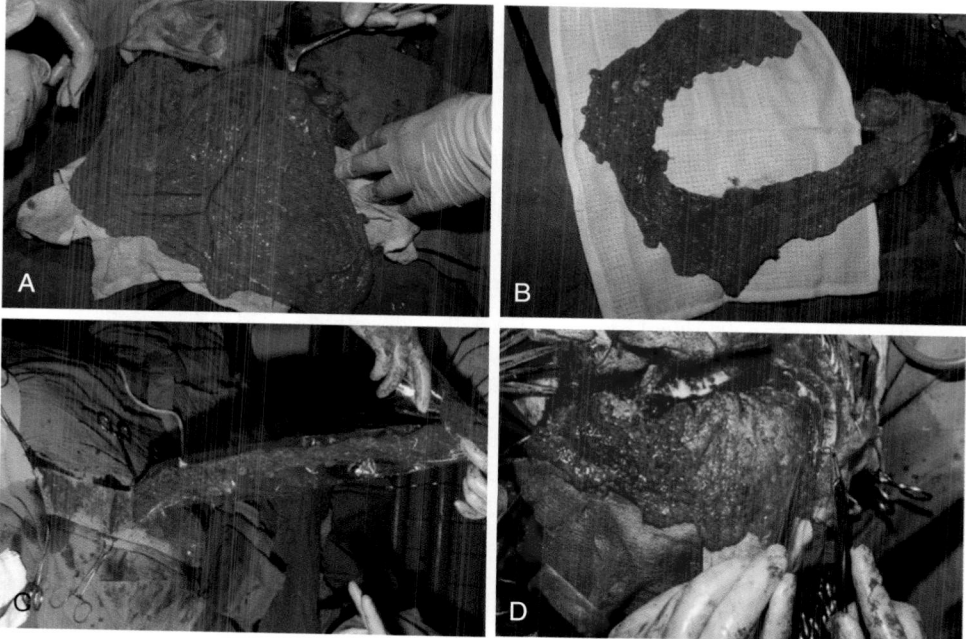

FIGURE 71-11 Transposition of omentum. A, Presentation of omentum through a midline supraumbilical laparotomy. B, Extension of the omentum through L-shaped incisions, preserving vascularization. C, Pass the omentum, tunneled through the subcutaneous tissue from the abdomen to the skull. D, Suture the edges of the omentum to the edges of the dura.

on the donor artery during venous anastomosis. After this set of anastomoses has been secured, the omentum is spread over the cerebral surface and under the edges of the exposed dura mater. The graft is sutured to the edges of the dura mater, and the craniotomy plate is fixed, taking care not to compress the vascular pedicle[30] (Fig. 71-9).

Omental Transposition

This surgical technique involves extending the omentum in order to reach the skull, while it remains attached to its natural vascular pedicle. Advantages to such an approach include preserving lymphatic drainage and avoiding an additional vascular anastomosis. The omentum's gastroepiploic pedicle is left to its normal anatomy and the omentum is able to reach the skull by dividing the elongated omentum with incisions in the form of an "L" (Fig. 71-10).

The omentum is then tunneled subcutaneously, passing through the subcutaneous chest, neck, and scalp, including behind the ear. The omentum, with its pedicle, must not be under tension after the tunneling, nor should it be angled in any segment of the subcutaneous tunnel. Thus, several incisions are made in the skin along the tunnel to facilitate graft passage. Once inside the skull, the omentum is placed on the brain surface under the edges of the exposed dura mater. The graft is sutured to the edges of the dura mater, and the craniotomy plate is fixed, taking care not to compress the vascular pedicle[31] (Fig. 71-11).

Multiple Burr-Holes Operation

This operation is performed under general anesthesia and is technically similar to the creation of burr holes for the placement of external ventricular drainage systems.

To avoid injury to the STA over the burr holes, the trajectory of the STA is located by Doppler. After creating two to four burr holes over each cerebral hemisphere, the dura mater and arachnoid are widely opened, preserving the meningeal arteries with the use of a microscope. Then, the

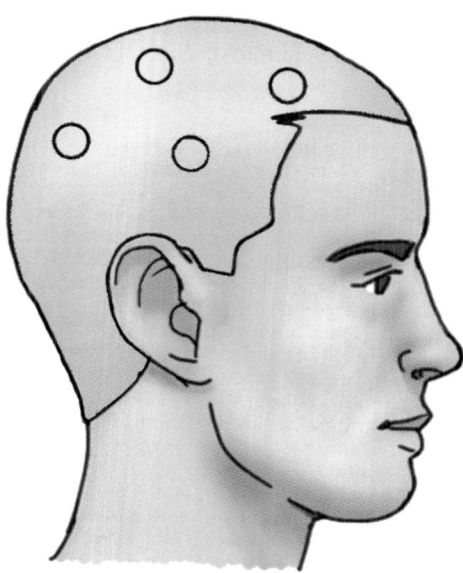

FIGURE 71-12 Revascularization through burr holes. Outline of the burr-hole sites (2 to 4) to achieve indirect revascularization.

skin is sutured tightly closed with 2-0 monofilament[28,29] (Fig. 71-12).

Surgical Complications

With the reviewed surgical techniques, the incidence of surgical complications is very low; however, the incidence of complications is not zero. Postoperative complications include bleeding from the surgical site (subcutaneous, epidural, subdural, and intracerebral), anemia, cerebral infarction (due to perioperative hypotension, hypocapnia due to hyperventilation, and prolonged, temporary clipping of arteries), transient ischemic attacks, scalp necrosis, surgical wound infection, and convulsive seizures.[19,23,33,35]

The benefits of sugery usually do not appear immediately. However, the frequency of ischemic events tends to gradually decline.[23,27,29,33-35] The postoperative course of patients is variable and depends on increase in cerebral blood flow and surgical method, among other factors.[15,19,22,24,27,35]

General anesthesia for moyamoya disease has been associated with a relatively low risk of a new stroke, both during bypass surgery as well as during cerebral angiography, in adults.[26,27,33-35]

GENERAL RESULTS OF SURGICAL BYPASS

The purpose of using surgical anastomoses, either directly or indirectly, is to prevent recurrent cerebrovascular disease, not to reverse the effects of already completed strokes. In cases of ischemic stroke, most neurosurgeons with experience in the field believe that bypass presents an important modifier of the natural history of moyamoya disease. Indeed, many moyamoya patients with a history of ischemic events experience a reduction or disappearance of symptoms following surgery, correlated in the majority of series with good to excellent revascularization on imaging.[15,19,23,24,33-35]

In cases of hemorrhagic stroke, the purpose of the anastomosis is to prevent re-bleeding. The benefits of surgery in such cases are more unclear and controversial compared to the benefits seen following surgical intervention for moyamoya patients with ischemic disease.

KEY REFERENCES

Endo M, Kawano N, Misayaka Y, Yada K. Cranial burr hole for revascularization in moyamoya disease. *J Neurosurg.* 1989;71: 180-185.

Fujiwara H, Momoshima S, Kuribayashi S. Leptomeningeal high signal intensity (ivy sign) on fluid-attenuated inversion-recovery (FLAIR) MR images in moyamoya disease. *Eur J Radiol.* 2005;55:224-230.

Goldsmith HS. Brain and spinal cord revascularization by omental transposition. *Neurolog Res.* 1994;16:159-162.

Hirano M, Sakurai S. Psychiatric symptoms and signs associated with spontaneous occlusion of the circle of Willis. A case report and studies of 379 cases in Japan. *Psychiatr Med (Tokyo).* 1972;14:329-338.

Houkin K, Ishikawa T, Yoshimoto T, Abe H. Direct and indirect revascularization for moyamoya disease—surgical techniques and perioperative complications. *Clin Neurol Neurosurg.* 1997;99(Suppl 2): 142-145.

Ikesayki K, Matsushima T, Kubawara Y, et al. Cerebral circulation and oxigen metabolism in childhood moyamoya disease: a perioperative positron emission tomography study. *J Neurosurg.* 1994;81:843-850.

Karasawa J, Kikuchi H, Furuse S, et al. A surgical treatment of "moyamoya" disease—encephalo-myo-synangiosis. *Neurol Med Chir.* 1977;17: 29-37.

Karasawa J, Touho H, Ohnishi H. Cerebral revascularization using omental transplantation for childhood moyamoya disease. *J Neurosurg.* 1993;79(2):192-196.

Kim SK, Wang KC, Kim IO, et al. Combined encephaloduroarteriosynangiosis and bifrontal encephalogaleo (periostial) synangiosis in pediatric moyamoya disease. *Neurosurgery.* 2002;50:88-96.

Kudo T. Spontaneous occlusion of the circle of Willis: a disease apparently confined to Japanese. *Neurology.* 1968;18:485-496.

Little JR, Salerno TA. Continuous suturing for microvascular anastomosis—technical note. *J Neurosurg.* 1978;48:1042-1045.

Matsushima T, Inoue T, Katsuta T, et al. An indirect revascularization method in the surgical treatment of moyamoya disease—various kinds of indirect procedures and a multiple combined indirect procedure. *Neurol Med Chir (Tokyo).* 1998;38(Suppl):297-302.

Matsushima Y, Inaba Y. Moyamoya disease in children and its surgical treatment. Introduction of a new surgical procedure and its follow-up angiograms. *Childs Brain.* 1984;11(3):155-170.

McDonald C, Carter BS. Medical management of increased intracranial pressure after spontaneous intracerebral hemorrhage. *Neurosurg Clin North Am..* 2002;13(3):335-338.

Quintana L. Experiencia de 20 años en el manejo de la enfermedad moyamoya. *Rev Chil Neurocirug.* 2004;23:30-36.

Scott RM, Smith ER. Moyamoya disease and moyamoya syndrome. *N Engl J Med.* 2009;19;360(12):1226-1237.

Suzuki J. Epidemiology and symptomatology. In: Suzuku J, ed. *Moyamoya Disease.* Berlin and Heidelberg: Springer-Verlag; 1986:7-16.

Suzuki J, Takaku A. Cerebrovascular "moyamoya" disease showing abnormal net-like vessels in base of brain. *Arch Neurol (Chicago).* 1969;20:288-299.

Takeuchi K, Shimizu K. Hypogenesis of bilateral internal carotid arteries. *No To Shinkei.* 1957;9:37-43.

Takeuchi S, Tanaka R, Ishii R, et al. Cerebral hemodynamics in patients with moyamoya disease. A study of regional cerebral blood flow by the Xe-133 inhalation method. *Surg Neurol.* 1985;23:468-474.

Yamada I, Matsushima Y, Suzuki S. Moyamoya disease: diagnosis with three-dimensional time-of-flight MR angiography. *Radiology.* 1992; 184:773-778.

Yamada I, Suzuki S, Matsushima Y. Moyamoya disease: comparison of assessment with MR angiography and MR imaging versus conventional angiography. *Radiology.* 1995;196:211-218.

Yasargil MG, Yonekawa Y. Results of microsurgical extra-intracranial arterial bypass in the treatment of cerebral ischemia. *Neurosurgery.* 1977; 1:22.

Yonekawa Y, Yasargil MG. Extra-intracranial arterial anastomosis: clinical and technical aspects. Results. In: Krayenbühl H, ed. *Advances and Technical Standards in Neurosurgery.* Zürich, Wien, and New York: Springer-Verlag; 1977:47-78.

Numbered references appear on Expert Consult.

CHAPTER 72

Surgical Treatment of Paraclinoid Aneurysms

EDGAR NATHAL • GABRIEL CASTILLO

The portion of the proximal intradural internal carotid artery (ICA) adjacent to the anterior clinoid process (ACP) is called the paraclinoid segment. Aneurysms arising from the ICA between the roof of the cavernous sinus and the origin of the posterior communicating artery (PComA) are defined as paraclinoid aneurysms.[1-5] These aneurysms are of considerable surgical interest due to their particular anatomic features and technical difficulties. Some of these aneurysms were considered in the past as unclippable or associated with very bad results when surgically approached.[6] Fortunately, with the progressive refinement of microsurgical techniques their management has changed from the very conservative surgery to direct neck clipping, with results surpassing those of the endovascular therapy in terms of total neck obliteration and long-term recanalization (Table 72-1).[4,5,7] The classification of these aneurysms according to the origin of their necks and projection of the aneurysms is particularly important to select the optimum microsurgical approach.[1,8-12]

Incidence

Reported incidence of paraclinoid aneurysms varies from 5% to 9% of anterior circulation aneurysms. They are more frequent in female sex and tend to occur in association with multiple aneurysms in more than 20% of the cases, including the so-called mirror aneurysms. They tend to increase their size to become large or giant, presenting in these cases with visual deficit rather than subarachnoid hemorrhage.

Anatomic Aspects

In 1938, Fisher[12a] published an anatomic nomenclature for the ICA based on the angiographic course of the artery, describing five segments designated C1 through C5. However, these segments were numbered opposite to the direction of blood flow and the extracranial ICA was excluded (Fig. 72-1A). Recently, other classifications have been published that include the extracranial and intracranial segments, and the carotid segments have been numbered according to the direction of the blood flow. Therefore, the paraclinoid segment of the ICA comprises the C2 and C3 segments of the original Fisher classification (1938), the distal C3 and Proximal C4 segment of Gibo et al. (1981),[13] and the C5 and C6 segment of the Bouthillier classification (1996)[14] (Fig. 72-1). Because of the close topographical vicinity of these aneurysms to osseous, fibrous, nervous and vascular

structures of the skull base they may present with clinical symptoms due to compression of the optic nerve or other surrounding structures instead of the classic subarachnoid hemorrhage frequently seen in aneurysms in other locations.[3,15] The anatomic structures of the paraclinoid area not only produce a limited space for expanding vascular lesions, but also for the neurosurgeon during operation, thus, sufficient proximal control and minimal manipulation of the vascular and nerve structures around are of utmost importance for the postoperative outcome.[1,2,4,5,7,16-18]

Classification

Given the variability in projection, size and origin of these aneurysms, various authors in the past have classified them. Most of the classifications are based on the site of origin of the neck, the projection of the dome and its relationship with branches arising from the ICA.[2,7-10,12,17] The vast majority of saccular aneurysms arise within the angle formed by the parent artery and a significant arterial branch. Therefore, aneurysms related to these arteries are called accordingly, for example, ophthalmic and superior hypophyseal artery aneurysms.[2,8] In addition, aneurysms unrelated to branches occur only rarely in this segment (distal ophthalmic aneurysms).[12] Ventral paraclinoid carotid aneurysms seem to belong to the same category as infraophthalmic aneurysms, which originate from the ventral surface of the ICA and in which the proximal aspect of the neck is located approximately at the level of the ophthalmic artery and the distal aspect of the neck is located proximal to the posterior communicating artery[19] (Fig. 72-2). These aneurysms also project straight or slightly medial and downward. Carotid cave aneurysms are another distinct type of aneurysm located at non-branching sites of this segment. This type of aneurysm arises from the medial wall of the proximal intradural ICA, and grows within a small dural recess, with the apex of the sac directed toward the cavernous sinus[10] (Fig. 72-3). All these denominations have contributed to create a rather complex view of these aneurysms. Another confusing characteristic is that they are not always related to a branching artery and may point in any direction, as laterally, medially, ventrally, or dorsally (Fig. 72-2).

In order to simplify the classification of these aneurysms, we prefer to name them according to their site of origin in relation to the circumference of the ICA and some branching artery (if any), because this is also relevant at the time of clipping. Thus, the paraclinoid aneurysms can be classified

Table 72-1   Comparative Results in Surgical Series of Paraclinoid Aneurysms

Author/Year	Number of Aneurysms/ Patients	Direct Clipping (%)	Good Outcome (%)	Fair Outcome (%)	Poor Outcome (%)	Mortality (%)
Drake et al.[6]/1968	14/14 (AS)	50	40	—	—	60
Day[8]/1990	54/54 (AS)	96	87	—	7	6
Batjer et al./1994	89/89 (AS)	—	87	9	3	1
Arnautovic et al.[16]/1998	16/16 (L-G)	94	88	6	—	6
De Jesús et al.[32]/1999	35/28 (AS)	88	89	7	—	3.5
Kattner et al.[3]/1998	29/29 (L-G)	96	89	—	7	3.5
Raco et al.[18]/2008	108/104 (AS)	81	83	7	5.7	3.8
Liu et al.[11]/2008	40/38 (AS)	76.3	76.3	—	18.4	5.3
Present Series/2008	137/91 (AS)	94	88	7.6	—	4

AS, all sizes; L-G, large and giants.

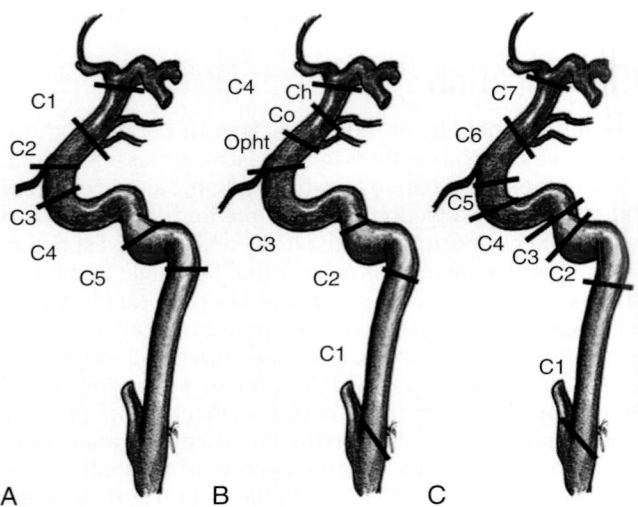

FIGURE 72-1 A, Classification of the internal carotid artery segments by Fisher (1938). B, Classification by Gibo et al. *(From Gibo H, Lenkey C, Rhoton AL Jr. Microsurgical anatomy of the supraclinoid portion of the internal carotid artery. J Neurosurg. 1981;55:560-574.)* C, Classification by Bouthillier et al. *(From Bouthillier A, van Loveren HR, Keller JT. Segments of the internal carotid artery: a new classification. Neurosurgery. 1996;38(3):425-433.)*

as follows: dorsal type aneurysms, ventral type aneurysms, carotid cave aneurysms, and global type aneurysms (Figs. 72-3 to 72-7).

DORSAL TYPE ANEURYSMS

These include the proximal dorsal type aneurysms that correspond to the carotid ophthalmic aneurysms. They arise from the ophthalmic segment of the ICA in close relationship with the ophthalmic artery.[7,9,11,15,18] On the lateral view of an angiogram the neck of the aneurysm is located just distal to the origin of this artery (Figs. 72-2A, 72-4, and 72-8). They grow upwards and cause compression of the optic nerve. As they have a

tendency to grow, many of these lesions are detected because of visual deficits. The second main type is the distal dorsal type aneurysm (also known as dorsal wall aneurysms). This aneurysm grows upward at the dorsal surface of the ICA (Fig. 72-5). They are located distal to the ophthalmic artery and seem not to origin from any branch of the ICA.[9,12] Whether they arise at bifurcations of vestigial arteries or because hemodynamic stress at the curvature of the carotid siphon is unknown.[20] The dorsal surface of the ICA is also a common site of blood blister–like aneurysms. These are dangerous small lesions with fragile walls consisting of normal adventitia or fibrin nets. Primary treatment in the acute stage is challenging due to the substantial risk of intraoperative bleeding, resulting in the formation of a large defect in the ICA. To treat these aneurysms, sometimes it is necessary to use especially designed encircling clips or some wrapping procedure, otherwise, a bypass procedure with trapping of the aneurysm can be used as an alternative.

VENTRAL TYPE ANEURYSMS

These aneurysms grow at the ventral or ventromedial surface of the ICA (Figs. 72-2B, 72-6, and 72-9). They are located opposite to the origin of the ophthalmic artery and in close relationship with the superior hypophyseal artery. As they increase in size, they are directed downward and medially. When large or giant, they produce an upward displacement of the ICA; however, visual disturbance is not as frequent as in dorsal type aneurysms.[1,2,5,8,19]

CAROTID CAVE ANEURYSMS

This is a special type of aneurysm originating between the proximal and distal carotid rings. They grow ventromedially proximal to the ophthalmic artery, and are visible mainly on the anterior or oblique angiographic views. On the lateral view, they remain hidden by the ICA (Figs. 72-3 and 72-10). Carotid cave aneurysms are transitional in type between paraclinoid intradural and cavernous sinus aneurysms. They may grow out of the cave into the intradural subarachnoid space. During surgery, they project ventrally at the level

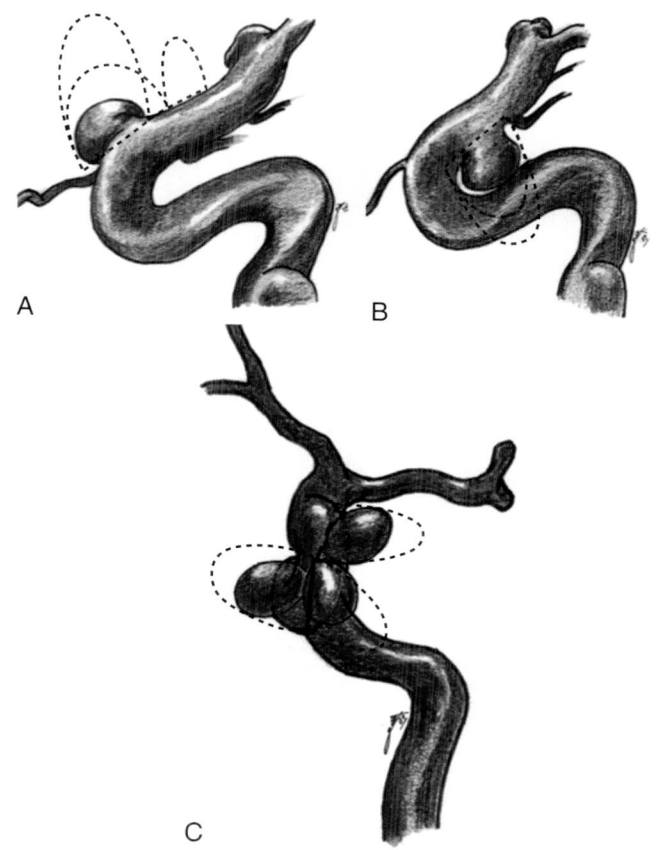

A   B

C

FIGURE 72-2 Projection and growth of paraclinoid aneurysms. A, Dorsal type aneurysms. Proximal type (ophthalmic) and distal dorsal type arise from the dorsal surface of the ICA between the ophthalmic artery and the ICA bifurcation. Growing produce a direct compression of the optic nerve causing visual acuity and field defects. B, Ventral type aneurysm. This aneurysm originates in the ventral or ventromedial surface of the ICA. When growing, they produce an upper displacement of the ICA with less optic compression than the dorsal type. They tend to occupy the space medial or lateral to the ICA, causing compression of surrounding structures (e.g., cranial nerve III). C, Paraclinoid aneurysms may increase in size according to the space around the site of origin. They may grow upward, medially, ventrally, laterally, or in a combination of these directions.

of the carotid genu[10] (Fig. 72-11). In this sense, the surgical genu is located more proximal than the angiographic genu, which roughly corresponds to the location of the dural ring.

GLOBAL TYPE ANEURYSMS

These aneurysms involve the entire circumference of the ICA; they are large or giant in size, and during angiography or surgery the origins of the neck are not as easy to identify as ventral or dorsal types even when the origin was surely at any of these points. Most cases are associated with degeneration of the carotid wall. The importance of this type of aneurysm is that the treatment is based on deconstructive techniques (parent artery obliteration and bypass surgery). This type of aneurysm should not be diagnosed only because of size and shape (Fig. 72-7).

It should be emphasized that during the growth process of a paraclinoid aneurysm, the dome could occupy anatomic spaces at the medial or lateral side of the ICA (Fig. 72-2). We do not believe that the medial or lateral sides of the ICA are

origin sites of such aneurysms. When we carefully analyze the angiographic videos and films or the intraoperative recordings (except for global type aneurysms), the origin can be traced to the dorsal or ventromedial surface of the ICA.

Surgical Technique

Even when the treatment of paraclinoid aneurysms seems to be more difficult than any other aneurysm of the anterior circulation, from the surgical point of view, however, clipping of these aneurysms requires essentially the same surgical technique; proximal control of the ICA, wide opening of the sylvian fissure, extensive microsurgical dissection of the subarachnoid cisterns, and according to the size of the aneurysm, complete removal of the ACP, unroofing the optic canal, complete opening of the proximal dural ring and exposure of the surgical genu and axilla of the ICA by opening the infraclinoid carotid groove sinus, and packing proximally along the wall of the ICA or injecting fibrin glue in the cavernous sinus to control venous bleeding. The great improvement in surgical results compared with the early efforts to treat these lesions has been due to the incorporation of these techniques and new tools. In this way, a systematic approach of these aneurysms should include the steps discussed in subsequent sections.

Preoperative Planning

A very careful preoperative plan should be obtained for every case, taking into account the size and position of neck and dome of the aneurysm and its relationship with surrounding structures, especially the optic nerve. In addition, the length of the ICA should be assessed as well as the position of the ophthalmic and posterior communicating arteries. The summary of all this information will provide important hints for selecting the craniotomy and the technique for drilling the ACP (extra or intradural), and to prepare the availability of proper instruments to be used in the operation including a complete set of ring (fenestrated) clips for ventral or carotid cave aneurysms. To prevent premature intraoperative rupture or prolonged ICA occlusion, the preoperative angiography should include a four-vessel angiography with a balloon or manual compressive test occlusion in the awake patient. This will provide information about the position of the aneurysm and the collateral circulation at the circle of Willis, especially from one side to the other through the anterior communicating artery and from the posterior to the anterior circulation. The results of this preoperative test allow for reliable estimation of the tolerance of temporary or even permanent ICA occlusion or to be prepared for a bypass procedure before attacking a complex aneurysm in case of poor collateral circulation[2,3,21] (Fig. 72-12).

PROXIMAL CONTROL OF THE ICA

Techniques to achieve proximal control of the ICA are briefly described in the following:

Proximal control at the neck. This is the simplest and safest method to obtain vascular control before beginning the craniotomy.[2] Exposure of the cervical ICA typically requires 15 minutes of operative time and secures the ICA early in the procedure, which is very important in the event of premature rupture of the aneurysm.

Exposure of the petrous ICA in the middle fossa.[22,23] In this technique, the middle fossa is approached extradurally

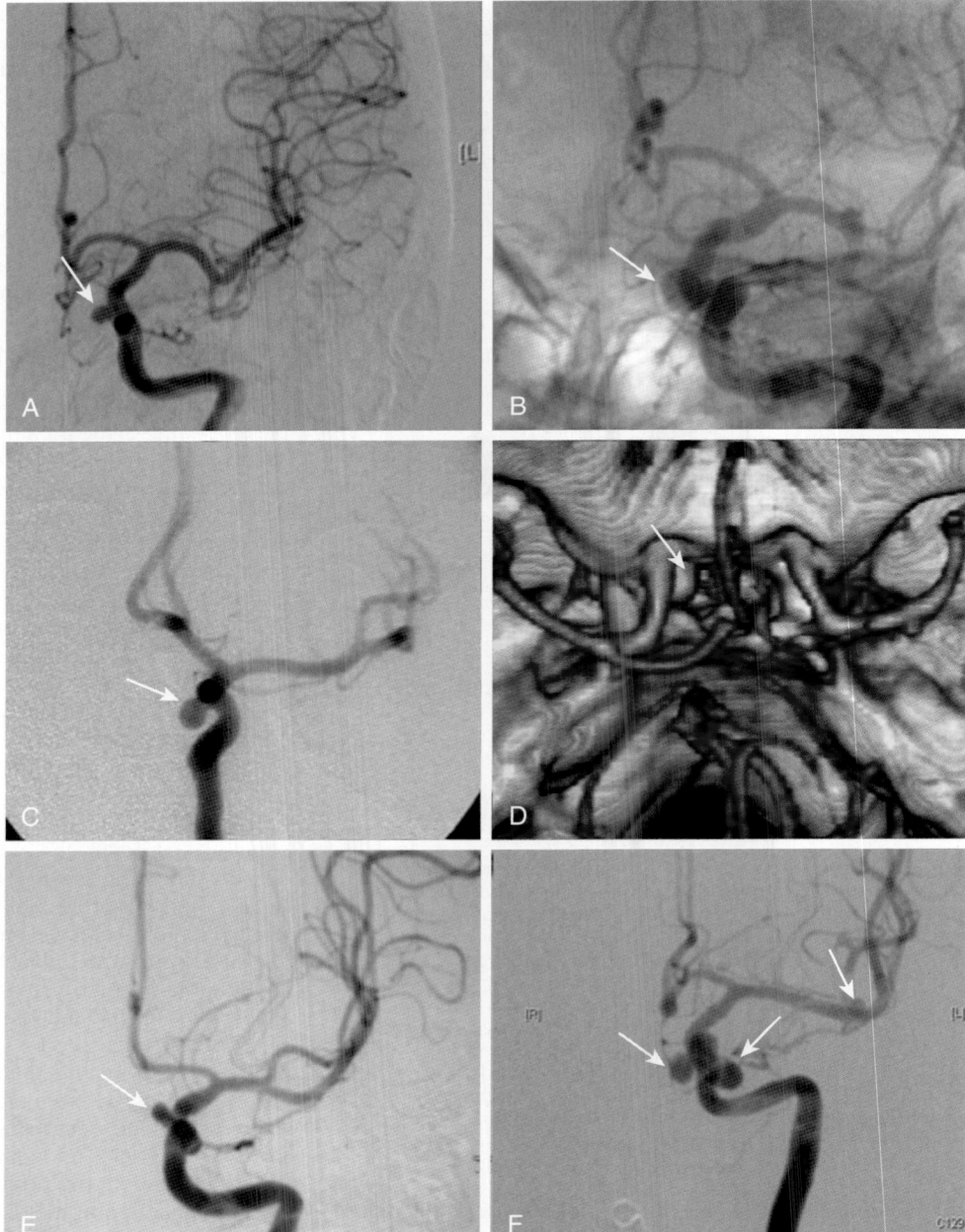

FIGURE 72-3 A to F, Carotid cave aneurysms. This aneurysm arises as transitional type of aneurysm between cavernous sinus and intradural paraclinoid. Located between proximal and distal carotid rings with ventromedial direction, they are found incidentally or because of subarachnoid hemorrhage. Most are <15 mm when discovered. Surgical approach should include opening of distal dural ring and packing cavernous sinus to avoid venous bleeding. Patient in panel F had multiple aneurysms (*arrows*) located at left middle cerebral artery, posterior communicating segment of the ICA, and carotid cave.

after the craniotomy is completed. The components of Glasscock's triangle are identified (arcuate eminence, foramen spinosum, and foramen ovale). The course of the greater superficial petrosal nerve is identified and the nerve is sectioned to avoid traction injury to the geniculate ganglion and facial nerve. The middle fossa floor is drilled along the course of the canal of the petrosal nerve. The bone covering the petrous carotid canal is usually thin, and sometimes a membranous layer covers the carotid. Unroofing the petrous bone over the ICA should not proceed caudally beyond the point where the ICA turns vertically if injury to the cochlea is to be avoided. Once identified, the petrous carotid should be dissected from its adherence to the petrous canal. Temporary occlusion of the ICA at this point can be obtained

by packing the carotid petrous segment with surgical patties (Fukushima's technique), by the introduction of a Fogarty catheter (Spetzler's technique), or by a standard clipping technique after 360-degree dissection of the carotid artery from the petrous wall. The main disadvantage of this technique is that the neurosurgeon should be very familiar with the anatomy of the floor of the middle fossa based on laboratory work and previous surgical experience.

Intracranial control of the ICA after opening the distal dural ring. This technique is feasible during clipping of small- or medium-size aneurysms; however, it is more difficult when dealing with large or giant aneurysms with a short intradural ICA.[4] It has the disadvantage of obtaining proximal control after the neurosurgeon faces the

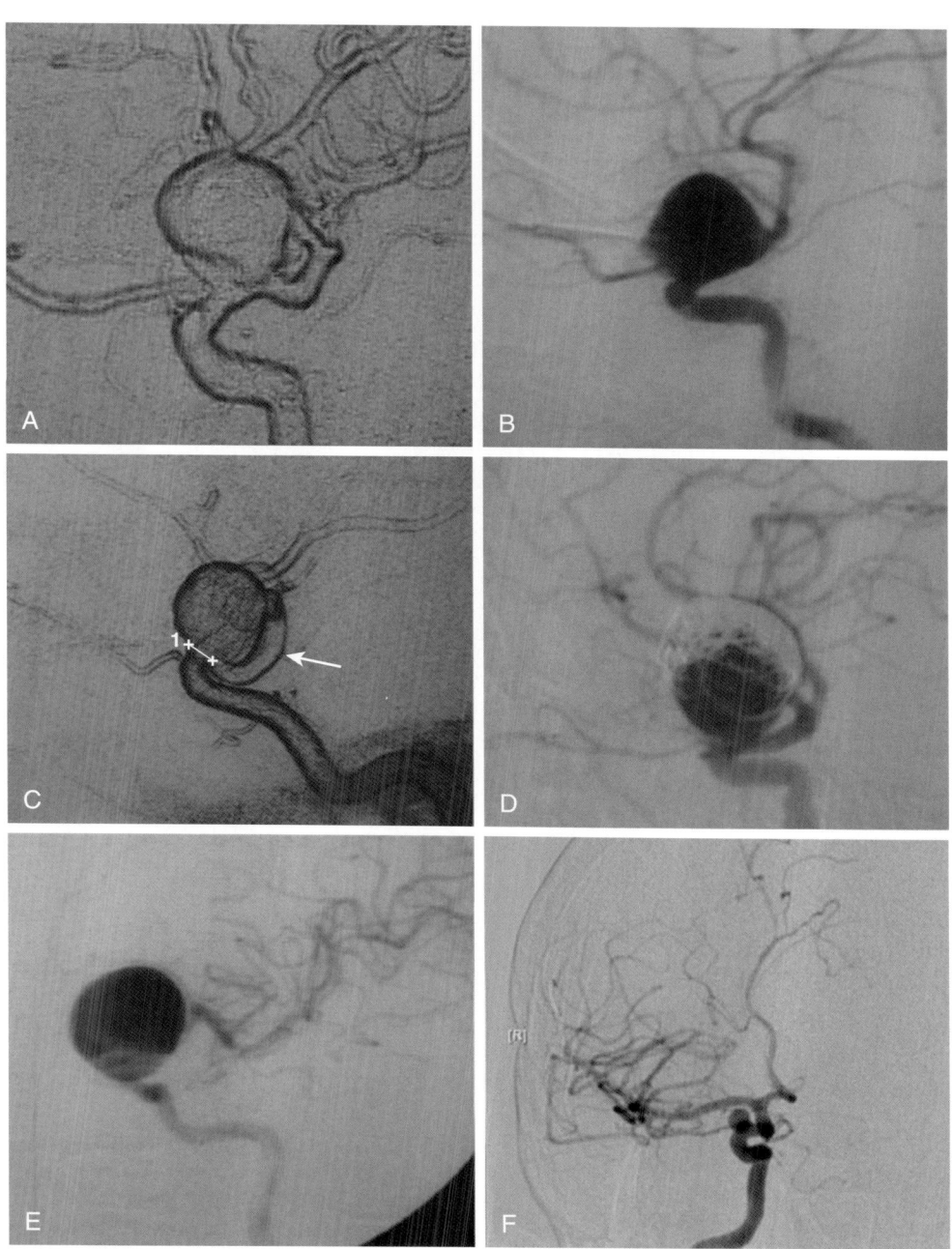

FIGURE 72-4 A to F, Proximal dorsal type aneurysms. Also defined as carotid-ophthalmic aneurysms, they grow at the dorsal surface of the ICA at close proximity with ophthalmic artery. They may reach giant size (>25 mm) before causing neurologic symptoms. The most common manifestation is visual deficit. Surgical technique include the anterior clinoid process resection to identify and preserve the ophthalmic artery. C, Ventral displacement of the ICA can be appreciated (*arrow*). D, This aneurysm had been coiled before, and showed recurrence in the 6 months following the endovascular procedure, suggesting heavy hemodynamic stress forces in this area.

aneurysm; therefore, if rupture occurs early, rapid proximal control is difficult.

Endovascular ICA occlusion via femoral artery catheter with the option to perform an intraoperative angiography. It has the advantage to perform a suction-decompression technique of large or giant aneurysms before clipping.[24] Another related endovascular technique is the Dallas maneuver. A deflated, double-lumen balloon catheter is placed in the appropriate ICA, 2 cm above the common carotid bifurcation. Proximal control is achieved by inflating the balloon. Temporary clipping just proximal to the origin of the posterior communicating artery then gains distal control. Retrograde suction decompression through the catheter collapses the aneurysm, which is then permanently clipped.[25] However, with

these techniques, it has been reported traumatic dissection and thromboembolism from the end of the catheter that caused patient injury. The technique to get proximal control of the ICA, however, should be selected according to experience of the neurosurgeon and local facilities.

PATIENT POSITIONING AND CRANIOTOMY

The patient is positioned supine with the head fixed with a three-point skeletal fixation device such as a Mayfield-Kees or Sugita. The head is directed 20 degrees vertex down and rotated about 30 degrees to the opposite side of the approach. The exact position of the head will allow a visual axis along the sphenoid ridge to the ACP and the parasellar area.

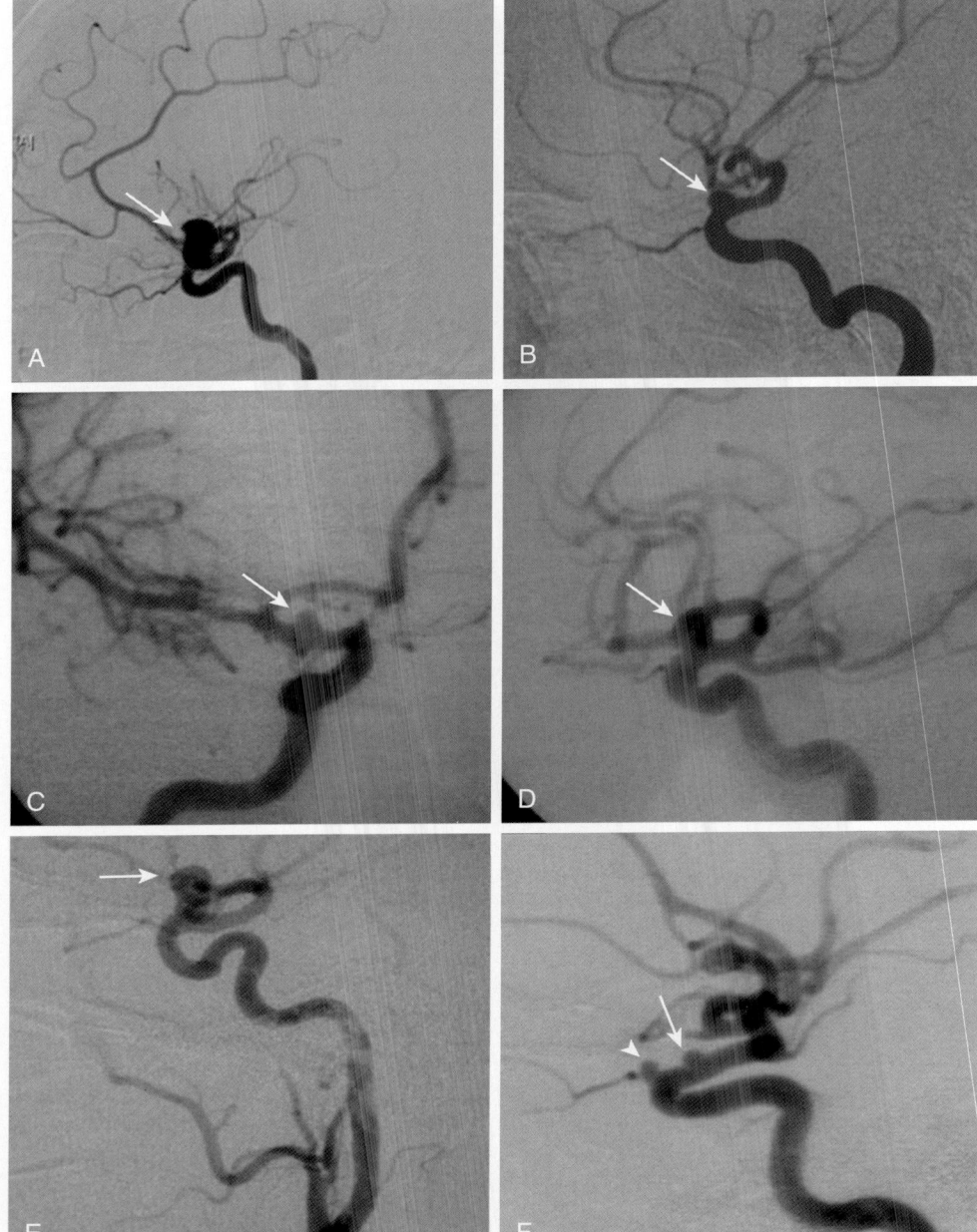

FIGURE 72-5 A to F, Distal dorsal type aneurysms. This type of aneurysm origin at the dorsal surface of the ICA, away from the origin of the ophthalmic artery (*arrows*). They usually do not progress to large or giant sizes, and present with subarachnoid hemorrhage as initial symptom. This is also a frequent site of location of the so-called blood blister–like aneurysms. In these cases, the resection of the anterior clinoid process may not be necessary to get proximal vascular control and expose the aneurysm. However, in case of blood blister–like aneurysms, special designed clips to encircle the ICA or a wrapping procedure may be necessary to treat these aneurysms. F, This patient had two dorsal type aneurysms, one proximal type (ophthalmic) (*arrowhead*) and one distal type (*arrow*).

A standard pterional craniotomy is performed for small- or medium-size aneurysms. Craniotomy should provide enough space to complete the ACP drilling and unroofing the optic nerve, to expose the ICA and the aneurysm, and to proceed to clip the aneurysm (Fig. 72-13). In cases of large or giant aneurysms, the extent of the craniotomy should be large enough to expose the aneurysm with minimal brain retraction, and to get the space for free hand movements to ensure a comfortable clipping without limitations.

A skin incision is made 1 cm in front of the tragus, at the level of the zygomatic arch, and carried behind the hairline after curving over the superior temporal line at the midpupilar level. The skin flap is reflected rostrally. Particular attention is paid to dissection of the superficial and deep fascia of the temporalis muscle to prevent injury to

the facial nerve and maintain the arterial vascularization to the muscle. The muscular flap in also reflected rostrally and fixed with sutures or hooks. A frontotemporal craniotomy is performed with one or more burr holes depending of the adherence of the dura to the bone. We start the first burr hole at the most caudal part of the craniotomy, at the level of the superior temporal line (Fig. 72-13). The bone flap is retired and bone hemostasis is completed with bone wax. If the proximal control will be obtained at the petrous carotid level, the craniotomy should be extended at the temporal side until the middle fossa floor level and the dura dissected from the orbital roof, the sphenoid ridge, and the middle fossa. Otherwise, the dura is only dissected around the sphenoid ridge down to the ACP. The sphenoid ridge is drilled with a diamond-tip drill until the ACP. If the

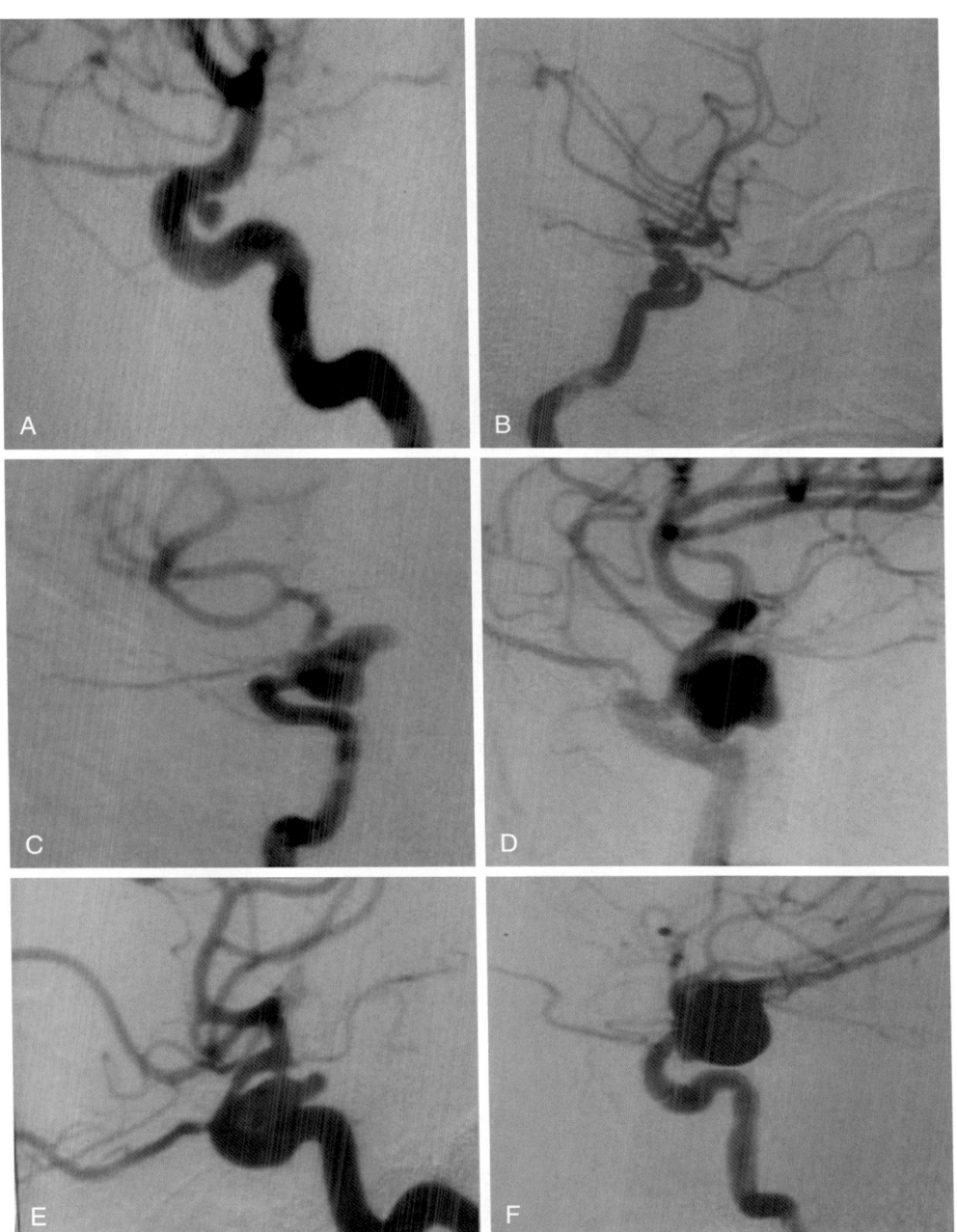

FIGURE 72-6 A to F, Ventral type aneurysms. Ventral type aneurysms originate opposite ophthalmic artery at ventral surface of ICA. They grow between distal dural ring and origin of posterior communicating artery and produce upper displacement of ICA. According to available anatomic space, they may grow medially or laterally. The most effective way to clip these aneurysms is using fenestrated clips.

aneurysm is of ventral type, the ACP could be resected extradurally.[4,26]

On the other hand, if the aneurysm is a dorsal type or the ACP is large, we stop at the base of the ACP and the drilling is completed intradurally. After the ACP is resected, drilling is continued over the optic canal until the dura covering the optic nerve is visible. Adequate water is used at this time to prevent thermal damage to the optic nerve. In cases of large or giant aneurysms, the orbital roof is also drilled to unlock all structures around the aneurysm.

Next we proceed to dissect the middle fossa separating the dura from the media fossa floor. At first it is identified as the foramen spinosum following the course of the middle meningeal artery that is usually visible at the dura surface. The foramen is expanded with a diamond tip drill to facilitate

the coagulation and cutting of the artery. The foramen ovale is then identified rostral and medial to the foramen spinosum. Afterward, the dura is dissected from the arcuate eminence in a caudal to rostral fashion to avoid stretching of the petrosal nerve. Once the greater superficial petrosal nerve is identified, it is separated from the adherent dural layer and followed until it reaches the lateral border of V3. The petrosal nerve is sectioned at its mid-portion avoiding any stretching that can be transmitted to the geniculate ganglion and facial nerve. The canal of the nerve is followed with a small diamond-tip drill until the petrous carotid is exposed. Sometimes, a thin layer of membranous tissue covers the petrous carotid, but in other cases it is located 2 to 3 mm from the surface of the middle fossa. During drilling you may find a soft tissue structure laterally, corresponding to

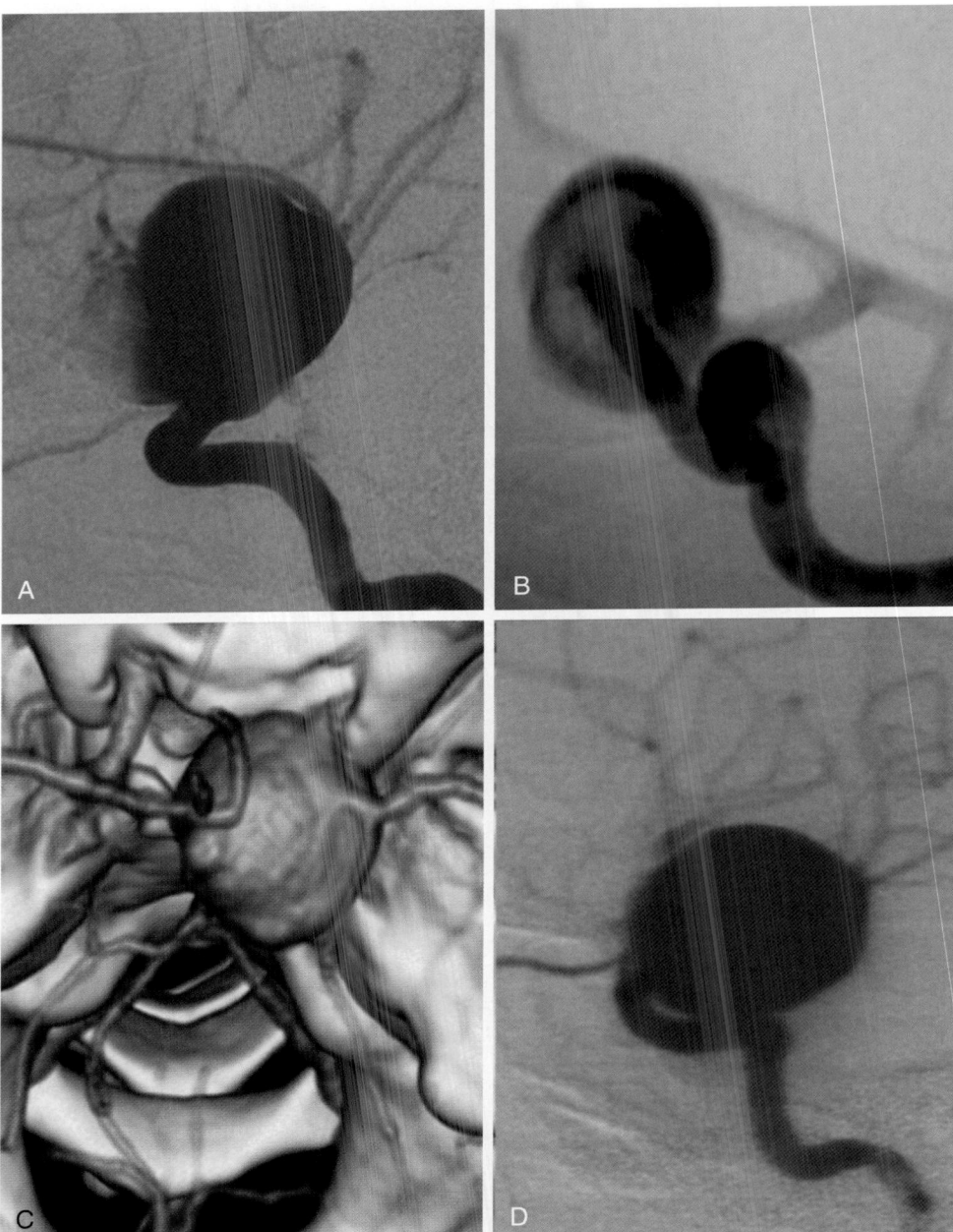

FIGURE 72-7 A to D, Global type aneurysms. This type of aneurysm represents technical challenge for reconstruction because site of origin cannot be well-defined as dorsal or ventral. In these cases, it is better to select a surgical technique based on proximal occlusion of the ICA if good collateral flow exists, or to perform bypass procedure to ensure blood flow distal to aneurysm.

the tensor tympani muscle. At this point you should direct the drilling medially, because lateral to the tensor tympani muscle is located the Eustachian tube. After exposure of the petrous carotid, the artery is dissected from the wall of the petrous canal to get space for the placement of surgical patties, Fogarty catheter, or temporary clip. If necessary, drilling can be extended medially to obtain more space through Kawase's triangle without harm to any structure.

SYLVIAN FISSURE AND BASAL CISTERNS

The dura is opened in a semi lunar fashion and reflected rostrally. The sylvian fissure is widely open to obtain a larger exposure with minimal brain retraction. Any unnecessary cutting of bridging veins should be avoided because of the risk of venous infarctions. The arachnoid space is open to include the sylvian fissure, carotid and chiasmatic cisterns,

and the Lilliequist membrane. This will expose the ACP, optic nerves and chiasm, lamina terminalis, and the ICA until the bifurcation (Fig. 72-14). In case of a recent bleeding, the lamina terminalis is open to release the maximal amount of cerebrospinal fluid (CSF) and to prevent hydrocephalus. In case of a contralateral paraclinoid aneurysm, the arachnoid tissue is further opened around the opposite optic nerve to expose the contralateral paraclinoid ICA.

ANTERIOR CLINOID PROCESS

The ACP should be removed in any case of paraclinoid aneurysm approached ipsilaterally independently of their size. This will provide enough space and vision of the neck and dome even in small aneurysms. Clipping one aneurysm with partial exposure has been one of the main causes of poor surgical results due to intraoperative rupture or neck

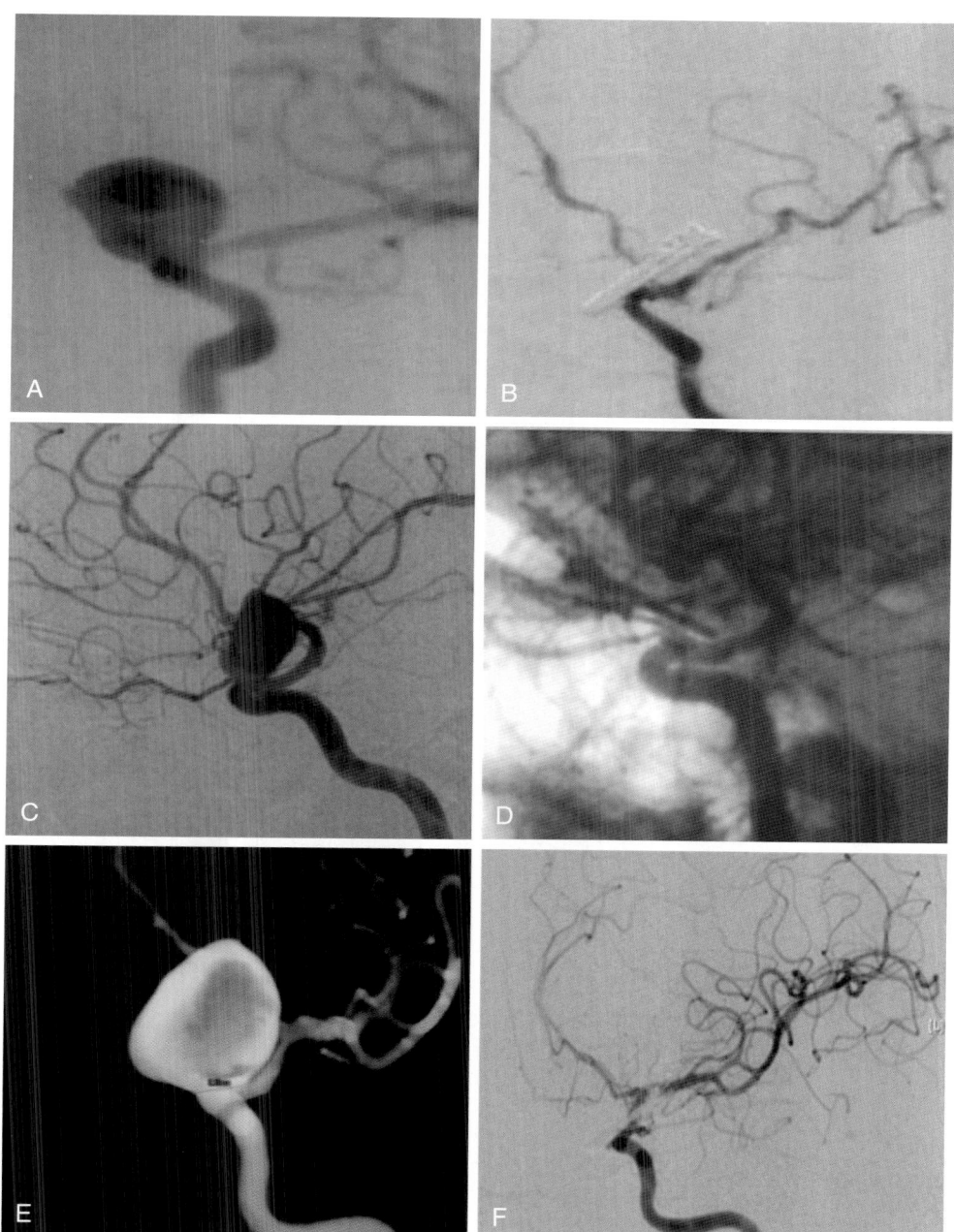

FIGURE 72-8 Demonstrative cases of dorsal type aneurysms. A and B, Pre- and post-operative angiograms show large aneurysm with medial extension. Postoperative image shows the clip position. Two straight 15-mm clips were used to obliterate the aneurysm. C and D, This aneurysm had a rather straight upward direction with a small neck. However, during surgery, it was noted that the aneurysm wall was thick. The neck was closed using a 11-mm straight clip and a miniclip for a small neck remnant. E and F, Giant aneurysm of dorsal type. The patient is a 40-year-old female admitted to the hospital because of visual deficit. At surgery we found a thin-walled aneurysm. The aneurysm could be obliterated using two 11-mm straight clips.

remnant. As mentioned previously, the ACP can be resected in an extradural or intradural fashion.[4,26] If an extradural resection could not be completed due to a large clinoid process or a dorsal type aneurysm in which the dome is close to the ACP or may have eroded it, a combined extradural-intradural technique is selected. In general, diamond drills are preferred to avoid damage to surrounding structures. In the case of intradural resection of the ACP, an incision is performed following the long axis of the ACP and curving the dura incision over the falciform ligament (Fig. 72-15). The ACP is drilled until the tip is reached and resected with the aid of a small rongeur or dissector. As an alternative, a bone ultrasonic aspirator can be used; unfortunately, this device is expensive and not available everywhere.[27] The resection of the ACP should be very careful in cases of dorsal type

aneurysms because of the risk of rupture. At this level of the operation the proximal control should be fully obtained. In addition, it is important to extend the level of bone resection to include the optic strut, which connects the ACP to the lateral wall of the sphenoid sinus and comprises the lateral and ventral border of the optic foramen (Fig. 72-16). Microsurgical resection of the optic strut is of paramount importance in visualizing the origin of the ophthalmic artery. The origin of the ophthalmic artery often demarcates the junction of the proximal aneurysm neck with normal ICA.

DISTAL DURAL RING AND OPTIC NERVE

Opening the dura of the optic nerve from the falciform fold along the entire length of the optic canal longitudinally allows slight but significant mobilization of the nerve and

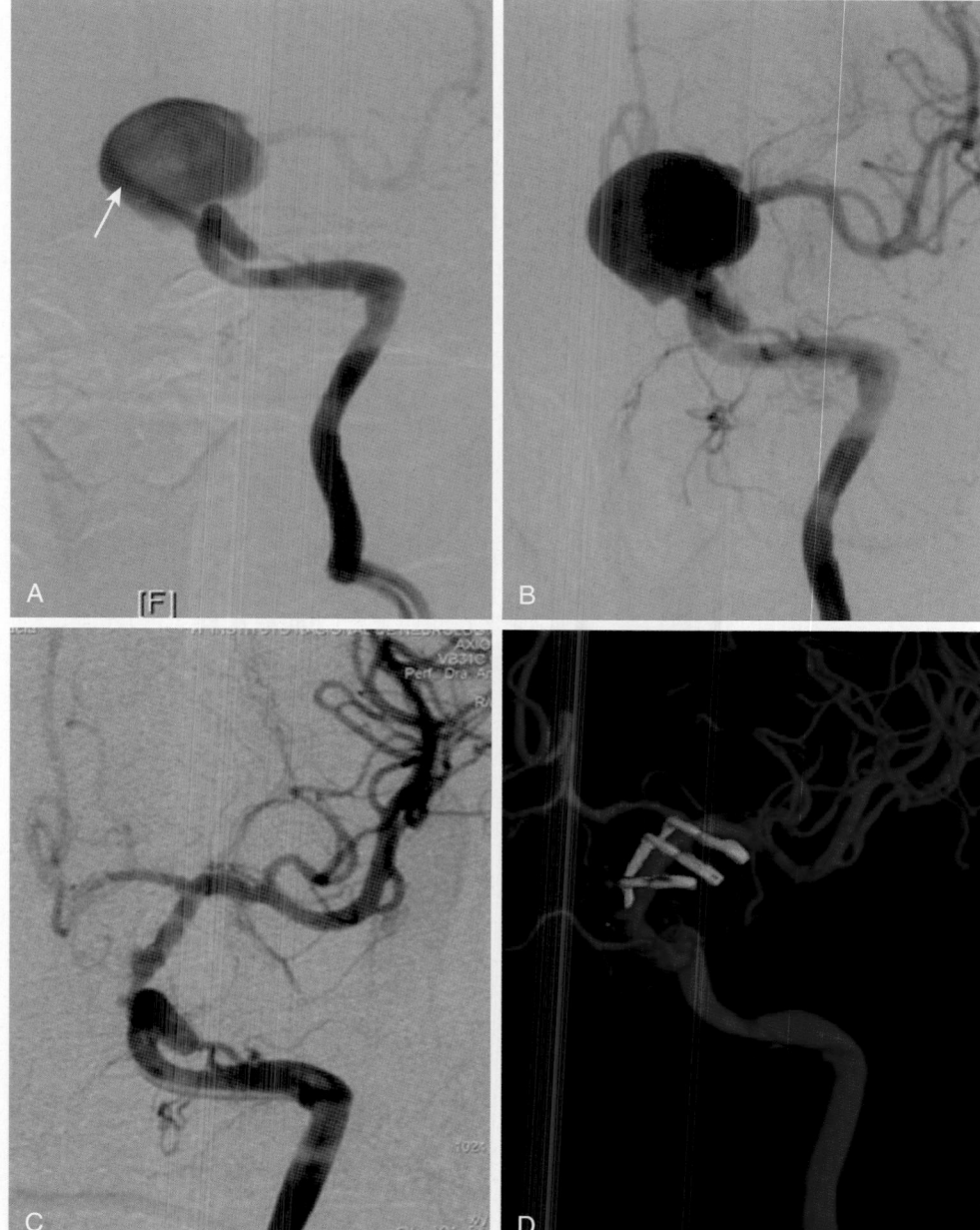

FIGURE 72-9 Demonstrative case of ventral type aneurysm. A, Even when aneurysm could be confused with dorsal type, at initial filling of sac, the course of ICA is visible over aneurysm dome (*arrow*). B, After sac of aneurysm is filled with contrast product, site of origin cannot be visualized. With this information, we expected to find aneurysm dome ventral to ICA. C, Postoperative anterior view shows total obliteration of aneurysm preserving course of ICA. D, Three-dimensional oblique view shows clip arrangement in tandem fashion to reconstruct ICA using ring clips.

dissection away from the aneurysm. Intermittent retraction of the optic nerve is preferred over single, protracted retraction. The origin of the ophthalmic artery is carefully dissected away from the aneurysm. Opening the distal dural ring anchoring the ICA reveals the proximal portion of the neck and the proximal ICA (Fig. 72-17). This opening is extended toward the third cranial nerve, and any resulting venous bleeding is easily controlled with packing with small pieces of Surgicel or injection of fibrin glue.[28] Stepwise dissection of the aneurysm from the surrounding structures follows. Papaverine or nimodipine is routinely applied to the ICA and its branches early in the surgical procedure and is repeated as necessary to avoid mechanical vasospasm.

DISSECTION AND CLIPPING OF THE ANEURYSM
Small- and Medium-Size Aneurysms
After the above–mentioned steps are completed and the ICA and aneurysm are brought into view, a space is created between the origin of the posterior communicating artery and the neck of the aneurysm for later placement of a distal temporary clip. The course of the anterior choroidal artery is also confirmed as well as all the branching arteries in the vicinity of the aneurysm. In small- and medium-size aneurysms, the wall can be thin and the blood flow could be seen through the wall of the aneurysm, warning the neurosurgeon to avoid aggressive movements over the dome of the aneurysm. On the other side, aneurysms with a thick or atherosclerotic wall could be gently compressed, as the

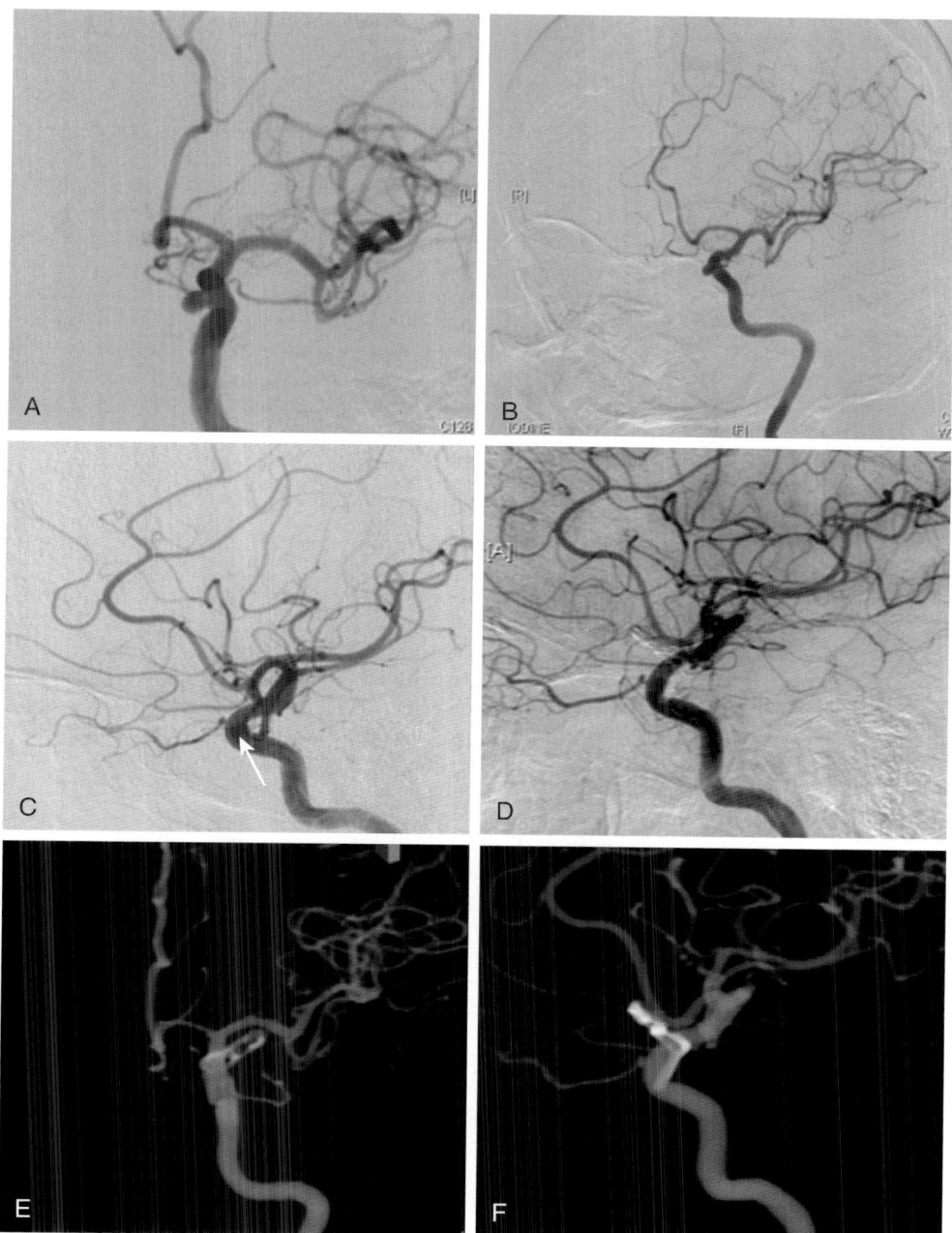

FIGURE 72-10 Carotid cave aneurysm, demonstrative case. This 32-year-old female patient arrived at the hospital with Hunt and Kosnik grade 2 subarachnoid hemorrhage. Angiogram showed a carotid cave aneurysm. A, Anterior view. Aneurysm is visible with medial and ventral directions. B, Oblique view shows the aneurysm projecting under genu of the ICA. C, In lateral view, aneurysm is usually hidden by genu of ICA (*arrow*). This is a very particular characteristic of small carotid cave aneurysms. D, Postoperative lateral view shows position of ring clip used to clip the aneurysm. Three-dimensional reconstruction image in the anterior and lateral views (E and F) shows clip position and elimination of the aneurysm.

aneurysm occasionally must be lifted to establish a plane between it and the ICA. At this stage, the aneurysm collapses and is carefully separated from the ICA. The neck of the aneurysm is dissected and permanently clipped. More than one clip may be necessary to exclude the aneurysm and to prevent circulation pressure from opening or pulsating the clip blades. Bipolar coagulation of the aneurismal sac does not have an effect in some patients because either the aneurysm wall or neck is thick with prominent atherosclerosis. After clipping the aneurysm, the blood flow is reestablished. Some additional aid, such as intraoperative angiography or microscope-based indocyanine green (ICG) video angiography could be used to confirm total obliteration of the aneurysm sac. Most paraclinoid aneurysms have a broad neck; therefore, neck occlusion will be difficult. The necessary

number of clips to secure complex aneurysms should be used (Figs. 72-8B, D, and F; 72-9D; and 72-10E).

GIANT ANEURYSMS

Treating giant or large paraclinoid aneurysms is more difficult than other anterior circulation aneurysms and demands particular operative technique. The risk of treatment is higher and is associated with greater operative hazards. Patients with giant aneurysms tend to be older, and have a higher risk for complications associated with a general anesthesia or systemic medical conditions. Giant aneurysms have also a higher rate of wall calcifications, atherosclerotic plaque, and intraluminal thrombus. All these aspects complicate direct clip reconstruction. Various techniques for conservative or indirect treatment have been

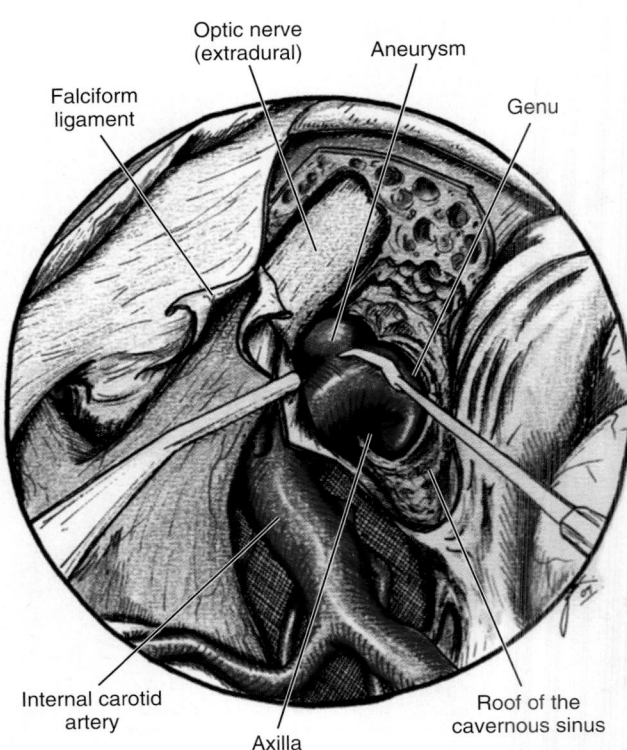

Falciform ligament
Optic nerve (extradural)
Aneurysm
Genu
Internal carotid artery
Axilla
Roof of the cavernous sinus

FIGURE 72-11 Surgical approach to carotid cave aneurysms. Drawing shows completed surgical steps to reach carotid cave region. At first clinoid region was exposed through sylvian fissure opening and dissection of basal cisterns around ICA and optic nerve. The anterior clinoid process has been drilled and optic nerve was unroofed. Dura along course of optic nerve has been opened including falciform ligament. Cavernous sinus has been packed with fibrin glue and genu and axilla of ICA have been exposed. At this time, ICA can be laterally mobilized to expose neck of aneurysm. Clipping using a fenestrated clip can then be completed.

advocated, including carotid occlusion, arterial extracranial-intracranial bypass, and subsequent ligation of the ICA with heparinization[3,21,22] (Fig. 72-12). However, most neurosurgeons agree that the best treatment for giant or large paraclinoid aneurysms is direct clipping. The goals should be to eliminate the risk of primary or recurrent subarachnoid hemorrhage, prevent further visual loss by decompressing the optic apparatus, and secure the hemodynamics by maintaining the patency of the ICA and its branches.

Perhaps the greatest technical difficulties in giant aneurysms are gaining proximal control and relieving the tension within the aneurysm to allow dissection and successful clipping. In this sense, Yasargil described the technique of trapping these aneurysms followed by puncture or excision of the dome, suction of the contents, deflation and coagulation of the sac, and finally clipping. Proximal vascular control and the suction decompression technique now comprise the best surgical adjunct to facilitate dissection and clipping of giant paraclinoid aneurysms. When this method is used, however, the duration of temporary occlusion of the ICA is an important issue. It is usually not possible to complete dissection and clipping of the aneurysm

within a few minutes. The occlusion time ranges from 10 to 60 minutes, with a mean of 30 minutes. Accordingly, a balloon occlusion test (BOT) should be performed routinely to select the best treatment. For patients at high risk from temporary arterial occlusion, the use of the retrograde suction decompression technique should be considered more carefully. Although the BOT is not perfect in predicting the tolerable occlusion time in each case, this test can select patients who cannot withstand even a short period of temporary occlusion. Such patients usually develop motor disturbance, aphasia, or loss of consciousness within 1 minute after test occlusion. For patients who are intolerant of the test occlusion, a combination of high-flow graft and proximal ICA occlusion (trapping technique) is used, or direct clipping using the suction decompression technique after performing a high flow bypass graft in the same operative session[22,23,29](Fig. 72-12).

CLIP SELECTION

Selection of the clip shape and size will depend on aneurysm size and direction. In this sense, it is important to take into consideration the main types of paraclinoid aneurysms described previously. Dorsal type aneurysms are in close relationship with the optic nerve and the anterior clinoid process and clinical presentation is very often with visual deficit more than with SAH.[15] In this case the resection of the anterior clinoid process and unroofing of the optic nerve should be more extensive because of the need of mobilization, especially in large aneurysms. Evacuation of the aneurismal sac permits immediate decompression of the optic pathway, and it may be the most effective method for the recovery of visual dysfunction caused by the aneurysm. Sometimes, however, despite a careful dissection of the sac away from the optic nerve, postoperative deterioration of visual acuity occurs. Nowadays, this remains as a significant problem related to the direct surgical clipping of large ophthalmic aneurysms. This kind of aneurysm is best clipped using straight or slightly curved clips because the course of the ICA remains under the sac of the aneurysm (Fig. 72-8). If necessary, according to the neurosurgeon's preference, clipping could be performed under temporary occlusion of the ICA to reduce the intraluminal pressure of a broad neck aneurysm. In giant aneurysms, proximal balloon occlusion and suction will facilitate clip positioning and will avoid intraoperative rupture.[24,25] If endovascular aid is not available, a proximal and distal temporary occlusion followed by direct puncture and suction of the dome will facilitate the clipping.

On the other side, ventral type aneurysms are located behind the circumference of the ICA. They grow downward and the optic nerve is not displaced in the same extent as with the dorsal type aneurysms. Therefore, the use of standard clips across the neck will produce stretching and kinking of the ICA or will left a remnant sac. For this type of aneurysm a combination of ring (fenestrated) clips should be used[2,3,8,16,18] (Fig. 72-9).

The carotid cave aneurysms are directed ventromedially between the proximal and distal dural rings at the level of the carotid genu. As this type of aneurysm projects ventral to the ICA circumference, they are best clipped using ring clips (Fig. 72-10). Kobayashi et al. have described a specially designed clip for these aneurysms taking into consideration the curve of the ICA when located on the left or right side.[10]

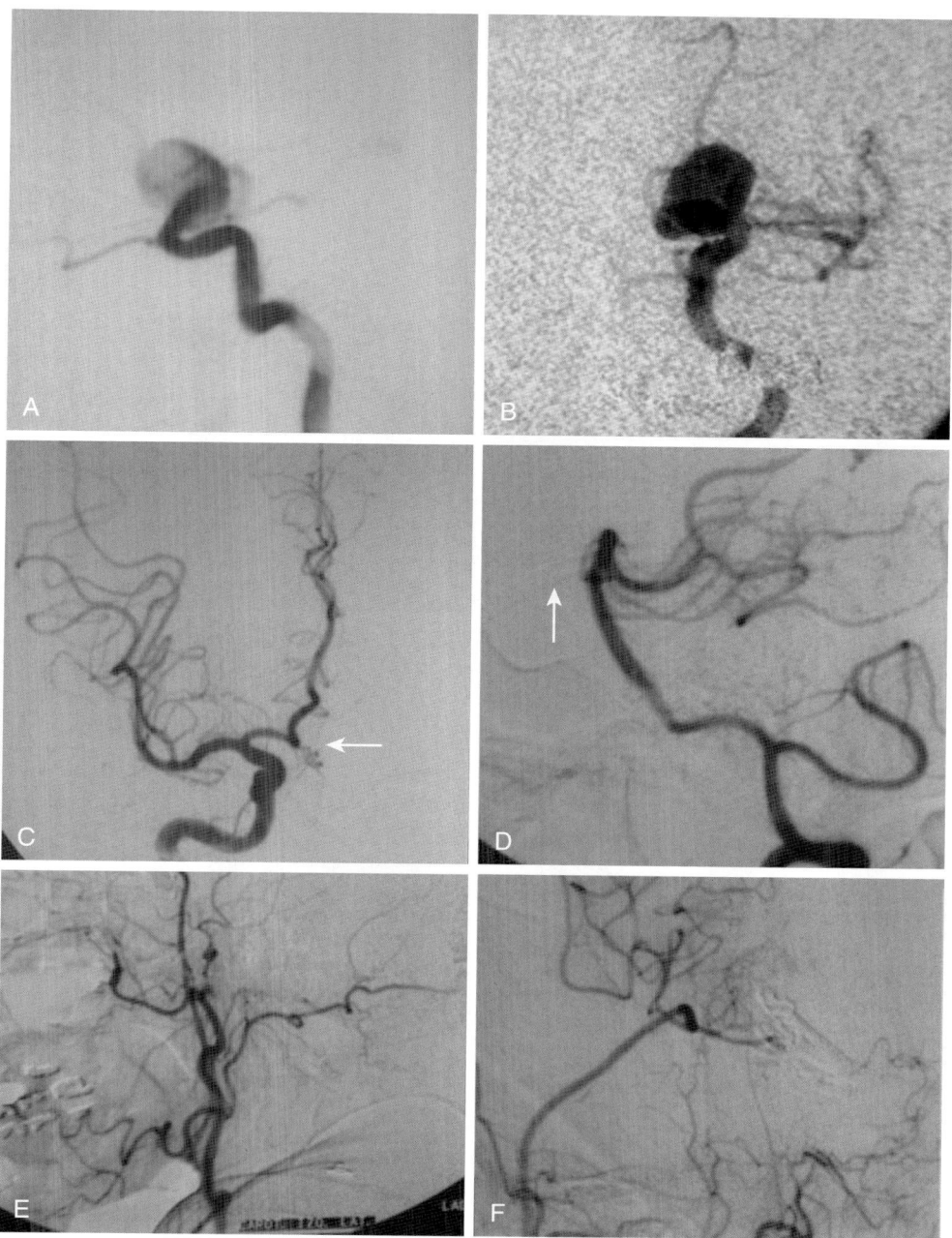

FIGURE 72-12 Global type aneurysm, demonstrative case. Angiogram shows initial filling of sac (A) without a clear definition of neck origin (B). Balloon occlusion test showed poor collateral circulation through anterior communicating artery (C) and posterior cerebral artery (D) (*arrows*). We decided to perform a high-flow bypass with a radial artery graft before attacking aneurysm. Aneurysm was trapped between origin of ICA and before origin of posterior communicating artery (E). Postoperative angiogram shows a good patency of bypass (F).

Again, use of standard (nonfenestrated) clips runs the risk of incomplete clipping.

Multiple Aneurysms

Paraclinoid region is a common site of location for mirror aneurysms. Optimally, all aneurysms should be clipped simultaneously. The frequency of multiple aneurysms also justifies an aggressive surgical approach. For patients with mirror aneurysms, the contralateral approach has been described without having visual obstruction caused by the ACP as when the aneurysm is approached through the same side.[30] In these cases, a wide opening of the arachnoid cisterns around the chiasmatic area will permit a proper visualization of the aneurysm as well as the ophthalmic and superior hypophyseal arteries. Therefore, clipping small- or medium-size

contralateral aneurysm could be performed with a high grade of efficiency.[31] In case of large or giant contralateral aneurysms, approaching the aneurysm from the side or origin in a second operation is recommended. On the other hand, in case of multiple nonmirror aneurysms, the possibility to clip them will depend on aneurysm location. For aneurysms located on the same side, including those at the anterior communicating artery or contralateral ICA bifurcation, they can be clipped starting from the deepest to the most superficial one in order to avoid visual limitation by the head of the clip.

ASSESSMENT OF BLOOD FLOW AT PARENT ARTERY

After the aneurysm is clipped, the patency of the ICA should be confirmed by visual inspection of the artery. In case of arteries with a thick-wall or broad-neck aneurysm, the

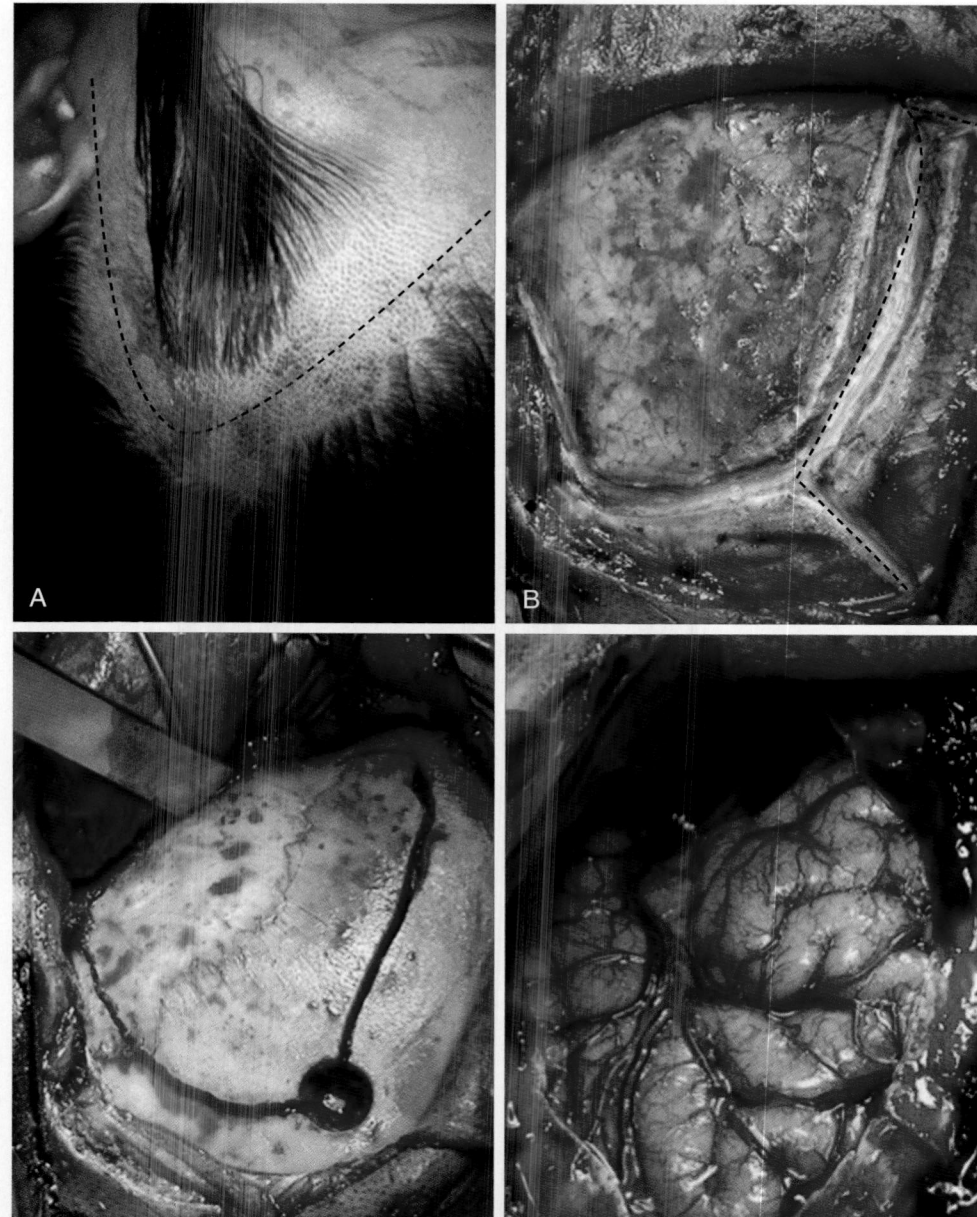

FIGURE 72-13 Craniotomy. A, Standard craniotomy for paraclinoid aneurysms includes an incision from root of zygomatic arch to midpupilar line over superior temporal line. B, Temporalis muscle is incised along superior temporal line (*dashed line*) and curved through zygomatic root. Two additional lines of incision (*dashed line*) are made at frontal side and most posterior part of exposition. This produces two flaps that increase area for craniotomy and will permit tight closure of temporalis muscle at end of operation. C, Burr-hole craniotomy positioned at most caudal part of superior temporal line. Bone chisel is used to complete cut between frontal and temporal lines of craniotomy at sphenoid ridge. D, Final exposure should give enough space for dissection, exposure, and clipping of aneurysm.

external inspection is not enough to confirm the patency of the ICA; using the intraoperative Doppler should then be mandatory. This device provides qualitative or quantitative information about blood flow. Other alternatives are the intraoperative angiography, or recently, use of intraoperative fluorescence-based angiography through the surgical microscope.

CLOSURE

After clipping is completed, the paraclinoid area should be sealed to avoid CSF leakage. The dural flaps at the region of the ACP are back to place and the use of some biologic sealant is recommended. The final position of the clip(s) is inspected in order to avoid any compression of the surrounding structures, specially the optic nerve and perforating arteries. If necessary, small pieces of surgical sponge

are left between the clip and the surrounding structures. The dura is closed watertight. The bone flap is positioned and the temporalis muscle is closed as tight as possible to prevent any leakage of CSF to the subgaleal space. A subcutaneous drainage could be left in place and the skin is sutured after the galea has been closed.

Results

The series of direct surgical treatment of paraclinoid aneurysms (among them giant and large ones) reported more than 2 decades ago had relatively high mortality rates, ranging from 20% to 60%.[6] Nonetheless, these authors should be credited for being the first to directly attack these difficult lesions. The postoperative mortality and morbidity decreased markedly over time, and the rate of direct surgical

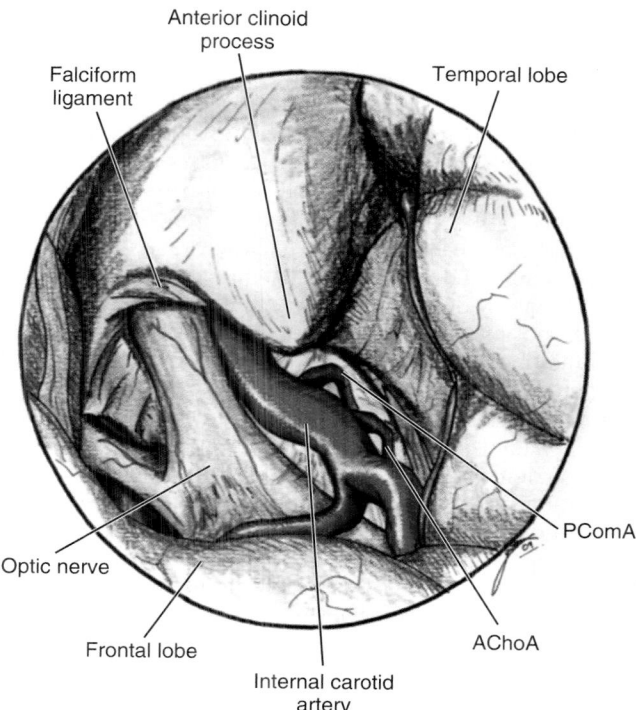

FIGURE 72-14 Initial exposure of paraclinoid area. After opening sylvian fissure and basal cisterns, operative view under microscope includes anterior clinoid process, temporal lobe tip, and basal part of frontal lobe, ICA until bifurcation and posterior communicating and choroidal arteries. Optic nerves and chiasm are also dissected and exposed.

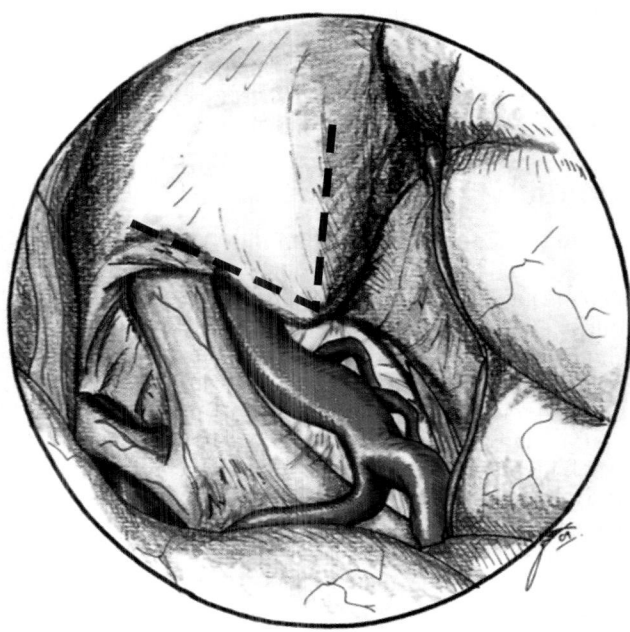

FIGURE 72-15 Anterior clinoid process (ACP) dural incision. Image shows line of incision to start drilling of ACP in an intradural fashion. After dural flap is incised with surgical blade, dural flap is separated to expose ACP body and tip. If some bleeding comes from dural border, bipolar coagulation is used to control bleeding. Dura around ACP is separated to facilitate bone drilling.

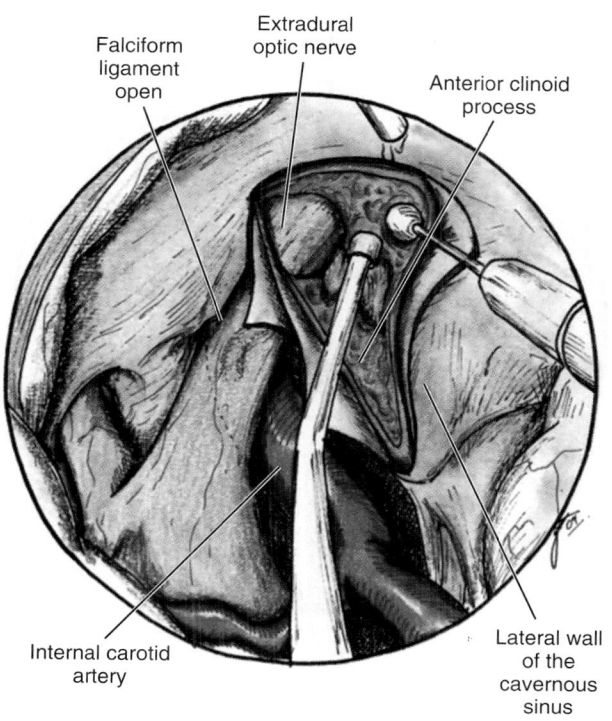

FIGURE 72-16 Drilling anterior clinoid process. After dural flap is separated, a diamond tip drill is used to start resection of clinoid. Drilling is extended medially until extradural optic nerve comes into view. At this point enough amount of water is used to avoid thermal damage to nerve. Drilling should not occur beyond medial optic nerve margin because of risk in penetrating ethmoid cells. Optic nerve is isolated and optic strut is drilled as much as possible. Resection extends to base of clinoid process and laterally until dura around bone is seen. Finally, clinoid tip is resected. Tip is sometimes adherent to dura and some force is necessary to separate it. This maneuver should be made very carefully in case of dorsal tip aneurysms close to undersurface of clinoid tip. If venous bleeding occurs, it can be controlled using bone wax mixed with small pieces of Surgicel.

approaches to these lesions increased, as did the rate of successful clipping of these giant and large aneurysms. In the recently reported series of giant and large paraclinoid aneurysms, the mortality rates of direct surgery are lowered to less than 10% in the majority of series[4,5,7,8,11,18,25] (Table 72-1). Furthermore, in his series, Batjer et al.[2] reported 59% good, 23% fair, and 14% poor outcomes, as well as permanent ICA occlusions in 14%; Day,[8] which also included small paraclinoid aneurysms, reported a 96% rate of successful clipping, with 87% good and 7% poor outcomes, and a 6% mortality rate. Overall, the direct surgery of giant aneurysms has recently increased, as has the rate of successful clipping. Furthermore, good outcomes range from 59% to 92%, and the number of patients with poor and fair outcomes is decreasing. Al-Mefty et al. reported a series of 16 large and giant aneurysms, with 88% good, 6% fair, and 6% mortality. In our personal experience in two reference centers, we have operated 992 aneurysms between 1992 and 2008. Of these, 137 (13.8%) were located at the paraclinoid

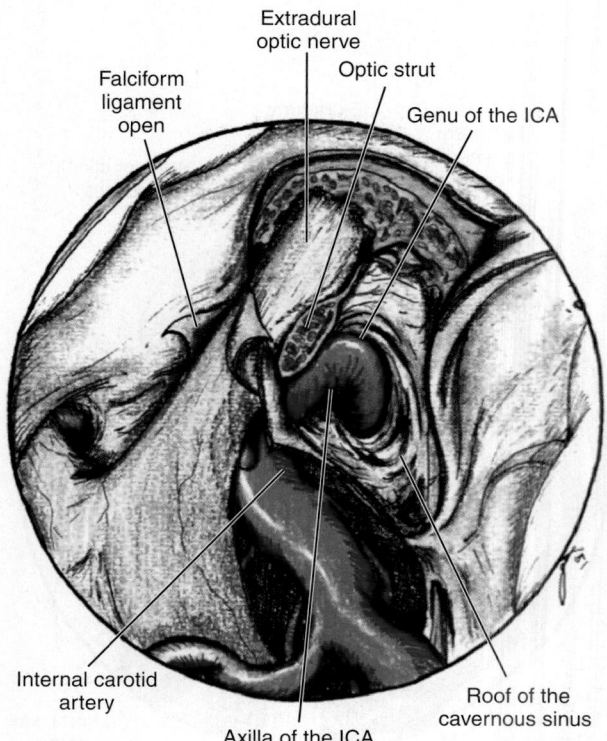

Falciform
ligament
open

Extradural
optic nerve

Optic strut

Genu of the ICA

Internal carotid
artery

Axilla of the ICA

Roof of the
cavernous sinus

FIGURE 72-17 Roof of cavernous sinus and dural folds. After anterior clinoid process is completely drilled, next step is packing cavernous sinus. This can be made with small pieces of Surgicel or using fibrin glue. If a biologic sealant is used, material is injected through roof of cavernous sinus. After bleeding stops, additional drilling of optic strut is attempted, taking care not to damage dura covering optic nerve. Afterward, dura covering optic nerve is incised along optic nerve axis. This will permit nerve mobilization and exposure of distal dural ring. After dural ring is opened, genu and axilla of ICA are dissected. At this stage, any paraclinoid aneurysm is visible as well as proximal parent vessel. Medial mobilization of optic nerve exposes ophthalmic artery and its origin from dorsal surface of ICA.

region. Nine (6.5%) of them were giants. Of 91 patients, 30 (27%) had multiple aneurysms. Our mortality rate was 4.3% (4 patients). The overall complications rate was 20% with a reduction to less than 8% after 3 months.

Complications

Surgery of paraclinoid aneurysms is not free of risks. Most common complications are related with the structures faced during the approach, mainly in cases of large or giant aneurysms and many of them are transitory. Among them have been reported a temporal lobe infarction due to the sacrifice of superficial sylvian veins and retraction of the temporal tip, transient and permanent third nerve palsy, ipsilateral occlusion of the ICA, subdural hygromas, transient cerebral edema, transitory neurologic deficits, and extensive cerebral infarctions due to parent artery occlusion in patients with poor collateral circulation.

VISUAL OUTCOME

Paraclinoid aneurysms may compress the optic apparatus and present clinically with visual deterioration. Also, the proximity of these aneurysms to the optic nerve accounts for the risk of visual deficit after surgical clipping. The risk

of this complication seems to occur in 5% to 10% of patients regardless of the treatment strategy, and is more common when treating large or giant aneurysms.[15] The risk to develop a new visual deficit is also related with the type of aneurysm. Proximal dorsal type aneurysms (true ophthalmic aneurysms) (Figs. 72-2A and 27-4) arise in close proximity to the ophthalmic artery, in contact with the undersurface of the optic nerve. When the aneurysm grows, direct compression of the optic nerve results, causing a progressive visual deficit. On the other hand, distal dorsal type aneurysms (Figs. 72-2A and 72-5) grow distal to the origin of the ophthalmic artery and do not produce a direct contact with the optic nerve until they become large or giant, situation that occurs less frequent when compared with the ophthalmic aneurysms. Ventral type aneurysms do not have a direct contact with the optic apparatus, and visual deficit may appear after upward displacement of the ICA in case of giant aneurysms (Fig. 72-9). After surgery, the main sources of optic nerve damage are (1) heat lesion caused by the drilling during the extradural unroofing of the nerve; (2) excessive mobilization of the nerve during clipping; (3) direct compression of the nerve caused by the clips, especially if large or multiple clips were used to treat a dorsal type aneurysm; and (4) sudden decompression of the nerve after clipping causing vascular damage.

The best way to avoid lesions to the optic nerve is unroofing the nerve with a diamond tip drill using large amounts of water to avoid heat damage, opening the dura along the nerve to increase the mobilization and working space around it. After clipping, the final position of the clips should be confirmed, and if necessary, a small piece of surgical sponge may be used to create a soft interface between the clips and the nerve. Patients with paraclinoid aneurysms should receive preoperative and postoperative neuro-ophthalmologic examinations. In general, 65% of the patients show improvement of the preoperative deficit, 25% do not show changes after surgery and 5% to 10% have deterioration after clipping. The risk of permanent deficit is higher in large or giant aneurysms especially if they belong to the proximal dorsal type.

Summary

Paraclinoid aneurysms have traditionally been considered difficult. The principal obstacles to safe clipping have been the initial poor view of the parent artery to get vascular control and the lack of exposition of the aneurysm dome. When one aneurysm is operated under these conditions, rupture during dissection or while clipping produces a very stressful scenario to the neurosurgeon. The life of the patient is put in danger or there exists the risk of an extensive and disabling infarction produced by the closure of the parent artery under desperate conditions. Past efforts by respectable neurosurgeons led to the present techniques and tools aimed at safe clipping of these lesions. The other important factor is that a wide variety of aneurysms and dome projections occur in only 1.5 to 2 cm of the ICA length, making the region a complex one. However, it is important to make the surgical approach a systematic one. The approach should include a good surgical planning evaluating the collateral blood flow conditions to anticipate the need for an indirect revascularization procedure if necessary. The type of the aneurysm should be identified because this will influence extension of the surgical approach and the kind of clips to be used. The surgical technique should include considerations about proximal control of the ICA, extent of the craniotomy, the need for an additional skull base approach (e.g., orbitozygomatic approach), dural opening, arachnoid cistern dissection, ACP resection technique, and aneurysm clipping. The availability of surgical tools should be checked (high-speed drill, set of clips, intraoperative Doppler, etc.). Even when this seems to be a very basic recommendation, having in mind all these aspects in a systematic way will permit the neurosurgeon to proceed to clip an aneurysm in this area with the highest rate of success.

ACKNOWLEDGMENT

The authors dedicate this chapter to the late Professor Humberto Matéos-Gómez. Professor Sergio Gómez–Llata Andrade.

KEY REFERENCES

Barami K, Hernandez VS, Diaz FG, Guthikonda M. Paraclinoid carotid aneurysms: surgical management, complications, and outcome based on a new classification scheme. *Skull Base*. 2003;13(1):31-41.

Batjer HH, Kopitnik TA, Giller CA, Samson DS. Surgery for paraclinoidal carotid artery aneurysms. *J Neurosurg*. 1994;80:650-658.

Batjer HH, Samson DS. Retrograde suction decompression of giant paraclinoidal aneurysms: technical note. *J Neurosurg*. 1990;73:305-306.

Bouthillier A, van Loveren HR, Keller JT. Segments of the internal carotid artery: a new classification. *Neurosurgery*. 1996;38(3):425-433.

Bulsara KR, Patel T, Fukushima T. Cerebral bypass surgery for skull base lesions: technical notes incorporating lessons learned over two decades. *Neurosurg Focus*. 2008;24(2):E11.

Day A. Aneurysms of the ophthalmic segment: a clinical and anatomical analysis. *J Neurosurg*. 1990;29:24-31.

De Jesús O, Sekhar LN, Riedel CJ. Clinoid and paraclinoid aneurysms: surgical anatomy, operative techniques, and outcome. *Surg Neurol*. 1999;51:477-488.

Dolenc V. A combined epi- and subdural direct approach to carotid-ophthalmic artery aneurysms. *J Neurosurg*. 1985;62:667-672.

Drake CG, Vanderlinded R, Amacher A. Carotid-ophthalmic aneurysm. *J Neurosurg*. 1968;29:24.

Fries G, Perneczky A, van Lindert E, Bahadori-Mortasawi F. Contralateral and ipsilateral microsurgical approaches to caroti-ophthalmic aneurysms. *Neurosurgery*. 1997;12:333-342.

Gibo H, Lenkey C, Rhoton Jr AL. Microsurgical anatomy of the supraclinoid portion of the internal carotid artery. *J Neurosurg*. 1981;55:560-574.

Hadeishi H, Suzuki A, Yasui N, Satou Y. Anterior clinoidectomy and opening of the internal auditory canal using an ultrasonic bone curette. *Neurosurgery*. 2003;52:867-871.

Kattner KA, Bailes J, Fukushima T. Direct surgical management of large bulbous and giant aneurysms involving the paraclinoid segment of the internal carotid artery: report of 29 cases. *Surg Neurol*. 1998;49:471-480.

Khan N, Yoshimura S, Roth P, et al. Conventional microsurgical treatment of paraclinoid aneurysms: state of the art with the use of the selective extradural anterior clinoidectomy SEAC. *Acta Neurochir Suppl*. 2005;94:23-29.

Kobayashi S, Kyoshima K, Gibo H, et al. Carotid cave aneurysms of the internal carotid artery. *J Neurosurg*. 1989;70:216-221.

Krayenbühl N, Hafez A, Hernesniemi JA, Krisht AF. Taming the cavernous sinus: technique of hemostasis using fibrin glue. *Neurosurgery*. 2007;61(Suppl 3):E-52.

Mastronardi L, Sameshima T, Ducati A, et al. Extradural middle fossa approach. Proposal of a learning method: the "rule of two fans." Technical note. *Skull Base*. 2006;16(3):181-184.

Nakagawa FF, Kobayashi S, Toshiki T, Sugita K. Aneurysms protruding from the dorsal wall of the internal carotid artery. *J Neurosurg*. 1986;65:303-308.

Nonaka T, Haraguchi K, Baba T, et al. Clinical manifestations and surgical results for paraclinoid cerebral aneurysms presenting with visual symptoms. *Surg Neurol*. 2007;67(6):612-619.

Nutik S. Subclinoid aneurysms. *J Neurosurg*. 2003;98:731-736.

Yasargil MG, Gasser JC, Hodosh RM, Rankin TV. Carotid-ophthalmic aneurysm: direct microsurgical approach. *Surg Neurol*. 1977;8:155-165.

Numbered references appear on Expert Consult.

CHAPTER 73

Surgical Management of Posterior Communicating, Anterior Choroidal, Carotid Bifurcation Aneurysms

KYRIAKOS PAPADIMITRIOU • JUDY HUANG

Aneurysms that arise from the supraclinoid internal carotid artery (ICA) in the subarachnoid space typically occur in association with the branches of the posterior communicating artery (PComA) and anterior choroidal artery (AChA) or at the ICA terminus where it bifurcates into the anterior cerebral artery (ACA) and middle cerebral artery (MCA). Rarely, supraclinoid ICA aneurysms may arise directly from the ICA wall without an associated branch vessel, and these are termed anterior wall and posterior wall ICA aneurysms. Supraclinoid ICA aneurysms that occur in each of these locations have unique features and warrant specific considerations in their surgical management.

Approximately 25% of all intracranial aneurysms are PComA aneurysms, making them the second most common overall after anterior communicating artery aneurysms. ICA bifurcation aneurysms account for about 4% to 15% of all intracranial aneurysms; those at the AChA are even more uncommon and comprise less than 5% of such aneurysms.[1,2] Although the incidence of intracranial aneurysms in the pediatric population is relatively low, the ICA termination is the most common location of intracranial aneurysms in this patient group.

The first described aneurysm clipping was of a PComA aneurysm by Dandy in 1938 at the Johns Hopkins Hospital. The patient presented with a complete third cranial nerve palsy and periorbital headaches. Dandy described complete obliteration of the aneurysm neck and preservation of the parent vessel with clip application. The patient recovered uneventfully with complete resolution of the third nerve palsy 7 months later.[3,4]

The presentation and diagnosis of aneurysms presenting with subarachnoid hemorrhage (SAH) is discussed elsewhere in this book. Similarly, the diagnosis and treatment planning for unruptured aneurysms is the focus of another chapter. This chapter focuses on specific considerations of ICA aneurysms arising at these specific locations.

Embryology of the ICA

The intracranial ICA is derived from the embryonic dorsal aorta. Around 28 to 30 days, the ICA has cranial and caudal divisions. The caudal divisions anastomose with the cranial ends of the longitudinal neural arteries. The AChA arises from the cranial division of the ICA, which subsequently also gives rise to the ACA and MCA by 41 to 48 days. The caudal divisions

of the ICA anastomose with the paired neural arteries located on the hindbrain that are the precursors of the basilar artery and regress to form the PComAs. Later, the embryologic anastomoses between the carotid and the basilar systems via the trigeminal, otic, and hypoglossal arteries regress.

FETAL POSTERIOR CEREBRAL ARTERY

The caudal division of the ICA continues to grow into the posterior cerebral artery (PCA) by 8 weeks, and the PComA regresses as the vertebrobasilar system develops. The caudal divisions also supply the stems of the PCAs. By 8 weeks, the PCAs may be identified as the posterior communication of the PComAs. If the embryonic PComA fails to regress, the dominant blood supply to the occipital lobes comes from the ICA via the fetal PCA instead of the vertebrobasilar system.[5] This occurs in approximately 20% to 30% of cases. A fetal PCA is defined as a variant of the PComA with the same caliber as the P2 segment of the PCA and is coupled with a hypoplastic P1 segment. In this configuration of the circle of Willis, the primary supply to the PCA territory is derived from the fetal PCA; therefore, clipping or coiling of PComA aneurysms must be achieved without jeopardizing flow to this artery.

Diagnosis, Preoperative Planning, and Patient Selection

The most common presentation of PComA, AChA, and ICA bifurcation aneurysms is SAH (Fig. 73-1A). While those presenting with SAH are considered for treatment on an emergency basis, preferably within 24 hours of presentation, to minimize the risk of rebleeding, those patients who are found to have symptomatic, unruptured aneurysms should also be considered for urgent treatment. The decision of whether to treat incidental unruptured aneurysms entails consideration of aneurysm- and patient-related factors, such as family history and prior history of aneurysmal SAH. Similarly, the complex choice of either microsurgical or endovascular therapy for any ruptured or unruptured aneurysm rests on multiple factors, such as the patient's age and medical condition; aneurysm size, location, and morphology; and operator experience. As greater understanding of the natural history continues, technological advances evolve, centralization of care to specialized

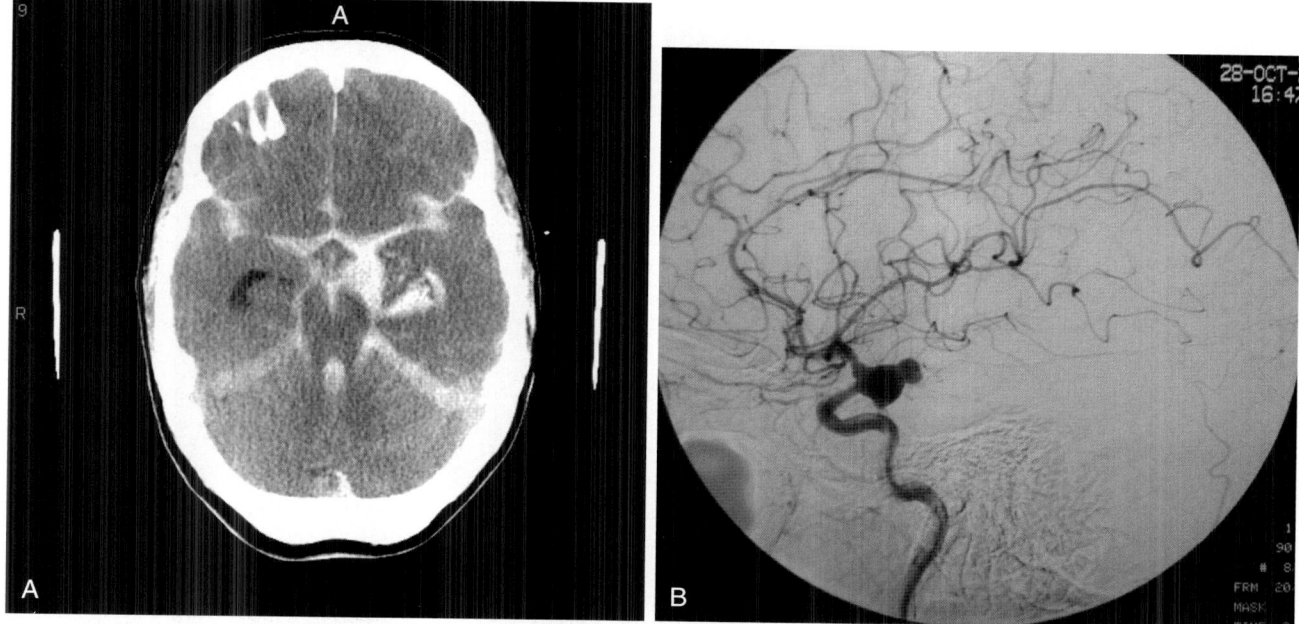

FIGURE 73-1 A, Head CT with a diffuse SAH, particularly in the left-sided basal cisterns, suspicious for a ruptured ICA aneurysm. B, Lateral view of a DSA of a left ICA injection showing a large, multilobulated PComA aneurysm.

centers with multidisciplinary capabilities expands, and refined microsurgical and endovascular techniques develop, an aneurysm-specific treatment strategy may be optimally tailored to the individual patient.

Presentation with symptoms caused by mass effect or hemorrhage other than SAH is also possible for these aneurysms. An enlarging unruptured or ruptured PComA aneurysm may also present with a partial or complete, non-pupil–sparing, third nerve palsy. The pupil dilates due to mechanical compression of the parasympathetic fibers that course on the outer surface of the oculomotor nerve. Since relief of the compressive effect caused by the aneurysm is readily accomplished with clipping, improvement in diplopia and ptosis is more often associated with clipping but remains possible with coiling. In univariate analysis,[6] the only variable that showed significant association with complete improvement of oculomotor nerve function following microsurgical clipping was severity of the third nerve palsy at admission. In this report, all patients with a partial third nerve palsy regained full oculomotor nerve function. Only 40% of patients with complete third nerve palsy demonstrated complete recovery. Furthermore, there is no statistically significant association between early surgery and improvement of the third nerve function.[6] Recovery of third nerve function after coiling has also been documented in case reports.[3]

Patients presenting with ruptured aneurysms at the PComA (Fig. 73-1B) and AChA (Fig. 73-2) locations may have, in addition to SAH, an associated temporal intracerebral hemorrhage (ICH) or an acute subdural hematoma for which evacuation may be accomplished, along with craniotomy for aneurysm clipping. Ruptured AChA aneurysms often are associated with intraventricular hemorrhage (IVH) and hydrocephalus. Occasionally, a ruptured ICA termination aneurysm manifests with a basal ganglia ICH, with or without IVH.

In addition, presentation with ischemic symptoms or stroke due to emboli from the aneurysm occurs in about 3.3% of patients. Although more frequently associated with anterior circulation aneurysms, ischemic events in the distal vascular territory attributable to the aneurysm can arise from aneurysms of all sizes, even small aneurysms.[7]

In patients presenting acutely with suspected SAH, computed tomography (CT) scanning remains the initial imaging modality for diagnosis. If the clinical suspicion remains high despite the absence of SAH on head CT, then lumbar puncture is warranted due to its greater sensitivity in detecting SAH. Computed tomography angiography (CTA) has gained increasing utility for aneurysm diagnosis and preoperative planning. Due to the wide availability of magnetic resonance angiography (MRA) and CTA, these noninvasive imaging studies are often the initial screening modality that establishes the diagnosis of an incidentally discovered, unruptured aneurysm (Fig. 73-3A).

The gold standard for diagnosis and preoperative planning remains the digital subtraction angiogram (DSA) (Fig. 73-3B), as this modality allows selective arterial injections, rotational views, three-dimensional (3D) reconstructions (Fig. 73-3C), and cross-compression testing, if necessary. When assessing the vasculature during the preoperative planning of PComA aneurysm treatment, a fetal PCA (Fig. 73-4A and B) is defined by absence of filling of the PCA or lack of visualization of the P1 segment with the vertebral artery injection (Fig. 73-4C).

In preoperative planning for ICA bifurcation aneurysms, the absence or presence of cross-filling of the ipsilateral ACA across the anterior communicating artery from the contralateral A1 is important to assess with a cross-compression test during the diagnostic angiogram. This maneuver entails compression of the ipsilateral ICA during contralateral ICA injection to determine whether the ipsilateral ACA territory can be supplied by the contralateral ICA.

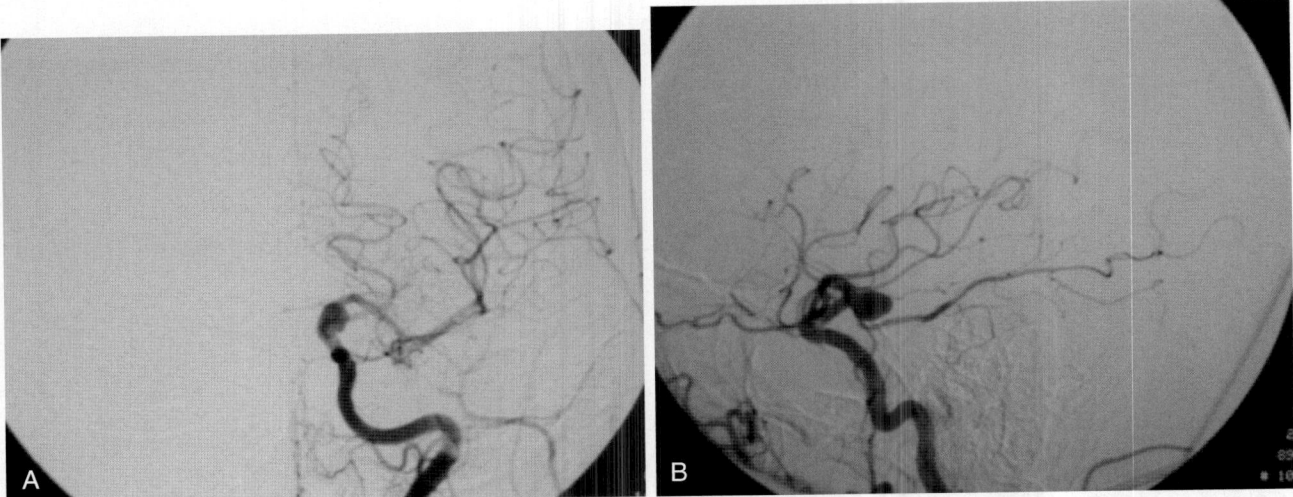

FIGURE 73-2 Left ICA injection on a DSA with an AChA aneurysm: anterior–posterior (A) and lateral (B) views.

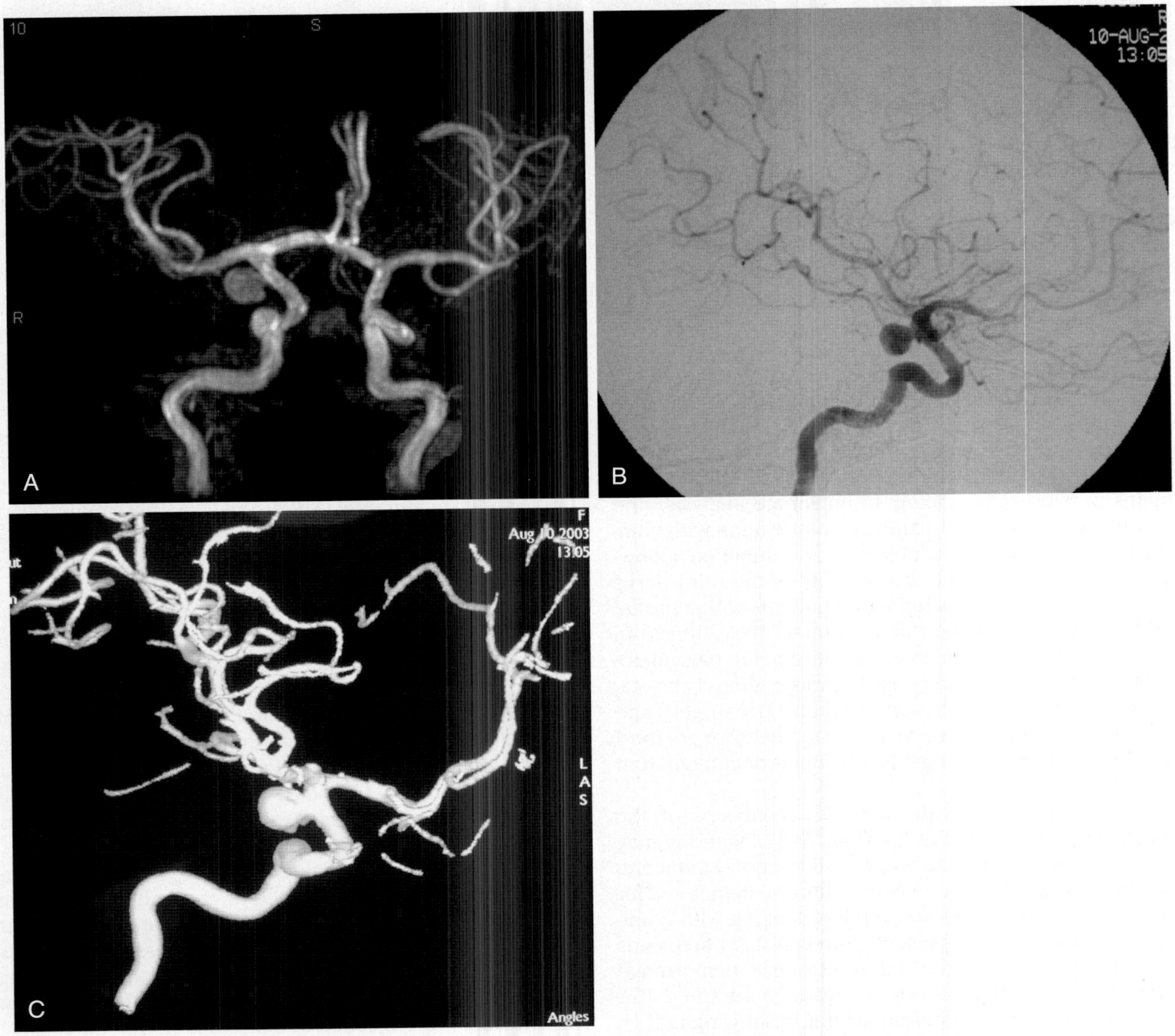

FIGURE 73-3 MRA (A), DSA (B), and 3D angiography (C) views of a right PComA-region aneurysm.

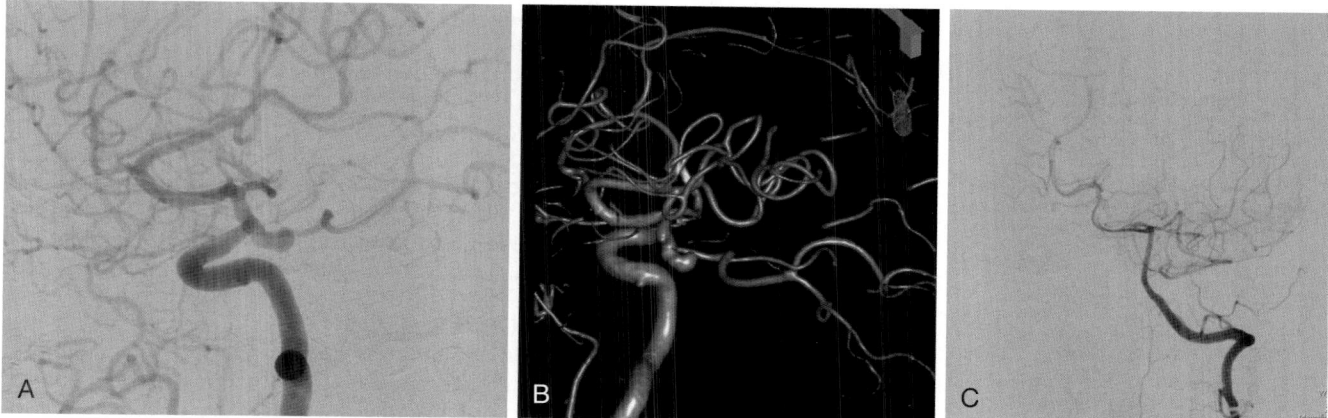

FIGURE 73-4 Lateral left ICA DSA (A) and 3D DSA (B) of a PComA aneurysm with a fetal PCA. Anterior–posterior view of a left vertebral artery DSA (C) in the same patient, with absence of a left PCA visualization, indicative of a fetal PCA configuration.

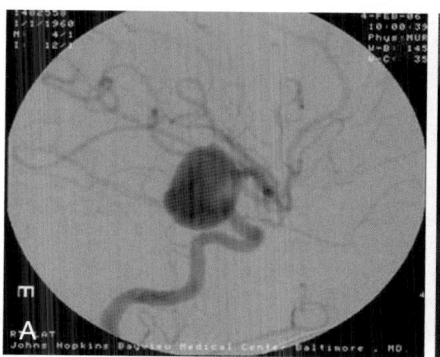

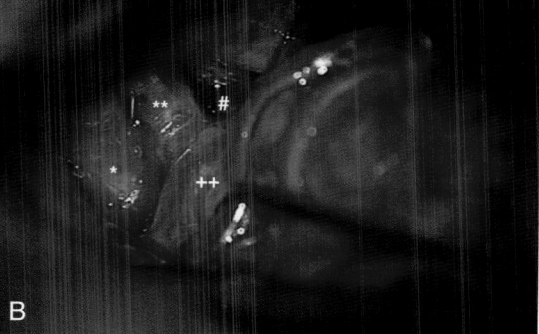

FIGURE 73-5 A, Lateral DSA of a right PComA aneurysm. B, Intraoperative view showing the optic nerve (*), supraclinoid ICA (**), PComA (#), and neck of the laterally projecting aneurysm (++).

The presence of cross-filling implies that compromise of the ipsilateral A1 during clip reconstruction of ICA bifurcation aneurysms may be compensated for by filling of the ipsilateral A2 via the contralateral A1 across the anterior communicating artery, rather than via the ipsilateral A1.

Anterior circulation aneurysms located at the posterior communicating segment (Fig. 73-5), anterior choroidal segment, and terminal ICA bifurcation are typically favorable for microsurgical clipping. Posterior communicating and anterior choroidal aneurysms are carotid wall aneurysms that frequently include the origin of the branch artery at the aneurysm base (Fig. 73-6A). Meticulous identification of the branch artery adjacent to the proximal neck of the aneurysm allows for clip application across the neck to be accomplished with simultaneous preservation of the origin of the branch artery and minimal brain retraction (Fig. 73-6B to E).

The ICA termination aneurysms that may be relatively more favorable for endovascular therapy than microsurgical clipping are those with heavily calcified walls or a primary posterior projection.[8] CT or CTA (Fig. 73-7) may be useful in treatment planning to determine the presence of calcification in the aneurysm walls. Using clip blades to gather the neck of a thick-walled aneurysm in the presence of severe atherosclerosis and calcification may risk hemodynamically significant stenosis of the proximal A1 or M1 segment at its origin from the terminal carotid bifurcation. A strategy of placing the clips more distally on the neck to avoid constriction of the origins of the A1 and M1 segments may be employed. Endovascular therapy may

be preferable for those ICA termination aneurysms that project posteriorly. Since the perforators originate from the distal ICA at its posterior wall, clipping of posteriorly projecting ICA termination aneurysm may be treacherous due to poor visualization of the perforating arteries.

In the treatment of patients with multiple aneurysms, clipping of a contralaterally located aneurysm via a unilateral pterional craniotomy is most often successful when the contralateral aneurysm is located at the ICA termination. Wide arachnoid opening of the chiasmatic, carotid, and lamina terminalis cisterns allows significant brain relaxation to permit perforator dissection and clip reconstruction of a contralateral ICA bifurcation aneurysm.

Anatomic and Clinical Considerations
POSTERIOR COMMUNICATING SEGMENT

The communicating segment of the ICA courses between the optic and the oculomotor nerves to the anterior perforated substance at the medial section of the sylvian fissure.[2] Angiographically, this segment extends from the origin of the PComA to the origin of the AChA. The PComA arises from the posteromedial or posterior surface of the ICA; courses medially and inferiorly, superior and medial to the oculomotor nerve, through the membrane of Liliequist; and joins the PCA at the junction of the P1 and P2 segments. Multiple, variable perforating arteries arise from the PComA, namely, the anterior thalamic perforators, which are at risk of compromise during aneurysm clipping.

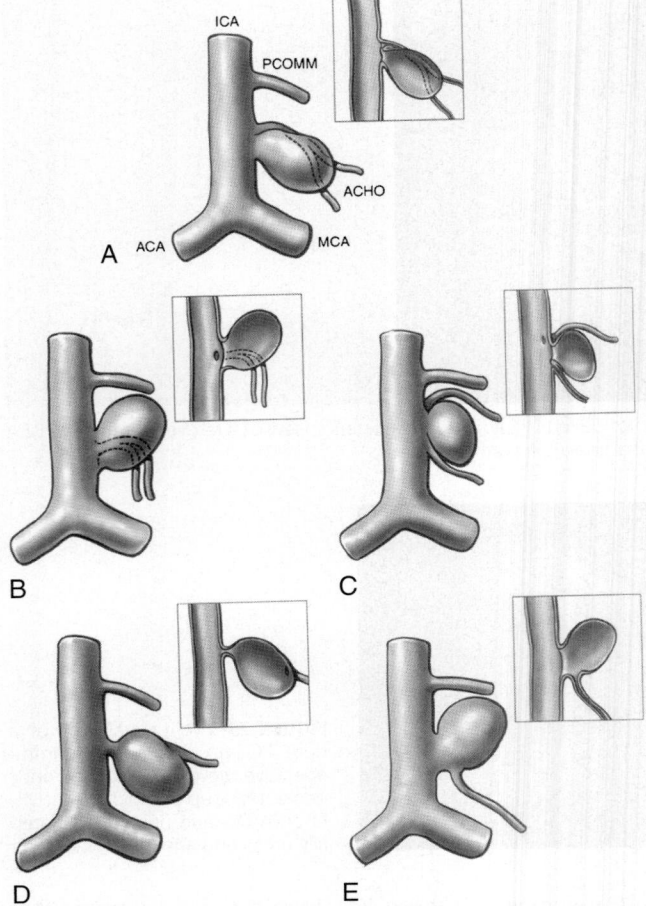

FIGURE 73-6 Schematic illustration of AChA arising from the proximal neck region of an AChA aneurysm (A) and various other configurations of branch artery origins (B-E).

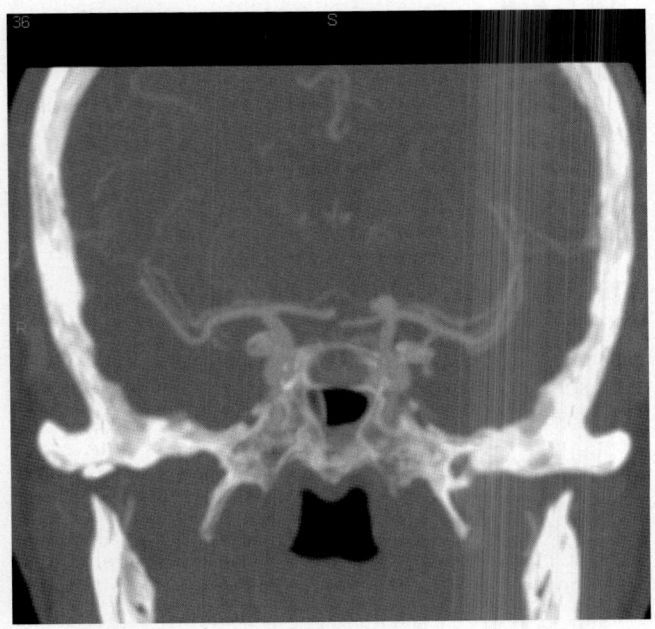

FIGURE 73-7 CTA of a left ICA termination aneurysm.

PComA aneurysms are most commonly ICA aneurysms that arise from the ICA and incorporate the origin of the PComA into its neck, rather than arising directly from the PComA. PComA aneurysms are considered relatively straightforward aneurysms for clipping, because their location is very proximal on the supraclinoid ICA. They comprise approximately 25% of all ruptured aneurysms.[9] The direction of the dome projection has significant implications for presentation and microsurgical treatment. Yasargil has described a classification system based on the direction of the dome.[10] When the dome projects anterolaterally, the origin of the PComA is likely to be obscured from view by the aneurysm. In addition, the aneurysm dome may adhere to the anterior clinoid process. This situation requires cautious dissection to mobilize the dome and visualize the origin of the PComA during clip placement. A superolateral dome is occasionally encountered in which the dome points toward the medial sphenoid ridge. Rupture of these aneurysms is likely associated with presentation with a subdural hematoma. Rare cases of a contralateral frontal ICH from PComA aneurysm rupture have been reported in the literature.[11] Aneurysms with a posterolateral superior projection point into the medial temporal lobe and are often associated with intraparenchymal hemorrhage or even hemorrhage into the temporal horn of the lateral ventricle. PComA aneurysms with a posterolateral dome projection may present with a dilated pupil and oculomotor paresis due to compression of the third cranial nerve. A posterolateral inferior fundus may penetrate the membrane of Liliequist with projection into the interpeduncular fossa. Comprising approximately 5% of all PComA aneurysms, the variant of a "true PComA aneurysm" refers to the configuration in which the neck of the aneurysm originates entirely from the PComA.[9,12-14] Essential for operative planning is review of the angiogram to determine whether the PCA is supplied by the posterior circulation and fills from the vertebral artery injection or is fetal in configuration and fills from the ICA injection. In the 4% to 25%[3,9,15,16] of patients who have a fetal PCA, the P1 segment of PCA is hypoplastic, and the PCA arises directly from the PComA. PComA aneurysms associated with a fetal PCA must be reconstructed either with clips or with coils in a manner that preserves the patency of the ICA and fetal PCA vessels. In contrast, a diminutive PComA may be sacrificed if necessary.

The origin of the PComA is usually found proximal and medial to the proximal neck of the aneurysm. PComA aneurysms typically project laterally and posteriorly; they rarely project medially.[2] The arachnoid of the sylvian fissure should be divided appropriately to reveal the medial border of the temporal lobe and to appreciate the PComA origin and the course and number of AChA vessels. The relationship between the dome of the aneurysm and the medial temporal lobe should not be disturbed before the arachnoid has been dissected adequately and proximal control of the ICA has been achieved. The dome of the aneurysm may adhere to the edge of the tentorium. If the dome is attached to the medial temporal lobe, temporal lobe retractors should be avoided or used cautiously. The two most common causes of intraoperative rupture are premature medial retraction of the supraclinoid ICA and retraction of the temporal lobe while the aneurysm dome remains adherent to the temporal lobe. In general, temporal lobe retraction should be avoided in ruptured cases.

In rare instances, a PComA aneurysm may be partially obscured by the anterior clinoid process.[17,18] In this situation, adequate proximal control of the ICA and visualization of the proximal neck of the aneurysm may necessitate partial removal of the anterior clinoid process, resection of the anterior petroclinoid fold, or exposure of the ICA in the neck. A predictor of the need for clinoidectomy is a short distance between the tip of the anterior clinoid process and the proximal neck of the aneurysm assessed using CTA.

Adequate dissection of the sylvian fissure facilitates identification and preservation of the AChA. This artery may travel medial to the aneurysm and adhere to the dome of the aneurysm at its cisternal segment, making it necessary to separate the vessel from the distal neck of the aneurysm. The AChA should be preserved in all instances. The AChA supplies the optic chiasm, optic tract, lateral geniculate nucleus, uncus and amygdala, middle third of the cerebral peduncle, caudate, globus pallidus, genu and posterior limb of internal capsule, anterior hippocampus and dentate gyrus, fornix, pulvinar, and choroid plexus.[19]

Exposure of the contralateral PComA and choroidal segment can be accomplished either through the interoptic space or through the contralateral opticocarotid space. Aneurysms at these locations are the most difficult aneurysms to expose via a contralateral approach. Boundaries of the triangular contralateral opticocarotid space are the lateral aspect of the contralateral optic nerve, chiasm, and tract; the medial aspect of the contralateral ICA; and the inferior aspect of the precommunicating segment of the contralateral ACA.[20] Since these aneurysms frequently project posterolaterally, the neck region and origins of the PComA and AChA may be partially obscured by the contralateral ICA and optic apparatus. Optic chiasm position can interfere with visualization.

As mentioned earlier, PComA aneurysms that project posteriorly, laterally, and slightly inferiorly may cause compression of the oculomotor nerve as it enters the dural fold of the cavernous sinus. Approximately 20% of PComA aneurysms present with oculomotor nerve palsy, and of aneurysms presenting with a third nerve palsy, 80% were located at the PComA region. Acute third nerve palsy can occur with an expanding PComA aneurysm; therefore, such a clinical presentation requires urgent evaluation and treatment.

INTERNAL CAROTID ARTERY

Rarely, internal carotid anterior or posterior wall aneurysms occur in communicating or choroidal segments of the ICA. These aneurysms are not associated with an arterial branch of the ICA. Anterior wall aneurysms are traditionally known as dorsal wall ICA aneurysms. These dorsal wall ICA aneurysms are often broad based and may be particularly treacherous if they harbor blister-type, thin walls. Wrap clipping has been reported in patients with a ruptured blister-type aneurysm of the supraclinoid ICA using materials such as a Silastic sheet coated with Dacron mesh, collagen-impregnated Dacron knitted fabric, and polytetrafluoroethylene. Encircling clips may be required for clip reconstruction. Clip-wrap techniques for treatment of fusiform and unclippable aneurysms is safe, and it can be associated with a low rate of acute or delayed postoperative complications.[21]

ANTERIOR CHOROIDAL SEGMENT

The choroidal segment of the ICA starts from the origin of the AChA and terminates at the ICA bifurcation. The AChA is the first branch from the supraclinoid ICA that is distal and lateral to the origin of the PComA. The cisternal segment of the AChA courses lateral initially and then posteriorly, following the optic tract and supplying the mesial temporal structures. Its main trunk then continues posteriorly, inferior to the optic tract, to enter the choroidal fissure. The choroidal segment supplies the choroid plexus of the temporal horn. The size of the artery is variable, from 0.5 to 2 mm, and duplication occurs in as many as 30% of the normal population.[22] In cases of duplicated AChA (Fig. 73-6C), each branch requires meticulous preservation, since occlusion may lead to contralateral hemiparesis, hemianopia, and hemisensory deficit. Adequate opening of the sylvian fissure facilitates vessel preservation by revealing the course of the AChA. In some cases, the AChA travels medial to the PComA aneurysm, making it necessary to separate the vessel from the neck of the aneurysm before clipping. Clear identification of the origin of the AChA should be made in all cases of PComA and AChA aneurysms. Compromise of the AChA may be inadvertent if the clip blades are placed on the distal neck of a wide-necked or large PComA aneurysm if the AChA origin is nearby and not first dissected away from the distal neck.

Operative repair of AChA aneurysms carries a risk of postoperative stroke as high as 16%, and the risk of stroke is associated with the anatomy of the aneurysm. Typically, the neck of an AChA aneurysm is relatively wider than the caliber of the AChA vessel, and compensatory clip placement more distally on the neck to preserve the origin of the AChA at the aneurysm base may be needed. Although judicious preservation of the AChA during aneurysm clipping is essential, many postoperative AChA-territory strokes occur several hours after surgery; these are thought to be related to delayed thrombosis of this small vessel. Although Buck and Cooper,[23] as well as others,[24,25] reported during the mid-20th century that the AChA might be safely occluded, contemporary experience suggests that AChA occlusion carries an associated risk of cerebral infarction and neurologic morbidity. In 1956, Diller et al. described 16 patients who underwent AChA occlusion for the treatment of Parkinson's disease. Tremor and rigidity improved in 10 of those patients, 3 remained the same, 1 died, 1 became hemiplegic, and 1 became hemiparetic.[24] It can be concluded that preservation of the AChA is a goal in optimizing outcomes after aneurysm treatment.

CAROTID BIFURCATION

Carotid bifurcation aneurysms are located at the terminal bifurcation of the ICA where it splits into the A1 segment of the ACA and the M1 segment of the MCA. Carotid bifurcation aneurysms comprise 4% to 15% of aneurysms. The ICA bifurcation is typically the highest point of the circle of Willis. The apex of the ICA bifurcation, similar to the MCA bifurcation or the apex of the basilar artery, is under particular hemodynamic stress and high wall shear stress. Some ICA bifurcation aneurysms arise preferentially from the A1 and others from the M1 portion of the ICA termination. It is important to identify this asymmetry and direction of dome projection in the planning of clip reconstruction. Most commonly, they project superiorly (medially), impinging on the orbitofrontal gyrus or olfactory tract, with the dome projecting along the A1 segment. Others project posteriorly, occupying the sylvian cistern and accompanying the MCA. It is crucial to identify the anatomy of the perforating vessels surrounding the neck of the aneurysm. The most critical perforators are the medial lenticulostriate arteries from the posterior aspect of A1 and M1 segments, and from the ICA bifurcation that course through the anterior perforated substance to the basal ganglia. Since these lenticulostriate vessels originate posteriorly, clipping of anteriorly projecting ICA bifurcation aneurysms is relatively more favorable than clipping of those that project posteriorly and thereby obscure the view of these perforators. Other vessels that often require identification and preservation are deep branches from the PComA and AChA and the recurrent artery of Heubner from the ACA.

Ruptured ICA bifurcation aneurysms typically present with primarily ICH and minimal SAH.[26] Isolated cranial nerve abnormalities are rare, but symptoms related to mass effect can arise from giant lesions. ICA bifurcation aneurysms tend to be larger than those detected at the PComA and AChA locations. The morbidity of carotid bifurcation aneurysms is higher than that of PComA or MCA aneurysms. Due to the relatively longer natural history of carotid bifurcation aneurysms before detection, there is a tendency for these to have calcification in the aneurysm walls at the time of presentation. Aneurysmal calcification can be detected with a CT scan. Calcium deposition may make clip obliteration challenging because of the rigidity of the neck of aneurysm. For this reason, endovascular therapy is the preferred strategy to treat those aneurysms with calcified walls.

Carotid bifurcation aneurysms are ideal for the contralateral approach in patients with multiple aneurysms. After the carotid termination is reached and the supracarotid space is opened, the contralateral sphenoidal segment of the MCA can be followed to the carotid bifurcation by dissecting along its inferior surface to avoid injury to the lateral lenticulostriate arteries as the contralateral frontal lobe is separated from the temporal lobe. Ease of access to these aneurysms is facilitated by the presence of a relatively short sphenoidal MCA segment. Laterally projecting aneurysms are more challenging to treat from the contralateral exposure because the visualization of aneurysmal neck may be obscured by the parent vessel.

Operative Procedure and Complication Avoidance

POSITIONING AND PTERIONAL CRANIOTOMY

The pterional craniotomy is ideal for PComA, AChA, and ICA termination aneurysms. With the patient in supine position, rigid head fixation with the radiolucent skull clamp is utilized in anticipation of intraoperative angiography, which is performed after each aneurysm treated with microsurgical clipping. The double pin is situated low at the ipsilateral retroauricular region, while the single pin is placed behind or at the contralateral hairline in the sagittal plane of the midpupillary line. The head is turned 15 to 30 degrees toward the side opposite to the planned craniotomy and extended so that the ipsilateral malar eminence is the highest point of the

operative field to allow gravity to facilitate brain retraction. A shoulder roll to elevate the ipsilateral shoulder and elevation of the head of the bed ensures good jugular venous return.

A strip shave located 2 cm behind the hairline to leave a cuff of hair or a shave extending for 3 cm behind the hairline, from the most anterior portion of the hairline at the midline (widow's peak) inferolaterally to the sideburn, is utilized to allow a curvilinear frontotemporal skin incision from the midline extending laterally to 1 cm anterior to the tragus and terminating within a skin crease. While creation of a cuff of temporalis muscle and fascia to prevent subsequent temporal muscle wasting is optional with the use of various cranioplasty materials, the myocutaneous flap is reflected anteriorly and inferiorly by subperiosteal dissection of temporalis muscle until the root of the zygoma, keyhole (located over the frontosphenoidal suture approximately 1 cm behind the frontozygomatic suture), and supraorbital ridge are identified. Bur holes are placed at the temporal squamosa and keyhole, and a frontosphenotemporal craniotomy flap is created.

To minimize brain retraction, maximize microscopic illumination for anatomic visualization, and enlarge the space for working corridors to the vessels, the greater and lesser medial sphenoid wings adjacent to the sylvian fissure are flattened with a high-speed drill to connect the lateral extent of the frontal fossa with the anterior extent of the temporal fossa. The landmark used to assess the adequacy of the medial extent of sphenoid wing removal is the dura of the superior orbital fissure.

After the dura is opened and tented flat anteriorly against the sphenoid wing, microdissection proceeds via either a subfrontal or a trans-sylvian approach. In cases of thick subarachnoid clot in the basal cisterns or hydrocephalus, in which brain relaxation is anticipated to be inadequate via cerebrospinal fluid (CSF) release from opening of the basal cisterns, a previously placed lumbar subarachnoid catheter or intraventricular catheter may be utilized for additional CSF drainage.

POSTERIOR COMMUNICATING ARTERY ANEURYSMS

A subfrontal approach to PComA aneurysms allows early proximal control. Frontal lobe retraction permits visualization of the proximal edge of the sylvian fissure, the optic nerve, and the supraclinoid ICA. Sharp arachnoid dissection begins over the optic nerve and proceeds laterally into the ipsilateral opticocarotid cistern. After the ipsilateral optic nerve is released from the inferior frontal lobe, the chiasmatic cistern is opened. The release of CSF from the basal cisterns allows brain relaxation, but if necessary, further brain relaxation may be accomplished by the release of CSF from the ventricular system with fenestration of the lamina terminalis.

The opticocarotid triangle is completely opened to expose the medial aspect of the ICA. Dissection continues on the anterior–superior surface of the supraclinoid ICA until proximal control is established. Arachnoid dissection proceeds with entry into the sylvian cistern at the region of the frontal operculum. Wide opening of the vertical portion of the sylvian fissure in a lateral to medial direction diminishes the need for vigorous frontal lobe retraction and offers an expansive corridor for dissection of the basal cisterns.

Coagulation of the temporopolar veins draining into the sphenoparietal sinus untethers the anterior temporal lobe. Retraction of the anteromedial temporal lobe is not typically required; it should be avoided in all ruptured cases and whenever the dome points laterally.

The PComA is the first branch arising from the lateral wall of the supraclinoid ICA. The PComA located proximal to the proximal neck of the aneurysm, the anterior thalamic perforators arising from the PComA, and the AChA located beyond the distal neck of the aneurysm should be clearly identified and preserved. When large aneurysms obstruct the visualization of the origin of the PComA, the vessel can be identified distally in the opticocarotid triangle and traced proximally to gain an appreciation of the location of its origin from the posterolateral ICA. Occasionally, identification of the PComA origin is possible only after clip placement, and clip adjustments may be necessary.

Anteromedial retraction of the ICA is avoided to prevent premature intraoperative rupture from inadvertent avulsion of the aneurysm dome from the medial temporal lobe, tentorial edge, or oculomotor nerve. If the aneurysm dome adheres to the third nerve, excessive traction of the oculomotor nerve should be minimized to avoid a postoperative third nerve palsy and improve prognosis for recovery in the event one occurs. Dissection of the aneurysm dome away from the adherent nerve is avoided because traction may result in irreversible oculomotor nerve damage. The decrease in arterial pulsations after aneurysm clipping is typically adequate for resolution of a partial third nerve palsy caused by mass effect from a PComA aneurysm. The use of a temporary clip on the proximal supraclinoid ICA facilitates neck dissection and clip placement with larger aneurysms. Intraoperative electophysiologic monitoring is useful in assuring the patient's tolerance of temporary flow arrest. If monitoring is not available, 3-minute periods of temporary occlusion alternating with 5-minute periods of reperfusion are generally safely tolerated. Once the aneurysm neck is clearly identified and cleared of surrounding vessels, clip reconstruction is typically accomplished with straight or slightly curved clips. The tips of the clip blades must be inspected to ensure complete obliteration across the aneurysm neck and patency of a fetal PCA, thalamoperforators, and the AChA. A small residual neck is acceptable to maintain the caliber of a fetal PCA. If the preoperative angiogram demonstrates the absence of a fetal PCA and confirms PCA filling from the vertebral injection, the PComA can be occluded by the clip if necessary. The PComA perforators will fill from the PCA, and potential backfilling of the aneurysm via the PComA is prevented with placement of a clip between the proximal neck of the aneurysm and the PComA or across the PComA before the first thalamoperforator vessel.

Relative to microsurgical treatment of aneurysms in other locations, neurologic morbidity from PComA aneurysms is the lowest. Wirth and co-workers report an operative morbidity of 5% compared to that associated with other anterior circulation aneurysms: MCA of 8%, ICA termination of 12%, and anterior communicating artery of 16%.[9,27]

ANTERIOR CHOROIDAL ARTERY ANEURYSMS

AChA aneurysms may be approached subfrontally utilizing a method of microdissection similar to that for PComA aneurysms. Early proximal control on the supraclinoid ICA

is readily established via this approach. Excessive temporal lobe retraction is best avoided due to the potential avulsion of the aneurysm dome that frequently adheres to the mesial temporal lobe. Identification of the origin of the AChA is critical. About one third of cases have a duplicated AChA and rarely a triplicated AChA.[28] If there is a duplicated AChA, the aneurysm typically arises from the largest branch. Preservation of all AChA vessels and choroidal perforators is critical to ensure a good outcome. An AChA infarct may result in hemiparesis, hemianopia, and hemisensory deficit,[23-25] but a range of deficits is possible after AChA occlusion due to the variability in collateral supply to the supplied structures.

Dissection proceeds on the medial wall of the supraclinoid ICA toward the proximal neck of the AChA aneurysm. Opening of the vertical, proximal portion of the sylvian fissure is necessary. Identification of the AChA and the corridor between the AChA origin and the proximal neck of the aneurysm is essential. In cases of large, superiorly projecting aneurysms, the recurrent artery of Heubner may be adjacent to the medial aspect of the aneurysm and must be preserved. Clip reconstruction with a straight clip perpendicular to the ICA is typical. Past pointing across the aneurysm neck with excessively long clip blades should be avoided to prevent injury to the nearby choroidal perforators, PComA, ICA perforators, recurrent artery of Heubner, and oculomotor nerve.

Microsurgical treatment of AChA aneurysms is associated with a risk of significant ischemic complications.[1,29] Due to the relatively small lumen of the AChA compared to the aneurysm neck, variations in the branches, and perforators of the AChA, an ischemic complication may occur even after blood flow had been confirmed after clip placement. Meticulous dissection and microsurgical technique are essential.

CAROTID BIFURCATION ANEURYSMS

Following pterional craniotomy as described earlier, the sylvian fissure is split widely in a distal to proximal direction in unruptured cases. In ruptured cases, microdissection begins first via the subfrontal approach, to establish proximal control over the supraclinoid ICA, before proceeding with the wide opening of the sylvian fissure. However, judicious frontal lobe retraction is critical to avoid compression of the aneurysm dome by the retractor. For isolated aneurysms, those at the ICA bifurcation aneurysms are approached from the ipsilateral side. In patients with multiple aneurysms, ICA bifurcation aneurysms are ideally suitable for a contralateral approach, particularly those with anterior or superior projections. Proximal control should be established prior to exposure of the carotid bifurcation aneurysm.

Dissection and clip reconstruction of ICA termination aneurysms may be challenging due to high position relative to the skull base, embedded dome in the brain parenchyma, and critical network of perforators adjacent to the neck and dome of the aneurysm. Posteriorly projecting carotid bifurcation aneurysms are most treacherous due to the location of the posteriorly projecting perforators arising from the proximal A1 and M1 segments and the ICA termination.

In addition to the prerequisite proximal control of the ICA, identification of both the M1 and the A1 segments originating from the base of the aneurysm is essential. Extensive arachnoid dissection of the carotid, optic, and sylvian cisterns to mobilize the supraclinoid ICA and the A1 and M1 segments is needed. Opening of the proximal third of the sylvian fissure is usually adequate for the majority of carotid bifurcation aneurysms. Large or giant carotid bifurcation aneurysms require a more extensive opening of the sylvian fissure. After the superficial arachnoid of the sylvian fissure is divided and access to the sylvian cistern is gained, the dissection proceeds proximally by gently spreading the fissure from the inside out. Small crossing veins may be cauterized and divided if necessary to allow frontal lobe retraction and decrease tension on the sylvian veins.[30,31] Minimal and cautious retraction of the frontal lobe is prudent, because the aneurysm dome is usually embedded in and adherent to the subfrontal cortex. Following identification of the proximal portion of the MCA (M1 segment), dissection proceeds along its lateral surface to identify the anterolateral wall of the ICA. Further medial dissection reveals the A1 segment. With carotid bifurcation aneurysms that project anteriorly, the A1 segment may be hidden behind the aneurysm dome. As the dissection of the ICA, M1, A1, and aneurysm neck proceeds, the objective is to identify and preserve all branches and perforators in the region of the carotid bifurcation so that their location and course are clear before applying temporary or permanent clips.

Temporary clip application facilitates complete circumferential dissection around the aneurysm neck. The ideal location for placement of the proximal temporary clip on the ICA is distal to the origin of the AChA in a segment that is clear of perforators. In certain instances, temporary clips on M1 and A1 may be helpful for clip reconstruction; such clipping decreases contralateral flow to the aneurysm. Particularly for posteriorly or superiorly projecting carotid bifurcation aneurysms, the dissection continues medially toward the olfactory and lamina terminalis cisterns to identify and protect the A1 segment and its perforators, including the recurrent artery of Heubner. For large aneurysms, the course of the PComA and the AChA and the relationship of their branches to the aneurysm dome should be elucidated. The temporopolar and the anterior temporal arteries should be mobilized to prevent them from injury sustained by retraction.

The final focus of dissection centers on identification and preservation of the ICA bifurcation perforators.[19] In small carotid bifurcation aneurysms, these perforators are usually free from the aneurysm base, but they may adhere to the dome of large or giant aneurysms. The dome of the carotid bifurcation aneurysms is typically buried in the orbitobasal frontal lobe, so cautious frontal lobe retraction should be utilized during the dissection. A limited resection of the frontobasal cortex may be necessary for adequate visualization in the situation of cerebral edema after acute SAH or when the carotid bifurcation aneurysm is embedded in the frontal lobe.

The length of the aneurysm clip should be one and a half times the width of the aneurysm neck. Proper clip selection to avoid kinking or stenosis of adjacent branches is essential. The technique of stepwise clipping of the aneurysm dome toward the base with further dissection facilitates complete occlusion in situations of large or complex carotid bifurcation aneurysms. An initial pilot clip may later be exchanged for a final clip after bipolar coagulation is used to reshape the dome and shrink the neck. Clip application is usually along the axis of M1 across the aneurysm neck, placing the blades between the neck of the aneurysm and the ACA and MCA, as well as their branches, to avoid stenosis of the carotid bifurcation. The surrounding arteries and perforators are inspected for patency as the clip is slowly closed. With the final clip in place, the whole aneurysm dome should be mobilized to allow direct confirmation of the absence of trapped perforators inside the final clip. Multiple (two or more) clips are typically required for wide-neck or thick-walled aneurysms.

In certain instances after clip application on the thick-walled neck of the aneurysm, the clip may slide down toward the proximal neck of the aneurysm and ICA termination where the vessel walls of the A1 and M1 origins are normal. This may lead to flow-limiting stenosis of the origins of the A1 and M1 segments and subsequent infarction. Occasionally, multiple parallel stacking clips must be applied proximally to distally along the aneurysm dome to close the neck of the aneurysm, with subsequent removal of the most proximal clips to ensure patency of the MCA and ACA origins.

Intraoperative angiography following clipping of ICA bifurcation aneurysms is especially helpful in assuring patency of the A1 and M1 segments, but preservation of the perforating medial lenticulostriate vessels in the region remains critical in achieving a good outcome.

KEY REFERENCES

Al-Yamani M, Wallace MC. Intracranial internal carotid artery aneurysms. In: Winn HR, ed. *Youman's Neurological Surgery II.* 5th Edition: Saunders; 2004, pp. 1915-1921.

Chang DJ. The "no-drill" technique of anterior clinoidectomy: a cranial base approach to the paraclinoid and parasellar region. *Neurosurgery.* 2009;64:96-105:discussion 105-106.

Chittiboina P, Cuellar H, Ballenilla F, et al. Two cases of ruptured cerebral aneurysms presenting with contralateral hematomas. *Emerg Radiol.* 2011;18:39-42.

Dandy WE. Intracranial aneurysm of the internal carotid artery: cured by operation. *Ann Surg.* 1938;107:654-659.

Dean BL, Wallace RC, Zabramski JM, et al. Incidence of superficial sylvian vein compromise and postoperative effects on CT imaging after surgical clipping of middle cerebral artery aneurysms. *AJNR Am J Neuroradiol.* 2005;26:2019-2026.

Diller L, Laszewski Z, Riklan M. Effects of anterior choroidal artery occlusion and of chemopallidectomy on the tremor and rigidity of Parkinson's disease: an independent appraisal. *J Am Geriatr Soc.* 1956;4:1246-1248.

Figueiredo EG, Foroni L, Monaco BA, et al. The clip-wrap technique in the treatment of intracranial unclippable aneurysms. *Arq Neuropsiquiatr.* 2010;68:115-118.

Friedman JA, Pichelmann MA, Piepgras DG, et al. Ischemic complications of surgery for anterior choroidal artery aneurysms. *J Neurosurg.* 2001;94:565-572.

Golshani K, Ferrell A, Zomorodi A, et al. A review of the management of posterior communicating artery aneurysms in the modern era. *Surg Neurol Int.* 2010;1:88.

Hammers R, Hacein-Bey L, Origitano TC. Anomalous medial origin of the anterior choroidal artery with associated aneurysm. *J Neurol Sci.* 2009;287:250-252.

Heros RC. Microneurosurgical management of anterior choroidal artery aneurysms. *World Neurosurg.* 2010;73:459-460.

Horikoshi T, Akiyama I, Yamagata Z, et al. Magnetic resonance angiographic evidence of sex-linked variations in the circle of Willis and the occurrence of cerebral aneurysms. *J Neurosurg.* 2002;96:697-703.

Javalkar V, Cardenas R, Nanda A. Recovery of third nerve palsy following surgical clipping of posterior communicating artery aneurysms. *World Neurosurg.* 73:353-356.

Jongen JC, Franke CL, Ramos LM, et al. Direction of flow in posterior communicating artery on magnetic resonance angiography in patients with occipital lobe infarcts. *Stroke.* 2004;35:104-108.

Lehecka M, Dashti R, Romani R, et al. Microneurosurgical management of internal carotid artery bifurcation aneurysms. *Surg Neurol.* 2009;71:649-667.

Liu X, Rinkel GJ. Aneurysmal and clinical characteristics as risk factors for intracerebral haematoma from aneurysmal rupture. *J Neurol.* 2011;258(5):862-865.

Macdonald RL. *Vascular Neurosurgery.* New York: Thieme; 2009.

Muneda K, Yoshizu H, Terada H. [True posterior communicating artery aneurysm]. *No Shinkei Geka.* 2001;29:163-168.

Park SK, Shin YS, Lim YC, et al. Preoperative predictive value of the necessity for anterior clinoidectomy in posterior communicating artery aneurysm clipping. *Neurosurgery.* 2009;65:281-285:discussion 285-286.

Pyysalo LM, Keski-Nisula LH, Niskakangas TT, et al. Long-term follow-up study of endovascularly treated intracranial aneurysms. *Interv Neuroradiol.* 2010;16:231-239.

Qureshi AI, Mohammad Y, Yahia AM, et al. Ischemic events associated with unruptured intracranial aneurysms: multicenter clinical study and review of the literature. *Neurosurgery.* 2000;46:282-289:discussion 289-290.

Tobenas-Dujardin AC, Duparc F, Ali N, et al. Embryology of the internal carotid artery dural crossing: apropos of a continuous series of 48 specimens. *Surg Radiol Anat.* 2005;27:495-501.

Uz A, Erbil KM, Esmer AF. The origin and relations of the anterior choroidal artery: an anatomical study. *Folia Morphol (Warsz).* 2005;64:269-272.

Wen HT, Rhoton Jr AL, de Oliveira E, et al. Microsurgical anatomy of the temporal lobe: part 2—sylvian fissure region and its clinical application. *Neurosurgery.* 2009;65:1-35:discussion 36.

Yasargil MG. Carotid-posterior communicating aneurysms. In: *Microneurosurgery II: Clinical Considerations, Surgery of the Intracranial Aneurysms and Results.* New York: Thieme; 1994, pp. 71-73.

Numbered references appear on Expert Consult.

CHAPTER 74

Surgical Management of Anterior Communicating and Anterior Cerebral Artery Aneurysms

MICHAEL T. LAWTON • ZAMAN MIRZADEH

The anterior communicating artery (ACoA) aneurysm is the most common aneurysm encountered in neurosurgical practice, accounting for one quarter to one third of all microsurgically treated aneurysms in published experiences[1-3] and 21% of the senior author's experience with 2320 aneurysms. This aneurysm has a propensity to hemorrhage, often at or below size limits considered safe for conservative management and often in younger patients for whom microsurgical clipping might be favored over endovascular coiling.[2,4] Consequently, neurosurgeons must be prepared to deal with this lesion. This particular aneurysm, more than any other, has an unusually wide variety of complexity and technical difficulty that depends on variations in parent artery anatomy, aneurysm projection, and clinical presentation. In addition, the ACoA complex is adjacent to the hypothalamus, optic apparatus, and cognitive/emotional centers in the basal frontal lobes, while arteries emanating from the ACoA complex affect the basal ganglia, internal capsule, and motor/sensory cortex. Therefore, surgery for ACoA aneurysms is associated with elevated risks. This chapter discusses the factors and techniques that facilitate surgical management of ACoA aneurysms and help improve patient outcome.

Anatomy

NOMENCLATURE

The anterior cerebral artery (ACA) is divided into five segments (Fig. 74-1). The A1 segment, also known as the precommunicating or horizontal segment of the ACA, originates with the ACA at the internal carotid artery (ICA) bifurcation and extends to the junction with the ACoA. The A2 segment, also known as the postcommunicating segment, originates at the ACoA and extends to the genu of the corpus callosum, following the contour of the rostrum. The A3 segment curves around the genu and extends to the body of the corpus callosum, where it assumes a posterior course. The A4 and A5 segments continue over the body of the corpus callosum, the division between them being located at the plane of the coronal suture. Contrary to popular opinion, this nomenclature is not defined by the bifurcation into pericallosal and callosomarginal arteries. This bifurcation is usually located along the A3 segment (approximately 60%

of patients), but it can be more proximal on the A2 segment (10%), it can be more distal on the A4 segment (12%), or the pericallosal artery can be absent (18%).[5]

NORMAL ANATOMY

The A1 segment courses medially and anteriorly over the optic tract and chiasm to the ACoA complex. Numerous penetrating branches (average 8, range 2-15)[5] originate from this segment and course superiorly to supply the anterior perforated substance, subfrontal area, dorsal surface of the optic apparatus, hypothalamus, anterior commissure, septum pellucidum, and paraolfactory structures. Collectively, these perforators are also known as the medial lenticulostriate arteries, as opposed to the lateral lenticulostriate arteries that originate from the M1 segment of the middle cerebral artery (MCA). The most important of these perforators is the recurrent artery of Heubner, which originates from the proximal A2 segment on its lateral wall, just distal to the ACoA. This artery can arise from the distal A1 segment, just proximal to the ACoA, in 14% of patients or at the level of the ACoA in 8% of patients but is within 4 mm of the ACoA in 95% of patients.[5] The artery is almost always present (98%) and can be duplicated (2%).[5] The artery follows a course parallel to the A1 segment, either superior (60%) or anterior (40%) to it.[5] The recurrent artery is typically seen before the A1 segment when the frontal lobe is retracted, making it a useful landmark to identify the A1 segment and the ACoA. The recurrent artery of Heubner supplies the head of the caudate nucleus, putamen, outer segment of the globus pallidus, and anterior limb of the internal capsule. Therefore, arterial injury can produce weakness involving the contralateral face and arm and expressive aphasia in the dominant hemisphere.[6]

The ACoA joins the two ACAs as they arrive in the interhemispheric fissure, completing the anterior part of the circle of Willis. Normally, the ACoA diameter is about half that of the A1 segments, but there is a direct correlation between asymmetry in the A1 segments and ACoA diameter. In other words, the ACoA diameter increases as the caliber of a hypoplastic A1 segment decreases, thereby compensating for the asymmetry in the A1 inflow.[7] The ACoA can be duplicated in one third of patients, and triplicated in 10% of patients, but is always present.[5] An ACoA that is not visualized angiographically is usually explained by an absence of cross-filling rather than an absence of the ACoA itself, and

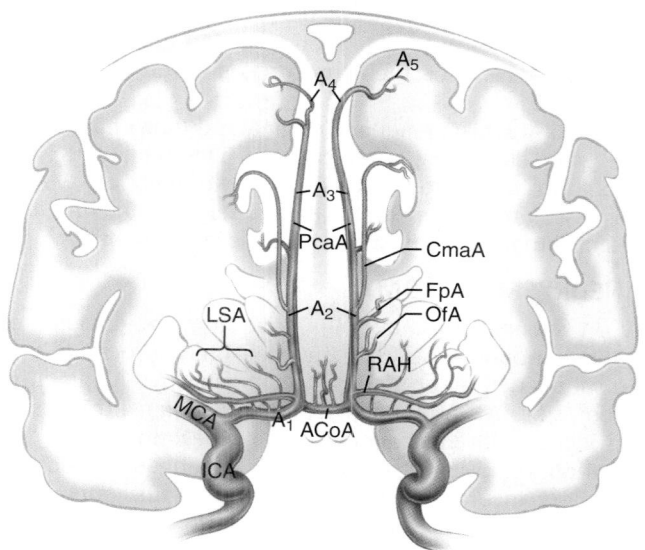

A Anterior cerebral arteries, anterior view

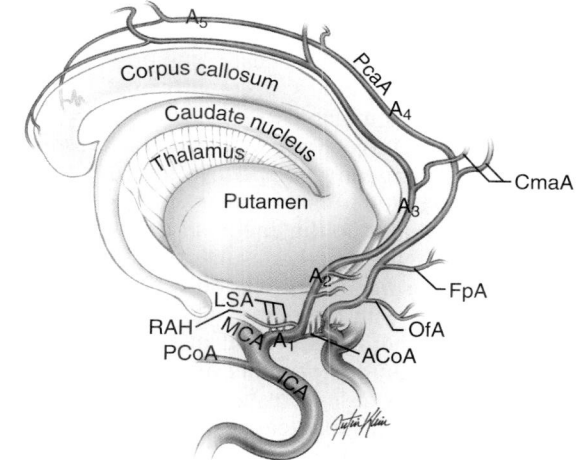

B Anterior cerebral arteries, lateral view

FIGURE 74-1 Microsurgical anatomy of the ACA. Anterior (A) and oblique (B) views, showing the five ACA segments and 12 arteries that can enter the surgical field around an ACoA aneurysm. The five ACA segments are: A1, precommunicating or horizontal segment; A2, postcommunicating or infracallosal segment; A3, precallosal segment; A4, supracallosal segment; and A5, postcallosal segment. CmaA, callosomarginal artery; FpA, frontopolar artery; LSA, lenticulostriate artery; OfA, orbitofrontal artery; PcaA, pericallosal artery; RAH, recurrent artery of Heubner. *(From Lawton, MT. Seven Aneurysms: Tenets and Techniques for Clipping. New York: Thieme, 2010.)*

fissure, coursing in front of the lamina terminalis and tracing the curvature of the genu. The branches arising from this segment are important more for correctly deciphering the anatomy of the ACoA complex than for their vascular supply. The orbitofrontal artery is the first cortical ACA branch, arising from the A2 segment approximately 5 mm distal to the ACoA from the anterolateral surface and coursing perpendicularly over the gyrus rectus and olfactory tract.[6] This artery supplies the gyrus rectus, orbital gyri (anterior, posterior, medial, and lateral), and olfactory bulb/tract. It is important to avoid mistaking the recurrent artery of Heubner for this orbitofrontal artery. Both can be seen on the medial aspect of the gyrus rectus, but their origins from the A2 segment are separated and their courses are different, with the recurrent artery of Heubner eventually rejoining the A1 segment, even if it meanders under the gyrus rectus along its more proximal course. Correctly identifying the recurrent artery is especially important when resecting gyrus rectus. The recurrent artery is also typically small in caliber, with a diameter of approximately 1 mm.[5] The orbitofrontal artery is often encountered draped over or adherent to the dome of a superiorly projecting aneurysm, which can tether the dome and make it more difficult to mobilize. The course of the orbitofrontal artery can also lead it across the neck of an ACoA aneurysm, requiring additional dissection before clipping.

The last relevant branch artery is the frontopolar artery, which originates from the A2 segment 14 mm, on average, from the ACoA near the genu.[5] This artery courses anteriorly in the interhemispheric fissure and supplies the ventromedial frontal lobes. Rarely, it can originate from a common trunk with the orbitofrontal artery. Like the orbitofrontal artery, the frontopolar artery can be draped over the dome of a superiorly projecting aneurysm and should not be misinterpreted.

The terminal branches of the ACA are the pericallosal and callosomarginal arteries, bifurcating at a variable point along the genu of the corpus callosum. The callosomarginal artery is usually the smaller of the two, and it runs across the cingulate gyrus to the cingulate sulcus, where it continues posteriorly. It gives rise to the anterior, middle, and posterior internal frontal arteries, which supply the medial frontal lobes back to the precentral gyrus. The pericallosal artery courses over the corpus callosum, giving rise to the paracentral, superior internal parietal (precuneal), and inferior internal parietal arteries. These cortical branches extend over the convexity to supply the superomedial surfaces of the hemisphere, anastomosing laterally with middle cerebral arteries and posteriorly with posterior cerebral arteries in these watershed areas.

VARIANT ANATOMY

Variations from the normal ACoA anatomy are common and probably contribute to the abnormal hemodynamic that forms aneurysms. While the effects of variant anatomy on aneurysm pathogenesis are poorly understood, the anatomy itself must be thoroughly understood by the neurosurgeon to correctly interpret the anatomy intraoperatively and safely clip an aneurysm. Variations can be categorized as involving the afferent arteries (A1 segments), efferent arteries (A2 segments), or the ACoA.

Asymmetry in the caliber of the A1 segments is seen in approximately 10% of patients, with a hypoplastic segment defined arbitrarily as having a diameter of 1.5 mm.[5] Smaller

it can be visualized by a carotid cross-compression maneuver during angiography. The ACoA gives rise to important perforating arteries, which originate from its superior (54%) and posterior (36%) surfaces.[5] These perforators course to the hypothalamus, median paraolfactory nuclei, genu, columns of the fornix, septum pellucidum, and anterior perforated substance. There can be perforators originating from the anterior and inferior aspects of the ACoA, supplying the dorsal optic chiasm, but these are few in number.

After making a right-angle turn from the horizontal A1 ACA, the A2 ACA runs superiorly in the interhemispheric diameters are observed less frequently, with approximately 2% of patients having an A1 segment diameter of 1 mm.[5] Aplastic A1 segments are rare, despite their suggestion on angiography with a contralateral A1 ACA that fills both distal ACAs. At surgery, a small A1 segment is typically found. The dominance of an A1 segment is relevant to aneurysm formation, projection of the dome, site of hematoma, and choice of side. Dominant A1 segments are frequently seen in association with ACoA aneurysms, which typically project in the direction of blood flow in that segment.[7] As discussed later, it is usually advantageous to surgically approach these aneurysms from the side of the dominant A1 ACA, both for easier proximal control of the aneurysm and for better clipping of the neck. One final variant, the duplicated A1 segment, is rare (2%) and almost always unilateral.[5]

Variations in ACoA anatomy include duplications, triplications, and fenestrations.[8,9] Accessory ACoAs are typically small and without significant perforators, making it important to recognize the primary ACoA and preserve both it and its perforators. Fenestrations can be the site of aneurysm formation and require special attention to differentiate the normal artery from the pathology. More important than these structural variations in the ACoA is its orientation. In only 18% of patients is the ACoA oriented in the transverse plane, as illustrated in anatomic textbooks.[5] Instead, the ACoA complex is usually rotated or tilted, causing the A2 ACAs to course obliquely to one another in the interhemispheric fissure. This variation in orientation can direct an A2 segment more posteriorly, making its visualization more difficult. Rotation of the ACoA can shift the location of perforators from posterior to lateral, again making visualization more difficult, particularly when the aneurysm lies between the neurosurgeon and the perforators. These subtle changes in angles can be misleading, particularly when visualization is compromised by factors such as a swollen brain, a large aneurysm, and thick hematoma.

Variant anatomy in the efferent arteries can be the most difficult to deal with and is best understood in terms of the classification by Baptista.[10] After analyzing 381 brain specimens, he defined three types of efferent artery anatomy. The type I anomaly, referred to as the azygos or "unpaired" ACA, is a single midline vessel arising from the confluence of the A1 segments (Fig. 74-2). Distally, the azygos ACA divides into pericallosal and callosomarginal arteries, with bifurcations, trifurcations, and quadrifurcations having been reported. This variant occurs in 0.3% to 2% of patients. The type II anomaly, referred to as the bihemispheric ACA, is an A2 ACA that transmits branches across the midline to supply both hemispheres, usually in the presence of a contralateral A2 segment that is hypoplastic or terminates early in its course toward the genu. This anomaly can be seen in as many as 12% of patients. The type III anomaly, referred to as an accessory ACA, is defined as a third artery originating from ACoA, in addition to the paired A2 segments and usually between them (Fig. 74-3). This accessory ACA variant is the most difficult one surgically because it results in some of the most unusual anatomic puzzles. If this variation is not appreciated, then a critical A2 ACA could be missed or, worse, sacrificed inadvertently during the aneurysm clipping (Fig. 74-4). The accessory ACA varies in caliber from a small remnant of the median artery of the corpus callosum (MACC) to a hyperplastic ACA that can resemble an azygos

ACA when the two A2 segments are small in caliber and terminate early. A careful analysis of the angiogram preoperatively can alert the neurosurgeon to this challenging variant.

The MACC just mentioned originates during embryogenesis when elongating ACAs coalesce in the midline to form plexiform anastomoses at 44 days.[11] Normally, the MACC regresses and disappears as the A2 segments mature, but vestigial remnants can account for the accessory ACA.

ANEURYSM ANATOMY

ACoA aneurysms, as a group, arise from the complex of arteries around the ACoA, but their precise location can be subdivided into true ACoA aneurysms, A1–A2 junction aneurysms, A1 ACA aneurysms, and variant aneurysms associated with the anatomic variants described earlier. In addition, the distal ACA aneurysms, notably the pericallosal artery aneurysms, are often included in this group.

The true ACoA aneurysm arises from ACoA and is defined further by the projection of its dome in an anterior, superior, posterior, or inferior direction. In Yasargil's experience with ACoA aneurysms, the superiorly and anteriorly projecting aneurysms were the most common (34% and 23%, respectively), while posteriorly and inferiorly projecting aneurysms were the least common (14% and 13%, respectively).[12] Some aneurysms (approximately 16%) have mixed projection or multiple lobes.

The anteriorly projecting aneurysm is a favorable one from the neurosurgeon's perspective because the parent arteries are separated from the aneurysm. The two A2 ACAs course at right angles to the aneurysm's axis, making their identification in the interhemispheric fissure straightforward. The neurosurgeon has a good view across the neck of the aneurysm, with the dome and its likely rupture site removed from where this critical dissection takes place. Posteriorly projecting perforators are well away from the aneurysm and are easily preserved. The anterior projection of the dome typically leaves room under the neck to view across to the contralateral A1 segment to complete the exposure for proximal control of the aneurysm. This orientation often adheres the dome to the frontal lobes, which can limit the mobility of the aneurysm, but the dome can be freed as a final step in the dissection if greater mobility is needed to see contralateral anatomy or to increase the aneurysm's maneuverability for clip application. In addition to their anterior projection, these aneurysms typically tilt to one side, most commonly away from the dominant A1 segment.

The superiorly projecting aneurysm is less favorable than the anterior projecting aneurysm, mainly because of the contralateral A2 ACA and the perforators (Fig. 74-5). Proximal control is straightforward, as the aneurysm is away from the A1 segments and the view to the contralateral side is unobstructed. However, the aneurysm is interposed between the neurosurgeon and the contralateral A2 ACA, requiring some manipulation of the aneurysm to locate this artery. Furthermore, larger aneurysms can displace perforators laterally or posteriorly, and their adherence to the aneurysm necessitates some delicate dissection. In addition, the A2 segments can be adherent, requiring aggressive dissection along the plane between this efferent artery and the fundus to fully expose the neck. Unlike the anteriorly

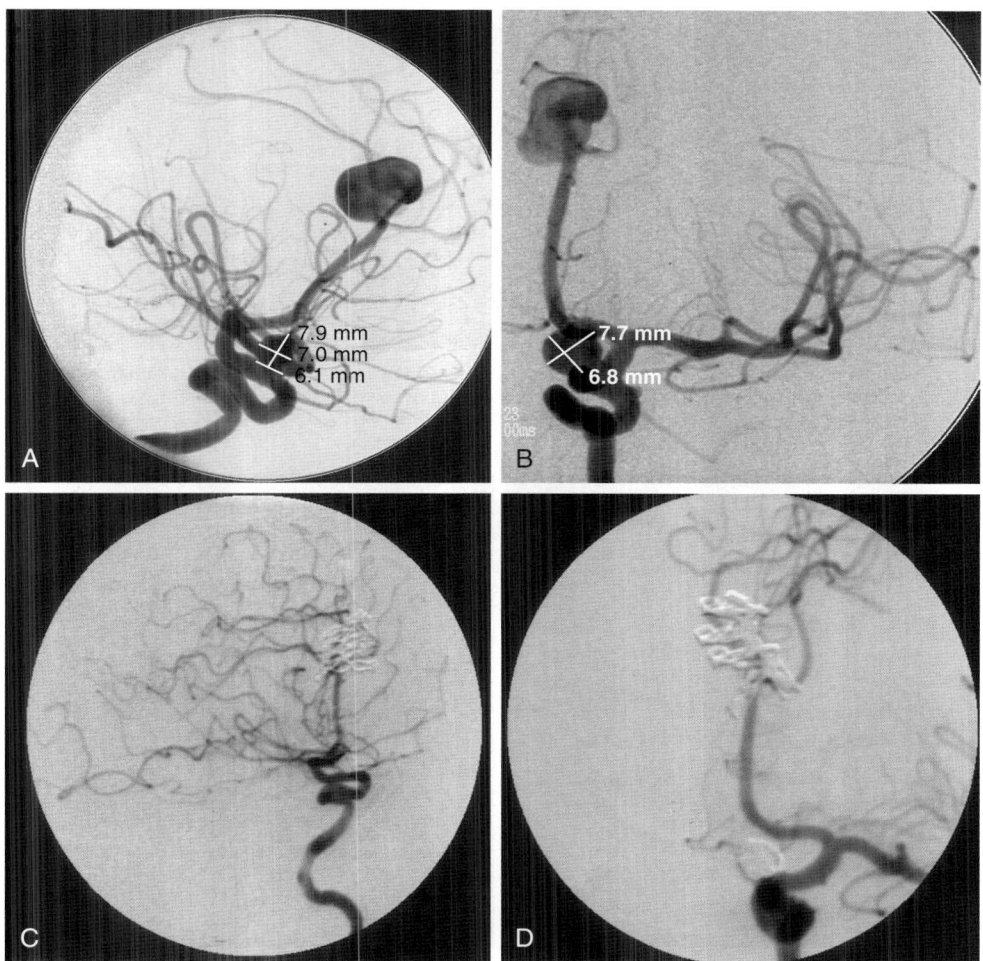

FIGURE 74-2 A 67-year-old woman, with chronic headaches, underwent left carotid artery angiography that demonstrated a 1.5-cm-diameter azygos ACA aneurysm and a 7-mm ophthalmic artery aneurysm in oblique (A) and anterior–posterior (AP) (B) views. The ophthalmic artery aneurysm was coiled, and the azygos ACA aneurysm was clipped through a bifrontal craniotomy and anterior interhemispheric approach. No residual aneurysms were seen on postoperative lateral (C) and AP (D) projection angiograms.

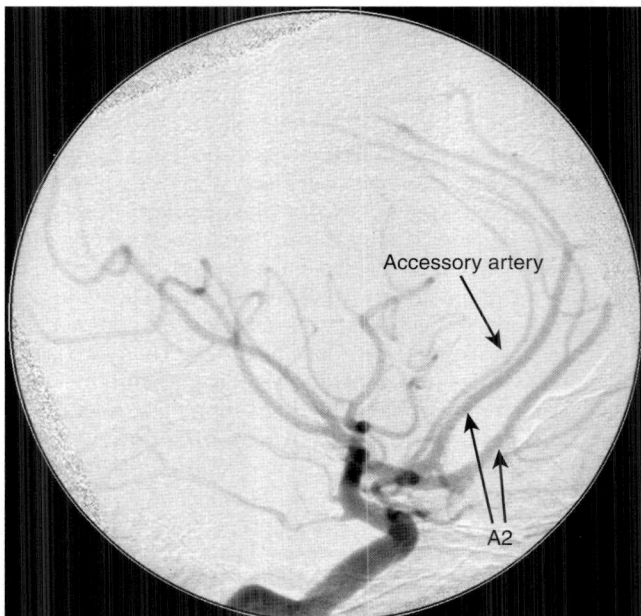

FIGURE 74-3 A 65-year-old male presented with severe headache and diffuse SAH. Two cerebral angiograms failed to reveal any aneurysms. His angiogram demonstrates a small accessory A2 ACA.

projecting aneurysms, where the view behind the aneurysm is panoramic, the view behind a superiorly projecting aneurysm requires more extensive dissection. The ipsilateral A2 ACA must be mobilized anteriorly and can require dissection of its branches (i.e., the orbitofrontal and frontopolar arteries). The clip application is often more complex with these aneurysms, sometimes requiring fenestrated clips that encircle the ipsilateral A2 ACA.

Posteriorly projecting ACoA aneurysms are arguably the most challenging to clip. With these lesions, the A1 and A2 segments can be identified readily, but the perforators are markedly more difficult to visualize and preserve. They are often displaced laterally, where they become obstacles to the clip blades during clip application, and/or they are displaced posteriorly, where they can easily elude detection. In addition, the parent arteries of the ACoA complex are interposed between the surgeon and the aneurysm neck, making it more difficult to dissect and apply the clips to the neck. Fortunately, these aneurysms are uncommon.[12]

The inferiorly projecting aneurysm is another favorable aneurysm, with the one caveat: its dome often adheres to the optic apparatus, making it susceptible to avulsion and rupture early in the dissection with frontal lobe retraction. From that standpoint, it can be treacherous, because at

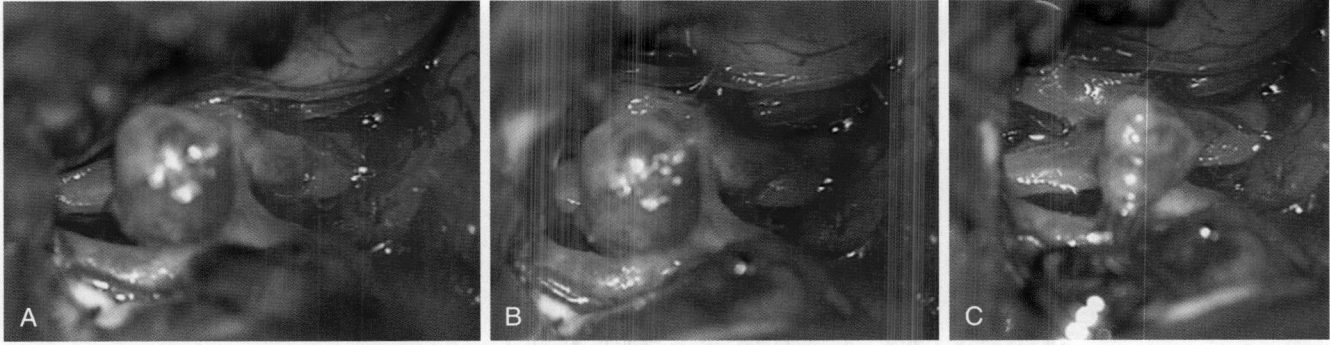

FIGURE 74-4 A, This small, ruptured anteriorly projecting ACoA aneurysm appeared to have classic anatomy at first glance. B, Additional dissection revealed an accessory A2 ACA. C, The neck was clipped with one straight clip that preserved flow through all three efferent A2 ACAs. *(From Lawton, MT. Seven Aneurysms: Tenets and Techniques for Clipping. New York: Thieme, 2010.)*

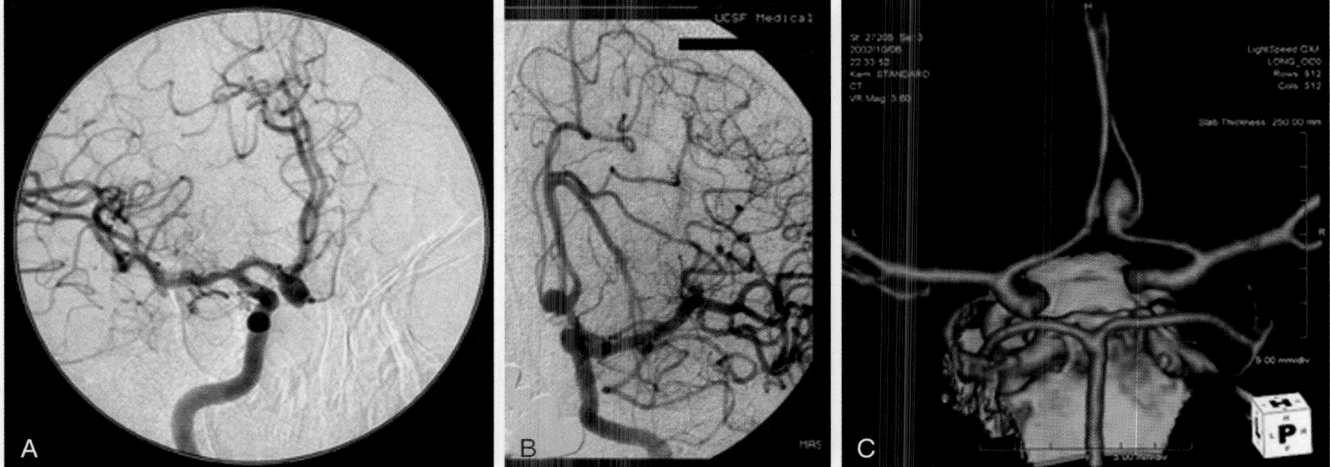

FIGURE 74-5 Cerebral angiograms demonstrate the different projections of ACoA aneurysms: inferiorly (A) and anteriorly (B) projecting aneurysms. C, A CTA demonstrates a superiorly projecting right A1–A2 junction aneurysm at the ACoA complex.

that point in the dissection, proximal control is inadequate and the aneurysm anatomy has not been analyzed or even exposed. However, care in retracting the frontal lobe can avert this complication, and the advantages of an inferior projection make it a relatively straightforward aneurysm. Like the anteriorly projecting aneurysm, the ipsilateral A1 and bilateral A2 segments are easily visualized. The contralateral A1 segment can be obscured, which could compromise proximal control of the aneurysm, but the other critical anatomy is accessible. Perforators are rarely a problem, and the necks of these aneurysms are easily closed. These aneurysms can be adherent to the optic nerves and/or chiasm, and often it is preferable to leave the dome undissected or amputate it after clipping the neck, rather than manipulating the optic nerves with unnecessary dissection.

A1–A2 junction aneurysms arise at the bifurcation of the A1 segment into the ACoA and A2 ACA, with a distinctly separate ACoA. These aneurysms have the same variability in their projection (anterior, superior, posterior, and inferior) but also tend to have a lateral projection leftward or rightward. This lateral deviation can result in rupture into frontal lobe parenchyma opposite from the dominant A1 ACA. The perforators tend to be more manageable with these aneurysms than with the ACoA aneurysms.

A1 segment aneurysms are uncommon and tend to be located more proximally toward the carotid bifurcation than the ACoA complex. They are associated with the perforators from this segment, or with curves and bends in the artery as it courses to the ACoA complex.

Variant aneurysms include aneurysms that arise from a fenestration, duplicated or accessory ACoA, accessory A2 ACA, or azygos ACA. Accessory anatomy can pose additional risks, because it can mislead the surgeon and result in inadvertent arterial occlusions if not carefully protected. For example, the neurosurgeon might erroneously clip an important accessory A2 segment if an ipsilateral and contralateral A2 segment have already been identified. Therefore, thorough preoperative review of the anatomy and intraoperative dissection is critical before the final clipping is performed. Infundibuli arising from the ACoA have been observed, particularly with other vascular lesions such as arteriovenous malformations. These infundibuli, like those at the posterior communicating artery and elsewhere, can appear on angiography like aneurysms but transmit normal arteries and must be preserved. Dissection along the course of these arteries distinguishes them from aneurysms. ACoA aneurysms can be giant, atherosclerotic, calcified, or thrombotic. Aneurysms at this location can also be nonsaccular and due to other causes, including infection, trauma, and dissection.

Clinical Presentation

Aneurysm rupture is the most common presentation of patients with ACoA aneurysms, with the classic headache characterized by its sudden onset and severity.[1] Patients can present in much worse neurologic condition, with obtundation or coma depending on the extent of hemorrhage and presence or absence of hydrocephalus. ACoA aneurysms are notoriously small, often rupturing at sizes smaller than those that would be considered a threshold for treatment. Therefore, advance symptoms are uncommon. When large or giant, ACoA aneurysms can produce symptoms from mass effect on the optic apparatus (visual field deficits), hypothalamus (endocrine dysfunction), hydrocephalus (obstruction of the foramen of Monro), or frontal lobes (cognitive dysfunction, memory impairment, and seizure).[13,14]

Diagnostic Imaging

The diagnosis of subarachnoid hemorrhage (SAH) requires the confirmation of blood in the subarachnoid space, which can be accomplished best with a computed tomography (CT) scan. Blood is easily seen on a noncontrast CT scan, with a sensitivity of greater than 95%.[15] CT can also pinpoint an aneurysm location based on SAH distribution, in addition to revealing the presence of intraparenchymal or intraventricular blood. Subarachnoid blood from a ruptured ACoA aneurysm tends to localize in the interhemispheric fissure.[16] The direction of aneurysm projection influences this pattern of blood distribution, with superior and posterior projecting aneurysms filling the interhemispheric fissure and anterior and inferior projecting aneurysms bleeding more diffusely. While interhemispheric SAH is the most common finding with ruptured ACoA aneurysms, intracerebral hemorrhage can be observed in the gyrus rectus with laterally projecting aneurysms and intraventricular hemorrhage can be observed with aneurysms that rupture through the lamina terminalis. Pericallosal artery aneurysms tend to have blood more distally located, such as over the genu or body of the corpus callosum. CT scanning is quick and definitive, can diagnose associated conditions such as hydrocephalus, and with an additional bolus of intravenous contrast, can generate a CT angiogram (Fig. 74-5C).

Ultimately, the diagnosis of an aneurysm depends on its identification with catheter angiography. A complete angiogram includes injections of all four major intracranial arteries (both ICAs and both vertebral arteries), filmed in two orthogonal views (anteroposterior and lateral). Additional views of the aneurysm (oblique, Townes, and Schuller views) are often needed to fully visualize its anatomy. Digital subtraction angiograms provide detailed information about the aneurysm location, anatomy, hemodynamics, other aneurysms, and collateral circulation. With ACoA aneurysms, balanced flow in symmetrical A1 segments may prevent opacification of the aneurysm, and cross-compression angiograms may be needed to visualize these aneurysms. Angiographic images show the internal anatomy of an aneurysm, which may be much smaller than the external diameter of the aneurysm seen on axial imaging studies if it is filled with thrombus or coil material or thickened with calcium or atherosclerotic changes.

While catheter angiography remains the gold standard for the diagnosis of aneurysms, it has disadvantages: it is invasive, time consuming, costly, and associated with some risk of dissection, embolization, and groin hematoma. Angiograms generated with CT or magnetic resonance data (computed tomography angiography, or CTA, and magnetic resonance angiography, respectively) are superb and, with computerized, three-dimensional reconstruction, can generate images with startlingly high resolution that are adequate for preoperative and intraoperative planning.[17,18] CTA in particular is noninvasive, easy to obtain, and fast, offering an alternative to catheter angiography in unstable patients with ruptured aneurysms that need to get to the operating room emergently.

Lumbar puncture is the only laboratory study that needs to be considered in the evaluation of an aneurysm patient and is used only when the patient's history is strongly suggestive of SAH but the CT scan is normal.[19] There are two explanations for this inconsistency. The first explanation is a sentinel hemorrhage has leaked so little blood that it is not radiographically apparent, in which case cerebrospinal fluid (CSF) may be blood tinged and will not clear in successive tubes. The second explanation is a delayed CT scan was performed days after the SAH. A delay in seeking medical attention or in ordering the CT scan allows subarachnoid blood to disperse, making it difficult to detect on the imaging study. CSF is thus xanthochromic. CSF from a lumbar puncture that is positive for new or old blood indicates further evaluation with an angiogram.

ACoA aneurysms have a rate of false-negative angiography that is higher than that observed with other aneurysms.[16,20] Patients with a characteristic aneurysmal SAH on CT scan and a negative angiogram should undergo repeat angiography within 1 week with careful attention focused on the ACoA region. This region is notorious for hiding small aneurysms that might elude detection due to intraluminal thrombus in the aneurysm, extraluminal thrombus compressing the aneurysm, or vasospasm in the afferent arteries.

Preoperative Management

After a ruptured aneurysm is diagnosed, the aneurysm is secured as quickly as possible, typically within 48 to 72 hours of the hemorrhage. In the meantime, efforts are made to stabilize the patient and minimize the risk of rerupture. There is a 4% risk of rehemorrhage in the first 24 hours after hemorrhage, with an associated mortality rate of 27% to 43%.[1] Most important is blood pressure control. Rebleeding is caused by absolute elevations and rapid variations in blood pressure. Blood pressure should be carefully monitored with invasive arterial lines in an intensive care unit (ICU) setting where intravenous agents or drips can be administered to keep the systolic blood pressure under 140 mm Hg. Hydrocephalus is present in approximately one fourth of SAH patients[21] and resolves with the insertion of a ventriculostomy. External ventricular drainage can improve the clinical status of patients dramatically and is recommended in all obtunded or comatose patients. In addition, ventriculostomy allows intracranial pressure (ICP) to be transduced and can guide preoperative management of increased pressures. In patients with a poor Hunt-Hess grade, intubation and mechanical ventilation are usually needed to protect the airway and sometimes to hyperventilate the patient for ICP management. Other comfort measures such as bed rest, sedation, and analgesics help minimize agitation that might precipitate rerupture. Seizures can precipitate rerupture, and anticonvulsants are given in the immediate post-SAH period when there is intraparenchymal hematoma.

Microsurgical Management

The successful treatment of an ACoA aneurysm depends on three critical elements: (1) adequate exposure of the aneurysm and its associated anatomy, (2) proper clipping technique, and (3) employing alternative techniques for complex aneurysms that are not amenable to conventional clipping.

EXPOSURE

The first decision in the surgical plan for an ACoA aneurysm is the choice of approach. For most aneurysms, a standard pterional craniotomy is sufficient. The alternative approach is the orbitozygomatic approach, which increases the exposure for large, giant, or complex ACoA aneurysms. The orbitozygomatic approach is, in essence, an application of skull base surgery principles, removing the orbital rim, roof, and inferior frontal skull to maximize the operating space under the brain and minimize retraction. The difference in exposure between the standard pterional and the orbitozygomatic approaches is well documented in cadaveric and clinical studies,[22,23] but the decision to remove the orbitozygomatic unit should be made judiciously. In the senior author's experience with 485 ACoA aneurysms, the orbitozygomatic approach was used in just 16% of patients. As with most maneuvers to expose ACoA aneurysms, the orbitozygomatic approach should be used only when necessary, since additional surgery adds to the patient's cumulative risk and impact from surgery.

The second decision in the surgical plan is the side of the craniotomy. In general, ACoA aneurysms are approached from the side of the dominant A1 segment, because this gives the neurosurgeon the best proximal control, avoids the dome of the aneurysm, and presents a more favorable vantage point for dissecting the aneurysm and applying the clips. When the A1 segments are symmetrical, the aneurysm is approached from the side of the nondominant hemisphere. With as many as 85% of ACoA aneurysms having asymmetrical or dominant A1 segments, this approach to choosing the craniotomy side results in a significant number of left-sided craniotomies. In the senior author's ACoA experience, exactly half of the craniotomies were left sided. While there is some theoretical concern about operating on the dominant hemisphere, in our experience there has been no observable difference in neurologic or cognitive outcomes based solely on the side of the craniotomy. Therefore, the real anatomic advantages of a craniotomy ipsilateral to the dominant A1 segment outweigh the theoretical disadvantages of a craniotomy on the patient's dominant hemisphere. In cases where there is intraparenchymal hematoma in the frontal lobe contralateral to the dominant A1 segment, there may be some inclination to approach the aneurysm from the side of the hematoma. However, in our experience, the hematoma connects to the aneurysm dome and can be easily evacuated from the contralateral side. In cases where there are multiple aneurysms, the choice of side may be influenced by the side of these other aneurysms to maximize the number of aneurysms that can be treated with a single craniotomy.

The technique of the pterional approach is well described and thus is not discussed in detail here, except for the critical aspects. The patient is positioned in the supine position and secured to the table with bolsters to enable extreme table tilting. The head is positioned in the Mayfield headrest with the midline rotated 30 degrees away from the operative side and the head extended to allow gravity to retract the frontal lobes. In this position, the malar eminence becomes the highest point in the surgical field. The skin incision extends from the zygomatic arch to the hair line in the midline, coursing in a semicircular arc. The CT scan and angiogram are reviewed preoperatively to determine the likelihood of encountering the frontal sinuses at the anterior–inferior edge of the craniotomy. In patients with large sinuses, the pericranium is harvested as a separate layer after just the scalp is reflected forward, because it is easiest at this point in the procedure to prepare a large and competent graft to cover the sinus during the closure. When the pericranium is dissected down from an elevated scalp flap at the end of the procedure, it is often more difficult to handle, smaller, and susceptible to perforations. The temporalis muscle is mobilized anteriorly after fashioning a cuff along the temporal line that is used to reattach the muscle during the closure. Fishhooks under tension retract and flatten this muscle to keep it from obscuring the operative field.

The pterional craniotomy is cut from a single bur hole in the temporal bone superior to the zygomatic arch. Extensive drilling of the greater and lesser wings of the sphenoid bone is essential to maximize the exposure. The inner table of the inferior frontal bone is drilled until flush with the anterior cranial fossa floor, and the ridges of the orbital roof are flattened. The temporal bone is drilled until flush with the middle fossa floor, and the anterior temporal bone is drilled until the exposure is contiguous with the lateral orbital wall. All intervening pterional bone is drilled away until the superior orbital fissure is identified and opened. Drilling is continued down the medial sphenoidal ridge to the base of the anterior clinoid process, which can leave a prominence in the surgical corridor if it is not flattened. Bleeding from the base of the anterior clinoid process can well up and run into the surgical field during microdissection, making absolute hemostasis mandatory. The dura is opened in a semicircular flap based on this hinge point at the anterior clinoid process. When reflected and tacked with suture, this dura flap should form a flat surface and afford an unobstructed view to the carotid cistern.

The orbitozygomatic approach differs only in the dissection of the temporalis muscle and in the osteotomies of the orbit and zygoma.[24] We prefer the subfascial dissection to expose the zygoma and lateral orbit, but an interfascial dissection can also be used.[25] The osteotomies are performed after the craniotomy, yielding a separate bone flap and orbitozygomatic unit that reassemble with excellent cosmetics postoperatively. The plates that replace the orbitozygomatic unit are applied and screw holes are predrilled before the unit is detached to ensure proper realignment. In addition, we prefer a reciprocating saw over a high-speed drill to make the osteotomies, and we prefer stepped cuts rather than linear cuts because they interlock the orbitozygomatic unit to the skull, enhancing the reconstruction.

A critical decision in the microdissection is whether to dissect the sylvian fissure. There is no need to expose the MCA or its branches, but the sylvian dissection separates the frontal and temporal lobes to open the corridor to the ACoA complex. The important maneuver is the gentle elevation of the frontal lobe to expose the recurrent artery of Heubner and the A1 ACA, and without splitting the sylvian fissure, the temporal lobe often is pulled into that corridor. Therefore, some degree of sylvian fissure dissection is required, sometimes just the proximal portion extending several centimeters from the carotid cistern but other times a full fissure split down to the limen insula. In older patients, this extensive dissection can be straightforward, but in younger patients with edematous brains after SAH, this dissection can be difficult. The neurosurgeon must weigh the facility of opening the fissure with its necessity in determining the extent of dissection.

With the proximal sylvian fissure dissected and the carotid bifurcation exposed, a retractor can be placed with its tip on the posterior portion of the medial orbital gyrus. This retractor gently elevates the frontal lobe and exposes the A1 segment. A site should be prepared along this segment early on to place a temporary clip for proximal control. The A1 segment can then be followed to the ACoA complex. The recurrent artery of Heubner can also be used as a guide to the ACoA complex and is often seen before the A1 ACA. The exposure of an ACoA aneurysm requires progressively shifting the frontal retraction forward, from the posterior medial orbital gyrus to the gyrus rectus. In anticipation of greater retraction and to optimize brain relaxation, the lamina terminalis is opened early in the dissection to release CSF. The arachnoid around the optic nerves is incised, extending the dissection into the chiasmatic cistern and across the chiasm to the contralateral optic nerve. The lamina terminalis is then identified posterior to the chiasm and beneath the ipsilateral A1 ACA and ACoA. Inferiorly projecting aneurysms and some anteriorly projecting aneurysms may impede access to the lamina terminalis, in which case this maneuver is best deferred until after the aneurysm is clipped.

The frontal retractor can then be advanced forward on the medial orbital gyrus, with the tip just lateral to the olfactory tract. The recurrent artery of Heubner is dissected away from the frontal lobe so that it lies with the A1 ACA. It is important to identify and mobilize this delicate artery to avoid inadvertent occlusion by the retractor blade or inadvertent injury with gyrus rectus resection. When the retractor is lateral to the olfactory tract, the gyrus rectus overlies the ACoA complex and the neurosurgeon can evaluate whether it should be resected or whether the interhemispheric fissure can be opened to elevate the gyrus rectus. Patients with unruptured aneurysms or atrophy often have interhemispheric fissures that can be opened widely to expose the ACoA complex without gyrus rectus resection. In others, gyrus rectus resection is the simplest, safest maneuver to expose the ipsilateral A2 ACA and proximal neck of the aneurysm.

The pia over the gyrus rectus is coagulated and incised, and brain is removed until the pia on the medial frontal lobe is reached. The orbitofrontal artery often courses across the gyrus rectus and should be avoided. When sufficient gyrus rectus has been removed, the retractor can be advanced again, with the tip of the blade within the resection cavity. The tip of the retractor should lie over the shoulder of the recurrent artery, as it originates from the ipsilateral A2 ACA, to protect this artery. The medial arachnoid is then incised to enter the interhemispheric fissure where the A2 ACA and its distal branches can be visualized.

CLIPPING

Successful clipping depends on thorough dissection and interpretation of the anatomy, which can be challenging at the ACoA complex (Fig. 74-6). In all, 11 arteries need to be identified: bilateral A1 ACAs, bilateral A2 ACAs, bilateral recurrent arteries of Heubner, ACoA, bilateral orbitofrontal arteries, and bilateral frontopolar arteries. The last two arteries are often outside the surgical field and are relevant only in rare cases where they course inferiorly into the surgical field. The first two arteries are the most important, because they provide the proximal control. Identification of the contralateral A1 ACA requires dissection across the region of the aneurysm, so its projection must be appreciated and the dissection should steer clear of the dome. Gyrus rectus resection or interhemispheric fissure dissection identifies the ipsilateral A2 ACA. The contralateral A2 ACA is the most difficult of the arteries to identify because it is the deepest artery in the surgical field and its visualization is usually

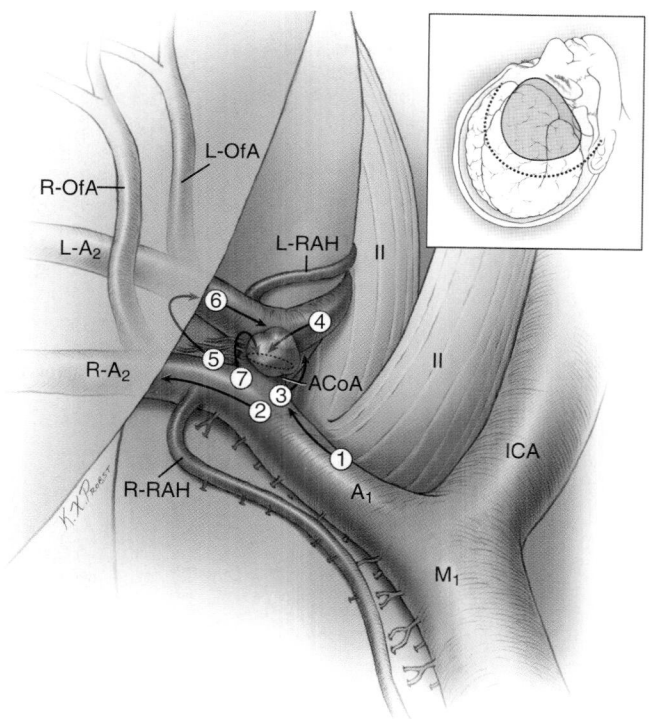

FIGURE 74-6 ACoA aneurysm dissection steps: (1) following the A1 segment and recurrent artery of Heubner, (2) identifying the A2 segment, (3) crossing the midline via the ACoA, (4) controlling the contralateral A1 segment, (5) entering the distal interhemispheric fissure, (6) tracing the contralateral A2 segment proximally, and (7) separating the perforators from the aneurysm neck. *(From Lawton, MT. Seven Aneurysms: Tenets and Techniques for Clipping. New York: Thieme, 2010.)*

obscured to some degree by the aneurysm. Therefore, the contralateral A2 ACA is typically the last of the five major arteries (two A1 ACAs, two A2 ACAs, and ACoA) to be found, often requiring some manipulation of the aneurysm. Alternatively, it can sometimes be seen in the interhemispheric fissure distal to the aneurysm and traced back to the ACoA complex. The orbitofrontal arteries are identified at their origin just distal to the recurrent artery and often course over the aneurysm or region of the dissection. Anatomic variations at the ACoA complex may add to or subtract from the 11 arteries.

After visualizing the parent arteries, attention is directed to the aneurysm neck and perforator dissection. ACoA aneurysms are notoriously adherent to surrounding structures. Aneurysms projecting superiorly typically adhere to the A2 ACAs, while those projecting inferiorly adhere to the optic apparatus. Posteriorly projecting aneurysms typically adhere to perforators, while anteriorly projecting aneurysms adhere to the frontal lobes. Therefore, the final steps in the dissection are often completed with the aneurysm softened with temporary clips on the A1 segments, mobilizing it from its surrounding adhesions and preparing it for clip application. For this, cerebroprotection with barbiturates is used, in conjunction with neurophysiologic monitoring.[26] Electroencephalography and somatosensory evoked potentials are monitored during administration of barbiturates, with the anesthetic dose titrated to achieve electroencephalogram burst suppression. Mild hypothermia is also used routinely for cerebroprotection. Temporary clips can then be applied, with neurophysiologic monitoring indicating the patient's tolerance to parent artery occlusion during the dissection. If changes in neurophysiologic monitoring are observed, temporary clips can be removed to reperfuse the ischemic territory, or the blood pressure can be elevated with vasopressor agents. Typically, only a few minutes are needed to complete the dissection and apply the clips. Minimizing temporary clip times requires maximizing the dissection that can be done beforehand, preselecting permanent clips, and having an experienced scrub nurse. Surgeon speed is of utmost importance during temporary clipping to reduce risk of ischemic injury. Temporary clipping relaxes the aneurysm to give the neurosurgeon the opportunity to perform the final, risky maneuvers, whether mobilizing the aneurysm to identify the remaining anatomy, clearing the perforators from the path of the clip blades, and/or establishing the cleavage planes between branch arteries and the aneurysm neck.

Permanent clipping depends on the aneurysm projection, size, and anatomy of the A1–A2 junction (Fig. 74-7). Aneurysms that project anteriorly and inferiorly can usually be clipped with a straight clip, since the aneurysm and the afferent/efferent arteries are on opposite sides of the ACoA. With these aneurysms, the viewing angle is along the length of the neck, parallel to the ACoA, with good visualization of

FIGURE 74-7 Clipping techniques for ACoA aneurysms projecting inferiorly (simple clipping, straight clip) (A), anteriorly (simple clipping, straight clip) (B), superiorly (tandem clipping) (C), and posteriorly (simple clipping, angled fenestrated clip) (D). *(From Lawton, MT. Seven Aneurysms: Tenets and Techniques for Clipping. New York: Thieme, 2010.)*

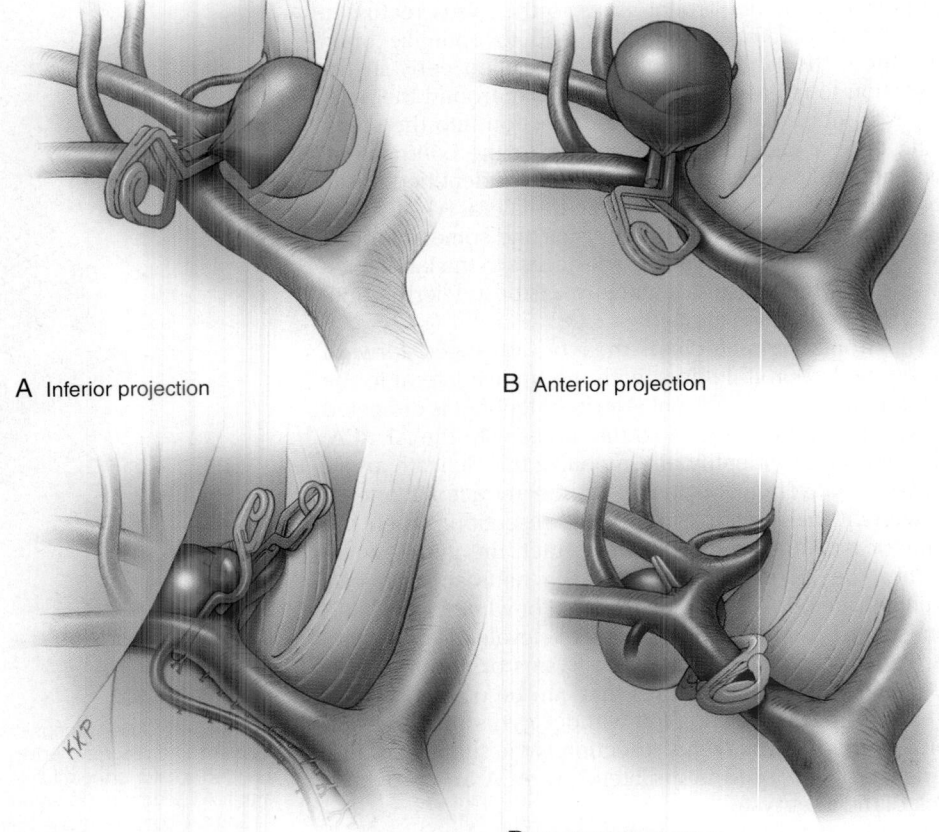

A Inferior projection

B Anterior projection

C Superior projection

D Posterior projection

posterior perforators and parent arteries. Aneurysms that project superiorly can be difficult because of the intimate relationship between the neck and the A2 segments. A clip that parallels the ACoA must be positioned so that its tips do not compromise the contralateral A2 ACA, with the tips either stopping just short of this segment or passing anterior or posterior to it. On the ipsilateral side, a fenestrated clip is often needed to close the proximal neck without compromising the ipsilateral A2 ACA. These requirements demand precise clip application, but fortunately the perforators are not as difficult to dissect as with posteriorly projecting aneurysms. Alternatively, a more posteriorly directed clip can sometimes be applied perpendicular to the ACoA. This clip application can produce a dog-ear remnant below the clip, which might require additional clips below the original one. Aneurysms that project posteriorly can be difficult because not only are the A2 segments intimately associated with the neck on its anterior aspect but so are the perforators on its posterior aspect. These aneurysms often require fenestrated clips such as the superiorly projecting aneurysms, because the clip blades pass through or around the ACA vessels. Most importantly, the back blade must course safely through a complex array of treacherous perforators.

The large and giant ACoA aneurysms have challenges associated with their size, as they do at other locations. Wide necks, fusiform morphology, or an atherosclerotic artery contribute to the complexity for endovascular and microsurgical treatment. These aneurysms often necessitate closure with multiple clips. Single straight clips on these aneurysms tend to fail, because tissue in the proximal blades prevents the distal tip from closing. Fenestrated clips address this problem, with the fenestration encircling only the proximal neck of the aneurysm rather than an A2 segment. Then, a second clip can close the proximal neck encircled by the first clip, thereby completing the repair and contouring the reconstruction. Some of the most challenging aneurysms are those with A2 ACAs originating from the base of the aneurysm (Fig. 74-8), with acute angles between the A1 and the A2 segments or, even worse, with A2 segments that leave the aneurysm parallel to the A1 segments. Clip reconstruction for this unusual anatomy is associated with a significant risk of efferent artery compromise and often requires intraoperative angiography.

Once the aneurysm is clipped, it is critical to carefully inspect the anatomy to be certain the aneurysm no longer fills, there is no neck remnant, and the parent arteries are patent. Gross inspection and palpation of the dome with a Rhoton No. 6 instrument can often indicate whether an aneurysm still fills, with persistent pulsations observed in those that are incompletely occluded. Incompletely occluded aneurysms typically have some neck remaining distal to the tips that may not have been appreciated during clip application, or the neck may have elongated as the blades closed. This situation requires advancement of the clip across this remnant. If the clips are across the neck completely but the aneurysm still fills, it may require an additional stacked clip to reinforce the closure. When the aneurysm appears completely closed, it is punctured and deflated to be sure. At this point, the dome can be transected or aggressively mobilized to visualize anatomy that might have been poorly appreciated prior to clipping. Sometimes additional dissection after

an aneurysm is clipped can confirm the interpretation of anatomy or proper clip application or can reveal technical errors. Therefore, it is critical to dissect beyond the point of aneurysm clipping. The neck beneath the clips along the ACoA is inspected next to ensure that no dog-ear remnants remain. These remnants are easily closed with additional microclips. Lastly, the 11 parent arteries are inspected for patency, often with a micro-Doppler probe and/or intraoperative angiography.

ALTERNATIVE TECHNIQUES

The ACoA complex is home to complex aneurysms that cannot be treated with conventional clipping, including giant aneurysms, thrombotic aneurysms, calcified/atherosclerotic aneurysms, fusiform aneurysms, and mycotic/infectious aneurysms. For these aneurysms, other techniques may be needed.

Giant aneurysms require techniques not unlike the ones already discussed. The additional room provided by the orbitozygomatic approach makes it routine for these aneurysms.[22] Temporary clipping is particularly valuable, because a giant aneurysm that no longer has antegrade filling is deflated and mobile, thereby opening the surgical field and facilitating the dissection and clipping.

With thrombotic aneurysms, the aneurysm does not respond to temporary clipping because thrombus transforms the aneurysm into a solid mass. Therefore, thrombectomy is needed to convert this mass into a deformable sac (Fig. 74-9). After trapping the aneurysm with temporary clips on both A1 and both A2 ACAs, it is entered by incising the wall. With some giant thrombotic aneurysms, complete control is not possible at the outset because the bulk of the aneurysm prevents visualization of contralateral anatomy. In these cases, bleeding can be controlled from inside the aneurysm with a Cottonoid over the orifice of the artery until the involved artery is isolated and temporarily clipped. A Cavitron ultrasonic surgical aspirator (CUSA) is typically used to break up thrombus and clean out the aneurysm lumen, with attention focused at the neck where the clip needs to be placed. Transecting the aneurysm can expedite thrombectomy by freeing the essential tissue needed to reconstruct a neck, rather than gutting the entire lumen and mobilizing the sac. This transaction maneuver can be important, because it minimizes ischemia time and risk of neurologic complication.

Previously coiled aneurysms that have residual filling or that recur are often managed like thrombotic aneurysms (Fig. 74-10). They too behave like a solid mass, and their intraluminal content is largely thrombus. Ideally, coils that have compacted create a neck beneath the coils that will accept a clip, thereby simplifying the management. In other cases, thrombectomy is required to mobilize the neck for clip reconstruction. The CUSA can be used as with purely thrombotic aneurysms, leaving the coil mass in place and clipping around the coils. Only rarely is it advisable to attempt to extract coils from the aneurysm.

Bypass techniques allow complex aneurysms to be proximally occluded or trapped with minimal risk of ischemic complications. However, revascularization of the distal ACA territory for ACoA aneurysms is more difficult than with other vascular territories and aneurysms. The superficial temporal artery (STA) and occipital artery, the two most commonly

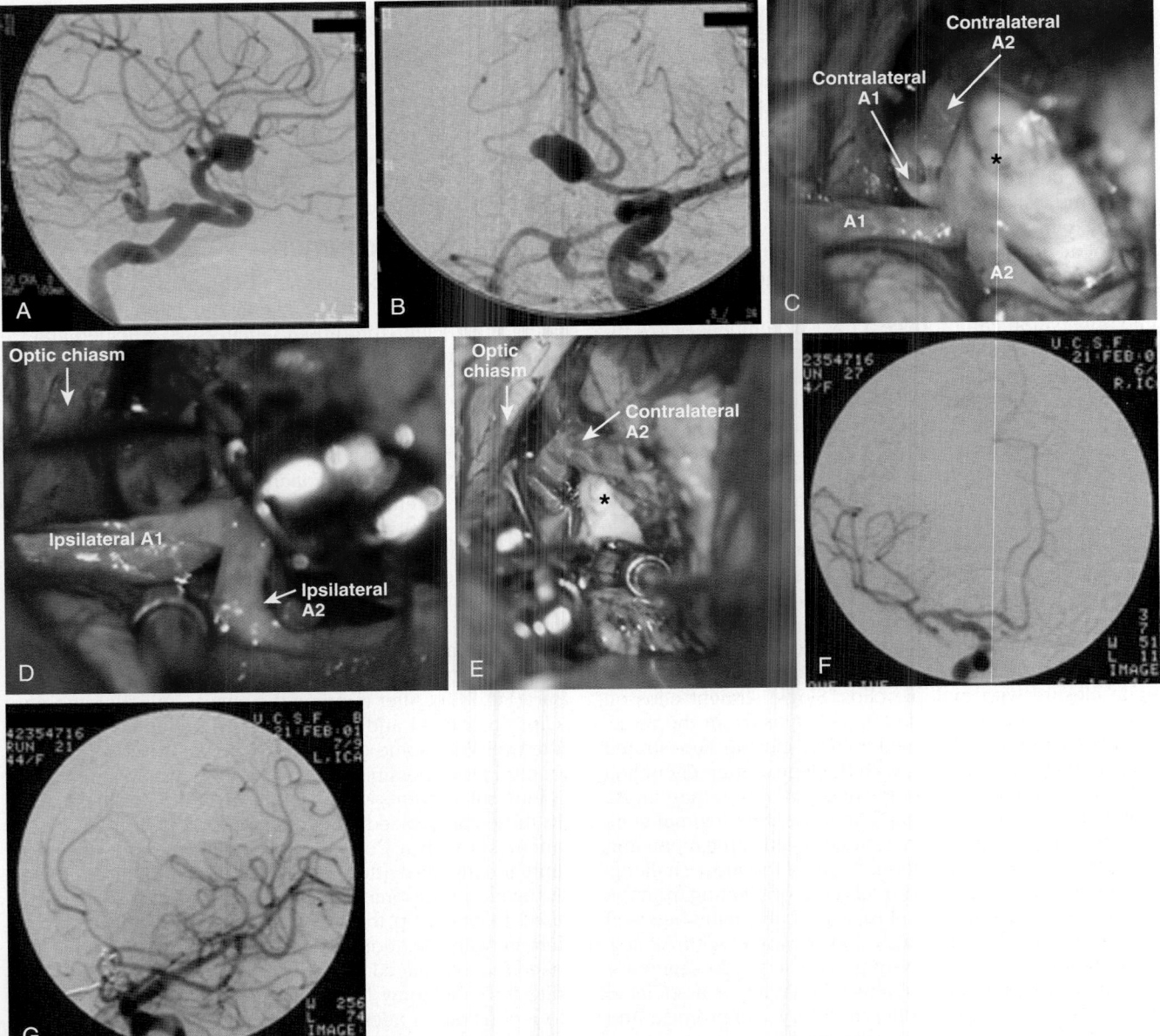

FIGURE 74-8 A 44-year-old woman with a family history of intracranial aneurysms underwent screening neuroimaging that revealed aneurysms. Lateral (A) and anterior–posterior (B) views of a left carotid artery angiogram demonstrated a large ACoA aneurysm measuring approximately 14 × 7 mm with an ill-define neck, as well as a small right superior hypophyseal artery (SHA) aneurysm (not shown). Note the incidental persistent left trigeminal artery. Endovascular coiling of the aneurysm was attempted, but the anatomy was not favorable for this modality. The patient then underwent a left orbitozygomatic–pterional craniotomy for clipping of the ACoA and right SHA aneurysms. The aneurysm anatomy is demonstrated before clipping (C) and after clipping, with views below the clips (D) and above them (E). The aneurysms are indicated by the asterisk. Postoperative cerebral angiography showed exclusion of both ACoA and SHA aneurysms and flow in bilateral ACA arteries (F, right carotid artery angiogram, anteroposterior view; G, left carotid artery angiogram, anterior oblique view).

used donor arteries for other extracranial-to-intracranial bypasses, are not long enough for a distal ACA bypass. Interposition grafts, such as the radial artery or saphenous vein, bridge from the carotid artery or STA to the ACA. They are long, require extensive exposure, and are prone to late occlusions. In situ bypasses that connect the A3 or A4 ACAs in the interhemispheric fissure with a side-to-side anastomosis can be used when blood flow in one of the efferent A2 arteries can be preserved during the aneurysm occlusion (Fig. 74-11). Most of these bypass procedures require an interhemispheric

approach, separate from the pterional approach used for the ACoA aneurysm. A multimodality approach that creates a surgical bypass first and then occludes the aneurysm endovascularly in a separate stage has appeal. It minimizes the extent of surgery, limiting the craniotomy to just an interhemispheric approach rather than a combined pterional–bifrontal approach. It also confirms bypass patency before arterial sacrifice and allows the patient's medical status and hemodynamics to be optimized for the second-stage procedure. This multimodality strategy has proved effective with

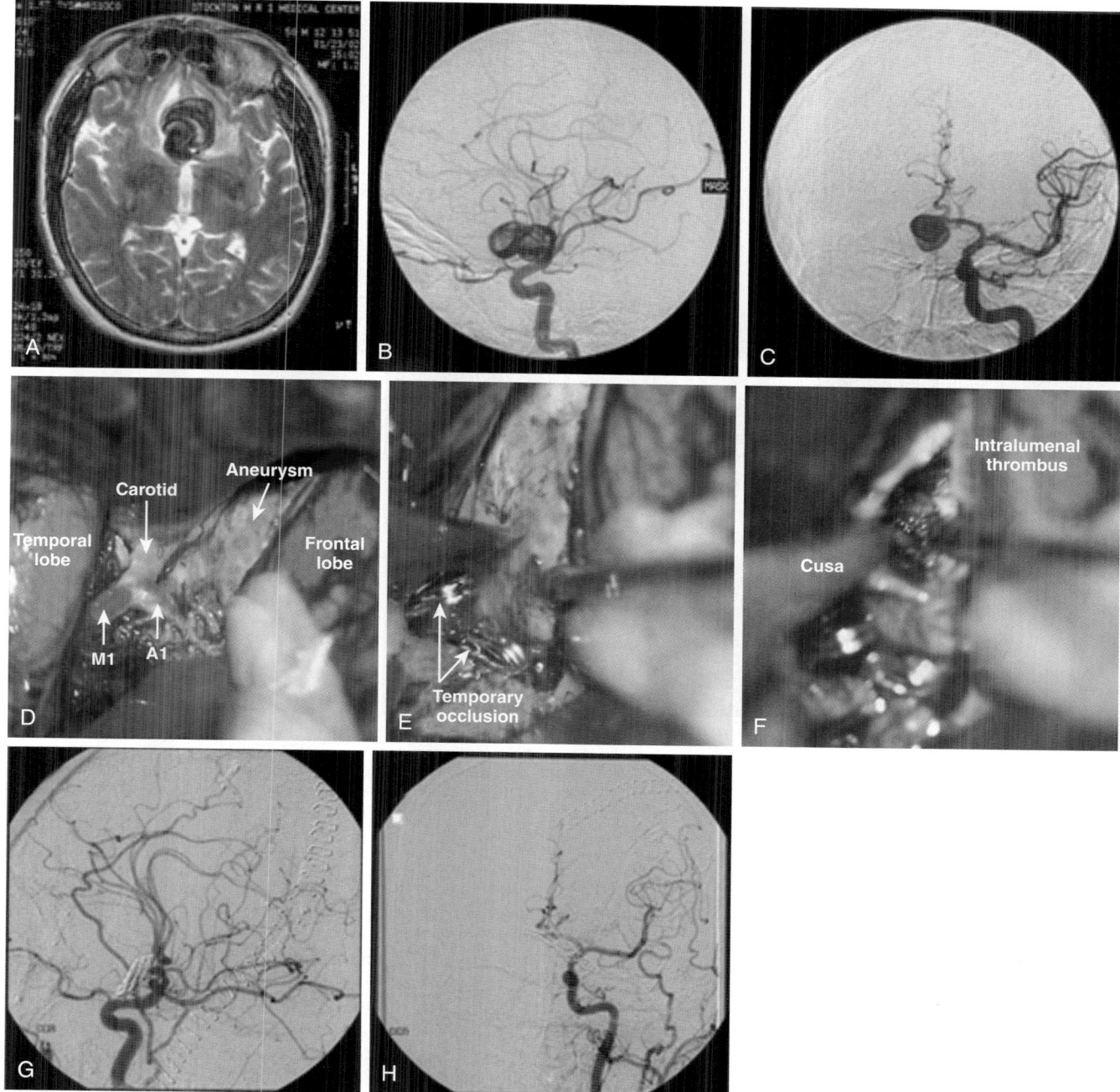

FIGURE 74-9 A 50-year-old man presented with a grand mal seizure and was diagnosed with an unruptured giant ACoA aneurysm. A, An axial T2-weighted magnetic resonance image revealed a giant, partially thrombosed aneurysm in the anterior interhemispheric fissure, with surrounding cerebral edema. Lateral (B) and anterior–posterior (C) views of the left carotid artery angiogram demonstrated an inferiorly and anteriorly projecting, bilobed aneurysm. D, The patient underwent a left orbitozygomatic craniotomy to widely expose the aneurysm. Before the aneurysm neck could be clipped, the aneurysm was incised (E) and the intraluminal thrombus was removed with a CUSA (F). Postoperative left carotid artery angiography revealed good flow in the A1 and A2 branches bilaterally and no residual aneurysm filling (G, lateral view; H, anteroposterior view).

atherosclerotic, fusiform, mycotic/infectious, and traumatic aneurysms involving the ACoA complex.[27]

Postoperative Management

Postoperatively, patients are assessed neurologically and radiographically with CT scan and digital subtraction angiogram. Angiography is essential in documenting complete aneurysm obliteration, patency of parent and branch arteries, and the presence of vasospasm. Patients at risk of developing vasospasm are monitored closely in an ICU. All patients are given nimodipine, starting within 4 days of SAH and continuing for 21 days, regardless of admission grade, at a dosage of 60 mg every 4 hours.[28,29] Vasospasm is detected with angiography, transcranial Doppler (TCD) ultrasonography, or changes in neurologic examination. Angiography is the optimal diagnostic study, but it is limited by its invasiveness. TCD ultrasonography is noninvasive

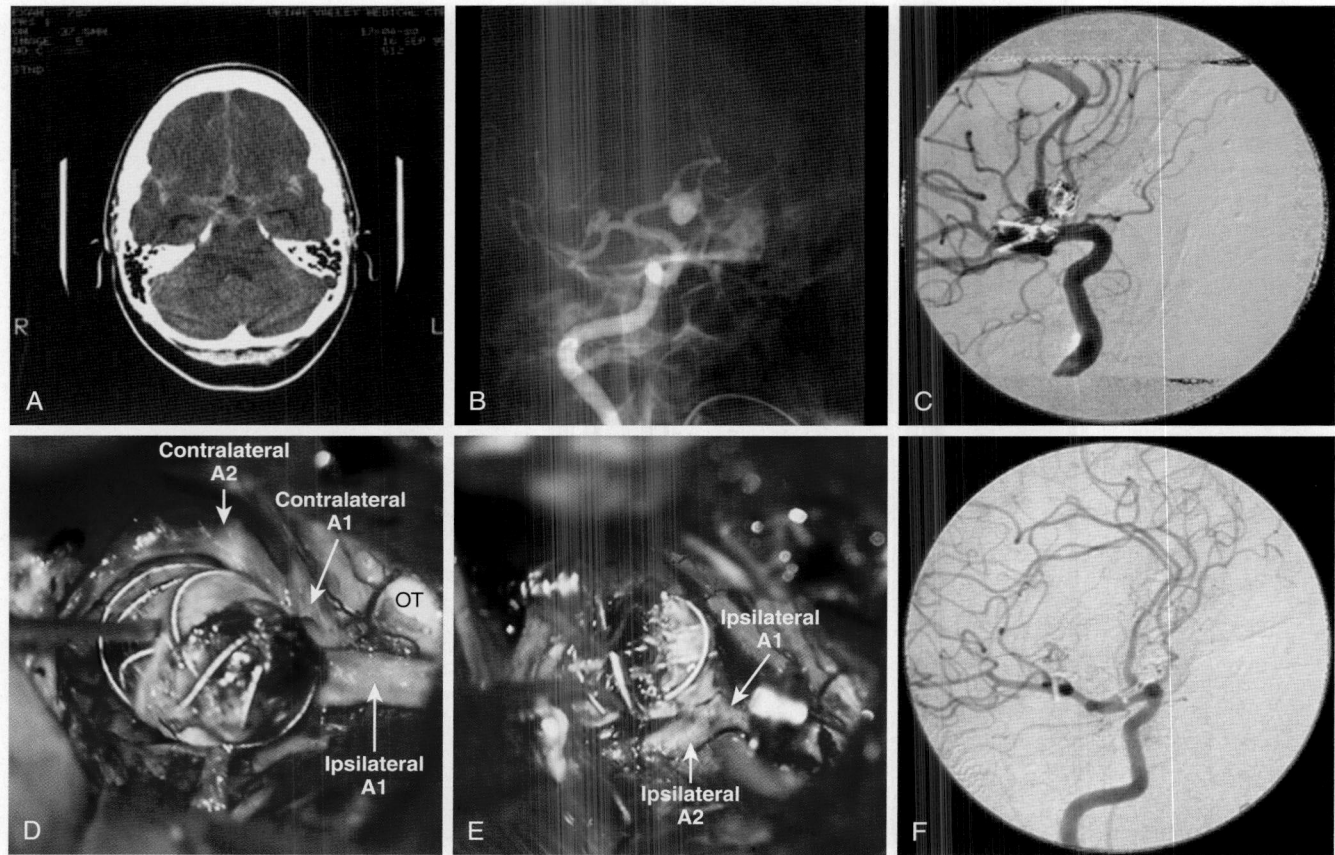

FIGURE 74-10 A, A 40-year-old woman presented to an outside hospital with SAH on an axial CT scan. B, She was found to have right MCA and ACoA aneurysms on a right carotid artery angiogram. She underwent a right pterional craniotomy to clip the right MCA aneurysm and was then referred to this institution for coiling of the ACoA aneurysm. C, Three years later, the ACoA aneurysm recurred and the patient was referred for microsurgical clipping. D, She underwent a right orbitozygomatic craniotomy, and the coiled anterior portion of the aneurysm could be visualized. E, The recurrent posterior portion of the aneurysm was located behind this coil mass and was occluded with a fenestrated clip that encircled the coils. F, Postoperative angiography revealed no residual filling of the aneurysm.

and can be done repeatedly to detect trends. Rising TCD velocities guide the timing of more aggressive measures, such as hypertensive therapy and angioplasty.

The mainstays of medical management are hypervolemia, hypertension, and hemodilution, collectively known as HHH therapy.[30] Volume expansion is achieved with packed red blood cells, albumin solution, or hypertonic saline solution. Invasive monitoring with either a central venous pressure line or a pulmonary artery catheter is required to guide fluid management. Volume expansion to central venous pressures greater than 8 mm Hg or diastolic pulmonary artery pressures greater than 14 mm Hg is usually enough to dilute the hematocrit to less than 35%. In addition, volume expansion may increase systolic blood pressure to desired end points. As the patient's clinical condition demands, the blood pressure is elevated further with pressor agents to systolic values between 180 and 220 mm Hg.[31]

Endovascular therapies for vasospasm are used when aggressive medical management fails, when TCD velocities rise, or when there are multiple risk factors for severe vasospasm. Transluminal balloon angioplasty (TBA) mechanically dilates segments of large cerebral arteries that are in spasm, restoring the normal caliber of the lumen, improving blood flow to ischemic brain, and resulting in clinical improvement.[32] Furthermore, the effects of angioplasty appear to

last up to a week, which corresponds to the duration of vasospasm.[33] The success of this intervention has largely to do with timing. Early angioplasty before or immediately after neurologic deterioration enhances its efficacy. TBA is limited to large cerebral arteries such as the ICA, MCA, and ACA. Smaller distal arteries, notably the A2 ACAs, are not amenable to angioplasty and instead are treated with an intra-arterial papaverine or verapamil infusion. Superselective infusion of a vasodilator can improve the caliber of vasospastic arteries, but the effects are short lived (less than 12 hours). Repeated treatments may be needed for severe distal vasospasm, which limits its utility.

Hydrocephalus is a common complication of SAH, especially when there is significant intraventricular hemorrhage. Up to 65% of all patients requiring an external ventricular drain for hydrocephalus or intraventricular hemorrhage also require permanent ventriculoperitoneal shunting.[34] Fenestration of the lamina terminalis during surgery appears to reduce the need for ventriculoperitoneal shunting.

Patients with ACoA aneurysms are susceptible to two postoperative entities: electrolyte abnormalities and the ACoA syndrome. Hyponatremia is frequently seen in SAH patients, with an incidence of around 18%, and lasts from 1 to 5 days.[35] This electrolyte abnormality is the result of cerebral salt wasting, a natriuresis and secondary water

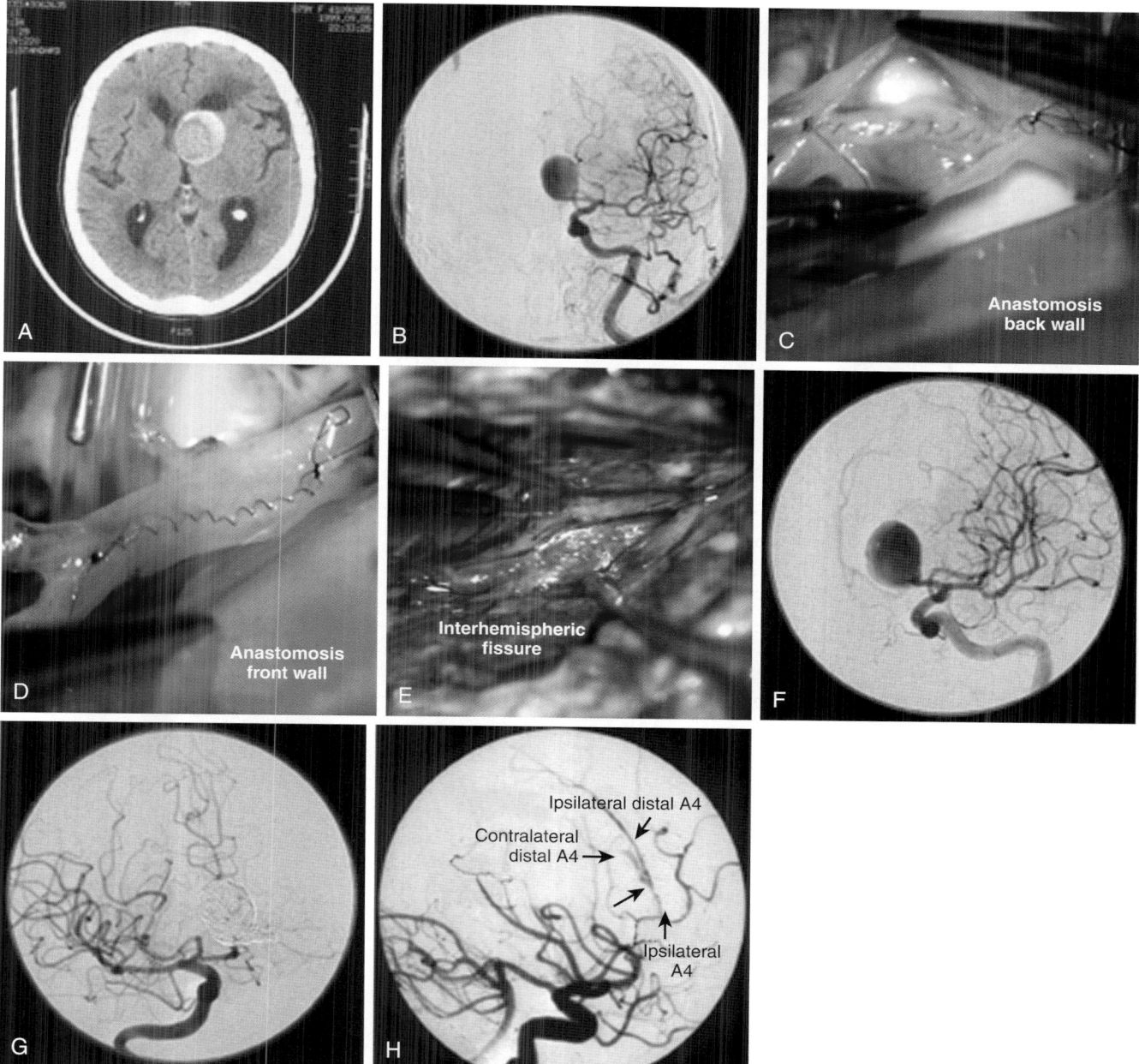

FIGURE 74-11 A, A 78-year-old woman presented with aphasia and headaches. Her head CT scan demonstrated obstructive hydrocephalus due to a giant, partially thrombosed ACoA aneurysm. B, Left carotid artery angiogram (anteroposterior view) revealed a superiorly projecting aneurysm without a discrete, clippable neck. The left A1 and A2 ACAs were separated by the base of the aneurysm, indicating a fusiform morphology. A multimodality treatment was planned, with a bypass to the distal ACA as a first stage and endovascular coil occlusion of the aneurysm as a second stage. She underwent bifrontal craniotomy, interhemispheric approach, and A3–A3 ACA side-to-side anastomosis to revascularize the ACA territory distal to the aneurysm. The back walls of the anastomosis are sutured from within the arterial lumen first (C), followed by the front walls (D). E, The depth of this surgical corridor is shown. F, Postoperative left carotid artery angiography demonstrated a patent bypass with good distal flow in bilateral ACA territories. G and H, The patient then underwent coil occlusion of the aneurysm and the proximal left A1 ACA, with right carotid artery angiography demonstrating obliteration of the aneurysm and blood flow in bilateral ACA territories that originates from the right A2 ACA and crosses to the left hemisphere through the bypass. H, The anastomosis site is indicated by the large black arrow.

loss due to the kidneys' inability to retain sodium. Clinically, cerebral salt wasting can mimic the ischemic neurologic deterioration observed in patients with vasospasm. The laboratory picture of cerebral salt wasting is similar to that of the syndrome of inappropriate antidiuretic hormone secretion (SIADH), except that extracellular fluid volumes are low with cerebral salt wasting and elevated with SIADH. The routine treatment of SIADH, namely, fluid restriction, can be dangerous in patients with cerebral salt wasting, since further dehydration can exacerbate the diminished cerebral blood flow and ischemia in patients with vasospasm. Instead, cerebral salt wasting is treated with normal saline infusion, supplemental salt intake, and sometimes hypertonic saline infusion. The ACoA syndrome after SAH is characterized by impaired memory, personality changes, and confabulation.[36]

KEY REFERENCES

Avci E, Fossett D, et al. Branches of the anterior cerebral artery near the anterior communicating artery complex: an anatomic study and surgical perspective. *Neurol Med Chir (Tokyo).* 2003;43(7):329-333:discussion 333.

Gonzalez LF, Crawford NR, et al. Working area and angle of attack in three cranial base approaches: pterional, orbitozygomatic, and maxillary extension of the orbitozygomatic approach. *Neurosurgery.* 2002;50(3):550-555:discussion 555–557.

Iwanaga H, Wakai S, et al. Ruptured cerebral aneurysms missed by initial angiographic study. *Neurosurgery.* 1990;27(1):45-51.

Kassell NF, Torner JC, et al. The international cooperative study on the timing of aneurysm surgery. Part 1: Overall management results. *J Neurosurg.* 1990;73(1):18-36.

Kerber CW, Imbesi SG, et al. Flow dynamics in a lethal anterior communicating artery aneurysm. *AJNR Am J Neuroradiol.* 1999;20(10):2000-2003.

Molyneux A, Kerr R, et al. International Subarachnoid Aneurysm Trial (ISAT) of neurosurgical clipping versus endovascular coiling in 2143 patients with ruptured intracranial aneurysms: a randomised trial. *Lancet.* 2002;360(9342):1267-1274.

Perlmutter D, Rhoton Jr AL. Microsurgical anatomy of the anterior cerebral-anterior communicating-recurrent artery complex. *J Neurosurg.* 1976;45(3):259-272.

Yasargil MG. *Microneurosurgery.* New York: Georg Thieme Verlag/Thieme Stratton; 1984.

Numbered references appear on Expert Consult.

Surgical Management of Aneurysms of the Middle Cerebral Artery

MARTIN LEHECKA • REZA DASHTI • JAAKKO RINNE • ROSSANA ROMANI • RIKU KIVISAARI • MIKA NIEMELÄ • JUHA HERNESNIEMI

The middle cerebral artery (MCA) is a very common site for aneurysm formation. In Finland, MCA aneurysms (MCAAs) represent 40% of all intracranial aneurysms.[1-3] MCAAs are more frequent among unruptured aneurysms (48%) than among ruptured aneurysms (34%).[4] Despite being so common, surprisingly few reports deal with MCA aneurysms, and especially the overall management outcome of this specific group of patients.[5-17] Most MCAAs are located distal to the circle of Willis, and they are often broad based and one or several branches originate from a base.[18] When ruptured, they present with intracerebral hematoma (ICH) in nearly half of all cases; many of these hematomas cause severe mass effect.[1-3] In his pioneering work on surgery for intracranial aneurysms (IAs), Dandy considered MCAAs hazardous for surgical management, and even inoperable.[19] Although currently only a few MCAAs are inoperable, they certainly still present striking problems as compared with other aneurysms in the anterior circulation. The main challenges when operating on MCA aneurysms is the lack of collateral circulation, so that inadvertent occlusion of the MCA or one of its branches can lead to calamitous infarctions and death, especially in acute subarachnoid hemorrhage (SAH). The MCAAs are less suitable for endovascular surgery than other anterior circulation aneurysms,[20-25] because of both their anatomy (broad neck with high recanalization rate) and their frequent association with expanding hematomas; thus neurosurgeons should focus on the safe treatment of these lesions.[17,26-32]

The purpose of this chapter is to review practical anatomy, preoperative planning, and avoidance of complications in the microsurgical dissection and clipping of MCAAs. This review is mainly based on the experience of the senior author (JH) in two of the five Finnish University Hospital neurosurgical departments (Helsinki and Kuopio), which serve, without selection, the catchment area of the entire southern and eastern Finland regions (population 3 million). These two centers have treated nearly 10,000 aneurysm patients since the beginning of the microneurosurgical era in the mid 1970s. Our aim is to present a consecutive, population-based series with as little selection bias as possible. The data presented is not reflective of the senior author's personal series alone. Most of the data is derived from the Kuopio Cerebral Aneurysm Database (1977–2005),

which contains information on all 3005 consecutive patients harboring 4253 aneurysms who were treated at Kuopio University Hospital, Finland, from 1977 to 2005.[1-3]

Aneurysms of the MCA

Middle cerebral artery aneurysms can be classified into three groups: proximal (M1As), bifurcation (MbifAs), or distal type (MdistAs) aneurysms (Table 75-1). The proximal MCA aneurysms or M1As are located on the main trunk (M1) of the MCA, between the bifurcation of the internal carotid artery (ICA) and the main bifurcation of MCA.[1] The MbifAs are located at the main bifurcation of the MCA.[2] The MdistAs, originate from the branches of the MCA distal to the main bifurcation inside the sylvian fissure.[3] Each of these aneurysms have special features due to anatomic location and general behavior that need to be taken into consideration when planning occlusive treatment. Assigning an MCAA into a particular group can sometimes be difficult since the length and caliber of the M1 segment often varies and there may be two or even three major branching sites along its course. Generally, we consider MCA bifurcation to be the first and major branching site of the MCA where two or more rather similarly sized arterial trunks divide at the limen insula level. Occasionally, a thick frontal or temporal cortical branch of the M1 trunk creates a more proximal "false bifurcation."[33]

Incidence of MCA Aneurysms

The MCA aneurysms represented 40% of all IAs in a consecutive and population-based series of 3005 patients with 4253 IAs from 1977 to 2005 in the Kuopio Cerebral Aneurysm Data Base.[1-4] Tables 75-2 through 75-5 present the clinical data on the 1456 patients with MCA aneurysms in this series. Of the 3005 patients, 1456 (48%) had 1704 MCA aneurysms (Table 75-2). The most frequent location for MCAAs was the MCA bifurcation, and 1166 patients had 1385 MbifAs (33% of all 4253 IAs and 81% of all MCAAs). This breakdown is similar to other MCAA series.[6,10-13,15,17,34,35] M1As comprised 14% of the MCAAs and MdistAs were the least frequent ones (5%) (Table 75-2). The right side dominated over the left side (55% vs. 45%) (Table 75-3).

Table 75-1 Three Categories of MCA Aneurysms

Category	Location
M1A	Main trunk of MCA, between ICA bifurcation and main MCA bifurcation
MbifA	Main MCA bifurcation
MdistA	Branches distal to main MCA bifurcation

ICA, internal carotid artery; MCA, middle cerebral artery.

Table 75-2 Patients with MCA Aneurysms in Consecutive and Population-Based Series of 3005 Patients with 4253 IAs from 1977 to 2005 in Kuopio Cerebral Aneurysm Database

	No. Patients	No. Aneurysms
Whole series	3005	4253
Patients with primary SAH	2365 (79%)	3325 (78%)
Patients without primary SAH	640 (21%)	928 (22%)
MCA aneurysms	1456	1704
M1As	221 (15%)	241 (14%)
MbifAs	1166 (80%)	1385 (81%)
MdistAs	69 (5%)	78 (5%)
Ruptured MCA aneurysms	802	802
M1As	73 (9%)	73 (9%)
MbifAs	711 (87%)	711 (87%)
MdistAs	18 (2%)	18 (2%)
Fusiform MCA aneurysms	18	18
Fusiform M1As	6 (33%)	6 (33%)
Fusiform MbifAs	8 (44%)	8 (44%)
Fusiform MdistAs	4 (22%)	4 (22%)

IA, intracranial aneurysm; MCA, middle cerebral artery; SAH, subarachnoid hemorrhage.

RUPTURED AND UNRUPTURED MCA ANEURYSMS

Of the 3005 patients, 2365 (79%) had a primary subarachnoid hemorrhage (SAH) from a ruptured IA. MCAAs were the cause of SAH in 802 (34%) of the 2365 patients. Again the MbifAs were the most frequent, comprising 87% of all the ruptured MCAAs (Table 75-2). M1As represented 9% of the ruptured MCAAs. There were only 18 patients with ruptured MdistA, less than 1% of all the ruptured IAs, and 2% of all the ruptured MCAAs. The median size for ruptured MbifAs was 10 mm (range 1 to 80 mm) (Table 75-3). Both the M1As and MdistAs were smaller than MbifAs in general, with median diameters of 4 mm (range 1–54 mm). Interestingly, 29% of the ruptured MbifAs, and as many as 51% of the ruptured M1As were smaller than 7 mm in diameter. This would indicate, that at least in the Finnish population, even small MCAAs are dangerous and the International Study of Unruptured Intracranial Aneurysms (ISUIA) results are controversial.[36] Among the 1704 MCAAs, 69 (4%) were giant, most of them (80%) located at the MCA bifurcation. Of the 69 giant MCAAs, 72% were ruptured. There were 18 fusiform MCAAs, only 1% of all the 1704 MCAAs. Unlike the giant aneurysms, fusiform aneurysms were distributed rather evenly along the whole course of the MCA (Table 75-2). The total number of unruptured IAs in this series was 1888. Among the unruptured IAs, the MCAAs were even more frequent than among the ruptured ones (n = 902, 48%). MbifAs were again the most common (75% of all the unruptured MCAAs). The unruptured MCAAs

were smaller in general than their ruptured counterparts, with median size ranging from 3 to 5 mm depending on the aneurysm location (Table 75-3).

INTRACEREBRAL HEMATOMA, INTRAVENTRICULAR HEMORRHAGE, AND PREOPERATIVE HYDROCEPHALUS

Ruptured MCAAs bleed frequently into the adjacent brain, and as many as 347 (43%) of the 802 patients with ruptured MCAAs presented with a space-occupying ICH (Table 75-4). ICHs were most often seen in MbifAs and MdistAs, 44% and 50%, respectively, and it were less frequently present in ruptured M1As (36%) (Fig. 75-1A to C). The higher risk for ICH in more distal MCAAs is probably due to a tighter cistern with the aneurysm more closely surrounded by the adjacent brain. The ICH was usually located in the temporal lobe (80%) and less frequently in the frontal lobe (20%) (Table 75-3). In the entire series, there was only one patient with a ruptured MCAA and parietal ICH. Intraventricular hemorrhage (IVH) was associated with the ICH in 15%, and isolated IVH without ICH was seen in only 5% of patients (Table 75-4). Rarely, ruptured MCAAs can also present with a subdural hematoma adding to the mass effect of an ICH (0.5% in our series) (Fig. 75-1B). Preoperative hydrocephalus was detected in 29% of the ruptured MCAAs (Table 75-4).

ASSOCIATED ANEURYSMS

Middle cerebral artery aneurysms are often associated with other aneurysms, accounting for 40% of cases in our series (Table 75-5). Of the 579 patients who had at least one associated aneurysm, 313 (54%) had an MCAA as an associated aneurysm and 46% had associated aneurysms at locations other than the MCA. The most common associated aneurysm was MbifA. The associated MCAAs were more often seen at the opposite MCA than at the same MCA as the primary aneurysm (58% vs. 29%); 13% of patients with multiple MCAAs had the associated MCAAs on both MCAs ("mirror aneurysms") (Table 75-5) (Fig. 75-2). MbifA was also the most frequently associated aneurysm among all 2365 patients with ruptured IAs in this series, and 12% had at least one associated MbifA.

Microsurgically Relevant Anatomy

MIDDLE CEREBRAL ARTERY

The middle cerebral artery (MCA) is the major terminal branch of the ICA supplying a large part of the cerebral hemisphere along with the insula, lentiform nucleus, and internal capsule.[37] The MCA is the most complex major cerebral artery owing to its anatomic and hemodynamic features. Microneurosurgical anatomy details of the MCA have been described by Yaşargil[13,33] and others.[37-42]

The MCA is generally divided into four segments: M1 (sphenoidal), M2 (insular), M3 (opercular), and M4 (cortical).[43] The M1 segment, the most proximal segment of the MCA, begins at the carotid bifurcation and extends to the bifurcation of the MCA, which is usually at the level of limen insula where it splits into two, sometimes three, major M2 branches. The M2s give rise to 8 to 12 branches before becoming the M3s at the peri-insular sulcus.[37] The M3s

Table 75-3   Characteristics of 1704 MCA Aneurysms

	RUPTURED				UNRUPTURED				TOTAL		
	M1As	MbifAs	MdistAs	M1As	M1As	MbifAs	MdistAs	M1As	M1As	MbifAs	MdistAs
No. of aneurysms	73	711	18	168	674	60	241	1385	78		
Median aneurysm size [mm]; median (range)	6 (2–48)	10 (1–80)	8 (2–25)	4 (1–54)	5 (1–65)	3 (1–25)	4 (1–54)	8 (1–80)	4 (1–25)		
Aneurysm Size											
Small (<7 mm)	37 (51%)	206 (29%)	8 (44%)	137 (82%)	390 (58%)	47 (78%)	174 (72%)	596 (43%)	55 (71%)		
Medium (7–14 mm)	27 (37%)	341 (48%)	8 (44%)	24 (14%)	241 (36%)	10 (17%)	51 (21%)	582 (42%)	18 (23%)		
Large (15–24 mm)	3 (4%)	121 (17%)	1 (6%)	1 (1%)	31 (5%)	2 (3%)	4 (2%)	152 (11%)	3 (4%)		
Giant (≥25 mm)	6 (8%)	43 (6%)	1 (6%)	6 (4%)	12 (2%)	1 (2%)	12 (5%)	55 (4%)	2 (3%)		
Aneurysm Side											
Right	34 (47%)	407 (57%)	8 (44%)	91 (54%)	367 (54%)	32 (53%)	125 (52%)	774 (56%)	40 (51%)		
Left	39 (53%)	304 (43%)	10 (56%)	77 (46%)	307 (46%)	28 (47%)	116 (48%)	611 (44%)	38 (49%)		
ICH	26 (36%)	312 (44%)	9 (50%)								
Frontal	5	50	1								
Temporal	21	261	8								
Parietal	0	1	0								
IVH	12 (16%)	138 (19%)	4 (22%)								
Preoperative hydrocephalus	23 (32%)	206 (29%)	4 (22%)								

Note: Data are given in number of aneurysms.
ICH, intracerebral hematoma; IVH, intraventricular hemorrhage; MCA, middle cerebral artery.

continue to the surface of the sylvian fissure at the lateral surface of the brain. The M4 segments are located on the parasylvian surface of the brain and supply the lateral cortical surface of the cerebral hemisphere.[13,33,37,38,43]

M1 SEGMENT

The M1 starts in the sylvian cistern at the carotid bifurcation, supralateral to the optic chiasm, inferior to the anterior perforated substance, and posterior to the division of olfactory tract. Thick arachnoid covers the M1 origin and bridging arachnoid fibers surround its proximal part. M1 travels laterally in the sylvian fissure until the bifurcation at the insular apex.[37] At the MCA bifurcation, the M1 splits usually into two (bifurcation) branches (M2s), the superior (frontal) and the inferior (temporal).[33,37] Türe et al. divided M1 branches into (1) the cortical branches (often named as temporopolar, frontotemporal, and orbitofrontal branches) and (2) the lateral lenticulostriate branches. In the surgical trajectory to the sylvian cistern, the cortical branches (one to three) mainly project toward the temporal lobe (75%) and less often toward the frontal lobe (25%). Variations include temporal only, temporal and frontal, frontal only, and no major cortical branches.[37,43] Lateral lenticulostriate arteries originate mainly from the M1 trunk (see below), and identification of their origin should help to distinguish the true MCA bifurcation. The preservation of M1 branches is of paramount importance in the occlusive therapy for M1As.

LATERAL LENTICULOSTRIATE ARTERIES

The lateral lenticulostriate arteries (LLAs) are quite variable in number (up to 20) and in sites of origin.[33,37,38,40,41,44] Lateral lenticulostriate arteries mainly arise from the frontal aspect or cortical branches of the M1. However, LLAs may also arise, in up to 23%, from the MCA bifurcation, the M2s, or an accessory M2.[37,40] The more proximal the bifurcation, the greater the number of postbifurcational LLA branches.[43] In the surgical trajectory, LLAs mainly arise from the frontal aspect of the M1 and they mainly turn toward the frontal lobe. LLAs enter the brain via central and lateral parts of the anterior perforating substance and supply the substantia innominata, putamen, globus pallidus, head and body of the caudate nucleus, internal capsule and adjacent corona radiata, and the central portion of the anterior commissure.[37] M1As and MbifAs may more or less involve LLAs at their branching sites,[13,40,43] and LLAs may be displaced, compressed, distorted, or stretched by M1As.[44] During dissection

Table 75-4 Intracerebral Hematoma, IVH, and Acute Hydrocephalus Associated with 802 Ruptured MCA Aneurysms

	M1As	MbifAs	MdistAs	Total
Ruptured aneurysms	73	711	18	802
ICH only	18 (25%)	207 (29%)	5 (28%)	230 (29%)
ICH with IVH component	8 (11%)	105 (15%)	4 (22%)	117 (15%)
IVH only	4 (5%)	33 (5%)	0	37 (5%)
Preoperative hydrocephalus	23 (32%)	206 (29%)	4 (22%)	233 (29%)

ICH, intracerebral hematoma; IVH, intraventricular hemorrhage; MCA, middle cerebral artery.

Table 75-5 Patients with MCAA and Possible Associated Aneurysms

	Ruptured MCAA	Unruptured MCAA	Total
Patients with MCAA	802	654	1456
Patients with single aneurysm	553 (69%)	324 (50%)	877 (60%)
Patients with multiple aneurysms	249 (31%)	330 (50%)	579 (40%)
Associated MCAAs	178	135	313
Same MCA	59	32	91
Opposite MCAA	99	83	182
Both MCAs	20	20	40
Associated aneurysms at other sites	110	156	266

Note: Data are given in number of patients.
MCA, middle cerebral artery; MCAA, middle cerebral artery aneurysm.

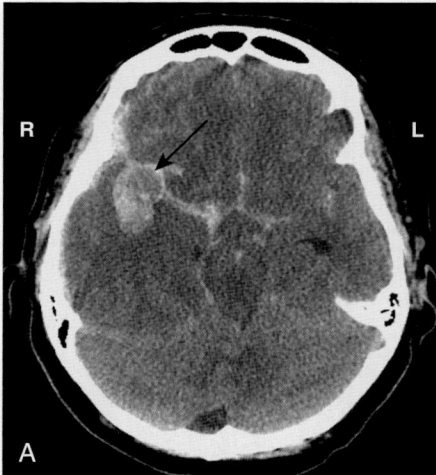 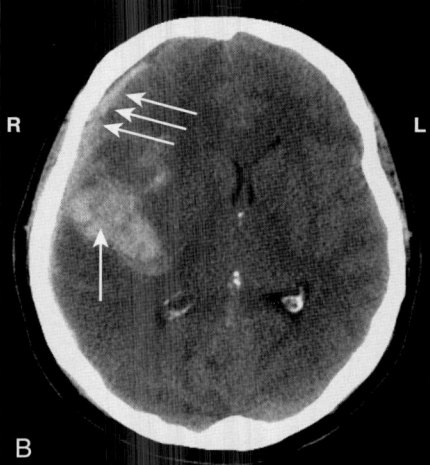 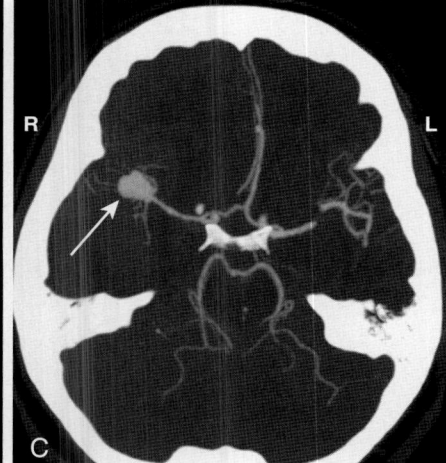

FIGURE 75-1 Deeply unconscious patient shown on initial computed tomography (CT). A, Subarachnoid hemorrhage and ruptured right-sided MbifA (*black arrow*), which caused intracerebral hematoma (*white arrow*). B, Subdural hematoma (*small arrows*) causing mass effect. C, CT angiography shows large, irregular, lateral projecting MbifA (*arrow*).

and clipping of M1As, the site and pattern of origin of the LLAs are of special concern. LLAs may arise from a single-stem branch of M1, and severing the stem branch causes infarct in the entire LLA supply area.[44] The arachnoid adhesions together with cortical and lateral lenticulostriate branches as well as very small pial branches, also originating from M1, limit the mobilization of M1 in the sylvian fissure.[33,37,41]

MCA BIFURCATION AND M2 SEGMENTS

The location of the bifurcational complex in the sylvian fissure varies considerably depending on the length of the M1, as well as the angioarchitecture of the bifurcation complex.[33,37,38,43] Occasionally, a thick frontal or temporal cortical branch of the M1 trunk creates a "false bifurcation" more proximal.[33] After their origin at the MCA bifurcation, the M2s run somewhat parallel and supply the insula.[37,41,43] The M2s are seldom of equal diameter (15%), and usually, the inferior (temporal) trunk is dominating (50%). In 55% of the hemispheres studied by Türe et al., the dominant M2 trunk bifurcated soon after the main bifurcation.[37] This gave an impression of trifurcation in 12.5%, and quadrifurcation was seen in 2.5% when both M2s bifurcated immediately. Umansky et al.[40] reported bifurcation in 66%, trifurcation in 26%, and quadrifurcation in 4%, and Gibo et al.[38] reported bifurcation in 78%, trifurcation in 12%, and multiple trunks in 10%.

The M2s give rise to 8 to 12 branches, mainly arising from the superior trunk, before becoming the M3s.[37] The superior (frontal) M2 is the origin of the prefrontal, precentral, and central arteries. Furthermore, 23% the anterior and posterior parietal arteries have their origin from the superior M2.[37] They mainly supply the inferior frontal cortex, the frontal opercular cortex, and also the cortex in parietal and central sulcus areas.[33,37,38,43] The inferior (temporal) M2 is the main origin of the posterior and middle temporal arteries, supplying mainly the middle and posterior temporal cortex and temporo-occipital, angular, and posterior parietal regions.[33,37,38,43]

DISTAL MCA BRANCHES (M3 AND M4)

The M3 (opercular) segments start at the peri-insular sulci, from where they rise toward the lateral surface of the brain at the surface of the sylvian fissure. The M3 branches run on

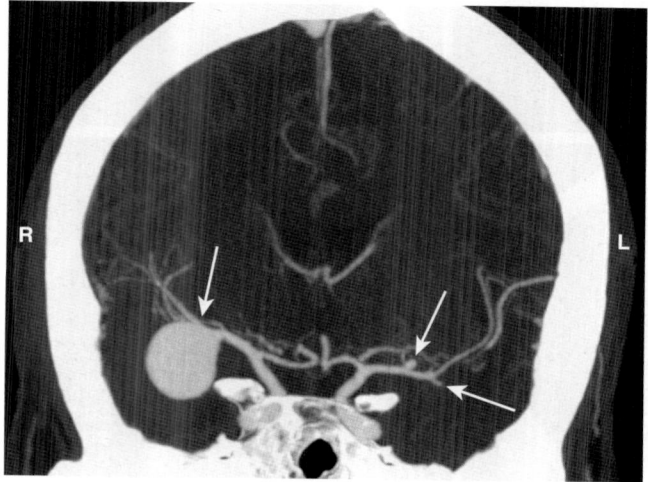

FIGURE 75-2 Patient with three middle cerebral artery aneurysms: giant right MbifA, left superior projecting M1A, and left lateral type MbifA.

either side (temporal or frontal) of the sylvian fissure, they do not generally cross over. The M3s mainly supply the medial opercular surface and, to a lesser extent (25%), the superior or inferior peri-insular sulcus.[37] The M4 segments are located on the cerebral cortex rising from inside the sylvian fissure.[33,37,38,43] They supply the 12 previously documented arterial territories of the lateral surface of the cerebral hemisphere: (1) the lateral orbitofrontal, (2) the prefrontal, (3) the precentral, (4) the central, (5) the anterior parietal, (6) the posterior parietal, (7) the angular, (8) the temporo-occipital, (9) the posterior temporal, (10) the middle temporal, (11) the anterior temporal, and (12) the temporopolar areas.[33,37,38,43]

CISTERNAL ANATOMY

The MCA (M1–M3) travels inside the sylvian fissure for most of its course. Only the proximal portion of the M1 segment is found inside the carotid cistern, which is limited by the proximal sylvian membrane from its lateral border.[45] After passing the proximal sylvian membrane the M1 enters into the anterior compartment of the sylvian cistern. It is usually in the anterior compartment of the sylvian cistern where most of the LLAs can be found.[45] The borderline between the anterior and posterior compartment of the sylvian cistern is the limen insula. The posterior compartment of the sylvian cistern is located behind the limen insulae where MCA, before or after bifurcating, makes a relatively sharp, almost 90-degree turn ("the genu of MCA").[46] The posterior compartment is further divided into the medial and lateral compartments by the intermediate sylvian membrane. The medial compartment contains the M2 trunks, whereas the M3 segments passing toward the cortical surface run for most of their course in the lateral compartment.[45] The width, depth, and folding of the sylvian fissure vary considerably.[33,46] In general, the portions of MCA that are the most difficult to reach are on the M1 segment once it has entered the sylvian cistern, as the cisternal space here is very deep and narrow and there is high risk of injuring the lateral lenticulostriate arteries.[1] The other challenging region is the very distal part of sylvian fissure, which is also narrow and there is risk of damage to cortical MCA branches. Fortunately, most MCA aneurysms are located at the MCA bifurcation, which can be found in most cases at the border of the anterior and posterior compartments of the sylvian cistern where the cistern is wider.

When opening the sylvian fissure for MCA aneurysms, the posterior compartment of the sylvian cistern is usually entered first. To enter the sylvian fissure, the frontotemporal arachnoid membrane covering the cortical surface above the sylvian fissure needs to be opened. Below that lies the lateral sylvian membrane, which needs to be opened as well. The superficial sylvian veins course between these two membranes. Entering still deeper into the sylvian fissure another arachnoid membrane is encountered, the intermediate sylvian membrane. Distal portion of the M3 trunks can be found already above the intermediate sylvian membrane, but the M2 trunks are deeper, below this level.

VENOUS ANATOMY

The most important vein encountered during surgery for MCA aneurysms is the superficial sylvian vein. It usually arises at the posterior end of the sylvian fissure as one or several trunks, and courses anteriorly and inferiorly along the fissure. The separate trunks often merge into a single large channel before emptying into the venous sinuses along the sphenoid ridge.[47] The superficial sylvian vein receives the frontosylvian, parietosylvian, and temporosylvian veins and commonly anastomoses with the veins of Trolard and Labbé. It penetrates the arachnoid covering of the anterior portion of the sylvian fissure and joins the sphenoparietal sinus as it courses just below the medial part of the sphenoid ridge, or it may pass directly to the cavernous sinus.[47] Anomalies of the venous configuration are common and sometimes the superficial sylvian vein may be absent altogether.[33,47] Most of the time the superficial sylvian vein courses mainly on the temporal side of the sylvian fissure so that arachnoid opening of the frontotemporal arachnoid membrane should be planned on the frontal-lobe side of the sylvian fissure. Venous crossover branches from one side of the sylvian fissure to the other are more frequent than in arteries. The main trunk of the superficial sylvian vein should always be left intact to prevent postoperative venous infarcts. Small crossover branch may need to be coagulated and cut to provide sufficient exposure of the deeper parts of the sylvian fissure. Deeper, inside the sylvian fissure the deep middle sylvian vein can be encountered. This collects venous outflow mainly from veins of the insular cortex and it terminates in the basal vein of Rosenthal.[48]

LOCATION AND ORIENTATION OF MCA ANEURYSMS

M1As can be found along the entire M1 segment, most often at the distal portion of the M1 segment at the origin of one of the cortical branches. On angiograms, the M1As are oriented with their dome pointing anterior, inferior, superior, or posterior (Fig. 75-3A to F). The superior or posterior projecting

M1As, also called frontally projecting, project toward the frontal lobe. They are considered the most challenging M1As for three main reasons: (1) heavy involvement with LLAs, (2) in the surgical view the M1 trunk is partially or completely obstructing the view toward the aneurysm base and the origin of the cortical branch(s), and (3) the dome is buried inside the inferior portion of the frontal lobe in the deepest and narrowest part of the proximal sylvian fissure. The M1As with anterior or inferior projection, also called temporally projecting, project toward the temporal lobe. They are usually easier to expose during dissection than the frontally projecting ones.

The orientation of *MbifAs* in the sylvian fissure depends on the depth of the fissure, the length and course of the M1, and the projection of the MbifA dome. We classify MbifAs into five groups based on their orientation (Fig. 75-4A to H):

1. Intertruncal MbifA: The dome projects superiorly in the coronal (AP) plane and posteriorly in the axial plane. Intertruncal MbifAs lie between the M2s, the base often more on the thicker M2, and the M2s are more or less involved in the base.
2. Inferior MbifA: The dome projects inferiorly in the coronal (AP) plane and anteriorly (toward the sphenoid ridge) in the axial plane.
3. Lateral MbifA: The dome projects laterally in the coronal (AP) plane and laterally in the axial plane, in the same direction as M1.
4. Insular MbifA: The dome projects medially (toward the insula) in the coronal (AP) plane and medially in the axial plane.
5. Complex MbifA: In some dysmorphic and large or giant aneurysms, the growth of the dome may be multidirectional and the relation with M1 and M2s may be a combination of the aforementioned types (Fig. 75-5). Types 2, 3, and 4 are

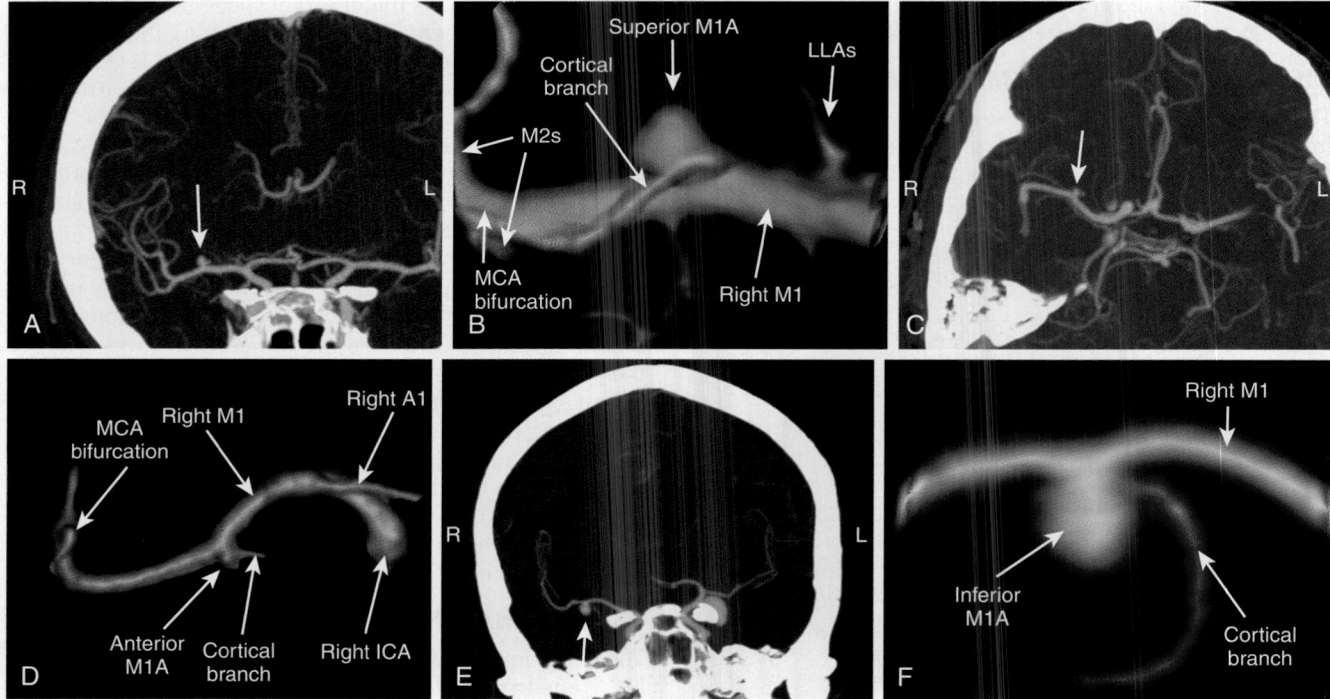

FIGURE 75-3 Different orientations for M1As (*arrow*) as seen in 2D and 3D computed tomography angiography projections. A and B, Right-sided superior projecting M1A. C and D, Anterior projecting right-sided M1A. E and F, Inferior projecting right-sided M1A.

not intertruncal and do not principally involve the M2s. The orientation may be distorted by a space-occupying ICH.

We divide *MdistAs* into aneurysms of the M2 trunk or at the M2–M3 junction (Fig. 75-6A and B), and those distal to the M2–M3 junction or of peripheral (M3) branches (Fig. 75-7). Location is more important than the dome orientation in MdistAs.

Imaging

In diagnostics, digital subtraction angiography (DSA) is still the "gold standard" in many centers. In our centers, multislice helical computed tomography (CT) angiography (CTA) is the primary modality for imaging of IAs for several reasons:

1. Noninvasive and quick imaging technique
2. Shows anatomy of the adjacent bony structures to help to plan the approach
3. Comparable sensitivity and specificity to DSA in aneurysms larger than 2 mm[49-56]
4. Disclosure of calcifications in the walls of arteries and aneurysm[57,58]

5. Quick reconstruction of three-dimensional (3D) images that, for example, show the surgeon's view of the origin of the MCA aneurysm

Some MCAAs may be difficult to visualize by routine 3D CTA,[50,57] usually due to very small size, so that subsequent rotational 3D DSA is required.

For intraoperative navigation, 3D CTA and/or DSA reconstructions should be rotated to illustrate the length, depth, and course of the M1 in the sylvian fissure; projection of the MCAA dome and its relationship to the MCA bifurcation and M2 trunks, distance from the ICA bifurcation along the M1, and possible involvement with cortical branches; and the site of possible rupture. Other lesions of the MCA should be differentiated and vascular anomalies of the region should be looked for. In giant and fusiform MCA aneurysms, magnetic resonance imaging (MRI) with different sequences, along with 3D CTA, helps to distinguish the true wall of the aneurysm and the intraluminal thrombosis.

At the workstation, 3D CTA images can be rotated accordingly to evaluate the surgeon's view to the MCA and the bifurcation, which is not standard but is tailored

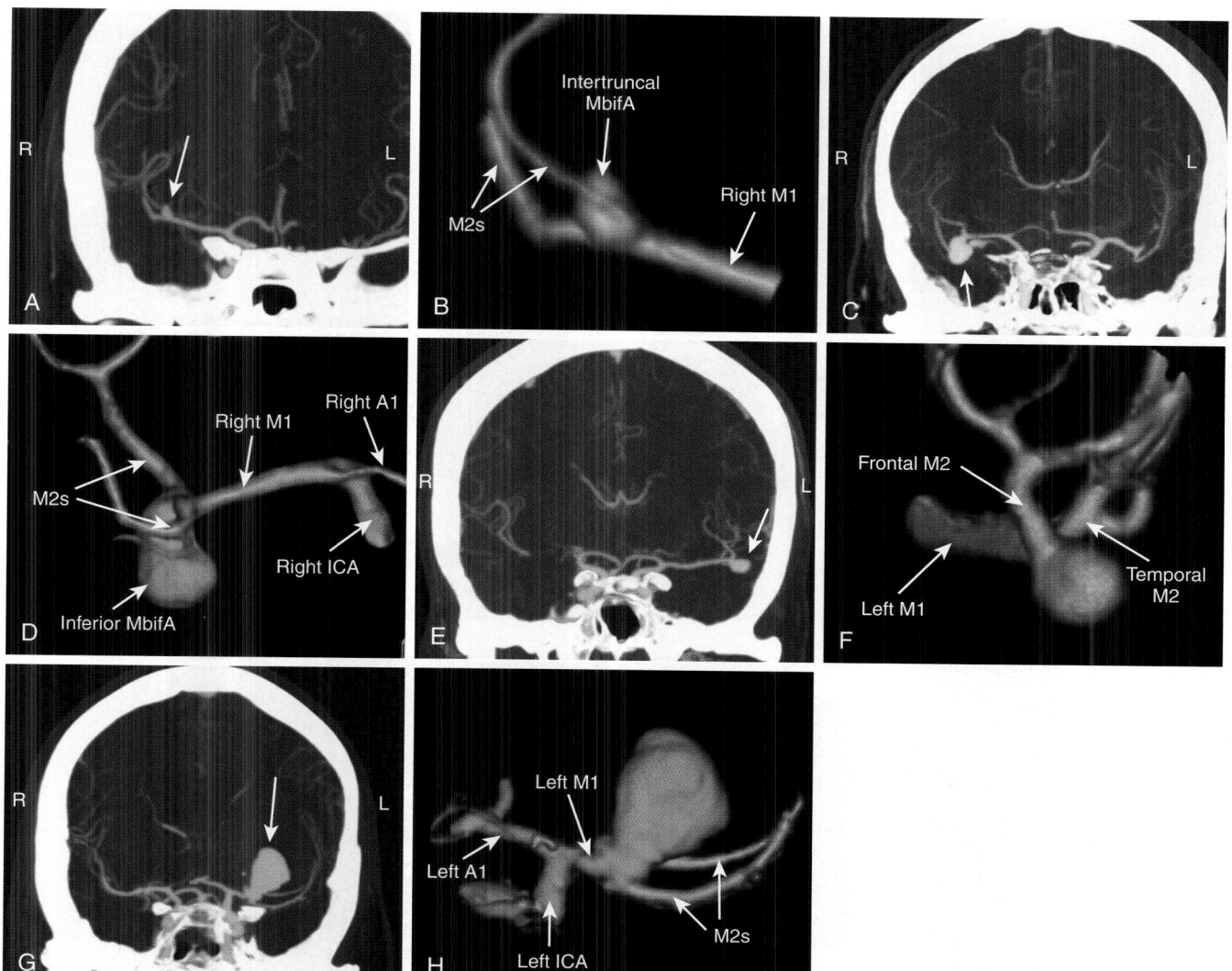

FIGURE 75-4 Different orientations for MbifAs (*arrow*) as seen on 2D and 3D computed tomography angiography projections. A and B, Right-sided intertruncal type MbifA. C and D, Right-sided inferior type MbifA. E and F, Left-sided lateral type MbifA. G and H, Left-sided insular type MbifA.

according to the aneurysm dome projection and relation to the MCA and its branches. The prime concern is to find a view that best helps to preserve the perforators around the base and the dome of the aneurysm.

Principles of Neuroanesthesia

A review of our neuroanesthesiologic principles in treatment of SAH patients has been published previously.[59] Here we present only some key points.

In all SAH patients, arterial blood pressure is measured invasively. Before the ruptured aneurysm has been secured, systolic blood pressure must be controlled, and blood pressures above 160 mm Hg should be treated, such as with labetalol. At the same time, too-low a systolic blood pressure will not provide sufficient perfusion pressure and should be prevented as well. In patients with an intracranial space-occupying hematoma, higher blood pressure can be allowed to secure adequate cerebral perfusion pressure. The transmural pressure of the aneurysm sac is one of the determinants of the risk of rebleeding, but as this cannot be measured, the accepted blood pressure remains to be determined individually.

In conscious patients, spontaneous breathing is usually adequate but in patients with Glasgow Coma Scale (GCS) 8 or less, an artificial airway and controlled ventilation are indicated. Adequate anesthesia is required before intubation to prevent rebleeding, since laryngoscopy and intubation induces a stress response with an increase in blood pressure. Sedation using propofol should be considered in patients under controlled ventilation.

Tranexamic acid (1 g intravenously every 6 hours for 3 days) is administered to prevent rebleeding until clipping.[60] Nimodipine (oral or intravenous) is given to all patients with ruptured aneurysms to prevent vasospasm.[61,62]

Postoperatively, all SAH patients are treated at the neurointensive care unit (NICU). Our general principles of postoperative treatment and monitoring are summarized in Table 75-6.

Patient Positioning and Craniotomy

All except those rare distal MCAAs can be reached through a standard pterional approach as described by Yaşargil.[13] At our institution we prefer the lateral supraorbital (LSO) approach, a more frontal and less invasive modification of the pterional approach.[63] The LSO approach has been used by the senior author (JH) in microsurgery of more than 3000 anterior circulation aneurysms over the past 20 years.

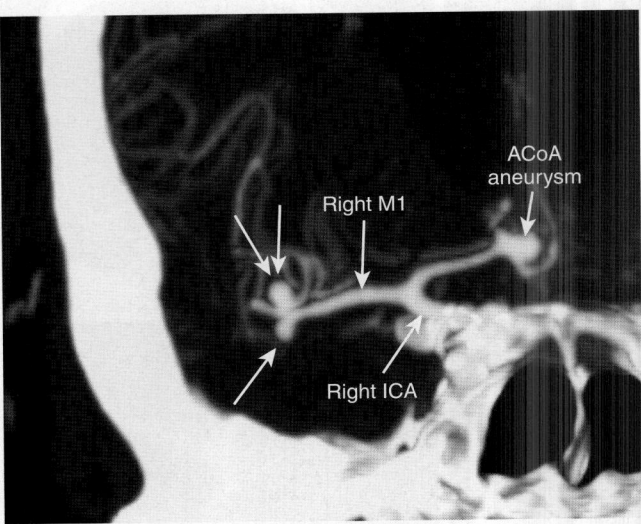

FIGURE 75-5 Complex type right-sided MbifA with two separate domes projecting in opposite directions, one inferiorly and the other superiorly. There is also an associated anterior communicating artery aneurysm.

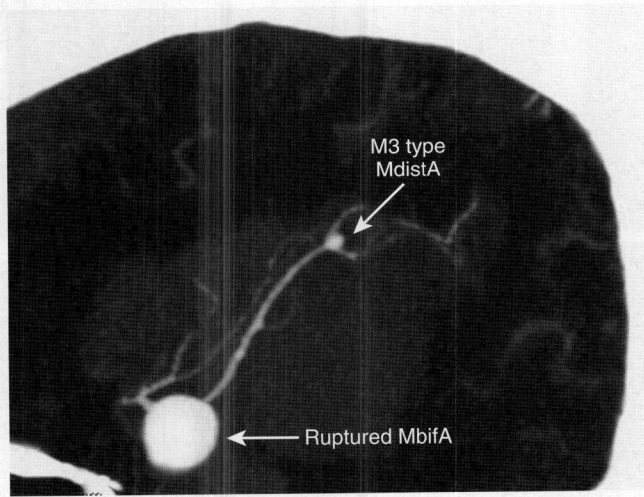

FIGURE 75-7 M3 type MdistA found in patient with ruptured MbifA as seen on sagittal computed tomography angiography.

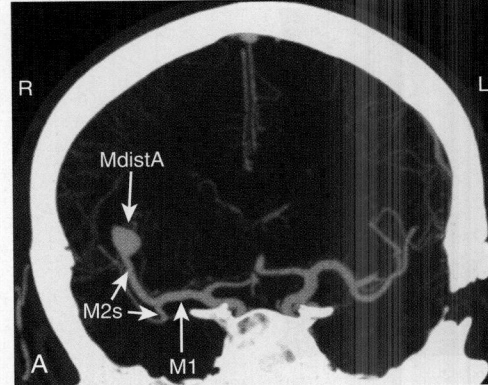

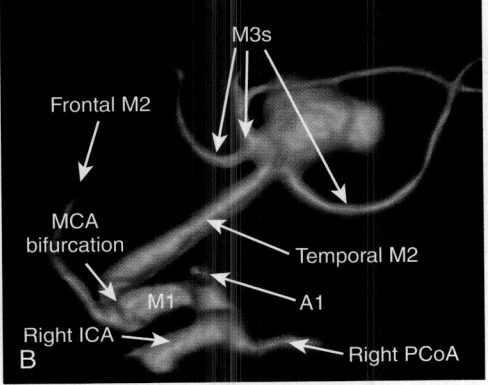

FIGURE 75-6 M2–M3 junction type MdistA as seen on 2D (A) and 3D (B) computed tomography angiography.

The pterional approach is reserved for selected cases with space occupying ICH or giant aneurysms. A detailed description of the LSO approach has been described elsewhere.[1,63]

Briefly, the head fixed to the head frame is elevated clearly above the cardiac level, rotated 20 degrees to 30 degrees toward the opposite side, tilted somewhat laterally for optimal visualization of the MCA and the aneurysm base, and minimally extended (Fig. 75-8). The lateral tilt is used to have the proximal part of the sylvian fissure almost vertical. It is an error to overturn the head so that the temporal lobe "covers" the sylvian fissure and the aneurysm in the surgeon's view requiring unnecessary retraction of the temporal lobe. It is our practice to adjust the position of the fixed head and body during the operation as needed.[64] We prefer to use a Sugita head frame with four-point fixation. Besides providing good retraction force by its fishhooks, the frame allows to be rotated during surgery. If this feature is not available, the table can be rotated as needed.

After minimal shaving, an oblique frontotemporal skin incision is made behind the hair line. The incision is short and stops 2 to 3 cm above the zygomatic arch. The incision

is partially opened by frontal spring hooks. The temporal muscle is split vertically by a short incision, and a single spring hook is placed in the incision to retract the muscle toward the zygomatic arch. The one-layer skin–muscle flap is retracted frontally by spring hooks until the superior orbital rim and the anterior zygomatic arch are exposed (Fig. 75-9). The extent of craniotomy depends on the surgeon's experience and preferences. Usually, a small LSO craniotomy is all that is necessary (the keyhole principle). A single burr hole is placed just under the temporal line in the bone, the superior insertion of the temporal muscle. The bone flap of 3×3 cm is detached mostly by the side-cutting drill, and the basal part can be drilled before lifting. In case of ICH or giant MCAA, a larger craniotomy is performed toward the zygomatic arch such as the classic pterional craniotomy. The vertical bone ridge and lateral sphenoid ridge are drilled to create an optimal view of the sylvian cistern (Fig. 75-10). Anterior clinoid is not removed.

The dura is incised curvilinearly with the base sphenoidally. Dural edges are elevated by multiple stitches, and extended over the craniotomy dressings. From this point on, all surgery is performed under the operating microscope, including the skin closure.

For MdistAs, the exposure of aneurysms on the M2s or at the M2–M3 junction depends on the location of the main bifurcation and the presence of ICH or associated aneurysms. These aneurysms are operated on using the LSO approach with little less of sphenoid ridge removal. Aneurysms located on the inferior (temporal) M2 trunk or its branches are usually hidden under the temporal operculum, so the head should be rotated less with minimal or no lateral tilt. Aneurysms located on the superior (frontal) M2 trunk are hidden under frontal operculum, so lateral tilt is usually helpful. The exposure in aneurysms distal to the M2–M3 junction depends on how distally they are in the sylvian fissure. Positioning of the head, and placement of the craniotomy and approach, should be tailored according to anatomic localization and projection of the aneurysm, and the presence of ICH or associated aneurysms. Usually,

Table 75-6 Postoperative Care of Patients with Aneurysmal SAH at Neurosurgical ICU in Helsinki

Prevention/Treatment of Vasospasm
Nimodipine oral/I.V.
Magnesium: 60 mmol/day (only in detected vasospasm)
Hypertension: phenylephrine, norepinephrine, or dopamine/dobutamine
Hemodilution: Hct 0.3. Ringer's acetate (+NaCl)/tetrastarch
Prevention of vasospasm:
HH: 1-2; Fischer: 1-2; sBP > 110–120 mm Hg, normovolemia
HH: 1-2; Fischer: 3-4; sBP > 140 mm Hg, normovolemia
HH: 3-5; Fischer: 3-4; sBP > 140–160 mm Hg, slight hypervolemia
Treatment of vasospasm:
"Triple H" (hypertension; hypervolemia; hemodilution): sBP > 160–180 mm Hg

Pulmonary/Airway Management
Oxygen/ventilatory support as needed: Normoventilation, SaO_2 > 95%, PaO_2 > 13 kPa
Pneumonia, aspiration: Antibiotics
Pulmonary edema: Noncardiogenic/cardiogenic, PEEP, furosemide, dobutamine

Seizures
Previous antiepileptic drugs (lorazepam or lavetiracetam)
No routine prophylaxis

Electrolytes and Glucose
Correct abnormalities
Hyponatremia: SIADH, CSW syndrome
B-gluc 5-8 mmol/L

Sedation, Postoperative Pain and Fever
Propofol and/or dexmedetomidine patients under mechanical ventilation
Benzodiatzepines
Opioids: Oxycodone
Paracetamol
Active cooling as needed
NSAIDs: 5–7 days post SAH

Thromboembolism
Antiembolic or pneumatic compression stockings
Individually LMWH 5–7 days postcraniotomy

CSW, cerebral salt wasting; HH, Hunt-Hess; LMWH, low molecular weight heparin; PEEP, positive end-expiratory pressure; SAH, subarachnoid hemorrhage; sBP, systolic blood pressure; SIADH, syndrome of inappropriate antidiuretic hormone hypersecretion.

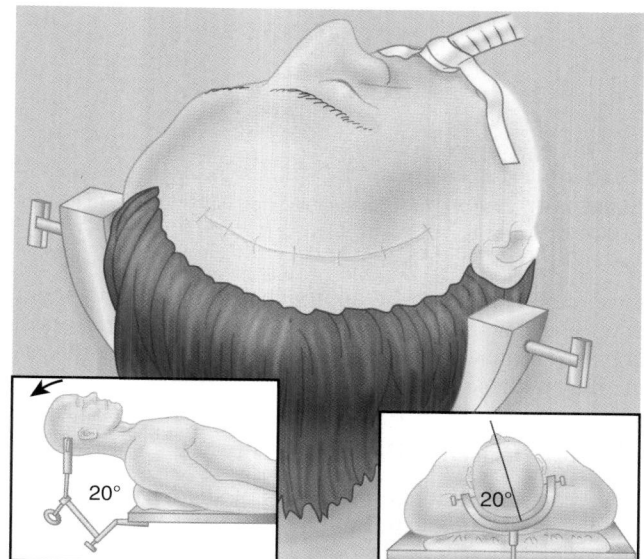

FIGURE 75-8 Positioning of the patient for right-sided lateral supraorbital approach.

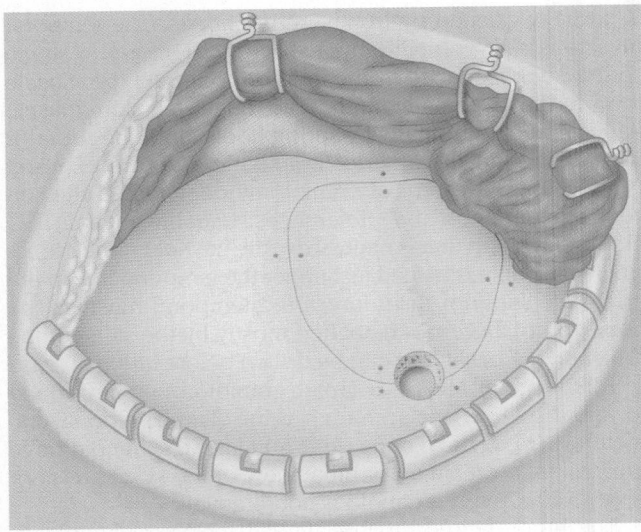

FIGURE 75-9 Location of the burr hole and the bone flap.

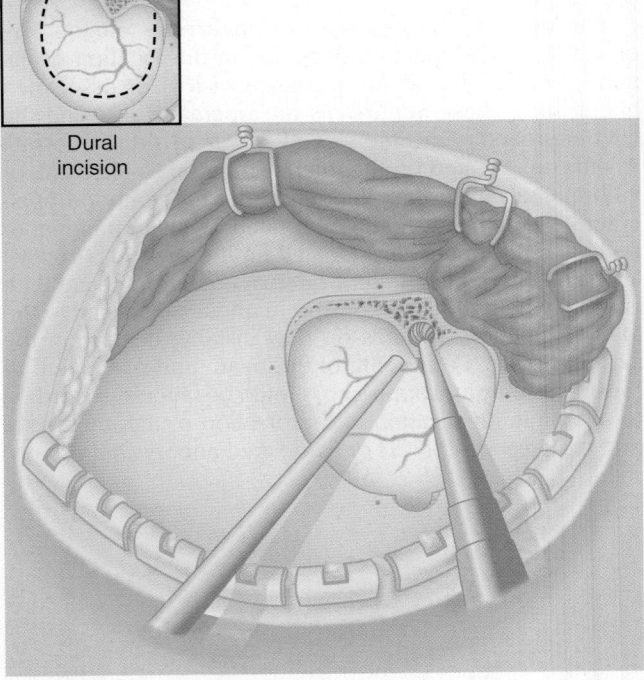

Dural incision

FIGURE 75-10 Removal of the sphenoid wing with high-speed drill and dural incision.

these aneurysms can be approached through a temporal craniotomy with the patient in lateral (park bench) position.[65] Neuronavigation may be of help in planning the craniotomy in these cases.

Intracerebral Hematoma

MbifAs are the most frequent cause of aneurysmal ICH that requires emergency removal (Fig. 75-1A to C).[17] In the Kuopio series, as many as 44% of the 711 ruptured MbifAs had bled into the adjacent brain tissue (Table 75-4). In our practice, patients with massive ICHs are transferred directly to the operating room from emergent CT/CTA for immediate evacuation of the ICH and clipping of the aneurysm(s). Early surgical removal of massive ICH is believed to improve the outcome with ruptured MCA aneurysms.[10,17,30,31,66-71] The propensity for ICH may explain higher-than-average management morbidity and mortality of patients with MbifA compared to other anterior circulation aneurysms.[17]

In case of large ICH and lack of space, after dissection of the proximal M1 to gain control, a small cortical incision is made accordingly in the temporal side of the sylvian fissure, or in the frontal side, avoiding the Broca's area. If the ICH is very large, a small part of it is removed via a cortical incision for more space, but care is taken not to cause inadvertent aneurysm rupture as this would be difficult to control through the ICH cavity. In removing the ICH clot, before or after clipping, only minor force should be applied so as not to sever the perforating arteries.

Dissection Toward the Aneurysm

For intrasylvian orientation, it is important to evaluate the preoperative images for the depth of the sylvian fissure, the length and course of the M1 and M2s, and the projection and size of the aneurysm dome. In addition, the CTA should be carefully reviewed for calcifications in the M1 trunk, the bifurcation, and the aneurysm wall. Calcified plaques in the M1 wall will interfere with temporary clipping, and those at the bifurcation area may risk rupture during clipping or result in incomplete closure of the neck.

The extent and placement of the arachnoid opening depends on whether the aneurysm is unruptured or ruptured, length of the M1, size of the aneurysm, and orientation of the dome with respect to the parent artery and the originating branches. Factors that would require more extensive and more distal opening of the sylvian fissure for better proximal control of the M1 or even the ICA bifurcation are ruptured aneurysm, secondary pouch in the aneurysm dome, intertruncal or lateral projection of the dome, and involvement of branches or the MCA bifurcation in the aneurysm. In small unruptured MCAAs when the dome is projecting toward the insula or inferiorly in the sylvian fissure, a more direct approach to the aneurysm is possible. In giant MCAAs, the sylvian fissure is opened widely, both from the carotid cistern and distal to the aneurysm. We measure the distance from the ICA bifurcation to the aneurysm along the M1 and also the vertical distance of the aneurysm from the zygomatic arch. Based on these two measurements, the exact site for a limited arachnoid opening and entering into the sylvian fissure is estimated. Our tactics are to enter the sylvian fissure and to go from distal to proximal toward the aneurysm. Only in some ruptured or complex aneurysms, where proximal control might be difficult to obtain through this route, we initially dissect the proximal M1 from the carotid cistern side to have control before entering the sylvian fissure. It is not necessary to open the whole sylvian fissure as most MCAAs can be clipped using only a 10- to 15-mm long arachnoid opening.

The best place to enter the sylvian fissure is usually where transparent arachnoid is present. The venous anatomy on the surface of the sylvian fissure is highly variable. Multiple large veins often follow the course of the sylvian fissure, draining into the sphenoparietal or cavernous sinuses. These veins are generally running on the temporal side of the sylvian fissure. Generally, we prefer to open the arachnoid covering the sylvian fissure on the frontal lobe side. However, in the presence of multiple large veins or anatomic variations the dissection plan should be tailored accordingly. Dissection of the sylvian fissure is more difficult with swollen brain tissue in acute SAH or with adhesions from previous SAH or microsurgery. Preservation of the dissection plane is mandatory.

The whole opening of the sylvian fissure should be performed under very high magnification (7–9×) of the microscope. First, we usually open a small window in the arachnoid with a pair of jeweler forceps or a sharp needle acting like an arachnoid knife. Then we expand the sylvian fissure by injecting saline using a handheld syringe, that is, the water dissection technique of Toth.[72] The idea is to get

relatively deep into the sylvian fissure to enter the sylvian cistern from this small arachnoid opening. There are two arachnoid membranes that need to be opened, a superficial one covering the cortex and a deeper one inside the fissure limiting the sylvian cistern (Fig. 75-11). Once inside the sylvian cistern, the dissection proceeds proximally by gently spreading the fissure in an inside-out manner. In our experience, this technique allows easier identification of the proper dissection plane. Bipolar forceps and suction act both as dissection instruments and delicate microretractors.[64] Cottonoids applied at the edges of the dissected space act as soft retractors, and pressure applied gently on both the walls of the fissure will stretch the overlying bridging tissues, facilitating their sharp dissection. All arachnoid attachments and strands are cut with microscissors, which can be also used as a dissector when the tips are closed. In order to preserve larger veins, some small bridging veins may have to be coagulated and cut.

Inside the sylvian cistern, the M3s and M2s are identified and followed proximally. The M2s should be covered by the intermediate sylvian membrane, another arachnoid membrane, which in some patients can be rather prominent and in others hardly identifiable. By following the M2s proximally, one should arrive at the MCA bifurcation where the most difficult task is to identify the M1 trunk for proximal control (Fig. 75-12A). In the surgical view the M1 is often hidden by the bifurcation and its course is often along the visual axis of the microscope making its identification quite difficult during the initial dissection of the MCA bifurcation. One of the M2 trunks with medial course is easily confused with the M1 unless one keeps this in mind. The M1 can be often more easily reached from behind and below the bifurcation than from in front and above. A more distal opening of the sylvian fissure provides a better angle to visualize and obtain control of the M1 just beneath the bifurcation. Also, both M2s should be prepared for temporary clips. For M1As, the dissection continues proximally along the M1 trunk in the deepest and often the narrowest part of the proximal sylvian fissure. Care is needed to avoid severing the LLAs during the various stages of dissection. To better expose the origin of the cortical branches and the M1A base, gentle retraction of the M1 trunk frontally by suction or bipolar may be necessary.

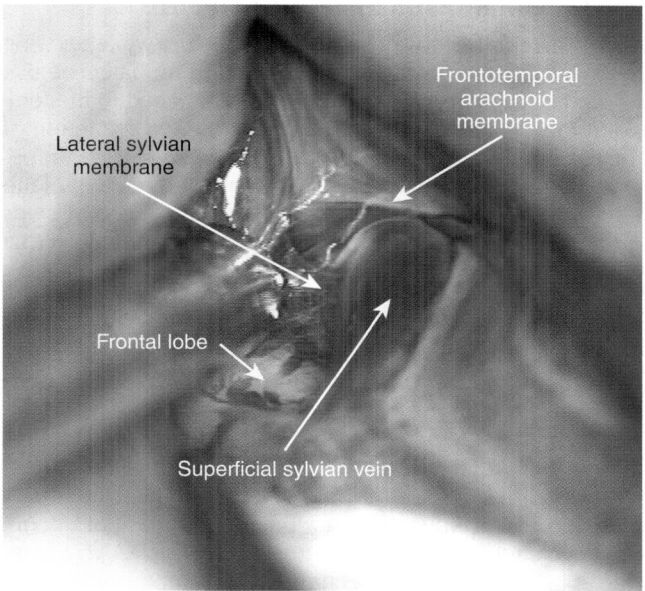

FIGURE 75-11 Intraoperative photograph showing the course of superficial sylvian vein between the two arachnoid membranes.

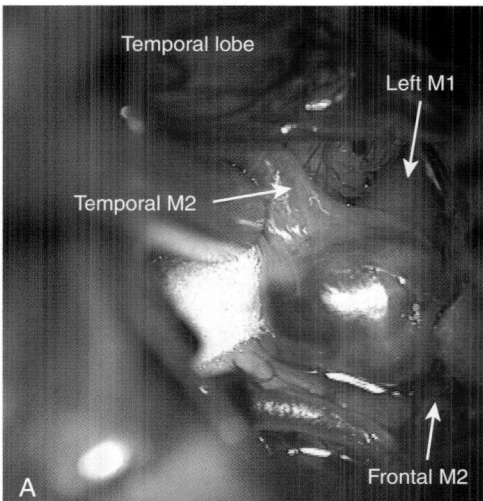

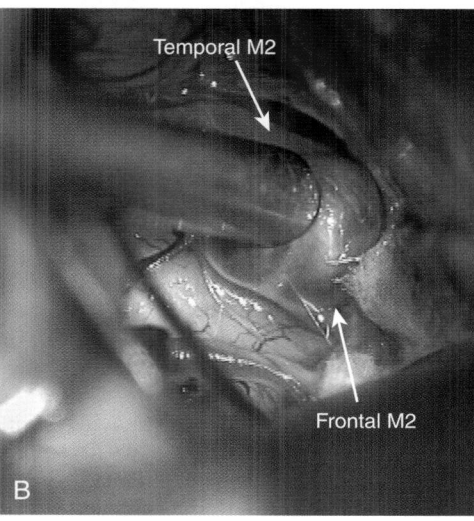

FIGURE 75-12 Intraoperative photograph. A, An unruptured left-sided intertruncal type MbifA. B, Origin of the frontal M2 branch can be seen only after the dome has been dislocated with suction.

Numerous arachnoid trabeculations around the proximal M1 trunk make dissection demanding, and we advocate sharp dissection.

Dissection and Clipping of MCA Aneurysms

Usually, dissecting the dome completely free before applying the so-called "pilot" clip is not recommended. Instead, the arteries around and adjacent to the base should be dissected free and the base cleared thoroughly. The M1, M2s, and adjacent and perforating branches should be unhurriedly, clearly, and painstakingly visualized before final clipping of the MCAA neck (Fig. 75-12B).

TEMPORARY CLIPPING

Frequent use of temporary clips on the M1 and the M2s allows for a safe and sharp dissection of MCAAs and the adjacent arteries. The duration of each temporary occlusion should be kept as short as possible (maximally 5 minutes). In elderly patients and those with very atherosclerotic arteries, temporary clipping should be used more sparingly. Curved temporary clips may be more suitable for proximal control and straight ones for distal control. Dissection and preparation of sites for temporary clips should be performed with bipolar forceps with blunt tips or with a microdissector. The proximal clip can be close to the aneurysm, but the distal ones should be at a distance so as not to interfere with the visualization and permanent clipping of the aneurysm neck. It is practical to gently press the temporary clip down by a small cottonoid to protect it from the dissecting instruments. Temporary clips should be removed from distal to proximal order. When removing the temporary clips, they are first opened in place to test for unwanted bleeding from the potentially incompletely clipped aneurysm. Quick removal can be followed by heavy bleeding and great difficulties in replacing the clip. While removing the temporary clips, even the slightest resistance should be noted as possible involvement of a small branch or a perforating artery in the clip or its applier.

FINAL CLIPPING

A proper selection of clips with different shapes and lengths of blades and applicators appropriate to the imaged MCAA anatomy should be ready for use. The optimal final clip closes the entire base but prevents kinking or occlusion of the adjacent branches. Typically, the smallest possible clip should be selected. The blade of a single occluding clip should be 1.5 times the width of the base as suggested by Drake. Frequent short-term application of temporary clips during the placement and replacement of aneurysm clips is routine in our practice. We prefer inserting first a pilot clip over the MCAA dome, often preferring Sugita clips for their wide opening and blunt tips. The pilot clip is finally exchanged for a smaller and lighter final clip. As the clip is slowly closed, the surrounding arteries and perforators are inspected for kinking, twisting, and compromised flow. Adequate dissection, proper sizes of clips, and careful checking that the clip blades are well placed up to their tips are required to preserve the adjacent branches. We use multiple clipping, two or more clips, for wide-based large

aneurysms, and often calcified, thick-walled aneurysms. In these cases, one should rather leave little neck to prevent occlusion of the parent artery by the clip. After the clipping, the dome of MCAA may be punctured and collapsed. It is important to inspect clip tips on both sides to ensure that they have not caught any branches or any of the perforators. The clip blades should completely close the neck of the aneurysm. Because the bifurcation may become kinked or occluded after removal of the retractors, the flow should be checked once more and papaverine applied. When appropriate, while not risking the surrounding branches, we resect the aneurysm dome for the final check of closure and for research purposes. This policy teaches one to dissect aneurysm domes more completely and thereby avoid closure of branching arteries. Opening of the aneurysm facilitates effective clipping by reducing intraluminal pressure and should be used in strong-walled, large, and giant aneurysms.

ANEURYSM RUPTURE BEFORE CLIPPING

Middle cerebral artery aneurysms may rupture while opening the sylvian fissure or dissecting the aneurysm base. The risk of rupture is highest for the aneurysms attached to the temporal lobe, where extensive manipulation and retraction of the temporal lobe may stretch the dome and cause intraoperative rupture of the aneurysm. This is why retraction of the temporal lobe should be avoided during the initial steps of the dissection. In case of rupture, control should be first attempted via suction and compression of the bleeding site with Cottonoids. One should not try to clip the aneurysm in haste directly as this could easily end up in tearing the aneurysm base or even the parent artery. Instead, the aneurysm should be isolated with temporary clips applied both proximally and distally. With the bleeding under control, the aneurysm neck is dissected free and the pilot clip applied. Short and sudden hypotension by cardiac arrest, induced by intravenous adenosine,[59] can be used to facilitate quick dissection and application of a pilot clip in case of uncontrolled bleeding. A small and thin walled MCAA may rupture at its neck during dissection. Under temporary clipping of arteries, reconstruction of the base by involving a part of the parent artery in the clip should be attempted. One option, hindered by the deep location inside the sylvian fissure, is to suture the rupture site with 8-0 or 9-0 running sutures or to repair the site using anastoclips,[73] followed by clipping and augmented by glue.

Acute Hydrocephalus and Cerebrospinal Fluid Drainage

In the Kuopio series, 29% of the SAH patients had hydrocephalus early in the treatment (Table 75-4). In few cases, an emergent extraventricular drain (EVD) can be life-saving to reduce the ICP, and thereby to lower the risk of brain damage. In most cases we do this after securing an acutely ruptured aneurysm, but we have not seen iatrogenic ruptures due to puncturing of the ventricles, either. Nowadays, leaving drainage via lamina terminalis after clipping of the aneurysm has almost completely replaced conventional EVDs.[74] In most unruptured MCAAs, we directly open the sylvian fissure. In ruptured MCAAs and in some unruptured ones, carotid and chiasmatic cisterns are first opened to gradually let cerebrospinal fluid (CSF) drain. In acute SAH, we usually continue the dissection subfrontally to open the lamina terminalis for additional CSF removal before clipping.[74] A catheter can be inserted into the third ventricle through the same opening in the lamina terminalis for postoperative ICP monitoring and CSF drainage. Intraoperative ventricular puncture is rarely adopted and may be technically challenging.

Special Considerations for Different Locations and Orientations of MCA Aneurysms

M1A

M1As are located deep and proximal inside the sylvian fissure where there is much less space for dissection than in more distal MCAAs. M1As are intimately connected to one or more branching arteries of the M1 and often in close proximity to LLAs (Fig. 75-3A to F). They are often wide-necked, small, and thin-walled, which makes their proper clipping tedious. There are few reports of M1A microsurgery.[1,8,9,13,75,76]

When M1A projects toward the temporal lobe, dissection can be started distally, first with the identification of arterial branches in the sylvian fissure, and continued toward M1 trunk for proximal control (see Hernesniemi, MCA Video 1 MCA Video 2). Dissection should be performed on the temporal side of M1 trunk, in anteroinferior direction, to avoid injury to LLAs and to identify cortical branches adjacent to M1A base. To better expose the origin of the cortical branches and M1A base, gentle retraction of the M1 trunk frontally by suction or bipolar may be necessary. When the M1A projects frontally, we advocate starting dissection medially from the ICA bifurcation. Numerous arachnoid trabeculations around the proximal M1 trunk make dissection demanding, and sharp dissection is advocated. In this type of M1A, thin and fragile branches adjacent to the M1A base are particularly vulnerable to injury. The deep location of M1As means much less room for manipulation.

In temporally oriented (inferior wall type) M1As, the aneurysm dome may prevent visualization and dissection of the M1 junction at the ICA bifurcation deep in the sylvian fissure, making temporary occlusion difficult. In frontally oriented M1As (superior wall type), it is always possible to prepare the proximal and distal parts of M1 for temporary clips. In this type, the efferent arteries may be attached to the M1A wall and difficult to dissect, requiring a delicate dissection technique not to damage them. Short temporary and final clips should be preferred for this group of aneurysms.

MBIFA

Of the MCA aneurysms, MbifAs are by far the most frequent (Table 75-2). In population-based services, MbifAs are frequent targets for elective surgery (unruptured), acute surgery (ruptured), emergency surgery (large ICH), and even advanced approaches (giant) (see Hernesniemi, MCA Video 5).[2] MbifAs are often broad-necked and may be dysmorphic in shape involving one or both branches of the

bifurcation (M2s). Other branches may be attached to their wall, and, less frequently, perforators may be at risk when originating from the bifurcational region. Exposure in MbifA surgery depends on the length of the M1, the size and projection of the aneurysm dome, and the existence of an ICH or associated aneurysms.

Intertruncal MbifAs project superiorly in the coronal (AP) and posteriorly in the axial plane (Fig. 75-4A and B). The dome projects to the same direction as the M2 trunks and lies between them. The base is often broad and involves the origin of one M2 (the thicker one) or both. The attachment of the M2s to the base and the proximal part of the dome makes intertruncal MbifAs demanding to clip adequately. The head is rotated 25 to 30 degrees with minimal extension and some lateral tilt. As the dome of the aneurysm lies between M2s, we prefer distal opening of the sylvian fissure and careful exposure of the frontal M2 at the beginning. Dissection is continued at the frontal side of the bifurcation, so as not to expose the aneurysm dome, and then turned below to search the M1. In intertruncal MbifAs, painstaking dissection of the base is required, with visualization of the M1 in the early phase of dissection for temporary clip placement.

Inferior MbifAs project inferiorly in the coronal (AP) and anteriorly toward the sphenoid ridge, in the axial plane (Fig. 75-4C and D). Consequently, the dome is projecting to the temporal aspect of the surgeon's view toward the surface of the sylvian fissure (Fig. 75-13). Minor flexion of the head plus normal rotation and increased lateral tilt provide a good view of the sphenoid ridge and proximal part of the M1. After proximal opening of the sylvian fissure, dissection is continued on the frontal side of the bifurcation, and, with slight retraction of the frontal lobe, the M1 and the frontal M2 are visualized and dissected (see Hernesniemi, MCA Video 3 and MCA Video 4). Any retraction on the temporal side would risk a rupture of the aneurysm. After sharp dissection of both the M1 and the frontal M2, the base of the aneurysm is exposed. Visualization of the temporal M2 requires further careful dissection on the distal side of the base. The base of this aneurysm type is usually free

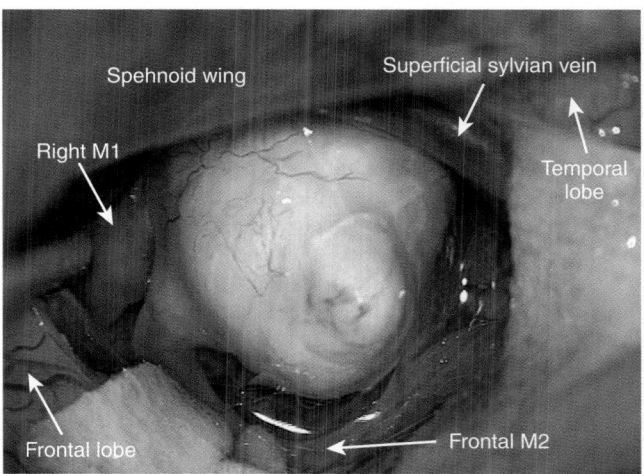

FIGURE 75-13 Intraoperative photograph showing a right-sided, heavily calcified and atherosclerotic inferior projecting MbifA. Note how the aneurysm dome is pointing toward the surface of the sylvian fissure. The other M2 is hidden behind the aneurysm dome.

Table 75-7   1-Year Outcome of 802 Ruptured MCAAs Compared to Initial HH Score

Initial HH score	Good Recovery	Moderate Disability	Severe Disability	Vegetative	Dead	Total
I	48 (79%)	9 (15%)	0	0	4 (7%)	61
II	228 (80%)	29 (10%)	10 (3%)	0	19 (7%)	286
III	91 (44%)	59 (29%)	20 (10%)	1 (0.5%)	34 (17%)	205
IV	25 (20%)	34 (27%)	16 (13%)	1 (1%)	52 (41%)	128
V	5 (4%)	6 (5%)	11 (9%)	0	100 (82%)	122
Total	397 (50%)	137 (17%)	57 (7%)	2 (0.2%)	209 (26%)	802

Note: Percentages are given for row.
HH, Hunt-Hess; MCAAs, middle cerebral artery aneurysms

of perforating arteries or branches, and the pilot clip can be placed easily under the control of temporary clips. Special attention must be paid to the origin of the temporal M2 trunk which easily becomes pinched or occluded by the distal tips of the clip blades.

Lateral MbifAs project laterally in the coronal (AP) plane and in the axial plane (Fig. 75-4E and F). In the surgeon's view, lateral MbifAs follow the same direction as the M1 trunk. Minor flexion of the head together with normal rotation (25–30 degrees) and more pronounced lateral tilt provide the best possible view of the base of the aneurysm and direct the tip of the aneurysm away from surgical trajectory. Lateral MbifAs are frequently attached to the arachnoid coverings of the sylvian fissure, risking premature rupture if the dissection of the coverings is started improperly. Sylvian dissection is started distally to find the frontal M2 which is then followed toward the bifurcation and the base of the aneurysm (see Hernesniemi, MCA Video 6). To prepare for a premature rupture, first the base of the aneurysm is carefully prepared for a pilot clip placement over the dome, and then the dissection is continued toward the M1 to find a proper place for proximal temporary clip. Special care must be taken to visualize the origin of the temporal M2. Coagulation and reshaping must be done with respect to the origins of the M2s. A final clip is placed along the largest diameter of the base.

Insular MbifAs project medially in the coronal (AP) plane and medially in the axial plane (Fig. 75-4G and H). In the surgeon's view, insular MbifAs project behind the bifurcation, toward the insular surface. The head is rotated more than normal (>25 to 30 degrees) so that the bifurcation is exposed to the surgeon, making proximal control and clipping most feasible. However, overturning may cause hiding of the sylvian fissure by the temporal lobe. Because the aneurysm dome projects behind the bifurcation, distal to proximal dissection of the M2s, the bifurcation and the M1 is safe. When the M1 and M2s are free, two to three temporary clips are applied, and with complete isolation of the blood flow, the base of the aneurysm is carefully dissected in its anterior and lateral parts. The shortest possible pilot clip is placed on the base and the temporary clips are removed. The position of the pilot clip is carefully checked with particular care for small perforating branches, which might easily be occluded, in the same way as during clipping of ICA and basilar tip aneurysms.

Complex MbifAs are a group of dysmorphic and large or giant aneurysms, where the growth of the dome is usually multidirectional and the relation of the base with the M1 and the M2s may be a combination of the other MbifA types

(Fig. 75-5). Head positioning and craniotomy should be tailored according to the 3D relation of aneurysm with the MCA bifurcation. Proper clipping of the aneurysm usually requires a combination of several clips.

MdistA

MdistAs are the least frequent of MCA aneurysms (Table 75-2). The greatest challenge in microneurosurgical treatment of MdistAs is to localize them, as they lie deep in the sylvian cistern, among the distal branches of the MCA.[3] Intraoperative navigation may be further complicated by the presence of SAHs and ICHs. Furthermore, MdistAs can be mycotic, inflammatory, or dissecting. The lack of collateral circulation makes occlusion more challenging, necessitating bypass and revascularization techniques. There are only few reports on management of MdistAs.[3,17,77-79]

The exposure in aneurysms on the M2 or at the M2–M3 junction depends on the location of the main bifurcation and the presence of ICH or associated aneurysms (Fig. 75-6A and B). In the proximity of the main MCA bifurcation, the same approach as for MbifAs will do. To expose more distal MdistAs, the approach must be more occipital over the sylvian fissure (see Hernesniemi, MCA Video 7). We measure the distance between the ICA and the MCA bifurcation (length of M1 segment) in CTA images, in both coronal and axial planes. This is important when selecting the proper site for the arachnoid opening and for intrasylvian orientation. The more distal the MdistAs are, the more difficult they are to localize. Bony landmarks in the CTA are of less value in the localization of MdistAs than in M1As or MbifAs. The sylvian fissure is opened at a proper site proximal to the aneurysm, and the dissection is performed from proximal to distal toward the aneurysm. After finding the aneurysm, the rest of the dissection and subsequent clipping are often straightforward. When the aneurysm site is identified, the parent artery is dissected free and a temporary clip is applied to allow final dissection of the aneurysm dome and clipping of its neck.

The exposure in aneurysms distal to the M2–M3 junction depends on how distally they are located in the sylvian fissure (Fig. 75-7). Positioning and placement of the craniotomy and approach should be tailored according to the anatomic localization and projection of the aneurysm, and the presence of an ICH or associated aneurysms. Typically, these aneurysms can be approached through a temporal craniotomy with the patient in lateral (park bench) position. When MdistAs originate from the branches distal to the M2–M3 junction, they are more difficult to find, especially when the sylvian fissure is filled with fresh blood in acute SAH. The parent artery and the aneurysm are usually deep and behind a corner in the T-shaped sylvian fissure, hidden behind the frontal (superior) or the temporal (inferior) operculum of the insula. Neuronavigation, intraoperative noninvasive indocyaninen green angiography (ICG),[80] or color Doppler ultrasound, should be considered for localizing the aneurysm. The actual clipping of the aneurysm is seldom a problem. A small and light final clip should be used when possible to prevent kinking of the arteries.

Postoperative Care and Imaging

Anesthesiologic principles for our postoperative management of patients after aneurysm surgery are summarized in Table 75-6. Postoperative imaging is performed in all patients; the aim is quality control to identify unexpected neck remnants and branch occlusions. In a previous analysis, we saw unexpected neck remnants in 10 (3%) and unexpected major branch occlusions in 11 (4%) of 306 clipped MCA aneurysms.[81] We perform CT and CTA routinely on all patients on the first postoperative day. Even though CTA has been considered less accurate than DSA for controlling neck remnants of clipped aneurysms, with modern devices and the use of titanium clips, accuracy has increased dramatically, and DSA can be reserved for complex aneurysms or situations where multiple clips prevent proper interpretation of the CTA images.[82] In general, the risk for rerupture of a previously clipped aneurysm is low and late imaging follow-up is not used routinely.[83,84] In young patients with familial history or multiple aneurysms, we recommend a more cautious approach with long-term angiographic follow-up.[85,86]

ASSOCIATED ANEURYSMS

Half of all patients with unruptured MCAAs and 31% of those with ruptured MCAAs have at least one additional aneurysm (Table 75-5). Multiple MCAAs were seen in as many as 54% of the patients with multiple aneurysms (Fig. 75-2). Our strategy is to clip all the aneurysms that can be exposed through the same craniotomy. This may not be advisable if the clipping of the ruptured aneurysm is difficult or the brain is swollen owing to an acute SAH.[87,88] We do not advocate multiple craniotomies in the acute stage of an SAH. The remaining unruptured aneurysms can be treated depending on the estimated rupture risk and patient's wishes in separate session(s) once the patient has recovered, such as 3 to 12 months after the initial SAH.

CONTRALATERAL APPROACH FOR MCA ANEURYSMS

Contralateral M1As close to the ICA bifurcation can be clipped via the contralateral approach irrespective of their orientation.[13,87,89-91] A contralateral MbifA can also be reached, but only if it projects downward in the sylvian fissure and the length of the M1 is reasonable (<20 mm). The contralateral approach for bilateral MCA aneurysms is not recommended at an early learning curve. Extensive dissection above the chiasm along the contralateral M1 risks overstretching of the medial lenticulostriate arteries, LLAs, and perforators to the chiasm, hypothalamus, and anterior perforating substance. A contralateral approach should be avoided if the brain is swollen due to an acute SAH. In

addition, extensive venous structures in the ICA bifurcation region and along the M1 may prevent proper visualization of the contralateral M1.

Special Subgroups of MCA Aneurysms

GIANT MCA ANEURYSMS

The MCA is the most frequent site for giant aneurysms. In the Kuopio series, 4% of all MCAAs and 6% of ruptured MCAAs were giant (≥25 mm) (Table 75-3). Combined 3D DSA, CTA, and MRI data are necessary for a complete view on the vascular anatomy, intraluminal thrombus, and thickness and calcifications of the wall.[92-94] In published series, direct clipping was possible in the majority of cases (38%–71%).[9,95-100] Cases considered for EC–IC or IC–IC bypass surgery are increasing.[101]

Giant MCAAs often protrude to the middle fossa, distorting the intrasylvian anatomy and shifting the bifurcation superiorly and medially. In these cases, clipping is considered, supported by a preoperative IC–IC or EC–IC bypass if necessary. Giant MbifAs of the inferior or lateral types can usually be resected and clipped, provided that M2s are not heavily involved in the base. Notably, some residual base may be accepted when the basal aneurysm wall appears strong. We prefer acute clipping in ruptured large/giant aneurysms if the calcified wall or complex neck anatomy is not an obstacle. The operative room setup and patient's positioning should allow intraoperative angiography- and endovascular-supporting approaches.

The head position is adjusted for a better view of the proximal M1. Classical pterional approach with a large enough bone flap, also to the medial frontobasal direction, is undertaken to allow specific neurovascular techniques. For adequate visualization of the aneurysm base, an extensive exposure of the sylvian fissure is needed. The ICA bifurcation and the proximal M1 and the M2s (distal to the aneurysm) should be exposed and prepared for temporary clipping. In patients with ICH, we prefer a combination of trans-sylvian and superior temporal approaches. Here, besides the removal of a part of the hematoma, a narrow cortical incision and subpial resection may provide a better view of the aneurysm base and branches. Lamina terminalis is opened to let CSF drain. Clips of proper lengths and configurations are selected. Temporary clips are inserted onto the proximal M1 and the M2s, and the aneurysm dome is incised with a knife for internal decompression, performed usually by suction or, in case of major thrombus, by ultrasonic aspirator. Intraluminal thrombus is carefully removed, and the decompressed dome, between the neck and the incision, is clamped by a DeBakey vascular clamp. The vascular clamp softens the base for aneurysm clips and also prevents slipping of the intraluminal thrombus inside the M2s.[102] The lumen is irrigated copiously by saline. Then the dome is usually reduced to allow for final dissection of the neck anatomy before deciding how to perform the final clipping. In case of extensive atheroma, it is dangerous to remove it down to the base and some part of it is left out of the clip so as not to occlude the origins of the M2s. Thick-walled and calcified large aneurysms usually require several clips (Fig. 75-13). If the first clip slides off from a broad base to occlude the parent artery or distally to leave a large neck remnant, a ring clip can be first inserted to compress a part of the neck, and a straight second clip is placed proximally to close the remaining neck inside the ring of the first clip (Drake's tandem-clipping technique).[103]

FUSIFORM AND DISSECTING MCA ANEURYSMS

Fusiform, dissecting, and mycotic aneurysms are longitudinal dilations of the cerebral arteries. We prefer microsurgery over endovascular procedures when there is a SAH or, in particular, a large ICH. With the new intra-arterial flow diverters, the situation might change in the future, but even with them there is the problem of postprocedural anticoagulation. In some fusiform aneurysms, it may be possible to find the so-called beer belly, which is tangentially clipped with a small straight or curved clip under temporary occlusion of the parent artery. In some distal aneurysms with good retrograde flow, it is often possible to sacrifice the parent artery without a bypass. In more proximal fusiform MCAAs bypass and proximal/distal occlusion or trapping is our treatment of choice. Wrapping may be reasonable in the absence of alternatives.[104]

Bypass Surgery for MCAAs

Preoperative high-flow EC–IC or IC–IC bypass using the high-flow or low-flow bypass may be considered in large or giant MCAAs, when the exclusion of the neck from the parent and branching arteries cannot be performed.[105,106] Each case must be evaluated individually and optimal configuration for the bypass depends on the angioarchitecture of the entire MCA. We prefer to use the most simple bypass strategy, utilizing the superficial temporal artery (STA) to the MCA direct arterial bypass whenever possible. Complex bypasses and proximal high-flow bypass with the ELANA technique[107] are limited to situations where other options are not possible. A comprehensive neurovascular team should be prepared to perform intraoperative arteriotomies—for example, to remove coils or thrombi—and intraoperative EC–IC or IC–IC bypasses, and in case of emergency as well. In clinical practice, bypass surgeries are relatively infrequent and they should be channeled into high-volume, dedicated neurovascular centers.

Outcome of Ruptured MCA Aneurysms

The outcome for ruptured MCAAs depends very much on the referral system of the particular institution. In centers with population responsibility where also poor-grade patients are also routinely admitted and treated, the management outcome is always going to be worse than in referral centers that treat mainly good-grade patients. In Suzuki's series (413 patients), 94% of the patients were in good or excellent condition 6 months after treatment.[11] Half of these patients had late surgery or their aneurysms were unruptured and/or had good grades (0 to I). In a Hungarian series of 289 patients with MCAAs, only 18% had poor outcome after surgery in a long-term follow-up.[10] Yaşargil reported unfavorable results in only 6% of his 231 patients with MCAAs who were not operated in the acute setting.[13] Excellent results were published also by Sundt et al., with a 14% frequency for poor results after surgery for MCAAs.[108] All these are surgical series, and reflect not only excellent surgical skills but

also selection and referral bias. Early surgery is now advocated to prevent early reruptures with high morbidity and mortality.[109]

Here we present results from the Kuopio Aneurysm Database in a patient population that is much less selected and where large numbers of poor-grade patients are admitted and treated. The department of neurosurgery at Kuopio is the only neurosurgical center for the entire eastern region of Finland with a catchment population of about 1 million. Between 1977 and 2005, there were 802 patients with ruptured MCAAs as mentioned earlier (see Incidence of MCA Aneurysm section). On admission, 346 (43%) of these patients were Hunt and Hess (HH) grade 1 or 2, 204 (26%) were HH 3, and 250 (31%) were HH grade 4 or 5. Of the 802 patients, 67% had favorable outcome (Glasgow Outcome Score [GOS] ≥ 4) at 1 year after the SAH, 7% were severely disabled (GOS 3), only two patients were in a vegetative state (GOS 2), and 26% were dead (GOS 1). These results represent total management outcome irrespective of the treatment method. Of the 346 HH 1 to 2 patients, 313 (90%) had favorable outcome at 1 year. In contrast, only 70 (28%) of the 250 HH 4 to 5 patients had favorable outcome, and 152 (61%) of them were dead (Table 75-7). These results show how management outcome strongly depends on patient selection and why comparison of different series is very difficult.

When compared to ruptured aneurysms at other locations, patients with MCAAs had slightly worse results. Among the 1562 patients with ruptured aneurysm other than MCAAs, 70% had a favorable outcome, 6% were severely disabled, and 23% were dead at 1 year. The overall management outcome was almost equal for all MCAA sites: 34% poor outcome (GOS ≤ 3) in patients with ruptured M1A, 32% with ruptured MbifA, and 30% for ruptured MdistA. Our earlier analysis of 561 MCAAs showed that in ruptured MCAAs, the patient's condition on admission, vasospasm, postoperative hematoma, and age are the most significant independent contributors to outcome.[17] Temporal ICHs, together with vasospasm and inadvertent occlusion of main vessel(s) or thalamostriate perforators, explain specific late disabilities seen in patients with MCAAs (see below).

Specific Late Disabilities Associated with Ruptured MCAAs

Epilepsy. The incidence of late epilepsy after SAH varies from 7% to 25% in different studies,[110-115] the risk depending on the exact aneurysm location, presence or absence of a temporal ICH, brain ischemia, and hypertension. Also, the existence of multiple IAs increases the risk for late epilepsy. In our series, late epilepsy occurred in 18% of the long-term survivors with a single MCAA. The frequencies were even higher in patients with MIA and one MCAA (20%) and with multiple MCAAs (27%). This is significantly higher than with any other ruptured aneurysms. Frequencies for late epilepsy were not significantly different according to MCAA location: M1A 22%, MbifA 24%, and MdistA 30%. ICH was a significant risk factor for the development of epilepsy. Half of the long-term survivors with ruptured MCAAs and epilepsy had an ICH on their initial CT scan, most often in the temporal lobe.

Hemiparesis. As a result of its feeding areas and the scarcity of the collateral circulation, as well as the frequent ICHs related to ruptured MCAAs, lesions (and spasm) of the MCA frequently cause hemiparesis and/or dysphasia. There were significantly more cases of severe hemiparesis among long-time survivors with ruptured MCAAs than among those with ruptured aneurysms at other sites. The M1As were associated with hemiparesis in 27% compared to 12% for MbifAs. This may be explained by technical difficulties associated with proper clipping of M1As, leading to occlusion or kinking of the anterior temporal artery, or the thalamoperforating arteries especially in superiorly projecting M1As.

Visual field deficit. Visual field deficits were more common in patients with MCAAs than in patients with any other types of aneurysm: 20% and 11%, respectively. There were no differences in the frequencies among different MCAA sites. In two thirds (69%) of the cases, visual field deficits were at least partly caused by the close anatomic relationship between the course of the optic tract and the temporal ICH.

Conclusions

The middle cerebral artery is a frequent site for intracranial aneurysms. MCAAs can be found along the entire course of the MCA, but in more than 80%, the aneurysm is at the MCA bifurcation. The MCAAs often have a broad base with several branches originating from or near the base. They are associated with multiple aneurysms in 30% to 50%. When ruptured, MCAAs present with ICH on the initial CT scan in 40% to 50%. The complex 3D anatomy, broad base with originating branches, frequent ICHs, and relatively superficial location often favor microsurgical clipping over endovascular coiling in treatment of MCAAs to prevent late recanalization and subsequent rupture risk. Exact aneurysm location and orientation with respect to the course of the MCA must be taken into account when planning the microsurgical approach to MCAAs. Good knowledge of microanatomy of the entire MCA region is mandatory for proper execution of the microsurgical clipping of MCAAs. Our belief is that only competent aneurysm surgeons should perform open aneurysm surgery.

KEY REFERENCES

Dashti R, Rinne J, Hernesniemi J, et al. Microneurosurgical management of proximal middle cerebral artery aneurysms. *Surg Neurol.* 2007;67:6-14.

Dashti R, Hernesniemi J, Niemela M, et al. Microneurosurgical management of middle cerebral artery bifurcation aneurysms. *Surg Neurol.* 2007;67:441-456.

Dashti R, Hernesniemi J, Niemela M, et al. Microneurosurgical management of distal middle cerebral artery aneurysms. *Surg Neurol.* 2007;67:553-563.

Dashti R, Laakso A, Niemela M, et al. Microscope-integrated near-infrared indocyanine green videoangiography during surgery of intracranial aneurysms: the Helsinki experience. *Surg Neurol.* 2009;71:543-550.

Heiskanen O, Poranen A, Kuurne T, et al. Acute surgery for intracerebral haematomas caused by rupture of an intracranial arterial aneurysm. A prospective randomized study. *Acta Neurochir (Wien).* 1988;90:81-83.

Hernesniemi J, Ishii K, Niemela M, et al. Lateral supraorbital approach as an alternative to the classical pterional approach. *Acta Neurochir Suppl.* 2005;94:17-21.

Hernesniemi J, Niemela M, Karatas A, et al. Some collected principles of microneurosurgery: simple and fast, while preserving normal anatomy: a review. *Surg Neurol.* 2005;64:195-200.

Heros RC. Aneurysms in the middle cerebral artery. In: Symon L, Thomas DG, Clarke K, eds. *Rob & Smith's Operative Surgery: Neurosurgery.* New York: Chapman and Hall; 1994:171-179.

Heros RC. Middle cerebral artery aneurysms. In: Wilkins RH, Rengachary SS, eds. *Neurosurgery.* New York: McGraw-Hill; 1985:1376-1382.

Inoue K, Seker A, Osawa S, et al. Microsurgical and endoscopic anatomy of the supratentorial arachnoidal membranes and cisterns. *Neurosurgery.* 2009;65:644-665.

Koivisto T, Vanninen R, Hurskainen H, et al. Outcomes of early endovascular versus surgical treatment of ruptured cerebral aneurysms. A prospective randomized study. *Stroke.* 2000;31:2369-2377.

Lawton MT, Spetzler RF. Surgical management of giant intracranial aneurysms: experience with 171 patients. *Clin Neurosurg.* 1995;42:245-266.

Lehecka M, Laakso A, Hernesniemi J. Helsinki Microneurosurgery: Basics and Tricks. Balgheim: Druckerei Hohl GmbH; 2011.

Lehto H, Dashti R, Karatas A, et al. Third ventriculostomy through the fenestrated lamina terminalis during microneurosurgical clipping of intracranial aneurysms: an alternative to conventional ventriculostomy. *Neurosurgery.* 2009;64:430-435.

Nagy L, Ishii K, Karatas A, et al. Water dissection technique of Toth for opening neurosurgical cleavage planes. *Surg Neurol.* 2006;65:38-41.

Ogilvy CS, Crowell RM, Heros RC. Surgical management of middle cerebral artery aneurysms: experience with transsylvian and superior temporal gyrus approaches. *Surg Neurol.* 1995;43:15-24.

Randell T, Niemela M, Kytta J, et al. Principles of neuroanesthesia in aneurysmal subarachnoid hemorrhage: the Helsinki experience. *Surg Neurol.* 2006;66:382-388.

Regli L, Dehdashti AR, Uske A, et al. Endovascular coiling compared with surgical clipping for the treatment of unruptured middle cerebral artery aneurysms: an update. *Acta Neurochir Suppl.* 2002;82:41-46.

Rhoton Jr AL. The supratentorial arteries. *Neurosurgery.* 2002;51:S53-S120.

Rhoton Jr AL. The cerebral veins. *Neurosurgery.* 2002;51:S159-S205.

Rinne J, Hernesniemi J, Niskanen M, et al. Analysis of 561 patients with 690 middle cerebral artery aneurysms: anatomic and clinical features as correlated to management outcome. *Neurosurgery.* 1996;38:2-11.

Suzuki J, Yoshimoto T, Kayama T. Surgical treatment of middle cerebral artery aneurysms. *J Neurosurg.* 1984;61:17-23.

Türe U, Yaşargil MG, Al-Mefty O, et al. Arteries of the insula. *J Neurosurg.* 2000;92:676-687.

Wen HT, Rhoton Jr AL, de Oliveira E, et al. Microsurgical anatomy of the temporal lobe: part 2—sylvian fissure region and its clinical application. *Neurosurgery.* 2009;65:1-36.

Yaşargil MG. Operative anatomy. In: Yaşargil MG, ed. *Microneurosurgery.* vol. 1. Stuttgart: Georg Thieme Verlag; 1984:165-168.

Yaşargil MG. Middle cerebral artery aneurysms. In: Yaşargil MG, ed. *Microneurosurgery.* vol. 2. Stuttgart: Thieme Verlag; 1984:124-164.

Numbered references appear on Expert Consult.

CHAPTER 76

Surgical Management of Terminal Basilar and Posterior Cerebral Artery Aneurysms

SCOTT Y. RAHIMI • MARK J. DANNENBAUM • C. MICHAEL CAWLEY • DANIEL L. BARROW

Background

In the early 1940s, following surgery for a posterior fossa aneurysm that ultimately took the life of the patient, Walter Dandy stated, "I know of no successful outcome from operative attack upon an aneurysm of the posterior cranial fossa, but for those upon the vertebral and posterior inferior cerebellar arteries, which afford good exposure, cures will certainly come in time."[1]

As time passed, Dandy's prediction came to fruition. Neurosurgeons overcame the obstacles that once challenged great surgeons who operated on posterior fossa aneurysms. Over the past several decades, outcomes in the surgical treatment of posterior circulation aneurysms have steadily improved. This success has been largely due to the development of the field of microsurgery with the advent of the surgical microscope and microinstruments. Success is also attributed to the numerous adjuncts to microsurgery, such as advances in neuroanesthesia and brain protection, modern aneurysm clips, intraoperative imaging, bypass techniques, skull base surgery, and specialty training of individuals allowing them to concentrate on cerebrovascular disease. Posterior circulation aneurysms, including those of the basilar apex (BA), have been among the most challenging to treat. Surgery in this area is especially treacherous due to the deep location, as well as the close proximity of perforators to the brain stem. Basilar tip aneurysms are also less frequently encountered than aneurysms of the anterior circulation, making it more difficult to master the nuances of their surgical treatment. The reduced exposure to basilar aneurysms has been exacerbated by the increasing utilization of endovascular therapy over the past decade.

The first description of a basilar aneurysm dates back to 1779, when Morgagni presented a case of an aneurysm involving the basilar artery and both posterior cerebral arteries (PCAs).[2] Little progress was made concerning the identification and treatment of posterior circulation aneurysms until the mid-20th century. In 1954, Herbert Olivecrona was the first surgeon to describe clipping of a basilar artery aneurysm through a subtemporal approach.[3] It was during this time that Charles Drake emerged as a pioneer in the surgical management of basilar tip aneurysms. In 1959, he presented his experience with four patients presenting with a

subarachnoid hemorrhage (SAH) from basilar bifurcation aneurysms at the American Academy of Neurological Surgeons in Pebble Beach, CA.[4] Although two of his patients succumbed to complications due to their initial hemorrhage, his case description laid the groundwork for standards of BA aneurysm treatment. Review of the literature over 2 decades prior to the publication of Drake's paper had identified 38 cases of aneurysms involving the vertebrobasilar (VB) circulation. Following Drake's publication, a plethora of literature were published concerning the treatment and outcome of basilar aneurysms. Kenneth Jamieson reviewed his operative experience of 19 patients with VB aneurysms.[5] Only four of those patients made sufficient recovery to return to work. As Drake's experience with basilar aneurysms grew, his results also improved in parallel.

Part of his success was also attributable to advances in microinstruments and microsurgical technique, including the use of the surgical microscope. Ultimately, these factors culminated in improved surgical outcome for Drake's patients harboring BA aneurysms. In a 1968 report, Drake described his experience after treating 17 basilar artery aneurysms with only one fatality.[6] One year later, Drake presented a review of 43 operative cases involving the VB circulation with 70% of patients attaining "satisfactory outcome."[7] As part of his legacy, Drake published his 25 years of experience treating 1767 aneurysms of the VB system 2 years prior to his death in 1998.[8] The vast majority of these patients (1286) harbored aneurysms at the basilar bifurcation or PCAs. Drake reported excellent outcomes in 70% to 80% of his patients who initially presented with a good-grade SAH and those who harbored nongiant BA aneurysms. Drake's 1996 chapter continues to be the standard that other series involving basilar artery aneurysms are judged against.

The approach to posterior circulation aneurysms has been significantly affected since the introduction of Guglielmi detachable coils (GDCs) in 1991. In the current era of minimally invasive procedures, the treatment of VB circulation aneurysms is different from what was encountered by Drake and his colleagues.

Neuroanesthesia

Improvements in the field of neuroanesthesia have allowed neurosurgeons to more safely attack aneurysm in the BA region. Our patients undergo a thorough preoperative evaluation by

---

Special thanks for the illustrations done by Eric Jablonowski.

the anesthesiology team that includes review of the patients' relevant medical history, as well as their general surgical risk factors. Most patients receive anxiolytic medications (e.g., benzodiazepines) prior to transport into the operating room. The patient may also receive light opioid sedation before insertion of a radial arterial line (many patients also receive a central venous catheter). After placement of standard monitors (pulse oximeters, electrocardiogram leads, noninvasive blood pressure cuff, and temperature probe), induction of anesthesia is performed. An intravenous anesthetic agent such as propofol or thiopental is typically administered, along with opioids and intravenous lidocaine, to blunt the hemodynamic response to intubation.

Neuromuscular blocking agents are also used to facilitate placement of the endotracheal tube. A deep plane of anesthesia is typically maintained with a volatile anesthetic such as isoflurane or sevoflurane in an O_2–air mixture. Brain relaxation is crucial for maximum exposure of the surgical site and minimization of retraction during the operation. In addition to CSF drainage following dural opening, intracranial relaxation is achieved by administration of 50 to 100 g of mannitol (0.5-2 g per kilogram of body weight) prior to entering the cranium. If further relaxation is necessary, furosemide (0.5-1 mg/kg) is given intravenously. If necessary, sympathetic agonists are used to maintain mean arterial pressure (MAP) within 20% of the patient's baseline pressure. Respiratory parameters are adjusted to keep the $PaCO_2$ between 32 and 44 mm Hg, with a PaO_2 target greater than 100 mm Hg. Continuous assessment of fluid status is facilitated by closely monitoring hourly urine output and central venous pressure. When the use of temporary clip occlusion of a parent vessel is necessary, a set of standard steps is initiated prior to clip placement. The MAP is kept above 90 mm Hg to augment collateral blood flow. Burst suppression for cerebral protection is achieved by supplementing the anesthetic with intravenous pentobarbital or propofol. Permissive hypothermia is closely monitored, and the patient is warmed to maintain a body temperature of at least 32°C. Temporary vessel occlusion is limited to 10-minute intervals to prevent ischemic injury. This technique softens the aneurysm sac, facilitating ease of clip placement at the neck. As the aneurysm sack softens, identification of perforator vessels is also achieved more easily. To lower the risk of recurrent hemorrhage prior to surgery, we routinely place our SAH patients on the lysine analogue, ε-aminocaproic acid (Amicar, Xanodyne Pharmaceuticals) with a 5-g intravenous bolus followed by 1 g/hr maintenance. We stop this infusion following clip placement.

We do not routinely perform electroencephalography or brain stem auditory evoked potentials (BAEPs) when treating BA aneurysms. An exception is made when we have treated "giants" or complex BA aneurysms using complete circulatory arrest. This technique has been shown to be a useful adjunct in the treatment of complex intracranial aneurysms, particularly when prolonged cerebral hypoperfusion is needed.[9,10] In these situations, we use electroencephalography, spontaneous somatosensory evoked potentials (SSEPs), and BAEPs, in conjunction with deep hypothermic (18°C) circulatory arrest. The suppression of electroencephalogram activity by barbiturates is used to titrate an effective dose for cerebral protection. The SSEPs are an indicator of intact sensory pathway conduction and

persist despite burst suppression. A BAEP is a useful tool, especially if manipulation of brain stem structures is anticipated during the procedure.

Surgical Strategies for BA Aneurysms

Surgical treatment of BA aneurysms is extremely challenging due to the complex anatomy in and around the interpeduncular cistern. Surgeons are forced to navigate through deep and narrow channels that make visualization of the anatomy in this region particularly difficult. The basilar tip and PCAs are located in the confined spaces of the interpeduncular cistern. They are enclosed by the posterior clinoids and clivus anteriorly, mesiotemporal lobes laterally, cerebral peduncles posteriorly, and mammillary bodies superiorly. The BA is approximately 15 mm posterior to the internal carotid artery (ICA).[11] The termination of the basilar artery gives rise to bilateral PCAs. The superior cerebellar arteries (SCAs) arise immediately proximal to the basilar bifurcation. The oculomotor nerve exits between the PCAs and the SCAs and is therefore vulnerable to injury during surgery. The segment of the PCA from its origin from the BA to the ostium of the posterior communicating artery (Pcomm) is referred to as the P1 segment of the PCA. The PCA distal to the Pcomm is also known as the P2 segment. The P2 segment extents from the Pcomm to the posterior edge of the midbrain. Flow to the PCA territory may be predominantly from the Pcomm in cases of a fetal Pcomm that occurs in 15% to 40% of the population. Anterior thalamoperforators typically arise from the Pcomm. These vessels supply a portion of the cerebral peduncles, posterior thalamus, subthalamic nucleus, optic chiasm, tuber cinereum, and mammillary bodies. The posterior thalamoperforators usually arise from the BA or the proximal P1 segments. These vessels supply the thalamus, hypothalamus, posterior limb of the internal capsule, and subthalamic nucleus. There may be considerable variation in the configuration and areas supplied by the anterior and posterior thalamoperforators. Due to the extent of the vascular territories supplied by these vessels, compromise of any of these perforators can lead to devastating results.

Approaches for BA Aneurysms

The approach to BA aneurysms largely relies on the relationship of the basilar bifurcation to the sella (Fig. 76-1). Multiple surgical approaches may be used to treat aneurysms in the BA region. These craniotomy routes include subtemporal, orbitozygomatic, and pterional craniotomies. These approaches describe an increasingly anterior trajectory to approaching basilar bifurcation aneurysms. Aneurysms arising at or below the middle depth of the sella are best approached via a subtemporal craniotomy, often combined with additional skull base techniques such as removal of the petrous apex (Kawase approach).[12] Aneurysms associated with a high bifurcation (more than 1 cm above the posterior clinoids) can be treated via an orbitozygomatic craniotomy that allows for better superior visualization due to more aggressive bone removal. Aneurysms that arise above the sella and up to 1 cm above the clinoids are accessible via a trans-sylvian pterional craniotomy. We have employed all three techniques in treating

BA aneurysms at our institution. However, we favor the use of a pterional trans-sylvian craniotomy, in combination with some elements of the subtemporal craniotomy (a half-and-half approach), when targeting lesions in this location.

SUBTEMPORAL APPROACH

The subtemporal approach was popularized by Peerless and Drake, who were pioneers in successfully treating aneurysms in the basilar bifurcation region.[13,14] This approach targets the aneurysm from a lateral trajectory as the temporal lobe is elevated. We utilize this approach for aneurysms originating from below the middle depth of the sella turcica and for posteriorly projecting aneurysms. Advantages to the subtemporal approach are many. Lateral trajectory facilitates visualization and dissection of posterior perforators, especially for posteriorly projecting aneurysms. Preservation of these perforators is perhaps the most crucial objective of these procedures. Proximal control is also easy to obtain with this approach. As the surgeon is working along the axis of the aneurysm neck, aneurysm clips can be placed with optimal visualization of the aneurysm neck as well as the thalamoperforators. Lastly, division of the tentorium and even removal of the petrous apex through this approach allows for exposure of the upper third of the clivus for access to low-lying bifurcations. The subtemporal craniotomy does have some disadvantages: there is poor visualization of the contralateral P1; cranial nerve III (CN III) is centered in the field, which often leads to postoperative oculomotor nerve palsies; and excessive retraction may lead to temporal lobe injury.

In most instances, a right-sided approach is used to avoid injury to a dominant temporal lobe. A left-sided approach is used when there is a preexisting left CN III palsy or right hemiparesis or if aneurysmal anatomy favors a left-sided approach.

Positioning and Scalp Incision

The patient is positioned supine with a shoulder roll placed on the right side. The head is fixed in a radiolucent Mayfield headrest. One pin is positioned over the forehead, and two pins are positioned over the occiput (Fig. 76-2). The head is

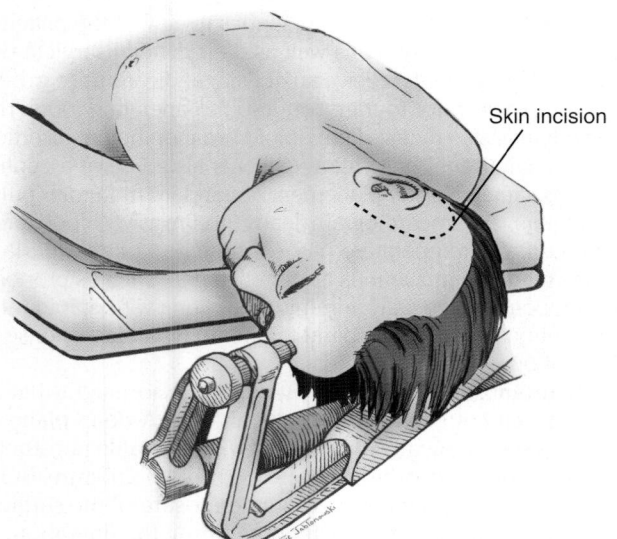

FIGURE 76-2 Patient positioning for a subtemporal approach.

rotated until the midline plane parallels the floor. The head is angled approximately 15 to 20 degrees until the floor of the middle cranial fossa is parallel to the line of sight. This maneuver also allows the temporal lobe to fall away from the middle cranial fossa, minimizing retraction during the procedure.

A question mark–shaped incision is made over the right temporal region (Fig. 76-3). The incision originates 1 cm anterior to the tragus and extends superiorly approximately 4 cm. The incision is then curved anteriorly to a point 1 cm behind the hairline. The line then follows the path of the superior temporal line, terminating just superior and

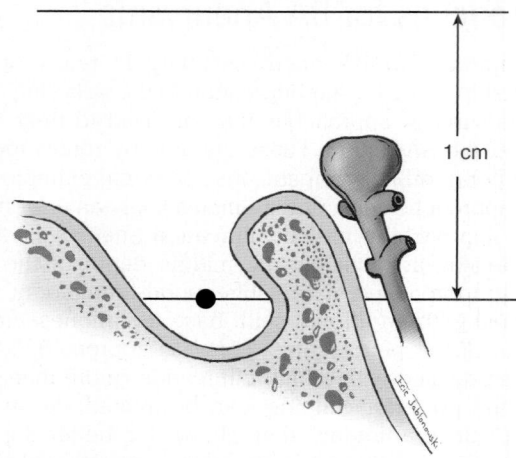

FIGURE 76-1 The approach to basilar tip aneurysms relies largely on the relationship of the aneurysm to a region between the midsella and 1 cm above the posterior clinoids. A majority of BA aneurysms are located in this region and can be approached by a half-and-half approach.

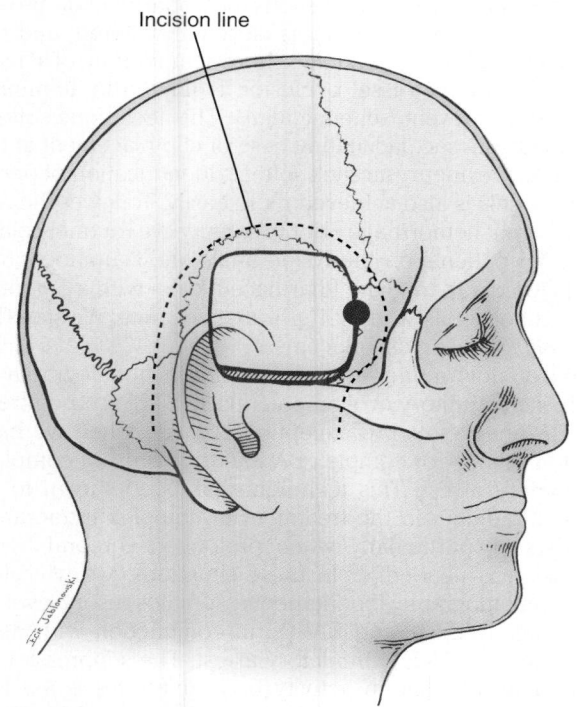

FIGURE 76-3 Skin incision and craniotomy for a subtemporal approach.

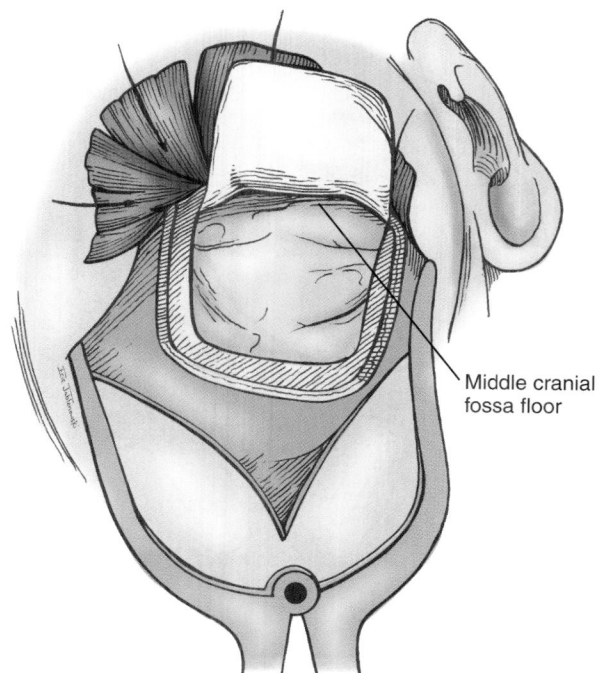

FIGURE 76-4 Subtemporal approach: dural opening and tack up, allowing for retraction of the temporal lobe.

posterior to the mastoid. The scalp flap is retracted anteriorly and secured with fishhooks connected to a Leyla bar. The temporalis muscle is divided and retracted anteriorly. An approximately 4 × 4 cm bone flap is made, based over the zygomatic root, using a high-speed pneumatic drill. Our craniotomies are slightly larger for patients with a SAH. We drill the temporal bone inferiorly and anteriorly until it is flush with the floor of the middle fossa to visualize the middle fossa floor, as well as the temporal tip. The dura is incised in a square based at the floor of the middle fossa (Fig. 76-4). The dura is retraced and secured to the overlying tissue using a 3-0 Vicryl suture. A ventricular catheter or lumbar drain, if present, is opened, allowing for

cerebrospinal fluid (CSF) drainage and brain relaxation. If sufficient brain relaxation is not achieved with CSF diversion, diuresis or hyperventilation subpial resection of the inferior temporal gyrus may be performed. The Budde Halo retraction system (Integra) is used to elevate the temporal gyrus, exposing the tentorial incisura. Incising the tentorium may be necessary for low-lying aneurysms. The surgical microscope is now brought into the field. It may be helpful at this point to place a 3-0 Vicryl suture into the free edge of the tentorium, anchoring it to the floor of the middle cranial fossa. This maneuver provides 3 to 4 mm of additional exposure in the surgical field.

Subarachnoid Dissection and Clip Application

Attention is now directed to dissecting through the subarachnoid space. The arachnoid between the third CN and the uncus is excised. The dissection is extended forward below the course of CN III. This arachnoid continues anteriorly, forming a band that runs medially across the interpeduncular fossa, known as the membrane of Liliequist. This membrane is sharply divided across the anterior aspect of the pons to allow for clot removal in the interpeduncular fossa if necessary. The SCA is identified and followed around the curve of the cerebral peduncle to the basilar artery. Arachnoid surrounding the basilar artery is cleared circumferentially in preparation for temporary clip placement. The inferior aspect of the ipsilateral P1 is identified. The P1 is followed medially across the basilar artery until the contralateral P1 is also identified. CN III can be seen passing between the SCAs and the PCAs. The dissection is now concentrated to the posterior aspect of the aneurysm complex. Perforators arising from the posterior aspect of the basilar artery often adhere to the neck and dome of the aneurysm. It is crucial to identify these vessels and dissect them off of the aneurysm (Fig. 76-5). The great advantage of the subtemporal approach arises from these important perforators potentially being easier to identify through a lateral approach. At this time, if temporary clip occlusion is needed, burst suppression is initiated by our anesthesiologists and the blood pressure is pharmacologically elevated. Temporary clipping of the basilar artery allows for

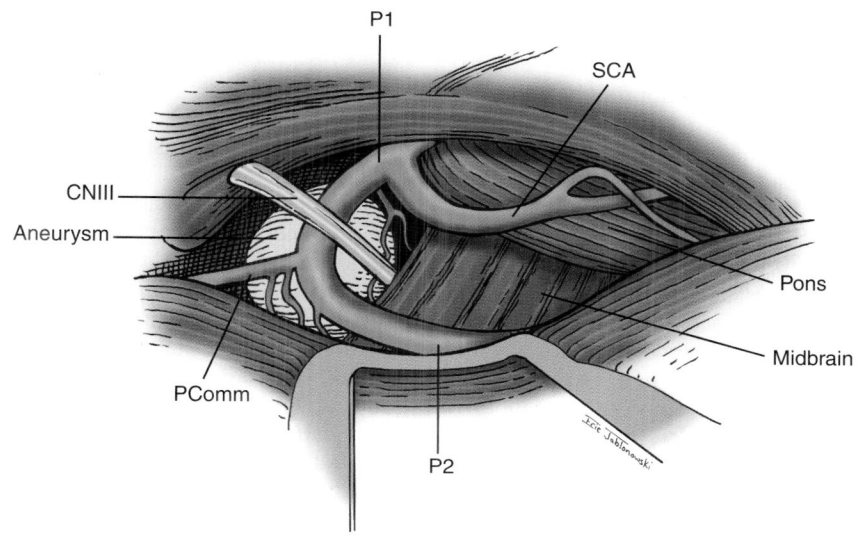

FIGURE 76-5 Microsurgical anatomy of the interpeduncular fossa. A subtemporal trajectory allows for visualization of the posterior perforating arteries.

more aggressive dissection of the aneurysm neck, perforators, and P1 arteries. Once the neck is well visualized, an aneurysm clip compatible with magnetic resonance imaging is placed across the neck of the aneurysm. A standard straight clip is used for anteriorly or posteriorly projecting aneurysms. However, most frequently, aneurysms in this location project superiorly. In these instances, a fenestrated clip is utilized. The aperture of the clip is used to enclose the P1 and any perforators, while the clip blades trap the neck of the aneurysm.

We typically use clips that are similar in size to the length of the aneurysm neck. Use of a longer clip may compromise perforators on the contralateral P1, which may be difficult to visualize with this approach. The use of a mouthpiece on the microscope allows subtle angle adjustments during the dissection that optimize visualization during clip application.

ORBITOZYGOMATIC APPROACH

The orbitozygomatic approach is similar to a pterional craniotomy with the additional removal of the superior and lateral portions of the orbit. The origins of the orbitozygomatic approach can be traced back to the description of the supraorbital craniotomy by Jane et al.[15] This approach subsequently evolved to its contemporary form through additional modifications by several authors.[16-18] The orbitozygomatic approach provides several advantages over the traditional trans-sylvian approach due to the increased bone removal at the skull base. The orbitozygomatic approach provides a better operative trajectory, provides a surgical field that is shallower than both the subtemporal and the trans-sylvian approaches, and requires less brain retraction. Due to the additional bone work, the orbitozygomatic approach may pose additional risks. These risks include frontalis nerve injury, extraocular muscle injury, and pulsatile enophthalmos. The orbitozygomatic approach offers extensive exposure of the anterior and middle cranial fossae by the removal of the superior and lateral portions of the orbit. As discussed previously, this exposure leads to a more anterior trajectory and a more upward view of the BA regions compared to the standard pterional approach. We utilize this approach for high-bifurcating aneurysms that are located 1 cm or more above the posterior clinoids. The orbitozygomatic craniotomy allows the surgeon's line of sight to pass from the globe and angle superiorly. We used a modified one-piece orbitozygomatic approach similar to that described by Lemole et al.[19]

Patient positioning is similar to that used for standard pterional craniotomies. Our scalp flap is a slight modification to the pterional flap. The scalp incision is extended across the midline to the contralateral midpupillary line adjacent to the hairline (Fig. 76-6). The temporalis muscle and fascia are dissected and retracted anteriorly, with the scalp flap connected to fishhooks and a Leyla bar. The orbitozygomatic modification poses little risk to injury of the frontalis branch of the facial nerve, since the malar eminence and the zygomatic root are not exposed. A standard pterional bone flap is made with a high-speed pneumatic drill (Fig. 76-7). The craniotomy stops at the orbital rim lateral to the supraorbital notch. An isolated area of bone remains between the supraorbital rim and the bur hole at the anatomic keyhole. The orbitotomy cuts must be made

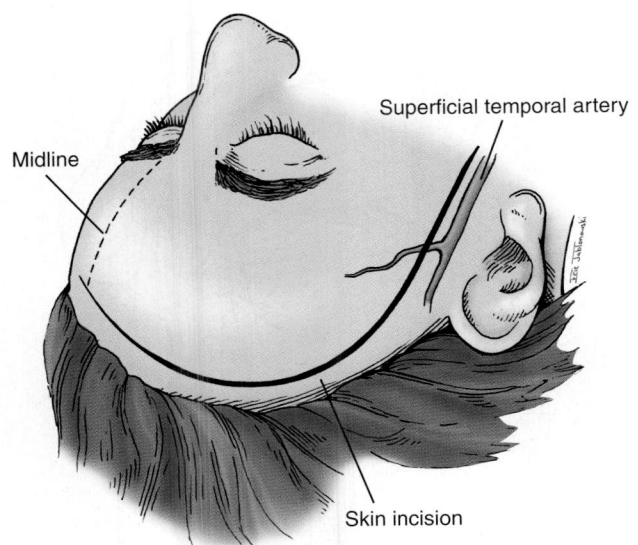

FIGURE 76-6 Modified pterional incision with the skin incision extended across the midline, allowing for more scalp retraction for modified orbitozygomatic and half-and-half approaches.

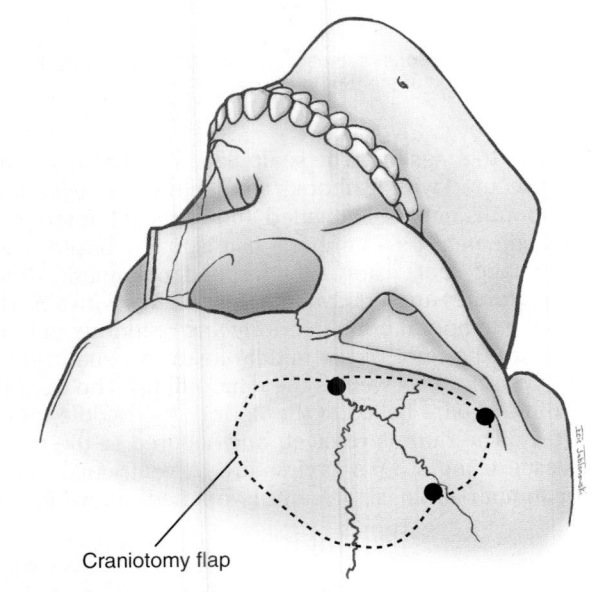

FIGURE 76-7 Standard pterional craniotomy in preparation for a modified orbitozygomatic approach.

from within the orbit, since the intracranial compartment has not been entered. Two additional cuts are made to the pterional craniotomy with a reciprocating saw for a modified one-piece orbitozygomatic approach. The first cut extends from the orbital rim lateral to the supraorbital notch and connects to the craniotomy superiorly. The second cut extends from the frontozygomatic suture over the orbital rim toward the bur hole at the pterion. Twisting and countertraction with a Penfield dissector may be necessary to extend fractures along the osteotomy lines to connect the cuts.

The intradural exposure of the modified orbitozygomatic approach is the same as in a standard pterional approach. The advantage with this approach is that the basilar region is viewed more easily due to the extra space created by the supraorbital osteotomy. The fulcrum of the trajectory is lower when the orbital roof is removed. This provides the surgeon with a higher view above the posterior clinoids.

EXTENDED LATERAL (HALF-AND-HALF) APPROACH

We employ a half-and-half approach for the vast majority of our basilar tip aneurysms. This approach represents a hybrid, combining the advantages of the trans-sylvian and subtemporal approaches while minimizing the limitations associated with each approach. Variations of the extended lateral approach have been previously described in the literature.[20]

There are many advantages to the trans-sylvian approach. The trans-sylvian approach is familiar to most neurosurgeons, since it is utilized for many standard aneurysms of the anterior circulation and tumors in the suprasellar region. Exposure of both the basilar trunk and the bilateral P1 segments is straightforward, allowing for temporary clip placement if needed for aneurysm trapping. The primary disadvantage of the trans-sylvian approach is that there is poor access to the posterior aspect of the interpeduncular fossa, where the thalamoperforators are located. By utilizing aspects of the subtemporal approach, the posterior perforators are more readily visualized than they are in a standard subtemporal approach. The primary disadvantages of the subtemporal approach are that the exposure is narrow, visualization of the contralateral P1 is suboptimal, and CN III is at risk for injury. These limitations are reduced by utilizing the trans-sylvian approach of the half-and-half craniotomy.

The half-and-half approach has many similarities to the standard pterional craniotomy pioneered by Yasargil.[21,22] In addition to the pterional craniotomy, an extensive subtemporal craniectomy is performed, providing exposure of the anterior temporal tip and the floor of the middle cranial fossa. The additional bone removal allows the surgeon to mobilize the temporal lobe superiorly and laterally, providing the surgeon with a wider corridor for approaching BA aneurysms.

Positioning and Scalp Incision

The procedure described here assumes a right-sided craniotomy, for reasons that have been previously described. In addition, for right-handed neurosurgeons, a right-sided trajectory is more familiar and intuitive.

The patient is placed supine on the operating room table, with the head placed in rigid pin fixation. We use a radiolucent headrest that allows unobstructed views during intraoperative angiography. A single pin is placed over the left frontal region, and two pins are placed in the right mastoid and occipital region. The head is rotated approximately 30 degrees to the left with slight neck extension, placing the malar eminence at the highest point of the operating field (Fig. 76-8). The Budde Halo retraction system is secured to the headrest in preparation for retraction once the craniotomy has been performed. The microscope and surgical chair are also draped and ready for use prior to skin incision. The incision begins 1 cm anterior to the tragus at the root of the zygomatic arch. The incision curves forward gently past the midline to where the hairline intersects with the contralateral midpupillary line. The scalp flap is elevated anteriorly with blunt and sharp dissection, leaving the fascia of the temporalis muscle intact. The skin flap is retracted

using fishhooks connected to a Leyla bar. The subgaleal fat pad is identified in the pterional region. The temporalis muscle and fascia are divided posterior to the fat pad and perpendicular to the zygomatic root to avoid injury to the frontalis branch of the facial nerve. The muscle is also divided along the superior temporal line, leaving a fascial cuff to facilitate reapproximation of the muscle later in the procedure. The posterior limb of the muscle is retracted posteriorly and is secured using a 2-0 Vicryl suture. The anterior limb of the dissected muscle is retracted anteriorly with the scalp flap and secured using the fishhook–Leyla construct (Fig. 76-9).

Craniotomy

A high-speed pneumatic drill is used to perform the craniotomy. Bur holes are placed at the posterior extent of the superior temporal line, the keyhole, and the root of the zygoma. A craniotome is used to connect the bur holes, making a circular bone flap with its superior edge extending to the level of the ipsilateral midpupillary line. The posterior edge extends to the edge of the scalp flap. The inferior edge is marked by the root of the zygoma, and the anterior border is marked by the sphenoid ridge. A round cutting bur is used to perform an extensive subtemporal craniectomy that allows us to visualize the anterior temporal tip. The same drill attachment is used to generously drill the lateral sphenoid wing flat to the level of the superior orbital fissure (Fig. 76-10). Once the bone work is complete, hemostasis is achieved using bone wax and oxidized cellulose.

Subarachnoid Dissection and Clip Application

The dura is opened in a curvilinear fashion with an anteriorly based flap and secured anteriorly using a 3-0 Vicryl suture. The dural opening extends from the anterior extent of the exposed frontal fossa, curves posteriorly around the proximal origin of the sylvian fissure, and terminates posteroinferiorly in the middle cranial fossa. If further relaxation is needed and a ventriculostomy is not in place, one is inserted at Paine's point, allowing CSF drainage from the lateral ventricles.[23] This technique typically provides the relaxation needed for proper brain mobilization (Fig. 76-11). The surgical microscope is brought into the field at this time. The operating table is lowered, and the operating chair is positioned for optimal comfort. The sylvian fissure is opened in a distal to proximal fashion, identifying the M2 branch of the middle cerebral artery. The dissection is continued medially until the anterior temporal branch is identified. A subfrontal brain retractor is used to elevate the frontal lobe, stretching the arachnoid of the deep sylvian fissure. The dissection is carried proximally and medially in the sylvian fissure until the optic nerve and supraclinoid ICA are visualized. Microdissectors and microscissors are used to dissect and clearly visualize the Pcomm, anterior choroidal artery, CN III, and ICA terminus (Fig. 76-12). The opticocarotid and prechiasmatic cisterns are opened sharply to free the frontal lobe further. Attention is then directed to elevating the temporal lobe posteriorly and laterally out of the middle cranial fossa. The bridging veins connecting the temporal lobe to the floor of the middle cranial fossa are coagulated and cut, avoiding potential bleeding during the critical clipping period. CN III is disconnected from its connection to the uncus. Retractors are

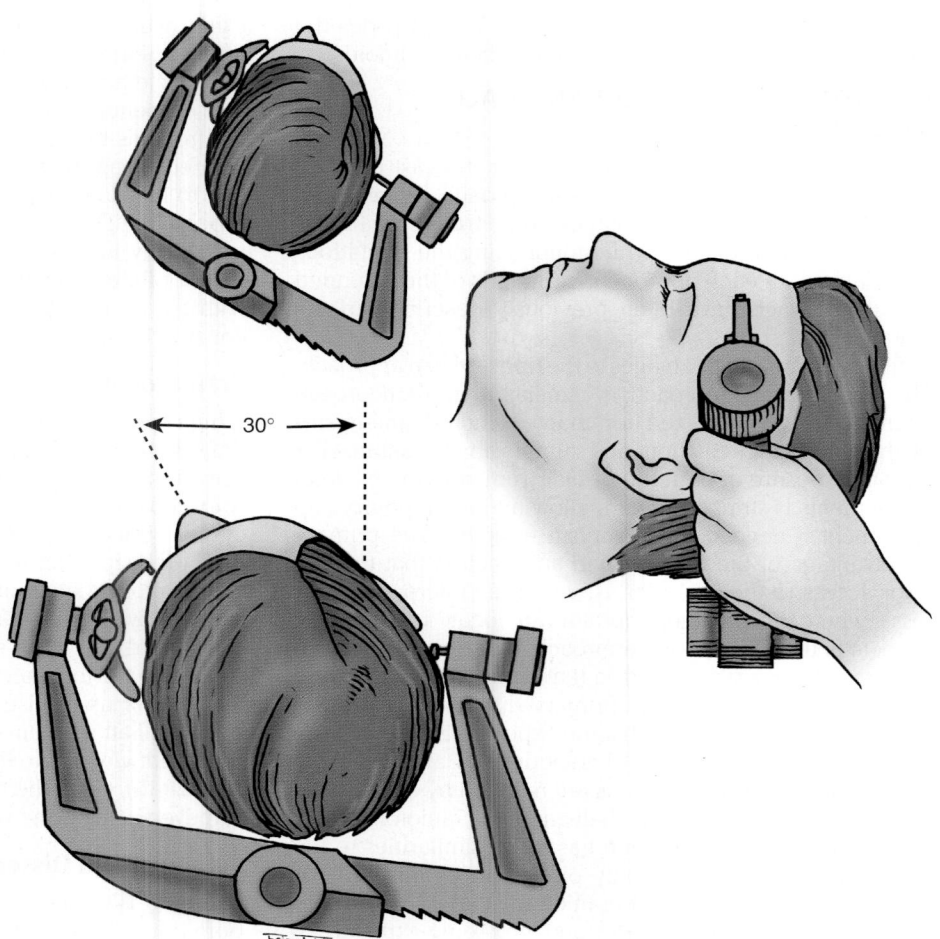

FIGURE 76-8 Head positioning for a half-and-half approach for BA aneurysms with the head slightly extended and turned 30 degrees to the left, placing the malar eminence at the highest point of the operating field.

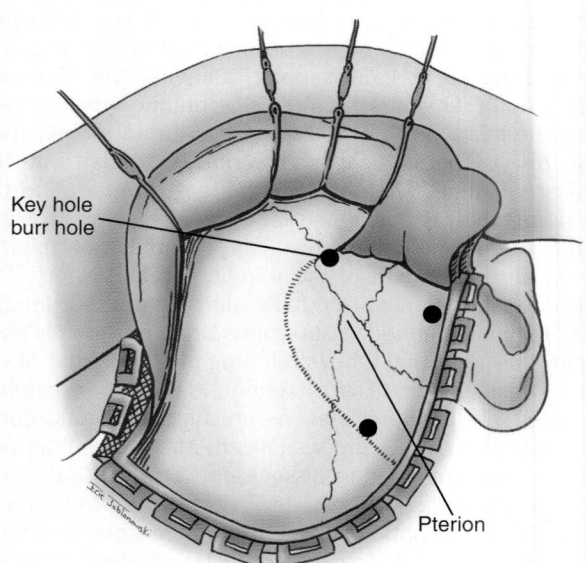

FIGURE 76-9 Bur hole locations for a half-and-half craniotomy. A bur hole is placed at the keyhole, a second hole is placed at the root of the zygoma, and a third is placed at the posterior extent of the superior temporal line.

used to elevate the frontal lobe medially and the temporal lobe laterally, providing a wide working corridor. Further arachnoid dissection is performed medial to the carotid, in the retrocarotid space along the Pcomm, and in the supracarotid region. The membrane of Liliequist is opened to provide clear visualization of the interpeduncular cistern. The Pcomm is followed to its junction with the PCA (P1–P2 junction). The SCA is identified and followed to its junction with the basilar trunk. The basilar artery is dissected free of its arachnoid adhesions in preparation for temporary clipping. The P1 segment is then identified above CN III and followed medially to the BA (Fig. 76-13). Dissection of the arachnoid around the BA also brings the contralateral P1 into view.

The surgeon can now work proximally from the basilar trunk and distally from the BA to identify the contralateral SCA. At times, it may be difficult to differentiate this vessel from the contralateral P1. This can be determined with certainty by establishing the relationship of the two arteries and CN III that runs between them. Review of the angiogram provides further information regarding the trajectory of each vessel. Visualization of the basilar trunk, bilateral P1 segments, and SCAs allows trapping of the aneurysm if needed.

Once these vessels are identified, attention is given to the posterior perforators that arise from the proximal P1 segments and the BA. We typically ask our anesthesiologist to initiate burst suppression at this time. A temporary clip is placed

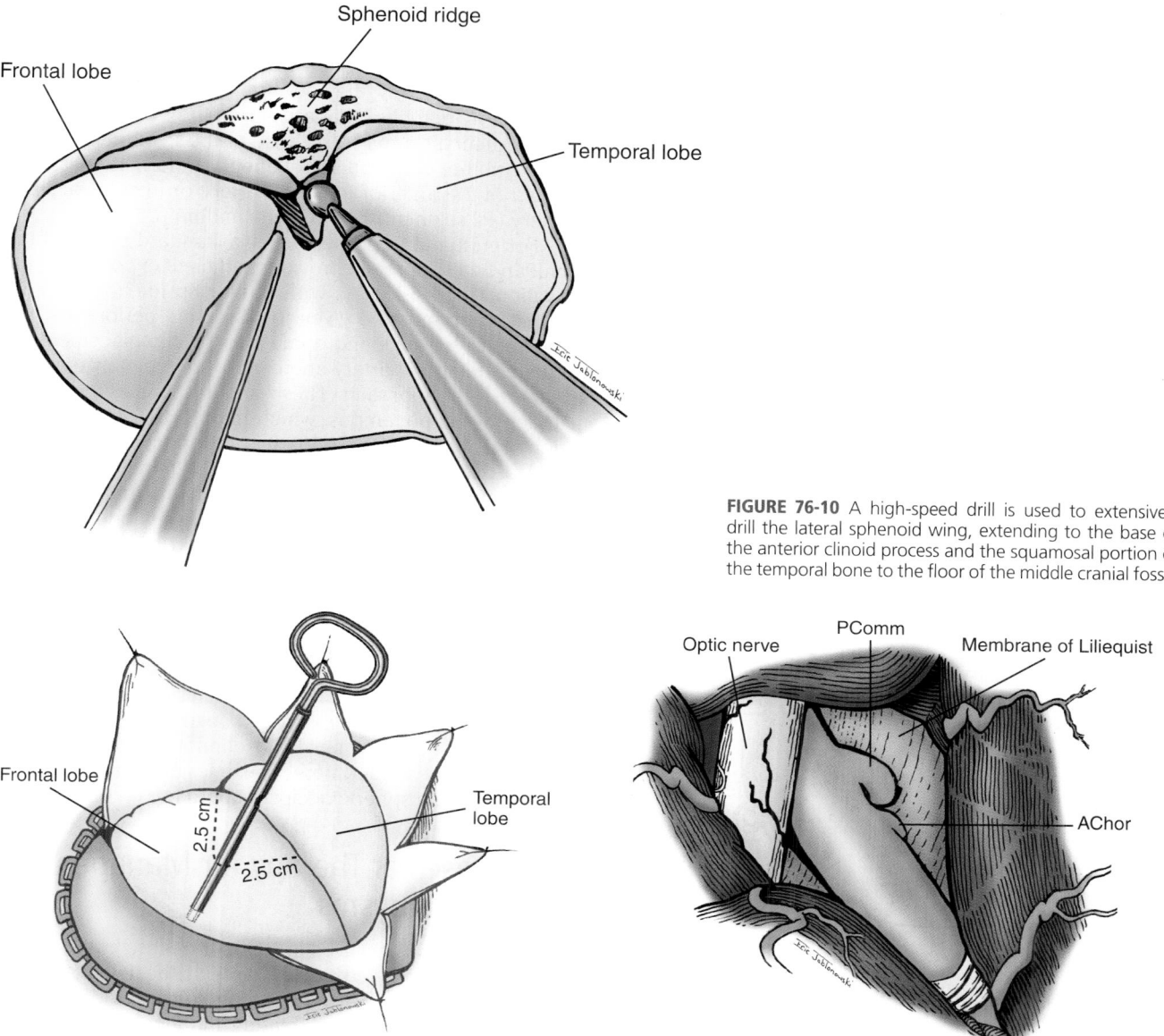

FIGURE 76-10 A high-speed drill is used to extensively drill the lateral sphenoid wing, extending to the base of the anterior clinoid process and the squamosal portion of the temporal bone to the floor of the middle cranial fossa.

FIGURE 76-11 Paine's point: Reliable access to the frontal horn of the lateral ventricle, employing an isosceles triangle with its base over the sylvian fissure, its anterior point extending to the drilled sphenoid ridge, and its apex marking the site of catheter insertion.

FIGURE 76-12 Microsurgical anatomy once the sylvian fissure is dissected, freeing the frontal and temporal lobes. The ICA is identified, along with the Pcomm and anterior choroidal artery. The membrane of Liliequist is identified lateral to the ICA.

across the basilar trunk lateral to CN III. From this point, the dissection can be more aggressive as the proximal and distal neck of the aneurysm is identified. Gentle traction with the microsuction can be placed on the fundus of the aneurysm to displace it anteriorly. This maneuver allows better visualization of the posterior thalamoperforators that need to be dissected off of the aneurysm and displaced posteriorly. Utilizing the half-and-half approach, dissection of the thalamoperforators occurs as it would during a subtemporal approach.

Several techniques can be used to clip aneurysm of the BA region (Fig. 76-14). It is typically necessary to use multiple clips to secure the neck of these aneurysms. Smaller aneurysm can typically be clipped using standard straight clips placed in tandem. Using the suction tip, the aneurysm is retracted anteriorly. The posterior blade of the clip is visualized first as

it passes across the neck above the contralateral P1. Once the posterior blade is in position, the anterior blade is closed to trap the distal neck of the aneurysm. Once the initial clip is applied, it may be necessary to place a second clip above the initial one to completely secure the aneurysm. We routinely use intraoperative indocyanine green videography and intraoperative angiography following clipping to evaluate perforators, larger vessels, and any residual aneurysm. Alternatively, for larger aneurysms with a wide neck, we initially use a fenestrated clip. The clip is often placed with its fenestration enclosing the ipsilateral P1 and the proximal neck. The blades are passed across the aneurysm to secure the distal neck. A second standard straight clip is then used to clip the remaining aneurysm, pushing the blades until they are adjacent to the fenestration of the first clip.

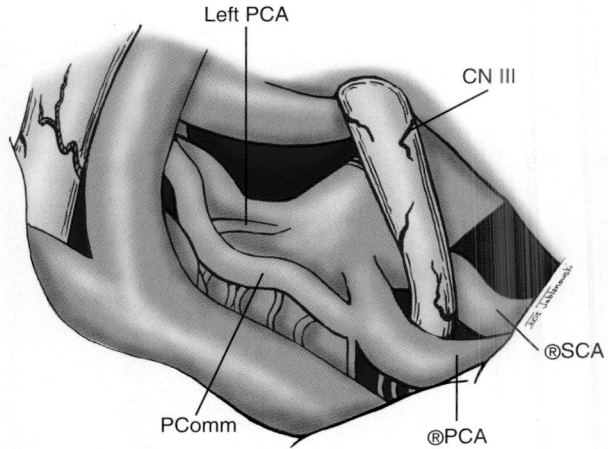

FIGURE 76-13 The Pcomm is followed to its junction with the PCA. The SCA is identified inferior to CN III. The basilar trunk is followed superiorly to the aneurysm neck.

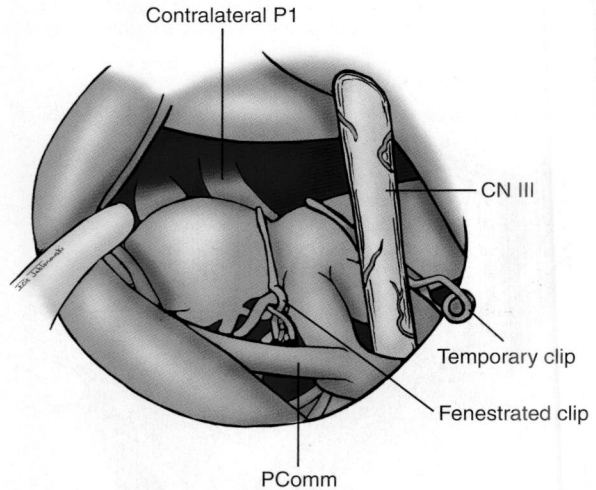

FIGURE 76-14 Temporary clip placement as more aggressive dissection of the aneurysm is performed. Using a retractor or the side of a suction tip, the Pcomm and overlying vessels can be retracted to allow better visualization of the aneurysm neck. Several techniques can be utilized to clip BA aneurysms. In this instance, a fenestrated clip is utilized to avoid compromising perforators adjacent to the neck of the aneurysm.

PCA Aneurysms

Aneurysms of the PCA may arise from several areas along its course. Typically, they develop at the origin of the large perforating branches that arise from the P1 segment of the PCA. Aneurysms may also arise at the Pcomm–PCA junction. Another common site of aneurysm formation is at the origin of the anterior temporal artery or internal occipital artery (P2 segment) lateral to the midbrain.

For proximal PCA aneurysms, a standard pterional or a half-and-half approach provides sufficient exposure for clip ligation (Fig. 76-15). As with basilar tip aneurysms, careful attention must be given to dissecting perforators from the aneurysm neck and dome prior to clip placement. For anterior temporal artery aneurysms, we typically employ a subtemporal approach. These aneurysms may be hidden under the hippocampus, which may require partial resection of that gyrus (Fig. 76-16). It is important to visualize the PCA proximally from the P1 and follow it laterally to avoid disorientation, which commonly occurs in this region. The trochlear nerve should be identified along the tentorial hiatus and moved laterally to avoid injury during the procedure. Large aneurysms in this location can be treated with parent vessel occlusion distal to the origin of the choroidal arteries. Thalamoperforators and thalamogeniculate arteries typically have originated prior to the origin of the anterior temporal artery. In addition, the PCA territory has a rich collateral supply, allowing occlusion of the distal P2 with only minor risk for ischemic injury. Aneurysm of the more distal PCA segment (P3) cannot be treated by the approaches described here. These lesions may be treated by an interhemispheric occipital approach.

Endovascular Therapy for Management of BA Aneurysms

The introduction of GDCs in 1990 for treatment of saccular aneurysms introduced a new chapter in the field of cerebrovascular surgery.[24] The GDC technology provided a completely new approach to treating intracranial aneurysms. No longer was it necessary to treat every aneurysm by a major craniotomy procedure, particularly challenging ones in the posterior circulation. The use of GDCs for aneurysms

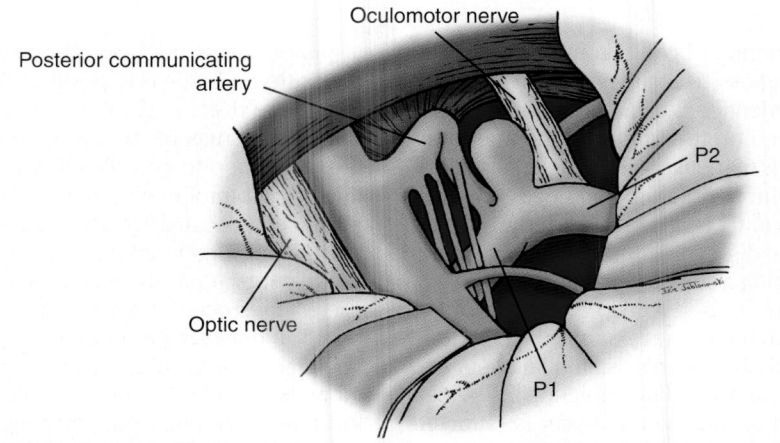

FIGURE 76-15 Standard half-and-half approach for proximal PCA (P1–P2) junction aneurysm.

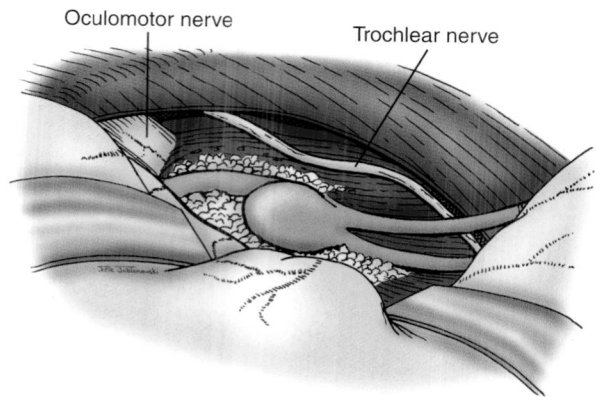

FIGURE 76-16 Subtemporal approach for a distal PCA aneurysm (P2–P3 segment).

did not gain wide acceptance until the milestone publication of the International Subarachnoid Aneurysm Trial (ISAT).[25] That study reported an absolute risk reduction of 6.9% for dependence or death when comparing patients who underwent endovascular therapy (23.7%) versus craniotomy (30.6%) for their aneurysms. Although the risk of rebleeding was higher in the endovascular group (4.2%) at 1 year and 7 years (seven patients) compared to the surgical group (3.6%) after 1 year and 7 years (two patients), the mortality rate after 7 years continued to be greater for the surgical group.[26] This data from ISAT helped mainstream the use of endovascular therapy for treatment of saccular aneurysms. The International Study of Unruptured Intracranial Aneurysms in 2003 further supported endovascular therapy as a treatment modality for cerebral aneurysms.[27] The investigators concluded that for any posterior circulation aneurysm 12 mm or larger, poor outcome was significantly greater in the surgical group compared to the endovascular group. Successful endovascular therapy for treatment of BA aneurysms has been well documented in the literature.[28-30] The procedural morbidity and mortality rates range from 3% to 9%. This has made coil embolization of these aneurysms the first line of treatment at many institutions. However, with reported recurrence rates as high as 17.5%, coiling of these aneurysms may not be the definitive treatment in every instance. In addition, with recurrence rates greater than 50% for large and giant BA aneurysms, endovascular therapy is not suitable for these larger lesions.

Wide-neck aneurysms of the BA have posed another challenge for neurointerventionalists. Initially, these aneurysms were difficult to embolize due to their poor dome-to-neck ratio (less than 2:1). In an effort to address some of these limitations, innovation led to new technology. The U.S. Food and Drug Administration approved the use of the Neuroform (Smart Therapeutics) and Enterprise (Cordis Endovascular) vascular construction devices (VCDs) under their Humanitarian Device Exemption in 2002 and 2007, respectively. These devices have enabled interventionalists to treat aneurysms that were not previously amenable to coil embolization. There have been limitations with the use of these devices as well. The use of these VCDs is limited in patients with SAHs. The Neuroform and Enterprise VCDs require the use of dual antiplatelet therapy for the prevention of in-stent stenosis. The use of antiplatelet medications

has been shown to have unacceptable complication rates associated with new hemorrhages when used in patients with ruptured aneurysms.[31]

Conclusions

The young history of basilar tip aneurysms is an interesting one. In the early 19th century, the diagnosis of a ruptured basilar tip aneurysm ultimately led to certain mortality. The pioneering work of Drake paved the way for the successful treatment of these treacherous aneurysms. With each passing decade, as microsurgical techniques and methods improved, so did patient outcomes. The presence of a BA aneurysm no longer carried the ominous prognosis it had borne just a few decades earlier. Another milestone in the late 20th century again revolutionized therapy for basilar terminus aneurysms: The successful use of GDCs provided a minimally invasive technique in treating aneurysms in this location. No longer was it necessary for neurosurgeons to navigate through eloquent tissue to treat every BA aneurysm. As with any technology, however, there have been limitations with endovascular therapy. Not every BA aneurysm is amenable to endovascular embolization. Therefore, preparation to navigate through the treacherous yet eloquent anatomy for these lesions is imperative for every cerebrovascular surgeon.

KEY REFERENCES

Baumgartner WA, Silverberg GD, Ream AK, et al. Reappraisal of cardiopulmonary bypass with deep hypothermia and circulatory arrest for complex neurosurgical operations. *Surgery.* 1983;94:242-249.

Bendok BR, Getch CC, Parkinson R, et al. Extended lateral transsylvian approach for basilar bifurcation aneurysms. *Neurosurgery.* 2004;55:174-178.

Drake CG. Bleeding aneurysms of the basilar artery: Direct surgical management in four cases. *J Neurosurg.* 1961;23:230.

Drake CG. Further experience with surgical treatment of aneurysms of the basilar artery. *J Neurosug.* 1968;29:372.

Drake CG. The surgical treatment of vertebral–basilar aneurysms. *Clin Neurosurg.* 1969;16:114-169.

Drake CG, Peerless SJ, Hernesniemi JA. Surgery of Vertebrobasilar Aneurysms: London, Ontario Experience on 1767 Patients. Vienna: Springer-Verlag; 1996:300-329.

Hakuba A, Liu S, Nishimura S. The orbitozygomatic infratemporal approach; a new surgical technique. *Surg Neurol.* 1986;26:271-276.

Jamieson KG. Aneurysms of the vertebrobasilar system: surgical intervention in 19 cases. *J Neurosurg.* 1964;21:781.

Kawase T, Toya S, Shiobara R, Mine T. Transpetrosal approach for aneurysms of the lower basilar artery. *J Neurosurg.* 1985;63:857-861.

Lemole Jr GM, Henn JS, Zabramski JM, et al. Modifications to the orbitozygomatic approach. Technical note. *J Neurosurg.* 2003;99:924-930.

Molyneux AJ, Kerr RS, Yu LM, et al. International Subarachnoid Aneurysm Trial (ISAT) Collaborative Group: International Subarachnoid Aneurysm Trial (ISAT) of neurosurgical clipping versus endovascular coiling in 2143 patients with ruptured intracranial aneurysms: a randomized comparison of effects on survival, dependency, seizures, rebleeding, subgroups, and aneurysm occlusion. *Lancet.* 2005;366:809-817.

Paine JT, Batjer HH, Samson D. Intraoperative ventricular puncture. *Neurosurgery.* 1988;22:1107-1109.

Peerless SJ, Drake CG. Management of aneurysms of the posterior circulation. In: Youmans JR, ed. *Neurological Surgery: A Comprehensive Guide to the Diagnosis and Management of Neurosurgical Problems.* Philadelphia: WB Saunders; 1990:1764-1806.

Peluso JP, van Rooij WJ, Sluzewski M, Beute GN. Coiling of basilar tip aneurysms: results in 154 consecutive patients with emphasis on recurrent hemorrhage and retreatment during mid and long term follow-up. *J Neurology, Neurosurg, and Psych.* 2008;79:706-711.

Samson DS, Hodosh RM, Clark WK. Microsurgical evaluation of the pterional approach to aneurysms of the distal basilar circulation. *Neurosurgery.* 1978;3:135-141.

Spetzler RF, Hadley MN, Rigamonti D, et al. Aneurysms of the basilar artery treated with circulatory arrest, hypothermia, and barbiturate cerebral protection. *J Neurosurg.* 1988;68:868-879.

Wiebers DO, Whisnant JP, Huston 3rd J, et al. International Study of Unruptured Intracranial Aneurysms Investigators: Unruptured intracranial aneurysms: natural history, clinical outcome, and risks of surgical and endovascular treatment. *Lancet.* 2003;362:103-110.

Yasargil M. Operative anatomy. In: Yasargil M, ed. *Microneurosurgery.* Stuttgart: George Thieme Verlag; 1984:5.

Yasargil MG, Antic J, Laciga R, et al. Microsurgical pterional approach to aneurysm of the basilar bifurcation. *Surg Neurol.* 1976;6:83-91.

Zabramski JM, Kiris T, Sankhla SK, et al. Orbitozygomatic craniotomy. Technical note. *J Neurosurg.* 1998;89:336-341.

Numbered references appear on Expert Consult.

CHAPTER 77

Surgical Management of Midbasilar and Lower Basilar Aneurysms

NADER SANAI • ALIM MITHA • ROBERT F. SPETZLER

Aneurysms of the midbasilar and lower basilar artery are located below the level of the superior cerebellar artery and involve the anteroinferior cerebellar artery (AICA), the inferior basilar artery trunk, and the vertebrobasilar junction.

Epidemiology

In most neurosurgical series, aneurysms of the midbasilar and lower basilar artery represent less than 1% of cerebral aneurysms. Yamaura[1] reported a frequency of 10 midbasilar and lower basilar artery aneurysms in 202 posterior circulation aneurysms (5%), whereas Sano and colleagues[2] reported that they accounted for 7 of 1480 (0.5%) total cerebral aneurysms and for 7 of 116 (6%) posterior circulation aneurysms. In their earlier work, Peerless and Drake[3] reported that midbasilar and lower basilar artery aneurysms accounted for 193 of all 1266 (15.2%) of their cases of posterior circulation aneurysms. In their more recent publication describing 1767 patients, aneurysms of the basilar trunk and vertebrobasilar junction were seen in 14.7% of patients.[4]

Recent large multicenter studies may overestimate the frequency of aneurysms in this anatomic location. In the original report from the International Study of Unruptured Intracranial Aneurysms, posterior circulation aneurysms (excluding basilar tip aneurysms) were seen in 6.2% of all patients.[5] In a subsequent report from this study, these lesions composed 5.1% of all patients with unruptured aneurysms, 3.9% of which were clipped surgically and 8.9% of which were treated with endovascular coiling.[6] Alternatively, the International Subarachnoid Aneurysm Trial probably incorporated a pre-established treatment bias in Europe, since only 2.7% of randomized patients had posterior circulation aneurysms and only one of the 2143 patients (0.05%) analyzed had a basilar trunk aneurysm.[7]

Presentation

The clinical features of subarachnoid hemorrhage (SAH) in patients with aneurysms located in this region of the posterior circulation are the same as those associated with other cerebral aneurysms. Giant unruptured aneurysms may produce neurologic symptoms specific to their anatomic location (i.e., brain stem, cranial nerves). The natural history of hemorrhage of aneurysms located in the midbasilar or lower basilar artery is also identical to that in cerebral aneurysms located in other areas. The basic principles of management are, therefore, not markedly different.

Principles of Management

Patients presenting with SAH and aneurysms located on the midbasilar and lower basilar artery are managed utilizing the same protocols previously established for other patients with SAH[8]: cardiorespiratory and basic neurologic supportive care, early ventriculostomy with cerebrospinal fluid (CSF) drainage in patients with Hunt-Hess[8] grade IV or V SAH,[9] early surgery in suitable cases,[9-11] prophylaxis, and, when appropriate, aggressive management of post SAH cerebral vasospasm associated with ischemic deficit[10,12,13] and aggressive management of increased intracranial pressure.[9,10] Patients with neurologic symptoms related to mass effect of the aneurysm are managed semiurgently. Typically, these patients present with signs of brain stem compression or cranial nerve deficits, and careful consideration of their deficits is required during planning of the treatment approach and of the timing of intervention.

Endovascular management of aneurysms of the middle and lower basilar artery is increasingly reported.[14-23] Although evidence of durability of treatment is still lacking, several recent reports have also described enhancements in surgical technique and outcomes associated with these improvements.[24-32] Notably, the Pipeline embolization device (Chestnut Medical Technologies, Menlo Park, CA) is a self-expanding, microcatheter-delivered, cylindrical mesh device composed of braided cobalt, chromium, and platinum strands.[19] The device, while not yet approved by the U.S. Food and Drug Administration (FDA), has a 30% to 35% metal surface area when fully deployed. Multiple devices can be deployed within each other (telescoped) to create a composite endovascular construct. The degree of metal surface area coverage can be manipulated by varying the technique of device deployment as well as by judiciously choosing the number of devices placed in a particular vascular segment. Evidence of its applicability for large midbasilar and lower basilar artery aneurysms is slowly becoming available—the device can be applied strategically to create an endovascular construct within a parent vessel that is rich with eloquent perforators.[19,20] However, the Pipeline device has not yet been approved by the FDA.

The general rules for the anesthetic management of patients undergoing surgical clipping involve the use of preoperative corticosteroids and prophylactic intravenous antibiotics. Intraoperative hypotension is prevented, and intraoperative blood pressure is allowed to run mildly hypertensive, especially during any temporary vessel clipping. During exposure and clipping of the aneurysm, all patients receive intravenous doses of a barbiturate (thiopental) titrated to achieve electroencephalographic (EEG) burst suppression.

PRINCIPLES OF MICROSURGERY

The general principles for treatment of aneurysms located on this part of the basilar artery are the same as for aneurysms located anywhere in the cerebral circulation. The objective is complete isolation of the aneurysm from cerebral circulation with preservation of the normal vasculature. Of particular importance when treating these aneurysms is preservation of the small perforating arteries from the basilar artery. This goal can be accomplished when maximum exposure of the basilar artery has been achieved with minimal brain retraction. With adequate visualization of the anatomic features and controlled application of an aneurysm clip of appropriate length and shape, the neck of the aneurysm can usually be obliterated and the parent vessels and perforators can be preserved.

HYPOTHERMIC CARDIAC STANDSTILL

In certain cases, the size of the aneurysm precludes adequate visualization of the parent vessel and perforators. This problem is often most difficult with basilar artery aneurysms. In such situations, additional exposure can be obtained through the use of hypothermic cardiac arrest with barbiturate cerebral protection.[33] During cardiac arrest, the aneurysm can be collapsed and the anatomic characteristics defined without the risk of hemorrhage. Since the original report from the Barrow Neurological Institute (BNI) in 1986,[33] hypothermic cardiac arrest has been used in many patients with posterior circulation aneurysms.

The successful use of hypothermic cardiac standstill requires an experienced cardiovascular and cerebrovascular team. The success of hypothermic cardiac arrest for clipping complex aneurysms is partially determined by four key variables: depth of hypothermia, duration of circulatory arrest, use of barbiturates, and hemostasis.[25] In the original BNI series, the mean brain temperature during standstill was 54°F, and the mean duration of standstill about 22 minutes (range, 3–72 minutes). The absolute maximum safe period of cerebral ischemia is unknown. The duration of cerebral ischemia that can be safely tolerated is significantly increased, however, by the utilization of profound hypothermia and precooling intravenous barbiturates administered to achieve burst suppression of EEG activity.

The major complication associated with hypothermic cardiac standstill has been postoperative hemorrhage (11% in the BNI series). Meticulous absolute hemostasis and close attention to the patient's clotting mechanisms are necessary. Therefore, the inherent morbidity involved with circulatory arrest stipulates that it be used only in patients for whom exposure and control of the parent vessels and aneurysm cannot be achieved with routine surgical techniques, including such measures as the application of multiple temporary aneurysm clips.

ANATOMIC ISSUES IN SURGICAL EXPOSURE

Aneurysms of the midbasilar and inferior basilar artery are located in a small, restricted area encased within thick dense bone, situated within a limited subarachnoid space and filled with the densest collection of vital cranial nerve and vascular structures in the nervous system. The general goals of aneurysm surgery therefore must be accomplished with a minimum of brain retraction: (1) proximal and distal vascular control; (2) preservation of the principal vessels, their branches, and the perforating vessels supplying the brain stem and cranial nerves; and (3) complete obliteration of the aneurysm.

Previously, aneurysms at this location were treated through a subtemporal-transtentorial approach or a suboccipital approach.[2,34-36] Although a transoral transclival or transmaxillary transclival approach has been used to expose the basilar artery by Peerless and Drake[3] and others,[2,37,38] they are associated with notable technical limitations of exposure and a significant risk of postoperative CSF leakage and meningitis.[3] These various techniques can provide access, but they do not meet the requirements of maximal exposure combined with minimal brain retraction. A number of techniques have been devised to maximize lateral bone removal and to provide a relatively short and flat route of access to the front of the brain stem and the basilar artery: the transpetrosal approach,[39,40] combined supratentorial-infratentorial approach,[41] far-lateral approach,[42-44] and far-lateral combined supratentorial-infratentorial approach.[39] Each of these techniques, when appropriately matched to the location and size of the aneurysm, can provide excellent access to almost any aneurysm located on the midbasilar and lower basilar artery (Table 77-1).

Table 77-1 Surgical Approaches to Midbasilar and Lower Basilar Artery
Transpetrosal Approaches
Retrolabyrinthine
Translabyrinthine
Transcochlear
Combined Supra- and Infra-Tentorial Approaches
Retrolabyrinthine
Translabyrinthine
Transcochlear
Far-Lateral Approach
Extreme Lateral Craniocervical Approach
Far Lateral: Combined Supra- and Infra-Tentorial ("Combined-Combined") Approaches
Retrolabyrinthine
Translabyrinthine
Transcochlear
Anterior Transclival Approaches
Transoral (transpalatal)
Transmaxillary
Transfacial
Other Approaches
Extended orbitozygomatic
Anterior petrosectomy
Subtemporal
Unilateral suboccipital

Transpetrosal Approaches

The anterior brain stem and clival regions can be reached through removal of portions of the petrosal bone with almost no brain or brain stem retraction.[45] There are three variations of the temporal (petrous) bone dissection. The retrolabyrinthine technique involves petrous bone resection and preserves hearing. The translabyrinthine technique increases the amount of petrous bone resected and sacrifices hearing. Finally, the transcochlear technique involves maximal petrous bone resection, sacrifices hearing, and requires transposition of the facial nerve.[41] Moving through these three variations represents a gradual increase in the amount of petrous bone resected and in the exposure of the brain stem and clivus.

For these exposures, the patient is positioned supine on the operating table with the head positioned parallel to the floor, inclined slightly downward, and fixed to the operating table in a Mayfield headrest. A soft roll is placed under the ipsilateral shoulder to provide support.

The skin incision begins 3 cm posterior to the pinna and continues in a gentle curving fashion around the ear to the inferior border of the mastoid. The ear is retracted inferiorly with fishhooks attached to a Leyla bar. This maneuver exposes part of the temporal squama, external auditory meatus, and mastoid region. The neuro-otologist performs the approach through the temporal (petrous) bone and exposes the sigmoid sinus and dura 1 to 2 cm posterior to the sinus, after which the neurosurgeon performs the intradural part of the procedure. The mastoidectomy portion of the temporal bone procedure is completed with a high-speed drill (Medtronic Midas Rex, Midas Rex Institute, Fort Worth, TX), whereas the Osteon system (Linvatec, Largo, FL) is used with the operating microscope for the more detailed bone removal. Suction irrigation is used continuously during the temporal bone drilling.

RETROLABYRINTHINE APPROACH

The retrolabyrinthine approach provides excellent access into the cerebellopontine angle but does not allow significant anterior visualization of the brain stem; therefore, it has a limited, isolated role in management of aneurysms of the midbasilar and lower basilar artery. If hearing is to be preserved, a retrolabyrinthine approach is used. The posterior and superior semicircular canals are skeletonized by drilling as far anteriorly as possible, both above and below the otic capsule, to expose as much dura as possible (Fig. 77-1A). The bone overlying the superior petrosal sinus and sigmoid sinus is removed with the drill. The endolymphatic sac and duct are preserved.

Recent studies describe a variation of the retrolabyrinthine approach designed to improve the surgical corridor to the midbasilar region but without necessarily jeopardizing hearing.[28,30] Incidental or accidental injuries to the semicircular canals are not universally associated with hearing loss. Consequently, the transmastoid partial labyrinthectomy has been described as a modification of the standard retrolabyrinthine approach. The posterior and superior semicircular canals are occluded and resected, but the vestibule and lateral semicircular canal are preserved. Serviceable hearing can be preserved in 80% of patients using this technique.[28]

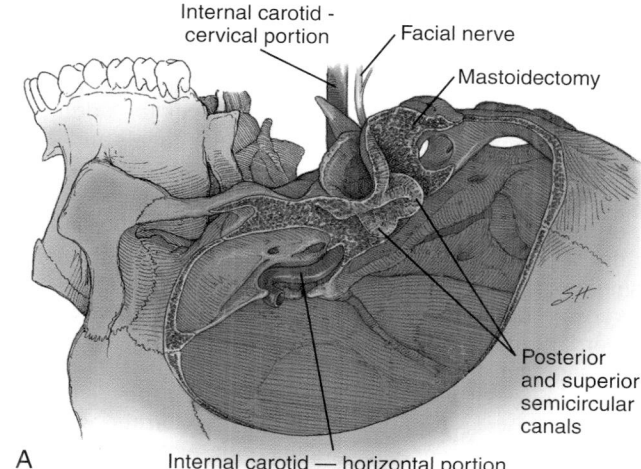

A — Internal carotid - cervical portion; Facial nerve; Mastoidectomy; Posterior and superior semicircular canals; Internal carotid — horizontal portion

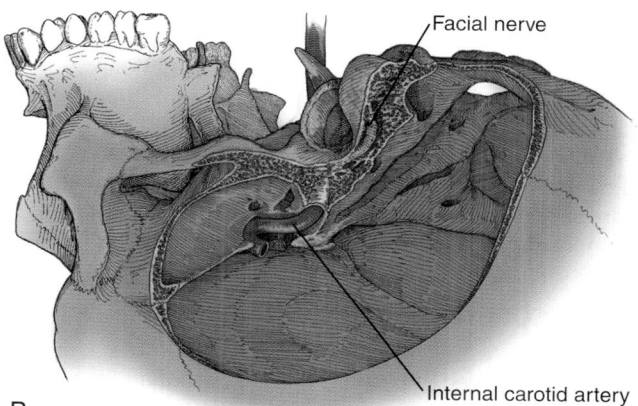

B — Facial nerve; Internal carotid artery

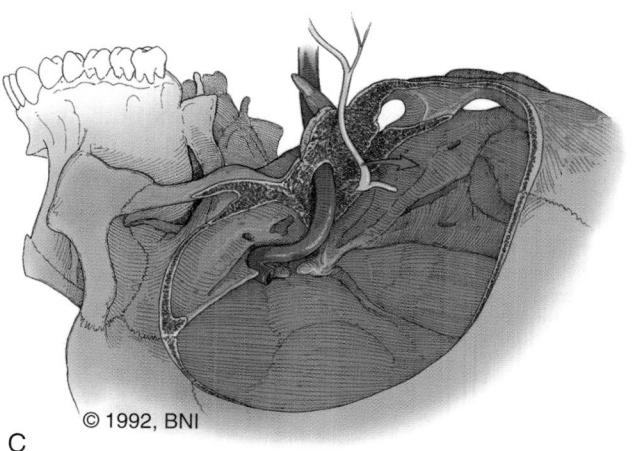

C — © 1992, BNI

FIGURE 77-1 The three variations in the combined supra- and infratentorial approach from the surgeon's viewpoint. (A) Extended retrolabyrinthine approach with skeletonized posterior and superior semicircular canals and mastoidectomy. (B) Translabyrinthine approach. Note that all three semicircular canals have been removed and a portion of the facial nerve has been skeletonized. (C) The transcochlear approach, which involves extending the translabyrinthine technique by posteriorly transposing the facial nerve and aggressively drilling away the medial aspect of the petrous bone. *(From Spetzler RF, Daspit CP, Pappas CT. The combined supra- and infratentorial approach for lesions of the petrous and clival regions: experience with 46 cases. J Neurosurg. 1992;76:588-599, with permission from Barrow Neurological Institute.)*

TRANSLABYRINTHINE APPROACH

If greater exposure is required, the standard translabyrinthine approach, which sacrifices hearing, can be used. The initial part of this approach is performed as described for the retrolabyrinthine approach but involves the additional complete removal of all three semicircular canals and skeletonization of the posterior half of the internal auditory canal (Fig. 77-1B). More bone is removed from the face of the petrous pyramid than is possible through the retrolabyrinthine technique. Removal of all bone overlying the sigmoid sinus and, if necessary, the jugular bulb provides greater exposure of the inferior aspect of the clivus. The posterior external auditory canal and the bone overlying the mastoid segment of the facial nerve should also be thinned to minimize the obstruction to visualization of the clivus. The distal end of the superior vestibular nerve in the vestibule is used as a reference for identification of the facial nerve as it exits the internal auditory canal. The bone overlying the labyrinthine segment of the facial nerve is also thinned with cautious drilling utilizing a diamond bit and continuous intraoperative monitoring of facial nerve function.

The translabyrinthine approach is a more direct, anterolateral approach to the cerebellopontine angle, allowing greater exposure of the anterolateral brain stem because of the removal of additional petrous bone. Although this exposure sacrifices ipsilateral hearing and is associated with an increased risk of CSF leakage, it is commonly required for these difficult aneurysms.

TRANSCOCHLEAR TECHNIQUE

For the greatest exposure of the clivus, the transcochlear technique is used (Fig. 77-1C). The external auditory canal is transected and oversewn in two layers. After the translabyrinthine exposure, the facial nerve is removed from its temporal bone canal,[46] the greater superficial petrosal nerve is sectioned, and the facial nerve is transposed posteriorly, utilizing the dura of the internal auditory canal to protect part of the nerve. The entire tympanic portion of the temporal bone is removed with exposure of the periosteum of the temporomandibular joint. The internal auditory canal and cochlea are then removed. The jugular bulb is exposed by removal of the bone that separates it from the internal carotid artery at the skull base. The bone surrounding the carotid artery is removed to the siphon.

If direct exposure of the internal carotid artery is unnecessary, a thin rim of bone can be left encasing the vessel. The option of extensive internal carotid artery exposure allows creation of a direct saphenous vein bypass graft from the petrous portion of the internal carotid artery to the subarachnoid internal carotid artery if necessary.[39,47] Bone is also removed from the floor of the plate of the middle fossa to the horizontal segment of the internal carotid artery. The difference in the amount of resection of the petrous ridge between the retrolabyrinthine and the transcochlear approaches can be appreciated on postoperative computed tomographic (CT) reconstruction scans (Fig. 77-2).

The transcochlear technique provides a very flat angle of approach to the clivus and excellent exposure of both the anterior and anterolateral aspects of the brain stem. This exposure is gained, however, at the expense of sacrificing hearing and increasing the risk of facial nerve paralysis. Furthermore, the chance of CSF leakage is high.

INTRADURAL EXPOSURE AND CLOSURE

Regardless of which of the previous extradural bony exposures is used, the dura mater is incised just inferior and parallel to the superior petrosal sinus and just superior to the jugular bulb. These two dural incisions meet at the sinodural angle and the porus acusticus. The dura mater of the internal auditory canal is opened, and the cerebellopontine angle is entered. The surgical procedure then proceeds according to the specific principles of aneurysm surgery as discussed earlier. After the aneurysm has been obliterated, the surgical field is closed in anatomic layers when possible. The temporal and occipital dura is reapproximated with 4-0 braided nylon suture. Abdominal adipose tissue, temporalis muscle, and fibrin glue are used to obliterate the eustachian tube in the translabyrinthine transcochlear approaches and to fill

FIGURE 77-2 Postoperative three-dimensional CT scans of bone window reconstruction comparing petrous bone resection by the retrolabyrinthine approach (A) with total petrous bone resection as performed with the transcochlear approach (B).

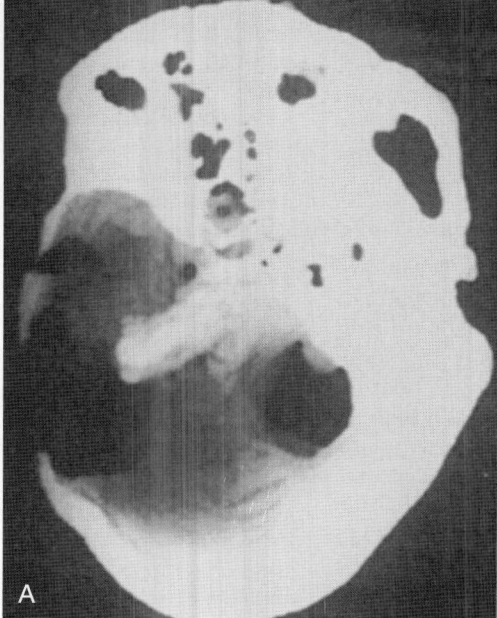
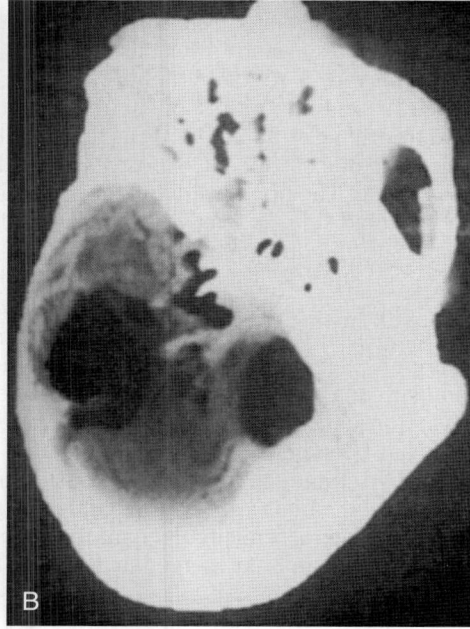

the void created by the temporal bone resection. Temporary lumbar spinal drainage of CSF is used for 3 to 5 days to prevent CSF leakage through the wound.

SELECTION OF SURGICAL APPROACH

The selection of the particular variation of the transpetrosal approaches for aneurysms of the midbasilar and lower basilar artery is based on (1) the location of the aneurysm, (2) the size of the aneurysm, and (3) an estimation of the amount of temporal bone that must be removed to expose the aneurysm adequately and to obtain proximal and distal vascular control.

The salient features of the various approaches can be summarized as follows:

- The retrolabyrinthine approach provides excellent exposure of the cerebellopontine angle but not of the anterior brain stem and preserves function of both hearing and the facial nerves.
- The translabyrinthine approach offers greater exposure of the cerebellopontine angle and significantly improves exposure of the anterolateral and anterior brain stem, but at the expense of hearing and with an increased risk of CSF leakage.
- The transcochlear technique achieves the maximal exposure possible but accomplishes it with not only the disadvantages associated with the translabyrinthine technique but also an increased risk of facial nerve paralysis.

Apart from the morbidity associated with bone removal, a problematic aspect of all the transpetrosal approaches is that the surgical corridor to the aneurysm is necessarily lateral to the lesion by the nature of the bony exposure. This geometry can increase the difficulty of clipping the aneurysm because the surgeon may need to explore around the dome of the aneurysm during dissection in preparation for clipping and also may need to manipulate the aneurysm to visualize the entire neck during clipping. The senior author (RFS) has explored the use of alternate approaches, specifically the extended orbitozygomatic approach for lesions involving the distal two-fifths of the basilar artery or the far-lateral approach for lesions of the proximal two fifths of the basilar artery and vertebrobasilar junction.[26] These approaches leave only the truly midbasilar (i.e., middle one fifth of the basilar artery) for transpetrosal approaches. The advantage of these alternate strategies, with or without hypothermic cardiac arrest, is that they allow visualization along the axis of the basilar artery, with good exposure of the neck and perforating vessels, facilitating aneurysm obliteration with a straight clip.

Using this more selected approach led to good scores on the Glasgow Outcome Scale (GOS)[48] in 75% of patients (GOS 4 and 5).[26] Only 11% had permanent treatment-related neurologic deficits. There were four deaths but only one occurred in the perioperative period.

Combined Supra- and Infra-Tentorial Approaches

The exposure of the basilar artery provided by a transpetrosal approach can be enhanced considerably when it is combined with a supratentorial approach. Using a combined supra- and infra-tentorial surgical approach, in conjunction with the operating microscope, provides exposure from the sphenoid ridge and cavernous sinus to the foramen magnum and anterior cervical spinal cord with minimal brain retraction. The combined approach requires the skills of both a neurosurgeon and a neuro-otologist, in that it utilizes (1) variable degrees of temporal bone removal, (2) a supra- and infra-tentorial craniotomy, and (3) division of the tentorium to connect the supra- and infra-tentorial compartments.

Variations of the combined approach have been described since the first report in 1905 by Borchardt. However, it was mostly abandoned, partially as a result of a high mortality rate and improvements in the suboccipital approach offered by Cushing and Dandy. In 1966 Hitselberger and House[40] described a combined suboccipital-petrosal approach for the removal of large cerebellopontine angle tumors and discussed how the wide exposure obtained with this technique overcame the individual limitations of the suboccipital and translabyrinthine approaches for dealing with extensive lesions. Their technique extended the translabyrinthine approach beyond the sigmoid sinus into the suboccipital areas, to achieve a wide view of the cerebellopontine angle with minimal brain retraction, and allowed the sigmoid sinus to be mobilized or divided to improve the surgical exposure.

Malis[49] popularized the idea of combining the subtemporal and posterior fossa (suboccipital) approaches to improve the surgical exposure when treating extensive lesions of the clivus or medial petrous region. In Malis's version, the petrosal bone is not extensively drilled, and the superior anastomotic vein (vein of Labbé) is preserved by ligation of the transverse sinus between the entrance of the superior anastomotic vein posteriorly and the sigmoid sinus and superior petrosal sinus anteriorly. After the transverse sinus is divided, the tentorium is split along the petrosal apex with sparing of the superior petrosal sinus. Elevation of the tentorium, transverse sinus, temporal lobe, and superior anastomotic vein allows exposure of the clivus down to the foramen magnum.

Morrison and King[50] also described a translabyrinthine transtemporal approach to provide extensive exposure by drilling the petrous bone from the cerebellopontine angle upward into the middle fossa. Exposure is increased by division of the superior petrosal sinus and tentorium. In 1977, Fisch[51] described the infratemporal fossa approach for extensive tumors of the temporal bone and base of the skull. Fisch combined a partial posterior and inferior petrosectomy with a cervicofacial approach. This approach provided good exposure of the jugular foramen but frequently required permanent anterior displacement of the facial nerve, resection of the zygomatic arch and mandibular condyle, and complete obliteration of the pneumatic spaces of the temporal bone. House and Hitselberger[52] modified the translabyrinthine approach by adding the transcochlear technique. Pellet and colleagues[53] combined the infratemporal approach of Fisch[51] and the transcochlear approach of House and Hitselberger[52] to create the widened transcochlear approach. This approach utilizes a petrosectomy to connect the posterior fossa to the superior carotid region, allowing for the single-stage removal of lesions that extend from the infratemporal region to the posterior fossa. The basic principles for the combined approach had thus been defined: variable amounts of petrous bone dissection with a supratentorial-infratentorial craniotomy and division of the tentorium. An important variable in the combined approach concerns the significance and fate of both the dural sinuses (superior petrosal, sigmoid, or transverse sinus) and the superior anastomotic vein.

A number of authors have also presented their experiences using variations of the combined infratemporal and posterior fossa approach for removal of large lesions involving the clivus and medial petrous region.[41,54-57] Some advocate preservation of the major dural sinus,[56,57] and others, with appropriate consideration for patency of the opposite transverse sinus, commonly sacrifice the sigmoid[41,54] or transverse sinus.[49]

SURGICAL TECHNIQUE

The patient is positioned supine on the operating table with the head positioned parallel to the floor, inclined slightly downward, and fixed to the operating table in a Mayfield headrest. A soft roll is placed under the ipsilateral shoulder to give appropriate support. The skin incision begins at the level of the zygoma, 1 cm anterior to the ear, and continues in a gentle curving fashion around the ear to just below the mastoid tip. To obtain greater exposure, the posterior part of the incision can be extended farther posteriorly. To obtain an exposure that includes the foramen magnum, this combined approach can be combined with the far-lateral suboccipital approach (discussed later).[39,42-44] The scalp flap is retracted inferiorly with fishhooks attached to a Leyla bar. This maneuver exposes the lateral aspect of the skull: the zygoma, lateral temporal bone, external auditory meatus, and mastoid region. The neuro-otologist performs the approach through the temporal (petrous) bone, after which the neurosurgeon performs a craniotomy with exposure of

the remaining sigmoid sinus and transverse sinus, followed by the intradural part of the procedure.

After the neuro-otologist has completed the petrous bone resection, the neurosurgeon proceeds with a subtemporal suboccipital craniotomy that crosses the transverse sinus and exposes the remainder of the sigmoid sinus. This craniotomy exposes a large dural surface. Brain relaxation, if required, is achieved initially with hyperventilation, administration of mannitol or barbiturates, or spinal drainage of CSF. Comprehensive electrophysiologic monitoring is routinely used: compressed spectral EEG, somatosensory-evoked potentials, brain stem auditory responses in both ears, or just the contralateral ear if ipsilateral hearing is to be sacrificed, and functional evaluation of facial and other appropriate cranial nerves. The anterior part of the dural incision (Fig. 77-3) is made over the temporal lobe and extends posteriorly to at least 1 cm below the site where the superior petrosal sinus enters the sigmoid sinus. Uncommonly, a low-lying superior anastomotic vein is found attached to the temporal dura or tentorium, and care must be exercised to prevent damaging this important vascular structure. If the sigmoid sinus is to be preserved, the dural incision crosses the superior petrosal sinus to join with a dural incision in front of the sigmoid sinus. The superior petrosal sinus can usually be cauterized or clipped and subsequently divided. Another incision can be made behind the sigmoid sinus (Fig. 77-3, inset)[56] to allow access, if necessary, in front of and behind the sinus.

SACRIFICE OF SIGMOID SINUS

Sacrifice of the sigmoid sinus can be considered if the contralateral transverse sinus and sigmoid sinus are patent (Fig. 77-4) and if these sinuses communicate with the sagittal sinus and ipsilateral transverse sinus through a patent confluence of the sinuses (confluens sinuum). To obtain

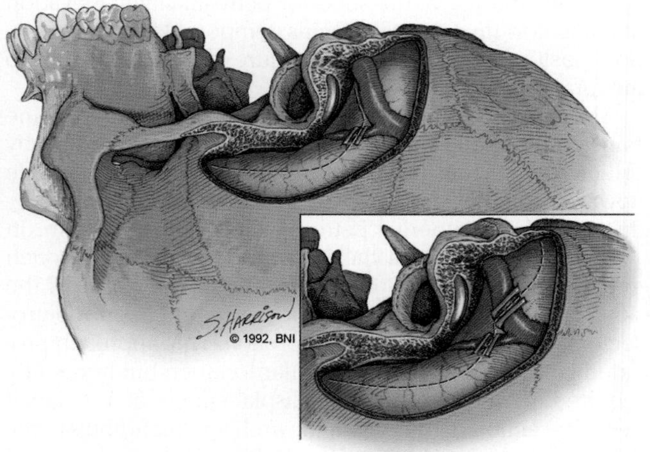

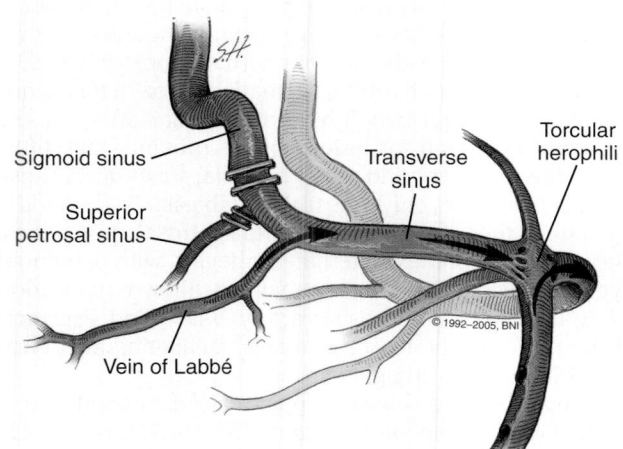

FIGURE 77-3 A right-side combined translabyrinthine approach. After the craniotomy and petrosal bone drilling have been completed, the dural opening is completed *(broken line)* along the floor of the middle fossa. The superior petrosal sinus is then divided between clips, and the dural opening is continued in the posterior fossa just anterior to the sigmoid sinus and the jugular bulb to the sinodural angle. An alternative dural incision (inset) crosses the sigmoid sinus. The sigmoid sinus can be sacrificed only if adequate collateral venous drainage can be demonstrated. *(From Spetzler RF, Daspit CP, Pappas CT. The combined supra- and infratentorial approach for lesions of the petrous and clival regions: experience with 46 cases. J Neurosurg. 1992;76:588-599, with permission from Barrow Neurological Institute.)*

FIGURE 77-4 The major veins and dural venous sinuses that must be considered in the combined approaches. Orientation is as seen by the surgeon: the top of the figure is inferior anatomically, and the right side corresponds to the posterior anatomically. Before the sigmoid sinus can be ligated, a widely patent torcular and contralateral jugular venous system must be demonstrated angiographically. If the sigmoid sinus is sacrificed, the ipsilateral superior anastomotic vein (vein of Labbé) will drain contralaterally through the medial transverse sinus, across the confluens sinuum (torcula) into the opposite jugular vein. *(From Spetzler RF, Daspit CP, Pappas CTS. The combined supra- and infratentorial approach for lesions of the petrous and clival regions: experience with 46 cases. J Neurosurg. 1992;76:588-599, with permission from Barrow Neurological Institute.)*

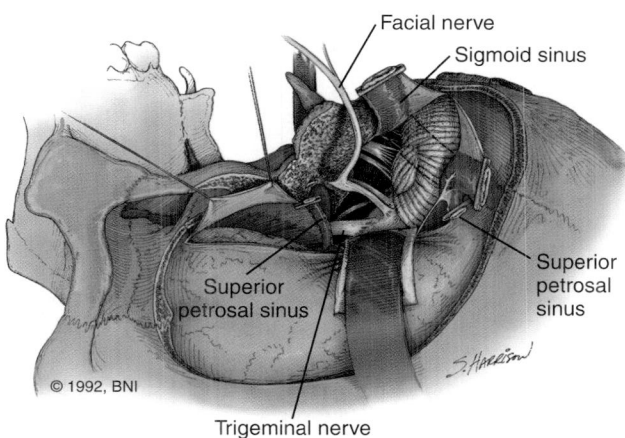

FIGURE 77-5 A right transcochlear combined approach after the dura has been opened, the superior petrosal and sigmoid sinuses have been divided, and the tentorium has been divided down to the incisura. Division of the tentorium allows the superior anastomotic vein (vein of Labbé) to be retracted superiorly with the tentorial leaflets. The resultant approach to the brain stem and clivus is very flat and extends from the cavernous sinus down to the foramen magnum. *(From Spetzler RF, Daspit CP, Pappas CT. The combined supra- and infratentorial approach for lesions of the petrous and clival regions: experience with 46 cases. J Neurosurg. 1992;76:588-599, with permission from Barrow Neurological Institute.)*

further assurance that the sigmoid sinus can be sacrificed, we assess intravascular pressure within the sigmoid sinus before and after temporary occlusion of the sinus. Once the superficial petrosal sinus has been divided, a no. 25 needle is inserted into the sigmoid sinus just proximal to the temporary clip location and pressure is recorded. In our experience when the sinuses are patent, intravascular pressure has not increased by more than 7 mm Hg after sigmoid sinus occlusion. Should pressure in the sigmoid sinus increase

more than 10 mm Hg with temporary occlusion, the sinus should be kept intact. If the sigmoid sinus is sacrificed, the ipsilateral superior anastomotic vein drains contralaterally, because it consistently and reliably enters the transverse sinus above the junction of the superior petrosal sinus and sigmoid sinus (Fig. 77-4). We now keep the sigmoid sinus intact in most patients.

INTRADURAL EXPOSURE

After the dural incisions have been completed, the superior petrosal sinus has been divided, and the fate of the sigmoid sinus has been determined, the dural incision is extended down through the tentorium (posterior to the fourth cranial nerve) to the tentorial hiatus, thus connecting the supra- and infra-tentorial compartments (Fig. 77-5). If the sigmoid sinus has been preserved, the posterior temporal lobe must be elevated, with care taken to protect the superior anastomotic vein, which is indirectly tethered to the skull base by the sigmoid sinus. The superior anastomotic vein can be mobilized by dissection from the cortical surface to minimize tension on the vessel.[57] These final maneuvers expose the ipsilateral petrous region, the entire clivus and brain stem, and the cranial nerves and major arterial vessels of the brain stem. With microscopic technique, tumors and vascular lesions can be resected or clipped between any pair of adjacent cranial nerves. These surgical approaches provide maximal angle of exposure along the base of the skull with minimal or no brain retraction (Figs. 77-5 and 77-6).

CLOSURE

When possible, the surgical field is closed in anatomic layers. The temporal and occipital dura is reapproximated with 4-0 braided nylon suture. Abdominal adipose tissue, temporalis muscle, and fibrin glue are used to obliterate the eustachian tube (translabyrinthine) and the void created

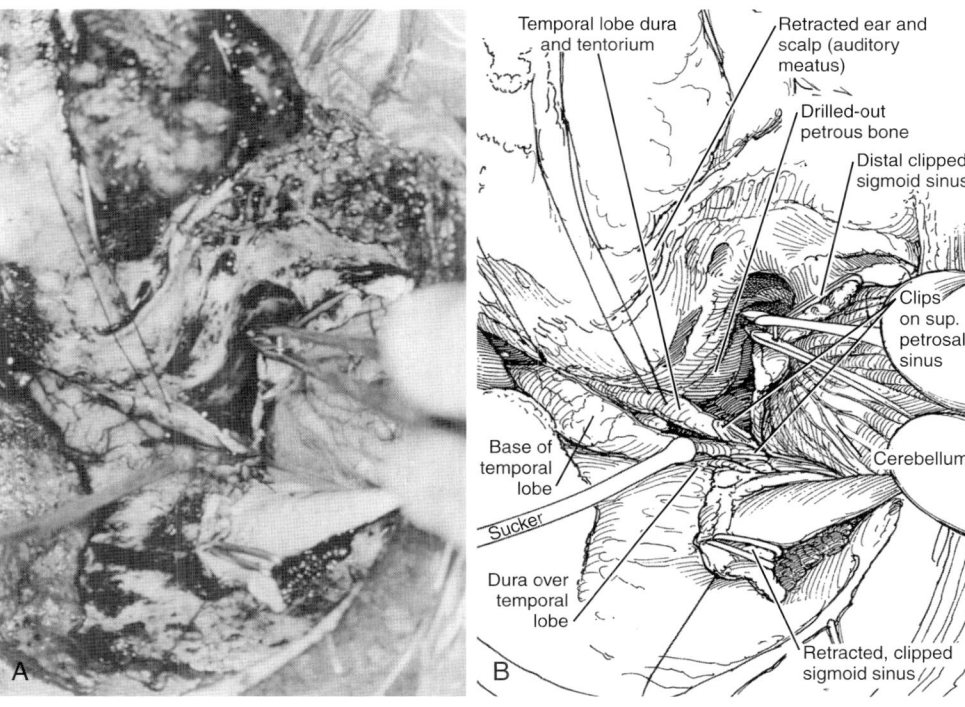

FIGURE 77-6 Translabyrinthine approach as illustrated by intraoperative photograph (A) and schematic drawing (B). The sigmoid sinus has been transected, and the dura of the temporal and posterior fossa has been opened. The tentorium will be divided along its entire length between the clips on the superior petrosal sinus. *(From Spetzler RF, Daspit CP, Pappas CT. The combined supra- and infratentorial approach for lesions of the petrous and clival regions: experience with 46 cases. J Neurosurg. 1992;76:588-599, with permission from American Association of Neurological Surgeons.)*

by temporal bone resection. Temporary lumbar drainage of CSF is used for 3 to 5 days to prevent CSF leakage through the wound. A standard closure of the fascial and skin layers is then undertaken.

SELECTION OF SURGICAL APPROACH

The selection of a particular variation of the combined approach for extensive lesions of the clivus and medial petrous region is based on the considerations outlined in the discussion concerning the transpetrosal approaches. Although sacrifice of the sigmoid sinus is optional, it provides further exposure, by permitting elevation of the temporal lobe, than is otherwise possible without stretching and potentially compromising the superior anastomotic vein. If the previously discussed procedure for verification of appropriate compensatory venous drainage is followed, no apparent risk appears to be associated with sacrifice of the sigmoid sinus.

TREATMENT COMPLICATIONS

A detailed analysis of 46 patients reported in 1992[41] summarizes the operative risks associated with the combined approach. There was no operative mortality in this series, and the postoperative morbidity and mortality data compare favorably with those of previously published reports for this approach. The incidence of facial nerve paralysis in our patient series has remained about 30%. The incidence of CSF leakage is about 13% and that of abducens paralysis is about 7%. The incidence of other operative complications (numbness, aphasia, sepsis, hemiparesis, pneumonia, and hematoma) ranges between 2% and 4% for each.

The senior author has found that the combined supra- and infra-tentorial approach, with its appropriate variations, permits exquisite surgical exposure for treating most aneurysms involving the midbasilar and lower basilar artery. These approaches permit the surgeon to treat these lesions safely and adequately with a minimum of brain retraction.

Far-Lateral Approach

The far-lateral approach to the inferior clivus and upper cervical region is a technical modification that achieves lateral extension to the unilateral suboccipital approach and has been a neurosurgical "standard" for more than a century.[42-44,58] This modification greatly enhances anterior exposure of this region (the inferior brain stem and clivus, upper cervical spine, and anterior spinal canal) and provides excellent access to the lower basilar artery and vertebrobasilar junction.

The main objective of the far-lateral approach is to achieve a flat exposure to the anterior aspect of the inferior brain stem or upper cervical cord and to the associated neurovascular structures and cranial nerves. This exposure is obtained by removing the inferior rim of the foramen magnum and part of the occipital condyle and the posterolateral arch of C1 to the level of the sulcus arteriosus of the vertebral artery. The dural opening obtained after this bony removal provides maximal exposure and requires minimal retraction of neurovascular structures.

PATIENT POSITIONING

The patient is placed in a modified park-bench position that is different from the standard park-bench position in two features (Figs. 77-7 and 77-8): the position of the body

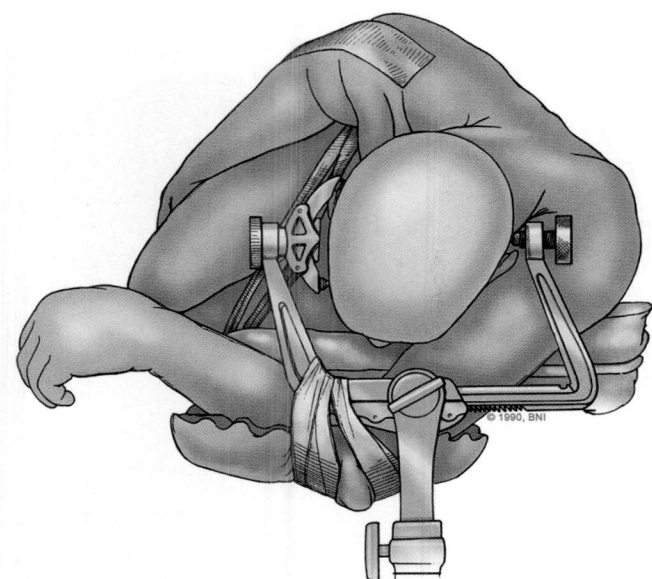

FIGURE 77-7 Schematic drawing of modified park-bench position for a right far-lateral approach viewed from the cranial vertex. The three maneuvers outlined in the text have been performed. Note that the dependent arm has been padded and cradled beneath the Mayfield headrest. A foam roll is placed under the axilla for extra protection (not shown). *(Used with permission from Barrow Neurological Institute.)*

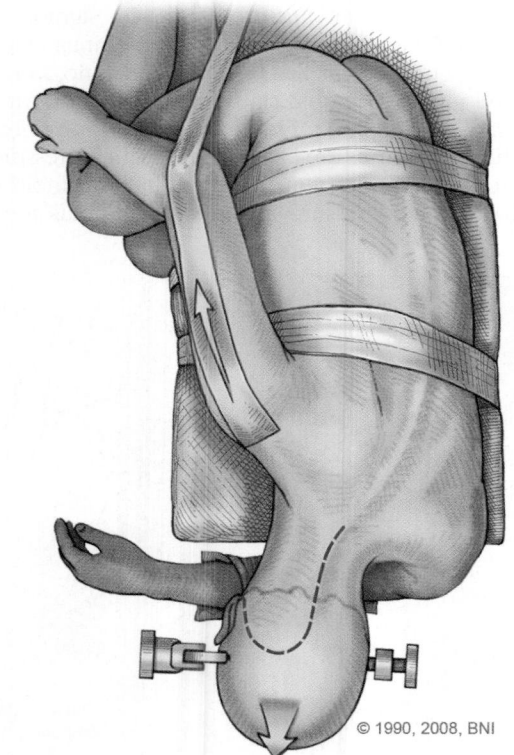

FIGURE 77-8 Schematic drawing of patient positioning for a right far-lateral position viewed from above. The right arm is pulled downward with tape to open the craniocervical angle, and the patient is taped securely to the operating table to allow the angle to be changed during the procedure. *(Used with permission from Barrow Neurological Institute.)*

and dependent arm, and the position of the head. Each of these features is critical to obtaining maximal exposure of the lesion with greatest ease for the surgeon and optimal safety for the patient.

The patient is placed in a Mayfield three-pin headrest (Fig. 77-7) and positioned laterally on the operating table with the side to be treated facing upward. The operating table is extended by placing a 34-inch plastic board under the mattress and pulling the mattress and board 15 to 20 cm beyond the end of the table. The patient's dependent arm is allowed to drop off the extended end of the operating table and is carefully cradled in foam underneath the edge of the table, within the gap between the Mayfield headrest and the table attachment (Figs. 77-7 and 77-8). A foam roll is placed in the axilla. This placement of the arm improves venous return and decreases the risk of brachial plexus compression. Furthermore, the amount of cranial rotation and flexion that can be achieved is maximized by allowing the dependent arm to drop.

The head is not positioned in the standard straight lateral position. The position of the head is achieved with a sequence of three maneuvers that places the inferior clivus perpendicular to the floor and that maximally opens the posterior cervical-suboccipital angle, thereby allowing greater movement of the operating microscope around the operative field. The head is positioned with the midline parallel to the floor. Then the head and neck are (1) flexed in the anteroposterior plane until the chin is one fingerbreadth from the sternum, (2) rotated 45 degrees downward (to the contralateral side, away from the lesion), and (3) laterally flexed 30 degrees downward toward the opposite shoulder. With the patient in this position, the ipsilateral mastoid process is at the highest point in the operative field. The upper shoulder is pulled down toward the feet and taped, thereby further enlarging the working space for the surgeon (Fig. 77-8). The knees and upper arm are well padded, and the entire body is secured with tape to allow for full rotation of the operating table.

SURGICAL TECHNIQUE

An inverted hockey-stick incision starts at the mastoid prominence and proceeds under the superior nuchal line to the midline. The incision follows the midline to the C3 or C4 spinous process (Fig. 77-9). A 1-cm edge of nuchal fascia and muscle is left at the upper incision to allow anatomic closure of the wound. This nuchal cuff is obtained by dissecting under the muscle with a narrow periosteal elevator, starting from the midline and ending at the mastoid prominence. The fascia and muscle are divided at the inferior edge of the instrument. At closure, the Mayfield headrest is temporarily loosened from the table attachment, and the neck is extended to help reapproximate the cervical musculature to the nuchal fascia. The paraspinal muscles are split along the midline ligament until the spinous processes of C1 and C2 are identified. Subperiosteal dissection is used to expose the occipital bone, spinous processes, and ipsilateral laminae of C1 and C2. The myocutaneous flap is retracted inferiorly and laterally with fishhooks attached to a Leyla bar. The midline part of the incision can be retracted contralaterally with fishhooks from a second Leyla bar.

The lateral mass of C1 and the vertebral artery from the sulcus of C1 to its point of posterior fossa dural entry are

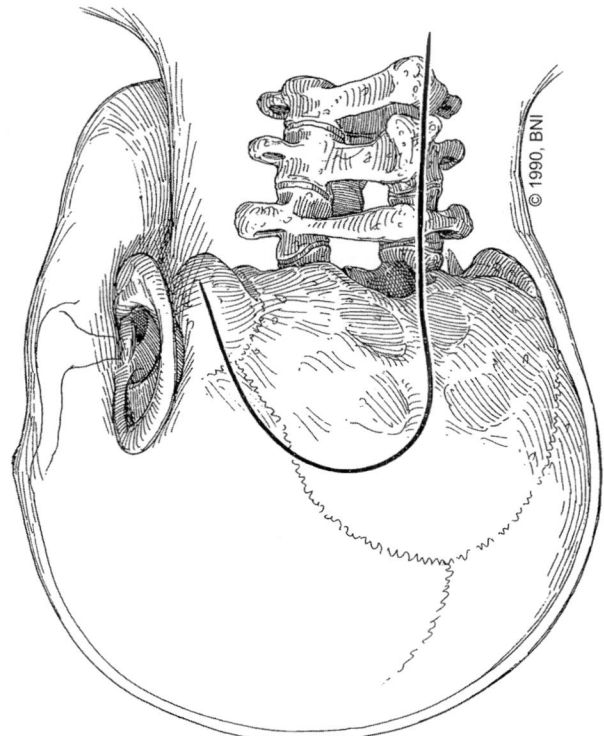

FIGURE 77-9 Close-up of the skin incision extending from the mastoid tip along the nuchal line to the midline, down to about C3 or C4 to allow for adequate muscle flap retraction. *(Used with permission from Barrow Neurological Institute.)*

exposed. Bleeding from the venous plexus surrounding the vertebral artery is controlled with bipolar coagulation or small pieces of hemostatic material (e.g., Gelfoam, Surgicel). The Midas Rex drill with the B1 bit and footplate is used to perform a C1 hemilaminectomy. The contralateral lamina is cut just across the midline, and the ipsilateral lamina is cut at the sulcus for the vertebral artery. The lamina can be replaced after the procedure is completed. A C2 hemilaminectomy can also be performed if additional caudal exposure is required.

A limited suboccipital, retrosigmoid craniotomy is performed with the same drill, extending from the contralateral margin of the foramen magnum (just past the midline) to as far lateral as possible and back down again to the foramen magnum, just medial to the level at which the vertebral artery enters the dura. The other dimension of the craniotomy—the height (the distance between the foramen magnum and the superior margin of the bone opening)—can extend to the level of the transverse sinus and is determined primarily by the location and size of the lesion (Fig. 77-10). Lesions confined to the foramen magnum do not require exposure to the transverse sinus. For access to clival lesions that extend beyond the reach of the far-lateral approach, the craniotomy can be expanded with a transpetrosal procedure or beyond the level of the transverse sinus and tentorium when it is combined with the combined approach (see section titled Far-Lateral Combined Supra- and Infra-Tentorial Approach).

The next stage involves removal of bone from the remaining ipsilateral lateral rim of the foramen magnum

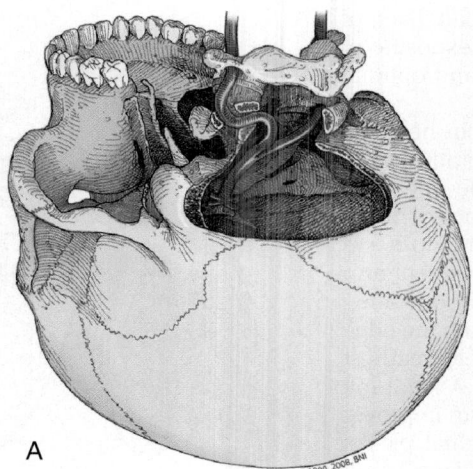

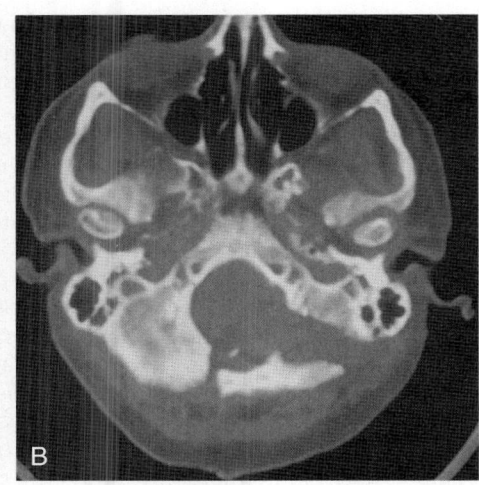

FIGURE 77-10 Illustration and post-operative CT scan illustrating the amount of bone resection. (A) Schematic illustration demonstrating the perspective of the skull and vessels in relation to the amount of bone resection. It is important to resect the occipital and C1 condylar interface so that a gap of 1 cm is present between the extradural vertebral artery and the bone. (B) Postoperative CT scan demonstrating the amount of bone removal that creates the lateral, extremely flat angle of approach to the clivus. *(Used with permission from Barrow Neurological Institute.)*

and occipital condyle. The rim of the foramen magnum is removed with rongeurs, and the posterior occipital condyle and the superior lateral mass and facet of C1 are removed with a high-speed drill. The inner portion of the condyle is drilled until only a thin shell of cortical bone remains. This "inside-out" approach, leaving a protective layer of cortical bone over the surrounding structures, facilitates safe removal in a restricted space. This shell is carefully removed with microcurettes. The extradural vertebral artery is protected with a small dissector while the condyle is drilled away.

Entry into the condylar veins usually indicates that sufficient anterior bone has been removed, typically about 1 cm anterior (deep) to the point at which the vertebral artery enters the dura. Bleeding from these condylar vessels can readily be controlled with bone wax and bipolar coagulation.

Because the hypoglossal canal is situated in the anterior medial third of the occipital condyle, it is not threatened by removal of the posterior lateral third of the condyle.[59] This extreme removal of lateral bone from the condyle and lateral mass of C1 is the crucial final step for approaching the anterior brain stem from an inferolateral angle with minimal brain retraction (Fig. 77-10). Even more extensive exposure can be obtained by drilling away the mastoid process and the occipitoatlantal articular facet; however, bony fusion of the craniocervical junction is then needed to maintain postoperative stability.[60]

The dura is opened in a curvilinear fashion with its base hinged laterally and pulled tight against the lateral aspect of the craniotomy with 4-0 braided nylon sutures. These tenting sutures are placed so that after passage of the needle through the dura, both limbs of the suture are on the inside surface of the dura, thereby aiding in retracting the dura tightly against the underlying bone. The extensive extradural removal of the lateral bone, without retraction, eliminates the last obstruction to direct vision of the inferior clivus, anteroinferior brain stem, and upper anterior cervical spinal cord (Fig. 77-11). With arachnoidal microdissection and minimal elevation of the cerebellar tonsil, visualization is improved as far rostrally as the pontomedullary junction. This approach also allows excellent proximal control of the vertebral artery and its branches.

When possible, the surgical field is closed in anatomic layers. The cervical and occipital dura is reapproximated with 4-0 braided nylon suture. The C1 hemilamina and the craniotomy segment are returned to their normal positions and secured with small plates and screws or 2-0 braided nylon suture. The muscle, fascia, and skin layers are then closed in standard fashion.

Salas and colleagues have recently described a variation of the far-lateral approach designed to improve exposure and visualization of aneurysms at the vertebrobasilar junction.[21] The transtubercular approach initially involves extradural resection of the posteromedial one third of the occipital condyle and C1 lateral mass. Partial resection of jugular tubercle is also performed extradurally. The

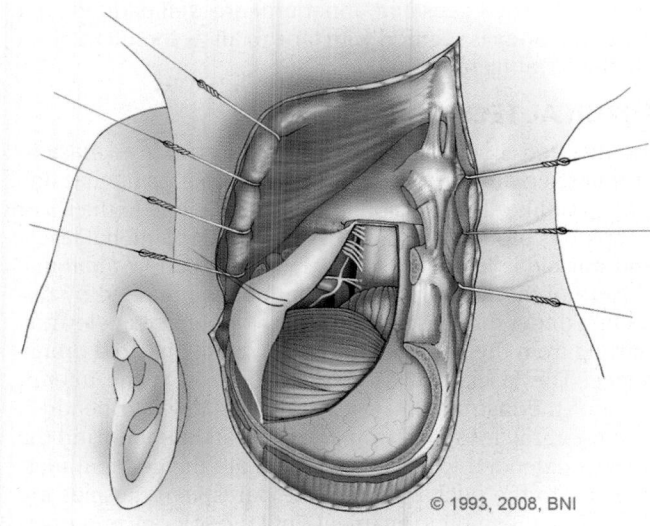

FIGURE 77-11 Schematic illustration demonstrating the dural opening and the amount of lateral exposure of the inferior clivus and associated neurovascular structures that can be obtained with the far-lateral exposure. It is very important to have the superior and inferior limbs of the dural incision perpendicular to the wound edge to allow maximum lateral retraction of the dural flap. *(Used with permission from Barrow Neurological Institute.)*

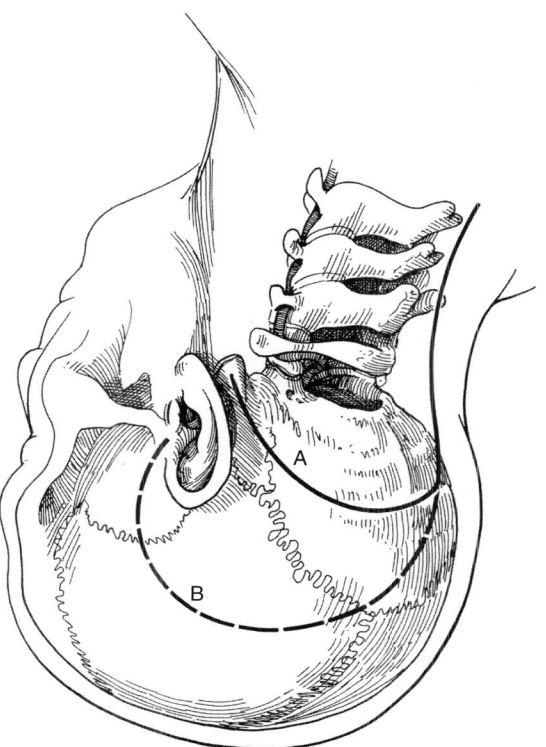

FIGURE 77-12 Schematic depiction of the skin incision used in the far-lateral exposure (A) and the modification utilized in the combined-combined exposure (B). *(From Baldwin HZ, Miller CG, Van Loveren HR, et al. The far lateral-combined supra- and infratentorial approach. A human cadaveric prosection model for routes of access to the petroclival region and ventral brain stem. J Neurosurg. 1994;81:60-68, with permission from AANS.)*

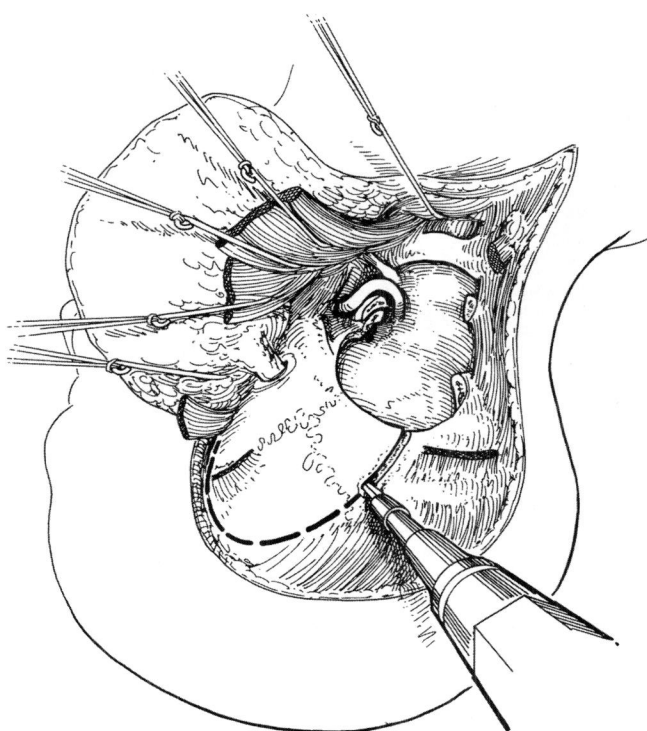

FIGURE 77-13 Schematic depiction of the craniotomy performed during the combined-combined procedure. In this illustration, the far-lateral craniotomy has already been performed, and the craniotomy for the combined craniotomy is being performed. An alternative would be to perform the craniotomy as one segment that crosses the transverse sinus. Though not depicted, the neuro-otologist typically performs the petrosal drilling before the craniotomy flaps are turned. *(From Baldwin HZ, Miller CG, Van Loveren HR,, et al. The far lateral-combined supra- and infratentorial approach. A human cadaveric prosection model for routes of access to the petroclival region and ventral brain stem. J Neurosurg. 1994;81:60-68, with permission from AANS.)*

remainder of the tubercle is craniectomized intradurally using a drill and working around the lower cranial nerves, with or without prior division of the sigmoid sinus (using similar principles for sinus division as described earlier).

Far-Lateral Combined Supra- and Infra-Tentorial Approach

Occasionally, a more extensive lateral exposure of the clivus is required to deal with giant aneurysms involving the midbasilar and lower basilar artery. Such exposure can be accomplished by combining the far-lateral approach with either a transpetrosal approach or the combined supra- and infratentorial approach.[39] This "combined-combined" approach offers a wide, flat route to the entire length of the clivus.

The combined-combined approach can be accomplished using the principles previously outlined for the individual procedures. The skin incision for the far-lateral approach is expanded to encompass the exposure needed for the transpetrosal or combined approach, thereby drawing the superior limb of the incision up over the ear, down to the level of the zygoma (Fig. 77-12). The transpetrosal drilling is completed by the neuro-otologist. The neurosurgeon follows with the far-lateral exposure. After the C1 hemilaminectomy has been completed, a craniotomy that starts at the foramen magnum and encompasses the suboccipital and temporal regions can be performed in two

sections (Fig. 77-13) or as a single unit. The dural opening for the far-lateral and transpetrosal or combined techniques is completed, and the two are joined if the sigmoid sinus is ligated and divided (Fig. 77-14). The exposure of the anterior brain stem and basilar artery that can be obtained is exquisite. The dural opening and wound are closed as previously described.

Anterior Transclival Approaches

The various transclival approaches are seldom used to treat aneurysms of the midbasilar and lower basilar artery. They are usually the subject of case reports or small institutional series. In general, the risks of CSF leakage and meningitis are higher than with the previously described approaches. There is also risk of palate dysfunction when the transpalatal route is used and when a transmaxillary approach Le Fort osteotomy is used. Ogilvy and colleagues developed the transfacial transclival approach through a lateral rhinotomy incision, an alternative to the other transclival approaches to optimize exposure without maxillotomy and to minimize complications.[25] Using this approach, they treated five patients with excellent surgical exposure, good cosmetic results, and no palatal dysfunction. Although three developed CSF leaks, none had any long-term sequelae of meningitis.

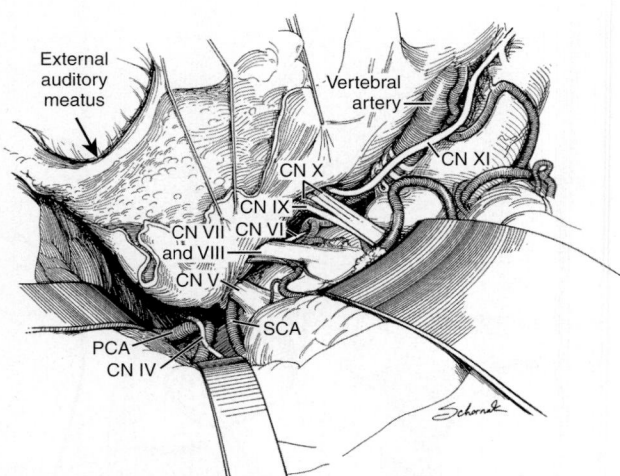

FIGURE 77-14 Schematic illustration of the amount of intradural exposure provided in the retrolabyrinthine combined-combined approach. Note that the lateral view extends from about C2 up to the top of the basilar artery. The lateral angle can be greatly augmented by removal of the labyrinths (translabyrinthine approach). CN, cranial nerve; PCA, posterior cerebral artery; SCA, superior cerebral artery. *(From Baldwin HZ, Miller CG, Van Loveren HR,, et al. The far lateral-combined supra- and infratentorial approach. A human cadaveric prosection model for routes of access to the petroclival region and ventral brain stem. J Neurosurg. 1994;81:60-68, with permission from AANS.)*

Summary and Conclusions

Aneurysms located on the midbasilar and lower basilar artery are uncommon, representing only a minority of cerebral aneurysms. They have the same natural history as aneurysms involving other cerebral vessels. Because of their location, however, midbasilar and lower basilar artery aneurysms remain among the most difficult neurosurgical challenges. The principles underlying management of these lesions require maximal surgical exposure with minimal brain retraction, and proximal and distal vascular control with preservation of the parent vessel and perforators, to achieve complete obliteration of the aneurysm. A number of surgical exposures have been developed that fulfill these requirements, allowing aneurysms of the midbasilar and lower basilar artery to be managed effectively. Continuing advances in surgical technique lead to improved patient outcomes. The mid- and lower basilar artery are relatively uncommon locations for cerebral aneurysms and the use of endovascular methods to treat such lesions is increasing. We therefore believe that there is also probably an increasing role for subspecialized management of these complex aneurysms at experienced cerebrovascular centers.

KEY REFERENCES

Baldwin HZ, Miller CG, van Loveren HR, et al. The far lateral/combined supra- and infratentorial approach. A human cadaveric prosection model for routes of access to the petroclival region and ventral brain stem. *J Neurosurg.* 1994;81(1):60-68.

Drake CG, Peerless SJ, Hernesniemi JA, et al. *Surgery of Vertebrobasilar Aneurysms: London, Ontario Experience on 1767 Patients.* Vienna: Springer-Verlag; 1996.

Fiorella D, Kelly ME, Albuquerque FC, Nelson PK. Curative reconstruction of a giant midbasilar trunk aneurysm with the pipeline embolization device. *Neurosurgery.* 2009;64(2):212-217.

Heros RC. Lateral suboccipital approach for vertebral and vertebrobasilar artery lesions. *J Neurosurg.* 1986;64(4):559-562.

Higa T, Ujiie H, Kato K, et al. Basilar artery trunk saccular aneurysms: morphological characteristics and management. *Neurosurg Rev.* 2009;32(2):181-191.

Hitselberger WE, House WF. A combined approach to the cerebellopontine angle: a suboccipital-petrosal approach. *Arch Otolaryngol.* 1966;84:49-67.

House WF. Translabyrinthine approach. In: House WF, Luetje CM, eds. *Acoustic Tumors II: Management.* Baltimore: University Park Press; 1979:43-87.

House WF, Hitselberger WE. The transcochlear approach to the skull base. *Arch Otolaryngol.* 1976;102(6):334-342.

Hunt WE, Hess RM. Surgical risk as related to time of intervention in the repair of intracranial aneurysms. *J Neurosurg.* 1968;28(1):14-20.

Lanzino G, Wakhloo AK, Fessler RD, et al. Efficacy and current limitations of intravascular stents for intracranial internal carotid, vertebral, and basilar artery aneurysms. *J Neurosurg.* 1999;91(4):538-546.

Molyneux A, Kerr R, Stratton I, et al. International Subarachnoid Aneurysm Trial (ISAT) of neurosurgical clipping versus endovascular coiling in 2143 patients with ruptured intracranial aneurysms: a randomised trial. *Lancet.* 2002;360(9342):1267-1274.

de Oliveira E, Rhoton Jr AL, Peace D, et al. Microsurgical anatomy of the region of the foramen magnum. *Surg Neurol.* 1985;24(3):293-352.

Peerless SJ, Drake CG. Surgical techniques of posterior circulation aneurysms. In: Schmidek HHS, Sweet WH, eds. *Operative Neurosurgical Techniques.* 2nd ed. Philadelphia: WB Saunders; 1988:973-989.

Sanai N, Tarapore P, Lee AC, et al. The current role of microsurgery for posterior circulation aneurysms: a selective approach in the endovascular era. *Neurosurgery.* 2008;62(6):1236-1249.

Seifert V, Raabe A, Zimmermann M. Conservative (labyrinth-preserving) transpetrosal approach to the clivus and petroclival region—indications, complications, results and lessons learned. *Acta Neurochir (Wien).* 2003;145(8):631-642.

Seifert V, Stolke D. Posterior transpetrosal approach to aneurysms of the basilar trunk and vertebrobasilar junction. *J Neurosurg.* 1996; 85(3):373-379.

Sen CN, Sekhar LN. An extreme lateral approach to intradural lesions of the cervical spine and foramen magnum. *Neurosurgery.* 1990;27(2):197-204.

Sen CN, Sekhar LN. Surgical management of anteriorly placed lesions at the craniocervical junction—an alternative approach. *Acta Neurochir (Wien).* 1991;108(1-2):70-77.

Spetzler RF, Daspit CP, Pappas CT. The combined supra- and infratentorial approach for lesions of the petrous and clival regions: experience with 46 cases. *J Neurosurg.* 1992;76(4):588-599.

Spetzler RF, Graham TF. The far lateral approach to the inferior clivus and the upper cervical region: technical note. *BNI Q.* 1990;6:35-38.

Uda K, Murayama Y, Gobin YP, et al. Endovascular treatment of basilar artery trunk aneurysms with Guglielmi detachable coils: clinical experience with 41 aneurysms in 39 patients. *J Neurosurg.* 2001;95(4): 624-632.

Unruptured intracranial aneurysms—risk of rupture and risks of surgical intervention. International Study of Unruptured Intracranial Aneurysms Investigators. *N Engl J Med.* 1998;339(24):1725-1733:10.

Van Rooij WJ, Sluzewski M, Menovsky T, Wijnalda D. Coiling of saccular basilar trunk aneurysms. *Neuroradiology.* 2003;45(1):19-21.

Wiebers DO, Whisnant JP, Huston III J, et al. Unruptured intracranial aneurysms: natural history, clinical outcome, and risks of surgical and endovascular treatment. *Lancet.* 2003;362(9378):103-110.

Yamaura A. Surgical management of posterior circulation aneurysms: Part I. *Contemp Neurosurg.* 1985;7:1-6.

Numbered references appear on Expert Consult.

Surgical Management of Aneurysms of the Vertebral and Posterior Inferior Cerebellar Artery Complex

HELMUT BERTALANFFY • LUDWIG BENES • STEFAN HEINZE • WUTTIPONG TIRAKOTAI • ULRICH SURE

Aneurysms of the vertebral artery–posterior inferior cerebellar artery (VA-PICA) complex originate from any portion of the intradural VA up to the vertebrobasilar junction and from one of the five PICA segments. During the past decade, the treatment of these aneurysms became more sophisticated due to significant developments in diagnostic methods, improvements in microsurgical technique, further development of skull base surgery, better understanding of the microsurgical anatomy of the vertebrobasilar arterial territory, and dramatic advances in endovascular therapy. However, despite such continuous improvements, management of these complex lesions remains a challenging task. Several characteristic features distinguish VA and VA-PICA aneurysms from those of the anterior circulation: (1) they are relatively uncommon, occurring approximately one tenth as frequently as aneurysms in the anterior circulation[1]; (2) they show great variability in size, location, and morphology; the percentage of dissecting and fusiform aneurysms is much higher than in the other intracranial compartments; and (3) most of them are located deeply in the posterior fossa having a close relationship to the lower brain stem, the lower cranial nerves, and the cerebellum, making them difficult to access. The anatomic variability of the VA, the PICA, and the skull base around the jugular tubercle add further to the complexity of these lesions and increase the risk of their management. The infrequency of these lesions is the main reason why many neurosurgeons have only limited personal experience with the surgical treatment of VA-PICA aneurysms. With the advent of modern endovascular therapy, the number of lesions available for surgery, particularly the number of less complex VA and VA-PICA aneurysms, has further decreased, a situation that also raises problems in neurosurgical training. On the other hand, recent treatment strategies have gradually changed toward combined endovascular and surgical management, especially in the acute phase of severe subarachnoid hemorrhage (SAH) or in high-risk patients. It is obvious that only a limited number of specialized neurovascular centers can offer sufficient expertise for the safe management of this subgroup of vascular lesions.

Epidemiology

Aneurysms of the VA-PICA complex comprise 0.5% to 3% of all intracranial aneurysms.[2-6] Approximately two thirds of these aneurysms are located at the bifurcation of the VAPICA junction, whereas distal PICA aneurysms account for approximately 0.3% to 1% of all aneurysms.[6-8] In a recently published series of 24 patients, distal PICA aneurysms accounted for only 0.3% of all intracranial aneurysms and for 3.7% of the vertebrobasilar lesions; 74% were saccular, 7% were fusiform, and 19% were dissecting.[7] Until 1992, only 140 patients harboring an aneurysm of the VA-PICA complex were reported in the literature[9]; of these, approximately 75% were VA or VA-PICA and 25% were distal PICA aneurysms. Multiple occurrence was occasionally reported.[4,10-13] Although the incidence of aneurysms arising in association with arteriovenous malformations may be as high as 46%, the combination of a VA-PICA aneurysm and an arteriovenous malformation is rarely reported in the literature.[14-16] With 85%, there is a clear predominance of female patients,[4,5,17,18] even more notable in saccular aneurysms.[19] Patients of virtually all ages may be affected, with an average age of 49.3 years.[20]

Aneurysm Characteristics

In contrast to intracranial aneurysms of other locations, only approximately 60% of VA-PICA aneurysms are saccular; approximately 30% are dissecting and 10% fusiform.[9,21,22] In Yamaura's[18] series, there were 60% saccular, 27% dissecting, and 13% arteriosclerotic fusiform aneurysms; moreover, he found three giant lesions with a diameter exceeding 25 mm and two partially thrombosed saccular aneurysms. Drs. Drake and Peerless and colleagues have treated the world's largest series of patients with vertebrobasilar aneurysms, comprising 1767 individual patients, of whom 217 (12.3%) harbored aneurysms of the VA-PICA complex.[19,20,23] One hundred sixty-six lesions were saccular (76.5%), 25 were dissecting (11%), 18 were fusiform (8%), 4 were atherosclerotic (1.8%), 3 were associated with an arteriovenous malformation (1.3%), and 1 was traumatic (0.4%). The majority (70%) were small (<12 mm); 27 aneurysms (12%) were large (13 to 24 mm) and 40 (18%) were giant (>25 mm). Left-sided origin was more common (55%). Forty-three aneurysms (19%) were unruptured.[19,23]

Fusiform aneurysms appear as spindle-shaped dilatations, the vertebrobasilar trunk being the most frequent location for fusiform aneurysms.[24] Due to a clear difference in natural history and optimal therapy, they must be clearly distinguished from dissecting aneurysms. More than two decades ago, nontraumatic dissecting aneurysms were considered to be extremely rare. However, improved neuroradiologic imaging techniques have demonstrated such lesions with increasing frequency, and during the past years, this type of aneurysm has received great attention in the pertinent literature.[10,22,25] On arteriography, such aneurysms appear as a saccular or spindle-shaped vascular dilatation, occasionally combined with proximal stenosis. The classic arteriographic features of dissecting arteries include the double-lumen sign, retention of contrast medium, the pearl-and-string sign,[26] and focal outpouching.[22,27] Usually, they are not related to vascular branches of the VA. Such dissecting aneurysms of the VA may occur proximal as well as distal to the origin of the PICA, but occasionally they may involve the origin of the PICA as well.[28] Yasui and colleagues[29] believe that a fusiform VA aneurysm is one predisposing condition for a dissecting lesion. The sudden disruption of the internal elastic lamina is the primary mechanism underlying the development of dissecting aneurysms. The plane of dissection extends through the media, and most aneurysms have one entrance to this pseudolumen.[30] Dissecting aneurysms of the VA often cause SAH by rupture of the adventitia and present a high risk of rebleeding.[28,31,32] These lesions are not confined to the VA but may be observed on the distal PICA as well.[7,33,34] Occasionally, a dissecting distal PICA aneurysm can develop as a traumatic lesion.[35]

Extreme dilations of the VA, termed "dolichoectasias," occur less frequently and are usually difficult to treat. The involved artery is elongated and tortuous. On histologic examination, large defects within the muscular and elastic lamina can be detected and sometimes also extensive arteriosclerotic changes.[30] Although dissecting aneurysms occur more frequently in male patients of younger age, dolichoectasias occur more frequently in the seventh decade.[9,22,36,37]

Historical Background

According to Hudgins and colleagues,[4] the first case description of a saccular VA-PICA aneurysm was given by Cruveilhier in 1829. Rizzoli and Hayes[38] were the first to surgically treat such an aneurysm in 1947 by interrupting the parent artery with two silver clips. Interestingly, the aneurysm was detected by these authors on a ventriculogram that showed a displaced fourth ventricle. Lewis and colleagues[33] mentioned that the first case of an aneurysm arising from the distal segment of the PICA was reported in 1864 by Fernet and that the first surgical treatment of a peripheral PICA aneurysm is accredited to Olivecrona. In the 1950s and 1960s, vertebrobasilar aneurysms were associated with the highest mortality rate.[39] Rizzoli and Hayes[38] treated a peripheral PICA aneurysm with trapping in 1953. Uihlein and Hughes[40] described in 1955 the nonsurgical treatment of 14 patients harboring a posterior fossa aneurysm; eight of these patients died after the aneurysm ruptured. After the introduction of routine vertebral angiography in patients with SAH, such aneurysms were detected with increasing frequency. In 1958, Desaussure and colleagues[41] reported the successful surgical obliteration of two PICA aneurysms found on vertebral angiograms. Further improvements of neuroradiologic techniques after the introduction of transfemoral catheter and subtraction angiography as well as the routine use of microsurgical techniques in neurosurgery have dramatically improved the outcome of surgical procedures for treatment of vertebrobasilar aneurysms.[42,43]

Neuroradiologic Imaging

A meticulous preoperative neuroradiologic assessment is indispensable for successful treatment of VA and VA-PICA aneurysms. Neuroradiologic investigations should clarify the following features: (1) the exact location and origin of the aneurysm with respect to the VA and the various segments of the PICA (Fig. 78-1); (2) the size, shape, extent, and limits of the lesion to differentiate between saccular, fusiform, and dissecting aneurysms; (3) the orientation of the neck and the dome of the aneurysm; (4) the presence or

FIGURE 78-1 The segmental nomenclature of the posterior inferior cerebellar artery (PICA) and the vertebral artery complex (VA) for possible localizations of aneurysm formation. 1, Anterior medullary segment; 2, lateral medullary segment; 3, tonsillomedullary segment; 4, telovelotonsillar segment; 5, cortical branch segments. *(Courtesy of Christoph Kappus.)*

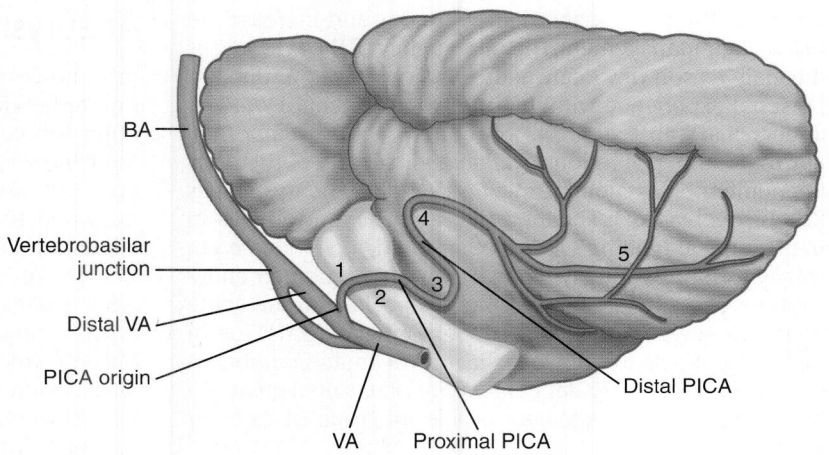

BA

Vertebrobasilar junction

Distal VA

PICA origin

VA   Proximal PICA

Distal PICA

absence of sufficient collateral circulation; (5) the patency of both VAs and the dominance of one of them, if present; (6) the presence or absence of multiple intracranial aneurysms or an associated arteriovenous malformation; (7) the precise relationship to the major surrounding anatomic structures as well as the degree of involvement of the brain stem and rootlets of the lower cranial nerves; and (8) the presence of hydrocephalus and/or intracerebral/intraventricular hemorrhage.

Neuroradiologic studies include high-quality arterial digital angiography as well as various techniques of coronal, sagittal, and axial magnetic resonance imaging, and computed tomography (CT). Digital subtraction angiography may be complemented by rotational angiography with 3-dimensional rendering. Yonekawa and colleagues[44] described three distances that can be measured on preoperative angiograms that are important predictors of the difficulty of operative access to VA-PICA aneurysms: the distance of the aneurysm from the midline, the distance from the most lateral point of the foramen magnum, and the distance from the clivus. According to these authors, optimal results are obtained when these distances are more than 5 to 10 mm, less than 10 to 21 mm, and less than 13 mm, respectively.

In a previous communication, we emphasized that high-resolution CT using a bone tissue algorithm is most useful to demonstrate the configuration of the skull base around the jugular foramen, in particular showing the size and shape of the jugular tubercle, the size of the posterior condylar canal, and the distance between the dural entrance of the vertebral artery and the hypoglossal canal or jugular tubercle.[45] Special sections or 3-dimensional reconstructions may further add to the understanding of the individual skull base configuration or presence of bony anomalies. When performed with a bolus of contrast medium, this 3-dimensional CT image may demonstrate the relationship between the lesion, brain stem, and skull base, adding important information required for the planning of the procedure.[45] Huynh-Le and colleagues[46] have confirmed the utility of 3-dimensional CT angiography for the surgical management of VA-PICA aneurysms; this diagnostic technique was most valuable in demonstrating not only the exact site and shape of the aneurysm but also the relationships between parent vessel and malformation on the one side and the bony structures of the skull base on the other side. CT is important to demonstrate the SAH, the blood distribution within the basal cisterns, an associated hydrocephalus, and an intraventricular or intracerebral hemorrhage. Intraventricular hemorrhage is present in as many as 82% of patients and associated hydrocephalus in approximately 75% of patients with ruptured aneurysms.[5,47,48] Magnetic resonance imaging is particularly valuable in fusiform, dissecting, or partially thrombosed aneurysms.[30,49] Magnetic resonance angiography can depict the aneurysm in relation to the brain stem, cerebellum, caudal cranial nerves, and skull base.

Clinical Presentation

The most frequent presenting symptom of patients with aneurysms of the VA-PICA complex is SAH. Rupture of these aneurysms occurs similarly to the rupture of aneurysms of the anterior circulation. However, the clinical consequences are far more disastrous. Although only a few patients experience intracerebellar hemorrhage or deficits of caudal cranial nerves, in some instances, prolonged coma, hemiparesis, or pulmonary embolism can occur.[50,51] Aneurysm rupture occurs more frequently in lesions smaller than 12 mm. Large and giant aneurysms rarely rupture; they become symptomatic more frequently by their compressive effect on the lower brain stem or the caudal cranial nerves. Ischemic complications such as Wallenberg's syndrome may occur in dissecting aneurysms due to occlusion of perforating arteries that supply the lateral aspect of the medulla. Patients with dolichoectatic VA and/or basilar artery may have ischemic stroke, brain stem compression, and occasionally hemifacial spasm or trigeminal neuralgia.[52] In the series of Drake and Peerless[53] of 221 patients, 178 had SAH (80.5%). Sixth nerve palsy, not lower cranial nerve paresis, was the most frequent preoperative cranial nerve dysfunction, as one might have expected. It was nearly always associated with SAH and recovered in 75% completely.

Management

The decision as to whether an aneurysm of the VA-PICA complex should be treated, as well as the timing and choice of treatment modality in case treatment appears indicated, depends on criteria such as the patient's age, actual clinical condition, and neurologic status; progression or resolution of initial symptoms and signs; presence or absence of SAH; the interval between SAH and time of decision making; aneurysm characteristics; medical history; and the presence or absence of hydrocephalus and intraventricular or intracerebral hemorrhage. Surgery, for instance, is preferable when a significant hematoma needs to be evacuated. For more than a decade, the concomitant availability of endovascular and microsurgical procedures has made possible a multimodal treatment of aneurysms of the VA-PICA complex.[54-57] Particularly, the technologic achievements in neurovascular instrumentation (i.e., coil technology, intracranial stent technique) of the recent years led to a continuing challenge for interventional neuroradiologists, enabling them to treat even previously "untreatable" aneurysms with a high success rate.[58-66] However, complications of the treatment such as brain stem infarction and hemorrhages are also reported for the interventional therapy of VA-PICA aneurysms.[61,67,68] For some rare complex cases, a combined interventional and microsurgical therapy may constitute a reasonable solution.[58]

In some aneurysms such as proximal PICA lesions, even in cases in which endovascular coil occlusion of the aneurysms seems possible, the direct microsurgical inspection of the affected segment of the PICA and of perforating brain stem-supplying arteries may offer significant advantages compared with endovascular therapy.[33] Considering the complexity and heterogeneity of VA and VA-PICA aneurysms, most lesions might require an individual case-by-case decision.

SURGICAL APPROACHES

To expose aneurysms of the VA-PICA complex surgically, a detailed analysis of aneurysm location, origin, extension, and orientation of the dome is necessary. Small saccular VA-PICA aneurysms may be exposed by a traditional suboccipital medial or lateral approach when they are located proximal to the rootlets of the lower cranial nerves. Aneurysms located more distally or even at the vertebrobasilar junction, as well as large or giant saccular or complex dissecting aneurysms, may require more extensive skull base approaches. Aneurysms of the third, fourth, and fifth PICA segments are best visualized via a suboccipital medial craniotomy. The patient is placed in either the sitting or prone position with the head flexed. The craniotomy includes the posterior rim of the foramen magnum. A number of lateral approaches are available to expose various aneurysms of the VA or the first two PICA segments.[2,9,69-72] For exposure of some proximal VA aneurysms, a traditional retrosigmoid approach may be sufficient.[73] However, several authors have underscored the necessity of extending the exposure more laterally.[69] The retrolabyrinthine transsigmoidal approach was described by Giannotta and Maceri[74] in 1988 and used to expose distal VA-PICA aneurysms or those of the vertebrobasilar junction.

It is a complex and more time-consuming skull base approach because large portions of the petrous bone must be drilled away and the ipsilateral sigmoid sinus is ligated, provided the contralateral sinus is intact. This approach, however, is rarely described in the literature for treatment of aneurysms of the VA-PICA complex. The transcondylar approach and several variations have been widely used by several authors in this context.[33,75-79] A detailed description of the technique as we use it is given later in this chapter. Aneurysms that are not suitable for either surgical clipping or endovascular procedure may require other surgical techniques such as coating,[5,80] external (surgical) trapping,[4] or one of the various procedures of revascularization.

SACCULAR ANEURYSMS

Hernesniemi[81] mentioned that most saccular nongiant aneurysms of the VA-PICA complex can be clipped. Today, most authors prefer an early treatment of these aneurysms after rupture, including distal PICA aneurysms,[33] and also when they are associated with an arteriovenous malformation.[15,82] The decision as to whether surgical clipping or endovascular coil occlusion is preferable should be made by an experienced neurovascular team. In the series of Horiuchi and colleagues[7] comprising 27 PICA aneurysms in 24 patients, 22 lesions were clipped (81%), 2 (7%) were wrapped, 1 (4%) was proximally ligated with occipital artery-PICA bypass, and only 1 (4%) was occluded endovascularly with Guglielmi detachable (GD) coils.

FUSIFORM ANEURYSMS

For fusiform aneurysms of the VA and PICA, there is no safe surgical technique without major risk of severe morbidity. Moreover, the natural history of unruptured fusiform aneurysms is not well known. The rebleeding rate of such aneurysms is estimated at 10% per year, which is remarkably minor when compared with saccular or dissecting aneurysms. Observation and conservative treatment appear justified in view of the favorable history of many of these aneurysms.

DISSECTING ANEURYSMS

With modern neuroimaging techniques, the diagnosis of dissecting aneurysms is now more precise than in the past.[49,83] Although a benign course has occasionally been documented,[84] the necessity of early treatment of dissecting aneurysms of the VA has been emphasized by many authors. An SAH from a dissecting aneurysm is considered a neurosurgical emergency because of a high incidence of rebleeding and a high mortality rate at the time of recurrent bleeding.[22,30,31,55] Conversely, the natural history of non-SAH cases is relatively benign and therefore the treatment remains controversial.[85-87] Despite early satisfactory results with a proximal occlusion of the VA,[88] it is now well recognized that proximal occlusion of the affected VA by clip placement or endovascular procedure may not be sufficient.[28] The primary goal of therapy is thus complete exclusion of the dissecting aneurysm from the circulation to avoid progression of the vascular dissection or a distal embolism with ischemic complications.[28] In most cases, clip occlusion is impossible and wrapping alone may not be efficient.[83] Test occlusion of the vertebral artery is performed, and thereafter either surgical or endovascular occlusion (internal trapping) is recommended.[54] According to Hamada and colleagues,[28] when occlusion of the VA is chosen as treatment option, patients should undergo a 20-minute occlusion tolerance test using a nondetachable balloon. Yoshimoto and Wakai[87] have questioned the necessity of this balloon test because they doubt its reliability; these authors believe that definitive unilateral VA occlusion can be performed safely unless the contralateral VA is hypoplastic. Kitanaka and colleagues[89] have mentioned that the choice of surgical technique depends on the location of the dissecting aneurysm in relation to the origin of the PICA. The VA can usually be occluded distal to the PICA origin, whereas a proximal occlusion of the VA may cause a secondary thrombosis of the PICA. A number of revascularization techniques have therefore been applied to occlude the VA with a consecutive reanastomosis of the PICA: PICA-PICA bypass at the level of the caudal loop,[90-92] occipital artery-PICA,[93-98] VA-PICA anastomosis with the superficial temporal artery or radial artery,[99-101] and VA-PICA transposition.[102]

GIANT ANEURYSMS

Despite the rare occurrence of giant aneurysms of the posterior circulation, these lesions have received much attention in the literature.[11,103-106]

The reasons for their frequent description are special characteristics of these lesions. The therapy of giant aneurysms is far more difficult that of those in the anterior circulation. Ausman and colleagues[93] have recommended surgical clip occlusion in cooperation with cardiosurgeons under hypothermia and circulatory arrest.[107] This method, however, has a specific morbidity and is associated with a certain mortality. The optimal therapy of giant aneurysms is the direct clip occlusion, which still bears a high risk for the patient. For this reason, the parent artery (VA) may be deliberately sacrificed or endovascularly occluded,[108] the same technique as that used for dissecting or fusiform aneurysms. According to Inamasu and colleagues[109] who treated six patients with giant VA and four patients with VA-PICA aneurysms surgically, more favorable results were

Table 78-1	Treatment Modalities for Patients with VA-PICA Aneurysms (Treated by the Authors)						
Therapeutic Procedure	No. of Patients (n)	Average Age, Sex (M/F)	VA	VA-PICA Complex	Distal PICA	VA-Basilar Junction	Surgical Approach
Clipping	23	52,0,7/16	6	10	6	1	Transcondylar (n = 13), medial suboccipital (n = 7), lateral suboccipital (n = 3)
Coating	1	55, M	1	—	—	—	Transcondylar
Coagulation	1	61, F	—	1	—	—	Lateral suboccipital
PICA end-to-end anastomosis	2	39.5, 1/1	—	—	2	—	Lateral suboccipital (n = 1), transcondylar (n = 1)
VA-PICA anastomosis	2	55.5, 1/1	2	—	—	—	Transcondylar (n = 1), lateral suboccipital (n = 1)
Aneurysm excision	1	56, F	—	—	1	—	Medial suboccipital
Conservative treatment	6	46.7, 2/4	1	3	—	2	—
Endovascular treatment	33	47.4, 15/18	3	19	9	2	Coiling (n = 32), stenting and coiling (n = 1)
Total (n)	69	51.6, 27/42	13	33	18	5	—

PICA, posterior inferior cerebellar artery; VA, vertebral artery.

obtained with surgical or endovascular rather than with conservative therapy.

The Authors' Series

A total of 69 patients with aneurysms of the VA-PICA complex were treated in the period 1992 to 2004. Thirty patients were treated surgically, 33 endovascularly and 6 conservatively. Patient data are summarized in Table 78-1.

AUTHORS' PREFERRED SURGICAL TECHNIQUE

Our preferred approach to VA and VA-PICA aneurysms, the suboccipital transcondylar approach, derives from the classic access route to the cerebellopontine angle and anterolateral aspect of the foramen magnum. The microsurgical exposure of these lesions usually requires extensive drilling of the bone around the jugular foramen. Among the pertinent anatomic structures of this area, the jugular tubercle plays a key role. When drilling the jugular tubercle, we must control a number of vital anatomic structures around the jugular foramen, which are described in more detail later in this chapter. Considering the great variability of the aneurysms to be treated, we do not advocate a rigid surgical approach. Instead, with a precise knowledge of all individual morphologic, pathomorphologic, and functional details, we design and perform the procedure in an individually tailored fashion, according to the guiding principle of minimal invasiveness. In our understanding, this principle as applied to skull base surgery means obtaining maximal microsurgical exposure with the least possible amount of surgical trauma. Apart from aneurysms of the distal PICA that can be treated via the median suboccipital or the telovelar route, we usually start the procedure with a limited suboccipital transcondylar approach. This procedure is then gradually extended according to the specific requirements of each case. It is obvious that our policy of minimal invasiveness has important implications on the planning of the procedure, the positioning of the patient on the surgical table, the skin incision and muscle opening, the removal of bone at the base of the skull, and the intradural microsurgical technique.

SURGICAL ANATOMY

The origin of the PICA at the VA varies from extradurally, below the foramen magnum, to the vertebrobasilar junction. The PICA arises from the posterior or lateral surfaces of the VA more often than from the anterior or medial surfaces.[110] The PICA is the artery with the most complex relationship to the cranial nerves of any artery.[111] By definition, the PICA originates from the VA. Although rarely encountered (5%), one must bear in mind the possibility of an extradural origin of the PICA and of an extracranial (intradural) site of distal PICA aneurysms.[110,112] In a few cases, the VA and the PICA are missing. If the PICA is present, it is the largest branch of the VA.[110] Lister and colleagues[113] have divided the artery into five segments based on its relationship to the medulla and the cerebellum. These five segments are the anterior medullary, the lateral medullary, the tonsillomedullary (includes the caudal loop), the telovelotonsillar (includes the cranial loop), and the cortical.[113] Each segment sometimes includes more than one trunk. The PICA is closely related to the cerebellomedullary fissure, the inferior half of the ventricular roof, the inferior peduncle, and the suboccipital surface.[110] The PICA supplies perforating branches to the medullar, choroidal arteries and cortical arteries. Perforating arteries arise from the medullary segment terminating into the brain stem.[110] Recently, Marinkovic and colleagues[114] gave a detailed description of the perforating branches of the VA providing valuable information for those performing aneurysm surgery in this region.

From the microsurgical point of view, a number of muscular and osseous anatomic landmarks are essential for successful dissection in this region. The following is a brief description of these anatomic landmarks and their significance for the surgical procedure.

The upper portion of the sternocleidomastoid muscle and its posterior border indicate the region for the skin incision and further muscular opening. The most important muscles of the deep layer are the rectus capitis posterior major and minor muscles and the superior and inferior oblique muscles. The area between the medial rim of the superior oblique muscle, the upper rim of the inferior oblique muscle, and the lateral rim of the rectus capitis posterior major muscle, called the suboccipital triangle, contains the posterior rim of the atlantal arch, the horizontal portion of the vertebral artery, and the C1 root between these two structures. The posterior atlantal arch also serves as an important landmark for early localization of the VA during the stage of muscular dissection. Once this structure has been identified by palpation, the artery can readily be exposed in the sulcus dorsal and medial to the lateral atlantal mass. A C1 hemilaminectomy may not always be necessary but can be helpful when mobilization of the VA is required. The posterior edge of the occipital condyle is located just lateral to the dural entrance of the VA. To better expose the proximal intradural VA, this portion of the occipital condyle must be drilled away.

The diameter of the posterior condylar canal that contains the posterior condylar emissary vein varies widely. This canal is a very important landmark because it opens into the posteromedial margin of the jugular foramen and indicates the direction of bony drilling to expose the jugular tubercle. The jugular tubercle is a rounded prominence located at the junction between the basal part (clivus) and the condylar part of the occipital bone (jugular process). The jugular tubercle is one of the most important landmarks being surrounded by a number of vital neurovascular structures that must be exposed partially or totally.[45,77] Medially and superiorly, the jugular tubercle is overcrossed by the cranial nerves IX, X, and XI intradurally. Laterally, the jugular tubercle has a close relationship with the jugular bulb, reaching the medial wall of the jugular foramen. Inferiorly, there is the hypoglossal canal containing the hypoglossal nerve surrounded by its venous plexus. Seeger[115] was the first to document the necessity of resecting the jugular tubercle for an adequate visualization of near-midline aneurysms of the VA-PICA complex, later underscored by Perneczky.[116]

POSITIONING OF THE PATIENT

Proper positioning of the patient on the surgical table is essential for adequate access to the condylar fossa. Ideally, the patient's positioning should fulfill the following criteria: it should allow for an optimal view of the intradural VA without being hampered, for instance, by the patient's shoulder. It should also allow a wide range of movement with the operative microscope to be able to visualize the surgical field from different angles. This is important particularly for a narrow and deep exposure as in aneurysms of the distal VA. It should also allow the surgeon to adopt a neutral, relaxed position because this may influence the surgical result. Finally, it should reduce venous congestion and thus venous bleeding, particularly in this area with abundant venous channels within a narrow surgical field. On the other hand, one has to bear in mind that exaggerated negative venous pressure may favor the occurrence of air embolism during surgery. In our opinion, these criteria are best accomplished by the sitting position of the patient so that the legs are level with the heart. A disadvantage of the sitting position worth mentioning is the loss of cerebrospinal fluid from all basal cisterns and even from the ventricles during surgery. Especially in the elderly, this may delay postoperative awakening from anesthesia. In some instances, we therefore use the lateral park bench position for the patient. In either position, the head of the patient should be mobilized in three planes: flexion, axial rotation to the ipsilateral side, and slight tilting to the contralateral side. Flexion of the head is important because it exposes the posterior articular facet of the occipital condyle.

ANESTHESIA AND MONITORING

The risk of air embolism in this position can be reduced to a minimum by an experienced neuroanesthetist who pays special attention to the blood volume and to normoventilation, particularly when carrying out the craniotomy and the bony drilling at the base of the skull. At present, all our procedures in the sitting position are performed with transesophageal Doppler monitoring, allowing for the early detection of very small amounts of air bubbles within the atrium. The source of air embolism is identified after bilateral compression of the jugular vein, which is done when necessary by the anesthetist. With this management, we have not encountered serious problems or hemodynamic complications due to air embolism over many years of neurosurgical procedures using the sitting position. In the majority of skull base procedures, standard techniques of monitoring of somatosensory and brain stem auditory evoked potentials are routinely used at our institution. Monitoring the accessory and hypoglossal nerves may increase the safety in some procedures, provided the function of these nerves is intact preoperatively.

SKIN INCISION

Before skin incision, the scalp is infiltrated with local anesthetic and epinephrine (1:200,000). A proper selection of the skin incision is important for sufficient deep exposure but also for adequately reducing the surgical trauma. To expose the distal intradural VA, we prefer a longitudinal, slightly curved skin incision with the convexity oriented medially, approximately 3 cm medial to the mastoid process. If the aneurysm is located more laterally (proximal VA, first or second segment of PICA), a straight-line skin incision is placed more medially to allow an additional medial-to-lateral viewing trajectory. Some authors advocate an inverse U-shaped (horseshoe) 24, 61, 64; an S-shaped 112, 145; a C-shaped 22, 24, 72; or a so-called hockey stick 60, 96 incision, which, in our opinion, offer no obvious advantages over the straight-line or curved incision.

EXPOSURE OF THE DEEP LATERAL SUBOCCIPITAL REGION

Basically, we have to deal with two muscular layers. The superficial muscle layer consists of the sternocleidomastoid and the splenius capitis muscles laterally, and the trapezius and the semispinalis capitis muscles medially. The occipital artery encountered either superficial or deep to the longissimus capitis and deep to the splenius capitis muscles is usually ligated and divided but may be preserved in case an occipital artery-PICA bypass is deemed necessary. From the deep muscle layer, the two oblique and the two rectus capitis posterior muscles deserve special attention. We start with freeing the attachment of the superficial and partially the deep muscles between the superior and inferior nuchal lines by using monopolar thermocautery. This instrument can be safely applied in this area when the tip of the instrument is permanently visualized and kept in contact with the occipital bone. The muscles are then divided in a craniocaudal direction layer by layer, as much as possible respecting the direction of the muscle fibers. Frequently, palpating the deep structures is helpful for avoiding injury to the VA, which sometimes may form a posterior loop that extends beyond the level of the atlantal arch. The surgeon should recognize this anatomic variation before surgery by carefully examining axial magnetic resonance imaging or CT slices taken at the C1 level. Instead of anatomically exposing the three suboccipital muscles that form the suboccipital triangle by extensive dissection, we prefer to identify the posterior arch of the atlas by palpation. The atlantal arch is then freed from its periosteal sheath using a sharp dissector, and the sulcus of the VA is thus exposed. The sulcus can easily be identified by observing the shape of the posterior rim of the atlantal arch. This structure is thick in its medial portion, changing into a thin and sharp osseous edge at the level of the sulcus more laterally. As the VA is surrounded by a venous plexus that may cause severe bleeding, it is advisable to identify the vessel at this stage by palpating its pulsations. Once the VA is identified, further detachment of the suboccipital muscles is continued and the posterior condylar fossa containing abundant fatty tissue is exposed together with the posterior aspect of the atlanto-occipital joint. It has proved favorable to perform this step under the operating microscope. The periarterial venous plexus may be coagulated or packed with collagen or Surgicel to control venous bleeding. Muscle and dural branches of the VA are coagulated and divided. Care is paid to the C1 root located beneath the horizontal portion of the VA. The fatty and connective tissue filling the condylar fossa is gradually removed and the posterior portion of the occipital condyle and lateral atlantal mass are exposed by subperiosteal dissection. When exposing the condylar fossa, the posterior condylar emissary vein is dissected free, coagulated, and then divided sharply. The remaining distal portion of the vein located within the posterior condylar canal is shrunk with bipolar forceps and serves as an important anatomic landmark, indicating the direction toward the posterior aspect of the jugular bulb (Fig. 78-2).

SUBOCCIPITAL CRANIECTOMY

Usually, we either perform a small bone flap or place several burr holes and preserve the bone dust for later wound closure. After placing the burr holes, the dura is gently detached from the bone. Craniectomy is continued step by step using a rongeur to preserve the bony fragments. The limits of the craniectomy are as follows: superiorly approximately 1 to 2 cm below the transverse sinus; medially and superiorly approximately 1 to 2 cm from the midline; medially and inferiorly the dorsolateral rim of the foramen magnum is completely opened from the midline to the dural entrance of the VA, thus reaching the posterior condylar fossa and posterior medial aspect of the jugular process; and laterally to the medial rim of the sigmoid sinus. This stage of the procedure is carried out without the aid of the operating microscope (see Fig. 78-2).

PARTIAL DRILLING OF THE OCCIPITAL CONDYLE AND JUGULAR TUBERCLE

The following surgical step is crucial for enabling direct access to the pathologic lesion at hand. It must be designed in great detail preoperatively because, on the one hand,

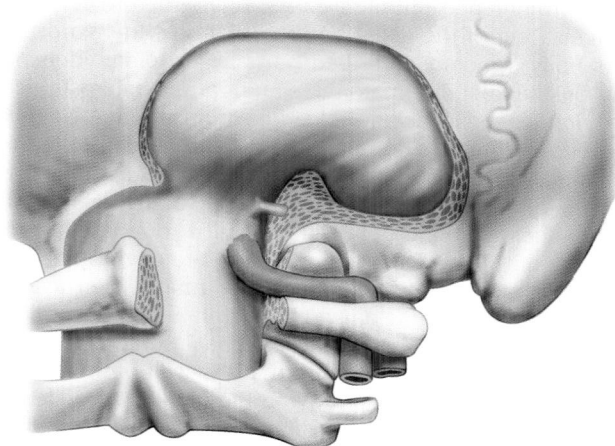

FIGURE 78-2 The bone resection of the approach. The suboccipital craniotomy exposes the inferior part of the cerebellum and edge of the jugular bulb. A resection of the medial part of the jugular tubercle and the occipital and C1 condylar interface has been done, producing a gap between the vertebral artery and the bone. Also a hemilaminectomy of C1 was performed for maximal lateral retraction of the dural flap. *(Courtesy of Christoph Kappus.)*

it offers the working space necessary for microsurgical manipulation around the intradural VA. On the other hand, unnecessary drilling in this area should be avoided because of the potential of damage to vital neurovascular structures. The amount of bony resection depends on the location, site, and extent of the aneurysm and on the specific anatomic configuration of the skull base.

Because drilling around the jugular foramen is a highly demanding procedure, it is carried out extradurally with the aid of a high-speed drill and under magnification. Before drilling, however, we gently separate the bone from the adjacent dura mater and distal sigmoid sinus that may firmly adhere to the bone. In the early stage, a cutting burr is used that never touches the dura. Thereafter, we use diamond burrs of different sizes under continuous irrigation with saline solution. Drilling begins with removing the medial aspect of the posterior wall of the distal sigmoid sinus and continues to the medial aspect of the jugular process of the occipital bone. At this stage, the point where the VA pierces the dura serves as an important landmark. By measuring the distance from this point to the area of drilling in the depth, we can estimate the remaining distance to the hypoglossal canal and jugular tubercle as known from preoperative neuroradiologic studies. To expose the dura lateral to the point of entrance of the VA, the posteromedial aspect of the occipital condyle is gradually removed, leaving the vast majority of the articular surface intact. Venous bleeding from the marginal sinus at the level of the foramen magnum is controlled with bipolar coagulation and packing with Surgicel. While using the high speed drill in this region, the VA is protected from damage with the suction tube or a self-retaining brain retractor. Drilling is continued to expose the posterior aspect of the hypoglossal canal. Because the dural sheet of the hypoglossal nerve is surrounded by a venous plexus, the exposure may require packing with Surgicel to achieve hemostasis. Once the hypoglossal canal is exposed, the dura overlying the jugular tubercle is gently detached. In many instances, the jugular tubercle is a very high prominence. In such cases, this structure hampers visualization of the distal VA. To obtain a wide exposure, this bony structure is drilled partially or totally, depending on the specific anatomic situation and microsurgical requirements. Occasional bleeding from the jugular bulb or venous channels draining into the bulb is controlled by packing small amounts of Surgicel, and, if necessary, fibrin glue is applied as well. It has proved advantageous to drill the cancellous bone until a thin shallow of cortical bone remains in place. This shallow is then removed piece by piece with a small rongeur. Such a technique is crucial to avoid injury to the jugular bulb or cranial nerves that traverse the jugular foramen. The skull base surgeon working in this area must bear in mind that the wall of the jugular bulb and also the dura overlying the jugular tubercle are thin and very vulnerable structures. Damaging the dura around the jugular tubercle may cause injury to the cranial nerves IX, X, and XI located immediately above this bony prominence or even premature aneurysm rupture. To avoid by all means such damage at this stage, we use very cautiously a conventional drill at low speed.

To enlarge the exposure, in most cases only small amounts of the occipital condyle must be drilled away in the posteromedial portion of this structure. We have always been able to preserve the function of the atlanto-occipital joint (see Fig. 78-2).

DURAL INCISION

The dura is opened in a longitudinal or Y-shaped fashion, usually medial to the dural entrance of the VA. The dural ring around the VA is left intact save for the cases with proximal artery involvement. Opening the dura exposes the lobulus biventer of the cerebellum rostrally and the medulla oblongata caudally. The dural edges are sutured to the muscles in the vicinity so that the dural entrance of the VA is gently reflected laterally together with the dura. This becomes possible only after sufficient resection of bone lateral to the dural entrance of the VA (Fig. 78-3).

INTRADURAL STAGE

The intradural procedure begins with opening the arachnoid membrane of the great cistern. Gentle elevation of the cerebellum gradually exposes the spinal root of the accessory nerve, the proximal intradural portion of the VA, the proximal PICA, the first dentate ligament, and the C1 root. To further retract the cerebellum, the arachnoid around cranial nerves IX through XI must be divided using microscissors. The rootlets of the caudal cranial nerves are then dissected free up to their origin from the antero-olivary and retro-olivary grooves. Anterior to these rootlets, the distal portion of the VA is visualized. The artery and aneurysm may be covered by the rootlets of the hypoglossal nerve, which may cross the PICA anteriorly as well as posteriorly. Close to the midline, the sixth nerve and the junction of both VAs become visible. Superior to the glossopharyngeal nerve, the exit zone of the statoacoustic and more anteriorly of the facial nerve can be seen. However, these anatomic structures may be covered, distorted, or displaced by the underlying aneurysm (Fig. 78-4).

Aneurysms located at the level of the jugular tubercle, such as proximal aneurysms of the VA at the origin of the PICA or true PICA aneurysms located at the anterior or posterior medullary portion of this artery, were readily visualized

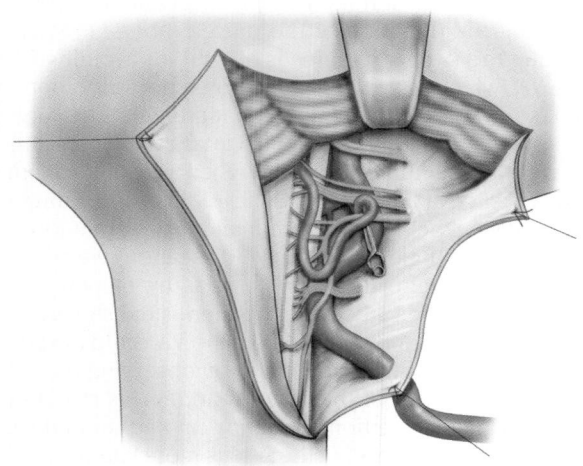

FIGURE 78-3 The dura opened by incision giving access to an aneurysm of the proximal posterior inferior cerebellar artery near its origin. A retractor is positioned to permit visualization of the caudal cranial nerves up to nerve VII. The lateral angle is augmented by partial removal of the jugular tubercle and the occipital and the C1 condylar interface. The remaining jugular tubercle appears as a bulge of the dura directly behind the aneurysm between the dural orifice of nerves XI and XII. *(Courtesy of Christoph Kappus.)*

with this technique. Apart from sufficient exposure of the vascular malformation, it was of great importance to obtain enough control of the VA distal to the aneurysm. Sufficient drilling of the jugular tubercle from extradurally was essential in these particular cases. Before applying an aneurysm clip, the rootlets of the lower cranial nerves including the 12th nerve were dissected free from the vascular malformation. After complete arachnoidal dissection, clipping was performed through a corridor between these rootlets. Only rarely, temporary clipping of the proximal and distal VA and/or PICA was necessary, usually to minimize the inner luminal pressure and shrink a larger aneurysm dome before definitive clipping. Dissecting aneurysms were wrapped or coated by either muscle or cottonoids. Before, during, and

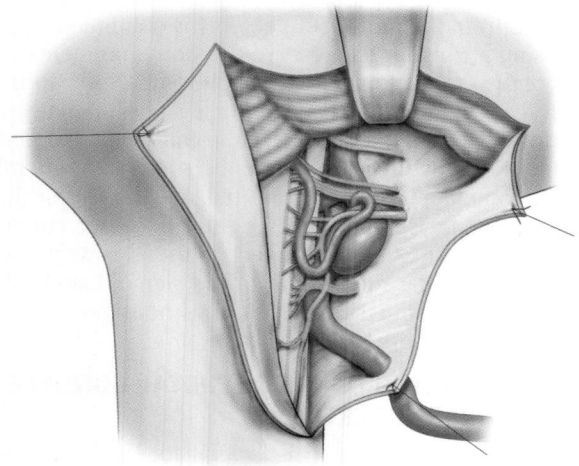

FIGURE 78-4 A clip positioned on the aneurysm. *(Courtesy of Christoph Kappus.)*

after aneurysm clipping, we routinely used a micro-Doppler probe for the control of vascular patency (see Fig. 78-4).

WOUND CLOSURE

One of the main purposes of wound closure is to avoid postoperative cerebrospinal fluid leak. A watertight dural suture or reconstruction is also essential to prevent postoperative meningitis and to avoid local hemorrhage, wound infection, and compression to the caudal cranial nerves. The bony contour of the suboccipital region is restored for cosmetic reasons. In the majority of cases, a primary watertight dural closure is possible without the necessity of dural graft, except for small pieces of muscle. When the proximal portion of the intradural VA is involved, a small amount of dura mater may have to be resected. In such cases, we use a small graft of muscle fascia taken from the nuchal region. The bone flap and bone dust obtained from craniectomy are replaced, if necessary using osteosynthetic microplates.

CLINICAL OUTCOME AND PERIOPERATIVE MORBIDITY AND MORTALITY

Both intra- and peri-operative conditions might influence the long-term outcome of patients. Intraoperatively, aneurysm rupture, perforating vessel injury, inadvertent arterial occlusion, or an inadequate arterial hypotension might cause postoperative new deficits. Perioperatively, a postoperative hematoma, postoperative significant vasospasm, rebleeding from a treated aneurysm, septicemia, meningitis, and bleeding diathesis were observed as negative outcome predictors along with further intensive care-related complications such as respiratory insufficiency or pulmonary embolism. However, most patients can be managed without such problems and thus can expect a favorable outcome.[45,71,117,118] Even for complex VA-PICA aneurysms,

good or excellent clinical results predominate in the larger surgical series.[33,34,45,71,78,117,118] One of the key issues for the management of these difficult lesions is the maintenance of cranial nerve function, which remains a challenging microsurgical problem during the treatment of VA-PICA aneurysms. In all major series, the most common postoperative neurologic deficit was a lower cranial nerve malfunction that can be observed in as many as 60% of the patients.[4,5,9,45,51,78,118-120] D'Ambrosio and colleagues[118] stated that the occurrence of lower cranial nerve dysfunction might be related to the extension of the approach. Our own data support this assumption.[45,78]

Severe morbidity or even mortality can be as high as 15% of the patients in the larger series, but is mostly related to a poor preoperative state of the patients.[78,117]

Generally, VA-PICA aneurysms can be treated with a fair degree of safety by an experienced neurovascular microsurgeon.

Illustrative Cases

CASE REPORT 1

A 37-year-old woman with a history of SAH Hunt and Hess grade III from a left-sided VA-PICA aneurysm was admitted to our department from another hospital primarily for endovascular treatment. During the intervention with a GD coil, both the aneurysm and the anterior medullary segment of the PICA were spontaneously occluded by a thrombus. Local lysis was not attempted due to the risk of rebleeding from the recently ruptured aneurysm. Instead, emergency surgery was carried out, the thrombus was removed, and the aneurysm was successfully clipped with a restored patency of the PICA. Postoperatively, there was no additional morbidity (Figs. 78-5 to 78-7).

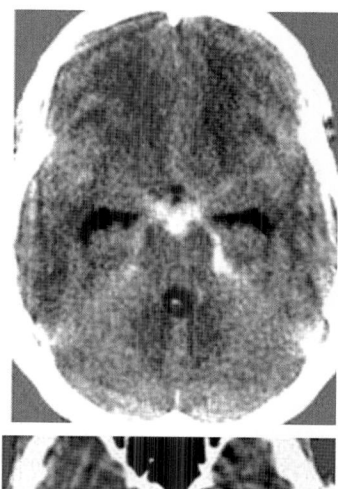
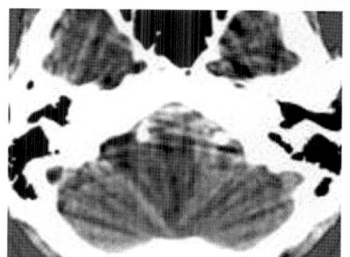
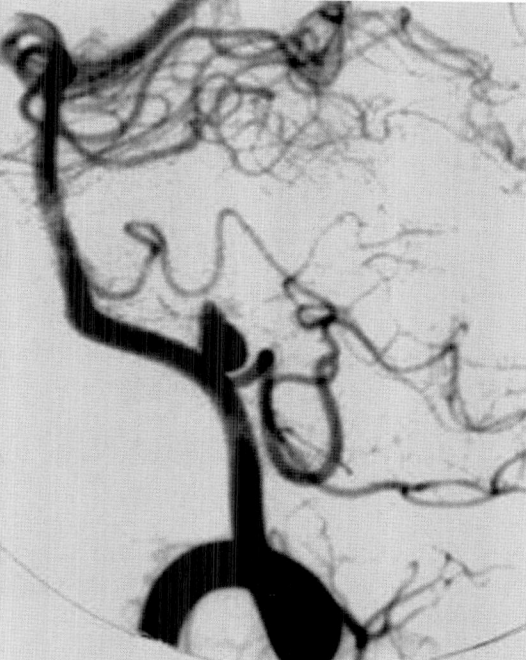
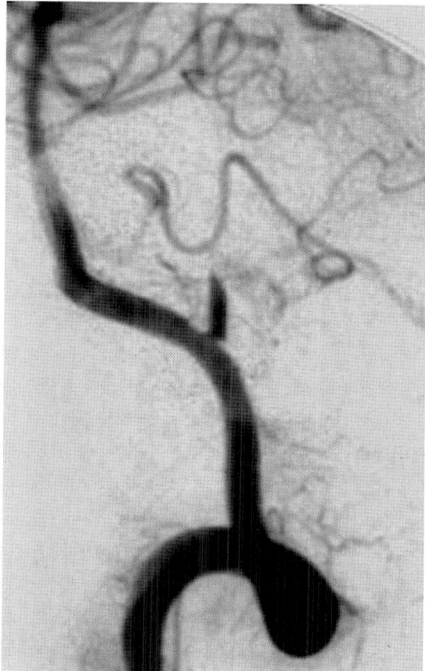

FIGURE 78-5 A 37-year-old woman with a subarachnoid hemorrhage (SAH) (Hunt and Hess grade III). Upper and lower left: Computed tomography scan demonstrates the SAH. Middle: Angiography reveals a left-sided vertebral artery-posterior inferior cerebellar artery (PICA) aneurysm. Right: During endovascular intervention before coiling, both the anterior medullary segment of the PICA and the aneurysm thrombosed.

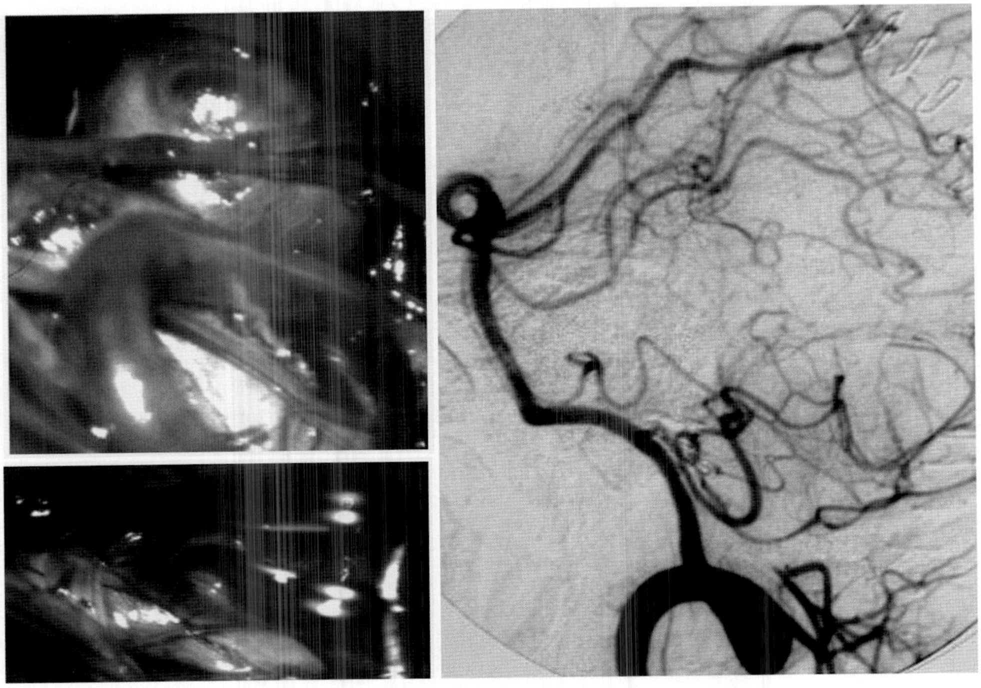

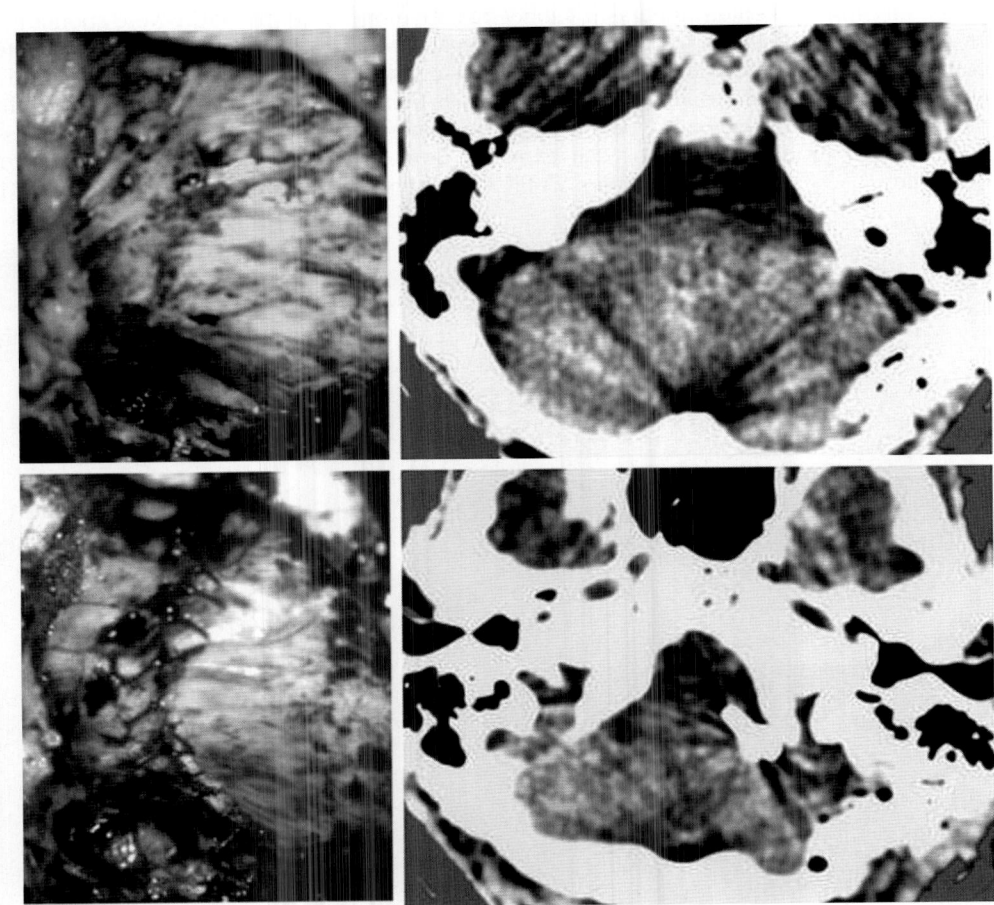

FIGURE 78-6 Intraoperative view and postoperative angiography of the same patient as shown in Fig. 78-5. Upper left: View of the thrombosed aneurysm and distal posterior inferior cerebellar artery (PICA) segment. Lower left: After thrombus removal from the aneurysm and the PICA, the aneurysm is clipped by two curved titanium clips. Right: Postoperative angiography reveals the patency of the PICA.

FIGURE 78-7 Intraoperative view and postoperative computed tomography (CT) of the same patient as shown in Figs. 85-5 and 85-6. Upper and lower left: Microscopic view before (upper) dural opening and after (lower) watertight dura closure. Upper and lower right: Postoperative CT shows the approach and clip artifacts (lower).

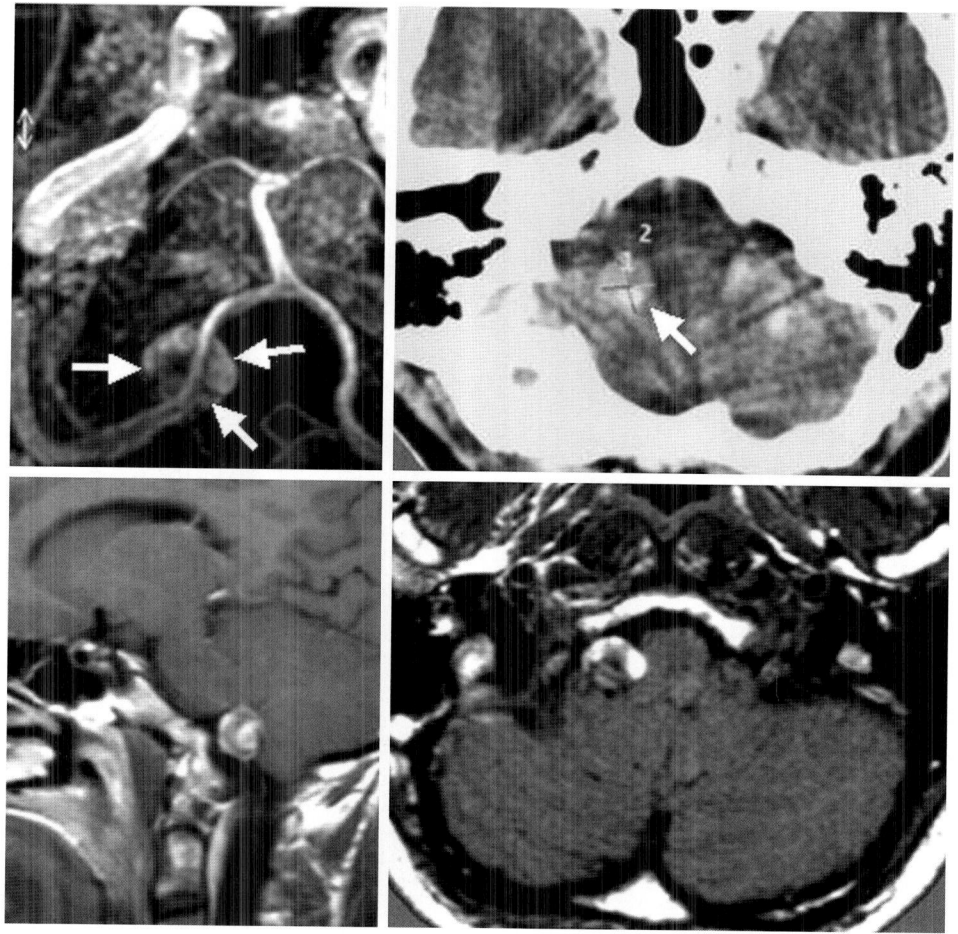

FIGURE 78-8 A 37-year-old man with recent history of occipital headache. Upper left: Magnetic resonance angiography displays a mass suspected to be a right vertebral artery aneurysm (arrows). Upper right: Plain computed tomography scan with a suspected mass within the right medullary cistern (arrow). Lower left and right: T1-weighted magnetic resonance imaging demonstrates a berry-like lesion within the medullary cistern.

CASE REPORT 2

A 37-year-old man was admitted to our hospital with a recent history of occipital headache. Magnetic resonance imaging showed a right perimedullary hyperintense signal compatible with a partially thrombosed aneurysm of the PICA located slightly above the foramen magnum level. Angiography revealed a saccular aneurysm of the tonsillomedullary segment of the right PICA with the dome oriented downward. Endovascular treatment was judged inadequate by the endovascular interventionalist because of the reduced vessel diameter. The aneurysm was surgically exposed via the transcondylar approach and could be clipped successfully after endovascular thrombectomy. Temporary vocal cord paresis occurred postoperatively. No additional cranial nerve deficit was found. The patient returned to work (Figs. 78-8 to 78-11).

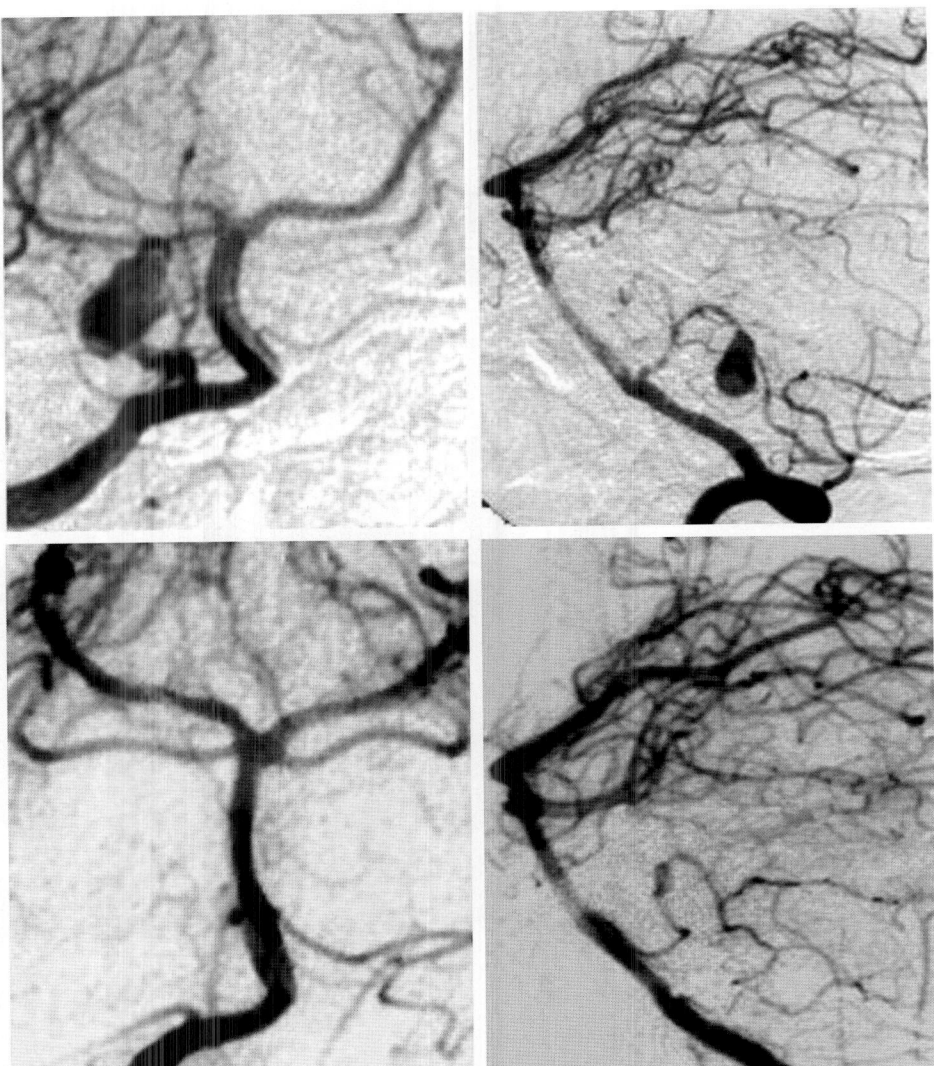

FIGURE 78-9 Pre- and post-operative angiography of the same patient as shown in Fig. 78-5. Angiography before (upper left and right) surgery reveals an aneurysm of the tonsillomedullary segment of the right posterior inferior cerebellar artery that could not be treated by coiling due to the small caliber of the parent vessel. Lower left and right: Postoperative angiography displays the complete clip occlusion of the aneurysm.

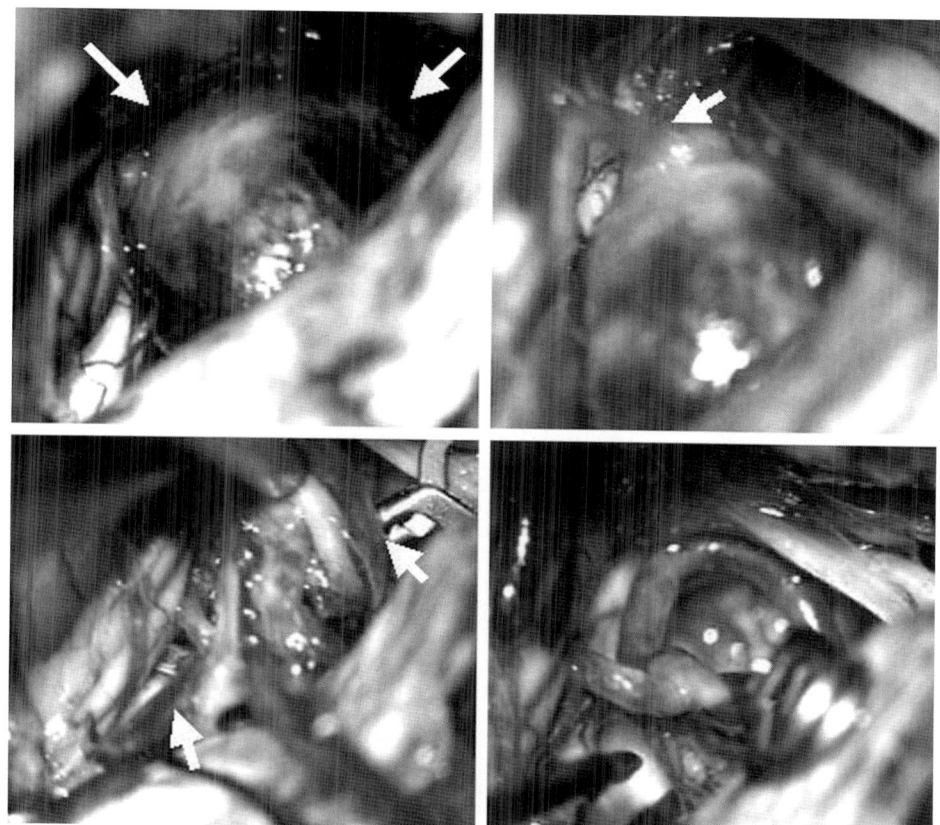

FIGURE 78-10 Intraoperative view of the same patient as shown in Figs. 78-8 and 78-9. The aneurysm was approached by the transcondylar route. Upper left: Aneurysm (arrows) after arachnoidal dissection. Upper right: Vision of the aneurysm neck (arrows). Note that the distal posterior inferior cerebellar artery cannot be observed during this state of dissection because it originates at the back of the aneurysm neck. Lower left: Proximal and distal clipping after (arrows) and removal of a thrombus inside the aneurysm. Lower right: Final clipping with parent vessel reconstruction.

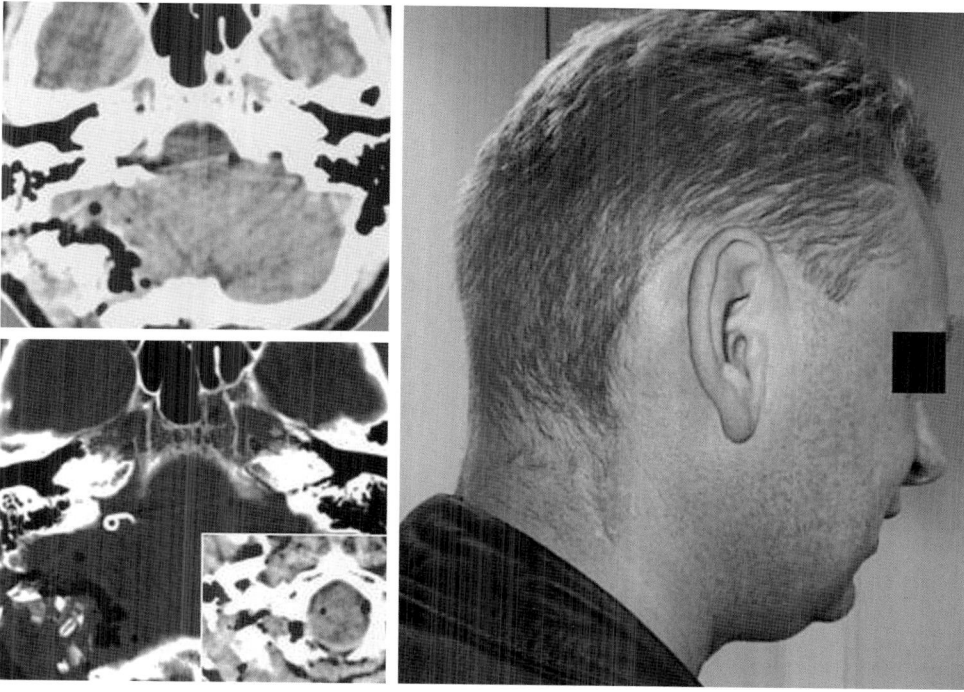

FIGURE 78-11 Postoperative computed tomography (CT) scans and photograph of the same patient as shown in Figs. 78-8 to 78-10. Upper and lower left: CT scan shows the transcondylar approach and the clip. Note the partial condylar drilling in the small image. Right: Cosmetic result after 1 year.

KEY REFERENCES

Andoh T, Shirakami S, Nakashima T, et al. Clinical analysis of a series of vertebral aneurysm cases. *Neurosurgery.* 1992;31:987-993.

Beyerl BD, Heros RC. Multiple peripheral aneurysms of the posterior inferior cerebellar artery. *Neurosurgery.* 1986;19:285-289.

Dernbach PD, Sila CA, Little JR. Giant and multiple aneurysms of the distal posterior inferior cerebellar artery. *Neurosurgery.* 1988;22:309-312.

Drake CG. The treatment of aneurysms of the posterior circulation. *Clin Neurosurg.* 1979;26:96-144.

Drake CG, Peerless SJ, Hernesniemi JA. *Surgery of Vertebrobasilar Aneurysms. London, Ontario, Experience on 1767 Patients.* Vienna: Springer-Verlag; 1996.

Friedman AH, Drake CG. Subarachnoid hemorrhage from intracranial dissecting aneurysm. *J Neurosurg.* 1984;60:325-334.

Gacs G, Vinuela F, Fox AJ, et al. Peripheral aneurysms of the cerebellar arteries. Review of 16 cases. *J Neurosurg.* 1983;58:63-68.

Hernesniemi J. Clinical and radiographic outcome in the management of posterior circulation aneurysms by use of direct surgical or endovascular techniques. *Neurosurgery.* 2003;52:1505-1506.

Hernesniemi J. Distal PICA aneurysms. *J Neurosurg.* 2003;98:1144.

Hiscott P, Crockard A. Multiple aneurysms of the distal posterior inferior cerebellar artery. *Neurosurgery.* 1982;10:101-102.

Horiuchi T, Tanaka Y, Hongo K, et al. Characteristics of distal posteroinferior cerebellar artery aneurysms. *Neurosurgery.* 2003;53:589-595.

Hudgins RJ, Day AL, Quisling RG, et al. Aneurysms of the posterior inferior cerebellar artery. A clinical and anatomical analysis. *J Neurosurg.* 1983;58:381-387.

Kai Y, Hamada JI, Morioka M, et al. Endovascular coil trapping for ruptured vertebral artery dissecting aneurysms by using double microcatheters technique in the acute stage. *Acta Neurochir (Wien).* 2003;145:447-451.

Kaptain GJ, Lanzino G, Do HM, et al. Posterior inferior cerebellar artery aneurysms associated with posterior fossa arteriovenous malformation. Report of five cases and literature review. *Surg Neurol.* 1999; 51:146-152.

Kassell NF, Torner JC. The International Cooperative Study on Timing of Aneurysm Surgery—an update. *Stroke.* 1984;15:566-570.

Lee KS, Gower DJ, Branch Jr CL, et al. Surgical repair of aneurysms of the posterior inferior cerebellar artery—a clinical series. *Surg Neurol.* 1989;31:85-91.

Meisel HJ, Mansmann U, Alvarez H, et al. Cerebral arteriovenous malformations and associated aneurysms. Analysis of 305 cases from a series of 662 patients. *Neurosurgery.* 2000;46:793-800.

Peerless SJ, Drake CG. Posterior circulation aneurysms. In: Wilkins RH, Rengachary SS, eds. *Neurosurgery.* New York: McGraw-Hill; 1985:1422-1436.

Rothman SL, zar-Kia B, Kier EL, et al. The angiography of posterior inferior cerebellar artery aneurysms. *Neuroradiology.* 1973;6:1-7.

Shokunbi MT, Vinters HV, Kaufmann JC. Fusiform intracranial aneurysms. Clinicopathologic features. *Surg Neurol.* 1988;29:263-270.

Tiyaworabun S, Wanis A, Schirmer M, et al. Aneurysms of the vertebrobasilar system. Clinical analysis and follow-up results. *Acta Neurochir (Wien).* 1982;63:221-229.

Westphal M, Grzyska U. Clinical significance of pedicle aneurysms on feeding vessels, especially those located in infratentorial arteriovenous malformations. *J Neurosurg.* 2000;92:995-1001.

Yamamoto I, Tsugane R, Ohya M, et al. Peripheral aneurysms of the posterior inferior cerebellar artery. *Neurosurgery.* 1984;15:839-845.

Yamaura A. Diagnosis and treatment of vertebral aneurysms. *J Neurosurg.* 1988;69:345-349.

Yamaura A, Watanabe Y, Saeki N. Dissecting aneurysms of the intracranial vertebral artery. *J Neurosurg.* 1990;72:183-188.

Numbered references appear on Expert Consult.

CHAPTER 79

Far Lateral Approach and Transcondylar and Supracondylar Extensions for Aneurysms of the Vertebrobasilar Junction

MOHAMED SAMY ELHAMMADY • ERIC C. PETERSON • ROBERTO C. HEROS • JACQUES J. MORCOS

Lesions of the anterior and anterolateral brain stem present special challenges to the neurologic surgeon. Unlike the posterior surface of the brain stem, the anterior surface is buried deep within several vital structures precluding easy anterior access. For this reason, lateral approaches have been proposed to access the anterolateral surface of the lower brain stem from a posterior incision. Heros[1] first described extensive removal of the lateral foramen magnum up to the condyle to approach these lesions. Later authors advocated progressive drilling of bony structures lateral to the foramen magnum such as the occipital condyle, jugular tubercle, atlanto-occipital joint, and mastoid. As each lateral structure is removed, the angle of approach to the anterolateral surface of the brain stem is increased and the surgical corridor widened. However, morbidity from damage to the vertebral artery (VA) and cranial nerves as well as frank instability of the craniocervical junction is also increased with each structure removed.

The far lateral approach refers to the lateral suboccipital craniotomy and removal of the lateral edge of the foramen magnum all the way to the condyle and lateral mass of C1. The two most common extensions of the far lateral, the transcondylar and the supracondylar, involve adding a resection of the occipital condyle and jugular tubercle, respectively. Other extensions of the far lateral such as the paracondylar and extreme lateral (ELITE) are rarely used for aneurysms and will not be discussed.

Anatomy

MUSCULAR ANATOMY

Despite our belief that separation of each individual muscle layer is unnecessary for the far lateral approach, an understanding of the upper cervical muscles and their attachments is an important aspect of performing the far lateral approach safely. The key to the exposure of the far lateral approach lies in the identification and preservation of the extradural vertebral artery, which lies within a triangle of muscles referred to as the suboccipital triangle (Fig. 79-1).

There are four superficial muscles that overlie the suboccipital triangle and three that comprise it. The former are the sternocleidomastoid, splenius capitis, longissimus capitis, and semispinalis capitis muscles in order from superficial to deep. The suboccipital triangle itself is formed by the rectus capitis posterior major medially, the superior oblique muscle superiorlaterally, and the inferior oblique muscle inferolaterally. The rectus capitis posterior major attaches to the spinous process of C2 and inserts on the occiput. The superior oblique muscle attaches to the transverse process of C1 and inserts on the occiput. The inferior oblique muscle attaches to the transverse process of C1 and inserts on the spinous process of C2. The floor of this triangle is comprised of the atlanto-occipital membrane and the posterior arch of the atlas. Practically speaking, the four muscles overlying the suboccipital triangle are often reflected as a single layer, regardless of the incision chosen.

EXTRADURAL ANATOMY

The anatomic keys to the extradural stage of the far lateral approach are twofold. The first is the location and course of the vertebral artery, variants of which can make the exposure dangerous if not recognized. As soon as the VA exits the transverse foramen of C1, it makes a sharp turn medially, running in a groove in the superior surface of the atlas known as the sulcus arteriosus. At this turn, it is immediately medial to the rectus capitis lateralis, an important landmark for the paracondylar extension for exposure of the jugular foramen. Medially, the VA turns cranially to enter the dura. Occasionally, the sulcus arteriosus is not just a sulcus but a circumferential bony canal enclosing the VA as it courses medially above C1. This variation places the VA at higher risk of injury due to torquing or laceration when the posterior arch of the atlas is removed with either the drill or a rongeur.

Three specific points regarding the extradural VA deserve mention. First, as it courses medially in the sulcus arteriosus, it may loop cranially near the occipital bone. This must be kept in mind during the muscular stage of the exposure—it is surprisingly easy to inadvertently bovie into the artery when attempting to separate the last bit of

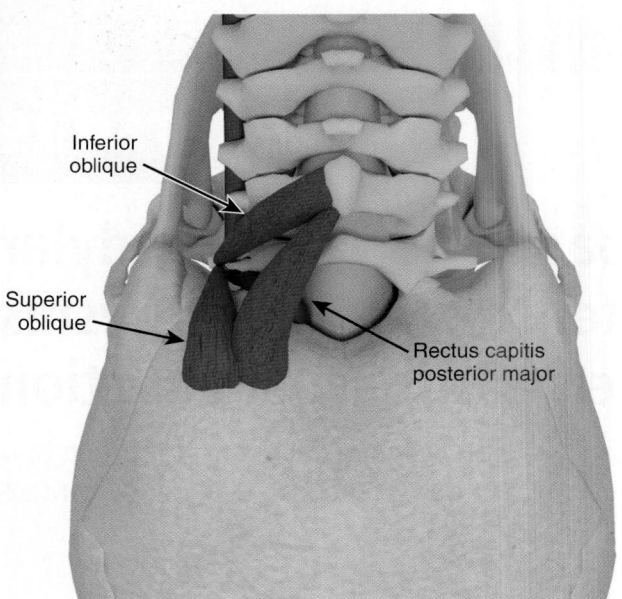

Inferior
oblique

Superior
oblique

Rectus capitis
posterior major

FIGURE 79-1 Schematic of the suboccipital muscular triangle.

cervical musculature off the suboccipital region. Second, while the posterior inferior cerebellar artery (PICA) usually arises from the VA intradurally, in approximately 5% to 20%[2] of specimens it arises extradurally and can be confused with a muscular branch off the VA. Third, the VA sits in a venous plexus as it courses in the sulcus arteriosus, which often leads to troublesome bleeding if one chooses to expose it.

The second anatomic key to the extradural stage of the far lateral approach is understanding the role that the bony protuberances of the occipital bone play in hindering access to different areas of the foramen magnum and anterolateral brain stem. The two most important of these bony protuberances are the occipital condyle and jugular tubercle.

The occipital condyle is an oval shaped structure that constitutes the occipital portion of the atlanto-occipital joint. The oval is pointed anteromedially as it is located on the anterolateral border of the foramen magnum at the level of the cervicomedullary junction. From an inferolateral point of view looking superomedially, it hinders access to the anterolateral medulla.

Running just above the occipital condyle almost perpendicular to its long axis is the hypoglossal nerve in the hypoglossal canal. This nerve represents the anterior limit to the condylar drilling, thus understanding of its course is vital to safely performing the transcondylar extension of the far lateral approach. Because the hypoglossal canal is oriented perpendicular to the long axis of the condyle, and because the canal runs in an anterolateral direction, more of the condyle can be drilled laterally before reaching the hypoglossal canal than can be drilled medially. The canal is surrounded by cortical bone, thus careful drilling of the cancellous bone of the condyle ensures its easy identification—the transcondylar extension has reached its limit when the cortical bone of the hypoglossal canal is reached. There is a prominent vein within the condyle which is often encountered in the course of the condylar drilling. This

vein, the condylar emissary vein, is simply a communication between the perivertebral venous plexus and the sigmoid sinus and can be routinely sacrificed.

The second bony protuberance that hinders exposure to the anterolateral brain stem is the jugular tubercle. The jugular tubercle is a medially projecting bump of the occipital bone anterior and rostral to the occipital condyle. It thus represents to exposure of the anterolateral pontomedullary junction what the occipital condyle represents to exposure of the anterolateral medulla—an obstruction. Like the occipital condyle, it also is associated with cranial nerves, specifically the 9th, 10th, and 11th, which wrap around the posterior aspect of the tubercle on their way to the jugular foramen. The hypoglossal nerve runs caudal to the jugular tubercle, so that drilling of the jugular tubercle is directed superior to the hypoglossal canal but inferior to cranial nerves 9, 10, and 11. This drilling of the jugular tubercle is the defining step in the supracondylar extension of the far lateral approach.

An interesting anatomic study quantified the benefit of removing these two structures in terms of visualization and surgical freedom.[3] The authors found that removing the occipital condyle up to the hypoglossal canal resulted in a mild improvement (21% to 28%) in visualization but a much larger improvement (18% to 40%) in surgical freedom (ability to manipulate surgical instruments within that space). Resection of the jugular tubercle on the other hand, had the opposite effect with a dramatic increase (28% to 71%) in visualization but only a modest (40% to 52%) increase in surgical freedom. This emphasizes the role the occipital condyle plays in narrowing the surgical spatial cone through which instruments are manipulated.

Anesthetic Technique and Neuroprotection

Several anesthetic maneuvers including hyperventilation and administrations of a bolus dose of 20% mannitol (0.5–1 mg/kg) can be implemented to achieve adequate brain relaxation. This minimizes cerebellar trauma due to excessive retraction while maximizing aneurysm exposure. Electrophysiologic monitoring using somatosensory and motor-evoked potentials and brain stem auditory-evoked potentials allows early detection of ischemia or excessive retraction and manipulation.

Surgical Technique

Various positions can be used including supine with the head rotated, lateral or half-lateral decubitus, and a three-quarter prone or park-bench position. At our institution we prefer a straight lateral position. The patient is placed on the operating table with the side of the lesion placed upward. The dependant arm hangs off the bed and is cradled in a padded sling between the table edge and the Mayfield head holder. The head is then secured in a three-pin Mayfield head clamp. Pin placement is crucial if an occipital artery bypass is contemplated as it may hinder the procedure if placed improperly. The pins are placed so that the single pin is 2 cm superior and anterior to the ear pinna ipsilateral to the lesion. The paired pins are positioned so that the

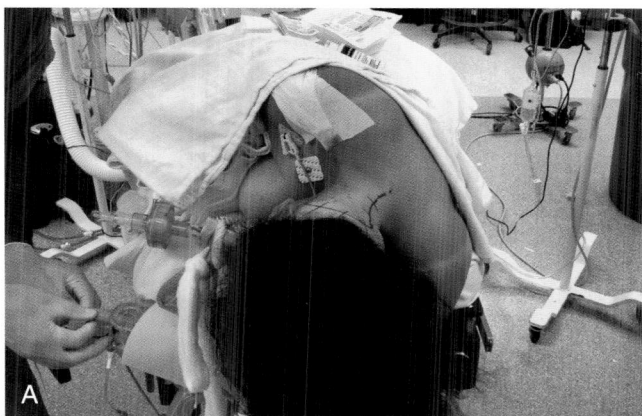

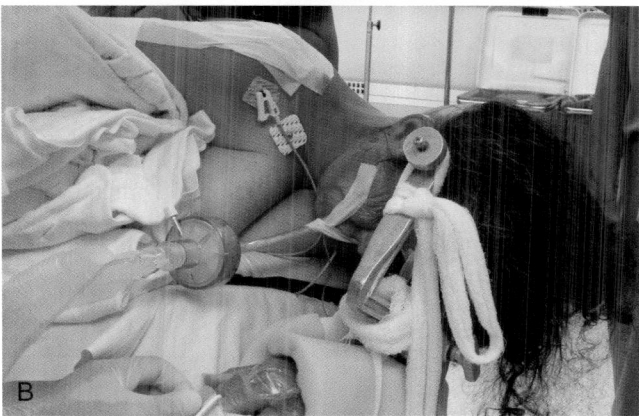

FIGURE 79-2 A, In the three quarter prone position, the head is flexed and tilted down. B, Additionally, the head is rotated facing toward the floor. The ipsilateral shoulder is taped caudally to augment the surgical space.

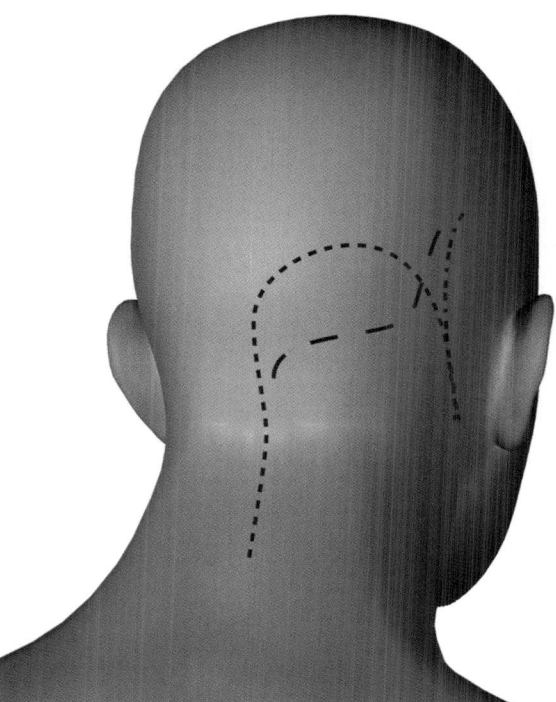

FIGURE 79-3 Types of skin incisions.

posterior pin is 2 cm above the contralateral ear pinna. The head is positioned with three or four movements:

1. Flexion in the anteroposterior plane with slight distraction until the chin is two finger breadths from the clavicle uncovers the suboccipital region.
2. Contralateral bending (approximately 30 degrees) increases the surgical space between the ipsilateral shoulder and the suboccipital region.
3. Upward translation partially and subtly subluxes the ipsilateral atlanto-occipital joint and facilitates possible condylar drilling.
4. Contralateral head rotation in order to bring the ipsilateral side uppermost in the surgical field. Although some authors have advocated this manuever,[4] the senior author (RCH) believes that this maneuver is not advisable as it results in rotation of the ventral surface of the brain stem and thus the vertebrobasilar junction away from the surgeon. In fact, upon completion of the bony drilling and opening of the dura, we routinely rotate the operating table toward the surgeon to allow a tangential view of the ventral brain stem. The operating table is placed in slight reverse Trendelenberg so as to position the patient's head above the level of the heart to reduce cerebral venous congestion. The patient's superior shoulder is retracted towards the patient's feet using adhesive tape to keep the cervical-suboccipital angle open (Fig. 79-2).

The surgical site is shaved. If the occipital artery is to be harvested, a portable Doppler probe is used to identify the course of the artery over the scalp from the mastoid to approximately 4 cm above the superior nuchal line. In such cases scalp infiltration solutions containing vasoconstrictive agents should not be used. The scalp is then prepped and draped in a standard fashion. Several skin incisions may be used including a linear or curvilinear retromastoid, S-shaped, or hockey-stick incision (Fig. 79-3). The linear or curvilinear retromastoid incision starts at about the level of the top of the ear approximately three finger-breadths medial to the mastoid process and extends straight down or a as a gentle curve to just below the mastoid tip. The S-shaped incision starts from the same point described above; however after an initial extension of the incision straight down toward the mastoid, the incision is curved sharply medially to the midline, and then straight downward to the spinous process of C3.

Advantages of the linear/curvilinear or S-shaped incisions include a more direct approach to the atlanto-occipital joint and vertebral artery, and because the incision is carried through the muscle there is less muscle bulk to retract laterally. Disadvantages include increased trauma to the muscles, sectioning of the occipital nerve and artery, and difficulty identifying bony landmarks, which in our opinion increases the risk of inadvertent vertebral artery injury.

The hockey-stick incision, which is currently preferred at our institution, is carried through the midline aponeurosis with minimal injury to the muscle mass and allows early identification of the spinous processes and lamina of C1 minimizing the risk of injury to vertebral artery. Superolaterally the muscle mass is cut along its attachment to the superior nuchal line leaving a small cuff of muscle and fascia for better anatomic closure. The main disadvantage to this incision is that the bulk of the musculature is retracted laterally.

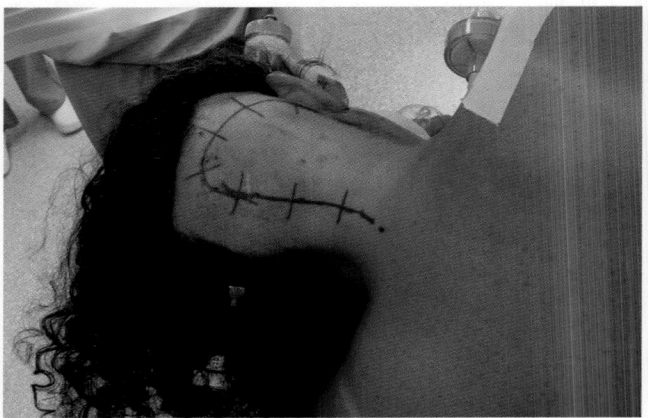

FIGURE 79-4 The skin incision is shaped like a hockey stick spanning the midline and extending to the mastoid tip.

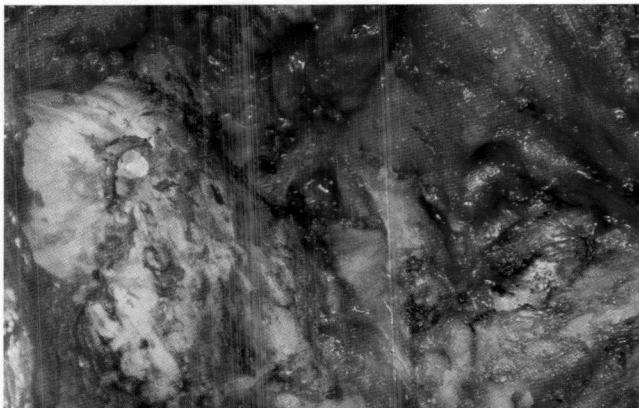

FIGURE 79-5 The muscle mass is retracted latero-caudally with fish hooks attached to the Leyla bar, leaving a 1-cm cuff on the superior nuchal line for resuturing during closure.

Since the angle of attack is lateral to medial, this can hinder access to the atlanto-occipital joint or obstruct the surgical view from an inferior direction under the cerebellar tonsil if not adequately retracted. The hockey-stick incision starts approximately at the level of the spinous process of C3 and extends superiorly in the avascular midline plane to approximately 2 cm above the superior nuchal line. The incision is then turned laterally parallel to the superior nuchal line. If the occipital artery is to be harvested, a curved hemostat is used to dissect over and protect the artery. The incision is then continued over the occipital artery to a point immediately superior to the mastoid process. Finally, the incision is curved inferiorly to end just inferior to the mastoid tip (Fig. 79-4).

The suboccipital muscles are cut leaving a cuff as stated above. This facilitates tight muscle closure at the end of the procedure and minimizes postoperative cerebrospinal fluid leaks. This is particularly important if an occipital artery bypass is to be performed as a watertight dural closure is not possible because of the necessity of creating an opening for passage of the occipital artery. The suboccipital musculature is then swept laterally in a subperiosteal fashion to expose the occiput as far laterally as the mastoid process as well as the arch of C1. The skin and muscle flap are retracted inferolaterally and held in position by fishhooks (Fig. 79-5). Adequate retraction of the cervical musculature is important (particularly if a hockey-stick incision is used) to avoid negating the advantage of a more lateral angle of vision achieved with the far lateral approach. An alternative method of layer-by-layer muscle dissection from lateral to medial has been described to avoid this problem.[5] The technique consists of cutting the muscles in layers leaving small cuffs of the sternomastoid, splenius capitis, and semispinalis muscle attached to the bone for later reattachment. The muscle mass is then elevated medially.

BASIC FAR LATERAL APPROACH

The basic far lateral approach consists of a suboccipital craniotomy and lateral removal of the bony rim of the foramen magnum up to the occipital condyle, which is left intact. The suboccipital craniotomy is performed extending from the junction of the transverse and sigmoid sinuses superiorlaterally to just beyond the midline through the foramen magnum in a teardrop fashion. After

the suboccipital craniotomy has been accomplished, the arch of C-1 is removed from just beyond the midline on the opposite side to the sulcus arteriosus underlying the vertebral artery (Fig. 79-6).

In the past, the senior author routinely exposed the vertebral artery. Currently we believe that for a basic far lateral approach, exposure of the vertebral artery is unnecessary and risks injuring the artery. In such cases the assistant retracts and protects the vertebral artery along with the perivertebral venous plexus inferiorly as the surgeon completes the bone removal.

The critical aspect of the basic far lateral approach is the radical removal of bone in the area of the foramen magnum. The resection should be carried as far laterally as the occipital condyle to a point lateral and superior to the entry of the vertebral artery into the dura. This allows an approach to the ventral aspect of the brain stem from an inferolateral angle with minimal or no brain stem retraction. Each extra millimeter removed from the lateral rim of the foramen magnum permits several extra degrees laterally in the angle of exposure. In this respect, the lateral rim of the foramen magnum represents to the suboccipital exposure what the pterion represents to the frontotemporal exposure. As the bone removal in the region of the foramen proceeds laterally, the bone edge becomes more vertical, and it becomes impossible to reach under the bone with the footplate of a Kerrison rongeur. A high-speed air drill is very useful for the removal of the final 3 to 4 mm of the exposure. It is not uncommon to encounter a posterior condylar emissary vein that runs through the condylar canal located in the condylar fossa. The emissary vein communicates the perivertebral venous plexus with the sigmoid sinus and can be controlled with bipolar coagulation and bone wax. This marks the lateral extent of the bone drilling for a basic far lateral approach. Any opened mastoid air cells must be thoroughly sealed with bone wax to avoid postoperative cerebrospinal fluid leaks.

TRANSCONDYLAR EXTENSION

The basic far lateral approach may be extended more laterally by resection of posterior aspect of the occipital condyle. This transcondylar approach allows a more lateral direction of view than that offered by the basic far lateral

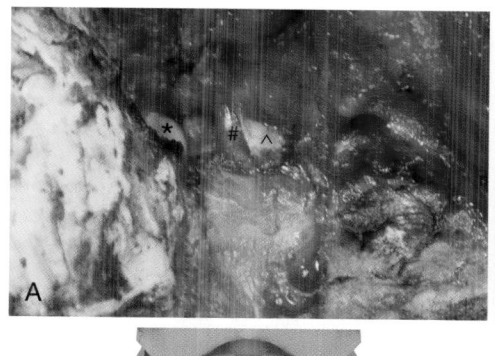
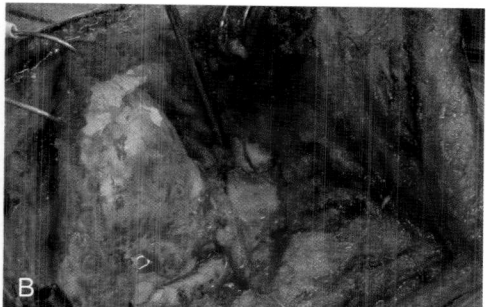

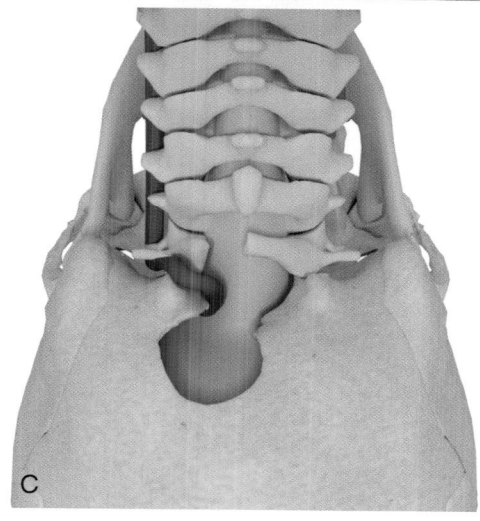

FIGURE 79-6 A, The right hemiarch of C1 has been removed to a point beyond the entrance of the vertebral artery through the dural (V3–V4 junction). Note the glistening white surface of the articular surface of the occipital condyle (*), made visible by the upward subtle translation of the head during positioning. The V3 segment (#) is well-delineated and dissected in the sulcus arteriosus for proximal control. The stump of C1 arch is easily visible (^). B, The suboccipital bone flap has been removed to just beyond the midline. C, Schematic of the craniotomy.

approach, thus providing improved exposure of the lower clivus and anterolateral medulla (Fig. 79-7).

The *occipital-transcondylar variant* involves removal of the occipital condyle without violating the atlanto-occipital joint. Initially the medial part of the posterior third of the occipital condyle is carefully drilled. After removal of the superficial cortical bone, the underlying cancellous bone is drilled until the cortical bone surrounding the hypoglossal canal is encountered. This marks the lateral aspect of the intracranial end of the hypoglossal canal. Because the hypoglossal canal is directed anterolaterally, further drilling of the lateral part of the posterior two thirds of the condyle may be performed without entering the hypoglossal canal. However, even though the hypoglossal nerve is intact, the further drilling of the condyle increases the risk of postoperative atlanto-occipital instability. From the practical point of view the senior author routinely adds this additional step of removing about one third of the condyle medially and posteriorly to the basic far lateral exposure. This suffices for management of most aneurysms of the vertebral artery and the vertebrobasilar junction. Incidentally the senior author also uses this exposure for a variety of tumors of this region including almost all meningiomas of the foramen magnum.

The *altanto-occipital transarticular variant* involves resection of the posterior occipital condyle as above, but adds resection of the adjoining superior articular facet of C1 and mobilization of the vertebral artery. The first step in this variant is removal of the posterior root of the C1 transverse foramen. The vertebral artery segment extending from the transverse foramen of C2 to its dural entrance is exposed by carefully coagulating the overlying perivertebral venous

plexus. Brisk venous bleeding is frequently encountered, but with patience this can be controlled with bipolar coagulation and packing with gel foam powder or Surgicel. The artery is then displaced medially and downward away from the atlanto-occipital joint. The occipital condyle along with the adjoining portion of the superior articular facet of C1 is then removed.

SUPRACONDYLAR EXTENSION

The supracondylar extension of the far lateral approach involves removal of the bone above the occipital condyle, specifically the jugular tubercle. This allows further visualization of the anterolateral surface of the brain stem. Extensive drilling of the bone below and above the hypoglossal canal allows transposition of the hypoglossal nerve. The supracondylar approach permits access to the clivus as well as the region medial to the hypoglossal canal. However, the jugular tubercle that lies above and anterior to the hypoglossal canal may obstruct visualization of the basal cisterns and the clivus anterior to the lower cranial nerves. The *trans-tubercular variant* of the supracondylar approach involves drilling of the jugular tubercle so that the dura covering the prominence can be pushed forward to gain access to the front of the medulla and pontomedullary junction. This is particularly useful for PICA aneurysms in patients in whom the PICA originates from the upper segment of the vertebral artery. Practically speaking, drilling the tubercle extradurally can be challenging because of the distance around the occipital bone one has to reach. One option is to shell out the tubercle extradurally, leaving a rim of cortical bone medially. Upon opening the dura, this shell of tubercle can be

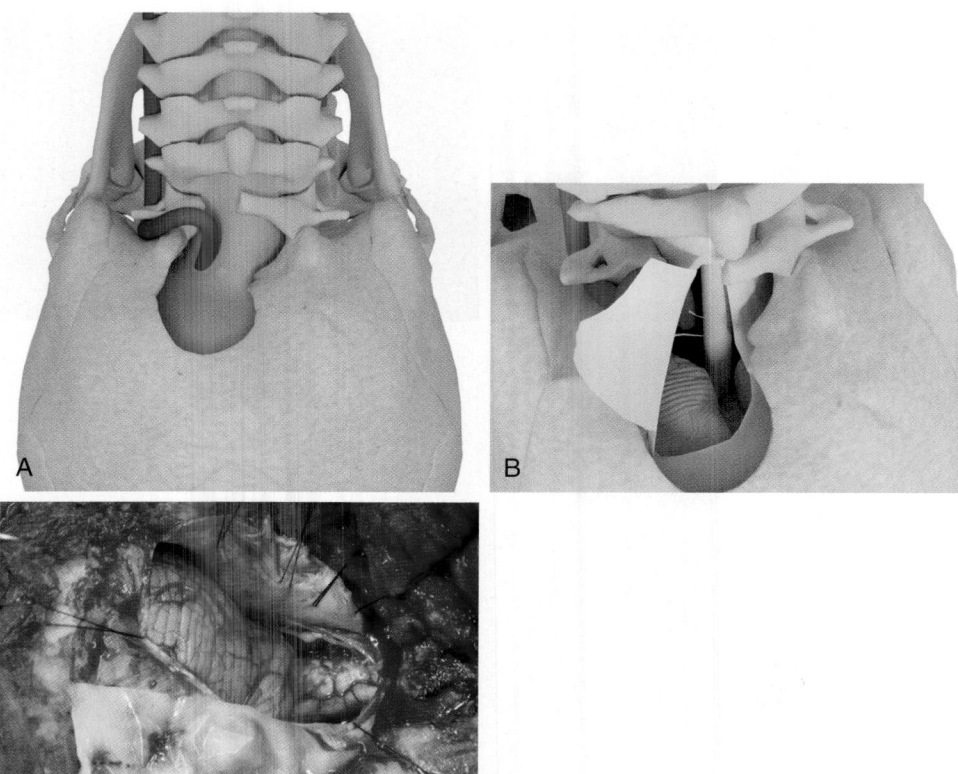

FIGURE 79-7 A, Schematic of the partial condylar resection. B, Schematic of the dural opening. C, Following partial drilling of the medial posterior portion of the occipital condyle, the dura was opened and retracted laterally. This provides a flatter view of the lateral intradural space at the cerebellomedullary cistern.

cracked laterally into the space created by the drilling. The other option is to drill the tubercle intradurally. This involves cutting the overlying dura and drilling the bone underneath, analogous to intradural anterior clinoid removal. The drilling is directed between the 10th and 11th nerves.

Complications

There are several potential complications inherent to the far-lateral approach and its extensions. These include arterial, cranial nerve, and brain stem injuries, craniocervical instability, and postoperative cerebrospinal fluid leaks.

The vertebral artery is at risk for injury during exposure or mobilization of the artery. Injuries may be prevented by careful sharp muscle dissection, stripping of the cervical musculature in a subperiosteal fashion, and avoiding the use of the bovie in the vicinity of the artery. In the event of an inadvertent vertebral artery injury it is much easier to repair a sharply made arteriotomy than that produced by a thermal injury. Preoperative knowledge of the anatomy and caliber of the contralateral vertebral artery is also helpful in guiding decisions regarding whether to repair or sacrifice the artery. The PICA is also vulnerable to injury at several stages of the procedure. Injuries may occur during the exposure if it originates extradurally as it may be mistaken for a muscular branch or for the posterior meningeal artery. The PICA and its perforators can also be injured or occluded intradurally during aneurysm dissection or clipping.

Inadvertent injury to the lower cranial nerves is a major cause of morbidity. Injuries usually result from manipulating the nerve rootlets during dissection and clipping of the aneurysm. These cranial nerves are very sensitive to

manipulation, necessitating very gentle retraction and sharp dissection. Lower cranial nerve injury may result in dysphagia, dysarthria, dysphonia, and inadequate airway protection, thus patients should be extubated and started on an oral diet only after a formal evaluation of lower cranial nerve function has been performed. In addition to the lower cranial nerves, injury to the seventh–eighth nerve complex may also occur during dissection of a high vertebrobasilar junction. Brain stem injury may result from either excessive retraction or vascular injury. Compromise of the PICA or its perforators may result in postoperative lateral medullary (Wallenberg) syndrome.

Extensive removal of the occipital condyle or C1 lateral mass may potentially result in atlanto-occipital instability. In a biomechanical study, it was found that occipitocervical mobility increased significantly as compared to baseline after removal of half of the occipital condyle.[6] A craniocervical fusion should therefore be strongly considered if greater than 50% of the occipital condyle is resected. As mentioned above, this extensive condylar resection is rarely indicated for vascular lesions.

Postoperative cerebrospinal fluid leaks and pseudomeningioceles can be prevented by thoroughly waxing any open mastoid air cells, closing the dura in a water-tight fashion, and by performing a careful multilayer closure of the muscles and fascia.

Conclusion

The basic far lateral suboccipital approach that we routinely extend by removing the posteromedial one fourth to one third of the occipital condyle provides an excellent surgical exposure that is adequate for managing almost all aneurysms of the intracranial portion of the vertebral artery, the proximal PICA, and the vertebral basilar junction. This approach, of course, is also excellent for many extra-axial tumors of this region, particularly meningiomas of the anterolateral rim of the foramen magnum. Intra-axial lesions of the anterolateral cervical medullary region can also be approached comfortably with this exposure. More complex exposures such as the transcondylar and supracondylar extensions are rarely required for vascular lesions, but can be quite useful for some complex extra-axial tumors of this region. The main complication specifically related to the cervical approach is injury to the vertebral artery or to the PICA when it has an extradural origin. This can be avoided by detailed knowledge of the anatomy and its variances and careful sharp dissection in the region of the vertebral artery. Intradural complications, which include not only vascular injuries but also injury to the lower cranial nerves, are usually related to the specific pathology, rather than to the surgical approach.

The senior author considers the far lateral approach with minimal removal of the posteromedial condyle as described above, together with the frontal or bifrontal approach with orbitotomy, the orbital zygomatic approach, and the retrolabryinthine presigmoid approach not to be specialized exposures within the exclusive domain of "skull base surgeons," but rather routine surgical exposures that should be part of the training of every competent neurosurgeon.

KEY REFERENCES

Babu RP, Sekhar LN, Wright DC. Extreme lateral transcondylar approach: technical improvements and lessons learned. *J Neurosurg.* 1994;81: 49-59.

Fine AD, Cardoso A, Rhoton Jr AL. Microsurgical anatomy of the extracranial-extradural origin of the posterior inferior cerebellar artery. *J Neurosurg.* 1999;91:645-652.

Heros RC. Lateral suboccipital approach for vertebral and vertebrobasilar artery lesions. *J Neurosurg.* 1986;64:559-562.

Lanzino G, Paolini S, Spetzler RF. Far-lateral approach to the craniocervical junction. *Neurosurgery.* 2005;57:367-371.

Spektor S, Anderson GJ, McMenomey SO, et al. Quantitative description of the far-lateral transcondylar transtubercular approach to the foramen magnum and clivus. *J Neurosurg.* 2000;92:824-831.

Vishteh AG, Crawford NR, Melton MS, et al. Stability of the cranioverterbral junction after unilateral occipital condyle resection: a biomechanical study. *J Neurosurg.* 1999;90:91-98.

Numbered references appear on Expert Consult.

CHAPTER 80

Surgical Management of Cranial Dural Arteriovenous Fistulas

MOHSEN JAVADPOUR • M. CHRISTOPHER WALLACE

Dural arteriovenous fistulas (DAVFs) are abnormal arteriovenous shunts within the dural leaflets. They are usually located within or near the wall of a dural venous sinus, which is often narrowed or obstructed. The nidus of arteriovenous shunting is contained solely within the dural leaflets, and this characteristic distinguishes DAVFs from pial arteriovenous malformations. The arterial supply is usually derived from dural arteries and less frequently from osseous branches. Venous drainage occurs via a dural venous sinus, retrogradely through leptomeningeal (cortical) veins, or both. Shunting of arterial blood from the meningeal arteries into venous sinuses and/or cortical veins results in venous hypertension, which is the main cause of clinical symptoms related to DAVFs. Drainage into cortical veins is referred to as cortical venous reflux (CVR).

DAVFs account for approximately 5% to 20% of all intracranial vascular malformations.[1,2] They can occur at any age, but the mean age at presentation in most studies lies between the sixth and seventh decades of life.[2,3] The term "dural arteriovenous malformation" has been applied by some authors to all types of DAVFs, both pediatric and adult. However, malformation implies a congenital origin. We prefer to use the term DAVF because, at least in adults, there is good evidence that these lesions are acquired rather than congenital.[4-6] The rare exception is in the pediatric age group in whom congenital malformations of dural venous sinuses are associated with high-flow arteriovenous fistulas.[7]

Pathogenesis

The etiologic factors and mechanisms involved in the pathogenesis of DAVFs are poorly understood. DAVFs are associated with several conditions including head injury, previous craniotomy, and dural venous sinus thrombosis, suggesting that they are acquired rather than congenital lesions.[4,7] According to the most popular theory, DAVFs are formed as a consequence of thrombosis and subsequent recanalization of dural venous sinuses.[8,9] Venous hypertension is thought to play an important role in this process. Indeed animal studies have shown that venous hypertension, even in the absence of sinus thrombosis, can elicit the formation of DAVFs.[6] Whether sinus thrombosis is in fact the initial event in the genesis of DAVFs is controversial.[8] Only a small number of patients with sinus thrombosis go on to develop DAVFs, and not all DAVFs are associated with sinus thrombosis.[4,10]

What follows sinus thrombosis and venous hypertension is also controversial. Two hypotheses have been proposed. The first suggests that DAVFs arise from opening up of preexisting microscopic vascular channels within the dura mater. These preexisting channels are thought to open up or enlarge as a result of venous hypertension secondary to sinus thrombosis.[7] The second hypothesis suggests that DAVFs result from the formation of new vascular channels in the dura, a process stimulated and regulated by angiogenic factors. To support this, surgical DAVF specimens have been shown to contain basic fibroblastic growth factor and vascular endothelial growth factor, which were absent in control specimens.[11,12] Angiogenic factors may originate either directly as part of the inflammatory process that occurs during organization and recanalization of a thrombosed sinus or indirectly as a result of cerebral ischemia secondary to venous hypertension.[13] If the angiogenic theory is true, antiangiogenic agents may provide an adjuvant therapy for patients with untreatable DAVFs.[8]

Many cranial DAVFs ultimately undergo spontaneous resolution. The exact mechanism for this is unknown, but it is thought to result from progressive thrombosis of the involved dural sinus. This is paradoxical in that the cause of the abnormality is also thought to be the curing process. In some cases, however, spontaneous resolution has occurred despite sinus patency.[14]

Classification

Ideally, a classification system should predict the clinical behavior of a lesion and aid in therapeutic decision making. Several classification schemes have been devised for DAVFs.[15-19] The most commonly used are those of Borden and colleagues[16] (Borden classification) and Cognard and colleagues[17] (Cognard classification) (Table 80-1 and Fig. 80-1). Both are based on the pattern of venous drainage of the lesion, the factor that best predicts the clinical presentation and natural history of DAVFs. The Cognard classification, which is a modification of the classification of Djindjian and colleagues,[18] divides cranial DAVFs into five types, based on the presence or absence of CVR, sinusal drainage, and direction of flow in the involved dural sinus.[17]

The Borden classification[16] is a more simplified scheme with three types based on the presence or absence of CVR

Table 80-1 Venous Drainage Pattern of Dural Arteriovenous Fistulas According to Borden and Cognard Classification Schemes

Borden Classification	Cognard Classification
Type I: Drainage into dural venous sinus or meningeal vein only	Type I: Drainage into dural venous sinus only, with normal antegrade flow Type IIa: Drainage into dural venous sinus only, with retrograde flow
Type II: Drainage into dural venous sinus or meningeal vein + CVR	Type IIb: Drainage into dural venous sinus (antegrade flow) + CVR Type IIa + b: Drainage into dural venous sinus (retrograde flow) + CVR
Type III: CVR only	Type III: CVR only without venous ectasia Type IV: CVR only with venous ectasia Type V: Drainage into spinal perimedullary veins

Data from Borden JA, Wu JK, Shucart WA. A proposed classification for spinal and cranial dural arteriovenous fistulous malformations and implications for treatment. J Neurosurg. 1995;82:166-179; Cognard C, Gobin YP, Pierot L, et al. Cerebral dural arteriovenous fistulas: clinical and angiographic correlation with a revised classification of venous drainage. Radiology. 1995;194:671-680. CVR, cortical venous reflux. This has also been referred to as cortical venous drainage,[3] retrograde leptomeningeal venous drainage,[20] and drainage into subarachnoid veins.[16]

and sinusal drainage, without taking into account the direction of flow in the venous sinus. In a study by the University of Toronto Brain Vascular Malformation Study Group, Davies and colleagues[19] validated the classification systems of Borden and of Cognard with respect to clinical presentation. Aggressive presentation (i.e., intracranial hemorrhage [ICH], focal neurologic deficit, or death) occurred in 2% of the Borden classification type I, 39% of type II, and 79% of type III cranial DAVFs. Similar correlation was found between the Cognard classification and clinical presentation (Table 80-2).[19] Subsequent studies by our group have demonstrated that the pattern of venous drainage and in particular the presence or absence of CVR also correlate with the natural history of DAVFs after the initial presentation.[3,20]

DAVFs were previously classified according to their anatomic location.[21] Anterior cranial fossa and tentorial lesions were associated with a higher risk of aggressive clinical behavior than lesions in other locations.[1,19] However, it was later shown that the poor prognosis of lesions in these "dangerous" locations was purely a function of their pattern of venous drainage.[19,22] It is the presence of CVR, not the anatomic location per se, that leads to aggressive clinical behavior.[1,19] Hemodynamically, DAVFs may be classified into high-flow or low-flow fistulas. The classification of Barrow and colleagues[23] is described later in the section on carotid cavernous fistulas. The classification of pediatric DAVFs is not discussed in this chapter.

Clinical Presentation

Other than pulsatile tinnitus, the symptoms of DAVFs are related to venous hypertension.[7,24] This may lead to venous congestion, cerebral edema, cerebral infarction, and ICH. The clinical features of cranial DAVFs are shown in Table 80-3. ICH, nonhemorrhagic neurologic deficit (NHND), and death are considered aggressive.[1,19] The most

significant risk factor for aggressive clinical presentation is the presence of CVR.[1,17,19] Therefore, type II and III lesions of the Borden classification are frequently associated with aggressive clinical behavior, whereas type I lesions are rarely so (see Table 80-2). ICH associated with DAVFs typically results from rupture of an arterialized cortical vein and is usually intraparenchymal but may also occur into the subarachnoid, subdural, and intraventricular spaces (Fig. 80-2). NHND is caused by cerebral ischemia secondary to venous congestion. This category does not include ophthalmoplegia secondary to cranial nerve dysfunction. The neurologic deficit may be focal or global.

Benign symptoms include pulsatile tinnitus and orbital symptoms. Pulsatile tinnitus is produced by turbulent flow in the diseased dural sinus.[4] Objective bruit is heard in 40% of patients with tinnitus. Ophthalmologic symptoms and signs are most commonly seen with cavernous sinus DAVFs, but they can also occur with lesions in other locations, if the venous drainage involves the cavernous sinus and ophthalmic veins.[25] The symptoms are caused by venous congestion.[4,26] The ophthalmologic symptoms may be progressive and disabling and may even lead to blindness and therefore may not be considered benign by the patient. In infants, heart failure and craniomegaly may occur.

Radiographic Evaluation

COMPUTED TOMOGRAPHY AND MAGNETIC RESONANCE

In cases of DAVF without CVR, computed tomography and magnetic resonance imaging (MRI) of the brain parenchyma are typically normal. However, MRI and magnetic resonance angiography may show the stenosis or occlusion of the dural sinuses.[7] Hydrocephalus may be seen in any DAVF that causes venous hypertension in the superior sagittal sinus. In cases of DAVF with CVR, computed tomography and MRI of the brain may show ICH, engorged pial vessels, and diffuse white matter edema secondary to venous congestion. The ICH is usually intraparenchymal but may also have subdural, subarachnoid, or intraventricular components (see Fig. 80-2). The pattern of hemorrhage is not specific to DAVFs, and a high index of suspicion is required. Dilated pial vessels and white matter edema are more likely to be seen on MRI than on computed tomography.[7] On T2-weighted MRI, dilated pial vessels are seen as flow voids on the surface of the brain, and diffuse white matter edema is seen as hyperintensity in the cerebral or cerebellar hemispheres, brain stem, or spinal cord (Fig. 80-3). Recent reports have demonstrated improvements in the ability of magnetic resonance angiography to diagnose DAVFs and to detect CVR.[27] However, these results have been reported in small selected series and require further study. At present, the diagnosis of DAVFs cannot be excluded with negative computed tomography, MRI, or magnetic resonance angiography. If clinically suspected, catheter angiography is required to confirm or exclude the presence of a DAVF.

INTRA-ARTERIAL CATHETER ANGIOGRAPHY

This is the gold standard method for diagnosis and evaluation of DAVFs. The characteristic angiographic feature of DAVFs is premature visualization of intracranial veins or

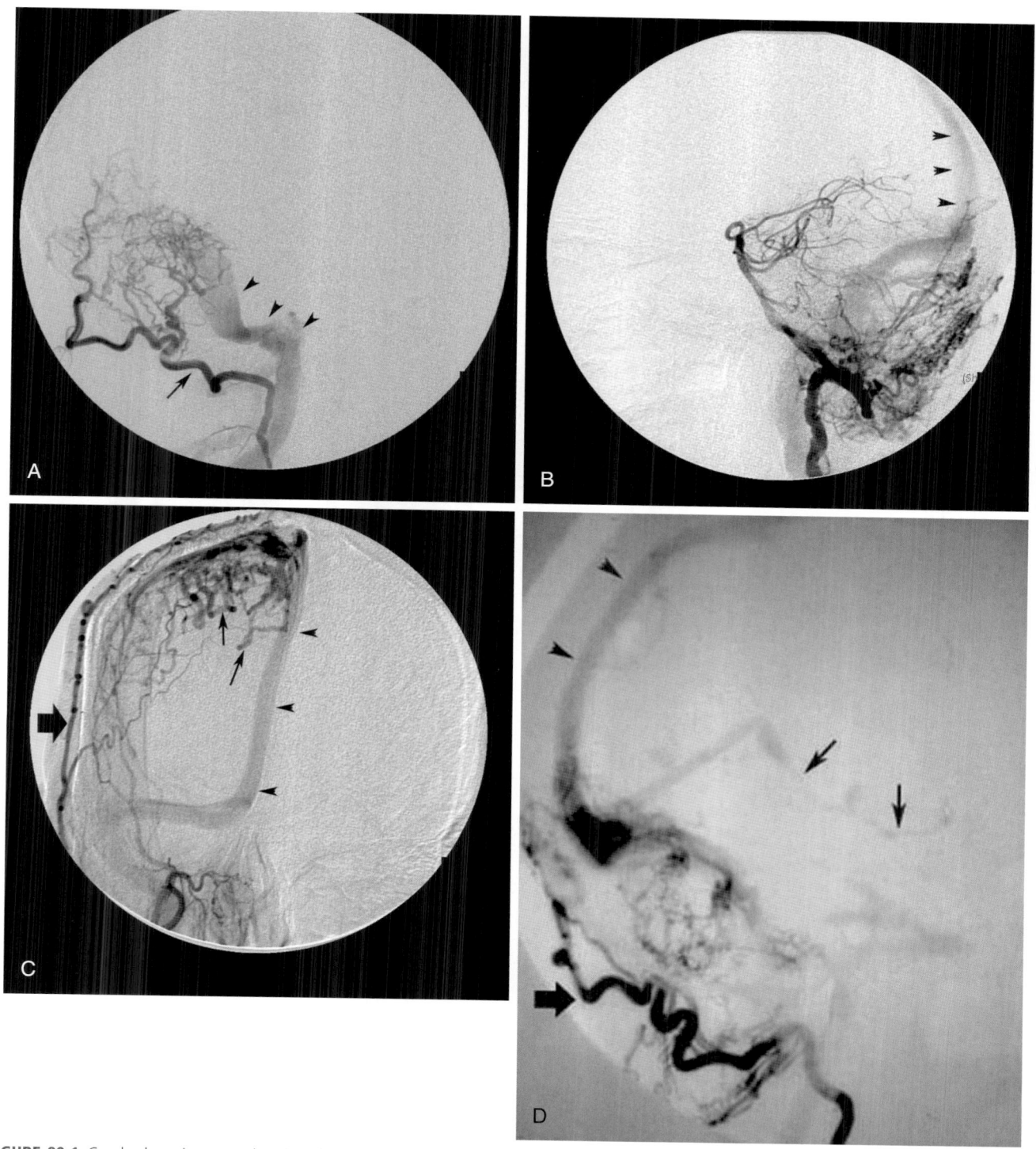

FIGURE 80-1 Cerebral angiograms showing the different types of DAVFs categorized according to the Borden and Cognard classifications. A, Borden type I/Cognard type I. Selective right occipital artery (*arrow*) angiogram, lateral projection, shows a right transverse/sigmoid sinus dural arteriovenous fistula (DAVF) with antegrade drainage into the transverse/sigmoid sinuses (*arrowheads*). B, Borden type I/Cognard type IIa. Left vertebral artery angiogram, lateral projection, shows a transverse/sigmoid sinus DAVF, with retrograde drainage into the transverse and superior sagittal sinuses (*arrowheads*). The direction of flow in the sinuses is retrograde. C, Borden type II/Cognard type IIb. Left external carotid artery (ECA) angiogram, anteroposterior projection, shows a superior sagittal sinus DAVF, fed by branches of the superficial temporal artery (*thick arrow*), with antegrade drainage into the superior sagittal sinus (*arrowheads*), and cortical venous reflux (*small arrows*). D, Borden type II/Cognard type IIa + b. Left ECA angiogram, lateral projection, shows a transverse sinus DAVF, fed by the posterior branch of the occipital artery (*thick arrow*), with retrograde drainage in the transverse sinus (*arrowheads*) and cortical venous reflux (*arrows*). The direction of flow in the sinuses is retrograde.

Continued

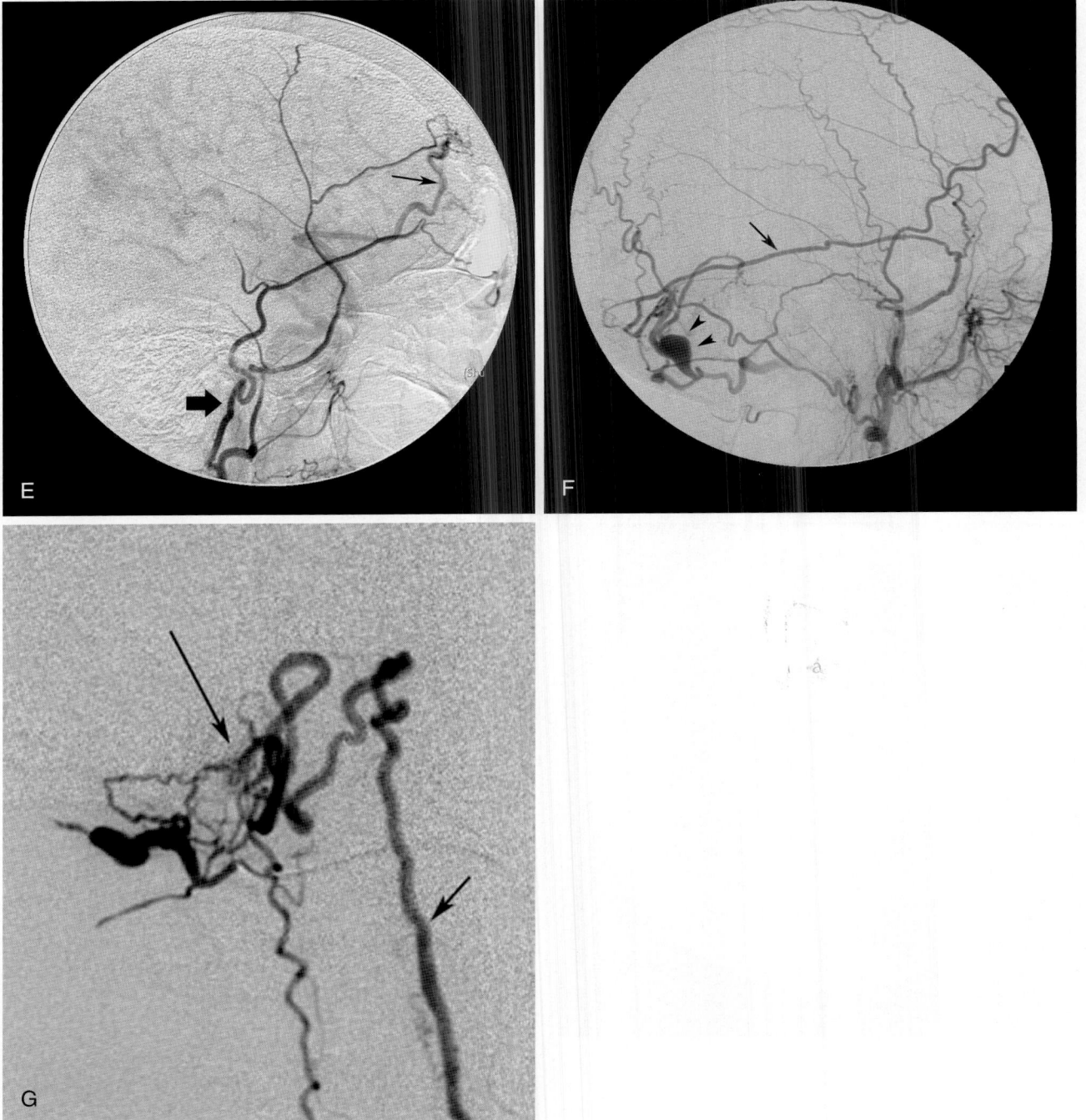

FIGURE 80-1, cont'd E, Borden type III/Cognard type III. Right ECA angiogram, lateral projection, shows a convexity DAVF fed by branches of the superficial temporal artery (*thick arrow*) and draining solely into a cortical vein (*small arrow*). F, Borden type III/Cognard type IV. Right ECA angiogram, lateral projection, shows a torcular DAVF, fed by the posterior branch of the middle meningeal artery (*small arrow*), and refluxing into an ectatic cortical vein (*arrowheads*). G, Borden type III/Cognard type V. Foramen magnum DAVF (*long arrow*) with cortical venous drainage via spinal cord (*arrow*).

venous sinuses during the arterial phase (see Fig. 80-3C; Fig. 80-4A).[28] This is caused by shunting of arterial blood into the venous system through the fistula. To obtain the necessary information regarding the arterial supply and venous drainage of the DAVF and the venous drainage of the brain, imaging must start in the ultraearly arterial phase and be carried well into the late venous phase. Selective angiography with magnification and subtraction techniques is essential.

The study should include injections of both internal carotid arteries (ICAs), both external carotid arteries (ECAs), and both vertebral arteries. This is because a single DAVF may have multiple feeding arteries (see Figs. 80-3 and 80-4) and also because 8% of patients have multiple DAVFs.[29] Detailed knowledge of dural arterial anatomy is essential in angiographic evaluation of DAVFs. Meningeal arteries that are invisible or difficult to see on normal angiograms may

Table 80-2 Relationship between Aggressive Clinical Presentation and Classification of 102 Cranial DAVFs

Classification and Type	% of DAVFs with Aggressive Clinical Presentation (i.e., ICH or NHND)
Borden type I (n = 55)	2
Cognard type I (n = 40)	0
Congard type IIa (n = 15)	7
Borden type II (n = 18)	39
Cognard type IIb (n = 8)	38
Cognard type IIa + b (n = 10)	40
Borden type III (n = 29)	79
Cognard type III (n = 13)	69
Cognard type IV (n = 12)	83
Cognard type V (n = 4)	100

From Davies MA, TerBrugge K, Willinsky R, et al. The validity of classification for the clinical presentation of intracranial dural arteriovenous fistulas. J Neurosurg. 1996;85:830-837.
DAVFs, dural arteriovenous fistulas; ICH, intracranial hemorrhage; NHND, nonhemorrhagic neurologic deficit.

be dilated and clearly visible when supplying a DAVF. For example, the tentorial branch of the meningohypophyseal trunk of the ICA (the artery of Bernasconi and Cassinari) or the meningeal branch of the posterior cerebral artery (the artery of Davidoff and Schecter) may be dilated and easily seen on the angiograms (see Fig. 80-3C).

The nidus of a DAVF is the site of arteriovenous shunting and refers to that part of the dura where there is convergence of all feeding arteries and the origin of venous draining channels. The best views of the nidus are often obtained during the ultraearly arterial phase of the angiogram and by injections of distant arterial feeders.[28] Images obtained when injecting the main arterial feeders, particularly in the later arterial phase or in the venous phase, are often obscured by engorged feeding arteries and draining veins.

Assessment of the venous drainage pattern of DAVFs is extremely important as this factor determines the natural history of the lesion and aids in selecting the most appropriate management strategy. The presence or absence of CVR, venous sinus occlusion, direction of flow in the venous sinuses, and the venous drainage pattern of the brain must be determined. The exact site of CVR must be determined

Table 80-3 Clinical Manifestations of Dural Arteriovenous Fistulas

Intracranial hemorrhage
Focal neurologic deficit (e.g., motor weakness, aphasia, cerebellar signs, progressive myelopathy)
Global neurologic deficit (e.g., dementia)
Pulsatile tinnitus, objective bruit
Proptosis, conjunctival injection, chemosis
Ophthalmoplegia (secondary to extraoccular muscle swelling, or compression of cranial nerves III, IV, VI)
Visual loss (secondary to orbital congestion and increased intraocular pressure, retinal hemorrhages, or optic neuropathy)
Glaucoma
Papilledema (secondary to hydrocephalus or pseudotumor cerebri caused by impaired venous drainage)
Facial pain (secondary to compression of the first and second divisions of trigeminal nerve in lateral wall of cavernous sinus)

to allow treatment planning.[7] At angiography, a delayed circulation time is compatible with venous congestion.[30] Focal areas of delayed venous drainage in the brain correspond to the site of CVR.[7] In some cases, tortuous, dilated pial veins may be seen that develop as a result of venous hypertension (see Fig. 80-3F). Willinsky and colleagues[30] have described this finding as the pseudophlebitic pattern, which is a sign of venous congestion of the brain and may be associated with an aggressive natural history.[7]

Natural History

The natural history of a disease refers to the disease course after presentation if left untreated. Knowledge of the natural history is essential in patient management. The results and complications of available treatment strategies must be compared with the outcome of the natural history of the disease. Recently, our group reported the results of the largest prospective natural history studies of patients with cranial DAVFs.[3,20] The results, summarized in the following, showed that the presence of CVR is the most significant predictive factor for an aggressive natural history.[3,20]

DURAL ARTERIOVENOUS FISTULAS WITH CORTICAL VENOUS REFLUX

Of 236 cranial DAVFs, 119 had CVR (Borden classification type II or III and Cognard classification type IIb, IIa + b, III, or IV). Of these, 96 patients successfully underwent curative treatment, and three patients were lost to follow-up. Van Dijk and colleagues[20] followed the remaining 20 patients with persistent CVR (14 patients who refused treatment and 6 who had partial treatment only) for a mean follow-up period of 4.3 years (86.9 patient-years). In these 20 patients, the annual risks of ICH and NHND (disregarding aggressive events at presentation) were found to be 8.1% and 6.9%, respectively, adding up to an annual event rate (i.e., ICH and NHND) of 15%. The annual mortality rate was 10.4%. These results demonstrate that DAVFs with CVR have an aggressive natural history.

DURAL ARTERIOVENOUS FISTULAS WITHOUT CORTICAL VENOUS REFLUX

Of the 236 cranial DAVFs, 117 had no CVR (Borden type I, Cognard type I or IIa). Five patients were lost to follow-up. The remaining 112 patients were followed up clinically for a median of 27.9 months (range, 1 month to 17.5 years), amounting to 348 patient-years. Of these, 68 underwent observation alone, and 44 underwent palliative treatment for symptomatic control (43 endovascular, 1 surgery). Palliative treatment, never aimed at cure, was performed if the patient had intolerable symptoms or if there was persistent high intraocular pressure or decreasing visual acuity. Using this conservative management strategy, 98% of patients had a benign and well-tolerated clinical course, without any ICH or NHND.[3] Long-term angiographic follow-up in 50 patients showed that DAVFs without CVR have a 2% to 3% risk of developing CVR.[3]

Indications for Treatment

Decisions regarding treatment of DAVFs should be guided by their natural history. Therefore, DAVFs with

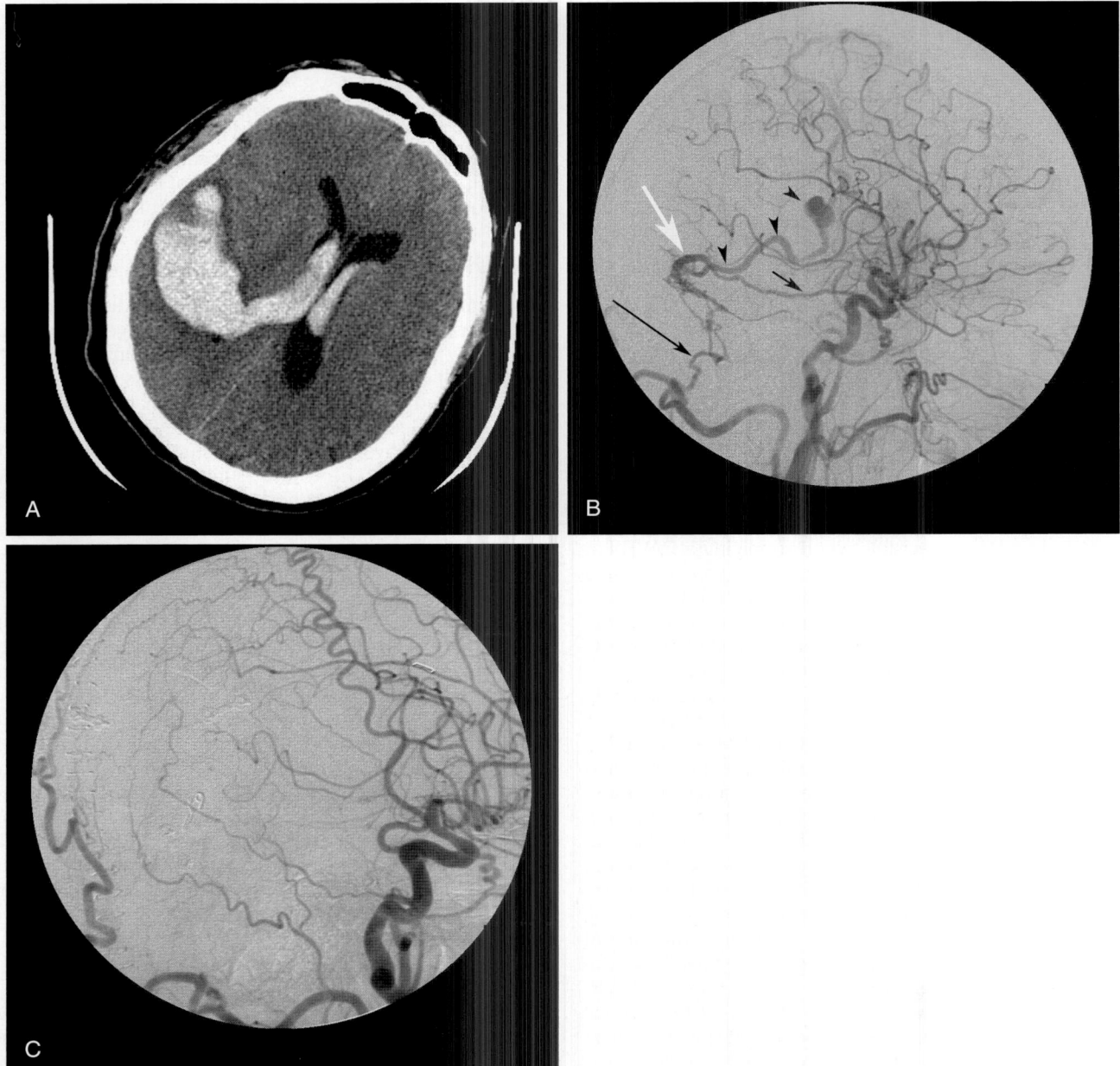

FIGURE 80-2 A, Axial computed tomography scan of a 56-year-old man who presented with sudden headache followed by loss of consciousness shows intracerebral and intraventricular hemorrhage. B, Right common carotid artery angiogram, lateral projection, shows a transverse sinus dural arteriovenous fistula (DAVF), fed by branches of the right middle meningeal artery (*arrow*) and the right occipital artery (*large arrow*). Venous drainage was by reflux into a cortical vein (*white arrow*) leading to an ectasia (*arrowheads*). There was no sinusal drainage, making this a Borden type III/Cognard type IV DAVF. In this patient, selective angiography was not possible because of severe atherosclerosis and tortuosity of the carotid arteries. C, Postoperative angiogram after right occipital craniotomy exposing the transverse sinus. The dura was opened and reflected inferiorly based on its attachment to the transverse sinus. The DAVF was treated by coagulation and division of this vein close to the transverse sinus, at the site shown by the white arrow in Figure 80-3B.

CVR should be treated to eliminate the risk of hemorrhage and neurologic deficit. The aim of treatment in these cases is elimination of CVR or complete cure if possible. Lesions without CVR do not require treatment unless they are associated with intolerable symptoms such as intolerable tinnitus and ophthalmologic symptoms including visual deterioration and pain. For these lesions, the aim of treatment is not cure, but palliative symptom control.

Management Options

Several options are available for the management of cranial DAVFs. In many cases, a combination of methods may be required.

OBSERVATION

DAVFs without CVR usually behave in a benign manner and are rarely associated with hemorrhage or neurologic

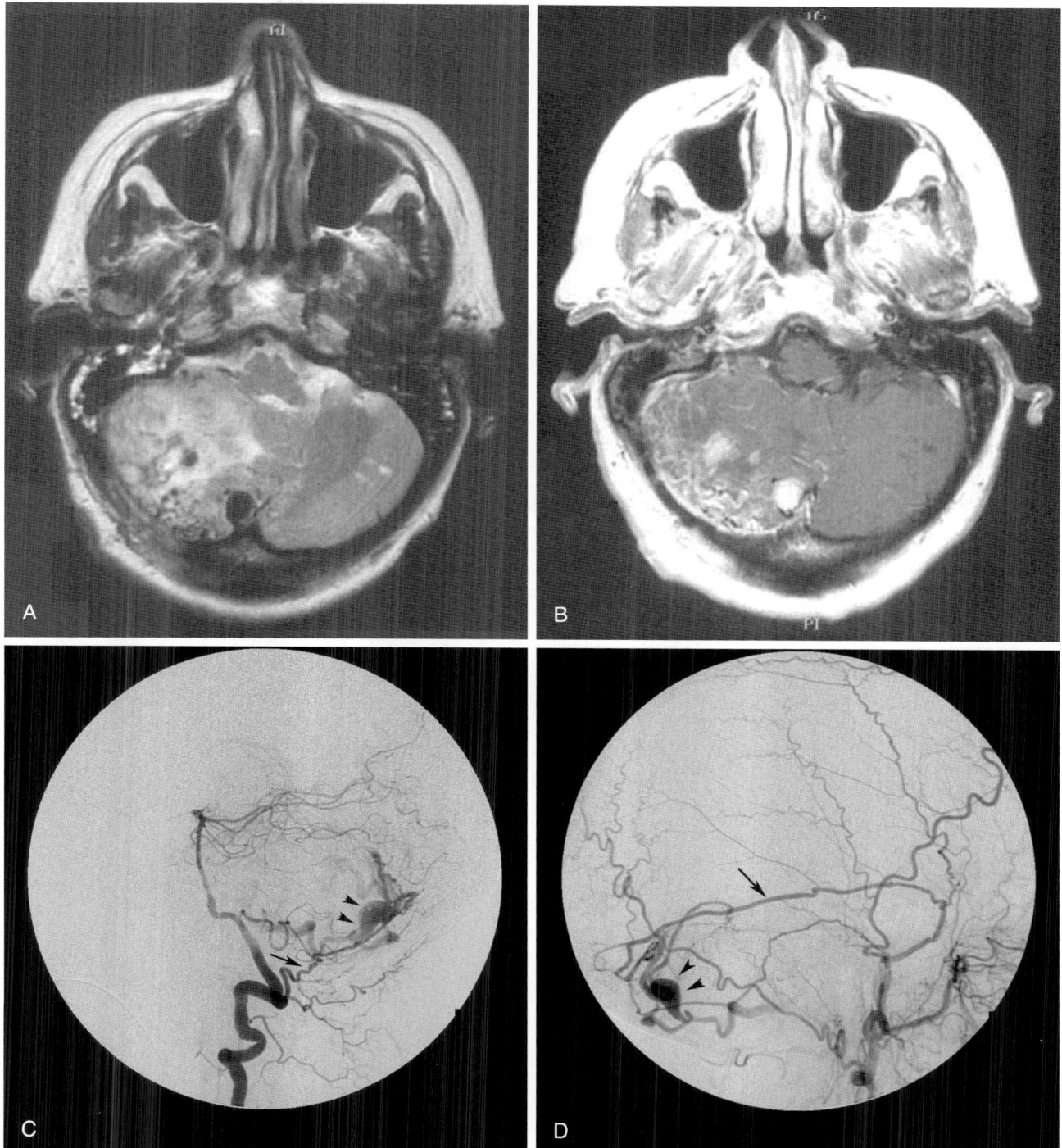

FIGURE 80-3 A 67-year-old woman presented with severe headache and subsequent deterioration in conscious level. Computed tomography scan showed a right cerebellar hematoma that was evacuated. A, Axial T2-weighted magnetic resonance imaging (MRI) shows a central area of hyperintensity in the right cerebellar hemisphere. Tortuous dilated vessels appearing as flow voids in the right cerebellar hemisphere indicate the presence of cortical venous reflux. B, Axial gadolinium-enhanced T1-weighted MRI shows peripheral enhancement surrounding the hyperintense region seen on the T2-weighted image. C, Left vertebral artery angiogram, lateral projection DAVF with ectasia (*arrowheads*) fed by dural branch of vertebral artery (*arrow*). D, Right external carotid artery (ECA) angiogram, lateral projection, same ectasia (*arrowheads*) fed by posterior branch of middle meningeal artery (*arrow*).

Continued

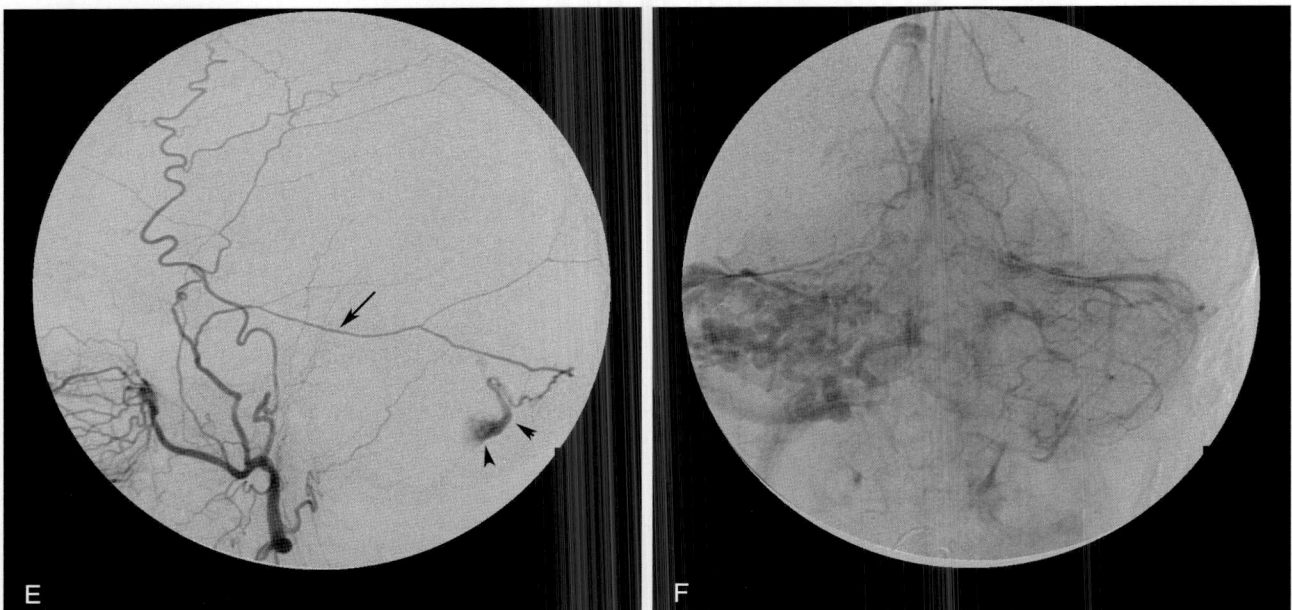

FIGURE 80-3, cont'd E, Show a torcular dural arteriovenous fistula (DAVF), fed by branches of the left vertebral artery (*arrow*), and right and left middle meningeal arteries (*arrowheads*). The fistula drains into a cortical vein (*curved arrows*), with a varix (*open curved arrow*), making this a Borden type III/Cognard type IV DAVF. F, The venous phase of the angiogram demonstrates tortuous, dilated pial veins, referred to as a pseudophlebitic pattern. This fistula was successfully cured by transarterial embolization.

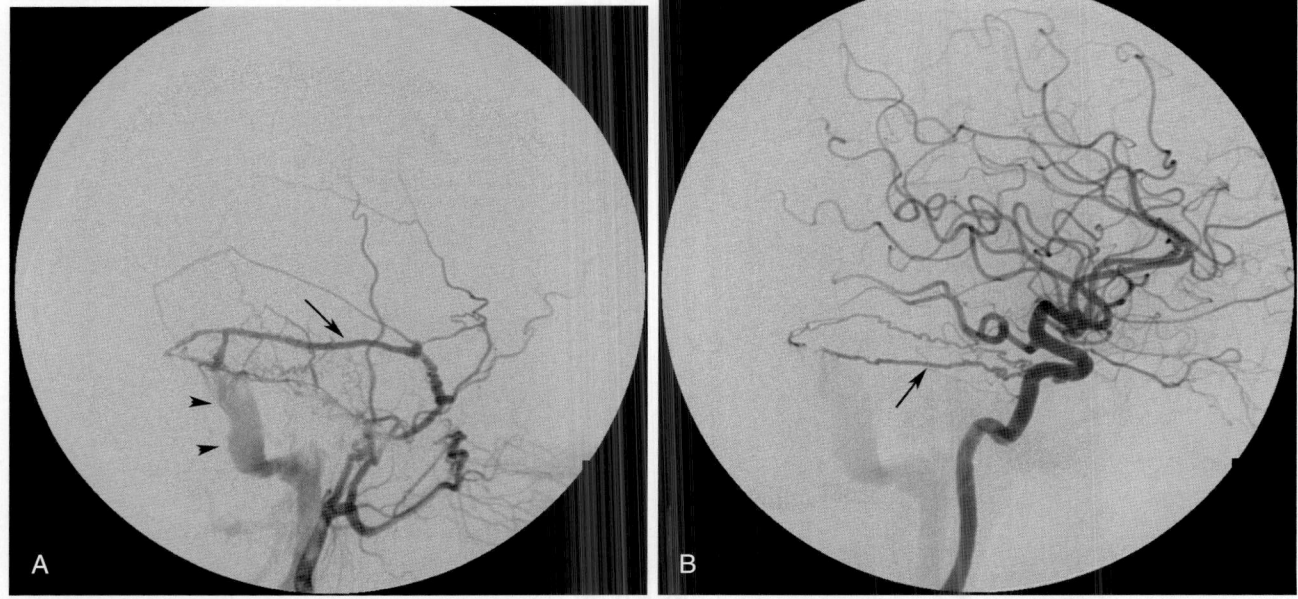

FIGURE 80-4 Angiograms of a 52-year-old woman who presented with pulsatile tinnitus and audible bruit behind the right ear. A, Right external carotid artery angiogram, lateral projection shows premature appearance of the sigmoid sinus (*arrowheads*) in the ultraearly arterial phase of the angiogram. A transverse sinus dural arteriovenous fistula (DAVF) is shown, fed by the posterior branch of the right middle meningeal artery (*arrow*) and draining antegradely into the transverse/sigmoid sinus (*arrowheads*) without any cortical venous reflux (CVR) (Borden type I, Cognard type I). The same DAVF is shown in Figure 80-1A being fed also by the right occipital artery. B, Right internal carotid artery angiogram, lateral projection, revealed a hypertrophied artery of Bernasconi and Cassinari, also supplying the DAVF (*arrow*). As there was no CVR, the patient was managed with observation alone.

deficit. Therefore, observation is the most appropriate management option for these patients if they are asymptomatic or are tolerating their symptoms.[4,7] As they have a 2% to 3% chance of developing CVR, all patients should be followed up clinically and radiographically. Any change in symptoms (worsening or improvement) may be a warning signal for development of CVR and should prompt repeat cerebral angiography.[3,7] In patients with a stable clinical condition, serial MRI and magnetic resonance angiography and a conventional angiogram after 3 years is advised.[7] Observation is not a valid treatment option for DAVFs with CVR.

COMPRESSION THERAPY

Intermittent manual carotid compression by the patient has been used by Halbach and colleagues,[8,31] to treat DAVFs of the cavernous sinus in patients with no evidence of carotid atherosclerosis. The patient is instructed to compress the carotid-jugular area ipsilateral to the DAVF, with the contralateral hand for as long as 30 minutes per session. The compression should be terminated if any weakness develops.[8] Halbach and colleagues[8,31] reported a cure rate of 27% with this technique after 4 to 6 weeks. However, this treatment has been the subject of debate because the 27% cure rate in the short term may reflect the natural history of the disease.[7]

TRANSARTERIAL EMBOLIZATION

Superselective embolization of the dural feeding vessels to a DAVF can be an effective treatment in some cases.[8] The ideal goal is to cure the DAVF by occluding the fistula itself. To achieve this from the arterial side, a microcatheter must be navigated into the distal part of a feeding artery and wedged, so that cyanoacrylate glue can be pushed through the nidus and into the most proximal venous outlet. This is essentially a venous treatment performed through the arterial side. Liquid adhesive agents (e.g., *n*-butyl cyanoacrylate), the rate of polymerization of which can be controlled, are the best agents to permanently occlude a fistula.[7] Successful occlusion of the fistula using this technique has been reported in a small number of patients.[7,32]

In most cases, transarterial embolization involves occlusion of the feeding arteries without occlusion of the fistula. This may decrease flow through the fistula but is rarely curative because most DAVFs have multiple small feeding arteries that are not amenable to transarterial embolization. Furthermore, in most cases, the lesion will continue to recruit feeding arteries from other sources, leading to recurrence.[8,32] Transarterial embolization is commonly used as an adjunct before surgical treatment or transvenous embolization of DAVFs. It is also used as palliative treatment for benign DAVFs with intolerable symptoms. Preoperative embolization of large feeding arteries, particularly in the external carotid territory, carries a relatively low risk and helps to reduce intraoperative blood loss. Particles (e.g., polyvinyl alcohol) may be used for this purpose.[7]

Endovascular therapy is not without risk. Knowledge of the important anastomoses between the external carotid, internal carotid, and vertebrobasilar systems is crucial for safe embolization.[33] Embolic agents can inadvertently travel through these anastomoses and lead to occlusion of important branches. Embolization of feeding arteries that arise directly from the ICA or vertebral artery may lead to reflux of embolic material into the parent artery and result in stroke. In the case of benign DAVFs, it is important to ensure that the embolic material does not flow past the fistula site and obstruct venous outflow. If this occurs, venous drainage may be diverted to cortical veins, thereby converting a benign fistula to an aggressive one.

TRANSVENOUS EMBOLIZATION

Transvenous embolization is increasingly used in the management of cranial DAVFs.[34,35] This involves a retrograde approach through the veins with deposition of materials such as coils into the venous compartment at the fistula site.

Usually the transfemoral route is employed. In the majority of cases, transvenous embolization involves sacrificing the involved dural venous sinus. This can only be performed if detailed study of the venous phase of the cerebral angiogram has shown that the involved dural sinus is not being used by the brain and that alternate pathways for venous drainage of the brain have developed.[7] In some cases it may be possible to use a retrograde transvenous approach to disconnect CVR without sacrificing the dural sinus. However, in most cases this is not possible because of the difficulty in access to the refluxing cortical veins and the tortuosity of these veins.

In some cases of transverse/sigmoid sinus DAVFs, the lesion may be draining into a venous pouch, parallel to and separate from the transverse sinus. The University of California-San Francisco interventional neuroradiology group have reported 10 such cases and named this entity the parallel venous channel. In their series, transvenous embolization was used to occlude the parallel venous channel and cure the fistula in all 10 cases while preserving the transverse/sigmoid sinus.[36] Identification of this separate venous channel is important as it may allow curative treatment of the fistula without sacrificing the transverse sinus. However, this type of channel has been identified in a small number of cases only.

The mainstay of transvenous embolization is occlusion of the affected venous sinus. Neurologic complications after embolization occur if outflow to normally draining veins is obstructed, resulting in venous hypertension and venous infarction. After embolization of cavernous sinus DAVFs, paradoxical worsening of ophthalmologic symptoms may develop secondary to excessive thrombosis and venous hypertension involving the ophthalmic veins. Other complications include guidewire injury to the wall of dural sinuses resulting in subarachnoid hemorrhage and injury to cranial nerves.[34]

SURGERY

Although endovascular therapy is increasingly used to treat intracranial DAVFs, surgery still plays an important role in the management of these lesions. We recommend surgery for DAVFs with CVR when endovascular therapy fails or is technically not feasible. Three different surgical strategies exist for treatment of intracranial DAVFs. The first is to obtain venous access for direct packing of the involved dural venous sinus. The second is complete excision of the DAVF. The third is to disconnect the arterialized leptomeningeal veins (CVR) only, without attempting to excise the entire lesion. These strategies are discussed in the following sections.

Surgery to Obtain Venous Access

In some cases, the usual venous access routes may not be available for transfemoral transvenous embolization. This can occur due to thrombosis or steno-occlusive disease of the dural venous sinuses. In these cases, access may be gained to the fistula by direct surgical exposure and catheterization of the involved sinus. Direct packing of the sinus can then be performed using coils or other thrombogenic materials such as Gelfoam and silk sutures.[37]

Surgical Excision

Traditionally, the goal of surgery for aggressive DAVFs has been complete excision of the lesion. This involves interruption of the arterial feeders, extensive coagulation, and excision of the pathologic dural leaflet, and disconnection of arterialized leptomeningeal veins (i.e., CVR). In some cases, the involved dural venous sinus is also excised if it is not participating in the venous drainage of normal brain. We use preoperative transarterial embolization of the arterial feeders whenever possible to reduce intraoperative blood loss. Prophylactic intravenous antibiotics are given at induction. Intraoperative mannitol and cerebrospinal fluid drainage using a lumbar spinal drain may be used when necessary to reduce the need for brain retraction. Under general endotracheal anesthesia, the scalp incision and craniotomy are fashioned in the appropriate location. Frameless or frame-based stereotaxy may be helpful in localizing the lesion, particularly if enlarged cortical veins or a venous varix can be visualized on computed tomography or MRI. Once the pathologic region of dura has been exposed, the involved dura and feeding arteries are extensively coagulated. If the involved venous sinus can be sacrificed, the dura is incised on both sides of, and parallel to, the sinus. Feeding arteries are coagulated or occluded using hemostatic clips as they are encountered. The involved segment of the venous sinus can then be ligated proximally and distally and excised together with the pathologic dura. All arterialized leptomeningeal veins are coagulated or clipped at their entrance into the sinus and divided. Intraoperative angiography is used to ensure complete obliteration of the fistula.

If the sinus is being used for normal venous drainage of the brain, it should be skeletonized and left in situ.[38] Skeletonization of the sinus involves interruption of the dural arterial supply to the fistula, and excision of dural segments on both sides of the sinus, while preserving the venous sinus and the nonarterialized cortical veins. In cases of transverse/sigmoid or superior sagittal sinus DAVFs, the tentorium or the falx adjacent to the sinus should also be coagulated and cut to ensure complete interruption of arterial supply to the fistula.

The extensive procedures used for total excision of DAVFs may be associated with significant complications. Access may be difficult when the lesion is in a deep location (e.g., tentorial and posterior fossa lesions) and may require extensive skull base procedures. Significant hemorrhage may occur at any stage of the procedure. Torrential hemorrhage may occur from engorged vessels when incising the scalp and from engorged osseous and dural vessels when performing the craniotomy.[39] Bleeding from bone should be controlled using bone wax. Bleeding from the enlarged dural arteries feeding the fistula should be controlled using extensive coagulation or hemostatic clips. Preoperative transarterial embolization of the feeding vessels is extremely helpful in reducing intraoperative hemorrhage.

DISCONNECTION OF CORTICAL VENOUS REFLUX ALONE

The goal of treatment for aggressive DAVFs is to eliminate the risk of ICH and neurologic deficit. Because CVR is the predisposing factor for aggressive natural history, it has been suggested that a procedure limited to disconnection of arterialized leptomeningeal veins (CVR) is sufficient in the treatment of aggressive lesions and that complete excision of the involved dural leaflet and the venous sinus is not necessary.[7,40-42] Disconnection of CVR is a simpler

procedure with less morbidity and changes the natural history of the lesion from aggressive to benign. There are now several reports showing that this technique is effective, and we now use it in preference to complete excision in most cases.[43]

The surgical procedure involves exposure of the pathologic dural leaflet as explained previously. Any dural feeding arteries are coagulated or occluded with hemostatic clips. The dura is then opened, and with careful dissection, the arterialized leptomeningeal veins are exposed. These veins are then coagulated or clipped and divided at their entrance into the dural venous sinus or as close to the fistula site as possible. It is important to ensure that the vein is adequately coagulated before division. The adjacent dural areas should be examined to ensure that all arterialized leptomeningeal veins have been disconnected. "Blue" nonarterialized cortical veins should be preserved. The dura is then closed, the bone flap replaced, and the wound closed in the usual manner.

STEREOTACTIC RADIOSURGERY

There is a limited number of reports on the radiosurgical treatment of intracranial DAVFs.[44-49] Pan and colleagues[47] reported complete angiographic resolution of the nidus in 47% of 19 transverse/sigmoid sinus DAVFs, after a median follow-up of 19 months. Pollock and colleagues[45,46] have used a combination of stereotactic radiosurgery and transarterial embolization. Although radiosurgery is effective in obliterating some DAVFs, its main disadvantage is the long interval between treatment and the expected therapeutic effects. In patients with CVR, this delay is not acceptable because of the high risk of ICH and neurologic deficit (15% per year) while waiting for obliteration of the lesion.[7,20,42] In patients without CVR, curative treatment is not required because of the benign natural history of these lesions. Most of these patients can be managed by observation alone or by palliative transarterial embolization. The risk of radiosurgery in these patients may not be acceptable, especially in view of the limited data available on the efficacy of this treatment.[3,7] Therefore, the role of radiosurgery in the management of intracranial DAVFs is currently unclear.

Comprehensive Management Strategy

This section outlines a comprehensive management strategy for the treatment of intracranial DAVFs. The specific features of individual DAVFs in different locations are dealt with later in the chapter. As a general principle, the management strategy is based on the pattern of venous drainage of the lesion because this determines the natural history of DAVFs.

DURAL ARTERIOVENOUS FISTULAS WITHOUT CORTICAL VENOUS REFLUX (BENIGN FISTULAS: BORDEN TYPE I, COGNARD TYPES I AND IIA)

For patients with DAVFs without CVR who are asymptomatic or have tolerable symptoms, observation is the most appropriate treatment option.[4,7] If the patient has intolerable symptoms, such as tinnitus or ophthalmologic symptoms, treatment may be indicated. In these cases, curative treatment is not necessary as the patient is not at risk of ICH or neurologic deficit. Palliative treatment in the form

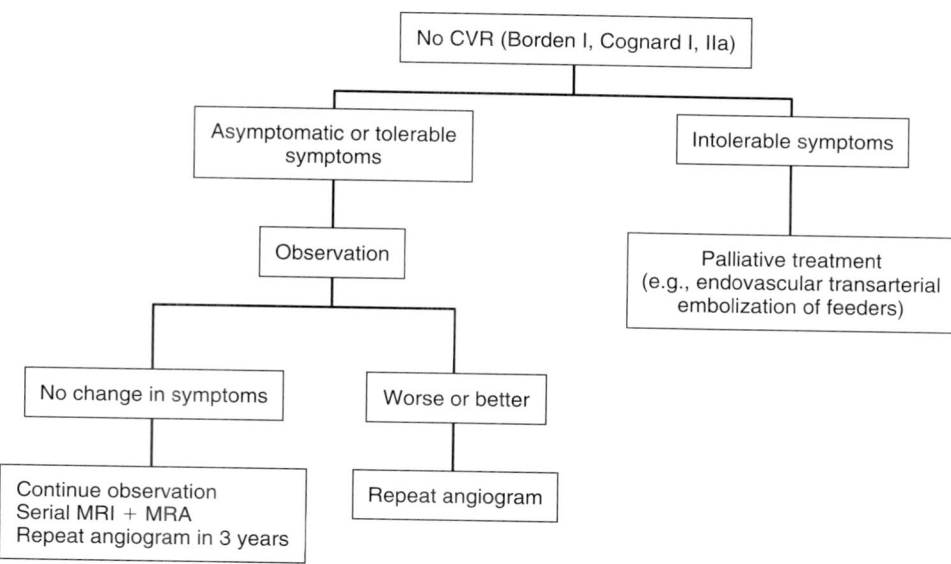

FIGURE 80-5 Management strategy for dural arteriovenous fistulas without cortical venous reflux (CVR) (benign dural arteriovenous fistulas, Borden type I and Cognard types I and IIa). MRA, magnetic resonance angiography; MRI, magnetic resonance imaging.

of transarterial embolization of the feeding arteries is usually effective in symptom control and is associated with fewer complications compared with curative transvenous embolization or surgery. All patients should be followed up clinically and radiographically, and any change in symptoms (deterioration or improvement) should prompt repeat conventional angiography to look for development of CVR (Fig. 80-5).

DURAL ARTERIOVENOUS FISTULAS WITH CORTICAL VENOUS REFLUX (AGGRESSIVE FISTULAS: BORDEN TYPES II AND III, COGNARD TYPES IIB THROUGH V)

These lesions must be treated aggressively because they are associated with a 15% annual risk of hemorrhage and neurologic deficit.[20] Treatment should be performed soon after the diagnosis has been made.[4] There is evidence that rebleeding may occur early after an initial hemorrhagic presentation. In one series, 35% of patients had a rebleed

within 2 weeks after the first hemorrhage.[50] Complete obliteration of the fistula is ideal but not critical because there is increasing evidence that disconnection of CVR alone results in long-term protection against hemorrhage and neurologic deficit.[4,40-43,51]

Treatment of cranial DAVFs with CVR requires a multidisciplinary approach. A combination of transarterial embolization, transvenous embolization, and surgery may be required in some cases. The primary goal of treatment, whether endovascular or surgical, is to eliminate CVR. Endovascular embolization is usually the primary treatment modality and often begins with transarterial embolization. This is rarely curative and is usually followed by transvenous embolization. If endovascular therapy is not feasible or fails, then surgery is indicated.

For lesions with CVR only without any sinusal drainage (Borden type III and Cognard types III, IV, and V), CVR disconnection alone is all that is required. Transvenous embolization is rarely successful in these cases because

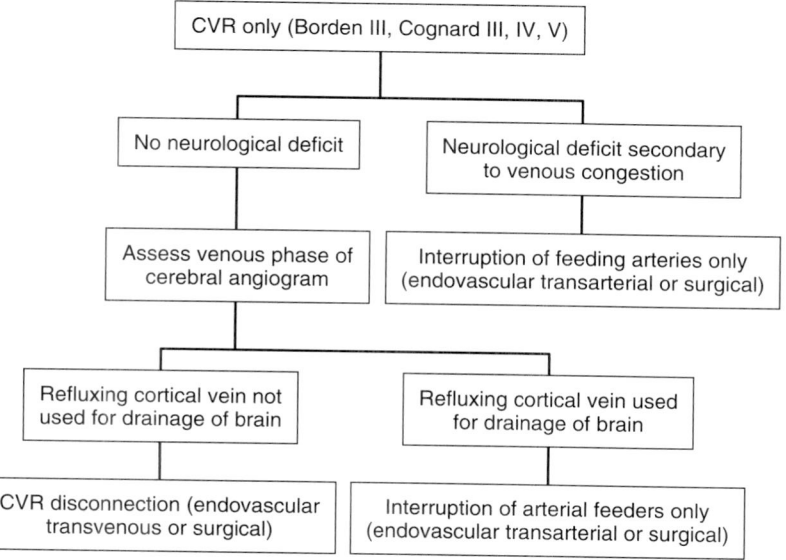

FIGURE 80-6 Management strategy for dural arteriovenous fistulas with cortical venous reflux (CVR) only (aggressive dural arteriovenous fistulas, Borden type III and Cognard types III, IV and V).

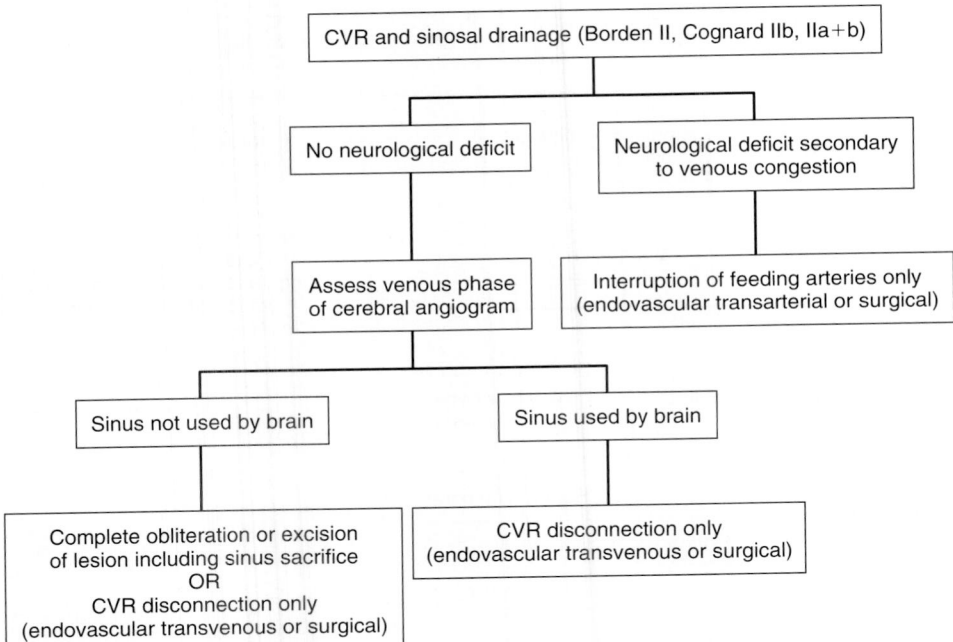

FIGURE 80-7 Management strategy for dural arteriovenous fistulas with cortical venous reflux (CVR) and sinusal drainage (aggressive dural arteriovenous fistulas, Borden type II and Cognard types IIb and IIa + b).

the adjacent venous sinus cannot be used for access to the refluxing cortical vein. Most of these cases therefore require surgical disconnection of CVR. Before disconnection, it must be decided whether it is safe to interrupt the veins involved in CVR. This is particularly important when the vein to be disconnected is a major cortical draining vein, such as the vein of Labbé. The venous phase of the cerebral angiograms must be studied in detail to ensure that normal brain is not draining into the concerned veins and that other venous routes are being used by the brain (Fig. 80-6).

The management of DAVFs that have both CVR and sinusal drainage (Borden type II and Cognard types IIb and IIa + b) is more complex. The management strategy for these lesions requires a detailed knowledge of the venous drainage of the brain as well as that of the fistula. If the involved dural sinus is being used only by the DAVF and is not being used for venous drainage of the brain, then it may be sacrificed. This can be achieved by transvenous embolization or by surgical packing or excision of the sinus. The decision regarding the safety of sinus sacrifice is based on preoperative clinical and angiographic assessment of the patient. If the patient is neurologically intact, and the venous phase of the cerebral angiogram shows that the involved venous sinus is not used for drainage of the brain and that other pathways have developed for venous drainage of the brain, the sinus may be sacrificed. However, if angiography shows that the sinus is used for venous drainage of the brain, treatment must be limited to CVR disconnection alone without obliteration or excision of the sinus. This converts Borden type II (Cognard types IIb and IIa + b) lesions to Borden type I (Cognard types I and IIa) lesions, which have a benign natural history.

The most difficult situation arises in patients with preoperative neurologic deficit. In these patients, an assumption that the sinus can be sacrificed, based solely on angiographic findings may be incorrect. In other words, the patient's neurologic deficit may be a consequence of the retrograde flow in the sinus and the resulting venous hypertension, which may improve if normal flow in the sinus can be reestablished. Occlusion of the sinus or the refluxing cortical veins in these cases would eliminate the chance of recovery of neurologic function and may lead to venous infarction. In these patients, the safest option may be to limit the procedure to the arterial side of the lesion. This can be achieved by extensive transarterial embolization of the feeding arteries or by surgical skeletonization of the sinus. All cortical veins and the venous sinuses should be left intact. Fortunately, this situation arises rarely (Fig. 80-7).

In all patients with DAVFs and CVR, treatment should continue until all CVR has been eliminated. Simply reducing the size of the nidus without eliminating CVR does not eradicate the risk of future hemorrhage or neurologic deficit. All patients, particularly those in whom complete obliteration of the fistula has not been achieved, require lifelong follow-up, with a routine delayed angiogram at 3 years to check for recurrence of CVR. Patients would also require an angiogram if there is any change (deterioration or improvement) in their symptoms.

ANATOMIC CONSIDERATIONS FOR DURAL ARTERIOVENOUS FISTULAS IN SPECIFIC LOCATIONS

In itself, anatomic location of a DAVF has no direct correlation with aggressive clinical events, although this has been suggested in the past.[3,19] DAVFs in any location can develop CVR (Table 80-4).[1,19] However, DAVFs in particular locations such as the anterior cranial fossa and the tentorium are more often associated with CVR and are therefore more likely to behave aggressively than are lesions in other locations. This reflects the pattern of regional venous anatomy in these locations. For example, anterior cranial fossa DAVFs cannot drain into any venous sinuses and can only

Table 80-4 Anatomic Location of 236 DAVFs Managed by University of Toronto Brain Vascular Malformation Study Group

Anatomic Location	No. (% of all DAVFs)	No. with CVR (% of DAVFs in This Location)
Transverse sigmoid	100 (42.4)	38 (38)
Cavernous sinus	79 (33.5)	29 (36.7)
Deep venous/tentorial incisural	20 (8.5)	20 (100)
Superior sagittal sinus and convexity	12 (5.1)	12 (100)
Foramen magnum	11 (4.6)	9 (81.8)
Anterior cranial fossa	9 (3.8)	9 (100)
Temporal fossa	4 (1.7)	1 (25)
Superior petrosal sinus	1 (0.4)	1 (100)

CVR, cortical venous reflux; DAVFs, dural arteriovenous fistulas.

drain into cortical veins and are therefore always associated with CVR.[19] Table 80-4 shows the anatomic location of intracranial DAVFs. They are named according to the dural sinus with which they are associated.[52] This section deals with the anatomy and surgical management of DAVFs in specific locations.

TRANSVERSE/SIGMOID SINUS DURAL ARTERIOVENOUS FISTULAS

Transverse/sigmoid sinus DAVFs are the most common intracranial DAVFs, accounting for 4% to 60% of cases (see Table 80-4).[28,36,43] Their arterial supply is derived mainly from branches of the ECA, namely, the transmastoid branches of the occipital artery, the posterior auricular artery, the posterior branch of the middle meningeal artery, and the neuromeningeal division of the ascending pharyngeal artery. They may also receive arterial supply from the posterior meningeal branch of the vertebral artery, the tentorial branch of the meningohypophyseal trunk of the ICA, and the petrous bone.[8,28] Venous drainage may be through the ipsilateral transverse/sigmoid sinuses or through the contralateral side if the ipsilateral sinus is occluded. Occasionally, these lesions drain into the diploic veins, which may lead to significant hemorrhage during craniotomy. CVR may occur through temporal, occipital, and cerebellar veins.[4,7]

If endovascular therapy fails, surgery should be performed in cases with CVR. Preoperative transarterial embolization is very helpful in reducing intraoperative bleeding and should be used whenever possible. The patient is placed in the park-bench position with the side of the lesion up. It is important to have access to the region between the inion and the mastoid. A lazy "S"-shaped incision is made two fingerbreadths behind the ear. The occipital and posterior auricular arteries, which are usually enlarged, should be doubly ligated and divided. In some cases, this interrupts the main arterial supply to the DAVF. The nuchal muscles are incised using monopolar cautery, leaving a small cuff of fascia at the superior nuchal line. The muscles are then scraped off the bone using subperiosteal dissection. A craniotomy is performed to expose the transverse sinus and the dura superior and inferior to it. Great care must be taken to prevent a dural

laceration while performing the craniotomy as this may lead to torrential hemorrhage from enlarged dural feeding arteries. The cutting bit of a high-speed drill may be used for performing the craniotomy. The bone is gradually removed along the margin of the bone plate until the dura can be seen through a thin layer of bone. The dura is gently separated from the bone flap, and the bone flap is elevated using a periosteal elevator.[39] Significant hemorrhage from the dura when elevating the bone flap may be controlled by placing a large piece of Gelfoam or Surgicel over the dura and applying pressure with a wet sponge for a few minutes. Dural feeders can be coagulated using bipolar cautery or occluded using hemostatic clips.

The remainder of the procedure depends on the goal of treatment, which should have been decided preoperatively. If the goal of treatment is CVR disconnection only, then the dura is incised above or below the transverse sinus depending on the location of CVR (i.e., temporal/occipital or cerebellar). The dural flap is reflected on a base along the transverse sinus. The arterialized leptomeningeal vein or veins should then be identified, coagulated or clipped, and divided as close to the fistula as possible. It is important to ensure that all arterialized leptomeningeal veins are disconnected. The dura is then closed in the usual manner. If the mastoid air cells have been entered, they should be obliterated using bone wax. The bone flap is then replaced, and muscle, fascia, and scalp are closed as usual.

If the goal of treatment is complete excision of the fistula and the sinus can be sacrificed, then after performing the craniotomy as described previously, the mastoid and posterolateral portion of the petrous bone are removed using a diamond burr on a high-speed drill to expose the dura lateral and anterior to the sigmoid sinus.[38,39] Knowledge of the anatomy of this region or assistance from an otolaryngologist is important to avoid damage to hearing or to the facial nerve during this stage of the procedure.[38] At this point, bleeding is mainly from arterial feeders contained within the petrous bone, which should be controlled using bone wax. The dura is incised above and below the transverse sinus and parallel to its long axis. Feeding arteries are coagulated or clipped as they are encountered. The transverse sinus is then occluded medially using two curved hemostats placed approximately 2 cm apart. The sinus is cut between the two hemostats, the ends are closed using 3-0 silk transfixion sutures, and the hemostats are removed. The dural incisions above and below the sinus are then continued laterally. Gentle retraction on the occipital lobe and the cerebellum exposes the tentorium, which should also be cut in a medial to lateral direction to interrupt any tentorial feeding arteries. All arterialized leptomeningeal veins are also coagulated and divided. The dural and tentorial incisions are extended laterally, distal to the junction of the transverse and sigmoid sinuses, which is usually the site of the fistula. The skeletonized sinus is resected distal to this site. The sigmoid sinus is then evaluated for patency. If there is a significant vein of Labbé, the sigmoid sinus should be left patent to drain it. However, if the vein of Labbé is arterialized and is not used for venous drainage of the brain, it can be clipped and divided, and the sigmoid sinus is then packed with Surgicel or Gelfoam and ligated. Duraplasty using fascia lata, pericranium, or synthetic dura is then performed to close the dural defect. The mastoid air cells are completely obliterated using bone wax, and the bone flap is replaced. The nuchal muscles and fascia are closed in multiple layers to prevent cerebrospinal fluid leak. The scalp is closed in the usual manner. Intraoperative angiography is used to ensure complete excision of the nidus.

CAVERNOUS SINUS DURAL ARTERIOVENOUS FISTULAS

These are the second most common intracranial DAVFs, accounting for a third of all lesions in our series (see Table 80-4).[8,28,43] They are supplied by branches from the ICAs, ECAs, or both. Venous drainage is via the cavernous sinus, with subsequent anterior drainage into the superior and inferior ophthalmic veins, posterior drainage into the superior and inferior petrosal sinuses (IPSs), or cortical venous drainage into the sphenoparietal sinus, sylvian, uncal, and anterior pontomesencephalic veins.[7,28] Barrow and colleagues[23] classified carotid cavernous fistulas into four categories based on the type of feeding arteries detected on angiography. Type A fistulas are direct fistulas between the ICA and the cavernous sinus. Types B, C, and D are DAVFs involving the cavernous sinus. Type B are fed by meningeal branches of the ICA, type C by meningeal branches of ECA, and type D by meningeal branches of both ICA and ECA. Type A fistulas are high-flow fistulas and usually result from a traumatic tear in the cavernous ICA or spontaneously from a rupture of an intracavernous ICA aneurysm. These high-flow fistulas rarely resolve spontaneously and require treatment to prevent progressive visual loss, intolerable bruit, or pain.[19] They are almost always treated by endovascular embolization and are not dealt with in this chapter. Most spontaneous carotid cavernous fistulas are of the low-flow types B, C, or D and are referred to as cavernous sinus DAVFs. They are usually idiopathic and occur most commonly in middle-aged women. They may present with proptosis, chemosis, diplopia, visual loss, pulsatile bruit, retro-orbital pain, and facial pain.[35] Cavernous sinus DAVFs may present with ophthalmologic symptoms on the contralateral side. Unlike type A fistulas, a significant proportion of these low-flow fistulas undergo spontaneous resolution.

Cavernous sinus DAVFs can also be classified according to the pattern of venous drainage based on the Borden or Cognard classification. As with other DAVFs, it is the presence or absence of CVR that determines the natural history of these lesions. CVR occurs in 19% to 37% of patients with cavernous sinus DAVFs (see Table 80-4).[35,53] CVR is more common in patients with bilateral orbital signs but can also occur in those with unilateral signs. In a study of 118 patients with cavernous sinus DAVFs, 43% of patients with bilateral orbital signs and 9% of those with unilateral orbital signs had CVR.[53] Cavernous sinus DAVFs without CVR usually have a benign clinical course. Many of these lesions undergo spontaneous involution, with symptom resolution over weeks or months.[28] The majority of patients can be managed conservatively but must be followed up closely by a neuro-ophthalmologist. Although these lesions have been referred to as benign, in some cases, spontaneous venous thrombosis and venous hypertension may result in increased intraocular pressure and progressive visual loss.[7] Medical therapy including topical agents, oral corticosteroids, and systemic anticoagulation may be used to prevent blindness. However, if medical therapy fails to control intraocular pressure and deteriorating vision, prompt endovascular treatment is indicated.[7] Transarterial embolization using particles may be tried first to slow down the flow through the fistula. If this fails, transvenous embolization is required.

If CVR exists, these DAVFs must be treated with the same aggressiveness as DAVFs in other locations. This is usually done using transvenous embolization. Before this, transarterial embolization may be performed, particularly if there is significant supply through ECA branches. For transvenous embolization, access to the cavernous sinus is usually obtained by the femoral route through the internal jugular vein and the IPS. This venous approach may be difficult or impossible in cases in which the IPS is partially or completely thrombosed. However, with improved materials and experience, some surgeons have successfully navigated an angiographic catheter, even through a thrombosed IPS.[54] If access through the IPS is not possible or has failed, other routes may be employed. These may involve endovascular and/or surgical techniques. The approach depends on the direction of venous drainage of the fistula and may use the superior ophthalmic vein (SOV), the facial and angular veins, the pterygoid plexus, the superior petrosal sinus, the refluxing cortical veins, or direct surgical puncture of the cavernous sinus.[34] The goal of transvenous embolization is to occlude the venous side of the lesion. This is usually achieved by placing coils into the cavernous sinus. Obliteration of the venous side of the lesion can result in the total disappearance of the fistula.[28] However, in some cases of successful treatment, thrombosis may extend into the orbital veins, and this may lead to venous hypertension and paradoxical visual deterioration.[7] This may require treatment with oral corticosteroids, antiplatelet therapy, or anticoagulation.

If endovascular therapy fails, surgery is indicated in cases with persistent CVR or when vision is at risk. The role of surgery in the treatment of cavernous sinus DAVFs is mainly in providing venous access to the cavernous sinus in cases in which access through the femoral route is not possible. Several options are available, including cannulation of the SOV, cannulation of refluxing intracranial veins such as the sylvian veins, or direct exposure of the cavernous sinus.[34]

The SOV approach is often performed by a team consisting of an ophthalmologist, a neurosurgeon, and a neuroradiologist.[55] The procedure is performed under general anesthesia and under fluoroscopic guidance. A sheath is placed in a common femoral artery to allow intraoperative angiography. The skin incision is made in the nasal part of the superior sulcus of the upper eyelid, under magnification provided by an operating microscope.[55] The incision is carried down through the orbicularis oculi muscle. The orbital septum is then opened, exposing the retroseptal orbital fat. The SOV is then identified and cleaned of the surrounding orbital fat to expose a segment of vein 5 to 20 mm in length. Two ligatures (2-0 silk suture) are placed around the vein approximately 1 cm apart. A sheath is then inserted into the vein between the ligatures, and thrombogenic material (such as platinum coils) is injected into the cavernous sinus under fluoroscopy. At the end of the procedure, an intraoperative angiogram is performed through the femoral sheath to ensure complete closure of the fistula. The SOV sheath is then removed, the vein is suture ligated, and the lid incision is closed. Alternatives to surgical exposure of the SOV have been reported and include direct percutaneous puncture of the SOV under angiographic guidance, direct percutaneous puncture of the facial vein under sonographic guidance, and transvenous transfemoral access to the facial vein.[34,35] In cases in which the facial vein is catheterized, the catheter is advanced into the angular vein, then into the SOV, and finally into the cavernous sinus.

In rare instances, a cavernous sinus DAVF may only drain by retrograde flow into cortical veins, and there may be no access through the IPSs, the ophthalmic veins, or the pterygoid plexus. In such cases, access to the cavernous sinus may be achieved via the refluxing cortical vein (e.g., a refluxing sylvian vein). This has been described using the percutaneous transfemoral technique and also by surgical exposure of the cortical vein.[34]

Direct microsurgery of cavernous sinus DAVFs has also been described,[9,56-58] but with advances in endovascular embolization, these techniques are rarely required. These procedures require surgical experience and detailed knowledge of the anatomy of the cavernous sinus. The cavernous sinus is approached through triangles that are formed by convergence and divergence of the cranial nerves in the region of the cavernous sinus and the middle fossa.[25] The selection of approach is determined by the pattern of venous drainage of the fistula, and the degree of familiarity of the surgeon. The two main approaches used are described below.

The anteroinferior extradural approach to the cavernous sinus is suitable for anteriorly draining fistulas and is performed through a standard pterional craniotomy. After administration of intravenous mannitol, the dura is reflected away from the anterior and anteromedial walls of the middle fossa to expose the lateral wall of the cavernous sinus. The posterior aspect of the orbital roof is then drilled all the way to the lateral aspect of the anterior clinoid process. The superior orbital fissure region is exposed, the periorbita is opened, and the cranial nerves are identified. The superior or inferior orbital vein is then identified. An intraoperative Doppler probe may be used to localize the high arterial flow in these veins.[58] An atraumatic intravenous cannula is then inserted into the vein, and a guidewire is directed posteriorly into the cavernous sinus. A catheter is then introduced over the guidewire into the cavernous sinus and used to introduce thrombogenic material such as coils to obliterate the fistula. An intraoperative angiogram is performed to confirm adequate obliteration of the sinus. It must be noted that it may be difficult to identify the ophthalmic veins in a low-flow fistula.[9]

The posterosuperior approach is appropriate for posteriorly draining fistulas. It is performed through a pterional craniotomy. After opening the dura, the sylvian fissure is split widely to allow gentle retraction of the frontal and temporal lobes. The oculomotor nerve is then identified as a landmark. Underneath the oculomotor nerve, the superior petrosal sinus is identified and followed proximally to its origin from the cavernous sinus. Thrombogenic material is injected through the superior petrosal sinus into the cavernous sinus.[9] If the superior petrosal sinus cannot be identified, the cavernous sinus can be packed through Parkinson's triangle, bounded by the lower margin of the trochlear nerve,

the upper margin of the ophthalmic division of trigeminal nerve, and a line connecting the point of entry of trochlear nerve into the dura to the point of entry of trigeminal nerve into Meckel's cave.[25] An intraoperative angiogram is performed to confirm complete occlusion of the fistula. The dura is closed as usual, the bone flap is repositioned, and the temporalis muscle, galea, and skin are closed in layers. Combined and more extensive approaches to the cavernous sinus, with opening and packing of all triangles, have been described but are rarely necessary.[56]

ANTERIOR CRANIAL FOSSA DURAL ARTERIOVENOUS FISTULAS

The arterial supply to the anterior cranial fossa dura is derived mainly from the ICA through the ophthalmic artery, which gives off the anterior and posterior ethmoidal arteries within the orbit. The ethmoidal arteries leave the orbit to enter the ethmoidal air cells. The smaller of the two, the posterior ethmoidal artery, supplies the dura in the region of planum sphenoidale. The anterior ethmoidal artery gives origin to the falcine artery and supplies the dura of the medial and inferior portions of the anterior cranial fossa. As well as supply from the ethmoidal arteries, DAVFs in this region may also recruit dural arterial supply via the anterior division of the middle meningeal arteries from both dural convexities and transcranial arterial supply via engorged scalp arteries.[28] The venous drainage of anterior cranial fossa DAVFs is always via cortical venous drainage through the frontal and olfactory veins.[4,7] The cortical veins may often be variceal. This constant presence of CVR explains the high incidence of aggressive clinical behavior for lesions in this location. They must therefore be treated aggressively to eliminate CVR. Anterior fossa DAVFs are rarely cured by endovascular means. Transarterial embolization is usually limited to ECA branches. Embolization of ophthalmic artery branches is usually avoided as it carries the risk of central retinal artery occlusion and visual compromise.[59] Transvenous embolization has been described in case reports[60] but is not possible for most lesions in this location due to lack of venous access. Surgery is associated with high cure rates and low complication rates and is the treatment of choice for most anterior fossa DAVFs.[59] This is performed through a low unilateral frontal craniotomy in the supine position with minimal retraction of the frontal lobes. A unilateral craniotomy allows disconnection of leptomeningeal veins on both sides via the transfalcine route. Alternatively, a bifrontal craniotomy may be performed. The next step is to disconnect the arterialized leptomeningeal veins, which should be coagulated and divided. Excision of the dura involved with the fistula is not necessary.[59]

SUPERIOR SAGITTAL SINUS (CONVEXITY) DURAL ARTERIOVENOUS FISTULAS

The arterial supply to these lesions is from the middle meningeal arteries. The venous drainage may be into the superior sagittal sinus, into cortical veins, or both. If CVR exists, the lesion must be treated to prevent future hemorrhage or neurologic deficit. Few cases of successful curative endovascular treatment have been reported.[8,61] Surgical treatment is therefore required in most cases and involves disconnection of CVR. The lesion is usually approached through a unilateral craniotomy on the side of the fistula.

Preoperative transarterial embolization is used to reduce the amount of hemorrhage from scalp and dura.

In some cases without CVR, there may be a high-flow fistula that shunts into a patent superior sagittal sinus. These lesions may be associated with papilledema.[28] These cases may be managed with extensive transarterial embolization or surgical skeletonization of the superior sagittal sinus to reduce the flow through the fistula. Other options include the use of lumboperitoneal shunting or optic nerve sheath decompression for treatment of papilledema.[28]

DEEP-SEATED AND POSTERIOR FOSSA DURAL ARTERIOVENOUS FISTULAS

This group consists of lesions associated with the deep veins (tentorial incisura), superior petrosal sinus, IPS, or the marginal sinus (foramen magnum). As with DAVFs in other locations, deep-seated and posterior fossa lesions without CVR can be observed or treated palliatively by transarterial embolization of the arterial feeders. Lesions with CVR should be treated aggressively until all CVR is disconnected. This may be achieved by endovascular or surgical means.[42,43,52] Extensive resection of the nidus, which was performed in the past, often requires complex skull base approaches, carries significant risk of morbidity, and is unnecessary. If endovascular treatment fails to eliminate CVR, surgical disconnection can be performed with relatively little risk to the patient.[42,43]

DEEP VENOUS (TENTORIAL INCISURA) DURAL ARTERIOVENOUS FISTULAS

These lesions are located at the tentorial incisura and involve the deep venous system. They may extend along the straight sinus to involve the falx. Their arterial supply may be bilateral and is derived from the tentorial dural branches of the ECA, ICA, and vertebral and posterior cerebral arteries. Angiography may reveal hypertrophy of embryonic dural arteries, including the artery of Bernasconi and Cassinari (tentorial branch of the meningohypophyseal trunk of the ICA) and the artery of Davidoff and Schecter (dural branch of the posterior cerebral artery).[28] Venous drainage is almost always leptomeningeal and involves the basal vein of Rosenthal, the lateral mesencephalic veins, and the vein of Galen.[7,8] Fistulas at this location may have infra- or supratentorial cortical venous drainage or drainage into spinal medullary veins.[42] The presence of CVR explains the high incidence of ICH and neurologic deficit with these lesions. Drainage into the spinal medullary veins may be associated with progressive quadriparesis.[62] Surgical exposure of these lesions may be performed using a posterior parasagittal craniotomy and interhemispheric approach with the trajectory posterior to the splenium of the corpus callosum.[63] Surgical treatment consists of CVR disconnection.

SUPERIOR PETROSAL SINUS DURAL ARTERIOVENOUS FISTULAS

These lesions are often included in the same group as the deep venous DAVFs and together are referred to as tentorial DAVFs. Other authors have grouped them separately because they are located at the petrous ridge and involve the superior petrosal sinus.[8,52] The arterial supply is from dural branches of the ECA, ICA, and the vertebrobasilar system. Most cases are associated with thrombosis of the

superior petrosal sinus on either side of the fistula site, with venous drainage diverted into cortical veins.[8,52] ICH is the most common mode of presentation. In a series of 18 patients reported by Ng and colleagues,[52] 17 (94%) had CVR and 9 (50%) presented with ICH. Ocular symptoms may occur if there is venous reflux into the cavernous sinus and the SOV. Trigeminal neuralgia may occur secondary to irritation of the trigeminal ganglion in Meckel's cave by dilated tortuous feeding arteries or compression of the trigeminal nerve at the root entry zone by a dilated petrosal vein. Surgical excision of this type of DAVF may require an extensive skull base approach consisting of subtemporal craniotomy, posterior petrosectomy, and suboccipital craniotomy.[63] These extensive procedures are usually unnecessary, and treatment should focus on disconnection of CVR only.

INFERIOR PETROSAL SINUS DURAL ARTERIOVENOUS FISTULAS

The main arterial supply to these lesions is usually from the dural and muscular branches of the vertebral arteries and dural branches from the ascending pharyngeal, middle meningeal, and occipital branches of the ECA. Venous drainage may be retrograde up the IPS and into the cavernous sinus. This may result in presentation with ocular symptoms similar to those of cavernous sinus DAVFs. Alternatively, venous drainage may flow into the ipsilateral jugular bulb, resulting in pulsatile tinnitus.[8] Retrograde flow up the ipsilateral sigmoid and transverse sinuses and into the contralateral transverse/sigmoid sinuses or into the straight and superior sagittal sinuses may also occur.[63] Surgical exposure may be performed using the far lateral suboccipital approach.[63] Treatment consists of CVR disconnection.

MARGINAL SINUS (FORAMEN MAGNUM REGION) DURAL ARTERIOVENOUS FISTULAS

These lesions are rare. The marginal sinus encircles the foramen magnum and communicates with the basal venous plexus of the clivus anteriorly and with the occipital sinus posteriorly. It normally drains to the sigmoid sinus or jugular bulb through a series of small sinuses.[64] Fistulas in this area have often been grouped together with posterior fossa DAVFs or referred to as foramen magnum region DAVFs. Their arterial supply is usually from the muscular branches of the vertebral artery, the transmastoid perforators of the occipital artery, the neuromeningeal division of the ascending pharyngeal artery, and the posterior clival dural branches of the meningohypophyseal trunk of the ICA.[64] Venous drainage may be into the sigmoid sinus/jugular vein, in which case the patient may complain of pulsatile tinnitus, or into the IPS, which may lead to venous engorgement in the ipsilateral cavernous sinus and ocular symptoms.[28,64] CVR may lead to ICH, and reflux into the spinal medullary veins may result in progressive myelopathy and quadriparesis.[65] These lesions are surgically approached through a posterior paramedian craniocervical exposure, with the patient in the semiprone position. The venous plexus surrounding the vertebral artery may be arterialized and require meticulous hemostasis during exposure. Suboccipital craniotomy and laminectomy at the appropriate levels are then performed. The dura is extensively coagulated and opened. Refluxing leptomeningeal veins communicate with arterialized tortuous posterior and/or anterior medullary veins. The refluxing leptomeningeal veins are coagulated or clipped and divided, whereas the anterior and posterior medullary veins should be left intact.

Outcome and Complications of Treatment

Between 1984 and 2001, 236 cranial DAVFs have been managed by the University of Toronto Brain Vascular Malformation Study Group. Of these, 117 did not have CVR (Borden type I and Cognard types I and IIa) and were managed by observation alone or by palliative treatment. Of these patients, 98% had a benign clinical course.[3] The other 119 patients had DAVFs with CVR (Borden types II and III, and Cognard type IIb, IIa + b, III, or IV). Three patients were lost to follow-up after initial assessment, and 14 patients declined treatment. The remaining 102 patients were treated.[43] Forty-seven patients (46.1%) were treated by disconnection of CVR, 49 (48%) had complete obliteration of the fistula, and 6 (5.9%) were partially treated. The six partially treated patients had persistent CVR but refused or were physically unable to undergo further treatment. Therefore, complete obliteration of the fistula or CVR disconnection was achieved in 94.1% of patients. This was achieved by endovascular treatment alone in 26 patients (25.5%), by surgery alone in 25 patients (24.5%), and by a combination of endovascular and surgical treatments in 45 patients (44%). Multiple treatment sessions were required in some patients, resulting in 120 endovascular and 74 surgical procedures. The complications of treatment were all transient and are outlined in Table 80-5. No deaths or permanent neurologic deficits occurred in this series. The mean follow-up period was 3.7 years (741 patient-years). Control angiography was performed in 93 patients (91.2%). CVR disconnection was equally effective in lowering the risk of aggressive events as total obliteration of the fistula.[43]

Summary

The clinical presentation and natural history of DAVFs are determined by their pattern of venous drainage. Lesions without CVR behave in a benign fashion and do not require curative treatment. Lesions with CVR have a 15% annual adverse event rate (ICH and NHND) and a 10% annual mortality rate and should be managed aggressively with the aim of eliminating all refluxing cortical veins. Treatment of DAVFs should be performed in a multidisciplinary setting and may consist of transarterial embolization, transvenous embolization, surgery, or a combination of these. Endovascular treatment should be tried first. If surgery is indicated, CVR disconnection is effective in eliminating the risk of future aggressive clinical events and carries less morbidity compared with complete excision of the lesion. All patients should be followed up for life, and any change in symptoms (deterioration or improvement) should be investigated with repeat cerebral angiography to look for development of CVR.

KEY REFERENCES

Al-Shahi R, Bhattacharya JJ, Currie DG, et al. Prospective, population-based detection of intracranial vascular malformations in adults: the Scottish Intracranial Vascular Malformation Study (SIVMS). *Stroke.* 2003;34:1163-1169.

Aminoff MJ. Vascular anomalies in the intracranial dura mater. *Brain.* 1973;96:601-612.

Awad IA, Little JR, Akarawi WP, et al. Intracranial dural arteriovenous malformations: factors predisposing to an aggressive neurological course. *J Neurosurg.* 1990;2:839-850.

Barrow DL, Spector RH, Braun IF, et al. Classification and treatment of spontaneous carotid-cavernous sinus fistulas. *J Neurosurg.* 1985;62:248-256.

Borden JA, Wu JK, Shucart WA. A proposed classification for spinal and cranial dural arteriovenous fistulous malformations and implications for treatment. *J Neurosurg.* 1995;82:166-179.

Cognard C, Gobin YP, Pierot L, et al. Cerebral dural arteriovenous fistulas: clinical and angiographic correlation with a revised classification of venous drainage. *Radiology.* 1995;194:671-680.

Davies MA, TerBrugge K, Willinsky R, et al. The validity of classification for the clinical presentation of intracranial dural arteriovenous fistulas. *J Neurosurg.* 1996;85:830-837.

Djindjian R, Merland JJ, Theron J. *Superselective Arteriography of the External Carotid Artery.* New York: Springer-Verlag; 1977.

Hamada Y, Goto K, Inoue T, et al. Histopathological aspects of dural arteriovenous fistulas in the transverse-sigmoid sinus region in nine patients. *Neurosurgery.* 1997;40:452-458.

Herman JM, Spetzler RF, Bederson JB, et al. Genesis of a dural arteriovenous malformation in a rat model. *J Neurosurg.* 1995;83:539-545.

Lalwani AK, Dowd CF, Halbach VV. Grading venous restrictive disease in patients with dural arteriovenous fistulas of the transverse/sigmoid sinus. *J Neurosurg.* 1993;79:11-15.

Lasjaunias P, Chiu M, ter Brugge K, et al. Neurological manifestations of intracranial dural arteriovenous malformations. *J Neurosurg.* 1986;64:724-730.

Lawton MT, Jacobowitz R, Spetzler RF. Redefined role of angiogenesis in the pathogenesis of dural arteriovenous malformations. *J Neurosurg.* 1997;87:267-274.

Luciani A, Houdart E, Mounayer C, et al. Spontaneous closure of dural arteriovenous fistulas: report of three cases and review of the literature. *AJNR Am J Neuroradiol.* 2001;22:992-996.

Malek AM, Halbach VV, Higashida RT, et al. Treatment of dural arteriovenous malformations and fistulas. *Neurosurg Clin North Am.* 2000;11:147-166.

Malik GM, Pearce JE, Ausman JI, et al. Dural arteriovenous malformations and intracranial hemorrhage. *Neurosurgery.* 1984;15:332-339.

Mullan S. Treatment of carotid-cavernous fistulas by cavernous sinus occlusion. *J Neurosurg.* 1979;50:131-144.

Rhoton Jr AL. The cavernous sinus, the cavernous venous plexus, and the carotid collar. *Neurosurgery.* 2002;51:S375-S410.

Sarma D, ter Brugge K. Management of intracranial dural arteriovenous shunts in adults. *Eur J Radiol.* 2003;46:206-220.

Table 80-5	Complications of Treatment in 102 Patients with Cranial Dural Arteriovenous Fistulas with Cortical Venous Reflux	
Complication	**Surgery (74 Procedures)**	**Endovascular Embolization (120 Procedures)**
Significant blood loss	8	0
Memory dysfunction	1	1
Seizures	1	0
Cranial nerve deficit	1	0
Hemorrhage	1	0
Meningitis	1	0
Embolic transient ischemic attack	0	1
Groin hematoma	0	1

From Van Dijk JM, Ter Brugge KG, Willinsky RA, Wallace MC. Selective disconnection of cortical venous reflux as treatment for cranial dural arteriovenous fistulas. J Neurosurg. 2004;101:31-35.

Satomi J, van Dijk JM, Terbrugge KG, et al. Benign cranial dural arterio-venous fistulas: outcome of conservative management based on the natural history of the lesion. *J Neurosurg.* 2002;97:767-770.

Terada T, Higashida RT, Halbach VV, et al. Development of acquired arteriovenous fistulas in rats due to venous hypertension. *J Neurosurg.* 1994;80:884-889.

Terada T, Tsuura M, Komai N, et al. The role of angiogenic factor bFGF in the development of dural AVFs. *Acta Neurochir (Wien).* 1996;138:877-883.

Uranishi R, Nakase H, Sakaki T. Expression of angiogenic growth factors in dural arteriovenous fistula. *J Neurosurg.* 1999;91:781-786.

van Dijk JM, terBrugge KG, Willinsky RA, et al. Clinical course of cranial dural arteriovenous fistulas with long-term persistent cortical venous reflux. *Stroke.* 2002;33:1233-1236.

van Dijk JM, Willinsky RA. Venous congestive encephalopathy related to cranial dural arteriovenous fistulas. *Neuroimaging Clin North Am.* 2003;13:55-72.

Numbered references appear on Expert Consult.

CHAPTER 81

Surgical Management Of Cavernous Malformations Of The Nervous System

ANOOP P. PATEL • SEPIDEH AMIN-HANJANI • CHRISTOPHER S. OGILVY

Cavernous malformations (CMs) have long been recognized as one of the major clinicopathologic categories of vascular malformations of the nervous system.[1-3] Because no abnormal vascularity is seen on angiography, CMs have been included in the descriptions of *cryptic* or *occult vascular malformations*, a term that has been used to describe any vascular malformation that cannot be seen on angiography.[4-9] The term *cavernous angioma* was used by Russell and Rubinstein[3] in their excellent description of the pathology of these lesions. CMs have also been called *cavernous hemangiomas* or *cavernomas*, but the term *cavernous malformation* has become more widely accepted, explicitly distinguishing these lesions from true vascular neoplasms as suggested by the term *angioma*.

Before computed tomography (CT), the diagnosis of CMs was rarely made before operation or autopsy. CT suggested the diagnosis in some patients; however, when high-field magnetic resonance imaging (MRI) became available, a picture characteristic of CMs was defined, allowing the diagnosis to be established in many cases. Furthermore, the advances in imaging not only have improved diagnosis of symptomatic lesions but also have resulted in increasing reports of incidental CMs.

The management of patients with CMs usually includes a consideration of surgical treatment or of observation. Rarely, radiosurgery is considered, but high complication rates and poor definition of end points for therapy have discouraged the use of this technique. With emerging knowledge of the natural history of CMs, the indications and guidelines for management decisions continue to evolve. This chapter reviews the surgical management of 121 cases of CMs that we saw at the Massachusetts General Hospital (MGH). From this information and from a review of the literature, recommendations are made for treating patients with this disorder.

Pathologic Features

CMs can occur throughout the brain or spinal cord parenchyma, as well as on cranial and spinal nerves.[10,11] The lesions, which may be multiple, can range in size from a few millimeters to several centimeters. Often, an associated venous malformation of the brain may be present; rarely, similar lesions may be found in other parts of the body.[3,12]

How a CM develops is unknown. In some patients, the lesions are clearly acquired, appearing in areas of brain that were normal on prior MRI studies.[9] These include patients with familial lesions and those in whom the CM has developed in an area of previously irradiated brain tissue or even developed sporadically.[13-17] Wilson[9] has proposed a possible pathogenesis for the development of acquired lesions.

The lesion is well defined and usually has a lobulated appearance. There is often a characteristic gross appearance that has been likened to a mulberry, characterized by a dark red or purple color. Inside the lesion is a honeycomb of thin-walled vascular spaces.[2] Small hemorrhages adjacent to or within the lesion may occur, but large hemorrhages are rare. A variable number of small blood vessels enter the lesion. Gliotic tissue surrounds the mass, and it is usually stained yellow. In some patients, the lesion may gradually enlarge as a result of small hemorrhages, progressive hyalinization, thickening of the vascular walls, or gradual thrombosis.[11,18]

Irregular sinusoidal spaces are visible on microscopic examination and many contain areas of thrombosis and organization with thin walls devoid of elastic tissue and muscle. These walls consist of a single layer of endothelium with varying amounts of extraluminal connective tissue. No intervening or neural tissue is present except that at the periphery, which is a layer of gliotic tissue that contains hemosiderin-packed macrophages adjacent to the lesion. There also may be seen hematomas of varying ages, extensive calcification, and on the surface, collections of capillaries.

Radiologic Features

High-quality CT scans suggest the diagnosis of CM in some patients. The characteristic findings are a roughly circular or irregularly shaped lesion located in the brain parenchyma; this lesion shows high density on the noncontrast scan and slight or no contrast enhancement. In some patients, extensive calcification is noted. Other types of occult vascular malformations, and some tumors associated with hemorrhage, also have the same CT appearance.

MRI accurately establishes the diagnosis in most cases and often is the only study needed. The criteria for MRI diagnosis is a well-circumscribed lesion with a combination of a reticulated or mottled core of mixed signal intensity and

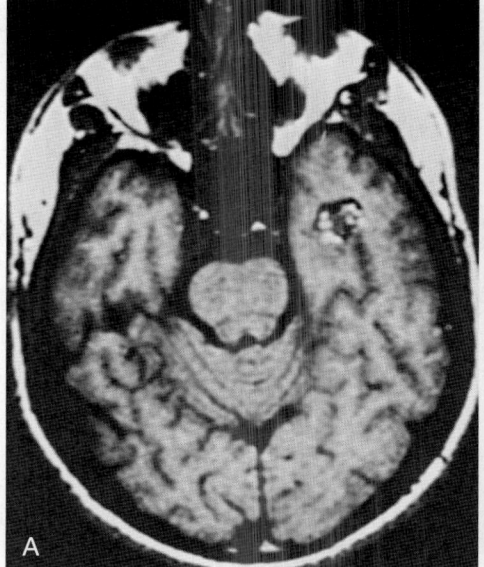
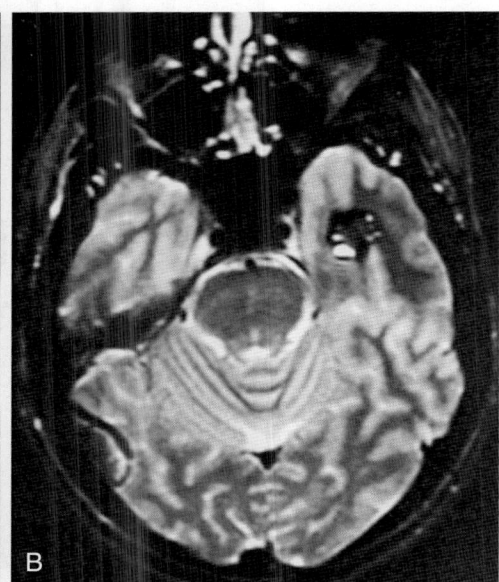

FIGURE 81-1 Temporal CM in a 34-year-old man presenting with a seizure. Removal of the lesion was followed by a normal recovery. Axial T1-weighted (A) and T2-weighted (B) MRI showed a well-circumscribed lesion in the left temporal lobe with a mottled core of mixed signal intensity and a surrounding rim of decreased signal intensity.

a prominent surrounding rim of decreased signal intensity (Fig. 81-1).[19] Hemorrhages of different ages may be seen within or around the lesion, and an associated venous anomaly may be seen. On T2-weighted images, an increased signal may be present in the adjacent brain as a result of edema. Usually little or no enhancement follows the administration of gadolinium. Although appearance on MRI has a high correlation with the diagnosis of CM, occasionally an occult arteriovenous malformation or a tumor can have a similar appearance.[9,20,21] Significant enhancement suggests the possibility of a tumor. Advances in MRI techniques have resulted in the use of susceptibility-weighted imaging as the gold standard for diagnosis of CMs. Head-to-head comparisons of susceptibility weighted imaging (SWI) against T2 gradient echo and other T2-weighted sequences have shown a significantly higher sensitivity for relatively small lesions that would have classically been considered occult.[22] This is particularly relevant in familial cases where multiple CMs are present and for locating otherwise-cryptogenic seizure foci in these patients.

The angiographic results are almost always normal because the lesion has small blood vessels with low flow and no hypertrophied feeding arteries or early draining veins. Rarely, an avascular mass or capillary blush can be identified.[19,23] Since the development of MRI, angiography is rarely indicated. Occasionally, angiography is needed to obtain information regarding the vascular anatomy to help plan a surgical approach. If the MRI scan suggests an association with another vascular malformation, or if the diagnosis is in doubt, angiography should be done.

Familial Occurrence and Genetics

CMs are known to be present in both sporadic and familial forms.[17,24,25] The familial form of the disease affects up to 30% to 50% of patients harboring a CM[19,24] and seems most common among Hispanic Americans.[17] Studies have shown that familial CMs are more prevalent than previously believed, and there is a greater incidence of multiple lesions (Fig. 81-2).[17] Rigamonti et al.[25] estimated a 73% familial incidence of multiple CMs of the brain, compared with a 10% to 15% incidence in the sporadic form. Further reports have indicated that familial CMs can be found in diverse ethnic groups, including the Japanese and French.[26,27] Familial and sporadic forms of the disease appear to be similar clinically[28]; however, as many as 75% of patients who present with multiple CMs likely harbor the hereditary form of the disease.[26]

An autosomal dominant pattern of inheritance with variable penetrance was first described in a 122-member Hispanic lineage, of whom 5 harbored symptomatic lesions.[24] This autosomal pattern of inheritance was confirmed by a subsequent description of 6 unrelated Hispanic families.[17] Subsequent study of other families utilizing MRI to detect silent lesions revealed a more complete expression than previously suspected.[26] The location of the responsible gene was mapped to the long arm of chromosome 7, to a locus named cerebral cavernous malformation 1 (CCM1).[29,30] CCM1 locus homogeneity was identified in an analysis of 14 Hispanic families with CMs[31] but did not extend to kindreds of different ethnicity. Investigation of 20 non-Hispanic Caucasian families revealed linkage to two additional loci: CCM2 at chromosome 7p and CCM3 at chromosome 3q.[32] The clinical, radiographic, and pathologic characteristics of the disease in kindreds mapping to these other loci does not appear to differ from those seen in kindreds mapping to the CCM1 locus. Linkage to one of these three loci (i.e., 7q, 7p, or 3q) accounted for inheritance in all 20 Caucasian kindreds studied. CCM1 was considered to be the locus involved in only 40% of non-Hispanic kindreds, with the remaining lineages linked to CCM2 (20%) or CCM3 (40%).[32] Subsequent analysis of further kindreds seems to confirm that about 40% of familial CMs are attributable to CCM1 mutations.[33] The discovery of genetic heterogeneity in familial CMs has important implications both for the ability to provide reliable genetic testing in presymptomatic diagnosis and for understanding the pathogenesis of the disease. It has been suggested that there may be locus-specific differences in the penetrance of the disease, although such differences may also be attributable to the particular mutation involved.[32]

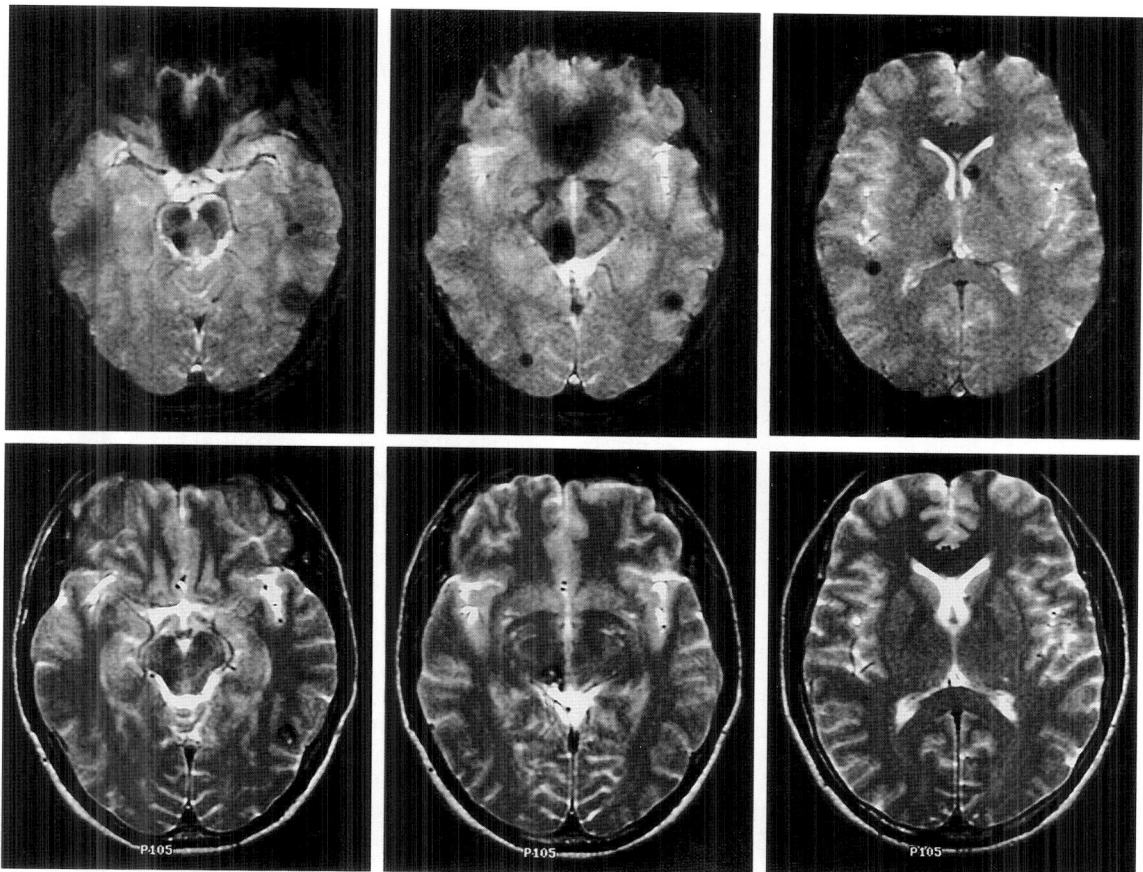

FIGURE 81-2 MRI in a middle-aged man with a family history of CMs who presented with seizures. T2-weighted images *(bottom panel)* revealed well-circumscribed lesions with a reticulated or mottled core of mixed signal intensity, typical for CMs. Susceptibility MRI *(top panel)* demonstrates further lesions showing the multiplicity of CMs. *(From Amin-Hanjani S. The genetics of cerebrovascular malformations. Seminars in Cerebrovascular Diseases and Stroke 2(1):73-81, 2002.)*

Given that the clinical phenotypes of mutations at all three loci are essentially identical, the presumption is that the involved proteins likely converge on a conserved pathway that is required for the regulation of endothelial development. This has been borne out in a series of detailed molecular studies aimed at identifying the molecular pathogenesis of the disease. The responsible gene associated with CCM1, at the chromosome 7q locus, has been identified as human Krev interaction trapped 1 (KRIT1). Mutations in KRIT1 were first identified in a study of 57 French kindreds with CMs; 12 different mutations were discovered.[34] Further KRIT1 mutations have been described in families of different ethnicities.[35,36] Although the exact function of KRIT1 remains unknown, its interaction with Krev/rap 1a (a ras family guanosine triphosphatase) and with integrin cytoplasmic domain-associated protein-1 alpha and evidence that KRIT1 is a microtubule-associated protein suggest a role in endothelial cell matrix interactions that in turn could play a role in abnormal vascular development.[37] Gene products associated with CCM2 have been recently reported as proteins with potential involvement in integrin signaling encoded by the gene MGC4607 (malcavernin, osmosensing scaffold for MEKK3).[38,39] Subsequent molecular studies have identified this gene as a key regulator of the Rho family of guanosine triphosphatases involved in

endothelial proliferation and migration through effects on microtubule stability and expression of cell adhesion molecules.[40] The most recent breakthrough was the identification of the gene product of the CCM3 locus, a protein known as programmed cell death 10 (PDC10).[41,42] While the exact mechanism has not been worked out, preliminary studies have shown that the CCM3 gene functions in the same Rho signaling pathway as its family members.[43] In a striking example of how the study of human disease has resulted in the advancement of our understanding of cellular biology, investigations into the CCM proteins have uncovered a signaling pathway that is fundamental to vascular biology.

Based on the identified genetic abnormalities, it could be proposed that familial CMs result from inherited mutations and that sporadic CMs result from either a germline mutation in an individual or a somatic mutation in a single cell. There are reports both for de novo germline mutations[44] and for somatic cell mutations in KRIT1 leading to sporadic CMs.[45] Support for the notion of somatic mutations may be found in the development of CMs following radiation therapy, where cerebral lesions have been described within the irradiated field and were not present prior to treatment.[14] The possibility of radiation-induced mutagenesis resulting in CM formation is one explanation for this observation.

Clinical Presentation

In 1976, Voigt and Yasargil[46] analyzed 163 cases reported up to 1974. They found that these lesions occurred in every age group and that the gender incidence was equal. In 1988, Simard et al.[47] reviewed 126 cases published since 1960 and added 12 of their own. The male-to-female ratio was 0.9:1, and the ages ranged from neonate to 75 years. In 1991, two publications were based on the analysis of consecutive MRI scans performed over several years.[48,49] In the report by Robinson et al.[48] of 66 patients, the male-to-female ratio was 1.2:1, and the ages ranged from 4 months to 84 years (mean 34.6 years). In the report of 32 patients by Curling et al.,[49] the male-to-female ratio was 1.1:1, the ages ranged from 16 to 72 years (mean 37.6 years), and multiple lesions were present in 6 patients (19%). Scott et al.[50] reported a series of 19 children ranging in age from 7 months to 17 years. In the MGH series of 116 patients, the ages ranged from 4 to 69 years (mean 35.5 years), with a male-to-female ratio of 1:1.2. Multiple lesions were present in 12 patients (10.3%) in this series, and associated venous malformations were present in 9 patients (7.8%).

Most CMs that come to attention are supratentorial in location[46]; the distribution of CMs within the central nervous system seems to reflect the volume of tissue, without specific predilection for any particular location. The locations of the 121 operated CMs in our series of 116 patients are listed in Table 81-1.

The four general categories of clinical presentation are seizures, headache, neurologic deficit, and asymptomatic presentation.[46-49] Seizure is the most common presenting symptom, affecting 35% to 55% of patients.[25,47-49,51,52] In many patients, more than one symptom is present. Within each of the symptomatic categories, some patients have had a hemorrhage into the adjacent brain parenchyma. The hemorrhages are usually small but on rare occasion can be large, with the patient having rapid deterioration.

In some patients, the CM gradually enlarges, and the lesion can act as a mass that causes a progressive neurologic deficit. The clinical symptoms arising from the 121 CMs in the MGH surgical series are presented in Table 81-2; among the intracranial lesions, seizures were the presenting symptom in 45%, followed by neurologic deficits (38%) and headaches (17%).

Natural History

In 1985, Wilkins[8] reviewed the natural history of vascular malformations. He concluded that not enough information was present in the literature to describe the natural history of cavernous angiomas. In 1991, two reports of CMs diagnosed in large consecutive series of MRI scans gave some information about the short-term natural history,[48,49] and data from familial cases have contributed to our knowledge.[17]

Most hemorrhages are noncatastrophic, but there are occasional exceptions. Zimmerman et al.[53] reported one patient who died from rehemorrhage of a tectal CM. There are consequences, however, even of repeated small hemorrhages.

Progressive deterioration with successive hemorrhages has been described,[6] and Robinson et al.[54] found a strong association between hemorrhage and neurologic disability in patients with CMs. Knowledge regarding the long-term risk of hemorrhage is of importance in management decisions, especially for CMs presenting incidentally or with minimal symptoms.

Overall, available estimates of the risks of initial hemorrhage from CMs have indicated low hemorrhage rates. In a retrospective study, Curling et al.[49] reported a 0.25% per person-year and 0.1% per lesion-year hemorrhage rate among 32 patients with 76 lesions. Robinson et al.[48] followed 57 symptomatic patients with 66 lesions for a mean of 26 months and observed only 1 hemorrhage in 143 lesion-years, resulting in a 0.7% per lesion-year hemorrhage rate. Porter et al.[52] reported a 1.6% per person-year hemorrhage rate among 110 patients followed for a mean of 46 months. For 68 prospectively followed patients, Moriarity et al. reported an overall 3.1% per person-year hemorrhage rate.[55] The risk of bleeding may be higher in deep or brain

Table 81-1   Location of CMs

Location	CMs	Percentage of Total CMs
Cerebrum	84	69.4
Frontal	36	
Parietal	16	
Temporal	28	
Occipital	4	
Brain stem	17	14.0
Mesencephalon	2	
Pontomesencephalon	4	
Pons	8	
Pontomedullary	2	
Medulla	1	
Cerebellum	8	6.6
Cranial nerves	4	3.3
Spinal cord	8	6.6
Cervicomedullary	2	
Cervical	3	
Thoracic	2	
Lumbar	1	
Total CMs	121	99.9

Table 81-2   Presenting Symptoms of CMs

Location	CMs	Presenting Symptoms	CMs by Presenting Symptom	Overt Hemorrhage*
Cerebrum	84	Seizure	51	28 (54.9%)
		Neurologic deficit	15	13 (86.6%)
		Headache	18	16 (88.9%)
Brain stem	17	Neurologic deficit	17	12 (70.6%)
Cerebellum	8	Neurologic deficit	7	7 (100%)
		Headache	1	0 (0%)
Cranial nerves	4	Neurologic deficit	4	1 (25%)
Spinal cord	8	Neurologic deficit	8	6 (75%)

*Percentage of patients with a particular clinical presentation who experienced overt hemorrhage.

stem CMs.[52] In their cohort of 110 prospectively followed patients, Porter et al.[52] found a 10-fold higher hemorrhage rate among infratentorial lesions at 3.8% per year compared with supratentorial lesions at 0.4% per year. This may reflect the eloquence of the surrounding tissue, with even small brain stem hemorrhages being more likely than lesions to be clinically manifest in the cerebral hemispheres.

The risk of hemorrhage in familial CMs appears to be similar to that in nonfamilial CMs, when considering the increased frequency of lesion multiplicity. In their follow-up of six families with familial CMs, Zabramski et al.[17] found a 1.1% per lesion-year (6.5% per person-year) rate of bleeding over a follow-up period of 26 months. In 40 patients with familial CMs, Labauge et al. reported a 2.5% per lesion-year hemorrhage risk.[56]

Several reports suggest a higher risk of bleeding after a first hemorrhage. Kondziolka et al.[57] followed 122 patients for 34 months and noted a low 0.6% per person-year hemorrhage rate among those without history of prior hemorrhage but a higher 4.5% per person-year rate among those with a previous hemorrhage. Kim et al. also reported a slightly higher recurrent hemorrhage rate of 3.8% per person-year compared with 2.3% per person-year for first hemorrhage.[58] For brain stem lesions, Kupersmith et al. reported a bleeding rate of 2.5% per person-year, with a rebleeding rate of 5.1% per person-year.[59] Tung et al.[6] reported recurrent hemorrhage occurring in 7 patients whose diagnosis of CM was confirmed at surgery. The median interval from the initial hemorrhage to the recurrent hemorrhage was 12 months, with only 2 months until a second rebleed. Aiba et al.[60] also found a much higher incidence of hemorrhage in those with prior bleeds at 22.9% per lesion-year versus 0.4% per lesion-year in those without prior bleeds. There is also evidence for temporal clustering of hemorrhages, with rates of rehemorrhage initially as high as 2% per month in a selected population but decreasing to less than 1% per month after 2 to 3 years.[61]

Information regarding the long-term risk of seizure development is scarce. Kondziolka et al.[57] reported that 4 of 94 patients without seizures developed seizures over the mean 34-month follow-up. Curling et al.[49] estimated the risk of seizure development to be 1.5% per person-year based on 32 patients. In Zabramski et al.'s[17] group of patients with familial CMs followed over a mean period of 2.2 years, 1 of 6 asymptomatic individuals developed seizures. The rate of new seizures in the 68 patients reported by Moriarity et al. was 2.4% per person-year.[55]

The natural history of familial CMs has been addressed in several reports. Zabramski et al.[17] reported six families with familial CMs; 31 patients among these families harbored CMs, 21 of whom were followed clinically and with serial imaging. A total of 128 CMs were identified radiographically in these patients. During the mean follow-up of 2.2 years, 5 lesions were found to change in size, 13 lesions showed changes in signal characteristics, and 17 new lesions were identified in 6 patients. Given the dynamic nature of the CMs, the report's authors recommended serial MRI at 12-month intervals for symptomatic individuals, in addition to screening of family members. This approach can clarify the risk of morbidity in these patients and the need for close radiographic and clinical follow-up while providing data regarding the natural history. Labauge et al.

noted 23 new lesions in 11 patients (27.5%) during follow-up of 40 patients with familial CM harboring 232 CMs over a mean follow-up of 3.2 years.[56] Nine lesions (3.9%) changed in size, and signal change was observed in 14 lesions (6%) over the same follow-up period.

De novo lesions have been described in nonfamilial cases of CMs as well. The primary risk factor identified has been radiation therapy, with reports of de novo development of CMs in the spinal cord[62] and the brain[14,15] years following irradiation. However, cases without an identifiable risk factor have also been documented.[63,64]

Little information is available about asymptomatic patients and their risks for developing symptoms. In the report by Robinson et al.,[48] four of nine asymptomatic patients developed symptoms related to the CM over a relatively short follow-up period of 6 months to 2 years (mean 18 months).

Management Considerations

Treatment for patients with CMs is based on careful comparison of the benefits and risks associated with the treatment options, usually either surgery or observation. Occasionally, radiosurgery has been used. The age and medical condition of the patient are considered in this decision. Because knowledge and experience are still in the cumulative stage, only guidelines can be offered.

OBSERVATION

Some patients with CMs should be followed conservatively. Almost all asymptomatic lesions are observed, because they can remain asymptomatic indefinitely and if a hemorrhage occurs, it is usually small and lacks a major neurologic deficit. Another group that may be observed consists of those with symptomatic lesions in a deep or critical area when the risks of surgery are judged to be significant and neither a recurrent hemorrhage nor an increasing neurologic deficit is present. Some patients with seizures or headache, in whom no hemorrhage has occurred, have been observed, but subsets of these patients are also candidates for surgery, as discussed in the following sections. The decision about which treatment is appropriate depends on a detailed evaluation of the clinical problem and on discussion with the patient.

No clear guidelines exist on how often the MRI scan should be repeated. We generally perform MRI on the patient at 6-month intervals for 2 years; then, if the lesion is stable, the scan is repeated once a year.

SURGERY

The current, well-established indications for surgical resection of CMs are recurrent hemorrhage, progressive neurologic deterioration, and intractable epilepsy, unless the location is associated with an unacceptably high surgical risk.[48,49,65] When the surgical risk is high, observation or radiosurgery should be considered. Because the risk of surgery is low for lesions in many locations, there are groups of patients (e.g., those with CMs of the cerebrum or cerebellum with a single overt hemorrhage, those with the onset of a seizure disorder, and those who are worried about the presence of the lesion) in whom surgery should be considered.[66] In children, Scott et al.[50] have a "policy to recommend surgery for patients with cavernous angiomas if the

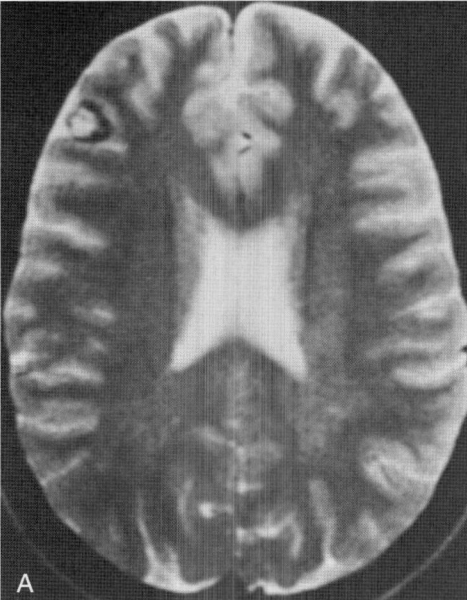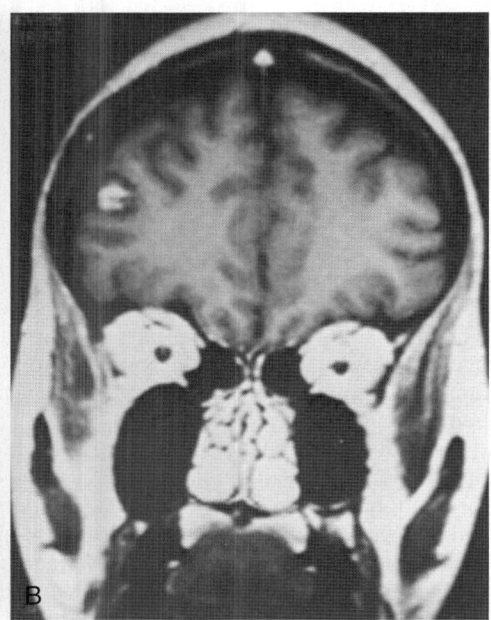

FIGURE 81-3 Frontal CM in a 34-year-old woman presenting with seizures. The seizures were controlled with medication, but she wanted to become pregnant and requested surgical excision. Removal of the lesion was followed by normal recovery. Axial T2-weighted (A) and coronal T1-weighted (B) MRI showed a superficial right frontal lesion with no parenchymal hemorrhage.

lesion is safely accessible, is currently symptomatic either by mass effect and/or hemorrhage or seizure, or shows evidence of having bled in the past."

In a special category is the young woman who wants to become pregnant (Fig. 81-3). Robinson et al.[48] noted that two of their six patients with acute hemorrhage were in the first trimester of pregnancy. They suggested that in women contemplating pregnancy, one of the indications for surgical excision was an accessible lesion. Other authors have also commented on the possible role of hormonal influences as a contributing factor.[16,60] Aiba et al.[60] reported that women predominated in the group of patients presenting with hemorrhage and that young women had a higher rate of subsequent hemorrhage.

When surgical excision of a CM is indicated, the lesion can usually be removed entirely with low morbidity. This procedure is facilitated by microsurgical dissection in the gliotic tissue that surrounds the lesion, allowing a distinct plane of cleavage to be developed through microsurgical techniques, bipolar coagulation, and the use of fine-regulated suction. When the lesion is exposed, internally decompressing the mass and retracting the capsule into the area of the decompression may help avoid pressure on the surrounding normal parenchyma. When the lesion is densely calcified, an ultrasonic surgical aspirator may be used for debulking. Bleeding is usually not a significant problem.

In some patients, splitting a cortical fissure may be possible rather than performing a full corticectomy to approach the lesion. For lesions in critical areas, cortical mapping and stimulation may be used. When removal of a CM in the deep portions of the cerebral hemispheres is indicated, the lesion is localized with stereotactic techniques and intraoperative ultrasound.[6,50,67] A comparison of microsurgical resection with or without neuronavigation demonstrated that the size of resection was significantly smaller when stereotaxy was used. While this study did not show a difference in outcome, it clearly demonstrated that neuronavigation can result in a safe, better-defined resection.[68] This is

particularly important for deeply seated lesions in the basal ganglia, thalamus, or brain stem. For brain stem lesions, special monitoring with evoked potential responses may be helpful, and arrangements for temporary cardiac pacing may be prudent.

RADIOSURGERY

Stereotactic radiosurgery has been used to treat patients with CMs thought to be inoperable and associated with progressive worsening of neurologic symptoms because of mass effect or recurrent hemorrhage. There is difficulty, however, in establishing valid end points for therapeutic success because the natural history is poorly understood, because complications can be related to either minor rebleeding or delayed radiation-induced injury, and because MRI results may not change significantly during the follow-up period.

Kondziolka et al.[69] reported on gamma knife use in the treatment of 47 patients with surgically inaccessible lesions with at least one prior hemorrhage. Over the mean follow-up of 3.6 years, they found a significant decline in the hemorrhage rate, from 32% per lesion-year pretreatment to 1.1% per lesion-year at 2 years after treatment. There was a high incidence of radiation-induced complications after treatment, with mean center doses of 32 Gy (range 20-40 Gy): 12 of the 42 patients (27%) were affected, although only 2 patients (4%) were reported to suffer permanent deficits. In a subsequent report from the same institution, 82 patients were analyzed. Again, a reduction in hemorrhage risk was reported from 33.9% to 12.3% during the first 2 years posttreatment and by 0.76% per patient-year thereafter.[70] Overall incidence of radiosurgical morbidity was 13.4%. Karlsson et al.[71] also reported experience with gamma knife, treating 22 patients with symptomatic CMs using maximum doses of 11 to 60 Gy (mean and median 33 Gy) and minimum doses of 9 to 35 Gy (mean and median 18 Gy). Over the mean follow-up of 6.5 years, they noted a decreasing trend in hemorrhages 4 years after treatment. However, they also found a high rate of morbidity, with 6 patients (27%) suffering radiation-related complications; in 5 of them (23%), these led to permanent deficits. Pollock et al. also noted a high incidence of radiation-related complications, occurring in 41% of their 17 patients with deep lesions, although hemorrhage rates did decline from 40.1% pretreatment to 2.9% more than 2 years after treatment.[72] Another series of gamma knife radiosurgery noted a reduced frequency of seizures following treatment, with 18 of 28 patients (64%) who had a chief complaint of seizure experiencing this benefit.[73]

More recent studies have shown similar results. Lunsford et al.recently published their results of a retrospective cohort of 103 patients who demonstrated propensity to bleed (more than two bleeds) and had CMs in locations deemed too risky for microsurgical resection. Their analysis again demonstrated a reduction in hemorrhage risk from 32.5% to 4.6%. Most of the risk of hemorrhage was in the first 2 years after surgery (10.8%), because the rate of hemorrhage after this initial latency period dropped to 1.06%.[74] The studies' authors commented that this latency period likely reflects the time period over which the endothelium undergoes progressive hyalinization and luminal obliteration, reminiscent of the mechanism of action on arteriovenous malformations. One report of histopathlogic analysis of a CM that was microsurgically resected 1 year after receiving 40 Gy of radiation supports this hypothesis.[75] Despite the use of a slightly lower mean dose (30.2 Gy, range 21.7-40 Gy) and confining the target volume to the hemosiderin ring as defined by high-resolution T2 images, the incidence of postradiation T2 signal change surrounding the CM was 18.4%. New neurologic deficit was noted in 13.5% of patients, though the report's authors commented that these deficits were all transient, with only 1 patient demonstrating persistent deficits.[74] Similar results were found by the same group looking at a cohort of 68 patients with hemorrhagic brain stem CMs that were also deemed surgically inaccessible.[76] Moreover, the authors bring up the point that previous studies demonstrating much higher and more permanent adverse radiation effects likely reflected treatment of CMs with associated developmental venous anomaly (DVAs), which are at intrinsically high risk for venous congestion and ischemic events if treated with stereotactic radiosurgery. As such, the authors advocate for better patient selection rather than abandonment of stereotactic radiosurgery for CMs in surgically high-risk areas.

Stereotactic charged-particle radiosurgery, both helium-ion radiosurgery and proton beam therapy, has also been used to treat cavernous angiomas. Fabrikant et al.[77] noted that the clinical results after helium-ion radiosurgery for cavernous angiomas were not as good as those for arteriovenous malformations. Radiosurgery using a linear accelerator has also been reported but with small numbers of patients treated and a lack of long-term data.[78] Chang et al.[79] summarized the results of 57 patients treated using helium ion (47 patients) or linear accelerator (10 patients). All patients harbored CMs that had bled previously and were treated with mean doses of 18 GyE. Hemorrhage rates decreased 3 years after treatment to 1.6% per patient-year. In this study, 5 patients (9%) suffered radiation-related edema or necrosis, resulting in permanent deficits in 2 patients (4%). Analysis of Kjellberg's experience at the Harvard Cyclotron Laboratory using proton beam therapy revealed a decline in hemorrhage rates from 17.3% per lesion-year before treatment

to 4.5% per lesion-year after a latency period of 2 years.[80] Among the 98 lesions treated with a median center dose of 18 Gy, 26 (26.5%) were associated with radiation-related complications, 16 of which were permanent and 3 of which resulted in mortality.

Because the long-term natural history of CMs is not well defined, current evidence favors expectant management, given the high rates of complications with radiosurgery. The risk of radiation-related complications appears to be significantly higher than that found for arteriovenous malformations of similar size and location[72]; although the basis for this is unknown, a role for the potential radiosensitizing properties of the hemosiderin ring around CMs has been proposed.[81] The decline in hemorrhage rates observed in most studies cannot definitively be ascribed to the treatment, because it may reflect the poorly characterized natural history of bleeding in these lesions.

Temporal clustering of hemorrhages, with a spontaneous 2.4-fold decline in hemorrhage rates after 2 years, has been observed and may affect the interpretation of hemorrhage risk reduction in radiosurgical series.[61] This modality is presently considered only rarely for deep, inaccessible lesions associated with repeated hemorrhage and progressive neurologic deficit.

CM of the Cerebrum

MANAGEMENT

Patients Presenting with Seizures

The treatment of patients with CMs presenting with seizures continues to evolve. With the good results of surgical removal, the indications for operation have expanded beyond conditions in which medical control of seizures is difficult and in which the diagnosis is in question (more common before the advent of MRI). Surgery is recommended in most patients who have had a parenchymal hemorrhage and in many patients who have not had a hemorrhage when the surgical risk is low. These patients are usually in their 20s to 40s but are sometimes younger, and they are often concerned about the presence of the lesion. Although the seizures can often be controlled with medication, the removal of the CM and the adjacent gliotic yellow-stained tissue may reduce the long-term frequency and severity of seizures and allow the patients to discontinue their medications.[2,48,49] Robinson et al.[48] reported that all 18 patients who did not have surgery continued to require medical control of their seizures. In the surgically treated group, 50% had no more seizures, and the others had a reduction in seizure frequency.

Rengachary and Kalyan-Raman[2] described a possible basis for recommending surgery. They suggest that slow lysis of red cells sequestrated in the cavernous spaces allows red cell pigment to diffuse out of the lesion into the adjacent tissue. This pigment seems to induce gliosis, which may contribute to the development of a seizure focus. The authors quote experimental studies that suggest chemical compounds containing iron play important roles in inducing a seizure focus.

In the MGH series, a seizure was the primary presenting symptom in 51 of 84 patients with lesions of the cerebrum (61%) (Table 81-2). Some of these patients had other symptoms (usually headache), and slightly more than half had an associated parenchymal hematoma. Patients with CMs presenting

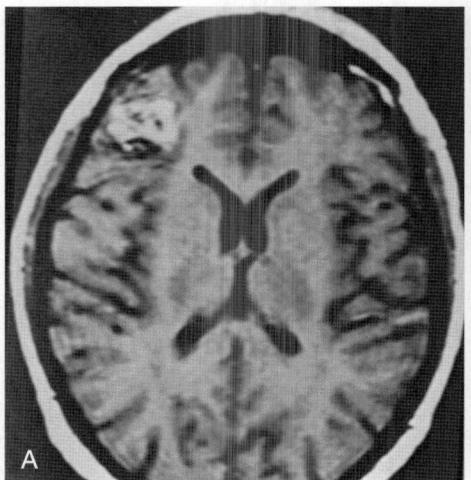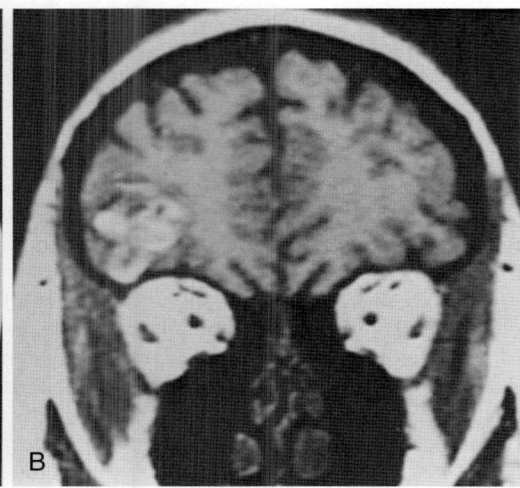

FIGURE 81-4 Frontal CM in a 45-year-old man with a history of mild frontal headache for several weeks who then presented with a seizure. After the malformation was removed, the patient had a normal recovery. Axial (A) and coronal (B) T1-weighted images showed findings consistent with a cavernous angioma but no hematoma in the adjacent parenchyma. These findings were confirmed at operation, but there was yellow staining in the adjacent cerebral tissue.

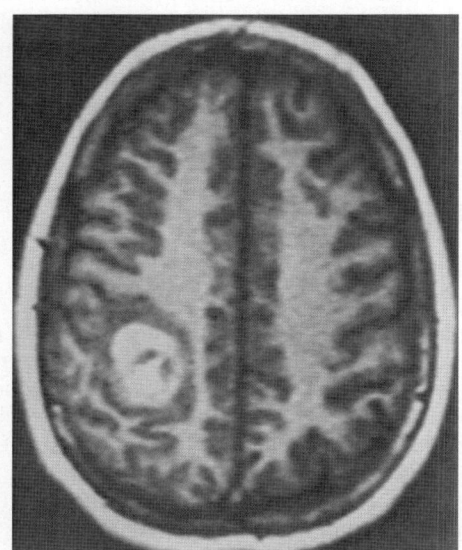

FIGURE 81-5 Parietal CM in a 19-year-old man who presented with a seizure. Removal of the lesion was followed by full recovery of the patient. Axial T1-weighted MRI showed the circumscribed mottled core with adjacent hematoma and edema.

with seizure are shown in Figs. 81-1 (temporal), 81-3 and 81-4 (frontal), 81-5 (parietal), and 81-6 (motor–sensory cortex).

Patients Presenting with Headache

If the headache is a new symptom or is recurrent, it can often be related to the CM. In these patients, MRI often shows a recent hemorrhage. In our series, 16 of 18 patients with headache (89%) had a parenchymal hemorrhage (Table 81-2). Surgery is indicated in most of these patients to avoid future neurologic disability from recurrent hemorrhage (except in patients with unacceptably high surgical risk because of a critical anatomic location). An example is illustrated in Fig. 81-7.

Patients Presenting with Neurologic Deficit

In most patients with a progressive or acute neurologic deficit, there is an associated hematoma, and surgical removal of the lesion is indicated to prevent further neurologic

damage and to help restore neurologic function. Some of these patients also have had headaches. In the patient whose deficit is improving, observation can be the initial strategy used. If the surgical risks are judged to be relatively low, however, the lesion should be electively removed to prevent the effects of rehemorrhage. These patients are generally younger than 60 years and are at risk for repeated hemorrhages and neurologic deficits.[6] Involvement of the speech or motor–sensory cortex should not preclude the consideration of surgery, but a final decision should include an assessment of the surgical accessibility of the lesion.

In our series, most patients (13 of 15, or 87%) presenting with a neurologic deficit had an associated acute hemorrhage. The indications for surgery were progressive neurologic deficit, sudden severe neurologic deficit, recurrent episodes of neurologic deficits lasting days to weeks, and history of a hemorrhage followed by recovery. An example is illustrated in Fig. 81-8.

RESULTS

Several reports documented good results in the surgical treatment of CMs of the cerebral hemispheres.[9,46,50,51,66,82-87] With accessible lesions, surgical morbidity is minimal and mortality is almost zero. Acciarri et al.[82] found a 90% incidence of good outcomes in 55 patients with hemispheric lesions, with 0% mortality. Smaller series have found similarly favorable results, with good results in 100% of patients.[51,85,86] Chadduck et al.[88] reviewed patients with intraventricular CMs. Although they found good outcomes, particularly in patients with lateral ventricular lesions, 2 of 15 surgically treated patients (13%) died, and 1 patient was rendered comatose. Acciarri et al.[82] reported two deaths among 4 patients with intraventricular lesions.

The treatment of CMs of the basal ganglia and thalamus has been controversial, and these lesions (along with brain stem lesions) may be considered dangerous to excise. Some practitioners suggest that surgery be considered when there are recurrent episodes of hemorrhage or progressive worsening neurologic deficit.[50,89] Lorenzana et al.[90] reported on a patient with a CM that involved the anterior third of the lentiform nucleus and a large part of white matter anterior to the nucleus. The patient was cured by use of CT-assisted stereotactic craniotomy with an approach through the second frontal

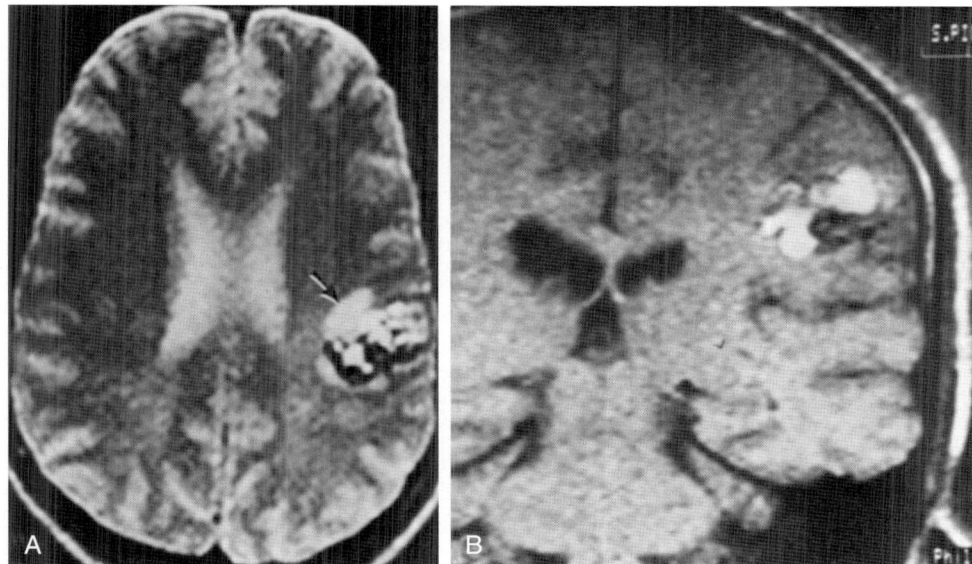

FIGURE 81-6 Frontoparietal CM in a 36-year-old neurosurgeon who had a focal seizure involving the right hand and right side of the face. After another seizure occurred 4 months later, axial T2-weighted (A) and coronal T1-weighted (B) MRI showed the cavernous angioma in the left inferior motor–sensory cortex and an area of new hemorrhage *(arrow)* that was not seen on the scan after the first seizure. The patient carefully considered the treatment options and concluded (as we had) that further hemorrhage entailed a risk of ending his career with damage to his dominant hand. Also, he wanted to reduce the probability of a seizure and to stop taking medications. Surgical removal was followed by the patient's complete recovery, with no focal neurologic deficit and with resumption of neurosurgical practice.

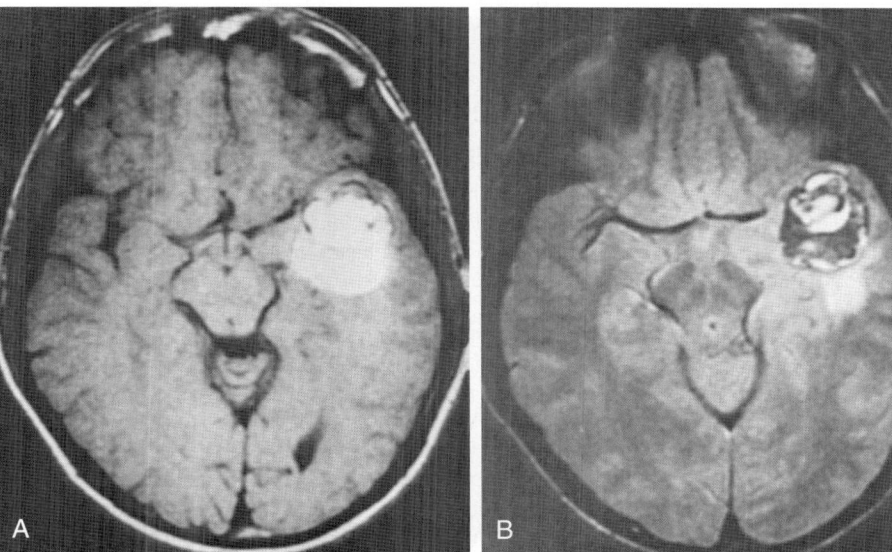

FIGURE 81-7 Temporal CM in a 26-year-old man who had the onset of headache with weight lifting. The headaches started to increase. An MRI scan showed a left temporal cavernous angioma with hemorrhage. Angiography showed no abnormal vascularity or stain. The patient was followed up, and his headaches persisted. The patient's neurologic examination remained normal, but repeat axial T1-weighted (A) and T2-weighted (B) MRI showed an increase in the size of the hematoma. Surgical removal of the left temporal CM and hematoma was followed by the patient's complete recovery with no speech difficulty.

sulcus. In other case reports, the results of treatment of CMs in the thalamus were discouraging.[86,91] Bertalanffy et al.[92] found permanent neurologic complications in 6 of 12 patients (50%) after resection of deep-seated lesions within the basal ganglia, thalamus, and insula. Steinberg et al. reported worsening in 16 of a group of 56 patients (29%) with deep or brain stem lesions, of which 15 were located in the basal ganglia or thalamus; long-term outcome, however, was improved condition in 52%, unchanged in 43%, and worse in 5%.[93]

The effects of resection on seizure control are pertinent given the frequency of seizures among supratentorial CMs. Lesionectomy alone has resulted in favorable results.[82,94,95] Despite the implication of iron products as potential seizure foci, there is considerable controversy as to whether removal of the surrounding hemosiderin ring should be a primary goal during microsurgical resection. Early studies did not show a correlation between removal of the hemosiderin-stained brain and improved outcome.[96,97] However, more recent literature seems to suggest the contrary: at least three recent studies have demonstrated a significantly higher proportion of patients classified as Engel class I (free from disabling seizures) after complete removal of the hemosiderin ring versus partial or no removal.[98-100] Length of seizure history and total number of seizures, however, do not seem to affect surgical outcome negatively.[95,97,101] Nevertheless, seizure control has obvious implications for long-term quality of life. Retrospective studies reveal that 75% to 100% of patients with fewer than five seizures or shorter than a 12-month history of seizures are

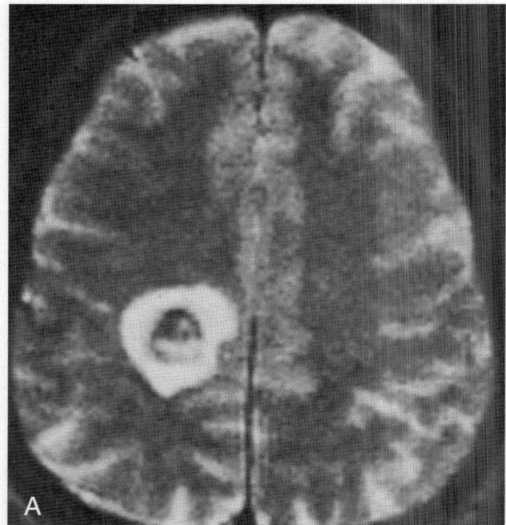
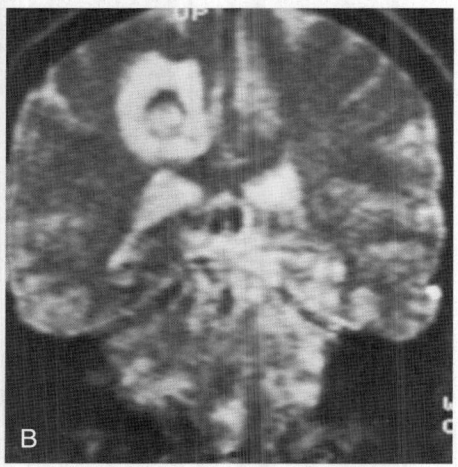

FIGURE 81-8 Parietal CM in a 42-year-old man who had a brief episode of weakness in his left lower extremity 2 weeks before being examined. Nine days before admission to the hospital, he developed a limp because of weakness in his left lower extremity. The next day, his foot became weaker, and then he noted weakness in his left upper extremity. The progression of the weakness stopped when he was given steroids. Axial (A) and coronal (B) T2-weighted MRI showed a hemorrhage associated with a cavernous angioma deep in the right parietal region. Stereotactic localization was performed, and the lesion was removed. The patient completely recovered except for a slight residual weakness in his foot.

seizure free after lesionectomy, compared with 50% to 62.5% of patients with more than five seizures or a seizure history longer than 1 year.[95,101] A newer study looked at 53 patients with epilepsy related to supratentorial CMs and demonstrated that complete microsurgical resection, along with the hemosiderin rim, resulted in 84.9% of patients being classified as Engel class I. This study also demonstrates a significant improvement in seizure control rate in patients with complete resection of the hemosiderin rim versus in those in whom the hemosiderin rim was left (77.8% vs. 65.7%, $p < 0.037$).[100]

In the MGH series of 84 patients with CMs of the cerebrum outside the basal ganglia and thalamus, operative mortality was zero, and all patients had complete removal of the lesion. Postoperatively, 81 of the 84 patients (96%) had an excellent or good outcome neurologically (i.e., were able to return to their previous level of activity) and, in most cases, had normal results on neurologic examination. Three patients (4%) were classified as fair because of residual disability. Neurologic outcome and comparison of presurgical and postsurgical neurologic status are shown in Table 81-3. Of the 52 patients presenting with seizures, 29 underwent surgery primarily for seizure control; the remainder underwent surgery to eliminate risk of further hemorrhage rather than primary treatment of the seizure disorder. Of the 52 patients, 50 (96%)

were seizure free on or off anticonvulsants after surgery. Of the 29 patients treated primarily for epilepsy, 26 (90%) experienced improvement in seizure control after surgery.

CM of the Brain Stem

MANAGEMENT

Based on their experiences with 8 patients (4 of whom had surgery), Falbusch et al.[102] recommended that CMs of the brain stem that are associated with recurrent episodes of hemorrhage, MRI-confirmed diagnosis, negative angiographic results, and progressive neurologic disability should be removed. Patients with recovery or stabilization of their neurologic deficit, or those who are asymptomatic, should be observed. The report by Zimmerman et al.[53] summarized 24 patients (16 of whom had surgery). They recommended that neurologically intact patients with CMs that did not touch the pial surface should be observed. When the lesion was associated with repeated hemorrhages or with progressive neurologic deficit and was close to the pial surface, surgery was performed. They also suggested that any symptomatic lesion of the brain stem located superficially be considered for surgery if eloquent tissue could be spared. Based on the poor

Table 81-3	Neurologic Outcome after Surgical Resection							
Location	CMs	Excellent	Good	Fair	Poor	Improved	Stable	Worse
Cerebrum	84	68 (80.9%)	13 (15.5%)	3 (3.6%)	0 (0%)	4 (4.8%)	76 (90.4%)	4 (4.8%)
Brain stem	17	1 (5.9%)	10 (58.8%)	4 (23.5%)	2 (11.7%)	5 (29.4%)	9 (52.9%)	3 (17.6%)
Cerebellum	8	2 (25%)	5 (62.5%)	1 (12.5%)	0 (0%)	2 (25%)	6 (75%)	0 (0%)
Cranial nerves	4	0 (0%)	4 (100%)	0 (0%)	0 (0%)	0 (0%)	4 (100%)	0 (0%)
Spinal cord	8	0 (0%)	6 (75%)	2 (25%)	0 (0%)	5 (62.5%)	3 (37.5%)	0 (0%)
Total	121	71 (58.7%)	38 (31.4%)	10 (8.3%)	2 (1.6%)	16 (13.2%)	98 (81%)	7 (5.8%)

Excellent, no neurologic deficit; good, free of major neurologic deficit and able to return to previous activity; fair, independent but some neurologic disability; poor, dependent with significant neurologic disability.

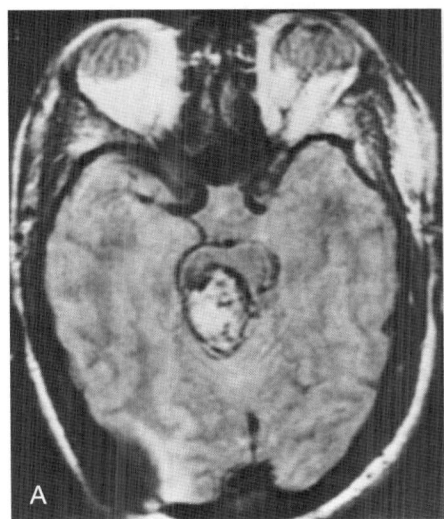
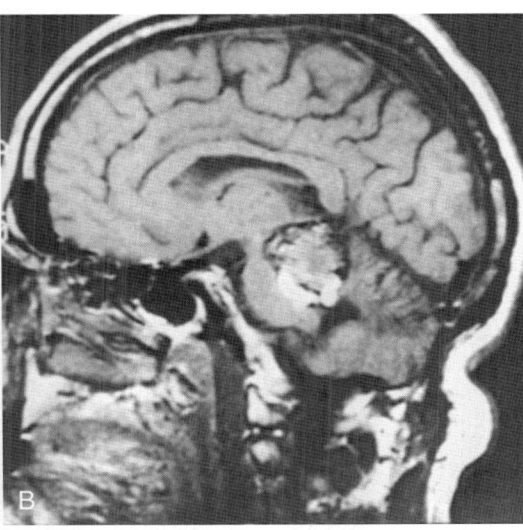

FIGURE 81-9 Brain stem cavernous angioma in a 27-year-old man treated with radiosurgery 4 years earlier, presenting with increased dysarthria and ataxia. Axial (A) and sagittal (B) T1-weighted MRI showed the lesion with new hemorrhage around the inferior margin. The patient declined to undergo surgery.

overall natural history of symptomatic CMs in a brain stem location, resection is advocated for lesions abutting a pial surface or surrounded by only a thin rim of tissue.[103-107] The optimal timing of surgery following hemorrhage is less well defined. Operation in the subacute phase following hemorrhage (several days to a few weeks) may be preferable.[107-109] This allows time to stabilize the patient's condition while conferring the benefit of earlier reduction of mass effect by evacuation of hematoma. Furthermore, the presence of a subacute hematoma may create a better surgical plane than would be present after delayed surgery following complete clot resorption, or with acute surgery with a firm clot.[93] Mathiesen et al. found better outcomes among their patients with brain stem cavernomas if surgery was performed within 1 month of the hemorrhagic ictus.[108] On the other hand, Samii et al. reported that there was no difference in long-term outcomes based on the timing of surgery in 36 patients.[106]

In the past, some CMs of the brain stem were treated with radiosurgery when recurrent hemorrhages and increased neurologic deficit were present. The patient whose MRI scan is illustrated in Fig. 81-9 was treated for this reason several years ago. The lesion did not become smaller, and recurrent hemorrhage with worsening symptoms occurred. The patient declined surgical management.

The indications for operation in our patients were progressive or recurrent neurologic symptoms. The risk of surgery is probably lower when the lesion comes to the surface, obviating pial incision. The risk of surgery is probably higher when the lesion is large without associated hemorrhage or when it is densely calcified, making removal more difficult.

Careful study of the MRI scan aids in planning of the precise corridor of exposure and resection. Neuronavigation can be of considerable help, especially for lesions that are covered by a thin rim of tissue and that are not directly visible on the surface.[109] Electrophysiologic monitoring (e.g., somatosensory evoked potentials, brain stem auditory evoked potentials, and cranial nerve V, IIV, and XII function monitoring) can be utilized in an effort to minimize complications.[93,109] While there is benefit to resecting the hemosiderin ring in supratentorial lesions with regard to seizure control, this is clearly not a concern in the brain stem. Moreover, high-resolution diffusion tensor imaging and tractography have shown that while the CM itself neatly displaces white matter tracts, the hemosiderin ring is often intimately involved with them. As such, resection of the hemosiderin ring should be avoided in cases of infratentorial CMs.[68]

Pontomedullary CMs can be approached through a midline suboccipital craniotomy and exposure of the fourth ventricle. Lesions in the pontomesencephalic region are more difficult to manage but may be treated by a subtemporal or combined subtemporal–suboccipital approach. Falbusch et al.[102] used a supracerebellar infratentorial approach for midline pontomesencephalic lesions.

In our patients, the approach to brain stem CMs is dictated by the relative rostral–caudal, as well as anterior–posterior, localization of the lesion (Table 81-4). Upper brain stem CMs were removed by a subtemporal approach (Fig. 81-10); in one patient, a laterally placed brain stem lesion was approached through the cerebellopontine angle between the fifth and seventh cranial nerves. In patients with lesions in the pons or medulla, a midline exposure through the floor of the fourth ventricle was used (Fig. 81-11).

RESULTS

Zimmerman et al.[53] reported that among 16 patients who underwent surgery, some had transient postoperative worsening, but the outcome in all except for 1 patient was the same or improved. Isamat and Louesa[110] had 6 patients with

Table 81-4	Approaches to CMs of the Brain Stem		
Lesion Location	Anterior	Lateral	Posterior
Midbrain	Pterional orbitozygomatic subtemporal	Lateral infratentorial/supracerebellar	Lateral infratentorial/supracerebellar
Pons	Pterional orbitozygomatic subtemporal	Far lateral suboccipital retrosigmoid	Midline suboccipital/fourth ventricular
Medulla	Subtemporal far lateral suboccipital transcondylar	Lateral suboccipital retrosigmoid	Midline suboccipital/fourth ventricular

Data from Asaad WF, Walcott BP, Nahed BV, Ogilvy CS. Operative management of brainstem cavernous malformations. *Neurosurg Focus.* 2010;29(3):E10.

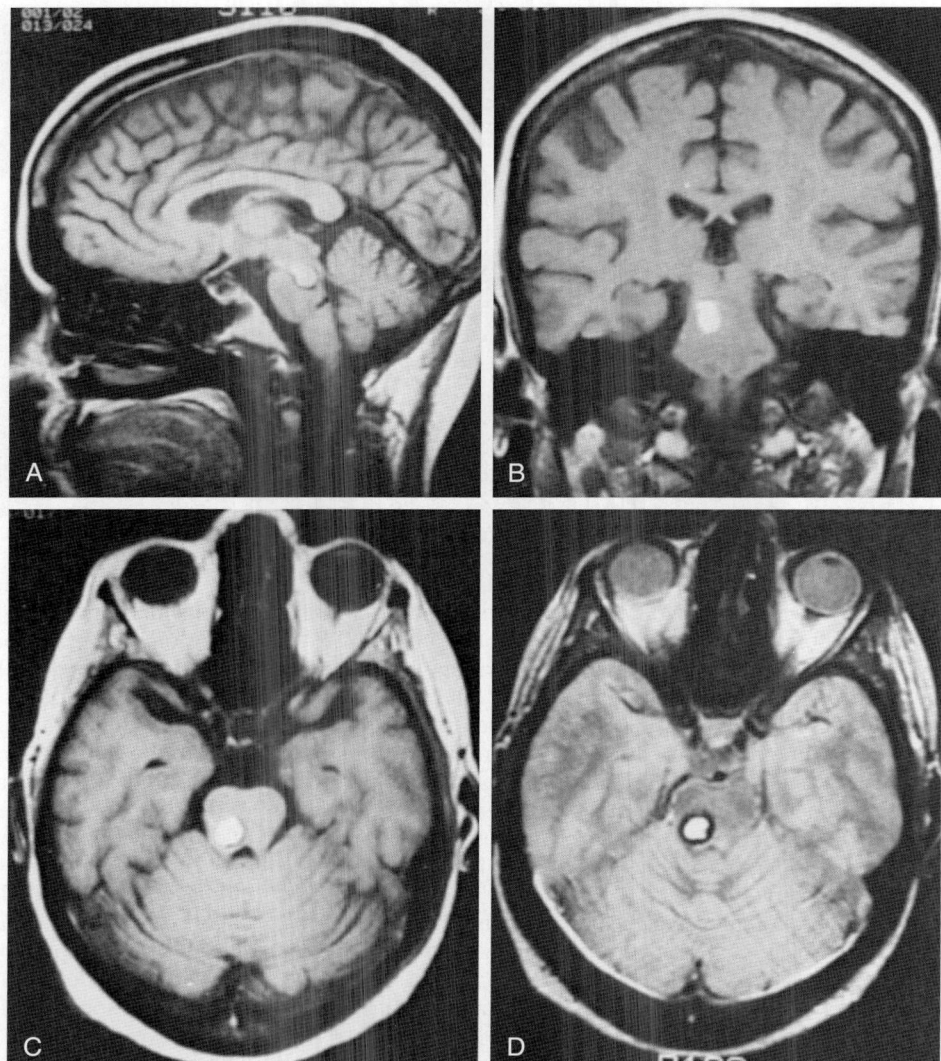

FIGURE 81-10 An upper brain stem CM in a 37-year-old woman. Because of recurrent symptoms (second hemorrhage and inability to walk), the lesion was removed using a right subtemporal approach. Sagittal (A), coronal (B), and axial (C) T1-weighted and axial T2-weighted (D) MRI. The lesion almost comes to the surface and is localized to one side.

CMs in the pons or medulla that were in contact with the floor of the fourth ventricle and were removed through the floor of the ventricle. All patients returned to their previous activities and had improvement in their neurologic deficits. Three other patients in their study are being followed because the lesion was completely surrounded by normal brain stem tissue.

Fritschi et al.[111] reviewed 93 cases of brain stem CMs treated operatively from their own experience and from the literature up to 1992. They found good outcomes in 84% of cases. The authors compared the surgical results with 30 patients treated conservatively without surgery. Although most nonoperative patients recovered completely or with minimal deficits (67%), 20% died, and 7% suffered poor outcomes. Porter et al. reported improved outcomes in 87% of 84 patients who underwent operation for brain stem CMs; 10% worsened postoperatively, and 4% died.[103] A 12% incidence of severe or permanent morbidity was reported. Despite successful resection of brain stem lesions, CMs within this location clearly carry a higher risk of operative morbidity and mortality. Rates of transient complications within the literature range from 25% to 70%,[53,92,104,108,112] rates of permanent complications are up to 25%,[92,103,104,112,113] and mortality rates are up to 6%.[53,92,103,111,114]

In the MGH series of 17 patients with CMs of the brain stem, 5 improved, but some residual neurologic deficits that had been present before surgery were usually persistent (see Table 81-3). Eight patients (47%) experienced transient postoperative neurologic deficits, all of which resolved to baseline within 1 month. Three patients (17.6%) experienced permanent postoperative deficits. One of these patients harbored a mesencephalic CM and initially presented with hemorrhage, in coma; clot evacuation and partial lesion resection was undertaken. He made a gradual recovery but had a small rehemorrhage 2 years later. He underwent reoperation, which resulted in poor outcome. Another patient presented with a progressive quadriparesis (Fig. 81-11), and at operation, the large lesion was calcified and difficult to remove. Complete resection was achieved, but the patient had further neurologic deficits postoperatively, leaving her bedridden. The third patient had a pontomedullary CM and presented with progressive diplopia and ataxia. Postoperatively, the patient's condition was worse, with difficulty swallowing and hoarseness that improved but with residual effect.

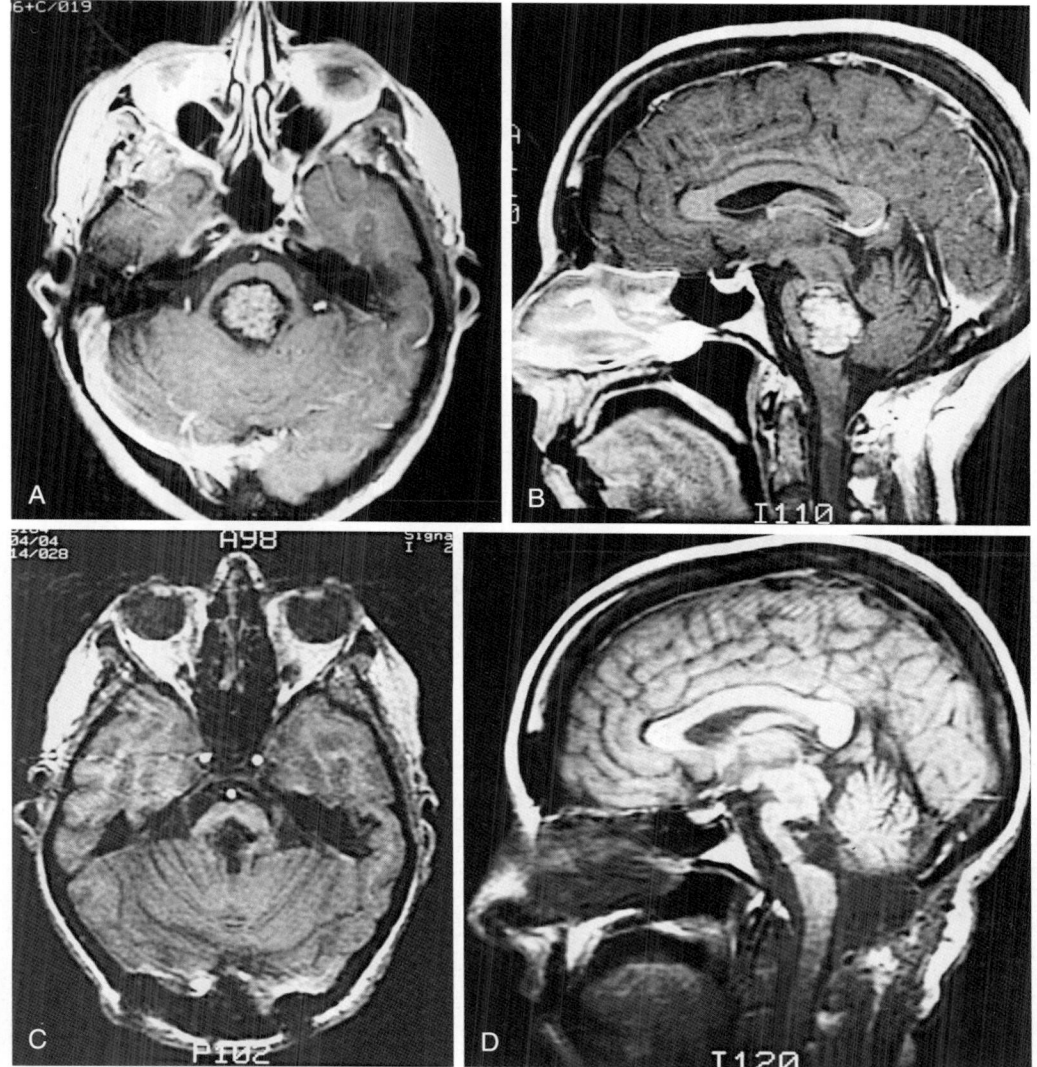

FIGURE 81-11 Pontomedullary CM in a 53-year-old woman who presented with progressive neurologic deficits; she was quadriparetic and wheel-chair-bound preoperatively. Axial and sagittal T1-weighted MRI revealed the large brain stem lesion preoperatively (A and B, respectively) and after complete resection (C and D, respectively). Postoperatively, the patient deteriorated neurologically and was bedridden. *(From Amin-Hanjani S, Ogilvy CS, Ojemann RG, et al: Risks of surgical management for CMs of the nervous system. Neurosurgery 42:1224, 1998.)*

Abla et al. recently published the largest series of brain stem CMs, in which they examine their experience with treating 300 patients between 1989 and 2005. Their data underscore the difficulty of operative management of these lesions, because the rate of postoperative neurologic deficit was approximately 51%, with 35% of patients having permanent deficits. Perioperative complications, most commonly from tracheostomy or feeding tube placement and cerebrospinal fluid leak, were noted in 28% of the cohort. Rehemorrhage was observed in 6.9% of patients, and the overall annual rate of rehemorrhage was 2.0%,[115] which represents a significant decrease compared to rates as high as 34%[116] that are quoted in the literature. The study spans a period during which dramatic improvements in microsurgical technique, MRI resolution, and intraoperative neuronavigation have been made. As such, it is not surprising that patients operated on at an earlier point in the study were more likely to have a poor outcome. However, this study reiterates the perils of operating in the brain stem and highlights the need for appropriate patient selection and serious consideration of the relative risks and benefits of surgery for brain stem CMs.

CM of the Cerebellum

MANAGEMENT

The general management guidelines for most cerebellar CMs are similar to those outlined for the cerebral hemisphere. Surgery is indicated because the patient has presented with a neurologic deficit, there is an associated hemorrhage, the morbidity of removal is low, and the risk of significant neurologic disability with repeat hemorrhage is high.

RESULTS

There were eight patients with CMs of the cerebellum in the MGH series: all made a good recovery and could be classified as having excellent or good outcomes

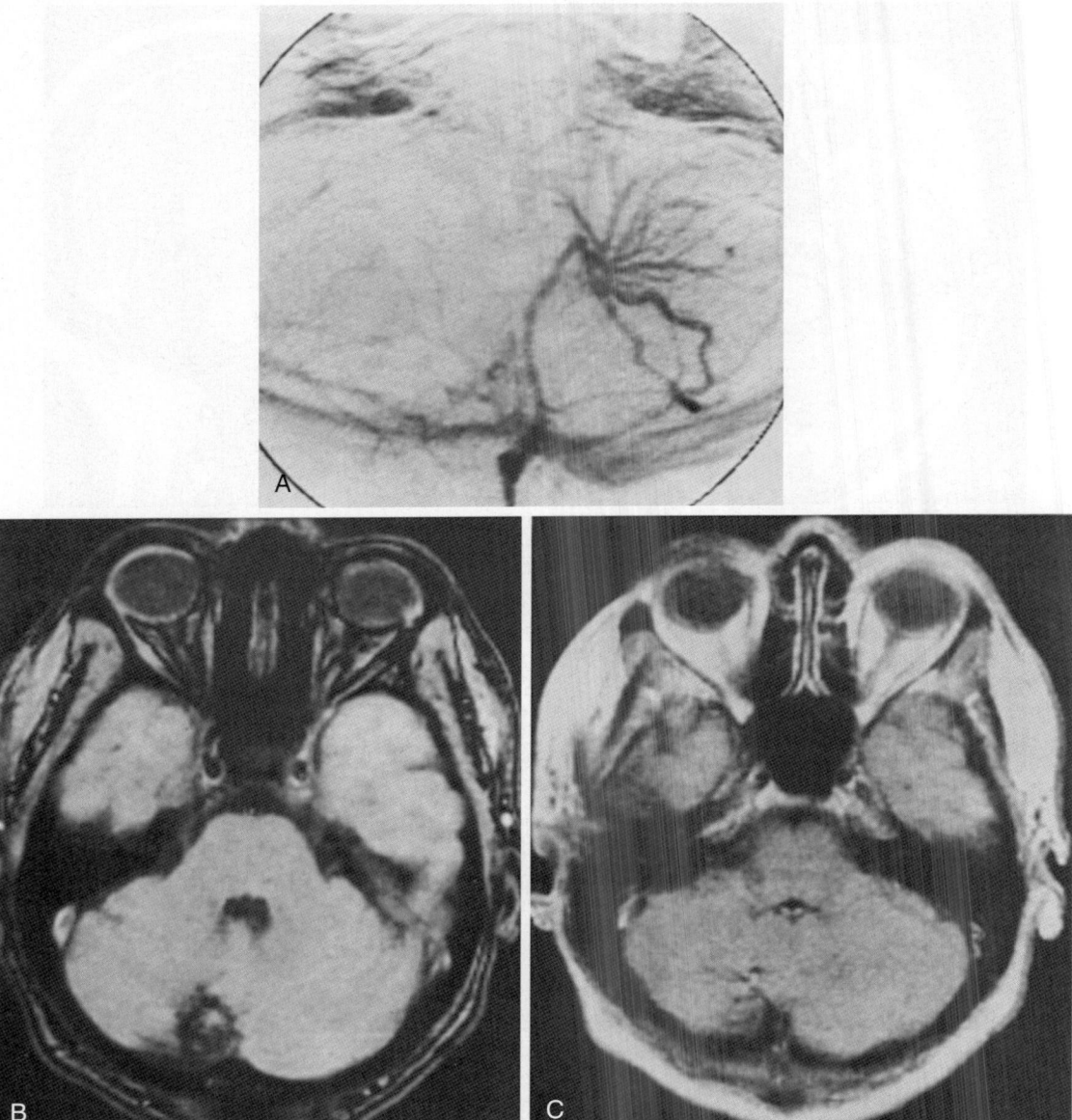

FIGURE 81-12 Cerebellar CM in a 32-year-old woman who had a sudden severe headache with nausea and vomiting and severe ataxia. At another hospital, a CT scan showed a right cerebellar hemorrhage. A, Angiography showed no early-filling veins but a large venous angioma. The patient recovered, and her neurologic examination was normal. B and C, Three months later, axial T1-weighted MRI showed evidence of the adjacent venous anomaly and the old hemorrhage with a mottled appearance within this area, supporting the diagnosis of CM. Surgery was recommended because of the serious disability that resulted from the first hemorrhage. The venous angioma was not treated, and the patient had a good recovery.

(see Table 81-3) except for one patient classified as a fair outcome secondary to persistence of a preoperative deficit. One patient had an associated venous anomaly (Fig. 81-12). At operation, a typical CM was resected, and the large venous angioma was carefully preserved. The patient made an uneventful recovery. Another patient with a cerebellar CM and associated venous anomaly developed a venous infarction 1 month postoperatively, despite efforts to leave the venous anomaly intact. This complication required reoperation for cerebellar decompression, but the patient ultimately regained her preoperative neurologic status.

CM of the Cranial Nerves

MANAGEMENT

CMs have been reported to involve cranial nerves in the following locations: optic nerves and chiasm, third nerve, seventh nerve in the temporal bone, and seventh and eighth nerves in the internal auditory canal (Table 81-5).[117-121] The presenting symptoms relate to the nerve involved with the lesion. The MRI scan usually suggests the diagnosis, but in some patients, the pathology may not be evident until surgery. Surgery does not usually restore function in the involved nerve, although some improvement in deficit can

Table 81-5 CMs of the Cranial Nerves

Age (years)/Sex	Location	Clinical Course	Outcome
33/F	Optic chiasm	Developed visual field deficit during pregnancy, second hemorrhage after delivery	Good: residual visual field deficit
25/M	Third nerve	Progressive third nerve palsy	Good: third nerve palsy
53/M	Seventh nerve	Progressive facial weakness	Good: facial nerve graft placed with some recovery
27/F	Seventh and eighth nerves in internal auditory canal and posterior fossa	Fullness in ear, facial twitch	Good: loss of hearing, facial nerve graft placed with some recovery

be observed.[121] Surgery is indicated to prevent hemorrhage into adjacent neural structures or, as in a patient with a facial nerve lesion, to remove the malformation and place a sural nerve graft, which may restore some function. Gross total resection of the lesion is required to prevent progression of the cranial nerve dysfunction.

RESULTS

Improvement in function has been documented with removal of cranial nerve CMs.[122] Others, however, report a low potential for restoration of function[118,119] and note that complete resection is difficult without incurring permanent nerve injury.[119,120]

In the MGH series of four patients (see Table 81-4), one patient had a CM in the optic chiasm. A field deficit developed during pregnancy as a result of hemorrhage and then improved, only to worsen after a second hemorrhage a few months after delivery. The field deficit improved somewhat after removal of the lesion. Malik et al.[118] reported the partial removal of a CM from the underside of the optic nerve and chiasm in one patient. Vision did not improve, but no further symptoms occurred. Shibuya et al.[122] reported visual improvement after resection of a chiasmal CM. Deshmukh et al. reported visual improvement in all four of their patients with chiasmal CMs.[121] A retrospective review of the literature on optic pathway CMs showed rates of vision preservation were highest in patients who underwent complete resection.[123] As such, resection is generally favored for preservation of vision and prevention of rehemorrhage.

One patient in the MGH series had a lesion involving the seventh and eighth nerves in the internal auditory canal. Involvement in the internal auditory canal has been reported in four patients, including the one in the MGH series.[119,124] The eighth nerve could not be saved in any patient, but reasonable facial nerve function remained in three patients. When the facial nerve cannot be saved, a nerve graft is placed at operation. One patient in the MGH series had a malformation involving the seventh nerve in the temporal bone. The malformation and nerve were removed, and a sural nerve graft was placed. The last patient in the series

had a lesion of the third cranial nerve[120] that was extensively involved and was resected to remove the malformation. The case reported by Scott[125] was treated in the same way.

CM of the Spinal Cord
CLINICAL PRESENTATION

Reviewing spinal cord CMs reported within the literature through 1991, Ogilvy et al.[11] described 36 patients with 37 spinal lesions, including 6 patients from the MGH series. The series included 25 (69%) women and 11 (31%) men. The locations of the lesions along the spinal axis were cervical medullary junction in 3 (8%), cervical in 12 (32%), thoracic in 20 (54%), lumbar spinal cord in 1 (3%), and conus medullaris in 1 (3%). The review found 2 patients had a history of familial CM, 4 had a CM at some other site in the central nervous system, and 1 had a second spinal lesion.

The ages ranged from 12 to 62 years, and the most common age range for the appearance of initial symptoms was in the 30s. Four clinical categories of symptoms were identified:

1. Thirteen patients presented with episodes of neurologic deterioration with variable degrees of neurologic recovery between episodes. The episodes lasted hours to days. The interval between events was often months to years.
2. Twelve patients had a clinical course characterized by slowly progressive neurologic deterioration. The duration of the progression was usually several years. Two patients had discrete episodes of gradual worsening separated by many years.
3. Eight patients had an acute onset of symptoms followed by neurologic worsening over several days.
4. Three patients had the acute onset of mild symptoms followed by weeks or months of deterioration of neurologic function.

Review of the brain imaging studies of 17 patients in a recent series of spinal CMs demonstrated a higher incidence of multiple neuraxis CMs, with 8 (47%) such patients harboring multiple CMs[126]; patients with spinal CMs may warrant complete neuraxis imaging to evaluate for additional lesions.

MANAGEMENT

The diagnosis of a CM of the spinal cord is established by the characteristic MRI appearance (Fig. 81-13). From the history obtained from symptomatic patients, it is evident that in some patients there can be intervals of several years between episodes of recurrent neurologic problems that presumably result from hemorrhage. In these intervals, a neurologic deficit is stable or the patient is symptom free. Also, in recurrent hemorrhages, the neurologic deficit often increases and does not always fully recover. Rehemorrhage rates as high as 66% per year have been reported, favoring resection of symptomatic lesions.[127] An alternative strategy has been proposed by Kharkar et al., who studied 14 symptomatic patients at their institution with a mean follow-up of 80 months. In this group, 10 patients were managed conservatively and did not demonstrate any new hemorrhage or neurologic deficit. They found that 2 of the patients showed significant improvement in neurologic status, while the rest

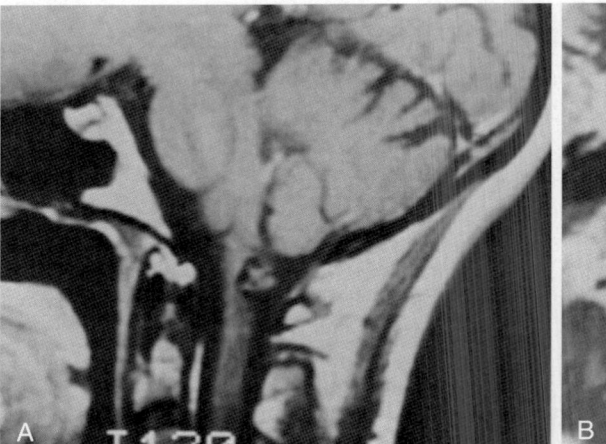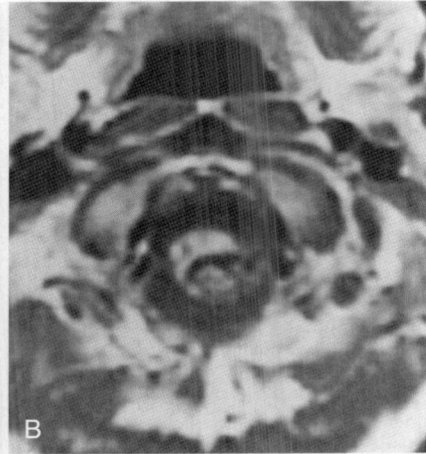

FIGURE 81-13 Cervical medullary junction CM in a 36-year-old woman who had the onset of generalized headache 4 months before surgery. Twenty-four hours later, she noted numbness in the left lateral leg that progressed over the next week to involve the entire left lower extremity; this condition improved. A CT scan of the head was normal. Two weeks later, the patient noted difficulty jogging because of discoordination in the left lower extremity. Sagittal (A) and axial (B) T1-weighted MRI showed a posteriorly placed lesion involving the midline and left side of the cervical medullary junction that is consistent with a cavernous angioma; the patient was followed. Ten days before she was admitted to the hospital, she had nausea and vomiting and increased numbness and weakness on the left side of her body. Complete excision of the lesion was followed by improvement in left lower extremity function, temporary worsening of position sense in the left hand, and numbness in the left upper extremity. Subsequently, she had a good recovery; she was able to jog, and she returned to work.

remained stable. In addition, 4 patients were treated surgically; 2 of these remained the same, 1 improved, and 1 deteriorated significantly.[128] While this is a relatively small study, the authors' conclusion was that observation of patients, even those with symptomatic intramedullary spinal cord malformations, is not unreasonable. Consensus on this issue is not available, and treatment must be tailored to the individual clinical scenario.

In most patients, lesions present on the dorsal or dorsolateral aspect of the spinal cord. We usually recommend surgery. The findings at operation are similar to those found at operation in CMs of the brain. A well-defined gliotic plane exists around the lesion, which aids in the microsurgical removal. The use of fine sutures in the pia to retract the spinal cord when the lesion is deep, fine-regulated suction, and microbipolar forceps facilitates the dissection. Gross total removal of the malformation should be the goal of surgical treatment.

RESULTS

Several small case series have shown favorable results with complete resection of intramedullary CMs.[129,130] Transient neurologic complications in the early postoperative period can be prominent, however.[130,131] Spetzger et al.[130] noted such complications in 5 of 9 patients (55%) but found that over long-term follow-up, 8 of 9 patients (88%) were normal or improved compared with preoperative status. Operative intervention for spinal cord CMs generally results in long-term improvement or stabilization of function.[11,127,129-133] Cantore et al.[134] found a correlation between surgical outcome and severity and length of preoperative symptoms in 6 patients, and Canavero et al.[135] found that preoperative status was the most important factor affecting outcome from surgery. Mitha et al. published the largest series to date of surgical outcomes in patients with spinal CMs. At 5-year follow-up, 10% of their cohort of 80 patients were worse, 68% were the same, and 23% were improved compared to

their preoperative status. Moreover, they noted an interesting correlation between outcome and anterior–posterior length of the lesion, but not with craniocaudal or transverse length. They surmise that this likely relates to the vast majority of the lesions operated on being posteriorly located. As lesions increased in anterior–posterior size, they extended more anteriorly, placing them in proximity with motor tracts.[136] With more frequent availability of MRI, a higher proportion of patients are being diagnosed with spinal CMs prior to neurologic deterioration, when the only symptom present is pain. Surgery for spinal CMs that are causing significant pain appears to be effective at reducing pain at 1 month and 1 year.[137]

In the MGH series of CMs involving the spinal cord, there were eight patients ranging in age from 31 to 61 years. The lesion was completely removed in all eight patients. On follow-up, all patients were ambulatory, and their conditions were as good as or better than before the operation. One patient had a previous subtotal removal at another institution and had a further small hemorrhage with a neurologic deficit that did not fully recover. In three patients, the CM protruded from the dorsal aspect of the spinal cord. In the others, a myelotomy was required; in three of these patients, the lesion projected more to one side and a myelotomy was placed in the dorsal root entry zone.

Conclusions

The management of patients with CMs continues to evolve. Current recommendations for management are as follows:
1. Patients who are asymptomatic are observed.
2. Patients with acute severe or progressive neurologic deficits undergo surgical resection.
3. Patients presenting with medically uncontrolled seizures undergo surgical resection; patients with new onset seizures may undergo resection, but some are observed, depending on the factors discussed in this chapter.

4. Patients with a single hemorrhage in the cerebrum, cerebellum, or spinal cord usually undergo surgical resection. When the hemorrhage is in the brain stem, thalamus, or basal ganglia, the patients are observed.

5. Patients with a recurrent hemorrhage usually undergo resection, but there are exceptions when the lesion is in a deep area with high surgical risk.

KEY REFERENCES

Abla AA, Lekovic GP, Turner J, et al. Advances in the Treatment and Outcome of Brain Stem Cavernous Malformation Surgery: a Case Series of 300 Surgically Treated Patients. *Neurosurgery*. 2010 Nov 25: [Epub ahead of print].

Amin-Hanjani S, Ogilvy CS, Candia GJ, et al. Stereotactic radiosurgery for cavernous malformations: Kjellberg's experience with proton beam therapy in 98 cases at the Harvard Cyclotron. *Neurosurgery*. 1998;42:1229-1238.

Asaad WF, Walcott BP, Nahed BV, Ogilvy CS. Operative management of brainstem cavernous malformations. *Neurosurg Focus*. 2010 Sep;29(3):E10.

Bertalanffy H, Benes L, Miyazawa T, et al. Cerebral cavernomas in the adult: review of the literature and analysis of 72 surgically treated patients. *Neurosurg Rev*. 2002;25:1-53.

Deshmukh VR, Albuquerque FC, Zabramski JM, et al. Surgical management of cavernous malformations involving the cranial nerves. *Neurosurgery*. 2003;53:352-357.

De Souza JM, Dominges RC, Cruz Jr LC, et al. Susceptibility-weighted imaging for the evaluation of patients with familial cerebral cavernous malformations: a comparison with T2-weighted fast spin-echo and gradient-echo sequences. *AJNR Am J Neuroradiol*. 2008 Jan;29(1):154-158.

Fabrikant JI, Levy RP, Steinberg GK, et al. Charged-particle radiosurgery for intracranial vascular malformations. *Neurosurg Clin N Am*. 1992;3:99-139.

Hammen T, Romstöck J, Dörfler A, et al. Prediction of postoperative outcome with special respect to removal of hemosiderin fringe: a study in patients with cavernous haemangiomas associated with symptomatic epilepsy. *Seizure*. 2007 Apr;16(3):248-253:Epub 2007 Feb 2.

Kharkar S, Shuck J, Conway J, et al. The natural history of conservatively managed symptomatic intramedullary spinal cord cavernomas. *Neurosurgery*. 2007 May;60(5):865-872:discussion 865–872.

Kondziolka D, Lunsford LD, Flickinger JC, et al. Reduction of hemorrhage risk after stereotactic radisourgery for cavernous malformations. *J Neurosurg*. 1995;83:825-831.

Kupersmith MJ, Kalish H, Epstein F, et al. Natural history of brain stem cavernous malformations. *Neurosurgery*. 2001;48:47-54.

Little JR, Awad IA, Jones SC, et al. Vascular pressures and cortical blood flow in cavernous angioma of the brain. *J Neurosurg*. 1990;73:555-559.

Louvi A, Chen L, Two AM, et al. Loss of cerebral cavernous malformation 3 (CCM3) in neuroglia leads to CCM and vascular pathology. *Proc Natl Acad Sci USA*. 2011 Mar 1;108(9):3737-3742.

Lunsford LD, Khan AA, Niranjan A, et al. Stereotactic radiosurgery for symptomatic solitary cerebral cavernous malformations considered high risk for resection. *J Neurosurg*. 2010 Jul;113(1):23-29.

Mitha AP, Turner JD, Abla AA, et al. Outcomes following resection of intramedullary spinal cord cavernous malformations: a 25-year experience. *J Neurosurg Spine*. 2011 May;14(5):605-611:Epub 2011 Feb 25.

Moriarity JL, Wetzel M, Clatterbuck RE, et al. The natural history of cavernous malformations: a prospective study of 68 patients. *Neurosurgery*. 1999;44:1166-1171.

Ogilvy CS, Heros RC, Ojemann RG, et al. Angiographically occult arteriovenous malformations. *J Neurosurg*. 1988;69:350-355.

Ojemann RG, Heros RG, Crowell RM. *Surgical Management of Cerebrovascular Disease*. Baltimore: Williams & Wilkins; 1988:401-403.

Rigamonti D, Hadley MN, Drayer BP, et al. Cerebral cavernous malformations: incidence and familial occurrence. *N Engl J Med*. 1988;19:343-347.

Roda JM, Alvarez F, Isla A, et al. Thalamic cavernous malformations. *J Neurosurg*. 1990;72:642-649.

Samii M, Eghbal R, Carvalho GA, et al. Surgical management of brain stem cavernomas. *J Neurosurg*. 2001;95:825-832.

Sandalcioglu IE, Wiedemayer H, Gasser T, et al. Intramedullary spinal cord cavernous malformations: clinical features and risk of hemorrhage. *Neurosurg Rev*. 2003;26:253-256.

Stavrou I, Baumgartner C, Frischer JM, et al. Long-term seizure control after resection of supratentorial cavernomas: a retrospective single-center study in 53 patients. *Neurosurgery*. 2008 Nov;63(5):888-896:discussion 897.

Whitehead KJ, Chan AC, Navankasattusas S, et al. The cerebral cavernous malformation signaling pathway promotes vascular integrity via Rho GTPases. *Nat Med*. 2009 Feb;15(2):177-184.

Zimmerman RS, Spetzler RF, Lee KS, et al. Cavernous malformations of the brain stem. *J Neurosurg*. 1991;75:32-39.

Numbered references appear on Expert Consult.

Surgical Management of Infratentorial Arteriovenous Malformations

TOMAS GÁRZÓN-MUVDI • GUSTAVO PRADILLA •
KIMON BEKELIS • PHILIPPE GAILLOUD • RAFAEL J. TAMARGO

Introduction

Brain stem and cerebellar arteriovenous malformations (AVMs) are rare vascular lesions that represent only a small fraction of all intracranial AVMs. Whereas brain stem AVMs are less likely to be appropriate for surgery, given their involvement of vital neural structures,[1] cerebellar AVMs are often treated surgically.[2-6] Olivecrona in 1932 performed the first successful resection of an infratentorial (cerebellar) AVM.[6,7] Current treatment algorithms for brain stem and cerebellar AVMs involve a multidisciplinary approach, where surgical resection, stereotactic radiosurgery (SRS), and endovascular embolization are used alone or in combination.[8-12]

Anatomy and Classification

Infratentorial AVMs consist of lesions located in the brain stem and the cerebellum. Given their location in the posterior fossa, AVMs in these locations are usually discussed together, despite their marked differences in clinical presentation, pathophysiology, and treatment options.[13] In this chapter we discuss them separately.

Brain stem AVMs encompass lesions in the midbrain, pons, and medulla. Angiography demonstrates the main arterial territories supplying the AVMs and facilitates their classification into three broad categories: (1) midbrain AVMs, supplied primarily by the superior cerebellar artery (SCA); (2) pontine AVMs, supplied primarily by the anterior inferior cerebellar artery (AICA); and (3) medullary AVMs, supplied primarily by the posterior inferior cerebellar artery (PICA) (Fig. 82-1).

Brain stem AVMs can then be subclassified according to the depth of their location into either superficial pial or parenchymal lesions. Pial brain stem AVMs are typically found in the anterolateral pons and are typically supplied by branches of an enlarged AICA, with venous drainage into the pontine-Galenic and petrosal systems,[14] the mesencephalic tectum, or the floor of the fourth ventricle. Parenchymal brain stem AVMs have variable locations within the brain stem and typically extend into the cerebellar peduncles. The most important difference between these two groups, however, lies on their potential resectability. Whereas superficial pial AVMs may be resectable—given early visualization and control of their superficial blood supply, as well as limited manipulation of critical structures—parenchymal AVMs have an arterial supply primarily consisting of perforating arteries, and they often require an approach through critical nuclei and fiber tracts.[14,15]

Cerebellar AVMs can be anatomically classified into hemispheric, vermian, and tonsillar lesions. Each of these locations has a characteristic arterial supply and a unique relationship to the fourth ventricle. Cerebellar hemispheric AVMs are typically supplied by SCA, AICA, and PICA branches and rarely involve the fourth ventricular ependyma. Vermian AVMs are most often supplied by the SCA and PICA and can extend into the fourth ventricular roof. Tonsilar AVMs are supplied by PICA branches and often project dorsally, away from the fourth ventricle (Fig. 82-1).

Although the Spetzler and Martin AVM classification[16] has been widely used and validated in supratentorial AVMs, this grading system, which takes into consideration size of the nidus, pattern of venous drainage, and location in eloquent areas, has been partially validated in infratentorial AVMs in only a few studies.[2,8,10]

Epidemiology

The annual incidence of brain AVMs has been estimated to be approximately 0.82 to 1.8 cases per 100,000 individuals.[17-19] The prevalence of AVMs is more difficult to ascertain, given that many are asymptomatic. In a total of 17 studies discussing the epidemiology of AVMs,[18-34] 11 were population studies[18-22,24,25,29,32-34] and 6 were autopsy studies.[23,26-28,30,31] These studies were conducted in centers across the United States,[19,23,24,30,32-34] Europe (Austria, Finland, Scotland, and Sweden),[20,25-28] the Caribbean Islands,[18] and Australia.[21] In these studies, the prevalence of AVMs ranged from 5 to 613 cases per 100,000 individuals. We then calculate the mean prevalence of AVMs to be 0.3% based on 284 cases per 100,000 individuals, with a 95% confidence interval (CI) of 108 to 461 cases per 100,000 individuals.

Infratentorial AVMs represent at most 20% of all intracranial AVMs.[9,14,35-37] However, because many of these

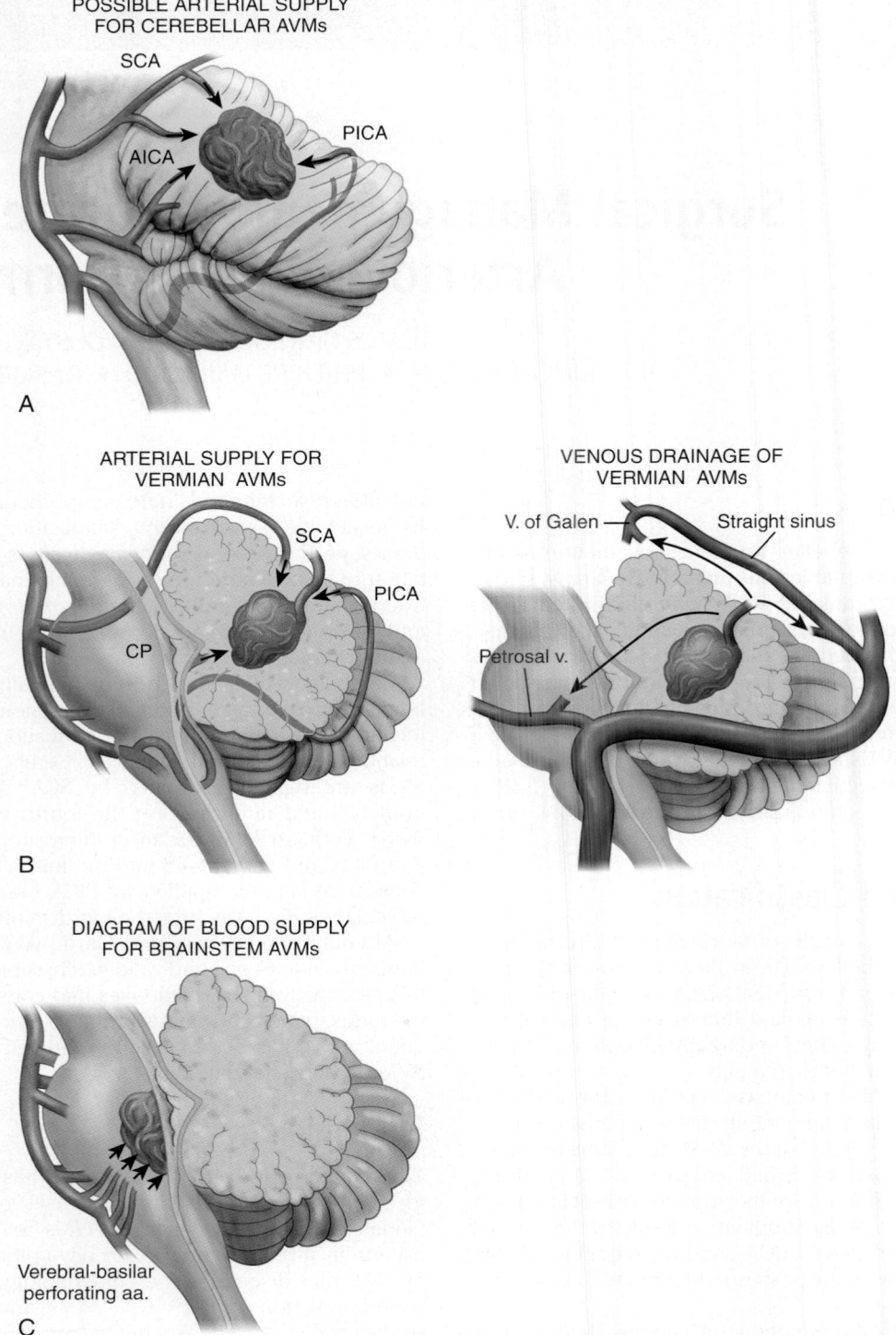

POSSIBLE ARTERIAL SUPPLY
FOR CEREBELLAR AVMs

SCA

PICA

AICA

A

ARTERIAL SUPPLY FOR
VERMIAN AVMs

SCA

PICA

CP

B

VENOUS DRAINAGE OF
VERMIAN AVMs

V. of Galen

Straight sinus

Petrosal v.

DIAGRAM OF BLOOD SUPPLY
FOR BRAINSTEM AVMs

Verebral-basilar
perforating aa.

C

FIGURE 82-1 Arterial blood supply for infratentorial AVMs according to their anatomic location. A, Possible arterial supply for cerebellar AVMs. B, Arterial supply (left) and venous drainage (right) for vermian AVMs. C, Diagram of blood supply for brain stem AVMs.

malformations remain asymptomatic, a true estimate of the prevalence of posterior fossa AVMs has not been formulated. Cerebellar AVMs constitute 12% to 16% of all intracranial AVMs and are four times more frequent that brain stem AVMs, which represent only 3% to 4% of all intracranial AVMs.[14,38]

Although patients with all infratentorial AVMs present at a mean age of 42 years,[39] those with brain stem AVMs present earlier, with their first symptoms occurring at a mean age of 32 years (range 9-65 years).[9] Patients diagnosed later in life with infratentorial AVMs tend to present with a hemorrhagic event.[39]

Although gender predominance has not been demonstrated in infratentorial AVMs, some studies report a slight female predominance.[9,12,39] Males with brain stem AVMs have a slightly higher risk of hemorrhage as opposed to females.[39]

Natural History

Infratentorial AVMs are rare entities that, in contrast to their supratentorial equivalents, present more commonly with hemorrhage (1.99 odds ratio, 1.07-3.69 95% CI).[39] The size of the AVM is a controversial risk factor for the first bleeding episode, since different analyses have yielded contradictory results.[40] Nevertheless, patients with small infratentorial AVMs may present more frequently with hemorrhage than those with large AVMs, given that small malformations otherwise remain asymptomatic.[40] Each episode of hemorrhage is accompanied by a 30% morbidity and a 10% mortality. Morbidity due to bleeding of posterior fossa AVMs is high given their critical location. Patients with posterior fossa AVMs have a high mortality associated with the first hemorrhagic episode (66.7%). In some studies, however, authors have found only a 27% mortality from the initial bleeding episode.[36] Subsequent hemorrhagic episodes often result in devastating neurologic deficits and have a mortality of 35.7%.[8,13] Risk factors for hemorrhage identified for all brain AVMs—but not necessarily for infratentorial AVMs—include young age, large size of the malformation, deep venous drainage, associated aneurysms, and infratentorial location.[1,40,41]

The annual risk of hemorrhage of infratentorial AVMs appears to be higher than that of all AVMs and ranges from 8.4% to 13%, but it is higher in patients with a prior hemorrhage.[2,8,39] After the first hemorrhagic episode and during the first 5 years after the same, infratentorial AVMs tend to hemorrhage repeatedly at a rate of 11.6% annually.[40] After this 5-year period, infratentorial AVMs carry an inherent risk of subsequent hemorrhage of 7.5% at 5 years and of 5% at 10 years.[42,43] Prospective studies have found that infratentorial AVMs have a higher annual rupture rate after the initial hemorrhage as compared to that of supratentorial AVMs.[40,41,44] Other studies have found an overall annual risk for subsequent hemorrhage of 8.4%, which increases to 9.4% in patients who initially presented with a hemorrhage.[8] The presence of associated aneurysms is another risk factor for poor outcome and subsequent hemorrhagic episodes. Hemodynamic factors that increase pressure gradients in the AVM, such as deep venous drainage, may also predispose patients to repeated hemorrhages.[35] Differences regarding the site of venous drainage or the location and degree of venous stenosis also affect bleeding rates of AVMs.[45,46]

Clinical Presentation

Patients with infratentorial AVMs can present with headaches, neurologic deficits, or pain.[38] Hemorrhage appears to be the most frequent clinical presentation and is more common in patients with small infratentorial AVMs (less than 2 cm in size).[47] Hemorrhagic episodes can be related to associated aneurysms on the feeding arteries of these lesions.[1] In patients with fourth ventricular hemorrhages, initial symptoms include those of obstructive hydrocephalus.

Less often, patients may present with progressive neurologic deficits but without hemorrhage. Under these circumstances, patients can present with a diverse array of symptoms, including headache, cranial nerve deficits, ataxia, dizziness, or hemiparesis. Although rare, infratentorial AVMs can cause mass effect and compression of important structures, especially in the confined space of the posterior fossa. While cerebellar compression may result in ataxia, dysmetria, and nystagmus, compression of the brain stem can affect different cranial nerve nuclei or traversing nerve fibers and may even present as trigeminal or glossopharyngeal neuralgia or as hemifacial spasm. Compression of the motor and sensory tracts may lead to hemiparesis and hemihypoalgesia.[12,15,48]

Preoperative Considerations

The three imaging studies needed to fully evaluate posterior fossa AVMs and plan their treatment are computed tomography (CT), magnetic resonance imaging (MRI), and digital subtraction angiography (DSA) (Fig. 82-3). CT scan best detects blood intraparenchymally, intraventricularly, or in the subarachnoid space, and is useful in identifying calcifications within the AVM. MRI reveals in detail the anatomic location of the AVM and its relationship to the surrounding structures. DSA provides critical information about feeding arteries and draining veins, as well as the structure of the nidus (i.e., compact vs. diffuse). All three studies are essential in the evaluation of an AVM.

CT scans are most useful in the initial evaluation of AVMs and in emergency settings in which the patient can quickly deteriorate as a result of intraparenchymal or intraventricular hemorrhage with hydrocephalus. CT scans detect approximately 95% of AVMs when contrast is used and about 84% when contrast is not used.[48] Hyperdense lesions are seen either intraparenchymally (i.e., after hemorrhage in the subarachnoid space), or intraventricularly.[48] Computed tomography angiography (CTA) may be useful in the initial evaluation of arterial supply and venous drainage of these lesions, and it may show enlarged arteries and draining veins, but CTA is not a substitute for DSA.[49]

MRI shows the anatomic relationship of the AVM to surrounding neural and vascular structures, either localizes the lesion entirely within the brain stem parenchyma or shows its pial representation, and can assist in determining previous bleeding episodes through hemosiderin-based sequences.[50] In T2 sequences, flow voids are evident and a hyperintense signal may be noted surrounding the lesion. Fluid-attenuated inversion recovery images show a hyperintense signal surrounding the AVM due to gliosis. Magnetic resonance angiography and venography can be misleading in AVMs because of the intermediate flow characteristics of the AVM vasculature (which is partially arterial and partially venous) and because turbulence and artifact from bony obstructions often encountered in the posterior fossa.[49]

The critical study for the diagnosis and evaluation of infratentorial AVMs is DSA with selective catheterization, which defines the arterial supply of the AVM, its venous drainage, and the size of the nidus.[49] In approximately 10% of posterior fossa AVMs, DSA shows a significant dural arterial component that originates from external carotid artery branches.[51] Also of critical importance are the presence of associated aneurysms and the visualization of *en passage* feeding arteries. These arteries do not connect directly to the malformation but go through and give branches to it, and they must be identified early on, since these vessels also supply critical structures in the brain stem.[3]

In preparation for surgery, size reduction of infratentorial AVMs may be possible using either endovascular embolization or SRS. The vascular supply to brain stem AVMs, however, makes endovascular therapies dangerous—particularly in parenchymal brain stem lesions, as perfusion through perforating arteries is frequently encountered and manipulation with a microcatheter and displacement of embolization materials can result in ischemia and stroke. The mortality and morbidity associated with embolization of brain stem AVMs can be high. In a series of cerebral AVMs treated with embolization, the authors found a mortality rate of 1.3% and a rate of moderate and severe complications of approximately 20%.[52]

SRS is often used in surgically inaccessible brain stem AVMs and has been shown to reduce the risk of hemorrhage.[10] In addition, SRS can be useful as a preoperative adjunct prior to microsurgical resection and in some series has minimized the need for embolization, decreased operative time, shortened hospital stay, and lowered morbidity.[53]

Timing of Surgery

Timing of surgery should be individualized by taking into consideration the general medical condition of the patient, age, and neurologic status, but in general we postpone surgery in patients with hemorrhagic presentations. Delaying surgery allows the patient to recover from the initial hemorrhage, facilitates hematoma organization or resolution, and allows for the evolution of dissection planes between the hematoma and the surrounding parenchyma.[3] In general, life-threatening hemorrhages and hematomas in the brain stem and cerebellum should be evacuated emergently to decrease mass effect and prevent acute hydrocephalus. In cases of acute intervention, it is often advisable to avoid the AVM nidus and to postpone surgical or radiologic treatment for at least 6 to 8 weeks.[14] A second angiogram should be obtained 6 to 8 weeks after the initial hemorrhagic episode and prior to microsurgical resection, since infratentorial AVMs may change overtime and even thrombose. Furthermore, the initial hematoma can prevent full visualization of compressed portions of the AVM.

Surgical Approaches

We favor the "park bench" position for all posterior fossa AVMs. This position is superior to the full prone position, because it decreases intrathoracic pressure (which minimizes ventilatory requirements and decreases venous congestion and intraoperative blood loss) and lowers intracranial pressure.

A large craniectomy and dural opening are important to gain full access to the vascular malformation within the limited space afforded by the posterior fossa. The craniectomy should expose the venous sinuses involved in drainage of the AVM. While access to cerebellar AVMs is easily obtained via midline, lateral, or combined suboccipital craniectomies, access to brain stem AVMs can be achieved through a variety of more complex corridors, depending on the location of the AVM. For instance, in ventrolateral pontine lesions, a lateral retrosigmoid exposure may not provide sufficient exposure and a far-lateral transcondylar approach may be required (Figure 82-2). The latter facilitates early visualization of the parent arterial feeders. Access to AVMs in the dorsal brain stem is dictated by their craniocaudal location and can be obtained via transvermian or telovelar exposures.

INCISION

For laterally located lesions, a "hockey stick" incision is used, which begins above the ear, descends to the superior nuchal line, reaches the midline, and continues down along the midline to the spinous process of C6 or C7. For vermian or tonsillar AVMs, a midline incision from the occiput to C3 is preferred.

CRANIECTOMY

A large suboccipital craniectomy should always be performed to allow exposure of the entire lesion, since complete visualization of feeding arteries, draining veins, and involved transverse or sigmoid sinuses is critical prior to resection of the nidus.[6] Careful dissection of the dura from the periosteal surface prior to elevation of the flap (if a craniotomy as opposed to a craniectomy is performed) is important to avoid injury to draining veins, since emissary veins and tributaries into the transverse, sigmoid, or petrosal sinuses or to the jugular bulb can be encountered. For lesions located in the midline along the cerebellar vermis, a large midline exposure is adequate; for lesions located in the lateral aspect of the cerebellum and brain stem, including the cerebellopontine angle, a lateral exposure via a suboccipital retrosigmoid approach or a far-lateral transcondylar approach (Fig. 82-2) can provide adequate visualization and if needed can be extended laterally to access the cerebellopontine angle cistern[14] and the ventrolateral brain stem. Removal of the lip of the foramen magnum is usually helpful.

INTRAOPERATIVE MONITORING

Brain stem auditory evoked potentials and somatosensory evoked potentials are used routinely during the resection of infratentorial AVMs. Electrophysiologic monitoring has proved useful in determining the extent of the resection of brain stem AVMs.[54,55]

Intraoperative angiography before conclusion of the case is essential to confirm obliteration of the AVM.[14] If residual malformation is identified, the resection can be completed and angiography repeated. The presence of a residual malformation can increase the risk for postoperative complications.[6]

LESION RESECTION

Early identification and interruption of the arterial supply as close to the nidus as possible and preservation of the draining veins until the final stages of the resection are critical. Resection of the AVM follows a standard technique of circumferential dissection. Feeding arteries and draining veins have aberrant morphology and are invariably arterialized, which often makes differentiation between arteries and veins challenging. For this reason, feeding arteries should be occluded preliminarily using temporary aneurysm clips to observe the response of the AVM. Darkening of the blood in the AVM and decreased turgidity are favorable signs. An increase in

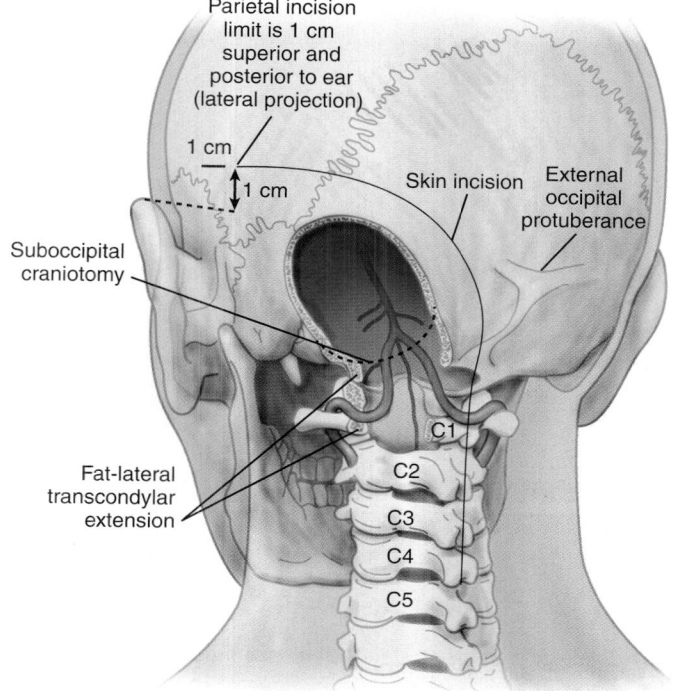

FIGURE 82-2 Artist's rendering of the far-lateral transcondylar approach to infratentorial AVMs.

AVM pulsation and turgidity indicate that the temporarily occluded vessel may be a draining vein. The dissection proceeds circumferentially from superficial to deep until all arterial vessels are ligated. Small hemostatic clips are preferred over aneurysm clips for permanent arterial ligation due to their lower profile and size. The disadvantage of hemostatic clips is that they are difficult to remove once applied. Special attention should be given to small vascular loops that are encountered in the periphery of the AVM. These loops that emerge from the AVM wall and reenter the lesion are almost always shunting vessels or draining venules that should be preserved until the arterial supply has been completely obliterated. Cumulative interruption of many of these loops can be equivalent to premature interruption of a major draining vein. After complete dissection and devascularization of the AVM, draining veins are ligated and divided and the remainder of the lesion is dissected from the surrounding parenchyma.

Although we do not typically use intraoperative ultrasound, some authors advocate its use to guide the resection of parenchymal AVMs and report that it can reduce operative time and decrease blood loss.[56,57]

Postoperative Management

Postoperatively, patients are admitted to the neurosurgical intensive care unit and monitored closely for signs of acute intracranial hypertension due to postoperative hemorrhage or thrombosis of the venous system. Surveillance of arterial pressure and maintenance of normotension or hypotension in the first 48 to 72 hours of the postoperative period may protect against bleeding in the surgical bed. It may also be necessary to implement measures to avoid obstructive hydrocephalus secondary to postoperative cerebellar edema, such as ventriculostomy and corticosteroids. If intraoperative electrophysiologic monitoring suggests possible injury of cranial nerves, affecting swallowing reflex or corneal sensation, measures may be taken to avoid further complications (i.e., tracheostomy, gastrostomy, temporary tarsorrhaphy, moisture chambers, and meticulous eye care). Intraoperative angiography may be complemented by postoperative angiography if a residual vascular malformation is suspected in the intraoperative angiogram.[3]

Complications

Intraoperatively, complications such as hemorrhage, edema, and ischemia can occur due to compromise of draining veins or injury to an *en passage* vessel. Disturbance of the normal venous drainage of the cerebellum can result in significant edema. Cerebellar and brain stem edema can also result from inadequate patient ventilation or obstructive hydrocephalus. Disturbance of arteriovenous shunts within the malformation during the resection can result in edema and hemorrhage of the parenchyma surrounding the AVM, but loss of autoregulation of the cerebral vasculature and obstruction of the venous drainage are also contributing factors.[58-61] Inadvertent occlusion or delayed thrombosis of normal veins during resection can similarly be problematic. Postoperatively, patients can develop a range of problems, including cranial neuropathies, ataxia and dysmetria secondary to cerebellar and peduncular injury, hemiplegia from corticospinal tract injury, and proprioceptive loss from injury to medial lemniscal fibers. Brain stem ischemia and strokes can also present after surgery due to lack of collateral vessels.[1,8,9,12,50]

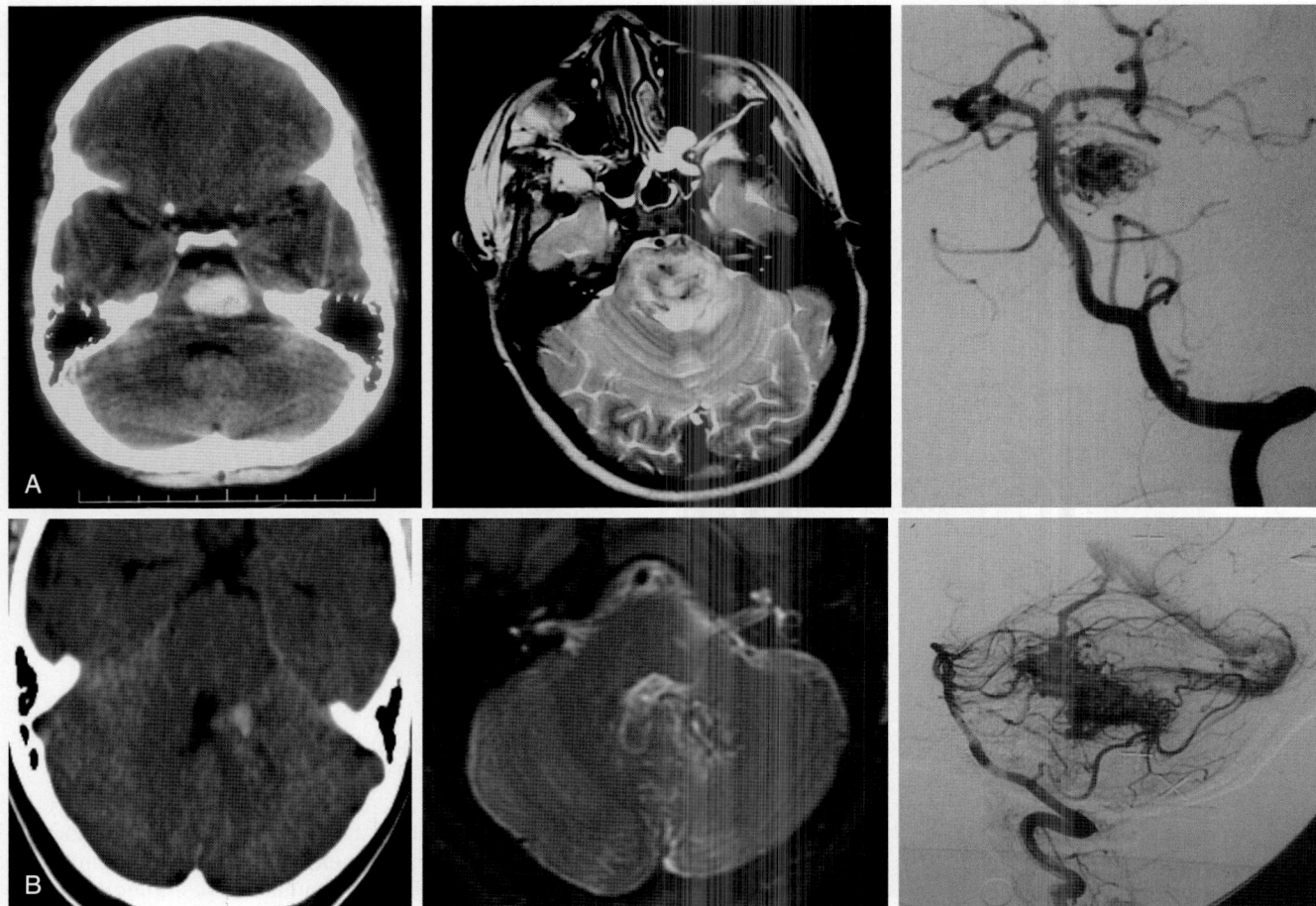

FIGURE 82-3 Radiologic characteristics of cerebellar and brain stem AVMs. A, MRI and DSA of a brain stem AVM. B, MRI and DSA of a cerebellar AVM.

Alternative Treatments

Stereotactic aspiration of the hematoma performed acutely to relieve mass effect from hemorrhage has been described.[62,63] This technique, however, has the risk of injury to vital brain stem structures as precise targeting and planning of the needle trajectory may be hindered by evolving edema and artifact from the acute hemorrhage. Furthermore, if the malformation vasculature is injured a bleeding episode may ensue, and hematoma evacuation would be suboptimal.[6,64]

ENDOVASCULAR THERAPY

As discussed previously, endovascular embolization of brain stem AVMs may be useful before surgical resection to decrease flow to the nidus and should target large vessels that are difficult to reach during the initial stages of the procedure, such as the ventricular branches of AICA and SCA. When the feeding arteries arise from PICA, embolization of large infratentorial malformations is often feasible. Proximal embolization of these vessels should be avoided to circumvent the possibility of cerebellar infarction, more so when the vessels are readily accessible during the surgical procedure. Complications due to embolization, such as brain stem and cerebellar infarcts and hemorrhage, can be significant and should be considered before utilizing this treatment method.[65] Combined surgical and endovascular treatment should be considered in superficial AVMs of the brain stem and cerebellum, since these may be safely resected.[8]

STEREOTACTIC RADIOSURGERY

Radiosurgery has evolved as the main treatment modality of brain stem AVMs and AVMs of the deep cerebellar nuclei. Parenchymal brain stem AVMs should be treated with radiosurgery alone. Radiosurgery has been extensively used to treat brain stem AVMs, with an obliteration rate of 73% at 3 years after treatment.[5] Complications due to radiosurgery have been seen in approximately 10% of patients in previous studies.[8] These complications include radiation necrosis of the brain stem and cerebellum, leading to cranial nerve palsies and hemiparesis.

Conclusions

Surgical treatment of infratentorial AVMs is challenging and carries significant risks. Cerebellar and brain stem AVMs have distinct clinical and pathophysiologic features, and they require different therapeutic approaches. While cerebellar AVMs are often resectable, brain stem AVMs are approached selectively based on their location, as pial malformations may be amenable for surgical resection but parenchymal malformations are rarely resected and instead are treated with SRS. Diagnostic evaluation requires CT and MRI scans and DSA. Microsurgical resection of selected superficial (mostly cerebellar) lesions is feasible and follows a standard technique of circumferential dissection with careful identification of feeding arteries and draining veins. Intraoperative angiography is critical to avoid incomplete resection. Finally, successful treatment of infratentorial AVMs requires a multimodality approach, combining diagnostic and interventional neuroradiology, microsurgical resection, and SRS in carefully selected patients.

KEY REFERENCES

Akdemir H, Oktem S, Menku A, et al. Image-guided microneurosurgical management of small arteriovenous malformation: role of neuronavigation and intraoperative Doppler sonography. *Minim Invasive Neurosurg.* 2007;50:163-169.

ApSimon HT, Reef H, Phadke RV, Popovic EA. A population-based study of brain arteriovenous malformation: long-term treatment outcomes. *Stroke.* 2002;33:2794-2800.

Arnaout OM, Gross BA, Eddleman CS, et al. Posterior fossa arteriovenous malformations. *Neurosurg Focus.* 2009;26:E12.

Batjer HH, Devous Sr MD, Meyer YJ, et al. Cerebrovascular hemodynamics in arteriovenous malformation complicated by normal perfusion pressure breakthrough. *Neurosurgery.* 1988;22:503-509.

Batjer H, Samson D. Arteriovenous malformations of the posterior fossa. Clinical presentation, diagnostic evaluation, and surgical treatment. *J Neurosurg.* 1986;64:849-856.

Chang SD, Lopez JR, Steinberg GK. The usefulness of electrophysiological monitoring during resection of central nervous system vascular malformations. *J Stroke Cerebrovasc Dis.* 1999;8:412-422.

da Costa L, Thines L, Dehdashti AR, et al. Management and clinical outcome of posterior fossa arteriovenous malformations: report on a single-centre 15-year experience. *J Neurol Neurosurg Psychiatry.* 2009;80:376-379.

da Costa L, Wallace MC, Ter Brugge KG, et al. The natural history and predictive features of hemorrhage from brain arteriovenous malformations. *Stroke.* 2009;40:100-105.

Guidetti B, Delitala A. Intracranial arteriovenous malformations. Conservative and surgical treatment. *J Neurosurg.* 1980;53:149-152.

Hernesniemi JA, Dashti R, Juvela S, et al. Natural history of brain arteriovenous malformations: a long-term follow-up study of risk of hemorrhage in 238 patients. *Neurosurgery.* 2008;63:823-829.

Hillman J. Population-based analysis of arteriovenous malformation treatment. *J Neurosurg.* 2001;95:633-637.

Jessurun GA, Kamphuis DJ, van der Zande FH, Nossent JC. Cerebral arteriovenous malformations in The Netherlands Antilles. High prevalence of hereditary hemorrhagic telangiectasia-related single and multiple cerebral arteriovenous malformations. *Clin Neurol Neurosurg.* 1993;95:193-198.

Kashiwagi S, van Loveren HR, Tew Jr JM, et al. Diagnosis and treatment of vascular brain-stem malformations. *J Neurosurg.* 1990;72:27-34.

Khaw AV, Mohr JP, Sciacca RR, et al. Association of infratentorial brain arteriovenous malformations with hemorrhage at initial presentation. *Stroke.* 2004;35:660-663.

Osborn A, Blaser S, Provenzale J, et al. Arteriovenous malformations. In: Osborn A, ed. *Diagnostic Imaging. Brain.* Altona, Manitoba: Amirsys; 2004:I5.

O'Shaughnessy BA, Getch CC, Bendok BR, Batjer HH. Microsurgical resection of infratentorial arteriovenous malformations. *Neurosurg Focus.* 2005;19:E5.

Pollock BE, Gorman DA, Brown PD. Radiosurgery for arteriovenous malformations of the basal ganglia, thalamus, and brainstem. *J Neurosurg.* 2004;100:210-214.

Samson D, Kopitnik Jr TA, Batjer H, Purdy PD. Technical Features of the Management of Arteriovenous Malformations of the Brainstem and Cerebellum. In: Batjer H, ed. *Cerebrovascular Disease.* Philadelphia: Lippincott-Raven Publishers; 1997:811-821.

Sanchez-Mejia RO, McDermott MW, Tan J, et al. Radiosurgery facilitates resection of brain arteriovenous malformations and reduces surgical morbidity. *Neurosurgery.* 2009;64:231-238.

Sinclair J, Kelly ME, Steinberg GK. Surgical management of posterior fossa arteriovenous malformations. *Neurosurgery.* 2006;58:189-201.

Spetzler RF, Martin NA. A proposed grading system for arteriovenous malformations. *J Neurosurg.* 1986;65:476-483.

Stapf C, Mast H, Sciacca RR, et al. Predictors of hemorrhage in patients with untreated brain arteriovenous malformation. *Neurology.* 2006;66:1350-1355.

Taylor CL, Dutton K, Rappard G, et al. Complications of preoperative embolization of cerebral arteriovenous malformations. *J Neurosurg.* 2004;100:810-812.

Unsgaard G, Ommedal S, Rygh OM, Lindseth F. Operation of arteriovenous malformations assisted by stereoscopic navigation-controlled display of preoperative magnetic resonance angiography and intraoperative ultrasound angiography. *Neurosurgery.* 2007;61:407-415.

Zabel-du Bois A, Milker-Zabel S, Huber P, et al. Stereotactic LINAC-based radiosurgery in the treatment of cerebral arteriovenous malformations located deep, involving corpus callosum, motor cortex, or brainstem. *Int J Radiat Oncol Biol Phys.* 2006;64:1044-1048.

Numbered references appear on Expert Consult.

CHAPTER 83

Surgical Management of Cerebral Arteriovenous Malformations

EDGARDO SPAGNUOLO

Talking or writing about the "surgical treatment" of cerebral arteriovenous malformations (AVMs) implies describing more than just opening the skull and resecting the nidus that constitutes the lesion. The surgical treatment involves everything concerning the endovascular surgery (or endovascular therapy); the radiation treatment, widely dominated by radiosurgery; and the classic surgical resection of the malformation.

The surgical treatment of an AVM is continually being updated. By the time this chapter is published, some innovations or changes may have already been carried out; hence, some guidelines given here may have become obsolete.

Advances in microneurosurgery, anesthetic techniques, endovascular surgery, and radiosurgery determine that some therapies proposed to date have to be changed or that some treatment protocols have to be modified.

History

AVM neurosurgery is a relatively recent innovation. Even though there have long been reports about the surgical management of this kind of lesion, only from 1960 onward has the veritable surgery become a reality. In the 1960s, endovascular treatments started to be performed as a way to assist neurosurgeons in the resection of such lesions. Since the first description of embolization by Luessenhop and Spence in 1960,[1] endovascular procedures have been improved, enabling a dramatic change in the direction of AVM treatments. In that same decade, with the appearance of the operating microscope, surgery took a 180-degree turn in everything regarding neurosurgery, including neurovascular surgery.[1] Permanent laboratory practice in microsurgery, better and continued training in neuroanatomy, and constant development of surgical instruments for microsurgery, together with the supraspecialization in vascular neurosurgery, have led neurosurgeons to acquire more practice in the resection of such lesions, with a consequent decrease in morbidity and mortality. Eventually, radiosurgery came up and started to become popular as an adjuvant treatment—or as the only treatment for some cerebral AVMs—in the 1980s.

Fifty years! Thanks to the appearance of the different procedures and technologies mentioned above, their improvement, and the combination of all of them, it can be said that such is the age of the AVM surgery.

Classification

As AVMs became known, particularly their characteristics and the difficulties they posed in each case, they started to be classified according to different factors. Such classifications sought and still seek to help neurosurgeons decide whether to treat a cerebral AVM and what therapeutic procedures would be most appropriate for each case.[2]

In 1977, Luessenhop and Gennarelli proposed a classification based on the arterial pedicles that supplied AVMs.[1,17] This classification did not take into account the draining veins or whether AVMs were located in eloquent areas. In 1984, Luessenhop, with Rosa's collaboration, published a grading scale based on AVM size.[4,18] Even though it was an easily applicable classification, it was not practical for surgery because it did not consider the venous drainage or whether it was in an eloquent area. Sugita also classified AVMs located at the sylvian fissure, taking into account whether they were directly in the fissure, lateral, medial, or deep seated.[3] In 1986, Shi and Chen published a classification that took into account size, location, depth, the feeding arteries, and the venous drainage.[4,18] It was a complex classification, one difficult to remember due to the various combinations therein (since it had seven grades), and the determination of eloquent or noneloquent areas was imprecise. But in that same year Spetzler and Martin's classification was published, which took into account size, location, and venous drainage.[4] This classification turned out to be the most practical one, and its diffusion and acceptance worldwide were fast and unanimous. As time went by, and with the application of this classification, it became evident that AVMs in grade III presented different difficulties in treatment and prognosis. This was motivated by the variability of the lesions included in this grade: for example, it included a small AVM with deep venous drainage located in an eloquent area, such as the brain stem, as well as a 6-cm-wide cortical lesion with superficial venous drainage located in a noneloquent area. This range led several authors to propose modifications to this grade of the classification. The most accepted ones are grades IIIA and IIIB, regarding location.[3-6]

Even though modifications are still being proposed, the Spetzler-Martin classification is the most commonly used at present, and treatment criteria are mostly based on it. Regardless, with the existing research possibilities on brain function, it is becoming increasingly difficult to speak of eloquent and noneloquent areas. In one way or another, practically the whole brain is "eloquent."

Based on my experience, as well as on the work that has been carried out in Uruguay for year, and the concepts given by Borovich in the 1980s,[6] I would add to the Spetzler-Martin classification the arterial territories involved in AVMs. They are grouped according to whether one, two, or three vascular territories are involved. Most AVMs are included in the groups for one or two vascular territories, which correspond, to a great extent, to grades I to III in the Spetzler-Martin classification.[6]

Treatment

In a publication about the management of AVMs in 1979, almost 20 years after the beginning of the AVM era, Drake proposed five options neurosurgeons could use when dealing with such a lesion[7]:

- Expectant behavior (which certainly refers to aggressive treatments, not to treatment symptoms, e.g., epilepsy)
- Surgery
- Endovascular therapy
- Radiotherapy (radiosurgery)
- Combination of the preceding options

What Drake proposed has never become obsolete. The five points suggested are still present in the neurosurgeons' considerations when dealing with cerebral AVMs.

After complete surgical resection of an AVM, with no evidence of remaining lesions in the angiographic control, the patient can be deemed cured. Although this happens in the vast majority of the cases, AVM relapses have been reported.[8] It is my opinion that in such cases the angiographic subtraction control study failed to reveal small pathologic pedicles, from which the lesion subsequently reproduced.

Better knowledge of the natural history of AVMs, their flow, the pressure at the nidus, and AVM functionality, as well as that of the surrounding brain, has permitted substantial improvement in the prognosis of such lesions in the last two decades. This has been achieved through the use of dynamic studies, such as supraselective digital angiographies, digital subtraction angiography combined with color scaling, diffusion and perfusion magnetic resonance imaging with flow study, magnetic resonance imaging tractography, magnetoencephalography, and positron emission tomography. All these techniques allow better knowledge of the malformation, its behavior, and the characteristics of the surrounding brain, thus enabling the surgical team to plan the best treatment or combination of treatments for each case.[9-16]

Constant advances in neuroanesthesia with brain protection allow complex surgeries, sometimes with transitory interruption of blood flow through the arteries (transitory clipping), to become less harmful. The association of neurophysiologic intraoperative monitoring with intraoperative control of the areas where the surgeon is working, as well as control of the remaining brain functions during transitory clipping, further increases the possibility for success in such surgeries. In turn, they permit surgeries that, due to the topography or complexity of the lesion, would have been impossible to perform in the past.

Arteriovenous Malformations

Vascular malformations of the brain (excluding aneurysms) constitute a heterogeneous group of lesions that includes AVMs, pial malformations, cavernous angiomas, venous malformations, dural fistulae, and telangiectasias. Therefore, AVMs widely dominate the spectrum of lesions.[17]

Cerebral AVMs are lesions of likely congenital origin or predisposition constituted by a conglomerate of abnormal vessels (both arterial and venous) of variable size and number. There is no intermediate capillary network; there is no parenchyma among vessels. Usually, AVMs are surrounded by a thin layer of nonfunctioning brain tissue (reactional gliosis).[6,17]

Independent of their classification, AVMs can be divided into one of two categories, superficial (also called "of the convexity," "cortical," or "corticosubcortical") or deep, when planning for their treatment.[6,18] Given the variability of these lesions, in both their anatomy and their physiology, there is no universal consensus about how to treat them, even those AVMs that a priori could be similar. Thus, there have long been attempts to establish standards and guidelines for the treatment of AVMs. The problem lies in rapid changes to the proposed guidelines arising from development in diagnostic techniques and knowledge about AVMs and their treatments.

Regardless, the guidelines are recommendations formulated by groups of professionals dedicated to a particular pathology and must be taken as a base for the treatment of AVMs. They are flexible and can be modified according to the results of the different possible treatments and to the appearance of new therapeutics.[19,20]

Through its chapter on vascular neurosurgery, the Latin American Federation of Neurosurgical Societies in 2003 formulated the first recommendations for the management of AVMs.[17] In 2009, I led a group of neurosurgeons dedicated to vascular surgery who published an updated version of those recommendations under the (translated) title "Recommendations for the Management of Brain Arteriovenous Malformations."[17] This publication aims to offer the specialist a guide for managing such lesions, but by no means is strict compliance necessary.[17,19]

In the last decade, several authors have published guides with the same objective (e.g., Vazquez and Larrea in 2000,[21] Ogilvy et al. in 2001,[19] and Starke et al. in 2009[22]). These guides do not substantially differ in their recommendations, proposing surgery for grades I and II, combination of treatment for grade III, and conservative treatment for grades IV and V. Starke et al. conclude that surgery is the ideal and curative treatment. They advocate surgery, endovascular surgery, radiosurgery, or combination therapies depending on various factors: angioarchitecture of the AVM, topography, experience of the surgical team, and so on.[19-22]

AVMs are lesions whose incidence ranges between 1.4% and 4.3% of the population.[23,24] The percentage of symptomatic AVMs is unknown, but it has been proved that they are "dynamic" lesions.[23,24] In other words, a cerebral AVM diagnosed but not treated can show in a high percentage of the cases, under a periodic follow-up, changes in its anatomy, size, and symptomatology.[23,24] Hence, the conservative (do nothing) treatment should not be considered in low-grade malformations or in high-grade AVMs that have shown important clinical aggressiveness, such as repeated bleeding and epilepsy that is difficult to control.

When a treatment for an AVM is proposed—which should be a curative one—it should have a lower morbidity and mortality than those accorded by the natural history of that particular malformation. The treatment or treatments to be carried out in each case issue from the discussion of a multidisciplinary group formed by neurosurgeons, neurointerventionists, neurophysiologists, neurointensivists, neuroanesthesiologists, and neurologists. With all the necessary studies that enable understanding of an AVM (computed tomography, magnetic resonance with functional components, digital angiography, etc.), the team can then decide whether to treat the lesion. If treatment is chosen, one or a combination of the previously mentioned options should be chosen. Every time the team decides to treat an AVM, a curative treatment should be sought, which means the elimination of the lesion. If the treatment was meant to be curative but a remnant of the lesion remained, the treatment is considered a failure. Frequently, palliative treatments are considered, for instance, when dealing with grade V AVMs with recurrent bleeding. In such cases, we know that the possibility of curing the patient is low, but a palliative treatment may significantly reduce the possibility of future bleeding.[25-28]

When and How to Treat a Cerebral AVM

Cerebral AVMs manifest clinically through bleeding in 50% of the cases, followed by epilepsy. When an AVM has bled, it must be treated. When we face epilepsy refractory to the medical treatment, it must also be treated. When we face an AVM with no bleeding or significant clinical manifestations but with studies that show it presents intranidal aneurysms, stenosis of the afferent vessels, or significant venous stasis, it also must be treated. If AVMs are small and deep seated, they also must be treated, since it is accepted that they have a greater chance of developing complications. Regardless, studies have not been able to demonstrate—based on levels of evidence—a clear correlation between the characteristics of the lesion and its chances of bleeding.[26,27,29,30]

Following the analysis of malformations according to the Spetzler-Martin grading scale, the following guidelines could be established.[17]

GRADE I AND II AVMS

Grade I AVMs should always, in principle, be treated. Due to their characteristics, they should not pose any difficulty for the surgeon. Direct surgery without prior endovascular treatment is the indicated, and curative, procedure. Morbidity and mortality rates are extremely low. If this malformation has not bled, the second option is radiosurgery. There is a period (perhaps up to 2 years) during which the malformation can bleed until its disappearance.

The endovascular option would be, for this group, in the third place. Even though they should not represent any difficulty for the endovascular surgeon, the angiographic disappearance of the lesions does not ensure they have been cured. Small, nonvisible pedicles may exist that may make

the nidus reappear.[2,5,6-19,21-23,25,31-37] Even though previous papers mentioned total and definitive occlusion with histo-acryl glue,[38] recent publications about treatment with Onyx reinforce that grade I AVMs can be cured with endovascular treatment (Fig. 83-1).[39,40]

GRADE I AVM

1. Surgery
2. Radiosurgery
3. Endovascular therapy
4. Do nothing

In principle, grade II AVMs should be treated. The natural risks are higher than those consequent to the treatment. As with grade I AVMs, surgery is the first therapeutic option for this group. It ensures the complete cure and, due to the characteristics that determine lesions' inclusion in this grade, they should not indicate a priori a major difficulty for a well-trained neurosurgeon. Endovascular therapy (endovascular neurosurgery) may be of help for the surgeon as treatment prior to surgery. However, it is not advisable as the sole therapeutic option. Although it is possible to achieve an "angiographic cure" by means of endovascular therapy, it is highly probable the presence of small pedicles not revealed in the studies that will determine the reappearance of the lesion, evidenced in early or later angiographic controls (1 or 2 years later) if it has not bled previously. Surgeons are well aware that when operating patients with this grade of AVM (with complete angiographic closure after the endovascular therapy), arterial open pedicles are always found and even some arterialized veins are seen. In surgery, as the nidus is being surrounded and these small pedicles are coagulated, the aspect of the lesion visibly changes.

Radiosurgery is not indicated as a stand-alone option in this group of lesions. It can be considered a second-line treatment after endovascular therapy has been carried out, but it has been proved (as in AVMs of higher volume) that the area to be radiated does not include the whole nidus and that areas treated by endovascular means may not be included, thus leading to lesion reproduction in the long term.[13,17,75] Even though the proposal to always treat grade I

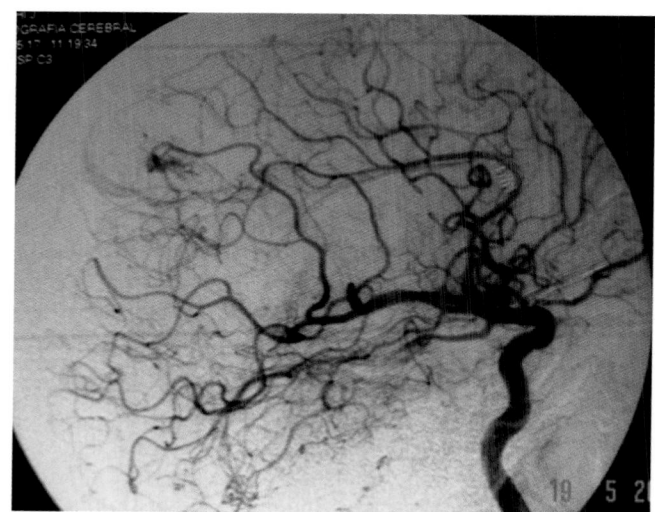

FIGURE 83-1 Grade I AVM. Only one pedicle, small size.

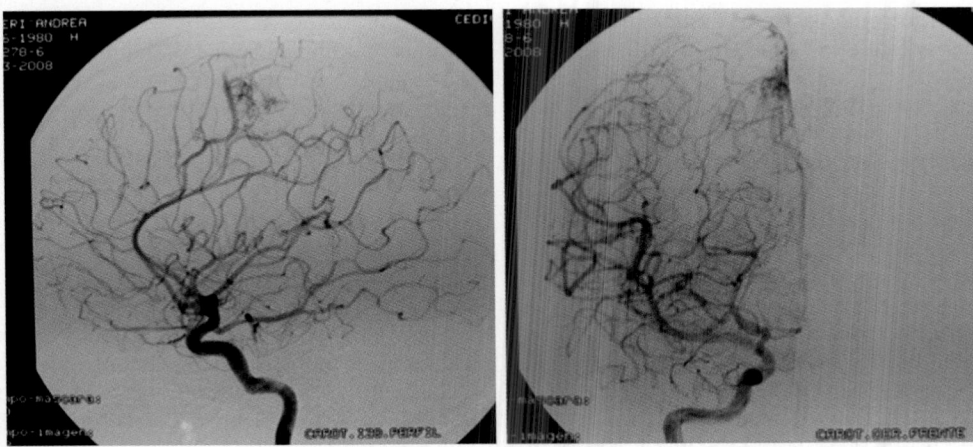

FIGURE 83-2 Grade II AVM. Two pedicles, small size, eloquent area.

and II AVMs may be controversial, the specialized bibliography supports my strong recommendation for surgery (Fig. 83-2).[2,5,6-19,21-23,25,29,31-37]

GRADE II AVM

1. Surgery
2. Endovascular therapy + surgery
3. Endovascular therapy
4. Radiosurgery
5. Surgery + radiosurgery

Grade I and II AVMs have with surgery (alone or combined) a cure rate close to 100%.[17,31,32,36,37,41,42]

GRADE III AVMS

Grade III AVMs must always be treated. They can become highly problematic due to the extensive number of variants that can appear within this group. AVMs that have a large nidus, are superficial (corticosubcortical), and involve one or two vascular territories must always be treated by means of combined techniques. Endovascular therapy is essential in these cases (in either one or two sessions) and is aimed at progressively occluding the afferent vessels (through which inversion of the flow is achieved) but not causing a sudden redistribution of it, which could be harmful. Endovascular therapy with Onyx offers excellent results in this group of AVMs as a treatment prior to surgery.[43,44] A prudent amount of time should elapse between this treatment and surgery (no less than 4 or 5 days). After the surgery, and by means of a control angiogram, the complete elimination of the nidus must be verified. If small remnants remain, the treatment can be complemented with radiosurgery.

Direct surgery can be performed in these AVMs, but a grade III malformation that was embolized beforehand clearly bleeds less, the surgery time diminishes significantly, and the possibility of sequelae lowers dramatically. Grade III AVMs, although small, are always deep seated. They pose technical and surgical difficulties, but not unsurpassable ones, as explained later. According to their topography, it is possible to plan the surgery with assistance (e.g., neuronavigation and stereotaxy).

Endovascular therapy (depending on the afferent pedicles) with radiosurgery and radiosurgery alone are valid options in these cases.

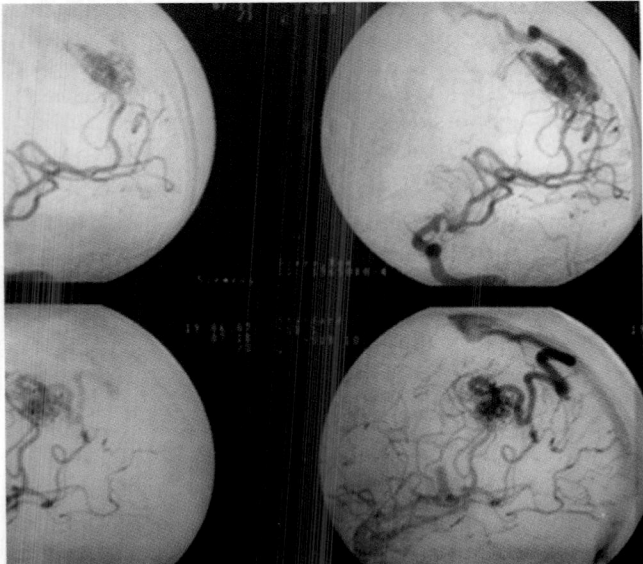

FIGURE 83-3 Grade III AVM. Eloquent area, superficial location, and deep venous drainage.

Most lesions within this grade, when treated, have a cure rate close to 100% but a morbidity rate close to 25%.[27,31,37] As with grades I and II, the preceding proposal may result in controversy, but the specialized bibliography recommends such treatment (Figs. 83-3 and 83-4).[17,21-23,25,31-37,45]

GRADE III AVM

1. Endovascular therapy + surgery
2. Surgery
3. Endovascular therapy + surgery + radiosurgery
4. Endovascular therapy + radiosurgery
5. Radiosurgery

GRADE IV AVMS

Grade IV AVMs that have not bled and do not have angiographic signs suggestive of complications (e.g., intranidal aneurysms) should be controlled with clinical and imagenologic evaluation.[19,22,33,34] The morbidity and mortality rates of the treatment are higher than those supplied by

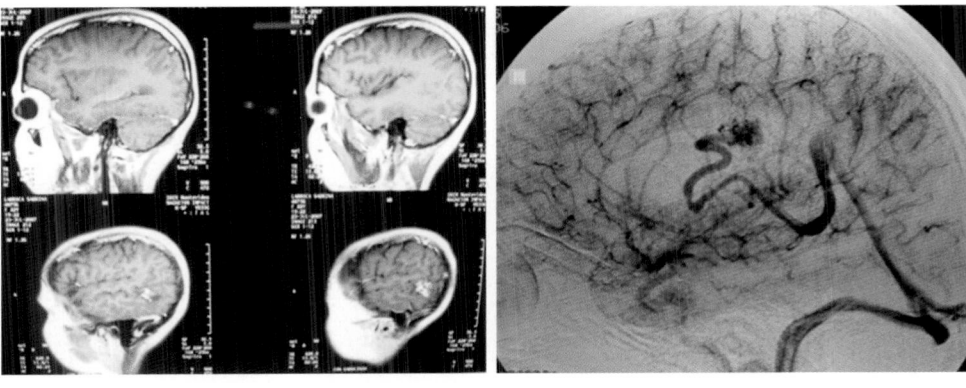

FIGURE 83-4 Grade III AVM. Small size, deep localization, and deep venous drainage.

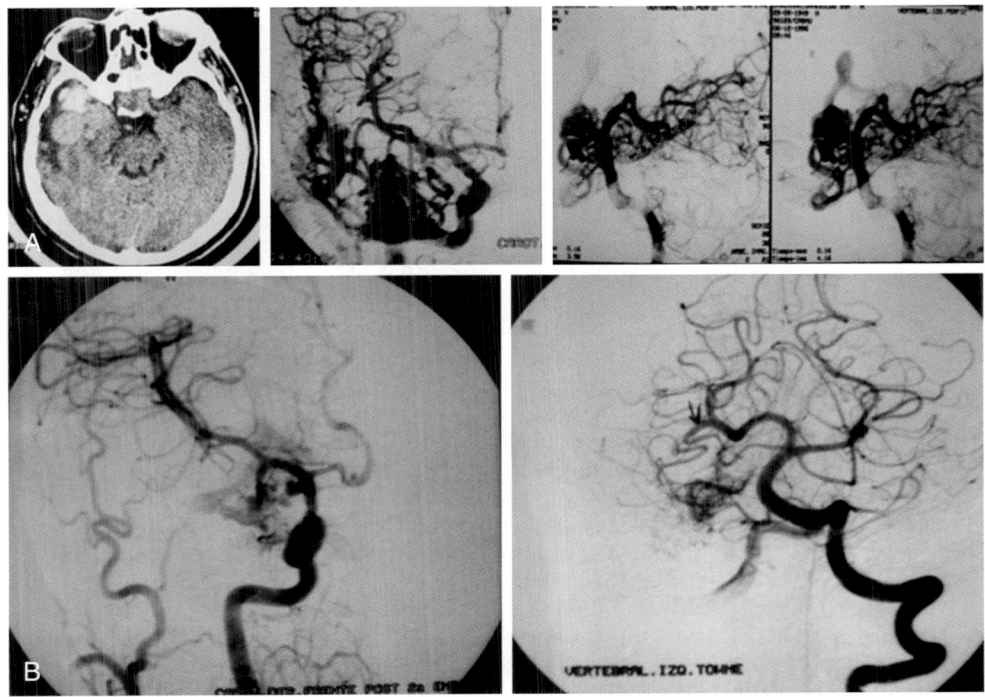

FIGURE 83-5 Grade IV AVM. A, Preembolization. B, Postembolization but before surgery.

spontaneous course. If there was hemorrhage, these AVMs must be treated, since it is well known that if a lesion of such characteristics has bled and the patient survived, the AVMs will bleed again. In addition, it is highly likely that after hemorrhage the patient will present with neurologic sequelae, which diminishes the rate of sequelae occurrence due to treatment.

If these lesions are treated, the treatment should always be a combination of techniques, starting with endovascular therapy. The number of sessions depends on the characteristics of the lesion, the number of pedicles, the compromised vascular territories, and the results of every session of endovascular therapy. There are always at least two sessions. Once the endovascular treatment has been completed, a prudent amount of time must elapse; this period should be decided on by the multidisciplinary team in charge of the treatment, because surgery is the next step. A posteriori, and if the angiographic control shows any remnant, the treatment is completed with radiosurgery.

When these cerebral vascular malformations are treated (using a combination of options), the cure rate is close to 100%, but the possibility of sequelae rises to almost 50%.[17,21,22,32-34]

Sometimes a palliative treatment will be proposed: endovascular surgery in association with radiosurgery or as a standalone option. With such treatment, the possibility of bleeding is reduced but the patient is not necessarily cured (Fig. 83-5).

GRADE IV AVM

1. Do nothing
2. Endovascular therapy + surgery
3. Endovascular therapy + surgery + radiosurgery
4. Endovascular therapy + radiosurgery
5. Endovascular therapy

GRADE V AVMS

In principle, grade V AVMs are not treated.[17,19,37] Risks are high; cure is possible, but at the cost of sequelae. If they are aggressive lesions, in the sense of presenting recurrent bleeding,

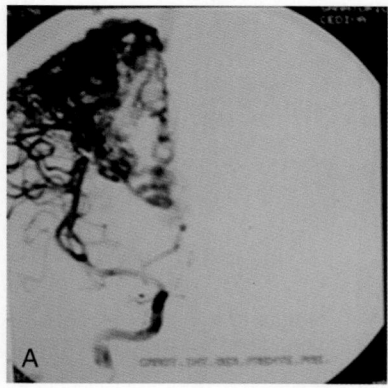
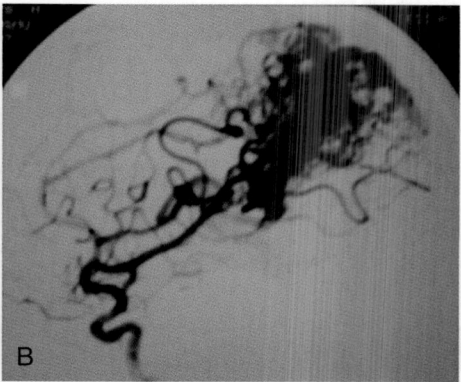
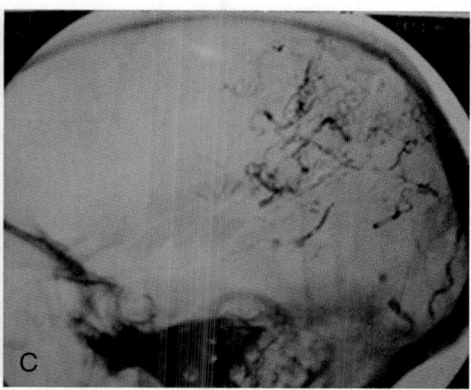

FIGURE 83-6 Grade V AVM. A and B, Preembolization; C, postembolization before surgery.

treatments must be tried. In my opinion, those treatments will always be palliative and will be dominated by endovascular surgery and the possibility of being completed with radiosurgery. Direct surgery should not be an option in malformations of this grade. Regardless, a grade V malformation can be operated on, but always with the prior endovascular therapy as an adjuvant. Surgery will always be difficult. The sequelae rate is high. In my opinion, surgery of grade V AVMs must be reserved exclusively for those cases in which there is recurrent bleeding and the patient, already with sequelae, has a life risk in case of new hemorrhage.[17,19,33,35,45-48] Some authors propose radiosurgery as the first step of treatment and then endovascular therapy. In all cases, it will be a palliative treatment (Fig. 83-6).[17,21,22,37,46-48]

GRADE V AVM

1. Do nothing
2. Endovascular therapy + radiosurgery
3. Endovascular therapy
4. Endovascular therapy + surgery
5. Endovascular therapy + surgery + radiosurgery
6. Radiosurgery + endovascular therapy

A recent publication[49] studied the safety of surgery in the treatment of AVMs. The conclusion was that in grades I and II the surgical risk (morbidity) is under 1%, while in grade III to V AVMs it varies according to the involvement of eloquent areas; surgical morbidity and mortality range from 17% to 21%. The comments of Batjer and Hernesniemi on this study support surgery as the best option in the treatment of the AVMs.[49]

The Surgeon

The specialist who is going to perform the surgical operation of an AVM must be a well-trained and experienced neurosurgeon. This surgeon must have training in microsurgery, which mean many hours of practice in a laboratory. The laboratory must be a continuous practice. Also, proper knowledge of anatomy is indispensable, with continual updates regarding cisterns, sulcus, circumvolutions, arteries, and veins.

Constantly updating knowledge of the brain's anatomy, as well as its vascular tree, allows the surgeon to better interpret angiographic imaging, magnetic resonance imaging, and so on. The laboratory practice allows the surgeon

to acquire more skill in the dissection of sulci and cisterns, indispensable points in any AVM surgery.

Preparation for Surgery

Unlike in other neurosurgical interventions, the preparation for AVM surgery requires the fulfillment of several indispensable steps that allow the surgical act to be performed with fewer risks. First, the surgical intervention of an AVM should always be scheduled. A patient with an AVM complicated by a hemorrhage may require an emergency operation—a case that supports such action. But the indicated action in these cases is to proceed exclusively to the hemorrhagic area evacuation and not seek the malformation in this urgent surgical act. A swollen brain, a distorted anatomy, vessels compressed by the hematoma, venous stasis, and associated ischemic phenomena due to several of these factors conspire in such conditions against the surgical attempt on the AVM, rendering it a surgical failure, not to mention affecting the vital and functional prognosis of the patient. The exception can lay in small malformations found in the wall of the hematoma. In such cases, the resection can be performed. Although a hemorrhagic lesion was evacuated and nothing was found on searching in its "walls," the pathologist may later report that a small AVM was found among the clots (Fig. 83-7).

Second, when a malformation is going to be operated on, the patient must be prepared for surgery. This implies complete studies and, if necessary, the performance of endovascular techniques. When occlusions of afferent pedicles and part of the malformation nidus have been carried out by endovascular means, surgery must be performed no fewer than 4 or 5 days after the treatment was carried out.[50,51] Apart from this requirement, the timing for the surgery depends on the characteristics of the AVM, its flow, its size, the afferents and efferents, and the grade of occlusion achieved. Most importantly, it depends on the patient's clinical condition after the procedure. An asymptomatic patient can be operated on prematurely, but those who start to present a neurologic deficit and whose imaging studies reveal an ischemic lesion must be differed until clinical stabilization is achieved. Therefore, the surgical team, taking into consideration these factors, should determine the best moment for surgery in each case. The existence of an AVM provokes an alteration in the brain's blood flow. The occlusion

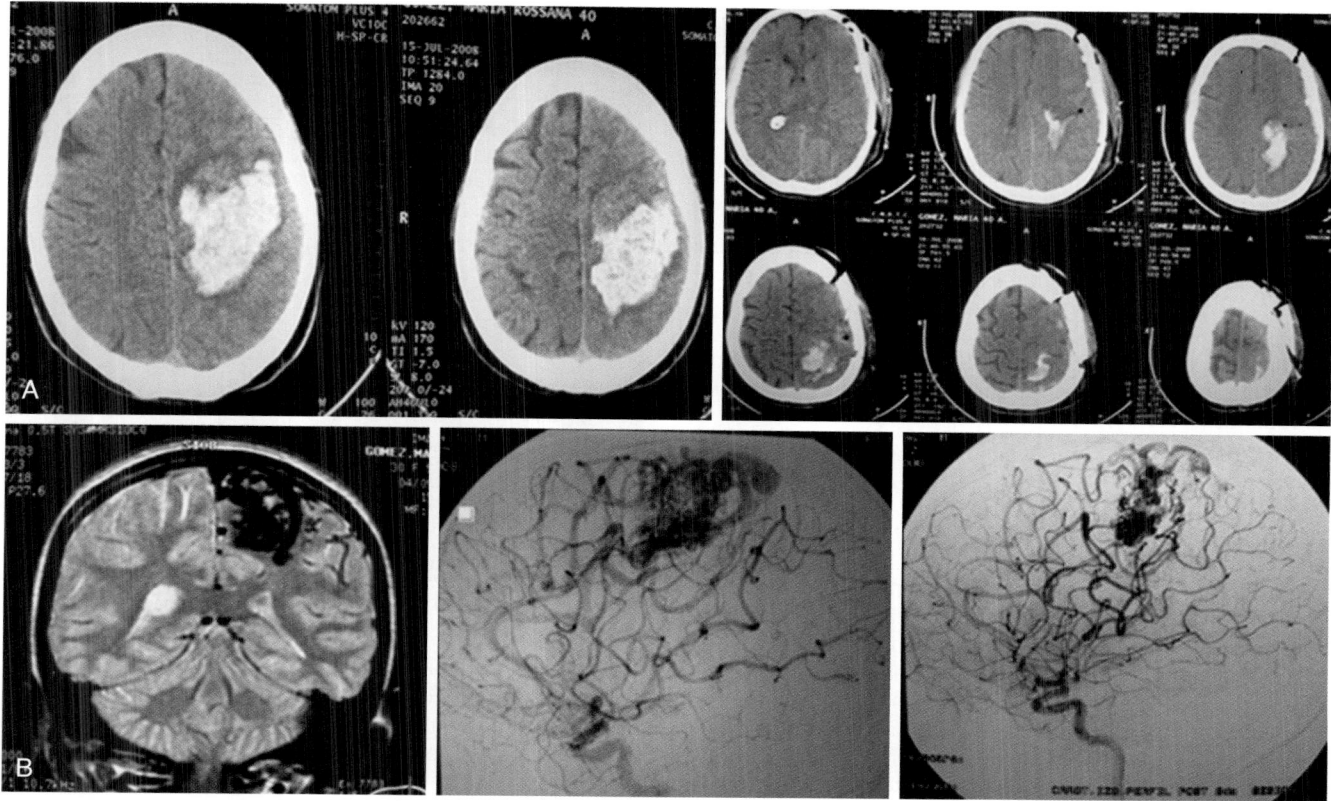

FIGURE 83-7 A, In an AVM treated 3 years prior solely with radiosurgery, hematoma is now seen (GCS 4). Angiography shows pre- and postemboliza-tion before surgery. Emergency surgery for evacuation of the hematoma is performed. B, The same case is shown on recovery after surgery (GCS 14) through magnetic resonance imaging. A, left: CT at admission; right: CT after emergency surgery. B, right: MRI postsurgery; middle: angiography preembolization; left: angiography postembolization.

determines a new redistribution of the brain's blood flow, regardless of the percentage occluded by endovascular means. Such modification, which has been progressive with the endovascular therapy, experiences an abrupt change with surgery. Thus, allowing time for the changes in blood flow to be induced by the therapy before surgery takes place reduces the possibility of associated morbidity.[51]

Third, every case must be discussed and surgery must be planned by the team that will work with the surgeon, that is, the assistant vascular surgeons, endovascular therapists, neuroanesthesiologists, neurologists, and neurophysiologists.

Operating Room

The surgery begins with the anesthetic act performed by a neuroanesthesiologist, who, knowledgeable about the pathology and well informed about the particular case, plans the appropriate anesthesia for that case. Due to the ongoing advances in anesthetic techniques and drugs, it is impossible to impose one anesthetic protocol. The use of a purely intravenous anesthesia or one in combination with inhalation agents depends on the particular case. It is necessary to count on a central venous line, as well as large peripheral venous catheters in case further access is needed. Monitoring the arterial pressure with an arterial line is indispensable, not to mention the classic monitoring of oxygen saturation, capnography, entropy, and so on. Next,

the neurophysiologist places the electrodes for the neuro-physiologic control of the cortical activity, peripheral motor response, cranial nerves, and so on. If necessary because of the lesion's topography, it is possible to then proceed to localization by means of a stereotactic frame or to start with neuronavigation to localize lesions in real time. The next step is fixing and positioning the head by means of a cranial fixation headrest, according to the lesion topography.

An operating microscope is essential for surgery. Regard-ing the surgical instruments, leaving aside all necessary implements to perform the craniotomy, little is needed for the AVM resection:

- Microscalpel or arachnoid knife.
- Two aspirators, one that is 5 or 6 French and another that is 8 French, for use in case of bleeding.
- Microsurgery scissors. In the case of a superficial AVM, straight 12- or 15-cm microscissors are enough. When dealing with a deep-seated AVM or subcortical compo-nents, 18-cm bayonet scissors may be necessary.
- Bipolar forceps for coagulation. For cortical lesions, short forceps no longer than 15 cm should suffice. As with microscissors, in deep-seated lesions, longer bayo-net forceps (18 cm) are needed.
- Microdissector, an accessory device that can be neces-sary to separate or dissect an arachnoid.
- Hemoclips and aneurysm or AVM clips, both transitory and definitive, together with their corresponding appli-cation forceps.

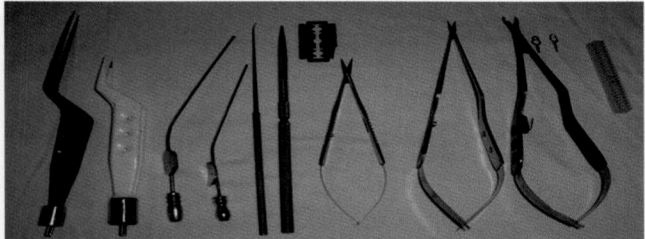

FIGURE 83-8 Surgical instruments for AVM resection.

Of these, the essential "tools" that surgeons use in most malformation dissections are the aspirator and the bipolar coagulator (Fig. 83-8).

Surgical Technique

SUPERFICIAL MALFORMATIONS

Regardless of whether the AVM to be resected was previously treated, either by endovascular treatment or by radiosurgery, the technique does not vary. The skin flap, as well as the bone flap, is determined by the lesion characteristics. The surgeon must always be focused on the malformation. The position of the head follows the same criteria as those previously described. It must always be fixed with a cranial fixation headrest, and care must be taken not to lateralize or flex the head significantly so as not to compress the veins at the neck level, since this could provoke a limitation in the venous return. Such a limitation can lead to surgical complications, with a tense brain and venous pressure in a malformation, which increases the risks of intra- and postoperative complications.

In interhemispheric lesions, which represent a significant amount of the supratentorial malformations, it is possible to choose the half-sitting position, with the head held by a cranial fixation headrest. It is possible to place the head in a medial position or slightly laterally toward the side of the malformation. When adhesions and so on fixing the brain to the midline are released, this permits the brain to droop slightly (i.e., to separate spontaneously), enhancing—without the use of retractors—the interhemispheric sight.

In superficial (corticosubcortical) AVMs, a large flap must be performed centered on the malformation. Even in lesions only a few centimeters wide, the best option is for the flap to include not only the lesion but also the surrounding area, giving the surgeon a view of the normal surrounding brain and thus allowing identification of the sulcus, the different circumvolutions, and the eloquent areas. This also enables the surgeon to assess the normal and not-so-normal vessels that supply and leave the malformation. Thus, the surgeon ensures control of the afferent arterial vessels and of veins, as well as the capacity to identify the arterialized veins. Once structures have been visualized and recognized, the anatomy is compared with the imaging, which must be carefully studied before and during the surgical act (Fig. 83-9).

Before starting the resection, the neurophysiologist has to place electrodes for corticography with identification of areas in the zones surrounding the lesion, which allows the surgeon to work more comfortably.

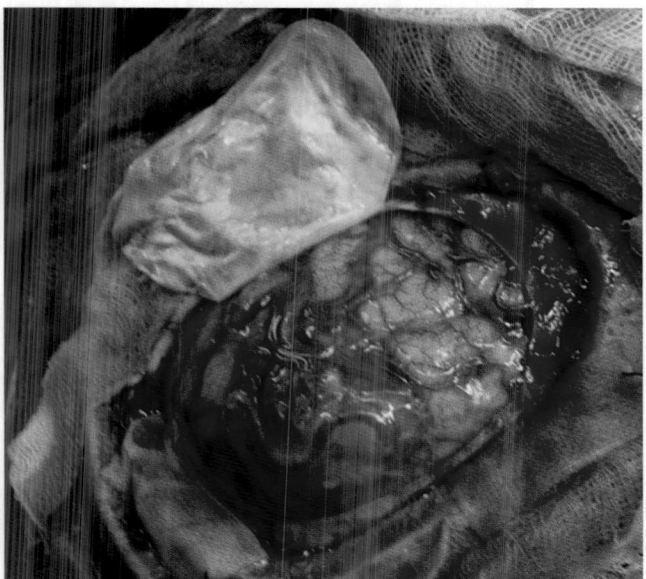

FIGURE 83-9 Big flap with the AVM in the center.

A technical detail in the approach, both for superficial AVMs and for subcortical ones, is the opening of the dura mater, but with venous drainage toward the surface. There is always the risk of vessels, especially venous ones, that have adhered to the dura mater. The dura mater must be opened slowly and with the proper care; otherwise, a vessel may be torn in the process, with consequent bleeding that in cortical AVMs may correspond to a hemorrhage of the core of the lesion. Both in these AVMs and in those that drain to the surface, a vein can be torn—even the main vein exiting the AVM. Thus, a previously planned surgery of a priori low risk can turn into a catastrophe. Therefore, the opening of the dura mater must be performed slowly, with the surgeon continually checking for adhesions to release them with extreme care. The use of magnification is even necessary in many cases at this stage, by means of magnifiers or operating microscopes (preferably the latter), so that the surgeon can adapt to the surgical field under the microscope after opening of the dura mater (i.e., before seeing the malformation), which avoids distractions.

It is well known that a significant portion of cerebral AVMs are superficial but with an interhemispheric component. In these cases, the bone flap must surpass the midline, and the opening of the dura mater must expose the interhemispheric fissure to have at sight (i.e., to be able to manage) the longitudinal sinus. These maneuvers can take several minutes and even delay the resection of the nidus, but we must take into consideration that good exposure and good control over the structures later results in a less complicated malformation surgery.

In addition to the previously described care that must be used at the opening of the dura mater, if the sinus and the interhemispheric fissure have to be exposed, the dural opening must be done slowly and cautiously. In a brain with no vascular lesions, like the ones dealt with in this chapter, there are usually thick veins and adhesions in the vicinity of the sinus. When there is an AVM, such situations become more frequent; hence, the dissection and separation of veins and dural adhesions must be performed carefully.

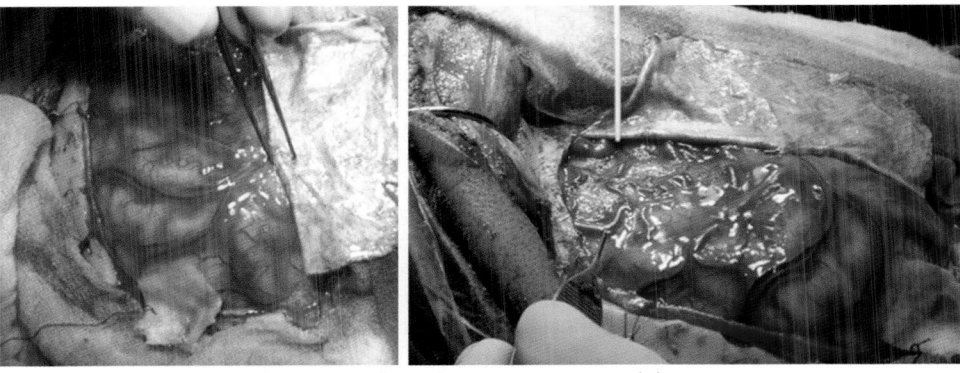

FIGURE 83-10 Relationship between veins and dura mater.

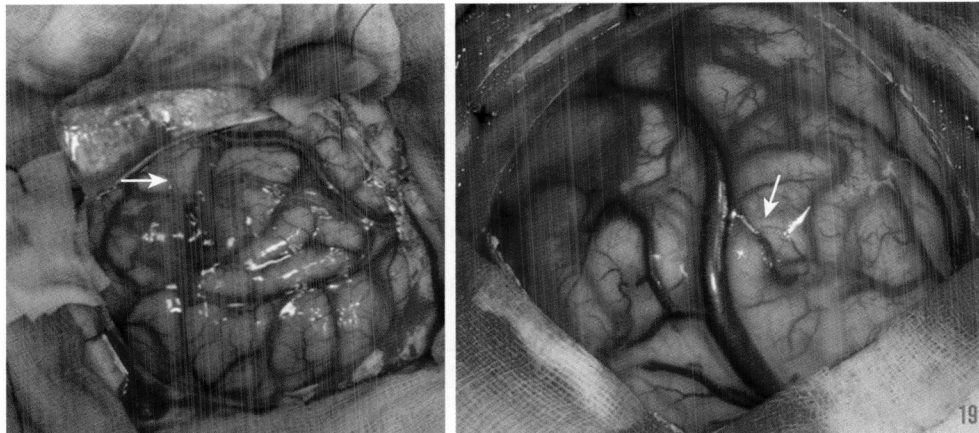

FIGURE 83-11 Arterialized veins, indicating the approach to the AVM.

Venous bleeding in the vicinity of the midline is not rare in such patients. Thus, it is recommended in these cases that the small dural vessels be coagulated and cut against the arachnoid and not against the dura. In case of tearing or bleeding of large-caliber vessels, they must not be coagulated, but a hemostasis must be performed by means of hemostatic materials and later compression with cottons. Trying to perform hemostasis with coagulation of large-caliber venous vessels is a technical mistake and will not solve the problem; on the contrary, the bleeding will increase and will lead the surgery to failure (Fig. 83-10).

Once the dura mater has been opened and the surgeon can see the malformation in the superficial lesions or its afferent vessels and draining veins—many of them arterialized in the subcortical lesions—it is necessary to identify the surrounding areas by means of direct cortical stimulation.

Afterward, and always with the corresponding magnification by means of an operating microscope, the area to be operated on is delimited. Arteries are studied as the surgeon tries to identify whether they are vessels heading to the malformation or *en passage* vessels; the process is repeated with veins. Usually, the veins that exit the nidus have an abnormal coloration, looking more like an artery, hence their designation as "arterialized veins" (Fig. 83-11).

Such veins can be mistaken sometimes for arteries. These veins must be looked after; the surgeon must try neither to injure them nor to coagulate them until the final stages of the nidus resection. The main draining vein is the last to be eliminated. Its early elimination brings about an important increase in the pressure inside the nidus, with resultant bleeding that, in this kind of situation, becomes difficult to control. One way of knowing whether the resection is being performed correctly and the arterial pedicles are being eliminated (either in previously treated or in untreated malformations) is that, during resection and coagulation of the arterial pedicles, veins change their tension and coloration, becoming darker. It is often difficult—even for an experienced surgeon—to identify which arteries correspond to the malformation and which do not.

The resection of a malformation is always performed from the outside inward. The nidus is surrounded but never entered. The opening of the arachnoid is started, usually from the sulcus delimiting the lesion. This maneuver is continued until the whole AVM is practically surrounded. In general, in superficial malformations, this maneuver stops when the thick draining vein is reached. Like most superficial malformations, the corticosubcortical ones are roughly conical with the apex at the deepest point, and the dissection follows this contour. It could be said that it is being surrounded and deepened step by step.

An essential step is to identify the plane between the nidus and the surrounding tissue. Because of the chronic ischemia that determines the malformation on the neighboring parenchyma, there is always at least a small layer of nonfunctioning tissue (gliotic or cicatricial) that surrounds the lesion. This tissue is the margin within which the surgeon has to work without provoking lesions for compression and/or coagulation. In each step, it is important to seek the pedicles and coagulate them. The thickest can be coagulated or clipped. The use of clips is reserved for thick vessels, where coagulation or placement of hemoclips is controversial regarding their efficiency. If they are used, they must always be small or miniature clips. The placement of transitory clips is reserved for those vessels that the surgeon wants to preserve, because it is uncertain whether they are *en passage* arteries, go to the malformation, or supply the nidus. However, clipping distal to the malformation is preferred to enable the surgeon to manage it better, identify the branches that come to the nidus, and eliminate them. The new clips for AVMs are useful at this point in the surgery.

The aspirator, resting on cotton, separates the nidus, and the bipolar coagulator performs the double function of dissection and coagulation. This must always be performed following a circumferential pattern. Every section left behind is covered with cotton, which allows not only hemostasis but also separation.

As this type of malformation is being deepened, the vessels become smaller. Close to the apex of the lesion, it becomes increasingly difficult to coagulate them since they are thin walled and they recoil from this maneuver. In such cases, it is recommended to not insist on coagulation but to persist with the placement of hemostatic materials covered with cotton. Only in exceptional cases do these maneuvers not lead to hemostasis. Usually, during the resection of a malformation, it is not considered good practice to reach the subcortical region or the apex of the malformation to start coagulating all small vessels of altered walls that appear in the white matter. This would only lead to increased bleeding and to entry of healthy zones of the brain that can thus be damaged.

During a dissection of AVMs performed in a circumferential pattern, it is possible to mistakenly enter the nidus, often because we have not been able to identify its boundaries. Such entry is manifested through bleeding, often profuse. In such cases, it is recommended to apply hemostatic material, cover the area with cottons, and compress with the second aspirator. This area should be left alone, and the plane in another zone of the lesion must be sought to continue the circumferential dissection step by step. As the surgeon comes back to the zone that caused bleeding problems, it is necessary to seek the plane from the outer part of the area where work had been undertaken. Once it is found, surgery proceeds in the customary way. Any time bleeding is difficult to stop, it is because we are inside the nidus and not in the plane between the nidus and the surrounding brain.

By the end of the resection, the surgeon may be weary, especially if dealing with large lesions. In such cases, more care must be taken. Sometimes weariness leads to incorrect maneuvers, such as thinking the whole nidus has been surrounded and there are no pedicles left in the depth and then proceeding to try to withdraw it, which can lead to arterial or venous tearing. From the beginning to the end of the resection, the same level of attention must be paid, and a meticulous inspection of the bed must be performed before withdrawing the nidus.

As soon as the dissection of the whole AVM is complete, the coagulation and the cutting of the main draining vein are undertaken. Only then can the nidus be removed. Often, the bed where the lesion lies presents small and multiple bleedings. In such a case, placing hemostatic material and covering it with cottons is the indicated procedure. Later, the surgeons wash with saline and wait for spontaneous hemostasis to take place.

Occasionally, there is a zone of major bleeding that cannot be controlled with these maneuvers. This usually indicates that remnants of the malformation were not removed. In such cases, and by means of higher magnification, the zone must be explored. This small, remaining nest must be surrounded and then resected in the same way as with the main nidus.[6,29,37,52-56]

DEEP-SEATED MALFORMATIONS

As their name indicates, deep-seated lesions are not visualized in the cortical inspection. At most, an arterialized vein can be seen "going out" of a sulcus, which would be a guide for dissection. But in most cases, and following the criterion that surgically treated deep-seated AVMs are usually small, help is needed to know the precise location of such lesions and their corresponding resection.

It is necessary to differentiate those malformations that bled from those that did not. If there are deep hematomas (e.g., in the basal ganglia or the insular region), a high percentage of these patients are already presenting a neurologic deficit determined by this bleeding. In such cases, the surgeon works in a relatively secure way, since the hematoma dramatically diminishes the possibility of adding morbidity. But malformations that did not bleed pose the problem that, due to their topography, will always be in an eloquent area.

Whatever the therapeutic maneuver, it entails life risk and especially a considerable morbidity risk. Therefore, in those lesions that did not bleed, abstention is probably the best choice. However, it is well known that deep-seated lesions have higher possibilities of bleeding than those located in other areas of the brain. Morbidity of these lesions has diminished significantly in recent years,[18,23,24,37] basically because of advances in neuroanesthesia, the practice of neurosurgeons in microsurgery of sulcus and cisterns, and the strict knowledge of gyri (Fig. 83-12).

Following Spetzler and Martin's classification, deep-seated AVMs with indication for surgery would be grades II and III. Rarely would surgery be performed on a grade IV AVM, not to mention a deep-seated grade V AVM. In such cases, both surgical morbidity and surgical mortality are very high, even higher than those of the natural evolution of the disease. But grade II and III lesions that undergo surgery would be, in most cases, of small nidus, with venous drainage to the depth exclusively or associated superficial drainage.

This subgroup of malformations poses an important challenge to neurosurgeons, and every case raises a dilemma about how to reach the final and curative solution. Prior to describing surgery of deep-seated AVMs, I must mention the usual topographies of this group of lesions. At the supratentorial level, they are localized in the region of the basal ganglia and the insula, periventricular and intraventricular. At an infratentorial level, it

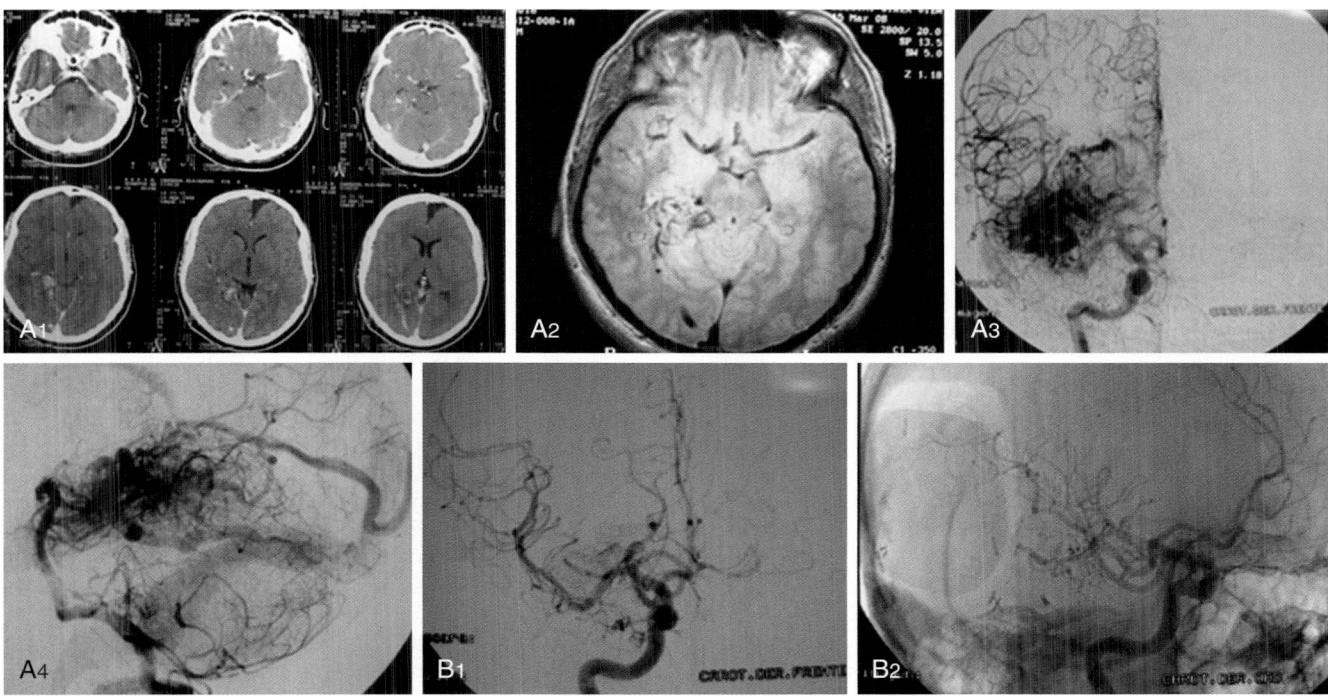

FIGURE 83-12 A, Deep grade III AVM preembolization. B, The same case after embolization and surgery.

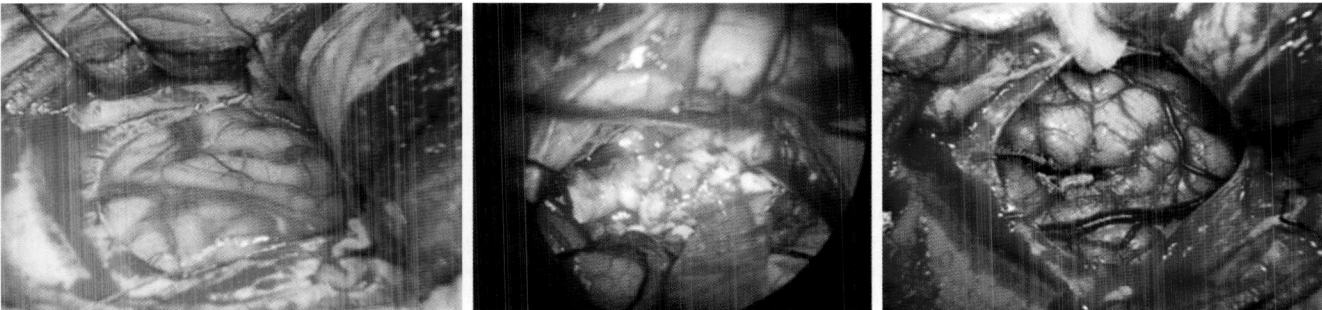

FIGURE 83-13 Deep AVM. Surgery by a sulcus.

is possible to find them along the brain stem, in the IV ventricle, or deep at the level of the vermis or cerebellar hemispheres.

Solomon and Stein[57] divide these malformations into three groups: the basal ganglia ones, especially the thalamocaudate; those of the brain stem; and those neighboring the tentorium. Among the first group, he includes those neighboring the atrium of the ventricle, and among the last group are those placed at the quadrigeminal cistern, mesencephalon, and cerebellar vermis.

Surgery

When lesions of small nidus are considered, which are generally irrigated by arteries of small caliber, it is possible to proceed directly to surgery, However, in those whose pedicles are thick and the nidus is not so small, preoperative endovascular treatment will be of great value to the surgeon. Depending on the lesion's topography, it is necessary to seek the proper approach, always following the criterion for dissection by cisterns, sulcus, or fissures.

For lesions of the hippocampus or of the insula, the transcisternal approach is ideal. In intraventricular or periventricular lesions, the interhemispheric callosal approach can be the best choice.

For external lesions of the basal ganglia, it is necessary to seek some sulcus that, due to its proximity, leads the surgeon to the lesion. It is always necessary to avoid injuring the parenchyma, so correct dissection of a cistern or sulcus permits the surgeon to make enough room to reach the malformation, with minimal or no brain compression. In this case, the head must be placed laterally toward the side opposite the lesion, always avoiding compressions of the neck. It is fixed with a cranial headrest (Fig. 83-13).

In deep-seated lesions of the basal ganglia, centered on the thalamus or the so-called thalamocaudate, an interhemispheric transcallous approach might be the most indicated. In these cases, the patient can be placed in a half-sitting position, with the head fixed with a cranial fixation headrest. The same position can be adopted for the intraventricular or subependymal lesions. This position has my preference. However, the patient could also be placed in lateral decubitus.

For those lesions neighboring the tentorium, it is possible to place the patient in lateral decubitus and use a subtemporal approach or to place the patient in a half-sitting position and use a supracerebellar, supratentorial, or infratentorial approach, depending on the lesion and its topography.

In lateral and subtemporal approaches, it is necessary to use special care in identifying and preserving the Labbé vein, independently of whether it is linked to the malformation, since the function of this vein in venous drainage is of the utmost importance, and damaging it not only can provoke swelling of the neighboring brain but also can lead to lesions by venous ischemia that endanger the patient's life or determine disabling sequelae.

For the interhemispheric approaches and the tentorial ones, it is possible to section the fold of the dura mater, either the falx cerebri or the tentorium, to have better control over the afferent branches, as well as the draining veins. Until recently, to perform such approaches, it was necessary to drain cerebrospinal fluid to permit a better retraction of the structures. At present, with neuroanesthesia performed in good conditions by a well-trained neuroanesthesiologist, a compliant brain is achieved without this maneuver. In subtemporal approaches, as well as in those of the posterior fossa, the liquid of the cistern can be extracted, which allows the surgeon to work without compression of the structures.

In malformations of the cerebellum, my preference is the half-sitting position with a cranial fixation headrest. This position requires correct monitoring by means of thoracic Doppler to search for embolisms and act in consequence. Other authors prefer to position the patient in ventral decubitus. Though this position is safer as concerns avoiding embolisms, there is a higher accumulation of blood in the bed as the surgeon goes forward through the different planes. Regardless, well-trained surgeons should never find difficulties in this position. I consider the ideal position to be the one to which the surgeon is accustomed and for which it is most comfortable for that surgeon to operate (Fig. 83-14).

In no case do I consider transcortical approaches proper. Anatomy should be preserved; the natural pathways that cisterns, fissures, and sulcus offer permit the surgeon to properly approach all brain sectors.

For these surgeries, the assistance of equipment that permits to the surgeon determine the topography of the lesion and to search (as explained earlier) for the sulcus or sector of the cistern or fissure through which to approach the malformation is indispensable.

At a minimum, localization by means of skull computed tomography–guided marking should be performed. This can be performed in the immediate preoperative stage or in those health centers with operating rooms equipped with tomography devices during operations. In such cases, it is possible to perform marking first and then, as dissection is started, to check whether the direction is correct.

The assistance with marking by means of stereotaxy is of much value. Surgery starts with the placement of the stereotactic frame. The corresponding localization is performed, and once the dura mater is opened, the surgeon checks the entry point and the direction with the help of the frame needle. This is highly valued help in the surgery of deep-seated AVMs. It has the advantage of permitting the surgeon to confirm the approach site, relate it to some sulcus or sector of the cistern or fissure, and know the depth at which the lesion should be.

Neuronavigation techniques, either with equipment that permits surgical team to locate and assist in real time or with the latest with Doppler technology, are of great value, not only to indicate where the lesion is but also to assist the surgeon in determining whether the resection was complete. Magnification by means of an operating microscope is also useful.

Finally, for this type of lesion, the assistance of an endoscope can be of great help. Its use may be necessary at different stages of the dissection. For instance, for intraventricular lesions or those in the ventricular wall, once the sinus of the ventricle is approached, direct visualization by means of an endoscope can help in locating the lesion. It is even possible to use it as an assistant, both for lighting and for magnification, during resection of AVMs. In other cases, after the surgical dissection has been completed under microscope—especially in small and deep-seated lesions—the inspection of the bed through the sulcus and cistern by means of a neuroendoscope can rule out the existence of any remaining malformation and help check the correct hemostasis.

Unlike what has been explained regarding superficial lesions (where wide flaps are my preference), in these cases

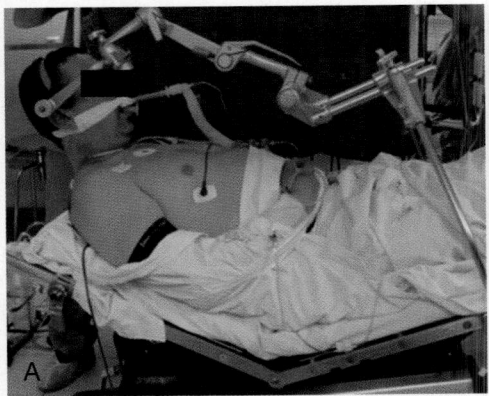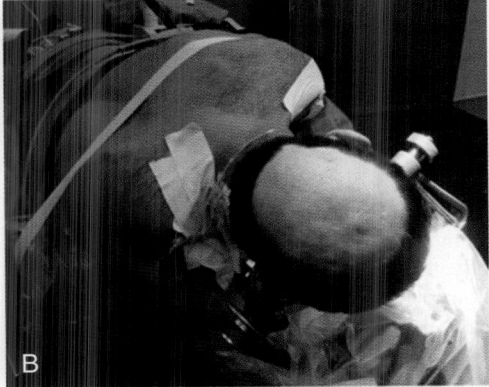

FIGURE 83-14 Half-sitting position (A) and park bench position (B), both for an interhemispheric approach.

and with corresponding assistance by means of the afore-mentioned equipment, small lesion–centered flaps can be performed.

Malformation dissections do not significantly differ from the previously described superficial lesion dissections. Unlike those dissections, malformation dissections do not have a conical aspect; rather, they stretch on a plane like a jellyfish. A direct dissection of the nidus should never be performed. It must be surrounded, while searching for pedicles that reach the lesion. Small afferents predominate, which often contrasts with a thick draining vein, especially in those of high flow.

The bipolar coagulation and the aspirator are again the surgeon's essential tools. The bed that is released must be covered with small cottons. The nidus is separated with the aspirator but always covered with cotton. Small, thin-walled vessels in the bed of the lesion are frequent. The hemostatic materials are of great help. It is necessary to avoid indiscriminate coagulation of the bed and of these small vessels, which, as has been described concerning the superficial ones, recoil to coagulation. The difference is the depth at which the surgeon is working and the small surgical field. Thus, it is necessary to be careful when coagulating and cutting the afferents that are clearly visualized; in the remaining ones, the surgeon must perform "indirect" hemostasis, that is, with hemostatic materials. The main draining vein is always left for the end. Once the lesion is dissected and liberated of all afferents, the surgeon proceeds to coagulation and cutting of the draining vein. Later, the bed is explored, either under microscope magnification or by means of an endoscope.

Eventually, the walls of the sulcus and/or of the cistern (through which the approach was performed) are covered with hemostatic materials to avoid bleeding of these walls, usually rich in vessels and congestive since it presents near a malformation and due to the neurosurgeon's work.[3,18,24,52,53,55-62]

Endovascular Surgery

For the treatment of an AVM, endovascular surgery, endovascular therapy, or neurointerventionism, a well-trained specialist in the management of such lesions is required. Before the treatment, correct planning of the surgery must be carried out by means of a throughout analysis of the imaging, widely dominated by the digital angiography of brain vessels. At present, it is also fundamental to have functional magnetic resonance, which permits the surgeon to delimit the areas of work.[9,11,12,14]

This method seeks the greatest occlusion of the nidus, as well as of its afferents and of the origin of the draining vein, without causing damage to the patient. Many of those who work in the area of endovascular surgery ponder the possibility of reaching complete endovascular occlusion of an AVM with this method. The permanent and complete occlusion of the nidus is posed.[63,64] I think that sometimes it is possible to achieve the complete radiologic occlusion, but this does not mean the complete disappearance of the AVM. In those cases in which complete closure of the lesion is ensured—and that later undergoes surgery—there may be small vessels that did not refill in the endovascular procedure and that eventually would make the lesion reappear

if surgery was not performed. In the cases of apparent complete endovascular occlusion with no surgery, it occasionally happens that in successive angiographic controls, which can be performed after 3, 6, or 9 months—or even later—pathologic vessels and draining veins reappear.[44] This is controversial, because endovascular surgeons consider complete and definitive occlusion to be achievable, especially in small AVMs and when Onyx is used.[39,40,43,44,64-66] In recent publications, Weber et al.[39,66] demonstrated that Onyx penetrates small vessels, achieving occlusion. Even as these authors stated that complete angiographic occlusion can be achieved, they remarked that some cases of recanalization have been found in long-term controls. However, in dural fistulae, complete occlusion was reported in another study, and at 5-year follow-up no recanalizations were found.[67]

Weber et al.[39] referred to the benefit of treatment with Onyx, achieving high occlusion rates, especially in cortical AVMs. Van Rooij et al.,[40] in a 5-year treatment series, referred to complete occlusion with Onyx in small AVMs. The authors recommended that several years of use of this method pass before the endovascular therapists' opinion is accepted as true. Up to now, there have been no papers with enough evidence to sustain that position.

Every case is different. It is necessary to have a complete notion of the angioarchitecture of the malformation, its flow; the pedicles that come to an end in the AVM; those that go to it, give branches to the lesion, and continue to the normal parenchyma; and the branches that are exclusively *en passage*. Special care must be taken by the endovascular neurosurgeon in ruling out possible intranidal aneurysms, since their occlusion is fundamental to diminishing the risks of bleeding. Another element to assess in the analysis of the angioarchitecture of an AVM is the presence of intranidal fistulas, since their elimination requires a special treatment.

In large lesions, neuromonitoring is fundamental, as well as the arterial occlusion tests. When the interventionist knows that navigating up to the origin of the nidus will not be possible, a test to assess the possible occlusion of proximal arterial branches or the stem, itself an important artery, is necessary. By means of administration of amobarbital sodium, Wada's test can be performed in arteries distant from the nidus, as well as in the distal vessels against the nidus. This is a highly valued test to determine the tolerance of a certain vessel to occlusion.[6,65]

The particles and histoacrylic glue were long the materials of choice for closure of the vessels of a malformation. Later, surgeons began to use some coils in some cases. Finally, the appearance of Onyx has been of great value in the treatment of such lesions. This material is administered in a liquid form that hardens when it comes into contact with blood, with scant risk of migration. At present, histoacrylic glue (*n*-butyl cyanoacrylate) and particularly Onyx are the materials of choice for the endovascular treatment of AVMs.[39,40,43,44,65,66,68-71]

The treatment must be always performed under general anesthesia. This allows the endovascular surgeon to work more comfortably and, if complications occur, enables the anesthesiologist to act rapidly, correcting parameters, improving oxygenation, controlling the capnography, provoking arterial hypertension if necessary, enabling delivery of volume and inotropes, and so on.

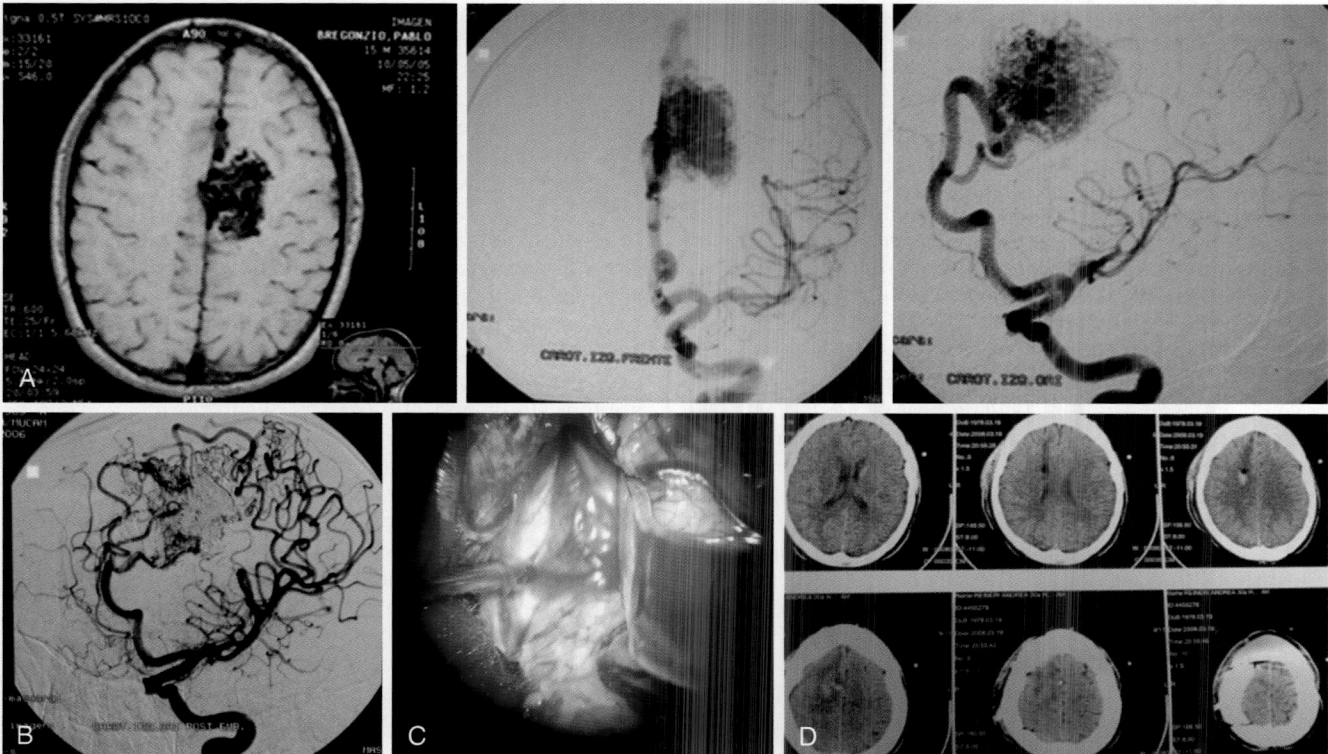

FIGURE 83-15 A, Interhemispheric AVM before treatment. B, The same case after endovascular therapy. C, The same case with an interhemispheric surgical approach. D, The same case shown on a computed tomography scan after surgery.

The femoral artery is the chosen route for catheterization. If difficulties or anatomic problems arise that prevent its use, it is possible to catheterize through the humeral artery. At present, direct carotid puncture is rare.

The procedure begins with the placement of a guiding catheter up to the carotid artery or the vertebral artery. Navigation continues by means of a microcatheter up to the nidus or its vicinity. The farther the microcatheter can be introduced into the nidus or into the arterial branches that feed it, the better the results. It is always necessary to try injection of the material to occlude (histoacrylic glue or Onyx) inside the nidus or in the clearly identified afferents that end in it. However, it may not be possible for the injection to reach the nidus due to difficulties with the catheterization, especially when afferent vessels are thin and tortuous. In such cases, those can be occluded after the patient has undergone a tolerance test.

If the injection is intranidal, there is practically no risk of migration of the embolization material. However, there is the slight possibility of such migration when the occlusion occurs in the vessels outside the nidus. It is important to identify the AVM flow and to plan the amount and intensity of the chosen embolic material to be injected so that it reaches as far as possible into the nidus and even to the draining vein or veins.

The percentage of the AVM to be occluded depends on its size, the flow, the afferents, and the functional status of the surrounding brain. In small malformations, it is possible to perform the total planned occlusion in just one session, but in larger malformations (grade III or higher), treatments must take at least two sessions. In these cases,

it is important not to cause an inversion of the flow due to an abrupt, massive occlusion, since this may provoke brain lesions, along with hemorrhages, ischemia, and intracranial hypertension, all of which can lead to sequelae—often permanent—and in some cases to the patient's death.

Never to proceed to surgery immediately after embolization; rather, allow time for the flow redistribution to be determined by the endovascular therapy. In this period, the patient can also recover from neurologic deficits that may have appeared due to the treatment. Even though endovascular therapies conducted by a well-trained surgeon usually exhibit low morbidity, if morbidity takes place, the surgeon can let several days or weeks to elapse before advising surgery. On the opposite end of the spectrum, there is the risk of adding morbidity to the surgery (Figs. 83-15 and 83-16).[72,73]

Radiosurgery

The therapeutic procedure of radiosurgery has been routinely used for the treatment of AVMs for more than 30 years. Technically, it consists of the administration of a high-radiation dose in only one session, locating the point of application where the lesion is concentrated with scant or no diffusion to the surrounding areas.

Radiosurgery has a widely spread use in neurosurgery, and the AVM is one of the pathologies to which it is frequently applied. In this application, the nidal thrombosis is sought. This is achieved through progressive hyperplasia of the tunica intima up to occlusion of the vessels. Although it is usually well tolerated, positive results are

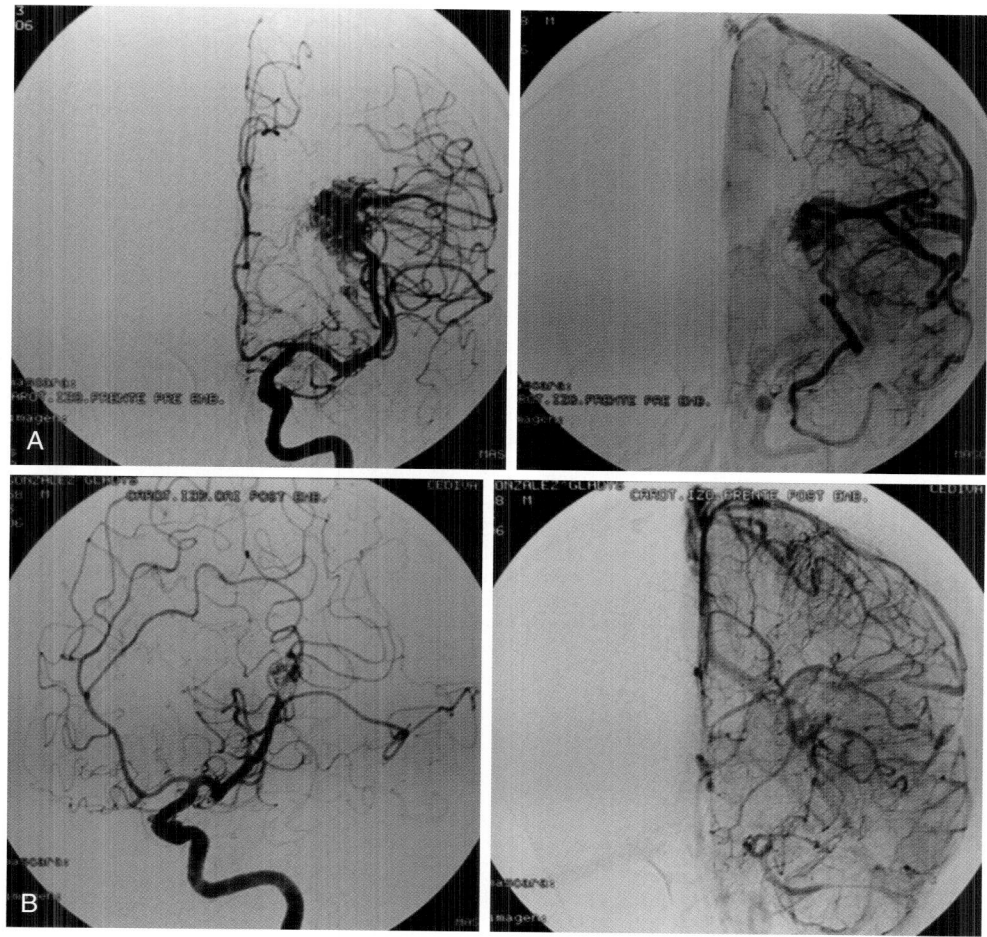

FIGURE 83-16 A, Deep AVM before endovascular therapy. B, The same case postembolization but before surgery.

never immediate.[74,75] On average, 2 years must elapse until complete sclerosis; thus, the AVM occlusion can be verified. Therefore, during the degenerative process that leads to closure of the nidus, the risk of bleeding persists. This is why radiosurgical therapy has some precautions. Such therapy is clearly indicated for some cases, whereas for other cases other options should be discussed; it is mostly indicated for AVMs that did not bleed and that have a volume below 8 cc. If we take the AVM as the integral dose (dose/volume relationship, expressed in millijoules) it would be 170 mJ. This is comparable with the 8-cc volume.[17] If the patient presented with bleeding due to an AVM, it is best to wait no less than 6 months before proceeding to treatment with radiation.

Deep-seated lesions, and especially those that compromise the brain stem, have a priori a higher indication for radiosurgery. In these cases, attention must be paid so that the lesion does not compromise more than 30% of the brain stem. Special care also must be taken when the AVM in question is near structures that can suffer the effects of the treatment, such as a malformation close to the optical chiasm.

The treatment must be planned by a well-trained physicist in these procedures. It is necessary to correctly define the target and the optimal dose to apply in each case. For planning, angioresonance, angiotomography, or angiography can be used, but planning always concludes with

stereotaxy. Hence, it is preferable to call it "stereotactic radiosurgery."

Recently published works refer to the benefits of radiosurgery as the only treatment for some AVMs but also refer to its value as an adjuvant to the surgery. It has been proposed that a malformation subjected to stereotactic radiosurgery can have better surgical management and fewer risks of intraoperative blood loss. However, it is also accepted that AVMs that underwent stereotactic radiosurgery but 2 years later have not yet disappeared should be operated on if are accessible to the surgeon. In all cases, when surgery has been performed after the radiant treatment, morbidity has been low.[74]

In 2008, a scale for radiosurgery and AVMs was proposed, with the aim of predicting the prognosis after the radiant treatment.[75] It needs to be used for some years before its value can be assessed.[76-89]

KEY REFERENCES

Awad JA, Magdinec M, Schubert A. Intracranial hypertension after resection of brain arteriovenous malformations: predisposing factors and management strategy. *Stroke.* 1994;25:611-620.

Brown R. Simple risk predictions for arteriovenous malformations hemorrhage. *Neurosurgery.* 2000;46:1024.

Brown R, Flemming K, Meyer F, et al. Natural history, evaluation and management of intracranial vascular malformations. *Mayo Clin Proc.* 2005;80:269-281.

Cood P, Mitha A, Ogilvy C. A recurrent brain malformation in an adult. *J. Neurosurg.* 2008;109(3):486-491.

Cover K, Lagerwaard F, Van den Berg R. Color intensity projection of digitally subtracted angiography for the visualization of brain arteriovenous malformations. *Neurosurgery.* 2007;60(3):511-515.

Davidson A, Morgan M. How safe is AVM surgery? A prospective observational study of surgery as first line treatment for brain arteriovenous malformations. *Neurosurgery.* 2010;66:498-505.

Drake C. Brain arteriovenous malformations: considerations for and experience with surgical treatment in 166 cases. *Clin Neurosurg.* 1979;26:145-208.

Guglielmi G. Analysis of the hemodynamic characteristics of brain arteriovenous malformations using electrical models: baseline setting, surgical extirpation, endovascular embolization and surgical bypass. *Neurosurgery.* 2008;63(1):1-11.

Hashimoto N, Nosaki N, Takogi Y. Surgery of arteriovenous malformations. *Neurosurgery.* 2007;61:375-389.

Hernesniemi A, Dashti R, Juvela S, et al. Natural history of brain arteriovenous malformations: a long-term follow-up study of risk of hemorrhage in 238 patients. *Neurosurgery.* 2008;63(5):823-831.

Heros RC. Spetzler-Martin grade IV and V arteriovenous malformations. *J Neursurg.* 2003;98:1-2.

Hoh BL, Chapman PH, Loeffler JS, et al. Results of multimodality treatment for 141 patients with brain arteriovenous malformations and seizures: factors associated with seizures incidence and seizures outcomes. *Neurosurgery.* 2002;51:303-309.

Kim L, Albuquerque F, Spetzler R. Postembolization neurological deficits in brain AVMs. *Neurosurgery.* 2006;59:53-59.

Laakso A, Dashti R, Seppänen J, et al. Long-term excess mortality in 623 patients with brain arteriovenous malformations. *Neurosurgery.* 2008;63(2):244-255.

Lawton MT. Spetzler-Martin grade III AVMs: surgical results and a modification of the grading scale. *Neurosurgery.* 2003;52:740-749.

Maruyama K, Shin M, Tago M, et al. Radiosurgery to reduce the risk hemorrhage from brain arteriovenous malformations. *Neurosurgery.* 2007;60(3):453-459.

Morgan M, Rochford A. Surgical risk associated with the management of grade I and II brain arteriovenous malformations. *Neurosurgery.* 2007;61:417-424.

Ogilvy CL, Awad I, Brown R, et al. Recommendations for the management of intracranial arteriovenous malformations: a statement for healthcare professionals from a special writing group of Stroke Council, American Stroke Association. *Stroke.* 2001;32:1458-1471.

Sanchez-Mejía R, McDermott M. Radiosurgery Facilitates Resection of Brain arteriovenous malformations and reduces surgical morbidity. *Neurosurgery.* 2009;64(2):231-240.

Sinclair J, Kelly M, Steinberg G. Surgical management of posterior fossa AVMs. *Neurosurgery.* 2006;58:189-201.

Spagnuolo E. Malformaciones arteriovenosas supratentoriales corticales. In: Pedroza A, Quintana L, Perilla T, eds. *Tratado de Neurocirugía Vascular Latinoamericana.* Bogotá: FLANC; 2008:412-423. Chap 29.

Spagnuolo E, Lemme-Plaghos L, Revilla F, et al. Recomendaciones para el manejo de las malformaciones arteriovenosas cerebrales. *Neurocirugía-Rev. Española de Neurociencias.* 2009;20:5-14.

Starke R, Komotor R, Hwang B. Treatment guidelines for arteriovenous malformations microsurgery. *BJNS.* 2009;23:376-385.

Weber W, Kis B, Siekmann R. Preoperative embolization of intracranial arteriovenous malformations with Onyx. *Neurosurgery.* 2007;61:244-254.

Weber W, Kis B, Siekman R, et al. Endovascular treatment of intracranial arteriovenous malformations with Onyx. Technical aspects. *AJNR.* 2007;28:371-377.

Numbered references appear on Expert Consult.

Endovascular Management of Intracranial Aneurysms

JOSEPH J. GEMMETE • ADITYA S. PANDEY • NEERAJ CHAUDHARY • B. GREGORY THOMPSON, JR.

Microsurgical clipping of intracranial aneurysms has been the historical definitive standard for treatment of intracranial aneurysms.[1] Today's surgical techniques routinely achieve complete exclusion of the aneurysm from the circulation without compromise of the parent vessel or arterial perforators in a large number of patients. However, several risk factors may put a patient at increased risk for morbidity and mortality. These factors include the aneurysm's size, its location, the patient's age, and the medical condition of the patient.[2] In addition, according to the International Subarachnoid Aneurysm Trial (ISAT), patients with subarachnoid hemorrhage fared better with endovascular coiling than with surgical clipping.[3] To overcome some of the limitations of surgical clipping, endovascular treatments were developed. They have grown considerably over the last 15 years, since U.S. Food and Drug Administration (FDA) approval of the Guglielmi detachable coil (GDC) in 1995.[4,5] This chapter discusses the basic techniques utilized in coiling of ruptured and nonruptured saccular intracranial aneurysms. After a brief discussion of each technique, we give a short review of the results of each form of treatment, concentrating on the large reported case series. Finally, we discuss specific complications related to endovascular treatment of saccular intracranial aneurysms.[6,7]

Conventional Coiling of a Simple Saccular Aneurysm

TECHNIQUE

At our institution, all intracranial aneurysm coiling procedures are performed under general anesthesia with neurologic monitoring. An arterial line is placed in the radial artery to closely monitor the patient's blood pressure. The anesthesiologist is aware of the need to avoid transient blood pressure spikes, especially when intubating or extubating the patient. This is particularly important in patients who have a ruptured aneurysm. The case can sometimes take a few hours; therefore, anesthesia is necessary to maintain immobility, because three-dimensional (3D) imaging and a fluoroscopic road map are very motion sensitive. A 6-French (Fr) sheath is inserted into the right common femoral artery. If balloon remodeling or additional microcatheters are needed, puncture of the left common femoral

artery may be necessary. Just after the sheath is inserted in the groin, a baseline activated clotting time (ACT) is drawn. Then, 6 to 10 international units (IUs) of heparin per kilogram of body weight are given intravenously as a bolus. For patients with unruptured aneurysms, the ACT is checked every 30 minutes throughout the procedure and heparin is given intermittently to keep the ACT between 250 to 300 seconds.[8] For patients with a ruptured aneurysm, 3000 IU of heparin are given after placement of framing coils; the patient is given additional heparin to maintain an ACT range of 250 to 300 seconds. A syringe of protamine is prepared in advance and readily available to be injected in case of aneurysm rupture. The usually dose is 10 mg of protamine per 1000 IU of heparin. The goal is to obtain an ACT of less than 150 seconds. Likewise, for patients with unruptured aneurysms who have been treated preoperatively with dual antiplatelet therapy, a five-pack of unpooled platelets are kept in preparation in case of rupture.

Patients who have not suffered a recent subarachnoid hemorrhage are preoperatively given 75 mg of clopidogrel (Plavix) and 81 mg of aspirin orally starting 7 days prior to the procedure to prevent thromboembolic complications. If emergent platelet inhibition is needed, the patient is loaded with a single dose of 600 mg of clopidogrel and 325 mg of aspirin. Full platelet inhibition occurs 2 hours afterward. If the procedure needs to be performed urgently, the patient may be given a glycoprotein IIb/IIIa inhibitor. A platelet inhibition assay is drawn for clopidogrel and aspirin prior to treatment, since approximately 25% of patients will have clopidogrel or aspirin resistance.[9,10]

A complete cerebral angiogram is performed prior to treatment with a 4- or 5-Fr catheter, including bilateral common carotid artery, internal carotid artery, and vertebral artery injections. Additional 3D rotational images are obtained to more accurately define the neck, dome, and size of the aneurysm. Once the diagnostic portion of the procedure is performed, the catheter is exchanged for a 6-Fr guide catheter, which is positioned as close as possible to the aneurysm. It is necessary to have a stable position of the guide catheter to be able to introduce a microcatheter safely into the aneurysm. Because of this, the guide catheter should be positioned as close to the aneurysm as possible. This gives optimal stability of the guide catheter and allows the operator to monitor the guide position on the same road map as the microcatheter during advancement of the coil into the aneurysm. New guide catheters that are more flexible, such as the Neuron (Penumbra, Alameda, CA), can be introduced farther into the intracranial circulation and can be routinely placed in the cavernous internal carotid artery or the basilar artery.[11] This allows more stability in advancing devices into the intracranial circulation. This has been a major innovation in the endovascular treatment of aneurysms over the last 3 years. If additional stability is needed to treat an aneurysm, a triple coaxial system consisting of a long sheath introduced into the origin of the great vessel followed by a guide catheter through this may offer enhanced stability in advancing devices through tortuous anatomy for the treatment of intracranial aneurysms. If an aneurysm cannot be treated from a femoral artery approach, a brachial, radial, direct carotid, or vertebral artery puncture is another option.[12-14]

MICROCATHETER PLACEMENT INTO THE ANEURYSM

All microcatheters have an outer hydrophilic coating; this reduces the friction between the catheters and the inner wall of the blood vessel, thus facilitating distal catheterization of the intracranial circulation. The microcatheter is advanced over a microwire into the aneurysm under road map. The microcatheter is never advanced into the aneurysm without using a wire, because doing so may perforate the aneurysm. Once the microcatheter is positioned within the aneurysm, the slack within the system is carefully removed and the wire is slowly withdrawn to prevent forward movement of the microcatheter tip. The best microcatheter position depends on the size and shape of the aneurysm; however, the best position is usually in the middle of the aneurysm or at the origin of the neck. This configuration usually allows the coil to form within the aneurysm with minimal resistance. Some operators in large aneurysms wrap the microcatheter around the dome of the aneurysm and placed the tip of the catheter at the neck. They claim this allows for placement of more coil loops across the neck of the aneurysm, thus limiting the possibility of prolapse of additional coils into the parent vessel during filling of the aneurysm.

COIL SELECTION

The choice of the coil is made based on the size and shape of the aneurysm as seen on the angiogram and 3D reconstruction. The purpose of the first coil (framing coil or complex shaped coil) is to create a support basket for the subsequent introduction of additional coils and to provide a bridge to prevent additional coils from migrating into the parent vessel. The first coil is sized to the largest dimension of the aneurysm sac. The first coil should be as large and long as possible to fully appose the aneurysm wall and provide a nice basket and stability, thus preventing the coil from prolapsing into the parent vessel. This also provides the maximum number of coil loops across the neck of the aneurysm, thus preventing herniation of additional coils placed into the aneurysm from compromising the parent vessel.

If the aneurysm sac has a sausage appearance, then the principles guiding the selection of the first coil are different. In such aneurysms, a helical coil is preferred to a complex shaped coil and the first coil is sized to the smallest sac diameter. The subsequent coils are similar in size and length, with the aneurysm coiled from the dome toward the neck.

COIL PLACEMENT

Through the microcatheter, the platinum portion of the coil is introduced into the aneurysm sac while still on the delivery wire. In the microcatheter, the coil assumes a straight configuration; however, as soon as the coil leaves the microcatheter, it assumes the manufactured memory shape. The coil is radiopaque under fluoroscopy and is visualized under live road map as it is placed into the aneurysm sac with the neck in profile. There should be limited resistance when introducing the coil into the aneurysm sac. If there is any resistance, the coil may be oversized. It is important to not force the coil into the aneurysm sac and thus to prevent possible rupture. If the coil is correctly sized, it will readily adapt to the shape of the aneurysm. If the coil is undersized, it will not be stable within the aneurysm sac and may herniate into the parent vessel. If the coil is oversized, it will not form with the aneurysm sac and will herniate into the parent vessel. Oversizing the coil may also cause excessive pressure on the wall of the aneurysm sac, possibly risking perforation.

Before detachment of the coil, an angiogram is performed to determine how the coil is confined within the aneurysm sac and to determine whether there is compromise of the parent vessel. Movement of the coil during the angiogram may indicate that the coil is undersized and may migrate out of the aneurysm sac after detachment. If the coil appears properly sized and there is no compromise of the parent vessel, the coil is detached under fluoroscopy. The detachment wire is then slowly pulled back through the microcatheter to make sure the coil has detached from the wire and does not move.

Additional coils of various sizes and shapes are subsequently introduced into the aneurysm sac until the aneurysm sac is densely packed and no longer filling with contrast or until the microcatheter is pushed outside the aneurysm sac. The first coils used for treatment of intracranial aneurysms were made out of platinum, but there were aneurysm recurrences after treatment; therefore, bioactive coils were introduced with the goal of inducing an exuberant healing response and improved filling volume of the coiled aneurysm. The first bioactive coil was the Matrix (Boston Scientific Neurovascular, Fremont, CA), introduced in 2002. The U.S. FDA approved the Matrix coil based on equivalency with the conventional GDC coil. Four bioactive coils are now available for clinical use: the Matrix, HydroCoil (Microvention, Aliso Viejo, CA), Cerecyte (Micrus, Sunnyvale, CA), and Nexus. The newer coils are manufactured so that the aneurysm sac is filled in a Russian nesting doll manner, from the periphery toward the center.[15] Filling coils are placed into the aneurysm sac after the placement of framing coils; once the aneurysm is nearly densely packed, the final coils usually placed into the aneurysm sac are finishing coils.[16] These coils are very short and soft. Once the aneurysm is densely packed, the microcatheter is removed slowly from the aneurysm, and a post-treatment angiogram is performed to assess the degree of aneurysm occlusion, parent vessel, and patency of the distal vasculature.

The heparin is reversed after the procedure with protamine and manual pressure, or a closure device is utilized to obtain hemostasis at the femoral puncture site.[17] Pressure is usually held on the puncture site for 20 to 30 minutes after removal of the sheath if manual compression is utilized, and the leg is immobilized for 6 hours to prevent groin complications. If a closure device is utilized, ambulation can occur as early as 2 hours after placement.[18,19] If there is compromise of the parent vessel, protrusion of coils, or thrombus formation during the coiling procedure, the heparin may be continued overnight with the sheath left in place. Antiplatelet therapy may also be given.

After endovascular treatment of nonruptured intracranial aneurysms, the patient is kept in the neurointensive care unit (NICU) for at least 24 hours for close monitoring of blood pressure, neurologic status, and puncture site. Subarachnoid hemorrhage patients are kept in the NICU for at least 14 days under close neuromonitoring and are prophalytically treated for vasospasm.

RESULTS OF ENDOVASCULAR TREATMENT FOR RUPTURED ANEURYSMS

Two prospective randomized trials have compared outcomes of endovascular coiling versus surgical clipping. The first study was performed in Finland[20] and randomized 109 patients with subarachnoid hemorrhage who were suitable for either surgery or endovascular coiling. Angiographic outcome in the posterior circulation was significantly better for endovascular coiling, whereas angiographic outcome in the anterior circulation was significantly better for surgery. Angiographic outcomes in the internal carotid artery and middle cerebral artery were similar in both groups. The Glasgow Outcome Scale was equivalent in both groups at 3 months. Mortality for technical reasons during surgery was twice that of the endovascular group (4% vs. 2%). One patient in the endovascular group suffered rebleeding following incomplete coiling of the aneurysm.

The second study was the ISAT,[3,21] in which nearly 2000 patients predominantly from Europe and with subarachnoid hemorrhage were randomized to surgery or endovascular coiling based on judgment of the treating team. Outcome analysis on the basis of death or dependence at 2 months and 1 year based on the modified Rankin Scale score was the primary parameter of interest in the first publication in 2002. At 1-year postprocedure, 250 of 1063 (23.5%) of the endovascular patients were dead or dependent, while 326 of 1055 (30.9%) of surgical patients were dead. This represents an absolute risk reduction of 7.4% by those treated from an endovascular approach. Delayed rebleeding was more common in the endovascular group; however, several cases were due to incomplete treatments. Seizures were also less common in the endovascular group.

RESULTS OF ENDOVASCULAR TREATMENT FOR UNRUPTURED ANEURYSMS

The data from endovascular treatment versus surgical clipping for unruptured aneurysms do not show a clear benefit for one form of treatment versus the other. A review of modern large clipping and coiling trials for unruptured aneurysms was published in 2005.[22] A majority of these trials were nonrandomized and retrospective. Adverse outcomes for endovascular coiling were estimated at 8.8% and for clipping were estimated at 17.8%. The International Study of Unruptured Intracranial Aneurysm[2] adverse outcomes were less common with endovascular treatment (9.3%) than with surgery (13.7%); however, the study was nonrandomized, and the endovascular treatment group included a higher number of elderly patients, larger aneurysms, and aneurysms within the posterior circulation. Surgical adverse outcomes in this study correlated with patient age greater than 50 years, aneurysm size greater than 12 mm, location in the posterior circulation, previous ischemic cerebrovascular disease, and symptoms of mass effect from the aneurysm. Endovascular outcomes were less influenced by these factors. Additional unruptured aneurysm trials are needed.

Coiling of Wide-Neck Aneurysms
BALLOON REMODELING TECHNIQUE
Sidewall Wide-Neck Aneurysm

The main feature that limits the endovascular treatment of aneurysms is the width of the neck. Other features that may limit treatment include the shape of the aneurysm. In 1992, Moret introduced the balloon remodeling technique for treatment of wide-neck intracranial aneurysms.[23,24] The technique involves placing a nondetachable balloon across the neck of the aneurysm during each coil placement. The coils remain molded around the balloon after deflation of the balloon, essentially "remodeling the arterial wall." The technique has been improved over the last 17 years with better coils and balloons. It is routinely used today to treat wide-neck aneurysms, particularly in patients with subarachnoid hemorrhage, thus eliminating stent placement and the use of antiplatelet agents. Most interventionalists consider an aneurysm neck to be wide when the ratio between the maximum diameter of the aneurysm sac and the size of the neck is 1 or less.

To treat sidewall wide-neck aneurysms at a location other than an arterial bifurcation, we routinely use the over-the-wire complaint HyperGlide balloon (Ev3, Irvine, CA). If distal catheterization of the neck of the aneurysm is difficult, we have utilized the less complaint gateway balloon (Boston Scientific Neurovascular) over a more torquable Synchro-14 wire (Boston Scientific Neurovascular) to perform balloon remodeling.

We prefer to perform the procedure using a 6-Fr shuttle sheath (Cook, Bloomington, IN) with a dual Y adaptor so that the microcatheter and balloon can be introduced separately. However, we have performed the procedure by puncturing both groins and introducing two separate guide catheters. With this technique, we usually introduce a 5- or 6-Fr guide catheter into the target vessel.

Under the road map, the balloon first is advanced across the neck of the aneurysm. The microcatheter is then advanced into the aneurysm. The balloon is inflated across the neck of the aneurysm, causing temporary occlusion of the neck and parent vessel. The first coil is positioned within the aneurysm sac. The balloon is deflated to test the stability of the coil within the aneurysm sac. If no movement of the coil is observed, the balloon is reinflated and the coil is detached. The coil is not detached if coil movement (meaning that the coil is not well anchored in the sac) is detected after balloon deflation. An angiogram is then performed. This is repeated multiple times until the aneurysm no longer fills with contrast or has a dense coil mass within the confines of its lumen.

The balloon acts as a temporary wall across the neck of the aneurysm, allowing coils to be deflected off the balloon back into the aneurysm sac during placement. The choice of the first coil is the most crucial decision in being able to treat a wide-neck aneurysm. The coil diameter should be large enough that it fully opposes the aneurysm wall and crosses the neck well. This provides friction between the coil and the wall, limiting migration of the coil outside of the aneurysm. The coil diameter should be the largest that will form within the aneurysm sac. The coil length should also be the longest that will fit within the aneurysm sac. This provides a large basket and allows the coils to be strongly anchored within the aneurysm sac. This also forms a bridge across the neck to help prevent additional coils from migrating into the parent vessel. The balloon occlusion should not last more than 5 minutes. The size of the balloon depends on the volume of a contrast and saline mixture introduced into the balloon; therefore, the balloon should only be inflated with the cadence syringe provided by the manufacturer. Overinflation of the balloon may cause rupture of the parent vessel or aneurysm. We feel the balloon is best inflated with a 60:40 contrast-to-saline mixture. This provides good visibility of the balloon under the road map and still leads to relative rapid deflation of the balloon. We test the balloon on the table before introducing it into the patient. We also inflate the balloon in the lower cervical carotid or vertebral artery prior to introducing into the intracranial circulation to determine whether the balloon is working properly and whether it can easily be seen under fluoroscopy. If the balloon will not deflate, the manufacturer recommends pulling negative pressure on the syringe connected to the Y adaptor. If all else fails, removing the wire from the balloon catheter will usually deflate the balloon; however, the entire system then has to be removed and prepped again prior to introducing it back into the body, because thrombus formation can occur within the balloon catheter, possibly making the balloon malfunction.

Bifurcation Wide-Neck Aneurysm

To treat a bifurcation aneurysm, we use a HyperForm balloon (Ev3). It is a compliant, low-pressure, over-the-wire balloon that can conform to the vasculature being treated. Most interventionalists believe this is the best-suited balloon for treating aneurysms located at arterial bifurcations or within small arteries. When the balloon is inflated, it may be partially herniated into the aneurysm neck or the origin of the arterial branches, emerging from the neck of the aneurysm. This allows the parent vessel and arterial branches emerging from the neck of the aneurysm to remain patent, with no compromise from the coils placed within the aneurysm sac.

Double Remodeling Technique

In certain bifurcation aneurysms, a single-balloon remodeling technique may not be able to treat patients from an endovascular technique. In these situations, another approach is to place two balloon catheters in a Y configuration, one beside the other, both beginning proximally in the parent artery, and both ending distally within each

of the branch vessels. The aneurysm is then coiled similar to the coiling of the single-balloon remodeling technique. This technique allows the operator to treat certain aneurysms that would otherwise not be treatable by coil embolization.

Results

Shapiro et al. in 2008 published a literature review with a meta-analysis of the safety and efficacy of adjunctive balloon remodeling during endovascular treatment of intracranial aneurysms.[25] They concluded that there was no higher incidence of thromboembolic events or iatrogenic rupture with the use of adjunctive balloon remodeling compared with unassisted coiling. They also commented that balloon remodeling appears to result in a higher initial and follow-up aneurysm occlusion rates. Mu et al. successfully treated 40 wide-neck aneurysms with the HyperForm balloon remodeling technique, with only 2 failed cases, in 2008.[26] Final results consisted of total occlusion in 34 cases (80.9%), subtotal occlusion in 4 cases (9.5%), and incomplete occlusion in 2 cases (4.8%). Nelson and Levy in 2001 treated 22 patients, with aneurysm occlusion on follow-up angiography at a mean of 19 months found in 17 of 20 patients.[27] The other two patients died prior to follow-up. Layton et al. treated 73 of 221 aneurysms over a 3-year period with balloon-assisted coiling.[28] They found no increased risk in thromboembolic complications when compared to simple coiling techniques. In conclusion, there appears to be no increased risk of complications with the balloon-remodeling technique. Aneurysm occlusion may be higher than with standard endovascular techniques; however, few studies report the results of this form of treatment.

STENT-ASSISTED COILING

Stent Characteristics

Certain wide-neck and dysplastic aneurysms may not be treated with simple coiling or balloon remodeling; however, with the current availability of stents made to navigate the intracranial circulation, treatment from an endovascular approach is now possible. The disadvantages are that a permanent implant is placed into the artery, there is a paucity of long-term patency data, and the patient is subjected to the risks associated with the long-term use of antiplatelet medication. The stent acts as a scaffold that prevents the coils placed in the aneurysm sac from herniation into the parent vessel. The stent may also reduce the inflow into the aneurysm, promoting stasis and thrombosis of the aneurysm. In addition, the struts of the stent may provide a matrix for the growth of endothelial cells across the neck of the aneurysm.

A standard cerebral angiogram is obtained, along with a 3D angiogram of the vessel in question. The dimensions of the artery above and below the aneurysm are measured, along with the size of the aneurysm and length of the neck. The targeted landing zone of the stent is determined. The self-expandable stent is sized to a nominal diameter 0.5 to 1.0 mm greater than the parent vessel at the targeted landing zone. The stent length should be centered on the aneurysm neck. The stent length is chosen to provide at least 5 mm of coverage proximal and distal to the aneurysm neck. If the parent vessel is tortuous, an attempt is made to place the distal and proximal aspect of the stent within a straight segment of the parent vessel.

Initially, balloon-expandable coronary stents were utilized; however, they were difficult to navigate into the intracranial circulation. Inflating the balloon also subjected the patient to possible rupture of the parent vessel, which is not possible with a self-expanding stent. Three self-expandable intracranial stents are currently available on the market: Neuroform (Boston Scientific Neurovascular), Leo (Balt Extrusion, Montmorency, France), and Enterprise (Codman Neurovascular, Raynham, MA). The Neuroform and Enterprise are only available in the United States. The major differences among these stents are the delivery system and whether they are closed or open cell. The Neuroform is an open cell stent, whereas the Enterprise and Leo stents are closed cell stents.

The self-expandable stent that comes preloaded into the delivery microcatheter is the Neuroform. The advantage is that the microwire remains within the lumen of the stent after its deployment. This may allow easier delivery of overlapping stents and catheterization of the aneurysm. The disadvantage is that navigating this system through the intracranial circulation can be difficult. This is due to the poor torquability of the microwire, because it is in contact with the stent. The system is also less flexible due to the stent being loaded into the microcatheter during navigation. To overcome these problems, many operators navigate a standard microcatheter and microwire into the distal intracranial circulation past the neck of the aneurysm. The wire is then exchanged for a 300-cm exchange-length microwire. This step is crucial, because during the exchange the distal tip of the microwire may produce a distal vessel perforation. The delivery microcatheter carrying the stent is then brought up over the exchange-length microwire, and the stent is deployed. This step of the procedure is also crucial in that the distal tip of the microwire should again be observed to prevent perforation. Because of these difficulties, the manufacturer has changed the platform for the delivery method so that it is similar to the method described next.

The self-expandable stents that are loaded into the delivery catheter only when it has reached its proper position are the Leo and Enterprise stents. The advantage of this system is that the delivery microcatheter is placed past the aneurysm without the necessity for an exchange wire, and without the stent in place in the microcatheter. This theoretically allows easier navigation through the vasculature because the operator can use the microwire of his or her choosing; the system is also not rigid due to the stent being absent from the microcatheter, and there is no friction on the wire from it contacting the stent, thus make it more readily torquable. Since there is no need for an exchange-length wire, the risk of distal perforation is greatly reduced. The disadvantage of this system is that the microwire must be removed prior to stent deployment, thus possibly making placement of overlapping stents or catherization of the aneurysm more difficult.

Technique of Coiling with Stent Assistance

The aneurysm may be coiled by three techniques utilizing stent assistant. With the first technique, the microcatheter is placed into the aneurysm sac and then the stent is placed across the aneurysm neck. This is called the jailed microcatheter technique. The second technique consists of placing the stent across the neck of the aneurysm and then navigating a microcatheter through the struts of the stent into the aneurysm sac. In the final technique, the aneurysm is first coiled utilizing the balloon remodeling technique and then the stent is placed across the neck of the aneurysm at the end of the procedure, with the idea that the stent struts will serve as a surface for endothelial cell growth across the neck of the aneurysm, thus preventing recanalization of the aneurysm. In a broad-neck dysplastic aneurysm or when the neck is not definable, the balloon may be inflated through the stent to define the parent vessel and prevent herniation of coils into the parent vessel.

Antiplatelet Treatment Regimen for Intracranial Stenting

A stent is a metallic foreign body; thus, introducing it into the cerebral vasculature may cause thrombus formation and platelet aggregation. To prevent this, it is important to administer antiplatelet agents prior to placement of an intracranial stent. This has been eloquently shown in the coronary literature, where placement of patients on a combination of aspirin and clopidogrel has been shown to prevent stent thrombosis and occlusion.[29] The optimal dosage and treatment regimen, however, have not been determined. Given that the average life span of a platelet is 7 days, we administer aspirin (81 mg/day orally) and clopidogrel (75 mg/day orally) for 7 days prior to the procedure. If a stent needs to be placed emergently, we load the patient with clopidogrel (600 mg orally) and aspirin (325 mg orally), wait 2 hours, and then perform the procedure. If a stent needs to be placed during the course of an endovascular procedure and the patient has not been preoperative treated with antiplatelet medications, we load the patient with the glycoprotein IIb/IIIa inhibitor abciximab. The patient is loaded with the cardiac dose of 0.25 mg/kg and then started on a 12-hour intravenous infusion at 0.125 µg/kg/min. The patient is also started on aspirin and clopidogrel. Most endovascular specialists avoid placement of a stent in patients with an acutely ruptured broad-neck aneurysm. This is because the patient will need to be placed on antiplatelet medications and will most likely need a ventriculostomy, given the subarachnoid hemorrhage. Also, if the patient develops vasospasm in the subacute period, intracranial balloon angioplasty can be more difficult with a stent placed in the intracranial circulation.

Results

Multiple articles have been published about the use of intracranial stents for treatment of wide-neck intracranial aneurysms. Given the limitations of space for this chapter, we briefly discuss the reports with a larger series of patients.

The use of the Enterprise stent was initially reported by Higashida et al.[30] All 5 cases were technically successful. The stent was well visualized, deployed easily, could be repositioned if needed, and was accurately placed without technical difficulties. Weber et al. in 2007 described the use of the stent in 31 saccular wide-neck aneurysms.[31] Follow-up angiography of 30 lesions after 6 months demonstrated 15 complete aneurysm occlusions, 8 aneurysm neck remnants, and 7 residual aneurysms. Two patients experienced possible device-related, serious adverse events. The Enterprise stent multicenter registry was published in 2009 and included 141 patients with 142 aneurysms who underwent 143 attempted stent deployments.[32] The use of stent assistance with aneurysm coiling was associated with a 76% rate of at least 90% occlusion. The stent could not be navigated to the desired location in 3% of cases, and there was a 2% occurrence of inaccurate deployment. Procedure data demonstrated a 6% temporary morbidity, 2.8% permanent morbidity, and 2% mortality.

Kis et al. in 2006 described the successful deployment of the Leo stent in 24 of 25 aneurysms.[33] There were 2 thromboembolic events related to the deployment of the Leo stent, 1 failure of stent deployment, difficulties in stent positioning in three cases, and 1 asymptomatic parent vessel occlusion after 7 months. Follow-up at an average of 5 months revealed aneurysm recurrence in 3 lesions, which were retreated.

The largest experience to date is with the Neuroform stent. This was the first intracranial stent available for the treatment of wide-neck aneurysms. The largest series to date is from China, reported by Liang et al. in 2009.[34] Their series included 110 wide-necked aneurysms. In all cases, the Neuroform stent system was delivered and deployed accurately. Procedure-related morbidity was 5.6%, and procedural-related mortality was 0.9%. Angiographic follow-up in 51 aneurysms at an average of 37 months showed an overall recanalization rate of 13.7%. In 2005, Lylyk et al. reported on 46 patients with 48 intracranial aneurysms treated using the Neuroform stent.[35] There was a 92% technical success rate. Approximately 19% of the stents were placed in a suboptimal location. In 31% of the cases, the stent was difficult to place. Procedure-related morbidity and mortality were 8.6% and 2.1%, respectively. Since this report, there have been at least two newer generations of the device, allowing easier placement of the stent. In 2007, Biondi et al. reported on 42 patients with 46 wide-neck aneurysms.[36] The balloon remodeling technique was performed in 77% of patients prior to stent placement. The stent was successfully deployed in 94% of the cases. Angiographic and clinical follow-up was available in 31 patients with 33 aneurysms. In the 30 aneurysms treated with stent-assisted coiling, there were 17 aneurysm occlusions (57%), 7 neck remnants (23%), and 6 residual aneurysms (20%). In 3 recanalized aneurysms treated with stent alone, 2 neck remnants remained unchanged (67%), and 1 neck remnant decreased in size (33%).

TRISPAN DEVICE

Characteristics of the Device

Another device used to treat a wide-neck intracranial aneurysm is the TriSpan device (Boston Scientific Neurovascular). This device was never marketed in the United States but is widely available in Asia, Canada, and Europe. The TriSpan device is composed of three loops of nitinol wire in the shape of a three-leaf clover. The device is delivered through a microcatheter into the aneurysm and deployed. It is held in place by its detachable wire. Once the TriSpan device is positioned to cover the neck of the aneurysm without compromise of the parent vessel, a microcatheter is placed through the device into the aneurysm, and the coils are delivered. After the aneurysm is adequately filled with coils, the TriSpan device is detached. Since the introduction of dedicated intracranial stents for wide-neck aneurysms,

the use of this device has decreased. We have no experience with the use of this device.

Results

The largest experience using the TriSpan for treating intracranial aneurysms has been in Montreal. In 2001, Raymond et al. reported on 25 patients with 19 basilar bifurcation and 6 anterior circulation aneurysms.[37] All aneurysms were wide neck except one. The procedure was successful in all patients, with complete obliteration of the aneurysm in 3 patients, residual necks in 13 patients, and a minimal sac in 7 patients. Follow-up angiogram in 16 patients reveal complete obliteration in 4 patients, a residual neck in 1 patient, a persistent residual neck in 4 patients, and recurrent aneurysm in 7 patients. De Keukeleire et al. in 2008 reported on 14 patients in whom 16 TriSpan devices were placed to assist coiling of wide-neck aneurysms in the anterior circulation.[38] TriSpan-assisted embolization was successful in 15 of the 16 procedures (93.8%), with complete occlusion in 2 procedures (12.5%), near-complete occlusion in 10 procedures (62.5%), and incomplete occlusion in 3 procedures (18.75%).

LIQUID EMBOLIC AGENTS

Technique Onyx 500

Numerous publications throughout the late 1980s and early 1990s described various techniques using liquid embolic agents to treat intracranial aneurysms. There were problems with the control of these agents during delivery into the aneurysm and nontarget embolization of the material distally into the intracranial circulation. Onyx (Ev3) is a liquid embolic agent designed for endovascular use. It is an ethylene–vinyl alcohol (EVOH) biocompatible copolymer used in conjunction with dimethyl sulfoxide (DMSO) as the solvent. Tantalum powder is added to the mixture to provide visualization under fluoroscopy. Onyx 500 used for aneurysm treatment contains 20% EVOH.

When the material comes in contact with an aqueous solution (i.e., blood or water), it precipitates and forms a soft spongy polymer cast, with the outer layer solidifying first and the central portion remaining in a semiliquid state. As further material is injected, it fills the space within the aneurysm. The material does not fragment during injection but remains in a cohesive semiliquid state similar to lava from a volcano.

In treatment of intracranial aneurysms, the material is kept within the aneurysm sac by placement of a DMSO-compatible balloon (HyperGlide or HyperForm) across the neck. The first step of the procedure consists of performing a seal test. During balloon inflation, contrast is injected through a DMSO-compatible microcatheter placed within the aneurysm sac to confirm any leakage of contrast into the parent vessel. If there is such leakage, patients are not treated with Onyx.

Depending on the therapeutic strategy, coils or a liquid embolic agent is delivered first to occlude the major part of the aneurysm sac. The dead space of the microcatheter is first filled with the solvent DMSO to prevent precipitation of the liquid embolic agent within the lumen of the microcatheter. The aneurysm is then obliterated slowly by injecting 0.1 to 0.2 ml/min of Onyx 500 with a cadence syringe. During each injection, the balloon remains inflated across the neck of the aneurysm. The balloon is deflated after about 5 minutes, allowing the polymer to solidify. Angiography is performed to confirm the polymer's location relative to the aneurysm, and this process is continued until the aneurysm is occluded. After the last injection, the material solidifies completely over a period of about 10 minutes, with diffusion of the solvent DMSO.

Results

Ev3 sponsored the Cerebral Aneurysm Multicenter European Onyx (CAMEO) trial in 20 centers.[39] CAMEO was a prospective, observational trial that enrolled 119 consecutive patients with 123 aneurysms. Follow-up results were reported for 100 of these patients. CAMEO reported complete occlusion in 79% of aneurysms, subtotal occlusion in 13%, and incomplete occlusion in 8%. Delayed occlusion of the parent vessel occurred in 9 patients, 5 of whom were asymptomatic. Piske et al. in 2009 treated 69 patients with 84 aneurysms.[40] All of the aneurysms had a wide neck. In this study, 50 aneurysms were small (less than 12 mm), 30 were large (12 to less than 25 mm), and 4 were giant. Angiographic follow-up was available for 65 of the 84 aneurysms at 6 months. Complete aneurysm occlusion was seen in 65.5% of aneurysms on immediate control and in 84.6% at 6 months. The rates of complete occlusion were 74% for small aneurysms and 80% for large aneurysms. Progression from incomplete to complete occlusion was seen in 68.2% of all aneurysms, with a higher percentage in small aneurysms (90.9%). Aneurysm recanalization was only observed in 3 patients (4.6%), with retreatment in 2 patients (3.3%).

Cekirge et al. presented the long-term clinical and angiographic follow-up results of 100 consecutive intracranial aneurysms treated with Onyx.[41] Intracranial stenting was used adjunctively in 25 aneurysms, including 19 during initial treatment and 6 during retreatment. Of the 100 aneurysms, 35 were giant or large/wide neck, and 65 were small. Follow-up angiography was performed in all 91 surviving patients (96 aneurysms) at 3 and/or 6 months. Overall, aneurysm recanalization was observed in 12 of 96 aneurysms with follow-up angiography (12.5%). All 12 were large or giant aneurysms, resulting in a 36% recanalization rate in the large and giant aneurysm group. The authors found that 1 aneurysm out of 25 treated with the combination of a stent and Onyx showed recanalization.

FLOW DIVERSION

Characteristics

A new generation of endovascular devices has appeared over the last 3 years. These devices are called flow divertors.[42] They have been developed to treat aneurysms from an endolumial rather than an endosaccular approach. These stentlike devices are designed to reconstruct the parent vessel and to divert flow from the aneurysm lumen without the use of coils. The device promotes thrombus formation within the aneurysm by decreasing the hemodynamic effects within the aneurysm sac, thus promoting stasis. It addition, the device has tighter scaffolding than a conventional intracranial stent, providing a means over which endothelial cells can grow to seal off the neck of the aneurysm. Kallmes et al. have characterized the effects of the pipeline embolization device (PED) in an experimental rabbit aneurysm model.[43,44] The PED (Ev3) is one of

the first flow-diversion devices used in humans, and it was approved by the U.S. FDA for treatment of aneurysms on April 10, 2011. The PED is a cylindrical, stentlike construct composed of 48 braided strands of cobalt chromium and platinum. Its appearance is similar to the Wallstent; however, there is a denser wire mesh. The Silk stent (Balt Extrusion) is another device. It is a braided, self-expanding, high metal surface area coverage construct that has Conformité Européenne marking approval in Europe. Other devices were in development as this chapter was being written. The flow divertors are delivered and placed in a similar fashion to current conventional intracranial stents described previously.

Results

Lylyk et al. reported their single-center results for a series of 53 patients treated with the PED.[45] No major procedure-related complications were reported in their series. On angiographic follow-up, there was a 93% and 95% rate of complete aneurysm occlusion observed at 6 and 12 months, respectively. Fiorella et al. reported two cases of fusiform vertebral artery aneurysms that were treated successfully with the PED.[46] Kadziolka et al. reported on 6 patients with intracranial aneurysms treated with the Silk stent.[47] The stent was deployed in all cases with no morbidity or mortality; however, the results were not commented upon in the abstract.

Complications of Endovascular Coiling and their Treatment

Every peri- or postprocedural complication needs to be examined thoroughly prior to a corrective action being taken. For example, further manipulation of a single malpositioned loop of coil in a parent vessel may lead to aneurysm rupture and death or further thrombus formation and a cerebral infarction. If a single loop of coil is within the parent vessel and there is no thrombus formation on the coil or compromise of antegrade flow within the parent vessel, it may be prudent to just watch the situation by placing the patient on intravenous heparin overnight and on antiplatelet medications and avoiding possible significant morbidity or mortality.

The advantages and disadvantages, along with the risks, of endovascular coiling should be weighed against the risks of surgical treatment or a conservative approach prior to treatment. This is to determine the best option for the most optimal clinical outcome.

Patients should be given their full options, along with extensive information prior to treatment. This information should be given whenever possible, in case of a ruptured aneurysm, to the patient's relatives as well. The information provided must include the natural history of the disease, goal of treatment, and potential risks.

COIL MALPOSITION

Deposition of a coil outside the aneurysm sac can occur. Most commonly, it is a single loop of coil protruding into the parent vessel. This seldom causes a thromboembolic complication. However, if thrombus forms around the loop of coil, a glycoprotein IIb/IIIa inhibitor can be given at the site of thrombus formation to dissolve the clot. The coil should then be removed with one of the retrieval devices. If this is not possible, then the single loop of coil should be pushed against the vessel wall by placement of a self-expanding intracranial stent. Malposition of a coil is infrequent and usually the result of a poor coil choice, poor catheter position, or poor technique. We commonly apply some minimal forward force on the microcatheter during coiling of the aneurysm in the late stages to prevent the microcatheter from being kicked out of the aneurysm and the coil loop being deposited outside of the aneurysm sac.

STRETCHED COIL

Stretching of a coil is one of the biggest fears for the endovascular neurosurgeon; however, the incidence of this occurring has decreased dramatically since the introduction of stretch-resistant coils. To avoid this, retraction of the coil under fluoroscopy must be one to one with the delivery wire and hand movements at the groin. If the coil is not responding one to one under fluoroscopy with hand movements at the groin or if difficulty is encountered repositioning the coil, it most likely has stretched. In this situation, the coil and microcatheter should be removed as a unit from the patient. If this is not possible, then the coil should be stretched as long as possible and positioned into the external carotid artery or descending thoracic aorta to prevent migration distally and to prevent a large coil mass from occluding the parent vessel. A majority of patients will tolerate stretching of a single loop of coil into the parent vessel without a thromboembolic event or vessel occlusion. If this occurs, the patient should be kept anticoagulated overnight in the NICU and should be placed on an antiplatelet agent. A layer on endothelial cells will form over the stretched coil in about 8 to 10 weeks.

BROKEN COIL

A broken coil usually occurs when a stretched coil is pushed to mechanical failure. If a large portion of the coil is left in the parent vessel, thrombus formation with platelet aggregation may occur rapidly. In these cases, it may be necessary to give a glycoprotein IIb/IIIa inhibitor at the site of thrombus formation and make sure the patient is fully anticoagulated. An attempt at retrieving the coil with a dedicated device such as a loop snare, alligator clip, or the Merci device (Concentric Medical, Mountain View, CA) can then be made. If this attempt cannot be performed and the coil is compromising antegrade flow within the parent vessel, the coil can be pushed against the vessel wall and trapped with a self-expanding stent.

RUPTURE OF ANEURYSM

Aneurysm rupture is the most dreaded complication. This can occur spontaneously due to the fragile nature of the aneurysm. It may also occur iatrogenically from the cerebral angiogram or placement of a microcatheter or coil into the aneurysm.[48] When this occurs, a rapid severe transient elevation of intracranial pressure causes severe elevation of the blood pressure. If electroencephalogram monitoring is being performed, electric activity will seize. The aneurysm needs to be secured quickly, since a ruptured aneurysm can easily cause death to the patient.[49,50]

If the patient is anticoagulated, this must be immediately reversed with protamine (i.e., 10 mg of protamine per 1000 IU of heparin given) so that the ACT is less than 150 seconds. If the patient has been premedicated with aspirin or clopidogrel, an attempt at reversal of platelet inhibition should be made with the infusion of platelets. We have a prepared, nonpooled, five-pack of platelets ready in the rooms prior to coil placement so as to be prepared for this event. The blood pressure should also be lower immediately by pharmaceutical means to try and prevent further extravasation of blood into the subarachnoid space. If a balloon is present within the parent vessel, this should be carefully inflated and the aneurysm should be rapidly packed with addition coils. If the microcatheter is within the subarachnoid space, this should not be removed, but coiling should be performed from the subarachnoid space into the aneurysm. Computed tomography of the head should be immediately performed after the aneurysm is secure to assess for hydrocephalus and the need for placement of a ventriculostomy catheter. Vasospasm should be treated by intra-arterial injection of a pharmacologic agent (verapamil, nicardipine, nimodipine, etc.) once the aneurysm is secure.

RUPTURE OF VESSEL

Perforation of a blood vessel by a microguidewire is rare. This may be self-limiting and seal or may lead to life-threatening hemorrhage. If life-threatening hemorrhage is identified, permanent occlusion of the vessel may be life saving. A liquid embolic agent or coils can be utilized.[51] Rarely, rupture of a blood vessel after placement of a balloon-expandable stent can be managed conservatively with prolonged balloon inflation across the area of rupture.[52]

PROCEDURAL THROMBUS FORMATION

A thromboembolic event is probably the most common complication related to endovascular management of an aneurysm. This has decreased over the last few years mainly due to better and more liberal use of antiplatelet agents. Patients are now routinely placed on clopidogrel and aspirin 7 days prior to treatment. This is based on the coronary intervention literature, which has shown a significant decrease in the risk of thromboembolic events in patients treated with this regimen. Furthermore, to prevent thrombus formation during the procedure, patients are fully anticoagulated so that the ACT range is between 250 and 300 seconds. Biliverdin is a direct thrombin inhibitor with a better anticoagulation profile and a shorter half-life when compared to heparin; however, it does not have a reversal agent, which limits its use in the cerebral vascular circulation. If thrombus forms on coils placed at the neck of the aneurysm, most interventionalists prefer local infusion of a glycoprotein IIb/IIIa receptor.[53] This is administered intra-arterially through the microcatheter at a dosage of 4 to 10 mg over 10 to 20 minutes.[54] This has also been shown to be effective in ruptured aneurysms with no increased risk of bleeding complications. Three glycoprotein IIb/IIIa receptor inhibitors are available on the market. The most common one utilized is abciximab, which is mainly used in our lab. However, eptifibatide (Integrilin) may be the preferred agent due to its shorter half-life and reversible binding to the glycoprotein IIb/IIIa receptor.

KEY REFERENCES

Biondi A, Janardhan V, Katz JM, et al. Neuroform stent-assisted coil embolization of wide-neck intracranial aneurysms: strategies in stent deployment and midterm follow-up. *Neurosurgery.* 2007;61(3): 460-468:discussion 468–469.

Cekirge HS, Saatci I, Ozturk MH, et al. Late angiographic and clinical follow-up results of 100 consecutive aneurysms treated with Onyx reconstruction: largest single-center experience. *Neuroradiology.* 2006;48(2):113-126.

Doerfler A, Wanke I, Egelhof T, et al. Aneurysmal rupture during embolization with Guglielmi detachable coils: causes, management, and outcome. *AJNR Am J Neuroradiol.* 2001;22(10):1825-1832.

Guglielmi G, Vinuela F, Dion J, Duckwiler G. Electrothrombosis of saccular aneurysms via endovascular approach. Part 2: preliminary clinical experience. *J Neurosurg.* 1991;75(1):8-14.

Guglielmi G, Vinuela F, Sepetka I, Macellari V. Electrothrombosis of saccular aneurysms via endovascular approach. Part 1: electrochemical basis, technique, and experimental results. *J Neurosurg.* 1991;75(1):1-7.

Layton KF, Cloft HJ, Gray LA, et al. Balloon-assisted coiling of intracranial aneurysms: evaluation of local thrombus formation and symptomatic thromboembolic complications. *AJNR Am J Neuroradiol.* 2007;28(6):1172-1175.

Lee T, Baytion M, Sciacca R, et al. Aggregate analysis of the literature for unruptured intracranial aneurysm treatment. *AJNR Am J Neuroradiol.* 2005;26(8):1902-1908.

Le Roux PD, Winn HR, Newell DW. *Management of cerebral aneurysms.* Philadelphia, Pa: Saunders; 2004.

Liang G, Gao X, Li Z, et al. Neuroform stent-assisted coiling of intracranial aneurysms: a 5 year single-center experience and follow-up. *Neurol Res.* 2010;32(7):721-727.

Lylyk P, Ferrario A, Pasbon B, et al. Buenos Aires experience with the Neuroform self-expanding stent for the treatment of intracranial aneurysms. *J Neurosurg.* 2005;102(2):235-241.

Lylyk P, Miranda C, Ceratto R, et al. Curative endovascular reconstruction of cerebral aneurysms with the pipeline embolization device: the Buenos Aires experience. *Neurosurgery.* 2009;64(4):632-642:discussion 642-643; quiz N6.

Mocco J, Snyder KV, Albuquerque FC, et al. Treatment of intracranial aneurysms with the Enterprise stent: a multicenter registry. *J Neurosurg.* 2009;110(1):35-39.

Molyneux AJ, Cekirge S, Saatci I, Gal G. Cerebral Aneurysm Multicenter European Onyx (CAMEO) trial: results of a prospective observational study in 20 European centers. *AJNR Am J Neuroradiol.* 2004;25(1): 39-51.

Molyneux AJ, Kerr R, Stratton I, et al. International Subarachnoid Aneurysm Trial (ISAT) of neurosurgical clipping versus endovascular coiling in 2143 patients with ruptured intracranial aneurysms: a randomised trial. *Lancet.* 2002;360(9342):1267-1274.

Molyneux AJ, Kerr RS, Yu LM, et al. International Subarachnoid Aneurysm Trial (ISAT) of neurosurgical clipping versus endovascular coiling in 2143 patients with ruptured intracranial aneurysms: a randomised comparison of effects on survival, dependency, seizures, rebleeding, subgroups, and aneurysm occlusion. *Lancet.* 2005;366(9488):809-817.

Moret J, Cognard C, Weill A, et al. Reconstruction technique in the treatment of wide-neck intracranial aneurysms. Long-term angiographic and clinical results. Apropos of 56 cases. *J Neuroradiol.* 1997;24(1): 30-44.

Mounayer C, Piotin M, Baldi S, et al. Intraarterial administration of abciximab for thromboembolic events occurring during aneurysm coil placement. *AJNR Am J Neuroradiol.* 2003;24(10):2039-2043.

Park MS, Stiefel MF, Fiorella D, et al. Intracranial placement of a new, compliant guide catheter: technical note. *Neurosurgery.* 2008;63(3): E616-E617:discussion E617.

Piotin M, Iijima A, Wada H, Moret J. Increasing the packing of small aneurysms with complex-shaped coils: an in vitro study. *AJNR Am J Neuroradiol.* 2003;24(7):1446-1448.

Piotin M, Liebig T, Feste CD, et al. Increasing the packing of small aneurysms with soft coils: an in vitro study. *Neuroradiology.* 2004;46(11): 935-939.

Raymond J, Guilbert F, Roy D. Neck-bridge device for endovascular treatment of wide-neck bifurcation aneurysms: initial experience. *Radiology.* 2001;221(2):318-326.

Shapiro M, Babb J, Becske T, Nelson PK. Safety and efficacy of adjunctive balloon remodeling during endovascular treatment of intracranial aneurysms: a literature review. *AJNR Am J Neuroradiol.* 2008;29(9):1777-1781.

Vanninen R, Koivisto T, Saari T, et al. Ruptured intracranial aneurysms: acute endovascular treatment with electrolytically detachable coils—a prospective randomized study. *Radiology.* 1999;211(2):325-336.

Wang TH, Bhatt DL, Topol EJ. Aspirin and clopidogrel resistance: an emerging clinical entity. *Eur Heart J.* 2006;27(6):647-654.

Wiebers DO, Whisnant JP, Huston 3rd J, et al. Unruptured intracranial aneurysms: natural history, clinical outcome, and risks of surgical and endovascular treatment. *Lancet.* 2003;362(9378):103-110.

Numbered references appear on Expert Consult.

CHAPTER 85

Endovascular Treatment of Stroke

KYLE M. FARGEN • GREGORY J. VELAT • MICHAEL F. WATERS •
BRIAN L. HOH • J. MOCCO

Stroke is the third leading cause of death in the United States, accounting for more than 143,000 deaths each year. The Centers for Disease Control and Prevention estimates approximately 795,000 strokes occur annually in the United States. Of these, 610,000 are sentinel events, with the remainder occurring in those who have suffered a prior stroke.[1] Stroke is a leading cause of long-term disability due to loss of independence, language, motor skills, and cognitive abilities.[1] The American Heart Association has estimated the financial burden of stroke to be nearly $70 billion in 2009 due to both direct and indirect costs.[2] Although acute stroke is dichotomized into both ischemic and hemorrhagic etiologies, the vast majority of strokes are secondary to ischemia. Roughly 80% to 85% of acute strokes are secondary to thromboembolic vessel occlusion, typically arising from cardiac, carotid, or intracranial artery pathology.[3]

Timely arterial recanalization and prevention of reocclusion after treatment have become integral foci of the modern management of acute stroke. Current therapeutic modalities include intravenous chemical thrombolysis, intra-arterial mechanical and chemical thrombolysis, and stenting. Rapid diagnosis and treatment of acute stroke have been shown to improve patient outcomes in multiple studies.[4-10] However, multiple barriers exist that may prevent patients from receiving timely revascularization, including delay in diagnosis, resource constraints, and lack of physicians trained in stroke management. Regionalization of stroke care has been popularized in recent years in the United States to combat such barriers. Despite these efforts, it is estimated that less than 1% of patients suffering an acute stroke receive intravenous thrombolytic therapy.[11] The recent results of the third European Cooperative Acute Stroke Study (ECASS), which showed benefit in patients who received intravenous recombinant tissue plasminogen activator (rtPA) within 4.5 hours of symptom onset,[12] may increase the number of patients eligible to receive intravenous thrombolytic therapy.

The only medical therapy approved by the U.S. Food and Drug Administration (FDA) for acute stroke remains intravenous rtPA. Recently, the Merci Retriever thrombectomy device (Concentric Medical, Mountain View, CA) and the Penumbra System thromboaspiration device (Alameda, CA) also gained FDA approval for the treatment of acute stroke.

Intravenous thrombolysis, intra-arterial chemical and mechanical thrombolytic therapies, and stenting for acute ischemic stroke are discussed in this chapter. Specific indications, methods, potential complications, and supportive evidence are presented for each of the modalities.

Occlusion and Recanalization

Integral to the endovascular treatment of acute ischemic stroke are the principles of arterial occlusion, recanalization, and reocclusion. Stroke onset typically correlates with acute occlusion of an intracranial artery by platelet- and/or fibrin-rich clot, resulting in reduced parenchymal perfusion. If perfusion is not restored in a timely fashion, a hypoxia-induced cellular cascade is triggered, resulting in cell vulnerability and potential cellular necrosis. Various factors may influence the extent of cellular necrosis, including potential collateral blood flow contingent upon the patency of the circle of Willis or anastomoses from external carotid or posterior circulation vessels, patient coagulation status, and platelet function, as well as other patient comorbidities. Irreversible neuronal death may occur within 3 to 4 minutes of ischemia. Potentially salvageable tissue on the verge of necrosis is referred to as the penumbra. The primary goal of endovascular stroke therapy is to restore blood flow to the brain tissue within the penumbra and territory at potential risk while avoiding hemorrhagic transformation of unsalvageable tissue.

Arterial recanalization is widely accepted as a surrogate marker of efficacy for stroke therapies. The Thrombolysis in Myocardial Infarction (TIMI) scale is accepted among neurointerventionalists as a semiquantitative measure of vessel recanalization (Table 85-1).[13] Transcranial Doppler ultrasonography has also shown promise in evaluating vessel recanalization.[14-16] Successful recanalization has been linked to improved clinical outcomes in many series.[17] Pretreatment residual flow has been shown to be predictive of both time to achieve recanalization and likelihood of a successful intervention.[15] In a meta-analysis of recanalization and outcome, Rha and Saver demonstrated a strong correlation between arterial recanalization and improved functional outcomes with reduced mortality.[17] Successful arterial recanalization at the time of intervention does not always correlate with lasting benefit, because some vessels may reocclude. Reocclusion rates as high as 34% have been reported in some studies following intra-arterial administration of rtPA.[18-20] In addition, distal propagation of thrombus has been reported in approximately 16% of patients undergoing pharmacologic or mechanical thrombolysis.[20] Potential reperfusion injury may

Table 85-1	TIMI Flow Grading System[13]	
TIMI Grade	**Classification**	**Criteria**
0	No perfusion	No recanalization of the primary occlusive lesion
1	Penetration without perfusion	Incomplete or partial recanalization with flow past the initial occlusion, but no distal branch filling
2	Partial perfusion	Partial recanalization with incomplete or slow distal branch filling
3	Complete perfusion	Full recanalization with filling of all distal branches

occur when the blood–brain barrier becomes destabilized. Secondary cerebral edema and/or intracranial hemorrhage may result, possibly necessitating operative intervention.

Goals of Therapy

The goals of endovascular treatment of stroke are: (1) obtain timely recanalization of the occluded vessel (TIMI grade 2 or 3 blood flow), (2) prevent reocclusion following recanalization, (3) minimize distal propagation of thrombus, and (4) avoid intractable cerebral edema and intracranial hemorrhage following reperfusion.

Presentation

Patients suffering an acute ischemic stroke most commonly present with sudden-onset neurologic deficit(s) that localize to the brain territory supplied by the affected vessel(s). It is imperative to perform a thorough but succinct history and neurologic examination to assess the extent of stroke. Physicians must gather information regarding the progression of neurologic deficit over time and any improvements that have occurred since onset, as spontaneous improvement

may indicate a transient ischemic attack or point to an alternative diagnosis, such as seizure. The National Institute of Health Stroke Scale (NIHSS) quantitatively rates the severity of the stroke and has demonstrated excellent reliability and clinical utility.[21-23] The scale ranges from 0 (no symptoms) to 42 and grades patient deficits in multiple functions, including motor, sensory, language, and alertness. Generally, scores of 1 to 5 represent mild stroke, 5 to 20 moderate to severe stroke, and greater than 20 very severe stroke. The NIHSS and its booklet are accessible online at the National Institute of Neurological Disorders and Stroke (NINDS) Web site (http://www.ninds.nih.gov/).

Imaging

All patients presenting with stroke symptoms should undergo brain imaging. Computed tomography (CT) is the most readily available and efficient imaging modality, although magnetic resonance imaging (MRI) may also be performed. Early noncontrasted CT scanning is critical for evaluation of intracranial hemorrhage and serves as the primary differentiator for standard of care therapies. In addition, noncontrasted CT scanning of the head may reveal hypodensities consistent with evolving territories of infarction, cerebral edema or herniation, loss of gray–white matter differentiation, or arterial occlusion referred to as the "hyperdense sign." At the University of Florida, computed tomography angiography (CTA) of the head and neck and cerebral CT perfusion are performed on all patients who present with acute stroke symptoms. It is imperative the aortic arch and major arteries of the head and neck be visualized to evaluate for arterial occlusion, flow-limiting stenosis, dissection, or other vessel anomalies. CT perfusion is used to assess the extent of stroke and the amount of potentially salvageable brain parenchyma. Tissue with preserved cerebral blood volume, despite reduced cerebral blood flow and increased mean transit time, represents the stroke penumbra (Fig. 85-1).[24,25] CT perfusion may be

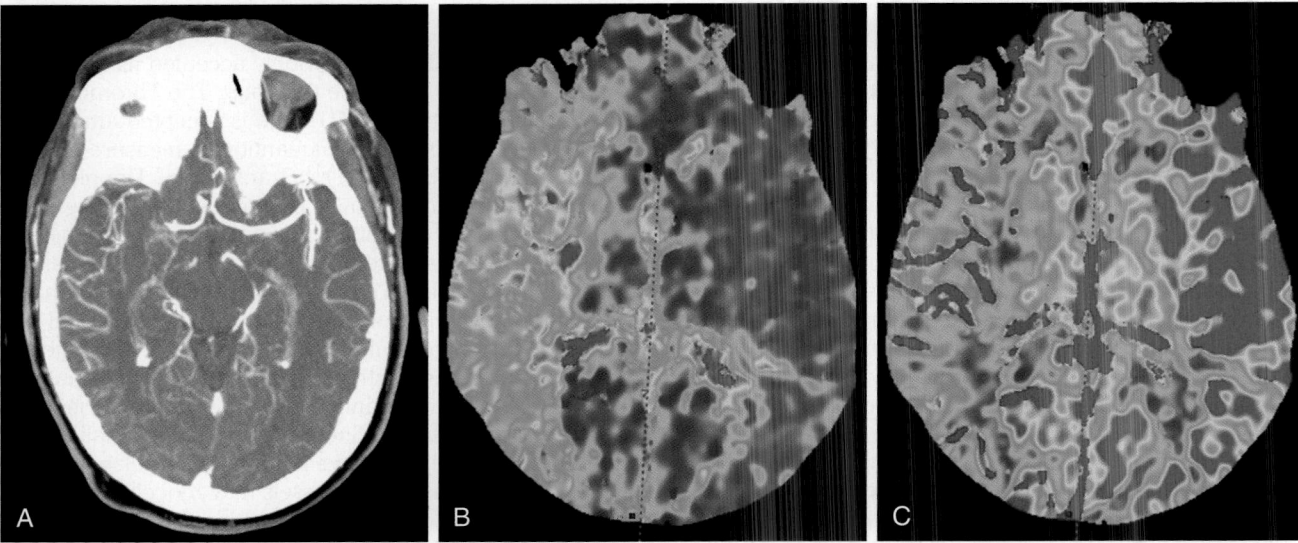

FIGURE 85-1 CTA of a patient presenting with symptoms of right MCA ischemia. A, CTA demonstrates right M1 segment occlusion from thrombus. B, Perfusion imaging reveals an elevated mean transit time in the right MCA distribution. C, Perfusion imaging demonstrates decreased cerebral blood flow within the right MCA distribution. If perfusion imaging demonstrates spared cerebral blood volume, these findings indicate a potential therapeutic target for intervention.

limited at visualizing the posterior fossa due to significant bone artifact and beam scatter; however, it is hoped that newer imaging technologies and techniques will ameliorate this difficulty. Alternatively, some institutions rely on diffusion-weighted MRI to evaluate the brain's physiologic state. Whichever modality is used, timely evaluation of actual brain physiology is rapidly becoming a new standard in the cutting-edge treatment of stroke.

Patient Selection

Indications and contraindications for intravenous thrombolysis are listed in Table 85-2. Intracranial hemorrhage is a direct contraindication for revascularization therapy. The therapeutic window for intravenous rtPA has been extended to 4.5 hours from the onset of symptoms based on results of the recent ECASS III trial.[12,26] Patients eligible for intravenous rtPA should undergo this treatment prior to attempts at endovascular therapy. If patients fail to improve neurologically with intravenous rtPA, present outside of the therapeutic window, or have a contraindication to intravenous rtPA, endovascular therapy may be considered, including the use of intra-arterial rtPA, mechanical disruption using the microwire, the use of mechanical thrombectomy/aspiration devices, angioplasty, stenting, or a combination of procedures in those with persistent occlusive thrombi.

The relative amount of ischemic parenchyma should be considered strongly when deciding to pursue endovascular treatment. Specifically, unsalvageable tissue (defined by regions with decreased cerebral blood volume in the setting of increased mean transit time and decreased cerebral blood flow on perfusion imaging) comprising greater than one third of the overall brain territory at risk of ischemia is a relative contraindication to endovascular therapy. In our experience, these patients are at high risk of hemorrhagic transformation following intra-arterial pharmacologic and/or mechanical thrombolysis or stenting, particularly if the nonsalvageable region involves the basal ganglia. Other factors linked to poor clinical outcomes in patients undergoing endovascular therapy include advanced age (greater than 75 years), presentation NIHSS score greater than 18, and admission glucose greater than 150 mg/dl.[9] While the conventional ideal therapeutic window for endovascular therapy is within 6 to 8 hours of symptom onset,[10,26,27] patients are increasingly being successfully treated outside of this time frame guided by physiologic imaging (CT perfusion or MRI perfusion).[28,29]

Intracerebral Hemorrhage

The major complication of endovascular therapies for stroke is intracranial hemorrhage, which is estimated to occur in roughly 5% to 10% of patients undergoing intravenous tissue plasminogen activator therapy.[7,30,31] Clinically significant intracerebral hematomas, so-called symptomatic intracerebral hemorrhage (SICH), develops in around 3% of patients. The frequency of SICH increases with the concomitant presence of early signs of infarction on CT scan prior to administration.[31,32] Furthermore, symptom severity, diabetes mellitus, and elevated blood glucose are well-demonstrated independent risk factors for SICH.[32,33] Other possible risk factors include high systolic blood pressure, low platelets, advanced age, and delay in treatment. Intra-arterial tissue plasminogen activator, in contrast to venous, has a slightly higher risk of SICH. Estimates of SICH in those receiving intra-arterial thrombolysis are approximately 6% to 12%, while those receiving both intravenous and intra-arterial administration are estimated to be roughly 9% to 20%.[10,31]

The pathophysiology of post-treatment SICH appears to be primarily the result of reperfusion injury with hemorrhagic transformation at ischemic sites.[34] Ischemia results in disruption of the blood–brain barrier, causing leakage from vessels, tissue edema, and loss of autoregulation secondary to increased free radical and matrix metalloproteinase activity.[35,36] Reperfusion of damaged vessels results in small ruptures with microhemorrhages that may ultimately enlarge into a hematoma due to disruption of the normal clotting cascade by the presence of thrombolytic agents.

Table 85-2	Indications and Contraindications to rtPA Administration
Indications	**Contraindications**
· Ischemic stroke onset within 4.5 hours of drug administration · Measurable deficit on NIHSS examination · No hemorrhage or nonstroke cause of deficit on CT · Age >18 years	· Minor or rapidly improving symptoms · Seizure at onset of stroke · Stroke or serious head trauma within the past 3 months · Major surgery within the last 2 weeks · Known history of intracranial hemorrhage · Sustained systolic blood pressure >185 mm Hg · Sustained diastolic blood pressure >110 mm Hg · Aggressive treatment needed to lower the patient's blood pressure · Symptoms suggestive of subarachnoid hemorrhage · Gastrointestinal or urinary tract hemorrhage within the last 3 weeks · Arterial puncture at noncompressible site within the last 7 days · Heparin received within the last 48 hours and elevated partial thromboplastin time · Prothrombin time >15 seconds · Platelet count <100,000 μl. · Serum glucose <50 or >400 mg/dl
Administration	
0.9 mg/kg infused intravenously over 60 minutes, with 10% of the initial dose given as a bolus over 1 minute	

Intravenous Thrombolytic Therapy

Intravenous thrombolytic therapy with rtPA was the first FDA-approved intervention for acute stroke. The NINDS trial, published in 1995, was a large, randomized, placebo-controlled study consisting of more than 600 patients randomized to rtPA versus placebo within 3 hours of stroke onset.[4] At 24 hours, no difference was seen in NIHSS improvement between those receiving rtPA and those receiving placebo. At 3 months, patients receiving rtPA had 1.7 times greater odds of a favorable outcome than did those receiving placebo. SICH occurred in 34 of the 312 patients receiving rtPA (20 were symptomatic, of which 9 were fatalities), compared to 11 of the 312 patients receiving placebo (2 symptomatic, 1 fatality). Two additional trials, ECASS I and II, demonstrated comparable results with improved functional outcomes but increased risk of hemorrhage.[7,8] These findings led to approval by the FDA of rtPA, at a dose of 0.9 mg/kg, in acute stroke patients presenting within 3 hours of symptom onset.

Recently, trials have focused on the benefits of rtPA beyond the 3-hour window. The Alteplase Thrombolysis for Acute Noninterventional Therapy in Ischemic Stroke (ATLANTIS) trial, published in 1999, evaluated the benefits of rtPA administration between 3 and 5 hours after symptom onset.[5] This trial demonstrated no benefit to the administration of rtPA beyond 3 hours. In 2004, published pooled data from the ATLANTIS, ECASS, and NINDS trials suggested a potential benefit in administration beyond the 3-hour window.[37] In 2008, Hacke et al. demonstrated significant benefit in clinical outcome at 90 days in patients receiving rtPA within 180 to 270 minutes after symptom onset.[12] In 2009, the FDA approved the use of rtPA in acute ischemic stroke in patients 3 to 4.5 hours after symptom onset.

Despite the recent temporal expansion, intravenous rtPA faces several important limitations. Research has demonstrated ineffectiveness in lysing thromboembolic obstruction of large proximal vessels as compared to more distal, smaller vessels.[16] One study of 349 patients undergoing intravenous rtPA for stroke revealed nearly one third with no recanalization, one third with partial recanalization, and only one third with complete recanalization.[38] In addition, early reocclusion has been demonstrated in up to 34% of patients receiving intravenous rtPA.[14,19] To combat these limitations, new endovascular therapies have been developed to provide better targeting of thrombolytic agents with improved recanalization and prevention of reocclusion. These therapies are described in the remaining sections of this chapter.

General Endovascular Procedure

The access area, typically the common femoral artery (the radial artery remains a secondary option), is prepped and draped sterilely. A 5- to 8-French (Fr) sheath is then placed depending on the anticipated device to be utilized. After confirmed, uncomplicated arterial access, a heparin bolus may be administered to maintain an activated coagulation time between 250 and 300 seconds. Some interventionalists aim for a lower activated coagulation time to compensate for planned dosing of intra-arterial thrombolytics

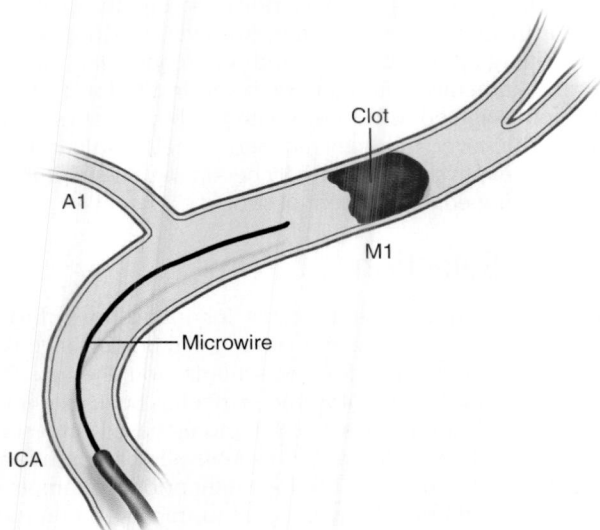

FIGURE 85-2 Schematic diagram illustrating an occlusive thrombus in the M1 segment of the MCA. The microcatheter is shown just proximal to the occlusion. At this juncture, the microwire is gently navigated across the occlusion with a twisting motion, followed by advancement of the microcatheter over the microwire to a position beyond the occlusion. A microcatheter angiographic run is then performed to define the distal aspect of the occlusion.

and antiplatelet agents and thus potentially reduce the theoretical risk of hemorrhagic transformation. If prior CTA or magnetic resonance angiography (MRA) has been performed (recommended), then selective catheterization of the target vessel can be performed. If CTA or MRA has not been completed, a diagnostic cerebral angiogram guided by patient symptomatology should be performed to localize the occlusion. The interventionalist then assesses the location of arterial occlusion and evaluates for additional arterial pathology (i.e., vessel dissection) prior to intracranial intervention. A microcatheter is then introduced over a microwire and is navigated to the site of arterial occlusion (Fig. 85-2). The microwire is then gently navigated across the occlusion with a twisting motion. Once this is done, the microcatheter is advanced over the microwire to a position beyond the occlusion. A microcatheter angiographic run should then be performed to define the distal aspect of the occlusion. At this juncture, the interventionalist must make a decision regarding the type of intra-arterial intervention that will be undertaken. There are no data published to definitively support the choice of one intervention modality over another. This decision should be guided by the comfort level and experience of the interventionalist with each technique and device, as well as the patient-specific anatomy. Following each endovascular intervention, angiography is performed to observe for vessel recanalization. All catheters and wires are removed upon conclusion of the intervention, and the arteriotomy puncture is sealed using a percutaneous closure device. Alternatively, a flexible sheath may be left in place until serum thrombolytic levels normalize. The patient should be monitored in an intensive care unit with frequent neurologic examinations and strict blood pressure and glucose control.

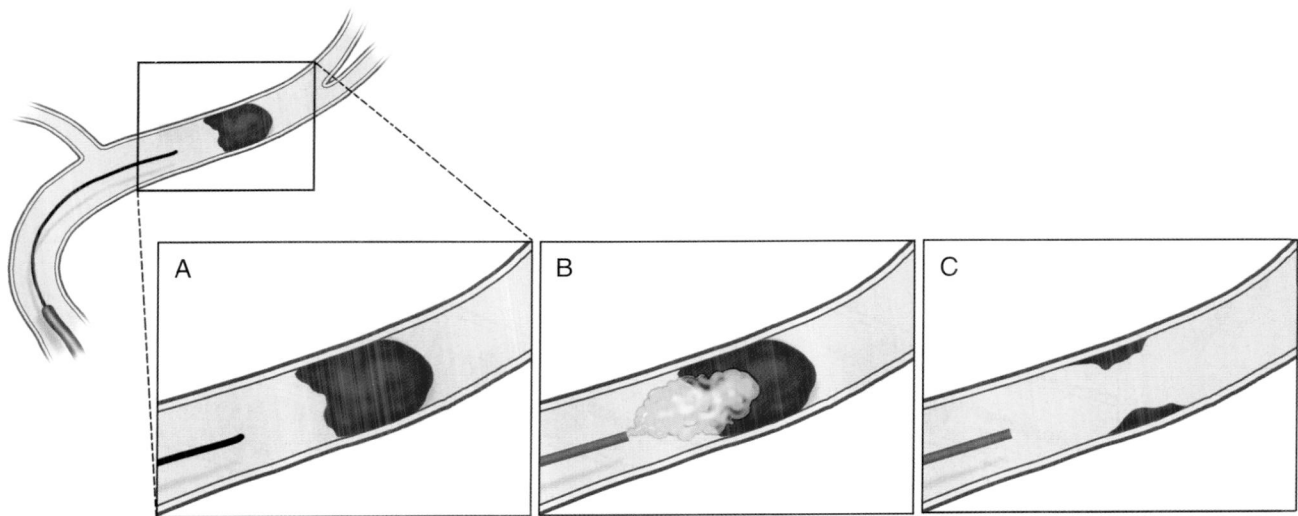

FIGURE 85-3 Schematic diagram depicting intra-arterial thrombolysis. A, The microwire is navigated just proximal to the occlusion. B, The microcatheter is passed over the wire to the occlusion, and intra-arterial thrombolytics are administered. C, Dissolution of the thrombus has occurred with restoration of vessel patency.

Intra-Arterial Thrombolytic Therapy

Intra-arterial thrombolysis utilizes precise localization for administration of thrombolytic agents while minimizing systemic exposure. The agent is administered through an endovascular microcatheter placed at the site of the occlusion. When the region of occlusion is approached, thrombolytics are administered in immediate proximity to the clot, maximizing the effect of the agent at the target while reducing the systemic consequences of circulating thrombolytic agent (Fig. 85-3). Intuitively, early series suggested improved recanalization rates.[39,40] These findings prompted the first randomized, controlled trial in intra-arterial thrombolysis, the Prolyse in Acute Cerebral Thromboembolism (PROACT) II trial.[6] Patients with middle cerebral artery (MCA) occlusion were randomized to 6 mg of intra-arterial recombinant prourokinase (rpro-UK) versus intra-arterial placebo. All patients received intravenous heparin. This trial demonstrated a significant improvement, following administration up to 6 hours after symptom onset, in both recanalization (66% vs. 18%) and functional independence following MCA occlusion. However, intra-arterial rpro-UK was associated with a twofold risk of SICH. Mortality was equivalent between groups. Unfortunately, at this time rpro-UK is unavailable in the United States. Therefore, while providing an exciting proof of concept, these data have not resulted in an available therapy for acute stroke therapy in the United States.

The Interventional Management of Stroke II (IMS II) study, published in 2007, was a pilot trial with a planned comparison of the 3-month outcomes of patients treated with a combined algorithm of intra-arterial and intravenous rtPA versus the NINDS intravenous rtPA trial cohorts as historical controls, placebo, and intravenous rtPA groups.[10] The IMS II protocol involved administration of 0.6 mg/kg of intravenous rtPA followed by up to 22 mg of intra-arterial rtPA administered at the site of thrombus by the EKOS

microinfusion or standard microcatheters. Outcomes and mortality were significantly better in the intra-arterial group compared to the NINDS placebo group in all categories and trended toward significance compared to the intravenous rtPA cohort in most categories (achieving significance in two global measures). The IMS III trial, a prospective, randomized, controlled trial to further investigate intra-arterial plus intravenous rtPA, is under way.

Mechanical Thrombectomy

The phase 1 results of the Mechanical Embolus Removal in Cerebral Ischemia (MERCI) 1 study were published in 2004,[41] demonstrating safety and efficacy of a new mechanical thrombectomy device. The Merci Retrieval System (Concentric Medical), a catheter-based retrieval device that physically ensnares the clot and then withdraws it from the site of occlusion, was further evaluated in the MERCI and Multi-MERCI trials that followed.[42] These studies were single arm and therefore did not allow direct comparison to other therapeutic modalities; however, they suggested improved recanalization rates over either intravenous or intra-arterial thrombolysis. The first-generation MERCI devices, such as the Merci Retrieval System, demonstrated recanalization rates of approximately 50% with clot retrieval alone and 60% when paired with intra-arterial thrombolysis. In addition, benefit was seen up to 8 hours after symptom onset, compared to the 4.5- or 6-hour windows of intravenous or intra-arterial rtPA, respectively. Unlike intravenous or intra-arterial rtPA, mechanical thrombectomy devices do not use potent thrombolytics and therefore represent a useful alternative treatment modality in those patients with thromboembolic stroke who have contraindications to systemic thrombolytic therapy. SICH was comparable to other treatment modalities and has been reported in roughly 7% to 10% of patients. Given its documented efficacy and relative safety, the FDA

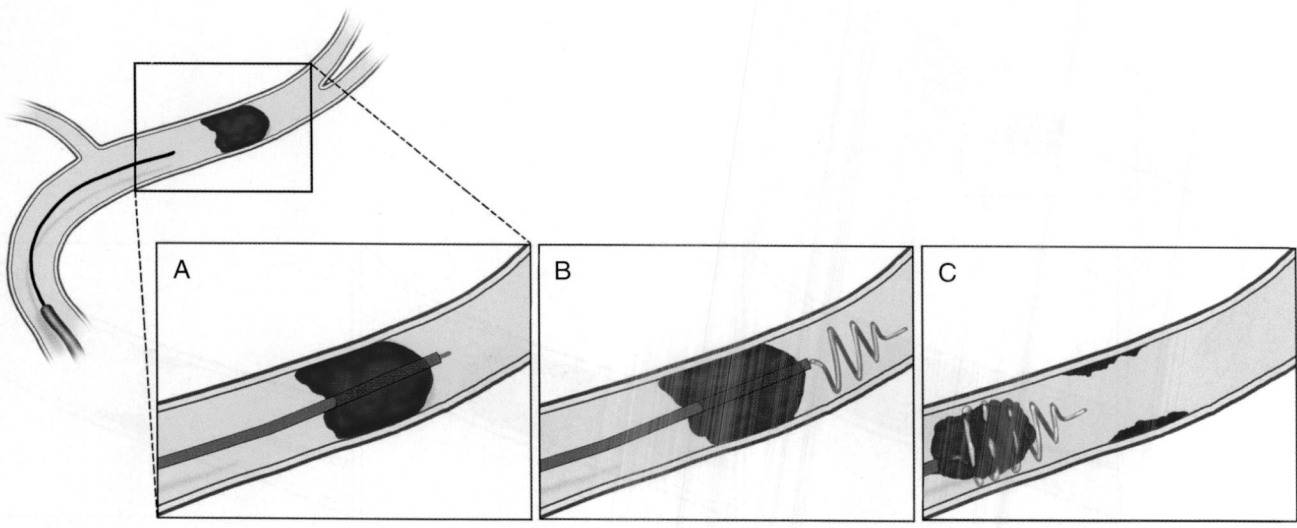

FIGURE 85-4 Schematic diagram depicting the action of the prototypical mechanical thrombectomy device. A, The microcatheter is navigated over a microwire into and beyond the occlusive thrombus. The microwire is then exchanged for the retriever device. B, The retriever device is deployed distal to and within the thrombus and acquires its coiled shape. When the clot is ensnared, the proximal balloon (not pictured) is inflated. C, The microcatheter, retriever device, and clot are withdrawn into the balloon catheter; subsequently, the balloon is deflated, restoring vessel patency.

approved the use of the Merci Retriever in 2004 for revascularization in acute ischemic stroke.

The Merci Retrieval System, the prototype for mechanical thrombectomy devices, is composed of five essential subunits: the balloon guide catheter, the distal access catheter, the microcatheter, the guidewire, and the retrieval device (Fig. 85-4). First, the balloon guide catheter is navigated into the distal cervical arterial vessel. The distal access catheter is then advanced over the microcatheter to a position of stability, preferably at least as distal as the origin of the target vessel. The microcatheter and guidewire are then advanced to the clot. The guidewire is then exchanged for the retriever device, and the retriever is deployed just beyond and within the clot. The retriever device has a natural coiled shape and, when deployed, acquires its coiled shape both distal and within the clot. When the clot is engaged by the retriever catheter, the balloon is inflated and the interventionalist then performs a slow pull and holds while maintaining the position of the distal access catheter relative to the clot. Next, the distal access catheter is secured relative to the microcatheter, and then all units are pulled proximally to the balloon catheter. While this maneuver is performed, aspiration through the balloon guide catheter is performed to minimize the likelihood of reembolization while the clot is withdrawn. Once all units and the clot have entered the balloon catheter, the elements are then removed from the system and angiography is performed to examine for adequacy of recanalization and distal perfusion.

Newer-generation MERCI thrombectomy devices utilize additional suture elements to improve clot retrieval. Such improvements have been demonstrated in the Multi-MERCI trial to provide roughly 60% recanalization rates when used alone and recanalization rates of nearly 70% when used with intra-arterial thrombolysis.[27,42] Trends of improved recanalization, lower mortality, and improved outcomes were demonstrated by the newer devices compared to the

prototype device, although these were not statistically significant. No differences in SICH were seen among devices, with all devices having a roughly 7% to 10% risk of clinically significant hemorrhage.

Thromboaspiration

A novel device utilizing a suction catheter was introduced several years after the success of the mechanical thrombectomy devices. The first thromboaspiration device tested, the Penumbra System, was designed for large-vessel intracranial occlusive thrombi. The Penumbra System utilizes a suction catheter and separator to debulk and remove the thrombus piecemeal (Fig. 85-5).

The procedure is initiated via standard endovascular cannulation techniques. A guidewire is passed just proximal to the arterial thrombus. Next, a suction catheter is passed over the wire to a position just proximal to the clot. Then, the wire is removed and replaced by a separator microwire. The separator is then passed forward into the thrombus. At this time, the suction is turned on and the separator is repeatedly withdrawn and advanced into the thrombus. As the separator is withdrawn, pieces of thrombus are aspirated into the suction catheter. Finally, after the clot is removed in its entirety, the suction is extinguished. The separator and the suction catheter are then withdrawn.

The initial phase I study of the Penumbra System thromboaspiration catheter demonstrated 100% efficacy in achieving revascularization to TIMI grade 2 or 3 in the 21 patients tested.[43] The phase III trial that followed, involving 125 patients from 24 centers, demonstrated an 82% revascularization rate, with 58% achieving an improvement in greater than or equal to 4 points on the NIHSS.[44] SICH occurred in 11% of patients. After review of the efficacy of this system, the Penumbra System achieved FDA approval in 2008 for revascularization in acute ischemic stroke.

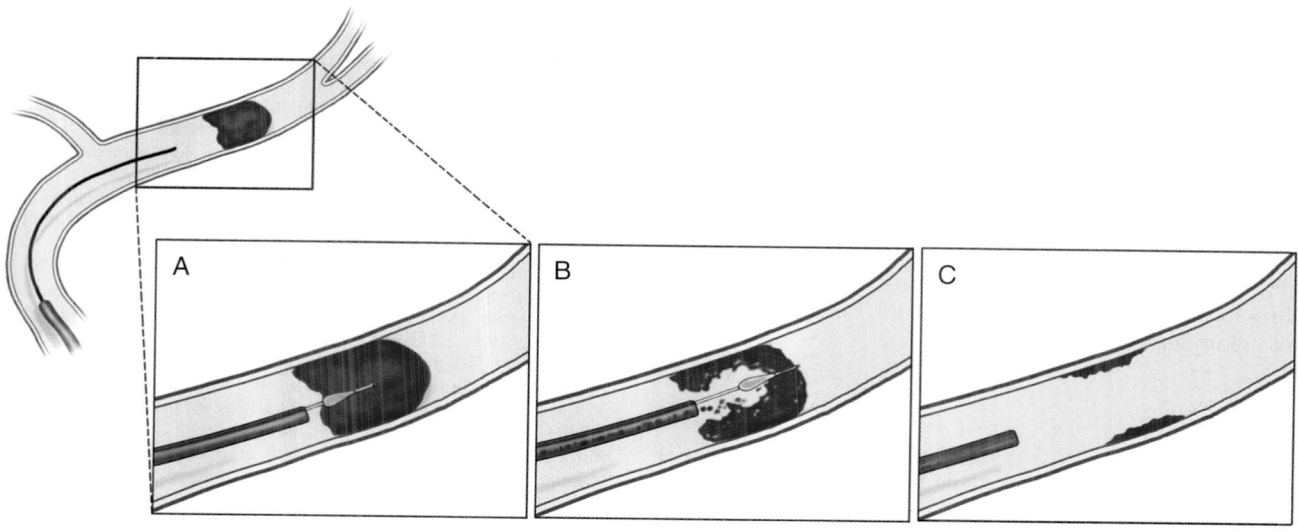

FIGURE 85-5 Schematic diagram depicting the prototypical thromboaspiration device. A, The suction microcatheter is guided over a microwire to the occlusive thrombus. The microwire is then exchanged for the separator device. B, The separator is passed distally into the thrombus, and suction is initiated. The separator is repeatedly advanced into, and withdrawn from, the thrombus. Pieces of freed clot are aspirated proximally into the suction catheter. C, Vessel patency has been restored, and the microcatheter is withdrawn.

Angioplasty

Angioplasty, alone or with other endovascular therapies, has also demonstrated effectiveness in patients presenting with acute stroke. A pilot study by Nakano et al. in 1998 demonstrated successful recanalization with percutaneous angioplasty (PTA) in 8 of 10 patients with acute MCA occlusion.[45] These findings led to a trial comparing PTA versus intra-arterial thrombolysis in patients with acute MCA trunk occlusion, in which 36 patients were treated with intra-arterial thrombolytic therapy alone (control group) and 34 patients underwent PTA.[46] Recanalization rates were 91% in the PTA group versus 64% in the intra-arterial group. In addition, the incidence of symptomatic intracranial hemorrhage was only 2.9% in the PTA group versus 19% in controls.[46] Other studies have since supported these findings, demonstrating high rates of recanalization, low rates of SICH or systemic bleeding, and significant improvement in neurologic function with combined angioplasty and thrombolysis.[47,48] In addition, many investigations have shown the technical feasibility and high efficacy of PTA in acute ischemic stroke,[46,49,50] and it seems to be particularly useful in cases of atherothrombotic disease, in which the residual stenosis may reduce flow sufficiently to lead to rethrombosis.[51]

Stenting

Stent placement as a treatment for acute ischemic stroke was introduced primarily as a rescue therapy in combination with other treatments. Investigations into the application of stents in this patient group focused on achieving the high recanalization rate of stenting seen in other physiologic settings while minimizing the risk of SICH through traumatic vessel injury. The development of self-expanding stents and innovations in delivery catheter design for neurointerventional applications has improved the overall safety and deliverability of stent deployment for stroke. One prospective study, the Stent-Assisted Recanalization in Acute Ischemic Stroke trial, analyzed outcomes for patients who underwent primary stenting for stroke.[52] Of 20 patients presenting within 8 hours of stroke onset, 100% achieved recanalization rates of TIMI 2 or 3. In addition, 60% of patients achieved a modified Rankin score of 3 or less and nearly 50% achieved a score of 0 or 1 at 1-month follow-up.

Temporary endovascular bypass is an attractive method of achieving arterial recanalization without permanent deployment of a stent. This technique involves temporary deployment of a retrievable stent into the affected artery to achieve recanalization, followed by removal of the stent once satisfactory blood flow has been restored. This is an attractive option for patients who cannot tolerate long-term antiplatelet therapy (i.e., active gastrointestinal bleeding). In addition, novel acute stroke treatment devices are in development based on this temporary stent model.

Currently, no phase III trials have been published in either primary stenting or stent-assisted therapy in acute ischemic stroke. However, several small series have been published documenting anywhere from 68% to 92% recanalization rates.[52-55] In addition, low SICH and in-stent stenosis rates have been reported. The theoretical benefits of stenting are well described but to this point have only been demonstrated in several small series. These benefits include immediate recanalization, reduced reocclusion rates compared to other techniques, and reduction of distal embolization through displacement of fragments against the vessel wall.

Future of Endovascular Techniques in Stroke

A prospective, randomized trial is under way to further evaluate the use of intra-arterial thrombolytics in conjunction with other modalities. In addition, numerous innovations to mechanical devices are actively being evaluated for efficacy. PROACT, the IMS trials, and the multiple mechanical device series all indicate that recanalization provides improved outcomes following acute stroke. As technological and pharmacologic therapies continue to improve and physician experience leads to increasingly refined technical abilities, an inflection point of maximal safety and efficacy must be reached. When this occurs, the endovascular treatment of acute stroke will rapidly become one of the most frequent and profound interventions performed by interventionalists. High-quality randomized trials are needed to demonstrate the successful achievement of this goal. Excitingly, such trials are under way.

KEY REFERENCES

Bose A, Henkes H, Alfke K, et al. The Penumbra System: a mechanical device for the treatment of acute stroke due to thromboembolism. *AJNR Am J Neuroradiol.* 2008;29:1409-1413.

Clark WM, Wissman S, Albers GW, et al. Recombinant tissue-type plasminogen activator (alteplase) for ischemic stroke 3 to 5 hours after symptom onset. The ATLANTIS Study: a randomized controlled trial. Alteplase Thrombolysis for Acute Noninterventional Therapy in Ischemic Stroke. *JAMA.* 1999;282:2019-2026.

Del Zoppo GJ, Saver JL, Jauch EC, et al. Expansion of the time window for treatment of acute ischemic stroke with intravenous tissue plasminogen activator: a science advisory from the American Heart Association/American Stroke Association. *Stroke.* 2009;40:2945-2948.

Flint AC, Duckwiler GR, Budzick RF, et al. Mechanical thrombectomy of intracranial internal carotid occlusion: pooled results of the MERCI and Multi MERCI Part I trials. *Stroke.* 2007;38:1274-1280.

Furlan A, Higashida R, Wechsler L, et al. Intra-arterial prourokinase for acute ischemic stroke. The PROACT II study: a randomized controlled trial. Prolyse in Acute Cerebral Thromboembolism. *JAMA.* 1999;282:2003-2011.

Gobin YP, Starkman S, Duckwiler GR, et al. MERCI 1: a phase 1 study of Mechanical Embolus Removal in Cerebral Ischemia. *Stroke.* 2004;35:2848-2854.

Hacke W, Donnan G, Fieschi C, et al. Association of outcome with early stroke treatment: pooled analysis of ATLANTIS, ECASS, and NINDS rt-PA stroke trials. *Lancet.* 2004;363:768-774.

Hacke W, Kaste M, Bluhmki E, et al. Thrombolysis with alteplase 3 to 4.5 hours after acute ischemic stroke. *N Engl J Med.* 2008;359:1317-1329.

Hacke W, Kaste M, Fieschi C, et al. Intravenous thrombolysis with recombinant tissue plasminogen activator for acute hemispheric stroke. The European Cooperative Acute Stroke Study (ECASS). *JAMA.* 1995;274:1017-1025.

Hacke W, Kaste M, Fieschi C, et al. Randomised double-blind placebo-controlled trial of thrombolytic therapy with intravenous alteplase in acute ischaemic stroke (ECASS II). Second European-Australasian Acute Stroke Study Investigators. *Lancet.* 1998;352:1245-1251.

Hallevi H, Barreto AD, Liebeskind DS, et al. Identifying patients at high risk for poor outcome after intra-arterial therapy for acute ischemic stroke. *Stroke.* 2009;40:1780-1785.

IMS II Trial Investigators. The Interventional Management of Stroke (IMS) II Study. *Stroke.* 2007;38:2127-2135.

Janjua N, El-Gengaihy A, Pile-Spellman J, et al. Late endovascular revascularization in acute ischemic stroke based on clinical-diffusion mismatch. *AJNR Am J Neuroradiol.* 2009;30:1024-1027.

Levy EI, Siddiqui AH, Crumlish A, et al. First Food and Drug Administration–approved prospective trial of primary intracranial stenting for acute stroke: SARIS (Stent-Assisted Recanalization in Acute Ischemic Stroke). *Stroke.* 2009;40:3552-3556.

Lloyd-Jones D, Adams R, Carnethon M, et al. Heart disease and stroke statistics—2009 update: a report from the American Heart Association Statistics Committee and Stroke Statistics Subcommittee. *Circulation.* 2009;119:e21-181.

Murphy BD, Fox AJ, Lee DH, et al. Identification of penumbra and infarct in acute ischemic stroke using computed tomography perfusion-derived blood flow and blood volume measurements. *Stroke.* 2006;37:1771-1777.

Nakano S, Iseda T, Yoneyama T, et al. Direct percutaneous transluminal angioplasty for acute middle cerebral artery trunk occlusion: an alternative option to intra-arterial thrombolysis. *Stroke.* 2002;33:2872-2876.

Nakano S, Yokogami K, Ohta H, et al. Direct percutaneous transluminal angioplasty for acute middle cerebral artery occlusion. *AJNR Am J Neuroradiol.* 1998;19:767-772.

Penumbra Pivotal Stroke Trial Investigators. The penumbra pivotal stroke trial: safety and effectiveness of a new generation of mechanical devices for clot removal in intracranial large vessel occlusive disease. *Stroke.* 2009;40:2761-2768.

Rha JH, Saver JL. The impact of recanalization on ischemic stroke outcome: a meta-analysis. *Stroke.* 2007;38:967-973.

Saqqur M, Molina CA, Salam A, et al. Clinical deterioration after intravenous recombinant tissue plasminogen activator treatment: a multicenter transcranial Doppler study. *Stroke.* 2007;38:69-74.

Saqqur M, Tsivgoulis G, Molina CA, et al. Symptomatic intracerebral hemorrhage and recanalization after IV rt-PA: a multicenter study. *Neurology.* 2008;71:1304-1312.

Smith WS, Sung G, Saver J, et al. Mechanical thrombectomy for acute ischemic stroke: final results of the Multi MERCI trial. *Stroke.* 2008;39:1205-1212.

TIMI Study Group. The Thrombolysis in Myocardial Infarction (TIMI) trial. Phase I findings. *N Engl J Med.* 1985;312:932-936.

Tissue plasminogen activator for acute ischemic stroke. The National Institute of Neurological Disorders and Stroke rt-PA Stroke Study Group. *N Engl J Med.* 1995;333:1581-1587.

Numbered references appear on Expert Consult.

Endovascular Treatment of Cerebral Arteriovenous Malformations

ROHAN CHITALE • PASCAL M. JABBOUR • L. FERNANDO GONZALEZ • ROBERT H. ROSENWASSER • STAVROPOULA I. TJOUMAKARIS

Significant developments in the management and treatment of cerebral arteriovenous malformations (AVMs) have been made over the last few years. While surgical resection remains the most definitive treatment option in selected patients, both endovascular and radiosurgical techniques have been added to the arsenal available for treatment of these lesions. These treatment modalities can be used individually or combined in a multimodality approach. This chapter takes a closer look at the endovascular role in the treatment of AVMs.

Pretherapeutic Evaluation

NONINVASIVE TECHNIQUES

Cerebral AVMs can be visualized with a variety of diagnostic modalities, including computed tomography (CT), computed tomography angiography (CTA), magnetic resonance imaging (MRI), and magnetic resonance angiography (MRA). Noncontrast CT scans have a low sensitivity but enable evaluation of acute hemorrhage. Prominent draining veins are often seen on noncontrast scans. CTA provides important vascular detail within the AVM, including the enlargement of feeding arteries, engorged cortical veins, or the presence of associated aneurysms. However, it provides lower definition of surrounding cerebral structures, which MRI and MRA can better show. MRI characterizes AVMs by exhibiting flow voids on T1 and T2 imaging, with occasional hemosiderin deposits suggesting prior hemorrhage.[1] Additional modalities have been used in preoperative evaluation of AVMs in efforts to understand the anatomic, as well as functional, relationship of the brain to the vascular malformation.

Functional MRI

Functional MRI quantifies the local increase in oxyhemoglobin concentration secondary to increased blood flow and volume that occurs after stimulation of eloquent cortex. The images enable the clinician to recognize the relationship of AVMs to eloquent brain structures, as well as elucidate cortical reorganization secondary to the AVM.[2-4] This information may help during preoperative planning and during patient counseling, because it could, in some measure, predict the development of post-therapy deficits in patients.

Diffusion-Tensor Imaging

Diffusion-tensor imaging is a developing technology that enables in vivo visualization of multiple white matter tracts and their relationship to an AVM. The ability to use this information can help minimize treatment risks and determine the best therapeutic modality for the patient.[2,5]

INVASIVE TECHNIQUES

Provocative Injection Testing (Wada's Test)

Prior to embolization of an AVM, Wada's testing of selective feeding vessels can be performed. Amobarbital sodium or propofol injections have been performed on vessels in or remote from the lesion.[6-8] This pharmacologic test helps predict the effect of occluding a feeding vessel. Due to their short half-life, their effect disappears rapidly. Such evaluation helps prevent embolization of pedicles that may result in focal neurologic deficit. This preoperative functional evaluation is helpful when supraselective intranidal microcatheter placement is not achieved and there is concern that vessels to adjacent normal brain may be compromised.

Angiography

Angiography remains the gold standard for defining arterial and venous anatomy of an AVM.[2] Such analysis of the angioarchitecture helps in evaluating the risk of hemorrhage and selecting the best therapeutic management of the AVM.[9] Angiographic characterization of the AVM includes identification of the main arterial feeders, size of the AVM, shape of the nidus (compact vs. diffuse, without clear borders that separate it from adjacent brain), drainage patterns (superficial drainage into cortical veins, deep drainage through deep venous system, or proximity to dural sinuses), and characteristics of outflow (presence of restriction from stenosis or sinus thrombosis). Anatomic characteristics of AVMs such as deep location, deep venous drainage pattern, presence of a single draining vein, venous stenosis, eloquent location, and small diameter are all related to increased risk of hemorrhage or neurologic deficit.[10-19]

Angiography helps elucidate the presence of associated aneurysms. These aneurysms are categorized by their location (i.e., feeding artery, intranidal, circle of Willis, or venous). Associated aneurysms are found in roughly 7% to 41% of patients with AVMs.[20-25] Studies evaluating hemorrhage risks for AVMs with associated aneurysms have shown conflicting results. A 2007 study from the Columbia study group described prospectively collected hemorrhage risk factors limited to the period between the initial AVM diagnosis and the start of treatment, calculating annual hemorrhage rates in 622 patients.[26] In the group's model, the presence of associated intranidal or feeding artery aneurysms did not have a significant effect on hemorrhage rates.[11] Other studies, however, have included intranidal aneurysms as important risk factors for hemorrhage in AVMs,[1,13-16,21,27,28] with increased size of the aneurysm related to increased risk of hemorrhage.[21,29] These aneurysms are exposed to the same intraluminal pressures as the arterial components of the AVM. Therefore, any pressure changes following AVM embolization could lead to associated aneurysm rupture. Thus, vessels that supply intranidal aneurysms should be recognized and treated early to reduce the risk of hemorrhage.[30]

Angiography further evaluates for the presence of pseudoaneurysms (false aneurysms), which may form in previously ruptured AVMs. These irregularly shaped cavities have abnormally structured vessel walls and are often located at the point where artery and vein make contact due to inherent weakness.[31] Previous rupture of an AVM is an independent predictor of future hemorrhage,[26] and recognizing the presence of posthemorrhage pseudoaneurysm formation can help reduce the risk of future hemorrhage.

AVM-associated arteriovenous fistulas are sometimes discovered in the nidus during angiographic evaluation. The presence of these high-flow AVFs is associated with increased risk of intra- and postoperative complications, including hemorrhage.[32,33] Prior endovascular treatment of these AVFs helps decrease the chance of this complication. Reducing the flow through the AVF also helps decrease the chances of undesired embolization of the AVMs' venous drainage, cerebral veins, dural sinuses, or pulmonary circulation.[33,34]

Timing of imaging after a hemorrhage must be considered. Performing an angiogram immediately after hemorrhage can result in a false negative secondary to compression of the nidus by the hematoma.[35-38] Therefore, a late angiogram, performed 3 months after the hemorrhage, remains the gold standard for detection of an AVM.[35]

Endovascular Technique

ANESTHETIC AND PERIOPERATIVE CONSIDERATIONS

The type of anesthesia is selected depending on the angioarchitecture of the AVM. If the target vessel is terminal, ending directly into the AVM, the procedure can be done under general anesthesia. This facilitates patient comfort and ensures a motionless patient during the procedure, enabling improved visualization of the AVM structures and minimizing patient risk associated with mobility during the procedure.[1] Because there is no functional intervening

tissue within the AVM, embolization of appropriate vessels should theoretically not cause any functional deficit. In our institution, general anesthesia and endotracheal intubation are utilized for all AVM embolizations. A brief period of apnea helps decrease the motion caused by the respiratory cycle in certain cases when rapid injection of embolic material and removal of microcatheter is necessary. Intraoperatively, the patient's neurologic status is monitored continuously via somatosensory evoked potentials and electroencephalography.

In some cases, it is necessary to assess the patient's functional status with provocative tests intraoperatively. This requires intravenous anesthesia with short-acting agents such as propofol and midazolam[39] and avoiding paralytic agents so that the patient's neurologic function can be assessed quickly during the procedure. Authors that favor this approach point to the wide variability and cortical reorganization described in patients with AVMs.[40,41]

Foley catheters and continuous transduction of arterial pressure are standard. Blood pressure transduction can be obtained through the femoral sheath or existing arterial line. This is especially important when vasoactive drugs must be given intraprocedurally.[1] Deliberate systemic hypotension through vasoactive agents, general anesthesia, or adenosine-induced cardiac pause may also be used to slow flow through the AVM and allow for more controlled deposition of embolic material.[42] In addition, a pulse oximeter is applied to the foot ipsilateral to the femoral sheath to monitor signs of early vessel obstruction, distal thromboemboli, or overcompression following sheath removal.[1] Foley catheters are typically used for fluid management, and supplemental oxygen or nasopharyngeal airways can be considered, especially in those patients under sedative–hypnotic agent.[1]

STANDARD PROCEDURE

The goals, expectations, risks, and benefits of endovascular treatment must be discussed with the patient and family prior to the procedure. Vascular access is obtained by inserting a No. 7 French gauge (Fr) sheath into the femoral artery via a Seldinger technique. Anticoagulation algorithms to prevent thromboembolic complications during and after the procedure remain controversial.[43-45] In our institution, continuous heparinized flush is used for the femoral sheath, guide catheter, and microcatheter. However, no additional heparin bolus is used during the procedure. A 6-Fr guiding catheter is advanced into the internal carotid or vertebral artery. Flow-directed microcatheters are used to reach the intranidal target. Their selection is based on the size of the vessel. The catheter is drawn through the vessels primarily through blood flow and contains a flexible distal tip to enable navigation through distant and tortuous neurovasculature. Some flow-directed catheters have a steam-formed distal tip to enable more selective tracking of the catheter into the desired vessels. Variations in microcatheters, including those in Prowler (Cordis Endovascular, Miami Lakes, FL), Spinnaker (Boston Scientific/Target Therapeutics, Fremont, CA), Marathon (ev3 Neurovascular, Irvine, CA), and Echelon (ev3 Neurovascular), allow for differences in flexibility, torque, maneuverability, and responsiveness.

IDENTIFICATION OF THE EMBOLIZATION POINT

The clinician requires a full understanding of the AVM's anatomy and architecture to identify pedicles that do not share supply with the adjacent normal brain. It is critical to identify *en passage* vessels that share supply with normal brain when en route to the nidus. In such a scenario, either a pretherapeutic or an intraoperative (Wada's test) functional evaluation must demonstrate lack of functional significance to avoid neurologic deficit from embolization.[34]

INJECTION OF EMBOLIC MATERIAL

A variety of embolic materials have been utilized for the treatment of AVMs. They include polyvinyl alcohol (PVA), n-butyl cyanoacrylate (n-BCA) (Cordis), Onyx (ev3 Neurovascular), ethibloc, silk, microcoils, liquid coils, or a combination of these. The most common embolic materials are described here.

n-Butyl Cyanoacrylate

n-BCA is a liquid monomer that permanently polymerizes to a solid compound after contact with solutions containing anions like blood.[46] This compound must be combined with Ethiodol, an iodine-based oil that serves as a radiopaque contrast agent. Tantalum powder can also be added to increase its opacity, although its use is not common currently. Embolization with n-BCA initiates an inflammatory endothelial response and subsequent occlusion of target vessels.[47] A variety of factors influence the effectiveness of n-BCA in treating AVMs, namely, viscosity and polymerization time. Increasing the concentration of Ethiodol in the mixture increases the viscosity, which delays the transit within the lesion. Increasing the concentration of Ethiodol delays the polymerization time, which is useful in lesions that exhibit slow flow. Temperature, homogeneity of the mixture, and changes in the pH of the solution also play a role in polymerization time.[48,49] The distance between the microcatheter and the nidus, tortuosity of the vessels, and intranidal flow are factors that influence the choice of n-BCA viscosity and polymerization time. Manipulation of viscosity and polymerization time allows for control of injection speed. Diluted glue permits prolonged injection times and dense casting of the nidus with less microcatheter retention risk.[34] In general, a 1:1 dilution of n-BCA to Ethiodol is used when the hemodynamic flow of the AVM is very fast and the catheter is close to the nidus. Different concentrations, such as 1:2 or 1:3, are used when the flow is slower. We frequently use a 1:2 or 1:3 n-BCA-to-Ethiodol ratio. Acid compounds such as glacial acetic acid have been used to decrease the pH, which delays polymerization time without compromising viscosity.[50] Dextrose 5% can also be used to improve distal progression of the n-BCA through small, tortuous feeders. In this technique, dextrose is injected through the guide catheter and n-BCA is simultaneously injected through the microcatheter. The dextrose injection delays the contact of the blood with the n-BCA and, in this way, delays its polymerization.[51] Sometimes, as the microcatheter tip reaches smaller distal vessels, it can potentially occlude blood flow. This technique is known as "flow control" and can be utilized to prevent blood from contacting the n-BCA, thus allowing for its prolonged distal penetration.[34] Injection of n-BCA is stopped when glue reaches the venous system through the nidus or if there is backflow toward the catheter. The microcatheter must be removed quickly to prevent catheter retention.[47-49,52]

Onyx

Onyx is a newer liquid embolic agent composed of ethylene–vinyl alcohol copolymer (EVOH) mixed in a dimethyl sulfoxide (DMSO) solvent. This nonadhesive, cohesive solution is mixed with micronized tantalum for radiopacity and must be shaken together for at least 20 minutes[53] to achieve homogeneity of the mixture. It is available in different concentrations of the EVOH polymer, with lower concentrations being associated with decreased viscosity and thus more distal penetration of the AVM.[54] When the mixture comes into contact with aqueous solutions, the polymer begins to precipitate on the surface while the core remains liquid. This produces what has been described as a "lavalike flow pattern" within blood vessels of a soft and nonadherent mass that does not fragment during the injection.[54] Similar to n-BCA, Onyx is a nonabsorbable agent. Therefore, theoretical permanent occlusion of the AVM can be achieved.[55] However, recent evidence suggests that there exists a risk of recanalization or reperfusion of the AVM following Onyx embolization.[56,57] Its nonadhesive nature enables longer, slower, and more controlled injections, which allow for the embolization of a larger percentage of the AVM from a single catheter position. However, only partial reflux around the catheter is permissible, because catheter withdrawal can become difficult. Its nonadhesive nature also enables cerebral angiography between injections to monitor the progress of embolization,[54,55,58,59] a big advantage over the use of n-BCA. Care must be taken to use slow infusion rates and thus avoid the angiotoxicity associated with DMSO.[60] Chaloupka et al., using a swine rete mirabilis embolization model, report that a DMSO injection of 0.5 to 0.8 ml over 30 to 90 seconds, while causing mild transient acute vasospasm, results in no adverse clinical sequelae and less angiotoxicity than reported in prior studies.[60] Separation of tantalum from the Onyx is another pitfall that can increase the difficulty of viewing smaller feeding pedicles.[59,61] Onyx injection is limited to DMSO-compatible microcatheters only, such as the Marathon and the Echelon.

Polyvinyl Alcohol

PVA consists of particles available in different diameters depending on the size of target vessels.[52,62-64] PVA produces slower occlusion than liquid embolic agents. PVA particles occlude low pressure shunts first, causing an increase in intranidal vessel pressure and subsequent immediate risk of hemorrhage prior to nidal obliteration.[65] In addition, PVA is associated with high recanalization rates, ranging from 12% to 43%.[66,67] The development of collateral feeders secondary to proximal occlusion of the AVM with large size particles may contribute to such high recanalization rates.[52,62-64] Given these characteristics of PVA, it has been used with success preoperatively to reduce AVM flow prior to open or radiosurgical treatment.

Goals of Treatment and Outcomes

There are four possible objectives of endovascular therapy.

Table 86-1 Curative Success of Embolization with Different Agents			
	Patients	**Embolization Agent**	**Rate of AVM Cure (%)**
Deruty et al.[68]	82	*n*-BCA	5
Vinuela et al.[69]	405	*n*-BCA	9.9
Lundqvist et al.[70]	150	*n*-BCA	13
Valavanis and Yasargil[58]	387	*n*-BCA	40
Gobin et al.[71]	125	*n*-BCA	11.2
Pérez-Higueras et al.[56]	45	Onyx	22
Pierot et al.[72]	48	Onyx	4.2
Leonardi et al.[73]	34	Onyx	5.9
van Rooij et al.[77]	44	Onyx	15.9
Weber et al.[121]	93	Onyx	20
Mounayer et al.[79]	94	Onyx, *n*-BCA, or combination	27.7
Panagiotopoulos et al.[57]	82	Onyx	24.4

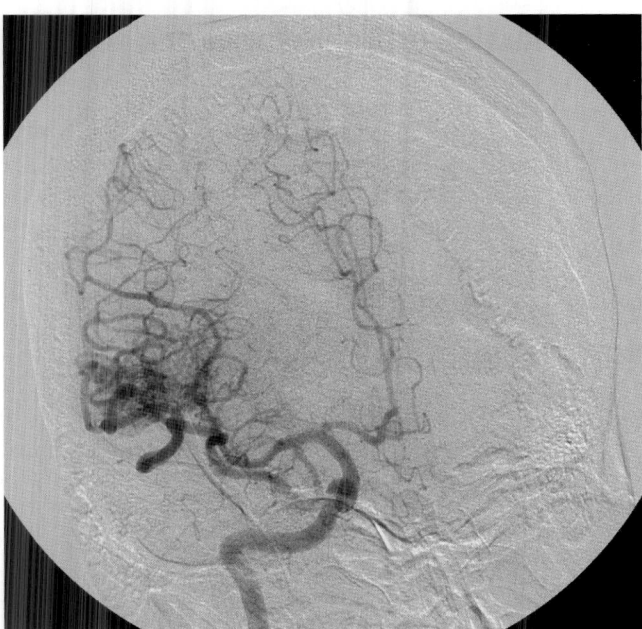

FIGURE 86-1 Subtracted cerebral angiogram of the right internal carotid artery, midarterial phase, frontal projection, demonstrating a right temporal AVM before treatment.

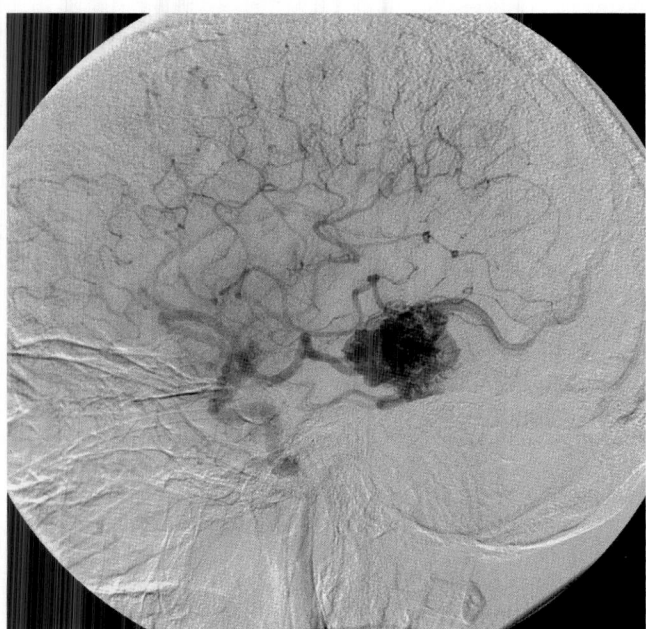

FIGURE 86-2 Subtracted cerebral angiogram of the right internal carotid artery, late arterial–capillary phase, lateral projection, demonstrating a right temporal AVM before treatment.

EMBOLIZATION FOR DEFINITIVE CURE

Liquid embolic agents, including *n*-BCA and Onyx, have been used for curative AVM embolization (Table 86-1). Varying rates of complete occlusion with *n*-BCA have been noted in the literature. Deruty et al. reported complete obliteration in 5% after embolization alone, done mostly in patients with high-grade AVMs.[68] Vinuela et al. reported 9.9% rate for embolization alone in small to medium AVMs with less than four pedicles among 405 patients treated.[69] Lundqvist et al. reported a 13% rate of occlusion.[70] Valavanis and Yasargil reported a rate of 40% angiographic cure in a study of 387 consecutive patients.[58] Gobin et al. reported a complete occlusion rate of 11.2% in patients after embolization prior to radiosurgery in a study of 125 patients who were poor surgical candidates.[71] Newer studies using Onyx or a combination of Onyx and *n*-BCA have shown variable cure rates from 15% to 53.9%.[54,56,57,59,72-83] Other studies have also shown evidence that embolization for cure of small, deep-seated, nonresectable AVMs offers immediate protection from new or recurrent hemorrhage.[32,58,84-86]

Figures 86-1 to 86-3 show a 26-year-old female with a past medical history of migraines who presented with seizures. Angiography reveal a right temporal AVM fed by multiple branches of the MCA and PCA, with superficial draining veins. Embolization using *n*-BCA over three sessions resulted in complete occlusion of the AVM.

EMBOLIZATION AS A PRECURSOR FOR DEFINITIVE OPERATIVE RESECTION

The goals of presurgical embolization are the reduction of the size of the nidus and the occlusion of deep arterial feeding vessels, which may be surgically inaccessible. Draining veins should be preserved, because restricting the venous outflow could result in increased risk of hemorrhage.[59,77,79,87] In addition, preoperative embolization can be used to treat intranidal aneurysms and high-flow fistulas to promote progressive thrombosis of the nidus.[1] Preoperative embolization may help reduce blood loss, improve operative time, and convert high-grade Spetzler-Martin AVMs to lower-grade lesions, and thereby reduce associated morbidity and mortality.[88-92] However, proximal embolization of feeding vessels may result in the development of collaterals[93] and thus result in a more treacherous open resection. Figure 86-4 reveals effective use of embolization prior to open surgical resection. In this example, a 32-year-old male with no past medical history presented with a new onset of seizure. Embolization

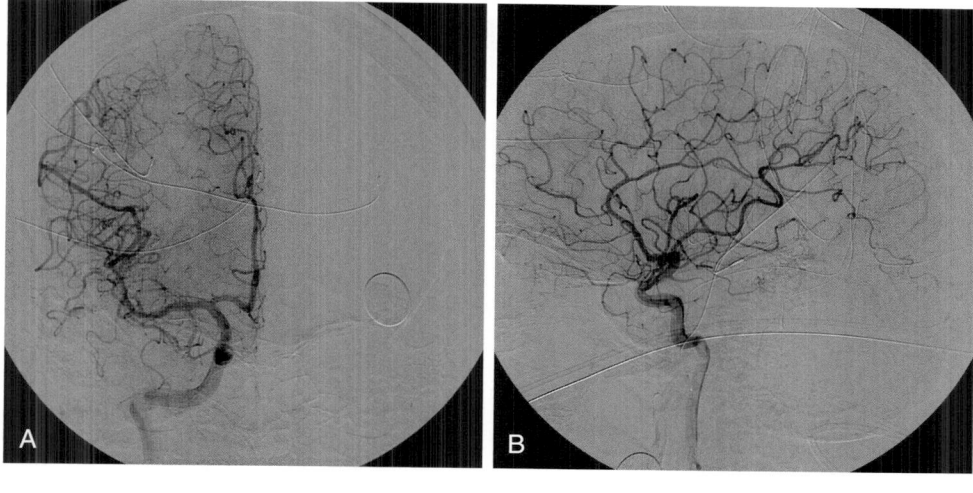

FIGURE 86-3 Subtracted cerebral angiogram of the right internal carotid artery, midarterial phase, frontal (A) and lateral (B) projections, following the third and final *n*-BCA treatment.

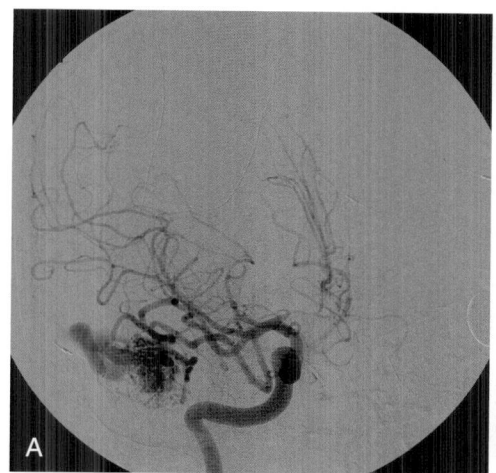
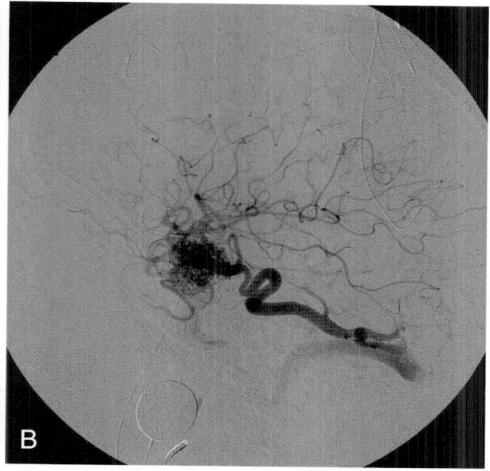

FIGURE 86-4 Subtracted cerebral angiogram of the right internal carotid artery, midarterial phase, frontal (A) and lateral (B) projections, demonstrating a right temporal AVM (pretreatment) fed by the right M4 pedicle and anterior temporal artery, with superficial draining veins.

of the right M4 and anterior temporal pedicles of the AVM with Onyx allowed for nearly 95% obliteration (Fig. 86-5) prior to the complete removal with craniotomy (Fig. 86-6). From a surgical perspective, lesions embolized with *n*-BCA intraoperatively exhibit a harder, less compliant mass in contrast to lesions embolized with Onyx, which is a softer agent.

EMBOLIZATION AS A PRECURSOR TO RADIOSURGERY

There are a few primary objectives of endovascular embolization prior to radiosurgery. Embolization decreases the target size of the AVM, which allows for a higher dose of radiation to be delivered to a smaller volume. This practice is associated with less morbidity (radiation necrosis) and higher cure rates following radiosurgery. Embolization can also reduce weakness in the AVM angioarchitecture by eliminating intranidal or venous aneurysms. This aims to reduce hemorrhage risk during the radiosurgery latency period. Embolization may also reduce symptoms related to venous hypertension.[71,94,95] However, delayed recanalization related to the use of PVA, as well as *n*-BCA, has been noted in AVMs treated with embolization prior to radiosurgery.[71,82,96,97] In addition, flow reduction alone without reduction of AVM volume has not been shown

to improve radiosurgical success. It may even challenge conformal dose planning for radiosurgery.[97] Recent studies with small series of patients have noted angiographic occlusion of AVMs with embolization followed by radiosurgery in some patients; however, more long-term clinical data are necessary for definitive analysis.[59,77,79] Figure 86-7 shows a 40 × 40-mm left parietal AVM fed by the left MCA and PCA. Staged embolizations over four sessions with *n*-BCA enabled reduction of AVM volume prior to radiosurgery (Figs. 86-8 and 86-9). The patient is currently undergoing linear accelerator treatment for the residual AVM.

EMBOLIZATION AS PALLIATION FOR PROGRESSIVE DEBILITATING SYMPTOMS AND TARGET EMBOLIZATION OF BLEEDING OR HIGH-RISK LESIONS

Palliative embolization is an alternative treatment for patients with large, nonresectable AVMs, medically intractable seizures, or progressive debilitating neurologic deficits secondary to arterial steal (due to preferential blood flow through the low-resistance AVM, causing ischemia of surrounding normal tissue), or venous hypertension that could cause headaches or local mass effect from engorged

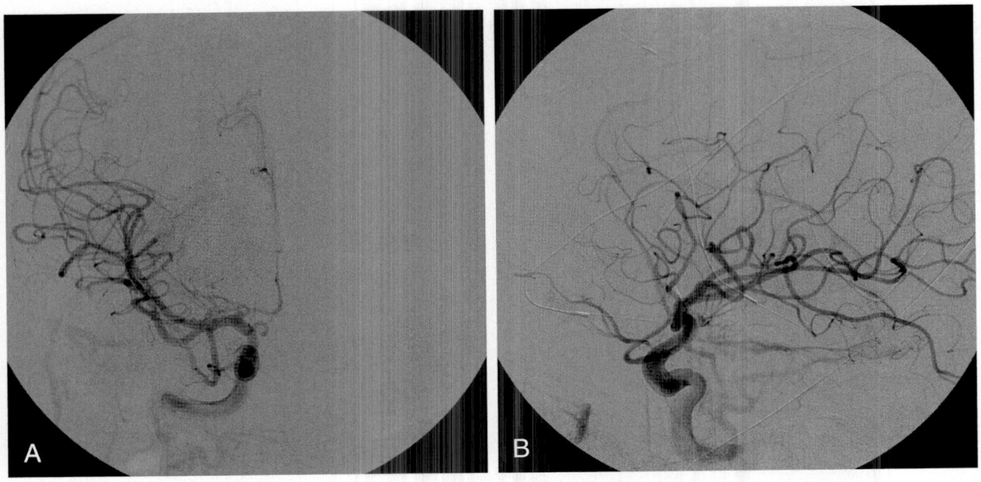

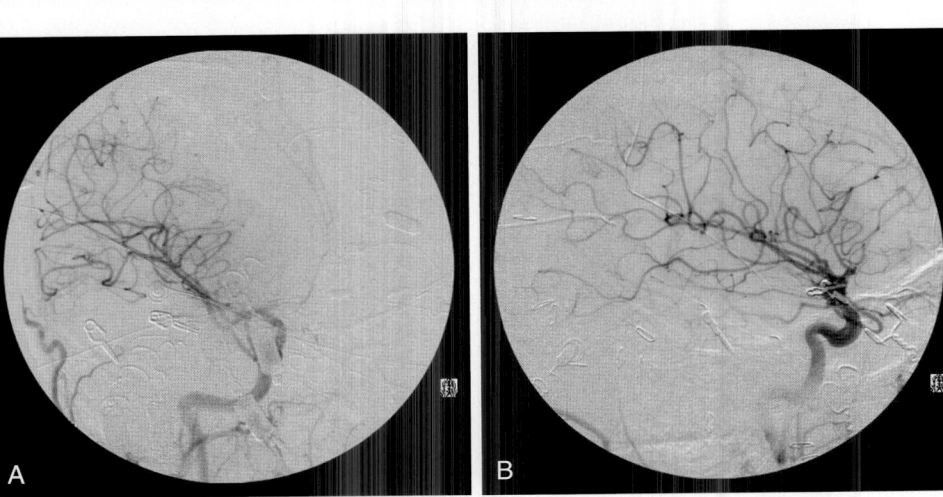

FIGURE 86-5 Subtracted cerebral angiogram of the right internal carotid artery, midarterial phase, frontal (A) and lateral (B) projections, following embolization of the M4 pedicle and anterior temporal pedicle.

FIGURE 86-6 Subtracted cerebral angiogram of the right internal carotid artery, midarterial phase, frontal (A) and lateral (B) projections, following craniotomy for complete excision of the remaining right temporal AVM.

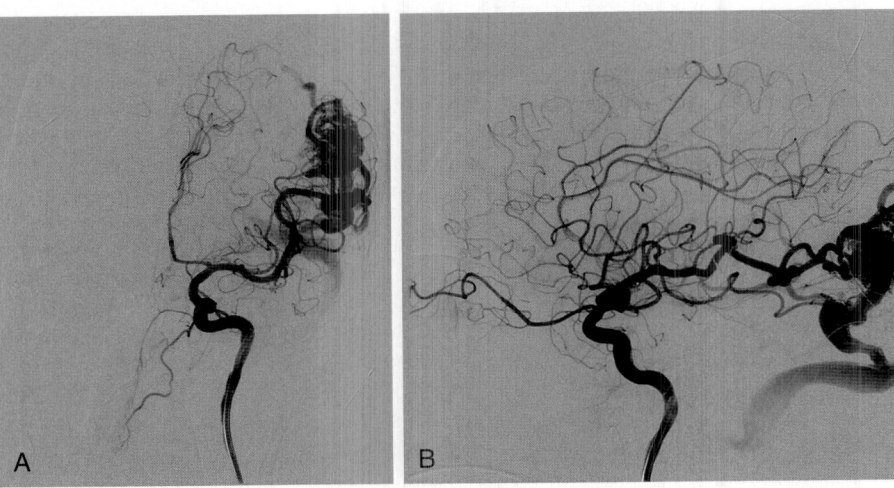

FIGURE 86-7 Subtracted cerebral angiogram of the left internal carotid artery, midarterial phase, frontal (A) and lateral (B) projections, demonstrating a 40 × 40-mm left parietal AVM.

veins.[98-101] It can also be used in a targeted approach or staged treatment to reduce the hemorrhagic risk from associated aneurysms or from increased pressure in veins that have an outflow restriction.[102] While partial embolization can be helpful in reversing neurologic deficit, the development of rapidly forming collaterals following embolization reduces the long-term effectiveness of this strategy.

Complications

Embolization of AVMs carries with it inherent risks, primarily hemorrhage, edema, infarction, and ischemia. The complications that occur can result in temporary or permanent neurologic morbidity of variable severity or even death.

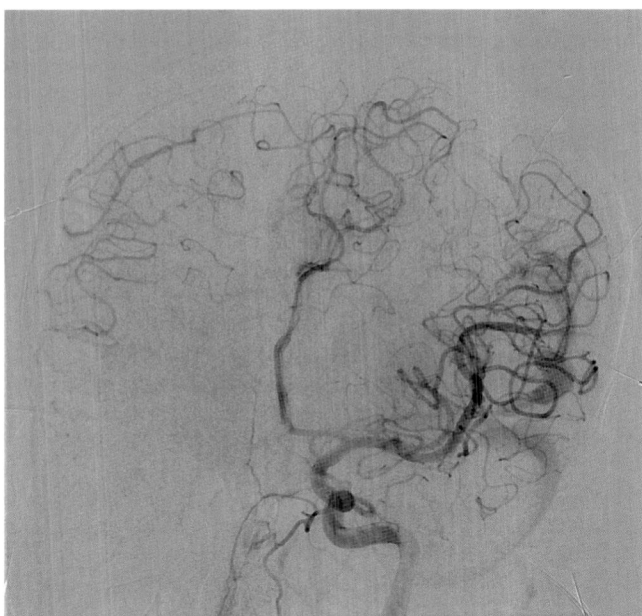

FIGURE 86-8 Subtracted cerebral angiogram of the left internal carotid artery, late arterial–capillary phase, frontal projection, following the fourth *n*-BCA treatment of the left M4 pedicle.

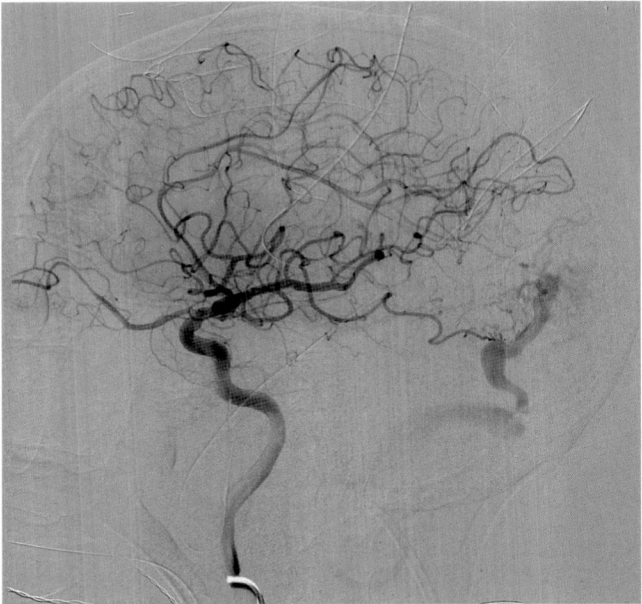

FIGURE 86-9 Subtracted cerebral angiogram of the left internal carotid artery, midarterial phase, lateral projection, following the fourth *n*-BCA treatment of the left M4 pedicle. Note the presence of residual AVM with a diffuse pattern and persistence of early venous drainage.

HEMORRHAGE AND EDEMA

Causes of embolization-associated hemorrhage include arterial perforation, intranidal aneurysm rupture, or disturbances in AVM drainage through occlusion of major draining veins.[45,88,103-105] Venous disturbances in areas of brain adjacent to the AVM result in passive engorgement of vessels, arterial stagnation, and subsequent cerebral edema and/or hemorrhage. This phenomenon may occur even with complete obliteration of the AVM and has been referred to as venous overload[106] or occlusive hyperemia.[107] Guglielmi in 2008 used a simple electric model to highlight the hemorrhagic risk. His study showed that occlusion of the venular part of the AVM nidus results in a 68% increase in blood pressure to the remaining proximal portion of the nidus, while occlusion of the drainage vein itself results in a 284% increase in blood pressure through the nidus.[108] Hemorrhage and edema may also occur secondary to loss of autoregulation in surrounding ischemic tissue following embolization. The loss of autoregulation around the AVM results in disruption of normal capillary beds. This is known as the normal perfusion pressure breakthrough theory.[109] Inflammatory reactions, mural necrosis induced by embolic material, and ischemic softening of tissue surrounding an abnormal blood vessel that bled under pressure are also potential causes of postembolization hemorrhage.[57,110] If periprocedural hemorrhage occurs, protamine must be administered immediately for reversal of anticoagulation.[111] Administration of steroids has been used to combat vasogenic edema related to AVM treatment.[107]

ISCHEMIA AND INFARCTION

Inadvertent embolization of normal blood vessels, thrombotic emboli, and retention of the microcatheter can result in ischemia and infarction. Immediate treatment with deliberate hypertension to open collateral circulation is indicated to help mitigate neurologic deficit.[111] In addition, intra-arterial administration of platelet glycoprotein IIb/IIIa antagonists can be used to combat the development of periprocedural thrombi.[57] Other specific hemodynamic complications can occur from the procedure itself and depend on the location and extension of the lesion. Angiographic data, as well as preprocedural noninvasive testing, are used to help minimize this risk.

Current literature estimates the morbidity rate associated with AVM embolization to be 10% for temporary neurologic deficits and 8% for permanent deficits. Mortality rates are documented as around 1%.[112] These complications occurred mainly in high-grade AVMs. Newer studies documenting embolization prior to the use of Onyx report rates ranging between 5.6% and 14% for overall morbidity and 2% to 12.8% for permanent morbidity. Mortality rates during this period vary from 0.6% to 3.7%.[23,32,71,113-119] Single- and multicenter studies have been performed to look at risks associated with embolization with Onyx. Overall morbidity rates have ranged from 7.1% to 10%, with 2% to 3% related to temporary morbidity and 1% to 15.5% related to permanent morbidity. Mortality rates have been quoted from 0% to 3%.[54,56,59,73,74,76-79,120,121] These studies have shown that curative embolization of AVMs in multiple sessions can achieve high rates of total or near-total occlusion with acceptable rates of morbidity and mortality.[101] A retrospective review of 153 patients by Kim et al. in 2006, looked at a variety of factors, including age, gender, AVM grade, location of lesion, number and location of embolized arteries, and number of embolization sessions. Analysis of these variables with respect to neurologic complications revealed that only the number of branches embolized was found to be related to neurologic deficit with statistical significance.[117] Risk of embolization by Spetzler-Martin grade was also evaluated. Immediate and long-term neurologic deficits were found to increase with increasing grade of AVM, demonstrating a trend—although it was not statistically significant. Long-term rates of deficit were 0%, 5%, 7%, 10%, and 18% for AVM grades I, II, III, IV, and V, respectively.[117]

Conclusions

Current advances in endovascular techniques enable the preoperative evaluation and treatment of AVMs. Embolic agents can be used in a variety of ways to help treat AVMs in a multimodality approach or to provide a complete cure. A promising ongoing clinical trial, called ARUBA for A Randomized Trial of Unruptured Brain Arteriovenous Malformations, investigates the outcome of unruptured AVMs based on type of treatment in comparison to natural history. Long-term data from this trial, as well as others, may help to formulate a framework for optimal management of AVM patients. Undoubtedly, endovascular management will play an integral role in future management of AVMs.

KEY REFERENCES

Berenstein A, Lasjaunias P. *Surgical Neuroangiography.* Vol 4. New York, NY: Springer-Verlag; 1987.

Brown Jr RD, et al. The natural history of unruptured intracranial arteriovenous malformations. *J Neurosurg.* 1988;68(3):352-357.

Friedlander RM. Clinical practice. Arteriovenous malformations of the brain. *N Engl J Med.* 2007;356(26):2704-2712.

Hartmann A, et al. Determinants of staged endovascular and surgical treatment outcome of brain arteriovenous malformations. *Stroke.* 2005;36(11):2431-2435.

Hartmann A, et al. Risk of endovascular treatment of brain arteriovenous malformations. *Stroke.* 2002;33(7):1816-1820.

Haw CS, et al. Complications of embolization of arteriovenous malformations of the brain. *J Neurosurg.* 2006;104(2):226-232.

Linfante I, Wakhloo AK. Brain aneurysms and arteriovenous malformations: advancements and emerging treatments in endovascular embolization. *Stroke.* 2007;38(4):1411-1417.

Lundqvist C, Wikholm G, Svendsen P. Embolization of cerebral arteriovenous malformations: part II—Aspects of complications and late outcome. *Neurosurgery.* 1996;39(3):460-467:discussion 467-469.

Muller-Forell W, Valavanis A. How angioarchitecture of cerebral arteriovenous malformations should influence the therapeutic considerations. *Minim Invasive Neurosurg.* 1995;38(1):32-40.

Ogilvy CS, et al. Recommendations for the management of intracranial arteriovenous malformations: a statement for healthcare professionals from a special writing group of the Stroke Council, American Stroke Association. *Circulation.* 2001;103(21):2644-2657.

Pérez-Higueras A, López RR, Tapia DQ. Endovascular treatment of cerebral AVM: our experience with Onyx. *Interventional Neuroradiology.* 2005(11):141-157.

Pierot L, et al. Endovascular treatment of brain arteriovenous malformations using onyx: results of a prospective, multicenter study. *J Neuroradiol.* 2009;36(3):147-152.

Stapf C, et al. Predictors of hemorrhage in patients with untreated brain arteriovenous malformation. *Neurology.* 2006;66(9):1350-1355.

Redekop G, et al. Arterial aneurysms associated with cerebral arteriovenous malformations: classification, incidence, and risk of hemorrhage. *J Neurosurg.* 1998;89(4):539-546.

Rosenwasser RH, Thomas JE, Gannon PM, et al. *Current Strategies for the Management of Cerebral Arteriovenous Malformations.* Rolling Meadows, Illinois: American Association of Neurological Surgeons; 1998.

Schaller C, Schramm J. Microsurgical results for small arteriovenous malformations accessible for radiosurgical or embolization treatment. *Neurosurgery.* 1997;40(4):664-672:discussion 672-674.

Schmidek HH, Roberts DW. *Schmidek & Sweet Operative Neurosurgical Techniques: Indications, Methods, and Results.* 5th ed. Philadelphia: Elsevier; 2006. 2 v. (xxxix, 2337, p.67).

Spetzler RF, Wilson CB, Weinstein P, et al. Normal perfusion pressure breakthrough theory. *Clin Neurosurg.* 1977;25:651-672.

Spetzler RF, et al. Surgical management of large AVM's by staged embolization and operative excision. *J Neurosurg.* 1987;67(1):17-28.

Spetzler RF, et al. Relationship of perfusion pressure and size to risk of hemorrhage from arteriovenous malformations. *J Neurosurg.* 1992;76(6):918-923.

Valavanis A, Christoforidis G. Endovascular management of cerebral arteriovenous malformations. *Neurointerventionist.* 1999(1):34-40.

Valavanis A, Yasargil MG. The endovascular treatment of brain arteriovenous malformations. *Adv Tech Stand Neurosurg.* 1998;24:131-214.

Vinuela F, Duckwiler G, Guglielmi G. Contribution of interventional neuroradiology in the therapeutic management of brain arteriovenous malformations. *J Stroke Cerebrovasc Dis.* 1997;6(4):268-271.

Vinuela F, et al. Combined endovascular embolization and surgery in the management of cerebral arteriovenous malformations: experience with 101 cases. *J Neurosurg.* 1991;75(6):856-864.

Wikholm G, Lundqvist C, Svendsen P. Embolization of cerebral arteriovenous malformations: part I—Technique, morphology, and complications. *Neurosurgery.* 1996;39(3):448-457:discussion 457-459.

Numbered references appear on Expert Consult.

Endovascular Treatment of Intracranial Occlusive Disease

SABAREESH K. NATARAJAN • ALEXANDER A. KHALESSI •
YUVAL KARMON • ADNAN H. SIDDIQUI •
L. NELSON HOPKINS • ELAD I. LEVY

Introduction

Most common among the causes of intracranial occlusive disease are atherosclerosis and moyamoya disease (MMD). In this chapter, we focus on endovascular approaches for the treatment of atherosclerotic arterial stenosis and MMD.

Intracranial Atherosclerotic Disease

Approximately 8% to 10% of ischemic strokes are attributable to intracranial atherosclerosis.[1,2] In the United States, it is estimated that 40,000 to 60,000 new strokes per year are due to intracranial atherosclerosis.[3] The most common intracranial location for stenosis is the middle cerebral artery (MCA) (33.9%), followed by the internal carotid artery (ICA) (20.3%), basilar artery (20.3%), vertebral arteries (VAs) (19.6%), and a combination of these arteries (5.9%).[4] Ischemic symptoms due to intracranial stenosis are believed to arise from (1) hypoperfusion[5]; (2) thrombosis at the site of stenosis due to plaque rupture, hemorrhage within the plaque, or occlusive growth of the plaque[5]; (3) thromboembolism distal to the stenosis; and (4) occlusion of small perforating arteries at the site of the plaque.[6,7]

RISK FACTORS

African Americans with transient ischemic attack (TIA) or stroke are more likely than Caucasian Americans to have intracranial stenosis, whereas the latter are more likely to have extracranial carotid atherosclerotic stenosis.[2] Asian Americans have a higher proportion of MCA stenosis compared with Caucasian and African Americans.[6] Hypertension is present in up to 75% of individuals with intracranial atherosclerosis.[8] Diabetes, coronary artery disease, cigarette smoking, hypercholesterolemia, and peripheral arterial occlusive disease are also strongly associated. Individuals without carotid bifurcation disease are more likely to demonstrate progression of intracranial stenosis than those with carotid bifurcation disease.[9] Metabolic syndrome is present in approximately 50% of individuals who have symptomatic intracranial atherosclerotic disease and is associated with a substantially higher risk of major vascular events.[10]

NATURAL HISTORY

In a study of patients with intracranial stenosis undergoing repeat angiography at an average interval of 26.7 months, 40% of lesions had stabilized, 20% had regressed, and 40% had progressed.[9] Stenosis progression, as detected by transcranial Doppler imaging, was an independent predictor of stroke recurrence.[11] Extracranial–intracranial (EC-IC) bypass surgery appears to promote progression of the lesion and occlusion of the MCA in patients with nonoccluded MCA stenosis.[12]

Asymptomatic intracranial stenosis is believed by some to be benign. In a series of 50 patients with asymptomatic MCA stenosis followed for a mean of 351 days, no patient had an ischemic stroke in the corresponding territory.[8]

The most definitive study of symptomatic intracranial stenosis thus far is the prospective Warfarin–Aspirin Symptomatic Intracranial Disease (WASID) trial, which found an 11% to 12% first-year risk of ischemic stroke in territory attributable to the patient's symptoms.[4] The majority of strokes (73%) in WASID patients were in the territory of the stenotic artery.[13] The risk of stroke in the territory of the stenotic artery was greatest in patients with severe (70%) stenosis ($p = 0.0025$) and among patients enrolled early (17 days) ($p = 0.028$). At 1 year, the stroke risk for patients with 50% to 69% stenosis was 6%, compared with 19% for those with 70% to 99% stenosis. The recent results of the WASID trial suggest that perhaps an indication for endovascular therapy can be extended to those patients who present with stroke (regardless of previous medical therapy) and have stenosis of a major intracranial artery exceeding 70%.[13]

The subset of patients in the EC-IC Bypass Study with MCA stenosis randomized to medical therapy had an annual ipsilateral ischemic stroke rate of 7.8% per year.[6,14] In the prospective, nonrandomized Groupe d'Etude des Sténoses Intra-Crâniennes Athéromateuses Symptomatiques study, 102 patients with more than 50% symptomatic intracranial stenosis had "optimal" medical therapy, with a follow-up of 23.4 months.[15] Risks in the territory of the affected artery were 12.6% for TIA and 7.0% for stroke.

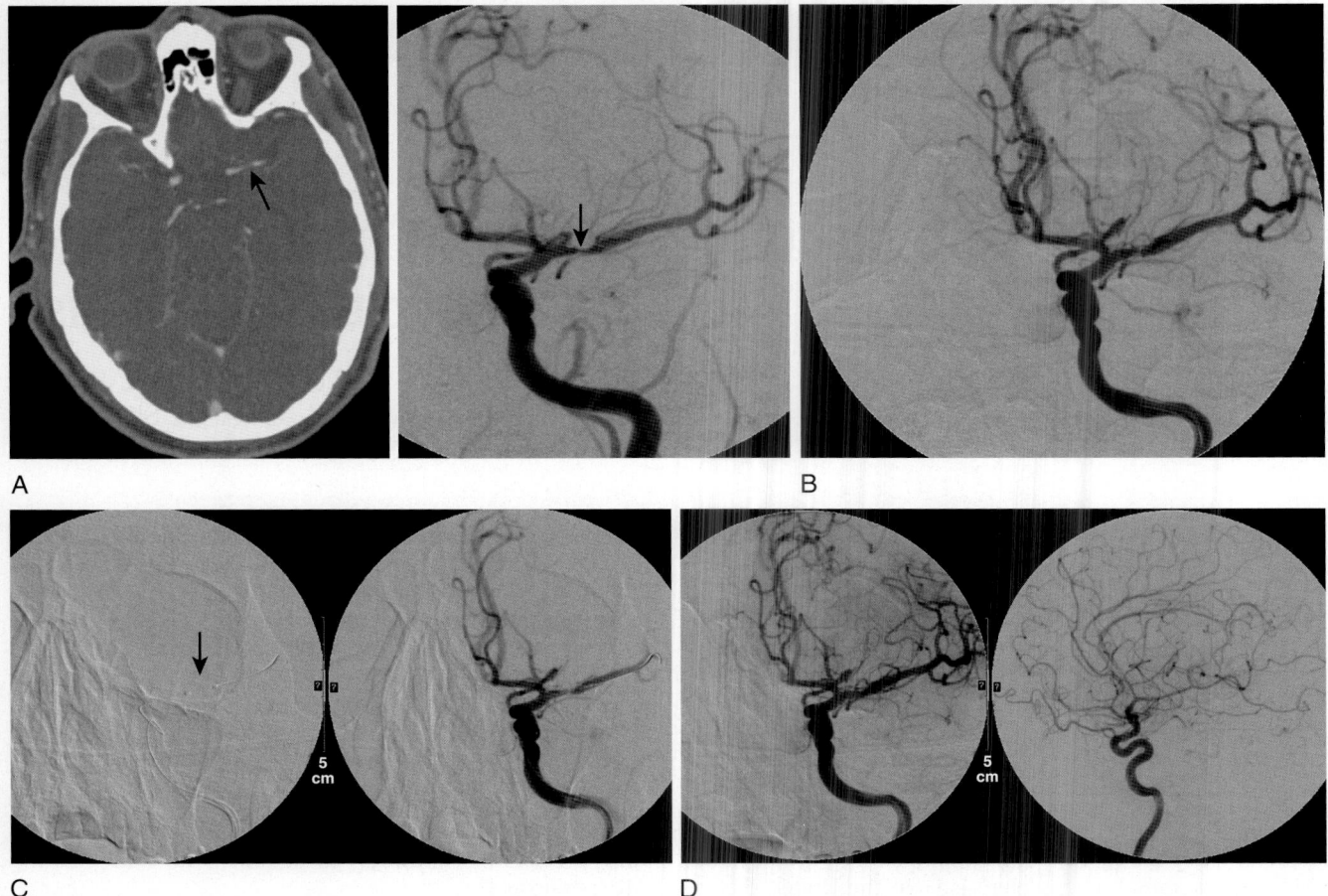

FIGURE 87-1 A 74-year-old who had two TIAs characterized by aphasia and right hemiparesis and left M1 stenosis by CT angiography (A) and digital subtraction angiography (B) (the *arrow* in each image depicts the stenosis). Episodes were refractory to aspirin–clopidogrel dual therapy. B and C, pre- and postangioplasty angiographic runs, respectively. C, Gateway balloon *(arrow)*. D, AP *(left)* and lateral *(right)* postprocedural runs. Notice the improved caliber of the M1 and normal filling of the MCA candelabra.

Evolution and Results of Endovascular Therapy

PRIMARY ANGIOPLASTY

Initially, coronary angioplasty balloons were used off-label to perform intracranial percutaneous transluminal angioplasty (PTA) (Fig. 87-1). In 1999, Connors and Wojak[16] published the report of their learning curve with a series of 70 patients who underwent angioplasty for intracranial atherosclerotic disease. Their technique progressed from directly sizing the balloon to the artery caliber with rapid balloon inflation to undersizing the balloon with slow inflation. The occurrence of acute vessel occlusion and dissection dropped from 75% to 14% with this technique. Currently, we utilize a technique of slow inflation (1 atmosphere, or atm, per minute) when performing angioplasty. In addition, we tend to undersize the balloon relative to the parent vessel.

Mori et al.[17,18] reported on angioplasty without stenting in 42 patients with more than 70% intracranial stenosis. The risk of recurrent stenosis was strongly associated with lesion length and complexity. Lesion types were categorized as follows: type A as 5 mm or less in length, concentric or moderately eccentric lesions that were less than

totally occlusive; type B as tubular, 5 to 10 mm in length, extremely eccentric or totally occluded lesions that were less than 3 months old; and type C as diffuse, more than 10 mm in length, extremely angulated (approximately 90 degrees) lesions with excessive tortuosity of the proximal segment or totally occluded lesions that were 3 months old. At the 1-year follow-up evaluation, restenosis rates associated with these lesion types were 0%, 33%, and 100%, respectively; the risk of major stroke or death was 8%, 26%, and 87%, respectively.

In 2006, Marks et al.[19] reported on 20 patients with 50% intracranial stenosis who were treated with angioplasty without stenting. A total of 116 patients were available for a mean follow-up duration of 42.3 months. The degree of stenosis was reduced by angioplasty from a mean of 82.2% to a mean of 36.0%. The combined 30-day periprocedural stroke and death rate was 5.8%. The annual postprocedure stroke rate in the territory of the treatment was 3.2%, and the annual overall stroke rate was 4.4%.

BALLOON-MOUNTED CORONARY STENTS

Angioplasty without stenting was associated with a significant risk of restenosis, which led to interest in angioplasty with stenting. Balloon-mounted coronary stents, however, are limited by the high inflation pressures needed for deployment in fragile intracranial vessels and the risk of shearing the stent from the balloon while navigating to the target lesion. These stents were associated with relatively high rates of technical failure due to the tortuosity of the intracranial circulation and the relative stiffness of coronary platforms; for successful procedures, the rates of periprocedural morbidity and mortality were acceptable.[20-22] Jiang et al.[22] reported a technical success rate (defined as equal to 20% residual stenosis) of 97.6%, with a 10% major complication rate in 40 patients with 42 symptomatic M1 stenotic lesions treated with angioplasty and balloon-mounted coronary stents.

BALLOON-MOUNTED INTRACRANIAL STENTS

The Stenting of Symptomatic Atherosclerotic Lesions in the Vertebral or Intracranial Arteries (SSYLVIA) trial was a multicenter, prospective, nonrandomized feasibility study involving the balloon-mounted Neurolink intracranial stent system (a product of the Guidant Corporation, which is now part of Boston Scientific, Natick, MA).[23] A total of 43 patients with symptomatic intracranial stenosis and 18 patients with extracranial VA stenosis were enrolled. Successful stent placement was achieved in 95% of cases. The 30-day periprocedural stroke rate was 6.6%. No deaths occurred. Two strokes occurred during the procedure. At the 6-month angiographic follow-up, more than 50% restenosis occurred in 32.4% of intracranial vessels and 42.9% of extracranial VAs; 39% of the recurrent stenoses were symptomatic. Strokes in the distribution of the target lesion occurring after 30 days but within 12 months were seen in 7.3% of patients. On the basis of the results of this study, the U.S. Food and Drug Administration (FDA) granted a humanitarian device exemption (HDE) to treat patients with significant intracranial and extracranial atherosclerotic disease via balloon angioplasty and stent placement. Boston Scientific is not currently marketing the Neurolink device in favor of its Wingspan system (discussed later).

The Pharos Vitesse intracranial stent (Micrus Endovascular, San Jose, CA) is a relatively new balloon-expandable stent developed for the treatment of intracranial stenosis. The first clinical experience of 21 patients with symptomatic intracranial stenoses (more than 70%) who were treated with the Pharos stent reported one stroke due to restenosis and one death during a median follow-up period of 7.3 months.[24] This pilot study was limited by the small sample size and severe morbidity of the included patients. The Pharos stent received Conformité Européen mark of approval in June 2008. The Vitesse Intracranial Stent Study for Ischemic Therapy clinical trial is currently under way to evaluate the efficacy of this stent. In our experience, this balloon-mounted stent navigates the intracranial circulation with relative ease.

STAGED SUBMAXIMAL ANGIOPLASTY WITH DELAYED STENTING

Because blood flow is directly proportional to the fourth power of the vessel radius (according to Poiseuille's law), small increases in luminal diameter increase blood flow significantly, thereby alleviating hemodynamic insufficiency and changing the milieu such that an embolism is less likely to form. A technique of submaximal angioplasty followed by delayed repeat angioplasty and, if necessary, stenting was developed for intracranial symptomatic atherosclerotic disease.[25] In this staged treatment approach, the patient returned for angiography approximately 4 to 6 weeks after angioplasty. If there was evidence of binary stenosis in the lesion (50% luminal-diameter stenosis), stenting was performed. The rationale for this approach is that during the weeks of delay, neointimal proliferation and scar formation after angioplasty result in a thickened fibrous lesion,[26,27] which may incur a lower risk for "snow-plowing" (stent struts pushing plaque into branch vessels), plaque embolization, and vessel dissection during a subsequent stenting procedure. With this strategy, the composite rate of mortality and permanent neurologic morbidity for the procedure dropped to below 5%, and 20% to 30% of patients did not require further intervention at follow-up.[28]

SELF-EXPANDING STENTS

The Wingspan stent system with a Gateway PTA balloon catheter (Boston Scientific) was designed for the treatment of intracranial atherosclerotic stenosis. Present dilation of the lesion is done with the angioplasty balloon; the stent, a self-expanding nitinol device, is then deployed (Fig. 87-2). The device received FDA approval as a new HDE device in August 2005. The approval was based on a 45-patient Wingspan HDE safety study that was conducted at 12 sites in Europe and Asia.[29] Patients who had a stroke caused by an intracranial lesion (stenosis of 50% or more) and for whom medical treatment was ineffective were enrolled in the study. Among the 45 patients, 44 patients subsequently underwent stent placement; in 1 patient, the lesion could not be traversed by the microwire. The procedural success rate was 98%, and a 4.4% incidence ($n = 2$) of death or ipsilateral stroke was observed 30 days after the procedure. The mean severity of angiographic stenosis decreased after the procedure from 75% to 32%. Among the 43 patients who completed the 6-month follow-up, the incidence of death or ipsilateral stroke was 7.0% ($n = 3$). Further lesion reduction was observed in 24 of 40 patients (mean severity 28%) who underwent follow-up angiography at 6 months. Angiograms in 3 patients (6.8%) showed more than 50% restenosis; all patients were asymptomatic. In contrast to SSYLVIA, which reported a rate of restenosis of more than 50% in 32.4% of patients at 6 months, the mean degree of stenosis at 6 months in the Wingspan study was not significantly different from the degree of stenosis immediately after the procedure.

In the U.S. Wingspan registry,[30-32] treatment with the stent system was attempted in 158 patients with 168 intracranial atheromatous lesions (updated statistics, Fiorella DJ, personal communication, November 2009). Of these, 161 lesions (96.0%) were successfully treated during the first treatment session. Of the 168 lesions in which treatment was attempted, there were 9 (5.4%) major periprocedural neurologic complications, 4 of which ultimately led to the death of the patient within 30 days of the procedure. The total periprocedural event rate was 12.5% (21 of 168 cases). Most postprocedure events (18 of 21) were related to definable (and potentially controllable) issues: early antiplatelet interruption ($n = 6$) and in-stent restenosis (ISR) ($n = 13$). There were 10 patients with strokes and 12 patients with TIAs that occurred 30 days after the procedure. Imaging follow-up was available for

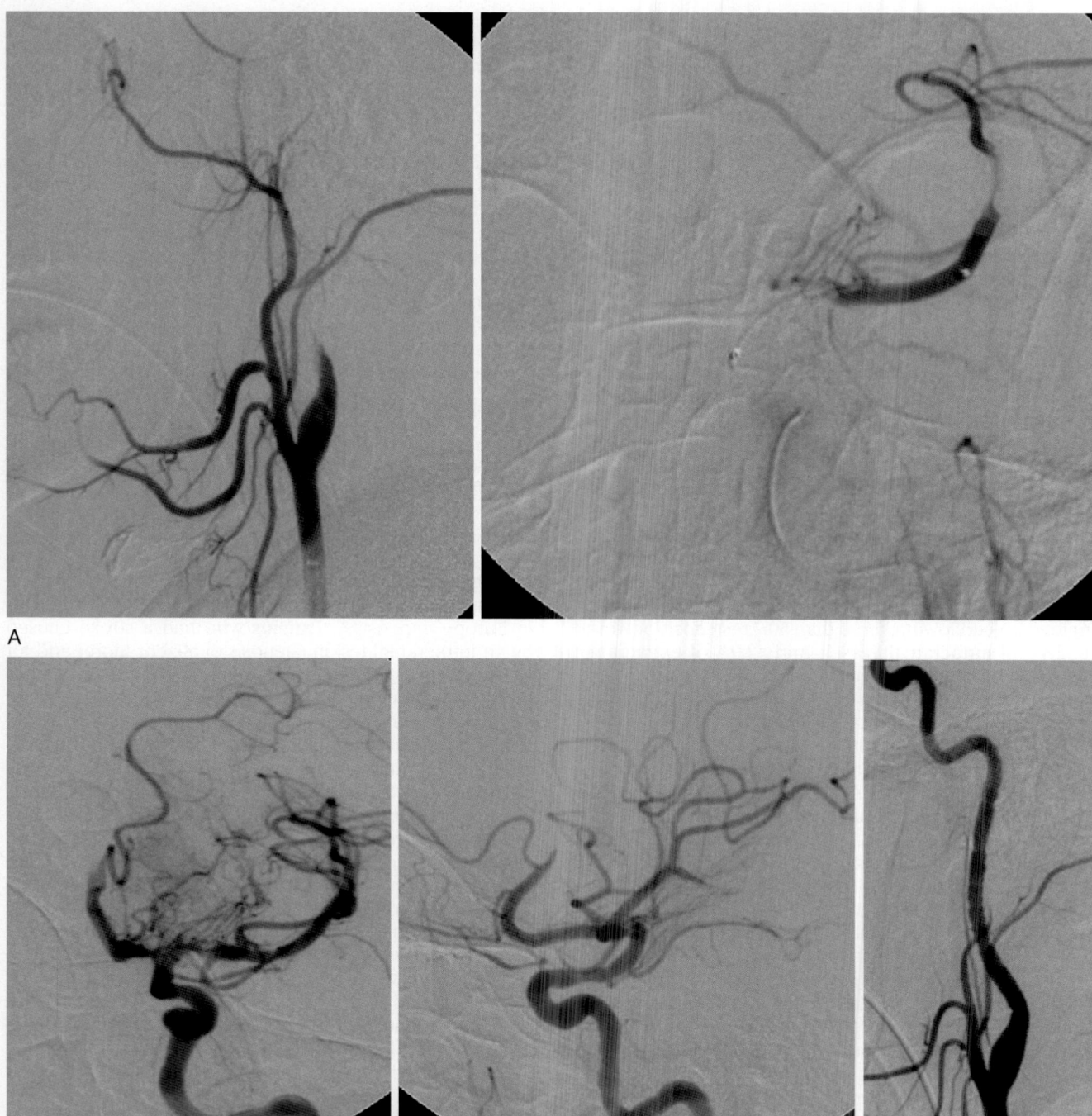

FIGURE 87-2 A 36-year-old with cardiomyopathy and atrial fibrillation (on warfarin therapy) presented with an NIH Stroke Scale score of 16. A, An angiogram *(left)* shows stasis of the contrast material in the ICA due to carotid terminus occlusion and (right) a Penumbra aspiration device in distal M1 after traversing the lesion into the M1 sequentially with a Nautica microcatheter (ev3)/Terumo gold-tipped microwire (Tokyo, Japan), and a Balance Middle Weight (Abbott Vascular) exchange wire, and a Penumbra aspiration device *(right)*. B, Combination endovascular therapy with the Merci retrieval device (Concentric Medical, Mountain View, CA), Penumbra device, and intra-arterial reteplase were successful *(left* = AP intracranial, *middle* = lateral intracranial, *right* = extracranial carotid) with reconstitution of the ICA, anterior cerebral artery, and MCA distributions. The patient experienced only mild, residual right-upper extremity numbness. Nine months later, the patient reported coincident worsening of his right-upper extremity numbness and new-onset insidious weakness.

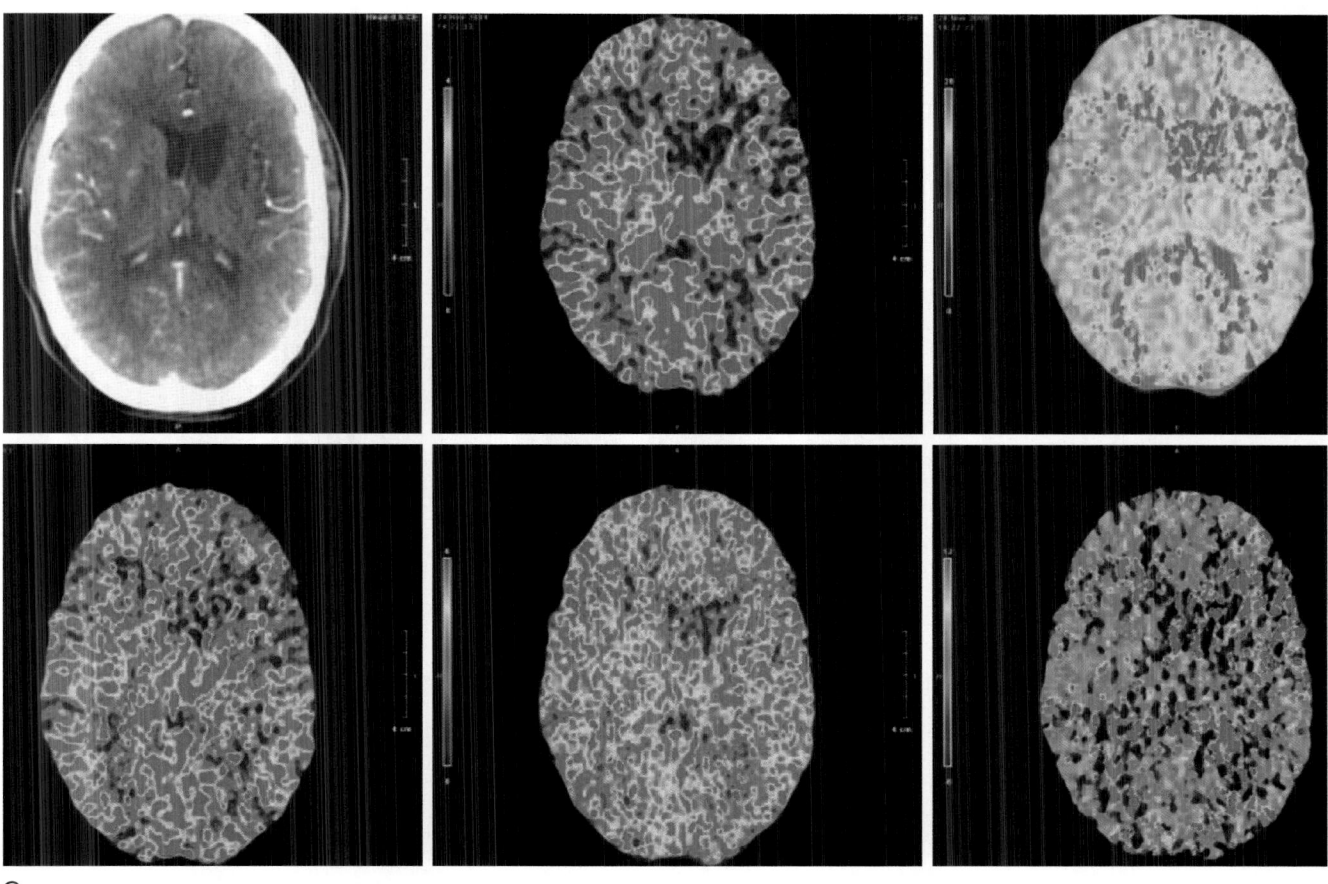

C

FIGURE 87-2, cont'd C, CT perfusion (color) images show increased left frontal time to peak *(upper right)*, slightly decreased cerebral blood flow *(lower left)*, and preserved cerebral blood volume *(upper middle)* in the same distribution.

129 treated lesions (75 anterior circulation and 54 posterior circulation). Post-Wingspan ISR was more common in patients younger than 55 years (2.6 odds ratio). This increased risk can be accounted for by a high prevalence of anterior circulation lesions in this population, specifically those affecting the supraclinoid segment. When patients of all ages were considered, much higher rates of both ISR (66.6% vs. 24.4%) and symptomatic ISR (40% vs. 3.9%) were associated with supraclinoid segment lesions, in comparison with all other locations. Of 129 patients with imaging follow-up of treated lesions, 36 patients (27.9%) experienced ISR. Of these 36, 29 patients (80.6%) underwent target lesion revascularization (TLR) with angioplasty alone ($n = 26$) or angioplasty with restenting ($n = 3$). Restenting was performed for in-stent dissections that occurred after the initial PTA. Among the retreated lesions, 23 were located within the anterior circulation (79.3%) versus 6 in the posterior circulation. ISR lesions selected for retreatment were often either symptomatic ($n = 4$), angiographically more severe (longer segment involved or greater percentage of stenosis) than the presenting stenosis ($n = 8$), or both ($n = 9$). In some cases ($n = 8$), however, retreatment was performed in the absence of any of these factors. When symptomatic ($n = 13$), approximately two thirds of patients presented with TIA ($n = 9$) and one third presented with

ipsilateral stroke ($n = 4$). Of the 29 patients undergoing primary TLR, 9 required 1 intervention for recurrent ISR, for a total of 42 TLR interventions. Only 1 major complication, a postprocedural reperfusion hemorrhage, was encountered during TLR (complication rates: 2.4% per procedure, 3.5% per patient). Angiographic follow-up was available for 22 of 29 patients after primary TLR. Of the 22 patients, 11 patients (50%) demonstrated recurrent ISR at follow-up angiography. Subsequently, 9 of these patients have undergone multiple retreatments (6 patients had two retreatments each, 2 had three retreatments each, and 1 had four retreatments) for recurrent ISR.

In the Wingspan National Institutes of Health (NIH) registry,[33] 129 patients with symptomatic 70% to 99% intracranial stenosis were enrolled from 16 medical centers. The rate of technical success rate (stent placement across the target lesion with less than 50% residual stenosis) was 97%. The rate of any stroke, intracerebral hemorrhage, or death within 30 days or ipsilateral stroke beyond 30 days was 14% at 6 months. The rate of 50% restenosis on follow-up angiography was 25% among 52 patients with follow-up. The NIH registry investigators published a post hoc analysis report of 158 of 160 patients who had successful placement for intracranial atherosclerotic lesion with 50% to 99% stenosis.[34] The primary endpoint

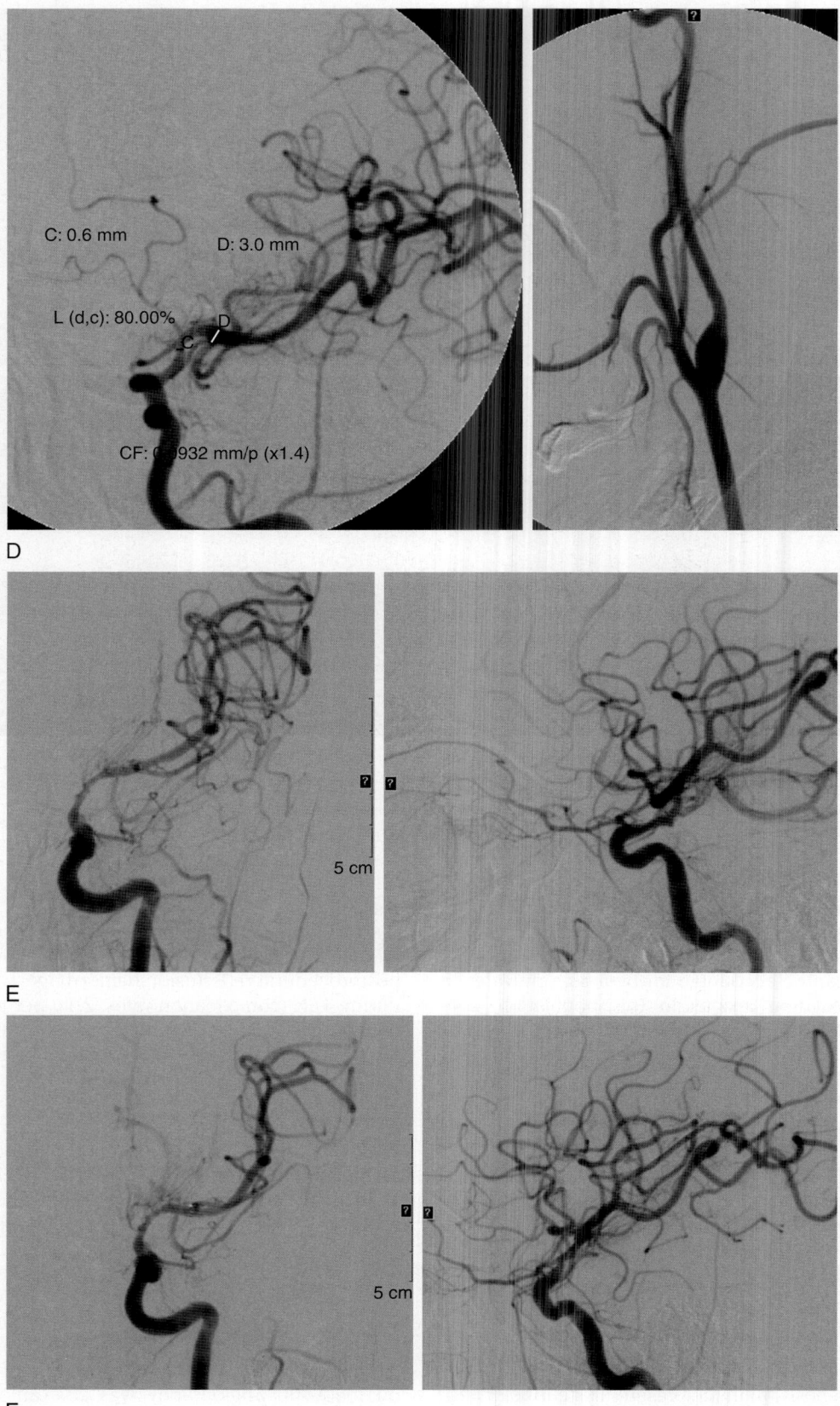

FIGURE 87-2, cont'd D, An angiogram shows supraclinoid ICA and M1 stenosis (left = intracranial, right = extracranial) of possible iatrogenic origin. E and F, Angiograms before (left = AP, right = lateral) and after (left = AP, right = lateral), respectively, placement of a self-expanding intracranial stent.

(any stroke or death within 30 days or stroke in the territory of the stented artery beyond 30 days) at 6 months occurred in 13.9%. In multivariable analysis, the primary endpoint was associated with posterior circulation stenosis (vs. anterior circulation), with a hazard ratio (HR) of 3.4 ($p = 0.018$); stenting at low enrollment sites with fewer than 10 patients each (vs. high enrollment sites) and an HR of 2.8 ($p = 0.038$); 10 days from the qualifying event to stenting (vs. 10 days), with an HR of 2.7 ($p = 0.058$); and stroke as a qualifying event (vs. TIA or another cerebral ischemic event, e.g., vertebrobasilar insufficiency), with an HR of 3.2 ($p = 0.064$).

DRUG-ELUTING STENTS

In a recent systematic review of 31 studies including 1177 procedures for symptomatic high-grade intracranial atheromatous disease, ISR occurred more frequently after the use of a self-expandable stent (16 of 92 cases, or 17.4%; mean follow-up period 5.4 months) than after use of a balloon-mounted stent (61 of 443 cases, or 13.8%; mean follow-up period 8.7 months; $p < 0.001$).[35] Thus, ISR is a major potential downfall of the predicate technologies that might be overcome with the implementation of drug-eluting stents (DESs) (Figs. 87-3 and 87-4). First-generation

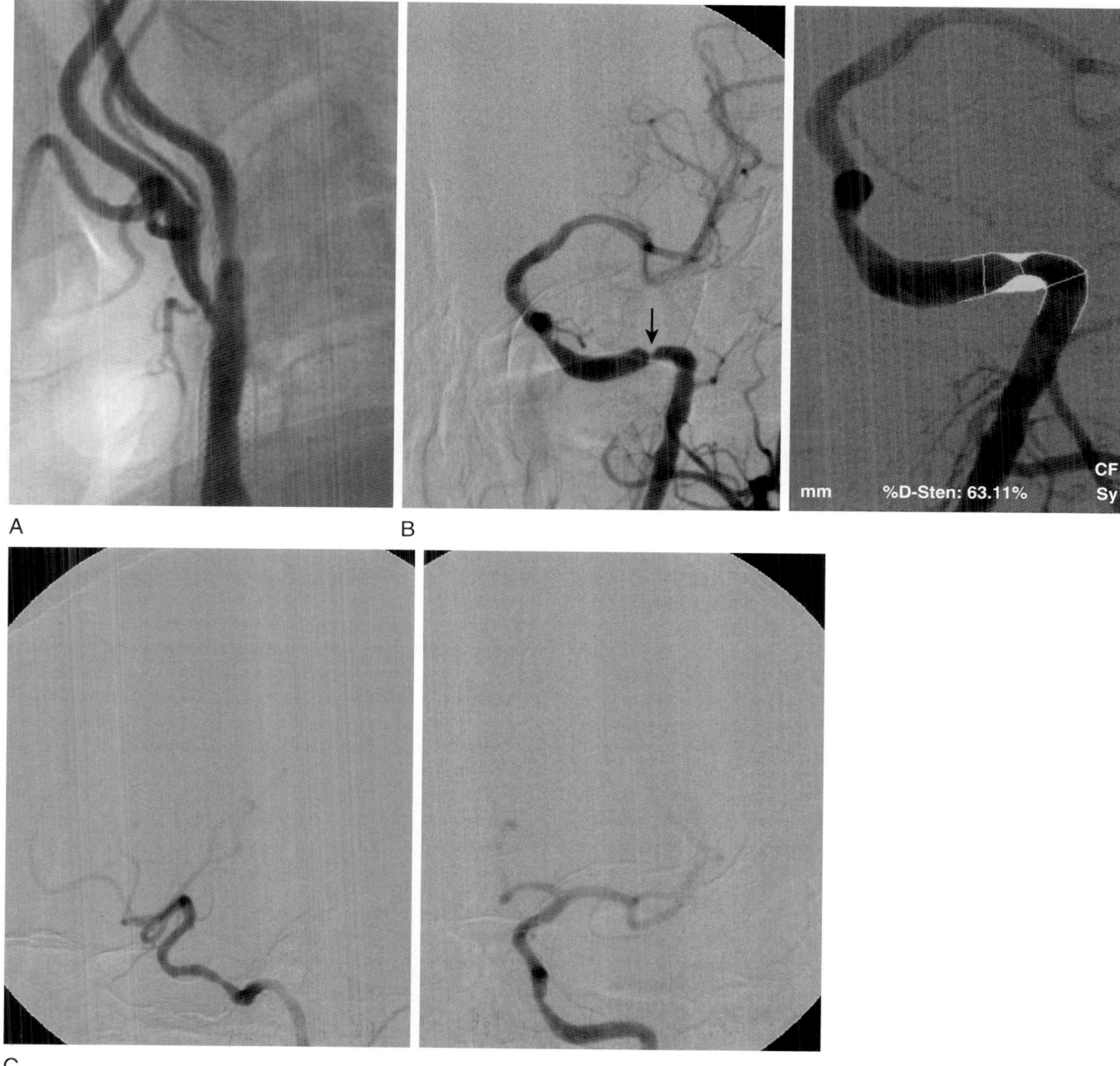

FIGURE 87-3 A 69-year-old with an old left MCA infarct due to ICA occlusion treated with carotid artery stenting (A, angiogram) with good recovery. B, A follow-up angiogram shows new severe left petrous ICA stenosis (*arrow* on left). CT perfusion imaging showed delayed hemispheric time to peak without acetazolamide augmentation (not shown). B and C, Postprocedural EES stent placement (left = AP, right = lateral).

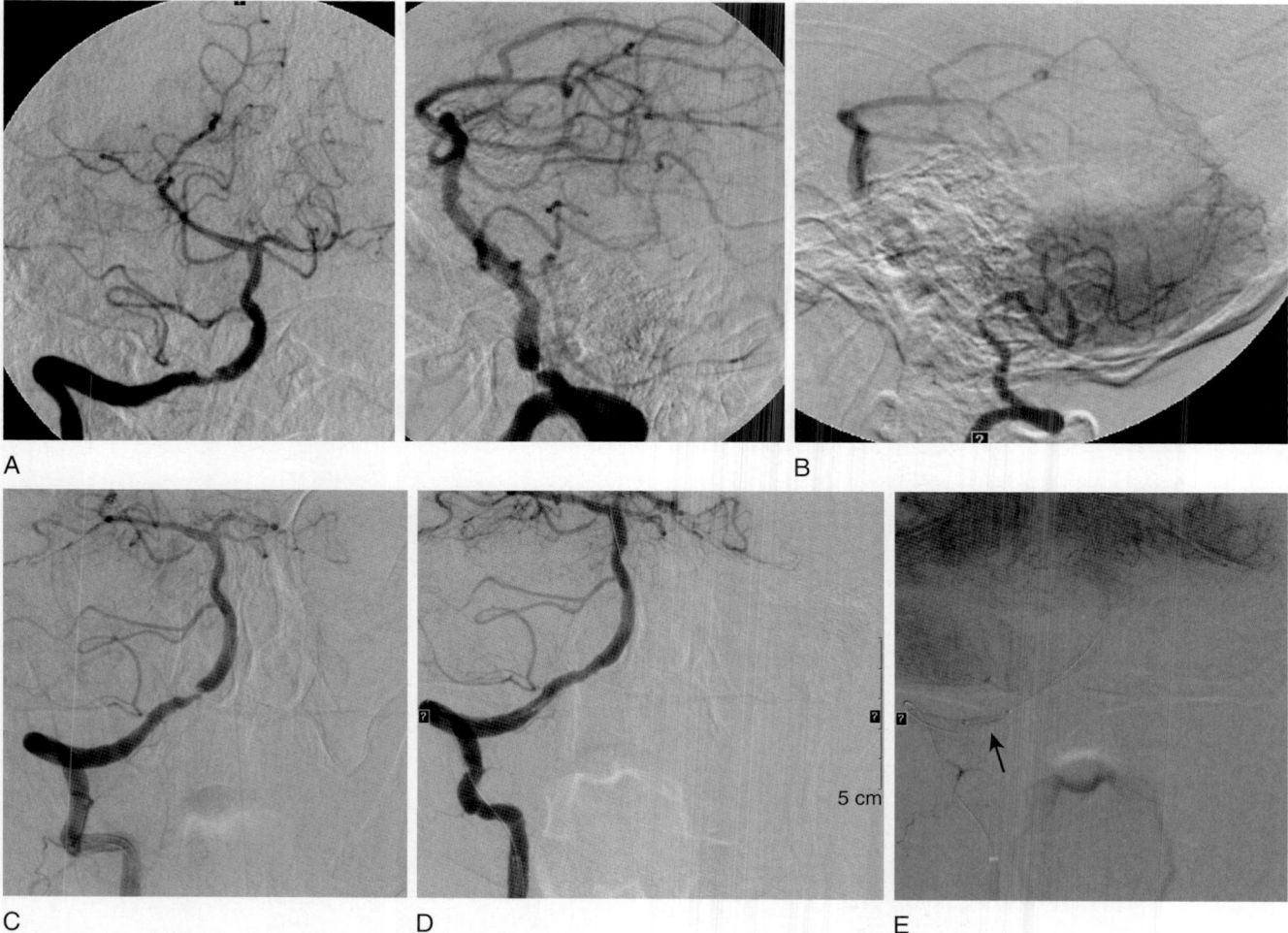

FIGURE 87-4 The patient has a 6-month history of substantial postural dizziness. A, Right V4 segment has severe 84% ulcerated stenosis (left = AP, right = lateral). B, Left VA ends in the posterior inferior cerebellar artery. C and D, Pre- and postangiographic runs, respectively, after placement of an EES, balloon-mounted stent. E, Stent with the deflated deployment balloon still in place *(arrow)*.

balloon-mounted coronary DESs coated with sirolimus or paclitaxel have reduced the coronary ISR rate to 10% from the 30% observed with bare-metal stents.[36] There have been a few reports of the use of the first-generation DESs in patients with intracranial arterial stenosis,[37-41] and the safety of implanting these devices has been studied in the intracranial vasculature of canine models.[42,43] The Xience V everolimus-eluting stent (EES) (Abbott Vascular, Abbott Park, IL) is a new second-generation DES that was approved by the FDA for coronary stenting in July 2008. This stent has a thin cobalt-chromium strut stent platform that allows greater deliverability in tortuous vasculature[44] and is coated with an antirestenotic drug, everolimus, that has proven ability to suppress ISR to a degree equivalent to that with sirolimus and more than that for paclitaxel-eluting stents.[45,46] The DESs may reduce the overall ISR rate if they can be used selectively in patients with lesions who have been identified to have a higher incidence of ISR. We have reported our initial experience with EES in patients with intracranial arterial stenosis.[47] These devices are used off-label in the intracranial vasculature.

Endovascular Therapy versus Best Medical Therapy

A comparison between 254 patients recruited in the WASID trial and 158 patients entered in the NIH Wingspan multicenter stenting registry matched by patient and lesion characteristics was performed to determine the differential rates of primary outcome of stroke or death within 30 days or ipsilateral stroke beyond 30 days.[48] The frequency of the primary outcome at 6 months in patients with 70% to 99% stenosis was 16% for WASID patients (treated with best medical therapy) and 13% for stent-treated Wingspan registry patients. The study concluded that stent placement may offer benefit in patients with 70% to 99% stenosis, but the benefit may not be seen in patients with 50% to 69% stenosis due to the low event rates in the medically treated patients.

In 2007, the NIH approved funding for the multicenter, prospective, randomized Stenting and Aggressive Medical Management for Preventing Recurrent Stroke in Intracranial Stenosis study.[49] The hypothesis of the study is that "Compared with intensive medical therapy alone, intracranial angioplasty and stenting combined with intensive medical therapy will decrease the risk of the primary endpoint by 35% over a mean follow-up of 2 years in high-risk patients (patients with 70% to 99% intracranial stenosis who had a TIA or stroke within 30 days prior to enrollment) with symptomatic stenosis of a major intracranial artery."[49] A total of 764 patients will be recruited within 30 days of TIA or stroke due to 70% to 99% stenosis of a major intracranial artery. The patients will be randomized to receive either (1) stent treatment with the Wingspan intracranial stent and Gateway balloon system plus intensive medical therapy with management of blood pressure, lipids, and other risk factors for vascular events or (2) intensive medical therapy with management of blood pressure, lipids, and other risk factors for vascular events. Each patient will be followed up for a minimum of 1 year and a maximum of 4 years after randomization.

Primary Angioplasty versus Stenting

Some controversy exists as to whether primary angioplasty is equivalent to intracranial stent placement for intracranial atherosclerotic disease. In a systematic review[50] of 69 studies (33 primary angioplasty studies with a total of 1027 patients and 36 stent-placement studies with a total of 1291 patients), the incidence of technical success (defined as 50% or less residual stenosis of the target vessel after angioplasty or stent treatment) was 80% in the angioplasty group and 95% in the stent-treated group (relative risk, or RR, of 0.84, $p < 0.0001$). A total of 91 strokes and deaths were reported in the angioplasty-treated group (9%), compared with 104 in the stent-treated group (8%) during the 1-month postprocedure period (RR 1.1, $p = 0.5$). The pooled incidence of 1-year stroke and death in the angioplasty group was 20%, compared with 14% in the stent-placement group (RR 1.39, $p = 0.009$). The pooled restenosis rate was 14% in the angioplasty group, compared with 11% in the stent-placement group (RR 1.28, $p = 0.04$).

Technique of Angioplasty or Stenting
PREOPERATIVE IMAGING

Catheter-based angiography, three-dimensional computed tomography (CT) examination, and magnetic resonance angiography (MRA) are helpful in confirming the diagnosis and/or planning the endovascular procedure. A cerebral blood flow study (e.g., positron emission tomography, xenon CT with acetazolamide challenge, or single-photon emission CT) can confirm a diagnosis of intracranial hemodynamic failure and identify cerebral territories at risk of ischemic injury. We prefer to have a CT/MRA image of the arch and supra-aortic vessel to plan the access approach and be prepared for difficulty with access.

ANESTHESIA

At our center, we prefer to perform these procedures in conscious patients after the administration of mild sedatives and local anesthetic agents so that we can perform intermittent neurologic examinations during the procedure. Avoidance of general anesthesia also reduces the cardiovascular risk of the overall procedure. However, if a complication does occur, the potential exists for further harm until the patient's airway can be secured and additional maneuvers (e.g., ventriculostomy and further embolization) can be performed. We must be prepared to intubate the patient on a moment's notice. Not all patients are candidates for conscious sedation because of poor neurologic status, young age, excessive anxiety, or inability to lie still. General anesthesia is routinely used at most centers and offers the advantages of control of the airway as well as reduction or elimination of patient movement during the procedure. In a report of 37 intracranial angioplasty and stenting cases performed with conscious sedation, technical success was achieved in all patients.[51] Approximately 61% of patients experienced intraprocedural symptoms that led to some alteration of the interventional technique. Headache was the most common symptom and, when persistent, signaled the occurrence of intracranial hemorrhage.

ANTIPLATELET THERAPY

Patients scheduled to undergo elective stent placement at our center receive aspirin (325 mg by mouth daily) and clopidogrel (75 mg by mouth daily) for a minimum of 4 days before the procedure. Those undergoing stenting more urgently receive aspirin (650 mg by mouth) and clopidogrel (600 mg by mouth) 4 hours before the procedure. If stenting is performed as an emergency bailout maneuver, we administer an intravenous bolus dose of a glycoprotein IIb/IIIa inhibitor (180 mg of eptifibatide per kilogram of body weight at our institution) and then clopidogrel (600 mg by mouth) and aspirin (650 mg by mouth) immediately after the procedure. Eptifibatide (2 mg/kg/min) is continued as an intravenous drip for 4 hours after the procedure to allow the clopidogrel to reach therapeutic levels of platelet inhibition.

ANTICOAGULATION THERAPY

We routinely administer heparin (an intravenous bolus of 50-70 units/kg) to obtain an activated coagulation time of 250 to 300 seconds before catheterization of intracranial vessels. The heparin is allowed to wear off after the procedure unless there is evidence that intraprocedural wire perforation or contrast extravasation has occurred. In such a case, the effect of the heparin is reversed with protamine sulfate during or after the procedure.

Before the endovascular procedure is performed, preferably on the previous day, the patient's neurologic status is assessed, and all available imaging studies are reviewed in preparation for the case. Decisions concerning the overall strategy should be made ahead of time to permit accurate device selection and smooth and efficient performance during the case. Considerations should include choice of access vessel, endovascular technique (i.e., primary angioplasty vs. stent-assisted angioplasty), and device types and sizes.

ACCESS SITE

For each case, the iliofemoral anatomy, arch anatomy, and supra-aortic vessel need to be assessed to decide on the access site and the devices that will facilitate safe access and provide a stable platform for intracranial therapies. (The brachial or radial artery may be chosen as the access site if there is a disease in the iliofemoral segments or descending aorta.) Patients with intracranial atherosclerotic disease have a higher chance of having an atherosclerotic arch or tortuous and elongated supra-aortic vessels. In such cases, special devices to access difficult arch anatomy, a carotid cut-down in the neck, or a cut-down of the extracranial VA as it traverses over the posterior arch of the C1 vertebra may be used to access the intracranial vasculature.

For transfemoral access, dorsalis pedis and posterior tibialis pulses are assessed and marked. The right or left groin is prepped, draped, and infiltrated with a local anesthetic (lidocaine). For conscious sedation, midazolam and fentanyl are intravenously administered. A 6-French (Fr) sheath is placed in the femoral artery. An angiogram is performed using a diagnostic catheter. Angiograms of the access vessel (carotid artery or VA) and anteroposterior (AP) and lateral views of the intracranial circulation are obtained immediately before the intervention. Examination of the carotid artery or VA is necessary for guide catheter selection and for evaluation of the presence of atherosclerosis or fibromuscular dysplasia.

GUIDE CATHETER SELECTION

Guide catheter support is more important for intracranial angioplasty procedures than for most other intracranial interventions. Angioplasty balloons and stents are relatively rigid and difficult to navigate; forward motion of these devices can cause unexpectedly high amounts of downward-directed force on the guide catheter. Therefore, due caution is warranted in guide catheter selection and positioning. High positioning of the guide catheter maximizes the stability of that catheter and improves control over the microcatheter and microwire. In a nontortuous, healthy carotid arterial system, we prefer to position the tip of the guide catheter in the vertical segment of the petrous ICA. In a cervical ICA with a significant curve in the vessel, the guide can be adequately positioned immediately proximal to the curve. Moderate curves in the vessel can be straightened out by guiding a relatively stiff hydrophilic wire (e.g., a 0.038-inch wire) through the affected segment, followed by the catheter. In the VA, the guide catheter is positioned in the distal extracranial VA, usually at the first curve (at the level of the C2 vertebra).

The Neuron Intracranial Access System (Penumbra, Alameda, CA) is increasingly used as the guide catheter at our center. These catheters are more stable the farther distally they are placed. The two guide catheters we used previously were the Envoy (Cordis Neurovascular, Miami Lakes, FL) and the Guider Softip XF (Boston Scientific). A 6-Fr, 90-cm Shuttle (Cook Inc., Bloomington, IN) also provides a large stable platform for intervention. The guide catheter can be placed directly or by an exchange method in patients with tortuous anatomy, atherosclerosis, or fibromuscular dysplasia. A 5-Fr guide catheter is used if the vessel caliber is small and collateral circulation is limited, for example, in a small VA when the contralateral vessel is hypoplastic. The main disadvantage of the Neuron System is that it is difficult to attain an angiogram with a microcatheter or balloon in place within the 5-Fr guide catheter.

DEVICE SELECTION

Essential devices for intracranial angioplasty include an exchange-length microwire, a microcatheter, and a balloon. Microwire properties that are most important for intracranial angioplasty are "beefiness," trackability, and

torque control. A relatively soft distal tip is helpful as well to minimize the chances of distal vessel vasospasm and perforation. We prefer to use the 0.014-inch, 300-cm Transend FloppyTip microwire (Boston Scientific), because it has superior torque control compared with other microwires. The 0.014-inch, 300-cm X-Celerator microwire (ev3, Irvine, CA) is another option; it has a soft tip, has a relatively supportive body, and is very lubricious. A low-profile, straight microcatheter, usually of any kind, is sufficient. The 1.7-Fr Echelon-10 microcatheter (ev3) can be pushed through tortuous and stenotic vessels better than other microcatheters.

GATEWAY PTA BALLOON CATHETER

The Gateway is a modified version of the Maverick 2 balloon catheter (Boston Scientific) with silicone coating on the balloon and hydrophilic coating on the catheter to facilitate access. Radiopaque markers on the balloon permit visualization of the proximal and distal ends of the balloon during fluoroscopic imaging. Available balloon diameters include 1.5, 2.0, 2.25, 2.75, 3.0, 3.25, 3.5, 3.75, and 4.0 mm; balloon lengths include 9, 15, and 20 mm. The normal inflation pressure is 6 atm, and rated burst pressures include 12 atm (14 atm for 2.25- to 3.25-mm balloons). Angioplasty is performed with the intent to achieve 80% dilation of the normal vessel diameter. If the target vessel has different diameters proximal and distal to the lesion, the balloon is sized to the smaller of the two.

The Gateway balloon may be taken up primarily, over a non-exchange-length microwire, if the anatomy is favorable. Alternatively, an exchange-length microwire can be advanced into a distal intracranial vessel within a microcatheter, which can be exchanged for the Gateway balloon. After flushing, the balloon catheter is advanced over the microwire into the guide catheter. When positioned at the rotating hemostatic valve, a marker on the balloon catheter shaft indicates the guide catheter tip. This feature saves fluoroscopy time. With road map guidance, the balloon is advanced until the balloon markers are across the lesion. A guide catheter angiogram is performed with the balloon in position to confirm proper positioning. The balloon is slowly inflated to nominal pressure, at a rate of approximately 1 atm every 10 seconds, under fluoroscopy. When the balloon is fully inflated, it is left inflated for another 10 to 20 seconds and then deflated. A guide catheter angiogram is obtained prior to removal of the balloon. For most cases, a single inflation is sufficient to achieve 80% dilation. Occasionally, a second inflation, at a slightly higher pressure (e.g., 8 atm) is helpful. If the balloon is difficult to inflate, it is removed and another balloon is used. If the balloon "watermelon seeds" (i.e., slips forward or backward during inflation), gentle traction is applied to the balloon catheter during inflation to stabilize the balloon and prevent it from migrating distally during inflation or a longer balloon is selected. After angioplasty, the balloon is removed and angiography is repeated.

WINGSPAN STENT (VIDEO)

The Wingspan is a 3.5-Fr, nitinol, over-the-wire self-expanding stent. The design of this stent is similar to that of the Neuroform2 stent (Boston Scientific); the Wingspan has four platinum markers at each end for visualization and is deployed from the delivery microcatheter (called the "outer body") with the "inner body"; the inner body is analogous to the "stabilizer" device that is used to deploy Neuroform stents. Available sizes include stent diameters of 2.5 to 4.5 mm in 0.5-mm increments, and stent lengths include 9, 15, and 20 mm. The stent length should extend a minimum of 3 mm on both sides of the lesion. If the target vessel has different diameters proximal and distal to the stenotic lesion, the stent is sized to the larger of the two.

The Wingspan system should be flushed with heparinized saline, as indicated in the diagram on the package in accordance with the manufacturer's directions. Continuous flushes with heparinized saline should be connected via stopcocks and rotating hemostatic valves to both the Wingspan deployment catheter (the outer body) and the inner body. The tapered tip of the inner body should be loosened slightly, with approximately 1 mm of space between the spearhead-shaped tip of the inner body and the distal end of the outer body, to allow adequate flushing and prevent "corking" or binding of the inner body tip to the outer body catheter. During flushing, heparinized saline should be seen dripping from the inner lumen and from between the inner and the outer bodies.

The rotating hemostatic valve is tightened on the inner body to prevent its migration, and the outer body of the Wingspan system is advanced over the exchange-length microwire. The delivery system is advanced by grasping the outer body and not the inner body. This avoids inadvertent advancement of the inner body and premature deployment of the stent. The tapered tip of the inner body extends for 10 to 12 mm past the distal tip of the outer body and is radiolucent. Care should be taken to avoid jamming the distal end of the system into a curving vessel. Once the stent catheter is advancing over the microwire, the surgeon can take advantage of the forward momentum and continue tracking to a site distal to the lesion. It is easier to move the system from distal to proximal than vice versa. The inner body is advanced just proximal to the stent using the marker bands to identify the position of the stent. The outer body is pulled back to bring the outer body tip into position just past the region of stenosis. This is the final maneuver prior to stent deployment. Holding the inner body in a stable position with the right hand, while slowly withdrawing the outer body with the left hand, results in deployment of the stent. The position of the stent should not be changed during deployment. Once the stent is deployed, the deployment system is brought into the proximal part of the vessel or into the guide catheter, while the microwire is left in position. A guide catheter angiogram is done to confirm the placement of the stent. If the stent is malpositioned during deployment, the placement of a second stent is considered.

POSTPROCEDURE MANAGEMENT

Patients are admitted to the intensive care unit or a stepdown unit. Neurologic status and access site are evaluated hourly. Most patients can be discharged from the hospital 1 or 2 days after the procedure. Aspirin is continued for life, and we prefer to continue clopidogrel (75 mg by mouth daily) for 3 to 6 months. Cardiologists are recently moving toward longer periods of dual antiplatelet therapy (3, 6, or 12 months) after coronary angioplasty and stenting.[52] It can be argued that atherosclerotic intracranial arteries are

similar in size and pathology to similarly diseased coronary arteries.

RECOGNITION AND MANAGEMENT OF INTRACRANIAL COMPLICATIONS

During the endovascular procedure, if an abrupt change in blood pressure or heart rate occurs, or if a neurologic change occurs in an awake patient, AP and lateral intracranial angiograms are obtained to look for contrast extravasation and other signs of vessel perforation (such as a wire tip in the wrong location), intraluminal thrombus, intracranial vessel dropout, or slowing of the passage of contrast material through distal intracranial vessels (which indicates a shower of emboli into multiple small branches) or intracranial dissection. Intravenous glycoprotein IIb/IIIa inhibitors or intra-arterial thrombolytics can be used if there is new clot formation. The glycoprotein IIb/IIIa inhibitors are more effective for the dissolution of fresh platelet-rich thrombi than are intra-arterially administered thrombolytic agents. If intracranial hemorrhage is identified, heparin is reversed with protamine (10 mg intravenously administered per 1000 units of heparin given). Tight control of blood pressure is maintained, and a platelet transfusion is administered (to reverse the effect of the antiplatelet medications). In patients with postprocedure neurologic changes, a cranial CT scan is obtained. The performance of a diagnostic angiogram and intra-arterial thrombolysis are considered. When angiography or CT imaging does not explain a neurologic change, magnetic resonance imaging with diffusion-weighted imaging can identify subtle ischemic changes.

Moyamoya Disease

MMD is a rare, progressive cerebrovascular disease with spontaneous occlusion or stenosis at the circle of Willis and its principal branches, along with the development of an aberrant network of collateral circulation that leads to hemorrhagic and ischemic strokes. Patients with unilateral disease are included in the cohort of moyamoya syndrome (MMS), even though they do not have any of the described associated risk factors for MMS.[53] MMD primarily affects Asians, with a prevalence of 3 to 6 per 100,000 people in Japan.[54-56] A less severe or less progressive form of the disease has been identified in the United States[57-59] with an incidence of 0.086 cases per 100,000 people. This form of the disease assumes a more benign course, predominates in adults between the third and fifth decade, and is associated with more ischemic than hemorrhagic strokes.

Traditionally, patients with MMD and ischemic symptoms are treated with direct (superficial temporal artery–MCA bypass) or indirect (encephaloduroarteriosynangiosis) surgical revascularization procedures. The largest surgical series, which is from Stanford University School of Medicine, reported on 233 adult patients, of whom 95.1% underwent direct revascularization procedures.[60] The cumulative 5-year risk of perioperative or subsequent stroke or death in this series was 5.5%.

There have been four single-case reports of treatment of endovascular therapy for MMD in the literature.[61-64] At our center, we treated six MMS patients (Figs. 87-5 to 87-7) with endovascular therapy between August 2005 and February

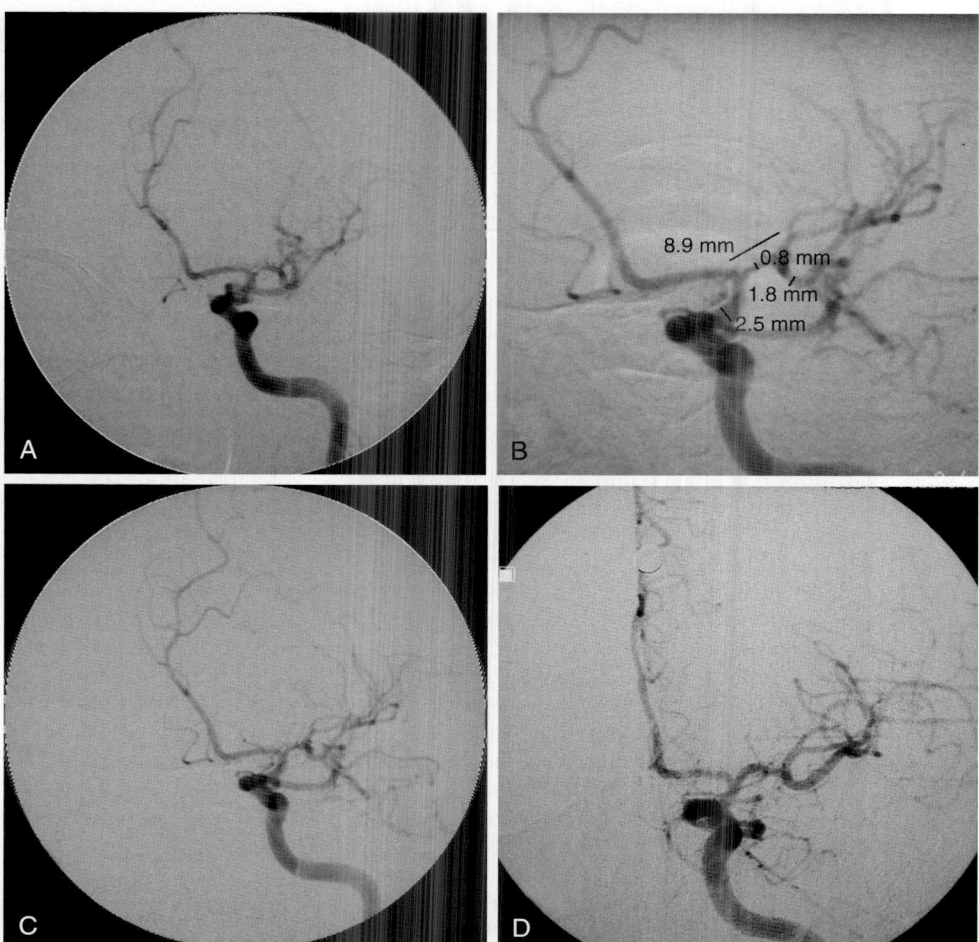

FIGURE 87-5 A and B, A 35-year-old presented with a more than 90%, symptomatic left M1 stenosis. C and D, The patient was taking aspirin and clopidogrel and had experienced a previous stroke with a complete recovery. Balloon angioplasty reduced the stenosis to 35%.

2009. All patients were women who were symptomatic, had a previous stroke or TIA, and were young (mean age 36.8 years). Stenotic lesion locations included a unilateral M1-segment lesion in five patients and, in the remaining patient, ipsilateral ICA-terminus, M1, and A1 lesions, in addition to contralateral supraclinoid carotid artery stenosis. The mean M1 stenosis was $77.3 \pm 14.3\%$. Five patients had balloon angioplasty for M1 stenosis. In the remaining patient, balloon angioplasty failed to relieve the M1 stenosis, and a Wingspan stent was deployed successfully. Among the six patients in our series, mean post-treatment M1 stenosis was $39.3 \pm 35\%$. Vessel rupture that occurred during angioplasty in one patient with near-complete M1 occlusion caused severe disability (modified Rankin score of 5). Of the five successfully treated patients, two were asymptomatic for 4 years and 6 months, respectively, after the primary treatment. Three of the remaining patients had retreatment 1, 2, and 5 months, respectively, after primary treatment. The first had repeat balloon angioplasty and has been asymptomatic for 6 months. The second underwent encephaloduroarteriosynangiosis after a failed balloon angioplasty and has been asymptomatic for 10 months. The third patient was asymptomatic but had angiographic restenosis (81%) and underwent Wingspan stent placement. She developed subsequent asymptomatic, severe in-stent restenosis that was treated with angioplasty at 3 months and has been asymptomatic for 4 months postangioplasty.

As we built our experience with these six patients, we realized that endovascular therapy was dangerous and was associated with a high rate of TLR when performed in patients with MMS who had severe (80%-100%) intracranial stenosis. The results were more sustainable in patients who had a single lesion that was forme fruste, minimally stenotic, and shorter. The goal of angioplasty in these patients was to achieve adequate distal perfusion with the use of a submaximal, slow inflation technique. We chose the shortest angioplasty balloon that would fully cover the lesion and inflated this balloon to approximately 50% to 75% of the parent vessel lumen. A slow inflation was used, as has been described by others.[16] The lesion need not be completely dilated because of the higher chance of reperfusion hemorrhage associated with a significant increase of flow in these patients. Excessive dilatation and the use of maximal balloon dilatation, especially for a tight stenosis, may be dangerous and lead to vessel rupture.

Intracranial stents were used only when the lesion narrowed or occluded after balloon angioplasty. The Wingspan intracranial self-expanding stent is our choice for these lesions. The stents were sized to exactly match the largest dimensions of both the proximal and the distal parts of the vessel. Present angioplasty with a Gateway balloon was always used, and poststent angioplasty was avoided, unless a flow-limiting lesion remained. Patients who had stent placement were placed on aspirin and clopidogrel for

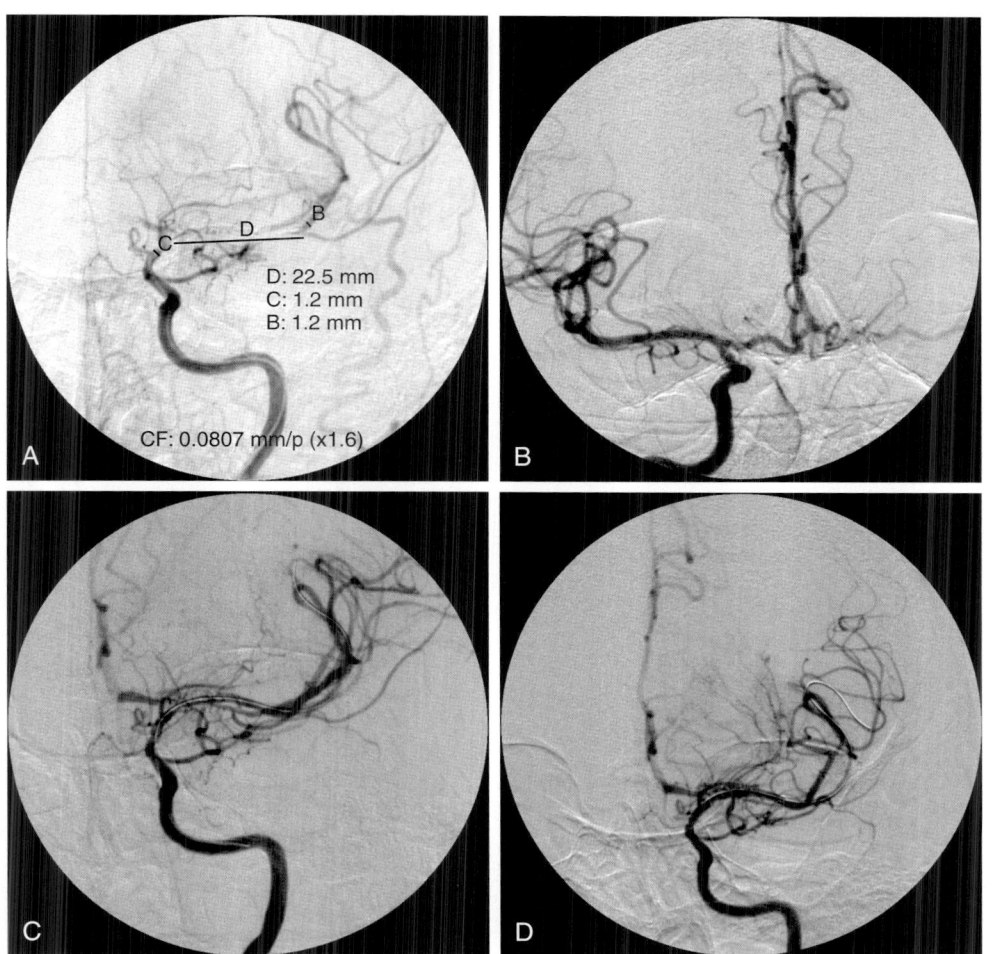

FIGURE 87-6 Same patient as prior figure. A, Severe, asymptomatic restenosis was evident on the 5-month follow-up angiogram. B, Right ICA injection and cross-flow through the anterior communicating artery into the left MCA. Repeat angioplasty with a Wingspan stent placement was performed after crossing the lesion (C) and after stent placement (D).

at least 1 year because of the high rate of reported asymptomatic ISR after stenting in intracranial atherosclerotic stenosis (especially in patients younger than 55 years in the anterior circulation and more so with ICA lesions).[32,33,65] For most patients with symptomatic MMD, we favor a surgical option over endovascular treatment.

Conclusions

Intracranial angioplasty with or without stent placement is an emerging technique with evolving technology. New data will provide additional information on appropriate patient selection, optimal timing of interventional therapy, and surgical and endovascular treatment options for intracranial occlusive disease. Development of more trackable, noncompliant balloons and stent systems and technology to avoid ISR and accelerate stent endothelialization may make endovascular therapy the primary and a safe treatment option for intracranial occlusive disease. Identification of patients who will benefit from therapy by physiologic imaging may increase the benefit of revascularization for these patients against the risk involved in the procedure.

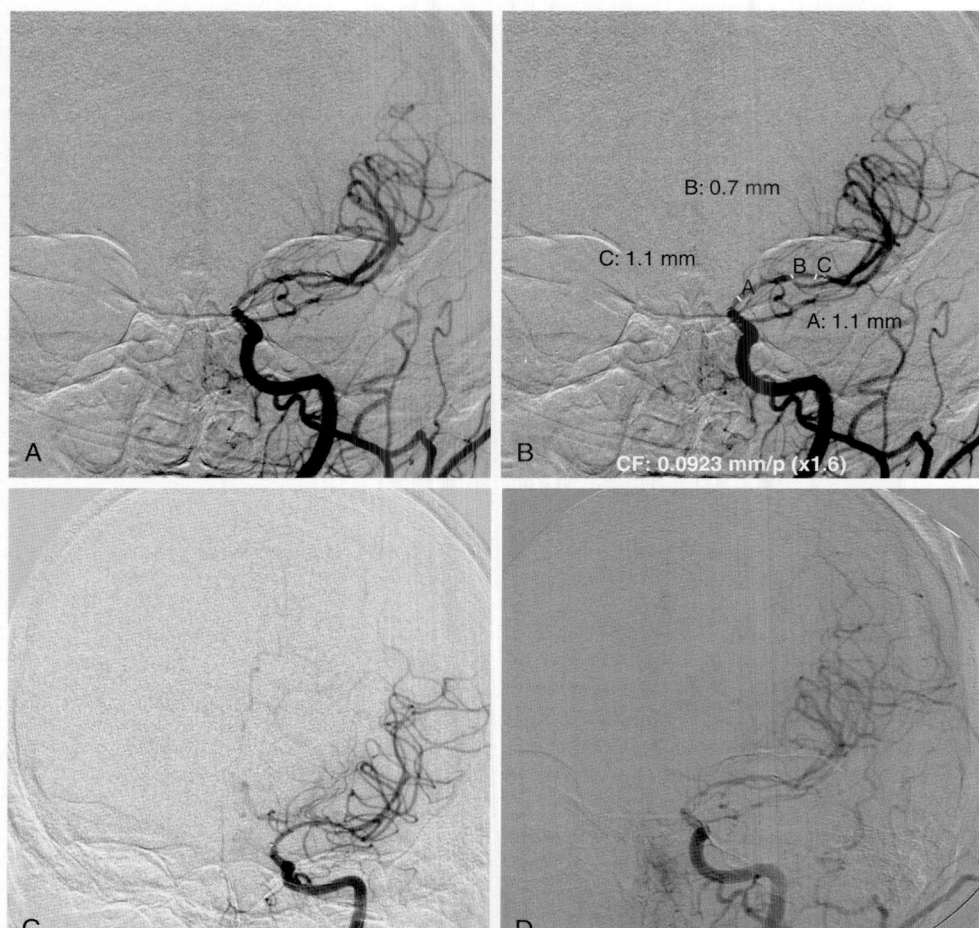

FIGURE 87-7 Same patient as prior figures. The patient developed severe in-stent restenosis 3 months later (A, B) that was relieved by balloon angioplasty (C). D, Follow-up angiogram 2 months after this angioplasty shows minimal narrowing (28%), good distal perfusion, and no in-stent restenosis.

KEY REFERENCES

Albuquerque FC, Levy EI, Turk AS, et al. Angiographic patterns of Wingspan in-stent restenosis. *Neurosurgery.* 2008;63:23-28.

Bose A, Hartmann M, Henkes H, et al. A novel, self-expanding, nitinol stent in medically refractory intracranial atherosclerotic stenoses: the Wingspan study. *Stroke.* 2007;38:1531-1537.

Chimowitz MI, Lynn MJ, Howlett-Smith H, et al. Comparison of warfarin and aspirin for symptomatic intracranial arterial stenosis. *N Engl J Med.* 2005;352:1305-1316.

Derdeyn CP, Chimowitz MI. Angioplasty and stenting for atherosclerotic intracranial stenosis: rationale for a randomized clinical trial. *Neuroimaging Clin N Am.* 2007;17:355-363:viii-ix.

EC/IC Bypass Study Group. Failure of extracranial–intracranial arterial bypass to reduce the risk of ischemic stroke. Results of an international randomized trial. *N Engl J Med.* 1985;313:1191-1200.

Fiorella D, Chow MM, Anderson M, et al. A 7-year experience with balloon-mounted coronary stents for the treatment of symptomatic vertebrobasilar intracranial atheromatous disease. *Neurosurgery.* 2007;61:236-243.

Fiorella DJ, Levy EI, Turk AS, et al. Target lesion revascularization after wingspan: assessment of safety and durability. *Stroke.* 2009;40:106-110.

Guzman R, Lee M, Achrol A, et al. Clinical outcome after 450 revascularization procedures for moyamoya disease. *J Neurosurg.* 2009;111:927-935.

Higashida RT, Meyers PM, Connors 3rd JJ, et al. Intracranial angioplasty & stenting for cerebral atherosclerosis: a position statement of the American Society of Interventional and Therapeutic Neuroradiology, Society of Interventional Radiology, and the American Society of Neuroradiology. *AJNR Am J Neuroradiol.* 2005;26:2323-2327.

Kasner SE, Chimowitz MI, Lynn MJ, et al. Predictors of ischemic stroke in the territory of a symptomatic intracranial arterial stenosis. *Circulation.* 2006;113:555-563.

Levy EI, Hanel RA, Bendok BR, et al. Staged stent-assisted angioplasty for symptomatic intracranial vertebrobasilar artery stenosis. *J Neurosurg.* 2002;97:1294-1301.

Levy EI, Hanel RA, Boulos AS, et al. Comparison of periprocedure complications resulting from direct stent placement compared with those due to conventional and staged stent placement in the basilar artery. *J Neurosurg.* 2003;99:653-660.

Levy EI, Turk AS, Albuquerque FC, et al. Wingspan in-stent restenosis and thrombosis: incidence, clinical presentation, and management. *Neurosurgery.* 2007;61:644-651.

Marks MP, Wojak JC, Al-Ali F, et al. Angioplasty for symptomatic intracranial stenosis: clinical outcome. *Stroke.* 2006;37:1016-1020.

Mori T, Fukuoka M, Kazita K, et al. Follow-up study after intracranial percutaneous transluminal cerebral balloon angioplasty. *AJNR Am J Neuroradiol.* 1998;19:1525.

Mori T, Mori K, Fukuoka M, et al. Percutaneous transluminal cerebral angioplasty: serial angiographic follow-up after successful dilatation. *Neuroradiology.* 1997;39:111-116.

Natarajan SK, Ogilvy CS, Hopkins LN, Siddiqui AH, Levy EI. Initial Experience with an Everolimus-Eluting, Second-Generation Drug-Eluting Stent for Treatment of Intracranial Atherosclerosis. *J Neurointervent Surg.* 2010;2:104-109.

Scott RM, Smith ER. Moyamoya disease and moyamoya syndrome. *N Engl J Med.* 2009;360:1226-1237.

SSYLVIA Study Investigators. Stenting of Symptomatic Atherosclerotic Lesions in the Vertebral or Intracranial Arteries (SSYLVIA): study results. *Stroke.* 2004;35:1388-1392.

Turk AS, Levy EI, Albuquerque FC, et al. Influence of patient age and stenosis location on Wingspan in-stent restenosis. *AJNR Am J Neuroradiol.* 2008;29:23-27.

Zaidat OO, Klucznik R, Alexander MJ, et al. The NIH registry on use of the Wingspan stent for symptomatic 70-99% intracranial arterial stenosis. *Neurology.* 2008;70:1518-1524.

Numbered references appear on Expert Consult.

CHAPTER 88

Endovascular Treatment of Extracranial Occlusive Disease

HENRY MOYLE • AMAN PATEL

Stroke is currently the third leading cause of death in the United States.[1] Carotid occlusive disease is the underlying pathology for 25% of the estimated 750,000 annual strokes.[2-4] The prevalence of carotid stenosis is 0.5% after age 60 and increases to 10% in the population older than 80 years.[5-7] There is a direct correlation between the degree of carotid artery stenosis and the risk of ipsilateral stroke.[8] The majority of cases of carotid stenosis are asymptomatic; however, symptomatic stroke treatment and lost productivity due to stroke account for an estimated annual cost of $74 billion.[9] The clinical and fiscal significance of stroke-related disabling morbidity has led to medical and surgical treatments for carotid occlusive disease, the goals of which lie in lowering the risk of stroke.

In the past, medical treatment for carotid occlusive disease was based on strategies stemming from studies directed at the treatment of general cardiovascular disease. However, more recently, prospective, randomized, controlled studies have proved a combination of surgical carotid revascularization by means of carotid endarterectomy (CEA) and medical management is highly successful in reducing the incidence of stroke among patients with moderate to severe symptomatic carotid stenosis[10] and among those with severe asymptomatic carotid stenosis.[3] CEA has been the standard of care for surgical revascularization for carotid occlusive disease; however, since the 1990s, carotid artery stenting (CAS) has evolved as an alternative treatment to CEA when dealing with patients deemed to be too high a surgical risk. High-risk patients account for up to one third of the patients undergoing CEA.[11,12] CAS is an attractive alternative to CEA because it is less invasive, has less risk for cranial nerve damage, and has the ability to treat lesions that are anatomically out of reach or too difficult for CEA.[12]

Indications and Patient Selection

There is irrefutable evidence that for certain patient populations CEA offers an advantage over best medical treatment (BMT) alone. The North American Symptomatic Carotid Endarterectomy Trial (NASCET) generated prospective, randomized data demonstrating symptomatic patients with carotid stenosis greater than 70% and a perioperative stroke or death rate below 6% are best treated by CEA over BMT alone.[13,14] The Veterans Affairs Cooperative Studies Program (VACSP) also found a beneficial effect of CEA when compared to BMT.[15] The Asymptomatic Carotid Atherosclerosis Study (ACAS) proved asymptomatic patients

with carotid stenosis of greater than 60% could benefit from CEA with a reduction in 5-year ipsilateral stroke risk, provided that their perioperative stroke or death rate was less than 3% and their modifiable risk factors were aggressively treated.[16] Based on the preceding results, the Stroke Council of the American Heart Association has published guidelines and indications for CEA.[17] However, these key trials excluded patients deemed to be high risk for CEA. The initial indications for CAS were some of the key exclusion criteria from NASCET, VACSP, and ACAS, including restenosis after CEA, contralateral internal carotid artery (ICA) occlusion, previous neck irradiation, advanced age, renal failure, chronic obstructive pulmonary disease, and severe cardiopulmonary disease. The increasing use of CAS has led investigators to question whether either revascularization procedure is more beneficial over the other. Over the last 10 years, multiple studies have attempted to answer that question; however, variability in study design, technology used, and patient selection have made a comparison between CAS and CEA difficult.[12,18-22] It is beyond the scope of this chapter to detail individual study design flaws, results, and criticisms; however, several study trials have helped influence patient selection for CAS in my practice. The trial that led to U.S. Food and Drug Administration approval for CAS was the Stenting and Angioplasty with Protection in Patients at High Risk for Endarterectomy (SAPPHIRE). The SAPPHIRE study led to a general sense that CAS was at least equivalent to CEA in high-risk patients. SAPPHIRE 30-day myocardial infarction (MI), stroke, and death rates were 4.8% in the CAS arm versus 9.8% in the CEA arm ($P = 0.09$).[12] One-year MI, ipsilateral stroke, and death rates were 12.2% in CAS versus 20.1% in CEA ($P = 0.048$).[12] The 3-year incidence of stroke was 7% for both CAS and CEA. The Carotid Revascularization Endarterectomy versus Stenting Trial (CREST) randomized 1326 symptomatic and 1196 asymptomatic patients to CAS or CEA with a median follow-up period of 2.5 years. This study recently concluded that among patients with symptomatic or asymptomatic carotid stenosis, the risk of the composite primary outcome of stroke, MI, or death did not differ significantly in the groups treated by CAS from those treated by CEA.[18] This study did find a higher risk of periprocedural stroke with stenting (4.1% vs. 2.3%, $P = 0.01$) and periprocedural MI with endarterectomy (1.1% vs. 2.3%, $P = 0.03$). Further, quality-of-life analyses among survivors at 1 year indicated that stroke had a greater adverse effect than did MI on a range of health-status domains. It is the current practice of my colleagues and I to offer CAS to asymptomatic or symptomatic patients who would benefit from CEA but are deemed to be too high a surgical risk for CEA.

Preoperative Preparation

All patients in our surgical practice undergoing CAS are reported in ongoing clinical registries. Pretreatment patient evaluation consists of a noninvasive study suggesting carotid stenosis and a neurologic assessment performed by a neurologist or neurosurgeon. On the day of the procedure, the patient's National Institutes of Health Stroke Scale is assessed and recorded. Preoperative laboratory results include hematocrit, hemoglobin, platelet count, white blood cell count, serum creatinine, prothrombin time, and activated partial prothrombin time obtained within a week of intervention. My colleagues and I also routinely obtain a baseline 12-lead electrocardiogram. Further cardiac or pulmonary evaluation is performed case by case as deemed medically necessary. MI is always a primary or secondary endpoint for clinical trials; thus, postprocedure creatine kinase, creatine kinase-MB, and troponin-I levels are routinely collected the morning after the procedure. All patients have a baseline brain computed tomography or magnetic resonance imaging to document preexisting infarctions.

In our practice, all patients considered for CAS are started on aspirin at a dosage of 325 mg daily at least 5 days prior to the procedure. My colleagues and I also start clopidogrel at least 24 hours prior to the procedure but preferably 3 to 5 days prior to intervention. Clopidogrel is loaded as a 300-mg dose the day before or 75 mg daily 5 days prior to intervention. Some evidence suggests the combination of aspirin and clopidogrel decreases restenosis by inhibiting myointimal proliferation.[23-25] In emergent cases in which patients are not pretreated, patients are loaded the day of surgery with aspirin at 325 mg and clopidogrel at 300 mg. After the angiogram is completed and the determination to proceed with CAS is made, 4000 U of heparin is administered intravenously and redosed at 1000 U every hour until completion of the stenting procedure. Although not a standard of care, many surgeons check activated coagulation times with the practice of anticoagulating to achieve the goal of doubling these times.

Anesthesia and Intraoperative Monitoring

CAS can be performed under monitored anesthesia care (MAC) or conscious sedation in the majority of cases, with only the rare need to convert to general endotracheal anesthesia. In my practice, my colleagues and I have not needed to convert to general anesthesia in any case. MAC allows us to monitor the patient's neurologic status throughout the case; thus, we have not found the need to use other physiologic monitoring, such as electroencephalogram or intraoperative transcranial Doppler. MAC is also preferable because many candidates we evaluate for CAS are high-risk surgical patients due to an underlying cardiopulmonary disease rather than an anatomic consideration. The decision on arterial line blood pressure monitoring is based on the patient's cardiopulmonary status, but all arterial lines are removed immediately after the procedure.

Procedure

Arterial access is gained through the femoral artery using the Seldinger technique to place a 6-French (Fr) sheath over a guidewire. Next, a 5-Fr diagnostic catheter is used to catheterize the common carotid artery (CCA). If needed, catheterization of the other vessels should be performed prior to the catheterization of the carotid artery needing treatment. Cervical carotid arteriography is performed to assess the degree of carotid stenosis. The intracranial circulation is also assessed at this point to characterize collateral flow, estimate delayed cranial perfusion secondary to stenosis, and identify any tandem lesions. Once measurements are performed and NASCET criteria are met for carotid stenting, a 0.035-inch exchange-length wire is passed under fluoroscopic road map guidance into the internal maxillary artery via the 5-Fr diagnostic catheter. The diagnostic catheter and femoral sheath are then removed over the exchange-length wire, and a 6-Fr, 90-cm sheath is passed under fluoroscopic guidance to a position 1 cm proximal to the cervical carotid bifurcation. If tortuous vessel anatomy does not allow the stiffer sheath to make the turn from the aortic arch into the right brachiocephalic or left CCA, a triaxial technique is used to advance the much stiffer sheath through this turn. This technique uses the 5-Fr diagnostic catheter over the exchange-length wire inside the 6-Fr sheath to give more support to the sheath through the turn. It is important on anteroposterior projections during positioning of the 90-cm sheath to visualize the projection over the chest. This ensures the sheath is taking a normal path through the turn from the aortic arch and not buckling.

The 0.035-inch exchange-length wire (and 5-Fr diagnostic catheter, if used) is removed, and more accurate measurements using a magnified cervical carotid arteriogram are performed using the 8-Fr outer diameter of the sheath as the measurement standard. The stenosis is determined according to NASCET criteria (Fig. 88-1A). The diameter of a straight portion of the ICA distal to the stenosis is determined to select the appropriate size of the distal protection device (DPD) and the appropriate diameter of the angioplasty balloon. The diameter of the CCA and the length of the stenosis are also determined to ensure selection of the appropriate length and diameter of the carotid stent. The carotid stent is sized so that it is 1 mm greater in diameter than the CCA.

Next, the DPD is mounted on a 0.014-inch wire and advanced past the stenosis into the distal ICA under fluoroscopic guidance. The filter basket is deployed, with the surgeon taking care to position the filter distal enough to the stenosis to allow for positioning of the stent (Fig. 88-1B). My colleagues and I have found a very gentle curve on the guidewire tip helps the surgeon manipulate the wire past the stenosis. At this stage, we prefer to position and deploy the self-expanding carotid stent (Fig. 88-1C and D) in cases where the degree of stenosis will allow this, but we predilate with angioplasty if the degree of stenosis is severe enough to make stent passage difficult. If the lesion cannot be crossed with the DPD, the options are to perform the procedure without distal protection or the use of a proximal protection device that relies on flow reversal.[26] Once the

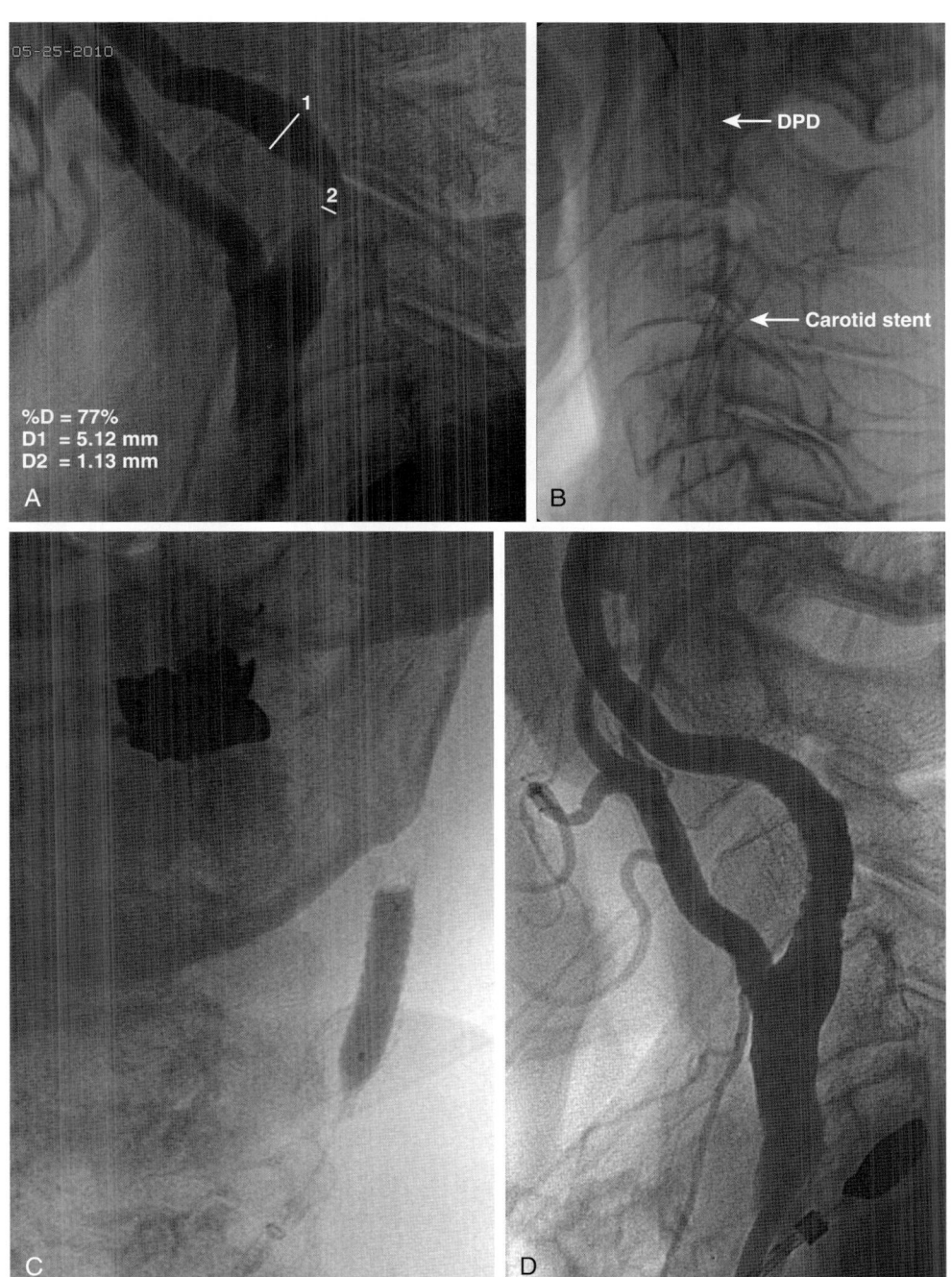

FIGURE 88-1 A, Lateral arteriogram showing a calculation of extracranial ICA stenosis. This is expressed as the ratio of residual ICA lumen (labeled 2) divided by the estimated normal extracranial ICA diameter (labeled 1). B, Lateral fluoroscopic image demonstrating correct positioning of the DPD distal to the stenosis in the extracranial ICA. C, Anteroposterior fluoroscopic image demonstrating inflation of the angioplasty balloon within the stented extracranial ICA. D, Lateral unsubtracted arteriogram of the extracranial carotid artery following stent deployment and angioplasty of the ICA.

stent is deployed and stent position is confirmed, the stent delivery system is removed over the 0.014-inch wire. Angioplasty is then performed under fluoroscopy (Fig. 88-1C). It is important to warn the anesthesia team prior to angioplasty, because this step can induce profound bradycardia, requiring treatment with atropine. This is particularly true when angioplasty involves the carotid bulb.

The final step is removal of the DPD with a DPD recapture catheter. Occasionally, if the stent extends around a turn in the carotid, it can be difficult to pass the retrieval catheter. In this case, removal is aided by straightening the stented section of the ICA by gentle external manipulation of the carotid artery or by the use of a second 0.014-inch wire as

a "buddy wire." The basket should be inspected for any debris. Prior to removal of the sheath, a poststent arteriogram is performed (Fig. 88-2). My colleagues and I routinely perform a poststent cerebral arteriogram and compare it to our initial prestent arteriogram to assess for any thromboembolic events during the stenting or angioplasty.

Postoperative Care

Following CAS, almost all postoperative patients are sent to monitored floor beds for overnight observation and discharged home the following day. If there was significant intraprocedural hemodynamic change or there continues

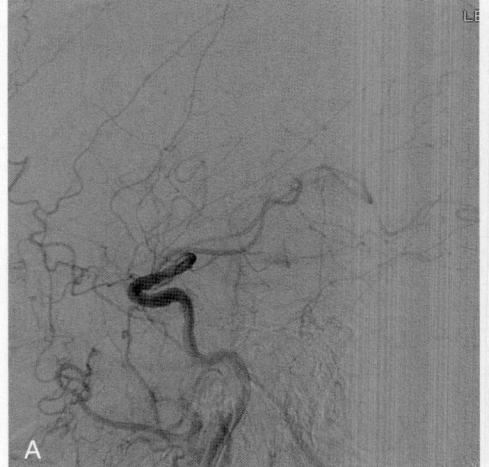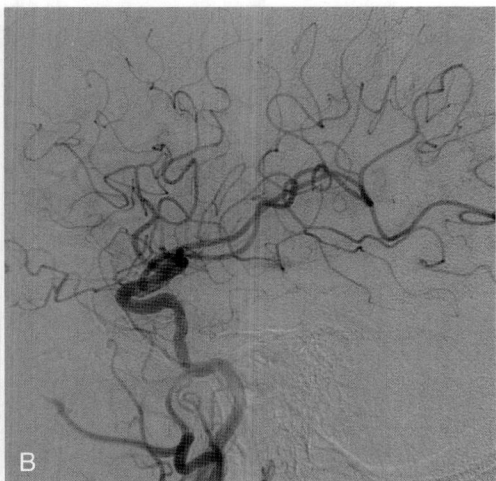

FIGURE 88-2 A, Lateral cerebral ICA arteriogram demonstrating poor intracranial flow in a symptomatic patient with severe extracranial ICA stenosis prior to CAS. B, Lateral cerebral ICA arteriogram demonstrating improved intracranial flow in the same patient following CAS and angioplasty.

to be profound hemodynamic aberrations postoperatively, my colleagues and I monitor the patient in an intensive care unit until hemodynamic instability has resolved.

The clopidogrel is discontinued 6 weeks after intervention, and patients are continued on an aspirin dosage of 81 to 325 mg daily indefinitely.

Patients undergoing CAS have carotid Doppler monitoring performed shortly after stenting to obtain a baseline and then are reassessed at 6-month intervals thereafter. If further follow-up noninvasive imaging is needed, my colleagues and I prefer computed tomography angiography because the stent artifact on magnetic resonance angiography makes the latter futile for assessing restenosis.

Complications

Following successful deployment of the carotid stent and removal of the DPD, a repeat cerebral arteriogram is performed and compared with the prestent cerebral arteriogram to assess for any large vessel occlusions. If a large vessel occlusion is identified, treatment options include intra-arterial tissue plasminogen activator or intra-arterial abciximab. Another option is mechanical thromboembolectomy using the Penumbra System (Penumbra, Alameda, CA).[27] In rare cases where thrombosis is seen in the stent, my colleagues and I have used intravenous abciximab, because the thrombus is felt to be an acute platelet aggregation (Fig. 88-3).

Another potential complication that can be identified on the poststent arteriogram is dissection of the artery at the ends of the stent. If a dissection is identified, it needs to be treated with a second stent across the dissection.

Outcome Data

The endovascular technique for CAS presented here has produced acceptable results in asymptomatic and symptomatic high-risk patients with carotid stenosis.[28] In a review of treatment outcomes found by my colleagues and I for 101 consecutive patients (109 stents), in which DPDs were used in 72% of the cases treated, the overall in-hospital adverse event rate was 8.3%. Periprocedural events included, 2 patients (1.8%) experienced a hemispheric transient ischemic attack, 2 patients (1.8%) had transiently symptomatic

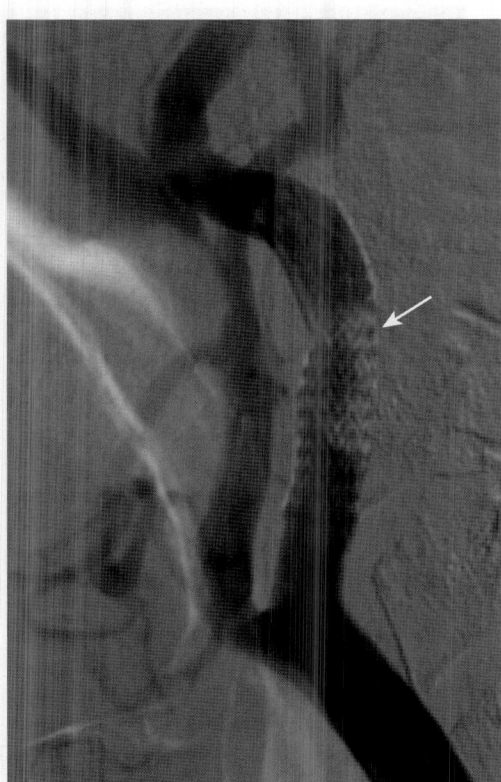

FIGURE 88-3 Lateral extracranial carotid arteriogram demonstrating acute thrombus *(arrow)* in a freshly deployed carotid stent.

acute reperfusion syndrome, and 1 patient (0.9%) died of an MI. The 30-day MI, stroke, and death outcome included 3 patients (2.7%) with minor strokes, defined as a modified Rankin score of less than 3, at 1-year follow-up and 1 patient (0.9%) with a major stroke, defined as a modified Rankin score of 3 or more, at 1-year follow-up.

Conclusions

We presented the technique and outcomes at our clinic for CAS treatment of high-risk patients with extracranial carotid disease. Despite the debate generated by several large trials attempting to compare CAS and CEA,[12,18-22] my colleagues and I feel that—with proper patient selection, evolving endovascular technology, and attention to interventional technique—CAS is a viable option for high-risk surgical patients. Improved periprocedural outcomes in both our data and the most recent CREST add credence to CAS for extracranial carotid disease in the high-surgical-risk population.

KEY REFERENCES

Bledsoe SL, et al. Effect of clopidogrel on platelet aggregation and intimal hyperplasia following carotid endarterectomy in the rat. *Vascular.* 2005;13(1):43-49.

Biller J, et al. Guidelines for carotid endarterectomy: a statement for healthcare professionals from a special writing group of the Stroke Council, American Heart Association. *Stroke.* 1998;29(2):554-562.

Brott TG, Hobson 2nd RW, Howard G, et al. Stenting versus endarterectomy for treatment of carotid-artery stenosis. *N Engl J Med.* 2010 Jul 1;363(1):1-23:Epub 2010 May 26.

Coppi G, et al. PRIAMUS—proximal flow blockage cerebral protection during carotid stenting: results from a multicenter Italian registry. *J Cardiovasc Surg (Torino).* 2005;46(3):219-227.

Eckstein HH, et al. Results of the Stent-Protected Angioplasty versus Carotid Endarterectomy (SPACE) study to treat symptomatic stenoses at 2 years: a multinational, prospective, randomised trial. *Lancet Neurol.* 2008;7(10):893-902.

Ederle J, et al. Endovascular treatment with angioplasty or stenting versus endarterectomy in patients with carotid artery stenosis in the Carotid and Vertebral Artery Transluminal Angioplasty Study (CAVATAS): long-term follow-up of a randomised trial. *Lancet Neurol.* 2009;8(10):898-907.

Goncu T, et al. Inhibitory effects of ticlopidine and clopidogrel on the intimal hyperplastic response after arterial injury. *Anadolu Kardiyol Derg* 2010;10(1):11–16.

Heart Disease and Stroke Statistics. *2010 Update At-A-Glance.* American Heart Association; 2010.

Herbert JM, et al. The antiaggregating and antithrombotic activity of clopidogrel is potentiated by aspirin in several experimental models in the rabbit. *Thromb Haemost.* 1998;80(3):512-518.

Mas JL, et al. Endarterectomy versus stenting in patients with symptomatic severe carotid stenosis. *N Engl J Med.* 2006;355(16):1660-1671.

Mayberg MR, et al. Carotid endarterectomy and prevention of cerebral ischemia in symptomatic carotid stenosis. Veterans Affairs Cooperative Studies Program 309 Trialist Group. *JAMA.* 1991;266(23):3289-3294.

Meyer SA, Gandhi CD, Johnson DM, Winn HR, Patel AB. Outcomes of carotid artery stenting in high-risk patients with carotid artery stenosis: A single neurovascular center retrospective review of 101 consecutive patients. *Neurosurgery.* 2010;66(3):448-453; discussion 453–454.

Moore WS, et al. Carotid endarterectomy: practice guidelines. Report of the Ad Hoc Committee to the Joint Council of the Society for Vascular Surgery and the North American Chapter of the International Society for Cardiovascular Surgery. *J Vasc Surg.* 1992;15(3):469-479.

North American Symptomatic Carotid Endarterectomy Trial. Methods, patient characteristics, and progress. *Stroke.* 1991;22(6):711-720.

North American Symptomatic Carotid Endarterectomy Trial Collaborators. Beneficial effect of carotid endarterectomy in symptomatic patients with high-grade carotid stenosis. *N Engl J Med.* 1991;325(7):445-453.

O'Leary DH, et al. Distribution and correlates of sonographically detected carotid artery disease in the Cardiovascular Health Study. The CHS Collaborative Research Group. *Stroke.* 1992;23(12):1752-1760.

Prati P, et al. Prevalence and determinants of carotid atherosclerosis in a general population. *Stroke.* 1992;23(12):1705-1711.

Ricci S, et al. (The prevalence of stenosis of the internal carotid in subjects over 49: a population study.) *Epidemiol Prev.* 1991;13(48-49): 173-176.

Ringleb PA, et al. 30 day results from the SPACE trial of stent-protected angioplasty versus carotid endarterectomy in symptomatic patients: a randomised non-inferiority trial. *Lancet.* 2006;368(9543):1239-1247.

Rosamond W, et al. Heart disease and stroke statistics—2007 update: a report from the American Heart Association Statistics Committee and Stroke Statistics Subcommittee. *Circulation.* 2007;115(5):e69-e171.

Rothwell PM, et al. Analysis of pooled data from the randomised controlled trials of endarterectomy for symptomatic carotid stenosis. *Lancet.* 2003;361(9352):107-116.

Wennberg DE, et al. Variation in carotid endarterectomy mortality in the Medicare population: trial hospitals, volume, and patient characteristics. *JAMA.* 1998;279(16):1278-1281.

Yadav JS, et al. Protected carotid-artery stenting versus endarterectomy in high-risk patients. *N Engl J Med.* 2004;351(15):1493-1501.

Young B, et al. An analysis of perioperative surgical mortality and morbidity in the Asymptomatic Carotid Atherosclerosis Study. *Stroke.* 1996;27(12):2216-2224.

Numbered references appear on Expert Consult.

CHAPTER 89

Embolization of Tumors: Brain, Head, Neck, and Spine

YIN C. HU • C. BENJAMIN NEWMAN • CAMERON G. MCDOUGALL • FELIPE C. ALBUQUERQUE

Hypervascular neoplasms of the central nervous system (CNS) can be formidable surgical challenges associated with significant morbidity and mortality. Vascular tumors can result in excessive intraoperative blood loss, prompting termination of the surgery before achieving its goals. Multiple reports have suggested preoperative embolization can reduce intraoperative blood loss, the need for transfusions, operative time, and the length of hospitalization.[1-4] Embolization also may reduce mass effect and alleviate pain.[5] Furthermore, preoperative embolization can facilitate a more complete surgical extirpation by clarifying the surgical field, enhancing tumor boundaries, and shrinking the tumor.

In most cases, preoperative embolization of arterial pedicles in various vascular CNS tumors is technically feasible, regardless of the tumor's origin and location (Table 89-1). The goals of tumor embolization are sacrificing the feeding vessels and obliterating the tumor capillary bed to the greatest extent possible. These goals must be balanced against the risks of embolization, which include occlusion of en passage vessels, pulmonary emboli, retained microcatheters, and compression of eloquent neural tissues by expanding intratumoral edema or hemorrhage.

Tumors of the Head

MENINGIOMAS

Meningiomas originate from arachnoid cap cells and can be hypervascular. They are slightly more common in females than in males and account for 13% to 18% of all intracranial tumors.[6] Typically, they are benign, with the potential for a surgical cure with complete resection. Recurrence rates are inversely proportional to the extent of surgical resection. Angiography and preoperative embolization of intracranial meningiomas are common practices used to improve the chances obtaining complete resection and a cure. The resection of many large meningiomas has been aborted due to heavy intraoperative blood loss, a complication that can be mitigated with judicious use of preoperative embolization. Angiography can also assist surgical planning by delineating the vascular supply to the tumor, the encasement and patency of vascular structures (arteries or dural venous sinuses), the degree of displacement of neuronal elements, and the site of dural attachment.

The blood supply to meningiomas is typically twofold: large arterial pedicles and pial and cortical arteries. Classically, large arteries supply the site of dural attachment and the center of the tumor, creating a "sunburst" appearance on angiography. The apex of the sunburst is usually the site of dural attachment. The pial and cortical vessels usually supply the tumor capsule, with their vascular contribution increasing as the tumor enlarges. Large arterial pedicles typically arise from branches of the external carotid artery (ECA), but they may also arise from the internal carotid artery (ICA). Dural pedicles arising from the ECA include the middle meningeal artery (MMA), accessory meningeal artery, neuromeningeal artery (arising from the ascending pharyngeal artery), and stylomastoid artery (arising from the occipital artery). The ICA occasionally supplies meningiomas via ethmoidal, cavernous, clival, or tentorial branches.

The location of the meningioma suggests which vessels warrant scrutiny during angiography. Anterior fossa meningiomas can be supplied by both the ICA and the ECA. Diaphragmatic or tuberculum sellae meningiomas frequently derive the majority of their blood supply from the ICA. High-convexity and parasagittal tumors tend to feed from the MMA, superficial temporal artery (STA), and artery of the falx cerebri and warrant angiography of the bilateral anterior circulation. Tumors of the anterior falx or frontal convexity frequently receive their blood supply from the meningeal branches of the ethmoidal artery and anterior falcine branches or, occasionally, from the anterior cerebral artery or a tentorial branch of the ophthalmic artery. Bilaterally, the anterior or posterior ethmoidal arteries often supply olfactory groove lesions, and evaluation of the ophthalmic and distal internal maxillary arteries must be meticulous.

Branches of the ECA, specifically the artery of the foramen rotundum, vidian arteries, or accessory meningeal artery, often supply middle fossa meningiomas. The vascular supply of meningiomas involving the sphenoid wing often derives from the recurrent meningeal branch of the ophthalmic artery or from branches of the MMA. Parasellar meningiomas tend to be fed by branches of the petrous, cavernous, or supraclinoid branches of the ICA; the artery of the foramen rotundum; the artery of the foramen ovale; or the neuromeningeal branch of the ascending pharyngeal artery.

The vascular supply of posterior fossa meningiomas is usually from the posterior meningeal artery, MMA, or

Table 89-1 Barrow Neurologic Institute Series of 169 Embolized CNS Tumors (1995-2009)

Tumors	No.
Meningiomas	
Olfactory groove	2
Convexity	10
Skull base	1
Parasagittal	3
Frontal	5
Sphenoid	3
Paraganglioma	
Glomus jugulare	17
Glomus tympanicum	1
Carotid body tumors	7
Hemangioblastoma	**12**
Juvenile Nasal Angiofibroma	**25**
Hemangiopericytoma	**3**
Others	
Plasmacytoma (spinal)	1
Aneurysmal bone cyst (spinal)	2
Thyroid carcinoma met (spinal)	1
Hemangioma (skull base)	1
Hemangioma (facial)	2
Hemangioma (spinal)	4
Renal carcinoma met (spinal)	12
Renal carcinoma met (cranial)	1
Giant cell tumor	3
Vestibular schwannoma	1
Jugular foramen nerve sheath tumor	1
Synovial cell sarcoma (spinal)	1
Osteogenic sarcoma (spinal)	1
Schwannoma (spinal)	2
Pharyngeal carcinoma	2
Chordoma (spinal)	1
Nasal polyp	1
Thyroid carcinoma	1
Melanoma (spinal)	1
Dural cavernous malformation	1
Total	**129**

accessory meningeal artery. Classically, tentorial meningiomas receive arterial feeders from the tentorial branch of the meningohypophyseal trunk (MHT), but they can be supplied by the infratentorial trunk, MMA, or accessory meningeal artery. Petroclival lesions are often supplied by the MMA (frequently from the petrosal, petrosquamosal, or occipital branches), transmastoid branches of the posterior auricular or occipital arteries, anterior inferior cerebellar artery (AICA, via the subarcuate branch), or neuromeningeal branch of the ascending pharyngeal artery.

The common vascular origins shared by posterior fossa meningiomas and cranial nerves require diligent attention when embolization of these lesions is considered. For example, cranial nerves III to VI share blood supply with tentorial meningiomas via the MMA, MHT, or accessory meningeal artery branches. Provocative testing before embolization can minimize the risks of inadvertently injuring the cranial nerves. Furthermore, extracranial-to-intracranial (EC-to-IC) arterial anastomoses, particularly between posterior

auricular or occipital arteries and the high cervical spino-laminar segment of the vertebral artery (VA), may be present.

Meningiomas commonly invade the dural venous sinuses. Patency of the adjacent sinus and surrounding cortical veins is an important consideration and should be evaluated to facilitate surgical planning. Complete occlusion of the venous sinus may allow aggressive surgical resection through excision of the involved portion of the sinus.

Outcomes

Many meningiomas do not require preoperative embolization because they often can be easily devascularized at surgery. At our institution, we recommend preoperative embolization of giant meningiomas, meningiomas involving the middle cranial fossa or skull base, falcine or parasagittal meningiomas, or meningiomas of the pineal region (Fig. 89-1). During surgery, the vascular supply to skull base meningiomas is frequently obscured until a substantial portion of the tumor has been excised, emphasizing the beneficial utility of embolization in these cases. In patients who are poor surgical candidates, embolization may be offered as a palliative measure to slow tumor growth.

Large, hypervascular skull base tumors whose vascular supply is not readily accessible via surgery should be evaluated for preoperative embolization. Embolization of deep-feeding arteries such as the inferolateral trunk and MHT can be technically challenging due to their small caliber and acute angle of origin. Technological advances in microcatheters and microguidewires have facilitated superselective catheterization of these blood vessels and expanded the range of treatable intracranial lesions through embolization. Even so, the potential for reflux of embolic material into the ICA remains a serious concern, and these lesions continue to present major challenges for even the most experienced neurointerventionalists. Abdel Kerim et al. described a technique of inflating a balloon in the MHT distal to the exit of a tumoral feeding artery to improve the penetration of Onyx (ev3 Endovascular, Irvine, CA) into the feeding vessel.[7] Several authors have successfully embolized middle fossa tumors with deep-feeding arteries with good surgical and radiographic outcomes.[8-10] The inferolateral trunk occasionally has collaterals with the ophthalmic artery via the deep recurrent ophthalmic artery. During embolization of the inferolateral trunk, extreme caution is warranted to minimize the risk of potential blindness.

Embolization of pial or ophthalmic branches is usually considered too perilous to undertake. However, Kaji et al. reported two cases in which distal cortical ICA branches were successfully embolized with Gelfoam (Pharmacia & Upjohn Company LLC, Peapack, NJ) before surgery.[11] Based on their experience, these authors recommend that embolization of pial or cortical vessels only be undertaken if the following conditions are met: (1) The tumor is supplied exclusively by the ICA. (2) The tumor is located in a noneloquent portion of the brain. (3) The patient has a negative sodium amytal test. (4) Superselective catheterization is performed with the catheter directly abutting the tumor capsule. (5) Particulate, rather than glue-based, embolisate is used.

Pineal region meningiomas are rare, accounting for 0.3% of intracranial meningiomas and 6% to 8% of pineal region tumors.[12] These uncommon lesions can draw their blood supply from a variety of sources, including meningeal

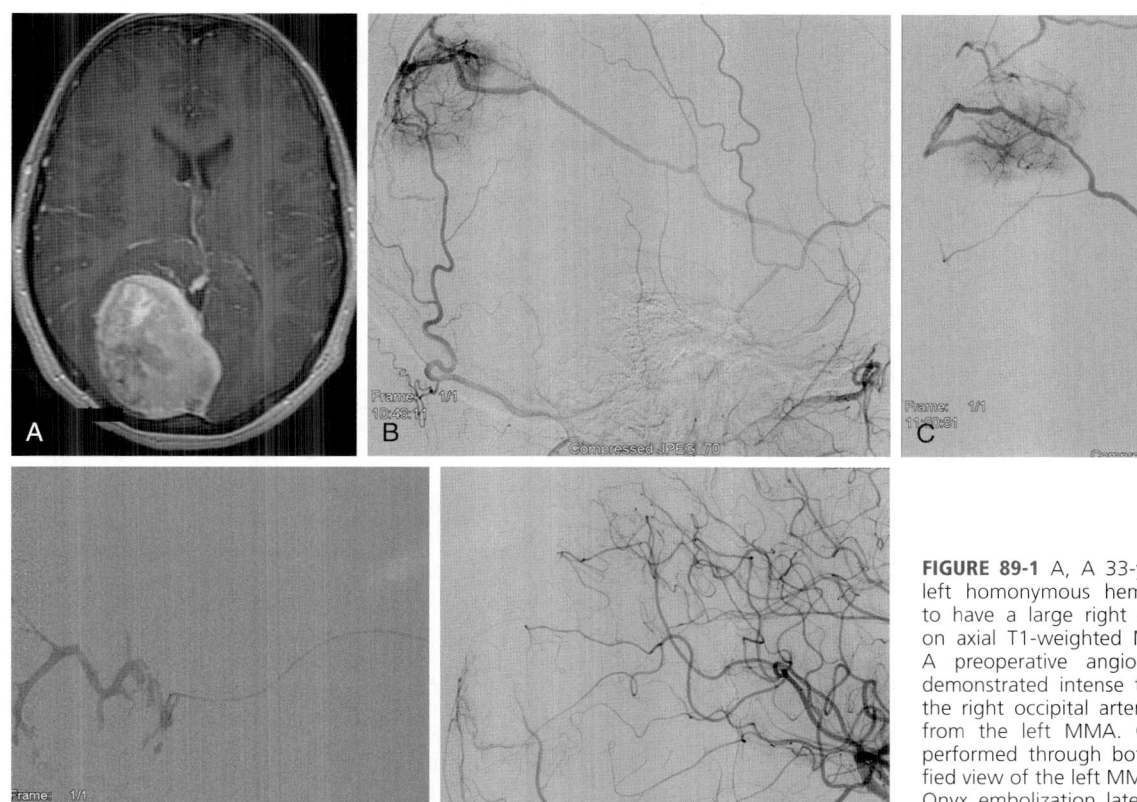

FIGURE 89-1 A, A 33-year-old woman with left homonymous hemianopsia was found to have a large right occipital meningioma on axial T1-weighted MRI with gadolinium. A preoperative angiographic lateral view demonstrated intense tumor blush (B) from the right occipital artery and MMA and (C) from the left MMA. Onyx injections were performed through both MMAs. D, Magnified view of the left MMA infusion. E, A post-Onyx embolization lateral view angiography showed significant tumor devascularization. (From Barrow Neurological Institute.)

branches of the ECA, the tentorial artery, medial or lateral posterior choroidal branches, branches of the superior vermian or superior cerebellar artery (SCA), meningeal branches of the posterior inferior cerebellar artery (PICA), or VAs. Sagoh et al. reported successful embolization of a pineal region meningioma with estrogen alcohol and polyvinyl alcohol (PVA) via the bilateral MMAs.[13]

Optic nerve meningiomas are seldom amenable to endovascular treatment because of the shared blood supply between the tumor and the optic nerve. Terada et al. concluded that if the microcatheter can be positioned distal to the origin of the central retinal artery, embolization is possible. However, the risk of causing blindness is high if reflux occurs into the central retinal artery.[14] In many cases, aggressive embolization of optic nerve meningiomas is neither beneficial nor advisable.

Indications for Embolization

In general, the primary rationale for the embolization of meningiomas is to reduce blood flow to the tumor, thereby facilitating a more complete surgical resection. Several studies have attempted to compare the risks associated with preoperative embolization for meningioma resection with its benefits. Bendszus et al. concluded that intraoperative blood loss was reduced only in patients who underwent complete tumor embolization as defined by absence of tumor blush on angiography.[15]

We performed a retrospective study to determine the risk-to-benefit profile of preoperative embolization of meningiomas. In the study, 33 patients underwent preoperative embolization followed by surgical resection. These patients were compared to an appropriately matched group of 193 nonembolized meningiomas that were extirpated. Preoperative embolization significantly reduced intraoperative blood loss and the need for transfusion. The operative time, total cost, length of stay, and rates of complication were similar in both groups. Other authors have found similar findings.[16,17]

Complications

The overall risk associated with endovascular embolization of meningiomas is low.[18,19] Major complications include stroke, blindness, intratumoral edema, or hemorrhage. Migration of embolic material via reflux or an unappreciated EC-to-IC anastomosis is the most common cause of major morbidity associated with embolization. The neurointerventionalist must have a working knowledge of the highly variable anatomy of EC-to-IC anastomoses and must constantly remain vigilant for the possibility of proximal reflux. Cataclysmic intratumoral swelling follows embolization, particularly if performed with particle embolisates, and can require emergent resection. Our practice is to resect meningiomas the day after embolization. Tumor swelling can sometimes be mitigated by the administration of corticosteroids.

Minor complications occur in as many as 30% of patients and include facial pain, trismus, or both.[19] These side effects can be managed symptomatically with corticosteroids or analgesics and are usually self-limited. Rare complications such as cranial nerve damage (thought to be related to occlusion of the vaso vasorum of the cranial nerves), subarachnoid hemorrhage, or retinal embolus have been reported.[20,21] Scalp necrosis is a rare but serious complication occasionally associated with embolization of ECA vessels. Several authors recommend preserving the STA as a donor vessel for a free tissue transfer in the event of massive scalp necrosis.[22,23]

Patients with skull base meningiomas often become symptomatic with some degree of cranial nerve dysfunction. Embolization can exacerbate this dysfunction, which should be emphasized during preoperative patient counseling. Embolization of the petrous branches of the MMA (which frequently supplies lesions of the posterior fossa or posterior parasellar region) can result in damage to the facial nerve. Embolization of branches of the ascending pharyngeal artery (which supplies clival or petroclival meningiomas) risks damage to the lower cranial nerves. The practice of superselection of tumor vessels as distally as possible, ideally with the microcatheter immediately adjacent to the tumor capsule, decreases the risk of inadvertent embolization of vessels supplying normal tissue. If there is any uncertainty, provocative testing may help define the shared vascular supply to the cranial nerves.

PARAGANGLIOMAS

Paragangliomas (PGGLs) are typically benign, slow-growing tumors arising from chemoreceptors located in blood vessel walls. Paragangliomas, which are highly vascular tumors, are often referred to a neurointerventionalist for presurgical embolization at the surgeon's request. In the head and neck, the most common location is at the carotid body, followed by the temporal bone (glomus jugulare or glomus tympanicum) and upper pharyngeal space (glomus vagale). Although histologically similar to pheochromocytomas, only 4% of paragangliomas of the head and neck are associated with catecholamine hypersecretion. Clinical evidence of paroxysmal catecholamine surges must be evaluated preoperatively with 24-hour urine fractionated catecholamine and metanephrine measurements.

Certain familial patterns or association with genetic syndromes (multiple endocrine neoplasia II, neurofibromatosis 1, von Hippel-Lindau (VHL) disease, familial paraganglioma, or Carney triad) have been associated with the diagnosis of paragangliomas. Multiple paragangliomas have been found in 22% and 87% of sporadic and familial paragangliomas, respectively.[24,25] Indium-111 octreotide, a radioisotope somatostatin analogue, has been used as a labeling tracer to selectively identify multiple or metastatic paragangliomas.[26]

Carotid body tumors arise from the carotid body, which is located at the posterior aspect of the carotid bifurcation. The chemoreceptive cells of the carotid body are located in the periadventitia of the carotid bifurcation and are primarily responsive to hypoxia. Conditions of chronic hypoxia, such as living in high altitudes (more than 1500 m above sea level), chronic obstructive pulmonary disease, and cyanotic heart disease are known risk factors for the development of carotid body tumors.

The most common presentation associated with carotid body tumors is a painless, slowly enlarging neck mass. These tumors can cause lower cranial nerve dysfunction (i.e., hoarseness, stridor, or hypoglossal palsy) due to local mass effect, but they rarely grow larger than 4 cm. The diagnosis of carotid body tumors can be confused with glomus

vagale. The latter lesions typically arise from paraganglionic tissue rests within the nodose ganglion and are found immediately rostral to the carotid bifurcation. The angiographic appearance of carotid body tumors and glomus vagale tumors differs in that carotid body tumors characteristically splay the ICA and ECA (Fig. 89-2), whereas vagal paragangliomas tend to displace the carotid arteries anteriorly and medially.[27]

Glomus jugulare tumors arise from glomus rests within the jugular foramen. Patients often complain of progressive unilateral hearing loss or pulse-synchronous tinnitus. Otoscopic examination of the external auditory canal may reveal a red or blue pulsatile mass. If seen on computed tomography (CT), bone-remodeling phenomena (e.g., demineralization, erosion, and destruction of bony structures) can be suggestive of the presence of a paraganglioma within the temporal bone. Gadolinium-enhanced magnetic resonance imaging (MRI) remains the predominant, noninvasive diagnostic imaging modality. On both T1- and T2-weighted sequences, these lesions typically appear as intensely gadolinium-enhancing masses with "salt-and-pepper" flow voids.

Angiography of these lesions must identify the intracranial and extracranial supply to the tumor, as well as the involvement of the dural venous sinus system. The patency of both transverse and sigmoid sinuses must be evaluated to determine whether sacrifice of the involved sinus is feasible without causing venous hypertension and infarction. The blood supply to a carotid body tumor is typically derived from proximal ECA branches or is derived directly from the bifurcation. The blood supply to tympanojugular tumors is almost uniformly derived from the ascending pharyngeal artery.[28] Glomus tympanicum tumors usually receive blood supply from the inferior tympanic branch of the ascending pharyngeal artery, while branches of the neuromeningeal trunk supply the hypoglossal canal and jugular fossa lesions. These lesions tend to be small and rarely require preoperative embolization. Glomus tumors within the temporal bone are often fed by branches of the petrous (via the vidian artery) or cavernous (clival branch of the MHT) segments of the ICA.

Glomus jugulare tumors, particularly those that extended into the intracranial compartment, require preoperative embolization.[29] These lesions frequently are multicompartmentalized, with a separate arterial supply to each compartment. To achieve complete embolization of a glomus jugulare tumor, the neurointerventionalist must selectively catheterize and embolize each arterial feeding vessel. In general, the ascending pharyngeal artery supplies the inferomedial compartment, while the stylomastoid branch of the occipital or posterior auricular artery contributes to the posterolateral compartment. The anterior compartment tends to be supplied by branches of the internal maxillary artery or the caroticotympanic artery. Branches of the MMA typically feed the superior compartment. If sacrifice of the jugular vein or sigmoid sinus will be necessary, the intracranial venous outflow system should be evaluated during angiography.

Superselective catheterization of the arterial pedicles is crucial for evaluating the angioarchitecture of the tumor and for identifying EC-to-IC anastomoses. Many such superselective microcatheterizations may be required to opacify or embolize the entire tumor. Tumors with substantial supply from the ICA or significant encasement of the ICA may

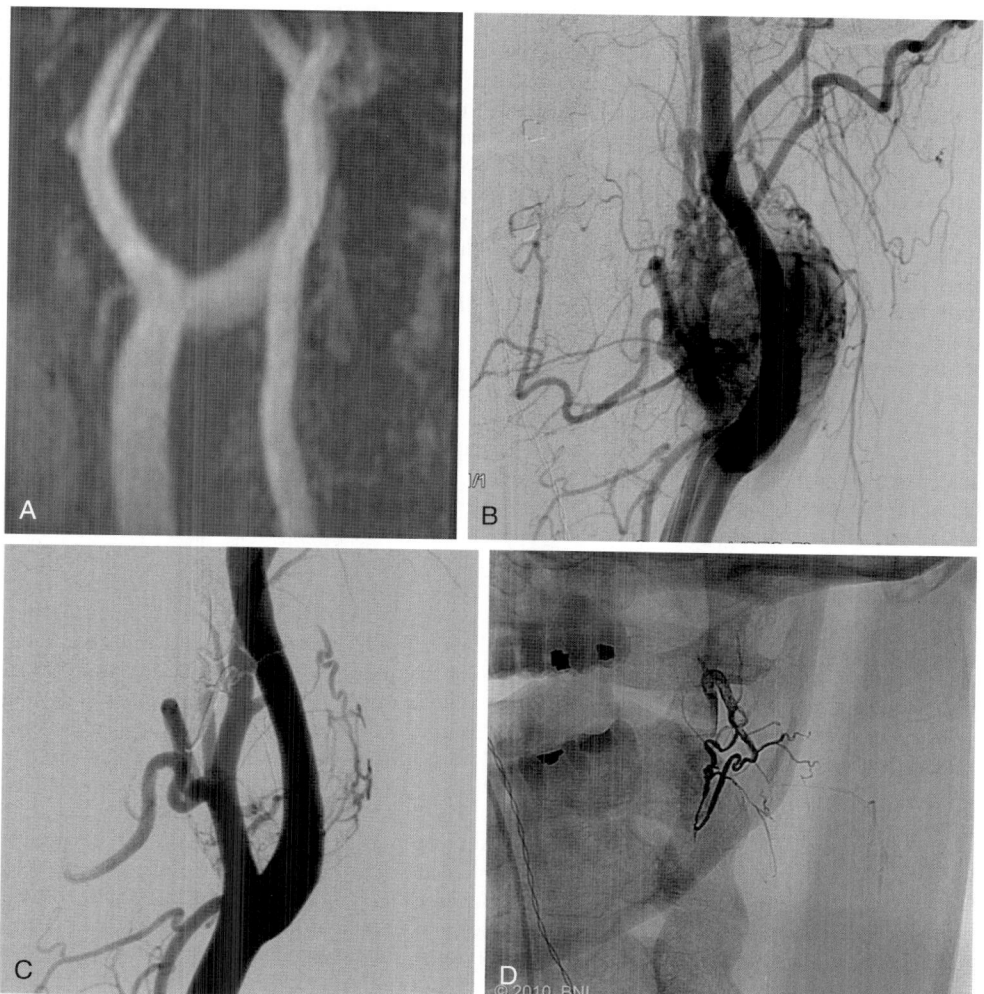

FIGURE 89-2 A 42-year-old woman presented with an enlarged mass on the left side of her neck. A, Magnetic resonance angiography of the neck showed splaying of the ECA and ICA, consistent with a carotid body tumor. A preoperative oblique angiographic view of the left common carotid artery injection demonstrated (B) an intense tumor blush at the carotid bifurcation and (C) a significant decrease in vascularity after Onyx embolization. D, A subtracted oblique angiographic view showed the amount of Onyx injected to complete the preoperative embolization. (From Barrow Neurological Institute.)

not be amenable to surgical resection and can be evaluated for possible vessel sacrifice with balloon test occlusion.

Embolization reduces operative time and intraoperative blood loss.[30,31] In the hands of an experienced neurointerventionalist, the risk of embolization for carotid body tumors is acceptably low, although the yield is probably too low to justify embolization of lesions smaller than 2 cm. Due to local soft-tissue inflammatory response, surgery within 48 hours of embolization is strongly recommended.

Complications

Most severe complications associated with embolization of head and neck paragangliomas are related to inadvertent migration of embolisate into the intracranial circulation, either through reflux or through the rich and highly variable EC-to-IC anastomotic network. Embolization of glomus jugulare tumors can cause lower cranial nerve palsies, presumably from embolization of the vaso vasorum supplying these nerves. Facial nerve palsies and even herniation syndromes have also been reported as rare complications of glomus jugulare tumor embolization.[32,33] Temporary facial nerve paresis is common after embolization because the facial nerve often receives its blood supply from the stylomastoid artery and the petrosal branches of the MMA or accessory meningeal artery. Recovery of facial nerve

paresis is more common when PVA is used as the embolic agent because the vessels tend to recanalize. Provocative testing should be undertaken before glue embolization because this embolisate is relatively permanent and may lead to irreversible deficits.

HEMANGIOBLASTOMAS

Hemangioblastomas are benign, hypervascular neoplasms primarily found in the cerebellum or spinal cord. They account for 1% to 2% of craniospinal tumors and occur most commonly within the cerebellar hemispheres, followed by the vermis, cerebellopontine angle, or brain stem.[6] Most hemangioblastomas are sporadic, but 20% are associated with VHL disease. The disease has an autosomal dominant inheritance pattern with incomplete penetrance. Multiple hemangioblastomas are common in patients with VHL disease.

Operative morbidity is high because of uncontrollable bleeding, so naturally these lesions have been targeted for preoperative embolization.[34] The blood supply to cerebellar hemangioblastomas is typically from PICA, but AICA or SCA branches can also contribute. Pontomedullary lesions often derive their blood supply from SCA branches, while cervicomedullary lesions are supplied by branches of the VA or anterior spinal artery. Superficial lesions can draw blood supply from dural branches of the VA (i.e., posterior meningeal artery). Due to the highly vascular nature of these lesions, the caliber of the feeding artery can exceed that of the basilar artery.

The risk associated with embolization of hemangioblastomas is high because the feeding arteries are often pial vessels. Suboptimal penetration of embolisate into the tumor nidus offers little in terms of reducing operative blood loss, particularly in posterior fossa lesions. The patient is thereby exposed to the risk of the embolization procedure without incurring any benefit.[35] Embolization of posterior fossa hemangioblastomas has been associated with complication rates as high as 50%, although some studies have shown preoperative embolization to be a helpful adjunct to resection.[36,37] Some authors postulate that postembolization hemorrhage is related to venous outflow obstruction.[38,39]

Between 1995 and 2009, we successfully embolized 13 posterior fossa hemangioblastomas. One patient suffered a nonfatal complication (stroke) as a result of embolization. Therefore, the morbidity rate was 7.7%. In 3 cases, embolization was aborted due to the lack of tumor vessels suitable for embolization. This underscores one of the tenets of safe embolization of posterior fossa hemangioblastomas: Judicious tumor selection is key to minimizing complications. Only a small percentage of hemangioblastomas resected at our institution are deemed suitable for preoperative embolization. Embolization is reserved for large lesions, lesions with arterial feeders that are difficult to access surgically, or lesions that cannot be resected due to intraoperative hemorrhage. By placing the microcatheter tip beyond normal vessels directly into the tumor vasculature, the risks associated with embolization can be mitigated. PVA and n-butyl cyanoacrylate (n-BCA) are the embolisates of choice for these lesions, although we have successfully used Onyx in two cases.

Clearly, the potential for postembolization hemorrhage or swelling exists and can be especially precipitous in the posterior fossa. However, we strongly believe that by meticulously adhering to the tenets of superselective catheterization and intracranial tumor embolization, hemangioblastomas of the posterior fossa can be safely embolized to aid surgical resection.

HEMANGIOPERICYTOMAS

Hemangiopericytomas are aggressive tumors arising from the contractile pericytes of Zimmerman, which are leiomyoblastic cells surrounding capillaries and postcapillary venules. These intracranial extra-axial neoplasms account for less than 1% of intracranial tumors. They are associated with high rates of recurrence and have the potential for metastasis.

Hemangiopericytomas are highly vascular lesions, and intraoperative hemorrhage can be significant. Hemorrhage is the most common cause for subtotal resection or operative morbidity. Embolization substantially reduces intraoperative bleeding and facilitates resection.[40-42] However, embolization can be technically difficult because these tumors tend to parasitize cortical vessels. Ethanol and direct surgical puncture have been successfully employed in the past, although we have had success with Onyx, n-BCA, and PVA. Postembolization swelling is common with these lesions; therefore, resection within 48 hours of embolization is recommended.

Juvenile Nasal Angiofibromas

Juvenile nasal angiofibromas (JNAs) are benign, extremely vascular, nonencapsulated neoplasms consisting of vascular and connective tissue. They usually arise from the superior posterior margin of the sphenopalatine foramen. JNAs are the most common benign tumor of the nasopharynx and account for 0.05% to 0.5% of all head and neck tumors.[43] These tumors almost exclusively affect adolescent boys; the mean age at diagnosis is 14 years. JNAs rarely metastasize but display locally malignant behavior and exhibit high rates of recurrence after subtotal resection.[44] Approximately 30% of JNAs manifest with intracranial extension.[45] The most common presenting symptoms are epistaxis and prolonged nasal obstruction.

The unique appearance of JNAs on CT and MRI eliminates the need for biopsy, which can result in uncontrollable bleeding. Angiography demonstrates multiple tortuous feeding vessels followed by a dense, homogeneous blush in the capillary phase (Fig. 89-3). Prominent draining veins are apparent immediately in the early venous phase. JNAs are typically supplied by branches of the internal maxillary artery, with contributions from the ascending pharyngeal artery in as many as 33% of cases.[46] Bilateral carotid angiography is mandatory in all cases, particularly if there is intracranial extension, because these tumors can recruit blood supply from the ophthalmic artery, contralateral internal maxillary artery, and branches of either ICA.

Surgical resection is regarded as the primary treatment modality.[47] JNAs are highly vascular, which can lead to significant intraoperative blood loss, increased morbidity, and incomplete resection. Preoperative embolization is an important adjunct to help reduce intraoperative blood loss and to facilitate surgical extirpation.[48-50] For embolization to be effective, the small distal vessels within the tumor must be obstructed. Failure of the embolisate to penetrate the tumor parenchyma results in inadequate devascularization and may lead to an unsatisfactory reduction in intraoperative blood loss.

Older case series recommend against embolization of JNAs, citing ineffective reduction of intraoperative blood loss or excessive risks of the procedure.[51,52] However, our experience has been positive. From 1995 to 2009, we successfully and safely embolized 30 JNAs without complications and with improvement in intraoperative blood loss based on the subjective opinion of the operators. We have successfully used PVA, n-BCA, and more recently, Onyx. Gay et al. reported an unusual case of postoperative palatal necrosis and oronasal fistula after a staged embolization followed by transpalatal resection of a JNA.[53] The authors believe that this complication was potentiated by the embolization but maintain that preoperative embolization is still warranted for these tumors.

After embolization of JNAs, the most common complications include fever and local pain. Fever is thought to arise from tissue ischemia and should not delay surgical resection. Bradycardia occasionally follows embolization of the internal maxillary artery or ascending pharyngeal artery. Intracranial embolization can arise as a result of unrecognized EC-to-IC collaterals or direct reflux of embolisate around the tip of the microcatheter.

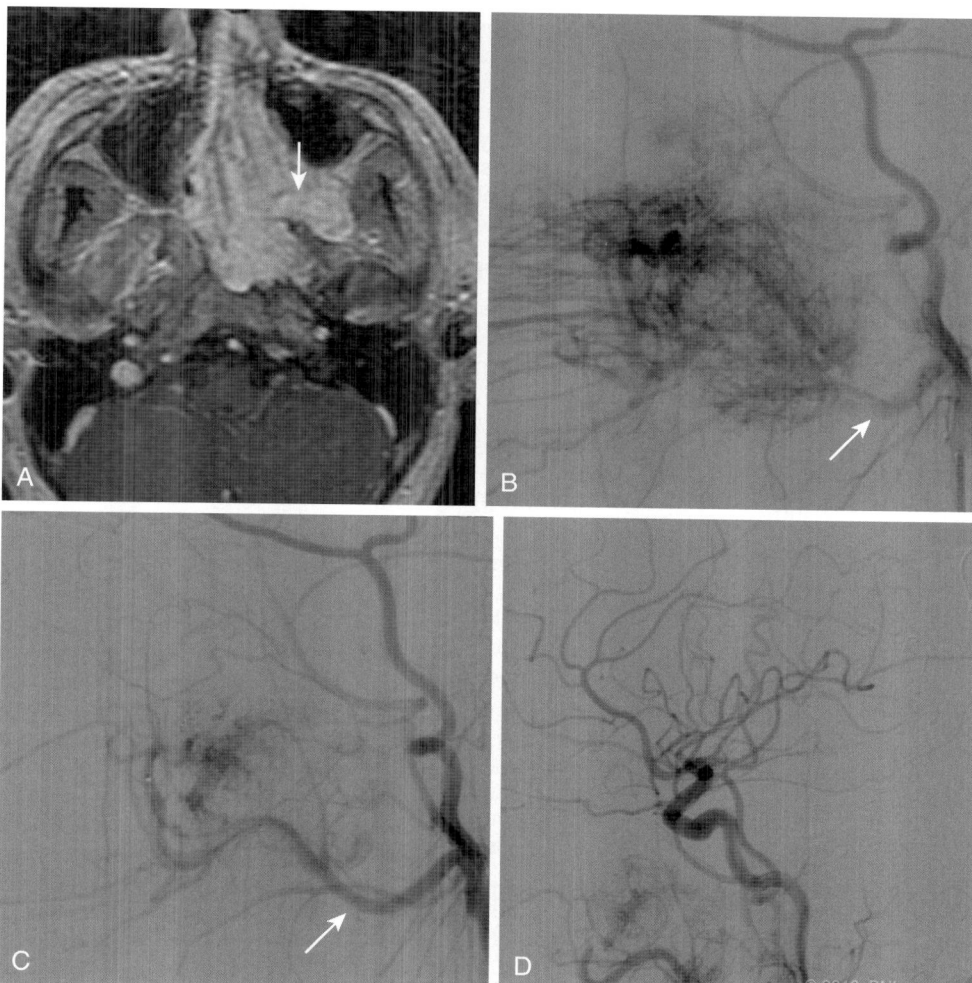

FIGURE 89-3 A 14-year-old boy presented with epistaxis. A, A T1-weighted MRI with gadolinium showed an enhanced tumor (JNA) in his nasal cavity. B, A lateral view, with a left ECA injection, showed an intense tumor blush with arterial feeders from the internal maxillary artery *(arrow)*. C, A lateral angiographic view, obtained after embolization with PVA particles, showed a significant decrease in the vascularity of the tumor. D, Additional embolization with *n*-BCA was performed in the distal internal maxillary artery. The lateral view on final angiography revealed minimal tumor opacification. (From Barrow Neurological Institute.)

MISCELLANEOUS LESIONS

Aneurysmal bone cysts are non-neoplastic expansile primary bone lesions that primarily affect individuals younger than 20 years. The pelvis and long bones are typically affected, but these lesions occasionally occur in the skull or spine. CT and MRI characteristically show multiple loculations within the cavity associated with perilesional sclerosis. Angiography shows prominent tumor blush on the outer aspect of the lesion, which is highly vascular and contrasts with the avascular core.

The treatment of choice is surgical excision. Preoperative embolization can be used for tumor devascularization or as the sole treatment modality in surgically inaccessible lesions.[54-56] Koci et al. described a patient treated with embolization as monotherapy for an aneurysmal bone cyst that regressed (characterized by involution of the soft-tissue component, sclerosis, and ossification) for 2 years.[57] However, a recurrence at 4 years led the authors to conclude that these lesions require continued surveillance. Successful preoperative embolization of large aneurysmal bone cysts of the skull base has also been reported.[58]

Embolization of metastatic disease to the skull has been reported in hepatocellular carcinoma and thyroid cancer (follicular and papillary histologic subtypes). These lesions tend to be supplied by branches of the ECA. Embolization can be used as a presurgical adjunct or as a palliative measure for pain control.[59] Lin et al. described the successful embolization of metastatic osteosarcoma to the orbit in a single patient.[60]

Bingaman et al. described presurgical embolization of an intracranial and extracranial mesenchymal chondrosarcoma of the right frontal region.[61] The lesion was supplied by branches of the ECA on both sides, and embolization was performed through the ipsilateral MMA. The authors emphasized the importance of gross total resection, as well as close surveillance of this potentially malignant tumor.

Avellino et al. described the embolization of a recurrent Masson's vegetant intravascular hemangioendothelioma involving the cerebellopontine angle and middle cranial fossa.[62] Despite attempted embolization followed by resection on two separate occasions, the lesion recurred. The tumor ultimately derived blood supply from the AICA, MHT, and bilateral occipital arteries. Embolization of the left occipital artery was initially successful, but angiography at the time of the recurrence demonstrated substantial contribution from the ECA and left MHT. The patient tolerated balloon test occlusion and ultimately underwent sacrifice of the left ICA.

Spinal Tumors

Spinal tumors are often managed surgically to preserve or improve neurologic function and to maintain spinal stability. The hypervascularity of certain tumors (i.e., renal cell carcinomas and hemangioblastomas) can make surgical resection extremely challenging and can even prompt early termination of the procedure when intraoperative bleeding is excessive.

Spinal tumors suspected to be hypervascular are potential candidates for presurgical tumor embolization, particularly when dorsal surgical approaches are used. Vascular spinal metastases often originate from renal cancer, thyroid cancer, sarcomas, or neuroendocrine tumors, while primary vascular tumors include giant cell tumors, hemangioblastomas, and paragangliomas.

Preoperative embolization serves two distinct therapeutic intentions. First, it may reduce excessive intraoperative blood loss, thereby improving surgical conditions and decreasing the surgical morbidity and mortality. Second, when surgery is considered unsafe or impossible, embolization can become the primary modality of treatment.

CT and MRI are the primary noninvasive diagnostic modalities used for evaluating for spinal tumors. MRI characteristics suggesting hypervascular spinal lesions include flow voids, hemorrhages, and intense contrast enhancement. It is also helpful if a systemic evaluation and a biopsy sample of the primary site or the spine can be obtained to confirm the histologic identity of the lesion. This information can help determine the need for preoperative embolization of a spinal tumor.

Presurgical embolization of vascular tumors has become common in many centers. Surgeons' experiences have been used to infer a definitive decrease in intraoperative blood loss associated with spinal tumors embolized before surgery. However, conflicting results regarding the benefits of preoperative embolization of vascular spinal tumors have also been reported. Multiple reports have suggested that preoperative embolization reduces intraoperative blood loss. Guzman et al. described their experience with preoperative embolization of vertebral metastases in 24 patients.[63] Two patients did not undergo embolization because the feeding pedicle branched from the artery of Adamkiewicz. The estimated operative blood loss was 5500 ml in those two patients compared to 1900 ml in the remaining patients whose tumors were successfully embolized.[63] Berkefeld et al. reported a median intraoperative blood loss of 4350 and 1800 ml in surgical cases of nonembolized and embolized spinal tumors using PVA particles, respectively.[64] In contrast, Jackson et al. found no significant reduction in intraoperative blood loss between embolized and nonembolized spinal tumors.[65] Empirically, however, they believed that embolization facilitated resection of renal cell carcinomas. King et al. also reported no significant differences in intraoperative blood loss between embolized and nonembolized spinal tumors.[66] However, they had to abort surgical resection due to excessive blood loss in three patients whose tumors were not embolized.

Certain biases, such as the lack of controls, small sample sizes, heterogenous spinal lesions, technical differences between procedures, and lack of randomization, have limited the conclusions that can be drawn about the utility of preoperative spinal tumor embolization. Given the near impossibility of conducting randomized trials from an ethical perspective, retrospective reviews may offer the only option for determining the outcome of preoperative embolization. Nevertheless, many centers practice preoperative embolization at the surgeon's request because experiences have led them to conclude that preoperative embolization of vascular spinal tumors is a necessity to minimize surgical complications.

PRIMARY SPINAL TUMORS

Preoperative embolization of intradural spinal tumors has rarely been reported. Paragangliomas and hemangioblastomas are the hypervascular intradural spinal tumors typically encountered by surgeons. Other primary tumors that have been treated with preoperative embolization include giant cell tumors, hemangiomas, and aneurysmal bone cysts.

Paragangliomas

As neuroendocrine tumors, paragangliomas most often arise in the intradural extramedullary compartment and in the lumbosacral segment when found in the spine. Patients usually develop symptoms consistent with cauda equina or spinal cord compression. Intracranial hypertension has been reported to be associated with paragangliomas.[67] On MRI, paragangliomas can be difficult to distinguish from other cauda equina tumors (i.e., ependymomas). Angiographically, paragangliomas are densely vascular with possible intratumoral arteriovenous shunting. Serpiginous vessels surrounding the tumor blush, which are often visible on angiograms, correspond to dilated veins.[68]

Hemangioblastomas

Hemangioblastomas compose 1% to 5% of all intramedullary spinal tumors. Most of these vascular lesions are sporadic; the remaining lesions are associated with VHL disease. Approximately 75% of these spinal lesions are intramedullary, and they are usually located in the posterior half of the spinal cord. Another 10% to 15% of hemangioblastomas have intradural intramedullary and intradural extramedullary components. Intradural extramedullary hemangioblastomas can also originate from nerve roots. They have a propensity to attach to the dorsal pia of the spinal cord. Intra- and extramedullary spinal hemangioblastomas are typically found in the cervical or thoracic regions, but a few cases have been reported in other locations of the spinal cord. Those found in the lower spinal cord can be extremely vascular because arterial feeders from the artery of Adamkiewicz are common.

The microsurgical resection of spinal hemangioblastomas can be challenging, especially large tumors extending beyond one spinal segment or in the lower spinal territory. The rate of surgical complications associated with hemangioblastomas in the CNS exceeds 15%.[69,70] Several investigators have described their successful experiences in embolizing spinal hemangioblastomas.[37,71] At our institution, we are rarely requested to perform preoperative embolization for spinal hemangioblastomas.

Giant Cell Tumors

Although usually considered benign tumors, 5% to 10% of giant cell tumors may undergo malignant degeneration and assume a more aggressive course.[72] These tumors have a predilection for the thoracolumbar and sacral regions. They can remain relatively asymptomatic until they grow to a significant size. Sacral giant cell tumors are difficult to manage, and their recurrence rate after initial therapy is higher than that of any other location. Treatment for these tumors includes surgical, radiation, and endovascular options.

Surgical management may be effective in treating some sacral giant cell tumors. Large space-occupying sacral giant cell tumors are seldom amenable to surgical resection without causing pelvic instability or neurologic dysfunctions. In a literature review of 159 patients with 166 lesions, Leggon et al. reported no recurrences after en bloc resection with a wide margin (0 of 8 patients).[73] The rate of local recurrence was 51% (25 of 49 lesions), 51% (18 of 31 lesions), and 49% (35 of 71 lesions) in patients treated with radiation, surgery with intralesional margins, and surgery with intralesional margins and radiation, respectively. The mortality rate attributable to the disease was 23%. When en bloc extirpation is infeasible, alternative forms of management should be considered with the understanding that the recurrence rate is relatively high.

By minimizing intraoperative blood loss, preoperative embolization can be a valuable adjuvant therapy for improving surgical safety, particularly for intralesional resections. In a number of small series, the results of embolization have been promising as the primary treatment modality. Lackman et al. treated four of five patients with sacral giant cell tumors exclusively with embolization and reported that symptoms resolved, tumor growth was arrested, and there were no recurrences.[74] Hosalkar et al. also reported their experiences in nine patients with sacral giant cell tumors treated with serial embolization as the primary modality.[5] No tumor progression was noted in seven of the nine patients with a mean follow-up of almost 9 years. All of Hosalkar et al.'s patients experienced significant pain relief.

Hemangiomas

Spinal hemangiomas are benign aggregates of hamartomatous proliferations of vascular tissue within endothelium-lined spaces that are found in about 11% of autopsy specimens.[75] Occasionally, hemangiomas can cause local pain or neurologic deficits related to nerve root compression. On CT, they have a polka-dot appearance with punctate sclerotic foci representing thickened vertical trabeculae. Bulging of the posterior cortex and paravertebral soft-tissue extension may be associated with aggressive hemangiomas.

Symptomatic spinal hemangiomas have been treated with a variety of modalities. For pain control, vertebroplasty, kyphoplasty, ethanol injection, radiotherapy, and transarterial embolization have been used with success.[76-80] For aggressive hemangiomas requiring surgical management, preoperative embolization can play a significant adjunctive role. Hurley et al. successfully used Onyx to embolize vertebral hemangiomas preoperatively in two cases, with a reported operative blood loss of 1500 and 100 ml.[81] Acosta et al. also found a significant reduction in blood loss after presurgical embolization of vertebral hemangiomas in their series.[76]

Aneurysmal Bone Cysts

Aneurysmal bone cysts are expansile lesions with blood-filled cavities separated by septa of trabeculae or fibrous tissue containing osteoblastic giant cells. The neoplastic

behavior of these lesions is debatable. Given the unpredictability of their progression, their natural history is difficult to predict. Some lesions resolve spontaneously, but most exhibit variable growth.

Preoperative embolization can play an important role before surgical resection or as a primary modality of treatment in selected nonsurgical cases.[82] Embolization of aneurysmal bone cysts causes involution of soft-tissue components, sclerosis, and ossification. However, these radiographic findings may not appear for months or years. A few investigators have reported diffuse involution and ossification after embolization of these lesions and claimed that surgical intervention is unnecessary.[57,83] However, continued surveillance is recommended because foci can reappear, and cystic changes have been observed as long as 2 years after embolization.[57]

METASTATIC SPINAL TUMORS

Metastatic vascular spinal tumors represent the largest group of spinal lesions that are often embolized before surgical resection. Hypervascular metastatic spinal tumors usually originate from renal cell carcinomas, sarcomas, thyroid cancer, and neuroendocrine tumors. Several retrospective studies reported a mean or median intraoperative blood loss that ranged between 1540 and 4300 ml after embolization of spinal tumors of various origins.[64,84,85]

Renal cell carcinomas represent the largest group of vertebral metastases that are treated with preoperative embolization (Fig. 89-4). Radical surgery is increasingly being used in the management of spinal metastatic renal cell carcinomas. Alternative methods of treatment, including chemotherapy and radiotherapy, offer limited benefit. The hypervascular nature of these tumors can result in life-threatening intraoperative blood loss.

Numerous investigators have suggested that preoperative embolization can facilitate radical extirpation of renal cell carcinoma in toto with a concomitant decrease in intraoperative blood loss.[3,64,84,86] Manke et al. reported a median intraoperative blood loss of 1500 ml in 19 embolized vertebral renal cell carcinomas and 5000 ml in 11 nonembolized renal cell carcinomas.[87] Even in patients with a partially embolized renal cell carcinoma, intraoperative blood loss was reduced compared to the control group. However, many other studies lacked control groups undergoing various degrees of embolization by different operators. Rehak et al. noted a greater-than-average amount of blood loss in their group undergoing embolization of renal cell carcinomas (4750 ml) compared to their nonembolized patients (1786 ml).[88] However, the groups differed in many respects, including the size of the tumor, the extent of metastases, and the complexity of the surgery. Tumors in the embolized group were twice as large as tumors in nonembolized group. An anterior approach was used twice as often in the embolized group as in the nonembolized group.

In selected cases, embolization offers palliative treatment of metastatic spinal lesions. Kuether et al. reported successful transarterial embolization of a T5 vertebral renal cell carcinoma metastasis in a patient with neurologic deficits.[89] They noted a dramatic reduction in spinal cord compression after embolization, and the patient improved neurologically. Four months later, her neurologic state deteriorated, and she was found to have a new sacral mass. The sacral

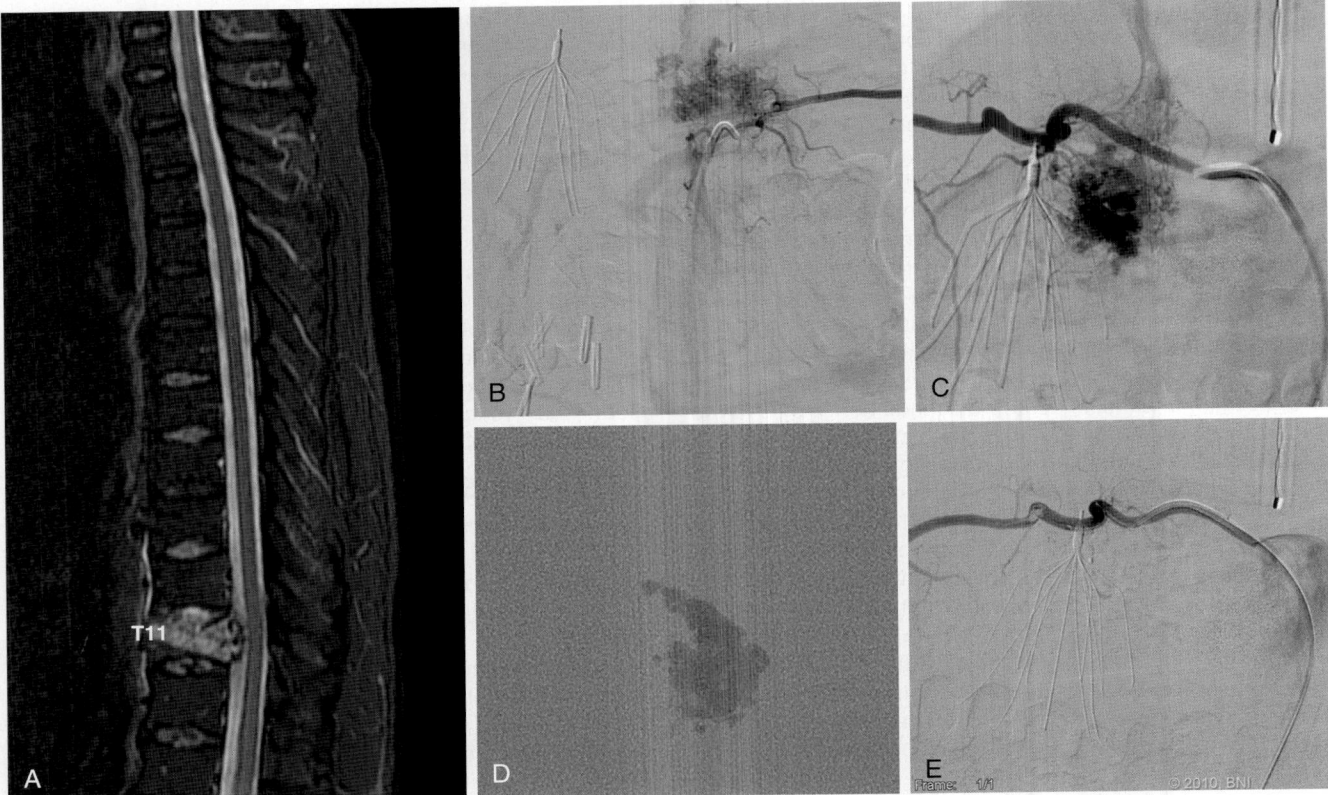

FIGURE 89-4 A 52-year-old man had a metastatic renal cell carcinoma at T11 that caused a burst fracture, spinal cord compression, and lower extremity weakness. A, Short τ-inversion recovery sagittal MRI showed the pathologic fracture. A preoperative anteroposterior (AP) angiogram of (B) the left T11 and (C) the right T10 segmental artery showed hypervascularity of the tumor. D, Blank road map showing a single Onyx injection from the left T11 segmental artery. E, Postembolization AP view of the right T10 after an Onyx injection showed satisfactory embolization. (From Barrow Neurological Institute.)

lesion was embolized, and the patient again improved after treatment. Smit et al. reported their experience with the embolization of four follicular thyroid carcinoma metastases to the spine in patients with neurologic deficits. After the procedure, the neurologic symptoms of all of the patients improved.[90] Other investigators have reported significant pain reduction in patients who underwent embolization of spinal metastases.[64,84]

Technical Nuances

The goal in tumor embolization is not only to sacrifice the feeding vessels but also to obliterate the tumor capillary bed to the greatest extent possible. These goals are balanced against the risks of embolization of *en passage* vessels, pulmonary emboli, retained microcatheters, and compression of spinal neural tissues by expanding necrotic tumors or hemorrhage.

At our institution, all craniospinal tumors are embolized while patients are under general anesthesia. Intraprocedural neurophysiologic monitoring, including brain stem auditory evoked potentials, somatosensory evoked potentials, and electroencephalography, is standard practice at our institution. We believe that a thorough evaluation of the angioarchitecture of the lesion and elimination of patient motion enhances the safety of the procedure. In patients with a complex vasculature, we use provocative testing (i.e., amobarbital and lidocaine)

to examine any change in neurophysiologic monitoring before proceeding.

Meticulous analysis of the angioarchitecture during spinal tumor embolization cannot be overemphasized. Complications often occur when attention to detail is lacking. For example, *en passage* vessels, particularly branches feeding into the anterior spinal artery, can be occluded. Unwanted neurologic complications can be minimized with fastidious techniques.

CRANIOSPINAL EMBOLIZATION

The arterial access site is guided by the most favorable guide catheter stabilization needed for treatment. A 6-French (Fr) sheath is used with a transfemoral approach. In rare instances, transbrachial or transradial access is required. The patient is then given intravenous heparin after the access site is obtained to achieve an activated clotting time between 200 and 300 seconds. Guide catheters (4, 5, or 6 Fr) are placed in the proximal parent ECA, ICA, VA, or spinal segmental artery, depending on the location of the pathology. A thorough understanding of the angioarchitecture of the feeding pedicles, *en passage* vessels, and EC-to-IC and anterior-to-posterior circulation anastomoses is needed. In spinal cases, diligent evaluation for potential anastomoses with the anterior spinal artery is essential to prevent embolic complications.

An over-the-wire or flow-directed microcatheter is used to perform superselective catheterization and angiography of the feeding pedicles. Meticulous evaluation of the superselective angiography for characteristics similar to those described earlier is needed before the next stage of intervention.

Embolization techniques vary, depending on the type of embolisate used. We use fastidious outside-the-body technique during the periembolization period. Fresh, sterile towels are laid over the patient's legs to create a working area isolated from extracorporeal blood and contrast medium. The gloves of the physician performing the embolization are replaced. Careful handling of the embolic agent may prevent unintended or premature precipitation of embolisates.

PVA has been used in many tumor embolization studies and has been the main embolic agent used by many interventionalists. At our center, there is a shift toward using liquid embolic agents, particularly Onyx. There are fundamental differences between PVA particles and liquid agents. PVA particles range from 50 to 1000 μm. For tumor embolization, we typically use PVA particles ranging between 200 and 350 μm. Since PVA is radiolucent, iodinated contrast is needed to create a suspension for fluoroscopic delivery. In certain cases, pushable, injectable, or detachable coils can be placed distally in selected large vessels to help inject a second embolisate such as PVA.

When PVA is used, the inner diameter of the delivery microcatheter must be bigger than the particles to prevent clumping and clogging. Typically, relatively large over-the-wire microcatheters, with their disadvantages of larger profile and less flexibility compared to smaller flow-directed microcatheters, are required when PVA is used. Superselective catheterization of pedicles feeding the nidus with such large microcatheters is labor intensive and associated with the risk of vessel perforation. Although iodinated contrast is mixed with the PVA, it may not be possible to identify where the embolisate is deposited.

PVA particles are injected under blank road map conditions to maximize visualization of the PVA contrast suspension. Angiographic runs are evaluated intermittently to determine the extent of embolization. When contrast reflux is noted proximally, injection of the embolisate is stopped and an angiography is again performed. If satisfactory embolization has been achieved, the procedure is terminated.

Two main types of liquid embolisates are used for tumor embolization: *n*-BCA and Onyx. There are fundamental differences in the techniques used with these two agents during craniospinal embolization. For most applications, we use a mixture of 1.5:1 to 3:1 Ethiodol–to–*n*-BCA for infusion. The suspended tantalum powder allows visualization of the solution during the injection. Infusion of *n*-BCA requires two experienced operators working in tandem. The microcatheter is cleared with 5% dextrose in water to flush all ionic catalysts from the lumen. The *n*-BCA is then injected under blank road map fluoroscopy, and apnea is prolonged until embolization is satisfactory. The embolization is usually performed fairly quickly. The microcatheter is then removed quickly under gentle traction and syringe aspiration.

The technique of infusing Onyx is completely different from injecting *n*-BCA. Before it is used, the Onyx solution must be shaken vigorously for 20 minutes to fully suspend the tantalum powder. Otherwise, sedimentation of the tantalum causes inadequate opacification during infusion. Once the microcatheter is in satisfactory position, as described previously, the dead space in the microcatheter is slowly purged with dimethyl sulfoxide (DMSO, 0.25 ml every 90 seconds). The Onyx is drawn into a DMSO-compatible 1-ml syringe and connected to the microcatheter.

The Onyx is injected slowly over 120 seconds to displace the DMSO, and subtracted fluoroscopic road map is initiated just before the injection is completed. The slow, steady injection should be about 0.1 ml/min and should not exceed 0.25 ml/min to avoid the effects from angiotoxicity of the solvent.

The Onyx injection can be stopped periodically to evaluate its progression. When reflux occurs proximally, the infusion is stopped for as long as 2 minutes to allow the Onyx to solidify around the catheter. This strategy allows a plug to form at the catheter tip, thereby increasing the probability of antegrade flow. Each time, a subtracted fluoroscopic road map is refreshed to prevent confusion regarding the progression of the Onyx injection. This process may need to be repeated multiple times. The goal is to establish forward flow into the capillary bed of the tumor.

This "plug and push" technique can cast additional areas of the tumor from a single pedicle through the rich capillary network within the tumor. Several milliliters of Onyx are often used for a single pedicle injection. However, the procedure is stopped when adequate Onyx casting is achieved or if retrograde reflux threatens to occlude proximal *en passage* branches.

After the embolization procedure, angiographic evaluation of the intracranial and spinal circulation is performed. Typically, heparinization is not reversed unless complications from intraprocedural bleeding are encountered. Patients are monitored in the intensive care unit before surgical intervention. Typically, surgery is performed the next day at our institution.

DIRECT TUMOR EMBOLIZATION

In carotid body tumors and selected JNAs, tumor embolization has been described by direct tumoral puncture with Onyx injection.[91,92] After angiography is performed in the appropriate common carotid artery, a 20-gauge spinal needle is inserted percutaneously into the lateral aspect of the neck. The needle is advanced under fluoroscopic road map guidance until arterial blood return is observed. Inadvertent puncture of the carotid artery must be avoided. Intratumoral angiography is performed through the spinal needle to confirm its location within the tumor. Potential dangerous anastomoses are also identified. Embolization then proceeds through the spinal needle. Postprocedural cerebral angiography is performed to rule out embolic events.

Types of Embolisates

The ideal embolisate is one that can penetrate deeply into the capillary bed while providing sufficient control over its injection to avoid occlusion of the normal arterial or venous vasculature. Other characteristics of an ideal embolisate include radiopacity for visualization, ease of surgical handling, and nontoxicity. Given that the treatment goal is surgical extirpation of the tumor, long-term durability of the embolisate is a less important consideration. Embolic materials can be divided into three major categories: solid occlusive devices, particles, and liquid embolic agents.

SOLID OCCLUSIVE DEVICES

Coils and balloons have been used to occlude large vessels. Liquid, fibered, and detachable coils are occasionally used in tumor embolization. Liquid coils are soft and injectable, while fibered coils are pushed mechanically through a coil pusher. Detachable coils are released mechanically, electrically, or hydrostatically. The primary role of coils is to augment the effects of a secondary embolisate by dampening the high arterial flow. Coils can eliminate dangerous EC-to-IC anastomoses to minimize embolic events before another occlusive agent is used.

PARTICLES

A variety of particles have been used with various degrees of success for tumor embolization. The embolisates include microfibrillar collagen, fibrin glue, Gelfoam, PVA, and microspheres.

Gelfoam

Gelfoam particles are typically 40 to 60 µm. Their advantages lie in their ease of use and deep tumoral penetration. However, innate proteolysis can easily disintegrate these agents, thereby causing occluded vessels to recanalize. Furthermore, the small caliber of these embolisates can potentially occlude the vaso vasorum of cranial nerves or cause other undesirable embolizations.

Polyvinyl Alcohol

PVA particles are the most commonly used agents for tumor embolization. The size of PVA particles ranges from 50 to 1000 µm. Smaller particles are more effective in penetrating tumors to facilitate tumor necrosis and reduce vascularity of the tumor. However, PVA is associated with an increased risk of inadvertent embolization of *en passage* vessels or the pulmonary capillary bed compared to larger particles. PVA is inert and insoluble; therefore, contrast is required to visualize it during injection. PVA can be long lasting, but it is not permanent; it degrades over weeks to months. With complete tumor resection, the durability of permanent occlusion of arterial feeders is not a major concern. However, if tumor resection is incomplete, the tumor can theoretically enlarge if the arterial feeders recanalize.

Embospheres

Embospheres (BioSphere Medical, Rockland, MA) are clear, radiolucent, acrylic microspheres composed of tri-sacryl gelatin microspheres. Unlike PVA, Embospheres have a uniform shape and size. Embospheres are compressible and may be associated with less clumping and clogging of microcatheters than PVA. They do not degrade and generate only a moderate inflammatory response.[93] Microspheres have been described to penetrate more distally than PVA during embolization and to result in significantly less operative blood loss.[94]

LIQUID EMBOLIC AGENTS

Alcohol

Alcohol is a potent sclerotic, devascularizing agent. It causes anoxic cellular damage and fibrinoid necrosis of the intimal lining.[95] Because of its low viscosity, alcohol can penetrate more deeply than other agents. However, the use of alcohol is associated with a high risk of cranial nerve deficits or normal tissue infarction.[96,97] Intraoperative intratumoral injections of ethanol have been performed with success. Lonser et al.[98] described their technique of injecting ethanol intratumorally in three spinal epidural lesions and one posterior fossa hemangioblastoma. They used a 28-gauge needle to inject alcohol into the tumors until the lesions blanched visibly. Although ethanol is a powerful embolisate, it must be used judiciously and with great caution to prevent infarction of normal tissue.

n-Butyl Cyanoacrylate

n-BCA is a nonabsorbable, adhesive liquid embolic agent that causes an inflammatory response in the endothelium and tumor. It must be mixed with Ethiodol and tantalum powder. When mixed with n-BCA, Ethiodol prolongs the polymerization time and promotes radiopacity. The embolisate promotes necrosis and fibrous ingrowth in the arterial feeders, leading to permanent durable occlusion.

n-BCA is used more frequently to treat arteriovenous malformations and fistulas of the CNS than to treat tumors. Even in tumor embolization, many interventionalists prefer PVA compared to n-BCA. The latter has a tendency to occlude both proximal and distal vessels, increasing the probability of injuring cranial nerves or causing infarctions. The adhesive nature of the polymer can make removal of the microcatheter difficult at the end of the procedure, causing it to break or be unmovable. The technical constraints associated with delivering n-BCA require extensive experience to use it successfully.

EVOH Copolymer–DMSO Solvent (Onyx)

In 2005, the U.S. Food and Drug Administration approved solvent ethylene–vinyl alcohol (EVOH) copolymer–DMSO for use in preoperative embolization of brain arteriovenous malformations. The compound is a mixture of EVOH, tantalum powder, and DMSO. It is sold in the United States as Onyx. Its applications continue to expand, and it is gaining popularity for preoperative embolization of tumors.

Unlike n-BCA, Onyx is a cohesive polymer. Although Onyx does not adhere to the endothelium, it can adhere to the microcatheter, making withdrawal of the catheter precarious. The DMSO solvent prevents polymerization of the Onyx. When Onyx is injected and contacts the aqueous solution, the DMSO diffuses away rapidly. The copolymer precipitates into a soft, spongy solid. The toxicity of DMSO in humans is well established. DMSO is angiotoxic, inducing vasospasm, angionecrosis, arterial thrombosis, and vascular rupture. However, these detrimental qualities are directly related to the volume of DMSO infused and its length of contact with the endothelium. Limiting the rate of DMSO infusion (less than 0.25 ml every 90 seconds) eliminates these undesirable side effects. An inadequate mixture of the solution before infusion can lead to sedimentation of

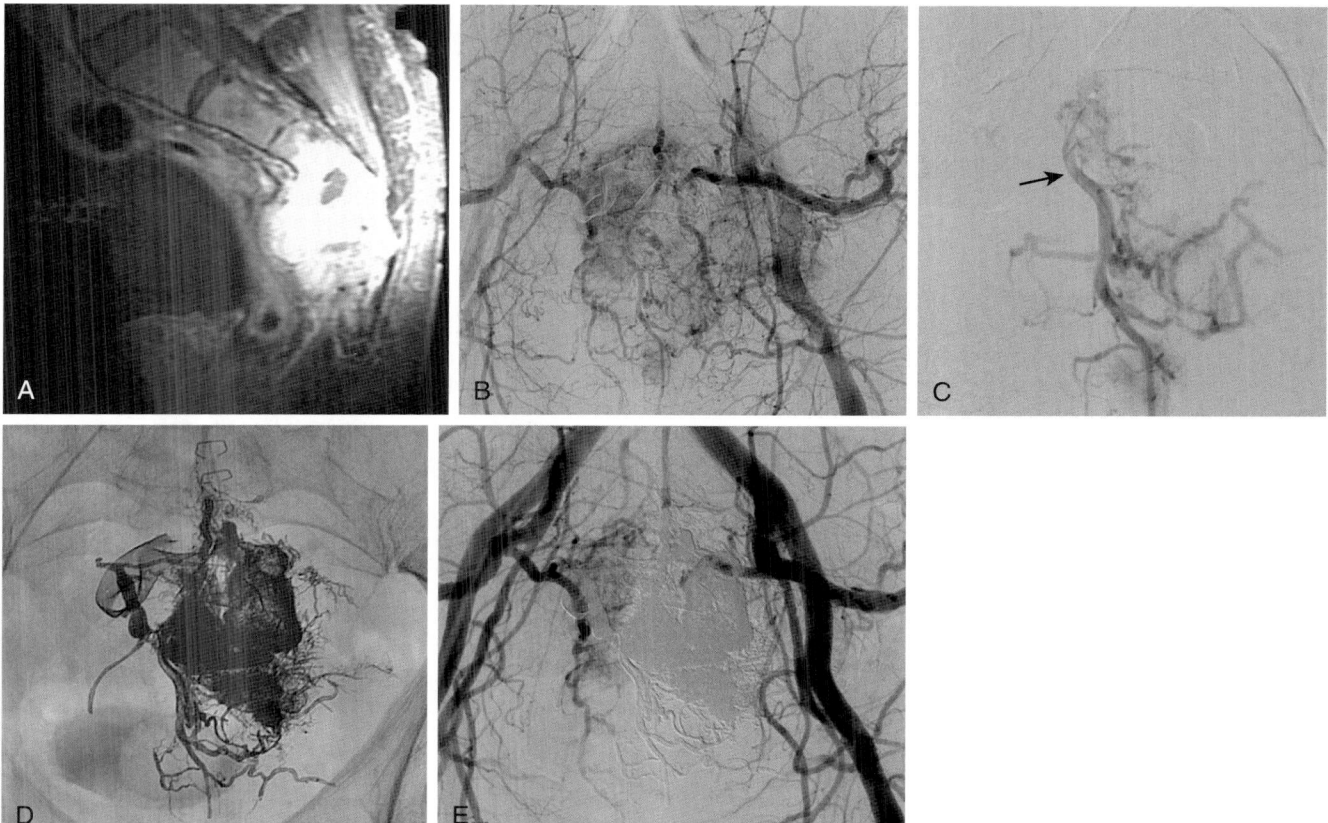

FIGURE 89-5 A, A T1-weighted sagittal MRI with gadolinium of a 74-year-old man with sacral pain showed a large sacral mass. Excessive blood loss was encountered intraoperatively. B, This prompted an urgent pelvic angiogram that delineated the hypervascularity of the sacral tumor. C, Catheterization of the median sacral artery *(arrowhead)* showed the increase in the caliber of the vessel and multiple arterial feeders supplying the tumor. D, A subtracted view demonstrated a significant amount of Onyx infused via a single arterial pedicle, the median sacral artery. E, Unsubtracted views of post-Onyx angiography illustrated the decreased vascularity of the tumor after embolization. (From Barrow Neurological Institute.)

the tantalum powder, producing suboptimal opacification and visualization.

The advantages of Onyx are that it can penetrate much deeper than other agents and that countless capillary networks can be occluded with a single pedicle injection. Unlike *n*-BCA, Onyx permits discontinuous injections on the order of minutes and allows continuous angiographic analysis of the angioarchitecture of the lesion. In particular, small collaterals not visualized on the initial angiogram may become apparent with progressive infusion of Onyx (Fig. 89-5). The ability to stop the infusion and analyze the progress of the Onyx can minimize complications from its unwanted diffusion into potentially dangerous anastomoses or collaterals. The ability of Onyx to penetrate enables progressive filling and deeper casting of the fine capillary network, and it can migrate in a retrograde fashion into arterial feeders from other vessels through a single pedicle. Venous filling can be stopped temporarily without the threat of unintended migration of Onyx into draining veins. These advantages allow exceptional control of Onyx flow and its progression to enable a large amount to be delivered via a single injection.

Another advantage of Onyx is the ease with which it can be manipulated during surgery. The black, embolized vessels are easy to see, divide, and cauterize. The microneurosurgeons in the study by Akin et al. reported that Onyx-embolized vessels have better handling characteristics than vessels that were embolized by *n*-BCA.[99] This finding was reported despite the endovascular interventionalist's belief that the *n*-BCA provided better angiographic embolization than Onyx in the same rete mirabile model of the swine.

COMPLICATIONS

Presurgical tumor embolization can cause significant morbidity and mortality. The most common complications from tumor embolization are fever and localized pain.[100] Other potential devastating complications include unintentional embolic events involving the craniospinal axis or pulmonary circulations, intratumoral hemorrhage, and cranial nerve injuries.

Unintended embolization most often occurs in unrecognized anastomoses. The rich vascular networks between the ECAs and the ICAs may not be visualized until certain feeders are occluded during the embolization procedure. The operator must have extensive knowledge and exert meticulous attention to avoid potential complications.

Embolization can injure cranial nerves by disrupting the vaso vasorum to the nerves. For example, the neuromeningeal branch of the ascending pharyngeal artery frequently supplies the spinal accessory and hypoglossal nerves. Provocative testing can be used to determine whether the potential embolized vessel supplies a cranial nerve.

The rates of false positives and false negatives associated with provocative testing are high, and reflux of lidocaine intracranially can cause seizures. These limitations prevent its widespread use as a standard procedure. Careful patient selection and meticulous techniques are essential tools for successful preoperative endovascular embolization of tumors.

Conclusion

Vascular craniospinal tumors can present formidable surgical challenges with high associated rates of operative morbidity and mortality. Preoperative embolization can effectively improve surgical outcomes by minimizing blood loss and transfusions, increasing tumor resection, and shortening operative times and hospital stays. Embolization may eventually become the primary modality of treatment of certain tumors. The techniques of tumor embolization continue to expand and improve as new innovations are developed.

KEY REFERENCES

Adler JR, Upton J, Wallman J, Winston KR. Management and prevention of necrosis of the scalp after embolization and surgery for meningioma. *Surg Neurol.* 1986 April;25(4):357-360.

Akin ED, Perkins E, Ross IB. Surgical handling characteristics of an ethylene–vinyl alcohol copolymer compared with *n*-butyl cyanoacrylate used for embolization of vessels in an arteriovenous malformation resection model in swine. *J Neurosurg.* 2003 February;98(2):366-370.

Alen JF, Lobato RD, Gomez PA, et al. Intracranial hemangiopericytoma: study of 12 cases. *Acta Neurochir (Wien).* 2001;143(6):575-586.

Bendszus M, Rao G, Burger R, et al. Is there a benefit of preoperative meningioma embolization? *Neurosurgery.* 2000 December;47(6):1306-1311.

Berkefeld J, Scale D, Kirchner J, et al. Hypervascular spinal tumors: influence of the embolization technique on perioperative hemorrhage. *AJNR Am J Neuroradiol.* 1999 May;20(5):757-763.

Breslau J, Eskridge JM. Preoperative embolization of spinal tumors. *J Vasc Interv Radiol.* 1995 November;6(6):871-875.

Cornelius JF, Saint-Maurice JP, Bresson D, et al. Hemorrhage after particle embolization of hemangioblastomas: comparison of outcomes in spinal and cerebellar lesions. *J Neurosurg.* 2007 June;106(6):994-998.

Dean BL, Flom RA, Wallace RC, et al. Efficacy of endovascular treatment of meningiomas: evaluation with matched samples. *AJNR Am J Neuroradiol.* 1994 October;15(9):1675-1680.

Deshmukh VR, Fiorella DJ, McDougall CG, et al. Preoperative embolization of central nervous system tumors. *Neurosurg Clin N Am.* 2005 April;16(2):411-432:xi.

Elhammady MS, Farhat H, Ziayee H, ziz-Sultan MA. Direct percutaneous embolization of a carotid body tumor with Onyx. *J Neurosurg.* 2009 January;110(1):124-127.

Elhammady MS, Wolfe SQ, Ashour R, et al. Safety and efficacy of vascular tumor embolization using Onyx: is angiographic devascularization sufficient? *J Neurosurg.* 2009 August 21.

Eskridge JM, McAuliffe W, Harris B, et al. Preoperative endovascular embolization of craniospinal hemangioblastomas. *AJNR Am J Neuroradiol.* 1996 March;17(3):525-531.

Gellad FE, Sadato N, Numaguchi Y, Levine AM. Vascular metastatic lesions of the spine: preoperative embolization. *Radiology.* 1990 September;176(3):683-686.

Gruber A, Bavinzski G, Killer M, Richling B. Preoperative embolization of hypervascular skull base tumors. *Minim Invasive Neurosurg.* 2000 June;43(2):62-71.

Hosalkar HS, Jones KJ, King JJ, Lackman RD. Serial arterial embolization for large sacral giant-cell tumors: mid- to long-term results. *Spine (Phila Pa 1976).* 2007 May 1;32(10):1107-1115.

Jacobsson M, Petruson B, Svendsen P, Berthelsen B. Juvenile nasopharyngeal angiofibroma. A report of eighteen cases. *Acta Otolaryngol.* 1988 January;105(1-2):132-139.

Kaji T, Hama Y, Iwasaki Y, et al. Preoperative embolization of meningiomas with pial supply: successful treatment of two cases. *Surg Neurol.* 1999 September;52(3):270-273.

Lackman RD, Khoury LD, Esmail A, Donthineni-Rao R. The treatment of sacral giant-cell tumours by serial arterial embolisation. *J Bone Joint Surg Br.* 2002 August;84(6):873-877.

Liapis CD, Evangelidakis EL, Papavassiliou VG, et al. Role of malignancy and preoperative embolization in the management of carotid body tumors. *World J Surg.* 2000 December;24(12):1526-1530.

Liu JK, Brockmeyer DL, Dailey AT, Schmidt MH. Surgical management of aneurysmal bone cysts of the spine. *Neurosurg Focus.* 2003 November 15;15(5):E4.

Murakami R, Baba Y, Furusawa M, et al. Short communication: the value of embolization therapy in painful osseous metastases from hepatocellular carcinomas; comparative study with radiation therapy. *Br J Radiol.* 1996 November;69(827):1042-1044.

Sundaresan N, Choi IS, Hughes JE, et al. Treatment of spinal metastases from kidney cancer by presurgical embolization and resection. *J Neurosurg.* 1990 October;73(4):548-554.

Tampieri D, Leblanc R, TerBrugge K. Preoperative embolization of brain and spinal hemangioblastomas. *Neurosurgery.* 1993 September;33(3):502-505.

Wang SJ, Wang MB, Barauskas TM, Calcaterra TC. Surgical management of carotid body tumors. *Otolaryngol Head Neck Surg.* 2000 September;123(3):202-206.

White JB, Link MJ. Endovascular embolization of paragangliomas: a safe adjunct to treatment. *J Vasc Interv Neurol.* 2008;1(2):37-41.

Numbered references appear on Expert Consult.

CHAPTER 90

Endovascular Management of Dural Arteriovenous Fistulas

GEOFFREY P. COLBY • ALEXANDRA R. PAUL • ELISA F. CICERI • ALEXANDER L. COON

Dural arteriovenous fistulas (DAVFs), also sometimes referred to as dural arteriovenous malformations, represent approximately 10% to 15% of all intracranial arteriovenous malformations. These lesions can occur in the brain and the spine and are characterized by abnormal arteriovenous shunts located within dural leaflets. Cranial DAVFs are most commonly located in the vicinity of dural venous sinuses and spinal DAVFs in the region where the radiculomedullary artery enters the dural root sleeve. The etiology of DAVFs is unknown, but many are acquired and can occur after trauma (e.g., skull fracture), surgery, sinus thrombosis, and venous channel stenosis.[1-4]

The pathophysiology and clinical significance of DAVFs stem from the location of the fistula or shunt and its effect on and disruption of normal venous drainage. Various classification systems have been published in the literature, with the key feature in each being the pattern of venous flow.[5-8] Borden et al. organized DAVFs into three groups: Type I DAVFs drain directly into meningeal veins or dural venous sinuses. Type II DAVFs also drain directly into dural sinuses or meningeal veins but have retrograde drainage into subarachnoid veins. Type III DAVFs do not have dural sinus or meningeal venous drainage; rather, they drain directly into subarachnoid veins.[8] Cognard et al. proposed a classification scheme with five main types: Type I DAVFs drain directly into dural venous sinuses or meningeal veins, and all venous flow is anterograde (in the normal direction). Type II DAVFs drain into dural sinuses or meningeal veins but have retrograde flow into the associated sinus (type IIa), cortical veins (type IIb), or both (type IIa+b). Type III and IV DAVFs drain directly into cortical veins either with (type III) or without (type IV) venous ectasia. Type V DAVFs include spinal venous drainage. DAVFs without cortical venous reflux (CVR) (Cognard types I or IIa or Borden type I) are generally considered benign.[7] Satomi et al. demonstrated that conservative management or palliative therapy is sufficient in 98% of cases of benign DAVFs; however, these patients have a 2% risk of developing CVR.[9] DAVFs with persistent CVR (Cognard types IIb-V or Borden types II and III) are much more aggressive, with an annual mortality of 10.4% and annual risk of hemorrhage or nonhemorrhagic neurologic deficit of 8.1% and 6.9%, respectively.[10] Symptomatic DAVFs are associated with variable clinical presentations, depending on the location of the shunt and the severity of venous hypertension secondary to retrograde leptomeningeal venous flow. Approximately 20% to 33% of symptomatic DAVFs present with intracranial hemorrhage.[4,10] Other presentations include pulsatile tinnitus (or bruit), headaches, visual changes, alterations in mental status, seizure, myelopathy, cranial nerve palsies, and motor or sensory deficits.

DAVFs can be treated by surgical techniques, endovascular techniques, a combination of surgical and endovascular techniques, or radiation therapy. For endovascular management, embolization targets are selected based on a thorough understanding of the fistula anatomy. The key is to obliterate the fistulous connections while limiting adverse outcomes, such as inadvertent worsening of cortical venous flow, closing external to internal carotid artery anastomoses, and embolizing external carotid artery branches with important arterial supply to cranial nerves. Transarterial and transvenous approaches are available for endovascular treatment of DAVFs. Embolic materials used in such procedures include n-butyl-2-cyanoacrylate (n-BCA) glue (Trufill, Cordis Neurovascular, Miami Lakes, FL), Onyx (ev3 Endovascular, Irvine, CA), detachable microcoils, and particles of polyvinyl alcohol. Particles are rarely used as a sole agent for DAVF embolization because of their temporary effects. Instead, they are used in certain circumstances as an adjuvant to reduce flow in collateral vessels and promote thrombosis.[11]

Transarterial Embolization

Transarterial embolization is ideally used for high-grade DAVFs, such as those with direct cortical venous drainage, or in situations in which venous access is limited. Nelson et al. listed the following advantages of transarterial procedures for DAVFs: (1) the arteriovenous fistula transition can be occluded through a transarterial approach, decreasing the possibility of flow diversion into an alternate venous pathway; (2) treatment is not limited by venous access (e.g., stenotic or thrombosed venous sinuses); (3) fistula treatment does not require sacrificing a functional venous pathway; (4) de novo DAVFs can develop at a secondary site following transvenous embolization, possibly as a result of venous hypertension; and (5) complications specific to transvenous routes can be avoided (e.g., abducens nerve palsy from catheterization of the superior petrosal sinus).[12]

Our practice has been to perform embolization procedures under general anesthesia with motor paralysis to decrease patient motion and obtain the best imaging and procedural results. Full systemic anticoagulation with heparin and catheters running continuous flush with heparinized saline are utilized to prevent blood embolic events. Advanced imaging techniques such as superselective microcatheter angiography; three-dimensional, rotational angiography; and a form of high-resolution flat-panel computed tomography (CT) known as DynaCT are quite helpful in defining the arterial and venous anatomy of a DAVF both before and after embolization. Embolic agents such as n-BCA and Onyx should be handled on a separate table when not in use to prevent premature polymerization and contamination of diagnostic catheters and solutions. A separate set of gloves should be used prior to handling these agents and at the end of the procedure prior to final diagnostic angiography.

Cyanoacrylic Glue Techniques

Cyanoacrylate adhesives have been used extensively for the embolization of high-flow cerebrovascular lesions,[13-15] including DAVFs.[11,12,16] n-BCA, a cyanoacrylate ester, is a clear, colorless liquid with a strong odor that is insoluble in water. This agent polymerizes rapidly when in contact with ionic substances, including blood or tissue fluids. Rapid polymerization and excellent tensile strength make n-BCA a highly effective embolic agent for endovascular procedures. However, it must be handled with great care to avoid the high risk of unintentional embolization of normal tissue. n-BCA is diluted with Ethiodol (ethiodized oil) to make the mixture radiopaque. Tantalum or tungsten powder can also be added to increase radiographic visibility.[17] The concentration of n-BCA in the mixture determines the migration, or penetration, of the embolic agent prior to polymerization. A high n-BCA-to-Ethiodol ratio (high concentration of glue) polymerizes more proximally in the arterial pedicle than a low n-BCA-to-Ethiodol ratio, which achieves more distal penetration. Glue concentrations of 25% to 33% are commonly used.

For transarterial glue embolization of DAVFs, the microcatheter should be positioned as close to the target fistula site as possible, because this increases the specificity of the injection and facilitates penetration of the embolic material to the fistula site. Wedging the microcatheter within a feeding artery creates a flow-arrest scenario that is thought to facilitate delivery of glue to the fistula site and its permeation into the extensive fistulous collateral network. In a series of 21 patients with 23 DAVFs, Nelson et al. demonstrated complete occlusion in all cases without complications using the wedge catheter technique.[12] Wedge catheterization also allows for arterioarterial reflex with occlusion of multiple arterial feeders from a single pedicle injection.[11]

Once the optimal catheter position is obtained, microcatheter angiography and test injections are used to determine fistula flow characteristics and the appropriate glue concentration for the procedure. Prior to the actual glue injection, the microcatheter must be flushed thoroughly with a nonionic solution, such as 5% dextrose, to ensure that the glue does not polymerize within the delivery catheter. The glue is then injected under direct digital subtraction angiography (DSA) guidance either as a continuous column or as a bolus followed by a column of nonionic flush.[17] If there is a suboptimal

catheter position (e.g., the catheter is too proximal along the pedicle or the neurointerventionalist is unable to wedge the catheter tip), simultaneous injection of 5% dextrose through the guide catheter can improve distal migration of the glue toward its target.[16] After adequate glue penetration, the microcatheter or the whole delivery system (microcatheter plus guide catheter) is rapidly removed from the patient. Communication among operators during a glue procedure is critical so that the catheter is pulled at the correct instant and not glued to the vessel. Examples of transarterial glue embolization of DAVFs are shown in Figs. 90-1 and 90-2.

Onyx Techniques

First reports describing the use of Onyx in vascular malformations were published in 1990.[18,19] Onyx has been commercially available in Europe since 1999 and was approved by the U.S. Food and Drug Administration in July 2005.

Onyx is a liquid agent composed of a mixture of ethylene–vinyl alcohol copolymer suspended in the solvent dimethyl sulfoxide (DMSO). Tantalum powder is added to the compound for radiopacity. To obtain homogeneous radiopacity of the mixture, Onyx must be shaken for at least 20 minutes before use. The potential angiotoxic effects of DMSO are negligible if the recommended dose and infusion rate are followed.[20-22] The polymer precipitates upon contact with aqueous solution, resulting in a soft, nonadherent material characterized by a "lavalike" flow pattern that is able to produce permanent vessel obliteration. Because of the presence of the solvent, all materials must be DMSO compatible, including syringes and microcatheters.

The therapeutic approach to cerebral DAVF mainly depends on the vascular drainage and CVR pattern of the malformation. In Cognard type II dural fistulas, with or without CVR, the best option, when feasible, remains the transvenous approach with coils or Onyx. However, this option entails the sacrifice of the sinus.[23-27] In the same setting, transarterial embolization could have the advantage of preserving the sinus when still functional.

In cases of DAVF with direct CVR Cognard type III to V, the transarterial embolization is the most advantageous technique. Several reports in the recent literature highlight the benefit of Onyx in these cases.[24,28-30] Compared to n-BCA glue injection, the Onyx technique has some technical advantages: it is less operator dependent, does not need a wedged microcatheter positioning, and has the capacity to occlude different feeders from a single pedicle with a single injection (Figs. 90-3 and 90-4). This last advantage is particularly relevant when the venous access is limited.[28-31] Onyx may also be used in the treatment of cavernous DAVFs. However, in these cases, the transvenous approach is recommended to avoid the risk of cranial nerve damage and penetration into extra- or intracranial anastomoses.[23,27]

We prefer to perform the embolization procedure under general anesthesia and full heparinization monitored with activating clotting time.[30] After a detailed diagnostic angiographic study, possibly including superselective injections of the vessels involved in the dural malformation, an accurate treatment strategy should be planned to select the cases that can benefit from intra-arterial Onyx injection. The strategy should be aimed at (1) locating the point, or points, of fistula; (2) recognizing the feeding arteries; (3) understanding the

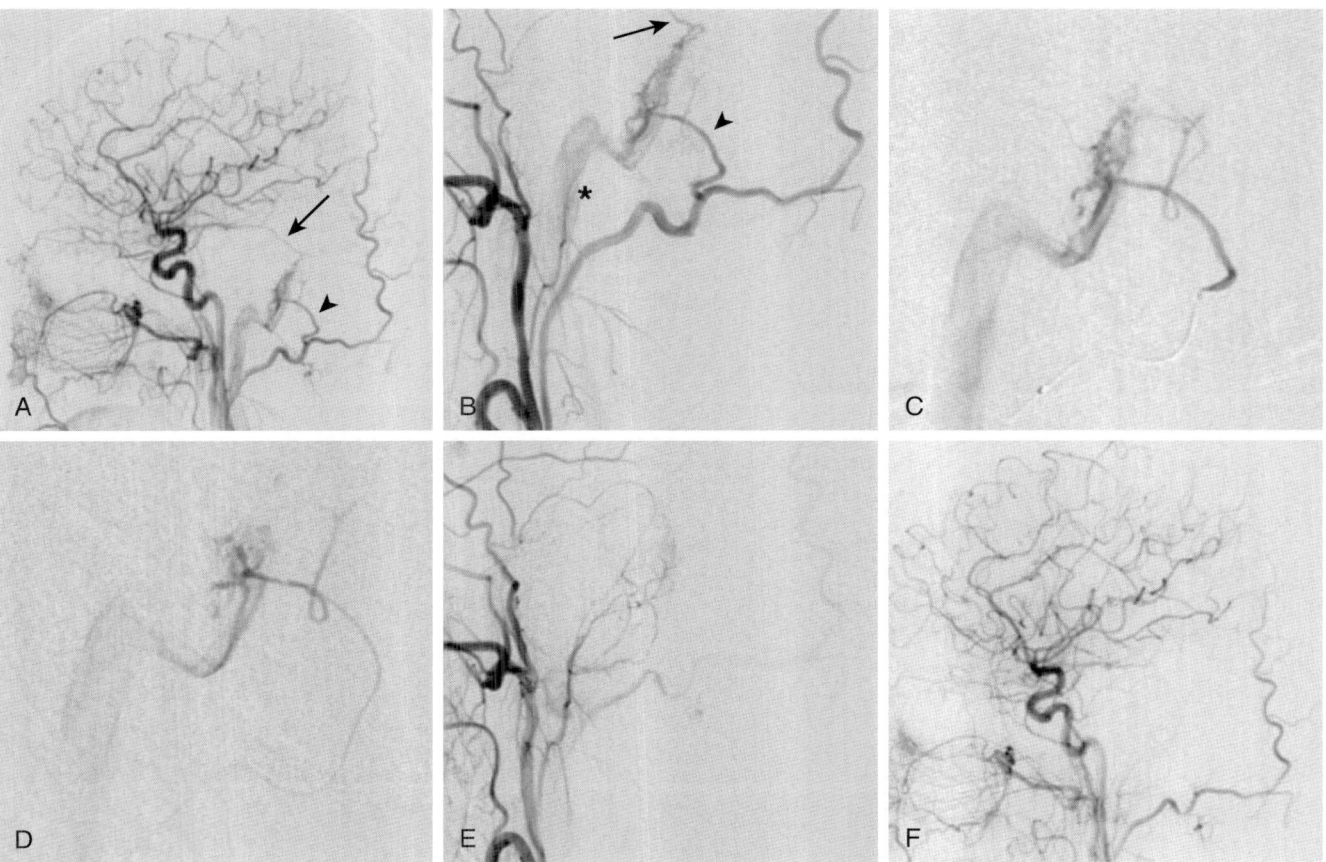

FIGURE 90-1 Transarterial *n*-BCA embolization of a Cognard type I DAVF. Lateral projections of right common carotid (A) and external carotid (B) angiograms of a 43-year-old woman who presented with right occipital pain and eventually developed a bruit. The angiograms demonstrate a type I DAVF of the right transverse and sigmoid sinuses fed primarily by a mastoid branch of the occipital artery *(arrowhead)* but with contributions from the middle meningeal artery *(arrow)* and the neuromeningeal branch of the ascending pharyngeal artery *(asterisk)*. The sinuses fill anterogradely. Pre-embolization microcatheter angiography of the mastoid branch of the occipital artery, both proximal (C) and distal (D) microcatheter positions, further demonstrating the fistulous connection. Post-*n*-BCA embolization angiograms of the right external carotid (E) and common carotid (F) arteries, demonstrating complete obliteration of the fistula.

venous drainage pattern; and (4) selecting the most promising pedicles to be injected based on navigability, expected efficacy, and safety. Biplanar angiography is mandatory. Tridimensional DSA reconstructions and pseudo-CT scans may be useful adjuncts.

When the microcatheter is in the desired position, before injecting Onyx, an initial flushing of the microcatheter with about 5 ml of normal saline is required, followed by injection of DMSO to fill the dead space of the microcatheter. Subsequently, Onyx can be slowly injected in 40 seconds to replace the DMSO. The entire procedure must be performed under double road map fluoroscopy to recognize any premature leakage of Onyx.[32] The injection speed can be adjusted according to vessel penetration and direction, as well as reflux conditions. If reflux is observed, however small, the procedure should be immediately stopped. It should be resumed within a few minutes to avoid plugging of the microcatheter with consequent risk of rupture. It is advisable to obtain a new road map prior to any injection to improve the visibility of the vessel penetration and reflux of Onyx. The control of the reflux is a crucial element for the success of the treatment; it is necessary to create a plug around the microcatheter that allows the Onyx to be pushed into the vascular malformation (Fig. 90-3F). On the other

hand, excessive reflux can determine retrograde filling of the feeder where the microcatheter is positioned up to the origin of the parent artery, causing unwanted obliteration of normal vessels. An additional risk is entrapment of the microcatheter so that it becomes difficult to retrieve at the end of the procedure.

The injection through a single pedicle can last more than 1 hour. During treatment, control angiograms can be performed from the main catheter to control the progression of the procedure. If necessary, more than one pedicle can be embolized during the same procedure or the treatment can be staged in different sessions.

At the end of the procedure, the microcatheter must be gently retracted, maintaining continuous and regular traction for a few minutes. If the microcatheter remains entrapped by the Onyx, it can be cut and left in place without further complications.[24] However, personal experience with two cases demonstrates that a microcatheter fixed to the arterial access can be safely retrieved 24 hours later.

Postembolization care includes medications for pain, which is caused by the dural involvement, and low-molecular-weight heparin for 1 to 4 weeks to prevent venous thrombosis. An immediate post-treatment CT scan is recommended,

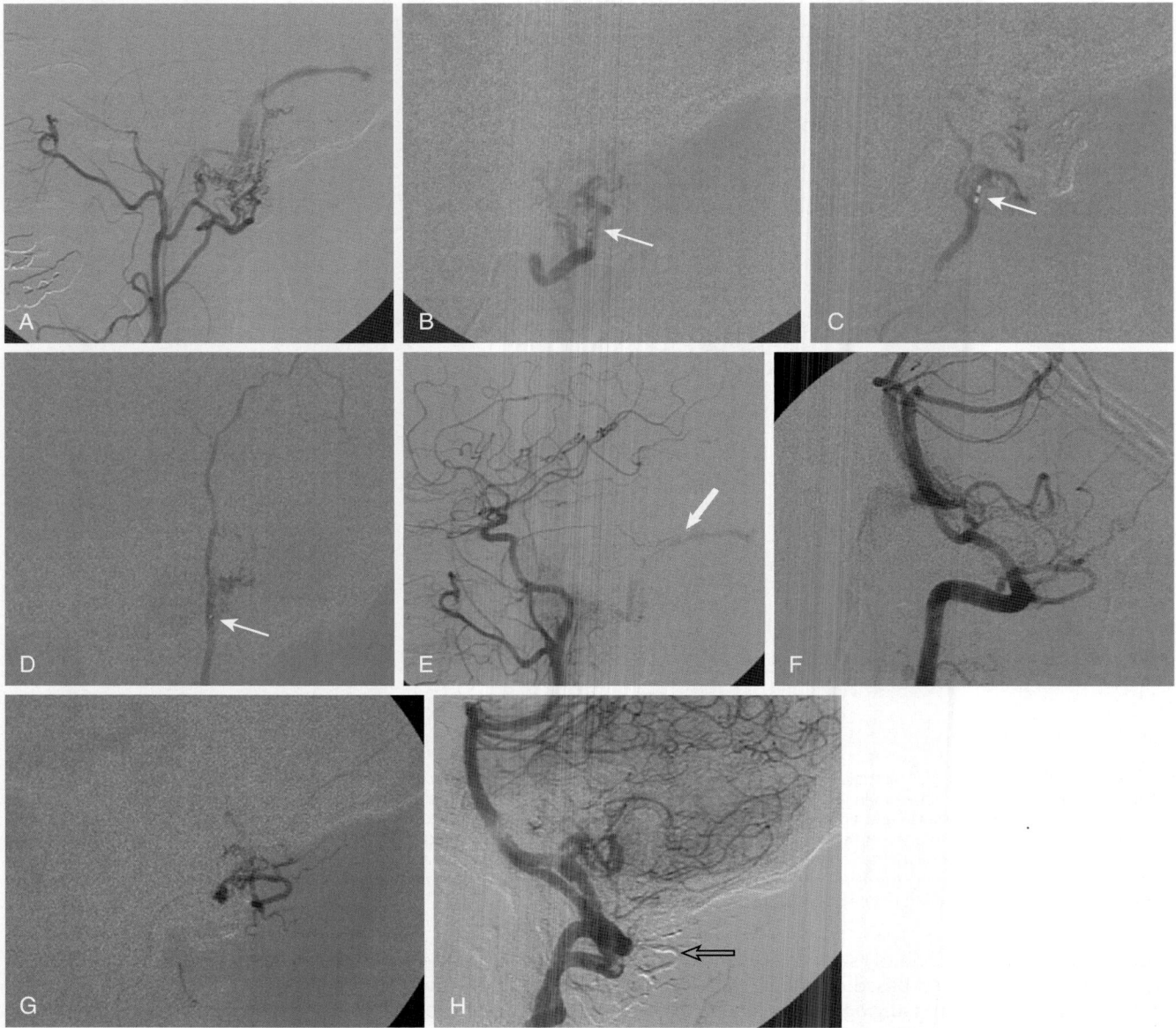

FIGURE 90-2 Transarterial *n*-BCA embolization of a Cognard type IIa DAVF. A, Lateral projections of right external carotid angiograms of a 50-year-old woman who had successful surgical excision of a right pontocerebellar meningioma and then a few months later developed right pulsatile tinnitus. Angiography demonstrates a type IIa DAVF with the arteriovenous shunt at the level of the sigmoid sinus that is fed by various branches of the external carotid artery (A) and a small muscular branch of the right vertebral artery (F). The venous flow course (A) is retrograde into the transverse sinus. Superselective *n*-BCA glue injections were performed in the occipital artery (B), posterior auricular artery (C), and ascending pharyngeal artery (D) (*open arrows* point to the tip of the microcatheters). E, Post-treatment common carotid artery angiography demonstrates the complete exclusion of the embolized arterial feeders, with a very small residual contribution to the fistula coming from the middle meningeal artery (*open arrow*). F to H, In the same session, a superselective *n*-BCA embolization procedure was performed in a muscular branch of the right vertebral artery. F, Pretreatment angiography. G, Superselective injection of the diluted glue. H, The post-treatment result (*open arrow* at the glue cast site).

followed by an angiographic study 3 to 6 months after the procedure to control the stability of the results (Fig. 90-4).[30]

Transvenous Embolization

The goal of endovascular DAVF treatment using a transvenous approach is to embolize the venous outlet of the fistula. Several approaches for transvenous embolization of DAVFs have been described[11,33]: catheterization of the involved sinus via a venous approach,[26,34] direct puncture of the affected sinus by a transcranial approach (used if endovascular navigation is not possible),[30,35] and selective transvenous embolization of veins with CVR without occlusion of the sinus.[36] The transvenous approach is favored when the main arterial feeders of a DAVF originate from the internal carotid artery or the vertebral artery, when sites of possible extracranial to intracranial anastomoses are involved, and when there is risk of compromising arterial supply to cranial nerves.[37]

Prior to transvenous occlusion of sinus for DAVF treatment, the venous drainage pathways of the normal brain must be clearly defined. Occlusion of a sinus that is necessary for

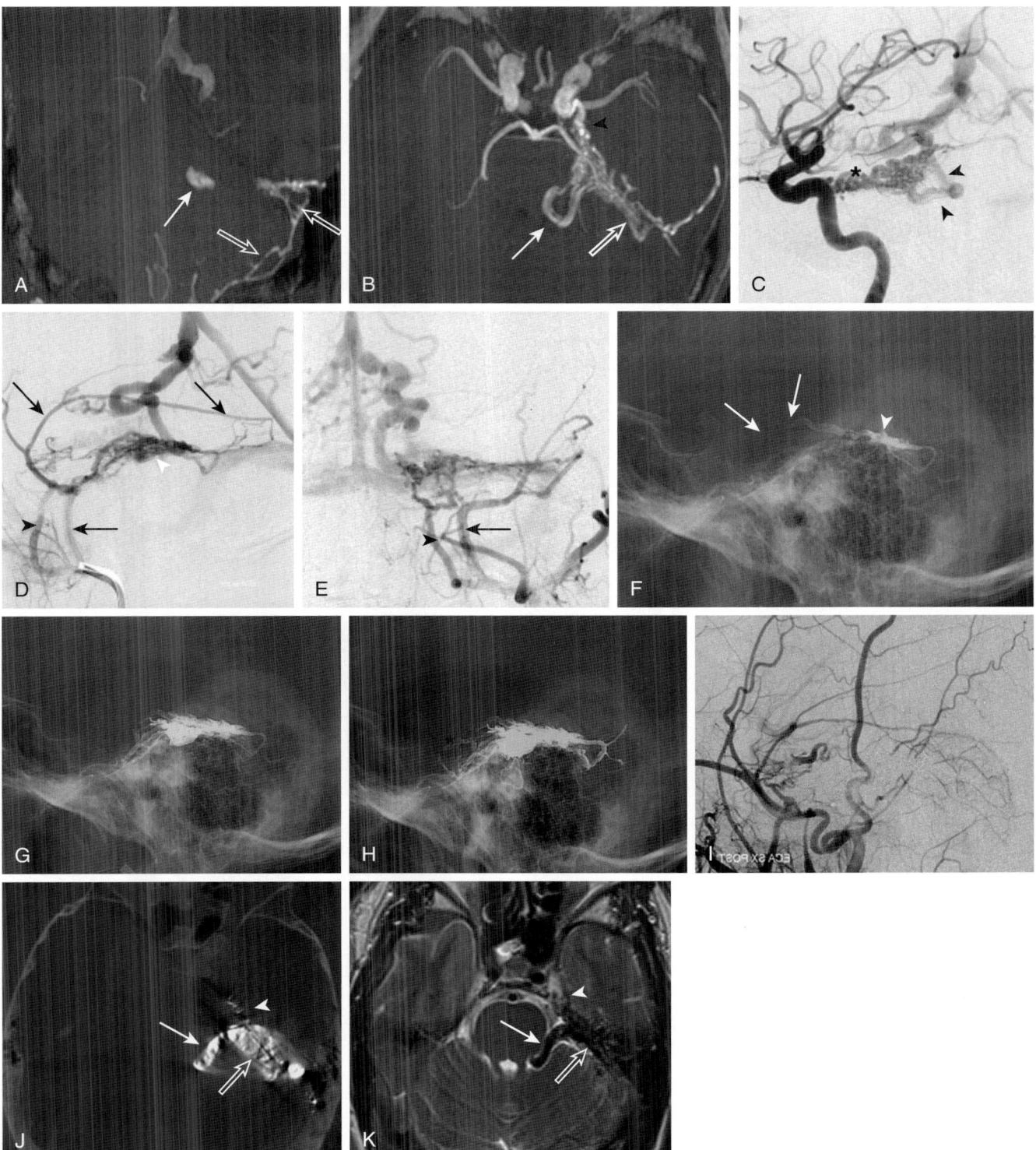

FIGURE 90-3 Onyx embolization of a DAVF of the left superior petrosal sinus. Pretreatment imaging studies: coronal (A) and axial (B) postcontrast magnetic resonance imaging (MRI) and cerebral angiogram with a left internal carotid artery lateral view (C) and left external carotid artery lateral (D) and anteroposterior (E) views. The thrombosis of the left transverse and sigmoid sinus (white open arrows in A) and the presence of numerous dysplastic vessels along the margin of the left petrous bone at the insertion of the tentorium (white open arrow in B) are suggestive for a dural fistula. Grossly dilated and tortuous marginal tentorial arteries (white arrow in B and asterisk in C) constitute the main anterior feeders. The left middle meningeal artery (black arrows in D and E) and the left accessory meningeal artery (black arrowhead in D and E) represent other important arterial feeders. A posterior inferior contribution originates from branches of the posterior meningeal artery of the left vertebral artery (not shown). The venous drainage is through the left superior petrosal vein, lateral mesencephalic vein, and basal Rosenthal vein to the Galen vein and straight sinus (white arrow in A and B and arrowhead in C). F to H, Unsubtracted lateral views during injection of Onyx. The microcatheter is positioned in a branch of the left accessory meningeal artery (arrows); its tip is marked by an arrowhead (F). The sequence of F to H demonstrates different embolization steps: early anterograde filling of the malformation and retrograde filling of the feeding artery (between the arrowhead and the first arrow in F); progressive filling of the whole malformation (G); and final cast of Onyx occluding the adjacent terminal segments of the different arterial feeders (H). Total injection time is 75 minutes. I, A postprocedural lateral view of the external carotid artery demonstrates complete obliteration of the fistula. No residual arteriovenous shunts were visible at injection of the other feeders (not shown). Post-treatment DynaCT (J) and axial T2-weighted MRI (K). The cast of Onyx that fills the whole malformation (open arrow) is hyperdense on CT and hypointense on all MRI sequences. The cast also fills the marginal tentorial branches of the left internal carotid artery (white arrow; see the corresponding arrow in B) and the petrosal vein (white arrow).

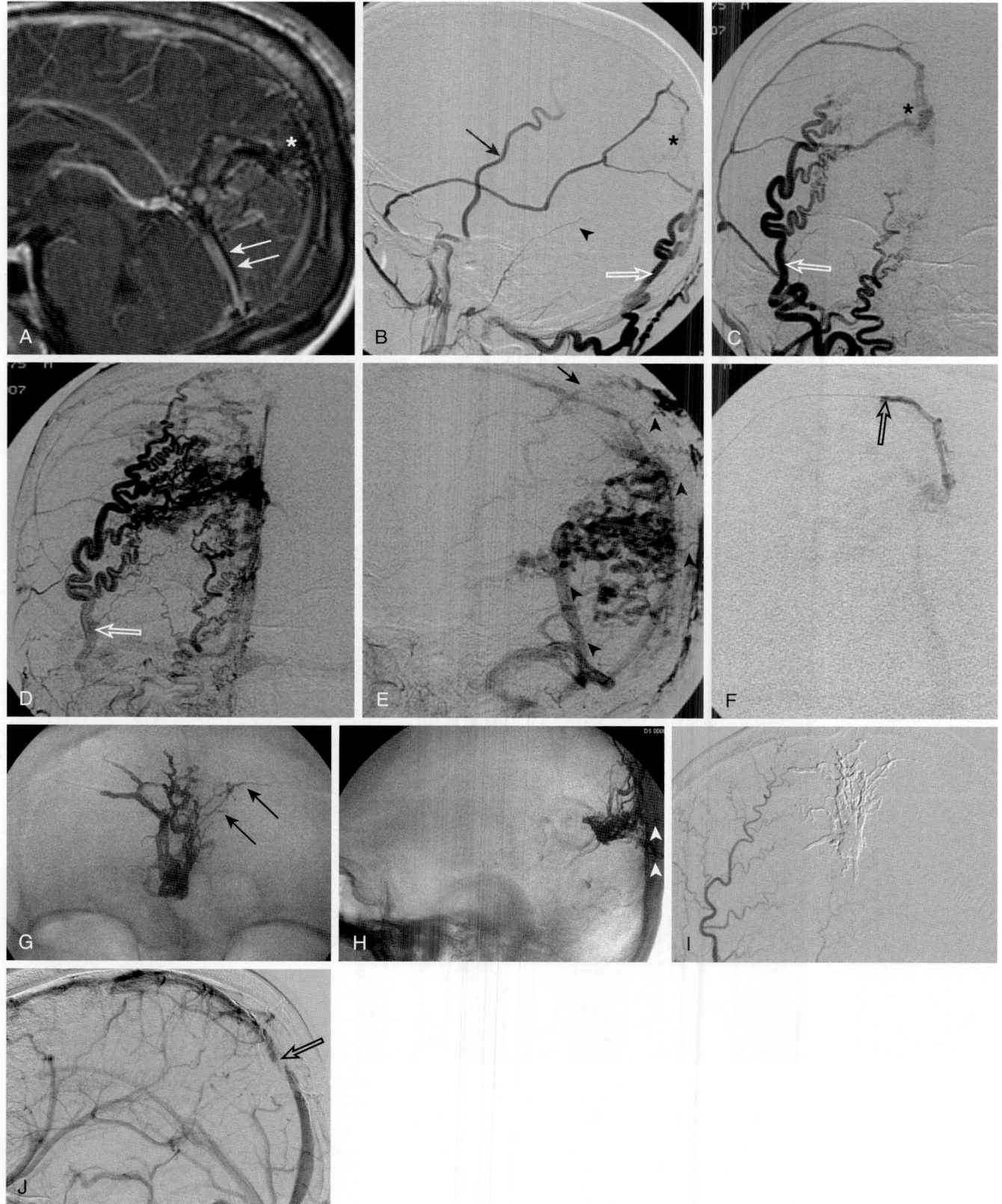

FIGURE 90-4 Onyx embolization of a DAVF involving the superior sagittal sinus. Pretreatment imaging studies: Midline sagittal postcontrast MRI (A) and right external carotid angiogram with lateral (B and E) and anteroposterior (C, D, and F) views. The MRI shows the presence of a falcine arteriovenous malformation (*asterisk*) draining into the straight sinus (*white arrows* in A and *black arrowheads* in E). The posterior branch of the middle meningeal artery runs over the convexity, reaching the falx before giving origin to the fistula (asterisk in B and C). A small meningeal retromastoid branch also reaches the fistula (*arrowhead* in B). Remarkable participation of extracranial vessels is present: The posterior branches of the superficial temporal artery (*black arrow* in B and E) and the external occipital artery (*open arrow* in B to D) are markedly dilated and tortuous; however, they contribute to the malformation only through tiny transosseous branches (*small arrowheads* in E). The same pattern is present on the left side (not shown). The posterior division of the right middle meningeal artery is superselectively catheterized with a microcatheter for Onyx injection (*arrow* in F). G to J, Post-treatment and follow-up studies. In the unsubstracted anteroposterior (G) and lateral views (H), the cast of Onyx fills the entire malformation, also occluding the contralateral arterial feeders (*arrows* in G) and the transosseous feeders (*arrowheads* in H). The 2-year follow-up right external carotid artery angiogram (anterior–posterior view in I) demonstrates persistent obliteration of the dural malformation. The lateral view of the right internal carotid angiogram (J) shows patency of the superior sagittal sinus. The false irregularities of the sinus profile (*arrow*) are due to superimposition of the Onyx cast.

normal venous drainage can lead to cerebral venous infarction and hemorrhage. Complete obliteration of the venous portion of the DAVF can lead to regression of the arterial feeders, which is in stark contrast to brain arteriovenous malformations, where occlusion of a draining vein can have serious consequences, including nidal rupture and bleeding.[17] However, care must be taken not to iatrogenically isolate the sinus involved in a DAVF, because this may worsen the CVR and increase the risk of hemorrhage. Sinus occlusion is safe if the affected region of the sinus is isolated, there is significant CVR, and the sinus segment is not responsible for venous drainage of normal brain.

Transvenous approaches are commonly used for fistulas involving the cavernous sinus, such as carotid–cavernous fistulas (CCFs). CCFs are categorized into direct (Barrow type A) and indirect (Barrow types B-D) types.[38] Indirect CCFs are dural fistulas with arterial feeders from the internal carotid artery (Barrow type B), external carotid artery (Barrow type C) (Fig. 90-5), or both (Barrow type D). For transvenous treatment of these lesions, numerous venous routes to the cavernous sinus are available: ipsilateral and contralateral inferior petrosal sinuses, basilar plexus, facial vein, superior ophthalmic vein (SOV), angular vein, and pterygoid plexus.[33] Selection of a transvenous route

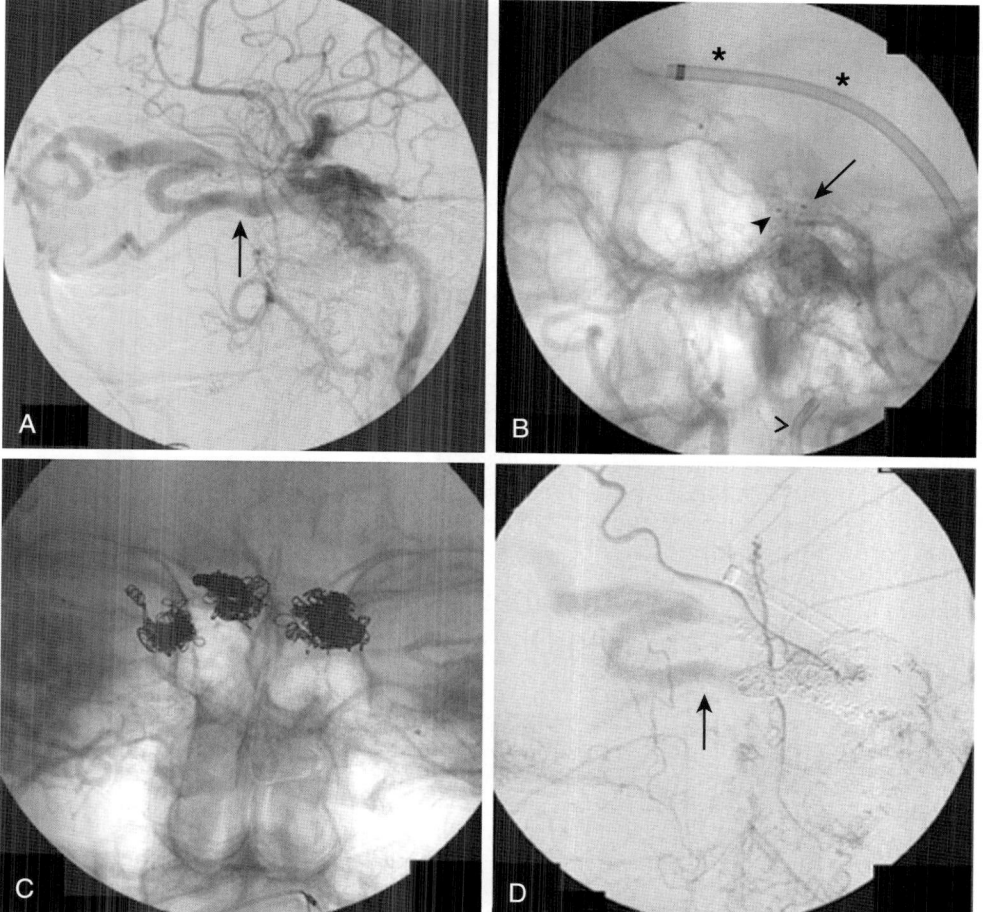

FIGURE 90-5 Transvenous microcoil embolization of an indirect CCF. A 45-year-old woman presented with progressive right-sided proptosis and ophthalmoplegia. A, Right common carotid injection (lateral view), demonstrating a Barrow type C CCF with venous reflux into the ophthalmic vein (*arrow*), SOV, and the inferior ophthalmic vein. B, Native lateral view demonstrating dual venous access to the cavernous sinus via the right superficial temporal vein (guide catheter labeled with *asterisks*) and SOV (microcatheter tip in cavernous sinus labeled with an *arrow*), as well as the left inferior petrosal sinus (guide catheter labeled with a > and microcatheter tip in the cavernous sinus labeled with an *arrowhead*). C, Native anterior–posterior view demonstrating coil masses in both sides of the cavernous sinus and the proximal right ophthalmic vein (42 coils total deployed). D, Right external carotid artery injection (lateral view) demonstrating near complete occlusion of the CCF with mild residual flow in the ophthalmic veins (*arrow*).

depends on the specific venous anatomy of the patient and the dominant venous outflow of the fistula. In general, percutaneous transfemoral–transvenous approaches should be attempted prior to other transvenous or combined surgical–transvenous approaches, such as the combined surgical–endovascular approach to the cavernous sinus via the SOV.[39] However, the latter techniques can be quite efficacious. The standard technique is to use retrograde catheterization along the internal jugular vein to approach the involved sinus.

Transvenous embolizations are commonly performed with similar equipment for access and catheterization as transarterial approaches. Yet arterial access and catheterization of the carotid or vertebral arteries is also helpful in transvenous procedures for visualization of the shunt site, road mapping, and control angiography during the embolization. Embolization agents commonly include microcoils, balloons, and liquid embolics.

A transvenous approach can be limited by sinus stenosis or occlusion, although recanalization is possible. Various techniques have been devised to accomplish transvenous embolization through an occluded sinus, such as embolization of a transverse sinus DAVF through an occluded sigmoid sinus. One method is recanalization of the occluded sinus with a stiff 0.035-inch guidewire, but perforation of the sinus is a potentially serious complication.[40,41] Recanalization using a microwire and microcatheter has also been successful and is presumed safer than using a stiff guidewire.[42] However, it is unknown whether true recanalization with a microwire versus navigation through existing small channels is being accomplished. Accessing the isolated sinus through a contralateral approach has also been described, but this technique is limited by the lengthy and tortuous route to the affected sinus.[43,44]

In cases where recanalization of a thrombosed sinus is unsuccessful, and the associated DAVF sinus is located close to the skin, a transcranial approach may be attempted.[35,45] Houdart et al.[35] reported a series of 10 patients who underwent craniectomy over the involved sinus in the operating room followed by sinus puncture with an 18-gauge angiocatheter, microcatheterization, and embolization. For the first case, catheterization was performed in the operating room immediately following the craniectomy; however, this case was complicated by a subdural hematoma. In all subsequent cases, the procedure was staged, with catheterization being done in the angiography suite under road map guidance 1 week after craniectomy. No further bleeding complications were reported. The authors note that a generous initial craniectomy is favorable, as 7 of the 10 patients in their series required enlargement of the craniectomy with repeat surgery. The craniectomy should allow distal sinus access to permit dense coil packing and an entry angle of 45 degrees for easy passage of the microcatheter.[35] As an alternative to the transcranial approach, novel venous routes to the involved sinus, such as the percutaneous transvenous approach through a mastoid emissary vein, have been described.[46]

Transvenous embolization procedures, such as those of the cavernous sinus, have certain risks, including dural dissection leading to hemorrhage and cranial nerve injury. Injury to cranial nerves III, V, and VI as they course through the cavernous sinus can occur secondary to thrombosis, elevated pressure, or coil/balloon overpacking in the cavernous sinus.[33] Similarly, navigation through the jugular foramen and inferior petrosal sinus could potentially result in damage to cranial nerves IX to XI. In addition, the SOV approach carries risks of visual loss, glaucoma, and acute exophthalmos.[47,48]

Follow-up angiography is recommended in patients following transvenous embolization of a DAVF, with resulting sinus occlusion to evaluate for recanalization of the treated DAVF and development of new DAVFs.[33] Sinus occlusion with microcoils and thrombosis might activate angiogenic factors, resulting in recurrence or de novo fistula formation.[49] Studies in rat models with experimentally induced venous hypertension have demonstrated increased dural angiogenesis and arteriovenous fistula formation, thought to be secondary to local cerebral hypoperfusion and ischemia.[50-51]

Outcomes of Transarterial Embolization with *n*-Butyl Cyanoacrylate

Transarterial embolization with *n*-BCA for DAVFs has a high cure rate, ranging from 64% to 100%, with some documented transient palsies but no permanent complications.[11,52,53] Guedin et al. treated 38 patients with DAVFs with CVR with solely transarterial cyanoacrylate glue (Histoacryl, B. Braun, Melsungen, Germany) or Glubran 2 (GEM, Viareggio, Italy) embolization. A complete cure was achieved after a single session in 76% (29/38) of patients. On average, 1.37 sessions per patient to complete treatment were required and 2.37 feeding vessels were embolized. The mean duration of injection was less than 1 minute. A cure rate of 89.5% (34/38) was reported with 29 patients achieving immediate cure and 5 patients demonstrating postembolization secondary thrombosis. Two transient cases of cerebellar syndrome were reported, but both patients recovered rapidly. The authors noted no permanent complications as well as no endovascular therapy related mortality.[11]

Agid et al. reported 11 patients with anterior cranial fossa DAVFs who were treated by transarterial catheterization through the ophthalmic artery and subsequent injection of *n*-BCA. Of these patients, 7 (63.6%) were completely cured with no reported complications.[52] Acrylic glue has proved effective and stable for use in endovascular procedures for more than 30 years. Some authors argue that glue compares advantageously, in terms of cost and long-term stability, to newer liquid agents such as Onyx.[11]

Outcomes of Transarterial Embolization with Onyx

Over the last several years, Onyx has been increasingly used in the endovascular treatment of DAVFs. Several large series have been published reporting cure rates between 61% and 91%, with complication rates between 0% and 16%. The volume of Onyx used per procedure ranged from 0.4 to 12.2 ml, and the duration of injection ranged from 7 to 100 minutes per pedicle.[24,29-31,54-58] Some authors have reported 100% cure rates of transarterial Onyx in small series, with no complications reported.[59,60]

In one series, the treatment of DAVF with CVR and transarterial Onyx in 30 patients was prospectively analyzed. Complete angiographic cure was observed in 80% (24/30) of cases, with 83% (20/24) of these cures achieved after a single procedure. The authors reported two complications: one postprocedure hemorrhage secondary to venous outlet thrombosis and one temporary cranial nerve palsy.[30]

The role of transarterial Onyx in patients with Cognard type I and II DAVFs has also been studied. Anatomic cure was achieved in 50% (13/26) patients, and clinical cure was achieved in 65.4% (17/26) patients. All anatomic cures were achieved in a single procedure, and follow-up angiography showed no recurrence. Complications included two cardiac Onyx migrations, two reflexive bradycardia episodes, one transient visual hallucination, two transient fifth nerve palsies, and one permanent seventh nerve palsy.[54] A rare side effect of Onyx embolization is trigeminocardiac reflex, which in one series had a reported rate of 10.7%.[61]

Outcomes of Transvenous Embolization of Indirect CCF

Since it was pioneered in the late 1970s by Mullan and Hosobuchi, the transvenous approach has become the preferred method of treatment of indirect CCFs.[62-64] The two largest series to date have demonstrated complete obliteration in 87% to 91% patients with indirect CCFs treated with transvenous coils and a procedure-related permanent morbidity of 0% to 2.3%.[65,66]

Studies analyzing the long-term outcome in patients who underwent coil embolization of CCFs have found a 44% rate of persistent cranial nerve deficits with disturbance of oculomotor and visual functions. Bink et al. noted a significant correlation between coil volume and persistent diplopia and persistent cranial nerve VI paresis.[67]

A major disadvantage of solely using coils is difficulty obtaining complete occlusion.[62] Wakhloo et al. evaluated the efficacy and safety of transvenous *n*-BCA alone or with coils in a series of 14 patients with indirect CCFs. Of the patients treated with *n*-BCA and coils, 88% (7/8) had complete angiographic obliteration of the CCF. Another 83% of patients (5/6) treated with *n*-BCA alone achieved immediate obliteration of the CCF. The remaining patient treated with *n*-BCA was noted to have thrombosed the residual internal carotid artery dural feeders at follow-up angiography 1 week later. One patient experienced a temporary worsening of clinical symptoms.[68]

Onyx has also been used as an adjunct to coils in transvenous embolization of indirect CCFs. Complete angiographic cure rates ranged from 67% to 100% with complications between 0% and 33%.[27,69-71] In one series, the authors prospectively studied eight patients with indirect CCFs who were treated with either transvenous Onyx alone (three patients) or a combination of Onyx and detachable coils (five patients). Complete fistula obliteration was achieved in all cases (100%) after a single session, as well as clinical resolution of the presenting symptoms in 100% of patients after 2 months. Some authors suggest the superiority of Onyx to coils alone or *n*-BCA because Onyx gradually permeates the sinus interstices and gradually precipitates from outside inward, allowing it to be injected more slowly and accurately. This allows interrupted injections, which in turn allow assessment of embolization patterns.[69] In addition, the procedure time and cost decrease significantly when Onyx is used with detachable coils as opposed to coils alone.[71]

The SOV has been described as an excellent and definitive alterative treatment in patients for whom traditional endovenous routes have failed. A rate of 90% embolization of CCFs that were previously unsuccessfully attempted has been reported.[72] Transorbital puncture has also been described in eight patients who underwent successful embolization of a CCF via the inferior ophthalmic vein.[73]

Conclusions

Endovascular management of DAVFs is a proven treatment technique. There are multiple approaches available to the surgeon, including a transvenous or transarterial approach. There are also a variety of agents available for use, including *n*-BCA, Onyx, and coils.

KEY REFERENCES

Agid R, Terbrugge K, Rodesch G, et al. Management strategies for anterior cranial fossa (ethmoidal) dural arteriovenous fistulas with an emphasis on endovascular treatment. *J Neurosurg.* 2009;110(1):79-84.

Arat A, Cekirge S, Saatci I, Ozgen B. Transvenous injection of Onyx for casting of the cavernous sinus for the treatment of a carotid–cavernous fistula. *Neuroradiology.* 2004;46:1012-1015.

Barrow DL, Spector RH, Braun IF, et al. Classification and treatment of spontaneous carotid–cavernous sinus fistulas. *J Neurosurg.* 1985; 62:248-256.

Bink A, Goller K, Luchtenberg M, et al. Long-term outcome after coil embolization of cavernous sinus arteriovenous fistulas. *AJNR Am J Neuroradiol.* 2010;31(7):1216-1221.

Borden JA, Wu JK, Shucart WA. A proposed classification for spinal and cranial dural arteriovenous fistulous malformations and implications for treatment. *J Neurosurg.* 1995;82:166-179.

Cognard C, Gobin YP, Pierot L, et al. Cerebral dural arteriovenous fistulas: clinical and angiographic correlation with a revised classification of venous drainage. *Radiology.* 1995;194:671-680.

Cognard C, Januel AC, Silva Jr NA, Tall P. Endovascular treatment of intracranial dural arteriovenous fistulas with cortical venous drainage: new management using Onyx. *AJNR Am J Neuroradiol.* 2008; 29:235-241.

Goddard AJ, Khangure MS. Multiple dural arteriovenous fistulas. Radiologic progression and endovascular cure. Case report. *Interv Neuroradiol.* 2002;8:183-191.

Guedin P, Gaillard S, Boulin A, et al. Therapeutic management of intracranial dural arteriovenous shunts with leptomeningeal venous drainage: report of 53 consecutive patients with emphasis on transarterial embolization with acrylic glue. *J Neurosurg.* 2010;112:603-610.

Houdart E, Saint-Maurice JP, Chapot R, et al. Transcranial approach for venous embolization of dural arteriovenous fistulas. *J Neurosurg.* 2002;97:280-286.

Jiang C, Lv X, Li Y, et al. Endovascular treatment of high-risk tentorial dural arteriovenous fistulas: clinical outcomes. *Neuroradiology.* 2009; 51:103-111.

Kirsch M, Liebig T, Kühne D, Henkes H. Endovascular management of dural arteriovenous fistulas of the transverse and sigmoid sinus in 150 patients. *Neuroradiology.* 2009;51:477-483.

Klisch J, Huppertz HJ, Spetzger U, et al. Transvenous treatment of carotid–cavernous and dural arteriovenous fistulae: results for 31 patients and review of the literature. *Neurosurgery.* 2003;53:836-856:discussion 856-857.

Lv X, Jiang C, Li Y, Wu Z. Results and complications of transarterial embolization of intracranial dural arteriovenous fistulas using Onyx-18. *J Neurosurg.* 2008;109:1083-1090.

Lv X, Jiang C, Li Y, et al. Intraarterial and intravenous treatment of transverse/sigmoid sinus dural arteriovenous fistulas. *Interv Neuroradiol.* 2009;15(3):291-300.

Macdonald JH, Millar JS, Barker CS. Endovascular treatment of cranial dural arteriovenous fistulae: a single-centre, 14-year experience and the impact of Onyx on local practise. *Neuroradiology.* 2009 Nov: [in press].

McConnell KA, Tjoumakaris SI, Allen J, et al. Neuroendovascular management of dural arteriovenous malformations. *Neurosurg Clin N Am.* 2009;20:431-439.

Meyers PM, Halbach VV, Dowd CF, et al. Dural carotid–cavernous fistula: definitive endovascular management and long-term follow-up. *Am J Ophthalmol.* 2002;134(1):85-92.

Moore C, Murphy K, Gailloud P. Improved distal distribution of *n*-butyl cyanoacrylate glue by simultaneous injection of dextrose 5% through the guiding catheter: technical note. *Neuroradiology.* 2006;48:327-332.

Morris P. *Practical Neuroangiography.* Philadelphia: Lippincott Williams & Wilkins; 2007.

Natarajan SK, Ghodke B, Kim LJ, et al. Multimodality treatment of intracranial dural arteriovenous fistulas in the Onyx era: a single center experience. *World Neurosurg.* 2010;73:365-379.

Nelson PK, Russell SM, Woo HH, et al. Use of a wedged microcatheter for curative transarterial embolization of complex intracranial dural arteriovenous fistulas: indications, endovascular technique, and outcome in 21 patients. *J Neurosurg.* 2003;98:498-506.

Nogueira RG, Dabus G, Rabinov JD, et al. Preliminary experience with Onyx embolization for the treatment of intracranial dural arteriovenous fistulas. *AJNR Am J Neuroradiol.* 2008;29:91-97.

Stiefel MF, Albuquerque FC, Park MS, et al. Endovascular treatment of intracranial dural arteriovenous fistulae using Onyx: a case series. *Neurosurgery.* 2009;65(Suppl 6):132-139:discussion 139-140.

Vinuela F, Dion JE, Duckwiler G, et al. Combined endovascular embolization and surgery in the management of cerebral arteriovenous malformations: experience with 101 cases. *J Neurosurg.* 1991;75: 856-864.

Numbered references appear on Expert Consult.

Endovascular Management of Spinal Vascular Malformations

ANITHA NIMMAGADDA • RUDY J. RAHME • ALI SHAIBANI •
GUILHERME DABUS • BERNARD R. BENDOK

Our knowledge of spinal vascular malformations has advanced significantly in the last century, and with this increased understanding of the anatomy and pathophysiology of this diverse group of lesions has come the advent of new classification schemes accompanied by a trend toward a multidisciplinary approach to the treatment of these rare disorders. Significant advances in spinal arteriography pioneered in the 1960s first allowed the detailed classification of these lesions based on their angiographic characteristics. The improved understanding of the anatomy of these lesions led to alterations in surgical technique and treatment. The last 2 decades have seen a gradual increase in the use of endovascular techniques as a primary treatment modality. This has been facilitated by advances in biplane imaging, embolic agents, microcatheters, and wires, and a more robust understanding of the pathophysiology and anatomy of these complex lesions. Despite these advances microsurgery and radiosurgery remain important tools in the multidisciplinary approach to these heterogeneous spinal pathologies. Moreover, advanced microcatheter angiography and sophisticated magnetic resonance imaging (MRI) and computed tomography (CT) axial imaging facilitate decision making and technique selection.

The first clinical report of a spinal vascular malformation was presented in 1890 by Berenbruch, who only recognized the lesion as a vascular malformation at autopsy.[1] Heboldt and Gaupp were the first to recognize that spinal vascular malformations could cause subarachnoid hemorrhage (SAH).[1] The first surgical treatment for a spinal vascular malformation was reported in 1916 by Elsberg.[2] In 1943, Wyburn-Mason described two distinct types of spinal vascular malformations: a venous type consisting of dilated, tortuous blue pial veins that was typically located posteriorly in the thoracic cord; and an arteriovenous type with a fistulous capillary bed located anteriorly in the cervical or lumbar enlargements. This was the first differentiation of spinal intramedullary arteriovenous malformations (AVMs) from spinal dural fistulas.[1] The first report of spinal angiography to characterize a spinal vascular malformation was published in 1962 by Djindjian and colleagues. Since that time, the use of spinal angiography as both a diagnostic and a therapeutic tool has become increasingly important in the management of spinal vascular malformations.

Spinal Vascular Anatomy

The arterial supply to the spine is primarily derived from the segmental arteries. There are 31 paired segmental arteries corresponding to the 31 somites into which the embryo divides (rostrocaudally) during the first few weeks of development. Each segmental artery provides blood supply to its corresponding metameric derivatives: muscle, skin, bone, spinal nerve, and spinal cord. At the start of embryologic development, each segmental artery has a branch that supplies the cord. Over time, most of these branches regress, so that by the completion of embryologic development, of the 62 segmental arteries, 4 to 8 supply the anterior spinal artery and 10 to 20 supply the posterior spinal arteries.

The anterior spinal artery extends along the ventral spinal axis for the entire length of the spinal cord. Its caudal extension is known as the artery of the filum terminale. It may be recognized angiographically by its characteristic midline hairpin appearance. The normal anterior spinal artery diameter is in the range of 110 to 340 μm. The anterior spinal artery gives origin to between 200 and 400 sulcocommissural arteries, which lie within the ventral sulcus of the spinal cord. From the ventral sulcus, the arteries enter the central gray matter, at which point they give off branches to the peripheral white matter. Each sulcocomissural artery supplies either the right or the left side of the spinal cord. The sulcocommissural arteries supply the ventral half of the cord and the gray matter. The dorsal half of the spinal cord is supplied by branches of the paired posterior spinal arteries. Angiographically the posterior spinal arteries may be recognized by a similar but smaller hairpin appearance located laterally.

Each segmental artery accompanies its corresponding nerve into the neural foramen. Each segmental artery divides into dural and radicular arteries. The radicular artery provides supply to the dorsal and ventral nerve roots. Some segmental arteries provide supply to the spinal cord via branches connecting to the pial/coronal arterial network and are designated radiculopial arteries. Some segmental arteries provide direct supply to the anterior spinal artery and are designated radiculomedullary arteries. The two most significant radiculomedullary arteries are the artery of cervical enlargement and the artery of lumbar enlargement, also known as the arteria radicularis magna or the artery of Adamkiewicz.[3]

Venous drainage occurs through the radial and coronal veins, which in turn drain into the primary dorsal and ventral longitudinal collecting veins, which drain into the radicular veins, which drain into the ventral epidural venous plexus. The radial veins are also connected by lateral longitudinal veins. The ventral epidural venous plexus is a valveless system in which the direction of flow depends on the outflow vein at each anatomic level. In the cervical spine, the epidural venous plexus drains into the vertebral veins, which empty into the innominate veins. In the thoracic spine, the epidural venous plexus drains into the intercostal veins, which then drain into the azygos and hemiazygos veins. In the lumbar spine, the epidural venous plexus drains into the ascending lumbar vein, the azygos and hemiazygos veins, and the left renal vein. In the sacral spine, the epidural venous plexus drains into the sacral veins, which eventually empty into the internal iliac veins.

Classification of Spinal Vascular Malformations

The classification of spinal vascular malformations has evolved significantly over the last 150 years as the understanding of the complex pathophysiology of these lesions has continued to improve. The initial classification schemes that were proposed failed to properly categorize the lesions based on their anatomy. The first classification scheme for spinal vascular lesions was proposed by Virchow in 1858.[4] Virchow subdivided vascular lesions into two types: angioma cavernosum (lesion without parenchyma between the blood vessels) and angioma racemosum (hamartoma: lesion with parenchyma between the blood vessels). Elsberg, in 1916, was the next to propose a classification scheme for spinal vascular lesions in which he divided them into three categories: aneurysm of spinal vessels, angioma in which a mass of dilated veins penetrates the spinal cord, and dilation of posterior spinal veins. In 1928, Cushing and Bailey proposed yet another classification system in which they divided spinal vascular lesions into two major groups: hemangioblastomas and vascular malformations. The broad group of vascular malformations included plexus of dilated veins, aneurismal varix, venous angioma, and telangiectasias.

Advances in neurointerventional surgery and microneurosurgery during the 1960s and 1970s combined with a clearer understanding of the true pathophysiology of spinal vascular lesions led to the development of a new classification system that divided spinal vascular malformations into types I to IV. This system, which is still widely used today, did not include neoplastic lesions (Table 91-1). The classification system proposed by Rodesch and colleagues divided spinal vascular malformations into three groups: AVMs, fistulas, and genetic classification of spinal cord arteriovenous shunts.[5] The last group was further subdivided into three groups: genetic hereditary lesions (macrofistulas and hereditary hemorrhagic telangectasia), genetic nonhereditary lesions (multiple lesions with metameric or myelomeric associations), and single lesions (incomplete associations of either of the first two categories). The classification system for spinal vascular lesions proposed by Spetzler and colleagues also subdivided the lesions into four large groups: neoplasms, spinal aneurysms,

---

Table 91-1 Common Classification of Spinal Vascular Malformations

Type I: Dural AVF
Type IA: Single arterial feeder
Type IB: Multiple arterial feeders
Type II: True AVMs of the Spinal Cord
Structurally similar to cerebral AVMs
Type III: Juvenile AVMs or Metameric AVMs
More diffuse lesions than type II
Type IV: Pial AVF
Perimedullary, intradural
High-flow fistulas
Type IV A: Solitary AVF fed by the ASA
Type IV B: Small group of AVFs
· Supplied by anterior and posterior spinal arteries
· Located at the conus
Type IV C: Single large AVF
· Supplied by the anterior and posterior spinal arteries
· Located in the cervical or thoracic spinal cord

AVF, Arteriovenous fistula; AVM, arteriovenous malformation; ASA, anterior spinal artery.

---

spinal AVMs, and spinal fistulas.[6] Arteriovenous fistulas (AVFs) were further subdivided into extradural and intradural (dorsal or ventral). AVMs were further classified into extradural-intradural or intradural. Intradural AVMs were further subclassified as intramedullary, compact, diffuse, and conus medullaris. This separate classification of conus medullaris AVMs is unique to the Spetzler system.[6]

Of these classification systems, the type I through IV system remains the most commonly used. Type 1 spinal vascular malformations are actually dorsal intradural AVFs with the fistulas located in the proximal dura of the nerve root sleeve. These malformations are the most common spinal vascular malformation. They are subdivided into type A, in which the malformation is supplied by a single arterial feeder, and type B, in which the malformation is supplied by multiple arterial feeders.[7] They occur most commonly in the lower thoracic and upper lumbar segments of the spinal cord, T4–L3, with the peak incidence between T7 and T12.[8]

In type IA malformations, the fistula is formed by an anastomosis of a dural branch of a radicular artery (very rarely a radiculomedullary artery) and a radiculomedullary vein.

In type IB malformations, there are anastomoses between branches of several adjacent radicular arteries and a radiculomedullary vein. The radiculomedullary vein becomes arterialized owing to increased flow and pressure, which it transmits to the valveless coronal plexus and the longitudinal veins. The radiculomedullary vein becomes enlarged and tortuous, leading to its classic angiographic appearance. Studies have shown that the mean intraluminal venous pressure is increased to 74% of the systemic arterial pressure.[9] The normal pressure in the coronal venous plexus is approximately twice that of the epidural venous plexus. This significant pressure gradient is necessary for normal venous drainage. When it is compromised, as in the case of type I spinal AVMs, venous hypertension develops. Venous hypertension then leads to the development of progressive myelopathy due to transmission of increased venous pressure to the spinal cord parenchyma, resulting in multiple pathologic changes including demyelination.

Type II spinal vascular malformations are true AVMs of the spinal cord with multiple arterial feeders, a nidus, and draining vein(s). They are structurally similar to cerebral AVMs. They are the second most common spinal vascular malformation. They are high-flow, low-resistance, high-pressure lesions.[6] The arterial feeders are usually branches of the anterior spinal artery or the posterior spinal arteries.

Type III spinal vascular malformations, also known as juvenile AVMs or metameric AVMs, are more diffuse lesions that can encircle the entire spinal cord. Involvement of all the derivatives of a metamere in the AVM (skin, bone, muscle, dura, nerve roots, and spinal cord) has been described as Cobb's syndrome.

Spinal artery aneurysms or venous aneurysms are found in 20% to 40% of patients with intramedullary AVMs. The presence of a spinal artery aneurysm has been associated with an increased risk of hemorrhage.[10]

Type IV spinal vascular malformations are actually perimedullary AVFs and were first described by Djindjian and colleagues. The fistula occurs ventrally and in the midline between the anterior spinal artery and the coronal venous plexus.[11] In contrast to type I dural AVFs, type IV lesions are high-flow fistulas. These lesions are further classified into three subtypes. Type A (Merland subtype I) is a solitary AVF fed by the anterior spinal artery (ASA) and located at the conus medullaris or the filum terminale. There is moderate venous hypertension without enlargement of the ASA. The ascending draining vein is only minimally dilated. Type B (Merland subtype II) is a small group of AVFs located at the conus and supplied by the anterior and posterior spinal arteries. The feeding arteries and draining veins are moderately dilated. Venous ectasia is present at the site of the fistula, and the ascending perimedullary veins are tortuous and enlarged. Type C (Merland subtype III) is a single large AVF supplied by the anterior and posterior spinal arteries and located in the cervical or thoracic spinal cord.[12] The draining vein is significantly dilated and ectatic and may be embedded within the spinal cord.

Clinical Presentation and Natural History

Type I spinal dural AVFs typically manifest with signs and symptoms of progressive myelopathy. They are more common in men and usually present in the sixth decade of life. Gradually worsening paraparesis accompanied by sensory loss is the most common presentation. Patients can also present with back pain, leg pain, sphincter dysfunction, and sexual dysfunction. Although gradual progression of symptoms is the most likely presentation, patients can present with acute exacerbation of their symptoms. Hemorrhage is very rare.

Type II spinal AVMs typically manifest with hemorrhage, intramedullary or subarachnoid, which results in acute myelopathy. Patients can also present with progressive myelopathy secondary to arterial steal. Pain may also be a presenting symptom. The majority of patients present before age 40 years. Type II spinal AVMs demonstrate no gender preference.

Type III spinal AVMs, similar to type II spinal AVMs, can manifest with hemorrhage resulting in acute neurologic deficit or with progressive myelopathy secondary to steal phenomenon. They occur more commonly in children.

Type IV spinal vascular malformations commonly manifest with progressive paraparesis secondary to myelopathy caused by venous congestion, but they can also manifest with acute neurologic deficit secondary to rupture of a feeding artery aneurysm. They occur more commonly in adults but can be seen in children.[10] Patients typically present before the age of 40 years.

Osler-Weber-Rendu syndrome (hereditary hemorrhagic telangectasisa) type 1 is an autosomal dominant disorder associated with spinal arteriovenous shunts. The syndrome is typically associated with type IV, subtype C intradural AVFs. Klippel-Trenaunay and Parkes-Weber syndromes are associated with vascular malformations of the lower limbs and can involve spinal cord vascular malformations.[3]

The pathophysiology of spinal vascular malformations was elegantly detailed by Aminoff and Logue[13] in a paper published in 1974 in which they refuted the previous theories of compression of the cord by the malformation being the primary cause of symptoms and argued that the most likely mechanism of neurologic deterioration was secondary to ischemia caused by venous hypertension. Aminoff and Logue further argued that support could be garnered for this theory by the fact most symptomatic spinal vascular malformations are located in the lower thoracic or thoracolumbar spine, where there are fewer large veins draining into the coronal plexus, compared to the cervical or upper thoracic spine. Histopathologic support for this theory has subsequently been provided by Matsuo and colleagues, who performed autopsies on three patients with progressive myelopathy and found evidence of venous congestive myelopathy. The spinal cord parenchyma at the affected levels demonstrated neuronal loss and gliosis with increased numbers of hyalinized vessels.[14] Autopsy also demonstrated tortuous, dilated venous vessels on the dorsal surface of the spinal cord at the affected levels.

Endovascular Management
TECHNIQUE

Spinal angiography is still the gold standard for the diagnosis of spinal vascular malformations, but recent advances in MRI and CT imaging have allowed diagnostic spinal angiograms to become more focused anatomically.[15] However, if a vascular lesion is suspected, and MRI does not provide localizing information, a thorough spinal angiogram including possible evaluation of the aortic arch, the descending aorta, the abdominal aorta, the pelvic vasculature including the iliac arteries and the median sacral artery, the vertebral arteries, the thyrocervical trunk, and the deep and ascending cervical arteries should be considered in addition to injection of the segmental arteries at each spinal level. The artery of Adamkiewicz should also be identified. An aortogram is occasionally helpful in the setting of an atherosclerotic or dilated aorta where segmental artery catheterization may be difficult and may be performed by using a pigtail catheter. Selective catheterization of the segmental arteries may be accomplished by a variety of catheters including but not limited to a 5-Fr H1, C1, or C2. Spinal angiograms are typically acquired in an anteroposterior projection, but biplane angiography can be used for three-dimensional localization of pathologic vasculature. It is especially important to study both the arterial and venous phases during evaluation for a spinal vascular malformation. Prolonged imaging in the venous phase of the angiogram may be necessary to diagnose fistulas with slower flow (e.g., type I).

At our institution, the majority of embolizations of spinal cord vascular malformations are performed under general anesthesia with neurophysiologic monitoring. The use of intraprocedural motor evoked potentials (MEPs) and somatosenory evoked potentials (SSEPs) to monitor spinal cord function during embolization of spinal cord vascular malformations has been studied in the literature with good results.[16,17] Intraprocedural neurophysiologic monitoring provides a method by which to assess the patient's neurologic function during embolization under general anesthesia. In 2004, Niimi and colleagues reported their experience with MEP and SSEP monitoring in conjunction with provocative testing with amytal and lidocaine during embolization of spinal cord AVMs. The group also monitored BCRs (bulbocavernosus reflexes) in patients with conus lesions. Niimi and colleagues performed 84 angiographic procedures in 52 patients and found that the use of neurophysiologic monitoring in conjunction with provocative testing had a high negative predictive value (97.6%).[16]

TYPE I FISTULAS

Surgical results are outstanding for this type of lesion; hence the bar for endovascular treatment is high. The first endovascular treatment of a spinal dural AVF was performed by Doppman and colleagues, who reported the embolization of a spinal dural AVF using metal pellets in 1968.[18] Since then many other embolic agents have been used with varying degrees of success. Polyvinyl alcohol (PVA) was one of the initial agents used but soon fell out of favor because of high recurrence rates and was quickly replaced by n-butyl cyanoacrylate (nBCA) (Codman, Raynham, MA), which became increasingly popular as an embolic agent. More recently, the use of Onyx (ev3 Inc, Plymouth, MN) for treatment of spinal dural AVFs has gained favor.

Narvid and colleagues[19] retrospectively reviewed their single institution experience over 20 years with the treatment of spinal dural AVFs. Between 1984 and 2005, they treated 63 patients for this condition. The diagnosis of spinal dural AVF was confirmed by spinal angiography in all patients. Thirty-nine patients underwent initial endovascular embolization, and 24 patients underwent surgical treatment initially. Of the 39 patients initially treated with embolization, 27 achieved complete obliteration of the fistula. Of the 12 patients who did not achieve complete obliteration, four were planned preoperative embolizations, and three were patients treated early in the series with PVA who required surgery for permanent obliteration. The remaining five patients demonstrated residual filling of the draining vein despite embolization. Of the 24 patients treated with surgery initially, 20 patients required no further treatment of their fistula. Of the four patients in the surgery group who required further treatment, one was successfully embolized and the other three required reoperation to obliterate the fistula. Embolization

was not attempted in patients who had common origin of the feeding artery and the anterior spinal artery. The first four patients treated endovascularly were treated with PVA. All subsequent treatments were performed with nBCA and lipiodol. If embolization failed to occlude the fistula, patients were referred for surgical treatment.

Aminoff-Logue scale (ALS) scores were used to clinically assess all patients before and after treatment. Significant improvements in ALS scores were seen in both endovascular and surgical groups, with no difference between the two groups in degree of improvement. Compared to the surgical group, a decrease in hospital stay was seen in the endovascular group. The mean hospital stay for patients in the endovascular group was 3.1 days, and in the surgical group the mean hospital stay was 9.8 days. The mean follow-up period was 49 months and improvement in ALS scores was preserved over the follow-up period. Based on these results, Narvid and colleagues concluded that treatment of spinal dural AVFs, whether endovascular or surgical, resulted in significant clinical improvement for patients that was maintained over a long-term follow-up period.

Niimi and colleagues[20] retrospectively reviewed 49 cases of spinal dural AVF treated by embolization at their institution between 1980 and 1995. The diagnosis of spinal dural AVF was made by spinal angiography in all cases. An acrylic material (isobutyl cyanoacrylate [IBCA] or nBCA) was used in 47 of the 49 cases, and variable stiffness microcatheters were used in 38 of the 49 cases. Initial embolization was deemed "adequate" in 39/49 cases (80%). Adequate embolization was defined as embolization with a liquid embolic agent in which the agent penetrated the fistula and draining vein with angiographic disappearance of the fistula without compromise of the venous drainage of the spinal cord. The initial success rate of embolization increased to 87% (33/38 cases) after variable stiffness microcatheters were introduced. Eight patients with initially "adequate" embolization required repeat embolization. Of the 10 cases that were initially "inadequately" embolized, 5 had been treated prior to the use of variable stiffness microcatheters and three demonstrated common origin of the arterial feeder and the ASA or posterior spinal artery (PSA), making "adequate" embolization difficult without incurring high risk. No patient developed neurologic complications as a result of embolization. No technical complications occurred after the introduction of variable stiffness microcatheters. Mean duration of follow-up post-treatment was 52 months for 29 patients. For 6 patients, follow-up was within 1 month of treatment, and for 14 patients follow-up was obtained between 1 and 12 months. No patient worsened clinically after treatment, and all except one improved clinically after treatment. A shorter duration of symptoms before treatment seemed to correlate with better clinical outcome, a finding that has since been noted in other similar studies.

Based on these results, Niimi and colleagues concluded that embolization with an acrylic material should be offered as the first-line treatment for spinal dural AVF unless there was common origin of the arterial feeder and the ASA or PSA and that patients should be followed long-term for potential recurrence. Niimi and colleagues argued that embolization was less invasive than surgery, that secondary to the advent of variable stiffness microcatheters and liquid embolic agents, embolization could be safely performed with a high cure rate, and that surgery could still be offered to a patient if embolization failed without increasing the difficulty or risk of the surgical procedure.

Ushikoshi and colleagues[21] performed a retrospective review of 13 patients with spinal dural AVFs treated at their institution with surgery, embolization, or embolization and surgery. Six patients were treated with surgery alone. Seven patients were initially treated with embolization. In six of these patients, nBCA was the embolic agent used. Four of the six patients treated with nBCA achieved complete occlusion. Embolization was unsuccessful in two patients treated with nBCA and these patients subsequently underwent surgery. One patient was treated with PVA and coils as planned preoperative embolization to decrease flow in a high-flow spinal dural AVF. Functional outcome was measured using the ALS score 6 months after treatment. In the surgical group, permanent neurologic complication occurred in one patient who suffered from brainstem hemorrhage 1 day after surgical treatment of a dural AVF fed by the left C1 segmental artery. Gait improvement was demonstrated in 6 of 10 patients who presented with gait disturbances. No patient experienced worsening of gait disturbance. Of the six patients who presented with bladder dysfunction, three experienced improvement in their symptoms after treatment. Based on these results, Ushikoshi and colleagues concluded that embolization should be offered as a first-line treatment for spinal dural AVF when the feeding artery did not share a common origin with the ASA or PSA. If embolization did not achieve complete obliteration, surgery should be undertaken without delay.

Andres and colleagues[22] performed a retrospective review of 21 patients at their institution who were treated for spinal dural AVFs with either surgery, embolization, or surgery after incomplete embolization. All patients underwent spinal angiography to confirm the presence of a spinal dural AVF. Thirteen patients were treated with embolization alone, four patients were treated with surgery, and four patients were treated with surgery after incomplete embolization. The four patients who were treated initially with surgery were deemed to be at high risk for endovascular treatment because of severe atherosclerosis, tortuous or small vessels that would be difficult to catheterize, or common origin of the anterior spinal artery and the feeding artery of the fistula. Median follow-up duration was 26 months after treatment. nBCA was the embolic agent employed. Patients were examined before and after treatment using the ALS score for myelopathy. Clinical outcome was also assessed using the modified Rankin scale (mRS). Patients treated with either embolization alone or surgery alone showed an improvement in both ALS and mRS scores after treatment. Patients treated with surgery after incomplete embolization showed improvement in only the ALS score after treatment. The failure rate of embolization was 23.5% (4/17). Based on these results, Andres and colleagues concluded that endovascular and surgical treatment both resulted in good, lasting clinical outcomes for patients and that the treatment modality for each patient should be determined by an interdisciplinary team after an initial spinal angiogram.

Sherif and colleagues[23] performed a retrospective review of 26 patients with spinal dural AVFs treated at their institution. All spinal dural AVFs were demonstrated on spinal angiogram after the diagnosis was suspected on MR imaging. Embolization was offered as the primary treatment in 19 cases. Seven patients underwent surgical treatment. Embolization was performed with a mixture of 33% Histoacryl and 66% Lipiodol, which was slowly injected until the material penetrated the draining vein or reflux occurred into the feeding artery. Surgery was offered to patients who had severe atheromatous disease, patients with recurrent dural AVF after embolization, patients with common origin of the feeding artery and the ASA or PSA, and patients in whom it was felt that endovascular embolization was likely to be unsuccessful based on the angioarchitecture of the fistula. Clinical examinations were performed before and after treatment using the ALS and mRS scores. All patients underwent follow-up spinal angiography and follow-up MR imaging. Mean duration of radiographic follow-up was 91.5 months. Of the 19 patients who were initially treated with embolization, two patients required retreatment. One patient developed collateral feeding arteries requiring reembolization. Another patient demonstrated recanalization of the fistula owing to incomplete occlusion of the draining vein and underwent surgical occlusion of the fistula. Neither of these patients suffered a setback in their long-term clinical outcome secondary to fistula recurrence.

Mean duration of clinical follow-up was 103.4 months. The mRS scale score did not worsen in any patient and improved in 13/17 patients (76.5%) after treatment. Gait scores improved in 21/26 patients (80.7%) after treatment, sensation improved in 13/21 patients (61.9%), and bladder and bowel dysfunction improved in 4/14 patients (28.6%). The improvements seen in the ALS scores and mRS scores after treatment were statistically significant ($p < 0.05$). Sherif and colleagues noted that their study demonstrated that patients who were treated with embolization had good long-term clinical results comparable to those achieved in surgical series with long-term results and that the recurrence of a spinal dural AVF after endovascular treatment did not adversely affect clinical outcome after retreatment. Based on these results, Sherif and colleagues recommended that a multidisciplinary approach should be applied to the treatment of spinal dural AVFs, with embolization being offered as first-line treatment when feasible.

Song and colleagues[24] performed a retrospective review of 30 patients with spinal dural AVFs treated at their institution between 1985 and 1999. Sixteen patients underwent embolization, seven patients underwent surgery, and seven patients underwent surgery after failed embolization. Of the seven patients who required surgery after embolization, two patients failed embolization during the initial treatment and were taken to surgery the next day. In the remaining five patients, the fistula recurred via collateral circulation as shown on follow-up angiography. nBCA was the embolic agent used in all procedures performed after 1990 (21/27 embolizations in 20/23 patients who underwent embolization). Before 1990, PVA, Gelfoam, or silicone were used as embolic agents. Twenty-six follow-up angiograms were performed in 19 patients. Seven of these angiograms demonstrated recurrence of the dural AVF, five of which were post-embolization and two of which were post-surgical. Mean clinical follow-up was 3.4 years. Clinical outcomes were assessed using the ALS score before and after treatment. Seventeen patients demonstrated improvement in gait, 12 were unchanged, and 1 demonstrated worsening of gait. There was no significant improvement in micturition scores unless treatment was initiated within 13 months of symptom onset. No significant differences in clinical outcome were noted between treatment groups: surgery alone, embolization alone, or combined embolization and surgery. Patients in all three groups demonstrated improvement in gait, which was sustained during the follow-up period.

ARTERIOVENOUS MALFORMATIONS

Konan and colleagues[25] reported five cases of embolization of spinal artery aneurysms associated with spinal cord AVMs in four patients. All four patients presented with hemorrhage: two with hematomyelia and two with SAH only. Three aneurysms were located on branches of the anterior spinal artery and two aneurysms were located in radiculopial arteries. All aneurysms were embolized with a mixture of nBCA and Lipiodol. Follow-up angiograms were obtained in all patients 3 to 6 months after treatment. No aneurysm recurrence was noted on follow-up angiography. Clinical follow-up ranged from 17 to 37 months. No rebleeding episodes or complications occurred during the follow-up period. Based on these results, Konan and colleagues concluded that aneurysms associated with spinal cord AVMs could be successfully embolized and that treatment of these aneurysms might decrease the risk of rebleeding in patients who could not be offered definitive surgical resection because of its high risk.

Spinal cord AVMs are notoriously difficult lesions to treat and often involve high risk of surgical morbidity. The poor natural history of these lesions combined with their relative high risk prompted neurointerventionalists to investigate possible endovascular approaches to the treatment of these lesions. In 1971, Doppman and colleagues reported on the use of percutaneous embolization for the treatment of seven patients.[26] Doppman and colleagues used metallic pellets, Gelfoam, and muscle fragments to occlude feeding arteries to the spinal cord AVM. The procedure was performed under local anesthesia. Percutaneous embolization was successful in five of the seven patients. The two patients who failed embolization were treated early in the series prior to the development of a system of coaxial catheters that allowed the use of larger pellets for embolization, providing proper occlusion of the feeding arteries. None of the seven patients experienced any neurologic decline, and three of the seven experienced progressive neurologic improvement. Based on these results, Doppman and colleagues concluded that percutaneous embolization of spinal cord AVMs was a reasonable option when total excision was not surgically feasible.

In 1990, Biondi and colleagues[27] reported their experience with particle embolization for the treatment of thoracic intramedullary AVMs. As expected with particle embolization, there were several instances of recanalization. They performed a retrospective review of 40 patients with thoracic intramedullary AVMs treated at their institution between 1978 and 1990. Of the 40 patients, 35 underwent embolization, 4 underwent surgery, and 1 did not receive either treatment. PVA particles were employed for the vast majority of the embolization procedures, but Gelfoam, silk threads, and microspheres were occasionally used. Follow-up angiography was performed 6 months after the initial embolization. The duration of mean follow-up after initial embolization

was 6 years. Twenty-nine of the 35 patients required multiple sessions of embolization. The number of embolizations in each patient ranged from 1 to 15 (mean, 4.5).

Before liquid embolic agents were introduced, the initial results of embolization for treatment of spinal cord vascular malformations were dismal, with significantly high rates of recurrence leading many to conclude that embolization was an unsuccessful treatment with a high rate of failure. Hall and colleagues[28] reported a series of three patients with spinal cord intramedullary glomus-type AVMs and three patients with spinal dural AVFs treated with PVA, five of whom demonstrated recurrence. Hall and colleagues concluded based on these results that embolization provided only temporary treatment and that surgery should be considered the treatment of choice when feasible. However, this study was conducted prior to the use of liquid embolic agents. More recent studies have demonstrated significantly better results for the treatment of spinal cord vascular malformations.[29-32]

The first report of the use of Onyx for treatment of a spinal vascular malformation was in 2000 from Molyneux and colleagues.[2,33] Corkill and colleagues subsequently reported on the use of Onyx in a larger series of patients.[2] In this retrospective review, Corkill and colleagues analyzed the records of 17 patients treated with Onyx embolization of spinal intramedullary AVMs. Thirteen patients underwent a single session of embolization and four patients underwent two sessions of embolization. There were two intraprocedural complications, which did not result in permanent neurologic sequelae. Mean follow-up interval was 24.3 months. Total obliteration of the AVM was achieved in six patients (37.5%), subtotal obliteration was achieved in five patients (31.25%), and partial obliteration was achieved in five patients (31.25%). Functional or neurologic status (or both) improved in 14 patients, resulting in a good clinical outcome for 82% of the study group. Based on these results, Corkill and colleagues concluded that Onyx embolization was a promising new treatment for spinal intramedullary AVMs.

Several studies have also examined the endovascular treatment of type IV spinal cord AVMs.[12,34] In 1993, Mourier and colleagues reported their experience with surgical and endovascular treatment of type IV spinal cord AVMs. Of the 35 patients they treated between 1970 and 1990, 4 patients were classified as Merland type I, 9 patients were classified as Merland type II, and 22 patients were classified as Merland type III.[12] Thirty-two of the patients presented with progressive neurologic symptoms and three patients presented with subarachnoid hemorrhage only. All of the Merland type III patients were treated with endovascular detachable silicone balloon occlusion of the fistula. Of the nine Merland type II patients, two were treated with embolization alone, and three were treated with surgery after incomplete embolization. One of the Merland type I patients was treated with endovascular embolization. Complete occlusion was achieved in all treated Merland type I and type II cases and in 15 of the type III cases. The 15 patients with Merland type III AVF that were completely embolized recovered completely. Two patients with Merland type III AVF worsened after incomplete occlusion, and one patient died after attempted endovascular obliteration of a cervical Merland type III AVF.

Halbach and colleagues also reported in 1993 on a series of 10 patients with Merland type II and type III perimedullary AVFs treated with embolization alone (three patients) or with embolization and surgical resection (seven patients).[34] Of the 10 patients, five presented with progressive myelopathy, four presented with subarachnoid hemorrhage, and one presented with acute paraplegia. Two patients had Merland type II perimedullary fistulas and the remaining eight patients had Merland type III perimedullary fistulas. Sixteen embolization procedures were performed: 14 via transarterial routes, and 2 via transvenous routes. Complete occlusion was achieved in seven of the patients, incomplete occlusion was achieved in two patients, and one patient refused follow-up angiography. One patient suffered transient worsening of paraplegia after rupture of the anterior spinal artery by a detachable balloon. The mean follow-up period was 44.8 months (range, 3 to 112 months).

Type II and type III spinal cord AVMs are characteristically difficult to treat via conventional microsurgical and endovascular techniques. Hence, there has been significant interest in the use of stereotactic radiosurgery to treat these lesions. Stereotactic radiosurgery is thought to induce gradual endothelial hyperplasia, which eventually causes vessel narrowing and occlusion. Initial reluctance to use stereotactic radiosurgery to treat spinal cord vascular malformations stemmed from concern for spinal cord injury secondary to radiation toxicity. Sinclair and colleagues reported a series of 15 patients with intramedullary spinal cord AVMs treated with multisession cyberknife radiosurgery.[35] Multisession radiosurgery was employed with the hope that allowing time between sessions would permit normal tissue repair, thus increasing the dose that could be administered to the AVM nidus because of increased radiation tolerance of the adjacent normal spinal cord. Patients were treated with an average marginal dose of 20.5 Gr over two to five sessions. Clinical and radiographic (MRI) follow-up were performed annually. Spinal angiography was repeated after 3 years. The mean follow-up period was 27.9 months (range, 3 to 59 months). Of the seven patients who were 3 years or more from treatment, six had significant reductions in the size of their lesions. Of the five patients who underwent post-treatment spinal angiograms, one patient showed complete obliteration of a conus medullaris AVM. No patient suffered a hemorrhage or neurologic deterioration after cyberknife treatment. Sinclair and colleagues were thus able to demonstrate that stereotactic radiosurgery for the treatment of intramedullary spinal cord AVMs is safe and feasible, but more studies are needed to further validate this approach.

Conclusion

Significant advances have been made in the treatment of spinal vascular malformations and fistulas during the last century. A more comprehensive understanding of the anatomy and pathophysiology of these lesions has led to a clearer classification system, which in turn has improved our ability to appropriately categorize these lesions. Advances in diagnostic neuroradiology have facilitated lesion classification and has reduced the need in many cases for extensive spinal angiograms. The current treatment of spinal dural AVFs involves the integration of multiple techniques including microsurgery, endovascular surgery, and radiosurgery. Future directions depend on further refinements in treatment technologies. In open surgery, minimally invasive

approaches might add benefit. For endovascular therapy, further refinements in biplane angiography and its integration with other modalities such as MRI hold great promise. Better embolic agents that might play a biological role or sensitize a lesion to radiation may be the next revolutionary advances. Radiosurgery is perhaps the least explored modality for spinal vascular malformations and will likely see a growing role in the next decade. Ultimately, continued thoughtful integration of all tools holds the greatest promise for patients who suffer from vascular malformations and fistulas of the spine and spinal cord.

Case Illustrations
CASE 1

A 40-year-old man with cervical spinal cord AVM detected incidentally after motor vehicle accident (Figs. 91-1 to 91-5) underwent radiosurgery cyberknife treatment. A repeat angiogram demonstrated persistent AVM nidus (Figs. 91-6 to 91-8). The patient underwent surgical resection 5 years later.

CASE 2

A 36-year-old woman with known Klippel-Trenaunay-Weber syndrome presented with increasing right lower extremity pain in March 2004. The patient was found to have a type IV arteriovenous pial fistula type B at the level of the conus, supplied by the anterior spinal artery, with two inferiorly draining veins and one superiorly draining vein arising from an anteriorly located venous varix (Figs. 91-9 to 91-11). She was treated with coil and glue embolization (Figs. 91-12 and 91-13).

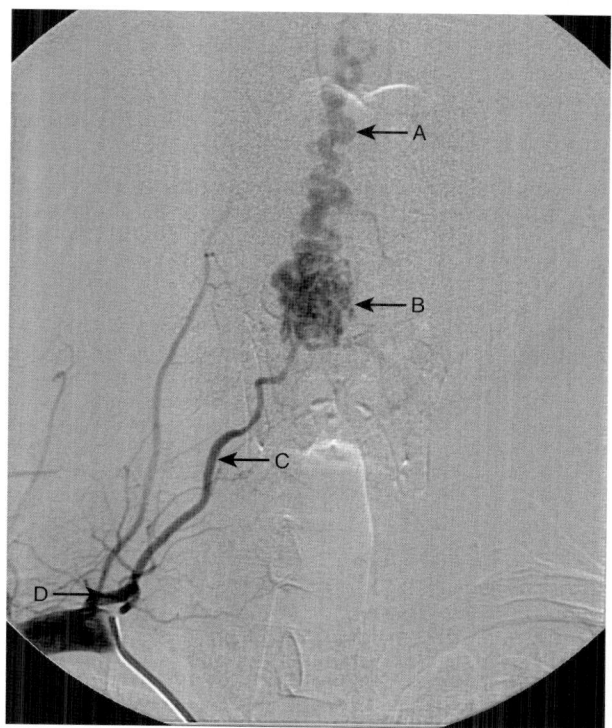

FIGURE 91-1 Anteroposterior view, right subclavian artery injection, initial angiogram. A, Draining vein. B, Arteriovenous malformation nidus. C, Radiculopial artery. D, Thyrocervical trunk.

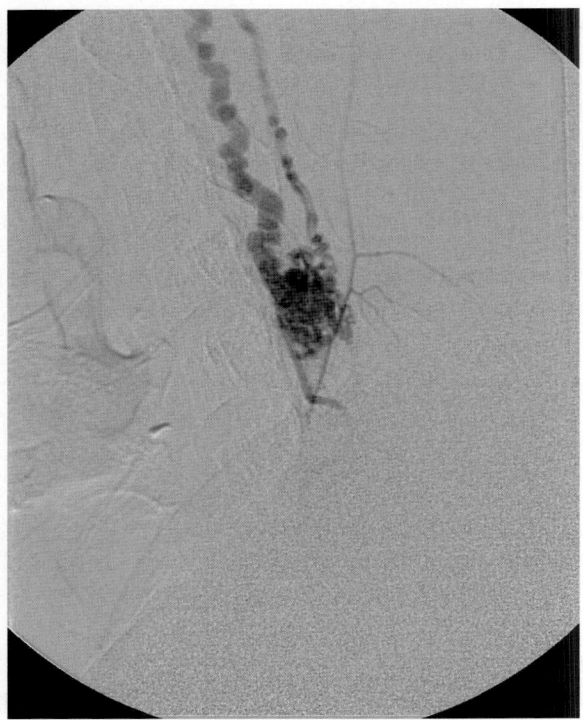

FIGURE 91-2 Lateral view, right subclavian artery injection, initial angiogram.

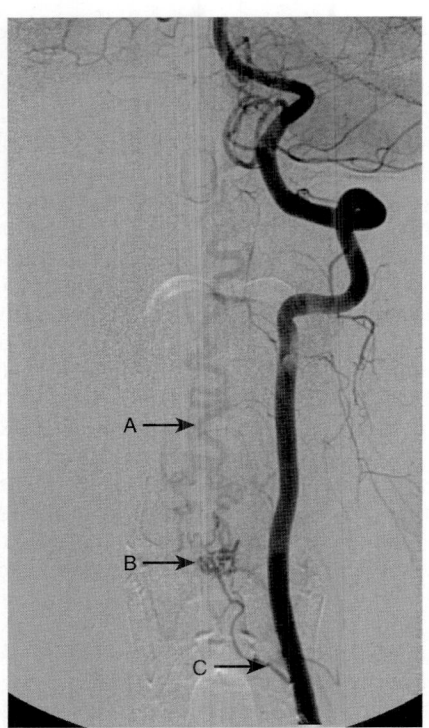

FIGURE 91-3 Oblique view, left vertebral artery injection, initial angiogram. A, Draining vein. B, Arteriovenous malformation nidus. C, Left C7 segmental artery.

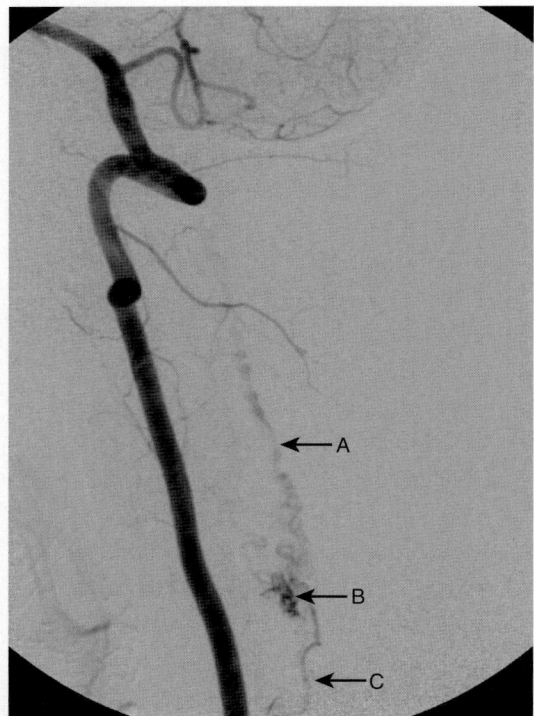

FIGURE 91-4 Lateral view, left vertebral artery injection, initial angiogram. A, Draining vein. B, Arteriovenous malformation nidus. C, Left C7 segmental artery.

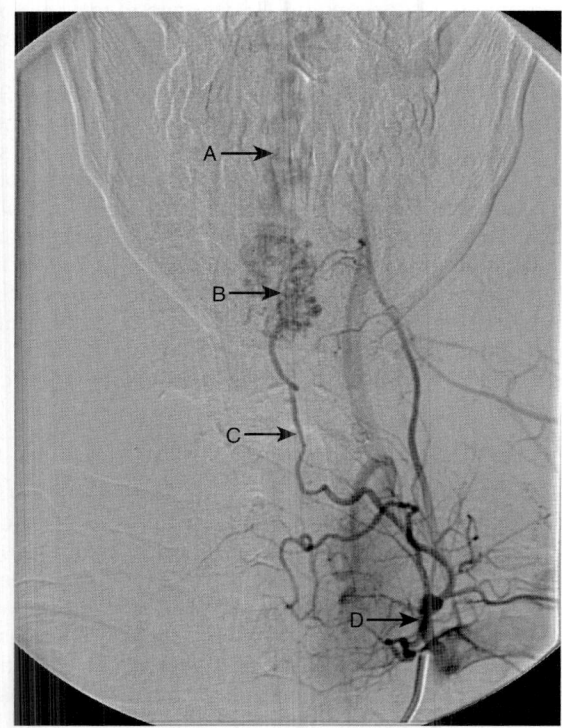

FIGURE 91-5 Anteroposterior view, left subclavian artery injection, initial angiogram. A, Draining vein. B, Arteriovenous malformation nidus. C, Left C8 segmental branch. D, Left thyrocervical trunk.

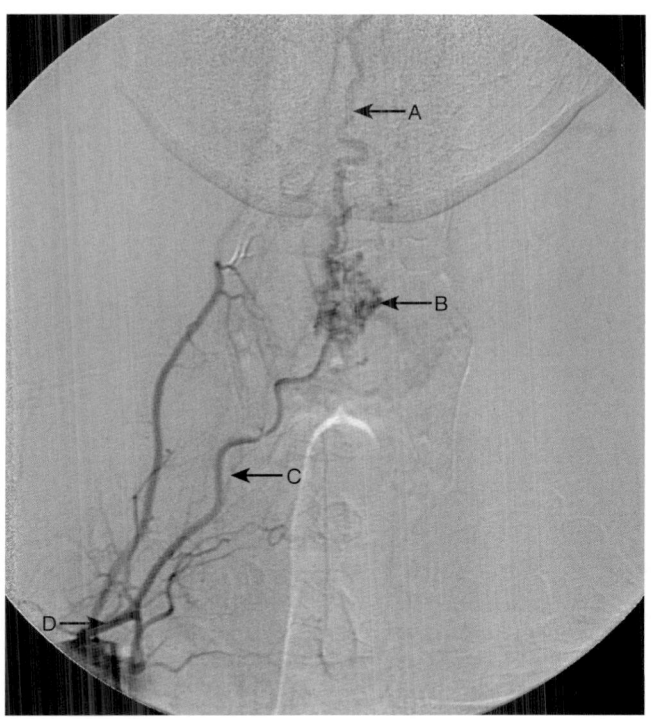

FIGURE 91-6 Anteroposterior view, right subclavian artery injection, preoperative angiogram. A, Draining vein. B, Arteriovenous malformation nidus. C, Radiculopial artery. D, Thyrocervical trunk.

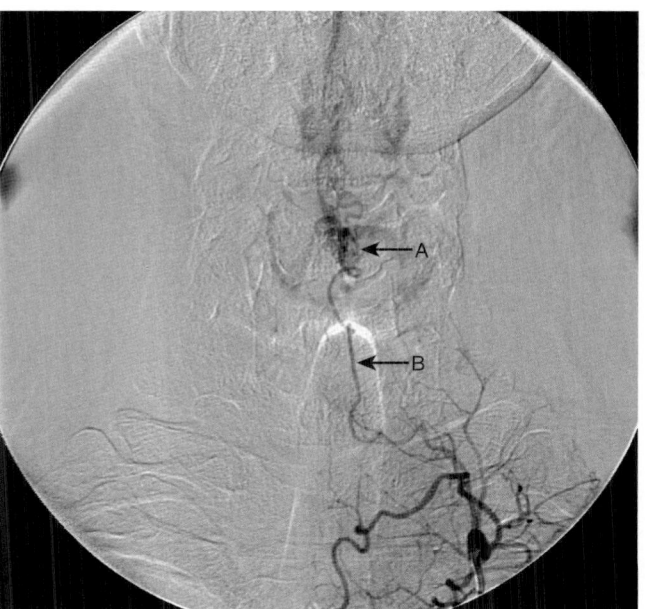

FIGURE 91-7 Anteroposterior view, left thryocervical trunk injection, preoperative angiogram. A, Arteriovenous malformation nidus. B, Left C8 segmental branch.

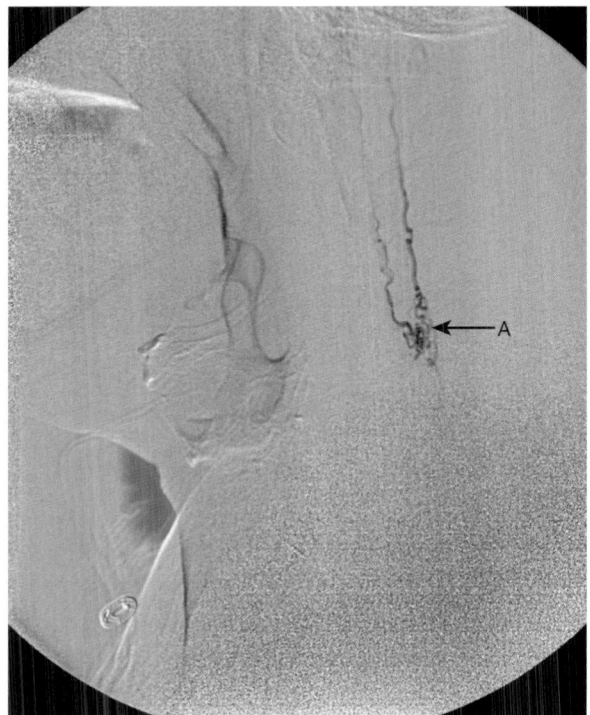

FIGURE 91-8 Lateral view, left vertebral artery injection, preoperative angiogram. A, Arteriovenous malformation nidus.

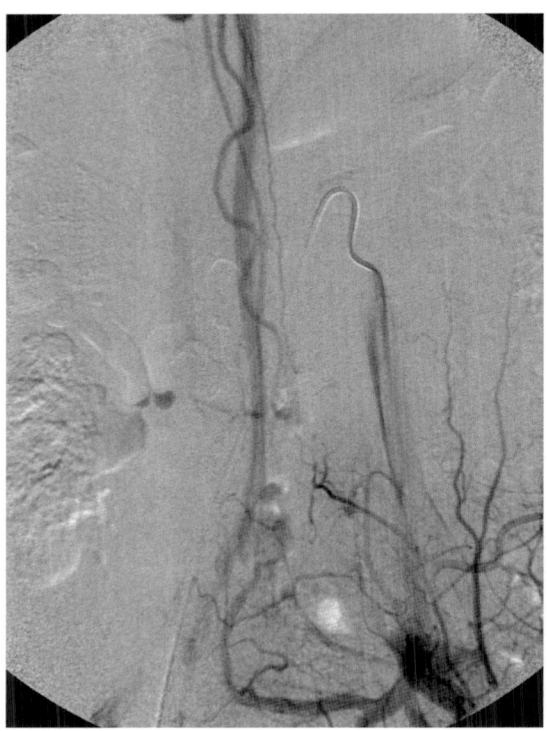

FIGURE 91-9 Anteroposterior view, left internal iliac artery injection, initial angiogram.

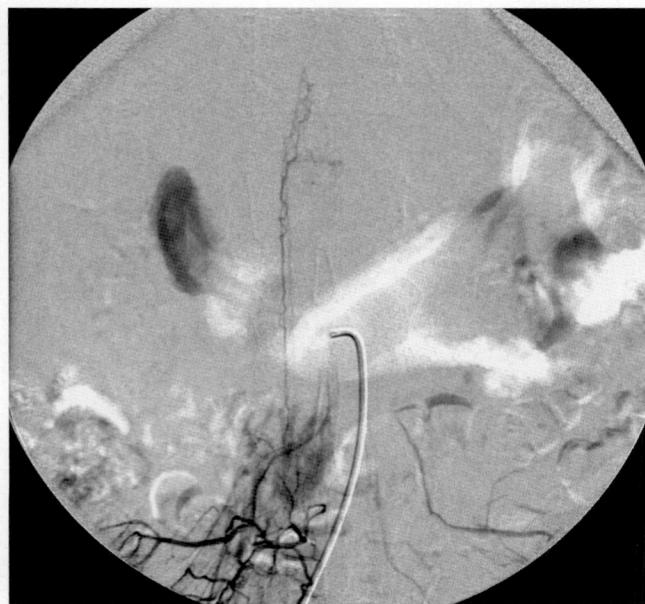

FIGURE 91-10 Anteroposterior view, right internal iliac artery injection, initial angiogram.

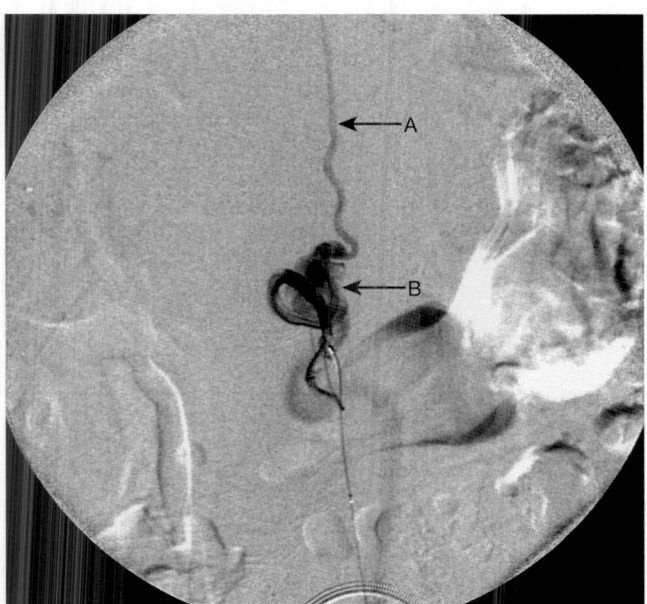

FIGURE 91-12 Anteroposterior view, microcatheter injection of the venous varix during embolization. A, Draining vein. B, Venous varix.

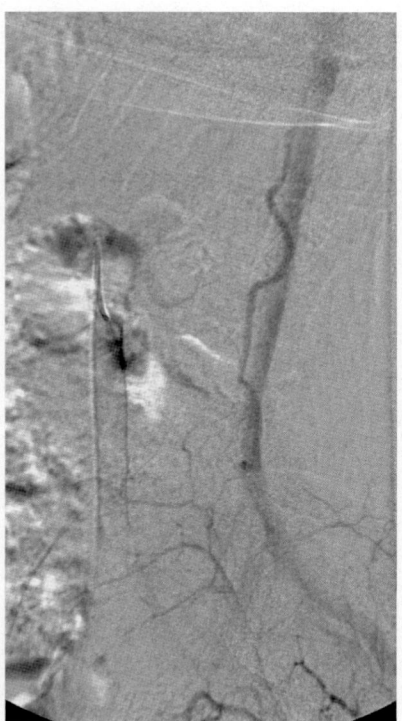

FIGURE 91-11 Lateral view, left internal iliac artery injection, initial angiogram.

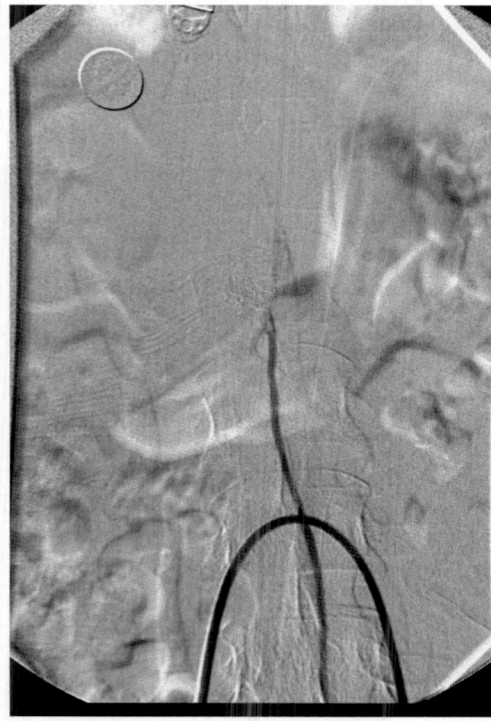

FIGURE 91-13 Anteroposterior view, left lateral sacral artery injection, after embolization.

Although the patient's symptoms continued to improve after embolization, follow-up MRI demonstrated residual fistula. The patient was brought back for repeat spinal angiography, which demonstrated that unlike previously thought, there were actually three type IV perimedullary fistulas: the previously embolized fistula at the conus and two other fistulas, which were centered at the inferior end plate of T11 (Figs. 91-14 and 91-15). These fistulas are supplied by the posterior spinal arteries and drain into short pial veins on the dorsal surface of the spinal cord and then subsequently converge into a large vein that drains inferiorly to the previously embolized venous varix at the conus.

The patient was taken to the operating room for surgical treatment of the fistula. Postoperative angiography demonstrated no residual fistula.

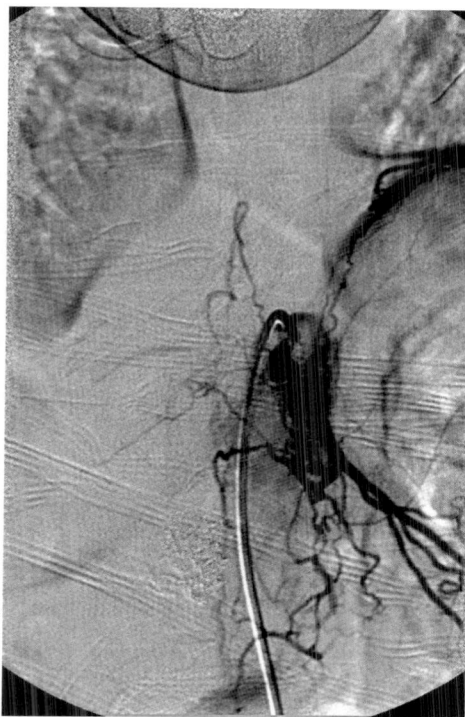

FIGURE 91-14 Anteroposterior view, left T12 segmental artery injection. Follow-up angiogram after embolization, demonstrating residual fistula.

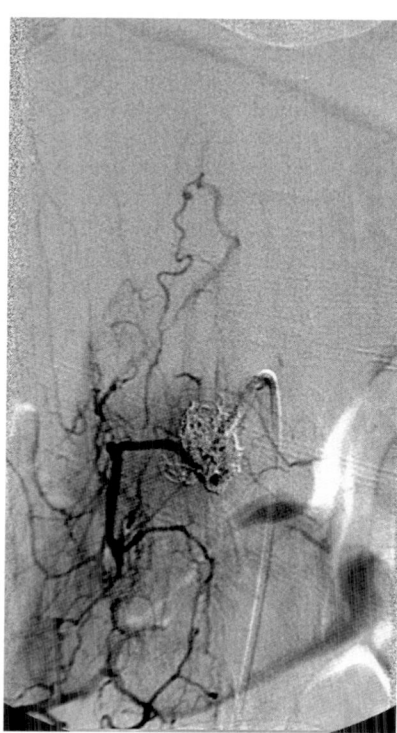

FIGURE 91-15 Anteroposterior view, right L1 segmental artery injection. Follow-up anigogram after embolization, demonstrating residual fistula.

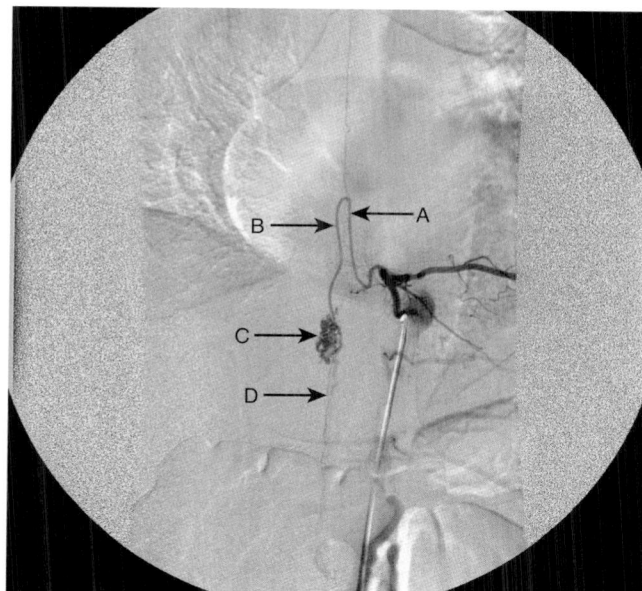

FIGURE 91-16 Anteroposterior view, right T9 segmental artery injection, initial angiogram. A, Artery of Adamkiewicz. B, Anterior spinal artery. C, Type 2 Arteriovenous malformation nidus. D, Draining vein.

CASE 3

A 43-year-old man presented with sudden-onset back pain followed by lower extremity numbness and weakness. Spinal angiogram demonstrated a type II glomus AVM centered at T10 with a compact nidus (Figs. 91-16 and 91-17).

The patient was taken to the operating room for surgical resection of the lesion. Postoperative angiography demonstrated no evidence of residual malformation (Fig. 91-18).

CASE 4

An 86-year-old woman was transferred from an outside institution with dense lower extremity paraparesis for several months. On workup she was found to have a left paraspinal mass and a spinal epidural AVF supplied primarily by the left L1 and L2 segmental arteries (Figs. 91-19 and 91-20). She was treated with Onyx embolization with mild residue filling. The patient and her family have not pursued further treatment options.

CASE 5

A 55-year-old man presented with SAH, Hunt/Hess grade 2. Angiography revealed an unusual spinal AVF at C2 with feeders from the right C2 segmental artery showing characteristics of a type 1 fistula and feeders from the anterior spinal artery arising from the left vertebral artery showing characteristics of a type 4A fistula (Figs. 91-21 to 91-23). Embolization (with nBCA) was performed via the right C2 segmental artery with extension of the nBCA into the draining vein. Angiography performed 4 days after embolization demonstrated complete occlusion of the fistula (Figs. 91-24 and 91-25).

CASE 6

A 70-year-old man presented with progressive lower extremity weakness. MRI demonstrated a dural AVF. Angiogram

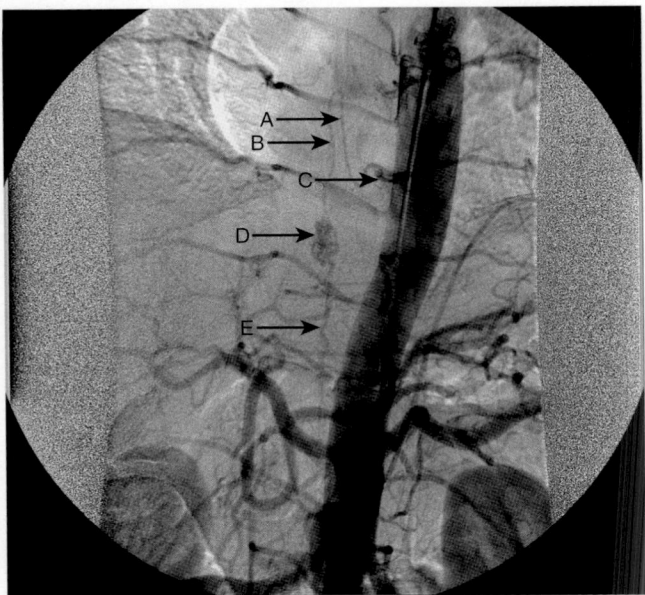

FIGURE 91-17 Anteroposterior view, descending aorta injection, initial angiogram. A, Artery of Adamkiewicz. B, Anterior spinal artery. C, Left T9 segmental artery. D, Arteriovenous malformation nidus. E, Draining vein.

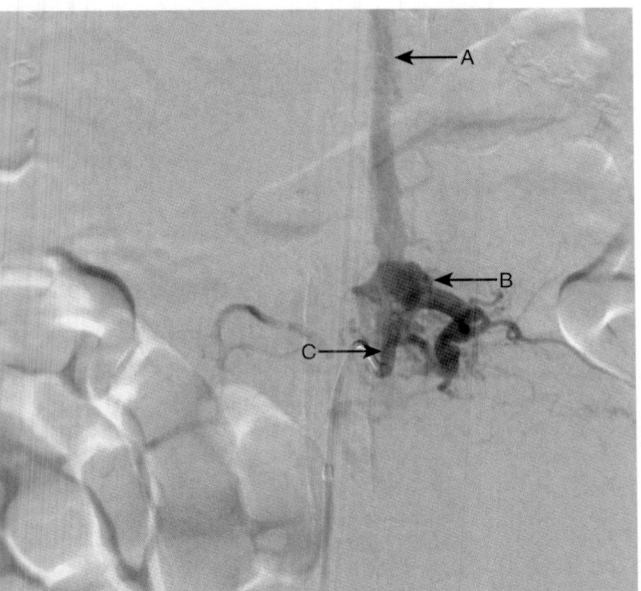

FIGURE 91-19 Anteroposterior view, left L2 segmental artery injection before embolization. A, Draining vein. B, Epidural arteriovenous fistula. C, Segmental artery.

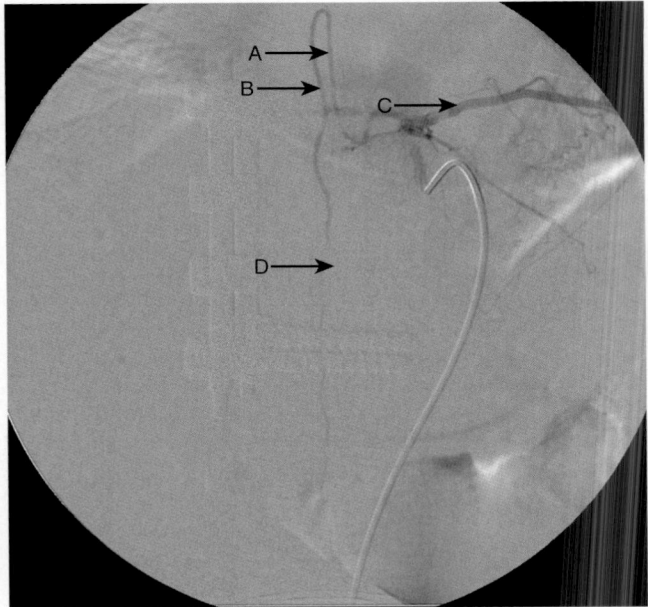

FIGURE 91-18 Anteroposterior view, left T9 segmental artery injection, postoperative angiogram. A, Artery of Adamkiewicz. B, Anterior spinal artery. C, Left T9 segmental artery. D, No residual arteriovenous malformation nidus.

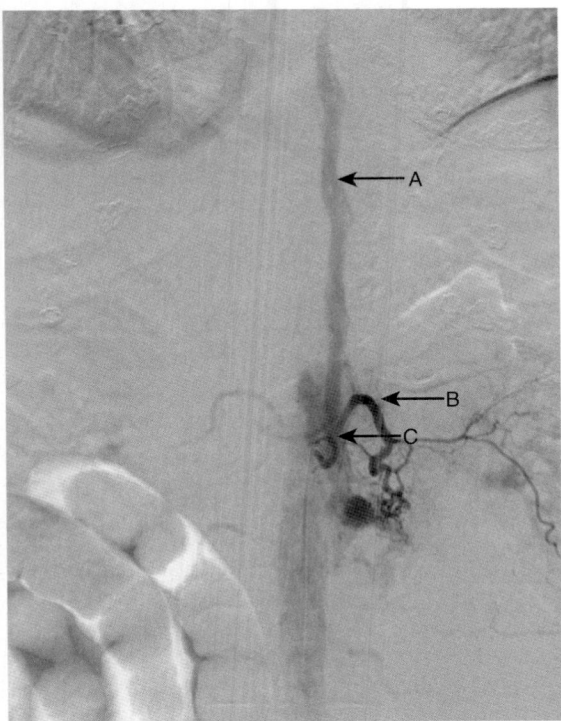

FIGURE 91-20 Anteroposterior view, left L1 segmental artery injection before embolization. A, Draining vein. B, Segmental artery. C, Fistulous point.

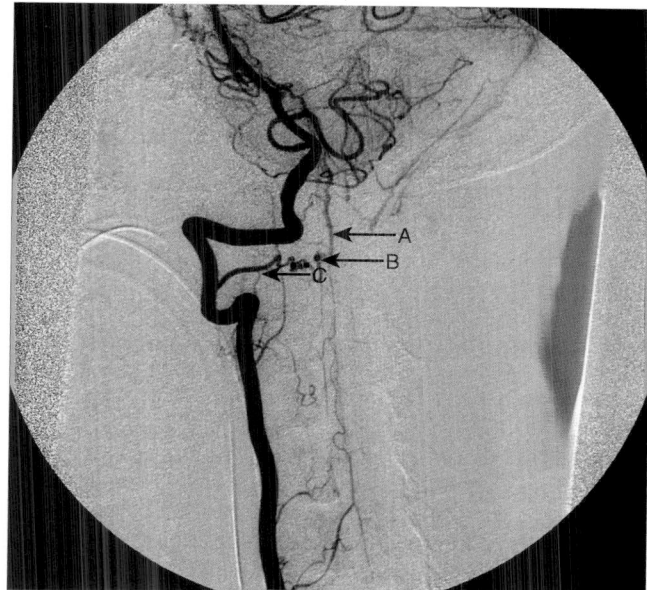

FIGURE 91-21 Anteroposterior view, right vertebral artery injection, initial angiogram. A, Perimesencephalic vein. B, Fistulous point. C, C2 segmental artery.

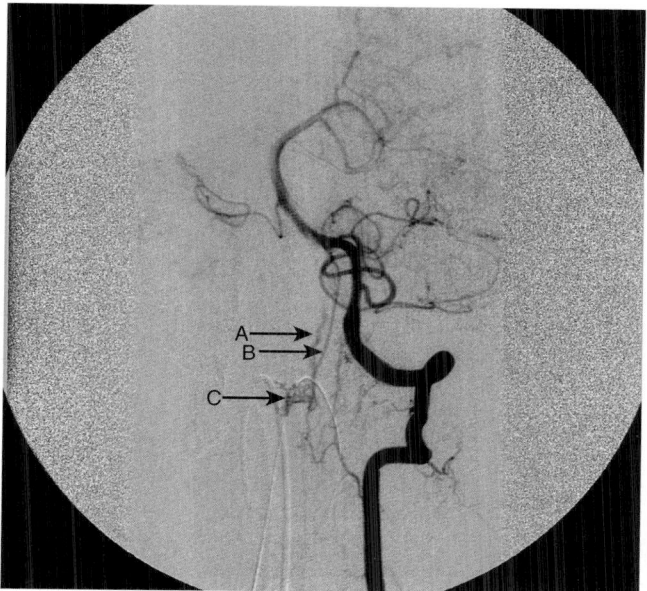

FIGURE 91-23 Anteroposterior view, left vertebral artery injection, initial angiogram. A, Draining vein. B, anterior spinal artery. C, Fistula.

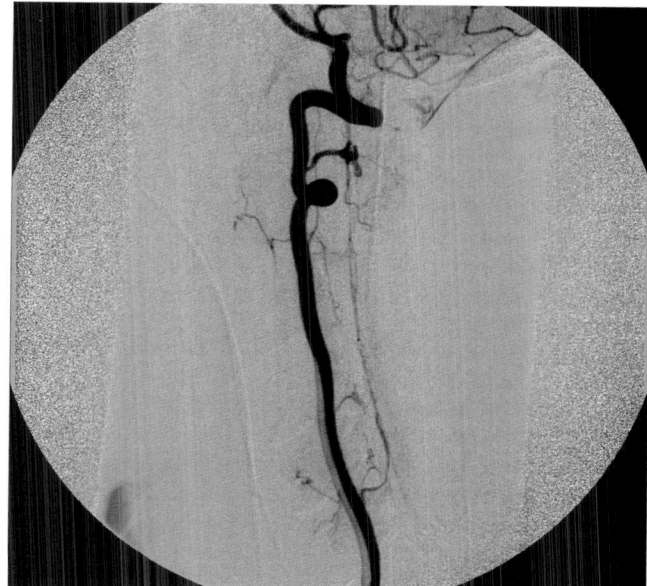

FIGURE 91-22 Anteroposterior view, right vertebral artery injection, Initial angiogram.

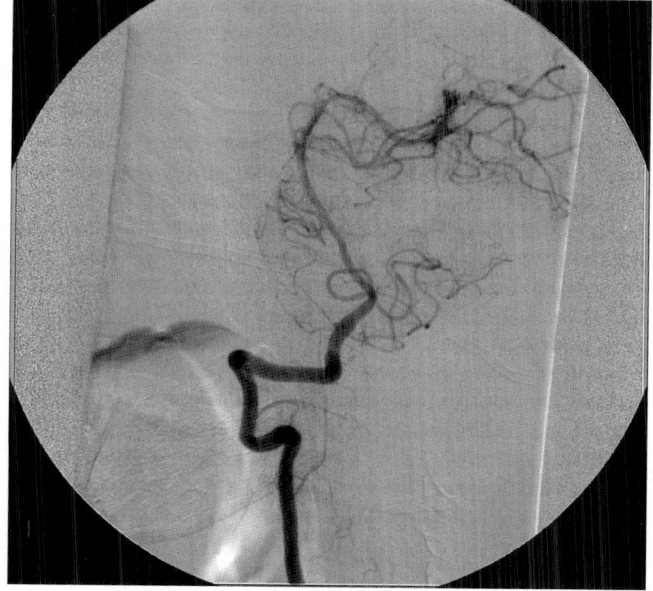

FIGURE 91-24 Oblique view, right vertebral artery injection, angiogram 4 days after embolization.

demonstrated type 1 dural AVF fed by the right L3 segmental artery (Fig. 91-26). The patient was successfully treated with nBCA embolization (Fig. 91-27).

CASE 7

A 67-year-old woman presented with progressive history of lower extremity weakness. Workup including diagnostic

spinal angiography demonstrated a type 1 spinal dural AVF supplied by the left L1 segmental artery (Fig. 91-28). The patient was treated with Onyx embolization of the spinal fistula with complete resolution of the fistula (Fig. 91-29).

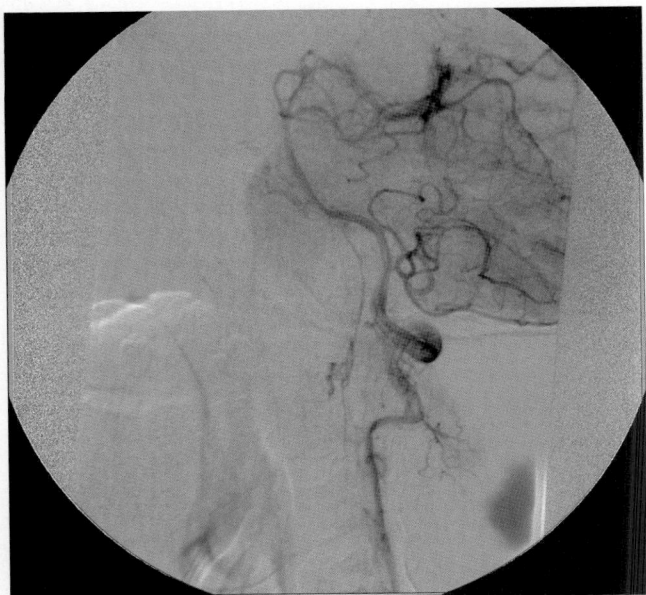

FIGURE 91-25 Lateral view, left vertebral artery injection, Angiogram 4 days after embolization.

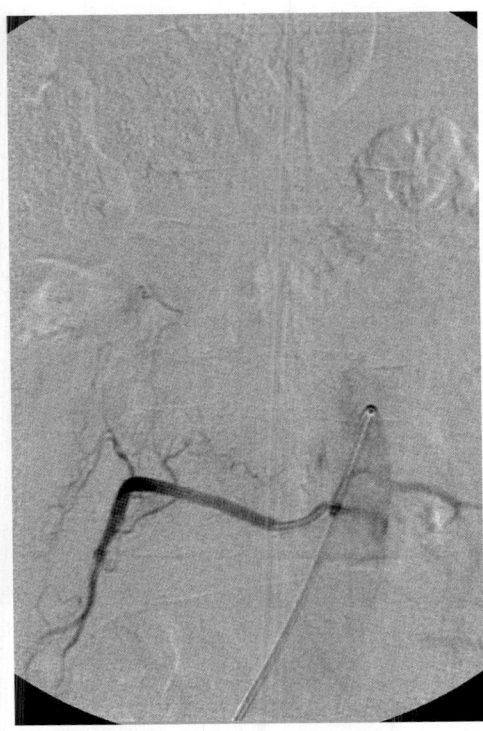

FIGURE 91-27 Anteroposterior view, right L3 segmental artery injection after embolization.

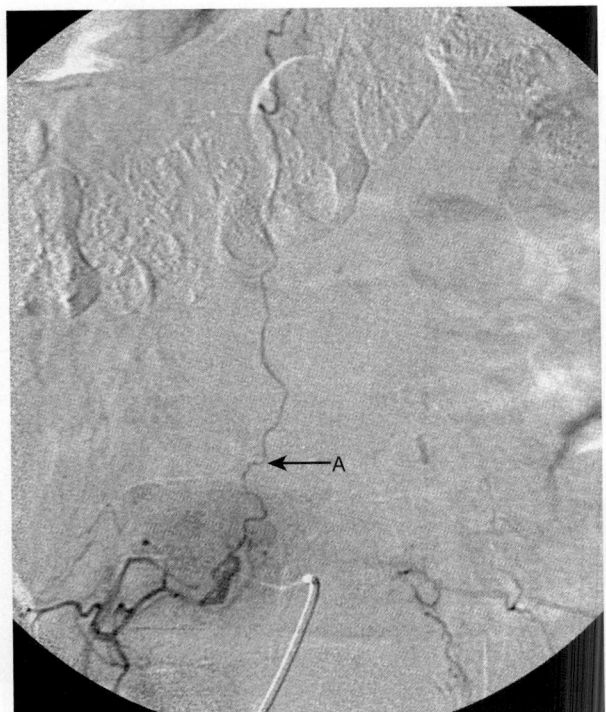

FIGURE 91-26 Anteroposterior view, right L3 segmental artery injection, type I dural arteriovenous fistula (AVF). A, Draining vein.

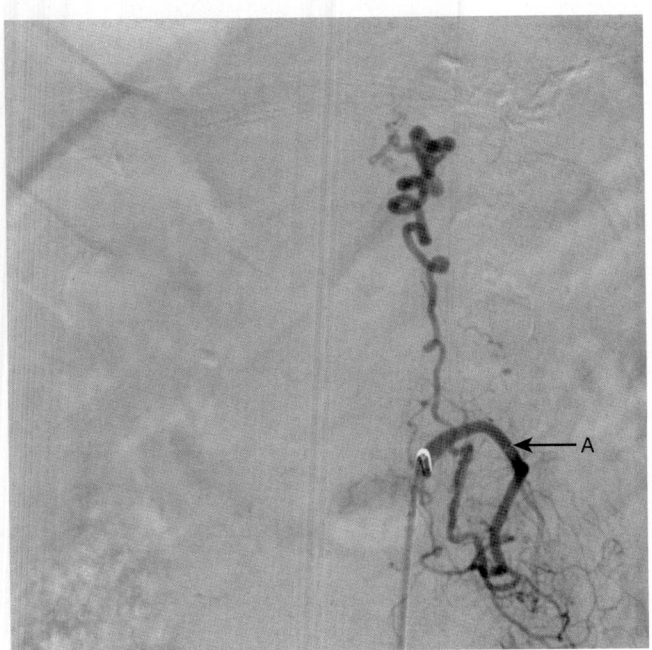

FIGURE 91-28 Anteroposterior view, left L1 segmental artery injection before embolization. A, Left L1 segmental artery.

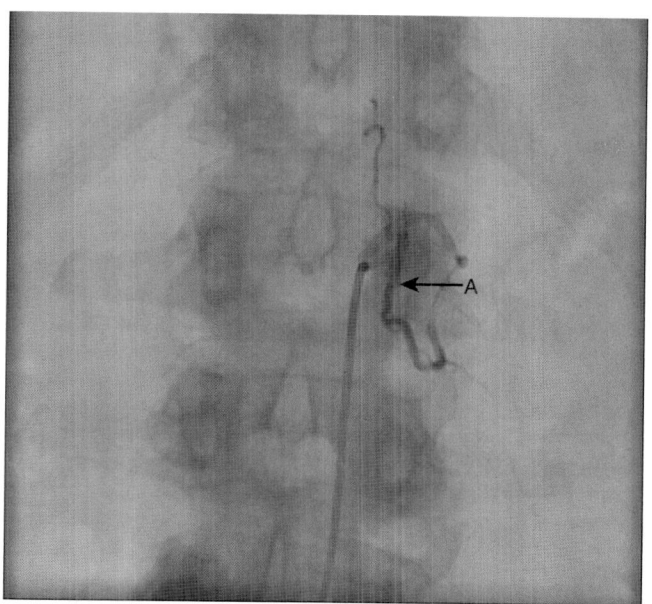

FIGURE 91-29 Anteroposterior view, left L1 segmental artery injection after embolization. A, Onyx cast.

KEY REFERENCES

Ali S, Cashen TA, Carroll TJ, et al. Time-resolved spinal MR angiography: initial clinical experience in the evaluation of spinal arteriovenous shunts. *AJNR Am J Neuroradiol.* 2007;28(9):1806-1810.

Aminoff MJ, Barnard RO, Logue V. The pathophysiology of spinal vascular malformations. *J Neurol Sci.* 1974;23(2):255-263.

Andres RH, Barth A, Guzman R, et al. Endovascular and surgical treatment of spinal dural arteriovenous fistulas. *Neuroradiology.* 2008;50(10):869-876.

Caragine Jr LP, Halbach VV, Ng PP, Dowd CF. Vascular myelopathies–vascular malformations of the spinal cord: presentation and endovascular surgical management. *Semin Neurol.* 2002;22(2):123-132.

Corkill RA, Mitsos AP, Molyneux AJ. Embolization of spinal intramedullary arteriovenous malformations using the liquid embolic agent, Onyx: a single-center experience in a series of 17 patients. *J Neurosurg Spine.* 2007;7(5):478-485.

da Costa L, Dehdashti AR, terBrugge KG. Spinal cord vascular shunts: spinal cord vascular malformations and dural arteriovenous fistulas. *Neurosurg Focus.* 2009;26(1):E6.

Dehdashti AR, Da Costa LB, terBrugge KG, et al. Overview of the current role of endovascular and surgical treatment in spinal dural arteriovenous fistulas. *Neurosurg Focus.* 2009;26(1):E8.

Doppman JL, Di Chiro G, Ommaya A. Obliteration of spinal-cord arteriovenous malformation by percutaneous embolisation. *Lancet.* 1968;1(7540):477.

Heros RC, Debrun GM, Ojemann RG, et al. Direct spinal arteriovenous fistula: a new type of spinal AVM. Case report. *J Neurosurg.* 1986;64(1):134-139.

Konan AV, Raymond J, Roy D. Transarterial embolization of aneurysms associated with spinal cord arteriovenous malformations. Report of four cases. *J Neurosurg.* 1999;90(Suppl 1):148-154.

Mathis JM, Shaibani A, Wakhloo AK. Spine anatomy. In: Mathis JM, ed. *Image-guided spine intervention.* New York: Springer-Verlag; 2004:1-26.

Matsuo K, Kakita A, Ishizu N, et al. Venous congestive myelopathy: three autopsy cases showing a variety of clinicopathologic features. *Neuropathology.* Jun 2008;28(3):303-308.

Medel R, Crowley RW, Dumont AS. Endovascular management of spinal vascular malformations: history and literature review. *Neurosurg Focus.* 2009;26(1):E7.

Molyneux AJ, Coley SC. Embolization of spinal cord arteriovenous malformations with an ethylene vinyl alcohol copolymer dissolved in dimethyl sulfoxide (Onyx liquid embolic system). Report of two cases. *J Neurosurg.* 2000;93(Suppl 2):304-308.

Mourier KL, Gobin YP, George B, et al. Intradural perimedullary arteriovenous fistulae: results of surgical and endovascular treatment in a series of 35 cases. *Neurosurgery.* 1993;32(6):885-891.

Narvid J, Hetts SW, Larsen D, et al. Spinal dural arteriovenous fistulae: clinical features and long-term results. *Neurosurgery.* 2008;62(1):159-166.

Niimi Y, Berenstein A, Setton A, Neophytides A. Embolization of spinal dural arteriovenous fistulae: results and follow-up. *Neurosurgery.* 1997;40(4):675-682.

Niimi Y, Sala F, Deletis V, et al. Neurophysiologic monitoring and pharmacologic provocative testing for embolization of spinal cord arteriovenous malformations. *AJNR Am J Neuroradiol.* 2004;25(7):1131-1138.

Rodesch G, Hurth M, Alvarez H, et al. Classification of spinal cord arteriovenous shunts: proposal for a reappraisal–the Bicetre experience with 155 consecutive patients treated between 1981 and 1999. *Neurosurgery.* 2002;51(2):374-379.

Shaibani A, Wakhloo AK. Endovascular therapy of the spine. In: Mathis JM, ed. *Image-guided spine intervention.* New York: Springer-Verlag; 2004:292-321.

Sherif C, Gruber A, Bavinzski G, et al. Long-term outcome of a multidisciplinary concept of spinal dural arteriovenous fistulae treatment. *Neuroradiology.* 2008;50(1):67-74.

Sinclair J, Chang SD, Gibbs IC, Adler Jr JR. Multisession CyberKnife radiosurgery for intramedullary spinal cord arteriovenous malformations. *Neurosurgery.* 2006;58(6):1081-1089.

Sivakumar W, Zada G, Yashar P, et al. Endovascular management of spinal dural arteriovenous fistulas. A review. *Neurosurg Focus.* 2009;26(5):E15.

Song JK, Vinuela F, Gobin YP, et al. Surgical and endovascular treatment of spinal dural arteriovenous fistulas: long-term disability assessment and prognostic factors. *J Neurosurg.* 2001;94(Suppl 2):199-204.

Spetzler RF, Detwiler PW, Riina HA, Porter RW. Modified classification of spinal cord vascular lesions. *J Neurosurg.* 2002;96(Suppl 2):145-156.

Numbered references appear on Expert Consult.

CHAPTER 92

Endovascular Treatment of Head and Neck Bleeding

ALEXANDROS D. ZOUZIAS • PAUL SCHMITT • CHIRAG D. GANDHI •
CHARLES J. PRESTIGIACOMO

The role of endovascular therapy in the treatment of neurologic disease has had a relatively short history. Since its initial introduction by Luessenhop and Spence in 1960, the technological improvements and subsequent indications for the use of endovascular techniques have evolved dramatically.[1] The advances in polymer science, device design, and technique development have resulted in the maturation of this specialty and its integration into neurosurgical management. Indeed, the last 20 years have demonstrated endovascular surgical neuroradiology's complementary role in several vascular disorders. One of the areas where this complementary relationship exists is in the treatment of traumatic injury to the vessels of the head and neck.

Though the incidence of blunt traumatic vascular injury is relatively rare—variably reported between 0.1% and 0.45% in trauma centers treating carotid injury—such injuries can be associated with high morbidity and mortality that have been reported from 20% to 40%.[2] Intracranial injury secondary to blunt trauma or penetrating trauma can range from subintimal dissection with possible ischemia, or pseudoaneurysm formation with potential rupture, to acute or delayed traumatic aneurysm formation and frank transection with subsequent hemorrhage or arteriovenous fistula formation. The role of endovascular therapy in the setting of these pathologic entities not only has grown but also has expanded into areas where previous treatment options were very high risk or unavailable. This chapter thus discusses the role of endovascular therapy as it relates to the multidisciplinary treatment of acute vascular injury of the head and neck.

Evaluating Effects of Ischemia

Basic principles of surgical management should be followed prior to advancing to therapeutic interventions. Control of airway and breathing, along with establishment of venous access for appropriate fluid resuscitation, are a priority.[3] The patient is usually under minimum sedation, allowing accurate neurologic assessment. If complete internal carotid artery (ICA) occlusion is necessary, collateral supply should be measured prior to occlusion to determine the effects of ischemia at the distal ICA segment. The standard procedure for assessing collateral sufficiency in the stable patient is balloon test occlusion (BTO), as introduced

by Serbinenko.[4-7] BTO of the ICA is designed to identify patients who are at risk for ischemic events following permanent ICA occlusion and to minimize the associated rates of complication.[8] The location of the balloon at the time of inflation depends on the location of the ICA lesion and the type of balloon, but the procedure should always be performed under road map guidance. Modern BTO implies simultaneous anatomic and physiologic assessment before and after inflation.

Anatomic testing consists of visualization of collateral circulation through the circle of Willis. Collateral circulation may be assessed in a number of ways, including transcranial Doppler sonography, electroencephalography, quantitative cerebral blood flow (CBF) analyses, and qualitative CBF analyses. Any of these studies represent an attempt to identify those patients with compromised hemodynamics despite a normal examination.[5,6] There has also been success with use of delayed venous phase protocols in assessing collateral adequacy.[8] A negative test occlusion, according to venous phase protocol, is when the delay of venous drainage between the territory of the injected artery and the occluded hemisphere is 2 to 3 seconds or less. The major advantages of relying on venous phase criteria are that the neurologic assessment is unnecessary and the patient may be placed under general anesthesia.

Physiologic testing traditionally includes a neurologic assessment (standard Wada) with or without electroencephalogram (EEG) monitoring.[5,9] EEG monitoring is primarily used for patients in whom the neurologic assessment may not be accurate. The addition of physiologic stressors—such as a hypotensive challenge, acetazolamide, or carbon dioxide challenge—represent an effort to identify patients who have a deficient circulatory reserve that would not be elucidated in a normal physical exam. A hypotensive challenge is performed with agents such as nitroprusside or labetalol, and blood pressure is brought down to 75% to 66% of baseline for 20 minutes. Confounding factors such as tumor-related deficits, hemorrhage- or vasospasm-related infarction, and embolic infarction have brought the predictive value of these challenges into question.[4] In patients who tolerate BTO, the surgeon can proceed to carotid occlusion. If technical problems occur, or if the patient demonstrates evidence of ischemic deficits, patency of the carotid artery must be maintained.[10]

Blunt and Penetrating Injuries of the Head

Blunt and penetrating trauma of the head can result in acute or delayed vascular injuries ranging from life-threatening hemorrhage, to infarction secondary to occlusion, to delayed hemorrhage from ruptured traumatic aneurysms. Because of this extreme variation in presentation, understanding the mechanisms of injury and anticipating and assessing for these injuries, whether acute or delayed, are critical in mitigating the potentially lethal sequelae.

Penetrating injuries of the head can result in a spectrum of vascular lesions, which partly depend on the anatomic structures involved, as well as the mechanism of injury. Laceration of an intracranial artery, such as the supraclinoid carotid artery, can be a fatal event, whereas a similar laceration of the cavernous portion of the ICA may result in a high-flow carotid–cavernous fistula (CCF) that is not uniformly fatal. Penetrating injuries to the more posterior regions of the skull or to the anterior portions of the face may result not only in exsanguinations but also in arteriovenous fistulas. Blast or cavitation injury from a gunshot wound can result in an occlusive dissection and subsequent cerebral infarction or in delayed formation of traumatic aneurysms. A keen awareness of the *potential* for these sequelae of trauma is important in determining the assessment and subsequent treatment paradigm.

CAROTID–CAVERNOUS FISTULAS

CCF or caroticocavernous fistula is the result of a tear of the ICA that allows it to form a high-flow, low-resistance fistula with the venous system of the cavernous sinus.[4,11] A CCF can be either direct or indirect. In a direct carotid–cavernous fistula (DCCF), blood is shunted from the ICA into the sinus; in an indirect carotid–cavernous fistula (ICCF), there is a dural arteriovenous communication and a slower flow rate. Barrow et al.[12] classified direct, trauma-induced, high-flow shunts between the ICA and the cavernous sinus as a type A fistula. In contrast to dural-based fistulas, spontaneous cure of a type A CCF is rare.[13,14] However, rare cases of spontaneous DCCF are found in cases of ruptured intracavernous ICA aneurysms and in patients with collagen vascular disease.[15] A comprehensive description of the dural CCF is beyond the scope of this chapter.

The pressure gradient in a DCCF results in reversal of flow into the superior ophthalmic vein and superficial middle cerebral vein, with concomitant rapid shunting to the inferior petrosal sinus and the pterygoid vein.[16,17] Classical presentation of DCCF is a pulsating exophthalmos with orbital bruit. Other symptoms may include visual changes, orbital pain, and proptosis. It is evident that most symptoms are a direct result of arterialization of the cavernous sinus and draining orbital veins.[18-20] Some common sequelae encountered include venous congestion, hemorrhage, headache, tinnitus, vertigo, and cranial nerve palsies.[21] In patients showing evidence of arterial steal phenomenon, such as cerebral hypoperfusion with subsequent focal neurologic deficits, urgent intervention is indicated.

Management of CCF depends on the stability of the patient, the anatomy of the fistula, and the hemodynamics involved in the system. Ideally, the focus of management should be on repair or obliteration of the tear or communication while preserving flow through the ICA.[5] Sometimes, complete occlusion of the artery may be necessary. In 1973, Parkinson described a direct surgical repair of a traumatic CCF with preservation of the ICA. While any procedure in this anatomic region is delicate, open repair in the acute setting amid potential polytrauma carries a significant risk of morbidity, so endovascular repair, if tolerated by the patient, is the method of choice.[22]

Approach of the CCF may be performed via transarterial or transvenous routes.[11,18] The transvenous approach consists of retrograde catheterization and embolization of the venous structure draining the fistula. A venous route is only appropriate if the diseased, venous portion of the system is permanently occluded—and only if occlusion of this venous outflow does not compromise the drainage of the surrounding neural structures. Transarterial routes are more selective. Using a microcatheter, access to the fistula is provided by the arterial branches supplying it, and these pedicles are selectively occluded.[23] The number of vessels occluded, and the route chosen to occlude them, are necessarily linked to the choice of embolic material. Today, the primary methods for endovascular embolization employ detachable coils or liquid embolic agents (Fig. 92-1).

Transarterial versus Transvenous Approach

Transvenous embolization is possible via the femoral vein or jugular vein and inferior petrosal sinus, or it may be possible by directly accessing the ophthalmic vein.[24] The goal of treatment is to thrombose the cavernous sinus, with the assumption that spontaneous resolution of fistula will follow. If the draining sinus is occluded but the upstream fistula is neglected, the high flow system forces drainage through other veins, potentially draining into the cortical venous system.[17,24-26] Cortical venous drainage in the setting of these shunts may result in potentially fatal intracranial hemorrhage.[27]

The transvenous approach for embolization, reported by Debrun in 1981, has become the treatment of choice for ICCF[28] and for some traumatic dural arteriovenous fistulas. However, for reasons already discussed, it is not ideal in the management of DCCF.[20] For instance, when treating traumatic dural fistulas of the cavernous sinus, the inferior petrosal sinus is the simplest and shortest venous route to the cavernous sinus. A guiding catheter is introduced via a femoral sheath and resides in the internal jugular vein near the inferior petrosal sinus. In cases of fistulas with feeders from the ICA, another guiding catheter is run through the ICA containing a balloon for BTO and a microcatheter for injection of the embolic.[29] The balloon may also be inflated during embolization to prevent inadvertent reflux of the embolic agent into the ICA. Alternative access points are the basilar plexus, the pterygoid plexus, or the facial and angular veins.[20] In cases of high-flow fistulas, coils may be placed at the confluence of the draining veins and within the cavernous sinus to act as a mesh, thus slowing the flow through the fistula and decreasing the efflux of embolic material through the veins.[20]

A transarterial approach allows the selective obliteration of individual pedicles feeding the CCF and makes the problem of venous rerouting less threatening.[5,23] Problems with a transarterial approach may include several feeding arteries, anastomotic connections to cortical or nervous arterial supplies, or tortuous vessels that limit microcatheter access.

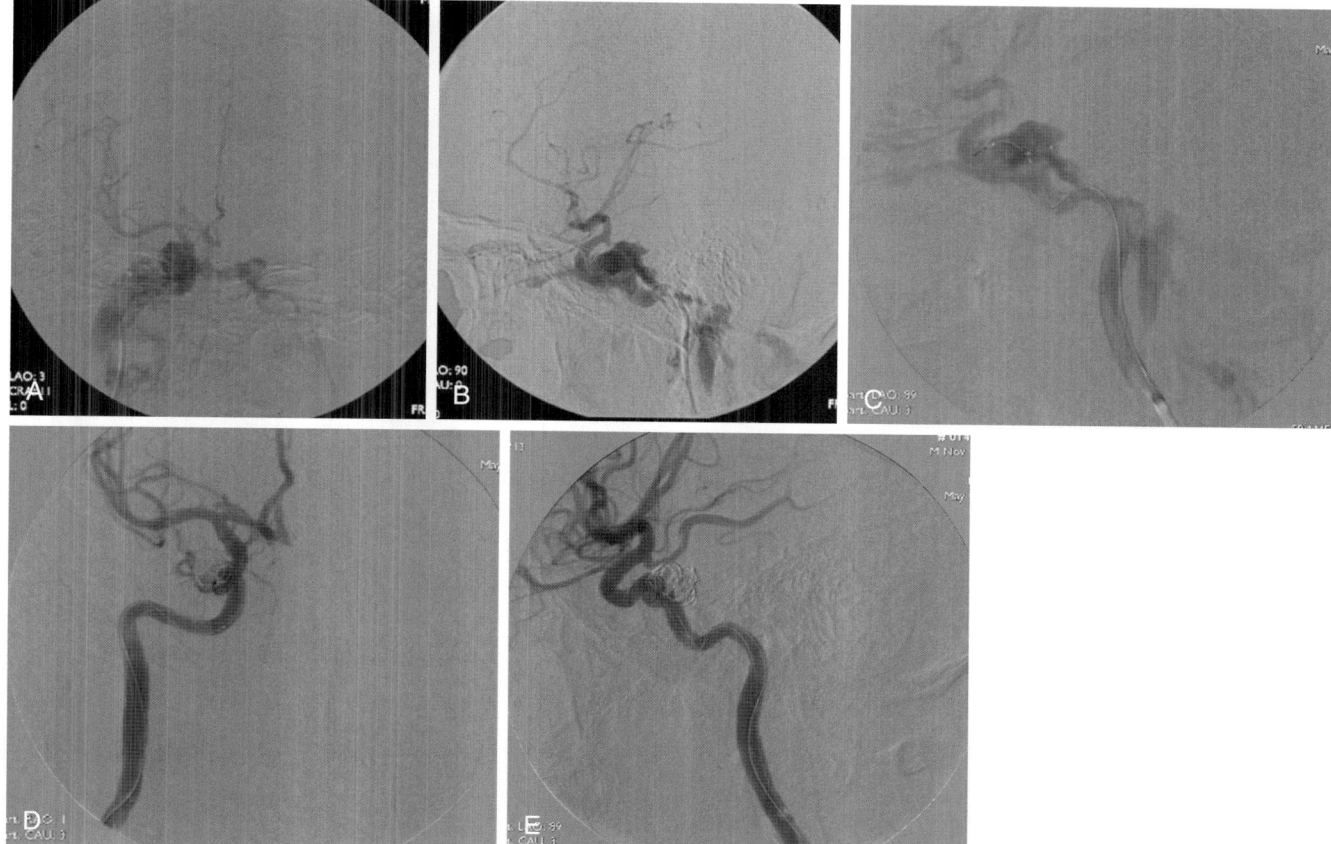

FIGURE 92-1 A 36-year-old man presenting 2 weeks after being struck in the head with a bat and with a proptotic, injected right eye; a pulse-synchronous bruit; and a right abducens palsy. A and B, A right ICA, anteroposterior (AP), and lateral angiogram demonstrating a type A CCF with opacification of both cavernous sinuses. There is also an associated 7-mm cavernous ICA aneurysm. C, A 4×10 mm Hyperglide (ev3 Neurovascular) is placed across the fistula site, and an Excelsior SL-10 microcatheter (Boston Scientific) is within the right cavernous sinus. D and E, A right ICA, AP, and lateral angiogram after the placement of coils into the cavernous sinus, showing no further filling of the fistula and no early venous phase. Symptoms resolved within 3 weeks of treatment.

For instance, catheterization of the small-caliber meningeal branches of ICCFs can be difficult or may supply several cranial nerves, thus limiting the success of this technique.[20,30]

In Barrow type A CCFs, a guide catheter is maneuvered into the ICA, followed by selective catheterization of feeding vessels. A microcatheter is navigated through the fistulous point into the cavernous sinus, and embolization is conducted. It may be necessary to simultaneously inflate a balloon in the cavernous ICA to prevent reflux into the parent artery.[20] Again, an angiogram should be performed to assess progress and screen for dangerous anastomoses.

In some instances, a combination of arterial and venous approaches may be used.[25,26] The transarterial component of therapy in this case decreases blood flow through the system, thus providing a less turbulent environment when deploying coils and allowing more precise targeting of the fistula from the venous side. During the procedure, the injection should be performed at a pace that allows the surgeon to monitor the evolving shape of the embolic. If a balloon is used, it should be deflated and any abnormal reflux should be noted prior to retrieval. Finally, a reference microguidewire should always be anchored in place to allow intraoperative navigation of the artery.[29]

Regardless of the route of approach, several principles apply: reflux of embolics into the parent vessel must be avoided. The ICA and the fistula have to be completely occluded, and the occlusion should be visually confirmed immediately after the procedure via angiography of the primary vascular tree, as well as potential collateral pathways.

Embolic Agents for Endovascular Occlusion

In choosing an embolic agent for CCF occlusion, consider what the desired properties of an ideal agent would be. The occlusion should be complete and permanent, and the delivery should be highly controllable. Radiopacity allows assessment of progress and precision of the occlusion. Finally, while some degree of proinflammatory properties may facilitate vessel occlusion, the material should not be antigenic. Modern embolics all attempt to strike a balance between these general themes, and some are more successful than others, depending on the task for which they were designed. Regardless of which embolic is chosen, all have inherent risks, including vessel rupture, vein occlusion, and embolization to normal parenchymal branches.[23,31]

The three broad categories of embolics are mechanical devices, such as balloons and detachable coils; particles; and liquids. Liquid embolics can further be divided into cyanoacrylates and polymers.[32] Coils are principally used in the occlusion of larger vessels and aneurysms. Liquid embolic agents include *n*-butyl-2-cyanoacrylate (*n*-BCA)

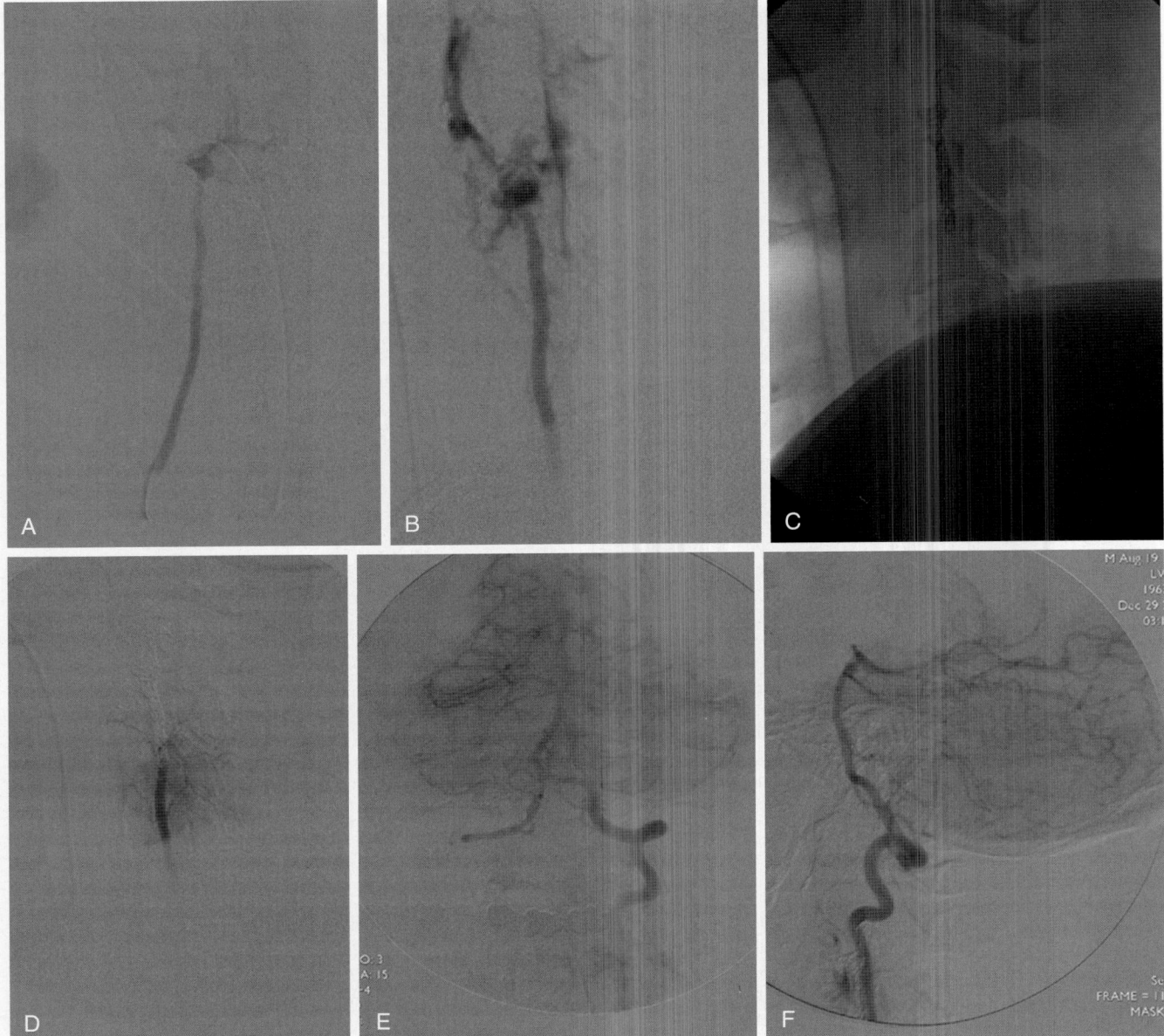

FIGURE 92-2 A 23-year-old man sustaining a single gunshot wound to the neck and brought to the emergency room alert and oriented. A and B, AP and lateral right vertebral angiogram, showing documented fistula of the vertebral artery with the epidural venous plexus at the C2 to C3 level. C and D, lateral, native image and subtraction status after vertebral artery occlusion with coils. E and F, AP early and late images of left vertebral angiogram status after right vertebral artery occlusion, demonstrating normal perfusion of the vertebrobasilar circulation with retrograde filling of the right vertebral artery to the level of occlusion. The patient remained asymptomatic postprocedure.

and ethylene–vinyl alcohol copolymer (Onyx, ev3 Neuro-vascular, Irvine, CA).

Balloons

For almost 30 years, the procedure of choice for the management and repair of type A CCFs was detachable balloon occlusion. While detachable balloons are no longer available in the United States, their description by Serbinenko in 1974 helped stimulate the growth of balloon technology in endovascular therapy.[6] The balloon had many advantages, including low cost, easy navigability to the fistula, and the ability to intermittently inflate and deflate the balloon, which allowed constant reassessment of fistula anatomy. However, some difficulties encountered with permanent balloon occlusion were early detachment or deflation, rupture by bone fragments, and iatrogenic dilation of the ostium of the fistula or the cavernous sinus proper, causing a delayed recurrence of the fistula.[33] If large balloons were used, or multiple balloons were deployed, de novo cranial nerve palsies sometimes resulted, or the resolution of preexisting palsies were sometimes hindered due to mass effect from the balloons.[13]

Particles

While particle embolic agents had been used for embolization of arteriovenous malformations,[1] the first use of a permanent particle for CCF embolization was by Kosary et al.

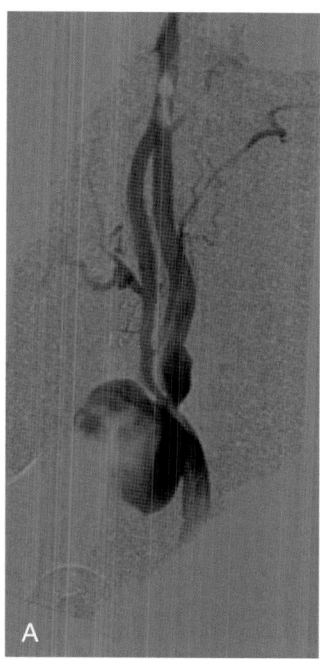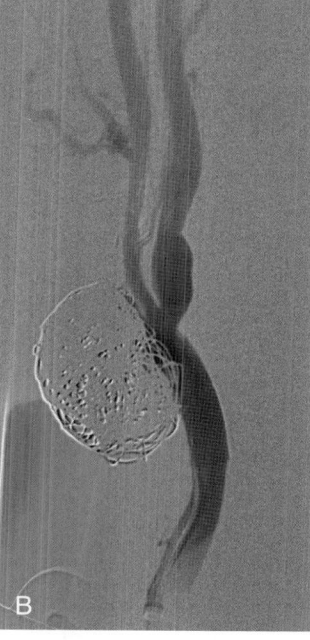

FIGURE 92-3 A 46-year-old man with squamous cell carcinoma status after radiation, chemotherapy, and laryngectomy with a 1-week history of intermittent hemorrhage and an enlarging neck mass on CT scan. A, Lateral angiographic projection of the right carotid artery demonstrating a large common carotid pseudoaneurysm. B, Right carotid angiogram after stent and coil placement with good short-term result.

in 1968.[34] Kosary et al. combined a porcelain bead with a Gelfoam technique described by Speakman in 1964.[35] The Gelfoam—used to quicken the clotting process in the sinus and prevent "downward displacement" of the bead—would herald the use of balloons in preventing reflux of liquid and particle embolics in later years. Gelfoam can be used as either a macro- or a microparticle, depending on how it is prepared, but in both cases it is a temporary embolic agent.[36] The choice of a porcelain bead was an important advancement, because it represented a rational choice of embolic particle size based on direct angiographic findings. Calibrated microparticles, such as Embospheres (BioSphere Medical, Rockland, MA) or polyvinyl alcohol particles of various sizes, now allow the physician to select a size based on the diameter of the vessels to be occluded, thus facilitating more accurate delivery of the embolics to the target vessel.

In the setting of high-flow CCF or trauma, where larger caliber vessels are directly involved, particle embolization would not be a consideration for treatment and is currently of historical interest only.

Coils

Detachable coils are easy to retrieve, reposition, or exchange when necessary, making them an appealing embolic agent. Endovascular treatment of CCF with coils is one of primary modes of treatment, with excellent results. In the setting of traumatic CCF, where the site of the fistula may be quite large, the coils may migrate or protrude into the ICA, thus risking carotid occlusion. Balloon-assist embolization, whereby the ICA is "protected" from coil migration and occlusion by the presence of a balloon that is inflated during coil delivery, has been quite efficacious in reducing this risk. Alternatively,

similar to the principle of balloon assist, combining the use of coils with stents can prevent or mitigate such a risk.[37] Complete obliteration of the fistula may be difficult, and there is a risk of impingement on the parent vessel and subsequent mass effects when excessive amounts of coil are packed.[13,37] However, certain coated coils, such as Hydrocoils, the coating of which expands when placed in contact with blood, seem to require fewer coils to achieve occlusion than others.

n-Butyl-Cyanoacrylate

The first description of n-BCA as an embolic material was by Brothers et al. in 1989.[38] This adhesive cyanoacrylate derivative polymerizes in the presence of anionic substances (e.g., blood) to form a solid cast that molds into the shape of the embolized region. The polymerization of n-BCA is immediate but can be prolonged by adding hydrophobic contrast agents (e.g., Ethiodol) or glacial acetic acid,[38] rendering this embolic agent more controllable when depositing it into the intravascular system. During long injection times, great care must be taken to avoid microcatheter retention, which may result from the polymerization of the n-BCA along the outer wall of the microcatheter.

Onyx

Onyx is an ethylene–vinyl alcohol copolymer suspended in dimethyl sulfoxide with tantalum added for radiopacity.[20,39,40] The first reported case of CCF embolization using Onyx was a type D fistula described by Arat et al. in 2004.[39] In contrast to n-BCA, which rapidly polymerizes, this cohesive embolic agent precipitates slowly from its outer surface as the dimethyl sulfoxide slowly diffuses into the circulation and the Onyx precipitates. The result is the formation of a cast in the embolized vessel. The slow speed of precipitation allows deep penetration of Onyx with a slow, controlled injection.[20,40] Because of these properties, Onyx permits the embolization of a venous sinus by a transarterial approach.[23] Unique to this liquid embolic agent, it is possible to interrupt the injection during the procedure to allow assessment of the degree of embolization and occlusion. In this way, the endovascular surgeon can recognize the presence of dangerous anastomoses and avoid occlusion of normal vascular anatomy.

In contrast to n-BCA, Onyx's nonadhesive characteristics allow a greater degree of reflux to be tolerated during embolization, leading to a reduced risk of catheter retention.[20,40] Some limitations exist with the use of Onyx. The current microcatheter technology is somewhat limited in provided access to very distal vasculature secondary to the inherent stiffness of the microcatheters approved for use with Onyx. Furthermore, the solvent, dimethyl sulfoxide, may cause painful necrosis in the vasculature if rapidly infused. Like n-BCA, occlusion of the vasa nervorum can result in cranial neuropathies.

Stents

As briefly discussed, the advent of neurospecific stents represents a novel approach to the treatment of CCF and vascular lesions in general. As a nonocclusive scaffold along the ostium of the fistula or an aneurysm, stents provide the necessary parent vessel protection without intermittent interruption of flow within the parent vessel. Made of various alloys, a number of the stents are self-expanding, and though not approved for use for this indication, they have proved quite

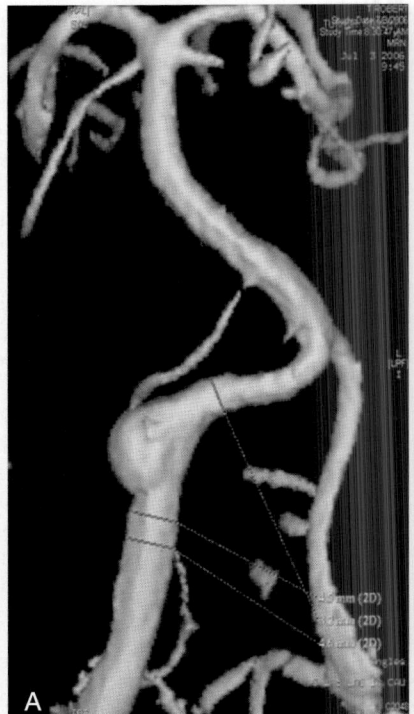
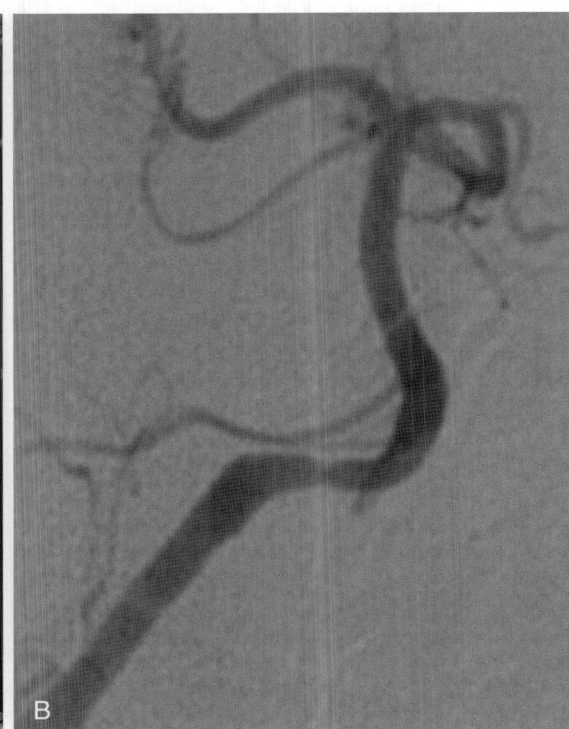

FIGURE 92-4 A 45-year-old man 3 months after a motor vehicle accident with persistent neck pain. A, Three-dimensional CT angiogram, demonstrating a traumatic pseudoaneurysm of the right vertebral artery. B, Follow-up angiogram 2 months after a single Neuroform stent is placed, demonstrating interval thrombosis of the aneurysm.

useful in specific situations. Coiling of the fistula can be performed in the same session as stent placement.[41]

The Pipeline embolization device (Chestnut Medical, Menlo Park, CA) is a flexible, self-expanding, stent used in the treatment of cerebral aneurysms. It is made out of platinum and cobalt chromium microfilaments in the form of a braided mesh cylinder. When deployed, the implants are designed to provide approximately 30% to 35% metal surface coverage at nominal expansion, which is a much higher percentage of coverage than that provided by uncovered intravascular stents.[42]

Covered stents may be used as an alternative to the combined use of coils and balloon-assist or stent placement. As in the peripheral vascular system, placement of covered stents allows for reconstruction of the ICA–cavernous sinus interface without occluding either. It essentially "patches" the traumatic tear in the ICA. Though elegant, this technology is somewhat limited when applied to the central nervous system vasculature. One of the major limitations in the successful delivery and deployment of covered stents is the relative tortuosity of the vessels and the stiffness of the stents. Newer models of stents are more flexible.

In addition to issues of flexibility, covered stents may occlude any small vessels in the region in which they are deployed. While this seriously limits their use in other areas of the neurovasculature, there seems to be little or no clinical significance to the occlusion of the perforators found within the cavernous sinus.[13] Several varieties of covered stents have been used in neurovascular procedures; there is currently only one that is specifically designed for intracranial endovascular procedures: the Willis covered stent.[13,43]

An important caveat in the use of the current stents is the need for adequate platelet inhibition to prevent acute or delayed stent occlusion and its clinical sequelae. Thus, in the setting of acute traumatic injury, this may represent

an absolute contraindication and should therefore not be considered. The benefits of stent use in the setting of traumatic CCF may best be realized in patients presenting in the subacute or chronic/delayed stages, when the hemorrhagic risk from the use of antiplatelet agents is minimal.

TRAUMATIC ANEURYSMS

The true incidence of traumatic intracranial aneurysm formation is unknown. Current reviews suggest that traumatic aneurysms after severe penetrating head trauma can have an incidence as high as 20% to 50%, though this literature may reflect severe injury secondary to military-grade weaponry.[44-46] There is further suggestion that a proportion of these lesions grows and can ultimately rupture in the subacute to chronic stage, with resultant mortality concomitant to the mortality associated with berry aneurysms of the circle of Willis.[44] Traumatic aneurysms have a higher propensity to form with penetrating injuries of the frontal or orbitobasilar region.[46]

Because of the propensity to bleed and the severe sequelae subsequent to hemorrhage, traumatic aneurysms, especially those with documented interval growth, should be treated. Surgical clipping, trapping, and bypass have been performed with variable results. The advent of endovascular techniques enables surgeons to approach these lesions in a minimally invasive fashion, which may be of some benefit in the acute phases of severe traumatic brain injury.

Blunt and Penetrating Injuries of the Neck

The treatment of injury to the arteries of the neck has a limited recorded history, with the majority of treatment advances occurring within the last 300 to 500 years.

The importance of the carotid artery was known since the days of the Greeks. Indeed, the term *carotid* is derived from the Greek *karos*, meaning "stupor," demonstrating the Greeks' knowledge of what happens when these arteries are compressed. Injury to these vessels was likely fatal the majority of times.

In 1522, Paré first reported the ligation of the common carotid artery and jugular vein in a soldier injured after a duel who tolerated common carotid occlusion for several days.[47] The literature hereafter is incomplete, and subsequent reports are nonexistent until the early 19th century, when the surgeon aboard the *HMS Tonnant* ligated the carotid of a suicidal sailor.[48] Soon thereafter, the first recorded treatment of an injured ICA was performed by Abernathy in 1804, when he tied the carotid artery of a man who had been gored by the horn of a cow.[49] This early literature, and the medical war literature up until World War I, attests to the relatively poor outcomes that come from deconstruction of the carotid artery in the setting of injury.[50]

PATHOPHYSIOLOGIC CORRELATES

Direct trauma to the intracranial and extracranial circulation can result from both blunt and penetrating forces. Blunt trauma to both the carotid and the vertebral circulations can result in dissection and in one series has been reported as high as 0.45% of neck traumas, with a high degree of associated morbidity and mortality.[51] Penetrating trauma can result in either complete transection of a vessel with concomitant extravasation or partial injury, which can then present immediately or after a delay. Injury to the tunica intima can result in dissection, intrusion of hematoma between layers of the vessel, and creation of true and false lumens. Compromise of all three arterial wall layers (the intima, media, and adventitia) can result in active extravasation and exsanguination in the field or containment of the hematoma by surrounding tissue planes. In this instance, a pseudoaneurysm results and can present with delayed bleeding subsequent to the inciting trauma. Penetrating trauma, particularly gunshot wounds, can also result in abnormal fistulas between native arteries and veins or venous sinuses (Fig. 92-2).

Cervical carotid injuries account for approximately 25% of all penetrating injuries to the neck, followed by the subclavian artery.[52] As such, understanding the role of open and endovascular techniques for the treatment of vascular injuries to the neck is important from the moment of initial evaluation. Most clinicians employ Saletta et al.'s original description of the three-zone model of cervical injury, though the treatment approaches may now differ.[53] Zone I injury is described as any vascular injury below the clavicle, which seems to be more akin to thoracic injury. Zone II is described as the region of the neck to the level of the angle of the mandible. Zone III is defined as the region above the angle of the mandible. Despite this model, penetrating or blunt injuries of the neck rarely present in isolation, with venous injury occurring in almost 30% of patients and tracheal or esophageal injury occurring in an additional 15%.

Noninvasive imaging has made substantial advances in the last 20 years and has been particularly useful in the diagnosis of cervical vascular injuries to the neck.[54] However, despite advances in both computed tomography

angiography (CTA) and magnetic resonance angiography, digital subtraction angiography remains the gold standard for diagnosis of traumatic vascular injuries to the vessels of the head and neck.[55] In addition to the obvious ability to evaluate both the venous and the arterial systems during time of flight, this modality offers the potential for immediate therapeutic intervention if warranted. However, certain caveats must be borne in mind for the neurointerventionalist. The majority of referred trauma patients have already undergone evaluation in the emergency department, by either the traumatologist or the emergency department physician, and quite possibly in subspecialties such as otolaryngology and maxillofacial surgery. By definition, these patients have failed conservative therapy and possibly basic surgical maneuvers. In addition, the trauma team has likely determined that surgical exploration and treatment are *not* indicated in this situation. As stated by Morris, odds therefore are that "those sent for endovascular management likely have an unusual set of prevailing circumstances, physiologic, anatomic, or otherwise."[56] A thorough history must be taken from the referring team, and the location of the bleeding must be pinpointed as accurately as possible; nasal laterality should be established in the case of traumatic epistaxis, and attention should then be focused on that side. When possible, a radiopaque marker should be affixed to the site of any visible bleeding. Unless the patient is actively extravasating, it may be difficult to identify the exact site of bleeding on angiographic runs.

Time constraints may rapidly prove a factor during treatment, and patients can either present in acute hemodynamic shock or decompensate during the course of treatment. For this reason, general anesthesia and close monitoring of vital signs are paramount during the case. Airway protection takes precedence, and blood should be available for transfusion before groin access. Should rebleeding and hemodynamic instability occur, rapid identification and sealing of the bleeding point take priority over normal concerns regarding sterility and line preparation, within reason.

Embolic and particulate agents may be used in the case of small distal vessels. Older agents such as Gelfoam pledgets and polyvinyl alcohol particles can be used as in epistaxis cases. Newer embolics such as Embospheres provide a uniformity of particulate size not assured with older agents, which can be useful should concern exist for anastomotic communication between the intracranial and the extracranial circulation. In general, the size of nonvisualized anastomotic arteries ranges from 50 to 80 μm; therefore, particles that are larger than 150 μm will not penetrate these anastomoses and will avoid potential embolic complications.[57]

Larger vessels with lacerations and pseudoaneurysms require more definitive therapy via either coil occlusion or liquid embolic agents. When vessel sacrifice is not an option, for instance, when dealing with the common carotid artery, ICA, or dominant vertebral artery, covered or uncovered stents with coils can preserve luminal patency while ensuring maintenance of CBF. Surgical options for these injuries, such as resection and reanastomosis procedures or patch grafting techniques, should always be considered, because they may be more efficacious and safe. In the setting of suspected or known injury to the trachea or esophagus (zone II), surgical exploration is indicated.

Vortex coils (Boston Scientific, Natick, MA) provide an excellent and inexpensive way to occlude larger vessels when coil retrieval is not a concern. Liquid embolics such as *n*-BCA and Onyx are useful for dealing with flow-directed anomalies such as fistulas, as well as for rapid elimination of tributaries off of the external carotid circulation. *n*-BCA augmentation may also be used with fibered coils that are not generating sufficient stagnation of flow within the vessel lumen. Care must be taken when utilizing liquid embolics, because they can open and enter small anastomotic channels that are not visualized on the initial angiograms. However, as previously mentioned, increasing uses are being found for liquid embolic agents in the case of CCFs, severe epistaxis secondary to facial fractures (where bilateral internal maxillary artery sacrifice is typically performed), and ICA transection.[58,59]

Stent placement is increasingly being favored over surgical repair as an initial modality of treatment for ICA pseudoaneurysms caused by both blunt and penetrating trauma.[60] Full anticoagulation is required during the procedure to minimize the risk of thromboembolic complications, and dual antiplatelet therapy is recommended postprocedure for 6 weeks while the stent endothelializes. While polytetrafluoroethylene-covered stents have traditionally been used for this purpose, data are emerging to support the use of specifically designed carotid artery stents. Stent-assisted vessel wall reconstruction may provide definitive treatment for traumatic pseudoaneurysms even if coil embolization proves unfeasible.[61]

EPISTAXIS

Endovascular treatment for control of epistaxis was first described in the literature by Sokoloff et al. in 1974 and then further refined by Lasjaunias et al., with particular emphasis on preoperative angiographic evaluation.[62,63] As has been previously stated, some caveats regarding patient selection must be held in mind. Bleeding from the anterior septal (Little's) area accounts for the majority of cases of epistaxis, a region that is vascularized by the Kiesselbach plexus and supplied primarily by the ethmoidal arteries, as well as branches off external carotid artery (sphenopalatine, descending palatine, and superior labial).[64] Hemorrhage from this region typically responds well to direct pressure, topical hemostatic or cauterizing agents, direct electrocautery, or anterior packing. These patients normally do well with conservative therapy and therefore are not referred for endovascular evaluation in the absence of confounding factors.

In approximately 5% of epistaxis cases, however, the origin of bleeding lies more posteriorly on the nasal cavity.[65] Posterior epistaxis typically presents with a more fulminant arterial bleeding and can result in a significant volume of blood loss in a short time. Causes can be varied and depend on individual patient comorbidities, but roughly 70% of cases are idiopathic.[66] Initial treatment usually involves application of anterior and posterior packing by the otolaryngology team, frequently with direct pressure maintained by a clamped balloon catheter. Despite these measures, one third of posterior epistaxis patients either continues bleeding or recommences hemorrhage with the

removal of tamponade.[67] Endovascular treatment of such patients can serve as an alternative to open surgical treatment, which involves transantral ligation of the internal maxillary and anterior ethmoidal arteries.

Goals of endovascular therapy include diminishing flow to the affected nasal mucosa while avoiding necrosis of treated tissues and inadvertent embolization of critical structures. Due to the potential for airway compromise and the ongoing risk of hemodynamic instability, general anesthesia is preferred for such cases. Bilateral preoperative angiographic evaluation of both external and internal carotid arteries is essential for multiple reasons. The internal carotid arteries must be assessed to ensure normal origin and distribution of the ophthalmic arteries, rule out an ICA source of bleeding, and check the extent of blood supply to the nasal mucosa via the ethmoidal arteries. The external carotid arteries require careful angiographic runs to map the territory of the internal maxillary artery, check for hazardous ECA-ICA anastomoses, and rule out nonidiopathic causes of epistaxis (e.g., vascular malformations, neoplasms or traumatic pseudoaneurysms).[68]

If no overt lesion is evident on angiography, particle embolization of both internal maxillary arteries is carried out. Polyvinyl alcohol particles or Embospheres are typically used, with sizes between 150 and 500 μm preferred to avoid the risk of entering dangerous anastomoses. Gelfoam pledgets can be used to occlude the internal maxillary artery at the origin once near-stagnation of flow is seen; coil occlusion is another option, but it prevents the possibility of a repeat embolization if hemorrhage recurs.[69] Light embolization of the facial artery ipsilateral to the bleeding can be carried out as well in cases of significant supply to the nasal mucosa via its angular branch. If embolization of the facial artery is to be performed, however, it should be carried out distal to the origin of the submandibular artery. In addition, the contralateral facial artery should not be embolized given the potential for nasal skin necrosis.

Technical success rates for bleeding control can range from 70% to 85% in selected patients.[67,70] Major complications from the procedure can include embolic stroke, cranial nerve palsies, septal perforation, facial skin or mucosal necrosis, and blindness (frequently from unappreciated anastomoses between the distal internal maxillary branches and the ophthalmic artery). Fortunately, the incidence of such adverse events is low: less than 2% in reported series.[69,71]

CAROTID BLOWOUT

Rupture of the extracranial carotid artery or its major branches, commonly referred to as carotid blowout, remains one of the most feared and life-threatening complications associated with head and neck cancer and its treatment. The reported incidence of this complication in patients who have undergone neck dissection with or without tumor resection is 3% to 4%.[72] While the morbidity and mortality associated with this condition were historically held to be quite high (60% and 40%, respectively), recent progress in diagnosis and management has resulted in a marked decrease.[72] Radiation therapy has been strongly associated with this condition due to the obliteration of the vasa vasorum and the weakening of the arterial wall as a sequelae of treatment. It is estimated that patients who have been irradiated previously have a sevenfold increase in the risk of carotid blowout.[73] Although traditionally associated with neoplastic processes, in particular squamous cell carcinoma, carotid blowout can result from direct blunt or penetrating trauma and may be iatrogenic as a result of endoscopic sinus surgery.

Carotid blowout is now considered to be a syndrome and can present as one of three separate entities: threatened, impending, and acute. Threatened carotid blowout is characterized by the suggestion of imminent hemorrhage, either due to exposure of the carotid artery via tissue necrosis or visualization of a pseudoaneurysm diagnostic angiography. Impending carotid blowout is indicated by the presence of a cervical or transoral sentinel hemorrhage that resolves spontaneously or with basic treatment. Acute carotid blowout is a life-threatening hemorrhage that cannot be controlled with packing or pressure and requires immediate surgical or endovascular intervention.[74]

The most common sites of hemorrhage on meta-analysis of multiple case studies were, in descending order of frequency, ICA (43.6%), external carotid artery (23.4%), common carotid artery (11.7%), buccal artery (3.2%), inferior thyroid artery (3.2%), superior thyroid artery (2.1%), internal mammary artery (2.1%), innominate artery (1.1%), facial artery (1.1%), and aorta (1.1%).[3]

Endovascular management of carotid blowout syndrome falls into two categories: constructive and deconstructive. Constructive management attempts to maintain the patency of the affected vasculature and can involve reconstruction with covered wall stents (polytetrafluoroethylene, Wallgraft), as well as stent-assisted coiling of associated pseudoaneurysms. Deconstructive management involves placement of embolic materials such as detachable balloons, coils, or liquid embolic agents with the goal of diseased vessel obliteration.

Retrospective case series have indicated that deconstructive management may be superior to constructive management. Stent occlusion in one series was 100% at 3 months, although technical issues and inadequate patient premedication with antiplatelet therapy may have accounted for this.[75] The incidence of rebleeding may also be higher with constructive management. Furthermore, extensive tissue necrosis and direct exposure of the fistula or the carotid artery make stent placement into a contaminated field a matter for concern, and intracranial abscesses likely secondary to septic emboli have been reported.[76] However, endovascular stent graft reconstruction may prove beneficial as a palliative measure, in patients who fail BTO in preparation for vessel sacrifice, or as an elective preventative measure for threatened blowout in the absence of active bleeding (Fig. 92-3).

VERTEBRAL ARTERY INJURY

Vertebral artery injury makes up less than 5% of all cervical arterial injuries, with penetrating trauma—most specifically, gunshot wounds—being the most common penetrating form of injury and motor vehicle accidents being the etiology of most blunt injuries to the vertebral artery. Almost 75% of injuries to the vertebral artery are asymptomatic because of its location and because the contralateral vertebral artery will most likely (85%) provide sufficient flow to the posterior circulation.[77] Furthermore, the anatomic proximity of

the epidural venous plexus along the C1 to C2 region, the most likely region of blunt vertebral artery injury, results in arteriovenous fistula formation. Physical and neurologic findings such as Horner syndrome, Wallenberg syndrome, cranial nerve palsies, and respiratory failure should lead the clinician to suspect possible vascular injury.[78]

Because of the relative rarity of this injury, management strategies for vertebral artery injury have largely been adopted from the carotid injury data. Though accessible, the surgical approaches to the vertebral artery can be challenging. Surgical ligation of the proximal vertebral artery (at its origin) can be considered and performed by vascular surgeons in the acute trauma setting, especially in the setting of a nondominant vertebral artery injury. However, endovascular options of ligation and reconstruction should be considered first if injury to the mid- or distal vertebral artery (V2 and V3 segments) occurs (Fig. 92-4).

It is somewhat difficult to determine the true outcomes of patients sustaining vertebral artery injury, because it is rare to have severe, isolated injury. It is estimated that though mortality ranges from 11% to 25%, only 5% of that mortality is directly attributable to injury of the vertebral artery.[77]

Conclusions

The role of endovascular therapy in traumatic vascular injury continues to mature. It has enabled surgeons to elegantly and definitively treat injuries that were previously untreatable while leaving the smallest of "footprints." Clinicians can now include this tool in the armamentarium of treatment options for complex vascular injury as a viable, safe, and effective technique in carefully selected patients. As the field continues to evolve, surgeons will continue to explore and apply innovative surgical and interventional techniques to save the lives of individuals sustaining devastating vascular injury through trauma or disease.

KEY REFERENCES

Aarabi B. Traumatic aneurysms of brain due to high velocity missile head wounds. *Neurosurgery.* 1988;22:1056-1063.

Barrow DL, Spector RH, Braun IF, et al. Classification and treatment of spontaneous carotid–cavernous sinus fistulas. *J Neurosurg.* 1985;62:248-256.

Brothers MF, Kaufmann JC, Fox AJ, Deveikis JP. n-Butyl 2-cyanoacrylate—substitute for IBCA in interventional neuroradiology: histopathologic and polymerization time studies. *AJNR Am J Neuroradiol.* 1989;10:777-786.

Cohen J, Rad I. Contemporary management of carotid blowout. *Curr Opin Otolaryngol Head Neck Surg.* 2004;12:110-115.

Fiorella D, Woo HH, Albuquerque FC, Nelson PK. Definitive reconstruction of circumferential, fusiform intracranial aneurysms with the pipeline embolization device. *Neurosurgery.* 2008;62:1115-1120.

Geibprasert S, Pongpech S, Armstrong D, et al. Dangerous Extracranial–Intracranial Anastomoses and Supply to the Cranial Nerves: Vessels the Neurointerventionalist Needs to Know. *American Journal of Neuroradiology.* 2009;30:1459-1468.

Houdart E, Gobin YP, Casasco A, et al. A proposed angiographic classification of intracranial arteriovenous fistulae and malformations. *Neuroradiology.* 1993;35:381-385.

Kosary IZ, Lerner MA, Mozes M, Lazar M. Artificial embolic occlusion of the terminal internal carotid artery in the treatment of carotid–cavernous fistula. Technical note. *J Neurosurg.* 1968;28:605-608.

Lasjaunias P, Marsot-Dupuch K, Doyon D. The radio-anatomic basis of arterial embolization for epistaxis. *J Neuroradiol.* 1979;6:45-53.

Luessenhop AJ, Spence WT. Artificial embolization of cerebral arteries. The report of use in a case of AV malformation. *JAMA.* 1960;172:1153-1155.

Morris PP. *Practical Neuroangiography.* 2nd ed. Philadelphia: Lippincott; 2007498-499.

Morrissey DD, Andersen PE, Nesbit GM, et al. Endovascular management of hemorrhage in patients with head and neck cancer. *Arch Otolaryngol Head Neck Surg.* 1997;123:15-19.

Mulloy JP, Flick PA, Gold RE. Blunt carotid injury: a review. *Radiology.* 1998;207:571-585.

Paré A. *The collected works of Ambroise Paré (translated out of the Latin by Thomas Johnson, London, first English edition, 1634).* Pound Ridge, NY: Milford House Inc; 1968.

Pearce WH, Whitehill Ta. Carotid and vertebral artery injuries. *Surg Clin North Am.* 1988;68:705-723.

Prestigiacomo CJ. Surgical endovascular neuroradiology in the 21st century: what lies ahead? *Neurosurgery.* 2006;59(5 Suppl 3):S48-S55.

Rubio PA, Reul GJ, Beall AC, et al. Acute carotid artery injury: 25 years' experience. *J Trauma.* 1974;14:967-973.

Saletta JD, Folk FA, Freeark RJ. Trauma to the neck region. *Surg Clin North Am.* 1973;53:73-85.

Schelhas KP, Latchaw RE, Wendling LR, Gold LHA. Vertebrobasilar injuries following cervical manipulation. *JAMA.* 1980;224:1450-1453.

Serbinenko FA. Balloon catheterization and occlusion of major cerebral vessels. *J Neurosurg.* 1974;41:125-145.

Sokoloff J, Wickbom I, McDonald D, et al. Therapeutic percutaneous embolization in intractable epistaxis. *Radiology.* 1974;111:285-287.

Stiefel MF, Albuquerque FC, Park MS, et al. Endovascular treatment of intracranial dural arteriovenous fistulae using Onyx: a case series. *Neurosurgery.* 2009;65(Suppl 6):132-139.

Willems PWA, Farb RI, Agid R. Endovascular treatment of epistaxis. *American Journal of Neuroradiology.* 2009;30:1637-1645.

Zenteno M, Santos-Franco J, Rodriguez-Parra V, et al. Management of direct carotid–cavernous sinus fistulas with the use of ethylene–vinyl alcohol (Onyx) only: preliminary results. *J Neurosurg.* 2009;112(3):595-602.

Numbered references appear on Expert Consult.

CHAPTER 93

Imaging Evaluation and Endovascular Treatment of Vasospasm

JAMES CHEN • SUDHIR KATHURIA • DHEERAJ GANDHI

The phenomenon of cerebral vasospasm following aneurysmal subarachnoid hemorrhage (aSAH) was first described in the 1950s by Ecker and Riemenschneider,[1] and substantial contributions have been made in subsequent decades to the clinical and pathophysiologic understanding of this debilitating condition. The traditional belief has been that subarachnoid blood products trigger vasospasm of the proximal, large-caliber cerebral vessels, which consequently leads to impaired cerebral perfusion and eventual infarction of the affected tissue. Modern investigations of this phenomenon, which has been termed delayed cerebral ischemia (DCI), have further implicated distal microvascular disease[2] and dysregulated proliferation of smooth muscle and endothelial cells in its pathophysiology.[3,4] While the complete picture of its pathogenesis remains to be fully elucidated, there is strong evidence that the presence of severe vasospasm correlates with the development of DCI and subsequent cerebral infarcts. Prompt diagnosis and treatment of vasospasm prior to the onset of permanent ischemic damage are therefore essential to improving survival and preventing secondary loss of neurologic function in the aSAH patient population.[5]

Historically, the most common cause of mortality following initial hemorrhage from aSAH was rebleeding. Advancements in surgical and endovascular techniques and a general trend toward more aggressive, early repair of aneurysm have led to a decrease in the incidence of this complication.[6] DCI from vasospasm has thus emerged as the most common cause of secondary morbidity and death. From literature and clinical experience, this reversible narrowing of cerebral vessels typically occurs between 3 and 14 days[7-9] following initial hemorrhage, with a peak incidence around day 7.[10] Up to 70% of patients demonstrate angiographically visible vasospasm within this time window, but only 20% to 30% of these cases develop clinical evidence of cerebral ischemia and consequently require acute therapy.[7,8,11,12] Of symptomatic patients, up to 50% suffer devastating neurologic deficits or death as a result of clinically significant vasospasm, highlighting the importance of prompt diagnosis and therapeutic management.[9,13]

To assess which patients are at highest risk of developing vasospasm, various groups have suggested clinical factors, including Hunt and Hess grading and characteristics of the subarachnoid clot on computed tomography (CT) (i.e., initial presence, volume, density, and duration) that associate with an increased risk of vasospasm.[6,7,8] Other clinical variables, including young patient age, poor neurologic grade, greater-than-normal thickness of the subarachnoid clot, intraventricular or intracerebral hemorrhage, and history of smoking, have been associated with the development of more severe vasospasm.[8,11,12] While these considerations can aid in the care of aSAH patients, no comprehensive prediction algorithm exists to determine which patients will suffer DCI. Therefore, there continues to be no substitute for vigilant clinical monitoring and careful decision making by an experienced, multidisciplinary care team to prevent or limit the neurologic injury from vasospasm.[14]

Clinical Assessment

Frequent neurologic evaluations play an essential role in the diagnosis of DCI. Common symptoms that should raise alarm include the development of confusion, delirium, decreased consciousness, or new, focal neurologic deficits. Symptoms can emerge acutely or fulminantly, and nonspecific signs such as headache or increasing neck stiffness can sometimes be the only notable findings during the onset of cerebral ischemia. Furthermore, alternative etiologies for altered mental status and focal neurologic deficits, including hydrocephalus, systemic infection, seizures, or ongoing delirium, must be ruled out. A meaningful neurologic examination may not be achievable in patients who have suffered severe neurologic impairment or are comatose at baseline. In such cases, imaging studies inevitably play a larger role in monitoring for symptomatic vasospasm.

Diagnostic Imaging
TRANSCRANIAL DOPPLER ULTRASONOGRAPHY

Transcranial Doppler (TCD) ultrasonography has been widely employed as the first-line modality for monitoring cerebral vasospasm in aSAH patients (Fig. 93-1). It is non-invasive, inexpensive, and easily performed at the bedside, making it particularly appropriate for daily evaluations. The sensitivity of TCD is highest for vasospasm in the proximal middle cerebral artery (MCA) but decreases in other vascular territories.[15] It also varies depending on the adequacy of vessel insonation.[16] The diagnostic value of TCD comes from its high specificity—detection of normal flow velocities can effectively exclude the presence of vasospasm.[17] It is thus an excellent modality for initial patient triage.

NONCONTRAST HEAD CT

For patients with changes in clinical exam or TCD findings, noncontrast head CT should be performed before any subsequent interventions are considered. This modality offers a rapid survey for infarctions in the territory of suspected vasospasm and rules out other etiologies of neurologic deterioration, including hydrocephalus and rehemorrhage. The identification of developing infarcts has important implications for subsequent treatment decision making, because the restoration of flow to these areas typically provides minimal recovery of neurologic function and can potentially lead to further decline as a result of reperfusion hemorrhage.[18,19]

COMPUTED TOMOGRAPHY ANGIOGRAPHY AND PERFUSION

Computed tomography angiography (CTA) and computed tomography perfusion (CTP) imaging have undergone significant advancements in recent years and have emerged as effective modalities for triaging vasospasm

patients toward endovascular therapy (Fig. 93-2). CTA has been shown to be highly accurate for detection of severe vasospasm (more than 50% luminal reduction) and has excellent negative predictive value.[20,21] The severity of vasospasm can be overestimated in certain vascular territories, and metallic artifacts from coils or clips can hinder the assessment of nearby territories. Despite these limitations, CTA provides an informative and practical assessment of cerebral vessel caliber in patients with concerning symptoms. The recent addition of CTP scans to the vasospasm imaging armamentarium has allowed insight into the hemodynamic implications of CTA findings. Stereotypical patterns of perfusion abnormality can indicate the presence of either reversible ischemia, which should be addressed promptly to maximize penumbral recovery, or irreversible ischemia, which is a contraindication to aggressive therapy. This distinction is essential for the appropriate triage of patients toward endovascular therapy, because the treatment of infarcted territories potentially leads to further morbidity. A combined, multimodality, CT-based approach has been implemented at many institutions, allowing acquisition of conventional CT, CTA, and CTP images in one setting. This protocol is

FIGURE 93-1 A patient with recent SAH demonstrated fluctuating right lower extremity weakness and aphasia. A, A screening color Doppler study reveals elevated flow velocities in the left MCA, suggestive of moderate vasospasm. B, A digital subtraction angiogram, with a anteroposterior view of left internal carotid injection, shows mild to moderate caliber reduction of the M2 branches (*arrows*). C, Given the predominantly distal location and moderate severity of the vasospasm, this patient was treated with IA nicardipine alone. The anteroposterior view of the left internal carotid injection following slow infusion of 5 mg of nicardipine demonstrates the augmented caliber of M2 branches and the improved filling of distal cortical branches.

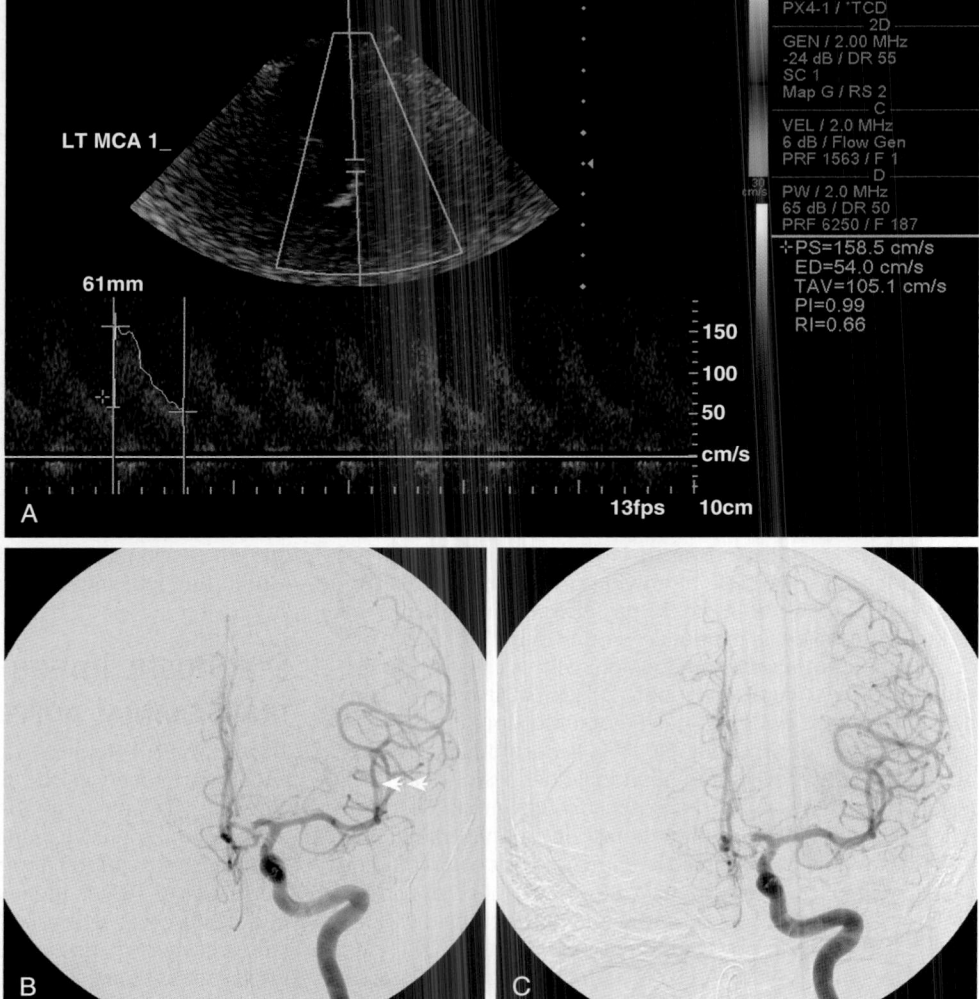

well suited for aSAH patients for whom lengthy transport or imaging studies may be unfeasible. Clinicians need to be wary of radiation exposure when ordering repeated CT studies; there have been reports of associated sequelae in the medical literature and lay press.[22]

MAGNETIC RESONANCE ANGIOGRAPHY AND PERFUSION-WEIGHTED MAGNETIC RESONANCE IMAGING

Magnetic resonance angiography and perfusion-weighted magnetic resonance imaging (MRI) have been used for detecting vasospasm (Fig. 93-2) but have failed to achieve wider adoption for vasospasm imaging due to logistical impracticability of MRI in acutely sick patients.

DIGITAL SUBTRACTION ANGIOGRAPHY

Digital subtraction angiography (DSA) remains the gold standard for evaluation of cerebral vasospasm and provides the foundation for all endovascular treatments. It is highly sensitive and specific for detection of proximal, as well as distal, lesions and provides real-time assessment of hemodynamic alterations. Because it is a costly and resource-intensive procedure with a small risk of procedural complications, patients should undergo noninvasive imaging first before receiving DSA.

Medical Therapies for Cerebral Vasospasm

Although the scope of this chapter is endovascular management for vasospasm, we must emphasize that medical therapy remains the first-line and mainstay treatment for a majority of patients. Hemodynamic therapy via induced hypervolemia, hypertension, and hemodilution (triple-H therapy) has achieved widespread use, and studies have demonstrated efficacy in improving cerebral perfusion, as well as clinical outcomes.[23] Patients who do not respond to this treatment or who cannot tolerate sufficient periods of hyperdynamic therapy due to underlying medical comorbidities are candidates for endovascular intervention.

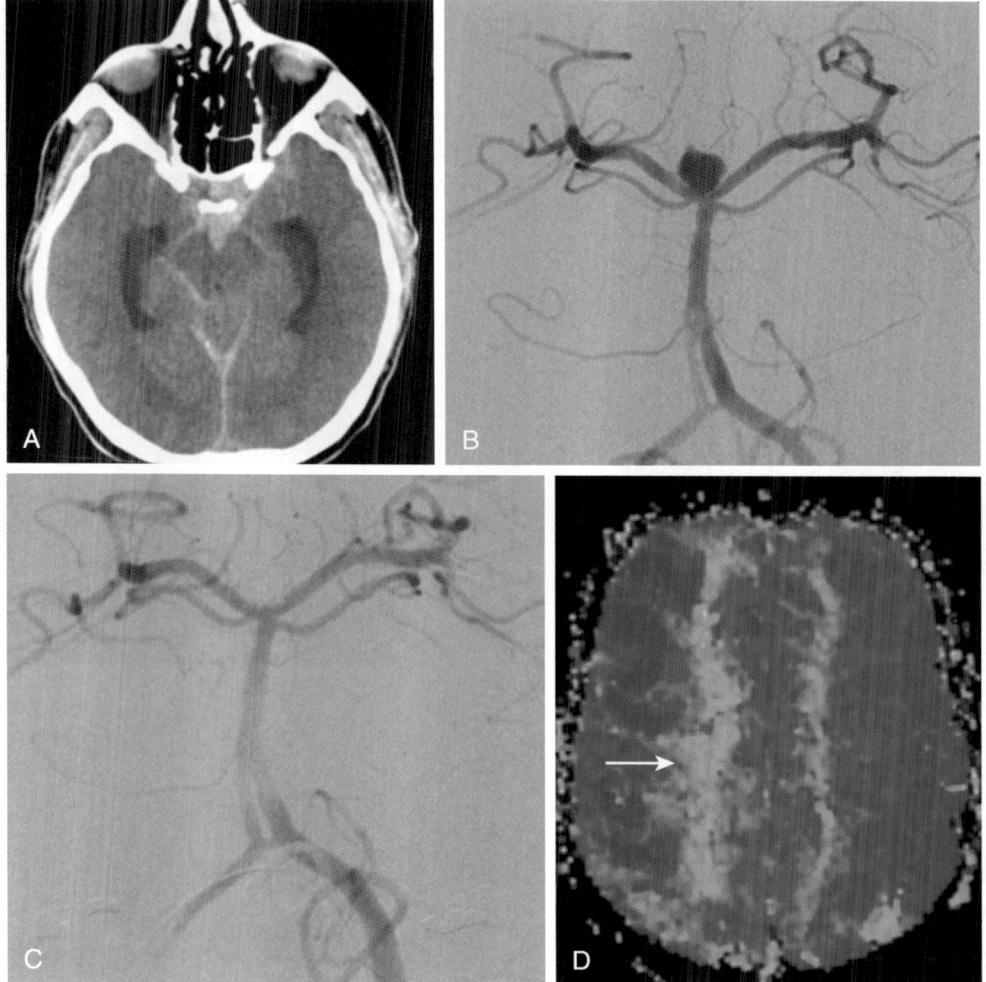

FIGURE 93-2 A 44-year-old male, 9 days status post-SAH and embolization, developed increasing drowsiness and stopped following commands. Doppler ultrasound was suspicious for severe vasospasm. A, Initial head CT demonstrating diffuse SAH. Note a more focal hemorrhage in the interpeduncular cistern. B, An irregular basilar tip aneurysm was the cause of the SAH. C, This was embolized, with complete occlusion of the aneurysm. D, MRI at this time showed small watershed infarcts. A perfusion image shown here reveals bilateral elevation in mean transit time, asymmetrically more so in the right hemisphere (arrow).

Continued

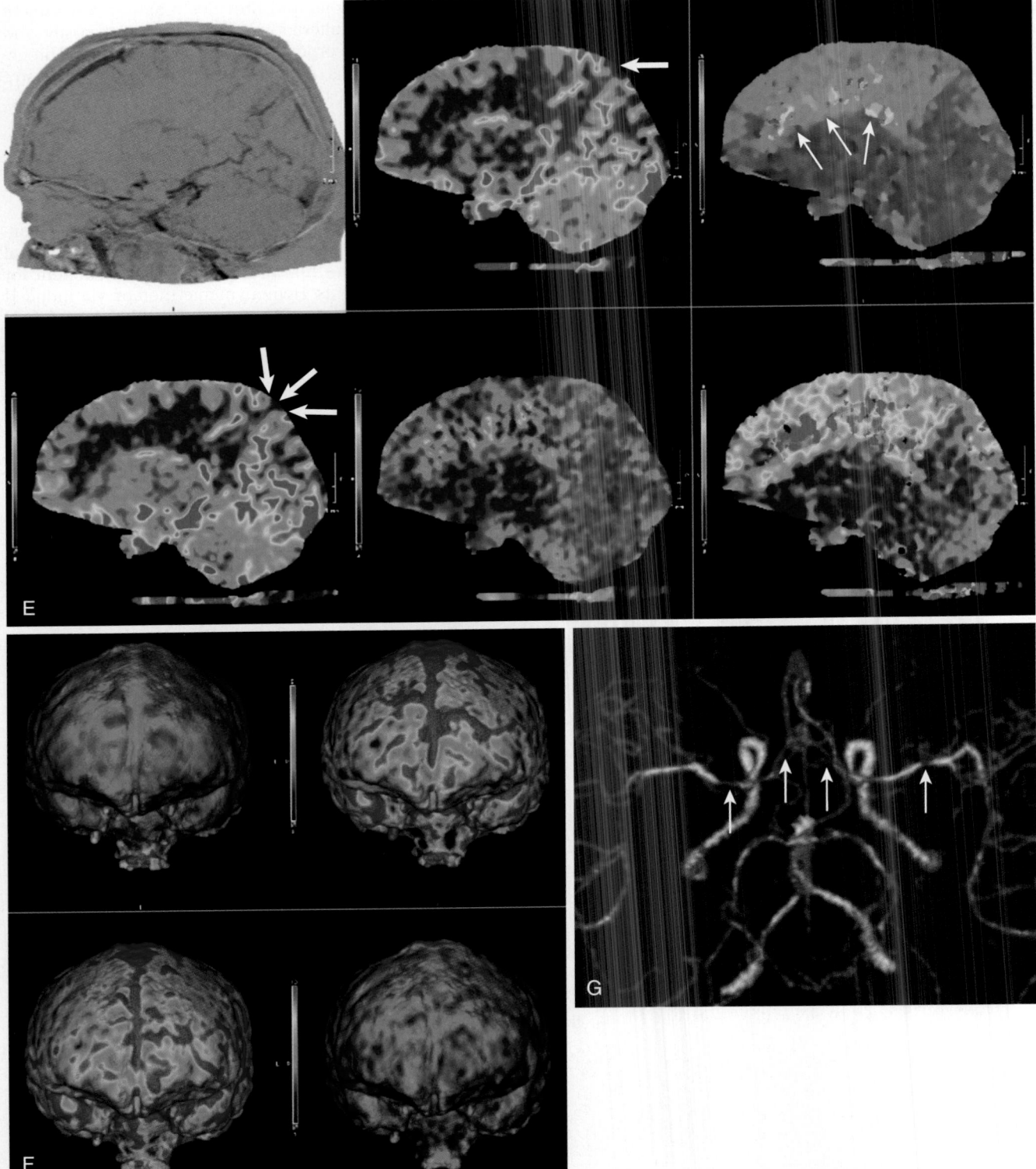

FIGURE 93-2, cont'd A CTP study in the sagittal (E) and coronal (F) planes confirms the perfusion abnormalities. Small matched defects on the cerebral blood flow (*arrow*) and cerebral blood volume maps in the watershed zones suggest small foci of irreversible ischemic injury. However, there is a large area of penumbra (*arrowheads*) that could be prevented with early intervention. G, A CTA shaded-surface image confirms bilateral MCA (right greater than left) and A1 spasm (*arrows*).

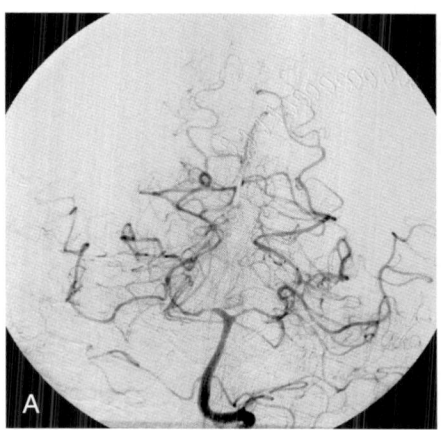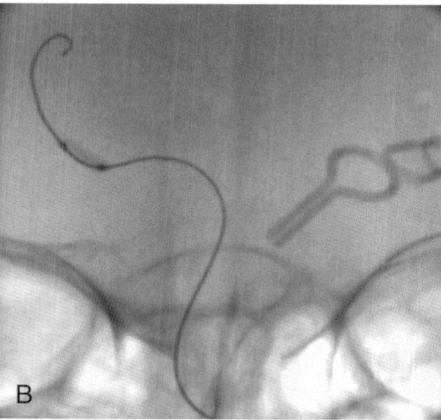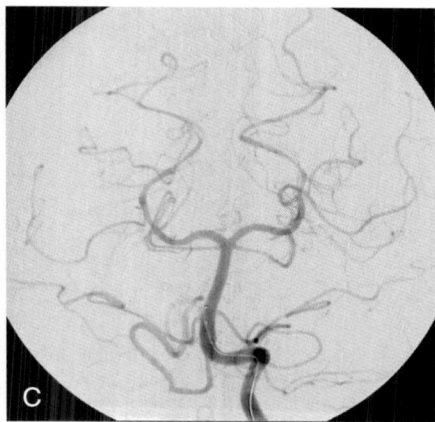

FIGURE 93-3 Improvements in endovascular semicompliant balloon technology have resulted in safer, more controlled angioplasty procedures. A, Left vertebral angiography in a patient with moderate spasm of the basilar artery and severe spasm of the bilateral P1 and P2 segments is demonstrated. B, This was treated with balloon angioplasty of all involved segments. This image shows an inflated Hyperform balloon in the right P2 segment. C, Note the markedly improved appearance of the basilar artery and the posterior cerebral arteries. There is some residual spasm in the cortical segments, but it was no longer restricting flow.

Overview of Endovascular Therapies for Cerebral Vasospasm

The goal of endovascular therapy for symptomatic cerebral vasospasm is to restore blood flow to ischemic parenchyma and salvage the penumbra region (Figs. 93-1, 93-3, and 93-4). These interventions are not the first-line treatment due to inherent procedural risks and intensive resource requirements, but when performed in appropriately selected patients, they can produce excellent angiographic and clinical outcomes.

The two classes of current endovascular therapies are intra-arterial (IA) vasodilator infusion and transluminal balloon angioplasty (TBA), which can be used in isolation or combination and are chosen depending on the location of vasospasm. Proximal lesions are ideally treated through mechanical balloon angioplasty with optional, complementary IA infusion, whereas distal lesions should be addressed with IA infusion alone.

IA Vasodilator Infusion

IA vasodilator infusions have been employed widely for the pharmacologic treatment of cerebral vasospasm, but the efficacy and duration of these agents remains modest. For distal vasospasm that cannot be readily accessed by mechanical angioplasty devices, IA vasodilator infusions nonetheless provide an important means to improve blood flow and prevent permanent ischemic damage (Fig. 93-1). Anecdotal reports have also suggested the use of IA vasodilator infusion as an adjunct to angioplasty to reduce the vasomotor tone of the vessel and potentially decrease the subsequent risk of acute vessel rupture during balloon dilation (Fig. 93-4).

PAPAVERINE

The first pharmacologic vasodilator that was employed broadly for treatment of cerebral vasospasm was papaverine, an alkaloid of the opium group with a half-life of 2 hours that acts as a nonspecific vasodilator by increasing cyclic adenosine monophosphate levels in smooth muscle cells.[24,25] Studies examining the efficacy of the drug demonstrated angiographic improvement in 75% of cases, but modest clinical improvements were achieved in only 25% to 52% of patients.[19,26,27] Furthermore, these improvements were often transient, and some patients required multiple treatments, which were associated with worsened complication profiles.[25] Described complications include raised intracranial pressure (ICP), seizures, hypotension, transient brain stem depression, worsening vasospasm, monocular blindness if infusion is performed proximal to the ophthalmic artery origin, and gray matter injury by direct neurotoxicity.[18,27,28] The combination of these risks with the papaverine's relatively short duration of action have led to the replacement of this drug by calcium channel blockers (CCBs) for IA treatment of vasospasm in modern practice.

CALCIUM CHANNEL BLOCKERS

As a class, CCBs have been met with the greatest recent investigational interest because of their excellent safety profiles and consistent efficacy. Their implementation as IA agents was logical, because there has been extensive experience with intravenous administration of these drugs to patients before and after definitive aneurysm therapy. Mechanistically, the benefit of these drugs have traditionally been attributed to inhibition of voltage-gated calcium channels in smooth muscle cells, but evidence that patients can demonstrate a positive clinical response without corresponding improvements to angiographic vasospasm have alluded to the presence of indirect benefits, such as neuroprotective effects.[29] Verapamil, nimodipine, and nicardipine have been the most studied of the CCBs, but randomized, controlled trials examining the use of these drugs for treatment of vasospasm remain to be conducted, and their use toward this application still remains off-label. As such, the optimal doses, infusion rates, and retreatment intervals remain to be definitively studied and vary substantially between groups.

Verapamil is a phenylalkylamine CCB with a half-life of approximately 7 hours. Preliminary studies have yielded

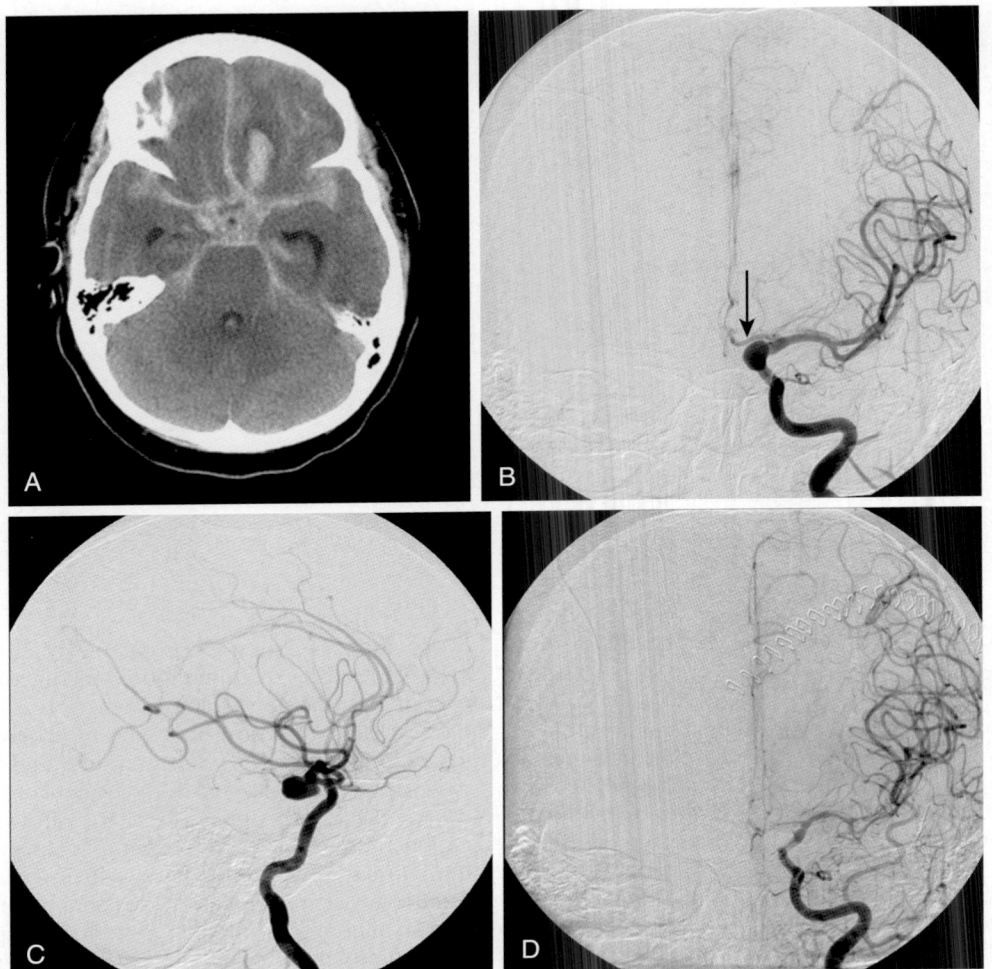

FIGURE 93-4 Combined therapy (IA verapamil and balloon angioplasty) of vasospasm. A, An initial CT scan shows diffuse SAH and a left frontal intraparenchymal hematoma. The cause of this SAH was believed to be a left-sided posterior communicating artery aneurysm, shown on antero-posterior (B) and lateral (C) projections. The aneurysm was clipped. In B, the left A1 segment is hypoplastic (*arrow*). D, The patient experienced symptomatic vasospasm. An angiogram reveals severe vasospasm of the left M1 segment and moderate spasm of the supraclinoid ICA.

mixed results, with some groups reporting angiographic and clinical improvement[30] while others have been unable to demonstrate statistically significant effects.[31] The ambiguity of these data may be due to the lack of quantified analysis and blinded radiographic review among some of these studies.[32] The appropriate dose to achieve therapeutic effects remains uncertain. On one hand, groups have reported the doses as high as 41 mg per procedure[33] but Feng et al. demonstrated increased vessel diameter in 44% of patients and neurologic improvement in 29% with only 3 mg per procedure.[30] The appropriate time course of administration also remains to be elucidated—most studies to date have employed bolus infusion strategies, but it has been suggested that prolonged infusions may offer greater clinical benefit. Albanese et al. recently examined the efficacy of long-term IA infusion (average of 7.8 hours) with an average dose per vessel of 164.6 mg in 12 patients and reported improved vessel caliber in 89% of treated vessels, with favorable clinical outcome at 8 to 12 months in 73% of patients.[34] As optimization of the treatment protocol improves through additional research, the potential for further improvements in angiographic and clinical outcomes is optimistic.

Nimodipine is a dihydropyridine CCB with a half-life of approximately 8 to 9 hours that works through mechanisms similar to those of verapamil and possesses a similar safety profile. It has not been available for use in the United States but has been adopted in Europe and Australasia. Biondi et al. reported clinical improvement 19 of 25 patients (76%) in the first 24 hours following IA nimodipine infusion.[35] At 3 to 6 months follow-up, 18 patients (72%) had a favorable clinical outcome. Successful dilation of infused vessels, however, occurred in only 13 out of 30 (43%) of procedures, so the results raise some uncertainty as to whether improvements in vessel caliber were truly responsible for the positive outcomes. Doses of up to 3 mg per vascular territory were used (for a total of 1-5 mg per session) at a rate of 1 mg over 10 to 15 minutes to minimize hypotension. No episodes of increased ICP or other complications were noted. The use of continuous nimodipine infusion for vasospasm that is refractory to bolus treatment has been reported in a series of 9 patients by Wolf et al.[36] The authors used a 2 mg per hour or 2 mg every 30 minutes for a three-times-daily infusion schedule and showed improvements in CTP patterns and positive long-term clinical outcomes in 3 patients (33%).

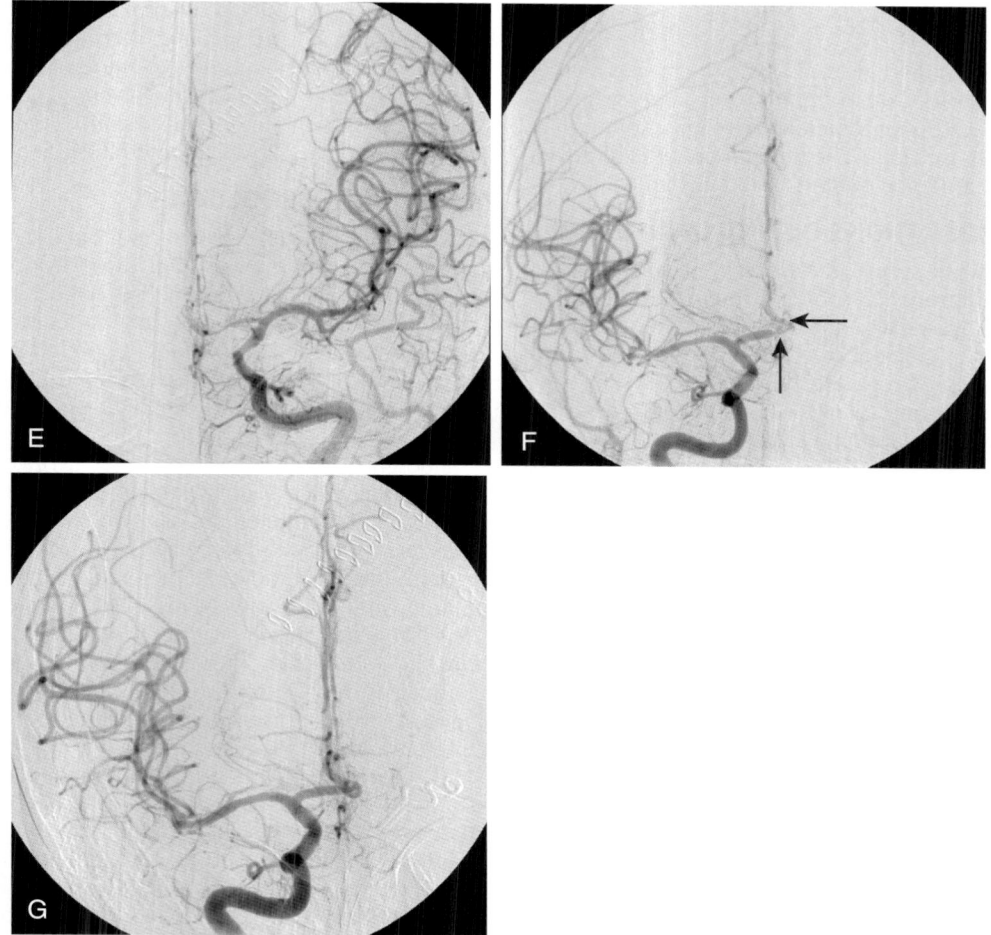

FIGURE 93-4, cont'd E, The left MCA and distal ICA were treated with angioplasty with good result. The A1 segment was intentionally not angioplastied since it was a congenitally hypoplastic vessel. Angioplasty of a hypoplastic vessel should be avoided to prevent the risk of vessel rupture. F, Restoration of anterior cerebral artery (ACA) perfusion was addressed from the contralateral, dominant right A1. This right ICA angiogram reveals vasospasm of the distal right A1 and proximal A2 segments (*arrows*). G, The spastic right A1 segment was treated with balloon angioplasty. A subsequent angiogram shows improved vessel caliber of the target segment and more robust filling of the distal ACA branches.

However, another 3 patients (33%) died from refractory vasospasm, so further investigations are necessary before definitive recommendations for the use of continuous infusions can be made.

Nicardipine is a dihydropyridine CCB that is more selective for vascular smooth muscle than for cardiac smooth muscle and possesses a half-life of approximately 16 hours (Fig. 93-1). In the series by Badjatia et al., 44 vessels were treated in 18 patients at doses of 0.5 to 6 mg per vessel.[37] DSA and TCD demonstrated reductions in vasospasm in all patients, and clinical improvement was observed in 42% of patients. Although the drug was generally well tolerated, 4 patients suffered transient increases in ICP and 1 had a persistent increase that necessitated termination of nicardipine infusion. In a subsequent paper, Tejada et al. reported a series of 20 treatments in 11 patients for which they attained effective angiographic responses of more than 60% increase in arterial diameter in all patients and clinical improvement in the Glasgow coma scale or resolution of focal symptoms in 10 of 11 patients (91%) following IA infusion of 10 to 40 mg of nicardipine.[38] Linfante et al. showed similarly promising results, with angiographic vasospasm improvement in 95% of cases following 2 to 25 mg of IA nicardipine infusion in 22 patients with symptomatic vasospasm, 50% of whom were functionally independent at the time of discharge.[39] Although retreatment is required in some patients, the current literature and experience suggest that the duration of effect of nicardipine is favorable when compared to other IA agents.

The benefits of IA nicardipine infusions may also extend to the microvascular and parenchymal levels, which may not be evidenced by angiographic examination of larger proximal vessel vasospasm.[40] In terms of complications, modest reductions in blood pressure of between 17 and 23 mm Hg have been reported with the use of IA nicardipine, and vasopressor support may occasionally be needed.[38,39,41]

OTHER PHARMACOLOGIC AGENTS UNDER INVESTIGATION

Aside from the previously mentioned drugs, agents including magnesium sulfate, 3-3-hydroxy-3-methylglutaryl–coenzyme A reductase inhibitors, nitric oxide donors, and endothelin-1 antagonists have been used, but their application remains limited.

INFUSION LOCATION

In general, infusions are performed from the proximal internal carotid artery (ICA) or vertebral artery depending on the target vessels, although superselective injections can be performed in certain cases. The clinical benefits of the latter approach remain to be demonstrated in studies.

SAFETY CONSIDERATIONS DURING IA INFUSION

Patient vitals must be monitored carefully during IA vasodilator infusion to prevent morbidity from associated complications. Cardiovascular parameters including arterial pressures, heart rate, electrocardiogram, and oxygen saturation should be assessed regularly during the course of treatment. Cerebrospinal fluid waveform and pressure should also be measured in patients with ventriculostomy catheters. Although the dose and infusion rate for the described infusion agents vary between studies, in our experience an infusion rate of 0.5 to 1 mg/min generally allows careful titration of arterial pressures during treatment. We closely monitor the arterial waveform and pressure and temporarily halt the infusion with drops in the mean arterial pressure of more than 15 mm Hg or systolic blood pressure of more than 25 mm Hg. The infusion is resumed when the pressures return to baseline values. A control angiogram can be obtained after 3 to 5 mg of the agent has been infused into the affected territory to assess for therapeutic effect. Poorly responsive, severe vasospasm causing flow limitation warrants urgent angioplasty to avoid imminent infarction.

Transluminal Balloon Angioplasty

INTRODUCTION AND VESSEL SELECTION

The use of TBA in cerebral vasospasm was first described in the 1980s by Zubkov et al.[42] and has been refined substantially in the decades since. The precise mechanisms by which mechanical angioplasty produces durable patency and resistance to recurrent vasospasm remains to be fully delineated but may include flattening of the smooth muscle and endothelial cells, disruption of the extracellular matrix, and separation of connections between cellular basement membranes.[43,44] Although the vessels seem to lose some responsiveness to pharmacologic vasodilators following angioplasty, there is no evidence that TBA causes significant structural damage to vessels when performed with appropriate safety considerations.[8,43]

All patients for whom the use of TBA is considered must undergo a detailed review of baseline angiographic findings. Assessment of vessel morphology and diameter is especially important as a means to differentiate congenitally hypoplastic vessels (most commonly seen in A1 segments, intradural vertebral arteries, P1 segments, and posterior communicating arteries) from vessels in acute spasm (Fig. 93-4). Attempts to angioplasty these hypoplastic segments can result in catastrophic, acute vessel rupture and must be avoided. In addition, vessels near the site of recent surgical clipping should be should be not be angioplastied, because fatal rupture has been reported under these circumstances.[45]

The segments that are traditionally considered amenable for angioplasty are the more proximal, large (more than 2 mm) vessels of the circle of Willis, including the vertebral,

basilar, and supraclinoid internal carotid arteries, as well as M1 segments. The adoption of dedicated neurovascular balloons, which have improved safety profiles and trackability, have allowed farther reach into the immediate distal branches of these vessels, including the posterior communicating arteries, A1, proximal A2, M2, P1, and P2 segments (Fig. 93-3).

BALLOON TECHNOLOGIES

Historically, the first endovascular balloons used for TBA in cerebral vasospasm were borrowed from the larger coronary interventional field. These balloons are composed of a stiff polyethylene or nylon membrane on a double-lumen shaft, which allows for balloon inflation and passage of a guidewire. Sizing decisions need to be conservative, because the rigid characteristics of these balloons can easily cause vessel rupture if the diameter of the chosen balloon is excessive—Eddleman et al. have suggested, as a general reference, 2-mm-diameter balloons for MCA spasm and 1.5-mm-diameter balloons for M2 or A1 segments.[14] Shorter coronary balloons such as the Maverick (Boston Scientific) have favorable characteristics, including improved maneuverability and less vessel straightening on inflation. The Gateway balloon (Boston Scientific) was more recently developed from coronary technologies for dedicated intracranial use and can be used for treatment of intracranial vasospasm, but it is primarily designed for the treatment of intracranial atherosclerotic stenoses.

The advent of intracranial balloon catheters has substantially improved the safety of TBA procedures, because these balloon systems are made of a softer, semipermeable silicone/elastomer membrane mounted on a flexible, single-lumen catheter shaft (Fig. 93-3). The single-lumen system is much softer than its coronary counterparts but has the slight disadvantage of lacking a continuous flush option. Examples of current neurovascular balloon catheter systems include the Hyperglide (ev3 Neurovascular) and Hyperform (ev3 Neurovascular), both of which come in a number of diameter and length configurations. The Hyperform is more compliant, but the Hyperglide has more length options and is thus better suited for angioplasty of longer arterial segments. Both are designed for navigation over an atraumatic, 0.010-inch X-Pedion guidewire. In occasional situations in which steerability in tortuous arteries with acute angles becomes cumbersome, a microcatheter can be placed into the target vessel first, followed by balloon exchange over a 0.010-inch exchange length X-Celerator microwire (ev3 Neurovascular).

BALLOON INFLATION

Balloons should be inflated with a 50/50 mixture of 300 mg/ml iodinated contrast and saline to facilitate precise fluoroscopic monitoring during balloon inflation. Because the catheter lumen narrows distal to the balloon, the guidewire effectively occludes this distal catheter position and diverts injected fluids into the balloon lumen. It is important to avoid retraction of the guidewire into the catheter once the system has been placed because backflow of blood into the balloon can cause reduced balloon opacification and result in consequent overinflation or difficult deflation.

We prefer to inflate the balloons with a threaded, precisely calibrated, 1-ml Cadence (ev3 Neurovascular) syringe that enables adjustment in the 0.01-ml range. To decrease the risk of acute vessel rupture, the goal of angioplasty should generally not be to achieve the projected normal caliber of the target vessel but rather to improve vessel caliber enough to augment flow to ischemic brain regions.

EFFICACY

A number of series have examined the efficacy of TBA for the treatment of subarachnoid hemorrhage (SAH)–related vasospasm. A review by Hoh and Ogilvy of the overall rate of clinical improvement among recent reports, which included a total of 530 patients, found an average rate of 62% with a range of 11% to 93%.[25] The studies analyzed in this review include that of Eskridge et al. (50 patients and 170 vessel segments, demonstrating 61% sustained neurologic improvement at 72 hours),[46] Bejjani et al. (31 patients with 72% neurologic improvement),[47] Higashida et al. (28 patients with 61% neurologic improvement),[19] and Fujii et al. (19 patients with 63% neurologic improvement).[48] These data were limited by the lack of matched controls, but further investigations comparing vascular territories treated with TBA to territories in the same patient that were not treated with TBA have shown decreased rates of infarction on CT following TBA (7% for treated vs. 38% for untreated).[49]

The timing of TBA for cerebral vasospasm is thought to be a critical component in achieving maximum clinical benefit in patients with symptomatic vasospasm, but the exact therapeutic window remains to be fully determined. Rosenwasser et al. published a retrospective study on vasospasm patients treated with TBA inside and outside of a 2-hour window and reported that the rate of angiographic improvement was not significantly different between the two groups (90% of patients treated within 2 hours vs. 88% of patients treated outside 2 hours) but that the rate of clinical improvement was significantly higher in patients treated sooner (70% of patients treated within 2 hours vs. 40% of patients treated outside 2 hours).[50] Although the use of prophylactic TBA has also been suggested, a recent phase II clinical trial for the prophylactic use of TBA in Fisher grade III SAH patients failed to show improvements in clinical outcome at 3 months follow-up, so this use cannot currently be recommended.[51]

COMPLICATIONS

Complications during TBA include vessel rupture, thromboembolism, and reperfusion hemorrhage and are essential considerations for the procedure, because each of these complications can be potentially devastating.[19,42,44,46,52] Vessel rupture is perhaps the most feared of these events, and reviews have cited rates between 0% and 7.7% with a mean occurrence of 1.1%.[25] With the wide adoption of dedicated neurovascular balloon systems and increased technical experience, the rate of rupture in current practice is likely trending toward the lower end of that spectrum. Particular care must still be taken in cases of severe vessel spasm in which limited distal visualization can be predisposed to wire- or catheter-induced perforation of small branch vessels. Thrombus formation can occur around the balloon or within the catheter lumen and should be prevented by appropriate patient heparinization unless contraindicated.

Reperfusion injury can be an uncommon complication of balloon angioplasty. This is believed to occur from reperfusion of the brain regions that have suffered prolonged ischemia. This can be prevented by careful analysis of cross-sectional imaging studies. For example, the surgeon should refrain from angioplasty in an arterial distribution that has already suffered a large area of infarction. If in doubt, we prefer to obtain MRI with evaluation of diffusion/perfusion mismatch to help guide our therapeutic decisions.

Combination Therapy

The use of current IA vasodilator agents in conjunction with TBA may possibly provide improvements in patient outcomes, but the evidence in literature remains limited. In theory, the use of IA agents prior to TBA can offer an initial improvement in proximal vessel diameter to facilitate safer subsequent navigation of endovascular balloon catheters. Alternatively, once proximal vessel spasm has been addressed with mechanical angioplasty, pharmacologic agents may be able to more easily access and treat distal and microvascular spasm (Fig. 93-3). Given the excellent safety profiles of the CCBs that are most commonly used for IA infusions today, the addition of pharmacologic agents to mechanical angioplasty is unlikely to add significant risk to the procedure and can be used at the discretion of the care team. Future studies investigating the benefit of modern IA vasodilators as an adjunct to TBA are needed before definitive recommendations can be made for practice.

Conclusions

Symptomatic cerebral vasospasm following aSAH remains a tremendous cause of morbidity and mortality for patients who survive the initial hemorrhagic event. Frequent neurologic examinations are essential in patients who are awake and alert as a means to monitor for the onset of delayed ischemic deficits. Imaging changes by TCD or CTP play a more significant role in early detection of vessel spasm in patients with a less reliable exam, particularly those with prolonged delirium or a comatose state. Once vasospasm has been identified, triple-H therapy should be instituted as the first-line management strategy, but patients who do not respond or cannot tolerate prolonged treatment based on cardiac or renal comorbidities should be promptly triaged to endovascular alternatives.

Perfusion scans, if available, should be interpreted carefully prior to aggressive endovascular therapy to identify evidence of significant, established, irreversible ischemia. Either CTA/CTP or MRI/magnetic resonance perfusion studies can be utilized based on institutional practices to help increase the safety and positive impact of endovascular therapeutic techniques. TBA is currently the most reliable option for durable treatment of proximal vasospasm and should be instituted for these vessel segments whenever technically possible. IA vasodilator infusions should be employed for distal vasospasm and can provide an adjunct to mechanical angioplasty. Although the safety profiles of these pharmacologic agents are favorable, patient vital signs and cerebrovascular parameters should be monitored closely to avoid additional morbidity from hypotension or elevated ICP. Because many of the technologies used for the modern diagnosis and treatment of symptomatic cerebral vasospasm remain to be fully investigated, further research will be important for clarification of the optimal role of endovascular therapies in managing patients within the post-SAH vasospasm window.

KEY REFERENCES

Albanese E, Russo A, Quiroga M, et al. Ultrahigh-dose intraarterial infusion of verapamil through an indwelling microcatheter for medically refractory severe vasospasm: initial experience. Clinical article. *J Neurosurg.* 2010;113:913-922.

Badjatia N, Topcuoglu MA, Pryor JC, et al. Preliminary experience with intra-arterial nicardipine as a treatment for cerebral vasospasm. *AJNR Am J Neuroradiol.* 2004;25:819-826.

Biondi A, Ricciardi GK, Puybasset L, et al. Intra-arterial nimodipine for the treatment of symptomatic cerebral vasospasm after aneurysmal subarachnoid hemorrhage: preliminary results. *AJNR Am J Neuroradiol.* 2004;25:1067-1076.

Dorsch N, King M. A review of cerebral vasospasm in aneurysmal subarachnoid hemorrhage. Part I: incidence and effects. *J Clinical Neuroscience.* 1994:19-26.

Ecker A, Riemenschneider PA. Arteriographic demonstration of spasm of the intracranial arteries, with special reference to saccular arterial aneurysms. *J Neurosurg.* 1951;8:660-667.

Eddleman CS, Hurley MC, Naidech AM, et al. Endovascular options in the treatment of delayed ischemic neurological deficits due to cerebral vasospasm. *Neurosurg Focus.* 2009;26:E6.

Eskridge JM, McAuliffe W, Song JK, et al. Balloon angioplasty for the treatment of vasospasm: results of first 50 cases. *Neurosurgery.* 1998;42:510-516:discussion 516–517.

Feng L, Fitzsimmons BF, Young WL, et al. Intraarterially administered verapamil as adjunct therapy for cerebral vasospasm: safety and 2-year experience. *AJNR Am J Neuroradiol.* 2002;23:1284-1290.

Fergusen S, Macdonald RL. Predictors of cerebral infarction in patients with aneurysmal subarachnoid hemorrhage. *Neurosurgery.* 2007;60:658-667:discussion 667.

Firlik KS, Kaufmann AM, Firlik AD, et al. Intra-arterial papaverine for the treatment of cerebral vasospasm following aneurysmal subarachnoid hemorrhage. *Surg Neurol.* 1999;51:66-74.

Frontera JA, Claassen J, Schmidt JM, et al. Prediction of symptomatic vasospasm after subarachnoid hemorrhage: the modified Fisher scale. *Neurosurgery.* 2006;59:21-27:discussion 21–27.

Fujii Y, Takahashi A, Yoshimoto T. Effect of balloon angioplasty on high grade symptomatic vasospasm after subarachnoid hemorrhage. *Neurosurg Rev.* 1995;18:7-13.

Higashida RT, Halbach VV, Dowd CF, et al. Intravascular balloon dilatation therapy for intracranial arterial vasospasm: patient selection, technique, and clinical results. *Neurosurg Rev.* 1992;15:89-95.

Hoh BL, Ogilvy CS. Endovascular treatment of cerebral vasospasm: transluminal balloon angioplasty, intra-arterial papaverine, and intra-arterial nicardipine. *Neurosurg Clin N Am.* 2005;16:501-516:vi.

Janardhan V, Biondi A, Riina HA, et al. Vasospasm in aneurysmal subarachnoid hemorrhage: diagnosis, prevention, and management. *Neuroimaging Clin N Am.* 2006;16:483-496:viii-ix.

Jestaedt L, Pham M, Bartsch AJ, et al. The impact of balloon angioplasty on the evolution of vasospasm-related infarction after aneurysmal subarachnoid hemorrhage. *Neurosurgery.* 2008;62:610-617:discussion 610–617.

Kassell NF, Helm G, Simmons N, et al. Treatment of cerebral vasospasm with intra-arterial papaverine. *J Neurosurg.* 1992;77:848-852.

Keuskamp J, Murali R, Chao KH. High-dose intraarterial verapamil in the treatment of cerebral vasospasm after aneurysmal subarachnoid hemorrhage. *J Neurosurg.* 2008;108:458-463.

Linfante I, Delgado-Mederos R, Andreone V, et al. Angiographic and hemodynamic effect of high concentration of intra-arterial nicardipine in cerebral vasospasm. *Neurosurgery.* 2008;63:1080-1086:discussion 1086–1087.

Macdonald RL, Pluta RM, Zhang JH. Cerebral vasospasm after subarachnoid hemorrhage: the emerging revolution. *Nat Clin Pract Neurol.* 2007;3:256-263.

Mazumdar A, Rivet DJ, Derdeyn CP, et al. Effect of intraarterial verapamil on the diameter of vasospastic intracranial arteries in patients with cerebral vasospasm. *Neurosurg Focus.* 2006;21:E15.

McGuinness B, Gandhi D. Endovascular management of cerebral vasospasm. *Neurosurg Clin N Am.* 2010;21:281-290.

Rosenwasser RH, Armonda RA, Thomas JE, et al. Therapeutic modalities for the management of cerebral vasospasm: timing of endovascular options. *Neurosurgery.* 1999;44:975-979:discussion 979–980.

Tejada JG, Taylor RA, Ugurel MS, et al. Safety and feasibility of intra-arterial nicardipine for the treatment of subarachnoid hemorrhage-associated vasospasm: initial clinical experience with high-dose infusions. *AJNR Am J Neuroradiol.* 2007;28:844-848.

Wolf S, Martin H, Landscheidt JF, et al. Continuous selective intraarterial infusion of nimodipine for therapy of refractory cerebral vasospasm. *Neurocrit Care.* 2010;12:346-351.

Numbered references appear on Expert Consult.

Section Four

HYDROCEPHALUS

DANIELE RIGAMONTI

CHAPTER 94

Surgical Management of Hydrocephalus in the Adult

DAVID M. FRIM • RICHARD PENN • MAUREEN LACY

Hydrocephalus, from the Greek word meaning "water in the head," is a general term used to describe many conditions of fluid collected in the intracranial space. For the purposes of this chapter, we define hydrocephalus as an inappropriate amount of cerebrospinal fluid (CSF) within the intracranial space at an inappropriate pressure. In this way, we can include a variety of both childhood and adult syndromes of abnormal CSF flow and absorption patterns and the sequelae of their treatments. This definition excludes syndromes such as the pseudotumor cerebri syndrome,[1,2] whose etiology and treatment may be somewhat different from those of hydrocephalus. Our definition would include low-pressure hydrocephalus syndromes in which the ventricles stay enlarged with relatively normal pressures, despite our lack of understanding of these syndromes.[3,4]

From a practical standpoint, the treatment of hydrocephalus in the adult can be divided into two broad categories: childhood onset and adult onset. The first situation revolves mostly around upkeep of shunting devices and monitoring of a care strategy already implemented to prevent or treat complications. The latter situation necessitates a standard approach of evaluation of a clinical entity, choice of intervention strategy, and then implementation of that intervention. We deal with these two situations separately.

Management of the Adult Treated for Hydrocephalus as a Child

As much as 40% of pediatric neurosurgical practice in most large centers involves the treatment of hydrocephalus. The most common etiologic factor is premature birth and intraventricular hemorrhage. The presumption is that blood in the CSF causes either scarring in the subarachnoid space or sclerosis from inflammation at the absorptive surface of the arachnoid villi. This situation decreases the absorption rate of fluid and causes hydrocephalus with four-ventricle dilatation. This condition has been referred to as communicating or absorptive hydrocephalus. Other etiologies for an absorptive defect in children can be a congenital incontinence of the arachnoid villi for a variety of etiologic reasons or an obstruction within the CSF pathways that will cause ventricular dilatation upstream from the obstruction. The most common situation that presents in this fashion is aqueductal stenosis from either scarring or a benign

tectal tumor. In children, obstructive hydrocephalus is first approached with the question of whether the obstruction can be removed or bypassed. Endoscopic third ventriculocisternostomy can be performed to bypass aqueductal obstruction with a high rate of success. At this stage in our ability to treat hydrocephalus, absorptive hydrocephalus causing dilatation of all four ventricles is almost always treated by an extracranial shunting device.

Children who have been treated with a third ventriculocisternostomy bypass need to be monitored into adulthood because there is risk of the ostomy closing many years after its initial placement. The true incidence of this is not yet known but is believed to be relatively low if the ostomy has survived several years. The adult who presents with a third ventriculocisternostomy bypass from childhood can be periodically evaluated by an imaging study such as magnetic resonance imaging with a cinematic gated flow study through the ostomy.[5] If the ostomy has begun to occlude, the lateral and third ventricles may slowly begin to enlarge, even in the absence of overt clinical symptoms. Options for treatment at this time include endoscopic re-exploration for reconstruction of the ostomy or placement of a shunting device.

The management of the majority of adult hydrocephalus that was first treated in childhood revolves around the upkeep of extracranial CSF shunting devices. The utility of yearly or biennially shunt checks for pediatric and adult patients is controversial. Our practice is to maintain a regimen of more or less yearly shunt check evaluations in all our adult patients with shunts to maintain contact with the patient and the patient's family, as well as to continually review the presentation and dangers of shunt malfunction. Where the upkeep of a shunting device in a child may concern issues of growth, such as ascertaining whether the extracranial portion of the shunt tubing is of adequate length during periods of growth or the ventricular catheter does not extrude from the ventricular system due to head growth, upkeep and management of shunting devices in adults are more straightforward. Shunt longevity is much longer in older children and adults than in infants,[6] presumably due to issues of growth. In the adult, as in the child, the most common overall complication of shunt placement is a malfunction due to catheter or valve occlusion or fracture.[7,8] The next most common complication is shunt infection, which is generally seen in an early phase after implantation.[9] Beyond that, issues of overdrainage and underdrainage may also need to be confronted.

Shunt malfunction in the adult, as generally seen in a child, presents with stereotypic symptoms more or less similar to past shunt malfunctions and consistent with the initial presentation of the hydrocephalus. In adulthood, cognitively high-functioning patients are often able to make the diagnosis on clinical grounds. The evaluation consists of the usual radiographic studies such as plain shunt radiographs and a head computed tomography scan after an adequate patient history has been taken and a physical examination has been performed. Oftentimes, the diagnosis of shunt malfunction is made due to either mechanical obstruction of the shunt tubing or enlargement of the ventricular system. In that situation, the shunt is explored operatively in the usual fashion.

We have generally opened the scalp incision first to determine the ventricular catheter patency versus malfunction of the components from the valve to the distal tubing. We then replace one portion of the shunt, either that in the brain or the extracranial space, in its entirety. Our experience, like that of others, has shown no benefit to replacing the entire shunt versus revision of the affected component.[6] Usually we replace a nonfunctioning valve with a valve of a similar type if the patient had done well for some time with that same valve. This may be different from the situation in the infant or child in whom, as the child grows, drainage needs may require a change to a valve type with other characteristics.

The advent of percutaneously programmable, differential pressure valves and programmable valves with fused antisiphoning components (Table 94-1) allows some flexibility in installing a valve that can provide dynamics similar to those of the one being replaced and retains the option of changing the shunting dynamics without operative intervention. With regard to shunt revision in the adult patient, generally we recommend replacing those components that are nonfunctional but not disturbing other components that appear to be functioning adequately.

Shunt infection in the adult patient almost always presents with some sign of systemic infection such as a fever, elevated serum leukocyte count, or frank meningitis, although the risk factors for infection, as well as many commonly used approaches to reduce infection rates in CSF shunts, remain insufficiently studied to determine significance.[10] The severity of symptoms depends on the infectious agent and may range from headache with minimal other signs of infection (for relatively benign organisms such as *Staphylococcus epidermidis* or *Corynebacterium*) to a more virulent picture of life-threatening meningitis (if the etiologic agent is *Staphylococcus aureus* or a gram-negative organism). A shunt infection needs to be treated as any foreign body infection would be in an adult, with removal of all infected foreign body material, which in general means removal of the entire shunt. Depending on the etiology of the hydrocephalus and the need for daily drainage, the shunt can be replaced with an external draining ventricular catheter or a lumbar drainage catheter for the period of the antibiotic treatment. Although the length of this period of temporary external drainage and antibiotic treatment can vary, most recommendations include at least several days of external drainage with negative CSF cultures before replacement of the shunting device in a new location, if possible.[10] Depending on the terminus of the shunt, whether it is in

Table 94-1	Currently Available Shunting Valves
Valve Type	**Examples**
Differential pressure (siphoning)	Contour (Medtronic Neurosurgery, Minneapolis, MN)
	Hakim (Integra Lifesciences, Plainsboro, NJ)
	Medos nonprogrammable (Codman/Johnson & Johnson, Randolf, MA)
Nonsiphoning, combination, differential pressure	Delta (Medtronic Neurosurgery)
	Equiflow (Radionics/Integra Lifesciences, Plainsboro, NJ)
	Novus (Integra Lifesciences)
Percutaneously programmable, differential variable pressure	Codman-Hakim programmable (Codman/Johnson & Johnson)
	Sophy (Sophysa, Orsay, France)
	Strata NSC (Medtronic Neurosurgery)
Percutaneously programmable, nonsiphoning or gravity compensating, variable pressure	Strata (Medtronic Neurosurgery)
	Aesculap-Miethke proGAV (Miethke/Aesculap, Center Valley, PA)
Flow dependent	Orbis-Sigma (Integra Lifesciences)
	Diamond (Phoenix Biomedical, Mississauga, Ontario, Canada)

the peritoneum, the pleura, or the cardiac atrium, the infection may spread or become loculated in those areas and require separate treatment. One other late complication of infection in the adult population that is more common than in the pediatric population is sclerosis of an absorbing surface from acute or chronic infection. In the peritoneum, this presents as a CSF pseudocyst or ascites, and in the pleural space this may present as CSF pleural effusion. In either situation, once recurrent infection is ruled out, the distal CSF catheter may be moved to another location or placed in the vascular tree through a large vein into the cardiac atrium where reabsorptive sclerosis is not present.

Shunt overdrainage and underdrainage in the adult can become a problem with age, in which presumably the brain may require lower pressure analogous to the normal-pressure hydrocephalus syndrome, which is described later. In that situation, the approach to the shunting dynamics is similar to that in the normal- or low-pressure hydrocephalus situation in that a trial of drainage at a low pressure may be appropriate or a programmable valve can be placed to allow percutaneous programming to lower pressures.

Our impression is that, in patients whom we have followed from childhood into adulthood, complications seem to be reduced as children reach adulthood. The etiologic basis for this is unclear but may have to do with cessation of growth and reduced physical activity. Upkeep and care of the adult who was treated for hydrocephalus as a child are quite rewarding and relatively straightforward.

Evaluation and Management of Hydrocephalus Presenting in Adulthood

The causes of hydrocephalus presenting in adulthood are the same and yet different from hydrocephalus presenting in childhood. Intraventricular and subarachnoid blood from aneurysmal subarachnoid hemorrhage or hemorrhage from intraparenchymal vascular malformations can cause chronic hydrocephalus via a mechanism believed to be similar to that seen in the absorptive hydrocephalus of prematurity. Similarly, bacterial meningitis can also cause inflammation and presumably scarring in the subarachnoid space or at the arachnoid villi that will cause an absorptive hydrocephalus. These entities present with four-ventricle enlargement as in childhood. Obstructive lesions such as tectal tumors or even congenital scarring at the sylvian aqueduct can cause triventricular enlargement and obstructive hydrocephalus, which present in adulthood.[11] The treatment of aqueductal stenosis in an adult, similar to that in a child, is third ventriculocisternostomy to bypass the obstruction.[12] Also, intraventricular tumors or large tumors abutting the ventricles can sometimes cause hydrocephalus from what is believed to be a CSF hyperprotein state that may reduce villus absorption of CSF. These causes of hydrocephalus and its presentation mirror similar situations in childhood and present with symptoms and signs of elevated intracranial pressure.

NORMAL-PRESSURE HYDROCEPHALUS (ADULT-ONSET CHRONIC HYDROCEPHALUS)

Unique to adults is the normal- or low-pressure hydrocephalus seen with advanced age. This syndrome, first described by Hakim and Adams[13] 40 years ago, has been undergoing continual reevaluation over the years. Classically, this syndrome presents as a triad of gait disorder, incontinence, and cognitive dysfunction, usually attention and short-term memory loss that can mimic a dementia.[14] The patient has CSF pressures measured in the normal range on lumbar puncture, and symptoms may often be reduced by large volume removal of CSF. The diagnosis of normal-pressure hydrocephalus syndrome is a subject of considerable controversy, as is the decision to treat the syndrome by CSF shunting.[3] A variety of diagnostic approaches have been described. These include imaging by computed tomography or magnetic resonance imaging, which show a characteristic pattern of ventricular enlargement with widening of the sylvian fissures and some cortical sulci.[15-17] One or several large-volume lumbar taps reducing CSF pressure and volume relieving or reducing the symptomatology has been advocated as an indication for treatment. An infusion test of fluid into either the lumbar or the ventricular CSF space while monitoring pressure response to a given volume has also been advocated as a test to predict outcome from shunting for this syndrome.[18] Bolus or continuous infusion can be used to measure compliance and outflow resistance. Long-term intracranial pressure measurements combined with magnetic resonance imaging to detect abnormal brain pressure waves have also been suggested.[19] Better results for shunting may be possible by using a high threshold for selection, but this may miss some patients who would benefit from, but are not selected for, surgery. The combination of protocols of temporary lumbar[20] or ventricular[21] drainage to tonically reduce CSF pressures to even less than would be the normal range, cognitive testing before and after several days of CSF drainage, and daily physical therapy evaluations to assess gait function has also been used as a predictor of outcome from shunting in this syndrome.[22] In our hands, such a protocol has had a 100%

Table 94-2 Testing Protocol Used to Assess Neurocognitive Responses to Long-Term Lumbar Drainage in the Patient with Normal-Pressure Hydrocephalus

Mini-Mental Status Examination
Repeatable Battery for the Assessment of Neuropsychological Status
Stroop Color–Word Test
Delis-Kaplan Executive Function System Sorting Test
Trail Making Test
Phonemic fluency
Clock-drawing test
Grooved Pegboard test
Geriatric Depression Scale (15 item)

positive predictive value in 23 consecutive patients for a good outcome with shunting when clear improvement in neurocognition or gait function is observed after temporary lumbar drainage. However, the false-negative rate in our cohort has not been investigated by shunt placement when no improvement with temporary drainage is seen. The neuropsychology testing protocol used at the University of Chicago is presented in Table 94-2. Unfortunately, there are not yet universally accepted diagnostic criteria for normal-pressure hydrocephalus or an agreed-upon set of predictors of outcome after shunt placement.

Deciding When to Treat Hydrocephalus in the Adult

In adult hydrocephalus, symptoms are primarily due to inappropriate pressure within the ventricular system. Compression of brain tissue by ventricular enlargement may produce problems in gait due to stretching of subcortical white matter tracts. The rate of development of hydrocephalus differs significantly and affects which symptoms occur. Slow progression may lead to subtle changes in cognition; rapid progression leads to headache and loss of consciousness. These symptoms can include headache, vomiting, mental status change, gait changes, extraocular movement deficit, visual changes, or cognitive changes. Hydrocephalus presenting after aneurysmal subarachnoid hemorrhage is diagnosed in the ongoing evaluation and treatment of the lesion that has caused the bleeding. Similarly, hydrocephalus developing after meningitis is recognized as the meningitis is treated. However, the exact threshold for treatment of hydrocephalus in the adult can sometimes be difficult to define. Clearly, symptoms such as headache or cognitive changes, which are interfering with life or lifestyle, would constitute indications for initiating treatment, regardless of whether the hydrocephalus is from a process of reducing absorption or one of obstruction. Radiographic evidence of enlarging ventricles in the absence of overt symptoms may also constitute indications for intervention, although in many cases it is difficult to discern whether a process, such as an infection, has begun to cause global brain atrophy or whether inappropriate pressure within the ventricular system is causing ventricular enlargement.

Using our definition of hydrocephalus as an inappropriate amount of CSF under an inappropriate pressure, a measurement of CSF pressure either by lumbar puncture (in the setting of communicating hydrocephalus) or by direct ventricular access (in the setting of triventricular enlargement from obstruction) is diagnostic when combined with imaging. A secondary criterion when CSF pressure is measured by lumbar puncture or ventricular tap is to observe a reduction in presenting symptoms by a reduction in CSF pressure. This is the analogous situation to the large-volume CSF removal that is often performed for the diagnosis of normal-pressure hydrocephalus syndrome. The exact limits of what is considered normal CSF pressure in adults are unclear. Many would consider pressures as high as 20 cm H_2O in the lumbar space with the patient in a supine position to be within the normal range. However, sometimes symptoms of elevated intracranial pressure can be witnessed when pressure is measured to be as low as 15 to 18 cm H_2O, and those symptoms can be ameliorated by reduction in the CSF pressure to less than 10 or even less than 5 cm H_2O. This situation begins to establish a continuum of inappropriate CSF pressures in the adult that begins in the clearly abnormal range above 20 or 25 cm H_2O but can end quite squarely in the middle of what most would consider a normal-pressure value. Similarly, pressures as high as mid-20 cm H_2O can be asymptomatic, with no change in ventricular size. Whether this defines compensated hydrocephalus or simply a variant of normal is unclear.

Regardless, when symptoms referable to elevated intracranial pressure in the presence of an enlarged ventricular space can be ameliorated or reduced by drainage of CSF, there exists a clear indication for treatment of hydrocephalus. In the absence of a pressure measurement, symptoms referable to elevated intracranial pressure that coincide with enlarged or enlarging ventricles also call for treatment. Precise indications for intervention are sometimes not possible, even considering ventricular size, CSF pressure, and the effect of drainage of CSF. Each case must be individually evaluated by the treating neurosurgeon. The goal of treatment is to restore a CSF pressure and dynamic that maximally reduces symptoms while maintaining the pressures within a range appropriate for cerebral profusion and reduces ventricular size to a normal range.

Choices of Techniques for Treating Hydrocephalus

The general approach to an individual presenting with symptomatic hydrocephalus or radiographic enlargement of ventricles depends on the etiology of the hydrocephalus. In practical terms, obstructive hydrocephalus should generally be considered for a bypass procedure or removal of obstruction before resorting to extracranial shunting. Hydrocephalus due to absorption or obstruction of the subarachnoid space with four-ventricle enlargement should be approached with extracranial shunting primarily. Aqueductal stenosis in a center where expertise is available should be treated by a third ventriculocisternostomy, which may avoid the need for permanently implanted hardware.[23] Still, extracranial shunting is certainly an option that will adequately treat this type of hydrocephalus. Extracranial shunting for obstruction or for four-ventricle hydrocephalus provides the additional possibility of fine-tuning CSF

drainage dynamics and pressures that a bypass procedure cannot accomplish.

Choices of Shunting Strategy and Shunting Hardware

Adults may be more sensitive to CSF dynamic pressure changes than children. This may be due to the decreased plasticity of the adult brain. Certainly, the existence of normal-pressure hydrocephalus syndrome in adults suggests that shunting in the adult may require obtaining a specific low CSF pressure or high flow rather than simply restoring elevated pressure to a normal range and allowing the brain to accommodate. Therefore, different shunting strategies may be of use in adult hydrocephalus.

The standard extracranial shunt operation now performed in this country is a ventricular catheter placed either frontally or occipitally and subcutaneously tunneled to an entry into the peritoneum. An intervening valve and often a tapping reservoir allow control of shunting pressure and access to the CSF space. The peritoneum provides little pressure of its own and allows drainage and reabsorption of a large volume of fluid. Alternative shunting strategies can rest on a different absorptive surface than the peritoneum. The cardiac atrium provides an egress for a very large volume of CSF. It can also handle high protein content that could cause malabsorption of spinal fluid in the peritoneal space. The pleural space also provides an alternative extracranial absorptive surface, but the pleural space generates its own negative pressure. This can be used to advantage in constructing a shunting system that provides less-than-normal pressure or even negative pressure if the valve is chosen appropriately.[24] Antisiphoning components, which prevent negative pressure in the shunt tubing, can be used to counteract the negative pressure "sink" of the pleural space. The gallbladder can also be used as an absorptive surface, and it provides a positive pressure postprandially that prevents overdrainage.[25] In addition, recipient sites such as the internal jugular vein in reverse orientation may be used in the adult more so than in the child because of easier access and a larger anatomy in which to place the distal shunting tube.[26]

Concerning placement of the catheter into the ventricular system, the larger head and larger ventricles of the adult provide better landmarks than those of the child. We have generally advocated a frontal approach in adults with small ventricles because of ease of ventricular access. An occipital approach is reasonable when the ventricles are large because it allows more catheter length to be placed within the ventricle and, particularly under endoscopic guidance, can allow the catheter tip to be placed as far as possible from the choroid plexus at the foramen of Monro.

A variety of shunting components are now available for use in constructing a shunting system. Although ventricular catheters and bur hole reservoirs are similar, shunt valves can be divided into three general groupings: differential pressure valves that siphon, differential pressure valves plus an antisiphoning or gravity-actuated resistance chamber that reduces siphoning, and valves designed to maintain constant flow of CSF called flow-control or flow-dependent valves (see Table 94-1). The differential pressure valves siphon when an adult stands upright and may cause low-pressure symptoms. However, this is a strategy that may be useful in a shunting system that drains CSF to a less-than-normal pressure. The antisiphoning shunt valves provide a more normal postural pressure dynamic but may underdrain in patients with normal-pressure hydrocephalus.[27] The flow-control valves are not free of complications of overdrainage in normal-pressure hydrocephalus[28] but are of value in patients who may require constant flow or flow that is more robust than that seen in the nonsiphoning combination valves. In any case, a thoughtful choice of an initial shunt system may prevent valve revision if the shunting system does not match an individual patient's needs. However, at times, two or even all three valve types will need to be tried if a patient remains symptomatic from initial valve placement.

There are currently four percutaneously programmable, differential pressure valves available for purchase. The valve setting mechanisms range in pressure from 3 to 20 cm H_2O by various increments. Only one of these valves, the Strata valve (Medtronic Neurosurgery) is manufactured with a fused antisiphoning chamber; a programmable valve from the Meithke Corporation contains a variable pressure differential component and a gravity-actuated resistance circuit in a single housing. To make the other two programmable valves (Codman-Hakim valve, Codman/Johnson & Johnson, and Sophy valve, Sophysa) into nonsiphoning valves, antisiphoning chambers need to be spliced inline distal to the valve mechanism. The Codman-Hakim valve is sold fused to a flow occlusive device; that device (called a siphon guard) can be of use in reducing the flow rate of the valve while allowing it to drain to a low pressure by a siphoning mechanism. The programmable valve can be of great use in the adult shunting system because adults may be less able to adapt to a fixed pressure than children, whose brains are more plastic.[29,30] Therefore, variable pressure settings may allow fine-tuning of shunting pressures to symptoms. In addition, there is the theoretical benefit with normal-pressure hydrocephalus or hydrocephalus with large ventricles and a small cortical mantle in initially placing a shunt in a patient with a high differential pressure setting on the valve and then slowly decreasing that pressure to a more normal or even less-than-normal one. This may allow better accommodation and prevent ventricular collapse from sudden overdrainage, with the attendant risk of subdural hematoma due to rupture of bridging subdural veins. In the future, hardware cost may dictate much of the decision making in shunt system construction. For now, the many choices of shunt valves and other accompanying hardware makes selecting shunting hardware difficult, particularly because no randomized studies show any system to be clearly superior.[12] Matching the shunt system to the patient's individual needs is, therefore, somewhat of an art.

Technical Aspects in the Treatment of Adult Hydrocephalus

TECHNIQUE OF ENDOSCOPIC THIRD VENTRICULOCISTERNOSTOMY

Endoscopic third ventriculocisternostomy is performed identically in adults and children. We recommend a coronal bur hole at the midpupillary line and dural opening to allow a 12.5- or 14-French (Fr) introducer with trocar. Once the ventricular space is entered, an endoscope, either rigid or flexible, is placed within the ventricular system and navigated through the foramen of Monro.

The landmarks for this navigation[31] are the choroid plexus in the choroidal fissure, which dives into the foramen, and the septal and thalamostriate veins, which enter medially and anterolaterally into foramen of Monro. Once the foramen is traversed, navigation through the third ventricle is based on identification of the paired mammillary bodies from which the surgeon can discern the midline and anteriorly the retrochiasmatic space. Frequently, behind the retrochiasmatic space, a small red stripe that corresponds to the infundibulum is seen. In the space between the retrochiasmatic recess and the mammillary bodies is the flat and often thinned anterior floor of the third ventricle. We use a point one third of the way back from the retrochiasmatic recess for our ostomy hole. This minimizes the risk of injury to the basilar artery, which is generally positioned beneath the anterior floor in the posterior half. A blunt 1-mm probe is used to gently traverse through the floor of the third ventricle. The probe is left in place for a moment to potentially tamponade bleeding in the floor. Then a Fogarty balloon dilator of either 3 or 4 mm in size is introduced. This can be placed through a working channel of the endoscope with or without concurrent irrigation. The ostomy is gently dilated by inflating the balloon within it. An alternative technique of inflating the balloon on the inferior side of the ostomy and pulling it through the hole to tear the tissue can be successful, though it may cause bleeding. Bleeding is controlled either with warm saline irrigation or with unipolar or bipolar cautery devices available for work through the endoscope. Once the bleeding is controlled, the endoscope can be navigated through the ostomy to inspect the prepontine cistern, where it is used to fenestrate leaflets of arachnoid if that can be safely done without injury to the basilar artery. Once there is free flow of CSF throughout the prepontine cistern and through the ostomy hole, the ventriculoscope is withdrawn into the third ventricle, which is inspected for bleeding, and then withdrawn into the lateral ventricle.

In adults, we leave a ventricular catheter placed under endoscopic guidance by withdrawing the endoscope into the introducer sheath and then placing the sheath approximately 1 cm from the foramen of Monro. The ventriculoscope is then removed, and a ventricular catheter is placed so that it is (by measured length) at the tip of the introducer, which is then peeled out of the hole. The catheter is cut and connected to a blunt-ended bur hole reservoir. This catheter and tapping reservoir provide emergency access to CSF should there be sudden catastrophic occlusion of the ostomy. The patency of a third ventriculocisternostomy after several months to years is between 60% and 80%. If the ostomy provides egress of CSF for several years, even if it occludes at that time, the procedure can be repeated safely. Early failure of the ostomy generally requires extracranial CSF shunting for a permanent solution.

TECHNIQUES FOR THE PLACEMENT OF AN EXTRACRANIAL SHUNTING DEVICE IN ADULTS

Ventriculoperitoneal shunts are placed identically in adults and children. As a rule, connections within the shunt devices should be minimized, and whenever possible connections should be orthogonal to the direction of tube movement, such as a right angle connection from a bur hole reservoir device into the proximal end of a ventricular catheter. Ample tubing must be placed into the peritoneal or pleural space for catheter movement; however, issues of selecting a shunt catheter of adequate length for growth no longer apply in adulthood.

The procedures for placement of a ventriculoperitoneal shunt begin with the patient being placed in the supine position with the head turned from the side of the ventricular access. Usually, we place the head in the lateral position with the falx parallel to the floor and a roll under the shoulder ipsilateral to the shunt placement. Hair can be shaved or not per the surgeon's preference.[32] The entry site is chosen to be either at the coronal suture in the midpupillary line for frontal access to the ventricle or approximately 5 or 6 cm above the inion and 4 to 5 cm lateral from the midline for occipital access. The surgical prep is continuous from the frontal or occipital region and down along a track to the neck, chest, and belly. The shunting device is tested to make sure that it closes at an appropriate pressure and that all connections are secured. The abdominal incision is in the upper midline or subcostal. Care is taken to cover all skin surfaces with iodine-impregnated adhesive drapery and to minimize the exposed skin surfaces. We have infused intravenous antibiotics within 45 minutes of placement of the skin incision.

An incision is made, and then layers are divided through fascia in the midline or through fascia and muscles in a subcostal incision until the peritoneum is identified below the linea alba in the midline or below the posterior rectus fascia in the subcostal position. The peritoneum is grasped and then opened. The scalp incision is made over the selected bur hole entry site. A skin flap is then elevated and retracted. A bur hole is made with a perforator using either a power or a hand drill. Before the dura is opened, a pocket is made inferior to the bur hole and then a shunt-tunneling device is used to tunnel from the bur hole to the peritoneum. In the case of a frontal entry site, an intermediate incision behind the ear is usually required to "turn the corner" with the tunneling device. Either a tunneling sheath or a long silk tie is then used to pull the shunting components from the head to the abdominal incision. Once in place with a bur hole reservoir or other connector over the bur hole, the dura is opened with unipolar cautery and the pia is opened with bipolar cautery. The trajectory into the ventricular system can be determined either by preoperative computed tomography scanning or by estimate for an occipital approach using the contralateral medial canthus at a level in the midforehead and for a frontal approach using lines from the frontal bur hole to the medial canthus and from the bur hole to halfway between the lateral canthus and the tragus. An additional option, using a stereotactic intraoperative image guidance system for catheter placement, is now available from several companies who have constructed such systems. However, with the generally enlarged ventricles seen in adult onset hydrocephalus, ventricular access is usually easily obtained utilizing surface landmarks only. This observation should not be construed as a recommendation against the use of intraoperative navigational guidance, which can reduce reoperation for catheter malpositioning.

Once the catheter is placed and CSF egress is seen, the connection is made to the connector at the bur hole and

is secured. The distal catheter is then placed in the peritoneum, and all incisions are closed in layers. For ventriculopleural access, we make an incision at the third or fourth rib off the midline in the same line that we would use for passage of the peritoneal catheter for a ventriculoperitoneal shunt. We then dissect down to the pleura through the muscles of the anterior chest wall and the intercostal muscles. Once the pleura is identified, it is not opened until the shunt is entirely connected. Analogous to the peritoneal catheter, which is placed in the peritoneum after the ventricular catheter is connected to the shunt, we also connect the ventricular catheter to the shunting device, visualize distal runoff of CSF, and then under direct vision make a pleural egress with a long hemostat and place approximately 20 cm of tubing into the pleural space. Alternatively, a trocar may be used for the catheter to be placed blindly. We recommend placement of a positive end–expiratory pressure valve in the anesthesia circuit to maintain lung inflation during placement of the pleural catheter and thus avoid pneumothorax.

For ventriculoatrial shunt placement, the procedure is best done with fluoroscopic or angiographic assistance. After the shunting device is connected either frontally or occipitally and a valve and distal tubing are in place, a tunnel is made either from the distal nipple of the valve (if placed occipitally) or from an intermediate incision behind the ear (if placed frontally) to a point over the internal jugular vein. This point is selected by placement of a "finding" needle and then a larger needle and J wire into the internal jugular vein on the neck lateral to the sternocleidomastoid muscle. The incision is enlarged with a stab wound, and adequate tubing is tunneled from the exposed distal valve nipple (or intermediate incision behind the ear) to the neck incision to allow the blunt-end catheter tubing into the cardiac atrium with an additional several centimeters for positioning. Once the wire is visualized in the cardiac atrium by fluoroscopy, a 10-Fr introducer sheath is placed over the wire, the wire is removed, and the tubing is threaded directly through the introducer sheath into the cardiac atrium under fluoroscopic guidance. If there is some kink in the venous system, a long, flexible guidance wire of a 0.038-inch diameter can be guided into the cardiac atrium and the atrial tubing can be threaded over the wire into the atrium. After wire removal, the tubing is then pulled back until it makes a straight connection to the shunting system, with the tip at the right atrium–superior vena cava junction. We have performed intraoperative cardiac angiography to confirm the placement of the catheter at the junction between the superior vena cava and the right atrium. Before connection, the atrial catheter is flushed with heparinized saline. Incisions are then closed in layers.

In our practice, other places for reabsorption of CSF, such as the gallbladder, are approached with the assistance of a general surgeon. Laparoscopic placement of peritoneal tubes also usually requires the assistance of a general surgeon until comfort is attained with that technique.

COMPLICATIONS OF TREATMENT OF ADULT HYDROCEPHALUS

Complications of a third ventriculostomy or other bypass procedures, whether they are fenestration of ventricular walls, cyst walls, or removal of obstructing tumors, are specific to the surgery for the bypass procedure. If the surgery proceeds without any immediate complications, the major long-term problem is whether the bypass ostomy occludes with time. This occurrence recapitulates the presenting symptoms of the hydrocephalus. If the ostomy fails, a decision needs to be made as to whether the ostomy can be reconstructed or whether the patient should proceed to placement of an extracranial shunting device.

Complications of extracranial shunting include shunt malfunction, shunt infection, and overdrainage and underdrainage of CSF, as well as complications relating to injury to the absorptive site by the distal shunting catheter.

Shunt Malfunction

Shunt malfunction is caused by occlusion or impedance to flow along the shunting device. The most common place for shunt malfunction occurs near the ventricular catheter from ingrowth of choroid plexus or other debris into the catheter, and this is true for both children and adults. Valve function can be degraded by particulate matter or protein within the CSF and necessitate valve replacement. Distal catheter occlusion in the peritoneal space can be precipitated by tissue ingrowth into the distal shunt tube. In all these situations, surgery must be performed to test the shunt components and to replace that which is malfunctioning.

The patient's history and physical findings most often suggest elevated intracranial pressure. The symptoms often recapitulate those that occurred at the time of initial presentation with hydrocephalus. The elevation in CSF pressure can be tested by lumbar puncture in absorptive hydrocephalus or by direct shunt tap if the shunt does not communicate with the lumbar CSF space. Once the diagnosis of shunt malfunction is established, the patient needs to be brought to the operating room for exploration.

We always prepare the entire length of the shunt. The incision overlying the ventricular bur hole is first opened, and then the proximal and distal components of the shunt are disconnected and tested individually. The component that is occluded or malfunctioning is replaced. Proximally, the ventricular catheter is frequently occluded and thus needs replacement. If distal function is compromised, the valve or tubing is occluded and needs to be removed. Sometimes the manipulation of the shunting components during exploration releases a site of impedance of CSF flow. In those situations, the ventricular catheter is the most likely culprit based on clinical experience. In some cases, if shunt function was demonstrated preoperatively to be nonoptimal, the entire shunting system may need to be replaced if no specific malfunction is found at the time of surgery.

Shunt Infection

Shunt infection is treated identically in the adult and the child. Suspicion for shunt infection is based on clinical presentation and CSF cultures. In our hands, there is a higher yield for positive culture in the setting of infection from fluid obtained directly by shunt tap than for that obtained by a lumbar puncture. Once laboratory investigation data support infection either by Gram stain or culture results, the entire shunt is removed and replaced by a temporary draining ventriculostomy or, in some cases, a lumbar drainage catheter. In cases of normal-pressure hydrocephalus in which the patient has no overt or dangerous symptoms

of hydrocephalus causing intracranial hypertension, the shunt may be removed in its entirety to have a period with no foreign body in the CSF space. Cultures are monitored daily from the external draining device when present. After several days of negative cultures, a new shunting device can be replaced at a site separate from the infected one. Few data provide a guideline for the length of temporary drainage before a new shunt is placed. Considerable variability in treatment of shunt infections is quite evident from the literature.[9,10] It seems that the standard of care encompasses both direct replacement of shunts under antibiotic coverage with no intermediate phase of external drainage or external drainage that can be anything from a few days to several weeks under antibiotic coverage.

Other Complications

The shunting complication of overdrainage or underdrainage is one that is difficult to treat. In general, overdrainage from shunting is diagnosed by a postural headache that improves with lying down. This can be approached by insertion of an antisiphoning device, if that is not yet in the shunting system, or by changing the valve to a higher pressure. The percutaneous programmable valves are particularly useful for finding a pressure that is appropriate. In some cases, the distal shunt tubing needs to be moved to a different location that decreases drainage, such as the gallbladder or the internal jugular vein in reverse orientation. Changes of valve type from a differential pressure valve or a differential pressure valve with an antisiphoning component to a flow-dependent valve sometimes alleviates symptoms. However, overdrainage is generally a problem that causes symptoms but as yet has not been described as having long-term effects on neurologic function beyond the symptoms. Underdrainage of extracranial CSF shunting devices is a problem encountered more often in adults than in children. In particular, normal-pressure hydrocephalus, which by definition calls for CSF drainage to a less-than-normal pressure, can be inadequately treated by underdrainage. Valve changes by removing an antisiphoning component or by replacing a differential pressure valve with a flow-regulated valve may sometimes provide additional drainage. Also, revising the terminus of the shunting device from the peritoneal space to the pleural space, which generates negative pressure, can improve drainage characteristics. One particular caveat of normal-pressure hydrocephalus syndrome is that in several of our patients we have observed that, with time, the syndrome requires ever-lower-pressure drainage to achieve therapeutic results. The etiology of this change is not known, nor is the reason that it only seems to affect a subset of the population. However, eventually manipulations to provide ever-lower pressure can be exhausted.

The one acute potential complication of overdrainage, particularly in the elderly, is ventricular collapse and disruption of the subdural bridging veins, causing subdural hematoma. This is a potentially catastrophic complication in individuals who have compromised brain function. In general, when the subdural collection is small, we have advocated placing an antisiphoning device, if one is not yet in the system, and increasing the valve pressure. Although this usually resolves a small subdural collection in the situation of normal-pressure hydrocephalus, it brings back the original symptoms. Usually, patients can tolerate several weeks of no symptomatic relief to resolve the subdural hematoma before gradually lowering valve pressure. The use of a percutaneous programmable valve has greatly simplified this process.[33] Another complication of overdrainage is the slit-ventricle syndrome. Thankfully, this is relatively rare in the adult population, but a variety of approaches to this problem have been advocated. They range from changes in valve pressure or the addition of an antisiphoning device to decompression of the intracranial space by craniectomy. Recently, we have found that the addition of a lumboperitoneal shunting system to the functioning ventricular shunting system can alleviate symptoms.[34] The slit-ventricle syndrome can be diagnosed by high CSF pressures in the presence of slitlike ventricles and a functioning ventriculoperitoneal shunt. Several more detailed discussions of its manifestations and treatment have been published.[35,36]

Conclusions

The treatment of an adult with hydrocephalus is similar and yet distinct from that of a child in many respects. Much of the treatment of adult hydrocephalus is the ongoing maintenance of shunting devices placed during childhood. Diagnosis of adult-onset hydrocephalus of any type is made based on evidence of an inappropriate amount of CSF at an inappropriate pressure in the intracranial space. However, the normal-pressure hydrocephalus syndrome in the adult population makes the determination of what is an appropriate pressure confusing. Hydrocephalus from an obstructive source can be bypassed, or the obstruction can be attacked directly, thereby resolving the symptomatology. For hydrocephalus due to abnormal absorption, shunting of CSF to an extracranial absorptive surface is needed. Various shunting systems with different valve types exist, and several potential absorptive surfaces are available. The choice of the best valve and the optimal absorptive surface must be individualized. Bypassing an obstruction and extracranial shunting can result in several types of surgical complications. However, shunt malfunction, shunt infection, overshunting, and undershunting can be treated successfully if approached thoughtfully. The treatment of hydrocephalus in the adult can be a rewarding exercise in the diagnosis of the syndrome and in the use of current technology to treat it.

KEY REFERENCES

Aschoff A, Kremer P, Hashemi B, Kunze S. The scientific history of hydrocephalus and its treatment. *Neurosurg Rev*. 1999;22:67-95.

Bergsneider M, Peacock WJ, Mazziotta JC, Becker DP. Beneficial effect of siphoning in treatment of adult hydrocephalus [see comment]. *Arch Neurol*. 1999;56:1224-1229.

Borgbjerg BM, Gjerris F, Albeck MJ, Borgesen SE. Risk of infection after cerebrospinal fluid shunt: an analysis of 884 first-time shunts. *Acta Neurochir*. 1995;136:1-7.

Bret P, Guyotat J, Chazal J. Is normal pressure hydrocephalus a valid concept in 2002? A reappraisal in five questions and proposal for a new designation of the syndrome as "chronic hydrocephalus" [see comment]. *J Neurol Neurosurg Psychiatry*. 2002;73:9-12.

Bruce DA, Weprin B. The slit ventricle syndrome. *Neurosurg Clin N Am*. 2001;12:709-717.

el-Shafei IL. Ventriculojugular shunt against the direction of blood flow. III. Operative technique and results. *Childs Nerv Syst*. 1987;3:342-349.

Frim DM, Lathrop D, Chwals WJ. Intraventricular pressure dynamics in ventriculocholecystic shunting: a telemetric study. *Pediatr Neurosurg*. 2001;33:237-242.

Fukuhara T, Luciano MG. Clinical features of late-onset idiopathic aqueductal stenosis. *Surg Neurol*. 2001;55:132-137.

Goumnerova LC, Frim DM. Treatment of hydrocephalus with third ventriculocisternostomy: outcome and CSF flow patterns. *Pediatr Neurosurg*. 1997;27:149-152.

Hebb AO, Cusimano MD. Idiopathic normal pressure hydrocephalus: a systematic review of diagnosis and outcome. *Neurosurgery*. 2001; 49:1166-1184.

Horgan MA, Piatt Jr JH. Shaving of the scalp may increase the rate of infection in CSF shunt surgery. *Pediatr Neurosurg*. 1997;26:180-184.

Hurley RA, Bradley Jr WG, Latifi HT, Taber KH. Normal pressure hydrocephalus: significance of MRI in a potentially treatable dementia. *J Neuropsychiatry Clin Neurosci*. 1999;11:297-300.

Kosmorsky G. Pseudotumor cerebri. *Neurosurg Clin N Am*. 2001;12: 775-797.

Krauss JK, Regel JP. The predictive value of ventricular CSF removal in normal pressure hydrocephalus. *Neurol Res*. 1997;19:357-360.

Le H, Yamini B, Frim DM. Lumboperitoneal shunting as a treatment for slit ventricle syndrome. *Pediatr Neurosurg*. 2002;36:178-182.

Mase M, Yamada K, Banno T, et al. Quantitative analysis of CSF flow dynamics using MRI in normal pressure hydrocephalus. *Acta Neurochir Suppl*. 1998;71:350-353.

Meier U, Bartels P. The importance of the intrathecal infusion test in the diagnosis of normal pressure hydrocephalus. *J Clin Neurosci*. 2002;9:260-267.

Meier U, Zeilinger FS, Kintzel D. Signs, symptoms and course of normal pressure hydrocephalus in comparison with cerebral atrophy. *Acta Neurochir*. 1999;141:1039-1048.

Munshi I, Lathrop D, Madsen JR, Frim DM. Intraventricular pressure dynamics in patients with ventriculopleural shunts: a telemetric study. *Pediatr Neurosurg*. 1998;28:67-69.

Piatt Jr JH, Carlson CV. A search for determinants of cerebrospinal fluid shunt survival: retrospective analysis of a 14-year institutional experience. *Pediatr Neurosurg*. 1993;19:233-242.

Qureshi AI, Williams MA, Razumovsky AY, Hanley DF. Magnetic resonance imaging, unstable intracranial pressure and clinical outcome in patients with normal pressure hydrocephalus. *Acta Neurochir Suppl*. 1998;71:354-356.

Savolainen S, Hurskainen H, Paljarvi L, et al. Five-year outcome of normal pressure hydrocephalus with or without a shunt: predictive value of the clinical signs, neuropsychological evaluation and infusion test. *Acta Neurochir*. 2002;144:515-523.

Tisell M, Almstrom O, Stephensen H, et al. How effective is endoscopic third ventriculostomy in treating adult hydrocephalus caused by primary aqueductal stenosis? *Neurosurgery*. 2000;46:104-111.

Walchenbach R, Geiger E, Thomeer RT, Vanneste JA. The value of temporary external lumbar CSF drainage in predicting the outcome of shunting on normal pressure hydrocephalus. *J Neurol Neurosurg Psychiatry*. 2002;72:503-506.

Zemack G, Romner B. Adjustable valves in normal-pressure hydrocephalus: a retrospective study of 218 patients. *Neurosurgery*. 2002;51: 1392-1402.

Numbered references appear on Expert Consult.

CHAPTER 95

Adult Pseudotumor Cerebri Syndrome

SACHIN BATRA • ABHAY MOGHEKAR • DAVID SOLOMON • ARI BLITZ •
DIEGO SAN MILLÁN RUÍZ • PHILIPPE GAILLOUD • PREM S. SUBRAMANIAN •
NEIL R. MILLER • DANIELE RIGAMONTI

Pseudotumor cerebri syndrome (PTCS) is characterized by (1) intracranial pressure (ICP) elevated to at least 250 mm H_2O, (2) normal or small-sized ventricles, (3) no evidence of an intracranial mass, and (4) normal cerebrospinal fluid (CSF) composition. Most patients also have papilledema on funduscopic examination.[1-3] About 10% of patients with PTCS have an identifiable cause for the condition; however, 90% of patients are young, obese women in whom no definite explanation can be found. Such individuals are said to have idiopathic intracranial hypertension (IIH). As implied by the term "pseudotumor cerebri," intracranial masses may present in a similar fashion. Patients with PTCS (including those with IIH) commonly present with headaches, tinnitus, horizontal diplopia, and progressive visual field defects. Headache, which is the most common symptom, is present in 94% patients and is dull in character and usually not localized.[4] Diurnal variations in headaches with early morning aggravation are common. Straining and maneuvers like Valsalva that elevate ICP also exacerbate headaches. Lhermitte sign (electric shock-like neck pain precipitated by neck flexion) has also been reported.[4,5] Pulsatile tinnitus is reported by up to 58% of patients.[4] Visual deterioration in patients with IIH occurs almost exclusively in the setting of severe papilledema, beginning with enlargement of the physiologic blind spot and then progressing to nasal constriction, followed by temporal constriction, and, eventually, loss of central vision and color vision. As this occurs, the papilledema resolves, leaving optic atrophy and blindness. Transient visual obscurations occur in about 68% of patients and can be monocular or binocular. They usually occur at the peak of headache and are often precipitated upon bending or stooping.[4] Metamorphopsia caused by distortion of the macula due to subretinal collections of fluid from a swollen optic disc usually occurs with very severe and chronic papilledema but may occur earlier in the course of IIH.[6]

Etiology and Causative Agents

Elevated dural venous pressures leading to disturbances in CSF absorption at the level of the arachnoid granulations is a widely proposed pathophysiology for IIH.[7] Secondary intracranial hypertension as a cause of PTCS has been reported to occur following cerebral venous thrombosis in thrombophilic states, such as systemic lupus erythematosus (SLE),[8] protein C and protein S deficiencies,[9,10] malignancies, oral contraceptive use,[11] pregnancy, polycystic ovary disease,[9] and from infections including meningitis and mastoiditis. Jugular valve insufficiency has also been found in association with PTCS/IIH.[12] Thrombophlebitis due to an indwelling central venous catheter has also been reported to cause PTCS.[13] Other associations with PTCS include metabolic and endocrine disturbances/conditions such as Addison disease, hyperthyroidism, hypothyroidism, menarche, and pregnancy. A variety of drugs have been implicated in the development of PTCS, most commonly tetracycline, vitamin A, and lithium carbonate (Table 95-1).

Diagnosis

Patients who present with headaches with features suggestive of elevated ICP should undergo a funduscopic examination to assess the optic discs for papilledema. Magnetic resonance imaging (MRI) or computed tomographic (CT) scanning should be performed in all patients with papilledema to evaluate for intracranial masses and to assess ventricular size. Patients with increased ICP may not only have normal or small-sized ventricles,[14] but those with long-standing increased ICP may have an empty appearance of the sella turcica (26.7% sensitive, 94.6% specific), and patients with severe papilledema may show flattening of the posterior aspect of the eye (43.3% sensitive, 100% specific) (Fig. 95-1).[15] The diagnosis of IIH thus should be suspected when no intracranial lesion is found and the ventricles are not dilated. In addition, MR or CT venography should be performed to determine if venous sinus stenosis or thrombosis is present, even if the patient appears to have a physical appearance typical of IIH. Neurologic examination in patients with PTCS/IIH usually reveals no focal deficits except for occasional unilateral or bilateral sixth nerve pareses.

A lumbar puncture to measure opening pressure and to assess CSF content is required to establish the diagnosis of PTCS/IIH. It is important however, that no patient undergoes lumbar puncture until an MRI or CT scan of the brain is performed to exclude an intracranial mass. CSF opening pressures greater than 250 mm H_2O and normal CSF composition and cytology are required for diagnosis.

Table 95-1   Causes of Pseudotumor Cerebri Syndrome

Metabolic Disorders and Endocrinopathies
Pseudohypoparathyroidism
Hypophosphatasia
Prolonged corticosteroid therapy or too rapid corticosteroid withdrawal
Addison disease
Galactosemia
Pregnancy
Oral Contraceptives
Anabolic Steroids
Norplant System (Levonorgestrel Implants)
Drug Toxicities
Nalidixic acid
Doxycycline
Minocycline
Hypervitaminosis A
Lithium
Clomiphene
Venous Sinus Thrombosis and Elevated Central Venous Pressures
Guillain-Barré syndrome
Chronic otitis media and mastoiditis
Sinusitis
Jugular venous thrombosis
Thrombophilic States (Including Hematologic Disorders and Hyperestrogenic States)
Systemic lupus erythematosus (SLE)
Chronic obstructive pulmonary disease (COPD)
Anemia
Iron deficiency anemia
Acquired aplastic anemia
Paroxysmal nocturnal hemoglobinuria
Megaloblastic anemia
Sickle cell disease
Wiskott-Aldrich syndrome
Other
Head injury
Sleep apnea

Lumbar opening pressures should be always be measured with patients lying in the lateral decubitus position with legs extended and relaxed. Patients lying prone during the insertion of the LP needle should be repositioned to the lateral decubitus position before opening pressures are measured to prevent falsely high measurements that result from an increase in abdominal pressure when patients lie prone.[1,3] This precaution should be observed especially when a lumbar drain is placed under fluoroscopic guidance during which patients are typically positioned prone. Similarly, patients whose lumbar puncture is performed with the patient sitting upright should be repositioned to the lateral decubitus position, as measurements of ICP in the sitting position are different from those in the lateral decubitus position, because of the relative positions of the heart and head.

Frequently, a single measurement of opening pressure and the presence of other clinical features fulfilling the criteria described above are sufficient to diagnose a patient with PTCS or IIH; however, patients with atypical presentations, such as chronic persistent headaches without papilledema and normal opening pressures, but in whom there is a high suspicion of IIH (obese patients or those with other conditions associated with IIH), require a 24- to 48-hour continuous recording of ICP, as intermittent elevations of ICP, mostly during sleep, can occur.[16,17]

In addition to neuroimaging and lumbar puncture, patients with suspected or proven PTCS should be evaluated for endocrine/metabolic disturbances, sleep apnea, and potential drug toxicities. When present, treatment of these entities may result in normalization of ICP and resolution of papilledema without surgery.

INVESTIGATIONS

Investigations typically include fundoscopic examination with assessment of visual acuity and visual fields, and lumbar puncture with CSF opening pressure following neuroimaging. Fluids typically sent for include glucose, protein, cells, tumor markers, and cytology for occult malignancies.

IMAGING

Magnetic resonance imaging or CT of the head (preferably with contrast) used to exclude a mass lesion or other etiology as the cause of increased ICP. In cases of unilateral papilledema or when initial imaging suggests the possibility of an abnormality of the region of the sella turcica, further imaging with dedicated orbital and/or pituitary protocol MRI should be considered for added sensitivity and specificity. MRV or CTV may demonstrate the presence or absence of sinovenous thrombosis and/or stenosis.

MANAGEMENT

The management of a patient with PTCS requires an attempt to identify and treat any underlying cause whenever possible. Patients should be weaned of all drugs that have been reported to cause PTCS. Medical conditions such as anemia, sarcoidosis, SLE, and Behçet disease should be treated, as should venous sinus thrombosis. Acetazolamide, a carbonic anhydrase inhibitor proven to lower ICP, should be started immediately in most patients; however, in patients with no identifiable cause of elevated ICP and in whom there has already been loss of visual acuity, visual field, or both, surgical management using optic nerve sheath fenestration (ONSF) or CSF diversion is crucial in preserving or restoring visual function.

The treatment approach to patients of IIH is determined based on assessment of visual function. Weight loss, salt restriction, and analgesics for headaches should be recommended to patients with mild-to-moderate papilledema, but without any decrease in visual acuity or impairment of visual fields other than enlargement of the blind spot. Although weight loss is often difficult to achieve, it is clearly beneficial in attaining control of headaches and visual symptoms. Kupersmith et al. reported improvement in headaches and papilledema in 58 obese females with IIH who lost 7% to 10% of their weight over a 3-month period, and others have reported similar results with surgically produced weight loss.[18,19] Acetazolamide should be initiated at doses of 250 mg QID or 500 mg (sequels) BID to lower ICP and decrease papilledema. Paresthesias, dizziness, dysgusia, and so on are common side effects

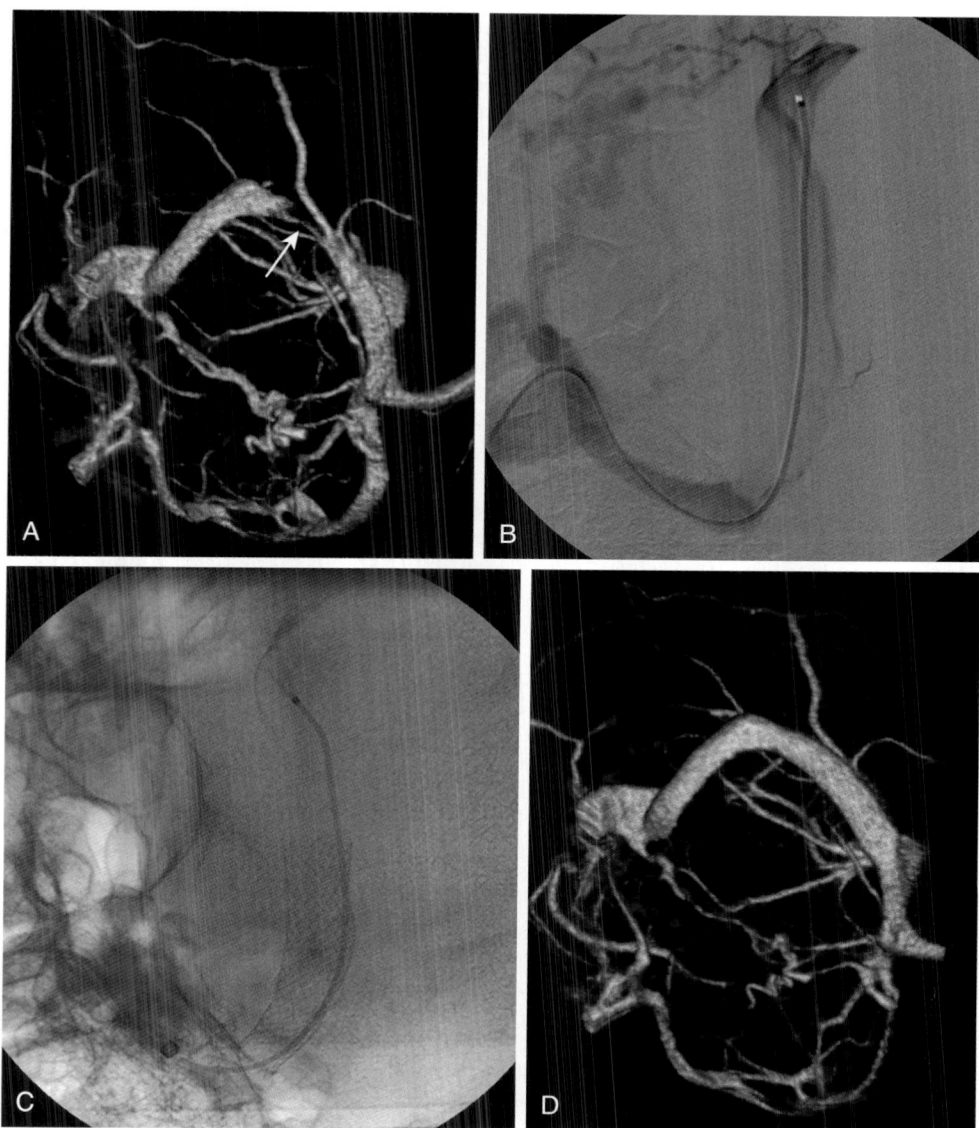

FIGURE 95-1 Thirty-seven-year-old patient with pseudotumor cerebri presenting with headache, papilledema, and a pulsatile tinnitus. A, CT venography, 3D reconstruction prior to stent placement, left posterior oblique projection. Bilateral transverse sinus stenoses initially suspected by MR venography are confirmed by this study performed after lumbar puncture. The *arrow* points at the left transverse sinus lesion that will be targeted during the endovascular procedure. B, Digital subtraction angiography, injection of the left transverse sinus proximal to the site of stenosis, right anterior oblique projection. The pressure gradient across the lesions was measured at 30 mm Hg. C, Same projection as B, unsubtracted image obtained after stent placement. Measurements performed after treatment showed no residual pressure gradient. D, CT venography, 3D reconstruction, left posterior oblique projection, obtained 6 months after stent placement. The study shows full patency of the stented segment. Clinically, the papilledema had completely resolved. Both the pulsatile tinnitus and the headache had disappeared immediately after treatment. The CSF opening pressure was measured at 42 cm of water before treatment and 20 cm of water after stenting. 3D, three-dimensional; CSF, cerebrospinal fluid; CT, computed tomography; MR, magnetic resonance.

of acetazolamide and may limit compliance or any increment in dose, particularly if patients are not warned about these effects before starting the drug. Visual function and fundus appearance should be monitored at regular intervals in all patients on medical treatment, so that any evidence of onset of progression of papilledema or development or progression of optic nerve dysfunction can be detected and treated with ONSF or shunt surgery. Patients with more severe papilledema or rapid decline in visual function should be monitored more frequently (e.g., every 1 to 2 weeks) than other patients. In such patients, the dose of acetazolamide may be increased up to 4 g/day. Some physicians are reluctant to use acetazolamide in patients with a sulfa allergy; however, this drug is not the same as typical sulfa drugs, and there is no evidence that patients allergic to sulfa drugs will have a similar allergic response to acetazolamide. For patients who cannot be treated with, cannot tolerate, or do not respond to acetazolamide, furosemide, triamterene or spironolactone may be used or added to the regimen. Topiramate is an antiepileptic agent

that is being increasingly used in patients with IIH for its ability to lower ICP, reduce weight, and control headache, but its efficacy is not yet proven. A single open-label study reported equivalent visual field outcomes for topiramate and acetazolamide.[32] Corticosteroids may be added to regimens of patients with autoimmune conditions such as sarcoidosis or SLE or in patients with recent venous sinus thrombosis; however, they have no place in the treatment of typical IIH and may, in fact, aggravate the condition by causing weight gain. In addition, withdrawal of steroids prescribed for other reasons has been associated with the development of PTCS.

In patients with moderate or severe papilledema who experience deterioration of visual acuity or worsening of their visual fields (other than enlargement of the blind spot) despite medical therapy or who cannot tolerate medical therapy, consideration should be given to more aggressive therapy. Surgical approaches to treatment of IIH include CSF diversion to lower ICP, ONSF, stenting of venous sinuses, and bariatric surgery for obese patients. Surgical treatment also should be considered in patients who are noncompliant with medications and in those with uncertain follow-up.

Shunt Surgery

Shunt surgery allows egress of CSF, thereby normalizing ICP, improving visual symptoms, and resolving papilledema. Reversible causes of PTCS should be investigated and treated before shunt surgery is considered. Shunt placement, in addition to preserving or improving vision, also benefits other symptoms of PTCS, particularly headache. This is not the case with ONSF, which, although it may result in resolution of papilledema, may not improve the headaches associated with PTCS. Lumboperitoneal (LP) shunts are preferred by some neurosurgeons, as it is relatively easier to access the lumbar subarachnoid space than to place a shunt in small or normal-sized ventricles as are present in patients with PTCS; however, several authors have reported a high incidence of tonsillar herniation following LP shunts, higher failure rates than occurring with other types of shunts,[20,21] and complication of the proximal end of the shunt, such as radiculopathy. LP shunts are also associated with other complications commonly associated with other types of shunts, such as infection and malposition.

Tulipan et al. reported that ventricular shunts can be accurately placed under stereotactic guidance in patients of IIH.[22] In their series, ventriculoperitoneal (VP) shunts were successfully placed in seven patients who had failed medical therapy for IIH without any complications. Papilledema resolved in five patients, and two patients had mild residual papilledema at last follow-up. Headaches resolved in all but one patient whose headache persisted despite a patent shunt. Bynke et al. reported successful insertion of a VP shunt in 17 patients without any stereotactic guidance.[23] Papilledema resolved within 0.6 to 7 months (mean, 3.1 months) in all patients, and visual field defects disappeared in 11 eyes, were better than prior to shunt placement in 11 eyes, and stabilized in 12 eyes. Over the follow-up period, seven patients required nine revisions, one because of peritoneal malposition, two due to suspected shunt infection, and six for shunt obstruction.

In our experience of 115 shunts placed in 42 patients between 1973 and 2003, 36 ventricular shunts were successfully placed under stereotactic guidance, with no procedure having to be aborted. Ventricular and lumbar shunts were equally efficacious in resolving headache and visual symptoms, with 95% of patients responding in 1 month. Headaches and visual symptoms responded to shunting best in patients with shorter duration of symptoms. Revision rates were higher for lumbar shunts (86%) than for ventricular shunts (44%) over a mean follow-up of 49 months. The risk of LP shunt revision due to obstruction was three times that for ventricular shunts, even though both shunt types were similar as regards other causes of malfunction. The overall incidence of shunt overdrainage was 14%, distal catheter migration was 5%, shunt infection was 3.5% and CSF leakage was 3%. Severe complications such as back pain (possibly due to radiculopathy) and tonsillar herniation were observed in 4% and 5% of patients, respectively.[24] We therefore prefer ventricular shunts over lumbar shunts as they are less likely to become obstructed and are free from severe complications such as tonsillar herniation.

Ventricular shunts can be placed in ventriculoatrial (VA) or ventriculoperitoneal configurations. VP shunts are preferred over VA shunts by some surgeons as the latter may cause complications such as arrhythmias, thromboembolism, pulmonary hypertension, and perforation. Furthermore, migration of the distal catheter or malposition of the catheter into the superior vena cava or innominate artery may also occur with VA shunts. VA shunt placement is therefore recommended primarily in patients in whom poor peritoneal absorption is suspected, such as patients with a history of peritonitis, abdominal surgery, or abdominal or pelvic masses. In our experience, however, VA shunts are safe and have acceptable rates of complications, including obstruction (22%), infection (5.5%), malposition/migration (5.5%), and CSF leakage (0.9%). VP shunts are associated with similar risks of obstruction and malposition,[23] as well as some uncommon complications such as abdominal pain due to peritoneal irritation and, rarely, perforation. Rare instances of delayed intra-cerebral hemorrhage following insertion of ventricular shunts have been reported from 5th to 18th postoperative day.[25-27] The site of hemorrhage is often in the parenchyma surrounding the catheter but may occur at any site. The hemorrhage can be caused by diverse etiologies such as bleeding disorders, anticoagulation, shunt-induced disseminated intravascular coagulopathy (DIC) related to the release of plasminogen activators from the choroid plexus in response to shunting, erosion of the parenchymal vessels by the catheter due to transmitted pulsations from the CSF, and arterial vasculature, bleeding from an occult vascular aneurysm, and so on.[25,28]

Excessive drainage/overdrainage of CSF through shunts lowers ICP below the physiologic limit (5 cm H_2O) and may cause symptoms such as headache, nausea, and vomiting. It is important that low-pressure headaches be distinguished from headaches caused by shunt obstruction, the latter being a condition that can cause rapid loss of vision if timely shunt revision is not performed. In addition, in many patients with IIH, headaches that occur despite apparently successful shunting are not due to increased ICP but to migraines or other non-related conditions. Thus, distinguishing low-pressure headaches from headaches caused by increased ICP or unrelated causes is crucial in preventing unwarranted shunt revisions. Low-pressure headaches show postural variances. They are aggravated with upright posture and mitigated upon lying down. Imaging in patients with IIH and postshunt low ICP may not show changes in ventricular size due to altered brain compliance in such patients but there may be pachymeningeal enhancement or subdural hygromas. Overdrainage occurs more often in VP or VA shunts than in LP shunts, but it can be prevented and treated by the use of valve or antisiphon devices in the shunt assembly. Low-pressure symptoms that occur in such cases may be treated by raising the adjustable valve settings to a higher level and following the patient's symptoms. Shunt malfunction in patients with fixed valves requires surgery to replace the fixed valve with an adjustable valve or with a fixed valve of a desired setting. An antisiphon device can treat symptoms of overdrainage and may be added to the shunt valve assembly when needed.

Despite the specific features of most low-pressure headaches, it often is difficult to distinguish low-pressure conditions from shunt obstruction using clinical assessment and results of imaging. Under such circumstances, it is important to perform a diagnostic procedure such as a radionuclide shunt patency study (described later) or ICP monitoring. Radionuclide studies can evaluate accurately the patency of the distal catheter; however, they cannot diagnose overdrainage, which often requires ICP monitoring. ICP recordings within the normal range suggest a normal-functioning shunt, in which case, other causes of headaches should be considered and evaluated. Alternatively, in an emergency setting where suspicion of shunt obstruction and visual deterioration is feared, a lumbar tap will not only aid diagnosis by measuring lumbar CSF opening pressure but also provide relief from symptoms until shunt revision is performed.

Optic Nerve Sheath Fenestration

Optic nerve sheath fenestration decompresses the optic nerve by making one or more openings (or a window) in the dura and arachnoid of the optic nerve, and usually results in resolution of papilledema.[29-32] Banta et al. described the outcomes of 158 ONSFs performed in 86 patients with IIH.[29] Improvement or stabilization of visual acuity and visual fields was observed in 94% and 88% patients, respectively. Complications were often self-limiting, the most common being diplopia (34.86%) and anisocoria (7.5%). One patient had total loss of vision and ophthalmoplegia following surgery, which resolved after a month with corticosteroid treatment, whereas another patient had worse vision postoperatively due to intraoperative damage to the optic nerve. Sergott et al.[32] reported the use of a modified ONSF wherein multiple longitudinal fenestrations were created and subarachnoid adhesions lysed. These authors noted improvement in 21 of 23 patients (91.3%) with IIH who underwent the procedure for progressive decline of vision in one or both eyes. Two patients who did not respond to initial surgery improved following the modified procedure. Interestingly, 12 of the patients had improvement in both eyes following unilateral ONSF,[32] presumably because the procedure resulted not only in decompression of the operated optic nerve but also reduction in ICP. It is therefore recommended that most patients with bilateral papilledema undergo unilateral surgery first, with the contralateral eye being operated on only after observing the response of both eyes to the first surgery.

Despite the observations described previously and although ONSF is usually an efficacious treatment for visual symptoms in patients with IIH, it does not always reduce ICP or relieve headaches. Thus, concurrent medical treatment with acetazolamide and analgesics or even shunt surgery may be required in some cases. As both ONSF and shunt surgery can prevent loss of vision, either of the two can be offered as treatment; however, ONSF is preferred in patients with predominantly visual manifestations and mild-to-moderate headaches that do not require treatment or that can be managed medically. Early failure of ONSF characterized by progressive loss of vision may occur immediately or within a month after surgery due to intraoperative bleeding into the sheath and formation of a fibrous plug that occludes the surgically made openings.[33] These can sometimes be treated with corticosteroids; however, in other cases, shunt placement is required. Mauriello et al.

described five patients who experienced loss of vision shortly after ONSF.[33] One patient who presented with loss of vision on the sixth postoperative day had restoration of normal vision after treatment with high-dose corticosteroids followed by LP shunt placement. A second patient presented with visual loss and conjunctival injection on the third postoperative day and recovered after treatment for presumed infectious optic neuropathy. The vision stabilized after insertion of an LP shunt in three patients who had gradual loss of vision. Progressive visual loss despite a functioning shunt also can be successfully treated with ONSF.[34] The complications of ONSF include blindness from damage to the optic nerve, diplopia, bleeding, and infection, among others. Feldon et al. performed a meta-analysis of the visual outcome of 423 eyes in 252 patients who underwent ONSF for IIH.[35] Visual improvement occurred in 80% of patients over a mean follow-up of 21.1 months. Specifically, visual acuity improved in 113 eyes (50%), and visual field deficits improved in 226 (72%) eyes. Worsening of vision was observed in 42 (10%) eyes. Further surgery was required in 50 (12%) eyes, including repeat ONSF in 26 (6%) cases, shunt surgery in 19 (4%) cases, and both ONSF and shunt surgery in four (1%) cases.

Long-term failure of ONSF is common due to occlusion of the openings by scarring and formation of subarachnoid adhesions. Spoor and McHenry reported a series of 75 eyes in 54 patients.[31] In their series, 24 (32%) eyes in 20 patients failed during 6 to 60 months of follow-up. The authors calculated a 35% failure rate within 5 years of surgery. All patients were treated with repeat procedures, resulting in visual improvement in 5 (21%) eyes, stabilization in 13 (54%) eyes, and deterioration in 6 (25%) eyes. Spoor and McHenry emphasized that such repeat procedures are difficult to perform with less favorable visual outcomes than occur with primary ONSF.[31] In addition, they pointed out that in rare cases, particularly those in which severe visual loss has been present for some time, visual function may not improve despite CSF diversion after a failed ONSF.[31]

Venous Sinus Stenting

Elevation of intracranial venous pressure is known to raise ICP by impeding CSF absorption. Stenosis of transverse venous sinuses and, to a lesser extent, the superior sagittal sinus, increasingly is being diagnosed in patients with otherwise typical IIH, and it is believed by many that stenting of such sinuses may directly address the primary pathology of IIH. Bussiere et al. reported transverse sinus stenosis in 13 patients with IIH, 10 of whom underwent stenting of the affected sinus.[36] Nine patients had successful stent placement via femoral access. One patient required a temporo-occipital craniectomy to place the stent after an unsuccessful attempt to stent via femoral route due to undue tortuosity of sigmoid-jugular junction. Immediate improvement in symptoms was observed in four patients whereas others improved gradually over subsequent 2 to 6 weeks. Almost complete resolution of papilledema was seen in eight patients and significantly improved in two others. Significant improvement of visual acuity occurred in three patients who had pretreatment decline in vision. One patient did not improve significantly due to pre-existing optic nerve atrophy.

Higgins et al. diagnosed venous sinus stenosis associated with an elevated, trans-stenosis pressure gradient in 12 patients with refractory IIH using MRV.[37] All 12 patients underwent dilation and stenting of the stenosed segment of the sinus. Complete resolution of clinical symptoms occurred in 5 patients, 2 patients improved, and 5 remained unchanged over the follow-up period. Furthermore, of 8 patients with papilledema at baseline, 4 (50%) had resolution of disc swelling and 2 had a decrease in swelling. No clinical response was noted in 4 patients whose papilledema failed to resolve after stenting even though measurements of sinus venous pressure before and after stenting showed resolution of venous hypertension in all 8 patients.

Similar to these findings, Owler et al. reported the presence of venous sinus stenosis in five of nine patients with presumed IIH who underwent direct retrograde cerebral venography.[38] Stenting of the stenosed segment was performed in four patients, all of whom experienced improvement in vision and other symptoms related to increased ICP. These and other series underscore the high prevalence of venous sinus stenosis and the potential utility of stenting these patients.

As noted above, we recommend either MRV, preferably contrast-enhanced, or CTV at the time of initial neuroimaging in all patients with presumed IIH to exclude venous sinus stenosis or thrombosis. If a stenosis is identified, direct measurement of venous pressure across the stenosis should be considered to determine if the stenosis is hemodynamically significant. Stenting of a hemodynamically significant stenosis by an experienced neurointerventionalist in such cases can be curative. All patients currently undergoing stenting on an investigational basis at our institution receive anticoagulation with clopidogrel and aspirin for at least 6 months after stenting to prevent thrombosis and occlusion of the stent while it epithelizes. Patients who fail to improve or who experience recurrence of symptoms after stenting must be evaluated with MRV or CTV to exclude loss of patency of the stent or residual stenosis in the contralateral transverse sinus.

Management of IIH in Pregnancy

Pregnancy may not only exacerbate IIH in some patients but also pose limitations with respect to treatment. Patients presenting with acute new onset of symptoms or sudden worsening of previously well-controlled symptoms during pregnancy or in the peripartum period should raise the suspicion of venous sinus thrombosis, particularly if they complain of sudden, very severe headache. In such patients, an MRV or CTV should be obtained and a coagulopathy evaluation should be performed. In addition, in women with IIH and a previously functioning shunt, a functional shunt obstruction may occur during pregnancy from increasing intra-abdominal pressure that prevents CSF flow through the shunt. A shunt revision from peritoneal to another configuration (e.g., VA) may be useful in such cases. In addition, acetazolamide may be used after the first trimester of pregnancy without fear of teratogenicity, although other drugs such as thiazide diuretics are contraindicated in this setting. Finally, serial lumbar punctures are required in some patients to adequately control symptoms and preserve or restore vision.

Conclusion

Appropriate and timely management of PTCS and its most common subtype, IIH, usually prevents irreversible loss of vision and often can restore visual function that has been lost. In all cases, once the diagnosis of PTCS has been made by neuroimaging and lumbar puncture, potential causes for the condition should be thoroughly investigated and treated. Regardless of whether a specific cause can be found or a diagnosis of IIH is made, medical therapy (combined with weight loss in obese patients with IIH) is often sufficient to cure the condition, whereas surgery should be offered to those who fail, cannot tolerate, or decline medical treatment, or who already have significant visual dysfunction when first diagnosed. Long-term monitoring with funduscopic and visual function examination is crucial while a patient is on medical management and after surgical treatment. Shunt placement or optic nerve sheath fenestration are efficacious treatments but not free from long-term morbidity.

KEY REFERENCES

Agid R, Farb R, Willinsky R, et al. Idiopathic intracranial hypertension: the validity of cross-sectional neuroimaging signs. *Neuroradiology.* 2006;48:521-527.

Banta J, Farris B. Pseudotumor cerebri and optic nerve sheath decompression. *Ophthalmology.* 2000;107:1907-1912.

Bynke G, Zemack G, Bynke H, Romner B. Ventriculoperitoneal shunting for idiopathic intracranial hypertension. *Neurology.* 2004;63:1314-1316.

Chumas P, et al. Tonsillar herniation: the rule rather than the exception after lumboperitoneal shunting in the pediatric population. *J Neurosurg.* 1993;78:568-573.

Corbett J, Mehta M. Cerebrospinal fluid pressure in normal obese subjects and patients with pseudotumor cerebri. *Neurology.* 1983;33:1386-1388.

Feldon S. Visual outcomes comparing surgical techniques for management of severe idiopathic intracranial hypertension. *Neurosurg Focus.* 2007;23:E6.

Friedman D, Jacobson D. Diagnostic criteria for idiopathic intracranial hypertension. *Neurology.* 2002;59:1492-1495.

Giuseffi V, Wall M, Siegel P, Rojas P. Symptoms and disease associations in idiopathic intracranial hypertension (pseudotumor cerebri): a case-control study. *Neurology.* 1991;41:239-244.

Higgins J, Cousins C, Owler B, et al. Idiopathic intracranial hypertension: 12 cases treated by venous sinus stenting. *J Neurol Neurosurg Psychiatry.* 2003;74:1662-1666.

Karabatsou K, Quigley G, Buxton N, et al. Lumboperitoneal shunts: are the complications acceptable? *Acta Neurochir (Wien).* 2004;146:1193-1197.

Karahalios D, Rekate H, Khayata M, Apostolides P. Elevated intracranial venous pressure as a universal mechanism in pseudotumor cerebri of varying etiologies. *Neurology.* 1996;46:198-202.

Kelman S, et al. Modified optic nerve decompression in patients with functioning lumboperitoneal shunts and progressive visual loss. *Ophthalmology.* 1991;98:1449-1453.

Kelman S, Heaps R, Wolf A, Elman M. Optic nerve decompression surgery improves visual function in patients with pseudotumor cerebri. *Neurosurgery.* 1992;30:391-395.

Kupersmith M, et al. Effects of weight loss on the course of idiopathic intracranial hypertension in women. *Neurology.* 1998;50:1094-1098.

Lim M, Pushparajah K, Jan W, et al. Magnetic resonance imaging changes in idiopathic intracranial hypertension in children. *J Child Neurol.* 2010;25(3):294-299.

Mascalchi M. Delayed intracerebral hemorrhage after CSF shunt for communicating "normal-pressure" hydrocephalus. Case report. *Ital J Neurol Sci.* 1991;12:109-112.

Mauriello JJ, Shaderowfsky P, Gizzi M, Frohman L. Management of visual loss after optic nerve sheath decompression in patients with pseudotumor cerebri. *Ophthalmology.* 1995;102:441-445.

McGirt M, et al. Cerebrospinal fluid shunt placement for pseudotumor cerebri-associated intractable headache: predictors of treatment response and an analysis of long-term outcomes. *J Neurosurg.* 2004; 101:627-632.

Owler B, et al. Pseudotumor cerebri syndrome: venous sinus obstruction and its treatment with stent placement. *J Neurosurg.* 2003;98: 1045-1055.

Sergott R, Savino P, Bosley T. Modified optic nerve sheath decompression provides long-term visual improvement for pseudotumor cerebri. *Arch Ophthalmol.* 1988;106:1384-1390.

Spence J, Amacher A, Willis N. Benign intracranial hypertension without papilledema: role of 24-hour cerebrospinal fluid pressure monitoring in diagnosis and management. *Neurosurgery.* 1980;7:326-336.

Spoor T, McHenry J. Long-term effectiveness of optic nerve sheath decompression for pseudotumor cerebri. *Arch Ophthalmol.* 1993; 111:632-635.

Sugerman H, Felton WR, Salvant JJ, et al. Effects of surgically induced weight loss on idiopathic intracranial hypertension in morbid obesity. *Neurology.* 1995;45:1655-1659.

Torbey M, Geocadin R, Razumovsky A, et al. Utility of CSF pressure monitoring to identify idiopathic intracranial hypertension without papilledema in patients with chronic daily headache. *Cephalalgia.* 2004;24:495-502.

Whiteley W, Al-Shahi R, Warlow C, et al. CSF opening pressure: reference interval and the effect of body mass index. *Neurology.* 2006;67: 1690-1691.

Numbered references appear on Expert Consult.

CHAPTER 96

Endoscopic Third Ventriculostomy

PABLO F. RECINOS • GEORGE I. JALLO • VIOLETTE RENARD RECINOS

Neuroendoscopy and minimally invasive techniques have played an increasing role in contemporary neurosurgery. Endoscopic third ventriculostomy, specifically, is a procedure that has experienced a resurgence in popularity in the last 30 years and has become the most commonly performed neuroendoscopic procedure.[1] However, endoscopy was present and utilized since the turn of the 20th century, when surgical interventions for hydrocephalus were first being developed.

Historical Background

The first neuroendoscopic procedure was performed in 1910 by Vincent Darwin L'Espinasse, a Chicago urologist, who used a cystoscope to fulgurate the choroid plexus in two infants with hydrocephalus.[2] One of the patients died; however, the other lived for 5 years. Walter Dandy performed several procedures for hydrocephalus. In 1918, he performed the first open ventriculostomy by fenestrating the lamina terminalis through a transfrontal approach.[3] In 1922, he unsuccessfully attempted a choroid plexectomy using the endoscope and at that time coined the terms "ventriculoscope" and "ventriculoscopy."[4] Fay and Grant were the first to photograph the inside of the ventricular system in 1923. Interestingly, the exposure time for their images ranged from 30 to 90 seconds, accentuating the extremely poor lighting and visualization of neuroendoscopy at that time.[5]

This first successful endoscopic third ventriculostomy (ETV) was performed in 1923 by William J. Mixter in a 9-month-old hydrocephalic patient. Utilizing a urethroscope, he was able to pass through the foramen of Monro, visualize the third ventricle and cerebral aqueduct, and make a hole in the floor of the third ventricle connecting it to the interpeduncular cistern. He subsequently enlarged the hole with side-to-side mechanical motion up to a diameter of 4 mm.[6] The next successful ETV did not appear in the literature until 1935, when Scharff reported his initial results using a novel endoscope. Scharff described several modifications including an irrigation system that kept the ventricles open, a mobile cautery tip, and a moveable operating tip that could perforate the floor of the third ventricle.[7] Around the same time, resection of the choroid plexus was still a popular treatment for hydrocephalus. Tracy Putnam modified a cystoscope for use in the ventricular system, specifically designing it to cauterize choroid plexus in order to treat children with hydrocephalus.[8] In one of his series of 42 patients, which was the largest at that time, 17 patients (40%) responded favorably while 10 patients (25%) died perioperatively.[9] In 1947, McNickle described a modified technique of performing a percutaneous

third ventriculostomy utilizing a 19-gauge needle to puncture the floor of the third ventricle. Although he initially used an endoscope for the procedure, he later abandoned its use in favor of using x-rays and tactile feedback for localization.[10]

Despite the advances made by a few pioneering surgeons, neuroendoscopic procedures were not widely adopted during the first half of the 20th century.[11-13] Technology was a significant limiting factor as lighting and visualization were very poor and the setup of the endoscopic lenses was complicated and cumbersome.[11,12] In 1952, Nulsen and Spitz first reported creation of a shunt diverting cerebrospinal fluid (CSF) from the ventricular system to the jugular vein to successfully treat communicating hydrocephalus.[14] This began a monumental shift in the hydrocephalus treatment paradigm toward shunt diversion. Although a select few surgeons would continue performing neuroendoscopic procedures to treat hydrocephalus, the majority of neurosurgeons adopted CSF shunt diversion as standard practice due to the low complexity and safety of the procedure.[12]

During this hiatus in the clinical use of neuroendoscopy, critical advances in technology would eventually lead to revisiting the role of neuroendoscopy in neurosurgery. First-generation endoscopes utilized conventional lenses, which had a fixed refractive index. This required the lenses of the endoscope to be carefully placed in series in order to relay an image. In 1966, Hopkins and Storz revolutionized lens technology by developing the SELFOC lens. These lenses used gradient-index glass, which allowed adjustment based on the lens radius.[15] Compared to conventional lenses, a wider field of vision could be viewed while preserving the illumination.[12,15,16] In 1969, Smith and Boyle developed the charge-coupled device, which allowed optical data to be converted into electrical current.[12] This precluded the need for large relay stations and allowed for the development of smaller endoscopes. Perhaps most important was the development and improvement of fiberoptic cables that occurred between the 1950s to 1970s. Using fiberoptic cable technology, light could be separated from the rest of the endoscope and emitted from the tip without emitting significant amounts of heat or losing luminescence.[12,15]

With improved technology, use of the endoscope was revisited for hydrocephalus treatment. In 1978, Vries reported a series of five patients who he had treated with ETV utilizing a fiberoptic endoscope.[17] Although all of his patients eventually required a shunt diversion procedure, the patients did well postoperatively demonstrating that ETV was technically feasible with current technology. In 1990, Jones et al. reported

50% successful outcome from ETV in 24 patients with non-communicating hydrocephalus with 8% morbidity and no mortality.[18] In 1994, the same group reported an even better success rate (61%) in a series of 103 patients.[19] Given the technological advances in endoscopic illumination and optics, the demonstrated safety of the procedure with second-generation endoscopes, and the clinical efficacy reported in the literature, ETV was widely adopted in the 1990's by the neurosurgical community to treat hydrocephalus.[1,12]

Patient Selection

Selection of the appropriate patient for ETV requires an understanding of CSF physiology, detailed study of radiographic anatomy, an appreciation for the location of CSF obstruction, and knowledge of results for various age groups and etiologies of hydrocephalus.[3,20] The CSF circulation is analogous to a hydraulic system. CSF flows sequentially through each chamber starting in the choroid plexus until being reabsorbed in the arachnoid villi. Pathologic obstruction can occur at any point in the circuit or at the end. ETV treats hydrocephalus by creating an internal shunt from the third ventricle to the interpeduncular cistern in the cortical subarachnoid space (Fig. 96-1). If the pathologic obstruction lies between the third ventricle and the cortical subarachnoid space, then ETV will likely be an effective treatment. If the pathologic obstruction lies downstream from the cortical subarachnoid space, then ETV will be of no benefit.[20]

Pathologic Considerations

The etiology of the pathologic obstruction should be determined when considering the most appropriate treatment for hydrocephalus. The most responsive etiologies of hydrocephalus to ETV are tumors of the tectal region and congenital aqueductal stenosis.[21,22] Tectal gliomas or pineal region tumors can compress the cerebral aqueduct, obstructing CSF flow from the third ventricle to the fourth ventricle. Likewise, congenital aqueductal stenosis also results in impaired flow from the third ventricle to the fourth ventricle. It can present in infants, children, adolescents, or adults.[23,24] The later it presents, the better chance that ETV will successfully treat the hydrocephalus. Care must be taken not to confuse congenital aqueductal stenosis with narrowing of the cerebral aqueduct that occurs secondary to inward displacement of the brainstem. This scenario can be present in infants or young children with increased pressure of the superior sagittal sinus leading to decreased terminal absorption of CSF. When the sutures are open, this can lead to global increases in CSF volume, including in the ventricular system and the basal cisterns. An increase in the CSF volume in the prepontine and interpeduncular cisterns can produce compression of the brainstem leading to secondary compression of the cerebral aqueduct, mimicking aqueductal stenosis.[20] In these cases, the site of obstruction lies distal to the interpeduncular cistern and placement of a ventricular shunt, not ETV, would be the indicated intervention.[20,25]

Nontectal/pineal region tumors producing hydrocephalus can also benefit from ETV if properly selected.[26-28] Prior to surgical intervention, the exact point of CSF obstruction needs to be determined. If the point of obstruction occurs along the course of CSF flow between the third ventricle and the interpeduncular cistern, then ETV may be useful. If the point of obstruction lies outside this course, then shunting should be considered. However, tumor resection may be the only treatment needed to cure the hydrocephalus.

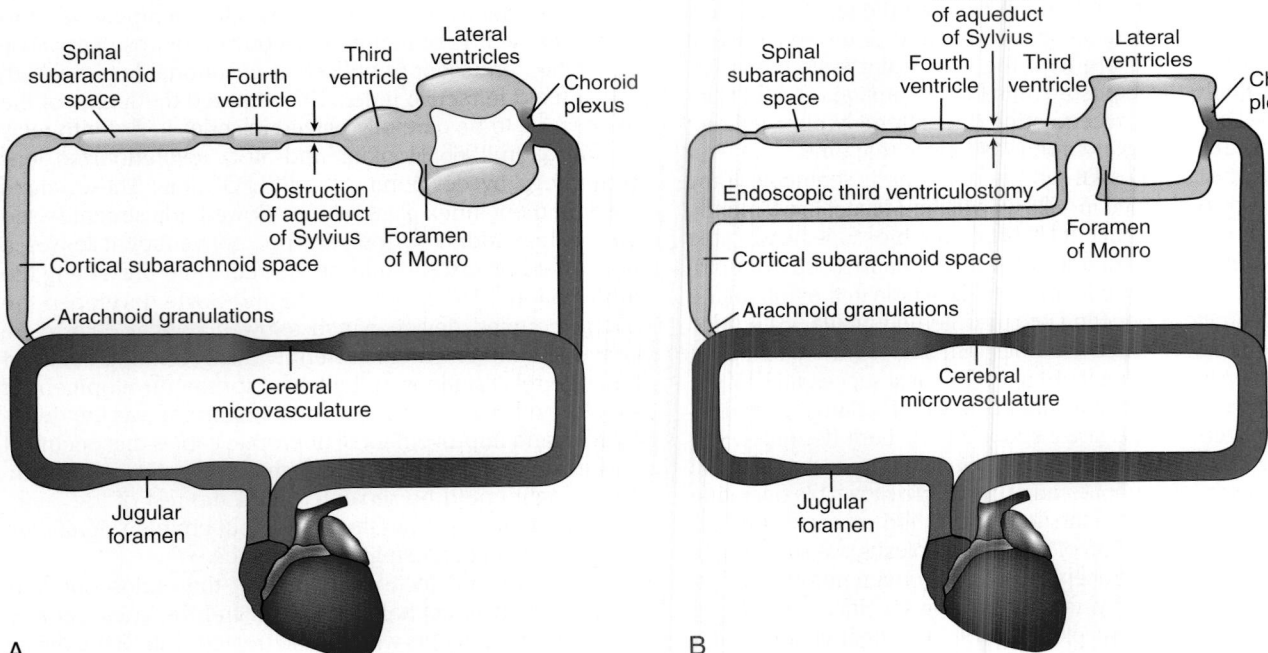

A

B

FIGURE 96-1 Schematic of bulk flow model of CSF hydraulics from the point of production in the choroid plexus until its absorption and incorporation into the systemic circulation. A, Aqueductal stenosis is portrayed along with the resultant triventriculomegaly. B, ETV creates a bypass from the third ventricle to the cortical subarachnoid space and results in resolution of the triventriculomegaly. (Adapted from Rekate H. Selecting patients for endoscopic third ventriculostomy. Neurosurg Clin North Am. 2004;15(1):39.)

For example, in patients with noncommunicating hydrocephalus secondary to mass effect from fourth ventricular tumors, we prefer surgical resection of the tumor to correct hydrocephalus. An intraventricular catheter can be placed for intracranial pressure monitoring and temporary CSF drainage as needed prior to the tumor resection. Others advocate performing an ETV prior to tumor resection.[29,30] Although this option bypasses the site of CSF obstruction, these patients need to be carefully selected due to the risk of upward herniation of the superior cerebellar vermis which can result in midbrain compression.[20]

Congenital abnormalities can be associated with hydrocephalus. Approximately 80% to 90% of patients with myelomeningocele have hydrocephalus requiring intervention.[31,32] The localization of CSF obstruction in these patients is often more complex than in patients with obstruction secondary to a tumor. For example, Chiari II patients can have up to four pathologic sites of obstruction.[33] If there are multiple sites of obstruction, ETV may not effectively bypass the entire site and hence be unsuccessful. However, not all Chiari II patients have the same patterns of obstruction. For example, ETV has been shown to be successful in a small cohort of adult Chiari II patients, implying a more simplified pattern of obstruction between the third ventricle and the interpeduncular cistern.[34] Thus, the role of ETV in cases of congenital malformations associated with hydrocephalus is not clear and consideration of intervention must be done on a case-by-case basis.

Vascular pathologies such as subarachnoid hemorrhage (SAH) and intraventricular hemorrhage (IVH) can produce hydrocephalus. The mechanism of hydrocephalus in the acute setting is usually decreased CSF absorption from obstruction in the arachnoid granulations and a mechanical outflow obstruction from clot within the ventricular system. However, over time as the blood resolves, obstruction at the level of arachnoid granulations and within the ventricles may not be the long-term cause of hydrocephalus. Once the inflammatory process progresses, the point of obstruction usually becomes localized to the basal cisterns, at the interface of the spinal subarachnoid/cranial subarachnoid spaces.[20] In the setting of SAH, external ventricular drainage is commonly performed to temporize the patient. In some SAH patients, there is minimal residual obstruction and the external ventricular drainage can be weaned off without further intervention. Other patients with SAH may require permanent CSF diversion. In patients without prior surgical intervention, ETV can be considered if there is no anatomic contraindication. In patients with a prior surgical intervention, ETV may be of more limited use.[35] For example, fenestration of the lamina terminalis during open surgery for a ruptured aneurysm is direct, safe, and potentially avoids the need for a repeat operation to treat hydrocephalus.[36] Patients with IVH can similarly show a clinically significant, time-dependent change in the localization of CSF obstruction. In the series by Siomin et al., a higher rate of ETV success was associated with previous history of ventriculoperitoneal shunt placement post-hemorrhage.[37]

Post-infectious hydrocephalus can also require CSF diversion. Obstruction resulting from infection can be localized to the basal cisterns or to the arachnoid granulations.[20]

If the obstruction is in the basal cisterns then ETV can be considered. If the obstruction is in the arachnoid granulations, then ETV would not be beneficial. However, determination of the exact site of obstruction in these patients can be challenging and is not always possible. Another consideration in post-infectious patients is that there can be significant meningeal thickening of the leptomeninges and third ventricular floor. Thus, creation of a hole in the floor of the third ventricle can be more challenging and have a higher risk of closure.[37] History of infection has been shown to be a negative predictor of ETV success.[22,38] However, in properly selected patients ETV can be successful in treating post-infectious hydrocephalus.[20,37]

The pathophysiology of idiopathic normal-pressure hydrocephalus (iNPH) has been the subject of much debate. Although some patients exhibit asymmetry between the third and fourth ventricles, suggestive of an associated late-onset idiopathic aqueductal stenosis, others exhibit global enlargement of the ventricular system. Indeed, the pathophysiology of iNPH is likely unrelated to a mechanical obstruction, but rather an abnormality of ventricular compliance and CSF flow.[37,39] It is known that certain patients with iNPH respond favorably to ETV. Gangemi and colleagues reported the largest series to date of iNPH patients treated with ETV. Out of 110 patients, improvement was seen in 69.1% of patients, no change in 21.8%, and continued deterioration was seen in 9.1%.[39] This compares favorably to other reported outcomes from shunting, although no randomized comparison has yet been performed.[39,40] ETV may be a more physiologic solution and the problems associated with overdrainage have not been seen, which make it a promising alternative to shunt diversion in select iNPH patients.[39]

Other Considerations

There are factors other than pathology that have been shown to impact success of ETV for hydrocephalus. Age is one of the most important factors in predicting success of ETV in the pediatric population. Kulkarni and co-workers performed a multicenter, retrospective analysis on 618 pediatric patients who had undergone ETV.[22] A training set of 455 patients was used to identify predictors of ETV success and the remaining 163 patients were used to internally validate those predictors. In their analysis, age was the most significant predictor of ETV success. Younger patients (<1 year old) had a higher chance of failure compared to older patients, and infants (<1 month old) in particular had the highest likelihood of failure.[22] This confirmed previous reports and added weight to those that discourage ETV in infant patients.[41,42] In adult patients, there does not appear to be an association between age and risk of failure.[39]

The presence of a previous shunt has different implications when considering treatment with ETV. In the prior analysis of 618 pediatric patients by Kulkarni et al., presence of a shunt was shown to increase risk of ETV failure, although to a lower degree than certain hydrocephalus etiologies (e.g., postinfectious and very young patient age).[22] However, the effect of treatment with shunting prior to ETV likely is different depending on the pathology. In the series reported by Siomin and colleagues, treatment with shunting prior to ETV was actually a positive predictor of ETV success. This difference was especially pronounced in the subset of patients with a history of premature birth.[43]

In chronically shunted patients with associated symptoms, conversion to an ETV from a shunt can be done by following an algorithm[20] (Fig. 96-2). The shunt is first removed and replaced with an external ventricular drain. The patient is placed in the intensive care unit for monitoring and the external ventricular drain subsequently clamped. If the ventricles enlarge and the intracranial pressure (ICP) rises, ETV is attempted. If there is subsequently no ventricular enlargement after ETV, patients are either observed for 48 hours (no change in ICP) or shunted (significant rise in ICP).[20]

Contraindications to Endoscopic Third Ventriculostomy

There are certain situations in which an ETV is contraindicated. Anatomically, the lateral and third ventricles can be too small to safely pass an endoscope. This occurs in situations of "normal volume hydrocephalus," when little to no change is observed in ventricular size when ICP rises such as in pseudotumor cerebri. In other cases, one of the anatomic structures can block the path to the floor of the third ventricle. For example, the massa intermedia in Chiari II patients can be so large as to prevent safe passage of the endoscope. Pathology, such as a tumor or other mass lesion can also block the

trajectory to the floor of the third ventricle. Physiologically, the CSF flow should be examined on preoperative imaging. If the obstruction is above the level of the third ventricle, distal to the interpeduncular cistern, or if no clear obstruction can be identified then the utility of ETV is limited.[20]

Preoperative Workup

Preoperative imaging is critical to selecting the appropriate patient for ETV and to prevent undue risk while performing the procedure. Magnetic resonance imaging (MRI) with constructive interface steady state (CISS) sequence is the modality of choice, preferably with cine sequences. MRI is the best modality for studying the anatomy, pathology, and localizing the point(s) of obstruction. Cine sequences are especially helpful in studying the flow of CSF. Particular attention should be placed on studying the relationship of the basilar artery to the floor of the third ventricle to avoid damaging it during the procedure. If MRI is contraindicated, computed tomography (CT) can also provide useful anatomic and pathologic information, although not to the degree of detail as MRI.

Surgical Equipment

There are several components to a functioning endoscopic setup: the endoscope, a light source, a video unit, and irrigation source. Familiarization with each piece of equipment is critical in order to ensure a smooth procedure. Additionally, it is not uncommon for an inexperienced scrub staff to be assisting an endoscopic procedure. In theses cases, the surgeon can guide troubleshooting should a problem arise.

There are three basic types of endoscopes: rigid, flexible, and semiflexible (Fig. 96-3). Rigid scopes offer the best

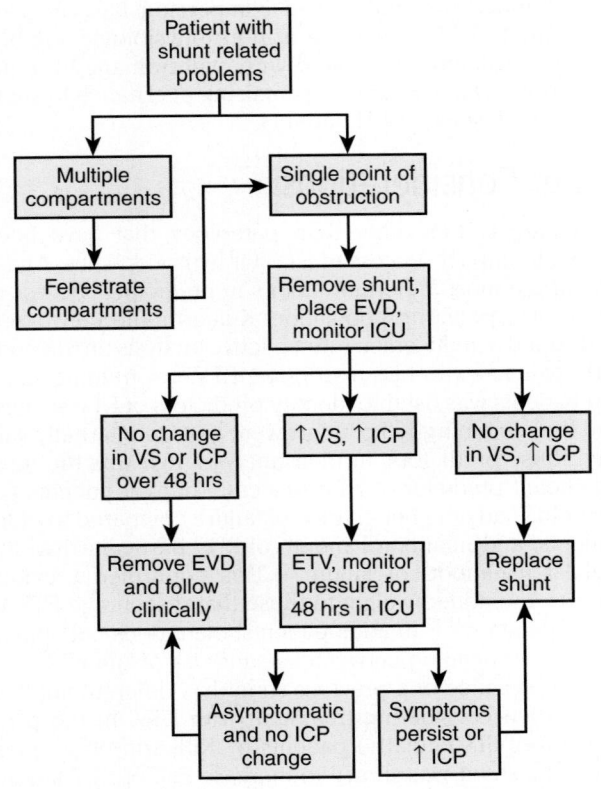

VS = Ventricular size, EVD = External ventricular drain, ICP = Intracranial pressure

FIGURE 96-2 Algorithm for the management of shunt-related problems to select patients appropriate for shunt removal. (Adapted from Rekate H. Selecting patients for endoscopic third ventriculostomy. Neurosurg Clin North Am. 2004;15(1):39.)

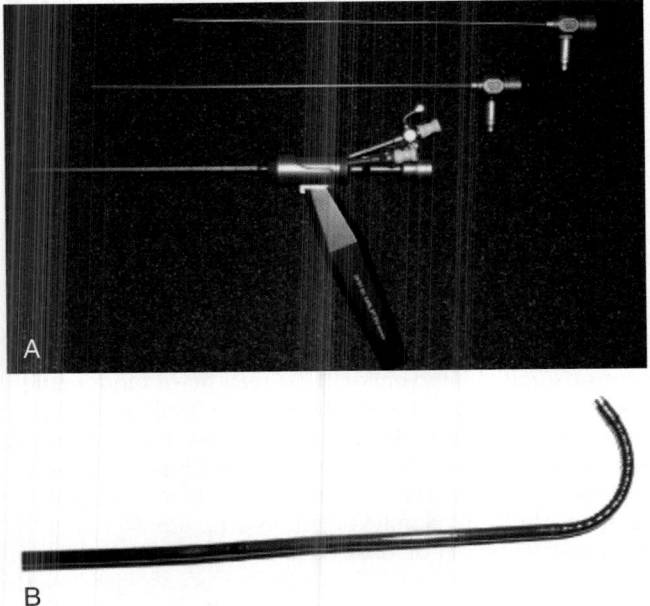

FIGURE 96-3 An example of a 0- and 30-degree rigid endoscope with sheath (A) and a flexible endoscope (B). (From Sciubba DM, Noggle JC, Jallo GI: Equipment for neuroendoscopic procedures. In: Jallo GI, Conway JE, Bognar L, eds., eds. Neuroendoscopy of the Central Nervous System. San Diego: Plural; 2008:13-22.)

optics, a wide-angled view, allow magnification without loss of resolution, and can have instruments passed through them. Flexible scopes allow a wide degree of bending, which allows the operator to look around corners. However, their resolution diminishes with magnification and they may not allow many instruments to be passed through them. Semiflexible scopes have better resolution and less flexibility compared to flexible scopes, but do not have the resolution or wide-angled view seen with rigid scopes.[44] We prefer rigid scopes with a 0- or 12-degree angle of view for ETV.

The light source provides bright, cold illumination and typically comes from a halogen, xenon, or metal-halide lamp. In particular, the color of the picture seen under illumination with xenon most closely resembles the color in natural sunlight.[15,44] The video unit is composed of a chip video camera, a camera control unit, video monitor, and a video documentation system. The video documentation system can include still-shot capture, video recording, a CD/DVD burner, and a printer (Fig. 96-4).

The irrigation source can either be manual or mechanical. Manual irrigation requires an assistant to continuously irrigate and intermittently change syringes. The pressure of irrigation can be adjusted, which can be helpful in achieving hemostasis and to test the flow once the ventriculostomy is made. Mechanical irrigation is automated precluding the need for an assistant to continuously irrigate. Some systems allow for variations in flow speed while in others, the pressure of irrigation is constant and cannot be adjusted. The solution used for irrigation should be slightly warmed Ringer solution at a flow rate of 15 ml/min.

Operative Technique

There are a variety of operative techniques that are in use for the treatment of hydrocephalus with ETV. Irrespective of technique employed, it is important to be comfortable and familiar with the components of the endoscopic system. As mentioned above, endoscopic equipment generally used for an ETV include the following: endoscope, control panel, irrigation pump with preference for slightly warmed Ringer solution at a flow rate less than 15 ml/min, ventricular cannula (usually no. 12.5 or 14 French peel-away sheath that cannulates the ventricular system and allows the endoscope to pass easily and safely down its lumen, while also providing for egress of CSF and irrigation fluid), an instrument to create the fenestration in the floor of the third ventricle, and a tool such as a balloon catheter to assist in the enlargement of the stoma (our preference is for a no. 3 French Fogarty). If using a balloon catheter, it is also advised that the surgeon verifies that the balloon inflates properly prior to starting the procedure.

The patient is first placed supine with the head in the neutral position on a doughnut pillow or in three-pin fixation when neuronavigation is used. The head of bed is placed at 30 degrees to prevent air entry and excessive loss of CSF. The monitor and neuroendoscopy tower should be placed at the foot of the bed so that the surgeon may directly visualize the monitor while operating (Fig. 96-5). Antibiotics are given within 1 hour prior to skin incision to reduce risk of infection. Site of entry will vary slightly depending on age, and side of surgery is determined preoperatively depending on the anatomy and pathology of the patient. If no contraindication is present, the nondominant side is selected.[45] A useful reference point superficially is the intersection between the midpupillary line and the coronal suture. A burr hole is made just anterior to the coronal suture. The dura is opened in a cruciate fashion and the dural leaflets and pia are coagulated with bipolar cautery. If a large cortical vein is present, it is important to make minor adjustments in the surgical tract in order to avoid unnecessary damage to the vein.

A peel-away catheter (12.5 or 14 French) is passed into the lateral ventricle by aiming medially toward the ipsilateral medial canthus and posteriorly toward the contralateral

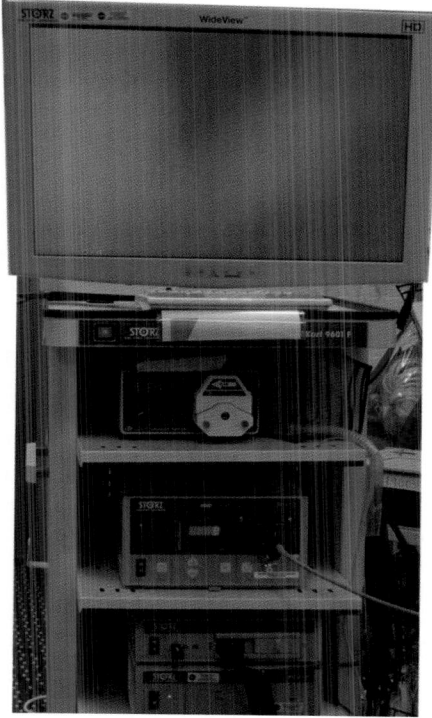

FIGURE 96-4 Neuroendoscopy tower which contains a monitor, light source, camera control unit, CD/DVD recording device, and printer.

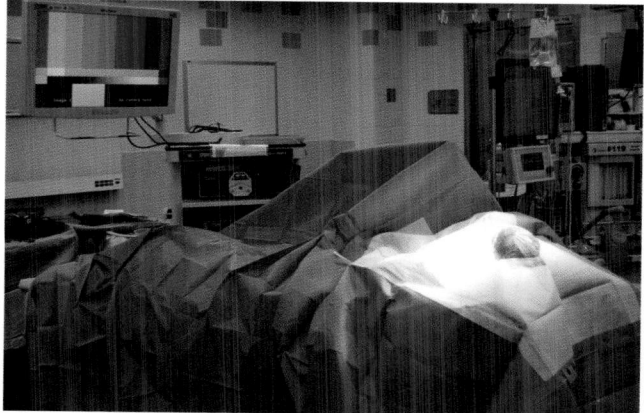

FIGURE 96-5 The monitor and neuroendoscopy tower are placed at the foot of the bed allowing the surgeon to work with direct visualization of the monitor and without unnecessary body movements.

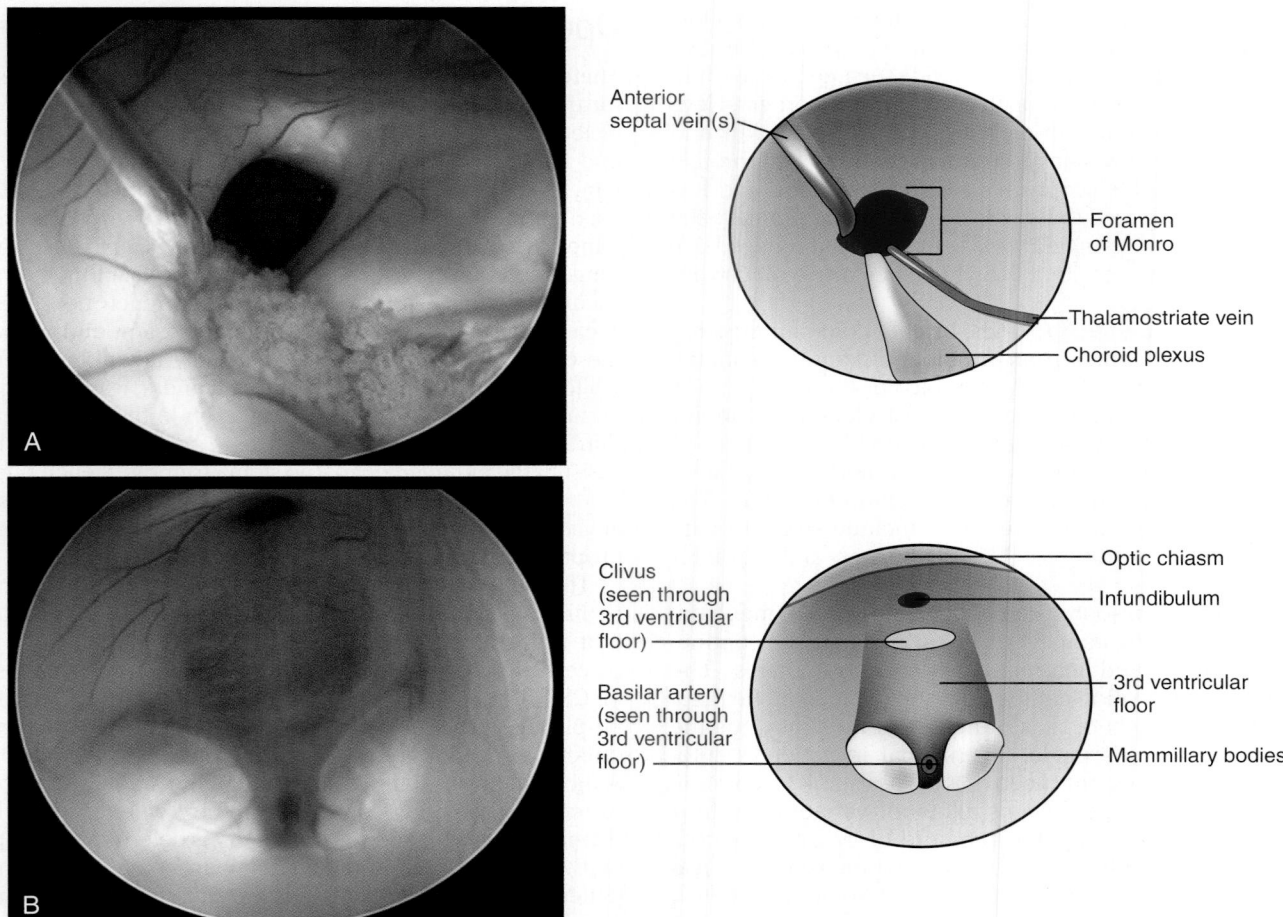

FIGURE 96-6 Intraoperative views and corresponding schematic representations. A, View of foramen of Monro from right lateral ventricle. The choroid plexus (center), anterior septal vein (medial), and thalamostriate vein (lateral) are seen. Care must be taken not to damage these structures when entering the foramen of Monro in order to prevent hemorrhage or venous infarcts. B, View of the floor of the third ventricle. From anterior to posterior, the optic chiasm, infundibulum, tuber cinereum, paired mammillary bodies are clearly seen. The basilar artery can also be seen between the mammillary arteries and must be avoided upon perforation of the third ventricular floor.

external acoustic meatus. Once CSF return is appreciated and the peel-away catheter is frankly in the lateral ventricle, the stylet is removed and the sheath is secured by peeling away its two sides. The sides are secured to the drapes with staples to avoid inadvertent deepening of the sheath. The endoscope is inserted through the sheath and the ventricle is inspected. The main landmarks including choroid plexus, fornix, posterior commissure, veins, and the foramen of Monro are identified[45,46] (Fig. 96-6A). In adults, the foramen of Monro sits 5 to 6 cm from the dura mater, however, in children this distance is less. Continuous irrigation is usually unnecessary during inspection. If bleeding is encountered, gentle irrigation clears the operative view. Most small hemorrhages tend to stop spontaneously after irrigating for several minutes. A bipolar probe may also be used if irrigation is unsuccessful. Once the foramen of Monro is clearly visualized, the endoscope is passed through until the third ventricle comes into view. On average, the floor of the third ventricle lies 7 cm deep to the dura, however, this can vary depending on the age of the patient and the extent of the hydrocephalus.[45]

Perforation of the floor of the third ventricle is the most dangerous step of an ETV. Inspection of the anatomic landmarks must be done to identify the safe zone in the floor of the third ventricle. These landmarks include the mammillary bodies, the tuber cinereum, the infundibular recess, and optic chiasm[45,46] (Fig. 96-6B). The target for the ventriculostomy lies between the mammillary bodies and the infundibular recess. Care must be taken not to injure the basilar artery, which lies just anterior and inferior to the mammillary bodies and can sometimes be visualized through the diaphanous floor of the third ventricle (Fig. 96-7). We prefer using the Bugbee wire to bluntly puncture the floor of the third ventricle. A 3-French Fogarty balloon catheter is passed into the opening in the floor of the third ventricle and the balloon is inflated with 0.2 ml of fluid. The inflating balloon widens the aperture and the process is repeated until the opening is sufficiently wide. It is not recommended to inflate the balloon under the floor and pull back through the stoma; rather, the balloon is inflated while its center is within the newly created fenestration. Doppler devices are also available to help locate the basilar artery prior to fenestration. While the technique described is the one we feel is the safest, several other techniques are used. Perforation of the floor of the third ventricle can be done using a variety of instruments including electrocautery,

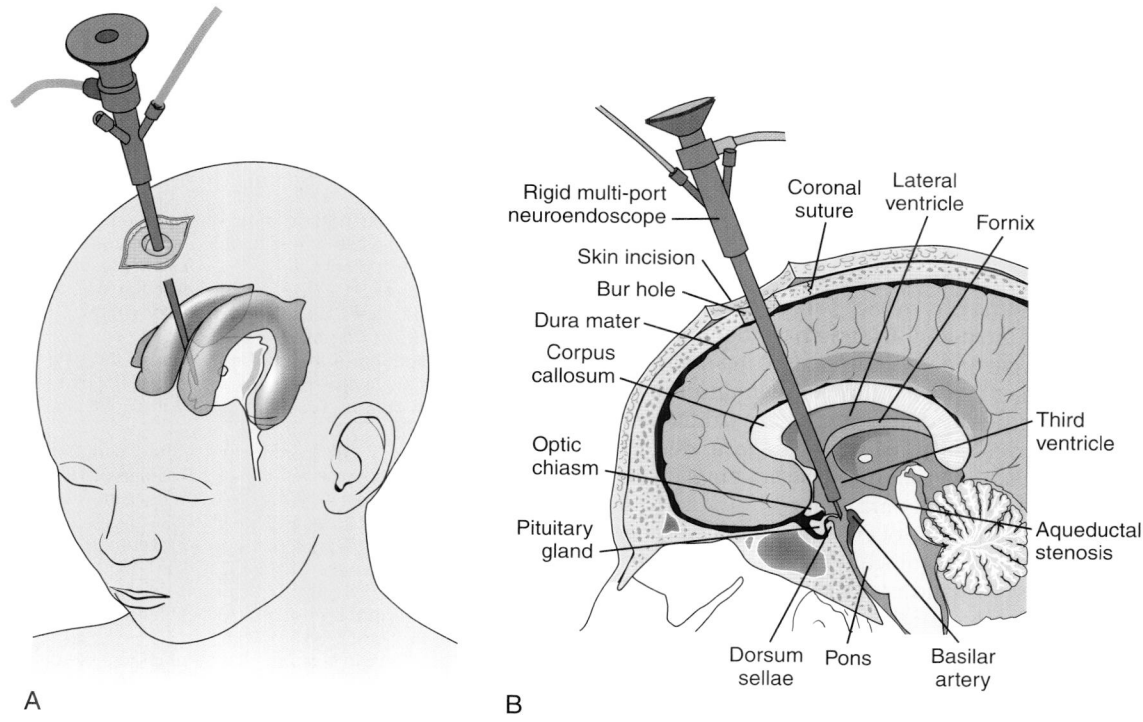

FIGURE 96-7 Schematics demonstrating the surgical trajectory for ETV using a rigid endoscope. A, Oblique view showing the endoscope passing through the lateral ventricle and foramen of Monro and into the third ventricle. B, Sagittal view depicting the perforation of the floor of the third ventricle. It is important to understand the close relationship of the floor of the third ventricle to the anterior structures (optic chiasm, infundibulum, and clivus) and posterior structures (basilar artery and brainstem) to avoid undesired complications.

ultrasonic microprobes, or laser devices. Likewise, enlarging the opening can be done using hooks, scissors, or by using blunt forceps.[45,47] The technique originally described by Mixter, which used the tip of the endoscope to bluntly perforate the floor of the third ventricle and widened it with a side-to-side motion, is still used by some surgeons today.[6,47] Each of these instruments has their advantages and limitations. Regardless of the technique used, care should be taken to avoid the structures within the interpeduncular cistern, which underlies the floor of the third ventricle. These include the basilar artery and its branches, and both oculomotor nerves.

With the fenestration enlarged, the endoscope is then carefully passed into the interpeduncular cistern. The membrane of Liliequist and any adhesions or arachnoid bands are bluntly dissected to further facilitate CSF flow. Aggressive exploration is not recommended for fear of injuring any arterial perforators. Once dissection is complete, the floor of the third ventricle is examined for pulsatile flow. If the ventricular floor oscillates back and forth, then good CSF communication has been established between the third ventricle and the interpeduncular cistern.

Upon completion of the fenestration, inspection of the ventricular system should be conducted on the way out to ensure that there are no active sites of bleeding. If the CSF is not clear due to residual blood, then an external ventricular drain is often left in place for 24 to 48 hours. If the ETV was performed to replace a previous shunt, an external ventricular drain should be left for monitoring of ICP. After the endoscope and sheath are removed, the burr hole is covered with a piece of Gelfoam. The incision is closed with galeal stitches followed by surgical staples or suture.

Postoperative Monitoring

The patient is observed for 24 hours in the intensive care unit or monitored setting. If an external ventricular drain was left due to bleeding, CSF is aggressively drained during this time period in order to clear the fluid and minimize the risk of intraventricular clot formation. If the external ventricular drain was left in because the ETV was to replace a previous shunt, the drain should remain clamped and ICP continuously monitored. In these patients, the ventricular drain needs to be weaned slowly as it has been noted to take up to 10 days for patients to tolerate the new absorption pathway.[45] Once the drain is removed, the patient may be sent home if ambulating and tolerating a diet. If the patient is having headaches, nausea, or vomiting, it is prudent to keep the patient in the hospital until symptoms have largely resolved. In infants, the fontanelle should be soft and sunken when in an upright position.

A postoperative CT scan is helpful prior to patient discharge. Although the initial change in ventricular size may be unimpressive, the subarachnoid space often appears less effaced. MRI is usually performed within 2 months of the procedure, which can show smaller ventricular size, decreased transependymal edema, and a flow void in the floor of the third ventricle. A cine-MRI with CISS sequence may be especially helpful in demonstrating flow from the third ventricle to the interpeduncular cistern.

Complications

The morbidity reported for ETV in modern series, in which contemporary endoscopic equipment and techniques were used, ranges from 6% to 21%.[48] Additionally, the procedure-abort rate varied from 0.4% to 26%.[48] Mortality rates are low following ETV and are usually related to fatal subarachnoid hemorrhage or late failure of the third ventriculostomy.

Hypothalamic injury can occur intraoperatively with a variety of effects. It is first important to remember that the floor of the third ventricle is in fact part of the hypothalamus. Serious bradycardia and asystole have been noted at the time of fenestration and upon reversal of the neuromuscular block. This may be caused by a mechanism involving distortion of the posterior hypothalamus. Additionally, increased appetite, loss of thirst, diabetes insipidus, and amenorrhea have also been reported postoperatively secondary to presumed hypothalamic injury.[49]

Vascular injury can also occur intraoperatively and ranges from clinically insignificant to devastating. In a series of 55 patients, Teo and coworkers reported a 10.9% incidence of "clinically insignificant" hemorrhage.[50] In most instances, minor intraventricular bleeding can be controlled with irrigation although it can result in aborting the procedure. Although extraordinarily rare, major vascular injury resulting in significant morbidity and mortality has been reported. This includes trauma to the basilar artery or one of its branches, subarachnoid, intraventricular, or intracerebral hemorrhage, pseudoaneurysm formation at the basilar tip, and arterial or venous infarcts.[51-53]

CSF leak after ETV is a rare, but known postoperative complication. In order to prevent CSF leak, it is important to perform a multilayered closure and to minimize the size of the dural opening used. However, CSF leak can be a sign of increased ICP, and ETV failure must not be ruled out.[49] Although fever in the first 24 to 48 hours postoperatively is common, ventriculitis is rare. The presence of blood in the ventricular system is the most common cause of perioperative fever.[49] However, any previous shunt hardware can harbor bacteria and should be completely removed in order to prevent late ventriculitis.[54] Other rare complications include overdrainage resulting in subdural hematoma or hygroma, symptomatic pneumoencephalus, and psychiatric or memory disorders caused by forniceal or mammillary body injury.[49]

Conclusion

Endoscopic third ventriculostomy has become a standard surgical treatment of hydrocephalus along with shunting. A rudimentary understanding of CSF physiology and etiologies of hydrocephalus is critical in appropriately selecting patients for ETV. At this time, evidence shows that both patient age and etiology affect long-term success of ETV. In addition, it is critical for the surgeon to be familiarized with the equipment and surgical anatomy to prevent complications. With appropriate patient selection, knowledge of surgical anatomy, and awareness of potential complications, ETV is a safe and effective procedure to treat hydrocephalus that avoids long-term complications that can occur with a shunt.

KEY REFERENCES

Abbott R. History of neuroendoscopy. *Neurosurg Clin North Am.* 2004; 15:1-7.

Bhatia R, Tahir M, Chandler CL. The management of hydrocephalus in children with posterior fossa tumours: the role of pre-resectional endoscopic third ventriculostomy. *Pediatr Neurosurg.* 2009;45:186-191.

Conway JE, Baird CJ, Li KW, et al. Ventricular anatomy. In: Jallo GI, Conway JE, Bognar L, eds. *Neuroendoscopy of the Central Nervous System.* San Diego: Plural; 2008:23-36.

Dandy W. Extirpation of the choroid plexus of the lateral ventricles in communicating hydrocephalus. *Ann Surg.* 1918;68:569.

Dandy WE. An operative procedure for hydrocephalus. *Bull Johns Hopkins Hosp.* 1922;33:189-190.

Drake JM, Iantosca MR. Cerebrospinal fluid shunting and management of pediatric hydrocephalus. In: Schmidek HH, Roberts DW, eds. *Schmidek and Sweet's Operative Techniques in Neurosurgery.* 5th ed. vol 1. Philadelphia: Elsevier; 2005:487-508.

Fay T, Grant FC. Ventriculoscopy and intraventricular photography in internal hydrocephalus. *JAMA.* 1923;80:461-463.

Gangemi M, Maiuri F, Naddeo M, et al. Endoscopic third ventriculostomy in idiopathic normal pressure hydrocephalus: an Italian multicenter study. *Neurosurgery.* 2008;63:62-69.

Grant JA. Victor Darwin Lespinasse: a biographical sketch. *Neurosurgery.* 1996;39:1232-1233.

Iantosca M, Hader W, Drake J. Results of endoscopic third ventriculostomy. *Neurosurg Clin North Am.* 2004;15:67.

Kulkarni AV, Drake JM, Mallucci CL, et al. Endoscopic third ventriculostomy in the treatment of childhood hydrocephalus. *J Pediatr.* 2009;155:254-259:e251.

Li KW, Nelson C, Suk I, Jallo GI. Neuroendoscopy: past, present, and future. *Neurosurgical Focus.* 2005;19:E1.

Mixter WJ. Ventriculoscopy and puncture of the floor of the third ventricle. *Boston Medical and Surgical Journal.* 1923;188:277-278.

Putnam TJ. Treatment of hydrocephalus by endoscopic coagulation of the choroid plexus: description of a new instrument and preliminary report of results. *New England Journal of Medicine.* 1934;210:1373-1376.

Rekate H. Selecting patients for endoscopic third ventriculostomy. *Neurosurg Clin North Am.* 2004;15:39.

Renard VM, Jallo GI. Endoscopic third ventriculostomy. In: Jallo GI, Conway JE, Bognar L, eds. *Neuroendoscopy of the Central Nervous System.* San Diego: Plural; 2008:43-50.

Sainte-Rose C, Cinalli G, Roux FE, et al. Management of hydrocephalus in pediatric patients with posterior fossa tumors: the role of endoscopic third ventriculostomy. *J Neurosurg.* 2001;95:791-797.

Scarff J. Endoscopic treatment of hydrocephalus: description of a ventriculoscope and preliminary report of cases. *Arch Neurol Psychiatry.* 1936;35:853.

Sciubba DM, Noggle JC, Jallo GI. Equipment for neuroendoscopic procedures. In: Jallo GI, Conway JE, Bognar L, eds. *Neuroendoscopy of the Central Nervous System.* San Diego: Plural; 2008:13-22.

Siomin V, Cinalli G, Grotenhuis A, et al. Endoscopic third ventriculostomy in patients with cerebrospinal fluid infection and/or hemorrhage. *J Neurosurg.* 2002;97:519-524.

Smyth MD, Tubbs RS, Wellons 3rd JC, et al. Endoscopic third ventriculostomy for hydrocephalus secondary to central nervous system infection or intraventricular hemorrhage in children. *Pediatr Neurosurg.* 2003;39:258-263.

Teo C, Rahman S, Boop FA, Cherny B. Complications of endoscopic neurosurgery. *Childs Nerv Syst.* 1996;12:248-253:discussion 253.

Yamini B, Refai D, Rubin CM, Frim DM. Initial endoscopic management of pineal region tumors and associated hydrocephalus: clinical series and literature review. *J Neurosurg.* 2004;100:437-441.

Numbered references appear on Expert Consult.

CHAPTER 97

Management of Shunt Infections

CLAUDIO YAMPOLSKY • PABLO AJLER

Hydrocephalus is one of the most common conditions in neurosurgical practice. Hydrocephalus prevalence in childhood ranges from 0.5 to 1 per 1,000 children.[1,2] In the adult population, initial diagnosis is rather uncommon, and incidence is approximately 3.4 per 100,000.[3]

Since the introduction of cerebrospinal fluid (CSF) shunts in the 1940s,[4] morbidity and mortality rates associated with shunt implantation have decreased significantly, from 50% to between 5% and 10%,[5] and many shunted patients can lead a normal life. Shunt malfunction and infection, however, are the most common complications in hydrocephalus management, often having serious sequelae. Furthermore, shunt complications represent a significant cost to healthcare systems and a serious problem. According to recent reports, approximately 27,800 shunt implantation or revision procedures were performed in the United States in 2000 alone.[6] Considering that each procedure costs the American healthcare system $35,000 on average and that infected patients represent an estimated 5% to 15% of shunted patients,[1,7-9] the number of cases potentially requiring reoperation could range from 1,393.5 to 4,181 and cost between $48.76 million and $146.34 million annually. These patients require longer hospital stays, multiple diagnostic and treatment procedures, and antibiotic therapy, all of which have an impact on the healthcare system and could be averted with the right preventative measures. Moreover, the aforementioned complications are associated with high morbidity and mortality rates and the subsequent sequelae affecting patients for life.[10]

Several studies have tried to establish why these patients develop infections, and in some cases, the use of strict surgical techniques has reduced the incidence of infections nearly to zero.[11]

Shunt malfunction is reportedly around 25% to 35% during the first postimplantation year.[12,13] Rates of infection are variable, ranging from 5% to 15% of all implanted shunts.[1,7-9] Shunt infection can be ascribed to various factors; reviewing them individually assists in understanding how to minimize the risks of serious complications and implement an appropriate treatment.

Etiology of Hydrocephalus

The etiology of hydrocephalus as a risk factor for the development of infections has not been clearly shown. An association between the causal agent and a higher risk for shunt infection has rarely been found,[11,14] although a recent review described an association between obstructive hydrocephalus and rate of complications.[15]

Hydrocephalus following perinatal bleeding has been associated with a higher incidence of infection,[16] but we could not establish such an association in our series of 964 operated patients.

Patient Age and Nutritional Status

Many reports stress the importance of age as a risk factor for infectious complications in patients who have a CSF shunt.[9,17] The risk of complications is mainly present in infants and elders. A multicenter study analyzing shunt complications in general found that younger children were at a higher risk of complications and malfunction; however, the study fails to specify whether these were infectious or obstructive.[18]

Nutritional status is yet another significant factor, as undernourished subjects seem to have a higher rate of infectious complications.[19] Infant nutrition may also play an important role, and a lower incidence of infection has been described in breastfed infants.[20]

Surgical Technique

The implantation technique of a ventriculoperitoneal or ventriculoatrial shunt is also extremely important. The absence of an appropriate strategy may turn a procedure normally representing low mortality and morbidity, and presumably requiring a short hospital stay, into a complicated procedure that eventually results in multiple reoperations, longer hospital stays, higher costs for the healthcare system, and potentially serious sequelae for the patient.

Shunt implantation is a procedure often performed by neurosurgical trainees who have inadequate experience in the technique; this factor may be critical for the development of postoperative infections.[21]

Many papers have shown that postoperative infection rates may be reduced by using a meticulous surgical technique.[7,11,22] Where possible, the procedure should be carried out in a dedicated neurosurgical operating room and be the first procedure of the day. The paramedic personnel involved in the procedure should be trained in prosthesis manipulation and instructed to maximally restrict circulation into and out of the operating room. Entrance to and exit from the operating room would only be allowed in emergency situations; where possible, the number of personnel within the operating room should be restricted to four professionals—an anesthesiologist, a nurse, a surgeon experienced in the management of hydrocephalus, and an assistant. Contaminated elements should be carefully placed away from the sterile sector of the operating room.

We recommend giving prophylactic antibiotic therapy at the time of anesthetic induction, as well as during the first 24 postoperative hours. A meta-analysis of recent reports showed the effectiveness of prophylactic antibiotic therapy in the reduction of infection rates.[23] The prophylactic antibiotic drugs scheme to be used should be designed after the bacterial flora prevailing in the healthcare site.

As far as individual patient care, the antiseptic procedure should be thorough; therefore, we recommend bathing the patient with povidone–iodine soap or a similar product 24 hours preoperatively. Immediately before the surgical procedure, the operating field must be washed three times with povidone–iodine soap using a nonsterile technique, and then the skin should be prepared another three times with povidone–iodine solution using a sterile technique. Placement of sterile fields should be meticulous and should try to expose the surgical area only, which should be covered with sterile drapes impregnated in iodoform (3M Ioban 2 Antimicrobial Incise Drapes EZ). Unnecessary surgical steps should be avoided to shorten the length of the procedure as much as possible.

The valve not only should suit the patient's needs but also should be a device with which the surgical team is accustomed to working.

Many studies have investigated the association between antibiotic-impregnated shunt catheters and risk of infection. In vitro results[24] reported antibiotic-impregnated catheters afford a lower colonization risk, but reports of studies conducted in humans showed controversial results. Some authors stress the contribution of these devices to lower postoperative infection rates and thus recommend them as an effective tool.[25,26] Other reports have found no significant infection rate differences in patients who underwent the implantation of antibiotic-impregnated catheters.[23,27] This kind of devices could be used in patients with a history of previous infection or in high-risk cases, but regardless of the circumstance, the previously described perioperative care steps should be followed carefully.

Silastic exposure to room air must be minimized. For this reason, the sterile container should be opened exactly at the moment of implantation.

We recommend using forceps for implantation to avoid manipulation of the shunt system. Intraoperative preparation with povidone–iodine is useful, and some authors suggest immersing the shunt in a gentamicin solution bath.[11] The implementation of this kind of protocol has already been described by other authors[7,11,22] and proved to have high efficacy in preventing infection.

Presentation and Clinical Features of Shunt Infection

Presentation of shunt infections is highly variable, depending on the causal agent, the site of infection, and patient age. Many patients remain asymptomatic,[28] whereas others are oligosymptomatic or show signs and symptoms of increased intracranial pressure due to shunt malfunction. In neonates, clinical features of shunt malfunction include bulging fontanelle, irritability, vomiting, fever, and feeding difficulty. In older children and adults, the signs and symptoms tend to be nonspecific, though fever, headache, vomiting, meningism, and abdominal pain may suggest shunt infection. Up to 50% of shunt malfunctions may be explained by an underlying infection.[29]

Occasionally, shunt infection signs are seen at the distal end, with abdominal symptoms that may vary from nontender focal peritoneal fluid collections to acute abdomen. The finding of abdominal fluid collections or pseudocysts is considered by many authors to be a sign suggestive of infection in patients with ventriculoperitoneal shunts,[30,31] although cystic fluid cultures often test negative.[32] Early diagnosis of this complication by means of an abdomen computed tomography (CT) scan (Fig. 97-1) affords an effective management by externalizing the catheter, removing the shunt or re-placing the peritoneal catheter laparoscopically.[33,34]

Infections associated with ventriculoatrial shunts are usually more severe and may cause bacteremia with a subsequent hemodynamic involvement on account of the close link between CSF and circulating blood flow, which could result in the formation of thrombi at the catheter tip and thus lead to endocarditis or thromboembolic events. Shunt nephritis is a glomerular disease produced by antibody deposits in the renal glomeruli and the production of complement, which is characterized by hematuria, anemia, liver and spleen enlargement, and nephrotic syndrome. Although shunt nephritis has a low incidence, it should be considered a potential diagnosis in patients who have a ventriculoatrial shunt.[35]

Infections caused by skin organisms may present with redness and edema along the length of the shunt, wound dehiscence and shunt exposure, or purulent discharge through the wound (Fig. 97-2). This kind of infection is

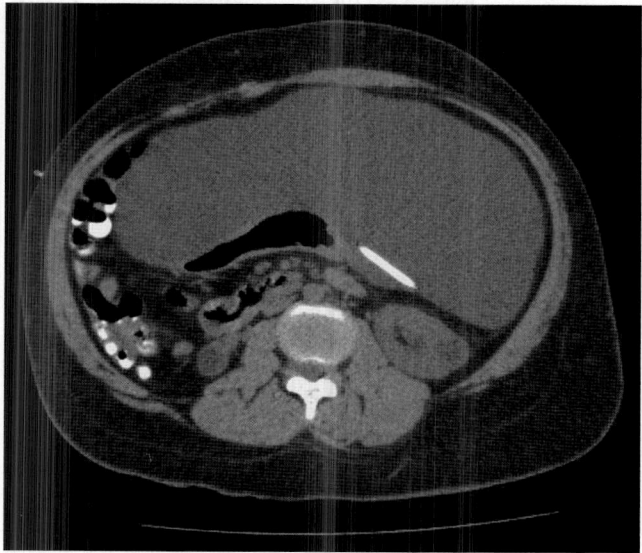

FIGURE 97-1 Oral and intravenous contrast-enhanced CT scan of the abdomen and pelvis. A large fluid collection (pseudocyst) is seen. Note the catheter inside the collection.

commonly external and occurs in neonates when CSF accumulates, particularly when CSF fistulas are present.[36] Thus, given the external nature of the infection in these cases, puncturing the valve would be inadvisable because it could lead to germ contamination of a sterile fluid.

Mechanisms for Entry of Bacteria Into Shunts

Because skin organisms are the most commonly identified causal agents in shunt infection, colonization of prosthetic materials by direct inoculation at the time of shunt implantation usually constitutes the infection mechanism. This accounts for the early presentation of infections postoperatively. Skin wounds may also cause shunt colonization. Blood spread may occur in the setting of bacteremia and become particularly important when there is a ventriculoatrial shunt; it may also be seen in patients with neurogenic bladder. Finally, infections by gram-negative organisms in particular may show a retrograde spread as a result of bowel perforation.[37]

Microbiology and Pathogenesis

CSF shunt infections are most commonly produced by certain low-virulence organisms present in skin flora. Common causal agents are coagulase-negative staphylococci, which are identified in 50% to 80% of shunt infections, together with coagulase-positive staphylococci.[38-40] Staphylococci can synthesize and secrete a mucoid substance called slime. Slime has been shown to be associated with vascular

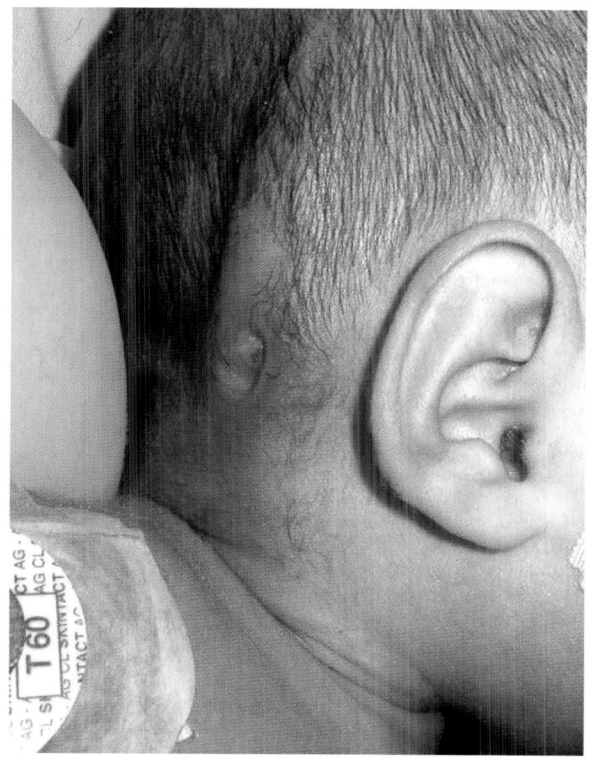

FIGURE 97-2 Skin redness, hardening, and ulceration with a purulent background along the length of the shunt.

catheter infections as it adheres to plastic or polymeric materials and induces organism growth. It may also act as a mechanical barrier to systemic antibiotic action.[39,40] Although they are less common, gram-negative organisms are clinically important because they lead to higher morbidity and mortality rates.[37,41] Such anaerobic diphtheroid agents as the *Propionibacterium acnes* are a less common source of infection but should be equally regarded as a potential causal agent, because they are usually found on the skin and can contaminate shunts with few signs and symptoms.[41]

Diagnosis

CSF sampling for culture is mandatory to establish the diagnosis of infection.

Diagnostic criteria for shunt infection include the following:[42-44]
1. Positive CSF culture with fluid obtained from the shunt in patients presenting clinically with acute bacterial meningitis or signs or symptoms of malfunction
2. At least one of the following parameters of bacterial inflammation of the CSF:
   a. A white blood cell count higher than 0.25×10^9 μl, with a predominance of polymorphonuclear neutrophil
   b. A CSF lactate level higher than 3.5 mmol/L
   c. A CSF-to-serum glucose ratio lower than 0.4 g/dl
   d. An absolute CSF glucose level lower than 2.5 mmol/L

Wherever possible, and depending on the type of shunt that has been implanted, the sample should be obtained from the valve reservoir. CSF culture is a key element for diagnosis; because of the common presence of low-virulence organisms, cultures should be kept for a long time to allow identification of slow-growing organisms.[45] CSF physical and chemical properties may raise clinical suspicion; CSF pleocytosis (particularly when neutrophils predominate), along with increased CSF protein levels and decreased CSF glucose levels, are suggestive of an ongoing bacterial infection.[46] Leukocytosis, erythrocyte sedimentation rate (ESR) elevation, and increased C-reactive protein levels may also prove useful for diagnosis (we found that ESR elevation is also useful in adults).

Infection may initially present with redness and/or skin hardening over the shunt area. In these cases, sampling from this area should be avoided.

Imaging techniques such as brain CT scans, as well as shunt x-rays and abdominal ultrasound or CT scans, are ancillary investigations that may prove useful to rule out malfunction or abdominal cysts.

Treatment

Controversy exists over what constitutes the best treatment for ventriculoperitoneal and ventriculoatrial shunt infections. Discussion is raised by whether the system should or should not be removed, since the ventricular catheter may adhere to the choroid plexus and removing the catheter may lead to intraventricular bleeding. Other factors to be taken into account when removing the shunt are patient dependence on the system and potential increase of intracranial pressure. CSF drainage should be ensured at the time of removal. Placement of an external ventricular drainage is associated with a risk for overinfection. Consequently, some authors suggest the implementation of less invasive treatment options, namely, intravenous and/or intrashunt antibiotic therapy.[47] Intravenous antibiotic therapy with shunt removal and CSF external drainage or ventricular punctures followed by reimplantation of the shunt when the CSF is sterilized has proved more effective in patients with shunt infection.[48] This is the most widely accepted procedure and the only one whose effectiveness has been demonstrated in a prospective randomized study comparing treatment options and a follow-up study.[49,50] Other studies have also shown the success of this treatment option,[51-54] which is reportedly close to 95%, with the lowest associated morbidity and mortality rates.[48]

Bacteria such as staphylococci produce vitronectin, a substance that mediates bacterial adhesion to the catheter, preventing antibiotic action and making shunt removal unavoidable.[55] Some reports have shown a high cure rate when direct replacement of the shunt is performed and no external drainage is used before the replacement procedure.[48]

Once a microbiologic diagnosis of infection has been established, management should consist of broad-spectrum systemic antibiotic agents, bactericides, and intravenous antibiotic agents; the shunt must be removed, and either an external ventricular drainage system must be placed or repeated ventricular punctures must be performed (in patients with bulging fontanelle). Once three CSF cultures test negative, the external drainage system should be removed and a new shunt should be implanted at a different location.

The duration of intravenous antibiotic therapy should be decided case by case because there are no defined protocols in this regard. In our experience, 14 days of intravenous antibiotic therapy are enough if there is no overinfection associated with the external ventricular drainage system.

When intravenous antibiotic therapy does not provide successful control of the infection (persistence of positive cultures), the intrathecal route may become an administration alternative (Fig. 97-3).

KEY REFERENCES

Brown E, Edwards R, Pople I. Conservative management of patients with cerebrospinal fluid shunt infections. *Neurosurgery.* 2006;58:657-665.

Brown EM, de Luvois J, Boyston R, et al. Distinguishing between chemical and bacterial meningitis in patients who have undergone neurosurgery. *Clin Infec Dis.* 2002;34:556-558.

Choksey MS, Malik A. Zero tolerance to shunt infections: can it be achieved? *J Neurol Neurosurg Psychiatry.* 2004;75:87-91.

Choux M, Genitori L, Lang D, et al. Shunt implantation: reducing the incidence of shunt infection. *J Neurosurg.* 1992;77:875-880.

Christiansen GD, Simpson WA, Bisno AL, et al. Adherence of slime-producing strains of Staphylococcus epidermidis to smooth surfaces. *Infect. Immunol.* 1982;37:318-325.

Cochrane DO, Kestle JR. The influence of surgical operative experience on the duration of first ventriculoperitoneal shunt function and infection. *Pediatr Neurosurg.* 2003;38:295-301.

Desai A, Lollis S, Missios S, et al. How long should cerebrospinal fluid cultures be held to detect shunt infections? *J Neurosurg Pediatrics.* 2009;4:184-189.

Garner JS, Jarvis WR, Emori TG, et al. CDC definition for nosocomial infection. *Am J Infect Control.* 1988;16:128-140.

James HE, Walsh JW, Wilson HD, et al. The management of CSF shunt infection: a clinical experience. *Acta Neurochir (Wien).* 1981;59: 157-166.

James HE, Walsh JW, Wilson HD, et al. Prospective randomized study of therapy in cerebrospinal fluid shunt infection. *Neurosurgery.* 1980;7:459-463.

Jeelani N, Kulkarni A, DeSilva P, et al. Postoperative cerebrospinal fluid wound leakage as a predictor of shunt infection: a prospective analysis of 205 cases. *J Neurosurg Pediatrics.* 2009;4:166-169.

Lan CC, Wong TT, Chen SJ, et al. Early diagnosis of ventriculoperitoneal shunt infections and malfunctions in children with hydrocephalus. *J Microbiol Immunol Infect.* 2003;36:47-50.

Li DQ, Lundberg F, Ljungh A. Characterization of vitronectin-binding proteins of *Staphylococcus epidermidis. Curr Microbiol.* 2001;42: 361-367.

Nejat F, Tajik P, Ghodsi SM, et al. Breastfeeding: a potential protective factor against ventriculoperitoneal shunt infection in young infants. *J Neurosurg Pediatr.* 2008;1:138-141.

Patwardhan R, Nanda A. Implanted ventricular shunts in the United States: the billion–dollar-a-year cost of hydrocephalus treatment. *Neurosurgery.* 2005;56:139-145.

Persson EK, Anderson S, Wiklund LM, et al. Hydrocephalus in children born in 1999-2002: epidemiology, outcome and ophthalmological findings. *Childs Nerv Syst.* 2007;23:1111-1118.

Persson EK, Hagberg G, Uvebrant P. Hydrocephalus prevalence and outcome in a population-based cohort of children born in 1989-1998. *Acta Paediatr.* 2005;94:726-732.

Pirotte B, Lubansu A, Bruneau M, et al. Sterile surgical technique for shunt placement reduces the shunt infection rate in children: preliminary analysis of a prospective protocol in 115 consecutive procedures. *Childs Nerv Syst.* 2007;23:1251-1261.

Ratilal B, Costa J, Sampaio C. Antibiotic prophylaxis for surgical introduction of intracranial ventricular shunts: a systematic review. *J Neurosurg Pediatrics.* 2008;1:48-56.

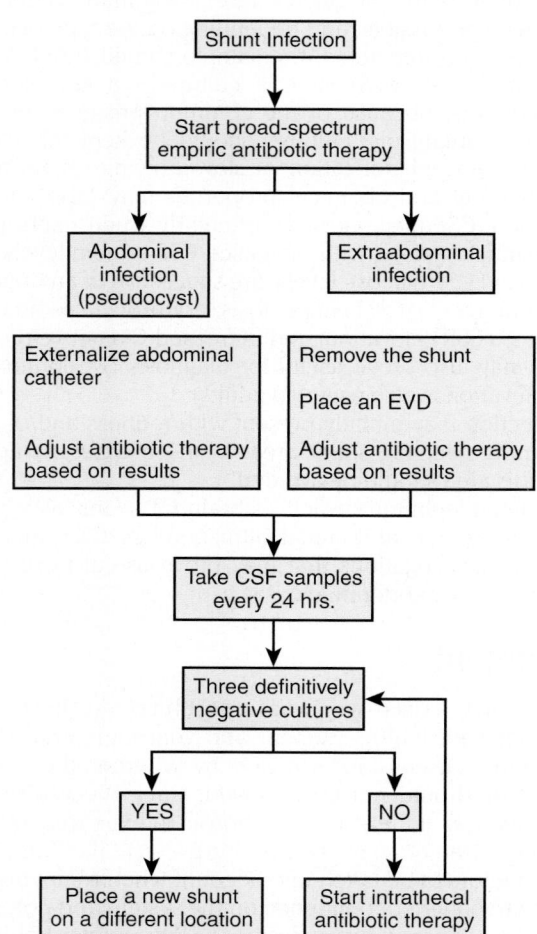

FIGURE 97-3 Treatment algorithm for shunt infections.

Richards HK, Seeley HM, Pickard JD. Efficacy of antibiotic impregnated shunt catheters in reducing shunt infection: data from the United Kingdom Shunt Registry. *J Neurosurg Pediatrics.* 2009;4:389-393.

Schreffler RT, Schreffler AJ, Wittler RR. Treatment of cerebrospinal fluid shunt infections: a decision analysis. *Pediatr Infect Dis J.* 2002;21: 632-636.

Shah S, Hall M, Slonim A, et al. A multicentric study of factors influencing cerebrospinal fluid shunt survival in infants and children. *Neurosurgery.* 2008;62:1095-1103.

Tisell M, Hoglund C, Wikkelso C. National and regional incidence of surgery for adult in Sweden. *Acta Neurol Scan.* 2005;112:72-75.

Vinchon M, Dhellemmes P. Cerebrospinal fluid shunt infection: risk factors and long-term follow-up. *Childs Nerv Syst.* 2006;22:692-697.

Wu Y, Green N, Wrensh M, et al. Ventriculoperitoneal shunt complications in California: 1990 to 2000. *Neurosurgery.* 2007;61:557-563.

Numbered references appear on Expert Consult.

Section Five

STEREOTACTIC RADIOSURGERY

DANIELE RIGAMONTI

CHAPTER 98

Interstitial and LINAC-Radiosurgery for Brain Metastases*

GUIDO NIKKHAH • JAROSLAW MACIACZYK •
THOMAS REITHMEIER • MICHAEL TRIPPEL •
MARCUS O. PINSKER

Brain metastases are diagnosed in approximately 20% to 40% of patients with neoplastic diseases[1-3] and thereby represent the most common intracranial malignancy, with lung, breast, and renal cancers, and melanoma as the most frequent primary tumors.[4,5] The incidence of brain metastatic lesions appears to be increasing, possibly due to an aging population, improved neuroimaging techniques, and more efficient treatment of the systemic disease, leading to a growing group of patients presenting multiple lesions within the central nervous system at the time of diagnosis. Brain metastatic tumors are predominantly encountered supratentorially within the cerebral hemispheres, followed by cerebellar and brain stem localization.[6] Despite the significant improvement of the management of intracranial metastases in the last decades, the overall prognosis remains relatively poor. Thorough assessment of the individual prognosis is, therefore, required to offer the best possible care while avoiding unnecessary and possibly debilitating treatment. The extensive analysis of various demographic and clinical variables, including age, performance status (determined as on the Karnofsky performance scale, or KPS), type of primary tumor, number of cerebral metastases, and activity of the extracranial disease, based on Radiation Therapy Oncology Group (RTOG) trials[7] using recursive partitioning analysis (RPA) led to the identification of prognostic groups (RPA groups 1-3 in modification of Lutterbach et al.;[8] for details, see Table 98-1), with age below 65 years, a KPS score of at least 70, and no extracranial disease, as well as a single metastatic tumor, as the most important positive predictive factors concerning favorable outcome.

Modern therapeutic management of brain metastases is based on approaches combining different therapeutic strategies (i.e., surgery or radiosurgery with whole brain radiation therapy [WBRT] or systemic chemotherapy). Surgical resection with adjuvant WBRT is considered the standard of treatment of brain metastases in many patients. However, in metastatic lesions localized in deep structures or in eloquent brain areas not amenable to surgery, patients may benefit from stereotactic radiosurgical (SRS) treatment. This chapter focuses exclusively on SRS, a fast-growing field that has been progressing over recent years from an experimental concept to an effective treatment modality for brain metastases.

SRS is based on focusing multiple, high-dose, ionizing radiation beams using stereotactic guidance on an intracranial target. It converges with the pioneering work of Leksell and Larsson,[9] inventors of the first gamma knife (GK) unit at the Karolinska Institute in Stockholm in 1967.[10] However, the growing importance of the SRS techniques has greatly benefited from the development of novel visualization methods—computed tomography (CT) and magnetic resonance imaging (MRI) based—that allow precise planning and safe execution of radiosurgical treatment. Classical radiosurgery requires application of either photon or charged particles radiation (usually proton beam radiation) using multiple cobalt-60 sources (GK), linear accelerators (LINACs) (XKnife or CyberKnife) or cyclotrons. The original definition of SRS has been significantly extended by application of ionized radiation.[11] Therefore, besides traditional SRS techniques based on external radiation sources, more invasive radiosurgical methods like iodine-125 (I-125) seeds implantation and the Photon Radiosurgery System for interstitial application of radiation in the case of metastatic brain lesions are discussed in this chapter.

Radiosurgical Techniques

Noninvasive radiosurgical treatment modalities consist of percutaneous or external irradiation using photon radiation technology (GK and LINACs). Current GK units use 201 cobalt-60 sources enclosed within a hemispheric vault, leading to the emission of gamma ray energy converged at the isocenter and allowing high-precision treatment of an intracranial target. The aperture of collimators differs from 4 to 18 mm, so the diameter of the radiation beam can be adapted to the size of the lesion. Due to high radiation activity (up to 300 TBq) the propagation of the dose reaches 2 Gy/min by 80 cm from the radiation source. However, during the therapy of irregular lesions, multiple spherical

---

*We dedicate this chapter to our esteemed academic and clinical teacher and mentor Prof. Christoph Ostertag for his 70th birthday. He has influenced and encouraged us through his high academic standards and his deep personal relationship with our patients. His vision is always to approach each target in the shortest and best way and continuously improve our understanding of the human brain, its function, anatomy, pathology, and novel treatment modalities.

Table 98-1	Stratification of Prognostic Factors by RPA Class
	Median Survival (months)
RPA Class 1	
KPS ≥ 70, age <65 years, controlled primary tumor, no extracranial disease	7.1
Single metastasis	13.5
Multiple metastases	6.0
RPA Class 2	
All others	4.2
Single metastasis	8.1
Multiple metastases	4.1
RPA Class 3	
KPS < 70	2.3

Modified from Kaal et al. 2005.[5]

isocenters have to be superimposed to allow conformal treatment, resulting in anatomic regions that receive much higher radiation dosage than the marginal dose. GK technology is limited exclusively to the treatment of intracranial lesions and high cervical lesions (when GK perfexion is available).

LINAC radiosurgery was introduced in the early 1980s following modifications of standard LINACs used for external beam radiotherapy to obtain high conformity of the radiation. The frequency of the electromagnetic field is about 3 GHz, and the accelerating energy is 4 to 25 MeV. X-ray photons are bundled to achieve a collimated beam of radiation. The advantages of LINAC devices compared to GK units are better penetration and homogeneity of radiation, steeper falloff of the dose at the margins of the irradiated lesion, and no problems with radioactive waste disposal. Moreover, application of the multileaf collimators enabled safe treatment of irregular intracranial lesions with an accuracy of less than 1 mm. Originally, the LINAC is mounted to a gantry that rotates over the patient's head fixed in a stereotactic apparatus. However, recent LINAC devices (i.e., CyberKnife) applying dynamic position adjustment of the rotating arm do not require head fixation to preserve high accuracy of the radiation.

Particle beam radiation therapy with protons or heavy helium nuclei based on the so-called Bragg peak phenomenon, applied in only few centers worldwide, are not discussed further due to the paucity of reliable clinical data.

Another important technique of radiosurgical brain metastases therapy is interstitial radiosurgery (brachytherapy), allowing direct intratumoral application of low-energy ionizing radiation (0.5-10 cGy/min). Following stereotactic serial biopsy that provides the confirmation of the histopathologic diagnosis, single or multiple radioactive sources are temporarily implanted, allowing optimal dose distribution

(e.g., I-125, iridium-192, and gold-198).[12] I-125 seeds (0.8 × 4.5 mm titanium cylinder) are fixed in a Teflon catheter, sterilized, and inserted into the center of the lesion, where they are left for 3 to 4 weeks (delivering a dose of 60 Gy to the tumor margins). The steep radial dose falloff is inversely proportional to the square of the distance from the radiation source, which provides minimal exposure to radiation of the healthy surrounding brain tissue.

At the beginning of 1990s, Photoelectron (Lexington, Waltham, MA) developed the Photon Radiosurgery System. It is a battery-powered, miniature x-ray generator capable of delivering low-energy radiation (soft x-rays) directly to small brain lesions in a single therapeutic session. Thus, it combines the direct dose application of brachytherapy with the advantages of short-time exposure typical for external radiosurgical techniques (GK and LINAC).[13] Brief characteristics of the physical parameters of the radiosurgical procedures discussed in this chapter are summarized in Table 98-2.

The rest of the chapter is devoted to the presentation of the clinical results of radiosurgical treatment of brain metastatic diseases, based on the literature data and the experience of the authors. Furthermore, algorithms of clinical decision making concerning treatment devices for brain metastases developed in University Medical Centre in Freiburg, Germany, are described.

Linac-Based Stereotactic Radiosurgery

Due to the pioneer work of Betti and Derechinsky,[14] Colombo et al.,[15] Winston and Lutz,[16] and others in the 1980s, precision and stability of LINAC radiosurgery systems was dramatically enhanced and became comparable to GK units. Nowadays, several techniques exist for LINAC systems that can be used to achieve an exact and highly conformal dose distribution. Target dose distribution can be adjusted by varying the collimator size, eliminating undesirable arcs, manipulating arc angles, using multiple isocenters, and differentially weighting the isocenters.[17] A highly conformal dose distribution can be achieved by generating nonspherical beam shapes that are conformal to the beam's eye view of the tumor with a multileaf collimator (Fig. 98-1A-C). Comparison of a modern LINAC radiosurgery system with GK units showed no differences in efficiency and safety.[18,19] The most important difference between these two systems is the number of metastases that can be irradiated in a single session. In GK units, up to 25 brain metastases can be treated simultaneously when the lesions are diffusely scattered and the total tumor volume is less than 15 to 30 cm³.[20] In contrast, LINAC radiosurgery systems can irradiate a

Table 98-2	Physical Parameters of the Radiosurgical Techniques			
	GK	**LINAC**	**Interstitial Radiosurgery**	**PRS**
Radiation source	Cobalt-60	Linear accelerator	Iodine-125/iridium-192	X-ray generator
Type of radiation	Photons (1.2 MeV)	Photons (4-15 MeV)	Photons (27-35 keV / 380 keV)	Photons (10-20 keV)
Dosimetry	±5 Gy/min	±5 Gy/min	±10 cGy/min	≤2 Gy/min
Application	External single time	External single time	Interstitial continuous	Interstitial single time
Application time	±20 min	±20 min	±25 day	±20 min

Modified from Ostertag 1994.[11]

maximum of 3 to 4 metastases as the multiple intersecting radiation arcs may cause a hot spot outside the target volume within normal brain tissue.[21]

Brain metastases are ideal targets for SRS, because these tumors are usually pseudospherical and show, in contrast to glioma, a noninfiltrative growth pattern with a sharp delineation to normal brain tissue. In addition, brain metastases occur often multifocally and have a diameter of less than 3.5 cm at the time of diagnosis. In Freiburg, we usually treat a maximum of three metastases during one session, and the prescribed dose for metastases with a diameter below 2.5 cm is 20 Gy calculated on the 80% isodose surrounding the outer tumor margin. Metastases with a diameter greater than 2.5 cm are treated with 18 Gy to prevent radiation necrosis. With nonspherical, irregularly shaped tumor margins, the application of one isocenter is not adequate to spare healthy brain tissue, especially when the metastasis is located within eloquent areas (e.g., the central region or brain stem). In these cases, we apply techniques like the use of multiple isocenters or a micromultileaf collimator to achieve a highly conformal target volume. Nataf et al.[22] showed the importance of an exact dose application to the target volume by comparison of patients with a 2-mm margin to patients without this additional radiation volume. In contrast to Nöel et al.,[23] who achieved improved local control with a 1-mm margin, the addition of a 2-mm margin resulted in more severe parenchymal complications, no increase in the 1- and 2-year local control rates, and no statistical significant difference in median overall survival (classic radiosurgery of 11.3 months vs. 2-mm margin radiosurgery of 19 months, $p = 0.34$).

Taking into account the usually limited life span of patients with brain metastases, SRS is a less invasive treatment method with the potential to treat several targets at one time and with the possibility to be repeated during the further course of the disease. In comparison to open surgery, the disadvantages of this method are that the diagnosis of a metastasis is not histologically proven, the mass effect is not relieved at once but over weeks or months, and the surrounding edema may be aggravated and become symptomatic.

For a solitary metastasis, one prospective[24] and four retrospective studies[25-28] compared stereotactic radiosurgery (SRS) with open tumor resection. Because they generally found no difference in overall survival, open surgery and radiosurgery are not concurrent but complementary methods in the treatment of brain metastases. Therefore, indication for SRS versus open surgery is based on individual aspects of the patients.

Singular or Solitary Metastasis

Radiosurgical treatment of brain lesions is usually based on a histopathologic diagnosis. For a solitary brain lesion, we recommend confirming diagnosis by either open surgery or stereotactic biopsy. When the location of the lesion or the general condition of the patient requires stereotactic biopsy, an intraoperative smear preparation may confirm the diagnosis of a metastasis. In this case, interstitial radiosurgery with I-125 seeds can be initiated during the same surgical procedure. This technique is discussed in detail later in this chapter. For a known tumor manifestation in other organ systems, histologic confirmation of a brain metastasis is not mandatory before SRS.

Number and Size of Metastases

Up to four metastases can be treated by SRS at once. However, a diameter of 3.5 cm is the upper limit for SRS, and metastases larger than 3.5 cm, especially with a pronounced perilesional edema, should be surgically resected. A combination of both techniques can also be performed by resecting the largest lesion, thereby relieving the mass effect, reducing the peritumoral edema, and treating afterward the remaining metastases by SRS.

Clinical Condition of the Patient

Patients with a pronounced comorbidity and a reduced general condition are usually treated by SRS as long as the patient is not threatened by the mass effect or surrounding edema of the lesion. In these patients, the possibility of not

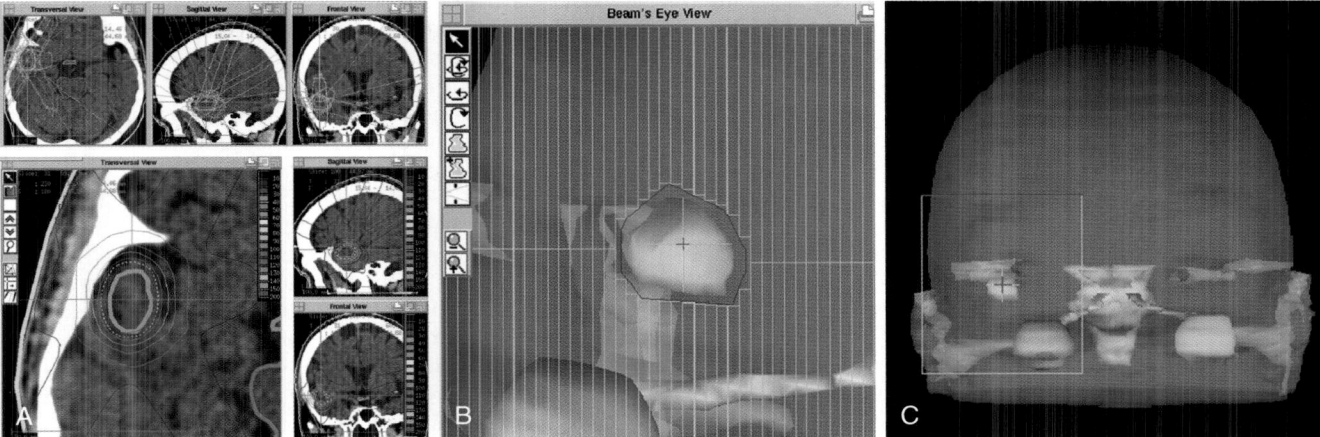

FIGURE 98-1 LINAC-based SRS with micromultileaf collimators (Virtuoso 3.4 planning software, Stryker Leibinger, Freiburg). A, Conformal application of 20 Gy to an irregularly shaped target volume (blue line). B, Beam's eye view. C, 3D reconstruction of target volume (blue) and rise structures (optic system and brain stem).

interrupting chemotherapy while treating brain metastases adds another reason in favor of SRS.

The risks for postoperative wound infections (leucopenia), healing problems, or bleeding complications (thrombocytopenia) are therefore eliminated without jeopardizing their optimal care.

Location of the Metastases

In general, deeply located or small metastases are ideal candidates for SRS, whereas superficially located lesions with a pronounced mass effect or peritumoral edema are preferentially treated by microsurgical resection. However, the clinical condition of the patient, as well as the expected life span, has to be considered.

Neurologic Symptoms Caused by Metastases

A symptomatic metastasis, when surgically accessible, should be resected to relieve the mass effect at once, reduce the surrounding edema, and thereby improve neurologic condition of the patients faster.

Prognosis

According to Lutterbach et al.,[8] prognosis of patients with up to three cerebral metastases treated by LINAC radiosurgery can be predicted accurately with the RPA classification. Median overall survival for patients is 13.4, 9.3, and 1.5 months in RPA classes 1, 2, and 3, respectively. Due to the poor prognosis of RPA class 3, patients with a KPS score below 70 should only be treated with SRS when their age is under 65 and have no signs of extracerebral tumor progression. These two factors are independent risk factors associated with an improved prognosis in RPA class 3 patients.

In summary, SRS achieves local tumor control rates at 1 year between 80% and 90%. Brain metastases from radio-resistant tumors (renal cell carcinoma, melanoma, and sarcoma) may also benefit from SRS.[29] Complication rates associated with SRS are low. However, the risk of radiation necrosis increases with larger tumor volumes and prior radiation therapy. Other risk factors for neurologic complications after SRS are the location in eloquent brain areas, SRS doses higher than 15 Gy, and progression of the primary cancer.[30]

Interstitial Radiosurgery with I-125 Seeds

Interstitial radiosurgery, a form of brachytherapy (from the Greek word *brachy,* meaning "short"), is an internal radiotherapy where a radiation source is placed inside or near a radiosensitive lesion. Brachytherapy can be used for the treatment of primary cancers of the prostate, cervix, breast, and skin. For intracranial lesions, brachytherapy is useful in the treatment of metastases and low-grade glioma with good clinical results.

In early procedures, permanent implants made from thin flexible wires of iridium-192 that could be cut to any length were implanted in a stereotactic procedure. Iridium-192 has a half-life of 73.83 days and a mean energy of 380 keV. Nowadays, mostly I-125 seeds are used, which are sized 4.5 × 0.8 mm with a half-life of 59.43 days and deliver lower photon energy of 27.4, 31.4, and 35.5 keV (Fig. 98-2A-D). These seeds contain I-125 adsorbed onto a radiopaque silver rod hermetically encapsulated in a welded titanium capsule. Typical radioactivities range from 1 to 25 mCi.

Temporary Versus Permanent Interstitial Radiosurgery

Interstitial radiosurgery can be done by temporary or permanent implantation of radiation sources, which is typically decided intraoperatively during the planning phase. A permanent seed has the advantage that no second surgical procedure is necessary, whereas the final explantation of the temporary seeds facilitates the macrophage activity and thereby accelerates the degradation of necrosis and repair processes.

Interstitial Radiosurgery Versus SRS

In contrast to external radiotherapy where a high-energy radiation beam (4-15 MeV) passes through brain tissue and the tumor, the much lower photon radiation energy (27.4-35.5 keV) of the I-125 seed is partially absorbed inside the tumor. For I-125, the half-value layer of tissue required to reduce the intensity of radiation by 50% is approximately 2 cm. This attenuation in tissue is superimposed by the inverse square law stating that dose delivery is inversely proportional to the square of the distance from the source, resulting in a steep dose decline on the surface in the treatment of small lesions.

Absorbed Dose Rates

In SRS, 18 to 20 Gy are administered in only a few minutes corresponding to a high absorbed dose rate of up to 10 Gy/min. In interstitial radiosurgery, 60 Gy are continuously delivered within 25 days, corresponding to mean absorbed dose rates of 0.1 Gy/hr or 1.67 mGy/min. This continuous dose delivery best corresponds biologically to a hyperfractionated radiation. Due to their physical properties with a sharp dose decline, I-125 seeds are well suited for the treatment of small (10-30 mm) intracranial lesions also near eloquent and radiosensitive areas, especially if the histopathologic diagnosis is going to be verified by a stereotactic biopsy during the same surgical procedure.

In our center, patients are proposed a stereotactic biopsy prior to radiosurgery to confirm the histopathologic diagnosis and to exclude misinterpretations of benign or inflammatory lesions if one of the following conditions is given: (1) missing extracranial proof of a primary tumor, (2) low probability for brain metastases of a known primary tumor (e.g., prostate carcinoma), (3) an interval longer than 3 years between the initial diagnosis of a primary tumor and a late cerebral lesion that is suspected to be a metastatic recurrence of this tumor, or (4) the presence of multiple and different primary tumors.

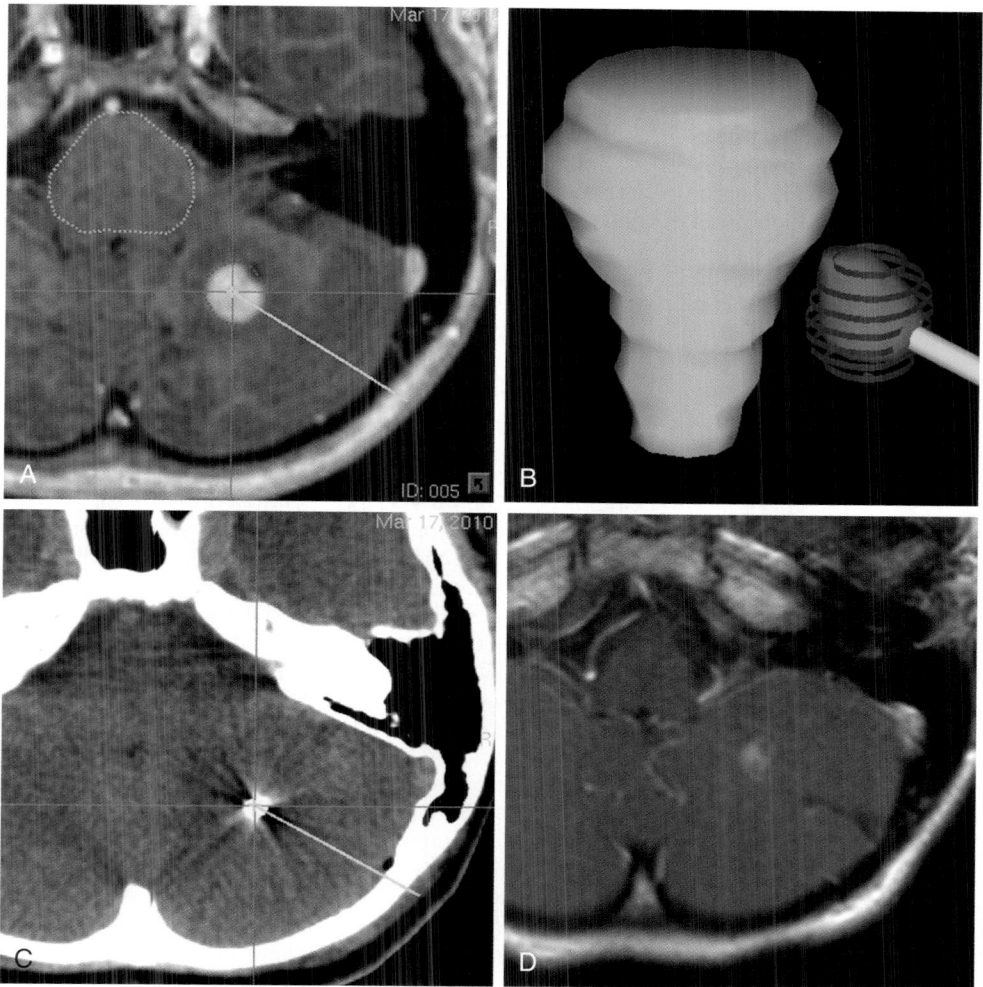

FIGURE 98-2 I-125 seed–based interstitial radiosurgery. A, Planning MRI showing the posterior fossa, the segmentation of the tumor (pink), the brain stem (turquoise), and the implantation tract (yellow). B, 3D model of these structures, including the 60-Gy isodose (red) surrounding the tumor. C, Postoperative CT for position control with the metallic artifact of the I-125 seed. D, MRI follow-up 7 months later. (STP-Workstation, Radio System 1.1-5, Stryker Leibinger, Freiburg.)

Treatment Planning

In our center, the patient is admitted to the ward the day before surgery. Frameless, nonreformatted magnetic resonance tomography imaging (T1 weighted 1 mm postgadolinium and T2 weighted 1 mm) and, if applicable, positron emission tomography (PET) are performed and transferred to the planning workstation. Next, the stereotactic base ring is fixed in local anesthesia, and a stereotactic CT scan postcontrast is acquired with fiducials fixed to the base ring. A stereotactic transformation with three-dimensional (3D) reconstruction is calculated, followed by fusions of the CT scan and the T1- and T2-weighted MRI using either anatomic landmark coregistration or fully automatic fusion. In the planning workstation, a spatial segmentation of the external contour, the tumor, and the organs of risk (e.g., eyes, chiasm, optical nerves and tracts, brain stem, and pituitary stalk) is done, and the dose at the tumor surface and the dose limitations at organs of risk are calculated. For brain metastases, a dose of 60 Gy to the surface of the lesion is applied. Then, the treatment using one or more seeds is planned. The seeds delivering the calculated dose in about 25 days are selected. The actual implantation time and stereotactic target coordinates are optimized using isodose diagrams and 3D surface modeling, respecting eloquent areas and blood vessels for the tracts. The appropriate I-125 seeds are taken from the radiation-protected vault, and the radiation activity is measured and documented. Each seed is heat shrunk into a Teflon catheter and autoclaved in a radiation-shielded container.

The stereotactic biopsy is done by a small skin incision and a 5-mm bur hole and typically following the tract of the seed catheter. The planned target position is retained by fluoroscopy, preferably in two plains, using a probe. The sterile seed within the catheter is exactly implanted at the planned target position under fluoroscopy control. The seed catheter is fixed in the bur hole using either fibrin foam or bone cement and a radiopaque hemoclip. The skin is closed by a suture. If high precision is required, the exact positioning of the seed can be controlled by a native CT scan and a fusion with the treatment plan. The radiation emission is measured and documented at distances of 0, 20, and 100 cm to the body's surface according to legal rules. If applicable, the patient is instructed to avoid long-lasting and close contact (less than 1 m) with pregnant women and children. The patient is dismissed the second day after seed implantation. We propose autoclaving of the seeds and using a single-shot antibiosis during the seed implantation. A possible reactive brain edema during the implantation time can be treated best with oral administration of a low-dose steroid such as dexamethasone.

In most patients, one seed is inserted; however, two or more seeds are applied when the size or shape of the metastases makes it necessary (9% in our series). The radiation at the surface of the head and at distances of 20 and 100 cm is measured and documented. Rules for surrounding people are given to ensure radiation exposure far below 1 mSv during total implantation time in compliance with legislation and regulations. Isolation of the implanted patients was never necessary.

At the end of the implantation period, preferably after an MRI control, the seed with the catheter and the hemoclip are removed by a small skin incision in local anesthesia; this takes only a few minutes. The explantation of the seed increases macrophage activity, inducing further shrinking and degradation of the tumor over the following months. This has to be taken into account in the interpretation of PET, CT, and MRI during this time.

Radiation Parameters for Temporary I-125 Seeds

The radiation parameters of the last consecutive 250 patients treated with I-125 seeds in our center are as follows: The mean diameter of the metastases was 20.72 ± 5.8 mm (median 20.86 mm); the mean volume of the lesions was 5.77 ml. The median dosage at the tumor margin was 60 Gy (mean 60.28 ± 2.74 Gy, range 60-65 Gy), biologically corresponding to hyperfractionated radiotherapy. The continuous dose delivery of 60.28 Gy in 26 ± 7.28 days resulted in a mean energy dose rate of 10.56 ± 2.48 cGy/hr, as compared to SRS delivering around 18 to 20 Gy in about 30 minutes to the metastasis and resulting in a much higher absorbed dose rate. At the time of implantation, the mean total activity of the seeds was 12.05 ± 7.19 mCi (median 11.4 mCi).

In summary, interstitial radiosurgery based on I-125 seeds is a safe, minimally invasive, well-tolerated, and efficient neurosurgical procedure with a low rate of morbidity and adverse events. It can be done in local anesthesia and offers the additional possibility of verifying the histopathologic diagnosis by a stereotactic biopsy with minimal additional effort.

Discussion

The annual incidence of intracranial metastases is about 8.3 per 100,000 population[31] and is present in up to 24% of cancer patients based on autopsy studies.[32] Approximately one third of the patients with cerebral metastases are candidates for microsurgical resection. The other patients are amenable to nonsurgical treatment options due to their medical comorbidities precluding surgery, multiple metastases (roughly 50%-63% of the patients have multiple lesions at initial presentation),[1,6] or location in surgically inaccessible regions.[33] Brain metastases usually are almost spherical and small; unlike the glioma, they have a clear border to the surrounding brain tissue. Therefore, they are regarded as perfect targets for SRS, provided they are causing only minimal mass effect (less than 1 cm of midline shift).

The number of brain metastases that can be treated in one session is still an issue of debate. In most centers, including ours, it is common to treat up to three lesions in one radiosurgery session. In 2006, the American Society for Therapeutic Radiology and Oncology, the American Association of Neurological Surgeons, and the Congress of Neurological Surgeons jointly agreed to define SRS in a way that includes both traditional single-dose SRS and multidose SRS for up to five doses (two to five doses).[34,35]

Both LINAC and GK radiosurgery have been used for the treatment of these lesions. There were no survival differences using either LINAC or GK radiosurgery, according to the RTOG 95-08 trial.[19] The CyberKnife, which is a recently commercially available LINAC-based system, combines a robotic arm with an image guidance system to track the patient's position, thereby obviating the need for application of a stereotactic frame.

SRS can be used alone or with surgical resection or WBRT.

SRS ALONE VERSUS WBRT+SRS

One prospective randomized, controlled trial (RCT) (class I evidence) with a companion paper has evaluated superior local control and an improved KPS alone versus WBRT+SRS for the initial management of patients with solid metastatic brain tumors.[36,37] There was no difference between study groups for median survival (8.0 vs. 7.5 months), one year local control rate (72.5% vs. 88.7%), neurologic cause of death, 1-year KPS score, acute or late neurotoxicity. The 1-year chance of recurrence locally (27.5% vs. 11.3%), at a distant site (63.7% vs. 41.5%), or anywhere in the brain (76.4% vs. 46.8%) was significantly greater for SRS alone.

Single-dose SRS alone may provide an equivalent survival advantage compared with WBRT+SRS. Since there is a class I evidence demonstrating a lower risk of distant metastases with WBRT, careful surveillance is warranted for patients treated with SRS alone to provide identification of local and distant recurrences as early as possible.

WBRT ALONE VERSUS WBRT+SRS

There are two prospective RCTs (class I evidence) on the topic of WBRT alone versus WBRT+SRS. The first is a RTOG multicenter trial published by Andrews et al. in 2004.[19] This trial showed significantly better survival for patients with single metastatic tumors, superior local control and an improved KPS score for patients with one to three metastatic tumors treated with WBRT+SRS. A shortcoming of this study is that there was no follow-up neuroimaging review on 43% of the patients, and tumors greater than 3 cm had been included, which are known to be less favorable for SRS. Therefore, no conclusion can be assured.

The second RCT is from a Pittsburgh group and was published by Kondziolka et al. in 1999.[38] This study was stopped at the 60% accrual point due to an overwhelming positive tumor control difference at interim analysis. There was a significantly better local control rate measured in terms of local failure at 1 year (8% vs. 100%) and median time to recurrence/progression at the original site (36 vs. 6 months) for patients treated with WBRT+SRS.

SURGICAL RESECTION+WBRT VERSUS WBRT+SRS

Both surgical resection+WBRT and WBRT+SRS represent effective treatment strategies, resulting in relatively equal survival times. SRS has not been evaluated for larger lesions (greater than 3 cm) or those with significant mass effect (greater than 1-cm midline shift).

SRS ALONE VERSUS WBRT ALONE

No RCTs were identified for the treatment comparison of SRS and WBRT alone. While both are effective, SRS alone seems to be superior to WBRT alone for patients with up to three metastatic brain tumors in terms of patients' survival.

Moriarty et al.[39] presented factors related to decreased survival and failure of local tumor control in uni- and multivariate analysis of their series. The only independent factors decreasing survival were ongoing systemic disease and age over 60 years. Failure of local tumor control was associated with infratentorial location, tumor volume greater than 3 cm^3, and recurrent lesions. Neither histology (radiosensitive vs. radioresistant lesions) nor number of lesions had an impact on survival or local tumor control rates.

Conclusions

Radiosurgery is effective in the treatment of single or multiple brain metastases that are smaller than 3 cm in diameter. The local control rates range from 85% to 100%. The incidence of side effects is low, from 2% to 5%. Radiation-induced edema and/or radiation necrosis was observed in 4% to 13% of the patients. Median survival ranged from 6 to 11 months. The results are comparable to those achieved with conventional therapy (microsurgical resection followed by whole brain radiotherapy). The advantages of radiosurgery are short hospitalization time (1-3 days), low morbidity, no delay of adjuvant therapy due to healing of surgical wounds, and favorable local control rates.

KEY REFERENCES

American Society for Radiation Oncology. Stereotactic radiosurgery definition. *Int J Radiat Oncol Biol Phys.* 2007;67:1280.

Andrews DW, Scott CB, Sperduto PW, et al. Whole brain radiation therapy with or without stereotactic radiosurgery boost for patients with one to three brain metastases: phase III results of the RTOG 1995-2008 randomised trial. *Lancet.* 2004;363:1665-1672.

Aoyama H, Shirato H, Tago M, et al. Stereotactic radiosurgery plus whole-brain radiation therapy vs. stereotactic radiosurgery alone for treatment of brain metastases: a randomized controlled trial. *JAMA.* 2006;295:2483-2491.

Aoyama H, Tago M, Kato N, et al. Neurocognitive function of patients with brain metastasis who received either whole brain radiotherapy plus stereotactic radiosurgery or radiosurgery alone. *Int J Radiat Oncol Biol Phys.* 2007;68:1388-1395.

Barnett GH, Linskey ME, Adler JR, et al. Stereotactic radiosurgery—an organized neurosurgery-sanctioned definition. *J Neurosurg.* 2007;106:1-5.

Bindal AK, Bindal RK, Hess KR, et al. Surgery versus radiosurgery in the treatment of brain metastasis. *J Neurosurg.* 1996;84:748-754.

Gaspar LE, Scott C, Murray K, Curran W. Validation of the RTOG recursive partitioning analysis (RPA) classification for brain metastases. *Int J Radiat Oncol Biol Phys.* 2000;47:1001-1006.

Kaal EC, Niel CG, Vecht CJ. Therapeutic management of brain metastasis. *Lancet Neurol.* 2005;4:289-298.

Kondziolka D, Patel A, Lunsford LD, et al. Stereotactic radiosurgery plus whole brain radiotherapy versus radiotherapy alone for patients with multiple brain metastases. *Int J Radiat Oncol Biol Phys.* 1999;45:427-434.

Lutterbach J, Cyron D, Henne K, Ostertag CB. Radiosurgery followed by planned observation in patients with one to three brain metastases. *Neurosurgery.* 2003;52:1066-1073.

Moriarty TM, et al. *Radiosurgery.* Basel: Karger; 1996.

Muacevic A, Kreth FW, Horstmann GA, et al. Surgery and radiotherapy compared with gamma knife radiosurgery in the treatment of solitary cerebral metastases of small diameter. *J Neurosurg.* 1999;91:35-43.

Muacevic A, Wowra B, Siefert A, et al. Microsurgery plus whole brain irradiation versus gamma knife surgery alone for treatment of single metastases to the brain: a randomized controlled multicentre phase III trial. *J Neurooncol.* 2008;87:299-307.

Muller-Riemenschneider F, Bockelbrink A, Ernst I, et al. Stereotactic radiosurgery for the treatment of brain metastases. *Radiother Oncol.* 2009;91:67-74.

Nataf F, Schlienger M, Liu Z, et al. Radiosurgery with or without a 2-mm margin for 93 single brain metastases. *Int J Radiat Oncol Biol Phys.* 2008;70:766-772.

Nöel G, Simon JM, Valery CA, et al. Radiosurgery for brain metastasis: impact of CTV on local control. *Radiother Oncol.* 2003;68:15-21.

O'Neill BP, Iturria NJ, Link MJ, et al. A comparison of surgical resection and stereotactic radiosurgery in the treatment of solitary brain metastases. *Int J Radiat Oncol Biol Phys.* 2003;55:1169-1176.

Ostertag CB. [Stereotaxic radiosurgery]. *Nervenarzt.* 1994;65:660-669.

Ostertag CB. Brachytherapy—interstitial implant radiosurgery. *Acta Neurochir Suppl (Wien).* 1993;58:79-84.

Pantazis G, Trippel M, Birg W, et al. Stereotactic interstitial radiosurgery with the Photon Radiosurgery System (PRS) for metastatic brain tumors: a prospective single-center clinical trial. *Int J Radiat Oncol Biol Phys.* 2009;75:1392-1400.

Schoggl A, Kitz K, Reddy M, et al. Defining the role of stereotactic radiosurgery versus microsurgery in the treatment of single brain metastases. *Acta Neurochir (Wien).* 2000;142:621-626.

Serizawa T. Radiosurgery for metastatic brain tumors. *Int J Clin Oncol.* 2009;14:289-298.

Serizawa T, Saeki N, Higuchi Y, et al. Gamma knife surgery for brain metastasis: indications for and limitations of a local treatment protocol. *Acta Neurochir (Wien).* 2005;147:721-726.

Sneed PK, Suh JH, Goetsch SJ, et al. A multi-institutional review of radiosurgery alone vs. radiosurgery with whole brain radiotherapy as the initial management of brain metastases. *Int J Radiat Oncol Biol Phys.* 2002;53:519-526.

Williams BJ, Suki D, Fox BD, et al. Stereotactic radiosurgery for metastatic brain tumors: a comprehensive review of complications. *J Neurosurg.* 2009;111:439-448.

Numbered references appear on Expert Consult.

CHAPTER 99

Stereotactic Radiosurgery for Trigeminal Neuralgia

PABLO F. RECINOS • TRANG NGUYEN • MICHAEL LIM

Trigeminal neuralgia (TN) has been defined as sudden, paroxysmal, recurring stabbing pains of one or more branches of the trigeminal nerve that are generally unilateral.[1] Classic TN is typically secondary to vascular compression or is idiopathic. Patients may recognize different pain triggers, such as chewing, talking, washing, shaving, smoking, or tooth brushing. Between pain episodes, patients tend to be asymptomatic, although a minority of patients continue to experience background pain.[2,3] Many interventions exist for the treatment of TN. Application of stereotactically delivered radiation to treat TN has become a useful, minimally to noninvasive treatment option.

Historical Background

Ionizing radiation for the treatment of TN dates to within a few years of when x-rays were discovered, but it eventually grew out of favor.[4] When stereotactic radiosurgery (SRS) was invented, the use of radiation for TN was revisited. In 1971, Leksell reported on two patients with classic TN whom he treated in 1953 with a single dose of ionizing radiation targeted on the gasserian ganglion and root entry zone.[5] Results were unsatisfactory until the target was moved from the gasserian ganglion to the proximal trigeminal root near the pons.[6] The effects of stereotactically delivered radiation at the root entry zone produces focal axonal degeneration and necrosis of the trigeminal nerve without affecting the gasserian ganglion, which is thought to be the mechanism resulting in pain relief in TN patients.[7] Use of SRS, usually with the gamma knife machine, became widely acceptable in 1996 after a multi-institutional study demonstrated favorable results.[8] Other technologies delivering stereotactic radiation to treat TN have also been reported. In 2003, Romanelli et al. reported the first use of the CyberKnife to treat TN.[9] In the same year, Smith et al. reported the first series of patients with TN treated with linear accelerator (LINAC) radiosurgery.[10]

Indications

The initial treatment for TN is medical therapy, with carbamazepine being the gold standard and oxcarbazepine, a keto derivative of carbamazepine, a suitable alternative with more tolerable side effects. SRS is recommended for patients with medically refractory TN who are not surgical candidates, since microvascular decompression

(MVD) has the highest rates of pain control in patients who are surgical candidates.[11] SRS is regarded as the safest minimally invasive therapy for TN and is particularly useful in patients who are older than 70 years, have significant medical comorbidities, or decide not to undergo MVD.[4,12] However, pain relief is not immediate and may take months.[13] Ideally, SRS should be performed in patients who can undergo magnetic resonance imaging (MRI) for treatment planning. For patients with MRI-incompatible pacemakers or defibrillators, computed tomography (CT) with contrast cisternography can be used.[14]

As with other surgical treatments for TN, patients with typical TN symptomatology fare the best after SRS. Therefore, an accurate diagnosis is critical, because SRS may not be the best treatment option for patients with atypical features. For example, TN pain related to multiple sclerosis can be satisfactorily treated with SRS but not with the same success as classic TN.[15] SRS can be used as a first-time interventional treatment and as repeat or salvage treatment for those who continue to have pain following SRS or other procedures.

Gamma Knife Technique

Gamma knife radiosurgery is a frame-based technique that delivers radiation from a fixed cobalt source. Planning and treatment occur the same day in a single session. On the day of treatment, the first step involves the placement of the stereotactic Leksell frame under local anesthesia. Typically, four points (two anterolateral and two occipital) are chosen to ensure appropriate fixation of the frame (Fig. 99-1). The insertion points are injected with a mixture of 2% lidocaine with sodium bicarbonate for local anesthesia. Bupivacaine can be injected concurrently for long-term analgesia. The screws are then inserted into the frame and skull. The appropriate screw should be selected so that it sits flush with the frame. If a screw is too long, it will lie outside of the frame, create additional artifact during the MRI, and possibly interfere with the treatment beams. It is also critical that the anterior screws be applied while the eyes of the patient are closed. If the screws are applied while the patient's eyes are open, complete eye closure may not be possible, making it uncomfortable for the patient and risking corneal ulceration.

After application of the Leksell frame is completed, a 1-mm-slice MRI with gadolinium is obtained. T1, T2, and fast imaging employing steady-state acquisition (FIESTA) sequences allow trigeminal nerve identification and its relationship to adjacent blood vessels to be examined.[16] The target is a single, 4-mm isocenter positioned at the trigeminal nerve root entry zone, 2 to 4 mm from the junction of the nerve and the pons[8,13,17] (Fig. 99-2). Maintenance of this buffer zone between the nerve and the pons keeps the radiation delivered to the brain stem between 20% and 30% of the isodose.[8] Final dose selection and calculation of the dosage delivery plans are done in conjunction with a radiation oncologist and a physicist.

Once the planning is complete, treatment can proceed. The patient is placed on the treatment bed, and the collimator helmet is affixed (Fig. 99-3). Once the target coordinates for the beam have been confirmed, the treatment commences. After the treatment is complete, the Leksell frame is taken off by sequentially removing the screws opposite each other. The pin site defects are covered with gauze and antibiotic ointment.

Linear Accelerator

Other frame-based technologies have emerged, such as LINAC radiosurgery. Similar to gamma knife radiosurgery, frame placement on the patient, treatment planning, and the radiosurgical treatment session take place in the same day. The dose fallout areas have been shown to be comparable to those of gamma knife.[18]

Cyberknife Technique

An MRI FIESTA sequence with 1.25-mm thin cuts and a CT with 1.25-mm thin cuts should be obtained. The MRI is used to localize and target the trigeminal nerve root entry zone.[19-21] The CT images are used as a template for localization during the treatment. The images from CT and MRI are fused together to combine the two data sets for treatment. The CT/MRI fusion technique has become standard practice at centers utilizing CyberKnife for the treatment of TN

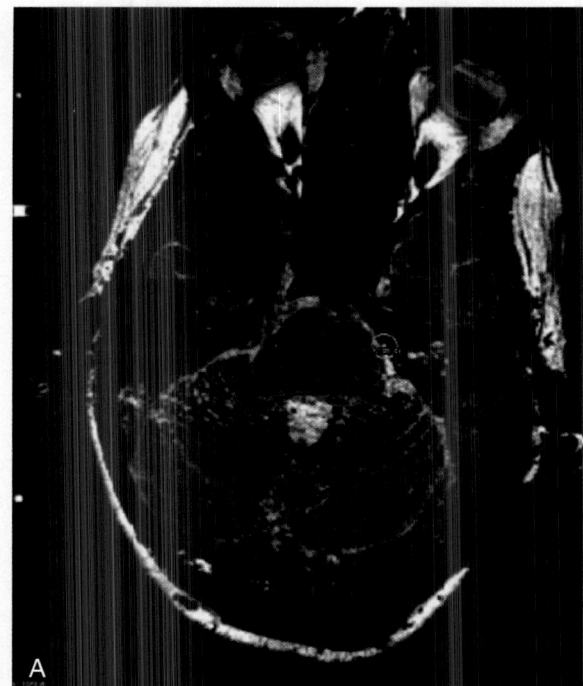
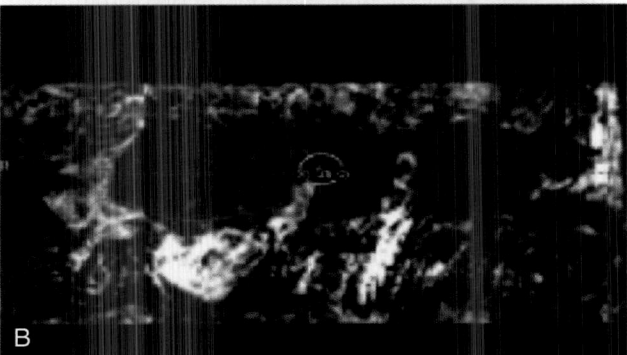

FIGURE 99-2 Typical gamma knife plan that was used to treat a patient with classic left-sided TN. A, A single, 4-mm isocenter is planned at the trigeminal nerve root entry zone. B, Keeping a 2- to 4-mm buffer zone between the isocenter and the pons reduces the radiation delivered to the brain stem to 20% to 30% of the maximum treatment dose.

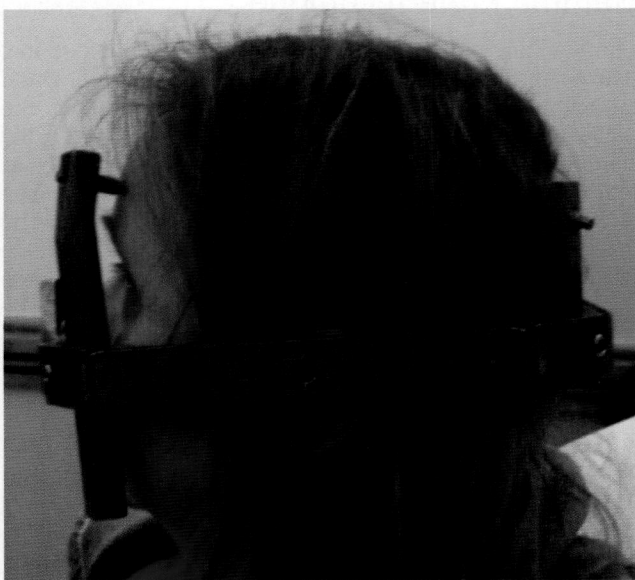

FIGURE 99-1 Side profile of a patient after application of the Leksell frame prior to SRS treatment with gamma knife. The patient is placed in a four-pin configuration with two anterolateral pins and two occipital pins.

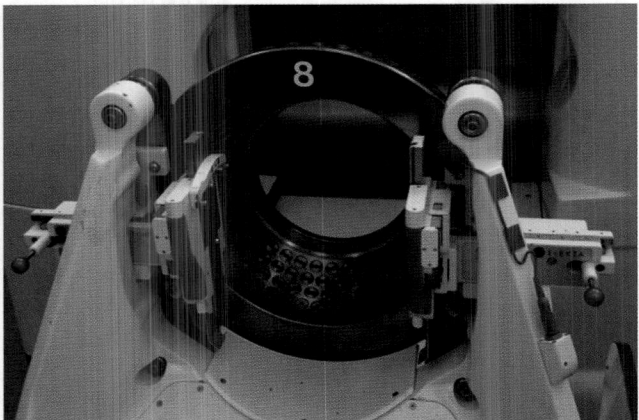

FIGURE 99-3 Collimator helmet of the gamma knife radiosurgery apparatus attached to the treatment bed. Once the Leksell frame is placed on the patient, the patient lies on the treatment bed and the frame is fixed to the collimator helmet.

and has obviated the need for obtaining a CT-cisternogram to localize and target the trigeminal nerve root entry zone.[20] As a result, treatment of TN with CyberKnife has become a noninvasive procedure.

Once the trigeminal nerve and its root entry zone have been identified, a segment of the nerve is targeted for treatment. The segment should be 2 to 3 mm from the dorsal root entry zone to minimize the dose delivered to the brain stem. At this distance, the brain stem receives between 30% and 50% of the maximum treatment dose[20] (Fig. 99-4). Likewise, extension into the gasserian ganglion in Meckel's cave should be avoided. To minimize hot spots and heterogenous radiation dosages delivered to the nerve, a nonisocentric plan is used.

Once the planning is complete, the patient is placed supine on the treatment bed and kept in place using a custom-made thermoplastic mask. During the treatment session, orthogonal cranial x-rays are taken between every three to five treatment shots. The x-ray films are analyzed with reference to the previously loaded CT data and compared during the session to detect patient movement. When patient movement has occurred, the target coordinates are recalculated and the movements of the robotic arm movements are adjusted accordingly.[22,23] Approximately 30 x-rays are taken during the treatment session, which is roughly equivalent to the radiation dose delivered during a routine CT scan.[20] Using a 1.25-mm-slice CT scan in the data set, the accuracy of the target is roughly within 1.1 mm.[24]

Ideal Dosage and Targeting

Several factors affect the outcomes and side effects from treatment of TN with radiosurgery. These include the specific portion of the nerve treated, the dose delivered, and the length of nerve treated. Targeting of the gasserian ganglion was shown by multiple groups to reduce pain in a select number of patients but had poor long-term results.[25,26] Improved short- and long-term results have been seen when the proximal nerve is targeted shortly after its takeoff from the pons. In this segment, the source of myelin of the nerve changes from oligodendrocytes (central) to Schwann cells (peripheral). It has been hypothesized that this zone is more sensitive to radiation.[17] At the same time, minimizing the radiation delivered to the brain stem is of paramount importance.

In the first multi-institutional study conducted by Kondziolka et al., the effect of different dosages delivered to the trigeminal nerve using the gamma knife was examined. A significantly higher number of patients (72% vs. 9%) had complete pain relief with treatment doses greater than 70 Gy compared to those treated with doses less than 70 Gy.[4,8] As the doses delivered increase above 70 Gy, the benefits are tempered by the associated morbidity. Pollock et al. examined the differences in treating patients with 70 and 90 Gy. A nonsignificant trend toward improved facial pain was seen. However, there was a significantly higher incidence of dysesthesias, corneal ulceration, and permanent trigeminal nerve dysfunction. Therefore, the dose delivered should be greater than 70 Gy but less than 90 Gy.[7,27]

The effect of radiating a longer length of the trigeminal nerve using the gamma knife was explored by Flickinger et al. In their study, 87 patients were randomized to either one isocenter or two isocenters on the proximal trigeminal nerve, receiving a maximum of 75 Gy to each isocenter. Pain control was equivalent in the two groups, and a significantly higher number of patients experienced complications (numbness or paresthesias) in the two-isocenter group.[28] Therefore, treating a longer segment of the trigeminal nerve is not recommended.

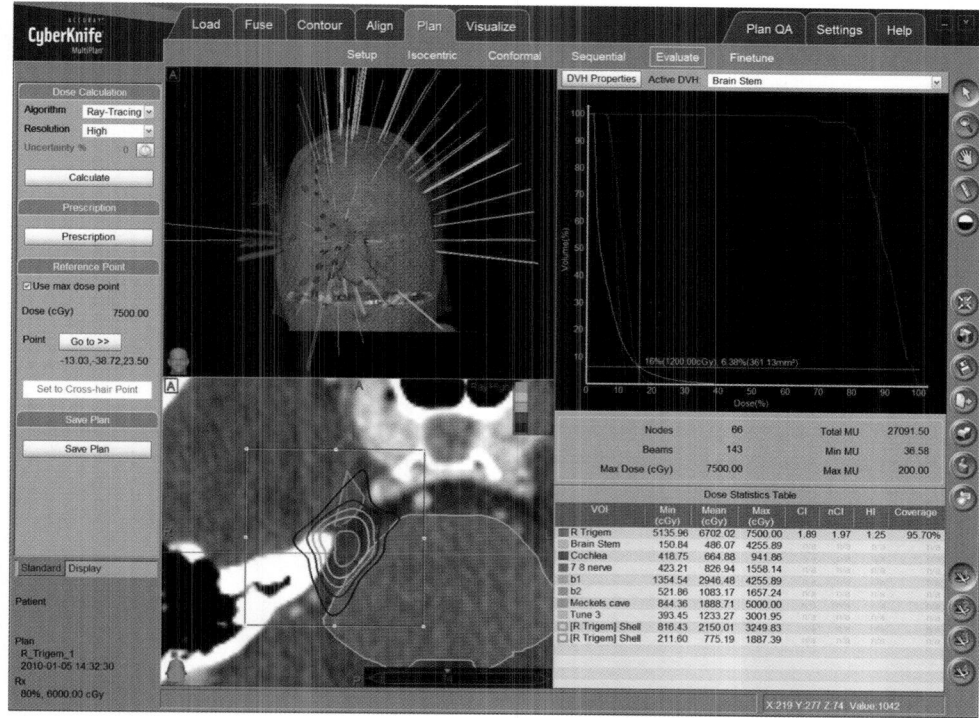

FIGURE 99-4 A typical CyberKnife plan that was used to treat a patient with classic right-sided TN. The treatment plan is mapped out on a CT/MRI fusion image. The nonisocentric plan allows the target to be shaped irregularly while still minimizing the radiation delivered to the brain stem.

The optimal dose and length of trigeminal nerve targeted for treatment by CyberKnife is still being refined. Lim et al. reported a series of 38 patients with TN treated with CyberKnife and divided them into two groups: Group 1 received a lower maximum dose (71.4 - 79.5 Gy), a lower minimum dose to the nerve margin (60 - 65.5 Gy), and had a shorter length of nerve treated; Group 2 received a higher maximum dose (80 - 86.3 Gy), a higher minimum dose to the nerve margin (66 - 70 Gy), and a longer length of nerve treated.[29] While there was also no difference in pain response or recurrence based on length of nerve treated, the mean degree of numbness was significantly less when a shorter length (5-6.5 mm; median 6 mm) than a longer length (7-12 mm; median 8 mm) of nerve was treated. A subsequent study of 95 patients demonstrated that using higher radiation doses and treating longer nerve segments resulted in better pain relief.[20] However, there was also a higher rate of numbness. This larger study suggested the treatment cohort with a median maximum dose of 78 Gy and a median treated nerve length of 6 mm had the optimal outcome of balancing pain relief with less numbness and side effects.

Outcomes

SRS is the least invasive treatment option, but pain relief is not as immediate as it is for other trigeminal rhizotomy procedures and MVD. Most studies on SRS have been retrospective case series with a large proportion of patients who had prior surgical interventions. Patients who underwent SRS as their first procedure had a longer duration without pain. The median time to pain relief is 2 weeks to 1 month, but relief can occur as fast as 1 day or as long as 6 months.[8,19,20,30] With gamma knife, initial pain relief occurs in about 75% of patients. Three years following treatment, approximately 50% have sustained pain relief.[12] However, reported results on treatment effectiveness vary widely among studies.[31]

All complications due to gamma knife radiation are related to trigeminal nerve dysfunction. The most common side effects are facial paresthesias, which occur in 6% to 13%. The risk of complications increases with higher doses, especially greater than 90 Gy.[27,32] Repeat gamma knife radiation at a lower dose has similar pain relief rates, but the risk of complications is greater than with first-time use.[33,34] Salvage gamma knife radiation for patients who have refractory TN following MVD provides pain relief for 50% and complete resolution for 20% at 5 years.[35] Gamma knife radiation is also useful to treat TN related to multiple sclerosis but less effective than treating patients without multiple sclerosis. Reasonable pain control is reported in 80% to 97.3% of these

patients overall and 82.6% at 1 year, 73.9% at 3 years, and 54.0% at 5 years after treatment in this patient population.[15,36]

In a large, prospective, controlled trial of gamma knife radiosurgery in 100 evaluable patients, initial pain relief occurred in 94% of patients at a median of 10 days. In this trial, 34 patients had pain recurrence at a median time of 6 months following treatment, with 17 patients undergoing additional surgeries. Overall, 83 patients were pain free at last follow-up, which was, at a minimum, 1 year after the procedure, and 69% were pain free without requiring another procedure. In addition, 10 patients had complications, all related to trigeminal nerve injury.[31]

The time to pain relief is arguably shorter by as much as 7 days with CyberKnife compared to gamma knife or LINAC radiation.[29] The rate of initial pain relief with CyberKnife is as great as 92% to 94%.[19,20,29] However, the proportion of patients with continous pain relief 3 years following treatment decreases by as much as 50%.[20] Better pain relief is achieved with higher radiation doses or with a longer segment of nerve treated—but with higher rates of hypesthesia.[20] Success of treatment is also improved when CyberKnife is used as the first treatment. For patients with no prior interventional treatment, 94% had initial pain relief, which was sustained in 78% at 1 year and 67% at 2 years after treatment.[19] The use of CyberKnife for atypical TN has not been as well studied. In a series of seven patients with atypical TN, four experienced complete pain at a mean follow-up time of 28 months.[21]

In addition to numbness, the main complication seen with radiosurgical treatment of TN is anesthesia dolorosa. It is defined as "painful numbness." Some have suggested that including the gasserian ganglion could increase the chances of anesthesia dolorosa. Others have suggested that patients who have had multiple procedures (i.e., rhizotomies) are at higher risk for anesthesia dolorosa. Unfortunately, there is little that can be done for this condition.

Comparison of Radiosurgery as Whole to Other Treatment Modalities

SRS is just one of many treatment options for medically refractory TN patients (Table 99-1). It is the newest treatment modality; therefore, long-term results have not been as extensively published as with the other modalities. It is an attractive option since it is the least invasive. However, patients who are surgical candidates are recommended to undergo MVD unless they prefer to avoid open surgery. In a prospective, nonrandomized cohort study of 80 consecutive patients comparing MVD and gamma knife radiosurgery,

Table 99-1	Outcome Comparison of Modalities Used to Treat Trigeminal Neuralgia*							
		ACTUARIAL PAIN RELIEF RATES			**COMPLICATIONS**			
Procedure	Initial Pain Relief	1 Year	3 Years	5 Years	Sensory	Dysesthesia	8th Nerve	AD
Gamma knife[31,40,41]	75%	69%	52%	NR	6.9%	0.3%	NR	0%
CyberKnife	92%	63%	50%	NR	47%	0.2%	0.2%	0.2%
Percutaneous procedures	90%	68%-85%	54%-64%	50%	45%	5.8%	2%	4.4%
MVD[42,43]	90%	80%	75%	73%	6.7%	3.8%	3.7%	0.1%

*From Villavicencio et al. 2008[20] and Gronseth et al. 2008.[39]
AD, anesthesia dolorosa, NR, not reported.

the actuarial pain-free rates were significantly higher with MVD initially (100% vs. 78%), at 2 years (88% vs. 50%), and at 5 years (80% vs. 33%).[11] The relative risk in this study of no longer being pain free at 5 years after treatment was 3.35 for MVD versus gamma knife. Compared to SRS, the other trigeminal rhizolysis treatments (glycerol rhizotomy, radiofrequency ablation, and balloon microcompression) require at least intravenous sedation and needle insertion to or past the foramen ovale. Gamma knife radiation can be performed with only local anesthesia for frame placement, whereas CyberKnife radiosurgery is frameless and noninvasive.

For patients who are not surgical candidates, the percutaneous ablative techniques, particularly radiofrequency thermocoagulation, seem to have better sustained pain relief compared to gamma knife but with a higher risk of complications. The complication rate with gamma knife is less than with the percutaneous procedures, and side effects are limited to trigeminal nerve dysfunction.[37] These conclusions have been made from systematic reviews, and a trial directly comparing SRS to the percutaneous procedures has yet to be completed.[37]

The literature thus far shows a higher rate of numbness with CyberKnife radiation.[20] As experience grows, this is likely to be reduced as dose and target selection is optimized to best balance treatment effectiveness and complications. When only 6 mm of the trigeminal nerve was treated with CyberKnife, 5 out of 30 patients (17%) experienced post-treatment numbness and 1 out of 30 patients (3.3%) had a decreased corneal reflex.[20] Complications not due to trigeminal nerve dysfunction, such as diplopia, decreased hearing, dry eyes, and right foot paresthesias, are reported with CyberKnife and are usually due to inadvertent excessive radiation of the brain stem.[20]

Rare complications such as meningitis, nontrigeminal cranial nerve dysfunction, accidental vascular injury, and decreased hearing can occur with the percutaneous rhizolysis techniques but should not occur with SRS if proper treatment planning is performed.[38] Therefore, SRS is preferable for the subset of patients with contralateral hearing loss, because there is no risk of hearing impairment. Patients who are considering SRS should be counseled that pain relief may not occur for weeks. Patients who need immediate relief from debilitating pain may prefer the percutaneous therapies. Overall, SRS appears to be the safest treatment option for TN.

KEY REFERENCES

Barker FG, Jannetta PJ, Bissonette DJ, et al. The long-term outcome of microvascular decompression for trigeminal neuralgia. *N Engl J Med.* 1996;334:1077-1083.

Chavez GD, De Salles AA, Solberg TD, et al. Three-dimensional fast imaging employing steady-state acquisition magnetic resonance imaging for stereotactic radiosurgery of trigeminal neuralgia. *Neurosurgery.* 2005;56:E628; discussion E.

de Lotbiniere A. Gamma knife surgery for trigeminal neuralgia and facial pain. In: Lozano AM, Gildenberg PL, Tasker RR, eds. *Textbook of Stereotactic and Functional Neurosurgery.* Berlin, Heidelberg: Springer Berlin Heidelberg; 2009:2475-2481.

Dhople AA, Adams JR, Maggio WW, et al. Long-term outcomes of gamma knife radiosurgery for classic trigeminal neuralgia: implications of treatment and critical review of the literature. *J Neurosurg.* 2009:111(2):351-358.

Fariselli L, Marras C, De Santis M, et al. CyberKnife radiosurgery as a first treatment for idiopathic trigeminal neuralgia. *Neurosurgery.* 2009; 64:A96-101.

Flickinger JC, Pollock BE, Kondziolka D, et al. Does increased nerve length within the treatment volume improve trigeminal neuralgia radiosurgery? A prospective double-blind, randomized study. *Int J Radiat Oncol Biol Phys.* 2001;51:449-454.

Gronseth G, Cruccu G, Alksne J, et al. Practice parameter: the diagnostic evaluation and treatment of trigeminal neuralgia (an evidence-based review): report of the Quality Standards Subcommittee of the American Academy of Neurology and the European Federation of Neurological Societies. *Neurology.* 2008;71:1183-1190.

Hasegawa T, Kondziolka D, Spiro R, et al. Repeat radiosurgery for refractory trigeminal neuralgia. *Neurosurgery.* 2002;50:494-500: discussion 500-502.

Kondziolka D, Flickinger JC, Lunsford LD, Habeck M. Trigeminal neuralgia radiosurgery: the University of Pittsburgh experience. *Stereotact Funct Neurosurg.* 1996;66(Suppl 1):343-348.

Kondziolka D, Lunsford LD, Flickinger JC, et al. Stereotactic radiosurgery for trigeminal neuralgia: a multiinstitutional study using the gamma unit. *J Neurosurg.* 1996;84:940-945.

Kondziolka D, Perez B, Flickinger JC, et al. Gamma knife radiosurgery for trigeminal neuralgia: results and expectations. *Arch Neurol.* 1998;55:1524-1529.

Lim M, Villavicencio AT, Burneikiene S, et al. CyberKnife radiosurgery for idiopathic trigeminal neuralgia. *Neurosurg Focus.* 2005;18:E9.

Linskey ME, Ratanatharathorn V, Peñagaricano J. A prospective cohort study of microvascular decompression and gamma knife surgery in patients with trigeminal neuralgia. *J Neurosurg.* 2008;109(Suppl):160-172.

Ma L, Kwok Y, Chin LS, et al. Comparative analyses of LINAC and gamma knife radiosurgery for trigeminal neuralgia treatments. *Phys Med Biol.* 2005;50:5217-5227.

Merskey H, Bogduk N. *Classification of Chronic Pain: Description of Chronic Pain Syndromes and Definition of Pain Terms.* 2nd ed. Seattle: IASP; 1994.

Nurmikko TJ, Eldridge PR. Trigeminal neuralgia—pathophysiology, diagnosis and current treatment. *British Journal of Anaesthesia.* 2001;87:117-132.

Patil CG, Veeravagu A, Bower RS, et al. CyberKnife radiosurgical rhizotomy for the treatment of atypical trigeminal nerve pain. *Neurosurg Focus.* 2007;23:E9.

Pollock BE, Phuong LK, Foote RL, et al. High-dose trigeminal neuralgia radiosurgery associated with increased risk of trigeminal nerve dysfunction. *Neurosurgery.* 2001;49:58-62:discussion -4.

Regis J, Metellus P, Hayashi M, et al. Prospective controlled trial of gamma knife surgery for essential trigeminal neuralgia. *J Neurosurg.* 2006;104:913-924.

Rogers CL, Shetter AG, Ponce FA, et al. Gamma knife radiosurgery for trigeminal neuralgia associated with multiple sclerosis. *J Neurosurg.* 2002;97:529-532.

Smith ZA, De Salles AA, Frighetto L, et al. Dedicated linear accelerator radiosurgery for the treatment of trigeminal neuralgia. *J Neurosurg.* 2003;99:511-516.

The International Classification of Headache Disorders: 2nd ed. *Cephalalgia.* 2004;24(Suppl 1):9-160.

Zakrzewska JM. Diagnosis and differential diagnosis of trigeminal neuralgia. *Clin J Pain.* 2002;18:14-21.

Zakrzewska JM, Lopez BC, Kim SE, Coakham HB. Patient reports of satisfaction after microvascular decompression and partial sensory rhizotomy for trigeminal neuralgia. *Neurosurgery.* 2005;56:1304-1311: discussion 1311-1312.

Zorro O, Lobato-Polo J, Kano H, et al. Gamma knife radiosurgery for multiple sclerosis–related trigeminal neuralgia. *Neurology.* 2009;73: 1149-1154.

Numbered references appear on Expert Consult.

CyberKnife Radiosurgery for Spinal Neoplasms

ROBERT E. LIEBERSON • AKE HANSASUTA • ROBERT DODD • STEVEN D. CHANG • JOHN R. ADLER, JR.

The successes of cranial stereotactic radiosurgery (SRS) inspired the development of spinal SRS.[1-4] In little more than a decade, spinal SRS has revolutionized the treatment of spinal tumors and vascular malformations. The introduction of CyberKnife™ has allowed the delivery of very large doses of radiation to small lesions while sparing adjacent normal structures. CyberKnife™ outcomes are comparable or superior to those obtained with conventional radiotherapy, frame-based stereotactic systems, or conventional surgery.[1-13] Since 1994, the CyberKnife™ has been used to treat over 10,000 spinal lesions at more than 200 sites worldwide.

Technology Overview

The CyberKnife system consists of a lightweight, 6-megavolt (MV) linear accelerator (LINAC) mounted on an industrial robot, a remotely repositionable treatment couch, orthogonally placed digital x-ray cameras, a treatment-delivery computer, and treatment planning stations (Fig. 100-1). During treatment, numerous images are obtained to optimally locate the target before the delivery of 100 to 150 individual treatment beams.[14] The CyberKnife can deliver individual beams to any part of a tumor from nearly any angle and provides highly conformal dosing to complex three-dimensional (3D) targets.[15]

Several conventional radiation therapy (RT) systems have recently been modified to provide SRS using techniques originally developed for the CyberKnife™. The BrainLab Novalis, with floor and ceiling mounted x-ray detectors, most directly emulates the CyberKnife™ localization system. The Elekta Synergy, Varian Trilogy, and Novalis TX systems use different combinations of cone-beam CT scanners and orthogonal x-ray cameras. These RT-based systems are constrained by the gimbal design of the gantry which only allows radiation to be delivered along two-dimensional arcs. Nevertheless, multileaf collimators can compensate for much of the constraints that stem from this gantry design.

Treatment Details

Spinal SRS is image guided and completely frameless. Individually molded masks or cradles are fashioned before the planning scans are completed. The patient rests in the mask or cradle during computed tomography (CT) scanning, magnetic resonance imaging (MRI), 3D angiography or positron emission tomography (PET) imaging, and again during treatment. The devices are comfortable, limit movement, and expedite positioning. At Stanford, we use an Aquaplast mask (WFR Corp., Wyckoff, NJ) for upper cervical lesions (Fig. 100-2A). Lower cervical, thoracic, lumbar, and sacral lesions are treated using an AlphaCradle (Smithers Medical Products, Akron, OH) (Fig. 100-2B). Most patients are treated supine but prone and lateral decubitus positioning is possible.

A high-resolution, fine-cut CT scan, most often with contrast, is required for all treatment plans. The CT is essential for its excellent spatial accuracy and is needed to calculate the digitally reconstructed radiographs (DRRs) used for real-time targeting. MRI scans may help with visualization but cannot be utilized alone because of the need to generate DRRs. Meanwhile, MRI often suffers from inherent limitations in spatial resolution. In the appropriate clinical situation, PET or angiogram images are also obtained. When a frame-less radiosurgical system is used, the patient does not need to remain in the facility while the treatment plan is developed.

Bony landmarks are used to target spinal lesions and those in adjacent structures. Spinal fusion hardware does not interfere with treatment. The accuracy of CyberKnife approaches ±0.5 mm.[7,16] For lesions not associated with bony landmarks, three or more gold seeds or titanium screws are implanted (Fig. 100-3).[13,15]

CyberKnife treatment plans use Accuray's MultiPlan software. BrainLab, Varian, and Elekta systems employ similar programs. After uploading the CT and other images to the planning station, the surgeon and radiotherapist "contour" the target and radiation-sensitive structures by tracing their outlines (Fig. 100-4). The dose and number of sessions, as well as dose limits for adjacent structures, are prescribed by the physicians (Fig. 100-5). Physicists then use the planning system, the contour data, and the dose prescriptions to create a 3D representation of the lesion geometry and define sets of treatment beams. An ideal treatment includes evenly distributed beams that target the dose uniformly while limiting exposure to sensitive structures (Fig. 100-6). The neurosurgeon and/or physicist will iteratively perfect the plan by adding or removing constraints, or re-positioning individual beams. A multidisciplinary team reviews and accepts each treatment plan before delivery.

During spinal radiosurgery, CyberKnife™ patients are placed on the operating table in their custom mask or cradle. Images are automatically obtained by the orthogonally placed x-ray cameras and compared with digitally reconstructed radiographs (DRRs) that were precalculated by the planning software. The table is aligned and the computer aims and delivers the first treatment beam. Additional images are obtained, automatic corrections for movement are made, and all planned treatment beams delivered in order. This process is automatic; after the initial targeting verification is performed by the treating neurosurgeon, radiation delivery is simply monitored by a radiation therapist. Not all commercially available systems permit periodic reimaging and beam retargeting. As a result, in the event of patient movement during treatment with such radiosurgical devices, accuracy may be compromised.

Indications

It cannot be emphasized enough that the indications for spinal SRS continue to evolve quickly; spinal SRS is a new subdiscipline within neurosurgery and only now are standardized procedures for its application being developed. At our institution, we most frequently treat metastases, small benign tumors, postoperative residuals, lesions that recur

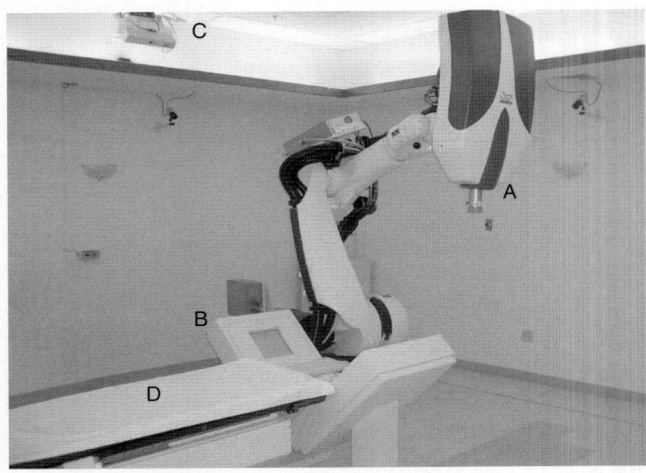

FIGURE 100-1 A, The CyberKnife frameless stereotactic system includes a modified 6-MV X-band LINAC mounted on a highly maneuverable robotic manipulator (KUKA Roboter GmbH, Augsburg, Germany). B, Two high-resolution x-ray cameras are mounted orthogonally to the headrest. C, One of the two x-ray sources is mounted in the ceiling projecting onto the camera. D, The treatment couch is mobile, allowing the x-ray sources to image targets at any point along the neuraxis.

following conventional surgery or radiation, vascular malformations, inoperable tumors, and lesions in those who decline surgery (Tables 100-1 and 100-2).[3,7,13] Spinal lesions appropriate for CyberKnife™ radiosurgery should be reasonably well circumscribed, clearly visible on CT or MRI, and smaller than approximately 5 cm in diameter. We do not insist on obtaining a biopsy in advance of treatment if the diagnosis is clear from preradiosurgical imaging studies.

Spinal SRS is contraindicated in the presence of significant spinal cord compression causing a severe neurologic deficit, especially when the treated lesion is relatively radioresistant. Radiographic evidence of spinal cord compression is not in itself a contraindication to spinal radiosurgery. Spinal SRS can be used as an adjunct if there is evidence of spinal instability. If the adjacent spinal cord has already received the maximum tolerated radiation dose, then surgery and/or chemotherapy may be more appropriate.

Extradural Metastases

The spine is the most common site for bony metastases, accounting for nearly 40% of osseous tumor spread.[17] Forty percent of cancer patients will develop at least 1 spinal metastasis.[18] Historically, spinal metastases have been managed with chemotherapy, radiopharmaceuticals, surgery, and external beam irradiation.[17,19] Conventional irradiation of spinal metastatic tumors is useful for palliation but its effectiveness is limited by spinal cord tolerance.[20] Moreover, relapses are common,[21-24] and retreatment with RT is generally impossible.[18] SRS enables much larger biologically effective doses to be delivered by utilizing a more highly conformal plan that protects the cord. Multiple courses of spinal SRS can control multiple asynchronous metastases, and SRS may be used to sterilize a vertebral body before vertebroplasty[25] or following a debulking procedure. The presence of spinal fusion hardware is not a contraindication.[26] SRS is ideal for those with limited life expectancies or those who need other treatment. Most SRS treatments are completed in a single 1-hour session.

Treatment protocols in the published literature vary greatly and there is significant debate regarding the most appropriate treatment margins.[27] For purely bony lesions, Amdur et al.[27] recommend treating visible tumor plus a 1-cm margin in bone or a 2-mm volume outside the external cortex. For lesions within the canal, the margins are not extended beyond the visible tumor. Many groups irradiate the entire affected vertebral body including the pedicles.

FIGURE 100-2 Simple immobilization devices used during CyberKnife treatment. A, The Aquaplast mask is used in patients with upper cervical lesions. B, AlphaCradle custom body mold is used in patients with lesions below the cervical spine.

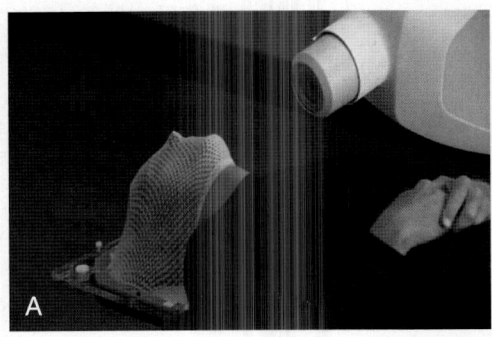
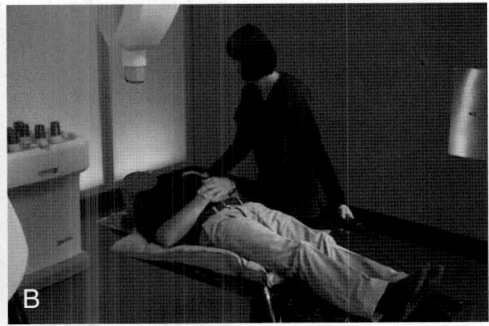

Chang et al.[18] recommend treating the pedicles for possible tumor extension, pointing out that 18% of recurrences occurred in the pedicles. At Stanford we typically treat the tumor volume as seen on CT or MRI.[17] There are no studies that show a clear benefit of one approach over the other, but those who treat smaller volumes argue that the cord dose is decreased and that recurrences can be retreated. Dose recommendations are variable with single-session prescriptions ranging from 8 to 24 Gy in the published literature.[27] At Stanford we have used from 16 to 25 Gy in up to five fractions, but usually opt to treat in the fewest possible sessions as dictated by the length and dose of irradiated spinal cord.[17]

Overall the efficacy of radiosurgery for spinal metastases appears roughly comparable to that for brain metastases.[2,3,17] Tumor growth is arrested by radiosurgery in up to 100% of cases and results are independent of histology (Table 100-3).[4,28] Pain relief ranged from 43% to 96% and unlike standard RT, is generally apparent within days of SRS.[27]

Because of the delay between SRS and the involution of the tumor, radiosurgery is almost never an alternative to emergency decompression. Neither generalized metastatic involvement of the axial skeleton nor epidural carcinomatosis is an indication for radiosurgery, as SRS cannot cover such broad areas effectively. In the presence of instability, radiosurgery may be used as an adjunct to a stabilization procedure such as vertebroplasty. Delayed post-SRS spinal instability can occur but is not common.

Intradural Metastases

Intramedullary spinal cord metastases, which are rarely seen clinically, are found in 0.9% to 2.1% of autopsies in cancer patients.[33] Such lesions comprise 8.5% of central nervous system metastases[34] and their frequency will likely increase with longer patient survival. Wowra et al.[29] review their results and the literature. They report that 96% of spinal metastases were well controlled with spinal SRS. The risk of myelopathy was less than 1%.

Primary Intramedullary Lesions

At Stanford, we have treated 92 hemangioblastomas in 31 patients. Sixteen were spinal intramedullary tumors. Patients were treated with a median radiosurgical dose of 23 Gy, and after a median 34 months of follow-up, 15 of the 16 spinal hemangioblastomas in this series either remained stable or decreased in size. Among all hemangioblastomas, those causing edema and those associated with cysts did less well. None of the patients developed radiation myelopathy.[35]

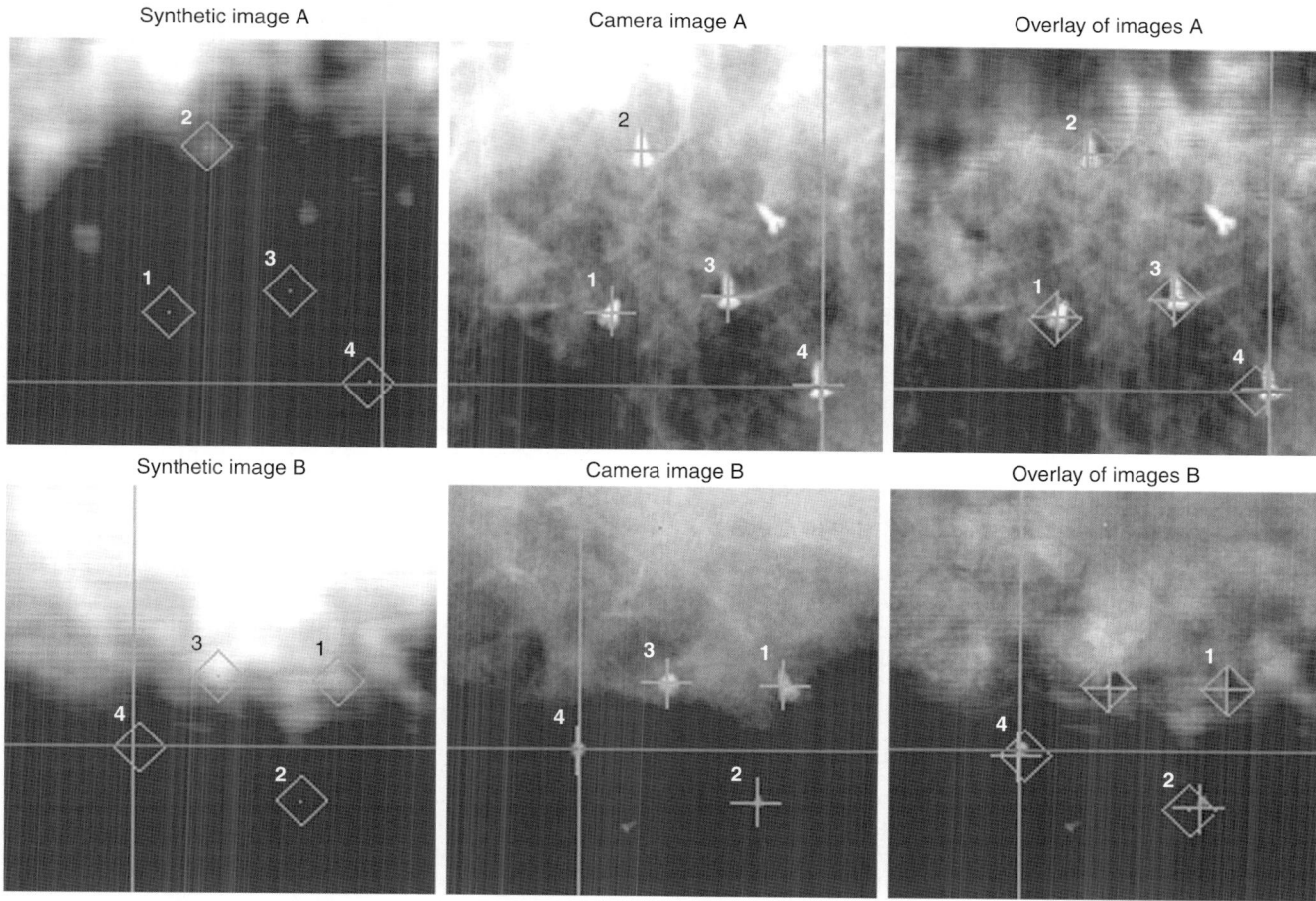

FIGURE 100-3 Implanted fiducials are marked and numbered. Left, Computed tomography-based digitally reconstructed images from the perspective of the two orthogonal CyberKnife mounted x-ray cameras (A and B). Center, Real-time x-ray images from the two x-ray cameras. Right, Overlay of the reconstructed and actual radiographic images.

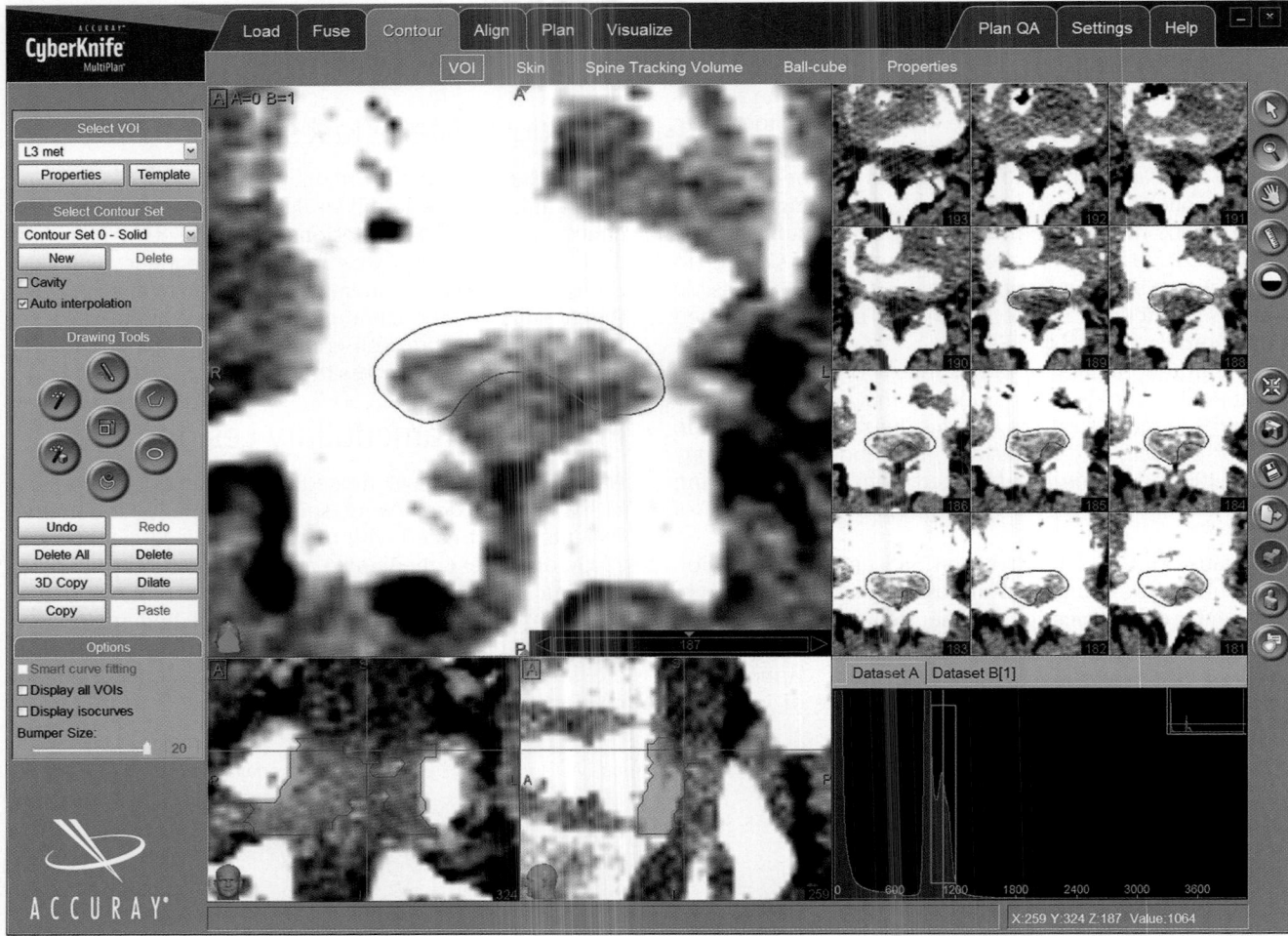

FIGURE 100-4 Contour of L3 metastasis in axial, saggital, and coronal projections. The epidural metastasis is in red.

Some spinal ependymomas prove difficult to resect for reasons of anatomy or associated medical comorbidities. Although not common, tumor recurrence also occurs. There is very little information available regarding SRS. Ependymomas, which may be controlled with conventional radiation therapy, have responded favorably to spinal SRS in the few cases that have been published.[3,36,37] The Stanford experience with CyberKnife radiosurgery has been quite favorable with good local control and no complications (unpublished data). We know even less about the treatment of spinal astrocytomas. For the occasional well-demarcated, biopsy-proven, newly diagnosed or recurrent spinal cord astrocytoma, spinal SRS may be a theoretical alternative if surgery is not possible.

Intradural, Extramedullary Lesions

Meningiomas, schwannomas, neurofibromas, and hemangioblastomas are the benign lesions most frequently considered for treatment with spinal SRS. However, microsurgical resection remains the most appropriate intervention for most patients. Surgical resection is generally curative and in the process, the surgeon both establishes a tissue diagnosis and immediately decompresses the spinal cord.[38] Nevertheless,

SRS is appropriate for benign lesions that are inaccessible, when lesions are numerous (as in neurofibromatosis or von Hippel-Lindau disease), in patients with significant medical comorbidities, or for patients who decline open surgery.[39-41] Moreover, spinal radiosurgery also has the virtue of posing little risk to the parent motor or sensory nerves in cases of nerve sheath tumors.

Short-term control rates for intradural, extramedullary spinal tumors appear comparable to those of similar intracranial lesions. At Stanford we have treated 110 patients with 117 lesions (unpublished data). Greater numbers and longer follow-up periods confirm earlier published observations.[42] Following SRS, 56% of schwannomas and meningiomas stabilized and 44% regressed radiographically. Neurofibromas did less well with 11% enlarging radiographically, over 50% causing increased pain, and 80% showing a worsening in at least one examination finding. Even including neurofibromas, most myelopathies and radiculopathies improved with SRS, whereas bowel and bladder dysfunction did not. Two of our patients eventually required surgery for tumor enlargement and three required surgery for persistent or progressing symptoms. Only one patient developed radiation myelopathy. Other centers have reported similar results.[39-41]

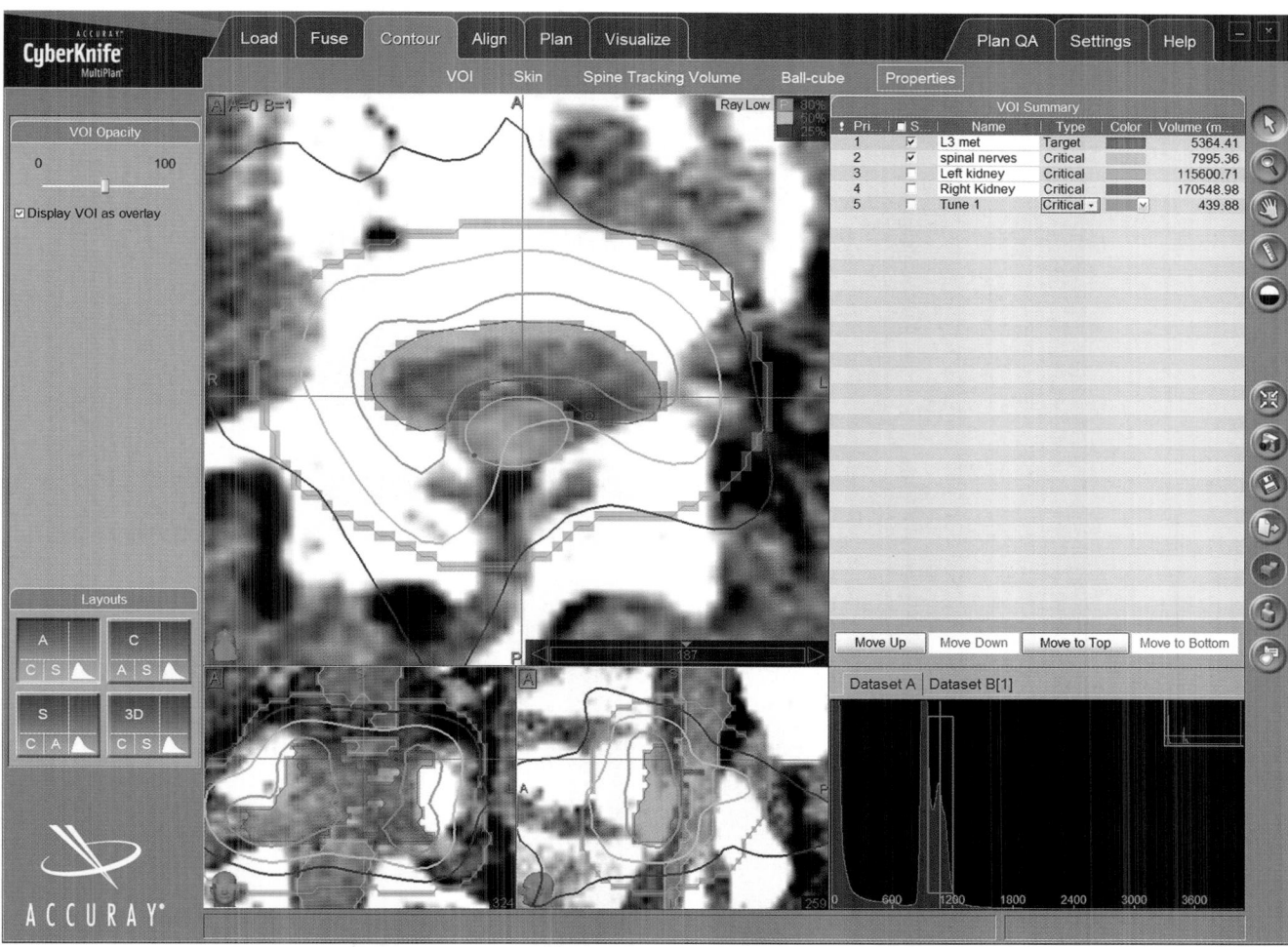

FIGURE 100-5 Contour of L3 metastasis and spinal roots with superimposed isodose lines from treatment plan in axial, saggital, and coronal projections. The epidural metastasis is in red, the spinal roots are blue, and the 80% isodose line is represented by the thin green line.

VASCULAR MALFORMATIONS

Steinter et al.[43] published the first description of SRS for cranial arteriovenous malformations (AVMs) in 1972. The successes in treating the intracranial AVMs inspired the use of SRS for spinal vascular malformations. Spinal AVMs have been described using various systems. Most commonly they have been divided into four types.[44] Types I and IV are dural and perimedullary fistulas and are better treated with embolization and resection. Most AVMs treated with SRS are type II, or glomus AVMs, with a well-defined nidus. Some type III, or juvenile AVMs, may be amenable to SRS when well-focal and well-defined (Fig. 100-7). SRS causes endothelial damage that leads to the obliteration of the vascular lumena.[45] Low-flow lesions, such as cavernous malformations, are rarely candidates for spinal SRS.[46] Of 29 patients treated at Stanford between 1997 and 2009, 22 were followed more than 24 months (unpublished data). Most had glomus AVMs and one had a type III lesion. Sixteen patients presented with hemorrhage and 8 had more than one bleed. Twelve lesions were cervical, 8 were thoracic, and 3 were in the conus. The usual treatment dose was 16 Gy in one session or 20 Gy in two sessions (with 10 Gy delivered to adjacent spinal cord). Ten patients (43%) were previously embolized. All postoperative MRIs in treated patients showed a reduction in volume. Of the 8 patients who had post-SRS angiography, 3 had complete obliteration. None of the treated patients suffered a rebleed, including those where the AVM was not obliterated by MRI or angiography. There was no mortality. Symptoms improved in over 50% and only 3 patients reported worsening of symptoms. There was only 1 case of radiation myelopathy (3%).

Treatment Failures and Complications

Treatment failures fall into several groups. "In-field failures" refer to tumor regrowth within the treated volume and may be related to inadequate dosing. "Marginal failures" involve regrowth at the edges of the treated volume and may be related to poor imaging, underestimation of the tumor volume, or inaccuracies in position or setup. "Distant failures" are not complications but rather involve new lesions in untreated areas. For vertebral metastases, the chance of an asynchronous metastasis in an adjacent level is only 5%.[47] Furthermore, neurologic damage can be divided into three groups: (1) acute complications that occur within 1 month are usually due to edema, are transient, and are treated with steroids; (2) subacute complications that occur 3 to 6 months after treatment, may be secondary to demyelination,

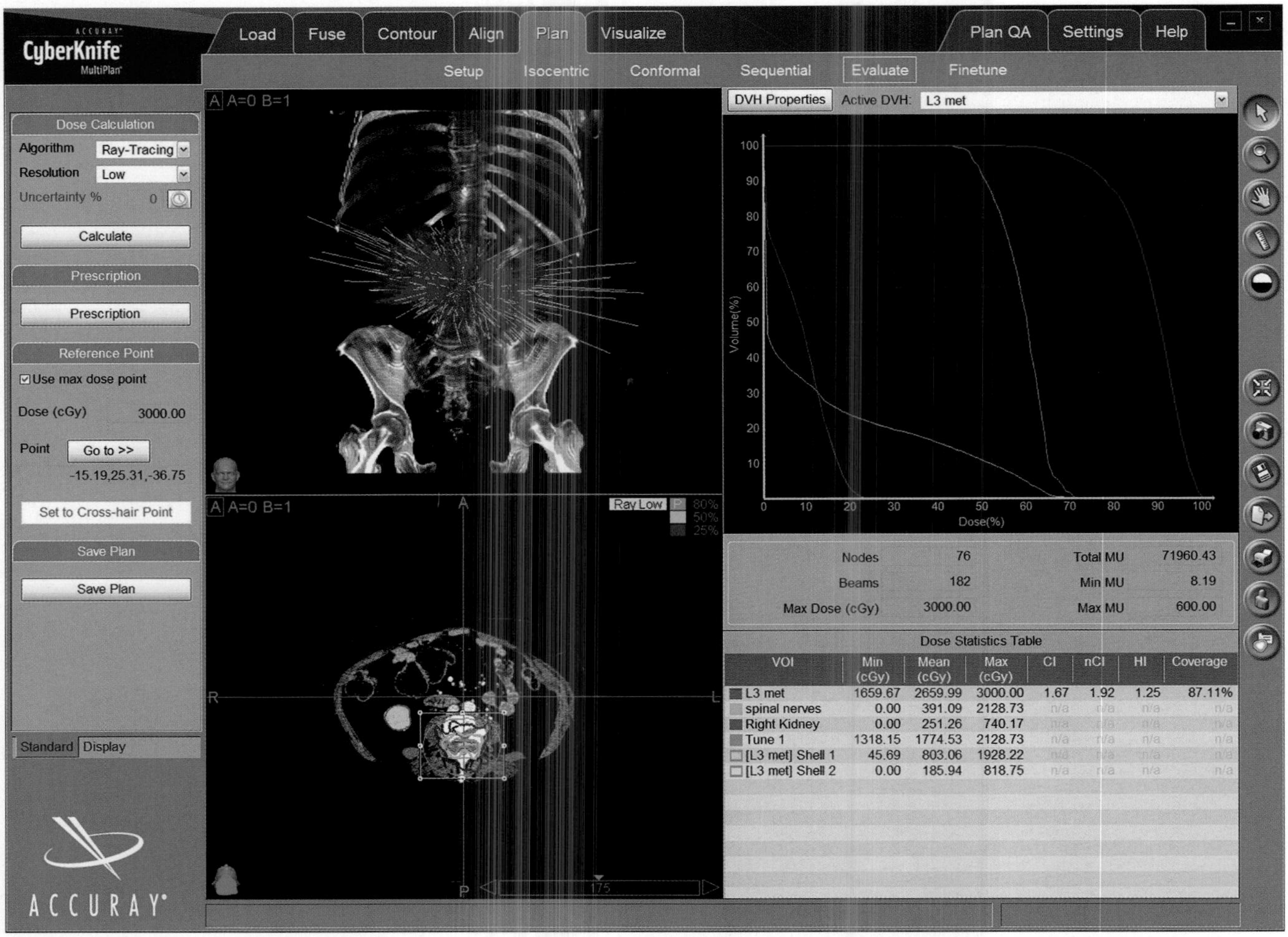

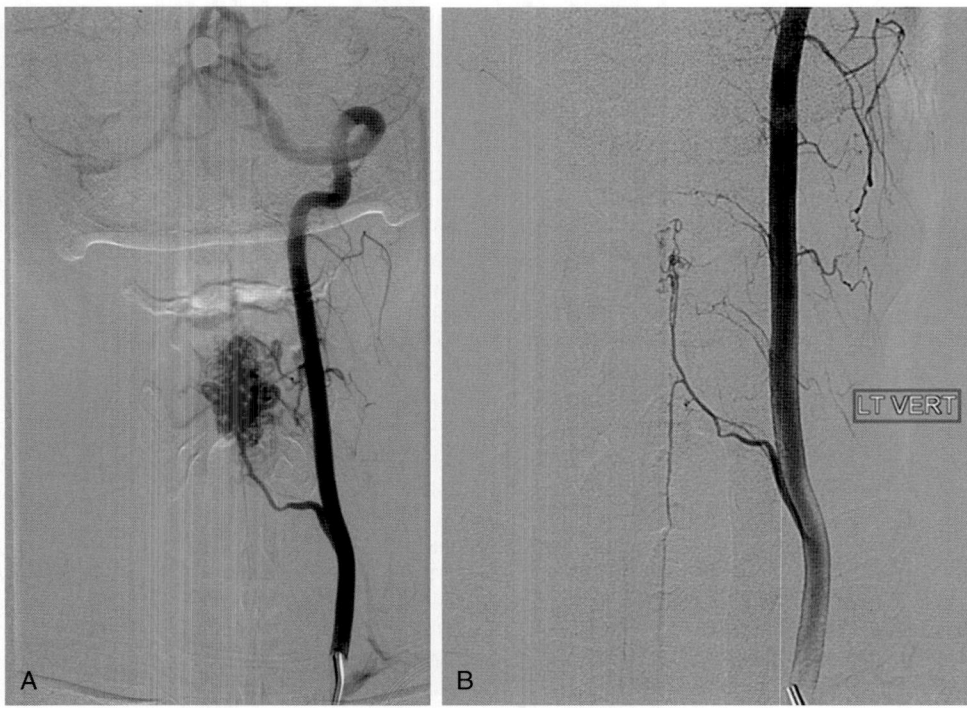

FIGURE 100-6 Contour of L3 metastasis and cauda equina with superimposed isodose lines from treatment plan in axial, saggital, and coronal projections. The epidural metastasis is in red, the spinal roots are blue, and the 80% isodose line is the smaller green line.

FIGURE 100-7 A, Spinal cord AVM prior to treatment. Note the compact nidus. B, Spinal cord AVM 3 years after SRS. Complete angiographic obliteration noted.

and usually recover; and (3) radiation myelopathy, which is the most feared complication and usually occurs after 6 months. The latter risk more than any other limits the radiosurgical dose used for most paraspinal lesions.[48] In conventional radiotherapy, it is generally believed that

treatment with 45 Gy in 22 to 25 fractions is associated with an incidence of myelopathy of only 0.2%. Meanwhile, among the first 1000 patients treated with the CyberKnife for spinal lesions at both Stanford and the University of Pittsburgh over the past decade, only 6 developed myelopathy (0.6%). In large part due to this 10-year track record with radiosurgery, a re-evaluation of the conventional wisdom and long-standing radiotherapy guidelines pertaining to spinal cord tolerance is taking place. Nevertheless, at Stanford we generally seek to avoid exposing more than 1 cm^3 of spinal cord to greater than 10 Gy in single-session plans.[49]

Other complications are rare and, fortunately, less severe. Skin reactions are seen most commonly when the posterior elements are radiated; nausea pharyngitis, esophagitis, and diarrhea are related to gastrointestinal tract exposure. Renal complications, occasionally related to thoracolumbar SRS, are rare.

Summary

While the complexity of spinal lesions and their close association with the cord make operative treatment difficult, it also makes them ideal candidates for spinal SRS. SRS, although a recent development, is supported by a rapidly expanding literature. For many lesions of the vertebral bodies, and some intradural, extramedullary lesions, CyberKnife radiosurgery is clearly both safe and effective. For vascular lesions, the treatment is superior to embolization and surgery for AVMs. Early results show that treatment of selected intramedullary lesions is also possible. It is likely that the indications will expand and the quality of the results will improve as our experience increases.

Table 100-1 Indications and Contraindications for Stereotactic Spinal Radiosurgery

Indications	Contraindications
Progressive but minimal neurologic deficit	Spinal instability (adjunctive treatment only)
Postresection or post-RT local irradiation (boost)	Neurologic deficit caused by bony compression
Disease progression after surgery and/or irradiation	Severe neurologic deficit due to cord compression
Inoperable lesions or high-risk lesion locations	Adjacent cord previously radiated to maximum dose
Medical comorbidities that preclude surgery	Very rare lesions not responsive to ionizing radiation
Lesions in patients who decline surgery	

Table 100-2 Treated/Treatable Lesions with CyberKnife Radiosurgery

Tumors

Benign

Neurofibroma, schwannoma, meningioma, hemangioblastoma, chordoma, paraganglioma, ependymoma, epidermoid

Malignant/Metastatic

Breast, renal, non–small-cell lung, colon, gastric and prostate metastases; squamous cell (laryngeal, esophageal, and lung) tumors; osteosarcoma; carcinoid; multiple myeloma; clear cell carcinoma; adenoid cystic carcinoma; malignant nerve sheath tumor; endometrial carcinoma; malignant neuroendocrine tumor

Vascular Malformations

Arteriovenous malformation (types 2 and 3)

Table 100-3 Literature Review: SRS for Spinal Vertebral Metastases

Site	Lesions/ Patients	Tumor Type	Modality	Dose/ Fractions	Contouring	Complications	Pain Reduced	Local Control	Overall Survival
Amdur, et al., 2009[27]	25/21	Various	LINAC/IMRT	15 Gy/1	Lesion with margin	No neurologic toxicity	43%	95%	25% at 1 year
Wowra, et al., 2009[29]	134/102	Various	CyberKnife	15–24 Gy/1	Not specified	No SRS-related neurologic deficits	86%	88%	Median survival 1.4 years
Yamada, et al., 2008[4]	103/93	Various	LINAC/IMRT	18–24 Gy/1	Entire vertebral body	No neurologic toxicity	Not reported	90%	36% at 3 years
Gibbs, et al., 2007[17]	102/74	Various	CyberKnife	14–25 Gy/1–5	Lesion only	3 cases myelopathy	84%	No symptom progression	46% at 1 year
Chang, et al., 2007[18]	74/63	Various	LINAC/IMRT	27–30 Gy/3–5	Entire vertebral body	No neurologic toxicity	60%	77%	70% at 1 year
Gerszten et al., 2007[30]	500/393	Various	CyberKnife	12.5–25 Gy/1	Lesion only	No neurologic toxicity	86%	90%	Not stated
Ryu, et al., 2006[31]	230/177	Various	LINAC/IMRT	8–18 Gy/1	Entire body with pedicles	1% risk of myelopathy	85%	96%	49% at 1 year
Milker-Zabel, et al., 2003[32]	19/18	Various	LINAC/IMRT or FCRT	24–45/ variable	Entire vertebral body	No neurologic toxicity	81%	95%	65% at 1 year

SRS, stereotactic radiosurgery.

KEY REFERENCES

Amdur RJ, Bennett J, Olivier K, et al. A prospective phase II study demonstrating the potential value and limitation of radiosurgery for spine metastases. *Am J Clin Oncol.* 2009;32:1-6.

Bhatnagar AK, Gerszten PC, Ozhasaglu C, et al. CyberKnife radiosurgery for the treatment of extracranial benign tumors. *Technol Cancer Res Treat.* 2005;4:571-576.

Chang SD, Le QT, Martin DP, et al. The CyberKnife. In: Fehlings MG, Gokaslan ZL, Dickman CA, eds. *Spinal Cord and Spinal Column Tumors: Principles and Practice.* New York: Thieme; 2006.

Chang EL, Shiu AS, Mendel E, et al. Phase I/II study of stereotactic body radiotherapy for spinal metastasis and its pattern of failure. *J Neurosurg Spine.* 2007;7:151-160.

Dodd RL, Ryu MR, Kamnerdsupaphon P, et al. CyberKnife radiosurgery for benign intradural extramedullary spinal tumors. *Neurosurgery.* 2006;58:674-685.

Gibbs IC, Kamnerdsupaphon P, Ryu MR, et al. Image-guided robotic radiosurgry for spinal metastases. *Radiother Oncol.* 2007;82:185-189.

Gerszten PC, Burton SA, Ozhasoglu C, et al. Radiosurgery for benign intradural spinal tumors. *Neurosurgery.* 2008;62:887-895.

Gerszten PC, Burton SA, Ozhasoglu C, Welch WC. Radiosurgery for spinal metastases. Clinical experience in 500 cases from a single institution. *Spine.* 2007;32:193-199.

Gerszten PC, Germanwala A, Burton SA, et al. Combination kyphoplasty and spinal radiosurgery: a new treatment paradigm for pathological fractures. *Neurosurg Focus.* 2005;18:E8.

Gerszten PC, Ozhasoglu C, Burton SA, et al. CyberKnife frameless real-time image-guided stereotactic radiosurgery for the treatment of spinal lesions. *Int J Radiat Oncol Biol Phys.* 2003;30:S370-S371.

Gibbs IC, Patil C, Gerszten PC, et al. Delayed radiation-induced myelopathy after spinal radiosurgery. *Neurosurgery.* 2009;64:A67-A72.

Kim LJ, Spetzler RF. Classification and surgical management of spinal arteriovenous lesions: arteriovenous fistulae and arteriovenous malformations. *Neurosurgery.* 2006;59:195-201.

Moss JM, Choi CY, Adler JR, et al. Stereotactic radiosurgical treatment of cranial and spinal hemangioblastomas. *Neurosurgery.* 2009;65:79-85.

Muacevic A, Staehler M, Drexler C, et al. Technical description, phantom accuracy, and clinical feasibility for fiducial free frameless real-time image-guided spinal radiosurgery. *J Neurosurg Spine.* 2006;5:303-312.

Murovic JA, Gibbs IC, Chang SD, et al. Foraminal nerve sheath tumors: intermediate follow-up after CyberKnife radiosurgery. *Neurosurgery.* 2009;64(Suppl):A33-A43.

Murphy MJ, Cox RS. The accuracy of dose localization for an image-guided frameless radiosurgery system. *Med Physics.* 1996;23:2043-2049.

Rampling R, Symonds P. Radiation myelopathy. *Curr Opin Neurol.* 1998;11:627-632.

Ryu SI, Chang SD, Kim DH, et al. Image-guided hypo-fractionated stereotactic radiosurgery to spinal lesions. *Neurosurgery.* 2001;49:838-846.

Ryu S, Jian-Yue J, Ryan J, et al. Partial volume tolerance of the spinal cord and complicationsof single-dose radiosurgery. *Cancer.* 2006;109:628-636.

Ryu S, Kim DH, Chang SD. Stereotactic radiosurgery for hemangioblastomas and ependymomas of the spinal cord. *Neurosurgery Focus.* 2003;15:1-5.

Ryu S, Rock J, Rosenblum M, et al. Pattern of failure after single dose radiosurgery for spinal metastasis. *Neurosurgery.* 2004;101:402-405.

Selch MT, Lin K, Agazaryan N, et al. Initial clinical experience with image-guided linear accelerator-based spinal radiosurgery for treatment of benign nerve sheath tumors. *Surg Neurol.* 2009;72:668-674.

Sinclair J, Chang SD, Gibbs IC, Adler JR. Multisession CyberKnife radiosurgery for intramedullary spinal cord arteriovenous malformations. *Neurosurgery.* 2006;58:1081-1089.

Yamada Y, Bilsky MH, Lovelock DM, et al. High-dose, single-fraction intensity-modulated radiotherapy for metastatic spinal lesions. *Int J Radiat Oncol Biol Phys.* 2008;71:484-490.

Yamada Y, Lovelock DM, Yenice KM, et al. Multifractionated image-guided and stereotactic intensity-modulated radiotherapy of paraspinal tumors: a preliminary report. *Int J Radiat Oncol Biol Phys.* 2005;62:53-61.

Numbered references appear on Expert Consult.

Stereotactic Radiosurgery for Pituitary Adenomas

DANIEL Q. SUN • SACHIN BATRA • JUAN JACKSON •
ROBERTO SALVATORI • DANIELE RIGAMONTI

This chapter focuses on the use of gamma knife stereotactic radiosurgery (GKSRS) in the treatment of secretory and non-functional pituitary adenomas (NFPAs). GKSRS is most often used as an adjuvant to surgical resection and medical management to induce biochemical remission of endocrinologically active adenomas or to halt tumor progression in NFPAs (Figs. 101-1 and 101-2). Other modalities of irradiation, such as fractionated radiosurgery (FSR), have also been used and continue to play a specific role in certain clinical scenarios. In many situations, however, the exact role of GKSRS is still incompletely understood, mostly due to lack of data with long-term follow-up. Therefore, the care of patients with pituitary adenomas necessitates an interdisciplinary approach with collaboration between endocrinologists, neurosurgeons, radiation oncologists, and ophthalmologists.

Adrenocorticotropic Hormone-Producing Tumors

Cushing's disease is associated with significant morbidity and premature death. Up to 30% of patients may experience persistent or recurrent disease after trans-sphenoidal surgery.[1] Most studies define remission as normalization of 24-hour, urine-free cortisol (UFC) in the absence of medical suppression. Remission rates after radiotherapy reported in literature vary widely from 17% to 83% due to varying indications for radiosurgery, dosing, definitions of remission, and follow-up length. The time to remission also varies widely, from 2 months to 8 years,[2] although the majority occur within 2 years of radiosurgery.[1]

Jagannathan et al.[3] reviewed the GK radiosurgery experience in 90 patients with Cushing's disease treated between 1990 and 2005, all of whom either had at least 12 months of follow-up postirradiation or experienced remission within 12 months of treatment. Patients presenting with Nelson's syndrome were not included in this study. Indication for GK radiosurgery in all patients was persistent elevation of 24-hour UFC following surgical resection. The mean follow-up length post-GK was 45 months (range 12–132 months), and the mean marginal dose was 23 Gy (median 25 Gy). At the time of treatment, only 49 patients (54%) had tumors that were visible on magnetic resonance imaging (MRI). Remission was defined as normalized 24-hour UFC without

concomitant medical therapy. Remission was achieved in 54% of patients at an average time of 13 months after radiosurgery (range 2–67 months). In patients with MRI-evident tumors, tumor volume decreased in 80%, remained constant in 14%, and increased in 6%. Of the patients who experienced biochemical remission, 20% suffered relapse at a mean time of 27 months (range, 6–60) after remission. Radiosurgical complications included hormone deficiencies in 22% of patients diagnosed at a mean time of 16 months (range, 4–36 months) after GKS and cranial nerve (CN) and visual field deficits in 5% of patients.

In the above study, no correlation between either maximum dose, marginal dose, or treatment volume and biochemical remission or tumor control was found, consistent with findings from another recent study.[4] In two other studies,[5,6] however, the authors found the maximum dose and prescription isodose volume to be significantly correlated with hormone response, although it is worth noting that when analyzing hormone response, these two studies lumped all functioning adenomas, and therefore the specific applicability of the conclusions to Cushing's disease may be brought into question. Indeed, as mentioned previously, functioning adenomas show differential responses to irradiation as reflected by their differential response rates.[7] To maximize the likelihood of treatment success, many authors[3,5] advocate the use of more than 20 Gy at the 50% prescription isodose line when safe to do so.

Endocrinologic relapse after initial remission is an important problem in Cushing's disease and, in some series,[3,4,7] occurs in approximately 20% of patients cured by radiosurgery. In the Jagannathan et al. study,[3] recurrence occurred at a mean time of 27 months after radiosurgery and 43% had their disease brought into remission again after a second radiosurgery treatment. In the study with the longest follow-up to date (mean follow-up of 94 months), Castinetti et al.[4] observed a 50% cure rate in 18 patients with Cushing's disease and recurrence in two patients (11%) at 6 and 8 years after initial treatment. Therefore, long-term endocrinologic follow-up is recommended.

Patients undergoing bilateral adrenalectomy due to persistent Cushing's disease risk the development of Nelson syndrome, characterized by aggressive growth of the residual ACTH-secreting adenoma due to a reduced feedback inhibition by cortisol. Periodic imaging and monitoring of

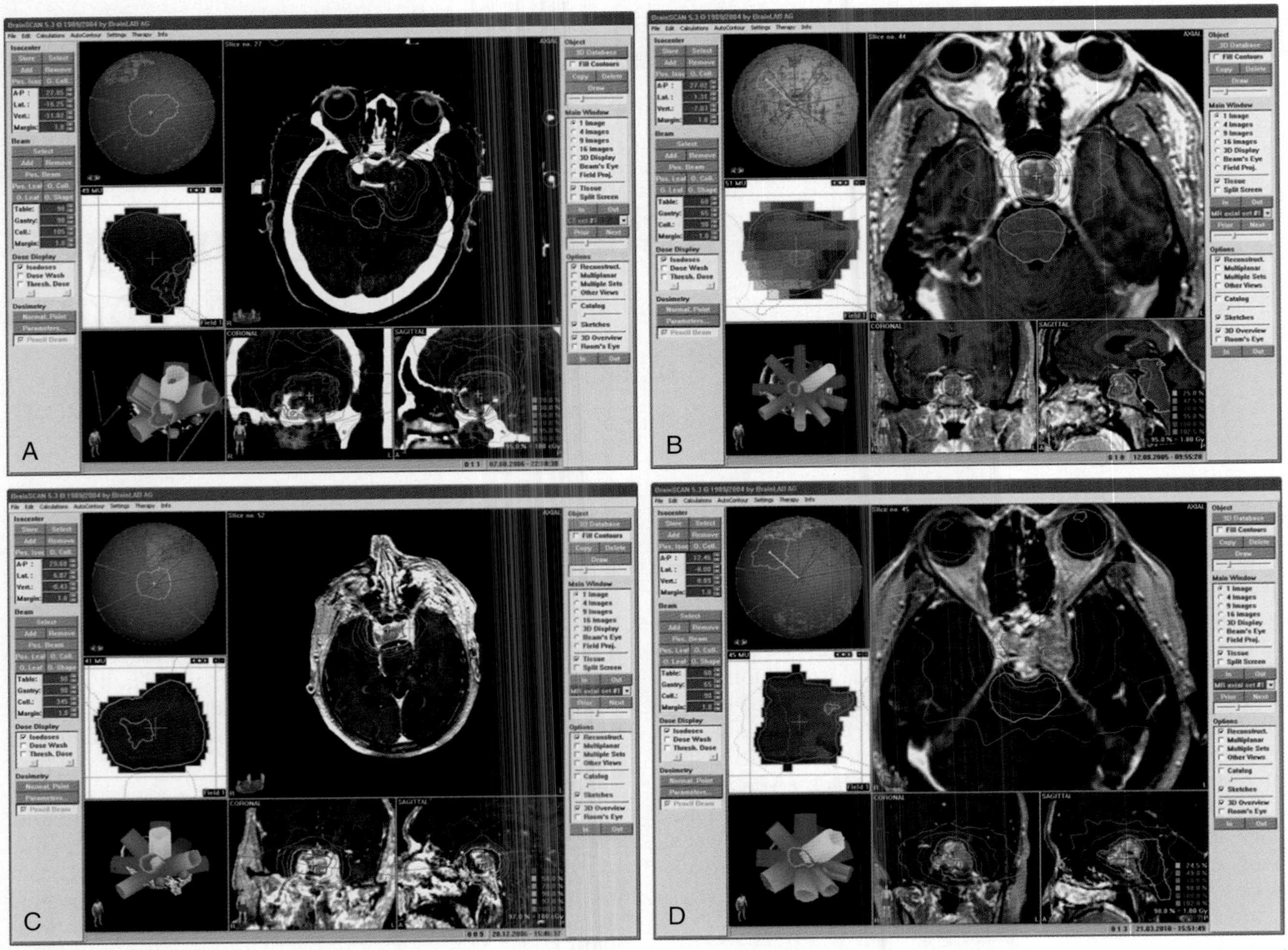

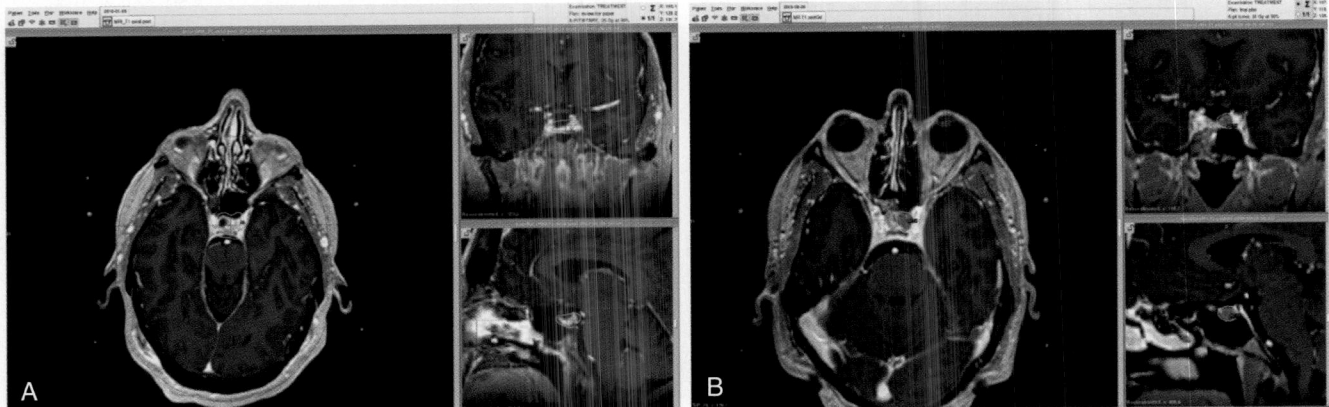

FIGURE 101-1 Image-guided radiosurgical planning for pituitary adenomas. A, A 53-year-old woman presenting with worsening headaches and galactorrhea found to have a 3.5-cm prolactinoma with left cavernous sinus extension. After subtotal transcranial resection, she received 25 Gy to the residual tumor that successfully induced biochemical remission. B, A 39-year-old man presenting with acromegaly and a 1.5-cm GH-secreting adenoma. After subtotal trans-sphenoidal resection, he received 18 Gy and experienced hypopituitarism and a moderate decrease in IGF-1, still necessitating medical therapy. C, An 81-year-old man presenting with a 1.6-cm NFPA treated with 16 Gy after subtotal resection. He has intact visual function without tumor progression or hypopituitarism. D, A 72-year-old male with a 3-cm NFPA with suprasellar and cavernous sinus extension and recurrence after multiple surgeries. He was treated with fractionated stereotactic radiosurgery (50.4 Gy over 28 fractions) due to proximity to the optic chiasm, which has been successful in halting tumor progression but complicated by decline in visual function and a sellar hematoma postradiation. NFPA, nonfunctional pituitary adenoma.

FIGURE 101-2 Image-guided radiosurgical planning for LGK. A, A 58-year-old woman with 1.1-cc growth hormone–releasing pituitary adenoma refractory to medical management and surgical resection treated with 25 Gy to the 50% isodose line using LGK. B, A 43-year-old man with 4.0-cc nonfunctional pituitary adenoma recurrent after gross total resection was treated with 20 Gy to the 50% isodose line using LGK. The optic chiasm received 2.2 Gy. LGK, Leksell Gamma Knife.

plasma ACTH levels have allowed early detection and treatment of these tumors. Corticotroph growth is rare in radiated patients, but may occur in up to 50% of nonradiated patients within 3 years of adrenalectomy.[8] Few studies have been conducted to specifically investigate the safety and efficacy of stereotactic radiosurgery for Nelson syndrome. Nonetheless, GKSRS seems to offer a favorable tumor control rate of 82% to 100% and some authors have reported endocrinologic remission rates of up to 36%.[9-11]

Growth Hormone–Producing Tumors

Biochemical remission for growth hormone (GH)–producing pituitary adenomas is commonly defined as normalization of age- and sex-adjusted serum level of insulin-like growth factor-1 (IGF-1) in the absence of medical therapy, as well as a basal GH level of less than 2.5 µg/L or less than 1 µg/L after glucose challenge (see Figs. 101B and 102A).[1,4,12-14] In general, GH-secreting adenomas are particularly resistant to the effects of radiation. In a retrospective study[13] of 83 patients with GH-secreting pituitary adenomas and acromegaly who received stereotactic radiosurgery as treatment for residual or recurrent disease following trans-sphenoidal surgery, biochemical remission was achieved in 60% of patients with a median follow-up of 69 months. The 5-year remission rate was 52%. Two patients experienced tumor progression, which occurred outside the treated volume. The median marginal dose at the 50% prescription isodose line was 21.5 Gy, no patients suffered CN toxicities, and hypopituitarism occurred in 8.5% of patients. Biochemical recurrence occurred in 1 patient and was managed medically. For patients with somatostatin analog-resistant tumors ($n = 13$), the authors found a much lower 16% remission rate.

In GH-secreting tumors lower basal GH levels are associated with increased rate of cure after radiosurgery. Losa et al.,[13] using multivariate analysis, found increased likelihood of remission when basal GH levels were below 7.0 µg/L and basal multiples of upper limit (mUNL) IGF-1 levels were below 1.83 times UNL, with hazard ratios of 2.7 (95% confidence interval [CI] = 1.4–5.3) and 2.6 (95% CI = 1.3–5.1), respectively. This finding has since been replicated by Castinetti et al.[4] in a series of 43 acromegalic patients with a mean follow-up of 102 months (42% remission). In these studies, radiation dose did not have a statistically significant impact.

There is emerging evidence that somatostatin analogs, when present at the time of radiosurgery, have a detrimental effect on achieving biochemical remission. In the initial study by Landolt et al.,[15] 9 patients treated with octreotide at time of radiosurgery were compared to 22 patients who did not receive octreotide at time of radiosurgery but had baseline characteristics with respect to age, sex, GH and IGF-1 levels at time of radiosurgery, treatment volume, and radiation dose. While patients who did not receive octreotide achieved a remission rate of 60%, patients who received octreotide achieved a remission rate of only 20% at 3-year follow-up. The radioprotective effect of octreotide has since been observed in other studies as well,[12,16] albeit inconsistently.[4,13] It is hypothesized[15] that antisecretory agents such as octreotide may exert a radioprotective effect by decreasing cell cycling and thereby render cells less vulnerable to radiation-induced DNA damage. Based on these data, it is recommended that patients undergoing stereotactic

radiosurgery for GH-releasing pituitary adenomas discontinue somatostatin-analogs at least 2 months prior to, and not resume them until 6 weeks after, radiosurgery. It is important to note however, that patients in these studies were not randomized and therefore selection biases, such as patients on octreotide were likely to have more severe and intractable disease, cannot be excluded.

Prolactin-Producing Tumors

Due to prolactin-secreting tumors' robust response to dopamine-agonists, radiosurgery is commonly the last-line treatment, reserved for tumors that fail medical management and trans-sphenoidal resection (see Fig. 101A). In a retrospective study[17] of 23 patients with medically and surgically refractory prolactinomas treated by GK, biochemical remission was achieved in 26% of patients with an average time of 24.5 months. Remission was defined as normalized serum prolactin without concomitant dopamine-agonist therapy. Volumetric control of tumors was achieved in 89% of patients with shrinkage in 46%. The mean marginal dose was 18.6 Gy. Pituitary insufficiency occurred in 28% of patients with an average time to onset of 44 months. Moreover, one patient developed a 3rd CN palsy and another patient a 6th CN palsy. Both patients suffered from tumors with cavernous sinus extension and were treated with a maximum dose of 50 Gy. The remission rate reported here is consistent with other series.[4,7,18,19] Among functional adenomas, prolactin-secreting tumors have been reported in a study to be the least responsive to irradiation.[7] However, the study with the longest follow-up[4] showed similar remission rates for secretory tumors (42%, 46%, and 50% of patients with GH-, PRL-, and ACTH-secreting adenomas, respectively). The difference was the mean time to remission (50, 24, and 28 months for GH-, PRL-, and ACTH-secreting adenomas, respectively), suggesting again that GH-secreting adenomas are more resistant to the effects of radiosurgery. Although no study has specifically addressed the issue of fertility after radiosurgery for prolactin-secreting adenomas, Landolt and Lomax[18] observed that 2 out of 11 patients with normalized serum prolactin became pregnant spontaneously.

It has been found[17] that biochemical remission was significantly associated with a tumor volume of less than 3 cc. Moreover, analogous to GH-secreting adenomas, dopamine-agonist therapy at the time of radiosurgery decreases the likelihood of achieving biochemical remission.[17,18] The investigation of factors important to remission is hampered by the small number of patients in each series, resulting in few series with sufficient statistical power to address this issue, and also increasing the likelihood of spurious associations due to selection bias. Moreover, it has been observed[2] that radiosurgery to the pituitary may cause an increase in serum prolactin, possibly via radiation-induced injury to the infundibulum, that may last several years and obscure its tumor-toxic effects.

Nonfunctional Adenomas

Stereotactic radiosurgery is a treatment option for nonfunctional pituitary adenomas (NFPAs) that exhibit parasellar extension and/or recurrent growth after surgical resection (see Figs. 101C and D and 101-2B). The primary goal of adjuvant radiosurgery is to halt tumor progression and preserve the integrity of CN function especially with respect to the optic apparatus. Losa et al.[20] conducted a retrospective study analyzing the outcomes of 54 patients who had undergone GKRS for residual tumor after surgical resection. Cavernous sinus extension was present in 77.8% of patients, 29.6% of patients had visual deficits, while 3.7% had oculomotor deficits. Treatment characteristics included mean target volume of 2.3 cc and marginal dose of 16.6 Gy at the 50% isodose line. The mean follow-up length was 41 months. Tumor control was achieved in all but 2 patients during the study period, with 42.3% of patients experiencing a tumor volume decrease of 20% or more. The recurrence-free interval at 5 years was 88.2% (95% CI 72.6–100%). Recurrence in 2 patients was detected at 40 and 49 months, occurring outside the treated volume in both cases. No patient in this series experienced new or worsened neurological deficits while 23.4% suffered some form of hypopituitarism during the study period.

Most series[21-25] have shown tumor growth control of at least 90% using radiosurgery with up to 25% risk of new-onset pituitary insufficiency and up to 5% risk of new visual deficits. Especially worth noting is the similar rate of success in the control of tumors with parasellar extension, which would otherwise be untreatable. For instance, in a series of 61 tumors with parasellar extension treated by radiosurgery,[1] volume reduction occurred in 63%, remained constant in 27%, and tumor growth occurred in 10%.

Chang et al.[26] specifically examined the indications for radiotherapy by retrospectively studying the outcomes of 663 patients who received surgical resection between 1975 and 1995 for NFPAs. Although patients were not randomized, changing practice patterns allowed the authors to analyze the relationship between extent of surgical resection, radiotherapy, and tumor control. Increased recurrence was correlated with subtotal resection without adjuvant radiotherapy, while radiotherapy after gross-total resection had no effect on recurrence. Therefore, radiation seems specifically indicated as adjuvant therapy in patients with subtotal resection of NFPAs and provides excellent tumor control rates with a moderate risk of pituitary insufficiency, necessitating long-term monitoring (see Fig. 101-2D). On the other hand, the natural history of residual pituitary adenomas without extrasellar remnant seems to show that not all of them will have clinically significant growth, and therefore a watchful waiting approach with periodic MRI imaging needs to be considered particularly in young patients who may desire fertility.[27]

Complications

CRANIAL NERVE DEFICITS

Damage to the optic apparatus is a major morbidity associated with irradiation of the sella while targeting parasellar tumors risks damage to CNs 3, 4, and 6. The rate of visual complications, defined as visual field defect or CN 3, 4, or 6 palsy, following radiosurgery for functional or nonfunctional pituitary adenomas is 0% to 7%.[3,13,17,23,24] The optic apparatus is especially sensitive to irradiation and it is recommended that the maximum dose to the chiasm not

exceed 8 to 10 Gy,[28,29] although some authors have advocated the use of up to 12 Gy.[30] Radiation toxicity may occur at any dosage however, and has been documented after as little as 0.7 Gy (Fig. 101-1C and D).[25] The tolerable dose likely varies from patient to patient, and is greatly affected by factors such as age, previous irradiation, degree of compression by the adenoma, and comorbidities such as diabetes. For adenomas located so close to the optic apparatus that a sufficient dose fall-off cannot be achieved to spare the optic chiasm, fractionated radiosurgery should be chosen to decrease the risk of visual deficits after radiosurgery. CN 3, 4, and 6 appear to be much more resistant to radiation toxicity. In a review of 35 studies involving 1621 patients, Sheehan et al.[25] identified only 21 patients with CN 3, 4, or 6 neuropathies, most of which were transient.

HYPOPITUITARISM

Radiation-induced pituitary insufficiency is a major risk for all patients undergoing sellar irradiation (see Fig. 101-1B). Currently, there is a lack of reliable data regarding the quantitative risk of developing hypopituitarism, defined as any new hormone deficiency, following radiosurgery. Most series have found a prevalence of 0%–36%[3,31,32] in treated patients, although these findings have been hampered by lack of long-term follow-up, variable means of evaluation of pituitary function, and heterogeneous tumor and treatment characteristics. Despite an earlier report of up to 76%[2] rate of hypopituitarism in patients followed for 17 years, Hoybye Rahn[21] recently found the rate of hypopituitarism to be surprisingly low in a group of 23 patients treated with GK and followed for a median of 97 months, with no new hormone deficiencies discovered. The study population was highly selected, however, with small tumor volumes and radiation targeting parasellar extensions, thereby hampering the generalizability of the results. Pollock et al.[23] found a significant association between tumor volume and the risk of developing hypopituitarism at 5 years. While 50% of patients with tumors larger than 4 cc developed hypopituitarism by 5 years, the prevalence was only 18% for patients with tumor volumes smaller than 4 cc.

RADIATION-INDUCED NEOPLASMS

The study of radiation-induced neoplasms is hampered by the long time scale over which lesions develop and the difficulty in causally linking any specific lesion to previous radiation. Therefore, although radiation-induced neoplasms are exceedingly rare, their true incidence is unknown. In order for a tumor to be considered causally linked to radiosurgery, the tumor must (1) occur within the previous radiation field, (2) not be present prior to radiosurgery, (3) be histologically distinct from any primary tumor, (4) not develop in the setting of a genetic predisposition in the host, and (5) develop during an expected latency period of roughly 5 years.[25] Only three cases[33-35] have been reported in the radiosurgery literature comprised of more than 200,000 patients that meet the above criteria. In one patient,[33] a malignant transformation of a vestibular schwannoma occurred 6 months following adjuvant GKSRS to treat residual tumor. The dose at the 50% isodose line was 15 Gy. In another patient with vestibular schwannoma treated by GKSRS (11 Gy at the 40% isodose line), a glioblastoma multiforme (GBM) occurred in the radiation scatter field

7.5 years after GKSRS.[35] In the third patient, a GBM occurred following GKSRS (20 Gy peripheral dose) for an arteriovenous malformation 6.5 years after radiosurgery.[34]

Summary

Gamma knife SRS is a safe and effective adjuvant treatment for patients with secretory or non-functional pituitary adenomas. Secretory adenomas show differential response to GKSRS based on tumor type.[7] The biochemical remission rates on long term follow-up are similar for patients with ACTH-, GH- or prolactin secreting adenomas, however the length of time to remission varies, with prolcatinomas having the longest time to remission. GKSRS is indicated for patients with NFPAs and subtotal surgical resection or parasellar extension. It offers an excellent tumor control rate of greater than 90%. Major complications from GKSRS include radiation-induced CN deficits and hypopituitarism. Up to 7% of patients may suffer visual field deficits due to radiation injury to the optic apparatus while CN 3, 4, and 6 appear to be much more resistant to irradiation. Hypopituitarism has been observed in approximately 36% of patients, although there is a lack of long-term data. Other complications, such as damage to the internal carotid artery in the cavernous sinus, brain parenchyma, and radiation-induced neoplasms have been shown to be extremely rare.[1]

KEY REFERENCES

Castinetti F, Nagai M, Morange I, et al. Long-term results of stereotactic radiosurgery in secretory pituitary adenomas. *J Clin Endocrinol Metab.* 2009;94:3400-3407.

Chang EF, Zada G, Kim S, et al. Long-term recurrence and mortality after surgery and adjuvant radiotherapy for nonfunctional pituitary adenomas. *J Neurosurg.* 2008;108:736-745.

Girkin C, Comey C, Lunsford L, et al. Radiation optic neuropathy after stereotactic radiosurgery. *Ophthalmology.* 1997;104:1634-1643.

Höybye C, Rähn T. Adjuvant gamma knife radiosurgery in non-functioning pituitary adenomas; low risk of long-term complications in selected patients. *Pituitary.* 2009;12:211-216.

Höybye C, Grenbäck E, Rähn T, et al. Adrenocorticotropic hormone-producing pituitary tumors: 12- to 22-year follow-up after treatment with stereotactic radiosurgery. *Neurosurgery.* 2001;49:284-292.

Jagannathan J, Sheehan J, Pouratian N, et al. Gamma knife radiosurgery for acromegaly: outcomes after failed transsphenoidal surgery. *Neurosurgery.* 2008;62:1262-1269.

Jagannathan J, Sheehan JP, Pouratian N, et al. Gamma knife surgery for Cushing's disease. *J Neurosurg.* 2007;106:980.

Jagannathan J, Yen C-P, Pouratian N, et al. Stereotactic radiosurgery for pituitary adenomas: a comprehensive review of indications, techniques and long-term results using the gamma knife. *J Neurooncol.* 2009;92:345-356.

Kim S, Huh R, Chang J, et al. Gamma knife radiosurgery for functioning pituitary adenomas. *Stereotact Funct Neurosurg.* 1999;72:101-110.

Landolt A, Lomax N. Gamma knife radiosurgery for prolactinomas. *J Neurosurg.* 2000;93:14-18.

Landolt AM, Haller D, Lomax N, et al. Octreotide may act as a radioprotective agent in acromegaly. *J Clin Endocrinol Metab.* 2000;85:1287-1289.

Losa M, Gioia L, Picozzi P, et al. The role of stereotactic radiotherapy in patients with growth hormone-secreting pituitary adenoma. *J Clin Endocrinol Metab.* 2008;93:2546-2552.

Mokry M, Ramschak-Schwarzer S, Simbrunner J, et al. A six year experience with the postoperative radiosurgical management of pituitary adenomas. *Stereotact Funct Neurosurg.* 1999;72:88-100.

O'Sullivan E, Woods C, Glynn N, et al. The natural history of surgically treated but radiotherapy-naïve nonfunctioning pituitary adenomas. *Clin Endocrinol (Oxf).* 2009;71:709-714.

Pollock B, Brown P, Nippoldt T, Young WJ. Pituitary tumor type affects the chance of biochemical remission after radiosurgery of hormone-secreting pituitary adenomas. *Neurosurgery.* 2008;62:1271-1276.

Pollock B, Nippoldt T, Stafford S, et al. Results of stereotactic radiosurgery in patients with hormone-producing pituitary adenomas: factors associated with endocrine normalization. *J Neurosurg.* 2002;97:525-530.

Pollock BE, Cochran J, Natt N, et al. Gamma knife radiosurgery for patients with nonfunctioning pituitary adenomas: results from a 15-year experience. *Int J Radiat Oncol Biol Phys.* 2008;70:1325-1329.

Pollock BE, Jacob JT, Brown PD, Nippoldt TB. Radiosurgery of growth hormone–producing pituitary adenomas: factors associated with biochemical remission. *J Neurosurg.* 2007;106:833.

Pollock BE, Young WF. Stereotactic radiosurgery for patients with ACTH-producing pituitary adenomas after prior adrenalectomy. *Int J Radiat Oncol Biol Phys.* 2002;54:839-841.

Pouratian N, Sheehan J, Jagannathan J, et al. Gamma knife radiosurgery for medically and surgically refractory prolactinomas. *Neurosurgery.* 2006;59:255-266.

Sheehan JP, Kondziolka D, Flickinger J, Lunsford LD. Radiosurgery for residual or recurrent nonfunctioning pituitary adenoma. *J Neurosurg.* 2002;97:408.

Sheehan JP, Niranjan A, Sheehan JM, et al. Stereotactic radiosurgery for pituitary adenomas: an intermediate review of its safety, efficacy, and role in the neurosurgical treatment armamentarium. *J Neurosurg.* 2005;102:678.

Stafford S, Pollock B, Leavitt J, et al. A study on the radiation tolerance of the optic nerves and chiasm after stereotactic radiosurgery. *Int J Radiat Oncol Biol Phys.* 2003;55:1177-1181.

Tishler R, Loeffler J, Lunsford L, et al. Tolerance of cranial nerves of the cavernous sinus to radiosurgery. *Int J Radiat Oncol Biol Phys.* 1993;27:215-221.

Numbered references appear on Expert Consult.

Radiation Therapy and Radiosurgery in the Management of Craniopharyngiomas

ANAND VEERAVAGU • MARCO LEE • BOWEN JIANG • JOHN R. ADLER, JR. • STEVEN D. CHANG

Craniopharyngiomas are benign extra-axial epithelial tumors that arise from squamous epithelial remnants of Rathke's pouch, near the pituitary gland.[1] These cells may extend from the nasopharynx to the tuber cinereum and may arise within the sphenoid bone, the sella, or the suprasellar region. Although craniopharyngiomas are rare, they are the most common suprasellar tumor in the pediatric age group, accounting for as many as 5% of all intracranial tumors or up to 10% of pediatric brain tumors.[2] Its incidence has been estimated to be about 1.5 per million persons per year,[3,4] but may be considerably higher in specific ethnic groups, such as Japanese children (5.25 per million).[5] Craniopharyngiomas have a bimodal age distribution, generally appearing in young patients between the ages of 5 and 14 years and in adults between 50 and 74 years.

Despite being histologically benign, craniopharyngiomas can cause severe and often permanent damage to nearby hypothalamic, visual, and endocrine apparatus. The presentation of these tumors may include symptoms related to endocrine derangement of the hypothalamic–pituitary axis, with severity dependent upon location, size, and rate of growth. Mass effect from the tumor may result in increased intracranial pressure presenting as headache, nausea, and vomiting. Cases with larger mass lesions may also present with hydrocephalus (seen more commonly in children than in adults), as a result of the obstruction of the cerebral aqueduct or the interventricular foramina.[6,7] Compression of the nearby optic apparatus typically results in visual field defects, such as chiasmal syndrome and papilledema. Endocrine disruption often manifest as amenorrhea, hypothyroidism, and diabetes insipidus.[8,9]

The structural composition of these tumors may include solid, cystic, mixed solid and cystic or calcified components. Traditionally, craniopharyngiomas have been separated into either the adamantinomatous or papillary variety. More commonly observed in the pediatric population, the adamantinomatous type is characterized as calcified with mixed composition. Papillary craniopharyngiomas seen in adults are often more solid.

Current treatment strategies include cystic drainage, intracavity chemotherapy, limited or gross total resection, and radiation therapy. These strategies are often combined in a patient-specific treatment plan based on age at presentation, tumor size, relation to optic chiasm and third ventricle, presence of hydrocephalus, and degree of pituitary endocrinopathy. If total excision can be safely performed with minimal risk to these structures, then surgery remains the treatment of choice as this allows rapid decompression, minimizes recurrence, and provides a histologic diagnosis. However, judgment of minimal risk is often unclear as some favor subtotal resection coupled with adjunctive therapy to achieve similar outcomes.[10-18] Although surgical approaches are often curative, they harbor high treatment-related morbidity and mortality due to the close proximity of crucial neurovascular structures. Recurrent craniopharyngiomas must be considered separately, as secondary surgery is associated with higher risk of complications and a lower cure rate.[16,19-23] More recently, stereotactic radiosurgery techniques have become increasingly utilized as either a primary or secondary treatment for craniopharyngioma patients.

Surgical Outcomes

Complete surgical resection is a primary objective and has curative potential. In a recent series by Shi et al., 284 patients (58 children) were treated surgically, without adjunctive therapy, between 1996 and 2006. Total, subtotal, and partial removal of the tumors were achieved in 237 (83.5%), 34 (12.0%), and 13 (4.5%) patients, respectively.[24,25] Upon follow-up, 23 (14.1%) patients experienced recurrence 1 to 3.5 years after total resection, and 24 (64.9%) recurred after 0.25 to 1.5 years after subtotal or partial resection. In this series, the early mortality rate was 4.2%. In another 25-year retrospective study by Van Effenterre and Boch, 122 patients underwent gross total (59%), subtotal (29%), or partial (12%) surgical resection. During the follow-up period, 29 patients (24%) experienced one or more recurrences. The delay to recurrence was 1 to 180 months (mean 42 months, median 12 months). Patients that underwent total, subtotal, or partial removal experienced 13%, 33%, and 69% recurrence, respectively. Radiotherapy was reserved only for cases of recurrence. The surgical mortality rate was 2.5% and overall survival was 95% at two years, 91% at 5 years, and 83% at 10 years.[26]

The comparison of surgical complications across various series produces a variable picture. Most of the recent large series report a total resection rate of 59% to 90%.[16,26-28]

The 10-year recurrence-free survival rates have been reported as 74% to 81% for gross total resection,[23,29,30] 41% to 42% after partial removal,[31,32] and 83% to 90% after combined surgery and radiotherapy.[18,42] Surgical mortality rates vary between 1.1% and 4.2%.[16,26,28,33] It is well documented that recurrent tumors are associated with significantly higher risk and poorer outcome, with overall mortality rates reported between 10.5% to 40.6%.[16, 28] Pituitary dysfunction may occur in 50% to 100% of patients, the most common being diabetes insipidus. Visual deterioration may occur in up to 50% of patients undergoing gross total resection.[34]

Radiation Therapy for Craniopharyngiomas

While surgical drainage or resection may be the initial step in management, the rate of complete obliteration is low with one modality alone. The fine balance between further neurologic deficit and complete tumor resection has led to the use of various noninvasive forms of therapy. Radiation therapy is often applied during the postoperative course in the event of subtotal resection or tumor recurrence. Frequently, external radiation therapy is the preferred strategy; however, in recent years endocavitary/intracavitary radiation and stereotactic radiosurgery have also demonstrated efficacy in tumor control.

ENDOCAVITARY RADIATION THERAPY

Endocavitary/intracavitary irradiation with a beta-emitter (^{186}Re, ^{32}P, ^{198}Au, ^{90}Y) or an antitumoral antibiotic (bleomycin) can be used to treat purely cystic or cystic components of craniopharyngiomas.[35] This treatment modality requires the use of stereotactic technique to achieve intracystic instillation of radioactive agents. In a recent retrospective study of endocavitary irradiation (^{186}Re) treatment by Derrey et al., of 48 patients treated, complete cystic resolution was achieved in 17 patients (44%) and partial resolution in another 17 patients (44%). Visual function improved in 12 patients, while baseline endocrine function was preserved.[35] Similarly, Julow and colleagues observed an 80% reduction in 47 patients and complete disappearance of cyst in 27 patients within 1 year after treatment with intracystic colloidal yttrium-90.[36] Across several studies, the response rate of tumors to endocavitary/intracavitary irradiation is 71% to 88%.[37,38] However, because intracavitary irradiation is limited to cystic tumors, recurrence, and survival rates with this type of therapy alone are considered inferior to surgery or external radiotherapy.[24,38] Additionally, the risk of visual deterioration is considerable, possibly due to unpredictable radiation dose to the optic pathway and radiation damage from leakage. In a review by Caceres, no change or improvement in visual acuity after intracavitary irradiation ranged from 42% to 99% while 31% to 58% experienced deterioration in visual function.[39]

EXTERNAL BEAM RADIATION THERAPY

Fractionated radiation therapy improves craniopharyngioma control and survival[32,40-44] and is the standard treatment for residual or recurrent tumor. Most series demonstrate that when combined with subtotal resection, adjuvant radiotherapy allows for greater tumor control and

survival than surgery alone.[31, 45-49] In a study by Varlotto et al.,[49] an 89% tumor control rate was seen in patients who received both subtotal resection and external beam irradiation.[39] Stripp and colleagues[48] compared 57 patients treated only with surgery to 18 treated with subtotal resection combined with radiation therapy, demonstrating a 10-year tumor control rate of 42% and 84%, respectively. The case for primary radiation therapy for recurrent craniopharyngioma is even stronger for lower risk and better outcome (30% vs. 90% 10-year progression-free survival).[12,50-52] Finally, Karavitaki and colleagues examined the records of 121 patients and subdivided the patients into four treatment categories: gross total removal, gross total removal with radiotherapy, partial removal, and partial removal with radiotherapy. The recurrence-free survival rate was 100% at 10 years in the gross total removal and gross total removal with radiotherapy groups, 38% in the partial removal group, and 77% in the partial removal with radiotherapy group.[34]

With radiotherapy, the risk of neurotoxicity from radiation injury should be considered alongside gains in potential tumor control. Conventionally fractionated focal radiation therapy around the sellar–suprasellar region is also associated with risks similar to surgery. Disruption of the hypothalamic-pituitary axis (30% to 70%) may result in diabetes insipidus, panhypopituitarism, hypogonadism, hypothalamic obesity, or sleep disturbance.[53-55] The normal optic apparatus is particularly sensitive to radiation, and optimized dose and fractionation regimes carry a 3% risk of optic neuropathy.[56-58] There is also considerable discussion about the effect of radiation on cognitive function, an issue particularly pertinent in the pediatric population. Additionally, radiation itself carries the risk of secondary malignancies,[59-61] radiation necrosis,[61,62] and vasculopathy, which also have end-neurodegenerative effects.

Typically, craniopharyngiomas are treated with doses between 45 and 60 Gy in 1.8- to 2-Gy fractions to prevent growth of tumor and minimize injury to the visual pathways. Long-term (10 years) local control ranges from 31% to 42% with surgery alone compared with 57% to 89% with surgery and radiotherapy.[31,32,45,47-49] However, there are limitations as the wide treatment field includes irradiating many structures, such as the optic apparatus, pituitary gland, hypothalamus, and medial temporal lobe. The risk may only manifest itself after a long delay, but this is particularly important since benign conditions such as craniopharyngiomas confer favorable long-term survival and its predilection for the pediatric population. Another limitation is when conventional radiotherapy fails, it almost inevitably precludes further radiotherapy treatment to the recurrent tumor. Finally, although of minor importance, conventional fractionated radiotherapy usually takes place over a 6-week course, which is less attractive to patients when compared to other shorter treatment courses. For these reasons, radiosurgery (particularly multisession radiosurgery) may present a more amenable option, especially to tumors surrounding the optic apparatus.

STEREOTACTIC RADIOSURGERY

Stereotactic radiosurgery (SRS) is a relatively recent therapeutic option that has significantly improved the effectiveness of and morbidity associated with radiation therapy. With SRS, one to five sessions of radiation are utilized to treat residual or recurrent lesions. The application of stereotaxis for target localization, treatment planning, and daily treatment immobilization allows for a more precise delivery of radiation dose with a steeper dose gradient between tumor and parenchymal tissue to prevent further neurologic deficit. The irradiation dose can be delivered using either a multiple cobalt-60, gamma radiation-emitting source such as a gamma knife (GK) or a modified linear accelerator (LINAC, CyberKnife). Most stereotactic systems can deliver a radiation beam with no more than approximately 1 mm of error. Historically, SRS for craniopharyngiomas was limited to tumors 3 cm or less that are 3 to 5 mm away from the optic chiasm and nerves. In the case of single-session radiosurgery, the optic chiasm becomes a limiting anatomic structure capable of only receiving 8 to 10 Gy per session before the incidence of optic neuropathy increases.[63,64] More recent multisession radiosurgery using image-guided radiosurgical techniques has allowed for treatment of craniopharyngiomas immediately adjacent to the anterior visual pathways.[65]

In the current literature, several studies have reported safe and effective long-term results with the application of SRS using a GK for the treatment of craniopharyngiomas.[66-69] Kobayashi et al. published the largest treatment and outcomes series with 98 cases. At a mean marginal dose of 11.5 Gy and a mean tumor size of 3.5 cm^3, Kobayashi and colleagues observed a tumor control rate of 79.6%, with a complete response in 19.4% and partial response in 67.4% of the cases.[70] The actuarial 5- and 10-year survival rates were 94.1% and 91% with respective progression-free survival rates of 60.8% and 53.8%. Yomo and colleagues demonstrated the outcomes of 18 patients with residual or recurrent craniopharyngioma who were treated by the Leksell Gamma Knife Model C. Tumor growth (mean tumor volume of 1.8 cm^3 and a mean marginal irradiation dose of 11.6 Gy) was controlled in 17 cases (94%), and volume reduction was attained in 13 cases (72%).[71] No new endocrinopathy was observed and 3 patients experienced substantial improvement of visual functions following shrinkage of the neoplasm. In another study by Chung et al., tumor control was achieved in 87% of the 31 patients and 84% had fair to excellent clinical outcome.[72] Finally, Minniti et al. completed a meta-analysis of eight published studies that includes 252 patients who underwent either unfractionated radiosurgery or GK therapy, demonstrating a tumor control rate of 69%. Taken together (Table 102-1), the published studies on GK therapy for craniopharyngiomas demonstrate an average control rate of 90% for solid tumors, 88% for cystic tumors, and 60% for mixed tumors.[73] Tumor control was achieved with a mean marginal dose of 12 Gy and recurrence of tumor was observed in 85% of cases that received a marginal dose of less than 6 Gy.

With the current advances in image-guided radiosurgical technology, the principle of multi-session delivery of radiosurgery can be incorporated with the anatomic precision and conformality of radiosurgery. This allows for the precise delivery of potentially safer radiation doses than encountered in single session radiosurgery, while exploiting the volume effect by applying higher and more effective doses than was possible with conventional radiation therapy. The multisession delivery approach is particularly pertinent in treating craniopharyngiomas, which are often located near delicate neurovascular structures. The tolerance of these critical structures to radiation depends on the amount of radiation being received, volume of tissue irradiated, previous insult, and prior radiotherapy. Due to the proximity of the tumors to the optic apparatus, single doses of 8 to 10 Gy appear tolerable to avoid damage to nearby structures.[24] Higher doses to optic nerve are associated with increasing rates of deficit. Leber et al. reported that optic neuropathy occurred in 22 (26.7%) patients who received 10 to 15 Gy and 13 (78%) of patients who received more than 15 Gy, while 31 patients who received less than 10 Gy were without optic insult.[64] Likewise, Stafford and colleagues observed optic neuropathy in <2% of patients who received 8 to 10 Gy and in 6.9% who received more than 12 Gy after treatment with RS for benign tumors of the sellar or parasellar region.[73,74]

Cyberknife SRS for Craniopharyngiomas: Our Experience

In a study by Lee et al.,[75] 11 patients with residual craniopharyngiomas within 2 mm of the optic apparatus or pituitary gland were treated with the CyberKnife SRS System (Accuray, Sunnyvale, CA). The clinical presentation, surgical history, radiation received, and outcome of these 5 male and 6 female patients with an average age of 34.5 years are documented in Tables 102-2 and 102-3. A mean marginal dose of 21.6 Gy prescribed to a mean isodose line of 75% was applied over multiple sessions (Figure 102.1). The mean maximum dose was 29.9 Gy and the mean target volume was 6 cm^3. Patient outcomes were quantified using magnetic resonance imaging (MRI) and formal Goldman visual field assessments at 6 months intervals for two years, then once every year. Prior to CyberKnife therapy, 10 patients suffered from a degree of visual loss while 5 had endocrine abnormalities requiring hormonal replacement. Ten patients had operative reports documenting a subtotal resection with radiologic confirmation and one had a complete resection with follow-up MRI demonstrating recurrence 1 year after surgery. Residual tumor was most often located in the suprasellar region and in 10 cases was found to be against or displacing the optic nerve or chiasm. The pituitary stalk alone was compressed in 1 patient.

The mean follow-up time was 15.4 months (range, 4 to 64 months). All 10 patients with visual field or acuity problems either improved or remained stable after CyberKnife radiosurgery. In this series, treatment plans were designed to keep the dose experienced by the optic apparatus less than 5 Gy during any single session. The volume of the optic apparatus that received 80% of the prescribed dose was less than 0.05 cm^3, whereas the volume that received 50% of the dose was less than 0.5 cm^3. Therefore, the actual volume of the optic segment that received 5 Gy would be small relative to the total volume of the optic apparatus. Preservation of baseline visual function is supported by our previous work which showed that the risk of visual loss with multi-session radiosurgery appears to be low for perioptic tumors.[65,76] Radiation-induced optic neuropathy is a known entity that tends to present over the course of several years; however, our study's short follow-up prevents definitive conclusions regarding the effect of multisession therapy.

Table 102-1   Published Series of Patients Who Underwent SRS for Craniopharyngioma

Authors & Year	Study Country	Intervention	Number of Patients	Mean Marginal Dose	Mean Size of Tumor	Outcome
Miyazaki et al., 2009[79]	Japan	CyberKnife RS	13	22.7 Gy	N/A	Tumor shrinkage in 6/13 patients, and tumor control in 5. 2 patients had cystic enlargement of the residual tumor followed by microsurgical resection.
Yomo et al., 2009[71]	Japan	Gamma knife RS	18	11.6 Gy	1.8 cm³	Tumor growth controlled in 17 (94%), with volume reduction in 13 (72%). 3 patients had improved visual symptoms after SRS.
Kobayashi et al., 2009[70]	Japan	Gamma knife RS	98	11.5 Gy	3.5 cm³	Complete 19.4% and partial 67.4% response. Tumor control 79.6% and progression rate 20.4%. Patient outcome was excellent in 45 cases, good in 23, fair in 4, and poor in 3. 16 patients died and deterioration of visual and endocrinologic functions occurred in 6 (6.1%) cases.
Lee et al., 2008[75]	United States	CyberKnife RS	11	21.6 Gy	5.9 cm³	Tumor shrinkage in 7/11 patients, and tumor control in 3. 1 patient had cystic enlargement of the residual tumor. Control or shrinkage of tumor in 91% of patients, with no visual or neuroendocrine complications.
Minniti et al., 2007[78]	United Kingdom	SCRT	39	50 Gy	10.2 cm³	3- and 5-year progression-free survival, 97% and 92%. 3- and 5-year survival 100%. 12 (30%) patients had acute clinical deterioration due to cystic enlargement post-SCRT and required cyst aspiration. 1 patient with post-SCRT visual deterioration. 7/10 patients no further endocrine deficits following treatment.
Combs et al., 2007[80]	Germany	FSRT	40	52.2 Gy	13.3 cm³	Local control 100% at 5 and 10 years. Survival rates at 5 and 10 years, 97% and 89%, respectively. Complete response in 4 and partial response in 25 cases. 11 patients had stable disease at follow-up.
Giller et al., 2005[81]	United States	CyberKnife RS	3	42 Gy	1.14 cm³	Tumor regression without visual changes was achieved in all three patients at 29, 39, and 40 months after treatment, respectively.
Albright et al., 2005[82]	United States	Gamma knife RS	5	N/A	6.5 cm³	There was no morbidity or mortality from gamma knife RS, which achieved tumor stabilization or shrinkage in 4/5 cases.
Amendola et al., 2003[83]	United States	Gamma knife RS	14	14 Gy	3.7 cm³	All patients alive and without evidence of recurrent disease 6–86 months after treatment.
Selch et al., 2002[68]	United States	FSRT	16	55 Gy	7.7 cm³	3-year actuarial survival 93% and rate of survival free of imaging evidence of progressive disease was 75%. 3-year actuarial survival rates free of solid tumor growth or cyst enlargement were 94% and 81%, respectively.
Ulfarsson et al., 2002[69]	Sweden	Gamma knife RS	21	3–25 Gy	7.8 cm³	5/22 tumors reduced in size, 3 unchanged, and 14 increased. 11/13 (85%) tumors that received <6 Gy to the margin increased in size, whereas only 3/9 (33%) of tumors that received 6 Gy increased. In 5/6 patients tumors that became smaller after gamma knife RS there were no recurrences within a mean follow-up period of 12 years. 9/11 (82%) tumors in children ultimately increased after gamma knife RS, compared to 5/10 (50%) in adults. 8 patients had deterioration of visual function. 4 patients developed pituitary deficiencies.
Chiou et al., 2001[66]	United States	Gamma knife RS	10	16 Gy	1.7 cm³	7/12 tumors became smaller or resolved within median 8.5 months. Prior visual defects improved in 6 patients. 1 patient with prior visual defect deteriorated further and lost vision 9 months after RS.
Yu et al., 2000[84]	China	Gamma knife RS	46	8–18 Gy	13.5 cm³	Tumor control rate was 90% in solid tumors, 85.7% in mixed tumors, 92.1% in the solid segment, and 89.5% in total.
Chung et al., 2000[72]	Taiwan	Gamma knife RS	31	12 Gy	8.9 cm³	Tumor control was achieved in 87% of patients and 84% had fair to excellent clinical outcome at 36 months follow-up. Treatment failure in 4 patients. Only 1 patient with restricted visual field; no additional endocrinologic impairment or neurologic deterioration. No treatment-related mortality.
Mokry et al., 1999[85]	Austria	Gamma knife RS	23	10.8 Gy	7.0 cm³	Volume reduction in 74% of cases. Smaller tumors and targets more likely to shrink. 5 patients with large multicystic residual or recurrent tumors showed further progression.
Prasad et al., 1995[86]	United States	Gamma knife RS	9	13 Gy	10 cm³	Decrease in solid component of tumor in 5 patients with no change in 2. 1 patient increase in solid tumor component. Clinical improvement in 6/8 cases.

FSRT, fractionated stereotactic radiotherapy; RS, radiosurgery; SCRT, stereotactically guided conformational radiotherapy; SRS, stereotactic radiosurgery.

Table 102-2   Patient Characteristics Undergoing CyberKnife Radiosurgery for Residual Craniopharyngioma between 2000 and 2007

Case No.	Age (yr), Sex	Presentation	No. of Surgery	Postoperative RT	Pre-SRS Visual Problems	Pre-SRS Endocrine Problems	No. of Sessions	Treatment Dose (Gy)	Mean Isodense line (%)	Max Dose (Gy)	Target Volume (cm³)
1	32, F	HA, VFD	3	N	Y	N	3	18	75	22.5	1.4
2	16, F	HA, VFD	2	Y	Y	N	3	19.5	80	24.3	12.7
3	71, M	N&V, VFD	1	N	Y	N	3	20	74	26.6	0.7
4	45, F	HPP, VFD	2	N	Y	Y	5	20	77	26	1.1
5	43, M	HPP, VFD	2	N	Y	Y	10	38	72	42.1	26.3
6	17, F	HA, VFD	1	N	Y	N	4	20	77	24.1	1.2
7	13, F	Weightt gain, HPP	3	N	N	Y	5	27.5	71	36.7	10.1
8	20, M	VFD, HPP	1	N	Y	Y	5	25	76	30.5	0.3
9	39, F	HA, VFD	2	N	Y	N	5	25	67	33.3	6.3
10	37, M	HA, VFD	3	N	Y	N	5	25	73	31.7	3.8
11	46, M	HPP, VFD	1	N	Y	Y	5	25	80	31.3	1.3

HA, headache; HPP, hypopituitarism; N&V, nausea and vomiting; VFD, visual field deficit

Table 102-3   Summary of 11 Patients and Treatment Planning Characteristics Included in Analysis

Gender (No.)	
Male	5
Female	6
Age (years)	
Mean	34.5 (range, 13–71)
Previous Surgery (No.)	
1	4
2	4
3	3
Previous Radiotherapy (No.)	1
Extent of Last Resection (No.)	
Complete	1
Subtotal	10
Site of residual or recurrent tumor	
Intrasellar	1
Suprasellar	9
Both	1
Against optic apparatus	8
Against pituitary stalk or gland	1
Both	2
CyberKnife Sessions (No.)	
3	3
4	1
5	6
10	1
Mean Target Volume (cm³)	6 (range, 0.3–26.3)
Mean Marginal Dose (Gy)	21.6 (range, 18–38)
Mean Maximal Dose (Gy)	29.9 (range, 24.1–42.1)

There were no new neuroendocrine problems and the five patients with endocrine derangement remained stable with no new deterioration after CyberKnife treatment. Tumor shrinkage was seen in seven patients, with three staying the same at 2 years post-treatment, resulting in

a 91% tumor control rate. One patient developed a cystic enlargement of the residual tumor without any worsening symptoms or signs. Irradiation of cystic craniopharyngiomas may result in cystic enlargement, which does not represent tumor recurrence and may later regress.[77] In our series, the patient's symptoms remained stable; however, rigorous clinical and radiologic including visual and neuroendocrine assessment is critical. We believe that multisession treatment regimens minimize the risk to the optic apparatus and pituitary gland while delivering an appropriate amount of radiation for disease control.

Conclusion

Optimal management of craniopharyngiomas remains controversial. Their location often implicates vital structures that may be subjected to undue harm. Because radical surgical resection is associated with a high rate of visual loss and impaired hormone function requiring replacement therapy, many authors recommend minimal surgery (subtotal resection or biopsy) followed by radiation therapy, given that extensive surgery is not required to decompress mass effect. As technology continues to improve, precision and delivery of radiotherapy increase its efficacy in tumor control. Our experience demonstrates that multisession therapy may spare unintended consequences to surrounding optic structures and provide significant disease control. Although further long-term studies are required to fully evaluate clinical outcome, current evidence suggests beneficial results may be obtained with sparing of critical neurovascular structures that often surround the tumor.

DISCLOSURE AND ACKNOWLEDGMENT

Drs. Adler and Chang are shareholders of Accuray, Inc. Steven D. Chang, MD, is supported in part by a research gift from Robert C. and Jeannette Powell.

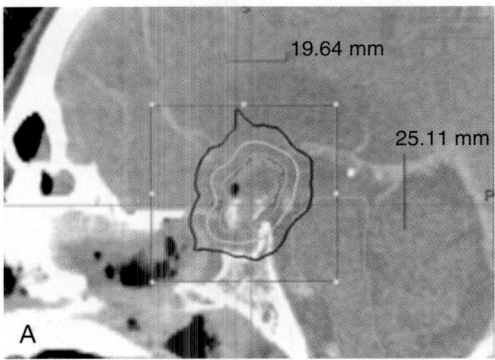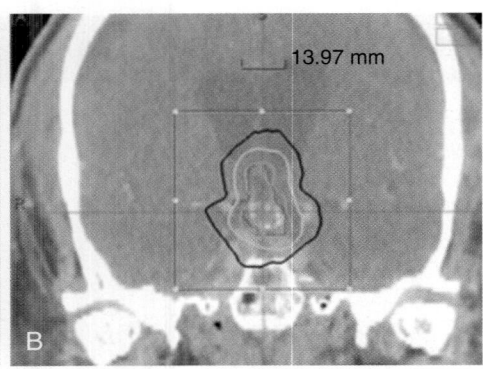

FIGURE 102-1 A typical CyberKnife treatment plan for a craniopharyngioma tumor shown in sagittal (A) and coronal (B) views.

KEY REFERENCES

Adler Jr JR, Gibbs IC, Puataweepong P, et al. Visual field preservation after multisession CyberKnife radiosurgery for perioptic lesions. *Neurosurgery.* 2006;59:244-254:discussion 244–254.

Derrey S, Blond S, Reyns N, et al. Management of cystic craniopharyngiomas with stereotactic endocavitary irradiation using colloidal 186. Re: a retrospective study of 48 consecutive patients. *Neurosurgery.* 2008;63:1045-1052:discussion 1052-1053.

Fisher BJ, Gaspar LE, Noone B. Radiation therapy of pituitary adenoma: delayed sequelae. *Radiology.* 1993;187:843-846.

Flickinger JC, Lunsford LD, Singer J, et al. Megavoltage external beam irradiation of craniopharyngiomas: analysis of tumor control and morbidity. *Int J Radiat Oncol Biol Phys.* 1990;19:117-122.

Garre ML, Cama A. Craniopharyngioma: modern concepts in pathogenesis and treatment. *Curr Opin Pediatr.* 2007;19:471-479.

Girkin CA, Comey CH, Lunsford LD, et al. Radiation optic neuropathy after stereotactic radiosurgery. *Ophthalmology.* 1997;104:1634-1643.

Gopalan R, Dassoulas K, Rainey J, et al. Evaluation of the role of gamma knife surgery in the treatment of craniopharyngiomas. *Neurosurg Focus.* 2008;24:E5.

Hetelekidis S, Barnes PD, Tao ML, et al. 20-year experience in childhood craniopharyngioma. *Int J Radiat Oncol Biol Phys.* 1993;27:189-195.

Honegger J, Buchfelder M, Fahlbusch R. Surgical treatment of craniopharyngiomas: endocrinological results. *J Neurosurg.* 1999;90:251-257.

Jane Jr JA, Laws ER. Craniopharyngioma. *Pituitary.* 2006;9:323-326.

Karavitaki N, Cudlip S, Adams CB, et al. Craniopharyngiomas. *Endocr Rev.* 2006;27:371-397.

Kobayashi T. Long-term results of gamma knife radiosurgery for 100 consecutive cases of craniopharyngioma and a treatment strategy. *Prog Neurol Surg.* 2009;22:63-76.

Leber KA, Bergloff J, Pendl G. Dose–response tolerance of the visual pathways and cranial nerves of the cavernous sinus to stereotactic radiosurgery. *J Neurosurg.* 1998;88:43-50.

Minniti G, Esposito V, Amichetti M, et al. The role of fractionated radiotherapy and radiosurgery in the management of patients with craniopharyngioma. *Neurosurg Rev.* 2009;32:125-132:discussion 132.

Moon SH, Kim IH, Park SW, et al. Early adjuvant radiotherapy toward long-term survival and better quality of life for craniopharyngiomas–a study in single institute. *Childs Nerv Syst.* 2005;21:799-807.

Pollock BE, Lunsford LD, Kondziolka D, et al. Phosphorus-32 intracavitary irradiation of cystic craniopharyngiomas: current technique and long-term results. *Int J Radiat Oncol Biol Phys.* 1995;33:437-446.

Rajan B, Ashley S, Gorman C, et al. Craniopharyngioma–long-term results following limited surgery and radiotherapy. *Radiother Oncol.* 1993;26:1-10.

Shi XE, Wu B, Zhou ZQ, et al. Microsurgical treatment of craniopharyngiomas: report of 284 patients. *Chin Med J (Engl).* 2006;119:1653-1663.

Stafford SL, Pollock BE, Leavitt JA, et al. A study on the radiation tolerance of the optic nerves and chiasm after stereotactic radiosurgery. *Int J Radiat Oncol Biol Phys.* 2003;55:1177-1181.

Stripp DC, Maity A, Janss AJ, et al. Surgery with or without radiation therapy in the management of craniopharyngiomas in children and young adults. *Int J Radiat Oncol Biol Phys.* 2004;58:714-720.

Ulfarsson E, Lindquist C, Roberts M, et al. Gamma knife radiosurgery for craniopharyngiomas: long-term results in the first Swedish patients. *J Neurosurg.* 2002;97:613-622.

Van Effenterre R, Boch AL. Craniopharyngioma in adults and children: a study of 122 surgical cases. *J Neurosurg.* 2002;97:3-11.

Varlotto JM, Flickinger JC, Kondziolka D, et al. External beam irradiation of craniopharyngiomas: long-term analysis of tumor control and morbidity. *Int J Radiat Oncol Biol Phys.* 2002;54:492-499.

Yasargil MG, Curcic M, Kis M, et al. Total removal of craniopharyngiomas. Approaches and long-term results in 144 patients. *J Neurosurg.* 1990;73:3-11.

Yomo S, Hayashi M, Chernov M, et al. Stereotactic radiosurgery of residual or recurrent craniopharyngioma: new treatment concept using Leksell Gamma Knife Model C with automatic positioning system. *Stereotact Funct Neurosurg.* 87:360-367, 2009.

Numbered references appear on Expert Consult.

Vestibular Schwannomas: The Role of Stereotactic Radiosurgery

DOUGLAS KONDZIOLKA • L. DADE LUNSFORD • AJAY NIRANJAN • HIDEYUKI KANO • JOHN C. FLICKINGER

Acoustic neuromas (vestibular schwannomas) are generally slow-growing, intracranial extra-axial benign tumors that usually develop from the vestibular portion of the eighth nerve.[1] Bilateral vestibular schwannomas are usually associated with neurofibromatosis 2 (NF2). Both unilateral and bilateral vestibular schwannomas may form due to malfunction of a gene on chromosome 22, which produces a protein (schwannomine/merlin) that controls the growth of Schwann cells. In NF2 patients, the faulty gene on chromosome 22 is inherited and is present in all or most somatic cells. However, in individuals with unilateral vestibular schwannoma, for unknown reasons this gene loses its ability to function properly and is present only in the schwannoma cells.[2]

A progressive unilateral hearing decline is the most common symptom that leads to the diagnosis of a vestibular schwannoma.[3] In years past it was rare for patients to present with intact hearing, but this is becoming more common due to earlier diagnosis and higher-quality magnetic resonance imaging (MRI). Overall, three separate growth patterns can be distinguished[1]: no or very slow growth,[2] slow growth (i.e., 2 mm/year linear growth on imaging studies),[3] and fast growth (i.e., >8 mm/year). Although most tumors grow slowly, some grow quickly and can double in volume within 6 months to a year.[4] Cystic vestibular schwannomas are sometimes capable of relatively rapid enlargement of their cystic component. Although rare, other tumors may hemorrhage spontaneously.[5] Stereotactic radiosurgery has greatly expanded the management options since patients no longer have to choose simply between resection and observation.

We believe that early diagnosis is crucial to preventing functional decline. In addition to the three primary options of surgical removal, radiosurgery, and observation with serial imaging studies, some centers suggest conformal fractionated radiation therapy using linear accelerators or proton beam irradiation.

Observation with Serial Imaging

In some cases, usually elderly or medically infirm patients or individuals with very small tumors, it may be reasonable to "watch" the tumor for potential growth.[6] Repeat MRI scans over time are used to carefully monitor the tumor for any growth.[7] The object of serial observation is to obviate treatment unless signs of growth are confirmed.[6,8] In our 20-year experience 70% of tumors under observation have measurable growth in 5 years and almost all by 10 years. Recent published series continue to note annual tumor growth rates in the 1 to 3 mm/year range, with some evidence that extracanalicular tumors grow at a faster rate. This could be due to an easier appreciation of volumetric growth with a larger lesion.

Considering Radiosurgery Versus Surgical Resection

Resection is indicated for larger tumors with disabling brainstem compression, hydrocephalus, intractable headache, or trigeminal neuralgia. The majority of patients have smaller tumors and do not have these problems. The three main surgical avenues include the retrosigmoid, translabyrinthine, and middle fossa approaches.[9,10] As discussed elsewhere in this text, several factors help in the decision on which approach is optimal. Although the outcomes of surgical removal at centers of excellence have improved markedly over the last two decades, patients increasingly seek lesser invasive options. It is important to understand the differences between approaches.

First, preservation of facial function varies according to tumor size and the surgeon's experience.[11] When tumors are smaller than 1.5 cm, good facial nerve function can be expected (House-Brackmann grades I–II) in more than 90% of patients who have surgery at centers of excellence. Only 3.2% to 6.7% of patients with smaller tumors have poor facial nerve outcomes (House-Brackmann grades III–V). In addition to tumor size, intraoperative electrophysiologic facial nerve monitoring assists the surgeon to save the nerve.[12] The overall facial nerve anatomic preservation rate is 80%.[13] However, facial nerve function (grades I and II) can be preserved in only 40% to 50% of patients with large (>4-cm diameter) tumors.[14] Injuries of the nervus intermedius are underestimated because this nerve is rarely assessed preoperatively.[15]

Second, hearing preservation rates have also improved. Depending on the criteria used for reporting successful hearing conservation, preservation has been reported in

30% to 80% of patients considered eligible for hearing preservation surgery.[16] A meta-analysis performed by Gardner and Robertson in 1988 revealed an overall average success rate of about 33%.[17] Delayed hearing deterioration may occur days to years after surgery in 30% to 50% of patients who originally had successful hearing preservation.[18-21] In various studies, serviceable hearing preservation rates vary from 8% to 57%[18,22,23] using the retrosigmoid approach and from 32% to 68%[23] using the middle fossa approach.

Tinnitus is a frequent symptom at presentation. It is reported to worsen in 6% to 20% of individuals after tumor removal. In the majority of individuals, tinnitus remains unchanged. Approximately 25% to 60% of patients experience a decrease in tinnitus. Of patients without preoperative tinnitus, 30% to 50% developed it in the immediate postoperative period. Tinnitus appears to mimic phantom limb pain in the sense that it may remain even in the absence of preserved hearing.

Cerebrospinal fluid leakage through either the surgical incision or the Eustachian tube and middle ear occurs in 2% to 20% of patients.[20,21,24-26] Although in individual published reports the cerebrospinal fluid leak rate appears higher with the retrosigmoid approach (2.9%–18%),[23] a recent meta analysis suggests similar rates of cerebrospinal fluid leak for all surgical approaches (10.6% of 2273 retrosigmoid surgeries; 9.5% of 3118 translabyrinthine surgeries; and 10.6% of 573 middle fossa surgeries). The adjunctive use of endoscopy may assist the surgeon to avoid or to detect a CSF leakage.[27] Other rarer perioperative complications include death (0%–3%),[28,29] intracranial hematomas (1%–2%), wound hematoma (3%), cerebellar and brainstem edema, hemiparesis, meningitis (1.2%), wound infections (1.2%), abducens nerve paresis (1%–2%), and other lower cranial nerve injuries.[25,29]

Overall, tumor recurrence rates of 5% to 10% are found in the published literature, although a few studies report no long term recurrence after translabyrinthine approach.[30] However, incomplete resection of vestibular schwannomas is associated with a significant risk of tumor progression requiring subsequent intervention.[31]

The Patients' Perspective on Resection

A variety of complications have been reported after vestibular schwannoma surgery.[32-38] Studies from the Acoustic Neuroma Association are a good resource.[39] Bateman et al., described patients' subjective condition after vestibular schwannoma surgery as impairment (141, 51%), disability (95, 34%) or handicap (43, 15%).[40] Most of the impairments were related to problems with facial nerve function. The other most common issues were "balance problems" (19/141, 13%) followed by "hearing loss" (17/141, 12%) and "difficulty with background noise" (14/141, 10%). Tinnitus accounted for 5 of 141 responses (4%). Disabilities resulting from facial nerve dysfunction accounted for most of the disabilities reported by patients. A significant number of disabilities were associated with balance problems (e.g., "unable to drive," "problems changing direction," "unable to swim, cycle, run, climb steps, do aerobics," and "problems bending down") and with hearing loss (e.g., "difficulty locating the source of sounds," "difficulty following conversations in a crowd," "unable to hear people to one side" and "unable to hear doorbell/telephone").

Some patients reported symptoms of social isolation after the surgery. Fifteen out of forty-three responses (35%) were "reluctance to attend large social gatherings." Employment-related problems were also important with 7 of 43 responses (16%).

Stereotactic Radiosurgery

Vestibular schwannoma stereotactic radiosurgery using the gamma knife was first performed by Leksell in 1969.[41] During the past two decades radiosurgery has emerged as an effective alternative to surgical removal of small- to moderate-sized vestibular schwannomas (Figs. 103-1 and 103-2). Long-term results have established radiosurgery as an important minimally invasive alternative to resection. Advanced multi-isocenter dose-planning software, high-resolution MRI for targeting, dose optimization, and robotic delivery reflect the evolution of this technology. Other image-guided linear accelerator (LINAC) devices (Trilogy, Synergy S, Novalis and CyberKnife) generally can be used to fractionate radiation delivery in 5 to 30 sessions. Proton beam technology is also used to deliver fractionated radiation therapy. The goals of vestibular schwannoma radiosurgery are to prevent further tumor growth, preserve neurologic function where possible, avoid the risks associated with open resection, and in selected patients to improve pre-existing symptoms.

RADIOSURGERY TECHNIQUE FOR VESTIBULAR SCHWANNOMAS

Patients with vestibular schwannomas are evaluated with high-resolution MRI (CT may be substituted in patients who cannot undergo MRI scans) and audiologic tests that include pure tone average (PTA) and speech discrimination score (SDS) measurements. Hearing is graded using the Gardner-Robertson modification of the Silverstein and Norell classification and/or the American Academy of Otolaryngology-Head and Neck Surgery guidelines, and facial nerve function is assessed according to the House-Brackmann grading system. "Serviceable" hearing (classes I and II) is defined as a PTA or speech reception threshold lower than 50 dB and speech discrimination score better than 50%. The Committee on Hearing and Equilibrium of the American Academy of Otolaryngology-Head and Neck Surgery has established guidelines for reporting vestibular schwannoma results. In this classification, hearing loss at a higher frequency (3000 Hz) is also included in calculating the PTA. "Serviceable" hearing (classes A and B) is similar to class I and II of Gardner-Robertson hearing classes. Every patient is counseled about the options and risks and benefit of microsurgical and radiosurgical management strategies. Modern reports on vestibular schwannoma outcomes should include these data.

Radiosurgery can be performed using the gamma knife, modified LINACs, or the proton beam. Techniques of head frame fixation, stereotactic imaging, dose planning, and dose delivery are different for these three modalities. In gamma knife radiosurgery the procedure begins with rigid fixation of an MRI-compatible Leksell stereotactic frame (Model G, Elekta Instruments, Atlanta, GA) to the patient's head. Local anesthetic scalp infiltration (5% Marcaine and 1% Xylocaine) is used, supplemented by mild intravenous sedation as needed. High-resolution images are acquired

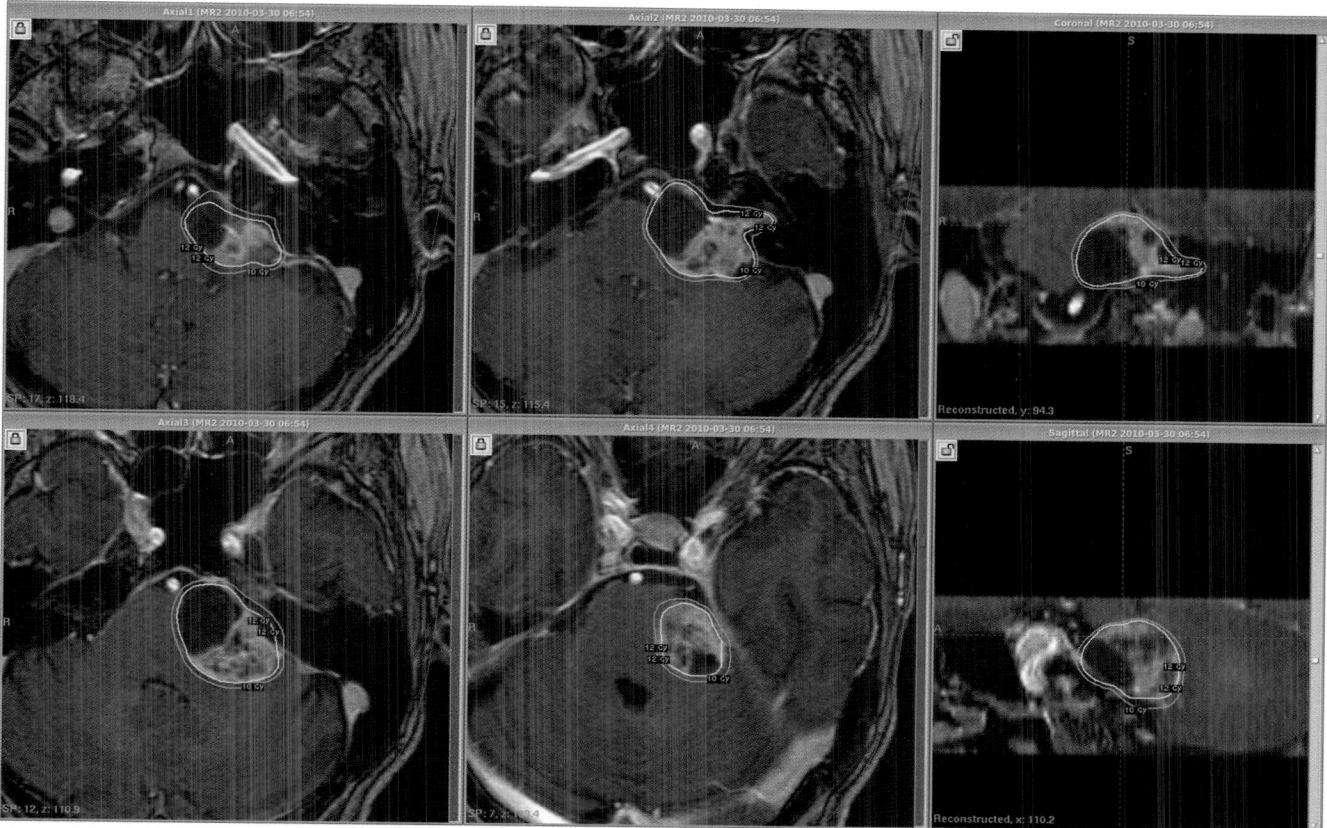

FIGURE 103-1 MR images at gamma knife radiosurgery in an 84-year-old woman with a vestibular schwannoma. The dose plan is shown using the Perfexion gamma knife to a margin dose of 12 Gy.

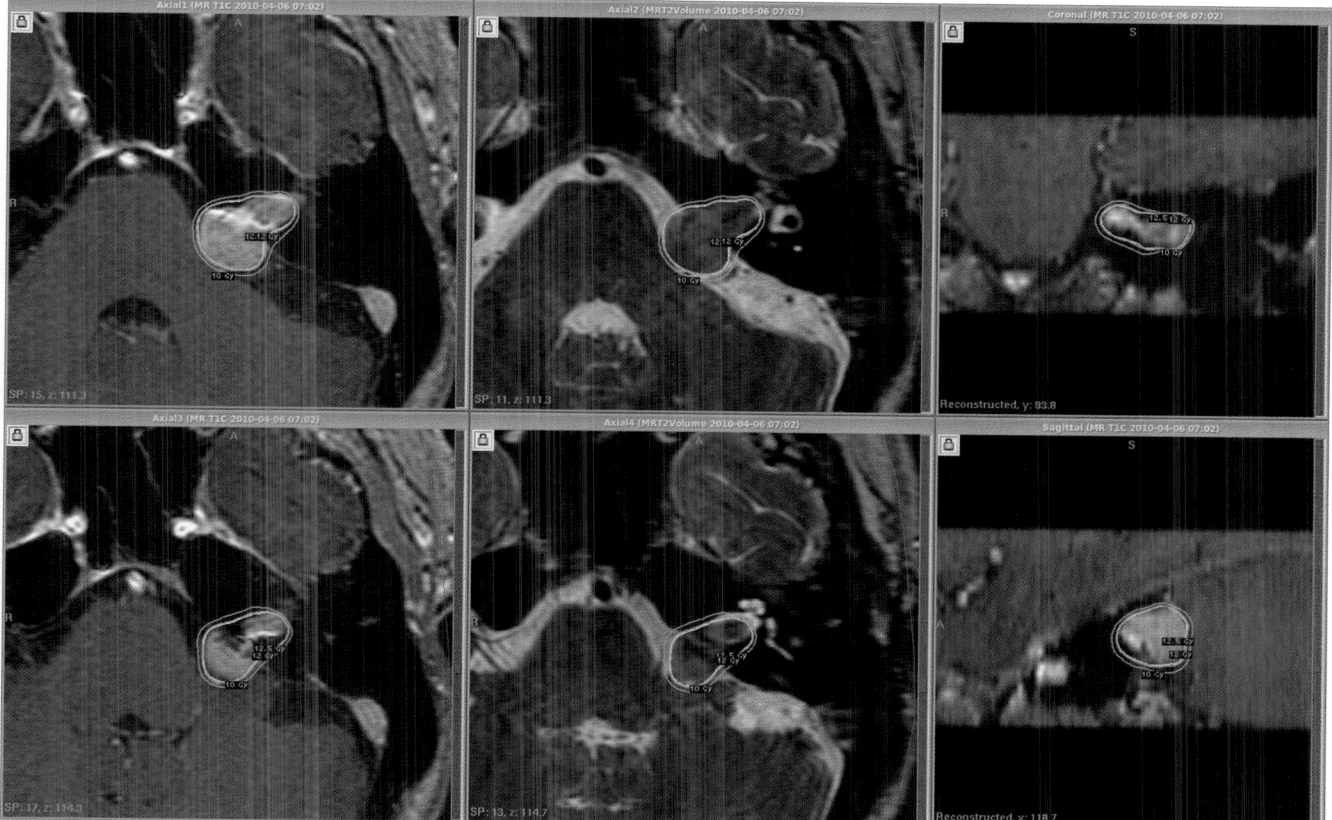

FIGURE 103-2 MR images at gamma knife radiosurgery in an 80-year-old woman with a vestibular schwannoma. The dose plan is shown using the Perfexion gamma knife to a margin dose of 12.5 Gy.

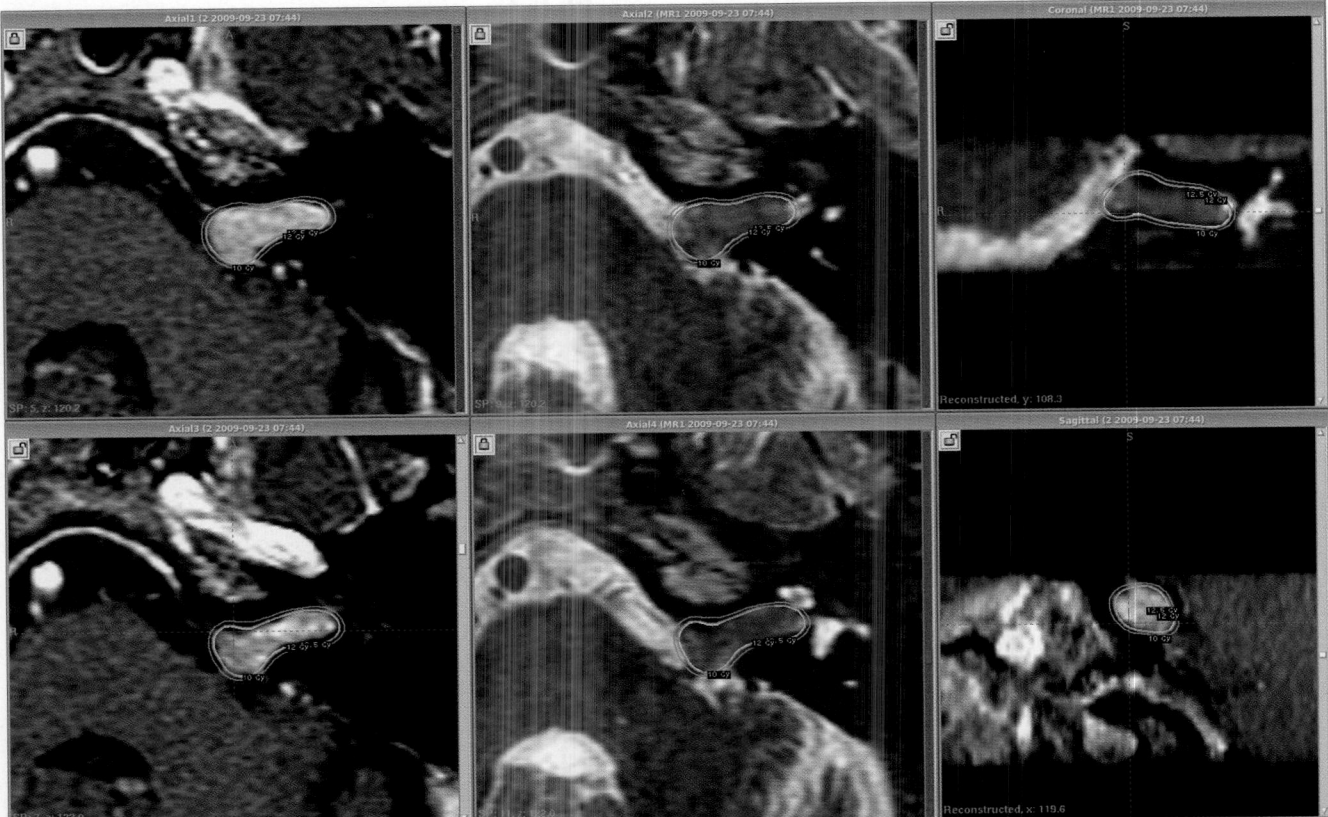

FIGURE 103-3 MR images at gamma knife radiosurgery in a 60-year-old man with a long intracanalicular vestibular schwannoma that caused hearing loss. The dose plan is shown using the Perfexion gamma knife to a margin dose of 12.5 Gy. Short- and long-relaxation time images help to define both the tumor and the cochlea.

with a fiducial system attached to the stereotactic frame. For vestibular schwannoma radiosurgery, a three-dimensional (3-D) volume acquisition MRI using a gradient pulse sequence (divided into 1- or 1.5-mm thick, 28–36 axial slices) is performed in order to cover the entire lesion and surrounding critical structures. A T2-weighted, 3-D volume sequence is performed to visualize cranial nerves and delineate inner ear structures (the cochlea and semicircular canals) (Figs. 103-3 and 103-4). Planning is performed on narrow-slice thickness, axial MR images with coronal and sagittal reconstructions. Centers using LINAC or proton-beam systems may use mask immobilization of the patient's head along with image guidance and typically deliver the radiation dose in five or more fractions over many days. CT is used for planning at most LINAC sites but may be fused to MRI scans.

RADIOSURGICAL DOSE PLANNING

Dose planning is a critical aspect of radiosurgery. Complete coverage of the tumor and preservation of facial, cochlear, and trigeminal nerve function is given priority during dose planning. For large tumors, preservation of brain-stem function is also a consideration. Conformality and selectivity is necessary for hearing and facial nerve preservation.[42] Specific gamma knife radiosurgery techniques include accurate definition of the tumor volume, use of multiple isocenters, beam weighting, and selective use of plug patterns to reduce dose to critical structures. This degree of conformality can be achieved through complex multi-isocenter

planning (see all figures). Vestibular schwannoma planning is usually performed using a combination of small-beam-diameter (4- and 8-mm) collimators. For large tumors, 14-, 16-, or 18-mm collimators are used. A series of 4-mm isocenters are used to create a tapered isodose plan to conform to the intracanalicular portion of the tumor.

DOSE SELECTION

After optimizing the plan, a maximum dose inside target is determined as well as the dose to the tumor edge. The treatment isodose, maximum dose, and dose to the margin (edge) are jointly decided by a neurosurgeon, radiation oncologist, and medical physicist and, in some centers, a neurotologist. In gamma knife radiosurgery, a dose of 12 to 13 Gy is typically prescribed to the 50% (or other) isodose line that conforms to the tumor margin. The commonest dose is 12.5 Gy, used for hearing preservation in smaller tumors. Larger tumors may receive 12 Gy, and in those with hearing loss or prior resection, 13 Gy. Dose prescription for vestibular schwannomas changed significantly during the first 10 years experience at our center. This margin dose range is associated with a low complication rate and yet maintains a high rate of tumor control as we have found in our most recent 10-years-plus experience using these doses. We suspect that further dose reduction is unwarranted. Most centers are reluctant to prescribe lower margin doses (such as 12 Gy) for vestibular schwannomas. Similar doses are also used for patients with bilateral (NF2 related)

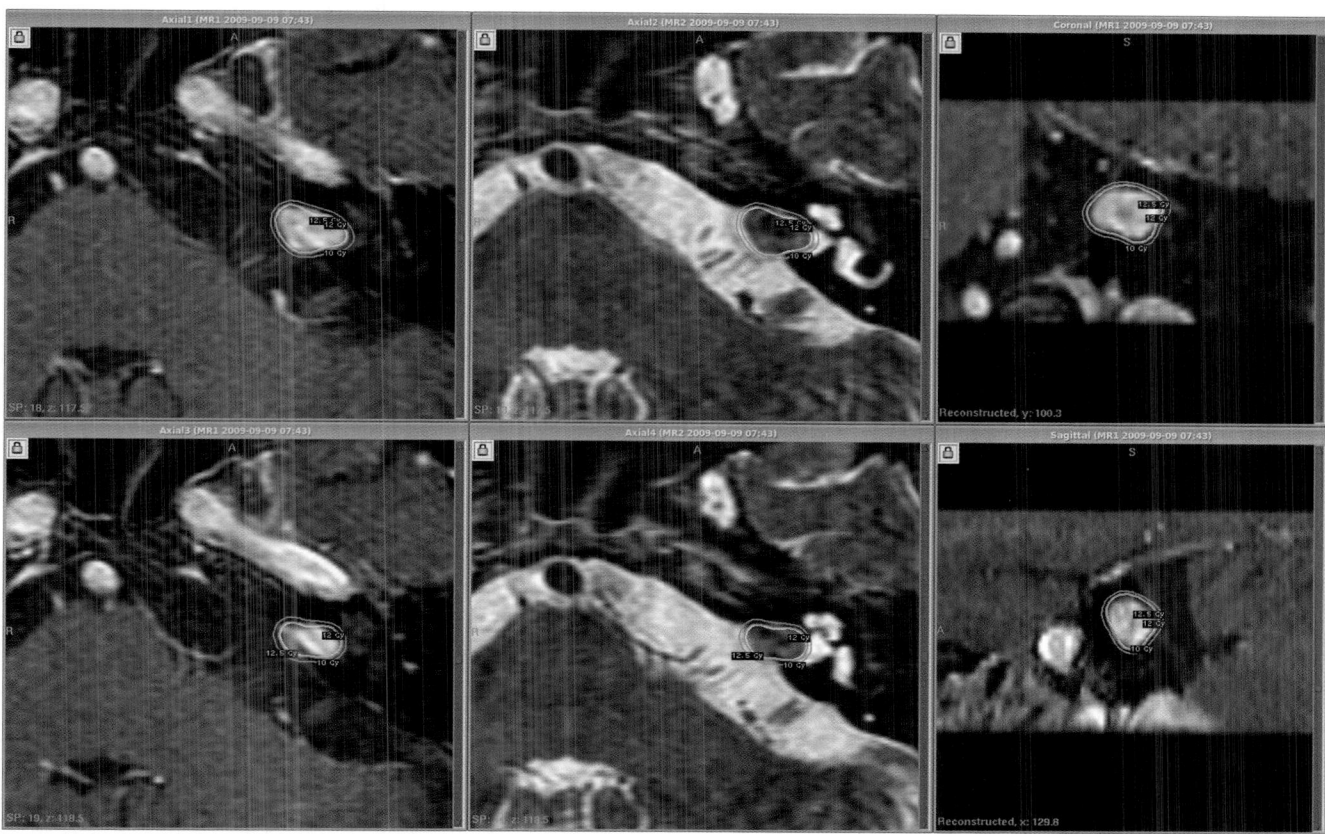

FIGURE 103-4 MR images at gamma knife radiosurgery in a man with an intracanalicular vestibular schwannoma. The dose plan is shown using the Perfexion gamma knife to a margin dose of 12.5 Gy. The relationship between the tumor and the inner ear structures are well seen using these imaging sequences.

vestibular schwannomas and for patients with contralateral deafness from other causes, for whom hearing preservation is highly desirable. After prescribing the margin dose, the mean dose to the cochlea, semicircular canals, and brain stem are assessed. A mean cochlear dose less than 4.2 Gy may be important for hearing preservation (Fig. 103-5). The majority of the tumor volume is receiving a radiobiologic dose in excess of a biologically equivalent dose delivered by fractionated image-guided radiation therapy. The maximum radiosurgical dose of 25 Gy may be radiobiologically equivalent to 100 Gy of fractionated radiation. While many radiosurgical centers have evolved toward similar dose selection parameters, the doses and regimens chosen for fractionated radiotherapy continue to vary widely.

After radiosurgery, all patients are followed up with serial contrast-enhanced, gadolinium-enhanced MRI scans, which are generally requested at 6 months, 12 months, and 2, 4, 8, 12, 16, and 20 years. All patients who have detectable hearing before radiosurgery are requested to obtain audiologic tests (PTA and SDS) near the time of their follow-up MRI.

Gamma Knife Radiosurgery: Clinical Results

Long-term results of gamma knife radiosurgery for vestibular schwannomas have been documented.[43-48] Recent reports suggest a tumor control rate of 93% to 100% after

radiosurgery.[42-64] Kondziolka et al. studied 5- to 10-year outcomes in 162 vestibular schwannoma patients who had radiosurgery at the University of Pittsburgh.[58] In this study a long-term 98% tumor control rate was reported. Sixty-two percent of tumors became smaller, 33% remained unchanged, and 6% became slightly larger. Some tumors initially enlarged 1 to 2 mm during the first 6 to 12 months after radiosurgery as they lost their central contrast enhancement. Such tumors generally regressed in volume compared to their preradiosurgery size. Only 2% of patients required tumor resection after radiosurgery. Norén, in his 28-year experience with vestibular schwannoma radiosurgery, reported a 95% long-term tumor control rate. Litvack et al. reported a 98% tumor control rate at a mean follow-up of 31 months after radiosurgery using a 12-Gy margin dose.[65] Niranjan et al. analyzed the outcome of intracanalicular tumor radiosurgery performed at the University of Pittsburgh.[66] All patients (100%) had imaging-documented tumor growth control.

Flickinger et al. performed an outcome analysis of acoustic neuroma patients treated between August 1992 and August 1997 at the University of Pittsburgh. The actuarial 5-year clinical tumor control rate (no requirement for surgical intervention) was 99.4 ± 0.6%.[44,50] The long-term (10–15 years) outcome of benign tumor radiosurgery also has been evaluated. In a study which included 157 patients with vestibular schwannomas, the median follow-up for the patients still living at the time of the study ($n = 136$) was

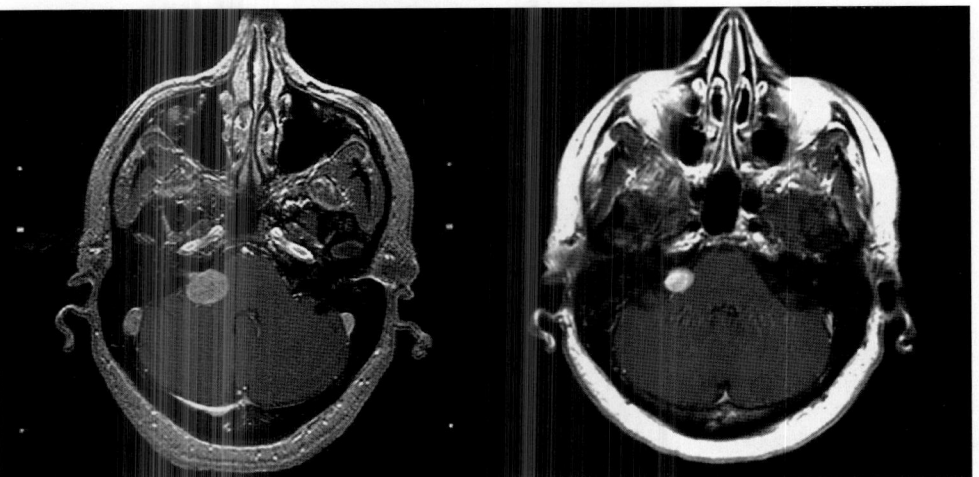

FIGURE 103-5 MR images (at radiosurgery, left) and 5 years later (right) in a 58-year-old woman with a right vestibular schwannoma. Tumor regression is noted. Her audiogram at presentation showed a speech discrimination score (SDS) of 100% and pure tone average (PTA) of 15 dB. At 5 years, her SDS was 100% and PTA was 20 dB.

10.2 years. Serial imaging studies after radiosurgery (n = 157) showed a decrease in tumor size in 114 patients (73%), no change in 40 patients (25.5%), and an increase in three patients who later had resection (1.9%).[47] No patient developed a radiation-associated malignant or benign tumor (defined as a histologically confirmed and distinct neoplasm arising in the initial radiation field after at least 2 years have passed). In patients under 40 years of age, with minimum 4-year follow-up, all remained employed and active.[65]

HEARING PRESERVATION

Preradiosurgery hearing can now be preserved in 60% to 90% of patients, with higher preservation rates found for smaller tumors. In a long-term (5–10-year follow-up) study conducted at the University of Pittsburgh, 51% of patients had no change in hearing ability.[50,58] All patients (100%) who were treated with a margin dose of 14 Gy or less maintained a serviceable level of hearing after intracanalicular tumor radiosurgery.[66] Among patients treated after 1992, the 5-year actuarial rates of hearing level preservation and speech preservation were 75.2% and 89.2%, respectively, for patients (n = 89) treated with a 13-Gy tumor margin dose. However, in a longer-term assessment at a median of 6 years, the same Gardner/Robertson level was preserved in 71%, serviceable hearing in 74%, and any testable hearing in 95%. For intracanalicular tumors, these rates were 84%, 92%, and 100%.

Our recent research has shown that the mean cochlear dose is important for hearing preservation. A dose of less than 4.2 Gy was associated with better hearing,[67] a finding similar to the dose of 4 Gy noted from Marseille. Age is also important, as those under 60 years old fare better.[67] Long-relaxation-time (T2) volumetric images are important to identify the cochlea for dose planning.

FACIAL NERVE AND TRIGEMINAL NERVE PRESERVATION

Facial and trigeminal nerve function can now be preserved in the majority of patients (>95%). In a study using MR-based dose planning, a 13-Gy tumor margin dose was associated with 0% risk of new facial weakness and 3.1% risk of facial numbness (5-year actuarial rates). A margin dose of greater than 14 Gy was associated with a 2.5% risk of new onset facial weakness and a 3.9% risk of facial numbness (5-year

actuarial rates).[44] None of the patients who had radiosurgery for intracanalicular tumors developed new facial or trigeminal neuropathies. At the current 12- to 13-Gy dose range, any degree of facial weakness is exceedingly rare.

NEUROFIBROMATOSIS 2

Patients with vestibular schwannomas associated with neurofibromatosis 2 represent a special challenge because of the risk of complete deafness. Unlike the solitary sporadic tumors that tend to displace the cochlear nerve, tumors associated with NF2 tend to form nodular clusters that engulf or even infiltrate the cochlear nerve. Complete resection may not always be possible. Radiosurgery has been performed for patients with NF2. Subach et al. studied our first 40 patients (with 45 tumors) who were treated with radiosurgery for NF2. Serviceable hearing was preserved in 6 of 14 patients (43%), and this rate improved to 67% after modifications made to the technique in 1992. The tumor control rate was 98%.[68] Only one patient showed imaging-documented growth. Normal facial nerve function and trigeminal nerve function were preserved in 81% and 94% of patients, respectively. In two recent series,[69,70] serviceable hearing was preserved in only 30%[69] and 40%[70] of cases, respectively. The tumor control rate was respectively 71%[69] and 79%.[70] Mathieu et al. updated outcomes of our NF2 series over the year 2007.[71] The tumor control rate was 87.5%. The rate of serviceable hearing preservation using current technique was 52.6%. It now appears that preservation of serviceable hearing in patients with NF2 is an attainable goal using gamma-knife radiosurgery. However, longer-term results from Sheffield showed a drop off in hearing over many years. We believe that early radiosurgery when the hearing level is still excellent may become an appropriate strategy in the future. At present we generally delay radiosurgery in NF2 patients until we see hearing deterioration or tumor growth.

Proton Beam Radiosurgery: Clinical Results

Weber et al. evaluated 88 patients with vestibular schwannomas treated with proton beam stereotactic radiosurgery, in which two to four convergent fixed beams of

160-MeV protons were applied.[72] A median dose of 12 cobalt Gy equivalents was prescribed to the 70% to 108% isodose lines (median, 70%). The median follow-up period was 38.7 months. The actuarial 2- and 5-year tumor control rates were 95.3% and 93.6%, respectively. Serviceable hearing was preserved in 33.3% of patients. Actuarial 5-year normal facial and trigeminal nerve function preservation rates were 91.1% and 89.4%, respectively. Harsh et al. evaluated 68 patients with vestibular schwannomas who were treated with proton beam using a marginal dose of only 12 Gy.[53] After a mean clinical follow-up of 44 months and imaging follow-up of 34 months, actuarial control rates of 94% at 2 years and 84% at 5 years were reported. Cranial neuropathies included persistent facial hypoesthesia (4.7%), intermittent facial paresthesias (9.4%), persistent facial weakness (4.7%) requiring oculoplasty, transient partial facial weakness (9.4%), and synkinesis (9.4%).

Linac Radiosurgery: Clinical Results

Suh et al. evaluated 29 patients treated with a modified linear accelerator stereotactic radiosurgery system.[73] The median margin dose was 1600 cGy. The 5-year local disease control rate was 94%. Long-term complications included new or progressive trigeminal and facial nerve deficits with estimated 5-year incidences of 15% and 32%, respectively. Subjective hearing reduction or loss occurred in 14 of the 19 patients (74%) who had useful hearing prior to treatment. Since there was a high risk of cranial nerve neuropathy, these authors did not recommend using only computed tomography-based planning and high prescription doses. Spiegelmann et al. reported their results of LINAC radiosurgery for 44 patients with vestibular schwannomas.[74] After a mean follow-up period of 32 months (range, 12–60 months), 98% of the tumors were controlled. The actuarial hearing preservation rate was 71%. New transient facial neuropathy developed in 24% of the patients and persisted to a mild degree in 8%. The University of Florida group published clinical outcomes in a series of 390 patients, with a high control rate and a facial neuropathy rate of 0.7% using current techniques and dose.[52]

Stereotactic Radiation Therapy: Clinical Results

Stereotactic radiation therapy (SRT) or fractionated stereotactic radiation therapy (FSRT) refers to the delivery of a standard fractionation scheme of radiation, used with rigidly applied or relocatable stereotactic-guiding devices. Some LINAC based radiosurgery centers (driven by the desire to reduce complication rates) have shifted to fractionated stereotactic radiotherapy for vestibular schwannomas.[56,73,75-80] Ishihara et al. reported 94% tumor control rate at a median follow-up of 31.9 months in a series of 38 patients who had CyberKnife SRT for vestibular schwannoma. One patient developed transient facial paresis (2.6%) and one developed trigeminal nerve neuropathy (2.6%).[56] Fuss et al. described 51 patients with vestibular schwannomas who were treated with SRT.[81] The mean follow-up was 42 months and the actuarial 5-year tumor control rate was 95%. One patient developed a

transient facial nerve paresis and two noted new trigeminal dysesthesias. Chung et al., using SRT for 25 patients with useful hearing, reported 57% hearing preservation at 2 years.[82] The mean pre- and post-SRT speech recognition threshold was 20 and 38 dB, respectively. The mean proportion of pre- and post-SRT speech discrimination was 91% and 59%, respectively.

Sawamura et al. treated 101 patients with vestibular schwannoma using fractionated SRT to a total dose of 40 to 50 Gy, administered in 20 to 25 fractions over a 5- to 6-week period.[78] The median follow-up period was 45 months, and the actuarial 5-year rate of tumor control was 91.4%. The actuarial 5-year rate of useful hearing preservation (Gardner-Robertson class I or II) was 71%. The complications of fractionated SRT included transient facial nerve palsy (4%), trigeminal neuropathy (14%), and balance disturbance (17%). Eleven patients (11%) who had progressive communicating hydrocephalus after FSRT required a shunt.

Meijer et al. performed a single-institution trial to study whether fractionated stereotactic radiation therapy is superior to single-session LINAC-based radiosurgery with respect to treatment-related toxicity and local control in patients with vestibular schwannomas.[83] These authors analyzed 129 vestibular schwannoma patients who were treated at a LINAC-based radiosurgery facility. Stereotactic radiation therapy was performed on 80 patients with a relocatable guidance device using 5 × 4 Gy and later 5 × 5 Gy at the 80% isodose. Forty-nine patients had stereotactic radiosurgery of 1 × 10 Gy and later 1 × 12.5 Gy at the 80% isodose using a stereotactic frame. There was no statistically significant difference between the single-fraction group and the fractionated group with respect to mean tumor diameter (2.6 vs. 2.5 cm) or mean follow-up time (both 33 months). Outcome differences between the single-session group and the fractionated treatment group with respect to 5-year local control probability (100% vs. 94%), 5-year facial nerve preservation probability (93% vs. 97%), and 5-year hearing preservation probability (75% vs. 61%) were not statistically significant. The difference in 5-year trigeminal nerve preservation (92% vs. 98%) reached statistical significance ($p = 0.048$). These authors concluded that LINAC-based radiosurgery was as good as LINAC-based fractionated stereotactic radiation therapy in vestibular schwannoma patients, except for a small difference in trigeminal nerve preservation rate in favor of a fractionated schedule.

Andrews et al. published their outcomes using stereotactic radiotherapy at total dose of 50.4 or 46.8 Gy. In patients with grade 1 or 2 hearing, the median follow-up was 65 weeks. Although no patient had later tumor growth, the hearing preservation rates were better at the lower dose. At 3 years, the hearing preservation rate was 55% to 60%, and no patient with grade 2 hearing preserved it at the 50-Gy dose.[84]

At the present time there are limited data on SRT for vestibular schwannomas.[85] There are no compelling radiobiological principles supporting the use of SRT over radiosurgery for achieving an optimal therapeutic response for the slowly proliferating, late-responding tissue of a schwannoma. The long-term results (5–10 years) of SRT are not yet available. For those centers who cannot achieve the necessary conformal plan to permit radiosurgery, SRT may be an option for vestibular schwannomas if they have a higher complication rate using LINAC radiosurgery.

Comparison of Radiosurgery and Microsurgery Options

It is likely that a randomized clinical trial will probably never be completed to compare surgical resection with radiosurgery for vestibular schwannoma.[86] However, there are several well-matched cohort studies that compare outcomes for patients with tumors less than 2.5 cm in extracanalicular diameter. Karpinos et al. analyzed 96 patients with unilateral acoustic neuromas treated with the Leksell gamma knife or microsurgery and concluded that radiosurgery was associated with a lower rate of immediate and long-term development of facial and trigeminal neuropathy, postoperative complications, and hospital stay. Radiosurgery yielded better measurable hearing preservation than microsurgery and equivalent serviceable hearing preservation rate and tumor growth control.[87]

Pollock et al. studied 87 patients with unilateral, previously unoperated vestibular schwannomas with an average diameter of less than 3 cm treated at the University of Pittsburgh between 1990 and 1991.[88] In this matched cohort trial preoperative patient characteristics and average tumor size were similar between the treatment groups. Microsurgical or radiosurgical techniques were used by experienced surgeons in both treatment groups. The treatment groups were compared based on cranial nerve preservation, tumor control, postoperative complications, patient symptomatology, length of hospital stay, total management charges, effect on employment status and overall patient satisfaction. Stereotactic radiosurgery was more effective in preserving normal postoperative facial function and hearing preservation with less treatment associated morbidity. Effects on preoperative symptoms were similar between

the treatment groups. Postoperative functional outcomes and patients' satisfaction were greater after radiosurgery when compared to microsurgery. Patients returned to independent functioning sooner after radiosurgery. Hospital length of stay and total management charges were less in the radiosurgical group.

In a similar study of vestibular schwannoma patients, Régis et al. used objective results and questionnaire answers to compare the results of radiosurgery (97 consecutive patients) with a microsurgery group (110 patients who fulfilled the inclusion criteria).[89] Questionnaire answers indicated that 100% of patients who underwent gamma knife® radiosurgery compared with 63% of patients who underwent microsurgery had no new facial motor disturbance. Ninety-one percent of patients treated with gamma knife® radiosurgery, and 61% in the microsurgery study, had no functional deterioration after treatment. The mean hospital stay was 3 days after gamma knife® radiosurgery and 23 days after microsurgery. All working patients who underwent gamma knife® radiosurgery kept the same professional activity, compared to 56% in the microsurgery arm. The mean time away from work was 7 days for gamma knife® radiosurgery compared to 130 days for the microsurgery group. Among patients whose preoperative hearing level was Class 1 according to the Gardner and Robertson scale, 70% had preserved functional hearing after gamma knife radiosurgery (class 1 or 2), compared with only 37.5% in the microsurgery group. At 4 years of follow-up, gamma knife radiosurgery provided better functional outcomes than microsurgery. It was concluded that stereotactic radiosurgery was an effective and less costly management strategy for unilateral vestibular schwannomas less than 3 cm in diameter, and should be considered a primary management option.

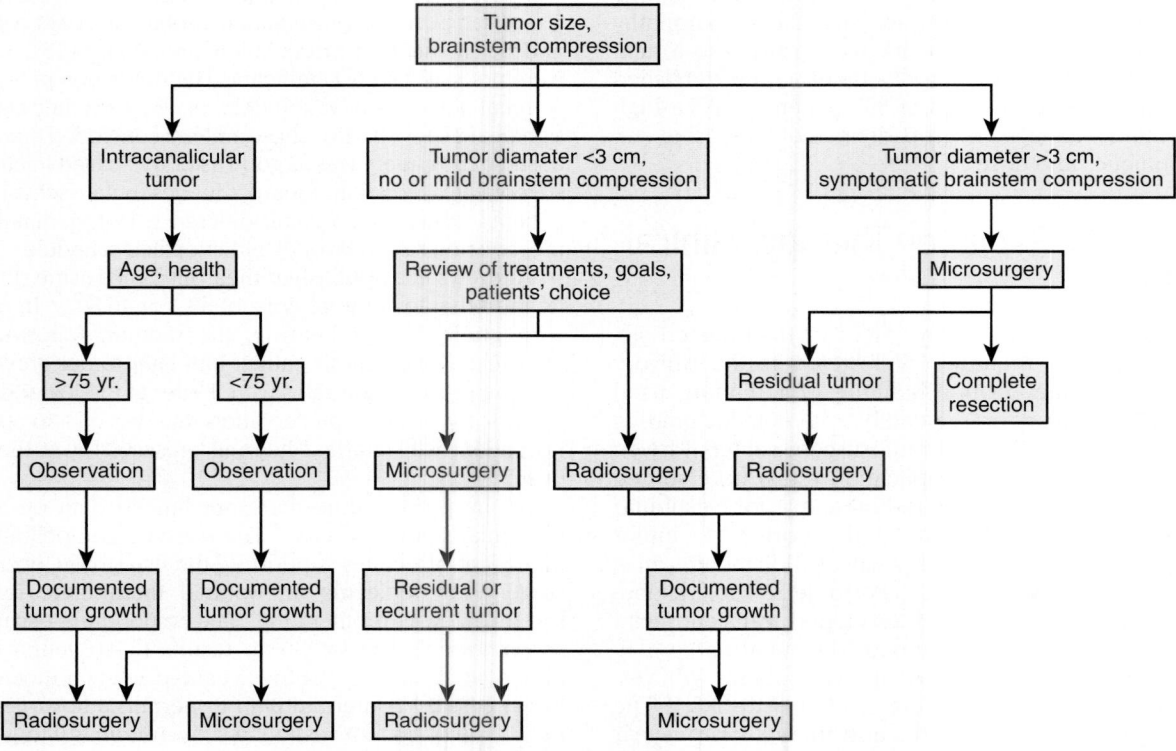

FIGURE 103-6 Management algorithm for acoustic tumors.

In a recently published study, Myrseth et al. compared the quality of life outcomes for 189 acoustic neuroma patients with tumors less than 30 mm in diameter who were treated with either microsurgery or radiosurgery.[13] The outcome analysis included assessments of tumor control, cranial nerve preservation rates, and complications. The results showed that cranial nerve function and overall patient outcomes were better in the radiosurgery group. The results reveal that from the patients' perspective, radiosurgery provides a more desirable outcome than microsurgery. Pollock et al. prospectively collected data on patients undergoing either resection or gamma knife radiosurgery and found similar or better outcomes after radiosurgery, including quality of life measures.[90]

Summary

Radiosurgery has become a well documented management option for patients with vestibular schwannomas. As a minimally invasive strategy, we now know the expected success rate and risks. Long-term data are now published, and for the first time, systematic, serially collected outcomes data are available on patients with this tumor. Like microsurgical resection, not all radiosurgery technologies are the same. The evolution of radiosurgery has led to enhanced outcomes for patients diagnosed with such tumors. It may currently be the most common treatment choice for patients. An algorithm for management is shown (Fig. 103-6).

KEY REFERENCES

Andrews D, Werner-Wasik M, Den R, et al. Toward dose optimization for fractionated stereotactic radiotherapy for acoustic neuromas: comparison of two dose cohorts. *Int J Radiat Oncol Biol Phys.* 2009; 74:419-426.

Chung WY, Liu KD, Shiau CY, et al. Gamma knife surgery for vestibular schwannoma: 10-year experience of 195 cases. *J Neurosurg.* 2005; 102(Suppl):87-96.

Delbrouck C, Hassid S, Massager N, et al. Preservation of hearing in vestibular schwannomas treated by radiosurgery using Leksell gamma knife: preliminary report of a prospective Belgian clinical study. *Acta Otorhinolaryngol Belg.* 2003;57:197-204.

Flickinger JC, Kondziolka D, Niranjan A, Lunsford LD. Results of acoustic neuroma radiosurgery: an analysis of 5 years' experience using current methods [see comment]. *J Neurosurg.* 2001;94:1-6.

Flickinger JC, Kondziolka D, Niranjan A, et al. Acoustic neuroma radiosurgery with marginal tumor doses of 12 to 13 Gy. *Int J Radiat Oncol Biol Phys.* 2004;60:225-230.

Friedman WA, Bradshaw P, Myers A, Bova FJ. Linear accelerator radiosurgery for vestibular schwannomas. *J Neurosurg.* 2006;105: 657-661.

Hasegawa T, Kida Y, Kobayashi T, Yoshimoto M, et al. Long-term outcomes in patients with vestibular schwannomas treated using gamma knife surgery: 10-year follow up. *J Neurosurg.* 2005;102:10-16.

Kano H, Kondziolka D, Flickinger JC, Lunsford LD. Predictors of hearing preservation after stereotactic radiosurgery for acoustic neuromas. *J Neurosurg.* 2009;111:863-873.

Kondziolka D, Lunsford LD, McLaughlin MR, Flickinger JC. Long-term outcomes after radiosurgery for acoustic neuromas [see comment]. *N Engl J Med.* 1998;339:1426-1433.

Kondziolka D, Nathoo N, Flickinger JC, et al. Long-term results after radiosurgery for benign intracranial tumors [see comment]. *Neurosurgery.* 2003;53:815-821:discussion 821-822.

Lee DJ, Westra WH, Staecker H, et al. Clinical and histopathologic features of recurrent vestibular schwannoma (acoustic neuroma) after stereotactic radiosurgery. *Otol Neurotol.* 2003;24:650-660:discussion 660.

Linskey ME, Johnstone PA. Radiation tolerance of normal temporal bone structures: implications for gamma knife stereotactic radiosurgery. *Int J Radiat Oncol Biol Phys.* 2003;57:196-200.

Lobato-Polo J, Kondziolka D, Zorro O, et al. Gamma knife radiosurgery in younger patients with vestibular schwannomas. *Neurosurgery.* 2009;65:294-301.

Lunsford LD, Niranjan A, Flickinger JC, et al. Radiosurgery of vestibular schwannomas: summary of experience in 829 cases. *J Neurosurg.* 2005;102(Suppl):195-199.

Mathieu D, Kondziolka D, Flickinger JC, et al. Stereotactic radiosurgery for vestibular schwannomas in patients with neurofibromatosis type 2: an analysis of tumor control, complications, and hearing preservation rates. *Neurosurgery.* 2007;60:460-468:discussion 468-470.

Matthies C, Samii M. Management of vestibular schwannomas (acoustic neuromas): the value of neurophysiology for intraoperative monitoring of auditory function in 200 cases. *Neurosurgery.* 1997;40:459-466:discussion 466-468.

McIver JI, Pollock BE. Radiation-induced tumor after stereotactic radiosurgery and whole brain radiotherapy: case report and literature review. *J Neurooncol.* 2004;66:301-305.

Myrseth E, Moller P, Pedersen PH, et al. Vestibular schwannomas: clinical results and quality of life after microsurgery or gamma knife radiosurgery. *Neurosurgery.* 2005;56:927-935:discussion 927-935.

Niranjan A, Lunsford LD, Flickinger JC, et al. Dose reduction improves hearing preservation rates after intracanalicular acoustic tumor radiosurgery. *Neurosurgery.* 1999;45:753-762:discussion 762-765.

Noren G. Long-term complications following gamma knife radiosurgery of vestibular schwannomas. *Stereotact Funct Neurosurg.* 1998; 70(Suppl 1):65-73.

Petit JH, Hudes RS, Chen TT, et al. Reduced-dose radiosurgery for vestibular schwannomas. *Neurosurgery.* 2001;49:1299-1306:discussion 1306-1307.

Pollock BE, Driscoll CL, Foote RL, et al. Patient outcomes after vestibular schwannoma management: a prospective comparison of microsurgical resection and stereotactic radiosurgery. *Neurosurgery.* 2006;59: 77-85.

Pollock BE, Lunsford LD, Flickinger JC, et al. Vestibular schwannoma management. Part I. Failed microsurgery and the role of delayed stereotactic radiosurgery. *J Neurosurg.* 1998;89:944-948.

Pollock BE, Lunsford LD, Kondziolka D, et al. Outcome analysis of acoustic neuroma management: a comparison of microsurgery and stereotactic radiosurgery. *Neurosurgery.* 1995;36:215-224:discussion 224-229 [erratum Neurosurgery. 1995;36:427].

Pollock BE, Lunsford LD, Kondziolka D, et al. Vestibular schwannoma management. Part II. Failed radiosurgery and the role of delayed microsurgery. *J Neurosurg.* 1998;89:949-955.

Regis J, Pellet W, Delsanti C, et al. Functional outcome after gamma knife surgery or microsurgery for vestibular schwannomas. *J Neurosurg.* 2002;97:1091-1100.

Rowe JG, Radatz MW, Walton L, et al. Clinical experience with gamma knife stereotactic radiosurgery in the management of vestibular schwannomas secondary to type 2 neurofibromatosis. *J Neurol Neurosurg Psychiatry.* 2003;74:1288-1293.

Numbered references appear on Expert Consult.

CHAPTER 104

Stereotactic Radiosurgery Meningiomas

MASSIMO GEROSA • BRUNO ZANOTTI • ANGELA VERLICCHI • ANTONIO NICOLATO

Meningiomas arise from the arachnoid cap cells, or "meningothelial" cells, and are the most frequently reported neuro-oncologic challenge, accounting for 16% to 30% of intracranial tumors,[1-6] and for 22% to 25% of spinal cord tumors.[7,8] Furthermore, a non-negligible percentage of them is diagnosed on the basis of imaging alone,[3,9,10] and an additional 2.3% in autopsy reports (Fig. 104-1).[3,11] With the growing contribution of imaging and necroptic observations the relative percentage might become higher.

Epidemiology

The average annual incidence is five to six new cases per 100,000,[1-6,12,13] with the age-related risk drastically increasing from the pediatric population to a peak during the sixth and seventh decades.[14,15] It is worth stressing that more aggressive clinical and histologic features have been observed in children and adolescents.[14] The female/male ratio is approximately 2:1 to 3:1,[3,16-18] and this prevalence is presumably related to as yet poorly known progesterone- and estrogen-receptor–mediated cytoactivation.[3,15,19]

As to their natural history, the few reported series of conservatively managed symptomatic meningiomas have documented a consistent trend to progression in one third of the patients, although with a wide spectrum of variability.[20-28] In fact, in a non-negligible percentage, either spontaneously or after subtotal resection, the annual growth rate may suddenly increase up to several millimeters documenting an unexpected aggressiveness.[29-32] The main factors associated with growth are younger age and T2-hyperintensity, and presence of calcifications.[20] Both growth and recurrence rates are higher in grades 2 and 3 meningiomas[29,33,34] and this justifies the advocated multidisciplinary treatments.[1-3] Finally, although in anecdotal cases, post-surgical or radiosurgical remnants of a "benign" meningioma have been shown to undergo spontaneous or "induced" malignant cytologic transformation, subsequently confirmed at reoperation.[30,35,36]

Citopathology

During the last decade, the pathologic criteria for the definition of "atypical" as well as of "anaplastic" meningiomas have been gradually expanded to include not only nuclear pleomorphism, mitoses, atypia, necrosis, and so on, but also other relevant landmarks of parenchymal invasion such as the formation of small cell infiltrates, arachnoidal disruption, sheeting, macronucleoli focal malignant macrodifferentiation (e.g., glial fibrillary acidic protein (GFAP) production, melanocytic foci, etc.), and extra-axial diffusion (Fig. 104-2).[2] According to the Mayo Clinic Scheme,[2,36,37] substantially endorsed by recent revisions of the World Health Organization (WHO) (Table 104-1),[2] these specific parameters may be associated with malignant behavior regardless of their histologic subtype.[2] In fact, the very peculiar metastatic potential of these tumors seems to confirm the mentioned cytobiological discrepancy, since histologically benign meningiomas have sometimes shown biological aggressiveness, not only in terms of craniospinal seedings, but also of extraneural colonization (lung, liver, bone, lymph nodes).[2,7,38,39] However, the vast majority of these tumors are considered benign or grade 1 in the WHO classification,[2,40] currently accounting for a 5-year survival rate exceeding 80%.[1,41,42] Atypical (grade 2, 4.7-7.2%, prototypes: clear cell and chordoid varieties) and anaplastic or malignant (grade 3, 1.0%-2.8%, prototypes papillary and rhabdoid) forms are rarer[2,40,43-45] and usually bear a worse prognosis, with reported 5-year survivals of 32% to 64%.[1,36,42,46-50] Monosomy of chromosome 22 is the most common cytogenetic alteration in the overall oncotype population.[51,52] Nearly all neurofibromatosis type 2 (NF2)–associated meningiomas have mutations of the NF2 gene on 22q12.[3,51] Moreover, a stepwise change in the genetic characteristics of benign meningiomas undergoing anaplastic transformation has been observed: The loss on 22q, 1p, 6q, 10, 14q, and a gain on 9q, 12q, 15q, 17q, may frequently parallel this evolution as well as amplification on 17q and loss on 9p (CDKN2 gene).[2,53-55] Such a theory of correlative clinical-pathologic malignant progression is supported by atypical or anaplastic recurrences of formerly benign lesions, but the oncologic rationale is still debated.[2,56]

Treatment Options

SURGERY

There is general agreement that the optimal treatment for these lesions, whenever feasible, should be a Simpson grade I resection of the tumor—carefully pre-embolyzed if necessary—providing definitive diagnosis, reducing immediately any mass effect, and alleviating clinical signs and symptoms.[2,57,59,60] Such a golden therapeutic standard is still the dominant option in the vast majority of convexity meningiomas in fronto-orbital and spinal locations, whereas

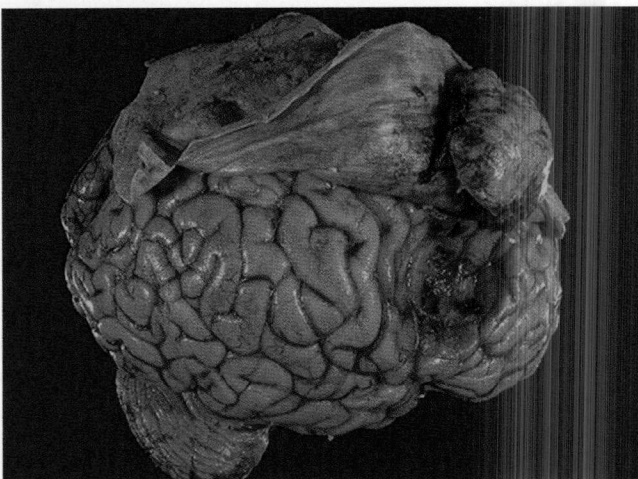

FIGURE 104-1 Autoptic finding, showing how meningioma are discrete, smooth-surfaced massed attached to the dura, with pushing of the leptomeninges. *(Courtesy of Prof. Felice Giangaspero and Dr. Manila Antonelli, Department of Experimental Medicine, University La Sapienza, Rome.)*

surgical results are less satisfactory in intraparenchymal or cranial base lesions[2,59-62] and particularly grim in grades 2 and 3.[3] Unfortunately, despite surgical advances, when these tumors are infiltrating the skull base, cranial nerves, or vascular structures, complete resection may not be feasible without unacceptable morbidity rates. Considering more recently published series, gross removal of basal meningiomas was achieved in 60% to 87.5% of the patients,[59-65] with 30% to 56% of severe complications,[58,60,65-67] mostly represented by newer or deteriorated pre-existing cranial nerve deficit, occurring temporarily in 20% to 44%, and permanently in 16% to 56% of the cases. Median postoperative mortality rate was 3.6% (range 0%–9%).[59-68] Moreover, local recurrence rates are strictly dependent on Simpson's grade[69]: at 10-year follow-up, 10% to 33% (average 20% to 25%) after complete resection (Simpson 1–2); and 55% to 75% (average 60%–62%) after partial resection, that is, Simpson >2 (Table 104-2).[20,32,70-74] The relevance of these findings may probably explain why, particularly in atypical-anaplastic varieties, adjuvant therapies and sometimes preplanned, combined multidisciplinary approaches may be advocated, to avoid early recurrences and repeat surgery, thereby reducing morbidity.[2,12,35]

FRACTIONATED RADIOTHERAPY

External beam radiation therapy (EBRT) has been used for decades, either as a primary or as an adjuvant treatment, with documented improvement in local control and rarely in recurrences (see Table 104-2).[12,41,42,75-80] In more aggressive cytotypes, most authors seem to favor administering EBRT—mostly Fractionated Stereotactic Radiotherapy (FSRT) early to patients who have undergone subtotal and even total resections.[2,3,12,42,43,45,81] FSRT has proven to be successful in primary (imaging defined) meningiomas,[12,82-87] particularly in all cases with crucial exposure of extremely radiosensitive structures such as the optic pathways.[12,88-91] Series reports comparing progression-free survival (PFS) for patients treated with gross/total removal and subtotal removal (STR), with or without EBRT, have consistently shown the best results with the radical surgery or STR plus radiation, whereas STR alone turned out to be less valuable.[3,32,33,41,42,45,70,71,76-78,85,92-107]

STEREOTACTIC RADIOSURGERY

According to the historical definition by Lars Leksell stereotactic radiosurgery (SRS) is "a technique of closed skull destruction of a predetermined intracranial target by a single-fraction high dose of ionizing radiation using a precision stereotactic apparatus".[108] In contrast with spatially less accurate conventional radiotherapy, radiosurgery has the capacity to maximize/optimize the dose exposure on the target volume, while minimizing the irradiation of surrounding critical structures, thereby reducing collateral damages. The concept of delivering a high dose of radiation energy to treat focal pathologic lesions fits all criteria for minimal invasiveness and has gradually become a powerful and attractive therapeutic strategy for many neurosurgical disorders. Recently the impressive advances in neuroimaging, stereotactic techniques, and robotic technology have further improved results, expanding the spectrum of applications. This approach may be increasingly considered not only as potentially adjuvant to microsurgery but also as a valuable alternative option.

Lars Leksell designed the first arc centered device in 1948,[109] and in 1951 he introduced the term and concept of radiosurgery.[108,109] His first stereotactic instruments were suitable for replacing a probe (needle electrode) by cross firing intracerebral structures with narrow beams of radiant energy. X-rays were first tried, but both gamma rays and ultrasonic rays were included as alternatives. In close collaboration with Borje Larsson, a physicist at the synchrocyclotron unit in Uppsala, Leksell performed the original experiments with highly focused high-energy proton irradiation of human malignancies.[110] As a rule, precise, well-limited lesions were produced, but the synchrocyclotron proved to be too complicated for widespread clinical use. This compelled Leksell to consider other radiation sources and he started designing a 179-source ^{60}Co gamma unit that was fully integrated into the stereotactic system; the first unit was inaugurated in 1967.[110] Radiosurgery was initially developed with the aim to offer a bloodless and less risky method, essentially for functional treatments. However, within a few years the machine proved to be extremely effective in a variety of intracranial lesions, provided that the rationale of the approach, that is, the fundamentals of the technique, had been respected. Briefly, the latter are limited target volume, well-defined imaging, compatible site, and adequate cytology. As shown in the following reported experiences, to date it is possible or nearly possible to overcome each of the following constraints: tackling larger volumes with lower dosages,[111,112] crucial locations with staged procedures, and, perhaps in the near future, radioresistant oncotypes by means of radiosensitizers.

In recent decades, SRS techniques, particularly gamma knife radiosurgery (GKR), have progressively gained an unquestionable momentum in the therapeutic armamentarium for most brain tumors, particularly for well defined lesions, such as meningiomas. The main reasons for this growing role may be summarized as follows: (1) targeting update, with the advent of computerized and coregistered, morphofunctional neuroimaging; (2) the availability of newer, more powerful and precise irradiation devices; (3) the introduction of computer-guided dose planning; and (4) a deeper radiobiological experience. To date, an estimated half a million people have

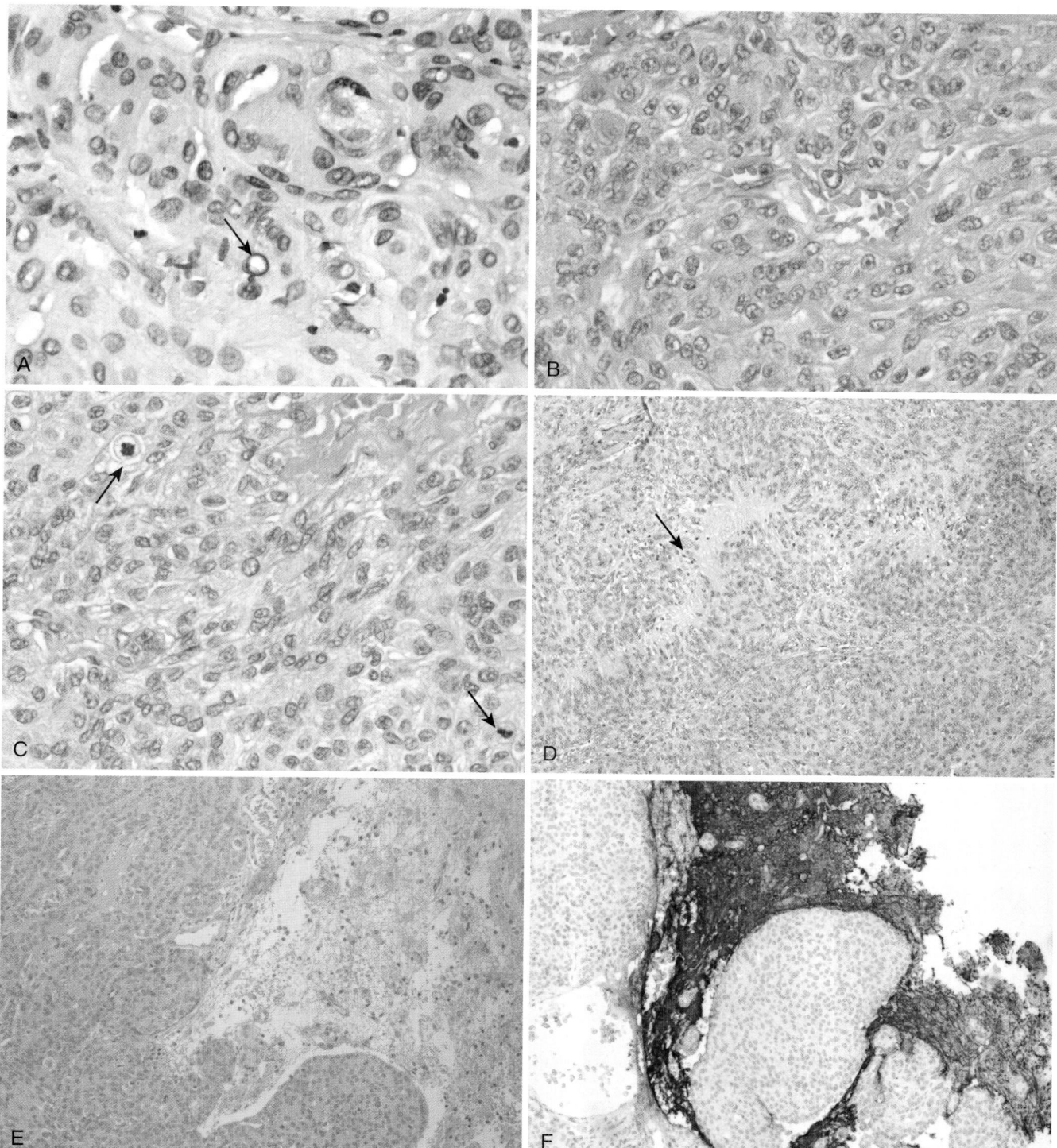

FIGURE 104-2 Histopathologic findings of meningiomas. In grade I meningioma: neoplastic cells have round and oval nuclei, delicate chromatin and small and solitary nucleoli; a classic finding is the presence of nuclear-cytoplasmic invagination, also termed pseudoinclusion (A) (40× EE). In atypical meningioma (grade II), nucleoli become prominent (B) and mitosis appears (C) (40× EE). Small foci of necrosis with pseudopalisading are common features in grade II meningioma (D) (20× EE). Invasion of the brain establishes grade II: islands of neoplastic cells invade the cerebral cortex (E); glial fibrillary acidic protein staining helps identify brain tissue between tongues of neoplasm (F) (10× EE).

Continued

been treated by GKR worldwide at a continuously increasing annual rate (in 2009, roughly 50,000 patients were treated). In addition, approximately 200,000 patients worldwide have experienced SRS with other dedicated machines. Elective indications currently include metastatic brain tumors, benign endocranial tumors (meningiomas, neuromas, pituitary adenomas, etc.), low-grade neuro-ectodermal tumors, vascular malformations, and some types of functional neurosurgery (e.g., trigeminal neuralgia). Finally, it is generally accepted that the putative mechanism of action of SRS is intimately

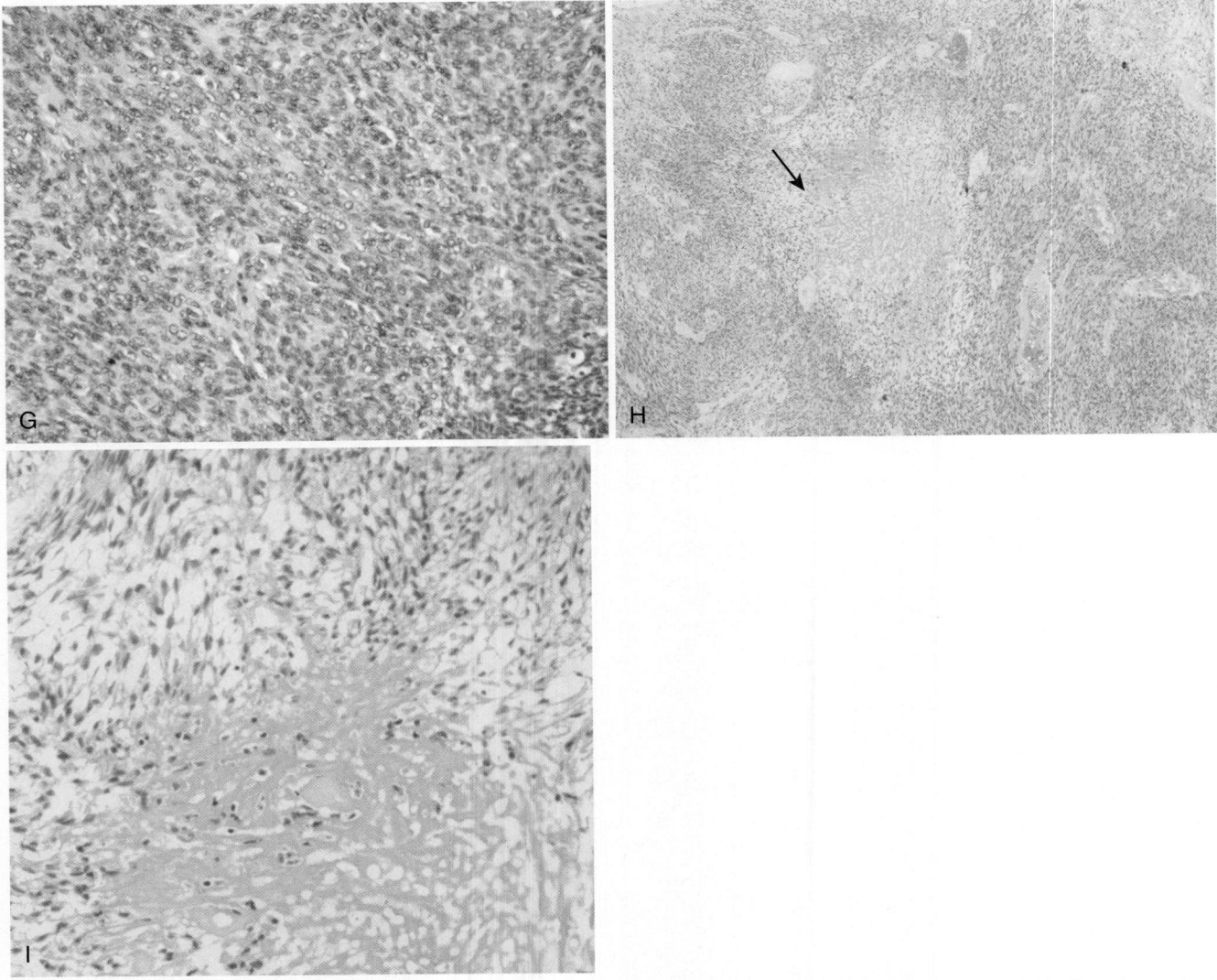

FIGURE 104-2, cont'd Loss of meningothelial phenotype and evidence of carcinoma or sarcoma-like features are classic findings in anaplastic meningioma (grade III) (G) (20× EE). Relapse of meningioma after radiotherapy: it is evident the meningothelial neoplasm (H), and inside the tumor a discrete area of coagulative necrosis (I), distinctive of radionecrosis (4× EE). *(Courtesy of Prof. Felice Giangaspero and Dr. Manila Antonelli, Department of Experimental Medicine, University La Sapienza, Rome.)*

Table 104-1   Meningiomas Grouped by Likelihood of Recurrence and World Health Organization Classification

Meningiomas with Low Risk of Recurrence and Aggressive Growth	Meningiomas with Greater Likelihood of Recurrence and/or Aggressive Behavior	
Grade I	Grade II	Grade III
Meningothelial	Atypical: Clear cell/chordoid[a]	Anaplastic (Malignant): Rhabdoid, Papillary, etc.
Fibrous (fibroblastic)	· ≥ 4 mitoses/10 HPF (≥2.5/mm²)	Papillary
Transitional (mixed)	· *Or at least three of the following four features:*	Anaplastic (malignant)[a]
Psammomatous	· Sheeting	· ≥20 mitotic figures/10 HPF (≥12.5/mm²)
Angiomatous	· Macronucleoli	· *Or:*
Microcystic	· Small cell formation	· Focal or diffuse loss of meningothelial differ-
Secretory	· Hypercellularity (≥53 nuclei/HPF, ≥118/mm²)	entiation resulting in carcinoma-, sarcoma-, or
Lymphoplasmacyte-rich	· Or Brain invasion	melanoma-like appearance
Metaplastic	Clear cell (intracranial)	Meningiomas of any subtype or grade exhibiting
	Chordoid	high proliferation indices or brain invasion

Note: World Health Organization meningioma grading according to aggressive behavior (i.e., probability of recurrence).
[a]Mayo Clinic meningioma grading scheme.
HPF, high-power microscopic fields.

Table 104-2 Neurosurgical Resection and Radiation Treatment for Intracranial Meningiomas: Series Summaries

Publication Year	Authors	Study Period	No. of Patients	Treatment Modality (%)	5-Year PFS (%)	10-Year PFS (%)	15-Year PFS (%)
Gross Total Resection							
1997	Condra et al.[32]	1964-1992	137		93	80	76
1998	Stafford et al.[71]	1978-1988	465		88	75	
1999	Ayerbe et al.[104]	1973-1994	242		90		
2004	Soyuer et al.[102]	1953-2001	48		77	61	
Subtotal Resection							
1997	Condra et al.[32]	1964-1992	92		53	40	30
1998	Stafford et al.[71]	1978-1988	116		61	39	
1999	Ayerbe et al.[104]	1973-1994	44		70		
2004	Soyuer et al.[102]	1953-2001	32		38		
External Beam Radiation Therapy							
1997	Condra et al.[32]	1964-1992	33	CRT (adjuvant 64 + primary 36)[a]	86 (primary)		87 (adjuvant)
1999	Connell et al.[105]	1984-1995	54	CRT (adjuvant 80 + primary 20)	76		
1999	Nutting et al.[95]	1962-1992	82	STR + CRT	92	83	
1999	Vendrely et al.[96]	1981-1996	156	CRT (adjuvant 51 + primary 49)	89[b]	76[b]	
2000	Wenkel et al.[97]	1981-1996	46	RT with PH and protons (adjuvant 83 + primary 17)	100	88	
2001	Debus et al.[98]	1985-1998	189	FSRT (adjuvant 69 + primary 31)	98		
2001	Pourel et al.[45]	1978-1997	26	CRT (adjuvant 80 + primary 20)	95		
2002	Uy et al.[100]	1994-1999	40	IMRT (adjuvant 62.5 + primary 27.5)	93		
2003	Mendenhall et al.[80]	1984-2001	101	CRT (adjuvant 35 + primary 65)	95	92	92
2003	Pirzkall et al.[101]	1998-1999	20	IMRT (adjuvant 80 + primary 20)	100		
2004	Soyuer et al.[102]	1953-2001	40	STR + FSRT[b]	91		
2005	Milker-Zabel et al.[86]	1985-2001	317	FSRT (adjuvant 69 + primary 31)[c]	90.5 (grade I)	89 (grade I)	
2006	Henzel et al.[87]	1997-2003	224	FSRT (adjuvant 58 + primary 42)[a]	96.9		
2007	Milker-Zabel et al.[103]	1998-2004	94	IMRT (adjuvant 72 + primary 28)	93.6		
2008	Hamm et al.[106]	1997-2003	183	FSRT (adjuvant 70 + primary 30)	96.9[a]		

Notes: Comparative progression-free survival (PFS) rates after gross total resection (GTR), subtotal resection (STR), and radiation therapy (RT), primary or adjuvant, of the largest series published in the last 15 years. Gross total resection corresponds to Simpson grades 1 and 2 (1, complete excision, including dura and bone; 2, complete excision plus coagulation of dural attachments). Subtotal resection summarizes all Simpson grades ≥3 (3, complete excision but insufficient dural coagulation or bone resection; 4, partial resection of tumor; 5, biopsy only). External beam radiation therapy includes conventional radiation therapy (CRT), fractionated stereotactic radiation therapy (FSRT), intensive modulated radiation therapy (IMRT), and radiotherapy with protons and photons (PH). In these series of patients, meningiomas were typically but nonexclusively of WHO grade 1. As a rule of thumb, tumor progression after STR is 30%, 60%, and 90% at 5, 10, and 15 years, respectively. STR alone is an inadequate therapeutic regimen, because it usually entails worse rates of local tumor control; STR must be associated with RT. The results after STR+RT or GTR are similar.[188] Therefore, extremely radical resections, which are often followed by neurologic complications, may be unnecessary.

[a]Radiosurgery for a few patients.
[b]Overall cause-specific-survival rates.
[c]At 4.4 years.

dependent on the main technical variables (dose–volume integral, timing, target cytology), as well as the goals that we are pursuing (tumor growth control [TGC], necrotic evolution, ephaptic block, etc.). Regarding meningiomas, routine protocols are focused on TGC, probably obtained through a combined mechanism, such as: 1, direct cytotoxicity, presumably promoting apoptosis; 2, damage to the vascular supply, mediated by inhibition of growth factors (vascular endothelial growth factor (VEGF), epidermal growth factor (EGF), factor 8, etc.); and 3, inactivation/destruction of hormonal receptors (e.g., octreotide [OCT] receptor).[113,114]

Targeting Update

The development of SRS has closely followed the impressive evolution of neuroradiologic techniques. The best example is perhaps the exponential increase of radiosurgical indications after the introduction of computerized imaging, particularly magnetic resonance imaging (MRI). Indeed, for routine SRS procedures, stereo-MRI remains a mainstay in target localization. Coregistered multimodality acquisitions (MRI, computed tomography [CT], angiography, positron emission tomography [PET] scan) have led on one side to the development of fusion algorithms based on contour definition, signal intensity, and voxel matching that allow detailed, interpolated 3D and 4D pictures, speeding up all the preoperative procedures. On the other, advances in computerized integration of stereotactic and nonstereotactic imaging,

including functional MRI and diffusion tensor imaging (DTI), are opening unexpected frontiers to SRS treatments.[115] Improving safety and efficacy of radiosurgical planning is now possible via fusing the conventional sequences of a stereotactic MRI with the three Tesla pictures of corticospinal, visual, or arcuate DTI, with the aim of preserving the specific tract from undue damage (Fig. 104-3).[116] CT and MRI scans sometimes may not adequately identify the regions of functional interest surrounding the planned target. Coregistration of functional MRI becomes mandatory, albeit sometimes still inadequate. Molecular imaging may be the appropriate integration. Using stereo-PET scan metabolic mapping, with FDG or a spectrum of amino acids, particularly fluorodopa and 11C-methionine,[117,118] can be merged with conventional pictures, thereby helping to identify the borders of the lesion as well as the metabolically active sites of the tumor or necrotic/radionecrotic foci on the basis of the differential uptake.[119,120] Moreover, PET techniques allow us to differentiate the usually octreotide-rich surfaces of meningiomas from other skull base tumors that generally lack these receptors.[113,114]

Irradiation Techniques and Modalities

Radiosurgery, in the absolute majority of cases, differs from conventional ab externo radiotherapy in various well-known aspects:
1. A single fractionated high dose is used, with very few exceptions, as opposed to multiple small daily fractions.

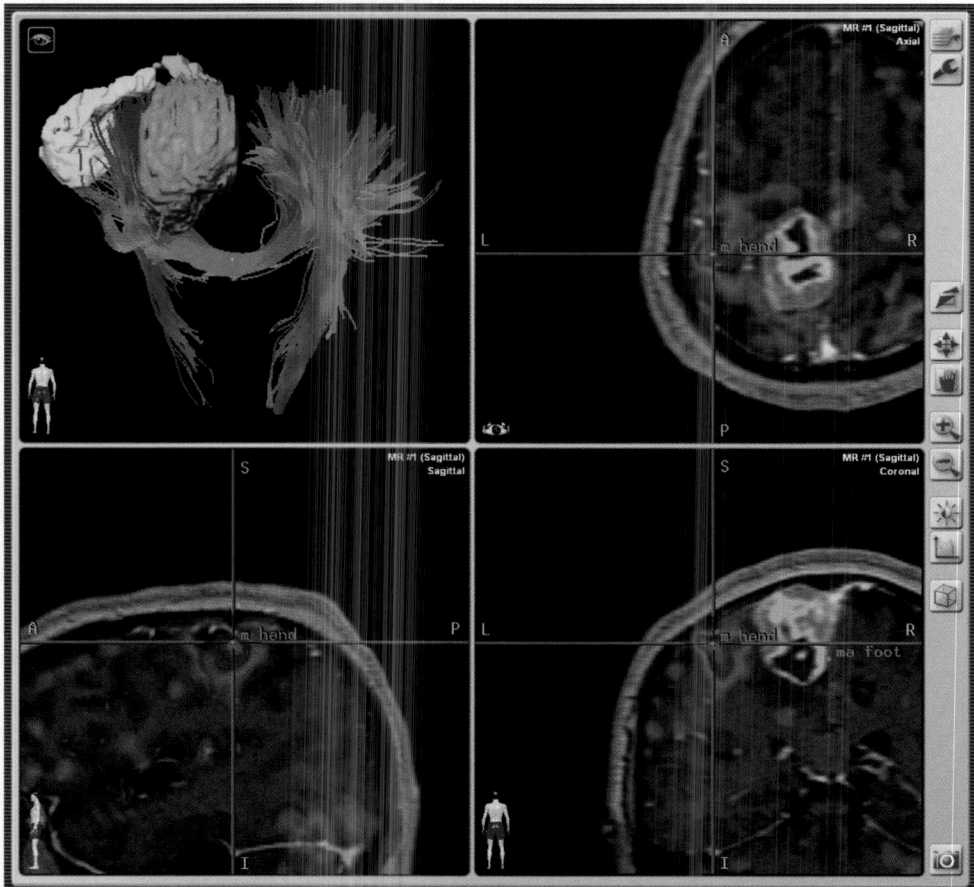

FIGURE 104-3 Parasagittal rolandic meningioma: functional magnetic resonance and integrated coregistered neuroimaging using diffusion tensor imaging.

2. The use of stereotactic technology entails considerable accuracy of the treatment (with a standard mechanical error of 0.3 mm).
3. The dose gradient is extremely steep; thus the resulting lesions are very sharply circumscribed. As a consequence, exposure outside of the target volume is minimized.
4. Radiotherapy relies on the difference in susceptibility between tumor tissue and normal brain tissue, whereas radiosurgery delivers an ablative dose to the target margin with a higher dose delivered centrally.

Currently stereotactic radiosurgery techniques may utilize different types of penetrating energy, including cyclotron- or synchrotron-generated particles such as protons or heavy-charged particles, and photon devices such as modified linear accelerators (LINACs) or the gamma knife (GK) (Fig. 104-4).

PROTON BEAM

High-energy protons represent an extremely important alternative option to photon and electron beams. In fact, proton beams offer the advantage to improve tumor control, especially for treating small volumes, where it is necessary to obtain a localized high-dose distribution in small deep-sited locations, while relatively sparing the surrounding normal tissue.[2,12] The tissue depth at which the Bragg ionization peak is maximal can be adjusted by cross-firing systems according to the target position.

Moreover, there is increasing evidence that a proton boost combined with more than 60-Gy photon therapy significantly improves mean survival and local tumor control (LTC) rates in atypical (5-year PFS, 89%) and anaplastic (5-year PFS, 51%) meningiomas. The drawbacks of

this technique include the great expense of building and maintaining these sites; some compromise in spatial accuracy because instead of a frame attached to the skull, the patient wears an immobilizing plastic mask or bite block in the mouth to achieve fixation; relatively time-consuming treatment planning; and the need for beam-modifying devices that must be customized for each patient, thereby increasing the time and cost of treatments. The use of these charged particles has developed rapidly in recent decades. Currently there are 20 hadron-therapy facilities worldwide (half of them in Europe).

LINEAR ACCELERATOR

Linear accelerator–based radiosurgery uses x-ray beams that are produced by the collision of accelerated electrons with a metal target (see Fig. 104-4). Multiple noncoplanar arcs converge at a single isocenter, where a nearly sphere-shaped dose distribution is created. These arcs are produced by gantry rotation during irradiation, and each is defined by a different couch angle. By adjusting the number, length, angles, and weights of individual arcs, irradiation of adjacent crucial structures can be reduced. Most LINAC radiosurgery units (e.g., Synergy and Axesse by Elekta, Stockholm; Trilogy by Varian, Palo Alto, CA; Novalis by Brain Lab, Feldkirchen, Germany) use tertiary circular collimators that further decrease beam divergence, thereby protecting normal tissues. For higher conformality while departing from a spherical shape, multiple isocenters are possible, at the cost of greater inhomogeneity and much longer treatment times. This technique has proved to be an effective, alternative radiosurgical option, particularly in cases of larger target volumes, or whenever fractionated radiosurgical procedures are required.[2,12,121] Comparative

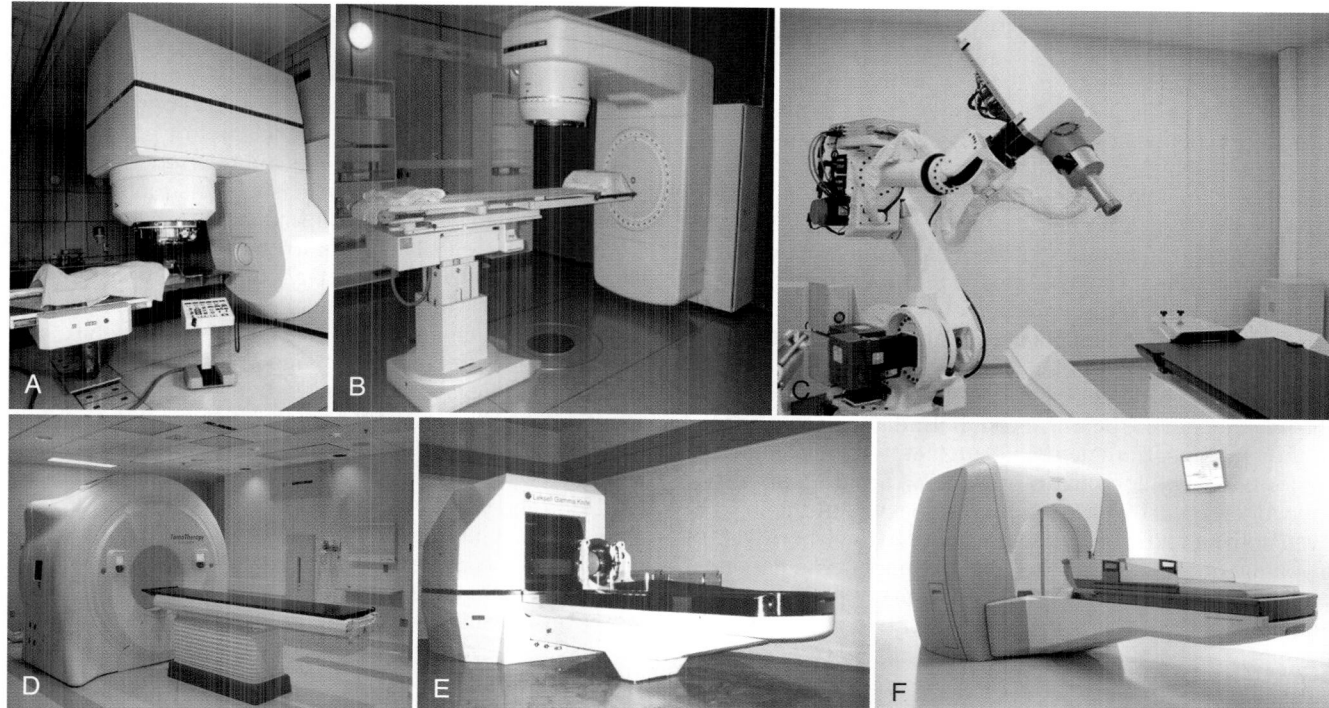

FIGURE 104-4 Stereotactic radiosurgery options: proton beam gantry (A); linear accelerator (B); CyberKnife (C); Tomotherapy Hi-Art System (D); first (1993) (model C) (E) and last (Perfexion model) (F) gamma knife of our center in Verona. *(Courtesy of Riv Med and new magazine edition.)*

analyses of the literature concerning LINAC versus GK results in meningiomas, however, still show on one side similar tumor control indexes, and on the other, much higher complication rates with LINAC, with comparable or shorter follow-up periods (Table 104-3).[9,29,42,58,63,122-159]

With the increasing use of SRS, the growing interest for highly sophisticated photon linear accelerators has led to micro-multileaf (MML) technology, potentially more competitive with GK and proton beam devices, and characterized by an easy patient setup and greater possibilities of reaching any irradiation position. Basic parameters that allow complex field shaping with the LINAC include the patient couch angle, gantry arc angle, isocenter position, and collimator size. Additional factors include beam weighting and the tissue depth through which various arc segments are delivered. Manipulation of these simple elements provides significant flexibility in the conformal three-dimensional dose distribution for a single isocenter. By using multiple isocenters, it is also possible to maximize the buffer exposure of the target, and of the adjacent critical structures.

CYBERKNIFE

This extremely refined instrument was conceived in the mid-1980s and manufactured within a decade. In its 15-year history, the CyberKnife (Accuray, Sunnyvale, CA), has clearly shown basic pros and cons of the technique.[121,155,160-163] Regarding the former, the main advantages include (1) easier fractionation, that is, increased protection of sensory cranial nerves,[162] and so on; (2) no need of general anesthesia even in young patients; and (3) flexibility to treat lesions throughout the body. Regarding the latter, the absence of a stereotactic frame, as well as the mobility of the radiation source should somehow entail a slightly superior error margin if compared to the gamma knife. It is well known that CyberKnife operative programs are essentially based on CT scan imaging recognition. For certain targets, this might involve less sophisticated imaging.

The CyberKnife (see Fig. 104-4) combines a lightweight 6-MeV LINAC designed for radiosurgery and mounted onto a highly maneuverable robotic arm that can position and point the LINAC. Internally controlled real-time image guidance eliminates the need of skeletal fixation for either positioning or rigid immobilization of the target. This system acquires radiographs of skeletal features associated with the treatment site, uses image registration techniques to determine the target's coordinates with respect to the LINAC and to the manipulator, which finally directs the beam to the planned point. Whenever the patient moves, internal controls detect the change, stop radiation, correct the trajectory of the beam, and start irradiating again nearly in the real time. Complex radiosurgical treatments may be performed, in which beams originate at arbitrary points in the workspace to target arbitrary points within the lesion. Even nonisocentric beams can be focused anywhere within a volume around the center. Total treatment time depends on the complexity of the plan and delivery paths but it is comparable to standard LINAC treatments.

TOMOTHERAPY

Helical tomotherapy unit is a new modality for radiation treatments, the first dedicated to intensity-modulated irradiation using a fully integrated image-guided radiotherapy machine with on-board megavoltage CT capability. The tomotherapy system (see Fig. 104-4) uses a 6-megavoltage accelerator, and a 64-leaf binary multileaf collimator and xenon image detector array mounted on a rotating gantry. Radiation is delivered in a helical way, obtained by concurrent gantry rotation and couch/patient movements. Altogether, these components allow continuous, intensity-modulated rotational irradiation with fan beam entry from 360 degrees. A megavoltage CT scan before the treatment (nominal energy of 3.5 megavoltages) can be fused with a planning CT scan to determine the correct patient setup every time that the radiotherapist needs to check it. Finally, ultimate dose calculation is refined by means of convolution/superimposition. Tomotherapy has been used for the treatment of benign brain tumors (meningiomas and neurinomas), resulting in good target coverage with high-dose homogeneity and respecting organs-at-risk constraints.[164] In addition, this technique allows treatment of larger brain lesions than GKS. Once again the most important difference seems to be that the latter still maintains a better conformity index, and non-negligible advantages in terms of the integral dose to the brain.

GAMMA KNIFE

Depending on the model, the gamma knife (GK) (Elekta, Sweden) contains an array of 201 (Model B or C) or 192 (Perfexion) (see Fig. 104-4) individual ^{60}Co sources aligned with a collimation system that directs each of the radiation beams to a very precise focal point. As a consequence, even very small targets can be treated by a high radiation dosage, whereas peripheral dose levels remain low. GK treatments are therefore quite heterogeneous in terms of dose distribution inside and outside of the target; tumor control and tissue sparing is achieved via the steep dose gradient at the periphery rather than exploiting the radiobiological differential between normal and pathologic tissue as in fractionated radiotherapy. At installation, GK units have an initial dose rate of approximately 4 Gy/min. Given that the ^{60}Co half-life of 5.28 years, the primary sources must be replaced every 6 to 7 years. Due to the low energy of the isotope sources, most treatments are referred to a normalization of 50%. With the multiple isocenters routinely used, GK plans tend to be more conformal but less homogeneous than LINAC-based plans. Due to the typically steep dose gradients of radiosurgery, an accurate alignment of the plan's isocenter with the physical isocenter of the machine is a quite challenging issue.[12] Details of the structure and operation of the central body and collimation system are among the biggest differences between the Perfexion Gamma Knife (GKPx) and earlier B and C models. While the external hemispheric helmet in the B and C models is fundamental in providing the final beam collimation, in the Perfexion model the central body and collimation system are somewhat more complex because the ^{60}Co sources are mobile and the conical collimator body is entirely internal to the unit, so that there are no external helmets (Fig. 104-5). Moreover the surgeon can modify the shooting collimator size using the sector drive motors that move the sources along their bushing to the correct position; the localization of each sector is monitored by linear and rotational encoders characterized by a positioning repeatability of less than 0.01 mm.[165,166] Critical structures such as optic pathways

Table 104-3 Stereotactic Radiosurgery for Meningiomas: Major Series of Patients (>100)

Publication Year	Authors	Group	Study Period	No. of Patients	Type of Meningiomas: A or B (% Patients)	Basic Modalities of SRS (GK, LINAC, or Protons)	Local Control (%)
1994	Goldsmith et al.[42]	San Francisco (USA)	1967-1990	140 (117 benign and 23 malignant)	B	Proton beam therapy	89 for benign and 48 for malignant meningiomas at 5 years
1996	Hudgins et al.[137]	Dallas (USA)	–	100	9 A and 91 B	GK	91
1998	Hakim et al.[138]	Boston (USA)	1988-1995	127 (155 tumors, of which 106 benign)	31 A and 69 B	LINAC	89.3 for benign tumors at 5 years
2001	Pendl et al.[134]	Graz (Austria)	1992-1998	197 (198 tumors)	53 A and 47 B	GK	98 (for 164 patients)
2001	Stafford et al.[139]	Rochester (USA)	1990-1998	190 (206 tumors)	41 A and 59 B	GK	93 for benign, 68 for atypical and 0 for malignant tumors at 5 years
2002	Eustacchio et al.[136]	Graz (Austria)	1992-1997	121	51 A and 49 B	GK	98.3
2002	Lee et al.[140]	Pittsburgh (USA)	1987-2000	159	52 A and 48 B	GK	93.1 at 5 years
2002	Nicolato et al.[217]	Verona (Italy)	1993-2002	122	51 A and 49 B	GK	96.5 at 5 years
2003	Chang et al.[142]	Seoul (Korea)	1992-2000	179 (194 tumors)	61 A and 39 B	GK	97.1 (radiologic control rate: >6 months and for 136 lesions)
2003	Flickinger et al.[10]	Pittsburgh (USA)	1987-2000	219	A	GK	93.2 at 5 years
2003	Pollock et al.[143]	Rochester (USA)	1990-2002	330 (356 tumors)	58 A and 42 B	GK	94% (radiologic control rate: >6 months and for 297 lesions)
2004	DiBiase et al.[9]	Camden (USA)	1992-2000	137	62 A and 38 B	GK	86.2 at 5 years
2004	Liscak et al.[145]	Prague (Czech Republic)	1992-1999	192 (197 tumors)	66 A and 34 B	GK	95
2005	Feigl et al.[146]	Hannover (Germany)	1999-2003	127 (142 tumors)	36 A and 64 B	GK	96.4
2005	Friedman et al.[147]	Gainesville (USA)	1989-2001	210	46 A and 54 B	LINAC	96 for benign, 77 for atypical, and 19 for malignant tumors at 5 years
2005	Kreil et al.[58]	Graz (Austria)	1992-1999	200	50.5 A and 49.5 B	GK	98.5 at 5 years
2005	Malik et al.[148]	Sheffield (United Kingdom)	1994-2000	277 (309 tumors)	44 tumor A and 56 tumor B	GK	87 for typical, 49 for atypical, and 0 for malignant meningiomas at 5 years
2007	Feigl et al.[158]	Hannover (Germany)	1999-2004	211 (243 tumors)	42 A and 58 B	GK	86.3 at 4 years
2007	Hasegawa et al.[149]	Komaki (Japan)	1991-2003	115	43 A and 57 B	GK	87 at 5 years (for 111 patients)
2007	Kollová et al.[150]	Prague (Czech Republic)	1992-1999	368 (400 tumors)	70 A and 30 B	GK	97.9 at 5 years
2007	Lee et al.[151]	Pittsburgh (USA)	1987-2004	964	54 A and 46 B	GK	93 for benign, 83 for atypical, and 72 for malignant meningiomas at 5 years
2008	Iwai et al.[152]	Osaka (Japan)	1994-2001	108	43 A and 57 B	GK	93 at 5 years
2008	Kondziolka et al.[153]	Pittsburgh (USA)	18-year interval	972 (1045 tumors)	51 tumor A and 49 tumor B	GK	97 for benign meningiomas at 5 years
2009	Bledsoe et al.[154]	Rochester (USA)	1990-2007	116	36 A and 64 B	GK	99 at 3 years
2009	Colombo et al.[155]	Vicenza (Italy)	2003-2007	199	43 A and 57 B	CyberKnife	93.6 at 5 years
2009	Flannery et al.[156]	Pittsburgh (USA)	21-year interval	168	58 A and 42 B	GK	91 at 5 years
2009	Kondziolka et al.[29]	Pittsburgh (USA)	18-year interval	125	51 A and 49 B	GK	71.6 at 5 years (For patients with benign tumors [Grade I] and those who had not undergone prior surgery, the actuarial tumor control rates were 95.3 and 85.8, respectively.)
2009	Takanashi et al.[157]	Sapporo (Japan)	1991-2003	101	56 A and 44 B	GK	95.5% in cavernous sinus meningiomas and 98.4% in posterior fossa meningiomas

Notes: GK, LINAC, and CyberKnife stereotactic radiosurgery for meningiomas. Synopsis of the largest series (over 100 patients) in the last 15 years comparing local tumor control. A, newly diagnosed meningioma. B, recurrent and/or previously resected meningiomas and/or other; GK, gamma knife; LINAC, linear accelerator.

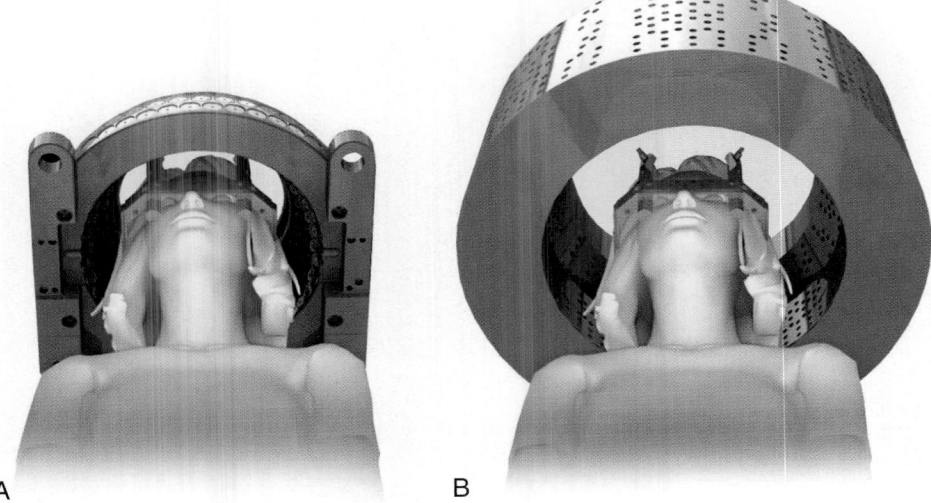

A

B

FIGURE 104-5 Schematic drawing of the original gamma knife "model C" helmet (A) and the new Perfexion helmet (B). The latter evidently covers a much wider volume allowing easier treatment of skull base lesions, reaching C1–C2 level.

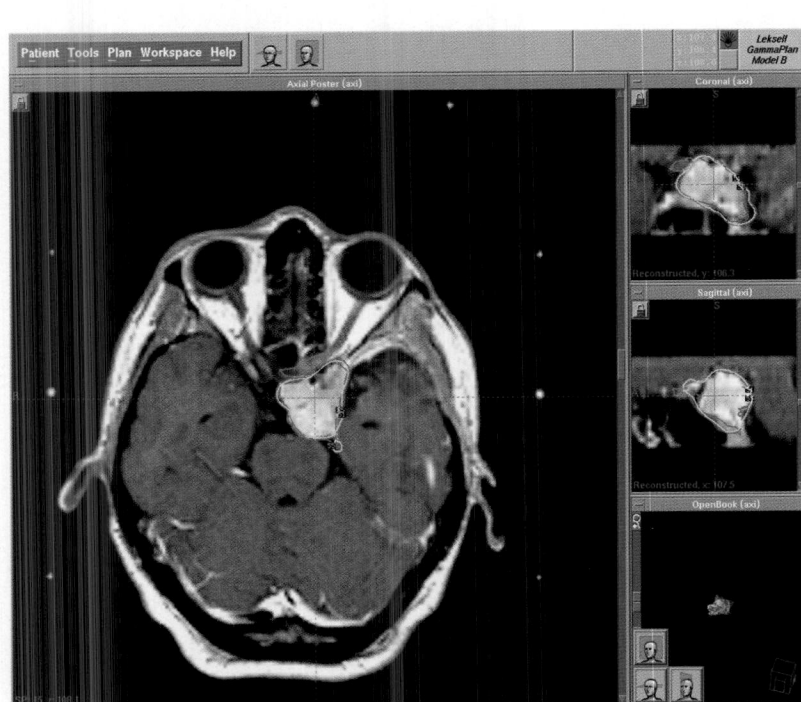

FIGURE 104-6 Gamma knife radiosurgery treatment of a left cavernous sinus meningioma. Note the highly conformal shape of the therapeutic isodose.

and cranial nerves may be shielded through the application of beam blocking patterns that minimize the contribution of possibly dangerous shots.

DOSE PLANNING

The goal of dose planning is to create an extremely conformal and selective isodose configuration, with complete covering of the tumor, and minimal exposure of the surrounding tissues (Fig. 104-6). Using a combination of multiple isocenters of different sizes, differential weighting of the crucial shots, selective blocking of the collimated beams and—typical of the Perfexion Gamma Knife—using hybrid shots,[165] it is possible to produce dose plans that closely conform not only to the main shape of the meningioma, but also to all the MRI-documented dural attachments (Fig. 104-7),

while sparing the neighboring neural structures. Probabilistic models, quadrature-sum analysis, and phantom studies have repeatedly confirmed the reliability of such operative models.[107,108,166] These newer approaches in treatment planning have consistently improved Paddick's conformity index,[167] meanwhile reducing treatment times for both GKR and GKPx[88,165,169] and for MML LINAC.[88,168] To date, the recommended surface (SD), edge (ED), or peripheral (PD) doses for meningiomas range from 11 to 15 Gy at the 50% isodose; the higher levels are currently reserved for more aggressive histotypes.[2,3] The "ideal"—that is, the most biologically justified—planning target volume, is still a matter of debate, with a spectrum of options, ranging from including the gross, T1 contrast–enhancing image plus a supposedly infiltrated margin of a few millimeters,[3,32,41,98,103,170] to the

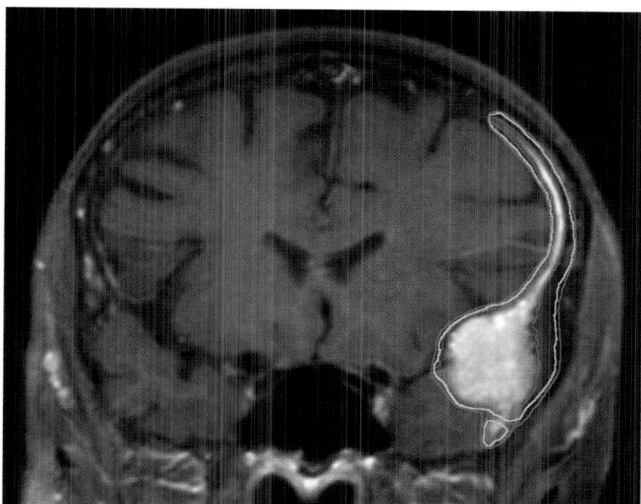

FIGURE 104-7 A multiple-isocenter conformal gamma plan for a Sylvian meningioma (*red line*) with dural attachment, the so-called "dural tail"; and bone reaction in the adjacent skull. The *yellow line* corresponds to the 55% isodose line and the green line indicates the 50% isodose curve.

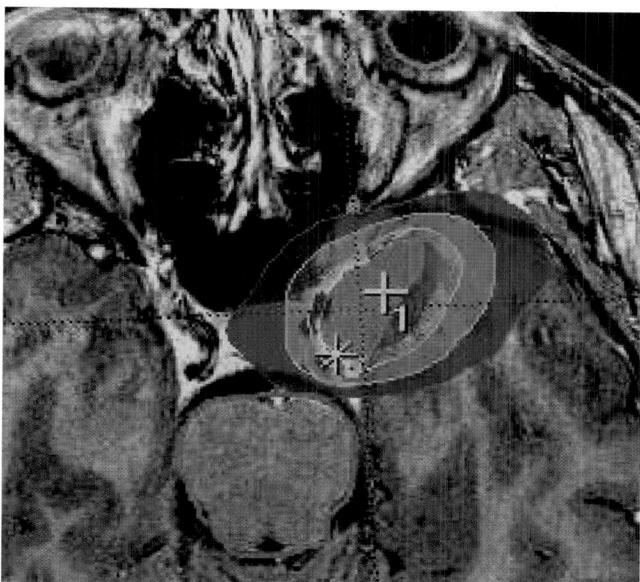

FIGURE 104-8 Gamma knife radiosurgery treatment of a left cavernous sinus meningioma. Paddick's conformity index is extremely rewarding, although at the price of a pronounced in homogeneity, with a too large, potentially dangerous hot spot (75%) covering the carotid artery and not far from the left optic nerve-hemichiasm. The dose plan needs modification. The *yellow line* corresponds to the 50% isodose line and the *blue line* indicates the 20% isodose curve.

controversial inclusion of the "dural tail" that—according to studies of extremely refined doses—should be essentially composed of hypervascular dura with none of the expected tumor colonies.[3,92,171,172] Another deceptive variable in the definition of the target volume is represented by hyperostosis,[3,173,174] particularly after the studies of Pieper et al.[174] showing that (in a series of 26 consecutively operated patients) hyperostotic bone was almost constantly (25/26) present, even without any imaging evidence. In these cases, ablative radiosurgery on the hyperostotic bone might have the same meaning of Simpson's grade 1 in surgical approaches. As mentioned previously, the novel and impressive advances in radiosurgical treatment strategies, particularly coregistration and fusion algorithms–dose-planning software, and automatic positioning systems are helping to overcome some of the major SRS, and specifically GKR, constraints. We can reasonably target unusually larger volumes, even in crucial sites, by using lower dosages or adopting "staged" SRS procedures, via means of dose and/or volume fractionation.[111,112]

Published results are interesting, and there is no evidence of increased adverse radiation effects (AREs).[111,112,152] In fact, the well-known relationship between the dose–volume integral and the risk of adverse radiation effects does not seem to apply at lower-dose regimens.[135,152,175,176] Nonetheless, in meningioma treatments, relevant limits, pitfalls, and risks remain to be tackled. An instructive example is represented by dosimetry planning for cavernous sinus meningiomas (Fig. 104-8). The dose heterogeneity of these treatments usually requires an extremely careful evaluation of dose-distribution algorithms,[177-179] because of the occasional reported cases of radio-induced vascular injury to the carotid arteries,[177-179] the still observed morbidity of this technique on sensory nerves,[151] and the sometimes disappointing results in atypical and anaplastic lesions.[2,151] Finally, a controversial issue in treatment planning pertains to the so-called "radiation-induced meningiomas.[180-182] These tumors usually appear at a variable interval from

radiation exposure, depending on the dose and timing. They are non-infrequently deep seated, multifocal in 4.6% to 18.7% of the cases.[180,181] Surgical resection is considered to be the best therapeutic option. However, when dealing with frail patients or with particularly crucial locations, radical surgery may be too risky, opening the question on the SRS alternative. The published literature is rather scanty.[180,182] Eligibility criteria (limited volume, well-defined imaging, etc.) adopted in these cases do not differ from standard protocols. Clinical-radiologic results—particularly the LTC (75% to 78%) and the 5-year PFS (similar)—are satisfactory, and only slightly inferior to the published data regarding regular meningiomas. Morbidity remains low (5%) with no reported cases of newer carcinogenesis.[180-182]

Radiobiology

Radiosurgery, like most radiation treatments, results in the formation of free radicals as electrons are freed from their atoms. Their main biological effect occurs at the DNA level: The transfer of energy results in breaks in the DNA strands (direct effect). Additional radiation damage to the DNA is mediated through reactive species of water (indirect effect). Whenever single-strand breaks occurs, the aberrations are of little eventual consequence, because the breaks are easily repaired. Conversely, lethal aberrations may occur leading to mutagenesis, or to cell death, due either to double-strand breaks or to chromosome breaks with the "sticky ends" rearranging and rejoining in grossly distorted, nonviable formations. The number of lethal aberrations and subsequent killed cells is closely related to several conditioning factors: the specific oncotype and a complex series of cellular parameters ("alpha–beta ratio," superoxide-enzyme characterization, etc.) defining the specific radiosensitivity, the radiation dose, the tumor volume, and the microscopic model of energy deposition. On the basis of these features, meningiomas mostly belong to relatively radiosensitive, late-responding tissues.

Effective dosages are in the lower range, not far from normal-cell thresholds, while the time interval for the effect is close to the maximum in-vivo doubling time.[21,22,183-185] Moreover, all kinds of ionizing radiations are currently identified, not only according to dose level, but also characteristic pattern of energy transfer and consequent relative biological effectiveness (RBE).[186] Linear energy transfer (LET) is defined as the average energy that is locally delivered by a particle in an absorbing medium divided by unit length of the crossed distance. Larger particles are correlated with higher LET values, with increasing ionization density and greater RBE. The differential cytotoxicity of low- versus high-LET radiation beams is particularly emphasized in hypoxic tumors. Indeed, some of the main reactive molecules produced by radiation beams (i.e., ion pairs and free radicals) are represented by superoxide compounds with unpaired valence electrons, breaking DNA-protein chemical bonds. Therefore, in most cases the permanent effect of this free radical–mediated injury is dependent on the presence of oxygen.

When tumor cells rapidly divide, they outgrow their vascular supply and become chronically hypoxic. With increased LET beams, this close dependence on oxygenation for biological effect decreases. On the contrary, low-LET sources such as x-rays and gamma-rays rely significantly on local oxygen levels for their biological effect. Hence, the importance sometimes associated with the radiosurgically typical dose inhomogeneity that may somehow compensate for this disadvantage is the hot spot in the "core" of a tumor, which may be desirable for several reasons. First, it offsets the relative protection offered by the poor oxygenation of the tumor core; second, it may increase the cell kill in the surrounding of the hot spot due to the "penumbra effect." Fractionated radiation results in the distribution of lethal and sublethal effects within a wider targeted field. In contrast, the typically small targeted size and sharp dose fall-off of radiosurgery allows the delivery of high radiation levels to a limited area.

Furthermore, comparing pathologic tissues with normal brain cells, the relative abundance of replicating nuclear materials in tumor tissues and the higher potential of DNA repair (sublethal damage [SLD]) of normal neural cells may explain the differential sensitivity threshold of these treatments. In SRS, the use of a single dose results in a higher incidence of lethal damage to cells, enhancing the biological efficacy of the beam. Additional factors may justify the spectrum of responses: (1) rate of cell proliferation, resulting in increased sensitivity of endothelial, glial and subependymal plate cells; (2) vascular obliteration also seems to play a role in the death of tumor cells as well; and (3) due to the steep dose gradient at the margin of the target volume, normal tissue is exposed to lower levels than the target periphery, and this explains why SLD is of little concern.

Radiosensitizers and radioenhancers are supposed to concurrently increase the toxicity of ionizing radiation on tumor cells reducing the required dose and therefore protecting peripheral brain tissues. The literature of the last decade apparently abounds in experimental—and a few clinical—reports analyzing the potentially beneficial role of a variety of radiosensitizers and radioenhancers in specific trials.[183,187]

To summarize, radiosensitizers are chemical or pharmacologic agents that should putatively increase the radiation effects if administered during the treatment. The historical example is hyperbaric oxygen. They are usually classified into the following three categories: hypoxic cell sensitizers, hypoxic cytotoxins, and nonhypoxic cell sensitizers.

1. Hypoxic cell sensitizers are able to increase the radiosensitivity of tumor cells deficient of oxygen by inducing the formation and stabilization of DNA-toxic radicals, mimicking the effect of oxygen. These drugs include nitroimidazole, misonidazole, etanidazole, nimorazole, and efaproxaril.
2. Hypoxic cytotoxins presumably play their role by selectively killing hypoxic cells, which are generally more resistant to radiation. This group includes three classes of drugs: quinone antibiotics, nitroaromatic compounds, and benzotriazine di-N-oxides.
3. Promising non-hypoxic sensitizers include the halogenated pyridines working as DNA base analogues, becoming incorporated in newly synthesized DNA, and rendering tumors more sensitive to ionizing radiations. Radioenhancers are agents aimed to reduce the amount of radiation required to kill a given population of tumor cells. More recently, interesting protocols using gene therapy–guided radiosurgical procedures (i.e., viral vectors) have further expanded the spectrum of radioenhancers available.[187]

Radiosurgery Treatment Results

Since the early 1990s, the role of radiosurgery in the spectrum of therapeutic options for intracranial meningiomas has been increasingly emphasized even as a primary treatment alternative, especially in the elderly, and in tumors in critical locations. Indeed, the impact of the significant surgical morbidity, mortality, and postoperative recurrences, on patient's and caregiver's quality of life, has triggered such dramatic change in the therapeutic paradigm. Skull base lesions are classic examples of this phenomenon. To date the majority of these tumors are treated with SRS procedures, limiting surgical approaches to the debulking of larger tumors. If we analyze the largest (over 100 patients) published radiosurgical series of the last decade, GKR is by far the most diffused technical option (4,608 reported patients) followed by MicroMultiLeaf LINAC (337) and CyberKnife (301) (see Table 104-3).[10,114,142,144,145,148,188-193] In terms of localization, meningiomas of the cranial base—and specifically of the cavernous sinus and of the petroclival region—are the most represented. As a rule the cytologic grading is the main determinant of the radiosurgical effectiveness.[2,3,12] It is generally accepted that for benign (grade 1) meningiomas, a similar, effective, and durable LTC may be obtained using lower SRS dosages of 11 to 16 Gy at the isodose prescription line (ED or SD), and slightly higher dosages with aggressive oncotypes. The overall neuroradiologic results are rewarding and stable. In spite of the fact that the available literature is mostly limited to Evidence Based Medicine class 3 Data, with only a few studies presenting class 2 information,[75] the overall neuroradiologic results seem rewarding. Given the definition of "local tumor control" as a post-treatment computerized target volume equal to or smaller than the original, the 5-year actuarial tumor control rates range from 86.2% to 97.9% both after GKR, and CyberKnife treatment.[155,161-163] In the former and larger group (GKR), primary or "imaging-diagnosed" meningiomas and recurrences show comparable 5-year PFS (93%–98%)[144,145,148,154] than recurrences (34%–97%[144,154]). Instead, patients with benign histotypes (grade 1) are usually characterized by 5-year actuarial tumor control rates (87%–96%) much higher than those with atypical (49%–77%) or anaplastic (0%–19%) lesions.[144,145,149-154] The still limited number of reports with a mean follow-up period of 7 to 10 years have consistently confirmed such findings.[58,144,154,156,176] Adopting the concept of clinical improvement as resolution or reduction of preoperative neurologic symptoms,[152] the vast majority of cases shows stable or improved KPS and neurologic gradings at 5 to 7 years or longer follow-up.[140] A recent review published by the Pittsburgh Gamma Knife Center confirms in a cohort of 972 patients, with a long-term follow-up (for some of them up to 20 years) an overall tumor control rate up to 97% and morbidity rate of 7.7%.[29,151,153] Morbidity rates are usually low, albeit slightly higher for crucial locations such as the cavernous sinus and petroclival region.[156,175]

Our experience in GK meningioma treatment (1993–2009) is briefly summarized in Table 104-4. Clinical radiologic results have been extremely rewarding (Figs. 104-9 and 104-10). A comparative analysis of LINAC-based radiosurgical experiences in meningiomas versus GKR experiences clearly shows that follow-up period is longer for GKR (as seen previously), with several reports reaching 6 to 7 years mean follow-up versus 3 to 4 years for the LINAC series, targeted tumor volumes are extremely variable with both approaches, whereas the relative marginal dosages (12–15 Gy) as well as the tumor control rates (usually over

90%) are quite similar. The incidence of sequelae with both techniques is quantitatively (3%–13%) and qualitatively reasonable,[58] with severe neurologic worsening extremely rare and no mortality.

Special Issues

SITE

Paraoptic Meningiomas

The group includes all meningiomas located in close proximity to, or in direct contact with, the anterior optic pathways (AOPs), that is, meningiomas of the optic nerve sheaths, spheno-orbital, clinoid, para- or supra-sellar lesions, and so on. There is no documented evidence that encasement of the optic nerve and chiasm by one of these tumors is an absolute contraindication to radiation therapy.[121] Instead, extremely valuable PFS rates, with stable or improved visual fields and acuity have been described in the vast majority of patients treated with definitive radiation therapy for tumors of these regions.[88-91,121,194] Dose ranges were at or above 50 to 53 Gy in conventional fractionation.[121] This seems to confirm that LTC is the primary factor in maintaining functional vision.[90,91,121,195] It is generally accepted that for benign (grade 1) meningiomas, a similar, effective and durable LTC may be obtained using SRS doses of 11 to 15 Gy at the isodose prescription line. However, AOPs currently represent, together with the cochlear region, the most radiosensitive intracranial structure.[90,121,196] As a consequence, meningiomas of this region require an extremely careful dosimetry planning to avoid any possible damage to the visual function that is documented at the time of the treatment. In fact, a radiosurgical dose exposure of more than 9 Gy to an AOP volume exceeding 10 cubic mm—even less in children—may eventually produce irreversible visual damage, particularly if administered on a previously suffering target.[121,196] NF2, with the complex imbalance of the visual function (neurotubular deficit, etc.), which is frequently bilateral, is a classic example of such situation.[197,198] In an accurate analysis of the risk for radiation optic neuropathy (RON), a series of 215 patients received in 73% of cases doses exceeding the 8- to 9-Gy threshold on a short segment of the AOP: Only 1.1% of the patients eventually developed a RON.[199] Several different alternatives have been recommended and used with rather successful results, including fractionated GKR[88] or CyberKnife[12,121,155,162] procedures, to fractionated STR to proton-photon therapy to Perfexion-guided hybrid shots.[61] The growing experience in this area is leading to an improved therapeutic ratio.[88,121,162,200,201]

Cavernous Sinus

The first published case of sphenocavernous meningioma dates back to 1910 with an autopsy report by Frotscher and Becker,[20,28] but systematic nosography of these challenging tumors came only in 1938 with the famous monograph by Cushing and Eisenhardt.[20,173] For decades they had been considered mostly inoperable and treatment options for these patients included simple observation, palliation, and fractionated radiation therapy, with aggressive and risky surgical attempts only in young patients with large progressing tumors.[20,75,202,203]

Table 104-4	Gamma Knife Radiosurgery in Meningiomas: Synopsis of Our Experience (1993-2009)
Total number of treated patients/treated lesions	1062/1207
Imaging-defined lesions (primary treatments)	58%
Remnants/recurrences	42%
Grade	
Benign (grade 1)	92%
Atypical (grade 2)	5.5%
Anaplastic (grade 3)	2.5%
Site	
Skull base	68%
· Cavernous sinus	31%
· Petroclival	18%
Other	32%
Dose Planning and Local Tumor Control	
Average tumor volume	8.4 cc (0.8–24)
Superficial dose	14.3 Gy (9–22)
Absorbed dose	23.7 Gy (14.6–31)
Integral dose	246 mJoule (42–475)
Number of isocenters	14 (1–34)
Local tumor control (overall)	91%
Mean follow-up	70 months

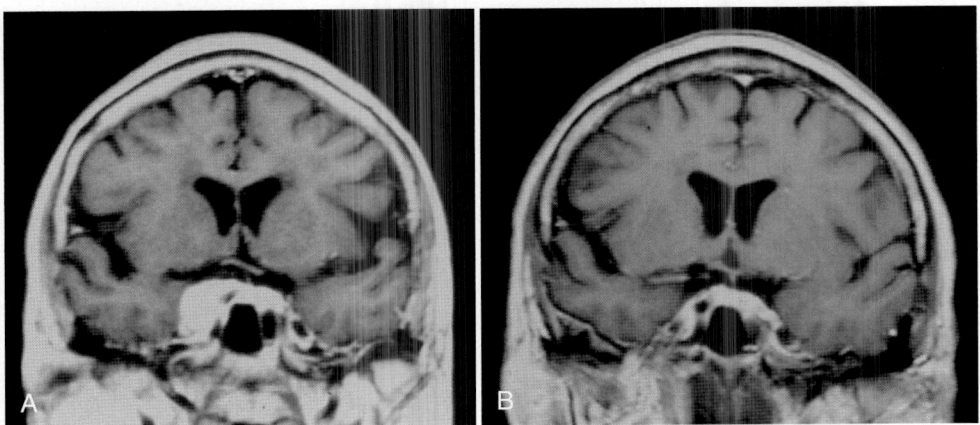

FIGURE 104-9 A, A right cavernous sinus meningioma. B, Substantial shrinkage after gamma knife radiosurgery.

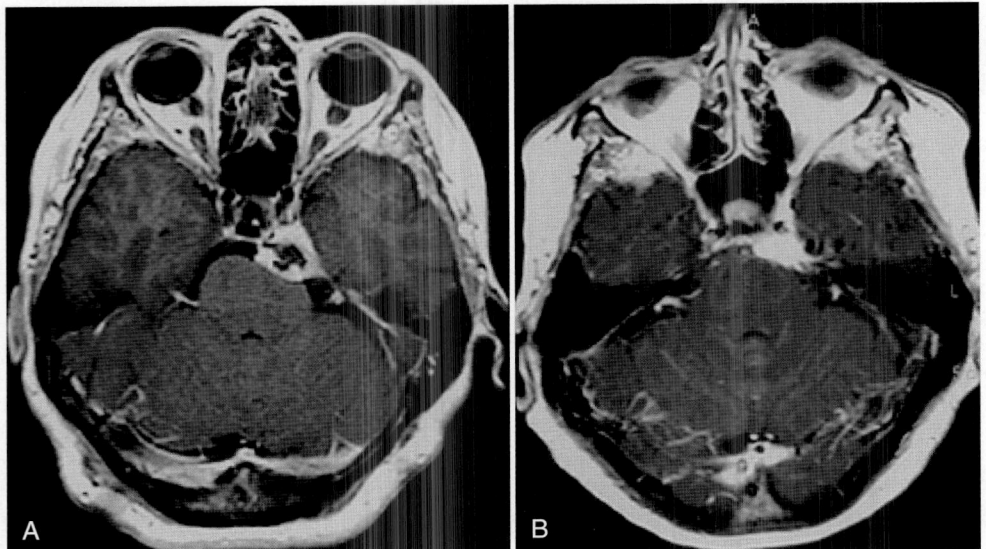

FIGURE 104-10 A, Relatively small petroclival-cavernous meningioma. B, Showing a slight shrinkage after gamma knife radiosurgery.

The intensive, multidimensional anatomic investigation of pioneer microsurgeons led in the 1970s and 1980s to newer, relatively safer, and more sophisticated surgical procedures, improving the chances for a better outcome.[20,61,62,204-206] Nonetheless, on the one hand, morbidity and mortality rates remained non-negligible, basically due to the almost constant infiltration, on the part of the tumor, of the carotid artery and its branches,[20,207-209] and to the encasement of the oculomotor and trigeminal nerves.[20,208,209] Furthermore, recurrence rates varied from 5% to 10% at 1- to 8-year follow-up, after radical resection; this rate is double that observed after partial resection.[20,61,62,205,206,210] These are the principal reasons that explain the growing role of radiotherapy and subsequently of SRS as a valid therapeutic option for these patients. Indeed, published results indicate for fractionated radiotherapy, at a mean follow-up of 30 to 70 months, progression rates of 0%–10%, and for cranial neuropathy, rates from 0% to 22%. Gamma knife results reported in the radiosurgical literature are yet more rewarding than those reported for LINAC[213] and proton therapy[218] (Table 104-5).[20,128,140,211-216] Clinical radiologic results in our experience support these findings.[141,217] LTC may vary from a slight-to-substantial reduction (Figs. 104-9

and 104-10), to—in a minority of cases—a dramatic shrinkage (Figs. 104-11 and 104-12). Furthermore, neurologic recovery, particularly of the oculomotor nerves, has been noted (Table 104-6), occurring more frequently in primary treatments. Finally, it is worth mentioning that in cavernous sinus meningiomas, SRS has shown to be effective (e.g., in restoring ocular motility), not only by reducing the tumor volume and its mechanical compression, but also via an octreotide receptor-mediated effect, that seems to prevent an anticolinergic activity of those lesions even without modifying the actual tumor size.[114,141,217] Once again, like in functional radiosurgery models, the clinical results of this technique cannot be classified as a mere mechanical consequence of a radiation-induced necrosis with volumetric shrinkage and decreased pressure on the neighboring cranial nerves, and an additional factor plays a role (Fig. 104-13).[2,50,217]

Petroclival Meningiomas

In these patients, during the last decade SRS treatments have gained an increasing role, either as a primary or as an adjuvant procedure. Microsurgery remains the basic option for the non-infrequent large petroclival lesions, sometimes

Table 104-5 Radiosurgical Treatment for Cavernous Sinus Meningiomas

Publication Year	Authors	Study Period	No. Patients	Adjuvant Treatment (%)	Mean Follow-up (Months)	5-Year PFS (%)	Cranial Nerve Complication Rate (%)
Linear Accelerator							
2002	Spiegelmann et al.[213]	1993-2001	42	26	38	97.5 (at 3 years)	7.1
2004	Selch et al.[85]	1997-2002	45	64.4	36	97.4 (at 3 years)	0
Gamma Knife							
2000	Roche et al.[212]	1992-1998	80	37.5	30.5	92.8	3.75
2001	Shin et al.[200]	1990-1999	40	70	42	86.4 (at 3 years)	20
2002	Lee et al.[140]	1987-2000	159	48	35	93.1	5
2002	Nicolato et al.[141]	1993-2002	122	49	48.9	96.5	1
2003	Iwai et al.[214]	1994-1999	42	52	49.4	92	4.8
2004	Maruyama et al.[215]	1997-2002	40	57.5	47	94.1	12.5
2005	Metellus et al.[216]	1994-1997	36	36.1	63.6	94.4	8.3
2006	Pollock et al.[178]	1992-2001	49	0	58	85 (at 3 years)	12.2
2007	Hasegawa et al.[149]	1991-2003	115	57	62	87	4.3

Notes: Stereotactic radiosurgery with gamma knife versus linear accelerator in cavernous sinus meningiomas. Major reported series of the last decade comparing follow-up, local tumor control, and cranial neuropathy incidence.

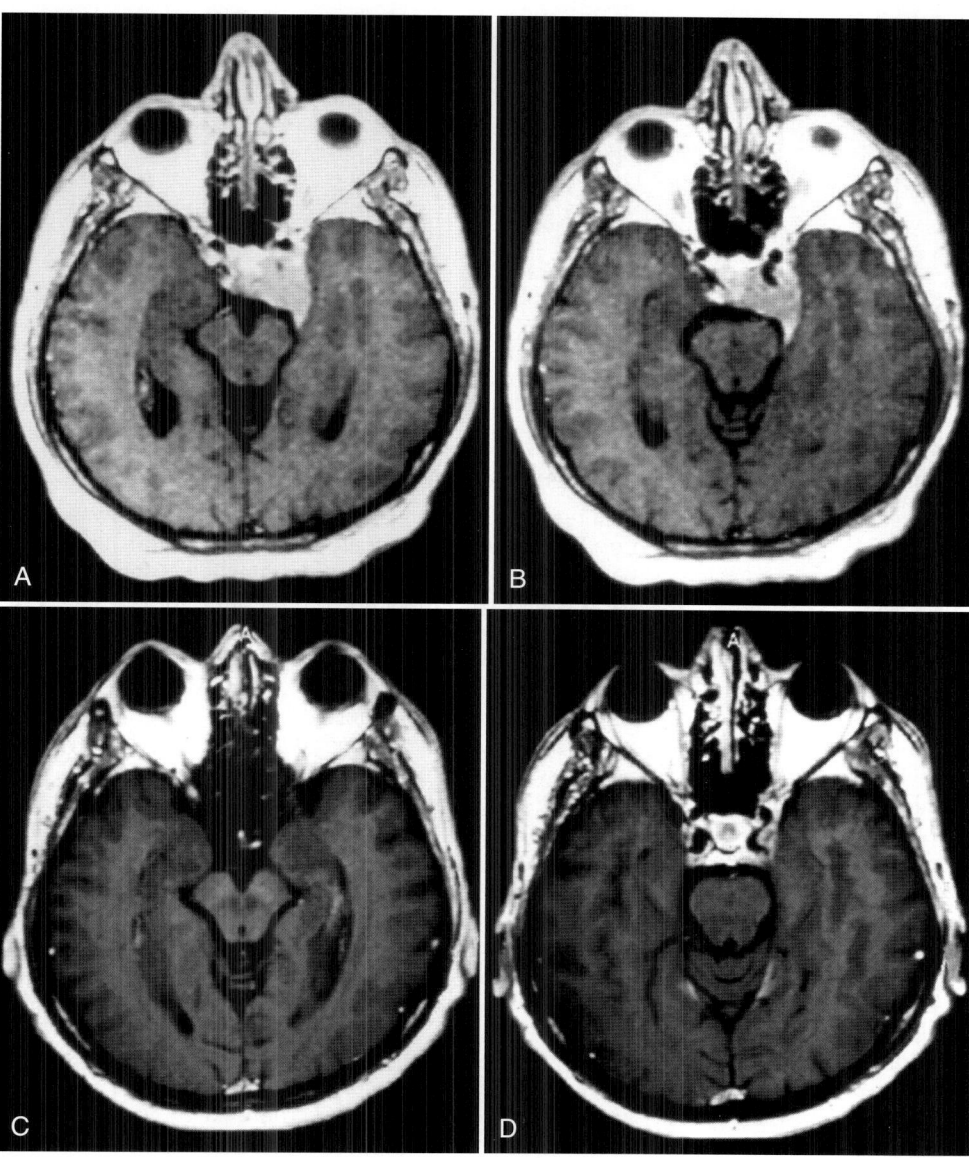

FIGURE 104-11 A and B, Left cavernous sinus meningioma. C and D, A rare example of substantial disappearance of the lesion after gamma knife radiosurgery.

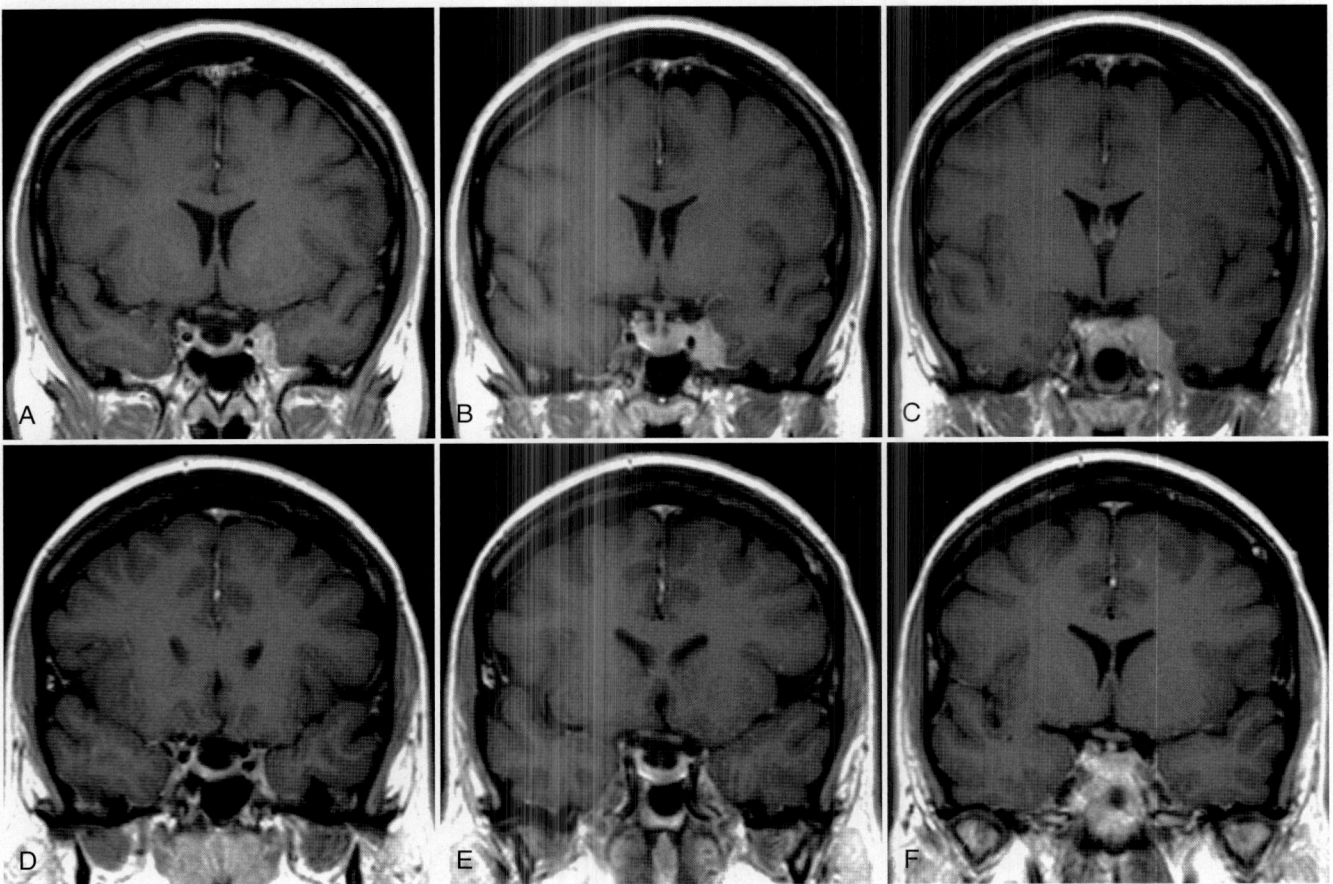

FIGURE 104-12 A to C, Left cavernous sinus meningioma, pretreatment. D to F, Seven months post–gamma knife radiosurgery. Tumor regression is evident as well as the improved visibility of the left carotid artery.

Table 104-6   Gamma Knife Radiosurgery in Cavernous Sinus Meningioma: Our Clinical Results in Primary versus Adjuvant Gamma Knife Radiosurgery

	% Improved			% Worsened		
Visual acuity	22.1	vs.	8.6	1.2	vs.	4.3
Visual field	35.7	vs.	17	3.8	vs.	5.7
Ocular motility	43	vs.	14.8	4.9	vs.	5.1
Ptosis	22.3	vs.	13.5	1.6	vs.	2.8
Facial pain	10.2	vs.	8.6	3.2	vs.	4.3

Note: The oculomotor deficit shows the best chances for recovery.

with the goal of a gross debulking giving substantial relief to intracranial pressure. Newer techniques, particularly via orbitozygomatic and retrosigmoid approaches, have gradually improved the surgical outcome, thanks to reduced morbidity.[57,219] Nevertheless, in small- to medium-sized tumors of this region, SRS has become an accepted alternative, both in terms of LTC in medium-to-long term follow-up and of reduced morbidity (Table 104-7).[10,156,176,220-224] This treatment is characterized by an absolute low rate of sequelae[10,156,176,220-224] and favorable symptomatic results often obtained on secondary trigeminal neuralgia.[225] We recently reviewed our series of GKR-treated petroclival meningiomas, updating previously published results,[221] to a longer mid-term follow-up. Preliminary, positive results

were confirmed on both outcome score and neuroradiologic pictures (see Table 104-7).

Intraventricular Meningiomas

Meningiomas growing within the ventricular system are rare, and probably originate from arachnoidal "buds" partially embedded in the choroid plexus.[226-228] Incidence has been reported as the 0.5% to 3.7% of all intracranial locations.[226-229] The rationale for primary SRS, as in several other instances, is closely related to the limitations and morbidity that frequently characterize radical removal of these lesions. However, as recently reported,[230] with the combined use of the most sophisticated operative techniques (advanced neuronavigation, third-generation ultrasonic aspirator, and molecular coagulation), total excision of these deep-seated and usually highly vascularized tumors may be safely accomplished. When planning primary SRS, it should be emphasized that dealing with "imaging-defined" lesions, a reliable diagnosis is extremely relevant. Current strategies include a clearly defined picture via MRI—typical site and morphology, homogeneous contrast enhancement, and hyperintense signal on T2-weighted images[226]—and a spectrum MRI analysis. However, SRS has been used in adjuvant protocols on surgical residual or—as an alternative to surgery—in recurrences. Considering the very peculiar localization of the target—surrounded by variably thick, cerebral spinal fluid (CSF) films—prescription doses higher

CS meningioma: pre-GKR

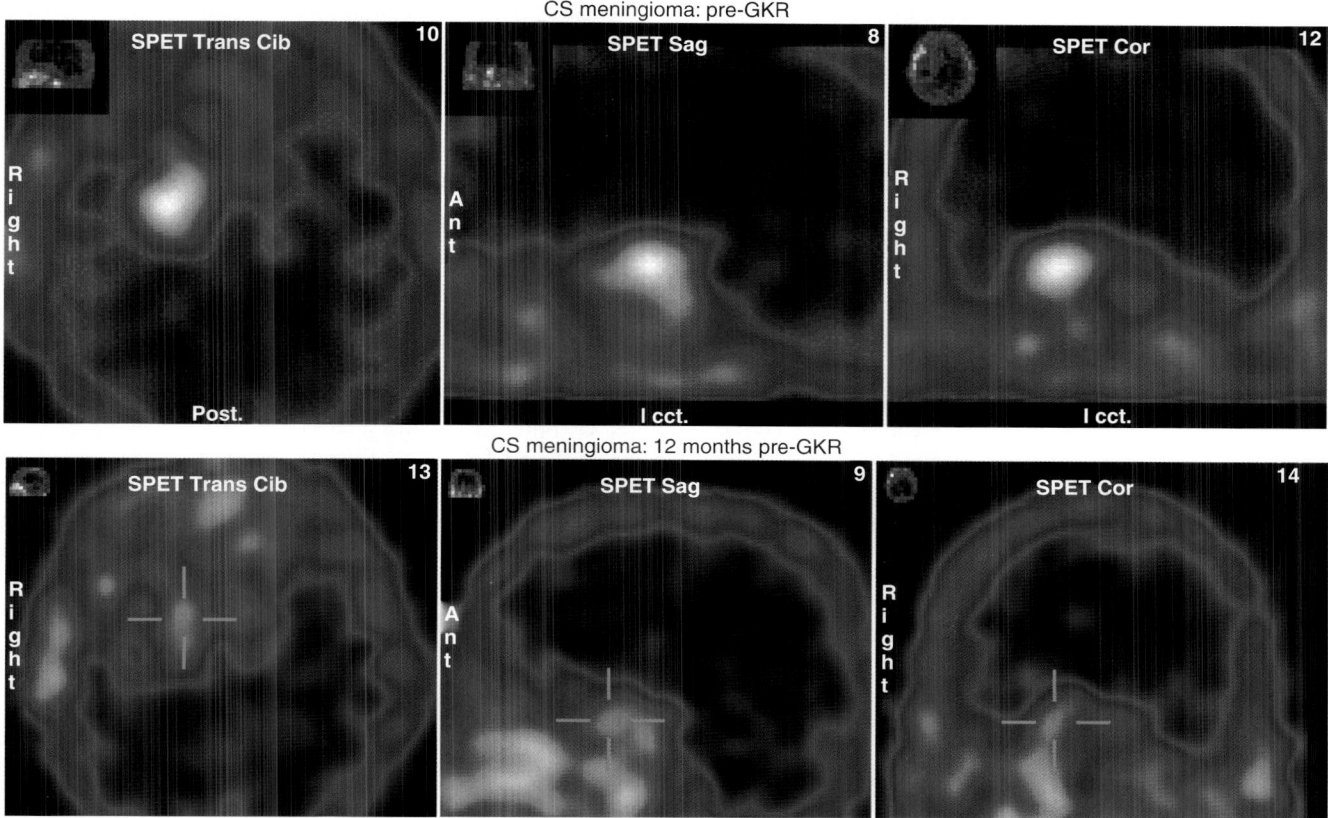

CS meningioma: 12 months pre-GKR

FIGURE 104-13 Octreotide single-photon-emission computed tomography image of a cavernous sinus meningioma, before and after gamma knife radiosurgery. Tumor volume was substantially unchanged but occular motility was normalized. The three examined sections clearly show the drastic reduction in positivity for the isotopic receptors.

Table 104-7 Gamma Knife Radiosurgery in Petroclival Meningiomas

Published Series of the Last Decade

Authors, Year	No. Patients	Primary (%)	Adjuvant (%)	Mean Fu (Months)	Tumor Volume (%)			Outcome (%)		
					Decreased	Unchanged	Increased	Improved	Unchanged	Worsened
Subach et al., 1998[223]	62	37	63	37	24	68	8	21	66	13
Iwai et al., 2000[240]	20	47	53	25	68	28	4	30	64.5	5.5
Nicolato et al., 2001[221]	23	56	44	29	55	40	5	30	63	2
Flickinger et al., 2003[10]	91	41	59	78	27	67	6	23	63	14
Roche et al., 2003[220]	32	75	25	56	12.5	87.5	—	40.5	53	6.5
Zachenhofer et al., 2006[176]	36	—	—	103	31	62	7	44	52	4
Flannery et al., 2009[156]	168	58	42	72	48	45	7	26	58	15
Summary of Our Series (1993-2008)										
Gerosa et al.	84	38	46	78 (12-162)	44[a] 13.3[b]	36.7	6	91.2%[c]		6.4%[c]

Note: Gamma knife radiosurgery in petroclival meningiomas: published series of the last decade and summary of our series (1993-2008).
FU, follow-up.
[a]Reduced up to 20%.
[b]Reduced by more than 20%.
[c]Dead for other causes (heart attack, accident), 2.4%.

(>20 Gy) than usual had been used before 1995.[150,226,230] The most recent literature has shown that reduced (12–15 Gy) dosages may obtain the same satisfactory results, while decreasing undue neurologic risks.[150,154]

Convexity and Parasagittal Meningiomas

Microsurgery still represents the major therapeutic option for meningiomas arising in these regions, because both the tumor mass and the involved dural attachment can be radically removed in most cases and with acceptable risks.[29,161,231,232] The role of SRS in convexity meningiomas is usually marginal, whereas in the parasagittal variety radiosurgery may be a relevant alternative—in deeply located small- to medium-sized lesions—either as a primary treatment for elderly patients (general anesthesia too dangerous or refused, etc.) or as an adjuvant to surgery in the case of residual tumors invading the sagittal sinus or aggressive recurrences.[29,161,232] In these special localizations, the SRS procedure appears to carry an increased risk of ARE, particularly brain edema and peritumoral imaging changes (PRICs).[3,75,161] These increased risks have also been confirmed in CyberKnife series[155,161] and extensively analyzed in the literature.[3,190,233-237] Indeed, parasagittal tumor location has been shown to be a potential predictor of peritumoral edema,[161] which is significantly more common in this location than in skull base radiosurgery, regardless of dose–volume influence.[161] Such peculiar, radio-induced "regional" sequelae presumably develop because of the crucial and "vulnerable" local venous drainage. Clinical consequences usually appear 3 to 6 months after treatment, and often require steroids, diuretics, and pentoxifylline.[3,29,75,161]

SEQUELAE: ADVERSE RADIATION EFFECTS

The variable (2.6%–9.6%)[29,111,142] occurrence of these AREs is essentially a function of the dose–volume integral, only marginally modulated by individual radiosensitivity thresholds.[9,10,111,142,238,239] As a consequence, in most treatment protocols, large tumors have been receiving lower doses than the smaller ones.[9,10,12,111,137,146,168,214,224,238,240,241] According to a broadly accepted notion, SRS should never treat targets exceeding 3 to 3.5 cm in diameter and 14 to 22.5 cm³ in volume. Violations of these principles might in time trigger the multistep process of AREs, starting with the formation or the worsening of perifocal edema, followed by the focal vasculopathy and by other, more severe sequelae.

Peritumoral Imaging Changes

"Satellite" edema, particularly common in the parasagittal or in the convexity region, is the dominant feature—together with minor vascular sequelae—in the early stages of the peritumoral imaging changes. Accurately reported series have shown the described influence of the dose–volume factor in determining the severity and the timing of these processes, at least in standard dosimetry protocols.[3,190,233,234,236,237] However, recent reports have extensively emphasized the chances for maintaining an adequate LTC without increasing side effects[9,111,128,136,146,214,224,238] by treating larger meningiomas with reduced dosages.[111,126,131,240] According to Ganz et al.,[111,137,178] at least in WHO grade 1 meningiomas, the straightforward relation between the dose–volume

integral and the incidence of AREs, may be too simplistic for lower-dose protocols.[111,112] Furthermore, the predominance of PRICs and AREs following SRS in non–skull-base meningiomas compared with basal tumors observed with GKS,[29] MML-LINAC,[168] and CyberKnife,[161] might be strictly dependent on the prescription dose adopted, becoming irrelevant at reduced dose regimens.[111,112]

Vasculopathy—Radiation Necrosis

These neuropathologic entities represent the next steps of the worsening AREs sequence, taking place in 1.5% to 4.6% of the cases during mid- to long-term follow-up.[242] The typical process is comparable to the parenchymal multistep damage described in irradiated arteriovenous *malformation* by Nataf et al.,[242] including the specific radiation-tolerance limits of the neural tissue.[243] The final pathophysiology of the radionecrotic stage is still poorly known. In a minority of cases, an obvious, solid fibromatous nodule further increases the edema—presumably related to vascular permeability factors. Surgical removal of the nodule is usually the most appropriate solution.[244]

Cranial Neuropathy

Various cranial nerves are characterized by a wide spectrum of radiosensitivity. As a rule, special sensory nerves—and especially their primary receptor fibers—such as those belonging to the cochlear (radiation threshold on 10–15 mm³ in single fraction, 5–6 Gy)[245] and to the optic nerve (same landmark, 8–9 Gy)[121,196,199] may be easily damaged. Somatic motor nerves like the oculomotor usually tolerate dose exposures superior to 20 Gy.[151,196,203]

Oncogenicity

In a very limited number of cases, putative cancerogenic mechanisms have been advocated to explain the rapid growth of previously small, quiescent meningiomas following SRS.[30,35] The surgically verified atypical-anaplastic oncotypes were the most reasonable explanation. The definition of radiation-induced tumors is still based on the indirect criteria devised by Cahan[246]: 5-year-plus latency time, localization overlapping the irradiated one, and different oncotype. The relative risk of carcinogenesis after radiosurgery in the central nervous system has been calculated by means of probabilistic methods,[247] and varies from 1.57 to 8.75 for a dose of 1 Gy, increasing in time up to 18.4 between 20 and 25 years. The long-term (30-year) risk of newer radiation-induced tumors in meningioma patients has been estimated in 1 per 1000 treated patients.[247] The natural incidence of new gliomas in the population (1/10,000 every year), and the number of meningiomas treated over three decades with SRS worldwide (75,000) must be the basic reference for any statistical evaluation. As a consequence, the thus far extremely rare (two cases) reported instances of malignant tumors diagnosed in SRS-treated meningioma patients are probably an underestimation of the real incidence; that, however, should not affect further development of this technique.

OTHER EFFECTS

Rare to extremely rare putative radiosurgical sequelae include persisting headache (2.5%),[29] seizures (7%),[29] and normal pressure[248] or hypertensive[29] hydrocephalus (1%).

In the few reported cases of ventricular dilatation, the trigger mechanism is reminiscent of vestibular schwannoma–related hydrocephalus, increased albumin concentration in the CSF.[29,248]

The Future

During the last decade the evolution of radiosurgical techniques has been essentially supported by serial advancements either in terms of stereotactic imaging—such as particularly high Tesla MRI, image-fusion algorithms, virtual "nonrigid" reproductions—and of computerized dosimetry, using multi-isocentric targeting allowing highly conformal and selective planning. The latter actually represents the most precise and recent form of intensity-modulated irradiation. Indeed, by 1994 several LINAC units were adopting multiple isocenter techniques, switching to multiple static conformal fields to improve conformality, or switching to fractionated techniques and lower radiation doses,[249] in order to limit radiotoxicity on normal brain. In fact, prescription doses for single-stage radiosurgery began to decrease in the early 1990s, and we still do not know how much further they will be lowered. In the near future, further improvements in clinical results may be reasonably expected from some of the main investigative trials presently in progress.

Tridimensional anatomofunctional coregistered imaging will presumably provide a better definition either of the target "core"—such as in secreting tumors like pituitary adenomas, or in large, octreotide positive meningiomas—or of the neoplastic peripheral borders, as in brain malignancies.

Management strategies for "oversized tumors" will probably routinely include planned neoplastic debulking followed by radiosurgery on the residual mass, with additional protection of normal brain structures.

Dosimetry programs seem consistently oriented toward lower levels, once again to meet the goal of stopping tumor progression while preserving neurologic functions. The introduction of novel radioenhancers might accelerate this process.

Additional therapeutic support should come from newer radioprotective agents presently under investigation—for instance, free radical scavengers, membrane stabilizers, 21-aminosteroids—as well as from compounds limiting the incidence of adverse radiation effects, such as cyclooxygenase 2 inhibitors.[250]

The mid- to long-term future of radiosurgical treatments will be totally or partially dominated by molecular, biological, and oncogenetic approaches modifying our present radiobiological knowledge, and putatively introducing the era of gene-guided therapy in several radiosurgical protocols.

KEY REFERENCES

Al-Mefty O, Kadri PA, Pravdenkova S, et al. Malignant progression in meningioma: documentation of a series and analysis of cytogenetic findings. *J Neurosurg.* 2004;101:210-218.
Elia AE, Shih HA, Loeffler JS. Stereotactic radiation treatment for benign meningiomas. *Neurosurg Focus.* 2007;23:E5.
Eustacchio S, Trummer M, Fuchs I, et al. Preservation of cranial nerve function following gamma knife radiosurgery for benign skull base meningiomas: experience in 121 patients with follow-up of 5 to 9.8 years. *Acta Neurochir.* 2002;84(Suppl):71-76.
Flickinger JC, Kondziolka D, Maitz AH, et al. Gamma knife radiosurgery of imaging-diagnosed intracranial meningioma. *Int J Radiat Oncol Biol Phys.* 2003;56:801-806.
Friedman WA, Murad GJ, Bradshaw P, et al. Linear accelerator surgery for meningiomas. *J Neurosurg.* 2005;103:206-209.
Ganz JC, Reda WA, Abdelkarim K. Adverse radiation effects after gamma knife surgery in relation to dose and volume. *Acta Neurochir.* 2009;151:9-19.
Kondziolka D, Mathieu D, Lunsford LD, et al. Radiosurgery as definitive management of intracranial meningiomas. *Neurosurgery.* 2008;62:53-58.
Kreil W, Luggin J, Fuchs I, et al. Long term experience of gamma knife radiosurgery for benign skull base meningiomas. *J Neurol Neurosurg Psychiatry.* 2005;76:1425-1430.
Malik I, Rowe JG, Walton L, et al. The use of stereotactic radiosurgery in the management of meningiomas. *Br J Neurosurg.* 2005;19:13-20.
Marosi C, Hassler M, Roessler K, et al. Meningioma. *Crit Rev Oncol Hematol.* 2008;67:153-171.
Minniti G, Amichetti M, Enrici RM. Radiotherapy and radiosurgery for benign skull base meningiomas. *Radiat Oncol.* 2009;4:42-53.
Modha A, Gutin PH. Diagnosis and treatment of atypical and anaplastic meningiomas: a review. *Neurosurgery.* 2005;57:538-550.
Nakamura M, Roser F, Michel J, et al. The natural history of incidental meningiomas. *Neurosurgery.* 2003;53:62-70.
Nicolato A, Foroni R, Alessandrini F, et al. Radiosurgical treatment of cavernous sinus meningiomas: experience with 122 treated patients. *Neurosurgery.* 2002;51:1153-1159.
Patil CG, Hoang S, Borchers 3rd DJ, et al. Predictors of peritumoral edema after stereotactic radiosurgery of supratentorial meningiomas. *Neurosurgery.* 2008;63:435-440.
Perry A, Dehner LP. Meningeal tumors of childhood and infancy. An update and literature review. *Brain Pathol.* 2003;13:386-408.
Perry A, Gutmann DH, Reifenberger G. Molecular pathogenesis of meningiomas. *J Neurooncol.* 2004;70:183-202.
Perry A, Louis DN, Scheithauer BW, et al. Meningeal tumors. In: Louis DN, Ohgaki H, Wiestler OD, Cavenee WK, eds. *World Health Organization Classification of Tumours of the Central Nervous System.* Lyon: International Agency for Research on Cancer; 2007, pp 164-172.
Pollock BE. Stereotactic radiosurgery of benign intracranial tumors. *J Neurooncol.* 2009;92:337-343.
Pollock BE. Stereotactic radiosurgery for intracranial meningiomas: indications and results. *Neurosurg Focus.* 2003;14:e4.
Rogers L, Mehta M. Role of radiation therapy in treating intracranial meningiomas. *Neurosurg Focus.* 2007;23:E4.
Stafford SL, Pollock BE, Foote RL, et al. Meningioma radiosurgery: tumor control, outcomes, and complications among 190 consecutive patients. *Neurosurgery.* 2001;49:1029-1037.
Stieber VW. Radiation therapy for visual pathway tumors. *J Neuroophthalmol.* 2008;28:222-230.
Takanashi M, Fukuoka S, Hojyo A, et al. Gamma knife radiosurgery for skull-base meningiomas. *Prog Neurol Surg.* 2009;22:96-111.
Walsh MT, Couldwell WT. Management options for cavernous sinus meningiomas. *J Neurooncol.* 2009;92:307-316.

Numbered references appear on Expert Consult.

CHAPTER 105

Role of Gamma Knife Radiosurgery in the Management of Arteriovenous Malformations

RAMIRO DEL-VALLE • MARCO ZENTENO

Following Roentgen's discovery of x-rays, there was early interest in the use of irradiation for arteriovenous malformation (AVM) treatment from 1914 to 1950.[1] In spite of occasional successes, until 1970, there was consensus among neurosurgeons that radiation had little practical use in the management of AVMs.[2]

Things began to change with the development of the concept of stereotactically guided treatment of intracranial lesions using a single high dose of ionizing beams by Lars Leksell.[3] He defined the term and initiated investigation, first using an orthovoltage x-ray tube combined with his initial rectilinear stereotactic coordinate frame. In 1951, working with Borje Larsson, a physicist, Leksell subsequently reported the first clinical use of stereotactic guidance linked with a cyclotron-generated proton beam.[4]

In 1968, continuing their work, Leksell built the first dedicated radiosurgical unit, the gamma knife.[4,5] The potential value of irradiation in the treatment of vascular malformations was subsequently reassessed. Encouraging factors were evidence that the vessels were radiosensitive and a long-term angiographic follow-up of a small series of AVMs treated with fractionated irradiation by Johnson in the 1950s confirming that the AVM was obliterated in 45% of cases.[6]

Stereotactic radiosurgery is the closed skull destruction of an intracranial target using ionizing beams of radiation, directed in a focused manner with the help of an extracranial guiding device.[7] The application of stereotactic radiosurgery for cerebral arteriovenous malformations began in earnest in the early 1970s.[10]

Radiosurgical Treatment of Arteriovenous Malformations

It has been estimated that as many as 500,000 people in the United States and Canada have AVMs.[8,9] During the last 40 years, the overall role of stereotactic radiosurgery has been established in the management of selected vascular malformations. Together with advances in microsurgical techniques, postoperative neurointensive care management,

and advances in intravascular microcatheter techniques for AVM characterization and embolization, radiosurgery alone or in combination represents a moderately low-risk and effective strategy for properly selected patients.[11,12]

A cure for every patient treated with radiosurgery has not yet been achieved. The obliteration rates at 3 years ("angiographic cure") range from 70% to 85%.[13-17] Several factors have been associated with the likelihood of obliteration, such as AVM volume, prescription dose, location, angioarchitecture, and patient age and lack of history of embolization. Radioresistance has been reported in some lesions that show no response, despite appropriate doses of radiation.[17,19]

Small treatment volume, a 23- to 25-Gy prescription dose, and a small number of draining veins[18-23] are factors associated with a more favorable prognosis. Conversely, factors such as a large AVM's volume, site, and the radiation dose to the exposed brain tissue, have been associated with the likelihood of complications, including bleeding during the latency period, cerebral edema, and/or radionecrosis.[23-34]

Some researchers, including Chang et al.,[35] have suggested that other factors in addition to volume should be considered when predicting obliteration results, such as the AVM's flow pattern and the number of draining veins. Furthermore, some lesions that appear to be similar in vessel architecture, location, and volume, respond differently or unexpectedly to treatment plans based on the dose–volume relationship. Some AVMs are obliterated within 2 years, whereas others do so after 3 or 4 years.

In terms of angiographic features associated with lower likelihood of obliteration, Meder et al.[36] reported that radiosurgery is less effective in AVMs with direct intranidal fistulas and single draining vessels and suggest that radiosurgery is more likely in patients with plexiform or compact-type AVMs.

Similarly, in a semiquantitative flow study using phase-contrast two-dimensional (2D) magnetic resonance angiography (MRA), Petereit et al.[37] reported a negative effect on the obliteration of AVMs by flow speeds greater than 100 ml/s. We reviewed our own experience by defining a critical zone for treatment, the high flow nidus excluding the perilesional draining veins in AVMs using dynamic analysis of circulation times through the AVMs.

Improved Imaging in Radiosurgery

The accuracy of radiosurgical treatment is dependent on the accuracy of target delineation by radiological studies performed with a stereotactic frame in place. In the management of vascular malformations, the primary imaging modality is angiography. Magnetic resonance imaging (MRI) examinations are also recommended for obtaining further information, to fully understand the topographic and tomographic anatomy of the malformation as well as the relationship between the targeted AVM and the non-targeted anatomical structures adjacent to the AVM. The gamma surgery planning program allows target outlines marked on the angiogram to be projected on the MRIs and vice versa (Fig. 105-1). Thus, both modalities can be used in the planning procedure.

With the goal of improving imaging, and therefore targeting of the AVM, our protocol focuses on the definition of the AVM's critical zone, which corresponds to the least-resistant portion of the lesion with the predominant flow draining to the main vein. Our experience in measuring the pedicular pressure in feeders, when treating malformations with superselective embolization, was taken into account in a dynamic study of malformations.[38] Pedicular pressures lower than 25 mm Hg are observed in direct AV fistulas, whereas plexiform AVM pressures increase gradually to nearly 50 mm Hg (Table 105-1).

Because the direct pressure measurement protocol is both time consuming and costly, it is impractical for routine radiosurgery planning. We have chosen, therefore, a more practical way to measure the arterial, nidal, and venous circulation times dynamically in a digital subtraction angiogram, frame by frame, using the digital counter of the angiography equipment.

The theoretical underpinning of our approach is that AVMs with fistulous patterns have shorter circulation times and those with plexiform patterns have longer circulation times. The dynamic study also allows us to characterize the AVM from the portion that is least radioresistant and has the fastest flow, ruling out the recruitment vessels, especially

in large malformations. Theoretically, with time, an AVM behaves as a waterfall, with the recruitment siphon effect of the vessels normally found around the original AVM. This secondary recruitment phenomenon is seen in perilesional tortuous normal vessels in an angiogram, which change their appearance as they participate in the steal phenomenon.

The recruitment phenomenon is more clearly seen once the flow in the dominant shunt zone decreases with embolization. This is the perinidal portion, with a diffuse appearance, and we have defined it as a "pseudonidus," which we do not believe it is absolutely necessary to include in the prescription dose. If the pseudonidus is not included, the treatment volume will be smaller and the dose to the critical zone may therefore be increased.

In our protocol, once the Leksell stereotaxic frame (Elekta) is in place on the patient's head, three-dimensional (3D) volume MRIs are acquired in T1 simple and gadolinium-enhanced sequences, together with axial T2 and coronal sequences for 3D images of the AVM. For digital subtraction angiography (DSA), Axiom Artis equipment is used with software for automated outline correction (Artis&Syngo, Siemens). Currently, images are obtained at 10.5 frames/seconds with a digital contrast injector (Mark V Pro Vis, Medrad), with contrast injected at 7 ml/s in the proximal portion of the carotid and vertebral arteries at the skull base. With superselective contrast injection, the volume is reduced to 3 ml/s. Several circulation times (Fig. 105-2) are then measured frame by frame in the angiography console: nidal filling time (NFT), time from the first frame with nidal staining to the corresponding frame at maximum arterial enhancement; nidal time (NT), includes NFT up to the last frame outlining the arterial nidus; draining time (DT), from the time of the first or predominant draining vein image, when venous draining is multiple, to the time when the abnormal draining vein or veins are no longer seen; total circulation time (TCT), time elapsed from the first frame of the nidal filling time to the last draining frame; and early shunt time (EST), time from the first frame of nidal filling to the first frame of venous draining time.

As the circulation times are studied and recorded, the various AVM components are defined, including the single or multiple compartments (Fig. 105-3), the type of venous drainage, and several flow patterns, depending on the

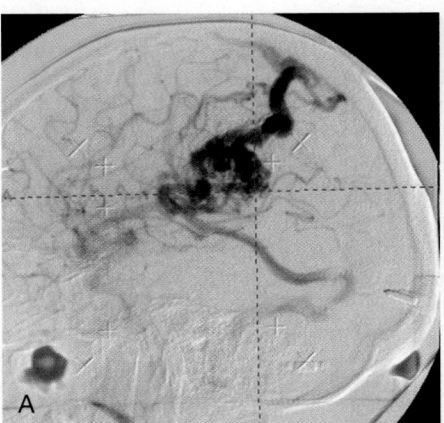
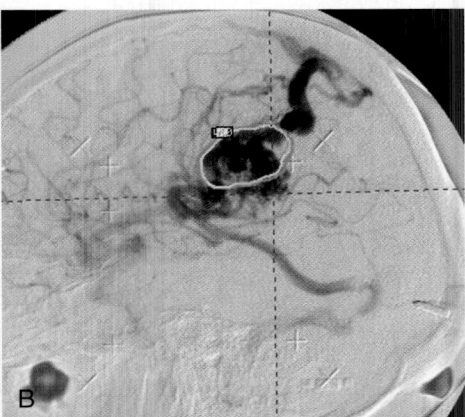
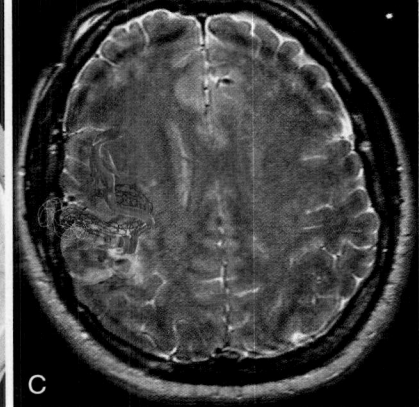

FIGURE 105-1 A, DSA pre-embolization. B, DSA postembolization. C, Three-dimensional angiography-magnetic resonance imaging planning for key target volume definition. DSA, digital subtraction angiography.

Table 105-1	Types of Pressure-Related Fistulas		
TYPE		**Flow Pattern**	**Pressure**
A		Fast flow, direct	8–17 mm Hg
B		Intermediate fast flow	18–29 mm Hg
C		Intermediate slow flow, moderate plexiform	30–45 mm Hg
D		Plexiform	>45 mm Hg

circulation time compatible with the three types of circulation: I-A direct fistulae, I-B predominantly fistulous, II-A mixed fistulous-plexiform without stenosis of the draining vein, II-B mixed with draining vein stenosis, and III predominantly plexiform (Table 105-2).

Associated factors that increase the risk of bleeding are also identified, such as perinidal and proximal aneurysms with high hyperflows, as well as aneurysms in the draining system and stenosis of the main draining vein. The dynamic anatomic definition of the nidus allows us to exclude the recruiting vessels from the pseudonidus.

Nidal circulation times (NTs) less than 2 seconds and a total circulation of less than 6 seconds correlate with the I-A and I-B fistulous flow patterns. Shunt (EST) times of less than 2 seconds and nidal filling times (NFTs) of 2 to 4 seconds and total circulation times of up to 8 seconds correlate with the mixed fistulous-plexiform flow pattern, and nidal times greater than 4 seconds and total circulation time greater than 9 seconds reflect predominantly plexiform flow. It is important to note that a patient with a II-B flow pattern with an early shunt time less than 1.5 seconds and a slow draining time greater than 7 seconds, resulting from stenosis of the predominant venous drainage, should

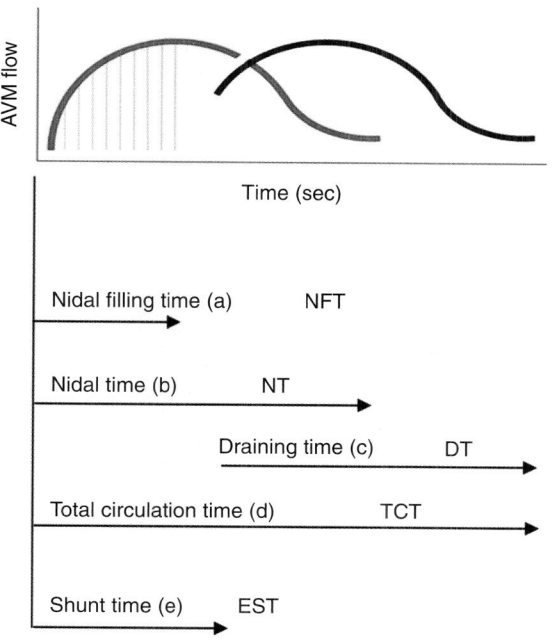

FIGURE 105-2 Circulation times.

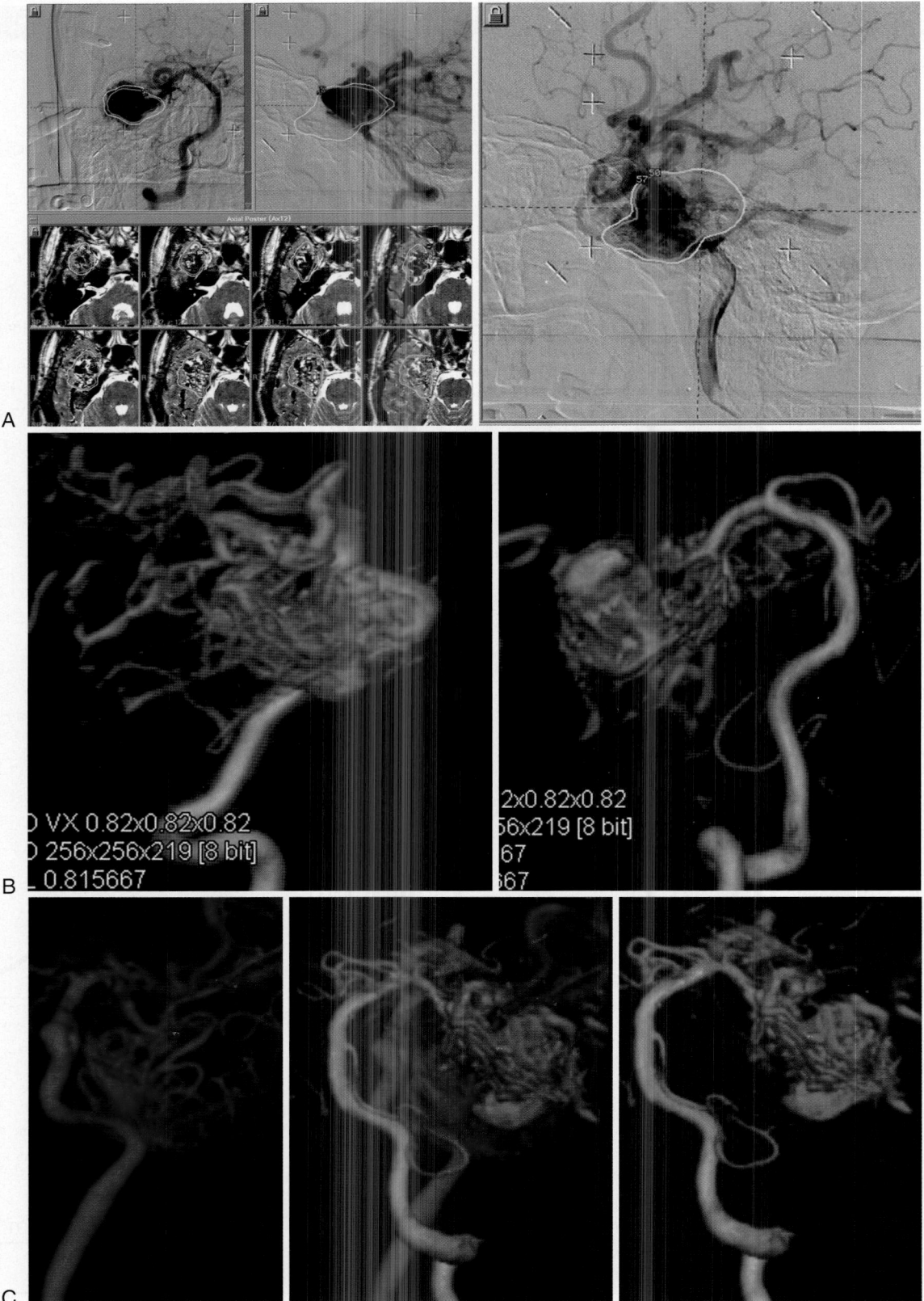

FIGURE 105-3 A to C, Thirty-eight-year-old man, arteriovenous malformation with two carotid and vertebral compartments, flow pattern type II-A, prescription treatment volume 16.1 ml,16 Gy/50% isodose line, radiosurgery-based grading system 2.37.

be considered a candidate for embolization to reduce the risk of bleeding.

The crucial stage in the definition of the critical zone is when the angiographic images are transferred to the workstation and correlated with 3D multiplanar MRIs, including topographic and volumetric target analysis related to functional perilesional eloquence, for proper adjustment of the prescription dose.

Our embolization protocol for radiosurgery depends on the volume of the AVM, the corresponding flow pattern, and the risk factors for bleeding. If the size of the pre-embolization target is less than 10 ml, the treatment volume should include all the original volume. If the pre-embolization volume is greater than 10 ml, the prescription dose is delivered to the residual volume in the critical zone. In terms of the flow pattern, it is advisable to use embolization to reduce the flow in patterns I and II-B. Endovascular therapy is also used to eliminate high-flow aneurysms or reduce volume in prospective staged protocols (Fig. 105-4).

Table 105-2	Circulation Time–Dependent Arteriovenous Malformation Flow Patterns				
	TIME IN SECONDS				
Type	**EST**	**NFT**	**DT**	**Flow Pattern**	
I-A	<1	<1	<4	Direct fistulae	Fast flow fistulae
I-B	<1	<2	<5	Predominantly fistulous	
II-A	<1.5	2–4	4–6	Mixed fistulous plexiform, nondraining vein stenosis	Intermediate mixed
II-B	<2	2–4	<7	Mixed fistulous plexiform with draining vein stenosis	
III	>2	>4	>7	Predominantly plexiform	Slow form plexiform

DT, draining time; EST, early shunt time; NFT, nidal filling time.

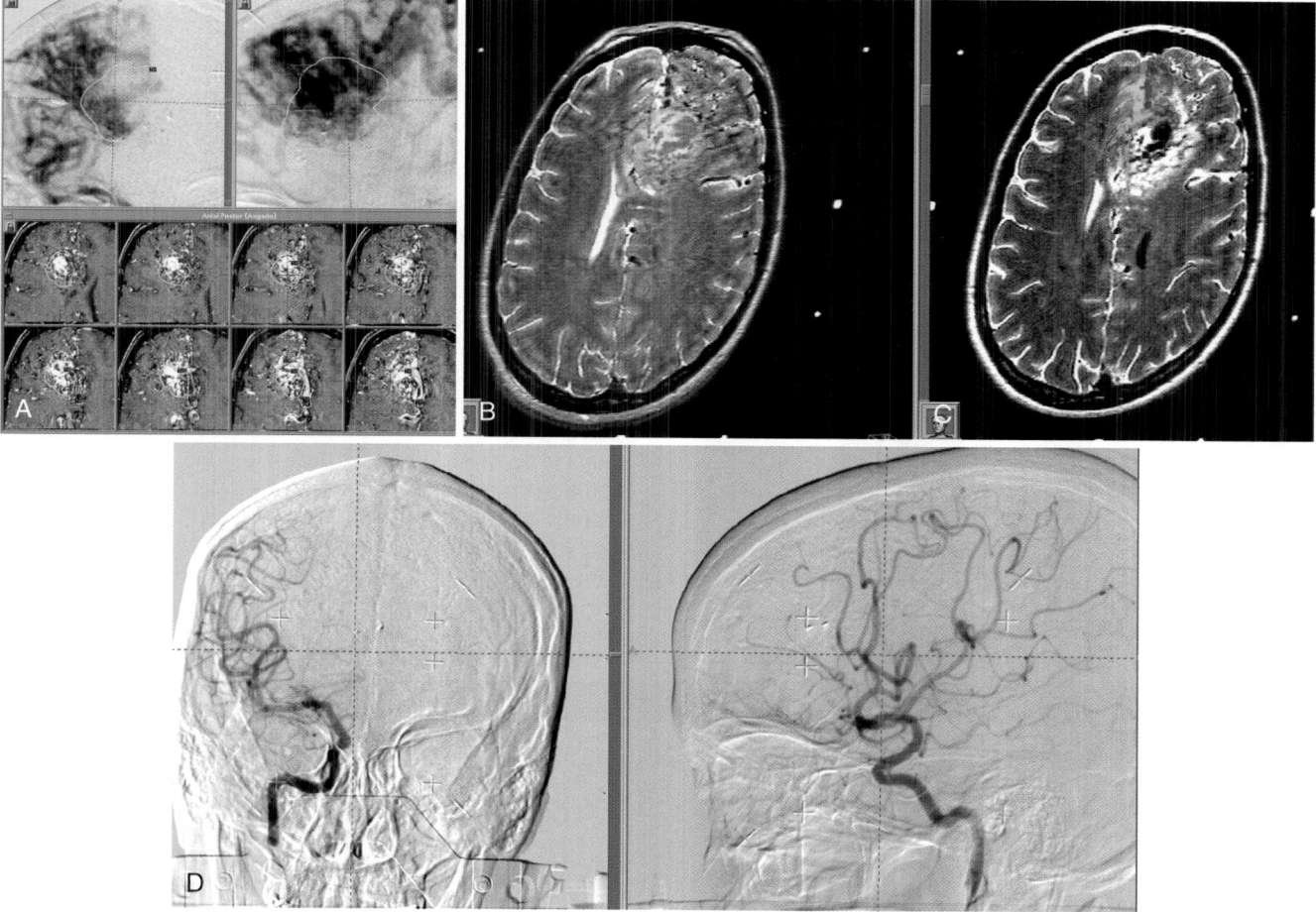

FIGURE 105-4 A, Staged radiosurgery. Thirty-eight-year-old woman, large arteriovenous malformation with two compartments, flow pattern type II-A and recruitment phenomena (pseudonidus). First GK treatment-embolization same day, PTV 14.9 ml off recruitment vessels, 18 Gy/50%, RGBS 2.25. B, First 3D GK plan. C, Second GK treatment 1 year after magnetic resonance imaging-3D treatment plan, PTV 10.7 ml, 18 Gy/57%, RGBS 1.87. D, Digital subtraction angiography showing complete obliteration 3 years after second treatment. GK, gamma knife; PTV, prescription treatment volume; RGBS, radiosurgery-based grading system.

Patients Characteristics

From 1995 to 2008, a total of 250 patients with AVMs underwent gamma knife (Elekta) radiosurgery. Of these, 75 patients were treated after dynamic measurement planning to accurately define the critical zone of the AVM, including the dynamic angiographic criteria that categorize the type of AVM: fistulous versus plexiform or mixed, and Spetzler-Martin (S-M) classification into grade III (55), IV (18), or V (2). According to radiosurgery-based grading system (RBGS) proposed by Pollock and Flickinger,[39] the minimum score was 0.6 and the maximum was 2.68, with a mean score of 1.64.

The clinical presentation was bleeding in 50% of patients, headache in 30%, seizure in 40%, and neurologic deficit in 10%. Most (70%) AVMs were located in the hemisphere and the rest were deepseated. Two patients had a lesion in the posterior fossa.

Endovascular therapy was performed in 56% of patients and superselective angiography without embolization in 29%. Radiosurgery was administered as a single treatment in 64 patients, repeat radiosurgery in 7 patients, or prospective staged radiosurgery in four patients (Tables 105-3 and 105-4). The AVM original volume was up to 120 ml, with a critical zone target volume of up to 15 ml in the single treatment group, a median target volume of 8.5 ml, and 28 ml in the prospective staged radiosurgery group. The marginal

dose of radiation to the AVM was 18 to 22 Gy, with a median dose of 20 Gy.

Results

In 55 patients, DSA was used to review the treatment response (Table 105-5). In 75 patients, the evaluation was performed with MRA at 12 to 40 months (mean follow-up 28 months). Obliteration was observed in 90%, 67%, and 50% of patients in groups with S-M grades III, IV, and V, respectively. In the single treatment group, obliteration was 84% and obliteration was complete in 5 out of 7 patients who underwent repeat radiosurgery. In 4 patients who underwent prospectively staged radiosurgery, the lesion was obliterated in 3. In 2 patients, this was confirmed by DSA, and in the other one by MRA. One patient displayed subtotal obliteration after 40 months of follow-up and was completely obliterated at 5 years. The overall MRA obliteration rate was 84%.

Complications

Permanent neurologic complications were found in 7.0% (5 of 75) of patients, and in 4 of 42 patients embolized during preradiosurgery endovascular therapy. Two patients had nonfatal bleeding during the latency period, 1 had a minor visual field defect, and 1 a lacunar and occipital infarct after embolization. There was no mortality.

Discussion

Inadequate characterization of the AVM nidus for radiosurgical treatment is one of the most common factors contributing to treatment failure. Therefore, we propose a protocol with dynamic characterization that includes the hemodynamic conditions of flow in a very close real-time collaboration between the neurosurgical and endovascular teams.

Some researchers, including Pan et al.,[23] Chang et al.,[35] Meder et al.,[36] and Petereit et al.,[37] among others, have suggested that flow pattern–related factors and even the fistulous type of AVM have a negative effect on obliteration. Frame-by-frame dynamic flow analysis and multiplanar MRI allow the identification of failure-related factors more objectively, including prenidal fistulas with early shunt times (<1 second; Fig. 105-5). The presence of a prenidal fistula could represent one of the factors related to the radiobiological resistance published by the Pittsburgh group.[17,19]

Table 105-3 Dynamic Protocol for Arteriovenous Malformations in 75 Patients

Spetzler-Martin Grade	Embolization plus Gamma Knife	Superselective Angiography for Gamma Knife Planning
III	20 (29%)	15
IV	20 (86%)	5 (4 staged)
V	2 (67%)	2
Total	42/75 (56)%	22/75 (29%)

Table 105-4 Spetzler-Martin Grades and Type of Treatment

Spetzler-Martin Grade	Single Treatment	Repeated Gamma Knife	Prospective Staged	Total
III	52	2	1	55
IV	11	5	2	18
V	1	0	1	2
Total	64	7	4	75

Table 105-5 Treatment Results

Spetzler-Martin Grade	DIGITAL SUBTRACTION ANGIOGRAPHY (55 PATIENTS)		ANGIOGRAPHY-MAGNETIC RESONANCE IMAGING FOLLOW-UP (75 PATIENTS)	
	Obliteration	Failure	Obliteration	Failure
III	34 (91%)	3	50 (90%)	5
IV	12 (75%)	4	12 (67%)	6
V	1 (50%)	1	1 (50%)	1
Single treatment	40 (89%)	5	55 (84%)	9
Repeated gamma knife	5 (72%)	2	5 (72%)	2
Prospective staged	2 (67%)	1	3 (75%)	1
Total patients	47 (85.5%)	8 (14.5)	63 (84%)	12 (16%)

The (Controversial) Role of Embolization

Luessenhop and Spence performed the first cerebral AVM embolization in 1959.[40] Flow-directed catheters have been most commonly used since 1990, and the most common complications are aberrant embolization, embolization of the normal proximal arteries, venous system occlusion, and arterial perforation.[41,42] Recommendations for embolization are supported by anecdotal case series and nonrandomized cohort studies.

The use of embolization to improve the results of radiosurgery has been controversial. Most publications concerning retrospective studies conclude that the procedure has a negative impact on outcome and that complications from endovascular therapy add to the complications of radiosurgery.

Andrade Souza et al.[43] addressed the question of whether preradiosurgical AVM embolization affects obliteration or clinical outcomes. They found that embolization reduced the obliteration rate and that outcomes were better in the nonembolized group, but the differences were not statistically significant. Obliteration was achieved in 70% of patients receiving radiosurgery alone and in 47% of patients treated with embolization before radiosurgery.

Unfortunately, there has been no standardization of the embolization technique. In reports of endovascular therapy, there are distinct outcomes from different groups.

Some series have combined the use of particles and cyanoacrylate. There is also no clear information about results and more specifically in terms of the volume of the AVM, flow patterns, risk factors for bleeding, or nidus fragmentation. Furthermore, it is usually not specified whether an endovascular therapist worked together with the neurosurgeon. There is also no systemization of the two-dimensional versus 3D volume measurements,[44] or of quantitative flow measurements before and after embolization.[45]

We are of the opinion that it is important in order to better understand the contribution of embolization, to define whether the radiosurgical treatment volume is based on the global initial volume before embolization or whether the radiation was targeted to the residual volume. We also recommend that neurosurgeons work very closely with endovascular therapists in real time. In some AVMs, stereotactically guided embolization and correlation with 3D topography of the pedicle on MRI using Gamma Plan (Elekta) can optimize the preradiosurgery results by estimating the objective volume and flow reduction, and by providing information about the hemodynamic factors that work against favorable radiosurgery outcomes (Fig. 105-6).

Ideally, the embolization procedure should be concentric to simulate the usual surgical approach, thus avoiding inconvenient postembolization fragmentation of the target. Furthermore, it should be recorded whether the treated area belongs to the early filling and dominant flow zone, which is related to predominantly venous drainage, while excluding pseudonidus (Fig. 105-7). Special attention must

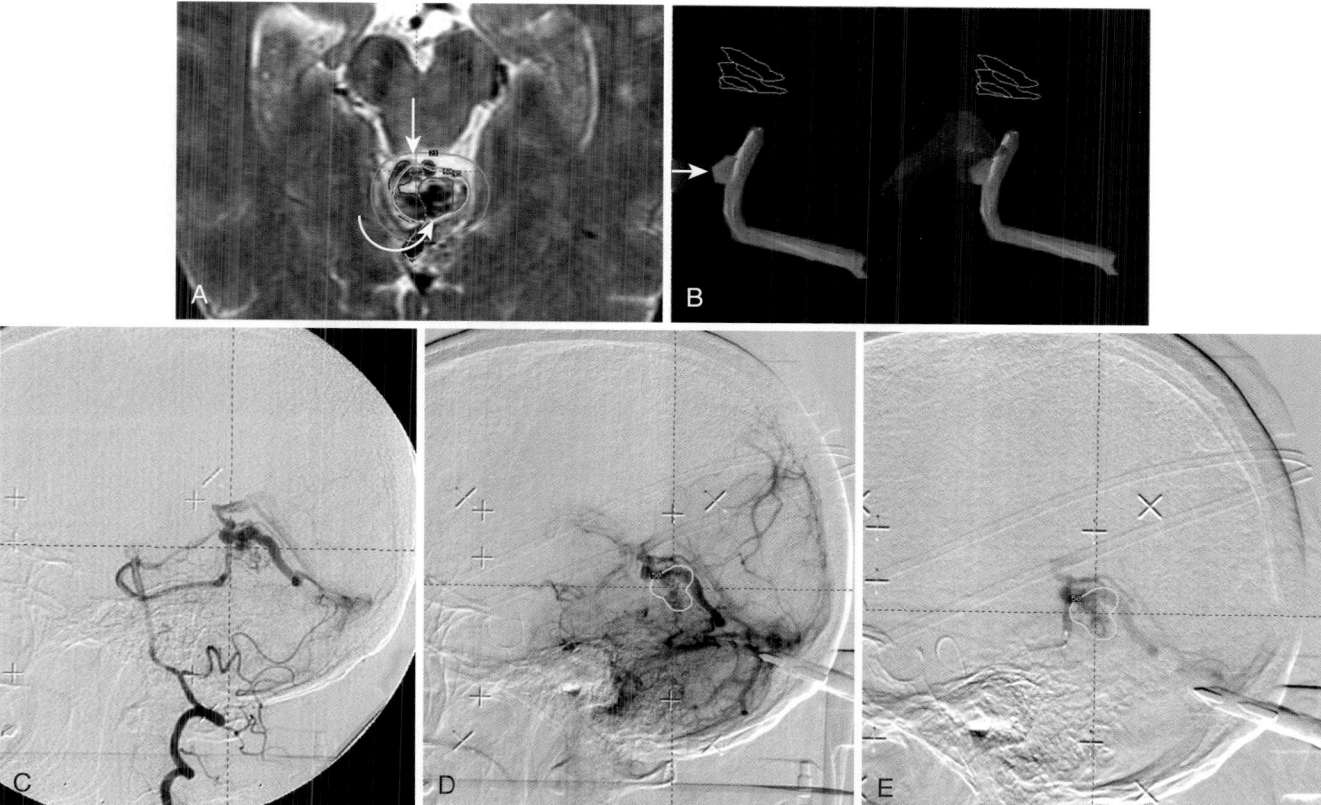

FIGURE 105-5 A and B, Prenidal direct fistula (straight arrow) plus nidal component (curved arrow): 58-year-old woman, type I-B, prescription treatment volume 1.1 ml, 24 Gy/50%, radiosurgery-based grading system 1.57. C, Four-year follow-up: failed treatment (radiobiological resistance). D and E, Repeated digital subtraction angiography treatment plan; direct prenidal fistula superselective embolization and gamma knife treatment, same day.

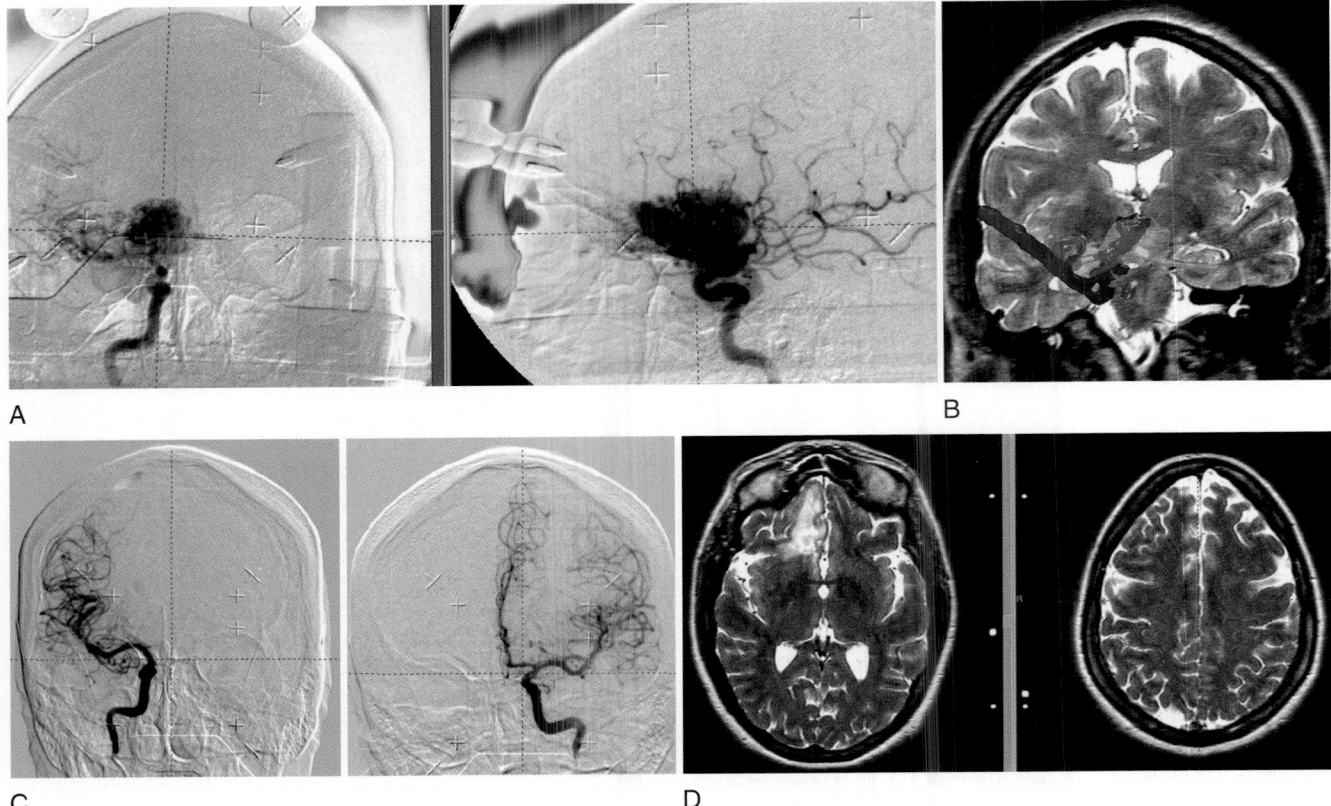

A

B

C

D

FIGURE 105-6 A and B, Forty-two-year-old woman, arteriovenous malformation type IIA, prescription treatment volume 5.4 ml, 21 Gy/50%, radiosurgery-based grading system 1.38. C and D, Digital subtraction angiography and magnetic resonance imaging, 2 years follow-up, complete obliteration, minor visual field impairment, seizure free, epileptic syndrome outcome Engel I.

FIGURE 105-7 A, Sixty-eight-year-old male, volume 10.2 ml, Pollock scale (RBGS) 2.68, obliteration rate probability <70%, demential syndrome, steal phenomenon. Pre-embolization: flow pattern type I-B. Early shunt time <1 sec: fast fistulae plus nidal component, which is why embolization is indicated. B, Postembolization. Modified flow pattern: type III plexiform slow-flow nidal filling time > 4 sec. Embolization plus gamma knife same day, prescription treatment volume 9.7 ml; 20 Gy/60%, RBGS 2.63.

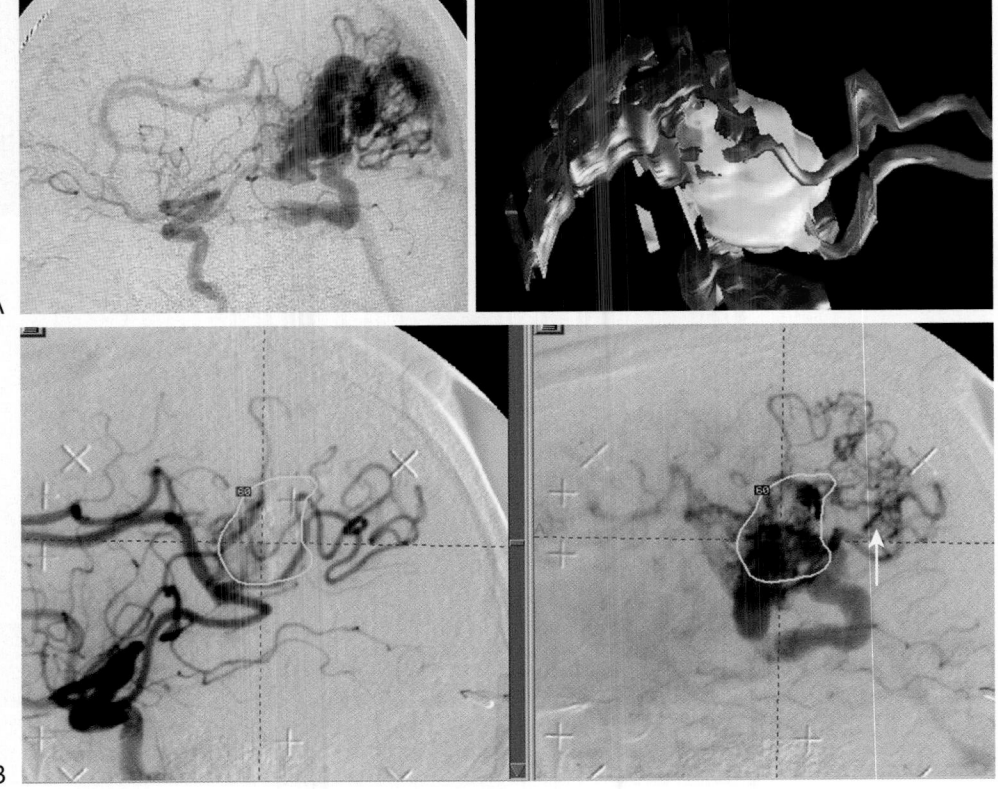

A

B

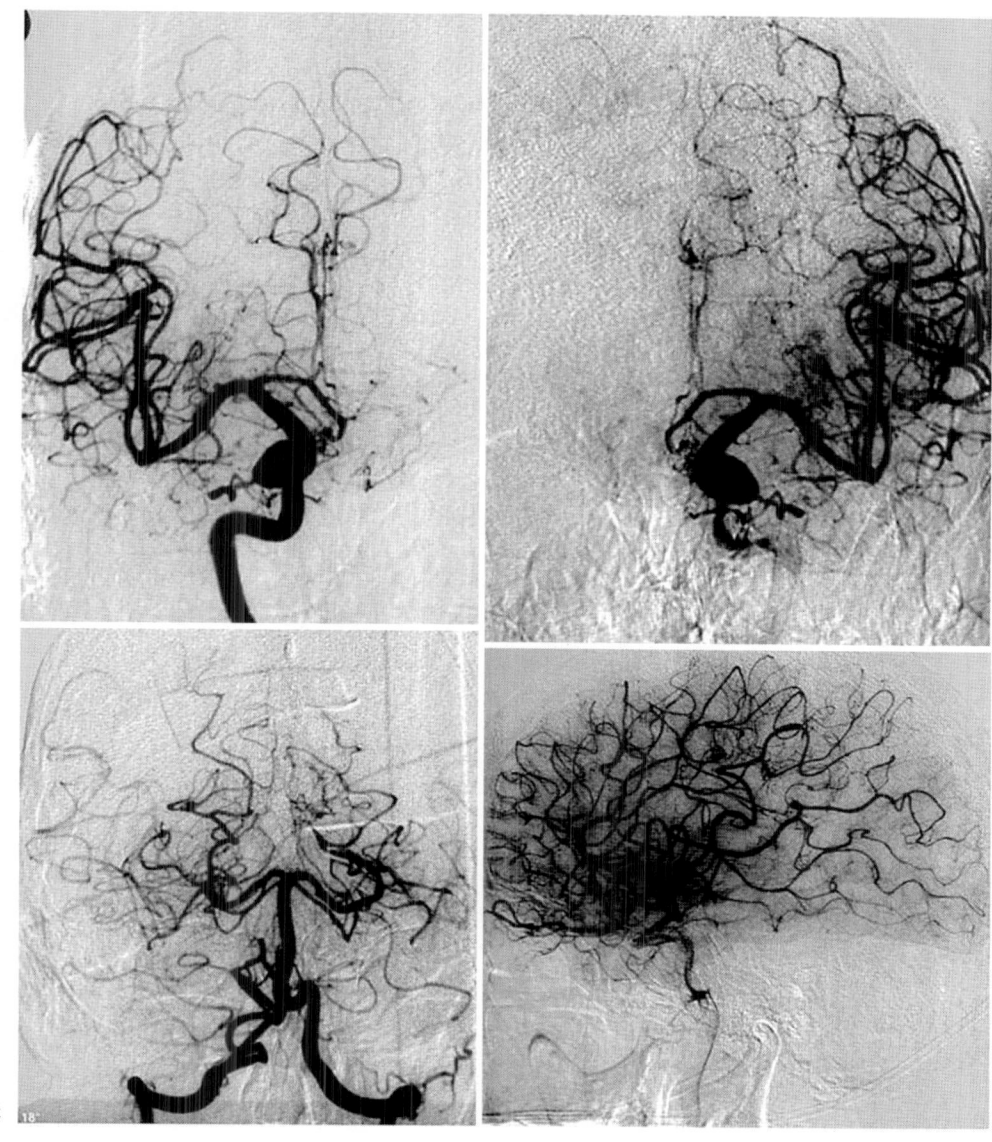

C

FIGURE 105-7, cont'd C, Digital subtraction angiography at 14 months follow-up. RBGS, radio-surgery-based grading system.

be paid to postembolization fragmentation, because the outcomes and complications are operator-dependent.

Embolization should be considered to reduce the bleeding risk in AVM with I-A, I-B, and II-B flow pattern, with an early shunt time less than 1.5 seconds and a slow draining time of more than 6 seconds, resulting from stenosis of the predominant venous drainage. The greatest benefit of embolization is obtained when the flow and concentric volume are reduced.

In our series, there was no negative effect of performing embolization and radiosurgery on the same day in 10 patients, although more intense asymptomatic signal changes were seen in the T2 sequences at 3 months in 60% of these patients, 2 of whom required temporary steroids as outpatients, without permanent sequelae.

Contrary to our expectations, 2 patients with complex AVMs and steroid treatment who underwent embolization and radiosurgery on the same day remained obliterated 10 years later (Fig. 105-8A and B). We cannot rule out a synergistic effect between radiation damage and the

inflammatory response due to embolization. Furthermore, in this series the mean RBGS of 1.64 would represent an expected 60% to 70% mean obliteration rate.

Conclusion

Critical decisions are required before therapy is undertaken for a patient with an AVM. It is reasonable to state that the total morbidity and mortality of embolization averages 9% in experienced hands. The benefits of embolization are yet to be established, particularly with regard to lowering surgical morbidity and mortality, as well as improving the cure rate of radiosurgery for large lesions and fistulous flow patterns.

The additional therapeutic benefits and financial considerations of multiple embolization procedures have not been addressed. These issues and others remain future challenges in defining the benefits of embolization in the treatment of AVMs.

In order to improve the outcomes of AVM radiosurgery, our protocol is designed to be easily followed by any

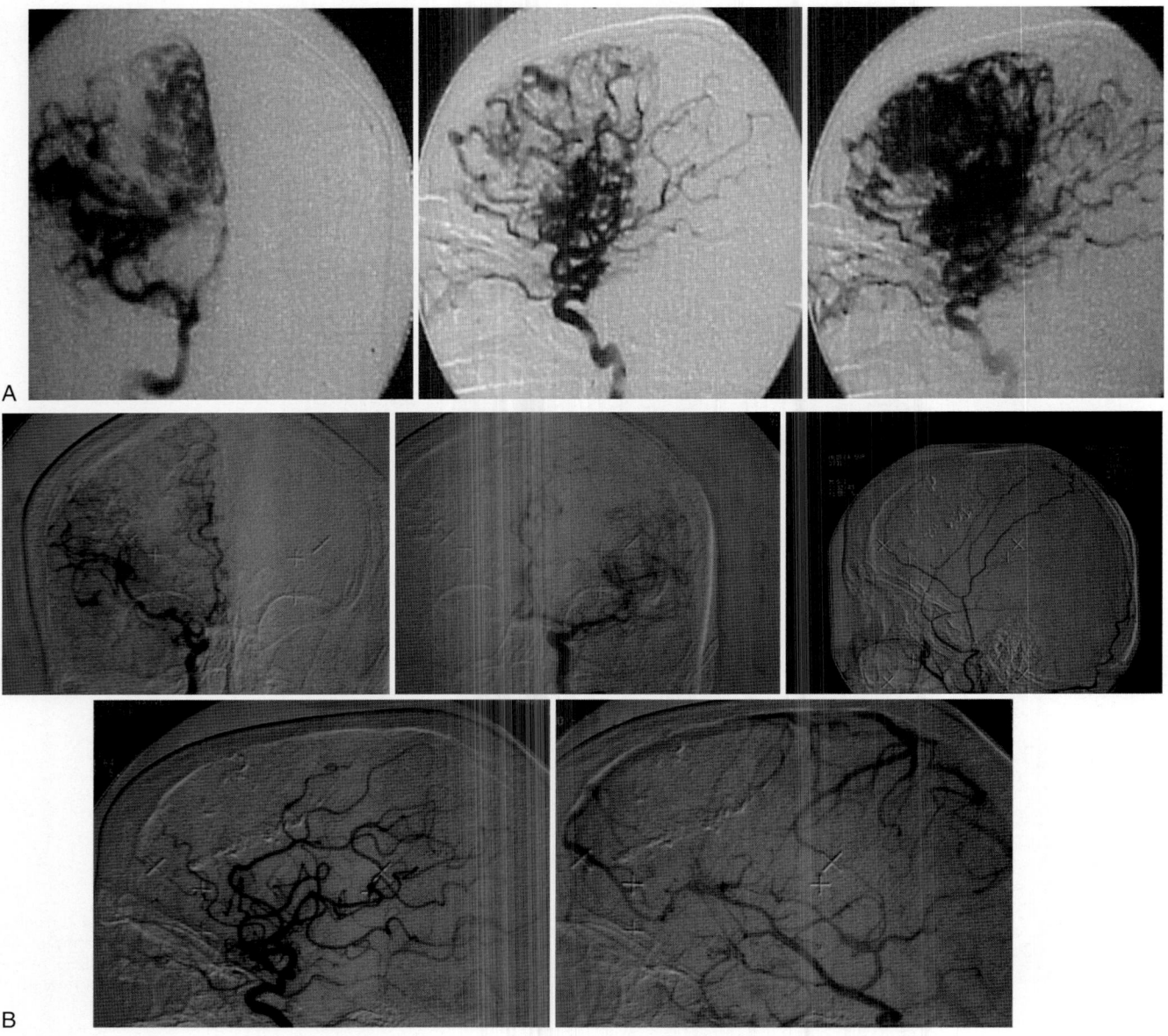

FIGURE 105-8 A, Seventeen-year-old female, epileptic syndrome, pre-embolization volume 120 ml, flow pattern pre-embolization II-A. Two embolizations preradiosurgery, last one the same radiosurgery treatment day. Arteriovenous malformation flow pattern, postembolization type III plexiform dominant component. Critical zone: prescription treatment volume 14.9 ml, 18 Gy/50%, radiosurgery-based grading system 1.83 B, Digital subtraction angiography at 10 years follow-up, epileptic syndrome outcome Engel I. The fiducials on follow-up studies mean noninvasive stereotactic volume protocol.

radiosurgical center. Instead of retrospectively, as has usually been suggested, our method can be prospectively and systematically used to evaluate hemodynamic variables of AVMs undergoing radiosurgery. Using digital quantitative methods to measure flow and volume, it is possible to obtain an objective measurement of the flow pattern and volume modifications in an embolized AVM, which will be a helpful tool in endovascular therapy. Building a clear and reliable database that includes data from other radiosurgery centers should help to standardize indications, and to analyze and share review and research results of endovascular therapy for AVMs, which until now have been anarchic and heterogeneous. A dynamic definition of the AVM critical

zone might increase the obliteration rate and decrease the treatment volume in big lesions by removing the pseudonidus from the target.

KEY REFERENCES

Andrade Souza YM, Ramani M, Scora D, et al. Embolization before radiosurgery reduces the obliteration rates of arteriovenous malformations. *Neurosurgery.* 2007;60:443-445.

Chang JH, Chang JW, Park YG, Chung SS. Factors related to complete occlusion of arteriovenous malformations after gamma knife radiosurgery. *J Neurosurg.* 2000;93:96-101.

Chang SD, Marcellus ML, Marks MP, et al. Multimodality treatment of giant intracranial arteriovenous malformations. *Neurosurgery.* 2003;53:1-13.

Del Valle R, Perez M, Ortiz J, et al. Stereotactic noninvasive volume measurement compared with geometric measurement for indications and evaluation of gamma knife treatment. *J Neurosurg.* 2005;102:140-142.

Del Valle R, Zenteno M, Jaramillo J, et al. Definition of the key target volume in radiosurgical management of arteriovenous malformations: a new dynamic concept based on angiographic circulation time. *J Neurosurg.* 2008;109:41-50.

Flickinger JC. An integrated logistic formula for prediction of complications from radiosurgery. *Int J Radiat Oncol Biol Phys.* 1989;17:879-885.

Flickinger JC, Pollock BE, Kondziolka D, Lunsford LD. A dose–response analysis of arteriovenous malformations obliteration after radiosurgery. *Int J Radiat Oncol Biol Phys.* 1996;36:873-879.

Friedman WA, Bova FJ, Bollampaly S, Bradshaw P. Analysis of factors predictive success or complications in arteriovenous malformation radiosurgery. *Neurosurgery.* 2003;52:296-308.

Haw CS, terBrugge K, Willinsky R, Tomlinson G. Complications of embolization of arteriovenous malformations of the brain. *J Neurosurg.* 2006;104:226-232.

Karlsson B, Lax I, Sodermann M. Risk for hemorrhage during the 2-year latency period following gamma knife radiosurgery for arteriovenous malformations. *Int J Radiat Oncol Biol Phys.* 2001;49:1045-1051.

Karlsson B, Lax I, Soderman M. Can the probability for obliteration after radiosurgery for arteriovenous malformations be accurately predicted. *Int J Radiat Oncol Biol Phys.* 1999;43:313-319.

Leksell L. The stereotaxic method and radiosurgery of the brain. *Acta Chir Scand.* 1951;102:316-319.

Leksell L. Stereotactic radiosurgery. *J Neurol Neurosurg Psychiatry.* 1983;46:797-803.

Lunsford LD. Stereotactic radiosurgery of intracranial arteriovenous malformations. In: Wilkins RH, Rengachary SS, eds. *Neurosurgery Update II: Vascular, Spinal, Pediatric and Functional Neurosurgery.* New York: McGraw Hill; 1991;175-185.

Maruyama K, Shin M, Tago M, et al. Radiosurgery to reduce the risk of first hemorrhage from brain arteriovenous malformations. *Neurosurgery.* 2007;60:453-459.

Meder JF, Oppenheim C, Blustajn J, et al. Cerebral arteriovenous malformations: the value of radiologic parameters in predicting response to radiosurgery. *AJNR Am J Neuroradiol.* 1997;18:1473-1483.

Pan HC. Gamma knife radiosurgery as a single treatment modality for large cerebral arteriovenous malformations. *J Neurosurg.* 2000;93: 113-119.

Petereit D, Metha M, Turski P, et al. Treatment of arteriovenous malformations with stereotactic radiosurgery employing both magnetic resonance angiography and standard angiography as a database. *Int J Radiat Oncol Biol Phys.* 1993;25:309-313.

Pollock BE, Flickinger JC. A proposed radiosurgery-based grading system for arteriovenous malformations. *J Neurosurg.* 2002;96:79-85.

Pollock BE, Flickinger JC, Lunsford LD, et al. Factors associated with successful arteriovenous malformations radiosurgery. *Neurosurgery.* 1998;42:1239-1244.

Pollock BE, Kondziolka D, Lunsford LD, et al. Repeat stereotactic radiosurgery of arteriovenous malformations: factors associated with incomplete obliteration. *Neurosurgery.* 1996;38:318-324.

Steiner L, Leksell L, Greitz T, et al. Stereotaxic radiosurgery for cerebral arteriovenous malformations. *Acta Chir Scand.* 1972;138:459-464.

Steiner L, Rankin PB, Prasad D, Steiner M. Gamma surgery for vascular disorders of the brain. In: Germano I, ed. *LINAC and Gamma Knife Radiosurgery. Neurosurgical Topics.* New York: Thieme/AANS; 2000;91-140.

Zenteno M, Jaramillo J. The predictive value of intrapedicle sodium amobarbital injection in conjunction with pressure recording. *AJNR Am J Neuroradiol.* 1991;12:1241-1249.

Numbered references appear on Expert Consult.

CHAPTER 106

Radiation Therapy of Epilepsy

ELLEN AIR • NICHOLAS BARBARO

History

Experience with stereotactic radiosurgery (SRS) over the 60 years since its development by Lars Leksell[1] has demonstrated its efficacy in the treatment of various central nervous system conditions. Although Leksell initially developed this technique to treat functional disorders such as pain and movement disorders, the earliest widespread uses of SRS focused on deep-seated tumors or arteriovenous malformations (AVMs) located in eloquent regions of the brain, using it as a means of treating these lesions while avoiding the risks associated with surgical resection.[2] Within these contexts, seizures were treated as secondary manifestations of the primary disorder, rather than as specific conditions. Subsequent to radiosurgical treatment, significant reduction, or even resolution, of the associated seizures has been documented.

The efficacy of SRS in secondary epilepsy has been most evident following the treatment of AVMs.[3-9] Several large series of patients with AVMs have found complete seizure remission in 50% to 80% of patients following SRS.[5,7-9] Small lesion size,[7] shorter duration of epilepsy,[5] and absence of prior hemorrhage[9] were associated with higher seizure-free outcomes. In contrast, seizure outcome appears to be independent of AVM obliteration.[3,4,6,8] Steiner et al. found 3 of 11 patients who became seizure free following SRS did so despite persistence of the AVM,[8] while Lim et al. found 40% of patients with partial AVM obliteration to be seizure free.[6] A similar phenomenon was described by Schrottner et al. in the treatment of 24 patients with tumor-related intractable epilepsy. Prolonged seizure control was achieved in 54% of patients in a dose-dependent manner, while tumor control was achieved in all patients.[10] These studies indicate that radiosurgery exerts an independent antiepileptic effect.

Animal studies have provided additional support for the use of radiosurgery in the treatment of seizures, as well as insight into the potential mechanism underlying its antiepileptic effect. One hypothesis has been that radiation causes destruction of epileptogenic tissue. Dose-dependent cell death and radiation necrosis develop in both normal and epileptic rat models in response to increasing doses of radiation.[11-15] Similarly, a dose-dependent effect of radiation on seizure control has been demonstrated in several rat models of epilepsy. However, seizure reduction occurred in the absence of necrosis,[11,13,14,16] suggesting necrosis may not be required for antiepileptic effects.

Another hypothesis has been that radiation inhibits seizure-induced neurogenesis and mitosis. In electrically kindled rats, radiation prevented kindling-associated neuroblast proliferation.[17,18] Similarly, radiation halted seizure-induced mitosis in flurothyl-kindled mice.[19] Despite the clear effect on neurogenesis and mitosis in these models, radiation did not inhibit mossy fiber synaptic reorganization,[20] kindling progression, or seizure threshold.[17,19] Alternatively, radiation may induce vascular and inflammatory changes that lead to seizure reduction.[21] Further animal studies will be critical to understanding the mechanisms underlying radiation-induced seizure control.

Modern Indications

HYPOTHALAMIC HAMARTOMAS

Hypothalamic hamartomas (HHs), though rare, are an important cause of debilitating epilepsy in childhood. HHs can cause a progressive epileptic encephalopathy characterized by seizures, endocrine dysfunction, cognitive and behavioral impairment, and developmental delay. Classically, HHs are associated with gelastic seizures, which appear as recurrent bouts of emotionless laughter or grimacing. In addition, most patients develop multiple seizure types, including tonic–clonic, partial complex, and drop attacks.[22,23] As devastating is the progressive cognitive decline that accompanies the medically refractory epilepsy.[24]

These heterotopic masses of mixed neuronal and glial cells arise from the floor of the third ventricle or mammillary bodies and present a significant therapeutic challenge due to their deep location and critical surrounding structures. Both open and endoscopic surgical approaches have been used in the resection of these lesions. While good seizure outcomes have been achieved, resection is associated with high morbidity and mortality.[25-27] SRS has therefore emerged as a primary treatment for HHs due to its ability to precisely target and treat HHs without the morbidity of surgical resection.

Arita et al. first applied gamma knife radiosurgery (GKS) to the treatment of a 25-year-old male with HH-associated epilepsy who remained seizure free 21 months after treatment.[28] Regis et al. have the largest experience with GKS treatment of HH. They reported seizure cessation in 40% of patients, with an additional 20% experiencing only rare, nondisabling seizures after 3 years.[29] Benefits extend to improved sleep, behavior, and learning; these have been documented independent of seizure remission.[29-34] No surgical mortality and limited morbidity have been reported in these patients. For these reasons, we advocate SRS as a valid option in the treatment in most patients with HHs, especially when the lesion is confined to the third ventricle.

MESIAL TEMPORAL LOBE EPILEPSY

The success with secondary epilepsies and HHs has prompted interest in the use of SRS for mesial temporal lobe epilepsy (MTLE) associated with mesial temporal sclerosis. In 1999, Regis et al. reported the first seven cases of amygdalohippocampectomy by GKS. All patients exhibited a reduction in seizure frequency, and all but one patient remained seizure free 2 years after the operation. In addition, magnetic resonance imaging (MRI) changes were noted, specifically in the amygdalohippocampal target, indicating focused destruction.[35] Since Regis et al.'s initial study, two large multicenter prospective trials have been completed. In the European trial a 24-Gy marginal dose was used, while in the U.S. trial 20- and 24-Gy marginal doses were compared. In both series, 51 patients in total, a significant reduction in seizure frequency was observed by 1 year and 65% of patients were seizure free at 2 years.[36,37] A multicenter prospective trial directly comparing GKS to open surgery (Radiosurgery or Open Surgery for Epilepsy, or the ROSE trial) is under way in the United States.

GKS has also shown efficacy in the treatment of recurrent seizures after incomplete temporal lobectomy. Yen et al. treated four such patients using GKS. This resulted in significant, persistent seizure reduction in all four patients without morbidity.[38]

SECONDARY EPILEPSIES

As discussed earlier, SRS has shown efficacy in the treatment of seizures secondary to AVMs and tumors. SRS has also been applied in the treatment of cavernous malformations (CMs). Seizure control following GKS is less than that found in the treatment of AVMs or tumors, with remission rates ranging from 25% to 53%.[39-41] In addition, GKS for CM is associated with an increased risk of radiation-induced complications, including hemorrhage.[42] Shih and Pan retrospectively compared surgical resection and GKS of CMs and noted seizure control and complication rates were better with open surgery.[40] We therefore feel strongly that the decision to treat seizures due to CMs, as well as due to AVMs or tumors, should be guided primarily by the natural history and the risk–benefit ratio of surgical resection in each particular case.

NONLESIONAL EPILEPSY

Currently, SRS does not offer any advantages over surgical resection in the treatment of nonlesional, cortical epilepsies because of the common need to perform invasive monitoring for seizure localization. Corpus callosotomy (CC), however, reduces the frequency or severity of generalized or multifocal seizures independent of seizure focus and may be a target for SRS. Eder et al. treated three children with SRS callosotomy, one with Lennox-Gastaut syndrome, and two following functional hemispherotomy for cortical dysplasia. The two children with persistent seizures after hemispherotomy became seizure free after GKS.[43]

Preoperative Evaluation

Patient selection and preoperative evaluation are the same as for patients considered for open resective surgery.[44] A complete medical and neurologic history, as well as a physical examination, is critical for understanding the scope of the patient's disease and identifying the risk factors that may affect treatment. Patients should be refractory to medical therapy. Patients with significant medical disorders (e.g., cardiac, pulmonary, or oncologic), progressive neurologic disorders (e.g., multiple sclerosis), psychiatric disorders, or a history of substance abuse or noncompliance should be excluded. Women of child-bearing age should have a negative pregnancy test and documented use of a reliable birth control method.

Complete clinical evaluation should include video-electroencephalogram recording sufficient for localization of the seizure focus, neuropsychological testing, and high-resolution (1.5 T) MRI. A thorough endocrine evaluation should be performed prior to treatment of patients with HH. For patients with MTLE, electrographic recordings should indicate the seizures, which may be simple and/or complex partial seizures with or without secondary generalization, arise from a single temporal lobe. Radiographic evidence of mesial temporal sclerosis (hippocampal atrophy or increased T2 signal) should be present in the same temporal lobe. Language and memory dominance should be determined using the intracarotid sodium Amytal test (Wada test) or functional MRI as guided by the clinical situation. A normal MRI, bilateral hippocampal pathology, or multifocal seizure onset is a contraindication for SRS treatment of MTLE.

Surgical Approaches

Radiosurgery can be performed under either general or local anesthesia, though typically we reserve general anesthesia for children. We recommend administering a small dose of a benzodiazepine sedative (e.g., lorazepam) to reduce the risk of seizures during the procedure. Pin sites are prepared with antiseptic solution, and local anesthetic is injected. The stereotactic frame must be affixed to the skull such that the base sits below the target. We then obtain a high-resolution MRI to include sequences that highlight the target (see specifics later). While the practices at individual centers vary, we find consultation among the neurosurgeon, radiation oncologist, and physicist beneficial in treatment planning. Advances in the gamma knife system and planning software (Leksell GammaPlan, Elekta, Stockholm, Sweden) allow more conformal radiation delivery using multiple isocenters. There is no predefined number of isocenters recommended for treatment. Treatment duration ranges from 1 to 2 hours, during which the patient's blood pressure, oxygen saturation, and neurologic status should be monitored. After treatment, the frame is removed. Most patients can be discharged to home within 2 hours of treatment completion, depending on their baseline neurologic function and the amount of sedatives given during the procedure.

HYPOTHALAMIC HAMARTOMAS

T2 and gadolinium-enhanced T1 coronal and axial magnetic resonance images must be carefully studied to delineate lesion boundaries and adjacent critical structures. HHs tend to be hyperintense on T2 and hypointense on T1 as compared to normal gray matter, and they do not enhance.[45] The planning software can be used to minimize radiation to the optic nerves and tracts, as well as normal hypothalamus, using a beam-blocking approach (Fig. 106-1). For most patients we set the 50% isodose line to be the marginal isodose line, corresponding to the tumor margin. As seizure remission is greater among patients receiving a marginal dose of at least 17 Gy,[30] every attempt should be made to achieve this marginal dose while preventing dosing greater than 8 Gy to the optic pathways. We typically use 18 or 19 Gy as our marginal dose.

MESIAL TEMPORAL LOBE EPILEPSY

Planning is most direct when the frame is applied with the base parallel to the long axis of the temporal horn. Coronal T2 fluid-attenuated inversion recovery, three-dimensional spoiled gradient recalled, and gadolinium-enhanced T1 magnetic resonance images are obtained, in addition to axial fast spin echo and gadolinium-enhanced T1 images. Planning software is then used to delineate the target defined as the head and anterior body of the hippocampus (approximately 2 cm), amygdala, and parahippocampal gyrus. As with HHs, the 50% isodose line is set to be the marginal dose (Fig. 106-2). Marginal doses ranging from 20 to 24 Gy have been reported to reduce seizure frequency,[36,37] though the optimal dose has yet to be clearly established. The optimal target volume also remains in debate.[46] The current multicenter ROSE trial uses 24 Gy for the margin and has a range of treatment volumes between

5.5 and 7.5 ml. Care must be taken to limit radiation to the neighboring brain stem and optic pathways (less than 10 and 8 Gy, respectively).

CORPUS CALLOSOTOMY

GKS for CC remains in the investigational phase, because few patients have been treated to date. The group from Austria has the largest experience, having treated both adults and children with GKS. They describe using two to five isocenters along the anterior or posterior corpus callosum with a marginal dose (equal to the 50% isodose line) of 55 to 85 Gy.[43,47,48] Future work will be necessary to define the optimal treatment parameters.

OTHER RADIOSURGICAL SYSTEMS

GKS has been the predominant technology applied to the radiosurgical treatment of epilepsy. While there is no reason to believe that other technologies cannot be utilized, experience has been limited thus far. Using linear accelerator particle accelerator (LINAC) technology, Liang et al. administered a total of 12 Gy (85% isodose line) in two fractions to seven patients with MTLE.[49] All patients in their cohort had poor seizure control at 2 years, including two patients who experienced a doubling of their seizure frequency. The maximum seizure reduction documented was 50% (two patients). Cmelak et al. also used LINAC to treated one patient with MTLE using a single fraction of 15 Gy. While the patient experienced good seizure control for 3 months after treatment, his seizure frequency then increased to the preceding pretreatment levels. He subsequently underwent surgical resection due to intractable seizures 1 year after SRS.[50] Poor seizure control in these studies is likely due to insufficient dosing, rather than limitations of the technology, as seizure outcome has been equivalent in the instances when LINAC or proton beam radiation were used to treat

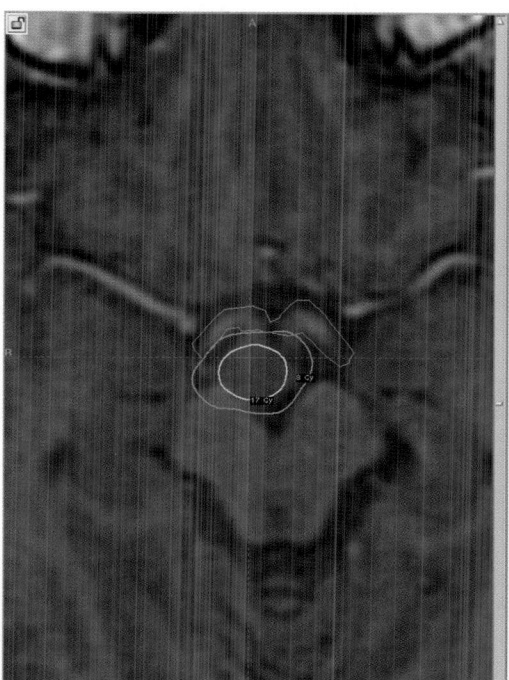

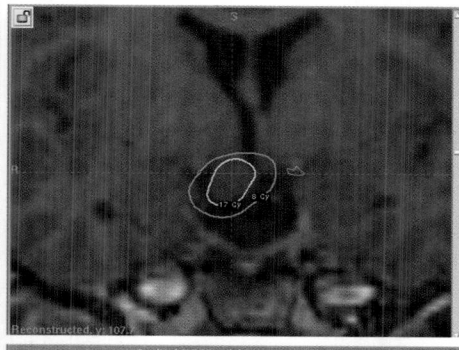

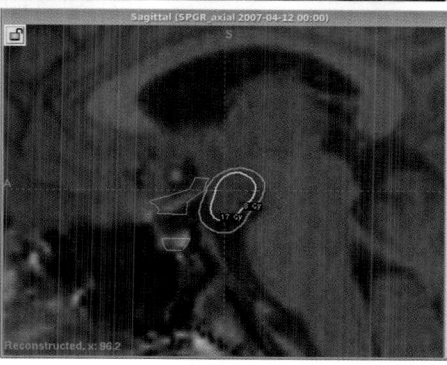

FIGURE 106-1 Example radiosurgical plan for HH. The green line delineates the 8-Gy isodose line, while the orange line highlights the optic tracts. Note the relative underdosing of the left portion of the HH due to limitations of the adjacent optic tracts.

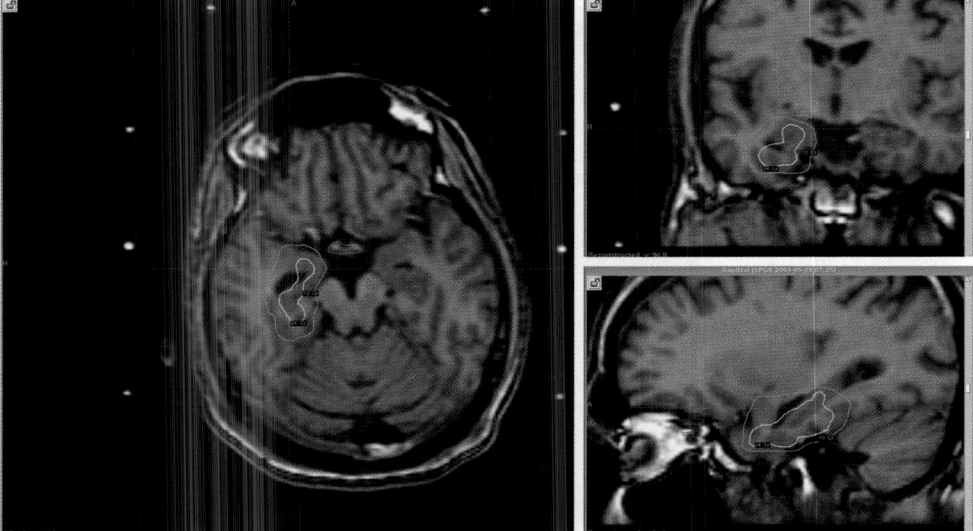

FIGURE 106-2 Example radiosurgical plan for MTLE. The green line delineates the 10-Gy isodose line. The optic apparatus is outlined in blue.

secondary epilepsies.[3,51,52] We recommend the specific SRS parameters be worked out for each system at each facility.

Surgical Morbidity

The most significant benefit of GKS in the treatment of epilepsies may be the avoidance of morbidity and mortality related to open surgical procedures. This benefit has already been documented in patients with HH. Several highly experienced centers have reported serious complications to occur in 30% to 60% of patients following open resection.[53] Such complications include ischemic stroke, endocrine dysfunction, cranial nerve damage, and a high rate of short-term memory impairment.[25,53-56] In contrast, morbidity associated with GKS treatment of HHs has been low. No deaths or serious neurologic deficits have been reported, though a few patients experienced transient poikilothermia.[29,31,32,34,53,57]

Data from two multicenter trials have indicated that GKS is also safe for the treatment of MTLE.[36,37] In our series of 30 patients, 1 patient developed headaches, papilledema, and blind spots associated with edema on MRI. As these symptoms progressed despite steroids, a temporal lobectomy was performed.[37] Regis et al. reported 1 case mortality due to myocardial infarction in their series of 21 patients that was deemed unrelated to GKS.[36] The most frequent side effect following GKS is headache (70%), often requiring steroid treatment.[37] In addition, 50% of patients were noted to have a quadranopsia identified by formal visual field testing, though less than 10% were symptomatic.[36,37] This is similar to the rate reported after surgical resection of the mesial temporal lobe structures.[58]

The risk of long-term, or delayed, complications must also be considered. Fractionated radiation treatment has been associated with gradual cognitive decline and secondary malignancies[59-62]; however, these complications have only rarely been reported with SRS.[63] Furthermore, the small, theoretical risk of cognitive decline due to SRS must be weighed against the well-documented association between uncontrolled seizures and cognitive function.[64]

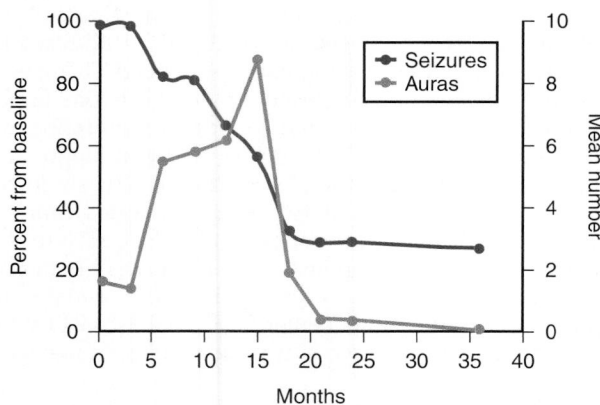

FIGURE 106-3 Time course of aura frequency relative to seizure frequency in MTLE. (*Courtesy of Edward F. Chang, Department of Neurosurgery, University of California–San Francisco.*)

Outcomes

SEIZURE CONTROL

Unlike the immediate effect of surgical resection, seizure remission following GKS is a process that takes months to years. Patients with HH often experience an immediate, though short-lived improvement, in seizures. This is followed by seizure return at pretreatment frequency (2-6 months after treatment). A third phase of acute increase in seizures lasts for days to weeks but seems to herald the progressive resolution of seizures.[53] Overall, at 3 years, 60% of patients have significant seizure reduction, as well as improved cognition and behavior.[53]

Patients with MTLE experience a dramatic increase in auras 9 to 15 months after GKS, coinciding with the reduction, or cessation, of complex partial seizures, as illustrated in Fig. 106-3.[36,37] Also during this period, MRI-documented temporal lobe edema reaches its peak (Fig. 106-4). Data from Chang et al. indicated that this process of radiation-induced temporal lobe damage is necessary for seizure

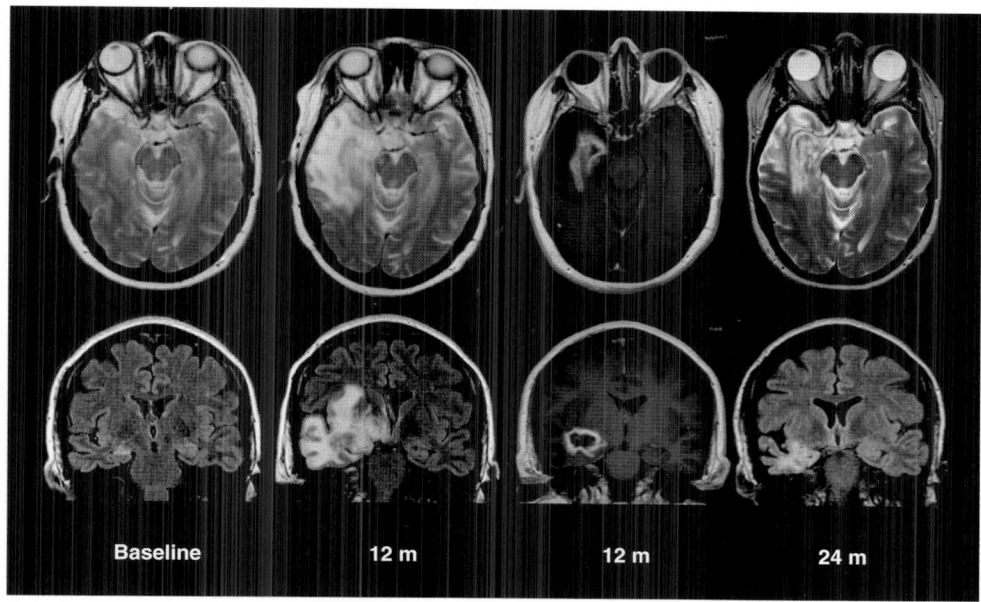

FIGURE 106-4 Progressive course of temporal lobe edema and subsequent resolution as revealed by MRI. Peak edema (T2 change) can be seen 9 to 15 months after treatment. (*Barbaro NM, Quigg M, Broshek DK, et al. A multicenter, prospective pilot study of gamma knife radiosurgery for mesial temporal lobe epilepsy: seizure response, adverse events, and verbal memory. Ann Neurology 65:167-175, 2009.*)

remission. Two MRI markers of edema (volume of T2 hyperintensity and contrast enhancement), when measured 12 months post-treatment, correlated with seizure remission documented 24 to 36 months post-treatment.[65] Though the edema and increased aura frequency may persist for several months, they subsequently resolve. After a minimum of 2 years follow-up, 65% to 67% of patients were seizure free,[36,37,66] with 60% seizure free at 5 years.[66] The ongoing multicenter trial direct comparison between radiosurgery and open surgery will offer the best determination of equivalence.

COGNITION AND MEMORY

As discussed previously, cognition and behavior significantly improve after SRS for HH, even before meaningful seizure reduction occurs.[29-34] This presents a major benefit of treatment, particularly given the severe epileptic encephalopathy caused by persistent gelastic seizures.[67]

In the case of MTLE, SRS may provide benefit with respect to verbal memory preservation. Open surgical resection presents a well-characterized risk of significant decline in verbal memory. Significant verbal memory decline is documented to occur in 38% of patients after temporal lobectomy.[68] Such decline is more consistent among patients who undergo dominant hemisphere resection.[69] Stroup et al. found that 60% of patients declined in at least one measure of verbal memory (either the Long Delay Free Recall score of the California Verbal Learning Test or the Rey Delay Recall score of the Wechsler Memory Scale) after dominant temporal lobe resection.[68] In contrast, only 25% of patients who underwent dominant temporal lobe SRS in the U.S. multicenter pilot study experienced a significant decline in either measure of verbal memory.[37]

Conclusions

SRS should be considered first-line therapy for the treatment of intractable epilepsy in the majority of HH lesions. Current literature supports a potential role in the treatment of MTLE,

though long-term study of efficacy and cognitive outcomes is necessary. Other indications for SRS in epilepsy require further study.

KEY REFERENCES

Barbaro NM, Quigg M, Broshek DK, et al. A multicenter, prospective pilot study of gamma knife radiosurgery for mesial temporal lobe epilepsy: seizure response, adverse events, and verbal memory. *Ann Neurol.* 2009;65(2):167-175.

Bartolomei F, Regis J, Kida Y, et al. Gamma knife radiosurgery for epilepsy associated with cavernous hemangiomas: a retrospective study of 49 cases. *Stereotact Funct Neurosurg.* 1999;72(Suppl 1):22-28.

Brisman JL, Cole AJ, Cosgrove GR, et al. Radiosurgery of the rat hippocampus: magnetic resonance imaging, neurophysiological, histological, and behavioral studies. *Neurosurgery.* 2003;53(4):951,61: discussion 961-962.

Chang EF, Quigg M, Oh MC, et al. Predictors of efficacy after stereotactic radiosurgery for medial temporal lobe epilepsy. *Neurology.* 2010;74(2):165-172.

Chen ZF, Kamiryo T, Henson SL, et al. Anticonvulsant effects of gamma surgery in a model of chronic spontaneous limbic epilepsy in rats. *J Neurosurg.* 2001;94(2):270-280.

Feichtinger M, Schrottner O, Eder H, et al. Efficacy and safety of radiosurgical callosotomy: a retrospective analysis. *Epilepsia.* 2006;47(7): 1184-1191.

Gerszten PC, Adelson PD, Kondziolka D, et al. Seizure outcome in children treated for arteriovenous malformations using gamma knife radiosurgery. *Pediatr Neurosurg.* 1996;24(3):139-144.

Heikkinen ER, Konnov B, Melnikov L, et al. Relief of epilepsy by radiosurgery of cerebral arteriovenous malformations. *Stereotact Funct Neurosurg.* 1989;53(3):157-166.

Kida Y, Kobayashi T, Tanaka T, et al. Seizure control after radiosurgery on cerebral arteriovenous malformations. *J Clin Neurosci.* 2000; 7(Suppl 1):6-9.

Kondziolka D, Lunsford LD, Flickinger JC. The application of stereotactic radiosurgery to disorders of the brain. *Neurosurgery.* 2008;62(Suppl 2): 707,19: discussion 719–720.

Leksell L. The stereotaxic method and radiosurgery of the brain. *Acta Chir Scand.* 1951;102(4):316-319.

Liang S, Liu T, Li A, et al. Long-term follow up of very low-dose LINAC-based stereotactic radiotherapy in temporal lobe epilepsy. *Epilepsy Res.* 2010;90(1-2):60-67.

Liscak R, Vladyka V, Novotny Jr J, et al. Leksell gamma knife lesioning of the rat hippocampus: the relationship between radiation dose and functional and structural damage. *J Neurosurg.* 2002;97(5 Suppl): 666-673.

Maesawa S, Kondziolka D, Dixon CE, et al. Subnecrotic stereotactic radiosurgery controlling epilepsy produced by kainic acid injection in rats. *J Neurosurg.* 2000;93(6):1033-1040.

Mathieu D, Kondziolka D, Niranjan A, et al. Gamma knife radiosurgery for refractory epilepsy caused by hypothalamic hamartomas. *Stereotact Funct Neurosurg.* 2006;84(2-3):82-87.

Mori Y, Kondziolka D, Balzer J, et al. Effects of stereotactic radiosurgery on an animal model of hippocampal epilepsy. *Neurosurgery.* 2000;46(1):157,65: discussion 165-168.

Quigg M, Barbaro NM. Stereotactic radiosurgery for treatment of epilepsy. *Arch Neurol.* 2008;65(2):177-183.

Raedt R, Boon P, Persson A, et al. Radiation of the rat brain suppresses seizure-induced neurogenesis and transiently enhances excitability during kindling acquisition. *Epilepsia.* 2007;48(10):1952-1963.

Regis J, Bartolomei F, de Toffol B, et al. Gamma knife surgery for epilepsy related to hypothalamic hamartomas. *Neurosurgery.* 2000;47(6):1343,51: discussion 1351-1352.

Regis J, Bartolomei F, Rey M, et al. Gamma knife surgery for mesial temporal lobe epilepsy. *Epilepsia.* 1999;40(11):1551-1556.

Regis J, Rey M, Bartolomei F, et al. Gamma knife surgery in mesial temporal lobe epilepsy: a prospective multicenter study. *Epilepsia.* 2004;45(5):504-515.

Rheims S, Fischer C, Ryvlin P, et al. Long-term outcome of gamma-knife surgery in temporal lobe epilepsy. *Epilepsy Res.* 2008;80(1):23-29.

Schrottner O, Eder HG, Unger F, et al. Radiosurgery in lesional epilepsy: brain tumors. *Stereotact Funct Neurosurg.* 1998;70(Suppl 1):50-56.

Schulze-Bonhage A, Trippel M, Wagner K, et al. Outcome and predictors of interstitial radiosurgery in the treatment of gelastic epilepsy. *Neurology.* 2008;71(4):277-282.

Yen DJ, Chung WY, Shih YH, et al. Gamma knife radiosurgery for the treatment of recurrent seizures after incomplete anterior temporal lobectomy. *Seizure.* 2009;18(7):511-514.

Numbered references appear on Expert Consult.

CHAPTER 107

Gamma Surgery for Functional Disorders

CHUN-PO YEN • LADISLAU STEINER

Leksell's original intention in designing the gamma knife was to use the tool to treat functional disorders such as Parkinson's diseases, pain, or psychiatric conditions. The collimators in the first gamma knife model were constructed to produce a discoid-shaped lesion to ablate the stereotactically targeted neuronal pathway or nuclei using a single high dose of gamma irradiation. However, the lack of neurophysiologic confirmation of the targets and the introduction of deep brain stimulation have made the radiosurgical procedures for functional disorders only indicated in patients who for some reason are unable to undergo an open stereotactic lesioning or insertion of deep brain stimulators.

Gamma Surgery for Pain

The lack of anatomic and pathophysiologic background knowledge of the mechanisms of pain makes management of pain by open or closed stereotactic techniques largely unsatisfactory. Early results using gamma surgery to produce thalamotomies for pain control were published by Steiner et al.[1] All 52 patients treated suffered from terminal cancer and were treated prior to the advent of computed tomography (CT) or magnetic resonance imaging (MRI). Pneumoencephalography was used to target the thalamic centrum medianum-parafasciculus (CM-Pf) complex. Good pain relief was obtained in 8 patients and moderate pain relief in 18. The patients had in general only temporary relief of pain. Of those with good pain relief, 5 died without recurrence of pain between 1 and 13 months after the procedure, and 3 had recurrence of pain at 3, 6, and 9 months. Doses between 100 and 250 Gy were tested. The collimators used were 3 × 5 and 3 × 7 mm. Observation of an actual lesion was only possible in 21 of 36 patients who had a postmortem examination. Not surprisingly, the presence of a lesion was associated with relief. Lesions were only reliably created with doses greater than 160 Gy. The most effective lesions were more medially located near the wall of the third ventricle, and the greatest relief was for face or arm pain.

These early results were not very encouraging. However, with improvements in neuroimaging and alternate target selection, it is possible that more effective lesions can be produced. Recent reports seem to support this expectation. Hayashi et al. reported significant pain reduction in patients with severe cancer pain and post-stroke thalamic pain after gamma knife lesioning of the hypophysis.[2,3] Using the 4-mm collimator and doses of 140 to 180 Gy, Young et al.

have published effective pain relief in patients with chronic, intractable pain following medial thalamotomy with the gamma knife.[4,5] In a series of 15 patients followed for more than 3 months after a radiosurgical medial thalamotomy, 4 (27%) were pain free, and 5 others (33%) had greater than 50% pain relief.[4] Additional investigation must be conducted before the role of the gamma knife for pain treatment can be fully defined.

Gamma Surgery for Trigeminal Neuralgia

The first time radiosurgery was used to treat trigeminal neuralgia, Leksell treated two patients with the stereotactic technique using orthovoltage x-rays.[16] The patients treated with this method were followed up for 17 years, during which time both remained pain free. With the introduction of the gamma knife, a series of 46 patients were treated in Stockholm with less encouraging results.[6] The target in these cases was the Gasserian ganglion, and targeting was by bony landmarks or cisternography. In the first 24 patients, where stereotactic cranial x-rays were used for targeting, 33% of patients were pain free at 6 months and 8.3% at a mean follow-up of 26 months. Transoral cisternography with tantalum dust suspended in glycerol was used in a group of 22 patients and 59% of the patients became pain free at 6 months and 18% at 26 months. A later report by Lindquist et al. stated that approximately 50% of the patients initially became pain free, but neuralgia recurred for most of them several years after radiosurgery.[7] With advances in neuroimaging, most notably MRI, gamma surgery for trigeminal neuralgia was revisited. However, the focus of treatment shifted from the ganglion to the nerve root entry zone or the cisternal segment of trigeminal nerve.[8]

A number of centers have since shown the safety and at least short-term pain relief with gamma surgery for trigeminal neuralgia (Fig. 107-1). Maesawa et al. reported complete pain relief without medication in 47.7% of patients at the initial follow-up and in 40% of patients at the last follow-up in 220 patients with a median follow-up of 22 months (range 6–78 months).[9] In a series of 117 consecutive patients who were followed up for an average of 26 months (range 1–48 months), Pollock et al. reported an actuarial rate of freedom from pain without medication in 57% and 55% of patients at 1 and 3 years, respectively.[10] Tawk et al. in a series of 38 patients followed up for a median of 24 months observed

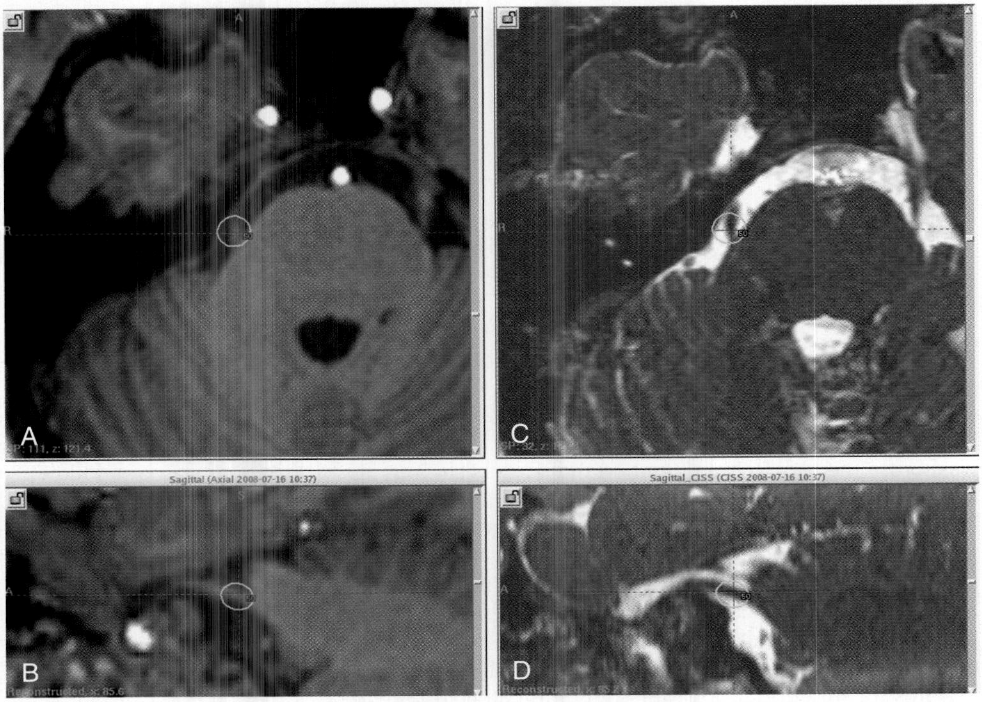

FIGURE 107-1 A gamma knife treatment plan illustrating the targeting of posterior root of trigeminal nerve on T1-weighted images (A, axial view; B, sagittal view) and constructive interference steady-state images (C, axial view; D, sagittal view). A 4-mm collimator was used. The circle represents the 50% isodose line and encircles the entry zone of the posterior root of the right trigeminal nerve.

Table 107-1   Published Radiosurgical Series for Typical Trigeminal Neuralgia

	Year	Patient No.	Follow-up Median/Mean[a] or Minimum (Months)	Pain-Free Condition without Medication	Trigeminal Dysfunction[b]	Recurrence
Han et al.[52]	2009	60	12	62%	13%	52%
Dellaretti et al.[53]	2008	76	12	83%	21%	26%
			24	71%		
			36	63%		
Jagannathan et al.[15]	2008	172	12	50%	22%	59%
			36	41%		
Longhi et al.[54]	2007	160	37[a]	61%	9.5%	18%
Regis et al.[8]	2006	100	12	58%	10%	34%
Fountas et al.[17]	2006	77	12	73%	16%	NA
			36	40%		
Brisman et al.[55]	2004	293	23[a]	22%	13%	24%
Petit et al.[56]	2003	96	30[a]	42%	7%	29%
Pollock et al.[10]	2002	117	12	57%	37%	23%
			36	55%		
Maesawa et al.[9]	2001	220	22[a]	40%	10%	14%

[a]Median/mean.
[b]Including any new or aggravated facial numbness, dysesthesia, hypothesia, hyperesthesia.
NA, not available.

pain relief without medication in 44% at the 3-month evaluation but in only 16% of patients at the 24-month follow-up visit.[11] Regis et al. reported a series of 100 patients with a minimum follow-up of 12 months. Fifty-eight patients were pain free without medication.[8]

The reported rates of recurrence following radiosurgery for trigeminal neuralgia have ranged from 5% to 42% and probably are related to incomplete radiation effects on the targeted tissues (Table 107-1).

Pain free outcomes were usually achieved within several weeks after the gamma procedure. Fountas et al. reported that most patients with no previous surgeries responded within 4 weeks after treatment.[12] Pollock et al. reported that complete pain relief occurred within a median of 3 weeks

(range 1–20 weeks).[10] According to Regis et al., initial pain relief occurred after a median delay of 10 days (range 2–5 weeks) in 94% of patients.[8]

The incidence of new trigeminal dysfunction varies in the literature from 6% to 66%. Pollock et al. reported new trigeminal dysfunction in 43 patients (37%) and demonstrated an association between greater radiation doses and the risk of trigeminal nerve dysfunction—90 Gy as a maximum dose caused numbness in 50% of patients, whereas in only 15% of patients who received 70 Gy.[13] They also reported a strong correlation between the development of new facial sensory loss and achievement and maintenance of pain relief—excellent pain-free outcome 4.5 times more likely in patients with new trigeminal deficits compared with those

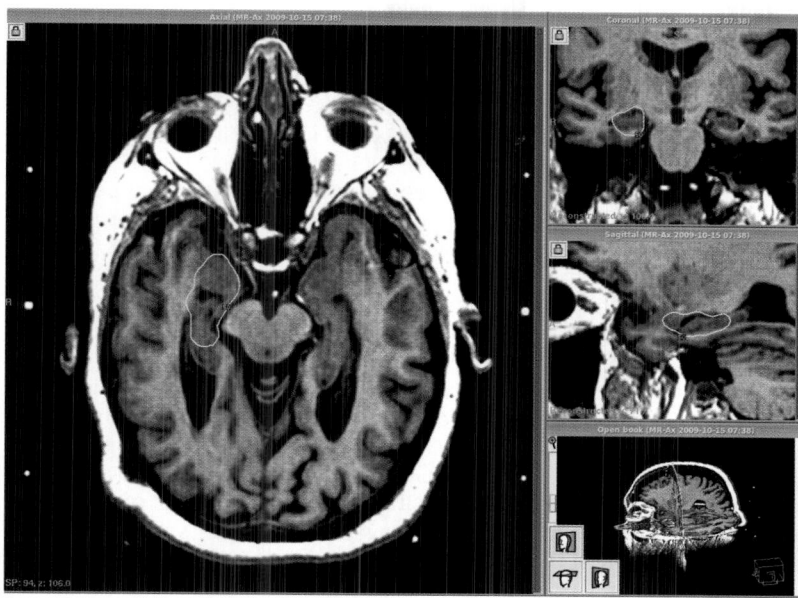

FIGURE 107-2 A gamma knife treatment plan illustrating the target for mesial temporal lobe epilepsy on T1-weighted images. The amygdala, anterior hippocampus, and parahippocampal gyrus are included in the 50% isodose line.

who had normal postradiosurgical trigeminal nerve function. Regis et al. reported that six patients in their series of 100 cases presented with facial paresthesia and four with facial hyperesthesia.[8] In Young's series, facial numbness occurred in 12%, 20%, and 29% of cases when a maximum dose of 70, 80, and 90 Gy, respectively, was used.[14]

At the University of Virginia, we have recently reviewed our treatment of 170 cases of typical trigeminal neuralgia with gamma surgery.[15] There were 67 males and 93 females with a mean age of 63.8 years (range 23–95 years). Prior to gamma surgery, 24 patients had prior microvascular decompression, 44 had one or more glycerol injections, radio-frequency thermocoagulation, balloon compression or neurectomy prior to radiosurgery. In each case, the radiosurgical target chosen was 2 to 4 mm anterior to the entry zone of the trigeminal nerve into the pons. A prescription dose of between 30 and 45 Gy to the 50% isodose line was used. The maximum dose ranged from 60 to 90 Gy (median 80 Gy). Excellent outcome was defined as complete pain-free condition without medication. Pain relief of a different degree with or without medication was considered palliative outcome. Follow-up ranged from 6 months to 12 years (mean 4.2 years) (Fig. 107-2).

Thirty-four patients (20%) never had any improvement of their pain following gamma surgery. Fifty-six percent of patients became pain free without medication at some point after treatment. At 1, 2, 3, and 5 years follow-up, 50%, 44%, 42%, and 30% of patients, respectively, were pain free without medication. Twenty patients remained pain free without medication more than 5 years after gamma surgery (range 62–111 months). Palliative results were obtained by 16%, 10%, 8%, and 6%, respectively, at 1, 2, 3, and 5 years follow-up. Patients with two or more percutaneous procedures or neurectomy prior to gamma surgery had less favorable outcome.

Thirty-eight patients (22%) developed postradiosurgical facial numbness. Two patients considered the numbness to be worse than the original facial pain. The fact that they did not have pain relief after gamma surgery presumably

contributed to their dissatisfaction. We also observed the association of facial numbness with higher rate of pain free outcome as reported by Pollock et al.[13] Forty-five patients (26.4%) including 32 who were pain free without medication and 13 who had palliative results after gamma surgery eventually had a recurrence of pain at some point during the follow-up. Twenty-three patients underwent a second gamma procedure. Of 17 patients who were completely pain free for two to 60 months following the initial procedure, 12 became pain free without medication again after retreatment. Four of six patients who had only palliative outcome after the initial procedure became pain free without medication following the second treatment.

Among the treatment alternatives for trigeminal neuralgia, microvascular decompression providing both immediate and long-lasting complete pain relief as well as relatively low incidence of trigeminal nerve dysfunction appears to come closest to what one would expect of a good treatment for trigeminal neuralgia. Although less effective than microvascular decompression, radiosurgery remains a reasonable treatment option for those patients who are unwilling or unable to undergo more invasive surgical approaches and it offers a low risk of mortality or major morbidity.

Gamma Surgery for Movement Disorders

Thalamotomy for tremor in Parkinson's disease remains one of the most gratifying procedures in functional neurosurgery and defends its place in the therapeutic armory for those common cases in which drugs fail to stop the tremor. To avoid the potential risks of open thalamotomies, the prototype of the gamma knife was used by Leksell[16] to produce thalamic lesions in five cases of tremor between 1968 and 1970. At that time, the intended target could not be visualized but was indirectly determined by using derived coordinates relative to the anterior and posterior commisures visualized by pneumoencephalography. Verification that a lesion had been produced could not be obtained because neither CT nor MRI was available. The fixation of the head of the patient for the radiosurgical procedure was also unsatisfactory, because the stereotactic frame used for target localization was too large to fit into the collimator helmet. Instead, fixation devices were applied onto a plaster-of-Paris helmet previously molded on the patient's head. It is therefore not surprising that beneficial results were lacking.

In 1986, MRI was introduced at Karolinska Hospital, and better anatomic visualization of the target volume became possible. A new stereotactic frame compatible with MRI that also served as the fixation device in the gamma knife was introduced.[16] These improvements paved the way for new attempts to relieve Parkinsonian tremor by gammathalamotomy, and two cases were treated using this improved methodology.[7] The first procedure was performed using an 8-mm collimator, and the volume of the resulting lesion was much larger than intended (1.5 cm³). The tremor began to dwindle after 2 months, but a transient hemiparesis and mild speech disturbance ensued secondary to edema. The eventual outcome was, however, satisfactory, and 4 years after the treatment the patient returned free of tremor contralateral to the side of the thalamic lesion, asking for a second procedure to stop the tremor that had developed on the other side. The second patient was treated using a 4-mm collimator, which gave a smaller volume to the thalamic lesion. In this case, the clinical result was not satisfactory. The patient was treated a second time without relief of tremor. It is not clear whether the lack of effect was due to the atypical clinical picture in this patient or to the lack of physiologic corroboration of the target. In spite of experience from centers active in this field indicating that modern imaging techniques, especially MRI, may obviate the need for physiologic target definition, this assertion remains controversial.

Pioneering work in neuroanatomy and neurophysiology by Hirai, Jones, and Ohye has shed much light on the position, anatomic organization, and physiologic significance of the thalamus as it pertains to tremor, rigidity, and dyskinesia.[17-19] MRI guidance for selective thalamotomy in the treatment of Parkinsonian or essential tremors has been well established. The correlations between neuroanatomic and electrophysiologic findings in the human ventrolateral thalamic nuclei (e.g., VLa, VLp, VPLa, VPLc) are better understood. For gamma surgery, the difficulty arises in identifying the VLp and VLa nuclei in the human thalamus purely by radiologic methods. As such, thin-slice MRI, Surgiplan, and a neuroanatomic atlas may be required to treat these nuclei with the gamma knife.

Rand treated 18 cases of movement disorder with radiosurgery (R. Rand, personal communication, 1994). Of the seven patients with resting tremor, four responded to a nucleus ventralis lateralis (NVL) lesion with marked improvement in the tremor, and in two patients, rigidity improved as well. Eight other patients underwent radiosurgical pallidotomy for rigidity, and four had significant improvement. Two of three patients treated with a NVL lesion for intention tremor showed dramatic improvement.

Ohye (C. Ohye, personal communications, 2004) has performed gammathalamotomies on 56 patients for Parkinson's disease, 21 with essential tremor, and 6 with intention tremor. Thalamotomies were performed using a single 4-mm shot and 130-Gy dose. Follow-up MRI revealed two different types of thalamic changes. One type was a round, punched-out lesion with a volume of less than 100 mm³, and the other was an irregular high-signal zone (volume up to 800 mm³) that may extend into the internal capsule and streak along the border of the thalamus. The efficacy of the procedure did not seem to correlate with the type of postoperative imaging observed. Ohye noted improvements in tremor and/or rigidity in 85% of patients. Hirai (T. Hirai, personal communications, 2004) has treated 14 patients with gamma surgery for movement disorders. Of these 14 patients, 8 had tremor-dominant Parkinson's disease, 4 rigidity and dyskinesia-dominant Parkinson's disease, and 2 had essential tremors. Hirai's target points were the VLp nucleus for control of tremor and the VLa nucleus for control of rigidity and dyskinesia. The maximum dose varied from 130 to 150 Gy; a single 4-mm isocenter was used to make each lesion. At the last follow-up, 13 out of 14 patients noted subjective improvement in their symptomatology. In 9 of these patients who had at least 1 year of follow-up, Hirai noted symptomatic improvement by 50% to 90% in the patients' Unified Parkinson's Disease Rating Scale for tremor, rigidity, and dyskinesia scores. On follow-up MRI, Hirai observed T2-weighted changes 3 months after gamma surgery, and these lesions gradually increased to 5 to 8 mm in diameter. In another series, Young et al. reported significant improvements in Unified Parkinson's Disease Rating Scale tremor and rigidity scores in 74 of 102 Parkinson's patients (73%) at 4 years or longer post–gamma knife thalamotomy; in 52 patients with essential tremor, 88.2% remained tremor free at 4 years or more postoperatively.[20] Two patients had permanent hemiparesis and facial paresthesias. One patient experienced transient deficit.

In general the outcome of gamma pallidotomy is less satisfactory and a high risk of complication has been reported.[18,21] The gamma knife was occasionally used to create a lesion in subthalamic nucleus, however, its efficacy and safety remain to be investigated.[22]

A significant change in the surgical management of movement disorders, particularly Parkinson's disease, was the introduction of deep brain stimulation (DBS), which allows the amelioration of symptoms without a destructive lesion. Good results have been obtained with this technique, and, at present, DBS has supplanted destructive lesions as the surgical procedure of choice in most patients.[23,24] The enthusiasm for deep brain stimulation may be lessened by the high rate of complications and cost.[19,25-27] As the benefits and risks for DBS become better defined, neurosurgeons will be able to counsel patients and select the more appropriate neurosurgical tool (i.e., gamma knife or DBS).

Gamma Surgery for Obsessive-Compulsive Neurosis

Despite therapeutic progress in recent years, conventional treatment of anxiety disorders fails or has only a temporary effect in 20% of patients. These disorders are often severely disabling and are associated with rates of suicide comparable to those of depression. First described by Leksell,[28] psychosurgery targeting the frontolimbic connections in both anterior internal capsules (capsulotomy) occasionally may be useful for selected severe cases. The first cases using the gamma knife to create the lesions were also performed by Leksell.

Mindus et al. at the Karolinska Institute[29] reported the effects of such procedures on the anxiety symptoms and personality characteristics presented in conjunction with results of imaging studies performed by MRI and PET. The patient material comprised two series of patients with a 15-year mean duration of psychiatric illness, in all of whom various extensive treatment trials had previously been made. One series consisted of 24 patients subjected to capsulotomy by a conventional thermocoagulation technique and followed for 1 year. The other series comprised 7 patients treated by gamma surgery and followed for 7 years. The clinical effects of these treatments were evaluated subjectively by two independent observers and also rated on the Comprehensive Psychopathological Rating Scale (CPRS). Ratings were performed 10 days before and 2, 6, and 12 months after surgery. The effects on the personality were evaluated by the Karolinska Scales of Personality (KSP). These scales have been developed to measure traits related to frontal lobe dysfunction and to reflect different dimensions of anxiety proneness. At the 12-month follow-up, statistically and clinically significant improvement was noted in all assessments of symptomatic and psychosocial function. Freedom from symptoms or considerable improvement was noted in 79% of patients, and none were worse after the operation. At the 1-year follow-up, seven patients reported fatigue, four poor memory, two carelessness, and two long-windedness. Behind these numbers are numerous examples of dramatic improvements in individual lifestyles. A number of patients were preoperatively unable to work or function socially owing to such problems as preoccupation with personal cleanliness and the inability to use public transportation, with resulting domestic confinement, aggravated psychological problems, deterioration of family relationships, and devastation of personal economy. Postoperatively, these patients could return to their previous occupation and to a normal social function. The results of gamma capsulotomy were found to be comparable to those of capsulotomy performed by the thermocoagulation technique. Only in five of the seven patients could a lesion be demonstrated by MRI, and those were the patients who benefited from the procedure. The lowest effective target dose was 160 Gy, whereas 100, 120, and 152 Gy failed to produce lesions.

Treatment of a new series of 10 patients was started in 1988, using stereotactic MRI for more accurate anatomic target localization and the new gamma knife model to produce the lesions. In this series, the lesions were produced by using a 4-mm collimator and three isocenters on each side for overlapping fields, creating a cylindrical lesion. The maximum dose within the target volume was 200 Gy. Development of lesions has been followed by MRI and CT scans every 3 months. On T2-weighted images, a high signal appears in the target area after approximately 3 months. This signal is most likely produced by local edema. The edema reaches a maximal volume at around 9 months and then progressively subsides. The edema is directly related to the dose and to the volume radiated. The preliminary results equal those obtained in the earlier series.

Ruck et al. in 2008 reported 25 obsessive-compulsive disorder (OCD) patients undergoing gamma- or thermocapsulotomy between 1988 and 2000 at the Karolinska Institute.[30] Among these patients were nine cases treated with bilateral gamma capsulotomy with long-term follow-up. Two hundred Gy with three 4-mm shots were used in five cases and 180 Gy with a single 4-mm shot at each side were performed in five (two of them had repeat bilateral gamma capsulotomy and one had retreatment with thermocapsulotomy). The mean Yale-Brown Obsessive-Compulsive Scale used to rate OCD severity decreased significantly from 33.4 preoperatively to 17 at 1-year follow-up and 14.2 at long-term follow-up. Fifty percent of patients display signs of apathy and dysexecutive function behavior. Cases showed these neurologic deficits were those who received high radiation doses or underwent a repeat procedure. There was no difference in outcome between patients who underwent gamma or thermocapsulotomy and the incidence of apathy and executive dysfunction were similar in both groups. The authors suggested that a small lesion would achieve an adequate outcome with fewer complications.

Gamma capsulotomy offers several important clinical advantages over capsulotomy via an open technique.[31] The most important is patient tolerance. This psychologically vulnerable group of patients seems to be much more willing to undergo a closed stereotactic procedure in contrast to open surgery. Theoretically, the gradual development of the radiolesion may also allow the patient better psychological adjustment to his new situation. The psychological rehabilitation phase is an important part of any psychosurgical procedure.

If it would be ethically acceptable, a control group of patients could be subjected to a sham gamma treatment. In a later stage, if this sham procedure is proven to give no result in comparison with the real procedure, the patients would receive the appropriate gamma treatment. Such a controlled study would probably be necessary before the real effect of gamma capsulotomy can be established. Further efforts should also be made to study the biology of the developing lesions. Important questions are: When does the functional effect of the radiation start and what are the characteristics of the MRI and CT images at this time? Even the issue of dose–volume relationships needs to be addressed further. PET or SPECT imaging may help to answer some of these questions, and pre- and posttreatment evaluation should be carried out before further series of patients are treated. The experience from multiple centers suggests a degree of optimism for the use of radiosurgery in the treatment of intractable OCD, and future research in psychiatric neurosurgery is proceeding in a cautious fashion.[32] Any such work necessitates the coordination and effort of a multidisciplinary team.

Gamma Surgery for Epilepsy

When the gamma knife was installed in Stockholm, Leksell always invited his colleagues and pupils to suggest indications for using the "gadget." None of them mentioned epilepsy as a possible indication. The interest in using gamma surgery for epilepsy was triggered by an early report that seizures were alleviated in a series of arteriovenous malformation (AVM) cases. In 59 of the 247 AVM patients with seizure as the presenting symptom treated by Steiner et al. using gamma surgery between 1970 and 1984, the treatment resulted in relief of some or all seizures in 52 of these patients.[33] Eleven were successfully taken off anticonvulsant medication. Interestingly, in three patients seizure disorder symptoms were eliminated, although the AVM itself was unaffected by the radiation. These observations and the observations made by others[34-36] prompted the idea of testing focal irradiation as a treatment modality for focal epilepsy.

At the University of Virginia, basic science research was done on changes in neuroexcitability after irradiation. The hippocampal slices from rats treated with the gamma knife were found to have a higher seizure threshold than those of controls when placed in solutions of varying concentrations of penicillin. This effect was lost at high concentrations (S.L. Henson, personal communication, 2001). Using single doses of either 20 or 40 Gy to the hippocampus in a rat model of chronic spontaneous limbic epilepsy, a reduction in both the frequency and duration of spontaneous seizures was observed.[37] Histologic evaluation of the targeted region revealed no signs of necrosis and hippocampal slice recordings revealed intact synaptically driven neuronal firing.[37] Subsequent work by the University of Pittsburgh group using a kainic acid–induced hippocampal epilepsy rat model revealed similarly efficacious results in terms of seizure control and the absence of behavioral impairment with subnecrotic doses of radiosurgery.[38,39]

Biochemical analysis of changes in rat brains after gamma surgery showed changes in the concentrations of excitatory and inhibitory amino acids, particularly gamma-amino butyric acid (GABA).[40] Warnke et al. showed that patients with low-grade astrocytomas and associated epilepsy had significant relief from seizures following interstitial radiosurgery. SPECT scanning showed a reduced number of GABA receptors prior to treatment in both the tumors and surrounding brain. Levels of these receptors increased following therapy.[41] These early studies show that functional changes may occur at the cellular level without gross structural damage. The implications of this for functional neurosurgery are intriguing.

Epilepsy has been treated with the gamma knife at many centers but there have been few published long-term results. Barcia Salorio et al. treated 11 patients with idiopathic epilepsy. Preoperative invasive electrodiagnostic confirmation of the epileptogenic focus was performed and treatment was with low-dose (10–20 Gy) radiosurgery.[34] Complete relief from seizures was obtained in four patients and significant reduction in seizure activity in five. The effect of the treatment was not seen for several months in most instances. Regis et al. reported the first radiosurgical amygadohippocampectomy in a case of mesial temporal lobe epilepsy (MTLE) treated with gamma surgery.[42] They used 25 Gy given to the 50% isodose line. The patient was seizure free after the treatment. At 10 months a lesion was evident on both CT and MRI that conformed to the 50% isodose line (amygdala and hippocampus). Whether actual gross structural lesioning with this method is associated with better results or more complications is unknown. Further results of 25 patients with medically intractable MTLE treated by Regis et al. (2000) showed that of the 16 patients with more than 2 years of follow-up, 13 are seizure free and two are improved.[43] In addition, they noted minimal morbidity

(only three cases of nonsymptomatic visual field deficit) and no mortality associated with the gamma surgery.

The potential of a less invasive, nondestructive therapy to treat epilepsy prompted the creation of prospective European and a National Institutes of Health (NIH)–sponsored multicenter studies of gamma surgery for temporal lobe epilepsy. In the European study, three centers enrolled 21 patients with MTLE. The anterior parahippocampal cortex, the basal and lateral portions of the amygdala, and the anterior hippocampus were targeted, and patients received a mean dose of 24 Gy. At 2 years postradiosurgery, 65% of the patients were seizure free. However, nine patients developed visual field deficits, and five suffered transient side effects, including depression, headache, nausea, vomiting, and imbalance.[44] The NIH sponsored study, in which our center also participated, was recently reported.[45] Thirty patients were randomized to have gamma surgery with a prescription dose of 20 or 24 Gy targeting the amygdala, hippocampus, and parahippocampus. At the 3-year follow-up, 67% were free of seizure. Ten of 13 patients (76.9%) receiving the high dose and 10 of 17 patients (58.8%) receiving low dose were seizure free. "A wide range of responses on serial MRI" was reported; however, when followed up over time, the edema resolved. One patient did require an urgent anterior temporal resection due to headache and visual field defect caused by brain edema. Twenty-one patients experienced new headaches at least once during the follow-up and 15 developed superior quadrantanopsias similar to those observed after temporal lobectomy. Verbal memory impairment was noticed in four of 26 patients (15%). The authors concluded that radiosurgery for MTLE offers seizure remission rates comparable with those reported for open microsurgery and there are no major safety concerns.

The long-term outcomes of a series of 14 patients who underwent gamma surgery for MTLE reported by Vojtech et al. are not promising.[46] A prescription dose of 18 Gy was used in six patients, 20 Gy in two, and 25 Gy in six. In the control group of seven patients, no patient was seizure free after a follow-up of 96 to 138 months. In the second group of seven patients, none of the patients became seizure free 40 to 105 months following radiosurgery and subsequently underwent microsurgical amygdalohippocampectomy. At 11 to 74 months following open surgery, four were seizure free, one had rare seizures, and one had nondisabling nocturnal seizures. Edema was observed in nine patients, of whom three presented signs of increased intracranial pressure. Two developed permanent visual field defects related to radiosurgery. Two had repeated psychotic episodes and two developed status epilepticus following radiosurgery. No significant memory changes occurred.

The safety and demonstrated short-term efficacy of gamma surgery for the treatment of epilepsies arising from space occupying lesions (e.g., low-grade gliomas, hypothalamic hamartomas, cavernous malformations, and arteriovenous malformations) make it an attractive option.[47,48] However, the gamma knife's long-term feasibility and effectiveness for MTLE need to be proved. Also, it is unclear what underlying mechanisms are responsible for amelioration of seizures following radiosurgery. Some have suggested a "neuromodulation" phenomenon following gamma surgery with accompanying glial cell reduction, stem cell migration, neuronal plasticity and sprouting, and biochemical changes.[49] Rigorous scientific studies evaluating the cellular and subcellular mechanisms responsible for improvements in epilepsy post-gamma surgery are thus far lacking. Furthermore, the need for physiologic monitoring (e.g., depth electrodes, cortical grids) to determine conclusively the epileptogenic focus cannot be entirely discarded.

Conclusions

The indications and usefulness of gamma surgery for functional disorders are being defined more carefully with the passage of time. The advances of neuroimaging in the past several decades have offered the identification of discrete thalamic, subthalamic, and basal ganglia nuclei with acceptable confidence, and allowed the use of gamma surgery in a wider variety of functional disorders. This will require a better understanding of the relationship of anatomy and function as well as improved spatial definition of these nuclei. The ongoing developments of noninvasive physiologic monitoring will influence the development of gamma surgery for epilepsy.[50,51] When everything is considered, one may contend that while gamma surgery may be used for functional diseases of the brain, the current efficacy of alternative methods significantly limits the role of gamma surgery in the management of these diseases.

KEY REFERENCES

Barbaro NM, Quigg M, Broshek DK, et al. A multicenter, prospective pilot study of gamma knife radiosurgery for mesial temporal lobe epilepsy: seizure response, adverse events, and verbal memory. *Ann Neurol.* 2009;65:167-175.

Chen ZF, Kamiryo T, Henson SL, et al. Anticonvulsant effects of gamma surgery in a model of chronic spontaneous limbic epilepsy in rats. *J Neurosurg.* 2001;94:270-280.

Fountas KN, Smith JR, Lee GP, et al. Gamma knife stereotactic radiosurgical treatment of idiopathic trigeminal neuralgia: long-term outcome and complications. *Neurosurg Focus.* 2007;23:E8.

Friehs GM, Park MC, Goldman MA, et al. Stereotactic radiosurgery for functional disorders. *Neurosurg Focus.* 2007;23:E3.

Han JH, Kim DG, Chung HT, et al. Long-term outcome of gamma knife radiosurgery for treatment of typical trigeminal neuralgia. *Int J Radiat Oncol Biol Phys.* 2009;75:822-827.

Hayashi M, Chernov MF, Taira T, et al. Outcome after pituitary radiosurgery for thalamic pain syndrome. *Int J Radiat Oncol Biol Phys.* 2007;69:852-857.

Hayashi M, Taira T, Chernov M, et al. Role of pituitary radiosurgery for the management of intractable pain and potential future applications. *Stereotact Funct Neurosurg.* 2003;81:75-83.

Jagannathan J, Yen CP, Steiner L. Gamma knife radiosurgery for idiopathic trigeminal neuralgia. *Contemp Neurosurg.* 2008;30:1-8.

Keep MF, Mastrofrancesco L, Erdman D, et al. Gamma knife subthalamotomy for Parkinson disease: the subthalamic nucleus as a new radiosurgical target. Case report. *J Neurosurg.* 2002;97:592-599.

Lindquist C, Kihlstrom L, Hellstrand E. Functional neurosurgery—a future for the gamma knife? *Stereotact Funct Neurosurg.* 1991;57:72-81.

Longhi M, Rizzo P, Nicolato A, et al. Gamma knife radiosurgery for trigeminal neuralgia: results and potentially predictive parameters. Part I: idiopathic trigeminal neuralgia. *Neurosurgery.* 2007;61:1254-1260:discussion 1260-1261.

Maesawa S, Kondziolka D, Dixon CE, et al. Subnecrotic stereotactic radiosurgery controlling epilepsy produced by kainic acid injection in rats. *J Neurosurg.* 2000;93:1033-1040.

Maesawa S, Salame C, Flickinger JC, et al. Clinical outcomes after stereotactic radiosurgery for idiopathic trigeminal neuralgia. *J Neurosurg.* 2001;94:14-20.

Mori Y, Kondziolka D, Balzer J, et al. Effects of stereotactic radiosurgery on an animal model of hippocampal epilepsy. *Neurosurgery.* 2000;46:157-165:discussion 165-168.

Pollock BE, Phuong LK, Foote RL, et al. High-dose trigeminal neuralgia radiosurgery associated with increased risk of trigeminal nerve dysfunction. *Neurosurgery.* 2001;49:58-62:discussion 62-64.

Pollock BE, Phuong LK, Gorman DA, et al. Stereotactic radiosurgery for idiopathic trigeminal neuralgia. *J Neurosurg.* 2002;97:347-353.

Regis J, Kerkerian-Legoff L, Rey M, et al. First biochemical evidence of differential functional effects following gamma knife surgery. *Stereotact Funct Neurosurg.* 1996;66(suppl 1):29-38.

Regis J, Metellus P, Hayashi M, et al. Prospective controlled trial of gamma knife surgery for essential trigeminal neuralgia. *J Neurosurg.* 2006;104:913-924.

Regis J, Rey M, Bartolomei F, et al. Gamma knife surgery in mesial temporal lobe epilepsy: a prospective multicenter study. *Epilepsia.* 2004;45:504-515.

Ruck C, Karlsson A, Steele JD, et al. Capsulotomy for obsessive-compulsive disorder: long-term follow-up of 25 patients. *Arch Gen Psychiatry.* 2008;65:914-921.

Steiner L, Forster D, Leksell L, et al. Gammathalamotomy in intractable pain. *Acta Neurochir (Wien).* 1980;52:173-184.

Vojtech Z, Vladyka V, Kalina M, et al. The use of radiosurgery for the treatment of mesial temporal lobe epilepsy and long-term results. *Epilepsia.* 2009;50:2061-2071.

Young RF, Jacques DS, Mark R, et al. Gamma knife radiosurgery for treatment of trigeminal neuralgia: long-term results. *Neurosurgery.* 2001;49:533-534.

Young RF, Jacques S, Mark R, et al. Gamma knife thalamotomy for treatment of tremor: long-term results. *J Neurosurg.* 2000;93(suppl 3):128-135.

Young RF, Vermeulen SS, Grimm P, et al. Gamma knife thalamotomy for the treatment of persistent pain. *Stereotact Funct Neurosurg.* 1995;64(suppl 1):172-181.

Numbered references appear on Expert Consult.

Cranioplasty (Continued)
  polyethylethylketone, 1628f
  synthetic materials for, 1608
Craniospinal embolization, 1074–1075
Craniospinal radiation
  ependymomas treated with, 665
  medulloblastomas treated with, 663
Craniosynostosis
  anterior plagiocephaly, 773–776, 785, 787
  Apert syndrome, 776f–777f, 778–780
  brachycephaly, 776
  Chiari malformation in, 783–788
  complications of, 790
  Crouzon syndrome, 776–777, 778f–779f
  endoscopically assisted suturectomies and osteotomies, 784–785
  history of, 768
  hydrocephalus in, 781–782
  incidence of, 768
  Kleeblattschädel, 780–781, 781f
  multiple suture, 776–781, 779f
  Pfeiffer syndrome, 780, 783
  prognosis for, 789–790
  recurrence of, 788–789
  scaphocephaly, 769, 770f–772f, 784–786
  surgical treatment of
    bicoronal approach, 787
    complications, 790
    fronto-orbital advancement, 787–788
    holocranial dismantling, 787–788
    posterior occipital advancement, 787
    reoperations, 790
    selection of procedure, 790
    techniques, 784–788
  trigonocephaly, 769–773, 785–787, 785f–786f
Craniotomy
  anterior skull base cerebrospinal fluid fistula treated with, 1570–1571
  anterior temporal, 493–494
  antimicrobial prophylaxis in, 1644
  awake, 107
  in basilar apex aneurysm treatment, 919
  bifrontal, 295, 296f
  brain abscess excision using, 1638–1639
  burr-hole, 1574–1576
  cavernous sinus tumors treated with, 457–460
  cerebellopontine angle meningiomas treated with, 511
  cerebrospinal fluid leaks treated with, 1586–1587
  chronic subdural hematoma treated with, 1576, 1577f
  epidural hematoma evacuation with, 1533f
  falcine meningiomas treated with, 413
  frameless stereotactic navigation during, 106
  frontosphenotemporal, 282–284
  frontotemporal, 457
  infections after
    aseptic meningitis, 1646
    bacterial meningitis, 1645–1646
    bone flap, 1647
    brain abscess, 1646
    central nervous system defenses against, 1644–1645
    cerebrospinal fluid leak as risk factor for, 1643–1644
    factors that affect, 1643
    incidence of, 1643, 1644t
    summary of, 1647
    wound, 1646–1647

Craniotomy (Continued)
  intracerebral hemorrhage treated with, 832–834
  miniorbitofrontal, 1590–1592
  orbitozygomatic, 284–286, 285f, 458, 458f
  in paraclinoid aneurysm repair, 859–862, 868f
  pial synangiosis, 738, 739f
  posterior fossa, 660f
  posterior fossa craniectomy and, 575
  pterional
    craniopharyngiomas treated with, 295–297
    description of, 282–284, 283f
    in paraclinoid aneurysm repair, 860
  skull base cerebrospinal fluid fistula treated with, 1570–1571
  sphenoid wing meningiomas treated with, 439–440
  subfrontal, 1589f
  suboccipital
    cerebellar tumors treated with, 174–176
    fourth ventricle tumors treated with, 372, 372f–373f
  supraorbital (keyhole)
    craniopharyngiomas treated with, 293–294
    description of, 288, 289f
    principle of, 428
  transblepharoplasty orbitofrontal, 1592f
  in transcallosal approach to third ventricle tumors, 342, 342f
  transzygomatic, 457, 458f
  twist-drill, 1576
Crankshaft phenomenon, 766
C-reactive protein, 1651
Cribriform fossa, 1589–1590
Crooke's hyaline change, 228
Crouzon syndrome, 769, 776–777, 778f–779f, 783
Cryptococcal meningitis, 1721–1722
Cryptococcomas, 1706
Cryptococcosis, 1704–1706, 1705f–1706f
Cryptococcus spp., 1693t, 1697t, 1704–1705
Cubital tunnel, 2288
Cubital tunnel syndrome, 2289–2290
Cushing, Harvey, 1, 280
Cushing's disease, 196–197
  ACTH-secreting pituitary adenoma as cause of, 197, 233f, 241
  adrenal inhibitors for, 212–213, 213t
  adrenalectomy for, 241
  chemical adrenalectomy for, 241
  in children, 229
  clinical manifestations of, 229
  corticotroph hyperplasia as cause of, 228
  cure and remission criteria, 212
  definition of, 196
  description of, 228
  dexamethasone suppression test for, 196–197, 233f–234f
  ectopic ACTH secretion versus, 230–232
  etiology of, 228, 229t
  experimental treatments in, 213–214
  gamma knife stereotactic radiosurgery in, 1181
  glucocorticoid excess as cause of, 228
  hypercortisolism in, 229–230, 230f, 235–237
  imaging of, 232–233, 236f
  life expectancy affected by, 229
  medical therapy for, 212, 241

Cushing's disease (Continued)
  microadenomas as cause of, 228
  morbidity rates, 1181
  pathology of, 228
  pathophysiology of, 228
  radiation therapy for, 239–241, 245f
  recurrent, 212, 237–239, 244f
  remission of, 244f–245f
  screening tests for, 196–197
  signs and symptoms of, 195t
  trans-sphenoidal surgery for, 212
  treatment of
    surgery, 233–239
    trans-sphenoidal microsurgery, 233
  urine-free cortisol testing, 229–230, 230f
Cushing's syndrome
  clinical manifestations of, 229
  corticotropin-releasing hormone stimulation test for, 230, 234f–235f
  definition of, 228
  diagnosis of, 229–233
  etiology of, 229t
  signs and symptoms of, 229, 229t
Cutaneous hemangiomas, 2082
Cyberkinetics, 1363
CyberKnife stereotactic radiosurgery
  accuracy of, 1173
  craniopharyngiomas treated with, 1189–1191
  illustration of, 1174f
  immobilization devices used with, 1174f
  lesions treated with, 1179t
  meningiomas treated with, 1209f, 1210
  overview of, 1173
  software for, 1173
  trigeminal neuralgia treated with, 1168–1169, 1169f, 1171
Cyst(s)
  aneurysmal bone, 1071, 1073, 2205
  arachnoid. See Arachnoid cysts
  cerebellopontine angle, 312
  cerebral convexity, 312
  dermoid. See Dermoid cysts
  endodermal, 392–393
  epidermoid, 391–393
  ganglion, 2325–2326
  intraparenchymal cerebral, 1723, 1724f–1725f
  intraventricular, 1677t
  neuroepithelial, 392–393
  parenchymal, 1677t
  Rathke's cleft. See Rathke's cleft cysts
  spinal, 1677t
  subarachnoid, 312f
  suprasellar. See Suprasellar cysts
  synovial, 1909f
Cysternal cysts, 1677t
Cystic adenomas, 199
Cystic craniopharyngiomas, 328, 329f
Cystic hemangioblastomas, 390f
Cysticercal encephalitis, 1670
Cysticercus cellulosae, 1667–1669, 1669f, 1675f
Cytoreduction
  glioma recurrence after, 129
  high-grade gliomas treated with, 105–106

D
D wave
  in children, 44–45
  description of, 40
  motor-evoked potentials and, 39
Dallas maneuver, 859

Extratemporal lobe epilepsy *(Continued)*
  stereoelectroencephalography, 1282, 1282f
  surgical technique for, 1284–1285, 1284f–1285f
  surgical treatment of, 1278–1279
Extratemporal resections, for pediatric epilepsy, 692–693, 693f
Extreme lateral interbody fusion, 2107
Extreme lateral transcondylar approach
  clival chordomas treated with, 491, 495f–496f
  clival meningiomas treated with, 498
Eyebrow incisions, 15

F
Facet degeneration, 1885
Facet dislocations
  bilateral, 1989, 1989f
  unilateral, 1988–1989, 1989f
Facetectomy, 1872f
  full, 1877
  medial, 1877
Facet–spinous process wiring technique, 2019, 2021f
Facial fractures, 1588, 2332
Facial nerve
  injury of, 2333–2335
  preservation of, during suboccipital retrosigmoid surgical approach for vestibular schwannoma, 551, 552t
  radiation sensitivity of, 49
  in translabyrinthine approach to vestibular schwannomas, 559–560, 562
Facial pain, 1407
Facial paralysis, after translabyrinthine approach to vestibular schwannomas, 562
Facial translocation, for skull base tumors, 618–619
Failed back surgery syndrome, 1461–1463, 1465–1466
Falcine meningiomas
  cerebral angiography of, 412
  classification of, 410
  clinical presentation of, 410
  craniotomy for, 413
  description of, 399
  magnetic resonance imaging of, 410, 411f–412f
  parasagittal meningiomas versus, 410
  radiographic findings, 410–413, 411f–412f
  sinus invasion of, 414–415
  surgical treatment of, 413–415
  symptoms of, 410
Far lateral approach
  anatomy of, 951–952
  anesthetic technique, 952
  atlanto-occipital instability secondary to, 956
  basic, 954, 955f, 956–957
  cerebrospinal fluid leaks after, 956
  clival meningiomas treated with, 498
  complications of, 956
  cranial nerve injuries caused by, 956
  extradural stage of, 951–952
  foramen magnum tumors treated with, 518–521
  infratentorial arteriovenous malformations treated with, 999f
  lower basilar and midbasilar aneurysms treated with, 932–935, 932f–934f

Far lateral approach *(Continued)*
  neuroprotection for, 952
  patient positioning for, 952–953, 953f
  skin incisions for, 953–954, 953f–954f
  summary of, 956–957
  supracondylar extension of, 955–956
  surgical technique for, 952–956
  transcondylar extension of, 954–955, 956f
  vertebral artery risks during, 956
Far lateral lumbar disc herniations, 1860–1861, 1860f
  anatomy of, 1872–1873
  cliniconeurologic parameters of, 1874
  computed tomography of, 1875–1877, 1876f
  conservative management of, 1877
  degenerative scoliosis, 1875
  degenerative spondylolisthesis, 1874–1875
  incidence of, 1873–1874
  location of, 1873–1874
  lumbar spinal stenosis and, 1874
  lumbar vertebral fractures, 1874
  magnetic resonance imaging of, 1875, 1875f
  myelo-computed tomography scans of, 1875–1877
  neurodiagnostic evaluations of, 1875–1877, 1875f–1876f
  prevalence of, 1871
  spondylosis and, 1874
  surgical management of
    adjuncts to, 1877
    anterior interbody fusion devices, 1879–1880
    anterolateral retroperitoneal approach, 1878–1879
    computed tomography before, 1880
    endoscopy, 1878
    errors in, 1881
    extraforaminal approach, 1878
    full facetectomy, 1877
    fusion, 1879–1880
    interbody fusion cages, 1879
    interbody fusion devices, 1879–1880
    intertransverse technique, 1871f, 1878
    magnetic resonance imaging before, 1880
    materials and methods for, 1872–1874
    medial facetectomy, 1877–1878
    outcomes, 1880–1882
    percutaneous pedicle screw fixation, 1879
    posterior interbody fusion devices, 1879
    preoperative testing, 1880
    techniques for, 1871
    trans-pars technique, 1873f, 1877
Fasciculus subcallosal medialis, 86
Femoral neurotomy, 1380–1382, 1381f
Fetal posterior cerebral artery, 872
Fetal surgery
  goal of, 702
  hysterotomy and exposure, 703
  myelomeningocele treated with, 702–705, 704f
  open neural tube defects treated with, 702–705
  rationale for, 702
  results of, 704–705
  steps involved in, 703
  timing of, 702–703

α-Fetoprotein, in pineal region tumors, 358, 676–677, 677t
^{18}F-fluorodeoxyglucose positron emission tomography, 153, 154f
Fiber tracts, 26
Fibrillary astrocytoma, 670
Fibroblast growth factor receptors, 768
Fibrous adenomas
  description of, 249
  magnetic resonance imaging of, 249, 250f
Fibrous dysplasia, 615–616
Fick equation, 1497
Filum terminale
  anatomy of, 2081, 2082f, 2085, 2202
  fatty, 2085, 2085f
  meningiomas of, 2133f
  tight, 2085, 2165f
  tumors of, 2132–2133, 2133f
Finger spasticity, 1382–1383, 1383f
Fisch classification, of glomus tumors, 535–536, 535t
Fistulas
  carotid–cavernous. *See* Carotid–cavernous fistulas
  cerebrospinal fluid. *See* Cerebrospinal fluid fistula
  dural arteriovenous. *See* Dural arteriovenous fistulas
  dural cutaneous, 1585
  prenidal direct, 1229f
  pressure-related, 1225t
"Fit-for-duty" examinations, 7–8
Flash visual-evoked potentials, 2330
Flow diversion, for intracranial aneurysms, 1025
Flow-regulated valves, for shunts, 638, 639f–640f
Fluconazole, 1730
Flucytosine, 1730
Fluent aphasia, 141–142
Fluoro-L-m-tyrosine, 1343–1344
Fluoroquinolones, 1646
Fluoroscopy
  intraoperative, 13, 19
  3D rotation, 13
Focal cortical dysplasia, 692, 693f
Focal dystonia, 1323
Focal epilepsy, 1262
Focal pontine astrocytomas, 388
Focal pontine glioma, 160, 162f
Focal traumatic brain injury, 1496, 1496t
Foix-Chavany-Marie syndrome, 84
Folate receptor, 252
Foot spasticity, 1380, 1381f
Foramen magnum
  anatomy of, 517
  dural arteriovenous fistulas of, 974–975
Foramen magnum meningiomas, 513–515
  classification of, 517
  extradural, 517–518
  fractionated radiation therapy for, 506f
  incidence of, 513
  intradural, 517, 527
  magnetic resonance imaging of, 514f
  surgical treatment of, 526
Foramen magnum tumors
  anatomy of, 517
  classification of, 517–518
  clinical presentation of, 517
  magnetic resonance imaging of, 524f
  meningiomas. *See* Foramen magnum meningiomas

Temozolomide
alkylating agents and, 133
anaplastic astrocytoma treated with, 100
description of, 95
glioblastoma treated with, 97, 132–133
low-grade gliomas treated with, 96
recurrent glioblastoma treated with, 132–133
Temporal bone fractures, 1563, 1564f, 2333, 2333f
Temporal ependymomas, 680f
Temporal language area resection, 90
Temporal lobe
cavernous malformations of, 985f
high-grade gliomas of, 108, 109f
resections of, for pediatric epilepsy, 690–692
seizures of, 684–685
Temporal oligodendrogliomas, 120f
Tendon transfer, 1386
Tentorial meningiomas, 509, 510f
Teratomas
characteristics of, 676t
in children, 2159
fourth ventricle, 396
intramedullary, 2139, 2143
sacrococcygeal, 2204
Teres major neurotomy, 1382
Terminal lipomas, 713, 714f, 716, 722, 2086
Terminal syrinx, 2088–2089, 2089f
Termination aneurysms, 875, 876f
Tethered cord syndrome
conus medullaris in, 2089
dermoid tumors as cause of, 2087–2088
detethering of, 2089
embryology of, 2081
epidemiology of, 2082
foot amputation secondary to, 2082f
intraoperative physiologic monitoring in, 2089–2090
lower extremity findings, 2084f
outcome of, 2090
pathophysiology of, 2081
physical examination of, 2082
spina bifida occulta associated with, 2083
surgical decision making in, 2089–2090
Thalamic glioma, 671–673
Thalamocaudate, 1013–1014
Thalamostriate vein, 330
Thalamus
arteriovenous malformation of, 50f
centromedian–parafascicular complex, 1333
intracerebral hemorrhage in, 826, 831, 833
Third ventricle
anatomy of, 334, 339–340, 341f
colloid cyst of, 353f
floor of, 340
lateral wall of, 334
Third ventricle tumors
anterior, 334–336
differential diagnosis of, 339
frequency of, 340t
hydrocephalus caused by, 337
magnetic resonance imaging of, 340, 352f
overview of, 330
posterior, 336
surgical treatment of
anatomy, 334
anterior interforniceal approach, 343–344, 349f

Third ventricle tumors (Continued)
complications of, 336–337
endoscopic approaches, 335–336
infratentorial supracerebellar approach, 336
interforniceal approach, 334, 343–344, 348f, 349t
lateral subfrontal approach, 334–335, 335f
mortality rate for, 336
occipital transtentorial approach, 336
outcomes, 337
pterional approach, 335
seizures secondary to, 337
summary of, 349–350
suprachoroidal approach, 342–343, 349t
transcallosal approach, 336, 339–347, 341f–349f, 349–350
transcavum interforniceal endoscopic approach, 352
transchoroidal approach, 342–343, 347, 347f, 349t
transforaminal approach, 334, 335f, 342, 346f, 349t
trans-sylvian approach, 342–343
Third ventriculostomy, endoscopic
description of, 353
hydrocephalus treated with, 646–652
choroid plexus cauterization with, 646, 649–650, 650f
complications of, 652
factors that affect, 647t
goal of, 650
history of, 646
outcome of, 650–652, 651t
patient selection, 646–647
success rates, 646t
technique, 647–649, 649f
Thoracic cavity, 1844–1846, 1845f
Thoracic disc disease, 1843–1844
Thoracic disc herniation
asymptomatic, 1833
computed tomography of, 1834f
description of, 1833
history of, 1843–1844
incidence of, 1843
localization of, 1835, 1836f
magnetic resonance imaging of, 1834f
natural history of, 1834
radiography of, 1833–1834
studies of, 1834t
surgical treatment of
advances in, 1843
anterior approaches, 1835, 1839
complications of, 1841–1842
costotransversectomy procedure, 1837–1838, 1838f
lateral extracavitary approach, 1838, 1839f
localization during, 1835, 1836f
mini-open procedures, 1838–1839
patient selection, 1834
posterior approaches, 1835–1838, 1836f–1838f
retropleural thoracotomy, 1840–1841, 1840f–1841f
transcostovertebral approach, 1836–1837, 1838f
transfacet pedicle-sparing procedure, 1836, 1837f
transpedicular approach, 1835–1836, 1837f
transpleural approach, 1843–1844

Thoracic disc herniation (Continued)
transsternal approach, 1841
transthoracic procedure, 1839–1840, 1840f, 1843–1844
symptomatic, 1833
Thoracic duct, 2181
Thoracic inlet, 2181
Thoracic outlet syndrome, 2240–2241
clinical presentation of, 2341–2342
complications of, 2347
conservative treatment of, 2344
definition of, 2339, 2347–2348
diagnosis of, 2341–2344
disputed, 2339
electrophysiologic evaluation of, 2343
historical description of, 2339
imaging of, 2343–2344
magnetic resonance imaging of, 2343
muscle hypertrophy caused by, 2339
neurogenic, 2339
pathogenesis of, 2340–2341
physical examination of, 2341–2342
predisposing factors for, 2339
provocative maneuvers for, 2342–2343, 2342f
radiographs of, 2343
recurrent, 2347
surgical anatomy of, 2340
surgical treatment of
anterior supraclavicular approach, 2344–2345, 2345f, 2347
approaches, 2344–2346
case study of, 2346
clinical outcomes after, 2346–2347
indications for, 2344
posterior subscapular approach, 2345–2347, 2345f
transaxillary approach, 2346–2347, 2346f
treatment of, 2340
vascular, 2339–2340
vascular insufficiency in, 2343
Thoracic spinal cord stimulation, 1462
Thoracic spine
anatomy of, 1846
instrumentation of, 763–765, 764f
stability of, 2182
Thoracic sympathectomy, for hyperhidrosis, 1374–1376, 1374f–1376f
Thoracic vertebrae, 1846
Thoracolumbar cages, 2032–2033
Thoracolumbar vertebral fractures
anterolateral approach for, 2030–2033, 2031f–2033f
description of, 2027
posterior stabilization of, 2028–2030, 2029f–2030f, 2033
Thoracoscopic discectomy, video-assisted
anesthesia for, 1847, 1848f
complications of, 1850–1851
contraindications, 1847
endoscopic instruments, 1848–1849, 1849f
indications for, 1847
operating room setup for, 1848, 1848f
outcomes of, 1850–1851
patient positioning for, 1848
portals for, 1848, 1848f
preoperative evaluation, 1846–1847
procedure, 1849–1850, 1850f
single-lung ventilation, 1847
smoking cessation before, 1846
surgical anatomy, 1844–1846